Mark frequently used sections in your code book with these color-coded flags.

2015 DRAFT

ICD-10-PCS Code Book

Anne B. Casto, RHIA, CCS
Consulting Editor

AHIMA
American Health Information Management Association®

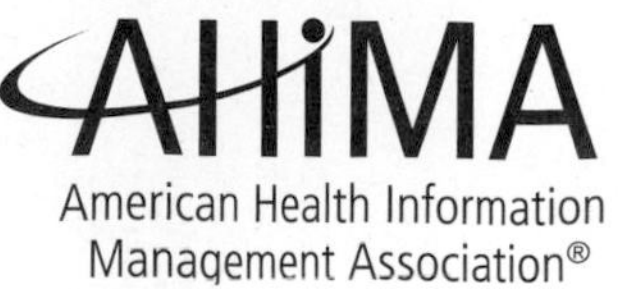

ISBN: 978-1-58426-439-2
AHIMA Product No.: AC222014

AHIMA Staff:
Angie Comfort, RHIA, CDIP, CCS, Technical Review
Katherine Greenock, MS, Production Development Editor
Megan Grennan, Production Development Editor
Jason O. Malley, Vice President, Business and Innovation
Caitlin Wilson, Assistant Editor
Pamela Woolf, Director of Publications

The websites listed in this book were current and valid as of the date of publication. However, webpage addresses and the information on them may change at any time. The user is encouraged to perform his or her own general web searches to locate any site addresses listed here that are no longer valid.

For more information about AHIMA Press publications, including updates, visit http://www.ahima.org/publications/updates.aspx.

American Health Information Management Association
233 North Michigan Avenue, 21st Floor
Chicago, Illinois 60601-5809
ahima.org

Contents

About the Consulting Editor

Anne B. Casto, RHIA, CCS, is the president of Casto Consulting, LLC. Casto Consulting, LLC is a consulting firm that provides services to hospitals and other healthcare stakeholders primarily in the areas of reimbursement and coding. Casto Consulting, LLC specializes in linking coding and billing practices to positive revenue cycle outcomes. Additionally, the firm provides guidance to consulting firms, healthcare organizations and healthcare insurers regarding reimbursement methodologies and Medicare regulations.

Prior to founding the firm, Ms. Casto was the program manager of the HIMS Division at The Ohio State University School of Allied Medical Professions. Ms. Casto taught healthcare reimbursement, ICD-9-CM coding, and CPT coding courses for several years. Additionally, Ms. Casto was responsible for curriculum revisions in the areas of chargemaster management, clinical data management, and healthcare reimbursement.

Additionally, Ms. Casto was the vice president of clinical information for Cleverley & Associates where she worked very closely with APC regulations and guidelines, preparing hospitals for the implementation of the Medicare OPPS. Ms. Casto was also the clinical information product manager for CHIPS/Ingenix. She joined CHIPS/Ingenix in 1998 and spent the majority of her time developing coding compliance products for the inpatient and outpatient settings.

Ms. Casto has been responsible for inpatient and outpatient coding activities in several large hospitals including Mt. Sinai Medical Center (NYC), Beth Israel Medical Center (NYC), and The Ohio State University. She worked extensively with CMI, quality measures, physician documentation, and coding accuracy efforts at these facilities.

Ms. Casto received her degree in Health Information Management at The Ohio State University in 1995. She received her Certified Coding Specialist credential in 1998 from the American Health Information Management Association. Ms. Casto is the co-author of an AHIMA-published text book entitled *Principles of Healthcare Reimbursement*. Additionally, Ms. Casto was a contributing author to the published AHIMA books: *Severity DRGs and Reimbursement; A MS-DRG Primer* and *Effective Management of Coding Services*. Most recently, Ms. Casto authored the AHIMA-published text entitled *The CDM Handbook*.

Ms. Casto received the AHIMA Legacy Award, part of the FORE Triumph Awards, in 2007 which honors a significant contribution to the knowledge base of the HIM field through an insightful publication. Additionally, Ms. Casto was honored with the Ohio Health Information Management Association's Distinguished Member Award in 2008 and the Ohio Health Information Management Association's Professional Achievement Award in 2011.

Acknowledgments

Many thanks to my family for their support during this project. Thanks to Dr. Susan White, The Ohio State University; your data manipulation skills are second to none. Thanks to Drew Beverick for providing valuable insight from the student perspective. I thank the reviewers for their thoughtful comments and suggestions. Many thanks to Linda Hyde for her very thorough technical review of the book.

ICD-10-PCS Overview

The International Classification of Diseases, Tenth Revision, Procedure Coding System (ICD-10-PCS) was created to accompany the World Health Organization's (WHO) ICD-10 diagnosis classification. This coding system was developed to replace ICD-9-CM procedure codes for reporting inpatient procedures. Unlike the ICD-9-CM classification, ICD-10-PCS was designed to enable each code to have a standard structure and be very descriptive, and yet flexible enough to accommodate future needs.

History of ICD-10-PCS

The WHO has maintained the International Classification of Diseases (ICD) for recording cause of death since 1893. It has updated the ICD periodically to reflect new discoveries in epidemiology and changes in medical understanding of disease. The International Classification of Diseases Tenth Revision (ICD-10), published in 1992, is the latest revision of the ICD. The WHO authorized the National Center for Health Statistics (NCHS) to develop a clinical modification of ICD-10 for use in the United States. This version of ICD-10 is called ICD-10-CM, and is intended to replace the previous US clinical modification, ICD-9-CM, that has been in use since 1979. ICD-9-CM contains a procedure classification; ICD-10-CM does not.

The Centers for Medicare and Medicaid Services (CMS), the agency responsible for maintaining the inpatient procedure code set in the United States, contracted with 3M Health Information Systems in 1993 to design and then develop a procedure classification system to replace Volume 3 of ICD-9-CM. ICD-10-PCS is the result. ICD-10-PCS was initially released in 1998. It has been updated annually since that time.

ICD-9-CM Volume 3 Compared with ICD-10-PCS

With ICD-10 implementation, the US clinical modification of the ICD will not include a procedure classification based on the same principles of organization as the diagnosis classification. Instead, a separate procedure coding system has been developed to meet the rigorous and varied demands that are made of coded data in the healthcare industry. This represents a significant step toward building a health information infrastructure that functions optimally in the electronic age. The following information highlights some of the basic differences between ICD-9-CM Volume 3 and ICD-10-PCS:

ICD-9-CM Volume 3

- Follows ICD structure (designed for diagnosis coding)
- Codes available as a fixed/finite set in list form
- Codes are numeric
- Codes are three or four digits long

ICD-10-PCS

- Designed and developed to meet healthcare needs for a procedure code system
- Codes constructed from flexible code components (values) using tables
- Codes are alphanumeric
- All codes are seven characters long

ICD-10-PCS Design

ICD-10-PCS is fundamentally different from ICD-9-CM in its structure, organization, and capabilities. It was designed and developed to adhere to recommendations made by the National Committee on Vital and Health Statistics (NCVHS). It also incorporates input from a wide range of organizations, individual physicians, healthcare professionals, and researchers. Several structural attributes were recommended for a new procedure coding system. These attributes include a multiaxial structure, completeness, and expandability.

Multiaxial Structure

The key attribute that provides the framework for all other structural attributes is multiaxial code structure. *Multiaxial code structure* makes it possible for the ICD-10-PCS to be complete, expandable, and provide a high degree of flexibility and functionality.

ICD-10-PCS codes are composed of seven characters. Each character represents a category of information that can be specified about the procedure performed. A character defines both the category of information and its physical position in the code. A character's position can be understood as a semi-independent axis of classification that allows different specific values to be inserted into that space, and whose physical position remains stable. Within a defined code range, a character retains the general meaning that it confers on any value in that position.

Completeness

Completeness is considered a key structural attribute for a new procedure coding system. The specific recommendation for completeness included that a unique code be available for each significant procedure, that each code retain its unique definition, and that codes that have been deleted are not reused.

In Volume 3 of ICD-9-CM, procedures performed on many different body parts using different approaches or devices may be assigned to the same procedure code. In ICD-10-PCS, a unique code is constructed for every significantly different procedure.

Within each section, a character defines a consistent component of a code, and contains all applicable values for that character. The values define individual expressions (Open, Percutaneous) of the character's general meaning (approach) that are then used to construct unique procedure codes. Because all approaches by which a procedure is performed are assigned a separate approach value, every procedure which uses a different approach will have its own unique code. This is true of the other characters as well. The same procedure performed on a different body part has its own unique code; the same procedure performed using a different device has its own unique code, and so on.

Because ICD-10-PCS codes are constructed of individual values rather than lists of fixed codes and text descriptions, the unique, stable definition of a code in the system is retained. New values may be added to the system to represent a specific new approach or device or qualifier, but whole codes by design cannot be given new meanings and reused.

Expandability

Expandability was also recommended as a key structural attribute. The specific recommendation for expandability included that the system be capable of accommodating new procedures and technology and that these new codes could be added to the system without disrupting the existing structure.

ICD-10-PCS is designed to be easily updated as new codes are required for new procedures and new techniques. Changes to ICD-10-PCS can all be made within the existing structure because whole codes are not added. Instead, a new value for a character can be added to the system as needed. Likewise, an existing value for a character can be added to a table(s) in the system.

ICD-10-PCS Additional Characteristics

ICD-10-PCS possesses several additional characteristics in response to government and industry recommendations. These characteristics are

- Standardized terminology within the coding system
- Standardized level of specificity
- No diagnostic information
- No explicit "not otherwise specified" (NOS) code options
- Limited use of "not elsewhere classified" (NEC) code options

Standardized Terminology

Words commonly used in clinical vocabularies may have multiple meanings. This can cause confusion and result in inaccurate data. ICD-10-PCS is standardized and self-contained. Characters and values used in the system are defined in the system. For example, the word *excision* is used to describe a wide variety of surgical procedures. In ICD-10-PCS, the word *excision* describes a single, precise surgical objective, defined as "cutting out or off, without replacement, a portion of a body part."

No Eponyms or Common Procedure Names

The terminology used in ICD-10-PCS is standardized to provide precise and stable definitions of all procedures performed. This standardized terminology is used in all ICD-10-PCS code descriptions. As a result, ICD-10-PCS code descriptions do not include eponyms or common procedure names. Two examples from ICD-9-CM are

22.61, Excision of lesion of maxillary sinus with Caldwell-Luc approach

51.10, Endoscopic retrograde cholangiopancreatography [ERCP]

In ICD-10-PCS, physicians' names are not included in a code description, nor are procedures identified by common terms or acronyms such as appendectomy or CABG. Instead, such procedures are coded to the root operation that accurately identifies the objective of the procedure.

The procedures described in the preceding paragraph by ICD-9-CM codes are coded in ICD-10-PCS according to the root operation that matches the objective of the procedure. Here, the ICD-10-PCS equivalents would be Excision and Inspection, respectively. By relying on the universal objectives defined in root operations rather than eponyms or specific procedure titles that change or become obsolete, ICD-10-PCS preserves the capacity to define past, present, and future procedures accurately using stable terminology in the form of characters and values.

No Combination Codes

With rare exceptions, ICD-10-PCS does not define multiple procedures with one code. This is to preserve standardized terminology and consistency across the system. Procedures that are typically performed together but are distinct procedures may be defined by a single *combination code* in ICD-9-CM. An example of a combination code in ICD-9-CM is 28.3, Tonsillectomy with adenoidectomy.

A procedure that meets the reporting criteria for a separate procedure is coded separately in ICD-10-PCS. This allows the system to respond to changes in technology and medical practice with the maximum degree of stability and flexibility.

Standardized Level of Specificity

In ICD-9-CM, one code with its description and includes notes may encompass a vast number of procedure variations while another code defines a single specific procedure. ICD-10-PCS provides a standardized level of specificity for each code, so each code represents a single procedure variation.

The ICD-9-CM code 39.31, Suture of artery, does not specify the artery, whereas the code range 38.40–38.49, Resection of artery with replacement, provides a fourth-digit subclassification for specifying the artery by anatomical region (Thoracic, Abdominal, etc.). In ICD-10-PCS, the codes identifying all artery suture and artery replacement procedures possess the same degree of specificity. The ICD-9-CM examples above coded to their ICD-10-PCS equivalents would use the same artery body part values in all codes identifying the respective procedures.

In general, ICD-10-PCS code descriptions are much more specific than their ICD-9-CM counterparts, but sometimes an ICD-10-PCS code description is actually less specific. In most cases this is because the ICD-9-CM code contains diagnosis information. The standardized level of code specificity in ICD-10-PCS cannot always take account of these fluctuations in ICD-9-CM level of specificity. Instead, ICD-10-PCS provides a standardized level of specificity that can be predicted across the system.

Diagnosis Information Excluded

Another key feature of ICD-10-PCS is that information pertaining to a diagnosis is excluded from the code descriptions. ICD-9-CM often contains information about the diagnosis in its procedure codes. Adding diagnosis information limits the flexibility and functionality of a procedure coding system. It has the effect of placing a code "off limits" because the diagnosis in the medical record does not match the diagnosis in the procedure code description. The code cannot be used even though the procedural part of the code description precisely matches the procedure performed. Diagnosis information is not contained in any ICD-10-PCS code. The diagnosis codes, not the procedure codes, will specify the reason the procedure is performed.

NOS Code Options Restricted

ICD-9-CM often designates codes as "unspecified" or "not otherwise specified" (NOS) codes. By contrast, the standardized level of specificity designed into ICD-10-PCS restricts the use of broadly applicable NOS or unspecified code options in the system. A minimal level of specificity is required to construct a valid code.

Limited NEC Code Options

ICD-9-CM often designates codes as "not elsewhere classified" (NEC) or "other specified" versions of a procedure throughout the code set. NEC options are also provided in ICD-10-PCS, but only for specific, limited use.

In the Medical and Surgical section, two significant NEC options are the root operation value Q, Repair, and the device value Y, Other Device. The root operation Repair is a true NEC value. It is used only when the procedure performed is not one of the other root operations in the Medical and Surgical section. Other Device, on the other hand, is intended to be used to temporarily define new devices that do not have a specific value assigned, until one can be added to the system. No categories of medical or surgical devices are permanently classified to Other Device.

ICD-10-PCS Code Structure

Undergirding ICD-10-PCS is a logical, consistent structure that informs the system as a whole, down to the level of a single code. This means the process of constructing codes in ICD-10-PCS is also logical and consistent: the spaces of the code, called *characters* are filled with individual letters and numbers, called *values*.

Characters

All codes in ICD-10-PCS are seven characters long. Each character in the seven-character code represents an aspect of the procedure. The following are two examples of the code structure: one from the Medical and Surgical section and one from the Ancillary section.

Medical and Surgical Code Structure

Character 1	Character 2	Character 3	Character 4	Character 5	Character 6	Character 7
Section	Body System	Operation	Body Part	Approach	Device	Qualifier

Imaging Section Code Structure

Character 1	Character 2	Character 3	Character 4	Character 5	Character 6	Character 7
Section	Body System	Type	Body Part	Contrast	Qualifier	Qualifier

An ICD-10-PCS code is best understood as the result of a process rather than as an isolated, fixed quantity. The process consists of assigning values from among the valid choices for that part of the system, according to the rules governing the construction of codes.

Values

One of 34 possible values can be assigned to each character in a code: the numbers 0 through 9 and the alphabet (except the letters I and O, because they are easily confused with the numbers 1 and 0). A finished code looks like this: 02103D4.

This code is derived by choosing a specific value for each of the seven characters. Based on details about the procedure performed, values for each character specifying the section, body system, root operation, body part, approach, device, and qualifier are assigned. Because the definition of each character is a function of its physical position in the code, the same value placed in a different position in the code means something different. The value 0 in the first character means something different than 0 in the second character, or 0 in the third character, and so on.

Code Structure Example

The following example defines each character using the code 0LB50ZZ, Excision of right lower arm and wrist tendon, Open approach. This example comes from the Medical and Surgical section of ICD-10-PCS.

Character 1: Section

The first character in the code determines the broad procedure category, or section, where the code is found. In this example, the section is Medical and Surgical. 0 is the value that represents Medical and Surgical in the first character.

Character 1	Character 2	Character 3	Character 4	Character 5	Character 6	Character 7
Section	**Body** System	**Root** Operation	**Body** Part	**Approach**	**Device**	**Qualifier**
0						

Character 2: Body System

The second character defines the body system—the general physiological system or anatomical region involved. Examples of body systems include Lower Arteries, Central Nervous System, and Respiratory System. In this example, the body system is Tendons, represented by the value L.

Character 1	Character 2	Character 3	Character 4	Character 5	Character 6	Character 7
Section	**Body System**	**Root** Operation	**Body** Part	**Approach**	**Device**	**Qualifier**
0	L					

Character 3: Root Operation

The third character defines the root operation, or the objective of the procedure. Some examples of root operations are Bypass, Drainage, and Reattachment. In this example code, the root operation is Excision. When used in the third character of the code, the value B represents Excision.

Character 1	Character 2	Character 3	Character 4	Character 5	Character 6	Character 7
Section	**Body** System	**Root Operation**	**Body** Part	**Approach**	**Device**	**Qualifier**
0	L	B				

Character 4: Body Part

The fourth character defines the body part or specific anatomical site where the procedure was performed. The body system (second character) provides only a general indication of the procedure site. The body part and body system values together provide a precise description of the procedure site. Examples of body parts are Kidney, Tonsils, and Thymus. In this example, the body part value is 5, Lower Arm and Wrist, Right. When the second character is L, the value 5 when used in the fourth character of the code represents the right lower arm and wrist tendon.

Character 1	Character 2	Character 3	Character 4	Character 5	Character 6	Character 7
Section	**Body** System	**Root** Operation	**Body Part**	**Approach**	**Device**	**Qualifier**
0	L	B	5			

Character 5: Approach

The fifth character defines the approach, or the technique used to reach the procedure site. Seven different approach values are used in the Medical and Surgical section to define the approach. Examples of approaches include Open and Percutaneous Endoscopic. In this example code, the approach is Open and is represented by the value 0.

Character 1	Character 2	Character 3	Character 4	Character 5	Character 6	Character 7
Section	**Body** System	**Root** Operation	**Body** Part	**Approach**	**Device**	**Qualifier**
0	L	B	5	0		

Character 6: Device

Depending on the procedure performed, there may be a device left in place at the end of the procedure. The sixth character defines the device. Device values fall into four basic categories:

- Grafts and Prostheses
- Implants
- Simple or Mechanical Appliances
- Electronic Appliances

In this example, there is no device used in the procedure. The value Z is used to represent No Device, as shown here:

Character 1	Character 2	Character 3	Character 4	Character 5	Character 6	Character 7
Section	**Body** System	**Operation**	**Body** Part	**Approach**	**Device**	**Qualifier**
0	L	B	5	0	Z	

Character 7: Qualifier

The seventh character defines a qualifier for the code. A qualifier specifies an additional attribute of the procedure, if applicable. Examples of qualifiers include Diagnostic and Stereotactic. Qualifier choices vary depending on the previous values selected. In this example, there is no specific qualifier applicable to this procedure, so the value is No Qualifier, represented by the letter Z.

Character 1	Character 2	Character 3	Character 4	Character 5	Character 6	Character 7
Section	**Body** System	**Operation**	**Body** Part	**Approach**	**Device**	**Qualifier**
0	L	B	5	0	Z	Z

0LB50ZZ is the complete specification of the procedure "Excision of right lower arm and wrist tendon, Open approach."

ICD-10-PCS Organization and Official Conventions

The *ICD-10-PCS Code Book, 2015 Draft* is based on the official draft of the International Classification of Diseases, Tenth Revision, Procedure Classification System, issued by the US Department of Health and Human Services (HHS) and CMS. This book is consistent with the content of the government's version of ICD-10-PCS and follows the official conventions.

Index

The Alphabetic Index is provided to assist the user with locating the appropriate table to construct procedure codes. Each table contains all the information required to construct valid procedure codes. Coders should not code from the PCS Index alone; the PCS code tables should always be consulted before assigning a PCS procedure code.

Main Terms

Main terms in the Alphabetic Index reflect the root operations, third character, of procedures. The Index includes not only root operation terms, but also other common procedural terms, anatomical sites, and device terms. The main terms are listed alphabetically. After the coder has located the correct main term and subterm in the Alphabetic Index, he or she is provided with the first three to four digits of the procedure code. The coder should then move to the Tables section of the code book and locate the appropriate table to complete the code construction. Even if the entire seven-digit code is provided in the Index, the coder should still reference the Tables to ensure the correct PCS code has been constructed.

See Reference

Common procedure terms are often listed with the *see* reference. The coder is instructed to follow the reference provided in order to locate the appropriate table to construct the code. For example, the *see* reference is present for the main term Colectomy. The Index excerpt is as follows:

Colectomy

see Excision, Gastrointestinal System 0DB

see Resection, Gastrointestinal System 0DT

In this example, the coder should review the definition of the root operations Excision and Resection to determine which is consistent with the medical record documentation. The coder should then proceed to the corresponding table as suggested by the *see* reference.

Use Reference

Anatomical site terms and device terms are often listed with the *use* reference. The coder is instructed to follow the reference provided in order to locate the appropriate main term for the procedure in question. For example, the *use* reference is present for the main term Inferior rectus muscle. The Index excerpt is as follows:

Inferior rectus muscle

use Muscle, Extraocular, Left

use Muscle, Extraocular, Right

In this example, the coder should identify the root operation for the procedure, and then look for the subterm that identifies the body part indicated in the *use* reference. For example, the procedure is excision of the inferior rectus muscle. The coder would locate the main term Excision. The Index excerpt is as follows:

Excision
Muscle
Extraocular
Left 08BM
Right 08BL

In this example, the coder knows that the Code Table 08B is the correct table because the previous review of the *use* reference identified that the inferior rectus muscle is and extraocular muscle. The coder can now proceed to the 08B Table to finish constructing the PCS code.

In addition to the *use* reference, the coder may also consult appendix D for Body Part Table or appendix E for the Device Table.

Code Tables

ICD-10-PCS contains 16 sections of Code Tables, represented by the numbers 0 through 9 and the letters B through D and F through H. The Tables are organized by general type of procedure. The three main sections of tables include:

1. **Medical and Surgical section**
   - Medical and Surgical (first character 0)
2. **Medical and Surgical Related sections**
   - Obstetrics (first character 1)
   - Placement (first character 2)
   - Administration (first character 3)
   - Measurement and Monitoring (first character 4)
   - Extracorporeal Assistance and Performance (first character 5)
   - Extracorporeal Therapies (first character 6)
   - Osteopathic (first character 7)
   - Other Procedures (first character 8)
   - Chiropractic (first character 9)
3. **Ancillary sections**
   - Imaging (first character B)
   - Nuclear Medicine (first character C)
   - Radiation Therapy (first character D)
   - Physical Rehabilitation and Diagnostic Audiology (first character F)
   - Mental Health (first character G)
   - Substance Abuse (first character H)

Each code table is defined by the first three characters of the PCS code. Each of these characters is displayed above the table. The table consists of all the options for characters 4 through 7. The root operation or root type, character 3, is present along with its official definition. Table 097 is provided here as an example of the table structure.

0 Medical and Surgical

9 Ear, Nose, Sinus

7 Dilation, Expanding an orifice or the lumen of a tubular body part

Body Part Character 4	Approach Character 5	Device Character 6	Qualifier Character 7
F Eustachian Tube, Right **G** Eustachian Tube, Left	**0** Open **7** Via Natural or Artificial Opening **8** Via Natural or Artificial Opening **Endoscopic**	**D** Intraluminal Device **Z** No Device	**Z** No Qualifier
F Eustachian Tube, Right **G** Eustachian Tube, Left	**3** Percutaneous **4** Percutaneous Endoscopic	**Z** No Device	**Z** No Qualifier

There can be multiple rows within the table for the first three characters, so the coder must carefully review all the applicable rows. Additionally, a table may cover multiple pages. Therefore, the coder must continue to review the code table options until the end of the table is reached to ensure the correct PCS code has been constructed.

Code Listing

Code Listings for the Medical and Surgical and Obstetrics sections are included in this manual to assist coders with ensuring that the intended code has been selected for reporting. The Code Listings are presented in alphanumeric order. Within the Code Listing, several additional conventions are included to assist coders with navigating the Medicare Code Editor (MCE) edits, official coding guidelines, and other reporting requirements such as the Inpatient Prospective Payment System (IPPS) Hospital-Acquired Conditions (HACs) related codes. The Code Listings are combined with the Tables section of the code book. In the Medical and Surgical section, the Code Listing appears after each body system. For the Obstetrics section, the Code Listing appears at the end of the section.

ICD-10-PCS Additional Conventions

The use of symbols has been added to this code book to alert the user to Medicare reimbursement logic and edits that are impacted by procedure coding. Some codes may be included in multiple reimbursement issues and, therefore, may have more than one symbol. For a quick reference review, the legend at the bottom of each page of the Code Listing (Medical/Surgical section and Obstetrics section) as well as the inside cover of the code book. The symbols are described in detail here.

Medicare Code Edits

Hospital inpatient Medicare claims paid under the IPPS are processed through the MCE prior to payment by the Medicare administrative contractor (MAC). The code edits are intended to ensure that all claims processed by the MAC are accurate and complete. Medicare has released an ICD-10 version of the MCE v31R and is provided to the general public as a tool to assist in the implementation of ICD-10-CM/PCS. The information in this manual is based on the MCE v31R.

Several of the MCE edits pertain to procedures. We have included identification of the codes included in these edits in this manual to assist users with preparing accurate and complete claims. The MCE edits included in this manual:

- Sex conflict
- Medicare non-covered procedures
- Medicare limited coverage procedures

Note: It is important to remember these edits are Medicare edits and may not apply to other third-party payers claim processing.

Sex Conflict Edit

The sex conflict edit is activated when the sex of the patient and the type of procedure performed does not match. The following symbols are used to identify female-only and male-only procedures.

♀ **Female-only** procedure: This symbol appears to the left of the applicable code in the code listing.

♂ **Male-only** procedure: This symbol appears to the left of the applicable code in the code listing.

Medicare Non-covered Procedure

Medicare does not reimburse for all ICD-10-PCS procedures. There are some procedures that are never reimbursed, and there are some procedures that are only reimbursed when certain specified diagnosis codes are also included on the claim. Non-covered procedures are designated by a red triangle symbol ▲ located next to the code description for the applicable code. If there is conditional logic for the non-coverage, it is provided to the right of the red triangle.

Medicare Limited Coverage Procedures

For certain procedures whose medical complexity and serious nature incur extraordinary associated costs, Medicare limits coverage to a portion of the cost. The limited coverage edit indicates this type of limited coverage. Limited coverage procedures are designated by a yellow triangle symbol located next to the code description for the applicable code. If there is conditional logic for the limited coverage, it is provided to the right of the yellow triangle.

MS-DRG Procedure Designations

The MS-DRG system is utilized within the IPPS to determine the unadjusted reimbursement amount for Medicare hospital inpatient claims. The MS-DRG Definitions Manual includes the logic for MS-DRG refinement and selection as well as logic based on the IPPS final rules released each August. CMS has released an ICD-10-CM/PCS version of the MS-DRG v31R. The information in this manual is based on the MS-DRG v31R. *Note:* It is important to remember that these edits are Medicare edits and may not apply to other third-party payers claim processing.

Non-Operating Room Procedures

Within the MS-DRG logic, CMS designates which procedures are operating room (OR) procedures and which procedures are non-OR procedures. Non-OR procedures do not impact the MS-DRG assignment; in the basic sense they do not covert medical MS-DRGs to surgical MS-DRGs. Once an encounter is determined as "surgical" specified OR procedures are utilized to refine the final MS-DRG assignment. Throughout the Medical and Surgical and Obstetrics sections, non-OR procedures are indicated with a purple dot ●. The purple dot symbol is located to the left of the applicable code in the code listing.

Hospital-Acquired Conditions Related Procedures

As part of the Medicare Value-Based Purchasing program, CMS has implemented a Paying for Value program entitled Hospital-Acquired Conditions (HACs). This program is designed to reduce reimbursements to facilities where value of the medical or surgical has been comprised due to preventable conditions. The HAC program identifies diagnosis and procedure codes that when reported as "not present on admission" activate the HAC reduced reimbursement logic. In this manual, the HAC-associated procedures are identified with an orange rectangle HAC with HAC. The orange rectangle is located below the code description in the code listing. If there is conditional logic for the procedure code, it is included to the right of the orange rectangle.

Combination Codes Required

Within the MS-DRG logic CMS has designated codes that must be reported with specified other codes in order to fully report a complete procedure. For such procedures, such as simultaneous pancreas and kidney transplants, if the correct combination of codes is not reported, the desired MS-DRG will not be calculated for the encounter. Combination codes are identified with a green box with a plus sign in the middle +. The green box with a code-specific note is located below the code description for applicable code in the code listing.

AHA Coding Clinic ® for ICD-10-CM and ICD-10-PCS

The American Hospital Association began publishing coding guidance for ICD-10-CM and ICD-10-PCS in the Fourth Quarter of 2012. In this code book we identify procedure codes that are discussed in the Coding Clinic guidance fourth quarter 2012 through second quarter 2014. Within the Code Listing the following sky blue note alerts the coder to review the AHA Coding Clinic prior to assignment of the code to ensure appropriate and accurate reporting. The quarter of publication, year and page number(s) are provided in the note.

AHA CC: 4Q; 2012; pg#-pg#

ICD-10-PCS Draft Coding Guidelines

The ICD-10-PCS Draft Coding Guidelines are presented throughout this manual. The Conventions and Selection of Principal Procedure sections are presented in the front of the manual prior to the start of the Alphabetical Index. The Medical and Surgical Section Guidelines are presented after the Introduction of the Medical and Surgical section. The Obstetric Section Guidelines are presented after the Introduction of the Obstetrics section.

Throughout the Code Listings, applicable guidelines are identified via an instruction note in order to remind users to reference the coding guidelines prior to code reporting. The instruction note *Review Coding Guideline…* followed by the guideline reference number is included after the section header for applicable sections or after the code description for applicable codes. It is imperative to review the ICD-10-PCS draft coding guidelines to ensure the procedure code being reported is accurate and complete.

ICD-10-PCS Official Guidelines for Coding and Reporting, 2015

The Centers for Medicare and Medicaid Services (CMS) and the National Center for Health Statistics (NCHS), two departments within the US federal government's Department of Health and Human Services (HHS) provide the following guidelines for coding and reporting using the International Classification of Diseases, 10th Revision, Procedure Coding System (ICD-10-PCS). These guidelines should be used as a companion document to the official version of the ICD-10-PCS as published on the CMS website. The ICD-10-PCS is a procedure classification published by the United States for classifying procedures performed in hospital inpatient health care settings.

These guidelines have been approved by the four organizations that make up the Cooperating Parties for the ICD-10-PCS: the American Hospital Association (AHA), the American Health Information Management Association (AHIMA), CMS, and NCHS.

These guidelines are a set of rules that have been developed to accompany and complement the official conventions and instructions provided within the ICD-10-PCS itself. The instructions and conventions of the classification take precedence over guidelines. These guidelines are based on the coding and sequencing instructions in the Tables, Index, and Definitions of ICD-10-PCS, but provide additional instruction. Adherence to these guidelines when assigning ICD-10-PCS procedure codes is required under the Health Insurance Portability and Accountability Act (HIPAA). The procedure codes have been adopted under HIPAA for hospital inpatient healthcare settings. A joint effort between the healthcare provider and the coder is essential to achieve complete and accurate documentation, code assignment, and reporting of diagnoses and procedures. These guidelines have been developed to assist both the healthcare provider and the coder in identifying those procedures that are to be reported. The importance of consistent, complete documentation in the medical record cannot be overemphasized. Without such documentation, accurate coding cannot be achieved.

Conventions

A1. ICD-10-PCS codes are composed of seven characters. Each character is an axis of classification that specifies information about the procedure performed. Within a defined code range, a character specifies the same type of information in that axis of classification.

Example: The fifth axis of classification specifies the approach in sections 0 through 4 and 7 through 9 of the system.

A2. One of 34 possible values can be assigned to each axis of classification in the seven-character code: they are the numbers 0 through 9 and the alphabet (except the letters I and O because they are easily confused with the numbers 1 and 0). The number of unique values used in an axis of classification differs as needed.

Example: Where the fifth axis of classification specifies the approach, seven different approach values are currently used to specify the approach.

A3. The valid values for an axis of classification can be added to as needed.

Example: If a significantly distinct type of device is used in a new procedure, a new device value can be added to the system.

A4. As with words in their context, the meaning of any single value is a combination of its axis of classification and any preceding values on which it may be dependent.

Example: The meaning of a body part value in the Medical and Surgical section is always dependent on the body system value. The body part value 0 in the Central Nervous body system specifies Brain and the body part value 0 in the Peripheral Nervous body system specifies Cervical Plexus.

A5. As the system is expanded to become increasingly detailed, more values will depend on preceding values for their meaning.

Example: In the Lower Joints body system, the device value 3 in the root operation Insertion specifies Infusion Device and the device value 3 in the root operation Replacement specifies Ceramic Synthetic Substitute.

A6. The purpose of the Alphabetic Index is to locate the appropriate table that contains all information necessary to construct a procedure code. The PCS Tables should always be consulted to find the most appropriate valid code.

A7. It is not required to consult the Index first before proceeding to the tables to complete the code. A valid code may be chosen directly from the Tables.

A8. All seven characters must be specified to be a valid code. If the documentation is incomplete for coding purposes, the physician should be queried for the necessary information.

A9. Within a PCS Table, valid codes include all combinations of choices in characters 4 through 7 contained in the same row of the table. In the example below, 0JHT3VZ is a valid code, and 0JHW3VZ is *not* a valid code.

Section: **0** **Medical and Surgical**
Body System: **J** **Subcutaneous Tissue and Fascia**
Operation: **H** **Insertion:** Putting in a nonbiological appliance that monitors, assists, performs, or prevents a physiological function but does not physically take the place of a body part

Body Part (4th)	Approach (5th)	Device (6th)	Qualifier (7th)
S Subcutaneous Tissue and Fascia, Head and Neck **V** Subcutaneous Tissue and Fascia, Upper Extremity **W** Subcutaneous Tissue and Fascia, Lower Extremity	**0** Open **3** Percutaneous	**1** Radioactive Element **3** Infusion Device	**Z** No Qualifier
T Subcutaneous Tissue and Fascia, Trunk	**0** Open **3** Percutaneous	**1** Radioactive Element **3** Infusion Device **V** Infusion Pump	**Z** No Qualifier

A10. "And," when used in a code description, means "and/or."

Example: Lower Arm and Wrist Muscle means lower arm and/or wrist muscle.

A11. Many of the terms used to construct PCS codes are defined within the system. It is the coder's responsibility to determine what the documentation in the medical record equates to in the PCS definitions. The physician is not expected to use the terms used in PCS code descriptions, nor is the coder required to query the physician when the correlation between the documentation and the defined PCS terms is clear.

Example: When the physician documents "partial resection" the coder can independently correlate "partial resection" to the root operation Excision without querying the physician for clarification.

Medical and Surgical Section Guidelines (section 0)

B2. Body System

General guidelines

B2.1a

The procedure codes in the general anatomical regions body systems should only be used when the procedure is performed on an anatomical region rather than a specific body part (e.g., root operations Control and Detachment, Drainage of a body cavity) or on the rare occasion when no information is available to support assignment of a code to a specific body part.

Example: Control of postoperative hemorrhage is coded to the root operation Control found in the general anatomical regions body systems.

B2.1b

Where the general body part values "upper" and "lower" are provided as an option in the Upper Arteries, Lower Arteries, Upper Veins, Lower Veins, Muscles and Tendons body systems, "upper" or "lower "specifies body parts located above or below the diaphragm respectively.

Example: Vein body parts above the diaphragm are found in the Upper Veins body system; vein body parts below the diaphragm are found in the Lower Veins body system.

B3. Root Operation

General guidelines

B3.1a

In order to determine the appropriate root operation, the full definition of the root operation as contained in the PCS Tables must be applied.

B3.1b

Components of a procedure specified in the root operation definition and explanation are not coded separately. Procedural steps necessary to reach the operative site and close the operative site, including anastomosis of a tubular body part, are also not coded separately.

Example: Resection of a joint as part of a joint replacement procedure is included in the root operation definition of Replacement and is not coded separately. Laparotomy performed to reach the site of an open liver biopsy is not coded separately. In a resection of sigmoid colon with anastomosis of descending colon to rectum, the anastomosis is not coded separately.

Multiple procedures

B3.2

During the same operative episode, multiple procedures are coded if:

a. The same root operation is performed on different body parts as defined by distinct values of the body part character.

   Example: Diagnostic excision of liver and pancreas are coded separately.

b. The same root operation is repeated at different body sites that are included in the same body part value.

   Example: Excision of the sartorius muscle and excision of the gracilis muscle are both included in the upper leg muscle body part value, and multiple procedures are coded.

c. Multiple root operations with distinct objectives are performed on the same body part.

   Example: Destruction of sigmoid lesion and bypass of sigmoid colon are coded separately.

d. The intended root operation is attempted using one approach, but is converted to a different approach.

   Example: Laparoscopic cholecystectomy converted to an open cholecystectomy is coded as percutaneous endoscopic Inspection and open Resection.

Discontinued procedures

B3.3

If the intended procedure is discontinued, code the procedure to the root operation performed. If a procedure is discontinued before any other root operation is performed, code the root operation Inspection of the body part or anatomical region inspected.

Example: A planned aortic valve replacement procedure is discontinued after the initial thoracotomy and before any incision is made in the heart muscle, when the patient becomes hemodynamically unstable. This procedure is coded as an open Inspection of the mediastinum.

Biopsy procedures

B3.4a

Biopsy procedures are coded using the root operations Excision, Extraction, or Drainage and the qualifier Diagnostic. The qualifier Diagnostic is used only for biopsies.

Examples: Fine needle aspiration biopsy of lung is coded to the root operation Drainage with the qualifier Diagnostic. Biopsy of bone marrow is coded to the root operation Extraction with the qualifier Diagnostic. Lymph node sampling for biopsy is coded to the root operation Excision with the qualifier Diagnostic.

Biopsy followed by more definitive treatment

B3.4b

If a diagnostic Excision, Extraction, or Drainage procedure (biopsy) is followed by a more definitive procedure, such as Destruction, Excision or Resection at the same procedure site, both the biopsy and the more definitive treatment are coded.

Example: Biopsy of breast followed by partial mastectomy at the same procedure site, both the biopsy and the partial mastectomy procedure are coded.

Overlapping body layers

B3.5

If the root operations Excision, Repair or Inspection are performed on overlapping layers of the musculoskeletal system, the body part specifying the deepest layer is coded.

Example: Excisional debridement that includes skin and subcutaneous tissue and muscle is coded to the muscle body part.

Bypass procedures

B3.6a

Bypass procedures are coded by identifying the body part bypassed "from" and the body part bypassed "to." The fourth character body part specifies the body part bypassed from, and the qualifier specifies the body part bypassed to.

Example: Bypass from stomach to jejunum, stomach is the body part and jejunum is the qualifier.

B3.6b

Coronary arteries are classified by number of distinct sites treated, rather than number of coronary arteries or anatomic name of a coronary artery (e.g., left anterior descending). Coronary artery bypass procedures are coded differently than other bypass procedures as described in the previous guideline. Rather than identifying the body part bypassed from, the body part identifies the number of coronary artery sites bypassed to, and the qualifier specifies the vessel bypassed from.

Example: Aortocoronary artery bypass of one site on the left anterior descending coronary artery and one site on the obtuse marginal coronary artery is classified in the body part axis of classification as two coronary artery sites and the qualifier specifies the aorta as the body part bypassed from.

B3.6c

If multiple coronary artery sites are bypassed, a separate procedure is coded for each coronary artery site that uses a different device and/or qualifier.

Example: Aortocoronary artery bypass and internal mammary coronary artery bypass are coded separately.

Control vs. more definitive root operations

B3.7

The root operation Control is defined as, "Stopping, or attempting to stop, postprocedural bleeding." If an attempt to stop postprocedural bleeding is initially unsuccessful, and to stop the bleeding requires performing any of the definitive root operations Bypass, Detachment, Excision, Extraction, Reposition, Replacement, or Resection, then that root operation is coded instead of Control.

Example: Resection of spleen to stop postprocedural bleeding is coded to Resection instead of Control.

Excision vs. Resection

B3.8

PCS contains specific body parts for anatomical subdivisions of a body part, such as lobes of the lungs or liver and regions of the intestine. Resection of the specific body part is coded whenever all of the body part is cut out or off, rather than coding Excision of a less specific body part.

Example: Left upper lung lobectomy is coded to Resection of Upper Lung Lobe, Left rather than Excision of Lung, Left.

Excision for graft

B3.9

If an autograft is obtained from a different body part in order to complete the objective of the procedure, a separate procedure is coded.

Example: Coronary bypass with excision of saphenous vein graft, excision of saphenous vein is coded separately.

Fusion procedures of the spine

B3.10a

The body part coded for a spinal vertebral joint(s) rendered immobile by a spinal fusion procedure is classified by the level of the spine (e.g. thoracic). There are distinct body part values for a single vertebral joint and for multiple vertebral joints at each spinal level.

Example: Body part values specify Lumbar Vertebral Joint, Lumbar Vertebral Joints, 2 or More and Lumbosacral Vertebral Joint.

B3.10b

If multiple vertebral joints are fused, a separate procedure is coded for each vertebral joint that uses a different device and/or qualifier.

Example: Fusion of lumbar vertebral joint, posterior approach, anterior column and fusion of lumbar vertebral joint, posterior approach, posterior column are coded separately.

B3.10c

Combinations of devices and materials are often used on a vertebral joint to render the joint immobile. When combinations of devices are used on the same vertebral joint, the device value coded for the procedure is as follows:

- If an interbody fusion device is used to render the joint immobile (alone or containing other material like bone graft), the procedure is coded with the device value Interbody Fusion Device
- If bone graft is the *only* device used to render the joint immobile, the procedure is coded with the device value Nonautologous Tissue Substitute or Autologous Tissue Substitute
- If a mixture of autologous and nonautologous bone graft (with or without biological or synthetic extenders or binders) is used to render the joint immobile, code the procedure with the device value Autologous Tissue Substitute

Examples: Fusion of a vertebral joint using a cage style interbody fusion device containing morsellized bone graft is coded to the device Interbody Fusion Device. Fusion of a vertebral joint using a bone dowel interbody fusion device made of cadaver bone and packed with a mixture of local morsellized bone and demineralized bone matrix is coded to the device Interbody Fusion Device.

Fusion of a vertebral joint using both autologous bone graft and bone bank bone graft is coded to the device Autologous Tissue Substitute.

Inspection procedures
B3.11a
Inspection of a body part(s) performed in order to achieve the objective of a procedure is not coded separately.

Example: Fiberoptic bronchoscopy performed for irrigation of bronchus, only the irrigation procedure is coded.

B3.11b
If multiple tubular body parts are inspected, the most distal body part inspected is coded. If multiple non-tubular body parts in a region are inspected, the body part that specifies the entire area inspected is coded.

Examples: Cystoureteroscopy with inspection of bladder and ureters is coded to the ureter body part value.

Exploratory laparotomy with general inspection of abdominal contents is coded to the peritoneal cavity body part value.

B3.11c
When both an Inspection procedure and another procedure are performed on the same body part during the same episode, if the Inspection procedure is performed using a different approach than the other procedure, the Inspection procedure is coded separately. *Example*: Endoscopic Inspection of the duodenum is coded separately when open Excision of the duodenum is performed during the same procedural episode.

Occlusion vs. Restriction for vessel embolization procedures
B3.12
If the objective of an embolization procedure is to completely close a vessel, the root operation Occlusion is coded. If the objective of an embolization procedure is to narrow the lumen of a vessel, the root operation Restriction is coded.

Examples: Tumor embolization is coded to the root operation Occlusion, because the objective of the procedure is to cut off the blood supply to the vessel.

Embolization of a cerebral aneurysm is coded to the root operation Restriction, because the objective of the procedure is not to close off the vessel entirely, but to narrow the lumen of the vessel at the site of the aneurysm where it is abnormally wide.

Release procedures
B3.13
In the root operation Release, the body part value coded is the body part being freed and not the tissue being manipulated or cut to free the body part.

Example: Lysis of intestinal adhesions is coded to the specific intestine body part value.

Release vs. Division
B3.14
If the sole objective of the procedure is freeing a body part without cutting the body part, the root operation is Release. If the sole objective of the procedure is separating or transecting a body part, the root operation is Division.

Examples: Freeing a nerve root from surrounding scar tissue to relieve pain is coded to the root operation Release. Severing a nerve root to relieve pain is coded to the root operation Division.

Reposition for fracture treatment
B3.15
Reduction of a displaced fracture is coded to the root operation Reposition and the application of a cast or splint in conjunction with the Reposition procedure is not coded separately. Treatment of a nondisplaced fracture is coded to the procedure performed.

Examples: Casting of a nondisplaced fracture is coded to the root operation Immobilization in the Placement section.

Putting a pin in a nondisplaced fracture is coded to the root operation Insertion.

Transplantation vs. Administration
B3.16
Putting in a mature and functioning living body part taken from another individual or animal is coded to the root operation Transplantation. Putting in autologous or nonautologous cells is coded to the Administration section.

Example: Putting in autologous or nonautologous bone marrow, pancreatic islet cells or stem cells is coded to the Administration section.

B4. Body Part
General guidelines
B4.1a
If a procedure is performed on a portion of a body part that does not have a separate body part value, code the body part value corresponding to the whole body part.

Example: A procedure performed on the alveolar process of the mandible is coded to the mandible body part.

B4.1b

If the prefix "peri" is combined with a body part to identify the site of the procedure, the procedure is coded to the body part named.

Example: A procedure site identified as perirenal is coded to the kidney body part.

Branches of body parts

B4.2

Where a specific branch of a body part does not have its own body part value in PCS, the body part is coded to the closest proximal branch that has a specific body part value.

Example: A procedure performed on the mandibular branch of the trigeminal nerve is coded to the trigeminal nerve body part value.

Bilateral body part values

B4.3

Bilateral body part values are available for a limited number of body parts. If the identical procedure is performed on contralateral body parts, and a bilateral body part value exists for that body part, a single procedure is coded using the bilateral body part value. If no bilateral body part value exists, each procedure is coded separately using the appropriate body part value.

Example: The identical procedure performed on both fallopian tubes is coded once using the body part value Fallopian Tube, Bilateral. The identical procedure performed on both knee joints is coded twice using the body part values Knee Joint, Right and Knee Joint, Left.

Coronary arteries

B4.4

The coronary arteries are classified as a single body part that is further specified by number of sites treated and not by name or number of arteries. Separate body part values are used to specify the number of sites treated when the same procedure is performed on multiple sites in the coronary arteries.

Examples: Angioplasty of two distinct sites in the left anterior descending coronary artery with placement of two stents is coded as Dilation of Coronary Arteries, Two Sites, with Intraluminal Device.

Angioplasty of two distinct sites in the left anterior descending coronary artery, one with stent placed and one without, is coded separately as Dilation of Coronary Artery, One Site with Intraluminal Device, and Dilation of Coronary Artery, One Site with no device.

Tendons, ligaments, bursae and fascia near a joint

B4.5

Procedures performed on tendons, ligaments, bursae and fascia supporting a joint are coded to the body part in the respective body system that is the focus of the procedure. Procedures performed on joint structures themselves are coded to the body part in the joint body systems.

Example: Repair of the anterior cruciate ligament of the knee is coded to the knee bursaand ligament body part in the bursae and ligaments body system. Knee arthroscopy with shaving of articular cartilage is coded to the knee joint body part in the Lower Joints body system.

Skin, subcutaneous tissue and fascia overlying a joint

B4.6

If a procedure is performed on the skin, subcutaneous tissue or fascia overlying a joint, the procedure is coded to the following body part:

- Shoulder is coded to Upper Arm
- Elbow is coded to Lower Arm
- Wrist is coded to Lower Arm
- Hip is coded to Upper Leg
- Knee is coded to Lower Leg
- Ankle is coded to Foot

Fingers and toes

B4.7

If a body system does not contain a separate body part value for fingers, procedures performed on the fingers are coded to the body part value for the hand. If a body system does not contain a separate body part value for toes, procedures performed on the toes are coded to the body part value for the foot.

Example: Excision of finger muscle is coded to one of the hand muscle body part values in the Muscles body system.

Upper and lower intestinal tract

B4.8

In the Gastrointestinal body system, the general body part values Upper Intestinal Tract and Lower Intestinal Tract are provided as an option for the root operations Change, Inspection, Removal and Revision. Upper Intestinal Tract includes the portion of the gastrointestinal tract from the esophagus down to and including the duodenum, and Lower Intestinal Tract includes the portion of the gastrointestinal tract from the jejunum down to and including the rectum and anus.

Example: In the root operation Change table, change of a device in the jejunum is coded using the body part Lower Intestinal Tract.

B5. Approach

Open approach with percutaneous endoscopic assistance

B5.2

Procedures performed using the open approach with percutaneous endoscopic assistance are coded to the approach Open.

Example: Laparoscopic-assisted sigmoidectomy is coded to the approach Open.

External approach

B5.3a

Procedures performed within an orifice on structures that are visible without the aid of any instrumentation are coded to the approach External.

Example: Resection of tonsils is coded to the approach External.

B5.3b

Procedures performed indirectly by the application of external force through the intervening body layers are coded to the approach External.

Example: Closed reduction of fracture is coded to the approach External.

Percutaneous procedure via device

B5.4

Procedures performed percutaneously via a device placed for the procedure are coded to the approach Percutaneous.

Example: Fragmentation of kidney stone performed via percutaneous nephrostomy is coded to the approach Percutaneous.

B6. Device

General guidelines

B6.1a

A device is coded only if a device remains after the procedure is completed. If no device remains, the device value No Device is coded.

B6.1b

Materials such as sutures, ligatures, radiological markers and temporary post-operative wound drains are considered integral to the performance of a procedure and are not coded as devices.

B6.1c

Procedures performed on a device only and not on a body part are specified in the root operations Change, Irrigation, Removal and Revision, and are coded to the procedure performed.

Example: Irrigation of percutaneous nephrostomy tube is coded to the root operation

Irrigation of indwelling device in the Administration section.

Drainage device

B6.2

A separate procedure to put in a drainage device is coded to the root operation Drainage with the device value Drainage Device.

Obstetric Section Guidelines (section 1)

C. Obstetrics Section

Products of conception

C1

Procedures performed on the products of conception are coded to the Obstetrics section. Procedures performed on the pregnant female other than the products of conception are coded to the appropriate root operation in the Medical and Surgical section.

Example: Amniocentesis is coded to the products of conception body part in the Obstetrics section. Repair of obstetric urethral laceration is coded to the urethra body part in the Medical and Surgical section.

Procedures following delivery or abortion

C2

Procedures performed following a delivery or abortion for curettage of the endometrium or evacuation of retained products of conception are all coded in the Obstetrics section, to the root operation Extraction and the body part Products of Conception, Retained. Diagnostic or therapeutic dilation and curettage performed during times other than the postpartum or post-abortion period are all coded in the Medical and Surgical section, to the root operation Extraction and the body part Endometrium.

Selection of Principal Procedure

The following instructions should be applied in the selection of principal procedure and clarification on the importance of the relation to the principal diagnosis when more than one procedure is performed:

1. Procedure performed for definitive treatment of both principal diagnosis and secondary diagnosis
   a. Sequence procedure performed for definitive treatment most related to principal diagnosis as principal procedure.
2. Procedure performed for definitive treatment and diagnostic procedures performed for both principal diagnosis and secondary diagnosis
   a. Sequence procedure performed for definitive treatment most related to principal diagnosis as principal procedure
3. A diagnostic procedure was performed for the principal diagnosis and a procedure is performed for definitive treatment of a secondary diagnosis.
   a. Sequence diagnostic procedure as principal procedure, since the procedure most related to the principal diagnosis takes precedence.
4. No procedures performed that are related to principal diagnosis; procedures performed for definitive treatment and diagnostic procedures were performed for secondary diagnosis
   a. Sequence procedure performed for definitive treatment of secondary diagnosis as principal procedure, since there are no procedures (definitive or nondefinitive treatment) related to principal diagnosis.

3

A

B

Beam Radiation *(continued)*
- Glands
  - Intraoperative D9063Z0
  - Salivary D906
- Head and Neck DW01
  - Intraoperative DW013Z0
- Hemibody DW04
  - Intraoperative DW043Z0
- Humerus DP06
  - Intraoperative DP063Z0
- Hypopharynx D903
  - Intraoperative D9033Z0
- Ileum DD04
  - Intraoperative DD043Z0
- Jejunum DD03
  - Intraoperative DD033Z0
- Kidney DT00
  - Intraoperative DT003Z0
- Larynx D90B
  - Intraoperative D90B3Z0
- Liver DF00
  - Intraoperative DF003Z0
- Lung DB02
  - Intraoperative DB023Z0
- Lymphatics
  - Abdomen D706
    - Intraoperative D7063Z0
  - Axillary D704
    - Intraoperative D7043Z0
  - Inguinal D708
    - Intraoperative D7083Z0
  - Neck D703
    - Intraoperative D7033Z0
  - Pelvis D707
    - Intraoperative D7073Z0
  - Thorax D705
    - Intraoperative D7053Z0
- Mandible DP03
  - Intraoperative DP033Z0
- Maxilla DP02
  - Intraoperative DP023Z0
- Mediastinum DB06
  - Intraoperative DB063Z0
- Mouth D904
  - Intraoperative D9043Z0
- Nasopharynx D90D
  - Intraoperative D90D3Z0
- Neck and Head DW01
  - Intraoperative DW013Z0
- Nerve
  - Intraoperative D0073Z0
  - Peripheral D007
- Nose D901
  - Intraoperative D9013Z0
- Oropharynx D90F
  - Intraoperative D90F3Z0
- Ovary DU00
  - Intraoperative DU003Z0
- Palate
  - Hard D908
    - Intraoperative D9083Z0
  - Soft D909
    - Intraoperative D9093Z0
- Pancreas DF03
  - Intraoperative DF033Z0
- Parathyroid Gland DG04
  - Intraoperative DG043Z0
- Pelvic Bones DP08
  - Intraoperative DP083Z0
- Pelvic Region DW06
  - Intraoperative DW063Z0
- Pineal Body DG01
  - Intraoperative DG013Z0
- Pituitary Gland DG00
  - Intraoperative DG003Z0
- Pleura DB05
  - Intraoperative DB053Z0
- Prostate DV00
  - Intraoperative DV003Z0
- Radius DP07
  - Intraoperative DP073Z0

Beam Radiation *(continued)*
- Rectum DD07
  - Intraoperative DD073Z0
- Rib DP05
  - Intraoperative DP053Z0
- Sinuses D907
  - Intraoperative D9073Z0
- Skin
  - Abdomen DH08
    - Intraoperative DH083Z0
  - Arm DH04
    - Intraoperative DH043Z0
  - Back DH07
    - Intraoperative DH073Z0
  - Buttock DH09
    - Intraoperative DH093Z0
  - Chest DH06
    - Intraoperative DH063Z0
  - Face DH02
    - Intraoperative DH023Z0
  - Leg DH0B
    - Intraoperative DH0B3Z0
  - Neck DH03
    - Intraoperative DH033Z0
- Skull DP00
  - Intraoperative DP003Z0
- Spinal Cord D006
  - Intraoperative D0063Z0
- Spleen D702
  - Intraoperative D7023Z0
- Sternum DP04
  - Intraoperative DP043Z0
- Stomach DD01
  - Intraoperative DD013Z0
- Testis DV01
  - Intraoperative DV013Z0
- Thymus D701
  - Intraoperative D7013Z0
- Thyroid Gland DG05
  - Intraoperative DG053Z0
- Tibia DP0B
  - Intraoperative DP0B3Z0
- Tongue D905
  - Intraoperative D9053Z0
- Trachea DB00
  - Intraoperative DB003Z0
- Ulna DP07
  - Intraoperative DP073Z0
- Ureter DT01
  - Intraoperative DT013Z0
- Urethra DT03
  - Intraoperative DT033Z0
- Uterus DU02
  - Intraoperative DU023Z0
- Whole Body DW05
  - Intraoperative DW053Z0

Bedside swallow F00ZJWZ

Berlin Heart Ventricular Assist Device
- *use* Implantable Heart Assist System in Heart and Great Vessels

Biceps brachii muscle
- *use* Muscle, Upper Arm, Left
- *use* Muscle, Upper Arm, Right

Biceps femoris muscle
- *use* Muscle, Upper Leg, Left
- *use* Muscle, Upper Leg, Right

Bicipital aponeurosis
- *use* Subcutaneous Tissue and Fascia, Lower Arm, Left
- *use* Subcutaneous Tissue and Fascia, Lower Arm, Right

Bicuspid valve
- *use* Valve, Mitral

Bililite therapy
- *see* Ultraviolet Light Therapy, Skin 6A80

Bioactive embolization coil(s)
- *use* Intraluminal Device, Bioactive in Upper Arteries

Biofeedback GZC9ZZZ

Biopsy
- *see* Drainage with qualifier Diagnostic
- *see* Excision with qualifier Diagnostic
- Bone Marrow
  - *see* Extraction with qualifier Diagnostic

BiPAP
- *see* Assistance, Respiratory v5A09

Bisection
- *see* Division

Biventricular external heart assist system
- *use* External Heart Assist System in Heart and Great Vessels

Blepharectomy
- *see* Excision, Eye 08B
- *see* Resection, Eye 08T

Blepharoplasty
- *see* Repair, Eye 08Q
- *see* Replacement, Eye 08R
- *see* Reposition, Eye 08S
- *see* Supplement, Eye 08U

Blepharorrhaphy
- *see* Repair, Eye 08Q

Blepharotomy
- *see* Drainage, Eye 089

Block, Nerve, anesthetic injection 3E0T3CZ

Blood glucose monitoring system
- *use* Monitoring Device

Blood pressure
- *see* Measurement, Arterial 4A03

BMR (basal metabolic rate)
- *see* Measurement, Physiological Systems 4A0Z

Body of femur
- *use* Femoral Shaft, Left
- *use* Femoral Shaft, Right

Body of fibula
- *use* Fibula, Left
- *use* Fibula, Right

Bone anchored hearing device
- *use* Hearing Device, Bone Conduction in 09H
- *use* Hearing Device in Head and Facial Bones

Bone bank bone graft
- *use* Nonautologous Tissue Substitute

Bone Growth Stimulator
- Insertion of device in
  - Bone
    - Facial 0NHW
    - Lower 0QHY
    - Nasal 0NHB
    - Upper 0PHY
  - Skull 0NH0
- Removal of device from
  - Bone
    - Facial 0NPW
    - Lower 0QPY
    - Nasal 0NPB
    - Upper 0PPY
  - Skull 0NP0
- Revision of device in
  - Bone
    - Facial 0NWW
    - Lower 0QWY
    - Nasal 0NWB
    - Upper 0PWY
  - Skull 0NW0

Bone marrow transplant
- *see* Transfusion

Bone morphogenetic protein 2 (BMP 2)
- *use* Recombinant Bone Morphogenetic Protein

Bone screw (interlocking)(lag)(pedicle)(recessed)
- *use* Internal Fixation Device in Head and Facial Bones

Bone screw *(continued)*
- *use* Internal Fixation Device in Lower Bones
- *use* Internal Fixation Device in Upper Bones

Bony labyrinth
- *use* Ear, Inner, Left
- *use* Ear, Inner, Right

Bony orbit
- *use* Orbit, Left
- *use* Orbit, Right

Bony vestibule
- *use* Ear, Inner, Left
- *use* Ear, Inner, Right

Botallo's duct
- *use* Artery, Pulmonary, Left

Bovine pericardial valve
- *use* Zooplastic Tissue in Heart and Great Vessels

Bovine pericardium graft
- *use* Zooplastic Tissue in Heart and Great Vessels

BP (blood pressure)
- *see* Measurement, Arterial 4A03

Brachial (lateral) lymph node
- *use* Lymphatic, Axillary, Left
- *use* Lymphatic, Axillary, Right

Brachialis muscle
- *use* Muscle, Upper Arm, Left
- *use* Muscle, Upper Arm, Right

Brachiocephalic artery
- *use* Artery, Innominate

Brachiocephalic trunk
- *use* Artery, Innominate

Brachiocephalic vein
- *use* Vein, Innominate, Left
- *use* Vein, Innominate, Right

Brachioradialis muscle
- *use* Muscle, Lower Arm and Wrist, Left
- *use* Muscle, Lower Arm and Wrist, Right

Brachytherapy
- Abdomen DW13
- Adrenal Gland DG12
- Bile Ducts DF12
- Bladder DT12
- Bone Marrow D710
- Brain D010
- Brain Stem D011
- Breast
  - Left DM10
  - Right DM11
- Bronchus DB11
- Cervix DU11
- Chest DW12
- Chest Wall DB17
- Colon DD15
- Diaphragm DB18
- Duodenum DD12
- Ear D910
- Esophagus DD10
- Eye D810
- Gallbladder DF11
- Gland
  - Adrenal DG12
  - Parathyroid DG14
  - Pituitary DG10
  - Thyroid DG15
- Glands, Salivary D916
- Head and Neck DW11
- Hypopharynx D913
- Ileum DD14
- Jejunum DD13
- Kidney DT10
- Larynx D91B
- Liver DF10
- Lung DB12
- Lymphatics
  - Abdomen D716
  - Axillary D714
  - Inguinal D718

C

Capsulorrhaphy, joint
- *see* Repair, Lower Joints 0SQ
- *see* Repair, Upper Joints 0RQ

Cardia
- *use* Esophagogastric Junction

Cardiac contractility modulation lead
- *use* Cardiac Lead in Heart and Great Vessels

Cardiac event recorder
- *use* Monitoring Device

Cardiac Lead
- Defibrillator
  - Atrium
    - Left 02H7
    - Right 02H6
  - Pericardium 02HN
  - Vein, Coronary 02H4
  - Ventricle
    - Left 02HL
    - Right 02HK
- Insertion of device in
  - Atrium
    - Left 02H7Z
    - Right 02H6
  - Pericardium 02HN
  - Vein, Coronary 02H4
  - Ventricle
    - Left 02HL
    - Right 02HK
- Pacemaker
  - Atrium
    - Left 02H7
    - Right 02H6
  - Pericardium 02HN
  - Vein, Coronary 02H4
  - Ventricle
    - Left 02HL
    - Right 02HK
- Removal of device from, Heart 02PA
- Revision of device in, Heart 02WA

Cardiac plexus
- *use* Nerve, Thoracic Sympathetic

Cardiac Resynchronization Defibrillator Pulse Generator
- Abdomen 0JH8
- Chest 0JH6

Cardiac Resynchronization Pacemaker Pulse Generator
- Abdomen 0JH8
- Chest 0JH6

Cardiac resynchronization therapy (CRT) lead
- *use* Cardiac Lead, Defibrillator in 02H
- *use* Cardiac Lead, Pacemaker in 02H

Cardiac Rhythm Related Device
- Insertion of device in
  - Abdomen 0JH8
  - Chest 0JH6
- Removal of device from, Subcutaneous Tissue and Fascia, Trunk 0JPT
- Revision of device in, Subcutaneous Tissue and Fascia, Trunk 0JWT

Cardiocentesis
- *see* Drainage, Pericardial Cavity 0W9D

Cardioesophageal junction
- *use* Esophagogastric Junction

Cardiolysis
- *see* Release, Heart and Great Vessels 02N

CardioMEMS® pressure sensor
- *use* Monitoring Device, Pressure Sensor in 02H

Cardiomyotomy
- *see* Division, Esophagogastric Junction 0D84

Cardioplegia
- *see* Introduction of substance in or on, Heart 3E08

Cardiorrhaphy
- *see* Repair, Heart and Great Vessels 02Q

Cardioversion 5A2204Z

Caregiver Training F0FZ

Caroticotympanic artery
- *use* Artery, Internal Carotid, Left
- *use* Artery, Internal Carotid, Right

Carotid (artery) sinus (baroreceptor) lead
- *use* Stimulator Lead in Upper Arteries

Carotid glomus
- *use* Carotid Bodies, Bilateral
- *use* Carotid Body, Left
- *use* Carotid Body, Right

Carotid sinus
- *use* Artery, Internal Carotid, Left
- *use* Artery, Internal Carotid, Right

Carotid sinus nerve
- *use* Nerve, Glossopharyngeal

Carotid WALLSTENT® Monorail® Endoprosthesis
- *use* Intraluminal Device

Carpectomy
- *see* Excision, Upper Bones 0PB
- *see* Resection, Upper Bones 0PT

Carpometacarpal (CMC) joint
- *use* Joint, Metacarpocarpal, Left
- *use* Joint, Metacarpocarpal, Right

Carpometacarpal ligament
- *use* Bursa and Ligament, Hand, Left
- *use* Bursa and Ligament, Hand, Right

Casting
- *see* Immobilization

CAT scan
- *see* Computerized Tomography (CT Scan)

Catheterization
- *see* Dilation
- *see* Drainage
- Heart
  - *see* Measurement, Cardiac 4A02
- *see* Irrigation
- *see* Insertion of device in
- Umbilical vein, for infusion 06H033T

Cauda equina
- *use* Spinal Cord, Lumbar

Cauterization
- *see* Destruction
- *see* Repair

Cavernous plexus
- *use* Nerve, Head and Neck Sympathetic

Cecectomy
- *see* Excision, Cecum 0DBH
- *see* Resection, Cecum 0DTH

Cecocolostomy
- *see* Bypass, Gastrointestinal System 0D1
- *see* Drainage, Gastrointestinal System 0D9

Cecopexy
- *see* Repair, Cecum 0DQH
- *see* Reposition, Cecum 0DSH

Cecoplication
- *see* Restriction, Cecum 0DVH

Cecorrhaphy
- *see* Repair, Cecum 0DQH

Cecostomy
- *see* Bypass, Cecum 0D1H
- *see* Drainage, Cecum 0D9H

Cecotomy
- *see* Drainage, Cecum 0D9H

Celiac (solar) plexus
- *use* Nerve, Abdominal Sympathetic

Celiac ganglion
- *use* Nerve, Abdominal Sympathetic

Celiac lymph node
- *use* Lymphatic, Aortic

Celiac trunk
- *use* Artery, Celiac

Central axillary lymph node
- *use* Lymphatic, Axillary, Left
- *use* Lymphatic, Axillary, Right

Central venous pressure
- *see* Measurement, Venous 4A04

Centrimag® Blood Pump
- *use* External Heart Assist System in Heart and Great Vessels

Cephalogram BN00ZZZ

Cerclage
- *see* Restriction

Cerebral aqueduct (Sylvius)
- *use* Cerebral Ventricle

Cerebrum
- *use* Brain

Cervical esophagus
- *use* Esophagus, Upper

Cervical facet joint
- *use* Joint, Cervical Vertebral
- *use* Joint, Cervical Vertebral, 2 or more

Cervical ganglion
- *use* Nerve, Head and Neck Sympathetic

Cervical interspinous ligament
- *use* Bursa and Ligament, Head and Neck

Cervical intertransverse ligament
- *use* Bursa and Ligament, Head and Neck

Cervical ligamentum flavum
- *use* Bursa and Ligament, Head and Neck

Cervical lymph node
- *use* Lymphatic, Neck, Left
- *use* Lymphatic, Neck, Right

Cervicectomy
- *see* Excision, Cervix 0UBC
- *see* Resection, Cervix 0UTC

Cervicothoracic facet joint
- *use* Joint, Cervicothoracic Vertebral

Cesarean section
- *see* Extraction, Products of Conception 10D0

Change device in
- Abdominal Wall 0W2FX
- Back
  - Lower 0W2LX
  - Upper 0W2KX
- Bladder 0T2BX
- Bone
  - Facial 0N2WX
  - Lower 0Q2YX
  - Nasal 0N2BX
  - Upper 0P2YX
- Bone Marrow 072TX
- Brain 0020X
- Breast
  - Left 0H2UX
  - Right 0H2TX
- Bursa and Ligament
  - Lower 0M2YX
  - Upper 0M2XX
- Cavity, Cranial 0W21X
- Chest Wall 0W28X
- Cisterna Chyli 072LX
- Diaphragm 0B2TX
- Duct
  - Hepatobiliary 0F2BX
  - Pancreatic 0F2DX
- Ear
  - Left 092JX
  - Right 092HX
- Epididymis and Spermatic Cord 0V2MX
- Extremity
  - Lower

Change device in *(continued)*
- Extremity *(continued)*
  - Lower *(continued)*
    - Left 0Y2BX
    - Right 0Y29X
  - Upper
    - Left 0X27X
    - Right 0X26X
- Eye
  - Left 0821X
  - Right 0820X
- Face 0W22X
- Fallopian Tube 0U28X
- Gallbladder 0F24X
- Gland
  - Adrenal 0G25X
  - Endocrine 0G2SX
  - Pituitary 0G20X
  - Salivary 0C2AX
- Head 0W20X
- Intestinal Tract
  - Lower 0D2DXUZ
  - Upper 0D20XUZ
- Jaw
  - Lower 0W25X
  - Upper 0W24X
- Joint
  - Lower 0S2YX
  - Upper 0R2YX
- Kidney 0T25X
- Larynx 0C2SX
- Liver 0F20X
- Lung
  - Left 0B2LX
  - Right 0B2KX
- Lymphatic 072NX
  - Thoracic Duct 072KX
- Mediastinum 0W2CX
- Mesentery 0D2VX
- Mouth and Throat 0C2YX
- Muscle
  - Lower 0K2YX
  - Upper 0K2XX
- Neck 0W26X
- Nerve
  - Cranial 002EX
  - Peripheral 012YX
- Nose 092KX
- Omentum 0D2UX
- Ovary 0U23X
- Pancreas 0F2GX
- Parathyroid Gland 0G2RX
- Pelvic Cavity 0W2JX
- Penis 0V2SX
- Pericardial Cavity 0W2DX
- Perineum
  - Female 0W2NX
  - Male 0W2MX
- Peritoneal Cavity 0W2GX
- Peritoneum 0D2WX
- Pineal Body 0G21X
- Pleura 0B2QX
- Pleural Cavity
  - Left 0W2BX
  - Right 0W29X
- Products of Conception 10207
- Prostate and Seminal Vesicles 0V24X
- Retroperitoneum 0W2HX
- Scrotum and Tunica Vaginalis 0V28X
- Sinus 092YX
- Skin 0H2PX
- Skull 0N20X
- Spinal Canal 002UX
- Spleen 072PX
- Subcutaneous Tissue and Fascia
  - Head and Neck 0J2SX
  - Lower Extremity 0J2WX
  - Trunk 0J2TX
  - Upper Extremity 0J2VX

Change device in *(continued)*
Tendon
Lower 0L2YX
Upper 0L2XX
Testis 0V2DX
Thymus 072MX
Thyroid Gland 0G2KX
Trachea 0B21
Tracheobronchial Tree 0B20X
Ureter 0T29X
Urethra 0T2DX
Uterus and Cervix 0U2DXHZ
Vagina and Cul-de-sac 0U2HXGZ
Vas Deferens 0V2RX
Vulva 0U2MX
Change device in or on
Abdominal Wall 2W03X
Anorectal 2Y03X5Z
Arm
Lower
Left 2W0DX
Right 2W0CX
Upper
Left 2W0BX
Right 2W0AX
Back 2W05X
Chest Wall 2W04X
Ear 2Y02X5Z
Extremity
Lower
Left 2W0MX
Right 2W0LX
Upper
Left 2W09X
Right 2W08X
Face 2W01X
Finger
Left 2W0KX
Right 2W0JX
Foot
Left 2W0TX
Right 2W0SX
Genital Tract, Female 2Y04X5Z
Hand
Left 2W0FX
Right 2W0EX
Head 2W00X
Inguinal Region
Left 2W07X
Right 2W06X
Leg
Lower
Left 2W0RX
Right 2W0QX
Upper
Left 2W0PX
Right 2W0NX
Mouth and Pharynx 2Y00X5Z
Nasal 2Y01X5Z
Neck 2W02X
Thumb
Left 2W0HX
Right 2W0GX
Toe
Left 2W0VX
Right 2W0UX
Urethra 2Y05X5Z
Chemoembolization
see Introduction of substance in or on
Chemosurgery, Skin 3E00XTZ
Chemothalamectomy
see Destruction, Thalamus 0059
Chemotherapy, Infusion for cancer
see Introduction of substance in or on
Chest x-ray
see Plain Radiography, Chest BW03
Chiropractic Manipulation
Abdomen 9WB9X
Cervical 9WB1X

Chiropractic Manipulation *(continued)*
Extremities
Lower 9WB6X
Upper 9WB7X
Head 9WB0X
Lumbar 9WB3X
Pelvis 9WB5X
Rib Cage 9WB8X
Sacrum 9WB4X
Thoracic 9WB2X
Choana
use Nasopharynx
Cholangiogram
see Plain Radiography, Hepatobiliary System and Pancreas BF0
see Fluoroscopy, Hepatobiliary System and Pancreas BF1
Cholecystectomy
see Excision, Gallbladder 0FB4
see Resection, Gallbladder 0FT4
Cholecystojejunostomy
see Bypass, Hepatobiliary System and Pancreas 0F1
see Drainage, Hepatobiliary System and Pancreas 0F9
Cholecystopexy
see Repair, Gallbladder 0FQ4
see Reposition, Gallbladder 0FS4
Cholecystoscopy 0FJ44ZZ
Cholecystostomy
see Drainage, Gallbladder 0F94
see Bypass, Gallbladder 0F14
Cholecystotomy
see Drainage, Gallbladder 0F94
Choledochectomy
see Excision, Hepatobiliary System and Pancreas 0FB
see Resection, Hepatobiliary System and Pancreas 0FT
Choledocholithotomy
see Extirpation, Duct, Common Bile 0FC9
Choledochoplasty
see Repair, Hepatobiliary System and Pancreas 0FQ
see Replacement, Hepatobiliary System and Pancreas 0FR
see Supplement, Hepatobiliary System and Pancreas 0FU
Choledochoscopy 0FJB8ZZ
Choledochotomy
see Drainage, Hepatobiliary System and Pancreas 0F9
Cholelithotomy
see Extirpation, Hepatobiliary System and Pancreas 0FC
Chondrectomy
see Excision, Lower Joints 0SB
see Excision, Upper Joints 0RB
Knee *see* Excision, Lower Joints 0SB
Semilunar cartilage
see Excision, Lower Joints 0SB
Chondroglossus muscle
use Muscle, Tongue, Palate, Pharynx
Chorda tympani
use Nerve, Facial
Chordotomy
see Division, Central Nervous System 008
Choroid plexus
use Cerebral Ventricle
Choroidectomy
see Excision, Eye 08B
see Resection, Eye 08T
Ciliary body
use Eye, Left
use Eye, Right
Ciliary ganglion
use Nerve, Head and Neck Sympathetic

Circle of Willis
use Artery, Intracranial
Circumflex iliac artery
use Artery, Femoral, Left
use Artery, Femoral, Right
Clamp and rod internal fixation system (CRIF)
use Internal Fixation Device in Lower Bones
use Internal Fixation Device in Upper Bones
Clamping
see Occlusion
Claustrum
use Basal Ganglia
Claviculectomy
see Excision, Upper Bones 0PB
see Resection, Upper Bones 0PT
Claviculotomy
see Division, Upper Bones 0P8
see Drainage, Upper Bones 0P9
Clipping, aneurysm
see Restriction using Extraluminal Device
Clitorectomy, clitoridectomy
see Excision, Clitoris 0UBJ
see Resection, Clitoris 0UTJ
Clolar
use Clofarabine
Closure
see Occlusion
see Repair
Clysis
see Introduction of substance in or on
Coagulation
see Destruction
CoAxia NeuroFlo catheter
use Intraluminal Device
Cobalt/chromium head and polyethylene socket
use Synthetic Substitute, Metal on Polyethylene in 0SR
Cobalt/chromium head and socket
use Synthetic Substitute, Metal in 0SR
Coccygeal body
use Coccygeal Glomus
Coccygeus muscle
use Muscle, Trunk, Left
use Muscle, Trunk, Right
Cochlea
use Ear, Inner, Left
use Ear, Inner, Right
Cochlear implant (CI), multiple channel (electrode)
use Hearing Device, Multiple Channel Cochlear Prosthesis in 09H
Cochlear implant (CI), single channel (electrode)
use Hearing Device, Single Channel Cochlear Prosthesis in 09H
Cochlear Implant Treatment F0BZ0
Cochlear nerve
use Nerve, Acoustic
COGNIS® CRT-D
use Cardiac Resynchronization Defibrillator Pulse Generator in 0JH
Colectomy
see Excision, Gastrointestinal System 0DB
see Resection, Gastrointestinal System 0DT
Collapse
see Occlusion
Collection from
Breast, Breast Milk 8E0HX62

Collection from *(continued)*
Indwelling Device
Circulatory System
Blood 8C02X6K
Other Fluid 8C02X6L
Nervous System
Cerebrospinal Fluid 8C01X6J
Other Fluid 8C01X6L
Integumentary System, Breast Milk 8E0HX62
Reproductive System, Male, Sperm 8E0VX63
Colocentesis
see Drainage, Gastrointestinal System 0D9
Colofixation
see Repair, Gastrointestinal System 0DQ
see Reposition, Gastrointestinal System 0DS
Cololysis
see Release, Gastrointestinal System 0DN
Colonic Z-Stent®
use Intraluminal Device
Colonoscopy 0DJD8ZZ
Colopexy
see Repair, Gastrointestinal System 0DQ
see Reposition, Gastrointestinal System 0DS
Coloplication
see Restriction, Gastrointestinal System 0DV
Coloproctectomy
see Excision, Gastrointestinal System 0DB
see Resection, Gastrointestinal System 0DT
Coloproctostomy
see Bypass, Gastrointestinal System 0D1
see Drainage, Gastrointestinal System 0D9
Colopuncture
see Drainage, Gastrointestinal System 0D9
Colorrhaphy
see Repair, Gastrointestinal System 0DQ
Colostomy
see Bypass, Gastrointestinal System 0D1
see Drainage, Gastrointestinal System 0D9
Colpectomy
see Excision, Vagina 0UBG
see Resection, Vagina 0UTG
Colpocentesis
see Drainage, Vagina 0U9G
Colpopexy
see Repair, Vagina 0UQG
see Reposition, Vagina 0USG
Colpoplasty
see Repair, Vagina 0UQG
see Supplement, Vagina 0UUG
Colporrhaphy
see Repair, Vagina 0UQG
Colposcopy 0UJH8ZZ
Columella
use Nose
Common digital vein
use Vein, Foot, Left
use Vein, Foot, Right
Common facial vein
use Vein, Face, Left
use Vein, Face, Right
Common fibular nerve
use Nerve, Peroneal
Common hepatic artery
use Artery, Hepatic

Computerized Tomography (CT Scan) *(continued)*
- Tibia
  - Left BQ2C
  - Right BQ2B
- Toe
  - Left BQ2Q
  - Right BQ2P
- Trachea BB2F
- Tracheobronchial Tree
  - Bilateral BB29
  - Left BB28
  - Right BB27
- Vein
  - Pelvic (Iliac)
    - Left B52G
      - Intravascular Optical Coherence B52GZ2Z
    - Right B52F
      - Intravascular Optical Coherence B52FZ2Z
  - Pelvic (Iliac) Bilateral B52H
    - Intravascular Optical Coherence B52HZ2Z
  - Portal B52T
    - Intravascular Optical Coherence B52TZ2Z
  - Pulmonary
    - Bilateral B52S
      - Intravascular Optical Coherence B52SZ2Z
    - Left B52R
      - Intravascular Optical Coherence B52RZ2Z
    - Right B52Q
      - Intravascular Optical Coherence B52QZ2Z
  - Renal
    - Bilateral B52L
      - Intravascular Optical Coherence B52LZ2Z
    - Left B52K
      - Intravascular Optical Coherence B52KZ2Z
    - Right B52J
      - Intravascular Optical Coherence B52JZ2Z
  - Spanchnic B52T
    - Intravascular Optical Coherence B52TZ2Z
- Vena Cava
  - Inferior B529
    - Intravascular Optical Coherence B529Z2Z
  - Superior B528
    - Intravascular Optical Coherence B528Z2Z
- Ventricle, Cerebral B028
- Wrist
  - Left BP2M
  - Right BP2L

Concerto II CRT-D
- *use* Cardiac Resynchronization Defibrillator Pulse Generator in 0JH

Condylectomy
- *see* Excision, Head and Facial Bones 0NB
- *see* Excision, Lower Bones 0QB
- *see* Excision, Upper Bones 0PB

Condyloid process
- *use* Mandible, Left
- *use* Mandible, Right

Condylotomy
- *see* Division, Head and Facial Bones 0N8
- *see* Division, Lower Bones 0Q8
- *see* Division, Upper Bones 0P8
- *see* Drainage, Head and Facial Bones 0N9
- *see* Drainage, Lower Bones 0Q9
- *see* Drainage, Upper Bones 0P9

Condylysis
- *see* Release, Head and Facial Bones 0NN
- *see* Release, Lower Bones 0QN
- *see* Release, Upper Bones 0PN

Conization, cervix
- *see* Excision, Uterus 0UB9

Conjunctivoplasty
- *see* Repair, Eye 08Q
- *see* Replacement, Eye 08R

CONSERVE® PLUS Total Resurfacing Hip System
- *use* Resurfacing Device in Lower Joints

Construction
- Auricle, ear
  - *see* Bypass, Urinary System 0T1
- Ileal conduit
  - *see* Replacement, Ear, Nose, Sinus 09R

Consulta CRT-D
- *use* Cardiac Resynchronization Defibrillator Pulse Generator in 0JH

Consulta CRT-P
- *use* Cardiac Resynchronization Pacemaker Pulse Generator in 0JH

Contact Radiation
- Abdomen DWY37ZZ
- Adrenal Gland DGY27ZZ
- Bile Ducts DFY27ZZ
- Bladder DTY27ZZ
- Bone, Other DPYC7ZZ
- Brain D0Y07ZZ
- Brain Stem D0Y17ZZ
- Breast
  - Left DMY07ZZ
  - Right DMY17ZZ
- Bronchus DBY17ZZ
- Cervix DUY17ZZ
- Chest DWY27ZZ
- Chest Wall DBY77ZZ
- Colon DDY57ZZ
- Diaphragm DBY87ZZ
- Duodenum DDY27ZZ
- Ear D9Y07ZZ
- Esophagus DDY07ZZ
- Eye D8Y07ZZ
- Femur DPY97ZZ
- Fibula DPYB7ZZ
- Gallbladder DFY17ZZ
- Gland
  - Adrenal DGY27ZZ
  - Parathyroid DGY47ZZ
  - Pituitary DGY07ZZ
  - Thyroid DGY57ZZ
- Glands, Salivary D9Y67ZZ
- Head and Neck DWY17ZZ
- Hemibody DWY47ZZ
- Humerus DPY67ZZ
- Hypopharynx D9Y37ZZ
- Ileum DDY47ZZ
- Jejunum DDY37ZZ
- Kidney DTY07ZZ
- Larynx D9YB7ZZ
- Liver DFY07ZZ
- Lung DBY27ZZ
- Mandible DPY37ZZ
- Maxilla DPY27ZZ
- Mediastinum DBY67ZZ
- Mouth D9Y47ZZ
- Nasopharynx D9YD7ZZ
- Neck and Head DWY17ZZ
- Nerve, Peripheral D0Y77ZZ
- Nose D9Y17ZZ
- Oropharynx D9YF7ZZ
- Ovary DUY07ZZ
- Palate
  - Hard D9Y87ZZ
  - Soft D9Y97ZZ
- Pancreas DFY37ZZ

Contact Radiation *(continued)*
- Parathyroid Gland DGY47ZZ
- Pelvic Bones DPY87ZZ
- Pelvic Region DWY67ZZ
- Pineal Body DGY17ZZ
- Pituitary Gland DGY07ZZ
- Pleura DBY57ZZ
- Prostate DVY07ZZ
- Radius DPY77ZZ
- Rectum DDY77ZZ
- Rib DPY57ZZ
- Sinuses D9Y77ZZ
- Skin
  - Abdomen DHY87ZZ
  - Arm DHY47ZZ
  - Back DHY77ZZ
  - Buttock DHY97ZZ
  - Chest DHY67ZZ
  - Face DHY27ZZ
  - Leg DHYB7ZZ
  - Neck DHY37ZZ
- Skull DPY07ZZ
- Spinal Cord D0Y67ZZ
- Sternum DPY47ZZ
- Stomach DDY17ZZ
- Testis DVY17ZZ
- Thyroid Gland DGY57ZZ
- Tibia DPYB7ZZ
- Tongue D9Y57ZZ
- Trachea DBY07ZZ
- Ulna DPY77ZZ
- Ureter DTY17ZZ
- Urethra DTY37ZZ
- Uterus DUY27ZZ
- Whole Body DWY57ZZ

CONTAK RENEWAL® 3 RF (HE) CRT-D
- *use* Cardiac Resynchronization Defibrillator Pulse Generator in 0JH

Contegra Pulmonary Valved Conduit
- *use* Zooplastic Tissue in Heart and Great Vessels

Continuous Glucose Monitoring (CGM) device
- *use* Monitoring Device

Continuous Negative Airway Pressure
- 24-96 Consecutive Hours, Ventilation 5A09459
- Greater than 96 Consecutive Hours, Ventilation 5A09559
- Less than 24 Consecutive Hours, Ventilation 5A09359

Continuous Positive Airway Pressure
- 24-96 Consecutive Hours, Ventilation 5A09457
- Greater than 96 Consecutive Hours, Ventilation 5A09557
- Less than 24 Consecutive Hours, Ventilation 5A09357

Contraceptive Device
- Change device in, Uterus and Cervix 0U2DXHZ
- Insertion of device in
  - Cervix 0UHC
  - Subcutaneous Tissue and Fascia
    - Abdomen 0JH8
    - Chest 0JH6
    - Lower Arm
      - Left 0JHH
      - Right 0JHG
    - Lower Leg
      - Left 0JHP
      - Right 0JHN
    - Upper Arm
      - Left 0JHF
      - Right 0JHD
    - Upper Leg
      - Left 0JHM
      - Right 0JHL
  - Uterus 0UH9

Contraceptive Device *(continued)*
- Removal of device from
  - Subcutaneous Tissue and Fascia
    - Lower Extremity 0JPW
    - Trunk 0JPT
    - Upper Extremity 0JPV
  - Uterus and Cervix 0UPD
- Revision of device in
  - Subcutaneous Tissue and Fascia
    - Lower Extremity 0JWW
    - Trunk 0JWT
    - Upper Extremity 0JWV
  - Uterus and Cervix 0UWD

Contractility Modulation Device
- Abdomen 0JH8
- Chest 0JH6

Control postprocedural bleeding in
- Abdominal Wall 0W3F
- Ankle Region
  - Left 0Y3L
  - Right 0Y3K
- Arm
  - Lower
    - Left 0X3F
    - Right 0X3D
  - Upper
    - Left 0X39
    - Right 0X38
- Axilla
  - Left 0X35
  - Right 0X34
- Back
  - Lower 0W3L
  - Upper 0W3K
- Buttock
  - Left 0Y31
  - Right 0Y30
- Cavity, Cranial 0W31
- Chest Wall 0W38
- Elbow Region
  - Left 0X3C
  - Right 0X3B
- Extremity
  - Lower
    - Left 0Y3B
    - Right 0Y39
  - Upper
    - Left 0X37
    - Right 0X36
- Face 0W32
- Femoral Region
  - Left 0Y38
  - Right 0Y37
- Foot
  - Left 0Y3N
  - Right 0Y3M
- Gastrointestinal Tract 0W3P
- Genitourinary Tract 0W3R
- Hand
  - Left 0X3K
  - Right 0X3J
- Head 0W30
- Inguinal Region
  - Left 0Y36
  - Right 0Y35
- Jaw
  - Lower 0W35
  - Upper 0W34
- Knee Region
  - Left 0Y3G
  - Right 0Y3F
- Leg
  - Lower
    - Left 0Y3J
    - Right 0Y3H
  - Upper
    - Left 0Y3D
    - Right 0Y3C
- Mediastinum 0W3C
- Neck 0W36
- Oral Cavity and Throat 0W33
- Pelvic Cavity 0W3J

Control postprocedural bleeding in *(continued)*
- Pericardial Cavity 0W3D
- Perineum
  - Female 0W3N
  - Male 0W3M
- Peritoneal Cavity 0W3G
- Pleural Cavity
  - Left 0W3B
  - Right 0W39
- Respiratory Tract 0W3Q
- Retroperitoneum 0W3H
- Shoulder Region
  - Left 0X33
  - Right 0X32
- Wrist Region
  - Left 0X3H
  - Right 0X3G

Conus arteriosus
- *use* Ventricle, Right

Conus medullaris
- *use* Spinal Cord, Lumbar

Conversion
- Cardiac rhythm 5A2204Z
- Gastrostomy to jejunostomy feeding device *see* Insertion of device in, Jejunum 0DHA

Coracoacromial ligament
- *use* Bursa and Ligament, Shoulder, Left
- *use* Bursa and Ligament, Shoulder, Right

Coracobrachialis muscle
- *use* Muscle, Upper Arm, Left
- *use* Muscle, Upper Arm, Right

Coracoclavicular ligament
- *use* Bursa and Ligament, Shoulder, Left
- *use* Bursa and Ligament, Shoulder, Right

Coracohumeral ligament
- *use* Bursa and Ligament, Shoulder, Left
- *use* Bursa and Ligament, Shoulder, Right

Coracoid process
- *use* Scapula, Left
- *use* Scapula, Right

Cordotomy
- *see* Division, Central Nervous System 008

Core needle biopsy
- *see* Excision with qualifier Diagnostic

CoreValve transcatheter aortic valve
- *use* Zooplastic Tissue in Heart and Great Vessels

Cormet Hip Resurfacing System
- *use* Resurfacing Device in Lower Joints

Corniculate cartilage
- *use* Larynx

CoRoent® XL
- *use* Interbody Fusion Device in Lower Joints

Coronary arteriography
- *see* Fluoroscopy, Heart B21
- *see* Plain Radiography, Heart B20

Corox (OTW) Bipolar Lead
- *use* Cardiac Lead, Defibrillator in 02H
- *use* Cardiac Lead, Pacemaker in 02H

Corpus callosum
- *use* Brain

Corpus cavernosum
- *use* Penis

Corpus spongiosum
- *use* Penis

Corpus striatum
- *use* Basal Ganglia

Corrugator supercilii muscle
- *use* Muscle, Facial

Cortical strip neurostimulator lead
- *use* Neurostimulator Lead in Central Nervous System

Costatectomy
- *see* Excision, Upper Bones 0PB
- *see* Resection, Upper Bones 0PT

Costectomy
- *see* Excision, Upper Bones 0PB
- *see* Resection, Upper Bones 0PT

Costocervical trunk
- *use* Artery, Subclavian, Left
- *use* Artery, Subclavian, Right

Costochondrectomy
- *see* Excision, Upper Bones 0PB
- *see* Resection, Upper Bones 0PT

Costoclavicular ligament
- *use* Bursa and Ligament, Shoulder, Left
- *use* Bursa and Ligament, Shoulder, Right

Costosternoplasty
- *see* Repair, Upper Bones 0PQ
- *see* Replacement, Upper Bones 0PR
- *see* Supplement, Upper Bones 0PU

Costotomy
- *see* Division, Upper Bones 0P8
- *see* Drainage, Upper Bones 0P9

Costotransverse joint
- *use* Joint, Thoracic Vertebral

Costotransverse ligament
- *use* Bursa and Ligament, Thorax, Left
- *use* Bursa and Ligament, Thorax, Right

Costovertebral joint
- *use* Joint, Thoracic Vertebral

Costoxiphoid ligament
- *use* Bursa and Ligament, Thorax, Left
- *use* Bursa and Ligament, Thorax, Right

Counseling
- Family, for substance abuse, Other Family Counseling HZ63ZZZ
- Group
  - 12-Step HZ43ZZZ
  - Behavioral HZ41ZZZ
  - Cognitive HZ40ZZZ
  - Cognitive-Behavioral HZ42ZZZ
  - Confrontational HZ48ZZZ
  - Continuing Care HZ49ZZZ
  - Infectious Disease
    - Post-Test HZ4CZZZ
    - Pre-Test HZ4CZZZ
  - Interpersonal HZ44ZZZ
  - Motivational Enhancement HZ47ZZZ
  - Psychoeducation HZ46ZZZ
  - Spiritual HZ4BZZZ
  - Vocational HZ45ZZZ
- Individual
  - 12-Step HZ33ZZZ
  - Behavioral HZ31ZZZ
  - Cognitive HZ30ZZZ
  - Cognitive-Behavioral HZ32ZZZ
  - Confrontational HZ38ZZZ
  - Continuing Care HZ39ZZZ
  - Infectious Disease
    - Post-Test HZ3CZZZ
    - Pre-Test HZ3CZZZ
  - Interpersonal HZ34ZZZ
  - Motivational Enhancement HZ37ZZZ
  - Psychoeducation HZ36ZZZ
  - Spiritual HZ3BZZZ
  - Vocational HZ35ZZZ
- Mental Health Services
  - Educational GZ60ZZZ
  - Other Counseling GZ63ZZZ
  - Vocational GZ61ZZZ

Countershock, cardiac 5A2204Z

Cowper's (bulbourethral) gland
- *use* Urethra

CPAP (continuous positive airway pressure)
- *see* Assistance, Respiratory 5A09

Cranial dura mater
- *use* Dura Mater

Cranial epidural space
- *use* Epidural Space

Cranial subarachnoid space
- *use* Subarachnoid Space

Cranial subdural space
- *use* Subdural Space

Craniectomy
- *see* Excision, Head and Facial Bones 0NB
- *see* Resection, Head and Facial Bones 0NT

Cranioplasty
- *see* Repair, Head and Facial Bones 0NQ
- *see* Replacement, Head and Facial Bones 0NR
- *see* Supplement, Head and Facial Bones 0NU

Craniotomy
- *see* Drainage, Central Nervous System 009
- *see* Division, Head and Facial Bones 0N8
- *see* Drainage, Head and Facial Bones 0N9

Creation
- Female 0W4N0
- Male 0W4M0

Cremaster muscle
- *use* Muscle, Perineum

Cribriform plate
- *use* Bone, Ethmoid, Left
- *use* Bone, Ethmoid, Right

Cricoid cartilage
- *use* Larynx

Cricoidectomy
- *see* Excision, Larynx 0CBS

Cricothyroid artery
- *use* Artery, Thyroid, Left
- *use* Artery, Thyroid, Right

Cricothyroid muscle
- *use* Muscle, Neck, Left
- *use* Muscle, Neck, Right

Crisis Intervention GZ2ZZZZ

Crural fascia
- *use* Subcutaneous Tissue and Fascia, Upper Leg, Left
- *use* Subcutaneous Tissue and Fascia, Upper Leg, Right

Crushing, nerve
- Cranial
  - *see* Destruction, Central Nervous System 005
- Peripheral
  - *see* Destruction, Peripheral Nervous System 015

Cryoablation
- *see* Destruction

Cryotherapy
- *see* Destruction

Cryptorchidectomy
- *see* Excision, Male Reproductive System 0VB
- *see* Resection, Male Reproductive System 0VT

Cryptorchiectomy
- *see* Excision, Male Reproductive System 0VB
- *see* Resection, Male Reproductive System 0VT

Cryptotomy
- *see* Division, Gastrointestinal System 0D8
- *see* Drainage, Gastrointestinal System 0D9

CT scan
- *see* Computerized Tomography (CT Scan)

CT sialogram
- *see* Computerized Tomography (CT Scan), Ear, Nose, Mouth and Throat B92

Cubital lymph node
- *use* Lymphatic, Upper Extremity, Left
- *use* Lymphatic, Upper Extremity, Right

Cubital nerve
- *use* Nerve, Ulnar

Cuboid bone
- *use* Tarsal, Left
- *use* Tarsal, Right

Cuboideonavicular joint
- *use* Joint, Tarsal, Left
- *use* Joint, Tarsal, Right

Culdocentesis
- *see* Drainage, Cul-de-sac 0U9F

Culdoplasty
- *see* Repair, Cul-de-sac 0UQF
- *see* Supplement, Cul-de-sac 0UUF

Culdoscopy 0UJH8ZZ

Culdotomy
- *see* Drainage, Cul-de-sac 0U9F

Culmen
- *use* Cerebellum

Cultured epidermal cell autograft
- *use* Autologous Tissue Substitute

Cuneiform cartilage
- *use* Larynx

Cuneonavicular joint
- *use* Joint, Tarsal, Left
- *use* Joint, Tarsal, Right

Cuneonavicular ligament
- *use* Bursa and Ligament, Foot, Left
- *use* Bursa and Ligament, Foot, Right

Curettage
- *see* Excision
- *see* Extraction

Cutaneous (transverse) cervical nerve
- *use* Nerve, Cervical Plexus

CVP (central venous pressure)
- *see* Measurement, Venous 4A04

Cyclodiathermy
- *see* Destruction, Eye 085

Cyclophotocoagulation
- *see* Destruction, Eye 085

CYPHER® Stent
- *use* Intraluminal Device, Drug-eluting in Heart and Great Vessels

Cystectomy
- *see* Excision, Bladder 0TBB
- *see* Resection, Bladder 0TTB

Cystocele repair
- *see* Repair, Subcutaneous Tissue and Fascia, Pelvic Region 0JQC

Cystography
- *see* Fluoroscopy, Urinary System BT1
- *see* Plain Radiography, Urinary System BT0

Cystolithotomy
- *see* Extirpation, Bladder 0TCB

Cystopexy
- *see* Repair, Bladder 0TQB
- *see* Reposition, Bladder 0TSB

Cystoplasty
- *see* Repair, Bladder 0TQB
- *see* Replacement, Bladder 0TRB
- *see* Supplement, Bladder 0TUB

Cystorrhaphy
- *see* Repair, Bladder 0TQB

Cystoscopy 0TJB8ZZ

Cystostomy
- *see* Bypass, Bladder 0T1B

Cystostomy tube
- *use* Drainage Device

Cystotomy
- *see* Drainage, Bladder 0T9B

Cystourethrography
- *see* Fluoroscopy, Urinary System BT1
- *see* Plain Radiography, Urinary System BT0

Cystourethroplasty
- *see* Repair, Urinary System 0TQ
- *see* Replacement, Urinary System 0TR
- *see* Supplement, Urinary System 0TU

D

DBS lead
- *use* Neurostimulator Lead in Central Nervous System

DeBakey Left Ventricular Assist Device
- *use* Implantable Heart Assist System in Heart and Great Vessels

Debridement
- Excisional
  - *see* Excision
- Non-excisional
  - *see* Extraction

Decompression, Circulatory 6A15

Decortication, lung
- *see* Extraction, Respiratory System 0BD

Deep brain neurostimulator lead
- *use* Neurostimulator Lead in Central Nervous System

Deep cervical fascia
- *use* Subcutaneous Tissue and Fascia, Neck, Anterior

Deep cervical vein
- *use* Vein, Vertebral, Left
- *use* Vein, Vertebral, Right

Deep circumflex iliac artery
- *use* Artery, External Iliac, Left
- *use* Artery, External Iliac, Right

Deep facial vein
- *use* Vein, Face, Left
- *use* Vein, Face, Right

Deep femoral (profunda femoris) vein
- *use* Vein, Femoral, Left
- *use* Vein, Femoral, Right

Deep femoral artery
- *use* Artery, Femoral, Left
- *use* Artery, Femoral, Right

Deep Inferior Epigastric Artery Perforator Flap
- Bilateral 0HRV077
- Left 0HRU077
- Right 0HRT077

Deep palmar arch
- *use* Artery, Hand, Left
- *use* Artery, Hand, Right

Deep transverse perineal muscle
- *use* Muscle, Perineum

Deferential artery
- *use* Artery, Internal Iliac, Left
- *use* Artery, Internal Iliac, Right

Defibrillator Generator
- Abdomen 0JH8
- Chest 0JH6

Delivery
- Cesarean
  - *see* Extraction, Products of Conception 10D0
- Forceps
  - *see* Extraction, Products of Conception 10D0
- Manually assisted 10E0XZZ

Delivery *(continued)*
- Products of Conception 10E0XZZ
- Vacuum assisted
  - *see* Extraction, Products of Conception 10D0

Delta frame external fixator
- *use* External Fixation Device, Hybrid in 0PH
- *use* External Fixation Device, Hybrid in 0PS
- *use* External Fixation Device, Hybrid in 0QH
- *use* External Fixation Device, Hybrid in 0QS

Delta III Reverse shoulder prosthesis
- *use* Synthetic Substitute, Reverse Ball and Socket in 0RR

Deltoid fascia
- *use* Subcutaneous Tissue and Fascia, Upper Arm, Left
- *use* Subcutaneous Tissue and Fascia, Upper Arm, Right

Deltoid ligament
- *use* Bursa and Ligament, Ankle, Left
- *use* Bursa and Ligament, Ankle, Right

Deltoid muscle
- *use* Muscle, Shoulder, Left
- *use* Muscle, Shoulder, Right

Deltopectoral (infraclavicular) lymph node
- *use* Lymphatic, Upper Extremity, Left
- *use* Lymphatic, Upper Extremity, Right

Denervation
- Cranial nerve
  - *see* Destruction, Central Nervous System 005
- Peripheral nerve
  - *see* Destruction, Peripheral Nervous System 015

Densitometry
- Plain Radiography
  - Femur
    - Left BQ04ZZ1
    - Right BQ03ZZ1
  - Hip
    - Left BQ01ZZ1
    - Right BQ00ZZ1
  - Spine
    - Cervical BR00ZZ1
    - Lumbar BR09ZZ1
    - Thoracic BR07ZZ1
    - Whole BR0GZZ1
- Ultrasonography
  - Elbow
    - Left BP4HZZ1
    - Right BP4GZZ1
  - Hand
    - Left BP4PZZ1
    - Right BP4NZZ1
  - Shoulder
    - Left BP49ZZ1
    - Right BP48ZZ1
  - Wrist
    - Left BP4MZZ1
    - Right BP4LZZ1

Dentate ligament
- *use* Dura Mater

Denticulate ligament
- *use* Spinal Meninges

Depressor anguli oris muscle
- *use* Muscle, Facial

Depressor labii inferioris muscle
- *use* Muscle, Facial

Depressor septi nasi muscle
- *use* Muscle, Facial

Depressor supercilii muscle
- *use* Muscle, Facial

Dermabrasion
- *see* Extraction, Skin and Breast 0HD

Dermis
- *use* Skin

Descending genicular artery
- *use* Artery, Femoral, Left
- *use* Artery, Femoral, Right

Destruction
- Acetabulum
  - Left 0Q55
  - Right 0Q54
- Adenoids 0C5Q
- Ampulla of Vater 0F5C
- Anal Sphincter 0D5R
- Anterior Chamber
  - Left 08533ZZ
  - Right 08523ZZ
- Anus 0D5Q
- Aorta
  - Abdominal 0450
  - Thoracic 025W
- Aortic Body 0G5D
- Appendix 0D5J
- Artery
  - Anterior Tibial
    - Left 045Q
    - Right 045P
  - Axillary
    - Left 0356
    - Right 0355
  - Brachial
    - Left 0358
    - Right 0357
  - Celiac 0451
  - Colic
    - Left 0457
    - Middle 0458
    - Right 0456
  - Common Carotid
    - Left 035J
    - Right 035H
  - Common Iliac
    - Left 045D
    - Right 045C
  - External Carotid
    - Left 035N
    - Right 035M
  - External Iliac
    - Left 045J
    - Right 045H
  - Face 035R
  - Femoral
    - Left 045L
    - Right 045K
  - Foot
    - Left 045W
    - Right 045V
  - Gastric 0452
  - Hand
    - Left 035F
    - Right 035D
  - Hepatic 0453
  - Inferior Mesenteric 045B
  - Innominate 0352
  - Internal Carotid
    - Left 035L
    - Right 035K
  - Internal Iliac
    - Left 045F
    - Right 045E
  - Internal Mammary
    - Left 0351
    - Right 0350
  - Intracranial 035G
  - Lower 045Y
  - Peroneal
    - Left 045U
    - Right 045T
  - Popliteal
    - Left 045N
    - Right 045M
  - Posterior Tibial
    - Left 045S
    - Right 045R

Destruction *(continued)*
- Artery *(continued)*
  - Pulmonary
    - Left 025R
    - Right 025Q
  - Pulmonary Trunk 025P
  - Radial
    - Left 035C
    - Right 035B
  - Renal
    - Left 045A
    - Right 0459
  - Splenic 0454
  - Subclavian
    - Left 0354
    - Right 0353
  - Superior Mesenteric 0455
  - Temporal
    - Left 035T
    - Right 035S
  - Thyroid
    - Left 035V
    - Right 035U
  - Ulnar
    - Left 035A
    - Right 0359
  - Upper 035Y
  - Vertebral
    - Left 035Q
    - Right 035P
- Atrium
  - Left 0257
  - Right 0256
- Auditory Ossicle
  - Left 095A0ZZ
  - Right 09590ZZ
- Basal Ganglia 0058
- Bladder 0T5B
- Bladder Neck 0T5C
- Bone
  - Ethmoid
    - Left 0N5G
    - Right 0N5F
  - Frontal
    - Left 0N52
    - Right 0N51
  - Hyoid 0N5X
  - Lacrimal
    - Left 0N5J
    - Right 0N5H
  - Nasal 0N5B
  - Occipital
    - Left 0N58
    - Right 0N57
  - Palatine
    - Left 0N5L
    - Right 0N5K
  - Parietal
    - Left 0N54
    - Right 0N53
  - Pelvic
    - Left 0Q53
    - Right 0Q52
  - Sphenoid
    - Left 0N5D
    - Right 0N5C
  - Temporal
    - Left 0N56
    - Right 0N55
  - Zygomatic
    - Left 0N5N
    - Right 0N5M
- Brain 0050
- Breast
  - Bilateral 0H5V
  - Left 0H5U
  - Right 0H5T
- Bronchus
  - Lingula 0B59
  - Lower Lobe
    - Left 0B5B
    - Right 0B56

Destruction *(continued)*
- Bronchus *(continued)*
  - Main
    - Left 0B57
    - Right 0B53
  - Middle Lobe, Right 0B55
  - Upper Lobe
    - Left 0B58
    - Right 0B54
- Buccal Mucosa 0C54
- Bursa and Ligament
  - Abdomen
    - Left 0M5J
    - Right 0M5H
  - Ankle
    - Left 0M5R
    - Right 0M5Q
  - Elbow
    - Left 0M54
    - Right 0M53
  - Foot
    - Left 0M5T
    - Right 0M5S
  - Hand
    - Left 0M58
    - Right 0M57
  - Head and Neck 0M50
  - Hip
    - Left 0M5M
    - Right 0M5L
  - Knee
    - Left 0M5P
    - Right 0M5N
  - Lower Extremity
    - Left 0M5W
    - Right 0M5V
  - Perineum 0M5K
  - Shoulder
    - Left 0M52
    - Right 0M51
  - Thorax
    - Left 0M5G
    - Right 0M5F
  - Trunk
    - Left 0M5D
    - Right 0M5C
  - Upper Extremity
    - Left 0M5B
    - Right 0M59
  - Wrist
    - Left 0M56
    - Right 0M55
- Carina 0B52
- Carotid Bodies, Bilateral 0G58
- Carotid Body
  - Left 0G56
  - Right 0G57
- Carpal
  - Left 0P5N
  - Right 0P5M
- Cecum 0D5H
- Cerebellum 005C
- Cerebral Hemisphere 0057
- Cerebral Meninges 0051
- Cerebral Ventricle 0056
- Cervix 0U5C
- Chordae Tendineae 0259
- Choroid
  - Left 085B
  - Right 085A
- Cisterna Chyli 075L
- Clavicle
  - Left 0P5B
  - Right 0P59
- Clitoris 0U5J
- Coccygeal Glomus 0G5B
- Coccyx 0Q5S
- Colon
  - Ascending 0D5K
  - Descending 0D5M
  - Sigmoid 0D5N
  - Transverse 0D5L

Destruction *(continued)*
- Conduction Mechanism 0258
- Conjunctiva
  - Left 085TXZZ
  - Right 085SXZZ
- Cord
  - Bilateral 0V5H
  - Left 0V5G
  - Right 0V5F
- Cornea
  - Left 0859XZZ
  - Right 0858XZZ
- Cul-de-sac 0U5F
- Diaphragm
  - Left 0B5S
  - Right 0B5R
- Disc
  - Cervical Vertebral 0R53
  - Cervicothoracic Vertebral 0R55
  - Lumbar Vertebral 0S52
  - Lumbosacral 0S54
  - Thoracic Vertebral 0R59
  - Thoracolumbar Vertebral 0R5B
- Duct
  - Common Bile 0F59
  - Cystic 0F58
  - Hepatic
    - Left 0F56
    - Right 0F55
  - Lacrimal
    - Left 085Y
    - Right 085X
  - Pancreatic 0F5D
    - Accessory 0F5F
  - Parotid
    - Left 0C5C
    - Right 0C5B
- Duodenum 0D59
- Dura Mater 0052
- Ear
  - External
    - Left 0951
    - Right 0950
  - External Auditory Canal
    - Left 0954
    - Right 0953
  - Inner
    - Left 095E0ZZ
    - Right 095D0ZZ
  - Middle
    - Left 09560ZZ
    - Right 09550ZZ
- Endometrium 0U5B
- Epididymis
  - Bilateral 0V5L
  - Left 0V5K
  - Right 0V5J
- Epiglottis 0C5R
- Esophagogastric Junction 0D54
- Esophagus 0D55
  - Lower 0D53
  - Middle 0D52
  - Upper 0D51
- Eustachian Tube
  - Left 095G
  - Right 095F
- Eye
  - Left 0851XZZ
  - Right 0850XZZ
- Eyelid
  - Lower
    - Left 085R
    - Right 085Q
  - Upper
    - Left 085P
    - Right 085N
- Fallopian Tube
  - Left 0U56
  - Right 0U55
- Fallopian Tubes, Bilateral 0U57

Destruction *(continued)*
- Femoral Shaft
  - Left 0Q59
  - Right 0Q58
- Femur
  - Lower
    - Left 0Q5C
    - Right 0Q5B
  - Upper
    - Left 0Q57
    - Right 0Q56
- Fibula
  - Left 0Q5K
  - Right 0Q5J
- Finger Nail 0H5QXZZ
- Gallbladder 0F54
- Gingiva
  - Lower 0C56
  - Upper 0C55
- Gland
  - Adrenal
    - Bilateral 0G54
    - Left 0G52
    - Right 0G53
  - Lacrimal
    - Left 085W
    - Right 085V
  - Minor Salivary 0C5J
  - Parotid
    - Left 0C59
    - Right 0C58
  - Pituitary 0G50
  - Sublingual
    - Left 0C5F
    - Right 0C5D
  - Submaxillary
    - Left 0C5H
    - Right 0C5G
  - Vestibular 0U5L
- Glenoid Cavity
  - Left 0P58
  - Right 0P57
- Glomus Jugulare 0G5C
- Humeral Head
  - Left 0P5D
  - Right 0P5C
- Humeral Shaft
  - Left 0P5G
  - Right 0P5F
- Hymen 0U5K
- Hypothalamus 005A
- Ileocecal Valve 0D5C
- Ileum 0D5B
- Intestine
  - Large 0D5E
    - Left 0D5G
    - Right 0D5F
  - Small 0D58
- Iris
  - Left 085D3ZZ
  - Right 085C3ZZ
- Jejunum 0D5A
- Joint
  - Acromioclavicular
    - Left 0R5H
    - Right 0R5G
  - Ankle
    - Left 0S5G
    - Right 0S5F
  - Carpal
    - Left 0R5R
    - Right 0R5Q
  - Cervical Vertebral 0R51
  - Cervicothoracic Vertebral 0R54
  - Coccygeal 0S56
  - Elbow
    - Left 0R5M
    - Right 0R5L
  - Finger Phalangeal
    - Left 0R5X
    - Right 0R5W

Destruction *(continued)*
- Joint *(continued)*
  - Hip
    - Left 0S5B
    - Right 0S59
  - Knee
    - Left 0S5D
    - Right 0S5C
  - Lumbar Vertebral 0S50
  - Lumbosacral 0S53
  - Metacarpocarpal
    - Left 0R5T
    - Right 0R5S
  - Metacarpophalangeal
    - Left 0R5V
    - Right 0R5U
  - Metatarsal-Phalangeal
    - Left 0S5N
    - Right 0S5M
  - Metatarsal-Tarsal
    - Left 0S5L
    - Right 0S5K
  - Occipital-cervical 0R50
  - Sacrococcygeal 0S55
  - Sacroiliac
    - Left 0S58
    - Right 0S57
  - Shoulder
    - Left 0R5K
    - Right 0R5J
  - Sternoclavicular
    - Left 0R5F
    - Right 0R5E
  - Tarsal
    - Left 0S5J
    - Right 0S5H
  - Temporomandibular
    - Left 0R5D
    - Right 0R5C
  - Thoracic Vertebral 0R56
  - Thoracolumbar Vertebral 0R5A
  - Toe Phalangeal
    - Left 0S5Q
    - Right 0S5P
  - Wrist
    - Left 0R5P
    - Right 0R5N
- Kidney
  - Left 0T51
  - Right 0T50
- Kidney Pelvis
  - Left 0T54
  - Right 0T53
- Larynx 0C5S
- Lens
  - Left 085K3ZZ
  - Right 085J3ZZ
- Lip
  - Lower 0C51
  - Upper 0C50
- Liver 0F50
  - Left Lobe 0F52
  - Right Lobe 0F51
- Lung
  - Bilateral 0B5M
  - Left 0B5L
  - Lower Lobe
    - Left 0B5J
    - Right 0B5F
  - Middle Lobe, Right 0B5D
  - Right 0B5K
  - Upper Lobe
    - Left 0B5G
    - Right 0B5C
- Lung Lingula 0B5H
- Lymphatic
  - Aortic 075D
  - Axillary
    - Left 0756
    - Right 0755
  - Head 0750

Destruction *(continued)*
- Tendon *(continued)*
  - Upper Arm *(continued)*
    - Right 0L53
  - Upper Leg
    - Left 0L5M
    - Right 0L5L
- Testis
  - Bilateral 0V5C
  - Left 0V5B
  - Right 0V59
- Thalamus 0059
- Thymus 075M
- Thyroid Gland 0G5K
  - Left Lobe 0G5G
  - Right Lobe 0G5H
- Tibia
  - Left 0Q5H
  - Right 0Q5G
- Toe Nail 0H5RXZZ
- Tongue 0C57
- Tonsils 0C5P
- Tooth
  - Lower 0C5X
  - Upper 0C5W
- Trachea 0B51
- Tunica Vaginalis
  - Left 0V57
  - Right 0V56
- Turbinate, Nasal 095L
- Tympanic Membrane
  - Left 0958
  - Right 0957
- Ulna
  - Left 0P5L
  - Right 0P5K
- Ureter
  - Left 0T57
  - Right 0T56
- Urethra 0T5D
- Uterine Supporting Structure 0U54
- Uterus 0U59
- Uvula 0C5N
- Vagina 0U5G
- Valve
  - Aortic 025F
  - Mitral 025G
  - Pulmonary 025H
  - Tricuspid 025J
- Vas Deferens
  - Bilateral 0V5Q
  - Left 0V5P
  - Right 0V5N
- Vein
  - Axillary
    - Left 0558
    - Right 0557
  - Azygos 0550
  - Basilic
    - Left 055C
    - Right 055B
  - Brachial
    - Left 055A
    - Right 0559
  - Cephalic
    - Left 055F
    - Right 055D
  - Colic 0657
  - Common Iliac
    - Left 065D
    - Right 065C
  - Coronary 0254
  - Esophageal 0653
  - External Iliac
    - Left 065G
    - Right 065F
  - External Jugular
    - Left 055Q
    - Right 055P
  - Face
    - Left 055V
    - Right 055T

Destruction *(continued)*
- Vein *(continued)*
  - Femoral
    - Left 065N
    - Right 065M
  - Foot
    - Left 065V
    - Right 065T
  - Gastric 0652
  - Greater Saphenous
    - Left 065Q
    - Right 065P
  - Hand
    - Left 055H
    - Right 055G
  - Hemiazygos 0551
  - Hepatic 0654
  - Hypogastric
    - Left 065J
    - Right 065H
  - Inferior Mesenteric 0656
  - Innominate
    - Left 0554
    - Right 0553
  - Internal Jugular
    - Left 055N
    - Right 055M
  - Intracranial 055L
  - Lesser Saphenous
    - Left 065S
    - Right 065R
  - Lower 065Y
  - Portal 0658
  - Pulmonary
    - Left 025T
    - Right 025S
  - Renal
    - Left 065B
    - Right 0659
  - Splenic 0651
  - Subclavian
    - Left 0556
    - Right 0555
  - Superior Mesenteric 0655
  - Upper 055Y
  - Vertebral
    - Left 055S
    - Right 055R
- Vena Cava
  - Inferior 0650
  - Superior 025V
- Ventricle
  - Left 025L
  - Right 025K
- Vertebra
  - Cervical 0P53
  - Lumbar 0Q50
  - Thoracic 0P54
- Vesicle
  - Bilateral 0V53
  - Left 0V52
  - Right 0V51
- Vitreous
  - Left 08553ZZ
  - Right 08543ZZ
- Vocal Cord
  - Left 0C5V
  - Right 0C5T
- Vulva 0U5M

Detachment
- Arm
  - Lower
    - Left 0X6F0Z
    - Right 0X6D0Z
  - Upper
    - Left 0X690Z
    - Right 0X680Z
- Elbow Region
  - Left 0X6C0ZZ
  - Right 0X6B0ZZ

Detachment *(continued)*
- Femoral Region
  - Left 0Y680ZZ
  - Right 0Y670ZZ
- Finger
  - Index
    - Left 0X6P0Z
    - Right 0X6N0Z
  - Little
    - Left 0X6W0Z
    - Right 0X6V0Z
  - Middle
    - Left 0X6R0Z
    - Right 0X6Q0Z
  - Ring
    - Left 0X6T0Z
    - Right 0X6S0Z
- Foot
  - Left 0Y6N0Z
  - Right 0Y6M0Z
- Forequarter
  - Left 0X610ZZ
  - Right 0X600ZZ
- Hand
  - Left 0X6K0Z
  - Right 0X6J0Z
- Hindquarter
  - Bilateral 0Y640ZZ
  - Left 0Y630ZZ
  - Right 0Y620ZZ
- Knee Region
  - Left 0Y6G0ZZ
  - Right 0Y6F0ZZ
- Leg
  - Lower
    - Left 0Y6J0Z
    - Right 0Y6H0Z
  - Upper
    - Left 0Y6D0Z
    - Right 0Y6C0Z
- Shoulder Region
  - Left 0X630ZZ
  - Right 0X620ZZ
- Thumb
  - Left 0X6M0Z
  - Right 0X6L0Z
- Toe
  - 1st
    - Left 0Y6Q0Z
    - Right 0Y6P0Z
  - 2nd
    - Left 0Y6S0Z
    - Right 0Y6R0Z
  - 3rd
    - Left 0Y6U0Z
    - Right 0Y6T0Z
  - 4th
    - Left 0Y6W0Z
    - Right 0Y6V0Z
  - 5th
    - Left 0Y6Y0Z
    - Right 0Y6X0Z

Determination, Mental status GZ14ZZZ

Detorsion
- *see* Release
- *see* Reposition

Detoxification Services, for substance abuse HZ2ZZZZ

Device Fitting F0DZ

Diagnostic Audiology
- *see* Audiology, Diagnostic

Diagnostic imaging
- *see* Imaging, Diagnostic

Diagnostic radiology
- *see* Imaging, Diagnostic

Dialysis
- Hemodialysis 5A1D00Z
- Peritoneal 3E1M39Z

Diaphragma sellae
- *use* Dura Mater

Diaphragmatic pacemaker generator
- *use* Stimulator Generator in Subcutaneous Tissue and Fascia

Diaphragmatic Pacemaker Lead
- Insertion of device in
  - Left 0BHS
  - Right 0BHR
- Removal of device from, Diaphragm 0BPT
- Revision of device in, Diaphragm 0BWT

Digital radiography, plain
- *see* Plain Radiography

Dilation
- Ampulla of Vater 0F7C
- Anus 0D7Q
- Aorta
  - Abdominal 0470
  - Thoracic 027W
- Artery
  - Anterior Tibial
    - Left 047Q
    - Right 047P
  - Axillary
    - Left 0376
    - Right 0375
  - Brachial
    - Left 0378
    - Right 0377
  - Celiac 0471
  - Colic
    - Left 0477
    - Middle 0478
    - Right 0476
  - Common Carotid
    - Left 037J
    - Right 037H
  - Common Iliac
    - Left 047D
    - Right 047C
  - Coronary
    - Four or More Sites 0273
    - One Site 0270
    - Three Sites 0272
    - Two Sites 0271
  - External Carotid
    - Left 037N
    - Right 037M
  - External Iliac
    - Left 047J
    - Right 047H
  - Face 037R
  - Femoral
    - Left 047L
    - Right 047K
  - Foot
    - Left 047W
    - Right 047V
  - Gastric 0472
  - Hand
    - Left 037F
    - Right 037D
  - Hepatic 0473
  - Inferior Mesenteric 047B
  - Innominate 0372
  - Internal Carotid
    - Left 037L
    - Right 037K
  - Internal Iliac
    - Left 047F
    - Right 047E
  - Internal Mammary
    - Left 0371
    - Right 0370
  - Intracranial 037G
  - Lower 047Y
  - Peroneal
    - Left 047U
    - Right 047T
  - Popliteal
    - Left 047N
    - Right 047M

Dilation *(continued)*
- Femoral Shaft
  - Left 0Q89
  - Right 0Q88
- Femur
  - Lower
    - Left 0Q8C
    - Right 0Q8B
  - Upper
    - Left 0Q87
    - Right 0Q86
- Fibula
  - Left 0Q8K
  - Right 0Q8J
- Gland, Pituitary 0G80
- Glenoid Cavity
  - Left 0P88
  - Right 0P87
- Humeral Head
  - Left 0P8D
  - Right 0P8C
- Humeral Shaft
  - Left 0P8G
  - Right 0P8F
- Hymen 0U8K
- Kidneys, Bilateral 0T82
- Mandible
  - Left 0N8V
  - Right 0N8T
- Maxilla
  - Left 0N8S
  - Right 0N8R
- Metacarpal
  - Left 0P8Q
  - Right 0P8P
- Metatarsal
  - Left 0Q8P
  - Right 0Q8N
- Muscle
  - Abdomen
    - Left 0K8L
    - Right 0K8K
  - Facial 0K81
  - Foot
    - Left 0K8W
    - Right 0K8V
  - Hand
    - Left 0K8D
    - Right 0K8C
  - Head 0K80
  - Hip
    - Left 0K8P
    - Right 0K8N
  - Lower Arm and Wrist
    - Left 0K8B
    - Right 0K89
  - Lower Leg
    - Left 0K8T
    - Right 0K8S
  - Neck
    - Left 0K83
    - Right 0K82
  - Papillary 028D
  - Perineum 0K8M
  - Shoulder
    - Left 0K86
    - Right 0K85
  - Thorax
    - Left 0K8J
    - Right 0K8H
  - Tongue, Palate, Pharynx 0K84
  - Trunk
    - Left 0K8G
    - Right 0K8F
  - Upper Arm
    - Left 0K88
    - Right 0K87
  - Upper Leg
    - Left 0K8R
    - Right 0K8Q
- Nerve
  - Abdominal Sympathetic 018M

Dilation *(continued)*
- Nerve *(continued)*
  - Abducens 008L
  - Accessory 008R
  - Acoustic 008N
  - Brachial Plexus 0183
  - Cervical 0181
  - Cervical Plexus 0180
  - Facial 008M
  - Femoral 018D
  - Glossopharyngeal 008P
  - Head and Neck Sympathetic 018K
  - Hypoglossal 008S
  - Lumbar 018B
  - Lumbar Plexus 0189
  - Lumbar Sympathetic 018N
  - Lumbosacral Plexus 018A
  - Median 0185
  - Oculomotor 008H
  - Olfactory 008F
  - Optic 008G
  - Peroneal 018H
  - Phrenic 0182
  - Pudendal 018C
  - Radial 0186
  - Sacral 018R
  - Sacral Plexus 018Q
  - Sacral Sympathetic 018P
  - Sciatic 018F
  - Thoracic 0188
  - Thoracic Sympathetic 018L
  - Tibial 018G
  - Trigeminal 008K
  - Trochlear 008J
  - Ulnar 0184
  - Vagus 008Q
- Orbit
  - Left 0N8Q
  - Right 0N8P
- Ovary
  - Bilateral 0U82
  - Left 0U81
  - Right 0U80
- Pancreas 0F8G
- Patella
  - Left 0Q8F
  - Right 0Q8D
- Perineum, Female 0W8NXZZ
- Phalanx
  - Finger
    - Left 0P8V
    - Right 0P8T
  - Thumb
    - Left 0P8S
    - Right 0P8R
  - Toe
    - Left 0Q8R
    - Right 0Q8Q
- Radius
  - Left 0P8J
  - Right 0P8H
- Rib
  - Left 0P82
  - Right 0P81
- Sacrum 0Q81
- Scapula
  - Left 0P86
  - Right 0P85
- Skin
  - Abdomen 0H87XZZ
  - Back 0H86XZZ
  - Buttock 0H88XZZ
  - Chest 0H85XZZ
  - Ear
    - Left 0H83XZZ
    - Right 0H82XZZ
  - Face 0H81XZZ
  - Foot
    - Left 0H8NXZZ
    - Right 0H8MXZZ
  - Genitalia 0H8AXZZ

Dilation *(continued)*
- Skin *(continued)*
  - Hand
    - Left 0H8GXZZ
    - Right 0H8FXZZ
  - Lower Arm
    - Left 0H8EXZZ
    - Right 0H8DXZZ
  - Lower Leg
    - Left 0H8LXZZ
    - Right 0H8KXZZ
  - Neck 0H84XZZ
  - Perineum 0H89XZZ
  - Scalp 0H80XZZ
  - Upper Arm
    - Left 0H8CXZZ
    - Right 0H8BXZZ
  - Upper Leg
    - Left 0H8JXZZ
    - Right 0H8HXZZ
- Skull 0N80
- Spinal Cord
  - Cervical 008W
  - Lumbar 008Y
  - Thoracic 008X
- Sternum 0P80
- Stomach, Pylorus 0D87
- Subcutaneous Tissue and Fascia
  - Abdomen 0J88
  - Back 0J87
  - Buttock 0J89
  - Chest 0J86
  - Face 0J81
  - Foot
    - Left 0J8R
    - Right 0J8Q
  - Hand
    - Left 0J8K
    - Right 0J8J
  - Head and Neck 0J8S
  - Lower Arm
    - Left 0J8H
    - Right 0J8G
  - Lower Extremity 0J8W
  - Lower Leg
    - Left 0J8P
    - Right 0J8N
  - Neck
    - Anterior 0J84
    - Posterior 0J85
  - Pelvic Region 0J8C
  - Perineum 0J8B
  - Scalp 0J80
  - Trunk 0J8T
  - Upper Arm
    - Left 0J8F
    - Right 0J8D
  - Upper Extremity 0J8V
  - Upper Leg
    - Left 0J8M
    - Right 0J8L
- Tarsal
  - Left 0Q8M
  - Right 0Q8L
- Tendon
  - Abdomen
    - Left 0L8G
    - Right 0L8F
  - Ankle
    - Left 0L8T
    - Right 0L8S
  - Foot
    - Left 0L8W
    - Right 0L8V
  - Hand
    - Left 0L88
    - Right 0L87
  - Head and Neck 0L80
  - Hip
    - Left 0L8K
    - Right 0L8J

Dilation *(continued)*
- Tendon *(continued)*
  - Knee
    - Left 0L8R
    - Right 0L8Q
  - Lower Arm and Wrist
    - Left 0L86
    - Right 0L85
  - Lower Leg
    - Left 0L8P
    - Right 0L8N
  - Perineum 0L8H
  - Shoulder
    - Left 0L82
    - Right 0L81
  - Thorax
    - Left 0L8D
    - Right 0L8C
  - Trunk
    - Left 0L8B
    - Right 0L89
  - Upper Arm
    - Left 0L84
    - Right 0L83
  - Upper Leg
    - Left 0L8M
    - Right 0L8L
- Thyroid Gland Isthmus 0G8J
- Tibia
  - Left 0Q8H
  - Right 0Q8G
- Turbinate, Nasal 098L
- Ulna
  - Left 0P8L
  - Right 0P8K
- Uterine Supporting Structure 0U84
- Vertebra
  - Cervical 0P83
  - Lumbar 0Q80
  - Thoracic 0P84

Doppler study
- *see* Ultrasonography

Dorsal digital nerve
- *use* Nerve, Radial

Dorsal metacarpal vein
- *use* Vein, Hand, Left
- *use* Vein, Hand, Right

Dorsal metatarsal artery
- *use* Artery, Foot, Left
- *use* Artery, Foot, Right

Dorsal metatarsal vein
- *use* Vein, Foot, Left
- *use* Vein, Foot, Right

Dorsal scapular artery
- *use* Artery, Subclavian, Left
- *use* Artery, Subclavian, Right

Dorsal scapular nerve
- *use* Nerve, Brachial Plexus

Dorsal venous arch
- *use* Vein, Foot, Left
- *use* Vein, Foot, Right

Dorsalis pedis artery
- *use* Artery, Anterior Tibial, Left
- *use* Artery, Anterior Tibial, Right

Drainage
- Abdominal Wall 0W9F
- Acetabulum
  - Left 0Q95
  - Right 0Q94
- Adenoids 0C9Q
- Ampulla of Vater 0F9C
- Anal Sphincter 0D9R
- Ankle Region
  - Left 0Y9L
  - Right 0Y9K
- Anterior Chamber
  - Left 0893
  - Right 0892
- Anus 0D9Q

Drainage *(continued)*
- Aorta, Abdominal 0490
- Aortic Body 0G9D
- Appendix 0D9J
- Arm
  - Lower
    - Left 0X9F
    - Right 0X9D
  - Upper
    - Left 0X99
    - Right 0X98
- Artery
  - Anterior Tibial
    - Left 049Q
    - Right 049P
  - Axillary
    - Left 0396
    - Right 0395
  - Brachial
    - Left 0398
    - Right 0397
  - Celiac 0491
  - Colic
    - Left 0497
    - Middle 0498
    - Right 0496
  - Common Carotid
    - Left 039J
    - Right 039H
  - Common Iliac
    - Left 049D
    - Right 049C
  - External Carotid
    - Left 039N
    - Right 039M
  - External Iliac
    - Left 049J
    - Right 049H
  - Face 039R
  - Femoral
    - Left 049L
    - Right 049K
  - Foot
    - Left 049W
    - Right 049V
  - Gastric 0492
  - Hand
    - Left 039F
    - Right 039D
  - Hepatic 0493
  - Inferior Mesenteric 049B
  - Innominate 0392
  - Internal Carotid
    - Left 039L
    - Right 039K
  - Internal Iliac
    - Left 049F
    - Right 049E
  - Internal Mammary
    - Left 0391
    - Right 0390
  - Intracranial 039G
  - Lower 049Y
  - Peroneal
    - Left 049U
    - Right 049T
  - Popliteal
    - Left 049N
    - Right 049M
  - Posterior Tibial
    - Left 049S
    - Right 049R
  - Radial
    - Left 039C
    - Right 039B
  - Renal
    - Left 049A
    - Right 0499
  - Splenic 0494
  - Subclavian
    - Left 0394
    - Right 0393

Drainage *(continued)*
- Artery *(continued)*
  - Superior Mesenteric 0495
  - Temporal
    - Left 039T
    - Right 039S
  - Thyroid
    - Left 039V
    - Right 039U
  - Ulnar
    - Left 039A
    - Right 0399
  - Upper 039Y
  - Vertebral
    - Left 039Q
    - Right 039P
- Auditory Ossicle
  - Left 099A
  - Right 0999
- Axilla
  - Left 0X95
  - Right 0X94
- Back
  - Lower 0W9L
  - Upper 0W9K
- Basal Ganglia 0098
- Bladder 0T9B
- Bladder Neck 0T9C
- Bone
  - Ethmoid
    - Left 0N9G
    - Right 0N9F
  - Frontal
    - Left 0N92
    - Right 0N91
  - Hyoid 0N9X
  - Lacrimal
    - Left 0N9J
    - Right 0N9H
  - Nasal 0N9B
  - Occipital
    - Left 0N98
    - Right 0N97
  - Palatine
    - Left 0N9L
    - Right 0N9K
  - Parietal
    - Left 0N94
    - Right 0N93
  - Pelvic
    - Left 0Q93
    - Right 0Q92
  - Sphenoid
    - Left 0N9D
    - Right 0N9C
  - Temporal
    - Left 0N96
    - Right 0N95
  - Zygomatic
    - Left 0N9N
    - Right 0N9M
- Bone Marrow 079T
- Brain 0090
- Breast
  - Bilateral 0H9V
  - Left 0H9U
  - Right 0H9T
- Bronchus
  - Lingula 0B99
  - Lower Lobe
    - Left 0B9B
    - Right 0B96
  - Main
    - Left 0B97
    - Right 0B93
  - Middle Lobe, Right 0B95
  - Upper Lobe
    - Left 0B98
    - Right 0B94
- Buccal Mucosa 0C94

Drainage *(continued)*
- Bursa and Ligament
  - Abdomen
    - Left 0M9J
    - Right 0M9H
  - Ankle
    - Left 0M9R
    - Right 0M9Q
  - Elbow
    - Left 0M94
    - Right 0M93
  - Foot
    - Left 0M9T
    - Right 0M9S
  - Hand
    - Left 0M98
    - Right 0M97
  - Head and Neck 200M90
  - Hip
    - Left 0M9M
    - Right 0M9L
  - Knee
    - Left 0M9P
    - Right 0M9N
  - Lower Extremity
    - Left 0M9W
    - Right 0M9V
  - Perineum 0M9K
  - Shoulder
    - Left 0M92
    - Right 0M91
  - Thorax
    - Left 0M9G
    - Right 0M9F
  - Trunk
    - Left 0M9D
    - Right 0M9C
  - Upper Extremity
    - Left 0M9B
    - Right 0M99
  - Wrist
    - Left 0M96
    - Right 0M95
- Buttock
  - Left 0Y91
  - Right 0Y90
- Carina 0B92
- Carotid Bodies, Bilateral 0G98
- Carotid Body
  - Left 0G96
  - Right 0G97
- Carpal
  - Left 0P9N
  - Right 0P9M
- Cavity, Cranial 0W91
- Cecum 0D9H
- Cerebellum 009C
- Cerebral Hemisphere 0097
- Cerebral Meninges 0091
- Cerebral Ventricle 0096
- Cervix 0U9C
- Chest Wall 0W98
- Choroid
  - Left 089B
  - Right 089A
- Cisterna Chyli 079L
- Clavicle
  - Left 0P9B
  - Right 0P99
- Clitoris 0U9J
- Coccygeal Glomus 0G9B
- Coccyx 0Q9S
- Colon
  - Ascending 0D9K
  - Descending 0D9M
  - Sigmoid 0D9N
  - Transverse 0D9L
- Conjunctiva
  - Left 089T
  - Right 089S
- Cord
  - Bilateral 0V9H

Drainage *(continued)*
- Cord *(continued)*
  - Left 0V9G
  - Right 0V9F
- Cornea
  - Left 0899
  - Right 0898
- Cul-de-sac 0U9F
- Diaphragm
  - Left 0B9S
  - Right 0B9R
- Disc
  - Cervical Vertebral 0R93
  - Cervicothoracic Vertebral 0R95
  - Lumbar Vertebral 0S92
  - Lumbosacral 0S94
  - Thoracic Vertebral 0R99
  - Thoracolumbar Vertebral 0R9B
- Duct
  - Common Bile 0F99
  - Cystic 0F98
  - Hepatic
    - Left 0F96
    - Right 0F95
  - Lacrimal
    - Left 089Y
    - Right 089X
  - Pancreatic 0F9D
    - Accessory 0F9F
  - Parotid
    - Left 0C9C
    - Right 0C9B
- Duodenum 0D99
- Dura Mater 0092
- Ear
  - External
    - Left 0991
    - Right 0990
  - External Auditory Canal
    - Left 0994
    - Right 0993
  - Inner
    - Left 099E
    - Right 099D
  - Middle
    - Left 0996
    - Right 0995
- Elbow Region
  - Left 0X9C
  - Right 0X9B
- Epididymis
  - Bilateral 0V9L
  - Left 0V9K
  - Right 0V9J
- Epidural Space 0093
- Epiglottis 0C9R
- Esophagogastric Junction 0D94
- Esophagus 0D95
  - Lower 0D93
  - Middle 0D92
  - Upper 0D91
- Eustachian Tube
  - Left 099G
  - Right 099F
- Extremity
  - Lower
    - Left 0Y9B
    - Right 0Y99
  - Upper
    - Left 0X97
    - Right 0X96
- Eye
  - Left 0891
  - Right 0890
- Eyelid
  - Lower
    - Left 089R
    - Right 089Q
  - Upper
    - Left 089P
    - Right 089N
- Face 0W92

Drainage *(continued)*
- Fallopian Tube
  - Left 0U96
  - Right 0U95
- Fallopian Tubes, Bilateral 0U97
- Femoral Region
  - Left 0Y98
  - Right 0Y97
- Femoral Shaft
  - Left 0Q99
  - Right 0Q98
- Femur
  - Lower
    - Left 0Q9C
    - Right 0Q9B
  - Upper
    - Left 0Q97
    - Right 0Q96
- Fibula
  - Left 0Q9K
  - Right 0Q9J
- Finger Nail 0H9Q
- Foot
  - Left 0Y9N
  - Right 0Y9M
- Gallbladder 0F94
- Gingiva
  - Lower 0C96
  - Upper 0C95
- Gland
  - Adrenal
    - Bilateral 0G94
    - Left 0G92
    - Right 0G93
  - Lacrimal
    - Left 089W
    - Right 089V
  - Minor Salivary 0C9J
  - Parotid
    - Left 0C99
    - Right 0C98
  - Pituitary 0G90
  - Sublingual
    - Left 0C9F
    - Right 0C9D
  - Submaxillary
    - Left 0C9H
    - Right 0C9G
  - Vestibular 0U9L
- Glenoid Cavity
  - Left 0P98
  - Right 0P97
- Glomus Jugulare 0G9C
- Hand
  - Left 0X9K
  - Right 0X9J
- Head 0W90
- Humeral Head
  - Left 0P9D
  - Right 0P9C
- Humeral Shaft
  - Left 0P9G
  - Right 0P9F
- Hymen 0U9K
- Hypothalamus 009A
- Ileocecal Valve 0D9C
- Ileum 0D9B
- Inguinal Region
  - Left 0Y96
  - Right 0Y95
- Intestine
  - Large 0D9E
    - Left 0D9G
    - Right 0D9F
  - Small 0D98
- Iris
  - Left 089D
  - Right 089C
- Jaw
  - Lower 0W95
  - Upper 0W94
- Jejunum 0D9A

Drainage *(continued)*
- Joint
  - Acromioclavicular
    - Left 0R9H
    - Right 0R9G
  - Ankle
    - Left 0S9G
    - Right 0S9F
  - Carpal
    - Left 0R9R
    - Right 0R9Q
  - Cervical Vertebral 0R91
  - Cervicothoracic Vertebral 0R94
  - Coccygeal 0S96
  - Elbow
    - Left 0R9M
    - Right 0R9L
  - Finger Phalangeal
    - Left 0R9X
    - Right 0R9W
  - Hip
    - Left 0S9B
    - Right 0S99
  - Knee
    - Left 0S9D
    - Right 0S9C
  - Lumbar Vertebral 0S90
  - Lumbosacral 0S93
  - Metacarpocarpal
    - Left 0R9T
    - Right 0R9S
  - Metacarpophalangeal
    - Left 0R9V
    - Right 0R9U
  - Metatarsal-Phalangeal
    - Left 0S9N
    - Right 0S9M
  - Metatarsal-Tarsal
    - Left 0S9L
    - Right 0S9K
  - Occipital-cervical 0R90
  - Sacrococcygeal 0S95
  - Sacroiliac
    - Left 0S98
    - Right 0S97
  - Shoulder
    - Left 0R9K
    - Right 0R9J
  - Sternoclavicular
    - Left 0R9F
    - Right 0R9E
  - Tarsal
    - Left 0S9J
    - Right 0S9H
  - Temporomandibular
    - Left 0R9D
    - Right 0R9C
  - Thoracic Vertebral 0R96
  - Thoracolumbar Vertebral 0R9A
  - Toe Phalangeal
    - Left 0S9Q
    - Right 0S9P
  - Wrist
    - Left 0R9P
    - Right 0R9N
- Kidney
  - Left 0T91
  - Right 0T90
- Kidney Pelvis
  - Left 0T94
  - Right 0T93
- Knee Region
  - Left 0Y9G
  - Right 0Y9F
- Larynx 0C9S
- Leg
  - Lower
    - Left 0Y9J
    - Right 0Y9H
  - Upper
    - Left 0Y9D
    - Right 0Y9C

Drainage *(continued)*
- Lens
  - Left 089K
  - Right 089J
- Lip
  - Lower 0C91
  - Upper 0C90
- Liver 0F90
  - Left Lobe 0F92
  - Right Lobe 0F91
- Lung
  - Bilateral 0B9M
  - Left 0B9L
  - Lower Lobe
    - Left 0B9J
    - Right 0B9F
  - Middle Lobe, Right 0B9D
  - Right 0B9K
  - Upper Lobe
    - Left 0B9G
    - Right 0B9C
- Lung Lingula 0B9H
- Lymphatic
  - Aortic 079D
  - Axillary
    - Left 0796
    - Right 0795
  - Head 0790
  - Inguinal
    - Left 079J
    - Right 079H
  - Internal Mammary
    - Left 0799
    - Right 0798
  - Lower Extremity
    - Left 079G
    - Right 079F
  - Mesenteric 079B
  - Neck
    - Left 0792
    - Right 0791
  - Pelvis 079C
  - Thoracic Duct 079K
  - Thorax 0797
  - Upper Extremity
    - Left 0794
    - Right 0793
- Mandible
  - Left 0N9V
  - Right 0N9T
- Maxilla
  - Left 0N9S
  - Right 0N9R
- Mediastinum 0W9C
- Medulla Oblongata 009D
- Mesentery 0D9V
- Metacarpal
  - Left 0P9Q
  - Right 0P9P
- Metatarsal
  - Left 0Q9P
  - Right 0Q9N
- Muscle
  - Abdomen
    - Left 0K9L
    - Right 0K9K
  - Extraocular
    - Left 089M
    - Right 089L
  - Facial 0K91
  - Foot
    - Left 0K9W
    - Right 0K9V
  - Hand
    - Left 0K9D
    - Right 0K9C
  - Head 0K90
  - Hip
    - Left 0K9P
    - Right 0K9N
  - Lower Arm and Wrist
    - Left 0K9B

Drainage *(continued)*
- Muscle *(continued)*
  - Lower Arm and Wrist *(continued)*
    - Right 0K99
  - Lower Leg
    - Left 0K9T
    - Right 0K9S
  - Neck
    - Left 0K93
    - Right 0K92
  - Perineum 0K9M
  - Shoulder
    - Left 0K96
    - Right 0K95
  - Thorax
    - Left 0K9J
    - Right 0K9H
  - Tongue, Palate, Pharynx 0K94
  - Trunk
    - Left 0K9G
    - Right 0K9F
  - Upper Arm
    - Left 0K98
    - Right 0K97
  - Upper Leg
    - Left 0K9R
    - Right 0K9Q
- Nasopharynx 099N
- Neck 0W96
- Nerve
  - Abdominal Sympathetic 019M
  - Abducens 009L
  - Accessory 009R
  - Acoustic 009N
  - Brachial Plexus 0193
  - Cervical 0191
  - Cervical Plexus 0190
  - Facial 009M
  - Femoral 019D
  - Glossopharyngeal 009P
  - Head and Neck Sympathetic 019K
  - Hypoglossal 009S
  - Lumbar 019B
  - Lumbar Plexus 0199
  - Lumbar Sympathetic 019N
  - Lumbosacral Plexus 019A
  - Median 0195
  - Oculomotor 009H
  - Olfactory 009F
  - Optic 009G
  - Peroneal 019H
  - Phrenic 0192
  - Pudendal 019C
  - Radial 0196
  - Sacral 019R
  - Sacral Plexus 019Q
  - Sacral Sympathetic 019P
  - Sciatic 019F
  - Thoracic 0198
  - Thoracic Sympathetic 019L
  - Tibial 019G
  - Trigeminal 009K
  - Trochlear 009J
  - Ulnar 0194
  - Vagus 009Q
- Nipple
  - Left 0H9X
  - Right 0H9W
- Nose 099K
- Omentum
  - Greater 0D9S
  - Lesser 0D9T
- Oral Cavity and Throat 0W93
- Orbit
  - Left 0N9Q
  - Right 0N9P
- Ovary
  - Bilateral 0U92
  - Left 0U91
  - Right 0U90

Drainage *(continued)*
- Palate
  - Hard 0C92
  - Soft 0C93
- Pancreas 0F9G
- Para-aortic Body 0G99
- Paraganglion Extremity 0G9F
- Parathyroid Gland 0G9R
  - Inferior
    - Left 0G9P
    - Right 0G9N
  - Multiple 0G9Q
  - Superior
    - Left 0G9M
    - Right 0G9L
- Patella
  - Left 0Q9F
  - Right 0Q9D
- Pelvic Cavity 0W9J
- Penis 0V9S
- Pericardial Cavity 0W9D
- Perineum
  - Female 0W9N
  - Male 0W9M
- Peritoneal Cavity 0W9G
- Peritoneum 0D9W
- Phalanx
  - Finger
    - Left 0P9V
    - Right 0P9T
  - Thumb
    - Left 0P9S
    - Right 0P9R
  - Toe
    - Left 0Q9R
    - Right 0Q9Q
- Pharynx 0C9M
- Pineal Body 0G91
- Pleura
  - Left 0B9P
  - Right 0B9N
- Pleural Cavity
  - Left 0W9B
  - Right 0W99
- Pons 009B
- Prepuce 0V9T
- Products of Conception
  - Amniotic Fluid
    - Diagnostic 1090
    - Therapeutic 1090
  - Fetal Blood 1090
  - Fetal Cerebrospinal Fluid 1090
  - Fetal Fluid, Other 1090
  - Fluid, Other 1090
- Prostate 0V90
- Radius
  - Left 0P9J
  - Right 0P9H
- Rectum 0D9P
- Retina
  - Left 089F
  - Right 089E
- Retinal Vessel
  - Left 089H
  - Right 089G
- Retroperitoneum 0W9H
- Rib
  - Left 0P92
  - Right 0P91
- Sacrum 0Q91
- Scapula
  - Left 0P96
  - Right 0P95
- Sclera
  - Left 0897
  - Right 0896
- Scrotum 0V95
- Septum, Nasal 099M
- Shoulder Region
  - Left 0X93
  - Right 0X92

Drainage *(continued)*
- Sinus
  - Accessory 099P
  - Ethmoid
    - Left 099V
    - Right 099U
  - Frontal
    - Left 099T
    - Right 099S
  - Mastoid
    - Left 099C
    - Right 099B
  - Maxillary
    - Left 099R
    - Right 099Q
  - Sphenoid
    - Left 099X
    - Right 099W
- Skin
  - Abdomen 0H97
  - Back 0H96
  - Buttock 0H98
  - Chest 0H95
  - Ear
    - Left 0H93
    - Right 0H92
  - Face 0H91
  - Foot
    - Left 0H9N
    - Right 0H9M
  - Genitalia 0H9A
  - Hand
    - Left 0H9G
    - Right 0H9F
  - Lower Arm
    - Left 0H9E
    - Right 0H9D
  - Lower Leg
    - Left 0H9L
    - Right 0H9K
  - Neck 0H94
  - Perineum 0H99
  - Scalp 0H90
  - Upper Arm
    - Left 0H9C
    - Right 0H9B
  - Upper Leg
    - Left 0H9J
    - Right 0H9H
- Skull 0N90
- Spinal Canal 009U
- Spinal Cord
  - Cervical 009W
  - Lumbar 009Y
  - Thoracic 009X
- Spinal Meninges 009T
- Spleen 079P
- Sternum 0P90
- Stomach 0D96
  - Pylorus 0D97
- Subarachnoid Space 0095
- Subcutaneous Tissue and Fascia
  - Abdomen 0J98
  - Back 0J97
  - Buttock 0J99
  - Chest 0J96
  - Face 0J91
  - Foot
    - Left 0J9R
    - Right 0J9Q
  - Hand
    - Left 0J9K
    - Right 0J9J
  - Lower Arm
    - Left 0J9H
    - Right 0J9G
  - Lower Leg
    - Left 0J9P
    - Right 0J9N
  - Neck
    - Anterior 0J94
    - Posterior 0J95

Drainage *(continued)*
- Subcutaneous Tissue and Fascia *(continued)*
  - Pelvic Region 0J9C
  - Perineum 0J9B
  - Scalp 0J90
  - Upper Arm
    - Left 0J9F
    - Right 0J9D
  - Upper Leg
    - Left 0J9M
    - Right 0J9L
- Subdural Space 0094
- Tarsal
  - Left 0Q9M
  - Right 0Q9L
- Tendon
  - Abdomen
    - Left 0L9G
    - Right 0L9F
  - Ankle
    - Left 0L9T
    - Right 0L9S
  - Foot
    - Left 0L9W
    - Right 0L9V
  - Hand
    - Left 0L98
    - Right 0L97
  - Head and Neck 0L90
  - Hip
    - Left 0L9K
    - Right 0L9J
  - Knee
    - Left 0L9R
    - Right 0L9Q
  - Lower Arm and Wrist
    - Left 0L96
    - Right 0L95
  - Lower Leg
    - Left 0L9P
    - Right 0L9N
  - Perineum 0L9H
  - Shoulder
    - Left 0L92
    - Right 0L91
  - Thorax
    - Left 0L9D
    - Right 0L9C
  - Electrocautery
    - Right 0L99
  - Upper Arm
    - Left 0L94
    - Right 0L93
  - Upper Leg
    - Left 0L9M
    - Right 0L9L
- Testis
  - Bilateral 0V9C
  - Left 0V9B
  - Right 0V99
- Thalamus 0099
- Thymus 079M
- Thyroid Gland 0G9K
  - Left Lobe 0G9G
  - Right Lobe 0G9H
- Tibia
  - Left 0Q9H
  - Right 0Q9G
- Toe Nail 0H9R
- Tongue 0C97
- Tonsils 0C9P
- Tooth
  - Lower 0C9X
  - Upper 0C9W
- Trachea 0B91
- Tunica Vaginalis
  - Left 0V97
  - Right 0V96
- Turbinate, Nasal 099L
- Tympanic Membrane
  - Left 0998

Drainage *(continued)*
- Tympanic Membrane *(continued)*
  - Right 0997
- Ulna
  - Left 0P9L
  - Right 0P9K
- Ureter
  - Left 0T97
  - Right 0T96
- Ureters, Bilateral 0T98
- Urethra 0T9D
- Uterine Supporting Structure 0U94
- Uterus 0U99
- Uvula 0C9N
- Vagina 0U9G
- Vas Deferens
  - Bilateral 0V9Q
  - Left 0V9P
  - Right 0V9N
- Vein
  - Axillary
    - Left 0598
    - Right 0597
  - Azygos 0590
  - Basilic
    - Left 059C
    - Right 059B
  - Brachial
    - Left 059A
    - Right 0599
  - Cephalic
    - Left 059F
    - Right 059D
  - Colic 0697
  - Common Iliac
    - Left 069D
    - Right 069C
  - Esophageal 0693
  - External Iliac
    - Left 069G
    - Right 069F
  - External Jugular
    - Left 059Q
    - Right 059P
  - Face
    - Left 059V
    - Right 059T
  - Femoral
    - Left 069N
    - Right 069M
  - Foot
    - Left 069V
    - Right 069T
  - Gastric 0692
  - Greater Saphenous
    - Left 069Q
    - Right 069P
  - Hand
    - Left 059H
    - Right 059G
  - Hemiazygos 0591
  - Hepatic 0694
  - Hypogastric
    - Left 069J
    - Right 069H
  - Inferior Mesenteric 0696
  - Innominate
    - Left 0594
    - Right 0593
  - Internal Jugular
    - Left 059N
    - Right 059M
  - Intracranial 059L
  - Lesser Saphenous
    - Left 069S
    - Right 069R
  - Lower 069Y
  - Portal 0698
  - Renal
    - Left 069B
    - Right 0699
  - Splenic 0691

E

Excision *(continued)*
- Bursa and Ligament *(continued)*
  - Thorax
    - Left 0MBG
    - Right 0MBF
  - Trunk
    - Left 0MBD
    - Right 0MBC
  - Upper Extremity
    - Left 0MBB
    - Right 0MB9
  - Wrist
    - Left 0MB6
    - Right 0MB5
- Buttock
  - Left 0YB1
  - Right 0YB0
- Carina 0BB2
- Carotid Bodies, Bilateral 0GB8
- Carotid Body
  - Left 0GB6
  - Right 0GB7
- Carpal
  - Left 0PBN
  - Right 0PBM
- Cecum 0DBH
- Cerebellum 00BC
- Cerebral Hemisphere 00B7
- Cerebral Meninges 00B1
- Cerebral Ventricle 00B6
- Cervix 0UBC
- Chest Wall 0WB8
- Chordae Tendineae 02B9
- Choroid
  - Left 08BB
  - Right 08BA
- Cisterna Chyli 07BL
- Clavicle
  - Left 0PBB
  - Right 0PB9
- Clitoris 0UBJ
- Coccygeal Glomus 0GBB
- Coccyx 0QBS
- Colon
  - Ascending 0DBK
  - Descending 0DBM
  - Sigmoid 0DBN
  - Transverse 0DBL
- Conduction Mechanism 02B8
- Conjunctiva
  - Left 08BTXZ
  - Right 08BSXZ
- Cord
  - Bilateral 0VBH
  - Left 0VBG
  - Right 0VBF
- Cornea
  - Left 08B9XZ
  - Right 08B8XZ
- Cul-de-sac 0UBF
- Diaphragm
  - Left 0BBS
  - Right 0BBR
- Disc
  - Cervical Vertebral 0RB3
  - Cervicothoracic Vertebral 0RB5
  - Lumbar Vertebral 0SB2
  - Lumbosacral 0SB4
  - Thoracic Vertebral 0RB9
  - Thoracolumbar Vertebral 0RBB
- Duct
  - Common Bile 0FB9
  - Cystic 0FB8
  - Hepatic
    - Left 0FB6
    - Right 0FB5
  - Lacrimal
    - Left 08BY
    - Right 08BX

Excision *(continued)*
- Duct *(continued)*
  - Pancreatic 0FBD
    - Accessory 0FBF
  - Parotid
    - Left 0CBC
    - Right 0CBB
- Duodenum 0DB9
- Dura Mater 00B2
- Ear
  - External
    - Left 09B1
    - Right 09B0
  - External Auditory Canal
    - Left 09B4
    - Right 09B3
  - Inner
    - Left 09BE0Z
    - Right 09BD0Z
  - Middle
    - Left 09B60Z
    - Right 09B50Z
- Elbow Region
  - Left 0XBC
  - Right 0XBB
- Epididymis
  - Bilateral 0VBL
  - Left 0VBK
  - Right 0VBJ
- Epiglottis 0CBR
- Esophagogastric Junction 0DB4
- Esophagus 0DB5
  - Lower 0DB3
  - Middle 0DB2
  - Upper 0DB1
- Eustachian Tube
  - Left 09BG
  - Right 09BF
- Extremity
  - Lower
    - Left 0YBB
    - Right 0YB9
  - Upper
    - Left 0XB7
    - Right 0XB6
- Eye
  - Left 08B1
  - Right 08B0
- Eyelid
  - Lower
    - Left 08BR
    - Right 08BQ
  - Upper
    - Left 08BP
    - Right 08BN
- Face 0WB2
- Fallopian Tube
  - Left 0UB6
  - Right 0UB5
- Fallopian Tubes, Bilateral 0UB7
- Femoral Region
  - Left 0YB8
  - Right 0YB7
- Femoral Shaft
  - Left 0QB9
  - Right 0QB8
- Femur
  - Lower
    - Left 0QBC
    - Right 0QBB
  - Upper
    - Left 0QB7
    - Right 0QB6
- Fibula
  - Left 0QBK
  - Right 0QBJ
- Finger Nail 0HBQXZ
- Foot
  - Left 0YBN
  - Right 0YBM
- Gallbladder 0FB4

Excision *(continued)*
- Gingiva
  - Lower 0CB6
  - Upper 0CB5
- Gland
  - Adrenal
    - Bilateral 0GB4
    - Left 0GB2
    - Right 0GB3
  - Lacrimal
    - Left 08BW
    - Right 08BV
  - Minor Salivary 0CBJ
  - Parotid
    - Left 0CB9
    - Right 0CB8
  - Pituitary 0GB0
  - Sublingual
    - Left 0CBF
    - Right 0CBD
  - Submaxillary
    - Left 0CBH
    - Right 0CBG
  - Vestibular 0UBL
- Glenoid Cavity
  - Left 0PB8
  - Right 0PB7
- Glomus Jugulare 0GBC
- Hand
  - Left 0XBK
  - Right 0XBJ
- Head 0WB0
- Humeral Head
  - Left 0PBD
  - Right 0PBC
- Humeral Shaft
  - Left 0PBG
  - Right 0PBF
- Hymen 0UBK
- Hypothalamus 00BA
- Ileocecal Valve 0DBC
- Ileum 0DBB
- Inguinal Region
  - Left 0YB6
  - Right 0YB5
- Intestine
  - Large 0DBE
    - Left 0DBG
    - Right 0DBF
  - Small 0DB8
- Iris
  - Left 08BD3Z
  - Right 08BC3Z
- Jaw
  - Lower 0WB5
  - Upper 0WB4
- Jejunum 0DBA
- Joint
  - Acromioclavicular
    - Left 0RBH
    - Right 0RBG
  - Ankle
    - Left 0SBG
    - Right 0SBF
  - Carpal
    - Left 0RBR
    - Right 0RBQ
  - Cervical Vertebral 0RB1
  - Cervicothoracic Vertebral 0RB4
  - Coccygeal 0SB6
  - Elbow
    - Left 0RBM
    - Right 0RBL
  - Finger Phalangeal
    - Left 0RBX
    - Right 0RBW
  - Hip
    - Left 0SBB
    - Right 0SB9
  - Knee
    - Left 0SBD
    - Right 0SBC

Excision *(continued)*
- Joint *(continued)*
  - Lumbar Vertebral 0SB0
  - Lumbosacral 0SB3
  - Metacarpocarpal
    - Left 0RBT
    - Right 0RBS
  - Metacarpophalangeal
    - Left 0RBV
    - Right 0RBU
  - Metatarsal-Phalangeal
    - Left 0SBN
    - Right 0SBM
  - Metatarsal-Tarsal
    - Left 0SBL
    - Right 0SBK
  - Occipital-cervical 0RB0
  - Sacrococcygeal 0SB5
  - Sacroiliac
    - Left 0SB8
    - Right 0SB7
  - Shoulder
    - Left 0RBK
    - Right 0RBJ
  - Sternoclavicular
    - Left 0RBF
    - Right 0RBE
  - Tarsal
    - Left 0SBJ
    - Right 0SBH
  - Temporomandibular
    - Left 0RBD
    - Right 0RBC
  - Thoracic Vertebral 0RB6
  - Thoracolumbar Vertebral 0RBA
  - Toe Phalangeal
    - Left 0SBQ
    - Right 0SBP
  - Wrist
    - Left 0RBP
    - Right 0RBN
- Kidney
  - Left 0TB1
  - Right 0TB0
- Kidney Pelvis
  - Left 0TB4
  - Right 0TB3
- Knee Region
  - Left 0YBG
  - Right 0YBF
- Larynx 0CBS
- Leg
  - Lower
    - Left 0YBJ
    - Right 0YBH
  - Upper
    - Left 0YBD
    - Right 0YBC
- Lens
  - Left 08BK3Z
  - Right 08BJ3Z
- Lip
  - Lower 0CB1
  - Upper 0CB0
- Liver 0FB0
  - Left Lobe 0FB2
  - Right Lobe 0FB1
- Lung
  - Bilateral 0BBM
  - Left 0BBL
  - Lower Lobe
    - Left 0BBJ
    - Right 0BBF
  - Middle Lobe, Right 0BBD
  - Right 0BBK
  - Upper Lobe
    - Left 0BBG
    - Right 0BBC
- Lung Lingula 0BBH
- Lymphatic
  - Aortic 07BD

Excision *(continued)*
- Lymphatic *(continued)*
  - Axillary
    - Left 07B6
    - Right 07B5
  - Head 07B0
  - Inguinal
    - Left 07BJ
    - Right 07BH
  - Internal Mammary
    - Left 07B9
    - Right 07B8
  - Lower Extremity
    - Left 07BG
    - Right 07BF
  - Mesenteric 07BB
  - Neck
    - Left 07B2
    - Right 07B1
  - Pelvis 07BC
  - Thoracic Duct 07BK
  - Thorax 07B7
  - Upper Extremity
    - Left 07B4
    - Right 07B3
- Mandible
  - Left 0NBV
  - Right 0NBT
- Maxilla
  - Left 0NBS
  - Right 0NBR
- Mediastinum 0WBC
- Medulla Oblongata 00BD
- Mesentery 0DBV
- Metacarpal
  - Left 0PBQ
  - Right 0PBP
- Metatarsal
  - Left 0QBP
  - Right 0QBN
- Muscle
  - Abdomen
    - Left 0KBL
    - Right 0KBK
  - Extraocular
    - Left 08BM
    - Right 08BL
  - Facial 0KB1
  - Foot
    - Left 0KBW
    - Right 0KBV
  - Hand
    - Left 0KBD
    - Right 0KBC
  - Head 0KB0
  - Hip
    - Left 0KBP
    - Right 0KBN
  - Lower Arm and Wrist
    - Left 0KBB
    - Right 0KB9
  - Lower Leg
    - Left 0KBT
    - Right 0KBS
  - Neck
    - Left 0KB3
    - Right 0KB2
  - Papillary 02BD
  - Perineum 0KBM
  - Shoulder
    - Left 0KB6
    - Right 0KB5
  - Thorax
    - Left 0KBJ
    - Right 0KBH
  - Tongue, Palate, Pharynx 0KB4
  - Trunk
    - Left 0KBG
    - Right 0KBF
  - Upper Arm
    - Left 0KB8
    - Right 0KB7

Excision *(continued)*
- Muscle *(continued)*
  - Upper Leg
    - Left 0KBR
    - Right 0KBQ
- Nasopharynx 09BN
- Neck 0WB6
- Nerve
  - Abdominal Sympathetic 01BM
  - Abducens 00BL
  - Accessory 00BR
  - Acoustic 00BN
  - Brachial Plexus 01B3
  - Cervical 01B1
  - Cervical Plexus 01B0
  - Facial 00BM
  - Femoral 01BD
  - Glossopharyngeal 00BP
  - Head and Neck Sympathetic 01BK
  - Hypoglossal 00BS
  - Lumbar 01BB
  - Lumbar Plexus 01B9
  - Lumbar Sympathetic 01BN
  - Lumbosacral Plexus 01BA
  - Median 01B5
  - Oculomotor 00BH
  - Olfactory 00BF
  - Optic 00BG
  - Peroneal 01BH
  - Phrenic 01B2
  - Pudendal 01BC
  - Radial 01B6
  - Sacral 01BR
  - Sacral Plexus 01BQ
  - Sacral Sympathetic 01BP
  - Sciatic 01BF
  - Thoracic 01B8
  - Thoracic Sympathetic 01BL
  - Tibial 01BG
  - Trigeminal 00BK
  - Trochlear 00BJ
  - Ulnar 01B4
  - Vagus 00BQ
- Nipple
  - Left 0HBX
  - Right 0HBW
- Nose 09BK
- Omentum
  - Greater 0DBS
  - Lesser 0DBT
- Orbit
  - Left 0NBQ
  - Right 0NBP
- Ovary
  - Bilateral 0UB2
  - Left 0UB1
  - Right 0UB0
- Palate
  - Hard 0CB2
  - Soft 0CB3
- Pancreas 0FBG
- Para-aortic Body 0GB9
- Paraganglion Extremity 0GBF
- Parathyroid Gland 0GBR
  - Inferior
    - Left 0GBP
    - Right 0GBN
  - Multiple 0GBQ
  - Superior
    - Left 0GBM
    - Right 0GBL
- Patella
  - Left 0QBF
  - Right 0QBD
- Penis 0VBS
- Pericardium 02BN
- Perineum
  - Female 0WBN
  - Male 0WBM
- Peritoneum 0DBW

Excision *(continued)*
- Phalanx
  - Finger
    - Left 0PBV
    - Right 0PBT
  - Thumb
    - Left 0PBS
    - Right 0PBR
  - Toe
    - Left 0QBR
    - Right 0QBQ
- Pharynx 0CBM
- Pineal Body 0GB1
- Pleura
  - Left 0BBP
  - Right 0BBN
- Pons 00BB
- Prepuce 0VBT
- Prostate 0VB0
- Radius
  - Left 0PBJ
  - Right 0PBH
- Rectum 0DBP
- Retina
  - Left 08BF3Z
  - Right 08BE3Z
- Retroperitoneum 0WBH
- Rib
  - Left 0PB2
  - Right 0PB1
- Sacrum 0QB1
- Scapula
  - Left 0PB6
  - Right 0PB5
- Sclera
  - Left 08B7XZ
  - Right 08B6XZ
- Scrotum 0VB5
- Septum
  - Atrial 02B5
  - Nasal 09BM
  - Ventricular 02BM
- Shoulder Region
  - Left 0XB3
  - Right 0XB2
- Sinus
  - Accessory 09BP
  - Ethmoid
    - Left 09BV
    - Right 09BU
  - Frontal
    - Left 09BT
    - Right 09BS
  - Mastoid
    - Left 09BC
    - Right 09BB
  - Maxillary
    - Left 09BR
    - Right 09BQ
  - Sphenoid
    - Left 09BX
    - Right 09BW
- Skin
  - Abdomen 0HB7XZ
  - Back 0HB6XZ
  - Buttock 0HB8XZ
  - Chest 0HB5XZ
  - Ear
    - Left 0HB3XZ
    - Right 0HB2XZ
  - Face 0HB1XZ
  - Foot
    - Left 0HBNXZ
    - Right 0HBMXZ
  - Genitalia 0HBAXZ
  - Hand
    - Left 0HBGXZ
    - Right 0HBFXZ
  - Lower Arm
    - Left 0HBEXZ
    - Right 0HBDXZ

Excision *(continued)*
- Skin *(continued)*
  - Lower Leg
    - Left 0HBLXZ
    - Right 0HBKXZ
  - Neck 0HB4XZ
  - Perineum 0HB9XZ
  - Scalp 0HB0XZ
  - Upper Arm
    - Left 0HBCXZ
    - Right 0HBBXZ
  - Upper Leg
    - Left 0HBJXZ
    - Right 0HBHXZ
- Skull 0NB0
- Spinal Cord
  - Cervical 00BW
  - Lumbar 00BY
  - Thoracic 00BX
- Spinal Meninges 00BT
- Spleen 07BP
- Sternum 0PB0
- Stomach 0DB6
  - Pylorus 0DB7
- Subcutaneous Tissue and Fascia
  - Abdomen 0JB8
  - Back 0JB7
  - Buttock 0JB9
  - Chest 0JB6
  - Face 0JB1
  - Foot
    - Left 0JBR
    - Right 0JBQ
  - Hand
    - Left 0JBK
    - Right 0JBJ
  - Lower Arm
    - Left 0JBH
    - Right 0JBG
  - Lower Leg
    - Left 0JBP
    - Right 0JBN
  - Neck
    - Anterior 0JB4
    - Posterior 0JB5
  - Pelvic Region 0JBC
  - Perineum 0JBB
  - Scalp 0JB0
  - Upper Arm
    - Left 0JBF
    - Right 0JBD
  - Upper Leg
    - Left 0JBM
    - Right 0JBL
- Tarsal
  - Left 0QBM
  - Right 0QBL
- Tendon
  - Abdomen
    - Left 0LBG
    - Right 0LBF
  - Ankle
    - Left 0LBT
    - Right 0LBS
  - Foot
    - Left 0LBW
    - Right 0LBV
  - Hand
    - Left 0LB8
    - Right 0LB7
  - Head and Neck 0LB0
  - Hip
    - Left 0LBK
    - Right 0LBJ
  - Knee
    - Left 0LBR
    - Right 0LBQ
  - Lower Arm and Wrist
    - Left 0LB6
    - Right 0LB5

Extirpation *(continued)*
Joint *(continued)*
Elbow
Left 0RCM
Right 0RCL
Finger Phalangeal
Left 0RCX
Right 0RCW
Hip
Left 0SCB
Right 0SC9
Knee
Left 0SCD
Right 0SCC
Lumbar Vertebral 0SC0
Lumbosacral 0SC3
Metacarpocarpal
Left 0RCT
Right 0RCS
Metacarpophalangeal
Left 0RCV
Right 0RCU
Metatarsal-Phalangeal
Left 0SCN
Right 0SCM
Metatarsal-Tarsal
Left 0SCL
Right 0SCK
Occipital-cervical 0RC0
Sacrococcygeal 0SC5
Sacroiliac
Left 0SC8
Right 0SC7
Shoulder
Left 0RCK
Right 0RCJ
Sternoclavicular
Left 0RCF
Right 0RCE
Tarsal
Left 0SCJ
Right 0SCH
Temporomandibular
Left 0RCD
Right 0RCC
Thoracic Vertebral 0RC6
Thoracolumbar Vertebral 0RCA
Toe Phalangeal
Left 0SCQ
Right 0SCP
Wrist
Left 0RCP
Right 0RCN
Kidney
Left 0TC1
Right 0TC0
Kidney Pelvis
Left 0TC4
Right 0TC3
Larynx 0CCS
Lens
Left 08CK
Right 08CJ
Lip
Lower 0CC1
Upper 0CC0
Liver 0FC0
Left Lobe 0FC2
Right Lobe 0FC1
Lung
Bilateral 0BCM
Left 0BCL
Lower Lobe
Left 0BCJ
Right 0BCF
Middle Lobe, Right 0BCD
Right 0BCK
Upper Lobe
Left 0BCG
Right 0BCC

Extirpation *(continued)*
Lung Lingula 0BCH
Lymphatic
Aortic 07CD
Axillary
Left 07C6
Right 07C5
Head 07C0
Inguinal
Left 07CJ
Right 07CH
Internal Mammary
Left 07C9
Right 07C8
Lower Extremity
Left 07CG
Right 07CF
Mesenteric 07CB
Neck
Left 07C2
Right 07C1
Pelvis 07CC
Thoracic Duct 07CK
Thorax 07C7
Upper Extremity
Left 07C4
Right 07C3
Mandible
Left 0NCV
Right 0NCT
Maxilla
Left 0NCS
Right 0NCR
Mediastinum 0WCC
Medulla Oblongata 00CD
Mesentery 0DCV
Metacarpal
Left 0PCQ
Right 0PCP
Metatarsal
Left 0QCP
Right 0QCN
Muscle
Abdomen
Left 0KCL
Right 0KCK
Extraocular
Left 08CM
Right 08CL
Facial 0KC1
Foot
Left 0KCW
Right 0KCV
Hand
Left 0KCD
Right 0KCC
Head 0KC0
Hip
Left 0KCP
Right 0KCN
Lower Arm and Wrist
Left 0KCB
Right 0KC9
Lower Leg
Left 0KCT
Right 0KCS
Neck
Left 0KC3
Right 0KC2
Papillary 02CD
Perineum 0KCM
Shoulder
Left 0KC6
Right 0KC5
Thorax
Left 0KCJ
Right 0KCH
Tongue, Palate, Pharynx 0KC4
Trunk
Left 0KCG
Right 0KCF

Extirpation *(continued)*
Muscle *(continued)*
Upper Arm
Left 0KC8
Right 0KC7
Upper Leg
Left 0KCR
Right 0KCQ
Nasopharynx 09CN
Nerve
Abdominal Sympathetic 01CM
Abducens 00CL
Accessory 00CR
Acoustic 00CN
Brachial Plexus 01C3
Cervical 01C1
Cervical Plexus 01C0
Facial 00CM
Femoral 01CD
Glossopharyngeal 00CP
Head and Neck Sympathetic 01CK
Hypoglossal 00CS
Lumbar 01CB
Lumbar Plexus 01C9
Lumbar Sympathetic 01CN
Lumbosacral Plexus 01CA
Median 01C5
Oculomotor 00CH
Olfactory 00CF
Optic 00CG
Peroneal 01CH
Phrenic 01C2
Pudendal 01CC
Radial 01C6
Sacral 01CR
Sacral Plexus 01CQ
Sacral Sympathetic 01CP
Sciatic 01CF
Thoracic 01C8
Thoracic Sympathetic 01CL
Tibial 01CG
Trigeminal 00CK
Trochlear 00CJ
Ulnar 01C4
Vagus 00CQ
Nipple
Left 0HCX
Right 0HCW
Nose 09CK
Omentum
Greater 0DCS
Lesser 0DCT
Oral Cavity and Throat 0WC3
Orbit
Left 0NCQ
Right 0NCP
Ovary
Bilateral 0UC2
Left 0UC1
Right 0UC0
Palate
Hard 0CC2
Soft 0CC3
Pancreas 0FCG
Para-aortic Body 0GC9
Paraganglion Extremity 0GCF
Parathyroid Gland 0GCR
Inferior
Left 0GCP
Right 0GCN
Multiple 0GCQ
Superior
Left 0GCM
Right 0GCL
Patella
Left 0QCF
Right 0QCD
Pelvic Cavity 0WCJ
Penis 0VCS
Pericardial Cavity 0WCD
Pericardium 02CN

Extirpation *(continued)*
Peritoneal Cavity 0WCG
Peritoneum 0DCW
Phalanx
Finger
Left 0PCV
Right 0PCT
Thumb
Left 0PCS
Right 0PCR
Toe
Left 0QCR
Right 0QCQ
Pharynx 0CCM
Pineal Body 0GC1
Pleura
Left 0BCP
Right 0BCN
Pleural Cavity
Left 0WCB
Right 0WC9
Pons 00CB
Prepuce 0VCT
Prostate 0VC0
Radius
Left 0PCJ
Right 0PCH
Rectum 0DCP
Respiratory Tract 0WCQ
Retina
Left 08CF
Right 08CE
Retinal Vessel
Left 08CH
Right 08CG
Rib
Left 0PC2
Right 0PC1
Sacrum 0QC1
Scapula
Left 0PC6
Right 0PC5
Sclera
Left 08C7XZZ
Right 08C6XZZ
Scrotum 0VC5
Septum
Atrial 02C5
Nasal 09CM
Ventricular 02CM
Sinus
Accessory 09CP
Ethmoid
Left 09CV
Right 09CU
Frontal
Left 09CT
Right 09CS
Mastoid
Left 09CC
Right 09CB
Maxillary
Left 09CR
Right 09CQ
Sphenoid
Left 09CX
Right 09CW
Skin
Abdomen 0HC7XZZ
Back 0HC6XZZ
Buttock 0HC8XZZ
Chest 0HC5XZZ
Ear
Left 0HC3XZZ
Right 0HC2XZZ
Face 0HC1XZZ
Foot
Left 0HCNXZZ
Right 0HCMXZZ
Genitalia 0HCAXZZ

Extirpation *(continued)*
- Skin *(continued)*
  - Hand
    - Left 0HCGXZZ
    - Right 0HCFXZZ
  - Lower Arm
    - Left 0HCEXZZ
    - Right 0HCDXZZ
  - Lower Leg
    - Left 0HCLXZZ
    - Right 0HCKXZZ
  - Neck 0HC4XZZ
  - Perineum 0HC9XZZ
  - Scalp 0HC0XZZ
  - Upper Arm
    - Left 0HCCXZZ
    - Right 0HCBXZZ
  - Upper Leg
    - Left 0HCJXZZ
    - Right 0HCHXZZ
- Spinal Cord
  - Cervical 00CW
  - Lumbar 00CY
  - Thoracic 00CX
- Spinal Meninges 00CT
- Spleen 07CP
- Sternum 0PC0
- Stomach 0DC6
  - Pylorus 0DC7
- Subarachnoid Space 00C5
- Subcutaneous Tissue and Fascia
  - Abdomen 0JC8
  - Back 0JC7
  - Buttock 0JC9
  - Chest 0JC6
  - Face 0JC1
  - Foot
    - Left 0JCR
    - Right 0JCQ
  - Hand
    - Left 0JCK
    - Right 0JCJ
  - Lower Arm
    - Left 0JCH
    - Right 0JCG
  - Lower Leg
    - Left 0JCP
    - Right 0JCN
  - Neck
    - Anterior 0JC4
    - Posterior 0JC5
  - Pelvic Region 0JCC
  - Perineum 0JCB
  - Scalp 0JC0
  - Upper Arm
    - Left 0JCF
    - Right 0JCD
  - Upper Leg
    - Left 0JCM
    - Right 0JCL
- Subdural Space 00C4
- Tarsal
  - Left 0QCM
  - Right 0QCL
- Tendon
  - Abdomen
    - Left 0LCG
    - Right 0LCF
  - Ankle
    - Left 0LCT
    - Right 0LCS
  - Foot
    - Left 0LCW
    - Right 0LCV
  - Hand
    - Left 0LC8
    - Right 0LC7
  - Head and Neck 0LC0
  - Hip
    - Left 0LCK
    - Right 0LCJ

Extirpation *(continued)*
- Tendon *(continued)*
  - Knee
    - Left 0LCR
    - Right 0LCQ
  - Lower Arm and Wrist
    - Left 0LC6
    - Right 0LC5
  - Lower Leg
    - Left 0LCP
    - Right 0LCN
  - Perineum 0LCH
  - Shoulder
    - Left 0LC2
    - Right 0LC1
  - Thorax
    - Left 0LCD
    - Right 0LCC
  - Trunk
    - Left 0LCB
    - Right 0LC9
  - Upper Arm
    - Left 0LC4
    - Right 0LC3
  - Upper Leg
    - Left 0LCM
    - Right 0LCL
- Testis
  - Bilateral 0VCC
  - Left 0VCB
  - Right 0VC9
- Thalamus 00C9
- Thymus 07CM
- Thyroid Gland 0GCK
  - Left Lobe 0GCG
  - Right Lobe 0GCH
- Tibia
  - Left 0QCH
  - Right 0QCG
- Toe Nail 0HCRXZZ
- Tongue 0CC7
- Tonsils 0CCP
- Tooth
  - Lower 0CCX
  - Upper 0CCW
- Trachea 0BC1
- Tunica Vaginalis
  - Left 0VC7
  - Right 0VC6
- Turbinate, Nasal 09CL
- Tympanic Membrane
  - Left 09C8
  - Right 09C7
- Ulna
  - Left 0PCL
  - Right 0PCK
- Ureter
  - Left 0TC7
  - Right 0TC6
- Urethra 0TCD
- Uterine Supporting Structure 0UC4
- Uterus 0UC9
- Uvula 0CCN
- Vagina 0UCG
- Valve
  - Aortic 02CF
  - Mitral 02CG
  - Pulmonary 02CH
  - Tricuspid 02CJ
- Vas Deferens
  - Bilateral 0VCQ
  - Left 0VCP
  - Right 0VCN
- Vein
  - Axillary
    - Left 05C8
    - Right 05C7
  - Azygos 05C0
  - Basilic
    - Left 05CC
    - Right 05CB

Extirpation *(continued)*
- Vein *(continued)*
  - Brachial
    - Left 05CA
    - Right 05C9
  - Cephalic
    - Left 05CF
    - Right 05CD
  - Colic 06C7
  - Common Iliac
    - Left 06CD
    - Right 06CC
  - Coronary 02C4
  - Esophageal 06C3
  - External Iliac
    - Left 06CG
    - Right 06CF
  - External Jugular
    - Left 05CQ
    - Right 05CP
  - Face
    - Left 05CV
    - Right 05CT
  - Femoral
    - Left 06CN
    - Right 06CM
  - Foot
    - Left 06CV
    - Right 06CT
  - Gastric 06C2
  - Greater Saphenous
    - Left 06CQ
    - Right 06CP
  - Hand
    - Left 05CH
    - Right 05CG
  - Hemiazygos 05C1
  - Hepatic 06C4
  - Hypogastric
    - Left 06CJ
    - Right 06CH
  - Inferior Mesenteric 06C6
  - Innominate
    - Left 05C4
    - Right 05C3
  - Internal Jugular
    - Left 05CN
    - Right 05CM
  - Intracranial 05CL
  - Lesser Saphenous
    - Left 06CS
    - Right 06CR
  - Lower 06CY
  - Portal 06C8
  - Pulmonary
    - Left 02CT
    - Right 02CS
  - Renal
    - Left 06CB
    - Right 06C9
  - Splenic 06C1
  - Subclavian
    - Left 05C6
    - Right 05C5
  - Superior Mesenteric 06C5
  - Upper 05CY
  - Vertebral
    - Left 05CS
    - Right 05CR
- Vena Cava
  - Inferior 06C0
  - Superior 02CV
- Ventricle
  - Left 02CL
  - Right 02CK
- Vertebra
  - Cervical 0PC3
  - Lumbar 0QC0
  - Thoracic 0PC4
- Vesicle
  - Bilateral 0VC3

Extirpation *(continued)*
- Vesicle *(continued)*
  - Left 0VC2
  - Right 0VC1
- Vitreous
  - Left 08C5
  - Right 08C4
- Vocal Cord
  - Left 0CCV
  - Right 0CCT
- Vulva 0UCM

Extracorporeal shock wave lithotripsy
- *see* Fragmentation

Extracranial-intracranial bypass (EC-IC)
- *see* Bypass, Upper Arteries 031

Extraction
- Auditory Ossicle
  - Left 09DA0ZZ
  - Right 09D90ZZ
- Bone Marrow
  - Iliac 07DR
  - Sternum 07DQ
  - Vertebral 07DS
- Bursa and Ligament
  - Abdomen
    - Left 0MDJ
    - Right 0MDH
  - Ankle
    - Left 0MDR
    - Right 0MDQ
  - Elbow
    - Left 0MD4
    - Right 0MD3
  - Foot
    - Left 0MDT
    - Right 0MDS
  - Hand
    - Left 0MD8
    - Right 0MD7
  - Head and Neck 0MD0
  - Hip
    - Left 0MDM
    - Right 0MDL
  - Knee
    - Left 0MDP
    - Right 0MDN
  - Lower Extremity
    - Left 0MDW
    - Right 0MDV
  - Perineum 0MDK
  - Shoulder
    - Left 0MD2
    - Right 0MD1
  - Thorax
    - Left 0MDG
    - Right 0MDF
  - Trunk
    - Left 0MDD
    - Right 0MDC
  - Upper Extremity
    - Left 0MDB
    - Right 0MD9
  - Wrist
    - Left 0MD6
    - Right 0MD5
- Cerebral Meninges 00D1
- Cornea
  - Left 08D9XZ
  - Right 08D8XZ
- Dura Mater 00D2
- Endometrium 0UDB
- Finger Nail 0HDQXZZ
- Hair 0HDSXZZ
- Kidney
  - Left 0TD1
  - Right 0TD0
- Lens
  - Left 08DK3ZZ
  - Right 08DJ3ZZ

Extraction *(continued)*
  Nerve
    Abdominal Sympathetic 01DM
    Abducens 00DL
    Accessory 00DR
    Acoustic 00DN
    Brachial Plexus 01D3
    Cervical 01D1
    Cervical Plexus 01D0
    Facial 00DM
    Femoral 01DD
    Glossopharyngeal 00DP
    Head and Neck Sympathetic 01DK
    Hypoglossal 00DS
    Lumbar 01DB
    Lumbar Plexus 01D9
    Lumbar Sympathetic 01DN
    Lumbosacral Plexus 01DA
    Median 01D5
    Oculomotor 00DH
    Olfactory 00DF
    Optic 00DG
    Peroneal 01DH
    Phrenic 01D2
    Pudendal 01DC
    Radial 01D6
    Sacral 01DR
    Sacral Plexus 01DQ
    Sacral Sympathetic 01DP
    Sciatic 01DF
    Thoracic 01D8
    Thoracic Sympathetic 01DL
    Tibial 01DG
    Trigeminal 00DK
    Trochlear 00DJ
    Ulnar 01D4
    Vagus 00DQ
  Ova 0UDN
  Pleura
    Left 0BDP
    Right 0BDN
  Products of Conception
    Classical 10D00Z0
    Ectopic 10D2
    Extraperitoneal 10D00Z2
    High Forceps 10D07Z5
    Internal Version 10D07Z7
    Low Cervical 10D00Z1
    Low Forceps 10D07Z3
    Mid Forceps 10D07Z4
    Other 10D07Z8
    Retained 10D1
    Vacuum 10D07Z6
  Septum, Nasal 09DM
  Sinus
    Accessory 09DP
    Ethmoid
      Left 09DV
      Right 09DU
    Frontal
      Left 09DT
      Right 09DS
    Mastoid
      Left 09DC
      Right 09DB
    Maxillary
      Left 09DR
      Right 09DQ
    Sphenoid
      Left 09DX
      Right 09DW
  Skin
    Abdomen 0HD7XZZ
    Back 0HD6XZZ
    Buttock 0HD8XZZ
  Skin
    Chest 0HD5XZZ
    Ear
      Left 0HD3XZZ
      Right 0HD2XZZ
    Face 0HD1XZZ

Extraction *(continued)*
  Skin *(continued)*
    Foot
      Left 0HDNXZZ
      Right 0HDMXZZ
    Genitalia 0HDAXZZ
    Hand
      Left 0HDGXZZ
      Right 0HDFXZZ
    Lower Arm
      Left 0HDEXZZ
      Right 0HDDXZZ
    Lower Leg
      Left 0HDLXZZ
      Right 0HDKXZZ
    Neck 0HD4XZZ
    Perineum 0HD9XZZ
    Scalp 0HD0XZZ
    Upper Arm
      Left 0HDCXZZ
      Right 0HDBXZZ
    Upper Leg
      Left 0HDJXZZ
      Right 0HDHXZZ
  Spinal Meninges 00DT
  Subcutaneous Tissue and Fascia
    Abdomen 0JD8
    Back 0JD7
    Buttock 0JD9
    Chest 0JD6
    Face 0JD1
    Foot
      Left 0JDR
      Right 0JDQ
    Hand
      Left 0JDK
      Right 0JDJ
    Lower Arm
      Left 0JDH
      Right 0JDG
    Lower Leg
      Left 0JDP
      Right 0JDN
    Neck
      Anterior 0JD4
      Posterior 0JD5
    Pelvic Region 0JDC
    Perineum 0JDB
    Scalp 0JD0
    Upper Arm
      Left 0JDF
      Right 0JDD
    Upper Leg
      Left 0JDM
      Right 0JDL
  Toe Nail 0HDRXZZ
  Tooth
    Lower 0CDXXZ
    Upper 0CDWXZ
  Turbinate, Nasal 09DL
  Tympanic Membrane
    Left 09D8
    Right 09D7
  Vein
    Basilic
      Left 05DC
      Right 05DB
    Brachial
      Left 05DA
      Right 05D9
    Cephalic
      Left 05DF
      Right 05DD
    Femoral
      Left 06DN
      Right 06DM
    Foot
      Left 06DV
      Right 06DT
    Greater Saphenous
      Left 06DQ
      Right 06DP

Extraction *(continued)*
  Vein *(continued)*
    Hand
      Left 05DH
      Right 05DG
    Lesser Saphenous
      Left 06DS
      Right 06DR
    Lower 06DY
    Upper 05DY
  Vocal Cord
    Left 0CDV
    Right 0CDT
Extradural space
  use Epidural Space
EXtreme Lateral Interbody Fusion (XLIF) device
  use Interbody Fusion Device in Lower Joints

F

Face lift
  see Alteration, Face 0W02
Facet replacement spinal stabilization device
  use Spinal Stabilization Device, Facet Replacement in 0RH
  use Spinal Stabilization Device, Facet Replacement in 0SH
Facial artery
  use Artery, Face
False vocal cord
  use Larynx
Falx cerebri
  use Dura Mater
Fascia lata
  use Subcutaneous Tissue and Fascia, Upper Leg, Left
  use Subcutaneous Tissue and Fascia, Upper Leg, Right
Fasciaplasty, fascioplasty
  see Repair, Subcutaneous Tissue and Fascia 0JQ
  see Replacement, Subcutaneous Tissue and Fascia 0JR
Fasciectomy
  see Excision, Subcutaneous Tissue and Fascia 0JB
Fasciorrhaphy
  see Repair, Subcutaneous Tissue and Fascia 0JQ
Fasciotomy
  see Division, Subcutaneous Tissue and Fascia 0J8
  see Drainage, Subcutaneous Tissue and Fascia 0J9
Feeding Device
  Change device in
    Lower 0D2DXUZ
    Upper 0D20XUZ
  Insertion of device in
    Duodenum 0DH9
    Esophagus 0DH5
    Ileum 0DHB
    Intestine, Small 0DH8
    Jejunum 0DHA
    Stomach 0DH6
  Removal of device from
    Esophagus 0DP5
    Intestinal Tract
      Lower 0DPD
      Upper 0DP0
    Stomach 0DP6
  Revision of device in
    Intestinal Tract
      Lower 0DWD
      Upper 0DW0
    Stomach 0DW6
Femoral head
  use Femur, Upper, Left
  use Femur, Upper, Right

Femoral lymph node
  use Lymphatic, Lower Extremity, Left
  use Lymphatic, Lower Extremity, Right
Femoropatellar joint
  use Joint, Knee, Left
  use Joint, Knee, Left, Femoral Surface
  use Joint, Knee, Right
  use Joint, Knee, Right, Femoral Surface
Femorotibial joint
  use Joint, Knee, Left
  use Joint, Knee, Left, Tibial Surface
  use Joint, Knee, Right
  use Joint, Knee, Right, Tibial Surface
Fibular artery
  use Artery, Peroneal, Left
  use Artery, Peroneal, Right
Fibularis brevis muscle
  use Muscle, Lower Leg, Left
  use Muscle, Lower Leg, Right
Fibularis longus muscle
  use Muscle, Lower Leg, Left
  use Muscle, Lower Leg, Right
Fifth cranial nerve
  use Nerve, Trigeminal
Fimbriectomy
  see Excision, Female Reproductive System 0UB
  see Resection, Female Reproductive System 0UT
First cranial nerve
  use Nerve, Olfactory
First intercostal nerve
  use Nerve, Brachial Plexus
Fistulization
  see Bypass
  see Drainage
  see Repair
Fitting
  Arch bars, for fracture reduction
    see Reposition, Mouth and Throat 0CS
  Arch bars, for immobilization
    see Immobilization, Face 2W31
  Artificial limb
    see Device Fitting, Rehabilitation F0D
  Hearing aid
    see Device Fitting, Rehabilitation F0D
  Ocular prosthesis F0DZ8UZ
  Prosthesis, limb
    see Device Fitting, Rehabilitation F0D
  Prosthesis, ocular F0DZ8UZ
Fixation, bone
  External, with fracture reduction
    see Reposition
  External, without fracture reduction
    see Insertion
  Internal, with fracture reduction
    see Reposition
  Internal, without fracture reduction
    see Insertion
FLAIR® Endovascular Stent Graft
  use Intraluminal Device
Flexible Composite Mesh
  use Synthetic Substitute
Flexor carpi radialis muscle
  use Muscle, Lower Arm and Wrist, Left
  use Muscle, Lower Arm and Wrist, Right
Flexor carpi ulnaris muscle
  use Muscle, Lower Arm and Wrist, Left
  use Muscle, Lower Arm and Wrist, Right

- **Flexor digitorum brevis muscle**
  - *use* Muscle, Foot, Left
  - *use* Muscle, Foot, Right
- **Flexor digitorum longus muscle**
  - *use* Muscle, Lower Leg, Left
  - *use* Muscle, Lower Leg, Right
- **Flexor hallucis brevis muscle**
  - *use* Muscle, Foot, Left
  - *use* Muscle, Foot, Right
- **Flexor hallucis longus muscle**
  - *use* Muscle, Lower Leg, Left
  - *use* Muscle, Lower Leg, Right
- **Flexor pollicis longus muscle**
  - *use* Muscle, Lower Arm and Wrist, Left
  - *use* Muscle, Lower Arm and Wrist, Right
- **Fluoroscopy**
  - Abdomen and Pelvis BW11
  - Airway, Upper BB1DZZZ
  - Ankle
    - Left BQ1
    - Right BQ1G
  - Aorta
    - Abdominal B410
      - Laser, Intraoperative B410
    - Thoracic B310
      - Laser, Intraoperative B310
    - Thoraco-Abdominal B31P
      - Laser, Intraoperative B31P
  - Aorta and Bilateral Lower Extremity Arteries B41D
    - Laser, Intraoperative B41D
  - Arm
    - Left BP1FZZZ
    - Right BP1EZZZ
  - Artery
    - Brachiocephalic-Subclavian
      - Right B311
        - Laser, Intraoperative B311
    - Bronchial B31L
      - Laser, Intraoperative B31L
    - Bypass Graft, Other B21F
    - Cervico-Cerebral Arch B31Q
      - Laser, Intraoperative B31Q
    - Common Carotid
      - Bilateral B315
        - Laser, Intraoperative B315
      - Left B314
        - Laser, Intraoperative B314
      - Right B313
        - Laser, Intraoperative B313
    - Coronary
      - Bypass Graft
        - Multiple B213
          - Laser, Intraoperative B213
        - Single B212
          - Laser, Intraoperative B212
      - Multiple B211
        - Laser, Intraoperative B211
      - Single B210
        - Laser, Intraoperative B210
    - External Carotid
      - Bilateral B31C
        - Laser, Intraoperative B31C
      - Left B31B
        - Laser, Intraoperative B31B
      - Right B319
        - Laser, Intraoperative B319
    - Hepatic B412
      - Laser, Intraoperative B412
    - Inferior Mesenteric B415
      - Laser, Intraoperative B415

- **Fluoroscopy** *(continued)*
  - Artery *(continued)*
    - Intercostal B31L
      - Laser, Intraoperative B31L
    - Internal Carotid
      - Bilateral B318
        - Laser, Intraoperative B318
      - Left B317
        - Laser, Intraoperative B317
      - Right B316
        - Laser, Intraoperative B316
    - Internal Mammary Bypass Graft
      - Left B218
      - Right B217
    - Intra-Abdominal
      - Laser, Intraoperative B41B
      - Other B41B
    - Intracranial B31R
      - Laser, Intraoperative B31R
    - Lower
      - Laser, Intraoperative B41J
      - Other B41J
    - Lower Extremity
      - Bilateral and Aorta B41D
        - Laser, Intraoperative B41D
      - Left B41G
        - Laser, Intraoperative B41G
      - Right B41F
        - Laser, Intraoperative B41F
    - Lumbar B419
      - Laser, Intraoperative B419
    - Pelvic B41C
      - Laser, Intraoperative B41C
    - Pulmonary
      - Left B31T
        - Laser, Intraoperative B31T
      - Right B31S
        - Laser, Intraoperative B31S
    - Renal
      - Bilateral B418
        - Laser, Intraoperative B418
      - Left B417
        - Laser, Intraoperative B417
      - Right B416
        - Laser, Intraoperative B416
    - Spinal B31M
      - Laser, Intraoperative B31M
    - Splenic B413
      - Laser, Intraoperative B413
    - Subclavian
      - Laser, Intraoperative B312
      - Left B312
    - Superior Mesenteric B414
      - Laser, Intraoperative B414
    - Upper
      - Laser, Intraoperative B31N
      - Other B31N
    - Upper Extremity
      - Bilateral B31K
        - Laser, Intraoperative B31K
      - Left B31J
        - Laser, Intraoperative B31J
      - Right B31H
        - Laser, Intraoperative B31H

- **Fluoroscopy** *(continued)*
  - Artery *(continued)*
    - Vertebral
      - Bilateral B31G
        - Laser, Intraoperative B31G
      - Left B31F
        - Laser, Intraoperative B31F
      - Right B31D
        - Laser, Intraoperative B31D
  - Bile Duct BF10
    - Pancreatic Duct and Gallbladder BF14
  - Bile Duct and Gallbladder BF13
  - Biliary Duct BF11
  - Bladder BT10
    - Kidney and Ureter BT14
      - Left BT1F
      - Right BT1D
  - Bladder and Urethra BT1B
  - Bowel, Small BD1
  - Calcaneus
    - Left BQ1KZZZ
    - Right BQ1JZZZ
  - Clavicle
    - Left BP15ZZZ
    - Right BP14ZZZ
  - Coccyx BR1F
  - Colon BD14
  - Corpora Cavernosa BV10
  - Dialysis Fistula B51W
  - Dialysis Shunt B51W
  - Diaphragm BB16ZZZ
  - Disc
    - Cervical BR11
    - Lumbar BR13
    - Thoracic BR12
  - Duodenum BD19
  - Elbow
    - Left BP1H
    - Right BP1G
  - Epiglottis B91G
  - Esophagus BD11
  - Extremity
    - Lower BW1C
    - Upper BW1J
  - Facet Joint
    - Cervical BR14
    - Lumbar BR16
    - Thoracic BR15
  - Fallopian Tube
    - Bilateral BU12
    - Left BU11
    - Right BU10
  - Fallopian Tube and Uterus BU18
  - Femur
    - Left BQ14ZZZ
    - Right BQ13ZZZ
  - Finger
    - Left BP1SZZZ
    - Right BP1RZZZ
  - Foot
    - Left BQ1MZZZ
    - Right BQ1LZZZ
  - Forearm
    - Left BP1KZZZ
    - Right BP1JZZZ
  - Gallbladder BF12
    - Bile Duct and Pancreatic Duct BF14
  - Gallbladder and Bile Duct BF13
  - Gastrointestinal, Upper BD1
  - Hand
    - Left BP1PZZZ
    - Right BP1NZZZ
  - Head and Neck BW19
  - Heart
    - Left B215
    - Right B214
    - Right and Left B216

- **Fluoroscopy** *(continued)*
  - Hip
    - Left BQ11
    - Right BQ10
  - Humerus
    - Left BP1BZZZ
    - Right BP1AZZZ
  - Ileal Diversion Loop BT1C
  - Ileal Loop, Ureters and Kidney BT1G
  - Intracranial Sinus B512
  - Joint
    - Acromioclavicular, Bilateral BP13ZZZ
    - Finger
      - Left BP1D
      - Right BP1C
    - Foot
      - Left BQ1Y
      - Right BQ1X
    - Hand
      - Left BP1D
      - Right BP1C
    - Lumbosacral BR1B
    - Sacroiliac BR1D
    - Sternoclavicular
      - Bilateral BP12ZZZ
      - Left BP11ZZZ
      - Right BP10ZZZ
    - Temporomandibular
      - Bilateral BN19
      - Left BN18
      - Right BN17
    - Thoracolumbar BR18
    - Toe
      - Left BQ1Y
      - Right BQ1X
  - Kidney
    - Bilateral BT13
    - Ileal Loop and Ureter BT1G
    - Left BT12
    - Right BT11
    - Ureter and Bladder BT14
      - Left BT1F
      - Right BT1D
  - Knee
    - Left BQ18
    - Right BQ17
  - Larynx B91J
  - Leg
    - Left BQ1FZZZ
    - Right BQ1DZZZ
  - Lung
    - Bilateral BB14ZZZ
    - Left BB13ZZZ
    - Right BB12ZZZ
  - Mediastinum BB1CZZZ
  - Mouth BD1B
  - Neck and Head BW19
  - Oropharynx BD1B
  - Pancreatic Duct BF1
    - Gallbladder and Bile Buct BF14
  - Patella
    - Left BQ1WZZZ
    - Right BQ1VZZZ
  - Pelvis BR1C
  - Pelvis and Abdomen BW11
  - Pharynix B91G
  - Ribs
    - Left BP1YZZZ
    - Right BP1XZZZ
  - Sacrum BR1F
  - Scapula
    - Left BP17ZZZ
    - Right BP16ZZZ
  - Shoulder
    - Left BP19
    - Right BP18
  - Sinus, Intracranial B512
  - Spinal Cord B01B

G

Gastric pacemaker lead
use Stimulator Lead in Gastrointestinal System
Gastric plexus
use Nerve, Abdominal Sympathetic
Gastrocnemius muscle
use Muscle, Lower Leg, Left
use Muscle, Lower Leg, Right
Gastrocolic ligament
use Omentum, Greater
Gastrocolic omentum
use Omentum, Greater
Gastrocolostomy
see Bypass, Gastrointestinal System 0D1
see Drainage, Gastrointestinal System 0D9
Gastroduodenal artery
use Artery, Hepatic
Gastroduodenectomy
see Excision, Gastrointestinal System 0DB
see Resection, Gastrointestinal System 0DT
Gastroduodenoscopy 0DJ08ZZ
Gastroenteroplasty
see Repair, Gastrointestinal System 0DQ
see Supplement, Gastrointestinal System 0DU
Gastroenterostomy
see Bypass, Gastrointestinal System 0D1
see Drainage, Gastrointestinal System 0D9
Gastroesophageal (GE) junction
use Esophagogastric Junction
Gastrogastrostomy
see Bypass, Stomach 0D16
see Drainage, Stomach 0D96
Gastrohepatic omentum
use Omentum, Lesser
Gastrojejunostomy
see Bypass, Stomach 0D16
see Drainage, Stomach 0D96
Gastrolysis
see Release, Stomach 0DN6
Gastropexy
see Repair, Stomach 0DQ6
see Reposition, Stomach 0DS6
Gastrophrenic ligament
use Omentum, Greater
Gastroplasty
see Repair, Stomach 0DQ6
see Supplement, Stomach 0DU6
Gastroplication
see Restriction, Stomach 0DV6
Gastropylorectomy
see Excision, Gastrointestinal System 0DB
Gastrorrhaphy
see Repair, Stomach 0DQ6
Gastroscopy 0DJ68ZZ
Gastrosplenic ligament
use Omentum, Greater
Gastrostomy
see Bypass, Stomach 0D16
see Drainage, Stomach 0D96
Gastrotomy
see Drainage, Stomach 0D96
Gemellus muscle
use Muscle, Hip, Left
use Muscle, Hip, Right
Geniculate ganglion
use Nerve, Facial
Geniculate nucleus
use Thalamus
Genioglossus muscle
use Muscle, Tongue, Palate, Pharynx
Genioplasty
see Alteration, Jaw, Lower 0W05
Genitofemoral nerve
use Nerve, Lumbar Plexus
Gingivectomy
see Excision, Mouth and Throat 0CB
Gingivoplasty
see Repair, Mouth and Throat 0CQ
see Replacement, Mouth and Throat 0CR
see Supplement, Mouth and Throat 0CU
Glans penis
use Prepuce
Glenohumeral joint
use Joint, Shoulder, Left
use Joint, Shoulder, Right
Glenohumeral ligament
use Bursa and Ligament, Shoulder, Left
use Bursa and Ligament, Shoulder, Right
Glenoid fossa (of scapula)
use Glenoid Cavity, Left
use Glenoid Cavity, Right
Glenoid ligament (labrum)
use Bursa and Ligament, Shoulder, Left
use Bursa and Ligament, Shoulder, Right
Globus pallidus
use Basal Ganglia
Glomectomy
see Excision, Endocrine System 0GB
see Resection, Endocrine System 0GT
Glossectomy
see Excision, Tongue 0CB7
see Resection, Tongue 0CT7
Glossoepiglottic fold
use Epiglottis
Glossopexy
see Repair, Tongue 0CQ7
see Reposition, Tongue 0CS7
Glossoplasty
see Repair, Tongue 0CQ7
see Replacement, Tongue 0CR7
see Supplement, Tongue 0CU7
Glossorrhaphy
see Repair, Tongue 0CQ7
Glossotomy
see Drainage, Tongue 0C97
Glottis
use Larynx
Gluteal Artery Perforator Flap
Bilateral 0HRV079
Left 0HRU079
Right 0HRT079
Gluteal lymph node
use Lymphatic, Pelvis
Gluteal vein
use Vein, Hypogastric, Left
use Vein, Hypogastric, Right
Gluteus maximus muscle
use Muscle, Hip, Left
use Muscle, Hip, Right
Gluteus medius muscle
use Muscle, Hip, Left
use Muscle, Hip, Right
Gluteus minimus muscle
use Muscle, Hip, Left
use Muscle, Hip, Right
GORE® DUALMESH®
use Synthetic Substitute
Gracilis muscle
use Muscle, Upper Leg, Left
use Muscle, Upper Leg, Right
Graft
see Replacement
see Supplement
Great auricular nerve
use Nerve, Cervical Plexus
Great cerebral vein
use Vein, Intracranial
Great saphenous vein
use Vein, Greater Saphenous, Left
use Vein, Greater Saphenous, Right
Greater alar cartilage
use Nose
Greater occipital nerve
use Nerve, Cervical
Greater splanchnic nerve
use Nerve, Thoracic Sympathetic
Greater superficial petrosal nerve
use Nerve, Facial
Greater trochanter
use Femur, Upper, Left
use Femur, Upper, Right
Greater tuberosity
use Humeral Head, Left
use Humeral Head, Right
Greater vestibular (Bartholin's) gland
use Gland, Vestibular
Greater wing
use Bone, Sphenoid, Left
use Bone, Sphenoid, Right
Guedel airway
use Intraluminal Device, Airway in Mouth and Throat
Guidance, catheter placement
EKG
see Measurement, Physiological Systems 4A0
Fluoroscopy
see Fluoroscopy, Veins B51
Ultrasound
see Ultrasonography, Veins B54

H

Hallux
use Toe, 1st, Left
use Toe, 1st, Right
Hamate bone
use Carpal, Left
use Carpal, Right
Hancock Bioprosthesis (aortic) (mitral) valve
use Zooplastic Tissue in Heart and Great Vessels
Hancock Bioprosthetic Valved Conduit
use Zooplastic Tissue in Heart and Great Vessels
Harvesting, stem cells
see Pheresis, Circulatory 6A55
Head of fibula
use Fibula, Left
use Fibula, Right
Hearing Aid Assessment F14Z
Hearing Assessment F13Z
Hearing Device
Bone Conduction
Left 09HE
Right 09HD
Insertion of device in
Left 0NH6
Right 0NH5
Multiple Channel Cochlear Prosthesis
Left 09HE
Right 09HD
Removal of device from, Skull 0NP0
Revision of device in, Skull 0NW0
Single Channel Cochlear Prosthesis
Left 09HE
Right 09HD
Hearing Treatment F09Z
Heart Assist System
External
Insertion of device in, Heart 02HA
Removal of device from, Heart 02PA
Heart Assist System *(continued)*
External *(continued)*
Revision of device in, Heart 02WA
Implantable
Insertion of device in, Heart 02HA
Removal of device from, Heart 02PA
Revision of device in, Heart 02WA
HeartMate II® Left Ventricular Assist Device (LVAD)
use Implantable Heart Assist System in Heart and Great Vessels
HeartMate XVE® Left Ventricular Assist Device (LVAD)
use Implantable Heart Assist System in Heart and Great Vessels
HeartMate® implantable heart assist system
see Insertion of device in, Heart 02HA
Helix
use Ear, External, Bilateral
use Ear, External, Left
use Ear, External, Right
Hemicolectomy
see Resection, Gastrointestinal System 0DT
Hemicystectomy
see Excision, Urinary System 0TB
Hemigastrectomy
see Excision, Gastrointestinal System 0DB
Hemiglossectomy
see Excision, Mouth and Throat 0CB
Hemilaminectomy
see Excision, Lower Bones 0QB
see Excision, Upper Bones 0PB
Hemilaminotomy
see Drainage, Lower Bones 0Q9
see Drainage, Upper Bones 0P9
see Excision, Lower Bones 0QB
see Excision, Upper Bones 0PB
see Release, Central Nervous System 00N
see Release, Lower Bones 0QN
see Release, Peripheral Nervous System 01N
see Release, Upper Bones 0PN
Hemilaryngectomy
see Excision, Larynx 0CBS
Hemimandibulectomy
see Excision, Head and Facial Bones 0NB
Hemimaxillectomy
see Excision, Head and Facial Bones 0NB
Hemipylorectomy
see Excision, Gastrointestinal System 0DB
Hemispherectomy
see Excision, Central Nervous System 00B
see Resection, Central Nervous System 00T
Hemithyroidectomy
see Resection, Endocrine System 0GT
see Excision, Endocrine System 0GB
Hemodialysis 5A1D00Z
Hepatectomy
see Excision, Hepatobiliary System and Pancreas 0FB
see Resection, Hepatobiliary System and Pancreas 0FT
Hepatic artery proper
use Artery, Hepatic

I

- **Imaging, diagnostic** *(continued)*
  - *see* Plain Radiography
  - *see* Ultrasonography
- **Immobilization**
  - Abdominal Wall 2W33X
  - Arm
    - Lower
      - Left 2W3DX
      - Right 2W3CX
    - Upper
      - Left 2W3BX
      - Right 2W3AX
  - Back 2W35X
  - Chest Wall 2W34X
  - Extremity
    - Lower
      - Left 2W3MX
      - Right 2W3LX
    - Upper
      - Left 2W39X
      - Right 2W38X
  - Face 2W31X
  - Finger
    - Left 2W3KX
    - Right 2W3JX
  - Foot
    - Left 2W3TX
    - Right 2W3SX
  - Hand
    - Left 2W3FX
    - Right 2W3EX
  - Head 2W30X
  - Inguinal Region
    - Left 2W37X
    - Right 2W36X
  - Leg
    - Lower
      - Left 2W3RX
      - Right 2W3QX
    - Upper
      - Left 2W3PX
      - Right 2W3NX
  - Neck 2W32X
  - Thumb
    - Left 2W3H
    - Right 2W3GX
  - Toe
    - Left 2W3VX
    - Right 2W3UX
- **Immunization**
  - *see* Introduction of Serum, Toxoid, and Vaccine
- **Immunotherapy**
  - *see* Introduction of Immunotherapeutic Substance
- **Immunotherapy, antineoplastic**
  - Interferon
    - *see* Introduction of Low-dose Interleukin-2
  - Interleukin-2, high-dose
    - *see* Introduction of High-dose Interleukin-2
  - Interleukin-2, low-dose
    - *see* Introduction of Low-dose Interleukin-2
  - Monoclonal antibody
    - *see* Introduction of Monoclonal Antibody
  - Proleukin, high-dose
    - *see* Introduction of High-dose Interleukin-2
  - Proleukin, low-dose
    - *see* Introduction of Low-dose Interleukin-2
- **Impeller Pump**
  - Continuous, Output 5A0221D
  - Intermittent, Output 5A0211D
- **Implantable cardioverter-defibrillator (ICD)**
  - *use* Defibrillator Generator in 0JH
- **Implantable drug infusion pump (anti-spasmodic) (chemotherapy)(pain)**
  - *use* Infusion Device, Pump in Subcutaneous Tissue and Fascia
- **Implantable glucose monitoring device**
  - *use* Monitoring Device
- **Implantable hemodynamic monitor (IHM)**
  - *use* Monitoring Device, Hemodynamic in 0JH
- **Implantable hemodynamic monitoring system (IHMS)**
  - *use* Monitoring Device, Hemodynamic in 0JH
- **Implantable Miniature Telescope™ (IMT)**
  - *use* Synthetic Substitute, Intraocular Telescope in 08R
- **Implantation**
  - *see* Insertion
  - *see* Replacement
- **Implanted (venous)(access) port**
  - *use* Vascular Access Device, Reservoir in Subcutaneous Tissue and Fascia
- **IMV (intermittent mandatory ventilation)**
  - *see* Assistance, Respiratory 5A09
- **In Vitro Fertilization** 8E0ZXY1
- **Incision, abscess**
  - *see* Drainage
- **Incudectomy**
  - *see* Excision, Ear, Nose, Sinus 09B
  - *see* Resection, Ear, Nose, Sinus 09T
- **Incudopexy**
  - *see* Reposition, Ear, Nose, Sinus 09S
  - *see* Repair, Ear, Nose, Sinus 09Q
- **Incus**
  - *use* Auditory Ossicle, Left
  - *use* Auditory Ossicle, Right
- **Induction of labor**
  - Artificial rupture of membranes
    - *see* Drainage, Pregnancy 109
  - Oxytocin
    - *see* Introduction of Hormone
- **InDura, intrathecal catheter (1P) (spinal)**
  - *use* Infusion Device
- **Inferior cardiac nerve**
  - *use* Nerve, Thoracic Sympathetic
- **Inferior cerebellar vein**
  - *use* Vein, Intracranial
- **Inferior cerebral vein**
  - *use* Vein, Intracranial
- **Inferior epigastric artery**
  - *use* Artery, External Iliac, Left
  - *use* Artery, External Iliac, Right
- **Inferior epigastric lymph node**
  - *use* Lymphatic, Pelvis
- **Inferior genicular artery**
  - *use* Artery, Popliteal, Left
  - *use* Artery, Popliteal, Right
- **Inferior gluteal artery**
  - *use* Artery, Internal Iliac, Left
  - *use* Artery, Internal Iliac, Right
- **Inferior gluteal nerve**
  - *use* Nerve, Sacral Plexus
- **Inferior hypogastric plexus**
  - *use* Nerve, Abdominal Sympathetic
- **Inferior labial artery**
  - *use* Artery, Face
- **Inferior longitudinal muscle**
  - *use* Muscle, Tongue, Palate, Pharynx
- **Inferior mesenteric ganglion**
  - *use* Nerve, Abdominal Sympathetic
- **Inferior mesenteric lymph node**
  - *use* Lymphatic, Mesenteric
- **Inferior mesenteric plexus**
  - *use* Nerve, Abdominal Sympathetic
- **Inferior oblique muscle**
  - *use* Muscle, Extraocular, Left
  - *use* Muscle, Extraocular, Right
- **Inferior pancreaticoduodenal artery**
  - *use* Artery, Superior Mesenteric
- **Inferior phrenic artery**
  - *use* Aorta, Abdominal
- **Inferior rectus muscle**
  - *use* Muscle, Extraocular, Left
  - *use* Muscle, Extraocular, Right
- **Inferior suprarenal artery**
  - *use* Artery, Renal, Left
  - *use* Artery, Renal, Right
- **Inferior tarsal plate**
  - *use* Eyelid, Lower, Left
  - *use* Eyelid, Lower, Right
- **Inferior thyroid vein**
  - *use* Vein, Innominate, Left
  - *use* Vein, Innominate, Right
- **Inferior tibiofibular joint**
  - *use* Joint, Ankle, Left
  - *use* Joint, Ankle, Right
- **Inferior turbinate**
  - *use* Turbinate, Nasal
- **Inferior ulnar collateral artery**
  - *use* Artery, Brachial, Left
  - *use* Artery, Brachial, Right
- **Inferior vesical artery**
  - *use* Artery, Internal Iliac, Left
  - *use* Artery, Internal Iliac, Right
- **Infraauricular lymph node**
  - *use* Lymphatic, Head
- **Infraclavicular (deltopectoral) lymph node**
  - *use* Lymphatic, Upper Extremity, Left
  - *use* Lymphatic, Upper Extremity, Right
- **Infrahyoid muscle**
  - *use* Muscle, Neck, Left
  - *use* Muscle, Neck, Right
- **Infraparotid lymph node**
  - *use* Lymphatic, Head
- **Infraspinatus fascia**
  - *use* Subcutaneous Tissue and Fascia, Upper Arm, Left
  - *use* Subcutaneous Tissue and Fascia, Upper Arm, Right
- **Infraspinatus muscle**
  - *use* Muscle, Shoulder, Left
  - *use* Muscle, Shoulder, Right
- **Infundibulopelvic ligament**
  - *use* Uterine Supporting Structure
- **Infusion**
  - *see* Introduction of substance in or on
- **Infusion Device, Pump**
  - Insertion of device in
    - Abdomen 0JH8
    - Back 0JH7
    - Chest 0JH6
    - Lower Arm
      - Left 0JHH
      - Right 0JHG
    - Lower Leg
      - Left 0JHP
      - Right 0JHN
    - Trunk 0JHT
    - Upper Arm
      - Left 0JHF
      - Right 0JHD
    - Upper Leg
      - Left 0JHM
      - Right 0JHL
  - Removal of device from
    - Lower Extremity 0JPW
    - Trunk 0JPT
    - Upper Extremity 0JPV
- **Infusion Device, Pump** *(continued)*
  - Revision of device in
    - Lower Extremity 0JWW
    - Trunk 0JWT
    - Upper Extremity 0JWV
- **Infusion, glucarpidase**
  - Central vein 3E043GQ
  - Peripheral vein 3E033GQ
- **Inguinal canal**
  - *use* Inguinal Region, Bilateral
  - *use* Inguinal Region, Left
  - *use* Inguinal Region, Right
  - **Inguinal triangle**
  - *use* Inguinal Region, Bilateral
  - *use* Inguinal Region, Left
  - *use* Inguinal Region, Right
- **Injection**
  - *see* Introduction of substance in or on
- **Injection reservoir, port**
  - *use* Vascular Access Device, Reservoir in Subcutaneous Tissue and Fascia
- **Injection reservoir, pump**
  - *use* Infusion Device, Pump in Subcutaneous Tissue and Fascia
- **Insemination, artificial** 3E0P7LZ
- **Insertion**
  - Antimicrobial envelope
    - *see* Introduction of Anti-infective
  - Aqueous drainage shunt
    - *see* Bypass, Eye 081
    - *see* Drainage, Eye 089
  - Products of Conception 10H0
  - Spinal Stabilization Device
    - *see* Insertion of device in, Upper Joints 0RH
    - *see* Insertion of device in, Lower Joints 0SH
- **Insertion of device in**
  - Abdominal Wall 0WHF
  - Acetabulum
    - Left 0QH5
    - Right 0QH4
  - Anal Sphincter 0DHR
  - Ankle Region
    - Left 0YHL
    - Right 0YHK
  - Anus 0DHQ
  - Aorta
    - Abdominal 04H0
    - Thoracic 02HW
  - Arm
    - Lower
      - Left 0XHF
      - Right 0XHD
    - Upper
      - Left 0XH9
      - Right 0XH8
  - Artery
    - Anterior Tibial
      - Left 04HQ
      - Right 04HP
    - Axillary
      - Left 03H6
      - Right 03H5
    - Brachial
      - Left 03H8
      - Right 03H7
    - Celiac 04H1
    - Colic
      - Left 04H7
      - Middle 04H8
      - Right 04H6
    - Common Carotid
      - Left 03HJ
      - Right 03HH
    - Common Iliac
      - Left 04HD
      - Right 04HC

Insertion of device in *(continued)*
- Artery *(continued)*
  - External Carotid
    - Left 03HN
    - Right 03HM
  - External Iliac
    - Left 04HJ
    - Right 04HH
  - Face 03HR
  - Femoral
    - Left 04HL
    - Right 04HK
  - Foot
    - Left 04HW
    - Right 04HV
  - Gastric 04H2
  - Hand
    - Left 03HF
    - Right 03HD
  - Hepatic 04H3
  - Inferior Mesenteric 04HB
  - Innominate 03H2
  - Internal Carotid
    - Left 03HL
    - Right 03HK
  - Internal Iliac
    - Left 04HF
    - Right 04HE
  - Internal Mammary
    - Left 03H1
    - Right 03H0
  - Intracranial 03HG
  - Lower 04HY
  - Peroneal
    - Left 04HU
    - Right 04HT
  - Popliteal
    - Left 04HN
    - Right 04HM
  - Posterior Tibial
    - Left 04HS
    - Right 04HR
  - Pulmonary
    - Left 02HR
    - Right 02HQ
  - Pulmonary Trunk 02HP
  - Radial
    - Left 03HC
    - Right 03HB
  - Renal
    - Left 04HA
    - Right 04H9
  - Splenic 04H4
  - Subclavian
    - Left 03H4
    - Right 03H3
  - Superior Mesenteric 04H5
  - Temporal
    - Left 03HT
    - Right 03HS
  - Thyroid
    - Left 03HV
    - Right 03HU
  - Ulnar
    - Left 03HA
    - Right 03H9
  - Upper 03HY
  - Vertebral
    - Left 03HQ
    - Right 03HP
- Atrium
  - Left 02H7
  - Right 02H6
- Axilla
  - Left 0XH5
  - Right 0XH4
- Back
  - Lower 0WHL
  - Upper 0WHK
- Bladder 0THB
- Bladder Neck 0THC

Insertion of device in *(continued)*
- Bone
  - Ethmoid
    - Left 0NHG
    - Right 0NHF
  - Facial 0NHW
  - Frontal
    - Left 0NH2
    - Right 0NH1
  - Hyoid 0NHX
  - Lacrimal
    - Left 0NHJ
    - Right 0NHH
  - Lower 0QHY
  - Nasal 0NHB
  - Occipital
    - Left 0NH8
    - Right 0NH7
  - Palatine
    - Left 0NHL
    - Right 0NHK
  - Parietal
    - Left 0NH4
    - Right 0NH3
  - Pelvic
    - Left 0QH3
    - Right 0QH2
  - Sphenoid
    - Left 0NHD
    - Right 0NHC
  - Temporal
    - Left 0NH6
    - Right 0NH5
  - Upper 0PHY
  - Zygomatic
    - Left 0NHN
    - Right 0NHM
- Brain 00H0
- Breast
  - Bilateral 0HHV
  - Left 0HHU
  - Right 0HHT
- Bronchus
  - Lingula 0BH9
  - Lower Lobe
    - Left 0BHB
    - Right 0BH6
  - Main
    - Left 0BH7
    - Right 0BH3
  - Middle Lobe, Right 0BH5
  - Upper Lobe
    - Left 0BH8
    - Right 0BH4
- Buttock
  - Left 0YH1
  - Right 0YH0
- Carpal
  - Left 0PHN
  - Right 0PHM
- Cavity, Cranial 0WH1
- Cerebral Ventricle 00H6
- Cervix 0UHC
- Chest Wall 0WH8
- Cisterna Chyli 07HL
- Clavicle
  - Left 0PHB
  - Right 0PH9
- Coccyx 0QHS
- Cul-de-sac 0UHF
- Diaphragm
  - Left 0BHS
  - Right 0BHR
- Disc
  - Cervical Vertebral 0RH3
  - Cervicothoracic Vertebral 0RH5
  - Lumbar Vertebral 0SH2
  - Lumbosacral 0SH4
  - Thoracic Vertebral 0RH9
  - Thoracolumbar Vertebral 0RHB

Insertion of device in *(continued)*
- Duct
  - Hepatobiliary 0FHB
  - Pancreatic 0FHD
- Duodenum 0DH9
- Ear
  - Left 09HE
  - Right 09HD
- Elbow Region
  - Left 0XHC
  - Right 0XHB
- Epididymis and Spermatic Cord 0VHM
- Esophagus 0DH5
- Extremity
  - Lower
    - Left 0YHB
    - Right 0YH9
  - Upper
    - Left 0XH7
    - Right 0XH6
- Eye
  - Left 08H1
  - Right 08H0
- Face 0WH2
- Fallopian Tube 0UH8
- Femoral Region
  - Left 0YH8
  - Right 0YH7
- Femoral Shaft
  - Left 0QH9
  - Right 0QH8
- Femur
  - Lower
    - Left 0QHC
    - Right 0QHB
  - Upper
    - Left 0QH7
    - Right 0QH6
- Fibula
  - Left 0QHK
  - Right 0QHJ
- Foot
  - Left 0YHN
  - Right 0YHM
- Gallbladder 0FH4
- Gastrointestinal Tract 0WHP
- Genitourinary Tract 0WHR
- Gland, Endocrine 0GHS
- Glenoid Cavity
  - Left 0PH8
  - Right 0PH7
- Hand
  - Left 0XHK
  - Right 0XHJ
- Head 0WH0
- Heart 02HA
- Humeral Head
  - Left 0PHD
  - Right 0PHC
- Humeral Shaft
  - Left 0PHG
  - Right 0PHF
- Ileum 0DHB
- Inguinal Region
  - Left 0YH6
  - Right 0YH5
- Intestine
  - Large 0DHE
  - Small 0DH8
- Jaw
  - Lower 0WH5
  - Upper 0WH4
- Jejunum 0DHA
- Joint
  - Acromioclavicular
    - Left 0RHH
    - Right 0RHG
  - Ankle
    - Left 0SHG
    - Right 0SHF

Insertion of device in *(continued)*
- Joint *(continued)*
  - Carpal
    - Left 0RHR
    - Right 0RHQ
  - Cervical Vertebral 0RH1
  - Cervicothoracic Vertebral 0RH4
  - Coccygeal 0SH6
  - Elbow
    - Left 0RHM
    - Right 0RHL
  - Finger Phalangeal
    - Left 0RHX
    - Right 0RHW
  - Hip
    - Left 0SHB
    - Right 0SH9
  - Knee
    - Left 0SHD
    - Right 0SHC
  - Lumbar Vertebral 0SH0
  - Lumbosacral 0SH3
  - Metacarpocarpal
    - Left 0RHT
    - Right 0RHS
  - Metacarpophalangeal
    - Left 0RHV
    - Right 0RHU
  - Metatarsal-Phalangeal
    - Left 0SHN
    - Right 0SHM
  - Metatarsal-Tarsal
    - Left 0SHL
    - Right 0SHK
  - Occipital-cervical 0RH0
  - Sacrococcygeal 0SH5
  - Sacroiliac
    - Left 0SH8
    - Right 0SH7
  - Shoulder
    - Left 0RHK
    - Right 0RHJ
  - Sternoclavicular
    - Left 0RHF
    - Right 0RHE
  - Tarsal
    - Left 0SHJ
    - Right 0SHH
  - Temporomandibular
    - Left 0RHD
    - Right 0RHC
  - Thoracic Vertebral 0RH6
  - Thoracolumbar Vertebral 0RHA
  - Toe Phalangeal
    - Left 0SHQ
    - Right 0SHP
  - Wrist
    - Left 0RHP
    - Right 0RHN
- Kidney 0TH5
- Knee Region
  - Left 0YHG
  - Right 0YHF
- Leg
  - Lower
    - Left 0YHJ
    - Right 0YHH
  - Upper
    - Left 0YHD
    - Right 0YHC
- Liver 0FH0
  - Left Lobe 0FH2
  - Right Lobe 0FH1
- Lung
  - Left 0BHL
  - Right 0BHK
- Lymphatic 07HN3
  - Thoracic Duct 07HK
- Mandible
  - Left 0NHV
  - Right 0NHT

Inspection *(continued)*
- Inguinal Region
  - Bilateral 0YJA
  - Left 0YJ6
  - Right 0YJ5
- Intestinal Tract
  - Lower 0DJD
  - Upper 0DJ0
- Jaw
  - Lower 0WJ5
  - Upper 0WJ4
- Joint
  - Acromioclavicular
    - Left 0RJH
    - Right 0RJG
  - Ankle
    - Left 0SJG
    - Right 0SJF
  - Carpal
    - Left 0RJR
    - Right 0RJQ
  - Cervical Vertebral 0RJ1
  - Cervicothoracic Vertebral 0RJ4
  - Coccygeal 0SJ6
  - Elbow
    - Left 0RJM
    - Right 0RJL
  - Finger Phalangeal
    - Left 0RJX
    - Right 0RJW
  - Hip
    - Left 0SJB
    - Right 0SJ9
  - Knee
    - Left 0SJD
    - Right 0SJC
  - Lumbar Vertebral 0SJ0
  - Lumbosacral 0SJ3
  - Metacarpocarpal
    - Left 0RJT
    - Right 0RJS
  - Metacarpophalangeal
    - Left 0RJV
    - Right 0RJU
  - Metatarsal-Phalangeal
    - Left 0SJN
    - Right 0SJM
  - Metatarsal-Tarsal
    - Left 0SJL
    - Right 0SJK
  - Occipital-cervical 0RJ0
  - Sacrococcygeal 0SJ5
  - Sacroiliac
    - Left 0SJ8
    - Right 0SJ7
  - Shoulder
    - Left 0RJK
    - Right 0RJJ
  - Sternoclavicular
    - Left 0RJF
    - Right 0RJE
  - Tarsal
    - Left 0SJJ
    - Right 0SJH
  - Temporomandibular
    - Left 0RJD
    - Right 0RJC
  - Thoracic Vertebral 0RJ6
  - Thoracolumbar Vertebral 0RJA
  - Toe Phalangeal
    - Left 0SJQ
    - Right 0SJP
  - Wrist
    - Left 0RJP
    - Right 0RJN
- Kidney 0TJ5
- Knee Region
  - Left 0YJG
  - Right 0YJF
- Larynx 0CJS

Inspection *(continued)*
- Leg
  - Lower
    - Left 0YJJ
    - Right 0YJH
  - Upper
    - Left 0YJD
    - Right 0YJC
- Lens
  - Left 08JKXZZ
  - Right 08JJXZZ
- Liver 0FJ0
- Lung
  - Left 0BJL
  - Right 0BJK
- Lymphatic 07JN
  - Thoracic Duct 07JK
- Mediastinum 0WJC
- Mesentery 0DJV
- Mouth and Throat 0CJY
- Muscle
  - Extraocular
    - Left 08JM
    - Right 08JL
  - Lower 0KJY
  - Upper 0KJX
- Neck 0WJ6
- Nerve
  - Cranial 00JE
  - Peripheral 01JY
- Nose 09JK
- Omentum 0DJU
- Oral Cavity and Throat 0WJ3
- Ovary 0UJ3
- Pancreas 0FJG
- Parathyroid Gland 0GJR
- Pelvic Cavity 0WJJ
- Penis 0VJS
- Pericardial Cavity 0WJD
- Perineum
  - Female 0WJN
  - Male 0WJM
- Peritoneal Cavity 0WJG
- Peritoneum 0DJW
- Pineal Body 0GJ1
- Pleura 0BJQ
- Pleural Cavity
  - Left 0WJB
  - Right 0WJ9
- Products of Conception 10J0
  - Ectopic 10J2
  - Retained 10J1
- Prostate and Seminal Vesicles 0VJ4
- Respiratory Tract 0WJQ
- Retroperitoneum 0WJH
- Scrotum and Tunica Vaginalis 0VJ8
- Shoulder Region
  - Left 0XJ3
  - Right 0XJ2
- Sinus 09JY
- Skin 0HJPXZZ
- Skull 0NJ0
- Spinal Canal 00JU
- Spinal Cord 00JV
- Spleen 07JP
- Stomach 0DJ6
- Subcutaneous Tissue and Fascia
  - Head and Neck 0JJS
  - Lower Extremity 0JJW
  - Trunk 0JJT
  - Upper Extremity 0JJV
- Tendon
  - Lower 0LJY
  - Upper 0LJX
- Testis 0VJD
- Thymus 07JM
- Thyroid Gland 0GJK
- Toe Nail 0HJRX
- Trachea 0BJ1
- Tracheobronchial Tree 0BJ0

Inspection *(continued)*
- Tympanic Membrane
  - Left 09J8
  - Right 09J7
- Ureter 0TJ9
- Urethra 0TJD
- Uterus and Cervix 0UJD
- Vagina and Cul-de-sac 0UJH
- Vas Deferens 0VJR
- Vein
  - Lower 06JY
  - Upper 05JY
- Vulva 0UJM
- Wrist Region
  - Left 0XJH
  - Right 0XJG

Instillation
- *see* Introduction of substance in or on

Insufflation
- *see* Introduction of substance in or on

Interatrial septum
- *use* Septum, Atrial

Interbody fusion (spine) cage
- *use* Interbody Fusion Device in Lower Joints
- *use* Interbody Fusion Device in Upper Joints

Intercarpal joint
- *use* Joint, Carpal, Left
- *use* Joint, Carpal, Right

Intercarpal ligament
- *use* Bursa and Ligament, Hand, Left
- *use* Bursa and Ligament, Hand, Right

Interclavicular ligament
- *use* Bursa and Ligament, Shoulder, Left
- *use* Bursa and Ligament, Shoulder, Right

Intercostal lymph node
- *use* Lymphatic, Thorax

Intercostal muscle
- *use* Muscle, Thorax, Left
- *use* Muscle, Thorax, Right

Intercostal nerve
- *use* Nerve, Thoracic

Intercostobrachial nerve
- *use* Nerve, Thoracic

Intercuneiform joint
- *use* Joint, Tarsal, Left
- *use* Joint, Tarsal, Right

Intercuneiform ligament
- *use* Bursa and Ligament, Foot, Left
- *use* Bursa and Ligament, Foot, Right

Intermediate cuneiform bone
- *use* Tarsal, Left
- *use* Tarsal, Right

Intermittent mandatory ventilation
- *see* Assistance, Respiratory 5A09

Intermittent Negative Airway Pressure
- 24-96 Consecutive Hours, Ventilation 5A0945B
- Greater than 96 Consecutive Hours, Ventilation 5A0955B
- Less than 24 Consecutive Hours, Ventilation 5A0935B

Intermittent Positive Airway Pressure
- 24-96 Consecutive Hours, Ventilation 5A09458
- Greater than 96 Consecutive Hours, Ventilation 5A09558
- Less than 24 Consecutive Hours, Ventilation 5A09358

Intermittent positive pressure breathing
- *see* Assistance, Respiratory 5A09

Internal anal sphincter
- *use* Anal Sphincter

Internal (basal) cerebral vein
- *use* Vein, Intracranial

Internal carotid plexus
- *use* Nerve, Head and Neck Sympathetic

Internal iliac vein
- *use* Vein, Hypogastric, Left
- *use* Vein, Hypogastric, Right

Internal maxillary artery
- *use* Artery, External Carotid, Left
- *use* Artery, External Carotid, Right

Internal naris
- *use* Nose

Internal oblique muscle
- *use* Muscle, Abdomen, Left
- *use* Muscle, Abdomen, Right

Internal pudendal artery
- *use* Artery, Internal Iliac, Left
- *use* Artery, Internal Iliac, Right

Internal pudendal vein
- *use* Vein, Hypogastric, Left
- *use* Vein, Hypogastric, Right

Internal thoracic artery
- *use* Artery, Internal Mammary, Left
- *use* Artery, Internal Mammary, Right
- *use* Artery, Subclavian, Left
- *use* Artery, Subclavian, Right

Internal urethral sphincter
- *use* Urethra

Interphalangeal (IP) joint
- *use* Joint, Finger Phalangeal, Left
- *use* Joint, Finger Phalangeal, Right
- *use* Joint, Toe Phalangeal, Left
- *use* Joint, Toe Phalangeal, Right

Interphalangeal ligament
- *use* Bursa and Ligament, Foot, Left
- *use* Bursa and Ligament, Foot, Right
- *use* Bursa and Ligament, Hand, Left
- *use* Bursa and Ligament, Hand, Right

Interrogation, cardiac rhythm related device
- Interrogation only
  - *see* Measurement, Cardiac 4B02
- With cardiac function testing
  - *see* Measurement, Cardiac 4A02

Interruption
- *see* Occlusion

Interspinalis muscle
- *use* Muscle, Trunk, Left
- *use* Muscle, Trunk, Right

Interspinous ligament
- *use* Bursa and Ligament, Trunk, Left
- *use* Bursa and Ligament, Trunk, Right

Interspinous process spinal stabilization device
- *use* Spinal Stabilization Device, Interspinous Process in 0RH
- *use* Spinal Stabilization Device, Interspinous Process in 0SH

InterStim® Therapy lead
- *use* Neurostimulator Lead in Peripheral Nervous System

InterStim® Therapy neurostimulator
- *use* Stimulator Generator, Single Array in 0JH

Intertransversarius muscle
- *use* Muscle, Trunk, Left
- *use* Muscle, Trunk, Right

Intertransverse ligament
- *use* Bursa and Ligament, Trunk, Left
- *use* Bursa and Ligament, Trunk, Right

Interventricular foramen (Monro)
- *use* Cerebral Ventricle

Interventricular septum
- *use* Septum, Ventricular

Intestinal lymphatic trunk
- *use* Cisterna Chyli

Introduction of substance in or on *(continued)*

Introduction of substance in or on *(continued)*

Introduction of substance in or on *(continued)*

- **Introduction of substance in or on** *(continued)*
  - Skin 3E00XGC *(continued)*
    - Sedatives 3E00XNZ
    - Serum 3E00X4Z
    - Toxoid 3E00X4Z
    - Vaccine 3E00X4Z
  - Spinal Canal 3E0R3GC
    - Analgesics 3E0R3NZ
    - Anesthetic
      - Local 3E0R3BZ
      - Regional 3E0R3CZ
    - Anti-infective 3E0R32
    - Anti-inflammatory 3E0R33Z
    - Antineoplastic 3E0R30
    - Destructive Agent 3E0R3TZ
    - Diagnostic Substance, Other 3E0R3KZ
    - Electrolytic Substance 3E0R37Z
    - Gas 3E0R
    - Hypnotics 3E0R3NZ
    - Nutritional Substance 3E0R36Z
    - Radioactive Substance 3E0R3HZ
    - Sedatives 3E0R3NZ
    - Stem Cells
      - Embryonic 3E0R
      - Somatic 3E0R
    - Water Balance Substance 3E0R37Z
  - Subcutaneous Tissue 3E013GC
    - Analgesics 3E013NZ
    - Anesthetic, Local 3E013BZ
    - Anti-infective 3E01
    - Anti-inflammatory 3E0133Z
    - Antineoplastic 3E0130
    - Destructive Agent 3E013TZ
    - Diagnostic Substance, Other 3E013KZ
    - Electrolytic Substance 3E0137Z
    - Hormone 3E013V
    - Hypnotics 3E013NZ
    - Nutritional Substance 3E0136Z
    - Radioactive Substance 3E013HZ
    - Sedatives 3E013NZ
    - Serum 3E0134Z
    - Toxoid 3E0134Z
    - Vaccine 3E0134Z
    - Water Balance Substance 3E0137Z
  - Vein
    - Central 3E04
      - Analgesics 3E04
      - Anesthetic, Intracirculatory 3E04
      - Anti-infective 3E04
      - Anti-inflammatory 3E04
      - Antiarrhythmic 3E04
      - Antineoplastic 3E04
      - Destructive Agent 3E04
      - Diagnostic Substance, Other 3E04
      - Electrolytic Substance 3E04
      - Hormone 3E04
      - Hypnotics 3E04
      - Immunotherapeutic 3E04
      - Nutritional Substance 3E04
      - Platelet Inhibitor 3E04
      - Radioactive Substance 3E04
      - Sedatives 3E04
      - Serum 3E04
      - Thrombolytic 3E04
      - Toxoid 3E04
      - Vaccine 3E04
      - Vasopressor 3E04
      - Water Balance Substance 3E04
    - Peripheral 3E03
      - Analgesics 3E03
      - Anesthetic, Intracirculatory 3E03
      - Anti-infective 3E03

- **Introduction of substance in or on** *(continued)*
  - Vein *(continued)*
    - Peripheral (continued)
      - Anti-inflammatory 3E03
      - Antiarrhythmic 3E03
      - Antineoplastic 3E03
      - Destructive Agent 3E03
      - Diagnostic Substance, Other 3E03
      - Electrolytic Substance 3E03
      - Hormone 3E03
      - Hypnotics 3E03
      - Immunotherapeutic 3E03
      - Islet Cells, Pancreatic 3E03
      - Nutritional Substance 3E03
      - Platelet Inhibitor 3E03
      - Radioactive Substance 3E03
      - Sedatives 3E03
      - Serum 3E03
      - Thrombolytic 3E03
      - Toxoid 3E03
      - Vaccine 3E03
      - Vasopressor 3E03
      - Water Balance Substance 3E03
- **Intubation**
  - Airway
    - *see* Insertion of device in, Esophagus 0DH5
    - *see* Insertion of device in, Mouth and Throat 0CHY
    - *see* Insertion of device in, Trachea 0BH1
  - Drainage device
    - *see* Drainage
  - Feeding Device
    - *see* Insertion of device in, Gastrointestinal System 0DH
- **IPPB (intermittent positive pressure breathing)**
  - *see* Assistance, Respiratory 5A09
- **Iridectomy**
  - *see* Excision, Eye 08B
  - *see* Resection, Eye 08T
- **Iridoplasty**
  - *see* Repair, Eye 08Q
  - *see* Replacement, Eye 08R
  - *see* Supplement, Eye 08U
- **Iridotomy**
  - *see* Drainage, Eye 089
- **Irrigation**
  - Biliary Tract, Irrigating Substance 3E1J
  - Brain, Irrigating Substance 3E1Q38Z
  - Cranial Cavity, Irrigating Substance 3E1Q38Z
  - Ear, Irrigating Substance 3E1B
  - Epidural Space, Irrigating Substance 3E1S38Z
  - Eye, Irrigating Substance 3E1C
  - Gastrointestinal Tract
    - Lower, Irrigating Substance 3E1H
    - Upper, Irrigating Substance 3E1G
  - Genitourinary Tract, Irrigating Substance 3E1K
  - Irrigating Substance 3C1ZX8Z
  - Joint, Irrigating Substance 3E1U38Z
  - Mucous Membrane, Irrigating Substance 3E10
  - Nose, Irrigating Substance 3E19
  - Pancreatic Tract, Irrigating Substance 3E1J
  - Pericardial Cavity, Irrigating Substance 3E1Y38Z
  - Peritoneal Cavity
    - Dialysate 3E1M39Z
    - Irrigating Substance 3E1M38Z
  - Pleural Cavity, Irrigating Substance 3E1L38Z

- **Irrigation** *(continued)*
  - Reproductive
    - Female, Irrigating Substance 3E1P
    - Male, Irrigating Substance 3E1N
  - Respiratory Tract, Irrigating Substance 3E1F
  - Skin, Irrigating Substance 3E10
  - Spinal Canal, Irrigating Substance 3E1R38Z
- **Ischiatic nerve**
  - *use* Nerve, Sciatic
- **Ischiocavernosus muscle**
  - *use* Muscle, Perineum
- **Ischiofemoral ligament**
  - *use* Bursa and Ligament, Hip, Left
  - *use* Bursa and Ligament, Hip, Right
- **Ischium**
  - *use* Bone, Pelvic, Left
  - *use* Bone, Pelvic, Right
- **Isolation** 8E0ZXY6
- **Isotope Administration, Whole Body** DWY5G
- **Itrel (3)(4) neurostimulator**
  - *use* Stimulator Generator, Single Array in 0JH

J

- **Jejunal artery**
  - *use* Artery, Superior Mesenteric
- **Jejunectomy**
  - *see* Excision, Jejunum 0DBA
  - *see* Resection, Jejunum 0DTA
- **Jejunocolostomy**
  - *see* Bypass, Gastrointestinal System 0D1
  - *see* Drainage, Gastrointestinal System 0D9
- **Jejunopexy**
  - *see* Repair, Jejunum 0DQA
  - *see* Reposition, Jejunum 0DSA
- **Jejunostomy**
  - *see* Bypass, Jejunum 0D1A
  - *see* Drainage, Jejunum 0D9A
- **Jejunotomy**
  - *see* Drainage, Jejunum 0D9A
- **Joint fixation plate**
  - *use* Internal Fixation Device in Lower Joints
  - *use* Internal Fixation Device in Upper Joints
- **Joint liner (insert)**
  - *use* Liner in Lower Joints
- **Joint spacer (antibiotic)**
  - *use* Spacer in Lower Joints
  - *use* Spacer in Upper Joints
- **Jugular body**
  - *use* Glomus Jugulare
- **Jugular lymph node**
  - *use* Lymphatic, Neck, Left
  - *use* Lymphatic, Neck, Right

K

- **Kappa**
  - *use* Pacemaker, Dual Chamber in 0JH
- **Kcentra**
  - *use* 4-Factor Prothrombin Complex Concentrate
- **Keratectomy, kerectomy**
  - *see* Excision, Eye 08B
  - *see* Resection, Eye 08T
- **Keratocentesis**
  - *see* Drainage, Eye 089
- **Keratoplasty**
  - *see* Repair, Eye 08Q
  - *see* Replacement, Eye 08R
  - *see* Supplement, Eye 08U
- **Keratotomy**
  - *see* Drainage, Eye 089
  - *see* Repair, Eye 08Q
- **Kirschner wire (K-wire)**
  - *use* Internal Fixation Device in Head and Facial Bones
  - *use* Internal Fixation Device in Lower Bones
  - *use* Internal Fixation Device in Lower Joints
  - *use* Internal Fixation Device in Upper Bones
  - *use* Internal Fixation Device in Upper Joints
- **Knee (implant) insert**
  - *use* Liner in Lower Joints
- **KUB x-ray**
  - *see* Plain Radiography, Kidney, Ureter and Bladder BT04
- **Kuntscher nail**
  - *use* Internal Fixation Device, Intramedullary in Lower Bones
  - *use* Internal Fixation Device, Intramedullary in Upper Bones

L

- **Labia majora**
  - *use* Vulva
- **Labia minora**
  - *use* Vulva
- **Labial gland**
  - *use* Lip, Lower
  - *use* Lip, Upper
- **Labiectomy**
  - *see* Excision, Female Reproductive System 0UB
  - *see* Resection, Female Reproductive System 0UT
- **Lacrimal canaliculus**
  - *use* Duct, Lacrimal, Left
  - *use* Duct, Lacrimal, Right
- **Lacrimal punctum**
  - *use* Duct, Lacrimal, Left
  - *use* Duct, Lacrimal, Right
- **Lacrimal sac**
  - *use* Duct, Lacrimal, Left
  - *use* Duct, Lacrimal, Right
- **Laminectomy**
  - *see* Excision, Lower Bones 0QB
  - *see* Excision, Upper Bones 0PB
- **Laminotomy**
  - *see* Drainage, Lower Bones 0Q9
  - *see* Drainage, Upper Bones 0P9
  - *see* Excision, Lower Bones 0QB
  - *see* Excision, Upper Bones 0PB
  - *see* Release, Central Nervous System 00N
  - *see* Release, Lower Bones 0QN
  - *see* Release, Peripheral Nervous System 01N
  - *see* Release, Upper Bones 0PN
- **LAP-BAND® adjustable gastric banding system**
  - *use* Extraluminal Device
- **Laparoscopy**
  - *see* Inspection
- **Laparotomy**
  - Drainage
    - *see* Drainage, Peritoneal Cavity 0W9G
  - Exploratory
    - *see* Inspection, Peritoneal Cavity 0WJG
- **Laryngectomy**
  - *see* Excision, Larynx 0CBS
  - *see* Resection, Larynx 0CTS
- **Laryngocentesis**
  - *see* Drainage, Larynx 0C9S
- **Laryngogram**
  - *see* Fluoroscopy, Larynx B91J

Lumbar lymph node
use Lymphatic, Aortic
Lumbar lymphatic trunk
use Cisterna Chyli
Lumbar splanchnic nerve
use Nerve, Lumbar Sympathetic
Lumbosacral facet joint
use Joint, Lumbosacral
Lumbosacral trunk
use Nerve, Lumbar
Lumpectomy
see Excision
Lunate bone
use Carpal, Left
use Carpal, Right
Lunotriquetral ligament
use Bursa and Ligament, Hand, Left
use Bursa and Ligament, Hand, Right
Lymphadenectomy
see Excision, Lymphatic and Hemic Systems 07B
see Resection, Lymphatic and Hemic Systems 07T
Lymphadenotomy
see Drainage, Lymphatic and Hemic Systems 079
Lymphangiectomy
see Excision, Lymphatic and Hemic Systems 07B
see Resection, Lymphatic and Hemic Systems 07T
Lymphangiogram
see Plain Radiography, Lymphatic System B70
Lymphangioplasty
see Repair, Lymphatic and Hemic Systems 07Q
see Supplement, Lymphatic and Hemic Systems 07U
Lymphangiorrhaphy
see Repair, Lymphatic and Hemic Systems 07Q
Lymphangiotomy
see Drainage, Lymphatic and Hemic Systems 079
Lysis
see Release

M

Macula
use Retina, Left
use Retina, Right
Magnet extraction, ocular foreign body
see Extirpation, Eye 08C
Magnetic Resonance Imaging (MRI)
Abdomen BW30
Ankle
Left BQ3H
Right BQ3G
Aorta
Abdominal B430
Thoracic B330
Arm
Left BP3F
Right BP3E
Artery
Celiac B431
Cervico-Cerebral Arch B33Q
Common Carotid, Bilateral B335
Coronary
Bypass Graft, Multiple B233
Multiple B231
Internal Carotid, Bilateral B338
Intracranial B33R
Lower Extremity
Bilateral B43H
Left B43G
Right B43F

Magnetic Resonance Imaging (MRI) *(continued)*
Artery *(continued)*
Pelvic B43C
Renal, Bilateral B438
Spinal B33M
Superior Mesenteric B434
Upper Extremity
Bilateral B33K
Left B33J
Right B33H
Vertebral, Bilateral B33G
Bladder BT30
Brachial Plexus BW3P
Brain B030
Breast
Bilateral BH32
Left BH31
Right BH30
Calcaneus
Left BQ3K
Right BQ3J
Chest BW33Y
Coccyx BR3F
Connective Tissue
Lower Extremity BL31
Upper Extremity BL30
Corpora Cavernosa BV30
Disc
Cervical BR31
Lumbar BR33
Thoracic BR32
Ear B930
Elbow
Left BP3H
Right BP3G
Eye
Bilateral B837
Left B836
Right B835
Femur
Left BQ34
Right BQ33
Fetal Abdomen BY33
Fetal Extremity BY35
Fetal Head BY30
Fetal Heart BY31
Fetal Spine BY34
Fetal Thorax BY32
Fetus, Whole BY36
Foot
Left BQ3M
Right BQ3L
Forearm
Left BP3K
Right BP3J
Gland
Adrenal, Bilateral BG32
Parathyroid BG33
Parotid, Bilateral B936
Salivary, Bilateral B93D
Submandibular, Bilateral B939
Thyroid BG34
Head BW38
Heart, Right and Left B236
Hip
Left BQ31
Right BQ30
Intracranial Sinus B532
Joint
Finger
Left BP3D
Right BP3C
Hand
Left BP3D
Right BP3C
Temporomandibular, Bilateral BN39
Kidney
Bilateral BT33
Left BT32

Magnetic Resonance Imaging (MRI) *(continued)*
Kidney *(continued)*
Right BT31
Transplant BT39
Knee
Left BQ38
Right BQ37
Larynx B93J
Leg
Left BQ3F
Right BQ3D
Liver BF35
Liver and Spleen BF36
Lung Apices BB3G
Nasopharynx B93F
Neck BW3F
Nerve
Acoustic B03C
Brachial Plexus BW3P
Oropharynx B93F
Ovary
Bilateral BU35
Left BU34
Right BU33
Ovary and Uterus BU3C
Pancreas BF37
Patella
Left BQ3W
Right BQ3V
Pelvic Region BW3G
Pelvis BR3C
Pituitary Gland B039
Plexus, Brachial BW3P
Prostate BV33
Retroperitoneum BW3H
Sacrum BR3F
Scrotum BV34
Sella Turcica B039
Shoulder
Left BP39
Right BP38
Sinus
Intracranial B532
Paranasal B932
Spinal Cord B03B
Spine
Cervical BR30
Lumbar BR39
Thoracic BR37
Spleen and Liver BF36
Subcutaneous Tissue
Abdomen BH3H
Extremity
Lower BH3J
Upper BH3F
Head BH3D
Neck BH3D
Pelvis BH3H
Thorax BH3G
Tendon
Lower Extremity BL33
Upper Extremity BL32
Testicle
Bilateral BV37
Left BV36
Right BV35
Toe
Left BQ3Q
Right BQ3P
Uterus BU36
Pregnant BU3B
Uterus and Ovary BU3C
Vagina BU39
Vein
Cerebellar B531
Cerebral B531
Jugular, Bilateral B535
Lower Extremity
Bilateral B53D
Left B53C
Right B53B

Magnetic Resonance Imaging (MRI) *(continued)*
Vein *(continued)*
Other B53V
Pelvic (Iliac) Bilateral B53H
Portal B53T
Pulmonary, Bilateral B53S
Renal, Bilateral B53L
Spanchnic B53T
Upper Extremity
Bilateral B53P
Left B53N
Right B53M
Vena Cava
Inferior B539
Superior B538
Wrist
Left BP3M
Right BP3L
Malleotomy
see Drainage, Ear, Nose, Sinus 099
Malleus
use Auditory Ossicle, Left
use Auditory Ossicle, Right
Mammaplasty, mammoplasty
see Alteration, Skin and Breast 0H0
see Repair, Skin and Breast 0HQ
see Replacement, Skin and Breast 0HR
see Supplement, Skin and Breast 0HU
Mammary duct
use Breast, Bilateral
use Breast, Left
use Breast, Right
Mammary gland
use Breast, Bilateral
use Breast, Left
use Breast, Right
Mammectomy
see Excision, Skin and Breast 0HB
see Resection, Skin and Breast 0HT
Mammillary body
use Hypothalamus
Mammography
see Plain Radiography, Skin, Subcutaneous Tissue and Breast BH0
Mammotomy
see Drainage, Skin and Breast 0H9
Mandibular nerve
use Nerve, Trigeminal
Mandibular notch
use Mandible, Left
use Mandible, Right
Mandibulectomy
see Excision, Head and Facial Bones 0NB
see Resection, Head and Facial Bones 0NT
Manipulation
Adhesions
see Release
Chiropractic
see Chiropractic Manipulation
Manubrium
use Sternum
Map
Basal Ganglia 00K8
Brain 00K0
Cerebellum 00KC
Cerebral Hemisphere 00K7
Conduction Mechanism 02K8
Hypothalamus 00KA
Medulla Oblongata 00KD
Pons 00KB
Thalamus 00K9
Mapping
Doppler ultrasound
see Ultrasonography
Electrocardiogram only
see Measurement, Cardiac 4A02

N

- **Neurostimulator generator, single channel**
  - *use* Stimulator Generator, Single Array in 0JH
- **Neurostimulator generator, single channel rechargeable**
  - *use* Stimulator Generator, Single Array Rechargeable in 0JH
- **Neurostimulator Lead**
  - Insertion of device in
    - Brain 00H0
    - Cerebral Ventricle 00H6
    - Nerve
      - Cranial 00HE
      - Peripheral 01HY
    - Spinal Canal 00HU
    - Spinal Cord 00HV
  - Removal of device from
    - Brain 00P0
    - Cerebral Ventricle 00P6
    - Nerve
      - Cranial 00PE
      - Peripheral 01PY
    - Spinal Canal 00PU
    - Spinal Cord 00PV
  - Revision of device in
    - Brain 00W0
    - Cerebral Ventricle 00W6
    - Nerve
      - Cranial 00WE
      - Peripheral 01WY
    - Spinal Canal 00WU
    - Spinal Cord 00WV
- **Neurotomy**
  - *see* Division, Central Nervous System 008
  - *see* Division, Peripheral Nervous System 018
- **Neurotripsy**
  - *see* Destruction, Central Nervous System 005
  - *see* Destruction, Peripheral Nervous System 015
- **Neutralization plate**
  - *use* Internal Fixation Device in Head and Facial Bones
  - *use* Internal Fixation Device in Lower Bones
  - *use* Internal Fixation Device in Upper Bones
- **Ninth cranial nerve**
  - *use* Nerve, Glossopharyngeal
- **Nitinol framed polymer mesh**
  - *use* Synthetic Substitute
- **Non-tunneled central venous catheter**
  - *use* Infusion Device
- **Nonimaging Nuclear Medicine Assay**
  - Bladder, Kidneys and Ureters CT63
  - Blood C763
  - Kidneys, Ureters and Bladder CT63
  - Lymphatics and Hematologic System C76YYZZ
  - Ureters, Kidneys and Bladder CT63
  - Urinary System CT6YYZZ
- **Nonimaging Nuclear Medicine Probe** CP5YYZZ
  - Abdomen CW50
  - Abdomen and Chest CW54
  - Abdomen and Pelvis CW51
  - Brain C050
  - Central Nervous System C05YYZZ
  - Chest CW53ZZ
  - Chest and Abdomen CW54
  - Chest and Neck CW56
  - Extremity
    - Lower CP5
    - Upper CP5
  - Head and Neck CW5B
  - Heart C25YYZZ
    - Right and Left C256
- **Nonimaging Nuclear Medicine Probe (continued)**
  - Lymphatics
    - Head C75J
    - Head and Neck C755
    - Lower Extremity C75P
    - Neck C75K
    - Pelvic C75D
    - Trunk C75M
    - Upper Chest C75L
    - Upper Extremity C75N
  - Lymphatics and Hematologic System C75YYZZ
  - Neck and Chest CW56
  - Neck and Head CW5B
  - Pelvic Region CW5J
  - Pelvis and Abdomen CW51
  - Spine CP55ZZZ
- **Nonimaging Nuclear Medicine Uptake**
  - Endocrine System CG4YYZZ
  - Gland, Thyroid CG42
- **Nostril**
  - *use* Nose
- **Novacor Left Ventricular Assist Device**
  - *use* Implantable Heart Assist System in Heart and Great Vessels
- **Novation® Ceramic AHS® (Articulation Hip System)**
  - *use* Synthetic Substitute, Ceramic in 0SR
- **Nuclear medicine**
  - *see* Nonimaging Nuclear Medicine Assay
  - *see* Nonimaging Nuclear Medicine Probe
  - *see* Nonimaging Nuclear Medicine Uptake
  - *see* Planar Nuclear Medicine Imaging
  - *see* Positron Emission Tomographic (PET) Imaging
  - *see* Systemic Nuclear Medicine Therapy
  - *see* Tomographic (Tomo) Nuclear Medicine Imaging
- **Nuclear scintigraphy**
  - *see* Nuclear Medicine
- **Nutrition, concentrated substances**
  - Enteral infusion 3E0G36Z
  - Parenteral (peripheral) infusion
  - *see* Introduction of Nutritional Substance

O

- **Obliteration**
  - *see* Destruction
- **Obturator artery**
  - *use* Artery, Internal Iliac, Left
  - *use* Artery, Internal Iliac, Right
- **Obturator lymph node**
  - *use* Lymphatic, Pelvis
- **Obturator muscle**
  - *use* Muscle, Hip, Left
  - *use* Muscle, Hip, Right
- **Obturator nerve**
  - *use* Nerve, Lumbar Plexus
- **Obturator vein**
  - *use* Vein, Hypogastric, Left
  - *use* Vein, Hypogastric, Right
- **Obtuse margin**
  - *use* Heart, Left
- **Occipital artery**
  - *use* Artery, External Carotid, Left
  - *use* Artery, External Carotid, Right
- **Occipital lobe**
  - *use* Cerebral Hemisphere
- **Occipital lymph node**
  - *use* Lymphatic, Neck, Left
  - *use* Lymphatic, Neck, Right
- **Occipitofrontalis muscle**
  - *use* Muscle, Facial
- **Occlusion**
  - Ampulla of Vater 0FLC
  - Anus 0DLQ
  - Aorta, Abdominal 04L0
  - Artery
    - Anterior Tibial
      - Left 04LQ
      - Right 04LP
    - Axillary
      - Left 03L6
      - Right 03L5
    - Brachial
      - Left 03L8
      - Right 03L7
    - Celiac 04L1
    - Colic
      - Left 04L7
      - Middle 04L8
      - Right 04L6
    - Common Carotid
      - Left 03LJ
      - Right 03LH
    - Common Iliac
      - Left 04LD
      - Right 04LC
    - External Carotid
      - Left 03LN
      - Right 03LM
    - External Iliac
      - Left 04LJ
      - Right 04LH
    - Face 03LR
    - Femoral
      - Left 04LL
      - Right 04LK
    - Foot
      - Left 04LW
      - Right 04LV
    - Gastric 04L2
    - Hand
      - Left 03LF
      - Right 03LD
    - Hepatic 04L3
    - Inferior Mesenteric 04LB
    - Innominate 03L2
    - Internal Carotid
      - Left 03LL
      - Right 03LK
    - Internal Iliac
      - Left, Uterine Artery, Left 04LF
      - Right, Uterine Artery, Right 04LE
    - Internal Mammary
      - Left 03L1
      - Right 03L0
    - Intracranial 03LG
    - Lower 04LY
    - Peroneal
      - Left 04LU
      - Right 04LT
    - Popliteal
      - Left 04LN
      - Right 04LM
    - Posterior Tibial
      - Left 04LS
      - Right 04LR
    - Pulmonary, Left 02LR
    - Radial
      - Left 03LC
      - Right 03LB
    - Renal
      - Left 04LA
      - Right 04L9
    - Splenic 04L4
    - Subclavian
      - Left 03L4
      - Right 03L3
- **Occlusion** *(continued)*
  - Artery *(continued)*
    - Superior Mesenteric 04L5
    - Temporal
      - Left 03LT
      - Right 03LS
    - Thyroid
      - Left 03LV
      - Right 03LU
    - Ulnar
      - Left 03LA
      - Right 03L9
    - Upper 03LY
    - Vertebral
      - Left 03LQ
      - Right 03LP
  - Atrium, Left 02L7
  - Bladder 0TLB
  - Bladder Neck 0TLC
  - Bronchus
    - Lingula 0BL9
    - Lower Lobe
      - Left 0BLB
      - Right 0BL6
    - Main
      - Left 0BL7
      - Right 0BL3
    - Middle Lobe, Right 0BL5
    - Upper Lobe
      - Left 0BL8
      - Right 0BL4
  - Carina 0BL2
  - Cecum 0DLH
  - Cisterna Chyli 07LL
  - Colon
    - Ascending 0DLK
    - Descending 0DLM
    - Sigmoid 0DLN
    - Transverse 0DLL
  - Cord
    - Bilateral 0VLH
    - Left 0VLG
    - Right 0VLF
  - Cul-de-sac 0ULF
  - Duct
    - Common Bile 0FL9
    - Cystic 0FL8
    - Hepatic
      - Left 0FL6
      - Right 0FL5
    - Lacrimal
      - Left 08LY
      - Right 08LX
    - Pancreatic 0FLD
      - Accessory 0FLF
    - Parotid
      - Left 0CLC
      - Right 0CLB
  - Duodenum 0DL9
  - Esophagogastric Junction 0DL4
  - Esophagus 0DL5
    - Lower 0DL3
    - Middle 0DL2
    - Upper 0DL1
  - Fallopian Tube
    - Left 0UL6
    - Right 0UL5
  - Fallopian Tubes, Bilateral 0UL7
  - Ileocecal Valve 0DLC
  - Ileum 0DLB
  - Intestine
    - Large 0DLE
      - Left 0DLG
      - Right 0DLF
    - Small 0DL8
  - Jejunum 0DLA
  - Kidney Pelvis
    - Left 0TL4
    - Right 0TL3
  - Left atrial appendage (LAA)
    - *see* Occlusion, Atrium, Left 02L7

P

Plain Radiography *(continued)*

Plain Radiography *(continued)*

Plain Radiography *(continued)*

Plain Radiography *(continued)*

Plain Radiography *(continued)*
- Vein *(continued)*
  - Subclavian
    - Left B507
    - Right B506
  - Upper Extremity
    - Bilateral B50P
    - Left B50N
    - Right B50M
- Vena Cava
  - Inferior B509
  - Superior B508
- Whole Body BW0KZZZ
  - Infant BW0MZZZ
- Whole Skeleton BW0LZZZ
- Wrist
  - Left BP0M
  - Right BP0L

Planar Nuclear Medicine Imaging CP1
- Abdomen CW10
- Abdomen and Chest CW14
- Abdomen and Pelvis CW11
- Anatomical Regions, Multiple CW1YYZZ
- Bladder, Kidneys and Ureters CT13
- Bladder and Ureters CT1H
- Blood C713
- Bone Marrow C710
- Brain C010
- Breast CH1YYZZ
  - Bilateral CH12
  - Left CH11
  - Right CH10
- Bronchi and Lungs CB12
- Central Nervous System C01YYZZ
- Cerebrospinal Fluid C015
- Chest CW13
- Chest and Abdomen CW14
- Chest and Neck CW16
- Digestive System CD1YYZZ
- Ducts, Lacrimal, Bilateral C819
- Ear, Nose, Mouth and Throat C91YYZZ
- Endocrine System CG1YYZZ
- Extremity
  - Lower CW1D
    - Bilateral CP1F
    - Left CP1D
    - Right CP1C
  - Upper CW1M
    - Bilateral CP1B
    - Left CP19
    - Right CP18
- Eye C81YYZZ
- Gallbladder CF14
- Gastrointestinal Tract CD17
  - Upper CD15
- Gland
  - Adrenal, Bilateral CG14
  - Parathyroid CG11
  - Thyroid CG12
- Glands, Salivary, Bilateral C91B
- Head and Neck CW1B
- Heart C21YYZZ
  - Right and Left C216
- Hepatobiliary System, All CF1C
- Hepatobiliary System and Pancreas CF1YYZZ
- Kidneys, Ureters and Bladder CT13
- Liver CF15
- Liver and Spleen CF16
- Lungs and Bronchi CB12
- Lymphatics
  - Head C71J
  - Head and Neck C715
  - Lower Extremity C71P
  - Neck C71K
  - Pelvic C71D
  - Trunk C71M
  - Upper Chest C71L
  - Upper Extremity C71N

Planar Nuclear Medicine Imaging CP1 *(continued)*
- Lymphatics and Hematologic System C71YYZZ
- Musculoskeletal System, All CP1Z
- Myocardium C21G
- Neck and Chest CW16
- Neck and Head CW1B
- Pancreas and Hepatobiliary System CF1YYZZ
- Pelvic Region CW1J
- Pelvis CP16
- Pelvis and Abdomen CW11
- Pelvis and Spine CP17
- Reproductive System, Male CV1YYZZ
- Respiratory System CB1YYZZ
- Skin CH1YYZZ
- Skull CP11
- Spine CP15
- Spine and Pelvis CP17
- Spleen C712
- Spleen and Liver CF16
- Subcutaneous Tissue CH1YYZZ
- Testicles, Bilateral CV19
- Thorax CP14
- Ureters, Kidneys and Bladder CT13
- Ureters and Bladder CT1H
- Urinary System CT1YYZZ
- Veins C51YYZZ
  - Central C51R
  - Lower Extremity
    - Bilateral C51D
    - Left C51C
    - Right C51B
  - Upper Extremity
    - Bilateral C51Q
    - Left C51P
    - Right C51N
- Whole Body CW1N

Plantar digital vein
- *use* Vein, Foot, Left
- *use* Vein, Foot, Right

Plantar fascia (aponeurosis)
- *use* Subcutaneous Tissue and Fascia, Foot, Left
- *use* Subcutaneous Tissue and Fascia, Foot, Right

Plantar metatarsal vein
- *use* Vein, Foot, Left
- *use* Vein, Foot, Right

Plantar venous arch
- *use* Vein, Foot, Left
- *use* Vein, Foot, Right

Plaque Radiation
- Abdomen DWY3FZZ
- Adrenal Gland DGY2FZZ
- Anus DDY8FZZ
- Bile Ducts DFY2FZZ
- Bladder DTY2FZZ
- Bone, Other DPYCFZZ
- Bone Marrow D7Y0FZZ
- Brain D0Y0FZZ
- Brain Stem D0Y1FZZ
- Breast
  - Left DMY0FZZ
  - Right DMY1FZZ
- Bronchus DBY1FZZ
- Cervix DUY1FZZ
- Chest DWY2FZZ
- Chest Wall DBY7FZZ
- Colon DDY5FZZ
- Diaphragm DBY8FZZ
- Duodenum DDY2FZZ
- Ear D9Y0FZZ
- Esophagus DDY0FZZ
- Eye D8Y0FZZ
- Femur DPY9FZZ
- Fibula DPYBFZZ
- Gallbladder DFY1FZZ

Plaque Radiation *(continued)*
- Gland
  - Adrenal DGY2FZZ
  - Parathyroid DGY4FZZ
  - Pituitary DGY0FZZ
  - Thyroid DGY5FZZ
- Glands, Salivary D9Y6FZZ
- Head and Neck DWY1FZZ
- Hemibody DWY4FZZ
- Humerus DPY6FZZ
- Ileum DDY4FZZ
- Jejunum DDY3FZZ
- Kidney DTY0FZZ
- Larynx D9YBFZZ
- Liver DFY0FZZ
- Lung DBY2FZZ
- Lymphatics
  - Abdomen D7Y6FZZ
  - Axillary D7Y4FZZ
  - Inguinal D7Y8FZZ
  - Neck D7Y3FZZ
  - Pelvis D7Y7FZZ
  - Thorax D7Y5FZZ
- Mandible DPY3FZZ
- Maxilla DPY2FZZ
- Mediastinum DBY6FZZ
- Mouth D9Y4FZZ
- Nasopharynx D9YDFZZ
- Neck and Head DWY1FZZ
- Nerve, Peripheral D0Y7FZZ
- Nose D9Y1FZZ
- Ovary DUY0FZZ
- Palate
  - Hard D9Y8FZZ
  - Soft D9Y9FZZ
- Pancreas DFY3FZZ
- Parathyroid Gland DGY4FZZ
- Pelvic Bones DPY8FZZ
- Pelvic Region DWY6FZZ
- Pharynx D9YCFZZ
- Pineal Body DGY1FZZ
- Pituitary Gland DGY0FZZ
- Pleura DBY5FZZ
- Prostate DVY0FZZ
- Radius DPY7FZZ
- Rectum DDY7FZZ
- Rib DPY5FZZ
- Sinuses D9Y7FZZ
- Skin
  - Abdomen DHY8FZZ
  - Arm DHY4FZZ
  - Back DHY7FZZ
  - Buttock DHY9FZZ
  - Chest DHY6FZZ
  - Face DHY2FZZ
  - Foot DHYCFZZ
  - Hand DHY5FZZ
  - Leg DHYBFZZ
  - Neck DHY3FZZ
- Skull DPY0FZZ
- Spinal Cord D0Y6FZZ
- Spleen D7Y2FZZ
- Sternum DPY4FZZ
- Stomach DDY1FZZ
- Testis DVY1FZZ
- Thymus D7Y1FZZ
- Thyroid Gland DGY5FZZ
- Tibia DPYBFZZ
- Tongue D9Y5FZZ
- Trachea DBY0FZZ
- Ulna DPY7FZZ
- Ureter DTY1FZZ
- Urethra DTY3FZZ
- Uterus DUY2FZZ
- Whole Body DWY5FZZ

Plasmapheresis, therapeutic 6A550Z3

Plateletpheresis, therapeutic 6A550Z2

Platysma muscle
- *use* Muscle, Neck, Left
- *use* Muscle, Neck, Right

Pleurectomy
- *see* Excision, Respiratory System 0BB
- *see* Resection, Respiratory System 0BT

Pleurocentesis
- *see* Drainage, Anatomical Regions, General 0W9

Pleurodesis, pleurosclerosis
- Chemical injection
  - *see* Introduction of substance in or on, Pleural Cavity 3E0L
- Surgical
  - *see* Destruction, Respiratory System 0B5

Pleurolysis
- *see* Release, Respiratory System 0BN

Pleuroscopy 0BJQ4ZZ

Pleurotomy
- *see* Drainage, Respiratory System 0B9

Plica semilunaris
- *use* Conjunctiva, Left
- *use* Conjunctiva, Right

Plication
- *see* Restriction

Pneumectomy
- *see* Excision, Respiratory System 0BB
- *see* Resection, Respiratory System 0BT

Pneumocentesis
- *see* Drainage, Respiratory System 0B9

Pneumogastric nerve
- *use* Nerve, Vagus

Pneumolysis
- *see* Release, Respiratory System 0BN

Pneumonectomy
- *see* Resection, Respiratory System 0BT

Pneumonolysis
- *see* Release, Respiratory System 0BN

Pneumonopexy
- *see* Repair, Respiratory System 0BQ
- *see* Reposition, Respiratory System 0BS

Pneumonorrhaphy
- *see* Repair, Respiratory System 0BQ

Pneumonotomy
- *see* Drainage, Respiratory System 0B9

Pneumotaxic center
- *use* Pons

Pneumotomy
- *see* Drainage, Respiratory System 0B9

Pollicization
- *see* Transfer, Anatomical Regions, Upper Extremities 0XX

Polyethylene socket
- *use* Synthetic Substitute, Polyethylene in 0SR

Polymethylmethacrylate (PMMA)
- *use* Synthetic Substitute

Polypectomy, gastrointestinal
- *see* Excision, Gastrointestinal System 0DB

Polypropylene mesh
- *use* Synthetic Substitute

Polysomnogram 4A1ZXQZ

Pontine tegmentum
- *use* Pons

Popliteal ligament
- *use* Bursa and Ligament, Knee, Left
- *use* Bursa and Ligament, Knee, Right

Puncture
- *see* Drainage

Puncture, lumbar
- *see* Drainage, Spinal Canal 009U

Pyelography
- *see* Fluoroscopy, Urinary System BT1
- *see* Plain Radiography, Urinary System BT0

Pyeloileostomy, urinary diversion
- *see* Bypass, Urinary System 0T1

Pyeloplasty
- *see* Repair, Urinary System 0TQ
- *see* Replacement, Urinary System 0TR
- *see* Supplement, Urinary System 0TU

Pyelorrhaphy
- *see* Repair, Urinary System 0TQ

Pyeloscopy 0TJ58ZZ

Pyelostomy
- *see* Drainage, Urinary System 0T9
- *see* Bypass, Urinary System 0T1

Pyelotomy
- *see* Drainage, Urinary System 0T9

Pylorectomy
- *see* Excision, Stomach, Pylorus 0DB7
- *see* Resection, Stomach, Pylorus 0DT7

Pyloric antrum
- *use* Stomach, Pylorus

Pyloric canal
- *use* Stomach, Pylorus

Pyloric sphincter
- *use* Stomach, Pylorus

Pylorodiosis
- *see* Dilation, Stomach, Pylorus 0D77

Pylorogastrectomy
- *see* Excision, Gastrointestinal System 0DB
- *see* Resection, Gastrointestinal System 0DT

Pyloroplasty
- *see* Repair, Stomach, Pylorus 0DQ7
- *see* Supplement, Stomach, Pylorus 0DU7

Pyloroscopy 0DJ68ZZ

Pylorotomy
- *see* Drainage, Stomach, Pylorus 0D97

Pyramidalis muscle
- *use* Muscle, Abdomen, Left
- *use* Muscle, Abdomen, Right

Q

Quadrangular cartilage
- *use* Septum, Nasal

Quadrant resection of breast
- *see* Excision, Skin and Breast 0HB

Quadrate lobe
- *use* Liver

Quadratus femoris muscle
- *use* Muscle, Hip, Left
- *use* Muscle, Hip, Right

Quadratus lumborum muscle
- *use* Muscle, Trunk, Left
- *use* Muscle, Trunk, Right

Quadratus plantae muscle
- *use* Muscle, Foot, Left
- *use* Muscle, Foot, Right

Quadriceps (femoris)
- *use* Muscle, Upper Leg, Left
- *use* Muscle, Upper Leg, Right

Quarantine 8E0ZXY6

R

Radial collateral carpal ligament
- *use* Bursa and Ligament, Wrist, Left
- *use* Bursa and Ligament, Wrist, Right

Radial collateral ligament
- *use* Bursa and Ligament, Elbow, Left
- *use* Bursa and Ligament, Elbow, Right

Radial notch
- *use* Ulna, Left
- *use* Ulna, Right

Radial recurrent artery
- *use* Artery, Radial, Left
- *use* Artery, Radial, Right

Radial vein
- *use* Vein, Brachial, Left
- *use* Vein, Brachial, Right

Radialis indicis
- *use* Artery, Hand, Left
- *use* Artery, Hand, Right

Radiation Therapy
- *see* Beam Radiation
- *see* Brachytherapy

Radiation treatment
- *see* Radiation Therapy

Radiocarpal joint
- *use* Joint, Wrist, Left
- *use* Joint, Wrist, Right

Radiocarpal ligament
- *use* Bursa and Ligament, Wrist, Left
- *use* Bursa and Ligament, Wrist, Right

Radiography
- *see* Plain Radiography

Radiology, analog
- *see* Plain Radiography

Radiology, diagnostic
- *see* Imaging, Diagnostic

Radioulnar ligament
- *use* Bursa and Ligament, Wrist, Left
- *use* Bursa and Ligament, Wrist, Right

Range of motion testing
- *see* Motor Function Assessment, Rehabilitation F01

REALIZE® Adjustable Gastric Band
- *use* Extraluminal Device

Reattachment
- Abdominal Wall 0WMF0ZZ
- Ampulla of Vater 0FMC
- Ankle Region
  - Left 0YML0ZZ
  - Right 0YMK0ZZ
- Arm
  - Lower
    - Left 0XMF0ZZ
    - Right 0XMD0ZZ
  - Upper
    - Left 0XM90ZZ
    - Right 0XM80ZZ
- Axilla
  - Left 0XM50ZZ
  - Right 0XM40ZZ
- Back
  - Lower 0WML0ZZ
  - Upper 0WMK0ZZ
- Bladder 0TMB
- Bladder Neck 0TMC
- Breast
  - Bilateral 0HMVXZZ
  - Left 0HMUXZZ
  - Right 0HMTXZZ
- Bronchus
  - Lingula 0BM90ZZ
  - Lower Lobe
    - Left 0BMB0ZZ
    - Right 0BM60ZZ
  - Main
    - Left 0BM70ZZ
    - Right 0BM30ZZ
  - Middle Lobe, Right 0BM50ZZ
  - Upper Lobe
    - Left 0BM80ZZ
    - Right 0BM40ZZ
- Bursa and Ligament

Reattachment *(continued)*
- Bursa and Ligament *(continued)*
  - Abdomen
    - Left 0MMJ
    - Right 0MMH
  - Ankle
    - Left 0MMR
    - Right 0MMQ
  - Elbow
    - Left 0MM4
    - Right 0MM3
  - Foot
    - Left 0MMT
    - Right 0MMS
  - Hand
    - Left 0MM8
    - Right 0MM7
  - Head and Neck 0MM0
  - Hip
    - Left 0MMM
    - Right 0MML
  - Knee
    - Left 0MMP
    - Right 0MMN
  - Lower Extremity
    - Left 0MMW
    - Right 0MMV
  - Perineum 0MMK
  - Shoulder
    - Left 0MM2
    - Right 0MM1
  - Thorax
    - Left 0MMG
    - Right 0MMF
  - Trunk
    - Left 0MMD
    - Right 0MMC
  - Upper Extremity
    - Left 0MMB
    - Right 0MM9
  - Wrist
    - Left 0MM6
    - Right 0MM5
- Buttock
  - Left 0YM10ZZ
  - Right 0YM00ZZ
- Carina 0BM20ZZ
- Cecum 0DMH
- Cervix 0UMC
- Chest Wall 0WM80ZZ
- Clitoris 0UMJXZZ
- Colon
  - Ascending 0DMK
  - Descending 0DMM
  - Sigmoid 0DMN
  - Transverse 0DML
- Cord
  - Bilateral 0VMH
  - Left 0VMG
  - Right 0VMF
- Cul-de-sac 0UMF
- Diaphragm
  - Left 0BMS0ZZ
  - Right 0BMR0ZZ
- Duct
  - Common Bile 0FM9
  - Cystic 0FM8
  - Hepatic
    - Left 0FM6
    - Right 0FM5
  - Pancreatic 0FMD
    - Accessory 0FMF
- Duodenum 0DM9
- Ear
  - Left 09M1XZZ
  - Right 09M0XZZ
- Elbow Region
  - Left 0XMC0ZZ
  - Right 0XMB0ZZ
- Esophagus 0DM5

Reattachment *(continued)*
- Extremity
  - Lower
    - Left 0YMB0ZZ
    - Right 0YM90ZZ
  - Upper
    - Left 0XM70ZZ
    - Right 0XM60ZZ
- Eyelid
  - Lower
    - Left 08MRXZZ
    - Right 08MQXZZ
  - Upper
    - Left 08MPXZZ
    - Right 08MNXZZ
- Face 0WM20ZZ
- Fallopian Tube
  - Left 0UM6
  - Right 0UM5
- Fallopian Tubes, Bilateral 0UM7
- Femoral Region
  - Left 0YM80ZZ
  - Right 0YM70ZZ
- Finger
  - Index
    - Left 0XMP0ZZ
    - Right 0XMN0ZZ
  - Little
    - Left 0XMW0ZZ
    - Right 0XMV0ZZ
  - Middle
    - Left 0XMR0ZZ
    - Right 0XMQ0ZZ
  - Ring
    - Left 0XMT0ZZ
    - Right 0XMS0ZZ
- Foot
  - Left 0YMN0ZZ
  - Right 0YMM0ZZ
- Forequarter
  - Left 0XM10ZZ
  - Right 0XM00ZZ
- Gallbladder 0FM4
- Gland
  - Left 0GM2
  - Right 0GM3
- Hand
  - Left 0XMK0ZZ
  - Right 0XMJ0ZZ
- Hindquarter
  - Bilateral 0YM40ZZ
  - Left 0YM30ZZ
  - Right 0YM20ZZ
- Hymen 0UMK
- Ileum 0DMB
- Inguinal Region
  - Left 0YM60ZZ
  - Right 0YM50ZZ
- Intestine
  - Large 0DME
    - Left 0DMG
    - Right 0DMF
  - Small 0DM8
- Jaw
  - Lower 0WM50ZZ
  - Upper 0WM40ZZ
- Jejunum 0DMA
- Kidney
  - Left 0TM1
  - Right 0TM0
- Kidney Pelvis
  - Left 0TM4
  - Right 0TM3
- Kidneys, Bilateral 0TM2
- Knee Region
  - Left 0YMG0ZZ
  - Right 0YMF0ZZ
- Leg
  - Lower
    - Left 0YMJ0ZZ
    - Right 0YMH0ZZ

Reattachment *(continued)*
- Leg *(continued)*
  - Upper
    - Left 0YMD0ZZ
    - Right 0YMC0ZZ
- Lip
  - Lower 0CM10ZZ
  - Upper 0CM00ZZ
- Liver 0FM0
  - Left Lobe 0FM2
  - Right Lobe 0FM1
- Lung
  - Left 0BML0ZZ
  - Lower Lobe
    - Left 0BMJ0ZZ
    - Right 0BMF0ZZ
  - Middle Lobe, Right 0BMD0ZZ
  - Right 0BMK0ZZ
  - Upper Lobe
    - Left 0BMG0ZZ
    - Right 0BMC0ZZ
- Lung Lingula 0BMH0ZZ
- Muscle
  - Abdomen
    - Left 0KML
    - Right 0KMK
  - Facial 0KM1
  - Foot
    - Left 0KMW
    - Right 0KMV
  - Hand
    - Left 0KMD
    - Right 0KMC
  - Head 0KM0
  - Hip
    - Left 0KMP
    - Right 0KMN
  - Lower Arm and Wrist
    - Left 0KMB
    - Right 0KM9
  - Lower Leg
    - Left 0KMT
    - Right 0KMS
  - Neck
    - Left 0KM3
    - Right 0KM2
  - Perineum 0KMM
  - Shoulder
    - Left 0KM6
    - Right 0KM5
  - Thorax
    - Left 0KMJ
    - Right 0KMH
  - Tongue, Palate, Pharynx 0KM4
  - Trunk
    - Left 0KMG
    - Right 0KMF
  - Upper Arm
    - Left 0KM8
    - Right 0KM7
  - Upper Leg
    - Left 0KMR
    - Right 0KMQ
- Neck 0WM60ZZ
- Nipple
  - Left 0HMXXZZ
  - Right 0HMWXZZ
- Nose 09MKXZZ
- Ovary
  - Bilateral 0UM2
  - Left 0UM1
  - Right 0UM0
- Palate, Soft 0CM30ZZ
- Pancreas 0FMG
- Parathyroid Gland 0GMR
  - Inferior
    - Left 0GMP
    - Right 0GMN
  - Multiple 0GMQ
  - Superior
    - Left 0GMM
    - Right 0GML

Reattachment *(continued)*
- Penis 0VMSXZZ
- Perineum
  - Female 0WMN0ZZ
  - Male 0WMM0ZZ
- Rectum 0DMP
- Scrotum 0VM5XZZ
- Shoulder Region
  - Left 0XM30ZZ
  - Right 0XM20ZZ
- Skin
  - Abdomen 0HM7XZZ
  - Back 0HM6XZZ
  - Buttock 0HM8XZZ
  - Chest 0HM5XZZ
  - Ear
    - Left 0HM3XZZ
    - Right 0HM2XZZ
  - Face 0HM1XZZ
  - Foot
    - Left 0HMNXZZ
    - Right 0HMMXZZ
  - Genitalia 0HMAXZZ
  - Hand
    - Left 0HMGXZZ
    - Right 0HMFXZZ
  - Lower Arm
    - Left 0HMEXZZ
    - Right 0HMDXZZ
  - Lower Leg
    - Left 0HMLXZZ
    - Right 0HMKXZZ
  - Neck 0HM4XZZ
  - Perineum 0HM9XZZ
  - Scalp 0HM0XZZ
  - Upper Arm
    - Left 0HMCXZZ
    - Right 0HMBXZZ
  - Upper Leg
    - Left 0HMJXZZ
    - Right 0HMHXZZ
- Stomach 0DM6
- Tendon
  - Abdomen
    - Left 0LMG
    - Right 0LMF
  - Ankle
    - Left 0LMT
    - Right 0LMS
  - Foot
    - Left 0LMW
    - Right 0LMV
  - Hand
    - Left 0LM8
    - Right 0LM7
  - Head and Neck 0LM0
  - Hip
    - Left 0LMK
    - Right 0LMJ
  - Knee
    - Left 0LMR
    - Right 0LMQ
  - Lower Arm and Wrist
    - Left 0LM6
    - Right 0LM5
  - Lower Leg
    - Left 0LMP
    - Right 0LMN
  - Perineum 0LMH
  - Shoulder
    - Left 0LM2
    - Right 0LM1
  - Thorax
    - Left 0LMD
    - Right 0LMC
  - Trunk
    - Left 0LMB
    - Right 0LM9
  - Upper Arm
    - Left 0LM4
    - Right 0LM3

Reattachment *(continued)*
- Tendon *(continued)*
  - Upper Leg
    - Left 0LMM
    - Right 0LML
- Testis
  - Bilateral 0VMC
  - Left 0VMB
  - Right 0VM9
- Thumb
  - Left 0XMM0ZZ
  - Right 0XML0ZZ
- Thyroid Gland
  - Left Lobe 0GMG
  - Right Lobe 0GMH
- Toe
  - 1st
    - Left 0YMQ0ZZ
    - Right 0YMP0ZZ
  - 2nd
    - Left 0YMS0ZZ
    - Right 0YMR0ZZ
  - 3rd
    - Left 0YMU0ZZ
    - Right 0YMT0ZZ
  - 4th
    - Left 0YMW0ZZ
    - Right 0YMV0ZZ
  - 5th
    - Left 0YMY0ZZ
    - Right 0YMX0ZZ
- Tongue 0CM70ZZ
- Tooth
  - Lower 0CMX
  - Upper 0CMW
- Trachea 0BM10ZZ
- Tunica Vaginalis
  - Left 0VM7
  - Right 0VM6
- Ureter
  - Left 0TM7
  - Right 0TM6
- Ureters, Bilateral 0TM8
- Urethra 0TMD
- Uterine Supporting Structure 0UM4
- Uterus 0UM9
- Uvula 0CMN0ZZ
- Vagina 0UMG
- Vulva 0UMMXZZ
- Wrist Region
  - Left 0XMH0ZZ
  - Right 0XMG0ZZ

Rebound HRD® (Hernia Repair Device)
- *use* Synthetic Substitute

Recession
- *see* Repair
- *see* Reposition

Reclosure, disrupted abdominal wall 0WQFXZZ

Reconstruction
- *see* Repair
- *see* Replacement
- *see* Supplement

Rectectomy
- *see* Excision, Rectum 0DBP
- *see* Resection, Rectum 0DTP

Rectocele repair
- *see* Repair, Subcutaneous Tissue and Fascia, Pelvic Region 0JQC

Rectopexy
- *see* Repair, Gastrointestinal System 0DQ
- *see* Reposition, Gastrointestinal System 0DS

Rectoplasty
- *see* Repair, Gastrointestinal System 0DQ
- *see* Supplement, Gastrointestinal System 0DU

Rectorrhaphy
- *see* Repair, Gastrointestinal System 0DQ

Rectoscopy 0DJD8ZZ

Rectosigmoid junction
- *use* Colon, Sigmoid

Rectosigmoidectomy
- *see* Excision, Gastrointestinal System 0DB
- *see* Resection, Gastrointestinal System 0DT

Rectostomy
- *see* Drainage, Rectum 0D9P

Rectotomy
- *see* Drainage, Rectum 0D9P

Rectus abdominis muscle
- *use* Muscle, Abdomen, Left
- *use* Muscle, Abdomen, Right

Rectus femoris muscle
- *use* Muscle, Upper Leg, Left
- *use* Muscle, Upper Leg, Right

Recurrent laryngeal nerve
- *use* Nerve, Vagus

Reduction
- Dislocation
  - *see* Reposition
- Fracture
  - *see* Reposition
- Intussusception, intestinal
  - *see* Reposition, Gastrointestinal System 0DS
- Mammoplasty
  - *see* Excision, Skin and Breast 0HB
- Prolapse
  - *see* Reposition
- Torsion
  - *see* Reposition
- Volvulus, gastrointestinal
  - *see* Reposition, Gastrointestinal System 0DS

Refusion
- *see* Fusion

Reimplantation
- *see* Reattachment
- *see* Reposition
- *see* Transfer

Reinforcement
- *see* Repair
- *see* Supplement

Relaxation, scar tissue
- *see* Release

Release
- Acetabulum
  - Left 0QN5
  - Right 0QN4
- Adenoids 0CNQ
- Ampulla of Vater 0FNC
- Anal Sphincter 0DNR
- Anterior Chamber
  - Left 08N33ZZ
  - Right 08N23ZZ
- Anus 0DNQ
- Aorta
  - Abdominal 04N0
  - Thoracic 02NW
- Aortic Body 0GND
- Appendix 0DNJ
- Artery
  - Anterior Tibial
    - Left 04NQ
    - Right 04NP
  - Axillary
    - Left 03N6
    - Right 03N5
  - Brachial
    - Left 03N8
    - Right 03N7
  - Celiac 04N1
  - Colic
    - Left 04N7
    - Middle 04N8

Release *(continued)*
- Artery *(continued)*
  - Colic *(continued)*
    - Right 04N6
  - Common Carotid
    - Left 03NJ
    - Right 03NH
  - Common Iliac
    - Left 04ND
    - Right 04NC
  - External Carotid
    - Left 03NN
    - Right 03NM
  - External Iliac
    - Left 04NJ
    - Right 04NH
  - Face 03NR
  - Femoral
    - Left 04NL
    - Right 04NK
  - Foot
    - Left 04NW
    - Right 04NV
  - Gastric 04N2
  - Hand
    - Left 03NF
    - Right 03ND
  - Hepatic 04N3
  - Inferior Mesenteric 04NB
  - Innominate 03N2
  - Internal Carotid
    - Left 03NL
    - Right 03NK
  - Internal Iliac
    - Left 04NF
    - Right 04NE
  - Internal Mammary
    - Left 03N1
    - Right 03N0
  - Intracranial 03NG
  - Lower 04NY
  - Peroneal
    - Left 04NU
    - Right 04NT
  - Popliteal
    - Left 04NN
    - Right 04NM
  - Posterior Tibial
    - Left 04NS
    - Right 04NR
  - Pulmonary
    - Left 02NR
    - Right 02NQ
  - Pulmonary Trunk 02NP
  - Radial
    - Left 03NC
    - Right 03NB
  - Renal
    - Left 04NA
    - Right 04N9
  - Splenic 04N4
  - Subclavian
    - Left 03N4
    - Right 03N3
  - Superior Mesenteric 04N5
  - Temporal
    - Left 03NT
    - Right 03NS
  - Thyroid
    - Left 03NV
    - Right 03NU
  - Ulnar
    - Left 03NA
    - Right 03N9
  - Upper 03NY
  - Vertebral
    - Left 03NQ
    - Right 03NP
- Atrium
  - Left 02N7
  - Right 02N6

Release *(continued)*
- Auditory Ossicle
  - Left 09NA0ZZ
  - Right 09N90ZZ
- Basal Ganglia 00N8
- Bladder 0TNB
- Bladder Neck 0TNC
- Bone
  - Ethmoid
    - Left 0NNG
    - Right 0NNF
  - Frontal
    - Left 0NN2
    - Right 0NN1
  - Hyoid 0NNX
  - Lacrimal
    - Left 0NNJ
    - Right 0NNH
  - Nasal 0NNB
  - Occipital
    - Left 0NN8
    - Right 0NN7
  - Palatine
    - Left 0NNL
    - Right 0NNK
  - Parietal
    - Left 0NN4
    - Right 0NN3
  - Pelvic
    - Left 0QN3
    - Right 0QN2
  - Sphenoid
    - Left 0NND
    - Right 0NNC
  - Temporal
    - Left 0NN6
    - Right 0NN5
  - Zygomatic
    - Left 0NNN
    - Right 0NNM
- Brain 00N0
- Breast
  - Bilateral 0HNV
  - Left 0HNU
  - Right 0HNT
- Bronchus
  - Lingula 0BN9
  - Lower Lobe
    - Left 0BNB
    - Right 0BN6
  - Main
    - Left 0BN7
    - Right 0BN3
  - Middle Lobe, Right 0BN5
  - Upper Lobe
    - Left 0BN8
    - Right 0BN4
- Buccal Mucosa 0CN4
- Bursa and Ligament
  - Abdomen
    - Left 0MNJ
    - Right 0MNH
  - Ankle
    - Left 0MNR
    - Right 0MNQ
  - Elbow
    - Left 0MN4
    - Right 0MN3
  - Foot
    - Left 0MNT
    - Right 0MNS
  - Hand
    - Left 0MN8
    - Right 0MN7
  - Head and Neck 0MN0
  - Hip
    - Left 0MNM
    - Right 0MNL
  - Knee
    - Left 0MNP
    - Right 0MNN

Release *(continued)*
- Bursa and Ligament *(continued)*
  - Lower Extremity
    - Left 0MNW
    - Right 0MNV
  - Perineum 0MNK
  - Shoulder
    - Left 0MN2
    - Right 0MN1
  - Thorax
    - Left 0MNG
    - Right 0MNF
  - Trunk
    - Left 0MND
    - Right 0MNC
  - Upper Extremity
    - Left 0MNB
    - Right 0MN9
  - Wrist
    - Left 0MN6
    - Right 0MN5
- Carina 0BN2
- Carotid Bodies, Bilateral 0GN8
- Carotid Body
  - Left 0GN6
  - Right 0GN7
- Carpal
  - Left 0PNN
  - Right 0PNM
- Cecum 0DNH
- Cerebellum 00NC
- Cerebral Hemisphere 00N7
- Cerebral Meninges 00N1
- Cerebral Ventricle 00N6
- Cervix 0UNC
- Chordae Tendineae 02N9
- Choroid
  - Left 08NB
  - Right 08NA
- Cisterna Chyli 07NL
- Clavicle
  - Left 0PNB
  - Right 0PN9
- Clitoris 0UNJ
- Coccygeal Glomus 0GNB
- Coccyx 0QNS
- Colon
  - Ascending 0DNK
  - Descending 0DNM
  - Sigmoid 0DNN
  - Transverse 0DNL
- Conduction Mechanism 02N8
- Conjunctiva
  - Left 08NTXZZ
  - Right 08NSXZZ
- Cord
  - Bilateral 0VNH
  - Left 0VNG
  - Right 0VNF
- Cornea
  - Left 08N9XZZ
  - Right 08N8XZZ
- Cul-de-sac 0UNF
- Diaphragm
  - Left 0BNS
  - Right 0BNR
- Disc
  - Cervical Vertebral 0RN3
  - Cervicothoracic Vertebral 0RN5
  - Lumbar Vertebral 0SN2
  - Lumbosacral 0SN4
  - Thoracic Vertebral 0RN9
  - Thoracolumbar Vertebral 0RNB
- Duct
  - Common Bile 0FN9
  - Cystic 0FN8
  - Hepatic
    - Left 0FN6
    - Right 0FN5
  - Lacrimal
    - Left 08NY
    - Right 08NX

Release *(continued)*
- Duct *(continued)*
  - Pancreatic 0FND
    - Accessory 0FNF
  - Parotid
    - Left 0CNC
    - Right 0CNB
- Duodenum 0DN9
- Dura Mater 00N2
- Ear
  - External
    - Left 09N1
    - Right 09N0
  - External Auditory Canal
    - Left 09N4
    - Right 09N3
  - Inner
    - Left 09NE0ZZ
    - Right 09ND0ZZ
  - Middle
    - Left 09N60ZZ
    - Right 09N50ZZ
- Epididymis
  - Bilateral 0VNL
  - Left 0VNK
  - Right 0VNJ
- Epiglottis 0CNR
- Esophagogastric Junction 0DN4
- Esophagus 0DN5
  - Lower 0DN3
  - Middle 0DN2
  - Upper 0DN1
- Eustachian Tube
  - Left 09NG
  - Right 09NF
- Eye
  - Left 08N1XZZ
  - Right 08N0XZZ
- Eyelid
  - Lower
    - Left 08NR
    - Right 08NQ
  - Upper
    - Left 08NP
    - Right 08NN
- Fallopian Tube
  - Left 0UN6
  - Right 0UN5
- Fallopian Tubes, Bilateral 0UN7
- Femoral Shaft
  - Left 0QN9
  - Right 0QN8
- Femur
  - Lower
    - Left 0QNC
    - Right 0QNB
  - Upper
    - Left 0QN7
    - Right 0QN6
- Fibula
  - Left 0QNK
  - Right 0QNJ
- Finger Nail 0HNQXZZ
- Gallbladder 0FN4
- Gingiva
  - Lower 0CN6
  - Upper 0CN5
- Gland
  - Adrenal
    - Bilateral 0GN4
    - Left 0GN2
    - Right 0GN3
  - Lacrimal
    - Left 08NW
    - Right 08NV
  - Minor Salivary 0CNJ
  - Parotid
    - Left 0CN9
    - Right 0CN8
  - Pituitary 0GN0

- **Release** *(continued)*
  - Gland *(continued)*
    - Sublingual
      - Left 0CNF
      - Right 0CND
    - Submaxillary
      - Left 0CNH
      - Right 0CNG
    - Vestibular 0UNL
  - Glenoid Cavity
    - Left 0PN8
    - Right 0PN7
  - Glomus Jugulare 0GNC
  - Humeral Head
    - Left 0PND
    - Right 0PNC
  - Humeral Shaft
    - Left 0PNG
    - Right 0PNF
  - Hymen 0UNK
  - Hypothalamus 00NA
  - Ileocecal Valve 0DNC
  - Ileum 0DNB
  - Intestine
    - Large 0DNE
      - Left 0DNG
      - Right 0DNF
    - Small 0DN8
  - Iris
    - Left 08ND3
    - Right 08NC3
  - Jejunum 0DNA
  - Joint
    - Acromioclavicular
      - Left 0RNH
      - Right 0RNG
    - Ankle
      - Left 0SNG
      - Right 0SNF
    - Carpal
      - Left 0RNR
      - Right 0RNQ
    - Cervical Vertebral 0RN1
    - Cervicothoracic Vertebral 0RN4
    - Coccygeal 0SN6
    - Elbow
      - Left 0RNM
      - Right 0RNL
    - Finger Phalangeal
      - Left 0RNX
      - Right 0RNW
    - Hip
      - Left 0SNB
      - Right 0SN9
    - Knee
      - Left 0SND
      - Right 0SNC
    - Lumbar Vertebral 0SN0
    - Lumbosacral 0SN3
    - Metacarpocarpal
      - Left 0RNT
      - Right 0RNS
    - Metacarpophalangeal
      - Left 0RNV
      - Right 0RNU
    - Metatarsal-Phalangeal
      - Left 0SNN
      - Right 0SNM
    - Metatarsal-Tarsal
      - Left 0SNL
      - Right 0SNK
    - Occipital-cervical 0RN0
    - Sacrococcygeal 0SN5
    - Sacroiliac
      - Left 0SN8
      - Right 0SN7
    - Shoulder
      - Left 0RNK
      - Right 0RNJ
    - Sternoclavicular
      - Left 0RNF
      - Right 0RNE

- **Release** *(continued)*
  - Joint *(continued)*
    - Tarsal
      - Left 0SNJ
      - Right 0SNH
    - Temporomandibular
      - Left 0RND
      - Right 0RNC
    - Thoracic Vertebral 0RN6
    - Thoracolumbar Vertebral 0RNA
    - Toe Phalangeal
      - Left 0SNQ
      - Right 0SNP
    - Wrist
      - Left 0RNP
      - Right 0RNN
  - Kidney
    - Left 0TN1
    - Right 0TN0
  - Kidney Pelvis
    - Left 0TN4
    - Right 0TN3
  - Larynx 0CNS
  - Lens
    - Left 08NK3ZZ
    - Right 08NJ3ZZ
  - Lip
    - Lower 0CN1
    - Upper 0CN0
  - Liver 0FN0
    - Left Lobe 0FN2
    - Right Lobe 0FN1
  - Lung
    - Bilateral 0BNM
    - Left 0BNL
    - Lower Lobe
      - Left 0BNJ
      - Right 0BNF
    - Middle Lobe, Right 0BND
    - Right 0BNK
    - Upper Lobe
      - Left 0BNG
      - Right 0BNC
  - Lung Lingula 0BNH
  - Lymphatic
    - Aortic 07ND
    - Axillary
      - Left 07N6
      - Right 07N5
    - Head 07N0
    - Inguinal
      - Left 07NJ
      - Right 07NH
    - Internal Mammary
      - Left 07N9
      - Right 07N8
    - Lower Extremity
      - Left 07NG
      - Right 07NF
    - Mesenteric 07NB
    - Neck
      - Left 07N2
      - Right 07N1
    - Pelvis 07NC
    - Thoracic Duct 07NK
    - Thorax 07N7
    - Upper Extremity
      - Left 07N4
      - Right 07N3
  - Mandible
    - Left 0NNV
    - Right 0NNT
  - Maxilla
    - Left 0NNS
    - Right 0NNR
  - Medulla Oblongata 00ND
  - Mesentery 0DNV
  - Metacarpal
    - Left 0PNQ
    - Right 0PNP

- **Release** *(continued)*
  - Metatarsal
    - Left 0QNP
    - Right 0QNN
  - Muscle
    - Abdomen
      - Left 0KNL
      - Right 0KNK
    - Extraocular
      - Left 08NM
      - Right 08NL
    - Facial 0KN1
    - Foot
      - Left 0KNW
      - Right 0KNV
    - Hand
      - Left 0KND
      - Right 0KNC
    - Head 0KN0
    - Hip
      - Left 0KNP
      - Right 0KNN
    - Lower Arm and Wrist
      - Left 0KNB
      - Right 0KN9
    - Lower Leg
      - Left 0KNT
      - Right 0KNS
    - Neck
      - Left 0KN3
      - Right 0KN2
    - Papillary 02ND
    - Perineum 0KNM
    - Shoulder
      - Left 0KN6
      - Right 0KN5
    - Thorax
      - Left 0KNJ
      - Right 0KNH
    - Tongue, Palate, Pharynx 0KN4
    - Trunk
      - Left 0KNG
      - Right 0KNF
    - Upper Arm
      - Left 0KN8
      - Right 0KN7
    - Upper Leg
      - Left 0KNR
      - Right 0KNQ
  - Nasopharynx 09NN
  - Nerve
    - Abdominal Sympathetic 01NM
    - Abducens 00NL
    - Accessory 00NR
    - Acoustic 00NN
    - Brachial Plexus 01N3
    - Cervical 01N1
    - Cervical Plexus 01N0
    - Facial 00NM
    - Femoral 01ND
    - Glossopharyngeal 00NP
    - Head and Neck Sympathetic 01NK
    - Hypoglossal 00NS
    - Lumbar 01NB
    - Lumbar Plexus 01N9
    - Lumbar Sympathetic 01NN
    - Lumbosacral Plexus 01NA
    - Median 01N5
    - Oculomotor 00NH
    - Olfactory 00NF
    - Optic 00NG
    - Peroneal 01NH
    - Phrenic 01N2
    - Pudendal 01NC
    - Radial 01N6
    - Sacral 01NR
    - Sacral Plexus 01NQ
    - Sacral Sympathetic 01NP
    - Sciatic 01NF
    - Thoracic 01N8
    - Thoracic Sympathetic 01NL

- **Release** *(continued)*
  - Nerve *(continued)*
    - Tibial 01NG
    - Trigeminal 00NK
    - Trochlear 00NJ
    - Ulnar 01N4
    - Vagus 00NQ
  - Nipple
    - Left 0HNX
    - Right 0HNW
  - Nose 09NKZZ
  - Omentum
    - Greater 0DNS
    - Lesser 0DNT
  - Orbit
    - Left 0NNQ
    - Right 0NNP
  - Ovary
    - Bilateral 0UN2
    - Left 0UN1
    - Right 0UN0
  - Palate
    - Hard 0CN2
    - Soft 0CN3
  - Pancreas 0FNG
  - Para-aortic Body 0GN9
  - Paraganglion Extremity 0GNF
  - Parathyroid Gland 0GNR
    - Inferior
      - Left 0GNP
      - Right 0GNN
    - Multiple 0GNQ
    - Superior
      - Left 0GNM
      - Right 0GNL
  - Patella
    - Left 0QNF
    - Right 0QND
  - Penis 0VNSZZ
  - Pericardium 02NN
  - Peritoneum 0DNW
  - Phalanx
    - Finger
      - Left 0PNV
      - Right 0PNT
    - Thumb
      - Left 0PNS
      - Right 0PNR
    - Toe
      - Left 0QNR
      - Right 0QNQ
  - Pharynx 0CNM
  - Pineal Body 0GN1
  - Pleura
    - Left 0BNP
    - Right 0BNN
  - Pons 00NB
  - Prepuce 0VNT
  - Prostate 0VN0
  - Radius
    - Left 0PNJ
    - Right 0PNH
  - Rectum 0DNP
  - Retina
    - Left 08NF3ZZ
    - Right 08NE3ZZ
  - Retinal Vessel
    - Left 08NH3ZZ
    - Right 08NG3ZZ
  - Rib
    - Left 0PN2
    - Right 0PN1
  - Sacrum 0QN1
  - Scapula
    - Left 0PN6
    - Right 0PN5
  - Sclera
    - Left 08N7XZZ
    - Right 08N6XZZ
  - Scrotum 0VN5
  - Septum
    - Atrial 02N5

Repair *(continued)*
- Duct *(continued)*
  - Hepatic
    - Left 0FQ6
    - Right 0FQ5
  - Lacrimal
    - Left 08QY
    - Right 08QX
  - Pancreatic 0FQD
    - Accessory 0FQF
  - Parotid
    - Left 0CQC
    - Right 0CQB
- Duodenum 0DQ9
- Dura Mater 00Q2
- Ear
  - External
    - Bilateral 09Q2
    - Left 09Q1
    - Right 09Q0
  - External Auditory Canal
    - Left 09Q4
    - Right 09Q3
  - Inner
    - Left 09QE0ZZ
    - Right 09QD0ZZ
  - Middle
    - Left 09Q60ZZ
    - Right 09Q50ZZ
- Elbow Region
  - Left 0XQC
  - Right 0XQB
- Epididymis
  - Bilateral 0VQL
  - Left 0VQK
  - Right 0VQJ
- Epiglottis 0CQR
- Esophagogastric Junction 0DQ4
- Esophagus 0DQ5
  - Lower 0DQ3
  - Middle 0DQ2
  - Upper 0DQ1
- Eustachian Tube
  - Left 09QG
  - Right 09QF
- Extremity
  - Lower
    - Left 0YQB
    - Right 0YQ9
  - Upper
    - Left 0XQ7
    - Right 0XQ6
- Eye
  - Left 08Q1XZZ
  - Right 08Q0XZZ
- Eyelid
  - Lower
    - Left 08QR
    - Right 08QQ
  - Upper
    - Left 08QP
    - Right 08QN
- Face 0WQ2
- Fallopian Tube
  - Left 0UQ6
  - Right 0UQ5
- Fallopian Tubes, Bilateral 0UQ7
- Femoral Region
  - Bilateral 0YQE
  - Left 0YQ8
  - Right 0YQ7
- Femoral Shaft
  - Left 0QQ9
  - Right 0QQ8
- Femur
  - Lower
    - Left 0QQC
    - Right 0QQB
  - Upper
    - Left 0QQ7
    - Right 0QQ6

Repair *(continued)*
- Fibula
  - Left 0QQK
  - Right 0QQJ
- Finger
  - Index
    - Left 0XQP
    - Right 0XQN
  - Little
    - Left 0XQW
    - Right 0XQV
  - Middle
    - Left 0XQR
    - Right 0XQQ
  - Ring
    - Left 0XQT
    - Right 0XQS
- Finger Nail 0HQQXZZ
- Foot
  - Left 0YQN
  - Right 0YQM
- Gallbladder 0FQ4
- Gingiva
  - Lower 0CQ6
  - Upper 0CQ5
- Gland
  - Adrenal
    - Bilateral 0GQ4
    - Left 0GQ2
    - Right 0GQ3
  - Lacrimal
    - Left 08QW
    - Right 08QV
  - Minor Salivary 0CQJ
  - Parotid
    - Left 0CQ9
    - Right 0CQ8
  - Pituitary 0GQ0
  - Sublingual
    - Left 0CQF
    - Right 0CQD
  - Submaxillary
    - Left 0CQH
    - Right 0CQG
  - Vestibular 0UQL
- Glenoid Cavity
  - Left 0PQ8
  - Right 0PQ7
- Glomus Jugulare 0GQC
- Hand
  - Left 0XQK
  - Right 0XQJ
- Head 0WQ0
- Heart 02QA
  - Left 02QC
  - Right 02QB
- Humeral Head
  - Left 0PQD
  - Right 0PQC
- Humeral Shaft
  - Left 0PQG
  - Right 0PQF
- Hymen 0UQK
- Hypothalamus 00QA
- Ileocecal Valve 0DQC
- Ileum 0DQB
- Inguinal Region
  - Bilateral 0YQA
  - Left 0YQ6
  - Right 0YQ5
- Intestine
  - Large 0DQE
    - Left 0DQG
    - Right 0DQF
  - Small 0DQ8
- Iris
  - Left 08QD3ZZ
  - Right 08QC3ZZ
- Jaw
  - Lower 0WQ5
  - Upper 0WQ4
- Jejunum 0DQA

Repair *(continued)*
- Joint
  - Acromioclavicular
    - Left 0RQH
    - Right 0RQG
  - Ankle
    - Left 0SQG
    - Right 0SQF
  - Carpal
    - Left 0RQR
    - Right 0RQQ
  - Cervical Vertebral 0RQ1
  - Cervicothoracic Vertebral 0RQ4
  - Coccygeal 0SQ6
  - Elbow
    - Left 0RQM
    - Right 0RQL
  - Finger Phalangeal
    - Left 0RQX
    - Right 0RQW
  - Hip
    - Left 0SQB
    - Right 0SQ9
  - Knee
    - Left 0SQD
    - Right 0SQC
  - Lumbar Vertebral 0SQ0
  - Lumbosacral 0SQ3
  - Metacarpocarpal
    - Left 0RQT
    - Right 0RQS
  - Metacarpophalangeal
    - Left 0RQV
    - Right 0RQU
  - Metatarsal-Phalangeal
    - Left 0SQN
    - Right 0SQM
  - Metatarsal-Tarsal
    - Left 0SQL
    - Right 0SQK
  - Occipital-cervical 0RQ0
  - Sacrococcygeal 0SQ5
  - Sacroiliac
    - Left 0SQ8
    - Right 0SQ7
  - Shoulder
    - Left 0RQK
    - Right 0RQJ
  - Sternoclavicular
    - Left 0RQF
    - Right 0RQE
  - Tarsal
    - Left 0SQJ
    - Right 0SQH
  - Temporomandibular
    - Left 0RQD
    - Right 0RQC
  - Thoracic Vertebral 0RQ6
  - Thoracolumbar Vertebral 0RQA
  - Toe Phalangeal
    - Left 0SQQ
    - Right 0SQP
  - Wrist
    - Left 0RQP
    - Right 0RQN
- Kidney
  - Left 0TQ1
  - Right 0TQ0
- Kidney Pelvis
  - Left 0TQ4
  - Right 0TQ3
- Knee Region
  - Left 0YQG
  - Right 0YQF
- Larynx 0CQS
- Leg
  - Lower
    - Left 0YQJ
    - Right 0YQH
  - Upper
    - Left 0YQD
    - Right 0YQC

Repair *(continued)*
- Lens
  - Left 08QK3ZZ
  - Right 08QJ3ZZ
- Lip
  - Lower 0CQ1
  - Upper 0CQ0
- Liver 0FQ0
  - Left Lobe 0FQ2
  - Right Lobe 0FQ1
- Lung
  - Bilateral 0BQM
  - Left 0BQL
  - Lower Lobe
    - Left 0BQJ
    - Right 0BQF
  - Middle Lobe, Right 0BQD
  - Right 0BQK
  - Upper Lobe
    - Left 0BQG
    - Right 0BQC
- Lung Lingula 0BQH
- Lymphatic
  - Aortic 07QD
  - Axillary
    - Left 07Q6
    - Right 07Q5
  - Head 07Q0
  - Inguinal
    - Left 07QJ
    - Right 07QH
  - Internal Mammary
    - Left 07Q9
    - Right 07Q8
  - Lower Extremity
    - Left 07QG
    - Right 07QF
  - Mesenteric 07QB
  - Neck
    - Left 07Q2
    - Right 07Q1
  - Pelvis 07QC
  - Thoracic Duct 07QK
  - Thorax 07Q7
  - Upper Extremity
    - Left 07Q4
    - Right 07Q3
- Mandible
  - Left 0NQV
  - Right 0NQT
- Maxilla
  - Left 0NQS
  - Right 0NQR
- Mediastinum 0WQC
- Medulla Oblongata 00QD
- Mesentery 0DQV
- Metacarpal
  - Left 0PQQ
  - Right 0PQP
- Metatarsal
  - Left 0QQP
  - Right 0QQN
- Muscle
  - Abdomen
    - Left 0KQL
    - Right 0KQK
  - Extraocular
    - Left 08QM
    - Right 08QL
  - Facial 0KQ1
  - Foot
    - Left 0KQW
    - Right 0KQV
  - Hand
    - Left 0KQD
    - Right 0KQC
  - Head 0KQ0
  - Hip
    - Left 0KQP
    - Right 0KQN

- **Repair** *(continued)*
  - Muscle *(continued)*
    - Lower Arm and Wrist
      - Left 0KQB
      - Right 0KQ9
    - Lower Leg
      - Left 0KQT
      - Right 0KQS
    - Neck
      - Left 0KQ3
      - Right 0KQ2
    - Papillary 02QD
    - Perineum 0KQM
    - Shoulder
      - Left 0KQ6
      - Right 0KQ5
    - Thorax
      - Left 0KQJ
      - Right 0KQH
    - Tongue, Palate, Pharynx 0KQ4
    - Trunk
      - Left 0KQG
      - Right 0KQF
    - Upper Arm
      - Left 0KQ8
      - Right 0KQ7
    - Upper Leg
      - Left 0KQR
      - Right 0KQQ
  - Nasopharynx 09QN
  - Neck 0WQ6
  - Nerve
    - Abdominal Sympathetic 01QM
    - Abducens 00QL
    - Accessory 00QR
    - Acoustic 00QN
    - Brachial Plexus 01Q3
    - Cervical 01Q1
    - Cervical Plexus 01Q0
    - Facial 00QM
    - Femoral 01QD
    - Glossopharyngeal 00QP
    - Head and Neck Sympathetic 01QK
    - Hypoglossal 00QS
    - Lumbar 01QB
    - Lumbar Plexus 01Q9
    - Lumbar Sympathetic 01QN
    - Lumbosacral Plexus 01QA
    - Median 01Q5
    - Oculomotor 00QH
    - Olfactory 00QF
    - Optic 00QG
    - Peroneal 01QH
    - Phrenic 01Q2
    - Pudendal 01QC
    - Radial 01Q6
    - Sacral 01QR
    - Sacral Plexus 01QQ
    - Sacral Sympathetic 01QP
    - Sciatic 01QF
    - Thoracic 01Q8
    - Thoracic Sympathetic 01QL
    - Tibial 01QG
    - Trigeminal 00QK
    - Trochlear 00QJ
    - Ulnar 01Q4
    - Vagus 00QQ
  - Nipple
    - Left 0HQX
    - Right 0HQW
  - Nose 09QK
  - Omentum
    - Greater 0DQS
    - Lesser 0DQT
  - Orbit
    - Left 0NQQ
    - Right 0NQP
  - Ovary
    - Bilateral 0UQ2
    - Left 0UQ1
    - Right 0UQ0

- **Repair** *(continued)*
  - Palate
    - Hard 0CQ2
    - Soft 0CQ3
  - Pancreas 0FQG
  - Para-aortic Body 0GQ9
  - Paraganglion Extremity 0GQF
  - Parathyroid Gland 0GQR
    - Inferior
      - Left 0GQP
      - Right 0GQN
    - Multiple 0GQQ
    - Superior
      - Left 0GQM
      - Right 0GQL
  - Patella
    - Left 0QQF
    - Right 0QQD
  - Penis 0VQS
  - Pericardium 02QN
  - Perineum
    - Female 0WQN
    - Male 0WQM
  - Peritoneum 0DQW
  - Phalanx
    - Finger
      - Left 0PQV
      - Right 0PQT
    - Thumb
      - Left 0PQS
      - Right 0PQR
    - Toe
      - Left 0QQR
      - Right 0QQQ
  - Pharynx 0CQM
  - Pineal Body 0GQ1
  - Pleura
    - Left 0BQP
    - Right 0BQN
  - Pons 00QB
  - Prepuce 0VQT
  - Products of Conception 10Q0
  - Prostate 0VQ0
  - Radius
    - Left 0PQJ
    - Right 0PQH
  - Rectum 0DQP
  - Retina
    - Left 08QF3ZZ
    - Right 08QE3ZZ
  - Retinal Vessel
    - Left 08QH3ZZ
    - Right 08QG3ZZ
  - Rib
    - Left 0PQ2
    - Right 0PQ1
  - Sacrum 0QQ1
  - Scapula
    - Left 0PQ6
    - Right 0PQ5
  - Sclera
    - Left 08Q7XZZ
    - Right 08Q6XZZ
  - Scrotum 0VQ5
  - Septum
    - Atrial 02Q5
    - Nasal 09QM
    - Ventricular 02QM
  - Shoulder Region
    - Left 0XQ3
    - Right 0XQ2
  - Sinus
    - Accessory 09QP
    - Ethmoid
      - Left 09QV
      - Right 09QU
    - Frontal
      - Left 09QT
      - Right 09QS
    - Mastoid
      - Left 09QC
      - Right 09QB

- **Repair** *(continued)*
  - Sinus *(continued)*
    - Maxillary
      - Left 09QR
      - Right 09QQ
    - Sphenoid
      - Left 09QX
      - Right 09QW
  - Skin
    - Abdomen 0HQ7XZZ
    - Back 0HQ6XZZ
    - Buttock 0HQ8XZZ
    - Chest 0HQ5XZZ
    - Ear
      - Left 0HQ3XZZ
      - Right 0HQ2XZZ
    - Face 0HQ1XZZ
    - Foot
      - Left 0HQNXZZ
      - Right 0HQMXZZ
    - Genitalia 0HQAXZZ
    - Hand
      - Left 0HQGXZZ
      - Right 0HQFXZZ
    - Lower Arm
      - Left 0HQEXZZ
      - Right 0HQDXZZ
    - Lower Leg
      - Left 0HQLXZZ
      - Right 0HQKXZZ
    - Neck 0HQ4XZZ
    - Perineum 0HQ9XZZ
    - Scalp 0HQ0XZZ
    - Upper Arm
      - Left 0HQCXZZ
      - Right 0HQBXZZ
    - Upper Leg
      - Left 0HQJXZZ
      - Right 0HQHXZZ
  - Skull 0NQ0
  - Spinal Cord
    - Cervical 00QW
    - Lumbar 00QY
    - Thoracic 00QX
  - Spinal Meninges 00QT
  - Spleen 07QP
  - Sternum 0PQ0
  - Stomach 0DQ6
    - Pylorus 0DQ7
  - Subcutaneous Tissue and Fascia
    - Abdomen 0JQ8
    - Back 0JQ7
    - Buttock 0JQ9
    - Chest 0JQ6
    - Face 0JQ1
    - Foot
      - Left 0JQR
      - Right 0JQQ
    - Hand
      - Left 0JQK
      - Right 0JQJ
    - Lower Arm
      - Left 0JQH
      - Right 0JQG
    - Lower Leg
      - Left 0JQP
      - Right 0JQN
    - Neck
      - Anterior 0JQ4
      - Posterior 0JQ5
    - Pelvic Region 0JQC
    - Perineum 0JQB
    - Scalp 0JQ0
    - Upper Arm
      - Left 0JQF
      - Right 0JQD
    - Upper Leg
      - Left 0JQM
      - Right 0JQL
  - Tarsal
    - Left 0QQM
    - Right 0QQL

- **Repair** *(continued)*
  - Tendon
    - Abdomen
      - Left 0LQG
      - Right 0LQF
    - Ankle
      - Left 0LQT
      - Right 0LQS
    - Foot
      - Left 0LQW
      - Right 0LQV
    - Hand
      - Left 0LQ8
      - Right 0LQ7
    - Head and Neck 0LQ0
    - Hip
      - Left 0LQK
      - Right 0LQJ
    - Knee
      - Left 0LQR
      - Right 0LQQ
    - Lower Arm and Wrist
      - Left 0LQ6
      - Right 0LQ5
    - Lower Leg
      - Left 0LQP
      - Right 0LQN
    - Perineum 0LQH
    - Shoulder
      - Left 0LQ2
      - Right 0LQ1
    - Thorax
      - Left 0LQD
      - Right 0LQC
    - Trunk
      - Left 0LQB
      - Right 0LQ9
    - Upper Arm
      - Left 0LQ4
      - Right 0LQ3
    - Upper Leg
      - Left 0LQM
      - Right 0LQL
  - Testis
    - Bilateral 0VQC
    - Left 0VQB
    - Right 0VQ9
  - Thalamus 00Q9
  - Thumb
    - Left 0XQM
    - Right 0XQL
  - Thymus 07QM
  - Thyroid Gland 0GQK
    - Left Lobe 0GQG
    - Right Lobe 0GQH
  - Thyroid Gland Isthmus 0GQJ
  - Tibia
    - Left 0QQH
    - Right 0QQG
  - Toe
    - 1st
      - Left 0YQQ
      - Right 0YQP
    - 2nd
      - Left 0YQS
      - Right 0YQR
    - 3rd
      - Left 0YQU
      - Right 0YQT
    - 4th
      - Left 0YQW
      - Right 0YQV
    - 5th
      - Left 0YQY
      - Right 0YQX
  - Toe Nail 0HQRXZZ
  - Tongue 0CQ7
  - Tonsils 0CQP
  - Tooth
    - Lower 0CQX
    - Upper 0CQW
  - Trachea 0BQ1

Repair *(continued)*
- Tunica Vaginalis
  - Left 0VQ7
  - Right 0VQ6
  - Turbinate, Nasal 09QL
- Tympanic Membrane
  - Left 09Q8
  - Right 09Q7
- Ulna
  - Left 0PQL
  - Right 0PQK
- Ureter
  - Left 0TQ7
  - Right 0TQ6
- Urethra 0TQD
- Uterine Supporting Structure 0UQ4
- Uterus 0UQ9
- Uvula 0CQN
- Vagina 0UQG
- Valve
  - Aortic 02QF
  - Mitral 02QG
  - Pulmonary 02QH
  - Tricuspid 02QJ
- Vas Deferens
  - Bilateral 0VQQ
  - Left 0VQP
  - Right 0VQN
- Vein
  - Axillary
    - Left 05Q8
    - Right 05Q7
  - Azygos 05Q0
  - Basilic
    - Left 05QC
    - Right 05QB
  - Brachial
    - Left 05QA
    - Right 05Q9
  - Cephalic
    - Left 05QF
    - Right 05QD
  - Colic 06Q7
  - Common Iliac
    - Left 06QD
    - Right 06QC
  - Coronary 02Q4
  - Esophageal 06Q3
  - External Iliac
    - Left 06QG
    - Right 06QF
  - External Jugular
    - Left 05QQ
    - Right 05QP
  - Face
    - Left 05QV
    - Right 05QT
  - Femoral
    - Left 06QN
    - Right 06QM
  - Foot
    - Left 06QV
    - Right 06QT
  - Gastric 06Q2
  - Greater Saphenous
    - Left 06QQ
    - Right 06QP
  - Hand
    - Left 05QH
    - Right 05QG
  - Hemiazygos 05Q1
  - Hepatic 06Q4
  - Hypogastric
    - Left 06QJ
    - Right 06QH
  - Inferior Mesenteric 06Q6
  - Innominate
    - Left 05Q4
    - Right 05Q3
  - Internal Jugular
    - Left 05QN
    - Right 05QM

Repair *(continued)*
- Vein *(continued)*
  - Intracranial 05QL
  - Lesser Saphenous
    - Left 06QS
    - Right 06QR
  - Lower 06QY
  - Portal 06Q8
  - Pulmonary
    - Left 02QT
    - Right 02QS
  - Renal
    - Left 06QB
    - Right 06Q9
  - Splenic 06Q1
  - Subclavian
    - Left 05Q6
    - Right 05Q5
  - Superior Mesenteric 06Q5
  - Upper 05QY
  - Vertebral
    - Left 05QS
    - Right 05QR
- Vena Cava
  - Inferior 06Q0
  - Superior 02QV
- Ventricle
  - Left 02QL
  - Right 02QK
- Vertebra
  - Cervical 0PQ3
  - Lumbar 0QQ0
  - Thoracic 0PQ4
- Vesicle
  - Bilateral 0VQ3
  - Left 0VQ2
  - Right 0VQ1
- Vitreous
  - Left 08Q53ZZ
  - Right 08Q43ZZ
- Vocal Cord
  - Left 0CQV
  - Right 0CQT
- Vulva 0UQM
- Wrist Region
  - Left 0XQH
  - Right 0XQG

Replacement
- Acetabulum
  - Left 0QR5
  - Right 0QR4
- Ampulla of Vater 0FRC
- Anal Sphincter 0DRR
- Aorta
  - Abdominal 04R0
  - Thoracic 02RW
- Artery
  - Anterior Tibial
    - Left 04RQ
    - Right 04RP
  - Axillary
    - Left 03R6
    - Right 03R5
  - Brachial
    - Left 03R8
    - Right 03R7
  - Celiac 04R1
  - Colic
    - Left 04R7
    - Middle 04R8
    - Right 04R6
  - Common Carotid
    - Left 03RJ
    - Right 03RH
  - Common Iliac
    - Left 04RD
    - Right 04RC
  - External Carotid
    - Left 03RN
    - Right 03RM

Replacement *(continued)*
- Artery *(continued)*
  - External Iliac
    - Left 04RJ
    - Right 04RH
  - Face 03RR
  - Femoral
    - Left 04RL
    - Right 04RK
  - Foot
    - Left 04RW
    - Right 04RV
  - Gastric 04R2
  - Hand
    - Left 03RF
    - Right 03RD
  - Hepatic 04R3
  - Inferior Mesenteric 04RB
  - Innominate 03R2
  - Internal Carotid
    - Left 03RL
    - Right 03RK
  - Internal Iliac
    - Left 04RF
    - Right 04RE
  - Internal Mammary
    - Left 03R1
    - Right 03R0
  - Intracranial 03RG
  - Lower 04RY
  - Peroneal
    - Left 04RU
    - Right 04RT
  - Popliteal
    - Left 04RN
    - Right 04RM
  - Posterior Tibial
    - Left 04RS
    - Right 04RR
  - Pulmonary
    - Left 02RR
    - Right 02RQ
  - Pulmonary Trunk 02RP
  - Radial
    - Left 03RC
    - Right 03RB
  - Renal
    - Left 04RA
    - Right 04R9
  - Splenic 04R4
  - Subclavian
    - Left 03R4
    - Right 03R3
  - Superior Mesenteric 04R5
  - Temporal
    - Left 03RT
    - Right 03RS
  - Thyroid
    - Left 03RV
    - Right 03RU
  - Ulnar
    - Left 03RA
    - Right 03R9
  - Upper 03RY
  - Vertebral
    - Left 03RQ
    - Right 03RP
- Atrium
  - Left 02R
  - Right 02R6
- Auditory Ossicle
  - Left 09RA0
  - Right 09R90
- Bladder 0TRB
- Bladder Neck 0TRC
- Bone
  - Ethmoid
    - Left 0NRG
    - Right 0NRF
  - Frontal
    - Left 0NR2
    - Right 0NR1

Replacement *(continued)*
- Bone *(continued)*
  - Hyoid 0NRX
  - Lacrimal
    - Left 0NRJ
    - Right 0NRH
  - Nasal 0NRB
  - Occipital
    - Left 0NR8
    - Right 0NR7
  - Palatine
    - Left 0NRL
    - Right 0NRK
  - Parietal
    - Left 0NR4
    - Right 0NR3
  - Pelvic
    - Left 0QR3
    - Right 0QR2
  - Sphenoid
    - Left 0NRD
    - Right 0NRC
  - Temporal
    - Left 0NR6
    - Right 0NR5
  - Zygomatic
    - Left 0NRN
    - Right 0NRM
- Breast
  - Bilateral 0HRV
  - Left 0HRU
  - Right 0HRT
- Buccal Mucosa 0CR4
- Carpal
  - Left 0PRN
  - Right 0PRM
- Chordae Tendineae 02R9
- Choroid
  - Left 08RB
  - Right 08RA
- Clavicle
  - Left 0PRB
  - Right 0PR9
- Coccyx 0QRS
- Conjunctiva
  - Left 08RTX
  - Right 08RSX
- Cornea
  - Left 08R9
  - Right 08R8
- Disc
  - Cervical Vertebral 0RR30
  - Cervicothoracic Vertebral 0RR50
  - Lumbar Vertebral 0SR20
  - Lumbosacral 0SR40
  - Thoracic Vertebral 0RR90
  - Thoracolumbar Vertebral 0RRB0
- Duct
  - Common Bile 0FR9
  - Cystic 0FR8
  - Hepatic
    - Left 0FR6
    - Right 0FR5
  - Lacrimal
    - Left 08RY
    - Right 08RX
  - Pancreatic 0FRD
    - Accessory 0FRF
  - Parotid
    - Left 0CRC
    - Right 0CRB
- Ear
  - External
    - Bilateral 09R2
    - Left 09R1
    - Right 09R0
  - Inner
    - Left 09RE0
    - Right 09RD0
  - Middle
    - Left 09R60
    - Right 09R50

Replacement *(continued)*
- Epiglottis 0CRR
- Esophagus 0DR5
- Eye
  - Left 08R1
  - Right 08R0
- Eyelid
  - Lower
    - Left 08RR
    - Right 08RQ
  - Upper
    - Left 08RP
    - Right 08RN
- Femoral Shaft
  - Left 0QR9
  - Right 0QR8
- Femur
  - Lower
    - Left 0QRC
    - Right 0QRB
  - Upper
    - Left 0QR7
    - Right 0QR6
- Fibula
  - Left 0QRK
  - Right 0QRJ
- Finger Nail 0HRQX
- Gingiva
  - Lower 0CR6
  - Upper 0CR5
- Glenoid Cavity
  - Left 0PR8
  - Right 0PR7
- Hair 0HRSX
- Humeral Head
  - Left 0PRD
  - Right 0PRC
- Humeral Shaft
  - Left 0PRG
  - Right 0PRF
- Iris
  - Left 08RD3
  - Right 08RC3
- Joint
  - Acromioclavicular
    - Left 0RRH0
    - Right 0RRG0
  - Ankle
    - Left 0SRG
    - Right 0SRF
  - Carpal
    - Left 0RRR0
    - Right 0RRQ0
  - Cervical Vertebral 0RR10
  - Cervicothoracic Vertebral 0RR40
  - Coccygeal 0SR60
  - Elbow
    - Left 0RRM0
    - Right 0RRL0
  - Finger Phalangeal
    - Left 0RRX0
    - Right 0RRW0
  - Hip
    - Left 0SRB
      - Acetabular Surface 0SRE
      - Femoral Surface 0SRS
    - Right 0SR9
      - Acetabular Surface 0SRA
      - Femoral Surface 0SRR
  - Knee
    - Left 0SRD
      - Femoral Surface 0SRU
      - Tibial Surface 0SRW
    - Right 0SRC
      - Femoral Surface 0SRT
      - Tibial Surface 0SRV
  - Lumbar Vertebral 0SR00
  - Lumbosacral 0SR30

Replacement *(continued)*
- Joint *(continued)*
  - Metacarpocarpal
    - Left 0RRT0
    - Right 0RRS0
  - Metacarpophalangeal
    - Left 0RRV0
    - Right 0RRU0
  - Metatarsal-Phalangeal
    - Left 0SRN0
    - Right 0SRM0
  - Metatarsal-Tarsal
    - Left 0SRL0
    - Right 0SRK0
  - Occipital-cervical 0RR00
  - Sacrococcygeal 0SR50
  - Sacroiliac
    - Left 0SR80
    - Right 0SR70
  - Shoulder
    - Left 0RRK
    - Right 0RRJ
  - Sternoclavicular
    - Left 0RRF0
    - Right 0RRE0
  - Tarsal
    - Left 0SRJ0
    - Right 0SRH0
  - Temporomandibular
    - Left 0RRD0
    - Right 0RRC0
  - Thoracic Vertebral 0RR60
  - Thoracolumbar Vertebral 0RRA0
  - Toe Phalangeal
    - Left 0SRQ0
    - Right 0SRP0
  - Wrist
    - Left 0RRP0
    - Right 0RRN0
- Kidney Pelvis
  - Left 0TR4
  - Right 0TR3
- Larynx 0CRS
- Lens
  - Left 08RK30Z
  - Right 08RJ30Z
- Lip
  - Lower 0CR1
  - Upper 0CR0
- Mandible
  - Left 0NRV
  - Right 0NRT
- Maxilla
  - Left 0NRS
  - Right 0NRR
- Mesentery 0DRV
- Metacarpal
  - Left 0PRQ
  - Right 0PRP
- Metatarsal
  - Left 0QRP
  - Right 0QR
- Muscle, Papillary 02RD
- Nasopharynx 09RN
- Nipple
  - Left 0HRX
  - Right 0HRW
- Nose 09RK
- Omentum
  - Greater 0DRS
  - Lesser 0DRT
- Orbit
  - Left 0NRQ
  - Right 0NRP
- Palate
  - Hard 0CR2
  - Soft 0CR3
- Patella
  - Left 0QRF
  - Right 0QRD

Replacement *(continued)*
- Pericardium 02RN
- Peritoneum 0DRW
- Phalanx
  - Finger
    - Left 0PRV
    - Right 0PRT
  - Thumb
    - Left 0PRS
    - Right 0PRR
  - Toe
    - Left 0QRR
    - Right 0QRQ
- Pharynx 0CRM
- Radius
  - Left 0PRJ
  - Right 0PRH
- Retinal Vessel
  - Left 08RH3
  - Right 08RG3
- Rib
  - Left 0PR2
  - Right 0PR1
- Sacrum 0QR1
- Scapula
  - Left 0PR6
  - Right 0PR5
- Sclera
  - Left 08R7X
  - Right 08R6X
- Septum
  - Atrial 02R5
  - Nasal 09RM
  - Ventricular 02RM
- Skin
  - Abdomen 0HR7
  - Back 0HR6
  - Buttock 0HR8
  - Chest 0HR5
  - Ear
    - Left 0HR3
    - Right 0HR2
  - Face 0HR1
  - Foot
    - Left 0HRN
    - Right 0HRM
  - Genitalia 0HRA
  - Hand
    - Left 0HRG
    - Right 0HRF
  - Lower Arm
    - Left 0HRE
    - Right 0HRD
  - Lower Leg
    - Left 0HRL
    - Right 0HRK
  - Neck 0HR4
  - Perineum 0HR9
  - Scalp 0HR0
  - Upper Arm
    - Left 0HRC
    - Right 0HRB
  - Upper Leg
    - Left 0HRJ
    - Right 0HRH
- Skull 0NR0
- Sternum 0PR0
- Subcutaneous Tissue and Fascia
  - Abdomen 0JR8
  - Back 0JR7
  - Buttock 0JR9
  - Chest 0JR6
  - Face 0JR1
  - Foot
    - Left 0JRR
    - Right 0JRQ
  - Hand
    - Left 0JRK
    - Right 0JRJ
  - Lower Arm
    - Left 0JRH
    - Right 0JRG

Replacement *(continued)*
- Subcutaneous Tissue and Fascia *(continued)*
  - Lower Leg
    - Left 0JRP
    - Right 0JRN
  - Neck
    - Anterior 0JR4
    - Posterior 0JR5
  - Pelvic Region 0JRC
  - Perineum 0JRB
  - Scalp 0JR0
  - Upper Arm
    - Left 0JRF
    - Right 0JRD
  - Upper Leg
    - Left 0JRM
    - Right 0JRL
- Tarsal
  - Left 0QRM
  - Right 0QRL
- Tendon
  - Abdomen
    - Left 0LRG
    - Right 0LRF
  - Ankle
    - Left 0LRT
    - Right 0LRS
  - Foot
    - Left 0LRW
    - Right 0LRV
  - Hand
    - Left 0LR8
    - Right 0LR7
  - Head and Neck 0LR0
  - Hip
    - Left 0LRK
    - Right 0LRJ
  - Knee
    - Left 0LRR
    - Right 0LRQ
  - Lower Arm and Wrist
    - Left 0LR6
    - Right 0LR5
  - Lower Leg
    - Left 0LRP
    - Right 0LRN
  - Perineum 0LRH
  - Shoulder
    - Left 0LR2
    - Right 0LR1
  - Thorax
    - Left 0LRD
    - Right 0LRC
  - Trunk
    - Left 0LRB
    - Right 0LR9
  - Upper Arm
    - Left 0LR4
    - Right 0LR3
  - Upper Leg
    - Left 0LRM
    - Right 0LRL
- Testis
  - Bilateral 0VRC0J
  - Left 0VRB0J
  - Right 0VR90J
- Thumb
  - Left 0XRM
  - Right 0XRL
- Tibia
  - Left 0QRH
  - Right 0QRG
- Toe Nail 0HRRX
- Tongue 0CR7
- Tooth
  - Lower 0CRX
  - Upper 0CRW
- Turbinate, Nasal 09RL
- Tympanic Membrane
  - Left 09R8
  - Right 09R7

Reposition *(continued)*
- Tendon
  - Abdomen
    - Left 0LSG
    - Right 0LSF
  - Ankle
    - Left 0LST
    - Right 0LSS
  - Foot
    - Left 0LSW
    - Right 0LSV
  - Hand
    - Left 0LS8
    - Right 0LS7
  - Head and Neck 0LS0
  - Hip
    - Left 0LSK
    - Right 0LSJ
  - Knee
    - Left 0LSR
    - Right 0LSQ
  - Lower Arm and Wrist
    - Left 0LS6
    - Right 0LS5
  - Lower Leg
    - Left 0LSP
    - Right 0LSN
  - Perineum 0LSH
  - Shoulder
    - Left 0LS2
    - Right 0LS1
  - Thorax
    - Left 0LSD
    - Right 0LSC
  - Trunk
    - Left 0LSB
    - Right 0LS9
  - Upper Arm
    - Left 0LS4
    - Right 0LS3
  - Upper Leg
    - Left 0LSM
    - Right 0LSL
- Testis
  - Bilateral 0VSC
  - Left 0VSB
  - Right 0VS9
- Thymus 07SM0ZZ
- Thyroid Gland
  - Left Lobe 0GSG
  - Right Lobe 0GSH
- Tibia
  - Left 0QSH
  - Right 0QSG
- Tongue 0CS7
- Tooth
  - Lower 0CSX
  - Upper 0CSW
- Trachea 0BS10ZZ
- Turbinate, Nasal 09SL
- Tympanic Membrane
  - Left 09S8
  - Right 09S7
- Ulna
  - Left 0PSL
  - Right 0PSK
- Ureter
  - Left 0TS7
  - Right 0TS6
- Ureters, Bilateral 0TS8
- Urethra 0TSD
- Uterine Supporting Structure 0US4
- Uterus 0US9
- Uvula 0CSN
- Vagina 0USG
- Vein
  - Axillary
    - Left 05S8
    - Right 05S7
  - Azygos 05S0
  - Basilic
    - Left 05SC

Reposition *(continued)*
- Vein *(continued)*
  - Basilic *(continued)*
    - Right 05SB
  - Brachial
    - Left 05SA
    - Right 05S9
  - Cephalic
    - Left 05SF
    - Right 05SD
  - Colic 06S7
  - Common Iliac
    - Left 06SD
    - Right 06SC
  - Esophageal 06S3
  - External Iliac
    - Left 06SG
    - Right 06SF
  - External Jugular
    - Left 05SQ
    - Right 05SP
  - Face
    - Left 05SV
    - Right 05ST
  - Femoral
    - Left 06SN
    - Right 06SM
  - Foot
    - Left 06SV
    - Right 06ST
  - Gastric 06S2
  - Greater Saphenous
    - Left 06SQ
    - Right 06SP
  - Hand
    - Left 05SH
    - Right 05SG
  - Hemiazygos 05S1
  - Hepatic 06S4
  - Hypogastric
    - Left 06SJ
    - Right 06SH
  - Inferior Mesenteric 06S6
  - Innominate
    - Left 05S4
    - Right 05S3
  - Internal Jugular
    - Left 05SN
    - Right 05SM
  - Intracranial 05SL
  - Lesser Saphenous
    - Left 06SS
    - Right 06SR
  - Lower 06SY
  - Portal 06S8
  - Pulmonary
    - Left 02ST0ZZ
    - Right 02SS0ZZ
  - Renal
    - Left 06SB
    - Right 06S9
  - Splenic 06S1
  - Subclavian
    - Left 05S6
    - Right 05S5
  - Superior Mesenteric 06S5
  - Upper 05SY
  - Vertebral
    - Left 05SS
    - Right 05SR
- Vena Cava
  - Inferior 06S0
  - Superior 02SV0ZZ
- Vertebra
  - Cervical 0PS3
  - Lumbar 0QS0
  - Thoracic 0PS4
- Vocal Cord
  - Left 0CSV
  - Right 0CST

Resection
- Acetabulum
  - Left 0QT50ZZ
  - Right 0QT40ZZ
- Adenoids 0CTQ
- Ampulla of Vater 0FTC
- Anal Sphincter 0DTR
- Anus 0DTQ
- Aortic Body 0GTD
- Appendix 0DTJ
- Auditory Ossicle
  - Left 09TA0ZZ
  - Right 09T90ZZ
- Bladder 0TTB
- Bladder Neck 0TTC
- Bone
  - Ethmoid
    - Left 0NTG0ZZ
    - Right 0NTF0ZZ
  - Frontal
    - Left 0NT20ZZ
    - Right 0NT10ZZ
  - Hyoid 0NTX0ZZ
  - Lacrimal
    - Left 0NTJ0ZZ
    - Right 0NTH0ZZ
  - Nasal 0NTB0ZZ
  - Occipital
    - Left 0NT80ZZ
    - Right 0NT70ZZ
  - Palatine
    - Left 0NTL0ZZ
    - Right 0NTK0ZZ
  - Parietal
    - Left 0NT40ZZ
    - Right 0NT30ZZ
  - Pelvic
    - Left 0QT30ZZ
    - Right 0QT20ZZ
  - Sphenoid
    - Left 0NTD0ZZ
    - Right 0NTC0ZZ
  - Temporal
    - Left 0NT60ZZ
    - Right 0NT50ZZ
  - Zygomatic
    - Left 0NTN0ZZ
    - Right 0NTM0ZZ
- Breast
  - Bilateral 0HTV0ZZ
  - Left 0HTU0ZZ
  - Right 0HTT0ZZ
  - Supernumerary 0HTY0ZZ
- Bronchus
  - Lingula 0BT9
  - Lower Lobe
    - Left 0BTB
    - Right 0BT6
  - Main
    - Left 0BT7
    - Right 0BT3
  - Middle Lobe, Right 0BT5
  - Upper Lobe
    - Left 0BT8
    - Right 0BT4
- Bursa and Ligament
  - Abdomen
    - Left 0MTJ
    - Right 0MTH
  - Ankle
    - Left 0MTR
    - Right 0MTQ
  - Elbow
    - Left 0MT4
    - Right 0MT3
  - Foot
    - Left 0MTT
    - Right 0MTS
  - Hand
    - Left 0MT8
    - Right 0MT7
  - Head and Neck 0MT0

Resection *(continued)*
- Bursa and Ligament *(continued)*
  - Hip
    - Left 0MTM
    - Right 0MTL
  - Knee
    - Left 0MTP
    - Right 0MTN
  - Lower Extremity
    - Left 0MTW
    - Right 0MTV
  - Perineum 0MTK
  - Shoulder
    - Left 0MT2
    - Right 0MT1
  - Thorax
    - Left 0MTG
    - Right 0MTF
  - Trunk
    - Left 0MTD
    - Right 0MTC
  - Upper Extremity
    - Left 0MTB
    - Right 0MT9
  - Wrist
    - Left 0MT6
    - Right 0MT5
- Carina 0BT2
- Carotid Bodies, Bilateral 0GT8
- Carotid Body
  - Left 0GT6
  - Right 0GT7
- Carpal
  - Left 0PTN0ZZ
  - Right 0PTM0ZZ
- Cecum 0DTH
- Cerebral Hemisphere 00T7
- Cervix 0UTC
- Chordae Tendineae 02T9
- Cisterna Chyli 07TL
- Clavicle
  - Left 0PTB0ZZ
  - Right 0PT90ZZ
- Clitoris 0UTJ
- Coccygeal Glomus 0GTB
- Coccyx 0QTS0ZZ
- Colon
  - Ascending 0DTK
  - Descending 0DTM
  - Sigmoid 0DTN
  - Transverse 0DTL
- Conduction Mechanism 02T8
- Cord
  - Bilateral 0VTH
  - Left 0VTG
  - Right 0VTF
- Cornea
  - Left 08T9XZZ
  - Right 08T8XZZ
- Cul-de-sac 0UTF
- Diaphragm
  - Left 0BTS
  - Right 0BTR
- Disc
  - Cervical Vertebral 0RT30ZZ
  - Cervicothoracic Vertebral 0RT50ZZ
  - Lumbar Vertebral 0ST20ZZ
  - Lumbosacral 0ST40ZZ
  - Thoracic Vertebral 0RT90ZZ
  - Thoracolumbar Vertebral 0RTB0ZZ
- Duct
  - Common Bile 0FT9
  - Cystic 0FT8
  - Hepatic
    - Left 0FT6
    - Right 0FT5
  - Lacrimal
    - Left 08TY
    - Right 08TX

Resection *(continued)*
- Duct *(continued)*
  - Pancreatic 0FTD
    - Accessory 0FTF
  - Parotid
    - Left 0CTC0ZZ
    - Right 0CTB0ZZ
- Duodenum 0DT9
- Ear
  - External
    - Left 09T1
    - Right 09T0
  - Inner
    - Left 09TE0
    - Right 09TD0
  - Middle
    - Left 09T60
    - Right 09T50
- Epididymis
  - Bilateral 0VTL
  - Left 0VTK
  - Right 0VTJ
- Epiglottis 0CTR
- Esophagogastric Junction 0DT4
- Esophagus 0DT5
  - Lower 0DT3
  - Middle 0DT2
  - Upper 0DT1
- Eustachian Tube
  - Left 09TG
  - Right 09TF
- Eye
  - Left 08T1XZZ
  - Right 08T0XZZ
- Eyelid
  - Lower
    - Left 08TR
    - Right 08TQ
  - Upper
    - Left 08TP
    - Right 08TN
- Fallopian Tube
  - Left 0UT6
  - Right 0UT5
- Fallopian Tubes, Bilateral 0UT7
- Femoral Shaft
  - Left 0QT90ZZ
  - Right 0QT80ZZ
- Femur
  - Lower
    - Left 0QTC0ZZ
    - Right 0QTB0ZZ
  - Upper
    - Left 0QT70ZZ
    - Right 0QT60ZZ
- Fibula
  - Left 0QTK0ZZ
  - Right 0QTJ0ZZ
- Finger Nail 0HTQXZZ
- Gallbladder 0FT4
- Gland
  - Adrenal
    - Bilateral 0GT4
    - Left 0GT2
    - Right 0GT3
  - Lacrimal
    - Left 08TW
    - Right 08TV
  - Minor Salivary 0CTJ0ZZ
  - Parotid
    - Left 0CT90ZZ
    - Right 0CT80ZZ
  - Pituitary 0GT0
  - Sublingual
    - Left 0CTF0ZZ
    - Right 0CTD0ZZ
  - Submaxillary
    - Left 0CTH0ZZ
    - Right 0CTG0ZZ
  - Vestibular 0UTL

Resection *(continued)*
- Glenoid Cavity
  - Left 0PT80ZZ
  - Right 0PT70ZZ
- Glomus Jugulare 0GTC
- Humeral Head
  - Left 0PTD0ZZ
  - Right 0PTC0ZZ
- Humeral Shaft
  - Left 0PTG0ZZ
  - Right 0PTF0ZZ
- Hymen 0UTK
- Ileocecal Valve 0DTC
- Ileum 0DTB
- Intestine
  - Large 0DTE
    - Left 0DTG
    - Right 0DTF
  - Small 0DT8
- Iris
  - Left 08TD3ZZ
  - Right 08TC3ZZ
- Jejunum 0DTA
- Joint
  - Acromioclavicular
    - Left 0RTH0ZZ
    - Right 0RTG0ZZ
  - Ankle
    - Left 0STG0ZZ
    - Right 0STF0ZZ
  - Carpal
    - Left 0RTR0ZZ
    - Right 0RTQ0ZZ
  - Cervicothoracic Vertebral 0RT40ZZ
  - Coccygeal 0ST60ZZ
  - Elbow
    - Left 0RTM0ZZ
    - Right 0RTL0ZZ
  - Finger Phalangeal
    - Left 0RTX0ZZ
    - Right 0RTW0ZZ
  - Hip
    - Left 0STB0ZZ
    - Right 0ST90ZZ
  - Knee
    - Left 0STD0ZZ
    - Right 0STC0ZZ
  - Metacarpocarpal
    - Left 0RTT0ZZ
    - Right 0RTS0ZZ
  - Metacarpophalangeal
    - Left 0RTV0ZZ
    - Right 0RTU0ZZ
  - Metatarsal-Phalangeal
    - Left 0STN0ZZ
    - Right 0STM0ZZ
  - Metatarsal-Tarsal
    - Left 0STL0ZZ
    - Right 0STK0ZZ
  - Sacrococcygeal 0ST50ZZ
  - Sacroiliac
    - Left 0ST80ZZ
    - Right 0ST70ZZ
  - Shoulder
    - Left 0RTK0ZZ
    - Right 0RTJ0ZZ
  - Sternoclavicular
    - Left 0RTF0ZZ
    - Right 0RTE0ZZ
  - Tarsal
    - Left 0STJ0ZZ
    - Right 0STH0ZZ
  - Temporomandibular
    - Left 0RTD0ZZ
    - Right 0RTC0ZZ
  - Toe Phalangeal
    - Left 0STQ0ZZ
    - Right 0STP0ZZ
  - Wrist
    - Left 0RTP0ZZ

Resection *(continued)*
- Joint *(continued)*
  - Wrist *(continued)*
    - Right 0RTN0ZZ
- Kidney
  - Left 0TT1
  - Right 0TT0
- Kidney Pelvis
  - Left 0TT4
  - Right 0TT3
- Kidneys, Bilateral 0TT2
- Larynx 0CTS
- Lens
  - Left 08TK3ZZ
  - Right 08TJ3ZZ
- Lip
  - Lower 0CT1
  - Upper 0CT0
- Liver 0FT0
  - Left Lobe 0FT2
  - Right Lobe 0FT1
- Lung
  - Bilateral 0BTM
  - Left 0BTL
  - Lower Lobe
    - Left 0BTJ
    - Right 0BTF
  - Middle Lobe, Right 0BTD
  - Right 0BTK
  - Upper Lobe
    - Left 0BTG
    - Right 0BTC
- Lung Lingula 0BTH
- Lymphatic
  - Aortic 07TD
  - Axillary
    - Left 07T6
    - Right 07T5
  - Head 07T0
  - Inguinal
    - Left 07TJ
    - Right 07TH
  - Internal Mammary
    - Left 07T9
    - Right 07T8
  - Lower Extremity
    - Left 07TG
    - Right 07TF
  - Mesenteric 07TB
  - Neck
    - Left 07T2
    - Right 07T1
  - Pelvis 07TC
  - Thoracic Duct 07TK
  - Thorax 07T7
  - Upper Extremity
    - Left 07T4
    - Right 07T3
- Mandible
  - Left 0NTV0ZZ
  - Right 0NTT0ZZ
- Maxilla
  - Left 0NTS0ZZ
  - Right 0NTR0ZZ
- Metacarpal
  - Left 0PTQ0ZZ
  - Right 0PTP0ZZ
- Metatarsal
  - Left 0QTP0ZZ
  - Right 0QTN0ZZ
- Muscle
  - Abdomen
    - Left 0KTL
    - Right 0KTK
  - Extraocular
    - Left 08TM
    - Right 08TL
  - Facial 0KT1
  - Foot
    - Left 0KTW
    - Right 0KTV

Resection *(continued)*
- Muscle *(continued)*
  - Hand
    - Left 0KTD
    - Right 0KTC
  - Head 0KT0
  - Hip
    - Left 0KTP
    - Right 0KTN
  - Lower Arm and Wrist
    - Left 0KTB
    - Right 0KT9
  - Lower Leg
    - Left 0KTT
    - Right 0KTS
  - Neck
    - Left 0KT3
    - Right 0KT2
  - Papillary 02TD
  - Perineum 0KTM
  - Shoulder
    - Left 0KT6
    - Right 0KT5
  - Thorax
    - Left 0KTJ
    - Right 0KTH
  - Tongue, Palate, Pharynx 0KT4
  - Trunk
    - Left 0KTG
    - Right 0KTF
  - Upper Arm
    - Left 0KT8
    - Right 0KT7
  - Upper Leg
    - Left 0KTR
    - Right 0KTQ
- Nasopharynx 09TN
- Nipple
  - Left 0HTXXZZ
  - Right 0HTWXZZ
- Nose 09TK
- Omentum
  - Greater 0DTS
  - Lesser 0DTT
- Orbit
  - Left 0NTQ0ZZ
  - Right 0NTP0ZZ
- Ovary
  - Bilateral 0UT2
  - Left 0UT1
  - Right 0UT0
- Palate
  - Hard 0CT2
  - Soft 0CT3
- Pancreas 0FTG
- Para-aortic Body 0GT9
- Paraganglion Extremity 0GTF
- Parathyroid Gland 0GTR
  - Inferior
    - Left 0GTP
    - Right 0GTN
  - Multiple 0GTQ
  - Superior
    - Left 0GTM
    - Right 0GTL
- Patella
  - Left 0QTF0ZZ
  - Right 0QTD0ZZ
- Penis 0VTS
- Pericardium 02TN
- Phalanx
  - Finger
    - Left 0PTV0ZZ
    - Right 0PTT0ZZ
  - Thumb
    - Left 0PTS0ZZ
    - Right 0PTR0ZZ
  - Toe
    - Left 0QTR0ZZ
    - Right 0QTQ0ZZ
- Pharynx 0CTM

Salpingotomy
see Drainage, Female Reproductive System 0U9
Salpinx
use Fallopian Tube, Left
use Fallopian Tube, Right
Saphenous nerve
use Nerve, Femoral
SAPIEN transcatheter aortic valve
use Zooplastic Tissue in Heart and Great Vessels
Sartorius muscle
use Muscle, Upper Leg, Left
use Muscle, Upper Leg, Right
Scalene muscle
use Muscle, Neck, Left
use Muscle, Neck, Right
Scan
Computerized Tomography (CT)
see Computerized Tomography (CT Scan)
Radioisotope
see Planar Nuclear Medicine Imaging
Scaphoid bone
use Carpal, Left
use Carpal, Right
Scapholunate ligament
use Bursa and Ligament, Hand, Left
use Bursa and Ligament, Hand, Right
Scaphotrapezium ligament
use Bursa and Ligament, Hand, Left
use Bursa and Ligament, Hand, Right
Scapulectomy
see Excision, Upper Bones 0PB
see Resection, Upper Bones 0PT
Scapulopexy
see Repair, Upper Bones 0PQ
see Reposition, Upper Bones 0PS
Scarpa's (vestibular) ganglion
use Nerve, Acoustic
Sclerectomy
see Excision, Eye 08B
Sclerotherapy, mechanical
see Destruction
Sclerotomy
see Drainage, Eye 089
Scrotectomy
see Excision, Male Reproductive System 0VB
see Resection, Male Reproductive System 0VT
Scrotoplasty
see Repair, Male Reproductive System 0VQ
see Supplement, Male Reproductive System 0VU
Scrotorrhaphy
see Repair, Male Reproductive System 0VQ
Scrototomy
see Drainage, Male Reproductive System 0V9
Sebaceous gland
use Skin
Second cranial nerve
use Nerve, Optic
Section, cesarean
see Extraction, Pregnancy 10D
Secura (DR) (VR)
use Defibrillator Generator in 0JH
Sella Turcica
use Bone, Sphenoid, Left
use Bone, Sphenoid, Right
Semicircular canal
use Ear, Inner, Left
use Ear, Inner, Right
Semimembranosus muscle
use Muscle, Upper Leg, Left
use Muscle, Upper Leg, Right
Semitendinosus muscle
use Muscle, Upper Leg, Left
use Muscle, Upper Leg, Right
Seprafilm
use Adhesion Barrier
Septal cartilage
use Septum, Nasal
Septectomy
see Excision, Ear, Nose, Sinus 09B
see Excision, Heart and Great Vessels 02B
see Resection, Ear, Nose, Sinus 09T
see Resection, Heart and Great Vessels 02T
Septoplasty
see Repair, Ear, Nose, Sinus 09Q
see Repair, Heart and Great Vessels 02Q
see Replacement, Ear, Nose, Sinus 09R
see Replacement, Heart and Great Vessels 02R
see Reposition, Ear, Nose, Sinus 09S
see Supplement, Ear, Nose, Sinus 09U
see Supplement, Heart and Great Vessels 02U
Septotomy
see Drainage, Ear, Nose, Sinus 099
Sequestrectomy, bone
see Extirpation
Serratus anterior muscle
use Muscle, Thorax, Left
use Muscle, Thorax, Right
Serratus posterior muscle
use Muscle, Trunk, Left
use Muscle, Trunk, Right
Seventh cranial nerve
use Nerve, Facial
Sheffield hybrid external fixator
use External Fixation Device, Hybrid in 0PH
use External Fixation Device, Hybrid in 0PS
use External Fixation Device, Hybrid in 0QH
use External Fixation Device, Hybrid in 0QS
Sheffield ring external fixator
use External Fixation Device, Ring in 0PH
use External Fixation Device, Ring in 0PS
use External Fixation Device, Ring in 0QH
use External Fixation Device, Ring in 0QS
Shirodkar cervical cerclage 0UVC7ZZ
Shock Wave Therapy, Musculoskeletal 6A93
Short gastric artery
use Artery, Splenic
Shortening
see Excision
see Repair
see Reposition
Shunt creation
see Bypass
Sialoadenectomy
Complete
see Resection, Mouth and Throat 0CT
Partial
see Excision, Mouth and Throat 0CB
Sialodochoplasty
see Repair, Mouth and Throat 0CQ
see Replacement, Mouth and Throat 0CR
see Supplement, Mouth and Throat 0CU
Sialoectomy
see Excision, Mouth and Throat 0CB
see Resection, Mouth and Throat 0CT
Sialography
see Plain Radiography, Ear, Nose, Mouth and Throat B90
Sialolithotomy
see Extirpation, Mouth and Throat 0CC
Sigmoid artery
use Artery, Inferior Mesenteric
Sigmoid flexure
use Colon, Sigmoid
Sigmoid vein
use Vein, Inferior Mesenteric
Sigmoidectomy
see Excision, Gastrointestinal System 0DB
see Resection, Gastrointestinal System 0DT
Sigmoidorrhaphy
see Repair, Gastrointestinal System 0DQ
Sigmoidoscopy 0DJD8ZZ
Sigmoidotomy
see Drainage, Gastrointestinal System 0D9
Single lead pacemaker (atrium) (ventricle)
use Pacemaker, Single Chamber in 0JH
Single lead rate responsive pacemaker (atrium)(ventricle)
use Pacemaker, Single Chamber Rate Responsive in 0JH
Sinoatrial node
use Conduction Mechanism
Sinogram
Abdominal Wall
see Fluoroscopy, Abdomen and Pelvis BW11
Chest Wall
see Plain Radiography, Chest BW03
Retroperitoneum
see Fluoroscopy, Abdomen and Pelvis BW11
Sinusectomy
see Excision, Ear, Nose, Sinus 09B
see Resection, Ear, Nose, Sinus 09T
Sinusoscopy 09JY4ZZ
Sinusotomy
see Drainage, Ear, Nose, Sinus 099
Sinus venosus
use Atrium, Right
Sirolimus-eluting coronary stent
use Intraluminal Device, Drug-eluting in Heart and Great Vessels
Sixth cranial nerve
use Nerve, Abducens
Size reduction, breast
see Excision, Skin and Breast 0HB
SJM Biocor® Stented Valve System
use Zooplastic Tissue in Heart and Great Vessels
Skene's (paraurethral) gland
use Gland, Vestibular
Sling
Fascial, orbicularis muscle (mouth)
see Supplement, Muscle, Facial 0KU1
Levator muscle, for urethral suspension
see Reposition, Bladder Neck 0TSC
Pubococcygeal, for urethral suspension
see Reposition, Bladder Neck 0TSC
Rectum
see Reposition, Rectum 0DSP
Small bowel series
see Fluoroscopy, Bowel, Small BD13
Small saphenous vein
use Vein, Lesser Saphenous, Left
use Vein, Lesser Saphenous, Right
Snaring, polyp, colon
see Excision, Gastrointestinal System 0DB
Solar (celiac) plexus
use Nerve, Abdominal Sympathetic
Soleus muscle
use Muscle, Lower Leg, Left
use Muscle, Lower Leg, Right
Spacer
Insertion of device in
Disc
Lumbar Vertebral 0SH2
Lumbosacral 0SH4
Joint
Acromioclavicular
Left 0RHH
Right 0RHG
Ankle
Left 0SHG
Right 0SHF
Carpal
Left 0RHR
Right 0RHQ
Cervical Vertebral 0RH1
Cervicothoracic Vertebral 0RH4
Coccygeal 0SH6
Elbow
Left 0RHM
Right 0RHL
Finger Phalangeal
Left 0RHX
Right 0RHW
Hip
Left 0SHB
Right 0SH9
Knee
Left 0SHD
Right 0SHC
Lumbar Vertebral 0SH0
Lumbosacral 0SH3
Metacarpocarpal
Left 0RHT
Right 0RHS
Metacarpophalangeal
Left 0RHV
Right 0RHU
Metatarsal-Phalangeal
Left 0SHN
Right 0SHM
Metatarsal-Tarsal
Left 0SHL
Right 0SHK
Occipital-cervical 0RH0
Sacrococcygeal 0SH5
Sacroiliac
Left 0SH8
Right 0SH7
Shoulder
Left 0RHK
Right 0RHJ
Sternoclavicular
Left 0RHF
Right 0RHE
Tarsal
Left 0SHJ
Right 0SHH
Temporomandibular
Left 0RHD
Right 0RHC
Thoracic Vertebral 0RH6
Thoracolumbar Vertebral 0RHA
Toe Phalangeal
Left 0SHQ
Right 0SHP

Supplement *(continued)*
- Artery *(continued)*
  - Internal Carotid
    - Left 03UL
    - Right 03UK
  - Internal Iliac
    - Left 04UF
    - Right 04UE
  - Internal Mammary
    - Left 03U1
    - Right 03U0
  - Intracranial 03UG
  - Lower 04UY
  - Peroneal
    - Left 04UU
    - Right 04UT
  - Popliteal
    - Left 04UN
    - Right 04UM
  - Posterior Tibial
    - Left 04US
    - Right 04UR
  - Pulmonary
    - Left 02UR
    - Right 02UQ
  - Pulmonary Trunk 02UP
  - Radial
    - Left 03UC
    - Right 03UB
  - Renal
    - Left 04UA
    - Right 04U9
  - Splenic 04U4
  - Subclavian
    - Left 03U4
    - Right 03U3
  - Superior Mesenteric 04U5
  - Temporal
    - Left 03UT
    - Right 03US
  - Thyroid
    - Left 03UV
    - Right 03UU
  - Ulnar
    - Left 03UA
    - Right 03U9
  - Upper 03UY
  - Vertebral
    - Left 03UQ
    - Right 03UP
- Atrium
  - Left 02U7
  - Right 02U6
- Auditory Ossicle
  - Left 09UA0
  - Right 09U90
- Axilla
  - Left 0XU5
  - Right 0XU4
- Back
  - Lower 0WUL
  - Upper 0WUK
- Bladder 0TUB
- Bladder Neck 0TUC
- Bone
  - Ethmoid
    - Left 0NUG
    - Right 0NUF
  - Frontal
    - Left 0NU2
    - Right 0NU1
  - Hyoid 0NUX
  - Lacrimal
    - Left 0NUJ
    - Right 0NUH
  - Nasal 0NUB
  - Occipital
    - Left 0NU8
    - Right 0NU7
  - Palatine
    - Left 0NUL
    - Right 0NUK

Supplement *(continued)*
- Bone *(continued)*
  - Parietal
    - Left 0NU4
    - Right 0NU3
  - Pelvic
    - Left 0QU3
    - Right 0QU2
  - Sphenoid
    - Left 0NUD
    - Right 0NUC
  - Temporal
    - Left 0NU6
    - Right 0NU5
  - Zygomatic
    - Left 0NUN
    - Right 0NUM
- Breast
  - Bilateral 0HUV
  - Left 0HUU
  - Right 0HUT
- Bronchus
  - Lingula 0BU9
  - Lower Lobe
    - Left 0BUB
    - Right 0BU6
  - Main
    - Left 0BU7
    - Right 0BU3
  - Middle Lobe, Right 0BU5
  - Upper Lobe
    - Left 0BU8
    - Right 0BU4
- Buccal Mucosa 0CU4
- Bursa and Ligament
  - Abdomen
    - Left 0MUJ
    - Right 0MUH
  - Ankle
    - Left 0MUR
    - Right 0MUQ
  - Elbow
    - Left 0MU4
    - Right 0MU3
  - Foot
    - Left 0MUT
    - Right 0MUS
  - Hand
    - Left 0MU8
    - Right 0MU7
  - Head and Neck 0MU0
  - Hip
    - Left 0MUM
    - Right 0MUL
  - Knee
    - Left 0MUP
    - Right 0MUN
  - Lower Extremity
    - Left 0MUW
    - Right 0MUV
  - Perineum 0MUK
  - Shoulder
    - Left 0MU2
    - Right 0MU1
  - Thorax
    - Left 0MUG
    - Right 0MUF
  - Trunk
    - Left 0MUD
    - Right 0MUC
  - Upper Extremity
    - Left 0MUB
    - Right 0MU9
  - Wrist
    - Left 0MU6
    - Right 0MU5
- Buttock
  - Left 0YU1
  - Right 0YU0
- Carina 0BU2

Supplement *(continued)*
- Carpal
  - Left 0PUN
  - Right 0PUM
- Cecum 0DUH
- Cerebral Meninges 00U1
- Chest Wall 0WU8
- Chordae Tendineae 02U9
- Cisterna Chyli 07UL
- Clavicle
  - Left 0PUB
  - Right 0PU9
- Clitoris 0UUJ
- Coccyx 0QUS
- Colon
  - Ascending 0DUK
  - Descending 0DUM
  - Sigmoid 0DUN
  - Transverse 0DUL
- Cord
  - Bilateral 0VUH
  - Left 0VUG
  - Right 0VUF
- Cornea
  - Left 08U9
  - Right 08U8
- Cul-de-sac 0UUF
- Diaphragm
  - Left 0BUS
  - Right 0BUR
- Disc
  - Cervical Vertebral 0RU3
  - Cervicothoracic Vertebral 0RU5
  - Lumbar Vertebral 0SU2
  - Lumbosacral 0SU4
  - Thoracic Vertebral 0RU9
  - Thoracolumbar Vertebral 0RUB
- Duct
  - Common Bile 0FU9
  - Cystic 0FU8
  - Hepatic
    - Left 0FU6
    - Right 0FU5
  - Lacrimal
    - Left 08UY
    - Right 08UX
  - Pancreatic 0FUD
    - Accessory 0FUF
- Duodenum 0DU9
- Dura Mater 00U2
- Ear
  - External
    - Bilateral 09U2
    - Left 09U1
    - Right 09U0
  - Inner
    - Left 09UE0
    - Right 09UD0
  - Middle
    - Left 09U60
    - Right 09U50
- Elbow Region
  - Left 0XUC
  - Right 0XUB
- Epididymis
  - Bilateral 0VUL
  - Left 0VUK
  - Right 0VUJ
- Epiglottis 0CUR
- Esophagogastric Junction 0DU4
- Esophagus 0DU5
  - Lower 0DU3
  - Middle 0DU2
  - Upper 0DU1
- Extremity
  - Lower
    - Left 0YUB
    - Right 0YU9
  - Upper
    - Left 0XU7
    - Right 0XU6

Supplement *(continued)*
- Eye
  - Left 08U1
  - Right 08U0
- Eyelid
  - Lower
    - Left 08UR
    - Right 08UQ
  - Upper
    - Left 08UP
    - Right 08UN
- Face 0WU2
- Fallopian Tube
  - Left 0UU6
  - Right 0UU5
- Fallopian Tubes, Bilateral 0UU7
- Femoral Region
  - Bilateral 0YUE
  - Left 0YU8
  - Right 0YU7
- Femoral Shaft
  - Left 0QU9
  - Right 0QU8
- Femur
  - Lower
    - Left 0QUC
    - Right 0QUB
  - Upper
    - Left 0QU7
    - Right 0QU6
- Fibula
  - Left 0QUK
  - Right 0QUJ
- Finger
  - Index
    - Left 0XUP
    - Right 0XUN
  - Little
    - Left 0XUW
    - Right 0XUV
  - Middle
    - Left 0XUR
    - Right 0XUQ
  - Ring
    - Left 0XUT
    - Right 0XUS
- Foot
  - Left 0YUN
  - Right 0YUM
- Gingiva
  - Lower 0CU6
  - Upper 0CU5
- Glenoid Cavity
  - Left 0PU8
  - Right 0PU7
- Hand
  - Left 0XUK
  - Right 0XUJ
- Head 0WU0
- Heart 02UA
- Humeral Head
  - Left 0PUD
  - Right 0PUC
- Humeral Shaft
  - Left 0PUG
  - Right 0PUF
- Hymen 0UUK
- Ileocecal Valve 0DUC
- Ileum 0DUB
- Inguinal Region
  - Bilateral 0YUA
  - Left 0YU6
  - Right 0YU5
- Intestine
  - Large 0DUE
    - Left 0DUG
    - Right 0DUF
  - Small 0DU8
- Iris
  - Left 08UD
  - Right 08UC

Supplement *(continued)*
- Tendon *(continued)*
  - Hip
    - Left 0LUK
    - Right 0LUJ
  - Knee
    - Left 0LUR
    - Right 0LUQ
  - Lower Arm and Wrist
    - Left 0LU6
    - Right 0LU5
  - Lower Leg
    - Left 0LUP
    - Right 0LUN
  - Perineum 0LUH
  - Shoulder
    - Left 0LU2
    - Right 0LU1
  - Thorax
    - Left 0LUD
    - Right 0LUC
  - Trunk
    - Left 0LUB
    - Right 0LU9
  - Upper Arm
    - Left 0LU4
    - Right 0LU3
  - Upper Leg
    - Left 0LUM
    - Right 0LUL
- Testis
  - Bilateral 0VUC0
  - Left 0VUB0
  - Right 0VU90
- Thumb
  - Left 0XUM
  - Right 0XUL
- Tibia
  - Left 0QUH
  - Right 0QUG
- Toe
  - 1st
    - Left 0YUQ
    - Right 0YUP
  - 2nd
    - Left 0YUS
    - Right 0YUR
  - 3rd
    - Left 0YUU
    - Right 0YUT
  - 4th
    - Left 0YUW
    - Right 0YUV
  - 5th
    - Left 0YUY
    - Right 0YUX
- Tongue 0CU7
- Trachea 0BU1
- Tunica Vaginalis
  - Left 0VU7
  - Right 0VU6
- Turbinate, Nasal 09UL
- Tympanic Membrane
  - Left 09U8
  - Right 09U7
- Ulna
  - Left 0PUL
  - Right 0PUK
- Ureter
  - Left 0TU7
  - Right 0TU6
- Urethra 0TUD
- Uterine Supporting Structure 0UU4
- Uvula 0CUN
- Vagina 0UUG
- Valve
  - Aortic 02UF
  - Mitral 02UG
  - Pulmonary 02UH
  - Tricuspid 02UJ
- Vas Deferens
  - Bilateral 0VUQ

Supplement *(continued)*
- Vas Deferens *(continued)*
  - Left 0VUP
  - Right 0VUN
- Vein
  - Axillary
    - Left 05U8
    - Right 05U7
  - Azygos 05U0
  - Basilic
    - Left 05UC
    - Right 05UB
  - Brachial
    - Left 05UA
    - Right 05U9
  - Cephalic
    - Left 05UF
    - Right 05UD
  - Colic 06U7
  - Common Iliac
    - Left 06UD
    - Right 06UC
  - Esophageal 06U3
  - External Iliac
    - Left 06UG
    - Right 06UF
  - External Jugular
    - Left 05UQ
    - Right 05UP
  - Face
    - Left 05UV
    - Right 05UT
  - Femoral
    - Left 06UN
    - Right 06UM
  - Foot
    - Left 06UV
    - Right 06UT
  - Gastric 06U2
  - Greater Saphenous
    - Left 06UQ
    - Right 06UP
  - Hand
    - Left 05UH
    - Right 05UG
  - Hemiazygos 05U1
  - Hepatic 06U4
  - Hypogastric
    - Left 06UJ
    - Right 06UH
  - Inferior Mesenteric 06U6
  - Innominate
    - Left 05U4
    - Right 05U3
  - Internal Jugular
    - Left 05UN
    - Right 05UM
  - Intracranial 05UL
  - Lesser Saphenous
    - Left 06US
    - Right 06UR
  - Lower 06UY
  - Portal 06U8
  - Pulmonary
    - Left 02UT
    - Right 02US
  - Renal
    - Left 06UB
    - Right 06U9
  - Splenic 06U1
  - Subclavian
    - Left 05U6
    - Right 05U5
  - Superior Mesenteric 06U5
  - Upper 05UY
  - Vertebral
    - Left 05US
    - Right 05UR
- Vena Cava
  - Inferior 06U0
  - Superior 02UV

Supplement *(continued)*
- Ventricle
  - Left 02UL
  - Right 02UK
- Vertebra
  - Cervical 0PU3
  - Lumbar 0QU0
  - Thoracic 0PU4
- Vesicle
  - Bilateral 0VU3
  - Left 0VU2
  - Right 0VU1
- Vocal Cord
  - Left 0CUV
  - Right 0CUT
- Vulva 0UUM
- Wrist Region
  - Left 0XUH
  - Right 0XUG

Supraclavicular (Virchow's) lymph node
- *use* Lymphatic, Neck, Left
- *use* Lymphatic, Neck, Right

Supraclavicular nerve
- *use* Nerve, Cervical Plexus

Suprahyoid lymph node
- *use* Lymphatic, Head

Suprahyoid muscle
- *use* Muscle, Neck, Left
- *use* Muscle, Neck, Right

Suprainguinal lymph node
- *use* Lymphatic, Pelvis

Supraorbital vein
- *use* Vein, Face, Left
- *use* Vein, Face, Right

Suprarenal gland
- *use* Gland, Adrenal
- *use* Gland, Adrenal, Bilateral
- *use* Gland, Adrenal, Left
- *use* Gland, Adrenal, Right

Suprarenal plexus
- *use* Nerve, Abdominal Sympathetic

Suprascapular nerve
- *use* Nerve, Brachial Plexus

Supraspinatus fascia
- *use* Subcutaneous Tissue and Fascia, Upper Arm, Left
- *use* Subcutaneous Tissue and Fascia, Upper Arm, Right

Supraspinatus muscle
- *use* Muscle, Shoulder, Left
- *use* Muscle, Shoulder, Right

Supraspinous ligament
- *use* Bursa and Ligament, Trunk, Left
- *use* Bursa and Ligament, Trunk, Right

Suprasternal notch
- *use* Sternum

Supratrochlear lymph node
- *use* Lymphatic, Upper Extremity, Left
- *use* Lymphatic, Upper Extremity, Right

Sural artery
- *use* Artery, Popliteal, Left
- *use* Artery, Popliteal, Right

Suspension
- Bladder Neck
  - *see* Reposition, Bladder Neck 0TSC
- Kidney
  - *see* Reposition, Urinary System 0TS
- Urethra
  - *see* Reposition, Urinary System 0TS
- Urethrovesical
  - *see* Reposition, Bladder Neck 0TSC
- Uterus
  - *see* Reposition, Uterus 0US9

Suspension *(continued)*
- Uterus *(continued)*
  - Vagina
  - *see* Reposition, Vagina 0USG

Suture
- Laceration repair
  - *see* Repair
- Ligation
  - *see* Occlusion

Suture Removal
- Extremity
  - Lower 8E0YXY8
  - Upper 8E0XXY8
- Head and Neck Region 8E09XY8
- Trunk Region 8E0WXY8

Sweat gland
- *use* Skin

Sympathectomy
- *see* Excision, Peripheral Nervous System 01B

SynCardia Total Artificial Heart
- *use* Synthetic Substitute

Synchra CRT-P
- *use* Cardiac Resynchronization Pacemaker Pulse Generator in 0JH

SynchroMed pump
- *use* Infusion Device, Pump in Subcutaneous Tissue and Fascia

Synechiotomy, iris
- *see* Release, Eye 08N

Synovectomy
- Lower joint
  - *see* Excision, Lower Joints 0SB
- Upper joint
  - *see* Excision, Upper Joints 0RB

Systemic Nuclear Medicine Therapy
- Abdomen CW70
- Anatomical Regions, Multiple CW7YYZZ
- Chest CW73
- Thyroid CW7G
- Whole Body CW7N

T

Takedown
- Arteriovenous shunt
  - *see* Removal of device from, Upper Arteries 03P
- Arteriovenous shunt, with creation of new shunt
  - *see* Bypass, Upper Arteries 031
- Stoma
  - *see* Repair

Talent® Converter
- *use* Intraluminal Device

Talent® Occluder
- *use* Intraluminal Device

Talent® Stent Graft (abdominal) (thoracic)
- *use* Intraluminal Device

Talocalcaneal (subtalar) joint
- *use* Joint, Tarsal, Left
- *use* Joint, Tarsal, Right

Talocalcaneal ligament
- *use* Bursa and Ligament, Foot, Left
- *use* Bursa and Ligament, Foot, Right

Talocalcaneonavicular joint
- *use* Joint, Tarsal, Left
- *use* Joint, Tarsal, Right

Talocalcaneonavicular ligament
- *use* Bursa and Ligament, Foot, Left
- *use* Bursa and Ligament, Foot, Right

Talocrural joint
- *use* Joint, Ankle, Left
- *use* Joint, Ankle, Right

V

Within each section of ICD-10-PCS the characters have different meanings. The seven character meanings for the Medical and Surgical section are illustrated here through the procedure example of *Percutaneous needle core biopsy of the right kidney*.

Section	Body System	Root Operation	Body Part	Approach	Device	Qualifier
Med/Surg	Urinary	Excision	Kidney, Right	Percutaneous	None	Diagnostic
0	T	B	0	3	Z	X

Section (Character 1)

All Medical and Surgical procedure codes have a first character value of 0.

Body System (Character 2)

The alphanumeric character for the body system is placed in the second position. The following are the body systems applicable to the Medical and Surgical section.

Character Value	Character Value Description
0	Central Nervous System
1	Peripheral Nervous System
2	Heart and Great Vessels
3	Upper Arteries
4	Lower Arteries
5	Upper Veins
6	Lower Veins
7	Lymphatic and Hemic Systems
8	Eye
9	Ear, Nose, Sinus
B	Respiratory System
C	Mouth and Throat
D	Gastrointestinal System
F	Hepatobiliary System and Pancreas
G	Endocrine System
H	Skin and Breast
J	Subcutaneous Tissue and Fascia
K	Muscles
L	Tendons
M	Bursae and Ligaments
N	Head and Facial Bones
P	Upper Bones
Q	Lower Bones
R	Upper Joints
S	Lower Joints
T	Urinary System
U	Female Reproductive System
V	Male Reproductive System
W	Anatomical Regions, General
X	Anatomical Regions, Upper Extremities
Y	Anatomical Regions, Lower Extremities

Root Operations (Character 3)

The alphanumeric character value for root operations is placed in the third position. Listed below are the root operations applicable to the Medical and Surgical section with their associated meaning. Note that the root operation definitions for ICD-10-PCS may differ from the terms that coders currently use today with ICD-9-CM Volume 3.

Character Value	Root Operation	Root Operation Definition
0	Alteration	Modifying the anatomic structure of a body part without affecting the function of the body part
1	Bypass	Altering the route of passage of the contents of a tubular body part
2	Change	Taking out or off a device from a body part and putting back an identical or similar device in or on the same body part without cutting or puncturing the skin or a mucous membrane
3	Control	Stopping, or attempting to stop, postprocedural bleeding
4	Creation	Making a new genital structure that does not take over the function of a body part
5	Destruction	Physical eradication of all or a portion of a body part by the direct use of energy, force, or a destructive agent
6	Detachment	Cutting off all or a portion of the upper or lower extremities
7	Dilation	Expanding an orifice or the lumen of a tubular body part
8	Division	Cutting into a body part, without draining fluids and/or gases from the body part, in order to separate or transect a body part
9	Drainage	Taking or letting out fluids and/or gases from a body part
B	Excision	Cutting out or off, without replacement, a portion of a body part
C	Extirpation	Taking or cutting out solid matter from a body part
D	Extraction	Pulling or stripping out or off all or a portion of a body part by the use of force
F	Fragmentation	Breaking solid matter in a body part into pieces
G	Fusion	Joining together portions of an articular body part rendering the articular body part immobile
H	Insertion	Putting in a nonbiological appliance that monitors, assists, performs, or prevents a physiological function but does not physically take the place of a body part
J	Inspection	Visually and/or manually exploring a body part
K	Map	Locating the route of passage of electrical impulses and/or locating functional areas in a body part
L	Occlusion	Completely closing an orifice or the lumen of a tubular body part
M	Reattachment	Putting back in or on all or a portion of a separated body part to its normal location or other suitable location
N	Release	Freeing a body part from an abnormal physical constraint by cutting or by the use of force
P	Removal	Taking out or off a device from a body part
Q	Repair	Restoring, to the extent possible, a body part to its normal anatomic structure and function
R	Replacement	Putting in or on biological or synthetic material that physically takes the place and/or function of all or a portion of a body part
S	Reposition	Moving to its normal location, or other suitable location, all or a portion of a body part
T	Resection	Cutting out or off, without replacement, all of a body part
V	Restriction	Partially closing an orifice or the lumen of a tubular body part
W	Revision	Correcting, to the extent possible, a portion of a malfunctioning device or the position of a displaced device
U	Supplement	Putting in or on biological or synthetic material that physically reinforces and/or augments the function of a portion of a body part
X	Transfer	Moving, without taking out, all or a portion of a body part to another location to take over the function of all or a portion of a body part
Y	Transplantation	Putting in or on all or a portion of a living body part taken from another individual or animal to physically take the place and/or function of all or a portion of a similar body part

Body Part (Character 4)

For each body system the applicable body part character values will be available for procedure code construction. An example of a body part for this section is the Large Intestines.

Approach (Character 5)

The approach is the technique used to reach the procedure site. The following are the approach character values for the Medical and Surgical section with the associated definitions.

Character Value	Approach	Approach Definition
0	Open	Cutting through the skin or mucous membrane and any other body layers necessary to expose the site of the procedure
3	Percutaneous	Entry, by puncture or minor incision, of instrumentation through the skin or mucous membrane and any other body layers necessary to reach the site of the procedure
4	Percutaneous Endoscopic	Entry, by puncture or minor incision, of instrumentation through the skin or mucous membrane and any other body layers necessary to reach and visualize the site of the procedure
7	Via Natural or Artificial Opening	Entry of instrumentation through a natural or artificial external opening to reach the site of the procedure
8	Via Natural or Artificial Opening Endoscopic	Entry of instrumentation through a natural or artificial external opening to reach and visualize the site of the procedure
F	Via Natural or Artificial Opening Percutaneous Endoscopic	Entry of instrumentation through a natural or artificial external opening to reach and visualize the site of the procedure, and entry, by puncture or minor incision, of instrumentation through the skin or mucous membrane and any other body layers necessary to aid in the performance of the procedure
X	External	Procedures performed directly on the skin or mucous membrane and procedures performed indirectly by the application of external force through the skin or mucous membrane

Device (Character 6)

Depending on the procedure performed there may or may not be a device used. There are several types of devices included in the Medical and Surgical section that fall into one of the four following categories.

- Electronic Appliances
- Grafts and Prostheses
- Implants
- Simple or Mechanical Appliances

When a device is not utilized during the procedure, the character value of Z should be reported.

If a coder is unsure of which option to select for the device utilized during the procedure, Appendix E can be used to guide the selection. For example, if the coder is in Table 02R (replacement of heart and great vessels) the coder can locate the device categories in Appendix E (Autologous Tissue Substitute, Zooplastic Tissue, Synthetic Substitute, and Nonautologous Tissue Substitue). For each of these categories brand name devices and other devices are listed. The coder should select the category in which the device utilized during the procedure is listed.

Qualifier (Character 7)

The qualifier represents an additional attribute for the procedure when applicable. In the preceding example of *Percutaneous needle core biopsy of the right kidney*, the qualifier of X was used to report that the biopsy procedure was diagnostic in nature. If there is no qualifier for a procedure, the Z character value should be reported.

Important Definitions for the Medical and Surgical Section

Medical Surgical Root Operation	Qualifier	Definition
Detachment of Upper and Lower Extremities (0X6 and 0Y6) Arms and Legs	1 – High	Amputation at the proximal portion of the shaft of the humerus or femur
	2 – Mid	Amputation at the middle portion of the shaft of the humerus or femur
	3 – Low	Amputation at the distal portion of the shaft of the humerus or femur
Detachment of Upper and Lower Extremities (0X6 and 0Y6) Fingers, Thumbs, and Toes	0 – Complete	Amputation at the metacarpophalangeal/metatarsal-phalangeal joint
	1 – High	Amputation anywhere along the proximal phalanx
	2 – Mid	Amputation through the proximal interphalangeal joint or anywhere along the middle phalanx
	3 – Low	Amputation through the distal interphalangeal joint or anywhere along the distal phalanx
Transplantation	0 – Allogeneic	Being genetically different although belonging to or obtained from the same species*
	1 – Syngeneic	Genetically identical or closely related, so as to allow tissue transplant; immunologically compatible*
	2 – Zooplastic	Surgical transfer of tissue from an animal to a human*

*Taken from The Free Dictionary by Farlex at www.thefreedictionary.com

Medical and Surgical Section Guidelines (section 0)

B2. Body System

General guidelines

B2.1a The procedure codes in the general anatomical regions body systems should only be used when the procedure is performed on an anatomical region rather than a specific body part (e.g., root operations Control and Detachment, Drainage of a body cavity) or on the rare occasion when no information is available to support assignment of a code to a specific body part.

Example: Control of postoperative hemorrhage is coded to the root operation Control found in the general anatomical regions body systems.

B2.1b Where the general body part values "upper" and "lower" are provided as an option in the Upper Arteries, Lower Arteries, Upper Veins, Lower Veins, Muscles and Tendons body systems, "upper" or "lower" specifies body parts located above or below the diaphragm respectively.

Example: Vein body parts above the diaphragm are found in the Upper Veins body system; vein body parts below the diaphragm are found in the Lower Veins body system.

B3. Root Operation

General guidelines

B3.1a In order to determine the appropriate root operation, the full definition of the root operation as contained in the PCS Tables must be applied.

B3.1b Components of a procedure specified in the root operation definition and explanation are not coded separately. Procedural steps necessary to reach the operative site and close the operative site, including anastomosis of a tubular body part, are also not coded separately.

Example: Resection of a joint as part of a joint replacement procedure is included in the root operation definition of Replacement and is not coded separately. Laparotomy performed to reach the site of an open liver biopsy is not coded separately. In a resection of sigmoid colon with anastomosis of descending colon to rectum, the anastomosis is not coded separately.

Multiple procedures

B3.2 During the same operative episode, multiple procedures are coded if:

a. The same root operation is performed on different body parts as defined by distinct values of the body part character.
   Example: Diagnostic excision of liver and pancreas are coded separately.
b. The same root operation is repeated at different body sites that are included in the same body part value.
   Example: Excision of the sartorius muscle and excision of the gracilis muscle are both included in the upper leg muscle body part value, and multiple procedures are coded.
c. Multiple root operations with distinct objectives are performed on the same body part.
   Example: Destruction of sigmoid lesion and bypass of sigmoid colon are coded separately.
d. The intended root operation is attempted using one approach, but is converted to a different approach.
   Example: Laparoscopic cholecystectomy converted to an open cholecystectomy is coded as percutaneous endoscopic Inspection and open Resection.

Discontinued procedures

B3.3 If the intended procedure is discontinued, code the procedure to the root operation performed. If a procedure is discontinued before any other root operation is performed, code the root operation Inspection of the body part or anatomical region inspected.

Example: A planned aortic valve replacement procedure is discontinued after the initial thoracotomy and before any incision is made in the heart muscle, when the patient becomes hemodynamically unstable. This procedure is coded as an open Inspection of the mediastinum.

Biopsy procedures

B3.4a Biopsy procedures are coded using the root operations Excision, Extraction, or Drainage and the qualifier Diagnostic. The qualifier Diagnostic is used only for biopsies.

Example: Fine needle aspiration biopsy of lung is coded to the root operation Drainage with the qualifier Diagnostic. Biopsy of bone marrow is coded to the root operation Extraction with the qualifier Diagnostic. Lymph node sampling for biopsy is coded to the root operation Excision with the qualifier Diagnostic.

Biopsy followed by more definitive treatment

B3.4b If a diagnostic Excision, Extraction, or Drainage procedure (biopsy) is followed by a more definitive procedure, such as Destruction, Excision or Resection at the same procedure site, both the biopsy and the more definitive treatment are coded.

Example: Biopsy of breast followed by partial mastectomy at the same procedure site, both the biopsy and the partial mastectomy procedure are coded.

Overlapping body layers

B3.5 If the root operations Excision, Repair or Inspection are performed on overlapping layers of the musculoskeletal system, the body part specifying the deepest layer is coded.

Example: Excisional debridement that includes skin and subcutaneous tissue and muscle is coded to the muscle body part.

Bypass procedures

B3.6a Bypass procedures are coded by identifying the body part bypassed "from" and the body part bypassed "to." The fourth character body part specifies the body part bypassed from, and the qualifier specifies the body part bypassed to.

Example: Bypass from stomach to jejunum, stomach is the body part and jejunum is the qualifier.

B3.6b Coronary arteries are classified by number of distinct sites treated, rather than number of coronary arteries or anatomic name of a coronary artery (e.g., left anterior descending). Coronary artery bypass procedures are coded differently than other bypass procedures as described in the previous guideline. Rather than identifying the body part bypassed from, the body part identifies the number of coronary artery sites bypassed to, and the qualifier specifies the vessel bypassed from.

Example: Aortocoronary artery bypass of one site on the left anterior descending coronary artery and one site on the obtuse marginal coronary artery is classified in the body part axis of classification as two coronary artery sites and the qualifier specifies the aorta as the body part bypassed from.

B3.6c If multiple coronary artery sites are bypassed, a separate procedure is coded for each coronary artery site that uses a different device and/or qualifier.

Example: Aortocoronary artery bypass and internal mammary coronary artery bypass are coded separately.

Control vs. more definitive root operations

B3.7 The root operation Control is defined as, "Stopping, or attempting to stop, postprocedural bleeding." If an attempt to stop postprocedural bleeding is initially unsuccessful, and to stop the bleeding requires performing any of the definitive root operations Bypass, Detachment, Excision, Extraction, Reposition, Replacement, or Resection, then that root operation is coded instead of Control.

Example: Resection of spleen to stop postprocedural bleeding is coded to Resection instead of Control.

Excision vs. Resection

B3.8 PCS contains specific body parts for anatomical subdivisions of a body part, such as lobes of the lungs or liver and regions of the intestine. Resection of the specific body part is coded whenever all of the body part is cut out or off, rather than coding Excision of a less specific body part.

Example: Left upper lung lobectomy is coded to Resection of Upper Lung Lobe, Left rather than Excision of Lung, Left.

Excision for graft

B3.9 If an autograft is obtained from a different body part in order to complete the objective of the procedure, a separate procedure is coded.

Example: Coronary bypass with excision of saphenous vein graft, excision of saphenous vein is coded separately.

Fusion procedures of the spine

B3.10a The body part coded for a spinal vertebral joint(s) rendered immobile by a spinal fusion procedure is classified by the level of the spine (e.g. thoracic). There are distinct body part values for a single vertebral joint and for multiple vertebral joints at each spinal level.

Example: Body part values specify Lumbar Vertebral Joint, Lumbar Vertebral Joints, 2 or More and Lumbosacral Vertebral Joint.

B3.10b If multiple vertebral joints are fused, a separate procedure is coded for each vertebral joint that uses a different device and/or qualifier.

Example: Fusion of lumbar vertebral joint, posterior approach, anterior column and fusion of lumbar vertebral joint, posterior approach, posterior column are coded separately.

B3.10c Combinations of devices and materials are often used on a vertebral joint to render the joint immobile. When combinations of devices are used on the same vertebral joint, the device value coded for the procedure is as follows:

- If an interbody fusion device is used to render the joint immobile (alone or containing other material like bone graft), the procedure is coded with the device value Interbody Fusion Device

- If bone graft is the only device used to render the joint immobile, the procedure is coded with the device value Nonautologous Tissue Substitute or Autologous Tissue Substitute
- If a mixture of autologous and nonautologous bone graft (with or without biological or synthetic extenders or binders) is used to render the joint immobile, code the procedure with the device value Autologous Tissue Substitute

Examples: Fusion of a vertebral joint using a cage style interbody fusion device containing morsellized bone graft is coded to the device Interbody Fusion Device.

Fusion of a vertebral joint using a bone dowel interbody fusion device made of cadaver bone and packed with a mixture of local morsellized bone and demineralized bone matrix is coded to the device Interbody Fusion Device.

Fusion of a vertebral joint using both autologous bone graft and bone bank bone graft is coded to the device Autologous Tissue Substitute.

Inspection procedures

B3.11a Inspection of a body part(s) performed in order to achieve the objective of a procedure is not coded separately.

Example: Fiberoptic bronchoscopy performed for irrigation of bronchus, only the irrigation procedure is coded.

B3.11b If multiple tubular body parts are inspected, the most distal body part inspected is coded. If multiple non-tubular body parts in a region are inspected, the body part that specifies the entire area inspected is coded.

Example: Cystoureteroscopy with inspection of bladder and ureters is coded to the ureter body part value.

Exploratory laparotomy with general inspection of abdominal contents is coded to the peritoneal cavity body part value.

B3.11c When both an Inspection procedure and another procedure are performed on the same body part during the same episode, if the Inspection procedure is performed using a different approach than the other procedure, the Inspection procedure is coded separately.

Example: Endoscopic Inspection of the duodenum is coded separately when open Excision of the duodenum is performed during the same procedural episode.

Occlusion vs. Restriction for vessel embolization procedures

B3.12 If the objective of an embolization procedure is to completely close a vessel, the root operation Occlusion is coded. If the objective of an embolization procedure is to narrow the lumen of a vessel, the root operation Restriction is coded.

Examples: Tumor embolization is coded to the root operation Occlusion, because the objective of the procedure is to cut off the blood supply to the vessel.

Embolization of a cerebral aneurysm is coded to the root operation Restriction, because the objective of the procedure is not to close off the vessel entirely, but to narrow the lumen of the vessel at the site of the aneurysm where it is abnormally wide.

Release procedures

B3.13 In the root operation Release, the body part value coded is the body part being freed and not the tissue being manipulated or cut to free the body part.

Example: Lysis of intestinal adhesions is coded to the specific intestine body part value.

Release vs. Division

B3.14 If the sole objective of the procedure is freeing a body part without cutting the body part, the root operation is Release. If the sole objective of the procedure is separating or transecting a body part, the root operation is Division.

Example: Freeing a nerve root from surrounding scar tissue to relieve pain is coded to the root operation Release. Severing a nerve root to relieve pain is coded to the root operation Division.

Reposition for fracture treatment

B3.15 Reduction of a displaced fracture is coded to the root operation Reposition and the application of a cast or splint in conjunction with the Reposition procedure is not coded separately. Treatment of a nondisplaced fracture is coded to the procedure performed.

Example: Putting a pin in a nondisplaced fracture is coded to the root operation Insertion.

Casting of a nondisplaced fracture is coded to the root operation Immobilization in the Placement section.

Transplantation vs. Administration

B3.16 Putting in a mature and functioning living body part taken from another individual or animal is coded to the root operation Transplantation. Putting in autologous or nonautologous cells is coded to the Administration section.

Example: Putting in autologous or nonautologous bone marrow, pancreatic islet cells or stem cells is coded to the Administration section.

B4. Body Part

General guidelines

B4.1a If a procedure is performed on a portion of a body part that does not have a separate body part value, code the body part value corresponding to the whole body part.

Example: A procedure performed on the alveolar process of the mandible is coded to the mandible body part.

B4.1b If the prefix "peri" is combined with a body part to identify the site of the procedure, the procedure is coded to the body part named.

Example: A procedure site identified as perirenal is coded to the kidney body part.

Branches of body parts

B4.2 Where a specific branch of a body part does not have its own body part value in PCS, the body part is coded to the closest proximal branch that has a specific body part value.

Example: A procedure performed on the mandibular branch of the trigeminal nerve is coded to the trigeminal nerve body part value.

Bilateral body part values

B4.3 Bilateral body part values are available for a limited number of body parts. If the identical procedure is performed on contralateral body parts, and a bilateral body part value exists for that body part, a single procedure is coded using the bilateral body part value. If no bilateral body part value exists, each procedure is coded separately using the appropriate body part value.

Example: The identical procedure performed on both fallopian tubes is coded once using the body part value Fallopian Tube, Bilateral. The identical procedure performed on both knee joints is coded twice using the body part values Knee Joint, Right and Knee Joint, Left.

Coronary arteries

B4.4 The coronary arteries are classified as a single body part that is further specified by number of sites treated and not by name or number of arteries. Separate body part values are used to specify the number of sites treated when the same procedure is performed on multiple sites in the coronary arteries.

Examples: Angioplasty of two distinct sites in the left anterior descending coronary artery with placement of two stents is coded as Dilation of Coronary Arteries, Two Sites, with Intraluminal Device.

Angioplasty of two distinct sites in the left anterior descending coronary artery, one with stent placed and one without, is coded separately as Dilation of Coronary Artery, One Site with Intraluminal Device, and Dilation of Coronary Artery, One Site with no device.

Tendons, ligaments, bursae and fascia near a joint

B4.5 Procedures performed on tendons, ligaments, bursae and fascia supporting a joint are coded to the body part in the respective body system that is the focus of the procedure. Procedures performed on joint structures themselves are coded to the body part in the joint body systems.

Example: Repair of the anterior cruciate ligament of the knee is coded to the knee bursae and ligament body part in the bursae and ligaments body system. Knee arthroscopy with shaving of articular cartilage is coded to the knee joint body part in the Lower Joints body system.

Skin, subcutaneous tissue and fascia overlying a joint

B4.6 If a procedure is performed on the skin, subcutaneous tissue or fascia overlying a joint, the procedure is coded to the following body part:

- Shoulder is coded to Upper Arm
- Elbow is coded to Lower Arm
- Wrist is coded to Lower Arm
- Hip is coded to Upper Leg
- Knee is coded to Lower Leg
- Ankle is coded to Foot

Fingers and toes

B4.7 If a body system does not contain a separate body part value for fingers, procedures performed on the fingers are coded to the body part value for the hand. If a body system does not contain a separate body part value for toes, procedures performed on the toes are coded to the body part value for the foot.

Example: Excision of finger muscle is coded to one of the hand muscle body part values in the Muscles body system.

Upper and lower intestinal tract

B4.8 In the Gastrointestinal body system, the general body part values Upper Intestinal Tract and Lower Intestinal Tract are provided as an option for the root operations Change, Inspection, Removal and Revision. Upper Intestinal Tract includes the portion of the gastrointestinal tract from the esophagus down to and including the duodenum, and Lower Intestinal Tract includes the portion of the gastrointestinal tract from the jejunum down to and including the rectum and anus.

Example: In the root operation Change table, change of a device in the jejunum is coded using the body part Lower Intestinal Tract.

B5. Approach

Open approach with percutaneous endoscopic assistance

B5.2 Procedures performed using the open approach with percutaneous endoscopic assistance are coded to the approach Open.

Example: Laparoscopic-assisted sigmoidectomy is coded to the approach Open.

External approach

B5.3a Procedures performed within an orifice on structures that are visible without the aid of any instrumentation are coded to the approach External.

Example: Resection of tonsils is coded to the approach External.

B5.3b Procedures performed indirectly by the application of external force through the intervening body layers are coded to the approach External.

Example: Closed reduction of fracture is coded to the approach External.

Percutaneous procedure via device

B5.4 Procedures performed percutaneously via a device placed for the procedure are coded to the approach Percutaneous.

Example: Fragmentation of kidney stone performed via percutaneous nephrostomy is coded to the approach Percutaneous.

B6. Device

General guidelines

B6.1a A device is coded only if a device remains after the procedure is completed. If no device remains, the device value No Device is coded.

B6.1b Materials such as sutures, ligatures, radiological markers and temporary post-operative wound drains are considered integral to the performance of a procedure and are not coded as devices.

B6.1c Procedures performed on a device only and not on a body part are specified in the root operations Change, Irrigation, Removal and Revision, and are coded to the procedure performed.

Example: Irrigation of percutaneous nephrostomy tube is coded to the root operation Irrigation of indwelling device in the Administration section.

Drainage device

B6.2 A separate procedure to put in a drainage device is coded to the root operation Drainage with the device value Drainage Device.

Brain

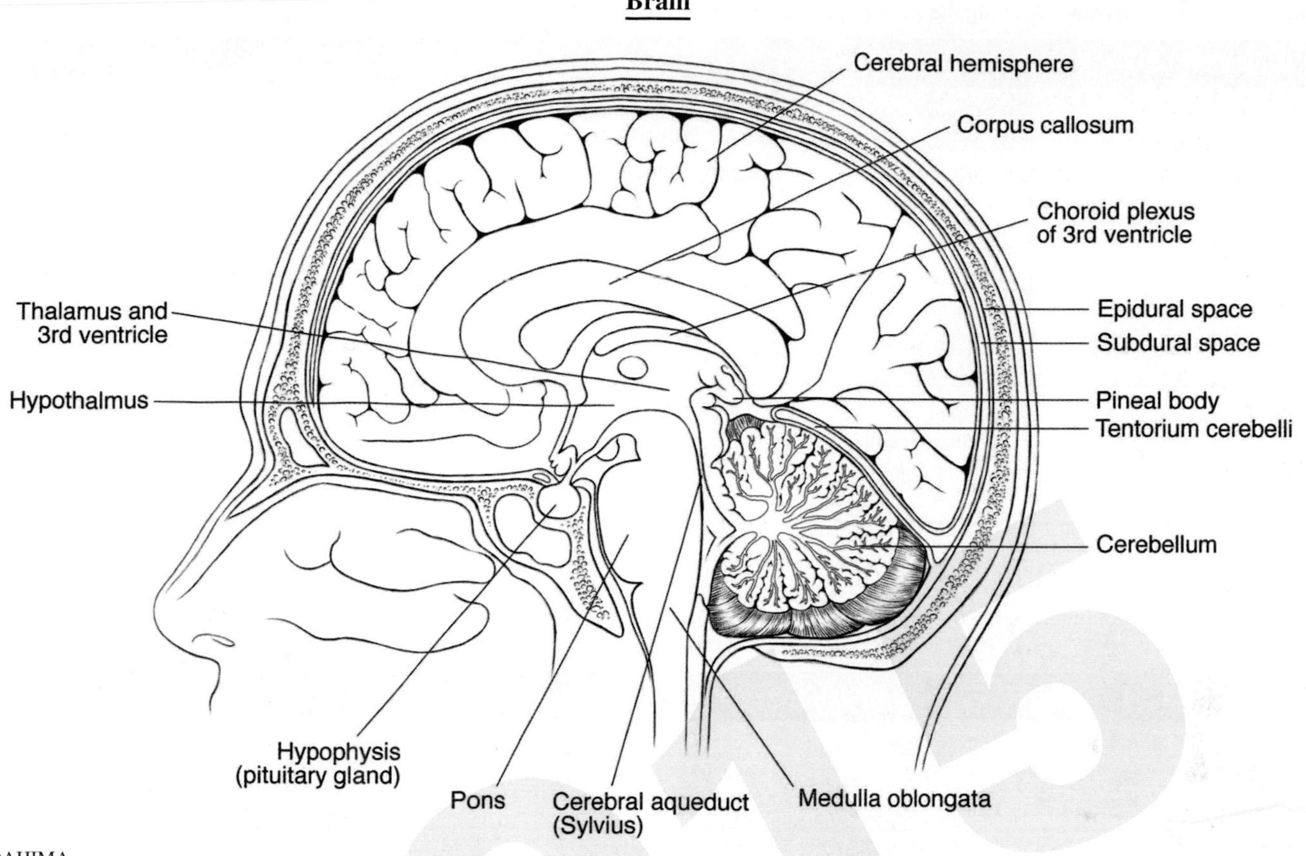
Cerebral hemisphere
Corpus callosum
Choroid plexus of 3rd ventricle
Epidural space
Subdural space
Pineal body
Tentorium cerebelli
Cerebellum
Thalamus and 3rd ventricle
Hypothalmus
Hypophysis (pituitary gland)
Pons
Cerebral aqueduct (Sylvius)
Medulla oblongata

Cranial Nerves

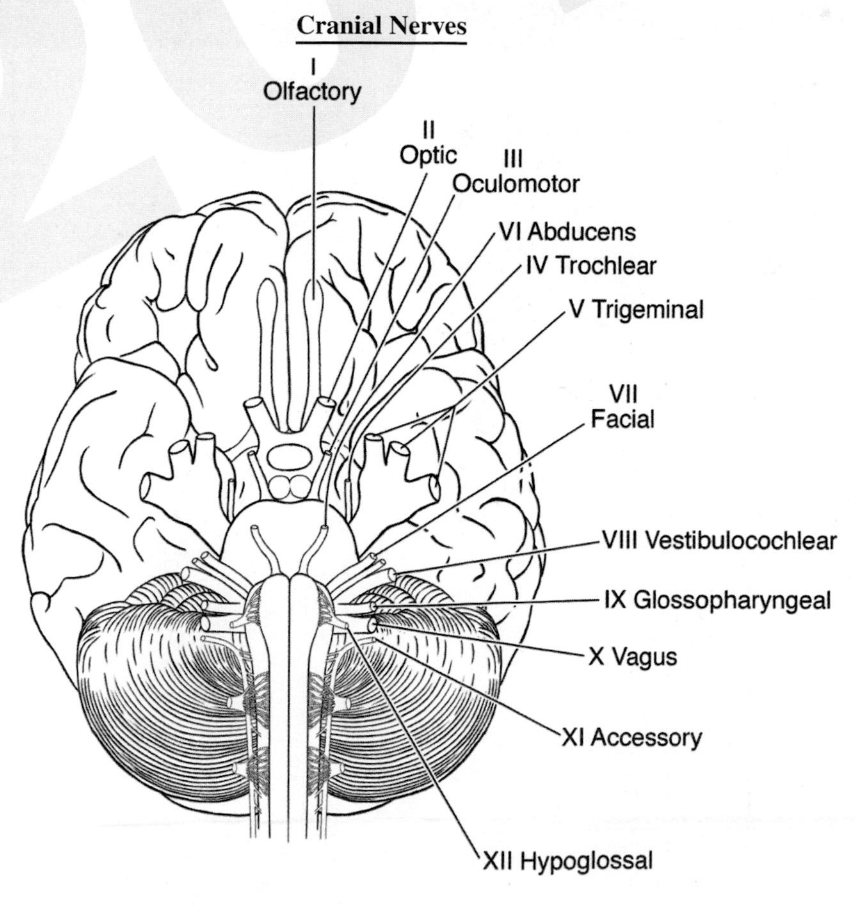
I Olfactory
II Optic
III Oculomotor
VI Abducens
IV Trochlear
V Trigeminal
VII Facial
VIII Vestibulocochlear
IX Glossopharyngeal
X Vagus
XI Accessory
XII Hypoglossal

Central Nervous System Tables 001–00X

Section 0 **Medical and Surgical**
Body System 0 **Central Nervous System**
Operation 1 **Bypass:** Altering the route of passage of the contents of a tubular body part

Body Part (4th)	Approach (5th)	Device (6th)	Qualifier (7th)
6 Cerebral Ventricle	**0** Open **3** Percutaneous	**7** Autologous Tissue Substitute **J** Synthetic Substitute **K** Nonautologous Tissue Substitute	**0** Nasopharynx **1** Mastoid Sinus **2** Atrium **3** Blood Vessel **4** Pleural Cavity **5** Intestine **6** Peritoneal Cavity **7** Urinary Tract **8** Bone Marrow **B** Cerebral Cisterns
U Spinal Canal	**0** Open **3** Percutaneous	**7** Autologous Tissue Substitute **J** Synthetic Substitute **K** Nonautologous Tissue Substitute	**4** Pleural Cavity **6** Peritoneal Cavity **7** Urinary Tract **9** Fallopian Tube

Section 0 **Medical and Surgical**
Body System 0 **Central Nervous System**
Operation 2 **Change:** Taking out or off a device from a body part and putting back an identical or similar device in or on the same body part without cutting or puncturing the skin or a mucous membrane

Body Part (4th)	Approach (5th)	Device (6th)	Qualifier (7th)
0 Brain **E** Cranial Nerve **U** Spinal Canal	**X** External	**0** Drainage Device **Y** Other Device	**Z** No Qualifier

Section 0 **Medical and Surgical**
Body System 0 **Central Nervous System**
Operation 5 **Destruction:** Physical eradication of all or a portion of a body part by the direct use of energy, force, or a destructive agent

Body Part (4th)	Approach (5th)	Device (6th)	Qualifier (7th)
0 Brain **1** Cerebral Meninges **2** Dura Mater **6** Cerebral Ventricle **7** Cerebral Hemisphere **8** Basal Ganglia **9** Thalamus **A** Hypothalamus **B** Pons **C** Cerebellum **D** Medulla Oblongata **F** Olfactory Nerve **G** Optic Nerve **H** Oculomotor Nerve **J** Trochlear Nerve **K** Trigeminal Nerve **L** Abducens Nerve **M** Facial Nerve **N** Acoustic Nerve **P** Glossopharyngeal Nerve **Q** Vagus Nerve **R** Accessory Nerve **S** Hypoglossal Nerve **T** Spinal Meninges **W** Cervical Spinal Cord **X** Thoracic Spinal Cord **Y** Lumbar Spinal Cord	**0** Open **3** Percutaneous **4** Percutaneous Endoscopic	**Z** No Device	**Z** No Qualifier

Section 0 **Medical and Surgical**
Body System 0 **Central Nervous System**
Operation 8 **Division:** Cutting into a body part, without draining fluids and/or gases from the body part, in order to separate or transect a body part

Body Part (4th)	Approach (5th)	Device (6th)	Qualifier (7th)
0 Brain **7** Cerebral Hemisphere **8** Basal Ganglia **F** Olfactory Nerve **G** Optic Nerve **H** Oculomotor Nerve **J** Trochlear Nerve **K** Trigeminal Nerve **L** Abducens Nerve **M** Facial Nerve **N** Acoustic Nerve **P** Glossopharyngeal Nerve **Q** Vagus Nerve **R** Accessory Nerve **S** Hypoglossal Nerve **W** Cervical Spinal Cord **X** Thoracic Spinal Cord **Y** Lumbar Spinal Cord	**0** Open **3** Percutaneous **4** Percutaneous Endoscopic	**Z** No Device	**Z** No Qualifier

Section 0 **Medical and Surgical**
Body System 0 **Central Nervous System**
Operation 9 **Drainage:** Taking or letting out fluids and/or gases from a body part

Body Part (4th)	Approach (5th)	Device (6th)	Qualifier (7th)
0 Brain **1** Cerebral Meninges **2** Dura Mater **3** Epidural Space **4** Subdural Space **5** Subarachnoid Space **6** Cerebral Ventricle **7** Cerebral Hemisphere **8** Basal Ganglia **9** Thalamus **A** Hypothalamus **B** Pons **C** Cerebellum **D** Medulla Oblongata **F** Olfactory Nerve **G** Optic Nerve **H** Oculomotor Nerve **J** Trochlear Nerve **K** Trigeminal Nerve **L** Abducens Nerve **M** Facial Nerve **N** Acoustic Nerve **P** Glossopharyngeal Nerve **Q** Vagus Nerve **R** Accessory Nerve **S** Hypoglossal Nerve **T** Spinal Meninges **U** Spinal Canal **W** Cervical Spinal Cord **X** Thoracic Spinal Cord **Y** Lumbar Spinal Cord	**0** Open **3** Percutaneous **4** Percutaneous Endoscopic	**0** Drainage Device	**Z** No Qualifier

Continued →

Section 0 **Medical and Surgical**
Body System 0 **Central Nervous System**
Operation 9 **Drainage:** Taking or letting out fluids and/or gases from a body part

Body Part (4th)	Approach (5th)	Device (6th)	Qualifier (7th)
0 Brain **1** Cerebral Meninges **2** Dura Mater **3** Epidural Space **4** Subdural Space **5** Subarachnoid Space **6** Cerebral Ventricle **7** Cerebral Hemisphere **8** Basal Ganglia **9** Thalamus **A** Hypothalamus **B** Pons **C** Cerebellum **D** Medulla Oblongata **F** Olfactory Nerve **G** Optic Nerve **H** Oculomotor Nerve **J** Trochlear Nerve **K** Trigeminal Nerve **L** Abducens Nerve **M** Facial Nerve **N** Acoustic Nerve **P** Glossopharyngeal Nerve **Q** Vagus Nerve **R** Accessory Nerve **S** Hypoglossal Nerve **T** Spinal Meninges **U** Spinal Canal **W** Cervical Spinal Cord **X** Thoracic Spinal Cord **Y** Lumbar Spinal Cord	**0** Open **3** Percutaneous **4** Percutaneous Endoscopic	**Z** No Device	**X** Diagnostic **Z** No Qualifier

Section 0 **Medical and Surgical**
Body System 0 **Central Nervous System**
Operation B **Excision:** Cutting out or off, without replacement, a portion of a body part

Body Part (4th)	Approach (5th)	Device (6th)	Qualifier (7th)
0 Brain **1** Cerebral Meninges **2** Dura Mater **6** Cerebral Ventricle **7** Cerebral Hemisphere **8** Basal Ganglia **9** Thalamus **A** Hypothalamus **B** Pons **C** Cerebellum **D** Medulla Oblongata **F** Olfactory Nerve **G** Optic Nerve **H** Oculomotor Nerve **J** Trochlear Nerve **K** Trigeminal Nerve **L** Abducens Nerve **M** Facial Nerve **N** Acoustic Nerve **P** Glossopharyngeal Nerve **Q** Vagus Nerve **R** Accessory Nerve **S** Hypoglossal Nerve **T** Spinal Meninges **W** Cervical Spinal Cord **X** Thoracic Spinal Cord **Y** Lumbar Spinal Cord	**0** Open **3** Percutaneous **4** Percutaneous Endoscopic	**Z** No Device	**X** Diagnostic **Z** No Qualifier

Section 0 **Medical and Surgical**
Body System 0 **Central Nervous System**
Operation C **Extirpation:** Taking or cutting out solid matter from a body part

Body Part (4th)	Approach (5th)	Device (6th)	Qualifier (7th)
0 Brain **1** Cerebral Meninges **2** Dura Mater **3** Epidural Space **4** Subdural Space **5** Subarachnoid Space **6** Cerebral Ventricle **7** Cerebral Hemisphere **8** Basal Ganglia **9** Thalamus **A** Hypothalamus **B** Pons **C** Cerebellum **D** Medulla Oblongata **F** Olfactory Nerve **G** Optic Nerve **H** Oculomotor Nerve **J** Trochlear Nerve **K** Trigeminal Nerve **L** Abducens Nerve **M** Facial Nerve **N** Acoustic Nerve **P** Glossopharyngeal Nerve **Q** Vagus Nerve **R** Accessory Nerve **S** Hypoglossal Nerve **T** Spinal Meninges **W** Cervical Spinal Cord **X** Thoracic Spinal Cord **Y** Lumbar Spinal Cord	**0** Open **3** Percutaneous **4** Percutaneous Endoscopic	**Z** No Device	**Z** No Qualifier

Section 0 **Medical and Surgical**
Body System 0 **Central Nervous System**
Operation D **Extraction:** Pulling or stripping out or off all or a portion of a body part by the use of force

Body Part (4th)	Approach (5th)	Device (6th)	Qualifier (7th)
1 Cerebral Meninges **2** Dura Mater **F** Olfactory Nerve **G** Optic Nerve **H** Oculomotor Nerve **J** Trochlear Nerve **K** Trigeminal Nerve **L** Abducens Nerve **M** Facial Nerve **N** Acoustic Nerve **P** Glossopharyngeal Nerve **Q** Vagus Nerve **R** Accessory Nerve **S** Hypoglossal Nerve **T** Spinal Meninges	**0** Open **3** Percutaneous **4** Percutaneous Endoscopic	**Z** No Device	**Z** No Qualifier

Section **0** **Medical and Surgical**
Body System **0** **Central Nervous System**
Operation **F** **Fragmentation:** Breaking solid matter in a body part into pieces

Body Part (4th)	Approach (5th)	Device (6th)	Qualifier (7th)
3 Epidural Space **4** Subdural Space **5** Subarachnoid Space **6** Cerebral Ventricle **U** Spinal Canal	**0** Open **3** Percutaneous **4** Percutaneous Endoscopic **X** External	**Z** No Device	**Z** No Qualifier

Section **0** **Medical and Surgical**
Body System **0** **Central Nervous System**
Operation **H** **Insertion:** Putting in a nonbiological appliance that monitors, assists, performs, or prevents a physiological function but does not physically take the place of a body part

Body Part (4th)	Approach (5th)	Device (6th)	Qualifier (7th)
0 Brain **6** Cerebral Ventricle **E** Cranial Nerve **U** Spinal Canal **V** Spinal Cord	**0** Open **3** Percutaneous **4** Percutaneous Endoscopic	**2** Monitoring Device **3** Infusion Device **M** Neurostimulator Lead	**Z** No Qualifier

Section **0** **Medical and Surgical**
Body System **0** **Central Nervous System**
Operation **J** **Inspection:** Visually and/or manually exploring a body part

Body Part (4th)	Approach (5th)	Device (6th)	Qualifier (7th)
0 Brain **E** Cranial Nerve **U** Spinal Canal **V** Spinal Cord	**0** Open **3** Percutaneous **4** Percutaneous Endoscopic	**Z** No Device	**Z** No Qualifier

Section **0** **Medical and Surgical**
Body System **0** **Central Nervous System**
Operation **K** **Map:** Locating the route of passage of electrical impulses and/or locating functional areas in a body part

Body Part (4th)	Approach (5th)	Device (6th)	Qualifier (7th)
0 Brain **7** Cerebral Hemisphere **8** Basal Ganglia **9** Thalamus **A** Hypothalamus **B** Pons **C** Cerebellum **D** Medulla Oblongata	**0** Open **3** Percutaneous **4** Percutaneous Endoscopic	**Z** No Device	**Z** No Qualifier

Section 0 Medical and Surgical
Body System 0 Central Nervous System
Operation N **Release:** Freeing a body part from an abnormal physical constraint by cutting or by the use of force

Body Part (4th)	Approach (5th)	Device (6th)	Qualifier (7th)
0 Brain **1** Cerebral Meninges **2** Dura Mater **6** Cerebral Ventricle **7** Cerebral Hemisphere **8** Basal Ganglia **9** Thalamus **A** Hypothalamus **B** Pons **C** Cerebellum **D** Medulla Oblongata **F** Olfactory Nerve **G** Optic Nerve **H** Oculomotor Nerve **J** Trochlear Nerve **K** Trigeminal Nerve **L** Abducens Nerve **M** Facial Nerve **N** Acoustic Nerve **P** Glossopharyngeal Nerve **Q** Vagus Nerve **R** Accessory Nerve **S** Hypoglossal Nerve **T** Spinal Meninges **W** Cervical Spinal Cord **X** Thoracic Spinal Cord **Y** Lumbar Spinal Cord	**0** Open **3** Percutaneous **4** Percutaneous Endoscopic	**Z** No Device	**Z** No Qualifier

Section 0 Medical and Surgical
Body System 0 Central Nervous System
Operation P **Removal:** Taking out or off a device from a body part

Body Part (4th)	Approach (5th)	Device (6th)	Qualifier (7th)
0 Brain **V** Spinal Cord	**0** Open **3** Percutaneous **4** Percutaneous Endoscopic	**0** Drainage Device **2** Monitoring Device **3** Infusion Device **7** Autologous Tissue Substitute **J** Synthetic Substitute **K** Nonautologous Tissue Substitute **M** Neurostimulator Lead	**Z** No Qualifier
0 Brain **V** Spinal Cord	**X** External	**0** Drainage Device **2** Monitoring Device **3** Infusion Device **M** Neurostimulator Lead	**Z** No Qualifier
6 Cerebral Ventricle **U** Spinal Canal	**0** Open **3** Percutaneous **4** Percutaneous Endoscopic	**0** Drainage Device **2** Monitoring Device **3** Infusion Device **J** Synthetic Substitute **M** Neurostimulator Lead	**Z** No Qualifier
6 Cerebral Ventricle **U** Spinal Canal	**X** External	**0** Drainage Device **2** Monitoring Device **3** Infusion Device **M** Neurostimulator Lead	**Z** No Qualifier
E Cranial Nerve	**0** Open **3** Percutaneous **4** Percutaneous Endoscopic	**0** Drainage Device **2** Monitoring Device **3** Infusion Device **7** Autologous Tissue Substitute **M** Neurostimulator Lead	**Z** No Qualifier

Continued →

Section 0 **Medical and Surgical**
Body System 0 **Central Nervous System**
Operation P **Removal:** Taking out or off a device from a body part

Body Part (4th)	Approach (5th)	Device (6th)	Qualifier (7th)
E Cranial Nerve	**X** External	**0** Drainage Device **2** Monitoring Device **3** Infusion Device **M** Neurostimulator Lead	**Z** No Qualifier

Section 0 **Medical and Surgical**
Body System 0 **Central Nervous System**
Operation Q **Repair:** Restoring, to the extent possible, a body part to its normal anatomic structure and function

Body Part (4th)	Approach (5th)	Device (6th)	Qualifier (7th)
0 Brain **1** Cerebral Meninges **2** Dura Mater **6** Cerebral Ventricle **7** Cerebral Hemisphere **8** Basal Ganglia **9** Thalamus **A** Hypothalamus **B** Pons **C** Cerebellum **D** Medulla Oblongata **F** Olfactory Nerve **G** Optic Nerve **H** Oculomotor Nerve **J** Trochlear Nerve **K** Trigeminal Nerve **L** Abducens Nerve **M** Facial Nerve **N** Acoustic Nerve **P** Glossopharyngeal Nerve **Q** Vagus Nerve **R** Accessory Nerve **S** Hypoglossal Nerve **T** Spinal Meninges **W** Cervical Spinal Cord **X** Thoracic Spinal Cord **Y** Lumbar Spinal Cord	**0** Open **3** Percutaneous **4** Percutaneous Endoscopic	**Z** No Device	**Z** No Qualifier

Section 0 **Medical and Surgical**
Body System 0 **Central Nervous System**
Operation S **Reposition:** Moving to its normal location, or other suitable location, all or a portion of a body part

Body Part (4th)	Approach (5th)	Device (6th)	Qualifier (7th)
F Olfactory Nerve **G** Optic Nerve **H** Oculomotor Nerve **J** Trochlear Nerve **K** Trigeminal Nerve **L** Abducens Nerve **M** Facial Nerve **N** Acoustic Nerve **P** Glossopharyngeal Nerve **Q** Vagus Nerve **R** Accessory Nerve **S** Hypoglossal Nerve **W** Cervical Spinal Cord **X** Thoracic Spinal Cord **Y** Lumbar Spinal Cord	**0** Open **3** Percutaneous **4** Percutaneous Endoscopic	**Z** No Device	**Z** No Qualifier

Section 0 **Medical and Surgical**
Body System 0 **Central Nervous System**
Operation T **Resection:** Cutting out or off, without replacement, all of a body part

Body Part (4th)	Approach (5th)	Device (6th)	Qualifier (7th)
7 Cerebral Hemisphere	**0** Open **3** Percutaneous **4** Percutaneous Endoscopic	**Z** No Device	**Z** No Qualifier

Section 0 **Medical and Surgical**
Body System 0 **Central Nervous System**
Operation U **Supplement:** Putting in or on biological or synthetic material that physically reinforces and/or augments the function of a portion of a body part

Body Part (4th)	Approach (5th)	Device (6th)	Qualifier (7th)
1 Cerebral Meninges **2** Dura Mater **T** Spinal Meninges	**0** Open **3** Percutaneous **4** Percutaneous Endoscopic	**7** Autologous Tissue Substitute **J** Synthetic Substitute **K** Nonautologous Tissue Substitute	**Z** No Qualifier
F Olfactory Nerve **G** Optic Nerve **H** Oculomotor Nerve **J** Trochlear Nerve **K** Trigeminal Nerve **L** Abducens Nerve **M** Facial Nerve **N** Acoustic Nerve **P** Glossopharyngeal Nerve **Q** Vagus Nerve **R** Accessory Nerve **S** Hypoglossal Nerve	**0** Open **3** Percutaneous **4** Percutaneous Endoscopic	**7** Autologous Tissue Substitute	**Z** No Qualifier

Section 0 **Medical and Surgical**
Body System 0 **Central Nervous System**
Operation W **Revision:** Correcting, to the extent possible, a portion of a malfunctioning device or the position of a displaced device

Body Part (4th)	Approach (5th)	Device (6th)	Qualifier (7th)
0 Brain **V** Spinal Cord	**0** Open **3** Percutaneous **4** Percutaneous Endoscopic **X** External	**0** Drainage Device **2** Monitoring Device **3** Infusion Device **7** Autologous Tissue Substitute **J** Synthetic Substitute **K** Nonautologous Tissue Substitute **M** Neurostimulator Lead	**Z** No Qualifier
6 Cerebral Ventricle **U** Spinal Canal	**0** Open **3** Percutaneous **4** Percutaneous Endoscopic **X** External	**0** Drainage Device **2** Monitoring Device **3** Infusion Device **J** Synthetic Substitute **M** Neurostimulator Lead	**Z** No Qualifier
E Cranial Nerve	**0** Open **3** Percutaneous **4** Percutaneous Endoscopic **X** External	**0** Drainage Device **2** Monitoring Device **3** Infusion Device **7** Autologous Tissue Substitute **M** Neurostimulator Lead	**Z** No Qualifier

Section 0 **Medical and Surgical**
Body System 0 **Central Nervous System**
Operation X **Transfer:** Moving, without taking out, all or a portion of a body part to another location to take over the function of all or a portion of a body part

Body Part (4th)	Approach (5th)	Device (6th)	Qualifier (7th)
F Olfactory Nerve **G** Optic Nerve **H** Oculomotor Nerve **J** Trochlear Nerve **K** Trigeminal Nerve **L** Abducens Nerve **M** Facial Nerve **N** Acoustic Nerve **P** Glossopharyngeal Nerve **Q** Vagus Nerve **R** Accessory Nerve **S** Hypoglossal Nerve	**0** Open **4** Percutaneous Endoscopic	**Z** No Device	**F** Olfactory Nerve **G** Optic Nerve **H** Oculomotor Nerve **J** Trochlear Nerve **K** Trigeminal Nerve **L** Abducens Nerve **M** Facial Nerve **N** Acoustic Nerve **P** Glossopharyngeal Nerve **Q** Vagus Nerve **R** Accessory Nerve **S** Hypoglossal Nerve

Central Nervous System Code Listing 001–00X

001 – Central Nervous System, Bypass

Review Coding Guideline B3.6a

0016070 Bypass Cerebral Ventricle to Nasopharynx with Autologous Tissue Substitute, Open Approach
0016071 Bypass Cerebral Ventricle to Mastoid Sinus with Autologous Tissue Substitute, Open Approach
0016072 Bypass Cerebral Ventricle to Atrium with Autologous Tissue Substitute, Open Approach
0016073 Bypass Cerebral Ventricle to Blood Vessel with Autologous Tissue Substitute, Open Approach
0016074 Bypass Cerebral Ventricle to Pleural Cavity with Autologous Tissue Substitute, Open Approach
0016075 Bypass Cerebral Ventricle to Intestine with Autologous Tissue Substitute, Open Approach
0016076 Bypass Cerebral Ventricle to Peritoneal Cavity with Autologous Tissue Substitute, Open Approach
0016077 Bypass Cerebral Ventricle to Urinary Tract with Autologous Tissue Substitute, Open Approach
0016078 Bypass Cerebral Ventricle to Bone Marrow with Autologous Tissue Substitute, Open Approach
001607B Bypass Cerebral Ventricle to Cerebral Cisterns with Autologous Tissue Substitute, Open Approach
00160J0 Bypass Cerebral Ventricle to Nasopharynx with Synthetic Substitute, Open Approach
00160J1 Bypass Cerebral Ventricle to Mastoid Sinus with Synthetic Substitute, Open Approach
00160J2 Bypass Cerebral Ventricle to Atrium with Synthetic Substitute, Open Approach
00160J3 Bypass Cerebral Ventricle to Blood Vessel with Synthetic Substitute, Open Approach
00160J4 Bypass Cerebral Ventricle to Pleural Cavity with Synthetic Substitute, Open Approach
00160J5 Bypass Cerebral Ventricle to Intestine with Synthetic Substitute, Open Approach
00160J6 Bypass Cerebral Ventricle to Peritoneal Cavity with Synthetic Substitute, Open Approach
00160J7 Bypass Cerebral Ventricle to Urinary Tract with Synthetic Substitute, Open Approach
00160J8 Bypass Cerebral Ventricle to Bone Marrow with Synthetic Substitute, Open Approach
00160JB Bypass Cerebral Ventricle to Cerebral Cisterns with Synthetic Substitute, Open Approach
00160K0 Bypass Cerebral Ventricle to Nasopharynx with Nonautologous Tissue Substitute, Open Approach
00160K1 Bypass Cerebral Ventricle to Mastoid Sinus with Nonautologous Tissue Substitute, Open Approach
00160K2 Bypass Cerebral Ventricle to Atrium with Nonautologous Tissue Substitute, Open Approach
00160K3 Bypass Cerebral Ventricle to Blood Vessel with Nonautologous Tissue Substitute, Open Approach
00160K4 Bypass Cerebral Ventricle to Pleural Cavity with Nonautologous Tissue Substitute, Open Approach
00160K5 Bypass Cerebral Ventricle to Intestine with Nonautologous Tissue Substitute, Open Approach
00160K6 Bypass Cerebral Ventricle to Peritoneal Cavity with Nonautologous Tissue Substitute, Open Approach
00160K7 Bypass Cerebral Ventricle to Urinary Tract with Nonautologous Tissue Substitute, Open Approach
00160K8 Bypass Cerebral Ventricle to Bone Marrow with Nonautologous Tissue Substitute, Open Approach
00160KB Bypass Cerebral Ventricle to Cerebral Cisterns with Nonautologous Tissue Substitute, Open Approach
0016370 Bypass Cerebral Ventricle to Nasopharynx with Autologous Tissue Substitute, Percutaneous Approach
0016371 Bypass Cerebral Ventricle to Mastoid Sinus with Autologous Tissue Substitute, Percutaneous Approach
0016372 Bypass Cerebral Ventricle to Atrium with Autologous Tissue Substitute, Percutaneous Approach
0016373 Bypass Cerebral Ventricle to Blood Vessel with Autologous Tissue Substitute, Percutaneous Approach
0016374 Bypass Cerebral Ventricle to Pleural Cavity with Autologous Tissue Substitute, Percutaneous Approach
0016375 Bypass Cerebral Ventricle to Intestine with Autologous Tissue Substitute, Percutaneous Approach
0016376 Bypass Cerebral Ventricle to Peritoneal Cavity with Autologous Tissue Substitute, Percutaneous Approach
0016377 Bypass Cerebral Ventricle to Urinary Tract with Autologous Tissue Substitute, Percutaneous Approach
0016378 Bypass Cerebral Ventricle to Bone Marrow with Autologous Tissue Substitute, Percutaneous Approach
001637B Bypass Cerebral Ventricle to Cerebral Cisterns with Autologous Tissue Substitute, Percutaneous Approach
00163J0 Bypass Cerebral Ventricle to Nasopharynx with Synthetic Substitute, Percutaneous Approach
00163J1 Bypass Cerebral Ventricle to Mastoid Sinus with Synthetic Substitute, Percutaneous Approach
00163J2 Bypass Cerebral Ventricle to Atrium with Synthetic Substitute, Percutaneous Approach
00163J3 Bypass Cerebral Ventricle to Blood Vessel with Synthetic Substitute, Percutaneous Approach
00163J4 Bypass Cerebral Ventricle to Pleural Cavity with Synthetic Substitute, Percutaneous Approach
00163J5 Bypass Cerebral Ventricle to Intestine with Synthetic Substitute, Percutaneous Approach
00163J6 Bypass Cerebral Ventricle to Peritoneal Cavity with Synthetic Substitute, Percutaneous Approach
AHA CC: 2Q, 2013, 36-37
00163J7 Bypass Cerebral Ventricle to Urinary Tract with Synthetic Substitute, Percutaneous Approach
00163J8 Bypass Cerebral Ventricle to Bone Marrow with Synthetic Substitute, Percutaneous Approach
00163JB Bypass Cerebral Ventricle to Cerebral Cisterns with Synthetic Substitute, Percutaneous Approach
00163K0 Bypass Cerebral Ventricle to Nasopharynx with Nonautologous Tissue Substitute, Percutaneous Approach

00163K1 Bypass Cerebral Ventricle to Mastoid Sinus with Nonautologous Tissue Substitute, Percutaneous Approach
00163K2 Bypass Cerebral Ventricle to Atrium with Nonautologous Tissue Substitute, Percutaneous Approach
00163K3 Bypass Cerebral Ventricle to Blood Vessel with Nonautologous Tissue Substitute, Percutaneous Approach
00163K4 Bypass Cerebral Ventricle to Pleural Cavity with Nonautologous Tissue Substitute, Percutaneous Approach
00163K5 Bypass Cerebral Ventricle to Intestine with Nonautologous Tissue Substitute, Percutaneous Approach
00163K6 Bypass Cerebral Ventricle to Peritoneal Cavity with Nonautologous Tissue Substitute, Percutaneous Approach
00163K7 Bypass Cerebral Ventricle to Urinary Tract with Nonautologous Tissue Substitute, Percutaneous Approach
00163K8 Bypass Cerebral Ventricle to Bone Marrow with Nonautologous Tissue Substitute, Percutaneous Approach
00163KB Bypass Cerebral Ventricle to Cerebral Cisterns with Nonautologous Tissue Substitute, Percutaneous Approach
001U074 Bypass Spinal Canal to Pleural Cavity with Autologous Tissue Substitute, Open Approach
001U076 Bypass Spinal Canal to Peritoneal Cavity with Autologous Tissue Substitute, Open Approach
001U077 Bypass Spinal Canal to Urinary Tract with Autologous Tissue Substitute, Open Approach
001U079 Bypass Spinal Canal to Fallopian Tube with Autologous Tissue Substitute, Open Approach
001U0J4 Bypass Spinal Canal to Pleural Cavity with Synthetic Substitute, Open Approach
001U0J6 Bypass Spinal Canal to Peritoneal Cavity with Synthetic Substitute, Open Approach
001U0J7 Bypass Spinal Canal to Urinary Tract with Synthetic Substitute, Open Approach
001U0J9 Bypass Spinal Canal to Fallopian Tube with Synthetic Substitute, Open Approach
001U0K4 Bypass Spinal Canal to Pleural Cavity with Nonautologous Tissue Substitute, Open Approach
001U0K6 Bypass Spinal Canal to Peritoneal Cavity with Nonautologous Tissue Substitute, Open Approach
001U0K7 Bypass Spinal Canal to Urinary Tract with Nonautologous Tissue Substitute, Open Approach
001U0K9 Bypass Spinal Canal to Fallopian Tube with Nonautologous Tissue Substitute, Open Approach
001U374 Bypass Spinal Canal to Pleural Cavity with Autologous Tissue Substitute, Percutaneous Approach
001U376 Bypass Spinal Canal to Peritoneal Cavity with Autologous Tissue Substitute, Percutaneous Approach
001U377 Bypass Spinal Canal to Urinary Tract with Autologous Tissue Substitute, Percutaneous Approach
001U379 Bypass Spinal Canal to Fallopian Tube with Autologous Tissue Substitute, Percutaneous Approach
001U3J4 Bypass Spinal Canal to Pleural Cavity with Synthetic Substitute, Percutaneous Approach
001U3J6 Bypass Spinal Canal to Peritoneal Cavity with Synthetic Substitute, Percutaneous Approach
001U3J7 Bypass Spinal Canal to Urinary Tract with Synthetic Substitute, Percutaneous Approach
001U3J9 Bypass Spinal Canal to Fallopian Tube with Synthetic Substitute, Percutaneous Approach
001U3K4 Bypass Spinal Canal to Pleural Cavity with Nonautologous Tissue Substitute, Percutaneous Approach
001U3K6 Bypass Spinal Canal to Peritoneal Cavity with Nonautologous Tissue Substitute, Percutaneous Approach
001U3K7 Bypass Spinal Canal to Urinary Tract with Nonautologous Tissue Substitute, Percutaneous Approach
001U3K9 Bypass Spinal Canal to Fallopian Tube with Nonautologous Tissue Substitute, Percutaneous Approach

002 – Central Nervous System, Change

Review Coding Guideline B6.1c

0020X0Z Change Drainage Device in Brain, External Approach
0020XYZ Change Other Device in Brain, External Approach
002EX0Z Change Drainage Device in Cranial Nerve, External Approach
002EXYZ Change Other Device in Cranial Nerve, External Approach
002UX0Z Change Drainage Device in Spinal Canal, External Approach
002UXYZ Change Other Device in Spinal Canal, External Approach

005 – Central Nervous System, Destruction

00500ZZ Destruction of Brain, Open Approach
00503ZZ Destruction of Brain, Percutaneous Approach
00504ZZ Destruction of Brain, Percutaneous Endoscopic Approach
00510ZZ Destruction of Cerebral Meninges, Open Approach
00513ZZ Destruction of Cerebral Meninges, Percutaneous Approach
00514ZZ Destruction of Cerebral Meninges, Percutaneous Endoscopic Approach
00520ZZ Destruction of Dura Mater, Open Approach
00523ZZ Destruction of Dura Mater, Percutaneous Approach
00524ZZ Destruction of Dura Mater, Percutaneous Endoscopic Approach
00560ZZ Destruction of Cerebral Ventricle, Open Approach
00563ZZ Destruction of Cerebral Ventricle, Percutaneous Approach
00564ZZ Destruction of Cerebral Ventricle, Percutaneous Endoscopic Approach
00570ZZ Destruction of Cerebral Hemisphere, Open Approach
00573ZZ Destruction of Cerebral Hemisphere, Percutaneous Approach
00574ZZ Destruction of Cerebral Hemisphere, Percutaneous Endoscopic Approach
00580ZZ Destruction of Basal Ganglia, Open Approach
00583ZZ Destruction of Basal Ganglia, Percutaneous Approach
00584ZZ Destruction of Basal Ganglia, Percutaneous Endoscopic Approach
00590ZZ Destruction of Thalamus, Open Approach
00593ZZ Destruction of Thalamus, Percutaneous Approach
00594ZZ Destruction of Thalamus, Percutaneous Endoscopic Approach
005A0ZZ Destruction of Hypothalamus, Open Approach
005A3ZZ Destruction of Hypothalamus, Percutaneous Approach
005A4ZZ Destruction of Hypothalamus, Percutaneous Endoscopic Approach
005B0ZZ Destruction of Pons, Open Approach
005B3ZZ Destruction of Pons, Percutaneous Approach
005B4ZZ Destruction of Pons, Percutaneous Endoscopic Approach
005C0ZZ Destruction of Cerebellum, Open Approach
005C3ZZ Destruction of Cerebellum, Percutaneous Approach
005C4ZZ Destruction of Cerebellum, Percutaneous Endoscopic Approach
005D0ZZ Destruction of Medulla Oblongata, Open Approach
005D3ZZ Destruction of Medulla Oblongata, Percutaneous Approach
005D4ZZ Destruction of Medulla Oblongata, Percutaneous Endoscopic Approach
005F0ZZ Destruction of Olfactory Nerve, Open Approach
005F3ZZ Destruction of Olfactory Nerve, Percutaneous Approach
005F4ZZ Destruction of Olfactory Nerve, Percutaneous Endoscopic Approach
005G0ZZ Destruction of Optic Nerve, Open Approach
005G3ZZ Destruction of Optic Nerve, Percutaneous Approach
005G4ZZ Destruction of Optic Nerve, Percutaneous Endoscopic Approach
005H0ZZ Destruction of Oculomotor Nerve, Open Approach
005H3ZZ Destruction of Oculomotor Nerve, Percutaneous Approach
005H4ZZ Destruction of Oculomotor Nerve, Percutaneous Endoscopic Approach
005J0ZZ Destruction of Trochlear Nerve, Open Approach
005J3ZZ Destruction of Trochlear Nerve, Percutaneous Approach
005J4ZZ Destruction of Trochlear Nerve, Percutaneous Endoscopic Approach
005K0ZZ Destruction of Trigeminal Nerve, Open Approach
005K3ZZ Destruction of Trigeminal Nerve, Percutaneous Approach
005K4ZZ Destruction of Trigeminal Nerve, Percutaneous Endoscopic Approach
005L0ZZ Destruction of Abducens Nerve, Open Approach
005L3ZZ Destruction of Abducens Nerve, Percutaneous Approach

005L4ZZ Destruction of Abducens Nerve, Percutaneous Endoscopic Approach
005M0ZZ Destruction of Facial Nerve, Open Approach
005M3ZZ Destruction of Facial Nerve, Percutaneous Approach
005M4ZZ Destruction of Facial Nerve, Percutaneous Endoscopic Approach
005N0ZZ Destruction of Acoustic Nerve, Open Approach
005N3ZZ Destruction of Acoustic Nerve, Percutaneous Approach
005N4ZZ Destruction of Acoustic Nerve, Percutaneous Endoscopic Approach
005P0ZZ Destruction of Glossopharyngeal Nerve, Open Approach
005P3ZZ Destruction of Glossopharyngeal Nerve, Percutaneous Approach
005P4ZZ Destruction of Glossopharyngeal Nerve, Percutaneous Endoscopic Approach
005Q0ZZ Destruction of Vagus Nerve, Open Approach
005Q3ZZ Destruction of Vagus Nerve, Percutaneous Approach
005Q4ZZ Destruction of Vagus Nerve, Percutaneous Endoscopic Approach
005R0ZZ Destruction of Accessory Nerve, Open Approach
005R3ZZ Destruction of Accessory Nerve, Percutaneous Approach
005R4ZZ Destruction of Accessory Nerve, Percutaneous Endoscopic Approach
005S0ZZ Destruction of Hypoglossal Nerve, Open Approach
005S3ZZ Destruction of Hypoglossal Nerve, Percutaneous Approach
005S4ZZ Destruction of Hypoglossal Nerve, Percutaneous Endoscopic Approach
005T0ZZ Destruction of Spinal Meninges, Open Approach
005T3ZZ Destruction of Spinal Meninges, Percutaneous Approach
005T4ZZ Destruction of Spinal Meninges, Percutaneous Endoscopic Approach
005W0ZZ Destruction of Cervical Spinal Cord, Open Approach
005W3ZZ Destruction of Cervical Spinal Cord, Percutaneous Approach
005W4ZZ Destruction of Cervical Spinal Cord, Percutaneous Endoscopic Approach
005X0ZZ Destruction of Thoracic Spinal Cord, Open Approach
005X3ZZ Destruction of Thoracic Spinal Cord, Percutaneous Approach
005X4ZZ Destruction of Thoracic Spinal Cord, Percutaneous Endoscopic Approach
005Y0ZZ Destruction of Lumbar Spinal Cord, Open Approach
005Y3ZZ Destruction of Lumbar Spinal Cord, Percutaneous Approach
005Y4ZZ Destruction of Lumbar Spinal Cord, Percutaneous Endoscopic Approach

008 – Central Nervous System, Division

Review Coding Guideline B3.14

00800ZZ Division of Brain, Open Approach
00803ZZ Division of Brain, Percutaneous Approach
00804ZZ Division of Brain, Percutaneous Endoscopic Approach
00870ZZ Division of Cerebral Hemisphere, Open Approach
00873ZZ Division of Cerebral Hemisphere, Percutaneous Approach
00874ZZ Division of Cerebral Hemisphere, Percutaneous Endoscopic Approach
00880ZZ Division of Basal Ganglia, Open Approach
00883ZZ Division of Basal Ganglia, Percutaneous Approach
00884ZZ Division of Basal Ganglia, Percutaneous Endoscopic Approach
008F0ZZ Division of Olfactory Nerve, Open Approach
008F3ZZ Division of Olfactory Nerve, Percutaneous Approach
008F4ZZ Division of Olfactory Nerve, Percutaneous Endoscopic Approach
008G0ZZ Division of Optic Nerve, Open Approach
008G3ZZ Division of Optic Nerve, Percutaneous Approach
008G4ZZ Division of Optic Nerve, Percutaneous Endoscopic Approach
008H0ZZ Division of Oculomotor Nerve, Open Approach
008H3ZZ Division of Oculomotor Nerve, Percutaneous Approach
008H4ZZ Division of Oculomotor Nerve, Percutaneous Endoscopic Approach
008J0ZZ Division of Trochlear Nerve, Open Approach
008J3ZZ Division of Trochlear Nerve, Percutaneous Approach
008J4ZZ Division of Trochlear Nerve, Percutaneous Endoscopic Approach
008K0ZZ Division of Trigeminal Nerve, Open Approach
008K3ZZ Division of Trigeminal Nerve, Percutaneous Approach
008K4ZZ Division of Trigeminal Nerve, Percutaneous Endoscopic Approach
008L0ZZ Division of Abducens Nerve, Open Approach
008L3ZZ Division of Abducens Nerve, Percutaneous Approach
008L4ZZ Division of Abducens Nerve, Percutaneous Endoscopic Approach
008M0ZZ Division of Facial Nerve, Open Approach
008M3ZZ Division of Facial Nerve, Percutaneous Approach
008M4ZZ Division of Facial Nerve, Percutaneous Endoscopic Approach
008N0ZZ Division of Acoustic Nerve, Open Approach
008N3ZZ Division of Acoustic Nerve, Percutaneous Approach
008N4ZZ Division of Acoustic Nerve, Percutaneous Endoscopic Approach
008P0ZZ Division of Glossopharyngeal Nerve, Open Approach
008P3ZZ Division of Glossopharyngeal Nerve, Percutaneous Approach
008P4ZZ Division of Glossopharyngeal Nerve, Percutaneous Endoscopic Approach
008Q0ZZ Division of Vagus Nerve, Open Approach
008Q3ZZ Division of Vagus Nerve, Percutaneous Approach
008Q4ZZ Division of Vagus Nerve, Percutaneous Endoscopic Approach
008R0ZZ Division of Accessory Nerve, Open Approach
008R3ZZ Division of Accessory Nerve, Percutaneous Approach
008R4ZZ Division of Accessory Nerve, Percutaneous Endoscopic Approach
008S0ZZ Division of Hypoglossal Nerve, Open Approach
008S3ZZ Division of Hypoglossal Nerve, Percutaneous Approach
008S4ZZ Division of Hypoglossal Nerve, Percutaneous Endoscopic Approach
008W0ZZ Division of Cervical Spinal Cord, Open Approach
008W3ZZ Division of Cervical Spinal Cord, Percutaneous Approach
008W4ZZ Division of Cervical Spinal Cord, Percutaneous Endoscopic Approach
008X0ZZ Division of Thoracic Spinal Cord, Open Approach
008X3ZZ Division of Thoracic Spinal Cord, Percutaneous Approach
008X4ZZ Division of Thoracic Spinal Cord, Percutaneous Endoscopic Approach
008Y0ZZ Division of Lumbar Spinal Cord, Open Approach
008Y3ZZ Division of Lumbar Spinal Cord, Percutaneous Approach
008Y4ZZ Division of Lumbar Spinal Cord, Percutaneous Endoscopic Approach

009 – Central Nervous System, Drainage

Review Coding Guidelines B3.4a and B3.4b

Review Coding Guideline B6.2

009000Z Drainage of Brain with Drainage Device, Open Approach
00900ZX Drainage of Brain, Open Approach, Diagnostic
00900ZZ Drainage of Brain, Open Approach
009030Z Drainage of Brain with Drainage Device, Percutaneous Approach
00903ZX Drainage of Brain, Percutaneous Approach, Diagnostic
00903ZZ Drainage of Brain, Percutaneous Approach
009040Z Drainage of Brain with Drainage Device, Percutaneous Endoscopic Approach
00904ZX Drainage of Brain, Percutaneous Endoscopic Approach, Diagnostic
00904ZZ Drainage of Brain, Percutaneous Endoscopic Approach
009100Z Drainage of Cerebral Meninges with Drainage Device, Open Approach
00910ZX Drainage of Cerebral Meninges, Open Approach, Diagnostic
00910ZZ Drainage of Cerebral Meninges, Open Approach
009130Z Drainage of Cerebral Meninges with Drainage Device, Percutaneous Approach
00913ZX Drainage of Cerebral Meninges, Percutaneous Approach, Diagnostic
00913ZZ Drainage of Cerebral Meninges, Percutaneous Approach

009140Z Drainage of Cerebral Meninges with Drainage Device, Percutaneous Endoscopic Approach
00914ZX Drainage of Cerebral Meninges, Percutaneous Endoscopic Approach, Diagnostic
00914ZZ Drainage of Cerebral Meninges, Percutaneous Endoscopic Approach
009200Z Drainage of Dura Mater with Drainage Device, Open Approach
00920ZX Drainage of Dura Mater, Open Approach, Diagnostic
00920ZZ Drainage of Dura Mater, Open Approach
009230Z Drainage of Dura Mater with Drainage Device, Percutaneous Approach
00923ZX Drainage of Dura Mater, Percutaneous Approach, Diagnostic
00923ZZ Drainage of Dura Mater, Percutaneous Approach
009240Z Drainage of Dura Mater with Drainage Device, Percutaneous Endoscopic Approach
00924ZX Drainage of Dura Mater, Percutaneous Endoscopic Approach, Diagnostic
00924ZZ Drainage of Dura Mater, Percutaneous Endoscopic Approach
009300Z Drainage of Epidural Space with Drainage Device, Open Approach
00930ZX Drainage of Epidural Space, Open Approach, Diagnostic
00930ZZ Drainage of Epidural Space, Open Approach
009330Z Drainage of Epidural Space with Drainage Device, Percutaneous Approach
00933ZX Drainage of Epidural Space, Percutaneous Approach, Diagnostic
00933ZZ Drainage of Epidural Space, Percutaneous Approach
009340Z Drainage of Epidural Space with Drainage Device, Percutaneous Endoscopic Approach
00934ZX Drainage of Epidural Space, Percutaneous Endoscopic Approach, Diagnostic
00934ZZ Drainage of Epidural Space, Percutaneous Endoscopic Approach
009400Z Drainage of Subdural Space with Drainage Device, Open Approach
00940ZX Drainage of Subdural Space, Open Approach, Diagnostic
00940ZZ Drainage of Subdural Space, Open Approach
009430Z Drainage of Subdural Space with Drainage Device, Percutaneous Approach
00943ZX Drainage of Subdural Space, Percutaneous Approach, Diagnostic
00943ZZ Drainage of Subdural Space, Percutaneous Approach
009440Z Drainage of Subdural Space with Drainage Device, Percutaneous Endoscopic Approach
00944ZX Drainage of Subdural Space, Percutaneous Endoscopic Approach, Diagnostic
00944ZZ Drainage of Subdural Space, Percutaneous Endoscopic Approach
009500Z Drainage of Subarachnoid Space with Drainage Device, Open Approach
00950ZX Drainage of Subarachnoid Space, Open Approach, Diagnostic
00950ZZ Drainage of Subarachnoid Space, Open Approach
009530Z Drainage of Subarachnoid Space with Drainage Device, Percutaneous Approach
00953ZX Drainage of Subarachnoid Space, Percutaneous Approach, Diagnostic
00953ZZ Drainage of Subarachnoid Space, Percutaneous Approach
009540Z Drainage of Subarachnoid Space with Drainage Device, Percutaneous Endoscopic Approach
00954ZX Drainage of Subarachnoid Space, Percutaneous Endoscopic Approach, Diagnostic
00954ZZ Drainage of Subarachnoid Space, Percutaneous Endoscopic Approach
009600Z Drainage of Cerebral Ventricle with Drainage Device, Open Approach
00960ZX Drainage of Cerebral Ventricle, Open Approach, Diagnostic
00960ZZ Drainage of Cerebral Ventricle, Open Approach
009630Z Drainage of Cerebral Ventricle with Drainage Device, Percutaneous Approach
00963ZX Drainage of Cerebral Ventricle, Percutaneous Approach, Diagnostic
00963ZZ Drainage of Cerebral Ventricle, Percutaneous Approach
009640Z Drainage of Cerebral Ventricle with Drainage Device, Percutaneous Endoscopic Approach
00964ZX Drainage of Cerebral Ventricle, Percutaneous Endoscopic Approach, Diagnostic
00964ZZ Drainage of Cerebral Ventricle, Percutaneous Endoscopic Approach
009700Z Drainage of Cerebral Hemisphere with Drainage Device, Open Approach
00970ZX Drainage of Cerebral Hemisphere, Open Approach, Diagnostic
00970ZZ Drainage of Cerebral Hemisphere, Open Approach
009730Z Drainage of Cerebral Hemisphere with Drainage Device, Percutaneous Approach
00973ZX Drainage of Cerebral Hemisphere, Percutaneous Approach, Diagnostic
00973ZZ Drainage of Cerebral Hemisphere, Percutaneous Approach
009740Z Drainage of Cerebral Hemisphere with Drainage Device, Percutaneous Endoscopic Approach
00974ZX Drainage of Cerebral Hemisphere, Percutaneous Endoscopic Approach, Diagnostic
00974ZZ Drainage of Cerebral Hemisphere, Percutaneous Endoscopic Approach
009800Z Drainage of Basal Ganglia with Drainage Device, Open Approach
00980ZX Drainage of Basal Ganglia, Open Approach, Diagnostic
00980ZZ Drainage of Basal Ganglia, Open Approach
009830Z Drainage of Basal Ganglia with Drainage Device, Percutaneous Approach
00983ZX Drainage of Basal Ganglia, Percutaneous Approach, Diagnostic
00983ZZ Drainage of Basal Ganglia, Percutaneous Approach
009840Z Drainage of Basal Ganglia with Drainage Device, Percutaneous Endoscopic Approach
00984ZX Drainage of Basal Ganglia, Percutaneous Endoscopic Approach, Diagnostic
00984ZZ Drainage of Basal Ganglia, Percutaneous Endoscopic Approach
009900Z Drainage of Thalamus with Drainage Device, Open Approach
00990ZX Drainage of Thalamus, Open Approach, Diagnostic
00990ZZ Drainage of Thalamus, Open Approach
009930Z Drainage of Thalamus with Drainage Device, Percutaneous Approach
00993ZX Drainage of Thalamus, Percutaneous Approach, Diagnostic
00993ZZ Drainage of Thalamus, Percutaneous Approach
009940Z Drainage of Thalamus with Drainage Device, Percutaneous Endoscopic Approach
00994ZX Drainage of Thalamus, Percutaneous Endoscopic Approach, Diagnostic
00994ZZ Drainage of Thalamus, Percutaneous Endoscopic Approach
009A00Z Drainage of Hypothalamus with Drainage Device, Open Approach
009A0ZX Drainage of Hypothalamus, Open Approach, Diagnostic
009A0ZZ Drainage of Hypothalamus, Open Approach
009A30Z Drainage of Hypothalamus with Drainage Device, Percutaneous Approach
009A3ZX Drainage of Hypothalamus, Percutaneous Approach, Diagnostic
009A3ZZ Drainage of Hypothalamus, Percutaneous Approach
009A40Z Drainage of Hypothalamus with Drainage Device, Percutaneous Endoscopic Approach
009A4ZX Drainage of Hypothalamus, Percutaneous Endoscopic Approach, Diagnostic
009A4ZZ Drainage of Hypothalamus, Percutaneous Endoscopic Approach
009B00Z Drainage of Pons with Drainage Device, Open Approach
009B0ZX Drainage of Pons, Open Approach, Diagnostic
009B0ZZ Drainage of Pons, Open Approach
009B30Z Drainage of Pons with Drainage Device, Percutaneous Approach
009B3ZX Drainage of Pons, Percutaneous Approach, Diagnostic
009B3ZZ Drainage of Pons, Percutaneous Approach
009B40Z Drainage of Pons with Drainage Device, Percutaneous Endoscopic Approach
009B4ZX Drainage of Pons, Percutaneous Endoscopic Approach, Diagnostic
009B4ZZ Drainage of Pons, Percutaneous Endoscopic Approach
009C00Z Drainage of Cerebellum with Drainage Device, Open Approach
009C0ZX Drainage of Cerebellum, Open Approach, Diagnostic
009C0ZZ Drainage of Cerebellum, Open Approach
009C30Z Drainage of Cerebellum with Drainage Device, Percutaneous Approach
009C3ZX Drainage of Cerebellum, Percutaneous Approach, Diagnostic
009C3ZZ Drainage of Cerebellum, Percutaneous Approach
009C40Z Drainage of Cerebellum with Drainage Device, Percutaneous Endoscopic Approach
009C4ZX Drainage of Cerebellum, Percutaneous Endoscopic Approach, Diagnostic
009C4ZZ Drainage of Cerebellum, Percutaneous Endoscopic Approach
009D00Z Drainage of Medulla Oblongata with Drainage Device, Open Approach
009D0ZX Drainage of Medulla Oblongata, Open Approach, Diagnostic
009D0ZZ Drainage of Medulla Oblongata, Open Approach
009D30Z Drainage of Medulla Oblongata with Drainage Device, Percutaneous Approach
009D3ZX Drainage of Medulla Oblongata, Percutaneous Approach, Diagnostic
009D3ZZ Drainage of Medulla Oblongata, Percutaneous Approach
009D40Z Drainage of Medulla Oblongata with Drainage Device, Percutaneous Endoscopic Approach
009D4ZX Drainage of Medulla Oblongata, Percutaneous Endoscopic Approach, Diagnostic

009D4ZZ Drainage of Medulla Oblongata, Percutaneous Endoscopic Approach
009F00Z Drainage of Olfactory Nerve with Drainage Device, Open Approach
009F0ZX Drainage of Olfactory Nerve, Open Approach, Diagnostic
009F0ZZ Drainage of Olfactory Nerve, Open Approach
009F30Z Drainage of Olfactory Nerve with Drainage Device, Percutaneous Approach
009F3ZX Drainage of Olfactory Nerve, Percutaneous Approach, Diagnostic
009F3ZZ Drainage of Olfactory Nerve, Percutaneous Approach
009F40Z Drainage of Olfactory Nerve with Drainage Device, Percutaneous Endoscopic Approach
009F4ZX Drainage of Olfactory Nerve, Percutaneous Endoscopic Approach, Diagnostic
009F4ZZ Drainage of Olfactory Nerve, Percutaneous Endoscopic Approach
009G00Z Drainage of Optic Nerve with Drainage Device, Open Approach
009G0ZX Drainage of Optic Nerve, Open Approach, Diagnostic
009G0ZZ Drainage of Optic Nerve, Open Approach
009G30Z Drainage of Optic Nerve with Drainage Device, Percutaneous Approach
009G3ZX Drainage of Optic Nerve, Percutaneous Approach, Diagnostic
009G3ZZ Drainage of Optic Nerve, Percutaneous Approach
009G40Z Drainage of Optic Nerve with Drainage Device, Percutaneous Endoscopic Approach
009G4ZX Drainage of Optic Nerve, Percutaneous Endoscopic Approach, Diagnostic
009G4ZZ Drainage of Optic Nerve, Percutaneous Endoscopic Approach
009H00Z Drainage of Oculomotor Nerve with Drainage Device, Open Approach
009H0ZX Drainage of Oculomotor Nerve, Open Approach, Diagnostic
009H0ZZ Drainage of Oculomotor Nerve, Open Approach
009H30Z Drainage of Oculomotor Nerve with Drainage Device, Percutaneous Approach
009H3ZX Drainage of Oculomotor Nerve, Percutaneous Approach, Diagnostic
009H3ZZ Drainage of Oculomotor Nerve, Percutaneous Approach
009H40Z Drainage of Oculomotor Nerve with Drainage Device, Percutaneous Endoscopic Approach
009H4ZX Drainage of Oculomotor Nerve, Percutaneous Endoscopic Approach, Diagnostic
009H4ZZ Drainage of Oculomotor Nerve, Percutaneous Endoscopic Approach
009J00Z Drainage of Trochlear Nerve with Drainage Device, Open Approach
009J0ZX Drainage of Trochlear Nerve, Open Approach, Diagnostic
009J0ZZ Drainage of Trochlear Nerve, Open Approach
009J30Z Drainage of Trochlear Nerve with Drainage Device, Percutaneous Approach
009J3ZX Drainage of Trochlear Nerve, Percutaneous Approach, Diagnostic
009J3ZZ Drainage of Trochlear Nerve, Percutaneous Approach
009J40Z Drainage of Trochlear Nerve with Drainage Device, Percutaneous Endoscopic Approach
009J4ZX Drainage of Trochlear Nerve, Percutaneous Endoscopic Approach, Diagnostic
009J4ZZ Drainage of Trochlear Nerve, Percutaneous Endoscopic Approach
009K00Z Drainage of Trigeminal Nerve with Drainage Device, Open Approach
009K0ZX Drainage of Trigeminal Nerve, Open Approach, Diagnostic
009K0ZZ Drainage of Trigeminal Nerve, Open Approach
009K30Z Drainage of Trigeminal Nerve with Drainage Device, Percutaneous Approach
009K3ZX Drainage of Trigeminal Nerve, Percutaneous Approach, Diagnostic
009K3ZZ Drainage of Trigeminal Nerve, Percutaneous Approach
009K40Z Drainage of Trigeminal Nerve with Drainage Device, Percutaneous Endoscopic Approach
009K4ZX Drainage of Trigeminal Nerve, Percutaneous Endoscopic Approach, Diagnostic
009K4ZZ Drainage of Trigeminal Nerve, Percutaneous Endoscopic Approach
009L00Z Drainage of Abducens Nerve with Drainage Device, Open Approach
009L0ZX Drainage of Abducens Nerve, Open Approach, Diagnostic
009L0ZZ Drainage of Abducens Nerve, Open Approach
009L30Z Drainage of Abducens Nerve with Drainage Device, Percutaneous Approach
009L3ZX Drainage of Abducens Nerve, Percutaneous Approach, Diagnostic
009L3ZZ Drainage of Abducens Nerve, Percutaneous Approach
009L40Z Drainage of Abducens Nerve with Drainage Device, Percutaneous Endoscopic Approach
009L4ZX Drainage of Abducens Nerve, Percutaneous Endoscopic Approach, Diagnostic
009L4ZZ Drainage of Abducens Nerve, Percutaneous Endoscopic Approach
009M00Z Drainage of Facial Nerve with Drainage Device, Open Approach
009M0ZX Drainage of Facial Nerve, Open Approach, Diagnostic
009M0ZZ Drainage of Facial Nerve, Open Approach
009M30Z Drainage of Facial Nerve with Drainage Device, Percutaneous Approach
009M3ZX Drainage of Facial Nerve, Percutaneous Approach, Diagnostic
009M3ZZ Drainage of Facial Nerve, Percutaneous Approach
009M40Z Drainage of Facial Nerve with Drainage Device, Percutaneous Endoscopic Approach
009M4ZX Drainage of Facial Nerve, Percutaneous Endoscopic Approach, Diagnostic
009M4ZZ Drainage of Facial Nerve, Percutaneous Endoscopic Approach
009N00Z Drainage of Acoustic Nerve with Drainage Device, Open Approach
009N0ZX Drainage of Acoustic Nerve, Open Approach, Diagnostic
009N0ZZ Drainage of Acoustic Nerve, Open Approach
009N30Z Drainage of Acoustic Nerve with Drainage Device, Percutaneous Approach
009N3ZX Drainage of Acoustic Nerve, Percutaneous Approach, Diagnostic
009N3ZZ Drainage of Acoustic Nerve, Percutaneous Approach
009N40Z Drainage of Acoustic Nerve with Drainage Device, Percutaneous Endoscopic Approach
009N4ZX Drainage of Acoustic Nerve, Percutaneous Endoscopic Approach, Diagnostic
009N4ZZ Drainage of Acoustic Nerve, Percutaneous Endoscopic Approach
009P00Z Drainage of Glossopharyngeal Nerve with Drainage Device, Open Approach
009P0ZX Drainage of Glossopharyngeal Nerve, Open Approach, Diagnostic
009P0ZZ Drainage of Glossopharyngeal Nerve, Open Approach
009P30Z Drainage of Glossopharyngeal Nerve with Drainage Device, Percutaneous Approach
009P3ZX Drainage of Glossopharyngeal Nerve, Percutaneous Approach, Diagnostic
009P3ZZ Drainage of Glossopharyngeal Nerve, Percutaneous Approach
009P40Z Drainage of Glossopharyngeal Nerve with Drainage Device, Percutaneous Endoscopic Approach
009P4ZX Drainage of Glossopharyngeal Nerve, Percutaneous Endoscopic Approach, Diagnostic
009P4ZZ Drainage of Glossopharyngeal Nerve, Percutaneous Endoscopic Approach
009Q00Z Drainage of Vagus Nerve with Drainage Device, Open Approach
009Q0ZX Drainage of Vagus Nerve, Open Approach, Diagnostic
009Q0ZZ Drainage of Vagus Nerve, Open Approach
009Q30Z Drainage of Vagus Nerve with Drainage Device, Percutaneous Approach
009Q3ZX Drainage of Vagus Nerve, Percutaneous Approach, Diagnostic
009Q3ZZ Drainage of Vagus Nerve, Percutaneous Approach
009Q40Z Drainage of Vagus Nerve with Drainage Device, Percutaneous Endoscopic Approach
009Q4ZX Drainage of Vagus Nerve, Percutaneous Endoscopic Approach, Diagnostic
009Q4ZZ Drainage of Vagus Nerve, Percutaneous Endoscopic Approach
009R00Z Drainage of Accessory Nerve with Drainage Device, Open Approach
009R0ZX Drainage of Accessory Nerve, Open Approach, Diagnostic
009R0ZZ Drainage of Accessory Nerve, Open Approach
009R30Z Drainage of Accessory Nerve with Drainage Device, Percutaneous Approach
009R3ZX Drainage of Accessory Nerve, Percutaneous Approach, Diagnostic
009R3ZZ Drainage of Accessory Nerve, Percutaneous Approach
009R40Z Drainage of Accessory Nerve with Drainage Device, Percutaneous Endoscopic Approach
009R4ZX Drainage of Accessory Nerve, Percutaneous Endoscopic Approach, Diagnostic
009R4ZZ Drainage of Accessory Nerve, Percutaneous Endoscopic Approach
009S00Z Drainage of Hypoglossal Nerve with Drainage Device, Open Approach
009S0ZX Drainage of Hypoglossal Nerve, Open Approach, Diagnostic
009S0ZZ Drainage of Hypoglossal Nerve, Open Approach
009S30Z Drainage of Hypoglossal Nerve with Drainage Device, Percutaneous Approach
009S3ZX Drainage of Hypoglossal Nerve, Percutaneous Approach, Diagnostic
009S3ZZ Drainage of Hypoglossal Nerve, Percutaneous Approach
009S40Z Drainage of Hypoglossal Nerve with Drainage Device, Percutaneous Endoscopic Approach
009S4ZX Drainage of Hypoglossal Nerve, Percutaneous Endoscopic Approach, Diagnostic
009S4ZZ Drainage of Hypoglossal Nerve, Percutaneous Endoscopic Approach
009T00Z Drainage of Spinal Meninges with Drainage Device, Open Approach

009T0ZX Drainage of Spinal Meninges, Open Approach, Diagnostic
009T0ZZ Drainage of Spinal Meninges, Open Approach
009T30Z Drainage of Spinal Meninges with Drainage Device, Percutaneous Approach
009T3ZX Drainage of Spinal Meninges, Percutaneous Approach, Diagnostic
009T3ZZ Drainage of Spinal Meninges, Percutaneous Approach
009T40Z Drainage of Spinal Meninges with Drainage Device, Percutaneous Endoscopic Approach
009T4ZX Drainage of Spinal Meninges, Percutaneous Endoscopic Approach, Diagnostic
009T4ZZ Drainage of Spinal Meninges, Percutaneous Endoscopic Approach
009U00Z Drainage of Spinal Canal with Drainage Device, Open Approach
009U0ZX Drainage of Spinal Canal, Open Approach, Diagnostic
009U0ZZ Drainage of Spinal Canal, Open Approach
009U30Z Drainage of Spinal Canal with Drainage Device, Percutaneous Approach
●**009U3ZX** Drainage of Spinal Canal, Percutaneous Approach, Diagnostic
AHA CC: 1Q, 2014, 8
009U3ZZ Drainage of Spinal Canal, Percutaneous Approach
009U40Z Drainage of Spinal Canal with Drainage Device, Percutaneous Endoscopic Approach
● **009U4ZX** Drainage of Spinal Canal, Percutaneous Endoscopic Approach, Diagnostic
009U4ZZ Drainage of Spinal Canal, Percutaneous Endoscopic Approach
009W00Z Drainage of Cervical Spinal Cord with Drainage Device, Open Approach
009W0ZX Drainage of Cervical Spinal Cord, Open Approach, Diagnostic
009W0ZZ Drainage of Cervical Spinal Cord, Open Approach
009W30Z Drainage of Cervical Spinal Cord with Drainage Device, Percutaneous Approach
009W3ZX Drainage of Cervical Spinal Cord, Percutaneous Approach, Diagnostic
009W3ZZ Drainage of Cervical Spinal Cord, Percutaneous Approach
009W40Z Drainage of Cervical Spinal Cord with Drainage Device, Percutaneous Endoscopic Approach
009W4ZX Drainage of Cervical Spinal Cord, Percutaneous Endoscopic Approach, Diagnostic
009W4ZZ Drainage of Cervical Spinal Cord, Percutaneous Endoscopic Approach
009X00Z Drainage of Thoracic Spinal Cord with Drainage Device, Open Approach
009X0ZX Drainage of Thoracic Spinal Cord, Open Approach, Diagnostic
009X0ZZ Drainage of Thoracic Spinal Cord, Open Approach
009X30Z Drainage of Thoracic Spinal Cord with Drainage Device, Percutaneous Approach
009X3ZX Drainage of Thoracic Spinal Cord, Percutaneous Approach, Diagnostic
009X3ZZ Drainage of Thoracic Spinal Cord, Percutaneous Approach
009X40Z Drainage of Thoracic Spinal Cord with Drainage Device, Percutaneous Endoscopic Approach
009X4ZX Drainage of Thoracic Spinal Cord, Percutaneous Endoscopic Approach, Diagnostic
009X4ZZ Drainage of Thoracic Spinal Cord, Percutaneous Endoscopic Approach
009Y00Z Drainage of Lumbar Spinal Cord with Drainage Device, Open Approach
009Y0ZX Drainage of Lumbar Spinal Cord, Open Approach, Diagnostic
009Y0ZZ Drainage of Lumbar Spinal Cord, Open Approach
009Y30Z Drainage of Lumbar Spinal Cord with Drainage Device, Percutaneous Approach
009Y3ZX Drainage of Lumbar Spinal Cord, Percutaneous Approach, Diagnostic
009Y3ZZ Drainage of Lumbar Spinal Cord, Percutaneous Approach
009Y40Z Drainage of Lumbar Spinal Cord with Drainage Device, Percutaneous Endoscopic Approach
009Y4ZX Drainage of Lumbar Spinal Cord, Percutaneous Endoscopic Approach, Diagnostic
009Y4ZZ Drainage of Lumbar Spinal Cord, Percutaneous Endoscopic Approach

00B – Central Nervous System, Excision

Review Coding Guidelines B3.4a and B3.4b

Review Coding Guideline B3.8

00B00ZX Excision of Brain, Open Approach, Diagnostic
00B00ZZ Excision of Brain, Open Approach
00B03ZX Excision of Brain, Percutaneous Approach, Diagnostic
00B03ZZ Excision of Brain, Percutaneous Approach
00B04ZX Excision of Brain, Percutaneous Endoscopic Approach, Diagnostic
00B04ZZ Excision of Brain, Percutaneous Endoscopic Approach
00B10ZX Excision of Cerebral Meninges, Open Approach, Diagnostic
00B10ZZ Excision of Cerebral Meninges, Open Approach
00B13ZX Excision of Cerebral Meninges, Percutaneous Approach, Diagnostic
00B13ZZ Excision of Cerebral Meninges, Percutaneous Approach
00B14ZX Excision of Cerebral Meninges, Percutaneous Endoscopic Approach, Diagnostic
00B14ZZ Excision of Cerebral Meninges, Percutaneous Endoscopic Approach
00B20ZX Excision of Dura Mater, Open Approach, Diagnostic
00B20ZZ Excision of Dura Mater, Open Approach
00B23ZX Excision of Dura Mater, Percutaneous Approach, Diagnostic
00B23ZZ Excision of Dura Mater, Percutaneous Approach
00B24ZX Excision of Dura Mater, Percutaneous Endoscopic Approach, Diagnostic
00B24ZZ Excision of Dura Mater, Percutaneous Endoscopic Approach
00B60ZX Excision of Cerebral Ventricle, Open Approach, Diagnostic
00B60ZZ Excision of Cerebral Ventricle, Open Approach
00B63ZX Excision of Cerebral Ventricle, Percutaneous Approach, Diagnostic
00B63ZZ Excision of Cerebral Ventricle, Percutaneous Approach
00B64ZX Excision of Cerebral Ventricle, Percutaneous Endoscopic Approach, Diagnostic
00B64ZZ Excision of Cerebral Ventricle, Percutaneous Endoscopic Approach
00B70ZX Excision of Cerebral Hemisphere, Open Approach, Diagnostic
00B70ZZ Excision of Cerebral Hemisphere, Open Approach
00B73ZX Excision of Cerebral Hemisphere, Percutaneous Approach, Diagnostic
00B73ZZ Excision of Cerebral Hemisphere, Percutaneous Approach
00B74ZX Excision of Cerebral Hemisphere, Percutaneous Endoscopic Approach, Diagnostic
00B74ZZ Excision of Cerebral Hemisphere, Percutaneous Endoscopic Approach
00B80ZX Excision of Basal Ganglia, Open Approach, Diagnostic
00B80ZZ Excision of Basal Ganglia, Open Approach
00B83ZX Excision of Basal Ganglia, Percutaneous Approach, Diagnostic
00B83ZZ Excision of Basal Ganglia, Percutaneous Approach
00B84ZX Excision of Basal Ganglia, Percutaneous Endoscopic Approach, Diagnostic
00B84ZZ Excision of Basal Ganglia, Percutaneous Endoscopic Approach
00B90ZX Excision of Thalamus, Open Approach, Diagnostic
00B90ZZ Excision of Thalamus, Open Approach
00B93ZX Excision of Thalamus, Percutaneous Approach, Diagnostic
00B93ZZ Excision of Thalamus, Percutaneous Approach
00B94ZX Excision of Thalamus, Percutaneous Endoscopic Approach, Diagnostic
00B94ZZ Excision of Thalamus, Percutaneous Endoscopic Approach
00BA0ZX Excision of Hypothalamus, Open Approach, Diagnostic
00BA0ZZ Excision of Hypothalamus, Open Approach
00BA3ZX Excision of Hypothalamus, Percutaneous Approach, Diagnostic
00BA3ZZ Excision of Hypothalamus, Percutaneous Approach
00BA4ZX Excision of Hypothalamus, Percutaneous Endoscopic Approach, Diagnostic
00BA4ZZ Excision of Hypothalamus, Percutaneous Endoscopic Approach
00BB0ZX Excision of Pons, Open Approach, Diagnostic
00BB0ZZ Excision of Pons, Open Approach
00BB3ZX Excision of Pons, Percutaneous Approach, Diagnostic
00BB3ZZ Excision of Pons, Percutaneous Approach
00BB4ZX Excision of Pons, Percutaneous Endoscopic Approach, Diagnostic
00BB4ZZ Excision of Pons, Percutaneous Endoscopic Approach
00BC0ZX Excision of Cerebellum, Open Approach, Diagnostic
00BC0ZZ Excision of Cerebellum, Open Approach
00BC3ZX Excision of Cerebellum, Percutaneous Approach, Diagnostic
00BC3ZZ Excision of Cerebellum, Percutaneous Approach

00BC4ZX Excision of Cerebellum, Percutaneous Endoscopic Approach, Diagnostic
00BC4ZZ Excision of Cerebellum, Percutaneous Endoscopic Approach
00BD0ZX Excision of Medulla Oblongata, Open Approach, Diagnostic
00BD0ZZ Excision of Medulla Oblongata, Open Approach
00BD3ZX Excision of Medulla Oblongata, Percutaneous Approach, Diagnostic
00BD3ZZ Excision of Medulla Oblongata, Percutaneous Approach
00BD4ZX Excision of Medulla Oblongata, Percutaneous Endoscopic Approach, Diagnostic
00BD4ZZ Excision of Medulla Oblongata, Percutaneous Endoscopic Approach
00BF0ZX Excision of Olfactory Nerve, Open Approach, Diagnostic
00BF0ZZ Excision of Olfactory Nerve, Open Approach
00BF3ZX Excision of Olfactory Nerve, Percutaneous Approach, Diagnostic
00BF3ZZ Excision of Olfactory Nerve, Percutaneous Approach
00BF4ZX Excision of Olfactory Nerve, Percutaneous Endoscopic Approach, Diagnostic
00BF4ZZ Excision of Olfactory Nerve, Percutaneous Endoscopic Approach
00BG0ZX Excision of Optic Nerve, Open Approach, Diagnostic
00BG0ZZ Excision of Optic Nerve, Open Approach
00BG3ZX Excision of Optic Nerve, Percutaneous Approach, Diagnostic
00BG3ZZ Excision of Optic Nerve, Percutaneous Approach
00BG4ZX Excision of Optic Nerve, Percutaneous Endoscopic Approach, Diagnostic
00BG4ZZ Excision of Optic Nerve, Percutaneous Endoscopic Approach
00BH0ZX Excision of Oculomotor Nerve, Open Approach, Diagnostic
00BH0ZZ Excision of Oculomotor Nerve, Open Approach
00BH3ZX Excision of Oculomotor Nerve, Percutaneous Approach, Diagnostic
00BH3ZZ Excision of Oculomotor Nerve, Percutaneous Approach
00BH4ZX Excision of Oculomotor Nerve, Percutaneous Endoscopic Approach, Diagnostic
00BH4ZZ Excision of Oculomotor Nerve, Percutaneous Endoscopic Approach
00BJ0ZX Excision of Trochlear Nerve, Open Approach, Diagnostic
00BJ0ZZ Excision of Trochlear Nerve, Open Approach
00BJ3ZX Excision of Trochlear Nerve, Percutaneous Approach, Diagnostic
00BJ3ZZ Excision of Trochlear Nerve, Percutaneous Approach
00BJ4ZX Excision of Trochlear Nerve, Percutaneous Endoscopic Approach, Diagnostic
00BJ4ZZ Excision of Trochlear Nerve, Percutaneous Endoscopic Approach
00BK0ZX Excision of Trigeminal Nerve, Open Approach, Diagnostic
00BK0ZZ Excision of Trigeminal Nerve, Open Approach
00BK3ZX Excision of Trigeminal Nerve, Percutaneous Approach, Diagnostic
00BK3ZZ Excision of Trigeminal Nerve, Percutaneous Approach
00BK4ZX Excision of Trigeminal Nerve, Percutaneous Endoscopic Approach, Diagnostic
00BK4ZZ Excision of Trigeminal Nerve, Percutaneous Endoscopic Approach
00BL0ZX Excision of Abducens Nerve, Open Approach, Diagnostic
00BL0ZZ Excision of Abducens Nerve, Open Approach
00BL3ZX Excision of Abducens Nerve, Percutaneous Approach, Diagnostic
00BL3ZZ Excision of Abducens Nerve, Percutaneous Approach
00BL4ZX Excision of Abducens Nerve, Percutaneous Endoscopic Approach, Diagnostic
00BL4ZZ Excision of Abducens Nerve, Percutaneous Endoscopic Approach
00BM0ZX Excision of Facial Nerve, Open Approach, Diagnostic
00BM0ZZ Excision of Facial Nerve, Open Approach
00BM3ZX Excision of Facial Nerve, Percutaneous Approach, Diagnostic
00BM3ZZ Excision of Facial Nerve, Percutaneous Approach
00BM4ZX Excision of Facial Nerve, Percutaneous Endoscopic Approach, Diagnostic
00BM4ZZ Excision of Facial Nerve, Percutaneous Endoscopic Approach
00BN0ZX Excision of Acoustic Nerve, Open Approach, Diagnostic
00BN0ZZ Excision of Acoustic Nerve, Open Approach
00BN3ZX Excision of Acoustic Nerve, Percutaneous Approach, Diagnostic
00BN3ZZ Excision of Acoustic Nerve, Percutaneous Approach
00BN4ZX Excision of Acoustic Nerve, Percutaneous Endoscopic Approach, Diagnostic
00BN4ZZ Excision of Acoustic Nerve, Percutaneous Endoscopic Approach
00BP0ZX Excision of Glossopharyngeal Nerve, Open Approach, Diagnostic
00BP0ZZ Excision of Glossopharyngeal Nerve, Open Approach
00BP3ZX Excision of Glossopharyngeal Nerve, Percutaneous Approach, Diagnostic
00BP3ZZ Excision of Glossopharyngeal Nerve, Percutaneous Approach
00BP4ZX Excision of Glossopharyngeal Nerve, Percutaneous Endoscopic Approach, Diagnostic
00BP4ZZ Excision of Glossopharyngeal Nerve, Percutaneous Endoscopic Approach
00BQ0ZX Excision of Vagus Nerve, Open Approach, Diagnostic
00BQ0ZZ Excision of Vagus Nerve, Open Approach
00BQ3ZX Excision of Vagus Nerve, Percutaneous Approach, Diagnostic
00BQ3ZZ Excision of Vagus Nerve, Percutaneous Approach
00BQ4ZX Excision of Vagus Nerve, Percutaneous Endoscopic Approach, Diagnostic
00BQ4ZZ Excision of Vagus Nerve, Percutaneous Endoscopic Approach
00BR0ZX Excision of Accessory Nerve, Open Approach, Diagnostic
00BR0ZZ Excision of Accessory Nerve, Open Approach
00BR3ZX Excision of Accessory Nerve, Percutaneous Approach, Diagnostic
00BR3ZZ Excision of Accessory Nerve, Percutaneous Approach
00BR4ZX Excision of Accessory Nerve, Percutaneous Endoscopic Approach, Diagnostic
00BR4ZZ Excision of Accessory Nerve, Percutaneous Endoscopic Approach
00BS0ZX Excision of Hypoglossal Nerve, Open Approach, Diagnostic
00BS0ZZ Excision of Hypoglossal Nerve, Open Approach
00BS3ZX Excision of Hypoglossal Nerve, Percutaneous Approach, Diagnostic
00BS3ZZ Excision of Hypoglossal Nerve, Percutaneous Approach
00BS4ZX Excision of Hypoglossal Nerve, Percutaneous Endoscopic Approach, Diagnostic
00BS4ZZ Excision of Hypoglossal Nerve, Percutaneous Endoscopic Approach
00BT0ZX Excision of Spinal Meninges, Open Approach, Diagnostic
00BT0ZZ Excision of Spinal Meninges, Open Approach
00BT3ZX Excision of Spinal Meninges, Percutaneous Approach, Diagnostic
00BT3ZZ Excision of Spinal Meninges, Percutaneous Approach
00BT4ZX Excision of Spinal Meninges, Percutaneous Endoscopic Approach, Diagnostic
00BT4ZZ Excision of Spinal Meninges, Percutaneous Endoscopic Approach
00BW0ZX Excision of Cervical Spinal Cord, Open Approach, Diagnostic
00BW0ZZ Excision of Cervical Spinal Cord, Open Approach
00BW3ZX Excision of Cervical Spinal Cord, Percutaneous Approach, Diagnostic
00BW3ZZ Excision of Cervical Spinal Cord, Percutaneous Approach
00BW4ZX Excision of Cervical Spinal Cord, Percutaneous Endoscopic Approach, Diagnostic
00BW4ZZ Excision of Cervical Spinal Cord, Percutaneous Endoscopic Approach
00BX0ZX Excision of Thoracic Spinal Cord, Open Approach, Diagnostic
00BX0ZZ Excision of Thoracic Spinal Cord, Open Approach
00BX3ZX Excision of Thoracic Spinal Cord, Percutaneous Approach, Diagnostic
00BX3ZZ Excision of Thoracic Spinal Cord, Percutaneous Approach
00BX4ZX Excision of Thoracic Spinal Cord, Percutaneous Endoscopic Approach, Diagnostic
00BX4ZZ Excision of Thoracic Spinal Cord, Percutaneous Endoscopic Approach
00BY0ZX Excision of Lumbar Spinal Cord, Open Approach, Diagnostic
00BY0ZZ Excision of Lumbar Spinal Cord, Open Approach
00BY3ZX Excision of Lumbar Spinal Cord, Percutaneous Approach, Diagnostic
00BY3ZZ Excision of Lumbar Spinal Cord, Percutaneous Approach
00BY4ZX Excision of Lumbar Spinal Cord, Percutaneous Endoscopic Approach, Diagnostic
00BY4ZZ Excision of Lumbar Spinal Cord, Percutaneous Endoscopic Approach

00C – Central Nervous System, Extirpation

00C00ZZ Extirpation of Matter from Brain, Open Approach
00C03ZZ Extirpation of Matter from Brain, Percutaneous Approach
00C04ZZ Extirpation of Matter from Brain, Percutaneous Endoscopic Approach

00C10ZZ Extirpation of Matter from Cerebral Meninges, Open Approach
00C13ZZ Extirpation of Matter from Cerebral Meninges, Percutaneous Approach
00C14ZZ Extirpation of Matter from Cerebral Meninges, Percutaneous Endoscopic Approach
00C20ZZ Extirpation of Matter from Dura Mater, Open Approach
00C23ZZ Extirpation of Matter from Dura Mater, Percutaneous Approach
00C24ZZ Extirpation of Matter from Dura Mater, Percutaneous Endoscopic Approach
00C30ZZ Extirpation of Matter from Epidural Space, Open Approach
00C33ZZ Extirpation of Matter from Epidural Space, Percutaneous Approach
00C34ZZ Extirpation of Matter from Epidural Space, Percutaneous Endoscopic Approach
00C40ZZ Extirpation of Matter from Subdural Space, Open Approach
00C43ZZ Extirpation of Matter from Subdural Space, Percutaneous Approach
00C44ZZ Extirpation of Matter from Subdural Space, Percutaneous Endoscopic Approach
00C50ZZ Extirpation of Matter from Subarachnoid Space, Open Approach
00C53ZZ Extirpation of Matter from Subarachnoid Space, Percutaneous Approach
00C54ZZ Extirpation of Matter from Subarachnoid Space, Percutaneous Endoscopic Approach
00C60ZZ Extirpation of Matter from Cerebral Ventricle, Open Approach
00C63ZZ Extirpation of Matter from Cerebral Ventricle, Percutaneous Approach
00C64ZZ Extirpation of Matter from Cerebral Ventricle, Percutaneous Endoscopic Approach
00C70ZZ Extirpation of Matter from Cerebral Hemisphere, Open Approach
00C73ZZ Extirpation of Matter from Cerebral Hemisphere, Percutaneous Approach
00C74ZZ Extirpation of Matter from Cerebral Hemisphere, Percutaneous Endoscopic Approach
00C80ZZ Extirpation of Matter from Basal Ganglia, Open Approach
00C83ZZ Extirpation of Matter from Basal Ganglia, Percutaneous Approach
00C84ZZ Extirpation of Matter from Basal Ganglia, Percutaneous Endoscopic Approach
00C90ZZ Extirpation of Matter from Thalamus, Open Approach
00C93ZZ Extirpation of Matter from Thalamus, Percutaneous Approach
00C94ZZ Extirpation of Matter from Thalamus, Percutaneous Endoscopic Approach
00CA0ZZ Extirpation of Matter from Hypothalamus, Open Approach
00CA3ZZ Extirpation of Matter from Hypothalamus, Percutaneous Approach
00CA4ZZ Extirpation of Matter from Hypothalamus, Percutaneous Endoscopic Approach
00CB0ZZ Extirpation of Matter from Pons, Open Approach
00CB3ZZ Extirpation of Matter from Pons, Percutaneous Approach
00CB4ZZ Extirpation of Matter from Pons, Percutaneous Endoscopic Approach
00CC0ZZ Extirpation of Matter from Cerebellum, Open Approach
00CC3ZZ Extirpation of Matter from Cerebellum, Percutaneous Approach
00CC4ZZ Extirpation of Matter from Cerebellum, Percutaneous Endoscopic Approach
00CD0ZZ Extirpation of Matter from Medulla Oblongata, Open Approach
00CD3ZZ Extirpation of Matter from Medulla Oblongata, Percutaneous Approach
00CD4ZZ Extirpation of Matter from Medulla Oblongata, Percutaneous Endoscopic Approach
00CF0ZZ Extirpation of Matter from Olfactory Nerve, Open Approach
00CF3ZZ Extirpation of Matter from Olfactory Nerve, Percutaneous Approach
00CF4ZZ Extirpation of Matter from Olfactory Nerve, Percutaneous Endoscopic Approach
00CG0ZZ Extirpation of Matter from Optic Nerve, Open Approach
00CG3ZZ Extirpation of Matter from Optic Nerve, Percutaneous Approach
00CG4ZZ Extirpation of Matter from Optic Nerve, Percutaneous Endoscopic Approach
00CH0ZZ Extirpation of Matter from Oculomotor Nerve, Open Approach
00CH3ZZ Extirpation of Matter from Oculomotor Nerve, Percutaneous Approach
00CH4ZZ Extirpation of Matter from Oculomotor Nerve, Percutaneous Endoscopic Approach
00CJ0ZZ Extirpation of Matter from Trochlear Nerve, Open Approach
00CJ3ZZ Extirpation of Matter from Trochlear Nerve, Percutaneous Approach
00CJ4ZZ Extirpation of Matter from Trochlear Nerve, Percutaneous Endoscopic Approach
00CK0ZZ Extirpation of Matter from Trigeminal Nerve, Open Approach
00CK3ZZ Extirpation of Matter from Trigeminal Nerve, Percutaneous Approach
00CK4ZZ Extirpation of Matter from Trigeminal Nerve, Percutaneous Endoscopic Approach
00CL0ZZ Extirpation of Matter from Abducens Nerve, Open Approach
00CL3ZZ Extirpation of Matter from Abducens Nerve, Percutaneous Approach
00CL4ZZ Extirpation of Matter from Abducens Nerve, Percutaneous Endoscopic Approach
00CM0ZZ Extirpation of Matter from Facial Nerve, Open Approach
00CM3ZZ Extirpation of Matter from Facial Nerve, Percutaneous Approach
00CM4ZZ Extirpation of Matter from Facial Nerve, Percutaneous Endoscopic Approach
00CN0ZZ Extirpation of Matter from Acoustic Nerve, Open Approach
00CN3ZZ Extirpation of Matter from Acoustic Nerve, Percutaneous Approach
00CN4ZZ Extirpation of Matter from Acoustic Nerve, Percutaneous Endoscopic Approach
00CP0ZZ Extirpation of Matter from Glossopharyngeal Nerve, Open Approach
00CP3ZZ Extirpation of Matter from Glossopharyngeal Nerve, Percutaneous Approach
00CP4ZZ Extirpation of Matter from Glossopharyngeal Nerve, Percutaneous Endoscopic Approach
00CQ0ZZ Extirpation of Matter from Vagus Nerve, Open Approach
00CQ3ZZ Extirpation of Matter from Vagus Nerve, Percutaneous Approach
00CQ4ZZ Extirpation of Matter from Vagus Nerve, Percutaneous Endoscopic Approach
00CR0ZZ Extirpation of Matter from Accessory Nerve, Open Approach
00CR3ZZ Extirpation of Matter from Accessory Nerve, Percutaneous Approach
00CR4ZZ Extirpation of Matter from Accessory Nerve, Percutaneous Endoscopic Approach
00CS0ZZ Extirpation of Matter from Hypoglossal Nerve, Open Approach
00CS3ZZ Extirpation of Matter from Hypoglossal Nerve, Percutaneous Approach
00CS4ZZ Extirpation of Matter from Hypoglossal Nerve, Percutaneous Endoscopic Approach
00CT0ZZ Extirpation of Matter from Spinal Meninges, Open Approach
00CT3ZZ Extirpation of Matter from Spinal Meninges, Percutaneous Approach
00CT4ZZ Extirpation of Matter from Spinal Meninges, Percutaneous Endoscopic Approach
00CW0ZZ Extirpation of Matter from Cervical Spinal Cord, Open Approach
00CW3ZZ Extirpation of Matter from Cervical Spinal Cord, Percutaneous Approach
00CW4ZZ Extirpation of Matter from Cervical Spinal Cord, Percutaneous Endoscopic Approach
00CX0ZZ Extirpation of Matter from Thoracic Spinal Cord, Open Approach
00CX3ZZ Extirpation of Matter from Thoracic Spinal Cord, Percutaneous Approach
00CX4ZZ Extirpation of Matter from Thoracic Spinal Cord, Percutaneous Endoscopic Approach
00CY0ZZ Extirpation of Matter from Lumbar Spinal Cord, Open Approach
00CY3ZZ Extirpation of Matter from Lumbar Spinal Cord, Percutaneous Approach
00CY4ZZ Extirpation of Matter from Lumbar Spinal Cord, Percutaneous Endoscopic Approach

00D – Central Nervous System, Extraction

00D10ZZ Extraction of Cerebral Meninges, Open Approach
00D13ZZ Extraction of Cerebral Meninges, Percutaneous Approach
00D14ZZ Extraction of Cerebral Meninges, Percutaneous Endoscopic Approach
00D20ZZ Extraction of Dura Mater, Open Approach
00D23ZZ Extraction of Dura Mater, Percutaneous Approach
00D24ZZ Extraction of Dura Mater, Percutaneous Endoscopic Approach
00DF0ZZ Extraction of Olfactory Nerve, Open Approach
00DF3ZZ Extraction of Olfactory Nerve, Percutaneous Approach
00DF4ZZ Extraction of Olfactory Nerve, Percutaneous Endoscopic Approach
00DG0ZZ Extraction of Optic Nerve, Open Approach
00DG3ZZ Extraction of Optic Nerve, Percutaneous Approach
00DG4ZZ Extraction of Optic Nerve, Percutaneous Endoscopic Approach
00DH0ZZ Extraction of Oculomotor Nerve, Open Approach
00DH3ZZ Extraction of Oculomotor Nerve, Percutaneous Approach
00DH4ZZ Extraction of Oculomotor Nerve, Percutaneous Endoscopic Approach
00DJ0ZZ Extraction of Trochlear Nerve, Open Approach
00DJ3ZZ Extraction of Trochlear Nerve, Percutaneous Approach

00DJ4ZZ Extraction of Trochlear Nerve, Percutaneous Endoscopic Approach
00DK0ZZ Extraction of Trigeminal Nerve, Open Approach
00DK3ZZ Extraction of Trigeminal Nerve, Percutaneous Approach
00DK4ZZ Extraction of Trigeminal Nerve, Percutaneous Endoscopic Approach
00DL0ZZ Extraction of Abducens Nerve, Open Approach
00DL3ZZ Extraction of Abducens Nerve, Percutaneous Approach
00DL4ZZ Extraction of Abducens Nerve, Percutaneous Endoscopic Approach
00DM0ZZ Extraction of Facial Nerve, Open Approach
00DM3ZZ Extraction of Facial Nerve, Percutaneous Approach
00DM4ZZ Extraction of Facial Nerve, Percutaneous Endoscopic Approach
00DN0ZZ Extraction of Acoustic Nerve, Open Approach
00DN3ZZ Extraction of Acoustic Nerve, Percutaneous Approach
00DN4ZZ Extraction of Acoustic Nerve, Percutaneous Endoscopic Approach
00DP0ZZ Extraction of Glossopharyngeal Nerve, Open Approach
00DP3ZZ Extraction of Glossopharyngeal Nerve, Percutaneous Approach
00DP4ZZ Extraction of Glossopharyngeal Nerve, Percutaneous Endoscopic Approach
00DQ0ZZ Extraction of Vagus Nerve, Open Approach
00DQ3ZZ Extraction of Vagus Nerve, Percutaneous Approach
00DQ4ZZ Extraction of Vagus Nerve, Percutaneous Endoscopic Approach
00DR0ZZ Extraction of Accessory Nerve, Open Approach
00DR3ZZ Extraction of Accessory Nerve, Percutaneous Approach
00DR4ZZ Extraction of Accessory Nerve, Percutaneous Endoscopic Approach
00DS0ZZ Extraction of Hypoglossal Nerve, Open Approach
00DS3ZZ Extraction of Hypoglossal Nerve, Percutaneous Approach
00DS4ZZ Extraction of Hypoglossal Nerve, Percutaneous Endoscopic Approach
00DT0ZZ Extraction of Spinal Meninges, Open Approach
00DT3ZZ Extraction of Spinal Meninges, Percutaneous Approach
00DT4ZZ Extraction of Spinal Meninges, Percutaneous Endoscopic Approach

00F – Central Nervous System, Fragmentation

00F30ZZ Fragmentation in Epidural Space, Open Approach
00F33ZZ Fragmentation in Epidural Space, Percutaneous Approach
00F34ZZ Fragmentation in Epidural Space, Percutaneous Endoscopic Approach
▲ **00F3XZZ** Fragmentation in Epidural Space, External Approach
00F40ZZ Fragmentation in Subdural Space, Open Approach
00F43ZZ Fragmentation in Subdural Space, Percutaneous Approach
00F44ZZ Fragmentation in Subdural Space, Percutaneous Endoscopic Approach
▲ **00F4XZZ** Fragmentation in Subdural Space, External Approach
00F50ZZ Fragmentation in Subarachnoid Space, Open Approach
00F53ZZ Fragmentation in Subarachnoid Space, Percutaneous Approach
00F54ZZ Fragmentation in Subarachnoid Space, Percutaneous Endoscopic Approach
▲ **00F5XZZ** Fragmentation in Subarachnoid Space, External Approach
00F60ZZ Fragmentation in Cerebral Ventricle, Open Approach
00F63ZZ Fragmentation in Cerebral Ventricle, Percutaneous Approach
00F64ZZ Fragmentation in Cerebral Ventricle, Percutaneous Endoscopic Approach
▲ **00F6XZZ** Fragmentation in Cerebral Ventricle, External Approach
00FU0ZZ Fragmentation in Spinal Canal, Open Approach
00FU3ZZ Fragmentation in Spinal Canal, Percutaneous Approach
00FU4ZZ Fragmentation in Spinal Canal, Percutaneous Endoscopic Approach
00FUXZZ Fragmentation in Spinal Canal, External Approach

Review Coding Guideline B4.6

00H – Central Nervous System, Insertion

00H002Z Insertion of Monitoring Device into Brain, Open Approach
00H003Z Insertion of Infusion Device into Brain, Open Approach
00H00MZ Insertion of Neurostimulator Lead into Brain, Open Approach
00H032Z Insertion of Monitoring Device into Brain, Percutaneous Approach
00H033Z Insertion of Infusion Device into Brain, Percutaneous Approach
00H03MZ Insertion of Neurostimulator Lead into Brain, Percutaneous Approach
00H042Z Insertion of Monitoring Device into Brain, Percutaneous Endoscopic Approach
00H043Z Insertion of Infusion Device into Brain, Percutaneous Endoscopic Approach
00H04MZ Insertion of Neurostimulator Lead into Brain, Percutaneous Endoscopic Approach
00H602Z Insertion of Monitoring Device into Cerebral Ventricle, Open Approach
00H603Z Insertion of Infusion Device into Cerebral Ventricle, Open Approach
00H60MZ Insertion of Neurostimulator Lead into Cerebral Ventricle, Open Approach
00H632Z Insertion of Monitoring Device into Cerebral Ventricle, Percutaneous Approach
00H633Z Insertion of Infusion Device into Cerebral Ventricle, Percutaneous Approach
00H63MZ Insertion of Neurostimulator Lead into Cerebral Ventricle, Percutaneous Approach
00H642Z Insertion of Monitoring Device into Cerebral Ventricle, Percutaneous Endoscopic Approach
00H643Z Insertion of Infusion Device into Cerebral Ventricle, Percutaneous Endoscopic Approach
00H64MZ Insertion of Neurostimulator Lead into Cerebral Ventricle, Percutaneous Endoscopic Approach
00HE02Z Insertion of Monitoring Device into Cranial Nerve, Open Approach
00HE03Z Insertion of Infusion Device into Cranial Nerve, Open Approach
00HE0MZ Insertion of Neurostimulator Lead into Cranial Nerve, Open Approach
00HE32Z Insertion of Monitoring Device into Cranial Nerve, Percutaneous Approach
00HE33Z Insertion of Infusion Device into Cranial Nerve, Percutaneous Approach
00HE3MZ Insertion of Neurostimulator Lead into Cranial Nerve, Percutaneous Approach
00HE42Z Insertion of Monitoring Device into Cranial Nerve, Percutaneous Endoscopic Approach
00HE43Z Insertion of Infusion Device into Cranial Nerve, Percutaneous Endoscopic Approach
00HE4MZ Insertion of Neurostimulator Lead into Cranial Nerve, Percutaneous Endoscopic Approach
00HU02Z Insertion of Monitoring Device into Spinal Canal, Open Approach
00HU03Z Insertion of Infusion Device into Spinal Canal, Open Approach
00HU0MZ Insertion of Neurostimulator Lead into Spinal Canal, Open Approach
00HU32Z Insertion of Monitoring Device into Spinal Canal, Percutaneous Approach
00HU33Z Insertion of Infusion Device into Spinal Canal, Percutaneous Approach
00HU3MZ Insertion of Neurostimulator Lead into Spinal Canal, Percutaneous Approach
00HU42Z Insertion of Monitoring Device into Spinal Canal, Percutaneous Endoscopic Approach
00HU43Z Insertion of Infusion Device into Spinal Canal, Percutaneous Endoscopic Approach
00HU4MZ Insertion of Neurostimulator Lead into Spinal Canal, Percutaneous Endoscopic Approach
00HV02Z Insertion of Monitoring Device into Spinal Cord, Open Approach
00HV03Z Insertion of Infusion Device into Spinal Cord, Open Approach
00HV0MZ Insertion of Neurostimulator Lead into Spinal Cord, Open Approach
00HV32Z Insertion of Monitoring Device into Spinal Cord, Percutaneous Approach
00HV33Z Insertion of Infusion Device into Spinal Cord, Percutaneous Approach
00HV3MZ Insertion of Neurostimulator Lead into Spinal Cord, Percutaneous Approach
00HV42Z Insertion of Monitoring Device into Spinal Cord, Percutaneous Endoscopic Approach
00HV43Z Insertion of Infusion Device into Spinal Cord, Percutaneous Endoscopic Approach
00HV4MZ Insertion of Neurostimulator Lead into Spinal Cord, Percutaneous Endoscopic Approach

00J – Central Nervous System, Inspection

Review Coding Guidelines B3.11a, B3.11b and B3.11c

00J00ZZ Inspection of Brain, Open Approach
00J03ZZ Inspection of Brain, Percutaneous Approach
00J04ZZ Inspection of Brain, Percutaneous Endoscopic Approach
00JE0ZZ Inspection of Cranial Nerve, Open Approach
00JE3ZZ Inspection of Cranial Nerve, Percutaneous Approach
00JE4ZZ Inspection of Cranial Nerve, Percutaneous Endoscopic Approach
00JU0ZZ Inspection of Spinal Canal, Open Approach
00JU3ZZ Inspection of Spinal Canal, Percutaneous Approach
00JU4ZZ Inspection of Spinal Canal, Percutaneous Endoscopic Approach
00JV0ZZ Inspection of Spinal Cord, Open Approach
00JV3ZZ Inspection of Spinal Cord, Percutaneous Approach
00JV4ZZ Inspection of Spinal Cord, Percutaneous Endoscopic Approach

00K – Central Nervous System, Map

00K00ZZ Map Brain, Open Approach
00K03ZZ Map Brain, Percutaneous Approach
00K04ZZ Map Brain, Percutaneous Endoscopic Approach
00K70ZZ Map Cerebral Hemisphere, Open Approach
00K73ZZ Map Cerebral Hemisphere, Percutaneous Approach
00K74ZZ Map Cerebral Hemisphere, Percutaneous Endoscopic Approach
00K80ZZ Map Basal Ganglia, Open Approach
00K83ZZ Map Basal Ganglia, Percutaneous Approach
00K84ZZ Map Basal Ganglia, Percutaneous Endoscopic Approach
00K90ZZ Map Thalamus, Open Approach
00K93ZZ Map Thalamus, Percutaneous Approach
00K94ZZ Map Thalamus, Percutaneous Endoscopic Approach
00KA0ZZ Map Hypothalamus, Open Approach
00KA3ZZ Map Hypothalamus, Percutaneous Approach
00KA4ZZ Map Hypothalamus, Percutaneous Endoscopic Approach
00KB0ZZ Map Pons, Open Approach
00KB3ZZ Map Pons, Percutaneous Approach
00KB4ZZ Map Pons, Percutaneous Endoscopic Approach
00KC0ZZ Map Cerebellum, Open Approach
00KC3ZZ Map Cerebellum, Percutaneous Approach
00KC4ZZ Map Cerebellum, Percutaneous Endoscopic Approach
00KD0ZZ Map Medulla Oblongata, Open Approach
00KD3ZZ Map Medulla Oblongata, Percutaneous Approach
00KD4ZZ Map Medulla Oblongata, Percutaneous Endoscopic Approach

00N – Central Nervous System, Release

Review Coding Guideline B3.13

Review Coding Guideline B3.14

00N00ZZ Release Brain, Open Approach
00N03ZZ Release Brain, Percutaneous Approach
00N04ZZ Release Brain, Percutaneous Endoscopic Approach
00N10ZZ Release Cerebral Meninges, Open Approach
00N13ZZ Release Cerebral Meninges, Percutaneous Approach
00N14ZZ Release Cerebral Meninges, Percutaneous Endoscopic Approach
00N20ZZ Release Dura Mater, Open Approach
00N23ZZ Release Dura Mater, Percutaneous Approach
00N24ZZ Release Dura Mater, Percutaneous Endoscopic Approach
00N60ZZ Release Cerebral Ventricle, Open Approach
00N63ZZ Release Cerebral Ventricle, Percutaneous Approach
00N64ZZ Release Cerebral Ventricle, Percutaneous Endoscopic Approach
00N70ZZ Release Cerebral Hemisphere, Open Approach
00N73ZZ Release Cerebral Hemisphere, Percutaneous Approach
00N74ZZ Release Cerebral Hemisphere, Percutaneous Endoscopic Approach
00N80ZZ Release Basal Ganglia, Open Approach
00N83ZZ Release Basal Ganglia, Percutaneous Approach
00N84ZZ Release Basal Ganglia, Percutaneous Endoscopic Approach
00N90ZZ Release Thalamus, Open Approach
00N93ZZ Release Thalamus, Percutaneous Approach
00N94ZZ Release Thalamus, Percutaneous Endoscopic Approach
00NA0ZZ Release Hypothalamus, Open Approach
00NA3ZZ Release Hypothalamus, Percutaneous Approach
00NA4ZZ Release Hypothalamus, Percutaneous Endoscopic Approach
00NB0ZZ Release Pons, Open Approach
00NB3ZZ Release Pons, Percutaneous Approach
00NB4ZZ Release Pons, Percutaneous Endoscopic Approach
00NC0ZZ Release Cerebellum, Open Approach
00NC3ZZ Release Cerebellum, Percutaneous Approach
00NC4ZZ Release Cerebellum, Percutaneous Endoscopic Approach
00ND0ZZ Release Medulla Oblongata, Open Approach
00ND3ZZ Release Medulla Oblongata, Percutaneous Approach
00ND4ZZ Release Medulla Oblongata, Percutaneous Endoscopic Approach
00NF0ZZ Release Olfactory Nerve, Open Approach
00NF3ZZ Release Olfactory Nerve, Percutaneous Approach
00NF4ZZ Release Olfactory Nerve, Percutaneous Endoscopic Approach
00NG0ZZ Release Optic Nerve, Open Approach
00NG3ZZ Release Optic Nerve, Percutaneous Approach
00NG4ZZ Release Optic Nerve, Percutaneous Endoscopic Approach
00NH0ZZ Release Oculomotor Nerve, Open Approach
00NH3ZZ Release Oculomotor Nerve, Percutaneous Approach
00NH4ZZ Release Oculomotor Nerve, Percutaneous Endoscopic Approach
00NJ0ZZ Release Trochlear Nerve, Open Approach
00NJ3ZZ Release Trochlear Nerve, Percutaneous Approach
00NJ4ZZ Release Trochlear Nerve, Percutaneous Endoscopic Approach
00NK0ZZ Release Trigeminal Nerve, Open Approach
00NK3ZZ Release Trigeminal Nerve, Percutaneous Approach
00NK4ZZ Release Trigeminal Nerve, Percutaneous Endoscopic Approach
00NL0ZZ Release Abducens Nerve, Open Approach
00NL3ZZ Release Abducens Nerve, Percutaneous Approach
00NL4ZZ Release Abducens Nerve, Percutaneous Endoscopic Approach
00NM0ZZ Release Facial Nerve, Open Approach
00NM3ZZ Release Facial Nerve, Percutaneous Approach
00NM4ZZ Release Facial Nerve, Percutaneous Endoscopic Approach
00NN0ZZ Release Acoustic Nerve, Open Approach
00NN3ZZ Release Acoustic Nerve, Percutaneous Approach
00NN4ZZ Release Acoustic Nerve, Percutaneous Endoscopic Approach
00NP0ZZ Release Glossopharyngeal Nerve, Open Approach
00NP3ZZ Release Glossopharyngeal Nerve, Percutaneous Approach
00NP4ZZ Release Glossopharyngeal Nerve, Percutaneous Endoscopic Approach
00NQ0ZZ Release Vagus Nerve, Open Approach
00NQ3ZZ Release Vagus Nerve, Percutaneous Approach
00NQ4ZZ Release Vagus Nerve, Percutaneous Endoscopic Approach
00NR0ZZ Release Accessory Nerve, Open Approach
00NR3ZZ Release Accessory Nerve, Percutaneous Approach
00NR4ZZ Release Accessory Nerve, Percutaneous Endoscopic Approach
00NS0ZZ Release Hypoglossal Nerve, Open Approach
00NS3ZZ Release Hypoglossal Nerve, Percutaneous Approach
00NS4ZZ Release Hypoglossal Nerve, Percutaneous Endoscopic Approach
00NT0ZZ Release Spinal Meninges, Open Approach
00NT3ZZ Release Spinal Meninges, Percutaneous Approach
00NT4ZZ Release Spinal Meninges, Percutaneous Endoscopic Approach
00NW0ZZ Release Cervical Spinal Cord, Open Approach

00NW3ZZ Release Cervical Spinal Cord, Percutaneous Approach
00NW4ZZ Release Cervical Spinal Cord, Percutaneous Endoscopic Approach
00NX0ZZ Release Thoracic Spinal Cord, Open Approach
00NX3ZZ Release Thoracic Spinal Cord, Percutaneous Approach
00NX4ZZ Release Thoracic Spinal Cord, Percutaneous Endoscopic Approach
00NY0ZZ Release Lumbar Spinal Cord, Open Approach
00NY3ZZ Release Lumbar Spinal Cord, Percutaneous Approach
00NY4ZZ Release Lumbar Spinal Cord, Percutaneous Endoscopic Approach

00P – Central Nervous System, Removal

Review Coding Guideline B6.1c

00P000Z Removal of Drainage Device from Brain, Open Approach
00P002Z Removal of Monitoring Device from Brain, Open Approach
00P003Z Removal of Infusion Device from Brain, Open Approach
00P007Z Removal of Autologous Tissue Substitute from Brain, Open Approach
00P00JZ Removal of Synthetic Substitute from Brain, Open Approach
00P00KZ Removal of Nonautologous Tissue Substitute from Brain, Open Approach
00P00MZ Removal of Neurostimulator Lead from Brain, Open Approach
00P030Z Removal of Drainage Device from Brain, Percutaneous Approach
00P032Z Removal of Monitoring Device from Brain, Percutaneous Approach
00P033Z Removal of Infusion Device from Brain, Percutaneous Approach
00P037Z Removal of Autologous Tissue Substitute from Brain, Percutaneous Approach
00P03JZ Removal of Synthetic Substitute from Brain, Percutaneous Approach
00P03KZ Removal of Nonautologous Tissue Substitute from Brain, Percutaneous Approach
00P03MZ Removal of Neurostimulator Lead from Brain, Percutaneous Approach
00P040Z Removal of Drainage Device from Brain, Percutaneous Endoscopic Approach
00P042Z Removal of Monitoring Device from Brain, Percutaneous Endoscopic Approach
00P043Z Removal of Infusion Device from Brain, Percutaneous Endoscopic Approach
00P047Z Removal of Autologous Tissue Substitute from Brain, Percutaneous Endoscopic Approach
00P04JZ Removal of Synthetic Substitute from Brain, Percutaneous Endoscopic Approach
00P04KZ Removal of Nonautologous Tissue Substitute from Brain, Percutaneous Endoscopic Approach
00P04MZ Removal of Neurostimulator Lead from Brain, Percutaneous Endoscopic Approach
00P0X0Z Removal of Drainage Device from Brain, External Approach
00P0X2Z Removal of Monitoring Device from Brain, External Approach
00P0X3Z Removal of Infusion Device from Brain, External Approach
00P0XMZ Removal of Neurostimulator Lead from Brain, External Approach
00P600Z Removal of Drainage Device from Cerebral Ventricle, Open Approach
00P602Z Removal of Monitoring Device from Cerebral Ventricle, Open Approach
00P603Z Removal of Infusion Device from Cerebral Ventricle, Open Approach
00P60JZ Removal of Synthetic Substitute from Cerebral Ventricle, Open Approach
00P60MZ Removal of Neurostimulator Lead from Cerebral Ventricle, Open Approach
00P630Z Removal of Drainage Device from Cerebral Ventricle, Percutaneous Approach
00P632Z Removal of Monitoring Device from Cerebral Ventricle, Percutaneous Approach
00P633Z Removal of Infusion Device from Cerebral Ventricle, Percutaneous Approach
00P63JZ Removal of Synthetic Substitute from Cerebral Ventricle, Percutaneous Approach
00P63MZ Removal of Neurostimulator Lead from Cerebral Ventricle, Percutaneous Approach
00P640Z Removal of Drainage Device from Cerebral Ventricle, Percutaneous Endoscopic Approach
00P642Z Removal of Monitoring Device from Cerebral Ventricle, Percutaneous Endoscopic Approach
00P643Z Removal of Infusion Device from Cerebral Ventricle, Percutaneous Endoscopic Approach
00P64JZ Removal of Synthetic Substitute from Cerebral Ventricle, Percutaneous Endoscopic Approach
00P64MZ Removal of Neurostimulator Lead from Cerebral Ventricle, Percutaneous Endoscopic Approach
00P6X0Z Removal of Drainage Device from Cerebral Ventricle, External Approach
00P6X2Z Removal of Monitoring Device from Cerebral Ventricle, External Approach
00P6X3Z Removal of Infusion Device from Cerebral Ventricle, External Approach
00P6XMZ Removal of Neurostimulator Lead from Cerebral Ventricle, External Approach
00PE00Z Removal of Drainage Device from Cranial Nerve, Open Approach
00PE02Z Removal of Monitoring Device from Cranial Nerve, Open Approach
00PE03Z Removal of Infusion Device from Cranial Nerve, Open Approach
00PE07Z Removal of Autologous Tissue Substitute from Cranial Nerve, Open Approach
00PE0MZ Removal of Neurostimulator Lead from Cranial Nerve, Open Approach
00PE30Z Removal of Drainage Device from Cranial Nerve, Percutaneous Approach
00PE32Z Removal of Monitoring Device from Cranial Nerve, Percutaneous Approach
00PE33Z Removal of Infusion Device from Cranial Nerve, Percutaneous Approach
00PE37Z Removal of Autologous Tissue Substitute from Cranial Nerve, Percutaneous Approach
00PE3MZ Removal of Neurostimulator Lead from Cranial Nerve, Percutaneous Approach
00PE40Z Removal of Drainage Device from Cranial Nerve, Percutaneous Endoscopic Approach
00PE42Z Removal of Monitoring Device from Cranial Nerve, Percutaneous Endoscopic Approach
00PE43Z Removal of Infusion Device from Cranial Nerve, Percutaneous Endoscopic Approach
00PE47Z Removal of Autologous Tissue Substitute from Cranial Nerve, Percutaneous Endoscopic Approach
00PE4MZ Removal of Neurostimulator Lead from Cranial Nerve, Percutaneous Endoscopic Approach
00PEX0Z Removal of Drainage Device from Cranial Nerve, External Approach
00PEX2Z Removal of Monitoring Device from Cranial Nerve, External Approach
00PEX3Z Removal of Infusion Device from Cranial Nerve, External Approach
00PEXMZ Removal of Neurostimulator Lead from Cranial Nerve, External Approach
00PU00Z Removal of Drainage Device from Spinal Canal, Open Approach
00PU02Z Removal of Monitoring Device from Spinal Canal, Open Approach
00PU03Z Removal of Infusion Device from Spinal Canal, Open Approach
00PU0JZ Removal of Synthetic Substitute from Spinal Canal, Open Approach
00PU0MZ Removal of Neurostimulator Lead from Spinal Canal, Open Approach
00PU30Z Removal of Drainage Device from Spinal Canal, Percutaneous Approach
00PU32Z Removal of Monitoring Device from Spinal Canal, Percutaneous Approach
00PU33Z Removal of Infusion Device from Spinal Canal, Percutaneous Approach
00PU3JZ Removal of Synthetic Substitute from Spinal Canal, Percutaneous Approach
00PU3MZ Removal of Neurostimulator Lead from Spinal Canal, Percutaneous Approach
00PU40Z Removal of Drainage Device from Spinal Canal, Percutaneous Endoscopic Approach
00PU42Z Removal of Monitoring Device from Spinal Canal, Percutaneous Endoscopic Approach
00PU43Z Removal of Infusion Device from Spinal Canal, Percutaneous Endoscopic Approach
00PU4JZ Removal of Synthetic Substitute from Spinal Canal, Percutaneous Endoscopic Approach
00PU4MZ Removal of Neurostimulator Lead from Spinal Canal, Percutaneous Endoscopic Approach
00PUX0Z Removal of Drainage Device from Spinal Canal, External Approach
00PUX2Z Removal of Monitoring Device from Spinal Canal, External Approach
00PUX3Z Removal of Infusion Device from Spinal Canal, External Approach
00PUXMZ Removal of Neurostimulator Lead from Spinal Canal, External Approach
00PV00Z Removal of Drainage Device from Spinal Cord, Open Approach
00PV02Z Removal of Monitoring Device from Spinal Cord, Open Approach
00PV03Z Removal of Infusion Device from Spinal Cord, Open Approach
00PV07Z Removal of Autologous Tissue Substitute from Spinal Cord, Open Approach
00PV0JZ Removal of Synthetic Substitute from Spinal Cord, Open Approach
00PV0KZ Removal of Nonautologous Tissue Substitute from Spinal Cord, Open Approach
00PV0MZ Removal of Neurostimulator Lead from Spinal Cord, Open Approach
00PV30Z Removal of Drainage Device from Spinal Cord, Percutaneous Approach

00PV32Z Removal of Monitoring Device from Spinal Cord, Percutaneous Approach
00PV33Z Removal of Infusion Device from Spinal Cord, Percutaneous Approach
00PV37Z Removal of Autologous Tissue Substitute from Spinal Cord, Percutaneous Approach
00PV3JZ Removal of Synthetic Substitute from Spinal Cord, Percutaneous Approach
00PV3KZ Removal of Nonautologous Tissue Substitute from Spinal Cord, Percutaneous Approach
00PV3MZ Removal of Neurostimulator Lead from Spinal Cord, Percutaneous Approach
00PV40Z Removal of Drainage Device from Spinal Cord, Percutaneous Endoscopic Approach
00PV42Z Removal of Monitoring Device from Spinal Cord, Percutaneous Endoscopic Approach
00PV43Z Removal of Infusion Device from Spinal Cord, Percutaneous Endoscopic Approach
00PV47Z Removal of Autologous Tissue Substitute from Spinal Cord, Percutaneous Endoscopic Approach
00PV4JZ Removal of Synthetic Substitute from Spinal Cord, Percutaneous Endoscopic Approach
00PV4KZ Removal of Nonautologous Tissue Substitute from Spinal Cord, Percutaneous Endoscopic Approach
00PV4MZ Removal of Neurostimulator Lead from Spinal Cord, Percutaneous Endoscopic Approach
00PVX0Z Removal of Drainage Device from Spinal Cord, External Approach
00PVX2Z Removal of Monitoring Device from Spinal Cord, External Approach
00PVX3Z Removal of Infusion Device from Spinal Cord, External Approach
00PVXMZ Removal of Neurostimulator Lead from Spinal Cord, External Approach

00Q – Central Nervous System, Repair

00Q00ZZ Repair Brain, Open Approach
00Q03ZZ Repair Brain, Percutaneous Approach
00Q04ZZ Repair Brain, Percutaneous Endoscopic Approach
00Q10ZZ Repair Cerebral Meninges, Open Approach
00Q13ZZ Repair Cerebral Meninges, Percutaneous Approach
00Q14ZZ Repair Cerebral Meninges, Percutaneous Endoscopic Approach
00Q20ZZ Repair Dura Mater, Open Approach
AHA CC: 3Q, 2013, 25
00Q23ZZ Repair Dura Mater, Percutaneous Approach
00Q24ZZ Repair Dura Mater, Percutaneous Endoscopic Approach
00Q60ZZ Repair Cerebral Ventricle, Open Approach
00Q63ZZ Repair Cerebral Ventricle, Percutaneous Approach
00Q64ZZ Repair Cerebral Ventricle, Percutaneous Endoscopic Approach
00Q70ZZ Repair Cerebral Hemisphere, Open Approach
00Q73ZZ Repair Cerebral Hemisphere, Percutaneous Approach
00Q74ZZ Repair Cerebral Hemisphere, Percutaneous Endoscopic Approach
00Q80ZZ Repair Basal Ganglia, Open Approach
00Q83ZZ Repair Basal Ganglia, Percutaneous Approach
00Q84ZZ Repair Basal Ganglia, Percutaneous Endoscopic Approach
00Q90ZZ Repair Thalamus, Open Approach
00Q93ZZ Repair Thalamus, Percutaneous Approach
00Q94ZZ Repair Thalamus, Percutaneous Endoscopic Approach
00QA0ZZ Repair Hypothalamus, Open Approach
00QA3ZZ Repair Hypothalamus, Percutaneous Approach
00QA4ZZ Repair Hypothalamus, Percutaneous Endoscopic Approach
00QB0ZZ Repair Pons, Open Approach
00QB3ZZ Repair Pons, Percutaneous Approach
00QB4ZZ Repair Pons, Percutaneous Endoscopic Approach
00QC0ZZ Repair Cerebellum, Open Approach
00QC3ZZ Repair Cerebellum, Percutaneous Approach
00QC4ZZ Repair Cerebellum, Percutaneous Endoscopic Approach
00QD0ZZ Repair Medulla Oblongata, Open Approach
00QD3ZZ Repair Medulla Oblongata, Percutaneous Approach
00QD4ZZ Repair Medulla Oblongata, Percutaneous Endoscopic Approach
00QF0ZZ Repair Olfactory Nerve, Open Approach
00QF3ZZ Repair Olfactory Nerve, Percutaneous Approach
00QF4ZZ Repair Olfactory Nerve, Percutaneous Endoscopic Approach
00QG0ZZ Repair Optic Nerve, Open Approach
00QG3ZZ Repair Optic Nerve, Percutaneous Approach
00QG4ZZ Repair Optic Nerve, Percutaneous Endoscopic Approach
00QH0ZZ Repair Oculomotor Nerve, Open Approach
00QH3ZZ Repair Oculomotor Nerve, Percutaneous Approach
00QH4ZZ Repair Oculomotor Nerve, Percutaneous Endoscopic Approach
00QJ0ZZ Repair Trochlear Nerve, Open Approach
00QJ3ZZ Repair Trochlear Nerve, Percutaneous Approach
00QJ4ZZ Repair Trochlear Nerve, Percutaneous Endoscopic Approach
00QK0ZZ Repair Trigeminal Nerve, Open Approach
00QK3ZZ Repair Trigeminal Nerve, Percutaneous Approach
00QK4ZZ Repair Trigeminal Nerve, Percutaneous Endoscopic Approach
00QL0ZZ Repair Abducens Nerve, Open Approach
00QL3ZZ Repair Abducens Nerve, Percutaneous Approach
00QL4ZZ Repair Abducens Nerve, Percutaneous Endoscopic Approach
00QM0ZZ Repair Facial Nerve, Open Approach
00QM3ZZ Repair Facial Nerve, Percutaneous Approach
00QM4ZZ Repair Facial Nerve, Percutaneous Endoscopic Approach
00QN0ZZ Repair Acoustic Nerve, Open Approach
00QN3ZZ Repair Acoustic Nerve, Percutaneous Approach
00QN4ZZ Repair Acoustic Nerve, Percutaneous Endoscopic Approach
00QP0ZZ Repair Glossopharyngeal Nerve, Open Approach
00QP3ZZ Repair Glossopharyngeal Nerve, Percutaneous Approach
00QP4ZZ Repair Glossopharyngeal Nerve, Percutaneous Endoscopic Approach
00QQ0ZZ Repair Vagus Nerve, Open Approach
00QQ3ZZ Repair Vagus Nerve, Percutaneous Approach
00QQ4ZZ Repair Vagus Nerve, Percutaneous Endoscopic Approach
00QR0ZZ Repair Accessory Nerve, Open Approach
00QR3ZZ Repair Accessory Nerve, Percutaneous Approach
00QR4ZZ Repair Accessory Nerve, Percutaneous Endoscopic Approach
00QS0ZZ Repair Hypoglossal Nerve, Open Approach
00QS3ZZ Repair Hypoglossal Nerve, Percutaneous Approach
00QS4ZZ Repair Hypoglossal Nerve, Percutaneous Endoscopic Approach
00QT0ZZ Repair Spinal Meninges, Open Approach
00QT3ZZ Repair Spinal Meninges, Percutaneous Approach
00QT4ZZ Repair Spinal Meninges, Percutaneous Endoscopic Approach
00QW0ZZ Repair Cervical Spinal Cord, Open Approach
00QW3ZZ Repair Cervical Spinal Cord, Percutaneous Approach
00QW4ZZ Repair Cervical Spinal Cord, Percutaneous Endoscopic Approach
00QX0ZZ Repair Thoracic Spinal Cord, Open Approach
00QX3ZZ Repair Thoracic Spinal Cord, Percutaneous Approach
00QX4ZZ Repair Thoracic Spinal Cord, Percutaneous Endoscopic Approach
00QY0ZZ Repair Lumbar Spinal Cord, Open Approach
00QY3ZZ Repair Lumbar Spinal Cord, Percutaneous Approach
00QY4ZZ Repair Lumbar Spinal Cord, Percutaneous Endoscopic Approach

00S – Central Nervous System, Reposition

00SF0ZZ Reposition Olfactory Nerve, Open Approach
00SF3ZZ Reposition Olfactory Nerve, Percutaneous Approach
00SF4ZZ Reposition Olfactory Nerve, Percutaneous Endoscopic Approach
00SG0ZZ Reposition Optic Nerve, Open Approach
00SG3ZZ Reposition Optic Nerve, Percutaneous Approach
00SG4ZZ Reposition Optic Nerve, Percutaneous Endoscopic Approach
00SH0ZZ Reposition Oculomotor Nerve, Open Approach
00SH3ZZ Reposition Oculomotor Nerve, Percutaneous Approach
00SH4ZZ Reposition Oculomotor Nerve, Percutaneous Endoscopic Approach
00SJ0ZZ Reposition Trochlear Nerve, Open Approach
00SJ3ZZ Reposition Trochlear Nerve, Percutaneous Approach
00SJ4ZZ Reposition Trochlear Nerve, Percutaneous Endoscopic Approach
00SK0ZZ Reposition Trigeminal Nerve, Open Approach
00SK3ZZ Reposition Trigeminal Nerve, Percutaneous Approach
00SK4ZZ Reposition Trigeminal Nerve, Percutaneous Endoscopic Approach
00SL0ZZ Reposition Abducens Nerve, Open Approach
00SL3ZZ Reposition Abducens Nerve, Percutaneous Approach

00SL4ZZ Reposition Abducens Nerve, Percutaneous Endoscopic Approach
00SM0ZZ Reposition Facial Nerve, Open Approach
00SM3ZZ Reposition Facial Nerve, Percutaneous Approach
00SM4ZZ Reposition Facial Nerve, Percutaneous Endoscopic Approach
00SN0ZZ Reposition Acoustic Nerve, Open Approach
00SN3ZZ Reposition Acoustic Nerve, Percutaneous Approach
00SN4ZZ Reposition Acoustic Nerve, Percutaneous Endoscopic Approach
00SP0ZZ Reposition Glossopharyngeal Nerve, Open Approach
00SP3ZZ Reposition Glossopharyngeal Nerve, Percutaneous Approach
00SP4ZZ Reposition Glossopharyngeal Nerve, Percutaneous Endoscopic Approach
00SQ0ZZ Reposition Vagus Nerve, Open Approach
00SQ3ZZ Reposition Vagus Nerve, Percutaneous Approach
00SQ4ZZ Reposition Vagus Nerve, Percutaneous Endoscopic Approach
00SR0ZZ Reposition Accessory Nerve, Open Approach
00SR3ZZ Reposition Accessory Nerve, Percutaneous Approach
00SR4ZZ Reposition Accessory Nerve, Percutaneous Endoscopic Approach
00SS0ZZ Reposition Hypoglossal Nerve, Open Approach
00SS3ZZ Reposition Hypoglossal Nerve, Percutaneous Approach
00SS4ZZ Reposition Hypoglossal Nerve, Percutaneous Endoscopic Approach
00SW0ZZ Reposition Cervical Spinal Cord, Open Approach
00SW3ZZ Reposition Cervical Spinal Cord, Percutaneous Approach
00SW4ZZ Reposition Cervical Spinal Cord, Percutaneous Endoscopic Approach
00SX0ZZ Reposition Thoracic Spinal Cord, Open Approach
00SX3ZZ Reposition Thoracic Spinal Cord, Percutaneous Approach
00SX4ZZ Reposition Thoracic Spinal Cord, Percutaneous Endoscopic Approach
00SY0ZZ Reposition Lumbar Spinal Cord, Open Approach
00SY3ZZ Reposition Lumbar Spinal Cord, Percutaneous Approach
00SY4ZZ Reposition Lumbar Spinal Cord, Percutaneous Endoscopic Approach

00T – Central Nervous System, Resection

Review Coding Guideline B3.8

00T70ZZ Resection of Cerebral Hemisphere, Open Approach
00T73ZZ Resection of Cerebral Hemisphere, Percutaneous Approach
00T74ZZ Resection of Cerebral Hemisphere, Percutaneous Endoscopic Approach

00U – Central Nervous System, Supplement

00U107Z Supplement Cerebral Meninges with Autologous Tissue Substitute, Open Approach
00U10JZ Supplement Cerebral Meninges with Synthetic Substitute, Open Approach
00U10KZ Supplement Cerebral Meninges with Nonautologous Tissue Substitute, Open Approach
00U137Z Supplement Cerebral Meninges with Autologous Tissue Substitute, Percutaneous Approach
00U13JZ Supplement Cerebral Meninges with Synthetic Substitute, Percutaneous Approach
00U13KZ Supplement Cerebral Meninges with Nonautologous Tissue Substitute, Percutaneous Approach
00U147Z Supplement Cerebral Meninges with Autologous Tissue Substitute, Percutaneous Endoscopic Approach
00U14JZ Supplement Cerebral Meninges with Synthetic Substitute, Percutaneous Endoscopic Approach
00U14KZ Supplement Cerebral Meninges with Nonautologous Tissue Substitute, Percutaneous Endoscopic Approach
00U207Z Supplement Dura Mater with Autologous Tissue Substitute, Open Approach
00U20JZ Supplement Dura Mater with Synthetic Substitute, Open Approach
00U20KZ Supplement Dura Mater with Nonautologous Tissue Substitute, Open Approach
00U237Z Supplement Dura Mater with Autologous Tissue Substitute, Percutaneous Approach
00U23JZ Supplement Dura Mater with Synthetic Substitute, Percutaneous Approach
00U23KZ Supplement Dura Mater with Nonautologous Tissue Substitute, Percutaneous Approach
00U247Z Supplement Dura Mater with Autologous Tissue Substitute, Percutaneous Endoscopic Approach
00U24JZ Supplement Dura Mater with Synthetic Substitute, Percutaneous Endoscopic Approach
00U24KZ Supplement Dura Mater with Nonautologous Tissue Substitute, Percutaneous Endoscopic Approach
00UF07Z Supplement Olfactory Nerve with Autologous Tissue Substitute, Open Approach
00UF37Z Supplement Olfactory Nerve with Autologous Tissue Substitute, Percutaneous Approach
00UF47Z Supplement Olfactory Nerve with Autologous Tissue Substitute, Percutaneous Endoscopic Approach
00UG07Z Supplement Optic Nerve with Autologous Tissue Substitute, Open Approach
00UG37Z Supplement Optic Nerve with Autologous Tissue Substitute, Percutaneous Approach
00UG47Z Supplement Optic Nerve with Autologous Tissue Substitute, Percutaneous Endoscopic Approach
00UH07Z Supplement Oculomotor Nerve with Autologous Tissue Substitute, Open Approach
00UH37Z Supplement Oculomotor Nerve with Autologous Tissue Substitute, Percutaneous Approach
00UH47Z Supplement Oculomotor Nerve with Autologous Tissue Substitute, Percutaneous Endoscopic Approach
00UJ07Z Supplement Trochlear Nerve with Autologous Tissue Substitute, Open Approach
00UJ37Z Supplement Trochlear Nerve with Autologous Tissue Substitute, Percutaneous Approach
00UJ47Z Supplement Trochlear Nerve with Autologous Tissue Substitute, Percutaneous Endoscopic Approach
00UK07Z Supplement Trigeminal Nerve with Autologous Tissue Substitute, Open Approach
00UK37Z Supplement Trigeminal Nerve with Autologous Tissue Substitute, Percutaneous Approach
00UK47Z Supplement Trigeminal Nerve with Autologous Tissue Substitute, Percutaneous Endoscopic Approach
00UL07Z Supplement Abducens Nerve with Autologous Tissue Substitute, Open Approach
00UL37Z Supplement Abducens Nerve with Autologous Tissue Substitute, Percutaneous Approach
00UL47Z Supplement Abducens Nerve with Autologous Tissue Substitute, Percutaneous Endoscopic Approach
00UM07Z Supplement Facial Nerve with Autologous Tissue Substitute, Open Approach
00UM37Z Supplement Facial Nerve with Autologous Tissue Substitute, Percutaneous Approach
00UM47Z Supplement Facial Nerve with Autologous Tissue Substitute, Percutaneous Endoscopic Approach
00UN07Z Supplement Acoustic Nerve with Autologous Tissue Substitute, Open Approach
00UN37Z Supplement Acoustic Nerve with Autologous Tissue Substitute, Percutaneous Approach
00UN47Z Supplement Acoustic Nerve with Autologous Tissue Substitute, Percutaneous Endoscopic Approach
00UP07Z Supplement Glossopharyngeal Nerve with Autologous Tissue Substitute, Open Approach
00UP37Z Supplement Glossopharyngeal Nerve with Autologous Tissue Substitute, Percutaneous Approach
00UP47Z Supplement Glossopharyngeal Nerve with Autologous Tissue Substitute, Percutaneous Endoscopic Approach
00UQ07Z Supplement Vagus Nerve with Autologous Tissue Substitute, Open Approach
00UQ37Z Supplement Vagus Nerve with Autologous Tissue Substitute, Percutaneous Approach
00UQ47Z Supplement Vagus Nerve with Autologous Tissue Substitute, Percutaneous Endoscopic Approach
00UR07Z Supplement Accessory Nerve with Autologous Tissue Substitute, Open Approach
00UR37Z Supplement Accessory Nerve with Autologous Tissue Substitute, Percutaneous Approach
00UR47Z Supplement Accessory Nerve with Autologous Tissue Substitute, Percutaneous Endoscopic Approach
00US07Z Supplement Hypoglossal Nerve with Autologous Tissue Substitute, Open Approach
00US37Z Supplement Hypoglossal Nerve with Autologous Tissue Substitute, Percutaneous Approach

00US47Z Supplement Hypoglossal Nerve with Autologous Tissue Substitute, Percutaneous Endoscopic Approach
00UT07Z Supplement Spinal Meninges with Autologous Tissue Substitute, Open Approach
00UT0JZ Supplement Spinal Meninges with Synthetic Substitute, Open Approach
00UT0KZ Supplement Spinal Meninges with Nonautologous Tissue Substitute, Open Approach
00UT37Z Supplement Spinal Meninges with Autologous Tissue Substitute, Percutaneous Approach
00UT3JZ Supplement Spinal Meninges with Synthetic Substitute, Percutaneous Approach
00UT3KZ Supplement Spinal Meninges with Nonautologous Tissue Substitute, Percutaneous Approach
00UT47Z Supplement Spinal Meninges with Autologous Tissue Substitute, Percutaneous Endoscopic Approach
00UT4JZ Supplement Spinal Meninges with Synthetic Substitute, Percutaneous Endoscopic Approach
00UT4KZ Supplement Spinal Meninges with Nonautologous Tissue Substitute, Percutaneous Endoscopic Approach

00W – Central Nervous System, Revision

Review Coding Guideline B6.1c

00W000Z Revision of Drainage Device in Brain, Open Approach
00W002Z Revision of Monitoring Device in Brain, Open Approach
00W003Z Revision of Infusion Device in Brain, Open Approach
00W007Z Revision of Autologous Tissue Substitute in Brain, Open Approach
00W00JZ Revision of Synthetic Substitute in Brain, Open Approach
00W00KZ Revision of Nonautologous Tissue Substitute in Brain, Open Approach
00W00MZ Revision of Neurostimulator Lead in Brain, Open Approach
00W030Z Revision of Drainage Device in Brain, Percutaneous Approach
00W032Z Revision of Monitoring Device in Brain, Percutaneous Approach
00W033Z Revision of Infusion Device in Brain, Percutaneous Approach
00W037Z Revision of Autologous Tissue Substitute in Brain, Percutaneous Approach
00W03JZ Revision of Synthetic Substitute in Brain, Percutaneous Approach
00W03KZ Revision of Nonautologous Tissue Substitute in Brain, Percutaneous Approach
00W03MZ Revision of Neurostimulator Lead in Brain, Percutaneous Approach
00W040Z Revision of Drainage Device in Brain, Percutaneous Endoscopic Approach
00W042Z Revision of Monitoring Device in Brain, Percutaneous Endoscopic Approach
00W043Z Revision of Infusion Device in Brain, Percutaneous Endoscopic Approach
00W047Z Revision of Autologous Tissue Substitute in Brain, Percutaneous Endoscopic Approach
00W04JZ Revision of Synthetic Substitute in Brain, Percutaneous Endoscopic Approach
00W04KZ Revision of Nonautologous Tissue Substitute in Brain, Percutaneous Endoscopic Approach
00W04MZ Revision of Neurostimulator Lead in Brain, Percutaneous Endoscopic Approach
00W0X0Z Revision of Drainage Device in Brain, External Approach
00W0X2Z Revision of Monitoring Device in Brain, External Approach
00W0X3Z Revision of Infusion Device in Brain, External Approach
00W0X7Z Revision of Autologous Tissue Substitute in Brain, External Approach
00W0XJZ Revision of Synthetic Substitute in Brain, External Approach
00W0XKZ Revision of Nonautologous Tissue Substitute in Brain, External Approach
00W0XMZ Revision of Neurostimulator Lead in Brain, External Approach
00W600Z Revision of Drainage Device in Cerebral Ventricle, Open Approach
00W602Z Revision of Monitoring Device in Cerebral Ventricle, Open Approach
00W603Z Revision of Infusion Device in Cerebral Ventricle, Open Approach
00W60JZ Revision of Synthetic Substitute in Cerebral Ventricle, Open Approach
00W60MZ Revision of Neurostimulator Lead in Cerebral Ventricle, Open Approach
00W630Z Revision of Drainage Device in Cerebral Ventricle, Percutaneous Approach
00W632Z Revision of Monitoring Device in Cerebral Ventricle, Percutaneous Approach
00W633Z Revision of Infusion Device in Cerebral Ventricle, Percutaneous Approach
00W63JZ Revision of Synthetic Substitute in Cerebral Ventricle, Percutaneous Approach
00W63MZ Revision of Neurostimulator Lead in Cerebral Ventricle, Percutaneous Approach
00W640Z Revision of Drainage Device in Cerebral Ventricle, Percutaneous Endoscopic Approach
00W642Z Revision of Monitoring Device in Cerebral Ventricle, Percutaneous Endoscopic Approach
00W643Z Revision of Infusion Device in Cerebral Ventricle, Percutaneous Endoscopic Approach
00W64JZ Revision of Synthetic Substitute in Cerebral Ventricle, Percutaneous Endoscopic Approach
00W64MZ Revision of Neurostimulator Lead in Cerebral Ventricle, Percutaneous Endoscopic Approach
00W6X0Z Revision of Drainage Device in Cerebral Ventricle, External Approach
00W6X2Z Revision of Monitoring Device in Cerebral Ventricle, External Approach
00W6X3Z Revision of Infusion Device in Cerebral Ventricle, External Approach
00W6XJZ Revision of Synthetic Substitute in Cerebral Ventricle, External Approach
00W6XMZ Revision of Neurostimulator Lead in Cerebral Ventricle, External Approach
00WE00Z Revision of Drainage Device in Cranial Nerve, Open Approach
00WE02Z Revision of Monitoring Device in Cranial Nerve, Open Approach
00WE03Z Revision of Infusion Device in Cranial Nerve, Open Approach
00WE07Z Revision of Autologous Tissue Substitute in Cranial Nerve, Open Approach
00WE0MZ Revision of Neurostimulator Lead in Cranial Nerve, Open Approach
00WE30Z Revision of Drainage Device in Cranial Nerve, Percutaneous Approach
00WE32Z Revision of Monitoring Device in Cranial Nerve, Percutaneous Approach
00WE33Z Revision of Infusion Device in Cranial Nerve, Percutaneous Approach
00WE37Z Revision of Autologous Tissue Substitute in Cranial Nerve, Percutaneous Approach
00WE3MZ Revision of Neurostimulator Lead in Cranial Nerve, Percutaneous Approach
00WE40Z Revision of Drainage Device in Cranial Nerve, Percutaneous Endoscopic Approach
00WE42Z Revision of Monitoring Device in Cranial Nerve, Percutaneous Endoscopic Approach
00WE43Z Revision of Infusion Device in Cranial Nerve, Percutaneous Endoscopic Approach
00WE47Z Revision of Autologous Tissue Substitute in Cranial Nerve, Percutaneous Endoscopic Approach
00WE4MZ Revision of Neurostimulator Lead in Cranial Nerve, Percutaneous Endoscopic Approach
00WEX0Z Revision of Drainage Device in Cranial Nerve, External Approach
00WEX2Z Revision of Monitoring Device in Cranial Nerve, External Approach
00WEX3Z Revision of Infusion Device in Cranial Nerve, External Approach
00WEX7Z Revision of Autologous Tissue Substitute in Cranial Nerve, External Approach
00WEXMZ Revision of Neurostimulator Lead in Cranial Nerve, External Approach
00WU00Z Revision of Drainage Device in Spinal Canal, Open Approach
00WU02Z Revision of Monitoring Device in Spinal Canal, Open Approach
00WU03Z Revision of Infusion Device in Spinal Canal, Open Approach
00WU0JZ Revision of Synthetic Substitute in Spinal Canal, Open Approach
00WU0MZ Revision of Neurostimulator Lead in Spinal Canal, Open Approach
00WU30Z Revision of Drainage Device in Spinal Canal, Percutaneous Approach
00WU32Z Revision of Monitoring Device in Spinal Canal, Percutaneous Approach
00WU33Z Revision of Infusion Device in Spinal Canal, Percutaneous Approach
00WU3JZ Revision of Synthetic Substitute in Spinal Canal, Percutaneous Approach
00WU3MZ Revision of Neurostimulator Lead in Spinal Canal, Percutaneous Approach
00WU40Z Revision of Drainage Device in Spinal Canal, Percutaneous Endoscopic Approach
00WU42Z Revision of Monitoring Device in Spinal Canal, Percutaneous Endoscopic Approach
00WU43Z Revision of Infusion Device in Spinal Canal, Percutaneous Endoscopic Approach
00WU4JZ Revision of Synthetic Substitute in Spinal Canal, Percutaneous Endoscopic Approach

00WU4MZ Revision of Neurostimulator Lead in Spinal Canal, Percutaneous Endoscopic Approach
00WUX0Z Revision of Drainage Device in Spinal Canal, External Approach
00WUX2Z Revision of Monitoring Device in Spinal Canal, External Approach
00WUX3Z Revision of Infusion Device in Spinal Canal, External Approach
00WUXJZ Revision of Synthetic Substitute in Spinal Canal, External Approach
00WUXMZ Revision of Neurostimulator Lead in Spinal Canal, External Approach
00WV00Z Revision of Drainage Device in Spinal Cord, Open Approach
00WV02Z Revision of Monitoring Device in Spinal Cord, Open Approach
00WV03Z Revision of Infusion Device in Spinal Cord, Open Approach
00WV07Z Revision of Autologous Tissue Substitute in Spinal Cord, Open Approach
00WV0JZ Revision of Synthetic Substitute in Spinal Cord, Open Approach
00WV0KZ Revision of Nonautologous Tissue Substitute in Spinal Cord, Open Approach
00WV0MZ Revision of Neurostimulator Lead in Spinal Cord, Open Approach
00WV30Z Revision of Drainage Device in Spinal Cord, Percutaneous Approach
00WV32Z Revision of Monitoring Device in Spinal Cord, Percutaneous Approach
00WV33Z Revision of Infusion Device in Spinal Cord, Percutaneous Approach
00WV37Z Revision of Autologous Tissue Substitute in Spinal Cord, Percutaneous Approach
00WV3JZ Revision of Synthetic Substitute in Spinal Cord, Percutaneous Approach
00WV3KZ Revision of Nonautologous Tissue Substitute in Spinal Cord, Percutaneous Approach
00WV3MZ Revision of Neurostimulator Lead in Spinal Cord, Percutaneous Approach
00WV40Z Revision of Drainage Device in Spinal Cord, Percutaneous Endoscopic Approach
00WV42Z Revision of Monitoring Device in Spinal Cord, Percutaneous Endoscopic Approach
00WV43Z Revision of Infusion Device in Spinal Cord, Percutaneous Endoscopic Approach
00WV47Z Revision of Autologous Tissue Substitute in Spinal Cord, Percutaneous Endoscopic Approach
00WV4JZ Revision of Synthetic Substitute in Spinal Cord, Percutaneous Endoscopic Approach
00WV4KZ Revision of Nonautologous Tissue Substitute in Spinal Cord, Percutaneous Endoscopic Approach
00WV4MZ Revision of Neurostimulator Lead in Spinal Cord, Percutaneous Endoscopic Approach
00WVX0Z Revision of Drainage Device in Spinal Cord, External Approach
00WVX2Z Revision of Monitoring Device in Spinal Cord, External Approach
00WVX3Z Revision of Infusion Device in Spinal Cord, External Approach
00WVX7Z Revision of Autologous Tissue Substitute in Spinal Cord, External Approach
00WVXJZ Revision of Synthetic Substitute in Spinal Cord, External Approach
00WVXKZ Revision of Nonautologous Tissue Substitute in Spinal Cord, External Approach
00WVXMZ Revision of Neurostimulator Lead in Spinal Cord, External Approach

00X – Central Nervous System, Transfer

00XF0ZF Transfer Olfactory Nerve to Olfactory Nerve, Open Approach
00XF0ZG Transfer Olfactory Nerve to Optic Nerve, Open Approach
00XF0ZH Transfer Olfactory Nerve to Oculomotor Nerve, Open Approach
00XF0ZJ Transfer Olfactory Nerve to Trochlear Nerve, Open Approach
00XF0ZK Transfer Olfactory Nerve to Trigeminal Nerve, Open Approach
00XF0ZL Transfer Olfactory Nerve to Abducens Nerve, Open Approach
00XF0ZM Transfer Olfactory Nerve to Facial Nerve, Open Approach
00XF0ZN Transfer Olfactory Nerve to Acoustic Nerve, Open Approach
00XF0ZP Transfer Olfactory Nerve to Glossopharyngeal Nerve, Open Approach
00XF0ZQ Transfer Olfactory Nerve to Vagus Nerve, Open Approach
00XF0ZR Transfer Olfactory Nerve to Accessory Nerve, Open Approach
00XF0ZS Transfer Olfactory Nerve to Hypoglossal Nerve, Open Approach
00XF4ZF Transfer Olfactory Nerve to Olfactory Nerve, Percutaneous Endoscopic Approach
00XF4ZG Transfer Olfactory Nerve to Optic Nerve, Percutaneous Endoscopic Approach
00XF4ZH Transfer Olfactory Nerve to Oculomotor Nerve, Percutaneous Endoscopic Approach
00XF4ZJ Transfer Olfactory Nerve to Trochlear Nerve, Percutaneous Endoscopic Approach
00XF4ZK Transfer Olfactory Nerve to Trigeminal Nerve, Percutaneous Endoscopic Approach
00XF4ZL Transfer Olfactory Nerve to Abducens Nerve, Percutaneous Endoscopic Approach
00XF4ZM Transfer Olfactory Nerve to Facial Nerve, Percutaneous Endoscopic Approach
00XF4ZN Transfer Olfactory Nerve to Acoustic Nerve, Percutaneous Endoscopic Approach
00XF4ZP Transfer Olfactory Nerve to Glossopharyngeal Nerve, Percutaneous Endoscopic Approach
00XF4ZQ Transfer Olfactory Nerve to Vagus Nerve, Percutaneous Endoscopic Approach
00XF4ZR Transfer Olfactory Nerve to Accessory Nerve, Percutaneous Endoscopic Approach
00XF4ZS Transfer Olfactory Nerve to Hypoglossal Nerve, Percutaneous Endoscopic Approach
00XG0ZF Transfer Optic Nerve to Olfactory Nerve, Open Approach
00XG0ZG Transfer Optic Nerve to Optic Nerve, Open Approach
00XG0ZH Transfer Optic Nerve to Oculomotor Nerve, Open Approach
00XG0ZJ Transfer Optic Nerve to Trochlear Nerve, Open Approach
00XG0ZK Transfer Optic Nerve to Trigeminal Nerve, Open Approach
00XG0ZL Transfer Optic Nerve to Abducens Nerve, Open Approach
00XG0ZM Transfer Optic Nerve to Facial Nerve, Open Approach
00XG0ZN Transfer Optic Nerve to Acoustic Nerve, Open Approach
00XG0ZP Transfer Optic Nerve to Glossopharyngeal Nerve, Open Approach
00XG0ZQ Transfer Optic Nerve to Vagus Nerve, Open Approach
00XG0ZR Transfer Optic Nerve to Accessory Nerve, Open Approach
00XG0ZS Transfer Optic Nerve to Hypoglossal Nerve, Open Approach
00XG4ZF Transfer Optic Nerve to Olfactory Nerve, Percutaneous Endoscopic Approach
00XG4ZG Transfer Optic Nerve to Optic Nerve, Percutaneous Endoscopic Approach
00XG4ZH Transfer Optic Nerve to Oculomotor Nerve, Percutaneous Endoscopic Approach
00XG4ZJ Transfer Optic Nerve to Trochlear Nerve, Percutaneous Endoscopic Approach
00XG4ZK Transfer Optic Nerve to Trigeminal Nerve, Percutaneous Endoscopic Approach
00XG4ZL Transfer Optic Nerve to Abducens Nerve, Percutaneous Endoscopic Approach
00XG4ZM Transfer Optic Nerve to Facial Nerve, Percutaneous Endoscopic Approach
00XG4ZN Transfer Optic Nerve to Acoustic Nerve, Percutaneous Endoscopic Approach
00XG4ZP Transfer Optic Nerve to Glossopharyngeal Nerve, Percutaneous Endoscopic Approach
00XG4ZQ Transfer Optic Nerve to Vagus Nerve, Percutaneous Endoscopic Approach
00XG4ZR Transfer Optic Nerve to Accessory Nerve, Percutaneous Endoscopic Approach
00XG4ZS Transfer Optic Nerve to Hypoglossal Nerve, Percutaneous Endoscopic Approach
00XH0ZF Transfer Oculomotor Nerve to Olfactory Nerve, Open Approach
00XH0ZG Transfer Oculomotor Nerve to Optic Nerve, Open Approach
00XH0ZH Transfer Oculomotor Nerve to Oculomotor Nerve, Open Approach
00XH0ZJ Transfer Oculomotor Nerve to Trochlear Nerve, Open Approach
00XH0ZK Transfer Oculomotor Nerve to Trigeminal Nerve, Open Approach
00XH0ZL Transfer Oculomotor Nerve to Abducens Nerve, Open Approach
00XH0ZM Transfer Oculomotor Nerve to Facial Nerve, Open Approach
00XH0ZN Transfer Oculomotor Nerve to Acoustic Nerve, Open Approach
00XH0ZP Transfer Oculomotor Nerve to Glossopharyngeal Nerve, Open Approach
00XH0ZQ Transfer Oculomotor Nerve to Vagus Nerve, Open Approach
00XH0ZR Transfer Oculomotor Nerve to Accessory Nerve, Open Approach
00XH0ZS Transfer Oculomotor Nerve to Hypoglossal Nerve, Open Approach
00XH4ZF Transfer Oculomotor Nerve to Olfactory Nerve, Percutaneous Endoscopic Approach

00XH4ZG Transfer Oculomotor Nerve to Optic Nerve, Percutaneous Endoscopic Approach
00XH4ZH Transfer Oculomotor Nerve to Oculomotor Nerve, Percutaneous Endoscopic Approach
00XH4ZJ Transfer Oculomotor Nerve to Trochlear Nerve, Percutaneous Endoscopic Approach
00XH4ZK Transfer Oculomotor Nerve to Trigeminal Nerve, Percutaneous Endoscopic Approach
00XH4ZL Transfer Oculomotor Nerve to Abducens Nerve, Percutaneous Endoscopic Approach
00XH4ZM Transfer Oculomotor Nerve to Facial Nerve, Percutaneous Endoscopic Approach
00XH4ZN Transfer Oculomotor Nerve to Acoustic Nerve, Percutaneous Endoscopic Approach
00XH4ZP Transfer Oculomotor Nerve to Glossopharyngeal Nerve, Percutaneous Endoscopic Approach
00XH4ZQ Transfer Oculomotor Nerve to Vagus Nerve, Percutaneous Endoscopic Approach
00XH4ZR Transfer Oculomotor Nerve to Accessory Nerve, Percutaneous Endoscopic Approach
00XH4ZS Transfer Oculomotor Nerve to Hypoglossal Nerve, Percutaneous Endoscopic Approach
00XJ0ZF Transfer Trochlear Nerve to Olfactory Nerve, Open Approach
00XJ0ZG Transfer Trochlear Nerve to Optic Nerve, Open Approach
00XJ0ZH Transfer Trochlear Nerve to Oculomotor Nerve, Open Approach
00XJ0ZJ Transfer Trochlear Nerve to Trochlear Nerve, Open Approach
00XJ0ZK Transfer Trochlear Nerve to Trigeminal Nerve, Open Approach
00XJ0ZL Transfer Trochlear Nerve to Abducens Nerve, Open Approach
00XJ0ZM Transfer Trochlear Nerve to Facial Nerve, Open Approach
00XJ0ZN Transfer Trochlear Nerve to Acoustic Nerve, Open Approach
00XJ0ZP Transfer Trochlear Nerve to Glossopharyngeal Nerve, Open Approach
00XJ0ZQ Transfer Trochlear Nerve to Vagus Nerve, Open Approach
00XJ0ZR Transfer Trochlear Nerve to Accessory Nerve, Open Approach
00XJ0ZS Transfer Trochlear Nerve to Hypoglossal Nerve, Open Approach
00XJ4ZF Transfer Trochlear Nerve to Olfactory Nerve, Percutaneous Endoscopic Approach
00XJ4ZG Transfer Trochlear Nerve to Optic Nerve, Percutaneous Endoscopic Approach
00XJ4ZH Transfer Trochlear Nerve to Oculomotor Nerve, Percutaneous Endoscopic Approach
00XJ4ZJ Transfer Trochlear Nerve to Trochlear Nerve, Percutaneous Endoscopic Approach
00XJ4ZK Transfer Trochlear Nerve to Trigeminal Nerve, Percutaneous Endoscopic Approach
00XJ4ZL Transfer Trochlear Nerve to Abducens Nerve, Percutaneous Endoscopic Approach
00XJ4ZM Transfer Trochlear Nerve to Facial Nerve, Percutaneous Endoscopic Approach
00XJ4ZN Transfer Trochlear Nerve to Acoustic Nerve, Percutaneous Endoscopic Approach
00XJ4ZP Transfer Trochlear Nerve to Glossopharyngeal Nerve, Percutaneous Endoscopic Approach
00XJ4ZQ Transfer Trochlear Nerve to Vagus Nerve, Percutaneous Endoscopic Approach
00XJ4ZR Transfer Trochlear Nerve to Accessory Nerve, Percutaneous Endoscopic Approach
00XJ4ZS Transfer Trochlear Nerve to Hypoglossal Nerve, Percutaneous Endoscopic Approach
00XK0ZF Transfer Trigeminal Nerve to Olfactory Nerve, Open Approach
00XK0ZG Transfer Trigeminal Nerve to Optic Nerve, Open Approach
00XK0ZH Transfer Trigeminal Nerve to Oculomotor Nerve, Open Approach
00XK0ZJ Transfer Trigeminal Nerve to Trochlear Nerve, Open Approach
00XK0ZK Transfer Trigeminal Nerve to Trigeminal Nerve, Open Approach
00XK0ZL Transfer Trigeminal Nerve to Abducens Nerve, Open Approach
00XK0ZM Transfer Trigeminal Nerve to Facial Nerve, Open Approach
00XK0ZN Transfer Trigeminal Nerve to Acoustic Nerve, Open Approach
00XK0ZP Transfer Trigeminal Nerve to Glossopharyngeal Nerve, Open Approach
00XK0ZQ Transfer Trigeminal Nerve to Vagus Nerve, Open Approach
00XK0ZR Transfer Trigeminal Nerve to Accessory Nerve, Open Approach
00XK0ZS Transfer Trigeminal Nerve to Hypoglossal Nerve, Open Approach
00XK4ZF Transfer Trigeminal Nerve to Olfactory Nerve, Percutaneous Endoscopic Approach
00XK4ZG Transfer Trigeminal Nerve to Optic Nerve, Percutaneous Endoscopic Approach
00XK4ZH Transfer Trigeminal Nerve to Oculomotor Nerve, Percutaneous Endoscopic Approach
00XK4ZJ Transfer Trigeminal Nerve to Trochlear Nerve, Percutaneous Endoscopic Approach
00XK4ZK Transfer Trigeminal Nerve to Trigeminal Nerve, Percutaneous Endoscopic Approach
00XK4ZL Transfer Trigeminal Nerve to Abducens Nerve, Percutaneous Endoscopic Approach
00XK4ZM Transfer Trigeminal Nerve to Facial Nerve, Percutaneous Endoscopic Approach
00XK4ZN Transfer Trigeminal Nerve to Acoustic Nerve, Percutaneous Endoscopic Approach
00XK4ZP Transfer Trigeminal Nerve to Glossopharyngeal Nerve, Percutaneous Endoscopic Approach
00XK4ZQ Transfer Trigeminal Nerve to Vagus Nerve, Percutaneous Endoscopic Approach
00XK4ZR Transfer Trigeminal Nerve to Accessory Nerve, Percutaneous Endoscopic Approach
00XK4ZS Transfer Trigeminal Nerve to Hypoglossal Nerve, Percutaneous Endoscopic Approach
00XL0ZF Transfer Abducens Nerve to Olfactory Nerve, Open Approach
00XL0ZG Transfer Abducens Nerve to Optic Nerve, Open Approach
00XL0ZH Transfer Abducens Nerve to Oculomotor Nerve, Open Approach
00XL0ZJ Transfer Abducens Nerve to Trochlear Nerve, Open Approach
00XL0ZK Transfer Abducens Nerve to Trigeminal Nerve, Open Approach
00XL0ZL Transfer Abducens Nerve to Abducens Nerve, Open Approach
00XL0ZM Transfer Abducens Nerve to Facial Nerve, Open Approach
00XL0ZN Transfer Abducens Nerve to Acoustic Nerve, Open Approach
00XL0ZP Transfer Abducens Nerve to Glossopharyngeal Nerve, Open Approach
00XL0ZQ Transfer Abducens Nerve to Vagus Nerve, Open Approach
00XL0ZR Transfer Abducens Nerve to Accessory Nerve, Open Approach
00XL0ZS Transfer Abducens Nerve to Hypoglossal Nerve, Open Approach
00XL4ZF Transfer Abducens Nerve to Olfactory Nerve, Percutaneous Endoscopic Approach
00XL4ZG Transfer Abducens Nerve to Optic Nerve, Percutaneous Endoscopic Approach
00XL4ZH Transfer Abducens Nerve to Oculomotor Nerve, Percutaneous Endoscopic Approach
00XL4ZJ Transfer Abducens Nerve to Trochlear Nerve, Percutaneous Endoscopic Approach
00XL4ZK Transfer Abducens Nerve to Trigeminal Nerve, Percutaneous Endoscopic Approach
00XL4ZL Transfer Abducens Nerve to Abducens Nerve, Percutaneous Endoscopic Approach
00XL4ZM Transfer Abducens Nerve to Facial Nerve, Percutaneous Endoscopic Approach
00XL4ZN Transfer Abducens Nerve to Acoustic Nerve, Percutaneous Endoscopic Approach
00XL4ZP Transfer Abducens Nerve to Glossopharyngeal Nerve, Percutaneous Endoscopic Approach
00XL4ZQ Transfer Abducens Nerve to Vagus Nerve, Percutaneous Endoscopic Approach
00XL4ZR Transfer Abducens Nerve to Accessory Nerve, Percutaneous Endoscopic Approach
00XL4ZS Transfer Abducens Nerve to Hypoglossal Nerve, Percutaneous Endoscopic Approach
00XM0ZF Transfer Facial Nerve to Olfactory Nerve, Open Approach
00XM0ZG Transfer Facial Nerve to Optic Nerve, Open Approach
00XM0ZH Transfer Facial Nerve to Oculomotor Nerve, Open Approach
00XM0ZJ Transfer Facial Nerve to Trochlear Nerve, Open Approach
00XM0ZK Transfer Facial Nerve to Trigeminal Nerve, Open Approach
00XM0ZL Transfer Facial Nerve to Abducens Nerve, Open Approach
00XM0ZM Transfer Facial Nerve to Facial Nerve, Open Approach
00XM0ZN Transfer Facial Nerve to Acoustic Nerve, Open Approach
00XM0ZP Transfer Facial Nerve to Glossopharyngeal Nerve, Open Approach
00XM0ZQ Transfer Facial Nerve to Vagus Nerve, Open Approach
00XM0ZR Transfer Facial Nerve to Accessory Nerve, Open Approach

00XM0ZS Transfer Facial Nerve to Hypoglossal Nerve, Open Approach
00XM4ZF Transfer Facial Nerve to Olfactory Nerve, Percutaneous Endoscopic Approach
00XM4ZG Transfer Facial Nerve to Optic Nerve, Percutaneous Endoscopic Approach
00XM4ZH Transfer Facial Nerve to Oculomotor Nerve, Percutaneous Endoscopic Approach
00XM4ZJ Transfer Facial Nerve to Trochlear Nerve, Percutaneous Endoscopic Approach
00XM4ZK Transfer Facial Nerve to Trigeminal Nerve, Percutaneous Endoscopic Approach
00XM4ZL Transfer Facial Nerve to Abducens Nerve, Percutaneous Endoscopic Approach
00XM4ZM Transfer Facial Nerve to Facial Nerve, Percutaneous Endoscopic Approach
00XM4ZN Transfer Facial Nerve to Acoustic Nerve, Percutaneous Endoscopic Approach
00XM4ZP Transfer Facial Nerve to Glossopharyngeal Nerve, Percutaneous Endoscopic Approach
00XM4ZQ Transfer Facial Nerve to Vagus Nerve, Percutaneous Endoscopic Approach
00XM4ZR Transfer Facial Nerve to Accessory Nerve, Percutaneous Endoscopic Approach
00XM4ZS Transfer Facial Nerve to Hypoglossal Nerve, Percutaneous Endoscopic Approach
00XN0ZF Transfer Acoustic Nerve to Olfactory Nerve, Open Approach
00XN0ZG Transfer Acoustic Nerve to Optic Nerve, Open Approach
00XN0ZH Transfer Acoustic Nerve to Oculomotor Nerve, Open Approach
00XN0ZJ Transfer Acoustic Nerve to Trochlear Nerve, Open Approach
00XN0ZK Transfer Acoustic Nerve to Trigeminal Nerve, Open Approach
00XN0ZL Transfer Acoustic Nerve to Abducens Nerve, Open Approach
00XN0ZM Transfer Acoustic Nerve to Facial Nerve, Open Approach
00XN0ZN Transfer Acoustic Nerve to Acoustic Nerve, Open Approach
00XN0ZP Transfer Acoustic Nerve to Glossopharyngeal Nerve, Open Approach
00XN0ZQ Transfer Acoustic Nerve to Vagus Nerve, Open Approach
00XN0ZR Transfer Acoustic Nerve to Accessory Nerve, Open Approach
00XN0ZS Transfer Acoustic Nerve to Hypoglossal Nerve, Open Approach
00XN4ZF Transfer Acoustic Nerve to Olfactory Nerve, Percutaneous Endoscopic Approach
00XN4ZG Transfer Acoustic Nerve to Optic Nerve, Percutaneous Endoscopic Approach
00XN4ZH Transfer Acoustic Nerve to Oculomotor Nerve, Percutaneous Endoscopic Approach
00XN4ZJ Transfer Acoustic Nerve to Trochlear Nerve, Percutaneous Endoscopic Approach
00XN4ZK Transfer Acoustic Nerve to Trigeminal Nerve, Percutaneous Endoscopic Approach
00XN4ZL Transfer Acoustic Nerve to Abducens Nerve, Percutaneous Endoscopic Approach
00XN4ZM Transfer Acoustic Nerve to Facial Nerve, Percutaneous Endoscopic Approach
00XN4ZN Transfer Acoustic Nerve to Acoustic Nerve, Percutaneous Endoscopic Approach
00XN4ZP Transfer Acoustic Nerve to Glossopharyngeal Nerve, Percutaneous Endoscopic Approach
00XN4ZQ Transfer Acoustic Nerve to Vagus Nerve, Percutaneous Endoscopic Approach
00XN4ZR Transfer Acoustic Nerve to Accessory Nerve, Percutaneous Endoscopic Approach
00XN4ZS Transfer Acoustic Nerve to Hypoglossal Nerve, Percutaneous Endoscopic Approach
00XP0ZF Transfer Glossopharyngeal Nerve to Olfactory Nerve, Open Approach
00XP0ZG Transfer Glossopharyngeal Nerve to Optic Nerve, Open Approach
00XP0ZH Transfer Glossopharyngeal Nerve to Oculomotor Nerve, Open Approach
00XP0ZJ Transfer Glossopharyngeal Nerve to Trochlear Nerve, Open Approach
00XP0ZK Transfer Glossopharyngeal Nerve to Trigeminal Nerve, Open Approach
00XP0ZL Transfer Glossopharyngeal Nerve to Abducens Nerve, Open Approach
00XP0ZM Transfer Glossopharyngeal Nerve to Facial Nerve, Open Approach
00XP0ZN Transfer Glossopharyngeal Nerve to Acoustic Nerve, Open Approach
00XP0ZP Transfer Glossopharyngeal Nerve to Glossopharyngeal Nerve, Open Approach
00XP0ZQ Transfer Glossopharyngeal Nerve to Vagus Nerve, Open Approach
00XP0ZR Transfer Glossopharyngeal Nerve to Accessory Nerve, Open Approach
00XP0ZS Transfer Glossopharyngeal Nerve to Hypoglossal Nerve, Open Approach
00XP4ZF Transfer Glossopharyngeal Nerve to Olfactory Nerve, Percutaneous Endoscopic Approach
00XP4ZG Transfer Glossopharyngeal Nerve to Optic Nerve, Percutaneous Endoscopic Approach
00XP4ZH Transfer Glossopharyngeal Nerve to Oculomotor Nerve, Percutaneous Endoscopic Approach
00XP4ZJ Transfer Glossopharyngeal Nerve to Trochlear Nerve, Percutaneous Endoscopic Approach
00XP4ZK Transfer Glossopharyngeal Nerve to Trigeminal Nerve, Percutaneous Endoscopic Approach
00XP4ZL Transfer Glossopharyngeal Nerve to Abducens Nerve, Percutaneous Endoscopic Approach
00XP4ZM Transfer Glossopharyngeal Nerve to Facial Nerve, Percutaneous Endoscopic Approach
00XP4ZN Transfer Glossopharyngeal Nerve to Acoustic Nerve, Percutaneous Endoscopic Approach
00XP4ZP Transfer Glossopharyngeal Nerve to Glossopharyngeal Nerve, Percutaneous Endoscopic Approach
00XP4ZQ Transfer Glossopharyngeal Nerve to Vagus Nerve, Percutaneous Endoscopic Approach
00XP4ZR Transfer Glossopharyngeal Nerve to Accessory Nerve, Percutaneous Endoscopic Approach
00XP4ZS Transfer Glossopharyngeal Nerve to Hypoglossal Nerve, Percutaneous Endoscopic Approach
00XQ0ZF Transfer Vagus Nerve to Olfactory Nerve, Open Approach
00XQ0ZG Transfer Vagus Nerve to Optic Nerve, Open Approach
00XQ0ZH Transfer Vagus Nerve to Oculomotor Nerve, Open Approach
00XQ0ZJ Transfer Vagus Nerve to Trochlear Nerve, Open Approach
00XQ0ZK Transfer Vagus Nerve to Trigeminal Nerve, Open Approach
00XQ0ZL Transfer Vagus Nerve to Abducens Nerve, Open Approach
00XQ0ZM Transfer Vagus Nerve to Facial Nerve, Open Approach
00XQ0ZN Transfer Vagus Nerve to Acoustic Nerve, Open Approach
00XQ0ZP Transfer Vagus Nerve to Glossopharyngeal Nerve, Open Approach
00XQ0ZQ Transfer Vagus Nerve to Vagus Nerve, Open Approach
00XQ0ZR Transfer Vagus Nerve to Accessory Nerve, Open Approach
00XQ0ZS Transfer Vagus Nerve to Hypoglossal Nerve, Open Approach
00XQ4ZF Transfer Vagus Nerve to Olfactory Nerve, Percutaneous Endoscopic Approach
00XQ4ZG Transfer Vagus Nerve to Optic Nerve, Percutaneous Endoscopic Approach
00XQ4ZH Transfer Vagus Nerve to Oculomotor Nerve, Percutaneous Endoscopic Approach
00XQ4ZJ Transfer Vagus Nerve to Trochlear Nerve, Percutaneous Endoscopic Approach
00XQ4ZK Transfer Vagus Nerve to Trigeminal Nerve, Percutaneous Endoscopic Approach
00XQ4ZL Transfer Vagus Nerve to Abducens Nerve, Percutaneous Endoscopic Approach
00XQ4ZM Transfer Vagus Nerve to Facial Nerve, Percutaneous Endoscopic Approach
00XQ4ZN Transfer Vagus Nerve to Acoustic Nerve, Percutaneous Endoscopic Approach
00XQ4ZP Transfer Vagus Nerve to Glossopharyngeal Nerve, Percutaneous Endoscopic Approach
00XQ4ZQ Transfer Vagus Nerve to Vagus Nerve, Percutaneous Endoscopic Approach
00XQ4ZR Transfer Vagus Nerve to Accessory Nerve, Percutaneous Endoscopic Approach
00XQ4ZS Transfer Vagus Nerve to Hypoglossal Nerve, Percutaneous Endoscopic Approach
00XR0ZF Transfer Accessory Nerve to Olfactory Nerve, Open Approach
00XR0ZG Transfer Accessory Nerve to Optic Nerve, Open Approach
00XR0ZH Transfer Accessory Nerve to Oculomotor Nerve, Open Approach
00XR0ZJ Transfer Accessory Nerve to Trochlear Nerve, Open Approach
00XR0ZK Transfer Accessory Nerve to Trigeminal Nerve, Open Approach
00XR0ZL Transfer Accessory Nerve to Abducens Nerve, Open Approach
00XR0ZM Transfer Accessory Nerve to Facial Nerve, Open Approach
00XR0ZN Transfer Accessory Nerve to Acoustic Nerve, Open Approach
00XR0ZP Transfer Accessory Nerve to Glossopharyngeal Nerve, Open Approach
00XR0ZQ Transfer Accessory Nerve to Vagus Nerve, Open Approach
00XR0ZR Transfer Accessory Nerve to Accessory Nerve, Open Approach
00XR0ZS Transfer Accessory Nerve to Hypoglossal Nerve, Open Approach
00XR4ZF Transfer Accessory Nerve to Olfactory Nerve, Percutaneous Endoscopic Approach
00XR4ZG Transfer Accessory Nerve to Optic Nerve, Percutaneous Endoscopic Approach
00XR4ZH Transfer Accessory Nerve to Oculomotor Nerve, Percutaneous Endoscopic Approach

00XR4ZJ Transfer Accessory Nerve to Trochlear Nerve, Percutaneous Endoscopic Approach

00XR4ZK Transfer Accessory Nerve to Trigeminal Nerve, Percutaneous Endoscopic Approach

00XR4ZL Transfer Accessory Nerve to Abducens Nerve, Percutaneous Endoscopic Approach

00XR4ZM Transfer Accessory Nerve to Facial Nerve, Percutaneous Endoscopic Approach

00XR4ZN Transfer Accessory Nerve to Acoustic Nerve, Percutaneous Endoscopic Approach

00XR4ZP Transfer Accessory Nerve to Glossopharyngeal Nerve, Percutaneous Endoscopic Approach

00XR4ZQ Transfer Accessory Nerve to Vagus Nerve, Percutaneous Endoscopic Approach

00XR4ZR Transfer Accessory Nerve to Accessory Nerve, Percutaneous Endoscopic Approach

00XR4ZS Transfer Accessory Nerve to Hypoglossal Nerve, Percutaneous Endoscopic Approach

00XS0ZF Transfer Hypoglossal Nerve to Olfactory Nerve, Open Approach

00XS0ZG Transfer Hypoglossal Nerve to Optic Nerve, Open Approach

00XS0ZH Transfer Hypoglossal Nerve to Oculomotor Nerve, Open Approach

00XS0ZJ Transfer Hypoglossal Nerve to Trochlear Nerve, Open Approach

00XS0ZK Transfer Hypoglossal Nerve to Trigeminal Nerve, Open Approach

00XS0ZL Transfer Hypoglossal Nerve to Abducens Nerve, Open Approach

00XS0ZM Transfer Hypoglossal Nerve to Facial Nerve, Open Approach

00XS0ZN Transfer Hypoglossal Nerve to Acoustic Nerve, Open Approach

00XS0ZP Transfer Hypoglossal Nerve to Glossopharyngeal Nerve, Open Approach

00XS0ZQ Transfer Hypoglossal Nerve to Vagus Nerve, Open Approach

00XS0ZR Transfer Hypoglossal Nerve to Accessory Nerve, Open Approach

00XS0ZS Transfer Hypoglossal Nerve to Hypoglossal Nerve, Open Approach

00XS4ZF Transfer Hypoglossal Nerve to Olfactory Nerve, Percutaneous Endoscopic Approach

00XS4ZG Transfer Hypoglossal Nerve to Optic Nerve, Percutaneous Endoscopic Approach

00XS4ZH Transfer Hypoglossal Nerve to Oculomotor Nerve, Percutaneous Endoscopic Approach

00XS4ZJ Transfer Hypoglossal Nerve to Trochlear Nerve, Percutaneous Endoscopic Approach

00XS4ZK Transfer Hypoglossal Nerve to Trigeminal Nerve, Percutaneous Endoscopic Approach

00XS4ZL Transfer Hypoglossal Nerve to Abducens Nerve, Percutaneous Endoscopic Approach

00XS4ZM Transfer Hypoglossal Nerve to Facial Nerve, Percutaneous Endoscopic Approach

00XS4ZN Transfer Hypoglossal Nerve to Acoustic Nerve, Percutaneous Endoscopic Approach

00XS4ZP Transfer Hypoglossal Nerve to Glossopharyngeal Nerve, Percutaneous Endoscopic Approach

00XS4ZQ Transfer Hypoglossal Nerve to Vagus Nerve, Percutaneous Endoscopic Approach

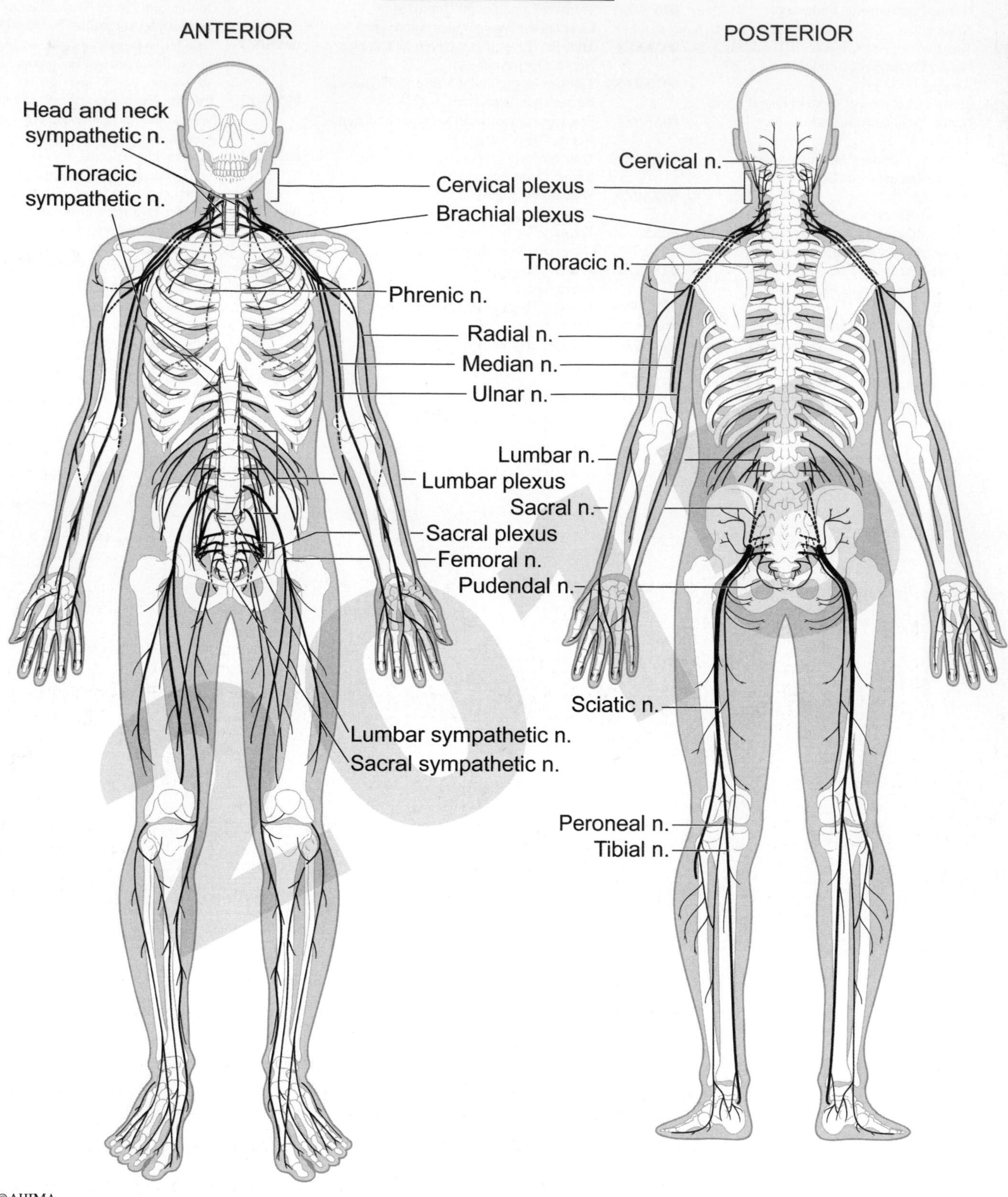
Peripheral Nervous System
ANTERIOR
POSTERIOR
Head and neck sympathetic n.
Thoracic sympathetic n.
Cervical n.
Cervical plexus
Brachial plexus
Thoracic n.
Phrenic n.
Radial n.
Median n.
Ulnar n.
Lumbar n.
Lumbar plexus
Sacral n.
Sacral plexus
Femoral n.
Pudendal n.
Sciatic n.
Lumbar sympathetic n.
Sacral sympathetic n.
Peroneal n.
Tibial n.

Spinal Column

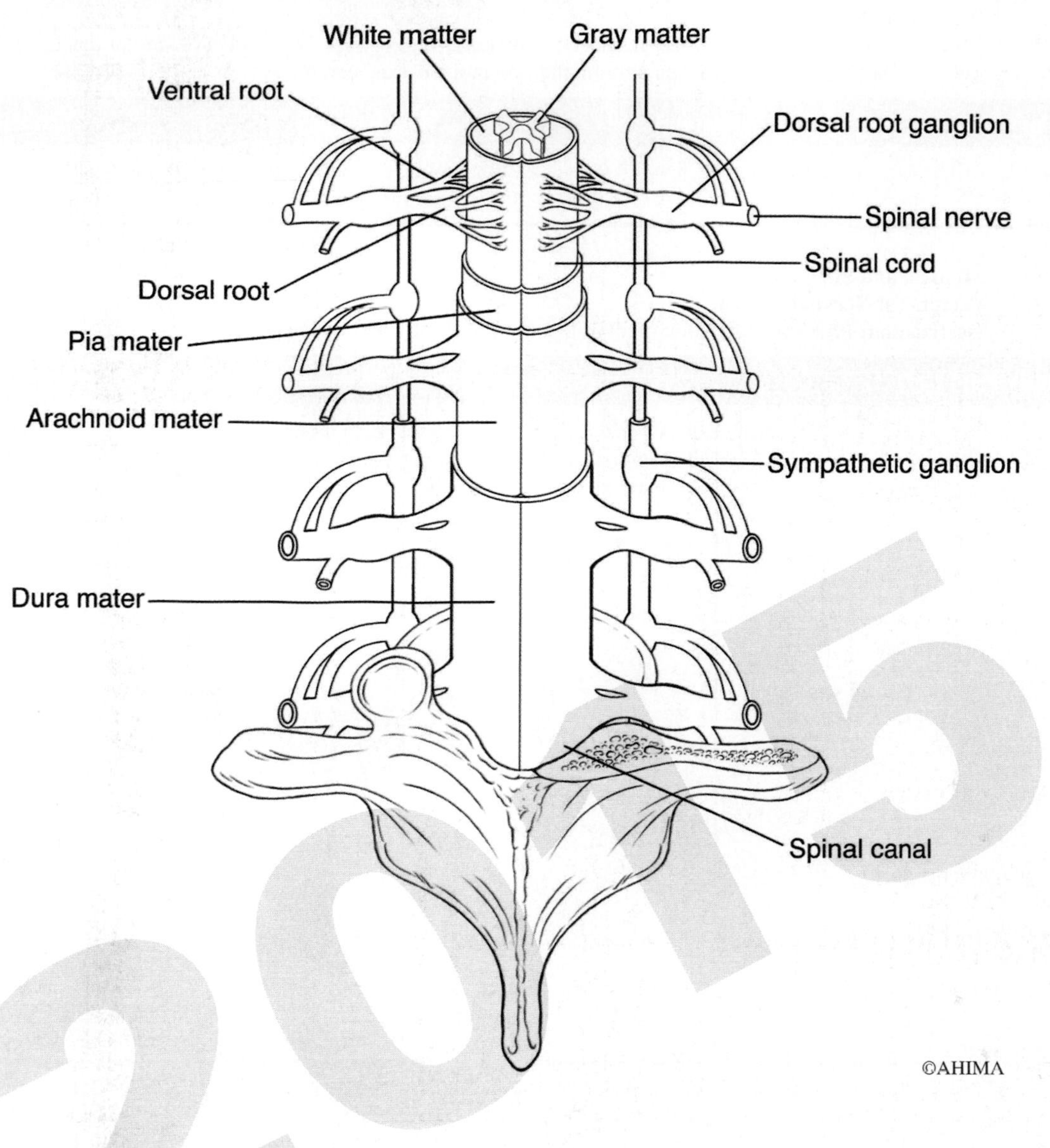

White matter
Gray matter
Ventral root
Dorsal root ganglion
Spinal nerve
Spinal cord
Dorsal root
Pia mater
Arachnoid mater
Sympathetic ganglion
Dura mater
Spinal canal

Peripheral Nervous System Tables 012–01X

Section 0 **Medical and Surgical**
Body System 1 **Peripheral Nervous System**
Operation 2 **Change:** Taking out or off a device from a body part and putting back an identical or similar device in or on the same body part without cutting or puncturing the skin or a mucous membrane

Body Part (4th)	Approach (5th)	Device (6th)	Qualifier (7th)
Y Peripheral Nerve	**X** External	**0** Drainage Device **Y** Other Device	**Z** No Qualifier

Section 0 **Medical and Surgical**
Body System 1 **Peripheral Nervous System**
Operation 5 **Destruction:** Physical eradication of all or a portion of a body part by the direct use of energy, force, or a destructive agent

Body Part (4th)	Approach (5th)	Device (6th)	Qualifier (7th)
0 Cervical Plexus **1** Cervical Nerve **2** Phrenic Nerve **3** Brachial Plexus **4** Ulnar Nerve **5** Median Nerve **6** Radial Nerve **8** Thoracic Nerve **9** Lumbar Plexus **A** Lumbosacral Plexus **B** Lumbar Nerve **C** Pudendal Nerve **D** Femoral Nerve **F** Sciatic Nerve **G** Tibial Nerve **H** Peroneal Nerve **K** Head and Neck Sympathetic Nerve **L** Thoracic Sympathetic Nerve **M** Abdominal Sympathetic Nerve **N** Lumbar Sympathetic Nerve **P** Sacral Sympathetic Nerve **Q** Sacral Plexus **R** Sacral Nerve	**0** Open **3** Percutaneous **4** Percutaneous Endoscopic	**Z** No Device	**Z** No Qualifier

Section 0 **Medical and Surgical**
Body System 1 **Peripheral Nervous System**
Operation 8 **Division:** Cutting into a body part, without draining fluids and/or gases from the body part, in order to separate or transect a body part

Body Part (4th)	Approach (5th)	Device (6th)	Qualifier (7th)
0 Cervical Plexus **1** Cervical Nerve **2** Phrenic Nerve **3** Brachial Plexus **4** Ulnar Nerve **5** Median Nerve **6** Radial Nerve **8** Thoracic Nerve **9** Lumbar Plexus **A** Lumbosacral Plexus **B** Lumbar Nerve **C** Pudendal Nerve **D** Femoral Nerve **F** Sciatic Nerve **G** Tibial Nerve **H** Peroneal Nerve **K** Head and Neck Sympathetic Nerve **L** Thoracic Sympathetic Nerve **M** Abdominal Sympathetic Nerve **N** Lumbar Sympathetic Nerve **P** Sacral Sympathetic Nerve **Q** Sacral Plexus **R** Sacral Nerve	**0** Open **3** Percutaneous **4** Percutaneous Endoscopic	**Z** No Device	**Z** No Qualifier

Section 0 **Medical and Surgical**
Body System 1 **Peripheral Nervous System**
Operation 9 **Drainage:** Taking or letting out fluids and/or gases from a body part

Body Part (4th)	Approach (5th)	Device (6th)	Qualifier (7th)
0 Cervical Plexus **1** Cervical Nerve **2** Phrenic Nerve **3** Brachial Plexus **4** Ulnar Nerve **5** Median Nerve **6** Radial Nerve **8** Thoracic Nerve **9** Lumbar Plexus **A** Lumbosacral Plexus **B** Lumbar Nerve **C** Pudendal Nerve **D** Femoral Nerve **F** Sciatic Nerve **G** Tibial Nerve **H** Peroneal Nerve **K** Head and Neck Sympathetic Nerve **L** Thoracic Sympathetic Nerve **M** Abdominal Sympathetic Nerve **N** Lumbar Sympathetic Nerve **P** Sacral Sympathetic Nerve **Q** Sacral Plexus **R** Sacral Nerve	**0** Open **3** Percutaneous **4** Percutaneous Endoscopic	**0** Drainage Device	**Z** No Qualifier

Continued →

Section 0 **Medical and Surgical**
Body System 1 **Peripheral Nervous System**
Operation 9 **Drainage:** Taking or letting out fluids and/or gases from a body part

Body Part (4th)	Approach (5th)	Device (6th)	Qualifier (7th)
0 Cervical Plexus **1** Cervical Nerve **2** Phrenic Nerve **3** Brachial Plexus **4** Ulnar Nerve **5** Median Nerve **6** Radial Nerve **8** Thoracic Nerve **9** Lumbar Plexus **A** Lumbosacral Plexus **B** Lumbar Nerve **C** Pudendal Nerve **D** Femoral Nerve **F** Sciatic Nerve **G** Tibial Nerve **H** Peroneal Nerve **K** Head and Neck Sympathetic Nerve **L** Thoracic Sympathetic Nerve **M** Abdominal Sympathetic Nerve **N** Lumbar Sympathetic Nerve **P** Sacral Sympathetic Nerve **Q** Sacral Plexus **R** Sacral Nerve	**0** Open **3** Percutaneous **4** Percutaneous Endoscopic	**Z** No Device	**X** Diagnostic **Z** No Qualifier

Section 0 **Medical and Surgical**
Body System 1 **Peripheral Nervous System**
Operation B **Excision:** Cutting out or off, without replacement, a portion of a body part

Body Part (4th)	Approach (5th)	Device (6th)	Qualifier (7th)
0 Cervical Plexus **1** Cervical Nerve **2** Phrenic Nerve **3** Brachial Plexus **4** Ulnar Nerve **5** Median Nerve **6** Radial Nerve **8** Thoracic Nerve **9** Lumbar Plexus **A** Lumbosacral Plexus **B** Lumbar Nerve **C** Pudendal Nerve **D** Femoral Nerve **F** Sciatic Nerve **G** Tibial Nerve **H** Peroneal Nerve **K** Head and Neck Sympathetic Nerve **L** Thoracic Sympathetic Nerve **M** Abdominal Sympathetic Nerve **N** Lumbar Sympathetic Nerve **P** Sacral Sympathetic Nerve **Q** Sacral Plexus **R** Sacral Nerve	**0** Open **3** Percutaneous **4** Percutaneous Endoscopic	**Z** No Device	**X** Diagnostic **Z** No Qualifier

Section 0 **Medical and Surgical**
Body System 1 **Peripheral Nervous System**
Operation C **Extirpation:** Taking or cutting out solid matter from a body part

Body Part (4th)	Approach (5th)	Device (6th)	Qualifier (7th)
0 Cervical Plexus **1** Cervical Nerve **2** Phrenic Nerve **3** Brachial Plexus **4** Ulnar Nerve **5** Median Nerve **6** Radial Nerve **8** Thoracic Nerve **9** Lumbar Plexus **A** Lumbosacral Plexus **B** Lumbar Nerve **C** Pudendal Nerve **D** Femoral Nerve **F** Sciatic Nerve **G** Tibial Nerve **H** Peroneal Nerve **K** Head and Neck Sympathetic Nerve **L** Thoracic Sympathetic Nerve **M** Abdominal Sympathetic Nerve **N** Lumbar Sympathetic Nerve **P** Sacral Sympathetic Nerve **Q** Sacral Plexus **R** Sacral Nerve	**0** Open **3** Percutaneous **4** Percutaneous Endoscopic	**Z** No Device	**Z** No Qualifier

Section 0 **Medical and Surgical**
Body System 1 **Peripheral Nervous System**
Operation D **Extraction:** Pulling or stripping out or off all or a portion of a body part by the use of force

Body Part (4th)	Approach (5th)	Device (6th)	Qualifier (7th)
0 Cervical Plexus **1** Cervical Nerve **2** Phrenic Nerve **3** Brachial Plexus **4** Ulnar Nerve **5** Median Nerve **6** Radial Nerve **8** Thoracic Nerve **9** Lumbar Plexus **A** Lumbosacral Plexus **B** Lumbar Nerve **C** Pudendal Nerve **D** Femoral Nerve **F** Sciatic Nerve **G** Tibial Nerve **H** Peroneal Nerve **K** Head and Neck Sympathetic Nerve **L** Thoracic Sympathetic Nerve **M** Abdominal Sympathetic Nerve **N** Lumbar Sympathetic Nerve **P** Sacral Sympathetic Nerve **Q** Sacral Plexus **R** Sacral Nerve	**0** Open **3** Percutaneous **4** Percutaneous Endoscopic	**Z** No Device	**Z** No Qualifier

Section 0 **Medical and Surgical**
Body System 1 **Peripheral Nervous System**
Operation H **Insertion:** Putting in a nonbiological appliance that monitors, assists, performs, or prevents a physiological function but does not physically take the place of a body part

Body Part (4th)	Approach (5th)	Device (6th)	Qualifier (7th)
Y Peripheral Nerve	**0** Open **3** Percutaneous **4** Percutaneous Endoscopic	**2** Monitoring Device **M** Neurostimulator Lead	**Z** No Qualifier

Section 0 **Medical and Surgical**
Body System 1 **Peripheral Nervous System**
Operation J **Inspection:** Visually and/or manually exploring a body part

Body Part (4th)	Approach (5th)	Device (6th)	Qualifier (7th)
Y Peripheral Nerve	**0** Open **3** Percutaneous **4** Percutaneous Endoscopic	**Z** No Device	**Z** No Qualifier

Section 0 **Medical and Surgical**
Body System 1 **Peripheral Nervous System**
Operation N **Release:** Freeing a body part from an abnormal physical constraint by cutting or by the use of force

Body Part (4th)	Approach (5th)	Device (6th)	Qualifier (7th)
0 Cervical Plexus **1** Cervical Nerve **2** Phrenic Nerve **3** Brachial Plexus **4** Ulnar Nerve **5** Median Nerve **6** Radial Nerve **8** Thoracic Nerve **9** Lumbar Plexus **A** Lumbosacral Plexus **B** Lumbar Nerve **C** Pudendal Nerve **D** Femoral Nerve **F** Sciatic Nerve **G** Tibial Nerve **H** Peroneal Nerve **K** Head and Neck Sympathetic Nerve **L** Thoracic Sympathetic Nerve **M** Abdominal Sympathetic Nerve **N** Lumbar Sympathetic Nerve **P** Sacral Sympathetic Nerve **Q** Sacral Plexus **R** Sacral Nerve	**0** Open **3** Percutaneous **4** Percutaneous Endoscopic	**Z** No Device	**Z** No Qualifier

Section 0 **Medical and Surgical**
Body System 1 **Peripheral Nervous System**
Operation P **Removal:** Taking out or off a device from a body part

Body Part (4th)	Approach (5th)	Device (6th)	Qualifier (7th)
Y Peripheral Nerve	**0** Open **3** Percutaneous **4** Percutaneous Endoscopic	**0** Drainage Device **2** Monitoring Device **7** Autologous Tissue Substitute **M** Neurostimulator Lead	**Z** No Qualifier
Y Peripheral Nerve	**X** External	**0** Drainage Device **2** Monitoring Device **M** Neurostimulator Lead	**Z** No Qualifier

Section 0 **Medical and Surgical**
Body System 1 **Peripheral Nervous System**
Operation Q **Repair:** Restoring, to the extent possible, a body part to its normal anatomic structure and function

Body Part (4th)	Approach (5th)	Device (6th)	Qualifier (7th)
0 Cervical Plexus **1** Cervical Nerve **2** Phrenic Nerve **3** Brachial Plexus **4** Ulnar Nerve **5** Median Nerve **6** Radial Nerve **8** Thoracic Nerve **9** Lumbar Plexus **A** Lumbosacral Plexus **B** Lumbar Nerve **C** Pudendal Nerve **D** Femoral Nerve **F** Sciatic Nerve **G** Tibial Nerve **H** Peroneal Nerve **K** Head and Neck Sympathetic Nerve **L** Thoracic Sympathetic Nerve **M** Abdominal Sympathetic Nerve **N** Lumbar Sympathetic Nerve **P** Sacral Sympathetic Nerve **Q** Sacral Plexus **R** Sacral Nerve	**0** Open **3** Percutaneous **4** Percutaneous Endoscopic	**Z** No Device	**Z** No Qualifier

Section 0 **Medical and Surgical**
Body System 1 **Peripheral Nervous System**
Operation S **Reposition:** Moving to its normal location, or other suitable location, all or a portion of a body part

Body Part (4th)	Approach (5th)	Device (6th)	Qualifier (7th)
0 Cervical Plexus **1** Cervical Nerve **2** Phrenic Nerve **3** Brachial Plexus **4** Ulnar Nerve **5** Median Nerve **6** Radial Nerve **8** Thoracic Nerve **9** Lumbar Plexus **A** Lumbosacral Plexus **B** Lumbar Nerve **C** Pudendal Nerve **D** Femoral Nerve **F** Sciatic Nerve **G** Tibial Nerve **H** Peroneal Nerve **Q** Sacral Plexus **R** Sacral Nerve	**0** Open **3** Percutaneous **4** Percutaneous Endoscopic	**Z** No Device	**Z** No Qualifier

Section 0 **Medical and Surgical**
Body System 1 **Peripheral Nervous System**
Operation U **Supplement:** Putting in or on biological or synthetic material that physically reinforces and/or augments the function of a portion of a body part

Body Part (4th)	Approach (5th)	Device (6th)	Qualifier (7th)
1 Cervical Nerve **2** Phrenic Nerve **4** Ulnar Nerve **5** Median Nerve **6** Radial Nerve **8** Thoracic Nerve **B** Lumbar Nerve **C** Pudendal Nerve **D** Femoral Nerve **F** Sciatic Nerve **G** Tibial Nerve **H** Peroneal Nerve **R** Sacral Nerve	**0** Open **3** Percutaneous **4** Percutaneous Endoscopic	**7** Autologous Tissue Substitute	**Z** No Qualifier

Section 0 **Medical and Surgical**
Body System 1 **Peripheral Nervous System**
Operation W **Revision:** Correcting, to the extent possible, a portion of a malfunctioning device or the position of a displaced device

Body Part (4th)	Approach (5th)	Device (6th)	Qualifier (7th)
Y Peripheral Nerve	**0** Open **3** Percutaneous **4** Percutaneous Endoscopic **X** External	**0** Drainage Device **2** Monitoring Device **7** Autologous Tissue Substitute **M** Neurostimulator Lead	**Z** No Qualifier

Section 0 **Medical and Surgical**
Body System 1 **Peripheral Nervous System**
Operation X **Transfer:** Moving, without taking out, all or a portion of a body part to another location to take over the function of all or a portion of a body part

Body Part (4th)	Approach (5th)	Device (6th)	Qualifier (7th)
1 Cervical Nerve **2** Phrenic Nerve	**0** Open **4** Percutaneous Endoscopic	**Z** No Device	**1** Cervical Nerve **2** Phrenic Nerve
4 Ulnar Nerve **5** Median Nerve **6** Radial Nerve	**0** Open **4** Percutaneous Endoscopic	**Z** No Device	**4** Ulnar Nerve **5** Median Nerve **6** Radial Nerve
8 Thoracic Nerve	**0** Open **4** Percutaneous Endoscopic	**Z** No Device	**8** Thoracic Nerve
B Lumbar Nerve **C** Pudendal Nerve	**0** Open **4** Percutaneous Endoscopic	**Z** No Device	**B** Lumbar Nerve **C** Perineal Nerve
D Femoral Nerve **F** Sciatic Nerve **G** Tibial Nerve **H** Peroneal Nerve	**0** Open **4** Percutaneous Endoscopic	**Z** No Device	**D** Femoral Nerve **F** Sciatic Nerve **G** Tibial Nerve **H** Peroneal Nerve

Peripheral Nervous System Code Listing 012–01X

012 – Peripheral Nervous System, Change

Review Coding Guideline B6.1c

012YX0Z Change Drainage Device in Peripheral Nerve, External Approach

012YXYZ Change Other Device in Peripheral Nerve, External Approach

015 – Peripheral Nervous System, Destruction

01500ZZ Destruction of Cervical Plexus, Open Approach

01503ZZ Destruction of Cervical Plexus, Percutaneous Approach

01504ZZ Destruction of Cervical Plexus, Percutaneous Endoscopic Approach

01510ZZ Destruction of Cervical Nerve, Open Approach
01513ZZ Destruction of Cervical Nerve, Percutaneous Approach
01514ZZ Destruction of Cervical Nerve, Percutaneous Endoscopic Approach
01520ZZ Destruction of Phrenic Nerve, Open Approach
01523ZZ Destruction of Phrenic Nerve, Percutaneous Approach
01524ZZ Destruction of Phrenic Nerve, Percutaneous Endoscopic Approach
01530ZZ Destruction of Brachial Plexus, Open Approach
01533ZZ Destruction of Brachial Plexus, Percutaneous Approach
01534ZZ Destruction of Brachial Plexus, Percutaneous Endoscopic Approach
01540ZZ Destruction of Ulnar Nerve, Open Approach
01543ZZ Destruction of Ulnar Nerve, Percutaneous Approach
01544ZZ Destruction of Ulnar Nerve, Percutaneous Endoscopic Approach
01550ZZ Destruction of Median Nerve, Open Approach
01553ZZ Destruction of Median Nerve, Percutaneous Approach
01554ZZ Destruction of Median Nerve, Percutaneous Endoscopic Approach
01560ZZ Destruction of Radial Nerve, Open Approach
01563ZZ Destruction of Radial Nerve, Percutaneous Approach
01564ZZ Destruction of Radial Nerve, Percutaneous Endoscopic Approach
01580ZZ Destruction of Thoracic Nerve, Open Approach
01583ZZ Destruction of Thoracic Nerve, Percutaneous Approach
01584ZZ Destruction of Thoracic Nerve, Percutaneous Endoscopic Approach
01590ZZ Destruction of Lumbar Plexus, Open Approach
01593ZZ Destruction of Lumbar Plexus, Percutaneous Approach
01594ZZ Destruction of Lumbar Plexus, Percutaneous Endoscopic Approach
015A0ZZ Destruction of Lumbosacral Plexus, Open Approach
015A3ZZ Destruction of Lumbosacral Plexus, Percutaneous Approach
015A4ZZ Destruction of Lumbosacral Plexus, Percutaneous Endoscopic Approach
015B0ZZ Destruction of Lumbar Nerve, Open Approach
015B3ZZ Destruction of Lumbar Nerve, Percutaneous Approach
015B4ZZ Destruction of Lumbar Nerve, Percutaneous Endoscopic Approach
015C0ZZ Destruction of Pudendal Nerve, Open Approach
015C3ZZ Destruction of Pudendal Nerve, Percutaneous Approach
015C4ZZ Destruction of Pudendal Nerve, Percutaneous Endoscopic Approach
015D0ZZ Destruction of Femoral Nerve, Open Approach
015D3ZZ Destruction of Femoral Nerve, Percutaneous Approach
015D4ZZ Destruction of Femoral Nerve, Percutaneous Endoscopic Approach
015F0ZZ Destruction of Sciatic Nerve, Open Approach
015F3ZZ Destruction of Sciatic Nerve, Percutaneous Approach
015F4ZZ Destruction of Sciatic Nerve, Percutaneous Endoscopic Approach
015G0ZZ Destruction of Tibial Nerve, Open Approach
015G3ZZ Destruction of Tibial Nerve, Percutaneous Approach
015G4ZZ Destruction of Tibial Nerve, Percutaneous Endoscopic Approach
015H0ZZ Destruction of Peroneal Nerve, Open Approach
015H3ZZ Destruction of Peroneal Nerve, Percutaneous Approach
015H4ZZ Destruction of Peroneal Nerve, Percutaneous Endoscopic Approach
015K0ZZ Destruction of Head and Neck Sympathetic Nerve, Open Approach
015K3ZZ Destruction of Head and Neck Sympathetic Nerve, Percutaneous Approach
015K4ZZ Destruction of Head and Neck Sympathetic Nerve, Percutaneous Endoscopic Approach
015L0ZZ Destruction of Thoracic Sympathetic Nerve, Open Approach
015L3ZZ Destruction of Thoracic Sympathetic Nerve, Percutaneous Approach
015L4ZZ Destruction of Thoracic Sympathetic Nerve, Percutaneous Endoscopic Approach
015M0ZZ Destruction of Abdominal Sympathetic Nerve, Open Approach
015M3ZZ Destruction of Abdominal Sympathetic Nerve, Percutaneous Approach
015M4ZZ Destruction of Abdominal Sympathetic Nerve, Percutaneous Endoscopic Approach
015N0ZZ Destruction of Lumbar Sympathetic Nerve, Open Approach
015N3ZZ Destruction of Lumbar Sympathetic Nerve, Percutaneous Approach
015N4ZZ Destruction of Lumbar Sympathetic Nerve, Percutaneous Endoscopic Approach
015P0ZZ Destruction of Sacral Sympathetic Nerve, Open Approach
015P3ZZ Destruction of Sacral Sympathetic Nerve, Percutaneous Approach
015P4ZZ Destruction of Sacral Sympathetic Nerve, Percutaneous Endoscopic Approach
015Q0ZZ Destruction of Sacral Plexus, Open Approach
015Q3ZZ Destruction of Sacral Plexus, Percutaneous Approach
015Q4ZZ Destruction of Sacral Plexus, Percutaneous Endoscopic Approach
015R0ZZ Destruction of Sacral Nerve, Open Approach
015R3ZZ Destruction of Sacral Nerve, Percutaneous Approach
015R4ZZ Destruction of Sacral Nerve, Percutaneous Endoscopic Approach

018 – Peripheral Nervous System, Division

Review Coding Guideline B3.14

01800ZZ Division of Cervical Plexus, Open Approach
01803ZZ Division of Cervical Plexus, Percutaneous Approach
01804ZZ Division of Cervical Plexus, Percutaneous Endoscopic Approach
01810ZZ Division of Cervical Nerve, Open Approach
01813ZZ Division of Cervical Nerve, Percutaneous Approach
01814ZZ Division of Cervical Nerve, Percutaneous Endoscopic Approach
01820ZZ Division of Phrenic Nerve, Open Approach
01823ZZ Division of Phrenic Nerve, Percutaneous Approach
01824ZZ Division of Phrenic Nerve, Percutaneous Endoscopic Approach
01830ZZ Division of Brachial Plexus, Open Approach
01833ZZ Division of Brachial Plexus, Percutaneous Approach
01834ZZ Division of Brachial Plexus, Percutaneous Endoscopic Approach
01840ZZ Division of Ulnar Nerve, Open Approach
01843ZZ Division of Ulnar Nerve, Percutaneous Approach
01844ZZ Division of Ulnar Nerve, Percutaneous Endoscopic Approach
01850ZZ Division of Median Nerve, Open Approach
01853ZZ Division of Median Nerve, Percutaneous Approach
01854ZZ Division of Median Nerve, Percutaneous Endoscopic Approach
01860ZZ Division of Radial Nerve, Open Approach
01863ZZ Division of Radial Nerve, Percutaneous Approach
01864ZZ Division of Radial Nerve, Percutaneous Endoscopic Approach
01880ZZ Division of Thoracic Nerve, Open Approach
01883ZZ Division of Thoracic Nerve, Percutaneous Approach
01884ZZ Division of Thoracic Nerve, Percutaneous Endoscopic Approach
01890ZZ Division of Lumbar Plexus, Open Approach
01893ZZ Division of Lumbar Plexus, Percutaneous Approach
01894ZZ Division of Lumbar Plexus, Percutaneous Endoscopic Approach
018A0ZZ Division of Lumbosacral Plexus, Open Approach
018A3ZZ Division of Lumbosacral Plexus, Percutaneous Approach
018A4ZZ Division of Lumbosacral Plexus, Percutaneous Endoscopic Approach
018B0ZZ Division of Lumbar Nerve, Open Approach
018B3ZZ Division of Lumbar Nerve, Percutaneous Approach
018B4ZZ Division of Lumbar Nerve, Percutaneous Endoscopic Approach
018C0ZZ Division of Pudendal Nerve, Open Approach
018C3ZZ Division of Pudendal Nerve, Percutaneous Approach
018C4ZZ Division of Pudendal Nerve, Percutaneous Endoscopic Approach
018D0ZZ Division of Femoral Nerve, Open Approach
018D3ZZ Division of Femoral Nerve, Percutaneous Approach
018D4ZZ Division of Femoral Nerve, Percutaneous Endoscopic Approach

018F0ZZ Division of Sciatic Nerve, Open Approach
018F3ZZ Division of Sciatic Nerve, Percutaneous Approach
018F4ZZ Division of Sciatic Nerve, Percutaneous Endoscopic Approach
018G0ZZ Division of Tibial Nerve, Open Approach
018G3ZZ Division of Tibial Nerve, Percutaneous Approach
018G4ZZ Division of Tibial Nerve, Percutaneous Endoscopic Approach
018H0ZZ Division of Peroneal Nerve, Open Approach
018H3ZZ Division of Peroneal Nerve, Percutaneous Approach
018H4ZZ Division of Peroneal Nerve, Percutaneous Endoscopic Approach
018K0ZZ Division of Head and Neck Sympathetic Nerve, Open Approach
018K3ZZ Division of Head and Neck Sympathetic Nerve, Percutaneous Approach
018K4ZZ Division of Head and Neck Sympathetic Nerve, Percutaneous Endoscopic Approach
018L0ZZ Division of Thoracic Sympathetic Nerve, Open Approach
018L3ZZ Division of Thoracic Sympathetic Nerve, Percutaneous Approach
018L4ZZ Division of Thoracic Sympathetic Nerve, Percutaneous Endoscopic Approach
018M0ZZ Division of Abdominal Sympathetic Nerve, Open Approach
018M3ZZ Division of Abdominal Sympathetic Nerve, Percutaneous Approach
018M4ZZ Division of Abdominal Sympathetic Nerve, Percutaneous Endoscopic Approach
018N0ZZ Division of Lumbar Sympathetic Nerve, Open Approach
018N3ZZ Division of Lumbar Sympathetic Nerve, Percutaneous Approach
018N4ZZ Division of Lumbar Sympathetic Nerve, Percutaneous Endoscopic Approach
018P0ZZ Division of Sacral Sympathetic Nerve, Open Approach
018P3ZZ Division of Sacral Sympathetic Nerve, Percutaneous Approach
018P4ZZ Division of Sacral Sympathetic Nerve, Percutaneous Endoscopic Approach
018Q0ZZ Division of Sacral Plexus, Open Approach
018Q3ZZ Division of Sacral Plexus, Percutaneous Approach
018Q4ZZ Division of Sacral Plexus, Percutaneous Endoscopic Approach
018R0ZZ Division of Sacral Nerve, Open Approach
018R3ZZ Division of Sacral Nerve, Percutaneous Approach
018R4ZZ Division of Sacral Nerve, Percutaneous Endoscopic Approach

019 – Peripheral Nervous System, Drainage

Review Coding Guidelines B3.4a and B3.4b

Review Coding Guideline B6.2

019000Z Drainage of Cervical Plexus with Drainage Device, Open Approach
01900ZX Drainage of Cervical Plexus, Open Approach, Diagnostic
01900ZZ Drainage of Cervical Plexus, Open Approach
019030Z Drainage of Cervical Plexus with Drainage Device, Percutaneous Approach
01903ZX Drainage of Cervical Plexus, Percutaneous Approach, Diagnostic
01903ZZ Drainage of Cervical Plexus, Percutaneous Approach
019040Z Drainage of Cervical Plexus with Drainage Device, Percutaneous Endoscopic Approach
01904ZX Drainage of Cervical Plexus, Percutaneous Endoscopic Approach, Diagnostic
01904ZZ Drainage of Cervical Plexus, Percutaneous Endoscopic Approach
019100Z Drainage of Cervical Nerve with Drainage Device, Open Approach
01910ZX Drainage of Cervical Nerve, Open Approach, Diagnostic
01910ZZ Drainage of Cervical Nerve, Open Approach
019130Z Drainage of Cervical Nerve with Drainage Device, Percutaneous Approach
01913ZX Drainage of Cervical Nerve, Percutaneous Approach, Diagnostic
01913ZZ Drainage of Cervical Nerve, Percutaneous Approach
019140Z Drainage of Cervical Nerve with Drainage Device, Percutaneous Endoscopic Approach
01914ZX Drainage of Cervical Nerve, Percutaneous Endoscopic Approach, Diagnostic
01914ZZ Drainage of Cervical Nerve, Percutaneous Endoscopic Approach
019200Z Drainage of Phrenic Nerve with Drainage Device, Open Approach
01920ZX Drainage of Phrenic Nerve, Open Approach, Diagnostic
01920ZZ Drainage of Phrenic Nerve, Open Approach
019230Z Drainage of Phrenic Nerve with Drainage Device, Percutaneous Approach
01923ZX Drainage of Phrenic Nerve, Percutaneous Approach, Diagnostic
01923ZZ Drainage of Phrenic Nerve, Percutaneous Approach
019240Z Drainage of Phrenic Nerve with Drainage Device, Percutaneous Endoscopic Approach
01924ZX Drainage of Phrenic Nerve, Percutaneous Endoscopic Approach, Diagnostic
01924ZZ Drainage of Phrenic Nerve, Percutaneous Endoscopic Approach
019300Z Drainage of Brachial Plexus with Drainage Device, Open Approach
01930ZX Drainage of Brachial Plexus, Open Approach, Diagnostic
01930ZZ Drainage of Brachial Plexus, Open Approach
019330Z Drainage of Brachial Plexus with Drainage Device, Percutaneous Approach
01933ZX Drainage of Brachial Plexus, Percutaneous Approach, Diagnostic
01933ZZ Drainage of Brachial Plexus, Percutaneous Approach
019340Z Drainage of Brachial Plexus with Drainage Device, Percutaneous Endoscopic Approach
01934ZX Drainage of Brachial Plexus, Percutaneous Endoscopic Approach, Diagnostic
01934ZZ Drainage of Brachial Plexus, Percutaneous Endoscopic Approach
019400Z Drainage of Ulnar Nerve with Drainage Device, Open Approach
01940ZX Drainage of Ulnar Nerve, Open Approach, Diagnostic
01940ZZ Drainage of Ulnar Nerve, Open Approach
019430Z Drainage of Ulnar Nerve with Drainage Device, Percutaneous Approach
01943ZX Drainage of Ulnar Nerve, Percutaneous Approach, Diagnostic
01943ZZ Drainage of Ulnar Nerve, Percutaneous Approach
019440Z Drainage of Ulnar Nerve with Drainage Device, Percutaneous Endoscopic Approach
01944ZX Drainage of Ulnar Nerve, Percutaneous Endoscopic Approach, Diagnostic
01944ZZ Drainage of Ulnar Nerve, Percutaneous Endoscopic Approach
019500Z Drainage of Median Nerve with Drainage Device, Open Approach
01950ZX Drainage of Median Nerve, Open Approach, Diagnostic
01950ZZ Drainage of Median Nerve, Open Approach
019530Z Drainage of Median Nerve with Drainage Device, Percutaneous Approach
01953ZX Drainage of Median Nerve, Percutaneous Approach, Diagnostic
01953ZZ Drainage of Median Nerve, Percutaneous Approach
019540Z Drainage of Median Nerve with Drainage Device, Percutaneous Endoscopic Approach
01954ZX Drainage of Median Nerve, Percutaneous Endoscopic Approach, Diagnostic
01954ZZ Drainage of Median Nerve, Percutaneous Endoscopic Approach
019600Z Drainage of Radial Nerve with Drainage Device, Open Approach
01960ZX Drainage of Radial Nerve, Open Approach, Diagnostic
01960ZZ Drainage of Radial Nerve, Open Approach
019630Z Drainage of Radial Nerve with Drainage Device, Percutaneous Approach
01963ZX Drainage of Radial Nerve, Percutaneous Approach, Diagnostic
01963ZZ Drainage of Radial Nerve, Percutaneous Approach
019640Z Drainage of Radial Nerve with Drainage Device, Percutaneous Endoscopic Approach
01964ZX Drainage of Radial Nerve, Percutaneous Endoscopic Approach, Diagnostic
01964ZZ Drainage of Radial Nerve, Percutaneous Endoscopic Approach
019800Z Drainage of Thoracic Nerve with Drainage Device, Open Approach
01980ZX Drainage of Thoracic Nerve, Open Approach, Diagnostic
01980ZZ Drainage of Thoracic Nerve, Open Approach
019830Z Drainage of Thoracic Nerve with Drainage Device, Percutaneous Approach
01983ZX Drainage of Thoracic Nerve, Percutaneous Approach, Diagnostic
01983ZZ Drainage of Thoracic Nerve, Percutaneous Approach
019840Z Drainage of Thoracic Nerve with Drainage Device, Percutaneous Endoscopic Approach
01984ZX Drainage of Thoracic Nerve, Percutaneous Endoscopic Approach, Diagnostic
01984ZZ Drainage of Thoracic Nerve, Percutaneous Endoscopic Approach

019900Z Drainage of Lumbar Plexus with Drainage Device, Open Approach
01990ZX Drainage of Lumbar Plexus, Open Approach, Diagnostic
01990ZZ Drainage of Lumbar Plexus, Open Approach
019930Z Drainage of Lumbar Plexus with Drainage Device, Percutaneous Approach
01993ZX Drainage of Lumbar Plexus, Percutaneous Approach, Diagnostic
01993ZZ Drainage of Lumbar Plexus, Percutaneous Approach
019940Z Drainage of Lumbar Plexus with Drainage Device, Percutaneous Endoscopic Approach
01994ZX Drainage of Lumbar Plexus, Percutaneous Endoscopic Approach, Diagnostic
01994ZZ Drainage of Lumbar Plexus, Percutaneous Endoscopic Approach
019A00Z Drainage of Lumbosacral Plexus with Drainage Device, Open Approach
019A0ZX Drainage of Lumbosacral Plexus, Open Approach, Diagnostic
019A0ZZ Drainage of Lumbosacral Plexus, Open Approach
019A30Z Drainage of Lumbosacral Plexus with Drainage Device, Percutaneous Approach
019A3ZX Drainage of Lumbosacral Plexus, Percutaneous Approach, Diagnostic
019A3ZZ Drainage of Lumbosacral Plexus, Percutaneous Approach
019A40Z Drainage of Lumbosacral Plexus with Drainage Device, Percutaneous Endoscopic Approach
019A4ZX Drainage of Lumbosacral Plexus, Percutaneous Endoscopic Approach, Diagnostic
019A4ZZ Drainage of Lumbosacral Plexus, Percutaneous Endoscopic Approach
019B00Z Drainage of Lumbar Nerve with Drainage Device, Open Approach
019B0ZX Drainage of Lumbar Nerve, Open Approach, Diagnostic
019B0ZZ Drainage of Lumbar Nerve, Open Approach
019B30Z Drainage of Lumbar Nerve with Drainage Device, Percutaneous Approach
019B3ZX Drainage of Lumbar Nerve, Percutaneous Approach, Diagnostic
019B3ZZ Drainage of Lumbar Nerve, Percutaneous Approach
019B40Z Drainage of Lumbar Nerve with Drainage Device, Percutaneous Endoscopic Approach
019B4ZX Drainage of Lumbar Nerve, Percutaneous Endoscopic Approach, Diagnostic
019B4ZZ Drainage of Lumbar Nerve, Percutaneous Endoscopic Approach
019C00Z Drainage of Pudendal Nerve with Drainage Device, Open Approach
019C0ZX Drainage of Pudendal Nerve, Open Approach, Diagnostic
019C0ZZ Drainage of Pudendal Nerve, Open Approach
019C30Z Drainage of Pudendal Nerve with Drainage Device, Percutaneous Approach
019C3ZX Drainage of Pudendal Nerve, Percutaneous Approach, Diagnostic
019C3ZZ Drainage of Pudendal Nerve, Percutaneous Approach
019C40Z Drainage of Pudendal Nerve with Drainage Device, Percutaneous Endoscopic Approach
019C4ZX Drainage of Pudendal Nerve, Percutaneous Endoscopic Approach, Diagnostic
019C4ZZ Drainage of Pudendal Nerve, Percutaneous Endoscopic Approach
019D00Z Drainage of Femoral Nerve with Drainage Device, Open Approach
019D0ZX Drainage of Femoral Nerve, Open Approach, Diagnostic
019D0ZZ Drainage of Femoral Nerve, Open Approach
019D30Z Drainage of Femoral Nerve with Drainage Device, Percutaneous Approach
019D3ZX Drainage of Femoral Nerve, Percutaneous Approach, Diagnostic
019D3ZZ Drainage of Femoral Nerve, Percutaneous Approach
019D40Z Drainage of Femoral Nerve with Drainage Device, Percutaneous Endoscopic Approach
019D4ZX Drainage of Femoral Nerve, Percutaneous Endoscopic Approach, Diagnostic
019D4ZZ Drainage of Femoral Nerve, Percutaneous Endoscopic Approach
019F00Z Drainage of Sciatic Nerve with Drainage Device, Open Approach
019F0ZX Drainage of Sciatic Nerve, Open Approach, Diagnostic
019F0ZZ Drainage of Sciatic Nerve, Open Approach
019F30Z Drainage of Sciatic Nerve with Drainage Device, Percutaneous Approach
019F3ZX Drainage of Sciatic Nerve, Percutaneous Approach, Diagnostic
019F3ZZ Drainage of Sciatic Nerve, Percutaneous Approach
019F40Z Drainage of Sciatic Nerve with Drainage Device, Percutaneous Endoscopic Approach
019F4ZX Drainage of Sciatic Nerve, Percutaneous Endoscopic Approach, Diagnostic
019F4ZZ Drainage of Sciatic Nerve, Percutaneous Endoscopic Approach
019G00Z Drainage of Tibial Nerve with Drainage Device, Open Approach
019G0ZX Drainage of Tibial Nerve, Open Approach, Diagnostic
019G0ZZ Drainage of Tibial Nerve, Open Approach
019G30Z Drainage of Tibial Nerve with Drainage Device, Percutaneous Approach
019G3ZX Drainage of Tibial Nerve, Percutaneous Approach, Diagnostic
019G3ZZ Drainage of Tibial Nerve, Percutaneous Approach
019G40Z Drainage of Tibial Nerve with Drainage Device, Percutaneous Endoscopic Approach
019G4ZX Drainage of Tibial Nerve, Percutaneous Endoscopic Approach, Diagnostic
019G4ZZ Drainage of Tibial Nerve, Percutaneous Endoscopic Approach
019H00Z Drainage of Peroneal Nerve with Drainage Device, Open Approach
019H0ZX Drainage of Peroneal Nerve, Open Approach, Diagnostic
019H0ZZ Drainage of Peroneal Nerve, Open Approach
019H30Z Drainage of Peroneal Nerve with Drainage Device, Percutaneous Approach
019H3ZX Drainage of Peroneal Nerve, Percutaneous Approach, Diagnostic
019H3ZZ Drainage of Peroneal Nerve, Percutaneous Approach
019H40Z Drainage of Peroneal Nerve with Drainage Device, Percutaneous Endoscopic Approach
019H4ZX Drainage of Peroneal Nerve, Percutaneous Endoscopic Approach, Diagnostic
019H4ZZ Drainage of Peroneal Nerve, Percutaneous Endoscopic Approach
019K00Z Drainage of Head and Neck Sympathetic Nerve with Drainage Device, Open Approach
019K0ZX Drainage of Head and Neck Sympathetic Nerve, Open Approach, Diagnostic
019K0ZZ Drainage of Head and Neck Sympathetic Nerve, Open Approach
019K30Z Drainage of Head and Neck Sympathetic Nerve with Drainage Device, Percutaneous Approach
019K3ZX Drainage of Head and Neck Sympathetic Nerve, Percutaneous Approach, Diagnostic
019K3ZZ Drainage of Head and Neck Sympathetic Nerve, Percutaneous Approach
019K40Z Drainage of Head and Neck Sympathetic Nerve with Drainage Device, Percutaneous Endoscopic Approach
019K4ZX Drainage of Head and Neck Sympathetic Nerve, Percutaneous Endoscopic Approach, Diagnostic
019K4ZZ Drainage of Head and Neck Sympathetic Nerve, Percutaneous Endoscopic Approach
019L00Z Drainage of Thoracic Sympathetic Nerve with Drainage Device, Open Approach
019L0ZX Drainage of Thoracic Sympathetic Nerve, Open Approach, Diagnostic
019L0ZZ Drainage of Thoracic Sympathetic Nerve, Open Approach
019L30Z Drainage of Thoracic Sympathetic Nerve with Drainage Device, Percutaneous Approach
019L3ZX Drainage of Thoracic Sympathetic Nerve, Percutaneous Approach, Diagnostic
019L3ZZ Drainage of Thoracic Sympathetic Nerve, Percutaneous Approach
019L40Z Drainage of Thoracic Sympathetic Nerve with Drainage Device, Percutaneous Endoscopic Approach
019L4ZX Drainage of Thoracic Sympathetic Nerve, Percutaneous Endoscopic Approach, Diagnostic
019L4ZZ Drainage of Thoracic Sympathetic Nerve, Percutaneous Endoscopic Approach
019M00Z Drainage of Abdominal Sympathetic Nerve with Drainage Device, Open Approach
019M0ZX Drainage of Abdominal Sympathetic Nerve, Open Approach, Diagnostic
019M0ZZ Drainage of Abdominal Sympathetic Nerve, Open Approach
019M30Z Drainage of Abdominal Sympathetic Nerve with Drainage Device, Percutaneous Approach
019M3ZX Drainage of Abdominal Sympathetic Nerve, Percutaneous Approach, Diagnostic
019M3ZZ Drainage of Abdominal Sympathetic Nerve, Percutaneous Approach
019M40Z Drainage of Abdominal Sympathetic Nerve with Drainage Device, Percutaneous Endoscopic Approach
019M4ZX Drainage of Abdominal Sympathetic Nerve, Percutaneous Endoscopic Approach, Diagnostic
019M4ZZ Drainage of Abdominal Sympathetic Nerve, Percutaneous Endoscopic Approach
019N00Z Drainage of Lumbar Sympathetic Nerve with Drainage Device, Open Approach
019N0ZX Drainage of Lumbar Sympathetic Nerve, Open Approach, Diagnostic
019N0ZZ Drainage of Lumbar Sympathetic Nerve, Open Approach
019N30Z Drainage of Lumbar Sympathetic Nerve with Drainage Device, Percutaneous Approach
019N3ZX Drainage of Lumbar Sympathetic Nerve, Percutaneous Approach, Diagnostic
019N3ZZ Drainage of Lumbar Sympathetic Nerve, Percutaneous Approach

019N40Z Drainage of Lumbar Sympathetic Nerve with Drainage Device, Percutaneous Endoscopic Approach
019N4ZX Drainage of Lumbar Sympathetic Nerve, Percutaneous Endoscopic Approach, Diagnostic
019N4ZZ Drainage of Lumbar Sympathetic Nerve, Percutaneous Endoscopic Approach
019P00Z Drainage of Sacral Sympathetic Nerve with Drainage Device, Open Approach
019P0ZX Drainage of Sacral Sympathetic Nerve, Open Approach, Diagnostic
019P0ZZ Drainage of Sacral Sympathetic Nerve, Open Approach
019P30Z Drainage of Sacral Sympathetic Nerve with Drainage Device, Percutaneous Approach
019P3ZX Drainage of Sacral Sympathetic Nerve, Percutaneous Approach, Diagnostic
019P3ZZ Drainage of Sacral Sympathetic Nerve, Percutaneous Approach
019P40Z Drainage of Sacral Sympathetic Nerve with Drainage Device, Percutaneous Endoscopic Approach
019P4ZX Drainage of Sacral Sympathetic Nerve, Percutaneous Endoscopic Approach, Diagnostic
019P4ZZ Drainage of Sacral Sympathetic Nerve, Percutaneous Endoscopic Approach
019Q00Z Drainage of Sacral Plexus with Drainage Device, Open Approach
019Q0ZX Drainage of Sacral Plexus, Open Approach, Diagnostic
019Q0ZZ Drainage of Sacral Plexus, Open Approach
019Q30Z Drainage of Sacral Plexus with Drainage Device, Percutaneous Approach
019Q3ZX Drainage of Sacral Plexus, Percutaneous Approach, Diagnostic
019Q3ZZ Drainage of Sacral Plexus, Percutaneous Approach
019Q40Z Drainage of Sacral Plexus with Drainage Device, Percutaneous Endoscopic Approach
019Q4ZX Drainage of Sacral Plexus, Percutaneous Endoscopic Approach, Diagnostic
019Q4ZZ Drainage of Sacral Plexus, Percutaneous Endoscopic Approach
019R00Z Drainage of Sacral Nerve with Drainage Device, Open Approach
019R0ZX Drainage of Sacral Nerve, Open Approach, Diagnostic
019R0ZZ Drainage of Sacral Nerve, Open Approach
019R30Z Drainage of Sacral Nerve with Drainage Device, Percutaneous Approach
019R3ZX Drainage of Sacral Nerve, Percutaneous Approach, Diagnostic
019R3ZZ Drainage of Sacral Nerve, Percutaneous Approach
019R40Z Drainage of Sacral Nerve with Drainage Device, Percutaneous Endoscopic Approach
019R4ZX Drainage of Sacral Nerve, Percutaneous Endoscopic Approach, Diagnostic
019R4ZZ Drainage of Sacral Nerve, Percutaneous Endoscopic Approach

01B – Peripheral Nervous System, Excision

Review Coding Guidelines B3.4a and B3.4b

Review Coding Guideline B3.8

01B00ZX Excision of Cervical Plexus, Open Approach, Diagnostic
01B00ZZ Excision of Cervical Plexus, Open Approach
01B03ZX Excision of Cervical Plexus, Percutaneous Approach, Diagnostic
01B03ZZ Excision of Cervical Plexus, Percutaneous Approach
01B04ZX Excision of Cervical Plexus, Percutaneous Endoscopic Approach, Diagnostic
01B04ZZ Excision of Cervical Plexus, Percutaneous Endoscopic Approach
01B10ZX Excision of Cervical Nerve, Open Approach, Diagnostic
01B10ZZ Excision of Cervical Nerve, Open Approach
01B13ZX Excision of Cervical Nerve, Percutaneous Approach, Diagnostic
01B13ZZ Excision of Cervical Nerve, Percutaneous Approach
01B14ZX Excision of Cervical Nerve, Percutaneous Endoscopic Approach, Diagnostic
01B14ZZ Excision of Cervical Nerve, Percutaneous Endoscopic Approach
01B20ZX Excision of Phrenic Nerve, Open Approach, Diagnostic
01B20ZZ Excision of Phrenic Nerve, Open Approach
01B23ZX Excision of Phrenic Nerve, Percutaneous Approach, Diagnostic
01B23ZZ Excision of Phrenic Nerve, Percutaneous Approach
01B24ZX Excision of Phrenic Nerve, Percutaneous Endoscopic Approach, Diagnostic
01B24ZZ Excision of Phrenic Nerve, Percutaneous Endoscopic Approach
01B30ZX Excision of Brachial Plexus, Open Approach, Diagnostic
01B30ZZ Excision of Brachial Plexus, Open Approach
01B33ZX Excision of Brachial Plexus, Percutaneous Approach, Diagnostic
01B33ZZ Excision of Brachial Plexus, Percutaneous Approach
01B34ZX Excision of Brachial Plexus, Percutaneous Endoscopic Approach, Diagnostic
01B34ZZ Excision of Brachial Plexus, Percutaneous Endoscopic Approach
01B40ZX Excision of Ulnar Nerve, Open Approach, Diagnostic
01B40ZZ Excision of Ulnar Nerve, Open Approach
01B43ZX Excision of Ulnar Nerve, Percutaneous Approach, Diagnostic
01B43ZZ Excision of Ulnar Nerve, Percutaneous Approach
01B44ZX Excision of Ulnar Nerve, Percutaneous Endoscopic Approach, Diagnostic
01B44ZZ Excision of Ulnar Nerve, Percutaneous Endoscopic Approach
01B50ZX Excision of Median Nerve, Open Approach, Diagnostic
01B50ZZ Excision of Median Nerve, Open Approach
01B53ZX Excision of Median Nerve, Percutaneous Approach, Diagnostic
01B53ZZ Excision of Median Nerve, Percutaneous Approach
01B54ZX Excision of Median Nerve, Percutaneous Endoscopic Approach, Diagnostic
01B54ZZ Excision of Median Nerve, Percutaneous Endoscopic Approach
01B60ZX Excision of Radial Nerve, Open Approach, Diagnostic
01B60ZZ Excision of Radial Nerve, Open Approach
01B63ZX Excision of Radial Nerve, Percutaneous Approach, Diagnostic
01B63ZZ Excision of Radial Nerve, Percutaneous Approach
01B64ZX Excision of Radial Nerve, Percutaneous Endoscopic Approach, Diagnostic
01B64ZZ Excision of Radial Nerve, Percutaneous Endoscopic Approach
01B80ZX Excision of Thoracic Nerve, Open Approach, Diagnostic
01B80ZZ Excision of Thoracic Nerve, Open Approach
01B83ZX Excision of Thoracic Nerve, Percutaneous Approach, Diagnostic
01B83ZZ Excision of Thoracic Nerve, Percutaneous Approach
01B84ZX Excision of Thoracic Nerve, Percutaneous Endoscopic Approach, Diagnostic
01B84ZZ Excision of Thoracic Nerve, Percutaneous Endoscopic Approach
01B90ZX Excision of Lumbar Plexus, Open Approach, Diagnostic
01B90ZZ Excision of Lumbar Plexus, Open Approach
01B93ZX Excision of Lumbar Plexus, Percutaneous Approach, Diagnostic
01B93ZZ Excision of Lumbar Plexus, Percutaneous Approach
01B94ZX Excision of Lumbar Plexus, Percutaneous Endoscopic Approach, Diagnostic
01B94ZZ Excision of Lumbar Plexus, Percutaneous Endoscopic Approach
01BA0ZX Excision of Lumbosacral Plexus, Open Approach, Diagnostic
01BA0ZZ Excision of Lumbosacral Plexus, Open Approach
01BA3ZX Excision of Lumbosacral Plexus, Percutaneous Approach, Diagnostic
01BA3ZZ Excision of Lumbosacral Plexus, Percutaneous Approach
01BA4ZX Excision of Lumbosacral Plexus, Percutaneous Endoscopic Approach, Diagnostic
01BA4ZZ Excision of Lumbosacral Plexus, Percutaneous Endoscopic Approach
01BB0ZX Excision of Lumbar Nerve, Open Approach, Diagnostic
01BB0ZZ Excision of Lumbar Nerve, Open Approach
01BB3ZX Excision of Lumbar Nerve, Percutaneous Approach, Diagnostic
01BB3ZZ Excision of Lumbar Nerve, Percutaneous Approach
01BB4ZX Excision of Lumbar Nerve, Percutaneous Endoscopic Approach, Diagnostic
01BB4ZZ Excision of Lumbar Nerve, Percutaneous Endoscopic Approach
01BC0ZX Excision of Pudendal Nerve, Open Approach, Diagnostic
01BC0ZZ Excision of Pudendal Nerve, Open Approach
01BC3ZX Excision of Pudendal Nerve, Percutaneous Approach, Diagnostic
01BC3ZZ Excision of Pudendal Nerve, Percutaneous Approach
01BC4ZX Excision of Pudendal Nerve, Percutaneous Endoscopic Approach, Diagnostic
01BC4ZZ Excision of Pudendal Nerve, Percutaneous Endoscopic Approach

01BD0ZX Excision of Femoral Nerve, Open Approach, Diagnostic
01BD0ZZ Excision of Femoral Nerve, Open Approach
01BD3ZX Excision of Femoral Nerve, Percutaneous Approach, Diagnostic
01BD3ZZ Excision of Femoral Nerve, Percutaneous Approach
01BD4ZX Excision of Femoral Nerve, Percutaneous Endoscopic Approach, Diagnostic
01BD4ZZ Excision of Femoral Nerve, Percutaneous Endoscopic Approach
01BF0ZX Excision of Sciatic Nerve, Open Approach, Diagnostic
01BF0ZZ Excision of Sciatic Nerve, Open Approach
01BF3ZX Excision of Sciatic Nerve, Percutaneous Approach, Diagnostic
01BF3ZZ Excision of Sciatic Nerve, Percutaneous Approach
01BF4ZX Excision of Sciatic Nerve, Percutaneous Endoscopic Approach, Diagnostic
01BF4ZZ Excision of Sciatic Nerve, Percutaneous Endoscopic Approach
01BG0ZX Excision of Tibial Nerve, Open Approach, Diagnostic
01BG0ZZ Excision of Tibial Nerve, Open Approach
01BG3ZX Excision of Tibial Nerve, Percutaneous Approach, Diagnostic
01BG3ZZ Excision of Tibial Nerve, Percutaneous Approach
01BG4ZX Excision of Tibial Nerve, Percutaneous Endoscopic Approach, Diagnostic
01BG4ZZ Excision of Tibial Nerve, Percutaneous Endoscopic Approach
01BH0ZX Excision of Peroneal Nerve, Open Approach, Diagnostic
01BH0ZZ Excision of Peroneal Nerve, Open Approach
01BH3ZX Excision of Peroneal Nerve, Percutaneous Approach, Diagnostic
01BH3ZZ Excision of Peroneal Nerve, Percutaneous Approach
01BH4ZX Excision of Peroneal Nerve, Percutaneous Endoscopic Approach, Diagnostic
01BH4ZZ Excision of Peroneal Nerve, Percutaneous Endoscopic Approach
01BK0ZX Excision of Head and Neck Sympathetic Nerve, Open Approach, Diagnostic
01BK0ZZ Excision of Head and Neck Sympathetic Nerve, Open Approach
01BK3ZX Excision of Head and Neck Sympathetic Nerve, Percutaneous Approach, Diagnostic
01BK3ZZ Excision of Head and Neck Sympathetic Nerve, Percutaneous Approach
01BK4ZX Excision of Head and Neck Sympathetic Nerve, Percutaneous Endoscopic Approach, Diagnostic
01BK4ZZ Excision of Head and Neck Sympathetic Nerve, Percutaneous Endoscopic Approach
01BL0ZX Excision of Thoracic Sympathetic Nerve, Open Approach, Diagnostic
01BL0ZZ Excision of Thoracic Sympathetic Nerve, Open Approach
01BL3ZX Excision of Thoracic Sympathetic Nerve, Percutaneous Approach, Diagnostic
01BL3ZZ Excision of Thoracic Sympathetic Nerve, Percutaneous Approach
01BL4ZX Excision of Thoracic Sympathetic Nerve, Percutaneous Endoscopic Approach, Diagnostic
01BL4ZZ Excision of Thoracic Sympathetic Nerve, Percutaneous Endoscopic Approach
01BM0ZX Excision of Abdominal Sympathetic Nerve, Open Approach, Diagnostic
01BM0ZZ Excision of Abdominal Sympathetic Nerve, Open Approach
01BM3ZX Excision of Abdominal Sympathetic Nerve, Percutaneous Approach, Diagnostic
01BM3ZZ Excision of Abdominal Sympathetic Nerve, Percutaneous Approach
01BM4ZX Excision of Abdominal Sympathetic Nerve, Percutaneous Endoscopic Approach, Diagnostic
01BM4ZZ Excision of Abdominal Sympathetic Nerve, Percutaneous Endoscopic Approach
01BN0ZX Excision of Lumbar Sympathetic Nerve, Open Approach, Diagnostic
01BN0ZZ Excision of Lumbar Sympathetic Nerve, Open Approach
01BN3ZX Excision of Lumbar Sympathetic Nerve, Percutaneous Approach, Diagnostic
01BN3ZZ Excision of Lumbar Sympathetic Nerve, Percutaneous Approach
01BN4ZX Excision of Lumbar Sympathetic Nerve, Percutaneous Endoscopic Approach, Diagnostic
01BN4ZZ Excision of Lumbar Sympathetic Nerve, Percutaneous Endoscopic Approach
01BP0ZX Excision of Sacral Sympathetic Nerve, Open Approach, Diagnostic
01BP0ZZ Excision of Sacral Sympathetic Nerve, Open Approach
01BP3ZX Excision of Sacral Sympathetic Nerve, Percutaneous Approach, Diagnostic
01BP3ZZ Excision of Sacral Sympathetic Nerve, Percutaneous Approach
01BP4ZX Excision of Sacral Sympathetic Nerve, Percutaneous Endoscopic Approach, Diagnostic
01BP4ZZ Excision of Sacral Sympathetic Nerve, Percutaneous Endoscopic Approach
01BQ0ZX Excision of Sacral Plexus, Open Approach, Diagnostic
01BQ0ZZ Excision of Sacral Plexus, Open Approach
01BQ3ZX Excision of Sacral Plexus, Percutaneous Approach, Diagnostic
01BQ3ZZ Excision of Sacral Plexus, Percutaneous Approach
01BQ4ZX Excision of Sacral Plexus, Percutaneous Endoscopic Approach, Diagnostic
01BQ4ZZ Excision of Sacral Plexus, Percutaneous Endoscopic Approach
01BR0ZX Excision of Sacral Nerve, Open Approach, Diagnostic
01BR0ZZ Excision of Sacral Nerve, Open Approach
01BR3ZX Excision of Sacral Nerve, Percutaneous Approach, Diagnostic
01BR3ZZ Excision of Sacral Nerve, Percutaneous Approach
01BR4ZX Excision of Sacral Nerve, Percutaneous Endoscopic Approach, Diagnostic
01BR4ZZ Excision of Sacral Nerve, Percutaneous Endoscopic Approach

01C – Peripheral Nervous System, Extirpation

01C00ZZ Extirpation of Matter from Cervical Plexus, Open Approach
01C03ZZ Extirpation of Matter from Cervical Plexus, Percutaneous Approach
01C04ZZ Extirpation of Matter from Cervical Plexus, Percutaneous Endoscopic Approach
01C10ZZ Extirpation of Matter from Cervical Nerve, Open Approach
01C13ZZ Extirpation of Matter from Cervical Nerve, Percutaneous Approach
01C14ZZ Extirpation of Matter from Cervical Nerve, Percutaneous Endoscopic Approach
01C20ZZ Extirpation of Matter from Phrenic Nerve, Open Approach
01C23ZZ Extirpation of Matter from Phrenic Nerve, Percutaneous Approach
01C24ZZ Extirpation of Matter from Phrenic Nerve, Percutaneous Endoscopic Approach
01C30ZZ Extirpation of Matter from Brachial Plexus, Open Approach
01C33ZZ Extirpation of Matter from Brachial Plexus, Percutaneous Approach
01C34ZZ Extirpation of Matter from Brachial Plexus, Percutaneous Endoscopic Approach
01C40ZZ Extirpation of Matter from Ulnar Nerve, Open Approach
01C43ZZ Extirpation of Matter from Ulnar Nerve, Percutaneous Approach
01C44ZZ Extirpation of Matter from Ulnar Nerve, Percutaneous Endoscopic Approach
01C50ZZ Extirpation of Matter from Median Nerve, Open Approach
01C53ZZ Extirpation of Matter from Median Nerve, Percutaneous Approach
01C54ZZ Extirpation of Matter from Median Nerve, Percutaneous Endoscopic Approach
01C60ZZ Extirpation of Matter from Radial Nerve, Open Approach
01C63ZZ Extirpation of Matter from Radial Nerve, Percutaneous Approach
01C64ZZ Extirpation of Matter from Radial Nerve, Percutaneous Endoscopic Approach
01C80ZZ Extirpation of Matter from Thoracic Nerve, Open Approach
01C83ZZ Extirpation of Matter from Thoracic Nerve, Percutaneous Approach
01C84ZZ Extirpation of Matter from Thoracic Nerve, Percutaneous Endoscopic Approach
01C90ZZ Extirpation of Matter from Lumbar Plexus, Open Approach
01C93ZZ Extirpation of Matter from Lumbar Plexus, Percutaneous Approach
01C94ZZ Extirpation of Matter from Lumbar Plexus, Percutaneous Endoscopic Approach
01CA0ZZ Extirpation of Matter from Lumbosacral Plexus, Open Approach
01CA3ZZ Extirpation of Matter from Lumbosacral Plexus, Percutaneous Approach
01CA4ZZ Extirpation of Matter from Lumbosacral Plexus, Percutaneous Endoscopic Approach
01CB0ZZ Extirpation of Matter from Lumbar Nerve, Open Approach
01CB3ZZ Extirpation of Matter from Lumbar Nerve, Percutaneous Approach
01CB4ZZ Extirpation of Matter from Lumbar Nerve, Percutaneous Endoscopic Approach
01CC0ZZ Extirpation of Matter from Pudendal Nerve, Open Approach
01CC3ZZ Extirpation of Matter from Pudendal Nerve, Percutaneous Approach
01CC4ZZ Extirpation of Matter from Pudendal Nerve, Percutaneous Endoscopic Approach
01CD0ZZ Extirpation of Matter from Femoral Nerve, Open Approach
01CD3ZZ Extirpation of Matter from Femoral Nerve, Percutaneous Approach
01CD4ZZ Extirpation of Matter from Femoral Nerve, Percutaneous Endoscopic Approach

01CF0ZZ Extirpation of Matter from Sciatic Nerve, Open Approach
01CF3ZZ Extirpation of Matter from Sciatic Nerve, Percutaneous Approach
01CF4ZZ Extirpation of Matter from Sciatic Nerve, Percutaneous Endoscopic Approach
01CG0ZZ Extirpation of Matter from Tibial Nerve, Open Approach
01CG3ZZ Extirpation of Matter from Tibial Nerve, Percutaneous Approach
01CG4ZZ Extirpation of Matter from Tibial Nerve, Percutaneous Endoscopic Approach
01CH0ZZ Extirpation of Matter from Peroneal Nerve, Open Approach
01CH3ZZ Extirpation of Matter from Peroneal Nerve, Percutaneous Approach
01CH4ZZ Extirpation of Matter from Peroneal Nerve, Percutaneous Endoscopic Approach
01CK0ZZ Extirpation of Matter from Head and Neck Sympathetic Nerve, Open Approach
01CK3ZZ Extirpation of Matter from Head and Neck Sympathetic Nerve, Percutaneous Approach
01CK4ZZ Extirpation of Matter from Head and Neck Sympathetic Nerve, Percutaneous Endoscopic Approach
01CL0ZZ Extirpation of Matter from Thoracic Sympathetic Nerve, Open Approach
01CL3ZZ Extirpation of Matter from Thoracic Sympathetic Nerve, Percutaneous Approach
01CL4ZZ Extirpation of Matter from Thoracic Sympathetic Nerve, Percutaneous Endoscopic Approach
01CM0ZZ Extirpation of Matter from Abdominal Sympathetic Nerve, Open Approach
01CM3ZZ Extirpation of Matter from Abdominal Sympathetic Nerve, Percutaneous Approach
01CM4ZZ Extirpation of Matter from Abdominal Sympathetic Nerve, Percutaneous Endoscopic Approach
01CN0ZZ Extirpation of Matter from Lumbar Sympathetic Nerve, Open Approach
01CN3ZZ Extirpation of Matter from Lumbar Sympathetic Nerve, Percutaneous Approach
01CN4ZZ Extirpation of Matter from Lumbar Sympathetic Nerve, Percutaneous Endoscopic Approach
01CP0ZZ Extirpation of Matter from Sacral Sympathetic Nerve, Open Approach
01CP3ZZ Extirpation of Matter from Sacral Sympathetic Nerve, Percutaneous Approach
01CP4ZZ Extirpation of Matter from Sacral Sympathetic Nerve, Percutaneous Endoscopic Approach
01CQ0ZZ Extirpation of Matter from Sacral Plexus, Open Approach
01CQ3ZZ Extirpation of Matter from Sacral Plexus, Percutaneous Approach
01CQ4ZZ Extirpation of Matter from Sacral Plexus, Percutaneous Endoscopic Approach
01CR0ZZ Extirpation of Matter from Sacral Nerve, Open Approach
01CR3ZZ Extirpation of Matter from Sacral Nerve, Percutaneous Approach
01CR4ZZ Extirpation of Matter from Sacral Nerve, Percutaneous Endoscopic Approach

01D – Peripheral Nervous System, Extraction

01D00ZZ Extraction of Cervical Plexus, Open Approach
01D03ZZ Extraction of Cervical Plexus, Percutaneous Approach
01D04ZZ Extraction of Cervical Plexus, Percutaneous Endoscopic Approach
01D10ZZ Extraction of Cervical Nerve, Open Approach
01D13ZZ Extraction of Cervical Nerve, Percutaneous Approach
01D14ZZ Extraction of Cervical Nerve, Percutaneous Endoscopic Approach
01D20ZZ Extraction of Phrenic Nerve, Open Approach
01D23ZZ Extraction of Phrenic Nerve, Percutaneous Approach
01D24ZZ Extraction of Phrenic Nerve, Percutaneous Endoscopic Approach
01D30ZZ Extraction of Brachial Plexus, Open Approach
01D33ZZ Extraction of Brachial Plexus, Percutaneous Approach
01D34ZZ Extraction of Brachial Plexus, Percutaneous Endoscopic Approach
01D40ZZ Extraction of Ulnar Nerve, Open Approach
01D43ZZ Extraction of Ulnar Nerve, Percutaneous Approach
01D44ZZ Extraction of Ulnar Nerve, Percutaneous Endoscopic Approach
01D50ZZ Extraction of Median Nerve, Open Approach
01D53ZZ Extraction of Median Nerve, Percutaneous Approach
01D54ZZ Extraction of Median Nerve, Percutaneous Endoscopic Approach
01D60ZZ Extraction of Radial Nerve, Open Approach
01D63ZZ Extraction of Radial Nerve, Percutaneous Approach
01D64ZZ Extraction of Radial Nerve, Percutaneous Endoscopic Approach
01D80ZZ Extraction of Thoracic Nerve, Open Approach
01D83ZZ Extraction of Thoracic Nerve, Percutaneous Approach
01D84ZZ Extraction of Thoracic Nerve, Percutaneous Endoscopic Approach
01D90ZZ Extraction of Lumbar Plexus, Open Approach
01D93ZZ Extraction of Lumbar Plexus, Percutaneous Approach
01D94ZZ Extraction of Lumbar Plexus, Percutaneous Endoscopic Approach
01DA0ZZ Extraction of Lumbosacral Plexus, Open Approach
01DA3ZZ Extraction of Lumbosacral Plexus, Percutaneous Approach
01DA4ZZ Extraction of Lumbosacral Plexus, Percutaneous Endoscopic Approach
01DB0ZZ Extraction of Lumbar Nerve, Open Approach
01DB3ZZ Extraction of Lumbar Nerve, Percutaneous Approach
01DB4ZZ Extraction of Lumbar Nerve, Percutaneous Endoscopic Approach
01DC0ZZ Extraction of Pudendal Nerve, Open Approach
01DC3ZZ Extraction of Pudendal Nerve, Percutaneous Approach
01DC4ZZ Extraction of Pudendal Nerve, Percutaneous Endoscopic Approach
01DD0ZZ Extraction of Femoral Nerve, Open Approach
01DD3ZZ Extraction of Femoral Nerve, Percutaneous Approach
01DD4ZZ Extraction of Femoral Nerve, Percutaneous Endoscopic Approach
01DF0ZZ Extraction of Sciatic Nerve, Open Approach
01DF3ZZ Extraction of Sciatic Nerve, Percutaneous Approach
01DF4ZZ Extraction of Sciatic Nerve, Percutaneous Endoscopic Approach
01DG0ZZ Extraction of Tibial Nerve, Open Approach
01DG3ZZ Extraction of Tibial Nerve, Percutaneous Approach
01DG4ZZ Extraction of Tibial Nerve, Percutaneous Endoscopic Approach
01DH0ZZ Extraction of Peroneal Nerve, Open Approach
01DH3ZZ Extraction of Peroneal Nerve, Percutaneous Approach
01DH4ZZ Extraction of Peroneal Nerve, Percutaneous Endoscopic Approach
01DK0ZZ Extraction of Head and Neck Sympathetic Nerve, Open Approach
01DK3ZZ Extraction of Head and Neck Sympathetic Nerve, Percutaneous Approach
01DK4ZZ Extraction of Head and Neck Sympathetic Nerve, Percutaneous Endoscopic Approach
01DL0ZZ Extraction of Thoracic Sympathetic Nerve, Open Approach
01DL3ZZ Extraction of Thoracic Sympathetic Nerve, Percutaneous Approach
01DL4ZZ Extraction of Thoracic Sympathetic Nerve, Percutaneous Endoscopic Approach
01DM0ZZ Extraction of Abdominal Sympathetic Nerve, Open Approach
01DM3ZZ Extraction of Abdominal Sympathetic Nerve, Percutaneous Approach
01DM4ZZ Extraction of Abdominal Sympathetic Nerve, Percutaneous Endoscopic Approach
01DN0ZZ Extraction of Lumbar Sympathetic Nerve, Open Approach
01DN3ZZ Extraction of Lumbar Sympathetic Nerve, Percutaneous Approach
01DN4ZZ Extraction of Lumbar Sympathetic Nerve, Percutaneous Endoscopic Approach
01DP0ZZ Extraction of Sacral Sympathetic Nerve, Open Approach
01DP3ZZ Extraction of Sacral Sympathetic Nerve, Percutaneous Approach
01DP4ZZ Extraction of Sacral Sympathetic Nerve, Percutaneous Endoscopic Approach
01DQ0ZZ Extraction of Sacral Plexus, Open Approach
01DQ3ZZ Extraction of Sacral Plexus, Percutaneous Approach
01DQ4ZZ Extraction of Sacral Plexus, Percutaneous Endoscopic Approach
01DR0ZZ Extraction of Sacral Nerve, Open Approach
01DR3ZZ Extraction of Sacral Nerve, Percutaneous Approach
01DR4ZZ Extraction of Sacral Nerve, Percutaneous Endoscopic Approach

01H – Peripheral Nervous System, Insertion

01HY02Z Insertion of Monitoring Device into Peripheral Nerve, Open Approach
01HY0MZ Insertion of Neurostimulator Lead into Peripheral Nerve, Open Approach
01HY32Z Insertion of Monitoring Device into Peripheral Nerve, Percutaneous Approach
01HY3MZ Insertion of Neurostimulator Lead into Peripheral Nerve, Percutaneous Approach
01HY42Z Insertion of Monitoring Device into Peripheral Nerve, Percutaneous Endoscopic Approach
01HY4MZ Insertion of Neurostimulator Lead into Peripheral Nerve, Percutaneous Endoscopic Approach

01J – Peripheral Nervous System, Inspection

Review Coding Guidelines B3.11a, B3.11b and B3.11c

01JY0ZZ Inspection of Peripheral Nerve, Open Approach
01JY3ZZ Inspection of Peripheral Nerve, Percutaneous Approach
01JY4ZZ Inspection of Peripheral Nerve, Percutaneous Endoscopic Approach

01N – Peripheral Nervous System, Release

Review Coding Guideline B3.13

Review Coding Guideline B3.14

01N00ZZ Release Cervical Plexus, Open Approach
01N03ZZ Release Cervical Plexus, Percutaneous Approach
01N04ZZ Release Cervical Plexus, Percutaneous Endoscopic Approach
01N10ZZ Release Cervical Nerve, Open Approach
01N13ZZ Release Cervical Nerve, Percutaneous Approach
01N14ZZ Release Cervical Nerve, Percutaneous Endoscopic Approach
01N20ZZ Release Phrenic Nerve, Open Approach
01N23ZZ Release Phrenic Nerve, Percutaneous Approach
01N24ZZ Release Phrenic Nerve, Percutaneous Endoscopic Approach
01N30ZZ Release Brachial Plexus, Open Approach
01N33ZZ Release Brachial Plexus, Percutaneous Approach
01N34ZZ Release Brachial Plexus, Percutaneous Endoscopic Approach
01N40ZZ Release Ulnar Nerve, Open Approach
01N43ZZ Release Ulnar Nerve, Percutaneous Approach
01N44ZZ Release Ulnar Nerve, Percutaneous Endoscopic Approach
01N50ZZ Release Median Nerve, Open Approach
01N53ZZ Release Median Nerve, Percutaneous Approach
01N54ZZ Release Median Nerve, Percutaneous Endoscopic Approach
01N60ZZ Release Radial Nerve, Open Approach
01N63ZZ Release Radial Nerve, Percutaneous Approach
01N64ZZ Release Radial Nerve, Percutaneous Endoscopic Approach
01N80ZZ Release Thoracic Nerve, Open Approach
01N83ZZ Release Thoracic Nerve, Percutaneous Approach
01N84ZZ Release Thoracic Nerve, Percutaneous Endoscopic Approach
01N90ZZ Release Lumbar Plexus, Open Approach
01N93ZZ Release Lumbar Plexus, Percutaneous Approach
01N94ZZ Release Lumbar Plexus, Percutaneous Endoscopic Approach
01NA0ZZ Release Lumbosacral Plexus, Open Approach
01NA3ZZ Release Lumbosacral Plexus, Percutaneous Approach
01NA4ZZ Release Lumbosacral Plexus, Percutaneous Endoscopic Approach
01NB0ZZ Release Lumbar Nerve, Open Approach
01NB3ZZ Release Lumbar Nerve, Percutaneous Approach
01NB4ZZ Release Lumbar Nerve, Percutaneous Endoscopic Approach
01NC0ZZ Release Pudendal Nerve, Open Approach
01NC3ZZ Release Pudendal Nerve, Percutaneous Approach
01NC4ZZ Release Pudendal Nerve, Percutaneous Endoscopic Approach
01ND0ZZ Release Femoral Nerve, Open Approach
01ND3ZZ Release Femoral Nerve, Percutaneous Approach
01ND4ZZ Release Femoral Nerve, Percutaneous Endoscopic Approach
01NF0ZZ Release Sciatic Nerve, Open Approach
01NF3ZZ Release Sciatic Nerve, Percutaneous Approach
01NF4ZZ Release Sciatic Nerve, Percutaneous Endoscopic Approach
01NG0ZZ Release Tibial Nerve, Open Approach
01NG3ZZ Release Tibial Nerve, Percutaneous Approach
01NG4ZZ Release Tibial Nerve, Percutaneous Endoscopic Approach
01NH0ZZ Release Peroneal Nerve, Open Approach
01NH3ZZ Release Peroneal Nerve, Percutaneous Approach
01NH4ZZ Release Peroneal Nerve, Percutaneous Endoscopic Approach
01NK0ZZ Release Head and Neck Sympathetic Nerve, Open Approach
01NK3ZZ Release Head and Neck Sympathetic Nerve, Percutaneous Approach
01NK4ZZ Release Head and Neck Sympathetic Nerve, Percutaneous Endoscopic Approach
01NL0ZZ Release Thoracic Sympathetic Nerve, Open Approach
01NL3ZZ Release Thoracic Sympathetic Nerve, Percutaneous Approach
01NL4ZZ Release Thoracic Sympathetic Nerve, Percutaneous Endoscopic Approach
01NM0ZZ Release Abdominal Sympathetic Nerve, Open Approach
01NM3ZZ Release Abdominal Sympathetic Nerve, Percutaneous Approach
01NM4ZZ Release Abdominal Sympathetic Nerve, Percutaneous Endoscopic Approach
01NN0ZZ Release Lumbar Sympathetic Nerve, Open Approach
01NN3ZZ Release Lumbar Sympathetic Nerve, Percutaneous Approach
01NN4ZZ Release Lumbar Sympathetic Nerve, Percutaneous Endoscopic Approach
01NP0ZZ Release Sacral Sympathetic Nerve, Open Approach
01NP3ZZ Release Sacral Sympathetic Nerve, Percutaneous Approach
01NP4ZZ Release Sacral Sympathetic Nerve, Percutaneous Endoscopic Approach
01NQ0ZZ Release Sacral Plexus, Open Approach
01NQ3ZZ Release Sacral Plexus, Percutaneous Approach
01NQ4ZZ Release Sacral Plexus, Percutaneous Endoscopic Approach
01NR0ZZ Release Sacral Nerve, Open Approach
01NR3ZZ Release Sacral Nerve, Percutaneous Approach
01NR4ZZ Release Sacral Nerve, Percutaneous Endoscopic Approach

01P – Peripheral Nervous System, Removal

Review Coding Guideline B6.1c

01PY00Z Removal of Drainage Device from Peripheral Nerve, Open Approach
01PY02Z Removal of Monitoring Device from Peripheral Nerve, Open Approach
01PY07Z Removal of Autologous Tissue Substitute from Peripheral Nerve, Open Approach
01PY0MZ Removal of Neurostimulator Lead from Peripheral Nerve, Open Approach
01PY30Z Removal of Drainage Device from Peripheral Nerve, Percutaneous Approach
01PY32Z Removal of Monitoring Device from Peripheral Nerve, Percutaneous Approach
01PY37Z Removal of Autologous Tissue Substitute from Peripheral Nerve, Percutaneous Approach
01PY3MZ Removal of Neurostimulator Lead from Peripheral Nerve, Percutaneous Approach
01PY40Z Removal of Drainage Device from Peripheral Nerve, Percutaneous Endoscopic Approach
01PY42Z Removal of Monitoring Device from Peripheral Nerve, Percutaneous Endoscopic Approach
01PY47Z Removal of Autologous Tissue Substitute from Peripheral Nerve, Percutaneous Endoscopic Approach
01PY4MZ Removal of Neurostimulator Lead from Peripheral Nerve, Percutaneous Endoscopic Approach

01PYX0Z Removal of Drainage Device from Peripheral Nerve, External Approach
01PYX2Z Removal of Monitoring Device from Peripheral Nerve, External Approach
01PYXMZ Removal of Neurostimulator Lead from Peripheral Nerve, External Approach

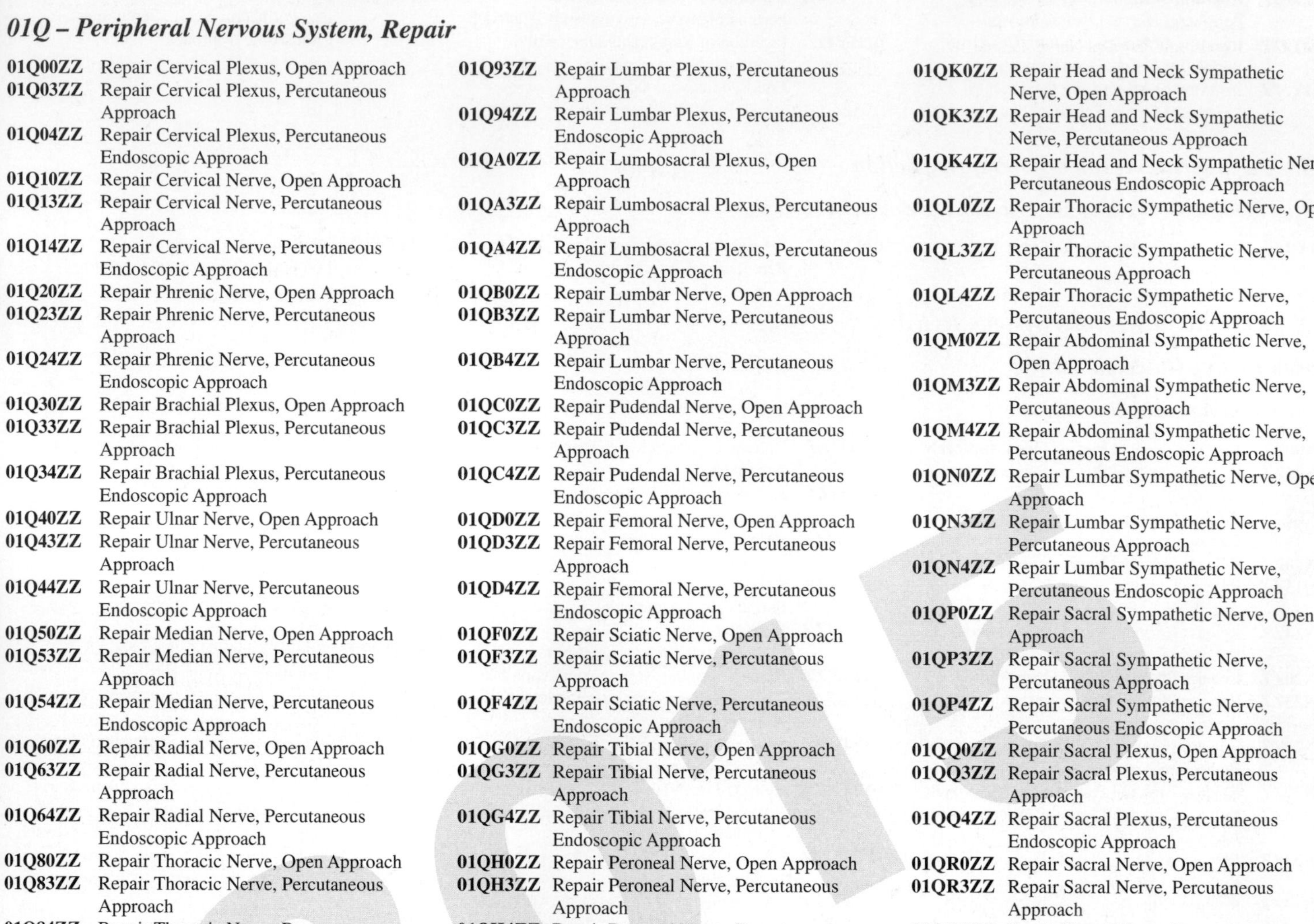

01Q – Peripheral Nervous System, Repair

01Q00ZZ Repair Cervical Plexus, Open Approach
01Q03ZZ Repair Cervical Plexus, Percutaneous Approach
01Q04ZZ Repair Cervical Plexus, Percutaneous Endoscopic Approach
01Q10ZZ Repair Cervical Nerve, Open Approach
01Q13ZZ Repair Cervical Nerve, Percutaneous Approach
01Q14ZZ Repair Cervical Nerve, Percutaneous Endoscopic Approach
01Q20ZZ Repair Phrenic Nerve, Open Approach
01Q23ZZ Repair Phrenic Nerve, Percutaneous Approach
01Q24ZZ Repair Phrenic Nerve, Percutaneous Endoscopic Approach
01Q30ZZ Repair Brachial Plexus, Open Approach
01Q33ZZ Repair Brachial Plexus, Percutaneous Approach
01Q34ZZ Repair Brachial Plexus, Percutaneous Endoscopic Approach
01Q40ZZ Repair Ulnar Nerve, Open Approach
01Q43ZZ Repair Ulnar Nerve, Percutaneous Approach
01Q44ZZ Repair Ulnar Nerve, Percutaneous Endoscopic Approach
01Q50ZZ Repair Median Nerve, Open Approach
01Q53ZZ Repair Median Nerve, Percutaneous Approach
01Q54ZZ Repair Median Nerve, Percutaneous Endoscopic Approach
01Q60ZZ Repair Radial Nerve, Open Approach
01Q63ZZ Repair Radial Nerve, Percutaneous Approach
01Q64ZZ Repair Radial Nerve, Percutaneous Endoscopic Approach
01Q80ZZ Repair Thoracic Nerve, Open Approach
01Q83ZZ Repair Thoracic Nerve, Percutaneous Approach
01Q84ZZ Repair Thoracic Nerve, Percutaneous Endoscopic Approach
01Q90ZZ Repair Lumbar Plexus, Open Approach
01Q93ZZ Repair Lumbar Plexus, Percutaneous Approach
01Q94ZZ Repair Lumbar Plexus, Percutaneous Endoscopic Approach
01QA0ZZ Repair Lumbosacral Plexus, Open Approach
01QA3ZZ Repair Lumbosacral Plexus, Percutaneous Approach
01QA4ZZ Repair Lumbosacral Plexus, Percutaneous Endoscopic Approach
01QB0ZZ Repair Lumbar Nerve, Open Approach
01QB3ZZ Repair Lumbar Nerve, Percutaneous Approach
01QB4ZZ Repair Lumbar Nerve, Percutaneous Endoscopic Approach
01QC0ZZ Repair Pudendal Nerve, Open Approach
01QC3ZZ Repair Pudendal Nerve, Percutaneous Approach
01QC4ZZ Repair Pudendal Nerve, Percutaneous Endoscopic Approach
01QD0ZZ Repair Femoral Nerve, Open Approach
01QD3ZZ Repair Femoral Nerve, Percutaneous Approach
01QD4ZZ Repair Femoral Nerve, Percutaneous Endoscopic Approach
01QF0ZZ Repair Sciatic Nerve, Open Approach
01QF3ZZ Repair Sciatic Nerve, Percutaneous Approach
01QF4ZZ Repair Sciatic Nerve, Percutaneous Endoscopic Approach
01QG0ZZ Repair Tibial Nerve, Open Approach
01QG3ZZ Repair Tibial Nerve, Percutaneous Approach
01QG4ZZ Repair Tibial Nerve, Percutaneous Endoscopic Approach
01QH0ZZ Repair Peroneal Nerve, Open Approach
01QH3ZZ Repair Peroneal Nerve, Percutaneous Approach
01QH4ZZ Repair Peroneal Nerve, Percutaneous Endoscopic Approach
01QK0ZZ Repair Head and Neck Sympathetic Nerve, Open Approach
01QK3ZZ Repair Head and Neck Sympathetic Nerve, Percutaneous Approach
01QK4ZZ Repair Head and Neck Sympathetic Nerve, Percutaneous Endoscopic Approach
01QL0ZZ Repair Thoracic Sympathetic Nerve, Open Approach
01QL3ZZ Repair Thoracic Sympathetic Nerve, Percutaneous Approach
01QL4ZZ Repair Thoracic Sympathetic Nerve, Percutaneous Endoscopic Approach
01QM0ZZ Repair Abdominal Sympathetic Nerve, Open Approach
01QM3ZZ Repair Abdominal Sympathetic Nerve, Percutaneous Approach
01QM4ZZ Repair Abdominal Sympathetic Nerve, Percutaneous Endoscopic Approach
01QN0ZZ Repair Lumbar Sympathetic Nerve, Open Approach
01QN3ZZ Repair Lumbar Sympathetic Nerve, Percutaneous Approach
01QN4ZZ Repair Lumbar Sympathetic Nerve, Percutaneous Endoscopic Approach
01QP0ZZ Repair Sacral Sympathetic Nerve, Open Approach
01QP3ZZ Repair Sacral Sympathetic Nerve, Percutaneous Approach
01QP4ZZ Repair Sacral Sympathetic Nerve, Percutaneous Endoscopic Approach
01QQ0ZZ Repair Sacral Plexus, Open Approach
01QQ3ZZ Repair Sacral Plexus, Percutaneous Approach
01QQ4ZZ Repair Sacral Plexus, Percutaneous Endoscopic Approach
01QR0ZZ Repair Sacral Nerve, Open Approach
01QR3ZZ Repair Sacral Nerve, Percutaneous Approach
01QR4ZZ Repair Sacral Nerve, Percutaneous Endoscopic Approach

01S – Peripheral Nervous System, Reposition

01S00ZZ Reposition Cervical Plexus, Open Approach
01S03ZZ Reposition Cervical Plexus, Percutaneous Approach
01S04ZZ Reposition Cervical Plexus, Percutaneous Endoscopic Approach
01S10ZZ Reposition Cervical Nerve, Open Approach
01S13ZZ Reposition Cervical Nerve, Percutaneous Approach
01S14ZZ Reposition Cervical Nerve, Percutaneous Endoscopic Approach
01S20ZZ Reposition Phrenic Nerve, Open Approach
01S23ZZ Reposition Phrenic Nerve, Percutaneous Approach
01S24ZZ Reposition Phrenic Nerve, Percutaneous Endoscopic Approach
01S30ZZ Reposition Brachial Plexus, Open Approach
01S33ZZ Reposition Brachial Plexus, Percutaneous Approach
01S34ZZ Reposition Brachial Plexus, Percutaneous Endoscopic Approach
01S40ZZ Reposition Ulnar Nerve, Open Approach
01S43ZZ Reposition Ulnar Nerve, Percutaneous Approach
01S44ZZ Reposition Ulnar Nerve, Percutaneous Endoscopic Approach
01S50ZZ Reposition Median Nerve, Open Approach
01S53ZZ Reposition Median Nerve, Percutaneous Approach
01S54ZZ Reposition Median Nerve, Percutaneous Endoscopic Approach
01S60ZZ Reposition Radial Nerve, Open Approach
01S63ZZ Reposition Radial Nerve, Percutaneous Approach
01S64ZZ Reposition Radial Nerve, Percutaneous Endoscopic Approach
01S80ZZ Reposition Thoracic Nerve, Open Approach
01S83ZZ Reposition Thoracic Nerve, Percutaneous Approach
01S84ZZ Reposition Thoracic Nerve, Percutaneous Endoscopic Approach
01S90ZZ Reposition Lumbar Plexus, Open Approach
01S93ZZ Reposition Lumbar Plexus, Percutaneous Approach
01S94ZZ Reposition Lumbar Plexus, Percutaneous Endoscopic Approach
01SA0ZZ Reposition Lumbosacral Plexus, Open Approach
01SA3ZZ Reposition Lumbosacral Plexus, Percutaneous Approach
01SA4ZZ Reposition Lumbosacral Plexus, Percutaneous Endoscopic Approach
01SB0ZZ Reposition Lumbar Nerve, Open Approach
01SB3ZZ Reposition Lumbar Nerve, Percutaneous Approach
01SB4ZZ Reposition Lumbar Nerve, Percutaneous Endoscopic Approach
01SC0ZZ Reposition Pudendal Nerve, Open Approach
01SC3ZZ Reposition Pudendal Nerve, Percutaneous Approach
01SC4ZZ Reposition Pudendal Nerve, Percutaneous Endoscopic Approach
01SD0ZZ Reposition Femoral Nerve, Open Approach
01SD3ZZ Reposition Femoral Nerve, Percutaneous Approach
01SD4ZZ Reposition Femoral Nerve, Percutaneous Endoscopic Approach
01SF0ZZ Reposition Sciatic Nerve, Open Approach
01SF3ZZ Reposition Sciatic Nerve, Percutaneous Approach
01SF4ZZ Reposition Sciatic Nerve, Percutaneous Endoscopic Approach
01SG0ZZ Reposition Tibial Nerve, Open Approach
01SG3ZZ Reposition Tibial Nerve, Percutaneous Approach
01SG4ZZ Reposition Tibial Nerve, Percutaneous Endoscopic Approach

01SH0ZZ Reposition Peroneal Nerve, Open Approach
01SH3ZZ Reposition Peroneal Nerve, Percutaneous Approach
01SH4ZZ Reposition Peroneal Nerve, Percutaneous Endoscopic Approach
01SQ0ZZ Reposition Sacral Plexus, Open Approach
01SQ3ZZ Reposition Sacral Plexus, Percutaneous Approach
01SQ4ZZ Reposition Sacral Plexus, Percutaneous Endoscopic Approach
01SR0ZZ Reposition Sacral Nerve, Open Approach
01SR3ZZ Reposition Sacral Nerve, Percutaneous Approach
01SR4ZZ Reposition Sacral Nerve, Percutaneous Endoscopic Approach

01U – Peripheral Nervous System, Supplement

01U107Z Supplement Cervical Nerve with Autologous Tissue Substitute, Open Approach
01U137Z Supplement Cervical Nerve with Autologous Tissue Substitute, Percutaneous Approach
01U147Z Supplement Cervical Nerve with Autologous Tissue Substitute, Percutaneous Endoscopic Approach
01U207Z Supplement Phrenic Nerve with Autologous Tissue Substitute, Open Approach
01U237Z Supplement Phrenic Nerve with Autologous Tissue Substitute, Percutaneous Approach
01U247Z Supplement Phrenic Nerve with Autologous Tissue Substitute, Percutaneous Endoscopic Approach
01U407Z Supplement Ulnar Nerve with Autologous Tissue Substitute, Open Approach
01U437Z Supplement Ulnar Nerve with Autologous Tissue Substitute, Percutaneous Approach
01U447Z Supplement Ulnar Nerve with Autologous Tissue Substitute, Percutaneous Endoscopic Approach
01U507Z Supplement Median Nerve with Autologous Tissue Substitute, Open Approach
01U537Z Supplement Median Nerve with Autologous Tissue Substitute, Percutaneous Approach
01U547Z Supplement Median Nerve with Autologous Tissue Substitute, Percutaneous Endoscopic Approach
01U607Z Supplement Radial Nerve with Autologous Tissue Substitute, Open Approach
01U637Z Supplement Radial Nerve with Autologous Tissue Substitute, Percutaneous Approach
01U647Z Supplement Radial Nerve with Autologous Tissue Substitute, Percutaneous Endoscopic Approach
01U807Z Supplement Thoracic Nerve with Autologous Tissue Substitute, Open Approach
01U837Z Supplement Thoracic Nerve with Autologous Tissue Substitute, Percutaneous Approach
01U847Z Supplement Thoracic Nerve with Autologous Tissue Substitute, Percutaneous Endoscopic Approach
01UB07Z Supplement Lumbar Nerve with Autologous Tissue Substitute, Open Approach
01UB37Z Supplement Lumbar Nerve with Autologous Tissue Substitute, Percutaneous Approach
01UB47Z Supplement Lumbar Nerve with Autologous Tissue Substitute, Percutaneous Endoscopic Approach
01UC07Z Supplement Pudendal Nerve with Autologous Tissue Substitute, Open Approach
01UC37Z Supplement Pudendal Nerve with Autologous Tissue Substitute, Percutaneous Approach
01UC47Z Supplement Pudendal Nerve with Autologous Tissue Substitute, Percutaneous Endoscopic Approach
01UD07Z Supplement Femoral Nerve with Autologous Tissue Substitute, Open Approach
01UD37Z Supplement Femoral Nerve with Autologous Tissue Substitute, Percutaneous Approach
01UD47Z Supplement Femoral Nerve with Autologous Tissue Substitute, Percutaneous Endoscopic Approach
01UF07Z Supplement Sciatic Nerve with Autologous Tissue Substitute, Open Approach
01UF37Z Supplement Sciatic Nerve with Autologous Tissue Substitute, Percutaneous Approach
01UF47Z Supplement Sciatic Nerve with Autologous Tissue Substitute, Percutaneous Endoscopic Approach
01UG07Z Supplement Tibial Nerve with Autologous Tissue Substitute, Open Approach
01UG37Z Supplement Tibial Nerve with Autologous Tissue Substitute, Percutaneous Approach
01UG47Z Supplement Tibial Nerve with Autologous Tissue Substitute, Percutaneous Endoscopic Approach
01UH07Z Supplement Peroneal Nerve with Autologous Tissue Substitute, Open Approach
01UH37Z Supplement Peroneal Nerve with Autologous Tissue Substitute, Percutaneous Approach
01UH47Z Supplement Peroneal Nerve with Autologous Tissue Substitute, Percutaneous Endoscopic Approach
01UR07Z Supplement Sacral Nerve with Autologous Tissue Substitute, Open Approach
01UR37Z Supplement Sacral Nerve with Autologous Tissue Substitute, Percutaneous Approach
01UR47Z Supplement Sacral Nerve with Autologous Tissue Substitute, Percutaneous Endoscopic Approach

01W – Peripheral Nervous System, Revision

Review Coding Guideline B6.1c

01WY00Z Revision of Drainage Device in Peripheral Nerve, Open Approach
01WY02Z Revision of Monitoring Device in Peripheral Nerve, Open Approach
01WY07Z Revision of Autologous Tissue Substitute in Peripheral Nerve, Open Approach
01WY0MZ Revision of Neurostimulator Lead in Peripheral Nerve, Open Approach
01WY30Z Revision of Drainage Device in Peripheral Nerve, Percutaneous Approach
01WY32Z Revision of Monitoring Device in Peripheral Nerve, Percutaneous Approach
01WY37Z Revision of Autologous Tissue Substitute in Peripheral Nerve, Percutaneous Approach
01WY3MZ Revision of Neurostimulator Lead in Peripheral Nerve, Percutaneous Approach
01WY40Z Revision of Drainage Device in Peripheral Nerve, Percutaneous Endoscopic Approach
01WY42Z Revision of Monitoring Device in Peripheral Nerve, Percutaneous Endoscopic Approach
01WY47Z Revision of Autologous Tissue Substitute in Peripheral Nerve, Percutaneous Endoscopic Approach
01WY4MZ Revision of Neurostimulator Lead in Peripheral Nerve, Percutaneous Endoscopic Approach
01WYX0Z Revision of Drainage Device in Peripheral Nerve, External Approach
01WYX2Z Revision of Monitoring Device in Peripheral Nerve, External Approach
01WYX7Z Revision of Autologous Tissue Substitute in Peripheral Nerve, External Approach
01WYXMZ Revision of Neurostimulator Lead in Peripheral Nerve, External Approach

01X – Peripheral Nervous System, Transfer

01X10Z1 Transfer Cervical Nerve to Cervical Nerve, Open Approach
01X10Z2 Transfer Cervical Nerve to Phrenic Nerve, Open Approach
01X14Z1 Transfer Cervical Nerve to Cervical Nerve, Percutaneous Endoscopic Approach
01X14Z2 Transfer Cervical Nerve to Phrenic Nerve, Percutaneous Endoscopic Approach
01X20Z1 Transfer Phrenic Nerve to Cervical Nerve, Open Approach
01X20Z2 Transfer Phrenic Nerve to Phrenic Nerve, Open Approach
01X24Z1 Transfer Phrenic Nerve to Cervical Nerve, Percutaneous Endoscopic Approach
01X24Z2 Transfer Phrenic Nerve to Phrenic Nerve, Percutaneous Endoscopic Approach
01X40Z4 Transfer Ulnar Nerve to Ulnar Nerve, Open Approach

01X40Z5 Transfer Ulnar Nerve to Median Nerve, Open Approach
01X40Z6 Transfer Ulnar Nerve to Radial Nerve, Open Approach
01X44Z4 Transfer Ulnar Nerve to Ulnar Nerve, Percutaneous Endoscopic Approach
01X44Z5 Transfer Ulnar Nerve to Median Nerve, Percutaneous Endoscopic Approach
01X44Z6 Transfer Ulnar Nerve to Radial Nerve, Percutaneous Endoscopic Approach
01X50Z4 Transfer Median Nerve to Ulnar Nerve, Open Approach
01X50Z5 Transfer Median Nerve to Median Nerve, Open Approach
01X50Z6 Transfer Median Nerve to Radial Nerve, Open Approach
01X54Z4 Transfer Median Nerve to Ulnar Nerve, Percutaneous Endoscopic Approach
01X54Z5 Transfer Median Nerve to Median Nerve, Percutaneous Endoscopic Approach
01X54Z6 Transfer Median Nerve to Radial Nerve, Percutaneous Endoscopic Approach
01X60Z4 Transfer Radial Nerve to Ulnar Nerve, Open Approach
01X60Z5 Transfer Radial Nerve to Median Nerve, Open Approach
01X60Z6 Transfer Radial Nerve to Radial Nerve, Open Approach
01X64Z4 Transfer Radial Nerve to Ulnar Nerve, Percutaneous Endoscopic Approach
01X64Z5 Transfer Radial Nerve to Median Nerve, Percutaneous Endoscopic Approach
01X64Z6 Transfer Radial Nerve to Radial Nerve, Percutaneous Endoscopic Approach
01X80Z8 Transfer Thoracic Nerve to Thoracic Nerve, Open Approach
01X84Z8 Transfer Thoracic Nerve to Thoracic Nerve, Percutaneous Endoscopic Approach
01XB0ZB Transfer Lumbar Nerve to Lumbar Nerve, Open Approach
01XB0ZC Transfer Lumbar Nerve to Perineal Nerve, Open Approach
01XB4ZB Transfer Lumbar Nerve to Lumbar Nerve, Percutaneous Endoscopic Approach
01XB4ZC Transfer Lumbar Nerve to Perineal Nerve, Percutaneous Endoscopic Approach
01XC0ZB Transfer Pudendal Nerve to Lumbar Nerve, Open Approach
01XC0ZC Transfer Pudendal Nerve to Perineal Nerve, Open Approach
01XC4ZB Transfer Pudendal Nerve to Lumbar Nerve, Percutaneous Endoscopic Approach
01XC4ZC Transfer Pudendal Nerve to Perineal Nerve, Percutaneous Endoscopic Approach
01XD0ZD Transfer Femoral Nerve to Femoral Nerve, Open Approach
01XD0ZF Transfer Femoral Nerve to Sciatic Nerve, Open Approach
01XD0ZG Transfer Femoral Nerve to Tibial Nerve, Open Approach
01XD0ZH Transfer Femoral Nerve to Peroneal Nerve, Open Approach
01XD4ZD Transfer Femoral Nerve to Femoral Nerve, Percutaneous Endoscopic Approach
01XD4ZF Transfer Femoral Nerve to Sciatic Nerve, Percutaneous Endoscopic Approach
01XD4ZG Transfer Femoral Nerve to Tibial Nerve, Percutaneous Endoscopic Approach
01XD4ZH Transfer Femoral Nerve to Peroneal Nerve, Percutaneous Endoscopic Approach
01XF0ZD Transfer Sciatic Nerve to Femoral Nerve, Open Approach
01XF0ZF Transfer Sciatic Nerve to Sciatic Nerve, Open Approach
01XF0ZG Transfer Sciatic Nerve to Tibial Nerve, Open Approach
01XF0ZH Transfer Sciatic Nerve to Peroneal Nerve, Open Approach
01XF4ZD Transfer Sciatic Nerve to Femoral Nerve, Percutaneous Endoscopic Approach
01XF4ZF Transfer Sciatic Nerve to Sciatic Nerve, Percutaneous Endoscopic Approach
01XF4ZG Transfer Sciatic Nerve to Tibial Nerve, Percutaneous Endoscopic Approach
01XF4ZH Transfer Sciatic Nerve to Peroneal Nerve, Percutaneous Endoscopic Approach
01XG0ZD Transfer Tibial Nerve to Femoral Nerve, Open Approach
01XG0ZF Transfer Tibial Nerve to Sciatic Nerve, Open Approach
01XG0ZG Transfer Tibial Nerve to Tibial Nerve, Open Approach
01XG0ZH Transfer Tibial Nerve to Peroneal Nerve, Open Approach
01XG4ZD Transfer Tibial Nerve to Femoral Nerve, Percutaneous Endoscopic Approach
01XG4ZF Transfer Tibial Nerve to Sciatic Nerve, Percutaneous Endoscopic Approach
01XG4ZG Transfer Tibial Nerve to Tibial Nerve, Percutaneous Endoscopic Approach
01XG4ZH Transfer Tibial Nerve to Peroneal Nerve, Percutaneous Endoscopic Approach
01XH0ZD Transfer Peroneal Nerve to Femoral Nerve, Open Approach
01XH0ZF Transfer Peroneal Nerve to Sciatic Nerve, Open Approach
01XH0ZG Transfer Peroneal Nerve to Tibial Nerve, Open Approach
01XH0ZH Transfer Peroneal Nerve to Peroneal Nerve, Open Approach
01XH4ZD Transfer Peroneal Nerve to Femoral Nerve, Percutaneous Endoscopic Approach
01XH4ZF Transfer Peroneal Nerve to Sciatic Nerve, Percutaneous Endoscopic Approach
01XH4ZG Transfer Peroneal Nerve to Tibial Nerve, Percutaneous Endoscopic Approach
01XH4ZH Transfer Peroneal Nerve to Peroneal Nerve, Percutaneous Endoscopic Approach

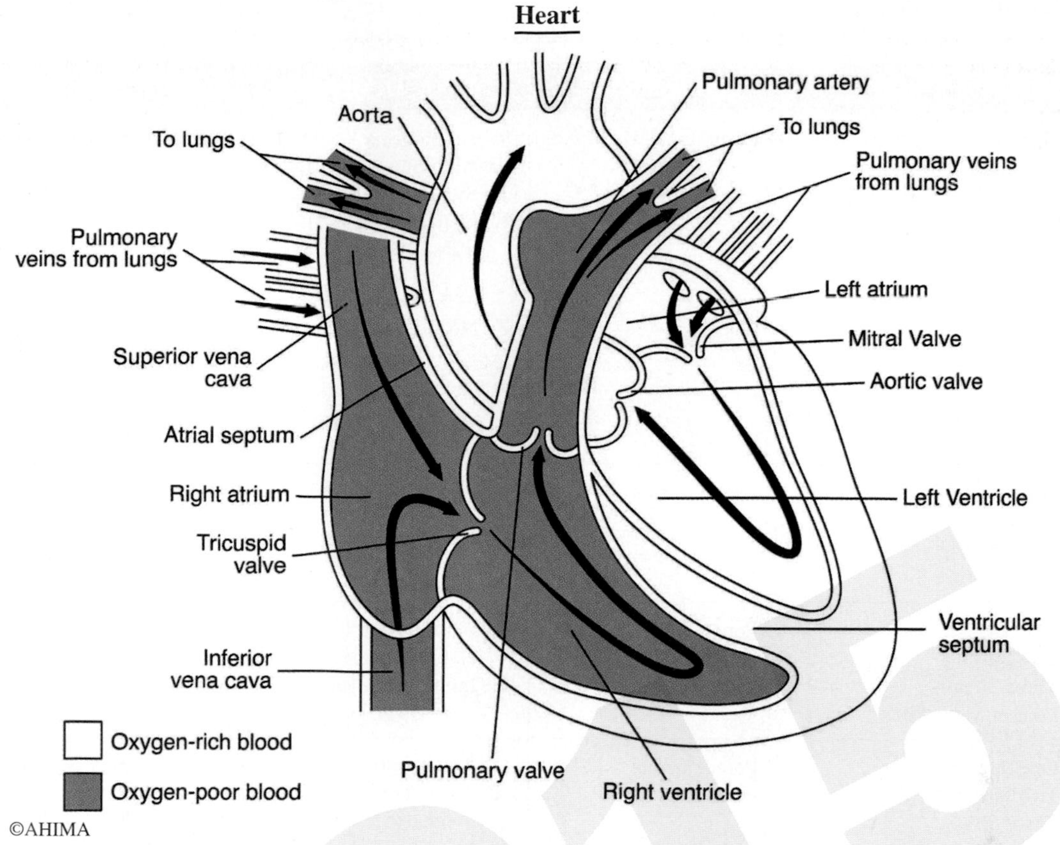
Heart
Aorta
Pulmonary artery
To lungs
To lungs
Pulmonary veins from lungs
Pulmonary veins from lungs
Left atrium
Mitral Valve
Superior vena cava
Aortic valve
Atrial septum
Right atrium
Left Ventricle
Tricuspid valve
Ventricular septum
Inferior vena cava
Oxygen-rich blood
Oxygen-poor blood
Pulmonary valve
Right ventricle
©AHIMA

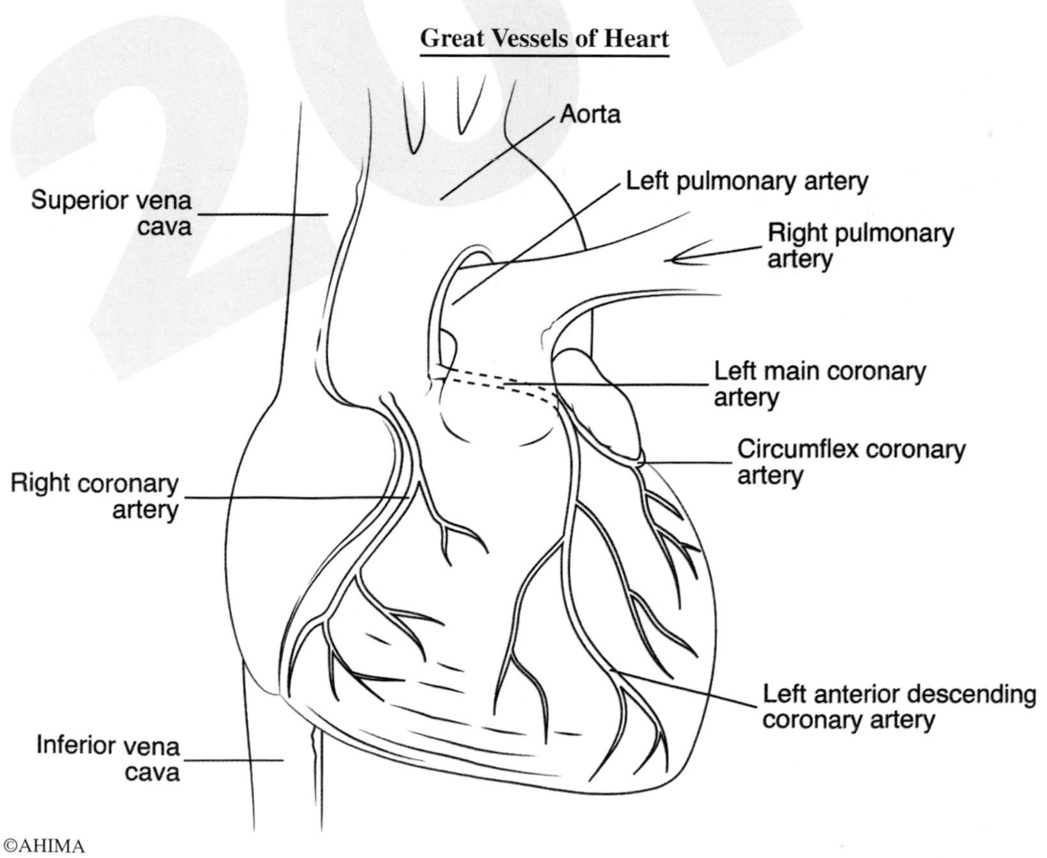
Great Vessels of Heart
Aorta
Superior vena cava
Left pulmonary artery
Right pulmonary artery
Left main coronary artery
Circumflex coronary artery
Right coronary artery
Left anterior descending coronary artery
Inferior vena cava
©AHIMA

Heart and Great Vessels Tables 021–02Y

Section 0 **Medical and Surgical**
Body System 2 **Heart and Great Vessels**
Operation 1 **Bypass:** Altering the route of passage of the contents of a tubular body part

Body Part (4th)	Approach (5th)	Device (6th)	Qualifier (7th)
0 Coronary Artery, One Site **1** Coronary Artery, Two Sites **2** Coronary Artery, Three Sites **3** Coronary Artery, Four or More Sites	**0** Open	**9** Autologous Venous Tissue **A** Autologous Arterial Tissue **J** Synthetic Substitute **K** Nonautologous Tissue Substitute	**3** Coronary Artery **8** Internal Mammary, Right **9** Internal Mammary, Left **C** Thoracic Artery **F** Abdominal Artery **W** Aorta
0 Coronary Artery, One Site **1** Coronary Artery, Two Sites **2** Coronary Artery, Three Sites **3** Coronary Artery, Four or More Sites	**0** Open	**Z** No Device	**3** Coronary Artery **8** Internal Mammary, Right **9** Internal Mammary, Left **C** Thoracic Artery **F** Abdominal Artery
0 Coronary Artery, One Site **1** Coronary Artery, Two Sites **2** Coronary Artery, Three Sites **3** Coronary Artery, Four or More Sites	**3** Percutaneous	**4** Intraluminal Device, Drug-eluting **D** Intraluminal Device	**4** Coronary Vein
0 Coronary Artery, One Site **1** Coronary Artery, Two Sites **2** Coronary Artery, Three Sites **3** Coronary Artery, Four or More Sites	**4** Percutaneous Endoscopic	**4** Intraluminal Device, Drug-eluting **D** Intraluminal Device	**4** Coronary Vein
0 Coronary Artery, One Site **1** Coronary Artery, Two Sites **2** Coronary Artery, Three Sites **3** Coronary Artery, Four or More Sites	**4** Percutaneous Endoscopic	**9** Autologous Venous Tissue **A** Autologous Arterial Tissue **J** Synthetic Substitute **K** Nonautologous Tissue Substitute	**3** Coronary Artery **8** Internal Mammary, Right **9** Internal Mammary, Left **C** Thoracic Artery **F** Abdominal Artery **W** Aorta
0 Coronary Artery, One Site **1** Coronary Artery, Two Sites **2** Coronary Artery, Three Sites **3** Coronary Artery, Four or More Sites	**4** Percutaneous Endoscopic	**Z** No Device	**3** Coronary Artery **8** Internal Mammary, Right **9** Internal Mammary, Left **C** Thoracic Artery **F** Abdominal Artery
6 Atrium, Right	**0** Open **4** Percutaneous Endoscopic	**9** Autologous Venous Tissue **A** Autologous Arterial Tissue **J** Synthetic Substitute **K** Nonautologous Tissue Substitute	**P** Pulmonary Trunk **Q** Pulmonary Artery, Right **R** Pulmonary Artery, Left
6 Atrium, Right	**0** Open **4** Percutaneous Endoscopic	**Z** No Device	**7** Atrium, Left **P** Pulmonary Trunk **Q** Pulmonary Artery, Right **R** Pulmonary Artery, Left
7 Atrium, Left **V** Superior Vena Cava	**0** Open **4** Percutaneous Endoscopic	**9** Autologous Venous Tissue **A** Autologous Arterial Tissue **J** Synthetic Substitute **K** Nonautologous Tissue Substitute **Z** No Device	**P** Pulmonary Trunk **Q** Pulmonary Artery, Right **R** Pulmonary Artery, Left
K Ventricle, Right **L** Ventricle, Left	**0** Open **4** Percutaneous Endoscopic	**9** Autologous Venous Tissue **A** Autologous Arterial Tissue **J** Synthetic Substitute **K** Nonautologous Tissue Substitute	**P** Pulmonary Trunk **Q** Pulmonary Artery, Right **R** Pulmonary Artery, Left

Continued →

Section 0 Medical and Surgical
Body System 2 Heart and Great Vessels
Operation 1 **Bypass:** Altering the route of passage of the contents of a tubular body part

Body Part (4th)	Approach (5th)	Device (6th)	Qualifier (7th)
K Ventricle, Right L Ventricle, Left	0 Open 4 Percutaneous Endoscopic	Z No Device	5 Coronary Circulation 8 Internal Mammary, Right 9 Internal Mammary, Left C Thoracic Artery F Abdominal Artery P Pulmonary Trunk Q Pulmonary Artery, Right R Pulmonary Artery, Left W Aorta
W Thoracic Aorta	0 Open 4 Percutaneous Endoscopic	9 Autologous Venous Tissue A Autologous Arterial Tissue J Synthetic Substitute K Nonautologous Tissue Substitute Z No Device	B Subclavian D Carotid P Pulmonary Trunk Q Pulmonary Artery, Right R Pulmonary Artery, Left

Section 0 Medical and Surgical
Body System 2 Heart and Great Vessels
Operation 5 **Destruction:** Physical eradication of all or a portion of a body part by the direct use of energy, force, or a destructive agent

Body Part (4th)	Approach (5th)	Device (6th)	Qualifier (7th)
4 Coronary Vein 5 Atrial Septum 6 Atrium, Right 8 Conduction Mechanism 9 Chordae Tendineae D Papillary Muscle F Aortic Valve G Mitral Valve H Pulmonary Valve J Tricuspid Valve K Ventricle, Right L Ventricle, Left M Ventricular Septum N Pericardium P Pulmonary Trunk Q Pulmonary Artery, Right R Pulmonary Artery, Left S Pulmonary Vein, Right T Pulmonary Vein, Left V Superior Vena Cava W Thoracic Aorta	0 Open 3 Percutaneous 4 Percutaneous Endoscopic	Z No Device	Z No Qualifier
7 Atrium, Left	0 Open 3 Percutaneous 4 Percutaneous Endoscopic	Z No Device	K Left Atrial Appendage Z No Qualifier

Section 0 Medical and Surgical
Body System 2 Heart and Great Vessels
Operation 7 **Dilation:** Expanding an orifice or the lumen of a tubular body part

Body Part (4th)	Approach (5th)	Device (6th)	Qualifier (7th)
0 Coronary Artery, One Site 1 Coronary Artery, Two Sites 2 Coronary Artery, Three Sites 3 Coronary Artery, Four or More Sites	0 Open 3 Percutaneous 4 Percutaneous Endoscopic	4 Intraluminal Device, Drug-eluting D Intraluminal Device T Intraluminal Device, Radioactive Z No Device	6 Bifurcation Z No Qualifier

Continued →

Section 0 **Medical and Surgical**
Body System 2 **Heart and Great Vessels**
Operation 7 **Dilation:** Expanding an orifice or the lumen of a tubular body part

Body Part (4th)	Approach (5th)	Device (6th)	Qualifier (7th)
F Aortic Valve **G** Mitral Valve **H** Pulmonary Valve **J** Tricuspid Valve **K** Ventricle, Right **P** Pulmonary Trunk **Q** Pulmonary Artery, Right **S** Pulmonary Vein, Right **T** Pulmonary Vein, Left **V** Superior Vena Cava **W** Thoracic Aorta	**0** Open **3** Percutaneous **4** Percutaneous Endoscopic	**4** Intraluminal Device, Drug-eluting **D** Intraluminal Device **Z** No Device	**Z** No Qualifier
R Pulmonary Artery, Left	**0** Open **3** Percutaneous **4** Percutaneous Endoscopic	**4** Intraluminal Device, Drug-eluting **D** Intraluminal Device **Z** No Device	**T** Ductus Arteriosus **Z** No Qualifier

Section 0 **Medical and Surgical**
Body System 2 **Heart and Great Vessels**
Operation 8 **Division:** Cutting into a body part, without draining fluids and/or gases from the body part, in order to separate or transect a body part

Body Part (4th)	Approach (5th)	Device (6th)	Qualifier (7th)
8 Conduction Mechanism **9** Chordae Tendineae **D** Papillary Muscle	**0** Open **3** Percutaneous **4** Percutaneous Endoscopic	**Z** No Device	**Z** No Qualifier

Section 0 **Medical and Surgical**
Body System 2 **Heart and Great Vessels**
Operation B **Excision:** Cutting out or off, without replacement, a portion of a body part

Body Part (4th)	Approach (5th)	Device (6th)	Qualifier (7th)
4 Coronary Vein **5** Atrial Septum **6** Atrium, Right **8** Conduction Mechanism **9** Chordae Tendineae **D** Papillary Muscle **F** Aortic Valve **G** Mitral Valve **H** Pulmonary Valve **J** Tricuspid Valve **K** Ventricle, Right **L** Ventricle, Left **M** Ventricular Septum **N** Pericardium **P** Pulmonary Trunk **Q** Pulmonary Artery, Right **R** Pulmonary Artery, Left **S** Pulmonary Vein, Right **T** Pulmonary Vein, Left **V** Superior Vena Cava **W** Thoracic Aorta	**0** Open **3** Percutaneous **4** Percutaneous Endoscopic	**Z** No Device	**X** Diagnostic **Z** No Qualifier
7 Atrium, Left	**0** Open **3** Percutaneous **4** Percutaneous Endoscopic	**Z** No Device	**K** Left Atrial Appendage **X** Diagnostic **Z** No Qualifier

Section 0 **Medical and Surgical**
Body System 2 **Heart and Great Vessels**
Operation C **Extirpation:** Taking or cutting out solid matter from a body part

Body Part (4th)	Approach (5th)	Device (6th)	Qualifier (7th)
0 Coronary Artery, One Site **1** Coronary Artery, Two Sites **2** Coronary Artery, Three Sites **3** Coronary Artery, Four or More Sites **4** Coronary Vein **5** Atrial Septum **6** Atrium, Right **7** Atrium, Left **8** Conduction Mechanism **9** Chordae Tendineae **D** Papillary Muscle **F** Aortic Valve **G** Mitral Valve **H** Pulmonary Valve **J** Tricuspid Valve **K** Ventricle, Right **L** Ventricle, Left **M** Ventricular Septum **N** Pericardium **P** Pulmonary Trunk **Q** Pulmonary Artery, Right **R** Pulmonary Artery, Left **S** Pulmonary Vein, Right **T** Pulmonary Vein, Left **V** Superior Vena Cava **W** Thoracic Aorta	**0** Open **3** Percutaneous **4** Percutaneous Endoscopic	**Z** No Device	**Z** No Qualifier

Section 0 **Medical and Surgical**
Body System 2 **Heart and Great Vessels**
Operation F **Fragmentation:** Breaking solid matter in a body part into pieces

Body Part (4th)	Approach (5th)	Device (6th)	Qualifier (7th)
N Pericardium	**0** Open **3** Percutaneous **4** Percutaneous Endoscopic **X** External	**Z** No Device	**Z** No Qualifier

Section 0 **Medical and Surgical**
Body System 2 **Heart and Great Vessels**
Operation H **Insertion:** Putting in a nonbiological appliance that monitors, assists, performs, or prevents a physiological function but does not physically take the place of a body part

Body Part (4th)	Approach (5th)	Device (6th)	Qualifier (7th)
4 Coronary Vein **6** Atrium, Right **7** Atrium, Left **K** Ventricle, Right **L** Ventricle, Left	**0** Open **3** Percutaneous **4** Percutaneous Endoscopic	**0** Monitoring Device, Pressure Sensor **2** Monitoring Device **3** Infusion Device **D** Intraluminal Device **J** Cardiac Lead, Pacemaker **K** Cardiac Lead, Defibrillator **M** Cardiac Lead	**Z** No Qualifier
A Heart	**0** Open **3** Percutaneous **4** Percutaneous Endoscopic	**Q** Implantable Heart Assist System	**Z** No Qualifier

Continued →

Section 0 **Medical and Surgical**
Body System 2 **Heart and Great Vessels**
Operation H **Insertion:** Putting in a nonbiological appliance that monitors, assists, performs, or prevents a physiological function but does not physically take the place of a body part

Body Part (4th)	Approach (5th)	Device (6th)	Qualifier (7th)
A Heart	0 Open 3 Percutaneous 4 Percutaneous Endoscopic	R External Heart Assist System	S Biventricular Z No Qualifier
N Pericardium	0 Open 3 Percutaneous 4 Percutaneous Endoscopic	0 Monitoring Device, Pressure Sensor 2 Monitoring Device J Cardiac Lead, Pacemaker K Cardiac Lead, Defibrillator M Cardiac Lead	Z No Qualifier
P Pulmonary Trunk Q Pulmonary Artery, Right R Pulmonary Artery, Left S Pulmonary Vein, Right T Pulmonary Vein, Left V Superior Vena Cava W Thoracic Aorta	0 Open 3 Percutaneous 4 Percutaneous Endoscopic	0 Monitoring Device, Pressure Sensor 2 Monitoring Device 3 Infusion Device D Intraluminal Device	Z No Qualifier

Section 0 **Medical and Surgical**
Body System 2 **Heart and Great Vessels**
Operation J **Inspection:** Visually and/or manually exploring a body part

Body Part (4th)	Approach (5th)	Device (6th)	Qualifier (7th)
A Heart Y Great Vessel	0 Open 3 Percutaneous 4 Percutaneous Endoscopic	Z No Device	Z No Qualifier

Section 0 **Medical and Surgical**
Body System 2 **Heart and Great Vessels**
Operation K **Map:** Locating the route of passage of electrical impulses and/or locating functional areas in a body part

Body Part (4th)	Approach (5th)	Device (6th)	Qualifier (7th)
8 Conduction Mechanism	0 Open 3 Percutaneous 4 Percutaneous Endoscopic	Z No Device	Z No Qualifier

Section 0 **Medical and Surgical**
Body System 2 **Heart and Great Vessels**
Operation L **Occlusion:** Completely closing an orifice or the lumen of a tubular body part

Body Part (4th)	Approach (5th)	Device (6th)	Qualifier (7th)
7 Atrium, Left	0 Open 3 Percutaneous 4 Percutaneous Endoscopic	C Extraluminal Device D Intraluminal Device Z No Device	K Left Atrial Appendage
R Pulmonary Artery, Left	0 Open 3 Percutaneous 4 Percutaneous Endoscopic	C Extraluminal Device D Intraluminal Device Z No Device	T Ductus Arteriosus
S Pulmonary Vein, Right T Pulmonary Vein, Left V Superior Vena Cava	0 Open 3 Percutaneous 4 Percutaneous Endoscopic	C Extraluminal Device D Intraluminal Device Z No Device	Z No Qualifier

Section 0 **Medical and Surgical**
Body System 2 **Heart and Great Vessels**
Operation N **Release:** Freeing a body part from an abnormal physical constraint by cutting or by the use of force

Body Part (4th)	Approach (5th)	Device (6th)	Qualifier (7th)
4 Coronary Vein **5** Atrial Septum **6** Atrium, Right **7** Atrium, Left **8** Conduction Mechanism **9** Chordae Tendineae **D** Papillary Muscle **F** Aortic Valve **G** Mitral Valve **H** Pulmonary Valve **J** Tricuspid Valve **K** Ventricle, Right **L** Ventricle, Left **M** Ventricular Septum **N** Pericardium **P** Pulmonary Trunk **Q** Pulmonary Artery, Right **R** Pulmonary Artery, Left **S** Pulmonary Vein, Right **T** Pulmonary Vein, Left **V** Superior Vena Cava **W** Thoracic Aorta	**0** Open **3** Percutaneous **4** Percutaneous Endoscopic	**Z** No Device	**Z** No Qualifier

Section 0 **Medical and Surgical**
Body System 2 **Heart and Great Vessels**
Operation P **Removal:** Taking out or off a device from a body part

Body Part (4th)	Approach (5th)	Device (6th)	Qualifier (7th)
A Heart	**0** Open **3** Percutaneous **4** Percutaneous Endoscopic	**2** Monitoring Device **3** Infusion Device **7** Autologous Tissue Substitute **8** Zooplastic Tissue **C** Extraluminal Device **D** Intraluminal Device **J** Synthetic Substitute **K** Nonautologous Tissue Substitute **M** Cardiac Lead **Q** Implantable Heart Assist System **R** External Heart Assist System	**Z** No Qualifier
A Heart	**X** External	**2** Monitoring Device **3** Infusion Device **D** Intraluminal Device **M** Cardiac Lead	**Z** No Qualifier
Y Great Vessel	**0** Open **3** Percutaneous **4** Percutaneous Endoscopic	**2** Monitoring Device **3** Infusion Device **7** Autologous Tissue Substitute **8** Zooplastic Tissue **C** Extraluminal Device **D** Intraluminal Device **J** Synthetic Substitute **K** Nonautologous Tissue Substitute	**Z** No Qualifier
Y Great Vessel	**X** External	**2** Monitoring Device **3** Infusion Device **D** Intraluminal Device	**Z** No Qualifier

Section 0 **Medical and Surgical**
Body System 2 **Heart and Great Vessels**
Operation Q **Repair:** Restoring, to the extent possible, a body part to its normal anatomic structure and function

Body Part (4th)	Approach (5th)	Device (6th)	Qualifier (7th)
0 Coronary Artery, One Site **1** Coronary Artery, Two Sites **2** Coronary Artery, Three Sites **3** Coronary Artery, Four or More Sites **4** Coronary Vein **5** Atrial Septum **6** Atrium, Right **7** Atrium, Left **8** Conduction Mechanism **9** Chordae Tendineae **A** Heart **B** Heart, Right **C** Heart, Left **D** Papillary Muscle **F** Aortic Valve **G** Mitral Valve **H** Pulmonary Valve **J** Tricuspid Valve **K** Ventricle, Right **L** Ventricle, Left **M** Ventricular Septum **N** Pericardium **P** Pulmonary Trunk **Q** Pulmonary Artery, Right **R** Pulmonary Artery, Left **S** Pulmonary Vein, Right **T** Pulmonary Vein, Left **V** Superior Vena Cava **W** Thoracic Aorta	**0** Open **3** Percutaneous **4** Percutaneous Endoscopic	**Z** No Device	**Z** No Qualifier

Section 0 **Medical and Surgical**
Body System 2 **Heart and Great Vessels**
Operation R **Replacement:** Putting in or on biological or synthetic material that physically takes the place and/or function of all or a portion of a body part

Body Part (4th)	Approach (5th)	Device (6th)	Qualifier (7th)
5 Atrial Septum **6** Atrium, Right **7** Atrium, Left **9** Chordae Tendineae **D** Papillary Muscle **J** Tricuspid Valve **K** Ventricle, Right **L** Ventricle, Left **M** Ventricular Septum **N** Pericardium **P** Pulmonary Trunk **Q** Pulmonary Artery, Right **R** Pulmonary Artery, Left **S** Pulmonary Vein, Right **T** Pulmonary Vein, Left **V** Superior Vena Cava **W** Thoracic Aorta	**0** Open **4** Percutaneous Endoscopic	**7** Autologous Tissue Substitute **8** Zooplastic Tissue **J** Synthetic Substitute **K** Nonautologous Tissue Substitute	**Z** No Qualifier
F Aortic Valve **G** Mitral Valve **H** Pulmonary Valve	**0** Open **4** Percutaneous Endoscopic	**7** Autologous Tissue Substitute **8** Zooplastic Tissue **J** Synthetic Substitute **K** Nonautologous Tissue Substitute	**Z** No Qualifier

Continued →

Section 0 **Medical and Surgical**
Body System 2 **Heart and Great Vessels**
Operation R **Replacement:** Putting in or on biological or synthetic material that physically takes the place and/or function of all or a portion of a body part

Body Part (4th)	Approach (5th)	Device (6th)	Qualifier (7th)
F Aortic Valve **G** Mitral Valve **H** Pulmonary Valve	**3** Percutaneous	**7** Autologous Tissue Substitute **8** Zooplastic Tissue **J** Synthetic Substitute **K** Nonautologous Tissue Substitute	**H** Transapical **Z** No Qualifier

Section 0 **Medical and Surgical**
Body System 2 **Heart and Great Vessels**
Operation S **Reposition:** Moving to its normal location, or other suitable location, all or a portion of a body part

Body Part (4th)	Approach (5th)	Device (6th)	Qualifier (7th)
P Pulmonary Trunk **Q** Pulmonary Artery, Right **R** Pulmonary Artery, Left **S** Pulmonary Vein, Right **T** Pulmonary Vein, Left **V** Superior Vena Cava **W** Thoracic Aorta	**0** Open	**Z** No Device	**Z** No Qualifier

Section 0 **Medical and Surgical**
Body System 2 **Heart and Great Vessels**
Operation T **Resection:** Cutting out or off, without replacement, all of a body part

Body Part (4th)	Approach (5th)	Device (6th)	Qualifier (7th)
5 Atrial Septum **8** Conduction Mechanism **9** Chordae Tendineae **D** Papillary Muscle **H** Pulmonary Valve **M** Ventricular Septum **N** Pericardium	**0** Open **3** Percutaneous **4** Percutaneous Endoscopic	**Z** No Device	**Z** No Qualifier

Section 0 **Medical and Surgical**
Body System 2 **Heart and Great Vessels**
Operation U **Supplement:** Putting in or on biological or synthetic material that physically reinforces and/or augments the function of a portion of a body part

Body Part (4th)	Approach (5th)	Device (6th)	Qualifier (7th)
5 Atrial Septum **6** Atrium, Right **7** Atrium, Left **9** Chordae Tendineae **A** Heart **D** Papillary Muscle **F** Aortic Valve **G** Mitral Valve **H** Pulmonary Valve **J** Tricuspid Valve **K** Ventricle, Right **L** Ventricle, Left **M** Ventricular Septum **N** Pericardium **P** Pulmonary Trunk **Q** Pulmonary Artery, Right **R** Pulmonary Artery, Left **S** Pulmonary Vein, Right **T** Pulmonary Vein, Left **V** Superior Vena Cava **W** Thoracic Aorta	**0** Open **3** Percutaneous **4** Percutaneous Endoscopic	**7** Autologous Tissue Substitute **8** Zooplastic Tissue **J** Synthetic Substitute **K** Nonautologous Tissue Substitute	**Z** No Qualifier

Section 0 **Medical and Surgical**
Body System 2 **Heart and Great Vessels**
Operation V **Restriction:** Partially closing an orifice or the lumen of a tubular body part

Body Part (4th)	Approach (5th)	Device (6th)	Qualifier (7th)
A Heart	**0** Open **3** Percutaneous **4** Percutaneous Endoscopic	**C** Extraluminal Device **Z** No Device	**Z** No Qualifier
P Pulmonary Trunk **Q** Pulmonary Artery, Right **S** Pulmonary Vein, Right **T** Pulmonary Vein, Left **V** Superior Vena Cava **W** Thoracic Aorta	**0** Open **3** Percutaneous **4** Percutaneous Endoscopic	**C** Extraluminal Device **D** Intraluminal Device **Z** No Device	**Z** No Qualifier
R Pulmonary Artery, Left	**0** Open **3** Percutaneous **4** Percutaneous Endoscopic	**C** Extraluminal Device **D** Intraluminal Device **Z** No Device	**T** Ductus Arteriosus **Z** No Qualifier

Section 0 **Medical and Surgical**
Body System 2 **Heart and Great Vessels**
Operation W **Revision:** Correcting, to the extent possible, a portion of a malfunctioning device or the position of a displaced device

Body Part (4th)	Approach (5th)	Device (6th)	Qualifier (7th)
5 Atrial Septum **M** Ventricular Septum	**0** Open **4** Percutaneous Endoscopic	**J** Synthetic Substitute	**Z** No Qualifier
A Heart	**0** Open **3** Percutaneous **4** Percutaneous Endoscopic **X** External	**2** Monitoring Device **3** Infusion Device **7** Autologous Tissue Substitute **8** Zooplastic Tissue **C** Extraluminal Device **D** Intraluminal Device **J** Synthetic Substitute **K** Nonautologous Tissue Substitute **M** Cardiac Lead **Q** Implantable Heart Assist System **R** External Heart Assist System	**Z** No Qualifier
F Aortic Valve **G** Mitral Valve **H** Pulmonary Valve **J** Tricuspid Valve	**0** Open **4** Percutaneous Endoscopic	**7** Autologous Tissue Substitute **8** Zooplastic Tissue **J** Synthetic Substitute **K** Nonautologous Tissue Substitute	**Z** No Qualifier
Y Great Vessel	**0** Open **3** Percutaneous **4** Percutaneous Endoscopic **X** External	**2** Monitoring Device **3** Infusion Device **7** Autologous Tissue Substitute **8** Zooplastic Tissue **C** Extraluminal Device **D** Intraluminal Device **J** Synthetic Substitute **K** Nonautologous Tissue Substitute	**Z** No Qualifier

Section 0 **Medical and Surgical**
Body System 2 **Heart and Great Vessels**
Operation Y **Transplantation:** Putting in or on all or a portion of a living body part taken from another individual or animal to physically take the place and/or function of all or a portion of a similar body part

Body Part (4th)	Approach (5th)	Device (6th)	Qualifier (7th)
A Heart	**0** Open	**Z** No Device	**0** Allogeneic **1** Syngeneic **2** Zooplastic

Heart and Great Vessels Code Listing 021–02Y

021 – Heart and Great Vessels, Bypass

Review Coding Guideline B3.6a

For Bypass procedures involving the coronary arteries, review Coding Guidelines B3.6b and B3.6c

For Bypass procedures involving the coronary arteries, review Coding Guideline B4.4

0210093 Bypass Coronary Artery, One Site from Coronary Artery with Autologous Venous Tissue, Open Approach
HAC When reported with secondary diagnosis code J98.5

0210098 Bypass Coronary Artery, One Site from Right Internal Mammary with Autologous Venous Tissue, Open Approach
HAC When reported with secondary diagnosis code J98.5

0210099 Bypass Coronary Artery, One Site from Left Internal Mammary with Autologous Venous Tissue, Open Approach
HAC When reported with secondary diagnosis code J98.5

021009C Bypass Coronary Artery, One Site from Thoracic Artery with Autologous Venous Tissue, Open Approach
HAC When reported with secondary diagnosis code J98.5

021009F Bypass Coronary Artery, One Site from Abdominal Artery with Autologous Venous Tissue, Open Approach
HAC When reported with secondary diagnosis code J98.5

021009W Bypass Coronary Artery, One Site from Aorta with Autologous Venous Tissue, Open Approach
HAC When reported with secondary diagnosis code J98.5
AHA CC: 1Q, 2014, 10-11

02100A3 Bypass Coronary Artery, One Site from Coronary Artery with Autologous Arterial Tissue, Open Approach
HAC When reported with secondary diagnosis code J98.5

02100A8 Bypass Coronary Artery, One Site from Right Internal Mammary with Autologous Arterial Tissue, Open Approach
HAC When reported with secondary diagnosis code J98.5

02100A9 Bypass Coronary Artery, One Site from Left Internal Mammary with Autologous Arterial Tissue, Open Approach
HAC When reported with secondary diagnosis code J98.5

02100AC Bypass Coronary Artery, One Site from Thoracic Artery with Autologous Arterial Tissue, Open Approach
HAC When reported with secondary diagnosis code J98.5

02100AF Bypass Coronary Artery, One Site from Abdominal Artery with Autologous Arterial Tissue, Open Approach
HAC When reported with secondary diagnosis code J98.5

02100AW Bypass Coronary Artery, One Site from Aorta with Autologous Arterial Tissue, Open Approach
HAC When reported with secondary diagnosis code J98.5

02100J3 Bypass Coronary Artery, One Site from Coronary Artery with Synthetic Substitute, Open Approach
HAC When reported with secondary diagnosis code J98.5

02100J8 Bypass Coronary Artery, One Site from Right Internal Mammary with Synthetic Substitute, Open Approach
HAC When reported with secondary diagnosis code J98.5

02100J9 Bypass Coronary Artery, One Site from Left Internal Mammary with Synthetic Substitute, Open Approach
HAC When reported with secondary diagnosis code J98.5

02100JC Bypass Coronary Artery, One Site from Thoracic Artery with Synthetic Substitute, Open Approach
HAC When reported with secondary diagnosis code J98.5

02100JF Bypass Coronary Artery, One Site from Abdominal Artery with Synthetic Substitute, Open Approach
HAC When reported with secondary diagnosis code J98.5

02100JW Bypass Coronary Artery, One Site from Aorta with Synthetic Substitute, Open Approach
HAC When reported with secondary diagnosis code J98.5

02100K3 Bypass Coronary Artery, One Site from Coronary Artery with Nonautologous Tissue Substitute, Open Approach
HAC When reported with secondary diagnosis code J98.5

02100K8 Bypass Coronary Artery, One Site from Right Internal Mammary with Nonautologous Tissue Substitute, Open Approach
HAC When reported with secondary diagnosis code J98.5

02100K9 Bypass Coronary Artery, One Site from Left Internal Mammary with Nonautologous Tissue Substitute, Open Approach
HAC When reported with secondary diagnosis code J98.5

02100KC Bypass Coronary Artery, One Site from Thoracic Artery with Nonautologous Tissue Substitute, Open Approach
HAC When reported with secondary diagnosis code J98.5

02100KF Bypass Coronary Artery, One Site from Abdominal Artery with Nonautologous Tissue Substitute, Open Approach
HAC When reported with secondary diagnosis code J98.5

02100KW Bypass Coronary Artery, One Site from Aorta with Nonautologous Tissue Substitute, Open Approach
HAC When reported with secondary diagnosis code J98.5

02100Z3 Bypass Coronary Artery, One Site from Coronary Artery, Open Approach
HAC When reported with secondary diagnosis code J98.5

02100Z8 Bypass Coronary Artery, One Site from Right Internal Mammary, Open Approach
HAC When reported with secondary diagnosis code J98.5

02100Z9 Bypass Coronary Artery, One Site from Left Internal Mammary, Open Approach
HAC When reported with secondary diagnosis code J98.5

02100ZC Bypass Coronary Artery, One Site from Thoracic Artery, Open Approach
HAC When reported with secondary diagnosis code J98.5

02100ZF Bypass Coronary Artery, One Site from Abdominal Artery, Open Approach
HAC When reported with secondary diagnosis code J98.5

0210344 Bypass Coronary Artery, One Site from Coronary Vein with Drug-eluting Intraluminal Device, Percutaneous Approach

02103D4 Bypass Coronary Artery, One Site from Coronary Vein with Intraluminal Device, Percutaneous Approach

0210444 Bypass Coronary Artery, One Site from Coronary Vein with Drug-eluting Intraluminal Device, Percutaneous Endoscopic Approach

0210493 Bypass Coronary Artery, One Site from Coronary Artery with Autologous Venous Tissue, Percutaneous Endoscopic Approach
HAC When reported with secondary diagnosis code J98.5

0210498 Bypass Coronary Artery, One Site from Right Internal Mammary with Autologous Venous Tissue, Percutaneous Endoscopic Approach
HAC When reported with secondary diagnosis code J98.5

0210499 Bypass Coronary Artery, One Site from Left Internal Mammary with Autologous Venous Tissue, Percutaneous Endoscopic Approach
HAC When reported with secondary diagnosis code J98.5

021049C Bypass Coronary Artery, One Site from Thoracic Artery with Autologous Venous Tissue, Percutaneous Endoscopic Approach
HAC When reported with secondary diagnosis code J98.5

021049F Bypass Coronary Artery, One Site from Abdominal Artery with Autologous Venous Tissue, Percutaneous Endoscopic Approach
HAC When reported with secondary diagnosis code J98.5

021049W Bypass Coronary Artery, One Site from Aorta with Autologous Venous Tissue, Percutaneous Endoscopic Approach
HAC When reported with secondary diagnosis code J98.5

02104A3 Bypass Coronary Artery, One Site from Coronary Artery with Autologous Arterial Tissue, Percutaneous Endoscopic Approach
HAC When reported with secondary diagnosis code J98.5

02104A8 Bypass Coronary Artery, One Site from Right Internal Mammary with Autologous Arterial Tissue, Percutaneous Endoscopic Approach
HAC When reported with secondary diagnosis code J98.5

02104A9 Bypass Coronary Artery, One Site from Left Internal Mammary with Autologous Arterial Tissue, Percutaneous Endoscopic Approach
HAC When reported with secondary diagnosis code J98.5

02104AC Bypass Coronary Artery, One Site from Thoracic Artery with Autologous Arterial Tissue, Percutaneous Endoscopic Approach
HAC When reported with secondary diagnosis code J98.5

02104AF Bypass Coronary Artery, One Site from Abdominal Artery with Autologous Arterial Tissue, Percutaneous Endoscopic Approach
HAC When reported with secondary diagnosis code J98.5

02104AW Bypass Coronary Artery, One Site from Aorta with Autologous Arterial Tissue, Percutaneous Endoscopic Approach
HAC When reported with secondary diagnosis code J98.5

02104D4 Bypass Coronary Artery, One Site from Coronary Vein with Intraluminal Device, Percutaneous Endoscopic Approach
HAC When reported with secondary diagnosis code J98.5

02104J3 Bypass Coronary Artery, One Site from Coronary Artery with Synthetic Substitute, Percutaneous Endoscopic Approach
HAC When reported with secondary diagnosis code J98.5

02104J8 Bypass Coronary Artery, One Site from Right Internal Mammary with Synthetic Substitute, Percutaneous Endoscopic Approach
HAC When reported with secondary diagnosis code J98.5

02104J9 Bypass Coronary Artery, One Site from Left Internal Mammary with Synthetic Substitute, Percutaneous Endoscopic Approach
HAC When reported with secondary diagnosis code J98.5

02104JC Bypass Coronary Artery, One Site from Thoracic Artery with Synthetic Substitute, Percutaneous Endoscopic Approach
HAC When reported with secondary diagnosis code J98.5

02104JF Bypass Coronary Artery, One Site from Abdominal Artery with Synthetic Substitute, Percutaneous Endoscopic Approach
HAC When reported with secondary diagnosis code J98.5

02104JW Bypass Coronary Artery, One Site from Aorta with Synthetic Substitute, Percutaneous Endoscopic Approach
HAC When reported with secondary diagnosis code J98.5

02104K3 Bypass Coronary Artery, One Site from Coronary Artery with Nonautologous Tissue Substitute, Percutaneous Endoscopic Approach
HAC When reported with secondary diagnosis code J98.5

02104K8 Bypass Coronary Artery, One Site from Right Internal Mammary with Nonautologous Tissue Substitute, Percutaneous Endoscopic Approach
HAC When reported with secondary diagnosis code J98.5

02104K9 Bypass Coronary Artery, One Site from Left Internal Mammary with Nonautologous Tissue Substitute, Percutaneous Endoscopic Approach
HAC When reported with secondary diagnosis code J98.5

02104KC Bypass Coronary Artery, One Site from Thoracic Artery with Nonautologous Tissue Substitute, Percutaneous Endoscopic Approach
HAC When reported with secondary diagnosis code J98.5

02104KF Bypass Coronary Artery, One Site from Abdominal Artery with Nonautologous Tissue Substitute, Percutaneous Endoscopic Approach
HAC When reported with secondary diagnosis code J98.5

02104KW Bypass Coronary Artery, One Site from Aorta with Nonautologous Tissue Substitute, Percutaneous Endoscopic Approach
HAC When reported with secondary diagnosis code J98.5

02104Z3 Bypass Coronary Artery, One Site from Coronary Artery, Percutaneous Endoscopic Approach
HAC When reported with secondary diagnosis code J98.5

02104Z8 Bypass Coronary Artery, One Site from Right Internal Mammary, Percutaneous Endoscopic Approach
HAC When reported with secondary diagnosis code J98.5

02104Z9 Bypass Coronary Artery, One Site from Left Internal Mammary, Percutaneous Endoscopic Approach
HAC When reported with secondary diagnosis code J98.5

02104ZC Bypass Coronary Artery, One Site from Thoracic Artery, Percutaneous Endoscopic Approach
HAC When reported with secondary diagnosis code J98.5

02104ZF Bypass Coronary Artery, One Site from Abdominal Artery, Percutaneous Endoscopic Approach
HAC When reported with secondary diagnosis code J98.5

0211093 Bypass Coronary Artery, Two Sites from Coronary Artery with Autologous Venous Tissue, Open Approach
HAC When reported with secondary diagnosis code J98.5

0211098 Bypass Coronary Artery, Two Sites from Right Internal Mammary with Autologous Venous Tissue, Open Approach
HAC When reported with secondary diagnosis code J98.5

0211099 Bypass Coronary Artery, Two Sites from Left Internal Mammary with Autologous Venous Tissue, Open Approach
HAC When reported with secondary diagnosis code J98.5

021109C Bypass Coronary Artery, Two Sites from Thoracic Artery with Autologous Venous Tissue, Open Approach
HAC When reported with secondary diagnosis code J98.5

021109F Bypass Coronary Artery, Two Sites from Abdominal Artery with Autologous Venous Tissue, Open Approach
HAC When reported with secondary diagnosis code J98.5

021109W Bypass Coronary Artery, Two Sites from Aorta with Autologous Venous Tissue, Open Approach
HAC When reported with secondary diagnosis code J98.5

02110A3 Bypass Coronary Artery, Two Sites from Coronary Artery with Autologous Arterial Tissue, Open Approach
HAC When reported with secondary diagnosis code J98.5

02110A8 Bypass Coronary Artery, Two Sites from Right Internal Mammary with Autologous Arterial Tissue, Open Approach
HAC When reported with secondary diagnosis code J98.5

02110A9 Bypass Coronary Artery, Two Sites from Left Internal Mammary with Autologous Arterial Tissue, Open Approach
HAC When reported with secondary diagnosis code J98.5

02110AC Bypass Coronary Artery, Two Sites from Thoracic Artery with Autologous Arterial Tissue, Open Approach
HAC When reported with secondary diagnosis code J98.5

02110AF Bypass Coronary Artery, Two Sites from Abdominal Artery with Autologous Arterial Tissue, Open Approach
HAC When reported with secondary diagnosis code J98.5

02110AW Bypass Coronary Artery, Two Sites from Aorta with Autologous Arterial Tissue, Open Approach
HAC When reported with secondary diagnosis code J98.5

02110J3 Bypass Coronary Artery, Two Sites from Coronary Artery with Synthetic Substitute, Open Approach
HAC When reported with secondary diagnosis code J98.5

02110J8 Bypass Coronary Artery, Two Sites from Right Internal Mammary with Synthetic Substitute, Open Approach
HAC When reported with secondary diagnosis code J98.5

02110J9 Bypass Coronary Artery, Two Sites from Left Internal Mammary with Synthetic Substitute, Open Approach
HAC When reported with secondary diagnosis code J98.5

02110JC Bypass Coronary Artery, Two Sites from Thoracic Artery with Synthetic Substitute, Open Approach
HAC When reported with secondary diagnosis code J98.5

02110JF Bypass Coronary Artery, Two Sites from Abdominal Artery with Synthetic Substitute, Open Approach
HAC When reported with secondary diagnosis code J98.5

02110JW Bypass Coronary Artery, Two Sites from Aorta with Synthetic Substitute, Open Approach
HAC When reported with secondary diagnosis code J98.5

02110K3 Bypass Coronary Artery, Two Sites from Coronary Artery with Nonautologous Tissue Substitute, Open Approach
HAC When reported with secondary diagnosis code J98.5

02110K8 Bypass Coronary Artery, Two Sites from Right Internal Mammary with Nonautologous Tissue Substitute, Open Approach
HAC When reported with secondary diagnosis code J98.5

02110K9 Bypass Coronary Artery, Two Sites from Left Internal Mammary with Nonautologous Tissue Substitute, Open Approach
HAC When reported with secondary diagnosis code J98.5

02110KC Bypass Coronary Artery, Two Sites from Thoracic Artery with Nonautologous Tissue Substitute, Open Approach
HAC When reported with secondary diagnosis code J98.5

02110KF Bypass Coronary Artery, Two Sites from Abdominal Artery with Nonautologous Tissue Substitute, Open Approach
HAC When reported with secondary diagnosis code J98.5

02110KW Bypass Coronary Artery, Two Sites from Aorta with Nonautologous Tissue Substitute, Open Approach
HAC When reported with secondary diagnosis code J98.5

02110Z3 Bypass Coronary Artery, Two Sites from Coronary Artery, Open Approach
HAC When reported with secondary diagnosis code J98.5

02110Z8 Bypass Coronary Artery, Two Sites from Right Internal Mammary, Open Approach
HAC When reported with secondary diagnosis code J98.5

02110Z9 Bypass Coronary Artery, Two Sites from Left Internal Mammary, Open Approach
HAC When reported with secondary diagnosis code J98.5

02110ZC Bypass Coronary Artery, Two Sites from Thoracic Artery, Open Approach
HAC When reported with secondary diagnosis code J98.5

02110ZF Bypass Coronary Artery, Two Sites from Abdominal Artery, Open Approach
HAC When reported with secondary diagnosis code J98.5

0211344 Bypass Coronary Artery, Two Sites from Coronary Vein with Drug-eluting Intraluminal Device, Percutaneous Approach

02113D4 Bypass Coronary Artery, Two Sites from Coronary Vein with Intraluminal Device, Percutaneous Approach

0211444 Bypass Coronary Artery, Two Sites from Coronary Vein with Drug-eluting Intraluminal Device, Percutaneous Endoscopic Approach
HAC When reported with secondary diagnosis code J98.5

0211493 Bypass Coronary Artery, Two Sites from Coronary Artery with Autologous Venous Tissue, Percutaneous Endoscopic Approach
HAC When reported with secondary diagnosis code J98.5

0211498 Bypass Coronary Artery, Two Sites from Right Internal Mammary with Autologous Venous Tissue, Percutaneous Endoscopic Approach
HAC When reported with secondary diagnosis code J98.5

0211499 Bypass Coronary Artery, Two Sites from Left Internal Mammary with Autologous Venous Tissue, Percutaneous Endoscopic Approach
HAC When reported with secondary diagnosis code J98.5

021149C Bypass Coronary Artery, Two Sites from Thoracic Artery with Autologous Venous Tissue, Percutaneous Endoscopic Approach
HAC When reported with secondary diagnosis code J98.5

021149F Bypass Coronary Artery, Two Sites from Abdominal Artery with Autologous Venous Tissue, Percutaneous Endoscopic Approach
HAC When reported with secondary diagnosis code J98.5

021149W Bypass Coronary Artery, Two Sites from Aorta with Autologous Venous Tissue, Percutaneous Endoscopic Approach
HAC When reported with secondary diagnosis code J98.5

02114A3 Bypass Coronary Artery, Two Sites from Coronary Artery with Autologous Arterial Tissue, Percutaneous Endoscopic Approach
HAC When reported with secondary diagnosis code J98.5

02114A8 Bypass Coronary Artery, Two Sites from Right Internal Mammary with Autologous Arterial Tissue, Percutaneous Endoscopic Approach
HAC When reported with secondary diagnosis code J98.5

02114A9 Bypass Coronary Artery, Two Sites from Left Internal Mammary with Autologous Arterial Tissue, Percutaneous Endoscopic Approach
HAC When reported with secondary diagnosis code J98.5

02114AC Bypass Coronary Artery, Two Sites from Thoracic Artery with Autologous Arterial Tissue, Percutaneous Endoscopic Approach
HAC When reported with secondary diagnosis code J98.5

02114AF Bypass Coronary Artery, Two Sites from Abdominal Artery with Autologous Arterial Tissue, Percutaneous Endoscopic Approach
HAC When reported with secondary diagnosis code J98.5

02114AW Bypass Coronary Artery, Two Sites from Aorta with Autologous Arterial Tissue, Percutaneous Endoscopic Approach
HAC When reported with secondary diagnosis code J98.5

02114D4 Bypass Coronary Artery, Two Sites from Coronary Vein with Intraluminal Device, Percutaneous Endoscopic Approach

02114J3 Bypass Coronary Artery, Two Sites from Coronary Artery with Synthetic Substitute, Percutaneous Endoscopic Approach
HAC When reported with secondary diagnosis code J98.5

02114J8 Bypass Coronary Artery, Two Sites from Right Internal Mammary with Synthetic Substitute, Percutaneous Endoscopic Approach
HAC When reported with secondary diagnosis code J98.5

02114J9 Bypass Coronary Artery, Two Sites from Left Internal Mammary with Synthetic Substitute, Percutaneous Endoscopic Approach
HAC When reported with secondary diagnosis code J98.5

02114JC Bypass Coronary Artery, Two Sites from Thoracic Artery with Synthetic Substitute, Percutaneous Endoscopic Approach
HAC When reported with secondary diagnosis code J98.5

02114JF Bypass Coronary Artery, Two Sites from Abdominal Artery with Synthetic Substitute, Percutaneous Endoscopic Approach
HAC When reported with secondary diagnosis code J98.5

02114JW Bypass Coronary Artery, Two Sites from Aorta with Synthetic Substitute, Percutaneous Endoscopic Approach
HAC When reported with secondary diagnosis code J98.5

02114K3 Bypass Coronary Artery, Two Sites from Coronary Artery with Nonautologous Tissue Substitute, Percutaneous Endoscopic Approach
HAC When reported with secondary diagnosis code J98.5

02114K8 Bypass Coronary Artery, Two Sites from Right Internal Mammary with Nonautologous Tissue Substitute, Percutaneous Endoscopic Approach
HAC When reported with secondary diagnosis code J98.5

02114K9 Bypass Coronary Artery, Two Sites from Left Internal Mammary with Nonautologous Tissue Substitute, Percutaneous Endoscopic Approach
HAC When reported with secondary diagnosis code J98.5

02114KC Bypass Coronary Artery, Two Sites from Thoracic Artery with Nonautologous Tissue Substitute, Percutaneous Endoscopic Approach
HAC When reported with secondary diagnosis code J98.5

02114KF Bypass Coronary Artery, Two Sites from Abdominal Artery with Nonautologous Tissue Substitute, Percutaneous Endoscopic Approach
HAC When reported with secondary diagnosis code J98.5

02114KW Bypass Coronary Artery, Two Sites from Aorta with Nonautologous Tissue Substitute, Percutaneous Endoscopic Approach
HAC When reported with secondary diagnosis code J98.5

02114Z3 Bypass Coronary Artery, Two Sites from Coronary Artery, Percutaneous Endoscopic Approach
HAC When reported with secondary diagnosis code J98.5

02114Z8 Bypass Coronary Artery, Two Sites from Right Internal Mammary, Percutaneous Endoscopic Approach
HAC When reported with secondary diagnosis code J98.5

02114Z9 Bypass Coronary Artery, Two Sites from Left Internal Mammary, Percutaneous Endoscopic Approach
HAC When reported with secondary diagnosis code J98.5

02114ZC Bypass Coronary Artery, Two Sites from Thoracic Artery, Percutaneous Endoscopic Approach
HAC When reported with secondary diagnosis code J98.5

02114ZF Bypass Coronary Artery, Two Sites from Abdominal Artery, Percutaneous Endoscopic Approach
HAC When reported with secondary diagnosis code J98.5

0212093 Bypass Coronary Artery, Three Sites from Coronary Artery with Autologous Venous Tissue, Open Approach
HAC When reported with secondary diagnosis code J98.5

0212098 Bypass Coronary Artery, Three Sites from Right Internal Mammary with Autologous Venous Tissue, Open Approach
HAC When reported with secondary diagnosis code J98.5

0212099 Bypass Coronary Artery, Three Sites from Left Internal Mammary with Autologous Venous Tissue, Open Approach
HAC When reported with secondary diagnosis code J98.5

021209C Bypass Coronary Artery, Three Sites from Thoracic Artery with Autologous Venous Tissue, Open Approach
HAC When reported with secondary diagnosis code J98.5

021209F Bypass Coronary Artery, Three Sites from Abdominal Artery with Autologous Venous Tissue, Open Approach
HAC When reported with secondary diagnosis code J98.5

021209W Bypass Coronary Artery, Three Sites from Aorta with Autologous Venous Tissue, Open Approach
HAC When reported with secondary diagnosis code J98.5

02120A3 Bypass Coronary Artery, Three Sites from Coronary Artery with Autologous Arterial Tissue, Open Approach
HAC When reported with secondary diagnosis code J98.5

02120A8 Bypass Coronary Artery, Three Sites from Right Internal Mammary with Autologous Arterial Tissue, Open Approach
HAC When reported with secondary diagnosis code J98.5

02120A9 Bypass Coronary Artery, Three Sites from Left Internal Mammary with Autologous Arterial Tissue, Open Approach
HAC When reported with secondary diagnosis code J98.5

02120AC Bypass Coronary Artery, Three Sites from Thoracic Artery with Autologous Arterial Tissue, Open Approach
HAC When reported with secondary diagnosis code J98.5

02120AF Bypass Coronary Artery, Three Sites from Abdominal Artery with Autologous Arterial Tissue, Open Approach
HAC When reported with secondary diagnosis code J98.5

02120AW Bypass Coronary Artery, Three Sites from Aorta with Autologous Arterial Tissue, Open Approach
HAC When reported with secondary diagnosis code J98.5

02120J3 Bypass Coronary Artery, Three Sites from Coronary Artery with Synthetic Substitute, Open Approach
HAC When reported with secondary diagnosis code J98.5

02120J8 Bypass Coronary Artery, Three Sites from Right Internal Mammary with Synthetic Substitute, Open Approach
HAC When reported with secondary diagnosis code J98.5

02120J9 Bypass Coronary Artery, Three Sites from Left Internal Mammary with Synthetic Substitute, Open Approach
HAC When reported with secondary diagnosis code J98.5

02120JC Bypass Coronary Artery, Three Sites from Thoracic Artery with Synthetic Substitute, Open Approach
HAC When reported with secondary diagnosis code J98.5

02120JF Bypass Coronary Artery, Three Sites from Abdominal Artery with Synthetic Substitute, Open Approach
HAC When reported with secondary diagnosis code J98.5

02120JW Bypass Coronary Artery, Three Sites from Aorta with Synthetic Substitute, Open Approach
HAC When reported with secondary diagnosis code J98.5

02120K3 Bypass Coronary Artery, Three Sites from Coronary Artery with Nonautologous Tissue Substitute, Open Approach
HAC When reported with secondary diagnosis code J98.5

02120K8 Bypass Coronary Artery, Three Sites from Right Internal Mammary with Nonautologous Tissue Substitute, Open Approach
HAC When reported with secondary diagnosis code J98.5

02120K9 Bypass Coronary Artery, Three Sites from Left Internal Mammary with Nonautologous Tissue Substitute, Open Approach
HAC When reported with secondary diagnosis code J98.5

02120KC Bypass Coronary Artery, Three Sites from Thoracic Artery with Nonautologous Tissue Substitute, Open Approach
HAC When reported with secondary diagnosis code J98.5

02120KF Bypass Coronary Artery, Three Sites from Abdominal Artery with Nonautologous Tissue Substitute, Open Approach
HAC When reported with secondary diagnosis code J98.5

02120KW Bypass Coronary Artery, Three Sites from Aorta with Nonautologous Tissue Substitute, Open Approach
HAC When reported with secondary diagnosis code J98.5

02120Z3 Bypass Coronary Artery, Three Sites from Coronary Artery, Open Approach
HAC When reported with secondary diagnosis code J98.5

02120Z8 Bypass Coronary Artery, Three Sites from Right Internal Mammary, Open Approach
HAC When reported with secondary diagnosis code J98.5

02120Z9 Bypass Coronary Artery, Three Sites from Left Internal Mammary, Open Approach
HAC When reported with secondary diagnosis code J98.5

02120ZC Bypass Coronary Artery, Three Sites from Thoracic Artery, Open Approach
HAC When reported with secondary diagnosis code J98.5

02120ZF Bypass Coronary Artery, Three Sites from Abdominal Artery, Open Approach
HAC When reported with secondary diagnosis code J98.5

0212344 Bypass Coronary Artery, Three Sites from Coronary Vein with Drug-eluting Intraluminal Device, Percutaneous Approach

02123D4 Bypass Coronary Artery, Three Sites from Coronary Vein with Intraluminal Device, Percutaneous Approach

0212444 Bypass Coronary Artery, Three Sites from Coronary Vein with Drug-eluting Intraluminal Device, Percutaneous Endoscopic Approach

0212493 Bypass Coronary Artery, Three Sites from Coronary Artery with Autologous Venous Tissue, Percutaneous Endoscopic Approach
HAC When reported with secondary diagnosis code J98.5

0212498 Bypass Coronary Artery, Three Sites from Right Internal Mammary with Autologous Venous Tissue, Percutaneous Endoscopic Approach
HAC When reported with secondary diagnosis code J98.5

0212499 Bypass Coronary Artery, Three Sites from Left Internal Mammary with Autologous Venous Tissue, Percutaneous Endoscopic Approach
HAC When reported with secondary diagnosis code J98.5

021249C Bypass Coronary Artery, Three Sites from Thoracic Artery with Autologous Venous Tissue, Percutaneous Endoscopic Approach
HAC When reported with secondary diagnosis code J98.5

021249F Bypass Coronary Artery, Three Sites from Abdominal Artery with Autologous Venous Tissue, Percutaneous Endoscopic Approach
HAC When reported with secondary diagnosis code J98.5

021249W Bypass Coronary Artery, Three Sites from Aorta with Autologous Venous Tissue, Percutaneous Endoscopic Approach
HAC When reported with secondary diagnosis code J98.5

02124A3 Bypass Coronary Artery, Three Sites from Coronary Artery with Autologous Arterial Tissue, Percutaneous Endoscopic Approach
HAC When reported with secondary diagnosis code J98.5

02124A8 Bypass Coronary Artery, Three Sites from Right Internal Mammary with Autologous Arterial Tissue, Percutaneous Endoscopic Approach
HAC When reported with secondary diagnosis code J98.5

02124A9 Bypass Coronary Artery, Three Sites from Left Internal Mammary with Autologous Arterial Tissue, Percutaneous Endoscopic Approach
HAC When reported with secondary diagnosis code J98.5

02124AC Bypass Coronary Artery, Three Sites from Thoracic Artery with Autologous Arterial Tissue, Percutaneous Endoscopic Approach
HAC When reported with secondary diagnosis code J98.5

02124AF Bypass Coronary Artery, Three Sites from Abdominal Artery with Autologous Arterial Tissue, Percutaneous Endoscopic Approach
HAC When reported with secondary diagnosis code J98.5

02124AW Bypass Coronary Artery, Three Sites from Aorta with Autologous Arterial Tissue, Percutaneous Endoscopic Approach
HAC When reported with secondary diagnosis code J98.5

02124D4 Bypass Coronary Artery, Three Sites from Coronary Vein with Intraluminal Device, Percutaneous Endoscopic Approach
HAC When reported with secondary diagnosis code J98.5

02124J3 Bypass Coronary Artery, Three Sites from Coronary Artery with Synthetic Substitute, Percutaneous Endoscopic Approach
HAC When reported with secondary diagnosis code J98.5

02124J8 Bypass Coronary Artery, Three Sites from Right Internal Mammary with Synthetic Substitute, Percutaneous Endoscopic Approach
HAC When reported with secondary diagnosis code J98.5

02124J9 Bypass Coronary Artery, Three Sites from Left Internal Mammary with Synthetic Substitute, Percutaneous Endoscopic Approach
HAC When reported with secondary diagnosis code J98.5

02124JC Bypass Coronary Artery, Three Sites from Thoracic Artery with Synthetic Substitute, Percutaneous Endoscopic Approach
HAC When reported with secondary diagnosis code J98.5

02124JF Bypass Coronary Artery, Three Sites from Abdominal Artery with Synthetic Substitute, Percutaneous Endoscopic Approach
HAC When reported with secondary diagnosis code J98.5

02124JW Bypass Coronary Artery, Three Sites from Aorta with Synthetic Substitute, Percutaneous Endoscopic Approach
HAC When reported with secondary diagnosis code J98.5

02124K3 Bypass Coronary Artery, Three Sites from Coronary Artery with Nonautologous Tissue Substitute, Percutaneous Endoscopic Approach
HAC When reported with secondary diagnosis code J98.5

02124K8 Bypass Coronary Artery, Three Sites from Right Internal Mammary with Nonautologous Tissue Substitute, Percutaneous Endoscopic Approach
HAC When reported with secondary diagnosis code J98.5

02124K9 Bypass Coronary Artery, Three Sites from Left Internal Mammary with Nonautologous Tissue Substitute, Percutaneous Endoscopic Approach
HAC When reported with secondary diagnosis code J98.5

02124KC Bypass Coronary Artery, Three Sites from Thoracic Artery with Nonautologous Tissue Substitute, Percutaneous Endoscopic Approach
HAC When reported with secondary diagnosis code J98.5

02124KF Bypass Coronary Artery, Three Sites from Abdominal Artery with Nonautologous Tissue Substitute, Percutaneous Endoscopic Approach
HAC When reported with secondary diagnosis code J98.5

02124KW Bypass Coronary Artery, Three Sites from Aorta with Nonautologous Tissue Substitute, Percutaneous Endoscopic Approach
HAC When reported with secondary diagnosis code J98.5

02124Z3 Bypass Coronary Artery, Three Sites from Coronary Artery, Percutaneous Endoscopic Approach
HAC When reported with secondary diagnosis code J98.5

02124Z8 Bypass Coronary Artery, Three Sites from Right Internal Mammary, Percutaneous Endoscopic Approach
HAC When reported with secondary diagnosis code J98.5

02124Z9 Bypass Coronary Artery, Three Sites from Left Internal Mammary, Percutaneous Endoscopic Approach
HAC When reported with secondary diagnosis code J98.5

02124ZC Bypass Coronary Artery, Three Sites from Thoracic Artery, Percutaneous Endoscopic Approach
HAC When reported with secondary diagnosis code J98.5

02124ZF Bypass Coronary Artery, Three Sites from Abdominal Artery, Percutaneous Endoscopic Approach
HAC When reported with secondary diagnosis code J98.5

0213093 Bypass Coronary Artery, Four or More Sites from Coronary Artery with Autologous Venous Tissue, Open Approach
HAC When reported with secondary diagnosis code J98.5

0213098 Bypass Coronary Artery, Four or More Sites from Right Internal Mammary with Autologous Venous Tissue, Open Approach
HAC When reported with secondary diagnosis code J98.5

0213099 Bypass Coronary Artery, Four or More Sites from Left Internal Mammary with Autologous Venous Tissue, Open Approach
HAC When reported with secondary diagnosis code J98.5

021309C Bypass Coronary Artery, Four or More Sites from Thoracic Artery with Autologous Venous Tissue, Open Approach
HAC When reported with secondary diagnosis code J98.5

021309F Bypass Coronary Artery, Four or More Sites from Abdominal Artery with Autologous Venous Tissue, Open Approach
HAC When reported with secondary diagnosis code J98.5

021309W Bypass Coronary Artery, Four or More Sites from Aorta with Autologous Venous Tissue, Open Approach
HAC When reported with secondary diagnosis code J98.5

02130A3 Bypass Coronary Artery, Four or More Sites from Coronary Artery with Autologous Arterial Tissue, Open Approach
HAC When reported with secondary diagnosis code J98.5

02130A8 Bypass Coronary Artery, Four or More Sites from Right Internal Mammary with Autologous Arterial Tissue, Open Approach
HAC When reported with secondary diagnosis code J98.5

02130A9 Bypass Coronary Artery, Four or More Sites from Left Internal Mammary with Autologous Arterial Tissue, Open Approach
HAC When reported with secondary diagnosis code J98.5

02130AC Bypass Coronary Artery, Four or More Sites from Thoracic Artery with Autologous Arterial Tissue, Open Approach
HAC When reported with secondary diagnosis code J98.5

02130AF Bypass Coronary Artery, Four or More Sites from Abdominal Artery with Autologous Arterial Tissue, Open Approach
HAC When reported with secondary diagnosis code J98.5

02130AW Bypass Coronary Artery, Four or More Sites from Aorta with Autologous Arterial Tissue, Open Approach
HAC When reported with secondary diagnosis code J98.5

02130J3 Bypass Coronary Artery, Four or More Sites from Coronary Artery with Synthetic Substitute, Open Approach
HAC When reported with secondary diagnosis code J98.5

02130J8 Bypass Coronary Artery, Four or More Sites from Right Internal Mammary with Synthetic Substitute, Open Approach
HAC When reported with secondary diagnosis code J98.5

02130J9 Bypass Coronary Artery, Four or More Sites from Left Internal Mammary with Synthetic Substitute, Open Approach
HAC When reported with secondary diagnosis code J98.5

02130JC Bypass Coronary Artery, Four or More Sites from Thoracic Artery with Synthetic Substitute, Open Approach
HAC When reported with secondary diagnosis code J98.5

02130JF Bypass Coronary Artery, Four or More Sites from Abdominal Artery with Synthetic Substitute, Open Approach
HAC When reported with secondary diagnosis code J98.5

02130JW Bypass Coronary Artery, Four or More Sites from Aorta with Synthetic Substitute, Open Approach
HAC When reported with secondary diagnosis code J98.5

02130K3 Bypass Coronary Artery, Four or More Sites from Coronary Artery with Nonautologous Tissue Substitute, Open Approach
HAC When reported with secondary diagnosis code J98.5

02130K8 Bypass Coronary Artery, Four or More Sites from Right Internal Mammary with Nonautologous Tissue Substitute, Open Approach
HAC When reported with secondary diagnosis code J98.5

02130K9 Bypass Coronary Artery, Four or More Sites from Left Internal Mammary with Nonautologous Tissue Substitute, Open Approach
HAC When reported with secondary diagnosis code J98.5

02130KC Bypass Coronary Artery, Four or More Sites from Thoracic Artery with Nonautologous Tissue Substitute, Open Approach
HAC When reported with secondary diagnosis code J98.5

02130KF Bypass Coronary Artery, Four or More Sites from Abdominal Artery with Nonautologous Tissue Substitute, Open Approach
HAC When reported with secondary diagnosis code J98.5

02130KW Bypass Coronary Artery, Four or More Sites from Aorta with Nonautologous Tissue Substitute, Open Approach
HAC When reported with secondary diagnosis code J98.5

02130Z3 Bypass Coronary Artery, Four or More Sites from Coronary Artery, Open Approach
HAC When reported with secondary diagnosis code J98.5

02130Z8 Bypass Coronary Artery, Four or More Sites from Right Internal Mammary, Open Approach
HAC When reported with secondary diagnosis code J98.5

02130Z9 Bypass Coronary Artery, Four or More Sites from Left Internal Mammary, Open Approach
HAC When reported with secondary diagnosis code J98.5

02130ZC Bypass Coronary Artery, Four or More Sites from Thoracic Artery, Open Approach
HAC When reported with secondary diagnosis code J98.5

02130ZF Bypass Coronary Artery, Four or More Sites from Abdominal Artery, Open Approach
HAC When reported with secondary diagnosis code J98.5

0213344 Bypass Coronary Artery, Four or More Sites from Coronary Vein with Drug-eluting Intraluminal Device, Percutaneous Approach
HAC When reported with secondary diagnosis code J98.5

02133D4 Bypass Coronary Artery, Four or More Sites from Coronary Vein with Intraluminal Device, Percutaneous Approach
HAC When reported with secondary diagnosis code J98.5

0213444 Bypass Coronary Artery, Four or More Sites from Coronary Vein with Drug-eluting Intraluminal Device, Percutaneous Endoscopic Approach
HAC When reported with secondary diagnosis code J98.5

0213493 Bypass Coronary Artery, Four or More Sites from Coronary Artery with Autologous Venous Tissue, Percutaneous Endoscopic Approach
HAC When reported with secondary diagnosis code J98.5

0213498 Bypass Coronary Artery, Four or More Sites from Right Internal Mammary with Autologous Venous Tissue, Percutaneous Endoscopic Approach
HAC When reported with secondary diagnosis code J98.5

0213499 Bypass Coronary Artery, Four or More Sites from Left Internal Mammary with Autologous Venous Tissue, Percutaneous Endoscopic Approach
HAC When reported with secondary diagnosis code J98.5

021349C Bypass Coronary Artery, Four or More Sites from Thoracic Artery with Autologous Venous Tissue, Percutaneous Endoscopic Approach
HAC When reported with secondary diagnosis code J98.5

021349F Bypass Coronary Artery, Four or More Sites from Abdominal Artery with Autologous Venous Tissue, Percutaneous Endoscopic Approach
HAC When reported with secondary diagnosis code J98.5

021349W Bypass Coronary Artery, Four or More Sites from Aorta with Autologous Venous Tissue, Percutaneous Endoscopic Approach
HAC When reported with secondary diagnosis code J98.5

02134A3 Bypass Coronary Artery, Four or More Sites from Coronary Artery with Autologous Arterial Tissue, Percutaneous Endoscopic Approach
HAC When reported with secondary diagnosis code J98.5

02134A8 Bypass Coronary Artery, Four or More Sites from Right Internal Mammary with Autologous Arterial Tissue, Percutaneous Endoscopic Approach
HAC When reported with secondary diagnosis code J98.5

02134A9 Bypass Coronary Artery, Four or More Sites from Left Internal Mammary with Autologous Arterial Tissue, Percutaneous Endoscopic Approach
HAC When reported with secondary diagnosis code J98.5

02134AC Bypass Coronary Artery, Four or More Sites from Thoracic Artery with Autologous Arterial Tissue, Percutaneous Endoscopic Approach
HAC When reported with secondary diagnosis code J98.5

02134AF Bypass Coronary Artery, Four or More Sites from Abdominal Artery with Autologous Arterial Tissue, Percutaneous Endoscopic Approach
HAC When reported with secondary diagnosis code J98.5

02134AW Bypass Coronary Artery, Four or More Sites from Aorta with Autologous Arterial Tissue, Percutaneous Endoscopic Approach
HAC When reported with secondary diagnosis code J98.5

02134D4 Bypass Coronary Artery, Four or More Sites from Coronary Vein with Intraluminal Device, Percutaneous Endoscopic Approach
HAC When reported with secondary diagnosis code J98.5

02134J3 Bypass Coronary Artery, Four or More Sites from Coronary Artery with Synthetic Substitute, Percutaneous Endoscopic Approach
HAC When reported with secondary diagnosis code J98.5

02134J8 Bypass Coronary Artery, Four or More Sites from Right Internal Mammary with Synthetic Substitute, Percutaneous Endoscopic Approach
HAC When reported with secondary diagnosis code J98.5

02134J9 Bypass Coronary Artery, Four or More Sites from Left Internal Mammary with Synthetic Substitute, Percutaneous Endoscopic Approach
HAC When reported with secondary diagnosis code J98.5

02134JC Bypass Coronary Artery, Four or More Sites from Thoracic Artery with Synthetic Substitute, Percutaneous Endoscopic Approach
HAC When reported with secondary diagnosis code J98.5

02134JF Bypass Coronary Artery, Four or More Sites from Abdominal Artery with Synthetic Substitute, Percutaneous Endoscopic Approach
HAC When reported with secondary diagnosis code J98.5

02134JW Bypass Coronary Artery, Four or More Sites from Aorta with Synthetic Substitute, Percutaneous Endoscopic Approach
HAC When reported with secondary diagnosis code J98.5

02134K3 Bypass Coronary Artery, Four or More Sites from Coronary Artery with Nonautologous Tissue Substitute, Percutaneous Endoscopic Approach
HAC When reported with secondary diagnosis code J98.5

02134K8 Bypass Coronary Artery, Four or More Sites from Right Internal Mammary with Nonautologous Tissue Substitute, Percutaneous Endoscopic Approach
HAC When reported with secondary diagnosis code J98.5

02134K9 Bypass Coronary Artery, Four or More Sites from Left Internal Mammary with Nonautologous Tissue Substitute, Percutaneous Endoscopic Approach
HAC When reported with secondary diagnosis code J98.5

02134KC Bypass Coronary Artery, Four or More Sites from Thoracic Artery with Nonautologous Tissue Substitute, Percutaneous Endoscopic Approach
HAC When reported with secondary diagnosis code J98.5

02134KF Bypass Coronary Artery, Four or More Sites from Abdominal Artery with Nonautologous Tissue Substitute, Percutaneous Endoscopic Approach
HAC When reported with secondary diagnosis code J98.5

02134KW Bypass Coronary Artery, Four or More Sites from Aorta with Nonautologous Tissue Substitute, Percutaneous Endoscopic Approach
HAC When reported with secondary diagnosis code J98.5

02134Z3 Bypass Coronary Artery, Four or More Sites from Coronary Artery, Percutaneous Endoscopic Approach
HAC When reported with secondary diagnosis code J98.5

02134Z8 Bypass Coronary Artery, Four or More Sites from Right Internal Mammary, Percutaneous Endoscopic Approach
HAC When reported with secondary diagnosis code J98.5

02134Z9 Bypass Coronary Artery, Four or More Sites from Left Internal Mammary, Percutaneous Endoscopic Approach
HAC When reported with secondary diagnosis code J98.5

02134ZC Bypass Coronary Artery, Four or More Sites from Thoracic Artery, Percutaneous Endoscopic Approach
HAC When reported with secondary diagnosis code J98.5

02134ZF Bypass Coronary Artery, Four or More Sites from Abdominal Artery, Percutaneous Endoscopic Approach
HAC When reported with secondary diagnosis code J98.5

021609P Bypass Right Atrium to Pulmonary Trunk with Autologous Venous Tissue, Open Approach

021609Q Bypass Right Atrium to Right Pulmonary Artery with Autologous Venous Tissue, Open Approach

021609R Bypass Right Atrium to Left Pulmonary Artery with Autologous Venous Tissue, Open Approach

02160AP Bypass Right Atrium to Pulmonary Trunk with Autologous Arterial Tissue, Open Approach

02160AQ Bypass Right Atrium to Right Pulmonary Artery with Autologous Arterial Tissue, Open Approach

02160AR Bypass Right Atrium to Left Pulmonary Artery with Autologous Arterial Tissue, Open Approach

02160JP Bypass Right Atrium to Pulmonary Trunk with Synthetic Substitute, Open Approach

02160JQ Bypass Right Atrium to Right Pulmonary Artery with Synthetic Substitute, Open Approach

02160JR Bypass Right Atrium to Left Pulmonary Artery with Synthetic Substitute, Open Approach

02160KP Bypass Right Atrium to Pulmonary Trunk with Nonautologous Tissue Substitute, Open Approach
02160KQ Bypass Right Atrium to Right Pulmonary Artery with Nonautologous Tissue Substitute, Open Approach
02160KR Bypass Right Atrium to Left Pulmonary Artery with Nonautologous Tissue Substitute, Open Approach
02160Z7 Bypass Right Atrium to Left Atrium, Open Approach
02160ZP Bypass Right Atrium to Pulmonary Trunk, Open Approach
02160ZQ Bypass Right Atrium to Right Pulmonary Artery, Open Approach
02160ZR Bypass Right Atrium to Left Pulmonary Artery, Open Approach
021649P Bypass Right Atrium to Pulmonary Trunk with Autologous Venous Tissue, Percutaneous Endoscopic Approach
021649Q Bypass Right Atrium to Right Pulmonary Artery with Autologous Venous Tissue, Percutaneous Endoscopic Approach
021649R Bypass Right Atrium to Left Pulmonary Artery with Autologous Venous Tissue, Percutaneous Endoscopic Approach
02164AP Bypass Right Atrium to Pulmonary Trunk with Autologous Arterial Tissue, Percutaneous Endoscopic Approach
02164AQ Bypass Right Atrium to Right Pulmonary Artery with Autologous Arterial Tissue, Percutaneous Endoscopic Approach
02164AR Bypass Right Atrium to Left Pulmonary Artery with Autologous Arterial Tissue, Percutaneous Endoscopic Approach
02164JP Bypass Right Atrium to Pulmonary Trunk with Synthetic Substitute, Percutaneous Endoscopic Approach
02164JQ Bypass Right Atrium to Right Pulmonary Artery with Synthetic Substitute, Percutaneous Endoscopic Approach
02164JR Bypass Right Atrium to Left Pulmonary Artery with Synthetic Substitute, Percutaneous Endoscopic Approach
02164KP Bypass Right Atrium to Pulmonary Trunk with Nonautologous Tissue Substitute, Percutaneous Endoscopic Approach
02164KQ Bypass Right Atrium to Right Pulmonary Artery with Nonautologous Tissue Substitute, Percutaneous Endoscopic Approach
02164KR Bypass Right Atrium to Left Pulmonary Artery with Nonautologous Tissue Substitute, Percutaneous Endoscopic Approach
02164Z7 Bypass Right Atrium to Left Atrium, Percutaneous Endoscopic Approach
02164ZP Bypass Right Atrium to Pulmonary Trunk, Percutaneous Endoscopic Approach
02164ZQ Bypass Right Atrium to Right Pulmonary Artery, Percutaneous Endoscopic Approach
02164ZR Bypass Right Atrium to Left Pulmonary Artery, Percutaneous Endoscopic Approach
021709P Bypass Left Atrium to Pulmonary Trunk with Autologous Venous Tissue, Open Approach
021709Q Bypass Left Atrium to Right Pulmonary Artery with Autologous Venous Tissue, Open Approach
021709R Bypass Left Atrium to Left Pulmonary Artery with Autologous Venous Tissue, Open Approach
02170AP Bypass Left Atrium to Pulmonary Trunk with Autologous Arterial Tissue, Open Approach
02170AQ Bypass Left Atrium to Right Pulmonary Artery with Autologous Arterial Tissue, Open Approach
02170AR Bypass Left Atrium to Left Pulmonary Artery with Autologous Arterial Tissue, Open Approach
02170JP Bypass Left Atrium to Pulmonary Trunk with Synthetic Substitute, Open Approach
02170JQ Bypass Left Atrium to Right Pulmonary Artery with Synthetic Substitute, Open Approach
02170JR Bypass Left Atrium to Left Pulmonary Artery with Synthetic Substitute, Open Approach
02170KP Bypass Left Atrium to Pulmonary Trunk with Nonautologous Tissue Substitute, Open Approach
02170KQ Bypass Left Atrium to Right Pulmonary Artery with Nonautologous Tissue Substitute, Open Approach
02170KR Bypass Left Atrium to Left Pulmonary Artery with Nonautologous Tissue Substitute, Open Approach
02170ZP Bypass Left Atrium to Pulmonary Trunk, Open Approach
02170ZQ Bypass Left Atrium to Right Pulmonary Artery, Open Approach
02170ZR Bypass Left Atrium to Left Pulmonary Artery, Open Approach
021749P Bypass Left Atrium to Pulmonary Trunk with Autologous Venous Tissue, Percutaneous Endoscopic Approach
021749Q Bypass Left Atrium to Right Pulmonary Artery with Autologous Venous Tissue, Percutaneous Endoscopic Approach
021749R Bypass Left Atrium to Left Pulmonary Artery with Autologous Venous Tissue, Percutaneous Endoscopic Approach
02174AP Bypass Left Atrium to Pulmonary Trunk with Autologous Arterial Tissue, Percutaneous Endoscopic Approach
02174AQ Bypass Left Atrium to Right Pulmonary Artery with Autologous Arterial Tissue, Percutaneous Endoscopic Approach
02174AR Bypass Left Atrium to Left Pulmonary Artery with Autologous Arterial Tissue, Percutaneous Endoscopic Approach
02174JP Bypass Left Atrium to Pulmonary Trunk with Synthetic Substitute, Percutaneous Endoscopic Approach
02174JQ Bypass Left Atrium to Right Pulmonary Artery with Synthetic Substitute, Percutaneous Endoscopic Approach
02174JR Bypass Left Atrium to Left Pulmonary Artery with Synthetic Substitute, Percutaneous Endoscopic Approach
02174KP Bypass Left Atrium to Pulmonary Trunk with Nonautologous Tissue Substitute, Percutaneous Endoscopic Approach
02174KQ Bypass Left Atrium to Right Pulmonary Artery with Nonautologous Tissue Substitute, Percutaneous Endoscopic Approach
02174KR Bypass Left Atrium to Left Pulmonary Artery with Nonautologous Tissue Substitute, Percutaneous Endoscopic Approach
02174ZP Bypass Left Atrium to Pulmonary Trunk, Percutaneous Endoscopic Approach
02174ZQ Bypass Left Atrium to Right Pulmonary Artery, Percutaneous Endoscopic Approach
02174ZR Bypass Left Atrium to Left Pulmonary Artery, Percutaneous Endoscopic Approach
021K09P Bypass Right Ventricle to Pulmonary Trunk with Autologous Venous Tissue, Open Approach
021K09Q Bypass Right Ventricle to Right Pulmonary Artery with Autologous Venous Tissue, Open Approach
021K09R Bypass Right Ventricle to Left Pulmonary Artery with Autologous Venous Tissue, Open Approach
021K0AP Bypass Right Ventricle to Pulmonary Trunk with Autologous Arterial Tissue, Open Approach
021K0AQ Bypass Right Ventricle to Right Pulmonary Artery with Autologous Arterial Tissue, Open Approach
021K0AR Bypass Right Ventricle to Left Pulmonary Artery with Autologous Arterial Tissue, Open Approach
021K0JP Bypass Right Ventricle to Pulmonary Trunk with Synthetic Substitute, Open Approach
021K0JQ Bypass Right Ventricle to Right Pulmonary Artery with Synthetic Substitute, Open Approach
021K0JR Bypass Right Ventricle to Left Pulmonary Artery with Synthetic Substitute, Open Approach
021K0KP Bypass Right Ventricle to Pulmonary Trunk with Nonautologous Tissue Substitute, Open Approach
021K0KQ Bypass Right Ventricle to Right Pulmonary Artery with Nonautologous Tissue Substitute, Open Approach
021K0KR Bypass Right Ventricle to Left Pulmonary Artery with Nonautologous Tissue Substitute, Open Approach
021K0Z5 Bypass Right Ventricle to Coronary Circulation, Open Approach
021K0Z8 Bypass Right Ventricle to Right Internal Mammary, Open Approach
021K0Z9 Bypass Right Ventricle to Left Internal Mammary, Open Approach
021K0ZC Bypass Right Ventricle to Thoracic Artery, Open Approach
021K0ZF Bypass Right Ventricle to Abdominal Artery, Open Approach
021K0ZP Bypass Right Ventricle to Pulmonary Trunk, Open Approach
021K0ZQ Bypass Right Ventricle to Right Pulmonary Artery, Open Approach
021K0ZR Bypass Right Ventricle to Left Pulmonary Artery, Open Approach
021K0ZW Bypass Right Ventricle to Aorta, Open Approach
021K49P Bypass Right Ventricle to Pulmonary Trunk with Autologous Venous Tissue, Percutaneous Endoscopic Approach
021K49Q Bypass Right Ventricle to Right Pulmonary Artery with Autologous Venous Tissue, Percutaneous Endoscopic Approach
021K49R Bypass Right Ventricle to Left Pulmonary Artery with Autologous Venous Tissue, Percutaneous Endoscopic Approach
021K4AP Bypass Right Ventricle to Pulmonary Trunk with Autologous Arterial Tissue, Percutaneous Endoscopic Approach
021K4AQ Bypass Right Ventricle to Right Pulmonary Artery with Autologous Arterial Tissue, Percutaneous Endoscopic Approach
021K4AR Bypass Right Ventricle to Left Pulmonary Artery with Autologous Arterial Tissue, Percutaneous Endoscopic Approach
021K4JP Bypass Right Ventricle to Pulmonary Trunk with Synthetic Substitute, Percutaneous Endoscopic Approach
021K4JQ Bypass Right Ventricle to Right Pulmonary Artery with Synthetic Substitute, Percutaneous Endoscopic Approach

021K4JR Bypass Right Ventricle to Left Pulmonary Artery with Synthetic Substitute, Percutaneous Endoscopic Approach
021K4KP Bypass Right Ventricle to Pulmonary Trunk with Nonautologous Tissue Substitute, Percutaneous Endoscopic Approach
021K4KQ Bypass Right Ventricle to Right Pulmonary Artery with Nonautologous Tissue Substitute, Percutaneous Endoscopic Approach
021K4KR Bypass Right Ventricle to Left Pulmonary Artery with Nonautologous Tissue Substitute, Percutaneous Endoscopic Approach
021K4Z5 Bypass Right Ventricle to Coronary Circulation, Percutaneous Endoscopic Approach
021K4Z8 Bypass Right Ventricle to Right Internal Mammary, Percutaneous Endoscopic Approach
021K4Z9 Bypass Right Ventricle to Left Internal Mammary, Percutaneous Endoscopic Approach
021K4ZC Bypass Right Ventricle to Thoracic Artery, Percutaneous Endoscopic Approach
021K4ZF Bypass Right Ventricle to Abdominal Artery, Percutaneous Endoscopic Approach
021K4ZP Bypass Right Ventricle to Pulmonary Trunk, Percutaneous Endoscopic Approach
021K4ZQ Bypass Right Ventricle to Right Pulmonary Artery, Percutaneous Endoscopic Approach
021K4ZR Bypass Right Ventricle to Left Pulmonary Artery, Percutaneous Endoscopic Approach
021K4ZW Bypass Right Ventricle to Aorta, Percutaneous Endoscopic Approach
021L09P Bypass Left Ventricle to Pulmonary Trunk with Autologous Venous Tissue, Open Approach
021L09Q Bypass Left Ventricle to Right Pulmonary Artery with Autologous Venous Tissue, Open Approach
021L09R Bypass Left Ventricle to Left Pulmonary Artery with Autologous Venous Tissue, Open Approach
021L0AP Bypass Left Ventricle to Pulmonary Trunk with Autologous Arterial Tissue, Open Approach
021L0AQ Bypass Left Ventricle to Right Pulmonary Artery with Autologous Arterial Tissue, Open Approach
021L0AR Bypass Left Ventricle to Left Pulmonary Artery with Autologous Arterial Tissue, Open Approach
021L0JP Bypass Left Ventricle to Pulmonary Trunk with Synthetic Substitute, Open Approach
021L0JQ Bypass Left Ventricle to Right Pulmonary Artery with Synthetic Substitute, Open Approach
021L0JR Bypass Left Ventricle to Left Pulmonary Artery with Synthetic Substitute, Open Approach
021L0KP Bypass Left Ventricle to Pulmonary Trunk with Nonautologous Tissue Substitute, Open Approach
021L0KQ Bypass Left Ventricle to Right Pulmonary Artery with Nonautologous Tissue Substitute, Open Approach
021L0KR Bypass Left Ventricle to Left Pulmonary Artery with Nonautologous Tissue Substitute, Open Approach
021L0Z5 Bypass Left Ventricle to Coronary Circulation, Open Approach
021L0Z8 Bypass Left Ventricle to Right Internal Mammary, Open Approach
021L0Z9 Bypass Left Ventricle to Left Internal Mammary, Open Approach
021L0ZC Bypass Left Ventricle to Thoracic Artery, Open Approach
021L0ZF Bypass Left Ventricle to Abdominal Artery, Open Approach
021L0ZP Bypass Left Ventricle to Pulmonary Trunk, Open Approach
021L0ZQ Bypass Left Ventricle to Right Pulmonary Artery, Open Approach
021L0ZR Bypass Left Ventricle to Left Pulmonary Artery, Open Approach
021L0ZW Bypass Left Ventricle to Aorta, Open Approach
021L49P Bypass Left Ventricle to Pulmonary Trunk with Autologous Venous Tissue, Percutaneous Endoscopic Approach
021L49Q Bypass Left Ventricle to Right Pulmonary Artery with Autologous Venous Tissue, Percutaneous Endoscopic Approach
021L49R Bypass Left Ventricle to Left Pulmonary Artery with Autologous Venous Tissue, Percutaneous Endoscopic Approach
021L4AP Bypass Left Ventricle to Pulmonary Trunk with Autologous Arterial Tissue, Percutaneous Endoscopic Approach
021L4AQ Bypass Left Ventricle to Right Pulmonary Artery with Autologous Arterial Tissue, Percutaneous Endoscopic Approach
021L4AR Bypass Left Ventricle to Left Pulmonary Artery with Autologous Arterial Tissue, Percutaneous Endoscopic Approach
021L4JP Bypass Left Ventricle to Pulmonary Trunk with Synthetic Substitute, Percutaneous Endoscopic Approach
021L4JQ Bypass Left Ventricle to Right Pulmonary Artery with Synthetic Substitute, Percutaneous Endoscopic Approach
021L4JR Bypass Left Ventricle to Left Pulmonary Artery with Synthetic Substitute, Percutaneous Endoscopic Approach
021L4KP Bypass Left Ventricle to Pulmonary Trunk with Nonautologous Tissue Substitute, Percutaneous Endoscopic Approach
021L4KQ Bypass Left Ventricle to Right Pulmonary Artery with Nonautologous Tissue Substitute, Percutaneous Endoscopic Approach
021L4KR Bypass Left Ventricle to Left Pulmonary Artery with Nonautologous Tissue Substitute, Percutaneous Endoscopic Approach
021L4Z5 Bypass Left Ventricle to Coronary Circulation, Percutaneous Endoscopic Approach
021L4Z8 Bypass Left Ventricle to Right Internal Mammary, Percutaneous Endoscopic Approach
021L4Z9 Bypass Left Ventricle to Left Internal Mammary, Percutaneous Endoscopic Approach
021L4ZC Bypass Left Ventricle to Thoracic Artery, Percutaneous Endoscopic Approach
021L4ZF Bypass Left Ventricle to Abdominal Artery, Percutaneous Endoscopic Approach
021L4ZP Bypass Left Ventricle to Pulmonary Trunk, Percutaneous Endoscopic Approach
021L4ZQ Bypass Left Ventricle to Right Pulmonary Artery, Percutaneous Endoscopic Approach
021L4ZR Bypass Left Ventricle to Left Pulmonary Artery, Percutaneous Endoscopic Approach
021L4ZW Bypass Left Ventricle to Aorta, Percutaneous Endoscopic Approach
021V09P Bypass Superior Vena Cava to Pulmonary Trunk with Autologous Venous Tissue, Open Approach
021V09Q Bypass Superior Vena Cava to Right Pulmonary Artery with Autologous Venous Tissue, Open Approach
021V09R Bypass Superior Vena Cava to Left Pulmonary Artery with Autologous Venous Tissue, Open Approach
021V0AP Bypass Superior Vena Cava to Pulmonary Trunk with Autologous Arterial Tissue, Open Approach
021V0AQ Bypass Superior Vena Cava to Right Pulmonary Artery with Autologous Arterial Tissue, Open Approach
021V0AR Bypass Superior Vena Cava to Left Pulmonary Artery with Autologous Arterial Tissue, Open Approach
021V0JP Bypass Superior Vena Cava to Pulmonary Trunk with Synthetic Substitute, Open Approach
021V0JQ Bypass Superior Vena Cava to Right Pulmonary Artery with Synthetic Substitute, Open Approach
021V0JR Bypass Superior Vena Cava to Left Pulmonary Artery with Synthetic Substitute, Open Approach
021V0KP Bypass Superior Vena Cava to Pulmonary Trunk with Nonautologous Tissue Substitute, Open Approach
021V0KQ Bypass Superior Vena Cava to Right Pulmonary Artery with Nonautologous Tissue Substitute, Open Approach
021V0KR Bypass Superior Vena Cava to Left Pulmonary Artery with Nonautologous Tissue Substitute, Open Approach
021V0ZP Bypass Superior Vena Cava to Pulmonary Trunk, Open Approach
021V0ZQ Bypass Superior Vena Cava to Right Pulmonary Artery, Open Approach
021V0ZR Bypass Superior Vena Cava to Left Pulmonary Artery, Open Approach
021V49P Bypass Superior Vena Cava to Pulmonary Trunk with Autologous Venous Tissue, Percutaneous Endoscopic Approach
021V49Q Bypass Superior Vena Cava to Right Pulmonary Artery with Autologous Venous Tissue, Percutaneous Endoscopic Approach
021V49R Bypass Superior Vena Cava to Left Pulmonary Artery with Autologous Venous Tissue, Percutaneous Endoscopic Approach
021V4AP Bypass Superior Vena Cava to Pulmonary Trunk with Autologous Arterial Tissue, Percutaneous Endoscopic Approach
021V4AQ Bypass Superior Vena Cava to Right Pulmonary Artery with Autologous Arterial Tissue, Percutaneous Endoscopic Approach
021V4AR Bypass Superior Vena Cava to Left Pulmonary Artery with Autologous Arterial Tissue, Percutaneous Endoscopic Approach
021V4JP Bypass Superior Vena Cava to Pulmonary Trunk with Synthetic Substitute, Percutaneous Endoscopic Approach
021V4JQ Bypass Superior Vena Cava to Right Pulmonary Artery with Synthetic Substitute, Percutaneous Endoscopic Approach
021V4JR Bypass Superior Vena Cava to Left Pulmonary Artery with Synthetic Substitute, Percutaneous Endoscopic Approach
021V4KP Bypass Superior Vena Cava to Pulmonary Trunk with Nonautologous Tissue Substitute, Percutaneous Endoscopic Approach
021V4KQ Bypass Superior Vena Cava to Right Pulmonary Artery with Nonautologous

Tissue Substitute, Percutaneous Endoscopic Approach

021V4KR Bypass Superior Vena Cava to Left Pulmonary Artery with Nonautologous Tissue Substitute, Percutaneous Endoscopic Approach

021V4ZP Bypass Superior Vena Cava to Pulmonary Trunk, Percutaneous Endoscopic Approach

021V4ZQ Bypass Superior Vena Cava to Right Pulmonary Artery, Percutaneous Endoscopic Approach

021V4ZR Bypass Superior Vena Cava to Left Pulmonary Artery, Percutaneous Endoscopic Approach

021W09B Bypass Thoracic Aorta to Subclavian with Autologous Venous Tissue, Open Approach

021W09D Bypass Thoracic Aorta to Carotid with Autologous Venous Tissue, Open Approach

021W09P Bypass Thoracic Aorta to Pulmonary Trunk with Autologous Venous Tissue, Open Approach

021W09Q Bypass Thoracic Aorta to Right Pulmonary Artery with Autologous Venous Tissue, Open Approach

021W09R Bypass Thoracic Aorta to Left Pulmonary Artery with Autologous Venous Tissue, Open Approach

021W0AB Bypass Thoracic Aorta to Subclavian with Autologous Arterial Tissue, Open Approach

021W0AD Bypass Thoracic Aorta to Carotid with Autologous Arterial Tissue, Open Approach

021W0AP Bypass Thoracic Aorta to Pulmonary Trunk with Autologous Arterial Tissue, Open Approach

021W0AQ Bypass Thoracic Aorta to Right Pulmonary Artery with Autologous Arterial Tissue, Open Approach

021W0AR Bypass Thoracic Aorta to Left Pulmonary Artery with Autologous Arterial Tissue, Open Approach

021W0JB Bypass Thoracic Aorta to Subclavian with Synthetic Substitute, Open Approach

021W0JD Bypass Thoracic Aorta to Carotid with Synthetic Substitute, Open Approach

021W0JP Bypass Thoracic Aorta to Pulmonary Trunk with Synthetic Substitute, Open Approach

021W0JQ Bypass Thoracic Aorta to Right Pulmonary Artery with Synthetic Substitute, Open Approach

021W0JR Bypass Thoracic Aorta to Left Pulmonary Artery with Synthetic Substitute, Open Approach

021W0KB Bypass Thoracic Aorta to Subclavian with Nonautologous Tissue Substitute, Open Approach

021W0KD Bypass Thoracic Aorta to Carotid with Nonautologous Tissue Substitute, Open Approach

021W0KP Bypass Thoracic Aorta to Pulmonary Trunk with Nonautologous Tissue Substitute, Open Approach

021W0KQ Bypass Thoracic Aorta to Right Pulmonary Artery with Nonautologous Tissue Substitute, Open Approach

021W0KR Bypass Thoracic Aorta to Left Pulmonary Artery with Nonautologous Tissue Substitute, Open Approach

021W0ZB Bypass Thoracic Aorta to Subclavian, Open Approach

021W0ZD Bypass Thoracic Aorta to Carotid, Open Approach

021W0ZP Bypass Thoracic Aorta to Pulmonary Trunk, Open Approach

021W0ZQ Bypass Thoracic Aorta to Right Pulmonary Artery, Open Approach

021W0ZR Bypass Thoracic Aorta to Left Pulmonary Artery, Open Approach

021W49B Bypass Thoracic Aorta to Subclavian with Autologous Venous Tissue, Percutaneous Endoscopic Approach

021W49D Bypass Thoracic Aorta to Carotid with Autologous Venous Tissue, Percutaneous Endoscopic Approach

021W49P Bypass Thoracic Aorta to Pulmonary Trunk with Autologous Venous Tissue, Percutaneous Endoscopic Approach

021W49Q Bypass Thoracic Aorta to Right Pulmonary Artery with Autologous Venous Tissue, Percutaneous Endoscopic Approach

021W49R Bypass Thoracic Aorta to Left Pulmonary Artery with Autologous Venous Tissue, Percutaneous Endoscopic Approach

021W4AB Bypass Thoracic Aorta to Subclavian with Autologous Arterial Tissue, Percutaneous Endoscopic Approach

021W4AD Bypass Thoracic Aorta to Carotid with Autologous Arterial Tissue, Percutaneous Endoscopic Approach

021W4AP Bypass Thoracic Aorta to Pulmonary Trunk with Autologous Arterial Tissue, Percutaneous Endoscopic Approach

021W4AQ Bypass Thoracic Aorta to Right Pulmonary Artery with Autologous Arterial Tissue, Percutaneous Endoscopic Approach

021W4AR Bypass Thoracic Aorta to Left Pulmonary Artery with Autologous Arterial Tissue, Percutaneous Endoscopic Approach

021W4JB Bypass Thoracic Aorta to Subclavian with Synthetic Substitute, Percutaneous Endoscopic Approach

021W4JD Bypass Thoracic Aorta to Carotid with Synthetic Substitute, Percutaneous Endoscopic Approach

021W4JP Bypass Thoracic Aorta to Pulmonary Trunk with Synthetic Substitute, Percutaneous Endoscopic Approach

021W4JQ Bypass Thoracic Aorta to Right Pulmonary Artery with Synthetic Substitute, Percutaneous Endoscopic Approach

021W4JR Bypass Thoracic Aorta to Left Pulmonary Artery with Synthetic Substitute, Percutaneous Endoscopic Approach

021W4KB Bypass Thoracic Aorta to Subclavian with Nonautologous Tissue Substitute, Percutaneous Endoscopic Approach

021W4KD Bypass Thoracic Aorta to Carotid with Nonautologous Tissue Substitute, Percutaneous Endoscopic Approach

021W4KP Bypass Thoracic Aorta to Pulmonary Trunk with Nonautologous Tissue Substitute, Percutaneous Endoscopic Approach

021W4KQ Bypass Thoracic Aorta to Right Pulmonary Artery with Nonautologous Tissue Substitute, Percutaneous Endoscopic Approach

021W4KR Bypass Thoracic Aorta to Left Pulmonary Artery with Nonautologous Tissue Substitute, Percutaneous Endoscopic Approach

021W4ZB Bypass Thoracic Aorta to Subclavian, Percutaneous Endoscopic Approach

021W4ZD Bypass Thoracic Aorta to Carotid, Percutaneous Endoscopic Approach

021W4ZP Bypass Thoracic Aorta to Pulmonary Trunk, Percutaneous Endoscopic Approach

021W4ZQ Bypass Thoracic Aorta to Right Pulmonary Artery, Percutaneous Endoscopic Approach

021W4ZR Bypass Thoracic Aorta to Left Pulmonary Artery, Percutaneous Endoscopic Approach

025 – Heart and Great Vessels, Destruction

02540ZZ Destruction of Coronary Vein, Open Approach

02543ZZ Destruction of Coronary Vein, Percutaneous Approach

02544ZZ Destruction of Coronary Vein, Percutaneous Endoscopic Approach

02550ZZ Destruction of Atrial Septum, Open Approach

02553ZZ Destruction of Atrial Septum, Percutaneous Approach

02554ZZ Destruction of Atrial Septum, Percutaneous Endoscopic Approach

02560ZZ Destruction of Right Atrium, Open Approach

02563ZZ Destruction of Right Atrium, Percutaneous Approach

02564ZZ Destruction of Right Atrium, Percutaneous Endoscopic Approach

● **02570ZK** Destruction of Left Atrial Appendage, Open Approach

02570ZZ Destruction of Left Atrium, Open Approach

● **02573ZK** Destruction of Left Atrial Appendage, Percutaneous Approach

02573ZZ Destruction of Left Atrium, Percutaneous Approach

● **02574ZK** Destruction of Left Atrial Appendage, Percutaneous Endoscopic Approach

02574ZZ Destruction of Left Atrium, Percutaneous Endoscopic Approach

02580ZZ Destruction of Conduction Mechanism, Open Approach

02583ZZ Destruction of Conduction Mechanism, Percutaneous Approach

02584ZZ Destruction of Conduction Mechanism, Percutaneous Endoscopic Approach

02590ZZ Destruction of Chordae Tendineae, Open Approach

02593ZZ Destruction of Chordae Tendineae, Percutaneous Approach

02594ZZ Destruction of Chordae Tendineae, Percutaneous Endoscopic Approach

025D0ZZ Destruction of Papillary Muscle, Open Approach

025D3ZZ Destruction of Papillary Muscle, Percutaneous Approach

025D4ZZ Destruction of Papillary Muscle, Percutaneous Endoscopic Approach

025F0ZZ Destruction of Aortic Valve, Open Approach

025F3ZZ Destruction of Aortic Valve, Percutaneous Approach

025F4ZZ Destruction of Aortic Valve, Percutaneous Endoscopic Approach

025G0ZZ Destruction of Mitral Valve, Open Approach

025G3ZZ Destruction of Mitral Valve, Percutaneous Approach

025G4ZZ Destruction of Mitral Valve, Percutaneous Endoscopic Approach

025H0ZZ Destruction of Pulmonary Valve, Open Approach

025H3ZZ Destruction of Pulmonary Valve, Percutaneous Approach

025H4ZZ Destruction of Pulmonary Valve, Percutaneous Endoscopic Approach
025J0ZZ Destruction of Tricuspid Valve, Open Approach
025J3ZZ Destruction of Tricuspid Valve, Percutaneous Approach
025J4ZZ Destruction of Tricuspid Valve, Percutaneous Endoscopic Approach
025K0ZZ Destruction of Right Ventricle, Open Approach
025K3ZZ Destruction of Right Ventricle, Percutaneous Approach
025K4ZZ Destruction of Right Ventricle, Percutaneous Endoscopic Approach
025L0ZZ Destruction of Left Ventricle, Open Approach
025L3ZZ Destruction of Left Ventricle, Percutaneous Approach
025L4ZZ Destruction of Left Ventricle, Percutaneous Endoscopic Approach
025M0ZZ Destruction of Ventricular Septum, Open Approach
025M3ZZ Destruction of Ventricular Septum, Percutaneous Approach
025M4ZZ Destruction of Ventricular Septum, Percutaneous Endoscopic Approach
025N0ZZ Destruction of Pericardium, Open Approach
025N3ZZ Destruction of Pericardium, Percutaneous Approach
025N4ZZ Destruction of Pericardium, Percutaneous Endoscopic Approach
025P0ZZ Destruction of Pulmonary Trunk, Open Approach
025P3ZZ Destruction of Pulmonary Trunk, Percutaneous Approach
025P4ZZ Destruction of Pulmonary Trunk, Percutaneous Endoscopic Approach
025Q0ZZ Destruction of Right Pulmonary Artery, Open Approach
025Q3ZZ Destruction of Right Pulmonary Artery, Percutaneous Approach
025Q4ZZ Destruction of Right Pulmonary Artery, Percutaneous Endoscopic Approach
025R0ZZ Destruction of Left Pulmonary Artery, Open Approach
025R3ZZ Destruction of Left Pulmonary Artery, Percutaneous Approach
025R4ZZ Destruction of Left Pulmonary Artery, Percutaneous Endoscopic Approach
025S0ZZ Destruction of Right Pulmonary Vein, Open Approach
025S3ZZ Destruction of Right Pulmonary Vein, Percutaneous Approach
AHA CC: 2Q, 2013, 38-39
025S4ZZ Destruction of Right Pulmonary Vein, Percutaneous Endoscopic Approach
025T0ZZ Destruction of Left Pulmonary Vein, Open Approach
025T3ZZ Destruction of Left Pulmonary Vein, Percutaneous Approach
AHA CC: 2Q, 2013, 38-39
025T4ZZ Destruction of Left Pulmonary Vein, Percutaneous Endoscopic Approach
025V0ZZ Destruction of Superior Vena Cava, Open Approach
025V3ZZ Destruction of Superior Vena Cava, Percutaneous Approach
025V4ZZ Destruction of Superior Vena Cava, Percutaneous Endoscopic Approach
025W0ZZ Destruction of Thoracic Aorta, Open Approach
025W3ZZ Destruction of Thoracic Aorta, Percutaneous Approach
025W4ZZ Destruction of Thoracic Aorta, Percutaneous Endoscopic Approach

027 – Heart and Great Vessels, Dilation

For Dilation procedures involving the coronary arteries, Review Coding Guideline B4.4

0270046 Dilation of Coronary Artery, One Site, Bifurcation, with Drug-eluting Intraluminal Device, Open Approach
027004Z Dilation of Coronary Artery, One Site with Drug-eluting Intraluminal Device, Open Approach
02700D6 Dilation of Coronary Artery, One Site, Bifurcation, with Intraluminal Device, Open Approach
02700DZ Dilation of Coronary Artery, One Site with Intraluminal Device, Open Approach
02700T6 Dilation of Coronary Artery, One Site, Bifurcation, with Radioactive Intraluminal Device, Open Approach
02700TZ Dilation of Coronary Artery, One Site with Radioactive Intraluminal Device, Open Approach
02700Z6 Dilation of Coronary Artery, One Site, Bifurcation, Open Approach
02700ZZ Dilation of Coronary Artery, One Site, Open Approach
0270346 Dilation of Coronary Artery, One Site, Bifurcation, with Drug-eluting Intraluminal Device, Percutaneous Approach
027034Z Dilation of Coronary Artery, One Site with Drug-eluting Intraluminal Device, Percutaneous Approach
AHA CC: 2Q, 2014, 4
02703D6 Dilation of Coronary Artery, One Site, Bifurcation, with Intraluminal Device, Percutaneous Approach
02703DZ Dilation of Coronary Artery, One Site with Intraluminal Device, Percutaneous Approach
02703T6 Dilation of Coronary Artery, One Site, Bifurcation, with Radioactive Intraluminal Device, Percutaneous Approach
02703TZ Dilation of Coronary Artery, One Site with Radioactive Intraluminal Device, Percutaneous Approach
02703Z6 Dilation of Coronary Artery, One Site, Bifurcation, Percutaneous Approach
02703ZZ Dilation of Coronary Artery, One Site, Percutaneous Approach
0270446 Dilation of Coronary Artery, One Site, Bifurcation, with Drug-eluting Intraluminal Device, Percutaneous Endoscopic Approach
027044Z Dilation of Coronary Artery, One Site with Drug-eluting Intraluminal Device, Percutaneous Endoscopic Approach
02704D6 Dilation of Coronary Artery, One Site, Bifurcation, with Intraluminal Device, Percutaneous Endoscopic Approach
02704DZ Dilation of Coronary Artery, One Site with Intraluminal Device, Percutaneous Endoscopic Approach
02704T6 Dilation of Coronary Artery, One Site, Bifurcation, with Radioactive Intraluminal Device, Percutaneous Endoscopic Approach
02704TZ Dilation of Coronary Artery, One Site with Radioactive Intraluminal Device, Percutaneous Endoscopic Approach
02704Z6 Dilation of Coronary Artery, One Site, Bifurcation, Percutaneous Endoscopic Approach
02704ZZ Dilation of Coronary Artery, One Site, Percutaneous Endoscopic Approach
0271046 Dilation of Coronary Artery, Two Sites, Bifurcation, with Drug-eluting Intraluminal Device, Open Approach
027104Z Dilation of Coronary Artery, Two Sites with Drug-eluting Intraluminal Device, Open Approach
02710D6 Dilation of Coronary Artery, Two Sites, Bifurcation, with Intraluminal Device, Open Approach
02710DZ Dilation of Coronary Artery, Two Sites with Intraluminal Device, Open Approach
02710T6 Dilation of Coronary Artery, Two Sites, Bifurcation, with Radioactive Intraluminal Device, Open Approach
02710TZ Dilation of Coronary Artery, Two Sites with Radioactive Intraluminal Device, Open Approach
02710Z6 Dilation of Coronary Artery, Two Sites, Bifurcation, Open Approach
02710ZZ Dilation of Coronary Artery, Two Sites, Open Approach
0271346 Dilation of Coronary Artery, Two Sites, Bifurcation, with Drug-eluting Intraluminal Device, Percutaneous Approach
027134Z Dilation of Coronary Artery, Two Sites with Drug-eluting Intraluminal Device, Percutaneous Approach
02713D6 Dilation of Coronary Artery, Two Sites, Bifurcation, with Intraluminal Device, Percutaneous Approach
02713DZ Dilation of Coronary Artery, Two Sites with Intraluminal Device, Percutaneous Approach
02713T6 Dilation of Coronary Artery, Two Sites, Bifurcation, with Radioactive Intraluminal Device, Percutaneous Approach
02713TZ Dilation of Coronary Artery, Two Sites with Radioactive Intraluminal Device, Percutaneous Approach
02713Z6 Dilation of Coronary Artery, Two Sites, Bifurcation, Percutaneous Approach
02713ZZ Dilation of Coronary Artery, Two Sites, Percutaneous Approach
0271446 Dilation of Coronary Artery, Two Sites, Bifurcation, with Drug-eluting Intraluminal Device, Percutaneous Endoscopic Approach
027144Z Dilation of Coronary Artery, Two Sites with Drug-eluting Intraluminal Device, Percutaneous Endoscopic Approach
02714D6 Dilation of Coronary Artery, Two Sites, Bifurcation, with Intraluminal Device, Percutaneous Endoscopic Approach
02714DZ Dilation of Coronary Artery, Two Sites with Intraluminal Device, Percutaneous Endoscopic Approach
02714T6 Dilation of Coronary Artery, Two Sites, Bifurcation, with Radioactive Intraluminal Device, Percutaneous Endoscopic Approach
02714TZ Dilation of Coronary Artery, Two Sites with Radioactive Intraluminal Device, Percutaneous Endoscopic Approach
02714Z6 Dilation of Coronary Artery, Two Sites, Bifurcation, Percutaneous Endoscopic Approach
02714ZZ Dilation of Coronary Artery, Two Sites, Percutaneous Endoscopic Approach
0272046 Dilation of Coronary Artery, Three Sites, Bifurcation, with Drug-eluting Intraluminal Device, Open Approach

027204Z Dilation of Coronary Artery, Three Sites with Drug-eluting Intraluminal Device, Open Approach

02720D6 Dilation of Coronary Artery, Three Sites, Bifurcation, with Intraluminal Device, Open Approach

02720DZ Dilation of Coronary Artery, Three Sites with Intraluminal Device, Open Approach

02720T6 Dilation of Coronary Artery, Three Sites, Bifurcation, with Radioactive Intraluminal Device, Open Approach

02720TZ Dilation of Coronary Artery, Three Sites with Radioactive Intraluminal Device, Open Approach

02720Z6 Dilation of Coronary Artery, Three Sites, Bifurcation, Open Approach

02720ZZ Dilation of Coronary Artery, Three Sites, Open Approach

0272346 Dilation of Coronary Artery, Three Sites, Bifurcation, with Drug-eluting Intraluminal Device, Percutaneous Approach

027234Z Dilation of Coronary Artery, Three Sites with Drug-eluting Intraluminal Device, Percutaneous Approach

02723D6 Dilation of Coronary Artery, Three Sites, Bifurcation, with Intraluminal Device, Percutaneous Approach

02723DZ Dilation of Coronary Artery, Three Sites with Intraluminal Device, Percutaneous Approach

02723T6 Dilation of Coronary Artery, Three Sites, Bifurcation, with Radioactive Intraluminal Device, Percutaneous Approach

02723TZ Dilation of Coronary Artery, Three Sites with Radioactive Intraluminal Device, Percutaneous Approach

02723Z6 Dilation of Coronary Artery, Three Sites, Bifurcation, Percutaneous Approach

02723ZZ Dilation of Coronary Artery, Three Sites, Percutaneous Approach

0272446 Dilation of Coronary Artery, Three Sites, Bifurcation, with Drug-eluting Intraluminal Device, Percutaneous Endoscopic Approach

027244Z Dilation of Coronary Artery, Three Sites with Drug-eluting Intraluminal Device, Percutaneous Endoscopic Approach

02724D6 Dilation of Coronary Artery, Three Sites, Bifurcation, with Intraluminal Device, Percutaneous Endoscopic Approach

02724DZ Dilation of Coronary Artery, Three Sites with Intraluminal Device, Percutaneous Endoscopic Approach

02724T6 Dilation of Coronary Artery, Three Sites, Bifurcation, with Radioactive Intraluminal Device, Percutaneous Endoscopic Approach

02724TZ Dilation of Coronary Artery, Three Sites with Radioactive Intraluminal Device, Percutaneous Endoscopic Approach

02724Z6 Dilation of Coronary Artery, Three Sites, Bifurcation, Percutaneous Endoscopic Approach

02724ZZ Dilation of Coronary Artery, Three Sites, Percutaneous Endoscopic Approach

0273046 Dilation of Coronary Artery, Four or More Sites, Bifurcation, with Drug-eluting Intraluminal Device, Open Approach

027304Z Dilation of Coronary Artery, Four or More Sites with Drug-eluting Intraluminal Device, Open Approach

02730D6 Dilation of Coronary Artery, Four or More Sites, Bifurcation, with Intraluminal Device, Open Approach

02730DZ Dilation of Coronary Artery, Four or More Sites with Intraluminal Device, Open Approach

02730T6 Dilation of Coronary Artery, Four or More Sites, Bifurcation, with Radioactive Intraluminal Device, Open Approach

02730TZ Dilation of Coronary Artery, Four or More Sites with Radioactive Intraluminal Device, Open Approach

02730Z6 Dilation of Coronary Artery, Four or More Sites, Bifurcation, Open Approach

02730ZZ Dilation of Coronary Artery, Four or More Sites, Open Approach

0273346 Dilation of Coronary Artery, Four or More Sites, Bifurcation, with Drug-eluting Intraluminal Device, Percutaneous Approach

027334Z Dilation of Coronary Artery, Four or More Sites with Drug-eluting Intraluminal Device, Percutaneous Approach

02733D6 Dilation of Coronary Artery, Four or More Sites, Bifurcation, with Intraluminal Device, Percutaneous Approach

02733DZ Dilation of Coronary Artery, Four or More Sites with Intraluminal Device, Percutaneous Approach

02733T6 Dilation of Coronary Artery, Four or More Sites, Bifurcation, with Radioactive Intraluminal Device, Percutaneous Approach

02733TZ Dilation of Coronary Artery, Four or More Sites with Radioactive Intraluminal Device, Percutaneous Approach

02733Z6 Dilation of Coronary Artery, Four or More Sites, Bifurcation, Percutaneous Approach

02733ZZ Dilation of Coronary Artery, Four or More Sites, Percutaneous Approach

0273446 Dilation of Coronary Artery, Four or More Sites, Bifurcation, with Drug-eluting Intraluminal Device, Percutaneous Endoscopic Approach

027344Z Dilation of Coronary Artery, Four or More Sites with Drug-eluting Intraluminal Device, Percutaneous Endoscopic Approach

02734D6 Dilation of Coronary Artery, Four or More Sites, Bifurcation, with Intraluminal Device, Percutaneous Endoscopic Approach

02734DZ Dilation of Coronary Artery, Four or More Sites with Intraluminal Device, Percutaneous Endoscopic Approach

02734T6 Dilation of Coronary Artery, Four or More Sites, Bifurcation, with Radioactive Intraluminal Device, Percutaneous Endoscopic Approach

02734TZ Dilation of Coronary Artery, Four or More Sites with Radioactive Intraluminal Device, Percutaneous Endoscopic Approach

02734Z6 Dilation of Coronary Artery, Four or More Sites, Bifurcation, Percutaneous Endoscopic Approach

02734ZZ Dilation of Coronary Artery, Four or More Sites, Percutaneous Endoscopic Approach

027F04Z Dilation of Aortic Valve with Drug-eluting Intraluminal Device, Open Approach

027F0DZ Dilation of Aortic Valve with Intraluminal Device, Open Approach

027F0ZZ Dilation of Aortic Valve, Open Approach

027F34Z Dilation of Aortic Valve with Drug-eluting Intraluminal Device, Percutaneous Approach

027F3DZ Dilation of Aortic Valve with Intraluminal Device, Percutaneous Approach

027F3ZZ Dilation of Aortic Valve, Percutaneous Approach

027F44Z Dilation of Aortic Valve with Drug-eluting Intraluminal Device, Percutaneous Endoscopic Approach

027F4DZ Dilation of Aortic Valve with Intraluminal Device, Percutaneous Endoscopic Approach

027F4ZZ Dilation of Aortic Valve, Percutaneous Endoscopic Approach

027G04Z Dilation of Mitral Valve with Drug-eluting Intraluminal Device, Open Approach

027G0DZ Dilation of Mitral Valve with Intraluminal Device, Open Approach

027G0ZZ Dilation of Mitral Valve, Open Approach

027G34Z Dilation of Mitral Valve with Drug-eluting Intraluminal Device, Percutaneous Approach

027G3DZ Dilation of Mitral Valve with Intraluminal Device, Percutaneous Approach

027G3ZZ Dilation of Mitral Valve, Percutaneous Approach

027G44Z Dilation of Mitral Valve with Drug-eluting Intraluminal Device, Percutaneous Endoscopic Approach

027G4DZ Dilation of Mitral Valve with Intraluminal Device, Percutaneous Endoscopic Approach

027G4ZZ Dilation of Mitral Valve, Percutaneous Endoscopic Approach

027H04Z Dilation of Pulmonary Valve with Drug-eluting Intraluminal Device, Open Approach

027H0DZ Dilation of Pulmonary Valve with Intraluminal Device, Open Approach

027H0ZZ Dilation of Pulmonary Valve, Open Approach

027H34Z Dilation of Pulmonary Valve with Drug-eluting Intraluminal Device, Percutaneous Approach

027H3DZ Dilation of Pulmonary Valve with Intraluminal Device, Percutaneous Approach

027H3ZZ Dilation of Pulmonary Valve, Percutaneous Approach

027H44Z Dilation of Pulmonary Valve with Drug-eluting Intraluminal Device, Percutaneous Endoscopic Approach

027H4DZ Dilation of Pulmonary Valve with Intraluminal Device, Percutaneous Endoscopic Approach

027H4ZZ Dilation of Pulmonary Valve, Percutaneous Endoscopic Approach

027J04Z Dilation of Tricuspid Valve with Drug-eluting Intraluminal Device, Open Approach

027J0DZ Dilation of Tricuspid Valve with Intraluminal Device, Open Approach

027J0ZZ Dilation of Tricuspid Valve, Open Approach

027J34Z Dilation of Tricuspid Valve with Drug-eluting Intraluminal Device, Percutaneous Approach

027J3DZ Dilation of Tricuspid Valve with Intraluminal Device, Percutaneous Approach

027J3ZZ Dilation of Tricuspid Valve, Percutaneous Approach

027J44Z Dilation of Tricuspid Valve with Drug-eluting Intraluminal Device, Percutaneous Endoscopic Approach

027J4DZ Dilation of Tricuspid Valve with Intraluminal Device, Percutaneous Endoscopic Approach

027J4ZZ Dilation of Tricuspid Valve, Percutaneous Endoscopic Approach

027K04Z Dilation of Right Ventricle with Drug-eluting Intraluminal Device, Open Approach

027K0DZ Dilation of Right Ventricle with Intraluminal Device, Open Approach

027K0ZZ Dilation of Right Ventricle, Open Approach

027K34Z Dilation of Right Ventricle with Drug-eluting Intraluminal Device, Percutaneous Approach
027K3DZ Dilation of Right Ventricle with Intraluminal Device, Percutaneous Approach
027K3ZZ Dilation of Right Ventricle, Percutaneous Approach
027K44Z Dilation of Right Ventricle with Drug-eluting Intraluminal Device, Percutaneous Endoscopic Approach
027K4DZ Dilation of Right Ventricle with Intraluminal Device, Percutaneous Endoscopic Approach
027K4ZZ Dilation of Right Ventricle, Percutaneous Endoscopic Approach
027P04Z Dilation of Pulmonary Trunk with Drug-eluting Intraluminal Device, Open Approach
027P0DZ Dilation of Pulmonary Trunk with Intraluminal Device, Open Approach
027P0ZZ Dilation of Pulmonary Trunk, Open Approach
027P34Z Dilation of Pulmonary Trunk with Drug-eluting Intraluminal Device, Percutaneous Approach
027P3DZ Dilation of Pulmonary Trunk with Intraluminal Device, Percutaneous Approach
027P3ZZ Dilation of Pulmonary Trunk, Percutaneous Approach
027P44Z Dilation of Pulmonary Trunk with Drug-eluting Intraluminal Device, Percutaneous Endoscopic Approach
027P4DZ Dilation of Pulmonary Trunk with Intraluminal Device, Percutaneous Endoscopic Approach
027P4ZZ Dilation of Pulmonary Trunk, Percutaneous Endoscopic Approach
027Q04Z Dilation of Right Pulmonary Artery with Drug-eluting Intraluminal Device, Open Approach
027Q0DZ Dilation of Right Pulmonary Artery with Intraluminal Device, Open Approach
027Q0ZZ Dilation of Right Pulmonary Artery, Open Approach
027Q34Z Dilation of Right Pulmonary Artery with Drug-eluting Intraluminal Device, Percutaneous Approach
027Q3DZ Dilation of Right Pulmonary Artery with Intraluminal Device, Percutaneous Approach
027Q3ZZ Dilation of Right Pulmonary Artery, Percutaneous Approach
027Q44Z Dilation of Right Pulmonary Artery with Drug-eluting Intraluminal Device, Percutaneous Endoscopic Approach
027Q4DZ Dilation of Right Pulmonary Artery with Intraluminal Device, Percutaneous Endoscopic Approach
027Q4ZZ Dilation of Right Pulmonary Artery, Percutaneous Endoscopic Approach
027R04T Dilation of Ductus Arteriosus with Drug-eluting Intraluminal Device, Open Approach
027R04Z Dilation of Left Pulmonary Artery with Drug-eluting Intraluminal Device, Open Approach
027R0DT Dilation of Ductus Arteriosus with Intraluminal Device, Open Approach
027R0DZ Dilation of Left Pulmonary Artery with Intraluminal Device, Open Approach
027R0ZT Dilation of Ductus Arteriosus, Open Approach
027R0ZZ Dilation of Left Pulmonary Artery, Open Approach
027R34T Dilation of Ductus Arteriosus with Drug-eluting Intraluminal Device, Percutaneous Approach
027R34Z Dilation of Left Pulmonary Artery with Drug-eluting Intraluminal Device, Percutaneous Approach
027R3DT Dilation of Ductus Arteriosus with Intraluminal Device, Percutaneous Approach
027R3DZ Dilation of Left Pulmonary Artery with Intraluminal Device, Percutaneous Approach
027R3ZT Dilation of Ductus Arteriosus, Percutaneous Approach
027R3ZZ Dilation of Left Pulmonary Artery, Percutaneous Approach
027R44T Dilation of Ductus Arteriosus with Drug-eluting Intraluminal Device, Percutaneous Endoscopic Approach
027R44Z Dilation of Left Pulmonary Artery with Drug-eluting Intraluminal Device, Percutaneous Endoscopic Approach
027R4DT Dilation of Ductus Arteriosus with Intraluminal Device, Percutaneous Endoscopic Approach
027R4DZ Dilation of Left Pulmonary Artery with Intraluminal Device, Percutaneous Endoscopic Approach
027R4ZT Dilation of Ductus Arteriosus, Percutaneous Endoscopic Approach
027R4ZZ Dilation of Left Pulmonary Artery, Percutaneous Endoscopic Approach
027S04Z Dilation of Right Pulmonary Vein with Drug-eluting Intraluminal Device, Open Approach
027S0DZ Dilation of Right Pulmonary Vein with Intraluminal Device, Open Approach
027S0ZZ Dilation of Right Pulmonary Vein, Open Approach
027S34Z Dilation of Right Pulmonary Vein with Drug-eluting Intraluminal Device, Percutaneous Approach
027S3DZ Dilation of Right Pulmonary Vein with Intraluminal Device, Percutaneous Approach
027S3ZZ Dilation of Right Pulmonary Vein, Percutaneous Approach
027S44Z Dilation of Right Pulmonary Vein with Drug-eluting Intraluminal Device, Percutaneous Endoscopic Approach
027S4DZ Dilation of Right Pulmonary Vein with Intraluminal Device, Percutaneous Endoscopic Approach
027S4ZZ Dilation of Right Pulmonary Vein, Percutaneous Endoscopic Approach
027T04Z Dilation of Left Pulmonary Vein with Drug-eluting Intraluminal Device, Open Approach
027T0DZ Dilation of Left Pulmonary Vein with Intraluminal Device, Open Approach
027T0ZZ Dilation of Left Pulmonary Vein, Open Approach
027T34Z Dilation of Left Pulmonary Vein with Drug-eluting Intraluminal Device, Percutaneous Approach
027T3DZ Dilation of Left Pulmonary Vein with Intraluminal Device, Percutaneous Approach
027T3ZZ Dilation of Left Pulmonary Vein, Percutaneous Approach
027T44Z Dilation of Left Pulmonary Vein with Drug-eluting Intraluminal Device, Percutaneous Endoscopic Approach
027T4DZ Dilation of Left Pulmonary Vein with Intraluminal Device, Percutaneous Endoscopic Approach
027T4ZZ Dilation of Left Pulmonary Vein, Percutaneous Endoscopic Approach
027V04Z Dilation of Superior Vena Cava with Drug-eluting Intraluminal Device, Open Approach
027V0DZ Dilation of Superior Vena Cava with Intraluminal Device, Open Approach
027V0ZZ Dilation of Superior Vena Cava, Open Approach
027V34Z Dilation of Superior Vena Cava with Drug-eluting Intraluminal Device, Percutaneous Approach
027V3DZ Dilation of Superior Vena Cava with Intraluminal Device, Percutaneous Approach
027V3ZZ Dilation of Superior Vena Cava, Percutaneous Approach
027V44Z Dilation of Superior Vena Cava with Drug-eluting Intraluminal Device, Percutaneous Endoscopic Approach
027V4DZ Dilation of Superior Vena Cava with Intraluminal Device, Percutaneous Endoscopic Approach
027V4ZZ Dilation of Superior Vena Cava, Percutaneous Endoscopic Approach
027W04Z Dilation of Thoracic Aorta with Drug-eluting Intraluminal Device, Open Approach
027W0DZ Dilation of Thoracic Aorta with Intraluminal Device, Open Approach
027W0ZZ Dilation of Thoracic Aorta, Open Approach
027W34Z Dilation of Thoracic Aorta with Drug-eluting Intraluminal Device, Percutaneous Approach
027W3DZ Dilation of Thoracic Aorta with Intraluminal Device, Percutaneous Approach
027W3ZZ Dilation of Thoracic Aorta, Percutaneous Approach
027W44Z Dilation of Thoracic Aorta with Drug-eluting Intraluminal Device, Percutaneous Endoscopic Approach
027W4DZ Dilation of Thoracic Aorta with Intraluminal Device, Percutaneous Endoscopic Approach
027W4ZZ Dilation of Thoracic Aorta, Percutaneous Endoscopic Approach

028 – Heart and Great Vessels, Division

Review Coding Guideline B3.14

02880ZZ Division of Conduction Mechanism, Open Approach
02883ZZ Division of Conduction Mechanism, Percutaneous Approach
02884ZZ Division of Conduction Mechanism, Percutaneous Endoscopic Approach
02890ZZ Division of Chordae Tendineae, Open Approach
02893ZZ Division of Chordae Tendineae, Percutaneous Approach
02894ZZ Division of Chordae Tendineae, Percutaneous Endoscopic Approach
028D0ZZ Division of Papillary Muscle, Open Approach
028D3ZZ Division of Papillary Muscle, Percutaneous Approach
028D4ZZ Division of Papillary Muscle, Percutaneous Endoscopic Approach

02B – Heart and Great Vessels, Excision

Review Coding Guidelines B3.4a and B3.4b

Review Coding Guideline B3.8

02B40ZX Excision of Coronary Vein, Open Approach, Diagnostic
02B40ZZ Excision of Coronary Vein, Open Approach
02B43ZX Excision of Coronary Vein, Percutaneous Approach, Diagnostic
02B43ZZ Excision of Coronary Vein, Percutaneous Approach
02B44ZX Excision of Coronary Vein, Percutaneous Endoscopic Approach, Diagnostic
02B44ZZ Excision of Coronary Vein, Percutaneous Endoscopic Approach
02B50ZX Excision of Atrial Septum, Open Approach, Diagnostic
02B50ZZ Excision of Atrial Septum, Open Approach
02B53ZX Excision of Atrial Septum, Percutaneous Approach, Diagnostic
02B53ZZ Excision of Atrial Septum, Percutaneous Approach
02B54ZX Excision of Atrial Septum, Percutaneous Endoscopic Approach, Diagnostic
02B54ZZ Excision of Atrial Septum, Percutaneous Endoscopic Approach
02B60ZX Excision of Right Atrium, Open Approach, Diagnostic
02B60ZZ Excision of Right Atrium, Open Approach
02B63ZX Excision of Right Atrium, Percutaneous Approach, Diagnostic
02B63ZZ Excision of Right Atrium, Percutaneous Approach
02B64ZX Excision of Right Atrium, Percutaneous Endoscopic Approach, Diagnostic
02B64ZZ Excision of Right Atrium, Percutaneous Endoscopic Approach
●**02B70ZK** Excision of Left Atrial Appendage, Open Approach
02B70ZX Excision of Left Atrium, Open Approach, Diagnostic
02B70ZZ Excision of Left Atrium, Open Approach
●**02B73ZK** Excision of Left Atrial Appendage, Percutaneous Approach
02B73ZX Excision of Left Atrium, Percutaneous Approach, Diagnostic
02B73ZZ Excision of Left Atrium, Percutaneous Approach
●**02B74ZK** Excision of Left Atrial Appendage, Percutaneous Endoscopic Approach
02B74ZX Excision of Left Atrium, Percutaneous Endoscopic Approach, Diagnostic
02B74ZZ Excision of Left Atrium, Percutaneous Endoscopic Approach
02B80ZX Excision of Conduction Mechanism, Open Approach, Diagnostic
02B80ZZ Excision of Conduction Mechanism, Open Approach
02B83ZX Excision of Conduction Mechanism, Percutaneous Approach, Diagnostic
02B83ZZ Excision of Conduction Mechanism, Percutaneous Approach
02B84ZX Excision of Conduction Mechanism, Percutaneous Endoscopic Approach, Diagnostic
02B84ZZ Excision of Conduction Mechanism, Percutaneous Endoscopic Approach
02B90ZX Excision of Chordae Tendineae, Open Approach, Diagnostic
02B90ZZ Excision of Chordae Tendineae, Open Approach
02B93ZX Excision of Chordae Tendineae, Percutaneous Approach, Diagnostic
02B93ZZ Excision of Chordae Tendineae, Percutaneous Approach
02B94ZX Excision of Chordae Tendineae, Percutaneous Endoscopic Approach, Diagnostic
02B94ZZ Excision of Chordae Tendineae, Percutaneous Endoscopic Approach
02BD0ZX Excision of Papillary Muscle, Open Approach, Diagnostic
02BD0ZZ Excision of Papillary Muscle, Open Approach
02BD3ZX Excision of Papillary Muscle, Percutaneous Approach, Diagnostic
02BD3ZZ Excision of Papillary Muscle, Percutaneous Approach
02BD4ZX Excision of Papillary Muscle, Percutaneous Endoscopic Approach, Diagnostic
02BD4ZZ Excision of Papillary Muscle, Percutaneous Endoscopic Approach
02BF0ZX Excision of Aortic Valve, Open Approach, Diagnostic
02BF0ZZ Excision of Aortic Valve, Open Approach
02BF3ZX Excision of Aortic Valve, Percutaneous Approach, Diagnostic
02BF3ZZ Excision of Aortic Valve, Percutaneous Approach
02BF4ZX Excision of Aortic Valve, Percutaneous Endoscopic Approach, Diagnostic
02BF4ZZ Excision of Aortic Valve, Percutaneous Endoscopic Approach
02BG0ZX Excision of Mitral Valve, Open Approach, Diagnostic
02BG0ZZ Excision of Mitral Valve, Open Approach
02BG3ZX Excision of Mitral Valve, Percutaneous Approach, Diagnostic
02BG3ZZ Excision of Mitral Valve, Percutaneous Approach
02BG4ZX Excision of Mitral Valve, Percutaneous Endoscopic Approach, Diagnostic
02BG4ZZ Excision of Mitral Valve, Percutaneous Endoscopic Approach
02BH0ZX Excision of Pulmonary Valve, Open Approach, Diagnostic
02BH0ZZ Excision of Pulmonary Valve, Open Approach
02BH3ZX Excision of Pulmonary Valve, Percutaneous Approach, Diagnostic
02BH3ZZ Excision of Pulmonary Valve, Percutaneous Approach
02BH4ZX Excision of Pulmonary Valve, Percutaneous Endoscopic Approach, Diagnostic
02BH4ZZ Excision of Pulmonary Valve, Percutaneous Endoscopic Approach
02BJ0ZX Excision of Tricuspid Valve, Open Approach, Diagnostic
02BJ0ZZ Excision of Tricuspid Valve, Open Approach
02BJ3ZX Excision of Tricuspid Valve, Percutaneous Approach, Diagnostic
02BJ3ZZ Excision of Tricuspid Valve, Percutaneous Approach
02BJ4ZX Excision of Tricuspid Valve, Percutaneous Endoscopic Approach, Diagnostic
02BJ4ZZ Excision of Tricuspid Valve, Percutaneous Endoscopic Approach
02BK0ZX Excision of Right Ventricle, Open Approach, Diagnostic
▲ **02BK0ZZ** Excision of Right Ventricle, Open Approach
02BK3ZX Excision of Right Ventricle, Percutaneous Approach, Diagnostic
▲ **02BK3ZZ** Excision of Right Ventricle, Percutaneous Approach
02BK4ZX Excision of Right Ventricle, Percutaneous Endoscopic Approach, Diagnostic
▲ **02BK4ZZ** Excision of Right Ventricle, Percutaneous Endoscopic Approach
02BL0ZX Excision of Left Ventricle, Open Approach, Diagnostic
▲ **02BL0ZZ** Excision of Left Ventricle, Open Approach
02BL3ZX Excision of Left Ventricle, Percutaneous Approach, Diagnostic
▲ **02BL3ZZ** Excision of Left Ventricle, Percutaneous Approach
02BL4ZX Excision of Left Ventricle, Percutaneous Endoscopic Approach, Diagnostic
▲ **02BL4ZZ** Excision of Left Ventricle, Percutaneous Endoscopic Approach
02BM0ZX Excision of Ventricular Septum, Open Approach, Diagnostic
02BM0ZZ Excision of Ventricular Septum, Open Approach
02BM3ZX Excision of Ventricular Septum, Percutaneous Approach, Diagnostic
02BM3ZZ Excision of Ventricular Septum, Percutaneous Approach
02BM4ZX Excision of Ventricular Septum, Percutaneous Endoscopic Approach, Diagnostic
02BM4ZZ Excision of Ventricular Septum, Percutaneous Endoscopic Approach
02BN0ZX Excision of Pericardium, Open Approach, Diagnostic
02BN0ZZ Excision of Pericardium, Open Approach
02BN3ZX Excision of Pericardium, Percutaneous Approach, Diagnostic
02BN3ZZ Excision of Pericardium, Percutaneous Approach
02BN4ZX Excision of Pericardium, Percutaneous Endoscopic Approach, Diagnostic
02BN4ZZ Excision of Pericardium, Percutaneous Endoscopic Approach
02BP0ZX Excision of Pulmonary Trunk, Open Approach, Diagnostic
02BP0ZZ Excision of Pulmonary Trunk, Open Approach
02BP3ZX Excision of Pulmonary Trunk, Percutaneous Approach, Diagnostic
02BP3ZZ Excision of Pulmonary Trunk, Percutaneous Approach
02BP4ZX Excision of Pulmonary Trunk, Percutaneous Endoscopic Approach, Diagnostic
02BP4ZZ Excision of Pulmonary Trunk, Percutaneous Endoscopic Approach
02BQ0ZX Excision of Right Pulmonary Artery, Open Approach, Diagnostic
02BQ0ZZ Excision of Right Pulmonary Artery, Open Approach
02BQ3ZX Excision of Right Pulmonary Artery, Percutaneous Approach, Diagnostic
02BQ3ZZ Excision of Right Pulmonary Artery, Percutaneous Approach
02BQ4ZX Excision of Right Pulmonary Artery, Percutaneous Endoscopic Approach, Diagnostic
02BQ4ZZ Excision of Right Pulmonary Artery, Percutaneous Endoscopic Approach
02BR0ZX Excision of Left Pulmonary Artery, Open Approach, Diagnostic
02BR0ZZ Excision of Left Pulmonary Artery, Open Approach

02BR3ZX Excision of Left Pulmonary Artery, Percutaneous Approach, Diagnostic
02BR3ZZ Excision of Left Pulmonary Artery, Percutaneous Approach
02BR4ZX Excision of Left Pulmonary Artery, Percutaneous Endoscopic Approach, Diagnostic
02BR4ZZ Excision of Left Pulmonary Artery, Percutaneous Endoscopic Approach
02BS0ZX Excision of Right Pulmonary Vein, Open Approach, Diagnostic
02BS0ZZ Excision of Right Pulmonary Vein, Open Approach
02BS3ZX Excision of Right Pulmonary Vein, Percutaneous Approach, Diagnostic
02BS3ZZ Excision of Right Pulmonary Vein, Percutaneous Approach
02BS4ZX Excision of Right Pulmonary Vein, Percutaneous Endoscopic Approach, Diagnostic
02BS4ZZ Excision of Right Pulmonary Vein, Percutaneous Endoscopic Approach
02BT0ZX Excision of Left Pulmonary Vein, Open Approach, Diagnostic
02BT0ZZ Excision of Left Pulmonary Vein, Open Approach
02BT3ZX Excision of Left Pulmonary Vein, Percutaneous Approach, Diagnostic
02BT3ZZ Excision of Left Pulmonary Vein, Percutaneous Approach
02BT4ZX Excision of Left Pulmonary Vein, Percutaneous Endoscopic Approach, Diagnostic
02BT4ZZ Excision of Left Pulmonary Vein, Percutaneous Endoscopic Approach
02BV0ZX Excision of Superior Vena Cava, Open Approach, Diagnostic
02BV0ZZ Excision of Superior Vena Cava, Open Approach
02BV3ZX Excision of Superior Vena Cava, Percutaneous Approach, Diagnostic
02BV3ZZ Excision of Superior Vena Cava, Percutaneous Approach
02BV4ZX Excision of Superior Vena Cava, Percutaneous Endoscopic Approach, Diagnostic
02BV4ZZ Excision of Superior Vena Cava, Percutaneous Endoscopic Approach
02BW0ZX Excision of Thoracic Aorta, Open Approach, Diagnostic
02BW0ZZ Excision of Thoracic Aorta, Open Approach
02BW3ZX Excision of Thoracic Aorta, Percutaneous Approach, Diagnostic
02BW3ZZ Excision of Thoracic Aorta, Percutaneous Approach
02BW4ZX Excision of Thoracic Aorta, Percutaneous Endoscopic Approach, Diagnostic
02BW4ZZ Excision of Thoracic Aorta, Percutaneous Endoscopic Approach

02C – Heart and Great Vessels, Extirpation

For Extirpation procedures involving coronary arteries, Review Coding Guideline B4.4

02C00ZZ Extirpation of Matter from Coronary Artery, One Site, Open Approach
02C03ZZ Extirpation of Matter from Coronary Artery, One Site, Percutaneous Approach
02C04ZZ Extirpation of Matter from Coronary Artery, One Site, Percutaneous Endoscopic Approach
02C10ZZ Extirpation of Matter from Coronary Artery, Two Sites, Open Approach
02C13ZZ Extirpation of Matter from Coronary Artery, Two Sites, Percutaneous Approach
02C14ZZ Extirpation of Matter from Coronary Artery, Two Sites, Percutaneous Endoscopic Approach
02C20ZZ Extirpation of Matter from Coronary Artery, Three Sites, Open Approach
02C23ZZ Extirpation of Matter from Coronary Artery, Three Sites, Percutaneous Approach
02C24ZZ Extirpation of Matter from Coronary Artery, Three Sites, Percutaneous Endoscopic Approach
02C30ZZ Extirpation of Matter from Coronary Artery, Four or More Sites, Open Approach
02C33ZZ Extirpation of Matter from Coronary Artery, Four or More Sites, Percutaneous Approach
02C34ZZ Extirpation of Matter from Coronary Artery, Four or More Sites, Percutaneous Endoscopic Approach
02C40ZZ Extirpation of Matter from Coronary Vein, Open Approach
02C43ZZ Extirpation of Matter from Coronary Vein, Percutaneous Approach
02C44ZZ Extirpation of Matter from Coronary Vein, Percutaneous Endoscopic Approach
02C50ZZ Extirpation of Matter from Atrial Septum, Open Approach
02C53ZZ Extirpation of Matter from Atrial Septum, Percutaneous Approach
02C54ZZ Extirpation of Matter from Atrial Septum, Percutaneous Endoscopic Approach
02C60ZZ Extirpation of Matter from Right Atrium, Open Approach
02C63ZZ Extirpation of Matter from Right Atrium, Percutaneous Approach
02C64ZZ Extirpation of Matter from Right Atrium, Percutaneous Endoscopic Approach
02C70ZZ Extirpation of Matter from Left Atrium, Open Approach
02C73ZZ Extirpation of Matter from Left Atrium, Percutaneous Approach
02C74ZZ Extirpation of Matter from Left Atrium, Percutaneous Endoscopic Approach
02C80ZZ Extirpation of Matter from Conduction Mechanism, Open Approach
02C83ZZ Extirpation of Matter from Conduction Mechanism, Percutaneous Approach
02C84ZZ Extirpation of Matter from Conduction Mechanism, Percutaneous Endoscopic Approach
02C90ZZ Extirpation of Matter from Chordae Tendineae, Open Approach
02C93ZZ Extirpation of Matter from Chordae Tendineae, Percutaneous Approach
02C94ZZ Extirpation of Matter from Chordae Tendineae, Percutaneous Endoscopic Approach
02CD0ZZ Extirpation of Matter from Papillary Muscle, Open Approach
02CD3ZZ Extirpation of Matter from Papillary Muscle, Percutaneous Approach
02CD4ZZ Extirpation of Matter from Papillary Muscle, Percutaneous Endoscopic Approach
02CF0ZZ Extirpation of Matter from Aortic Valve, Open Approach
02CF3ZZ Extirpation of Matter from Aortic Valve, Percutaneous Approach
02CF4ZZ Extirpation of Matter from Aortic Valve, Percutaneous Endoscopic Approach
02CG0ZZ Extirpation of Matter from Mitral Valve, Open Approach
02CG3ZZ Extirpation of Matter from Mitral Valve, Percutaneous Approach
02CG4ZZ Extirpation of Matter from Mitral Valve, Percutaneous Endoscopic Approach
02CH0ZZ Extirpation of Matter from Pulmonary Valve, Open Approach
02CH3ZZ Extirpation of Matter from Pulmonary Valve, Percutaneous Approach
02CH4ZZ Extirpation of Matter from Pulmonary Valve, Percutaneous Endoscopic Approach
02CJ0ZZ Extirpation of Matter from Tricuspid Valve, Open Approach
02CJ3ZZ Extirpation of Matter from Tricuspid Valve, Percutaneous Approach
02CJ4ZZ Extirpation of Matter from Tricuspid Valve, Percutaneous Endoscopic Approach
02CK0ZZ Extirpation of Matter from Right Ventricle, Open Approach
02CK3ZZ Extirpation of Matter from Right Ventricle, Percutaneous Approach
02CK4ZZ Extirpation of Matter from Right Ventricle, Percutaneous Endoscopic Approach
02CL0ZZ Extirpation of Matter from Left Ventricle, Open Approach
02CL3ZZ Extirpation of Matter from Left Ventricle, Percutaneous Approach
02CL4ZZ Extirpation of Matter from Left Ventricle, Percutaneous Endoscopic Approach
02CM0ZZ Extirpation of Matter from Ventricular Septum, Open Approach
02CM3ZZ Extirpation of Matter from Ventricular Septum, Percutaneous Approach
02CM4ZZ Extirpation of Matter from Ventricular Septum, Percutaneous Endoscopic Approach
02CN0ZZ Extirpation of Matter from Pericardium, Open Approach
02CN3ZZ Extirpation of Matter from Pericardium, Percutaneous Approach
02CN4ZZ Extirpation of Matter from Pericardium, Percutaneous Endoscopic Approach
02CP0ZZ Extirpation of Matter from Pulmonary Trunk, Open Approach
02CP3ZZ Extirpation of Matter from Pulmonary Trunk, Percutaneous Approach
02CP4ZZ Extirpation of Matter from Pulmonary Trunk, Percutaneous Endoscopic Approach
02CQ0ZZ Extirpation of Matter from Right Pulmonary Artery, Open Approach
02CQ3ZZ Extirpation of Matter from Right Pulmonary Artery, Percutaneous Approach
02CQ4ZZ Extirpation of Matter from Right Pulmonary Artery, Percutaneous Endoscopic Approach
02CR0ZZ Extirpation of Matter from Left Pulmonary Artery, Open Approach
02CR3ZZ Extirpation of Matter from Left Pulmonary Artery, Percutaneous Approach
02CR4ZZ Extirpation of Matter from Left Pulmonary Artery, Percutaneous Endoscopic Approach
02CS0ZZ Extirpation of Matter from Right Pulmonary Vein, Open Approach
02CS3ZZ Extirpation of Matter from Right Pulmonary Vein, Percutaneous Approach
02CS4ZZ Extirpation of Matter from Right Pulmonary Vein, Percutaneous Endoscopic Approach
02CT0ZZ Extirpation of Matter from Left Pulmonary Vein, Open Approach
02CT3ZZ Extirpation of Matter from Left Pulmonary Vein, Percutaneous Approach
02CT4ZZ Extirpation of Matter from Left Pulmonary Vein, Percutaneous Endoscopic Approach

02CV0ZZ Extirpation of Matter from Superior Vena Cava, Open Approach

02CV3ZZ Extirpation of Matter from Superior Vena Cava, Percutaneous Approach

02CV4ZZ Extirpation of Matter from Superior Vena Cava, Percutaneous Endoscopic Approach

02CW0ZZ Extirpation of Matter from Thoracic Aorta, Open Approach

02CW3ZZ Extirpation of Matter from Thoracic Aorta, Percutaneous Approach

02CW4ZZ Extirpation of Matter from Thoracic Aorta, Percutaneous Endoscopic Approach

02F – Heart and Great Vessels, Fragmentation

02FN0ZZ Fragmentation in Pericardium, Open Approach

02FN3ZZ Fragmentation in Pericardium, Percutaneous Approach

02FN4ZZ Fragmentation in Pericardium, Percutaneous Endoscopic Approach

▲ 02FNXZZ Fragmentation in Pericardium, External Approach

02H – Heart and Great Vessels, Insertion

02H400Z Insertion of Pressure Sensor Monitoring Device into Coronary Vein, Open Approach

02H402Z Insertion of Monitoring Device into Coronary Vein, Open Approach

02H403Z Insertion of Infusion Device into Coronary Vein, Open Approach

02H40DZ Insertion of Intraluminal Device into Coronary Vein, Open Approach

●02H40JZ Insertion of Pacemaker Lead into Coronary Vein, Open Approach

+ Lead device when reported with an Insertion of a pacemaker device or cardiac rhythm related device (6th character 4, 5, 6 or P) into the chest or abdomen subcutaneous tissue and fascia. *See table 0JH to construct the Insertion code.* When a device is replaced, also report the Removal of a cardiac rhythm related device (6th character P) from the trunk subcutaneous tissue and fascia. *See table 0JP to construct the Removal code.*

02H40KZ Insertion of Defibrillator Lead into Coronary Vein, Open Approach

●02H40MZ Insertion of Cardiac Lead into Coronary Vein, Open Approach

+ Lead device when reported with an Insertion of a pacemaker device or cardiac rhythm related device (6th character 4, 5, 6 or P) into the chest or abdomen subcutaneous tissue and fascia. *See table 0JH to construct the Insertion code.* When a device is replaced, also report the Removal of a cardiac rhythm related device (6th character P) from the trunk subcutaneous tissue and fascia. *See table 0JP to construct the Removal code.*

02H430Z Insertion of Pressure Sensor Monitoring Device into Coronary Vein, Percutaneous Approach

02H432Z Insertion of Monitoring Device into Coronary Vein, Percutaneous Approach

02H433Z Insertion of Infusion Device into Coronary Vein, Percutaneous Approach

02H43DZ Insertion of Intraluminal Device into Coronary Vein, Percutaneous Approach

02H43JZ Insertion of Pacemaker Lead into Coronary Vein, Percutaneous Approach

HAC With a secondary diagnosis code of K68.11, T81.4XXA, T82.6XXA, T82.7XXA

02H43KZ Insertion of Defibrillator Lead into Coronary Vein, Percutaneous Approach

HAC With a secondary diagnosis code of K68.11, T81.4XXA, T82.6XXA, T82.7XXA

02H43MZ Insertion of Cardiac Lead into Coronary Vein, Percutaneous Approach

HAC With a secondary diagnosis code of K68.11, T81.4XXA, T82.6XXA, T82.7XXA

02H440Z Insertion of Pressure Sensor Monitoring Device into Coronary Vein, Percutaneous Endoscopic Approach

02H442Z Insertion of Monitoring Device into Coronary Vein, Percutaneous Endoscopic Approach

02H443Z Insertion of Infusion Device into Coronary Vein, Percutaneous Endoscopic Approach

02H44DZ Insertion of Intraluminal Device into Coronary Vein, Percutaneous Endoscopic Approach

● 02H44JZ Insertion of Pacemaker Lead into Coronary Vein, Percutaneous Endoscopic Approach

+ Lead device when reported with an Insertion of a pacemaker device or cardiac rhythm related device (6th character 4, 5, 6 or P) into the chest or abdomen subcutaneous tissue and fascia. *See table 0JH to construct the Insertion code.* When a device is replaced, also report the Removal of a cardiac rhythm related device (6th character P) from the trunk subcutaneous tissue and fascia. *See table 0JP to construct the Removal code.*

02H44KZ Insertion of Defibrillator Lead into Coronary Vein, Percutaneous Endoscopic Approach

● 02H44MZ Insertion of Cardiac Lead into Coronary Vein, Percutaneous Endoscopic Approach

+ Lead device when reported with an Insertion of a pacemaker device or cardiac rhythm related device (6th character 4, 5, 6 or P) into the chest or abdomen subcutaneous tissue and fascia. *See table 0JH to construct the Insertion code.* When a device is replaced, also report the Removal of a cardiac rhythm related device (6th character P) from the trunk subcutaneous tissue and fascia. *See table 0JP to construct the Removal code.*

02H600Z Insertion of Pressure Sensor Monitoring Device into Right Atrium, Open Approach

02H602Z Insertion of Monitoring Device into Right Atrium, Open Approach

02H603Z Insertion of Infusion Device into Right Atrium, Open Approach

02H60DZ Insertion of Intraluminal Device into Right Atrium, Open Approach

● 02H60JZ Insertion of Pacemaker Lead into Right Atrium, Open Approach

+ Lead device when reported with an Insertion of a pacemaker device or cardiac rhythm related device (6th character 4, 5, 6 or P) into the chest or abdomen subcutaneous tissue and fascia. *See table 0JH to construct the Insertion code.* When a device is replaced, also report the Removal of a cardiac rhythm related device (6th character P) from the trunk subcutaneous tissue and fascia. *See table 0JP to construct the Removal code.*

02H60KZ Insertion of Defibrillator Lead into Right Atrium, Open Approach

+ Lead device when reported with an Insertion of a defibrillator generator (6th character 8) into the chest or abdomen subcutaneous tissue and fascia. *See table 0JH to construct the Insertion code.*

● 02H60MZ Insertion of Cardiac Lead into Right Atrium, Open Approach

+ Lead device when reported with an Insertion of a pacemaker device or cardiac rhythm related device (6th character 4, 5, 6 or P) into the chest or abdomen subcutaneous tissue and fascia. *See table 0JH to construct the Insertion code.* When a device is replaced, also report the Removal of a cardiac rhythm related device (6th character P) from the trunk subcutaneous tissue and fascia. *See table 0JP to construct the Removal code.*

02H630Z Insertion of Pressure Sensor Monitoring Device into Right Atrium, Percutaneous Approach

02H632Z Insertion of Monitoring Device into Right Atrium, Percutaneous Approach

● 02H633Z Insertion of Infusion Device into Right Atrium, Percutaneous Approach

02H63DZ Insertion of Intraluminal Device into Right Atrium, Percutaneous Approach

● 02H63JZ Insertion of Pacemaker Lead into Right Atrium, Percutaneous Approach

HAC With a secondary diagnosis code of K68.11, T81.4XXA, T82.6XXA, T82.7XXA

+ Lead device when reported with an Insertion of a pacemaker device or cardiac rhythm related device (6th character 4, 5, 6 or P) into the chest or abdomen subcutaneous tissue and fascia. *See table 0JH to construct the Insertion code.* When a device is replaced, also report the removal of a cardiac rhythm related device (6th character P) from the trunk subcutaneous tissue and fascia. *See table 0JP to construct the Removal code.* When a cardiac lead is replaced, also report the removal of cardiac lead (6th character M) from the heart. *See table 02P to construct the Removal code.*

02H63KZ Insertion of Defibrillator Lead into Right Atrium, Percutaneous Approach

+ Lead device when reported with an Insertion of a defibrillator generator (6th character 8) into the chest or abdomen subcutaneous tissue and fascia. *See table 0JH to construct the Insertion code.*

02H63MZ Insertion of Cardiac Lead into Right Atrium, Percutaneous Approach

+ Lead device when reported with an Insertion of a pacemaker device or cardiac rhythm related device (6th character 4, 5, 6 or P) into the chest or abdomen subcutaneous tissue and fascia. *See table 0JH to construct the Insertion code.* When a device is replaced, also report the Removal of a cardiac rhythm related device (6th character P) from the trunk subcutaneous tissue and fascia. *See table 0JP to construct the Removal code.*

HAC With a secondary diagnosis code of K68.11, T81.4XXA, T82.6XXA, T82.7XXA

02H640Z Insertion of Pressure Sensor Monitoring Device into Right Atrium, Percutaneous Endoscopic Approach

02H642Z Insertion of Monitoring Device into Right Atrium, Percutaneous Endoscopic Approach

02H643Z Insertion of Infusion Device into Right Atrium, Percutaneous Endoscopic Approach

02H64DZ Insertion of Intraluminal Device into Right Atrium, Percutaneous Endoscopic Approach

● **02H64JZ** Insertion of Pacemaker Lead into Right Atrium, Percutaneous Endoscopic Approach

+ Lead device when reported with an Insertion of a pacemaker device or cardiac rhythm related device (6th character 4, 5, 6 or P) into the chest or abdomen subcutaneous tissue and fascia. *See table 0JH to construct the Insertion code*. When a device is replaced, also report the Removal of a cardiac rhythm related device (6th character P) from the trunk subcutaneous tissue and fascia. *See table 0JP to construct the Removal code*.

02H64KZ Insertion of Defibrillator Lead into Right Atrium, Percutaneous Endoscopic Approach

+ Lead device when reported with an Insertion of a defibrillator generator (6th character 8) into the chest or abdomen subcutaneous tissue and fascia. *See table 0JH to construct the Insertion code*.

● **02H64MZ** Insertion of Cardiac Lead into Right Atrium, Percutaneous Endoscopic Approach

+ Lead device when reported with an Insertion of a pacemaker device or cardiac rhythm related device (6th character 4, 5, 6 or P) into the chest or abdomen subcutaneous tissue and fascia. *See table 0JH to construct the Insertion code*. When a device is replaced, also report the Removal of a cardiac rhythm related device (6th character P) from the trunk subcutaneous tissue and fascia. *See table 0JP to construct the Removal code*.

02H700Z Insertion of Pressure Sensor Monitoring Device into Left Atrium, Open Approach

02H702Z Insertion of Monitoring Device into Left Atrium, Open Approach

02H703Z Insertion of Infusion Device into Left Atrium, Open Approach

02H70DZ Insertion of Intraluminal Device into Left Atrium, Open Approach

● **02H70JZ** Insertion of Pacemaker Lead into Left Atrium, Open Approach

+ Lead device when reported with an Insertion of a pacemaker device or cardiac rhythm related device (6th character 4, 5, 6 or P) into the chest or abdomen subcutaneous tissue and fascia. *See table 0JH to construct the Insertion code*. When a device is replaced, also report the Removal of a cardiac rhythm related device (6th character P) from the trunk subcutaneous tissue and fascia. *See table 0JP to construct the Removal code*.

02H70KZ Insertion of Defibrillator Lead into Left Atrium, Open Approach

+ Lead device when reported with an Insertion of a defibrillator generator (6th character 8) into the chest or abdomen subcutaneous tissue and fascia. *See table 0JH to construct the Insertion code*.

● **02H70MZ** Insertion of Cardiac Lead into Left Atrium, Open Approach

+ Lead device when reported with an Insertion of a pacemaker device or cardiac rhythm related device (6th character 4, 5, 6 or P) into the chest or abdomen subcutaneous tissue and fascia. *See table 0JH to construct the Insertion code*. When a device is replaced, also report the Removal of a cardiac rhythm related device (6th character P) from the trunk subcutaneous tissue and fascia. *See table 0JP to construct the Removal code*.

02H730Z Insertion of Pressure Sensor Monitoring Device into Left Atrium, Percutaneous Approach

02H732Z Insertion of Monitoring Device into Left Atrium, Percutaneous Approach

02H733Z Insertion of Infusion Device into Left Atrium, Percutaneous Approach

02H73DZ Insertion of Intraluminal Device into Left Atrium, Percutaneous Approach

● **02H73JZ** Insertion of Pacemaker Lead into Left Atrium, Percutaneous Approach

HAC With a secondary diagnosis code of K68.11, T81.4XXA, T82.6XXA, T82.7XXA

+ Lead device when reported with an Insertion of a pacemaker device or cardiac rhythm related device (6th character 4, 5, 6 or P) into the chest or abdomen subcutaneous tissue and fascia. *See table 0JH to construct the Insertion code*. When a device is replaced, also report the removal of a cardiac rhythm related device (6th character P) from the trunk subcutaneous tissue and fascia. *See table 0JP to construct the Removal code*. When a cardiac lead is replaced, also report the removal of cardiac lead (6th character M) from the heart. *See table 02P to construct the Removal code*.

02H73KZ Insertion of Defibrillator Lead into Left Atrium, Percutaneous Approach

+ Lead device when reported with an Insertion of a defibrillator generator (6th character 8) into the chest or abdomen subcutaneous tissue and fascia. *See table 0JH to construct the Insertion code*.

02H73MZ Insertion of Cardiac Lead into Left Atrium, Percutaneous Approach

HAC With a secondary diagnosis code of K68.11, T81.4XXA, T82.6XXA, T82.7XXA

+ Lead device when reported with an Insertion of a pacemaker device or cardiac rhythm related device (6th character 4, 5, 6 or P) into the chest or abdomen subcutaneous tissue and fascia. *See table 0JH to construct the Insertion code*. When a device is replaced, also report the Removal of a cardiac rhythm related device (6th character P) from the trunk subcutaneous tissue and fascia. *See table 0JP to construct the Removal code*.

02H740Z Insertion of Pressure Sensor Monitoring Device into Left Atrium, Percutaneous Endoscopic Approach

02H742Z Insertion of Monitoring Device into Left Atrium, Percutaneous Endoscopic Approach

02H743Z Insertion of Infusion Device into Left Atrium, Percutaneous Endoscopic Approach

02H74DZ Insertion of Intraluminal Device into Left Atrium, Percutaneous Endoscopic Approach

● **02H74JZ** Insertion of Pacemaker Lead into Left Atrium, Percutaneous Endoscopic Approach

+ Lead device when reported with an Insertion of a pacemaker device or cardiac rhythm related device (6th character 4, 5, 6 or P) into the chest or abdomen subcutaneous tissue and fascia. *See table 0JH to construct the Insertion code*. When a device is replaced, also report the Removal of a cardiac rhythm related device (6th character P) from the trunk subcutaneous tissue and fascia. *See table 0JP to construct the Removal code*.

02H74KZ Insertion of Defibrillator Lead into Left Atrium, Percutaneous Endoscopic Approach

+ Lead device when reported with an Insertion of a defibrillator generator (6th character 8) into the chest or abdomen subcutaneous tissue and fascia. *See table 0JH to construct the Insertion code*.

● **02H74MZ** Insertion of Cardiac Lead into Left Atrium, Percutaneous Endoscopic Approach

+ Lead device when reported with an Insertion of a pacemaker device or cardiac rhythm related device (6th character 4, 5, 6 or P) into the chest or abdomen subcutaneous tissue and fascia. *See table 0JH to construct the Insertion code*. When a device is replaced, also report the Removal of a cardiac rhythm related device (6th character P) from the trunk subcutaneous tissue and fascia. *See table 0JP to construct the Removal code*.

▲ **02HA0QZ** Insertion of Implantable Heart Assist System into Heart, Open Approach

02HA0RS Insertion of Biventricular External Heart Assist System into Heart, Open Approach

+ Heart assist system replacement when reported with a removal of an external heart assist system (6th character R) from the heart. *See table 02P to construct the Removal code*.

02HA0RZ Insertion of External Heart Assist System into Heart, Open Approach

+ Heart assist system replacement when reported with a removal of an external heart assist system (6th character R) from the heart. *See table 02P to construct the Removal code*.

▲ **02HA3QZ** Insertion of Implantable Heart Assist System into Heart, Percutaneous Approach

02HA3RS Insertion of Biventricular External Heart Assist System into Heart, Percutaneous Approach

+ Heart assist system replacement when reported with a removal of an external heart assist system (6th character R) from the heart. *See table 02P to construct the Removal code*.

02HA3RZ Insertion of External Heart Assist System into Heart, Percutaneous Approach

+ Heart assist system replacement when reported with a removal of an external heart assist system (6th character R) from the heart. *See table 02P to construct the Removal code*.

▲ **02HA4QZ** Insertion of Implantable Heart Assist System into Heart, Percutaneous Endoscopic Approach

02HA4RS Insertion of Biventricular External Heart Assist System into Heart, Percutaneous Endoscopic Approach

+ Heart assist system replacement when reported with a removal of an external heart assist system (6th character R) from the heart. *See table 02P to construct the Removal code*.

02HA4RZ Insertion of External Heart Assist System into Heart, Percutaneous Endoscopic Approach

[+] Heart assist system replacement when reported with a removal of an external heart assist system (6th character R) from the heart. *See table 02P to construct the Removal code.*

02HK00Z Insertion of Pressure Sensor Monitoring Device into Right Ventricle, Open Approach

[+] Intracardiac lead device when reported with an Insertion of a hemodynamic monitoring device (6th character 0) into the chest or abdomen sucutaneous tissue and fascia. *See table 0JH to construct the Insertion code.*

02HK02Z Insertion of Monitoring Device into Right Ventricle, Open Approach

[+] Intracardiac lead device when reported with an Insertion of a hemodynamic monitoring device (6th character 0) into the chest or abdomen sucutaneous tissue and fascia. *See table 0JH to construct the Insertion code.*

02HK03Z Insertion of Infusion Device into Right Ventricle, Open Approach

02HK0DZ Insertion of Intraluminal Device into Right Ventricle, Open Approach

● **02HK0JZ** Insertion of Pacemaker Lead into Right Ventricle, Open Approach

[+] Lead device when reported with an Insertion of a pacemaker device or cardiac rhythm related device (6th character 4, 5, 6 or P) into the chest or abdomen subcutaneous tissue and fascia. *See table 0JH to construct the Insertion code.* When a device is replaced, also report the Removal of a cardiac rhythm related device (6th character P) from the trunk subcutaneous tissue and fascia. *See table 0JP to construct the Removal code.*

02HK0KZ Insertion of Defibrillator Lead into Right Ventricle, Open Approach

[+] Lead device when reported with an Insertion of a defibrillator generator (6th character 8 or 9) into the chest or abdomen subcutaneous tissue and fascia. *See table 0JH to construct the Insertion code.*

● **02HK0MZ** Insertion of Cardiac Lead into Right Ventricle, Open Approach

[+] Lead device when reported with an Insertion of a pacemaker device or cardiac rhythm related device (6th character 4, 5, 6 or P) into the chest or abdomen subcutaneous tissue and fascia. *See table 0JH to construct the Insertion code.* When a device is replaced, also report the Removal of a cardiac rhythm related device (6th character P) from the trunk subcutaneous tissue and fascia. *See table 0JP to construct the Removal code.*

02HK30Z Insertion of Pressure Sensor Monitoring Device into Right Ventricle, Percutaneous Approach

[+] Intracardiac lead device when reported with an Insertion of a hemodynamic monitoring device (6th character 0) into the chest or abdomen sucutaneous tissue and fascia. *See table 0JH to construct the Insertion code.*

02HK32Z Insertion of Monitoring Device into Right Ventricle, Percutaneous Approach

[+] Intracardiac lead device when reported with an Insertion of a hemodynamic monitoring device (6th character 0) into the chest or abdomen sucutaneous tissue and fascia. *See table 0JH to construct the Insertion code.*

● **02HK33Z** Insertion of Infusion Device into Right Ventricle, Percutaneous Approach

02HK3DZ Insertion of Intraluminal Device into Right Ventricle, Percutaneous Approach

● **02HK3JZ** Insertion of Pacemaker Lead into Right Ventricle, Percutaneous Approach

HAC With a secondary diagnosis code of K68.11, T81.4XXA, T82.6XXA, T82.7XXA

[+] Lead device when reported with an Insertion of a pacemaker device or cardiac rhythm related device (6th character 4, 5, 6 or P) into the chest or abdomen subcutaneous tissue and fascia. See table 0JH to construct the Insertion code. When a device is replaced, also report the removal of a cardiac rhythm related device (6th character P) from the trunk subcutaneous tissue and fascia. See table 0JP to construct the Removal code. When a cardiac lead is replaced, also report the removal of cardiac lead (6th character M) from the heart. *See table 02P to construct the Removal code.*

02HK3KZ Insertion of Defibrillator Lead into Right Ventricle, Percutaneous Approach

[+] Lead device when reported with an Insertion of a defibrillator generator (6th character 8 or 9) into the chest or abdomen subcutaneous tissue and fascia. *See table 0JH to construct the Insertion code.*

● **02HK3MZ** Insertion of Cardiac Lead into Right Ventricle, Percutaneous Approach

[+] Lead device when reported with an Insertion of a pacemaker device or cardiac rhythm related device (6th character 4, 5, 6 or P) into the chest or abdomen subcutaneous tissue and fascia. *See table 0JH to construct the Insertion code.* When a device is replaced, also report the Removal of a cardiac rhythm related device (6th character P) from the trunk subcutaneous tissue and fascia. *See table 0JP to construct the Removal code.*

02HK40Z Insertion of Pressure Sensor Monitoring Device into Right Ventricle, Percutaneous Endoscopic Approach

[+] Intracardiac lead device when reported with an Insertion of a hemodynamic monitoring device (6th character 0) into the chest or abdomen sucutaneous tissue and fascia. *See table 0JH to construct the Insertion code.*

02HK42Z Insertion of Monitoring Device into Right Ventricle, Percutaneous Endoscopic Approach

[+] Intracardiac lead device when reported with an Insertion of a hemodynamic monitoring device (6th character 0) into the chest or abdomen sucutaneous tissue and fascia. *See table 0JH to construct the Insertion code.*

02HK43Z Insertion of Infusion Device into Right Ventricle, Percutaneous Endoscopic Approach

02HK4DZ Insertion of Intraluminal Device into Right Ventricle, Percutaneous Endoscopic Approach

● **02HK4JZ** Insertion of Pacemaker Lead into Right Ventricle, Percutaneous Endoscopic Approach

[+] Lead device when reported with an Insertion of a pacemaker device or cardiac rhythm related device (6th character 4, 5, 6 or P) into the chest or abdomen subcutaneous tissue and fascia. *See table 0JH to construct the Insertion code.* When a device is replaced, also report the Removal of a cardiac rhythm related device (6th character P) from the trunk subcutaneous tissue and fascia. *See table 0JP to construct the Removal code.*

02HK4KZ Insertion of Defibrillator Lead into Right Ventricle, Percutaneous Endoscopic Approach

[+] Lead device when reported with an Insertion of a defibrillator generator (6th character 8 or 9) into the chest or abdomen subcutaneous tissue and fascia. *See table 0JH to construct the Insertion code.*

● **02HK4MZ** Insertion of Cardiac Lead into Right Ventricle, Percutaneous Endoscopic Approach

[+] Lead device when reported with an Insertion of a pacemaker device or cardiac rhythm related device (6th character 4, 5, 6 or P) into the chest or abdomen subcutaneous tissue and fascia. *See table 0JH to construct the Insertion code.* When a device is replaced, also report the Removal of a cardiac rhythm related device (6th character P) from the trunk subcutaneous tissue and fascia. *See table 0JP to construct the Removal code.*

02HL00Z Insertion of Pressure Sensor Monitoring Device into Left Ventricle, Open Approach

02HL02Z Insertion of Monitoring Device into Left Ventricle, Open Approach

02HL03Z Insertion of Infusion Device into Left Ventricle, Open Approach

02HL0DZ Insertion of Intraluminal Device into Left Ventricle, Open Approach

● **02HL0JZ** Insertion of Pacemaker Lead into Left Ventricle, Open Approach

[+] Lead device when reported with an Insertion of a pacemaker device or cardiac rhythm related device (6th character 4, 5, 6 or P) into the chest or abdomen subcutaneous tissue and fascia. *See table 0JH to construct the Insertion code.* When a device is replaced, also report the Removal of a cardiac rhythm related device (6th character P) from the trunk subcutaneous tissue and fascia. *See table 0JP to construct the Removal code.*

02HL0KZ Insertion of Defibrillator Lead into Left Ventricle, Open Approach

[+] Lead device when reported with an Insertion of a defibrillator generator (6th character 8 or 9) into the chest or abdomen subcutaneous tissue and fascia. *See table 0JH to construct the Insertion code.*

● **02HL0MZ** Insertion of Cardiac Lead into Left Ventricle, Open Approach

[+] Lead device when reported with an Insertion of a pacemaker device, cardiac rhythm related device or contractility modulation device (6th character 4, 5, 6, M or P) into the chest or abdomen subcutaneous tissue and fascia. *See table 0JH to construct the Insertion code.* When a device is replaced, also report the Removal of a cardiac rhythm related device (6th character P) from the trunk subcutaneous tissue and fascia. *See table 0JP to construct the Removal code.*

02HL30Z Insertion of Pressure Sensor Monitoring Device into Left Ventricle, Percutaneous Approach

02HL32Z Insertion of Monitoring Device into Left Ventricle, Percutaneous Approach

02HL33Z Insertion of Infusion Device into Left Ventricle, Percutaneous Approach

02HL3DZ Insertion of Intraluminal Device into Left Ventricle, Percutaneous Approach

● **02HL3JZ** Insertion of Pacemaker Lead into Left Ventricle, Percutaneous Approach

HAC With a secondary diagnosis code of K68.11, T81.4XXA, T82.6XXA, T82.7XXA

\+ Lead device when reported with an Insertion of a pacemaker device or cardiac rhythm related device (6th character 4, 5, 6 or P) into the chest or abdomen subcutaneous tissue and fascia. *See table 0JH to construct the Insertion code.* When a device is replaced, also report the removal of a cardiac rhythm related device (6th character P) from the trunk subcutaneous tissue and fascia. *See table 0JP to construct the Removal code.* When a cardiac lead is replaced, also report the removal of cardiac lead (6th character M) from the heart. *See table 02P to construct the Removal code.*

02HL3KZ Insertion of Defibrillator Lead into Left Ventricle, Percutaneous Approach

\+ Lead device when reported with an Insertion of a defibrillator generator (6th character 8 or 9) into the chest or abdomen subcutaneous tissue and fascia. *See table 0JH to construct the Insertion code.*

● **02HL3MZ** Insertion of Cardiac Lead into Left Ventricle, Percutaneous Approach

\+ Lead device when reported with an Insertion of a pacemaker device, cardiac rhythm related device or contractility modulation device (6th character 4, 5, 6, M or P) into the chest or abdomen subcutaneous tissue and fascia. *See table 0JH to construct the Insertion code.* When a device is replaced, also report the Removal of a cardiac rhythm related device (6th character P) from the trunk subcutaneous tissue and fascia. *See table 0JP to construct the Removal code.*

02HL40Z Insertion of Pressure Sensor Monitoring Device into Left Ventricle, Percutaneous Endoscopic Approach

02HL42Z Insertion of Monitoring Device into Left Ventricle, Percutaneous Endoscopic Approach

02HL43Z Insertion of Infusion Device into Left Ventricle, Percutaneous Endoscopic Approach

02HL4DZ Insertion of Intraluminal Device into Left Ventricle, Percutaneous Endoscopic Approach

● **02HL4JZ** Insertion of Pacemaker Lead into Left Ventricle, Percutaneous Endoscopic Approach

\+ Lead device when reported with an Insertion of a pacemaker device or cardiac rhythm related device (6th character 4, 5, 6 or P) into the chest or abdomen subcutaneous tissue and fascia. *See table 0JH to construct the Insertion code.* When a device is replaced, also report the Removal of a cardiac rhythm related device (6th character P) from the trunk subcutaneous tissue and fascia. *See table 0JP to construct the Removal code.*

02HL4KZ Insertion of Defibrillator Lead into Left Ventricle, Percutaneous Endoscopic Approach

● **02HL4MZ** Insertion of Cardiac Lead into Left Ventricle, Percutaneous Endoscopic Approach

\+ Lead device when reported with an Insertion of a pacemaker device or cardiac rhythm related device (6th character 4, 5, 6 or P) into the chest or abdomen subcutaneous tissue and fascia. *See table 0JH to construct the Insertion code.* When a device is replaced, also report the Removal of a cardiac rhythm related device (6th character P) from the trunk subcutaneous tissue and fascia. *See table 0JP to construct the Removal code.*

02HN00Z Insertion of Pressure Sensor Monitoring Device into Pericardium, Open Approach

02HN02Z Insertion of Monitoring Device into Pericardium, Open Approach

02HN0JZ Insertion of Pacemaker Lead into Pericardium, Open Approach

HAC With a secondary diagnosis code of K68.11, T81.4XXA, T82.6XXA, T82.7XXA

\+ Lead device when reported with an Insertion of a pacemaker device or cardiac rhythm related device (6th character 4, 5, 6 or P) into the chest or abdomen subcutaneous tissue and fascia. *See table 0JH to construct the Insertion code.* When a device is replaced, also report the Removal of a cardiac rhythm related device (6th character P) from the trunk subcutaneous tissue and fascia. *See table 0JP to construct the Removal code.*

02HN0KZ Insertion of Defibrillator Lead into Pericardium, Open Approach

02HN0MZ Insertion of Cardiac Lead into Pericardium, Open Approach

HAC With a secondary diagnosis code of K68.11, T81.4XXA, T82.6XXA, T82.7XXA

\+ Lead device when reported with an Insertion of a pacemaker device, cardiac rhythm related device or contractility modulation device (6th character 4, 5, 6, M or P) into the chest or abdomen subcutaneous tissue and fascia. *See table 0JH to construct the Insertion code.* When a device is replaced, also report the Removal of a cardiac rhythm related device (6th character P) from the trunk subcutaneous tissue and fascia. *See table 0JP to construct the Removal code.*

02HN30Z Insertion of Pressure Sensor Monitoring Device into Pericardium, Percutaneous Approach

02HN32Z Insertion of Monitoring Device into Pericardium, Percutaneous Approach

02HN3JZ Insertion of Pacemaker Lead into Pericardium, Percutaneous Approach

HAC With a secondary diagnosis code of K68.11, T81.4XXA, T82.6XXA, T82.7XXA

\+ Lead device when reported with an Insertion of a pacemaker device or cardiac rhythm related device (6th character 4, 5, 6 or P) into the chest or abdomen subcutaneous tissue and fascia. *See table 0JH to construct the Insertion code.* When a device is replaced, also report the Removal of a cardiac rhythm related device (6th character P) from the trunk subcutaneous tissue and fascia. *See table 0JP to construct the Removal code.*

02HN3KZ Insertion of Defibrillator Lead into Pericardium, Percutaneous Approach

02HN3MZ Insertion of Cardiac Lead into Pericardium, Percutaneous Approach

HAC With a secondary diagnosis code of K68.11, T81.4XXA, T82.6XXA, T82.7XXA

\+ Lead device when reported with an Insertion of a pacemaker device or cardiac rhythm related device (6th character 4, 5, 6 or P) into the chest or abdomen subcutaneous tissue and fascia. *See table 0JH to construct the Insertion code.* When a device is replaced, also report the Removal of a cardiac rhythm related device (6th character P) from the trunk subcutaneous tissue and fascia. *See table 0JP to construct the Removal code.*

02HN40Z Insertion of Pressure Sensor Monitoring Device into Pericardium, Percutaneous Endoscopic Approach

02HN42Z Insertion of Monitoring Device into Pericardium, Percutaneous Endoscopic Approach

02HN4JZ Insertion of Pacemaker Lead into Pericardium, Percutaneous Endoscopic Approach

HAC With a secondary diagnosis code of K68.11, T81.4XXA, T82.6XXA, T82.7XXA

\+ Lead device when reported with an Insertion of a pacemaker device or cardiac rhythm related device (6th character 4, 5, 6 or P) into the chest or abdomen subcutaneous tissue and fascia. *See table 0JH to construct the Insertion code.* When a device is replaced, also report the Removal of a cardiac rhythm related device (6th character P) from the trunk subcutaneous tissue and fascia. *See table 0JP to construct the Removal code.*

02HN4KZ Insertion of Defibrillator Lead into Pericardium, Percutaneous Endoscopic Approach

02HN4MZ Insertion of Cardiac Lead into Pericardium, Percutaneous Endoscopic Approach

HAC With a secondary diagnosis code of K68.11, T81.4XXA, T82.6XXA, T82.7XXA

\+ Lead device when reported with an Insertion of a pacemaker device or cardiac rhythm related device (6th character 4, 5, 6 or P) into the chest or abdomen subcutaneous tissue and fascia. *See table 0JH to construct the Insertion code.* When a device is replaced, also report the Removal of a cardiac rhythm related device (6th character P) from the trunk subcutaneous tissue and fascia. *See table 0JP to construct the Removal code.*

02HP00Z Insertion of Pressure Sensor Monitoring Device into Pulmonary Trunk, Open Approach

02HP02Z Insertion of Monitoring Device into Pulmonary Trunk, Open Approach

02HP03Z Insertion of Infusion Device into Pulmonary Trunk, Open Approach

02HP0DZ Insertion of Intraluminal Device into Pulmonary Trunk, Open Approach

02HP30Z Insertion of Pressure Sensor Monitoring Device into Pulmonary Trunk, Percutaneous Approach

02HP32Z Insertion of Monitoring Device into Pulmonary Trunk, Percutaneous Approach

02HP33Z Insertion of Infusion Device into Pulmonary Trunk, Percutaneous Approach

02HP3DZ Insertion of Intraluminal Device into Pulmonary Trunk, Percutaneous Approach

02HP40Z Insertion of Pressure Sensor Monitoring Device into Pulmonary Trunk, Percutaneous Endoscopic Approach

02HP42Z Insertion of Monitoring Device into Pulmonary Trunk, Percutaneous Endoscopic Approach

02HP43Z Insertion of Infusion Device into Pulmonary Trunk, Percutaneous Endoscopic Approach
02HP4DZ Insertion of Intraluminal Device into Pulmonary Trunk, Percutaneous Endoscopic Approach
02HQ00Z Insertion of Pressure Sensor Monitoring Device into Right Pulmonary Artery, Open Approach
02HQ02Z Insertion of Monitoring Device into Right Pulmonary Artery, Open Approach
02HQ03Z Insertion of Infusion Device into Right Pulmonary Artery, Open Approach
02HQ0DZ Insertion of Intraluminal Device into Right Pulmonary Artery, Open Approach
02HQ30Z Insertion of Pressure Sensor Monitoring Device into Right Pulmonary Artery, Percutaneous Approach
02HQ32Z Insertion of Monitoring Device into Right Pulmonary Artery, Percutaneous Approach
02HQ33Z Insertion of Infusion Device into Right Pulmonary Artery, Percutaneous Approach
02HQ3DZ Insertion of Intraluminal Device into Right Pulmonary Artery, Percutaneous Approach
02HQ40Z Insertion of Pressure Sensor Monitoring Device into Right Pulmonary Artery, Percutaneous Endoscopic Approach
02HQ42Z Insertion of Monitoring Device into Right Pulmonary Artery, Percutaneous Endoscopic Approach
02HQ43Z Insertion of Infusion Device into Right Pulmonary Artery, Percutaneous Endoscopic Approach
02HQ4DZ Insertion of Intraluminal Device into Right Pulmonary Artery, Percutaneous Endoscopic Approach
02HR00Z Insertion of Pressure Sensor Monitoring Device into Left Pulmonary Artery, Open Approach
02HR02Z Insertion of Monitoring Device into Left Pulmonary Artery, Open Approach
02HR03Z Insertion of Infusion Device into Left Pulmonary Artery, Open Approach
02HR0DZ Insertion of Intraluminal Device into Left Pulmonary Artery, Open Approach
02HR30Z Insertion of Pressure Sensor Monitoring Device into Left Pulmonary Artery, Percutaneous Approach
02HR32Z Insertion of Monitoring Device into Left Pulmonary Artery, Percutaneous Approach
02HR33Z Insertion of Infusion Device into Left Pulmonary Artery, Percutaneous Approach
02HR3DZ Insertion of Intraluminal Device into Left Pulmonary Artery, Percutaneous Approach
02HR40Z Insertion of Pressure Sensor Monitoring Device into Left Pulmonary Artery, Percutaneous Endoscopic Approach
02HR42Z Insertion of Monitoring Device into Left Pulmonary Artery, Percutaneous Endoscopic Approach
02HR43Z Insertion of Infusion Device into Left Pulmonary Artery, Percutaneous Endoscopic Approach
02HR4DZ Insertion of Intraluminal Device into Left Pulmonary Artery, Percutaneous Endoscopic Approach
02HS00Z Insertion of Pressure Sensor Monitoring Device into Right Pulmonary Vein, Open Approach
02HS02Z Insertion of Monitoring Device into Right Pulmonary Vein, Open Approach
02HS03Z Insertion of Infusion Device into Right Pulmonary Vein, Open Approach
02HS0DZ Insertion of Intraluminal Device into Right Pulmonary Vein, Open Approach
02HS30Z Insertion of Pressure Sensor Monitoring Device into Right Pulmonary Vein, Percutaneous Approach
02HS32Z Insertion of Monitoring Device into Right Pulmonary Vein, Percutaneous Approach
02HS33Z Insertion of Infusion Device into Right Pulmonary Vein, Percutaneous Approach
02HS3DZ Insertion of Intraluminal Device into Right Pulmonary Vein, Percutaneous Approach
02HS40Z Insertion of Pressure Sensor Monitoring Device into Right Pulmonary Vein, Percutaneous Endoscopic Approach
02HS42Z Insertion of Monitoring Device into Right Pulmonary Vein, Percutaneous Endoscopic Approach
02HS43Z Insertion of Infusion Device into Right Pulmonary Vein, Percutaneous Endoscopic Approach
02HS4DZ Insertion of Intraluminal Device into Right Pulmonary Vein, Percutaneous Endoscopic Approach
02HT00Z Insertion of Pressure Sensor Monitoring Device into Left Pulmonary Vein, Open Approach
02HT02Z Insertion of Monitoring Device into Left Pulmonary Vein, Open Approach
02HT03Z Insertion of Infusion Device into Left Pulmonary Vein, Open Approach
02HT0DZ Insertion of Intraluminal Device into Left Pulmonary Vein, Open Approach
02HT30Z Insertion of Pressure Sensor Monitoring Device into Left Pulmonary Vein, Percutaneous Approach
02HT32Z Insertion of Monitoring Device into Left Pulmonary Vein, Percutaneous Approach
02HT33Z Insertion of Infusion Device into Left Pulmonary Vein, Percutaneous Approach
02HT3DZ Insertion of Intraluminal Device into Left Pulmonary Vein, Percutaneous Approach
02HT40Z Insertion of Pressure Sensor Monitoring Device into Left Pulmonary Vein, Percutaneous Endoscopic Approach
02HT42Z Insertion of Monitoring Device into Left Pulmonary Vein, Percutaneous Endoscopic Approach
02HT43Z Insertion of Infusion Device into Left Pulmonary Vein, Percutaneous Endoscopic Approach
02HT4DZ Insertion of Intraluminal Device into Left Pulmonary Vein, Percutaneous Endoscopic Approach
02HV00Z Insertion of Pressure Sensor Monitoring Device into Superior Vena Cava, Open Approach
02HV02Z Insertion of Monitoring Device into Superior Vena Cava, Open Approach
02HV03Z Insertion of Infusion Device into Superior Vena Cava, Open Approach
02HV0DZ Insertion of Intraluminal Device into Superior Vena Cava, Open Approach
02HV30Z Insertion of Pressure Sensor Monitoring Device into Superior Vena Cava, Percutaneous Approach
02HV32Z Insertion of Monitoring Device into Superior Vena Cava, Percutaneous Approach
02HV33Z Insertion of Infusion Device into Superior Vena Cava, Percutaneous Approach
AHA CC: 3Q, 2013, 18
02HV3DZ Insertion of Intraluminal Device into Superior Vena Cava, Percutaneous Approach
02HV40Z Insertion of Pressure Sensor Monitoring Device into Superior Vena Cava, Percutaneous Endoscopic Approach
02HV42Z Insertion of Monitoring Device into Superior Vena Cava, Percutaneous Endoscopic Approach
02HV43Z Insertion of Infusion Device into Superior Vena Cava, Percutaneous Endoscopic Approach
02HV4DZ Insertion of Intraluminal Device into Superior Vena Cava, Percutaneous Endoscopic Approach
02HW00Z Insertion of Pressure Sensor Monitoring Device into Thoracic Aorta, Open Approach
02HW02Z Insertion of Monitoring Device into Thoracic Aorta, Open Approach
02HW03Z Insertion of Infusion Device into Thoracic Aorta, Open Approach
02HW0DZ Insertion of Intraluminal Device into Thoracic Aorta, Open Approach
02HW30Z Insertion of Pressure Sensor Monitoring Device into Thoracic Aorta, Percutaneous Approach
02HW32Z Insertion of Monitoring Device into Thoracic Aorta, Percutaneous Approach
02HW33Z Insertion of Infusion Device into Thoracic Aorta, Percutaneous Approach
02HW3DZ Insertion of Intraluminal Device into Thoracic Aorta, Percutaneous Approach

02J – Heart and Great Vessels, Inspection

Review Coding Guidelines B3.11a, B3.11b and B3.11c

02JA0ZZ Inspection of Heart, Open Approach
02JA3ZZ Inspection of Heart, Percutaneous Approach
02JA4ZZ Inspection of Heart, Percutaneous Endoscopic Approach
02JY0ZZ Inspection of Great Vessel, Open Approach
02JY3ZZ Inspection of Great Vessel, Percutaneous Approach
02JY4ZZ Inspection of Great Vessel, Percutaneous Endoscopic Approach

02K – Heart and Great Vessels, Map

● **02K80ZZ** Map Conduction Mechanism, Open Approach
● **02K83ZZ** Map Conduction Mechanism, Percutaneous Approach
● **02K84ZZ** Map Conduction Mechanism, Percutaneous Endoscopic Approach

02L – Heart and Great Vessels, Occlusion

● **02L70CK** Occlusion of Left Atrial Appendage with Extraluminal Device, Open Approach
● **02L70DK** Occlusion of Left Atrial Appendage with Intraluminal Device, Open Approach
● **02L70ZK** Occlusion of Left Atrial Appendage, Open Approach
● **02L73CK** Occlusion of Left Atrial Appendage with Extraluminal Device, Percutaneous Approach
● **02L73DK** Occlusion of Left Atrial Appendage with Intraluminal Device, Percutaneous Approach
● **02L73ZK** Occlusion of Left Atrial Appendage, Percutaneous Approach
● **02L74CK** Occlusion of Left Atrial Appendage with Extraluminal Device, Percutaneous Endoscopic Approach
● **02L74DK** Occlusion of Left Atrial Appendage with Intraluminal Device, Percutaneous Endoscopic Approach
● **02L74ZK** Occlusion of Left Atrial Appendage, Percutaneous Endoscopic Approach
02LR0CT Occlusion of Ductus Arteriosus with Extraluminal Device, Open Approach
02LR0DT Occlusion of Ductus Arteriosus with Intraluminal Device, Open Approach
02LR0ZT Occlusion of Ductus Arteriosus, Open Approach
02LR3CT Occlusion of Ductus Arteriosus with Extraluminal Device, Percutaneous Approach
02LR3DT Occlusion of Ductus Arteriosus with Intraluminal Device, Percutaneous Approach
02LR3ZT Occlusion of Ductus Arteriosus, Percutaneous Approach
02LR4CT Occlusion of Ductus Arteriosus with Extraluminal Device, Percutaneous Endoscopic Approach
02LR4DT Occlusion of Ductus Arteriosus with Intraluminal Device, Percutaneous Endoscopic Approach
02LR4ZT Occlusion of Ductus Arteriosus, Percutaneous Endoscopic Approach
02LS0CZ Occlusion of Right Pulmonary Vein with Extraluminal Device, Open Approach
02LS0DZ Occlusion of Right Pulmonary Vein with Intraluminal Device, Open Approach
02LS0ZZ Occlusion of Right Pulmonary Vein, Open Approach
02LS3CZ Occlusion of Right Pulmonary Vein with Extraluminal Device, Percutaneous Approach
02LS3DZ Occlusion of Right Pulmonary Vein with Intraluminal Device, Percutaneous Approach
02LS3ZZ Occlusion of Right Pulmonary Vein, Percutaneous Approach
02LS4CZ Occlusion of Right Pulmonary Vein with Extraluminal Device, Percutaneous Endoscopic Approach
02LS4DZ Occlusion of Right Pulmonary Vein with Intraluminal Device, Percutaneous Endoscopic Approach
02LS4ZZ Occlusion of Right Pulmonary Vein, Percutaneous Endoscopic Approach
02LT0CZ Occlusion of Left Pulmonary Vein with Extraluminal Device, Open Approach
02LT0DZ Occlusion of Left Pulmonary Vein with Intraluminal Device, Open Approach
02LT0ZZ Occlusion of Left Pulmonary Vein, Open Approach
02LT3CZ Occlusion of Left Pulmonary Vein with Extraluminal Device, Percutaneous Approach
02LT3DZ Occlusion of Left Pulmonary Vein with Intraluminal Device, Percutaneous Approach
02LT3ZZ Occlusion of Left Pulmonary Vein, Percutaneous Approach
02LT4CZ Occlusion of Left Pulmonary Vein with Extraluminal Device, Percutaneous Endoscopic Approach
02LT4DZ Occlusion of Left Pulmonary Vein with Intraluminal Device, Percutaneous Endoscopic Approach
02LT4ZZ Occlusion of Left Pulmonary Vein, Percutaneous Endoscopic Approach
02LV0CZ Occlusion of Superior Vena Cava with Extraluminal Device, Open Approach
02LV0DZ Occlusion of Superior Vena Cava with Intraluminal Device, Open Approach
02LV0ZZ Occlusion of Superior Vena Cava, Open Approach
02LV3CZ Occlusion of Superior Vena Cava with Extraluminal Device, Percutaneous Approach
02LV3DZ Occlusion of Superior Vena Cava with Intraluminal Device, Percutaneous Approach
02LV3ZZ Occlusion of Superior Vena Cava, Percutaneous Approach
02LV4CZ Occlusion of Superior Vena Cava with Extraluminal Device, Percutaneous Endoscopic Approach
02LV4DZ Occlusion of Superior Vena Cava with Intraluminal Device, Percutaneous Endoscopic Approach
02LV4ZZ Occlusion of Superior Vena Cava, Percutaneous Endoscopic Approach

02N – Heart and Great Vessels, Release

Review Coding Guideline B3.13

Review Coding Guideline B3.14

02N40ZZ Release Coronary Vein, Open Approach
02N43ZZ Release Coronary Vein, Percutaneous Approach
02N44ZZ Release Coronary Vein, Percutaneous Endoscopic Approach
02N50ZZ Release Atrial Septum, Open Approach
02N53ZZ Release Atrial Septum, Percutaneous Approach
02N54ZZ Release Atrial Septum, Percutaneous Endoscopic Approach
02N60ZZ Release Right Atrium, Open Approach
02N63ZZ Release Right Atrium, Percutaneous Approach
02N64ZZ Release Right Atrium, Percutaneous Endoscopic Approach
02N70ZZ Release Left Atrium, Open Approach
02N73ZZ Release Left Atrium, Percutaneous Approach
02N74ZZ Release Left Atrium, Percutaneous Endoscopic Approach
02N80ZZ Release Conduction Mechanism, Open Approach
02N83ZZ Release Conduction Mechanism, Percutaneous Approach
02N84ZZ Release Conduction Mechanism, Percutaneous Endoscopic Approach
02N90ZZ Release Chordae Tendineae, Open Approach
02N93ZZ Release Chordae Tendineae, Percutaneous Approach
02N94ZZ Release Chordae Tendineae, Percutaneous Endoscopic Approach
02ND0ZZ Release Papillary Muscle, Open Approach
02ND3ZZ Release Papillary Muscle, Percutaneous Approach
02ND4ZZ Release Papillary Muscle, Percutaneous Endoscopic Approach
02NF0ZZ Release Aortic Valve, Open Approach
02NF3ZZ Release Aortic Valve, Percutaneous Approach
02NF4ZZ Release Aortic Valve, Percutaneous Endoscopic Approach
02NG0ZZ Release Mitral Valve, Open Approach
02NG3ZZ Release Mitral Valve, Percutaneous Approach
02NG4ZZ Release Mitral Valve, Percutaneous Endoscopic Approach
02NH0ZZ Release Pulmonary Valve, Open Approach
02NH3ZZ Release Pulmonary Valve, Percutaneous Approach
02NH4ZZ Release Pulmonary Valve, Percutaneous Endoscopic Approach
02NJ0ZZ Release Tricuspid Valve, Open Approach
02NJ3ZZ Release Tricuspid Valve, Percutaneous Approach
02NJ4ZZ Release Tricuspid Valve, Percutaneous Endoscopic Approach
02NK0ZZ Release Right Ventricle, Open Approach
02NK3ZZ Release Right Ventricle, Percutaneous Approach
02NK4ZZ Release Right Ventricle, Percutaneous Endoscopic Approach
02NL0ZZ Release Left Ventricle, Open Approach
02NL3ZZ Release Left Ventricle, Percutaneous Approach
02NL4ZZ Release Left Ventricle, Percutaneous Endoscopic Approach
02NM0ZZ Release Ventricular Septum, Open Approach
02NM3ZZ Release Ventricular Septum, Percutaneous Approach
02NM4ZZ Release Ventricular Septum, Percutaneous Endoscopic Approach
02NN0ZZ Release Pericardium, Open Approach
02NN3ZZ Release Pericardium, Percutaneous Approach
02NN4ZZ Release Pericardium, Percutaneous Endoscopic Approach
02NP0ZZ Release Pulmonary Trunk, Open Approach
02NP3ZZ Release Pulmonary Trunk, Percutaneous Approach
02NP4ZZ Release Pulmonary Trunk, Percutaneous Endoscopic Approach
02NQ0ZZ Release Right Pulmonary Artery, Open Approach
02NQ3ZZ Release Right Pulmonary Artery, Percutaneous Approach
02NQ4ZZ Release Right Pulmonary Artery, Percutaneous Endoscopic Approach

02NR0ZZ Release Left Pulmonary Artery, Open Approach
02NR3ZZ Release Left Pulmonary Artery, Percutaneous Approach
02NR4ZZ Release Left Pulmonary Artery, Percutaneous Endoscopic Approach
02NS0ZZ Release Right Pulmonary Vein, Open Approach
02NS3ZZ Release Right Pulmonary Vein, Percutaneous Approach
02NS4ZZ Release Right Pulmonary Vein, Percutaneous Endoscopic Approach
02NT0ZZ Release Left Pulmonary Vein, Open Approach
02NT3ZZ Release Left Pulmonary Vein, Percutaneous Approach
02NT4ZZ Release Left Pulmonary Vein, Percutaneous Endoscopic Approach
02NV0ZZ Release Superior Vena Cava, Open Approach
02NV3ZZ Release Superior Vena Cava, Percutaneous Approach
02NV4ZZ Release Superior Vena Cava, Percutaneous Endoscopic Approach
02NW0ZZ Release Thoracic Aorta, Open Approach
02NW3ZZ Release Thoracic Aorta, Percutaneous Approach
02NW4ZZ Release Thoracic Aorta, Percutaneous Endoscopic Approach

02P – Heart and Great Vessels, Removal

Review Coding Guideline B6.1c

02PA02Z Removal of Monitoring Device from Heart, Open Approach
02PA03Z Removal of Infusion Device from Heart, Open Approach
02PA07Z Removal of Autologous Tissue Substitute from Heart, Open Approach
02PA08Z Removal of Zooplastic Tissue from Heart, Open Approach
02PA0CZ Removal of Extraluminal Device from Heart, Open Approach
02PA0DZ Removal of Intraluminal Device from Heart, Open Approach
02PA0JZ Removal of Synthetic Substitute from Heart, Open Approach
02PA0KZ Removal of Nonautologous Tissue Substitute from Heart, Open Approach
02PA0MZ Removal of Cardiac Lead from Heart, Open Approach
HAC With a secondary diagnosis code of K68.11, T81.4XXA, T82.6XXA, T82.7XXA
02PA0QZ Removal of Implantable Heart Assist System from Heart, Open Approach
02PA0RZ Removal of External Heart Assist System from Heart, Open Approach
02PA32Z Removal of Monitoring Device from Heart, Percutaneous Approach
02PA33Z Removal of Infusion Device from Heart, Percutaneous Approach
02PA37Z Removal of Autologous Tissue Substitute from Heart, Percutaneous Approach
02PA38Z Removal of Zooplastic Tissue from Heart, Percutaneous Approach
02PA3CZ Removal of Extraluminal Device from Heart, Percutaneous Approach
02PA3DZ Removal of Intraluminal Device from Heart, Percutaneous Approach
02PA3JZ Removal of Synthetic Substitute from Heart, Percutaneous Approach
02PA3KZ Removal of Nonautologous Tissue Substitute from Heart, Percutaneous Approach
02PA3MZ Removal of Cardiac Lead from Heart, Percutaneous Approach
HAC With a secondary diagnosis code of K68.11, T81.4XXA, T82.6XXA, T82.7XXA
02PA3QZ Removal of Implantable Heart Assist System from Heart, Percutaneous Approach
02PA3RZ Removal of External Heart Assist System from Heart, Percutaneous Approach
02PA42Z Removal of Monitoring Device from Heart, Percutaneous Endoscopic Approach
02PA43Z Removal of Infusion Device from Heart, Percutaneous Endoscopic Approach
02PA47Z Removal of Autologous Tissue Substitute from Heart, Percutaneous Endoscopic Approach
02PA48Z Removal of Zooplastic Tissue from Heart, Percutaneous Endoscopic Approach
02PA4CZ Removal of Extraluminal Device from Heart, Percutaneous Endoscopic Approach
02PA4DZ Removal of Intraluminal Device from Heart, Percutaneous Endoscopic Approach
02PA4JZ Removal of Synthetic Substitute from Heart, Percutaneous Endoscopic Approach
02PA4KZ Removal of Nonautologous Tissue Substitute from Heart, Percutaneous Endoscopic Approach
02PA4MZ Removal of Cardiac Lead from Heart, Percutaneous Endoscopic Approach
HAC With a secondary diagnosis code of K68.11, T81.4XXA, T82.6XXA, T82.7XXA
02PA4QZ Removal of Implantable Heart Assist System from Heart, Percutaneous Endoscopic Approach
02PA4RZ Removal of External Heart Assist System from Heart, Percutaneous Endoscopic Approach
02PAX2Z Removal of Monitoring Device from Heart, External Approach
02PAX3Z Removal of Infusion Device from Heart, External Approach
02PAXDZ Removal of Intraluminal Device from Heart, External Approach
02PAXMZ Removal of Cardiac Lead from Heart, External Approach
HAC With a secondary diagnosis code of K68.11, T81.4XXA, T82.6XXA, T82.7XXA
02PY02Z Removal of Monitoring Device from Great Vessel, Open Approach
02PY03Z Removal of Infusion Device from Great Vessel, Open Approach
02PY07Z Removal of Autologous Tissue Substitute from Great Vessel, Open Approach
02PY08Z Removal of Zooplastic Tissue from Great Vessel, Open Approach
02PY0CZ Removal of Extraluminal Device from Great Vessel, Open Approach
02PY0DZ Removal of Intraluminal Device from Great Vessel, Open Approach
02PY0JZ Removal of Synthetic Substitute from Great Vessel, Open Approach
02PY0KZ Removal of Nonautologous Tissue Substitute from Great Vessel, Open Approach
02PY32Z Removal of Monitoring Device from Great Vessel, Percutaneous Approach
02PY33Z Removal of Infusion Device from Great Vessel, Percutaneous Approach
02PY37Z Removal of Autologous Tissue Substitute from Great Vessel, Percutaneous Approach
02PY38Z Removal of Zooplastic Tissue from Great Vessel, Percutaneous Approach
02PY3CZ Removal of Extraluminal Device from Great Vessel, Percutaneous Approach
02PY3DZ Removal of Intraluminal Device from Great Vessel, Percutaneous Approach
02PY3JZ Removal of Synthetic Substitute from Great Vessel, Percutaneous Approach
02PY3KZ Removal of Nonautologous Tissue Substitute from Great Vessel, Percutaneous Approach
02PY42Z Removal of Monitoring Device from Great Vessel, Percutaneous Endoscopic Approach
02PY43Z Removal of Infusion Device from Great Vessel, Percutaneous Endoscopic Approach
02PY47Z Removal of Autologous Tissue Substitute from Great Vessel, Percutaneous Endoscopic Approach
02PY48Z Removal of Zooplastic Tissue from Great Vessel, Percutaneous Endoscopic Approach
02PY4CZ Removal of Extraluminal Device from Great Vessel, Percutaneous Endoscopic Approach
02PY4DZ Removal of Intraluminal Device from Great Vessel, Percutaneous Endoscopic Approach
02PY4JZ Removal of Synthetic Substitute from Great Vessel, Percutaneous Endoscopic Approach
02PY4KZ Removal of Nonautologous Tissue Substitute from Great Vessel, Percutaneous Endoscopic Approach
02PYX2Z Removal of Monitoring Device from Great Vessel, External Approach
02PYX3Z Removal of Infusion Device from Great Vessel, External Approach
02PYXDZ Removal of Intraluminal Device from Great Vessel, External Approach

02Q – Heart and Great Vessels, Repair

For Repair of coronary arteries, Review Coding Guideline B4.4

02Q00ZZ Repair Coronary Artery, One Site, Open Approach
02Q03ZZ Repair Coronary Artery, One Site, Percutaneous Approach
02Q04ZZ Repair Coronary Artery, One Site, Percutaneous Endoscopic Approach
02Q10ZZ Repair Coronary Artery, Two Sites, Open Approach
02Q13ZZ Repair Coronary Artery, Two Sites, Percutaneous Approach
02Q14ZZ Repair Coronary Artery, Two Sites, Percutaneous Endoscopic Approach

02Q20ZZ Repair Coronary Artery, Three Sites, Open Approach
02Q23ZZ Repair Coronary Artery, Three Sites, Percutaneous Approach
02Q24ZZ Repair Coronary Artery, Three Sites, Percutaneous Endoscopic Approach
02Q30ZZ Repair Coronary Artery, Four or More Sites, Open Approach
02Q33ZZ Repair Coronary Artery, Four or More Sites, Percutaneous Approach
02Q34ZZ Repair Coronary Artery, Four or More Sites, Percutaneous Endoscopic Approach
02Q40ZZ Repair Coronary Vein, Open Approach
02Q43ZZ Repair Coronary Vein, Percutaneous Approach
02Q44ZZ Repair Coronary Vein, Percutaneous Endoscopic Approach
02Q50ZZ Repair Atrial Septum, Open Approach
02Q53ZZ Repair Atrial Septum, Percutaneous Approach
02Q54ZZ Repair Atrial Septum, Percutaneous Endoscopic Approach
02Q60ZZ Repair Right Atrium, Open Approach
02Q63ZZ Repair Right Atrium, Percutaneous Approach
02Q64ZZ Repair Right Atrium, Percutaneous Endoscopic Approach
02Q70ZZ Repair Left Atrium, Open Approach
02Q73ZZ Repair Left Atrium, Percutaneous Approach
02Q74ZZ Repair Left Atrium, Percutaneous Endoscopic Approach
02Q80ZZ Repair Conduction Mechanism, Open Approach
02Q83ZZ Repair Conduction Mechanism, Percutaneous Approach
02Q84ZZ Repair Conduction Mechanism, Percutaneous Endoscopic Approach
02Q90ZZ Repair Chordae Tendineae, Open Approach
02Q93ZZ Repair Chordae Tendineae, Percutaneous Approach
02Q94ZZ Repair Chordae Tendineae, Percutaneous Endoscopic Approach
02QA0ZZ Repair Heart, Open Approach
02QA3ZZ Repair Heart, Percutaneous Approach
02QA4ZZ Repair Heart, Percutaneous Endoscopic Approach
02QB0ZZ Repair Right Heart, Open Approach
02QB3ZZ Repair Right Heart, Percutaneous Approach
02QB4ZZ Repair Right Heart, Percutaneous Endoscopic Approach
02QC0ZZ Repair Left Heart, Open Approach
02QC3ZZ Repair Left Heart, Percutaneous Approach
02QC4ZZ Repair Left Heart, Percutaneous Endoscopic Approach
02QD0ZZ Repair Papillary Muscle, Open Approach
02QD3ZZ Repair Papillary Muscle, Percutaneous Approach
02QD4ZZ Repair Papillary Muscle, Percutaneous Endoscopic Approach
02QF0ZZ Repair Aortic Valve, Open Approach
02QF3ZZ Repair Aortic Valve, Percutaneous Approach
02QF4ZZ Repair Aortic Valve, Percutaneous Endoscopic Approach
02QG0ZZ Repair Mitral Valve, Open Approach
02QG3ZZ Repair Mitral Valve, Percutaneous Approach
02QG4ZZ Repair Mitral Valve, Percutaneous Endoscopic Approach
02QH0ZZ Repair Pulmonary Valve, Open Approach
02QH3ZZ Repair Pulmonary Valve, Percutaneous Approach
02QH4ZZ Repair Pulmonary Valve, Percutaneous Endoscopic Approach
02QJ0ZZ Repair Tricuspid Valve, Open Approach
02QJ3ZZ Repair Tricuspid Valve, Percutaneous Approach
02QJ4ZZ Repair Tricuspid Valve, Percutaneous Endoscopic Approach
02QK0ZZ Repair Right Ventricle, Open Approach
02QK3ZZ Repair Right Ventricle, Percutaneous Approach
02QK4ZZ Repair Right Ventricle, Percutaneous Endoscopic Approach
02QL0ZZ Repair Left Ventricle, Open Approach
02QL3ZZ Repair Left Ventricle, Percutaneous Approach
02QL4ZZ Repair Left Ventricle, Percutaneous Endoscopic Approach
02QM0ZZ Repair Ventricular Septum, Open Approach
02QM3ZZ Repair Ventricular Septum, Percutaneous Approach
02QM4ZZ Repair Ventricular Septum, Percutaneous Endoscopic Approach
02QN0ZZ Repair Pericardium, Open Approach
02QN3ZZ Repair Pericardium, Percutaneous Approach
02QN4ZZ Repair Pericardium, Percutaneous Endoscopic Approach
02QP0ZZ Repair Pulmonary Trunk, Open Approach
02QP3ZZ Repair Pulmonary Trunk, Percutaneous Approach
02QP4ZZ Repair Pulmonary Trunk, Percutaneous Endoscopic Approach
02QQ0ZZ Repair Right Pulmonary Artery, Open Approach
02QQ3ZZ Repair Right Pulmonary Artery, Percutaneous Approach
02QQ4ZZ Repair Right Pulmonary Artery, Percutaneous Endoscopic Approach
02QR0ZZ Repair Left Pulmonary Artery, Open Approach
02QR3ZZ Repair Left Pulmonary Artery, Percutaneous Approach
02QR4ZZ Repair Left Pulmonary Artery, Percutaneous Endoscopic Approach
02QS0ZZ Repair Right Pulmonary Vein, Open Approach
02QS3ZZ Repair Right Pulmonary Vein, Percutaneous Approach
02QS4ZZ Repair Right Pulmonary Vein, Percutaneous Endoscopic Approach
02QT0ZZ Repair Left Pulmonary Vein, Open Approach
02QT3ZZ Repair Left Pulmonary Vein, Percutaneous Approach
02QT4ZZ Repair Left Pulmonary Vein, Percutaneous Endoscopic Approach
02QV0ZZ Repair Superior Vena Cava, Open Approach
02QV3ZZ Repair Superior Vena Cava, Percutaneous Approach
02QV4ZZ Repair Superior Vena Cava, Percutaneous Endoscopic Approach
02QW0ZZ Repair Thoracic Aorta, Open Approach
02QW3ZZ Repair Thoracic Aorta, Percutaneous Approach
02QW4ZZ Repair Thoracic Aorta, Percutaneous Endoscopic Approach

02R – Heart and Great Vessels, Replacement

02R507Z Replacement of Atrial Septum with Autologous Tissue Substitute, Open Approach
02R508Z Replacement of Atrial Septum with Zooplastic Tissue, Open Approach
02R50JZ Replacement of Atrial Septum with Synthetic Substitute, Open Approach
02R50KZ Replacement of Atrial Septum with Nonautologous Tissue Substitute, Open Approach
02R547Z Replacement of Atrial Septum with Autologous Tissue Substitute, Percutaneous Endoscopic Approach
02R548Z Replacement of Atrial Septum with Zooplastic Tissue, Percutaneous Endoscopic Approach
02R54JZ Replacement of Atrial Septum with Synthetic Substitute, Percutaneous Endoscopic Approach
02R54KZ Replacement of Atrial Septum with Nonautologous Tissue Substitute, Percutaneous Endoscopic Approach
02R607Z Replacement of Right Atrium with Autologous Tissue Substitute, Open Approach
02R608Z Replacement of Right Atrium with Zooplastic Tissue, Open Approach
02R60JZ Replacement of Right Atrium with Synthetic Substitute, Open Approach
02R60KZ Replacement of Right Atrium with Nonautologous Tissue Substitute, Open Approach
02R647Z Replacement of Right Atrium with Autologous Tissue Substitute, Percutaneous Endoscopic Approach
02R648Z Replacement of Right Atrium with Zooplastic Tissue, Percutaneous Endoscopic Approach
02R64JZ Replacement of Right Atrium with Synthetic Substitute, Percutaneous Endoscopic Approach
02R64KZ Replacement of Right Atrium with Nonautologous Tissue Substitute, Percutaneous Endoscopic Approach
02R707Z Replacement of Left Atrium with Autologous Tissue Substitute, Open Approach
02R708Z Replacement of Left Atrium with Zooplastic Tissue, Open Approach
02R70JZ Replacement of Left Atrium with Synthetic Substitute, Open Approach
02R70KZ Replacement of Left Atrium with Nonautologous Tissue Substitute, Open Approach
02R747Z Replacement of Left Atrium with Autologous Tissue Substitute, Percutaneous Endoscopic Approach
02R748Z Replacement of Left Atrium with Zooplastic Tissue, Percutaneous Endoscopic Approach
02R74JZ Replacement of Left Atrium with Synthetic Substitute, Percutaneous Endoscopic Approach
02R74KZ Replacement of Left Atrium with Nonautologous Tissue Substitute, Percutaneous Endoscopic Approach
02R907Z Replacement of Chordae Tendineae with Autologous Tissue Substitute, Open Approach
02R908Z Replacement of Chordae Tendineae with Zooplastic Tissue, Open Approach
02R90JZ Replacement of Chordae Tendineae with Synthetic Substitute, Open Approach
02R90KZ Replacement of Chordae Tendineae with Nonautologous Tissue Substitute, Open Approach
02R947Z Replacement of Chordae Tendineae with Autologous Tissue Substitute, Percutaneous Endoscopic Approach

02R948Z Replacement of Chordae Tendineae with Zooplastic Tissue, Percutaneous Endoscopic Approach

02R94JZ Replacement of Chordae Tendineae with Synthetic Substitute, Percutaneous Endoscopic Approach

02R94KZ Replacement of Chordae Tendineae with Nonautologous Tissue Substitute, Percutaneous Endoscopic Approach

02RD07Z Replacement of Papillary Muscle with Autologous Tissue Substitute, Open Approach

02RD08Z Replacement of Papillary Muscle with Zooplastic Tissue, Open Approach

02RD0JZ Replacement of Papillary Muscle with Synthetic Substitute, Open Approach

02RD0KZ Replacement of Papillary Muscle with Nonautologous Tissue Substitute, Open Approach

02RD47Z Replacement of Papillary Muscle with Autologous Tissue Substitute, Percutaneous Endoscopic Approach

02RD48Z Replacement of Papillary Muscle with Zooplastic Tissue, Percutaneous Endoscopic Approach

02RD4JZ Replacement of Papillary Muscle with Synthetic Substitute, Percutaneous Endoscopic Approach

02RD4KZ Replacement of Papillary Muscle with Nonautologous Tissue Substitute, Percutaneous Endoscopic Approach

02RF07Z Replacement of Aortic Valve with Autologous Tissue Substitute, Open Approach

02RF08Z Replacement of Aortic Valve with Zooplastic Tissue, Open Approach

02RF0JZ Replacement of Aortic Valve with Synthetic Substitute, Open Approach

02RF0KZ Replacement of Aortic Valve with Nonautologous Tissue Substitute, Open Approach

02RF37H Replacement of Aortic Valve with Autologous Tissue Substitute, Transapical, Percutaneous Approach

02RF37Z Replacement of Aortic Valve with Autologous Tissue Substitute, Percutaneous Approach

02RF38H Replacement of Aortic Valve with Zooplastic Tissue, Transapical, Percutaneous Approach

02RF38Z Replacement of Aortic Valve with Zooplastic Tissue, Percutaneous Approach

02RF3JH Replacement of Aortic Valve with Synthetic Substitute, Transapical, Percutaneous Approach

02RF3JZ Replacement of Aortic Valve with Synthetic Substitute, Percutaneous Approach

02RF3KH Replacement of Aortic Valve with Nonautologous Tissue Substitute, Transapical, Percutaneous Approach

02RF3KZ Replacement of Aortic Valve with Nonautologous Tissue Substitute, Percutaneous Approach

02RF47Z Replacement of Aortic Valve with Autologous Tissue Substitute, Percutaneous Endoscopic Approach

02RF48Z Replacement of Aortic Valve with Zooplastic Tissue, Percutaneous Endoscopic Approach

02RF4JZ Replacement of Aortic Valve with Synthetic Substitute, Percutaneous Endoscopic Approach

02RF4KZ Replacement of Aortic Valve with Nonautologous Tissue Substitute, Percutaneous Endoscopic Approach

02RG07Z Replacement of Mitral Valve with Autologous Tissue Substitute, Open Approach

02RG08Z Replacement of Mitral Valve with Zooplastic Tissue, Open Approach

02RG0JZ Replacement of Mitral Valve with Synthetic Substitute, Open Approach

02RG0KZ Replacement of Mitral Valve with Nonautologous Tissue Substitute, Open Approach

02RG37H Replacement of Mitral Valve with Autologous Tissue Substitute, Transapical, Percutaneous Approach

02RG37Z Replacement of Mitral Valve with Autologous Tissue Substitute, Percutaneous Approach

02RG38H Replacement of Mitral Valve with Zooplastic Tissue, Transapical, Percutaneous Approach

02RG38Z Replacement of Mitral Valve with Zooplastic Tissue, Percutaneous Approach

02RG3JH Replacement of Mitral Valve with Synthetic Substitute, Transapical, Percutaneous Approach

02RG3JZ Replacement of Mitral Valve with Synthetic Substitute, Percutaneous Approach

02RG3KH Replacement of Mitral Valve with Nonautologous Tissue Substitute, Transapical, Percutaneous Approach

02RG3KZ Replacement of Mitral Valve with Nonautologous Tissue Substitute, Percutaneous Approach

02RG47Z Replacement of Mitral Valve with Autologous Tissue Substitute, Percutaneous Endoscopic Approach

02RG48Z Replacement of Mitral Valve with Zooplastic Tissue, Percutaneous Endoscopic Approach

02RG4JZ Replacement of Mitral Valve with Synthetic Substitute, Percutaneous Endoscopic Approach

02RG4KZ Replacement of Mitral Valve with Nonautologous Tissue Substitute, Percutaneous Endoscopic Approach

02RH07Z Replacement of Pulmonary Valve with Autologous Tissue Substitute, Open Approach

02RH08Z Replacement of Pulmonary Valve with Zooplastic Tissue, Open Approach

02RH0JZ Replacement of Pulmonary Valve with Synthetic Substitute, Open Approach

02RH0KZ Replacement of Pulmonary Valve with Nonautologous Tissue Substitute, Open Approach

02RH37H Replacement of Pulmonary Valve with Autologous Tissue Substitute, Transapical, Percutaneous Approach

02RH37Z Replacement of Pulmonary Valve with Autologous Tissue Substitute, Percutaneous Approach

02RH38H Replacement of Pulmonary Valve with Zooplastic Tissue, Transapical, Percutaneous Approach

02RH38Z Replacement of Pulmonary Valve with Zooplastic Tissue, Percutaneous Approach

02RH3JH Replacement of Pulmonary Valve with Synthetic Substitute, Transapical, Percutaneous Approach

02RH3JZ Replacement of Pulmonary Valve with Synthetic Substitute, Percutaneous Approach

02RH3KH Replacement of Pulmonary Valve with Nonautologous Tissue Substitute, Transapical, Percutaneous Approach

02RH3KZ Replacement of Pulmonary Valve with Nonautologous Tissue Substitute, Percutaneous Approach

02RH47Z Replacement of Pulmonary Valve with Autologous Tissue Substitute, Percutaneous Endoscopic Approach

02RH48Z Replacement of Pulmonary Valve with Zooplastic Tissue, Percutaneous Endoscopic Approach

02RH4JZ Replacement of Pulmonary Valve with Synthetic Substitute, Percutaneous Endoscopic Approach

02RH4KZ Replacement of Pulmonary Valve with Nonautologous Tissue Substitute, Percutaneous Endoscopic Approach

02RJ07Z Replacement of Tricuspid Valve with Autologous Tissue Substitute, Open Approach

02RJ08Z Replacement of Tricuspid Valve with Zooplastic Tissue, Open Approach

02RJ0JZ Replacement of Tricuspid Valve with Synthetic Substitute, Open Approach

02RJ0KZ Replacement of Tricuspid Valve with Nonautologous Tissue Substitute, Open Approach

02RJ47Z Replacement of Tricuspid Valve with Autologous Tissue Substitute, Percutaneous Endoscopic Approach

02RJ48Z Replacement of Tricuspid Valve with Zooplastic Tissue, Percutaneous Endoscopic Approach

02RJ4JZ Replacement of Tricuspid Valve with Synthetic Substitute, Percutaneous Endoscopic Approach

02RJ4KZ Replacement of Tricuspid Valve with Nonautologous Tissue Substitute, Percutaneous Endoscopic Approach

02RK07Z Replacement of Right Ventricle with Autologous Tissue Substitute, Open Approach

02RK08Z Replacement of Right Ventricle with Zooplastic Tissue, Open Approach

02RK0JZ Replacement of Right Ventricle with Synthetic Substitute, Open Approach
When reported with 02RL0JZ and diagnosis code Z00.6

02RK0KZ Replacement of Right Ventricle with Nonautologous Tissue Substitute, Open Approach

02RK47Z Replacement of Right Ventricle with Autologous Tissue Substitute, Percutaneous Endoscopic Approach

02RK48Z Replacement of Right Ventricle with Zooplastic Tissue, Percutaneous Endoscopic Approach

02RK4JZ Replacement of Right Ventricle with Synthetic Substitute, Percutaneous Endoscopic Approach

02RK4KZ Replacement of Right Ventricle with Nonautologous Tissue Substitute, Percutaneous Endoscopic Approach

02RL07Z Replacement of Left Ventricle with Autologous Tissue Substitute, Open Approach

02RL08Z Replacement of Left Ventricle with Zooplastic Tissue, Open Approach

02RL0JZ Replacement of Left Ventricle with Synthetic Substitute, Open Approach
When reported with 02RK0JZ and diagnosis code Z00.6

02RL0KZ Replacement of Left Ventricle with Nonautologous Tissue Substitute, Open Approach

02RL47Z Replacement of Left Ventricle with Autologous Tissue Substitute, Percutaneous Endoscopic Approach

02RL48Z Replacement of Left Ventricle with Zooplastic Tissue, Percutaneous Endoscopic Approach

02RL4JZ Replacement of Left Ventricle with Synthetic Substitute, Percutaneous Endoscopic Approach
02RL4KZ Replacement of Left Ventricle with Nonautologous Tissue Substitute, Percutaneous Endoscopic Approach
02RM07Z Replacement of Ventricular Septum with Autologous Tissue Substitute, Open Approach
02RM08Z Replacement of Ventricular Septum with Zooplastic Tissue, Open Approach
02RM0JZ Replacement of Ventricular Septum with Synthetic Substitute, Open Approach
02RM0KZ Replacement of Ventricular Septum with Nonautologous Tissue Substitute, Open Approach
02RM47Z Replacement of Ventricular Septum with Autologous Tissue Substitute, Percutaneous Endoscopic Approach
02RM48Z Replacement of Ventricular Septum with Zooplastic Tissue, Percutaneous Endoscopic Approach
02RM4JZ Replacement of Ventricular Septum with Synthetic Substitute, Percutaneous Endoscopic Approach
02RM4KZ Replacement of Ventricular Septum with Nonautologous Tissue Substitute, Percutaneous Endoscopic Approach
02RN07Z Replacement of Pericardium with Autologous Tissue Substitute, Open Approach
02RN08Z Replacement of Pericardium with Zooplastic Tissue, Open Approach
02RN0JZ Replacement of Pericardium with Synthetic Substitute, Open Approach
02RN0KZ Replacement of Pericardium with Nonautologous Tissue Substitute, Open Approach
02RN47Z Replacement of Pericardium with Autologous Tissue Substitute, Percutaneous Endoscopic Approach
02RN48Z Replacement of Pericardium with Zooplastic Tissue, Percutaneous Endoscopic Approach
02RN4JZ Replacement of Pericardium with Synthetic Substitute, Percutaneous Endoscopic Approach
02RN4KZ Replacement of Pericardium with Nonautologous Tissue Substitute, Percutaneous Endoscopic Approach
02RP07Z Replacement of Pulmonary Trunk with Autologous Tissue Substitute, Open Approach
02RP08Z Replacement of Pulmonary Trunk with Zooplastic Tissue, Open Approach
02RP0JZ Replacement of Pulmonary Trunk with Synthetic Substitute, Open Approach
02RP0KZ Replacement of Pulmonary Trunk with Nonautologous Tissue Substitute, Open Approach
02RP47Z Replacement of Pulmonary Trunk with Autologous Tissue Substitute, Percutaneous Endoscopic Approach
02RP48Z Replacement of Pulmonary Trunk with Zooplastic Tissue, Percutaneous Endoscopic Approach
02RP4JZ Replacement of Pulmonary Trunk with Synthetic Substitute, Percutaneous Endoscopic Approach
02RP4KZ Replacement of Pulmonary Trunk with Nonautologous Tissue Substitute, Percutaneous Endoscopic Approach
02RQ07Z Replacement of Right Pulmonary Artery with Autologous Tissue Substitute, Open Approach
02RQ08Z Replacement of Right Pulmonary Artery with Zooplastic Tissue, Open Approach
02RQ0JZ Replacement of Right Pulmonary Artery with Synthetic Substitute, Open Approach
02RQ0KZ Replacement of Right Pulmonary Artery with Nonautologous Tissue Substitute, Open Approach
02RQ47Z Replacement of Right Pulmonary Artery with Autologous Tissue Substitute, Percutaneous Endoscopic Approach
02RQ48Z Replacement of Right Pulmonary Artery with Zooplastic Tissue, Percutaneous Endoscopic Approach
02RQ4JZ Replacement of Right Pulmonary Artery with Synthetic Substitute, Percutaneous Endoscopic Approach
02RQ4KZ Replacement of Right Pulmonary Artery with Nonautologous Tissue Substitute, Percutaneous Endoscopic Approach
02RR07Z Replacement of Left Pulmonary Artery with Autologous Tissue Substitute, Open Approach
02RR08Z Replacement of Left Pulmonary Artery with Zooplastic Tissue, Open Approach
02RR0JZ Replacement of Left Pulmonary Artery with Synthetic Substitute, Open Approach
02RR0KZ Replacement of Left Pulmonary Artery with Nonautologous Tissue Substitute, Open Approach
02RR47Z Replacement of Left Pulmonary Artery with Autologous Tissue Substitute, Percutaneous Endoscopic Approach
02RR48Z Replacement of Left Pulmonary Artery with Zooplastic Tissue, Percutaneous Endoscopic Approach
02RR4JZ Replacement of Left Pulmonary Artery with Synthetic Substitute, Percutaneous Endoscopic Approach
02RR4KZ Replacement of Left Pulmonary Artery with Nonautologous Tissue Substitute, Percutaneous Endoscopic Approach
02RS07Z Replacement of Right Pulmonary Vein with Autologous Tissue Substitute, Open Approach
02RS08Z Replacement of Right Pulmonary Vein with Zooplastic Tissue, Open Approach
02RS0JZ Replacement of Right Pulmonary Vein with Synthetic Substitute, Open Approach
02RS0KZ Replacement of Right Pulmonary Vein with Nonautologous Tissue Substitute, Open Approach
02RS47Z Replacement of Right Pulmonary Vein with Autologous Tissue Substitute, Percutaneous Endoscopic Approach
02RS48Z Replacement of Right Pulmonary Vein with Zooplastic Tissue, Percutaneous Endoscopic Approach
02RS4JZ Replacement of Right Pulmonary Vein with Synthetic Substitute, Percutaneous Endoscopic Approach
02RS4KZ Replacement of Right Pulmonary Vein with Nonautologous Tissue Substitute, Percutaneous Endoscopic Approach
02RT07Z Replacement of Left Pulmonary Vein with Autologous Tissue Substitute, Open Approach
02RT08Z Replacement of Left Pulmonary Vein with Zooplastic Tissue, Open Approach
02RT0JZ Replacement of Left Pulmonary Vein with Synthetic Substitute, Open Approach
02RT0KZ Replacement of Left Pulmonary Vein with Nonautologous Tissue Substitute, Open Approach
02RT47Z Replacement of Left Pulmonary Vein with Autologous Tissue Substitute, Percutaneous Endoscopic Approach
02RT48Z Replacement of Left Pulmonary Vein with Zooplastic Tissue, Percutaneous Endoscopic Approach
02RT4JZ Replacement of Left Pulmonary Vein with Synthetic Substitute, Percutaneous Endoscopic Approach
02RT4KZ Replacement of Left Pulmonary Vein with Nonautologous Tissue Substitute, Percutaneous Endoscopic Approach
02RV07Z Replacement of Superior Vena Cava with Autologous Tissue Substitute, Open Approach
02RV08Z Replacement of Superior Vena Cava with Zooplastic Tissue, Open Approach
02RV0JZ Replacement of Superior Vena Cava with Synthetic Substitute, Open Approach
02RV0KZ Replacement of Superior Vena Cava with Nonautologous Tissue Substitute, Open Approach
02RV47Z Replacement of Superior Vena Cava with Autologous Tissue Substitute, Percutaneous Endoscopic Approach
02RV48Z Replacement of Superior Vena Cava with Zooplastic Tissue, Percutaneous Endoscopic Approach
02RV4JZ Replacement of Superior Vena Cava with Synthetic Substitute, Percutaneous Endoscopic Approach
02RV4KZ Replacement of Superior Vena Cava with Nonautologous Tissue Substitute, Percutaneous Endoscopic Approach
02RW07Z Replacement of Thoracic Aorta with Autologous Tissue Substitute, Open Approach
02RW08Z Replacement of Thoracic Aorta with Zooplastic Tissue, Open Approach
02RW0JZ Replacement of Thoracic Aorta with Synthetic Substitute, Open Approach
02RW0KZ Replacement of Thoracic Aorta with Nonautologous Tissue Substitute, Open Approach
AHA CC: 1Q, 2014, 10-11
02RW47Z Replacement of Thoracic Aorta with Autologous Tissue Substitute, Percutaneous Endoscopic Approach
02RW48Z Replacement of Thoracic Aorta with Zooplastic Tissue, Percutaneous Endoscopic Approach
02RW4JZ Replacement of Thoracic Aorta with Synthetic Substitute, Percutaneous Endoscopic Approach
02RW4KZ Replacement of Thoracic Aorta with Nonautologous Tissue Substitute, Percutaneous Endoscopic Approach

02S – Heart and Great Vessels, Reposition

02SP0ZZ Reposition Pulmonary Trunk, Open Approach
02SQ0ZZ Reposition Right Pulmonary Artery, Open Approach
02SR0ZZ Reposition Left Pulmonary Artery, Open Approach
02SS0ZZ Reposition Right Pulmonary Vein, Open Approach
02ST0ZZ Reposition Left Pulmonary Vein, Open Approach
02SV0ZZ Reposition Superior Vena Cava, Open Approach
02SW0ZZ Reposition Thoracic Aorta, Open Approach

02T – Heart and Great Vessels, Resection

Review Coding Guideline B3.8

02T50ZZ Resection of Atrial Septum, Open Approach
02T53ZZ Resection of Atrial Septum, Percutaneous Approach
02T54ZZ Resection of Atrial Septum, Percutaneous Endoscopic Approach
02T80ZZ Resection of Conduction Mechanism, Open Approach
02T83ZZ Resection of Conduction Mechanism, Percutaneous Approach
02T84ZZ Resection of Conduction Mechanism, Percutaneous Endoscopic Approach
02T90ZZ Resection of Chordae Tendineae, Open Approach
02T93ZZ Resection of Chordae Tendineae, Percutaneous Approach
02T94ZZ Resection of Chordae Tendineae, Percutaneous Endoscopic Approach
02TD0ZZ Resection of Papillary Muscle, Open Approach
02TD3ZZ Resection of Papillary Muscle, Percutaneous Approach
02TD4ZZ Resection of Papillary Muscle, Percutaneous Endoscopic Approach
02TH0ZZ Resection of Pulmonary Valve, Open Approach
02TH3ZZ Resection of Pulmonary Valve, Percutaneous Approach
02TH4ZZ Resection of Pulmonary Valve, Percutaneous Endoscopic Approach
02TM0ZZ Resection of Ventricular Septum, Open Approach
02TM3ZZ Resection of Ventricular Septum, Percutaneous Approach
02TM4ZZ Resection of Ventricular Septum, Percutaneous Endoscopic Approach
02TN0ZZ Resection of Pericardium, Open Approach
02TN3ZZ Resection of Pericardium, Percutaneous Approach
02TN4ZZ Resection of Pericardium, Percutaneous Endoscopic Approach

02U – Heart and Great Vessels, Supplement

02U507Z Supplement Atrial Septum with Autologous Tissue Substitute, Open Approach
02U508Z Supplement Atrial Septum with Zooplastic Tissue, Open Approach
02U50JZ Supplement Atrial Septum with Synthetic Substitute, Open Approach
02U50KZ Supplement Atrial Septum with Nonautologous Tissue Substitute, Open Approach
02U537Z Supplement Atrial Septum with Autologous Tissue Substitute, Percutaneous Approach
02U538Z Supplement Atrial Septum with Zooplastic Tissue, Percutaneous Approach
02U53JZ Supplement Atrial Septum with Synthetic Substitute, Percutaneous Approach
02U53KZ Supplement Atrial Septum with Nonautologous Tissue Substitute, Percutaneous Approach
02U547Z Supplement Atrial Septum with Autologous Tissue Substitute, Percutaneous Endoscopic Approach
02U548Z Supplement Atrial Septum with Zooplastic Tissue, Percutaneous Endoscopic Approach
02U54JZ Supplement Atrial Septum with Synthetic Substitute, Percutaneous Endoscopic Approach
02U54KZ Supplement Atrial Septum with Nonautologous Tissue Substitute, Percutaneous Endoscopic Approach
02U607Z Supplement Right Atrium with Autologous Tissue Substitute, Open Approach
02U608Z Supplement Right Atrium with Zooplastic Tissue, Open Approach
02U60JZ Supplement Right Atrium with Synthetic Substitute, Open Approach
02U60KZ Supplement Right Atrium with Nonautologous Tissue Substitute, Open Approach
02U637Z Supplement Right Atrium with Autologous Tissue Substitute, Percutaneous Approach
02U638Z Supplement Right Atrium with Zooplastic Tissue, Percutaneous Approach
02U63JZ Supplement Right Atrium with Synthetic Substitute, Percutaneous Approach
02U63KZ Supplement Right Atrium with Nonautologous Tissue Substitute, Percutaneous Approach
02U647Z Supplement Right Atrium with Autologous Tissue Substitute, Percutaneous Endoscopic Approach
02U648Z Supplement Right Atrium with Zooplastic Tissue, Percutaneous Endoscopic Approach
02U64JZ Supplement Right Atrium with Synthetic Substitute, Percutaneous Endoscopic Approach
02U64KZ Supplement Right Atrium with Nonautologous Tissue Substitute, Percutaneous Endoscopic Approach
02U707Z Supplement Left Atrium with Autologous Tissue Substitute, Open Approach
02U708Z Supplement Left Atrium with Zooplastic Tissue, Open Approach
02U70JZ Supplement Left Atrium with Synthetic Substitute, Open Approach
02U70KZ Supplement Left Atrium with Nonautologous Tissue Substitute, Open Approach
02U737Z Supplement Left Atrium with Autologous Tissue Substitute, Percutaneous Approach
02U738Z Supplement Left Atrium with Zooplastic Tissue, Percutaneous Approach
● **02U73JZ** Supplement Left Atrium with Synthetic Substitute, Percutaneous Approach
02U73KZ Supplement Left Atrium with Nonautologous Tissue Substitute, Percutaneous Approach
02U747Z Supplement Left Atrium with Autologous Tissue Substitute, Percutaneous Endoscopic Approach
02U748Z Supplement Left Atrium with Zooplastic Tissue, Percutaneous Endoscopic Approach
● **02U74JZ** Supplement Left Atrium with Synthetic Substitute, Percutaneous Endoscopic Approach
02U74KZ Supplement Left Atrium with Nonautologous Tissue Substitute, Percutaneous Endoscopic Approach
02U907Z Supplement Chordae Tendineae with Autologous Tissue Substitute, Open Approach
02U908Z Supplement Chordae Tendineae with Zooplastic Tissue, Open Approach
02U90JZ Supplement Chordae Tendineae with Synthetic Substitute, Open Approach
02U90KZ Supplement Chordae Tendineae with Nonautologous Tissue Substitute, Open Approach
02U937Z Supplement Chordae Tendineae with Autologous Tissue Substitute, Percutaneous Approach
02U938Z Supplement Chordae Tendineae with Zooplastic Tissue, Percutaneous Approach
02U93JZ Supplement Chordae Tendineae with Synthetic Substitute, Percutaneous Approach
02U93KZ Supplement Chordae Tendineae with Nonautologous Tissue Substitute, Percutaneous Approach
02U947Z Supplement Chordae Tendineae with Autologous Tissue Substitute, Percutaneous Endoscopic Approach
02U948Z Supplement Chordae Tendineae with Zooplastic Tissue, Percutaneous Endoscopic Approach
02U94JZ Supplement Chordae Tendineae with Synthetic Substitute, Percutaneous Endoscopic Approach
02U94KZ Supplement Chordae Tendineae with Nonautologous Tissue Substitute, Percutaneous Endoscopic Approach
02UA07Z Supplement Heart with Autologous Tissue Substitute, Open Approach
02UA08Z Supplement Heart with Zooplastic Tissue, Open Approach
02UA0JZ Supplement Heart with Synthetic Substitute, Open Approach
02UA0KZ Supplement Heart with Nonautologous Tissue Substitute, Open Approach
02UA37Z Supplement Heart with Autologous Tissue Substitute, Percutaneous Approach
02UA38Z Supplement Heart with Zooplastic Tissue, Percutaneous Approach
02UA3JZ Supplement Heart with Synthetic Substitute, Percutaneous Approach
02UA3KZ Supplement Heart with Nonautologous Tissue Substitute, Percutaneous Approach
02UA47Z Supplement Heart with Autologous Tissue Substitute, Percutaneous Endoscopic Approach
02UA48Z Supplement Heart with Zooplastic Tissue, Percutaneous Endoscopic Approach
02UA4JZ Supplement Heart with Synthetic Substitute, Percutaneous Endoscopic Approach
02UA4KZ Supplement Heart with Nonautologous Tissue Substitute, Percutaneous Endoscopic Approach
02UD07Z Supplement Papillary Muscle with Autologous Tissue Substitute, Open Approach
02UD08Z Supplement Papillary Muscle with Zooplastic Tissue, Open Approach
02UD0JZ Supplement Papillary Muscle with Synthetic Substitute, Open Approach
02UD0KZ Supplement Papillary Muscle with Nonautologous Tissue Substitute, Open Approach
02UD37Z Supplement Papillary Muscle with Autologous Tissue Substitute, Percutaneous Approach
02UD38Z Supplement Papillary Muscle with Zooplastic Tissue, Percutaneous Approach
02UD3JZ Supplement Papillary Muscle with Synthetic Substitute, Percutaneous Approach

02UD3KZ Supplement Papillary Muscle with Nonautologous Tissue Substitute, Percutaneous Approach
02UD47Z Supplement Papillary Muscle with Autologous Tissue Substitute, Percutaneous Endoscopic Approach
02UD48Z Supplement Papillary Muscle with Zooplastic Tissue, Percutaneous Endoscopic Approach
02UD4JZ Supplement Papillary Muscle with Synthetic Substitute, Percutaneous Endoscopic Approach
02UD4KZ Supplement Papillary Muscle with Nonautologous Tissue Substitute, Percutaneous Endoscopic Approach
02UF07Z Supplement Aortic Valve with Autologous Tissue Substitute, Open Approach
02UF08Z Supplement Aortic Valve with Zooplastic Tissue, Open Approach
02UF0JZ Supplement Aortic Valve with Synthetic Substitute, Open Approach
02UF0KZ Supplement Aortic Valve with Nonautologous Tissue Substitute, Open Approach
02UF37Z Supplement Aortic Valve with Autologous Tissue Substitute, Percutaneous Approach
02UF38Z Supplement Aortic Valve with Zooplastic Tissue, Percutaneous Approach
02UF3JZ Supplement Aortic Valve with Synthetic Substitute, Percutaneous Approach
02UF3KZ Supplement Aortic Valve with Nonautologous Tissue Substitute, Percutaneous Approach
02UF47Z Supplement Aortic Valve with Autologous Tissue Substitute, Percutaneous Endoscopic Approach
02UF48Z Supplement Aortic Valve with Zooplastic Tissue, Percutaneous Endoscopic Approach
02UF4JZ Supplement Aortic Valve with Synthetic Substitute, Percutaneous Endoscopic Approach
02UF4KZ Supplement Aortic Valve with Nonautologous Tissue Substitute, Percutaneous Endoscopic Approach
02UG07Z Supplement Mitral Valve with Autologous Tissue Substitute, Open Approach
02UG08Z Supplement Mitral Valve with Zooplastic Tissue, Open Approach
02UG0JZ Supplement Mitral Valve with Synthetic Substitute, Open Approach
02UG0KZ Supplement Mitral Valve with Nonautologous Tissue Substitute, Open Approach
02UG37Z Supplement Mitral Valve with Autologous Tissue Substitute, Percutaneous Approach
02UG38Z Supplement Mitral Valve with Zooplastic Tissue, Percutaneous Approach
02UG3JZ Supplement Mitral Valve with Synthetic Substitute, Percutaneous Approach
02UG3KZ Supplement Mitral Valve with Nonautologous Tissue Substitute, Percutaneous Approach
02UG47Z Supplement Mitral Valve with Autologous Tissue Substitute, Percutaneous Endoscopic Approach
02UG48Z Supplement Mitral Valve with Zooplastic Tissue, Percutaneous Endoscopic Approach
02UG4JZ Supplement Mitral Valve with Synthetic Substitute, Percutaneous Endoscopic Approach
02UG4KZ Supplement Mitral Valve with Nonautologous Tissue Substitute, Percutaneous Endoscopic Approach
02UH07Z Supplement Pulmonary Valve with Autologous Tissue Substitute, Open Approach
02UH08Z Supplement Pulmonary Valve with Zooplastic Tissue, Open Approach
02UH0JZ Supplement Pulmonary Valve with Synthetic Substitute, Open Approach
02UH0KZ Supplement Pulmonary Valve with Nonautologous Tissue Substitute, Open Approach
02UH37Z Supplement Pulmonary Valve with Autologous Tissue Substitute, Percutaneous Approach
02UH38Z Supplement Pulmonary Valve with Zooplastic Tissue, Percutaneous Approach
02UH3JZ Supplement Pulmonary Valve with Synthetic Substitute, Percutaneous Approach
02UH3KZ Supplement Pulmonary Valve with Nonautologous Tissue Substitute, Percutaneous Approach
02UH47Z Supplement Pulmonary Valve with Autologous Tissue Substitute, Percutaneous Endoscopic Approach
02UH48Z Supplement Pulmonary Valve with Zooplastic Tissue, Percutaneous Endoscopic Approach
02UH4JZ Supplement Pulmonary Valve with Synthetic Substitute, Percutaneous Endoscopic Approach
02UH4KZ Supplement Pulmonary Valve with Nonautologous Tissue Substitute, Percutaneous Endoscopic Approach
02UJ07Z Supplement Tricuspid Valve with Autologous Tissue Substitute, Open Approach
02UJ08Z Supplement Tricuspid Valve with Zooplastic Tissue, Open Approach
02UJ0JZ Supplement Tricuspid Valve with Synthetic Substitute, Open Approach
02UJ0KZ Supplement Tricuspid Valve with Nonautologous Tissue Substitute, Open Approach
02UJ37Z Supplement Tricuspid Valve with Autologous Tissue Substitute, Percutaneous Approach
02UJ38Z Supplement Tricuspid Valve with Zooplastic Tissue, Percutaneous Approach
02UJ3JZ Supplement Tricuspid Valve with Synthetic Substitute, Percutaneous Approach
02UJ3KZ Supplement Tricuspid Valve with Nonautologous Tissue Substitute, Percutaneous Approach
02UJ47Z Supplement Tricuspid Valve with Autologous Tissue Substitute, Percutaneous Endoscopic Approach
02UJ48Z Supplement Tricuspid Valve with Zooplastic Tissue, Percutaneous Endoscopic Approach
02UJ4JZ Supplement Tricuspid Valve with Synthetic Substitute, Percutaneous Endoscopic Approach
02UJ4KZ Supplement Tricuspid Valve with Nonautologous Tissue Substitute, Percutaneous Endoscopic Approach
02UK07Z Supplement Right Ventricle with Autologous Tissue Substitute, Open Approach
02UK08Z Supplement Right Ventricle with Zooplastic Tissue, Open Approach
02UK0JZ Supplement Right Ventricle with Synthetic Substitute, Open Approach
02UK0KZ Supplement Right Ventricle with Nonautologous Tissue Substitute, Open Approach
02UK37Z Supplement Right Ventricle with Autologous Tissue Substitute, Percutaneous Approach
02UK38Z Supplement Right Ventricle with Zooplastic Tissue, Percutaneous Approach
02UK3JZ Supplement Right Ventricle with Synthetic Substitute, Percutaneous Approach
02UK3KZ Supplement Right Ventricle with Nonautologous Tissue Substitute, Percutaneous Approach
02UK47Z Supplement Right Ventricle with Autologous Tissue Substitute, Percutaneous Endoscopic Approach
02UK48Z Supplement Right Ventricle with Zooplastic Tissue, Percutaneous Endoscopic Approach
02UK4JZ Supplement Right Ventricle with Synthetic Substitute, Percutaneous Endoscopic Approach
02UK4KZ Supplement Right Ventricle with Nonautologous Tissue Substitute, Percutaneous Endoscopic Approach
02UL07Z Supplement Left Ventricle with Autologous Tissue Substitute, Open Approach
02UL08Z Supplement Left Ventricle with Zooplastic Tissue, Open Approach
02UL0JZ Supplement Left Ventricle with Synthetic Substitute, Open Approach
02UL0KZ Supplement Left Ventricle with Nonautologous Tissue Substitute, Open Approach
02UL37Z Supplement Left Ventricle with Autologous Tissue Substitute, Percutaneous Approach
02UL38Z Supplement Left Ventricle with Zooplastic Tissue, Percutaneous Approach
02UL3JZ Supplement Left Ventricle with Synthetic Substitute, Percutaneous Approach
02UL3KZ Supplement Left Ventricle with Nonautologous Tissue Substitute, Percutaneous Approach
02UL47Z Supplement Left Ventricle with Autologous Tissue Substitute, Percutaneous Endoscopic Approach
02UL48Z Supplement Left Ventricle with Zooplastic Tissue, Percutaneous Endoscopic Approach
02UL4JZ Supplement Left Ventricle with Synthetic Substitute, Percutaneous Endoscopic Approach
02UL4KZ Supplement Left Ventricle with Nonautologous Tissue Substitute, Percutaneous Endoscopic Approach
02UM07Z Supplement Ventricular Septum with Autologous Tissue Substitute, Open Approach
02UM08Z Supplement Ventricular Septum with Zooplastic Tissue, Open Approach
02UM0JZ Supplement Ventricular Septum with Synthetic Substitute, Open Approach
02UM0KZ Supplement Ventricular Septum with Nonautologous Tissue Substitute, Open Approach
02UM37Z Supplement Ventricular Septum with Autologous Tissue Substitute, Percutaneous Approach
02UM38Z Supplement Ventricular Septum with Zooplastic Tissue, Percutaneous Approach
02UM3JZ Supplement Ventricular Septum with Synthetic Substitute, Percutaneous Approach
02UM3KZ Supplement Ventricular Septum with Nonautologous Tissue Substitute, Percutaneous Approach
02UM47Z Supplement Ventricular Septum with Autologous Tissue Substitute, Percutaneous Endoscopic Approach

02UM48Z Supplement Ventricular Septum with Zooplastic Tissue, Percutaneous Endoscopic Approach
02UM4JZ Supplement Ventricular Septum with Synthetic Substitute, Percutaneous Endoscopic Approach
02UM4KZ Supplement Ventricular Septum with Nonautologous Tissue Substitute, Percutaneous Endoscopic Approach
02UN07Z Supplement Pericardium with Autologous Tissue Substitute, Open Approach
02UN08Z Supplement Pericardium with Zooplastic Tissue, Open Approach
02UN0JZ Supplement Pericardium with Synthetic Substitute, Open Approach
02UN0KZ Supplement Pericardium with Nonautologous Tissue Substitute, Open Approach
02UN37Z Supplement Pericardium with Autologous Tissue Substitute, Percutaneous Approach
02UN38Z Supplement Pericardium with Zooplastic Tissue, Percutaneous Approach
02UN3JZ Supplement Pericardium with Synthetic Substitute, Percutaneous Approach
02UN3KZ Supplement Pericardium with Nonautologous Tissue Substitute, Percutaneous Approach
02UN47Z Supplement Pericardium with Autologous Tissue Substitute, Percutaneous Endoscopic Approach
02UN48Z Supplement Pericardium with Zooplastic Tissue, Percutaneous Endoscopic Approach
02UN4JZ Supplement Pericardium with Synthetic Substitute, Percutaneous Endoscopic Approach
02UN4KZ Supplement Pericardium with Nonautologous Tissue Substitute, Percutaneous Endoscopic Approach
02UP07Z Supplement Pulmonary Trunk with Autologous Tissue Substitute, Open Approach
02UP08Z Supplement Pulmonary Trunk with Zooplastic Tissue, Open Approach
02UP0JZ Supplement Pulmonary Trunk with Synthetic Substitute, Open Approach
02UP0KZ Supplement Pulmonary Trunk with Nonautologous Tissue Substitute, Open Approach
02UP37Z Supplement Pulmonary Trunk with Autologous Tissue Substitute, Percutaneous Approach
02UP38Z Supplement Pulmonary Trunk with Zooplastic Tissue, Percutaneous Approach
02UP3JZ Supplement Pulmonary Trunk with Synthetic Substitute, Percutaneous Approach
02UP3KZ Supplement Pulmonary Trunk with Nonautologous Tissue Substitute, Percutaneous Approach
02UP47Z Supplement Pulmonary Trunk with Autologous Tissue Substitute, Percutaneous Endoscopic Approach
02UP48Z Supplement Pulmonary Trunk with Zooplastic Tissue, Percutaneous Endoscopic Approach
02UP4JZ Supplement Pulmonary Trunk with Synthetic Substitute, Percutaneous Endoscopic Approach
02UP4KZ Supplement Pulmonary Trunk with Nonautologous Tissue Substitute, Percutaneous Endoscopic Approach
02UQ07Z Supplement Right Pulmonary Artery with Autologous Tissue Substitute, Open Approach
02UQ08Z Supplement Right Pulmonary Artery with Zooplastic Tissue, Open Approach
02UQ0JZ Supplement Right Pulmonary Artery with Synthetic Substitute, Open Approach
02UQ0KZ Supplement Right Pulmonary Artery with Nonautologous Tissue Substitute, Open Approach
02UQ37Z Supplement Right Pulmonary Artery with Autologous Tissue Substitute, Percutaneous Approach
02UQ38Z Supplement Right Pulmonary Artery with Zooplastic Tissue, Percutaneous Approach
02UQ3JZ Supplement Right Pulmonary Artery with Synthetic Substitute, Percutaneous Approach
02UQ3KZ Supplement Right Pulmonary Artery with Nonautologous Tissue Substitute, Percutaneous Approach
02UQ47Z Supplement Right Pulmonary Artery with Autologous Tissue Substitute, Percutaneous Endoscopic Approach
02UQ48Z Supplement Right Pulmonary Artery with Zooplastic Tissue, Percutaneous Endoscopic Approach
02UQ4JZ Supplement Right Pulmonary Artery with Synthetic Substitute, Percutaneous Endoscopic Approach
02UQ4KZ Supplement Right Pulmonary Artery with Nonautologous Tissue Substitute, Percutaneous Endoscopic Approach
02UR07Z Supplement Left Pulmonary Artery with Autologous Tissue Substitute, Open Approach
02UR08Z Supplement Left Pulmonary Artery with Zooplastic Tissue, Open Approach
02UR0JZ Supplement Left Pulmonary Artery with Synthetic Substitute, Open Approach
02UR0KZ Supplement Left Pulmonary Artery with Nonautologous Tissue Substitute, Open Approach
02UR37Z Supplement Left Pulmonary Artery with Autologous Tissue Substitute, Percutaneous Approach
02UR38Z Supplement Left Pulmonary Artery with Zooplastic Tissue, Percutaneous Approach
02UR3JZ Supplement Left Pulmonary Artery with Synthetic Substitute, Percutaneous Approach
02UR3KZ Supplement Left Pulmonary Artery with Nonautologous Tissue Substitute, Percutaneous Approach
02UR47Z Supplement Left Pulmonary Artery with Autologous Tissue Substitute, Percutaneous Endoscopic Approach
02UR48Z Supplement Left Pulmonary Artery with Zooplastic Tissue, Percutaneous Endoscopic Approach
02UR4JZ Supplement Left Pulmonary Artery with Synthetic Substitute, Percutaneous Endoscopic Approach
02UR4KZ Supplement Left Pulmonary Artery with Nonautologous Tissue Substitute, Percutaneous Endoscopic Approach
02US07Z Supplement Right Pulmonary Vein with Autologous Tissue Substitute, Open Approach
02US08Z Supplement Right Pulmonary Vein with Zooplastic Tissue, Open Approach
02US0JZ Supplement Right Pulmonary Vein with Synthetic Substitute, Open Approach
02US0KZ Supplement Right Pulmonary Vein with Nonautologous Tissue Substitute, Open Approach
02US37Z Supplement Right Pulmonary Vein with Autologous Tissue Substitute, Percutaneous Approach
02US38Z Supplement Right Pulmonary Vein with Zooplastic Tissue, Percutaneous Approach
02US3JZ Supplement Right Pulmonary Vein with Synthetic Substitute, Percutaneous Approach
02US3KZ Supplement Right Pulmonary Vein with Nonautologous Tissue Substitute, Percutaneous Approach
02US47Z Supplement Right Pulmonary Vein with Autologous Tissue Substitute, Percutaneous Endoscopic Approach
02US48Z Supplement Right Pulmonary Vein with Zooplastic Tissue, Percutaneous Endoscopic Approach
02US4JZ Supplement Right Pulmonary Vein with Synthetic Substitute, Percutaneous Endoscopic Approach
02US4KZ Supplement Right Pulmonary Vein with Nonautologous Tissue Substitute, Percutaneous Endoscopic Approach
02UT07Z Supplement Left Pulmonary Vein with Autologous Tissue Substitute, Open Approach
02UT08Z Supplement Left Pulmonary Vein with Zooplastic Tissue, Open Approach
02UT0JZ Supplement Left Pulmonary Vein with Synthetic Substitute, Open Approach
02UT0KZ Supplement Left Pulmonary Vein with Nonautologous Tissue Substitute, Open Approach
02UT37Z Supplement Left Pulmonary Vein with Autologous Tissue Substitute, Percutaneous Approach
02UT38Z Supplement Left Pulmonary Vein with Zooplastic Tissue, Percutaneous Approach
02UT3JZ Supplement Left Pulmonary Vein with Synthetic Substitute, Percutaneous Approach
02UT3KZ Supplement Left Pulmonary Vein with Nonautologous Tissue Substitute, Percutaneous Approach
02UT47Z Supplement Left Pulmonary Vein with Autologous Tissue Substitute, Percutaneous Endoscopic Approach
02UT48Z Supplement Left Pulmonary Vein with Zooplastic Tissue, Percutaneous Endoscopic Approach
02UT4JZ Supplement Left Pulmonary Vein with Synthetic Substitute, Percutaneous Endoscopic Approach
02UT4KZ Supplement Left Pulmonary Vein with Nonautologous Tissue Substitute, Percutaneous Endoscopic Approach
02UV07Z Supplement Superior Vena Cava with Autologous Tissue Substitute, Open Approach
02UV08Z Supplement Superior Vena Cava with Zooplastic Tissue, Open Approach
02UV0JZ Supplement Superior Vena Cava with Synthetic Substitute, Open Approach
02UV0KZ Supplement Superior Vena Cava with Nonautologous Tissue Substitute, Open Approach
02UV37Z Supplement Superior Vena Cava with Autologous Tissue Substitute, Percutaneous Approach
02UV38Z Supplement Superior Vena Cava with Zooplastic Tissue, Percutaneous Approach
02UV3JZ Supplement Superior Vena Cava with Synthetic Substitute, Percutaneous Approach
02UV3KZ Supplement Superior Vena Cava with Nonautologous Tissue Substitute, Percutaneous Approach
02UV47Z Supplement Superior Vena Cava with Autologous Tissue Substitute, Percutaneous Endoscopic Approach
02UV48Z Supplement Superior Vena Cava with Zooplastic Tissue, Percutaneous Endoscopic Approach
02UV4JZ Supplement Superior Vena Cava with Synthetic Substitute, Percutaneous Endoscopic Approach

02UV4KZ Supplement Superior Vena Cava with Nonautologous Tissue Substitute, Percutaneous Endoscopic Approach
02UW07Z Supplement Thoracic Aorta with Autologous Tissue Substitute, Open Approach
02UW08Z Supplement Thoracic Aorta with Zooplastic Tissue, Open Approach
02UW0JZ Supplement Thoracic Aorta with Synthetic Substitute, Open Approach
02UW0KZ Supplement Thoracic Aorta with Nonautologous Tissue Substitute, Open Approach
02UW37Z Supplement Thoracic Aorta with Autologous Tissue Substitute, Percutaneous Approach
02UW38Z Supplement Thoracic Aorta with Zooplastic Tissue, Percutaneous Approach
02UW3JZ Supplement Thoracic Aorta with Synthetic Substitute, Percutaneous Approach
02UW3KZ Supplement Thoracic Aorta with Nonautologous Tissue Substitute, Percutaneous Approach
02UW47Z Supplement Thoracic Aorta with Autologous Tissue Substitute, Percutaneous Endoscopic Approach
02UW48Z Supplement Thoracic Aorta with Zooplastic Tissue, Percutaneous Endoscopic Approach
02UW4JZ Supplement Thoracic Aorta with Synthetic Substitute, Percutaneous Endoscopic Approach
02UW4KZ Supplement Thoracic Aorta with Nonautologous Tissue Substitute, Percutaneous Endoscopic Approach

02V – Heart and Great Vessels, Restriction

02VA0CZ Restriction of Heart with Extraluminal Device, Open Approach
02VA0ZZ Restriction of Heart, Open Approach
02VA3CZ Restriction of Heart with Extraluminal Device, Percutaneous Approach
02VA3ZZ Restriction of Heart, Percutaneous Approach
02VA4CZ Restriction of Heart with Extraluminal Device, Percutaneous Endoscopic Approach
02VA4ZZ Restriction of Heart, Percutaneous Endoscopic Approach
02VP0CZ Restriction of Pulmonary Trunk with Extraluminal Device, Open Approach
02VP0DZ Restriction of Pulmonary Trunk with Intraluminal Device, Open Approach
02VP0ZZ Restriction of Pulmonary Trunk, Open Approach
02VP3CZ Restriction of Pulmonary Trunk with Extraluminal Device, Percutaneous Approach
02VP3DZ Restriction of Pulmonary Trunk with Intraluminal Device, Percutaneous Approach
02VP3ZZ Restriction of Pulmonary Trunk, Percutaneous Approach
02VP4CZ Restriction of Pulmonary Trunk with Extraluminal Device, Percutaneous Endoscopic Approach
02VP4DZ Restriction of Pulmonary Trunk with Intraluminal Device, Percutaneous Endoscopic Approach
02VP4ZZ Restriction of Pulmonary Trunk, Percutaneous Endoscopic Approach
02VQ0CZ Restriction of Right Pulmonary Artery with Extraluminal Device, Open Approach
02VQ0DZ Restriction of Right Pulmonary Artery with Intraluminal Device, Open Approach
02VQ0ZZ Restriction of Right Pulmonary Artery, Open Approach
02VQ3CZ Restriction of Right Pulmonary Artery with Extraluminal Device, Percutaneous Approach
02VQ3DZ Restriction of Right Pulmonary Artery with Intraluminal Device, Percutaneous Approach
02VQ3ZZ Restriction of Right Pulmonary Artery, Percutaneous Approach
02VQ4CZ Restriction of Right Pulmonary Artery with Extraluminal Device, Percutaneous Endoscopic Approach
02VQ4DZ Restriction of Right Pulmonary Artery with Intraluminal Device, Percutaneous Endoscopic Approach
02VQ4ZZ Restriction of Right Pulmonary Artery, Percutaneous Endoscopic Approach
02VR0CT Restriction of Ductus Arteriosus with Extraluminal Device, Open Approach
02VR0CZ Restriction of Left Pulmonary Artery with Extraluminal Device, Open Approach
02VR0DT Restriction of Ductus Arteriosus with Intraluminal Device, Open Approach
02VR0DZ Restriction of Left Pulmonary Artery with Intraluminal Device, Open Approach
02VR0ZT Restriction of Ductus Arteriosus, Open Approach
02VR0ZZ Restriction of Left Pulmonary Artery, Open Approach
02VR3CT Restriction of Ductus Arteriosus with Extraluminal Device, Percutaneous Approach
02VR3CZ Restriction of Left Pulmonary Artery with Extraluminal Device, Percutaneous Approach
02VR3DT Restriction of Ductus Arteriosus with Intraluminal Device, Percutaneous Approach
02VR3DZ Restriction of Left Pulmonary Artery with Intraluminal Device, Percutaneous Approach
02VR3ZT Restriction of Ductus Arteriosus, Percutaneous Approach
02VR3ZZ Restriction of Left Pulmonary Artery, Percutaneous Approach
02VR4CT Restriction of Ductus Arteriosus with Extraluminal Device, Percutaneous Endoscopic Approach
02VR4CZ Restriction of Left Pulmonary Artery with Extraluminal Device, Percutaneous Endoscopic Approach
02VR4DT Restriction of Ductus Arteriosus with Intraluminal Device, Percutaneous Endoscopic Approach
02VR4DZ Restriction of Left Pulmonary Artery with Intraluminal Device, Percutaneous Endoscopic Approach
02VR4ZT Restriction of Ductus Arteriosus, Percutaneous Endoscopic Approach
02VR4ZZ Restriction of Left Pulmonary Artery, Percutaneous Endoscopic Approach
02VS0CZ Restriction of Right Pulmonary Vein with Extraluminal Device, Open Approach
02VS0DZ Restriction of Right Pulmonary Vein with Intraluminal Device, Open Approach
02VS0ZZ Restriction of Right Pulmonary Vein, Open Approach
02VS3CZ Restriction of Right Pulmonary Vein with Extraluminal Device, Percutaneous Approach
02VS3DZ Restriction of Right Pulmonary Vein with Intraluminal Device, Percutaneous Approach
02VS3ZZ Restriction of Right Pulmonary Vein, Percutaneous Approach
02VS4CZ Restriction of Right Pulmonary Vein with Extraluminal Device, Percutaneous Endoscopic Approach
02VS4DZ Restriction of Right Pulmonary Vein with Intraluminal Device, Percutaneous Endoscopic Approach
02VS4ZZ Restriction of Right Pulmonary Vein, Percutaneous Endoscopic Approach
02VT0CZ Restriction of Left Pulmonary Vein with Extraluminal Device, Open Approach
02VT0DZ Restriction of Left Pulmonary Vein with Intraluminal Device, Open Approach
02VT0ZZ Restriction of Left Pulmonary Vein, Open Approach
02VT3CZ Restriction of Left Pulmonary Vein with Extraluminal Device, Percutaneous Approach
02VT3DZ Restriction of Left Pulmonary Vein with Intraluminal Device, Percutaneous Approach
02VT3ZZ Restriction of Left Pulmonary Vein, Percutaneous Approach
02VT4CZ Restriction of Left Pulmonary Vein with Extraluminal Device, Percutaneous Endoscopic Approach
02VT4DZ Restriction of Left Pulmonary Vein with Intraluminal Device, Percutaneous Endoscopic Approach
02VT4ZZ Restriction of Left Pulmonary Vein, Percutaneous Endoscopic Approach
02VV0CZ Restriction of Superior Vena Cava with Extraluminal Device, Open Approach
02VV0DZ Restriction of Superior Vena Cava with Intraluminal Device, Open Approach
02VV0ZZ Restriction of Superior Vena Cava, Open Approach
02VV3CZ Restriction of Superior Vena Cava with Extraluminal Device, Percutaneous Approach
02VV3DZ Restriction of Superior Vena Cava with Intraluminal Device, Percutaneous Approach
02VV3ZZ Restriction of Superior Vena Cava, Percutaneous Approach
02VV4CZ Restriction of Superior Vena Cava with Extraluminal Device, Percutaneous Endoscopic Approach
02VV4DZ Restriction of Superior Vena Cava with Intraluminal Device, Percutaneous Endoscopic Approach
02VV4ZZ Restriction of Superior Vena Cava, Percutaneous Endoscopic Approach
02VW0CZ Restriction of Thoracic Aorta with Extraluminal Device, Open Approach
02VW0DZ Restriction of Thoracic Aorta with Intraluminal Device, Open Approach
02VW0ZZ Restriction of Thoracic Aorta, Open Approach
02VW3CZ Restriction of Thoracic Aorta with Extraluminal Device, Percutaneous Approach
02VW3DZ Restriction of Thoracic Aorta with Intraluminal Device, Percutaneous Approach
02VW3ZZ Restriction of Thoracic Aorta, Percutaneous Approach
02VW4CZ Restriction of Thoracic Aorta with Extraluminal Device, Percutaneous Endoscopic Approach
02VW4DZ Restriction of Thoracic Aorta with Intraluminal Device, Percutaneous Endoscopic Approach
02VW4ZZ Restriction of Thoracic Aorta, Percutaneous Endoscopic Approach

02W – Heart and Great Vessels, Revision

Review Coding Guideline B6.1c

- 02W50JZ Revision of Synthetic Substitute in Atrial Septum, Open Approach
- 02W54JZ Revision of Synthetic Substitute in Atrial Septum, Percutaneous Endoscopic Approach
- 02WA02Z Revision of Monitoring Device in Heart, Open Approach
- 02WA03Z Revision of Infusion Device in Heart, Open Approach
- 02WA07Z Revision of Autologous Tissue Substitute in Heart, Open Approach
- 02WA08Z Revision of Zooplastic Tissue in Heart, Open Approach
- 02WA0CZ Revision of Extraluminal Device in Heart, Open Approach
- 02WA0DZ Revision of Intraluminal Device in Heart, Open Approach
- 02WA0JZ Revision of Synthetic Substitute in Heart, Open Approach
- 02WA0KZ Revision of Nonautologous Tissue Substitute in Heart, Open Approach
- 02WA0MZ Revision of Cardiac Lead in Heart, Open Approach
  - HAC With a secondary diagnosis code of K68.11, T81.4XXA, T82.6XXA, T82.7XXA
- 02WA0QZ Revision of Implantable Heart Assist System in Heart, Open Approach
  - + Heart assist system replacement when reported with a removal of an external heart assist system (6th character R) from the heart. *See table 02P to construct the Removal code.*
- 02WA0RZ Revision of External Heart Assist System in Heart, Open Approach
  - + Heart assist system replacement when reported with a removal of an external heart assist system (6th character R) from the heart. *See table 02P to construct the Removal code.*
- 02WA32Z Revision of Monitoring Device in Heart, Percutaneous Approach
- 02WA33Z Revision of Infusion Device in Heart, Percutaneous Approach
- 02WA37Z Revision of Autologous Tissue Substitute in Heart, Percutaneous Approach
- 02WA38Z Revision of Zooplastic Tissue in Heart, Percutaneous Approach
- 02WA3CZ Revision of Extraluminal Device in Heart, Percutaneous Approach
- 02WA3DZ Revision of Intraluminal Device in Heart, Percutaneous Approach
- 02WA3JZ Revision of Synthetic Substitute in Heart, Percutaneous Approach
- 02WA3KZ Revision of Nonautologous Tissue Substitute in Heart, Percutaneous Approach
- 02WA3MZ Revision of Cardiac Lead in Heart, Percutaneous Approach
  - HAC With a secondary diagnosis code of K68.11, T81.4XXA, T82.6XXA, T82.7XXA
- 02WA3QZ Revision of Implantable Heart Assist System in Heart, Percutaneous Approach
  - + Heart assist system replacement when reported with a removal of an external heart assist system (6th character R) from the heart. *See table 02P to construct the Removal code.*
- 02WA3RZ Revision of External Heart Assist System in Heart, Percutaneous Approach
  - + Heart assist system replacement when reported with a removal of an external heart assist system (6th character R) from the heart. *See table 02P to construct the Removal code.*
- 02WA42Z Revision of Monitoring Device in Heart, Percutaneous Endoscopic Approach
- 02WA43Z Revision of Infusion Device in Heart, Percutaneous Endoscopic Approach
- 02WA47Z Revision of Autologous Tissue Substitute in Heart, Percutaneous Endoscopic Approach
- 02WA48Z Revision of Zooplastic Tissue in Heart, Percutaneous Endoscopic Approach
- 02WA4CZ Revision of Extraluminal Device in Heart, Percutaneous Endoscopic Approach
- 02WA4DZ Revision of Intraluminal Device in Heart, Percutaneous Endoscopic Approach
- 02WA4JZ Revision of Synthetic Substitute in Heart, Percutaneous Endoscopic Approach
- 02WA4KZ Revision of Nonautologous Tissue Substitute in Heart, Percutaneous Endoscopic Approach
- 02WA4MZ Revision of Cardiac Lead in Heart, Percutaneous Endoscopic Approach
  - HAC With a secondary diagnosis code of K68.11, T81.4XXA, T82.6XXA, T82.7XXA
- ▲ 02WA4QZ Revision of Implantable Heart Assist System in Heart, Percutaneous Endoscopic Approach
  - + Heart assist system replacement when reported with a removal of an external heart assist system (6th character R) from the heart. *See table 02P to construct the Removal code.*
- 02WA4RZ Revision of External Heart Assist System in Heart, Percutaneous Endoscopic Approach
  - + Heart assist system replacement when reported with a removal of an external heart assist system (6th character R) from the heart. *See table 02P to construct the Removal code.*
- 02WAX2Z Revision of Monitoring Device in Heart, External Approach
- 02WAX3Z Revision of Infusion Device in Heart, External Approach
- 02WAX7Z Revision of Autologous Tissue Substitute in Heart, External Approach
- 02WAX8Z Revision of Zooplastic Tissue in Heart, External Approach
- 02WAXCZ Revision of Extraluminal Device in Heart, External Approach
- 02WAXDZ Revision of Intraluminal Device in Heart, External Approach
- 02WAXJZ Revision of Synthetic Substitute in Heart, External Approach
- 02WAXKZ Revision of Nonautologous Tissue Substitute in Heart, External Approach
- 02WAXMZ Revision of Cardiac Lead in Heart, External Approach
- 02WAXQZ Revision of Implantable Heart Assist System in Heart, External Approach
- 02WAXRZ Revision of External Heart Assist System in Heart, External Approach
- 02WF07Z Revision of Autologous Tissue Substitute in Aortic Valve, Open Approach
- 02WF08Z Revision of Zooplastic Tissue in Aortic Valve, Open Approach
- 02WF0JZ Revision of Synthetic Substitute in Aortic Valve, Open Approach
- 02WF0KZ Revision of Nonautologous Tissue Substitute in Aortic Valve, Open Approach
- 02WF47Z Revision of Autologous Tissue Substitute in Aortic Valve, Percutaneous Endoscopic Approach
- 02WF48Z Revision of Zooplastic Tissue in Aortic Valve, Percutaneous Endoscopic Approach
- 02WF4JZ Revision of Synthetic Substitute in Aortic Valve, Percutaneous Endoscopic Approach
- 02WF4KZ Revision of Nonautologous Tissue Substitute in Aortic Valve, Percutaneous Endoscopic Approach
- 02WG07Z Revision of Autologous Tissue Substitute in Mitral Valve, Open Approach
- 02WG08Z Revision of Zooplastic Tissue in Mitral Valve, Open Approach
- 02WG0JZ Revision of Synthetic Substitute in Mitral Valve, Open Approach
- 02WG0KZ Revision of Nonautologous Tissue Substitute in Mitral Valve, Open Approach
- 02WG47Z Revision of Autologous Tissue Substitute in Mitral Valve, Percutaneous Endoscopic Approach
- 02WG48Z Revision of Zooplastic Tissue in Mitral Valve, Percutaneous Endoscopic Approach
- 02WG4JZ Revision of Synthetic Substitute in Mitral Valve, Percutaneous Endoscopic Approach
- 02WG4KZ Revision of Nonautologous Tissue Substitute in Mitral Valve, Percutaneous Endoscopic Approach
- 02WH07Z Revision of Autologous Tissue Substitute in Pulmonary Valve, Open Approach
- 02WH08Z Revision of Zooplastic Tissue in Pulmonary Valve, Open Approach
- 02WH0JZ Revision of Synthetic Substitute in Pulmonary Valve, Open Approach
- 02WH0KZ Revision of Nonautologous Tissue Substitute in Pulmonary Valve, Open Approach
- 02WH47Z Revision of Autologous Tissue Substitute in Pulmonary Valve, Percutaneous Endoscopic Approach
- 02WH48Z Revision of Zooplastic Tissue in Pulmonary Valve, Percutaneous Endoscopic Approach
- 02WH4JZ Revision of Synthetic Substitute in Pulmonary Valve, Percutaneous Endoscopic Approach
- 02WH4KZ Revision of Nonautologous Tissue Substitute in Pulmonary Valve, Percutaneous Endoscopic Approach
- 02WJ07Z Revision of Autologous Tissue Substitute in Tricuspid Valve, Open Approach
- 02WJ08Z Revision of Zooplastic Tissue in Tricuspid Valve, Open Approach
- 02WJ0JZ Revision of Synthetic Substitute in Tricuspid Valve, Open Approach
- 02WJ0KZ Revision of Nonautologous Tissue Substitute in Tricuspid Valve, Open Approach
- 02WJ47Z Revision of Autologous Tissue Substitute in Tricuspid Valve, Percutaneous Endoscopic Approach
- 02WJ48Z Revision of Zooplastic Tissue in Tricuspid Valve, Percutaneous Endoscopic Approach
- 02WJ4JZ Revision of Synthetic Substitute in Tricuspid Valve, Percutaneous Endoscopic Approach
- 02WJ4KZ Revision of Nonautologous Tissue Substitute in Tricuspid Valve, Percutaneous Endoscopic Approach
- 02WM0JZ Revision of Synthetic Substitute in Ventricular Septum, Open Approach

02WM4JZ Revision of Synthetic Substitute in Ventricular Septum, Percutaneous Endoscopic Approach

02WY02Z Revision of Monitoring Device in Great Vessel, Open Approach

02WY03Z Revision of Infusion Device in Great Vessel, Open Approach

02WY07Z Revision of Autologous Tissue Substitute in Great Vessel, Open Approach

02WY08Z Revision of Zooplastic Tissue in Great Vessel, Open Approach

02WY0CZ Revision of Extraluminal Device in Great Vessel, Open Approach

02WY0DZ Revision of Intraluminal Device in Great Vessel, Open Approach

02WY0JZ Revision of Synthetic Substitute in Great Vessel, Open Approach

02WY0KZ Revision of Nonautologous Tissue Substitute in Great Vessel, Open Approach

02WY32Z Revision of Monitoring Device in Great Vessel, Percutaneous Approach

02WY33Z Revision of Infusion Device in Great Vessel, Percutaneous Approach

02WY37Z Revision of Autologous Tissue Substitute in Great Vessel, Percutaneous Approach

02WY38Z Revision of Zooplastic Tissue in Great Vessel, Percutaneous Approach

02WY3CZ Revision of Extraluminal Device in Great Vessel, Percutaneous Approach

02WY3DZ Revision of Intraluminal Device in Great Vessel, Percutaneous Approach

02WY3JZ Revision of Synthetic Substitute in Great Vessel, Percutaneous Approach

02WY3KZ Revision of Nonautologous Tissue Substitute in Great Vessel, Percutaneous Approach

02WY42Z Revision of Monitoring Device in Great Vessel, Percutaneous Endoscopic Approach

02WY43Z Revision of Infusion Device in Great Vessel, Percutaneous Endoscopic Approach

02WY47Z Revision of Autologous Tissue Substitute in Great Vessel, Percutaneous Endoscopic Approach

02WY48Z Revision of Zooplastic Tissue in Great Vessel, Percutaneous Endoscopic Approach

02WY4CZ Revision of Extraluminal Device in Great Vessel, Percutaneous Endoscopic Approach

02WY4DZ Revision of Intraluminal Device in Great Vessel, Percutaneous Endoscopic Approach

02WY4JZ Revision of Synthetic Substitute in Great Vessel, Percutaneous Endoscopic Approach

02WY4KZ Revision of Nonautologous Tissue Substitute in Great Vessel, Percutaneous Endoscopic Approach

02WYX2Z Revision of Monitoring Device in Great Vessel, External Approach

02WYX3Z Revision of Infusion Device in Great Vessel, External Approach

02WYX7Z Revision of Autologous Tissue Substitute in Great Vessel, External Approach

02WYX8Z Revision of Zooplastic Tissue in Great Vessel, External Approach

02WYXCZ Revision of Extraluminal Device in Great Vessel, External Approach

02WYXDZ Revision of Intraluminal Device in Great Vessel, External Approach

02WYXJZ Revision of Synthetic Substitute in Great Vessel, External Approach

02WYXKZ Revision of Nonautologous Tissue Substitute in Great Vessel, External Approach

02Y – Heart and Great Vessels, Transplantation

Review Coding Guideline B3.16

02YA0Z0 Transplantation of Heart, Allogeneic, Open Approach
AHA CC: 3Q, 2013, 18-19

02YA0Z1 Transplantation of Heart, Syngeneic, Open Approach

02YA0Z2 Transplantation of Heart, Zooplastic, Open Approach

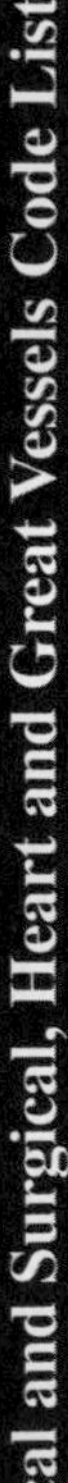

Arteries

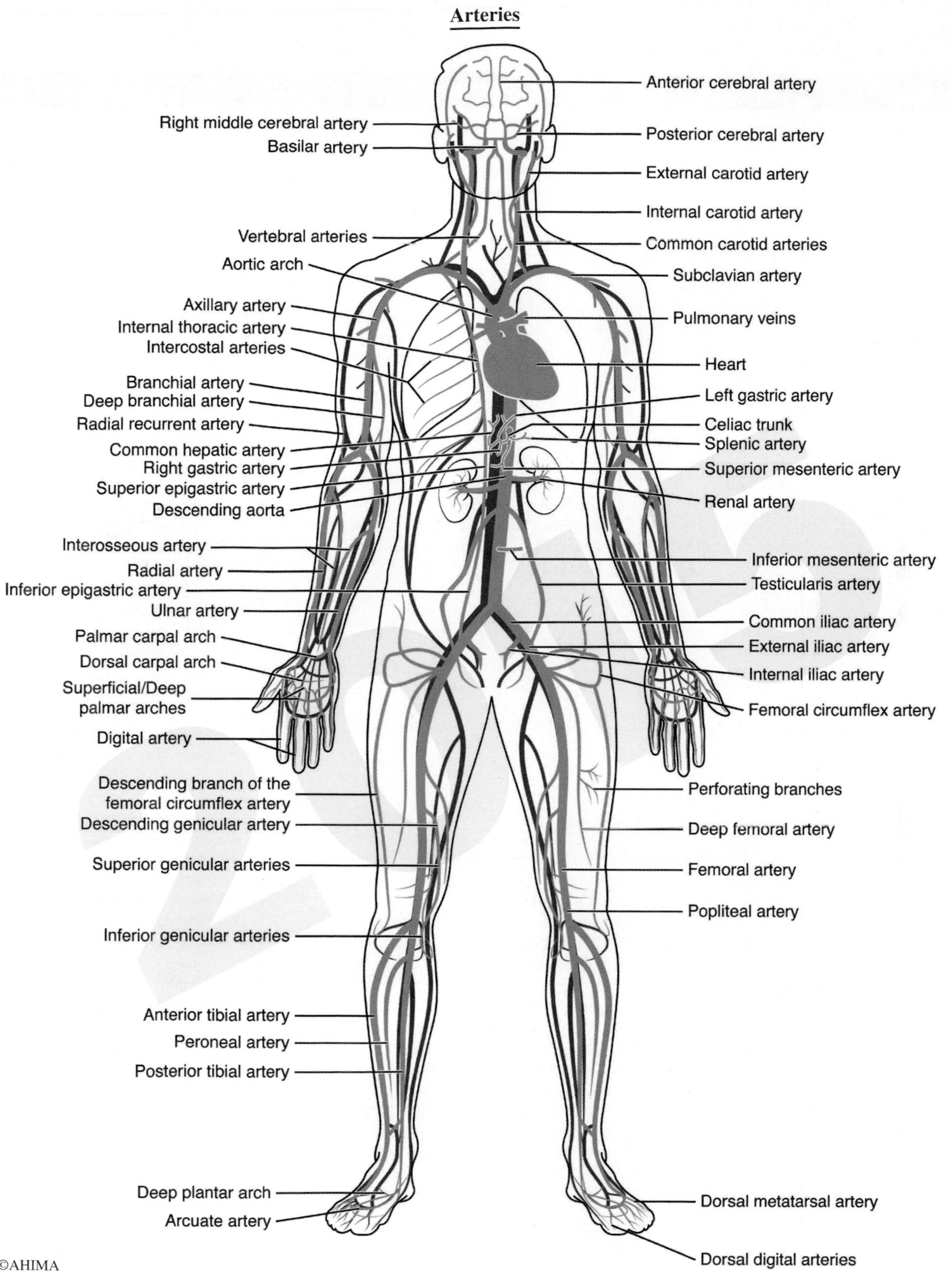
Anterior cerebral artery
Right middle cerebral artery
Posterior cerebral artery
Basilar artery
External carotid artery
Internal carotid artery
Vertebral arteries
Common carotid arteries
Aortic arch
Subclavian artery
Axillary artery
Pulmonary veins
Internal thoracic artery
Intercostal arteries
Heart
Branchial artery
Deep branchial artery
Left gastric artery
Radial recurrent artery
Celiac trunk
Common hepatic artery
Splenic artery
Right gastric artery
Superior mesenteric artery
Superior epigastric artery
Descending aorta
Renal artery
Interosseous artery
Inferior mesenteric artery
Radial artery
Testicularis artery
Inferior epigastric artery
Ulnar artery
Common iliac artery
Palmar carpal arch
External iliac artery
Dorsal carpal arch
Internal iliac artery
Superficial/Deep
palmar arches
Femoral circumflex artery
Digital artery
Descending branch of the
femoral circumflex artery
Perforating branches
Descending genicular artery
Deep femoral artery
Superior genicular arteries
Femoral artery
Popliteal artery
Inferior genicular arteries
Anterior tibial artery
Peroneal artery
Posterior tibial artery
Deep plantar arch
Dorsal metatarsal artery
Arcuate artery
Dorsal digital arteries

Section 0 **Medical and Surgical**
Body System 3 **Upper Arteries**
Operation 1 **Bypass:** Altering the route of passage of the contents of a tubular body part

Body Part (4th)	Approach (5th)	Device (6th)	Qualifier (7th)
2 Innominate Artery **5** Axillary Artery, Right **6** Axillary Artery, Left	**0** Open	**9** Autologous Venous Tissue **A** Autologous Arterial Tissue **J** Synthetic Substitute **K** Nonautologous Tissue Substitute **Z** No Device	**0** Upper Arm Artery, Right **1** Upper Arm Artery, Left **2** Upper Arm Artery, Bilateral **3** Lower Arm Artery, Right **4** Lower Arm Artery, Left **5** Lower Arm Artery, Bilateral **6** Upper Leg Artery, Right **7** Upper Leg Artery, Left **8** Upper Leg Artery, Bilateral **9** Lower Leg Artery, Right **B** Lower Leg Artery, Left **C** Lower Leg Artery, Bilateral **D** Upper Arm Vein **F** Lower Arm Vein **J** Extracranial Artery, Right **K** Extracranial Artery, Left
3 Subclavian Artery, Right **4** Subclavian Artery, Left	**0** Open	**9** Autologous Venous Tissue **A** Autologous Arterial Tissue **J** Synthetic Substitute **K** Nonautologous Tissue Substitute **Z** No Device	**0** Upper Arm Artery, Right **1** Upper Arm Artery, Left **2** Upper Arm Artery, Bilateral **3** Lower Arm Artery, Right **4** Lower Arm Artery, Left **5** Lower Arm Artery, Bilateral **6** Upper Leg Artery, Right **7** Upper Leg Artery, Left **8** Upper Leg Artery, Bilateral **9** Lower Leg Artery, Right **B** Lower Leg Artery, Left **C** Lower Leg Artery, Bilateral **D** Upper Arm Vein **F** Lower Arm Vein **J** Extracranial Artery, Right **K** Extracranial Artery, Left **M** Pulmonary Artery, Right **N** Pulmonary Artery, Left
7 Brachial Artery, Right	**0** Open	**9** Autologous Venous Tissue **A** Autologous Arterial Tissue **J** Synthetic Substitute **K** Nonautologous Tissue Substitute **Z** No Device	**0** Upper Arm Artery, Right **3** Lower Arm Artery, Right **D** Upper Arm Vein **F** Lower Arm Vein
8 Brachial Artery, Left	**0** Open	**9** Autologous Venous Tissue **A** Autologous Arterial Tissue **J** Synthetic Substitute **K** Nonautologous Tissue Substitute **Z** No Device	**1** Upper Arm Artery, Left **4** Lower Arm Artery, Left **D** Upper Arm Vein **F** Lower Arm Vein
9 Ulnar Artery, Right **B** Radial Artery, Right	**0** Open	**9** Autologous Venous Tissue **A** Autologous Arterial Tissue **J** Synthetic Substitute **K** Nonautologous Tissue Substitute **Z** No Device	**3** Lower Arm Artery, Right **F** Lower Arm Vein
A Ulnar Artery, Left **C** Radial Artery, Left	**0** Open	**9** Autologous Venous Tissue **A** Autologous Arterial Tissue **J** Synthetic Substitute **K** Nonautologous Tissue Substitute **Z** No Device	**4** Lower Arm Artery, Left **F** Lower Arm Vein

Continued →

Section 0 Medical and Surgical
Body System 3 Upper Arteries
Operation 1 **Bypass:** Altering the route of passage of the contents of a tubular body part

Body Part (4th)	Approach (5th)	Device (6th)	Qualifier (7th)
G Intracranial Artery **S** Temporal Artery, Right **T** Temporal Artery, Left	**0** Open	**9** Autologous Venous Tissue **A** Autologous Arterial Tissue **J** Synthetic Substitute **K** Nonautologous Tissue Substitute **Z** No Device	**G** Intracranial Artery
H Common Carotid Artery, Right	**0** Open	**9** Autologous Venous Tissue **A** Autologous Arterial Tissue **J** Synthetic Substitute **K** Nonautologous Tissue Substitute **Z** No Device	**G** Intracranial Artery **J** Extracranial Artery, Right
J Common Carotid Artery, Left	**0** Open	**9** Autologous Venous Tissue **A** Autologous Arterial Tissue **J** Synthetic Substitute **K** Nonautologous Tissue Substitute **Z** No Device	**G** Intracranial Artery **K** Extracranial Artery, Left
K Internal Carotid Artery, Right **M** External Carotid Artery, Right	**0** Open	**9** Autologous Venous Tissue **A** Autologous Arterial Tissue **J** Synthetic Substitute **K** Nonautologous Tissue Substitute **Z** No Device	**J** Extracranial Artery, Right
L Internal Carotid Artery, Left **N** External Carotid Artery, Left	**0** Open	**9** Autologous Venous Tissue **A** Autologous Arterial Tissue **J** Synthetic Substitute **K** Nonautologous Tissue Substitute **Z** No Device	**K** Extracranial Artery, Left

Section 0 Medical and Surgical
Body System 3 Upper Arteries
Operation 5 **Destruction:** Physical eradication of all or a portion of a body part by the direct use of energy, force, or a destructive agent

Body Part (4th)	Approach (5th)	Device (6th)	Qualifier (7th)
0 Internal Mammary Artery, Right **1** Internal Mammary Artery, Left **2** Innominate Artery **3** Subclavian Artery, Right **4** Subclavian Artery, Left **5** Axillary Artery, Right **6** Axillary Artery, Left **7** Brachial Artery, Right **8** Brachial Artery, Left **9** Ulnar Artery, Right **A** Ulnar Artery, Left **B** Radial Artery, Right **C** Radial Artery, Left **D** Hand Artery, Right **F** Hand Artery, Left **G** Intracranial Artery **H** Common Carotid Artery, Right **J** Common Carotid Artery, Left **K** Internal Carotid Artery, Right **L** Internal Carotid Artery, Left **M** External Carotid Artery, Right **N** External Carotid Artery, Left **P** Vertebral Artery, Right	**0** Open **3** Percutaneous **4** Percutaneous Endoscopic	**Z** No Device	**Z** No Qualifier

Continued →

Section 0 **Medical and Surgical**
Body System 3 **Upper Arteries**
Operation 5 **Destruction:** Physical eradication of all or a portion of a body part by the direct use of energy, force, or a destructive agent

Body Part (4th)	Approach (5th)	Device (6th)	Qualifier (7th)
Q Vertebral Artery, Left **R** Face Artery **S** Temporal Artery, Right **T** Temporal Artery, Left **U** Thyroid Artery, Right **V** Thyroid Artery, Left **Y** Upper Artery			

Section 0 **Medical and Surgical**
Body System 3 **Upper Arteries**
Operation 7 **Dilation:** Expanding an orifice or the lumen of a tubular body part

Body Part (4th)	Approach (5th)	Device (6th)	Qualifier (7th)
0 Internal Mammary Artery, Right **1** Internal Mammary Artery, Left **2** Innominate Artery **3** Subclavian Artery, Right **4** Subclavian Artery, Left **5** Axillary Artery, Right **6** Axillary Artery, Left **7** Brachial Artery, Right **8** Brachial Artery, Left **9** Ulnar Artery, Right **A** Ulnar Artery, Left **B** Radial Artery, Right **C** Radial Artery, Left **D** Hand Artery, Right **F** Hand Artery, Left **G** Intracranial Artery **H** Common Carotid Artery, Right **J** Common Carotid Artery, Left **K** Internal Carotid Artery, Right **L** Internal Carotid Artery, Left **M** External Carotid Artery, Right **N** External Carotid Artery, Left **P** Vertebral Artery, Right **Q** Vertebral Artery, Left **R** Face Artery **S** Temporal Artery, Right **T** Temporal Artery, Left **U** Thyroid Artery, Right **V** Thyroid Artery, Left **Y** Upper Artery	**0** Open **3** Percutaneous **4** Percutaneous Endoscopic	**4** Intraluminal Device, Drug-eluting **D** Intraluminal Device **Z** No Device	**Z** No Qualifier

Section 0 **Medical and Surgical**
Body System 3 **Upper Arteries**
Operation 9 **Drainage:** Taking or letting out fluids and/or gases from a body part

Body Part (4th)	Approach (5th)	Device (6th)	Qualifier (7th)
0 Internal Mammary Artery, Right **1** Internal Mammary Artery, Left **2** Innominate Artery **3** Subclavian Artery, Right **4** Subclavian Artery, Left **5** Axillary Artery, Right **6** Axillary Artery, Left **7** Brachial Artery, Right **8** Brachial Artery, Left **9** Ulnar Artery, Right **A** Ulnar Artery, Left **B** Radial Artery, Right **C** Radial Artery, Left **D** Hand Artery, Right **F** Hand Artery, Left **G** Intracranial Artery **H** Common Carotid Artery, Right **J** Common Carotid Artery, Left **K** Internal Carotid Artery, Right **L** Internal Carotid Artery, Left **M** External Carotid Artery, Right **N** External Carotid Artery, Left **P** Vertebral Artery, Right **Q** Vertebral Artery, Left **R** Face Artery **S** Temporal Artery, Right **T** Temporal Artery, Left **U** Thyroid Artery, Right **V** Thyroid Artery, Left **Y** Upper Artery	**0** Open **3** Percutaneous **4** Percutaneous Endoscopic	**0** Drainage Device	**Z** No Qualifier
0 Internal Mammary Artery, Right **1** Internal Mammary Artery, Left **2** Innominate Artery **3** Subclavian Artery, Right **4** Subclavian Artery, Left **5** Axillary Artery, Right **6** Axillary Artery, Left **7** Brachial Artery, Right **8** Brachial Artery, Left **9** Ulnar Artery, Right **A** Ulnar Artery, Left **B** Radial Artery, Right **C** Radial Artery, Left **D** Hand Artery, Right **F** Hand Artery, Left **G** Intracranial Artery **H** Common Carotid Artery, Right **J** Common Carotid Artery, Left **K** Internal Carotid Artery, Right **L** Internal Carotid Artery, Left **M** External Carotid Artery, Right **N** External Carotid Artery, Left **P** Vertebral Artery, Right **Q** Vertebral Artery, Left **R** Face Artery **S** Temporal Artery, Right **T** Temporal Artery, Left **U** Thyroid Artery, Right **V** Thyroid Artery, Left **Y** Upper Artery	**0** Open **3** Percutaneous **4** Percutaneous Endoscopic	**Z** No Device	**X** Diagnostic **Z** No Qualifier

Section 0 **Medical and Surgical**
Body System 3 **Upper Arteries**
Operation B **Excision:** Cutting out or off, without replacement, a portion of a body part

Body Part (4th)	Approach (5th)	Device (6th)	Qualifier (7th)
0 Internal Mammary Artery, Right	**0** Open	**Z** No Device	**X** Diagnostic
1 Internal Mammary Artery, Left	**3** Percutaneous		**Z** No Qualifier
2 Innominate Artery	**4** Percutaneous Endoscopic		
3 Subclavian Artery, Right			
4 Subclavian Artery, Left			
5 Axillary Artery, Right			
6 Axillary Artery, Left			
7 Brachial Artery, Right			
8 Brachial Artery, Left			
9 Ulnar Artery, Right			
A Ulnar Artery, Left			
B Radial Artery, Right			
C Radial Artery, Left			
D Hand Artery, Right			
F Hand Artery, Left			
G Intracranial Artery			
H Common Carotid Artery, Right			
J Common Carotid Artery, Left			
K Internal Carotid Artery, Right			
L Internal Carotid Artery, Left			
M External Carotid Artery, Right			
N External Carotid Artery, Left			
P Vertebral Artery, Right			
Q Vertebral Artery, Left			
R Face Artery			
S Temporal Artery, Right			
T Temporal Artery, Left			
U Thyroid Artery, Right			
V Thyroid Artery, Left			
Y Upper Artery			

Section 0 **Medical and Surgical**
Body System 3 **Upper Arteries**
Operation C **Extirpation:** Taking or cutting out solid matter from a body part

Body Part (4th)	Approach (5th)	Device (6th)	Qualifier (7th)
0 Internal Mammary Artery, Right	**0** Open	**Z** No Device	**Z** No Qualifier
1 Internal Mammary Artery, Left	**3** Percutaneous		
2 Innominate Artery	**4** Percutaneous Endoscopic		
3 Subclavian Artery, Right			
4 Subclavian Artery, Left			
5 Axillary Artery, Right			
6 Axillary Artery, Left			
7 Brachial Artery, Right			
8 Brachial Artery, Left			
9 Ulnar Artery, Right			
A Ulnar Artery, Left			
B Radial Artery, Right			
C Radial Artery, Left			
D Hand Artery, Right			
F Hand Artery, Left			
G Intracranial Artery			
H Common Carotid Artery, Right			
J Common Carotid Artery, Left			
K Internal Carotid Artery, Right			
L Internal Carotid Artery, Left			
M External Carotid Artery, Right			
N External Carotid Artery, Left			
P Vertebral Artery, Right			
Q Vertebral Artery, Left			
R Face Artery			
S Temporal Artery, Right			
T Temporal Artery, Left			
U Thyroid Artery, Right			
V Thyroid Artery, Left			
Y Upper Artery			

Section 0 **Medical and Surgical**
Body System 3 **Upper Arteries**
Operation H **Insertion:** Putting in a nonbiological appliance that monitors, assists, performs, or prevents a physiological function but does not physically take the place of a body part

Body Part (4th)	Approach (5th)	Device (6th)	Qualifier (7th)
0 Internal Mammary Artery, Right **1** Internal Mammary Artery, Left **2** Innominate Artery **3** Subclavian Artery, Right **4** Subclavian Artery, Left **5** Axillary Artery, Right **6** Axillary Artery, Left **7** Brachial Artery, Right **8** Brachial Artery, Left **9** Ulnar Artery, Right **A** Ulnar Artery, Left **B** Radial Artery, Right **C** Radial Artery, Left **D** Hand Artery, Right **F** Hand Artery, Left **G** Intracranial Artery **H** Common Carotid Artery, Right **J** Common Carotid Artery, Left **M** External Carotid Artery, Right **N** External Carotid Artery, Left **P** Vertebral Artery, Right **Q** Vertebral Artery, Left **R** Face Artery **S** Temporal Artery, Right **T** Temporal Artery, Left **U** Thyroid Artery, Right **V** Thyroid Artery, Left	**0** Open **3** Percutaneous **4** Percutaneous Endoscopic	**3** Infusion Device **D** Intraluminal Device	**Z** No Qualifier
K Internal Carotid Artery, Right **L** Internal Carotid Artery, Left	**0** Open **3** Percutaneous **4** Percutaneous Endoscopic	**3** Infusion Device **D** Intraluminal Device **M** Stimulator Lead	**Z** No Qualifier
Y Upper Artery	**0** Open **3** Percutaneous **4** Percutaneous Endoscopic	**2** Monitoring Device **3** Infusion Device **D** Intraluminal Device	**Z** No Qualifier

Section 0 **Medical and Surgical**
Body System 3 **Upper Arteries**
Operation J **Inspection:** Visually and/or manually exploring a body part

Body Part (4th)	Approach (5th)	Device (6th)	Qualifier (7th)
Y Upper Artery	**0** Open **3** Percutaneous **4** Percutaneous Endoscopic **X** External	**Z** No Device	**Z** No Qualifier

Section 0 **Medical and Surgical**
Body System 3 **Upper Arteries**
Operation L **Occlusion:** Completely closing an orifice or the lumen of a tubular body part

Body Part (4th)	Approach (5th)	Device (6th)	Qualifier (7th)
0 Internal Mammary Artery, Right **1** Internal Mammary Artery, Left **2** Innominate Artery **3** Subclavian Artery, Right **4** Subclavian Artery, Left **5** Axillary Artery, Right **6** Axillary Artery, Left **7** Brachial Artery, Right **8** Brachial Artery, Left **9** Ulnar Artery, Right **A** Ulnar Artery, Left **B** Radial Artery, Right **C** Radial Artery, Left **D** Hand Artery, Right **F** Hand Artery, Left **R** Face Artery **S** Temporal Artery, Right **T** Temporal Artery, Left **U** Thyroid Artery, Right **V** Thyroid Artery, Left **Y** Upper Artery	**0** Open **3** Percutaneous **4** Percutaneous Endoscopic	**C** Extraluminal Device **D** Intraluminal Device **Z** No Device	**Z** No Qualifier
G Intracranial Artery **H** Common Carotid Artery, Right **J** Common Carotid Artery, Left **K** Internal Carotid Artery, Right **L** Internal Carotid Artery, Left **M** External Carotid Artery, Right **N** External Carotid Artery, Left **P** Vertebral Artery, Right **Q** Vertebral Artery, Left	**0** Open **3** Percutaneous **4** Percutaneous Endoscopic	**B** Intraluminal Device, Bioactive **C** Extraluminal Device **D** Intraluminal Device **Z** No Device	**Z** No Qualifier

Section 0 **Medical and Surgical**
Body System 3 **Upper Arteries**
Operation N **Release:** Freeing a body part from an abnormal physical constraint by cutting or by the use of force

Body Part (4th)	Approach (5th)	Device (6th)	Qualifier (7th)
0 Internal Mammary Artery, Right **1** Internal Mammary Artery, Left **2** Innominate Artery **3** Subclavian Artery, Right **4** Subclavian Artery, Left **5** Axillary Artery, Right **6** Axillary Artery, Left **7** Brachial Artery, Right **8** Brachial Artery, Left **9** Ulnar Artery, Right **A** Ulnar Artery, Left **B** Radial Artery, Right **C** Radial Artery, Left **D** Hand Artery, Right **F** Hand Artery, Left **G** Intracranial Artery **H** Common Carotid Artery, Right **J** Common Carotid Artery, Left **K** Internal Carotid Artery, Right **L** Internal Carotid Artery, Left **M** External Carotid Artery, Right **N** External Carotid Artery, Left **P** Vertebral Artery, Right **Q** Vertebral Artery, Left **R** Face Artery **S** Temporal Artery, Right **T** Temporal Artery, Left **U** Thyroid Artery, Right **V** Thyroid Artery, Left **Y** Upper Artery	**0** Open **3** Percutaneous **4** Percutaneous Endoscopic	**Z** No Device	**Z** No Qualifier

Section 0 **Medical and Surgical**
Body System 3 **Upper Arteries**
Operation P **Removal:** Taking out or off a device from a body part

Body Part (4th)	Approach (5th)	Device (6th)	Qualifier (7th)
Y Upper Artery	**0** Open **3** Percutaneous **4** Percutaneous Endoscopic	**0** Drainage Device **2** Monitoring Device **3** Infusion Device **7** Autologous Tissue Substitute **C** Extraluminal Device **D** Intraluminal Device **J** Synthetic Substitute **K** Nonautologous Tissue Substitute **M** Stimulator Lead	**Z** No Qualifier
Y Upper Artery	**X** External	**0** Drainage Device **2** Monitoring Device **3** Infusion Device **D** Intraluminal Device **M** Stimulator Lead	**Z** No Qualifier

Section 0 **Medical and Surgical**
Body System 3 **Upper Arteries**
Operation Q **Repair:** Restoring, to the extent possible, a body part to its normal anatomic structure and function

Body Part (4th)	Approach (5th)	Device (6th)	Qualifier (7th)
0 Internal Mammary Artery, Right **1** Internal Mammary Artery, Left **2** Innominate Artery **3** Subclavian Artery, Right **4** Subclavian Artery, Left **5** Axillary Artery, Right **6** Axillary Artery, Left **7** Brachial Artery, Right **8** Brachial Artery, Left **9** Ulnar Artery, Right **A** Ulnar Artery, Left **B** Radial Artery, Right **C** Radial Artery, Left **D** Hand Artery, Right **F** Hand Artery, Left **G** Intracranial Artery **H** Common Carotid Artery, Right **J** Common Carotid Artery, Left **K** Internal Carotid Artery, Right **L** Internal Carotid Artery, Left **M** External Carotid Artery, Right **N** External Carotid Artery, Left **P** Vertebral Artery, Right **Q** Vertebral Artery, Left **R** Face Artery **S** Temporal Artery, Right **T** Temporal Artery, Left **U** Thyroid Artery, Right **V** Thyroid Artery, Left **Y** Upper Artery	**0** Open **3** Percutaneous **4** Percutaneous Endoscopic	**Z** No Device	**Z** No Qualifier

Section 0 **Medical and Surgical**
Body System 3 **Upper Arteries**
Operation R **Replacement:** Putting in or on biological or synthetic material that physically takes the place and/or function of all or a portion of a body part

Body Part (4th)	Approach (5th)	Device (6th)	Qualifier (7th)
0 Internal Mammary Artery, Right **1** Internal Mammary Artery, Left **2** Innominate Artery **3** Subclavian Artery, Right **4** Subclavian Artery, Left **5** Axillary Artery, Right **6** Axillary Artery, Left **7** Brachial Artery, Right **8** Brachial Artery, Left **9** Ulnar Artery, Right **A** Ulnar Artery, Left **B** Radial Artery, Right **C** Radial Artery, Left **D** Hand Artery, Right **F** Hand Artery, Left **G** Intracranial Artery **H** Common Carotid Artery, Right **J** Common Carotid Artery, Left **K** Internal Carotid Artery, Right **L** Internal Carotid Artery, Left **M** External Carotid Artery, Right **N** External Carotid Artery, Left **P** Vertebral Artery, Right **Q** Vertebral Artery, Left **R** Face Artery **S** Temporal Artery, Right **T** Temporal Artery, Left **U** Thyroid Artery, Right **V** Thyroid Artery, Left **Y** Upper Artery	**0** Open **4** Percutaneous Endoscopic	**7** Autologous Tissue Substitute **J** Synthetic Substitute **K** Nonautologous Tissue Substitute	**Z** No Qualifier

Section 0 **Medical and Surgical**
Body System 3 **Upper Arteries**
Operation S **Reposition:** Moving to its normal location, or other suitable location, all or a portion of a body part

Body Part (4th)	Approach (5th)	Device (6th)	Qualifier (7th)
0 Internal Mammary Artery, Right **1** Internal Mammary Artery, Left **2** Innominate Artery **3** Subclavian Artery, Right **4** Subclavian Artery, Left **5** Axillary Artery, Right **6** Axillary Artery, Left **7** Brachial Artery, Right **8** Brachial Artery, Left **9** Ulnar Artery, Right **A** Ulnar Artery, Left **B** Radial Artery, Right **C** Radial Artery, Left **D** Hand Artery, Right **F** Hand Artery, Left **G** Intracranial Artery **H** Common Carotid Artery, Right **J** Common Carotid Artery, Left **K** Internal Carotid Artery, Right **L** Internal Carotid Artery, Left **M** External Carotid Artery, Right **N** External Carotid Artery, Left **P** Vertebral Artery, Right **Q** Vertebral Artery, Left **R** Face Artery **S** Temporal Artery, Right **T** Temporal Artery, Left **U** Thyroid Artery, Right **V** Thyroid Artery, Left **Y** Upper Artery	**0** Open **3** Percutaneous **4** Percutaneous Endoscopic	**Z** No Device	**Z** No Qualifier

Section 0 **Medical and Surgical**
Body System 3 **Upper Arteries**
Operation U **Supplement:** Putting in or on biological or synthetic material that physically reinforces and/or augments the function of a portion of a body part

Body Part (4th)	Approach (5th)	Device (6th)	Qualifier (7th)
0 Internal Mammary Artery, Right **1** Internal Mammary Artery, Left **2** Innominate Artery **3** Subclavian Artery, Right **4** Subclavian Artery, Left **5** Axillary Artery, Right **6** Axillary Artery, Left **7** Brachial Artery, Right **8** Brachial Artery, Left **9** Ulnar Artery, Right **A** Ulnar Artery, Left **B** Radial Artery, Right **C** Radial Artery, Left **D** Hand Artery, Right **F** Hand Artery, Left **G** Intracranial Artery **H** Common Carotid Artery, Right **J** Common Carotid Artery, Left **K** Internal Carotid Artery, Right **L** Internal Carotid Artery, Left **M** External Carotid Artery, Right **N** External Carotid Artery, Left **P** Vertebral Artery, Right **Q** Vertebral Artery, Left **R** Face Artery **S** Temporal Artery, Right **T** Temporal Artery, Left **U** Thyroid Artery, Right **V** Thyroid Artery, Left **Y** Upper Artery	**0** Open **3** Percutaneous **4** Percutaneous Endoscopic	**7** Autologous Tissue Substitute **J** Synthetic Substitute **K** Nonautologous Tissue Substitute	**Z** No Qualifier

Section 0 **Medical and Surgical**
Body System 3 **Upper Arteries**
Operation V **Restriction:** Partially closing an orifice or the lumen of a tubular body part

Body Part (4th)	Approach (5th)	Device (6th)	Qualifier (7th)
0 Internal Mammary Artery, Right **1** Internal Mammary Artery, Left **2** Innominate Artery **3** Subclavian Artery, Right **4** Subclavian Artery, Left **5** Axillary Artery, Right **6** Axillary Artery, Left **7** Brachial Artery, Right **8** Brachial Artery, Left **9** Ulnar Artery, Right **A** Ulnar Artery, Left **B** Radial Artery, Right **C** Radial Artery, Left **D** Hand Artery, Right **F** Hand Artery, Left **R** Face Artery **S** Temporal Artery, Right **T** Temporal Artery, Left **U** Thyroid Artery, Right **V** Thyroid Artery, Left **Y** Upper Artery	**0** Open **3** Percutaneous **4** Percutaneous Endoscopic	**C** Extraluminal Device **D** Intraluminal Device **Z** No Device	**Z** No Qualifier
G Intracranial Artery **H** Common Carotid Artery, Right **J** Common Carotid Artery, Left **K** Internal Carotid Artery, Right **L** Internal Carotid Artery, Left **M** External Carotid Artery, Right **N** External Carotid Artery, Left **P** Vertebral Artery, Right **Q** Vertebral Artery, Left	**0** Open **3** Percutaneous **4** Percutaneous Endoscopic	**B** Intraluminal Device, Bioactive **C** Extraluminal Device **D** Intraluminal Device **Z** No Device	**Z** No Qualifier

Section 0 **Medical and Surgical**
Body System 3 **Upper Arteries**
Operation W **Revision:** Correcting, to the extent possible, a portion of a malfunctioning device or the position of a displaced device

Body Part (4th)	Approach (5th)	Device (6th)	Qualifier (7th)
Y Upper Artery	**0** Open **3** Percutaneous **4** Percutaneous Endoscopic **X** External	**0** Drainage Device **2** Monitoring Device **3** Infusion Device **7** Autologous Tissue Substitute **C** Extraluminal Device **D** Intraluminal Device **J** Synthetic Substitute **K** Nonautologous Tissue Substitute **M** Stimulator Lead	**Z** No Qualifier

Upper Arteries Code Listing 031–03W

031 – Upper Arteries, Bypass

Review Coding Guideline B3.6a

0312090 Bypass Innominate Artery to Right Upper Arm Artery with Autologous Venous Tissue, Open Approach

0312091 Bypass Innominate Artery to Left Upper Arm Artery with Autologous Venous Tissue, Open Approach

0312092 Bypass Innominate Artery to Bilateral Upper Arm Artery with Autologous Venous Tissue, Open Approach

0312093 Bypass Innominate Artery to Right Lower Arm Artery with Autologous Venous Tissue, Open Approach

0312094 Bypass Innominate Artery to Left Lower Arm Artery with Autologous Venous Tissue, Open Approach

0312095 Bypass Innominate Artery to Bilateral Lower Arm Artery with Autologous Venous Tissue, Open Approach

0312096 Bypass Innominate Artery to Right Upper Leg Artery with Autologous Venous Tissue, Open Approach

0312097 Bypass Innominate Artery to Left Upper Leg Artery with Autologous Venous Tissue, Open Approach

0312098 Bypass Innominate Artery to Bilateral Upper Leg Artery with Autologous Venous Tissue, Open Approach

0312099 Bypass Innominate Artery to Right Lower Leg Artery with Autologous Venous Tissue, Open Approach
031209B Bypass Innominate Artery to Left Lower Leg Artery with Autologous Venous Tissue, Open Approach
031209C Bypass Innominate Artery to Bilateral Lower Leg Artery with Autologous Venous Tissue, Open Approach
031209D Bypass Innominate Artery to Upper Arm Vein with Autologous Venous Tissue, Open Approach
031209F Bypass Innominate Artery to Lower Arm Vein with Autologous Venous Tissue, Open Approach
031209J Bypass Innominate Artery to Right Extracranial Artery with Autologous Venous Tissue, Open Approach
031209K Bypass Innominate Artery to Left Extracranial Artery with Autologous Venous Tissue, Open Approach
03120A0 Bypass Innominate Artery to Right Upper Arm Artery with Autologous Arterial Tissue, Open Approach
03120A1 Bypass Innominate Artery to Left Upper Arm Artery with Autologous Arterial Tissue, Open Approach
03120A2 Bypass Innominate Artery to Bilateral Upper Arm Artery with Autologous Arterial Tissue, Open Approach
03120A3 Bypass Innominate Artery to Right Lower Arm Artery with Autologous Arterial Tissue, Open Approach
03120A4 Bypass Innominate Artery to Left Lower Arm Artery with Autologous Arterial Tissue, Open Approach
03120A5 Bypass Innominate Artery to Bilateral Lower Arm Artery with Autologous Arterial Tissue, Open Approach
03120A6 Bypass Innominate Artery to Right Upper Leg Artery with Autologous Arterial Tissue, Open Approach
03120A7 Bypass Innominate Artery to Left Upper Leg Artery with Autologous Arterial Tissue, Open Approach
03120A8 Bypass Innominate Artery to Bilateral Upper Leg Artery with Autologous Arterial Tissue, Open Approach
03120A9 Bypass Innominate Artery to Right Lower Leg Artery with Autologous Arterial Tissue, Open Approach
03120AB Bypass Innominate Artery to Left Lower Leg Artery with Autologous Arterial Tissue, Open Approach
03120AC Bypass Innominate Artery to Bilateral Lower Leg Artery with Autologous Arterial Tissue, Open Approach
03120AD Bypass Innominate Artery to Upper Arm Vein with Autologous Arterial Tissue, Open Approach
03120AF Bypass Innominate Artery to Lower Arm Vein with Autologous Arterial Tissue, Open Approach
03120AJ Bypass Innominate Artery to Right Extracranial Artery with Autologous Arterial Tissue, Open Approach
03120AK Bypass Innominate Artery to Left Extracranial Artery with Autologous Arterial Tissue, Open Approach
03120J0 Bypass Innominate Artery to Right Upper Arm Artery with Synthetic Substitute, Open Approach
03120J1 Bypass Innominate Artery to Left Upper Arm Artery with Synthetic Substitute, Open Approach
03120J2 Bypass Innominate Artery to Bilateral Upper Arm Artery with Synthetic Substitute, Open Approach
03120J3 Bypass Innominate Artery to Right Lower Arm Artery with Synthetic Substitute, Open Approach
03120J4 Bypass Innominate Artery to Left Lower Arm Artery with Synthetic Substitute, Open Approach
03120J5 Bypass Innominate Artery to Bilateral Lower Arm Artery with Synthetic Substitute, Open Approach
03120J6 Bypass Innominate Artery to Right Upper Leg Artery with Synthetic Substitute, Open Approach
03120J7 Bypass Innominate Artery to Left Upper Leg Artery with Synthetic Substitute, Open Approach
03120J8 Bypass Innominate Artery to Bilateral Upper Leg Artery with Synthetic Substitute, Open Approach
03120J9 Bypass Innominate Artery to Right Lower Leg Artery with Synthetic Substitute, Open Approach
03120JB Bypass Innominate Artery to Left Lower Leg Artery with Synthetic Substitute, Open Approach
03120JC Bypass Innominate Artery to Bilateral Lower Leg Artery with Synthetic Substitute, Open Approach
03120JD Bypass Innominate Artery to Upper Arm Vein with Synthetic Substitute, Open Approach
03120JF Bypass Innominate Artery to Lower Arm Vein with Synthetic Substitute, Open Approach
03120JJ Bypass Innominate Artery to Right Extracranial Artery with Synthetic Substitute, Open Approach
03120JK Bypass Innominate Artery to Left Extracranial Artery with Synthetic Substitute, Open Approach
03120K0 Bypass Innominate Artery to Right Upper Arm Artery with Nonautologous Tissue Substitute, Open Approach
03120K1 Bypass Innominate Artery to Left Upper Arm Artery with Nonautologous Tissue Substitute, Open Approach
03120K2 Bypass Innominate Artery to Bilateral Upper Arm Artery with Nonautologous Tissue Substitute, Open Approach
03120K3 Bypass Innominate Artery to Right Lower Arm Artery with Nonautologous Tissue Substitute, Open Approach
03120K4 Bypass Innominate Artery to Left Lower Arm Artery with Nonautologous Tissue Substitute, Open Approach
03120K5 Bypass Innominate Artery to Bilateral Lower Arm Artery with Nonautologous Tissue Substitute, Open Approach
03120K6 Bypass Innominate Artery to Right Upper Leg Artery with Nonautologous Tissue Substitute, Open Approach
03120K7 Bypass Innominate Artery to Left Upper Leg Artery with Nonautologous Tissue Substitute, Open Approach
03120K8 Bypass Innominate Artery to Bilateral Upper Leg Artery with Nonautologous Tissue Substitute, Open Approach
03120K9 Bypass Innominate Artery to Right Lower Leg Artery with Nonautologous Tissue Substitute, Open Approach
03120KB Bypass Innominate Artery to Left Lower Leg Artery with Nonautologous Tissue Substitute, Open Approach
03120KC Bypass Innominate Artery to Bilateral Lower Leg Artery with Nonautologous Tissue Substitute, Open Approach
03120KD Bypass Innominate Artery to Upper Arm Vein with Nonautologous Tissue Substitute, Open Approach
03120KF Bypass Innominate Artery to Lower Arm Vein with Nonautologous Tissue Substitute, Open Approach
03120KJ Bypass Innominate Artery to Right Extracranial Artery with Nonautologous Tissue Substitute, Open Approach
03120KK Bypass Innominate Artery to Left Extracranial Artery with Nonautologous Tissue Substitute, Open Approach
03120Z0 Bypass Innominate Artery to Right Upper Arm Artery, Open Approach
03120Z1 Bypass Innominate Artery to Left Upper Arm Artery, Open Approach
03120Z2 Bypass Innominate Artery to Bilateral Upper Arm Artery, Open Approach
03120Z3 Bypass Innominate Artery to Right Lower Arm Artery, Open Approach
03120Z4 Bypass Innominate Artery to Left Lower Arm Artery, Open Approach
03120Z5 Bypass Innominate Artery to Bilateral Lower Arm Artery, Open Approach
03120Z6 Bypass Innominate Artery to Right Upper Leg Artery, Open Approach
03120Z7 Bypass Innominate Artery to Left Upper Leg Artery, Open Approach
03120Z8 Bypass Innominate Artery to Bilateral Upper Leg Artery, Open Approach
03120Z9 Bypass Innominate Artery to Right Lower Leg Artery, Open Approach
03120ZB Bypass Innominate Artery to Left Lower Leg Artery, Open Approach
03120ZC Bypass Innominate Artery to Bilateral Lower Leg Artery, Open Approach
03120ZD Bypass Innominate Artery to Upper Arm Vein, Open Approach
03120ZF Bypass Innominate Artery to Lower Arm Vein, Open Approach
03120ZJ Bypass Innominate Artery to Right Extracranial Artery, Open Approach
03120ZK Bypass Innominate Artery to Left Extracranial Artery, Open Approach
0313090 Bypass Right Subclavian Artery to Right Upper Arm Artery with Autologous Venous Tissue, Open Approach
0313091 Bypass Right Subclavian Artery to Left Upper Arm Artery with Autologous Venous Tissue, Open Approach
0313092 Bypass Right Subclavian Artery to Bilateral Upper Arm Artery with Autologous Venous Tissue, Open Approach
0313093 Bypass Right Subclavian Artery to Right Lower Arm Artery with Autologous Venous Tissue, Open Approach
0313094 Bypass Right Subclavian Artery to Left Lower Arm Artery with Autologous Venous Tissue, Open Approach
0313095 Bypass Right Subclavian Artery to Bilateral Lower Arm Artery with Autologous Venous Tissue, Open Approach
0313096 Bypass Right Subclavian Artery to Right Upper Leg Artery with Autologous Venous Tissue, Open Approach
0313097 Bypass Right Subclavian Artery to Left Upper Leg Artery with Autologous Venous Tissue, Open Approach
0313098 Bypass Right Subclavian Artery to Bilateral Upper Leg Artery with Autologous Venous Tissue, Open Approach

0313099 Bypass Right Subclavian Artery to Right Lower Leg Artery with Autologous Venous Tissue, Open Approach
031309B Bypass Right Subclavian Artery to Left Lower Leg Artery with Autologous Venous Tissue, Open Approach
031309C Bypass Right Subclavian Artery to Bilateral Lower Leg Artery with Autologous Venous Tissue, Open Approach
031309D Bypass Right Subclavian Artery to Upper Arm Vein with Autologous Venous Tissue, Open Approach
031309F Bypass Right Subclavian Artery to Lower Arm Vein with Autologous Venous Tissue, Open Approach
031309J Bypass Right Subclavian Artery to Right Extracranial Artery with Autologous Venous Tissue, Open Approach
031309K Bypass Right Subclavian Artery to Left Extracranial Artery with Autologous Venous Tissue, Open Approach
031309M Bypass Right Subclavian Artery to Right Pulmonary Artery with Autologous Venous Tissue, Open Approach
031309N Bypass Right Subclavian Artery to Left Pulmonary Artery with Autologous Venous Tissue, Open Approach
03130A0 Bypass Right Subclavian Artery to Right Upper Arm Artery with Autologous Arterial Tissue, Open Approach
03130A1 Bypass Right Subclavian Artery to Left Upper Arm Artery with Autologous Arterial Tissue, Open Approach
03130A2 Bypass Right Subclavian Artery to Bilateral Upper Arm Artery with Autologous Arterial Tissue, Open Approach
03130A3 Bypass Right Subclavian Artery to Right Lower Arm Artery with Autologous Arterial Tissue, Open Approach
03130A4 Bypass Right Subclavian Artery to Left Lower Arm Artery with Autologous Arterial Tissue, Open Approach
03130A5 Bypass Right Subclavian Artery to Bilateral Lower Arm Artery with Autologous Arterial Tissue, Open Approach
03130A6 Bypass Right Subclavian Artery to Right Upper Leg Artery with Autologous Arterial Tissue, Open Approach
03130A7 Bypass Right Subclavian Artery to Left Upper Leg Artery with Autologous Arterial Tissue, Open Approach
03130A8 Bypass Right Subclavian Artery to Bilateral Upper Leg Artery with Autologous Arterial Tissue, Open Approach
03130A9 Bypass Right Subclavian Artery to Right Lower Leg Artery with Autologous Arterial Tissue, Open Approach
03130AB Bypass Right Subclavian Artery to Left Lower Leg Artery with Autologous Arterial Tissue, Open Approach
03130AC Bypass Right Subclavian Artery to Bilateral Lower Leg Artery with Autologous Arterial Tissue, Open Approach
03130AD Bypass Right Subclavian Artery to Upper Arm Vein with Autologous Arterial Tissue, Open Approach
03130AF Bypass Right Subclavian Artery to Lower Arm Vein with Autologous Arterial Tissue, Open Approach
03130AJ Bypass Right Subclavian Artery to Right Extracranial Artery with Autologous Arterial Tissue, Open Approach
03130AK Bypass Right Subclavian Artery to Left Extracranial Artery with Autologous Arterial Tissue, Open Approach
03130AM Bypass Right Subclavian Artery to Right Pulmonary Artery with Autologous Arterial Tissue, Open Approach
03130AN Bypass Right Subclavian Artery to Left Pulmonary Artery with Autologous Arterial Tissue, Open Approach
03130J0 Bypass Right Subclavian Artery to Right Upper Arm Artery with Synthetic Substitute, Open Approach
03130J1 Bypass Right Subclavian Artery to Left Upper Arm Artery with Synthetic Substitute, Open Approach
03130J2 Bypass Right Subclavian Artery to Bilateral Upper Arm Artery with Synthetic Substitute, Open Approach
03130J3 Bypass Right Subclavian Artery to Right Lower Arm Artery with Synthetic Substitute, Open Approach
03130J4 Bypass Right Subclavian Artery to Left Lower Arm Artery with Synthetic Substitute, Open Approach
03130J5 Bypass Right Subclavian Artery to Bilateral Lower Arm Artery with Synthetic Substitute, Open Approach
03130J6 Bypass Right Subclavian Artery to Right Upper Leg Artery with Synthetic Substitute, Open Approach
03130J7 Bypass Right Subclavian Artery to Left Upper Leg Artery with Synthetic Substitute, Open Approach
03130J8 Bypass Right Subclavian Artery to Bilateral Upper Leg Artery with Synthetic Substitute, Open Approach
03130J9 Bypass Right Subclavian Artery to Right Lower Leg Artery with Synthetic Substitute, Open Approach
03130JB Bypass Right Subclavian Artery to Left Lower Leg Artery with Synthetic Substitute, Open Approach
03130JC Bypass Right Subclavian Artery to Bilateral Lower Leg Artery with Synthetic Substitute, Open Approach
03130JD Bypass Right Subclavian Artery to Upper Arm Vein with Synthetic Substitute, Open Approach
03130JF Bypass Right Subclavian Artery to Lower Arm Vein with Synthetic Substitute, Open Approach
03130JJ Bypass Right Subclavian Artery to Right Extracranial Artery with Synthetic Substitute, Open Approach
03130JK Bypass Right Subclavian Artery to Left Extracranial Artery with Synthetic Substitute, Open Approach
03130JM Bypass Right Subclavian Artery to Right Pulmonary Artery with Synthetic Substitute, Open Approach
03130JN Bypass Right Subclavian Artery to Left Pulmonary Artery with Synthetic Substitute, Open Approach
03130K0 Bypass Right Subclavian Artery to Right Upper Arm Artery with Nonautologous Tissue Substitute, Open Approach
03130K1 Bypass Right Subclavian Artery to Left Upper Arm Artery with Nonautologous Tissue Substitute, Open Approach
03130K2 Bypass Right Subclavian Artery to Bilateral Upper Arm Artery with Nonautologous Tissue Substitute, Open Approach
03130K3 Bypass Right Subclavian Artery to Right Lower Arm Artery with Nonautologous Tissue Substitute, Open Approach
03130K4 Bypass Right Subclavian Artery to Left Lower Arm Artery with Nonautologous Tissue Substitute, Open Approach
03130K5 Bypass Right Subclavian Artery to Bilateral Lower Arm Artery with Nonautologous Tissue Substitute, Open Approach
03130K6 Bypass Right Subclavian Artery to Right Upper Leg Artery with Nonautologous Tissue Substitute, Open Approach
03130K7 Bypass Right Subclavian Artery to Left Upper Leg Artery with Nonautologous Tissue Substitute, Open Approach
03130K8 Bypass Right Subclavian Artery to Bilateral Upper Leg Artery with Nonautologous Tissue Substitute, Open Approach
03130K9 Bypass Right Subclavian Artery to Right Lower Leg Artery with Nonautologous Tissue Substitute, Open Approach
03130KB Bypass Right Subclavian Artery to Left Lower Leg Artery with Nonautologous Tissue Substitute, Open Approach
03130KC Bypass Right Subclavian Artery to Bilateral Lower Leg Artery with Nonautologous Tissue Substitute, Open Approach
03130KD Bypass Right Subclavian Artery to Upper Arm Vein with Nonautologous Tissue Substitute, Open Approach
03130KF Bypass Right Subclavian Artery to Lower Arm Vein with Nonautologous Tissue Substitute, Open Approach
03130KJ Bypass Right Subclavian Artery to Right Extracranial Artery with Nonautologous Tissue Substitute, Open Approach
03130KK Bypass Right Subclavian Artery to Left Extracranial Artery with Nonautologous Tissue Substitute, Open Approach
03130KM Bypass Right Subclavian Artery to Right Pulmonary Artery with Nonautologous Tissue Substitute, Open Approach
03130KN Bypass Right Subclavian Artery to Left Pulmonary Artery with Nonautologous Tissue Substitute, Open Approach
03130Z0 Bypass Right Subclavian Artery to Right Upper Arm Artery, Open Approach
03130Z1 Bypass Right Subclavian Artery to Left Upper Arm Artery, Open Approach
03130Z2 Bypass Right Subclavian Artery to Bilateral Upper Arm Artery, Open Approach
03130Z3 Bypass Right Subclavian Artery to Right Lower Arm Artery, Open Approach
03130Z4 Bypass Right Subclavian Artery to Left Lower Arm Artery, Open Approach
03130Z5 Bypass Right Subclavian Artery to Bilateral Lower Arm Artery, Open Approach
03130Z6 Bypass Right Subclavian Artery to Right Upper Leg Artery, Open Approach
03130Z7 Bypass Right Subclavian Artery to Left Upper Leg Artery, Open Approach
03130Z8 Bypass Right Subclavian Artery to Bilateral Upper Leg Artery, Open Approach
03130Z9 Bypass Right Subclavian Artery to Right Lower Leg Artery, Open Approach
03130ZB Bypass Right Subclavian Artery to Left Lower Leg Artery, Open Approach
03130ZC Bypass Right Subclavian Artery to Bilateral Lower Leg Artery, Open Approach
03130ZD Bypass Right Subclavian Artery to Upper Arm Vein, Open Approach
03130ZF Bypass Right Subclavian Artery to Lower Arm Vein, Open Approach
03130ZJ Bypass Right Subclavian Artery to Right Extracranial Artery, Open Approach

03130ZK Bypass Right Subclavian Artery to Left Extracranial Artery, Open Approach
03130ZM Bypass Right Subclavian Artery to Right Pulmonary Artery, Open Approach
03130ZN Bypass Right Subclavian Artery to Left Pulmonary Artery, Open Approach
0314090 Bypass Left Subclavian Artery to Right Upper Arm Artery with Autologous Venous Tissue, Open Approach
0314091 Bypass Left Subclavian Artery to Left Upper Arm Artery with Autologous Venous Tissue, Open Approach
0314092 Bypass Left Subclavian Artery to Bilateral Upper Arm Artery with Autologous Venous Tissue, Open Approach
0314093 Bypass Left Subclavian Artery to Right Lower Arm Artery with Autologous Venous Tissue, Open Approach
0314094 Bypass Left Subclavian Artery to Left Lower Arm Artery with Autologous Venous Tissue, Open Approach
0314095 Bypass Left Subclavian Artery to Bilateral Lower Arm Artery with Autologous Venous Tissue, Open Approach
0314096 Bypass Left Subclavian Artery to Right Upper Leg Artery with Autologous Venous Tissue, Open Approach
0314097 Bypass Left Subclavian Artery to Left Upper Leg Artery with Autologous Venous Tissue, Open Approach
0314098 Bypass Left Subclavian Artery to Bilateral Upper Leg Artery with Autologous Venous Tissue, Open Approach
0314099 Bypass Left Subclavian Artery to Right Lower Leg Artery with Autologous Venous Tissue, Open Approach
031409B Bypass Left Subclavian Artery to Left Lower Leg Artery with Autologous Venous Tissue, Open Approach
031409C Bypass Left Subclavian Artery to Bilateral Lower Leg Artery with Autologous Venous Tissue, Open Approach
031409D Bypass Left Subclavian Artery to Upper Arm Vein with Autologous Venous Tissue, Open Approach
031409F Bypass Left Subclavian Artery to Lower Arm Vein with Autologous Venous Tissue, Open Approach
031409J Bypass Left Subclavian Artery to Right Extracranial Artery with Autologous Venous Tissue, Open Approach
031409K Bypass Left Subclavian Artery to Left Extracranial Artery with Autologous Venous Tissue, Open Approach
031409M Bypass Left Subclavian Artery to Right Pulmonary Artery with Autologous Venous Tissue, Open Approach
031409N Bypass Left Subclavian Artery to Left Pulmonary Artery with Autologous Venous Tissue, Open Approach
03140A0 Bypass Left Subclavian Artery to Right Upper Arm Artery with Autologous Arterial Tissue, Open Approach
03140A1 Bypass Left Subclavian Artery to Left Upper Arm Artery with Autologous Arterial Tissue, Open Approach
03140A2 Bypass Left Subclavian Artery to Bilateral Upper Arm Artery with Autologous Arterial Tissue, Open Approach
03140A3 Bypass Left Subclavian Artery to Right Lower Arm Artery with Autologous Arterial Tissue, Open Approach
03140A4 Bypass Left Subclavian Artery to Left Lower Arm Artery with Autologous Arterial Tissue, Open Approach
03140A5 Bypass Left Subclavian Artery to Bilateral Lower Arm Artery with Autologous Arterial Tissue, Open Approach
03140A6 Bypass Left Subclavian Artery to Right Upper Leg Artery with Autologous Arterial Tissue, Open Approach
03140A7 Bypass Left Subclavian Artery to Left Upper Leg Artery with Autologous Arterial Tissue, Open Approach
03140A8 Bypass Left Subclavian Artery to Bilateral Upper Leg Artery with Autologous Arterial Tissue, Open Approach
03140A9 Bypass Left Subclavian Artery to Right Lower Leg Artery with Autologous Arterial Tissue, Open Approach
03140AB Bypass Left Subclavian Artery to Left Lower Leg Artery with Autologous Arterial Tissue, Open Approach
03140AC Bypass Left Subclavian Artery to Bilateral Lower Leg Artery with Autologous Arterial Tissue, Open Approach
03140AD Bypass Left Subclavian Artery to Upper Arm Vein with Autologous Arterial Tissue, Open Approach
03140AF Bypass Left Subclavian Artery to Lower Arm Vein with Autologous Arterial Tissue, Open Approach
03140AJ Bypass Left Subclavian Artery to Right Extracranial Artery with Autologous Arterial Tissue, Open Approach
03140AK Bypass Left Subclavian Artery to Left Extracranial Artery with Autologous Arterial Tissue, Open Approach
03140AM Bypass Left Subclavian Artery to Right Pulmonary Artery with Autologous Arterial Tissue, Open Approach
03140AN Bypass Left Subclavian Artery to Left Pulmonary Artery with Autologous Arterial Tissue, Open Approach
03140J0 Bypass Left Subclavian Artery to Right Upper Arm Artery with Synthetic Substitute, Open Approach
03140J1 Bypass Left Subclavian Artery to Left Upper Arm Artery with Synthetic Substitute, Open Approach
03140J2 Bypass Left Subclavian Artery to Bilateral Upper Arm Artery with Synthetic Substitute, Open Approach
03140J3 Bypass Left Subclavian Artery to Right Lower Arm Artery with Synthetic Substitute, Open Approach
03140J4 Bypass Left Subclavian Artery to Left Lower Arm Artery with Synthetic Substitute, Open Approach
03140J5 Bypass Left Subclavian Artery to Bilateral Lower Arm Artery with Synthetic Substitute, Open Approach
03140J6 Bypass Left Subclavian Artery to Right Upper Leg Artery with Synthetic Substitute, Open Approach
03140J7 Bypass Left Subclavian Artery to Left Upper Leg Artery with Synthetic Substitute, Open Approach
03140J8 Bypass Left Subclavian Artery to Bilateral Upper Leg Artery with Synthetic Substitute, Open Approach
03140J9 Bypass Left Subclavian Artery to Right Lower Leg Artery with Synthetic Substitute, Open Approach
03140JB Bypass Left Subclavian Artery to Left Lower Leg Artery with Synthetic Substitute, Open Approach
03140JC Bypass Left Subclavian Artery to Bilateral Lower Leg Artery with Synthetic Substitute, Open Approach
03140JD Bypass Left Subclavian Artery to Upper Arm Vein with Synthetic Substitute, Open Approach
03140JF Bypass Left Subclavian Artery to Lower Arm Vein with Synthetic Substitute, Open Approach
03140JJ Bypass Left Subclavian Artery to Right Extracranial Artery with Synthetic Substitute, Open Approach
03140JK Bypass Left Subclavian Artery to Left Extracranial Artery with Synthetic Substitute, Open Approach
03140JM Bypass Left Subclavian Artery to Right Pulmonary Artery with Synthetic Substitute, Open Approach
03140JN Bypass Left Subclavian Artery to Left Pulmonary Artery with Synthetic Substitute, Open Approach
03140K0 Bypass Left Subclavian Artery to Right Upper Arm Artery with Nonautologous Tissue Substitute, Open Approach
03140K1 Bypass Left Subclavian Artery to Left Upper Arm Artery with Nonautologous Tissue Substitute, Open Approach
03140K2 Bypass Left Subclavian Artery to Bilateral Upper Arm Artery with Nonautologous Tissue Substitute, Open Approach
03140K3 Bypass Left Subclavian Artery to Right Lower Arm Artery with Nonautologous Tissue Substitute, Open Approach
03140K4 Bypass Left Subclavian Artery to Left Lower Arm Artery with Nonautologous Tissue Substitute, Open Approach
03140K5 Bypass Left Subclavian Artery to Bilateral Lower Arm Artery with Nonautologous Tissue Substitute, Open Approach
03140K6 Bypass Left Subclavian Artery to Right Upper Leg Artery with Nonautologous Tissue Substitute, Open Approach
03140K7 Bypass Left Subclavian Artery to Left Upper Leg Artery with Nonautologous Tissue Substitute, Open Approach
03140K8 Bypass Left Subclavian Artery to Bilateral Upper Leg Artery with Nonautologous Tissue Substitute, Open Approach
03140K9 Bypass Left Subclavian Artery to Right Lower Leg Artery with Nonautologous Tissue Substitute, Open Approach
03140KB Bypass Left Subclavian Artery to Left Lower Leg Artery with Nonautologous Tissue Substitute, Open Approach
03140KC Bypass Left Subclavian Artery to Bilateral Lower Leg Artery with Nonautologous Tissue Substitute, Open Approach
03140KD Bypass Left Subclavian Artery to Upper Arm Vein with Nonautologous Tissue Substitute, Open Approach
03140KF Bypass Left Subclavian Artery to Lower Arm Vein with Nonautologous Tissue Substitute, Open Approach
03140KJ Bypass Left Subclavian Artery to Right Extracranial Artery with Nonautologous Tissue Substitute, Open Approach
03140KK Bypass Left Subclavian Artery to Left Extracranial Artery with Nonautologous Tissue Substitute, Open Approach
03140KM Bypass Left Subclavian Artery to Right Pulmonary Artery with Nonautologous Tissue Substitute, Open Approach
03140KN Bypass Left Subclavian Artery to Left Pulmonary Artery with Nonautologous Tissue Substitute, Open Approach
03140Z0 Bypass Left Subclavian Artery to Right Upper Arm Artery, Open Approach
03140Z1 Bypass Left Subclavian Artery to Left Upper Arm Artery, Open Approach
03140Z2 Bypass Left Subclavian Artery to Bilateral Upper Arm Artery, Open Approach
03140Z3 Bypass Left Subclavian Artery to Right Lower Arm Artery, Open Approach
03140Z4 Bypass Left Subclavian Artery to Left Lower Arm Artery, Open Approach
03140Z5 Bypass Left Subclavian Artery to Bilateral Lower Arm Artery, Open Approach

03140Z6 Bypass Left Subclavian Artery to Right Upper Leg Artery, Open Approach
03140Z7 Bypass Left Subclavian Artery to Left Upper Leg Artery, Open Approach
03140Z8 Bypass Left Subclavian Artery to Bilateral Upper Leg Artery, Open Approach
03140Z9 Bypass Left Subclavian Artery to Right Lower Leg Artery, Open Approach
03140ZB Bypass Left Subclavian Artery to Left Lower Leg Artery, Open Approach
03140ZC Bypass Left Subclavian Artery to Bilateral Lower Leg Artery, Open Approach
03140ZD Bypass Left Subclavian Artery to Upper Arm Vein, Open Approach
03140ZF Bypass Left Subclavian Artery to Lower Arm Vein, Open Approach
03140ZJ Bypass Left Subclavian Artery to Right Extracranial Artery, Open Approach
03140ZK Bypass Left Subclavian Artery to Left Extracranial Artery, Open Approach
03140ZM Bypass Left Subclavian Artery to Right Pulmonary Artery, Open Approach
03140ZN Bypass Left Subclavian Artery to Left Pulmonary Artery, Open Approach
0315090 Bypass Right Axillary Artery to Right Upper Arm Artery with Autologous Venous Tissue, Open Approach
0315091 Bypass Right Axillary Artery to Left Upper Arm Artery with Autologous Venous Tissue, Open Approach
0315092 Bypass Right Axillary Artery to Bilateral Upper Arm Artery with Autologous Venous Tissue, Open Approach
0315093 Bypass Right Axillary Artery to Right Lower Arm Artery with Autologous Venous Tissue, Open Approach
0315094 Bypass Right Axillary Artery to Left Lower Arm Artery with Autologous Venous Tissue, Open Approach
0315095 Bypass Right Axillary Artery to Bilateral Lower Arm Artery with Autologous Venous Tissue, Open Approach
0315096 Bypass Right Axillary Artery to Right Upper Leg Artery with Autologous Venous Tissue, Open Approach
0315097 Bypass Right Axillary Artery to Left Upper Leg Artery with Autologous Venous Tissue, Open Approach
0315098 Bypass Right Axillary Artery to Bilateral Upper Leg Artery with Autologous Venous Tissue, Open Approach
0315099 Bypass Right Axillary Artery to Right Lower Leg Artery with Autologous Venous Tissue, Open Approach
031509B Bypass Right Axillary Artery to Left Lower Leg Artery with Autologous Venous Tissue, Open Approach
031509C Bypass Right Axillary Artery to Bilateral Lower Leg Artery with Autologous Venous Tissue, Open Approach
031509D Bypass Right Axillary Artery to Upper Arm Vein with Autologous Venous Tissue, Open Approach
031509F Bypass Right Axillary Artery to Lower Arm Vein with Autologous Venous Tissue, Open Approach
031509J Bypass Right Axillary Artery to Right Extracranial Artery with Autologous Venous Tissue, Open Approach
031509K Bypass Right Axillary Artery to Left Extracranial Artery with Autologous Venous Tissue, Open Approach
03150A0 Bypass Right Axillary Artery to Right Upper Arm Artery with Autologous Arterial Tissue, Open Approach
03150A1 Bypass Right Axillary Artery to Left Upper Arm Artery with Autologous Arterial Tissue, Open Approach
03150A2 Bypass Right Axillary Artery to Bilateral Upper Arm Artery with Autologous Arterial Tissue, Open Approach
03150A3 Bypass Right Axillary Artery to Right Lower Arm Artery with Autologous Arterial Tissue, Open Approach
03150A4 Bypass Right Axillary Artery to Left Lower Arm Artery with Autologous Arterial Tissue, Open Approach
03150A5 Bypass Right Axillary Artery to Bilateral Lower Arm Artery with Autologous Arterial Tissue, Open Approach
03150A6 Bypass Right Axillary Artery to Right Upper Leg Artery with Autologous Arterial Tissue, Open Approach
03150A7 Bypass Right Axillary Artery to Left Upper Leg Artery with Autologous Arterial Tissue, Open Approach
03150A8 Bypass Right Axillary Artery to Bilateral Upper Leg Artery with Autologous Arterial Tissue, Open Approach
03150A9 Bypass Right Axillary Artery to Right Lower Leg Artery with Autologous Arterial Tissue, Open Approach
03150AB Bypass Right Axillary Artery to Left Lower Leg Artery with Autologous Arterial Tissue, Open Approach
03150AC Bypass Right Axillary Artery to Bilateral Lower Leg Artery with Autologous Arterial Tissue, Open Approach
03150AD Bypass Right Axillary Artery to Upper Arm Vein with Autologous Arterial Tissue, Open Approach
03150AF Bypass Right Axillary Artery to Lower Arm Vein with Autologous Arterial Tissue, Open Approach
03150AJ Bypass Right Axillary Artery to Right Extracranial Artery with Autologous Arterial Tissue, Open Approach
03150AK Bypass Right Axillary Artery to Left Extracranial Artery with Autologous Arterial Tissue, Open Approach
03150J0 Bypass Right Axillary Artery to Right Upper Arm Artery with Synthetic Substitute, Open Approach
03150J1 Bypass Right Axillary Artery to Left Upper Arm Artery with Synthetic Substitute, Open Approach
03150J2 Bypass Right Axillary Artery to Bilateral Upper Arm Artery with Synthetic Substitute, Open Approach
03150J3 Bypass Right Axillary Artery to Right Lower Arm Artery with Synthetic Substitute, Open Approach
03150J4 Bypass Right Axillary Artery to Left Lower Arm Artery with Synthetic Substitute, Open Approach
03150J5 Bypass Right Axillary Artery to Bilateral Lower Arm Artery with Synthetic Substitute, Open Approach
03150J6 Bypass Right Axillary Artery to Right Upper Leg Artery with Synthetic Substitute, Open Approach
03150J7 Bypass Right Axillary Artery to Left Upper Leg Artery with Synthetic Substitute, Open Approach
03150J8 Bypass Right Axillary Artery to Bilateral Upper Leg Artery with Synthetic Substitute, Open Approach
03150J9 Bypass Right Axillary Artery to Right Lower Leg Artery with Synthetic Substitute, Open Approach
03150JB Bypass Right Axillary Artery to Left Lower Leg Artery with Synthetic Substitute, Open Approach
03150JC Bypass Right Axillary Artery to Bilateral Lower Leg Artery with Synthetic Substitute, Open Approach
03150JD Bypass Right Axillary Artery to Upper Arm Vein with Synthetic Substitute, Open Approach
03150JF Bypass Right Axillary Artery to Lower Arm Vein with Synthetic Substitute, Open Approach
03150JJ Bypass Right Axillary Artery to Right Extracranial Artery with Synthetic Substitute, Open Approach
03150JK Bypass Right Axillary Artery to Left Extracranial Artery with Synthetic Substitute, Open Approach
03150K0 Bypass Right Axillary Artery to Right Upper Arm Artery with Nonautologous Tissue Substitute, Open Approach
03150K1 Bypass Right Axillary Artery to Left Upper Arm Artery with Nonautologous Tissue Substitute, Open Approach
03150K2 Bypass Right Axillary Artery to Bilateral Upper Arm Artery with Nonautologous Tissue Substitute, Open Approach
03150K3 Bypass Right Axillary Artery to Right Lower Arm Artery with Nonautologous Tissue Substitute, Open Approach
03150K4 Bypass Right Axillary Artery to Left Lower Arm Artery with Nonautologous Tissue Substitute, Open Approach
03150K5 Bypass Right Axillary Artery to Bilateral Lower Arm Artery with Nonautologous Tissue Substitute, Open Approach
03150K6 Bypass Right Axillary Artery to Right Upper Leg Artery with Nonautologous Tissue Substitute, Open Approach
03150K7 Bypass Right Axillary Artery to Left Upper Leg Artery with Nonautologous Tissue Substitute, Open Approach
03150K8 Bypass Right Axillary Artery to Bilateral Upper Leg Artery with Nonautologous Tissue Substitute, Open Approach
03150K9 Bypass Right Axillary Artery to Right Lower Leg Artery with Nonautologous Tissue Substitute, Open Approach
03150KB Bypass Right Axillary Artery to Left Lower Leg Artery with Nonautologous Tissue Substitute, Open Approach
03150KC Bypass Right Axillary Artery to Bilateral Lower Leg Artery with Nonautologous Tissue Substitute, Open Approach
03150KD Bypass Right Axillary Artery to Upper Arm Vein with Nonautologous Tissue Substitute, Open Approach
03150KF Bypass Right Axillary Artery to Lower Arm Vein with Nonautologous Tissue Substitute, Open Approach
03150KJ Bypass Right Axillary Artery to Right Extracranial Artery with Nonautologous Tissue Substitute, Open Approach
03150KK Bypass Right Axillary Artery to Left Extracranial Artery with Nonautologous Tissue Substitute, Open Approach
03150Z0 Bypass Right Axillary Artery to Right Upper Arm Artery, Open Approach
03150Z1 Bypass Right Axillary Artery to Left Upper Arm Artery, Open Approach
03150Z2 Bypass Right Axillary Artery to Bilateral Upper Arm Artery, Open Approach
03150Z3 Bypass Right Axillary Artery to Right Lower Arm Artery, Open Approach
03150Z4 Bypass Right Axillary Artery to Left Lower Arm Artery, Open Approach
03150Z5 Bypass Right Axillary Artery to Bilateral Lower Arm Artery, Open Approach
03150Z6 Bypass Right Axillary Artery to Right Upper Leg Artery, Open Approach
03150Z7 Bypass Right Axillary Artery to Left Upper Leg Artery, Open Approach

03150Z8 Bypass Right Axillary Artery to Bilateral Upper Leg Artery, Open Approach
03150Z9 Bypass Right Axillary Artery to Right Lower Leg Artery, Open Approach
03150ZB Bypass Right Axillary Artery to Left Lower Leg Artery, Open Approach
03150ZC Bypass Right Axillary Artery to Bilateral Lower Leg Artery, Open Approach
03150ZD Bypass Right Axillary Artery to Upper Arm Vein, Open Approach
03150ZF Bypass Right Axillary Artery to Lower Arm Vein, Open Approach
03150ZJ Bypass Right Axillary Artery to Right Extracranial Artery, Open Approach
03150ZK Bypass Right Axillary Artery to Left Extracranial Artery, Open Approach
0316090 Bypass Left Axillary Artery to Right Upper Arm Artery with Autologous Venous Tissue, Open Approach
0316091 Bypass Left Axillary Artery to Left Upper Arm Artery with Autologous Venous Tissue, Open Approach
0316092 Bypass Left Axillary Artery to Bilateral Upper Arm Artery with Autologous Venous Tissue, Open Approach
0316093 Bypass Left Axillary Artery to Right Lower Arm Artery with Autologous Venous Tissue, Open Approach
0316094 Bypass Left Axillary Artery to Left Lower Arm Artery with Autologous Venous Tissue, Open Approach
0316095 Bypass Left Axillary Artery to Bilateral Lower Arm Artery with Autologous Venous Tissue, Open Approach
0316096 Bypass Left Axillary Artery to Right Upper Leg Artery with Autologous Venous Tissue, Open Approach
0316097 Bypass Left Axillary Artery to Left Upper Leg Artery with Autologous Venous Tissue, Open Approach
0316098 Bypass Left Axillary Artery to Bilateral Upper Leg Artery with Autologous Venous Tissue, Open Approach
0316099 Bypass Left Axillary Artery to Right Lower Leg Artery with Autologous Venous Tissue, Open Approach
031609B Bypass Left Axillary Artery to Left Lower Leg Artery with Autologous Venous Tissue, Open Approach
031609C Bypass Left Axillary Artery to Bilateral Lower Leg Artery with Autologous Venous Tissue, Open Approach
031609D Bypass Left Axillary Artery to Upper Arm Vein with Autologous Venous Tissue, Open Approach
031609F Bypass Left Axillary Artery to Lower Arm Vein with Autologous Venous Tissue, Open Approach
031609J Bypass Left Axillary Artery to Right Extracranial Artery with Autologous Venous Tissue, Open Approach
031609K Bypass Left Axillary Artery to Left Extracranial Artery with Autologous Venous Tissue, Open Approach
03160A0 Bypass Left Axillary Artery to Right Upper Arm Artery with Autologous Arterial Tissue, Open Approach
03160A1 Bypass Left Axillary Artery to Left Upper Arm Artery with Autologous Arterial Tissue, Open Approach
03160A2 Bypass Left Axillary Artery to Bilateral Upper Arm Artery with Autologous Arterial Tissue, Open Approach
03160A3 Bypass Left Axillary Artery to Right Lower Arm Artery with Autologous Arterial Tissue, Open Approach
03160A4 Bypass Left Axillary Artery to Left Lower Arm Artery with Autologous Arterial Tissue, Open Approach
03160A5 Bypass Left Axillary Artery to Bilateral Lower Arm Artery with Autologous Arterial Tissue, Open Approach
03160A6 Bypass Left Axillary Artery to Right Upper Leg Artery with Autologous Arterial Tissue, Open Approach
03160A7 Bypass Left Axillary Artery to Left Upper Leg Artery with Autologous Arterial Tissue, Open Approach
03160A8 Bypass Left Axillary Artery to Bilateral Upper Leg Artery with Autologous Arterial Tissue, Open Approach
03160A9 Bypass Left Axillary Artery to Right Lower Leg Artery with Autologous Arterial Tissue, Open Approach
03160AB Bypass Left Axillary Artery to Left Lower Leg Artery with Autologous Arterial Tissue, Open Approach
03160AC Bypass Left Axillary Artery to Bilateral Lower Leg Artery with Autologous Arterial Tissue, Open Approach
03160AD Bypass Left Axillary Artery to Upper Arm Vein with Autologous Arterial Tissue, Open Approach
03160AF Bypass Left Axillary Artery to Lower Arm Vein with Autologous Arterial Tissue, Open Approach
03160AJ Bypass Left Axillary Artery to Right Extracranial Artery with Autologous Arterial Tissue, Open Approach
03160AK Bypass Left Axillary Artery to Left Extracranial Artery with Autologous Arterial Tissue, Open Approach
03160J0 Bypass Left Axillary Artery to Right Upper Arm Artery with Synthetic Substitute, Open Approach
03160J1 Bypass Left Axillary Artery to Left Upper Arm Artery with Synthetic Substitute, Open Approach
03160J2 Bypass Left Axillary Artery to Bilateral Upper Arm Artery with Synthetic Substitute, Open Approach
03160J3 Bypass Left Axillary Artery to Right Lower Arm Artery with Synthetic Substitute, Open Approach
03160J4 Bypass Left Axillary Artery to Left Lower Arm Artery with Synthetic Substitute, Open Approach
03160J5 Bypass Left Axillary Artery to Bilateral Lower Arm Artery with Synthetic Substitute, Open Approach
03160J6 Bypass Left Axillary Artery to Right Upper Leg Artery with Synthetic Substitute, Open Approach
03160J7 Bypass Left Axillary Artery to Left Upper Leg Artery with Synthetic Substitute, Open Approach
03160J8 Bypass Left Axillary Artery to Bilateral Upper Leg Artery with Synthetic Substitute, Open Approach
03160J9 Bypass Left Axillary Artery to Right Lower Leg Artery with Synthetic Substitute, Open Approach
03160JB Bypass Left Axillary Artery to Left Lower Leg Artery with Synthetic Substitute, Open Approach
03160JC Bypass Left Axillary Artery to Bilateral Lower Leg Artery with Synthetic Substitute, Open Approach
03160JD Bypass Left Axillary Artery to Upper Arm Vein with Synthetic Substitute, Open Approach
03160JF Bypass Left Axillary Artery to Lower Arm Vein with Synthetic Substitute, Open Approach
03160JJ Bypass Left Axillary Artery to Right Extracranial Artery with Synthetic Substitute, Open Approach
03160JK Bypass Left Axillary Artery to Left Extracranial Artery with Synthetic Substitute, Open Approach
03160K0 Bypass Left Axillary Artery to Right Upper Arm Artery with Nonautologous Tissue Substitute, Open Approach
03160K1 Bypass Left Axillary Artery to Left Upper Arm Artery with Nonautologous Tissue Substitute, Open Approach
03160K2 Bypass Left Axillary Artery to Bilateral Upper Arm Artery with Nonautologous Tissue Substitute, Open Approach
03160K3 Bypass Left Axillary Artery to Right Lower Arm Artery with Nonautologous Tissue Substitute, Open Approach
03160K4 Bypass Left Axillary Artery to Left Lower Arm Artery with Nonautologous Tissue Substitute, Open Approach
03160K5 Bypass Left Axillary Artery to Bilateral Lower Arm Artery with Nonautologous Tissue Substitute, Open Approach
03160K6 Bypass Left Axillary Artery to Right Upper Leg Artery with Nonautologous Tissue Substitute, Open Approach
03160K7 Bypass Left Axillary Artery to Left Upper Leg Artery with Nonautologous Tissue Substitute, Open Approach
03160K8 Bypass Left Axillary Artery to Bilateral Upper Leg Artery with Nonautologous Tissue Substitute, Open Approach
03160K9 Bypass Left Axillary Artery to Right Lower Leg Artery with Nonautologous Tissue Substitute, Open Approach
03160KB Bypass Left Axillary Artery to Left Lower Leg Artery with Nonautologous Tissue Substitute, Open Approach
03160KC Bypass Left Axillary Artery to Bilateral Lower Leg Artery with Nonautologous Tissue Substitute, Open Approach
03160KD Bypass Left Axillary Artery to Upper Arm Vein with Nonautologous Tissue Substitute, Open Approach
03160KF Bypass Left Axillary Artery to Lower Arm Vein with Nonautologous Tissue Substitute, Open Approach
03160KJ Bypass Left Axillary Artery to Right Extracranial Artery with Nonautologous Tissue Substitute, Open Approach
03160KK Bypass Left Axillary Artery to Left Extracranial Artery with Nonautologous Tissue Substitute, Open Approach
03160Z0 Bypass Left Axillary Artery to Right Upper Arm Artery, Open Approach
03160Z1 Bypass Left Axillary Artery to Left Upper Arm Artery, Open Approach
03160Z2 Bypass Left Axillary Artery to Bilateral Upper Arm Artery, Open Approach
03160Z3 Bypass Left Axillary Artery to Right Lower Arm Artery, Open Approach
03160Z4 Bypass Left Axillary Artery to Left Lower Arm Artery, Open Approach
03160Z5 Bypass Left Axillary Artery to Bilateral Lower Arm Artery, Open Approach
03160Z6 Bypass Left Axillary Artery to Right Upper Leg Artery, Open Approach
03160Z7 Bypass Left Axillary Artery to Left Upper Leg Artery, Open Approach
03160Z8 Bypass Left Axillary Artery to Bilateral Upper Leg Artery, Open Approach
03160Z9 Bypass Left Axillary Artery to Right Lower Leg Artery, Open Approach
03160ZB Bypass Left Axillary Artery to Left Lower Leg Artery, Open Approach

03160ZC Bypass Left Axillary Artery to Bilateral Lower Leg Artery, Open Approach
03160ZD Bypass Left Axillary Artery to Upper Arm Vein, Open Approach
03160ZF Bypass Left Axillary Artery to Lower Arm Vein, Open Approach
03160ZJ Bypass Left Axillary Artery to Right Extracranial Artery, Open Approach
03160ZK Bypass Left Axillary Artery to Left Extracranial Artery, Open Approach
0317090 Bypass Right Brachial Artery to Right Upper Arm Artery with Autologous Venous Tissue, Open Approach
0317093 Bypass Right Brachial Artery to Right Lower Arm Artery with Autologous Venous Tissue, Open Approach
031709D Bypass Right Brachial Artery to Upper Arm Vein with Autologous Venous Tissue, Open Approach
031709F Bypass Right Brachial Artery to Lower Arm Vein with Autologous Venous Tissue, Open Approach
03170A0 Bypass Right Brachial Artery to Right Upper Arm Artery with Autologous Arterial Tissue, Open Approach
03170A3 Bypass Right Brachial Artery to Right Lower Arm Artery with Autologous Arterial Tissue, Open Approach
03170AD Bypass Right Brachial Artery to Upper Arm Vein with Autologous Arterial Tissue, Open Approach
03170AF Bypass Right Brachial Artery to Lower Arm Vein with Autologous Arterial Tissue, Open Approach
03170J0 Bypass Right Brachial Artery to Right Upper Arm Artery with Synthetic Substitute, Open Approach
03170J3 Bypass Right Brachial Artery to Right Lower Arm Artery with Synthetic Substitute, Open Approach
03170JD Bypass Right Brachial Artery to Upper Arm Vein with Synthetic Substitute, Open Approach
03170JF Bypass Right Brachial Artery to Lower Arm Vein with Synthetic Substitute, Open Approach
03170K0 Bypass Right Brachial Artery to Right Upper Arm Artery with Nonautologous Tissue Substitute, Open Approach
03170K3 Bypass Right Brachial Artery to Right Lower Arm Artery with Nonautologous Tissue Substitute, Open Approach
03170KD Bypass Right Brachial Artery to Upper Arm Vein with Nonautologous Tissue Substitute, Open Approach
03170KF Bypass Right Brachial Artery to Lower Arm Vein with Nonautologous Tissue Substitute, Open Approach
03170Z0 Bypass Right Brachial Artery to Right Upper Arm Artery, Open Approach
03170Z3 Bypass Right Brachial Artery to Right Lower Arm Artery, Open Approach
03170ZD Bypass Right Brachial Artery to Upper Arm Vein, Open Approach
AHA CC: 4Q, 2013, 125-126
03170ZF Bypass Right Brachial Artery to Lower Arm Vein, Open Approach
0318091 Bypass Left Brachial Artery to Left Upper Arm Artery with Autologous Venous Tissue, Open Approach
0318094 Bypass Left Brachial Artery to Left Lower Arm Artery with Autologous Venous Tissue, Open Approach
031809D Bypass Left Brachial Artery to Upper Arm Vein with Autologous Venous Tissue, Open Approach
031809F Bypass Left Brachial Artery to Lower Arm Vein with Autologous Venous Tissue, Open Approach
03180A1 Bypass Left Brachial Artery to Left Upper Arm Artery with Autologous Arterial Tissue, Open Approach
03180A4 Bypass Left Brachial Artery to Left Lower Arm Artery with Autologous Arterial Tissue, Open Approach
03180AD Bypass Left Brachial Artery to Upper Arm Vein with Autologous Arterial Tissue, Open Approach
03180AF Bypass Left Brachial Artery to Lower Arm Vein with Autologous Arterial Tissue, Open Approach
03180J1 Bypass Left Brachial Artery to Left Upper Arm Artery with Synthetic Substitute, Open Approach
03180J4 Bypass Left Brachial Artery to Left Lower Arm Artery with Synthetic Substitute, Open Approach
03180JD Bypass Left Brachial Artery to Upper Arm Vein with Synthetic Substitute, Open Approach
03180JF Bypass Left Brachial Artery to Lower Arm Vein with Synthetic Substitute, Open Approach
03180K1 Bypass Left Brachial Artery to Left Upper Arm Artery with Nonautologous Tissue Substitute, Open Approach
03180K4 Bypass Left Brachial Artery to Left Lower Arm Artery with Nonautologous Tissue Substitute, Open Approach
03180KD Bypass Left Brachial Artery to Upper Arm Vein with Nonautologous Tissue Substitute, Open Approach
03180KF Bypass Left Brachial Artery to Lower Arm Vein with Nonautologous Tissue Substitute, Open Approach
03180Z1 Bypass Left Brachial Artery to Left Upper Arm Artery, Open Approach
03180Z4 Bypass Left Brachial Artery to Left Lower Arm Artery, Open Approach
03180ZD Bypass Left Brachial Artery to Upper Arm Vein, Open Approach
03180ZF Bypass Left Brachial Artery to Lower Arm Vein, Open Approach
0319093 Bypass Right Ulnar Artery to Right Lower Arm Artery with Autologous Venous Tissue, Open Approach
031909F Bypass Right Ulnar Artery to Lower Arm Vein with Autologous Venous Tissue, Open Approach
03190A3 Bypass Right Ulnar Artery to Right Lower Arm Artery with Autologous Arterial Tissue, Open Approach
03190AF Bypass Right Ulnar Artery to Lower Arm Vein with Autologous Arterial Tissue, Open Approach
03190J3 Bypass Right Ulnar Artery to Right Lower Arm Artery with Synthetic Substitute, Open Approach
03190JF Bypass Right Ulnar Artery to Lower Arm Vein with Synthetic Substitute, Open Approach
03190K3 Bypass Right Ulnar Artery to Right Lower Arm Artery with Nonautologous Tissue Substitute, Open Approach
03190KF Bypass Right Ulnar Artery to Lower Arm Vein with Nonautologous Tissue Substitute, Open Approach
03190Z3 Bypass Right Ulnar Artery to Right Lower Arm Artery, Open Approach
03190ZF Bypass Right Ulnar Artery to Lower Arm Vein, Open Approach
031A094 Bypass Left Ulnar Artery to Left Lower Arm Artery with Autologous Venous Tissue, Open Approach
031A09F Bypass Left Ulnar Artery to Lower Arm Vein with Autologous Venous Tissue, Open Approach
031A0A4 Bypass Left Ulnar Artery to Left Lower Arm Artery with Autologous Arterial Tissue, Open Approach
031A0AF Bypass Left Ulnar Artery to Lower Arm Vein with Autologous Arterial Tissue, Open Approach
031A0J4 Bypass Left Ulnar Artery to Left Lower Arm Artery with Synthetic Substitute, Open Approach
031A0JF Bypass Left Ulnar Artery to Lower Arm Vein with Synthetic Substitute, Open Approach
031A0K4 Bypass Left Ulnar Artery to Left Lower Arm Artery with Nonautologous Tissue Substitute, Open Approach
031A0KF Bypass Left Ulnar Artery to Lower Arm Vein with Nonautologous Tissue Substitute, Open Approach
031A0Z4 Bypass Left Ulnar Artery to Left Lower Arm Artery, Open Approach
031A0ZF Bypass Left Ulnar Artery to Lower Arm Vein, Open Approach
031B093 Bypass Right Radial Artery to Right Lower Arm Artery with Autologous Venous Tissue, Open Approach
031B09F Bypass Right Radial Artery to Lower Arm Vein with Autologous Venous Tissue, Open Approach
031B0A3 Bypass Right Radial Artery to Right Lower Arm Artery with Autologous Arterial Tissue, Open Approach
031B0AF Bypass Right Radial Artery to Lower Arm Vein with Autologous Arterial Tissue, Open Approach
031B0J3 Bypass Right Radial Artery to Right Lower Arm Artery with Synthetic Substitute, Open Approach
031B0JF Bypass Right Radial Artery to Lower Arm Vein with Synthetic Substitute, Open Approach
031B0K3 Bypass Right Radial Artery to Right Lower Arm Artery with Nonautologous Tissue Substitute, Open Approach
031B0KF Bypass Right Radial Artery to Lower Arm Vein with Nonautologous Tissue Substitute, Open Approach
031B0Z3 Bypass Right Radial Artery to Right Lower Arm Artery, Open Approach
031B0ZF Bypass Right Radial Artery to Lower Arm Vein, Open Approach
031C094 Bypass Left Radial Artery to Left Lower Arm Artery with Autologous Venous Tissue, Open Approach
031C09F Bypass Left Radial Artery to Lower Arm Vein with Autologous Venous Tissue, Open Approach
031C0A4 Bypass Left Radial Artery to Left Lower Arm Artery with Autologous Arterial Tissue, Open Approach
031C0AF Bypass Left Radial Artery to Lower Arm Vein with Autologous Arterial Tissue, Open Approach
031C0J4 Bypass Left Radial Artery to Left Lower Arm Artery with Synthetic Substitute, Open Approach
031C0JF Bypass Left Radial Artery to Lower Arm Vein with Synthetic Substitute, Open Approach

031C0K4 Bypass Left Radial Artery to Left Lower Arm Artery with Nonautologous Tissue Substitute, Open Approach

031C0KF Bypass Left Radial Artery to Lower Arm Vein with Nonautologous Tissue Substitute, Open Approach

031C0Z4 Bypass Left Radial Artery to Left Lower Arm Artery, Open Approach

031C0ZF Bypass Left Radial Artery to Lower Arm Vein, Open Approach
AHA CC: 1Q, 2013, 27-28

031G09G Bypass Intracranial Artery to Intracranial Artery with Autologous Venous Tissue, Open Approach

031G0AG Bypass Intracranial Artery to Intracranial Artery with Autologous Arterial Tissue, Open Approach

031G0JG Bypass Intracranial Artery to Intracranial Artery with Synthetic Substitute, Open Approach

031G0KG Bypass Intracranial Artery to Intracranial Artery with Nonautologous Tissue Substitute, Open Approach

031G0ZG Bypass Intracranial Artery to Intracranial Artery, Open Approach

▲031H09G Bypass Right Common Carotid Artery to Intracranial Artery with Autologous Venous Tissue, Open Approach

031H09J Bypass Right Common Carotid Artery to Right Extracranial Artery with Autologous Venous Tissue, Open Approach

▲031H0AG Bypass Right Common Carotid Artery to Intracranial Artery with Autologous Arterial Tissue, Open Approach

031H0AJ Bypass Right Common Carotid Artery to Right Extracranial Artery with Autologous Arterial Tissue, Open Approach

▲031H0JG Bypass Right Common Carotid Artery to Intracranial Artery with Synthetic Substitute, Open Approach

031H0JJ Bypass Right Common Carotid Artery to Right Extracranial Artery with Synthetic Substitute, Open Approach

▲031H0KG Bypass Right Common Carotid Artery to Intracranial Artery with Nonautologous Tissue Substitute, Open Approach

031H0KJ Bypass Right Common Carotid Artery to Right Extracranial Artery with Nonautologous Tissue Substitute, Open Approach

▲031H0ZG Bypass Right Common Carotid Artery to Intracranial Artery, Open Approach

031H0ZJ Bypass Right Common Carotid Artery to Right Extracranial Artery, Open Approach

▲031J09G Bypass Left Common Carotid Artery to Intracranial Artery with Autologous Venous Tissue, Open Approach

031J09K Bypass Left Common Carotid Artery to Left Extracranial Artery with Autologous Venous Tissue, Open Approach

▲ 031J0AG Bypass Left Common Carotid Artery to Intracranial Artery with Autologous Arterial Tissue, Open Approach

031J0AK Bypass Left Common Carotid Artery to Left Extracranial Artery with Autologous Arterial Tissue, Open Approach

▲ 031J0JG Bypass Left Common Carotid Artery to Intracranial Artery with Synthetic Substitute, Open Approach

031J0JK Bypass Left Common Carotid Artery to Left Extracranial Artery with Synthetic Substitute, Open Approach

▲ 031J0KG Bypass Left Common Carotid Artery to Intracranial Artery with Nonautologous Tissue Substitute, Open Approach

031J0KK Bypass Left Common Carotid Artery to Left Extracranial Artery with Nonautologous Tissue Substitute, Open Approach

▲ 031J0ZG Bypass Left Common Carotid Artery to Intracranial Artery, Open Approach

031J0ZK Bypass Left Common Carotid Artery to Left Extracranial Artery, Open Approach

031K09J Bypass Right Internal Carotid Artery to Right Extracranial Artery with Autologous Venous Tissue, Open Approach

031K0AJ Bypass Right Internal Carotid Artery to Right Extracranial Artery with Autologous Arterial Tissue, Open Approach

031K0JJ Bypass Right Internal Carotid Artery to Right Extracranial Artery with Synthetic Substitute, Open Approach

031K0KJ Bypass Right Internal Carotid Artery to Right Extracranial Artery with Nonautologous Tissue Substitute, Open Approach

031K0ZJ Bypass Right Internal Carotid Artery to Right Extracranial Artery, Open Approach

031L09K Bypass Left Internal Carotid Artery to Left Extracranial Artery with Autologous Venous Tissue, Open Approach

031L0AK Bypass Left Internal Carotid Artery to Left Extracranial Artery with Autologous Arterial Tissue, Open Approach

031L0JK Bypass Left Internal Carotid Artery to Left Extracranial Artery with Synthetic Substitute, Open Approach

031L0KK Bypass Left Internal Carotid Artery to Left Extracranial Artery with Nonautologous Tissue Substitute, Open Approach

031L0ZK Bypass Left Internal Carotid Artery to Left Extracranial Artery, Open Approach

031M09J Bypass Right External Carotid Artery to Right Extracranial Artery with Autologous Venous Tissue, Open Approach

031M0AJ Bypass Right External Carotid Artery to Right Extracranial Artery with Autologous Arterial Tissue, Open Approach

031M0JJ Bypass Right External Carotid Artery to Right Extracranial Artery with Synthetic Substitute, Open Approach

031M0KJ Bypass Right External Carotid Artery to Right Extracranial Artery with Nonautologous Tissue Substitute, Open Approach

031M0ZJ Bypass Right External Carotid Artery to Right Extracranial Artery, Open Approach

031N09K Bypass Left External Carotid Artery to Left Extracranial Artery with Autologous Venous Tissue, Open Approach

031N0AK Bypass Left External Carotid Artery to Left Extracranial Artery with Autologous Arterial Tissue, Open Approach

031N0JK Bypass Left External Carotid Artery to Left Extracranial Artery with Synthetic Substitute, Open Approach

031N0KK Bypass Left External Carotid Artery to Left Extracranial Artery with Nonautologous Tissue Substitute, Open Approach

031N0ZK Bypass Left External Carotid Artery to Left Extracranial Artery, Open Approach

▲ 031S09G Bypass Right Temporal Artery to Intracranial Artery with Autologous Venous Tissue, Open Approach

▲ 031S0AG Bypass Right Temporal Artery to Intracranial Artery with Autologous Arterial Tissue, Open Approach

▲ 031S0JG Bypass Right Temporal Artery to Intracranial Artery with Synthetic Substitute, Open Approach

▲ 031S0KG Bypass Right Temporal Artery to Intracranial Artery with Nonautologous Tissue Substitute, Open Approach

▲ 031S0ZG Bypass Right Temporal Artery to Intracranial Artery, Open Approach

▲ 031T09G Bypass Left Temporal Artery to Intracranial Artery with Autologous Venous Tissue, Open Approach

▲ 031T0AG Bypass Left Temporal Artery to Intracranial Artery with Autologous Arterial Tissue, Open Approach

▲ 031T0JG Bypass Left Temporal Artery to Intracranial Artery with Synthetic Substitute, Open Approach

▲ 031T0KG Bypass Left Temporal Artery to Intracranial Artery with Nonautologous Tissue Substitute, Open Approach

▲ 031T0ZG Bypass Left Temporal Artery to Intracranial Artery, Open Approach

035 – Upper Arteries, Destruction

03500ZZ Destruction of Right Internal Mammary Artery, Open Approach

03503ZZ Destruction of Right Internal Mammary Artery, Percutaneous Approach

03504ZZ Destruction of Right Internal Mammary Artery, Percutaneous Endoscopic Approach

03510ZZ Destruction of Left Internal Mammary Artery, Open Approach

03513ZZ Destruction of Left Internal Mammary Artery, Percutaneous Approach

03514ZZ Destruction of Left Internal Mammary Artery, Percutaneous Endoscopic Approach

03520ZZ Destruction of Innominate Artery, Open Approach

03523ZZ Destruction of Innominate Artery, Percutaneous Approach

03524ZZ Destruction of Innominate Artery, Percutaneous Endoscopic Approach

03530ZZ Destruction of Right Subclavian Artery, Open Approach

03533ZZ Destruction of Right Subclavian Artery, Percutaneous Approach

03534ZZ Destruction of Right Subclavian Artery, Percutaneous Endoscopic Approach

03540ZZ Destruction of Left Subclavian Artery, Open Approach

03543ZZ Destruction of Left Subclavian Artery, Percutaneous Approach

03544ZZ Destruction of Left Subclavian Artery, Percutaneous Endoscopic Approach

03550ZZ Destruction of Right Axillary Artery, Open Approach
03553ZZ Destruction of Right Axillary Artery, Percutaneous Approach
03554ZZ Destruction of Right Axillary Artery, Percutaneous Endoscopic Approach
03560ZZ Destruction of Left Axillary Artery, Open Approach
03563ZZ Destruction of Left Axillary Artery, Percutaneous Approach
03564ZZ Destruction of Left Axillary Artery, Percutaneous Endoscopic Approach
03570ZZ Destruction of Right Brachial Artery, Open Approach
03573ZZ Destruction of Right Brachial Artery, Percutaneous Approach
03574ZZ Destruction of Right Brachial Artery, Percutaneous Endoscopic Approach
03580ZZ Destruction of Left Brachial Artery, Open Approach
03583ZZ Destruction of Left Brachial Artery, Percutaneous Approach
03584ZZ Destruction of Left Brachial Artery, Percutaneous Endoscopic Approach
03590ZZ Destruction of Right Ulnar Artery, Open Approach
03593ZZ Destruction of Right Ulnar Artery, Percutaneous Approach
03594ZZ Destruction of Right Ulnar Artery, Percutaneous Endoscopic Approach
035A0ZZ Destruction of Left Ulnar Artery, Open Approach
035A3ZZ Destruction of Left Ulnar Artery, Percutaneous Approach
035A4ZZ Destruction of Left Ulnar Artery, Percutaneous Endoscopic Approach
035B0ZZ Destruction of Right Radial Artery, Open Approach
035B3ZZ Destruction of Right Radial Artery, Percutaneous Approach
035B4ZZ Destruction of Right Radial Artery, Percutaneous Endoscopic Approach
035C0ZZ Destruction of Left Radial Artery, Open Approach
035C3ZZ Destruction of Left Radial Artery, Percutaneous Approach
035C4ZZ Destruction of Left Radial Artery, Percutaneous Endoscopic Approach
035D0ZZ Destruction of Right Hand Artery, Open Approach
035D3ZZ Destruction of Right Hand Artery, Percutaneous Approach
035D4ZZ Destruction of Right Hand Artery, Percutaneous Endoscopic Approach
035F0ZZ Destruction of Left Hand Artery, Open Approach
035F3ZZ Destruction of Left Hand Artery, Percutaneous Approach
035F4ZZ Destruction of Left Hand Artery, Percutaneous Endoscopic Approach
035G0ZZ Destruction of Intracranial Artery, Open Approach
035G3ZZ Destruction of Intracranial Artery, Percutaneous Approach
035G4ZZ Destruction of Intracranial Artery, Percutaneous Endoscopic Approach
035H0ZZ Destruction of Right Common Carotid Artery, Open Approach
035H3ZZ Destruction of Right Common Carotid Artery, Percutaneous Approach
035H4ZZ Destruction of Right Common Carotid Artery, Percutaneous Endoscopic Approach
035J0ZZ Destruction of Left Common Carotid Artery, Open Approach
035J3ZZ Destruction of Left Common Carotid Artery, Percutaneous Approach
035J4ZZ Destruction of Left Common Carotid Artery, Percutaneous Endoscopic Approach
035K0ZZ Destruction of Right Internal Carotid Artery, Open Approach
035K3ZZ Destruction of Right Internal Carotid Artery, Percutaneous Approach
035K4ZZ Destruction of Right Internal Carotid Artery, Percutaneous Endoscopic Approach
035L0ZZ Destruction of Left Internal Carotid Artery, Open Approach
035L3ZZ Destruction of Left Internal Carotid Artery, Percutaneous Approach
035L4ZZ Destruction of Left Internal Carotid Artery, Percutaneous Endoscopic Approach
035M0ZZ Destruction of Right External Carotid Artery, Open Approach
035M3ZZ Destruction of Right External Carotid Artery, Percutaneous Approach
035M4ZZ Destruction of Right External Carotid Artery, Percutaneous Endoscopic Approach
035N0ZZ Destruction of Left External Carotid Artery, Open Approach
035N3ZZ Destruction of Left External Carotid Artery, Percutaneous Approach
035N4ZZ Destruction of Left External Carotid Artery, Percutaneous Endoscopic Approach
035P0ZZ Destruction of Right Vertebral Artery, Open Approach
035P3ZZ Destruction of Right Vertebral Artery, Percutaneous Approach
035P4ZZ Destruction of Right Vertebral Artery, Percutaneous Endoscopic Approach
035Q0ZZ Destruction of Left Vertebral Artery, Open Approach
035Q3ZZ Destruction of Left Vertebral Artery, Percutaneous Approach
035Q4ZZ Destruction of Left Vertebral Artery, Percutaneous Endoscopic Approach
035R0ZZ Destruction of Face Artery, Open Approach
035R3ZZ Destruction of Face Artery, Percutaneous Approach
035R4ZZ Destruction of Face Artery, Percutaneous Endoscopic Approach
035S0ZZ Destruction of Right Temporal Artery, Open Approach
035S3ZZ Destruction of Right Temporal Artery, Percutaneous Approach
035S4ZZ Destruction of Right Temporal Artery, Percutaneous Endoscopic Approach
035T0ZZ Destruction of Left Temporal Artery, Open Approach
035T3ZZ Destruction of Left Temporal Artery, Percutaneous Approach
035T4ZZ Destruction of Left Temporal Artery, Percutaneous Endoscopic Approach
035U0ZZ Destruction of Right Thyroid Artery, Open Approach
035U3ZZ Destruction of Right Thyroid Artery, Percutaneous Approach
035U4ZZ Destruction of Right Thyroid Artery, Percutaneous Endoscopic Approach
035V0ZZ Destruction of Left Thyroid Artery, Open Approach
035V3ZZ Destruction of Left Thyroid Artery, Percutaneous Approach
035V4ZZ Destruction of Left Thyroid Artery, Percutaneous Endoscopic Approach
035Y0ZZ Destruction of Upper Artery, Open Approach
035Y3ZZ Destruction of Upper Artery, Percutaneous Approach
035Y4ZZ Destruction of Upper Artery, Percutaneous Endoscopic Approach

037 – Upper Arteries, Dilation

037004Z Dilation of Right Internal Mammary Artery with Drug-eluting Intraluminal Device, Open Approach
03700DZ Dilation of Right Internal Mammary Artery with Intraluminal Device, Open Approach
03700ZZ Dilation of Right Internal Mammary Artery, Open Approach
037034Z Dilation of Right Internal Mammary Artery with Drug-eluting Intraluminal Device, Percutaneous Approach
03703DZ Dilation of Right Internal Mammary Artery with Intraluminal Device, Percutaneous Approach
03703ZZ Dilation of Right Internal Mammary Artery, Percutaneous Approach
037044Z Dilation of Right Internal Mammary Artery with Drug-eluting Intraluminal Device, Percutaneous Endoscopic Approach
03704DZ Dilation of Right Internal Mammary Artery with Intraluminal Device, Percutaneous Endoscopic Approach
03704ZZ Dilation of Right Internal Mammary Artery, Percutaneous Endoscopic Approach
037104Z Dilation of Left Internal Mammary Artery with Drug-eluting Intraluminal Device, Open Approach
03710DZ Dilation of Left Internal Mammary Artery with Intraluminal Device, Open Approach
03710ZZ Dilation of Left Internal Mammary Artery, Open Approach
037134Z Dilation of Left Internal Mammary Artery with Drug-eluting Intraluminal Device, Percutaneous Approach
03713DZ Dilation of Left Internal Mammary Artery with Intraluminal Device, Percutaneous Approach
03713ZZ Dilation of Left Internal Mammary Artery, Percutaneous Approach
037144Z Dilation of Left Internal Mammary Artery with Drug-eluting Intraluminal Device, Percutaneous Endoscopic Approach
03714DZ Dilation of Left Internal Mammary Artery with Intraluminal Device, Percutaneous Endoscopic Approach
03714ZZ Dilation of Left Internal Mammary Artery, Percutaneous Endoscopic Approach
037204Z Dilation of Innominate Artery with Drug-eluting Intraluminal Device, Open Approach
03720DZ Dilation of Innominate Artery with Intraluminal Device, Open Approach
03720ZZ Dilation of Innominate Artery, Open Approach
037234Z Dilation of Innominate Artery with Drug-eluting Intraluminal Device, Percutaneous Approach

03723DZ Dilation of Innominate Artery with Intraluminal Device, Percutaneous Approach
03723ZZ Dilation of Innominate Artery, Percutaneous Approach
037244Z Dilation of Innominate Artery with Drug-eluting Intraluminal Device, Percutaneous Endoscopic Approach
03724DZ Dilation of Innominate Artery with Intraluminal Device, Percutaneous Endoscopic Approach
03724ZZ Dilation of Innominate Artery, Percutaneous Endoscopic Approach
037304Z Dilation of Right Subclavian Artery with Drug-eluting Intraluminal Device, Open Approach
03730DZ Dilation of Right Subclavian Artery with Intraluminal Device, Open Approach
03730ZZ Dilation of Right Subclavian Artery, Open Approach
037334Z Dilation of Right Subclavian Artery with Drug-eluting Intraluminal Device, Percutaneous Approach
03733DZ Dilation of Right Subclavian Artery with Intraluminal Device, Percutaneous Approach
03733ZZ Dilation of Right Subclavian Artery, Percutaneous Approach
037344Z Dilation of Right Subclavian Artery with Drug-eluting Intraluminal Device, Percutaneous Endoscopic Approach
03734DZ Dilation of Right Subclavian Artery with Intraluminal Device, Percutaneous Endoscopic Approach
03734ZZ Dilation of Right Subclavian Artery, Percutaneous Endoscopic Approach
037404Z Dilation of Left Subclavian Artery with Drug-eluting Intraluminal Device, Open Approach
03740DZ Dilation of Left Subclavian Artery with Intraluminal Device, Open Approach
03740ZZ Dilation of Left Subclavian Artery, Open Approach
037434Z Dilation of Left Subclavian Artery with Drug-eluting Intraluminal Device, Percutaneous Approach
03743DZ Dilation of Left Subclavian Artery with Intraluminal Device, Percutaneous Approach
03743ZZ Dilation of Left Subclavian Artery, Percutaneous Approach
037444Z Dilation of Left Subclavian Artery with Drug-eluting Intraluminal Device, Percutaneous Endoscopic Approach
03744DZ Dilation of Left Subclavian Artery with Intraluminal Device, Percutaneous Endoscopic Approach
03744ZZ Dilation of Left Subclavian Artery, Percutaneous Endoscopic Approach
037504Z Dilation of Right Axillary Artery with Drug-eluting Intraluminal Device, Open Approach
03750DZ Dilation of Right Axillary Artery with Intraluminal Device, Open Approach
03750ZZ Dilation of Right Axillary Artery, Open Approach
037534Z Dilation of Right Axillary Artery with Drug-eluting Intraluminal Device, Percutaneous Approach
03753DZ Dilation of Right Axillary Artery with Intraluminal Device, Percutaneous Approach
03753ZZ Dilation of Right Axillary Artery, Percutaneous Approach
037544Z Dilation of Right Axillary Artery with Drug-eluting Intraluminal Device, Percutaneous Endoscopic Approach
03754DZ Dilation of Right Axillary Artery with Intraluminal Device, Percutaneous Endoscopic Approach
03754ZZ Dilation of Right Axillary Artery, Percutaneous Endoscopic Approach
037604Z Dilation of Left Axillary Artery with Drug-eluting Intraluminal Device, Open Approach
03760DZ Dilation of Left Axillary Artery with Intraluminal Device, Open Approach
03760ZZ Dilation of Left Axillary Artery, Open Approach
037634Z Dilation of Left Axillary Artery with Drug-eluting Intraluminal Device, Percutaneous Approach
03763DZ Dilation of Left Axillary Artery with Intraluminal Device, Percutaneous Approach
03763ZZ Dilation of Left Axillary Artery, Percutaneous Approach
037644Z Dilation of Left Axillary Artery with Drug-eluting Intraluminal Device, Percutaneous Endoscopic Approach
03764DZ Dilation of Left Axillary Artery with Intraluminal Device, Percutaneous Endoscopic Approach
03764ZZ Dilation of Left Axillary Artery, Percutaneous Endoscopic Approach
037704Z Dilation of Right Brachial Artery with Drug-eluting Intraluminal Device, Open Approach
03770DZ Dilation of Right Brachial Artery with Intraluminal Device, Open Approach
03770ZZ Dilation of Right Brachial Artery, Open Approach
037734Z Dilation of Right Brachial Artery with Drug-eluting Intraluminal Device, Percutaneous Approach
03773DZ Dilation of Right Brachial Artery with Intraluminal Device, Percutaneous Approach
03773ZZ Dilation of Right Brachial Artery, Percutaneous Approach
037744Z Dilation of Right Brachial Artery with Drug-eluting Intraluminal Device, Percutaneous Endoscopic Approach
03774DZ Dilation of Right Brachial Artery with Intraluminal Device, Percutaneous Endoscopic Approach
03774ZZ Dilation of Right Brachial Artery, Percutaneous Endoscopic Approach
037804Z Dilation of Left Brachial Artery with Drug-eluting Intraluminal Device, Open Approach
03780DZ Dilation of Left Brachial Artery with Intraluminal Device, Open Approach
03780ZZ Dilation of Left Brachial Artery, Open Approach
037834Z Dilation of Left Brachial Artery with Drug-eluting Intraluminal Device, Percutaneous Approach
03783DZ Dilation of Left Brachial Artery with Intraluminal Device, Percutaneous Approach
03783ZZ Dilation of Left Brachial Artery, Percutaneous Approach
037844Z Dilation of Left Brachial Artery with Drug-eluting Intraluminal Device, Percutaneous Endoscopic Approach
03784DZ Dilation of Left Brachial Artery with Intraluminal Device, Percutaneous Endoscopic Approach
03784ZZ Dilation of Left Brachial Artery, Percutaneous Endoscopic Approach
037904Z Dilation of Right Ulnar Artery with Drug-eluting Intraluminal Device, Open Approach
03790DZ Dilation of Right Ulnar Artery with Intraluminal Device, Open Approach
03790ZZ Dilation of Right Ulnar Artery, Open Approach
037934Z Dilation of Right Ulnar Artery with Drug-eluting Intraluminal Device, Percutaneous Approach
03793DZ Dilation of Right Ulnar Artery with Intraluminal Device, Percutaneous Approach
03793ZZ Dilation of Right Ulnar Artery, Percutaneous Approach
037944Z Dilation of Right Ulnar Artery with Drug-eluting Intraluminal Device, Percutaneous Endoscopic Approach
03794DZ Dilation of Right Ulnar Artery with Intraluminal Device, Percutaneous Endoscopic Approach
03794ZZ Dilation of Right Ulnar Artery, Percutaneous Endoscopic Approach
037A04Z Dilation of Left Ulnar Artery with Drug-eluting Intraluminal Device, Open Approach
037A0DZ Dilation of Left Ulnar Artery with Intraluminal Device, Open Approach
037A0ZZ Dilation of Left Ulnar Artery, Open Approach
037A34Z Dilation of Left Ulnar Artery with Drug-eluting Intraluminal Device, Percutaneous Approach
037A3DZ Dilation of Left Ulnar Artery with Intraluminal Device, Percutaneous Approach
037A3ZZ Dilation of Left Ulnar Artery, Percutaneous Approach
037A44Z Dilation of Left Ulnar Artery with Drug-eluting Intraluminal Device, Percutaneous Endoscopic Approach
037A4DZ Dilation of Left Ulnar Artery with Intraluminal Device, Percutaneous Endoscopic Approach
037A4ZZ Dilation of Left Ulnar Artery, Percutaneous Endoscopic Approach
037B04Z Dilation of Right Radial Artery with Drug-eluting Intraluminal Device, Open Approach
037B0DZ Dilation of Right Radial Artery with Intraluminal Device, Open Approach
037B0ZZ Dilation of Right Radial Artery, Open Approach
037B34Z Dilation of Right Radial Artery with Drug-eluting Intraluminal Device, Percutaneous Approach
037B3DZ Dilation of Right Radial Artery with Intraluminal Device, Percutaneous Approach
037B3ZZ Dilation of Right Radial Artery, Percutaneous Approach
037B44Z Dilation of Right Radial Artery with Drug-eluting Intraluminal Device, Percutaneous Endoscopic Approach
037B4DZ Dilation of Right Radial Artery with Intraluminal Device, Percutaneous Endoscopic Approach
037B4ZZ Dilation of Right Radial Artery, Percutaneous Endoscopic Approach
037C04Z Dilation of Left Radial Artery with Drug-eluting Intraluminal Device, Open Approach
037C0DZ Dilation of Left Radial Artery with Intraluminal Device, Open Approach
037C0ZZ Dilation of Left Radial Artery, Open Approach
037C34Z Dilation of Left Radial Artery with Drug-eluting Intraluminal Device, Percutaneous Approach

037C3DZ Dilation of Left Radial Artery with Intraluminal Device, Percutaneous Approach
037C3ZZ Dilation of Left Radial Artery, Percutaneous Approach
037C44Z Dilation of Left Radial Artery with Drug-eluting Intraluminal Device, Percutaneous Endoscopic Approach
037C4DZ Dilation of Left Radial Artery with Intraluminal Device, Percutaneous Endoscopic Approach
037C4ZZ Dilation of Left Radial Artery, Percutaneous Endoscopic Approach
037D04Z Dilation of Right Hand Artery with Drug-eluting Intraluminal Device, Open Approach
037D0DZ Dilation of Right Hand Artery with Intraluminal Device, Open Approach
037D0ZZ Dilation of Right Hand Artery, Open Approach
037D34Z Dilation of Right Hand Artery with Drug-eluting Intraluminal Device, Percutaneous Approach
037D3DZ Dilation of Right Hand Artery with Intraluminal Device, Percutaneous Approach
037D3ZZ Dilation of Right Hand Artery, Percutaneous Approach
037D44Z Dilation of Right Hand Artery with Drug-eluting Intraluminal Device, Percutaneous Endoscopic Approach
037D4DZ Dilation of Right Hand Artery with Intraluminal Device, Percutaneous Endoscopic Approach
037D4ZZ Dilation of Right Hand Artery, Percutaneous Endoscopic Approach
037F04Z Dilation of Left Hand Artery with Drug-eluting Intraluminal Device, Open Approach
037F0DZ Dilation of Left Hand Artery with Intraluminal Device, Open Approach
037F0ZZ Dilation of Left Hand Artery, Open Approach
037F34Z Dilation of Left Hand Artery with Drug-eluting Intraluminal Device, Percutaneous Approach
037F3DZ Dilation of Left Hand Artery with Intraluminal Device, Percutaneous Approach
037F3ZZ Dilation of Left Hand Artery, Percutaneous Approach
037F44Z Dilation of Left Hand Artery with Drug-eluting Intraluminal Device, Percutaneous Endoscopic Approach
037F4DZ Dilation of Left Hand Artery with Intraluminal Device, Percutaneous Endoscopic Approach
037F4ZZ Dilation of Left Hand Artery, Percutaneous Endoscopic Approach
037G04Z Dilation of Intracranial Artery with Drug-eluting Intraluminal Device, Open Approach
037G0DZ Dilation of Intracranial Artery with Intraluminal Device, Open Approach
037G0ZZ Dilation of Intracranial Artery, Open Approach
037G34Z Dilation of Intracranial Artery with Drug-eluting Intraluminal Device, Percutaneous Approach
037G3DZ Dilation of Intracranial Artery with Intraluminal Device, Percutaneous Approach
▲ **037G3ZZ** Dilation of Intracranial Artery, Percutaneous Approach
037G44Z Dilation of Intracranial Artery with Drug-eluting Intraluminal Device, Percutaneous Endoscopic Approach
037G4DZ Dilation of Intracranial Artery with Intraluminal Device, Percutaneous Endoscopic Approach
▲ **037G4ZZ** Dilation of Intracranial Artery, Percutaneous Endoscopic Approach
037H04Z Dilation of Right Common Carotid Artery with Drug-eluting Intraluminal Device, Open Approach
037H0DZ Dilation of Right Common Carotid Artery with Intraluminal Device, Open Approach
037H0ZZ Dilation of Right Common Carotid Artery, Open Approach
037H34Z Dilation of Right Common Carotid Artery with Drug-eluting Intraluminal Device, Percutaneous Approach
037H3DZ Dilation of Right Common Carotid Artery with Intraluminal Device, Percutaneous Approach
037H3ZZ Dilation of Right Common Carotid Artery, Percutaneous Approach
037H44Z Dilation of Right Common Carotid Artery with Drug-eluting Intraluminal Device, Percutaneous Endoscopic Approach
037H4DZ Dilation of Right Common Carotid Artery with Intraluminal Device, Percutaneous Endoscopic Approach
037H4ZZ Dilation of Right Common Carotid Artery, Percutaneous Endoscopic Approach
037J04Z Dilation of Left Common Carotid Artery with Drug-eluting Intraluminal Device, Open Approach
037J0DZ Dilation of Left Common Carotid Artery with Intraluminal Device, Open Approach
037J0ZZ Dilation of Left Common Carotid Artery, Open Approach
037J34Z Dilation of Left Common Carotid Artery with Drug-eluting Intraluminal Device, Percutaneous Approach
037J3DZ Dilation of Left Common Carotid Artery with Intraluminal Device, Percutaneous Approach
037J3ZZ Dilation of Left Common Carotid Artery, Percutaneous Approach
037J44Z Dilation of Left Common Carotid Artery with Drug-eluting Intraluminal Device, Percutaneous Endoscopic Approach
037J4DZ Dilation of Left Common Carotid Artery with Intraluminal Device, Percutaneous Endoscopic Approach
037J4ZZ Dilation of Left Common Carotid Artery, Percutaneous Endoscopic Approach
037K04Z Dilation of Right Internal Carotid Artery with Drug-eluting Intraluminal Device, Open Approach
037K0DZ Dilation of Right Internal Carotid Artery with Intraluminal Device, Open Approach
037K0ZZ Dilation of Right Internal Carotid Artery, Open Approach
037K34Z Dilation of Right Internal Carotid Artery with Drug-eluting Intraluminal Device, Percutaneous Approach
037K3DZ Dilation of Right Internal Carotid Artery with Intraluminal Device, Percutaneous Approach
037K3ZZ Dilation of Right Internal Carotid Artery, Percutaneous Approach
037K44Z Dilation of Right Internal Carotid Artery with Drug-eluting Intraluminal Device, Percutaneous Endoscopic Approach
037K4DZ Dilation of Right Internal Carotid Artery with Intraluminal Device, Percutaneous Endoscopic Approach
037K4ZZ Dilation of Right Internal Carotid Artery, Percutaneous Endoscopic Approach
037L04Z Dilation of Left Internal Carotid Artery with Drug-eluting Intraluminal Device, Open Approach
037L0DZ Dilation of Left Internal Carotid Artery with Intraluminal Device, Open Approach
037L0ZZ Dilation of Left Internal Carotid Artery, Open Approach
037L34Z Dilation of Left Internal Carotid Artery with Drug-eluting Intraluminal Device, Percutaneous Approach
037L3DZ Dilation of Left Internal Carotid Artery with Intraluminal Device, Percutaneous Approach
037L3ZZ Dilation of Left Internal Carotid Artery, Percutaneous Approach
037L44Z Dilation of Left Internal Carotid Artery with Drug-eluting Intraluminal Device, Percutaneous Endoscopic Approach
037L4DZ Dilation of Left Internal Carotid Artery with Intraluminal Device, Percutaneous Endoscopic Approach
037L4ZZ Dilation of Left Internal Carotid Artery, Percutaneous Endoscopic Approach
037M04Z Dilation of Right External Carotid Artery with Drug-eluting Intraluminal Device, Open Approach
037M0DZ Dilation of Right External Carotid Artery with Intraluminal Device, Open Approach
037M0ZZ Dilation of Right External Carotid Artery, Open Approach
037M34Z Dilation of Right External Carotid Artery with Drug-eluting Intraluminal Device, Percutaneous Approach
037M3DZ Dilation of Right External Carotid Artery with Intraluminal Device, Percutaneous Approach
037M3ZZ Dilation of Right External Carotid Artery, Percutaneous Approach
037M44Z Dilation of Right External Carotid Artery with Drug-eluting Intraluminal Device, Percutaneous Endoscopic Approach
037M4DZ Dilation of Right External Carotid Artery with Intraluminal Device, Percutaneous Endoscopic Approach
037M4ZZ Dilation of Right External Carotid Artery, Percutaneous Endoscopic Approach
037N04Z Dilation of Left External Carotid Artery with Drug-eluting Intraluminal Device, Open Approach
037N0DZ Dilation of Left External Carotid Artery with Intraluminal Device, Open Approach
037N0ZZ Dilation of Left External Carotid Artery, Open Approach
037N34Z Dilation of Left External Carotid Artery with Drug-eluting Intraluminal Device, Percutaneous Approach
037N3DZ Dilation of Left External Carotid Artery with Intraluminal Device, Percutaneous Approach
037N3ZZ Dilation of Left External Carotid Artery, Percutaneous Approach
037N44Z Dilation of Left External Carotid Artery with Drug-eluting Intraluminal Device, Percutaneous Endoscopic Approach
037N4DZ Dilation of Left External Carotid Artery with Intraluminal Device, Percutaneous Endoscopic Approach
037N4ZZ Dilation of Left External Carotid Artery, Percutaneous Endoscopic Approach
037P04Z Dilation of Right Vertebral Artery with Drug-eluting Intraluminal Device, Open Approach
037P0DZ Dilation of Right Vertebral Artery with Intraluminal Device, Open Approach
037P0ZZ Dilation of Right Vertebral Artery, Open Approach
037P34Z Dilation of Right Vertebral Artery with Drug-eluting Intraluminal Device, Percutaneous Approach

037P3DZ Dilation of Right Vertebral Artery with Intraluminal Device, Percutaneous Approach
037P3ZZ Dilation of Right Vertebral Artery, Percutaneous Approach
037P44Z Dilation of Right Vertebral Artery with Drug-eluting Intraluminal Device, Percutaneous Endoscopic Approach
037P4DZ Dilation of Right Vertebral Artery with Intraluminal Device, Percutaneous Endoscopic Approach
037P4ZZ Dilation of Right Vertebral Artery, Percutaneous Endoscopic Approach
037Q04Z Dilation of Left Vertebral Artery with Drug-eluting Intraluminal Device, Open Approach
037Q0DZ Dilation of Left Vertebral Artery with Intraluminal Device, Open Approach
037Q0ZZ Dilation of Left Vertebral Artery, Open Approach
037Q34Z Dilation of Left Vertebral Artery with Drug-eluting Intraluminal Device, Percutaneous Approach
037Q3DZ Dilation of Left Vertebral Artery with Intraluminal Device, Percutaneous Approach
037Q3ZZ Dilation of Left Vertebral Artery, Percutaneous Approach
037Q44Z Dilation of Left Vertebral Artery with Drug-eluting Intraluminal Device, Percutaneous Endoscopic Approach
037Q4DZ Dilation of Left Vertebral Artery with Intraluminal Device, Percutaneous Endoscopic Approach
037Q4ZZ Dilation of Left Vertebral Artery, Percutaneous Endoscopic Approach
037R04Z Dilation of Face Artery with Drug-eluting Intraluminal Device, Open Approach
037R0DZ Dilation of Face Artery with Intraluminal Device, Open Approach
037R0ZZ Dilation of Face Artery, Open Approach
037R34Z Dilation of Face Artery with Drug-eluting Intraluminal Device, Percutaneous Approach
037R3DZ Dilation of Face Artery with Intraluminal Device, Percutaneous Approach
037R3ZZ Dilation of Face Artery, Percutaneous Approach
037R44Z Dilation of Face Artery with Drug-eluting Intraluminal Device, Percutaneous Endoscopic Approach
037R4DZ Dilation of Face Artery with Intraluminal Device, Percutaneous Endoscopic Approach
037R4ZZ Dilation of Face Artery, Percutaneous Endoscopic Approach
037S04Z Dilation of Right Temporal Artery with Drug-eluting Intraluminal Device, Open Approach
037S0DZ Dilation of Right Temporal Artery with Intraluminal Device, Open Approach
037S0ZZ Dilation of Right Temporal Artery, Open Approach
037S34Z Dilation of Right Temporal Artery with Drug-eluting Intraluminal Device, Percutaneous Approach
037S3DZ Dilation of Right Temporal Artery with Intraluminal Device, Percutaneous Approach
037S3ZZ Dilation of Right Temporal Artery, Percutaneous Approach
037S44Z Dilation of Right Temporal Artery with Drug-eluting Intraluminal Device, Percutaneous Endoscopic Approach
037S4DZ Dilation of Right Temporal Artery with Intraluminal Device, Percutaneous Endoscopic Approach
037S4ZZ Dilation of Right Temporal Artery, Percutaneous Endoscopic Approach
037T04Z Dilation of Left Temporal Artery with Drug-eluting Intraluminal Device, Open Approach
037T0DZ Dilation of Left Temporal Artery with Intraluminal Device, Open Approach
037T0ZZ Dilation of Left Temporal Artery, Open Approach
037T34Z Dilation of Left Temporal Artery with Drug-eluting Intraluminal Device, Percutaneous Approach
037T3DZ Dilation of Left Temporal Artery with Intraluminal Device, Percutaneous Approach
037T3ZZ Dilation of Left Temporal Artery, Percutaneous Approach
037T44Z Dilation of Left Temporal Artery with Drug-eluting Intraluminal Device, Percutaneous Endoscopic Approach
037T4DZ Dilation of Left Temporal Artery with Intraluminal Device, Percutaneous Endoscopic Approach
037T4ZZ Dilation of Left Temporal Artery, Percutaneous Endoscopic Approach
037U04Z Dilation of Right Thyroid Artery with Drug-eluting Intraluminal Device, Open Approach
037U0DZ Dilation of Right Thyroid Artery with Intraluminal Device, Open Approach
037U0ZZ Dilation of Right Thyroid Artery, Open Approach
037U34Z Dilation of Right Thyroid Artery with Drug-eluting Intraluminal Device, Percutaneous Approach
037U3DZ Dilation of Right Thyroid Artery with Intraluminal Device, Percutaneous Approach
037U3ZZ Dilation of Right Thyroid Artery, Percutaneous Approach
037U44Z Dilation of Right Thyroid Artery with Drug-eluting Intraluminal Device, Percutaneous Endoscopic Approach
037U4DZ Dilation of Right Thyroid Artery with Intraluminal Device, Percutaneous Endoscopic Approach
037U4ZZ Dilation of Right Thyroid Artery, Percutaneous Endoscopic Approach
037V04Z Dilation of Left Thyroid Artery with Drug-eluting Intraluminal Device, Open Approach
037V0DZ Dilation of Left Thyroid Artery with Intraluminal Device, Open Approach
037V0ZZ Dilation of Left Thyroid Artery, Open Approach
037V34Z Dilation of Left Thyroid Artery with Drug-eluting Intraluminal Device, Percutaneous Approach
037V3DZ Dilation of Left Thyroid Artery with Intraluminal Device, Percutaneous Approach
037V3ZZ Dilation of Left Thyroid Artery, Percutaneous Approach
037V44Z Dilation of Left Thyroid Artery with Drug-eluting Intraluminal Device, Percutaneous Endoscopic Approach
037V4DZ Dilation of Left Thyroid Artery with Intraluminal Device, Percutaneous Endoscopic Approach
037V4ZZ Dilation of Left Thyroid Artery, Percutaneous Endoscopic Approach
037Y04Z Dilation of Upper Artery with Drug-eluting Intraluminal Device, Open Approach
037Y0DZ Dilation of Upper Artery with Intraluminal Device, Open Approach
037Y0ZZ Dilation of Upper Artery, Open Approach
037Y34Z Dilation of Upper Artery with Drug-eluting Intraluminal Device, Percutaneous Approach
037Y3DZ Dilation of Upper Artery with Intraluminal Device, Percutaneous Approach
037Y3ZZ Dilation of Upper Artery, Percutaneous Approach
037Y44Z Dilation of Upper Artery with Drug-eluting Intraluminal Device, Percutaneous Endoscopic Approach
037Y4DZ Dilation of Upper Artery with Intraluminal Device, Percutaneous Endoscopic Approach
037Y4ZZ Dilation of Upper Artery, Percutaneous Endoscopic Approach

039 – Upper Arteries, Drainage

Review Coding Guidelines B3.4a and B3.4b

Review Coding Guideline B6.2

039000Z Drainage of Right Internal Mammary Artery with Drainage Device, Open Approach
03900ZX Drainage of Right Internal Mammary Artery, Open Approach, Diagnostic
03900ZZ Drainage of Right Internal Mammary Artery, Open Approach
039030Z Drainage of Right Internal Mammary Artery with Drainage Device, Percutaneous Approach
03903ZX Drainage of Right Internal Mammary Artery, Percutaneous Approach, Diagnostic
03903ZZ Drainage of Right Internal Mammary Artery, Percutaneous Approach
039040Z Drainage of Right Internal Mammary Artery with Drainage Device, Percutaneous Endoscopic Approach
03904ZX Drainage of Right Internal Mammary Artery, Percutaneous Endoscopic Approach, Diagnostic
03904ZZ Drainage of Right Internal Mammary Artery, Percutaneous Endoscopic Approach
039100Z Drainage of Left Internal Mammary Artery with Drainage Device, Open Approach
03910ZX Drainage of Left Internal Mammary Artery, Open Approach, Diagnostic
03910ZZ Drainage of Left Internal Mammary Artery, Open Approach
039130Z Drainage of Left Internal Mammary Artery with Drainage Device, Percutaneous Approach
03913ZX Drainage of Left Internal Mammary Artery, Percutaneous Approach, Diagnostic
03913ZZ Drainage of Left Internal Mammary Artery, Percutaneous Approach

039140Z Drainage of Left Internal Mammary Artery with Drainage Device, Percutaneous Endoscopic Approach
03914ZX Drainage of Left Internal Mammary Artery, Percutaneous Endoscopic Approach, Diagnostic
03914ZZ Drainage of Left Internal Mammary Artery, Percutaneous Endoscopic Approach
039200Z Drainage of Innominate Artery with Drainage Device, Open Approach
03920ZX Drainage of Innominate Artery, Open Approach, Diagnostic
03920ZZ Drainage of Innominate Artery, Open Approach
039230Z Drainage of Innominate Artery with Drainage Device, Percutaneous Approach
03923ZX Drainage of Innominate Artery, Percutaneous Approach, Diagnostic
03923ZZ Drainage of Innominate Artery, Percutaneous Approach
039240Z Drainage of Innominate Artery with Drainage Device, Percutaneous Endoscopic Approach
03924ZX Drainage of Innominate Artery, Percutaneous Endoscopic Approach, Diagnostic
03924ZZ Drainage of Innominate Artery, Percutaneous Endoscopic Approach
039300Z Drainage of Right Subclavian Artery with Drainage Device, Open Approach
03930ZX Drainage of Right Subclavian Artery, Open Approach, Diagnostic
03930ZZ Drainage of Right Subclavian Artery, Open Approach
039330Z Drainage of Right Subclavian Artery with Drainage Device, Percutaneous Approach
03933ZX Drainage of Right Subclavian Artery, Percutaneous Approach, Diagnostic
03933ZZ Drainage of Right Subclavian Artery, Percutaneous Approach
039340Z Drainage of Right Subclavian Artery with Drainage Device, Percutaneous Endoscopic Approach
03934ZX Drainage of Right Subclavian Artery, Percutaneous Endoscopic Approach, Diagnostic
03934ZZ Drainage of Right Subclavian Artery, Percutaneous Endoscopic Approach
039400Z Drainage of Left Subclavian Artery with Drainage Device, Open Approach
03940ZX Drainage of Left Subclavian Artery, Open Approach, Diagnostic
03940ZZ Drainage of Left Subclavian Artery, Open Approach
039430Z Drainage of Left Subclavian Artery with Drainage Device, Percutaneous Approach
03943ZX Drainage of Left Subclavian Artery, Percutaneous Approach, Diagnostic
03943ZZ Drainage of Left Subclavian Artery, Percutaneous Approach
039440Z Drainage of Left Subclavian Artery with Drainage Device, Percutaneous Endoscopic Approach
03944ZX Drainage of Left Subclavian Artery, Percutaneous Endoscopic Approach, Diagnostic
03944ZZ Drainage of Left Subclavian Artery, Percutaneous Endoscopic Approach
039500Z Drainage of Right Axillary Artery with Drainage Device, Open Approach
03950ZX Drainage of Right Axillary Artery, Open Approach, Diagnostic
03950ZZ Drainage of Right Axillary Artery, Open Approach
039530Z Drainage of Right Axillary Artery with Drainage Device, Percutaneous Approach
03953ZX Drainage of Right Axillary Artery, Percutaneous Approach, Diagnostic
03953ZZ Drainage of Right Axillary Artery, Percutaneous Approach
039540Z Drainage of Right Axillary Artery with Drainage Device, Percutaneous Endoscopic Approach
03954ZX Drainage of Right Axillary Artery, Percutaneous Endoscopic Approach, Diagnostic
03954ZZ Drainage of Right Axillary Artery, Percutaneous Endoscopic Approach
039600Z Drainage of Left Axillary Artery with Drainage Device, Open Approach
03960ZX Drainage of Left Axillary Artery, Open Approach, Diagnostic
03960ZZ Drainage of Left Axillary Artery, Open Approach
039630Z Drainage of Left Axillary Artery with Drainage Device, Percutaneous Approach
03963ZX Drainage of Left Axillary Artery, Percutaneous Approach, Diagnostic
03963ZZ Drainage of Left Axillary Artery, Percutaneous Approach
039640Z Drainage of Left Axillary Artery with Drainage Device, Percutaneous Endoscopic Approach
03964ZX Drainage of Left Axillary Artery, Percutaneous Endoscopic Approach, Diagnostic
03964ZZ Drainage of Left Axillary Artery, Percutaneous Endoscopic Approach
039700Z Drainage of Right Brachial Artery with Drainage Device, Open Approach
03970ZX Drainage of Right Brachial Artery, Open Approach, Diagnostic
03970ZZ Drainage of Right Brachial Artery, Open Approach
039730Z Drainage of Right Brachial Artery with Drainage Device, Percutaneous Approach
03973ZX Drainage of Right Brachial Artery, Percutaneous Approach, Diagnostic
03973ZZ Drainage of Right Brachial Artery, Percutaneous Approach
039740Z Drainage of Right Brachial Artery with Drainage Device, Percutaneous Endoscopic Approach
03974ZX Drainage of Right Brachial Artery, Percutaneous Endoscopic Approach, Diagnostic
03974ZZ Drainage of Right Brachial Artery, Percutaneous Endoscopic Approach
039800Z Drainage of Left Brachial Artery with Drainage Device, Open Approach
03980ZX Drainage of Left Brachial Artery, Open Approach, Diagnostic
03980ZZ Drainage of Left Brachial Artery, Open Approach
039830Z Drainage of Left Brachial Artery with Drainage Device, Percutaneous Approach
03983ZX Drainage of Left Brachial Artery, Percutaneous Approach, Diagnostic
03983ZZ Drainage of Left Brachial Artery, Percutaneous Approach
039840Z Drainage of Left Brachial Artery with Drainage Device, Percutaneous Endoscopic Approach
03984ZX Drainage of Left Brachial Artery, Percutaneous Endoscopic Approach, Diagnostic
03984ZZ Drainage of Left Brachial Artery, Percutaneous Endoscopic Approach
039900Z Drainage of Right Ulnar Artery with Drainage Device, Open Approach
03990ZX Drainage of Right Ulnar Artery, Open Approach, Diagnostic
03990ZZ Drainage of Right Ulnar Artery, Open Approach
039930Z Drainage of Right Ulnar Artery with Drainage Device, Percutaneous Approach
03993ZX Drainage of Right Ulnar Artery, Percutaneous Approach, Diagnostic
03993ZZ Drainage of Right Ulnar Artery, Percutaneous Approach
039940Z Drainage of Right Ulnar Artery with Drainage Device, Percutaneous Endoscopic Approach
03994ZX Drainage of Right Ulnar Artery, Percutaneous Endoscopic Approach, Diagnostic
03994ZZ Drainage of Right Ulnar Artery, Percutaneous Endoscopic Approach
039A00Z Drainage of Left Ulnar Artery with Drainage Device, Open Approach
039A0ZX Drainage of Left Ulnar Artery, Open Approach, Diagnostic
039A0ZZ Drainage of Left Ulnar Artery, Open Approach
039A30Z Drainage of Left Ulnar Artery with Drainage Device, Percutaneous Approach
039A3ZX Drainage of Left Ulnar Artery, Percutaneous Approach, Diagnostic
039A3ZZ Drainage of Left Ulnar Artery, Percutaneous Approach
039A40Z Drainage of Left Ulnar Artery with Drainage Device, Percutaneous Endoscopic Approach
039A4ZX Drainage of Left Ulnar Artery, Percutaneous Endoscopic Approach, Diagnostic
039A4ZZ Drainage of Left Ulnar Artery, Percutaneous Endoscopic Approach
039B00Z Drainage of Right Radial Artery with Drainage Device, Open Approach
039B0ZX Drainage of Right Radial Artery, Open Approach, Diagnostic
039B0ZZ Drainage of Right Radial Artery, Open Approach
039B30Z Drainage of Right Radial Artery with Drainage Device, Percutaneous Approach
039B3ZX Drainage of Right Radial Artery, Percutaneous Approach, Diagnostic
039B3ZZ Drainage of Right Radial Artery, Percutaneous Approach
039B40Z Drainage of Right Radial Artery with Drainage Device, Percutaneous Endoscopic Approach
039B4ZX Drainage of Right Radial Artery, Percutaneous Endoscopic Approach, Diagnostic
039B4ZZ Drainage of Right Radial Artery, Percutaneous Endoscopic Approach
039C00Z Drainage of Left Radial Artery with Drainage Device, Open Approach
039C0ZX Drainage of Left Radial Artery, Open Approach, Diagnostic
039C0ZZ Drainage of Left Radial Artery, Open Approach
039C30Z Drainage of Left Radial Artery with Drainage Device, Percutaneous Approach
039C3ZX Drainage of Left Radial Artery, Percutaneous Approach, Diagnostic
039C3ZZ Drainage of Left Radial Artery, Percutaneous Approach
039C40Z Drainage of Left Radial Artery with Drainage Device, Percutaneous Endoscopic Approach
039C4ZX Drainage of Left Radial Artery, Percutaneous Endoscopic Approach, Diagnostic
039C4ZZ Drainage of Left Radial Artery, Percutaneous Endoscopic Approach
039D00Z Drainage of Right Hand Artery with Drainage Device, Open Approach
039D0ZX Drainage of Right Hand Artery, Open Approach, Diagnostic

39D0ZZ Drainage of Right Hand Artery, Open Approach
39D30Z Drainage of Right Hand Artery with Drainage Device, Percutaneous Approach
39D3ZX Drainage of Right Hand Artery, Percutaneous Approach, Diagnostic
39D3ZZ Drainage of Right Hand Artery, Percutaneous Approach
39D40Z Drainage of Right Hand Artery with Drainage Device, Percutaneous Endoscopic Approach
39D4ZX Drainage of Right Hand Artery, Percutaneous Endoscopic Approach, Diagnostic
39D4ZZ Drainage of Right Hand Artery, Percutaneous Endoscopic Approach
39F00Z Drainage of Left Hand Artery with Drainage Device, Open Approach
39F0ZX Drainage of Left Hand Artery, Open Approach, Diagnostic
39F0ZZ Drainage of Left Hand Artery, Open Approach
39F30Z Drainage of Left Hand Artery with Drainage Device, Percutaneous Approach
39F3ZX Drainage of Left Hand Artery, Percutaneous Approach, Diagnostic
39F3ZZ Drainage of Left Hand Artery, Percutaneous Approach
39F40Z Drainage of Left Hand Artery with Drainage Device, Percutaneous Endoscopic Approach
39F4ZX Drainage of Left Hand Artery, Percutaneous Endoscopic Approach, Diagnostic
39F4ZZ Drainage of Left Hand Artery, Percutaneous Endoscopic Approach
39G00Z Drainage of Intracranial Artery with Drainage Device, Open Approach
39G0ZX Drainage of Intracranial Artery, Open Approach, Diagnostic
39G0ZZ Drainage of Intracranial Artery, Open Approach
39G30Z Drainage of Intracranial Artery with Drainage Device, Percutaneous Approach
39G3ZX Drainage of Intracranial Artery, Percutaneous Approach, Diagnostic
39G3ZZ Drainage of Intracranial Artery, Percutaneous Approach
39G40Z Drainage of Intracranial Artery with Drainage Device, Percutaneous Endoscopic Approach
39G4ZX Drainage of Intracranial Artery, Percutaneous Endoscopic Approach, Diagnostic
39G4ZZ Drainage of Intracranial Artery, Percutaneous Endoscopic Approach
39H00Z Drainage of Right Common Carotid Artery with Drainage Device, Open Approach
39H0ZX Drainage of Right Common Carotid Artery, Open Approach, Diagnostic
39H0ZZ Drainage of Right Common Carotid Artery, Open Approach
39H30Z Drainage of Right Common Carotid Artery with Drainage Device, Percutaneous Approach
39H3ZX Drainage of Right Common Carotid Artery, Percutaneous Approach, Diagnostic
039H3ZZ Drainage of Right Common Carotid Artery, Percutaneous Approach
039H40Z Drainage of Right Common Carotid Artery with Drainage Device, Percutaneous Endoscopic Approach
039H4ZX Drainage of Right Common Carotid Artery, Percutaneous Endoscopic Approach, Diagnostic
039H4ZZ Drainage of Right Common Carotid Artery, Percutaneous Endoscopic Approach
039J00Z Drainage of Left Common Carotid Artery with Drainage Device, Open Approach
039J0ZX Drainage of Left Common Carotid Artery, Open Approach, Diagnostic
039J0ZZ Drainage of Left Common Carotid Artery, Open Approach
039J30Z Drainage of Left Common Carotid Artery with Drainage Device, Percutaneous Approach
039J3ZX Drainage of Left Common Carotid Artery, Percutaneous Approach, Diagnostic
039J3ZZ Drainage of Left Common Carotid Artery, Percutaneous Approach
039J40Z Drainage of Left Common Carotid Artery with Drainage Device, Percutaneous Endoscopic Approach
039J4ZX Drainage of Left Common Carotid Artery, Percutaneous Endoscopic Approach, Diagnostic
039J4ZZ Drainage of Left Common Carotid Artery, Percutaneous Endoscopic Approach
039K00Z Drainage of Right Internal Carotid Artery with Drainage Device, Open Approach
039K0ZX Drainage of Right Internal Carotid Artery, Open Approach, Diagnostic
039K0ZZ Drainage of Right Internal Carotid Artery, Open Approach
039K30Z Drainage of Right Internal Carotid Artery with Drainage Device, Percutaneous Approach
039K3ZX Drainage of Right Internal Carotid Artery, Percutaneous Approach, Diagnostic
039K3ZZ Drainage of Right Internal Carotid Artery, Percutaneous Approach
039K40Z Drainage of Right Internal Carotid Artery with Drainage Device, Percutaneous Endoscopic Approach
039K4ZX Drainage of Right Internal Carotid Artery, Percutaneous Endoscopic Approach, Diagnostic
039K4ZZ Drainage of Right Internal Carotid Artery, Percutaneous Endoscopic Approach
039L00Z Drainage of Left Internal Carotid Artery with Drainage Device, Open Approach
039L0ZX Drainage of Left Internal Carotid Artery, Open Approach, Diagnostic
039L0ZZ Drainage of Left Internal Carotid Artery, Open Approach
039L30Z Drainage of Left Internal Carotid Artery with Drainage Device, Percutaneous Approach
039L3ZX Drainage of Left Internal Carotid Artery, Percutaneous Approach, Diagnostic
039L3ZZ Drainage of Left Internal Carotid Artery, Percutaneous Approach
039L40Z Drainage of Left Internal Carotid Artery with Drainage Device, Percutaneous Endoscopic Approach
039L4ZX Drainage of Left Internal Carotid Artery, Percutaneous Endoscopic Approach, Diagnostic
039L4ZZ Drainage of Left Internal Carotid Artery, Percutaneous Endoscopic Approach
039M00Z Drainage of Right External Carotid Artery with Drainage Device, Open Approach
039M0ZX Drainage of Right External Carotid Artery, Open Approach, Diagnostic
039M0ZZ Drainage of Right External Carotid Artery, Open Approach
039M30Z Drainage of Right External Carotid Artery with Drainage Device, Percutaneous Approach
039M3ZX Drainage of Right External Carotid Artery, Percutaneous Approach, Diagnostic
039M3ZZ Drainage of Right External Carotid Artery, Percutaneous Approach
039M40Z Drainage of Right External Carotid Artery with Drainage Device, Percutaneous Endoscopic Approach
039M4ZX Drainage of Right External Carotid Artery, Percutaneous Endoscopic Approach, Diagnostic
039M4ZZ Drainage of Right External Carotid Artery, Percutaneous Endoscopic Approach
039N00Z Drainage of Left External Carotid Artery with Drainage Device, Open Approach
039N0ZX Drainage of Left External Carotid Artery, Open Approach, Diagnostic
039N0ZZ Drainage of Left External Carotid Artery, Open Approach
039N30Z Drainage of Left External Carotid Artery with Drainage Device, Percutaneous Approach
039N3ZX Drainage of Left External Carotid Artery, Percutaneous Approach, Diagnostic
039N3ZZ Drainage of Left External Carotid Artery, Percutaneous Approach
039N40Z Drainage of Left External Carotid Artery with Drainage Device, Percutaneous Endoscopic Approach
039N4ZX Drainage of Left External Carotid Artery, Percutaneous Endoscopic Approach, Diagnostic
039N4ZZ Drainage of Left External Carotid Artery, Percutaneous Endoscopic Approach
039P00Z Drainage of Right Vertebral Artery with Drainage Device, Open Approach
039P0ZX Drainage of Right Vertebral Artery, Open Approach, Diagnostic
039P0ZZ Drainage of Right Vertebral Artery, Open Approach
039P30Z Drainage of Right Vertebral Artery with Drainage Device, Percutaneous Approach
039P3ZX Drainage of Right Vertebral Artery, Percutaneous Approach, Diagnostic
039P3ZZ Drainage of Right Vertebral Artery, Percutaneous Approach
039P40Z Drainage of Right Vertebral Artery with Drainage Device, Percutaneous Endoscopic Approach
039P4ZX Drainage of Right Vertebral Artery, Percutaneous Endoscopic Approach, Diagnostic
039P4ZZ Drainage of Right Vertebral Artery, Percutaneous Endoscopic Approach
039Q00Z Drainage of Left Vertebral Artery with Drainage Device, Open Approach
039Q0ZX Drainage of Left Vertebral Artery, Open Approach, Diagnostic
039Q0ZZ Drainage of Left Vertebral Artery, Open Approach
039Q30Z Drainage of Left Vertebral Artery with Drainage Device, Percutaneous Approach
039Q3ZX Drainage of Left Vertebral Artery, Percutaneous Approach, Diagnostic
039Q3ZZ Drainage of Left Vertebral Artery, Percutaneous Approach
039Q40Z Drainage of Left Vertebral Artery with Drainage Device, Percutaneous Endoscopic Approach
039Q4ZX Drainage of Left Vertebral Artery, Percutaneous Endoscopic Approach, Diagnostic
039Q4ZZ Drainage of Left Vertebral Artery, Percutaneous Endoscopic Approach
039R00Z Drainage of Face Artery with Drainage Device, Open Approach
039R0ZX Drainage of Face Artery, Open Approach, Diagnostic
039R0ZZ Drainage of Face Artery, Open Approach
039R30Z Drainage of Face Artery with Drainage Device, Percutaneous Approach
039R3ZX Drainage of Face Artery, Percutaneous Approach, Diagnostic

039R3ZZ Drainage of Face Artery, Percutaneous Approach
039R40Z Drainage of Face Artery with Drainage Device, Percutaneous Endoscopic Approach
039R4ZX Drainage of Face Artery, Percutaneous Endoscopic Approach, Diagnostic
039R4ZZ Drainage of Face Artery, Percutaneous Endoscopic Approach
039S00Z Drainage of Right Temporal Artery with Drainage Device, Open Approach
039S0ZX Drainage of Right Temporal Artery, Open Approach, Diagnostic
039S0ZZ Drainage of Right Temporal Artery, Open Approach
039S30Z Drainage of Right Temporal Artery with Drainage Device, Percutaneous Approach
039S3ZX Drainage of Right Temporal Artery, Percutaneous Approach, Diagnostic
039S3ZZ Drainage of Right Temporal Artery, Percutaneous Approach
039S40Z Drainage of Right Temporal Artery with Drainage Device, Percutaneous Endoscopic Approach
039S4ZX Drainage of Right Temporal Artery, Percutaneous Endoscopic Approach, Diagnostic
039S4ZZ Drainage of Right Temporal Artery, Percutaneous Endoscopic Approach
039T00Z Drainage of Left Temporal Artery with Drainage Device, Open Approach
039T0ZX Drainage of Left Temporal Artery, Open Approach, Diagnostic
039T0ZZ Drainage of Left Temporal Artery, Open Approach
039T30Z Drainage of Left Temporal Artery with Drainage Device, Percutaneous Approach
039T3ZX Drainage of Left Temporal Artery, Percutaneous Approach, Diagnostic
039T3ZZ Drainage of Left Temporal Artery, Percutaneous Approach
039T40Z Drainage of Left Temporal Artery with Drainage Device, Percutaneous Endoscopic Approach
039T4ZX Drainage of Left Temporal Artery, Percutaneous Endoscopic Approach, Diagnostic
039T4ZZ Drainage of Left Temporal Artery, Percutaneous Endoscopic Approach
039U00Z Drainage of Right Thyroid Artery with Drainage Device, Open Approach
039U0ZX Drainage of Right Thyroid Artery, Open Approach, Diagnostic
039U0ZZ Drainage of Right Thyroid Artery, Open Approach
039U30Z Drainage of Right Thyroid Artery with Drainage Device, Percutaneous Approach
039U3ZX Drainage of Right Thyroid Artery, Percutaneous Approach, Diagnostic
039U3ZZ Drainage of Right Thyroid Artery, Percutaneous Approach
039U40Z Drainage of Right Thyroid Artery with Drainage Device, Percutaneous Endoscopic Approach
039U4ZX Drainage of Right Thyroid Artery, Percutaneous Endoscopic Approach, Diagnostic
039U4ZZ Drainage of Right Thyroid Artery, Percutaneous Endoscopic Approach
039V00Z Drainage of Left Thyroid Artery with Drainage Device, Open Approach
039V0ZX Drainage of Left Thyroid Artery, Open Approach, Diagnostic
039V0ZZ Drainage of Left Thyroid Artery, Open Approach
039V30Z Drainage of Left Thyroid Artery with Drainage Device, Percutaneous Approach
039V3ZX Drainage of Left Thyroid Artery, Percutaneous Approach, Diagnostic
039V3ZZ Drainage of Left Thyroid Artery, Percutaneous Approach
039V40Z Drainage of Left Thyroid Artery with Drainage Device, Percutaneous Endoscopic Approach
039V4ZX Drainage of Left Thyroid Artery, Percutaneous Endoscopic Approach, Diagnostic
039V4ZZ Drainage of Left Thyroid Artery, Percutaneous Endoscopic Approach
039Y00Z Drainage of Upper Artery with Drainage Device, Open Approach
039Y0ZX Drainage of Upper Artery, Open Approach, Diagnostic
039Y0ZZ Drainage of Upper Artery, Open Approach
039Y30Z Drainage of Upper Artery with Drainage Device, Percutaneous Approach
039Y3ZX Drainage of Upper Artery, Percutaneous Approach, Diagnostic
039Y3ZZ Drainage of Upper Artery, Percutaneous Approach
039Y40Z Drainage of Upper Artery with Drainage Device, Percutaneous Endoscopic Approach
039Y4ZX Drainage of Upper Artery, Percutaneous Endoscopic Approach, Diagnostic
039Y4ZZ Drainage of Upper Artery, Percutaneous Endoscopic Approach

03B – Upper Arteries, Excision

Review Coding Guidelines B3.4a and B3.4b

Review Coding Guideline B3.8

03B00ZX Excision of Right Internal Mammary Artery, Open Approach, Diagnostic
03B00ZZ Excision of Right Internal Mammary Artery, Open Approach
03B03ZX Excision of Right Internal Mammary Artery, Percutaneous Approach, Diagnostic
03B03ZZ Excision of Right Internal Mammary Artery, Percutaneous Approach
03B04ZX Excision of Right Internal Mammary Artery, Percutaneous Endoscopic Approach, Diagnostic
03B04ZZ Excision of Right Internal Mammary Artery, Percutaneous Endoscopic Approach
03B10ZX Excision of Left Internal Mammary Artery, Open Approach, Diagnostic
03B10ZZ Excision of Left Internal Mammary Artery, Open Approach
03B13ZX Excision of Left Internal Mammary Artery, Percutaneous Approach, Diagnostic
03B13ZZ Excision of Left Internal Mammary Artery, Percutaneous Approach
03B14ZX Excision of Left Internal Mammary Artery, Percutaneous Endoscopic Approach, Diagnostic
03B14ZZ Excision of Left Internal Mammary Artery, Percutaneous Endoscopic Approach
03B20ZX Excision of Innominate Artery, Open Approach, Diagnostic
03B20ZZ Excision of Innominate Artery, Open Approach
03B23ZX Excision of Innominate Artery, Percutaneous Approach, Diagnostic
03B23ZZ Excision of Innominate Artery, Percutaneous Approach
03B24ZX Excision of Innominate Artery, Percutaneous Endoscopic Approach, Diagnostic
03B24ZZ Excision of Innominate Artery, Percutaneous Endoscopic Approach
03B30ZX Excision of Right Subclavian Artery, Open Approach, Diagnostic
03B30ZZ Excision of Right Subclavian Artery, Open Approach
03B33ZX Excision of Right Subclavian Artery, Percutaneous Approach, Diagnostic
03B33ZZ Excision of Right Subclavian Artery, Percutaneous Approach
03B34ZX Excision of Right Subclavian Artery, Percutaneous Endoscopic Approach, Diagnostic
03B34ZZ Excision of Right Subclavian Artery, Percutaneous Endoscopic Approach
03B40ZX Excision of Left Subclavian Artery, Open Approach, Diagnostic
03B40ZZ Excision of Left Subclavian Artery, Open Approach
03B43ZX Excision of Left Subclavian Artery, Percutaneous Approach, Diagnostic
03B43ZZ Excision of Left Subclavian Artery, Percutaneous Approach
03B44ZX Excision of Left Subclavian Artery, Percutaneous Endoscopic Approach, Diagnostic
03B44ZZ Excision of Left Subclavian Artery, Percutaneous Endoscopic Approach
03B50ZX Excision of Right Axillary Artery, Open Approach, Diagnostic
03B50ZZ Excision of Right Axillary Artery, Open Approach
03B53ZX Excision of Right Axillary Artery, Percutaneous Approach, Diagnostic
03B53ZZ Excision of Right Axillary Artery, Percutaneous Approach
03B54ZX Excision of Right Axillary Artery, Percutaneous Endoscopic Approach, Diagnostic
03B54ZZ Excision of Right Axillary Artery, Percutaneous Endoscopic Approach
03B60ZX Excision of Left Axillary Artery, Open Approach, Diagnostic
03B60ZZ Excision of Left Axillary Artery, Open Approach
03B63ZX Excision of Left Axillary Artery, Percutaneous Approach, Diagnostic
03B63ZZ Excision of Left Axillary Artery, Percutaneous Approach
03B64ZX Excision of Left Axillary Artery, Percutaneous Endoscopic Approach, Diagnostic
03B64ZZ Excision of Left Axillary Artery, Percutaneous Endoscopic Approach
03B70ZX Excision of Right Brachial Artery, Open Approach, Diagnostic
03B70ZZ Excision of Right Brachial Artery, Open Approach
03B73ZX Excision of Right Brachial Artery, Percutaneous Approach, Diagnostic

B73ZZ Excision of Right Brachial Artery, Percutaneous Approach
B74ZX Excision of Right Brachial Artery, Percutaneous Endoscopic Approach, Diagnostic
B74ZZ Excision of Right Brachial Artery, Percutaneous Endoscopic Approach
B80ZX Excision of Left Brachial Artery, Open Approach, Diagnostic
3B80ZZ Excision of Left Brachial Artery, Open Approach
3B83ZX Excision of Left Brachial Artery, Percutaneous Approach, Diagnostic
3B83ZZ Excision of Left Brachial Artery, Percutaneous Approach
3B84ZX Excision of Left Brachial Artery, Percutaneous Endoscopic Approach, Diagnostic
3B84ZZ Excision of Left Brachial Artery, Percutaneous Endoscopic Approach
3B90ZX Excision of Right Ulnar Artery, Open Approach, Diagnostic
3B90ZZ Excision of Right Ulnar Artery, Open Approach
3B93ZX Excision of Right Ulnar Artery, Percutaneous Approach, Diagnostic
3B93ZZ Excision of Right Ulnar Artery, Percutaneous Approach
3B94ZX Excision of Right Ulnar Artery, Percutaneous Endoscopic Approach, Diagnostic
3B94ZZ Excision of Right Ulnar Artery, Percutaneous Endoscopic Approach
3BA0ZX Excision of Left Ulnar Artery, Open Approach, Diagnostic
3BA0ZZ Excision of Left Ulnar Artery, Open Approach
3BA3ZX Excision of Left Ulnar Artery, Percutaneous Approach, Diagnostic
3BA3ZZ Excision of Left Ulnar Artery, Percutaneous Approach
3BA4ZX Excision of Left Ulnar Artery, Percutaneous Endoscopic Approach, Diagnostic
3BA4ZZ Excision of Left Ulnar Artery, Percutaneous Endoscopic Approach
3BB0ZX Excision of Right Radial Artery, Open Approach, Diagnostic
3BB0ZZ Excision of Right Radial Artery, Open Approach
3BB3ZX Excision of Right Radial Artery, Percutaneous Approach, Diagnostic
3BB3ZZ Excision of Right Radial Artery, Percutaneous Approach
3BB4ZX Excision of Right Radial Artery, Percutaneous Endoscopic Approach, Diagnostic
3BB4ZZ Excision of Right Radial Artery, Percutaneous Endoscopic Approach
3BC0ZX Excision of Left Radial Artery, Open Approach, Diagnostic
3BC0ZZ Excision of Left Radial Artery, Open Approach
3BC3ZX Excision of Left Radial Artery, Percutaneous Approach, Diagnostic
3BC3ZZ Excision of Left Radial Artery, Percutaneous Approach
3BC4ZX Excision of Left Radial Artery, Percutaneous Endoscopic Approach, Diagnostic
3BC4ZZ Excision of Left Radial Artery, Percutaneous Endoscopic Approach
3BD0ZX Excision of Right Hand Artery, Open Approach, Diagnostic
3BD0ZZ Excision of Right Hand Artery, Open Approach
3BD3ZX Excision of Right Hand Artery, Percutaneous Approach, Diagnostic
03BD3ZZ Excision of Right Hand Artery, Percutaneous Approach
03BD4ZX Excision of Right Hand Artery, Percutaneous Endoscopic Approach, Diagnostic
03BD4ZZ Excision of Right Hand Artery, Percutaneous Endoscopic Approach
03BF0ZX Excision of Left Hand Artery, Open Approach, Diagnostic
03BF0ZZ Excision of Left Hand Artery, Open Approach
03BF3ZX Excision of Left Hand Artery, Percutaneous Approach, Diagnostic
03BF3ZZ Excision of Left Hand Artery, Percutaneous Approach
03BF4ZX Excision of Left Hand Artery, Percutaneous Endoscopic Approach, Diagnostic
03BF4ZZ Excision of Left Hand Artery, Percutaneous Endoscopic Approach
03BG0ZX Excision of Intracranial Artery, Open Approach, Diagnostic
03BG0ZZ Excision of Intracranial Artery, Open Approach
03BG3ZX Excision of Intracranial Artery, Percutaneous Approach, Diagnostic
03BG3ZZ Excision of Intracranial Artery, Percutaneous Approach
03BG4ZX Excision of Intracranial Artery, Percutaneous Endoscopic Approach, Diagnostic
03BG4ZZ Excision of Intracranial Artery, Percutaneous Endoscopic Approach
03BH0ZX Excision of Right Common Carotid Artery, Open Approach, Diagnostic
03BH0ZZ Excision of Right Common Carotid Artery, Open Approach
03BH3ZX Excision of Right Common Carotid Artery, Percutaneous Approach, Diagnostic
03BH3ZZ Excision of Right Common Carotid Artery, Percutaneous Approach
03BH4ZX Excision of Right Common Carotid Artery, Percutaneous Endoscopic Approach, Diagnostic
03BH4ZZ Excision of Right Common Carotid Artery, Percutaneous Endoscopic Approach
03BJ0ZX Excision of Left Common Carotid Artery, Open Approach, Diagnostic
03BJ0ZZ Excision of Left Common Carotid Artery, Open Approach
03BJ3ZX Excision of Left Common Carotid Artery, Percutaneous Approach, Diagnostic
03BJ3ZZ Excision of Left Common Carotid Artery, Percutaneous Approach
03BJ4ZX Excision of Left Common Carotid Artery, Percutaneous Endoscopic Approach, Diagnostic
03BJ4ZZ Excision of Left Common Carotid Artery, Percutaneous Endoscopic Approach
03BK0ZX Excision of Right Internal Carotid Artery, Open Approach, Diagnostic
03BK0ZZ Excision of Right Internal Carotid Artery, Open Approach
03BK3ZX Excision of Right Internal Carotid Artery, Percutaneous Approach, Diagnostic
03BK3ZZ Excision of Right Internal Carotid Artery, Percutaneous Approach
03BK4ZX Excision of Right Internal Carotid Artery, Percutaneous Endoscopic Approach, Diagnostic
03BK4ZZ Excision of Right Internal Carotid Artery, Percutaneous Endoscopic Approach
03BL0ZX Excision of Left Internal Carotid Artery, Open Approach, Diagnostic
03BL0ZZ Excision of Left Internal Carotid Artery, Open Approach
03BL3ZX Excision of Left Internal Carotid Artery, Percutaneous Approach, Diagnostic
03BL3ZZ Excision of Left Internal Carotid Artery, Percutaneous Approach
03BL4ZX Excision of Left Internal Carotid Artery, Percutaneous Endoscopic Approach, Diagnostic
03BL4ZZ Excision of Left Internal Carotid Artery, Percutaneous Endoscopic Approach
03BM0ZX Excision of Right External Carotid Artery, Open Approach, Diagnostic
03BM0ZZ Excision of Right External Carotid Artery, Open Approach
03BM3ZX Excision of Right External Carotid Artery, Percutaneous Approach, Diagnostic
03BM3ZZ Excision of Right External Carotid Artery, Percutaneous Approach
03BM4ZX Excision of Right External Carotid Artery, Percutaneous Endoscopic Approach, Diagnostic
03BM4ZZ Excision of Right External Carotid Artery, Percutaneous Endoscopic Approach
03BN0ZX Excision of Left External Carotid Artery, Open Approach, Diagnostic
03BN0ZZ Excision of Left External Carotid Artery, Open Approach
03BN3ZX Excision of Left External Carotid Artery, Percutaneous Approach, Diagnostic
03BN3ZZ Excision of Left External Carotid Artery, Percutaneous Approach
03BN4ZX Excision of Left External Carotid Artery, Percutaneous Endoscopic Approach, Diagnostic
03BN4ZZ Excision of Left External Carotid Artery, Percutaneous Endoscopic Approach
03BP0ZX Excision of Right Vertebral Artery, Open Approach, Diagnostic
03BP0ZZ Excision of Right Vertebral Artery, Open Approach
03BP3ZX Excision of Right Vertebral Artery, Percutaneous Approach, Diagnostic
03BP3ZZ Excision of Right Vertebral Artery, Percutaneous Approach
03BP4ZX Excision of Right Vertebral Artery, Percutaneous Endoscopic Approach, Diagnostic
03BP4ZZ Excision of Right Vertebral Artery, Percutaneous Endoscopic Approach
03BQ0ZX Excision of Left Vertebral Artery, Open Approach, Diagnostic
03BQ0ZZ Excision of Left Vertebral Artery, Open Approach
03BQ3ZX Excision of Left Vertebral Artery, Percutaneous Approach, Diagnostic
03BQ3ZZ Excision of Left Vertebral Artery, Percutaneous Approach
03BQ4ZX Excision of Left Vertebral Artery, Percutaneous Endoscopic Approach, Diagnostic
03BQ4ZZ Excision of Left Vertebral Artery, Percutaneous Endoscopic Approach
03BR0ZX Excision of Face Artery, Open Approach, Diagnostic
03BR0ZZ Excision of Face Artery, Open Approach
03BR3ZX Excision of Face Artery, Percutaneous Approach, Diagnostic
03BR3ZZ Excision of Face Artery, Percutaneous Approach
03BR4ZX Excision of Face Artery, Percutaneous Endoscopic Approach, Diagnostic
03BR4ZZ Excision of Face Artery, Percutaneous Endoscopic Approach
03BS0ZX Excision of Right Temporal Artery, Open Approach, Diagnostic
03BS0ZZ Excision of Right Temporal Artery, Open Approach
03BS3ZX Excision of Right Temporal Artery, Percutaneous Approach, Diagnostic

03BS3ZZ Excision of Right Temporal Artery, Percutaneous Approach
03BS4ZX Excision of Right Temporal Artery, Percutaneous Endoscopic Approach, Diagnostic
03BS4ZZ Excision of Right Temporal Artery, Percutaneous Endoscopic Approach
03BT0ZX Excision of Left Temporal Artery, Open Approach, Diagnostic
03BT0ZZ Excision of Left Temporal Artery, Open Approach
03BT3ZX Excision of Left Temporal Artery, Percutaneous Approach, Diagnostic
03BT3ZZ Excision of Left Temporal Artery, Percutaneous Approach
03BT4ZX Excision of Left Temporal Artery, Percutaneous Endoscopic Approach, Diagnostic
03BT4ZZ Excision of Left Temporal Artery, Percutaneous Endoscopic Approach
03BU0ZX Excision of Right Thyroid Artery, Open Approach, Diagnostic
03BU0ZZ Excision of Right Thyroid Artery, Open Approach
03BU3ZX Excision of Right Thyroid Artery, Percutaneous Approach, Diagnostic
03BU3ZZ Excision of Right Thyroid Artery, Percutaneous Approach
03BU4ZX Excision of Right Thyroid Artery, Percutaneous Endoscopic Approach, Diagnostic
03BU4ZZ Excision of Right Thyroid Artery, Percutaneous Endoscopic Approach
03BV0ZX Excision of Left Thyroid Artery, Open Approach, Diagnostic
03BV0ZZ Excision of Left Thyroid Artery, Open Approach
03BV3ZX Excision of Left Thyroid Artery, Percutaneous Approach, Diagnostic
03BV3ZZ Excision of Left Thyroid Artery, Percutaneous Approach
03BV4ZX Excision of Left Thyroid Artery, Percutaneous Endoscopic Approach, Diagnostic
03BV4ZZ Excision of Left Thyroid Artery, Percutaneous Endoscopic Approach
03BY0ZX Excision of Upper Artery, Open Approac Diagnostic
03BY0ZZ Excision of Upper Artery, Open Approac
03BY3ZX Excision of Upper Artery, Percutaneous Approach, Diagnostic
03BY3ZZ Excision of Upper Artery, Percutaneous Approach
03BY4ZX Excision of Upper Artery, Percutaneous Endoscopic Approach, Diagnostic
03BY4ZZ Excision of Upper Artery, Percutaneous Endoscopic Approach

03C – Upper Arteries, Extirpation

03C00ZZ Extirpation of Matter from Right Internal Mammary Artery, Open Approach
03C03ZZ Extirpation of Matter from Right Internal Mammary Artery, Percutaneous Approach
03C04ZZ Extirpation of Matter from Right Internal Mammary Artery, Percutaneous Endoscopic Approach
03C10ZZ Extirpation of Matter from Left Internal Mammary Artery, Open Approach
03C13ZZ Extirpation of Matter from Left Internal Mammary Artery, Percutaneous Approach
03C14ZZ Extirpation of Matter from Left Internal Mammary Artery, Percutaneous Endoscopic Approach
03C20ZZ Extirpation of Matter from Innominate Artery, Open Approach
03C23ZZ Extirpation of Matter from Innominate Artery, Percutaneous Approach
03C24ZZ Extirpation of Matter from Innominate Artery, Percutaneous Endoscopic Approach
03C30ZZ Extirpation of Matter from Right Subclavian Artery, Open Approach
03C33ZZ Extirpation of Matter from Right Subclavian Artery, Percutaneous Approach
03C34ZZ Extirpation of Matter from Right Subclavian Artery, Percutaneous Endoscopic Approach
03C40ZZ Extirpation of Matter from Left Subclavian Artery, Open Approach
03C43ZZ Extirpation of Matter from Left Subclavian Artery, Percutaneous Approach
03C44ZZ Extirpation of Matter from Left Subclavian Artery, Percutaneous Endoscopic Approach
03C50ZZ Extirpation of Matter from Right Axillary Artery, Open Approach
03C53ZZ Extirpation of Matter from Right Axillary Artery, Percutaneous Approach
03C54ZZ Extirpation of Matter from Right Axillary Artery, Percutaneous Endoscopic Approach
03C60ZZ Extirpation of Matter from Left Axillary Artery, Open Approach
03C63ZZ Extirpation of Matter from Left Axillary Artery, Percutaneous Approach
03C64ZZ Extirpation of Matter from Left Axillary Artery, Percutaneous Endoscopic Approach
03C70ZZ Extirpation of Matter from Right Brachial Artery, Open Approach
03C73ZZ Extirpation of Matter from Right Brachial Artery, Percutaneous Approach
03C74ZZ Extirpation of Matter from Right Brachial Artery, Percutaneous Endoscopic Approach
03C80ZZ Extirpation of Matter from Left Brachial Artery, Open Approach
03C83ZZ Extirpation of Matter from Left Brachial Artery, Percutaneous Approach
03C84ZZ Extirpation of Matter from Left Brachial Artery, Percutaneous Endoscopic Approach
03C90ZZ Extirpation of Matter from Right Ulnar Artery, Open Approach
03C93ZZ Extirpation of Matter from Right Ulnar Artery, Percutaneous Approach
03C94ZZ Extirpation of Matter from Right Ulnar Artery, Percutaneous Endoscopic Approach
03CA0ZZ Extirpation of Matter from Left Ulnar Artery, Open Approach
03CA3ZZ Extirpation of Matter from Left Ulnar Artery, Percutaneous Approach
03CA4ZZ Extirpation of Matter from Left Ulnar Artery, Percutaneous Endoscopic Approach
03CB0ZZ Extirpation of Matter from Right Radial Artery, Open Approach
03CB3ZZ Extirpation of Matter from Right Radial Artery, Percutaneous Approach
03CB4ZZ Extirpation of Matter from Right Radial Artery, Percutaneous Endoscopic Approach
03CC0ZZ Extirpation of Matter from Left Radial Artery, Open Approach
03CC3ZZ Extirpation of Matter from Left Radial Artery, Percutaneous Approach
03CC4ZZ Extirpation of Matter from Left Radial Artery, Percutaneous Endoscopic Approach
03CD0ZZ Extirpation of Matter from Right Hand Artery, Open Approach
03CD3ZZ Extirpation of Matter from Right Hand Artery, Percutaneous Approach
03CD4ZZ Extirpation of Matter from Right Hand Artery, Percutaneous Endoscopic Approach
03CF0ZZ Extirpation of Matter from Left Hand Artery, Open Approach
03CF3ZZ Extirpation of Matter from Left Hand Artery, Percutaneous Approach
03CF4ZZ Extirpation of Matter from Left Hand Artery, Percutaneous Endoscopic Approach
03CG0ZZ Extirpation of Matter from Intracranial Artery, Open Approach
▲ **03CG3ZZ** Extirpation of Matter from Intracranial Artery, Percutaneous Approach
▲ **03CG4ZZ** Extirpation of Matter from Intracranial Artery, Percutaneous Endoscopic Approach
03CH0ZZ Extirpation of Matter from Right Commo Carotid Artery, Open Approach
03CH3ZZ Extirpation of Matter from Right Commo Carotid Artery, Percutaneous Approach
03CH4ZZ Extirpation of Matter from Right Commo Carotid Artery, Percutaneous Endoscopic Approach
03CJ0ZZ Extirpation of Matter from Left Common Carotid Artery, Open Approach
03CJ3ZZ Extirpation of Matter from Left Common Carotid Artery, Percutaneous Approach
03CJ4ZZ Extirpation of Matter from Left Common Carotid Artery, Percutaneous Endoscopic Approach
03CK0ZZ Extirpation of Matter from Right Internal Carotid Artery, Open Approach
03CK3ZZ Extirpation of Matter from Right Internal Carotid Artery, Percutaneous Approach
03CK4ZZ Extirpation of Matter from Right Internal Carotid Artery, Percutaneous Endoscopic Approach
03CL0ZZ Extirpation of Matter from Left Internal Carotid Artery, Open Approach
03CL3ZZ Extirpation of Matter from Left Internal Carotid Artery, Percutaneous Approach
03CL4ZZ Extirpation of Matter from Left Internal Carotid Artery, Percutaneous Endoscopic Approach
03CM0ZZ Extirpation of Matter from Right External Carotid Artery, Open Approach
03CM3ZZ Extirpation of Matter from Right External Carotid Artery, Percutaneous Approach
03CM4ZZ Extirpation of Matter from Right External Carotid Artery, Percutaneous Endoscopic Approach
03CN0ZZ Extirpation of Matter from Left External Carotid Artery, Open Approach
03CN3ZZ Extirpation of Matter from Left External Carotid Artery, Percutaneous Approach
03CN4ZZ Extirpation of Matter from Left External Carotid Artery, Percutaneous Endoscopic Approach
03CP0ZZ Extirpation of Matter from Right Vertebra Artery, Open Approach
03CP3ZZ Extirpation of Matter from Right Vertebra Artery, Percutaneous Approach
03CP4ZZ Extirpation of Matter from Right Vertebra Artery, Percutaneous Endoscopic Approach

3CQ0ZZ Extirpation of Matter from Left Vertebral Artery, Open Approach
3CQ3ZZ Extirpation of Matter from Left Vertebral Artery, Percutaneous Approach
3CQ4ZZ Extirpation of Matter from Left Vertebral Artery, Percutaneous Endoscopic Approach
3CR0ZZ Extirpation of Matter from Face Artery, Open Approach
3CR3ZZ Extirpation of Matter from Face Artery, Percutaneous Approach
3CR4ZZ Extirpation of Matter from Face Artery, Percutaneous Endoscopic Approach
3CS0ZZ Extirpation of Matter from Right Temporal Artery, Open Approach
03CS3ZZ Extirpation of Matter from Right Temporal Artery, Percutaneous Approach
03CS4ZZ Extirpation of Matter from Right Temporal Artery, Percutaneous Endoscopic Approach
03CT0ZZ Extirpation of Matter from Left Temporal Artery, Open Approach
03CT3ZZ Extirpation of Matter from Left Temporal Artery, Percutaneous Approach
03CT4ZZ Extirpation of Matter from Left Temporal Artery, Percutaneous Endoscopic Approach
03CU0ZZ Extirpation of Matter from Right Thyroid Artery, Open Approach
03CU3ZZ Extirpation of Matter from Right Thyroid Artery, Percutaneous Approach
03CU4ZZ Extirpation of Matter from Right Thyroid Artery, Percutaneous Endoscopic Approach
03CV0ZZ Extirpation of Matter from Left Thyroid Artery, Open Approach
03CV3ZZ Extirpation of Matter from Left Thyroid Artery, Percutaneous Approach
03CV4ZZ Extirpation of Matter from Left Thyroid Artery, Percutaneous Endoscopic Approach
03CY0ZZ Extirpation of Matter from Upper Artery, Open Approach
03CY3ZZ Extirpation of Matter from Upper Artery, Percutaneous Approach
03CY4ZZ Extirpation of Matter from Upper Artery, Percutaneous Endoscopic Approach

3H – Upper Arteries, Insertion

3H003Z Insertion of Infusion Device into Right Internal Mammary Artery, Open Approach
3H00DZ Insertion of Intraluminal Device into Right Internal Mammary Artery, Open Approach
3H033Z Insertion of Infusion Device into Right Internal Mammary Artery, Percutaneous Approach
3H03DZ Insertion of Intraluminal Device into Right Internal Mammary Artery, Percutaneous Approach
3H043Z Insertion of Infusion Device into Right Internal Mammary Artery, Percutaneous Endoscopic Approach
3H04DZ Insertion of Intraluminal Device into Right Internal Mammary Artery, Percutaneous Endoscopic Approach
3H103Z Insertion of Infusion Device into Left Internal Mammary Artery, Open Approach
3H10DZ Insertion of Intraluminal Device into Left Internal Mammary Artery, Open Approach
3H133Z Insertion of Infusion Device into Left Internal Mammary Artery, Percutaneous Approach
3H13DZ Insertion of Intraluminal Device into Left Internal Mammary Artery, Percutaneous Approach
3H143Z Insertion of Infusion Device into Left Internal Mammary Artery, Percutaneous Endoscopic Approach
3H14DZ Insertion of Intraluminal Device into Left Internal Mammary Artery, Percutaneous Endoscopic Approach
3H203Z Insertion of Infusion Device into Innominate Artery, Open Approach
3H20DZ Insertion of Intraluminal Device into Innominate Artery, Open Approach
3H233Z Insertion of Infusion Device into Innominate Artery, Percutaneous Approach
3H23DZ Insertion of Intraluminal Device into Innominate Artery, Percutaneous Approach
3H243Z Insertion of Infusion Device into Innominate Artery, Percutaneous Endoscopic Approach
3H24DZ Insertion of Intraluminal Device into Innominate Artery, Percutaneous Endoscopic Approach
3H303Z Insertion of Infusion Device into Right Subclavian Artery, Open Approach
3H30DZ Insertion of Intraluminal Device into Right Subclavian Artery, Open Approach
3H333Z Insertion of Infusion Device into Right Subclavian Artery, Percutaneous Approach
3H33DZ Insertion of Intraluminal Device into Right Subclavian Artery, Percutaneous Approach
3H343Z Insertion of Infusion Device into Right Subclavian Artery, Percutaneous Endoscopic Approach
03H34DZ Insertion of Intraluminal Device into Right Subclavian Artery, Percutaneous Endoscopic Approach
03H403Z Insertion of Infusion Device into Left Subclavian Artery, Open Approach
03H40DZ Insertion of Intraluminal Device into Left Subclavian Artery, Open Approach
03H433Z Insertion of Infusion Device into Left Subclavian Artery, Percutaneous Approach
03H43DZ Insertion of Intraluminal Device into Left Subclavian Artery, Percutaneous Approach
03H443Z Insertion of Infusion Device into Left Subclavian Artery, Percutaneous Endoscopic Approach
03H44DZ Insertion of Intraluminal Device into Left Subclavian Artery, Percutaneous Endoscopic Approach
03H503Z Insertion of Infusion Device into Right Axillary Artery, Open Approach
03H50DZ Insertion of Intraluminal Device into Right Axillary Artery, Open Approach
03H533Z Insertion of Infusion Device into Right Axillary Artery, Percutaneous Approach
03H53DZ Insertion of Intraluminal Device into Right Axillary Artery, Percutaneous Approach
03H543Z Insertion of Infusion Device into Right Axillary Artery, Percutaneous Endoscopic Approach
03H54DZ Insertion of Intraluminal Device into Right Axillary Artery, Percutaneous Endoscopic Approach
03H603Z Insertion of Infusion Device into Left Axillary Artery, Open Approach
03H60DZ Insertion of Intraluminal Device into Left Axillary Artery, Open Approach
03H633Z Insertion of Infusion Device into Left Axillary Artery, Percutaneous Approach
03H63DZ Insertion of Intraluminal Device into Left Axillary Artery, Percutaneous Approach
03H643Z Insertion of Infusion Device into Left Axillary Artery, Percutaneous Endoscopic Approach
03H64DZ Insertion of Intraluminal Device into Left Axillary Artery, Percutaneous Endoscopic Approach
03H703Z Insertion of Infusion Device into Right Brachial Artery, Open Approach
03H70DZ Insertion of Intraluminal Device into Right Brachial Artery, Open Approach
03H733Z Insertion of Infusion Device into Right Brachial Artery, Percutaneous Approach
03H73DZ Insertion of Intraluminal Device into Right Brachial Artery, Percutaneous Approach
03H743Z Insertion of Infusion Device into Right Brachial Artery, Percutaneous Endoscopic Approach
03H74DZ Insertion of Intraluminal Device into Right Brachial Artery, Percutaneous Endoscopic Approach
03H803Z Insertion of Infusion Device into Left Brachial Artery, Open Approach
03H80DZ Insertion of Intraluminal Device into Left Brachial Artery, Open Approach
03H833Z Insertion of Infusion Device into Left Brachial Artery, Percutaneous Approach
03H83DZ Insertion of Intraluminal Device into Left Brachial Artery, Percutaneous Approach
03H843Z Insertion of Infusion Device into Left Brachial Artery, Percutaneous Endoscopic Approach
03H84DZ Insertion of Intraluminal Device into Left Brachial Artery, Percutaneous Endoscopic Approach
03H903Z Insertion of Infusion Device into Right Ulnar Artery, Open Approach
03H90DZ Insertion of Intraluminal Device into Right Ulnar Artery, Open Approach
03H933Z Insertion of Infusion Device into Right Ulnar Artery, Percutaneous Approach
03H93DZ Insertion of Intraluminal Device into Right Ulnar Artery, Percutaneous Approach
03H943Z Insertion of Infusion Device into Right Ulnar Artery, Percutaneous Endoscopic Approach
03H94DZ Insertion of Intraluminal Device into Right Ulnar Artery, Percutaneous Endoscopic Approach
03HA03Z Insertion of Infusion Device into Left Ulnar Artery, Open Approach
03HA0DZ Insertion of Intraluminal Device into Left Ulnar Artery, Open Approach
03HA33Z Insertion of Infusion Device into Left Ulnar Artery, Percutaneous Approach
03HA3DZ Insertion of Intraluminal Device into Left Ulnar Artery, Percutaneous Approach
03HA43Z Insertion of Infusion Device into Left Ulnar Artery, Percutaneous Endoscopic Approach
03HA4DZ Insertion of Intraluminal Device into Left Ulnar Artery, Percutaneous Endoscopic Approach
03HB03Z Insertion of Infusion Device into Right Radial Artery, Open Approach
03HB0DZ Insertion of Intraluminal Device into Right Radial Artery, Open Approach
03HB33Z Insertion of Infusion Device into Right Radial Artery, Percutaneous Approach
03HB3DZ Insertion of Intraluminal Device into Right Radial Artery, Percutaneous Approach
03HB43Z Insertion of Infusion Device into Right Radial Artery, Percutaneous Endoscopic Approach
03HB4DZ Insertion of Intraluminal Device into Right Radial Artery, Percutaneous Endoscopic Approach
03HC03Z Insertion of Infusion Device into Left Radial Artery, Open Approach

03HC0DZ Insertion of Intraluminal Device into Left Radial Artery, Open Approach
03HC33Z Insertion of Infusion Device into Left Radial Artery, Percutaneous Approach
03HC3DZ Insertion of Intraluminal Device into Left Radial Artery, Percutaneous Approach
03HC43Z Insertion of Infusion Device into Left Radial Artery, Percutaneous Endoscopic Approach
03HC4DZ Insertion of Intraluminal Device into Left Radial Artery, Percutaneous Endoscopic Approach
03HD03Z Insertion of Infusion Device into Right Hand Artery, Open Approach
03HD0DZ Insertion of Intraluminal Device into Right Hand Artery, Open Approach
03HD33Z Insertion of Infusion Device into Right Hand Artery, Percutaneous Approach
03HD3DZ Insertion of Intraluminal Device into Right Hand Artery, Percutaneous Approach
03HD43Z Insertion of Infusion Device into Right Hand Artery, Percutaneous Endoscopic Approach
03HD4DZ Insertion of Intraluminal Device into Right Hand Artery, Percutaneous Endoscopic Approach
03HF03Z Insertion of Infusion Device into Left Hand Artery, Open Approach
03HF0DZ Insertion of Intraluminal Device into Left Hand Artery, Open Approach
03HF33Z Insertion of Infusion Device into Left Hand Artery, Percutaneous Approach
03HF3DZ Insertion of Intraluminal Device into Left Hand Artery, Percutaneous Approach
03HF43Z Insertion of Infusion Device into Left Hand Artery, Percutaneous Endoscopic Approach
03HF4DZ Insertion of Intraluminal Device into Left Hand Artery, Percutaneous Endoscopic Approach
03HG03Z Insertion of Infusion Device into Intracranial Artery, Open Approach
03HG0DZ Insertion of Intraluminal Device into Intracranial Artery, Open Approach
03HG33Z Insertion of Infusion Device into Intracranial Artery, Percutaneous Approach
03HG3DZ Insertion of Intraluminal Device into Intracranial Artery, Percutaneous Approach
03HG43Z Insertion of Infusion Device into Intracranial Artery, Percutaneous Endoscopic Approach
03HG4DZ Insertion of Intraluminal Device into Intracranial Artery, Percutaneous Endoscopic Approach
03HH03Z Insertion of Infusion Device into Right Common Carotid Artery, Open Approach
03HH0DZ Insertion of Intraluminal Device into Right Common Carotid Artery, Open Approach
03HH33Z Insertion of Infusion Device into Right Common Carotid Artery, Percutaneous Approach
03HH3DZ Insertion of Intraluminal Device into Right Common Carotid Artery, Percutaneous Approach
03HH43Z Insertion of Infusion Device into Right Common Carotid Artery, Percutaneous Endoscopic Approach
03HH4DZ Insertion of Intraluminal Device into Right Common Carotid Artery, Percutaneous Endoscopic Approach
03HJ03Z Insertion of Infusion Device into Left Common Carotid Artery, Open Approach
03HJ0DZ Insertion of Intraluminal Device into Left Common Carotid Artery, Open Approach
03HJ33Z Insertion of Infusion Device into Left Common Carotid Artery, Percutaneous Approach
03HJ3DZ Insertion of Intraluminal Device into Left Common Carotid Artery, Percutaneous Approach
03HJ43Z Insertion of Infusion Device into Left Common Carotid Artery, Percutaneous Endoscopic Approach
03HJ4DZ Insertion of Intraluminal Device into Left Common Carotid Artery, Percutaneous Endoscopic Approach
03HK03Z Insertion of Infusion Device into Right Internal Carotid Artery, Open Approach
03HK0DZ Insertion of Intraluminal Device into Right Internal Carotid Artery, Open Approach
03HK0MZ Insertion of Stimulator Lead into Right Internal Carotid Artery, Open Approach
03HK33Z Insertion of Infusion Device into Right Internal Carotid Artery, Percutaneous Approach
03HK3DZ Insertion of Intraluminal Device into Right Internal Carotid Artery, Percutaneous Approach
03HK3MZ Insertion of Stimulator Lead into Right Internal Carotid Artery, Percutaneous Approach
03HK43Z Insertion of Infusion Device into Right Internal Carotid Artery, Percutaneous Endoscopic Approach
03HK4DZ Insertion of Intraluminal Device into Right Internal Carotid Artery, Percutaneous Endoscopic Approach
03HK4MZ Insertion of Stimulator Lead into Right Internal Carotid Artery, Percutaneous Endoscopic Approach
03HL03Z Insertion of Infusion Device into Left Internal Carotid Artery, Open Approach
03HL0DZ Insertion of Intraluminal Device into Left Internal Carotid Artery, Open Approach
03HL0MZ Insertion of Stimulator Lead into Left Internal Carotid Artery, Open Approach
03HL33Z Insertion of Infusion Device into Left Internal Carotid Artery, Percutaneous Approach
03HL3DZ Insertion of Intraluminal Device into Left Internal Carotid Artery, Percutaneous Approach
03HL3MZ Insertion of Stimulator Lead into Left Internal Carotid Artery, Percutaneous Approach
03HL43Z Insertion of Infusion Device into Left Internal Carotid Artery, Percutaneous Endoscopic Approach
03HL4DZ Insertion of Intraluminal Device into Left Internal Carotid Artery, Percutaneous Endoscopic Approach
03HL4MZ Insertion of Stimulator Lead into Left Internal Carotid Artery, Percutaneous Endoscopic Approach
03HM03Z Insertion of Infusion Device into Right External Carotid Artery, Open Approach
03HM0DZ Insertion of Intraluminal Device into Right External Carotid Artery, Open Approach
03HM33Z Insertion of Infusion Device into Right External Carotid Artery, Percutaneous Approach
03HM3DZ Insertion of Intraluminal Device into Right External Carotid Artery, Percutaneous Approach
03HM43Z Insertion of Infusion Device into Right External Carotid Artery, Percutaneous Endoscopic Approach
03HM4DZ Insertion of Intraluminal Device into Right External Carotid Artery, Percutaneous Endoscopic Approach
03HN03Z Insertion of Infusion Device into Left External Carotid Artery, Open Approach
03HN0DZ Insertion of Intraluminal Device into Left External Carotid Artery, Open Approach
03HN33Z Insertion of Infusion Device into Left External Carotid Artery, Percutaneous Approach
03HN3DZ Insertion of Intraluminal Device into Left External Carotid Artery, Percutaneous Approach
03HN43Z Insertion of Infusion Device into Left External Carotid Artery, Percutaneous Endoscopic Approach
03HN4DZ Insertion of Intraluminal Device into Left External Carotid Artery, Percutaneous Endoscopic Approach
03HP03Z Insertion of Infusion Device into Right Vertebral Artery, Open Approach
03HP0DZ Insertion of Intraluminal Device into Right Vertebral Artery, Open Approach
03HP33Z Insertion of Infusion Device into Right Vertebral Artery, Percutaneous Approach
03HP3DZ Insertion of Intraluminal Device into Right Vertebral Artery, Percutaneous Approach
03HP43Z Insertion of Infusion Device into Right Vertebral Artery, Percutaneous Endoscopic Approach
03HP4DZ Insertion of Intraluminal Device into Right Vertebral Artery, Percutaneous Endoscopic Approach
03HQ03Z Insertion of Infusion Device into Left Vertebral Artery, Open Approach
03HQ0DZ Insertion of Intraluminal Device into Left Vertebral Artery, Open Approach
03HQ33Z Insertion of Infusion Device into Left Vertebral Artery, Percutaneous Approach
03HQ3DZ Insertion of Intraluminal Device into Left Vertebral Artery, Percutaneous Approach
03HQ43Z Insertion of Infusion Device into Left Vertebral Artery, Percutaneous Endoscopic Approach
03HQ4DZ Insertion of Intraluminal Device into Left Vertebral Artery, Percutaneous Endoscopic Approach
03HR03Z Insertion of Infusion Device into Face Artery, Open Approach
03HR0DZ Insertion of Intraluminal Device into Face Artery, Open Approach
03HR33Z Insertion of Infusion Device into Face Artery, Percutaneous Approach
03HR3DZ Insertion of Intraluminal Device into Face Artery, Percutaneous Approach
03HR43Z Insertion of Infusion Device into Face Artery, Percutaneous Endoscopic Approach
03HR4DZ Insertion of Intraluminal Device into Face Artery, Percutaneous Endoscopic Approach
03HS03Z Insertion of Infusion Device into Right Temporal Artery, Open Approach
03HS0DZ Insertion of Intraluminal Device into Right Temporal Artery, Open Approach
03HS33Z Insertion of Infusion Device into Right Temporal Artery, Percutaneous Approach
03HS3DZ Insertion of Intraluminal Device into Right Temporal Artery, Percutaneous Approach
03HS43Z Insertion of Infusion Device into Right Temporal Artery, Percutaneous Endoscopic Approach
03HS4DZ Insertion of Intraluminal Device into Right Temporal Artery, Percutaneous Endoscopic Approach
03HT03Z Insertion of Infusion Device into Left Temporal Artery, Open Approach
03HT0DZ Insertion of Intraluminal Device into Left Temporal Artery, Open Approach
03HT33Z Insertion of Infusion Device into Left Temporal Artery, Percutaneous Approach
03HT3DZ Insertion of Intraluminal Device into Left Temporal Artery, Percutaneous Approach

HT43Z Insertion of Infusion Device into Left Temporal Artery, Percutaneous Endoscopic Approach
HT4DZ Insertion of Intraluminal Device into Left Temporal Artery, Percutaneous Endoscopic Approach
HU03Z Insertion of Infusion Device into Right Thyroid Artery, Open Approach
HU0DZ Insertion of Intraluminal Device into Right Thyroid Artery, Open Approach
HU33Z Insertion of Infusion Device into Right Thyroid Artery, Percutaneous Approach
HU3DZ Insertion of Intraluminal Device into Right Thyroid Artery, Percutaneous Approach
HU43Z Insertion of Infusion Device into Right Thyroid Artery, Percutaneous Endoscopic Approach
03HU4DZ Insertion of Intraluminal Device into Right Thyroid Artery, Percutaneous Endoscopic Approach
03HV03Z Insertion of Infusion Device into Left Thyroid Artery, Open Approach
03HV0DZ Insertion of Intraluminal Device into Left Thyroid Artery, Open Approach
03HV33Z Insertion of Infusion Device into Left Thyroid Artery, Percutaneous Approach
03HV3DZ Insertion of Intraluminal Device into Left Thyroid Artery, Percutaneous Approach
03HV43Z Insertion of Infusion Device into Left Thyroid Artery, Percutaneous Endoscopic Approach
03HV4DZ Insertion of Intraluminal Device into Left Thyroid Artery, Percutaneous Endoscopic Approach
03HY02Z Insertion of Monitoring Device into Upper Artery, Open Approach
03HY03Z Insertion of Infusion Device into Upper Artery, Open Approach
03HY0DZ Insertion of Intraluminal Device into Upper Artery, Open Approach
03HY32Z Insertion of Monitoring Device into Upper Artery, Percutaneous Approach
03HY33Z Insertion of Infusion Device into Upper Artery, Percutaneous Approach
03HY3DZ Insertion of Intraluminal Device into Upper Artery, Percutaneous Approach
03HY42Z Insertion of Monitoring Device into Upper Artery, Percutaneous Endoscopic Approach
03HY43Z Insertion of Infusion Device into Upper Artery, Percutaneous Endoscopic Approach
03HY4DZ Insertion of Intraluminal Device into Upper Artery, Percutaneous Endoscopic Approach

3J – Upper Arteries, Inspection

eview Coding Guidelines B3.11a, B3.11b and B3.11c

3JY0ZZ Inspection of Upper Artery, Open Approach
3JY3ZZ Inspection of Upper Artery, Percutaneous Approach
03JY4ZZ Inspection of Upper Artery, Percutaneous Endoscopic Approach
03JYXZZ Inspection of Upper Artery, External Approach

3L – Upper Arteries, Occlusion

eview Coding Guideline B3.12

3L00CZ Occlusion of Right Internal Mammary Artery with Extraluminal Device, Open Approach
3L00DZ Occlusion of Right Internal Mammary Artery with Intraluminal Device, Open Approach
3L00ZZ Occlusion of Right Internal Mammary Artery, Open Approach
3L03CZ Occlusion of Right Internal Mammary Artery with Extraluminal Device, Percutaneous Approach
3L03DZ Occlusion of Right Internal Mammary Artery with Intraluminal Device, Percutaneous Approach
3L03ZZ Occlusion of Right Internal Mammary Artery, Percutaneous Approach
3L04CZ Occlusion of Right Internal Mammary Artery with Extraluminal Device, Percutaneous Endoscopic Approach
3L04DZ Occlusion of Right Internal Mammary Artery with Intraluminal Device, Percutaneous Endoscopic Approach
3L04ZZ Occlusion of Right Internal Mammary Artery, Percutaneous Endoscopic Approach
3L10CZ Occlusion of Left Internal Mammary Artery with Extraluminal Device, Open Approach
3L10DZ Occlusion of Left Internal Mammary Artery with Intraluminal Device, Open Approach
3L10ZZ Occlusion of Left Internal Mammary Artery, Open Approach
3L13CZ Occlusion of Left Internal Mammary Artery with Extraluminal Device, Percutaneous Approach
3L13DZ Occlusion of Left Internal Mammary Artery with Intraluminal Device, Percutaneous Approach
3L13ZZ Occlusion of Left Internal Mammary Artery, Percutaneous Approach
3L14CZ Occlusion of Left Internal Mammary Artery with Extraluminal Device, Percutaneous Endoscopic Approach
03L14DZ Occlusion of Left Internal Mammary Artery with Intraluminal Device, Percutaneous Endoscopic Approach
03L14ZZ Occlusion of Left Internal Mammary Artery, Percutaneous Endoscopic Approach
03L20CZ Occlusion of Innominate Artery with Extraluminal Device, Open Approach
03L20DZ Occlusion of Innominate Artery with Intraluminal Device, Open Approach
03L20ZZ Occlusion of Innominate Artery, Open Approach
03L23CZ Occlusion of Innominate Artery with Extraluminal Device, Percutaneous Approach
03L23DZ Occlusion of Innominate Artery with Intraluminal Device, Percutaneous Approach
03L23ZZ Occlusion of Innominate Artery, Percutaneous Approach
03L24CZ Occlusion of Innominate Artery with Extraluminal Device, Percutaneous Endoscopic Approach
03L24DZ Occlusion of Innominate Artery with Intraluminal Device, Percutaneous Endoscopic Approach
03L24ZZ Occlusion of Innominate Artery, Percutaneous Endoscopic Approach
03L30CZ Occlusion of Right Subclavian Artery with Extraluminal Device, Open Approach
03L30DZ Occlusion of Right Subclavian Artery with Intraluminal Device, Open Approach
03L30ZZ Occlusion of Right Subclavian Artery, Open Approach
03L33CZ Occlusion of Right Subclavian Artery with Extraluminal Device, Percutaneous Approach
03L33DZ Occlusion of Right Subclavian Artery with Intraluminal Device, Percutaneous Approach
03L33ZZ Occlusion of Right Subclavian Artery, Percutaneous Approach
03L34CZ Occlusion of Right Subclavian Artery with Extraluminal Device, Percutaneous Endoscopic Approach
03L34DZ Occlusion of Right Subclavian Artery with Intraluminal Device, Percutaneous Endoscopic Approach
03L34ZZ Occlusion of Right Subclavian Artery, Percutaneous Endoscopic Approach
03L40CZ Occlusion of Left Subclavian Artery with Extraluminal Device, Open Approach
03L40DZ Occlusion of Left Subclavian Artery with Intraluminal Device, Open Approach
03L40ZZ Occlusion of Left Subclavian Artery, Open Approach
03L43CZ Occlusion of Left Subclavian Artery with Extraluminal Device, Percutaneous Approach
03L43DZ Occlusion of Left Subclavian Artery with Intraluminal Device, Percutaneous Approach
03L43ZZ Occlusion of Left Subclavian Artery, Percutaneous Approach
03L44CZ Occlusion of Left Subclavian Artery with Extraluminal Device, Percutaneous Endoscopic Approach
03L44DZ Occlusion of Left Subclavian Artery with Intraluminal Device, Percutaneous Endoscopic Approach
03L44ZZ Occlusion of Left Subclavian Artery, Percutaneous Endoscopic Approach
03L50CZ Occlusion of Right Axillary Artery with Extraluminal Device, Open Approach
03L50DZ Occlusion of Right Axillary Artery with Intraluminal Device, Open Approach
03L50ZZ Occlusion of Right Axillary Artery, Open Approach
03L53CZ Occlusion of Right Axillary Artery with Extraluminal Device, Percutaneous Approach
03L53DZ Occlusion of Right Axillary Artery with Intraluminal Device, Percutaneous Approach
03L53ZZ Occlusion of Right Axillary Artery, Percutaneous Approach
03L54CZ Occlusion of Right Axillary Artery with Extraluminal Device, Percutaneous Endoscopic Approach

03L54DZ Occlusion of Right Axillary Artery with Intraluminal Device, Percutaneous Endoscopic Approach
03L54ZZ Occlusion of Right Axillary Artery, Percutaneous Endoscopic Approach
03L60CZ Occlusion of Left Axillary Artery with Extraluminal Device, Open Approach
03L60DZ Occlusion of Left Axillary Artery with Intraluminal Device, Open Approach
03L60ZZ Occlusion of Left Axillary Artery, Open Approach
03L63CZ Occlusion of Left Axillary Artery with Extraluminal Device, Percutaneous Approach
03L63DZ Occlusion of Left Axillary Artery with Intraluminal Device, Percutaneous Approach
03L63ZZ Occlusion of Left Axillary Artery, Percutaneous Approach
03L64CZ Occlusion of Left Axillary Artery with Extraluminal Device, Percutaneous Endoscopic Approach
03L64DZ Occlusion of Left Axillary Artery with Intraluminal Device, Percutaneous Endoscopic Approach
03L64ZZ Occlusion of Left Axillary Artery, Percutaneous Endoscopic Approach
03L70CZ Occlusion of Right Brachial Artery with Extraluminal Device, Open Approach
03L70DZ Occlusion of Right Brachial Artery with Intraluminal Device, Open Approach
03L70ZZ Occlusion of Right Brachial Artery, Open Approach
03L73CZ Occlusion of Right Brachial Artery with Extraluminal Device, Percutaneous Approach
03L73DZ Occlusion of Right Brachial Artery with Intraluminal Device, Percutaneous Approach
03L73ZZ Occlusion of Right Brachial Artery, Percutaneous Approach
03L74CZ Occlusion of Right Brachial Artery with Extraluminal Device, Percutaneous Endoscopic Approach
03L74DZ Occlusion of Right Brachial Artery with Intraluminal Device, Percutaneous Endoscopic Approach
03L74ZZ Occlusion of Right Brachial Artery, Percutaneous Endoscopic Approach
03L80CZ Occlusion of Left Brachial Artery with Extraluminal Device, Open Approach
03L80DZ Occlusion of Left Brachial Artery with Intraluminal Device, Open Approach
03L80ZZ Occlusion of Left Brachial Artery, Open Approach
03L83CZ Occlusion of Left Brachial Artery with Extraluminal Device, Percutaneous Approach
03L83DZ Occlusion of Left Brachial Artery with Intraluminal Device, Percutaneous Approach
03L83ZZ Occlusion of Left Brachial Artery, Percutaneous Approach
03L84CZ Occlusion of Left Brachial Artery with Extraluminal Device, Percutaneous Endoscopic Approach
03L84DZ Occlusion of Left Brachial Artery with Intraluminal Device, Percutaneous Endoscopic Approach
03L84ZZ Occlusion of Left Brachial Artery, Percutaneous Endoscopic Approach
03L90CZ Occlusion of Right Ulnar Artery with Extraluminal Device, Open Approach
03L90DZ Occlusion of Right Ulnar Artery with Intraluminal Device, Open Approach
03L90ZZ Occlusion of Right Ulnar Artery, Open Approach
03L93CZ Occlusion of Right Ulnar Artery with Extraluminal Device, Percutaneous Approach
03L93DZ Occlusion of Right Ulnar Artery with Intraluminal Device, Percutaneous Approach
03L93ZZ Occlusion of Right Ulnar Artery, Percutaneous Approach
03L94CZ Occlusion of Right Ulnar Artery with Extraluminal Device, Percutaneous Endoscopic Approach
03L94DZ Occlusion of Right Ulnar Artery with Intraluminal Device, Percutaneous Endoscopic Approach
03L94ZZ Occlusion of Right Ulnar Artery, Percutaneous Endoscopic Approach
03LA0CZ Occlusion of Left Ulnar Artery with Extraluminal Device, Open Approach
03LA0DZ Occlusion of Left Ulnar Artery with Intraluminal Device, Open Approach
03LA0ZZ Occlusion of Left Ulnar Artery, Open Approach
03LA3CZ Occlusion of Left Ulnar Artery with Extraluminal Device, Percutaneous Approach
03LA3DZ Occlusion of Left Ulnar Artery with Intraluminal Device, Percutaneous Approach
03LA3ZZ Occlusion of Left Ulnar Artery, Percutaneous Approach
03LA4CZ Occlusion of Left Ulnar Artery with Extraluminal Device, Percutaneous Endoscopic Approach
03LA4DZ Occlusion of Left Ulnar Artery with Intraluminal Device, Percutaneous Endoscopic Approach
03LA4ZZ Occlusion of Left Ulnar Artery, Percutaneous Endoscopic Approach
03LB0CZ Occlusion of Right Radial Artery with Extraluminal Device, Open Approach
03LB0DZ Occlusion of Right Radial Artery with Intraluminal Device, Open Approach
03LB0ZZ Occlusion of Right Radial Artery, Open Approach
03LB3CZ Occlusion of Right Radial Artery with Extraluminal Device, Percutaneous Approach
03LB3DZ Occlusion of Right Radial Artery with Intraluminal Device, Percutaneous Approach
03LB3ZZ Occlusion of Right Radial Artery, Percutaneous Approach
03LB4CZ Occlusion of Right Radial Artery with Extraluminal Device, Percutaneous Endoscopic Approach
03LB4DZ Occlusion of Right Radial Artery with Intraluminal Device, Percutaneous Endoscopic Approach
03LB4ZZ Occlusion of Right Radial Artery, Percutaneous Endoscopic Approach
03LC0CZ Occlusion of Left Radial Artery with Extraluminal Device, Open Approach
03LC0DZ Occlusion of Left Radial Artery with Intraluminal Device, Open Approach
03LC0ZZ Occlusion of Left Radial Artery, Open Approach
03LC3CZ Occlusion of Left Radial Artery with Extraluminal Device, Percutaneous Approach
03LC3DZ Occlusion of Left Radial Artery with Intraluminal Device, Percutaneous Approach
03LC3ZZ Occlusion of Left Radial Artery, Percutaneous Approach
03LC4CZ Occlusion of Left Radial Artery with Extraluminal Device, Percutaneous Endoscopic Approach
03LC4DZ Occlusion of Left Radial Artery with Intraluminal Device, Percutaneous Endoscopic Approach
03LC4ZZ Occlusion of Left Radial Artery, Percutaneous Endoscopic Approach
03LD0CZ Occlusion of Right Hand Artery with Extraluminal Device, Open Approach
03LD0DZ Occlusion of Right Hand Artery with Intraluminal Device, Open Approach
03LD0ZZ Occlusion of Right Hand Artery, Open Approach
03LD3CZ Occlusion of Right Hand Artery with Extraluminal Device, Percutaneous Approach
03LD3DZ Occlusion of Right Hand Artery with Intraluminal Device, Percutaneous Approach
03LD3ZZ Occlusion of Right Hand Artery, Percutaneous Approach
03LD4CZ Occlusion of Right Hand Artery with Extraluminal Device, Percutaneous Endoscopic Approach
03LD4DZ Occlusion of Right Hand Artery with Intraluminal Device, Percutaneous Endoscopic Approach
03LD4ZZ Occlusion of Right Hand Artery, Percutaneous Endoscopic Approach
03LF0CZ Occlusion of Left Hand Artery with Extraluminal Device, Open Approach
03LF0DZ Occlusion of Left Hand Artery with Intraluminal Device, Open Approach
03LF0ZZ Occlusion of Left Hand Artery, Open Approach
03LF3CZ Occlusion of Left Hand Artery with Extraluminal Device, Percutaneous Approach
03LF3DZ Occlusion of Left Hand Artery with Intraluminal Device, Percutaneous Approach
03LF3ZZ Occlusion of Left Hand Artery, Percutaneous Approach
03LF4CZ Occlusion of Left Hand Artery with Extraluminal Device, Percutaneous Endoscopic Approach
03LF4DZ Occlusion of Left Hand Artery with Intraluminal Device, Percutaneous Endoscopic Approach
03LF4ZZ Occlusion of Left Hand Artery, Percutaneous Endoscopic Approach
03LG0BZ Occlusion of Intracranial Artery with Bioactive Intraluminal Device, Open Approach
03LG0CZ Occlusion of Intracranial Artery with Extraluminal Device, Open Approach
03LG0DZ Occlusion of Intracranial Artery with Intraluminal Device, Open Approach
03LG0ZZ Occlusion of Intracranial Artery, Open Approach
03LG3BZ Occlusion of Intracranial Artery with Bioactive Intraluminal Device, Percutaneous Approach
03LG3CZ Occlusion of Intracranial Artery with Extraluminal Device, Percutaneous Approach
03LG3DZ Occlusion of Intracranial Artery with Intraluminal Device, Percutaneous Approach
03LG3ZZ Occlusion of Intracranial Artery, Percutaneous Approach
03LG4BZ Occlusion of Intracranial Artery with Bioactive Intraluminal Device, Percutaneous Endoscopic Approach
03LG4CZ Occlusion of Intracranial Artery with Extraluminal Device, Percutaneous Endoscopic Approach
03LG4DZ Occlusion of Intracranial Artery with Intraluminal Device, Percutaneous Endoscopic Approach

LG4ZZ Occlusion of Intracranial Artery, Percutaneous Endoscopic Approach
LH0BZ Occlusion of Right Common Carotid Artery with Bioactive Intraluminal Device, Open Approach
LH0CZ Occlusion of Right Common Carotid Artery with Extraluminal Device, Open Approach
LH0DZ Occlusion of Right Common Carotid Artery with Intraluminal Device, Open Approach
LH0ZZ Occlusion of Right Common Carotid Artery, Open Approach
LH3BZ Occlusion of Right Common Carotid Artery with Bioactive Intraluminal Device, Percutaneous Approach
LH3CZ Occlusion of Right Common Carotid Artery with Extraluminal Device, Percutaneous Approach
LH3DZ Occlusion of Right Common Carotid Artery with Intraluminal Device, Percutaneous Approach
LH3ZZ Occlusion of Right Common Carotid Artery, Percutaneous Approach
LH4BZ Occlusion of Right Common Carotid Artery with Bioactive Intraluminal Device, Percutaneous Endoscopic Approach
LH4CZ Occlusion of Right Common Carotid Artery with Extraluminal Device, Percutaneous Endoscopic Approach
3LH4DZ Occlusion of Right Common Carotid Artery with Intraluminal Device, Percutaneous Endoscopic Approach
3LH4ZZ Occlusion of Right Common Carotid Artery, Percutaneous Endoscopic Approach
3LJ0BZ Occlusion of Left Common Carotid Artery with Bioactive Intraluminal Device, Open Approach
3LJ0CZ Occlusion of Left Common Carotid Artery with Extraluminal Device, Open Approach
3LJ0DZ Occlusion of Left Common Carotid Artery with Intraluminal Device, Open Approach
3LJ0ZZ Occlusion of Left Common Carotid Artery, Open Approach
3LJ3BZ Occlusion of Left Common Carotid Artery with Bioactive Intraluminal Device, Percutaneous Approach
3LJ3CZ Occlusion of Left Common Carotid Artery with Extraluminal Device, Percutaneous Approach
3LJ3DZ Occlusion of Left Common Carotid Artery with Intraluminal Device, Percutaneous Approach
3LJ3ZZ Occlusion of Left Common Carotid Artery, Percutaneous Approach
3LJ4BZ Occlusion of Left Common Carotid Artery with Bioactive Intraluminal Device, Percutaneous Endoscopic Approach
3LJ4CZ Occlusion of Left Common Carotid Artery with Extraluminal Device, Percutaneous Endoscopic Approach
3LJ4DZ Occlusion of Left Common Carotid Artery with Intraluminal Device, Percutaneous Endoscopic Approach
3LJ4ZZ Occlusion of Left Common Carotid Artery, Percutaneous Endoscopic Approach
3LK0BZ Occlusion of Right Internal Carotid Artery with Bioactive Intraluminal Device, Open Approach
3LK0CZ Occlusion of Right Internal Carotid Artery with Extraluminal Device, Open Approach
3LK0DZ Occlusion of Right Internal Carotid Artery with Intraluminal Device, Open Approach
3LK0ZZ Occlusion of Right Internal Carotid Artery, Open Approach
03LK3BZ Occlusion of Right Internal Carotid Artery with Bioactive Intraluminal Device, Percutaneous Approach
03LK3CZ Occlusion of Right Internal Carotid Artery with Extraluminal Device, Percutaneous Approach
03LK3DZ Occlusion of Right Internal Carotid Artery with Intraluminal Device, Percutaneous Approach
03LK3ZZ Occlusion of Right Internal Carotid Artery, Percutaneous Approach
03LK4BZ Occlusion of Right Internal Carotid Artery with Bioactive Intraluminal Device, Percutaneous Endoscopic Approach
03LK4CZ Occlusion of Right Internal Carotid Artery with Extraluminal Device, Percutaneous Endoscopic Approach
03LK4DZ Occlusion of Right Internal Carotid Artery with Intraluminal Device, Percutaneous Endoscopic Approach
03LK4ZZ Occlusion of Right Internal Carotid Artery, Percutaneous Endoscopic Approach
03LL0BZ Occlusion of Left Internal Carotid Artery with Bioactive Intraluminal Device, Open Approach
03LL0CZ Occlusion of Left Internal Carotid Artery with Extraluminal Device, Open Approach
03LL0DZ Occlusion of Left Internal Carotid Artery with Intraluminal Device, Open Approach
03LL0ZZ Occlusion of Left Internal Carotid Artery, Open Approach
03LL3BZ Occlusion of Left Internal Carotid Artery with Bioactive Intraluminal Device, Percutaneous Approach
03LL3CZ Occlusion of Left Internal Carotid Artery with Extraluminal Device, Percutaneous Approach
03LL3DZ Occlusion of Left Internal Carotid Artery with Intraluminal Device, Percutaneous Approach
03LL3ZZ Occlusion of Left Internal Carotid Artery, Percutaneous Approach
03LL4BZ Occlusion of Left Internal Carotid Artery with Bioactive Intraluminal Device, Percutaneous Endoscopic Approach
03LL4CZ Occlusion of Left Internal Carotid Artery with Extraluminal Device, Percutaneous Endoscopic Approach
03LL4DZ Occlusion of Left Internal Carotid Artery with Intraluminal Device, Percutaneous Endoscopic Approach
03LL4ZZ Occlusion of Left Internal Carotid Artery, Percutaneous Endoscopic Approach
03LM0BZ Occlusion of Right External Carotid Artery with Bioactive Intraluminal Device, Open Approach
03LM0CZ Occlusion of Right External Carotid Artery with Extraluminal Device, Open Approach
03LM0DZ Occlusion of Right External Carotid Artery with Intraluminal Device, Open Approach
03LM0ZZ Occlusion of Right External Carotid Artery, Open Approach
03LM3BZ Occlusion of Right External Carotid Artery with Bioactive Intraluminal Device, Percutaneous Approach
03LM3CZ Occlusion of Right External Carotid Artery with Extraluminal Device, Percutaneous Approach
03LM3DZ Occlusion of Right External Carotid Artery with Intraluminal Device, Percutaneous Approach
03LM3ZZ Occlusion of Right External Carotid Artery, Percutaneous Approach
03LM4BZ Occlusion of Right External Carotid Artery with Bioactive Intraluminal Device, Percutaneous Endoscopic Approach
03LM4CZ Occlusion of Right External Carotid Artery with Extraluminal Device, Percutaneous Endoscopic Approach
03LM4DZ Occlusion of Right External Carotid Artery with Intraluminal Device, Percutaneous Endoscopic Approach
03LM4ZZ Occlusion of Right External Carotid Artery, Percutaneous Endoscopic Approach
03LN0BZ Occlusion of Left External Carotid Artery with Bioactive Intraluminal Device, Open Approach
03LN0CZ Occlusion of Left External Carotid Artery with Extraluminal Device, Open Approach
03LN0DZ Occlusion of Left External Carotid Artery with Intraluminal Device, Open Approach
03LN0ZZ Occlusion of Left External Carotid Artery, Open Approach
03LN3BZ Occlusion of Left External Carotid Artery with Bioactive Intraluminal Device, Percutaneous Approach
03LN3CZ Occlusion of Left External Carotid Artery with Extraluminal Device, Percutaneous Approach
03LN3DZ Occlusion of Left External Carotid Artery with Intraluminal Device, Percutaneous Approach
03LN3ZZ Occlusion of Left External Carotid Artery, Percutaneous Approach
03LN4BZ Occlusion of Left External Carotid Artery with Bioactive Intraluminal Device, Percutaneous Endoscopic Approach
03LN4CZ Occlusion of Left External Carotid Artery with Extraluminal Device, Percutaneous Endoscopic Approach
03LN4DZ Occlusion of Left External Carotid Artery with Intraluminal Device, Percutaneous Endoscopic Approach
03LN4ZZ Occlusion of Left External Carotid Artery, Percutaneous Endoscopic Approach
03LP0BZ Occlusion of Right Vertebral Artery with Bioactive Intraluminal Device, Open Approach
03LP0CZ Occlusion of Right Vertebral Artery with Extraluminal Device, Open Approach
03LP0DZ Occlusion of Right Vertebral Artery with Intraluminal Device, Open Approach
03LP0ZZ Occlusion of Right Vertebral Artery, Open Approach
03LP3BZ Occlusion of Right Vertebral Artery with Bioactive Intraluminal Device, Percutaneous Approach
03LP3CZ Occlusion of Right Vertebral Artery with Extraluminal Device, Percutaneous Approach
03LP3DZ Occlusion of Right Vertebral Artery with Intraluminal Device, Percutaneous Approach
03LP3ZZ Occlusion of Right Vertebral Artery, Percutaneous Approach
03LP4BZ Occlusion of Right Vertebral Artery with Bioactive Intraluminal Device, Percutaneous Endoscopic Approach
03LP4CZ Occlusion of Right Vertebral Artery with Extraluminal Device, Percutaneous Endoscopic Approach
03LP4DZ Occlusion of Right Vertebral Artery with Intraluminal Device, Percutaneous Endoscopic Approach
03LP4ZZ Occlusion of Right Vertebral Artery, Percutaneous Endoscopic Approach
03LQ0BZ Occlusion of Left Vertebral Artery with Bioactive Intraluminal Device, Open Approach
03LQ0CZ Occlusion of Left Vertebral Artery with Extraluminal Device, Open Approach
03LQ0DZ Occlusion of Left Vertebral Artery with Intraluminal Device, Open Approach

03LQ0ZZ Occlusion of Left Vertebral Artery, Open Approach
03LQ3BZ Occlusion of Left Vertebral Artery with Bioactive Intraluminal Device, Percutaneous Approach
03LQ3CZ Occlusion of Left Vertebral Artery with Extraluminal Device, Percutaneous Approach
03LQ3DZ Occlusion of Left Vertebral Artery with Intraluminal Device, Percutaneous Approach
03LQ3ZZ Occlusion of Left Vertebral Artery, Percutaneous Approach
03LQ4BZ Occlusion of Left Vertebral Artery with Bioactive Intraluminal Device, Percutaneous Endoscopic Approach
03LQ4CZ Occlusion of Left Vertebral Artery with Extraluminal Device, Percutaneous Endoscopic Approach
03LQ4DZ Occlusion of Left Vertebral Artery with Intraluminal Device, Percutaneous Endoscopic Approach
03LQ4ZZ Occlusion of Left Vertebral Artery, Percutaneous Endoscopic Approach
03LR0CZ Occlusion of Face Artery with Extraluminal Device, Open Approach
03LR0DZ Occlusion of Face Artery with Intraluminal Device, Open Approach
03LR0ZZ Occlusion of Face Artery, Open Approach
03LR3CZ Occlusion of Face Artery with Extraluminal Device, Percutaneous Approach
03LR3DZ Occlusion of Face Artery with Intraluminal Device, Percutaneous Approach
03LR3ZZ Occlusion of Face Artery, Percutaneous Approach
03LR4CZ Occlusion of Face Artery with Extraluminal Device, Percutaneous Endoscopic Approach
03LR4DZ Occlusion of Face Artery with Intraluminal Device, Percutaneous Endoscopic Approach
03LR4ZZ Occlusion of Face Artery, Percutaneous Endoscopic Approach
03LS0CZ Occlusion of Right Temporal Artery with Extraluminal Device, Open Approach
03LS0DZ Occlusion of Right Temporal Artery with Intraluminal Device, Open Approach
03LS0ZZ Occlusion of Right Temporal Artery, Open Approach
03LS3CZ Occlusion of Right Temporal Artery with Extraluminal Device, Percutaneous Approach
03LS3DZ Occlusion of Right Temporal Artery with Intraluminal Device, Percutaneous Approach
03LS3ZZ Occlusion of Right Temporal Artery, Percutaneous Approach
03LS4CZ Occlusion of Right Temporal Artery with Extraluminal Device, Percutaneous Endoscopic Approach
03LS4DZ Occlusion of Right Temporal Artery with Intraluminal Device, Percutaneous Endoscopic Approach
03LS4ZZ Occlusion of Right Temporal Artery, Percutaneous Endoscopic Approach
03LT0CZ Occlusion of Left Temporal Artery with Extraluminal Device, Open Approach
03LT0DZ Occlusion of Left Temporal Artery with Intraluminal Device, Open Approach
03LT0ZZ Occlusion of Left Temporal Artery, Open Approach
03LT3CZ Occlusion of Left Temporal Artery with Extraluminal Device, Percutaneous Approach
03LT3DZ Occlusion of Left Temporal Artery with Intraluminal Device, Percutaneous Approach
03LT3ZZ Occlusion of Left Temporal Artery, Percutaneous Approach
03LT4CZ Occlusion of Left Temporal Artery with Extraluminal Device, Percutaneous Endoscopic Approach
03LT4DZ Occlusion of Left Temporal Artery with Intraluminal Device, Percutaneous Endoscopic Approach
03LT4ZZ Occlusion of Left Temporal Artery, Percutaneous Endoscopic Approach
03LU0CZ Occlusion of Right Thyroid Artery with Extraluminal Device, Open Approach
03LU0DZ Occlusion of Right Thyroid Artery with Intraluminal Device, Open Approach
03LU0ZZ Occlusion of Right Thyroid Artery, Open Approach
03LU3CZ Occlusion of Right Thyroid Artery with Extraluminal Device, Percutaneous Approach
03LU3DZ Occlusion of Right Thyroid Artery with Intraluminal Device, Percutaneous Approach
03LU3ZZ Occlusion of Right Thyroid Artery, Percutaneous Approach
03LU4CZ Occlusion of Right Thyroid Artery with Extraluminal Device, Percutaneous Endoscopic Approach
03LU4DZ Occlusion of Right Thyroid Artery with Intraluminal Device, Percutaneous Endoscopic Approach
03LU4ZZ Occlusion of Right Thyroid Artery, Percutaneous Endoscopic Approach
03LV0CZ Occlusion of Left Thyroid Artery with Extraluminal Device, Open Approach
03LV0DZ Occlusion of Left Thyroid Artery with Intraluminal Device, Open Approach
03LV0ZZ Occlusion of Left Thyroid Artery, Open Approach
03LV3CZ Occlusion of Left Thyroid Artery with Extraluminal Device, Percutaneous Approach
03LV3DZ Occlusion of Left Thyroid Artery with Intraluminal Device, Percutaneous Approach
03LV3ZZ Occlusion of Left Thyroid Artery, Percutaneous Approach
03LV4CZ Occlusion of Left Thyroid Artery with Extraluminal Device, Percutaneous Endoscopic Approach
03LV4DZ Occlusion of Left Thyroid Artery with Intraluminal Device, Percutaneous Endoscopic Approach
03LV4ZZ Occlusion of Left Thyroid Artery, Percutaneous Endoscopic Approach
03LY0CZ Occlusion of Upper Artery with Extraluminal Device, Open Approach
03LY0DZ Occlusion of Upper Artery with Intraluminal Device, Open Approach
03LY0ZZ Occlusion of Upper Artery, Open Approach
03LY3CZ Occlusion of Upper Artery with Extraluminal Device, Percutaneous Approach
03LY3DZ Occlusion of Upper Artery with Intraluminal Device, Percutaneous Approach
03LY3ZZ Occlusion of Upper Artery, Percutaneous Approach
03LY4CZ Occlusion of Upper Artery with Extraluminal Device, Percutaneous Endoscopic Approach
03LY4DZ Occlusion of Upper Artery with Intraluminal Device, Percutaneous Endoscopic Approach
03LY4ZZ Occlusion of Upper Artery, Percutaneous Endoscopic Approach

03N – Upper Arteries, Release

Review Coding Guidelines B3.13 and B3.14

03N00ZZ Release Right Internal Mammary Artery, Open Approach
03N03ZZ Release Right Internal Mammary Artery, Percutaneous Approach
03N04ZZ Release Right Internal Mammary Artery, Percutaneous Endoscopic Approach
03N10ZZ Release Left Internal Mammary Artery, Open Approach
03N13ZZ Release Left Internal Mammary Artery, Percutaneous Approach
03N14ZZ Release Left Internal Mammary Artery, Percutaneous Endoscopic Approach
03N20ZZ Release Innominate Artery, Open Approach
03N23ZZ Release Innominate Artery, Percutaneous Approach
03N24ZZ Release Innominate Artery, Percutaneous Endoscopic Approach
03N30ZZ Release Right Subclavian Artery, Open Approach
03N33ZZ Release Right Subclavian Artery, Percutaneous Approach
03N34ZZ Release Right Subclavian Artery, Percutaneous Endoscopic Approach
03N40ZZ Release Left Subclavian Artery, Open Approach
03N43ZZ Release Left Subclavian Artery, Percutaneous Approach
03N44ZZ Release Left Subclavian Artery, Percutaneous Endoscopic Approach
03N50ZZ Release Right Axillary Artery, Open Approach
03N53ZZ Release Right Axillary Artery, Percutaneous Approach
03N54ZZ Release Right Axillary Artery, Percutaneous Endoscopic Approach
03N60ZZ Release Left Axillary Artery, Open Approach
03N63ZZ Release Left Axillary Artery, Percutaneous Approach
03N64ZZ Release Left Axillary Artery, Percutaneous Endoscopic Approach
03N70ZZ Release Right Brachial Artery, Open Approach
03N73ZZ Release Right Brachial Artery, Percutaneous Approach
03N74ZZ Release Right Brachial Artery, Percutaneous Endoscopic Approach
03N80ZZ Release Left Brachial Artery, Open Approach
03N83ZZ Release Left Brachial Artery, Percutaneous Approach
03N84ZZ Release Left Brachial Artery, Percutaneous Endoscopic Approach
03N90ZZ Release Right Ulnar Artery, Open Approach
03N93ZZ Release Right Ulnar Artery, Percutaneous Approach
03N94ZZ Release Right Ulnar Artery, Percutaneous Endoscopic Approach

NA0ZZ Release Left Ulnar Artery, Open Approach
NA3ZZ Release Left Ulnar Artery, Percutaneous Approach
NA4ZZ Release Left Ulnar Artery, Percutaneous Endoscopic Approach
NB0ZZ Release Right Radial Artery, Open Approach
NB3ZZ Release Right Radial Artery, Percutaneous Approach
NB4ZZ Release Right Radial Artery, Percutaneous Endoscopic Approach
NC0ZZ Release Left Radial Artery, Open Approach
NC3ZZ Release Left Radial Artery, Percutaneous Approach
NC4ZZ Release Left Radial Artery, Percutaneous Endoscopic Approach
ND0ZZ Release Right Hand Artery, Open Approach
ND3ZZ Release Right Hand Artery, Percutaneous Approach
ND4ZZ Release Right Hand Artery, Percutaneous Endoscopic Approach
3NF0ZZ Release Left Hand Artery, Open Approach
3NF3ZZ Release Left Hand Artery, Percutaneous Approach
3NF4ZZ Release Left Hand Artery, Percutaneous Endoscopic Approach
3NG0ZZ Release Intracranial Artery, Open Approach
3NG3ZZ Release Intracranial Artery, Percutaneous Approach
3NG4ZZ Release Intracranial Artery, Percutaneous Endoscopic Approach
3NH0ZZ Release Right Common Carotid Artery, Open Approach
3NH3ZZ Release Right Common Carotid Artery, Percutaneous Approach
03NH4ZZ Release Right Common Carotid Artery, Percutaneous Endoscopic Approach
03NJ0ZZ Release Left Common Carotid Artery, Open Approach
03NJ3ZZ Release Left Common Carotid Artery, Percutaneous Approach
03NJ4ZZ Release Left Common Carotid Artery, Percutaneous Endoscopic Approach
03NK0ZZ Release Right Internal Carotid Artery, Open Approach
03NK3ZZ Release Right Internal Carotid Artery, Percutaneous Approach
03NK4ZZ Release Right Internal Carotid Artery, Percutaneous Endoscopic Approach
03NL0ZZ Release Left Internal Carotid Artery, Open Approach
03NL3ZZ Release Left Internal Carotid Artery, Percutaneous Approach
03NL4ZZ Release Left Internal Carotid Artery, Percutaneous Endoscopic Approach
03NM0ZZ Release Right External Carotid Artery, Open Approach
03NM3ZZ Release Right External Carotid Artery, Percutaneous Approach
03NM4ZZ Release Right External Carotid Artery, Percutaneous Endoscopic Approach
03NN0ZZ Release Left External Carotid Artery, Open Approach
03NN3ZZ Release Left External Carotid Artery, Percutaneous Approach
03NN4ZZ Release Left External Carotid Artery, Percutaneous Endoscopic Approach
03NP0ZZ Release Right Vertebral Artery, Open Approach
03NP3ZZ Release Right Vertebral Artery, Percutaneous Approach
03NP4ZZ Release Right Vertebral Artery, Percutaneous Endoscopic Approach
03NQ0ZZ Release Left Vertebral Artery, Open Approach
03NQ3ZZ Release Left Vertebral Artery, Percutaneous Approach
03NQ4ZZ Release Left Vertebral Artery, Percutaneous Endoscopic Approach
03NR0ZZ Release Face Artery, Open Approach
03NR3ZZ Release Face Artery, Percutaneous Approach
03NR4ZZ Release Face Artery, Percutaneous Endoscopic Approach
03NS0ZZ Release Right Temporal Artery, Open Approach
03NS3ZZ Release Right Temporal Artery, Percutaneous Approach
03NS4ZZ Release Right Temporal Artery, Percutaneous Endoscopic Approach
03NT0ZZ Release Left Temporal Artery, Open Approach
03NT3ZZ Release Left Temporal Artery, Percutaneous Approach
03NT4ZZ Release Left Temporal Artery, Percutaneous Endoscopic Approach
03NU0ZZ Release Right Thyroid Artery, Open Approach
03NU3ZZ Release Right Thyroid Artery, Percutaneous Approach
03NU4ZZ Release Right Thyroid Artery, Percutaneous Endoscopic Approach
03NV0ZZ Release Left Thyroid Artery, Open Approach
03NV3ZZ Release Left Thyroid Artery, Percutaneous Approach
03NV4ZZ Release Left Thyroid Artery, Percutaneous Endoscopic Approach
03NY0ZZ Release Upper Artery, Open Approach
03NY3ZZ Release Upper Artery, Percutaneous Approach
03NY4ZZ Release Upper Artery, Percutaneous Endoscopic Approach

3P – Upper Arteries, Removal

eview Coding Guideline B6.1c

3PY00Z Removal of Drainage Device from Upper Artery, Open Approach
3PY02Z Removal of Monitoring Device from Upper Artery, Open Approach
3PY03Z Removal of Infusion Device from Upper Artery, Open Approach
3PY07Z Removal of Autologous Tissue Substitute from Upper Artery, Open Approach
3PY0CZ Removal of Extraluminal Device from Upper Artery, Open Approach
3PY0DZ Removal of Intraluminal Device from Upper Artery, Open Approach
3PY0JZ Removal of Synthetic Substitute from Upper Artery, Open Approach
3PY0KZ Removal of Nonautologous Tissue Substitute from Upper Artery, Open Approach
3PY0MZ Removal of Stimulator Lead from Upper Artery, Open Approach
3PY30Z Removal of Drainage Device from Upper Artery, Percutaneous Approach
3PY32Z Removal of Monitoring Device from Upper Artery, Percutaneous Approach
3PY33Z Removal of Infusion Device from Upper Artery, Percutaneous Approach
03PY37Z Removal of Autologous Tissue Substitute from Upper Artery, Percutaneous Approach
03PY3CZ Removal of Extraluminal Device from Upper Artery, Percutaneous Approach
03PY3DZ Removal of Intraluminal Device from Upper Artery, Percutaneous Approach
03PY3JZ Removal of Synthetic Substitute from Upper Artery, Percutaneous Approach
03PY3KZ Removal of Nonautologous Tissue Substitute from Upper Artery, Percutaneous Approach
03PY3MZ Removal of Stimulator Lead from Upper Artery, Percutaneous Approach
03PY40Z Removal of Drainage Device from Upper Artery, Percutaneous Endoscopic Approach
03PY42Z Removal of Monitoring Device from Upper Artery, Percutaneous Endoscopic Approach
03PY43Z Removal of Infusion Device from Upper Artery, Percutaneous Endoscopic Approach
03PY47Z Removal of Autologous Tissue Substitute from Upper Artery, Percutaneous Endoscopic Approach
03PY4CZ Removal of Extraluminal Device from Upper Artery, Percutaneous Endoscopic Approach
03PY4DZ Removal of Intraluminal Device from Upper Artery, Percutaneous Endoscopic Approach
03PY4JZ Removal of Synthetic Substitute from Upper Artery, Percutaneous Endoscopic Approach
03PY4KZ Removal of Nonautologous Tissue Substitute from Upper Artery, Percutaneous Endoscopic Approach
03PY4MZ Removal of Stimulator Lead from Upper Artery, Percutaneous Endoscopic Approach
03PYX0Z Removal of Drainage Device from Upper Artery, External Approach
03PYX2Z Removal of Monitoring Device from Upper Artery, External Approach
03PYX3Z Removal of Infusion Device from Upper Artery, External Approach
03PYXDZ Removal of Intraluminal Device from Upper Artery, External Approach
03PYXMZ Removal of Stimulator Lead from Upper Artery, External Approach

3Q – Upper Arteries, Repair

3Q00ZZ Repair Right Internal Mammary Artery, Open Approach
3Q03ZZ Repair Right Internal Mammary Artery, Percutaneous Approach
03Q04ZZ Repair Right Internal Mammary Artery, Percutaneous Endoscopic Approach
03Q10ZZ Repair Left Internal Mammary Artery, Open Approach
03Q13ZZ Repair Left Internal Mammary Artery, Percutaneous Approach
03Q14ZZ Repair Left Internal Mammary Artery, Percutaneous Endoscopic Approach

03Q20ZZ Repair Innominate Artery, Open Approach
03Q23ZZ Repair Innominate Artery, Percutaneous Approach
03Q24ZZ Repair Innominate Artery, Percutaneous Endoscopic Approach
03Q30ZZ Repair Right Subclavian Artery, Open Approach
03Q33ZZ Repair Right Subclavian Artery, Percutaneous Approach
03Q34ZZ Repair Right Subclavian Artery, Percutaneous Endoscopic Approach
03Q40ZZ Repair Left Subclavian Artery, Open Approach
03Q43ZZ Repair Left Subclavian Artery, Percutaneous Approach
03Q44ZZ Repair Left Subclavian Artery, Percutaneous Endoscopic Approach
03Q50ZZ Repair Right Axillary Artery, Open Approach
03Q53ZZ Repair Right Axillary Artery, Percutaneous Approach
03Q54ZZ Repair Right Axillary Artery, Percutaneous Endoscopic Approach
03Q60ZZ Repair Left Axillary Artery, Open Approach
03Q63ZZ Repair Left Axillary Artery, Percutaneous Approach
03Q64ZZ Repair Left Axillary Artery, Percutaneous Endoscopic Approach
03Q70ZZ Repair Right Brachial Artery, Open Approach
03Q73ZZ Repair Right Brachial Artery, Percutaneous Approach
03Q74ZZ Repair Right Brachial Artery, Percutaneous Endoscopic Approach
03Q80ZZ Repair Left Brachial Artery, Open Approach
03Q83ZZ Repair Left Brachial Artery, Percutaneous Approach
03Q84ZZ Repair Left Brachial Artery, Percutaneous Endoscopic Approach
03Q90ZZ Repair Right Ulnar Artery, Open Approach
03Q93ZZ Repair Right Ulnar Artery, Percutaneous Approach
03Q94ZZ Repair Right Ulnar Artery, Percutaneous Endoscopic Approach
03QA0ZZ Repair Left Ulnar Artery, Open Approach
03QA3ZZ Repair Left Ulnar Artery, Percutaneous Approach
03QA4ZZ Repair Left Ulnar Artery, Percutaneous Endoscopic Approach
03QB0ZZ Repair Right Radial Artery, Open Approach
03QB3ZZ Repair Right Radial Artery, Percutaneous Approach
03QB4ZZ Repair Right Radial Artery, Percutaneous Endoscopic Approach
03QC0ZZ Repair Left Radial Artery, Open Approach
03QC3ZZ Repair Left Radial Artery, Percutaneous Approach
03QC4ZZ Repair Left Radial Artery, Percutaneous Endoscopic Approach
03QD0ZZ Repair Right Hand Artery, Open Approach
03QD3ZZ Repair Right Hand Artery, Percutaneous Approach
03QD4ZZ Repair Right Hand Artery, Percutaneous Endoscopic Approach
03QF0ZZ Repair Left Hand Artery, Open Approach
03QF3ZZ Repair Left Hand Artery, Percutaneous Approach
03QF4ZZ Repair Left Hand Artery, Percutaneous Endoscopic Approach
03QG0ZZ Repair Intracranial Artery, Open Approach
03QG3ZZ Repair Intracranial Artery, Percutaneous Approach
03QG4ZZ Repair Intracranial Artery, Percutaneous Endoscopic Approach
03QH0ZZ Repair Right Common Carotid Artery, Open Approach
03QH3ZZ Repair Right Common Carotid Artery, Percutaneous Approach
03QH4ZZ Repair Right Common Carotid Artery, Percutaneous Endoscopic Approach
03QJ0ZZ Repair Left Common Carotid Artery, Open Approach
03QJ3ZZ Repair Left Common Carotid Artery, Percutaneous Approach
03QJ4ZZ Repair Left Common Carotid Artery, Percutaneous Endoscopic Approach
03QK0ZZ Repair Right Internal Carotid Artery, Open Approach
03QK3ZZ Repair Right Internal Carotid Artery, Percutaneous Approach
03QK4ZZ Repair Right Internal Carotid Artery, Percutaneous Endoscopic Approach
03QL0ZZ Repair Left Internal Carotid Artery, Open Approach
03QL3ZZ Repair Left Internal Carotid Artery, Percutaneous Approach
03QL4ZZ Repair Left Internal Carotid Artery, Percutaneous Endoscopic Approach
03QM0ZZ Repair Right External Carotid Artery, Open Approach
03QM3ZZ Repair Right External Carotid Artery, Percutaneous Approach
03QM4ZZ Repair Right External Carotid Artery, Percutaneous Endoscopic Approach
03QN0ZZ Repair Left External Carotid Artery, Ope[n] Approach
03QN3ZZ Repair Left External Carotid Artery, Percutaneous Approach
03QN4ZZ Repair Left External Carotid Artery, Percutaneous Endoscopic Approach
03QP0ZZ Repair Right Vertebral Artery, Open Approach
03QP3ZZ Repair Right Vertebral Artery, Percutaneous Approach
03QP4ZZ Repair Right Vertebral Artery, Percutaneous Endoscopic Approach
03QQ0ZZ Repair Left Vertebral Artery, Open Approach
03QQ3ZZ Repair Left Vertebral Artery, Percutaneou[s] Approach
03QQ4ZZ Repair Left Vertebral Artery, Percutaneou[s] Endoscopic Approach
03QR0ZZ Repair Face Artery, Open Approach
03QR3ZZ Repair Face Artery, Percutaneous Approach
03QR4ZZ Repair Face Artery, Percutaneous Endoscopic Approach
03QS0ZZ Repair Right Temporal Artery, Open Approach
03QS3ZZ Repair Right Temporal Artery, Percutaneous Approach
03QS4ZZ Repair Right Temporal Artery, Percutaneous Endoscopic Approach
03QT0ZZ Repair Left Temporal Artery, Open Approach
03QT3ZZ Repair Left Temporal Artery, Percutaneou[s] Approach
03QT4ZZ Repair Left Temporal Artery, Percutaneou[s] Endoscopic Approach
03QU0ZZ Repair Right Thyroid Artery, Open Approach
03QU3ZZ Repair Right Thyroid Artery, Percutaneou[s] Approach
03QU4ZZ Repair Right Thyroid Artery, Percutaneou[s] Endoscopic Approach
03QV0ZZ Repair Left Thyroid Artery, Open Approach
03QV3ZZ Repair Left Thyroid Artery, Percutaneous Approach
03QV4ZZ Repair Left Thyroid Artery, Percutaneous Endoscopic Approach
03QY0ZZ Repair Upper Artery, Open Approach
03QY3ZZ Repair Upper Artery, Percutaneous Approach
03QY4ZZ Repair Upper Artery, Percutaneous Endoscopic Approach

03R – Upper Arteries, Replacement

03R007Z Replacement of Right Internal Mammary Artery with Autologous Tissue Substitute, Open Approach
03R00JZ Replacement of Right Internal Mammary Artery with Synthetic Substitute, Open Approach
03R00KZ Replacement of Right Internal Mammary Artery with Nonautologous Tissue Substitute, Open Approach
03R047Z Replacement of Right Internal Mammary Artery with Autologous Tissue Substitute, Percutaneous Endoscopic Approach
03R04JZ Replacement of Right Internal Mammary Artery with Synthetic Substitute, Percutaneous Endoscopic Approach
03R04KZ Replacement of Right Internal Mammary Artery with Nonautologous Tissue Substitute, Percutaneous Endoscopic Approach
03R107Z Replacement of Left Internal Mammary Artery with Autologous Tissue Substitute, Open Approach
03R10JZ Replacement of Left Internal Mammary Artery with Synthetic Substitute, Open Approach
03R10KZ Replacement of Left Internal Mammary Artery with Nonautologous Tissue Substitute, Open Approach
03R147Z Replacement of Left Internal Mammary Artery with Autologous Tissue Substitute, Percutaneous Endoscopic Approach
03R14JZ Replacement of Left Internal Mammary Artery with Synthetic Substitute, Percutaneous Endoscopic Approach
03R14KZ Replacement of Left Internal Mammary Artery with Nonautologous Tissue Substitute, Percutaneous Endoscopic Approach
03R207Z Replacement of Innominate Artery with Autologous Tissue Substitute, Open Approach
03R20JZ Replacement of Innominate Artery with Synthetic Substitute, Open Approach
03R20KZ Replacement of Innominate Artery with Nonautologous Tissue Substitute, Open Approach
03R247Z Replacement of Innominate Artery with Autologous Tissue Substitute, Percutaneous Endoscopic Approach
03R24JZ Replacement of Innominate Artery with Synthetic Substitute, Percutaneous Endoscopic Approach
03R24KZ Replacement of Innominate Artery with Nonautologous Tissue Substitute, Percutaneous Endoscopic Approach
03R307Z Replacement of Right Subclavian Artery with Autologous Tissue Substitute, Open Approach
03R30JZ Replacement of Right Subclavian Artery with Synthetic Substitute, Open Approach
03R30KZ Replacement of Right Subclavian Artery with Nonautologous Tissue Substitute, Open Approach

3R347Z Replacement of Right Subclavian Artery with Autologous Tissue Substitute, Percutaneous Endoscopic Approach

3R34JZ Replacement of Right Subclavian Artery with Synthetic Substitute, Percutaneous Endoscopic Approach

3R34KZ Replacement of Right Subclavian Artery with Nonautologous Tissue Substitute, Percutaneous Endoscopic Approach

3R407Z Replacement of Left Subclavian Artery with Autologous Tissue Substitute, Open Approach

3R40JZ Replacement of Left Subclavian Artery with Synthetic Substitute, Open Approach

3R40KZ Replacement of Left Subclavian Artery with Nonautologous Tissue Substitute, Open Approach

3R447Z Replacement of Left Subclavian Artery with Autologous Tissue Substitute, Percutaneous Endoscopic Approach

3R44JZ Replacement of Left Subclavian Artery with Synthetic Substitute, Percutaneous Endoscopic Approach

3R44KZ Replacement of Left Subclavian Artery with Nonautologous Tissue Substitute, Percutaneous Endoscopic Approach

3R507Z Replacement of Right Axillary Artery with Autologous Tissue Substitute, Open Approach

3R50JZ Replacement of Right Axillary Artery with Synthetic Substitute, Open Approach

3R50KZ Replacement of Right Axillary Artery with Nonautologous Tissue Substitute, Open Approach

3R547Z Replacement of Right Axillary Artery with Autologous Tissue Substitute, Percutaneous Endoscopic Approach

3R54JZ Replacement of Right Axillary Artery with Synthetic Substitute, Percutaneous Endoscopic Approach

3R54KZ Replacement of Right Axillary Artery with Nonautologous Tissue Substitute, Percutaneous Endoscopic Approach

3R607Z Replacement of Left Axillary Artery with Autologous Tissue Substitute, Open Approach

3R60JZ Replacement of Left Axillary Artery with Synthetic Substitute, Open Approach

3R60KZ Replacement of Left Axillary Artery with Nonautologous Tissue Substitute, Open Approach

3R647Z Replacement of Left Axillary Artery with Autologous Tissue Substitute, Percutaneous Endoscopic Approach

3R64JZ Replacement of Left Axillary Artery with Synthetic Substitute, Percutaneous Endoscopic Approach

3R64KZ Replacement of Left Axillary Artery with Nonautologous Tissue Substitute, Percutaneous Endoscopic Approach

3R707Z Replacement of Right Brachial Artery with Autologous Tissue Substitute, Open Approach

3R70JZ Replacement of Right Brachial Artery with Synthetic Substitute, Open Approach

3R70KZ Replacement of Right Brachial Artery with Nonautologous Tissue Substitute, Open Approach

3R747Z Replacement of Right Brachial Artery with Autologous Tissue Substitute, Percutaneous Endoscopic Approach

3R74JZ Replacement of Right Brachial Artery with Synthetic Substitute, Percutaneous Endoscopic Approach

3R74KZ Replacement of Right Brachial Artery with Nonautologous Tissue Substitute, Percutaneous Endoscopic Approach

03R807Z Replacement of Left Brachial Artery with Autologous Tissue Substitute, Open Approach

03R80JZ Replacement of Left Brachial Artery with Synthetic Substitute, Open Approach

03R80KZ Replacement of Left Brachial Artery with Nonautologous Tissue Substitute, Open Approach

03R847Z Replacement of Left Brachial Artery with Autologous Tissue Substitute, Percutaneous Endoscopic Approach

03R84JZ Replacement of Left Brachial Artery with Synthetic Substitute, Percutaneous Endoscopic Approach

03R84KZ Replacement of Left Brachial Artery with Nonautologous Tissue Substitute, Percutaneous Endoscopic Approach

03R907Z Replacement of Right Ulnar Artery with Autologous Tissue Substitute, Open Approach

03R90JZ Replacement of Right Ulnar Artery with Synthetic Substitute, Open Approach

03R90KZ Replacement of Right Ulnar Artery with Nonautologous Tissue Substitute, Open Approach

03R947Z Replacement of Right Ulnar Artery with Autologous Tissue Substitute, Percutaneous Endoscopic Approach

03R94JZ Replacement of Right Ulnar Artery with Synthetic Substitute, Percutaneous Endoscopic Approach

03R94KZ Replacement of Right Ulnar Artery with Nonautologous Tissue Substitute, Percutaneous Endoscopic Approach

03RA07Z Replacement of Left Ulnar Artery with Autologous Tissue Substitute, Open Approach

03RA0JZ Replacement of Left Ulnar Artery with Synthetic Substitute, Open Approach

03RA0KZ Replacement of Left Ulnar Artery with Nonautologous Tissue Substitute, Open Approach

03RA47Z Replacement of Left Ulnar Artery with Autologous Tissue Substitute, Percutaneous Endoscopic Approach

03RA4JZ Replacement of Left Ulnar Artery with Synthetic Substitute, Percutaneous Endoscopic Approach

03RA4KZ Replacement of Left Ulnar Artery with Nonautologous Tissue Substitute, Percutaneous Endoscopic Approach

03RB07Z Replacement of Right Radial Artery with Autologous Tissue Substitute, Open Approach

03RB0JZ Replacement of Right Radial Artery with Synthetic Substitute, Open Approach

03RB0KZ Replacement of Right Radial Artery with Nonautologous Tissue Substitute, Open Approach

03RB47Z Replacement of Right Radial Artery with Autologous Tissue Substitute, Percutaneous Endoscopic Approach

03RB4JZ Replacement of Right Radial Artery with Synthetic Substitute, Percutaneous Endoscopic Approach

03RB4KZ Replacement of Right Radial Artery with Nonautologous Tissue Substitute, Percutaneous Endoscopic Approach

03RC07Z Replacement of Left Radial Artery with Autologous Tissue Substitute, Open Approach

03RC0JZ Replacement of Left Radial Artery with Synthetic Substitute, Open Approach

03RC0KZ Replacement of Left Radial Artery with Nonautologous Tissue Substitute, Open Approach

03RC47Z Replacement of Left Radial Artery with Autologous Tissue Substitute, Percutaneous Endoscopic Approach

03RC4JZ Replacement of Left Radial Artery with Synthetic Substitute, Percutaneous Endoscopic Approach

03RC4KZ Replacement of Left Radial Artery with Nonautologous Tissue Substitute, Percutaneous Endoscopic Approach

03RD07Z Replacement of Right Hand Artery with Autologous Tissue Substitute, Open Approach

03RD0JZ Replacement of Right Hand Artery with Synthetic Substitute, Open Approach

03RD0KZ Replacement of Right Hand Artery with Nonautologous Tissue Substitute, Open Approach

03RD47Z Replacement of Right Hand Artery with Autologous Tissue Substitute, Percutaneous Endoscopic Approach

03RD4JZ Replacement of Right Hand Artery with Synthetic Substitute, Percutaneous Endoscopic Approach

03RD4KZ Replacement of Right Hand Artery with Nonautologous Tissue Substitute, Percutaneous Endoscopic Approach

03RF07Z Replacement of Left Hand Artery with Autologous Tissue Substitute, Open Approach

03RF0JZ Replacement of Left Hand Artery with Synthetic Substitute, Open Approach

03RF0KZ Replacement of Left Hand Artery with Nonautologous Tissue Substitute, Open Approach

03RF47Z Replacement of Left Hand Artery with Autologous Tissue Substitute, Percutaneous Endoscopic Approach

03RF4JZ Replacement of Left Hand Artery with Synthetic Substitute, Percutaneous Endoscopic Approach

03RF4KZ Replacement of Left Hand Artery with Nonautologous Tissue Substitute, Percutaneous Endoscopic Approach

03RG07Z Replacement of Intracranial Artery with Autologous Tissue Substitute, Open Approach

03RG0JZ Replacement of Intracranial Artery with Synthetic Substitute, Open Approach

03RG0KZ Replacement of Intracranial Artery with Nonautologous Tissue Substitute, Open Approach

03RG47Z Replacement of Intracranial Artery with Autologous Tissue Substitute, Percutaneous Endoscopic Approach

03RG4JZ Replacement of Intracranial Artery with Synthetic Substitute, Percutaneous Endoscopic Approach

03RG4KZ Replacement of Intracranial Artery with Nonautologous Tissue Substitute, Percutaneous Endoscopic Approach

03RH07Z Replacement of Right Common Carotid Artery with Autologous Tissue Substitute, Open Approach

03RH0JZ Replacement of Right Common Carotid Artery with Synthetic Substitute, Open Approach

03RH0KZ Replacement of Right Common Carotid Artery with Nonautologous Tissue Substitute, Open Approach

03RH47Z Replacement of Right Common Carotid Artery with Autologous Tissue Substitute, Percutaneous Endoscopic Approach

03RH4JZ Replacement of Right Common Carotid Artery with Synthetic Substitute, Percutaneous Endoscopic Approach

03RH4KZ Replacement of Right Common Carotid Artery with Nonautologous Tissue Substitute, Percutaneous Endoscopic Approach
03RJ07Z Replacement of Left Common Carotid Artery with Autologous Tissue Substitute, Open Approach
03RJ0JZ Replacement of Left Common Carotid Artery with Synthetic Substitute, Open Approach
03RJ0KZ Replacement of Left Common Carotid Artery with Nonautologous Tissue Substitute, Open Approach
03RJ47Z Replacement of Left Common Carotid Artery with Autologous Tissue Substitute, Percutaneous Endoscopic Approach
03RJ4JZ Replacement of Left Common Carotid Artery with Synthetic Substitute, Percutaneous Endoscopic Approach
03RJ4KZ Replacement of Left Common Carotid Artery with Nonautologous Tissue Substitute, Percutaneous Endoscopic Approach
03RK07Z Replacement of Right Internal Carotid Artery with Autologous Tissue Substitute, Open Approach
03RK0JZ Replacement of Right Internal Carotid Artery with Synthetic Substitute, Open Approach
03RK0KZ Replacement of Right Internal Carotid Artery with Nonautologous Tissue Substitute, Open Approach
03RK47Z Replacement of Right Internal Carotid Artery with Autologous Tissue Substitute, Percutaneous Endoscopic Approach
03RK4JZ Replacement of Right Internal Carotid Artery with Synthetic Substitute, Percutaneous Endoscopic Approach
03RK4KZ Replacement of Right Internal Carotid Artery with Nonautologous Tissue Substitute, Percutaneous Endoscopic Approach
03RL07Z Replacement of Left Internal Carotid Artery with Autologous Tissue Substitute, Open Approach
03RL0JZ Replacement of Left Internal Carotid Artery with Synthetic Substitute, Open Approach
03RL0KZ Replacement of Left Internal Carotid Artery with Nonautologous Tissue Substitute, Open Approach
03RL47Z Replacement of Left Internal Carotid Artery with Autologous Tissue Substitute, Percutaneous Endoscopic Approach
03RL4JZ Replacement of Left Internal Carotid Artery with Synthetic Substitute, Percutaneous Endoscopic Approach
03RL4KZ Replacement of Left Internal Carotid Artery with Nonautologous Tissue Substitute, Percutaneous Endoscopic Approach
03RM07Z Replacement of Right External Carotid Artery with Autologous Tissue Substitute, Open Approach
03RM0JZ Replacement of Right External Carotid Artery with Synthetic Substitute, Open Approach
03RM0KZ Replacement of Right External Carotid Artery with Nonautologous Tissue Substitute, Open Approach
03RM47Z Replacement of Right External Carotid Artery with Autologous Tissue Substitute, Percutaneous Endoscopic Approach
03RM4JZ Replacement of Right External Carotid Artery with Synthetic Substitute, Percutaneous Endoscopic Approach
03RM4KZ Replacement of Right External Carotid Artery with Nonautologous Tissue Substitute, Percutaneous Endoscopic Approach
03RN07Z Replacement of Left External Carotid Artery with Autologous Tissue Substitute, Open Approach
03RN0JZ Replacement of Left External Carotid Artery with Synthetic Substitute, Open Approach
03RN0KZ Replacement of Left External Carotid Artery with Nonautologous Tissue Substitute, Open Approach
03RN47Z Replacement of Left External Carotid Artery with Autologous Tissue Substitute, Percutaneous Endoscopic Approach
03RN4JZ Replacement of Left External Carotid Artery with Synthetic Substitute, Percutaneous Endoscopic Approach
03RN4KZ Replacement of Left External Carotid Artery with Nonautologous Tissue Substitute, Percutaneous Endoscopic Approach
03RP07Z Replacement of Right Vertebral Artery with Autologous Tissue Substitute, Open Approach
03RP0JZ Replacement of Right Vertebral Artery with Synthetic Substitute, Open Approach
03RP0KZ Replacement of Right Vertebral Artery with Nonautologous Tissue Substitute, Open Approach
03RP47Z Replacement of Right Vertebral Artery with Autologous Tissue Substitute, Percutaneous Endoscopic Approach
03RP4JZ Replacement of Right Vertebral Artery with Synthetic Substitute, Percutaneous Endoscopic Approach
03RP4KZ Replacement of Right Vertebral Artery with Nonautologous Tissue Substitute, Percutaneous Endoscopic Approach
03RQ07Z Replacement of Left Vertebral Artery with Autologous Tissue Substitute, Open Approach
03RQ0JZ Replacement of Left Vertebral Artery with Synthetic Substitute, Open Approach
03RQ0KZ Replacement of Left Vertebral Artery with Nonautologous Tissue Substitute, Open Approach
03RQ47Z Replacement of Left Vertebral Artery with Autologous Tissue Substitute, Percutaneous Endoscopic Approach
03RQ4JZ Replacement of Left Vertebral Artery with Synthetic Substitute, Percutaneous Endoscopic Approach
03RQ4KZ Replacement of Left Vertebral Artery with Nonautologous Tissue Substitute, Percutaneous Endoscopic Approach
03RR07Z Replacement of Face Artery with Autologous Tissue Substitute, Open Approach
03RR0JZ Replacement of Face Artery with Synthetic Substitute, Open Approach
03RR0KZ Replacement of Face Artery with Nonautologous Tissue Substitute, Open Approach
03RR47Z Replacement of Face Artery with Autologous Tissue Substitute, Percutaneous Endoscopic Approach
03RR4JZ Replacement of Face Artery with Synthetic Substitute, Percutaneous Endoscopic Approach
03RR4KZ Replacement of Face Artery with Nonautologous Tissue Substitute, Percutaneous Endoscopic Approach
03RS07Z Replacement of Right Temporal Artery with Autologous Tissue Substitute, Open Approach
03RS0JZ Replacement of Right Temporal Artery with Synthetic Substitute, Open Approach
03RS0KZ Replacement of Right Temporal Artery with Nonautologous Tissue Substitute, Open Approach
03RS47Z Replacement of Right Temporal Artery with Autologous Tissue Substitute, Percutaneous Endoscopic Approach
03RS4JZ Replacement of Right Temporal Artery with Synthetic Substitute, Percutaneous Endoscopic Approach
03RS4KZ Replacement of Right Temporal Artery with Nonautologous Tissue Substitute, Percutaneous Endoscopic Approach
03RT07Z Replacement of Left Temporal Artery with Autologous Tissue Substitute, Open Approach
03RT0JZ Replacement of Left Temporal Artery with Synthetic Substitute, Open Approach
03RT0KZ Replacement of Left Temporal Artery with Nonautologous Tissue Substitute, Open Approach
03RT47Z Replacement of Left Temporal Artery with Autologous Tissue Substitute, Percutaneous Endoscopic Approach
03RT4JZ Replacement of Left Temporal Artery with Synthetic Substitute, Percutaneous Endoscopic Approach
03RT4KZ Replacement of Left Temporal Artery with Nonautologous Tissue Substitute, Percutaneous Endoscopic Approach
03RU07Z Replacement of Right Thyroid Artery with Autologous Tissue Substitute, Open Approach
03RU0JZ Replacement of Right Thyroid Artery with Synthetic Substitute, Open Approach
03RU0KZ Replacement of Right Thyroid Artery with Nonautologous Tissue Substitute, Open Approach
03RU47Z Replacement of Right Thyroid Artery with Autologous Tissue Substitute, Percutaneous Endoscopic Approach
03RU4JZ Replacement of Right Thyroid Artery with Synthetic Substitute, Percutaneous Endoscopic Approach
03RU4KZ Replacement of Right Thyroid Artery with Nonautologous Tissue Substitute, Percutaneous Endoscopic Approach
03RV07Z Replacement of Left Thyroid Artery with Autologous Tissue Substitute, Open Approach
03RV0JZ Replacement of Left Thyroid Artery with Synthetic Substitute, Open Approach
03RV0KZ Replacement of Left Thyroid Artery with Nonautologous Tissue Substitute, Open Approach
03RV47Z Replacement of Left Thyroid Artery with Autologous Tissue Substitute, Percutaneous Endoscopic Approach
03RV4JZ Replacement of Left Thyroid Artery with Synthetic Substitute, Percutaneous Endoscopic Approach
03RV4KZ Replacement of Left Thyroid Artery with Nonautologous Tissue Substitute, Percutaneous Endoscopic Approach
03RY07Z Replacement of Upper Artery with Autologous Tissue Substitute, Open Approach
03RY0JZ Replacement of Upper Artery with Synthetic Substitute, Open Approach
03RY0KZ Replacement of Upper Artery with Nonautologous Tissue Substitute, Open Approach

3RY47Z Replacement of Upper Artery with Autologous Tissue Substitute, Percutaneous Endoscopic Approach

03RY4JZ Replacement of Upper Artery with Synthetic Substitute, Percutaneous Endoscopic Approach

03RY4KZ Replacement of Upper Artery with Nonautologous Tissue Substitute, Percutaneous Endoscopic Approach

3S – Upper Arteries, Reposition

3S00ZZ Reposition Right Internal Mammary Artery, Open Approach

3S03ZZ Reposition Right Internal Mammary Artery, Percutaneous Approach

3S04ZZ Reposition Right Internal Mammary Artery, Percutaneous Endoscopic Approach

3S10ZZ Reposition Left Internal Mammary Artery, Open Approach

3S13ZZ Reposition Left Internal Mammary Artery, Percutaneous Approach

3S14ZZ Reposition Left Internal Mammary Artery, Percutaneous Endoscopic Approach

3S20ZZ Reposition Innominate Artery, Open Approach

3S23ZZ Reposition Innominate Artery, Percutaneous Approach

3S24ZZ Reposition Innominate Artery, Percutaneous Endoscopic Approach

3S30ZZ Reposition Right Subclavian Artery, Open Approach

3S33ZZ Reposition Right Subclavian Artery, Percutaneous Approach

3S34ZZ Reposition Right Subclavian Artery, Percutaneous Endoscopic Approach

3S40ZZ Reposition Left Subclavian Artery, Open Approach

3S43ZZ Reposition Left Subclavian Artery, Percutaneous Approach

3S44ZZ Reposition Left Subclavian Artery, Percutaneous Endoscopic Approach

3S50ZZ Reposition Right Axillary Artery, Open Approach

3S53ZZ Reposition Right Axillary Artery, Percutaneous Approach

3S54ZZ Reposition Right Axillary Artery, Percutaneous Endoscopic Approach

3S60ZZ Reposition Left Axillary Artery, Open Approach

3S63ZZ Reposition Left Axillary Artery, Percutaneous Approach

3S64ZZ Reposition Left Axillary Artery, Percutaneous Endoscopic Approach

3S70ZZ Reposition Right Brachial Artery, Open Approach

3S73ZZ Reposition Right Brachial Artery, Percutaneous Approach

3S74ZZ Reposition Right Brachial Artery, Percutaneous Endoscopic Approach

3S80ZZ Reposition Left Brachial Artery, Open Approach

3S83ZZ Reposition Left Brachial Artery, Percutaneous Approach

3S84ZZ Reposition Left Brachial Artery, Percutaneous Endoscopic Approach

3S90ZZ Reposition Right Ulnar Artery, Open Approach

3S93ZZ Reposition Right Ulnar Artery, Percutaneous Approach

03S94ZZ Reposition Right Ulnar Artery, Percutaneous Endoscopic Approach

03SA0ZZ Reposition Left Ulnar Artery, Open Approach

03SA3ZZ Reposition Left Ulnar Artery, Percutaneous Approach

03SA4ZZ Reposition Left Ulnar Artery, Percutaneous Endoscopic Approach

03SB0ZZ Reposition Right Radial Artery, Open Approach

03SB3ZZ Reposition Right Radial Artery, Percutaneous Approach

03SB4ZZ Reposition Right Radial Artery, Percutaneous Endoscopic Approach

03SC0ZZ Reposition Left Radial Artery, Open Approach

03SC3ZZ Reposition Left Radial Artery, Percutaneous Approach

03SC4ZZ Reposition Left Radial Artery, Percutaneous Endoscopic Approach

03SD0ZZ Reposition Right Hand Artery, Open Approach

03SD3ZZ Reposition Right Hand Artery, Percutaneous Approach

03SD4ZZ Reposition Right Hand Artery, Percutaneous Endoscopic Approach

03SF0ZZ Reposition Left Hand Artery, Open Approach

03SF3ZZ Reposition Left Hand Artery, Percutaneous Approach

03SF4ZZ Reposition Left Hand Artery, Percutaneous Endoscopic Approach

03SG0ZZ Reposition Intracranial Artery, Open Approach

03SG3ZZ Reposition Intracranial Artery, Percutaneous Approach

03SG4ZZ Reposition Intracranial Artery, Percutaneous Endoscopic Approach

03SH0ZZ Reposition Right Common Carotid Artery, Open Approach

03SH3ZZ Reposition Right Common Carotid Artery, Percutaneous Approach

03SH4ZZ Reposition Right Common Carotid Artery, Percutaneous Endoscopic Approach

03SJ0ZZ Reposition Left Common Carotid Artery, Open Approach

03SJ3ZZ Reposition Left Common Carotid Artery, Percutaneous Approach

03SJ4ZZ Reposition Left Common Carotid Artery, Percutaneous Endoscopic Approach

03SK0ZZ Reposition Right Internal Carotid Artery, Open Approach

03SK3ZZ Reposition Right Internal Carotid Artery, Percutaneous Approach

03SK4ZZ Reposition Right Internal Carotid Artery, Percutaneous Endoscopic Approach

03SL0ZZ Reposition Left Internal Carotid Artery, Open Approach

03SL3ZZ Reposition Left Internal Carotid Artery, Percutaneous Approach

03SL4ZZ Reposition Left Internal Carotid Artery, Percutaneous Endoscopic Approach

03SM0ZZ Reposition Right External Carotid Artery, Open Approach

03SM3ZZ Reposition Right External Carotid Artery, Percutaneous Approach

03SM4ZZ Reposition Right External Carotid Artery, Percutaneous Endoscopic Approach

03SN0ZZ Reposition Left External Carotid Artery, Open Approach

03SN3ZZ Reposition Left External Carotid Artery, Percutaneous Approach

03SN4ZZ Reposition Left External Carotid Artery, Percutaneous Endoscopic Approach

03SP0ZZ Reposition Right Vertebral Artery, Open Approach

03SP3ZZ Reposition Right Vertebral Artery, Percutaneous Approach

03SP4ZZ Reposition Right Vertebral Artery, Percutaneous Endoscopic Approach

03SQ0ZZ Reposition Left Vertebral Artery, Open Approach

03SQ3ZZ Reposition Left Vertebral Artery, Percutaneous Approach

03SQ4ZZ Reposition Left Vertebral Artery, Percutaneous Endoscopic Approach

03SR0ZZ Reposition Face Artery, Open Approach

03SR3ZZ Reposition Face Artery, Percutaneous Approach

03SR4ZZ Reposition Face Artery, Percutaneous Endoscopic Approach

03SS0ZZ Reposition Right Temporal Artery, Open Approach

03SS3ZZ Reposition Right Temporal Artery, Percutaneous Approach

03SS4ZZ Reposition Right Temporal Artery, Percutaneous Endoscopic Approach

03ST0ZZ Reposition Left Temporal Artery, Open Approach

03ST3ZZ Reposition Left Temporal Artery, Percutaneous Approach

03ST4ZZ Reposition Left Temporal Artery, Percutaneous Endoscopic Approach

03SU0ZZ Reposition Right Thyroid Artery, Open Approach

03SU3ZZ Reposition Right Thyroid Artery, Percutaneous Approach

03SU4ZZ Reposition Right Thyroid Artery, Percutaneous Endoscopic Approach

03SV0ZZ Reposition Left Thyroid Artery, Open Approach

03SV3ZZ Reposition Left Thyroid Artery, Percutaneous Approach

03SV4ZZ Reposition Left Thyroid Artery, Percutaneous Endoscopic Approach

03SY0ZZ Reposition Upper Artery, Open Approach

03SY3ZZ Reposition Upper Artery, Percutaneous Approach

03SY4ZZ Reposition Upper Artery, Percutaneous Endoscopic Approach

03U – Upper Arteries, Supplement

3U007Z Supplement Right Internal Mammary Artery with Autologous Tissue Substitute, Open Approach

3U00JZ Supplement Right Internal Mammary Artery with Synthetic Substitute, Open Approach

3U00KZ Supplement Right Internal Mammary Artery with Nonautologous Tissue Substitute, Open Approach

03U037Z Supplement Right Internal Mammary Artery with Autologous Tissue Substitute, Percutaneous Approach

03U03JZ Supplement Right Internal Mammary Artery with Synthetic Substitute, Percutaneous Approach

03U03KZ Supplement Right Internal Mammary Artery with Nonautologous Tissue Substitute, Percutaneous Approach

03U047Z Supplement Right Internal Mammary Artery with Autologous Tissue Substitute, Percutaneous Endoscopic Approach

03U04JZ Supplement Right Internal Mammary Artery with Synthetic Substitute, Percutaneous Endoscopic Approach

03U04KZ Supplement Right Internal Mammary Artery with Nonautologous Tissue Substitute, Percutaneous Endoscopic Approach
03U107Z Supplement Left Internal Mammary Artery with Autologous Tissue Substitute, Open Approach
03U10JZ Supplement Left Internal Mammary Artery with Synthetic Substitute, Open Approach
03U10KZ Supplement Left Internal Mammary Artery with Nonautologous Tissue Substitute, Open Approach
03U137Z Supplement Left Internal Mammary Artery with Autologous Tissue Substitute, Percutaneous Approach
03U13JZ Supplement Left Internal Mammary Artery with Synthetic Substitute, Percutaneous Approach
03U13KZ Supplement Left Internal Mammary Artery with Nonautologous Tissue Substitute, Percutaneous Approach
03U147Z Supplement Left Internal Mammary Artery with Autologous Tissue Substitute, Percutaneous Endoscopic Approach
03U14JZ Supplement Left Internal Mammary Artery with Synthetic Substitute, Percutaneous Endoscopic Approach
03U14KZ Supplement Left Internal Mammary Artery with Nonautologous Tissue Substitute, Percutaneous Endoscopic Approach
03U207Z Supplement Innominate Artery with Autologous Tissue Substitute, Open Approach
03U20JZ Supplement Innominate Artery with Synthetic Substitute, Open Approach
03U20KZ Supplement Innominate Artery with Nonautologous Tissue Substitute, Open Approach
03U237Z Supplement Innominate Artery with Autologous Tissue Substitute, Percutaneous Approach
03U23JZ Supplement Innominate Artery with Synthetic Substitute, Percutaneous Approach
03U23KZ Supplement Innominate Artery with Nonautologous Tissue Substitute, Percutaneous Approach
03U247Z Supplement Innominate Artery with Autologous Tissue Substitute, Percutaneous Endoscopic Approach
03U24JZ Supplement Innominate Artery with Synthetic Substitute, Percutaneous Endoscopic Approach
03U24KZ Supplement Innominate Artery with Nonautologous Tissue Substitute, Percutaneous Endoscopic Approach
03U307Z Supplement Right Subclavian Artery with Autologous Tissue Substitute, Open Approach
03U30JZ Supplement Right Subclavian Artery with Synthetic Substitute, Open Approach
03U30KZ Supplement Right Subclavian Artery with Nonautologous Tissue Substitute, Open Approach
03U337Z Supplement Right Subclavian Artery with Autologous Tissue Substitute, Percutaneous Approach
03U33JZ Supplement Right Subclavian Artery with Synthetic Substitute, Percutaneous Approach
03U33KZ Supplement Right Subclavian Artery with Nonautologous Tissue Substitute, Percutaneous Approach
03U347Z Supplement Right Subclavian Artery with Autologous Tissue Substitute, Percutaneous Endoscopic Approach
03U34JZ Supplement Right Subclavian Artery with Synthetic Substitute, Percutaneous Endoscopic Approach
03U34KZ Supplement Right Subclavian Artery with Nonautologous Tissue Substitute, Percutaneous Endoscopic Approach
03U407Z Supplement Left Subclavian Artery with Autologous Tissue Substitute, Open Approach
03U40JZ Supplement Left Subclavian Artery with Synthetic Substitute, Open Approach
03U40KZ Supplement Left Subclavian Artery with Nonautologous Tissue Substitute, Open Approach
03U437Z Supplement Left Subclavian Artery with Autologous Tissue Substitute, Percutaneous Approach
03U43JZ Supplement Left Subclavian Artery with Synthetic Substitute, Percutaneous Approach
03U43KZ Supplement Left Subclavian Artery with Nonautologous Tissue Substitute, Percutaneous Approach
03U447Z Supplement Left Subclavian Artery with Autologous Tissue Substitute, Percutaneous Endoscopic Approach
03U44JZ Supplement Left Subclavian Artery with Synthetic Substitute, Percutaneous Endoscopic Approach
03U44KZ Supplement Left Subclavian Artery with Nonautologous Tissue Substitute, Percutaneous Endoscopic Approach
03U507Z Supplement Right Axillary Artery with Autologous Tissue Substitute, Open Approach
03U50JZ Supplement Right Axillary Artery with Synthetic Substitute, Open Approach
03U50KZ Supplement Right Axillary Artery with Nonautologous Tissue Substitute, Open Approach
03U537Z Supplement Right Axillary Artery with Autologous Tissue Substitute, Percutaneous Approach
03U53JZ Supplement Right Axillary Artery with Synthetic Substitute, Percutaneous Approach
03U53KZ Supplement Right Axillary Artery with Nonautologous Tissue Substitute, Percutaneous Approach
03U547Z Supplement Right Axillary Artery with Autologous Tissue Substitute, Percutaneous Endoscopic Approach
03U54JZ Supplement Right Axillary Artery with Synthetic Substitute, Percutaneous Endoscopic Approach
03U54KZ Supplement Right Axillary Artery with Nonautologous Tissue Substitute, Percutaneous Endoscopic Approach
03U607Z Supplement Left Axillary Artery with Autologous Tissue Substitute, Open Approach
03U60JZ Supplement Left Axillary Artery with Synthetic Substitute, Open Approach
03U60KZ Supplement Left Axillary Artery with Nonautologous Tissue Substitute, Open Approach
03U637Z Supplement Left Axillary Artery with Autologous Tissue Substitute, Percutaneous Approach
03U63JZ Supplement Left Axillary Artery with Synthetic Substitute, Percutaneous Approach
03U63KZ Supplement Left Axillary Artery with Nonautologous Tissue Substitute, Percutaneous Approach
03U647Z Supplement Left Axillary Artery with Autologous Tissue Substitute, Percutaneous Endoscopic Approach
03U64JZ Supplement Left Axillary Artery with Synthetic Substitute, Percutaneous Endoscopic Approach
03U64KZ Supplement Left Axillary Artery with Nonautologous Tissue Substitute, Percutaneous Endoscopic Approach
03U707Z Supplement Right Brachial Artery with Autologous Tissue Substitute, Open Approach
03U70JZ Supplement Right Brachial Artery with Synthetic Substitute, Open Approach
03U70KZ Supplement Right Brachial Artery with Nonautologous Tissue Substitute, Open Approach
03U737Z Supplement Right Brachial Artery with Autologous Tissue Substitute, Percutaneous Approach
03U73JZ Supplement Right Brachial Artery with Synthetic Substitute, Percutaneous Approach
03U73KZ Supplement Right Brachial Artery with Nonautologous Tissue Substitute, Percutaneous Approach
03U747Z Supplement Right Brachial Artery with Autologous Tissue Substitute, Percutaneous Endoscopic Approach
03U74JZ Supplement Right Brachial Artery with Synthetic Substitute, Percutaneous Endoscopic Approach
03U74KZ Supplement Right Brachial Artery with Nonautologous Tissue Substitute, Percutaneous Endoscopic Approach
03U807Z Supplement Left Brachial Artery with Autologous Tissue Substitute, Open Approach
03U80JZ Supplement Left Brachial Artery with Synthetic Substitute, Open Approach
03U80KZ Supplement Left Brachial Artery with Nonautologous Tissue Substitute, Open Approach
03U837Z Supplement Left Brachial Artery with Autologous Tissue Substitute, Percutaneous Approach
03U83JZ Supplement Left Brachial Artery with Synthetic Substitute, Percutaneous Approach
03U83KZ Supplement Left Brachial Artery with Nonautologous Tissue Substitute, Percutaneous Approach
03U847Z Supplement Left Brachial Artery with Autologous Tissue Substitute, Percutaneous Endoscopic Approach
03U84JZ Supplement Left Brachial Artery with Synthetic Substitute, Percutaneous Endoscopic Approach
03U84KZ Supplement Left Brachial Artery with Nonautologous Tissue Substitute, Percutaneous Endoscopic Approach
03U907Z Supplement Right Ulnar Artery with Autologous Tissue Substitute, Open Approach
03U90JZ Supplement Right Ulnar Artery with Synthetic Substitute, Open Approach
03U90KZ Supplement Right Ulnar Artery with Nonautologous Tissue Substitute, Open Approach
03U937Z Supplement Right Ulnar Artery with Autologous Tissue Substitute, Percutaneous Approach
03U93JZ Supplement Right Ulnar Artery with Synthetic Substitute, Percutaneous Approach
03U93KZ Supplement Right Ulnar Artery with Nonautologous Tissue Substitute, Percutaneous Approach
03U947Z Supplement Right Ulnar Artery with Autologous Tissue Substitute, Percutaneous Endoscopic Approach

03U94JZ Supplement Right Ulnar Artery with Synthetic Substitute, Percutaneous Endoscopic Approach

03U94KZ Supplement Right Ulnar Artery with Nonautologous Tissue Substitute, Percutaneous Endoscopic Approach

03UA07Z Supplement Left Ulnar Artery with Autologous Tissue Substitute, Open Approach

03UA0JZ Supplement Left Ulnar Artery with Synthetic Substitute, Open Approach

03UA0KZ Supplement Left Ulnar Artery with Nonautologous Tissue Substitute, Open Approach

03UA37Z Supplement Left Ulnar Artery with Autologous Tissue Substitute, Percutaneous Approach

03UA3JZ Supplement Left Ulnar Artery with Synthetic Substitute, Percutaneous Approach

03UA3KZ Supplement Left Ulnar Artery with Nonautologous Tissue Substitute, Percutaneous Approach

03UA47Z Supplement Left Ulnar Artery with Autologous Tissue Substitute, Percutaneous Endoscopic Approach

03UA4JZ Supplement Left Ulnar Artery with Synthetic Substitute, Percutaneous Endoscopic Approach

03UA4KZ Supplement Left Ulnar Artery with Nonautologous Tissue Substitute, Percutaneous Endoscopic Approach

03UB07Z Supplement Right Radial Artery with Autologous Tissue Substitute, Open Approach

03UB0JZ Supplement Right Radial Artery with Synthetic Substitute, Open Approach

03UB0KZ Supplement Right Radial Artery with Nonautologous Tissue Substitute, Open Approach

03UB37Z Supplement Right Radial Artery with Autologous Tissue Substitute, Percutaneous Approach

03UB3JZ Supplement Right Radial Artery with Synthetic Substitute, Percutaneous Approach

03UB3KZ Supplement Right Radial Artery with Nonautologous Tissue Substitute, Percutaneous Approach

03UB47Z Supplement Right Radial Artery with Autologous Tissue Substitute, Percutaneous Endoscopic Approach

03UB4JZ Supplement Right Radial Artery with Synthetic Substitute, Percutaneous Endoscopic Approach

03UB4KZ Supplement Right Radial Artery with Nonautologous Tissue Substitute, Percutaneous Endoscopic Approach

03UC07Z Supplement Left Radial Artery with Autologous Tissue Substitute, Open Approach

03UC0JZ Supplement Left Radial Artery with Synthetic Substitute, Open Approach

03UC0KZ Supplement Left Radial Artery with Nonautologous Tissue Substitute, Open Approach

03UC37Z Supplement Left Radial Artery with Autologous Tissue Substitute, Percutaneous Approach

03UC3JZ Supplement Left Radial Artery with Synthetic Substitute, Percutaneous Approach

03UC3KZ Supplement Left Radial Artery with Nonautologous Tissue Substitute, Percutaneous Approach

03UC47Z Supplement Left Radial Artery with Autologous Tissue Substitute, Percutaneous Endoscopic Approach

03UC4JZ Supplement Left Radial Artery with Synthetic Substitute, Percutaneous Endoscopic Approach

03UC4KZ Supplement Left Radial Artery with Nonautologous Tissue Substitute, Percutaneous Endoscopic Approach

03UD07Z Supplement Right Hand Artery with Autologous Tissue Substitute, Open Approach

03UD0JZ Supplement Right Hand Artery with Synthetic Substitute, Open Approach

03UD0KZ Supplement Right Hand Artery with Nonautologous Tissue Substitute, Open Approach

03UD37Z Supplement Right Hand Artery with Autologous Tissue Substitute, Percutaneous Approach

03UD3JZ Supplement Right Hand Artery with Synthetic Substitute, Percutaneous Approach

03UD3KZ Supplement Right Hand Artery with Nonautologous Tissue Substitute, Percutaneous Approach

03UD47Z Supplement Right Hand Artery with Autologous Tissue Substitute, Percutaneous Endoscopic Approach

03UD4JZ Supplement Right Hand Artery with Synthetic Substitute, Percutaneous Endoscopic Approach

03UD4KZ Supplement Right Hand Artery with Nonautologous Tissue Substitute, Percutaneous Endoscopic Approach

03UF07Z Supplement Left Hand Artery with Autologous Tissue Substitute, Open Approach

03UF0JZ Supplement Left Hand Artery with Synthetic Substitute, Open Approach

03UF0KZ Supplement Left Hand Artery with Nonautologous Tissue Substitute, Open Approach

03UF37Z Supplement Left Hand Artery with Autologous Tissue Substitute, Percutaneous Approach

03UF3JZ Supplement Left Hand Artery with Synthetic Substitute, Percutaneous Approach

03UF3KZ Supplement Left Hand Artery with Nonautologous Tissue Substitute, Percutaneous Approach

03UF47Z Supplement Left Hand Artery with Autologous Tissue Substitute, Percutaneous Endoscopic Approach

03UF4JZ Supplement Left Hand Artery with Synthetic Substitute, Percutaneous Endoscopic Approach

03UF4KZ Supplement Left Hand Artery with Nonautologous Tissue Substitute, Percutaneous Endoscopic Approach

03UG07Z Supplement Intracranial Artery with Autologous Tissue Substitute, Open Approach

03UG0JZ Supplement Intracranial Artery with Synthetic Substitute, Open Approach

03UG0KZ Supplement Intracranial Artery with Nonautologous Tissue Substitute, Open Approach

03UG37Z Supplement Intracranial Artery with Autologous Tissue Substitute, Percutaneous Approach

03UG3JZ Supplement Intracranial Artery with Synthetic Substitute, Percutaneous Approach

03UG3KZ Supplement Intracranial Artery with Nonautologous Tissue Substitute, Percutaneous Approach

03UG47Z Supplement Intracranial Artery with Autologous Tissue Substitute, Percutaneous Endoscopic Approach

03UG4JZ Supplement Intracranial Artery with Synthetic Substitute, Percutaneous Endoscopic Approach

03UG4KZ Supplement Intracranial Artery with Nonautologous Tissue Substitute, Percutaneous Endoscopic Approach

03UH07Z Supplement Right Common Carotid Artery with Autologous Tissue Substitute, Open Approach

03UH0JZ Supplement Right Common Carotid Artery with Synthetic Substitute, Open Approach

03UH0KZ Supplement Right Common Carotid Artery with Nonautologous Tissue Substitute, Open Approach

03UH37Z Supplement Right Common Carotid Artery with Autologous Tissue Substitute, Percutaneous Approach

03UH3JZ Supplement Right Common Carotid Artery with Synthetic Substitute, Percutaneous Approach

03UH3KZ Supplement Right Common Carotid Artery with Nonautologous Tissue Substitute, Percutaneous Approach

03UH47Z Supplement Right Common Carotid Artery with Autologous Tissue Substitute, Percutaneous Endoscopic Approach

03UH4JZ Supplement Right Common Carotid Artery with Synthetic Substitute, Percutaneous Endoscopic Approach

03UH4KZ Supplement Right Common Carotid Artery with Nonautologous Tissue Substitute, Percutaneous Endoscopic Approach

03UJ07Z Supplement Left Common Carotid Artery with Autologous Tissue Substitute, Open Approach

03UJ0JZ Supplement Left Common Carotid Artery with Synthetic Substitute, Open Approach

03UJ0KZ Supplement Left Common Carotid Artery with Nonautologous Tissue Substitute, Open Approach

03UJ37Z Supplement Left Common Carotid Artery with Autologous Tissue Substitute, Percutaneous Approach

03UJ3JZ Supplement Left Common Carotid Artery with Synthetic Substitute, Percutaneous Approach

03UJ3KZ Supplement Left Common Carotid Artery with Nonautologous Tissue Substitute, Percutaneous Approach

03UJ47Z Supplement Left Common Carotid Artery with Autologous Tissue Substitute, Percutaneous Endoscopic Approach

03UJ4JZ Supplement Left Common Carotid Artery with Synthetic Substitute, Percutaneous Endoscopic Approach

03UJ4KZ Supplement Left Common Carotid Artery with Nonautologous Tissue Substitute, Percutaneous Endoscopic Approach

03UK07Z Supplement Right Internal Carotid Artery with Autologous Tissue Substitute, Open Approach

03UK0JZ Supplement Right Internal Carotid Artery with Synthetic Substitute, Open Approach

03UK0KZ Supplement Right Internal Carotid Artery with Nonautologous Tissue Substitute, Open Approach

03UK37Z Supplement Right Internal Carotid Artery with Autologous Tissue Substitute, Percutaneous Approach

03UK3JZ Supplement Right Internal Carotid Artery with Synthetic Substitute, Percutaneous Approach

03UK3KZ Supplement Right Internal Carotid Artery with Nonautologous Tissue Substitute, Percutaneous Approach

03UK47Z Supplement Right Internal Carotid Artery with Autologous Tissue Substitute, Percutaneous Endoscopic Approach
03UK4JZ Supplement Right Internal Carotid Artery with Synthetic Substitute, Percutaneous Endoscopic Approach
03UK4KZ Supplement Right Internal Carotid Artery with Nonautologous Tissue Substitute, Percutaneous Endoscopic Approach
03UL07Z Supplement Left Internal Carotid Artery with Autologous Tissue Substitute, Open Approach
03UL0JZ Supplement Left Internal Carotid Artery with Synthetic Substitute, Open Approach
03UL0KZ Supplement Left Internal Carotid Artery with Nonautologous Tissue Substitute, Open Approach
03UL37Z Supplement Left Internal Carotid Artery with Autologous Tissue Substitute, Percutaneous Approach
03UL3JZ Supplement Left Internal Carotid Artery with Synthetic Substitute, Percutaneous Approach
03UL3KZ Supplement Left Internal Carotid Artery with Nonautologous Tissue Substitute, Percutaneous Approach
03UL47Z Supplement Left Internal Carotid Artery with Autologous Tissue Substitute, Percutaneous Endoscopic Approach
03UL4JZ Supplement Left Internal Carotid Artery with Synthetic Substitute, Percutaneous Endoscopic Approach
03UL4KZ Supplement Left Internal Carotid Artery with Nonautologous Tissue Substitute, Percutaneous Endoscopic Approach
03UM07Z Supplement Right External Carotid Artery with Autologous Tissue Substitute, Open Approach
03UM0JZ Supplement Right External Carotid Artery with Synthetic Substitute, Open Approach
03UM0KZ Supplement Right External Carotid Artery with Nonautologous Tissue Substitute, Open Approach
03UM37Z Supplement Right External Carotid Artery with Autologous Tissue Substitute, Percutaneous Approach
03UM3JZ Supplement Right External Carotid Artery with Synthetic Substitute, Percutaneous Approach
03UM3KZ Supplement Right External Carotid Artery with Nonautologous Tissue Substitute, Percutaneous Approach
03UM47Z Supplement Right External Carotid Artery with Autologous Tissue Substitute, Percutaneous Endoscopic Approach
03UM4JZ Supplement Right External Carotid Artery with Synthetic Substitute, Percutaneous Endoscopic Approach
03UM4KZ Supplement Right External Carotid Artery with Nonautologous Tissue Substitute, Percutaneous Endoscopic Approach
03UN07Z Supplement Left External Carotid Artery with Autologous Tissue Substitute, Open Approach
03UN0JZ Supplement Left External Carotid Artery with Synthetic Substitute, Open Approach
03UN0KZ Supplement Left External Carotid Artery with Nonautologous Tissue Substitute, Open Approach
03UN37Z Supplement Left External Carotid Artery with Autologous Tissue Substitute, Percutaneous Approach
03UN3JZ Supplement Left External Carotid Artery with Synthetic Substitute, Percutaneous Approach
03UN3KZ Supplement Left External Carotid Artery with Nonautologous Tissue Substitute, Percutaneous Approach
03UN47Z Supplement Left External Carotid Artery with Autologous Tissue Substitute, Percutaneous Endoscopic Approach
03UN4JZ Supplement Left External Carotid Artery with Synthetic Substitute, Percutaneous Endoscopic Approach
03UN4KZ Supplement Left External Carotid Artery with Nonautologous Tissue Substitute, Percutaneous Endoscopic Approach
03UP07Z Supplement Right Vertebral Artery with Autologous Tissue Substitute, Open Approach
03UP0JZ Supplement Right Vertebral Artery with Synthetic Substitute, Open Approach
03UP0KZ Supplement Right Vertebral Artery with Nonautologous Tissue Substitute, Open Approach
03UP37Z Supplement Right Vertebral Artery with Autologous Tissue Substitute, Percutaneous Approach
03UP3JZ Supplement Right Vertebral Artery with Synthetic Substitute, Percutaneous Approach
03UP3KZ Supplement Right Vertebral Artery with Nonautologous Tissue Substitute, Percutaneous Approach
03UP47Z Supplement Right Vertebral Artery with Autologous Tissue Substitute, Percutaneous Endoscopic Approach
03UP4JZ Supplement Right Vertebral Artery with Synthetic Substitute, Percutaneous Endoscopic Approach
03UP4KZ Supplement Right Vertebral Artery with Nonautologous Tissue Substitute, Percutaneous Endoscopic Approach
03UQ07Z Supplement Left Vertebral Artery with Autologous Tissue Substitute, Open Approach
03UQ0JZ Supplement Left Vertebral Artery with Synthetic Substitute, Open Approach
03UQ0KZ Supplement Left Vertebral Artery with Nonautologous Tissue Substitute, Open Approach
03UQ37Z Supplement Left Vertebral Artery with Autologous Tissue Substitute, Percutaneous Approach
03UQ3JZ Supplement Left Vertebral Artery with Synthetic Substitute, Percutaneous Approach
03UQ3KZ Supplement Left Vertebral Artery with Nonautologous Tissue Substitute, Percutaneous Approach
03UQ47Z Supplement Left Vertebral Artery with Autologous Tissue Substitute, Percutaneous Endoscopic Approach
03UQ4JZ Supplement Left Vertebral Artery with Synthetic Substitute, Percutaneous Endoscopic Approach
03UQ4KZ Supplement Left Vertebral Artery with Nonautologous Tissue Substitute, Percutaneous Endoscopic Approach
03UR07Z Supplement Face Artery with Autologous Tissue Substitute, Open Approach
03UR0JZ Supplement Face Artery with Synthetic Substitute, Open Approach
03UR0KZ Supplement Face Artery with Nonautologous Tissue Substitute, Open Approach
03UR37Z Supplement Face Artery with Autologous Tissue Substitute, Percutaneous Approach
03UR3JZ Supplement Face Artery with Synthetic Substitute, Percutaneous Approach
03UR3KZ Supplement Face Artery with Nonautologous Tissue Substitute, Percutaneous Approach
03UR47Z Supplement Face Artery with Autologous Tissue Substitute, Percutaneous Endoscopic Approach
03UR4JZ Supplement Face Artery with Synthetic Substitute, Percutaneous Endoscopic Approach
03UR4KZ Supplement Face Artery with Nonautologous Tissue Substitute, Percutaneous Endoscopic Approach
03US07Z Supplement Right Temporal Artery with Autologous Tissue Substitute, Open Approach
03US0JZ Supplement Right Temporal Artery with Synthetic Substitute, Open Approach
03US0KZ Supplement Right Temporal Artery with Nonautologous Tissue Substitute, Open Approach
03US37Z Supplement Right Temporal Artery with Autologous Tissue Substitute, Percutaneous Approach
03US3JZ Supplement Right Temporal Artery with Synthetic Substitute, Percutaneous Approach
03US3KZ Supplement Right Temporal Artery with Nonautologous Tissue Substitute, Percutaneous Approach
03US47Z Supplement Right Temporal Artery with Autologous Tissue Substitute, Percutaneous Endoscopic Approach
03US4JZ Supplement Right Temporal Artery with Synthetic Substitute, Percutaneous Endoscopic Approach
03US4KZ Supplement Right Temporal Artery with Nonautologous Tissue Substitute, Percutaneous Endoscopic Approach
03UT07Z Supplement Left Temporal Artery with Autologous Tissue Substitute, Open Approach
03UT0JZ Supplement Left Temporal Artery with Synthetic Substitute, Open Approach
03UT0KZ Supplement Left Temporal Artery with Nonautologous Tissue Substitute, Open Approach
03UT37Z Supplement Left Temporal Artery with Autologous Tissue Substitute, Percutaneous Approach
03UT3JZ Supplement Left Temporal Artery with Synthetic Substitute, Percutaneous Approach
03UT3KZ Supplement Left Temporal Artery with Nonautologous Tissue Substitute, Percutaneous Approach
03UT47Z Supplement Left Temporal Artery with Autologous Tissue Substitute, Percutaneous Endoscopic Approach
03UT4JZ Supplement Left Temporal Artery with Synthetic Substitute, Percutaneous Endoscopic Approach
03UT4KZ Supplement Left Temporal Artery with Nonautologous Tissue Substitute, Percutaneous Endoscopic Approach
03UU07Z Supplement Right Thyroid Artery with Autologous Tissue Substitute, Open Approach
03UU0JZ Supplement Right Thyroid Artery with Synthetic Substitute, Open Approach
03UU0KZ Supplement Right Thyroid Artery with Nonautologous Tissue Substitute, Open Approach
03UU37Z Supplement Right Thyroid Artery with Autologous Tissue Substitute, Percutaneous Approach
03UU3JZ Supplement Right Thyroid Artery with Synthetic Substitute, Percutaneous Approach
03UU3KZ Supplement Right Thyroid Artery with Nonautologous Tissue Substitute, Percutaneous Approach
03UU47Z Supplement Right Thyroid Artery with Autologous Tissue Substitute, Percutaneous Endoscopic Approach

03UU4JZ Supplement Right Thyroid Artery with Synthetic Substitute, Percutaneous Endoscopic Approach
03UU4KZ Supplement Right Thyroid Artery with Nonautologous Tissue Substitute, Percutaneous Endoscopic Approach
03UV07Z Supplement Left Thyroid Artery with Autologous Tissue Substitute, Open Approach
03UV0JZ Supplement Left Thyroid Artery with Synthetic Substitute, Open Approach
03UV0KZ Supplement Left Thyroid Artery with Nonautologous Tissue Substitute, Open Approach
03UV37Z Supplement Left Thyroid Artery with Autologous Tissue Substitute, Percutaneous Approach
03UV3JZ Supplement Left Thyroid Artery with Synthetic Substitute, Percutaneous Approach
03UV3KZ Supplement Left Thyroid Artery with Nonautologous Tissue Substitute, Percutaneous Approach
03UV47Z Supplement Left Thyroid Artery with Autologous Tissue Substitute, Percutaneous Endoscopic Approach
03UV4JZ Supplement Left Thyroid Artery with Synthetic Substitute, Percutaneous Endoscopic Approach
03UV4KZ Supplement Left Thyroid Artery with Nonautologous Tissue Substitute, Percutaneous Endoscopic Approach
03UY07Z Supplement Upper Artery with Autologous Tissue Substitute, Open Approach
03UY0JZ Supplement Upper Artery with Synthetic Substitute, Open Approach
03UY0KZ Supplement Upper Artery with Nonautologous Tissue Substitute, Open Approach
03UY37Z Supplement Upper Artery with Autologous Tissue Substitute, Percutaneous Approach
03UY3JZ Supplement Upper Artery with Synthetic Substitute, Percutaneous Approach
03UY3KZ Supplement Upper Artery with Nonautologous Tissue Substitute, Percutaneous Approach
03UY47Z Supplement Upper Artery with Autologous Tissue Substitute, Percutaneous Endoscopic Approach
03UY4JZ Supplement Upper Artery with Synthetic Substitute, Percutaneous Endoscopic Approach
03UY4KZ Supplement Upper Artery with Nonautologous Tissue Substitute, Percutaneous Endoscopic Approach

03V – Upper Arteries, Restriction

Review Coding Guideline B3.12

03V00CZ Restriction of Right Internal Mammary Artery with Extraluminal Device, Open Approach
03V00DZ Restriction of Right Internal Mammary Artery with Intraluminal Device, Open Approach
03V00ZZ Restriction of Right Internal Mammary Artery, Open Approach
03V03CZ Restriction of Right Internal Mammary Artery with Extraluminal Device, Percutaneous Approach
03V03DZ Restriction of Right Internal Mammary Artery with Intraluminal Device, Percutaneous Approach
03V03ZZ Restriction of Right Internal Mammary Artery, Percutaneous Approach
03V04CZ Restriction of Right Internal Mammary Artery with Extraluminal Device, Percutaneous Endoscopic Approach
03V04DZ Restriction of Right Internal Mammary Artery with Intraluminal Device, Percutaneous Endoscopic Approach
03V04ZZ Restriction of Right Internal Mammary Artery, Percutaneous Endoscopic Approach
03V10CZ Restriction of Left Internal Mammary Artery with Extraluminal Device, Open Approach
03V10DZ Restriction of Left Internal Mammary Artery with Intraluminal Device, Open Approach
03V10ZZ Restriction of Left Internal Mammary Artery, Open Approach
03V13CZ Restriction of Left Internal Mammary Artery with Extraluminal Device, Percutaneous Approach
03V13DZ Restriction of Left Internal Mammary Artery with Intraluminal Device, Percutaneous Approach
03V13ZZ Restriction of Left Internal Mammary Artery, Percutaneous Approach
03V14CZ Restriction of Left Internal Mammary Artery with Extraluminal Device, Percutaneous Endoscopic Approach
03V14DZ Restriction of Left Internal Mammary Artery with Intraluminal Device, Percutaneous Endoscopic Approach
03V14ZZ Restriction of Left Internal Mammary Artery, Percutaneous Endoscopic Approach
03V20CZ Restriction of Innominate Artery with Extraluminal Device, Open Approach
03V20DZ Restriction of Innominate Artery with Intraluminal Device, Open Approach
03V20ZZ Restriction of Innominate Artery, Open Approach
03V23CZ Restriction of Innominate Artery with Extraluminal Device, Percutaneous Approach
03V23DZ Restriction of Innominate Artery with Intraluminal Device, Percutaneous Approach
03V23ZZ Restriction of Innominate Artery, Percutaneous Approach
03V24CZ Restriction of Innominate Artery with Extraluminal Device, Percutaneous Endoscopic Approach
03V24DZ Restriction of Innominate Artery with Intraluminal Device, Percutaneous Endoscopic Approach
03V24ZZ Restriction of Innominate Artery, Percutaneous Endoscopic Approach
03V30CZ Restriction of Right Subclavian Artery with Extraluminal Device, Open Approach
03V30DZ Restriction of Right Subclavian Artery with Intraluminal Device, Open Approach
03V30ZZ Restriction of Right Subclavian Artery, Open Approach
03V33CZ Restriction of Right Subclavian Artery with Extraluminal Device, Percutaneous Approach
03V33DZ Restriction of Right Subclavian Artery with Intraluminal Device, Percutaneous Approach
03V33ZZ Restriction of Right Subclavian Artery, Percutaneous Approach
03V34CZ Restriction of Right Subclavian Artery with Extraluminal Device, Percutaneous Endoscopic Approach
03V34DZ Restriction of Right Subclavian Artery with Intraluminal Device, Percutaneous Endoscopic Approach
03V34ZZ Restriction of Right Subclavian Artery, Percutaneous Endoscopic Approach
03V40CZ Restriction of Left Subclavian Artery with Extraluminal Device, Open Approach
03V40DZ Restriction of Left Subclavian Artery with Intraluminal Device, Open Approach
03V40ZZ Restriction of Left Subclavian Artery, Open Approach
03V43CZ Restriction of Left Subclavian Artery with Extraluminal Device, Percutaneous Approach
03V43DZ Restriction of Left Subclavian Artery with Intraluminal Device, Percutaneous Approach
03V43ZZ Restriction of Left Subclavian Artery, Percutaneous Approach
03V44CZ Restriction of Left Subclavian Artery with Extraluminal Device, Percutaneous Endoscopic Approach
03V44DZ Restriction of Left Subclavian Artery with Intraluminal Device, Percutaneous Endoscopic Approach
03V44ZZ Restriction of Left Subclavian Artery, Percutaneous Endoscopic Approach
03V50CZ Restriction of Right Axillary Artery with Extraluminal Device, Open Approach
03V50DZ Restriction of Right Axillary Artery with Intraluminal Device, Open Approach
03V50ZZ Restriction of Right Axillary Artery, Open Approach
03V53CZ Restriction of Right Axillary Artery with Extraluminal Device, Percutaneous Approach
03V53DZ Restriction of Right Axillary Artery with Intraluminal Device, Percutaneous Approach
03V53ZZ Restriction of Right Axillary Artery, Percutaneous Approach
03V54CZ Restriction of Right Axillary Artery with Extraluminal Device, Percutaneous Endoscopic Approach
03V54DZ Restriction of Right Axillary Artery with Intraluminal Device, Percutaneous Endoscopic Approach
03V54ZZ Restriction of Right Axillary Artery, Percutaneous Endoscopic Approach
03V60CZ Restriction of Left Axillary Artery with Extraluminal Device, Open Approach
03V60DZ Restriction of Left Axillary Artery with Intraluminal Device, Open Approach
03V60ZZ Restriction of Left Axillary Artery, Open Approach
03V63CZ Restriction of Left Axillary Artery with Extraluminal Device, Percutaneous Approach
03V63DZ Restriction of Left Axillary Artery with Intraluminal Device, Percutaneous Approach
03V63ZZ Restriction of Left Axillary Artery, Percutaneous Approach
03V64CZ Restriction of Left Axillary Artery with Extraluminal Device, Percutaneous Endoscopic Approach
03V64DZ Restriction of Left Axillary Artery with Intraluminal Device, Percutaneous Endoscopic Approach
03V64ZZ Restriction of Left Axillary Artery, Percutaneous Endoscopic Approach
03V70CZ Restriction of Right Brachial Artery with Extraluminal Device, Open Approach

03V70DZ Restriction of Right Brachial Artery with Intraluminal Device, Open Approach
03V70ZZ Restriction of Right Brachial Artery, Open Approach
03V73CZ Restriction of Right Brachial Artery with Extraluminal Device, Percutaneous Approach
03V73DZ Restriction of Right Brachial Artery with Intraluminal Device, Percutaneous Approach
03V73ZZ Restriction of Right Brachial Artery, Percutaneous Approach
03V74CZ Restriction of Right Brachial Artery with Extraluminal Device, Percutaneous Endoscopic Approach
03V74DZ Restriction of Right Brachial Artery with Intraluminal Device, Percutaneous Endoscopic Approach
03V74ZZ Restriction of Right Brachial Artery, Percutaneous Endoscopic Approach
03V80CZ Restriction of Left Brachial Artery with Extraluminal Device, Open Approach
03V80DZ Restriction of Left Brachial Artery with Intraluminal Device, Open Approach
03V80ZZ Restriction of Left Brachial Artery, Open Approach
03V83CZ Restriction of Left Brachial Artery with Extraluminal Device, Percutaneous Approach
03V83DZ Restriction of Left Brachial Artery with Intraluminal Device, Percutaneous Approach
03V83ZZ Restriction of Left Brachial Artery, Percutaneous Approach
03V84CZ Restriction of Left Brachial Artery with Extraluminal Device, Percutaneous Endoscopic Approach
03V84DZ Restriction of Left Brachial Artery with Intraluminal Device, Percutaneous Endoscopic Approach
03V84ZZ Restriction of Left Brachial Artery, Percutaneous Endoscopic Approach
03V90CZ Restriction of Right Ulnar Artery with Extraluminal Device, Open Approach
03V90DZ Restriction of Right Ulnar Artery with Intraluminal Device, Open Approach
03V90ZZ Restriction of Right Ulnar Artery, Open Approach
03V93CZ Restriction of Right Ulnar Artery with Extraluminal Device, Percutaneous Approach
03V93DZ Restriction of Right Ulnar Artery with Intraluminal Device, Percutaneous Approach
03V93ZZ Restriction of Right Ulnar Artery, Percutaneous Approach
03V94CZ Restriction of Right Ulnar Artery with Extraluminal Device, Percutaneous Endoscopic Approach
03V94DZ Restriction of Right Ulnar Artery with Intraluminal Device, Percutaneous Endoscopic Approach
03V94ZZ Restriction of Right Ulnar Artery, Percutaneous Endoscopic Approach
03VA0CZ Restriction of Left Ulnar Artery with Extraluminal Device, Open Approach
03VA0DZ Restriction of Left Ulnar Artery with Intraluminal Device, Open Approach
03VA0ZZ Restriction of Left Ulnar Artery, Open Approach
03VA3CZ Restriction of Left Ulnar Artery with Extraluminal Device, Percutaneous Approach
03VA3DZ Restriction of Left Ulnar Artery with Intraluminal Device, Percutaneous Approach
03VA3ZZ Restriction of Left Ulnar Artery, Percutaneous Approach
03VA4CZ Restriction of Left Ulnar Artery with Extraluminal Device, Percutaneous Endoscopic Approach
03VA4DZ Restriction of Left Ulnar Artery with Intraluminal Device, Percutaneous Endoscopic Approach
03VA4ZZ Restriction of Left Ulnar Artery, Percutaneous Endoscopic Approach
03VB0CZ Restriction of Right Radial Artery with Extraluminal Device, Open Approach
03VB0DZ Restriction of Right Radial Artery with Intraluminal Device, Open Approach
03VB0ZZ Restriction of Right Radial Artery, Open Approach
03VB3CZ Restriction of Right Radial Artery with Extraluminal Device, Percutaneous Approach
03VB3DZ Restriction of Right Radial Artery with Intraluminal Device, Percutaneous Approach
03VB3ZZ Restriction of Right Radial Artery, Percutaneous Approach
03VB4CZ Restriction of Right Radial Artery with Extraluminal Device, Percutaneous Endoscopic Approach
03VB4DZ Restriction of Right Radial Artery with Intraluminal Device, Percutaneous Endoscopic Approach
03VB4ZZ Restriction of Right Radial Artery, Percutaneous Endoscopic Approach
03VC0CZ Restriction of Left Radial Artery with Extraluminal Device, Open Approach
03VC0DZ Restriction of Left Radial Artery with Intraluminal Device, Open Approach
03VC0ZZ Restriction of Left Radial Artery, Open Approach
03VC3CZ Restriction of Left Radial Artery with Extraluminal Device, Percutaneous Approach
03VC3DZ Restriction of Left Radial Artery with Intraluminal Device, Percutaneous Approach
03VC3ZZ Restriction of Left Radial Artery, Percutaneous Approach
03VC4CZ Restriction of Left Radial Artery with Extraluminal Device, Percutaneous Endoscopic Approach
03VC4DZ Restriction of Left Radial Artery with Intraluminal Device, Percutaneous Endoscopic Approach
03VC4ZZ Restriction of Left Radial Artery, Percutaneous Endoscopic Approach
03VD0CZ Restriction of Right Hand Artery with Extraluminal Device, Open Approach
03VD0DZ Restriction of Right Hand Artery with Intraluminal Device, Open Approach
03VD0ZZ Restriction of Right Hand Artery, Open Approach
03VD3CZ Restriction of Right Hand Artery with Extraluminal Device, Percutaneous Approach
03VD3DZ Restriction of Right Hand Artery with Intraluminal Device, Percutaneous Approach
03VD3ZZ Restriction of Right Hand Artery, Percutaneous Approach
03VD4CZ Restriction of Right Hand Artery with Extraluminal Device, Percutaneous Endoscopic Approach
03VD4DZ Restriction of Right Hand Artery with Intraluminal Device, Percutaneous Endoscopic Approach
03VD4ZZ Restriction of Right Hand Artery, Percutaneous Endoscopic Approach
03VF0CZ Restriction of Left Hand Artery with Extraluminal Device, Open Approach
03VF0DZ Restriction of Left Hand Artery with Intraluminal Device, Open Approach
03VF0ZZ Restriction of Left Hand Artery, Open Approach
03VF3CZ Restriction of Left Hand Artery with Extraluminal Device, Percutaneous Approach
03VF3DZ Restriction of Left Hand Artery with Intraluminal Device, Percutaneous Approach
03VF3ZZ Restriction of Left Hand Artery, Percutaneous Approach
03VF4CZ Restriction of Left Hand Artery with Extraluminal Device, Percutaneous Endoscopic Approach
03VF4DZ Restriction of Left Hand Artery with Intraluminal Device, Percutaneous Endoscopic Approach
03VF4ZZ Restriction of Left Hand Artery, Percutaneous Endoscopic Approach
03VG0BZ Restriction of Intracranial Artery with Bioactive Intraluminal Device, Open Approach
03VG0CZ Restriction of Intracranial Artery with Extraluminal Device, Open Approach
03VG0DZ Restriction of Intracranial Artery with Intraluminal Device, Open Approach
03VG0ZZ Restriction of Intracranial Artery, Open Approach
03VG3BZ Restriction of Intracranial Artery with Bioactive Intraluminal Device, Percutaneous Approach
03VG3CZ Restriction of Intracranial Artery with Extraluminal Device, Percutaneous Approach
03VG3DZ Restriction of Intracranial Artery with Intraluminal Device, Percutaneous Approach
03VG3ZZ Restriction of Intracranial Artery, Percutaneous Approach
03VG4BZ Restriction of Intracranial Artery with Bioactive Intraluminal Device, Percutaneous Endoscopic Approach
03VG4CZ Restriction of Intracranial Artery with Extraluminal Device, Percutaneous Endoscopic Approach
03VG4DZ Restriction of Intracranial Artery with Intraluminal Device, Percutaneous Endoscopic Approach
03VG4ZZ Restriction of Intracranial Artery, Percutaneous Endoscopic Approach
03VH0BZ Restriction of Right Common Carotid Artery with Bioactive Intraluminal Device, Open Approach
03VH0CZ Restriction of Right Common Carotid Artery with Extraluminal Device, Open Approach
03VH0DZ Restriction of Right Common Carotid Artery with Intraluminal Device, Open Approach
03VH0ZZ Restriction of Right Common Carotid Artery, Open Approach
03VH3BZ Restriction of Right Common Carotid Artery with Bioactive Intraluminal Device, Percutaneous Approach
03VH3CZ Restriction of Right Common Carotid Artery with Extraluminal Device, Percutaneous Approach
03VH3DZ Restriction of Right Common Carotid Artery with Intraluminal Device, Percutaneous Approach
03VH3ZZ Restriction of Right Common Carotid Artery, Percutaneous Approach
03VH4BZ Restriction of Right Common Carotid Artery with Bioactive Intraluminal Device, Percutaneous Endoscopic Approach
03VH4CZ Restriction of Right Common Carotid Artery with Extraluminal Device, Percutaneous Endoscopic Approach

03VH4DZ Restriction of Right Common Carotid Artery with Intraluminal Device, Percutaneous Endoscopic Approach

03VH4ZZ Restriction of Right Common Carotid Artery, Percutaneous Endoscopic Approach

03VJ0BZ Restriction of Left Common Carotid Artery with Bioactive Intraluminal Device, Open Approach

03VJ0CZ Restriction of Left Common Carotid Artery with Extraluminal Device, Open Approach

03VJ0DZ Restriction of Left Common Carotid Artery with Intraluminal Device, Open Approach

03VJ0ZZ Restriction of Left Common Carotid Artery, Open Approach

03VJ3BZ Restriction of Left Common Carotid Artery with Bioactive Intraluminal Device, Percutaneous Approach

03VJ3CZ Restriction of Left Common Carotid Artery with Extraluminal Device, Percutaneous Approach

03VJ3DZ Restriction of Left Common Carotid Artery with Intraluminal Device, Percutaneous Approach

03VJ3ZZ Restriction of Left Common Carotid Artery, Percutaneous Approach

03VJ4BZ Restriction of Left Common Carotid Artery with Bioactive Intraluminal Device, Percutaneous Endoscopic Approach

03VJ4CZ Restriction of Left Common Carotid Artery with Extraluminal Device, Percutaneous Endoscopic Approach

03VJ4DZ Restriction of Left Common Carotid Artery with Intraluminal Device, Percutaneous Endoscopic Approach

03VJ4ZZ Restriction of Left Common Carotid Artery, Percutaneous Endoscopic Approach

03VK0BZ Restriction of Right Internal Carotid Artery with Bioactive Intraluminal Device, Open Approach

03VK0CZ Restriction of Right Internal Carotid Artery with Extraluminal Device, Open Approach

03VK0DZ Restriction of Right Internal Carotid Artery with Intraluminal Device, Open Approach

03VK0ZZ Restriction of Right Internal Carotid Artery, Open Approach

03VK3BZ Restriction of Right Internal Carotid Artery with Bioactive Intraluminal Device, Percutaneous Approach

03VK3CZ Restriction of Right Internal Carotid Artery with Extraluminal Device, Percutaneous Approach

03VK3DZ Restriction of Right Internal Carotid Artery with Intraluminal Device, Percutaneous Approach

03VK3ZZ Restriction of Right Internal Carotid Artery, Percutaneous Approach

03VK4BZ Restriction of Right Internal Carotid Artery with Bioactive Intraluminal Device, Percutaneous Endoscopic Approach

03VK4CZ Restriction of Right Internal Carotid Artery with Extraluminal Device, Percutaneous Endoscopic Approach

03VK4DZ Restriction of Right Internal Carotid Artery with Intraluminal Device, Percutaneous Endoscopic Approach

03VK4ZZ Restriction of Right Internal Carotid Artery, Percutaneous Endoscopic Approach

03VL0BZ Restriction of Left Internal Carotid Artery with Bioactive Intraluminal Device, Open Approach

03VL0CZ Restriction of Left Internal Carotid Artery with Extraluminal Device, Open Approach

03VL0DZ Restriction of Left Internal Carotid Artery with Intraluminal Device, Open Approach

03VL0ZZ Restriction of Left Internal Carotid Artery, Open Approach

03VL3BZ Restriction of Left Internal Carotid Artery with Bioactive Intraluminal Device, Percutaneous Approach

03VL3CZ Restriction of Left Internal Carotid Artery with Extraluminal Device, Percutaneous Approach

03VL3DZ Restriction of Left Internal Carotid Artery with Intraluminal Device, Percutaneous Approach

03VL3ZZ Restriction of Left Internal Carotid Artery, Percutaneous Approach

03VL4BZ Restriction of Left Internal Carotid Artery with Bioactive Intraluminal Device, Percutaneous Endoscopic Approach

03VL4CZ Restriction of Left Internal Carotid Artery with Extraluminal Device, Percutaneous Endoscopic Approach

03VL4DZ Restriction of Left Internal Carotid Artery with Intraluminal Device, Percutaneous Endoscopic Approach

03VL4ZZ Restriction of Left Internal Carotid Artery, Percutaneous Endoscopic Approach

03VM0BZ Restriction of Right External Carotid Artery with Bioactive Intraluminal Device, Open Approach

03VM0CZ Restriction of Right External Carotid Artery with Extraluminal Device, Open Approach

03VM0DZ Restriction of Right External Carotid Artery with Intraluminal Device, Open Approach

03VM0ZZ Restriction of Right External Carotid Artery, Open Approach

03VM3BZ Restriction of Right External Carotid Artery with Bioactive Intraluminal Device, Percutaneous Approach

03VM3CZ Restriction of Right External Carotid Artery with Extraluminal Device, Percutaneous Approach

03VM3DZ Restriction of Right External Carotid Artery with Intraluminal Device, Percutaneous Approach

03VM3ZZ Restriction of Right External Carotid Artery, Percutaneous Approach

03VM4BZ Restriction of Right External Carotid Artery with Bioactive Intraluminal Device, Percutaneous Endoscopic Approach

03VM4CZ Restriction of Right External Carotid Artery with Extraluminal Device, Percutaneous Endoscopic Approach

03VM4DZ Restriction of Right External Carotid Artery with Intraluminal Device, Percutaneous Endoscopic Approach

03VM4ZZ Restriction of Right External Carotid Artery, Percutaneous Endoscopic Approach

03VN0BZ Restriction of Left External Carotid Artery with Bioactive Intraluminal Device, Open Approach

03VN0CZ Restriction of Left External Carotid Artery with Extraluminal Device, Open Approach

03VN0DZ Restriction of Left External Carotid Artery with Intraluminal Device, Open Approach

03VN0ZZ Restriction of Left External Carotid Artery, Open Approach

03VN3BZ Restriction of Left External Carotid Artery with Bioactive Intraluminal Device, Percutaneous Approach

03VN3CZ Restriction of Left External Carotid Artery with Extraluminal Device, Percutaneous Approach

03VN3DZ Restriction of Left External Carotid Artery with Intraluminal Device, Percutaneous Approach

03VN3ZZ Restriction of Left External Carotid Artery, Percutaneous Approach

03VN4BZ Restriction of Left External Carotid Artery with Bioactive Intraluminal Device, Percutaneous Endoscopic Approach

03VN4CZ Restriction of Left External Carotid Artery with Extraluminal Device, Percutaneous Endoscopic Approach

03VN4DZ Restriction of Left External Carotid Artery with Intraluminal Device, Percutaneous Endoscopic Approach

03VN4ZZ Restriction of Left External Carotid Artery, Percutaneous Endoscopic Approach

03VP0BZ Restriction of Right Vertebral Artery with Bioactive Intraluminal Device, Open Approach

03VP0CZ Restriction of Right Vertebral Artery with Extraluminal Device, Open Approach

03VP0DZ Restriction of Right Vertebral Artery with Intraluminal Device, Open Approach

03VP0ZZ Restriction of Right Vertebral Artery, Open Approach

03VP3BZ Restriction of Right Vertebral Artery with Bioactive Intraluminal Device, Percutaneous Approach

03VP3CZ Restriction of Right Vertebral Artery with Extraluminal Device, Percutaneous Approach

03VP3DZ Restriction of Right Vertebral Artery with Intraluminal Device, Percutaneous Approach

03VP3ZZ Restriction of Right Vertebral Artery, Percutaneous Approach

03VP4BZ Restriction of Right Vertebral Artery with Bioactive Intraluminal Device, Percutaneous Endoscopic Approach

03VP4CZ Restriction of Right Vertebral Artery with Extraluminal Device, Percutaneous Endoscopic Approach

03VP4DZ Restriction of Right Vertebral Artery with Intraluminal Device, Percutaneous Endoscopic Approach

03VP4ZZ Restriction of Right Vertebral Artery, Percutaneous Endoscopic Approach

03VQ0BZ Restriction of Left Vertebral Artery with Bioactive Intraluminal Device, Open Approach

03VQ0CZ Restriction of Left Vertebral Artery with Extraluminal Device, Open Approach

03VQ0DZ Restriction of Left Vertebral Artery with Intraluminal Device, Open Approach

03VQ0ZZ Restriction of Left Vertebral Artery, Open Approach

03VQ3BZ Restriction of Left Vertebral Artery with Bioactive Intraluminal Device, Percutaneous Approach

03VQ3CZ Restriction of Left Vertebral Artery with Extraluminal Device, Percutaneous Approach

03VQ3DZ Restriction of Left Vertebral Artery with Intraluminal Device, Percutaneous Approach

03VQ3ZZ Restriction of Left Vertebral Artery, Percutaneous Approach

03VQ4BZ Restriction of Left Vertebral Artery with Bioactive Intraluminal Device, Percutaneous Endoscopic Approach

03VQ4CZ Restriction of Left Vertebral Artery with Extraluminal Device, Percutaneous Endoscopic Approach

03VQ4DZ Restriction of Left Vertebral Artery with Intraluminal Device, Percutaneous Endoscopic Approach

03VQ4ZZ Restriction of Left Vertebral Artery, Percutaneous Endoscopic Approach
03VR0CZ Restriction of Face Artery with Extraluminal Device, Open Approach
03VR0DZ Restriction of Face Artery with Intraluminal Device, Open Approach
03VR0ZZ Restriction of Face Artery, Open Approach
03VR3CZ Restriction of Face Artery with Extraluminal Device, Percutaneous Approach
03VR3DZ Restriction of Face Artery with Intraluminal Device, Percutaneous Approach
03VR3ZZ Restriction of Face Artery, Percutaneous Approach
03VR4CZ Restriction of Face Artery with Extraluminal Device, Percutaneous Endoscopic Approach
03VR4DZ Restriction of Face Artery with Intraluminal Device, Percutaneous Endoscopic Approach
03VR4ZZ Restriction of Face Artery, Percutaneous Endoscopic Approach
03VS0CZ Restriction of Right Temporal Artery with Extraluminal Device, Open Approach
03VS0DZ Restriction of Right Temporal Artery with Intraluminal Device, Open Approach
03VS0ZZ Restriction of Right Temporal Artery, Open Approach
03VS3CZ Restriction of Right Temporal Artery with Extraluminal Device, Percutaneous Approach
03VS3DZ Restriction of Right Temporal Artery with Intraluminal Device, Percutaneous Approach
03VS3ZZ Restriction of Right Temporal Artery, Percutaneous Approach
03VS4CZ Restriction of Right Temporal Artery with Extraluminal Device, Percutaneous Endoscopic Approach
03VS4DZ Restriction of Right Temporal Artery with Intraluminal Device, Percutaneous Endoscopic Approach
03VS4ZZ Restriction of Right Temporal Artery, Percutaneous Endoscopic Approach
03VT0CZ Restriction of Left Temporal Artery with Extraluminal Device, Open Approach
03VT0DZ Restriction of Left Temporal Artery with Intraluminal Device, Open Approach
03VT0ZZ Restriction of Left Temporal Artery, Open Approach
03VT3CZ Restriction of Left Temporal Artery with Extraluminal Device, Percutaneous Approach
03VT3DZ Restriction of Left Temporal Artery with Intraluminal Device, Percutaneous Approach
03VT3ZZ Restriction of Left Temporal Artery, Percutaneous Approach
03VT4CZ Restriction of Left Temporal Artery with Extraluminal Device, Percutaneous Endoscopic Approach
03VT4DZ Restriction of Left Temporal Artery with Intraluminal Device, Percutaneous Endoscopic Approach
03VT4ZZ Restriction of Left Temporal Artery, Percutaneous Endoscopic Approach
03VU0CZ Restriction of Right Thyroid Artery with Extraluminal Device, Open Approach
03VU0DZ Restriction of Right Thyroid Artery with Intraluminal Device, Open Approach
03VU0ZZ Restriction of Right Thyroid Artery, Open Approach
03VU3CZ Restriction of Right Thyroid Artery with Extraluminal Device, Percutaneous Approach
03VU3DZ Restriction of Right Thyroid Artery with Intraluminal Device, Percutaneous Approach
03VU3ZZ Restriction of Right Thyroid Artery, Percutaneous Approach
03VU4CZ Restriction of Right Thyroid Artery with Extraluminal Device, Percutaneous Endoscopic Approach
03VU4DZ Restriction of Right Thyroid Artery with Intraluminal Device, Percutaneous Endoscopic Approach
03VU4ZZ Restriction of Right Thyroid Artery, Percutaneous Endoscopic Approach
03VV0CZ Restriction of Left Thyroid Artery with Extraluminal Device, Open Approach
03VV0DZ Restriction of Left Thyroid Artery with Intraluminal Device, Open Approach
03VV0ZZ Restriction of Left Thyroid Artery, Open Approach
03VV3CZ Restriction of Left Thyroid Artery with Extraluminal Device, Percutaneous Approach
03VV3DZ Restriction of Left Thyroid Artery with Intraluminal Device, Percutaneous Approach
03VV3ZZ Restriction of Left Thyroid Artery, Percutaneous Approach
03VV4CZ Restriction of Left Thyroid Artery with Extraluminal Device, Percutaneous Endoscopic Approach
03VV4DZ Restriction of Left Thyroid Artery with Intraluminal Device, Percutaneous Endoscopic Approach
03VV4ZZ Restriction of Left Thyroid Artery, Percutaneous Endoscopic Approach
03VY0CZ Restriction of Upper Artery with Extraluminal Device, Open Approach
03VY0DZ Restriction of Upper Artery with Intraluminal Device, Open Approach
03VY0ZZ Restriction of Upper Artery, Open Approach
03VY3CZ Restriction of Upper Artery with Extraluminal Device, Percutaneous Approach
03VY3DZ Restriction of Upper Artery with Intraluminal Device, Percutaneous Approach
03VY3ZZ Restriction of Upper Artery, Percutaneous Approach
03VY4CZ Restriction of Upper Artery with Extraluminal Device, Percutaneous Endoscopic Approach
03VY4DZ Restriction of Upper Artery with Intraluminal Device, Percutaneous Endoscopic Approach
03VY4ZZ Restriction of Upper Artery, Percutaneous Endoscopic Approach

03W – Upper Arteries, Revision

Review Coding Guideline B6.1c

03WY00Z Revision of Drainage Device in Upper Artery, Open Approach
03WY02Z Revision of Monitoring Device in Upper Artery, Open Approach
03WY03Z Revision of Infusion Device in Upper Artery, Open Approach
03WY07Z Revision of Autologous Tissue Substitute in Upper Artery, Open Approach
03WY0CZ Revision of Extraluminal Device in Upper Artery, Open Approach
03WY0DZ Revision of Intraluminal Device in Upper Artery, Open Approach
03WY0JZ Revision of Synthetic Substitute in Upper Artery, Open Approach
03WY0KZ Revision of Nonautologous Tissue Substitute in Upper Artery, Open Approach
03WY0MZ Revision of Stimulator Lead in Upper Artery, Open Approach
03WY30Z Revision of Drainage Device in Upper Artery, Percutaneous Approach
03WY32Z Revision of Monitoring Device in Upper Artery, Percutaneous Approach
03WY33Z Revision of Infusion Device in Upper Artery, Percutaneous Approach
03WY37Z Revision of Autologous Tissue Substitute in Upper Artery, Percutaneous Approach
03WY3CZ Revision of Extraluminal Device in Upper Artery, Percutaneous Approach
03WY3DZ Revision of Intraluminal Device in Upper Artery, Percutaneous Approach
03WY3JZ Revision of Synthetic Substitute in Upper Artery, Percutaneous Approach
03WY3KZ Revision of Nonautologous Tissue Substitute in Upper Artery, Percutaneous Approach
03WY3MZ Revision of Stimulator Lead in Upper Artery, Percutaneous Approach
03WY40Z Revision of Drainage Device in Upper Artery, Percutaneous Endoscopic Approach
03WY42Z Revision of Monitoring Device in Upper Artery, Percutaneous Endoscopic Approach
03WY43Z Revision of Infusion Device in Upper Artery, Percutaneous Endoscopic Approach
03WY47Z Revision of Autologous Tissue Substitute in Upper Artery, Percutaneous Endoscopic Approach
03WY4CZ Revision of Extraluminal Device in Upper Artery, Percutaneous Endoscopic Approach
03WY4DZ Revision of Intraluminal Device in Upper Artery, Percutaneous Endoscopic Approach
03WY4JZ Revision of Synthetic Substitute in Upper Artery, Percutaneous Endoscopic Approach
03WY4KZ Revision of Nonautologous Tissue Substitute in Upper Artery, Percutaneous Endoscopic Approach
03WY4MZ Revision of Stimulator Lead in Upper Artery, Percutaneous Endoscopic Approach
03WYX0Z Revision of Drainage Device in Upper Artery, External Approach
03WYX2Z Revision of Monitoring Device in Upper Artery, External Approach
03WYX3Z Revision of Infusion Device in Upper Artery, External Approach
03WYX7Z Revision of Autologous Tissue Substitute in Upper Artery, External Approach
03WYXCZ Revision of Extraluminal Device in Upper Artery, External Approach
03WYXDZ Revision of Intraluminal Device in Upper Artery, External Approach
03WYXJZ Revision of Synthetic Substitute in Upper Artery, External Approach
03WYXKZ Revision of Nonautologous Tissue Substitute in Upper Artery, External Approach
03WYXMZ Revision of Stimulator Lead in Upper Artery, External Approach

Arteries

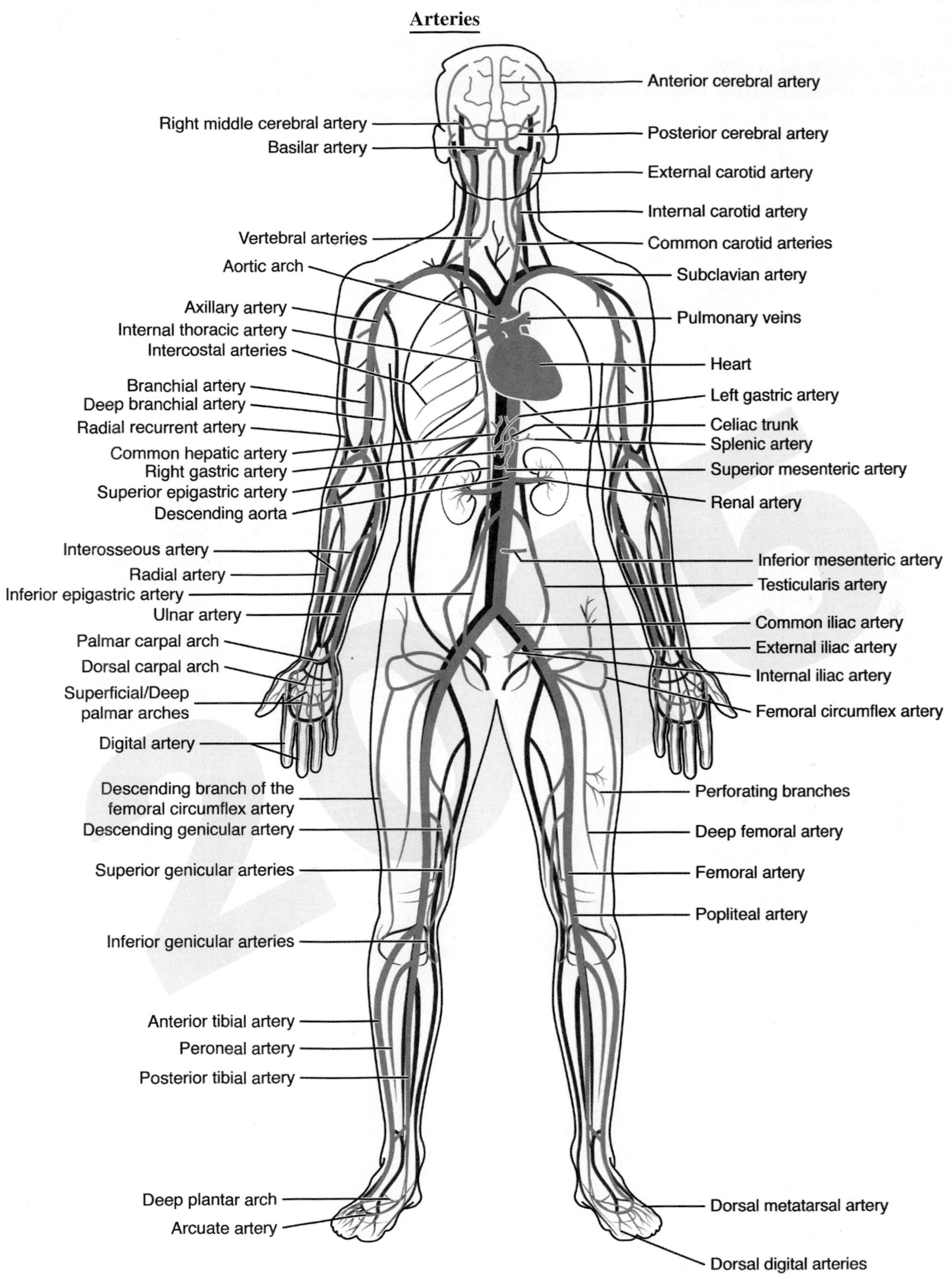
Anterior cerebral artery
Right middle cerebral artery
Posterior cerebral artery
Basilar artery
External carotid artery
Internal carotid artery
Vertebral arteries
Common carotid arteries
Aortic arch
Subclavian artery
Axillary artery
Pulmonary veins
Internal thoracic artery
Intercostal arteries
Heart
Branchial artery
Left gastric artery
Deep branchial artery
Radial recurrent artery
Celiac trunk
Common hepatic artery
Splenic artery
Right gastric artery
Superior mesenteric artery
Superior epigastric artery
Descending aorta
Renal artery
Interosseous artery
Inferior mesenteric artery
Radial artery
Testicularis artery
Inferior epigastric artery
Ulnar artery
Common iliac artery
Palmar carpal arch
External iliac artery
Dorsal carpal arch
Internal iliac artery
Superficial/Deep palmar arches
Femoral circumflex artery
Digital artery
Descending branch of the femoral circumflex artery
Perforating branches
Descending genicular artery
Deep femoral artery
Superior genicular arteries
Femoral artery
Popliteal artery
Inferior genicular arteries
Anterior tibial artery
Peroneal artery
Posterior tibial artery
Deep plantar arch
Dorsal metatarsal artery
Arcuate artery
Dorsal digital arteries

Lower Arteries Tables 041–04W

Section 0 **Medical and Surgical**
Body System 4 **Lower Arteries**
Operation 1 **Bypass:** Altering the route of passage of the contents of a tubular body part

Body Part (4th)	Approach (5th)	Device (6th)	Qualifier (7th)
0 Abdominal Aorta **C** Common Iliac Artery, Right **D** Common Iliac Artery, Left	**0** Open **4** Percutaneous Endoscopic	**9** Autologous Venous Tissue **A** Autologous Arterial Tissue **J** Synthetic Substitute **K** Nonautologous Tissue Substitute **Z** No Device	**0** Abdominal Aorta **1** Celiac Artery **2** Mesenteric Artery **3** Renal Artery, Right **4** Renal Artery, Left **5** Renal Artery, Bilateral **6** Common Iliac Artery, Right **7** Common Iliac Artery, Left **8** Common Iliac Arteries, Bilateral **9** Internal Iliac Artery, Right **B** Internal Iliac Artery, Left **C** Internal Iliac Arteries, Bilateral **D** External Iliac Artery, Right **F** External Iliac Artery, Left **G** External Iliac Arteries, Bilateral **H** Femoral Artery, Right **J** Femoral Artery, Left **K** Femoral Arteries, Bilateral **Q** Lower Extremity Artery **R** Lower Artery
4 Splenic Artery	**0** Open **4** Percutaneous Endoscopic	**9** Autologous Venous Tissue **A** Autologous Arterial Tissue **J** Synthetic Substitute **K** Nonautologous Tissue Substitute **Z** No Device	**3** Renal Artery, Right **4** Renal Artery, Left **5** Renal Artery, Bilateral
E Internal Iliac Artery, Right **F** Internal Iliac Artery, Left **H** External Iliac Artery, Right **J** External Iliac Artery, Left	**0** Open **4** Percutaneous Endoscopic	**9** Autologous Venous Tissue **A** Autologous Arterial Tissue **J** Synthetic Substitute **K** Nonautologous Tissue Substitute **Z** No Device	**9** Internal Iliac Artery, Right **B** Internal Iliac Artery, Left **C** Internal Iliac Arteries, Bilateral **D** External Iliac Artery, Right **F** External Iliac Artery, Left **G** External Iliac Arteries, Bilateral **H** Femoral Artery, Right **J** Femoral Artery, Left **K** Femoral Arteries, Bilateral **P** Foot Artery **Q** Lower Extremity Artery
K Femoral Artery, Right **L** Femoral Artery, Left	**0** Open **4** Percutaneous Endoscopic	**9** Autologous Venous Tissue **A** Autologous Arterial Tissue **J** Synthetic Substitute **K** Nonautologous Tissue Substitute **Z** No Device	**H** Femoral Artery, Right **J** Femoral Artery, Left **K** Femoral Arteries, Bilateral **L** Popliteal Artery **M** Peroneal Artery **N** Posterior Tibial Artery **P** Foot Artery **Q** Lower Extremity Artery **S** Lower Extremity Vein
M Popliteal Artery, Right **N** Popliteal Artery, Left	**0** Open **4** Percutaneous Endoscopic	**9** Autologous Venous Tissue **A** Autologous Arterial Tissue **J** Synthetic Substitute **K** Nonautologous Tissue Substitute **Z** No Device	**L** Popliteal Artery **M** Peroneal Artery **P** Foot Artery **Q** Lower Extremity Artery **S** Lower Extremity Vein

Section 0 **Medical and Surgical**
Body System 4 **Lower Arteries**
Operation 5 **Destruction:** Physical eradication of all or a portion of a body part by the direct use of energy, force, or a destructive agent

Body Part (4th)	Approach (5th)	Device (6th)	Qualifier (7th)
0 Abdominal Aorta **1** Celiac Artery **2** Gastric Artery **3** Hepatic Artery **4** Splenic Artery **5** Superior Mesenteric Artery **6** Colic Artery, Right **7** Colic Artery, Left **8** Colic Artery, Middle **9** Renal Artery, Right **A** Renal Artery, Left **B** Inferior Mesenteric Artery **C** Common Iliac Artery, Right **D** Common Iliac Artery, Left **E** Internal Iliac Artery, Right **F** Internal Iliac Artery, Left **H** External Iliac Artery, Right **J** External Iliac Artery, Left **K** Femoral Artery, Right **L** Femoral Artery, Left **M** Popliteal Artery, Right **N** Popliteal Artery, Left **P** Anterior Tibial Artery, Right **Q** Anterior Tibial Artery, Left **R** Posterior Tibial Artery, Right **S** Posterior Tibial Artery, Left **T** Peroneal Artery, Right **U** Peroneal Artery, Left **V** Foot Artery, Right **W** Foot Artery, Left **Y** Lower Artery	**0** Open **3** Percutaneous **4** Percutaneous Endoscopic	**Z** No Device	**Z** No Qualifier

Section 0 **Medical and Surgical**
Body System 4 **Lower Arteries**
Operation 7 **Dilation:** Expanding an orifice or the lumen of a tubular body part

Body Part (4th)	Approach (5th)	Device (6th)	Qualifier (7th)
0 Abdominal Aorta **1** Celiac Artery **2** Gastric Artery **3** Hepatic Artery **4** Splenic Artery **5** Superior Mesenteric Artery **6** Colic Artery, Right **7** Colic Artery, Left **8** Colic Artery, Middle **9** Renal Artery, Right **A** Renal Artery, Left **B** Inferior Mesenteric Artery **C** Common Iliac Artery, Right **D** Common Iliac Artery, Left **E** Internal Iliac Artery, Right **F** Internal Iliac Artery, Left **H** External Iliac Artery, Right **J** External Iliac Artery, Left **K** Femoral Artery, Right **L** Femoral Artery, Left **M** Popliteal Artery, Right **N** Popliteal Artery, Left **P** Anterior Tibial Artery, Right **Q** Anterior Tibial Artery, Left **R** Posterior Tibial Artery, Right **S** Posterior Tibial Artery, Left **T** Peroneal Artery, Right **U** Peroneal Artery, Left **V** Foot Artery, Right **W** Foot Artery, Left **Y** Lower Artery	**0** Open **3** Percutaneous **4** Percutaneous Endoscopic	**4** Intraluminal Device, Drug-eluting **D** Intraluminal Device **Z** No Device	**Z** No Qualifier

Section 0 **Medical and Surgical**
Body System 4 **Lower Arteries**
Operation 9 **Drainage:** Taking or letting out fluids and/or gases from a body part

Body Part (4th)	Approach (5th)	Device (6th)	Qualifier (7th)
0 Abdominal Aorta **1** Celiac Artery **2** Gastric Artery **3** Hepatic Artery **4** Splenic Artery **5** Superior Mesenteric Artery **6** Colic Artery, Right **7** Colic Artery, Left **8** Colic Artery, Middle **9** Renal Artery, Right **A** Renal Artery, Left **B** Inferior Mesenteric Artery **C** Common Iliac Artery, Right **D** Common Iliac Artery, Left **E** Internal Iliac Artery, Right **F** Internal Iliac Artery, Left **H** External Iliac Artery, Right **J** External Iliac Artery, Left **K** Femoral Artery, Right **L** Femoral Artery, Left **M** Popliteal Artery, Right **N** Popliteal Artery, Left **P** Anterior Tibial Artery, Right **Q** Anterior Tibial Artery, Left **R** Posterior Tibial Artery, Right **S** Posterior Tibial Artery, Left **T** Peroneal Artery, Right **U** Peroneal Artery, Left **V** Foot Artery, Right **W** Foot Artery, Left **Y** Lower Artery	**0** Open **3** Percutaneous **4** Percutaneous Endoscopic	**0** Drainage Device	**Z** No Qualifier
0 Abdominal Aorta **1** Celiac Artery **2** Gastric Artery **3** Hepatic Artery **4** Splenic Artery **5** Superior Mesenteric Artery **6** Colic Artery, Right **7** Colic Artery, Left **8** Colic Artery, Middle **9** Renal Artery, Right **A** Renal Artery, Left **B** Inferior Mesenteric Artery **C** Common Iliac Artery, Right **D** Common Iliac Artery, Left **E** Internal Iliac Artery, Right **F** Internal Iliac Artery, Left **H** External Iliac Artery, Right **J** External Iliac Artery, Left **K** Femoral Artery, Right **L** Femoral Artery, Left **M** Popliteal Artery, Right **N** Popliteal Artery, Left **P** Anterior Tibial Artery, Right **Q** Anterior Tibial Artery, Left **R** Posterior Tibial Artery, Right **S** Posterior Tibial Artery, Left **T** Peroneal Artery, Right **U** Peroneal Artery, Left **V** Foot Artery, Right **W** Foot Artery, Left **Y** Lower Artery	**0** Open **3** Percutaneous **4** Percutaneous Endoscopic	**Z** No Device	**X** Diagnostic **Z** No Qualifier

Section	0	Medical and Surgical
Body System	4	Lower Arteries
Operation	B	**Excision:** Cutting out or off, without replacement, a portion of a body part

Body Part (4th)	Approach (5th)	Device (6th)	Qualifier (7th)
0 Abdominal Aorta **1** Celiac Artery **2** Gastric Artery **3** Hepatic Artery **4** Splenic Artery **5** Superior Mesenteric Artery **6** Colic Artery, Right **7** Colic Artery, Left **8** Colic Artery, Middle **9** Renal Artery, Right **A** Renal Artery, Left **B** Inferior Mesenteric Artery **C** Common Iliac Artery, Right **D** Common Iliac Artery, Left **E** Internal Iliac Artery, Right **F** Internal Iliac Artery, Left **H** External Iliac Artery, Right **J** External Iliac Artery, Left **K** Femoral Artery, Right **L** Femoral Artery, Left **M** Popliteal Artery, Right **N** Popliteal Artery, Left **P** Anterior Tibial Artery, Right **Q** Anterior Tibial Artery, Left **R** Posterior Tibial Artery, Right **S** Posterior Tibial Artery, Left **T** Peroneal Artery, Right **U** Peroneal Artery, Left **V** Foot Artery, Right **W** Foot Artery, Left **Y** Lower Artery	**0** Open **3** Percutaneous **4** Percutaneous Endoscopic	**Z** No Device	**X** Diagnostic **Z** No Qualifier

Section **0** **Medical and Surgical**
Body System **4** **Lower Arteries**
Operation **C** **Extirpation:** Taking or cutting out solid matter from a body part

Body Part (4th)	Approach (5th)	Device (6th)	Qualifier (7th)
0 Abdominal Aorta **1** Celiac Artery **2** Gastric Artery **3** Hepatic Artery **4** Splenic Artery **5** Superior Mesenteric Artery **6** Colic Artery, Right **7** Colic Artery, Left **8** Colic Artery, Middle **9** Renal Artery, Right **A** Renal Artery, Left **B** Inferior Mesenteric Artery **C** Common Iliac Artery, Right **D** Common Iliac Artery, Left **E** Internal Iliac Artery, Right **F** Internal Iliac Artery, Left **H** External Iliac Artery, Right **J** External Iliac Artery, Left **K** Femoral Artery, Right **L** Femoral Artery, Left **M** Popliteal Artery, Right **N** Popliteal Artery, Left **P** Anterior Tibial Artery, Right **Q** Anterior Tibial Artery, Left **R** Posterior Tibial Artery, Right **S** Posterior Tibial Artery, Left **T** Peroneal Artery, Right **U** Peroneal Artery, Left **V** Foot Artery, Right **W** Foot Artery, Left **Y** Lower Artery	**0** Open **3** Percutaneous **4** Percutaneous Endoscopic	**Z** No Device	**Z** No Qualifier

Section **0** **Medical and Surgical**
Body System **4** **Lower Arteries**
Operation **H** **Insertion:** Putting in a nonbiological appliance that monitors, assists, performs, or prevents a physiological function but does not physically take the place of a body part

Body Part (4th)	Approach (5th)	Device (6th)	Qualifier (7th)
0 Abdominal Aorta **Y** Lower Artery	**0** Open **3** Percutaneous **4** Percutaneous Endoscopic	**2** Monitoring Device **3** Infusion Device **D** Intraluminal Device	**Z** No Qualifier

Continued →

Section 0 **Medical and Surgical**
Body System 4 **Lower Arteries**
Operation H **Insertion:** Putting in a nonbiological appliance that monitors, assists, performs, or prevents a physiological function but does not physically take the place of a body part

Body Part (4th)	Approach (5th)	Device (6th)	Qualifier (7th)
1 Celiac Artery **2** Gastric Artery **3** Hepatic Artery **4** Splenic Artery **5** Superior Mesenteric Artery **6** Colic Artery, Right **7** Colic Artery, Left **8** Colic Artery, Middle **9** Renal Artery, Right **A** Renal Artery, Left **B** Inferior Mesenteric Artery **C** Common Iliac Artery, Right **D** Common Iliac Artery, Left **E** Internal Iliac Artery, Right **F** Internal Iliac Artery, Left **H** External Iliac Artery, Right **J** External Iliac Artery, Left **K** Femoral Artery, Right **L** Femoral Artery, Left **M** Popliteal Artery, Right **N** Popliteal Artery, Left **P** Anterior Tibial Artery, Right **Q** Anterior Tibial Artery, Left **R** Posterior Tibial Artery, Right **S** Posterior Tibial Artery, Left **T** Peroneal Artery, Right **U** Peroneal Artery, Left **V** Foot Artery, Right **W** Foot Artery, Left	**0** Open **3** Percutaneous **4** Percutaneous Endoscopic	**3** Infusion Device **D** Intraluminal Device	**Z** No Qualifier

Section 0 **Medical and Surgical**
Body System 4 **Lower Arteries**
Operation J **Inspection:** Visually and/or manually exploring a body part

Body Part (4th)	Approach (5th)	Device (6th)	Qualifier (7th)
Y Lower Artery	**0** Open **3** Percutaneous **4** Percutaneous Endoscopic **X** External	**Z** No Device	**Z** No Qualifier

Section 0 Medical and Surgical
Body System 4 Lower Arteries
Operation L **Occlusion:** Completely closing an orifice or the lumen of a tubular body part

Body Part (4th)	Approach (5th)	Device (6th)	Qualifier (7th)
0 Abdominal Aorta **1** Celiac Artery **2** Gastric Artery **3** Hepatic Artery **4** Splenic Artery **5** Superior Mesenteric Artery **6** Colic Artery, Right **7** Colic Artery, Left **8** Colic Artery, Middle **9** Renal Artery, Right **A** Renal Artery, Left **B** Inferior Mesenteric Artery **C** Common Iliac Artery, Right **D** Common Iliac Artery, Left **H** External Iliac Artery, Right **J** External Iliac Artery, Left **K** Femoral Artery, Right **L** Femoral Artery, Left **M** Popliteal Artery, Right **N** Popliteal Artery, Left **P** Anterior Tibial Artery, Right **Q** Anterior Tibial Artery, Left **R** Posterior Tibial Artery, Right **S** Posterior Tibial Artery, Left **T** Peroneal Artery, Right **U** Peroneal Artery, Left **V** Foot Artery, Right **W** Foot Artery, Left **Y** Lower Artery	**0** Open **3** Percutaneous **4** Percutaneous Endoscopic	**C** Extraluminal Device **D** Intraluminal Device **Z** No Device	**Z** No Qualifier
E Internal Iliac Artery, Right	**0** Open **3** Percutaneous **4** Percutaneous Endoscopic	**C** Extraluminal Device **D** Intraluminal Device **Z** No Device	**T** Uterine Artery, Right **Z** No Qualifier
F Internal Iliac Artery, Left	**0** Open **3** Percutaneous **4** Percutaneous Endoscopic	**C** Extraluminal Device **D** Intraluminal Device **Z** No Device	**U** Uterine Artery, Left **Z** No Qualifier

Section 0 **Medical and Surgical**
Body System 4 **Lower Arteries**
Operation N **Release:** Freeing a body part from an abnormal physical constraint by cutting or by the use of force

Body Part (4th)	Approach (5th)	Device (6th)	Qualifier (7th)
0 Abdominal Aorta **1** Celiac Artery **2** Gastric Artery **3** Hepatic Artery **4** Splenic Artery **5** Superior Mesenteric Artery **6** Colic Artery, Right **7** Colic Artery, Left **8** Colic Artery, Middle **9** Renal Artery, Right **A** Renal Artery, Left **B** Inferior Mesenteric Artery **C** Common Iliac Artery, Right **D** Common Iliac Artery, Left **E** Internal Iliac Artery, Right **F** Internal Iliac Artery, Left **H** External Iliac Artery, Right **J** External Iliac Artery, Left **K** Femoral Artery, Right **L** Femoral Artery, Left **M** Popliteal Artery, Right **N** Popliteal Artery, Left **P** Anterior Tibial Artery, Right **Q** Anterior Tibial Artery, Left **R** Posterior Tibial Artery, Right **S** Posterior Tibial Artery, Left **T** Peroneal Artery, Right **U** Peroneal Artery, Left **V** Foot Artery, Right **W** Foot Artery, Left **Y** Lower Artery	**0** Open **3** Percutaneous **4** Percutaneous Endoscopic	**Z** No Device	**Z** No Qualifier

Section 0 **Medical and Surgical**
Body System 4 **Lower Arteries**
Operation P **Removal:** Taking out or off a device from a body part

Body Part (4th)	Approach (5th)	Device (6th)	Qualifier (7th)
Y Lower Artery	**0** Open **3** Percutaneous **4** Percutaneous Endoscopic	**0** Drainage Device **2** Monitoring Device **3** Infusion Device **7** Autologous Tissue Substitute **C** Extraluminal Device **D** Intraluminal Device **J** Synthetic Substitute **K** Nonautologous Tissue Substitute	**Z** No Qualifier
Y Lower Artery	**X** External	**0** Drainage Device **1** Radioactive Element **2** Monitoring Device **3** Infusion Device **D** Intraluminal Device	**Z** No Qualifier

Section 0 Medical and Surgical
Body System 4 Lower Arteries
Operation Q **Repair:** Restoring, to the extent possible, a body part to its normal anatomic structure and function

Body Part (4th)	Approach (5th)	Device (6th)	Qualifier (7th)
0 Abdominal Aorta **1** Celiac Artery **2** Gastric Artery **3** Hepatic Artery **4** Splenic Artery **5** Superior Mesenteric Artery **6** Colic Artery, Right **7** Colic Artery, Left **8** Colic Artery, Middle **9** Renal Artery, Right **A** Renal Artery, Left **B** Inferior Mesenteric Artery **C** Common Iliac Artery, Right **D** Common Iliac Artery, Left **E** Internal Iliac Artery, Right **F** Internal Iliac Artery, Left **H** External Iliac Artery, Right **J** External Iliac Artery, Left **K** Femoral Artery, Right **L** Femoral Artery, Left **M** Popliteal Artery, Right **N** Popliteal Artery, Left **P** Anterior Tibial Artery, Right **Q** Anterior Tibial Artery, Left **R** Posterior Tibial Artery, Right **S** Posterior Tibial Artery, Left **T** Peroneal Artery, Right **U** Peroneal Artery, Left **V** Foot Artery, Right **W** Foot Artery, Left **Y** Lower Artery	**0** Open **3** Percutaneous **4** Percutaneous Endoscopic	**Z** No Device	**Z** No Qualifier

Section 0 **Medical and Surgical**
Body System 4 **Lower Arteries**
Operation R **Replacement:** Putting in or on biological or synthetic material that physically takes the place and/or function of all or a portion of a body part

Body Part (4th)	Approach (5th)	Device (6th)	Qualifier (7th)
0 Abdominal Aorta **1** Celiac Artery **2** Gastric Artery **3** Hepatic Artery **4** Splenic Artery **5** Superior Mesenteric Artery **6** Colic Artery, Right **7** Colic Artery, Left **8** Colic Artery, Middle **9** Renal Artery, Right **A** Renal Artery, Left **B** Inferior Mesenteric Artery **C** Common Iliac Artery, Right **D** Common Iliac Artery, Left **E** Internal Iliac Artery, Right **F** Internal Iliac Artery, Left **H** External Iliac Artery, Right **J** External Iliac Artery, Left **K** Femoral Artery, Right **L** Femoral Artery, Left **M** Popliteal Artery, Right **N** Popliteal Artery, Left **P** Anterior Tibial Artery, Right **Q** Anterior Tibial Artery, Left **R** Posterior Tibial Artery, Right **S** Posterior Tibial Artery, Left **T** Peroneal Artery, Right **U** Peroneal Artery, Left **V** Foot Artery, Right **W** Foot Artery, Left **Y** Lower Artery	**0** Open **4** Percutaneous Endoscopic	**7** Autologous Tissue Substitute **J** Synthetic Substitute **K** Nonautologous Tissue Substitute	**Z** No Qualifier

Section 0 **Medical and Surgical**
Body System 4 **Lower Arteries**
Operation S **Reposition:** Moving to its normal location, or other suitable location, all or a portion of a body part

Body Part (4th)	Approach (5th)	Device (6th)	Qualifier (7th)
0 Abdominal Aorta **1** Celiac Artery **2** Gastric Artery **3** Hepatic Artery **4** Splenic Artery **5** Superior Mesenteric Artery **6** Colic Artery, Right **7** Colic Artery, Left **8** Colic Artery, Middle **9** Renal Artery, Right **A** Renal Artery, Left **B** Inferior Mesenteric Artery **C** Common Iliac Artery, Right **D** Common Iliac Artery, Left **E** Internal Iliac Artery, Right **F** Internal Iliac Artery, Left **H** External Iliac Artery, Right **J** External Iliac Artery, Left **K** Femoral Artery, Right **L** Femoral Artery, Left **M** Popliteal Artery, Right **N** Popliteal Artery, Left **P** Anterior Tibial Artery, Right **Q** Anterior Tibial Artery, Left **R** Posterior Tibial Artery, Right **S** Posterior Tibial Artery, Left **T** Peroneal Artery, Right **U** Peroneal Artery, Left **V** Foot Artery, Right **W** Foot Artery, Left **Y** Lower Artery	**0** Open **3** Percutaneous **4** Percutaneous Endoscopic	**Z** No Device	**Z** No Qualifier

Section 0 **Medical and Surgical**
Body System 4 **Lower Arteries**
Operation U **Supplement:** Putting in or on biological or synthetic material that physically reinforces and/or augments the function of a portion of a body part

Body Part (4th)	Approach (5th)	Device (6th)	Qualifier (7th)
0 Abdominal Aorta **1** Celiac Artery **2** Gastric Artery **3** Hepatic Artery **4** Splenic Artery **5** Superior Mesenteric Artery **6** Colic Artery, Right **7** Colic Artery, Left **8** Colic Artery, Middle **9** Renal Artery, Right **A** Renal Artery, Left **B** Inferior Mesenteric Artery **C** Common Iliac Artery, Right **D** Common Iliac Artery, Left **E** Internal Iliac Artery, Right **F** Internal Iliac Artery, Left **H** External Iliac Artery, Right **J** External Iliac Artery, Left **K** Femoral Artery, Right **L** Femoral Artery, Left **M** Popliteal Artery, Right **N** Popliteal Artery, Left **P** Anterior Tibial Artery, Right **Q** Anterior Tibial Artery, Left **R** Posterior Tibial Artery, Right **S** Posterior Tibial Artery, Left **T** Peroneal Artery, Right **U** Peroneal Artery, Left **V** Foot Artery, Right **W** Foot Artery, Left **Y** Lower Artery	**0** Open **3** Percutaneous **4** Percutaneous Endoscopic	**7** Autologous Tissue Substitute **J** Synthetic Substitute **K** Nonautologous Tissue Substitute	**Z** No Qualifier

Section 0 **Medical and Surgical**
Body System 4 **Lower Arteries**
Operation V **Restriction:** Partially closing an orifice or the lumen of a tubular body part

Body Part (4th)	Approach (5th)	Device (6th)	Qualifier (7th)
0 Abdominal Aorta	**0** Open **3** Percutaneous **4** Percutaneous Endoscopic	**C** Extraluminal Device **Z** No Device	**Z** No Qualifier
0 Abdominal Aorta	**0** Open **3** Percutaneous **4** Percutaneous Endoscopic	**D** Intraluminal Device	**J** Temporary **Z** No Qualifier

Continued →

ection 0 **Medical and Surgical**
ody System 4 **Lower Arteries**
peration V **Restriction:** Partially closing an orifice or the lumen of a tubular body part

Body Part (4th)	Approach (5th)	Device (6th)	Qualifier (7th)
1 Celiac Artery **2** Gastric Artery **3** Hepatic Artery **4** Splenic Artery **5** Superior Mesenteric Artery **6** Colic Artery, Right **7** Colic Artery, Left **8** Colic Artery, Middle **9** Renal Artery, Right **A** Renal Artery, Left **B** Inferior Mesenteric Artery **C** Common Iliac Artery, Right **D** Common Iliac Artery, Left **E** Internal Iliac Artery, Right **F** Internal Iliac Artery, Left **H** External Iliac Artery, Right **J** External Iliac Artery, Left **K** Femoral Artery, Right **L** Femoral Artery, Left **M** Popliteal Artery, Right **N** Popliteal Artery, Left **P** Anterior Tibial Artery, Right **Q** Anterior Tibial Artery, Left **R** Posterior Tibial Artery, Right **S** Posterior Tibial Artery, Left **T** Peroneal Artery, Right **U** Peroneal Artery, Left **V** Foot Artery, Right **W** Foot Artery, Left **Y** Lower Artery	**0** Open **3** Percutaneous **4** Percutaneous Endoscopic	**C** Extraluminal Device **D** Intraluminal Device **Z** No Device	**Z** No Qualifier

ection 0 **Medical and Surgical**
ody System 4 **Lower Arteries**
peration W **Revision:** Correcting, to the extent possible, a portion of a malfunctioning device or the position of a displaced device

Body Part (4th)	Approach (5th)	Device (6th)	Qualifier (7th)
Y Lower Artery	**0** Open **3** Percutaneous **4** Percutaneous Endoscopic **X** External	**0** Drainage Device **2** Monitoring Device **3** Infusion Device **7** Autologous Tissue Substitute **C** Extraluminal Device **D** Intraluminal Device **J** Synthetic Substitute **K** Nonautologous Tissue Substitute	**Z** No Qualifier

ower Arteries Code Listing 041–04W

41 – Lower Arteries, Bypass

eview Coding Guideline B3.6a

410090 Bypass Abdominal Aorta to Abdominal Aorta with Autologous Venous Tissue, Open Approach

410091 Bypass Abdominal Aorta to Celiac Artery with Autologous Venous Tissue, Open Approach

410092 Bypass Abdominal Aorta to Mesenteric Artery with Autologous Venous Tissue, Open Approach

410093 Bypass Abdominal Aorta to Right Renal Artery with Autologous Venous Tissue, Open Approach

0410094 Bypass Abdominal Aorta to Left Renal Artery with Autologous Venous Tissue, Open Approach

0410095 Bypass Abdominal Aorta to Bilateral Renal Artery with Autologous Venous Tissue, Open Approach

0410096 Bypass Abdominal Aorta to Right Common Iliac Artery with Autologous Venous Tissue, Open Approach

0410097 Bypass Abdominal Aorta to Left Common Iliac Artery with Autologous Venous Tissue, Open Approach

0410098 Bypass Abdominal Aorta to Bilateral Common Iliac Arteries with Autologous Venous Tissue, Open Approach

0410099 Bypass Abdominal Aorta to Right Internal Iliac Artery with Autologous Venous Tissue, Open Approach

041009B Bypass Abdominal Aorta to Left Internal Iliac Artery with Autologous Venous Tissue, Open Approach

041009C Bypass Abdominal Aorta to Bilateral Internal Iliac Arteries with Autologous Venous Tissue, Open Approach

041009D Bypass Abdominal Aorta to Right External Iliac Artery with Autologous Venous Tissue, Open Approach

041009F Bypass Abdominal Aorta to Left External Iliac Artery with Autologous Venous Tissue, Open Approach

041009G Bypass Abdominal Aorta to Bilateral External Iliac Arteries with Autologous Venous Tissue, Open Approach

041009H Bypass Abdominal Aorta to Right Femoral Artery with Autologous Venous Tissue, Open Approach

041009J Bypass Abdominal Aorta to Left Femoral Artery with Autologous Venous Tissue, Open Approach

041009K Bypass Abdominal Aorta to Bilateral Femoral Arteries with Autologous Venous Tissue, Open Approach

041009Q Bypass Abdominal Aorta to Lower Extremity Artery with Autologous Venous Tissue, Open Approach

041009R Bypass Abdominal Aorta to Lower Artery with Autologous Venous Tissue, Open Approach

04100A0 Bypass Abdominal Aorta to Abdominal Aorta with Autologous Arterial Tissue, Open Approach

04100A1 Bypass Abdominal Aorta to Celiac Artery with Autologous Arterial Tissue, Open Approach

04100A2 Bypass Abdominal Aorta to Mesenteric Artery with Autologous Arterial Tissue, Open Approach

04100A3 Bypass Abdominal Aorta to Right Renal Artery with Autologous Arterial Tissue, Open Approach

04100A4 Bypass Abdominal Aorta to Left Renal Artery with Autologous Arterial Tissue, Open Approach

04100A5 Bypass Abdominal Aorta to Bilateral Renal Artery with Autologous Arterial Tissue, Open Approach

04100A6 Bypass Abdominal Aorta to Right Common Iliac Artery with Autologous Arterial Tissue, Open Approach

04100A7 Bypass Abdominal Aorta to Left Common Iliac Artery with Autologous Arterial Tissue, Open Approach

04100A8 Bypass Abdominal Aorta to Bilateral Common Iliac Arteries with Autologous Arterial Tissue, Open Approach

04100A9 Bypass Abdominal Aorta to Right Internal Iliac Artery with Autologous Arterial Tissue, Open Approach

04100AB Bypass Abdominal Aorta to Left Internal Iliac Artery with Autologous Arterial Tissue, Open Approach

04100AC Bypass Abdominal Aorta to Bilateral Internal Iliac Arteries with Autologous Arterial Tissue, Open Approach

04100AD Bypass Abdominal Aorta to Right External Iliac Artery with Autologous Arterial Tissue, Open Approach

04100AF Bypass Abdominal Aorta to Left External Iliac Artery with Autologous Arterial Tissue, Open Approach

04100AG Bypass Abdominal Aorta to Bilateral External Iliac Arteries with Autologous Arterial Tissue, Open Approach

04100AH Bypass Abdominal Aorta to Right Femoral Artery with Autologous Arterial Tissue, Open Approach

04100AJ Bypass Abdominal Aorta to Left Femoral Artery with Autologous Arterial Tissue, Open Approach

04100AK Bypass Abdominal Aorta to Bilateral Femoral Arteries with Autologous Arterial Tissue, Open Approach

04100AQ Bypass Abdominal Aorta to Lower Extremity Artery with Autologous Arterial Tissue, Open Approach

04100AR Bypass Abdominal Aorta to Lower Artery with Autologous Arterial Tissue, Open Approach

04100J0 Bypass Abdominal Aorta to Abdominal Aorta with Synthetic Substitute, Open Approach

04100J1 Bypass Abdominal Aorta to Celiac Artery with Synthetic Substitute, Open Approach

04100J2 Bypass Abdominal Aorta to Mesenteric Artery with Synthetic Substitute, Open Approach

04100J3 Bypass Abdominal Aorta to Right Renal Artery with Synthetic Substitute, Open Approach

04100J4 Bypass Abdominal Aorta to Left Renal Artery with Synthetic Substitute, Open Approach

04100J5 Bypass Abdominal Aorta to Bilateral Renal Artery with Synthetic Substitute, Open Approach

04100J6 Bypass Abdominal Aorta to Right Common Iliac Artery with Synthetic Substitute, Open Approach

04100J7 Bypass Abdominal Aorta to Left Common Iliac Artery with Synthetic Substitute, Open Approach

04100J8 Bypass Abdominal Aorta to Bilateral Common Iliac Arteries with Synthetic Substitute, Open Approach

04100J9 Bypass Abdominal Aorta to Right Internal Iliac Artery with Synthetic Substitute, Open Approach

04100JB Bypass Abdominal Aorta to Left Internal Iliac Artery with Synthetic Substitute, Open Approach

04100JC Bypass Abdominal Aorta to Bilateral Internal Iliac Arteries with Synthetic Substitute, Open Approach

04100JD Bypass Abdominal Aorta to Right External Iliac Artery with Synthetic Substitute, Open Approach

04100JF Bypass Abdominal Aorta to Left External Iliac Artery with Synthetic Substitute, Open Approach

04100JG Bypass Abdominal Aorta to Bilateral External Iliac Arteries with Synthetic Substitute, Open Approach

04100JH Bypass Abdominal Aorta to Right Femoral Artery with Synthetic Substitute, Open Approach

04100JJ Bypass Abdominal Aorta to Left Femoral Artery with Synthetic Substitute, Open Approach

04100JK Bypass Abdominal Aorta to Bilateral Femoral Arteries with Synthetic Substitute, Open Approach

04100JQ Bypass Abdominal Aorta to Lower Extremity Artery with Synthetic Substitute, Open Approach

04100JR Bypass Abdominal Aorta to Lower Artery with Synthetic Substitute, Open Approach

04100K0 Bypass Abdominal Aorta to Abdominal Aorta with Nonautologous Tissue Substitute, Open Approach

04100K1 Bypass Abdominal Aorta to Celiac Artery with Nonautologous Tissue Substitute, Open Approach

04100K2 Bypass Abdominal Aorta to Mesenteric Artery with Nonautologous Tissue Substitute, Open Approach

04100K3 Bypass Abdominal Aorta to Right Renal Artery with Nonautologous Tissue Substitute, Open Approach

04100K4 Bypass Abdominal Aorta to Left Renal Artery with Nonautologous Tissue Substitute, Open Approach

04100K5 Bypass Abdominal Aorta to Bilateral Renal Artery with Nonautologous Tissue Substitute, Open Approach

04100K6 Bypass Abdominal Aorta to Right Common Iliac Artery with Nonautologou Tissue Substitute, Open Approach

04100K7 Bypass Abdominal Aorta to Left Commo Iliac Artery with Nonautologous Tissue Substitute, Open Approach

04100K8 Bypass Abdominal Aorta to Bilateral Common Iliac Arteries with Nonautologous Tissue Substitute, Open Approach

04100K9 Bypass Abdominal Aorta to Right Interna Iliac Artery with Nonautologous Tissue Substitute, Open Approach

04100KB Bypass Abdominal Aorta to Left Internal Iliac Artery with Nonautologous Tissue Substitute, Open Approach

04100KC Bypass Abdominal Aorta to Bilateral Internal Iliac Arteries with Nonautologous Tissue Substitute, Open Approach

04100KD Bypass Abdominal Aorta to Right Extern Iliac Artery with Nonautologous Tissue Substitute, Open Approach

04100KF Bypass Abdominal Aorta to Left External Iliac Artery with Nonautologous Tissue Substitute, Open Approach

04100KG Bypass Abdominal Aorta to Bilateral External Iliac Arteries with Nonautologou Tissue Substitute, Open Approach

04100KH Bypass Abdominal Aorta to Right Femora Artery with Nonautologous Tissue Substitute, Open Approach

04100KJ Bypass Abdominal Aorta to Left Femoral Artery with Nonautologous Tissue Substitute, Open Approach

04100KK Bypass Abdominal Aorta to Bilateral Femoral Arteries with Nonautologous Tissue Substitute, Open Approach

04100KQ Bypass Abdominal Aorta to Lower Extremity Artery with Nonautologous Tissue Substitute, Open Approach

04100KR Bypass Abdominal Aorta to Lower Artery with Nonautologous Tissue Substitute, Open Approach

04100Z0 Bypass Abdominal Aorta to Abdominal Aorta, Open Approach

04100Z1 Bypass Abdominal Aorta to Celiac Artery Open Approach

04100Z2 Bypass Abdominal Aorta to Mesenteric Artery, Open Approach

04100Z3 Bypass Abdominal Aorta to Right Renal Artery, Open Approach

04100Z4 Bypass Abdominal Aorta to Left Renal Artery, Open Approach

04100Z5 Bypass Abdominal Aorta to Bilateral Renal Artery, Open Approach

04100Z6 Bypass Abdominal Aorta to Right Common Iliac Artery, Open Approach

04100Z7 Bypass Abdominal Aorta to Left Commor Iliac Artery, Open Approach

04100Z8 Bypass Abdominal Aorta to Bilateral Common Iliac Arteries, Open Approach

04100Z9 Bypass Abdominal Aorta to Right Internal Iliac Artery, Open Approach

04100ZB Bypass Abdominal Aorta to Left Internal Iliac Artery, Open Approach

04100ZC Bypass Abdominal Aorta to Bilateral Internal Iliac Arteries, Open Approach

4100ZD Bypass Abdominal Aorta to Right External Iliac Artery, Open Approach

4100ZF Bypass Abdominal Aorta to Left External Iliac Artery, Open Approach

4100ZG Bypass Abdominal Aorta to Bilateral External Iliac Arteries, Open Approach

4100ZH Bypass Abdominal Aorta to Right Femoral Artery, Open Approach

4100ZJ Bypass Abdominal Aorta to Left Femoral Artery, Open Approach

4100ZK Bypass Abdominal Aorta to Bilateral Femoral Arteries, Open Approach

4100ZQ Bypass Abdominal Aorta to Lower Extremity Artery, Open Approach

4100ZR Bypass Abdominal Aorta to Lower Artery, Open Approach

410490 Bypass Abdominal Aorta to Abdominal Aorta with Autologous Venous Tissue, Percutaneous Endoscopic Approach

410491 Bypass Abdominal Aorta to Celiac Artery with Autologous Venous Tissue, Percutaneous Endoscopic Approach

410492 Bypass Abdominal Aorta to Mesenteric Artery with Autologous Venous Tissue, Percutaneous Endoscopic Approach

410493 Bypass Abdominal Aorta to Right Renal Artery with Autologous Venous Tissue, Percutaneous Endoscopic Approach

410494 Bypass Abdominal Aorta to Left Renal Artery with Autologous Venous Tissue, Percutaneous Endoscopic Approach

410495 Bypass Abdominal Aorta to Bilateral Renal Artery with Autologous Venous Tissue, Percutaneous Endoscopic Approach

410496 Bypass Abdominal Aorta to Right Common Iliac Artery with Autologous Venous Tissue, Percutaneous Endoscopic Approach

410497 Bypass Abdominal Aorta to Left Common Iliac Artery with Autologous Venous Tissue, Percutaneous Endoscopic Approach

410498 Bypass Abdominal Aorta to Bilateral Common Iliac Arteries with Autologous Venous Tissue, Percutaneous Endoscopic Approach

410499 Bypass Abdominal Aorta to Right Internal Iliac Artery with Autologous Venous Tissue, Percutaneous Endoscopic Approach

41049B Bypass Abdominal Aorta to Left Internal Iliac Artery with Autologous Venous Tissue, Percutaneous Endoscopic Approach

41049C Bypass Abdominal Aorta to Bilateral Internal Iliac Arteries with Autologous Venous Tissue, Percutaneous Endoscopic Approach

41049D Bypass Abdominal Aorta to Right External Iliac Artery with Autologous Venous Tissue, Percutaneous Endoscopic Approach

41049F Bypass Abdominal Aorta to Left External Iliac Artery with Autologous Venous Tissue, Percutaneous Endoscopic Approach

41049G Bypass Abdominal Aorta to Bilateral External Iliac Arteries with Autologous Venous Tissue, Percutaneous Endoscopic Approach

41049H Bypass Abdominal Aorta to Right Femoral Artery with Autologous Venous Tissue, Percutaneous Endoscopic Approach

41049J Bypass Abdominal Aorta to Left Femoral Artery with Autologous Venous Tissue, Percutaneous Endoscopic Approach

041049K Bypass Abdominal Aorta to Bilateral Femoral Arteries with Autologous Venous Tissue, Percutaneous Endoscopic Approach

041049Q Bypass Abdominal Aorta to Lower Extremity Artery with Autologous Venous Tissue, Percutaneous Endoscopic Approach

041049R Bypass Abdominal Aorta to Lower Artery with Autologous Venous Tissue, Percutaneous Endoscopic Approach

04104A0 Bypass Abdominal Aorta to Abdominal Aorta with Autologous Arterial Tissue, Percutaneous Endoscopic Approach

04104A1 Bypass Abdominal Aorta to Celiac Artery with Autologous Arterial Tissue, Percutaneous Endoscopic Approach

04104A2 Bypass Abdominal Aorta to Mesenteric Artery with Autologous Arterial Tissue, Percutaneous Endoscopic Approach

04104A3 Bypass Abdominal Aorta to Right Renal Artery with Autologous Arterial Tissue, Percutaneous Endoscopic Approach

04104A4 Bypass Abdominal Aorta to Left Renal Artery with Autologous Arterial Tissue, Percutaneous Endoscopic Approach

04104A5 Bypass Abdominal Aorta to Bilateral Renal Artery with Autologous Arterial Tissue, Percutaneous Endoscopic Approach

04104A6 Bypass Abdominal Aorta to Right Common Iliac Artery with Autologous Arterial Tissue, Percutaneous Endoscopic Approach

04104A7 Bypass Abdominal Aorta to Left Common Iliac Artery with Autologous Arterial Tissue, Percutaneous Endoscopic Approach

04104A8 Bypass Abdominal Aorta to Bilateral Common Iliac Arteries with Autologous Arterial Tissue, Percutaneous Endoscopic Approach

04104A9 Bypass Abdominal Aorta to Right Internal Iliac Artery with Autologous Arterial Tissue, Percutaneous Endoscopic Approach

04104AB Bypass Abdominal Aorta to Left Internal Iliac Artery with Autologous Arterial Tissue, Percutaneous Endoscopic Approach

04104AC Bypass Abdominal Aorta to Bilateral Internal Iliac Arteries with Autologous Arterial Tissue, Percutaneous Endoscopic Approach

04104AD Bypass Abdominal Aorta to Right External Iliac Artery with Autologous Arterial Tissue, Percutaneous Endoscopic Approach

04104AF Bypass Abdominal Aorta to Left External Iliac Artery with Autologous Arterial Tissue, Percutaneous Endoscopic Approach

04104AG Bypass Abdominal Aorta to Bilateral External Iliac Arteries with Autologous Arterial Tissue, Percutaneous Endoscopic Approach

04104AH Bypass Abdominal Aorta to Right Femoral Artery with Autologous Arterial Tissue, Percutaneous Endoscopic Approach

04104AJ Bypass Abdominal Aorta to Left Femoral Artery with Autologous Arterial Tissue, Percutaneous Endoscopic Approach

04104AK Bypass Abdominal Aorta to Bilateral Femoral Arteries with Autologous Arterial Tissue, Percutaneous Endoscopic Approach

04104AQ Bypass Abdominal Aorta to Lower Extremity Artery with Autologous Arterial Tissue, Percutaneous Endoscopic Approach

04104AR Bypass Abdominal Aorta to Lower Artery with Autologous Arterial Tissue, Percutaneous Endoscopic Approach

04104J0 Bypass Abdominal Aorta to Abdominal Aorta with Synthetic Substitute, Percutaneous Endoscopic Approach

04104J1 Bypass Abdominal Aorta to Celiac Artery with Synthetic Substitute, Percutaneous Endoscopic Approach

04104J2 Bypass Abdominal Aorta to Mesenteric Artery with Synthetic Substitute, Percutaneous Endoscopic Approach

04104J3 Bypass Abdominal Aorta to Right Renal Artery with Synthetic Substitute, Percutaneous Endoscopic Approach

04104J4 Bypass Abdominal Aorta to Left Renal Artery with Synthetic Substitute, Percutaneous Endoscopic Approach

04104J5 Bypass Abdominal Aorta to Bilateral Renal Artery with Synthetic Substitute, Percutaneous Endoscopic Approach

04104J6 Bypass Abdominal Aorta to Right Common Iliac Artery with Synthetic Substitute, Percutaneous Endoscopic Approach

04104J7 Bypass Abdominal Aorta to Left Common Iliac Artery with Synthetic Substitute, Percutaneous Endoscopic Approach

04104J8 Bypass Abdominal Aorta to Bilateral Common Iliac Arteries with Synthetic Substitute, Percutaneous Endoscopic Approach

04104J9 Bypass Abdominal Aorta to Right Internal Iliac Artery with Synthetic Substitute, Percutaneous Endoscopic Approach

04104JB Bypass Abdominal Aorta to Left Internal Iliac Artery with Synthetic Substitute, Percutaneous Endoscopic Approach

04104JC Bypass Abdominal Aorta to Bilateral Internal Iliac Arteries with Synthetic Substitute, Percutaneous Endoscopic Approach

04104JD Bypass Abdominal Aorta to Right External Iliac Artery with Synthetic Substitute, Percutaneous Endoscopic Approach

04104JF Bypass Abdominal Aorta to Left External Iliac Artery with Synthetic Substitute, Percutaneous Endoscopic Approach

04104JG Bypass Abdominal Aorta to Bilateral External Iliac Arteries with Synthetic Substitute, Percutaneous Endoscopic Approach

04104JH Bypass Abdominal Aorta to Right Femoral Artery with Synthetic Substitute, Percutaneous Endoscopic Approach

04104JJ Bypass Abdominal Aorta to Left Femoral Artery with Synthetic Substitute, Percutaneous Endoscopic Approach

04104JK Bypass Abdominal Aorta to Bilateral Femoral Arteries with Synthetic Substitute, Percutaneous Endoscopic Approach

04104JQ Bypass Abdominal Aorta to Lower Extremity Artery with Synthetic Substitute, Percutaneous Endoscopic Approach

04104JR Bypass Abdominal Aorta to Lower Artery with Synthetic Substitute, Percutaneous Endoscopic Approach

04104K0 Bypass Abdominal Aorta to Abdominal Aorta with Nonautologous Tissue Substitute, Percutaneous Endoscopic Approach

04104K1 Bypass Abdominal Aorta to Celiac Artery with Nonautologous Tissue Substitute, Percutaneous Endoscopic Approach

04104K2 Bypass Abdominal Aorta to Mesenteric Artery with Nonautologous Tissue Substitute, Percutaneous Endoscopic Approach

04104K3 Bypass Abdominal Aorta to Right Renal Artery with Nonautologous Tissue Substitute, Percutaneous Endoscopic Approach

04104K4 Bypass Abdominal Aorta to Left Renal Artery with Nonautologous Tissue Substitute, Percutaneous Endoscopic Approach

04104K5 Bypass Abdominal Aorta to Bilateral Renal Artery with Nonautologous Tissue Substitute, Percutaneous Endoscopic Approach

04104K6 Bypass Abdominal Aorta to Right Common Iliac Artery with Nonautologous Tissue Substitute, Percutaneous Endoscopic Approach

04104K7 Bypass Abdominal Aorta to Left Common Iliac Artery with Nonautologous Tissue Substitute, Percutaneous Endoscopic Approach

04104K8 Bypass Abdominal Aorta to Bilateral Common Iliac Arteries with Nonautologous Tissue Substitute, Percutaneous Endoscopic Approach

04104K9 Bypass Abdominal Aorta to Right Internal Iliac Artery with Nonautologous Tissue Substitute, Percutaneous Endoscopic Approach

04104KB Bypass Abdominal Aorta to Left Internal Iliac Artery with Nonautologous Tissue Substitute, Percutaneous Endoscopic Approach

04104KC Bypass Abdominal Aorta to Bilateral Internal Iliac Arteries with Nonautologous Tissue Substitute, Percutaneous Endoscopic Approach

04104KD Bypass Abdominal Aorta to Right External Iliac Artery with Nonautologous Tissue Substitute, Percutaneous Endoscopic Approach

04104KF Bypass Abdominal Aorta to Left External Iliac Artery with Nonautologous Tissue Substitute, Percutaneous Endoscopic Approach

04104KG Bypass Abdominal Aorta to Bilateral External Iliac Arteries with Nonautologous Tissue Substitute, Percutaneous Endoscopic Approach

04104KH Bypass Abdominal Aorta to Right Femoral Artery with Nonautologous Tissue Substitute, Percutaneous Endoscopic Approach

04104KJ Bypass Abdominal Aorta to Left Femoral Artery with Nonautologous Tissue Substitute, Percutaneous Endoscopic Approach

04104KK Bypass Abdominal Aorta to Bilateral Femoral Arteries with Nonautologous Tissue Substitute, Percutaneous Endoscopic Approach

04104KQ Bypass Abdominal Aorta to Lower Extremity Artery with Nonautologous Tissue Substitute, Percutaneous Endoscopic Approach

04104KR Bypass Abdominal Aorta to Lower Artery with Nonautologous Tissue Substitute, Percutaneous Endoscopic Approach

04104Z0 Bypass Abdominal Aorta to Abdominal Aorta, Percutaneous Endoscopic Approach

04104Z1 Bypass Abdominal Aorta to Celiac Artery, Percutaneous Endoscopic Approach

04104Z2 Bypass Abdominal Aorta to Mesenteric Artery, Percutaneous Endoscopic Approach

04104Z3 Bypass Abdominal Aorta to Right Renal Artery, Percutaneous Endoscopic Approach

04104Z4 Bypass Abdominal Aorta to Left Renal Artery, Percutaneous Endoscopic Approach

04104Z5 Bypass Abdominal Aorta to Bilateral Renal Artery, Percutaneous Endoscopic Approach

04104Z6 Bypass Abdominal Aorta to Right Common Iliac Artery, Percutaneous Endoscopic Approach

04104Z7 Bypass Abdominal Aorta to Left Common Iliac Artery, Percutaneous Endoscopic Approach

04104Z8 Bypass Abdominal Aorta to Bilateral Common Iliac Arteries, Percutaneous Endoscopic Approach

04104Z9 Bypass Abdominal Aorta to Right Internal Iliac Artery, Percutaneous Endoscopic Approach

04104ZB Bypass Abdominal Aorta to Left Internal Iliac Artery, Percutaneous Endoscopic Approach

04104ZC Bypass Abdominal Aorta to Bilateral Internal Iliac Arteries, Percutaneous Endoscopic Approach

04104ZD Bypass Abdominal Aorta to Right External Iliac Artery, Percutaneous Endoscopic Approach

04104ZF Bypass Abdominal Aorta to Left External Iliac Artery, Percutaneous Endoscopic Approach

04104ZG Bypass Abdominal Aorta to Bilateral External Iliac Arteries, Percutaneous Endoscopic Approach

04104ZH Bypass Abdominal Aorta to Right Femoral Artery, Percutaneous Endoscopic Approach

04104ZJ Bypass Abdominal Aorta to Left Femoral Artery, Percutaneous Endoscopic Approach

04104ZK Bypass Abdominal Aorta to Bilateral Femoral Arteries, Percutaneous Endoscopic Approach

04104ZQ Bypass Abdominal Aorta to Lower Extremity Artery, Percutaneous Endoscopic Approach

04104ZR Bypass Abdominal Aorta to Lower Artery, Percutaneous Endoscopic Approach

0414093 Bypass Splenic Artery to Right Renal Artery with Autologous Venous Tissue, Open Approach

0414094 Bypass Splenic Artery to Left Renal Artery with Autologous Venous Tissue, Open Approach

0414095 Bypass Splenic Artery to Bilateral Renal Artery with Autologous Venous Tissue, Open Approach

04140A3 Bypass Splenic Artery to Right Renal Artery with Autologous Arterial Tissue, Open Approach

04140A4 Bypass Splenic Artery to Left Renal Artery with Autologous Arterial Tissue, Open Approach

04140A5 Bypass Splenic Artery to Bilateral Renal Artery with Autologous Arterial Tissue, Open Approach

04140J3 Bypass Splenic Artery to Right Renal Artery with Synthetic Substitute, Open Approach

04140J4 Bypass Splenic Artery to Left Renal Artery with Synthetic Substitute, Open Approach

04140J5 Bypass Splenic Artery to Bilateral Renal Artery with Synthetic Substitute, Open Approach

04140K3 Bypass Splenic Artery to Right Renal Artery with Nonautologous Tissue Substitute, Open Approach

04140K4 Bypass Splenic Artery to Left Renal Artery with Nonautologous Tissue Substitute, Open Approach

04140K5 Bypass Splenic Artery to Bilateral Renal Artery with Nonautologous Tissue Substitute, Open Approach

04140Z3 Bypass Splenic Artery to Right Renal Artery, Open Approach

04140Z4 Bypass Splenic Artery to Left Renal Artery, Open Approach

04140Z5 Bypass Splenic Artery to Bilateral Renal Artery, Open Approach

414493 Bypass Splenic Artery to Right Renal Artery with Autologous Venous Tissue, Percutaneous Endoscopic Approach

0414494 Bypass Splenic Artery to Left Renal Artery with Autologous Venous Tissue, Percutaneous Endoscopic Approach

0414495 Bypass Splenic Artery to Bilateral Renal Artery with Autologous Venous Tissue, Percutaneous Endoscopic Approach

04144A3 Bypass Splenic Artery to Right Renal Artery with Autologous Arterial Tissue, Percutaneous Endoscopic Approach

04144A4 Bypass Splenic Artery to Left Renal Artery with Autologous Arterial Tissue, Percutaneous Endoscopic Approach

04144A5 Bypass Splenic Artery to Bilateral Renal Artery with Autologous Arterial Tissue, Percutaneous Endoscopic Approach

04144J3 Bypass Splenic Artery to Right Renal Artery with Synthetic Substitute, Percutaneous Endoscopic Approach

04144J4 Bypass Splenic Artery to Left Renal Artery with Synthetic Substitute, Percutaneous Endoscopic Approach

04144J5 Bypass Splenic Artery to Bilateral Renal Artery with Synthetic Substitute, Percutaneous Endoscopic Approach

04144K3 Bypass Splenic Artery to Right Renal Artery with Nonautologous Tissue Substitute, Percutaneous Endoscopic Approach

04144K4 Bypass Splenic Artery to Left Renal Artery with Nonautologous Tissue Substitute, Percutaneous Endoscopic Approach

04144K5 Bypass Splenic Artery to Bilateral Renal Artery with Nonautologous Tissue Substitute, Percutaneous Endoscopic Approach

04144Z3 Bypass Splenic Artery to Right Renal Artery, Percutaneous Endoscopic Approach

04144Z4 Bypass Splenic Artery to Left Renal Artery, Percutaneous Endoscopic Approach

04144Z5 Bypass Splenic Artery to Bilateral Renal Artery, Percutaneous Endoscopic Approach

041C090 Bypass Right Common Iliac Artery to Abdominal Aorta with Autologous Venous Tissue, Open Approach

041C091 Bypass Right Common Iliac Artery to Celiac Artery with Autologous Venous Tissue, Open Approach

041C092 Bypass Right Common Iliac Artery to Mesenteric Artery with Autologous Venous Tissue, Open Approach

041C093 Bypass Right Common Iliac Artery to Right Renal Artery with Autologous Venous Tissue, Open Approach

041C094 Bypass Right Common Iliac Artery to Left Renal Artery with Autologous Venous Tissue, Open Approach

41C095 Bypass Right Common Iliac Artery to Bilateral Renal Artery with Autologous Venous Tissue, Open Approach

41C096 Bypass Right Common Iliac Artery to Right Common Iliac Artery with Autologous Venous Tissue, Open Approach

41C097 Bypass Right Common Iliac Artery to Left Common Iliac Artery with Autologous Venous Tissue, Open Approach

41C098 Bypass Right Common Iliac Artery to Bilateral Common Iliac Arteries with Autologous Venous Tissue, Open Approach

41C099 Bypass Right Common Iliac Artery to Right Internal Iliac Artery with Autologous Venous Tissue, Open Approach

41C09B Bypass Right Common Iliac Artery to Left Internal Iliac Artery with Autologous Venous Tissue, Open Approach

41C09C Bypass Right Common Iliac Artery to Bilateral Internal Iliac Arteries with Autologous Venous Tissue, Open Approach

41C09D Bypass Right Common Iliac Artery to Right External Iliac Artery with Autologous Venous Tissue, Open Approach

41C09F Bypass Right Common Iliac Artery to Left External Iliac Artery with Autologous Venous Tissue, Open Approach

41C09G Bypass Right Common Iliac Artery to Bilateral External Iliac Arteries with Autologous Venous Tissue, Open Approach

41C09H Bypass Right Common Iliac Artery to Right Femoral Artery with Autologous Venous Tissue, Open Approach

41C09J Bypass Right Common Iliac Artery to Left Femoral Artery with Autologous Venous Tissue, Open Approach

41C09K Bypass Right Common Iliac Artery to Bilateral Femoral Arteries with Autologous Venous Tissue, Open Approach

41C09Q Bypass Right Common Iliac Artery to Lower Extremity Artery with Autologous Venous Tissue, Open Approach

41C09R Bypass Right Common Iliac Artery to Lower Artery with Autologous Venous Tissue, Open Approach

41C0A0 Bypass Right Common Iliac Artery to Abdominal Aorta with Autologous Arterial Tissue, Open Approach

41C0A1 Bypass Right Common Iliac Artery to Celiac Artery with Autologous Arterial Tissue, Open Approach

41C0A2 Bypass Right Common Iliac Artery to Mesenteric Artery with Autologous Arterial Tissue, Open Approach

41C0A3 Bypass Right Common Iliac Artery to Right Renal Artery with Autologous Arterial Tissue, Open Approach

41C0A4 Bypass Right Common Iliac Artery to Left Renal Artery with Autologous Arterial Tissue, Open Approach

41C0A5 Bypass Right Common Iliac Artery to Bilateral Renal Artery with Autologous Arterial Tissue, Open Approach

41C0A6 Bypass Right Common Iliac Artery to Right Common Iliac Artery with Autologous Arterial Tissue, Open Approach

41C0A7 Bypass Right Common Iliac Artery to Left Common Iliac Artery with Autologous Arterial Tissue, Open Approach

41C0A8 Bypass Right Common Iliac Artery to Bilateral Common Iliac Arteries with Autologous Arterial Tissue, Open Approach

041C0A9 Bypass Right Common Iliac Artery to Right Internal Iliac Artery with Autologous Arterial Tissue, Open Approach

041C0AB Bypass Right Common Iliac Artery to Left Internal Iliac Artery with Autologous Arterial Tissue, Open Approach

041C0AC Bypass Right Common Iliac Artery to Bilateral Internal Iliac Arteries with Autologous Arterial Tissue, Open Approach

041C0AD Bypass Right Common Iliac Artery to Right External Iliac Artery with Autologous Arterial Tissue, Open Approach

041C0AF Bypass Right Common Iliac Artery to Left External Iliac Artery with Autologous Arterial Tissue, Open Approach

041C0AG Bypass Right Common Iliac Artery to Bilateral External Iliac Arteries with Autologous Arterial Tissue, Open Approach

041C0AH Bypass Right Common Iliac Artery to Right Femoral Artery with Autologous Arterial Tissue, Open Approach

041C0AJ Bypass Right Common Iliac Artery to Left Femoral Artery with Autologous Arterial Tissue, Open Approach

041C0AK Bypass Right Common Iliac Artery to Bilateral Femoral Arteries with Autologous Arterial Tissue, Open Approach

041C0AQ Bypass Right Common Iliac Artery to Lower Extremity Artery with Autologous Arterial Tissue, Open Approach

041C0AR Bypass Right Common Iliac Artery to Lower Artery with Autologous Arterial Tissue, Open Approach

041C0J0 Bypass Right Common Iliac Artery to Abdominal Aorta with Synthetic Substitute, Open Approach

041C0J1 Bypass Right Common Iliac Artery to Celiac Artery with Synthetic Substitute, Open Approach

041C0J2 Bypass Right Common Iliac Artery to Mesenteric Artery with Synthetic Substitute, Open Approach

041C0J3 Bypass Right Common Iliac Artery to Right Renal Artery with Synthetic Substitute, Open Approach

041C0J4 Bypass Right Common Iliac Artery to Left Renal Artery with Synthetic Substitute, Open Approach

041C0J5 Bypass Right Common Iliac Artery to Bilateral Renal Artery with Synthetic Substitute, Open Approach

041C0J6 Bypass Right Common Iliac Artery to Right Common Iliac Artery with Synthetic Substitute, Open Approach

041C0J7 Bypass Right Common Iliac Artery to Left Common Iliac Artery with Synthetic Substitute, Open Approach

041C0J8 Bypass Right Common Iliac Artery to Bilateral Common Iliac Arteries with Synthetic Substitute, Open Approach

041C0J9 Bypass Right Common Iliac Artery to Right Internal Iliac Artery with Synthetic Substitute, Open Approach

041C0JB Bypass Right Common Iliac Artery to Left Internal Iliac Artery with Synthetic Substitute, Open Approach

041C0JC Bypass Right Common Iliac Artery to Bilateral Internal Iliac Arteries with Synthetic Substitute, Open Approach

041C0JD Bypass Right Common Iliac Artery to Right External Iliac Artery with Synthetic Substitute, Open Approach

041C0JF Bypass Right Common Iliac Artery to Left External Iliac Artery with Synthetic Substitute, Open Approach

041C0JG Bypass Right Common Iliac Artery to Bilateral External Iliac Arteries with Synthetic Substitute, Open Approach

041C0JH Bypass Right Common Iliac Artery to Right Femoral Artery with Synthetic Substitute, Open Approach

041C0JJ Bypass Right Common Iliac Artery to Left Femoral Artery with Synthetic Substitute, Open Approach

041C0JK Bypass Right Common Iliac Artery to Bilateral Femoral Arteries with Synthetic Substitute, Open Approach

041C0JQ Bypass Right Common Iliac Artery to Lower Extremity Artery with Synthetic Substitute, Open Approach

041C0JR Bypass Right Common Iliac Artery to Lower Artery with Synthetic Substitute, Open Approach

041C0K0 Bypass Right Common Iliac Artery to Abdominal Aorta with Nonautologous Tissue Substitute, Open Approach

041C0K1 Bypass Right Common Iliac Artery to Celiac Artery with Nonautologous Tissue Substitute, Open Approach

041C0K2 Bypass Right Common Iliac Artery to Mesenteric Artery with Nonautologous Tissue Substitute, Open Approach

041C0K3 Bypass Right Common Iliac Artery to Right Renal Artery with Nonautologous Tissue Substitute, Open Approach

041C0K4 Bypass Right Common Iliac Artery to Left Renal Artery with Nonautologous Tissue Substitute, Open Approach

041C0K5 Bypass Right Common Iliac Artery to Bilateral Renal Artery with Nonautologous Tissue Substitute, Open Approach

041C0K6 Bypass Right Common Iliac Artery to Right Common Iliac Artery with Nonautologous Tissue Substitute, Open Approach

041C0K7 Bypass Right Common Iliac Artery to Left Common Iliac Artery with Nonautologous Tissue Substitute, Open Approach

041C0K8 Bypass Right Common Iliac Artery to Bilateral Common Iliac Arteries with Nonautologous Tissue Substitute, Open Approach

041C0K9 Bypass Right Common Iliac Artery to Right Internal Iliac Artery with Nonautologous Tissue Substitute, Open Approach

041C0KB Bypass Right Common Iliac Artery to Left Internal Iliac Artery with Nonautologous Tissue Substitute, Open Approach

041C0KC Bypass Right Common Iliac Artery to Bilateral Internal Iliac Arteries with Nonautologous Tissue Substitute, Open Approach

041C0KD Bypass Right Common Iliac Artery to Right External Iliac Artery with Nonautologous Tissue Substitute, Open Approach

041C0KF Bypass Right Common Iliac Artery to Left External Iliac Artery with Nonautologous Tissue Substitute, Open Approach

041C0KG Bypass Right Common Iliac Artery to Bilateral External Iliac Arteries with Nonautologous Tissue Substitute, Open Approach

041C0KH Bypass Right Common Iliac Artery to Right Femoral Artery with Nonautologous Tissue Substitute, Open Approach

041C0KJ Bypass Right Common Iliac Artery to Left Femoral Artery with Nonautologous Tissue Substitute, Open Approach

041C0KK Bypass Right Common Iliac Artery to Bilateral Femoral Arteries with Nonautologous Tissue Substitute, Open Approach

041C0KQ Bypass Right Common Iliac Artery to Lower Extremity Artery with Nonautologous Tissue Substitute, Open Approach

041C0KR Bypass Right Common Iliac Artery to Lower Artery with Nonautologous Tissue Substitute, Open Approach

041C0Z0 Bypass Right Common Iliac Artery to Abdominal Aorta, Open Approach

041C0Z1 Bypass Right Common Iliac Artery to Celiac Artery, Open Approach

041C0Z2 Bypass Right Common Iliac Artery to Mesenteric Artery, Open Approach

041C0Z3 Bypass Right Common Iliac Artery to Right Renal Artery, Open Approach

041C0Z4 Bypass Right Common Iliac Artery to Left Renal Artery, Open Approach

041C0Z5 Bypass Right Common Iliac Artery to Bilateral Renal Artery, Open Approach

041C0Z6 Bypass Right Common Iliac Artery to Right Common Iliac Artery, Open Approach

041C0Z7 Bypass Right Common Iliac Artery to Left Common Iliac Artery, Open Approach

041C0Z8 Bypass Right Common Iliac Artery to Bilateral Common Iliac Arteries, Open Approach

041C0Z9 Bypass Right Common Iliac Artery to Right Internal Iliac Artery, Open Approach

041C0ZB Bypass Right Common Iliac Artery to Left Internal Iliac Artery, Open Approach

041C0ZC Bypass Right Common Iliac Artery to Bilateral Internal Iliac Arteries, Open Approach

041C0ZD Bypass Right Common Iliac Artery to Right External Iliac Artery, Open Approach

041C0ZF Bypass Right Common Iliac Artery to Left External Iliac Artery, Open Approach

041C0ZG Bypass Right Common Iliac Artery to Bilateral External Iliac Arteries, Open Approach

041C0ZH Bypass Right Common Iliac Artery to Right Femoral Artery, Open Approach

041C0ZJ Bypass Right Common Iliac Artery to Left Femoral Artery, Open Approach

041C0ZK Bypass Right Common Iliac Artery to Bilateral Femoral Arteries, Open Approach

041C0ZQ Bypass Right Common Iliac Artery to Lower Extremity Artery, Open Approach

041C0ZR Bypass Right Common Iliac Artery to Lower Artery, Open Approach

041C490 Bypass Right Common Iliac Artery to Abdominal Aorta with Autologous Venous Tissue, Percutaneous Endoscopic Approach

041C491 Bypass Right Common Iliac Artery to Celiac Artery with Autologous Venous Tissue, Percutaneous Endoscopic Approach

041C492 Bypass Right Common Iliac Artery to Mesenteric Artery with Autologous Venous Tissue, Percutaneous Endoscopic Approach

041C493 Bypass Right Common Iliac Artery to Right Renal Artery with Autologous Venous Tissue, Percutaneous Endoscopic Approach

041C494 Bypass Right Common Iliac Artery to Left Renal Artery with Autologous Venous Tissue, Percutaneous Endoscopic Approach

041C495 Bypass Right Common Iliac Artery to Bilateral Renal Artery with Autologous Venous Tissue, Percutaneous Endoscopic Approach

041C496 Bypass Right Common Iliac Artery to Right Common Iliac Artery with Autologous Venous Tissue, Percutaneous Endoscopic Approach

041C497 Bypass Right Common Iliac Artery to Left Common Iliac Artery with Autologous Venous Tissue, Percutaneous Endoscopic Approach

041C498 Bypass Right Common Iliac Artery to Bilateral Common Iliac Arteries with Autologous Venous Tissue, Percutaneous Endoscopic Approach

041C499 Bypass Right Common Iliac Artery to Right Internal Iliac Artery with Autologous Venous Tissue, Percutaneous Endoscopic Approach

041C49B Bypass Right Common Iliac Artery to Left Internal Iliac Artery with Autologous Venous Tissue, Percutaneous Endoscopic Approach

041C49C Bypass Right Common Iliac Artery to Bilateral Internal Iliac Arteries with Autologous Venous Tissue, Percutaneous Endoscopic Approach

041C49D Bypass Right Common Iliac Artery to Right External Iliac Artery with Autologous Venous Tissue, Percutaneous Endoscopic Approach

041C49F Bypass Right Common Iliac Artery to Left External Iliac Artery with Autologous Venous Tissue, Percutaneous Endoscopic Approach

041C49G Bypass Right Common Iliac Artery to Bilateral External Iliac Arteries with Autologous Venous Tissue, Percutaneous Endoscopic Approach

041C49H Bypass Right Common Iliac Artery to Right Femoral Artery with Autologous Venous Tissue, Percutaneous Endoscopic Approach

041C49J Bypass Right Common Iliac Artery to Left Femoral Artery with Autologous Venous Tissue, Percutaneous Endoscopic Approach

041C49K Bypass Right Common Iliac Artery to Bilateral Femoral Arteries with Autologous Venous Tissue, Percutaneous Endoscopic Approach

041C49Q Bypass Right Common Iliac Artery to Lower Extremity Artery with Autologous Venous Tissue, Percutaneous Endoscopic Approach

041C49R Bypass Right Common Iliac Artery to Lower Artery with Autologous Venous Tissue, Percutaneous Endoscopic Approach

041C4A0 Bypass Right Common Iliac Artery to Abdominal Aorta with Autologous Arterial Tissue, Percutaneous Endoscopic Approach

041C4A1 Bypass Right Common Iliac Artery to Celiac Artery with Autologous Arterial Tissue, Percutaneous Endoscopic Approach

041C4A2 Bypass Right Common Iliac Artery to Mesenteric Artery with Autologous Arterial Tissue, Percutaneous Endoscopic Approach

041C4A3 Bypass Right Common Iliac Artery to Right Renal Artery with Autologous Arterial Tissue, Percutaneous Endoscopic Approach

041C4A4 Bypass Right Common Iliac Artery to Left Renal Artery with Autologous Arterial Tissue, Percutaneous Endoscopic Approach

041C4A5 Bypass Right Common Iliac Artery to Bilateral Renal Artery with Autologous Arterial Tissue, Percutaneous Endoscopic Approach

041C4A6 Bypass Right Common Iliac Artery to Right Common Iliac Artery with Autologous Arterial Tissue, Percutaneous Endoscopic Approach

041C4A7 Bypass Right Common Iliac Artery to Left Common Iliac Artery with Autologous Arterial Tissue, Percutaneous Endoscopic Approach

041C4A8 Bypass Right Common Iliac Artery to Bilateral Common Iliac Arteries with Autologous Arterial Tissue, Percutaneous Endoscopic Approach

041C4A9 Bypass Right Common Iliac Artery to Right Internal Iliac Artery with Autologous Arterial Tissue, Percutaneous Endoscopic Approach

041C4AB Bypass Right Common Iliac Artery to Left Internal Iliac Artery with Autologous Arterial Tissue, Percutaneous Endoscopic Approach

041C4AC Bypass Right Common Iliac Artery to Bilateral Internal Iliac Arteries with Autologous Arterial Tissue, Percutaneous Endoscopic Approach

041C4AD Bypass Right Common Iliac Artery to Right External Iliac Artery with Autologous Arterial Tissue, Percutaneous Endoscopic Approach

041C4AF Bypass Right Common Iliac Artery to Left External Iliac Artery with Autologous Arterial Tissue, Percutaneous Endoscopic Approach

041C4AG Bypass Right Common Iliac Artery to Bilateral External Iliac Arteries with Autologous Arterial Tissue, Percutaneous Endoscopic Approach

041C4AH Bypass Right Common Iliac Artery to Right Femoral Artery with Autologous Arterial Tissue, Percutaneous Endoscopic Approach

041C4AJ Bypass Right Common Iliac Artery to Left Femoral Artery with Autologous Arterial Tissue, Percutaneous Endoscopic Approach

041C4AK Bypass Right Common Iliac Artery to Bilateral Femoral Arteries with Autologous Arterial Tissue, Percutaneous Endoscopic Approach

041C4AQ Bypass Right Common Iliac Artery to Lower Extremity Artery with Autologous Arterial Tissue, Percutaneous Endoscopic Approach

041C4AR Bypass Right Common Iliac Artery to Lower Artery with Autologous Arterial Tissue, Percutaneous Endoscopic Approach

041C4J0 Bypass Right Common Iliac Artery to Abdominal Aorta with Synthetic Substitute, Percutaneous Endoscopic Approach

041C4J1 Bypass Right Common Iliac Artery to Celiac Artery with Synthetic Substitute, Percutaneous Endoscopic Approach

41C4J2 Bypass Right Common Iliac Artery to Mesenteric Artery with Synthetic Substitute, Percutaneous Endoscopic Approach

41C4J3 Bypass Right Common Iliac Artery to Right Renal Artery with Synthetic Substitute, Percutaneous Endoscopic Approach

41C4J4 Bypass Right Common Iliac Artery to Left Renal Artery with Synthetic Substitute, Percutaneous Endoscopic Approach

41C4J5 Bypass Right Common Iliac Artery to Bilateral Renal Artery with Synthetic Substitute, Percutaneous Endoscopic Approach

41C4J6 Bypass Right Common Iliac Artery to Right Common Iliac Artery with Synthetic Substitute, Percutaneous Endoscopic Approach

41C4J7 Bypass Right Common Iliac Artery to Left Common Iliac Artery with Synthetic Substitute, Percutaneous Endoscopic Approach

41C4J8 Bypass Right Common Iliac Artery to Bilateral Common Iliac Arteries with Synthetic Substitute, Percutaneous Endoscopic Approach

41C4J9 Bypass Right Common Iliac Artery to Right Internal Iliac Artery with Synthetic Substitute, Percutaneous Endoscopic Approach

41C4JB Bypass Right Common Iliac Artery to Left Internal Iliac Artery with Synthetic Substitute, Percutaneous Endoscopic Approach

41C4JC Bypass Right Common Iliac Artery to Bilateral Internal Iliac Arteries with Synthetic Substitute, Percutaneous Endoscopic Approach

41C4JD Bypass Right Common Iliac Artery to Right External Iliac Artery with Synthetic Substitute, Percutaneous Endoscopic Approach

41C4JF Bypass Right Common Iliac Artery to Left External Iliac Artery with Synthetic Substitute, Percutaneous Endoscopic Approach

41C4JG Bypass Right Common Iliac Artery to Bilateral External Iliac Arteries with Synthetic Substitute, Percutaneous Endoscopic Approach

41C4JH Bypass Right Common Iliac Artery to Right Femoral Artery with Synthetic Substitute, Percutaneous Endoscopic Approach

41C4JJ Bypass Right Common Iliac Artery to Left Femoral Artery with Synthetic Substitute, Percutaneous Endoscopic Approach

41C4JK Bypass Right Common Iliac Artery to Bilateral Femoral Arteries with Synthetic Substitute, Percutaneous Endoscopic Approach

41C4JQ Bypass Right Common Iliac Artery to Lower Extremity Artery with Synthetic Substitute, Percutaneous Endoscopic Approach

41C4JR Bypass Right Common Iliac Artery to Lower Artery with Synthetic Substitute, Percutaneous Endoscopic Approach

41C4K0 Bypass Right Common Iliac Artery to Abdominal Aorta with Nonautologous Tissue Substitute, Percutaneous Endoscopic Approach

41C4K1 Bypass Right Common Iliac Artery to Celiac Artery with Nonautologous Tissue Substitute, Percutaneous Endoscopic Approach

041C4K2 Bypass Right Common Iliac Artery to Mesenteric Artery with Nonautologous Tissue Substitute, Percutaneous Endoscopic Approach

041C4K3 Bypass Right Common Iliac Artery to Right Renal Artery with Nonautologous Tissue Substitute, Percutaneous Endoscopic Approach

041C4K4 Bypass Right Common Iliac Artery to Left Renal Artery with Nonautologous Tissue Substitute, Percutaneous Endoscopic Approach

041C4K5 Bypass Right Common Iliac Artery to Bilateral Renal Artery with Nonautologous Tissue Substitute, Percutaneous Endoscopic Approach

041C4K6 Bypass Right Common Iliac Artery to Right Common Iliac Artery with Nonautologous Tissue Substitute, Percutaneous Endoscopic Approach

041C4K7 Bypass Right Common Iliac Artery to Left Common Iliac Artery with Nonautologous Tissue Substitute, Percutaneous Endoscopic Approach

041C4K8 Bypass Right Common Iliac Artery to Bilateral Common Iliac Arteries with Nonautologous Tissue Substitute, Percutaneous Endoscopic Approach

041C4K9 Bypass Right Common Iliac Artery to Right Internal Iliac Artery with Nonautologous Tissue Substitute, Percutaneous Endoscopic Approach

041C4KB Bypass Right Common Iliac Artery to Left Internal Iliac Artery with Nonautologous Tissue Substitute, Percutaneous Endoscopic Approach

041C4KC Bypass Right Common Iliac Artery to Bilateral Internal Iliac Arteries with Nonautologous Tissue Substitute, Percutaneous Endoscopic Approach

041C4KD Bypass Right Common Iliac Artery to Right External Iliac Artery with Nonautologous Tissue Substitute, Percutaneous Endoscopic Approach

041C4KF Bypass Right Common Iliac Artery to Left External Iliac Artery with Nonautologous Tissue Substitute, Percutaneous Endoscopic Approach

041C4KG Bypass Right Common Iliac Artery to Bilateral External Iliac Arteries with Nonautologous Tissue Substitute, Percutaneous Endoscopic Approach

041C4KH Bypass Right Common Iliac Artery to Right Femoral Artery with Nonautologous Tissue Substitute, Percutaneous Endoscopic Approach

041C4KJ Bypass Right Common Iliac Artery to Left Femoral Artery with Nonautologous Tissue Substitute, Percutaneous Endoscopic Approach

041C4KK Bypass Right Common Iliac Artery to Bilateral Femoral Arteries with Nonautologous Tissue Substitute, Percutaneous Endoscopic Approach

041C4KQ Bypass Right Common Iliac Artery to Lower Extremity Artery with Nonautologous Tissue Substitute, Percutaneous Endoscopic Approach

041C4KR Bypass Right Common Iliac Artery to Lower Artery with Nonautologous Tissue Substitute, Percutaneous Endoscopic Approach

041C4Z0 Bypass Right Common Iliac Artery to Abdominal Aorta, Percutaneous Endoscopic Approach

041C4Z1 Bypass Right Common Iliac Artery to Celiac Artery, Percutaneous Endoscopic Approach

041C4Z2 Bypass Right Common Iliac Artery to Mesenteric Artery, Percutaneous Endoscopic Approach

041C4Z3 Bypass Right Common Iliac Artery to Right Renal Artery, Percutaneous Endoscopic Approach

041C4Z4 Bypass Right Common Iliac Artery to Left Renal Artery, Percutaneous Endoscopic Approach

041C4Z5 Bypass Right Common Iliac Artery to Bilateral Renal Artery, Percutaneous Endoscopic Approach

041C4Z6 Bypass Right Common Iliac Artery to Right Common Iliac Artery, Percutaneous Endoscopic Approach

041C4Z7 Bypass Right Common Iliac Artery to Left Common Iliac Artery, Percutaneous Endoscopic Approach

041C4Z8 Bypass Right Common Iliac Artery to Bilateral Common Iliac Arteries, Percutaneous Endoscopic Approach

041C4Z9 Bypass Right Common Iliac Artery to Right Internal Iliac Artery, Percutaneous Endoscopic Approach

041C4ZB Bypass Right Common Iliac Artery to Left Internal Iliac Artery, Percutaneous Endoscopic Approach

041C4ZC Bypass Right Common Iliac Artery to Bilateral Internal Iliac Arteries, Percutaneous Endoscopic Approach

041C4ZD Bypass Right Common Iliac Artery to Right External Iliac Artery, Percutaneous Endoscopic Approach

041C4ZF Bypass Right Common Iliac Artery to Left External Iliac Artery, Percutaneous Endoscopic Approach

041C4ZG Bypass Right Common Iliac Artery to Bilateral External Iliac Arteries, Percutaneous Endoscopic Approach

041C4ZH Bypass Right Common Iliac Artery to Right Femoral Artery, Percutaneous Endoscopic Approach

041C4ZJ Bypass Right Common Iliac Artery to Left Femoral Artery, Percutaneous Endoscopic Approach

041C4ZK Bypass Right Common Iliac Artery to Bilateral Femoral Arteries, Percutaneous Endoscopic Approach

041C4ZQ Bypass Right Common Iliac Artery to Lower Extremity Artery, Percutaneous Endoscopic Approach

041C4ZR Bypass Right Common Iliac Artery to Lower Artery, Percutaneous Endoscopic Approach

041D090 Bypass Left Common Iliac Artery to Abdominal Aorta with Autologous Venous Tissue, Open Approach

041D091 Bypass Left Common Iliac Artery to Celiac Artery with Autologous Venous Tissue, Open Approach

041D092 Bypass Left Common Iliac Artery to Mesenteric Artery with Autologous Venous Tissue, Open Approach

041D093 Bypass Left Common Iliac Artery to Right Renal Artery with Autologous Venous Tissue, Open Approach

041D094 Bypass Left Common Iliac Artery to Left Renal Artery with Autologous Venous Tissue, Open Approach

041D095 Bypass Left Common Iliac Artery to Bilateral Renal Artery with Autologous Venous Tissue, Open Approach

041D096 Bypass Left Common Iliac Artery to Right Common Iliac Artery with Autologous Venous Tissue, Open Approach

041D097 Bypass Left Common Iliac Artery to Left Common Iliac Artery with Autologous Venous Tissue, Open Approach

041D098 Bypass Left Common Iliac Artery to Bilateral Common Iliac Arteries with Autologous Venous Tissue, Open Approach
041D099 Bypass Left Common Iliac Artery to Right Internal Iliac Artery with Autologous Venous Tissue, Open Approach
041D09B Bypass Left Common Iliac Artery to Left Internal Iliac Artery with Autologous Venous Tissue, Open Approach
041D09C Bypass Left Common Iliac Artery to Bilateral Internal Iliac Arteries with Autologous Venous Tissue, Open Approach
041D09D Bypass Left Common Iliac Artery to Right External Iliac Artery with Autologous Venous Tissue, Open Approach
041D09F Bypass Left Common Iliac Artery to Left External Iliac Artery with Autologous Venous Tissue, Open Approach
041D09G Bypass Left Common Iliac Artery to Bilateral External Iliac Arteries with Autologous Venous Tissue, Open Approach
041D09H Bypass Left Common Iliac Artery to Right Femoral Artery with Autologous Venous Tissue, Open Approach
041D09J Bypass Left Common Iliac Artery to Left Femoral Artery with Autologous Venous Tissue, Open Approach
041D09K Bypass Left Common Iliac Artery to Bilateral Femoral Arteries with Autologous Venous Tissue, Open Approach
041D09Q Bypass Left Common Iliac Artery to Lower Extremity Artery with Autologous Venous Tissue, Open Approach
041D09R Bypass Left Common Iliac Artery to Lower Artery with Autologous Venous Tissue, Open Approach
041D0A0 Bypass Left Common Iliac Artery to Abdominal Aorta with Autologous Arterial Tissue, Open Approach
041D0A1 Bypass Left Common Iliac Artery to Celiac Artery with Autologous Arterial Tissue, Open Approach
041D0A2 Bypass Left Common Iliac Artery to Mesenteric Artery with Autologous Arterial Tissue, Open Approach
041D0A3 Bypass Left Common Iliac Artery to Right Renal Artery with Autologous Arterial Tissue, Open Approach
041D0A4 Bypass Left Common Iliac Artery to Left Renal Artery with Autologous Arterial Tissue, Open Approach
041D0A5 Bypass Left Common Iliac Artery to Bilateral Renal Artery with Autologous Arterial Tissue, Open Approach
041D0A6 Bypass Left Common Iliac Artery to Right Common Iliac Artery with Autologous Arterial Tissue, Open Approach
041D0A7 Bypass Left Common Iliac Artery to Left Common Iliac Artery with Autologous Arterial Tissue, Open Approach
041D0A8 Bypass Left Common Iliac Artery to Bilateral Common Iliac Arteries with Autologous Arterial Tissue, Open Approach
041D0A9 Bypass Left Common Iliac Artery to Right Internal Iliac Artery with Autologous Arterial Tissue, Open Approach
041D0AB Bypass Left Common Iliac Artery to Left Internal Iliac Artery with Autologous Arterial Tissue, Open Approach
041D0AC Bypass Left Common Iliac Artery to Bilateral Internal Iliac Arteries with Autologous Arterial Tissue, Open Approach
041D0AD Bypass Left Common Iliac Artery to Right External Iliac Artery with Autologous Arterial Tissue, Open Approach
041D0AF Bypass Left Common Iliac Artery to Left External Iliac Artery with Autologous Arterial Tissue, Open Approach
041D0AG Bypass Left Common Iliac Artery to Bilateral External Iliac Arteries with Autologous Arterial Tissue, Open Approach
041D0AH Bypass Left Common Iliac Artery to Right Femoral Artery with Autologous Arterial Tissue, Open Approach
041D0AJ Bypass Left Common Iliac Artery to Left Femoral Artery with Autologous Arterial Tissue, Open Approach
041D0AK Bypass Left Common Iliac Artery to Bilateral Femoral Arteries with Autologous Arterial Tissue, Open Approach
041D0AQ Bypass Left Common Iliac Artery to Lower Extremity Artery with Autologous Arterial Tissue, Open Approach
041D0AR Bypass Left Common Iliac Artery to Lower Artery with Autologous Arterial Tissue, Open Approach
041D0J0 Bypass Left Common Iliac Artery to Abdominal Aorta with Synthetic Substitute, Open Approach
041D0J1 Bypass Left Common Iliac Artery to Celiac Artery with Synthetic Substitute, Open Approach
041D0J2 Bypass Left Common Iliac Artery to Mesenteric Artery with Synthetic Substitute, Open Approach
041D0J3 Bypass Left Common Iliac Artery to Right Renal Artery with Synthetic Substitute, Open Approach
041D0J4 Bypass Left Common Iliac Artery to Left Renal Artery with Synthetic Substitute, Open Approach
041D0J5 Bypass Left Common Iliac Artery to Bilateral Renal Artery with Synthetic Substitute, Open Approach
041D0J6 Bypass Left Common Iliac Artery to Right Common Iliac Artery with Synthetic Substitute, Open Approach
041D0J7 Bypass Left Common Iliac Artery to Left Common Iliac Artery with Synthetic Substitute, Open Approach
041D0J8 Bypass Left Common Iliac Artery to Bilateral Common Iliac Arteries with Synthetic Substitute, Open Approach
041D0J9 Bypass Left Common Iliac Artery to Right Internal Iliac Artery with Synthetic Substitute, Open Approach
041D0JB Bypass Left Common Iliac Artery to Left Internal Iliac Artery with Synthetic Substitute, Open Approach
041D0JC Bypass Left Common Iliac Artery to Bilateral Internal Iliac Arteries with Synthetic Substitute, Open Approach
041D0JD Bypass Left Common Iliac Artery to Right External Iliac Artery with Synthetic Substitute, Open Approach
041D0JF Bypass Left Common Iliac Artery to Left External Iliac Artery with Synthetic Substitute, Open Approach
041D0JG Bypass Left Common Iliac Artery to Bilateral External Iliac Arteries with Synthetic Substitute, Open Approach
041D0JH Bypass Left Common Iliac Artery to Right Femoral Artery with Synthetic Substitute, Open Approach
041D0JJ Bypass Left Common Iliac Artery to Left Femoral Artery with Synthetic Substitute, Open Approach
041D0JK Bypass Left Common Iliac Artery to Bilateral Femoral Arteries with Synthetic Substitute, Open Approach
041D0JQ Bypass Left Common Iliac Artery to Lower Extremity Artery with Synthetic Substitute, Open Approach
041D0JR Bypass Left Common Iliac Artery to Lower Artery with Synthetic Substitute, Open Approach
041D0K0 Bypass Left Common Iliac Artery to Abdominal Aorta with Nonautologous Tissue Substitute, Open Approach
041D0K1 Bypass Left Common Iliac Artery to Celiac Artery with Nonautologous Tissue Substitute, Open Approach
041D0K2 Bypass Left Common Iliac Artery to Mesenteric Artery with Nonautologous Tissue Substitute, Open Approach
041D0K3 Bypass Left Common Iliac Artery to Right Renal Artery with Nonautologous Tissue Substitute, Open Approach
041D0K4 Bypass Left Common Iliac Artery to Left Renal Artery with Nonautologous Tissue Substitute, Open Approach
041D0K5 Bypass Left Common Iliac Artery to Bilateral Renal Artery with Nonautologous Tissue Substitute, Open Approach
041D0K6 Bypass Left Common Iliac Artery to Right Common Iliac Artery with Nonautologous Tissue Substitute, Open Approach
041D0K7 Bypass Left Common Iliac Artery to Left Common Iliac Artery with Nonautologous Tissue Substitute, Open Approach
041D0K8 Bypass Left Common Iliac Artery to Bilateral Common Iliac Arteries with Nonautologous Tissue Substitute, Open Approach
041D0K9 Bypass Left Common Iliac Artery to Right Internal Iliac Artery with Nonautologous Tissue Substitute, Open Approach
041D0KB Bypass Left Common Iliac Artery to Left Internal Iliac Artery with Nonautologous Tissue Substitute, Open Approach
041D0KC Bypass Left Common Iliac Artery to Bilateral Internal Iliac Arteries with Nonautologous Tissue Substitute, Open Approach
041D0KD Bypass Left Common Iliac Artery to Right External Iliac Artery with Nonautologous Tissue Substitute, Open Approach
041D0KF Bypass Left Common Iliac Artery to Left External Iliac Artery with Nonautologous Tissue Substitute, Open Approach
041D0KG Bypass Left Common Iliac Artery to Bilateral External Iliac Arteries with Nonautologous Tissue Substitute, Open Approach
041D0KH Bypass Left Common Iliac Artery to Right Femoral Artery with Nonautologous Tissue Substitute, Open Approach
041D0KJ Bypass Left Common Iliac Artery to Left Femoral Artery with Nonautologous Tissue Substitute, Open Approach
041D0KK Bypass Left Common Iliac Artery to Bilateral Femoral Arteries with Nonautologous Tissue Substitute, Open Approach
041D0KQ Bypass Left Common Iliac Artery to Lower Extremity Artery with Nonautologous Tissue Substitute, Open Approach
041D0KR Bypass Left Common Iliac Artery to Lower Artery with Nonautologous Tissue Substitute, Open Approach
041D0Z0 Bypass Left Common Iliac Artery to Abdominal Aorta, Open Approach
041D0Z1 Bypass Left Common Iliac Artery to Celiac Artery, Open Approach

41D0Z2 Bypass Left Common Iliac Artery to Mesenteric Artery, Open Approach

41D0Z3 Bypass Left Common Iliac Artery to Right Renal Artery, Open Approach

41D0Z4 Bypass Left Common Iliac Artery to Left Renal Artery, Open Approach

41D0Z5 Bypass Left Common Iliac Artery to Bilateral Renal Artery, Open Approach

41D0Z6 Bypass Left Common Iliac Artery to Right Common Iliac Artery, Open Approach

41D0Z7 Bypass Left Common Iliac Artery to Left Common Iliac Artery, Open Approach

41D0Z8 Bypass Left Common Iliac Artery to Bilateral Common Iliac Arteries, Open Approach

41D0Z9 Bypass Left Common Iliac Artery to Right Internal Iliac Artery, Open Approach

41D0ZB Bypass Left Common Iliac Artery to Left Internal Iliac Artery, Open Approach

41D0ZC Bypass Left Common Iliac Artery to Bilateral Internal Iliac Arteries, Open Approach

41D0ZD Bypass Left Common Iliac Artery to Right External Iliac Artery, Open Approach

41D0ZF Bypass Left Common Iliac Artery to Left External Iliac Artery, Open Approach

41D0ZG Bypass Left Common Iliac Artery to Bilateral External Iliac Arteries, Open Approach

41D0ZH Bypass Left Common Iliac Artery to Right Femoral Artery, Open Approach

41D0ZJ Bypass Left Common Iliac Artery to Left Femoral Artery, Open Approach

41D0ZK Bypass Left Common Iliac Artery to Bilateral Femoral Arteries, Open Approach

41D0ZQ Bypass Left Common Iliac Artery to Lower Extremity Artery, Open Approach

41D0ZR Bypass Left Common Iliac Artery to Lower Artery, Open Approach

41D490 Bypass Left Common Iliac Artery to Abdominal Aorta with Autologous Venous Tissue, Percutaneous Endoscopic Approach

41D491 Bypass Left Common Iliac Artery to Celiac Artery with Autologous Venous Tissue, Percutaneous Endoscopic Approach

41D492 Bypass Left Common Iliac Artery to Mesenteric Artery with Autologous Venous Tissue, Percutaneous Endoscopic Approach

41D493 Bypass Left Common Iliac Artery to Right Renal Artery with Autologous Venous Tissue, Percutaneous Endoscopic Approach

41D494 Bypass Left Common Iliac Artery to Left Renal Artery with Autologous Venous Tissue, Percutaneous Endoscopic Approach

41D495 Bypass Left Common Iliac Artery to Bilateral Renal Artery with Autologous Venous Tissue, Percutaneous Endoscopic Approach

41D496 Bypass Left Common Iliac Artery to Right Common Iliac Artery with Autologous Venous Tissue, Percutaneous Endoscopic Approach

41D497 Bypass Left Common Iliac Artery to Left Common Iliac Artery with Autologous Venous Tissue, Percutaneous Endoscopic Approach

41D498 Bypass Left Common Iliac Artery to Bilateral Common Iliac Arteries with Autologous Venous Tissue, Percutaneous Endoscopic Approach

41D499 Bypass Left Common Iliac Artery to Right Internal Iliac Artery with Autologous Venous Tissue, Percutaneous Endoscopic Approach

041D49B Bypass Left Common Iliac Artery to Left Internal Iliac Artery with Autologous Venous Tissue, Percutaneous Endoscopic Approach

041D49C Bypass Left Common Iliac Artery to Bilateral Internal Iliac Arteries with Autologous Venous Tissue, Percutaneous Endoscopic Approach

041D49D Bypass Left Common Iliac Artery to Right External Iliac Artery with Autologous Venous Tissue, Percutaneous Endoscopic Approach

041D49F Bypass Left Common Iliac Artery to Left External Iliac Artery with Autologous Venous Tissue, Percutaneous Endoscopic Approach

041D49G Bypass Left Common Iliac Artery to Bilateral External Iliac Arteries with Autologous Venous Tissue, Percutaneous Endoscopic Approach

041D49H Bypass Left Common Iliac Artery to Right Femoral Artery with Autologous Venous Tissue, Percutaneous Endoscopic Approach

041D49J Bypass Left Common Iliac Artery to Left Femoral Artery with Autologous Venous Tissue, Percutaneous Endoscopic Approach

041D49K Bypass Left Common Iliac Artery to Bilateral Femoral Arteries with Autologous Venous Tissue, Percutaneous Endoscopic Approach

041D49Q Bypass Left Common Iliac Artery to Lower Extremity Artery with Autologous Venous Tissue, Percutaneous Endoscopic Approach

041D49R Bypass Left Common Iliac Artery to Lower Artery with Autologous Venous Tissue, Percutaneous Endoscopic Approach

041D4A0 Bypass Left Common Iliac Artery to Abdominal Aorta with Autologous Arterial Tissue, Percutaneous Endoscopic Approach

041D4A1 Bypass Left Common Iliac Artery to Celiac Artery with Autologous Arterial Tissue, Percutaneous Endoscopic Approach

041D4A2 Bypass Left Common Iliac Artery to Mesenteric Artery with Autologous Arterial Tissue, Percutaneous Endoscopic Approach

041D4A3 Bypass Left Common Iliac Artery to Right Renal Artery with Autologous Arterial Tissue, Percutaneous Endoscopic Approach

041D4A4 Bypass Left Common Iliac Artery to Left Renal Artery with Autologous Arterial Tissue, Percutaneous Endoscopic Approach

041D4A5 Bypass Left Common Iliac Artery to Bilateral Renal Artery with Autologous Arterial Tissue, Percutaneous Endoscopic Approach

041D4A6 Bypass Left Common Iliac Artery to Right Common Iliac Artery with Autologous Arterial Tissue, Percutaneous Endoscopic Approach

041D4A7 Bypass Left Common Iliac Artery to Left Common Iliac Artery with Autologous Arterial Tissue, Percutaneous Endoscopic Approach

041D4A8 Bypass Left Common Iliac Artery to Bilateral Common Iliac Arteries with Autologous Arterial Tissue, Percutaneous Endoscopic Approach

041D4A9 Bypass Left Common Iliac Artery to Right Internal Iliac Artery with Autologous Arterial Tissue, Percutaneous Endoscopic Approach

041D4AB Bypass Left Common Iliac Artery to Left Internal Iliac Artery with Autologous Arterial Tissue, Percutaneous Endoscopic Approach

041D4AC Bypass Left Common Iliac Artery to Bilateral Internal Iliac Arteries with Autologous Arterial Tissue, Percutaneous Endoscopic Approach

041D4AD Bypass Left Common Iliac Artery to Right External Iliac Artery with Autologous Arterial Tissue, Percutaneous Endoscopic Approach

041D4AF Bypass Left Common Iliac Artery to Left External Iliac Artery with Autologous Arterial Tissue, Percutaneous Endoscopic Approach

041D4AG Bypass Left Common Iliac Artery to Bilateral External Iliac Arteries with Autologous Arterial Tissue, Percutaneous Endoscopic Approach

041D4AH Bypass Left Common Iliac Artery to Right Femoral Artery with Autologous Arterial Tissue, Percutaneous Endoscopic Approach

041D4AJ Bypass Left Common Iliac Artery to Left Femoral Artery with Autologous Arterial Tissue, Percutaneous Endoscopic Approach

041D4AK Bypass Left Common Iliac Artery to Bilateral Femoral Arteries with Autologous Arterial Tissue, Percutaneous Endoscopic Approach

041D4AQ Bypass Left Common Iliac Artery to Lower Extremity Artery with Autologous Arterial Tissue, Percutaneous Endoscopic Approach

041D4AR Bypass Left Common Iliac Artery to Lower Artery with Autologous Arterial Tissue, Percutaneous Endoscopic Approach

041D4J0 Bypass Left Common Iliac Artery to Abdominal Aorta with Synthetic Substitute, Percutaneous Endoscopic Approach

041D4J1 Bypass Left Common Iliac Artery to Celiac Artery with Synthetic Substitute, Percutaneous Endoscopic Approach

041D4J2 Bypass Left Common Iliac Artery to Mesenteric Artery with Synthetic Substitute, Percutaneous Endoscopic Approach

041D4J3 Bypass Left Common Iliac Artery to Right Renal Artery with Synthetic Substitute, Percutaneous Endoscopic Approach

041D4J4 Bypass Left Common Iliac Artery to Left Renal Artery with Synthetic Substitute, Percutaneous Endoscopic Approach

041D4J5 Bypass Left Common Iliac Artery to Bilateral Renal Artery with Synthetic Substitute, Percutaneous Endoscopic Approach

041D4J6 Bypass Left Common Iliac Artery to Right Common Iliac Artery with Synthetic Substitute, Percutaneous Endoscopic Approach

041D4J7 Bypass Left Common Iliac Artery to Left Common Iliac Artery with Synthetic Substitute, Percutaneous Endoscopic Approach

041D4J8 Bypass Left Common Iliac Artery to Bilateral Common Iliac Arteries with Synthetic Substitute, Percutaneous Endoscopic Approach

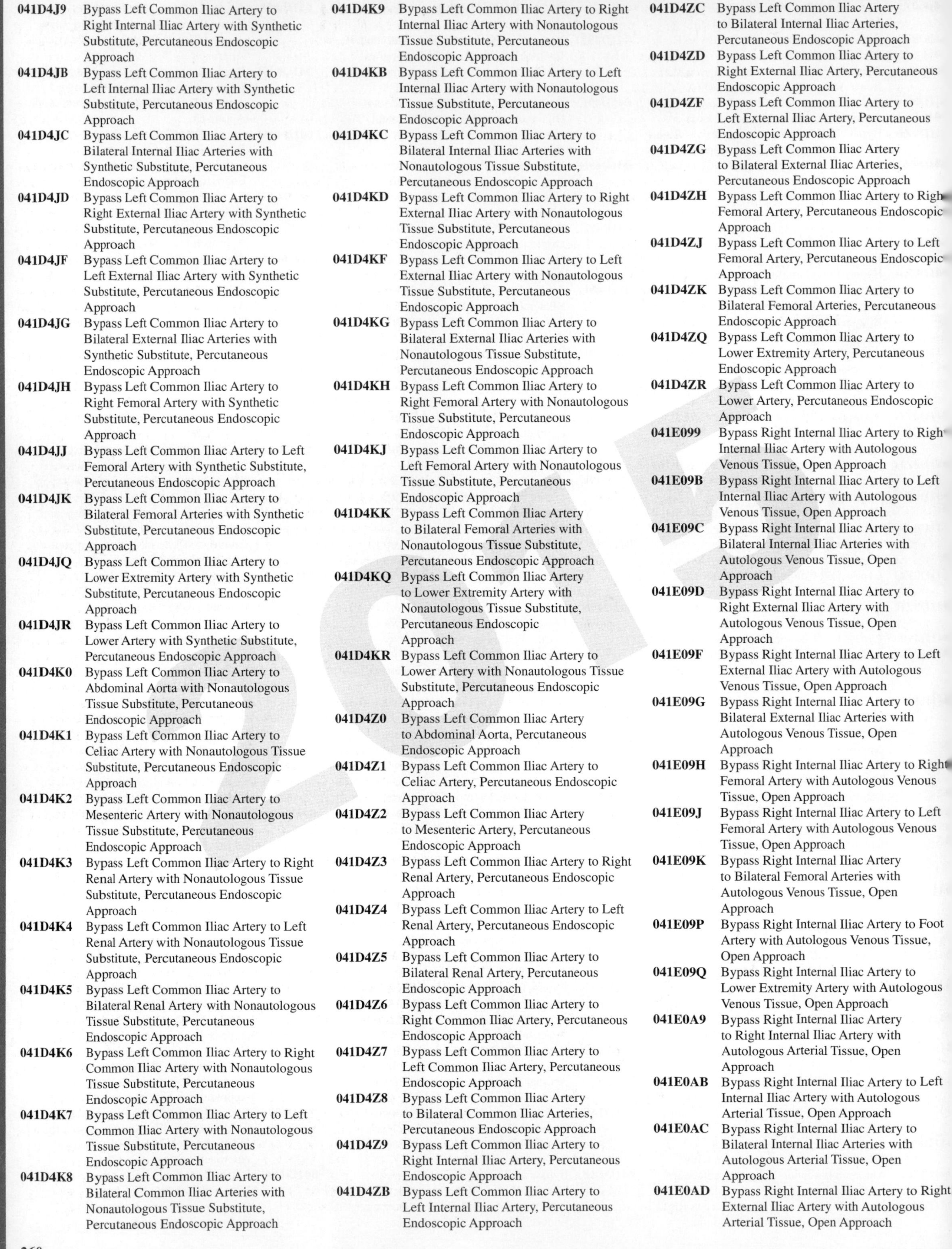

041D4J9 Bypass Left Common Iliac Artery to Right Internal Iliac Artery with Synthetic Substitute, Percutaneous Endoscopic Approach

041D4JB Bypass Left Common Iliac Artery to Left Internal Iliac Artery with Synthetic Substitute, Percutaneous Endoscopic Approach

041D4JC Bypass Left Common Iliac Artery to Bilateral Internal Iliac Arteries with Synthetic Substitute, Percutaneous Endoscopic Approach

041D4JD Bypass Left Common Iliac Artery to Right External Iliac Artery with Synthetic Substitute, Percutaneous Endoscopic Approach

041D4JF Bypass Left Common Iliac Artery to Left External Iliac Artery with Synthetic Substitute, Percutaneous Endoscopic Approach

041D4JG Bypass Left Common Iliac Artery to Bilateral External Iliac Arteries with Synthetic Substitute, Percutaneous Endoscopic Approach

041D4JH Bypass Left Common Iliac Artery to Right Femoral Artery with Synthetic Substitute, Percutaneous Endoscopic Approach

041D4JJ Bypass Left Common Iliac Artery to Left Femoral Artery with Synthetic Substitute, Percutaneous Endoscopic Approach

041D4JK Bypass Left Common Iliac Artery to Bilateral Femoral Arteries with Synthetic Substitute, Percutaneous Endoscopic Approach

041D4JQ Bypass Left Common Iliac Artery to Lower Extremity Artery with Synthetic Substitute, Percutaneous Endoscopic Approach

041D4JR Bypass Left Common Iliac Artery to Lower Artery with Synthetic Substitute, Percutaneous Endoscopic Approach

041D4K0 Bypass Left Common Iliac Artery to Abdominal Aorta with Nonautologous Tissue Substitute, Percutaneous Endoscopic Approach

041D4K1 Bypass Left Common Iliac Artery to Celiac Artery with Nonautologous Tissue Substitute, Percutaneous Endoscopic Approach

041D4K2 Bypass Left Common Iliac Artery to Mesenteric Artery with Nonautologous Tissue Substitute, Percutaneous Endoscopic Approach

041D4K3 Bypass Left Common Iliac Artery to Right Renal Artery with Nonautologous Tissue Substitute, Percutaneous Endoscopic Approach

041D4K4 Bypass Left Common Iliac Artery to Left Renal Artery with Nonautologous Tissue Substitute, Percutaneous Endoscopic Approach

041D4K5 Bypass Left Common Iliac Artery to Bilateral Renal Artery with Nonautologous Tissue Substitute, Percutaneous Endoscopic Approach

041D4K6 Bypass Left Common Iliac Artery to Right Common Iliac Artery with Nonautologous Tissue Substitute, Percutaneous Endoscopic Approach

041D4K7 Bypass Left Common Iliac Artery to Left Common Iliac Artery with Nonautologous Tissue Substitute, Percutaneous Endoscopic Approach

041D4K8 Bypass Left Common Iliac Artery to Bilateral Common Iliac Arteries with Nonautologous Tissue Substitute, Percutaneous Endoscopic Approach

041D4K9 Bypass Left Common Iliac Artery to Right Internal Iliac Artery with Nonautologous Tissue Substitute, Percutaneous Endoscopic Approach

041D4KB Bypass Left Common Iliac Artery to Left Internal Iliac Artery with Nonautologous Tissue Substitute, Percutaneous Endoscopic Approach

041D4KC Bypass Left Common Iliac Artery to Bilateral Internal Iliac Arteries with Nonautologous Tissue Substitute, Percutaneous Endoscopic Approach

041D4KD Bypass Left Common Iliac Artery to Right External Iliac Artery with Nonautologous Tissue Substitute, Percutaneous Endoscopic Approach

041D4KF Bypass Left Common Iliac Artery to Left External Iliac Artery with Nonautologous Tissue Substitute, Percutaneous Endoscopic Approach

041D4KG Bypass Left Common Iliac Artery to Bilateral External Iliac Arteries with Nonautologous Tissue Substitute, Percutaneous Endoscopic Approach

041D4KH Bypass Left Common Iliac Artery to Right Femoral Artery with Nonautologous Tissue Substitute, Percutaneous Endoscopic Approach

041D4KJ Bypass Left Common Iliac Artery to Left Femoral Artery with Nonautologous Tissue Substitute, Percutaneous Endoscopic Approach

041D4KK Bypass Left Common Iliac Artery to Bilateral Femoral Arteries with Nonautologous Tissue Substitute, Percutaneous Endoscopic Approach

041D4KQ Bypass Left Common Iliac Artery to Lower Extremity Artery with Nonautologous Tissue Substitute, Percutaneous Endoscopic Approach

041D4KR Bypass Left Common Iliac Artery to Lower Artery with Nonautologous Tissue Substitute, Percutaneous Endoscopic Approach

041D4Z0 Bypass Left Common Iliac Artery to Abdominal Aorta, Percutaneous Endoscopic Approach

041D4Z1 Bypass Left Common Iliac Artery to Celiac Artery, Percutaneous Endoscopic Approach

041D4Z2 Bypass Left Common Iliac Artery to Mesenteric Artery, Percutaneous Endoscopic Approach

041D4Z3 Bypass Left Common Iliac Artery to Right Renal Artery, Percutaneous Endoscopic Approach

041D4Z4 Bypass Left Common Iliac Artery to Left Renal Artery, Percutaneous Endoscopic Approach

041D4Z5 Bypass Left Common Iliac Artery to Bilateral Renal Artery, Percutaneous Endoscopic Approach

041D4Z6 Bypass Left Common Iliac Artery to Right Common Iliac Artery, Percutaneous Endoscopic Approach

041D4Z7 Bypass Left Common Iliac Artery to Left Common Iliac Artery, Percutaneous Endoscopic Approach

041D4Z8 Bypass Left Common Iliac Artery to Bilateral Common Iliac Arteries, Percutaneous Endoscopic Approach

041D4Z9 Bypass Left Common Iliac Artery to Right Internal Iliac Artery, Percutaneous Endoscopic Approach

041D4ZB Bypass Left Common Iliac Artery to Left Internal Iliac Artery, Percutaneous Endoscopic Approach

041D4ZC Bypass Left Common Iliac Artery to Bilateral Internal Iliac Arteries, Percutaneous Endoscopic Approach

041D4ZD Bypass Left Common Iliac Artery to Right External Iliac Artery, Percutaneous Endoscopic Approach

041D4ZF Bypass Left Common Iliac Artery to Left External Iliac Artery, Percutaneous Endoscopic Approach

041D4ZG Bypass Left Common Iliac Artery to Bilateral External Iliac Arteries, Percutaneous Endoscopic Approach

041D4ZH Bypass Left Common Iliac Artery to Righ Femoral Artery, Percutaneous Endoscopic Approach

041D4ZJ Bypass Left Common Iliac Artery to Left Femoral Artery, Percutaneous Endoscopic Approach

041D4ZK Bypass Left Common Iliac Artery to Bilateral Femoral Arteries, Percutaneous Endoscopic Approach

041D4ZQ Bypass Left Common Iliac Artery to Lower Extremity Artery, Percutaneous Endoscopic Approach

041D4ZR Bypass Left Common Iliac Artery to Lower Artery, Percutaneous Endoscopic Approach

041E099 Bypass Right Internal Iliac Artery to Righ Internal Iliac Artery with Autologous Venous Tissue, Open Approach

041E09B Bypass Right Internal Iliac Artery to Left Internal Iliac Artery with Autologous Venous Tissue, Open Approach

041E09C Bypass Right Internal Iliac Artery to Bilateral Internal Iliac Arteries with Autologous Venous Tissue, Open Approach

041E09D Bypass Right Internal Iliac Artery to Right External Iliac Artery with Autologous Venous Tissue, Open Approach

041E09F Bypass Right Internal Iliac Artery to Left External Iliac Artery with Autologous Venous Tissue, Open Approach

041E09G Bypass Right Internal Iliac Artery to Bilateral External Iliac Arteries with Autologous Venous Tissue, Open Approach

041E09H Bypass Right Internal Iliac Artery to Right Femoral Artery with Autologous Venous Tissue, Open Approach

041E09J Bypass Right Internal Iliac Artery to Left Femoral Artery with Autologous Venous Tissue, Open Approach

041E09K Bypass Right Internal Iliac Artery to Bilateral Femoral Arteries with Autologous Venous Tissue, Open Approach

041E09P Bypass Right Internal Iliac Artery to Foot Artery with Autologous Venous Tissue, Open Approach

041E09Q Bypass Right Internal Iliac Artery to Lower Extremity Artery with Autologous Venous Tissue, Open Approach

041E0A9 Bypass Right Internal Iliac Artery to Right Internal Iliac Artery with Autologous Arterial Tissue, Open Approach

041E0AB Bypass Right Internal Iliac Artery to Left Internal Iliac Artery with Autologous Arterial Tissue, Open Approach

041E0AC Bypass Right Internal Iliac Artery to Bilateral Internal Iliac Arteries with Autologous Arterial Tissue, Open Approach

041E0AD Bypass Right Internal Iliac Artery to Right External Iliac Artery with Autologous Arterial Tissue, Open Approach

41E0AF Bypass Right Internal Iliac Artery to Left External Iliac Artery with Autologous Arterial Tissue, Open Approach

41E0AG Bypass Right Internal Iliac Artery to Bilateral External Iliac Arteries with Autologous Arterial Tissue, Open Approach

41E0AH Bypass Right Internal Iliac Artery to Right Femoral Artery with Autologous Arterial Tissue, Open Approach

41E0AJ Bypass Right Internal Iliac Artery to Left Femoral Artery with Autologous Arterial Tissue, Open Approach

41E0AK Bypass Right Internal Iliac Artery to Bilateral Femoral Arteries with Autologous Arterial Tissue, Open Approach

41E0AP Bypass Right Internal Iliac Artery to Foot Artery with Autologous Arterial Tissue, Open Approach

41E0AQ Bypass Right Internal Iliac Artery to Lower Extremity Artery with Autologous Arterial Tissue, Open Approach

41E0J9 Bypass Right Internal Iliac Artery to Right Internal Iliac Artery with Synthetic Substitute, Open Approach

41E0JB Bypass Right Internal Iliac Artery to Left Internal Iliac Artery with Synthetic Substitute, Open Approach

41E0JC Bypass Right Internal Iliac Artery to Bilateral Internal Iliac Arteries with Synthetic Substitute, Open Approach

41E0JD Bypass Right Internal Iliac Artery to Right External Iliac Artery with Synthetic Substitute, Open Approach

41E0JF Bypass Right Internal Iliac Artery to Left External Iliac Artery with Synthetic Substitute, Open Approach

41E0JG Bypass Right Internal Iliac Artery to Bilateral External Iliac Arteries with Synthetic Substitute, Open Approach

41E0JH Bypass Right Internal Iliac Artery to Right Femoral Artery with Synthetic Substitute, Open Approach

41E0JJ Bypass Right Internal Iliac Artery to Left Femoral Artery with Synthetic Substitute, Open Approach

41E0JK Bypass Right Internal Iliac Artery to Bilateral Femoral Arteries with Synthetic Substitute, Open Approach

41E0JP Bypass Right Internal Iliac Artery to Foot Artery with Synthetic Substitute, Open Approach

41E0JQ Bypass Right Internal Iliac Artery to Lower Extremity Artery with Synthetic Substitute, Open Approach

41E0K9 Bypass Right Internal Iliac Artery to Right Internal Iliac Artery with Nonautologous Tissue Substitute, Open Approach

41E0KB Bypass Right Internal Iliac Artery to Left Internal Iliac Artery with Nonautologous Tissue Substitute, Open Approach

41E0KC Bypass Right Internal Iliac Artery to Bilateral Internal Iliac Arteries with Nonautologous Tissue Substitute, Open Approach

41E0KD Bypass Right Internal Iliac Artery to Right External Iliac Artery with Nonautologous Tissue Substitute, Open Approach

41E0KF Bypass Right Internal Iliac Artery to Left External Iliac Artery with Nonautologous Tissue Substitute, Open Approach

41E0KG Bypass Right Internal Iliac Artery to Bilateral External Iliac Arteries with Nonautologous Tissue Substitute, Open Approach

041E0KH Bypass Right Internal Iliac Artery to Right Femoral Artery with Nonautologous Tissue Substitute, Open Approach

041E0KJ Bypass Right Internal Iliac Artery to Left Femoral Artery with Nonautologous Tissue Substitute, Open Approach

041E0KK Bypass Right Internal Iliac Artery to Bilateral Femoral Arteries with Nonautologous Tissue Substitute, Open Approach

041E0KP Bypass Right Internal Iliac Artery to Foot Artery with Nonautologous Tissue Substitute, Open Approach

041E0KQ Bypass Right Internal Iliac Artery to Lower Extremity Artery with Nonautologous Tissue Substitute, Open Approach

041E0Z9 Bypass Right Internal Iliac Artery to Right Internal Iliac Artery, Open Approach

041E0ZB Bypass Right Internal Iliac Artery to Left Internal Iliac Artery, Open Approach

041E0ZC Bypass Right Internal Iliac Artery to Bilateral Internal Iliac Arteries, Open Approach

041E0ZD Bypass Right Internal Iliac Artery to Right External Iliac Artery, Open Approach

041E0ZF Bypass Right Internal Iliac Artery to Left External Iliac Artery, Open Approach

041E0ZG Bypass Right Internal Iliac Artery to Bilateral External Iliac Arteries, Open Approach

041E0ZH Bypass Right Internal Iliac Artery to Right Femoral Artery, Open Approach

041E0ZJ Bypass Right Internal Iliac Artery to Left Femoral Artery, Open Approach

041E0ZK Bypass Right Internal Iliac Artery to Bilateral Femoral Arteries, Open Approach

041E0ZP Bypass Right Internal Iliac Artery to Foot Artery, Open Approach

041E0ZQ Bypass Right Internal Iliac Artery to Lower Extremity Artery, Open Approach

041E499 Bypass Right Internal Iliac Artery to Right Internal Iliac Artery with Autologous Venous Tissue, Percutaneous Endoscopic Approach

041E49B Bypass Right Internal Iliac Artery to Left Internal Iliac Artery with Autologous Venous Tissue, Percutaneous Endoscopic Approach

041E49C Bypass Right Internal Iliac Artery to Bilateral Internal Iliac Arteries with Autologous Venous Tissue, Percutaneous Endoscopic Approach

041E49D Bypass Right Internal Iliac Artery to Right External Iliac Artery with Autologous Venous Tissue, Percutaneous Endoscopic Approach

041E49F Bypass Right Internal Iliac Artery to Left External Iliac Artery with Autologous Venous Tissue, Percutaneous Endoscopic Approach

041E49G Bypass Right Internal Iliac Artery to Bilateral External Iliac Arteries with Autologous Venous Tissue, Percutaneous Endoscopic Approach

041E49H Bypass Right Internal Iliac Artery to Right Femoral Artery with Autologous Venous Tissue, Percutaneous Endoscopic Approach

041E49J Bypass Right Internal Iliac Artery to Left Femoral Artery with Autologous Venous Tissue, Percutaneous Endoscopic Approach

041E49K Bypass Right Internal Iliac Artery to Bilateral Femoral Arteries with Autologous Venous Tissue, Percutaneous Endoscopic Approach

041E49P Bypass Right Internal Iliac Artery to Foot Artery with Autologous Venous Tissue, Percutaneous Endoscopic Approach

041E49Q Bypass Right Internal Iliac Artery to Lower Extremity Artery with Autologous Venous Tissue, Percutaneous Endoscopic Approach

041E4A9 Bypass Right Internal Iliac Artery to Right Internal Iliac Artery with Autologous Arterial Tissue, Percutaneous Endoscopic Approach

041E4AB Bypass Right Internal Iliac Artery to Left Internal Iliac Artery with Autologous Arterial Tissue, Percutaneous Endoscopic Approach

041E4AC Bypass Right Internal Iliac Artery to Bilateral Internal Iliac Arteries with Autologous Arterial Tissue, Percutaneous Endoscopic Approach

041E4AD Bypass Right Internal Iliac Artery to Right External Iliac Artery with Autologous Arterial Tissue, Percutaneous Endoscopic Approach

041E4AF Bypass Right Internal Iliac Artery to Left External Iliac Artery with Autologous Arterial Tissue, Percutaneous Endoscopic Approach

041E4AG Bypass Right Internal Iliac Artery to Bilateral External Iliac Arteries with Autologous Arterial Tissue, Percutaneous Endoscopic Approach

041E4AH Bypass Right Internal Iliac Artery to Right Femoral Artery with Autologous Arterial Tissue, Percutaneous Endoscopic Approach

041E4AJ Bypass Right Internal Iliac Artery to Left Femoral Artery with Autologous Arterial Tissue, Percutaneous Endoscopic Approach

041E4AK Bypass Right Internal Iliac Artery to Bilateral Femoral Arteries with Autologous Arterial Tissue, Percutaneous Endoscopic Approach

041E4AP Bypass Right Internal Iliac Artery to Foot Artery with Autologous Arterial Tissue, Percutaneous Endoscopic Approach

041E4AQ Bypass Right Internal Iliac Artery to Lower Extremity Artery with Autologous Arterial Tissue, Percutaneous Endoscopic Approach

041E4J9 Bypass Right Internal Iliac Artery to Right Internal Iliac Artery with Synthetic Substitute, Percutaneous Endoscopic Approach

041E4JB Bypass Right Internal Iliac Artery to Left Internal Iliac Artery with Synthetic Substitute, Percutaneous Endoscopic Approach

041E4JC Bypass Right Internal Iliac Artery to Bilateral Internal Iliac Arteries with Synthetic Substitute, Percutaneous Endoscopic Approach

041E4JD Bypass Right Internal Iliac Artery to Right External Iliac Artery with Synthetic Substitute, Percutaneous Endoscopic Approach

041E4JF Bypass Right Internal Iliac Artery to Left External Iliac Artery with Synthetic Substitute, Percutaneous Endoscopic Approach

041E4JG Bypass Right Internal Iliac Artery to Bilateral External Iliac Arteries with Synthetic Substitute, Percutaneous Endoscopic Approach

041E4JH Bypass Right Internal Iliac Artery to Right Femoral Artery with Synthetic Substitute, Percutaneous Endoscopic Approach

041E4JJ Bypass Right Internal Iliac Artery to Left Femoral Artery with Synthetic Substitute, Percutaneous Endoscopic Approach

041E4JK Bypass Right Internal Iliac Artery to Bilateral Femoral Arteries with Synthetic Substitute, Percutaneous Endoscopic Approach

041E4JP Bypass Right Internal Iliac Artery to Foot Artery with Synthetic Substitute, Percutaneous Endoscopic Approach

041E4JQ Bypass Right Internal Iliac Artery to Lower Extremity Artery with Synthetic Substitute, Percutaneous Endoscopic Approach

041E4K9 Bypass Right Internal Iliac Artery to Right Internal Iliac Artery with Nonautologous Tissue Substitute, Percutaneous Endoscopic Approach

041E4KB Bypass Right Internal Iliac Artery to Left Internal Iliac Artery with Nonautologous Tissue Substitute, Percutaneous Endoscopic Approach

041E4KC Bypass Right Internal Iliac Artery to Bilateral Internal Iliac Arteries with Nonautologous Tissue Substitute, Percutaneous Endoscopic Approach

041E4KD Bypass Right Internal Iliac Artery to Right External Iliac Artery with Nonautologous Tissue Substitute, Percutaneous Endoscopic Approach

041E4KF Bypass Right Internal Iliac Artery to Left External Iliac Artery with Nonautologous Tissue Substitute, Percutaneous Endoscopic Approach

041E4KG Bypass Right Internal Iliac Artery to Bilateral External Iliac Arteries with Nonautologous Tissue Substitute, Percutaneous Endoscopic Approach

041E4KH Bypass Right Internal Iliac Artery to Right Femoral Artery with Nonautologous Tissue Substitute, Percutaneous Endoscopic Approach

041E4KJ Bypass Right Internal Iliac Artery to Left Femoral Artery with Nonautologous Tissue Substitute, Percutaneous Endoscopic Approach

041E4KK Bypass Right Internal Iliac Artery to Bilateral Femoral Arteries with Nonautologous Tissue Substitute, Percutaneous Endoscopic Approach

041E4KP Bypass Right Internal Iliac Artery to Foot Artery with Nonautologous Tissue Substitute, Percutaneous Endoscopic Approach

041E4KQ Bypass Right Internal Iliac Artery to Lower Extremity Artery with Nonautologous Tissue Substitute, Percutaneous Endoscopic Approach

041E4Z9 Bypass Right Internal Iliac Artery to Right Internal Iliac Artery, Percutaneous Endoscopic Approach

041E4ZB Bypass Right Internal Iliac Artery to Left Internal Iliac Artery, Percutaneous Endoscopic Approach

041E4ZC Bypass Right Internal Iliac Artery to Bilateral Internal Iliac Arteries, Percutaneous Endoscopic Approach

041E4ZD Bypass Right Internal Iliac Artery to Right External Iliac Artery, Percutaneous Endoscopic Approach

041E4ZF Bypass Right Internal Iliac Artery to Left External Iliac Artery, Percutaneous Endoscopic Approach

041E4ZG Bypass Right Internal Iliac Artery to Bilateral External Iliac Arteries, Percutaneous Endoscopic Approach

041E4ZH Bypass Right Internal Iliac Artery to Right Femoral Artery, Percutaneous Endoscopic Approach

041E4ZJ Bypass Right Internal Iliac Artery to Left Femoral Artery, Percutaneous Endoscopic Approach

041E4ZK Bypass Right Internal Iliac Artery to Bilateral Femoral Arteries, Percutaneous Endoscopic Approach

041E4ZP Bypass Right Internal Iliac Artery to Foot Artery, Percutaneous Endoscopic Approach

041E4ZQ Bypass Right Internal Iliac Artery to Lower Extremity Artery, Percutaneous Endoscopic Approach

041F099 Bypass Left Internal Iliac Artery to Right Internal Iliac Artery with Autologous Venous Tissue, Open Approach

041F09B Bypass Left Internal Iliac Artery to Left Internal Iliac Artery with Autologous Venous Tissue, Open Approach

041F09C Bypass Left Internal Iliac Artery to Bilateral Internal Iliac Arteries with Autologous Venous Tissue, Open Approach

041F09D Bypass Left Internal Iliac Artery to Right External Iliac Artery with Autologous Venous Tissue, Open Approach

041F09F Bypass Left Internal Iliac Artery to Left External Iliac Artery with Autologous Venous Tissue, Open Approach

041F09G Bypass Left Internal Iliac Artery to Bilateral External Iliac Arteries with Autologous Venous Tissue, Open Approach

041F09H Bypass Left Internal Iliac Artery to Right Femoral Artery with Autologous Venous Tissue, Open Approach

041F09J Bypass Left Internal Iliac Artery to Left Femoral Artery with Autologous Venous Tissue, Open Approach

041F09K Bypass Left Internal Iliac Artery to Bilateral Femoral Arteries with Autologous Venous Tissue, Open Approach

041F09P Bypass Left Internal Iliac Artery to Foot Artery with Autologous Venous Tissue, Open Approach

041F09Q Bypass Left Internal Iliac Artery to Lower Extremity Artery with Autologous Venous Tissue, Open Approach

041F0A9 Bypass Left Internal Iliac Artery to Right Internal Iliac Artery with Autologous Arterial Tissue, Open Approach

041F0AB Bypass Left Internal Iliac Artery to Left Internal Iliac Artery with Autologous Arterial Tissue, Open Approach

041F0AC Bypass Left Internal Iliac Artery to Bilateral Internal Iliac Arteries with Autologous Arterial Tissue, Open Approach

041F0AD Bypass Left Internal Iliac Artery to Right External Iliac Artery with Autologous Arterial Tissue, Open Approach

041F0AF Bypass Left Internal Iliac Artery to Left External Iliac Artery with Autologous Arterial Tissue, Open Approach

041F0AG Bypass Left Internal Iliac Artery to Bilateral External Iliac Arteries with Autologous Arterial Tissue, Open Approach

041F0AH Bypass Left Internal Iliac Artery to Right Femoral Artery with Autologous Arterial Tissue, Open Approach

041F0AJ Bypass Left Internal Iliac Artery to Left Femoral Artery with Autologous Arterial Tissue, Open Approach

041F0AK Bypass Left Internal Iliac Artery to Bilateral Femoral Arteries with Autologous Arterial Tissue, Open Approach

041F0AP Bypass Left Internal Iliac Artery to Foot Artery with Autologous Arterial Tissue, Open Approach

041F0AQ Bypass Left Internal Iliac Artery to Lower Extremity Artery with Autologous Arterial Tissue, Open Approach

041F0J9 Bypass Left Internal Iliac Artery to Right Internal Iliac Artery with Synthetic Substitute, Open Approach

041F0JB Bypass Left Internal Iliac Artery to Left Internal Iliac Artery with Synthetic Substitute, Open Approach

041F0JC Bypass Left Internal Iliac Artery to Bilateral Internal Iliac Arteries with Synthetic Substitute, Open Approach

041F0JD Bypass Left Internal Iliac Artery to Right External Iliac Artery with Synthetic Substitute, Open Approach

041F0JF Bypass Left Internal Iliac Artery to Left External Iliac Artery with Synthetic Substitute, Open Approach

041F0JG Bypass Left Internal Iliac Artery to Bilateral External Iliac Arteries with Synthetic Substitute, Open Approach

041F0JH Bypass Left Internal Iliac Artery to Right Femoral Artery with Synthetic Substitute, Open Approach

041F0JJ Bypass Left Internal Iliac Artery to Left Femoral Artery with Synthetic Substitute, Open Approach

041F0JK Bypass Left Internal Iliac Artery to Bilateral Femoral Arteries with Synthetic Substitute, Open Approach

041F0JP Bypass Left Internal Iliac Artery to Foot Artery with Synthetic Substitute, Open Approach

041F0JQ Bypass Left Internal Iliac Artery to Lower Extremity Artery with Synthetic Substitute, Open Approach

041F0K9 Bypass Left Internal Iliac Artery to Right Internal Iliac Artery with Nonautologous Tissue Substitute, Open Approach

041F0KB Bypass Left Internal Iliac Artery to Left Internal Iliac Artery with Nonautologous Tissue Substitute, Open Approach

041F0KC Bypass Left Internal Iliac Artery to Bilateral Internal Iliac Arteries with Nonautologous Tissue Substitute, Open Approach

041F0KD Bypass Left Internal Iliac Artery to Right External Iliac Artery with Nonautologous Tissue Substitute, Open Approach

041F0KF Bypass Left Internal Iliac Artery to Left External Iliac Artery with Nonautologous Tissue Substitute, Open Approach

041F0KG Bypass Left Internal Iliac Artery to Bilateral External Iliac Arteries with Nonautologous Tissue Substitute, Open Approach

041F0KH Bypass Left Internal Iliac Artery to Right Femoral Artery with Nonautologous Tissue Substitute, Open Approach

041F0KJ Bypass Left Internal Iliac Artery to Left Femoral Artery with Nonautologous Tissue Substitute, Open Approach

041F0KK Bypass Left Internal Iliac Artery to Bilateral Femoral Arteries with Nonautologous Tissue Substitute, Open Approach

041F0KP Bypass Left Internal Iliac Artery to Foot Artery with Nonautologous Tissue Substitute, Open Approach

041F0KQ Bypass Left Internal Iliac Artery to Lower Extremity Artery with Nonautologous Tissue Substitute, Open Approach

041F0Z9 Bypass Left Internal Iliac Artery to Right Internal Iliac Artery, Open Approach

041F0ZB Bypass Left Internal Iliac Artery to Left Internal Iliac Artery, Open Approach

041F0ZC Bypass Left Internal Iliac Artery to Bilateral Internal Iliac Arteries, Open Approach

041F0ZD Bypass Left Internal Iliac Artery to Right External Iliac Artery, Open Approach

041F0ZF Bypass Left Internal Iliac Artery to Left External Iliac Artery, Open Approach

041F0ZG Bypass Left Internal Iliac Artery to Bilateral External Iliac Arteries, Open Approach

041F0ZH Bypass Left Internal Iliac Artery to Right Femoral Artery, Open Approach

041F0ZJ Bypass Left Internal Iliac Artery to Left Femoral Artery, Open Approach

041F0ZK Bypass Left Internal Iliac Artery to Bilateral Femoral Arteries, Open Approach

041F0ZP Bypass Left Internal Iliac Artery to Foot Artery, Open Approach

041F0ZQ Bypass Left Internal Iliac Artery to Lower Extremity Artery, Open Approach

041F499 Bypass Left Internal Iliac Artery to Right Internal Iliac Artery with Autologous Venous Tissue, Percutaneous Endoscopic Approach

041F49B Bypass Left Internal Iliac Artery to Left Internal Iliac Artery with Autologous Venous Tissue, Percutaneous Endoscopic Approach

041F49C Bypass Left Internal Iliac Artery to Bilateral Internal Iliac Arteries with Autologous Venous Tissue, Percutaneous Endoscopic Approach

041F49D Bypass Left Internal Iliac Artery to Right External Iliac Artery with Autologous Venous Tissue, Percutaneous Endoscopic Approach

041F49F Bypass Left Internal Iliac Artery to Left External Iliac Artery with Autologous Venous Tissue, Percutaneous Endoscopic Approach

041F49G Bypass Left Internal Iliac Artery to Bilateral External Iliac Arteries with Autologous Venous Tissue, Percutaneous Endoscopic Approach

041F49H Bypass Left Internal Iliac Artery to Right Femoral Artery with Autologous Venous Tissue, Percutaneous Endoscopic Approach

041F49J Bypass Left Internal Iliac Artery to Left Femoral Artery with Autologous Venous Tissue, Percutaneous Endoscopic Approach

041F49K Bypass Left Internal Iliac Artery to Bilateral Femoral Arteries with Autologous Venous Tissue, Percutaneous Endoscopic Approach

041F49P Bypass Left Internal Iliac Artery to Foot Artery with Autologous Venous Tissue, Percutaneous Endoscopic Approach

041F49Q Bypass Left Internal Iliac Artery to Lower Extremity Artery with Autologous Venous Tissue, Percutaneous Endoscopic Approach

041F4A9 Bypass Left Internal Iliac Artery to Right Internal Iliac Artery with Autologous Arterial Tissue, Percutaneous Endoscopic Approach

041F4AB Bypass Left Internal Iliac Artery to Left Internal Iliac Artery with Autologous Arterial Tissue, Percutaneous Endoscopic Approach

041F4AC Bypass Left Internal Iliac Artery to Bilateral Internal Iliac Arteries with Autologous Arterial Tissue, Percutaneous Endoscopic Approach

041F4AD Bypass Left Internal Iliac Artery to Right External Iliac Artery with Autologous Arterial Tissue, Percutaneous Endoscopic Approach

041F4AF Bypass Left Internal Iliac Artery to Left External Iliac Artery with Autologous Arterial Tissue, Percutaneous Endoscopic Approach

041F4AG Bypass Left Internal Iliac Artery to Bilateral External Iliac Arteries with Autologous Arterial Tissue, Percutaneous Endoscopic Approach

041F4AH Bypass Left Internal Iliac Artery to Right Femoral Artery with Autologous Arterial Tissue, Percutaneous Endoscopic Approach

041F4AJ Bypass Left Internal Iliac Artery to Left Femoral Artery with Autologous Arterial Tissue, Percutaneous Endoscopic Approach

041F4AK Bypass Left Internal Iliac Artery to Bilateral Femoral Arteries with Autologous Arterial Tissue, Percutaneous Endoscopic Approach

041F4AP Bypass Left Internal Iliac Artery to Foot Artery with Autologous Arterial Tissue, Percutaneous Endoscopic Approach

041F4AQ Bypass Left Internal Iliac Artery to Lower Extremity Artery with Autologous Arterial Tissue, Percutaneous Endoscopic Approach

041F4J9 Bypass Left Internal Iliac Artery to Right Internal Iliac Artery with Synthetic Substitute, Percutaneous Endoscopic Approach

041F4JB Bypass Left Internal Iliac Artery to Left Internal Iliac Artery with Synthetic Substitute, Percutaneous Endoscopic Approach

041F4JC Bypass Left Internal Iliac Artery to Bilateral Internal Iliac Arteries with Synthetic Substitute, Percutaneous Endoscopic Approach

041F4JD Bypass Left Internal Iliac Artery to Right External Iliac Artery with Synthetic Substitute, Percutaneous Endoscopic Approach

041F4JF Bypass Left Internal Iliac Artery to Left External Iliac Artery with Synthetic Substitute, Percutaneous Endoscopic Approach

041F4JG Bypass Left Internal Iliac Artery to Bilateral External Iliac Arteries with Synthetic Substitute, Percutaneous Endoscopic Approach

041F4JH Bypass Left Internal Iliac Artery to Right Femoral Artery with Synthetic Substitute, Percutaneous Endoscopic Approach

041F4JJ Bypass Left Internal Iliac Artery to Left Femoral Artery with Synthetic Substitute, Percutaneous Endoscopic Approach

041F4JK Bypass Left Internal Iliac Artery to Bilateral Femoral Arteries with Synthetic Substitute, Percutaneous Endoscopic Approach

041F4JP Bypass Left Internal Iliac Artery to Foot Artery with Synthetic Substitute, Percutaneous Endoscopic Approach

041F4JQ Bypass Left Internal Iliac Artery to Lower Extremity Artery with Synthetic Substitute, Percutaneous Endoscopic Approach

041F4K9 Bypass Left Internal Iliac Artery to Right Internal Iliac Artery with Nonautologous Tissue Substitute, Percutaneous Endoscopic Approach

041F4KB Bypass Left Internal Iliac Artery to Left Internal Iliac Artery with Nonautologous Tissue Substitute, Percutaneous Endoscopic Approach

041F4KC Bypass Left Internal Iliac Artery to Bilateral Internal Iliac Arteries with Nonautologous Tissue Substitute, Percutaneous Endoscopic Approach

041F4KD Bypass Left Internal Iliac Artery to Right External Iliac Artery with Nonautologous Tissue Substitute, Percutaneous Endoscopic Approach

041F4KF Bypass Left Internal Iliac Artery to Left External Iliac Artery with Nonautologous Tissue Substitute, Percutaneous Endoscopic Approach

041F4KG Bypass Left Internal Iliac Artery to Bilateral External Iliac Arteries with Nonautologous Tissue Substitute, Percutaneous Endoscopic Approach

041F4KH Bypass Left Internal Iliac Artery to Right Femoral Artery with Nonautologous Tissue Substitute, Percutaneous Endoscopic Approach

041F4KJ Bypass Left Internal Iliac Artery to Left Femoral Artery with Nonautologous Tissue Substitute, Percutaneous Endoscopic Approach

041F4KK Bypass Left Internal Iliac Artery to Bilateral Femoral Arteries with Nonautologous Tissue Substitute, Percutaneous Endoscopic Approach

041F4KP Bypass Left Internal Iliac Artery to Foot Artery with Nonautologous Tissue Substitute, Percutaneous Endoscopic Approach

041F4KQ Bypass Left Internal Iliac Artery to Lower Extremity Artery with Nonautologous Tissue Substitute, Percutaneous Endoscopic Approach

041F4Z9 Bypass Left Internal Iliac Artery to Right Internal Iliac Artery, Percutaneous Endoscopic Approach

041F4ZB Bypass Left Internal Iliac Artery to Left Internal Iliac Artery, Percutaneous Endoscopic Approach

041F4ZC Bypass Left Internal Iliac Artery to Bilateral Internal Iliac Arteries, Percutaneous Endoscopic Approach

041F4ZD Bypass Left Internal Iliac Artery to Right External Iliac Artery, Percutaneous Endoscopic Approach

041F4ZF Bypass Left Internal Iliac Artery to Left External Iliac Artery, Percutaneous Endoscopic Approach

041F4ZG Bypass Left Internal Iliac Artery to Bilateral External Iliac Arteries, Percutaneous Endoscopic Approach

041F4ZH Bypass Left Internal Iliac Artery to Right Femoral Artery, Percutaneous Endoscopic Approach

041F4ZJ Bypass Left Internal Iliac Artery to Left Femoral Artery, Percutaneous Endoscopic Approach

041F4ZK Bypass Left Internal Iliac Artery to Bilateral Femoral Arteries, Percutaneous Endoscopic Approach

041F4ZP Bypass Left Internal Iliac Artery to Foot Artery, Percutaneous Endoscopic Approach

041F4ZQ Bypass Left Internal Iliac Artery to Lower Extremity Artery, Percutaneous Endoscopic Approach

041H099 Bypass Right External Iliac Artery to Right Internal Iliac Artery with Autologous Venous Tissue, Open Approach
041H09B Bypass Right External Iliac Artery to Left Internal Iliac Artery with Autologous Venous Tissue, Open Approach
041H09C Bypass Right External Iliac Artery to Bilateral Internal Iliac Arteries with Autologous Venous Tissue, Open Approach
041H09D Bypass Right External Iliac Artery to Right External Iliac Artery with Autologous Venous Tissue, Open Approach
041H09F Bypass Right External Iliac Artery to Left External Iliac Artery with Autologous Venous Tissue, Open Approach
041H09G Bypass Right External Iliac Artery to Bilateral External Iliac Arteries with Autologous Venous Tissue, Open Approach
041H09H Bypass Right External Iliac Artery to Right Femoral Artery with Autologous Venous Tissue, Open Approach
041H09J Bypass Right External Iliac Artery to Left Femoral Artery with Autologous Venous Tissue, Open Approach
041H09K Bypass Right External Iliac Artery to Bilateral Femoral Arteries with Autologous Venous Tissue, Open Approach
041H09P Bypass Right External Iliac Artery to Foot Artery with Autologous Venous Tissue, Open Approach
041H09Q Bypass Right External Iliac Artery to Lower Extremity Artery with Autologous Venous Tissue, Open Approach
041H0A9 Bypass Right External Iliac Artery to Right Internal Iliac Artery with Autologous Arterial Tissue, Open Approach
041H0AB Bypass Right External Iliac Artery to Left Internal Iliac Artery with Autologous Arterial Tissue, Open Approach
041H0AC Bypass Right External Iliac Artery to Bilateral Internal Iliac Arteries with Autologous Arterial Tissue, Open Approach
041H0AD Bypass Right External Iliac Artery to Right External Iliac Artery with Autologous Arterial Tissue, Open Approach
041H0AF Bypass Right External Iliac Artery to Left External Iliac Artery with Autologous Arterial Tissue, Open Approach
041H0AG Bypass Right External Iliac Artery to Bilateral External Iliac Arteries with Autologous Arterial Tissue, Open Approach
041H0AH Bypass Right External Iliac Artery to Right Femoral Artery with Autologous Arterial Tissue, Open Approach
041H0AJ Bypass Right External Iliac Artery to Left Femoral Artery with Autologous Arterial Tissue, Open Approach
041H0AK Bypass Right External Iliac Artery to Bilateral Femoral Arteries with Autologous Arterial Tissue, Open Approach
041H0AP Bypass Right External Iliac Artery to Foot Artery with Autologous Arterial Tissue, Open Approach
041H0AQ Bypass Right External Iliac Artery to Lower Extremity Artery with Autologous Arterial Tissue, Open Approach
041H0J9 Bypass Right External Iliac Artery to Right Internal Iliac Artery with Synthetic Substitute, Open Approach
041H0JB Bypass Right External Iliac Artery to Left Internal Iliac Artery with Synthetic Substitute, Open Approach
041H0JC Bypass Right External Iliac Artery to Bilateral Internal Iliac Arteries with Synthetic Substitute, Open Approach
041H0JD Bypass Right External Iliac Artery to Right External Iliac Artery with Synthetic Substitute, Open Approach
041H0JF Bypass Right External Iliac Artery to Left External Iliac Artery with Synthetic Substitute, Open Approach
041H0JG Bypass Right External Iliac Artery to Bilateral External Iliac Arteries with Synthetic Substitute, Open Approach
041H0JH Bypass Right External Iliac Artery to Right Femoral Artery with Synthetic Substitute, Open Approach
041H0JJ Bypass Right External Iliac Artery to Left Femoral Artery with Synthetic Substitute, Open Approach
041H0JK Bypass Right External Iliac Artery to Bilateral Femoral Arteries with Synthetic Substitute, Open Approach
041H0JP Bypass Right External Iliac Artery to Foot Artery with Synthetic Substitute, Open Approach
041H0JQ Bypass Right External Iliac Artery to Lower Extremity Artery with Synthetic Substitute, Open Approach
041H0K9 Bypass Right External Iliac Artery to Right Internal Iliac Artery with Nonautologous Tissue Substitute, Open Approach
041H0KB Bypass Right External Iliac Artery to Left Internal Iliac Artery with Nonautologous Tissue Substitute, Open Approach
041H0KC Bypass Right External Iliac Artery to Bilateral Internal Iliac Arteries with Nonautologous Tissue Substitute, Open Approach
041H0KD Bypass Right External Iliac Artery to Right External Iliac Artery with Nonautologous Tissue Substitute, Open Approach
041H0KF Bypass Right External Iliac Artery to Left External Iliac Artery with Nonautologous Tissue Substitute, Open Approach
041H0KG Bypass Right External Iliac Artery to Bilateral External Iliac Arteries with Nonautologous Tissue Substitute, Open Approach
041H0KH Bypass Right External Iliac Artery to Right Femoral Artery with Nonautologous Tissue Substitute, Open Approach
041H0KJ Bypass Right External Iliac Artery to Left Femoral Artery with Nonautologous Tissue Substitute, Open Approach
041H0KK Bypass Right External Iliac Artery to Bilateral Femoral Arteries with Nonautologous Tissue Substitute, Open Approach
041H0KP Bypass Right External Iliac Artery to Foot Artery with Nonautologous Tissue Substitute, Open Approach
041H0KQ Bypass Right External Iliac Artery to Lower Extremity Artery with Nonautologous Tissue Substitute, Open Approach
041H0Z9 Bypass Right External Iliac Artery to Right Internal Iliac Artery, Open Approach
041H0ZB Bypass Right External Iliac Artery to Left Internal Iliac Artery, Open Approach
041H0ZC Bypass Right External Iliac Artery to Bilateral Internal Iliac Arteries, Open Approach
041H0ZD Bypass Right External Iliac Artery to Right External Iliac Artery, Open Approach
041H0ZF Bypass Right External Iliac Artery to Left External Iliac Artery, Open Approach
041H0ZG Bypass Right External Iliac Artery to Bilateral External Iliac Arteries, Open Approach
041H0ZH Bypass Right External Iliac Artery to Right Femoral Artery, Open Approach
041H0ZJ Bypass Right External Iliac Artery to Left Femoral Artery, Open Approach
041H0ZK Bypass Right External Iliac Artery to Bilateral Femoral Arteries, Open Approach
041H0ZP Bypass Right External Iliac Artery to Foot Artery, Open Approach
041H0ZQ Bypass Right External Iliac Artery to Lower Extremity Artery, Open Approach
041H499 Bypass Right External Iliac Artery to Right Internal Iliac Artery with Autologous Venous Tissue, Percutaneous Endoscopic Approach
041H49B Bypass Right External Iliac Artery to Left Internal Iliac Artery with Autologous Venous Tissue, Percutaneous Endoscopic Approach
041H49C Bypass Right External Iliac Artery to Bilateral Internal Iliac Arteries with Autologous Venous Tissue, Percutaneous Endoscopic Approach
041H49D Bypass Right External Iliac Artery to Right External Iliac Artery with Autologous Venous Tissue, Percutaneous Endoscopic Approach
041H49F Bypass Right External Iliac Artery to Left External Iliac Artery with Autologous Venous Tissue, Percutaneous Endoscopic Approach
041H49G Bypass Right External Iliac Artery to Bilateral External Iliac Arteries with Autologous Venous Tissue, Percutaneous Endoscopic Approach
041H49H Bypass Right External Iliac Artery to Right Femoral Artery with Autologous Venous Tissue, Percutaneous Endoscopic Approach
041H49J Bypass Right External Iliac Artery to Left Femoral Artery with Autologous Venous Tissue, Percutaneous Endoscopic Approach
041H49K Bypass Right External Iliac Artery to Bilateral Femoral Arteries with Autologous Venous Tissue, Percutaneous Endoscopic Approach
041H49P Bypass Right External Iliac Artery to Foot Artery with Autologous Venous Tissue, Percutaneous Endoscopic Approach
041H49Q Bypass Right External Iliac Artery to Lower Extremity Artery with Autologous Venous Tissue, Percutaneous Endoscopic Approach
041H4A9 Bypass Right External Iliac Artery to Right Internal Iliac Artery with Autologous Arterial Tissue, Percutaneous Endoscopic Approach
041H4AB Bypass Right External Iliac Artery to Left Internal Iliac Artery with Autologous Arterial Tissue, Percutaneous Endoscopic Approach
041H4AC Bypass Right External Iliac Artery to Bilateral Internal Iliac Arteries with Autologous Arterial Tissue, Percutaneous Endoscopic Approach
041H4AD Bypass Right External Iliac Artery to Right External Iliac Artery with

Autologous Arterial Tissue, Percutaneous Endoscopic Approach

041H4AF Bypass Right External Iliac Artery to Left External Iliac Artery with Autologous Arterial Tissue, Percutaneous Endoscopic Approach

041H4AG Bypass Right External Iliac Artery to Bilateral External Iliac Arteries with Autologous Arterial Tissue, Percutaneous Endoscopic Approach

041H4AH Bypass Right External Iliac Artery to Right Femoral Artery with Autologous Arterial Tissue, Percutaneous Endoscopic Approach

041H4AJ Bypass Right External Iliac Artery to Left Femoral Artery with Autologous Arterial Tissue, Percutaneous Endoscopic Approach

041H4AK Bypass Right External Iliac Artery to Bilateral Femoral Arteries with Autologous Arterial Tissue, Percutaneous Endoscopic Approach

041H4AP Bypass Right External Iliac Artery to Foot Artery with Autologous Arterial Tissue, Percutaneous Endoscopic Approach

041H4AQ Bypass Right External Iliac Artery to Lower Extremity Artery with Autologous Arterial Tissue, Percutaneous Endoscopic Approach

041H4J9 Bypass Right External Iliac Artery to Right Internal Iliac Artery with Synthetic Substitute, Percutaneous Endoscopic Approach

041H4JB Bypass Right External Iliac Artery to Left Internal Iliac Artery with Synthetic Substitute, Percutaneous Endoscopic Approach

041H4JC Bypass Right External Iliac Artery to Bilateral Internal Iliac Arteries with Synthetic Substitute, Percutaneous Endoscopic Approach

041H4JD Bypass Right External Iliac Artery to Right External Iliac Artery with Synthetic Substitute, Percutaneous Endoscopic Approach

041H4JF Bypass Right External Iliac Artery to Left External Iliac Artery with Synthetic Substitute, Percutaneous Endoscopic Approach

041H4JG Bypass Right External Iliac Artery to Bilateral External Iliac Arteries with Synthetic Substitute, Percutaneous Endoscopic Approach

041H4JH Bypass Right External Iliac Artery to Right Femoral Artery with Synthetic Substitute, Percutaneous Endoscopic Approach

041H4JJ Bypass Right External Iliac Artery to Left Femoral Artery with Synthetic Substitute, Percutaneous Endoscopic Approach

041H4JK Bypass Right External Iliac Artery to Bilateral Femoral Arteries with Synthetic Substitute, Percutaneous Endoscopic Approach

041H4JP Bypass Right External Iliac Artery to Foot Artery with Synthetic Substitute, Percutaneous Endoscopic Approach

041H4JQ Bypass Right External Iliac Artery to Lower Extremity Artery with Synthetic Substitute, Percutaneous Endoscopic Approach

041H4K9 Bypass Right External Iliac Artery to Right Internal Iliac Artery with Nonautologous Tissue Substitute, Percutaneous Endoscopic Approach

041H4KB Bypass Right External Iliac Artery to Left Internal Iliac Artery with Nonautologous Tissue Substitute, Percutaneous Endoscopic Approach

041H4KC Bypass Right External Iliac Artery to Bilateral Internal Iliac Arteries with Nonautologous Tissue Substitute, Percutaneous Endoscopic Approach

041H4KD Bypass Right External Iliac Artery to Right External Iliac Artery with Nonautologous Tissue Substitute, Percutaneous Endoscopic Approach

041H4KF Bypass Right External Iliac Artery to Left External Iliac Artery with Nonautologous Tissue Substitute, Percutaneous Endoscopic Approach

041H4KG Bypass Right External Iliac Artery to Bilateral External Iliac Arteries with Nonautologous Tissue Substitute, Percutaneous Endoscopic Approach

041H4KH Bypass Right External Iliac Artery to Right Femoral Artery with Nonautologous Tissue Substitute, Percutaneous Endoscopic Approach

041H4KJ Bypass Right External Iliac Artery to Left Femoral Artery with Nonautologous Tissue Substitute, Percutaneous Endoscopic Approach

041H4KK Bypass Right External Iliac Artery to Bilateral Femoral Arteries with Nonautologous Tissue Substitute, Percutaneous Endoscopic Approach

041H4KP Bypass Right External Iliac Artery to Foot Artery with Nonautologous Tissue Substitute, Percutaneous Endoscopic Approach

041H4KQ Bypass Right External Iliac Artery to Lower Extremity Artery with Nonautologous Tissue Substitute, Percutaneous Endoscopic Approach

041H4Z9 Bypass Right External Iliac Artery to Right Internal Iliac Artery, Percutaneous Endoscopic Approach

041H4ZB Bypass Right External Iliac Artery to Left Internal Iliac Artery, Percutaneous Endoscopic Approach

041H4ZC Bypass Right External Iliac Artery to Bilateral Internal Iliac Arteries, Percutaneous Endoscopic Approach

041H4ZD Bypass Right External Iliac Artery to Right External Iliac Artery, Percutaneous Endoscopic Approach

041H4ZF Bypass Right External Iliac Artery to Left External Iliac Artery, Percutaneous Endoscopic Approach

041H4ZG Bypass Right External Iliac Artery to Bilateral External Iliac Arteries, Percutaneous Endoscopic Approach

041H4ZH Bypass Right External Iliac Artery to Right Femoral Artery, Percutaneous Endoscopic Approach

041H4ZJ Bypass Right External Iliac Artery to Left Femoral Artery, Percutaneous Endoscopic Approach

041H4ZK Bypass Right External Iliac Artery to Bilateral Femoral Arteries, Percutaneous Endoscopic Approach

041H4ZP Bypass Right External Iliac Artery to Foot Artery, Percutaneous Endoscopic Approach

041H4ZQ Bypass Right External Iliac Artery to Lower Extremity Artery, Percutaneous Endoscopic Approach

041J099 Bypass Left External Iliac Artery to Right Internal Iliac Artery with Autologous Venous Tissue, Open Approach

041J09B Bypass Left External Iliac Artery to Left Internal Iliac Artery with Autologous Venous Tissue, Open Approach

041J09C Bypass Left External Iliac Artery to Bilateral Internal Iliac Arteries with Autologous Venous Tissue, Open Approach

041J09D Bypass Left External Iliac Artery to Right External Iliac Artery with Autologous Venous Tissue, Open Approach

041J09F Bypass Left External Iliac Artery to Left External Iliac Artery with Autologous Venous Tissue, Open Approach

041J09G Bypass Left External Iliac Artery to Bilateral External Iliac Arteries with Autologous Venous Tissue, Open Approach

041J09H Bypass Left External Iliac Artery to Right Femoral Artery with Autologous Venous Tissue, Open Approach

041J09J Bypass Left External Iliac Artery to Left Femoral Artery with Autologous Venous Tissue, Open Approach

041J09K Bypass Left External Iliac Artery to Bilateral Femoral Arteries with Autologous Venous Tissue, Open Approach

041J09P Bypass Left External Iliac Artery to Foot Artery with Autologous Venous Tissue, Open Approach

041J09Q Bypass Left External Iliac Artery to Lower Extremity Artery with Autologous Venous Tissue, Open Approach

041J0A9 Bypass Left External Iliac Artery to Right Internal Iliac Artery with Autologous Arterial Tissue, Open Approach

041J0AB Bypass Left External Iliac Artery to Left Internal Iliac Artery with Autologous Arterial Tissue, Open Approach

041J0AC Bypass Left External Iliac Artery to Bilateral Internal Iliac Arteries with Autologous Arterial Tissue, Open Approach

041J0AD Bypass Left External Iliac Artery to Right External Iliac Artery with Autologous Arterial Tissue, Open Approach

041J0AF Bypass Left External Iliac Artery to Left External Iliac Artery with Autologous Arterial Tissue, Open Approach

041J0AG Bypass Left External Iliac Artery to Bilateral External Iliac Arteries with Autologous Arterial Tissue, Open Approach

041J0AH Bypass Left External Iliac Artery to Right Femoral Artery with Autologous Arterial Tissue, Open Approach

041J0AJ Bypass Left External Iliac Artery to Left Femoral Artery with Autologous Arterial Tissue, Open Approach

041J0AK Bypass Left External Iliac Artery to Bilateral Femoral Arteries with Autologous Arterial Tissue, Open Approach

041J0AP Bypass Left External Iliac Artery to Foot Artery with Autologous Arterial Tissue, Open Approach

041J0AQ Bypass Left External Iliac Artery to Lower Extremity Artery with Autologous Arterial Tissue, Open Approach

041J0J9 Bypass Left External Iliac Artery to Right Internal Iliac Artery with Synthetic Substitute, Open Approach

041J0JB Bypass Left External Iliac Artery to Left Internal Iliac Artery with Synthetic Substitute, Open Approach

041J0JC Bypass Left External Iliac Artery to Bilateral Internal Iliac Arteries with Synthetic Substitute, Open Approach

041J0JD Bypass Left External Iliac Artery to Right External Iliac Artery with Synthetic Substitute, Open Approach

041J0JF Bypass Left External Iliac Artery to Left External Iliac Artery with Synthetic Substitute, Open Approach

041J0JG Bypass Left External Iliac Artery to Bilateral External Iliac Arteries with Synthetic Substitute, Open Approach

041J0JH Bypass Left External Iliac Artery to Right Femoral Artery with Synthetic Substitute, Open Approach

041J0JJ Bypass Left External Iliac Artery to Left Femoral Artery with Synthetic Substitute, Open Approach

041J0JK Bypass Left External Iliac Artery to Bilateral Femoral Arteries with Synthetic Substitute, Open Approach

041J0JP Bypass Left External Iliac Artery to Foot Artery with Synthetic Substitute, Open Approach

041J0JQ Bypass Left External Iliac Artery to Lower Extremity Artery with Synthetic Substitute, Open Approach

041J0K9 Bypass Left External Iliac Artery to Right Internal Iliac Artery with Nonautologous Tissue Substitute, Open Approach

041J0KB Bypass Left External Iliac Artery to Left Internal Iliac Artery with Nonautologous Tissue Substitute, Open Approach

041J0KC Bypass Left External Iliac Artery to Bilateral Internal Iliac Arteries with Nonautologous Tissue Substitute, Open Approach

041J0KD Bypass Left External Iliac Artery to Right External Iliac Artery with Nonautologous Tissue Substitute, Open Approach

041J0KF Bypass Left External Iliac Artery to Left External Iliac Artery with Nonautologous Tissue Substitute, Open Approach

041J0KG Bypass Left External Iliac Artery to Bilateral External Iliac Arteries with Nonautologous Tissue Substitute, Open Approach

041J0KH Bypass Left External Iliac Artery to Right Femoral Artery with Nonautologous Tissue Substitute, Open Approach

041J0KJ Bypass Left External Iliac Artery to Left Femoral Artery with Nonautologous Tissue Substitute, Open Approach

041J0KK Bypass Left External Iliac Artery to Bilateral Femoral Arteries with Nonautologous Tissue Substitute, Open Approach

041J0KP Bypass Left External Iliac Artery to Foot Artery with Nonautologous Tissue Substitute, Open Approach

041J0KQ Bypass Left External Iliac Artery to Lower Extremity Artery with Nonautologous Tissue Substitute, Open Approach

041J0Z9 Bypass Left External Iliac Artery to Right Internal Iliac Artery, Open Approach

041J0ZB Bypass Left External Iliac Artery to Left Internal Iliac Artery, Open Approach

041J0ZC Bypass Left External Iliac Artery to Bilateral Internal Iliac Arteries, Open Approach

041J0ZD Bypass Left External Iliac Artery to Right External Iliac Artery, Open Approach

041J0ZF Bypass Left External Iliac Artery to Left External Iliac Artery, Open Approach

041J0ZG Bypass Left External Iliac Artery to Bilateral External Iliac Arteries, Open Approach

041J0ZH Bypass Left External Iliac Artery to Right Femoral Artery, Open Approach

041J0ZJ Bypass Left External Iliac Artery to Left Femoral Artery, Open Approach

041J0ZK Bypass Left External Iliac Artery to Bilateral Femoral Arteries, Open Approach

041J0ZP Bypass Left External Iliac Artery to Foot Artery, Open Approach

041J0ZQ Bypass Left External Iliac Artery to Lower Extremity Artery, Open Approach

041J499 Bypass Left External Iliac Artery to Right Internal Iliac Artery with Autologous Venous Tissue, Percutaneous Endoscopic Approach

041J49B Bypass Left External Iliac Artery to Left Internal Iliac Artery with Autologous Venous Tissue, Percutaneous Endoscopic Approach

041J49C Bypass Left External Iliac Artery to Bilateral Internal Iliac Arteries with Autologous Venous Tissue, Percutaneous Endoscopic Approach

041J49D Bypass Left External Iliac Artery to Right External Iliac Artery with Autologous Venous Tissue, Percutaneous Endoscopic Approach

041J49F Bypass Left External Iliac Artery to Left External Iliac Artery with Autologous Venous Tissue, Percutaneous Endoscopic Approach

041J49G Bypass Left External Iliac Artery to Bilateral External Iliac Arteries with Autologous Venous Tissue, Percutaneous Endoscopic Approach

041J49H Bypass Left External Iliac Artery to Right Femoral Artery with Autologous Venous Tissue, Percutaneous Endoscopic Approach

041J49J Bypass Left External Iliac Artery to Left Femoral Artery with Autologous Venous Tissue, Percutaneous Endoscopic Approach

041J49K Bypass Left External Iliac Artery to Bilateral Femoral Arteries with Autologous Venous Tissue, Percutaneous Endoscopic Approach

041J49P Bypass Left External Iliac Artery to Foot Artery with Autologous Venous Tissue, Percutaneous Endoscopic Approach

041J49Q Bypass Left External Iliac Artery to Lower Extremity Artery with Autologous Venous Tissue, Percutaneous Endoscopic Approach

041J4A9 Bypass Left External Iliac Artery to Right Internal Iliac Artery with Autologous Arterial Tissue, Percutaneous Endoscopic Approach

041J4AB Bypass Left External Iliac Artery to Left Internal Iliac Artery with Autologous Arterial Tissue, Percutaneous Endoscopic Approach

041J4AC Bypass Left External Iliac Artery to Bilateral Internal Iliac Arteries with Autologous Arterial Tissue, Percutaneous Endoscopic Approach

041J4AD Bypass Left External Iliac Artery to Right External Iliac Artery with Autologous Arterial Tissue, Percutaneous Endoscopic Approach

041J4AF Bypass Left External Iliac Artery to Left External Iliac Artery with Autologous Arterial Tissue, Percutaneous Endoscopic Approach

041J4AG Bypass Left External Iliac Artery to Bilateral External Iliac Arteries with Autologous Arterial Tissue, Percutaneous Endoscopic Approach

041J4AH Bypass Left External Iliac Artery to Right Femoral Artery with Autologous Arterial Tissue, Percutaneous Endoscopic Approach

041J4AJ Bypass Left External Iliac Artery to Left Femoral Artery with Autologous Arterial Tissue, Percutaneous Endoscopic Approach

041J4AK Bypass Left External Iliac Artery to Bilateral Femoral Arteries with Autologous Arterial Tissue, Percutaneous Endoscopic Approach

041J4AP Bypass Left External Iliac Artery to Foot Artery with Autologous Arterial Tissue, Percutaneous Endoscopic Approach

041J4AQ Bypass Left External Iliac Artery to Lower Extremity Artery with Autologous Arterial Tissue, Percutaneous Endoscopic Approach

041J4J9 Bypass Left External Iliac Artery to Right Internal Iliac Artery with Synthetic Substitute, Percutaneous Endoscopic Approach

041J4JB Bypass Left External Iliac Artery to Left Internal Iliac Artery with Synthetic Substitute, Percutaneous Endoscopic Approach

041J4JC Bypass Left External Iliac Artery to Bilateral Internal Iliac Arteries with Synthetic Substitute, Percutaneous Endoscopic Approach

041J4JD Bypass Left External Iliac Artery to Right External Iliac Artery with Synthetic Substitute, Percutaneous Endoscopic Approach

041J4JF Bypass Left External Iliac Artery to Left External Iliac Artery with Synthetic Substitute, Percutaneous Endoscopic Approach

041J4JG Bypass Left External Iliac Artery to Bilateral External Iliac Arteries with Synthetic Substitute, Percutaneous Endoscopic Approach

041J4JH Bypass Left External Iliac Artery to Right Femoral Artery with Synthetic Substitute, Percutaneous Endoscopic Approach

041J4JJ Bypass Left External Iliac Artery to Left Femoral Artery with Synthetic Substitute, Percutaneous Endoscopic Approach

041J4JK Bypass Left External Iliac Artery to Bilateral Femoral Arteries with Synthetic Substitute, Percutaneous Endoscopic Approach

041J4JP Bypass Left External Iliac Artery to Foot Artery with Synthetic Substitute, Percutaneous Endoscopic Approach

041J4JQ Bypass Left External Iliac Artery to Lower Extremity Artery with Synthetic Substitute, Percutaneous Endoscopic Approach

041J4K9 Bypass Left External Iliac Artery to Right Internal Iliac Artery with Nonautologous Tissue Substitute, Percutaneous Endoscopic Approach

041J4KB Bypass Left External Iliac Artery to Left Internal Iliac Artery with Nonautologous Tissue Substitute, Percutaneous Endoscopic Approach

041J4KC Bypass Left External Iliac Artery to Bilateral Internal Iliac Arteries with Nonautologous Tissue Substitute, Percutaneous Endoscopic Approach

041J4KD Bypass Left External Iliac Artery to Right External Iliac Artery with Nonautologous Tissue Substitute, Percutaneous Endoscopic Approach

041J4KF Bypass Left External Iliac Artery to Left External Iliac Artery with Nonautologous Tissue Substitute, Percutaneous Endoscopic Approach

041J4KG Bypass Left External Iliac Artery to Bilateral External Iliac Arteries with Nonautologous Tissue Substitute, Percutaneous Endoscopic Approach
041J4KH Bypass Left External Iliac Artery to Right Femoral Artery with Nonautologous Tissue Substitute, Percutaneous Endoscopic Approach
041J4KJ Bypass Left External Iliac Artery to Left Femoral Artery with Nonautologous Tissue Substitute, Percutaneous Endoscopic Approach
041J4KK Bypass Left External Iliac Artery to Bilateral Femoral Arteries with Nonautologous Tissue Substitute, Percutaneous Endoscopic Approach
041J4KP Bypass Left External Iliac Artery to Foot Artery with Nonautologous Tissue Substitute, Percutaneous Endoscopic Approach
041J4KQ Bypass Left External Iliac Artery to Lower Extremity Artery with Nonautologous Tissue Substitute, Percutaneous Endoscopic Approach
041J4Z9 Bypass Left External Iliac Artery to Right Internal Iliac Artery, Percutaneous Endoscopic Approach
041J4ZB Bypass Left External Iliac Artery to Left Internal Iliac Artery, Percutaneous Endoscopic Approach
041J4ZC Bypass Left External Iliac Artery to Bilateral Internal Iliac Arteries, Percutaneous Endoscopic Approach
041J4ZD Bypass Left External Iliac Artery to Right External Iliac Artery, Percutaneous Endoscopic Approach
041J4ZF Bypass Left External Iliac Artery to Left External Iliac Artery, Percutaneous Endoscopic Approach
041J4ZG Bypass Left External Iliac Artery to Bilateral External Iliac Arteries, Percutaneous Endoscopic Approach
041J4ZH Bypass Left External Iliac Artery to Right Femoral Artery, Percutaneous Endoscopic Approach
041J4ZJ Bypass Left External Iliac Artery to Left Femoral Artery, Percutaneous Endoscopic Approach
041J4ZK Bypass Left External Iliac Artery to Bilateral Femoral Arteries, Percutaneous Endoscopic Approach
041J4ZP Bypass Left External Iliac Artery to Foot Artery, Percutaneous Endoscopic Approach
041J4ZQ Bypass Left External Iliac Artery to Lower Extremity Artery, Percutaneous Endoscopic Approach
041K09H Bypass Right Femoral Artery to Right Femoral Artery with Autologous Venous Tissue, Open Approach
041K09J Bypass Right Femoral Artery to Left Femoral Artery with Autologous Venous Tissue, Open Approach
041K09K Bypass Right Femoral Artery to Bilateral Femoral Arteries with Autologous Venous Tissue, Open Approach
041K09L Bypass Right Femoral Artery to Popliteal Artery with Autologous Venous Tissue, Open Approach
041K09M Bypass Right Femoral Artery to Peroneal Artery with Autologous Venous Tissue, Open Approach
041K09N Bypass Right Femoral Artery to Posterior Tibial Artery with Autologous Venous Tissue, Open Approach
041K09P Bypass Right Femoral Artery to Foot Artery with Autologous Venous Tissue, Open Approach
041K09Q Bypass Right Femoral Artery to Lower Extremity Artery with Autologous Venous Tissue, Open Approach
041K09S Bypass Right Femoral Artery to Lower Extremity Vein with Autologous Venous Tissue, Open Approach
041K0AH Bypass Right Femoral Artery to Right Femoral Artery with Autologous Arterial Tissue, Open Approach
041K0AJ Bypass Right Femoral Artery to Left Femoral Artery with Autologous Arterial Tissue, Open Approach
041K0AK Bypass Right Femoral Artery to Bilateral Femoral Arteries with Autologous Arterial Tissue, Open Approach
041K0AL Bypass Right Femoral Artery to Popliteal Artery with Autologous Arterial Tissue, Open Approach
041K0AM Bypass Right Femoral Artery to Peroneal Artery with Autologous Arterial Tissue, Open Approach
041K0AN Bypass Right Femoral Artery to Posterior Tibial Artery with Autologous Arterial Tissue, Open Approach
041K0AP Bypass Right Femoral Artery to Foot Artery with Autologous Arterial Tissue, Open Approach
041K0AQ Bypass Right Femoral Artery to Lower Extremity Artery with Autologous Arterial Tissue, Open Approach
041K0AS Bypass Right Femoral Artery to Lower Extremity Vein with Autologous Arterial Tissue, Open Approach
041K0JH Bypass Right Femoral Artery to Right Femoral Artery with Synthetic Substitute, Open Approach
041K0JJ Bypass Right Femoral Artery to Left Femoral Artery with Synthetic Substitute, Open Approach
041K0JK Bypass Right Femoral Artery to Bilateral Femoral Arteries with Synthetic Substitute, Open Approach
041K0JL Bypass Right Femoral Artery to Popliteal Artery with Synthetic Substitute, Open Approach
041K0JM Bypass Right Femoral Artery to Peroneal Artery with Synthetic Substitute, Open Approach
041K0JN Bypass Right Femoral Artery to Posterior Tibial Artery with Synthetic Substitute, Open Approach
041K0JP Bypass Right Femoral Artery to Foot Artery with Synthetic Substitute, Open Approach
041K0JQ Bypass Right Femoral Artery to Lower Extremity Artery with Synthetic Substitute, Open Approach
041K0JS Bypass Right Femoral Artery to Lower Extremity Vein with Synthetic Substitute, Open Approach
041K0KH Bypass Right Femoral Artery to Right Femoral Artery with Nonautologous Tissue Substitute, Open Approach
041K0KJ Bypass Right Femoral Artery to Left Femoral Artery with Nonautologous Tissue Substitute, Open Approach
041K0KK Bypass Right Femoral Artery to Bilateral Femoral Arteries with Nonautologous Tissue Substitute, Open Approach
041K0KL Bypass Right Femoral Artery to Popliteal Artery with Nonautologous Tissue Substitute, Open Approach
041K0KM Bypass Right Femoral Artery to Peroneal Artery with Nonautologous Tissue Substitute, Open Approach
041K0KN Bypass Right Femoral Artery to Posterior Tibial Artery with Nonautologous Tissue Substitute, Open Approach
041K0KP Bypass Right Femoral Artery to Foot Artery with Nonautologous Tissue Substitute, Open Approach
041K0KQ Bypass Right Femoral Artery to Lower Extremity Artery with Nonautologous Tissue Substitute, Open Approach
041K0KS Bypass Right Femoral Artery to Lower Extremity Vein with Nonautologous Tissue Substitute, Open Approach
041K0ZH Bypass Right Femoral Artery to Right Femoral Artery, Open Approach
041K0ZJ Bypass Right Femoral Artery to Left Femoral Artery, Open Approach
041K0ZK Bypass Right Femoral Artery to Bilateral Femoral Arteries, Open Approach
041K0ZL Bypass Right Femoral Artery to Popliteal Artery, Open Approach
041K0ZM Bypass Right Femoral Artery to Peroneal Artery, Open Approach
041K0ZN Bypass Right Femoral Artery to Posterior Tibial Artery, Open Approach
041K0ZP Bypass Right Femoral Artery to Foot Artery, Open Approach
041K0ZQ Bypass Right Femoral Artery to Lower Extremity Artery, Open Approach
041K0ZS Bypass Right Femoral Artery to Lower Extremity Vein, Open Approach
041K49H Bypass Right Femoral Artery to Right Femoral Artery with Autologous Venous Tissue, Percutaneous Endoscopic Approach
041K49J Bypass Right Femoral Artery to Left Femoral Artery with Autologous Venous Tissue, Percutaneous Endoscopic Approach
041K49K Bypass Right Femoral Artery to Bilateral Femoral Arteries with Autologous Venous Tissue, Percutaneous Endoscopic Approach
041K49L Bypass Right Femoral Artery to Popliteal Artery with Autologous Venous Tissue, Percutaneous Endoscopic Approach
041K49M Bypass Right Femoral Artery to Peroneal Artery with Autologous Venous Tissue, Percutaneous Endoscopic Approach
041K49N Bypass Right Femoral Artery to Posterior Tibial Artery with Autologous Venous Tissue, Percutaneous Endoscopic Approach
041K49P Bypass Right Femoral Artery to Foot Artery with Autologous Venous Tissue, Percutaneous Endoscopic Approach
041K49Q Bypass Right Femoral Artery to Lower Extremity Artery with Autologous Venous Tissue, Percutaneous Endoscopic Approach
041K49S Bypass Right Femoral Artery to Lower Extremity Vein with Autologous Venous Tissue, Percutaneous Endoscopic Approach
041K4AH Bypass Right Femoral Artery to Right Femoral Artery with Autologous Arterial Tissue, Percutaneous Endoscopic Approach
041K4AJ Bypass Right Femoral Artery to Left Femoral Artery with Autologous Arterial Tissue, Percutaneous Endoscopic Approach
041K4AK Bypass Right Femoral Artery to Bilateral Femoral Arteries with Autologous Arterial Tissue, Percutaneous Endoscopic Approach
041K4AL Bypass Right Femoral Artery to Popliteal Artery with Autologous Arterial Tissue, Percutaneous Endoscopic Approach
041K4AM Bypass Right Femoral Artery to Peroneal Artery with Autologous Arterial Tissue, Percutaneous Endoscopic Approach

041K4AN Bypass Right Femoral Artery to Posterior Tibial Artery with Autologous Arterial Tissue, Percutaneous Endoscopic Approach
041K4AP Bypass Right Femoral Artery to Foot Artery with Autologous Arterial Tissue, Percutaneous Endoscopic Approach
041K4AQ Bypass Right Femoral Artery to Lower Extremity Artery with Autologous Arterial Tissue, Percutaneous Endoscopic Approach
041K4AS Bypass Right Femoral Artery to Lower Extremity Vein with Autologous Arterial Tissue, Percutaneous Endoscopic Approach
041K4JH Bypass Right Femoral Artery to Right Femoral Artery with Synthetic Substitute, Percutaneous Endoscopic Approach
041K4JJ Bypass Right Femoral Artery to Left Femoral Artery with Synthetic Substitute, Percutaneous Endoscopic Approach
041K4JK Bypass Right Femoral Artery to Bilateral Femoral Arteries with Synthetic Substitute, Percutaneous Endoscopic Approach
041K4JL Bypass Right Femoral Artery to Popliteal Artery with Synthetic Substitute, Percutaneous Endoscopic Approach
041K4JM Bypass Right Femoral Artery to Peroneal Artery with Synthetic Substitute, Percutaneous Endoscopic Approach
041K4JN Bypass Right Femoral Artery to Posterior Tibial Artery with Synthetic Substitute, Percutaneous Endoscopic Approach
041K4JP Bypass Right Femoral Artery to Foot Artery with Synthetic Substitute, Percutaneous Endoscopic Approach
041K4JQ Bypass Right Femoral Artery to Lower Extremity Artery with Synthetic Substitute, Percutaneous Endoscopic Approach
041K4JS Bypass Right Femoral Artery to Lower Extremity Vein with Synthetic Substitute, Percutaneous Endoscopic Approach
041K4KH Bypass Right Femoral Artery to Right Femoral Artery with Nonautologous Tissue Substitute, Percutaneous Endoscopic Approach
041K4KJ Bypass Right Femoral Artery to Left Femoral Artery with Nonautologous Tissue Substitute, Percutaneous Endoscopic Approach
041K4KK Bypass Right Femoral Artery to Bilateral Femoral Arteries with Nonautologous Tissue Substitute, Percutaneous Endoscopic Approach
041K4KL Bypass Right Femoral Artery to Popliteal Artery with Nonautologous Tissue Substitute, Percutaneous Endoscopic Approach
041K4KM Bypass Right Femoral Artery to Peroneal Artery with Nonautologous Tissue Substitute, Percutaneous Endoscopic Approach
041K4KN Bypass Right Femoral Artery to Posterior Tibial Artery with Nonautologous Tissue Substitute, Percutaneous Endoscopic Approach
041K4KP Bypass Right Femoral Artery to Foot Artery with Nonautologous Tissue Substitute, Percutaneous Endoscopic Approach
041K4KQ Bypass Right Femoral Artery to Lower Extremity Artery with Nonautologous Tissue Substitute, Percutaneous Endoscopic Approach
041K4KS Bypass Right Femoral Artery to Lower Extremity Vein with Nonautologous Tissue Substitute, Percutaneous Endoscopic Approach
041K4ZH Bypass Right Femoral Artery to Right Femoral Artery, Percutaneous Endoscopic Approach
041K4ZJ Bypass Right Femoral Artery to Left Femoral Artery, Percutaneous Endoscopic Approach
041K4ZK Bypass Right Femoral Artery to Bilateral Femoral Arteries, Percutaneous Endoscopic Approach
041K4ZL Bypass Right Femoral Artery to Popliteal Artery, Percutaneous Endoscopic Approach
041K4ZM Bypass Right Femoral Artery to Peroneal Artery, Percutaneous Endoscopic Approach
041K4ZN Bypass Right Femoral Artery to Posterior Tibial Artery, Percutaneous Endoscopic Approach
041K4ZP Bypass Right Femoral Artery to Foot Artery, Percutaneous Endoscopic Approach
041K4ZQ Bypass Right Femoral Artery to Lower Extremity Artery, Percutaneous Endoscopic Approach
041K4ZS Bypass Right Femoral Artery to Lower Extremity Vein, Percutaneous Endoscopic Approach
041L09H Bypass Left Femoral Artery to Right Femoral Artery with Autologous Venous Tissue, Open Approach
041L09J Bypass Left Femoral Artery to Left Femoral Artery with Autologous Venous Tissue, Open Approach
041L09K Bypass Left Femoral Artery to Bilateral Femoral Arteries with Autologous Venous Tissue, Open Approach
041L09L Bypass Left Femoral Artery to Popliteal Artery with Autologous Venous Tissue, Open Approach
041L09M Bypass Left Femoral Artery to Peroneal Artery with Autologous Venous Tissue, Open Approach
041L09N Bypass Left Femoral Artery to Posterior Tibial Artery with Autologous Venous Tissue, Open Approach
041L09P Bypass Left Femoral Artery to Foot Artery with Autologous Venous Tissue, Open Approach
041L09Q Bypass Left Femoral Artery to Lower Extremity Artery with Autologous Venous Tissue, Open Approach
041L09S Bypass Left Femoral Artery to Lower Extremity Vein with Autologous Venous Tissue, Open Approach
041L0AH Bypass Left Femoral Artery to Right Femoral Artery with Autologous Arterial Tissue, Open Approach
041L0AJ Bypass Left Femoral Artery to Left Femoral Artery with Autologous Arterial Tissue, Open Approach
041L0AK Bypass Left Femoral Artery to Bilateral Femoral Arteries with Autologous Arterial Tissue, Open Approach
041L0AL Bypass Left Femoral Artery to Popliteal Artery with Autologous Arterial Tissue, Open Approach
041L0AM Bypass Left Femoral Artery to Peroneal Artery with Autologous Arterial Tissue, Open Approach
041L0AN Bypass Left Femoral Artery to Posterior Tibial Artery with Autologous Arterial Tissue, Open Approach
041L0AP Bypass Left Femoral Artery to Foot Artery with Autologous Arterial Tissue, Open Approach
041L0AQ Bypass Left Femoral Artery to Lower Extremity Artery with Autologous Arterial Tissue, Open Approach
041L0AS Bypass Left Femoral Artery to Lower Extremity Vein with Autologous Arterial Tissue, Open Approach
041L0JH Bypass Left Femoral Artery to Right Femoral Artery with Synthetic Substitute, Open Approach
041L0JJ Bypass Left Femoral Artery to Left Femoral Artery with Synthetic Substitute, Open Approach
041L0JK Bypass Left Femoral Artery to Bilateral Femoral Arteries with Synthetic Substitute, Open Approach
041L0JL Bypass Left Femoral Artery to Popliteal Artery with Synthetic Substitute, Open Approach
041L0JM Bypass Left Femoral Artery to Peroneal Artery with Synthetic Substitute, Open Approach
041L0JN Bypass Left Femoral Artery to Posterior Tibial Artery with Synthetic Substitute, Open Approach
041L0JP Bypass Left Femoral Artery to Foot Artery with Synthetic Substitute, Open Approach
041L0JQ Bypass Left Femoral Artery to Lower Extremity Artery with Synthetic Substitute, Open Approach
041L0JS Bypass Left Femoral Artery to Lower Extremity Vein with Synthetic Substitute, Open Approach
041L0KH Bypass Left Femoral Artery to Right Femoral Artery with Nonautologous Tissue Substitute, Open Approach
041L0KJ Bypass Left Femoral Artery to Left Femoral Artery with Nonautologous Tissue Substitute, Open Approach
041L0KK Bypass Left Femoral Artery to Bilateral Femoral Arteries with Nonautologous Tissue Substitute, Open Approach
041L0KL Bypass Left Femoral Artery to Popliteal Artery with Nonautologous Tissue Substitute, Open Approach
041L0KM Bypass Left Femoral Artery to Peroneal Artery with Nonautologous Tissue Substitute, Open Approach
041L0KN Bypass Left Femoral Artery to Posterior Tibial Artery with Nonautologous Tissue Substitute, Open Approach
041L0KP Bypass Left Femoral Artery to Foot Artery with Nonautologous Tissue Substitute, Open Approach
041L0KQ Bypass Left Femoral Artery to Lower Extremity Artery with Nonautologous Tissue Substitute, Open Approach
041L0KS Bypass Left Femoral Artery to Lower Extremity Vein with Nonautologous Tissue Substitute, Open Approach
041L0ZH Bypass Left Femoral Artery to Right Femoral Artery, Open Approach
041L0ZJ Bypass Left Femoral Artery to Left Femoral Artery, Open Approach
041L0ZK Bypass Left Femoral Artery to Bilateral Femoral Arteries, Open Approach
041L0ZL Bypass Left Femoral Artery to Popliteal Artery, Open Approach
041L0ZM Bypass Left Femoral Artery to Peroneal Artery, Open Approach
041L0ZN Bypass Left Femoral Artery to Posterior Tibial Artery, Open Approach
041L0ZP Bypass Left Femoral Artery to Foot Artery, Open Approach
041L0ZQ Bypass Left Femoral Artery to Lower Extremity Artery, Open Approach

041L0ZS Bypass Left Femoral Artery to Lower Extremity Vein, Open Approach
041L49H Bypass Left Femoral Artery to Right Femoral Artery with Autologous Venous Tissue, Percutaneous Endoscopic Approach
041L49J Bypass Left Femoral Artery to Left Femoral Artery with Autologous Venous Tissue, Percutaneous Endoscopic Approach
041L49K Bypass Left Femoral Artery to Bilateral Femoral Arteries with Autologous Venous Tissue, Percutaneous Endoscopic Approach
041L49L Bypass Left Femoral Artery to Popliteal Artery with Autologous Venous Tissue, Percutaneous Endoscopic Approach
041L49M Bypass Left Femoral Artery to Peroneal Artery with Autologous Venous Tissue, Percutaneous Endoscopic Approach
041L49N Bypass Left Femoral Artery to Posterior Tibial Artery with Autologous Venous Tissue, Percutaneous Endoscopic Approach
041L49P Bypass Left Femoral Artery to Foot Artery with Autologous Venous Tissue, Percutaneous Endoscopic Approach
041L49Q Bypass Left Femoral Artery to Lower Extremity Artery with Autologous Venous Tissue, Percutaneous Endoscopic Approach
041L49S Bypass Left Femoral Artery to Lower Extremity Vein with Autologous Venous Tissue, Percutaneous Endoscopic Approach
041L4AH Bypass Left Femoral Artery to Right Femoral Artery with Autologous Arterial Tissue, Percutaneous Endoscopic Approach
041L4AJ Bypass Left Femoral Artery to Left Femoral Artery with Autologous Arterial Tissue, Percutaneous Endoscopic Approach
041L4AK Bypass Left Femoral Artery to Bilateral Femoral Arteries with Autologous Arterial Tissue, Percutaneous Endoscopic Approach
041L4AL Bypass Left Femoral Artery to Popliteal Artery with Autologous Arterial Tissue, Percutaneous Endoscopic Approach
041L4AM Bypass Left Femoral Artery to Peroneal Artery with Autologous Arterial Tissue, Percutaneous Endoscopic Approach
041L4AN Bypass Left Femoral Artery to Posterior Tibial Artery with Autologous Arterial Tissue, Percutaneous Endoscopic Approach
041L4AP Bypass Left Femoral Artery to Foot Artery with Autologous Arterial Tissue, Percutaneous Endoscopic Approach
041L4AQ Bypass Left Femoral Artery to Lower Extremity Artery with Autologous Arterial Tissue, Percutaneous Endoscopic Approach
041L4AS Bypass Left Femoral Artery to Lower Extremity Vein with Autologous Arterial Tissue, Percutaneous Endoscopic Approach
041L4JH Bypass Left Femoral Artery to Right Femoral Artery with Synthetic Substitute, Percutaneous Endoscopic Approach
041L4JJ Bypass Left Femoral Artery to Left Femoral Artery with Synthetic Substitute, Percutaneous Endoscopic Approach
041L4JK Bypass Left Femoral Artery to Bilateral Femoral Arteries with Synthetic Substitute, Percutaneous Endoscopic Approach
041L4JL Bypass Left Femoral Artery to Popliteal Artery with Synthetic Substitute, Percutaneous Endoscopic Approach
041L4JM Bypass Left Femoral Artery to Peroneal Artery with Synthetic Substitute, Percutaneous Endoscopic Approach
041L4JN Bypass Left Femoral Artery to Posterior Tibial Artery with Synthetic Substitute, Percutaneous Endoscopic Approach
041L4JP Bypass Left Femoral Artery to Foot Artery with Synthetic Substitute, Percutaneous Endoscopic Approach
041L4JQ Bypass Left Femoral Artery to Lower Extremity Artery with Synthetic Substitute, Percutaneous Endoscopic Approach
041L4JS Bypass Left Femoral Artery to Lower Extremity Vein with Synthetic Substitute, Percutaneous Endoscopic Approach
041L4KH Bypass Left Femoral Artery to Right Femoral Artery with Nonautologous Tissue Substitute, Percutaneous Endoscopic Approach
041L4KJ Bypass Left Femoral Artery to Left Femoral Artery with Nonautologous Tissue Substitute, Percutaneous Endoscopic Approach
041L4KK Bypass Left Femoral Artery to Bilateral Femoral Arteries with Nonautologous Tissue Substitute, Percutaneous Endoscopic Approach
041L4KL Bypass Left Femoral Artery to Popliteal Artery with Nonautologous Tissue Substitute, Percutaneous Endoscopic Approach
041L4KM Bypass Left Femoral Artery to Peroneal Artery with Nonautologous Tissue Substitute, Percutaneous Endoscopic Approach
041L4KN Bypass Left Femoral Artery to Posterior Tibial Artery with Nonautologous Tissue Substitute, Percutaneous Endoscopic Approach
041L4KP Bypass Left Femoral Artery to Foot Artery with Nonautologous Tissue Substitute, Percutaneous Endoscopic Approach
041L4KQ Bypass Left Femoral Artery to Lower Extremity Artery with Nonautologous Tissue Substitute, Percutaneous Endoscopic Approach
041L4KS Bypass Left Femoral Artery to Lower Extremity Vein with Nonautologous Tissue Substitute, Percutaneous Endoscopic Approach
041L4ZH Bypass Left Femoral Artery to Right Femoral Artery, Percutaneous Endoscopic Approach
041L4ZJ Bypass Left Femoral Artery to Left Femoral Artery, Percutaneous Endoscopic Approach
041L4ZK Bypass Left Femoral Artery to Bilateral Femoral Arteries, Percutaneous Endoscopic Approach
041L4ZL Bypass Left Femoral Artery to Popliteal Artery, Percutaneous Endoscopic Approach
041L4ZM Bypass Left Femoral Artery to Peroneal Artery, Percutaneous Endoscopic Approach
041L4ZN Bypass Left Femoral Artery to Posterior Tibial Artery, Percutaneous Endoscopic Approach
041L4ZP Bypass Left Femoral Artery to Foot Artery, Percutaneous Endoscopic Approach
041L4ZQ Bypass Left Femoral Artery to Lower Extremity Artery, Percutaneous Endoscopic Approach
041L4ZS Bypass Left Femoral Artery to Lower Extremity Vein, Percutaneous Endoscopic Approach
041M09L Bypass Right Popliteal Artery to Popliteal Artery with Autologous Venous Tissue, Open Approach
041M09M Bypass Right Popliteal Artery to Peroneal Artery with Autologous Venous Tissue, Open Approach
041M09P Bypass Right Popliteal Artery to Foot Artery with Autologous Venous Tissue, Open Approach
041M09Q Bypass Right Popliteal Artery to Lower Extremity Artery with Autologous Venous Tissue, Open Approach
041M09S Bypass Right Popliteal Artery to Lower Extremity Vein with Autologous Venous Tissue, Open Approach
041M0AL Bypass Right Popliteal Artery to Popliteal Artery with Autologous Arterial Tissue, Open Approach
041M0AM Bypass Right Popliteal Artery to Peroneal Artery with Autologous Arterial Tissue, Open Approach
041M0AP Bypass Right Popliteal Artery to Foot Artery with Autologous Arterial Tissue, Open Approach
041M0AQ Bypass Right Popliteal Artery to Lower Extremity Artery with Autologous Arterial Tissue, Open Approach
041M0AS Bypass Right Popliteal Artery to Lower Extremity Vein with Autologous Arterial Tissue, Open Approach
041M0JL Bypass Right Popliteal Artery to Popliteal Artery with Synthetic Substitute, Open Approach
041M0JM Bypass Right Popliteal Artery to Peroneal Artery with Synthetic Substitute, Open Approach
041M0JP Bypass Right Popliteal Artery to Foot Artery with Synthetic Substitute, Open Approach
041M0JQ Bypass Right Popliteal Artery to Lower Extremity Artery with Synthetic Substitute, Open Approach
041M0JS Bypass Right Popliteal Artery to Lower Extremity Vein with Synthetic Substitute, Open Approach
041M0KL Bypass Right Popliteal Artery to Popliteal Artery with Nonautologous Tissue Substitute, Open Approach
041M0KM Bypass Right Popliteal Artery to Peroneal Artery with Nonautologous Tissue Substitute, Open Approach
041M0KP Bypass Right Popliteal Artery to Foot Artery with Nonautologous Tissue Substitute, Open Approach
041M0KQ Bypass Right Popliteal Artery to Lower Extremity Artery with Nonautologous Tissue Substitute, Open Approach
041M0KS Bypass Right Popliteal Artery to Lower Extremity Vein with Nonautologous Tissue Substitute, Open Approach
041M0ZL Bypass Right Popliteal Artery to Popliteal Artery, Open Approach
041M0ZM Bypass Right Popliteal Artery to Peroneal Artery, Open Approach
041M0ZP Bypass Right Popliteal Artery to Foot Artery, Open Approach
041M0ZQ Bypass Right Popliteal Artery to Lower Extremity Artery, Open Approach
041M0ZS Bypass Right Popliteal Artery to Lower Extremity Vein, Open Approach
041M49L Bypass Right Popliteal Artery to Popliteal Artery with Autologous Venous

Tissue, Percutaneous Endoscopic Approach

041M49M Bypass Right Popliteal Artery to Peroneal Artery with Autologous Venous Tissue, Percutaneous Endoscopic Approach

041M49P Bypass Right Popliteal Artery to Foot Artery with Autologous Venous Tissue, Percutaneous Endoscopic Approach

041M49Q Bypass Right Popliteal Artery to Lower Extremity Artery with Autologous Venous Tissue, Percutaneous Endoscopic Approach

041M49S Bypass Right Popliteal Artery to Lower Extremity Vein with Autologous Venous Tissue, Percutaneous Endoscopic Approach

041M4AL Bypass Right Popliteal Artery to Popliteal Artery with Autologous Arterial Tissue, Percutaneous Endoscopic Approach

041M4AM Bypass Right Popliteal Artery to Peroneal Artery with Autologous Arterial Tissue, Percutaneous Endoscopic Approach

041M4AP Bypass Right Popliteal Artery to Foot Artery with Autologous Arterial Tissue, Percutaneous Endoscopic Approach

041M4AQ Bypass Right Popliteal Artery to Lower Extremity Artery with Autologous Arterial Tissue, Percutaneous Endoscopic Approach

041M4AS Bypass Right Popliteal Artery to Lower Extremity Vein with Autologous Arterial Tissue, Percutaneous Endoscopic Approach

041M4JL Bypass Right Popliteal Artery to Popliteal Artery with Synthetic Substitute, Percutaneous Endoscopic Approach

041M4JM Bypass Right Popliteal Artery to Peroneal Artery with Synthetic Substitute, Percutaneous Endoscopic Approach

041M4JP Bypass Right Popliteal Artery to Foot Artery with Synthetic Substitute, Percutaneous Endoscopic Approach

041M4JQ Bypass Right Popliteal Artery to Lower Extremity Artery with Synthetic Substitute, Percutaneous Endoscopic Approach

041M4JS Bypass Right Popliteal Artery to Lower Extremity Vein with Synthetic Substitute, Percutaneous Endoscopic Approach

041M4KL Bypass Right Popliteal Artery to Popliteal Artery with Nonautologous Tissue Substitute, Percutaneous Endoscopic Approach

041M4KM Bypass Right Popliteal Artery to Peroneal Artery with Nonautologous Tissue Substitute, Percutaneous Endoscopic Approach

041M4KP Bypass Right Popliteal Artery to Foot Artery with Nonautologous Tissue Substitute, Percutaneous Endoscopic Approach

041M4KQ Bypass Right Popliteal Artery to Lower Extremity Artery with Nonautologous Tissue Substitute, Percutaneous Endoscopic Approach

041M4KS Bypass Right Popliteal Artery to Lower Extremity Vein with Nonautologous Tissue Substitute, Percutaneous Endoscopic Approach

041M4ZL Bypass Right Popliteal Artery to Popliteal Artery, Percutaneous Endoscopic Approach

041M4ZM Bypass Right Popliteal Artery to Peroneal Artery, Percutaneous Endoscopic Approach

041M4ZP Bypass Right Popliteal Artery to Foot Artery, Percutaneous Endoscopic Approach

041M4ZQ Bypass Right Popliteal Artery to Lower Extremity Artery, Percutaneous Endoscopic Approach

041M4ZS Bypass Right Popliteal Artery to Lower Extremity Vein, Percutaneous Endoscopic Approach

041N09L Bypass Left Popliteal Artery to Popliteal Artery with Autologous Venous Tissue, Open Approach

041N09M Bypass Left Popliteal Artery to Peroneal Artery with Autologous Venous Tissue, Open Approach

041N09P Bypass Left Popliteal Artery to Foot Artery with Autologous Venous Tissue, Open Approach

041N09Q Bypass Left Popliteal Artery to Lower Extremity Artery with Autologous Venous Tissue, Open Approach

041N09S Bypass Left Popliteal Artery to Lower Extremity Vein with Autologous Venous Tissue, Open Approach

041N0AL Bypass Left Popliteal Artery to Popliteal Artery with Autologous Arterial Tissue, Open Approach

041N0AM Bypass Left Popliteal Artery to Peroneal Artery with Autologous Arterial Tissue, Open Approach

041N0AP Bypass Left Popliteal Artery to Foot Artery with Autologous Arterial Tissue, Open Approach

041N0AQ Bypass Left Popliteal Artery to Lower Extremity Artery with Autologous Arterial Tissue, Open Approach

041N0AS Bypass Left Popliteal Artery to Lower Extremity Vein with Autologous Arterial Tissue, Open Approach

041N0JL Bypass Left Popliteal Artery to Popliteal Artery with Synthetic Substitute, Open Approach

041N0JM Bypass Left Popliteal Artery to Peroneal Artery with Synthetic Substitute, Open Approach

041N0JP Bypass Left Popliteal Artery to Foot Artery with Synthetic Substitute, Open Approach

041N0JQ Bypass Left Popliteal Artery to Lower Extremity Artery with Synthetic Substitute, Open Approach

041N0JS Bypass Left Popliteal Artery to Lower Extremity Vein with Synthetic Substitute, Open Approach

041N0KL Bypass Left Popliteal Artery to Popliteal Artery with Nonautologous Tissue Substitute, Open Approach

041N0KM Bypass Left Popliteal Artery to Peroneal Artery with Nonautologous Tissue Substitute, Open Approach

041N0KP Bypass Left Popliteal Artery to Foot Artery with Nonautologous Tissue Substitute, Open Approach

041N0KQ Bypass Left Popliteal Artery to Lower Extremity Artery with Nonautologous Tissue Substitute, Open Approach

041N0KS Bypass Left Popliteal Artery to Lower Extremity Vein with Nonautologous Tissue Substitute, Open Approach

041N0ZL Bypass Left Popliteal Artery to Popliteal Artery, Open Approach

041N0ZM Bypass Left Popliteal Artery to Peroneal Artery, Open Approach

041N0ZP Bypass Left Popliteal Artery to Foot Artery, Open Approach

041N0ZQ Bypass Left Popliteal Artery to Lower Extremity Artery, Open Approach

041N0ZS Bypass Left Popliteal Artery to Lower Extremity Vein, Open Approach

041N49L Bypass Left Popliteal Artery to Popliteal Artery with Autologous Venous Tissue, Percutaneous Endoscopic Approach

041N49M Bypass Left Popliteal Artery to Peroneal Artery with Autologous Venous Tissue, Percutaneous Endoscopic Approach

041N49P Bypass Left Popliteal Artery to Foot Artery with Autologous Venous Tissue, Percutaneous Endoscopic Approach

041N49Q Bypass Left Popliteal Artery to Lower Extremity Artery with Autologous Venous Tissue, Percutaneous Endoscopic Approach

041N49S Bypass Left Popliteal Artery to Lower Extremity Vein with Autologous Venous Tissue, Percutaneous Endoscopic Approach

041N4AL Bypass Left Popliteal Artery to Popliteal Artery with Autologous Arterial Tissue, Percutaneous Endoscopic Approach

041N4AM Bypass Left Popliteal Artery to Peroneal Artery with Autologous Arterial Tissue, Percutaneous Endoscopic Approach

041N4AP Bypass Left Popliteal Artery to Foot Artery with Autologous Arterial Tissue, Percutaneous Endoscopic Approach

041N4AQ Bypass Left Popliteal Artery to Lower Extremity Artery with Autologous Arterial Tissue, Percutaneous Endoscopic Approach

041N4AS Bypass Left Popliteal Artery to Lower Extremity Vein with Autologous Arterial Tissue, Percutaneous Endoscopic Approach

041N4JL Bypass Left Popliteal Artery to Popliteal Artery with Synthetic Substitute, Percutaneous Endoscopic Approach

041N4JM Bypass Left Popliteal Artery to Peroneal Artery with Synthetic Substitute, Percutaneous Endoscopic Approach

041N4JP Bypass Left Popliteal Artery to Foot Artery with Synthetic Substitute, Percutaneous Endoscopic Approach

041N4JQ Bypass Left Popliteal Artery to Lower Extremity Artery with Synthetic Substitute, Percutaneous Endoscopic Approach

041N4JS Bypass Left Popliteal Artery to Lower Extremity Vein with Synthetic Substitute, Percutaneous Endoscopic Approach

041N4KL Bypass Left Popliteal Artery to Popliteal Artery with Nonautologous Tissue Substitute, Percutaneous Endoscopic Approach

041N4KM Bypass Left Popliteal Artery to Peroneal Artery with Nonautologous Tissue Substitute, Percutaneous Endoscopic Approach

041N4KP Bypass Left Popliteal Artery to Foot Artery with Nonautologous Tissue Substitute, Percutaneous Endoscopic Approach

041N4KQ Bypass Left Popliteal Artery to Lower Extremity Artery with Nonautologous Tissue Substitute, Percutaneous Endoscopic Approach

041N4KS Bypass Left Popliteal Artery to Lower Extremity Vein with Nonautologous Tissue Substitute, Percutaneous Endoscopic Approach

041N4ZL Bypass Left Popliteal Artery to Popliteal Artery, Percutaneous Endoscopic Approach

041N4ZM Bypass Left Popliteal Artery to Peroneal Artery, Percutaneous Endoscopic Approach

041N4ZP Bypass Left Popliteal Artery to Foot Artery, Percutaneous Endoscopic Approach
041N4ZQ Bypass Left Popliteal Artery to Lower Extremity Artery, Percutaneous Endoscopic Approach
041N4ZS Bypass Left Popliteal Artery to Lower Extremity Vein, Percutaneous Endoscopic Approach

045 – Lower Arteries, Destruction

04500ZZ Destruction of Abdominal Aorta, Open Approach
04503ZZ Destruction of Abdominal Aorta, Percutaneous Approach
04504ZZ Destruction of Abdominal Aorta, Percutaneous Endoscopic Approach
04510ZZ Destruction of Celiac Artery, Open Approach
04513ZZ Destruction of Celiac Artery, Percutaneous Approach
04514ZZ Destruction of Celiac Artery, Percutaneous Endoscopic Approach
04520ZZ Destruction of Gastric Artery, Open Approach
04523ZZ Destruction of Gastric Artery, Percutaneous Approach
04524ZZ Destruction of Gastric Artery, Percutaneous Endoscopic Approach
04530ZZ Destruction of Hepatic Artery, Open Approach
04533ZZ Destruction of Hepatic Artery, Percutaneous Approach
04534ZZ Destruction of Hepatic Artery, Percutaneous Endoscopic Approach
04540ZZ Destruction of Splenic Artery, Open Approach
04543ZZ Destruction of Splenic Artery, Percutaneous Approach
04544ZZ Destruction of Splenic Artery, Percutaneous Endoscopic Approach
04550ZZ Destruction of Superior Mesenteric Artery, Open Approach
04553ZZ Destruction of Superior Mesenteric Artery, Percutaneous Approach
04554ZZ Destruction of Superior Mesenteric Artery, Percutaneous Endoscopic Approach
04560ZZ Destruction of Right Colic Artery, Open Approach
04563ZZ Destruction of Right Colic Artery, Percutaneous Approach
04564ZZ Destruction of Right Colic Artery, Percutaneous Endoscopic Approach
04570ZZ Destruction of Left Colic Artery, Open Approach
04573ZZ Destruction of Left Colic Artery, Percutaneous Approach
04574ZZ Destruction of Left Colic Artery, Percutaneous Endoscopic Approach
04580ZZ Destruction of Middle Colic Artery, Open Approach
04583ZZ Destruction of Middle Colic Artery, Percutaneous Approach
04584ZZ Destruction of Middle Colic Artery, Percutaneous Endoscopic Approach
04590ZZ Destruction of Right Renal Artery, Open Approach
04593ZZ Destruction of Right Renal Artery, Percutaneous Approach
04594ZZ Destruction of Right Renal Artery, Percutaneous Endoscopic Approach
045A0ZZ Destruction of Left Renal Artery, Open Approach
045A3ZZ Destruction of Left Renal Artery, Percutaneous Approach
045A4ZZ Destruction of Left Renal Artery, Percutaneous Endoscopic Approach
045B0ZZ Destruction of Inferior Mesenteric Artery, Open Approach
045B3ZZ Destruction of Inferior Mesenteric Artery, Percutaneous Approach
045B4ZZ Destruction of Inferior Mesenteric Artery, Percutaneous Endoscopic Approach
045C0ZZ Destruction of Right Common Iliac Artery, Open Approach
045C3ZZ Destruction of Right Common Iliac Artery, Percutaneous Approach
045C4ZZ Destruction of Right Common Iliac Artery, Percutaneous Endoscopic Approach
045D0ZZ Destruction of Left Common Iliac Artery, Open Approach
045D3ZZ Destruction of Left Common Iliac Artery, Percutaneous Approach
045D4ZZ Destruction of Left Common Iliac Artery, Percutaneous Endoscopic Approach
045E0ZZ Destruction of Right Internal Iliac Artery, Open Approach
045E3ZZ Destruction of Right Internal Iliac Artery, Percutaneous Approach
045E4ZZ Destruction of Right Internal Iliac Artery, Percutaneous Endoscopic Approach
045F0ZZ Destruction of Left Internal Iliac Artery, Open Approach
045F3ZZ Destruction of Left Internal Iliac Artery, Percutaneous Approach
045F4ZZ Destruction of Left Internal Iliac Artery, Percutaneous Endoscopic Approach
045H0ZZ Destruction of Right External Iliac Artery, Open Approach
045H3ZZ Destruction of Right External Iliac Artery, Percutaneous Approach
045H4ZZ Destruction of Right External Iliac Artery, Percutaneous Endoscopic Approach
045J0ZZ Destruction of Left External Iliac Artery, Open Approach
045J3ZZ Destruction of Left External Iliac Artery, Percutaneous Approach
045J4ZZ Destruction of Left External Iliac Artery, Percutaneous Endoscopic Approach
045K0ZZ Destruction of Right Femoral Artery, Open Approach
045K3ZZ Destruction of Right Femoral Artery, Percutaneous Approach
045K4ZZ Destruction of Right Femoral Artery, Percutaneous Endoscopic Approach
045L0ZZ Destruction of Left Femoral Artery, Open Approach
045L3ZZ Destruction of Left Femoral Artery, Percutaneous Approach
045L4ZZ Destruction of Left Femoral Artery, Percutaneous Endoscopic Approach
045M0ZZ Destruction of Right Popliteal Artery, Open Approach
045M3ZZ Destruction of Right Popliteal Artery, Percutaneous Approach
045M4ZZ Destruction of Right Popliteal Artery, Percutaneous Endoscopic Approach
045N0ZZ Destruction of Left Popliteal Artery, Open Approach
045N3ZZ Destruction of Left Popliteal Artery, Percutaneous Approach
045N4ZZ Destruction of Left Popliteal Artery, Percutaneous Endoscopic Approach
045P0ZZ Destruction of Right Anterior Tibial Artery, Open Approach
045P3ZZ Destruction of Right Anterior Tibial Artery, Percutaneous Approach
045P4ZZ Destruction of Right Anterior Tibial Artery, Percutaneous Endoscopic Approach
045Q0ZZ Destruction of Left Anterior Tibial Artery, Open Approach
045Q3ZZ Destruction of Left Anterior Tibial Artery, Percutaneous Approach
045Q4ZZ Destruction of Left Anterior Tibial Artery, Percutaneous Endoscopic Approach
045R0ZZ Destruction of Right Posterior Tibial Artery, Open Approach
045R3ZZ Destruction of Right Posterior Tibial Artery, Percutaneous Approach
045R4ZZ Destruction of Right Posterior Tibial Artery, Percutaneous Endoscopic Approach
045S0ZZ Destruction of Left Posterior Tibial Artery, Open Approach
045S3ZZ Destruction of Left Posterior Tibial Artery, Percutaneous Approach
045S4ZZ Destruction of Left Posterior Tibial Artery, Percutaneous Endoscopic Approach
045T0ZZ Destruction of Right Peroneal Artery, Open Approach
045T3ZZ Destruction of Right Peroneal Artery, Percutaneous Approach
045T4ZZ Destruction of Right Peroneal Artery, Percutaneous Endoscopic Approach
045U0ZZ Destruction of Left Peroneal Artery, Open Approach
045U3ZZ Destruction of Left Peroneal Artery, Percutaneous Approach
045U4ZZ Destruction of Left Peroneal Artery, Percutaneous Endoscopic Approach
045V0ZZ Destruction of Right Foot Artery, Open Approach
045V3ZZ Destruction of Right Foot Artery, Percutaneous Approach
045V4ZZ Destruction of Right Foot Artery, Percutaneous Endoscopic Approach
045W0ZZ Destruction of Left Foot Artery, Open Approach
045W3ZZ Destruction of Left Foot Artery, Percutaneous Approach
045W4ZZ Destruction of Left Foot Artery, Percutaneous Endoscopic Approach
045Y0ZZ Destruction of Lower Artery, Open Approach
045Y3ZZ Destruction of Lower Artery, Percutaneous Approach
045Y4ZZ Destruction of Lower Artery, Percutaneous Endoscopic Approach

047 – Lower Arteries, Dilation

047004Z Dilation of Abdominal Aorta with Drug-eluting Intraluminal Device, Open Approach
04700DZ Dilation of Abdominal Aorta with Intraluminal Device, Open Approach
04700ZZ Dilation of Abdominal Aorta, Open Approach
047034Z Dilation of Abdominal Aorta with Drug-eluting Intraluminal Device, Percutaneous Approach
04703DZ Dilation of Abdominal Aorta with Intraluminal Device, Percutaneous Approach
04703ZZ Dilation of Abdominal Aorta, Percutaneous Approach

047044Z Dilation of Abdominal Aorta with Drug-eluting Intraluminal Device, Percutaneous Endoscopic Approach
04704DZ Dilation of Abdominal Aorta with Intraluminal Device, Percutaneous Endoscopic Approach
04704ZZ Dilation of Abdominal Aorta, Percutaneous Endoscopic Approach
047104Z Dilation of Celiac Artery with Drug-eluting Intraluminal Device, Open Approach
04710DZ Dilation of Celiac Artery with Intraluminal Device, Open Approach
04710ZZ Dilation of Celiac Artery, Open Approach
047134Z Dilation of Celiac Artery with Drug-eluting Intraluminal Device, Percutaneous Approach
04713DZ Dilation of Celiac Artery with Intraluminal Device, Percutaneous Approach
04713ZZ Dilation of Celiac Artery, Percutaneous Approach
047144Z Dilation of Celiac Artery with Drug-eluting Intraluminal Device, Percutaneous Endoscopic Approach
04714DZ Dilation of Celiac Artery with Intraluminal Device, Percutaneous Endoscopic Approach
04714ZZ Dilation of Celiac Artery, Percutaneous Endoscopic Approach
047204Z Dilation of Gastric Artery with Drug-eluting Intraluminal Device, Open Approach
04720DZ Dilation of Gastric Artery with Intraluminal Device, Open Approach
04720ZZ Dilation of Gastric Artery, Open Approach
047234Z Dilation of Gastric Artery with Drug-eluting Intraluminal Device, Percutaneous Approach
04723DZ Dilation of Gastric Artery with Intraluminal Device, Percutaneous Approach
04723ZZ Dilation of Gastric Artery, Percutaneous Approach
047244Z Dilation of Gastric Artery with Drug-eluting Intraluminal Device, Percutaneous Endoscopic Approach
04724DZ Dilation of Gastric Artery with Intraluminal Device, Percutaneous Endoscopic Approach
04724ZZ Dilation of Gastric Artery, Percutaneous Endoscopic Approach
047304Z Dilation of Hepatic Artery with Drug-eluting Intraluminal Device, Open Approach
04730DZ Dilation of Hepatic Artery with Intraluminal Device, Open Approach
04730ZZ Dilation of Hepatic Artery, Open Approach
047334Z Dilation of Hepatic Artery with Drug-eluting Intraluminal Device, Percutaneous Approach
04733DZ Dilation of Hepatic Artery with Intraluminal Device, Percutaneous Approach
04733ZZ Dilation of Hepatic Artery, Percutaneous Approach
047344Z Dilation of Hepatic Artery with Drug-eluting Intraluminal Device, Percutaneous Endoscopic Approach
04734DZ Dilation of Hepatic Artery with Intraluminal Device, Percutaneous Endoscopic Approach
04734ZZ Dilation of Hepatic Artery, Percutaneous Endoscopic Approach
047404Z Dilation of Splenic Artery with Drug-eluting Intraluminal Device, Open Approach
04740DZ Dilation of Splenic Artery with Intraluminal Device, Open Approach
04740ZZ Dilation of Splenic Artery, Open Approach
047434Z Dilation of Splenic Artery with Drug-eluting Intraluminal Device, Percutaneous Approach
04743DZ Dilation of Splenic Artery with Intraluminal Device, Percutaneous Approach
04743ZZ Dilation of Splenic Artery, Percutaneous Approach
047444Z Dilation of Splenic Artery with Drug-eluting Intraluminal Device, Percutaneous Endoscopic Approach
04744DZ Dilation of Splenic Artery with Intraluminal Device, Percutaneous Endoscopic Approach
04744ZZ Dilation of Splenic Artery, Percutaneous Endoscopic Approach
047504Z Dilation of Superior Mesenteric Artery with Drug-eluting Intraluminal Device, Open Approach
04750DZ Dilation of Superior Mesenteric Artery with Intraluminal Device, Open Approach
04750ZZ Dilation of Superior Mesenteric Artery, Open Approach
047534Z Dilation of Superior Mesenteric Artery with Drug-eluting Intraluminal Device, Percutaneous Approach
04753DZ Dilation of Superior Mesenteric Artery with Intraluminal Device, Percutaneous Approach
04753ZZ Dilation of Superior Mesenteric Artery, Percutaneous Approach
047544Z Dilation of Superior Mesenteric Artery with Drug-eluting Intraluminal Device, Percutaneous Endoscopic Approach
04754DZ Dilation of Superior Mesenteric Artery with Intraluminal Device, Percutaneous Endoscopic Approach
04754ZZ Dilation of Superior Mesenteric Artery, Percutaneous Endoscopic Approach
047604Z Dilation of Right Colic Artery with Drug-eluting Intraluminal Device, Open Approach
04760DZ Dilation of Right Colic Artery with Intraluminal Device, Open Approach
04760ZZ Dilation of Right Colic Artery, Open Approach
047634Z Dilation of Right Colic Artery with Drug-eluting Intraluminal Device, Percutaneous Approach
04763DZ Dilation of Right Colic Artery with Intraluminal Device, Percutaneous Approach
04763ZZ Dilation of Right Colic Artery, Percutaneous Approach
047644Z Dilation of Right Colic Artery with Drug-eluting Intraluminal Device, Percutaneous Endoscopic Approach
04764DZ Dilation of Right Colic Artery with Intraluminal Device, Percutaneous Endoscopic Approach
04764ZZ Dilation of Right Colic Artery, Percutaneous Endoscopic Approach
047704Z Dilation of Left Colic Artery with Drug-eluting Intraluminal Device, Open Approach
04770DZ Dilation of Left Colic Artery with Intraluminal Device, Open Approach
04770ZZ Dilation of Left Colic Artery, Open Approach
047734Z Dilation of Left Colic Artery with Drug-eluting Intraluminal Device, Percutaneous Approach
04773DZ Dilation of Left Colic Artery with Intraluminal Device, Percutaneous Approach
04773ZZ Dilation of Left Colic Artery, Percutaneous Approach
047744Z Dilation of Left Colic Artery with Drug-eluting Intraluminal Device, Percutaneous Endoscopic Approach
04774DZ Dilation of Left Colic Artery with Intraluminal Device, Percutaneous Endoscopic Approach
04774ZZ Dilation of Left Colic Artery, Percutaneous Endoscopic Approach
047804Z Dilation of Middle Colic Artery with Drug-eluting Intraluminal Device, Open Approach
04780DZ Dilation of Middle Colic Artery with Intraluminal Device, Open Approach
04780ZZ Dilation of Middle Colic Artery, Open Approach
047834Z Dilation of Middle Colic Artery with Drug-eluting Intraluminal Device, Percutaneous Approach
04783DZ Dilation of Middle Colic Artery with Intraluminal Device, Percutaneous Approach
04783ZZ Dilation of Middle Colic Artery, Percutaneous Approach
047844Z Dilation of Middle Colic Artery with Drug-eluting Intraluminal Device, Percutaneous Endoscopic Approach
04784DZ Dilation of Middle Colic Artery with Intraluminal Device, Percutaneous Endoscopic Approach
04784ZZ Dilation of Middle Colic Artery, Percutaneous Endoscopic Approach
047904Z Dilation of Right Renal Artery with Drug-eluting Intraluminal Device, Open Approach
04790DZ Dilation of Right Renal Artery with Intraluminal Device, Open Approach
04790ZZ Dilation of Right Renal Artery, Open Approach
047934Z Dilation of Right Renal Artery with Drug-eluting Intraluminal Device, Percutaneous Approach
04793DZ Dilation of Right Renal Artery with Intraluminal Device, Percutaneous Approach
04793ZZ Dilation of Right Renal Artery, Percutaneous Approach
047944Z Dilation of Right Renal Artery with Drug-eluting Intraluminal Device, Percutaneous Endoscopic Approach
04794DZ Dilation of Right Renal Artery with Intraluminal Device, Percutaneous Endoscopic Approach
04794ZZ Dilation of Right Renal Artery, Percutaneous Endoscopic Approach
047A04Z Dilation of Left Renal Artery with Drug-eluting Intraluminal Device, Open Approach
047A0DZ Dilation of Left Renal Artery with Intraluminal Device, Open Approach
047A0ZZ Dilation of Left Renal Artery, Open Approach
047A34Z Dilation of Left Renal Artery with Drug-eluting Intraluminal Device, Percutaneous Approach
047A3DZ Dilation of Left Renal Artery with Intraluminal Device, Percutaneous Approach
047A3ZZ Dilation of Left Renal Artery, Percutaneous Approach
047A44Z Dilation of Left Renal Artery with Drug-eluting Intraluminal Device, Percutaneous Endoscopic Approach
047A4DZ Dilation of Left Renal Artery with Intraluminal Device, Percutaneous Endoscopic Approach

047A4ZZ	Dilation of Left Renal Artery, Percutaneous Endoscopic Approach
047B04Z	Dilation of Inferior Mesenteric Artery with Drug-eluting Intraluminal Device, Open Approach
047B0DZ	Dilation of Inferior Mesenteric Artery with Intraluminal Device, Open Approach
047B0ZZ	Dilation of Inferior Mesenteric Artery, Open Approach
047B34Z	Dilation of Inferior Mesenteric Artery with Drug-eluting Intraluminal Device, Percutaneous Approach
047B3DZ	Dilation of Inferior Mesenteric Artery with Intraluminal Device, Percutaneous Approach
047B3ZZ	Dilation of Inferior Mesenteric Artery, Percutaneous Approach
047B44Z	Dilation of Inferior Mesenteric Artery with Drug-eluting Intraluminal Device, Percutaneous Endoscopic Approach
047B4DZ	Dilation of Inferior Mesenteric Artery with Intraluminal Device, Percutaneous Endoscopic Approach
047B4ZZ	Dilation of Inferior Mesenteric Artery, Percutaneous Endoscopic Approach
047C04Z	Dilation of Right Common Iliac Artery with Drug-eluting Intraluminal Device, Open Approach
047C0DZ	Dilation of Right Common Iliac Artery with Intraluminal Device, Open Approach
047C0ZZ	Dilation of Right Common Iliac Artery, Open Approach
047C34Z	Dilation of Right Common Iliac Artery with Drug-eluting Intraluminal Device, Percutaneous Approach
047C3DZ	Dilation of Right Common Iliac Artery with Intraluminal Device, Percutaneous Approach
047C3ZZ	Dilation of Right Common Iliac Artery, Percutaneous Approach
047C44Z	Dilation of Right Common Iliac Artery with Drug-eluting Intraluminal Device, Percutaneous Endoscopic Approach
047C4DZ	Dilation of Right Common Iliac Artery with Intraluminal Device, Percutaneous Endoscopic Approach
047C4ZZ	Dilation of Right Common Iliac Artery, Percutaneous Endoscopic Approach
047D04Z	Dilation of Left Common Iliac Artery with Drug-eluting Intraluminal Device, Open Approach
047D0DZ	Dilation of Left Common Iliac Artery with Intraluminal Device, Open Approach
047D0ZZ	Dilation of Left Common Iliac Artery, Open Approach
047D34Z	Dilation of Left Common Iliac Artery with Drug-eluting Intraluminal Device, Percutaneous Approach
047D3DZ	Dilation of Left Common Iliac Artery with Intraluminal Device, Percutaneous Approach
047D3ZZ	Dilation of Left Common Iliac Artery, Percutaneous Approach
047D44Z	Dilation of Left Common Iliac Artery with Drug-eluting Intraluminal Device, Percutaneous Endoscopic Approach
047D4DZ	Dilation of Left Common Iliac Artery with Intraluminal Device, Percutaneous Endoscopic Approach
047D4ZZ	Dilation of Left Common Iliac Artery, Percutaneous Endoscopic Approach
047E04Z	Dilation of Right Internal Iliac Artery with Drug-eluting Intraluminal Device, Open Approach
047E0DZ	Dilation of Right Internal Iliac Artery with Intraluminal Device, Open Approach
047E0ZZ	Dilation of Right Internal Iliac Artery, Open Approach
047E34Z	Dilation of Right Internal Iliac Artery with Drug-eluting Intraluminal Device, Percutaneous Approach
047E3DZ	Dilation of Right Internal Iliac Artery with Intraluminal Device, Percutaneous Approach
047E3ZZ	Dilation of Right Internal Iliac Artery, Percutaneous Approach
047E44Z	Dilation of Right Internal Iliac Artery with Drug-eluting Intraluminal Device, Percutaneous Endoscopic Approach
047E4DZ	Dilation of Right Internal Iliac Artery with Intraluminal Device, Percutaneous Endoscopic Approach
047E4ZZ	Dilation of Right Internal Iliac Artery, Percutaneous Endoscopic Approach
047F04Z	Dilation of Left Internal Iliac Artery with Drug-eluting Intraluminal Device, Open Approach
047F0DZ	Dilation of Left Internal Iliac Artery with Intraluminal Device, Open Approach
047F0ZZ	Dilation of Left Internal Iliac Artery, Open Approach
047F34Z	Dilation of Left Internal Iliac Artery with Drug-eluting Intraluminal Device, Percutaneous Approach
047F3DZ	Dilation of Left Internal Iliac Artery with Intraluminal Device, Percutaneous Approach
047F3ZZ	Dilation of Left Internal Iliac Artery, Percutaneous Approach
047F44Z	Dilation of Left Internal Iliac Artery with Drug-eluting Intraluminal Device, Percutaneous Endoscopic Approach
047F4DZ	Dilation of Left Internal Iliac Artery with Intraluminal Device, Percutaneous Endoscopic Approach
047F4ZZ	Dilation of Left Internal Iliac Artery, Percutaneous Endoscopic Approach
047H04Z	Dilation of Right External Iliac Artery with Drug-eluting Intraluminal Device, Open Approach
047H0DZ	Dilation of Right External Iliac Artery with Intraluminal Device, Open Approach
047H0ZZ	Dilation of Right External Iliac Artery, Open Approach
047H34Z	Dilation of Right External Iliac Artery with Drug-eluting Intraluminal Device, Percutaneous Approach
047H3DZ	Dilation of Right External Iliac Artery with Intraluminal Device, Percutaneous Approach
047H3ZZ	Dilation of Right External Iliac Artery, Percutaneous Approach
047H44Z	Dilation of Right External Iliac Artery with Drug-eluting Intraluminal Device, Percutaneous Endoscopic Approach
047H4DZ	Dilation of Right External Iliac Artery with Intraluminal Device, Percutaneous Endoscopic Approach
047H4ZZ	Dilation of Right External Iliac Artery, Percutaneous Endoscopic Approach
047J04Z	Dilation of Left External Iliac Artery with Drug-eluting Intraluminal Device, Open Approach
047J0DZ	Dilation of Left External Iliac Artery with Intraluminal Device, Open Approach
047J0ZZ	Dilation of Left External Iliac Artery, Open Approach
047J34Z	Dilation of Left External Iliac Artery with Drug-eluting Intraluminal Device, Percutaneous Approach
047J3DZ	Dilation of Left External Iliac Artery with Intraluminal Device, Percutaneous Approach
047J3ZZ	Dilation of Left External Iliac Artery, Percutaneous Approach
047J44Z	Dilation of Left External Iliac Artery with Drug-eluting Intraluminal Device, Percutaneous Endoscopic Approach
047J4DZ	Dilation of Left External Iliac Artery with Intraluminal Device, Percutaneous Endoscopic Approach
047J4ZZ	Dilation of Left External Iliac Artery, Percutaneous Endoscopic Approach
047K04Z	Dilation of Right Femoral Artery with Drug-eluting Intraluminal Device, Open Approach
047K0DZ	Dilation of Right Femoral Artery with Intraluminal Device, Open Approach
047K0ZZ	Dilation of Right Femoral Artery, Open Approach
047K34Z	Dilation of Right Femoral Artery with Drug-eluting Intraluminal Device, Percutaneous Approach
047K3DZ	Dilation of Right Femoral Artery with Intraluminal Device, Percutaneous Approach
047K3ZZ	Dilation of Right Femoral Artery, Percutaneous Approach
047K44Z	Dilation of Right Femoral Artery with Drug-eluting Intraluminal Device, Percutaneous Endoscopic Approach
047K4DZ	Dilation of Right Femoral Artery with Intraluminal Device, Percutaneous Endoscopic Approach
047K4ZZ	Dilation of Right Femoral Artery, Percutaneous Endoscopic Approach
047L04Z	Dilation of Left Femoral Artery with Drug-eluting Intraluminal Device, Open Approach
047L0DZ	Dilation of Left Femoral Artery with Intraluminal Device, Open Approach
047L0ZZ	Dilation of Left Femoral Artery, Open Approach
047L34Z	Dilation of Left Femoral Artery with Drug-eluting Intraluminal Device, Percutaneous Approach
047L3DZ	Dilation of Left Femoral Artery with Intraluminal Device, Percutaneous Approach
047L3ZZ	Dilation of Left Femoral Artery, Percutaneous Approach
047L44Z	Dilation of Left Femoral Artery with Drug-eluting Intraluminal Device, Percutaneous Endoscopic Approach
047L4DZ	Dilation of Left Femoral Artery with Intraluminal Device, Percutaneous Endoscopic Approach
047L4ZZ	Dilation of Left Femoral Artery, Percutaneous Endoscopic Approach
047M04Z	Dilation of Right Popliteal Artery with Drug-eluting Intraluminal Device, Open Approach
047M0DZ	Dilation of Right Popliteal Artery with Intraluminal Device, Open Approach
047M0ZZ	Dilation of Right Popliteal Artery, Open Approach
047M34Z	Dilation of Right Popliteal Artery with Drug-eluting Intraluminal Device, Percutaneous Approach
047M3DZ	Dilation of Right Popliteal Artery with Intraluminal Device, Percutaneous Approach
047M3ZZ	Dilation of Right Popliteal Artery, Percutaneous Approach
047M44Z	Dilation of Right Popliteal Artery with Drug-eluting Intraluminal Device, Percutaneous Endoscopic Approach
047M4DZ	Dilation of Right Popliteal Artery with Intraluminal Device, Percutaneous Endoscopic Approach
047M4ZZ	Dilation of Right Popliteal Artery, Percutaneous Endoscopic Approach

047N04Z Dilation of Left Popliteal Artery with Drug-eluting Intraluminal Device, Open Approach
047N0DZ Dilation of Left Popliteal Artery with Intraluminal Device, Open Approach
047N0ZZ Dilation of Left Popliteal Artery, Open Approach
047N34Z Dilation of Left Popliteal Artery with Drug-eluting Intraluminal Device, Percutaneous Approach
047N3DZ Dilation of Left Popliteal Artery with Intraluminal Device, Percutaneous Approach
047N3ZZ Dilation of Left Popliteal Artery, Percutaneous Approach
047N44Z Dilation of Left Popliteal Artery with Drug-eluting Intraluminal Device, Percutaneous Endoscopic Approach
047N4DZ Dilation of Left Popliteal Artery with Intraluminal Device, Percutaneous Endoscopic Approach
047N4ZZ Dilation of Left Popliteal Artery, Percutaneous Endoscopic Approach
047P04Z Dilation of Right Anterior Tibial Artery with Drug-eluting Intraluminal Device, Open Approach
047P0DZ Dilation of Right Anterior Tibial Artery with Intraluminal Device, Open Approach
047P0ZZ Dilation of Right Anterior Tibial Artery, Open Approach
047P34Z Dilation of Right Anterior Tibial Artery with Drug-eluting Intraluminal Device, Percutaneous Approach
047P3DZ Dilation of Right Anterior Tibial Artery with Intraluminal Device, Percutaneous Approach
047P3ZZ Dilation of Right Anterior Tibial Artery, Percutaneous Approach
047P44Z Dilation of Right Anterior Tibial Artery with Drug-eluting Intraluminal Device, Percutaneous Endoscopic Approach
047P4DZ Dilation of Right Anterior Tibial Artery with Intraluminal Device, Percutaneous Endoscopic Approach
047P4ZZ Dilation of Right Anterior Tibial Artery, Percutaneous Endoscopic Approach
047Q04Z Dilation of Left Anterior Tibial Artery with Drug-eluting Intraluminal Device, Open Approach
047Q0DZ Dilation of Left Anterior Tibial Artery with Intraluminal Device, Open Approach
047Q0ZZ Dilation of Left Anterior Tibial Artery, Open Approach
047Q34Z Dilation of Left Anterior Tibial Artery with Drug-eluting Intraluminal Device, Percutaneous Approach
047Q3DZ Dilation of Left Anterior Tibial Artery with Intraluminal Device, Percutaneous Approach
047Q3ZZ Dilation of Left Anterior Tibial Artery, Percutaneous Approach
047Q44Z Dilation of Left Anterior Tibial Artery with Drug-eluting Intraluminal Device, Percutaneous Endoscopic Approach
047Q4DZ Dilation of Left Anterior Tibial Artery with Intraluminal Device, Percutaneous Endoscopic Approach
047Q4ZZ Dilation of Left Anterior Tibial Artery, Percutaneous Endoscopic Approach
047R04Z Dilation of Right Posterior Tibial Artery with Drug-eluting Intraluminal Device, Open Approach
047R0DZ Dilation of Right Posterior Tibial Artery with Intraluminal Device, Open Approach
047R0ZZ Dilation of Right Posterior Tibial Artery, Open Approach
047R34Z Dilation of Right Posterior Tibial Artery with Drug-eluting Intraluminal Device, Percutaneous Approach
047R3DZ Dilation of Right Posterior Tibial Artery with Intraluminal Device, Percutaneous Approach
047R3ZZ Dilation of Right Posterior Tibial Artery, Percutaneous Approach
047R44Z Dilation of Right Posterior Tibial Artery with Drug-eluting Intraluminal Device, Percutaneous Endoscopic Approach
047R4DZ Dilation of Right Posterior Tibial Artery with Intraluminal Device, Percutaneous Endoscopic Approach
047R4ZZ Dilation of Right Posterior Tibial Artery, Percutaneous Endoscopic Approach
047S04Z Dilation of Left Posterior Tibial Artery with Drug-eluting Intraluminal Device, Open Approach
047S0DZ Dilation of Left Posterior Tibial Artery with Intraluminal Device, Open Approach
047S0ZZ Dilation of Left Posterior Tibial Artery, Open Approach
047S34Z Dilation of Left Posterior Tibial Artery with Drug-eluting Intraluminal Device, Percutaneous Approach
047S3DZ Dilation of Left Posterior Tibial Artery with Intraluminal Device, Percutaneous Approach
047S3ZZ Dilation of Left Posterior Tibial Artery, Percutaneous Approach
047S44Z Dilation of Left Posterior Tibial Artery with Drug-eluting Intraluminal Device, Percutaneous Endoscopic Approach
047S4DZ Dilation of Left Posterior Tibial Artery with Intraluminal Device, Percutaneous Endoscopic Approach
047S4ZZ Dilation of Left Posterior Tibial Artery, Percutaneous Endoscopic Approach
047T04Z Dilation of Right Peroneal Artery with Drug-eluting Intraluminal Device, Open Approach
047T0DZ Dilation of Right Peroneal Artery with Intraluminal Device, Open Approach
047T0ZZ Dilation of Right Peroneal Artery, Open Approach
047T34Z Dilation of Right Peroneal Artery with Drug-eluting Intraluminal Device, Percutaneous Approach
047T3DZ Dilation of Right Peroneal Artery with Intraluminal Device, Percutaneous Approach
047T3ZZ Dilation of Right Peroneal Artery, Percutaneous Approach
047T44Z Dilation of Right Peroneal Artery with Drug-eluting Intraluminal Device, Percutaneous Endoscopic Approach
047T4DZ Dilation of Right Peroneal Artery with Intraluminal Device, Percutaneous Endoscopic Approach
047T4ZZ Dilation of Right Peroneal Artery, Percutaneous Endoscopic Approach
047U04Z Dilation of Left Peroneal Artery with Drug-eluting Intraluminal Device, Open Approach
047U0DZ Dilation of Left Peroneal Artery with Intraluminal Device, Open Approach
047U0ZZ Dilation of Left Peroneal Artery, Open Approach
047U34Z Dilation of Left Peroneal Artery with Drug-eluting Intraluminal Device, Percutaneous Approach
047U3DZ Dilation of Left Peroneal Artery with Intraluminal Device, Percutaneous Approach
047U3ZZ Dilation of Left Peroneal Artery, Percutaneous Approach
047U44Z Dilation of Left Peroneal Artery with Drug-eluting Intraluminal Device, Percutaneous Endoscopic Approach
047U4DZ Dilation of Left Peroneal Artery with Intraluminal Device, Percutaneous Endoscopic Approach
047U4ZZ Dilation of Left Peroneal Artery, Percutaneous Endoscopic Approach
047V04Z Dilation of Right Foot Artery with Drug-eluting Intraluminal Device, Open Approach
047V0DZ Dilation of Right Foot Artery with Intraluminal Device, Open Approach
047V0ZZ Dilation of Right Foot Artery, Open Approach
047V34Z Dilation of Right Foot Artery with Drug-eluting Intraluminal Device, Percutaneous Approach
047V3DZ Dilation of Right Foot Artery with Intraluminal Device, Percutaneous Approach
047V3ZZ Dilation of Right Foot Artery, Percutaneous Approach
047V44Z Dilation of Right Foot Artery with Drug-eluting Intraluminal Device, Percutaneous Endoscopic Approach
047V4DZ Dilation of Right Foot Artery with Intraluminal Device, Percutaneous Endoscopic Approach
047V4ZZ Dilation of Right Foot Artery, Percutaneous Endoscopic Approach
047W04Z Dilation of Left Foot Artery with Drug-eluting Intraluminal Device, Open Approach
047W0DZ Dilation of Left Foot Artery with Intraluminal Device, Open Approach
047W0ZZ Dilation of Left Foot Artery, Open Approach
047W34Z Dilation of Left Foot Artery with Drug-eluting Intraluminal Device, Percutaneous Approach
047W3DZ Dilation of Left Foot Artery with Intraluminal Device, Percutaneous Approach
047W3ZZ Dilation of Left Foot Artery, Percutaneous Approach
047W44Z Dilation of Left Foot Artery with Drug-eluting Intraluminal Device, Percutaneous Endoscopic Approach
047W4DZ Dilation of Left Foot Artery with Intraluminal Device, Percutaneous Endoscopic Approach
047W4ZZ Dilation of Left Foot Artery, Percutaneous Endoscopic Approach
047Y04Z Dilation of Lower Artery with Drug-eluting Intraluminal Device, Open Approach
047Y0DZ Dilation of Lower Artery with Intraluminal Device, Open Approach
047Y0ZZ Dilation of Lower Artery, Open Approach
047Y34Z Dilation of Lower Artery with Drug-eluting Intraluminal Device, Percutaneous Approach
047Y3DZ Dilation of Lower Artery with Intraluminal Device, Percutaneous Approach
047Y3ZZ Dilation of Lower Artery, Percutaneous Approach
047Y44Z Dilation of Lower Artery with Drug-eluting Intraluminal Device, Percutaneous Endoscopic Approach
047Y4DZ Dilation of Lower Artery with Intraluminal Device, Percutaneous Endoscopic Approach
047Y4ZZ Dilation of Lower Artery, Percutaneous Endoscopic Approach

049 – Lower Arteries, Drainage

Review Coding Guidelines B3.4a and B3.4b

Review Coding Guideline B6.2

049000Z Drainage of Abdominal Aorta with Drainage Device, Open Approach
04900ZX Drainage of Abdominal Aorta, Open Approach, Diagnostic
04900ZZ Drainage of Abdominal Aorta, Open Approach
049030Z Drainage of Abdominal Aorta with Drainage Device, Percutaneous Approach
04903ZX Drainage of Abdominal Aorta, Percutaneous Approach, Diagnostic
04903ZZ Drainage of Abdominal Aorta, Percutaneous Approach
049040Z Drainage of Abdominal Aorta with Drainage Device, Percutaneous Endoscopic Approach
04904ZX Drainage of Abdominal Aorta, Percutaneous Endoscopic Approach, Diagnostic
04904ZZ Drainage of Abdominal Aorta, Percutaneous Endoscopic Approach
049100Z Drainage of Celiac Artery with Drainage Device, Open Approach
04910ZX Drainage of Celiac Artery, Open Approach, Diagnostic
04910ZZ Drainage of Celiac Artery, Open Approach
049130Z Drainage of Celiac Artery with Drainage Device, Percutaneous Approach
04913ZX Drainage of Celiac Artery, Percutaneous Approach, Diagnostic
04913ZZ Drainage of Celiac Artery, Percutaneous Approach
049140Z Drainage of Celiac Artery with Drainage Device, Percutaneous Endoscopic Approach
04914ZX Drainage of Celiac Artery, Percutaneous Endoscopic Approach, Diagnostic
04914ZZ Drainage of Celiac Artery, Percutaneous Endoscopic Approach
049200Z Drainage of Gastric Artery with Drainage Device, Open Approach
04920ZX Drainage of Gastric Artery, Open Approach, Diagnostic
04920ZZ Drainage of Gastric Artery, Open Approach
049230Z Drainage of Gastric Artery with Drainage Device, Percutaneous Approach
04923ZX Drainage of Gastric Artery, Percutaneous Approach, Diagnostic
04923ZZ Drainage of Gastric Artery, Percutaneous Approach
049240Z Drainage of Gastric Artery with Drainage Device, Percutaneous Endoscopic Approach
04924ZX Drainage of Gastric Artery, Percutaneous Endoscopic Approach, Diagnostic
04924ZZ Drainage of Gastric Artery, Percutaneous Endoscopic Approach
049300Z Drainage of Hepatic Artery with Drainage Device, Open Approach
04930ZX Drainage of Hepatic Artery, Open Approach, Diagnostic
04930ZZ Drainage of Hepatic Artery, Open Approach
049330Z Drainage of Hepatic Artery with Drainage Device, Percutaneous Approach
04933ZX Drainage of Hepatic Artery, Percutaneous Approach, Diagnostic
04933ZZ Drainage of Hepatic Artery, Percutaneous Approach
049340Z Drainage of Hepatic Artery with Drainage Device, Percutaneous Endoscopic Approach
04934ZX Drainage of Hepatic Artery, Percutaneous Endoscopic Approach, Diagnostic
04934ZZ Drainage of Hepatic Artery, Percutaneous Endoscopic Approach
049400Z Drainage of Splenic Artery with Drainage Device, Open Approach
04940ZX Drainage of Splenic Artery, Open Approach, Diagnostic
04940ZZ Drainage of Splenic Artery, Open Approach
049430Z Drainage of Splenic Artery with Drainage Device, Percutaneous Approach
04943ZX Drainage of Splenic Artery, Percutaneous Approach, Diagnostic
04943ZZ Drainage of Splenic Artery, Percutaneous Approach
049440Z Drainage of Splenic Artery with Drainage Device, Percutaneous Endoscopic Approach
04944ZX Drainage of Splenic Artery, Percutaneous Endoscopic Approach, Diagnostic
04944ZZ Drainage of Splenic Artery, Percutaneous Endoscopic Approach
049500Z Drainage of Superior Mesenteric Artery with Drainage Device, Open Approach
04950ZX Drainage of Superior Mesenteric Artery, Open Approach, Diagnostic
04950ZZ Drainage of Superior Mesenteric Artery, Open Approach
049530Z Drainage of Superior Mesenteric Artery with Drainage Device, Percutaneous Approach
04953ZX Drainage of Superior Mesenteric Artery, Percutaneous Approach, Diagnostic
04953ZZ Drainage of Superior Mesenteric Artery, Percutaneous Approach
049540Z Drainage of Superior Mesenteric Artery with Drainage Device, Percutaneous Endoscopic Approach
04954ZX Drainage of Superior Mesenteric Artery, Percutaneous Endoscopic Approach, Diagnostic
04954ZZ Drainage of Superior Mesenteric Artery, Percutaneous Endoscopic Approach
049600Z Drainage of Right Colic Artery with Drainage Device, Open Approach
04960ZX Drainage of Right Colic Artery, Open Approach, Diagnostic
04960ZZ Drainage of Right Colic Artery, Open Approach
049630Z Drainage of Right Colic Artery with Drainage Device, Percutaneous Approach
04963ZX Drainage of Right Colic Artery, Percutaneous Approach, Diagnostic
04963ZZ Drainage of Right Colic Artery, Percutaneous Approach
049640Z Drainage of Right Colic Artery with Drainage Device, Percutaneous Endoscopic Approach
04964ZX Drainage of Right Colic Artery, Percutaneous Endoscopic Approach, Diagnostic
04964ZZ Drainage of Right Colic Artery, Percutaneous Endoscopic Approach
049700Z Drainage of Left Colic Artery with Drainage Device, Open Approach
04970ZX Drainage of Left Colic Artery, Open Approach, Diagnostic
04970ZZ Drainage of Left Colic Artery, Open Approach
049730Z Drainage of Left Colic Artery with Drainage Device, Percutaneous Approach
04973ZX Drainage of Left Colic Artery, Percutaneous Approach, Diagnostic
04973ZZ Drainage of Left Colic Artery, Percutaneous Approach
049740Z Drainage of Left Colic Artery with Drainage Device, Percutaneous Endoscopic Approach
04974ZX Drainage of Left Colic Artery, Percutaneous Endoscopic Approach, Diagnostic
04974ZZ Drainage of Left Colic Artery, Percutaneous Endoscopic Approach
049800Z Drainage of Middle Colic Artery with Drainage Device, Open Approach
04980ZX Drainage of Middle Colic Artery, Open Approach, Diagnostic
04980ZZ Drainage of Middle Colic Artery, Open Approach
049830Z Drainage of Middle Colic Artery with Drainage Device, Percutaneous Approach
04983ZX Drainage of Middle Colic Artery, Percutaneous Approach, Diagnostic
04983ZZ Drainage of Middle Colic Artery, Percutaneous Approach
049840Z Drainage of Middle Colic Artery with Drainage Device, Percutaneous Endoscopic Approach
04984ZX Drainage of Middle Colic Artery, Percutaneous Endoscopic Approach, Diagnostic
04984ZZ Drainage of Middle Colic Artery, Percutaneous Endoscopic Approach
049900Z Drainage of Right Renal Artery with Drainage Device, Open Approach
04990ZX Drainage of Right Renal Artery, Open Approach, Diagnostic
04990ZZ Drainage of Right Renal Artery, Open Approach
049930Z Drainage of Right Renal Artery with Drainage Device, Percutaneous Approach
04993ZX Drainage of Right Renal Artery, Percutaneous Approach, Diagnostic
04993ZZ Drainage of Right Renal Artery, Percutaneous Approach
049940Z Drainage of Right Renal Artery with Drainage Device, Percutaneous Endoscopic Approach
04994ZX Drainage of Right Renal Artery, Percutaneous Endoscopic Approach, Diagnostic
04994ZZ Drainage of Right Renal Artery, Percutaneous Endoscopic Approach
049A00Z Drainage of Left Renal Artery with Drainage Device, Open Approach
049A0ZX Drainage of Left Renal Artery, Open Approach, Diagnostic
049A0ZZ Drainage of Left Renal Artery, Open Approach
049A30Z Drainage of Left Renal Artery with Drainage Device, Percutaneous Approach
049A3ZX Drainage of Left Renal Artery, Percutaneous Approach, Diagnostic
049A3ZZ Drainage of Left Renal Artery, Percutaneous Approach
049A40Z Drainage of Left Renal Artery with Drainage Device, Percutaneous Endoscopic Approach
049A4ZX Drainage of Left Renal Artery, Percutaneous Endoscopic Approach, Diagnostic
049A4ZZ Drainage of Left Renal Artery, Percutaneous Endoscopic Approach

049B00Z Drainage of Inferior Mesenteric Artery with Drainage Device, Open Approach
049B0ZX Drainage of Inferior Mesenteric Artery, Open Approach, Diagnostic
049B0ZZ Drainage of Inferior Mesenteric Artery, Open Approach
049B30Z Drainage of Inferior Mesenteric Artery with Drainage Device, Percutaneous Approach
049B3ZX Drainage of Inferior Mesenteric Artery, Percutaneous Approach, Diagnostic
049B3ZZ Drainage of Inferior Mesenteric Artery, Percutaneous Approach
049B40Z Drainage of Inferior Mesenteric Artery with Drainage Device, Percutaneous Endoscopic Approach
049B4ZX Drainage of Inferior Mesenteric Artery, Percutaneous Endoscopic Approach, Diagnostic
049B4ZZ Drainage of Inferior Mesenteric Artery, Percutaneous Endoscopic Approach
049C00Z Drainage of Right Common Iliac Artery with Drainage Device, Open Approach
049C0ZX Drainage of Right Common Iliac Artery, Open Approach, Diagnostic
049C0ZZ Drainage of Right Common Iliac Artery, Open Approach
049C30Z Drainage of Right Common Iliac Artery with Drainage Device, Percutaneous Approach
049C3ZX Drainage of Right Common Iliac Artery, Percutaneous Approach, Diagnostic
049C3ZZ Drainage of Right Common Iliac Artery, Percutaneous Approach
049C40Z Drainage of Right Common Iliac Artery with Drainage Device, Percutaneous Endoscopic Approach
049C4ZX Drainage of Right Common Iliac Artery, Percutaneous Endoscopic Approach, Diagnostic
049C4ZZ Drainage of Right Common Iliac Artery, Percutaneous Endoscopic Approach
049D00Z Drainage of Left Common Iliac Artery with Drainage Device, Open Approach
049D0ZX Drainage of Left Common Iliac Artery, Open Approach, Diagnostic
049D0ZZ Drainage of Left Common Iliac Artery, Open Approach
049D30Z Drainage of Left Common Iliac Artery with Drainage Device, Percutaneous Approach
049D3ZX Drainage of Left Common Iliac Artery, Percutaneous Approach, Diagnostic
049D3ZZ Drainage of Left Common Iliac Artery, Percutaneous Approach
049D40Z Drainage of Left Common Iliac Artery with Drainage Device, Percutaneous Endoscopic Approach
049D4ZX Drainage of Left Common Iliac Artery, Percutaneous Endoscopic Approach, Diagnostic
049D4ZZ Drainage of Left Common Iliac Artery, Percutaneous Endoscopic Approach
049E00Z Drainage of Right Internal Iliac Artery with Drainage Device, Open Approach
049E0ZX Drainage of Right Internal Iliac Artery, Open Approach, Diagnostic
049E0ZZ Drainage of Right Internal Iliac Artery, Open Approach
049E30Z Drainage of Right Internal Iliac Artery with Drainage Device, Percutaneous Approach
049E3ZX Drainage of Right Internal Iliac Artery, Percutaneous Approach, Diagnostic
049E3ZZ Drainage of Right Internal Iliac Artery, Percutaneous Approach
049E40Z Drainage of Right Internal Iliac Artery with Drainage Device, Percutaneous Endoscopic Approach
049E4ZX Drainage of Right Internal Iliac Artery, Percutaneous Endoscopic Approach, Diagnostic
049E4ZZ Drainage of Right Internal Iliac Artery, Percutaneous Endoscopic Approach
049F00Z Drainage of Left Internal Iliac Artery with Drainage Device, Open Approach
049F0ZX Drainage of Left Internal Iliac Artery, Open Approach, Diagnostic
049F0ZZ Drainage of Left Internal Iliac Artery, Open Approach
049F30Z Drainage of Left Internal Iliac Artery with Drainage Device, Percutaneous Approach
049F3ZX Drainage of Left Internal Iliac Artery, Percutaneous Approach, Diagnostic
049F3ZZ Drainage of Left Internal Iliac Artery, Percutaneous Approach
049F40Z Drainage of Left Internal Iliac Artery with Drainage Device, Percutaneous Endoscopic Approach
049F4ZX Drainage of Left Internal Iliac Artery, Percutaneous Endoscopic Approach, Diagnostic
049F4ZZ Drainage of Left Internal Iliac Artery, Percutaneous Endoscopic Approach
049H00Z Drainage of Right External Iliac Artery with Drainage Device, Open Approach
049H0ZX Drainage of Right External Iliac Artery, Open Approach, Diagnostic
049H0ZZ Drainage of Right External Iliac Artery, Open Approach
049H30Z Drainage of Right External Iliac Artery with Drainage Device, Percutaneous Approach
049H3ZX Drainage of Right External Iliac Artery, Percutaneous Approach, Diagnostic
049H3ZZ Drainage of Right External Iliac Artery, Percutaneous Approach
049H40Z Drainage of Right External Iliac Artery with Drainage Device, Percutaneous Endoscopic Approach
049H4ZX Drainage of Right External Iliac Artery, Percutaneous Endoscopic Approach, Diagnostic
049H4ZZ Drainage of Right External Iliac Artery, Percutaneous Endoscopic Approach
049J00Z Drainage of Left External Iliac Artery with Drainage Device, Open Approach
049J0ZX Drainage of Left External Iliac Artery, Open Approach, Diagnostic
049J0ZZ Drainage of Left External Iliac Artery, Open Approach
049J30Z Drainage of Left External Iliac Artery with Drainage Device, Percutaneous Approach
049J3ZX Drainage of Left External Iliac Artery, Percutaneous Approach, Diagnostic
049J3ZZ Drainage of Left External Iliac Artery, Percutaneous Approach
049J40Z Drainage of Left External Iliac Artery with Drainage Device, Percutaneous Endoscopic Approach
049J4ZX Drainage of Left External Iliac Artery, Percutaneous Endoscopic Approach, Diagnostic
049J4ZZ Drainage of Left External Iliac Artery, Percutaneous Endoscopic Approach
049K00Z Drainage of Right Femoral Artery with Drainage Device, Open Approach
049K0ZX Drainage of Right Femoral Artery, Open Approach, Diagnostic
049K0ZZ Drainage of Right Femoral Artery, Open Approach
049K30Z Drainage of Right Femoral Artery with Drainage Device, Percutaneous Approach
049K3ZX Drainage of Right Femoral Artery, Percutaneous Approach, Diagnostic
049K3ZZ Drainage of Right Femoral Artery, Percutaneous Approach
049K40Z Drainage of Right Femoral Artery with Drainage Device, Percutaneous Endoscopic Approach
049K4ZX Drainage of Right Femoral Artery, Percutaneous Endoscopic Approach, Diagnostic
049K4ZZ Drainage of Right Femoral Artery, Percutaneous Endoscopic Approach
049L00Z Drainage of Left Femoral Artery with Drainage Device, Open Approach
049L0ZX Drainage of Left Femoral Artery, Open Approach, Diagnostic
049L0ZZ Drainage of Left Femoral Artery, Open Approach
049L30Z Drainage of Left Femoral Artery with Drainage Device, Percutaneous Approach
049L3ZX Drainage of Left Femoral Artery, Percutaneous Approach, Diagnostic
049L3ZZ Drainage of Left Femoral Artery, Percutaneous Approach
049L40Z Drainage of Left Femoral Artery with Drainage Device, Percutaneous Endoscopic Approach
049L4ZX Drainage of Left Femoral Artery, Percutaneous Endoscopic Approach, Diagnostic
049L4ZZ Drainage of Left Femoral Artery, Percutaneous Endoscopic Approach
049M00Z Drainage of Right Popliteal Artery with Drainage Device, Open Approach
049M0ZX Drainage of Right Popliteal Artery, Open Approach, Diagnostic
049M0ZZ Drainage of Right Popliteal Artery, Open Approach
049M30Z Drainage of Right Popliteal Artery with Drainage Device, Percutaneous Approach
049M3ZX Drainage of Right Popliteal Artery, Percutaneous Approach, Diagnostic
049M3ZZ Drainage of Right Popliteal Artery, Percutaneous Approach
049M40Z Drainage of Right Popliteal Artery with Drainage Device, Percutaneous Endoscopic Approach
049M4ZX Drainage of Right Popliteal Artery, Percutaneous Endoscopic Approach, Diagnostic
049M4ZZ Drainage of Right Popliteal Artery, Percutaneous Endoscopic Approach
049N00Z Drainage of Left Popliteal Artery with Drainage Device, Open Approach
049N0ZX Drainage of Left Popliteal Artery, Open Approach, Diagnostic
049N0ZZ Drainage of Left Popliteal Artery, Open Approach
049N30Z Drainage of Left Popliteal Artery with Drainage Device, Percutaneous Approach
049N3ZX Drainage of Left Popliteal Artery, Percutaneous Approach, Diagnostic
049N3ZZ Drainage of Left Popliteal Artery, Percutaneous Approach
049N40Z Drainage of Left Popliteal Artery with Drainage Device, Percutaneous Endoscopic Approach
049N4ZX Drainage of Left Popliteal Artery, Percutaneous Endoscopic Approach, Diagnostic
049N4ZZ Drainage of Left Popliteal Artery, Percutaneous Endoscopic Approach
049P00Z Drainage of Right Anterior Tibial Artery with Drainage Device, Open Approach
049P0ZX Drainage of Right Anterior Tibial Artery, Open Approach, Diagnostic
049P0ZZ Drainage of Right Anterior Tibial Artery, Open Approach

49P30Z Drainage of Right Anterior Tibial Artery with Drainage Device, Percutaneous Approach
49P3ZX Drainage of Right Anterior Tibial Artery, Percutaneous Approach, Diagnostic
49P3ZZ Drainage of Right Anterior Tibial Artery, Percutaneous Approach
49P40Z Drainage of Right Anterior Tibial Artery with Drainage Device, Percutaneous Endoscopic Approach
49P4ZX Drainage of Right Anterior Tibial Artery, Percutaneous Endoscopic Approach, Diagnostic
49P4ZZ Drainage of Right Anterior Tibial Artery, Percutaneous Endoscopic Approach
49Q00Z Drainage of Left Anterior Tibial Artery with Drainage Device, Open Approach
49Q0ZX Drainage of Left Anterior Tibial Artery, Open Approach, Diagnostic
49Q0ZZ Drainage of Left Anterior Tibial Artery, Open Approach
49Q30Z Drainage of Left Anterior Tibial Artery with Drainage Device, Percutaneous Approach
49Q3ZX Drainage of Left Anterior Tibial Artery, Percutaneous Approach, Diagnostic
49Q3ZZ Drainage of Left Anterior Tibial Artery, Percutaneous Approach
49Q40Z Drainage of Left Anterior Tibial Artery with Drainage Device, Percutaneous Endoscopic Approach
49Q4ZX Drainage of Left Anterior Tibial Artery, Percutaneous Endoscopic Approach, Diagnostic
49Q4ZZ Drainage of Left Anterior Tibial Artery, Percutaneous Endoscopic Approach
49R00Z Drainage of Right Posterior Tibial Artery with Drainage Device, Open Approach
49R0ZX Drainage of Right Posterior Tibial Artery, Open Approach, Diagnostic
49R0ZZ Drainage of Right Posterior Tibial Artery, Open Approach
49R30Z Drainage of Right Posterior Tibial Artery with Drainage Device, Percutaneous Approach
49R3ZX Drainage of Right Posterior Tibial Artery, Percutaneous Approach, Diagnostic
49R3ZZ Drainage of Right Posterior Tibial Artery, Percutaneous Approach
49R40Z Drainage of Right Posterior Tibial Artery with Drainage Device, Percutaneous Endoscopic Approach
49R4ZX Drainage of Right Posterior Tibial Artery, Percutaneous Endoscopic Approach, Diagnostic
49R4ZZ Drainage of Right Posterior Tibial Artery, Percutaneous Endoscopic Approach
049S00Z Drainage of Left Posterior Tibial Artery with Drainage Device, Open Approach
049S0ZX Drainage of Left Posterior Tibial Artery, Open Approach, Diagnostic
049S0ZZ Drainage of Left Posterior Tibial Artery, Open Approach
049S30Z Drainage of Left Posterior Tibial Artery with Drainage Device, Percutaneous Approach
049S3ZX Drainage of Left Posterior Tibial Artery, Percutaneous Approach, Diagnostic
049S3ZZ Drainage of Left Posterior Tibial Artery, Percutaneous Approach
049S40Z Drainage of Left Posterior Tibial Artery with Drainage Device, Percutaneous Endoscopic Approach
049S4ZX Drainage of Left Posterior Tibial Artery, Percutaneous Endoscopic Approach, Diagnostic
049S4ZZ Drainage of Left Posterior Tibial Artery, Percutaneous Endoscopic Approach
049T00Z Drainage of Right Peroneal Artery with Drainage Device, Open Approach
049T0ZX Drainage of Right Peroneal Artery, Open Approach, Diagnostic
049T0ZZ Drainage of Right Peroneal Artery, Open Approach
049T30Z Drainage of Right Peroneal Artery with Drainage Device, Percutaneous Approach
049T3ZX Drainage of Right Peroneal Artery, Percutaneous Approach, Diagnostic
049T3ZZ Drainage of Right Peroneal Artery, Percutaneous Approach
049T40Z Drainage of Right Peroneal Artery with Drainage Device, Percutaneous Endoscopic Approach
049T4ZX Drainage of Right Peroneal Artery, Percutaneous Endoscopic Approach, Diagnostic
049T4ZZ Drainage of Right Peroneal Artery, Percutaneous Endoscopic Approach
049U00Z Drainage of Left Peroneal Artery with Drainage Device, Open Approach
049U0ZX Drainage of Left Peroneal Artery, Open Approach, Diagnostic
049U0ZZ Drainage of Left Peroneal Artery, Open Approach
049U30Z Drainage of Left Peroneal Artery with Drainage Device, Percutaneous Approach
049U3ZX Drainage of Left Peroneal Artery, Percutaneous Approach, Diagnostic
049U3ZZ Drainage of Left Peroneal Artery, Percutaneous Approach
049U40Z Drainage of Left Peroneal Artery with Drainage Device, Percutaneous Endoscopic Approach
049U4ZX Drainage of Left Peroneal Artery, Percutaneous Endoscopic Approach, Diagnostic
049U4ZZ Drainage of Left Peroneal Artery, Percutaneous Endoscopic Approach
049V00Z Drainage of Right Foot Artery with Drainage Device, Open Approach
049V0ZX Drainage of Right Foot Artery, Open Approach, Diagnostic
049V0ZZ Drainage of Right Foot Artery, Open Approach
049V30Z Drainage of Right Foot Artery with Drainage Device, Percutaneous Approach
049V3ZX Drainage of Right Foot Artery, Percutaneous Approach, Diagnostic
049V3ZZ Drainage of Right Foot Artery, Percutaneous Approach
049V40Z Drainage of Right Foot Artery with Drainage Device, Percutaneous Endoscopic Approach
049V4ZX Drainage of Right Foot Artery, Percutaneous Endoscopic Approach, Diagnostic
049V4ZZ Drainage of Right Foot Artery, Percutaneous Endoscopic Approach
049W00Z Drainage of Left Foot Artery with Drainage Device, Open Approach
049W0ZX Drainage of Left Foot Artery, Open Approach, Diagnostic
049W0ZZ Drainage of Left Foot Artery, Open Approach
049W30Z Drainage of Left Foot Artery with Drainage Device, Percutaneous Approach
049W3ZX Drainage of Left Foot Artery, Percutaneous Approach, Diagnostic
049W3ZZ Drainage of Left Foot Artery, Percutaneous Approach
049W40Z Drainage of Left Foot Artery with Drainage Device, Percutaneous Endoscopic Approach
049W4ZX Drainage of Left Foot Artery, Percutaneous Endoscopic Approach, Diagnostic
049W4ZZ Drainage of Left Foot Artery, Percutaneous Endoscopic Approach
049Y00Z Drainage of Lower Artery with Drainage Device, Open Approach
049Y0ZX Drainage of Lower Artery, Open Approach, Diagnostic
049Y0ZZ Drainage of Lower Artery, Open Approach
049Y30Z Drainage of Lower Artery with Drainage Device, Percutaneous Approach
049Y3ZX Drainage of Lower Artery, Percutaneous Approach, Diagnostic
049Y3ZZ Drainage of Lower Artery, Percutaneous Approach
049Y40Z Drainage of Lower Artery with Drainage Device, Percutaneous Endoscopic Approach
049Y4ZX Drainage of Lower Artery, Percutaneous Endoscopic Approach, Diagnostic
049Y4ZZ Drainage of Lower Artery, Percutaneous Endoscopic Approach

04B – Lower Arteries, Excision

Review Coding Guidelines B3.4a and B3.4b

Review Coding Guideline B3.8

04B00ZX Excision of Abdominal Aorta, Open Approach, Diagnostic
04B00ZZ Excision of Abdominal Aorta, Open Approach
04B03ZX Excision of Abdominal Aorta, Percutaneous Approach, Diagnostic
04B03ZZ Excision of Abdominal Aorta, Percutaneous Approach
04B04ZX Excision of Abdominal Aorta, Percutaneous Endoscopic Approach, Diagnostic
04B04ZZ Excision of Abdominal Aorta, Percutaneous Endoscopic Approach
04B10ZX Excision of Celiac Artery, Open Approach, Diagnostic
04B10ZZ Excision of Celiac Artery, Open Approach
04B13ZX Excision of Celiac Artery, Percutaneous Approach, Diagnostic
04B13ZZ Excision of Celiac Artery, Percutaneous Approach
04B14ZX Excision of Celiac Artery, Percutaneous Endoscopic Approach, Diagnostic
04B14ZZ Excision of Celiac Artery, Percutaneous Endoscopic Approach
04B20ZX Excision of Gastric Artery, Open Approach, Diagnostic
04B20ZZ Excision of Gastric Artery, Open Approach
04B23ZX Excision of Gastric Artery, Percutaneous Approach, Diagnostic
04B23ZZ Excision of Gastric Artery, Percutaneous Approach
04B24ZX Excision of Gastric Artery, Percutaneous Endoscopic Approach, Diagnostic

♀ Female-only ♂ Male-only Limited Coverage ● Non-OR HAC-associated procedure ▲ Non-covered procedures Combination

04B24ZZ Excision of Gastric Artery, Percutaneous Endoscopic Approach
04B30ZX Excision of Hepatic Artery, Open Approach, Diagnostic
04B30ZZ Excision of Hepatic Artery, Open Approach
04B33ZX Excision of Hepatic Artery, Percutaneous Approach, Diagnostic
04B33ZZ Excision of Hepatic Artery, Percutaneous Approach
04B34ZX Excision of Hepatic Artery, Percutaneous Endoscopic Approach, Diagnostic
04B34ZZ Excision of Hepatic Artery, Percutaneous Endoscopic Approach
04B40ZX Excision of Splenic Artery, Open Approach, Diagnostic
04B40ZZ Excision of Splenic Artery, Open Approach
04B43ZX Excision of Splenic Artery, Percutaneous Approach, Diagnostic
04B43ZZ Excision of Splenic Artery, Percutaneous Approach
04B44ZX Excision of Splenic Artery, Percutaneous Endoscopic Approach, Diagnostic
04B44ZZ Excision of Splenic Artery, Percutaneous Endoscopic Approach
04B50ZX Excision of Superior Mesenteric Artery, Open Approach, Diagnostic
04B50ZZ Excision of Superior Mesenteric Artery, Open Approach
04B53ZX Excision of Superior Mesenteric Artery, Percutaneous Approach, Diagnostic
04B53ZZ Excision of Superior Mesenteric Artery, Percutaneous Approach
04B54ZX Excision of Superior Mesenteric Artery, Percutaneous Endoscopic Approach, Diagnostic
04B54ZZ Excision of Superior Mesenteric Artery, Percutaneous Endoscopic Approach
04B60ZX Excision of Right Colic Artery, Open Approach, Diagnostic
04B60ZZ Excision of Right Colic Artery, Open Approach
04B63ZX Excision of Right Colic Artery, Percutaneous Approach, Diagnostic
04B63ZZ Excision of Right Colic Artery, Percutaneous Approach
04B64ZX Excision of Right Colic Artery, Percutaneous Endoscopic Approach, Diagnostic
04B64ZZ Excision of Right Colic Artery, Percutaneous Endoscopic Approach
04B70ZX Excision of Left Colic Artery, Open Approach, Diagnostic
04B70ZZ Excision of Left Colic Artery, Open Approach
04B73ZX Excision of Left Colic Artery, Percutaneous Approach, Diagnostic
04B73ZZ Excision of Left Colic Artery, Percutaneous Approach
04B74ZX Excision of Left Colic Artery, Percutaneous Endoscopic Approach, Diagnostic
04B74ZZ Excision of Left Colic Artery, Percutaneous Endoscopic Approach
04B80ZX Excision of Middle Colic Artery, Open Approach, Diagnostic
04B80ZZ Excision of Middle Colic Artery, Open Approach
04B83ZX Excision of Middle Colic Artery, Percutaneous Approach, Diagnostic
04B83ZZ Excision of Middle Colic Artery, Percutaneous Approach
04B84ZX Excision of Middle Colic Artery, Percutaneous Endoscopic Approach, Diagnostic
04B84ZZ Excision of Middle Colic Artery, Percutaneous Endoscopic Approach
04B90ZX Excision of Right Renal Artery, Open Approach, Diagnostic
04B90ZZ Excision of Right Renal Artery, Open Approach
04B93ZX Excision of Right Renal Artery, Percutaneous Approach, Diagnostic
04B93ZZ Excision of Right Renal Artery, Percutaneous Approach
04B94ZX Excision of Right Renal Artery, Percutaneous Endoscopic Approach, Diagnostic
04B94ZZ Excision of Right Renal Artery, Percutaneous Endoscopic Approach
04BA0ZX Excision of Left Renal Artery, Open Approach, Diagnostic
04BA0ZZ Excision of Left Renal Artery, Open Approach
04BA3ZX Excision of Left Renal Artery, Percutaneous Approach, Diagnostic
04BA3ZZ Excision of Left Renal Artery, Percutaneous Approach
04BA4ZX Excision of Left Renal Artery, Percutaneous Endoscopic Approach, Diagnostic
04BA4ZZ Excision of Left Renal Artery, Percutaneous Endoscopic Approach
04BB0ZX Excision of Inferior Mesenteric Artery, Open Approach, Diagnostic
04BB0ZZ Excision of Inferior Mesenteric Artery, Open Approach
04BB3ZX Excision of Inferior Mesenteric Artery, Percutaneous Approach, Diagnostic
04BB3ZZ Excision of Inferior Mesenteric Artery, Percutaneous Approach
04BB4ZX Excision of Inferior Mesenteric Artery, Percutaneous Endoscopic Approach, Diagnostic
04BB4ZZ Excision of Inferior Mesenteric Artery, Percutaneous Endoscopic Approach
04BC0ZX Excision of Right Common Iliac Artery, Open Approach, Diagnostic
04BC0ZZ Excision of Right Common Iliac Artery, Open Approach
04BC3ZX Excision of Right Common Iliac Artery, Percutaneous Approach, Diagnostic
04BC3ZZ Excision of Right Common Iliac Artery, Percutaneous Approach
04BC4ZX Excision of Right Common Iliac Artery, Percutaneous Endoscopic Approach, Diagnostic
04BC4ZZ Excision of Right Common Iliac Artery, Percutaneous Endoscopic Approach
04BD0ZX Excision of Left Common Iliac Artery, Open Approach, Diagnostic
04BD0ZZ Excision of Left Common Iliac Artery, Opcn Approach
04BD3ZX Excision of Left Common Iliac Artery, Percutaneous Approach, Diagnostic
04BD3ZZ Excision of Left Common Iliac Artery, Percutaneous Approach
04BD4ZX Excision of Left Common Iliac Artery, Percutaneous Endoscopic Approach, Diagnostic
04BD4ZZ Excision of Left Common Iliac Artery, Percutaneous Endoscopic Approach
04BE0ZX Excision of Right Internal Iliac Artery, Open Approach, Diagnostic
04BE0ZZ Excision of Right Internal Iliac Artery, Open Approach
04BE3ZX Excision of Right Internal Iliac Artery, Percutaneous Approach, Diagnostic
04BE3ZZ Excision of Right Internal Iliac Artery, Percutaneous Approach
04BE4ZX Excision of Right Internal Iliac Artery, Percutaneous Endoscopic Approach, Diagnostic
04BE4ZZ Excision of Right Internal Iliac Artery, Percutaneous Endoscopic Approach
04BF0ZX Excision of Left Internal Iliac Artery, Open Approach, Diagnostic
04BF0ZZ Excision of Left Internal Iliac Artery, Open Approach
04BF3ZX Excision of Left Internal Iliac Artery, Percutaneous Approach, Diagnostic
04BF3ZZ Excision of Left Internal Iliac Artery, Percutaneous Approach
04BF4ZX Excision of Left Internal Iliac Artery, Percutaneous Endoscopic Approach, Diagnostic
04BF4ZZ Excision of Left Internal Iliac Artery, Percutaneous Endoscopic Approach
04BH0ZX Excision of Right External Iliac Artery, Open Approach, Diagnostic
04BH0ZZ Excision of Right External Iliac Artery, Open Approach
04BH3ZX Excision of Right External Iliac Artery, Percutaneous Approach, Diagnostic
04BH3ZZ Excision of Right External Iliac Artery, Percutaneous Approach
04BH4ZX Excision of Right External Iliac Artery, Percutaneous Endoscopic Approach, Diagnostic
04BH4ZZ Excision of Right External Iliac Artery, Percutaneous Endoscopic Approach
04BJ0ZX Excision of Left External Iliac Artery, Open Approach, Diagnostic
04BJ0ZZ Excision of Left External Iliac Artery, Open Approach
04BJ3ZX Excision of Left External Iliac Artery, Percutaneous Approach, Diagnostic
04BJ3ZZ Excision of Left External Iliac Artery, Percutaneous Approach
04BJ4ZX Excision of Left External Iliac Artery, Percutaneous Endoscopic Approach, Diagnostic
04BJ4ZZ Excision of Left External Iliac Artery, Percutaneous Endoscopic Approach
04BK0ZX Excision of Right Femoral Artery, Open Approach, Diagnostic
04BL4ZZ Excision of Left Femoral Artery, Percutaneous Endoscopic Approach
04BM0ZX Excision of Right Popliteal Artery, Open Approach, Diagnostic
04BM0ZZ Excision of Right Popliteal Artery, Open Approach
04BM3ZX Excision of Right Popliteal Artery, Percutaneous Approach, Diagnostic
04BM3ZZ Excision of Right Popliteal Artery, Percutaneous Approach
04BM4ZX Excision of Right Popliteal Artery, Percutaneous Endoscopic Approach, Diagnostic
04BM4ZZ Excision of Right Popliteal Artery, Percutaneous Endoscopic Approach
04BN0ZX Excision of Left Popliteal Artery, Open Approach, Diagnostic
04BN0ZZ Excision of Left Popliteal Artery, Open Approach
04BN3ZX Excision of Left Popliteal Artery, Percutaneous Approach, Diagnostic
04BN3ZZ Excision of Left Popliteal Artery, Percutaneous Approach
04BN4ZX Excision of Left Popliteal Artery, Percutaneous Endoscopic Approach, Diagnostic
04BN4ZZ Excision of Left Popliteal Artery, Percutaneous Endoscopic Approach
04BP0ZX Excision of Right Anterior Tibial Artery, Open Approach, Diagnostic
04BP0ZZ Excision of Right Anterior Tibial Artery, Open Approach
04BP3ZX Excision of Right Anterior Tibial Artery, Percutaneous Approach, Diagnostic
04BP3ZZ Excision of Right Anterior Tibial Artery, Percutaneous Approach

4BP4ZX Excision of Right Anterior Tibial Artery, Percutaneous Endoscopic Approach, Diagnostic
4BP4ZZ Excision of Right Anterior Tibial Artery, Percutaneous Endoscopic Approach
4BQ0ZX Excision of Left Anterior Tibial Artery, Open Approach, Diagnostic
4BQ0ZZ Excision of Left Anterior Tibial Artery, Open Approach
4BQ3ZX Excision of Left Anterior Tibial Artery, Percutaneous Approach, Diagnostic
4BQ3ZZ Excision of Left Anterior Tibial Artery, Percutaneous Approach
4BQ4ZX Excision of Left Anterior Tibial Artery, Percutaneous Endoscopic Approach, Diagnostic
4BQ4ZZ Excision of Left Anterior Tibial Artery, Percutaneous Endoscopic Approach
4BR0ZX Excision of Right Posterior Tibial Artery, Open Approach, Diagnostic
4BR0ZZ Excision of Right Posterior Tibial Artery, Open Approach
4BR3ZX Excision of Right Posterior Tibial Artery, Percutaneous Approach, Diagnostic
4BR3ZZ Excision of Right Posterior Tibial Artery, Percutaneous Approach
4BR4ZX Excision of Right Posterior Tibial Artery, Percutaneous Endoscopic Approach, Diagnostic
4BR4ZZ Excision of Right Posterior Tibial Artery, Percutaneous Endoscopic Approach
4BS0ZX Excision of Left Posterior Tibial Artery, Open Approach, Diagnostic
4BS0ZZ Excision of Left Posterior Tibial Artery, Open Approach
04BS3ZX Excision of Left Posterior Tibial Artery, Percutaneous Approach, Diagnostic
04BS3ZZ Excision of Left Posterior Tibial Artery, Percutaneous Approach
04BS4ZX Excision of Left Posterior Tibial Artery, Percutaneous Endoscopic Approach, Diagnostic
04BS4ZZ Excision of Left Posterior Tibial Artery, Percutaneous Endoscopic Approach
04BT0ZX Excision of Right Peroneal Artery, Open Approach, Diagnostic
04BT0ZZ Excision of Right Peroneal Artery, Open Approach
04BT3ZX Excision of Right Peroneal Artery, Percutaneous Approach, Diagnostic
04BT3ZZ Excision of Right Peroneal Artery, Percutaneous Approach
04BT4ZX Excision of Right Peroneal Artery, Percutaneous Endoscopic Approach, Diagnostic
04BT4ZZ Excision of Right Peroneal Artery, Percutaneous Endoscopic Approach
04BU0ZX Excision of Left Peroneal Artery, Open Approach, Diagnostic
04BU0ZZ Excision of Left Peroneal Artery, Open Approach
04BU3ZX Excision of Left Peroneal Artery, Percutaneous Approach, Diagnostic
04BU3ZZ Excision of Left Peroneal Artery, Percutaneous Approach
04BU4ZX Excision of Left Peroneal Artery, Percutaneous Endoscopic Approach, Diagnostic
04BU4ZZ Excision of Left Peroneal Artery, Percutaneous Endoscopic Approach
04BV0ZX Excision of Right Foot Artery, Open Approach, Diagnostic
04BV0ZZ Excision of Right Foot Artery, Open Approach
04BV3ZX Excision of Right Foot Artery, Percutaneous Approach, Diagnostic
04BV3ZZ Excision of Right Foot Artery, Percutaneous Approach
04BV4ZX Excision of Right Foot Artery, Percutaneous Endoscopic Approach, Diagnostic
04BV4ZZ Excision of Right Foot Artery, Percutaneous Endoscopic Approach
04BW0ZX Excision of Left Foot Artery, Open Approach, Diagnostic
04BW0ZZ Excision of Left Foot Artery, Open Approach
04BW3ZX Excision of Left Foot Artery, Percutaneous Approach, Diagnostic
04BW3ZZ Excision of Left Foot Artery, Percutaneous Approach
04BW4ZX Excision of Left Foot Artery, Percutaneous Endoscopic Approach, Diagnostic
04BW4ZZ Excision of Left Foot Artery, Percutaneous Endoscopic Approach
04BY0ZX Excision of Lower Artery, Open Approach, Diagnostic
04BY0ZZ Excision of Lower Artery, Open Approach
04BY3ZX Excision of Lower Artery, Percutaneous Approach, Diagnostic
04BY3ZZ Excision of Lower Artery, Percutaneous Approach
04BY4ZX Excision of Lower Artery, Percutaneous Endoscopic Approach, Diagnostic
04BY4ZZ Excision of Lower Artery, Percutaneous Endoscopic Approach

4C – Lower Arteries, Extirpation

4C00ZZ Extirpation of Matter from Abdominal Aorta, Open Approach
4C03ZZ Extirpation of Matter from Abdominal Aorta, Percutaneous Approach
4C04ZZ Extirpation of Matter from Abdominal Aorta, Percutaneous Endoscopic Approach
4C10ZZ Extirpation of Matter from Celiac Artery, Open Approach
4C13ZZ Extirpation of Matter from Celiac Artery, Percutaneous Approach
4C14ZZ Extirpation of Matter from Celiac Artery, Percutaneous Endoscopic Approach
4C20ZZ Extirpation of Matter from Gastric Artery, Open Approach
4C23ZZ Extirpation of Matter from Gastric Artery, Percutaneous Approach
4C24ZZ Extirpation of Matter from Gastric Artery, Percutaneous Endoscopic Approach
4C30ZZ Extirpation of Matter from Hepatic Artery, Open Approach
4C33ZZ Extirpation of Matter from Hepatic Artery, Percutaneous Approach
4C34ZZ Extirpation of Matter from Hepatic Artery, Percutaneous Endoscopic Approach
4C40ZZ Extirpation of Matter from Splenic Artery, Open Approach
4C43ZZ Extirpation of Matter from Splenic Artery, Percutaneous Approach
4C44ZZ Extirpation of Matter from Splenic Artery, Percutaneous Endoscopic Approach
4C50ZZ Extirpation of Matter from Superior Mesenteric Artery, Open Approach
4C53ZZ Extirpation of Matter from Superior Mesenteric Artery, Percutaneous Approach
4C54ZZ Extirpation of Matter from Superior Mesenteric Artery, Percutaneous Endoscopic Approach
4C60ZZ Extirpation of Matter from Right Colic Artery, Open Approach
04C63ZZ Extirpation of Matter from Right Colic Artery, Percutaneous Approach
04C64ZZ Extirpation of Matter from Right Colic Artery, Percutaneous Endoscopic Approach
04C70ZZ Extirpation of Matter from Left Colic Artery, Open Approach
04C73ZZ Extirpation of Matter from Left Colic Artery, Percutaneous Approach
04C74ZZ Extirpation of Matter from Left Colic Artery, Percutaneous Endoscopic Approach
04C80ZZ Extirpation of Matter from Middle Colic Artery, Open Approach
04C83ZZ Extirpation of Matter from Middle Colic Artery, Percutaneous Approach
04C84ZZ Extirpation of Matter from Middle Colic Artery, Percutaneous Endoscopic Approach
04C90ZZ Extirpation of Matter from Right Renal Artery, Open Approach
04C93ZZ Extirpation of Matter from Right Renal Artery, Percutaneous Approach
04C94ZZ Extirpation of Matter from Right Renal Artery, Percutaneous Endoscopic Approach
04CA0ZZ Extirpation of Matter from Left Renal Artery, Open Approach
04CA3ZZ Extirpation of Matter from Left Renal Artery, Percutaneous Approach
04CA4ZZ Extirpation of Matter from Left Renal Artery, Percutaneous Endoscopic Approach
04CB0ZZ Extirpation of Matter from Inferior Mesenteric Artery, Open Approach
04CB3ZZ Extirpation of Matter from Inferior Mesenteric Artery, Percutaneous Approach
04CB4ZZ Extirpation of Matter from Inferior Mesenteric Artery, Percutaneous Endoscopic Approach
04CC0ZZ Extirpation of Matter from Right Common Iliac Artery, Open Approach
04CC3ZZ Extirpation of Matter from Right Common Iliac Artery, Percutaneous Approach
04CC4ZZ Extirpation of Matter from Right Common Iliac Artery, Percutaneous Endoscopic Approach
04CD0ZZ Extirpation of Matter from Left Common Iliac Artery, Open Approach
04CD3ZZ Extirpation of Matter from Left Common Iliac Artery, Percutaneous Approach
04CD4ZZ Extirpation of Matter from Left Common Iliac Artery, Percutaneous Endoscopic Approach
04CE0ZZ Extirpation of Matter from Right Internal Iliac Artery, Open Approach
04CE3ZZ Extirpation of Matter from Right Internal Iliac Artery, Percutaneous Approach
04CE4ZZ Extirpation of Matter from Right Internal Iliac Artery, Percutaneous Endoscopic Approach
04CF0ZZ Extirpation of Matter from Left Internal Iliac Artery, Open Approach
04CF3ZZ Extirpation of Matter from Left Internal Iliac Artery, Percutaneous Approach
04CF4ZZ Extirpation of Matter from Left Internal Iliac Artery, Percutaneous Endoscopic Approach
04CH0ZZ Extirpation of Matter from Right External Iliac Artery, Open Approach
04CH3ZZ Extirpation of Matter from Right External Iliac Artery, Percutaneous Approach
04CH4ZZ Extirpation of Matter from Right External Iliac Artery, Percutaneous Endoscopic Approach

04CJ0ZZ Extirpation of Matter from Left External Iliac Artery, Open Approach
04CJ3ZZ Extirpation of Matter from Left External Iliac Artery, Percutaneous Approach
04CJ4ZZ Extirpation of Matter from Left External Iliac Artery, Percutaneous Endoscopic Approach
04CK0ZZ Extirpation of Matter from Right Femoral Artery, Open Approach
04CK3ZZ Extirpation of Matter from Right Femoral Artery, Percutaneous Approach
04CK4ZZ Extirpation of Matter from Right Femoral Artery, Percutaneous Endoscopic Approach
04CL0ZZ Extirpation of Matter from Left Femoral Artery, Open Approach
04CL3ZZ Extirpation of Matter from Left Femoral Artery, Percutaneous Approach
04CL4ZZ Extirpation of Matter from Left Femoral Artery, Percutaneous Endoscopic Approach
04CM0ZZ Extirpation of Matter from Right Popliteal Artery, Open Approach
04CM3ZZ Extirpation of Matter from Right Popliteal Artery, Percutaneous Approach
04CM4ZZ Extirpation of Matter from Right Popliteal Artery, Percutaneous Endoscopic Approach
04CN0ZZ Extirpation of Matter from Left Popliteal Artery, Open Approach
04CN3ZZ Extirpation of Matter from Left Popliteal Artery, Percutaneous Approach
04CN4ZZ Extirpation of Matter from Left Popliteal Artery, Percutaneous Endoscopic Approach
04CP0ZZ Extirpation of Matter from Right Anterior Tibial Artery, Open Approach
04CP3ZZ Extirpation of Matter from Right Anterior Tibial Artery, Percutaneous Approach
04CP4ZZ Extirpation of Matter from Right Anterior Tibial Artery, Percutaneous Endoscopic Approach
04CQ0ZZ Extirpation of Matter from Left Anterior Tibial Artery, Open Approach
04CQ3ZZ Extirpation of Matter from Left Anterior Tibial Artery, Percutaneous Approach
04CQ4ZZ Extirpation of Matter from Left Anterior Tibial Artery, Percutaneous Endoscopic Approach
04CR0ZZ Extirpation of Matter from Right Posterior Tibial Artery, Open Approach
04CR3ZZ Extirpation of Matter from Right Posterior Tibial Artery, Percutaneous Approach
04CR4ZZ Extirpation of Matter from Right Posterior Tibial Artery, Percutaneous Endoscopic Approach
04CS0ZZ Extirpation of Matter from Left Posterior Tibial Artery, Open Approach
04CS3ZZ Extirpation of Matter from Left Posterior Tibial Artery, Percutaneous Approach
04CS4ZZ Extirpation of Matter from Left Posterior Tibial Artery, Percutaneous Endoscopic Approach
04CT0ZZ Extirpation of Matter from Right Peroneal Artery, Open Approach
04CT3ZZ Extirpation of Matter from Right Perone Artery, Percutaneous Approach
04CT4ZZ Extirpation of Matter from Right Perone Artery, Percutaneous Endoscopic Approach
04CU0ZZ Extirpation of Matter from Left Peroneal Artery, Open Approach
04CU3ZZ Extirpation of Matter from Left Peroneal Artery, Percutaneous Approach
04CU4ZZ Extirpation of Matter from Left Peroneal Artery, Percutaneous Endoscopic Approach
04CV0ZZ Extirpation of Matter from Right Foot Artery, Open Approach
04CV3ZZ Extirpation of Matter from Right Foot Artery, Percutaneous Approach
04CV4ZZ Extirpation of Matter from Right Foot Artery, Percutaneous Endoscopic Approach
04CW0ZZ Extirpation of Matter from Left Foot Artery, Open Approach
04CW3ZZ Extirpation of Matter from Left Foot Artery, Percutaneous Approach
04CW4ZZ Extirpation of Matter from Left Foot Artery, Percutaneous Endoscopic Approach
04CY0ZZ Extirpation of Matter from Lower Artery, Open Approach
04CY3ZZ Extirpation of Matter from Lower Artery, Percutaneous Approach
04CY4ZZ Extirpation of Matter from Lower Artery, Percutaneous Endoscopic Approach

04H – Lower Arteries, Insertion

04H002Z Insertion of Monitoring Device into Abdominal Aorta, Open Approach
04H003Z Insertion of Infusion Device into Abdominal Aorta, Open Approach
04H00DZ Insertion of Intraluminal Device into Abdominal Aorta, Open Approach
04H032Z Insertion of Monitoring Device into Abdominal Aorta, Percutaneous Approach
04H033Z Insertion of Infusion Device into Abdominal Aorta, Percutaneous Approach
04H03DZ Insertion of Intraluminal Device into Abdominal Aorta, Percutaneous Approach
04H042Z Insertion of Monitoring Device into Abdominal Aorta, Percutaneous Endoscopic Approach
04H043Z Insertion of Infusion Device into Abdominal Aorta, Percutaneous Endoscopic Approach
04H04DZ Insertion of Intraluminal Device into Abdominal Aorta, Percutaneous Endoscopic Approach
04H103Z Insertion of Infusion Device into Celiac Artery, Open Approach
04H10DZ Insertion of Intraluminal Device into Celiac Artery, Open Approach
04H133Z Insertion of Infusion Device into Celiac Artery, Percutaneous Approach
04H13DZ Insertion of Intraluminal Device into Celiac Artery, Percutaneous Approach
04H143Z Insertion of Infusion Device into Celiac Artery, Percutaneous Endoscopic Approach
04H14DZ Insertion of Intraluminal Device into Celiac Artery, Percutaneous Endoscopic Approach
04H203Z Insertion of Infusion Device into Gastric Artery, Open Approach
04H20DZ Insertion of Intraluminal Device into Gastric Artery, Open Approach
04H233Z Insertion of Infusion Device into Gastric Artery, Percutaneous Approach
04H23DZ Insertion of Intraluminal Device into Gastric Artery, Percutaneous Approach
04H243Z Insertion of Infusion Device into Gastric Artery, Percutaneous Endoscopic Approach
04H24DZ Insertion of Intraluminal Device into Gastric Artery, Percutaneous Endoscopic Approach
04H303Z Insertion of Infusion Device into Hepatic Artery, Open Approach
04H30DZ Insertion of Intraluminal Device into Hepatic Artery, Open Approach
04H333Z Insertion of Infusion Device into Hepatic Artery, Percutaneous Approach
04H33DZ Insertion of Intraluminal Device into Hepatic Artery, Percutaneous Approach
04H343Z Insertion of Infusion Device into Hepatic Artery, Percutaneous Endoscopic Approach
04H34DZ Insertion of Intraluminal Device into Hepatic Artery, Percutaneous Endoscopic Approach
04H403Z Insertion of Infusion Device into Splenic Artery, Open Approach
04H40DZ Insertion of Intraluminal Device into Splenic Artery, Open Approach
04H433Z Insertion of Infusion Device into Splenic Artery, Percutaneous Approach
04H43DZ Insertion of Intraluminal Device into Splenic Artery, Percutaneous Approach
04H443Z Insertion of Infusion Device into Splenic Artery, Percutaneous Endoscopic Approach
04H44DZ Insertion of Intraluminal Device into Splenic Artery, Percutaneous Endoscopic Approach
04H503Z Insertion of Infusion Device into Superior Mesenteric Artery, Open Approach
04H50DZ Insertion of Intraluminal Device into Superior Mesenteric Artery, Open Approach
04H533Z Insertion of Infusion Device into Superior Mesenteric Artery, Percutaneous Approac
04H53DZ Insertion of Intraluminal Device into Superior Mesenteric Artery, Percutaneous Approach
04H543Z Insertion of Infusion Device into Superior Mesenteric Artery, Percutaneous Endoscopic Approach
04H54DZ Insertion of Intraluminal Device into Superior Mesenteric Artery, Percutaneous Endoscopic Approach
04H603Z Insertion of Infusion Device into Right Colic Artery, Open Approach
04H60DZ Insertion of Intraluminal Device into Righ Colic Artery, Open Approach
04H633Z Insertion of Infusion Device into Right Colic Artery, Percutaneous Approach
04H63DZ Insertion of Intraluminal Device into Righ Colic Artery, Percutaneous Approach
04H643Z Insertion of Infusion Device into Right Colic Artery, Percutaneous Endoscopic Approach
04H64DZ Insertion of Intraluminal Device into Righ Colic Artery, Percutaneous Endoscopic Approach
04H703Z Insertion of Infusion Device into Left Colic Artery, Open Approach
04H70DZ Insertion of Intraluminal Device into Left Colic Artery, Open Approach
04H733Z Insertion of Infusion Device into Left Colic Artery, Percutaneous Approach
04H73DZ Insertion of Intraluminal Device into Left Colic Artery, Percutaneous Approach
04H743Z Insertion of Infusion Device into Left Colic Artery, Percutaneous Endoscopic Approach
04H74DZ Insertion of Intraluminal Device into Left Colic Artery, Percutaneous Endoscopic Approach
04H803Z Insertion of Infusion Device into Middle Colic Artery, Open Approach

H80DZ Insertion of Intraluminal Device into Middle Colic Artery, Open Approach
H833Z Insertion of Infusion Device into Middle Colic Artery, Percutaneous Approach
H83DZ Insertion of Intraluminal Device into Middle Colic Artery, Percutaneous Approach
H843Z Insertion of Infusion Device into Middle Colic Artery, Percutaneous Endoscopic Approach
H84DZ Insertion of Intraluminal Device into Middle Colic Artery, Percutaneous Endoscopic Approach
H903Z Insertion of Infusion Device into Right Renal Artery, Open Approach
H90DZ Insertion of Intraluminal Device into Right Renal Artery, Open Approach
H933Z Insertion of Infusion Device into Right Renal Artery, Percutaneous Approach
H93DZ Insertion of Intraluminal Device into Right Renal Artery, Percutaneous Approach
H943Z Insertion of Infusion Device into Right Renal Artery, Percutaneous Endoscopic Approach
H94DZ Insertion of Intraluminal Device into Right Renal Artery, Percutaneous Endoscopic Approach
4HA03Z Insertion of Infusion Device into Left Renal Artery, Open Approach
4HA0DZ Insertion of Intraluminal Device into Left Renal Artery, Open Approach
4HA33Z Insertion of Infusion Device into Left Renal Artery, Percutaneous Approach
4HA3DZ Insertion of Intraluminal Device into Left Renal Artery, Percutaneous Approach
4HA43Z Insertion of Infusion Device into Left Renal Artery, Percutaneous Endoscopic Approach
4HA4DZ Insertion of Intraluminal Device into Left Renal Artery, Percutaneous Endoscopic Approach
4HB03Z Insertion of Infusion Device into Inferior Mesenteric Artery, Open Approach
4HB0DZ Insertion of Intraluminal Device into Inferior Mesenteric Artery, Open Approach
4HB33Z Insertion of Infusion Device into Inferior Mesenteric Artery, Percutaneous Approach
4HB3DZ Insertion of Intraluminal Device into Inferior Mesenteric Artery, Percutaneous Approach
4HB43Z Insertion of Infusion Device into Inferior Mesenteric Artery, Percutaneous Endoscopic Approach
4HB4DZ Insertion of Intraluminal Device into Inferior Mesenteric Artery, Percutaneous Endoscopic Approach
4HC03Z Insertion of Infusion Device into Right Common Iliac Artery, Open Approach
4HC0DZ Insertion of Intraluminal Device into Right Common Iliac Artery, Open Approach
4HC33Z Insertion of Infusion Device into Right Common Iliac Artery, Percutaneous Approach
4HC3DZ Insertion of Intraluminal Device into Right Common Iliac Artery, Percutaneous Approach
4HC43Z Insertion of Infusion Device into Right Common Iliac Artery, Percutaneous Endoscopic Approach
4HC4DZ Insertion of Intraluminal Device into Right Common Iliac Artery, Percutaneous Endoscopic Approach
4HD03Z Insertion of Infusion Device into Left Common Iliac Artery, Open Approach
4HD0DZ Insertion of Intraluminal Device into Left Common Iliac Artery, Open Approach
04HD33Z Insertion of Infusion Device into Left Common Iliac Artery, Percutaneous Approach
04HD3DZ Insertion of Intraluminal Device into Left Common Iliac Artery, Percutaneous Approach
04HD43Z Insertion of Infusion Device into Left Common Iliac Artery, Percutaneous Endoscopic Approach
04HD4DZ Insertion of Intraluminal Device into Left Common Iliac Artery, Percutaneous Endoscopic Approach
04HE03Z Insertion of Infusion Device into Right Internal Iliac Artery, Open Approach
04HE0DZ Insertion of Intraluminal Device into Right Internal Iliac Artery, Open Approach
04HE33Z Insertion of Infusion Device into Right Internal Iliac Artery, Percutaneous Approach
04HE3DZ Insertion of Intraluminal Device into Right Internal Iliac Artery, Percutaneous Approach
04HE43Z Insertion of Infusion Device into Right Internal Iliac Artery, Percutaneous Endoscopic Approach
04HE4DZ Insertion of Intraluminal Device into Right Internal Iliac Artery, Percutaneous Endoscopic Approach
04HF03Z Insertion of Infusion Device into Left Internal Iliac Artery, Open Approach
04HF0DZ Insertion of Intraluminal Device into Left Internal Iliac Artery, Open Approach
04HF33Z Insertion of Infusion Device into Left Internal Iliac Artery, Percutaneous Approach
04HF3DZ Insertion of Intraluminal Device into Left Internal Iliac Artery, Percutaneous Approach
04HF43Z Insertion of Infusion Device into Left Internal Iliac Artery, Percutaneous Endoscopic Approach
04HF4DZ Insertion of Intraluminal Device into Left Internal Iliac Artery, Percutaneous Endoscopic Approach
04HH03Z Insertion of Infusion Device into Right External Iliac Artery, Open Approach
04HH0DZ Insertion of Intraluminal Device into Right External Iliac Artery, Open Approach
04HH33Z Insertion of Infusion Device into Right External Iliac Artery, Percutaneous Approach
04HH3DZ Insertion of Intraluminal Device into Right External Iliac Artery, Percutaneous Approach
04HH43Z Insertion of Infusion Device into Right External Iliac Artery, Percutaneous Endoscopic Approach
04HH4DZ Insertion of Intraluminal Device into Right External Iliac Artery, Percutaneous Endoscopic Approach
04HJ03Z Insertion of Infusion Device into Left External Iliac Artery, Open Approach
04HJ0DZ Insertion of Intraluminal Device into Left External Iliac Artery, Open Approach
04HJ33Z Insertion of Infusion Device into Left External Iliac Artery, Percutaneous Approach
04HJ3DZ Insertion of Intraluminal Device into Left External Iliac Artery, Percutaneous Approach
04HJ43Z Insertion of Infusion Device into Left External Iliac Artery, Percutaneous Endoscopic Approach
04HJ4DZ Insertion of Intraluminal Device into Left External Iliac Artery, Percutaneous Endoscopic Approach
04HK03Z Insertion of Infusion Device into Right Femoral Artery, Open Approach
04HK0DZ Insertion of Intraluminal Device into Right Femoral Artery, Open Approach
04HK33Z Insertion of Infusion Device into Right Femoral Artery, Percutaneous Approach
04HK3DZ Insertion of Intraluminal Device into Right Femoral Artery, Percutaneous Approach
04HK43Z Insertion of Infusion Device into Right Femoral Artery, Percutaneous Endoscopic Approach
04HK4DZ Insertion of Intraluminal Device into Right Femoral Artery, Percutaneous Endoscopic Approach
04HL03Z Insertion of Infusion Device into Left Femoral Artery, Open Approach
04HL0DZ Insertion of Intraluminal Device into Left Femoral Artery, Open Approach
04HL33Z Insertion of Infusion Device into Left Femoral Artery, Percutaneous Approach
04HL3DZ Insertion of Intraluminal Device into Left Femoral Artery, Percutaneous Approach
04HL43Z Insertion of Infusion Device into Left Femoral Artery, Percutaneous Endoscopic Approach
04HL4DZ Insertion of Intraluminal Device into Left Femoral Artery, Percutaneous Endoscopic Approach
04HM03Z Insertion of Infusion Device into Right Popliteal Artery, Open Approach
04HM0DZ Insertion of Intraluminal Device into Right Popliteal Artery, Open Approach
04HM33Z Insertion of Infusion Device into Right Popliteal Artery, Percutaneous Approach
04HM3DZ Insertion of Intraluminal Device into Right Popliteal Artery, Percutaneous Approach
04HM43Z Insertion of Infusion Device into Right Popliteal Artery, Percutaneous Endoscopic Approach
04HM4DZ Insertion of Intraluminal Device into Right Popliteal Artery, Percutaneous Endoscopic Approach
04HN03Z Insertion of Infusion Device into Left Popliteal Artery, Open Approach
04HN0DZ Insertion of Intraluminal Device into Left Popliteal Artery, Open Approach
04HN33Z Insertion of Infusion Device into Left Popliteal Artery, Percutaneous Approach
04HN3DZ Insertion of Intraluminal Device into Left Popliteal Artery, Percutaneous Approach
04HN43Z Insertion of Infusion Device into Left Popliteal Artery, Percutaneous Endoscopic Approach
04HN4DZ Insertion of Intraluminal Device into Left Popliteal Artery, Percutaneous Endoscopic Approach
04HP03Z Insertion of Infusion Device into Right Anterior Tibial Artery, Open Approach
04HP0DZ Insertion of Intraluminal Device into Right Anterior Tibial Artery, Open Approach
04HP33Z Insertion of Infusion Device into Right Anterior Tibial Artery, Percutaneous Approach
04HP3DZ Insertion of Intraluminal Device into Right Anterior Tibial Artery, Percutaneous Approach
04HP43Z Insertion of Infusion Device into Right Anterior Tibial Artery, Percutaneous Endoscopic Approach
04HP4DZ Insertion of Intraluminal Device into Right Anterior Tibial Artery, Percutaneous Endoscopic Approach
04HQ03Z Insertion of Infusion Device into Left Anterior Tibial Artery, Open Approach
04HQ0DZ Insertion of Intraluminal Device into Left Anterior Tibial Artery, Open Approach
04HQ33Z Insertion of Infusion Device into Left Anterior Tibial Artery, Percutaneous Approach

04HQ3DZ Insertion of Intraluminal Device into Left Anterior Tibial Artery, Percutaneous Approach
04HQ43Z Insertion of Infusion Device into Left Anterior Tibial Artery, Percutaneous Endoscopic Approach
04HQ4DZ Insertion of Intraluminal Device into Left Anterior Tibial Artery, Percutaneous Endoscopic Approach
04HR03Z Insertion of Infusion Device into Right Posterior Tibial Artery, Open Approach
04HR0DZ Insertion of Intraluminal Device into Right Posterior Tibial Artery, Open Approach
04HR33Z Insertion of Infusion Device into Right Posterior Tibial Artery, Percutaneous Approach
04HR3DZ Insertion of Intraluminal Device into Right Posterior Tibial Artery, Percutaneous Approach
04HR43Z Insertion of Infusion Device into Right Posterior Tibial Artery, Percutaneous Endoscopic Approach
04HR4DZ Insertion of Intraluminal Device into Right Posterior Tibial Artery, Percutaneous Endoscopic Approach
04HS03Z Insertion of Infusion Device into Left Posterior Tibial Artery, Open Approach
04HS0DZ Insertion of Intraluminal Device into Left Posterior Tibial Artery, Open Approach
04HS33Z Insertion of Infusion Device into Left Posterior Tibial Artery, Percutaneous Approach
04HS3DZ Insertion of Intraluminal Device into Left Posterior Tibial Artery, Percutaneous Approach
04HS43Z Insertion of Infusion Device into Left Posterior Tibial Artery, Percutaneous Endoscopic Approach
04HS4DZ Insertion of Intraluminal Device into Left Posterior Tibial Artery, Percutaneous Endoscopic Approach
04HT03Z Insertion of Infusion Device into Right Peroneal Artery, Open Approach
04HT0DZ Insertion of Intraluminal Device into Right Peroneal Artery, Open Approach
04HT33Z Insertion of Infusion Device into Right Peroneal Artery, Percutaneous Approach
04HT3DZ Insertion of Intraluminal Device into Right Peroneal Artery, Percutaneous Approach
04HT43Z Insertion of Infusion Device into Right Peroneal Artery, Percutaneous Endoscopic Approach
04HT4DZ Insertion of Intraluminal Device into Right Peroneal Artery, Percutaneous Endoscopic Approach
04HU03Z Insertion of Infusion Device into Left Peroneal Artery, Open Approach
04HU0DZ Insertion of Intraluminal Device into Left Peroneal Artery, Open Approach
04HU33Z Insertion of Infusion Device into Left Peroneal Artery, Percutaneous Approach
04HU3DZ Insertion of Intraluminal Device into Left Peroneal Artery, Percutaneous Approach
04HU43Z Insertion of Infusion Device into Left Peroneal Artery, Percutaneous Endoscopic Approach
04HU4DZ Insertion of Intraluminal Device into Left Peroneal Artery, Percutaneous Endoscopic Approach
04HV03Z Insertion of Infusion Device into Right Foot Artery, Open Approach
04HV0DZ Insertion of Intraluminal Device into Right Foot Artery, Open Approach
04HV33Z Insertion of Infusion Device into Right Foot Artery, Percutaneous Approach
04HV3DZ Insertion of Intraluminal Device into Right Foot Artery, Percutaneous Approach
04HV43Z Insertion of Infusion Device into Right Foot Artery, Percutaneous Endoscopic Approach
04HV4DZ Insertion of Intraluminal Device into Rig Foot Artery, Percutaneous Endoscopic Approach
04HW03Z Insertion of Infusion Device into Left Fo Artery, Open Approach
04HW0DZ Insertion of Intraluminal Device into Lef Foot Artery, Open Approach
04HW33Z Insertion of Infusion Device into Left Fo Artery, Percutaneous Approach
04HW3DZ Insertion of Intraluminal Device into Lef Foot Artery, Percutaneous Approach
04HW43Z Insertion of Infusion Device into Left Foot Artery, Percutaneous Endoscopic Approach
04HW4DZ Insertion of Intraluminal Device into Lef Foot Artery, Percutaneous Endoscopic Approach
04HY02Z Insertion of Monitoring Device into Low Artery, Open Approach
04HY03Z Insertion of Infusion Device into Lower Artery, Open Approach
04HY0DZ Insertion of Intraluminal Device into Lower Artery, Open Approach
04HY32Z Insertion of Monitoring Device into Low Artery, Percutaneous Approach
04HY33Z Insertion of Infusion Device into Lower Artery, Percutaneous Approach
04HY3DZ Insertion of Intraluminal Device into Lower Artery, Percutaneous Approach
04HY42Z Insertion of Monitoring Device into Lower Artery, Percutaneous Endoscopic Approach
04HY43Z Insertion of Infusion Device into Lower Artery, Percutaneous Endoscopic Approach
04HY4DZ Insertion of Intraluminal Device into Lower Artery, Percutaneous Endoscopic Approach

04J – Lower Arteries, Inspection

Review Coding Guidelines B3.11a, B3.11b and B3.11c

04JY0ZZ Inspection of Lower Artery, Open Approach
04JY3ZZ Inspection of Lower Artery, Percutaneous Approach
04JY4ZZ Inspection of Lower Artery, Percutaneous Endoscopic Approach
04JYXZZ Inspection of Lower Artery, External Approach

04L – Lower Arteries, Occlusion

Review Coding Guideline B3.12

04L00CZ Occlusion of Abdominal Aorta with Extraluminal Device, Open Approach
04L00DZ Occlusion of Abdominal Aorta with Intraluminal Device, Open Approach
04L00ZZ Occlusion of Abdominal Aorta, Open Approach
04L03CZ Occlusion of Abdominal Aorta with Extraluminal Device, Percutaneous Approach
04L03DZ Occlusion of Abdominal Aorta with Intraluminal Device, Percutaneous Approach
04L03ZZ Occlusion of Abdominal Aorta, Percutaneous Approach
04L04CZ Occlusion of Abdominal Aorta with Extraluminal Device, Percutaneous Endoscopic Approach
04L04DZ Occlusion of Abdominal Aorta with Intraluminal Device, Percutaneous Endoscopic Approach
04L04ZZ Occlusion of Abdominal Aorta, Percutaneous Endoscopic Approach
04L10CZ Occlusion of Celiac Artery with Extraluminal Device, Open Approach
04L10DZ Occlusion of Celiac Artery with Intraluminal Device, Open Approach
04L10ZZ Occlusion of Celiac Artery, Open Approach
04L13CZ Occlusion of Celiac Artery with Extraluminal Device, Percutaneous Approach
04L13DZ Occlusion of Celiac Artery with Intraluminal Device, Percutaneous Approach
04L13ZZ Occlusion of Celiac Artery, Percutaneous Approach
04L14CZ Occlusion of Celiac Artery with Extraluminal Device, Percutaneous Endoscopic Approach
04L14DZ Occlusion of Celiac Artery with Intraluminal Device, Percutaneous Endoscopic Approach
04L14ZZ Occlusion of Celiac Artery, Percutaneous Endoscopic Approach
04L20CZ Occlusion of Gastric Artery with Extraluminal Device, Open Approach
04L20DZ Occlusion of Gastric Artery with Intraluminal Device, Open Approach
04L20ZZ Occlusion of Gastric Artery, Open Approach
04L23CZ Occlusion of Gastric Artery with Extraluminal Device, Percutaneous Approach
04L23DZ Occlusion of Gastric Artery with Intraluminal Device, Percutaneous Approach
04L23ZZ Occlusion of Gastric Artery, Percutaneous Approach
04L24CZ Occlusion of Gastric Artery with Extraluminal Device, Percutaneous Endoscopic Approach
04L24DZ Occlusion of Gastric Artery with Intraluminal Device, Percutaneous Endoscopic Approach
04L24ZZ Occlusion of Gastric Artery, Percutaneous Endoscopic Approach

L30CZ Occlusion of Hepatic Artery with Extraluminal Device, Open Approach
L30DZ Occlusion of Hepatic Artery with Intraluminal Device, Open Approach
L30ZZ Occlusion of Hepatic Artery, Open Approach
L33CZ Occlusion of Hepatic Artery with Extraluminal Device, Percutaneous Approach
L33DZ Occlusion of Hepatic Artery with Intraluminal Device, Percutaneous Approach
L33ZZ Occlusion of Hepatic Artery, Percutaneous Approach
L34CZ Occlusion of Hepatic Artery with Extraluminal Device, Percutaneous Endoscopic Approach
L34DZ Occlusion of Hepatic Artery with Intraluminal Device, Percutaneous Endoscopic Approach
L34ZZ Occlusion of Hepatic Artery, Percutaneous Endoscopic Approach
L40CZ Occlusion of Splenic Artery with Extraluminal Device, Open Approach
L40DZ Occlusion of Splenic Artery with Intraluminal Device, Open Approach
L40ZZ Occlusion of Splenic Artery, Open Approach
L43CZ Occlusion of Splenic Artery with Extraluminal Device, Percutaneous Approach
L43DZ Occlusion of Splenic Artery with Intraluminal Device, Percutaneous Approach
L43ZZ Occlusion of Splenic Artery, Percutaneous Approach
L44CZ Occlusion of Splenic Artery with Extraluminal Device, Percutaneous Endoscopic Approach
L44DZ Occlusion of Splenic Artery with Intraluminal Device, Percutaneous Endoscopic Approach
L44ZZ Occlusion of Splenic Artery, Percutaneous Endoscopic Approach
L50CZ Occlusion of Superior Mesenteric Artery with Extraluminal Device, Open Approach
L50DZ Occlusion of Superior Mesenteric Artery with Intraluminal Device, Open Approach
L50ZZ Occlusion of Superior Mesenteric Artery, Open Approach
L53CZ Occlusion of Superior Mesenteric Artery with Extraluminal Device, Percutaneous Approach
L53DZ Occlusion of Superior Mesenteric Artery with Intraluminal Device, Percutaneous Approach
L53ZZ Occlusion of Superior Mesenteric Artery, Percutaneous Approach
L54CZ Occlusion of Superior Mesenteric Artery with Extraluminal Device, Percutaneous Endoscopic Approach
L54DZ Occlusion of Superior Mesenteric Artery with Intraluminal Device, Percutaneous Endoscopic Approach
L54ZZ Occlusion of Superior Mesenteric Artery, Percutaneous Endoscopic Approach
4L60CZ Occlusion of Right Colic Artery with Extraluminal Device, Open Approach
4L60DZ Occlusion of Right Colic Artery with Intraluminal Device, Open Approach
4L60ZZ Occlusion of Right Colic Artery, Open Approach
4L63CZ Occlusion of Right Colic Artery with Extraluminal Device, Percutaneous Approach
4L63DZ Occlusion of Right Colic Artery with Intraluminal Device, Percutaneous Approach
04L63ZZ Occlusion of Right Colic Artery, Percutaneous Approach
04L64CZ Occlusion of Right Colic Artery with Extraluminal Device, Percutaneous Endoscopic Approach
04L64DZ Occlusion of Right Colic Artery with Intraluminal Device, Percutaneous Endoscopic Approach
04L64ZZ Occlusion of Right Colic Artery, Percutaneous Endoscopic Approach
04L70CZ Occlusion of Left Colic Artery with Extraluminal Device, Open Approach
04L70DZ Occlusion of Left Colic Artery with Intraluminal Device, Open Approach
04L70ZZ Occlusion of Left Colic Artery, Open Approach
04L73CZ Occlusion of Left Colic Artery with Extraluminal Device, Percutaneous Approach
04L73DZ Occlusion of Left Colic Artery with Intraluminal Device, Percutaneous Approach
04L73ZZ Occlusion of Left Colic Artery, Percutaneous Approach
04L74CZ Occlusion of Left Colic Artery with Extraluminal Device, Percutaneous Endoscopic Approach
04L74DZ Occlusion of Left Colic Artery with Intraluminal Device, Percutaneous Endoscopic Approach
04L74ZZ Occlusion of Left Colic Artery, Percutaneous Endoscopic Approach
04L80CZ Occlusion of Middle Colic Artery with Extraluminal Device, Open Approach
04L80DZ Occlusion of Middle Colic Artery with Intraluminal Device, Open Approach
04L80ZZ Occlusion of Middle Colic Artery, Open Approach
04L83CZ Occlusion of Middle Colic Artery with Extraluminal Device, Percutaneous Approach
04L83DZ Occlusion of Middle Colic Artery with Intraluminal Device, Percutaneous Approach
04L83ZZ Occlusion of Middle Colic Artery, Percutaneous Approach
04L84CZ Occlusion of Middle Colic Artery with Extraluminal Device, Percutaneous Endoscopic Approach
04L84DZ Occlusion of Middle Colic Artery with Intraluminal Device, Percutaneous Endoscopic Approach
04L84ZZ Occlusion of Middle Colic Artery, Percutaneous Endoscopic Approach
04L90CZ Occlusion of Right Renal Artery with Extraluminal Device, Open Approach
04L90DZ Occlusion of Right Renal Artery with Intraluminal Device, Open Approach
04L90ZZ Occlusion of Right Renal Artery, Open Approach
04L93CZ Occlusion of Right Renal Artery with Extraluminal Device, Percutaneous Approach
04L93DZ Occlusion of Right Renal Artery with Intraluminal Device, Percutaneous Approach
04L93ZZ Occlusion of Right Renal Artery, Percutaneous Approach
04L94CZ Occlusion of Right Renal Artery with Extraluminal Device, Percutaneous Endoscopic Approach
04L94DZ Occlusion of Right Renal Artery with Intraluminal Device, Percutaneous Endoscopic Approach
04L94ZZ Occlusion of Right Renal Artery, Percutaneous Endoscopic Approach
04LA0CZ Occlusion of Left Renal Artery with Extraluminal Device, Open Approach
04LA0DZ Occlusion of Left Renal Artery with Intraluminal Device, Open Approach
04LA0ZZ Occlusion of Left Renal Artery, Open Approach
04LA3CZ Occlusion of Left Renal Artery with Extraluminal Device, Percutaneous Approach
04LA3DZ Occlusion of Left Renal Artery with Intraluminal Device, Percutaneous Approach
04LA3ZZ Occlusion of Left Renal Artery, Percutaneous Approach
04LA4CZ Occlusion of Left Renal Artery with Extraluminal Device, Percutaneous Endoscopic Approach
04LA4DZ Occlusion of Left Renal Artery with Intraluminal Device, Percutaneous Endoscopic Approach
04LA4ZZ Occlusion of Left Renal Artery, Percutaneous Endoscopic Approach
04LB0CZ Occlusion of Inferior Mesenteric Artery with Extraluminal Device, Open Approach
04LB0DZ Occlusion of Inferior Mesenteric Artery with Intraluminal Device, Open Approach
04LB0ZZ Occlusion of Inferior Mesenteric Artery, Open Approach
04LB3CZ Occlusion of Inferior Mesenteric Artery with Extraluminal Device, Percutaneous Approach
04LB3DZ Occlusion of Inferior Mesenteric Artery with Intraluminal Device, Percutaneous Approach
04LB3ZZ Occlusion of Inferior Mesenteric Artery, Percutaneous Approach
04LB4CZ Occlusion of Inferior Mesenteric Artery with Extraluminal Device, Percutaneous Endoscopic Approach
04LB4DZ Occlusion of Inferior Mesenteric Artery with Intraluminal Device, Percutaneous Endoscopic Approach
04LB4ZZ Occlusion of Inferior Mesenteric Artery, Percutaneous Endoscopic Approach
04LC0CZ Occlusion of Right Common Iliac Artery with Extraluminal Device, Open Approach
04LC0DZ Occlusion of Right Common Iliac Artery with Intraluminal Device, Open Approach
04LC0ZZ Occlusion of Right Common Iliac Artery, Open Approach
04LC3CZ Occlusion of Right Common Iliac Artery with Extraluminal Device, Percutaneous Approach
04LC3DZ Occlusion of Right Common Iliac Artery with Intraluminal Device, Percutaneous Approach
04LC3ZZ Occlusion of Right Common Iliac Artery, Percutaneous Approach
04LC4CZ Occlusion of Right Common Iliac Artery with Extraluminal Device, Percutaneous Endoscopic Approach
04LC4DZ Occlusion of Right Common Iliac Artery with Intraluminal Device, Percutaneous Endoscopic Approach
04LC4ZZ Occlusion of Right Common Iliac Artery, Percutaneous Endoscopic Approach
04LD0CZ Occlusion of Left Common Iliac Artery with Extraluminal Device, Open Approach
04LD0DZ Occlusion of Left Common Iliac Artery with Intraluminal Device, Open Approach
04LD0ZZ Occlusion of Left Common Iliac Artery, Open Approach
04LD3CZ Occlusion of Left Common Iliac Artery with Extraluminal Device, Percutaneous Approach
04LD3DZ Occlusion of Left Common Iliac Artery with Intraluminal Device, Percutaneous Approach
04LD3ZZ Occlusion of Left Common Iliac Artery, Percutaneous Approach

04LD4CZ Occlusion of Left Common Iliac Artery with Extraluminal Device, Percutaneous Endoscopic Approach
04LD4DZ Occlusion of Left Common Iliac Artery with Intraluminal Device, Percutaneous Endoscopic Approach
04LD4ZZ Occlusion of Left Common Iliac Artery, Percutaneous Endoscopic Approach
♀ **04LE0CT** Occlusion of Right Uterine Artery with Extraluminal Device, Open Approach
04LE0CZ Occlusion of Right Internal Iliac Artery with Extraluminal Device, Open Approach
♀ **04LE0DT** Occlusion of Right Uterine Artery with Intraluminal Device, Open Approach
04LE0DZ Occlusion of Right Internal Iliac Artery with Intraluminal Device, Open Approach
♀ **04LE0ZT** Occlusion of Right Uterine Artery, Open Approach
04LE0ZZ Occlusion of Right Internal Iliac Artery, Open Approach
♀ **04LE3CT** Occlusion of Right Uterine Artery with Extraluminal Device, Percutaneous Approach
04LE3CZ Occlusion of Right Internal Iliac Artery with Extraluminal Device, Percutaneous Approach
♀ **04LE3DT** Occlusion of Right Uterine Artery with Intraluminal Device, Percutaneous Approach
04LE3DZ Occlusion of Right Internal Iliac Artery with Intraluminal Device, Percutaneous Approach
♀ **04LE3ZT** Occlusion of Right Uterine Artery, Percutaneous Approach
04LE3ZZ Occlusion of Right Internal Iliac Artery, Percutaneous Approach
♀ **04LE4CT** Occlusion of Right Uterine Artery with Extraluminal Device, Percutaneous Endoscopic Approach
04LE4CZ Occlusion of Right Internal Iliac Artery with Extraluminal Device, Percutaneous Endoscopic Approach
♀ **04LE4DT** Occlusion of Right Uterine Artery with Intraluminal Device, Percutaneous Endoscopic Approach
04LE4DZ Occlusion of Right Internal Iliac Artery with Intraluminal Device, Percutaneous Endoscopic Approach
♀ **04LE4ZT** Occlusion of Right Uterine Artery, Percutaneous Endoscopic Approach
04LE4ZZ Occlusion of Right Internal Iliac Artery, Percutaneous Endoscopic Approach
♀ **04LF0CU** Occlusion of Left Uterine Artery with Extraluminal Device, Open Approach
04LF0CZ Occlusion of Left Internal Iliac Artery with Extraluminal Device, Open Approach
♀ **04LF0DU** Occlusion of Left Uterine Artery with Intraluminal Device, Open Approach
04LF0DZ Occlusion of Left Internal Iliac Artery with Intraluminal Device, Open Approach
♀ **04LF0ZU** Occlusion of Left Uterine Artery, Open Approach
04LF0ZZ Occlusion of Left Internal Iliac Artery, Open Approach
♀ **04LF3CU** Occlusion of Left Uterine Artery with Extraluminal Device, Percutaneous Approach
04LF3CZ Occlusion of Left Internal Iliac Artery with Extraluminal Device, Percutaneous Approach
♀ **04LF3DU** Occlusion of Left Uterine Artery with Intraluminal Device, Percutaneous Approach
04LF3DZ Occlusion of Left Internal Iliac Artery with Intraluminal Device, Percutaneous Approach
♀ **04LF3ZU** Occlusion of Left Uterine Artery, Percutaneous Approach
04LF3ZZ Occlusion of Left Internal Iliac Artery, Percutaneous Approach
♀ **04LF4CU** Occlusion of Left Uterine Artery with Extraluminal Device, Percutaneous Endoscopic Approach
04LF4CZ Occlusion of Left Internal Iliac Artery with Extraluminal Device, Percutaneous Endoscopic Approach
♀ **04LF4DU** Occlusion of Left Uterine Artery with Intraluminal Device, Percutaneous Endoscopic Approach
04LF4DZ Occlusion of Left Internal Iliac Artery with Intraluminal Device, Percutaneous Endoscopic Approach
♀ **04LF4ZU** Occlusion of Left Uterine Artery, Percutaneous Endoscopic Approach
04LF4ZZ Occlusion of Left Internal Iliac Artery, Percutaneous Endoscopic Approach
04LH0CZ Occlusion of Right External Iliac Artery with Extraluminal Device, Open Approach
04LH0DZ Occlusion of Right External Iliac Artery with Intraluminal Device, Open Approach
04LH0ZZ Occlusion of Right External Iliac Artery, Open Approach
04LH3CZ Occlusion of Right External Iliac Artery with Extraluminal Device, Percutaneous Approach
04LH3DZ Occlusion of Right External Iliac Artery with Intraluminal Device, Percutaneous Approach
04LH3ZZ Occlusion of Right External Iliac Artery, Percutaneous Approach
04LH4CZ Occlusion of Right External Iliac Artery with Extraluminal Device, Percutaneous Endoscopic Approach
04LH4DZ Occlusion of Right External Iliac Artery with Intraluminal Device, Percutaneous Endoscopic Approach
04LH4ZZ Occlusion of Right External Iliac Artery, Percutaneous Endoscopic Approach
04LJ0CZ Occlusion of Left External Iliac Artery with Extraluminal Device, Open Approach
04LJ0DZ Occlusion of Left External Iliac Artery with Intraluminal Device, Open Approach
04LJ0ZZ Occlusion of Left External Iliac Artery, Open Approach
04LJ3CZ Occlusion of Left External Iliac Artery with Extraluminal Device, Percutaneous Approach
04LJ3DZ Occlusion of Left External Iliac Artery with Intraluminal Device, Percutaneous Approach
04LJ3ZZ Occlusion of Left External Iliac Artery, Percutaneous Approach
04LJ4CZ Occlusion of Left External Iliac Artery with Extraluminal Device, Percutaneous Endoscopic Approach
04LJ4DZ Occlusion of Left External Iliac Artery with Intraluminal Device, Percutaneous Endoscopic Approach
04LJ4ZZ Occlusion of Left External Iliac Artery, Percutaneous Endoscopic Approach
04LK0CZ Occlusion of Right Femoral Artery with Extraluminal Device, Open Approach
04LK0DZ Occlusion of Right Femoral Artery with Intraluminal Device, Open Approach
04LK0ZZ Occlusion of Right Femoral Artery, Open Approach
04LK3CZ Occlusion of Right Femoral Artery with Extraluminal Device, Percutaneous Approach
04LK3DZ Occlusion of Right Femoral Artery with Intraluminal Device, Percutaneous Approach
04LK3ZZ Occlusion of Right Femoral Artery, Percutaneous Approach
04LK4CZ Occlusion of Right Femoral Artery with Extraluminal Device, Percutaneous Endoscopic Approach
04LK4DZ Occlusion of Right Femoral Artery with Intraluminal Device, Percutaneous Endoscopic Approach
04LK4ZZ Occlusion of Right Femoral Artery, Percutaneous Endoscopic Approach
04LL0CZ Occlusion of Left Femoral Artery with Extraluminal Device, Open Approach
04LL0DZ Occlusion of Left Femoral Artery with Intraluminal Device, Open Approach
04LL0ZZ Occlusion of Left Femoral Artery, Open Approach
04LL3CZ Occlusion of Left Femoral Artery with Extraluminal Device, Percutaneous Approach
04LL3DZ Occlusion of Left Femoral Artery with Intraluminal Device, Percutaneous Approach
04LL3ZZ Occlusion of Left Femoral Artery, Percutaneous Approach
04LL4CZ Occlusion of Left Femoral Artery with Extraluminal Device, Percutaneous Endoscopic Approach
04LL4DZ Occlusion of Left Femoral Artery with Intraluminal Device, Percutaneous Endoscopic Approach
04LL4ZZ Occlusion of Left Femoral Artery, Percutaneous Endoscopic Approach
04LM0CZ Occlusion of Right Popliteal Artery with Extraluminal Device, Open Approach
04LM0DZ Occlusion of Right Popliteal Artery with Intraluminal Device, Open Approach
04LM0ZZ Occlusion of Right Popliteal Artery, Open Approach
04LM3CZ Occlusion of Right Popliteal Artery with Extraluminal Device, Percutaneous Approach
04LM3DZ Occlusion of Right Popliteal Artery with Intraluminal Device, Percutaneous Approach
04LM3ZZ Occlusion of Right Popliteal Artery, Percutaneous Approach
04LM4CZ Occlusion of Right Popliteal Artery with Extraluminal Device, Percutaneous Endoscopic Approach
04LM4DZ Occlusion of Right Popliteal Artery with Intraluminal Device, Percutaneous Endoscopic Approach
04LM4ZZ Occlusion of Right Popliteal Artery, Percutaneous Endoscopic Approach
04LN0CZ Occlusion of Left Popliteal Artery with Extraluminal Device, Open Approach
04LN0DZ Occlusion of Left Popliteal Artery with Intraluminal Device, Open Approach
04LN0ZZ Occlusion of Left Popliteal Artery, Open Approach
04LN3CZ Occlusion of Left Popliteal Artery with Extraluminal Device, Percutaneous Approach
04LN3DZ Occlusion of Left Popliteal Artery with Intraluminal Device, Percutaneous Approach
04LN3ZZ Occlusion of Left Popliteal Artery, Percutaneous Approach
04LN4CZ Occlusion of Left Popliteal Artery with Extraluminal Device, Percutaneous Endoscopic Approach
04LN4DZ Occlusion of Left Popliteal Artery with Intraluminal Device, Percutaneous Endoscopic Approach
04LN4ZZ Occlusion of Left Popliteal Artery, Percutaneous Endoscopic Approach
04LP0CZ Occlusion of Right Anterior Tibial Artery with Extraluminal Device, Open Approach
04LP0DZ Occlusion of Right Anterior Tibial Artery with Intraluminal Device, Open Approach

LP0ZZ Occlusion of Right Anterior Tibial Artery, Open Approach
LP3CZ Occlusion of Right Anterior Tibial Artery with Extraluminal Device, Percutaneous Approach
LP3DZ Occlusion of Right Anterior Tibial Artery with Intraluminal Device, Percutaneous Approach
LP3ZZ Occlusion of Right Anterior Tibial Artery, Percutaneous Approach
LP4CZ Occlusion of Right Anterior Tibial Artery with Extraluminal Device, Percutaneous Endoscopic Approach
LP4DZ Occlusion of Right Anterior Tibial Artery with Intraluminal Device, Percutaneous Endoscopic Approach
LP4ZZ Occlusion of Right Anterior Tibial Artery, Percutaneous Endoscopic Approach
LQ0CZ Occlusion of Left Anterior Tibial Artery with Extraluminal Device, Open Approach
LQ0DZ Occlusion of Left Anterior Tibial Artery with Intraluminal Device, Open Approach
LQ0ZZ Occlusion of Left Anterior Tibial Artery, Open Approach
LQ3CZ Occlusion of Left Anterior Tibial Artery with Extraluminal Device, Percutaneous Approach
LQ3DZ Occlusion of Left Anterior Tibial Artery with Intraluminal Device, Percutaneous Approach
LQ3ZZ Occlusion of Left Anterior Tibial Artery, Percutaneous Approach
LQ4CZ Occlusion of Left Anterior Tibial Artery with Extraluminal Device, Percutaneous Endoscopic Approach
LQ4DZ Occlusion of Left Anterior Tibial Artery with Intraluminal Device, Percutaneous Endoscopic Approach
LQ4ZZ Occlusion of Left Anterior Tibial Artery, Percutaneous Endoscopic Approach
LR0CZ Occlusion of Right Posterior Tibial Artery with Extraluminal Device, Open Approach
LR0DZ Occlusion of Right Posterior Tibial Artery with Intraluminal Device, Open Approach
LR0ZZ Occlusion of Right Posterior Tibial Artery, Open Approach
LR3CZ Occlusion of Right Posterior Tibial Artery with Extraluminal Device, Percutaneous Approach
LR3DZ Occlusion of Right Posterior Tibial Artery with Intraluminal Device, Percutaneous Approach
LR3ZZ Occlusion of Right Posterior Tibial Artery, Percutaneous Approach
LR4CZ Occlusion of Right Posterior Tibial Artery with Extraluminal Device, Percutaneous Endoscopic Approach
LR4DZ Occlusion of Right Posterior Tibial Artery with Intraluminal Device, Percutaneous Endoscopic Approach
LR4ZZ Occlusion of Right Posterior Tibial Artery, Percutaneous Endoscopic Approach
LS0CZ Occlusion of Left Posterior Tibial Artery with Extraluminal Device, Open Approach
LS0DZ Occlusion of Left Posterior Tibial Artery with Intraluminal Device, Open Approach
04LS0ZZ Occlusion of Left Posterior Tibial Artery, Open Approach
04LS3CZ Occlusion of Left Posterior Tibial Artery with Extraluminal Device, Percutaneous Approach
04LS3DZ Occlusion of Left Posterior Tibial Artery with Intraluminal Device, Percutaneous Approach
04LS3ZZ Occlusion of Left Posterior Tibial Artery, Percutaneous Approach
04LS4CZ Occlusion of Left Posterior Tibial Artery with Extraluminal Device, Percutaneous Endoscopic Approach
04LS4DZ Occlusion of Left Posterior Tibial Artery with Intraluminal Device, Percutaneous Endoscopic Approach
04LS4ZZ Occlusion of Left Posterior Tibial Artery, Percutaneous Endoscopic Approach
04LT0CZ Occlusion of Right Peroneal Artery with Extraluminal Device, Open Approach
04LT0DZ Occlusion of Right Peroneal Artery with Intraluminal Device, Open Approach
04LT0ZZ Occlusion of Right Peroneal Artery, Open Approach
04LT3CZ Occlusion of Right Peroneal Artery with Extraluminal Device, Percutaneous Approach
04LT3DZ Occlusion of Right Peroneal Artery with Intraluminal Device, Percutaneous Approach
04LT3ZZ Occlusion of Right Peroneal Artery, Percutaneous Approach
04LT4CZ Occlusion of Right Peroneal Artery with Extraluminal Device, Percutaneous Endoscopic Approach
04LT4DZ Occlusion of Right Peroneal Artery with Intraluminal Device, Percutaneous Endoscopic Approach
04LT4ZZ Occlusion of Right Peroneal Artery, Percutaneous Endoscopic Approach
04LU0CZ Occlusion of Left Peroneal Artery with Extraluminal Device, Open Approach
04LU0DZ Occlusion of Left Peroneal Artery with Intraluminal Device, Open Approach
04LU0ZZ Occlusion of Left Peroneal Artery, Open Approach
04LU3CZ Occlusion of Left Peroneal Artery with Extraluminal Device, Percutaneous Approach
04LU3DZ Occlusion of Left Peroneal Artery with Intraluminal Device, Percutaneous Approach
04LU3ZZ Occlusion of Left Peroneal Artery, Percutaneous Approach
04LU4CZ Occlusion of Left Peroneal Artery with Extraluminal Device, Percutaneous Endoscopic Approach
04LU4DZ Occlusion of Left Peroneal Artery with Intraluminal Device, Percutaneous Endoscopic Approach
04LU4ZZ Occlusion of Left Peroneal Artery, Percutaneous Endoscopic Approach
04LV0CZ Occlusion of Right Foot Artery with Extraluminal Device, Open Approach
04LV0DZ Occlusion of Right Foot Artery with Intraluminal Device, Open Approach
04LV0ZZ Occlusion of Right Foot Artery, Open Approach
04LV3CZ Occlusion of Right Foot Artery with Extraluminal Device, Percutaneous Approach
04LV3DZ Occlusion of Right Foot Artery with Intraluminal Device, Percutaneous Approach
04LV3ZZ Occlusion of Right Foot Artery, Percutaneous Approach
04LV4CZ Occlusion of Right Foot Artery with Extraluminal Device, Percutaneous Endoscopic Approach
04LV4DZ Occlusion of Right Foot Artery with Intraluminal Device, Percutaneous Endoscopic Approach
04LV4ZZ Occlusion of Right Foot Artery, Percutaneous Endoscopic Approach
04LW0CZ Occlusion of Left Foot Artery with Extraluminal Device, Open Approach
04LW0DZ Occlusion of Left Foot Artery with Intraluminal Device, Open Approach
04LW0ZZ Occlusion of Left Foot Artery, Open Approach
04LW3CZ Occlusion of Left Foot Artery with Extraluminal Device, Percutaneous Approach
04LW3DZ Occlusion of Left Foot Artery with Intraluminal Device, Percutaneous Approach
04LW3ZZ Occlusion of Left Foot Artery, Percutaneous Approach
04LW4CZ Occlusion of Left Foot Artery with Extraluminal Device, Percutaneous Endoscopic Approach
04LW4DZ Occlusion of Left Foot Artery with Intraluminal Device, Percutaneous Endoscopic Approach
04LW4ZZ Occlusion of Left Foot Artery, Percutaneous Endoscopic Approach
04LY0CZ Occlusion of Lower Artery with Extraluminal Device, Open Approach
04LY0DZ Occlusion of Lower Artery with Intraluminal Device, Open Approach
04LY0ZZ Occlusion of Lower Artery, Open Approach
04LY3CZ Occlusion of Lower Artery with Extraluminal Device, Percutaneous Approach
04LY3DZ Occlusion of Lower Artery with Intraluminal Device, Percutaneous Approach
04LY3ZZ Occlusion of Lower Artery, Percutaneous Approach
04LY4CZ Occlusion of Lower Artery with Extraluminal Device, Percutaneous Endoscopic Approach
04LY4DZ Occlusion of Lower Artery with Intraluminal Device, Percutaneous Endoscopic Approach
04LY4ZZ Occlusion of Lower Artery, Percutaneous Endoscopic Approach

4N – Lower Arteries, Release

eview Coding Guidelines B3.13 and B3.14

4N00ZZ Release Abdominal Aorta, Open Approach
4N03ZZ Release Abdominal Aorta, Percutaneous Approach
4N04ZZ Release Abdominal Aorta, Percutaneous Endoscopic Approach
4N10ZZ Release Celiac Artery, Open Approach
04N13ZZ Release Celiac Artery, Percutaneous Approach
04N14ZZ Release Celiac Artery, Percutaneous Endoscopic Approach
04N20ZZ Release Gastric Artery, Open Approach
04N23ZZ Release Gastric Artery, Percutaneous Approach
04N24ZZ Release Gastric Artery, Percutaneous Endoscopic Approach
04N30ZZ Release Hepatic Artery, Open Approach
04N33ZZ Release Hepatic Artery, Percutaneous Approach
04N34ZZ Release Hepatic Artery, Percutaneous Endoscopic Approach

04N40ZZ Release Splenic Artery, Open Approach
04N43ZZ Release Splenic Artery, Percutaneous Approach
04N44ZZ Release Splenic Artery, Percutaneous Endoscopic Approach
04N50ZZ Release Superior Mesenteric Artery, Open Approach
04N53ZZ Release Superior Mesenteric Artery, Percutaneous Approach
04N54ZZ Release Superior Mesenteric Artery, Percutaneous Endoscopic Approach
04N60ZZ Release Right Colic Artery, Open Approach
04N63ZZ Release Right Colic Artery, Percutaneous Approach
04N64ZZ Release Right Colic Artery, Percutaneous Endoscopic Approach
04N70ZZ Release Left Colic Artery, Open Approach
04N73ZZ Release Left Colic Artery, Percutaneous Approach
04N74ZZ Release Left Colic Artery, Percutaneous Endoscopic Approach
04N80ZZ Release Middle Colic Artery, Open Approach
04N83ZZ Release Middle Colic Artery, Percutaneous Approach
04N84ZZ Release Middle Colic Artery, Percutaneous Endoscopic Approach
04N90ZZ Release Right Renal Artery, Open Approach
04N93ZZ Release Right Renal Artery, Percutaneous Approach
04N94ZZ Release Right Renal Artery, Percutaneous Endoscopic Approach
04NA0ZZ Release Left Renal Artery, Open Approach
04NA3ZZ Release Left Renal Artery, Percutaneous Approach
04NA4ZZ Release Left Renal Artery, Percutaneous Endoscopic Approach
04NB0ZZ Release Inferior Mesenteric Artery, Open Approach
04NB3ZZ Release Inferior Mesenteric Artery, Percutaneous Approach
04NB4ZZ Release Inferior Mesenteric Artery, Percutaneous Endoscopic Approach
04NC0ZZ Release Right Common Iliac Artery, Open Approach
04NC3ZZ Release Right Common Iliac Artery, Percutaneous Approach
04NC4ZZ Release Right Common Iliac Artery, Percutaneous Endoscopic Approach
04ND0ZZ Release Left Common Iliac Artery, Open Approach
04ND3ZZ Release Left Common Iliac Artery, Percutaneous Approach
04ND4ZZ Release Left Common Iliac Artery, Percutaneous Endoscopic Approach
04NE0ZZ Release Right Internal Iliac Artery, Open Approach
04NE3ZZ Release Right Internal Iliac Artery, Percutaneous Approach
04NE4ZZ Release Right Internal Iliac Artery, Percutaneous Endoscopic Approach
04NF0ZZ Release Left Internal Iliac Artery, Open Approach
04NF3ZZ Release Left Internal Iliac Artery, Percutaneous Approach
04NF4ZZ Release Left Internal Iliac Artery, Percutaneous Endoscopic Approach
04NH0ZZ Release Right External Iliac Artery, Open Approach
04NH3ZZ Release Right External Iliac Artery, Percutaneous Approach
04NH4ZZ Release Right External Iliac Artery, Percutaneous Endoscopic Approach
04NJ0ZZ Release Left External Iliac Artery, Open Approach
04NJ3ZZ Release Left External Iliac Artery, Percutaneous Approach
04NJ4ZZ Release Left External Iliac Artery, Percutaneous Endoscopic Approach
04NK0ZZ Release Right Femoral Artery, Open Approach
04NK3ZZ Release Right Femoral Artery, Percutaneous Approach
04NK4ZZ Release Right Femoral Artery, Percutaneous Endoscopic Approach
04NL0ZZ Release Left Femoral Artery, Open Approach
04NL3ZZ Release Left Femoral Artery, Percutaneous Approach
04NL4ZZ Release Left Femoral Artery, Percutaneous Endoscopic Approach
04NM0ZZ Release Right Popliteal Artery, Open Approach
04NM3ZZ Release Right Popliteal Artery, Percutaneous Approach
04NM4ZZ Release Right Popliteal Artery, Percutaneous Endoscopic Approach
04NN0ZZ Release Left Popliteal Artery, Open Approach
04NN3ZZ Release Left Popliteal Artery, Percutaneous Approach
04NN4ZZ Release Left Popliteal Artery, Percutaneous Endoscopic Approach
04NP0ZZ Release Right Anterior Tibial Artery, Open Approach
04NP3ZZ Release Right Anterior Tibial Artery, Percutaneous Approach
04NP4ZZ Release Right Anterior Tibial Artery, Percutaneous Endoscopic Approach
04NQ0ZZ Release Left Anterior Tibial Artery, Open Approach
04NQ3ZZ Release Left Anterior Tibial Artery, Percutaneous Approach
04NQ4ZZ Release Left Anterior Tibial Artery, Percutaneous Endoscopic Approach
04NR0ZZ Release Right Posterior Tibial Artery, Open Approach
04NR3ZZ Release Right Posterior Tibial Artery, Percutaneous Approach
04NR4ZZ Release Right Posterior Tibial Artery, Percutaneous Endoscopic Approach
04NS0ZZ Release Left Posterior Tibial Artery, Open Approach
04NS3ZZ Release Left Posterior Tibial Artery, Percutaneous Approach
04NS4ZZ Release Left Posterior Tibial Artery, Percutaneous Endoscopic Approach
04NT0ZZ Release Right Peroneal Artery, Open Approach
04NT3ZZ Release Right Peroneal Artery, Percutaneous Approach
04NT4ZZ Release Right Peroneal Artery, Percutaneous Endoscopic Approach
04NU0ZZ Release Left Peroneal Artery, Open Approach
04NU3ZZ Release Left Peroneal Artery, Percutaneous Approach
04NU4ZZ Release Left Peroneal Artery, Percutaneous Endoscopic Approach
04NV0ZZ Release Right Foot Artery, Open Approach
04NV3ZZ Release Right Foot Artery, Percutaneous Approach
04NV4ZZ Release Right Foot Artery, Percutaneous Endoscopic Approach
04NW0ZZ Release Left Foot Artery, Open Approach
04NW3ZZ Release Left Foot Artery, Percutaneous Approach
04NW4ZZ Release Left Foot Artery, Percutaneous Endoscopic Approach
04NY0ZZ Release Lower Artery, Open Approach
04NY3ZZ Release Lower Artery, Percutaneous Approach
04NY4ZZ Release Lower Artery, Percutaneous Endoscopic Approach

04P – Lower Arteries, Removal

Review Coding Guideline B6.1c

04PY00Z Removal of Drainage Device from Lower Artery, Open Approach
04PY02Z Removal of Monitoring Device from Lower Artery, Open Approach
04PY03Z Removal of Infusion Device from Lower Artery, Open Approach
04PY07Z Removal of Autologous Tissue Substitute from Lower Artery, Open Approach
04PY0CZ Removal of Extraluminal Device from Lower Artery, Open Approach
04PY0DZ Removal of Intraluminal Device from Lower Artery, Open Approach
04PY0JZ Removal of Synthetic Substitute from Lower Artery, Open Approach
04PY0KZ Removal of Nonautologous Tissue Substitute from Lower Artery, Open Approach
04PY30Z Removal of Drainage Device from Lower Artery, Percutaneous Approach
04PY32Z Removal of Monitoring Device from Lower Artery, Percutaneous Approach
04PY33Z Removal of Infusion Device from Lower Artery, Percutaneous Approach
04PY37Z Removal of Autologous Tissue Substitute from Lower Artery, Percutaneous Approach
04PY3CZ Removal of Extraluminal Device from Lower Artery, Percutaneous Approach
04PY3DZ Removal of Intraluminal Device from Lower Artery, Percutaneous Approach
04PY3JZ Removal of Synthetic Substitute from Lower Artery, Percutaneous Approach
04PY3KZ Removal of Nonautologous Tissue Substitute from Lower Artery, Percutaneous Approach
04PY40Z Removal of Drainage Device from Lower Artery, Percutaneous Endoscopic Approach
04PY42Z Removal of Monitoring Device from Lower Artery, Percutaneous Endoscopic Approach
04PY43Z Removal of Infusion Device from Lower Artery, Percutaneous Endoscopic Approach
04PY47Z Removal of Autologous Tissue Substitute from Lower Artery, Percutaneous Endoscopic Approach
04PY4CZ Removal of Extraluminal Device from Lower Artery, Percutaneous Endoscopic Approach
04PY4DZ Removal of Intraluminal Device from Lower Artery, Percutaneous Endoscopic Approach
04PY4JZ Removal of Synthetic Substitute from Lower Artery, Percutaneous Endoscopic Approach

PY4KZ Removal of Nonautologous Tissue Substitute from Lower Artery, Percutaneous Endoscopic Approach
PYX0Z Removal of Drainage Device from Lower Artery, External Approach
04PYX1Z Removal of Radioactive Element from Lower Artery, External Approach
04PYX2Z Removal of Monitoring Device from Lower Artery, External Approach
04PYX3Z Removal of Infusion Device from Lower Artery, External Approach
04PYXDZ Removal of Intraluminal Device from Lower Artery, External Approach

Q – Lower Arteries, Repair

Q00ZZ Repair Abdominal Aorta, Open Approach
Q03ZZ Repair Abdominal Aorta, Percutaneous Approach
Q04ZZ Repair Abdominal Aorta, Percutaneous Endoscopic Approach
Q10ZZ Repair Celiac Artery, Open Approach
Q13ZZ Repair Celiac Artery, Percutaneous Approach
Q14ZZ Repair Celiac Artery, Percutaneous Endoscopic Approach
Q20ZZ Repair Gastric Artery, Open Approach
Q23ZZ Repair Gastric Artery, Percutaneous Approach
Q24ZZ Repair Gastric Artery, Percutaneous Endoscopic Approach
Q30ZZ Repair Hepatic Artery, Open Approach
Q33ZZ Repair Hepatic Artery, Percutaneous Approach
Q34ZZ Repair Hepatic Artery, Percutaneous Endoscopic Approach
Q40ZZ Repair Splenic Artery, Open Approach
Q43ZZ Repair Splenic Artery, Percutaneous Approach
Q44ZZ Repair Splenic Artery, Percutaneous Endoscopic Approach
Q50ZZ Repair Superior Mesenteric Artery, Open Approach
Q53ZZ Repair Superior Mesenteric Artery, Percutaneous Approach
Q54ZZ Repair Superior Mesenteric Artery, Percutaneous Endoscopic Approach
Q60ZZ Repair Right Colic Artery, Open Approach
Q63ZZ Repair Right Colic Artery, Percutaneous Approach
Q64ZZ Repair Right Colic Artery, Percutaneous Endoscopic Approach
Q70ZZ Repair Left Colic Artery, Open Approach
Q73ZZ Repair Left Colic Artery, Percutaneous Approach
Q74ZZ Repair Left Colic Artery, Percutaneous Endoscopic Approach
4Q80ZZ Repair Middle Colic Artery, Open Approach
4Q83ZZ Repair Middle Colic Artery, Percutaneous Approach
4Q84ZZ Repair Middle Colic Artery, Percutaneous Endoscopic Approach
4Q90ZZ Repair Right Renal Artery, Open Approach
4Q93ZZ Repair Right Renal Artery, Percutaneous Approach
4Q94ZZ Repair Right Renal Artery, Percutaneous Endoscopic Approach
4QA0ZZ Repair Left Renal Artery, Open Approach
4QA3ZZ Repair Left Renal Artery, Percutaneous Approach
4QA4ZZ Repair Left Renal Artery, Percutaneous Endoscopic Approach
04QB0ZZ Repair Inferior Mesenteric Artery, Open Approach
04QB3ZZ Repair Inferior Mesenteric Artery, Percutaneous Approach
04QB4ZZ Repair Inferior Mesenteric Artery, Percutaneous Endoscopic Approach
04QC0ZZ Repair Right Common Iliac Artery, Open Approach
04QC3ZZ Repair Right Common Iliac Artery, Percutaneous Approach
04QC4ZZ Repair Right Common Iliac Artery, Percutaneous Endoscopic Approach
04QD0ZZ Repair Left Common Iliac Artery, Open Approach
04QD3ZZ Repair Left Common Iliac Artery, Percutaneous Approach
04QD4ZZ Repair Left Common Iliac Artery, Percutaneous Endoscopic Approach
04QE0ZZ Repair Right Internal Iliac Artery, Open Approach
04QE3ZZ Repair Right Internal Iliac Artery, Percutaneous Approach
04QE4ZZ Repair Right Internal Iliac Artery, Percutaneous Endoscopic Approach
04QF0ZZ Repair Left Internal Iliac Artery, Open Approach
04QF3ZZ Repair Left Internal Iliac Artery, Percutaneous Approach
04QF4ZZ Repair Left Internal Iliac Artery, Percutaneous Endoscopic Approach
04QH0ZZ Repair Right External Iliac Artery, Open Approach
04QH3ZZ Repair Right External Iliac Artery, Percutaneous Approach
04QH4ZZ Repair Right External Iliac Artery, Percutaneous Endoscopic Approach
04QJ0ZZ Repair Left External Iliac Artery, Open Approach
04QJ3ZZ Repair Left External Iliac Artery, Percutaneous Approach
04QJ4ZZ Repair Left External Iliac Artery, Percutaneous Endoscopic Approach
04QK0ZZ Repair Right Femoral Artery, Open Approach
04QK3ZZ Repair Right Femoral Artery, Percutaneous Approach
04QK4ZZ Repair Right Femoral Artery, Percutaneous Endoscopic Approach
04QL0ZZ Repair Left Femoral Artery, Open Approach
04QL3ZZ Repair Left Femoral Artery, Percutaneous Approach
04QL4ZZ Repair Left Femoral Artery, Percutaneous Endoscopic Approach
04QM0ZZ Repair Right Popliteal Artery, Open Approach
04QM3ZZ Repair Right Popliteal Artery, Percutaneous Approach
04QM4ZZ Repair Right Popliteal Artery, Percutaneous Endoscopic Approach
04QN0ZZ Repair Left Popliteal Artery, Open Approach
04QN3ZZ Repair Left Popliteal Artery, Percutaneous Approach
04QN4ZZ Repair Left Popliteal Artery, Percutaneous Endoscopic Approach
04QP0ZZ Repair Right Anterior Tibial Artery, Open Approach
04QP3ZZ Repair Right Anterior Tibial Artery, Percutaneous Approach
04QP4ZZ Repair Right Anterior Tibial Artery, Percutaneous Endoscopic Approach
04QQ0ZZ Repair Left Anterior Tibial Artery, Open Approach
04QQ3ZZ Repair Left Anterior Tibial Artery, Percutaneous Approach
04QQ4ZZ Repair Left Anterior Tibial Artery, Percutaneous Endoscopic Approach
04QR0ZZ Repair Right Posterior Tibial Artery, Open Approach
04QR3ZZ Repair Right Posterior Tibial Artery, Percutaneous Approach
04QR4ZZ Repair Right Posterior Tibial Artery, Percutaneous Endoscopic Approach
04QS0ZZ Repair Left Posterior Tibial Artery, Open Approach
04QS3ZZ Repair Left Posterior Tibial Artery, Percutaneous Approach
04QS4ZZ Repair Left Posterior Tibial Artery, Percutaneous Endoscopic Approach
04QT0ZZ Repair Right Peroneal Artery, Open Approach
04QT3ZZ Repair Right Peroneal Artery, Percutaneous Approach
04QT4ZZ Repair Right Peroneal Artery, Percutaneous Endoscopic Approach
04QU0ZZ Repair Left Peroneal Artery, Open Approach
04QU3ZZ Repair Left Peroneal Artery, Percutaneous Approach
04QU4ZZ Repair Left Peroneal Artery, Percutaneous Endoscopic Approach
04QV0ZZ Repair Right Foot Artery, Open Approach
04QV3ZZ Repair Right Foot Artery, Percutaneous Approach
04QV4ZZ Repair Right Foot Artery, Percutaneous Endoscopic Approach
04QW0ZZ Repair Left Foot Artery, Open Approach
04QW3ZZ Repair Left Foot Artery, Percutaneous Approach
04QW4ZZ Repair Left Foot Artery, Percutaneous Endoscopic Approach
04QY0ZZ Repair Lower Artery, Open Approach
04QY3ZZ Repair Lower Artery, Percutaneous Approach
04QY4ZZ Repair Lower Artery, Percutaneous Endoscopic Approach

4R – Lower Arteries, Replacement

4R007Z Replacement of Abdominal Aorta with Autologous Tissue Substitute, Open Approach
4R00JZ Replacement of Abdominal Aorta with Synthetic Substitute, Open Approach
4R00KZ Replacement of Abdominal Aorta with Nonautologous Tissue Substitute, Open Approach
04R047Z Replacement of Abdominal Aorta with Autologous Tissue Substitute, Percutaneous Endoscopic Approach
04R04JZ Replacement of Abdominal Aorta with Synthetic Substitute, Percutaneous Endoscopic Approach
04R04KZ Replacement of Abdominal Aorta with Nonautologous Tissue Substitute, Percutaneous Endoscopic Approach
04R107Z Replacement of Celiac Artery with Autologous Tissue Substitute, Open Approach
04R10JZ Replacement of Celiac Artery with Synthetic Substitute, Open Approach

04R10KZ Replacement of Celiac Artery with Nonautologous Tissue Substitute, Open Approach
04R147Z Replacement of Celiac Artery with Autologous Tissue Substitute, Percutaneous Endoscopic Approach
04R14JZ Replacement of Celiac Artery with Synthetic Substitute, Percutaneous Endoscopic Approach
04R14KZ Replacement of Celiac Artery with Nonautologous Tissue Substitute, Percutaneous Endoscopic Approach
04R207Z Replacement of Gastric Artery with Autologous Tissue Substitute, Open Approach
04R20JZ Replacement of Gastric Artery with Synthetic Substitute, Open Approach
04R20KZ Replacement of Gastric Artery with Nonautologous Tissue Substitute, Open Approach
04R247Z Replacement of Gastric Artery with Autologous Tissue Substitute, Percutaneous Endoscopic Approach
04R24JZ Replacement of Gastric Artery with Synthetic Substitute, Percutaneous Endoscopic Approach
04R24KZ Replacement of Gastric Artery with Nonautologous Tissue Substitute, Percutaneous Endoscopic Approach
04R307Z Replacement of Hepatic Artery with Autologous Tissue Substitute, Open Approach
04R30JZ Replacement of Hepatic Artery with Synthetic Substitute, Open Approach
04R30KZ Replacement of Hepatic Artery with Nonautologous Tissue Substitute, Open Approach
04R347Z Replacement of Hepatic Artery with Autologous Tissue Substitute, Percutaneous Endoscopic Approach
04R34JZ Replacement of Hepatic Artery with Synthetic Substitute, Percutaneous Endoscopic Approach
04R34KZ Replacement of Hepatic Artery with Nonautologous Tissue Substitute, Percutaneous Endoscopic Approach
04R407Z Replacement of Splenic Artery with Autologous Tissue Substitute, Open Approach
04R40JZ Replacement of Splenic Artery with Synthetic Substitute, Open Approach
04R40KZ Replacement of Splenic Artery with Nonautologous Tissue Substitute, Open Approach
04R447Z Replacement of Splenic Artery with Autologous Tissue Substitute, Percutaneous Endoscopic Approach
04R44JZ Replacement of Splenic Artery with Synthetic Substitute, Percutaneous Endoscopic Approach
04R44KZ Replacement of Splenic Artery with Nonautologous Tissue Substitute, Percutaneous Endoscopic Approach
04R507Z Replacement of Superior Mesenteric Artery with Autologous Tissue Substitute, Open Approach
04R50JZ Replacement of Superior Mesenteric Artery with Synthetic Substitute, Open Approach
04R50KZ Replacement of Superior Mesenteric Artery with Nonautologous Tissue Substitute, Open Approach
04R547Z Replacement of Superior Mesenteric Artery with Autologous Tissue Substitute, Percutaneous Endoscopic Approach
04R54JZ Replacement of Superior Mesenteric Artery with Synthetic Substitute, Percutaneous Endoscopic Approach
04R54KZ Replacement of Superior Mesenteric Artery with Nonautologous Tissue Substitute, Percutaneous Endoscopic Approach
04R607Z Replacement of Right Colic Artery with Autologous Tissue Substitute, Open Approach
04R60JZ Replacement of Right Colic Artery with Synthetic Substitute, Open Approach
04R60KZ Replacement of Right Colic Artery with Nonautologous Tissue Substitute, Open Approach
04R647Z Replacement of Right Colic Artery with Autologous Tissue Substitute, Percutaneous Endoscopic Approach
04R64JZ Replacement of Right Colic Artery with Synthetic Substitute, Percutaneous Endoscopic Approach
04R64KZ Replacement of Right Colic Artery with Nonautologous Tissue Substitute, Percutaneous Endoscopic Approach
04R707Z Replacement of Left Colic Artery with Autologous Tissue Substitute, Open Approach
04R70JZ Replacement of Left Colic Artery with Synthetic Substitute, Open Approach
04R70KZ Replacement of Left Colic Artery with Nonautologous Tissue Substitute, Open Approach
04R747Z Replacement of Left Colic Artery with Autologous Tissue Substitute, Percutaneous Endoscopic Approach
04R74JZ Replacement of Left Colic Artery with Synthetic Substitute, Percutaneous Endoscopic Approach
04R74KZ Replacement of Left Colic Artery with Nonautologous Tissue Substitute, Percutaneous Endoscopic Approach
04R807Z Replacement of Middle Colic Artery with Autologous Tissue Substitute, Open Approach
04R80JZ Replacement of Middle Colic Artery with Synthetic Substitute, Open Approach
04R80KZ Replacement of Middle Colic Artery with Nonautologous Tissue Substitute, Open Approach
04R847Z Replacement of Middle Colic Artery with Autologous Tissue Substitute, Percutaneous Endoscopic Approach
04R84JZ Replacement of Middle Colic Artery with Synthetic Substitute, Percutaneous Endoscopic Approach
04R84KZ Replacement of Middle Colic Artery with Nonautologous Tissue Substitute, Percutaneous Endoscopic Approach
04R907Z Replacement of Right Renal Artery with Autologous Tissue Substitute, Open Approach
04R90JZ Replacement of Right Renal Artery with Synthetic Substitute, Open Approach
04R90KZ Replacement of Right Renal Artery with Nonautologous Tissue Substitute, Open Approach
04R947Z Replacement of Right Renal Artery with Autologous Tissue Substitute, Percutaneous Endoscopic Approach
04R94JZ Replacement of Right Renal Artery with Synthetic Substitute, Percutaneous Endoscopic Approach
04R94KZ Replacement of Right Renal Artery with Nonautologous Tissue Substitute, Percutaneous Endoscopic Approach
04RA07Z Replacement of Left Renal Artery with Autologous Tissue Substitute, Open Approach
04RA0JZ Replacement of Left Renal Artery with Synthetic Substitute, Open Approach
04RA0KZ Replacement of Left Renal Artery with Nonautologous Tissue Substitute, Open Approach
04RA47Z Replacement of Left Renal Artery with Autologous Tissue Substitute, Percutaneous Endoscopic Approach
04RA4JZ Replacement of Left Renal Artery with Synthetic Substitute, Percutaneous Endoscopic Approach
04RA4KZ Replacement of Left Renal Artery with Nonautologous Tissue Substitute, Percutaneous Endoscopic Approach
04RB07Z Replacement of Inferior Mesenteric Arte with Autologous Tissue Substitute, Open Approach
04RB0JZ Replacement of Inferior Mesenteric Arte with Synthetic Substitute, Open Approac
04RB0KZ Replacement of Inferior Mesenteric Arte with Nonautologous Tissue Substitute, Open Approach
04RB47Z Replacement of Inferior Mesenteric Artery with Autologous Tissue Substitute Percutaneous Endoscopic Approach
04RB4JZ Replacement of Inferior Mesenteric Arte with Synthetic Substitute, Percutaneous Endoscopic Approach
04RB4KZ Replacement of Inferior Mesenteric Arter with Nonautologous Tissue Substitute, Percutaneous Endoscopic Approach
04RC07Z Replacement of Right Common Iliac Artery with Autologous Tissue Substitute Open Approach
04RC0JZ Replacement of Right Common Iliac Artery with Synthetic Substitute, Open Approach
04RC0KZ Replacement of Right Common Iliac Artery with Nonautologous Tissue Substitute, Open Approach
04RC47Z Replacement of Right Common Iliac Artery with Autologous Tissue Substitute Percutaneous Endoscopic Approach
04RC4JZ Replacement of Right Common Iliac Artery with Synthetic Substitute, Percutaneous Endoscopic Approach
04RC4KZ Replacement of Right Common Iliac Artery with Nonautologous Tissue Substitute, Percutaneous Endoscopic Approach
04RD07Z Replacement of Left Common Iliac Arter with Autologous Tissue Substitute, Open Approach
04RD0JZ Replacement of Left Common Iliac Artery with Synthetic Substitute, Open Approach
04RD0KZ Replacement of Left Common Iliac Artery with Nonautologous Tissue Substitute, Open Approach
04RD47Z Replacement of Left Common Iliac Artery with Autologous Tissue Substitute Percutaneous Endoscopic Approach
04RD4JZ Replacement of Left Common Iliac Artery with Synthetic Substitute, Percutaneous Endoscopic Approach
04RD4KZ Replacement of Left Common Iliac Artery with Nonautologous Tissue Substitute, Percutaneous Endoscopic Approach
04RE07Z Replacement of Right Internal Iliac Artery with Autologous Tissue Substitute, Open Approach
04RE0JZ Replacement of Right Internal Iliac Artery with Synthetic Substitute, Open Approach
04RE0KZ Replacement of Right Internal Iliac Artery with Nonautologous Tissue Substitute, Open Approach
04RE47Z Replacement of Right Internal Iliac Artery with Autologous Tissue Substitute, Percutaneous Endoscopic Approach

RE4JZ Replacement of Right Internal Iliac Artery with Synthetic Substitute, Percutaneous Endoscopic Approach
RE4KZ Replacement of Right Internal Iliac Artery with Nonautologous Tissue Substitute, Percutaneous Endoscopic Approach
RF07Z Replacement of Left Internal Iliac Artery with Autologous Tissue Substitute, Open Approach
RF0JZ Replacement of Left Internal Iliac Artery with Synthetic Substitute, Open Approach
RF0KZ Replacement of Left Internal Iliac Artery with Nonautologous Tissue Substitute, Open Approach
RF47Z Replacement of Left Internal Iliac Artery with Autologous Tissue Substitute, Percutaneous Endoscopic Approach
RF4JZ Replacement of Left Internal Iliac Artery with Synthetic Substitute, Percutaneous Endoscopic Approach
RF4KZ Replacement of Left Internal Iliac Artery with Nonautologous Tissue Substitute, Percutaneous Endoscopic Approach
RH07Z Replacement of Right External Iliac Artery with Autologous Tissue Substitute, Open Approach
RH0JZ Replacement of Right External Iliac Artery with Synthetic Substitute, Open Approach
RH0KZ Replacement of Right External Iliac Artery with Nonautologous Tissue Substitute, Open Approach
RH47Z Replacement of Right External Iliac Artery with Autologous Tissue Substitute, Percutaneous Endoscopic Approach
RH4JZ Replacement of Right External Iliac Artery with Synthetic Substitute, Percutaneous Endoscopic Approach
RH4KZ Replacement of Right External Iliac Artery with Nonautologous Tissue Substitute, Percutaneous Endoscopic Approach
RJ07Z Replacement of Left External Iliac Artery with Autologous Tissue Substitute, Open Approach
RJ0JZ Replacement of Left External Iliac Artery with Synthetic Substitute, Open Approach
4RJ0KZ Replacement of Left External Iliac Artery with Nonautologous Tissue Substitute, Open Approach
4RJ47Z Replacement of Left External Iliac Artery with Autologous Tissue Substitute, Percutaneous Endoscopic Approach
4RJ4JZ Replacement of Left External Iliac Artery with Synthetic Substitute, Percutaneous Endoscopic Approach
4RJ4KZ Replacement of Left External Iliac Artery with Nonautologous Tissue Substitute, Percutaneous Endoscopic Approach
4RK07Z Replacement of Right Femoral Artery with Autologous Tissue Substitute, Open Approach
4RK0JZ Replacement of Right Femoral Artery with Synthetic Substitute, Open Approach
4RK0KZ Replacement of Right Femoral Artery with Nonautologous Tissue Substitute, Open Approach
4RK47Z Replacement of Right Femoral Artery with Autologous Tissue Substitute, Percutaneous Endoscopic Approach
4RK4JZ Replacement of Right Femoral Artery with Synthetic Substitute, Percutaneous Endoscopic Approach
4RK4KZ Replacement of Right Femoral Artery with Nonautologous Tissue Substitute, Percutaneous Endoscopic Approach
4RL07Z Replacement of Left Femoral Artery with Autologous Tissue Substitute, Open Approach
04RL0JZ Replacement of Left Femoral Artery with Synthetic Substitute, Open Approach
04RL0KZ Replacement of Left Femoral Artery with Nonautologous Tissue Substitute, Open Approach
04RL47Z Replacement of Left Femoral Artery with Autologous Tissue Substitute, Percutaneous Endoscopic Approach
04RL4JZ Replacement of Left Femoral Artery with Synthetic Substitute, Percutaneous Endoscopic Approach
04RL4KZ Replacement of Left Femoral Artery with Nonautologous Tissue Substitute, Percutaneous Endoscopic Approach
04RM07Z Replacement of Right Popliteal Artery with Autologous Tissue Substitute, Open Approach
04RM0JZ Replacement of Right Popliteal Artery with Synthetic Substitute, Open Approach
04RM0KZ Replacement of Right Popliteal Artery with Nonautologous Tissue Substitute, Open Approach
04RM47Z Replacement of Right Popliteal Artery with Autologous Tissue Substitute, Percutaneous Endoscopic Approach
04RM4JZ Replacement of Right Popliteal Artery with Synthetic Substitute, Percutaneous Endoscopic Approach
04RM4KZ Replacement of Right Popliteal Artery with Nonautologous Tissue Substitute, Percutaneous Endoscopic Approach
04RN07Z Replacement of Left Popliteal Artery with Autologous Tissue Substitute, Open Approach
04RN0JZ Replacement of Left Popliteal Artery with Synthetic Substitute, Open Approach
04RN0KZ Replacement of Left Popliteal Artery with Nonautologous Tissue Substitute, Open Approach
04RN47Z Replacement of Left Popliteal Artery with Autologous Tissue Substitute, Percutaneous Endoscopic Approach
04RN4JZ Replacement of Left Popliteal Artery with Synthetic Substitute, Percutaneous Endoscopic Approach
04RN4KZ Replacement of Left Popliteal Artery with Nonautologous Tissue Substitute, Percutaneous Endoscopic Approach
04RP07Z Replacement of Right Anterior Tibial Artery with Autologous Tissue Substitute, Open Approach
04RP0JZ Replacement of Right Anterior Tibial Artery with Synthetic Substitute, Open Approach
04RP0KZ Replacement of Right Anterior Tibial Artery with Nonautologous Tissue Substitute, Open Approach
04RP47Z Replacement of Right Anterior Tibial Artery with Autologous Tissue Substitute, Percutaneous Endoscopic Approach
04RP4JZ Replacement of Right Anterior Tibial Artery with Synthetic Substitute, Percutaneous Endoscopic Approach
04RP4KZ Replacement of Right Anterior Tibial Artery with Nonautologous Tissue Substitute, Percutaneous Endoscopic Approach
04RQ07Z Replacement of Left Anterior Tibial Artery with Autologous Tissue Substitute, Open Approach
04RQ0JZ Replacement of Left Anterior Tibial Artery with Synthetic Substitute, Open Approach
04RQ0KZ Replacement of Left Anterior Tibial Artery with Nonautologous Tissue Substitute, Open Approach
04RQ47Z Replacement of Left Anterior Tibial Artery with Autologous Tissue Substitute, Percutaneous Endoscopic Approach
04RQ4JZ Replacement of Left Anterior Tibial Artery with Synthetic Substitute, Percutaneous Endoscopic Approach
04RQ4KZ Replacement of Left Anterior Tibial Artery with Nonautologous Tissue Substitute, Percutaneous Endoscopic Approach
04RR07Z Replacement of Right Posterior Tibial Artery with Autologous Tissue Substitute, Open Approach
04RR0JZ Replacement of Right Posterior Tibial Artery with Synthetic Substitute, Open Approach
04RR0KZ Replacement of Right Posterior Tibial Artery with Nonautologous Tissue Substitute, Open Approach
04RR47Z Replacement of Right Posterior Tibial Artery with Autologous Tissue Substitute, Percutaneous Endoscopic Approach
04RR4JZ Replacement of Right Posterior Tibial Artery with Synthetic Substitute, Percutaneous Endoscopic Approach
04RR4KZ Replacement of Right Posterior Tibial Artery with Nonautologous Tissue Substitute, Percutaneous Endoscopic Approach
04RS07Z Replacement of Left Posterior Tibial Artery with Autologous Tissue Substitute, Open Approach
04RS0JZ Replacement of Left Posterior Tibial Artery with Synthetic Substitute, Open Approach
04RS0KZ Replacement of Left Posterior Tibial Artery with Nonautologous Tissue Substitute, Open Approach
04RS47Z Replacement of Left Posterior Tibial Artery with Autologous Tissue Substitute, Percutaneous Endoscopic Approach
04RS4JZ Replacement of Left Posterior Tibial Artery with Synthetic Substitute, Percutaneous Endoscopic Approach
04RS4KZ Replacement of Left Posterior Tibial Artery with Nonautologous Tissue Substitute, Percutaneous Endoscopic Approach
04RT07Z Replacement of Right Peroneal Artery with Autologous Tissue Substitute, Open Approach
04RT0JZ Replacement of Right Peroneal Artery with Synthetic Substitute, Open Approach
04RT0KZ Replacement of Right Peroneal Artery with Nonautologous Tissue Substitute, Open Approach
04RT47Z Replacement of Right Peroneal Artery with Autologous Tissue Substitute, Percutaneous Endoscopic Approach
04RT4JZ Replacement of Right Peroneal Artery with Synthetic Substitute, Percutaneous Endoscopic Approach
04RT4KZ Replacement of Right Peroneal Artery with Nonautologous Tissue Substitute, Percutaneous Endoscopic Approach
04RU07Z Replacement of Left Peroneal Artery with Autologous Tissue Substitute, Open Approach
04RU0JZ Replacement of Left Peroneal Artery with Synthetic Substitute, Open Approach
04RU0KZ Replacement of Left Peroneal Artery with Nonautologous Tissue Substitute, Open Approach
04RU47Z Replacement of Left Peroneal Artery with Autologous Tissue Substitute, Percutaneous Endoscopic Approach
04RU4JZ Replacement of Left Peroneal Artery with Synthetic Substitute, Percutaneous Endoscopic Approach
04RU4KZ Replacement of Left Peroneal Artery with Nonautologous Tissue Substitute, Percutaneous Endoscopic Approach

04RV07Z Replacement of Right Foot Artery with Autologous Tissue Substitute, Open Approach
04RV0JZ Replacement of Right Foot Artery with Synthetic Substitute, Open Approach
04RV0KZ Replacement of Right Foot Artery with Nonautologous Tissue Substitute, Open Approach
04RV47Z Replacement of Right Foot Artery with Autologous Tissue Substitute, Percutaneous Endoscopic Approach
04RV4JZ Replacement of Right Foot Artery with Synthetic Substitute, Percutaneous Endoscopic Approach
04RV4KZ Replacement of Right Foot Artery with Nonautologous Tissue Substitute, Percutaneous Endoscopic Approach
04RW07Z Replacement of Left Foot Artery with Autologous Tissue Substitute, Open Approach
04RW0JZ Replacement of Left Foot Artery with Synthetic Substitute, Open Approach
04RW0KZ Replacement of Left Foot Artery with Nonautologous Tissue Substitute, Open Approach
04RW47Z Replacement of Left Foot Artery with Autologous Tissue Substitute, Percutaneous Endoscopic Approach
04RW4JZ Replacement of Left Foot Artery with Synthetic Substitute, Percutaneous Endoscopic Approach
04RW4KZ Replacement of Left Foot Artery with Nonautologous Tissue Substitute, Percutaneous Endoscopic Approach
04RY07Z Replacement of Lower Artery with Autologous Tissue Substitute, Open Approach
04RY0JZ Replacement of Lower Artery with Synthetic Substitute, Open Approach
04RY0KZ Replacement of Lower Artery with Nonautologous Tissue Substitute, Open Approach
04RY47Z Replacement of Lower Artery with Autologous Tissue Substitute, Percutaneous Endoscopic Approach
04RY4JZ Replacement of Lower Artery with Synthetic Substitute, Percutaneous Endoscopic Approach
04RY4KZ Replacement of Lower Artery with Nonautologous Tissue Substitute, Percutaneous Endoscopic Approach

04S – Lower Arteries, Reposition

04S00ZZ Reposition Abdominal Aorta, Open Approach
04S03ZZ Reposition Abdominal Aorta, Percutaneous Approach
04S04ZZ Reposition Abdominal Aorta, Percutaneous Endoscopic Approach
04S10ZZ Reposition Celiac Artery, Open Approach
04S13ZZ Reposition Celiac Artery, Percutaneous Approach
04S14ZZ Reposition Celiac Artery, Percutaneous Endoscopic Approach
04S20ZZ Reposition Gastric Artery, Open Approach
04S23ZZ Reposition Gastric Artery, Percutaneous Approach
04S24ZZ Reposition Gastric Artery, Percutaneous Endoscopic Approach
04S30ZZ Reposition Hepatic Artery, Open Approach
04S33ZZ Reposition Hepatic Artery, Percutaneous Approach
04S34ZZ Reposition Hepatic Artery, Percutaneous Endoscopic Approach
04S40ZZ Reposition Splenic Artery, Open Approach
04S43ZZ Reposition Splenic Artery, Percutaneous Approach
04S44ZZ Reposition Splenic Artery, Percutaneous Endoscopic Approach
04S50ZZ Reposition Superior Mesenteric Artery, Open Approach
04S53ZZ Reposition Superior Mesenteric Artery, Percutaneous Approach
04S54ZZ Reposition Superior Mesenteric Artery, Percutaneous Endoscopic Approach
04S60ZZ Reposition Right Colic Artery, Open Approach
04S63ZZ Reposition Right Colic Artery, Percutaneous Approach
04S64ZZ Reposition Right Colic Artery, Percutaneous Endoscopic Approach
04S70ZZ Reposition Left Colic Artery, Open Approach
04S73ZZ Reposition Left Colic Artery, Percutaneous Approach
04S74ZZ Reposition Left Colic Artery, Percutaneous Endoscopic Approach
04S80ZZ Reposition Middle Colic Artery, Open Approach
04S83ZZ Reposition Middle Colic Artery, Percutaneous Approach
04S84ZZ Reposition Middle Colic Artery, Percutaneous Endoscopic Approach
04S90ZZ Reposition Right Renal Artery, Open Approach
04S93ZZ Reposition Right Renal Artery, Percutaneous Approach
04S94ZZ Reposition Right Renal Artery, Percutaneous Endoscopic Approach
04SA0ZZ Reposition Left Renal Artery, Open Approach
04SA3ZZ Reposition Left Renal Artery, Percutaneous Approach
04SA4ZZ Reposition Left Renal Artery, Percutaneous Endoscopic Approach
04SB0ZZ Reposition Inferior Mesenteric Artery, Open Approach
04SB3ZZ Reposition Inferior Mesenteric Artery, Percutaneous Approach
04SB4ZZ Reposition Inferior Mesenteric Artery, Percutaneous Endoscopic Approach
04SC0ZZ Reposition Right Common Iliac Artery, Open Approach
04SC3ZZ Reposition Right Common Iliac Artery, Percutaneous Approach
04SC4ZZ Reposition Right Common Iliac Artery, Percutaneous Endoscopic Approach
04SD0ZZ Reposition Left Common Iliac Artery, Open Approach
04SD3ZZ Reposition Left Common Iliac Artery, Percutaneous Approach
04SD4ZZ Reposition Left Common Iliac Artery, Percutaneous Endoscopic Approach
04SE0ZZ Reposition Right Internal Iliac Artery, Open Approach
04SE3ZZ Reposition Right Internal Iliac Artery, Percutaneous Approach
04SE4ZZ Reposition Right Internal Iliac Artery, Percutaneous Endoscopic Approach
04SF0ZZ Reposition Left Internal Iliac Artery, Open Approach
04SF3ZZ Reposition Left Internal Iliac Artery, Percutaneous Approach
04SF4ZZ Reposition Left Internal Iliac Artery, Percutaneous Endoscopic Approach
04SH0ZZ Reposition Right External Iliac Artery, Open Approach
04SH3ZZ Reposition Right External Iliac Artery, Percutaneous Approach
04SH4ZZ Reposition Right External Iliac Artery, Percutaneous Endoscopic Approach
04SJ0ZZ Reposition Left External Iliac Artery, Open Approach
04SJ3ZZ Reposition Left External Iliac Artery, Percutaneous Approach
04SJ4ZZ Reposition Left External Iliac Artery, Percutaneous Endoscopic Approach
04SK0ZZ Reposition Right Femoral Artery, Open Approach
04SK3ZZ Reposition Right Femoral Artery, Percutaneous Approach
04SK4ZZ Reposition Right Femoral Artery, Percutaneous Endoscopic Approach
04SL0ZZ Reposition Left Femoral Artery, Open Approach
04SL3ZZ Reposition Left Femoral Artery, Percutaneous Approach
04SL4ZZ Reposition Left Femoral Artery, Percutaneous Endoscopic Approach
04SM0ZZ Reposition Right Popliteal Artery, Open Approach
04SM3ZZ Reposition Right Popliteal Artery, Percutaneous Approach
04SM4ZZ Reposition Right Popliteal Artery, Percutaneous Endoscopic Approach
04SN0ZZ Reposition Left Popliteal Artery, Open Approach
04SN3ZZ Reposition Left Popliteal Artery, Percutaneous Approach
04SN4ZZ Reposition Left Popliteal Artery, Percutaneous Endoscopic Approach
04SP0ZZ Reposition Right Anterior Tibial Artery, Open Approach
04SP3ZZ Reposition Right Anterior Tibial Artery, Percutaneous Approach
04SP4ZZ Reposition Right Anterior Tibial Artery, Percutaneous Endoscopic Approach
04SQ0ZZ Reposition Left Anterior Tibial Artery, Open Approach
04SQ3ZZ Reposition Left Anterior Tibial Artery, Percutaneous Approach
04SQ4ZZ Reposition Left Anterior Tibial Artery, Percutaneous Endoscopic Approach
04SR0ZZ Reposition Right Posterior Tibial Artery, Open Approach
04SR3ZZ Reposition Right Posterior Tibial Artery, Percutaneous Approach
04SR4ZZ Reposition Right Posterior Tibial Artery, Percutaneous Endoscopic Approach
04SS0ZZ Reposition Left Posterior Tibial Artery, Open Approach
04SS3ZZ Reposition Left Posterior Tibial Artery, Percutaneous Approach
04SS4ZZ Reposition Left Posterior Tibial Artery, Percutaneous Endoscopic Approach
04ST0ZZ Reposition Right Peroneal Artery, Open Approach
04ST3ZZ Reposition Right Peroneal Artery, Percutaneous Approach
04ST4ZZ Reposition Right Peroneal Artery, Percutaneous Endoscopic Approach
04SU0ZZ Reposition Left Peroneal Artery, Open Approach
04SU3ZZ Reposition Left Peroneal Artery, Percutaneous Approach
04SU4ZZ Reposition Left Peroneal Artery, Percutaneous Endoscopic Approach
04SV0ZZ Reposition Right Foot Artery, Open Approach
04SV3ZZ Reposition Right Foot Artery, Percutaneous Approach
04SV4ZZ Reposition Right Foot Artery, Percutaneous Endoscopic Approach
04SW0ZZ Reposition Left Foot Artery, Open Approach
04SW3ZZ Reposition Left Foot Artery, Percutaneous Approach

SW4ZZ Reposition Left Foot Artery, Percutaneous Endoscopic Approach
SY0ZZ Reposition Lower Artery, Open Approach
04SY3ZZ Reposition Lower Artery, Percutaneous Approach
04SY4ZZ Reposition Lower Artery, Percutaneous Endoscopic Approach

4U – Lower Arteries, Supplement

U007Z Supplement Abdominal Aorta with Autologous Tissue Substitute, Open Approach
U00JZ Supplement Abdominal Aorta with Synthetic Substitute, Open Approach
U00KZ Supplement Abdominal Aorta with Nonautologous Tissue Substitute, Open Approach
U037Z Supplement Abdominal Aorta with Autologous Tissue Substitute, Percutaneous Approach
U03JZ Supplement Abdominal Aorta with Synthetic Substitute, Percutaneous Approach
4U03KZ Supplement Abdominal Aorta with Nonautologous Tissue Substitute, Percutaneous Approach
4U047Z Supplement Abdominal Aorta with Autologous Tissue Substitute, Percutaneous Endoscopic Approach
4U04JZ Supplement Abdominal Aorta with Synthetic Substitute, Percutaneous Endoscopic Approach
4U04KZ Supplement Abdominal Aorta with Nonautologous Tissue Substitute, Percutaneous Endoscopic Approach
4U107Z Supplement Celiac Artery with Autologous Tissue Substitute, Open Approach
4U10JZ Supplement Celiac Artery with Synthetic Substitute, Open Approach
4U10KZ Supplement Celiac Artery with Nonautologous Tissue Substitute, Open Approach
4U137Z Supplement Celiac Artery with Autologous Tissue Substitute, Percutaneous Approach
4U13JZ Supplement Celiac Artery with Synthetic Substitute, Percutaneous Approach
4U13KZ Supplement Celiac Artery with Nonautologous Tissue Substitute, Percutaneous Approach
4U147Z Supplement Celiac Artery with Autologous Tissue Substitute, Percutaneous Endoscopic Approach
4U14JZ Supplement Celiac Artery with Synthetic Substitute, Percutaneous Endoscopic Approach
4U14KZ Supplement Celiac Artery with Nonautologous Tissue Substitute, Percutaneous Endoscopic Approach
4U207Z Supplement Gastric Artery with Autologous Tissue Substitute, Open Approach
4U20JZ Supplement Gastric Artery with Synthetic Substitute, Open Approach
4U20KZ Supplement Gastric Artery with Nonautologous Tissue Substitute, Open Approach
4U237Z Supplement Gastric Artery with Autologous Tissue Substitute, Percutaneous Approach
4U23JZ Supplement Gastric Artery with Synthetic Substitute, Percutaneous Approach
4U23KZ Supplement Gastric Artery with Nonautologous Tissue Substitute, Percutaneous Approach
4U247Z Supplement Gastric Artery with Autologous Tissue Substitute, Percutaneous Endoscopic Approach
04U24JZ Supplement Gastric Artery with Synthetic Substitute, Percutaneous Endoscopic Approach
04U24KZ Supplement Gastric Artery with Nonautologous Tissue Substitute, Percutaneous Endoscopic Approach
04U307Z Supplement Hepatic Artery with Autologous Tissue Substitute, Open Approach
04U30JZ Supplement Hepatic Artery with Synthetic Substitute, Open Approach
04U30KZ Supplement Hepatic Artery with Nonautologous Tissue Substitute, Open Approach
04U337Z Supplement Hepatic Artery with Autologous Tissue Substitute, Percutaneous Approach
04U33JZ Supplement Hepatic Artery with Synthetic Substitute, Percutaneous Approach
04U33KZ Supplement Hepatic Artery with Nonautologous Tissue Substitute, Percutaneous Approach
04U347Z Supplement Hepatic Artery with Autologous Tissue Substitute, Percutaneous Endoscopic Approach
04U34JZ Supplement Hepatic Artery with Synthetic Substitute, Percutaneous Endoscopic Approach
04U34KZ Supplement Hepatic Artery with Nonautologous Tissue Substitute, Percutaneous Endoscopic Approach
04U407Z Supplement Splenic Artery with Autologous Tissue Substitute, Open Approach
04U40JZ Supplement Splenic Artery with Synthetic Substitute, Open Approach
04U40KZ Supplement Splenic Artery with Nonautologous Tissue Substitute, Open Approach
04U437Z Supplement Splenic Artery with Autologous Tissue Substitute, Percutaneous Approach
04U43JZ Supplement Splenic Artery with Synthetic Substitute, Percutaneous Approach
04U43KZ Supplement Splenic Artery with Nonautologous Tissue Substitute, Percutaneous Approach
04U447Z Supplement Splenic Artery with Autologous Tissue Substitute, Percutaneous Endoscopic Approach
04U44JZ Supplement Splenic Artery with Synthetic Substitute, Percutaneous Endoscopic Approach
04U44KZ Supplement Splenic Artery with Nonautologous Tissue Substitute, Percutaneous Endoscopic Approach
04U507Z Supplement Superior Mesenteric Artery with Autologous Tissue Substitute, Open Approach
04U50JZ Supplement Superior Mesenteric Artery with Synthetic Substitute, Open Approach
04U50KZ Supplement Superior Mesenteric Artery with Nonautologous Tissue Substitute, Open Approach
04U537Z Supplement Superior Mesenteric Artery with Autologous Tissue Substitute, Percutaneous Approach
04U53JZ Supplement Superior Mesenteric Artery with Synthetic Substitute, Percutaneous Approach
04U53KZ Supplement Superior Mesenteric Artery with Nonautologous Tissue Substitute, Percutaneous Approach
04U547Z Supplement Superior Mesenteric Artery with Autologous Tissue Substitute, Percutaneous Endoscopic Approach
04U54JZ Supplement Superior Mesenteric Artery with Synthetic Substitute, Percutaneous Endoscopic Approach
04U54KZ Supplement Superior Mesenteric Artery with Nonautologous Tissue Substitute, Percutaneous Endoscopic Approach
04U607Z Supplement Right Colic Artery with Autologous Tissue Substitute, Open Approach
04U60JZ Supplement Right Colic Artery with Synthetic Substitute, Open Approach
04U60KZ Supplement Right Colic Artery with Nonautologous Tissue Substitute, Open Approach
04U637Z Supplement Right Colic Artery with Autologous Tissue Substitute, Percutaneous Approach
04U63JZ Supplement Right Colic Artery with Synthetic Substitute, Percutaneous Approach
04U63KZ Supplement Right Colic Artery with Nonautologous Tissue Substitute, Percutaneous Approach
04U647Z Supplement Right Colic Artery with Autologous Tissue Substitute, Percutaneous Endoscopic Approach
04U64JZ Supplement Right Colic Artery with Synthetic Substitute, Percutaneous Endoscopic Approach
04U64KZ Supplement Right Colic Artery with Nonautologous Tissue Substitute, Percutaneous Endoscopic Approach
04U707Z Supplement Left Colic Artery with Autologous Tissue Substitute, Open Approach
04U70JZ Supplement Left Colic Artery with Synthetic Substitute, Open Approach
04U70KZ Supplement Left Colic Artery with Nonautologous Tissue Substitute, Open Approach
04U737Z Supplement Left Colic Artery with Autologous Tissue Substitute, Percutaneous Approach
04U73JZ Supplement Left Colic Artery with Synthetic Substitute, Percutaneous Approach
04U73KZ Supplement Left Colic Artery with Nonautologous Tissue Substitute, Percutaneous Approach
04U747Z Supplement Left Colic Artery with Autologous Tissue Substitute, Percutaneous Endoscopic Approach
04U74JZ Supplement Left Colic Artery with Synthetic Substitute, Percutaneous Endoscopic Approach
04U74KZ Supplement Left Colic Artery with Nonautologous Tissue Substitute, Percutaneous Endoscopic Approach
04U807Z Supplement Middle Colic Artery with Autologous Tissue Substitute, Open Approach
04U80JZ Supplement Middle Colic Artery with Synthetic Substitute, Open Approach
04U80KZ Supplement Middle Colic Artery with Nonautologous Tissue Substitute, Open Approach

04U837Z Supplement Middle Colic Artery with Autologous Tissue Substitute, Percutaneous Approach
04U83JZ Supplement Middle Colic Artery with Synthetic Substitute, Percutaneous Approach
04U83KZ Supplement Middle Colic Artery with Nonautologous Tissue Substitute, Percutaneous Approach
04U847Z Supplement Middle Colic Artery with Autologous Tissue Substitute, Percutaneous Endoscopic Approach
04U84JZ Supplement Middle Colic Artery with Synthetic Substitute, Percutaneous Endoscopic Approach
04U84KZ Supplement Middle Colic Artery with Nonautologous Tissue Substitute, Percutaneous Endoscopic Approach
04U907Z Supplement Right Renal Artery with Autologous Tissue Substitute, Open Approach
04U90JZ Supplement Right Renal Artery with Synthetic Substitute, Open Approach
04U90KZ Supplement Right Renal Artery with Nonautologous Tissue Substitute, Open Approach
04U937Z Supplement Right Renal Artery with Autologous Tissue Substitute, Percutaneous Approach
04U93JZ Supplement Right Renal Artery with Synthetic Substitute, Percutaneous Approach
04U93KZ Supplement Right Renal Artery with Nonautologous Tissue Substitute, Percutaneous Approach
04U947Z Supplement Right Renal Artery with Autologous Tissue Substitute, Percutaneous Endoscopic Approach
04U94JZ Supplement Right Renal Artery with Synthetic Substitute, Percutaneous Endoscopic Approach
04U94KZ Supplement Right Renal Artery with Nonautologous Tissue Substitute, Percutaneous Endoscopic Approach
04UA07Z Supplement Left Renal Artery with Autologous Tissue Substitute, Open Approach
04UA0JZ Supplement Left Renal Artery with Synthetic Substitute, Open Approach
04UA0KZ Supplement Left Renal Artery with Nonautologous Tissue Substitute, Open Approach
04UA37Z Supplement Left Renal Artery with Autologous Tissue Substitute, Percutaneous Approach
04UA3JZ Supplement Left Renal Artery with Synthetic Substitute, Percutaneous Approach
04UA3KZ Supplement Left Renal Artery with Nonautologous Tissue Substitute, Percutaneous Approach
04UA47Z Supplement Left Renal Artery with Autologous Tissue Substitute, Percutaneous Endoscopic Approach
04UA4JZ Supplement Left Renal Artery with Synthetic Substitute, Percutaneous Endoscopic Approach
04UA4KZ Supplement Left Renal Artery with Nonautologous Tissue Substitute, Percutaneous Endoscopic Approach
04UB07Z Supplement Inferior Mesenteric Artery with Autologous Tissue Substitute, Open Approach
04UB0JZ Supplement Inferior Mesenteric Artery with Synthetic Substitute, Open Approach
04UB0KZ Supplement Inferior Mesenteric Artery with Nonautologous Tissue Substitute, Open Approach
04UB37Z Supplement Inferior Mesenteric Artery with Autologous Tissue Substitute, Percutaneous Approach
04UB3JZ Supplement Inferior Mesenteric Artery with Synthetic Substitute, Percutaneous Approach
04UB3KZ Supplement Inferior Mesenteric Artery with Nonautologous Tissue Substitute, Percutaneous Approach
04UB47Z Supplement Inferior Mesenteric Artery with Autologous Tissue Substitute, Percutaneous Endoscopic Approach
04UB4JZ Supplement Inferior Mesenteric Artery with Synthetic Substitute, Percutaneous Endoscopic Approach
04UB4KZ Supplement Inferior Mesenteric Artery with Nonautologous Tissue Substitute, Percutaneous Endoscopic Approach
04UC07Z Supplement Right Common Iliac Artery with Autologous Tissue Substitute, Open Approach
04UC0JZ Supplement Right Common Iliac Artery with Synthetic Substitute, Open Approach
04UC0KZ Supplement Right Common Iliac Artery with Nonautologous Tissue Substitute, Open Approach
04UC37Z Supplement Right Common Iliac Artery with Autologous Tissue Substitute, Percutaneous Approach
04UC3JZ Supplement Right Common Iliac Artery with Synthetic Substitute, Percutaneous Approach
04UC3KZ Supplement Right Common Iliac Artery with Nonautologous Tissue Substitute, Percutaneous Approach
04UC47Z Supplement Right Common Iliac Artery with Autologous Tissue Substitute, Percutaneous Endoscopic Approach
04UC4JZ Supplement Right Common Iliac Artery with Synthetic Substitute, Percutaneous Endoscopic Approach
04UC4KZ Supplement Right Common Iliac Artery with Nonautologous Tissue Substitute, Percutaneous Endoscopic Approach
04UD07Z Supplement Left Common Iliac Artery with Autologous Tissue Substitute, Open Approach
04UD0JZ Supplement Left Common Iliac Artery with Synthetic Substitute, Open Approach
04UD0KZ Supplement Left Common Iliac Artery with Nonautologous Tissue Substitute, Open Approach
04UD37Z Supplement Left Common Iliac Artery with Autologous Tissue Substitute, Percutaneous Approach
04UD3JZ Supplement Left Common Iliac Artery with Synthetic Substitute, Percutaneous Approach
04UD3KZ Supplement Left Common Iliac Artery with Nonautologous Tissue Substitute, Percutaneous Approach
04UD47Z Supplement Left Common Iliac Artery with Autologous Tissue Substitute, Percutaneous Endoscopic Approach
04UD4JZ Supplement Left Common Iliac Artery with Synthetic Substitute, Percutaneous Endoscopic Approach
04UD4KZ Supplement Left Common Iliac Artery with Nonautologous Tissue Substitute, Percutaneous Endoscopic Approach
04UE07Z Supplement Right Internal Iliac Artery with Autologous Tissue Substitute, Open Approach
04UE0JZ Supplement Right Internal Iliac Artery with Synthetic Substitute, Open Approach
04UE0KZ Supplement Right Internal Iliac Artery with Nonautologous Tissue Substitute, Open Approach
04UE37Z Supplement Right Internal Iliac Artery with Autologous Tissue Substitute, Percutaneous Approach
04UE3JZ Supplement Right Internal Iliac Artery with Synthetic Substitute, Percutaneous Approach
04UE3KZ Supplement Right Internal Iliac Artery with Nonautologous Tissue Substitute, Percutaneous Approach
04UE47Z Supplement Right Internal Iliac Artery with Autologous Tissue Substitute, Percutaneous Endoscopic Approach
04UE4JZ Supplement Right Internal Iliac Artery with Synthetic Substitute, Percutaneous Endoscopic Approach
04UE4KZ Supplement Right Internal Iliac Artery with Nonautologous Tissue Substitute, Percutaneous Endoscopic Approach
04UF07Z Supplement Left Internal Iliac Artery with Autologous Tissue Substitute, Open Approach
04UF0JZ Supplement Left Internal Iliac Artery with Synthetic Substitute, Open Approach
04UF0KZ Supplement Left Internal Iliac Artery with Nonautologous Tissue Substitute, Open Approach
04UF37Z Supplement Left Internal Iliac Artery with Autologous Tissue Substitute, Percutaneous Approach
04UF3JZ Supplement Left Internal Iliac Artery with Synthetic Substitute, Percutaneous Approach
04UF3KZ Supplement Left Internal Iliac Artery with Nonautologous Tissue Substitute, Percutaneous Approach
04UF47Z Supplement Left Internal Iliac Artery with Autologous Tissue Substitute, Percutaneous Endoscopic Approach
04UF4JZ Supplement Left Internal Iliac Artery with Synthetic Substitute, Percutaneous Endoscopic Approach
04UF4KZ Supplement Left Internal Iliac Artery with Nonautologous Tissue Substitute, Percutaneous Endoscopic Approach
04UH07Z Supplement Right External Iliac Artery with Autologous Tissue Substitute, Open Approach
04UH0JZ Supplement Right External Iliac Artery with Synthetic Substitute, Open Approach
04UH0KZ Supplement Right External Iliac Artery with Nonautologous Tissue Substitute, Open Approach
04UH37Z Supplement Right External Iliac Artery with Autologous Tissue Substitute, Percutaneous Approach
04UH3JZ Supplement Right External Iliac Artery with Synthetic Substitute, Percutaneous Approach
04UH3KZ Supplement Right External Iliac Artery with Nonautologous Tissue Substitute, Percutaneous Approach
04UH47Z Supplement Right External Iliac Artery with Autologous Tissue Substitute, Percutaneous Endoscopic Approach
04UH4JZ Supplement Right External Iliac Artery with Synthetic Substitute, Percutaneous Endoscopic Approach
04UH4KZ Supplement Right External Iliac Artery with Nonautologous Tissue Substitute, Percutaneous Endoscopic Approach
04UJ07Z Supplement Left External Iliac Artery with Autologous Tissue Substitute, Open Approach
04UJ0JZ Supplement Left External Iliac Artery with Synthetic Substitute, Open Approach
04UJ0KZ Supplement Left External Iliac Artery with Nonautologous Tissue Substitute, Open Approach

4UJ37Z Supplement Left External Iliac Artery with Autologous Tissue Substitute, Percutaneous Approach

4UJ3JZ Supplement Left External Iliac Artery with Synthetic Substitute, Percutaneous Approach

4UJ3KZ Supplement Left External Iliac Artery with Nonautologous Tissue Substitute, Percutaneous Approach

4UJ47Z Supplement Left External Iliac Artery with Autologous Tissue Substitute, Percutaneous Endoscopic Approach

4UJ4JZ Supplement Left External Iliac Artery with Synthetic Substitute, Percutaneous Endoscopic Approach

4UJ4KZ Supplement Left External Iliac Artery with Nonautologous Tissue Substitute, Percutaneous Endoscopic Approach

4UK07Z Supplement Right Femoral Artery with Autologous Tissue Substitute, Open Approach

4UK0JZ Supplement Right Femoral Artery with Synthetic Substitute, Open Approach

4UK0KZ Supplement Right Femoral Artery with Nonautologous Tissue Substitute, Open Approach

4UK37Z Supplement Right Femoral Artery with Autologous Tissue Substitute, Percutaneous Approach

4UK3JZ Supplement Right Femoral Artery with Synthetic Substitute, Percutaneous Approach
AHA CC: 1Q, 2014, 22-23

4UK3KZ Supplement Right Femoral Artery with Nonautologous Tissue Substitute, Percutaneous Approach

4UK47Z Supplement Right Femoral Artery with Autologous Tissue Substitute, Percutaneous Endoscopic Approach

4UK4JZ Supplement Right Femoral Artery with Synthetic Substitute, Percutaneous Endoscopic Approach

4UK4KZ Supplement Right Femoral Artery with Nonautologous Tissue Substitute, Percutaneous Endoscopic Approach

4UL07Z Supplement Left Femoral Artery with Autologous Tissue Substitute, Open Approach

4UL0JZ Supplement Left Femoral Artery with Synthetic Substitute, Open Approach

4UL0KZ Supplement Left Femoral Artery with Nonautologous Tissue Substitute, Open Approach

4UL37Z Supplement Left Femoral Artery with Autologous Tissue Substitute, Percutaneous Approach

4UL3JZ Supplement Left Femoral Artery with Synthetic Substitute, Percutaneous Approach

4UL3KZ Supplement Left Femoral Artery with Nonautologous Tissue Substitute, Percutaneous Approach

4UL47Z Supplement Left Femoral Artery with Autologous Tissue Substitute, Percutaneous Endoscopic Approach

4UL4JZ Supplement Left Femoral Artery with Synthetic Substitute, Percutaneous Endoscopic Approach

4UL4KZ Supplement Left Femoral Artery with Nonautologous Tissue Substitute, Percutaneous Endoscopic Approach

4UM07Z Supplement Right Popliteal Artery with Autologous Tissue Substitute, Open Approach

4UM0JZ Supplement Right Popliteal Artery with Synthetic Substitute, Open Approach

4UM0KZ Supplement Right Popliteal Artery with Nonautologous Tissue Substitute, Open Approach

04UM37Z Supplement Right Popliteal Artery with Autologous Tissue Substitute, Percutaneous Approach

04UM3JZ Supplement Right Popliteal Artery with Synthetic Substitute, Percutaneous Approach

04UM3KZ Supplement Right Popliteal Artery with Nonautologous Tissue Substitute, Percutaneous Approach

04UM47Z Supplement Right Popliteal Artery with Autologous Tissue Substitute, Percutaneous Endoscopic Approach

04UM4JZ Supplement Right Popliteal Artery with Synthetic Substitute, Percutaneous Endoscopic Approach

04UM4KZ Supplement Right Popliteal Artery with Nonautologous Tissue Substitute, Percutaneous Endoscopic Approach

04UN07Z Supplement Left Popliteal Artery with Autologous Tissue Substitute, Open Approach

04UN0JZ Supplement Left Popliteal Artery with Synthetic Substitute, Open Approach

04UN0KZ Supplement Left Popliteal Artery with Nonautologous Tissue Substitute, Open Approach

04UN37Z Supplement Left Popliteal Artery with Autologous Tissue Substitute, Percutaneous Approach

04UN3JZ Supplement Left Popliteal Artery with Synthetic Substitute, Percutaneous Approach

04UN3KZ Supplement Left Popliteal Artery with Nonautologous Tissue Substitute, Percutaneous Approach

04UN47Z Supplement Left Popliteal Artery with Autologous Tissue Substitute, Percutaneous Endoscopic Approach

04UN4JZ Supplement Left Popliteal Artery with Synthetic Substitute, Percutaneous Endoscopic Approach

04UN4KZ Supplement Left Popliteal Artery with Nonautologous Tissue Substitute, Percutaneous Endoscopic Approach

04UP07Z Supplement Right Anterior Tibial Artery with Autologous Tissue Substitute, Open Approach

04UP0JZ Supplement Right Anterior Tibial Artery with Synthetic Substitute, Open Approach

04UP0KZ Supplement Right Anterior Tibial Artery with Nonautologous Tissue Substitute, Open Approach

04UP37Z Supplement Right Anterior Tibial Artery with Autologous Tissue Substitute, Percutaneous Approach

04UP3JZ Supplement Right Anterior Tibial Artery with Synthetic Substitute, Percutaneous Approach

04UP3KZ Supplement Right Anterior Tibial Artery with Nonautologous Tissue Substitute, Percutaneous Approach

04UP47Z Supplement Right Anterior Tibial Artery with Autologous Tissue Substitute, Percutaneous Endoscopic Approach

04UP4JZ Supplement Right Anterior Tibial Artery with Synthetic Substitute, Percutaneous Endoscopic Approach

04UP4KZ Supplement Right Anterior Tibial Artery with Nonautologous Tissue Substitute, Percutaneous Endoscopic Approach

04UQ07Z Supplement Left Anterior Tibial Artery with Autologous Tissue Substitute, Open Approach

04UQ0JZ Supplement Left Anterior Tibial Artery with Synthetic Substitute, Open Approach

04UQ0KZ Supplement Left Anterior Tibial Artery with Nonautologous Tissue Substitute, Open Approach

04UQ37Z Supplement Left Anterior Tibial Artery with Autologous Tissue Substitute, Percutaneous Approach

04UQ3JZ Supplement Left Anterior Tibial Artery with Synthetic Substitute, Percutaneous Approach

04UQ3KZ Supplement Left Anterior Tibial Artery with Nonautologous Tissue Substitute, Percutaneous Approach

04UQ47Z Supplement Left Anterior Tibial Artery with Autologous Tissue Substitute, Percutaneous Endoscopic Approach

04UQ4JZ Supplement Left Anterior Tibial Artery with Synthetic Substitute, Percutaneous Endoscopic Approach

04UQ4KZ Supplement Left Anterior Tibial Artery with Nonautologous Tissue Substitute, Percutaneous Endoscopic Approach

04UR07Z Supplement Right Posterior Tibial Artery with Autologous Tissue Substitute, Open Approach

04UR0JZ Supplement Right Posterior Tibial Artery with Synthetic Substitute, Open Approach

04UR0KZ Supplement Right Posterior Tibial Artery with Nonautologous Tissue Substitute, Open Approach

04UR37Z Supplement Right Posterior Tibial Artery with Autologous Tissue Substitute, Percutaneous Approach

04UR3JZ Supplement Right Posterior Tibial Artery with Synthetic Substitute, Percutaneous Approach

04UR3KZ Supplement Right Posterior Tibial Artery with Nonautologous Tissue Substitute, Percutaneous Approach

04UR47Z Supplement Right Posterior Tibial Artery with Autologous Tissue Substitute, Percutaneous Endoscopic Approach

04UR4JZ Supplement Right Posterior Tibial Artery with Synthetic Substitute, Percutaneous Endoscopic Approach

04UR4KZ Supplement Right Posterior Tibial Artery with Nonautologous Tissue Substitute, Percutaneous Endoscopic Approach

04US07Z Supplement Left Posterior Tibial Artery with Autologous Tissue Substitute, Open Approach

04US0JZ Supplement Left Posterior Tibial Artery with Synthetic Substitute, Open Approach

04US0KZ Supplement Left Posterior Tibial Artery with Nonautologous Tissue Substitute, Open Approach

04US37Z Supplement Left Posterior Tibial Artery with Autologous Tissue Substitute, Percutaneous Approach

04US3JZ Supplement Left Posterior Tibial Artery with Synthetic Substitute, Percutaneous Approach

04US3KZ Supplement Left Posterior Tibial Artery with Nonautologous Tissue Substitute, Percutaneous Approach

04US47Z Supplement Left Posterior Tibial Artery with Autologous Tissue Substitute, Percutaneous Endoscopic Approach

04US4JZ Supplement Left Posterior Tibial Artery with Synthetic Substitute, Percutaneous Endoscopic Approach

04US4KZ Supplement Left Posterior Tibial Artery with Nonautologous Tissue Substitute, Percutaneous Endoscopic Approach

04UT07Z Supplement Right Peroneal Artery with Autologous Tissue Substitute, Open Approach

04UT0JZ Supplement Right Peroneal Artery with Synthetic Substitute, Open Approach

04UT0KZ Supplement Right Peroneal Artery with Nonautologous Tissue Substitute, Open Approach

04UT37Z Supplement Right Peroneal Artery with Autologous Tissue Substitute, Percutaneous Approach

04UT3JZ Supplement Right Peroneal Artery with Synthetic Substitute, Percutaneous Approach

04UT3KZ Supplement Right Peroneal Artery with Nonautologous Tissue Substitute, Percutaneous Approach

04UT47Z Supplement Right Peroneal Artery with Autologous Tissue Substitute, Percutaneous Endoscopic Approach

04UT4JZ Supplement Right Peroneal Artery with Synthetic Substitute, Percutaneous Endoscopic Approach

04UT4KZ Supplement Right Peroneal Artery with Nonautologous Tissue Substitute, Percutaneous Endoscopic Approach

04UU07Z Supplement Left Peroneal Artery with Autologous Tissue Substitute, Open Approach

04UU0JZ Supplement Left Peroneal Artery with Synthetic Substitute, Open Approach

04UU0KZ Supplement Left Peroneal Artery with Nonautologous Tissue Substitute, Open Approach

04UU37Z Supplement Left Peroneal Artery with Autologous Tissue Substitute, Percutaneous Approach

04UU3JZ Supplement Left Peroneal Artery with Synthetic Substitute, Percutaneous Approach

04UU3KZ Supplement Left Peroneal Artery with Nonautologous Tissue Substitute, Percutaneous Approach

04UU47Z Supplement Left Peroneal Artery with Autologous Tissue Substitute, Percutaneous Endoscopic Approach

04UU4JZ Supplement Left Peroneal Artery with Synthetic Substitute, Percutaneous Endoscopic Approach

04UU4KZ Supplement Left Peroneal Artery with Nonautologous Tissue Substitute, Percutaneous Endoscopic Approach

04UV07Z Supplement Right Foot Artery with Autologous Tissue Substitute, Open Approach

04UV0JZ Supplement Right Foot Artery with Synthetic Substitute, Open Approach

04UV0KZ Supplement Right Foot Artery with Nonautologous Tissue Substitute, Open Approach

04UV37Z Supplement Right Foot Artery with Autologous Tissue Substitute, Percutaneous Approach

04UV3JZ Supplement Right Foot Artery with Synthetic Substitute, Percutaneous Approach

04UV3KZ Supplement Right Foot Artery with Nonautologous Tissue Substitute, Percutaneous Approach

04UV47Z Supplement Right Foot Artery with Autologous Tissue Substitute, Percutaneous Endoscopic Approach

04UV4JZ Supplement Right Foot Artery with Synthetic Substitute, Percutaneous Endoscopic Approach

04UV4KZ Supplement Right Foot Artery with Nonautologous Tissue Substitute, Percutaneous Endoscopic Approach

04UW07Z Supplement Left Foot Artery with Autologous Tissue Substitute, Open Approach

04UW0JZ Supplement Left Foot Artery with Synthetic Substitute, Open Approach

04UW0KZ Supplement Left Foot Artery with Nonautologous Tissue Substitute, Open Approach

04UW37Z Supplement Left Foot Artery with Autologous Tissue Substitute, Percutaneous Approach

04UW3JZ Supplement Left Foot Artery with Synthetic Substitute, Percutaneous Approach

04UW3KZ Supplement Left Foot Artery with Nonautologous Tissue Substitute, Percutaneous Approach

04UW47Z Supplement Left Foot Artery with Autologous Tissue Substitute, Percutaneous Endoscopic Approach

04UW4JZ Supplement Left Foot Artery with Synthetic Substitute, Percutaneous Endoscopic Approach

04UW4KZ Supplement Left Foot Artery with Nonautologous Tissue Substitute, Percutaneous Endoscopic Approach

04UY07Z Supplement Lower Artery with Autologous Tissue Substitute, Open Approach

04UY0JZ Supplement Lower Artery with Synthetic Substitute, Open Approach

04UY0KZ Supplement Lower Artery with Nonautologous Tissue Substitute, Open Approach

04UY37Z Supplement Lower Artery with Autologous Tissue Substitute, Percutaneous Approach

04UY3JZ Supplement Lower Artery with Synthetic Substitute, Percutaneous Approach

04UY3KZ Supplement Lower Artery with Nonautologous Tissue Substitute, Percutaneous Approach

04UY47Z Supplement Lower Artery with Autologous Tissue Substitute, Percutaneous Endoscopic Approach

04UY4JZ Supplement Lower Artery with Synthetic Substitute, Percutaneous Endoscopic Approach

04UY4KZ Supplement Lower Artery with Nonautologous Tissue Substitute, Percutaneous Endoscopic Approach

04V – Lower Arteries, Restriction

Review Coding Guideline B3.12

04V00CZ Restriction of Abdominal Aorta with Extraluminal Device, Open Approach

04V00DJ Restriction of Abdominal Aorta with Intraluminal Device, Temporary, Open Approach

04V00DZ Restriction of Abdominal Aorta with Intraluminal Device, Open Approach

04V00ZZ Restriction of Abdominal Aorta, Open Approach

04V03CZ Restriction of Abdominal Aorta with Extraluminal Device, Percutaneous Approach

04V03DJ Restriction of Abdominal Aorta with Intraluminal Device, Temporary, Percutaneous Approach

04V03DZ Restriction of Abdominal Aorta with Intraluminal Device, Percutaneous Approach
AHA CC: 1Q, 2014, 9

04V03ZZ Restriction of Abdominal Aorta, Percutaneous Approach

04V04CZ Restriction of Abdominal Aorta with Extraluminal Device, Percutaneous Endoscopic Approach

04V04DJ Restriction of Abdominal Aorta with Intraluminal Device, Temporary, Percutaneous Endoscopic Approach

04V04DZ Restriction of Abdominal Aorta with Intraluminal Device, Percutaneous Endoscopic Approach

04V04ZZ Restriction of Abdominal Aorta, Percutaneous Endoscopic Approach

04V10CZ Restriction of Celiac Artery with Extraluminal Device, Open Approach

04V10DZ Restriction of Celiac Artery with Intraluminal Device, Open Approach

04V10ZZ Restriction of Celiac Artery, Open Approach

04V13CZ Restriction of Celiac Artery with Extraluminal Device, Percutaneous Approach

04V13DZ Restriction of Celiac Artery with Intraluminal Device, Percutaneous Approach

04V13ZZ Restriction of Celiac Artery, Percutaneous Approach

04V14CZ Restriction of Celiac Artery with Extraluminal Device, Percutaneous Endoscopic Approach

04V14DZ Restriction of Celiac Artery with Intraluminal Device, Percutaneous Endoscopic Approach

04V14ZZ Restriction of Celiac Artery, Percutaneous Endoscopic Approach

04V20CZ Restriction of Gastric Artery with Extraluminal Device, Open Approach

04V20DZ Restriction of Gastric Artery with Intraluminal Device, Open Approach

04V20ZZ Restriction of Gastric Artery, Open Approach

04V23CZ Restriction of Gastric Artery with Extraluminal Device, Percutaneous Approach

04V23DZ Restriction of Gastric Artery with Intraluminal Device, Percutaneous Approach

04V23ZZ Restriction of Gastric Artery, Percutaneous Approach

04V24CZ Restriction of Gastric Artery with Extraluminal Device, Percutaneous Endoscopic Approach

04V24DZ Restriction of Gastric Artery with Intraluminal Device, Percutaneous Endoscopic Approach

04V24ZZ Restriction of Gastric Artery, Percutaneous Endoscopic Approach

04V30CZ Restriction of Hepatic Artery with Extraluminal Device, Open Approach

04V30DZ Restriction of Hepatic Artery with Intraluminal Device, Open Approach

04V30ZZ Restriction of Hepatic Artery, Open Approach

04V33CZ Restriction of Hepatic Artery with Extraluminal Device, Percutaneous Approach

04V33DZ Restriction of Hepatic Artery with Intraluminal Device, Percutaneous Approach

04V33ZZ Restriction of Hepatic Artery, Percutaneous Approach

04V34CZ Restriction of Hepatic Artery with Extraluminal Device, Percutaneous Endoscopic Approach

04V34DZ Restriction of Hepatic Artery with Intraluminal Device, Percutaneous Endoscopic Approach

04V34ZZ Restriction of Hepatic Artery, Percutaneous Endoscopic Approach

4V40CZ Restriction of Splenic Artery with Extraluminal Device, Open Approach

4V40DZ Restriction of Splenic Artery with Intraluminal Device, Open Approach

4V40ZZ Restriction of Splenic Artery, Open Approach

4V43CZ Restriction of Splenic Artery with Extraluminal Device, Percutaneous Approach

4V43DZ Restriction of Splenic Artery with Intraluminal Device, Percutaneous Approach

4V43ZZ Restriction of Splenic Artery, Percutaneous Approach

4V44CZ Restriction of Splenic Artery with Extraluminal Device, Percutaneous Endoscopic Approach

4V44DZ Restriction of Splenic Artery with Intraluminal Device, Percutaneous Endoscopic Approach

4V44ZZ Restriction of Splenic Artery, Percutaneous Endoscopic Approach

4V50CZ Restriction of Superior Mesenteric Artery with Extraluminal Device, Open Approach

4V50DZ Restriction of Superior Mesenteric Artery with Intraluminal Device, Open Approach

4V50ZZ Restriction of Superior Mesenteric Artery, Open Approach

4V53CZ Restriction of Superior Mesenteric Artery with Extraluminal Device, Percutaneous Approach

4V53DZ Restriction of Superior Mesenteric Artery with Intraluminal Device, Percutaneous Approach

4V53ZZ Restriction of Superior Mesenteric Artery, Percutaneous Approach

4V54CZ Restriction of Superior Mesenteric Artery with Extraluminal Device, Percutaneous Endoscopic Approach

4V54DZ Restriction of Superior Mesenteric Artery with Intraluminal Device, Percutaneous Endoscopic Approach

4V54ZZ Restriction of Superior Mesenteric Artery, Percutaneous Endoscopic Approach

4V60CZ Restriction of Right Colic Artery with Extraluminal Device, Open Approach

4V60DZ Restriction of Right Colic Artery with Intraluminal Device, Open Approach

4V60ZZ Restriction of Right Colic Artery, Open Approach

4V63CZ Restriction of Right Colic Artery with Extraluminal Device, Percutaneous Approach

4V63DZ Restriction of Right Colic Artery with Intraluminal Device, Percutaneous Approach

4V63ZZ Restriction of Right Colic Artery, Percutaneous Approach

4V64CZ Restriction of Right Colic Artery with Extraluminal Device, Percutaneous Endoscopic Approach

4V64DZ Restriction of Right Colic Artery with Intraluminal Device, Percutaneous Endoscopic Approach

4V64ZZ Restriction of Right Colic Artery, Percutaneous Endoscopic Approach

4V70CZ Restriction of Left Colic Artery with Extraluminal Device, Open Approach

4V70DZ Restriction of Left Colic Artery with Intraluminal Device, Open Approach

4V70ZZ Restriction of Left Colic Artery, Open Approach

4V73CZ Restriction of Left Colic Artery with Extraluminal Device, Percutaneous Approach

4V73DZ Restriction of Left Colic Artery with Intraluminal Device, Percutaneous Approach

04V73ZZ Restriction of Left Colic Artery, Percutaneous Approach

04V74CZ Restriction of Left Colic Artery with Extraluminal Device, Percutaneous Endoscopic Approach

04V74DZ Restriction of Left Colic Artery with Intraluminal Device, Percutaneous Endoscopic Approach

04V74ZZ Restriction of Left Colic Artery, Percutaneous Endoscopic Approach

04V80CZ Restriction of Middle Colic Artery with Extraluminal Device, Open Approach

04V80DZ Restriction of Middle Colic Artery with Intraluminal Device, Open Approach

04V80ZZ Restriction of Middle Colic Artery, Open Approach

04V83CZ Restriction of Middle Colic Artery with Extraluminal Device, Percutaneous Approach

04V83DZ Restriction of Middle Colic Artery with Intraluminal Device, Percutaneous Approach

04V83ZZ Restriction of Middle Colic Artery, Percutaneous Approach

04V84CZ Restriction of Middle Colic Artery with Extraluminal Device, Percutaneous Endoscopic Approach

04V84DZ Restriction of Middle Colic Artery with Intraluminal Device, Percutaneous Endoscopic Approach

04V84ZZ Restriction of Middle Colic Artery, Percutaneous Endoscopic Approach

04V90CZ Restriction of Right Renal Artery with Extraluminal Device, Open Approach

04V90DZ Restriction of Right Renal Artery with Intraluminal Device, Open Approach

04V90ZZ Restriction of Right Renal Artery, Open Approach

04V93CZ Restriction of Right Renal Artery with Extraluminal Device, Percutaneous Approach

04V93DZ Restriction of Right Renal Artery with Intraluminal Device, Percutaneous Approach

04V93ZZ Restriction of Right Renal Artery, Percutaneous Approach

04V94CZ Restriction of Right Renal Artery with Extraluminal Device, Percutaneous Endoscopic Approach

04V94DZ Restriction of Right Renal Artery with Intraluminal Device, Percutaneous Endoscopic Approach

04V94ZZ Restriction of Right Renal Artery, Percutaneous Endoscopic Approach

04VA0CZ Restriction of Left Renal Artery with Extraluminal Device, Open Approach

04VA0DZ Restriction of Left Renal Artery with Intraluminal Device, Open Approach

04VA0ZZ Restriction of Left Renal Artery, Open Approach

04VA3CZ Restriction of Left Renal Artery with Extraluminal Device, Percutaneous Approach

04VA3DZ Restriction of Left Renal Artery with Intraluminal Device, Percutaneous Approach

04VA3ZZ Restriction of Left Renal Artery, Percutaneous Approach

04VA4CZ Restriction of Left Renal Artery with Extraluminal Device, Percutaneous Endoscopic Approach

04VA4DZ Restriction of Left Renal Artery with Intraluminal Device, Percutaneous Endoscopic Approach

04VA4ZZ Restriction of Left Renal Artery, Percutaneous Endoscopic Approach

04VB0CZ Restriction of Inferior Mesenteric Artery with Extraluminal Device, Open Approach

04VB0DZ Restriction of Inferior Mesenteric Artery with Intraluminal Device, Open Approach

04VB0ZZ Restriction of Inferior Mesenteric Artery, Open Approach

04VB3CZ Restriction of Inferior Mesenteric Artery with Extraluminal Device, Percutaneous Approach

04VB3DZ Restriction of Inferior Mesenteric Artery with Intraluminal Device, Percutaneous Approach

04VB3ZZ Restriction of Inferior Mesenteric Artery, Percutaneous Approach

04VB4CZ Restriction of Inferior Mesenteric Artery with Extraluminal Device, Percutaneous Endoscopic Approach

04VB4DZ Restriction of Inferior Mesenteric Artery with Intraluminal Device, Percutaneous Endoscopic Approach

04VB4ZZ Restriction of Inferior Mesenteric Artery, Percutaneous Endoscopic Approach

04VC0CZ Restriction of Right Common Iliac Artery with Extraluminal Device, Open Approach

04VC0DZ Restriction of Right Common Iliac Artery with Intraluminal Device, Open Approach

04VC0ZZ Restriction of Right Common Iliac Artery, Open Approach

04VC3CZ Restriction of Right Common Iliac Artery with Extraluminal Device, Percutaneous Approach

04VC3DZ Restriction of Right Common Iliac Artery with Intraluminal Device, Percutaneous Approach

04VC3ZZ Restriction of Right Common Iliac Artery, Percutaneous Approach

04VC4CZ Restriction of Right Common Iliac Artery with Extraluminal Device, Percutaneous Endoscopic Approach

04VC4DZ Restriction of Right Common Iliac Artery with Intraluminal Device, Percutaneous Endoscopic Approach

04VC4ZZ Restriction of Right Common Iliac Artery, Percutaneous Endoscopic Approach

04VD0CZ Restriction of Left Common Iliac Artery with Extraluminal Device, Open Approach

04VD0DZ Restriction of Left Common Iliac Artery with Intraluminal Device, Open Approach

04VD0ZZ Restriction of Left Common Iliac Artery, Open Approach

04VD3CZ Restriction of Left Common Iliac Artery with Extraluminal Device, Percutaneous Approach

04VD3DZ Restriction of Left Common Iliac Artery with Intraluminal Device, Percutaneous Approach

04VD3ZZ Restriction of Left Common Iliac Artery, Percutaneous Approach

04VD4CZ Restriction of Left Common Iliac Artery with Extraluminal Device, Percutaneous Endoscopic Approach

04VD4DZ Restriction of Left Common Iliac Artery with Intraluminal Device, Percutaneous Endoscopic Approach

04VD4ZZ Restriction of Left Common Iliac Artery, Percutaneous Endoscopic Approach

04VE0CZ Restriction of Right Internal Iliac Artery with Extraluminal Device, Open Approach

04VE0DZ Restriction of Right Internal Iliac Artery with Intraluminal Device, Open Approach

04VE0ZZ Restriction of Right Internal Iliac Artery, Open Approach

04VE3CZ Restriction of Right Internal Iliac Artery with Extraluminal Device, Percutaneous Approach

04VE3DZ Restriction of Right Internal Iliac Artery with Intraluminal Device, Percutaneous Approach

04VE3ZZ Restriction of Right Internal Iliac Artery, Percutaneous Approach

04VE4CZ Restriction of Right Internal Iliac Artery with Extraluminal Device, Percutaneous Endoscopic Approach
04VE4DZ Restriction of Right Internal Iliac Artery with Intraluminal Device, Percutaneous Endoscopic Approach
04VE4ZZ Restriction of Right Internal Iliac Artery, Percutaneous Endoscopic Approach
04VF0CZ Restriction of Left Internal Iliac Artery with Extraluminal Device, Open Approach
04VF0DZ Restriction of Left Internal Iliac Artery with Intraluminal Device, Open Approach
04VF0ZZ Restriction of Left Internal Iliac Artery, Open Approach
04VF3CZ Restriction of Left Internal Iliac Artery with Extraluminal Device, Percutaneous Approach
04VF3DZ Restriction of Left Internal Iliac Artery with Intraluminal Device, Percutaneous Approach
04VF3ZZ Restriction of Left Internal Iliac Artery, Percutaneous Approach
04VF4CZ Restriction of Left Internal Iliac Artery with Extraluminal Device, Percutaneous Endoscopic Approach
04VF4DZ Restriction of Left Internal Iliac Artery with Intraluminal Device, Percutaneous Endoscopic Approach
04VF4ZZ Restriction of Left Internal Iliac Artery, Percutaneous Endoscopic Approach
04VH0CZ Restriction of Right External Iliac Artery with Extraluminal Device, Open Approach
04VH0DZ Restriction of Right External Iliac Artery with Intraluminal Device, Open Approach
04VH0ZZ Restriction of Right External Iliac Artery, Open Approach
04VH3CZ Restriction of Right External Iliac Artery with Extraluminal Device, Percutaneous Approach
04VH3DZ Restriction of Right External Iliac Artery with Intraluminal Device, Percutaneous Approach
04VH3ZZ Restriction of Right External Iliac Artery, Percutaneous Approach
04VH4CZ Restriction of Right External Iliac Artery with Extraluminal Device, Percutaneous Endoscopic Approach
04VH4DZ Restriction of Right External Iliac Artery with Intraluminal Device, Percutaneous Endoscopic Approach
04VH4ZZ Restriction of Right External Iliac Artery, Percutaneous Endoscopic Approach
04VJ0CZ Restriction of Left External Iliac Artery with Extraluminal Device, Open Approach
04VJ0DZ Restriction of Left External Iliac Artery with Intraluminal Device, Open Approach
04VJ0ZZ Restriction of Left External Iliac Artery, Open Approach
04VJ3CZ Restriction of Left External Iliac Artery with Extraluminal Device, Percutaneous Approach
04VJ3DZ Restriction of Left External Iliac Artery with Intraluminal Device, Percutaneous Approach
04VJ3ZZ Restriction of Left External Iliac Artery, Percutaneous Approach
04VJ4CZ Restriction of Left External Iliac Artery with Extraluminal Device, Percutaneous Endoscopic Approach
04VJ4DZ Restriction of Left External Iliac Artery with Intraluminal Device, Percutaneous Endoscopic Approach
04VJ4ZZ Restriction of Left External Iliac Artery, Percutaneous Endoscopic Approach
04VK0CZ Restriction of Right Femoral Artery with Extraluminal Device, Open Approach
04VK0DZ Restriction of Right Femoral Artery with Intraluminal Device, Open Approach
04VK0ZZ Restriction of Right Femoral Artery, Open Approach
04VK3CZ Restriction of Right Femoral Artery with Extraluminal Device, Percutaneous Approach
04VK3DZ Restriction of Right Femoral Artery with Intraluminal Device, Percutaneous Approach
04VK3ZZ Restriction of Right Femoral Artery, Percutaneous Approach
04VK4CZ Restriction of Right Femoral Artery with Extraluminal Device, Percutaneous Endoscopic Approach
04VK4DZ Restriction of Right Femoral Artery with Intraluminal Device, Percutaneous Endoscopic Approach
04VK4ZZ Restriction of Right Femoral Artery, Percutaneous Endoscopic Approach
04VL0CZ Restriction of Left Femoral Artery with Extraluminal Device, Open Approach
04VL0DZ Restriction of Left Femoral Artery with Intraluminal Device, Open Approach
04VL0ZZ Restriction of Left Femoral Artery, Open Approach
04VL3CZ Restriction of Left Femoral Artery with Extraluminal Device, Percutaneous Approach
04VL3DZ Restriction of Left Femoral Artery with Intraluminal Device, Percutaneous Approach
04VL3ZZ Restriction of Left Femoral Artery, Percutaneous Approach
04VL4CZ Restriction of Left Femoral Artery with Extraluminal Device, Percutaneous Endoscopic Approach
04VL4DZ Restriction of Left Femoral Artery with Intraluminal Device, Percutaneous Endoscopic Approach
04VL4ZZ Restriction of Left Femoral Artery, Percutaneous Endoscopic Approach
04VM0CZ Restriction of Right Popliteal Artery with Extraluminal Device, Open Approach
04VM0DZ Restriction of Right Popliteal Artery with Intraluminal Device, Open Approach
04VM0ZZ Restriction of Right Popliteal Artery, Open Approach
04VM3CZ Restriction of Right Popliteal Artery with Extraluminal Device, Percutaneous Approach
04VM3DZ Restriction of Right Popliteal Artery with Intraluminal Device, Percutaneous Approach
04VM3ZZ Restriction of Right Popliteal Artery, Percutaneous Approach
04VM4CZ Restriction of Right Popliteal Artery with Extraluminal Device, Percutaneous Endoscopic Approach
04VM4DZ Restriction of Right Popliteal Artery with Intraluminal Device, Percutaneous Endoscopic Approach
04VM4ZZ Restriction of Right Popliteal Artery, Percutaneous Endoscopic Approach
04VN0CZ Restriction of Left Popliteal Artery with Extraluminal Device, Open Approach
04VN0DZ Restriction of Left Popliteal Artery with Intraluminal Device, Open Approach
04VN0ZZ Restriction of Left Popliteal Artery, Open Approach
04VN3CZ Restriction of Left Popliteal Artery with Extraluminal Device, Percutaneous Approach
04VN3DZ Restriction of Left Popliteal Artery with Intraluminal Device, Percutaneous Approach
04VN3ZZ Restriction of Left Popliteal Artery, Percutaneous Approach
04VN4CZ Restriction of Left Popliteal Artery with Extraluminal Device, Percutaneous Endoscopic Approach
04VN4DZ Restriction of Left Popliteal Artery with Intraluminal Device, Percutaneous Endoscopic Approach
04VN4ZZ Restriction of Left Popliteal Artery, Percutaneous Endoscopic Approach
04VP0CZ Restriction of Right Anterior Tibial Artery with Extraluminal Device, Open Approach
04VP0DZ Restriction of Right Anterior Tibial Artery with Intraluminal Device, Open Approach
04VP0ZZ Restriction of Right Anterior Tibial Artery, Open Approach
04VP3CZ Restriction of Right Anterior Tibial Artery with Extraluminal Device, Percutaneous Approach
04VP3DZ Restriction of Right Anterior Tibial Artery with Intraluminal Device, Percutaneous Approach
04VP3ZZ Restriction of Right Anterior Tibial Artery, Percutaneous Approach
04VP4CZ Restriction of Right Anterior Tibial Artery with Extraluminal Device, Percutaneous Endoscopic Approach
04VP4DZ Restriction of Right Anterior Tibial Artery with Intraluminal Device, Percutaneous Endoscopic Approach
04VP4ZZ Restriction of Right Anterior Tibial Artery, Percutaneous Endoscopic Approach
04VQ0CZ Restriction of Left Anterior Tibial Artery with Extraluminal Device, Open Approach
04VQ0DZ Restriction of Left Anterior Tibial Artery with Intraluminal Device, Open Approach
04VQ0ZZ Restriction of Left Anterior Tibial Artery, Open Approach
04VQ3CZ Restriction of Left Anterior Tibial Artery with Extraluminal Device, Percutaneous Approach
04VQ3DZ Restriction of Left Anterior Tibial Artery with Intraluminal Device, Percutaneous Approach
04VQ3ZZ Restriction of Left Anterior Tibial Artery, Percutaneous Approach
04VQ4CZ Restriction of Left Anterior Tibial Artery with Extraluminal Device, Percutaneous Endoscopic Approach
04VQ4DZ Restriction of Left Anterior Tibial Artery with Intraluminal Device, Percutaneous Endoscopic Approach
04VQ4ZZ Restriction of Left Anterior Tibial Artery, Percutaneous Endoscopic Approach
04VR0CZ Restriction of Right Posterior Tibial Artery with Extraluminal Device, Open Approach
04VR0DZ Restriction of Right Posterior Tibial Artery with Intraluminal Device, Open Approach
04VR0ZZ Restriction of Right Posterior Tibial Artery, Open Approach
04VR3CZ Restriction of Right Posterior Tibial Artery with Extraluminal Device, Percutaneous Approach
04VR3DZ Restriction of Right Posterior Tibial Artery with Intraluminal Device, Percutaneous Approach
04VR3ZZ Restriction of Right Posterior Tibial Artery, Percutaneous Approach
04VR4CZ Restriction of Right Posterior Tibial Artery with Extraluminal Device, Percutaneous Endoscopic Approach
04VR4DZ Restriction of Right Posterior Tibial Artery with Intraluminal Device, Percutaneous Endoscopic Approach
04VR4ZZ Restriction of Right Posterior Tibial Artery, Percutaneous Endoscopic Approach

04VS0CZ Restriction of Left Posterior Tibial Artery with Extraluminal Device, Open Approach
04VS0DZ Restriction of Left Posterior Tibial Artery with Intraluminal Device, Open Approach
04VS0ZZ Restriction of Left Posterior Tibial Artery, Open Approach
04VS3CZ Restriction of Left Posterior Tibial Artery with Extraluminal Device, Percutaneous Approach
04VS3DZ Restriction of Left Posterior Tibial Artery with Intraluminal Device, Percutaneous Approach
04VS3ZZ Restriction of Left Posterior Tibial Artery, Percutaneous Approach
04VS4CZ Restriction of Left Posterior Tibial Artery with Extraluminal Device, Percutaneous Endoscopic Approach
04VS4DZ Restriction of Left Posterior Tibial Artery with Intraluminal Device, Percutaneous Endoscopic Approach
04VS4ZZ Restriction of Left Posterior Tibial Artery, Percutaneous Endoscopic Approach
04VT0CZ Restriction of Right Peroneal Artery with Extraluminal Device, Open Approach
04VT0DZ Restriction of Right Peroneal Artery with Intraluminal Device, Open Approach
04VT0ZZ Restriction of Right Peroneal Artery, Open Approach
04VT3CZ Restriction of Right Peroneal Artery with Extraluminal Device, Percutaneous Approach
04VT3DZ Restriction of Right Peroneal Artery with Intraluminal Device, Percutaneous Approach
04VT3ZZ Restriction of Right Peroneal Artery, Percutaneous Approach
04VT4CZ Restriction of Right Peroneal Artery with Extraluminal Device, Percutaneous Endoscopic Approach
04VT4DZ Restriction of Right Peroneal Artery with Intraluminal Device, Percutaneous Endoscopic Approach
04VT4ZZ Restriction of Right Peroneal Artery, Percutaneous Endoscopic Approach
04VU0CZ Restriction of Left Peroneal Artery with Extraluminal Device, Open Approach
04VU0DZ Restriction of Left Peroneal Artery with Intraluminal Device, Open Approach
04VU0ZZ Restriction of Left Peroneal Artery, Open Approach
04VU3CZ Restriction of Left Peroneal Artery with Extraluminal Device, Percutaneous Approach
04VU3DZ Restriction of Left Peroneal Artery with Intraluminal Device, Percutaneous Approach
04VU3ZZ Restriction of Left Peroneal Artery, Percutaneous Approach
04VU4CZ Restriction of Left Peroneal Artery with Extraluminal Device, Percutaneous Endoscopic Approach
04VU4DZ Restriction of Left Peroneal Artery with Intraluminal Device, Percutaneous Endoscopic Approach
04VU4ZZ Restriction of Left Peroneal Artery, Percutaneous Endoscopic Approach
04VV0CZ Restriction of Right Foot Artery with Extraluminal Device, Open Approach
04VV0DZ Restriction of Right Foot Artery with Intraluminal Device, Open Approach
04VV0ZZ Restriction of Right Foot Artery, Open Approach
04VV3CZ Restriction of Right Foot Artery with Extraluminal Device, Percutaneous Approach
04VV3DZ Restriction of Right Foot Artery with Intraluminal Device, Percutaneous Approach
04VV3ZZ Restriction of Right Foot Artery, Percutaneous Approach
04VV4CZ Restriction of Right Foot Artery with Extraluminal Device, Percutaneous Endoscopic Approach
04VV4DZ Restriction of Right Foot Artery with Intraluminal Device, Percutaneous Endoscopic Approach
04VV4ZZ Restriction of Right Foot Artery, Percutaneous Endoscopic Approach
04VW0CZ Restriction of Left Foot Artery with Extraluminal Device, Open Approach
04VW0DZ Restriction of Left Foot Artery with Intraluminal Device, Open Approach
04VW0ZZ Restriction of Left Foot Artery, Open Approach
04VW3CZ Restriction of Left Foot Artery with Extraluminal Device, Percutaneous Approach
04VW3DZ Restriction of Left Foot Artery with Intraluminal Device, Percutaneous Approach
04VW3ZZ Restriction of Left Foot Artery, Percutaneous Approach
04VW4CZ Restriction of Left Foot Artery with Extraluminal Device, Percutaneous Endoscopic Approach
04VW4DZ Restriction of Left Foot Artery with Intraluminal Device, Percutaneous Endoscopic Approach
04VW4ZZ Restriction of Left Foot Artery, Percutaneous Endoscopic Approach
04VY0CZ Restriction of Lower Artery with Extraluminal Device, Open Approach
04VY0DZ Restriction of Lower Artery with Intraluminal Device, Open Approach
04VY0ZZ Restriction of Lower Artery, Open Approach
04VY3CZ Restriction of Lower Artery with Extraluminal Device, Percutaneous Approach
04VY3DZ Restriction of Lower Artery with Intraluminal Device, Percutaneous Approach
04VY3ZZ Restriction of Lower Artery, Percutaneous Approach
04VY4CZ Restriction of Lower Artery with Extraluminal Device, Percutaneous Endoscopic Approach
04VY4DZ Restriction of Lower Artery with Intraluminal Device, Percutaneous Endoscopic Approach
04VY4ZZ Restriction of Lower Artery, Percutaneous Endoscopic Approach

04W – Lower Arteries, Revision

Review Coding Guideline B6.1c

04WY00Z Revision of Drainage Device in Lower Artery, Open Approach
04WY02Z Revision of Monitoring Device in Lower Artery, Open Approach
04WY03Z Revision of Infusion Device in Lower Artery, Open Approach
04WY07Z Revision of Autologous Tissue Substitute in Lower Artery, Open Approach
04WY0CZ Revision of Extraluminal Device in Lower Artery, Open Approach
04WY0DZ Revision of Intraluminal Device in Lower Artery, Open Approach
04WY0JZ Revision of Synthetic Substitute in Lower Artery, Open Approach
04WY0KZ Revision of Nonautologous Tissue Substitute in Lower Artery, Open Approach
04WY30Z Revision of Drainage Device in Lower Artery, Percutaneous Approach
04WY32Z Revision of Monitoring Device in Lower Artery, Percutaneous Approach
04WY33Z Revision of Infusion Device in Lower Artery, Percutaneous Approach
04WY37Z Revision of Autologous Tissue Substitute in Lower Artery, Percutaneous Approach
AHA CC: 1Q, 2014, 26
04WY3CZ Revision of Extraluminal Device in Lower Artery, Percutaneous Approach
04WY3DZ Revision of Intraluminal Device in Lower Artery, Percutaneous Approach
AHA CC: 1Q, 2014, 9-10
04WY3JZ Revision of Synthetic Substitute in Lower Artery, Percutaneous Approach
04WY3KZ Revision of Nonautologous Tissue Substitute in Lower Artery, Percutaneous Approach
04WY40Z Revision of Drainage Device in Lower Artery, Percutaneous Endoscopic Approach
04WY42Z Revision of Monitoring Device in Lower Artery, Percutaneous Endoscopic Approach
04WY43Z Revision of Infusion Device in Lower Artery, Percutaneous Endoscopic Approach
04WY47Z Revision of Autologous Tissue Substitute in Lower Artery, Percutaneous Endoscopic Approach
04WY4CZ Revision of Extraluminal Device in Lower Artery, Percutaneous Endoscopic Approach
04WY4DZ Revision of Intraluminal Device in Lower Artery, Percutaneous Endoscopic Approach
04WY4JZ Revision of Synthetic Substitute in Lower Artery, Percutaneous Endoscopic Approach
04WY4KZ Revision of Nonautologous Tissue Substitute in Lower Artery, Percutaneous Endoscopic Approach
04WYX0Z Revision of Drainage Device in Lower Artery, External Approach
04WYX2Z Revision of Monitoring Device in Lower Artery, External Approach
04WYX3Z Revision of Infusion Device in Lower Artery, External Approach
04WYX7Z Revision of Autologous Tissue Substitute in Lower Artery, External Approach
04WYXCZ Revision of Extraluminal Device in Lower Artery, External Approach
04WYXDZ Revision of Intraluminal Device in Lower Artery, External Approach
04WYXJZ Revision of Synthetic Substitute in Lower Artery, External Approach
04WYXKZ Revision of Nonautologous Tissue Substitute in Lower Artery, External Approach

Veins

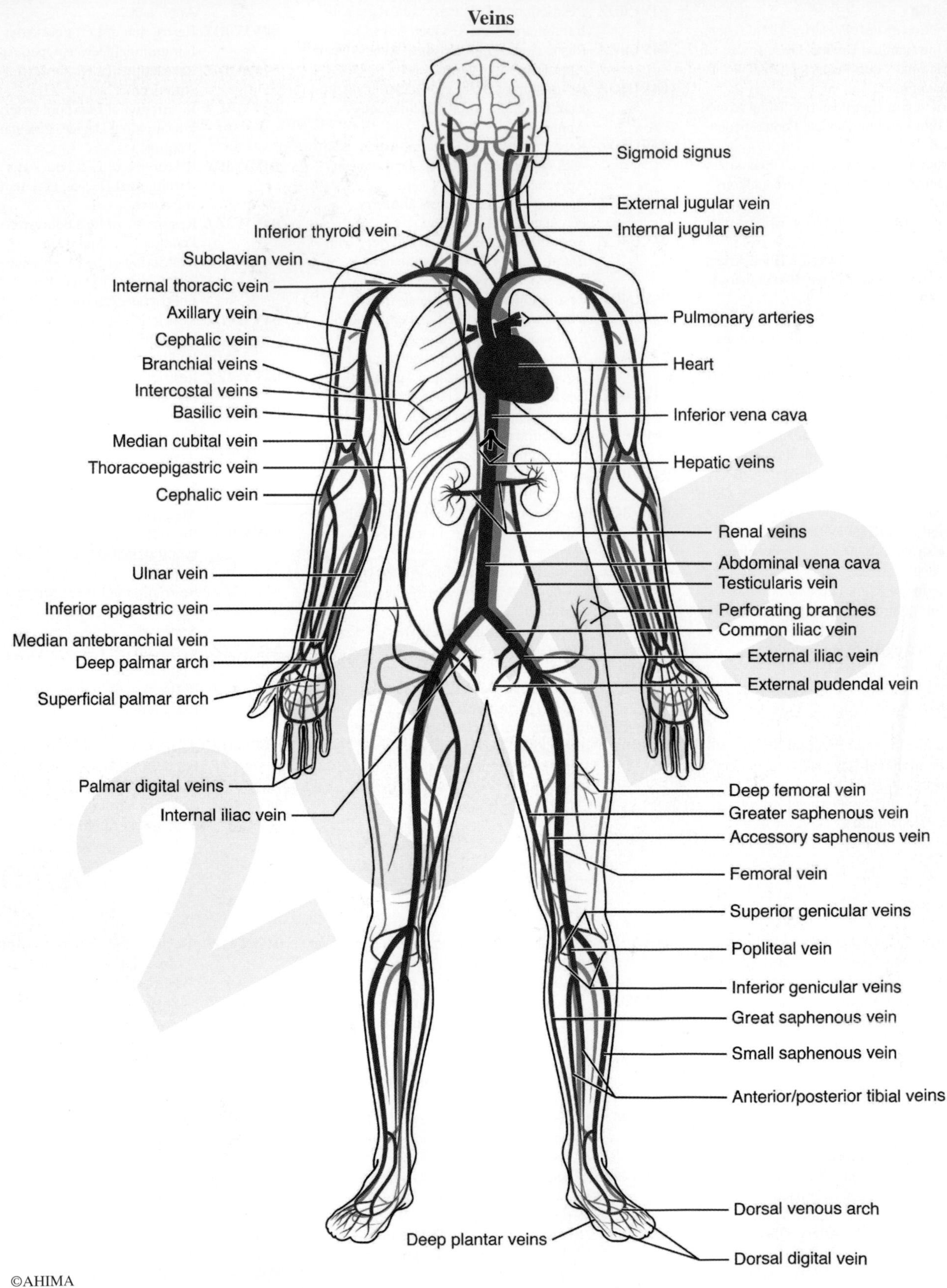
Sigmoid signus
External jugular vein
Internal jugular vein
Inferior thyroid vein
Subclavian vein
Internal thoracic vein
Axillary vein
Cephalic vein
Branchial veins
Intercostal veins
Basilic vein
Median cubital vein
Thoracoepigastric vein
Cephalic vein
Pulmonary arteries
Heart
Inferior vena cava
Hepatic veins
Renal veins
Abdominal vena cava
Testicularis vein
Perforating branches
Common iliac vein
External iliac vein
External pudendal vein
Ulnar vein
Inferior epigastric vein
Median antebranchial vein
Deep palmar arch
Superficial palmar arch
Palmar digital veins
Internal iliac vein
Deep femoral vein
Greater saphenous vein
Accessory saphenous vein
Femoral vein
Superior genicular veins
Popliteal vein
Inferior genicular veins
Great saphenous vein
Small saphenous vein
Anterior/posterior tibial veins
Dorsal venous arch
Deep plantar veins
Dorsal digital vein

Section	**0**	**Medical and Surgical**
Body System	**5**	**Upper Veins**
Operation	**1**	**Bypass:** Altering the route of passage of the contents of a tubular body part

Body Part (4th)	Approach (5th)	Device (6th)	Qualifier (7th)
0 Azygos Vein **1** Hemiazygos Vein **3** Innominate Vein, Right **4** Innominate Vein, Left **5** Subclavian Vein, Right **6** Subclavian Vein, Left **7** Axillary Vein, Right **8** Axillary Vein, Left **9** Brachial Vein, Right **A** Brachial Vein, Left **B** Basilic Vein, Right **C** Basilic Vein, Left **D** Cephalic Vein, Right **F** Cephalic Vein, Left **G** Hand Vein, Right **H** Hand Vein, Left **L** Intracranial Vein **M** Internal Jugular Vein, Right **N** Internal Jugular Vein, Left **P** External Jugular Vein, Right **Q** External Jugular Vein, Left **R** Vertebral Vein, Right **S** Vertebral Vein, Left **T** Face Vein, Right **V** Face Vein, Left	**0** Open **4** Percutaneous Endoscopic	**7** Autologous Tissue Substitute **9** Autologous Venous Tissue **A** Autologous Arterial Tissue **J** Synthetic Substitute **K** Nonautologous Tissue Substitute **Z** No Device	**Y** Upper Vein

Section	**0**	**Medical and Surgical**
Body System	**5**	**Upper Veins**
Operation	**5**	**Destruction:** Physical eradication of all or a portion of a body part by the direct use of energy, force, or a destructive agent

Body Part (4th)	Approach (5th)	Device (6th)	Qualifier (7th)
0 Azygos Vein **1** Hemiazygos Vein **3** Innominate Vein, Right **4** Innominate Vein, Left **5** Subclavian Vein, Right **6** Subclavian Vein, Left **7** Axillary Vein, Right **8** Axillary Vein, Left **9** Brachial Vein, Right **A** Brachial Vein, Left **B** Basilic Vein, Right **C** Basilic Vein, Left **D** Cephalic Vein, Right **F** Cephalic Vein, Left **G** Hand Vein, Right **H** Hand Vein, Left **L** Intracranial Vein **M** Internal Jugular Vein, Right **N** Internal Jugular Vein, Left **P** External Jugular Vein, Right **Q** External Jugular Vein, Left **R** Vertebral Vein, Right **S** Vertebral Vein, Left **T** Face Vein, Right **V** Face Vein, Left **Y** Upper Vein	**0** Open **3** Percutaneous **4** Percutaneous Endoscopic	**Z** No Device	**Z** No Qualifier

Section 0 Medical and Surgical
Body System 5 Upper Veins
Operation 7 **Dilation:** Expanding an orifice or the lumen of a tubular body part

Body Part (4th)	Approach (5th)	Device (6th)	Qualifier (7th)
0 Azygos Vein **1** Hemiazygos Vein **3** Innominate Vein, Right **4** Innominate Vein, Left **5** Subclavian Vein, Right **6** Subclavian Vein, Left **7** Axillary Vein, Right **8** Axillary Vein, Left **9** Brachial Vein, Right **A** Brachial Vein, Left **B** Basilic Vein, Right **C** Basilic Vein, Left **D** Cephalic Vein, Right **F** Cephalic Vein, Left **G** Hand Vein, Right **H** Hand Vein, Left **L** Intracranial Vein **M** Internal Jugular Vein, Right **N** Internal Jugular Vein, Left **P** External Jugular Vein, Right **Q** External Jugular Vein, Left **R** Vertebral Vein, Right **S** Vertebral Vein, Left **T** Face Vein, Right **V** Face Vein, Left **Y** Upper Vein	**0** Open **3** Percutaneous **4** Percutaneous Endoscopic	**D** Intraluminal Device **Z** No Device	**Z** No Qualifier

Section 0 Medical and Surgical
Body System 5 Upper Veins
Operation 9 **Drainage:** Taking or letting out fluids and/or gases from a body part

Body Part (4th)	Approach (5th)	Device (6th)	Qualifier (7th)
0 Azygos Vein **1** Hemiazygos Vein **3** Innominate Vein, Right **4** Innominate Vein, Left **5** Subclavian Vein, Right **6** Subclavian Vein, Left **7** Axillary Vein, Right **8** Axillary Vein, Left **9** Brachial Vein, Right **A** Brachial Vein, Left **B** Basilic Vein, Right **C** Basilic Vein, Left **D** Cephalic Vein, Right **F** Cephalic Vein, Left **G** Hand Vein, Right **H** Hand Vein, Left **L** Intracranial Vein **M** Internal Jugular Vein, Right **N** Internal Jugular Vein, Left **P** External Jugular Vein, Right **Q** External Jugular Vein, Left **R** Vertebral Vein, Right **S** Vertebral Vein, Left **T** Face Vein, Right **V** Face Vein, Left **Y** Upper Vein	**0** Open **3** Percutaneous **4** Percutaneous Endoscopic	**0** Drainage Device	**Z** No Qualifier

Continued →

Section 0 **Medical and Surgical**
Body System 5 **Upper Veins**
Operation 9 **Drainage:** Taking or letting out fluids and/or gases from a body part

Body Part (4th)	Approach (5th)	Device (6th)	Qualifier (7th)
0 Azygos Vein	**0** Open	**Z** No Device	**X** Diagnostic
1 Hemiazygos Vein	**3** Percutaneous		**Z** No Qualifier
3 Innominate Vein, Right	**4** Percutaneous Endoscopic		
4 Innominate Vein, Left			
5 Subclavian Vein, Right			
6 Subclavian Vein, Left			
7 Axillary Vein, Right			
8 Axillary Vein, Left			
9 Brachial Vein, Right			
A Brachial Vein, Left			
B Basilic Vein, Right			
C Basilic Vein, Left			
D Cephalic Vein, Right			
F Cephalic Vein, Left			
G Hand Vein, Right			
H Hand Vein, Left			
L Intracranial Vein			
M Internal Jugular Vein, Right			
N Internal Jugular Vein, Left			
P External Jugular Vein, Right			
Q External Jugular Vein, Left			
R Vertebral Vein, Right			
S Vertebral Vein, Left			
T Face Vein, Right			
V Face Vein, Left			
Y Upper Vein			

Section 0 **Medical and Surgical**
Body System 5 **Upper Veins**
Operation B **Excision:** Cutting out or off, without replacement, a portion of a body part

Body Part (4th)	Approach (5th)	Device (6th)	Qualifier (7th)
0 Azygos Vein	**0** Open	**Z** No Device	**X** Diagnostic
1 Hemiazygos Vein	**3** Percutaneous		**Z** No Qualifier
3 Innominate Vein, Right	**4** Percutaneous Endoscopic		
4 Innominate Vein, Left			
5 Subclavian Vein, Right			
6 Subclavian Vein, Left			
7 Axillary Vein, Right			
8 Axillary Vein, Left			
9 Brachial Vein, Right			
A Brachial Vein, Left			
B Basilic Vein, Right			
C Basilic Vein, Left			
D Cephalic Vein, Right			
F Cephalic Vein, Left			
G Hand Vein, Right			
H Hand Vein, Left			
L Intracranial Vein			
M Internal Jugular Vein, Right			
N Internal Jugular Vein, Left			
P External Jugular Vein, Right			
Q External Jugular Vein, Left			
R Vertebral Vein, Right			
S Vertebral Vein, Left			
T Face Vein, Right			
V Face Vein, Left			
Y Upper Vein			

Section 0 **Medical and Surgical**
Body System 5 **Upper Veins**
Operation C **Extirpation:** Taking or cutting out solid matter from a body part

Body Part (4th)	Approach (5th)	Device (6th)	Qualifier (7th)
0 Azygos Vein **1** Hemiazygos Vein **3** Innominate Vein, Right **4** Innominate Vein, Left **5** Subclavian Vein, Right **6** Subclavian Vein, Left **7** Axillary Vein, Right **8** Axillary Vein, Left **9** Brachial Vein, Right **A** Brachial Vein, Left **B** Basilic Vein, Right **C** Basilic Vein, Left **D** Cephalic Vein, Right **F** Cephalic Vein, Left **G** Hand Vein, Right **H** Hand Vein, Left **L** Intracranial Vein **M** Internal Jugular Vein, Right **N** Internal Jugular Vein, Left **P** External Jugular Vein, Right **Q** External Jugular Vein, Left **R** Vertebral Vein, Right **S** Vertebral Vein, Left **T** Face Vein, Right **V** Face Vein, Left **Y** Upper Vein	**0** Open **3** Percutaneous **4** Percutaneous Endoscopic	**Z** No Device	**Z** No Qualifier

Section 0 **Medical and Surgical**
Body System 5 **Upper Veins**
Operation D **Extraction:** Pulling or stripping out or off all or a portion of a body part by the use of force

Body Part (4th)	Approach (5th)	Device (6th)	Qualifier (7th)
9 Brachial Vein, Right **A** Brachial Vein, Left **B** Basilic Vein, Right **C** Basilic Vein, Left **D** Cephalic Vein, Right **F** Cephalic Vein, Left **G** Hand Vein, Right **H** Hand Vein, Left **Y** Upper Vein	**0** Open **3** Percutaneous	**Z** No Device	**Z** No Qualifier

Section 0 Medical and Surgical
Body System 5 Upper Veins
Operation H **Insertion:** Putting in a nonbiological appliance that monitors, assists, performs, or prevents a physiological function but does not physically take the place of a body part

Body Part (4th)	Approach (5th)	Device (6th)	Qualifier (7th)
0 Azygos Vein **1** Hemiazygos Vein **3** Innominate Vein, Right **4** Innominate Vein, Left **5** Subclavian Vein, Right **6** Subclavian Vein, Left **7** Axillary Vein, Right **8** Axillary Vein, Left **9** Brachial Vein, Right **A** Brachial Vein, Left **B** Basilic Vein, Right **C** Basilic Vein, Left **D** Cephalic Vein, Right **F** Cephalic Vein, Left **G** Hand Vein, Right **H** Hand Vein, Left **L** Intracranial Vein **M** Internal Jugular Vein, Right **N** Internal Jugular Vein, Left **P** External Jugular Vein, Right **Q** External Jugular Vein, Left **R** Vertebral Vein, Right **S** Vertebral Vein, Left **T** Face Vein, Right **V** Face Vein, Left	**0** Open **3** Percutaneous **4** Percutaneous Endoscopic	**3** Infusion Device **D** Intraluminal Device	**Z** No Qualifier
Y Upper Vein	**0** Open **3** Percutaneous **4** Percutaneous Endoscopic	**2** Monitoring Device **3** Infusion Device **D** Intraluminal Device	**Z** No Qualifier

Section 0 Medical and Surgical
Body System 5 Upper Veins
Operation J **Inspection:** Visually and/or manually exploring a body part

Body Part (4th)	Approach (5th)	Device (6th)	Qualifier (7th)
Y Upper Vein	**0** Open **3** Percutaneous **4** Percutaneous Endoscopic **X** External	**Z** No Device	**Z** No Qualifier

Section 0 **Medical and Surgical**
Body System 5 **Upper Veins**
Operation L **Occlusion:** Completely closing an orifice or the lumen of a tubular body part

Body Part (4th)	Approach (5th)	Device (6th)	Qualifier (7th)
0 Azygos Vein **1** Hemiazygos Vein **3** Innominate Vein, Right **4** Innominate Vein, Left **5** Subclavian Vein, Right **6** Subclavian Vein, Left **7** Axillary Vein, Right **8** Axillary Vein, Left **9** Brachial Vein, Right **A** Brachial Vein, Left **B** Basilic Vein, Right **C** Basilic Vein, Left **D** Cephalic Vein, Right **F** Cephalic Vein, Left **G** Hand Vein, Right **H** Hand Vein, Left **L** Intracranial Vein **M** Internal Jugular Vein, Right **N** Internal Jugular Vein, Left **P** External Jugular Vein, Right **Q** External Jugular Vein, Left **R** Vertebral Vein, Right **S** Vertebral Vein, Left **T** Face Vein, Right **V** Face Vein, Left **Y** Upper Vein	**0** Open **3** Percutaneous **4** Percutaneous Endoscopic	**C** Extraluminal Device **D** Intraluminal Device **Z** No Device	**Z** No Qualifier

Section 0 **Medical and Surgical**
Body System 5 **Upper Veins**
Operation N **Release:** Freeing a body part from an abnormal physical constraint by cutting or by the use of force

Body Part (4th)	Approach (5th)	Device (6th)	Qualifier (7th)
0 Azygos Vein **1** Hemiazygos Vein **3** Innominate Vein, Right **4** Innominate Vein, Left **5** Subclavian Vein, Right **6** Subclavian Vein, Left **7** Axillary Vein, Right **8** Axillary Vein, Left **9** Brachial Vein, Right **A** Brachial Vein, Left **B** Basilic Vein, Right **C** Basilic Vein, Left **D** Cephalic Vein, Right **F** Cephalic Vein, Left **G** Hand Vein, Right **H** Hand Vein, Left **L** Intracranial Vein **M** Internal Jugular Vein, Right **N** Internal Jugular Vein, Left **P** External Jugular Vein, Right **Q** External Jugular Vein, Left **R** Vertebral Vein, Right **S** Vertebral Vein, Left **T** Face Vein, Right **V** Face Vein, Left **Y** Upper Vein	**0** Open **3** Percutaneous **4** Percutaneous Endoscopic	**Z** No Device	**Z** No Qualifier

Section 0 Medical and Surgical
Body System 5 Upper Veins
Operation P **Removal:** Taking out or off a device from a body part

Body Part (4th)	Approach (5th)	Device (6th)	Qualifier (7th)
Y Upper Vein	**0** Open **3** Percutaneous **4** Percutaneous Endoscopic	**0** Drainage Device **2** Monitoring Device **3** Infusion Device **7** Autologous Tissue Substitute **C** Extraluminal Device **D** Intraluminal Device **J** Synthetic Substitute **K** Nonautologous Tissue Substitute	**Z** No Qualifier
Y Upper Vein	**X** External	**0** Drainage Device **2** Monitoring Device **3** Infusion Device **D** Intraluminal Device	**Z** No Qualifier

Section 0 Medical and Surgical
Body System 5 Upper Veins
Operation Q **Repair:** Restoring, to the extent possible, a body part to its normal anatomic structure and function

Body Part (4th)	Approach (5th)	Device (6th)	Qualifier (7th)
0 Azygos Vein **1** Hemiazygos Vein **3** Innominate Vein, Right **4** Innominate Vein, Left **5** Subclavian Vein, Right **6** Subclavian Vein, Left **7** Axillary Vein, Right **8** Axillary Vein, Left **9** Brachial Vein, Right **A** Brachial Vein, Left **B** Basilic Vein, Right **C** Basilic Vein, Left **D** Cephalic Vein, Right **F** Cephalic Vein, Left **G** Hand Vein, Right **H** Hand Vein, Left **L** Intracranial Vein **M** Internal Jugular Vein, Right **N** Internal Jugular Vein, Left **P** External Jugular Vein, Right **Q** External Jugular Vein, Left **R** Vertebral Vein, Right **S** Vertebral Vein, Left **T** Face Vein, Right **V** Face Vein, Left **Y** Upper Vein	**0** Open **3** Percutaneous **4** Percutaneous Endoscopic	**Z** No Device	**Z** No Qualifier

Section 0 **Medical and Surgical**
Body System 5 **Upper Veins**
Operation R **Replacement:** Putting in or on biological or synthetic material that physically takes the place and/or function of all or a portion of a body part

Body Part (4th)	Approach (5th)	Device (6th)	Qualifier (7th)
0 Azygos Vein 1 Hemiazygos Vein 3 Innominate Vein, Right 4 Innominate Vein, Left 5 Subclavian Vein, Right 6 Subclavian Vein, Left 7 Axillary Vein, Right 8 Axillary Vein, Left 9 Brachial Vein, Right A Brachial Vein, Left B Basilic Vein, Right C Basilic Vein, Left D Cephalic Vein, Right F Cephalic Vein, Left G Hand Vein, Right H Hand Vein, Left L Intracranial Vein M Internal Jugular Vein, Right N Internal Jugular Vein, Left P External Jugular Vein, Right Q External Jugular Vein, Left R Vertebral Vein, Right S Vertebral Vein, Left T Face Vein, Right V Face Vein, Left Y Upper Vein	0 Open 4 Percutaneous Endoscopic	7 Autologous Tissue Substitute J Synthetic Substitute K Nonautologous Tissue Substitute	Z No Qualifier

Section 0 **Medical and Surgical**
Body System 5 **Upper Veins**
Operation S **Reposition:** Moving to its normal location, or other suitable location, all or a portion of a body part

Body Part (4th)	Approach (5th)	Device (6th)	Qualifier (7th)
0 Azygos Vein 1 Hemiazygos Vein 3 Innominate Vein, Right 4 Innominate Vein, Left 5 Subclavian Vein, Right 6 Subclavian Vein, Left 7 Axillary Vein, Right 8 Axillary Vein, Left 9 Brachial Vein, Right A Brachial Vein, Left B Basilic Vein, Right C Basilic Vein, Left D Cephalic Vein, Right F Cephalic Vein, Left G Hand Vein, Right H Hand Vein, Left L Intracranial Vein M Internal Jugular Vein, Right N Internal Jugular Vein, Left P External Jugular Vein, Right Q External Jugular Vein, Left R Vertebral Vein, Right S Vertebral Vein, Left T Face Vein, Right V Face Vein, Left Y Upper Vein	0 Open 3 Percutaneous 4 Percutaneous Endoscopic	Z No Device	Z No Qualifier

Section 0 **Medical and Surgical**
Body System 5 **Upper Veins**
Operation U **Supplement:** Putting in or on biological or synthetic material that physically reinforces and/or augments the function of a portion of a body part

Body Part (4th)	Approach (5th)	Device (6th)	Qualifier (7th)
0 Azygos Vein **1** Hemiazygos Vein **3** Innominate Vein, Right **4** Innominate Vein, Left **5** Subclavian Vein, Right **6** Subclavian Vein, Left **7** Axillary Vein, Right **8** Axillary Vein, Left **9** Brachial Vein, Right **A** Brachial Vein, Left **B** Basilic Vein, Right **C** Basilic Vein, Left **D** Cephalic Vein, Right **F** Cephalic Vein, Left **G** Hand Vein, Right **H** Hand Vein, Left **L** Intracranial Vein **M** Internal Jugular Vein, Right **N** Internal Jugular Vein, Left **P** External Jugular Vein, Right **Q** External Jugular Vein, Left **R** Vertebral Vein, Right **S** Vertebral Vein, Left **T** Face Vein, Right **V** Face Vein, Left **Y** Upper Vein	**0** Open **3** Percutaneous **4** Percutaneous Endoscopic	**7** Autologous Tissue Substitute **J** Synthetic Substitute **K** Nonautologous Tissue Substitute	**Z** No Qualifier

Section 0 **Medical and Surgical**
Body System 5 **Upper Veins**
Operation V **Restriction:** Partially closing an orifice or the lumen of a tubular body part

Body Part (4th)	Approach (5th)	Device (6th)	Qualifier (7th)
0 Azygos Vein **1** Hemiazygos Vein **3** Innominate Vein, Right **4** Innominate Vein, Left **5** Subclavian Vein, Right **6** Subclavian Vein, Left **7** Axillary Vein, Right **8** Axillary Vein, Left **9** Brachial Vein, Right **A** Brachial Vein, Left **B** Basilic Vein, Right **C** Basilic Vein, Left **D** Cephalic Vein, Right **F** Cephalic Vein, Left **G** Hand Vein, Right **H** Hand Vein, Left **L** Intracranial Vein **M** Internal Jugular Vein, Right **N** Internal Jugular Vein, Left **P** External Jugular Vein, Right **Q** External Jugular Vein, Left **R** Vertebral Vein, Right **S** Vertebral Vein, Left **T** Face Vein, Right **V** Face Vein, Left **Y** Upper Vein	**0** Open **3** Percutaneous **4** Percutaneous Endoscopic	**C** Extraluminal Device **D** Intraluminal Device **Z** No Device	**Z** No Qualifier

Section 0 **Medical and Surgical**
Body System 5 **Upper Veins**
Operation W **Revision:** Correcting, to the extent possible, a portion of a malfunctioning device or the position of a displaced device

Body Part (4th)	Approach (5th)	Device (6th)	Qualifier (7th)
Y Upper Vein	0 Open 3 Percutaneous 4 Percutaneous Endoscopic X External	0 Drainage Device 2 Monitoring Device 3 Infusion Device 7 Autologous Tissue Substitute C Extraluminal Device D Intraluminal Device J Synthetic Substitute K Nonautologous Tissue Substitute	Z No Qualifier

Upper Veins Code Listing 051–05W

051 – Upper Veins, Bypass

Review Coding Guideline B3.6a

051007Y Bypass Azygos Vein to Upper Vein with Autologous Tissue Substitute, Open Approach
051009Y Bypass Azygos Vein to Upper Vein with Autologous Venous Tissue, Open Approach
05100AY Bypass Azygos Vein to Upper Vein with Autologous Arterial Tissue, Open Approach
05100JY Bypass Azygos Vein to Upper Vein with Synthetic Substitute, Open Approach
05100KY Bypass Azygos Vein to Upper Vein with Nonautologous Tissue Substitute, Open Approach
05100ZY Bypass Azygos Vein to Upper Vein, Open Approach
051047Y Bypass Azygos Vein to Upper Vein with Autologous Tissue Substitute, Percutaneous Endoscopic Approach
051049Y Bypass Azygos Vein to Upper Vein with Autologous Venous Tissue, Percutaneous Endoscopic Approach
05104AY Bypass Azygos Vein to Upper Vein with Autologous Arterial Tissue, Percutaneous Endoscopic Approach
05104JY Bypass Azygos Vein to Upper Vein with Synthetic Substitute, Percutaneous Endoscopic Approach
05104KY Bypass Azygos Vein to Upper Vein with Nonautologous Tissue Substitute, Percutaneous Endoscopic Approach
05104ZY Bypass Azygos Vein to Upper Vein, Percutaneous Endoscopic Approach
051107Y Bypass Hemiazygos Vein to Upper Vein with Autologous Tissue Substitute, Open Approach
051109Y Bypass Hemiazygos Vein to Upper Vein with Autologous Venous Tissue, Open Approach
05110AY Bypass Hemiazygos Vein to Upper Vein with Autologous Arterial Tissue, Open Approach
05110JY Bypass Hemiazygos Vein to Upper Vein with Synthetic Substitute, Open Approach
05110KY Bypass Hemiazygos Vein to Upper Vein with Nonautologous Tissue Substitute, Open Approach
05110ZY Bypass Hemiazygos Vein to Upper Vein, Open Approach
051147Y Bypass Hemiazygos Vein to Upper Vein with Autologous Tissue Substitute, Percutaneous Endoscopic Approach
051149Y Bypass Hemiazygos Vein to Upper Vein with Autologous Venous Tissue, Percutaneous Endoscopic Approach
05114AY Bypass Hemiazygos Vein to Upper Vein with Autologous Arterial Tissue, Percutaneous Endoscopic Approach
05114JY Bypass Hemiazygos Vein to Upper Vein with Synthetic Substitute, Percutaneous Endoscopic Approach
05114KY Bypass Hemiazygos Vein to Upper Vein with Nonautologous Tissue Substitute, Percutaneous Endoscopic Approach
05114ZY Bypass Hemiazygos Vein to Upper Vein, Percutaneous Endoscopic Approach
051307Y Bypass Right Innominate Vein to Upper Vein with Autologous Tissue Substitute, Open Approach
051309Y Bypass Right Innominate Vein to Upper Vein with Autologous Venous Tissue, Open Approach
05130AY Bypass Right Innominate Vein to Upper Vein with Autologous Arterial Tissue, Open Approach
05130JY Bypass Right Innominate Vein to Upper Vein with Synthetic Substitute, Open Approach
05130KY Bypass Right Innominate Vein to Upper Vein with Nonautologous Tissue Substitute, Open Approach
05130ZY Bypass Right Innominate Vein to Upper Vein, Open Approach
051347Y Bypass Right Innominate Vein to Upper Vein with Autologous Tissue Substitute, Percutaneous Endoscopic Approach
051349Y Bypass Right Innominate Vein to Upper Vein with Autologous Venous Tissue, Percutaneous Endoscopic Approach
05134AY Bypass Right Innominate Vein to Upper Vein with Autologous Arterial Tissue, Percutaneous Endoscopic Approach
05134JY Bypass Right Innominate Vein to Upper Vein with Synthetic Substitute, Percutaneous Endoscopic Approach
05134KY Bypass Right Innominate Vein to Upper Vein with Nonautologous Tissue Substitute, Percutaneous Endoscopic Approach
05134ZY Bypass Right Innominate Vein to Upper Vein, Percutaneous Endoscopic Approach
051407Y Bypass Left Innominate Vein to Upper Vein with Autologous Tissue Substitute, Open Approach
051409Y Bypass Left Innominate Vein to Upper Vein with Autologous Venous Tissue, Open Approach
05140AY Bypass Left Innominate Vein to Upper Vein with Autologous Arterial Tissue, Open Approach
05140JY Bypass Left Innominate Vein to Upper Vein with Synthetic Substitute, Open Approach
05140KY Bypass Left Innominate Vein to Upper Vein with Nonautologous Tissue Substitute, Open Approach
05140ZY Bypass Left Innominate Vein to Upper Vein, Open Approach
051447Y Bypass Left Innominate Vein to Upper Vein with Autologous Tissue Substitute, Percutaneous Endoscopic Approach
051449Y Bypass Left Innominate Vein to Upper Vein with Autologous Venous Tissue, Percutaneous Endoscopic Approach
05144AY Bypass Left Innominate Vein to Upper Vein with Autologous Arterial Tissue, Percutaneous Endoscopic Approach
05144JY Bypass Left Innominate Vein to Upper Vein with Synthetic Substitute, Percutaneous Endoscopic Approach
05144KY Bypass Left Innominate Vein to Upper Vein with Nonautologous Tissue Substitute, Percutaneous Endoscopic Approach
05144ZY Bypass Left Innominate Vein to Upper Vein, Percutaneous Endoscopic Approach
051507Y Bypass Right Subclavian Vein to Upper Vein with Autologous Tissue Substitute, Open Approach
051509Y Bypass Right Subclavian Vein to Upper Vein with Autologous Venous Tissue, Open Approach
05150AY Bypass Right Subclavian Vein to Upper Vein with Autologous Arterial Tissue, Open Approach
05150JY Bypass Right Subclavian Vein to Upper Vein with Synthetic Substitute, Open Approach
05150KY Bypass Right Subclavian Vein to Upper Vein with Nonautologous Tissue Substitute, Open Approach
05150ZY Bypass Right Subclavian Vein to Upper Vein, Open Approach
051547Y Bypass Right Subclavian Vein to Upper Vein with Autologous Tissue Substitute, Percutaneous Endoscopic Approach
051549Y Bypass Right Subclavian Vein to Upper Vein with Autologous Venous Tissue, Percutaneous Endoscopic Approach
05154AY Bypass Right Subclavian Vein to Upper Vein with Autologous Arterial Tissue, Percutaneous Endoscopic Approach
05154JY Bypass Right Subclavian Vein to Upper Vein with Synthetic Substitute, Percutaneous Endoscopic Approach

5154KY Bypass Right Subclavian Vein to Upper Vein with Nonautologous Tissue Substitute, Percutaneous Endoscopic Approach

5154ZY Bypass Right Subclavian Vein to Upper Vein, Percutaneous Endoscopic Approach

51607Y Bypass Left Subclavian Vein to Upper Vein with Autologous Tissue Substitute, Open Approach

51609Y Bypass Left Subclavian Vein to Upper Vein with Autologous Venous Tissue, Open Approach

5160AY Bypass Left Subclavian Vein to Upper Vein with Autologous Arterial Tissue, Open Approach

5160JY Bypass Left Subclavian Vein to Upper Vein with Synthetic Substitute, Open Approach

5160KY Bypass Left Subclavian Vein to Upper Vein with Nonautologous Tissue Substitute, Open Approach

5160ZY Bypass Left Subclavian Vein to Upper Vein, Open Approach

51647Y Bypass Left Subclavian Vein to Upper Vein with Autologous Tissue Substitute, Percutaneous Endoscopic Approach

51649Y Bypass Left Subclavian Vein to Upper Vein with Autologous Venous Tissue, Percutaneous Endoscopic Approach

5164AY Bypass Left Subclavian Vein to Upper Vein with Autologous Arterial Tissue, Percutaneous Endoscopic Approach

5164JY Bypass Left Subclavian Vein to Upper Vein with Synthetic Substitute, Percutaneous Endoscopic Approach

5164KY Bypass Left Subclavian Vein to Upper Vein with Nonautologous Tissue Substitute, Percutaneous Endoscopic Approach

5164ZY Bypass Left Subclavian Vein to Upper Vein, Percutaneous Endoscopic Approach

51707Y Bypass Right Axillary Vein to Upper Vein with Autologous Tissue Substitute, Open Approach

51709Y Bypass Right Axillary Vein to Upper Vein with Autologous Venous Tissue, Open Approach

5170AY Bypass Right Axillary Vein to Upper Vein with Autologous Arterial Tissue, Open Approach

5170JY Bypass Right Axillary Vein to Upper Vein with Synthetic Substitute, Open Approach

5170KY Bypass Right Axillary Vein to Upper Vein with Nonautologous Tissue Substitute, Open Approach

5170ZY Bypass Right Axillary Vein to Upper Vein, Open Approach

51747Y Bypass Right Axillary Vein to Upper Vein with Autologous Tissue Substitute, Percutaneous Endoscopic Approach

051749Y Bypass Right Axillary Vein to Upper Vein with Autologous Venous Tissue, Percutaneous Endoscopic Approach

05174AY Bypass Right Axillary Vein to Upper Vein with Autologous Arterial Tissue, Percutaneous Endoscopic Approach

05174JY Bypass Right Axillary Vein to Upper Vein with Synthetic Substitute, Percutaneous Endoscopic Approach

05174KY Bypass Right Axillary Vein to Upper Vein with Nonautologous Tissue Substitute, Percutaneous Endoscopic Approach

05174ZY Bypass Right Axillary Vein to Upper Vein, Percutaneous Endoscopic Approach

051807Y Bypass Left Axillary Vein to Upper Vein with Autologous Tissue Substitute, Open Approach

051809Y Bypass Left Axillary Vein to Upper Vein with Autologous Venous Tissue, Open Approach

05180AY Bypass Left Axillary Vein to Upper Vein with Autologous Arterial Tissue, Open Approach

05180JY Bypass Left Axillary Vein to Upper Vein with Synthetic Substitute, Open Approach

05180KY Bypass Left Axillary Vein to Upper Vein with Nonautologous Tissue Substitute, Open Approach

05180ZY Bypass Left Axillary Vein to Upper Vein, Open Approach

051847Y Bypass Left Axillary Vein to Upper Vein with Autologous Tissue Substitute, Percutaneous Endoscopic Approach

051849Y Bypass Left Axillary Vein to Upper Vein with Autologous Venous Tissue, Percutaneous Endoscopic Approach

05184AY Bypass Left Axillary Vein to Upper Vein with Autologous Arterial Tissue, Percutaneous Endoscopic Approach

05184JY Bypass Left Axillary Vein to Upper Vein with Synthetic Substitute, Percutaneous Endoscopic Approach

05184KY Bypass Left Axillary Vein to Upper Vein with Nonautologous Tissue Substitute, Percutaneous Endoscopic Approach

05184ZY Bypass Left Axillary Vein to Upper Vein, Percutaneous Endoscopic Approach

051907Y Bypass Right Brachial Vein to Upper Vein with Autologous Tissue Substitute, Open Approach

051909Y Bypass Right Brachial Vein to Upper Vein with Autologous Venous Tissue, Open Approach

05190AY Bypass Right Brachial Vein to Upper Vein with Autologous Arterial Tissue, Open Approach

05190JY Bypass Right Brachial Vein to Upper Vein with Synthetic Substitute, Open Approach

05190KY Bypass Right Brachial Vein to Upper Vein with Nonautologous Tissue Substitute, Open Approach

05190ZY Bypass Right Brachial Vein to Upper Vein, Open Approach

051947Y Bypass Right Brachial Vein to Upper Vein with Autologous Tissue Substitute, Percutaneous Endoscopic Approach

051949Y Bypass Right Brachial Vein to Upper Vein with Autologous Venous Tissue, Percutaneous Endoscopic Approach

05194AY Bypass Right Brachial Vein to Upper Vein with Autologous Arterial Tissue, Percutaneous Endoscopic Approach

05194JY Bypass Right Brachial Vein to Upper Vein with Synthetic Substitute, Percutaneous Endoscopic Approach

05194KY Bypass Right Brachial Vein to Upper Vein with Nonautologous Tissue Substitute, Percutaneous Endoscopic Approach

05194ZY Bypass Right Brachial Vein to Upper Vein, Percutaneous Endoscopic Approach

051A07Y Bypass Left Brachial Vein to Upper Vein with Autologous Tissue Substitute, Open Approach

051A09Y Bypass Left Brachial Vein to Upper Vein with Autologous Venous Tissue, Open Approach

051A0AY Bypass Left Brachial Vein to Upper Vein with Autologous Arterial Tissue, Open Approach

051A0JY Bypass Left Brachial Vein to Upper Vein with Synthetic Substitute, Open Approach

051A0KY Bypass Left Brachial Vein to Upper Vein with Nonautologous Tissue Substitute, Open Approach

051A0ZY Bypass Left Brachial Vein to Upper Vein, Open Approach

051A47Y Bypass Left Brachial Vein to Upper Vein with Autologous Tissue Substitute, Percutaneous Endoscopic Approach

051A49Y Bypass Left Brachial Vein to Upper Vein with Autologous Venous Tissue, Percutaneous Endoscopic Approach

051A4AY Bypass Left Brachial Vein to Upper Vein with Autologous Arterial Tissue, Percutaneous Endoscopic Approach

051A4JY Bypass Left Brachial Vein to Upper Vein with Synthetic Substitute, Percutaneous Endoscopic Approach

051A4KY Bypass Left Brachial Vein to Upper Vein with Nonautologous Tissue Substitute, Percutaneous Endoscopic Approach

051A4ZY Bypass Left Brachial Vein to Upper Vein, Percutaneous Endoscopic Approach

051B07Y Bypass Right Basilic Vein to Upper Vein with Autologous Tissue Substitute, Open Approach

051B09Y Bypass Right Basilic Vein to Upper Vein with Autologous Venous Tissue, Open Approach

051B0AY Bypass Right Basilic Vein to Upper Vein with Autologous Arterial Tissue, Open Approach

051B0JY Bypass Right Basilic Vein to Upper Vein with Synthetic Substitute, Open Approach

051B0KY Bypass Right Basilic Vein to Upper Vein with Nonautologous Tissue Substitute, Open Approach

051B0ZY Bypass Right Basilic Vein to Upper Vein, Open Approach

051B47Y Bypass Right Basilic Vein to Upper Vein with Autologous Tissue Substitute, Percutaneous Endoscopic Approach

051B49Y Bypass Right Basilic Vein to Upper Vein with Autologous Venous Tissue, Percutaneous Endoscopic Approach

051B4AY Bypass Right Basilic Vein to Upper Vein with Autologous Arterial Tissue, Percutaneous Endoscopic Approach

051B4JY Bypass Right Basilic Vein to Upper Vein with Synthetic Substitute, Percutaneous Endoscopic Approach

051B4KY Bypass Right Basilic Vein to Upper Vein with Nonautologous Tissue Substitute, Percutaneous Endoscopic Approach

051B4ZY Bypass Right Basilic Vein to Upper Vein, Percutaneous Endoscopic Approach

051C07Y Bypass Left Basilic Vein to Upper Vein with Autologous Tissue Substitute, Open Approach

051C09Y Bypass Left Basilic Vein to Upper Vein with Autologous Venous Tissue, Open Approach

051C0AY Bypass Left Basilic Vein to Upper Vein with Autologous Arterial Tissue, Open Approach

051C0JY Bypass Left Basilic Vein to Upper Vein with Synthetic Substitute, Open Approach

051C0KY Bypass Left Basilic Vein to Upper Vein with Nonautologous Tissue Substitute, Open Approach

051C0ZY Bypass Left Basilic Vein to Upper Vein, Open Approach

051C47Y Bypass Left Basilic Vein to Upper Vein with Autologous Tissue Substitute, Percutaneous Endoscopic Approach

051C49Y Bypass Left Basilic Vein to Upper Vein with Autologous Venous Tissue, Percutaneous Endoscopic Approach

051C4AY Bypass Left Basilic Vein to Upper Vein with Autologous Arterial Tissue, Percutaneous Endoscopic Approach

051C4JY Bypass Left Basilic Vein to Upper Vein with Synthetic Substitute, Percutaneous Endoscopic Approach

051C4KY Bypass Left Basilic Vein to Upper Vein with Nonautologous Tissue Substitute, Percutaneous Endoscopic Approach
051C4ZY Bypass Left Basilic Vein to Upper Vein, Percutaneous Endoscopic Approach
051D07Y Bypass Right Cephalic Vein to Upper Vein with Autologous Tissue Substitute, Open Approach
051D09Y Bypass Right Cephalic Vein to Upper Vein with Autologous Venous Tissue, Open Approach
051D0AY Bypass Right Cephalic Vein to Upper Vein with Autologous Arterial Tissue, Open Approach
051D0JY Bypass Right Cephalic Vein to Upper Vein with Synthetic Substitute, Open Approach
051D0KY Bypass Right Cephalic Vein to Upper Vein with Nonautologous Tissue Substitute, Open Approach
051D0ZY Bypass Right Cephalic Vein to Upper Vein, Open Approach
051D47Y Bypass Right Cephalic Vein to Upper Vein with Autologous Tissue Substitute, Percutaneous Endoscopic Approach
051D49Y Bypass Right Cephalic Vein to Upper Vein with Autologous Venous Tissue, Percutaneous Endoscopic Approach
051D4AY Bypass Right Cephalic Vein to Upper Vein with Autologous Arterial Tissue, Percutaneous Endoscopic Approach
051D4JY Bypass Right Cephalic Vein to Upper Vein with Synthetic Substitute, Percutaneous Endoscopic Approach
051D4KY Bypass Right Cephalic Vein to Upper Vein with Nonautologous Tissue Substitute, Percutaneous Endoscopic Approach
051D4ZY Bypass Right Cephalic Vein to Upper Vein, Percutaneous Endoscopic Approach
051F07Y Bypass Left Cephalic Vein to Upper Vein with Autologous Tissue Substitute, Open Approach
051F09Y Bypass Left Cephalic Vein to Upper Vein with Autologous Venous Tissue, Open Approach
051F0AY Bypass Left Cephalic Vein to Upper Vein with Autologous Arterial Tissue, Open Approach
051F0JY Bypass Left Cephalic Vein to Upper Vein with Synthetic Substitute, Open Approach
051F0KY Bypass Left Cephalic Vein to Upper Vein with Nonautologous Tissue Substitute, Open Approach
051F0ZY Bypass Left Cephalic Vein to Upper Vein, Open Approach
051F47Y Bypass Left Cephalic Vein to Upper Vein with Autologous Tissue Substitute, Percutaneous Endoscopic Approach
051F49Y Bypass Left Cephalic Vein to Upper Vein with Autologous Venous Tissue, Percutaneous Endoscopic Approach
051F4AY Bypass Left Cephalic Vein to Upper Vein with Autologous Arterial Tissue, Percutaneous Endoscopic Approach
051F4JY Bypass Left Cephalic Vein to Upper Vein with Synthetic Substitute, Percutaneous Endoscopic Approach
051F4KY Bypass Left Cephalic Vein to Upper Vein with Nonautologous Tissue Substitute, Percutaneous Endoscopic Approach
051F4ZY Bypass Left Cephalic Vein to Upper Vein, Percutaneous Endoscopic Approach
051G07Y Bypass Right Hand Vein to Upper Vein with Autologous Tissue Substitute, Open Approach
051G09Y Bypass Right Hand Vein to Upper Vein with Autologous Venous Tissue, Open Approach
051G0AY Bypass Right Hand Vein to Upper Vein with Autologous Arterial Tissue, Open Approach
051G0JY Bypass Right Hand Vein to Upper Vein with Synthetic Substitute, Open Approach
051G0KY Bypass Right Hand Vein to Upper Vein with Nonautologous Tissue Substitute, Open Approach
051G0ZY Bypass Right Hand Vein to Upper Vein, Open Approach
051G47Y Bypass Right Hand Vein to Upper Vein with Autologous Tissue Substitute, Percutaneous Endoscopic Approach
051G49Y Bypass Right Hand Vein to Upper Vein with Autologous Venous Tissue, Percutaneous Endoscopic Approach
051G4AY Bypass Right Hand Vein to Upper Vein with Autologous Arterial Tissue, Percutaneous Endoscopic Approach
051G4JY Bypass Right Hand Vein to Upper Vein with Synthetic Substitute, Percutaneous Endoscopic Approach
051G4KY Bypass Right Hand Vein to Upper Vein with Nonautologous Tissue Substitute, Percutaneous Endoscopic Approach
051G4ZY Bypass Right Hand Vein to Upper Vein, Percutaneous Endoscopic Approach
051H07Y Bypass Left Hand Vein to Upper Vein with Autologous Tissue Substitute, Open Approach
051H09Y Bypass Left Hand Vein to Upper Vein with Autologous Venous Tissue, Open Approach
051H0AY Bypass Left Hand Vein to Upper Vein with Autologous Arterial Tissue, Open Approach
051H0JY Bypass Left Hand Vein to Upper Vein with Synthetic Substitute, Open Approach
051H0KY Bypass Left Hand Vein to Upper Vein with Nonautologous Tissue Substitute, Open Approach
051H0ZY Bypass Left Hand Vein to Upper Vein, Open Approach
051H47Y Bypass Left Hand Vein to Upper Vein with Autologous Tissue Substitute, Percutaneous Endoscopic Approach
051H49Y Bypass Left Hand Vein to Upper Vein with Autologous Venous Tissue, Percutaneous Endoscopic Approach
051H4AY Bypass Left Hand Vein to Upper Vein with Autologous Arterial Tissue, Percutaneous Endoscopic Approach
051H4JY Bypass Left Hand Vein to Upper Vein with Synthetic Substitute, Percutaneous Endoscopic Approach
051H4KY Bypass Left Hand Vein to Upper Vein with Nonautologous Tissue Substitute, Percutaneous Endoscopic Approach
051H4ZY Bypass Left Hand Vein to Upper Vein, Percutaneous Endoscopic Approach
051L07Y Bypass Intracranial Vein to Upper Vein with Autologous Tissue Substitute, Open Approach
051L09Y Bypass Intracranial Vein to Upper Vein with Autologous Venous Tissue, Open Approach
051L0AY Bypass Intracranial Vein to Upper Vein with Autologous Arterial Tissue, Open Approach
051L0JY Bypass Intracranial Vein to Upper Vein with Synthetic Substitute, Open Approach
051L0KY Bypass Intracranial Vein to Upper Vein with Nonautologous Tissue Substitute, Open Approach
051L0ZY Bypass Intracranial Vein to Upper Vein, Open Approach
051L47Y Bypass Intracranial Vein to Upper Vein with Autologous Tissue Substitute, Percutaneous Endoscopic Approach
051L49Y Bypass Intracranial Vein to Upper Vein with Autologous Venous Tissue, Percutaneous Endoscopic Approach
051L4AY Bypass Intracranial Vein to Upper Vein with Autologous Arterial Tissue, Percutaneous Endoscopic Approach
051L4JY Bypass Intracranial Vein to Upper Vein with Synthetic Substitute, Percutaneous Endoscopic Approach
051L4KY Bypass Intracranial Vein to Upper Vein with Nonautologous Tissue Substitute, Percutaneous Endoscopic Approach
051L4ZY Bypass Intracranial Vein to Upper Vein, Percutaneous Endoscopic Approach
051M07Y Bypass Right Internal Jugular Vein to Upper Vein with Autologous Tissue Substitute, Open Approach
051M09Y Bypass Right Internal Jugular Vein to Upper Vein with Autologous Venous Tissue, Open Approach
051M0AY Bypass Right Internal Jugular Vein to Upper Vein with Autologous Arterial Tissue, Open Approach
051M0JY Bypass Right Internal Jugular Vein to Upper Vein with Synthetic Substitute, Open Approach
051M0KY Bypass Right Internal Jugular Vein to Upper Vein with Nonautologous Tissue Substitute, Open Approach
051M0ZY Bypass Right Internal Jugular Vein to Upper Vein, Open Approach
051M47Y Bypass Right Internal Jugular Vein to Upper Vein with Autologous Tissue Substitute, Percutaneous Endoscopic Approach
051M49Y Bypass Right Internal Jugular Vein to Upper Vein with Autologous Venous Tissue, Percutaneous Endoscopic Approach
051M4AY Bypass Right Internal Jugular Vein to Upper Vein with Autologous Arterial Tissue, Percutaneous Endoscopic Approach
051M4JY Bypass Right Internal Jugular Vein to Upper Vein with Synthetic Substitute, Percutaneous Endoscopic Approach
051M4KY Bypass Right Internal Jugular Vein to Upper Vein with Nonautologous Tissue Substitute, Percutaneous Endoscopic Approach
051M4ZY Bypass Right Internal Jugular Vein to Upper Vein, Percutaneous Endoscopic Approach
051N07Y Bypass Left Internal Jugular Vein to Upper Vein with Autologous Tissue Substitute, Open Approach
051N09Y Bypass Left Internal Jugular Vein to Upper Vein with Autologous Venous Tissue, Open Approach
051N0AY Bypass Left Internal Jugular Vein to Upper Vein with Autologous Arterial Tissue, Open Approach
051N0JY Bypass Left Internal Jugular Vein to Upper Vein with Synthetic Substitute, Open Approach
051N0KY Bypass Left Internal Jugular Vein to Upper Vein with Nonautologous Tissue Substitute, Open Approach
051N0ZY Bypass Left Internal Jugular Vein to Upper Vein, Open Approach
051N47Y Bypass Left Internal Jugular Vein to Upper Vein with Autologous Tissue Substitute, Percutaneous Endoscopic Approach

1N49Y Bypass Left Internal Jugular Vein to Upper Vein with Autologous Venous Tissue, Percutaneous Endoscopic Approach

1N4AY Bypass Left Internal Jugular Vein to Upper Vein with Autologous Arterial Tissue, Percutaneous Endoscopic Approach

1N4JY Bypass Left Internal Jugular Vein to Upper Vein with Synthetic Substitute, Percutaneous Endoscopic Approach

1N4KY Bypass Left Internal Jugular Vein to Upper Vein with Nonautologous Tissue Substitute, Percutaneous Endoscopic Approach

1N4ZY Bypass Left Internal Jugular Vein to Upper Vein, Percutaneous Endoscopic Approach

51P07Y Bypass Right External Jugular Vein to Upper Vein with Autologous Tissue Substitute, Open Approach

51P09Y Bypass Right External Jugular Vein to Upper Vein with Autologous Venous Tissue, Open Approach

51P0AY Bypass Right External Jugular Vein to Upper Vein with Autologous Arterial Tissue, Open Approach

51P0JY Bypass Right External Jugular Vein to Upper Vein with Synthetic Substitute, Open Approach

51P0KY Bypass Right External Jugular Vein to Upper Vein with Nonautologous Tissue Substitute, Open Approach

51P0ZY Bypass Right External Jugular Vein to Upper Vein, Open Approach

51P47Y Bypass Right External Jugular Vein to Upper Vein with Autologous Tissue Substitute, Percutaneous Endoscopic Approach

51P49Y Bypass Right External Jugular Vein to Upper Vein with Autologous Venous Tissue, Percutaneous Endoscopic Approach

51P4AY Bypass Right External Jugular Vein to Upper Vein with Autologous Arterial Tissue, Percutaneous Endoscopic Approach

51P4JY Bypass Right External Jugular Vein to Upper Vein with Synthetic Substitute, Percutaneous Endoscopic Approach

51P4KY Bypass Right External Jugular Vein to Upper Vein with Nonautologous Tissue Substitute, Percutaneous Endoscopic Approach

51P4ZY Bypass Right External Jugular Vein to Upper Vein, Percutaneous Endoscopic Approach

51Q07Y Bypass Left External Jugular Vein to Upper Vein with Autologous Tissue Substitute, Open Approach

51Q09Y Bypass Left External Jugular Vein to Upper Vein with Autologous Venous Tissue, Open Approach

51Q0AY Bypass Left External Jugular Vein to Upper Vein with Autologous Arterial Tissue, Open Approach

51Q0JY Bypass Left External Jugular Vein to Upper Vein with Synthetic Substitute, Open Approach

51Q0KY Bypass Left External Jugular Vein to Upper Vein with Nonautologous Tissue Substitute, Open Approach

51Q0ZY Bypass Left External Jugular Vein to Upper Vein, Open Approach

51Q47Y Bypass Left External Jugular Vein to Upper Vein with Autologous Tissue Substitute, Percutaneous Endoscopic Approach

051Q49Y Bypass Left External Jugular Vein to Upper Vein with Autologous Venous Tissue, Percutaneous Endoscopic Approach

051Q4AY Bypass Left External Jugular Vein to Upper Vein with Autologous Arterial Tissue, Percutaneous Endoscopic Approach

051Q4JY Bypass Left External Jugular Vein to Upper Vein with Synthetic Substitute, Percutaneous Endoscopic Approach

051Q4KY Bypass Left External Jugular Vein to Upper Vein with Nonautologous Tissue Substitute, Percutaneous Endoscopic Approach

051Q4ZY Bypass Left External Jugular Vein to Upper Vein, Percutaneous Endoscopic Approach

051R07Y Bypass Right Vertebral Vein to Upper Vein with Autologous Tissue Substitute, Open Approach

051R09Y Bypass Right Vertebral Vein to Upper Vein with Autologous Venous Tissue, Open Approach

051R0AY Bypass Right Vertebral Vein to Upper Vein with Autologous Arterial Tissue, Open Approach

051R0JY Bypass Right Vertebral Vein to Upper Vein with Synthetic Substitute, Open Approach

051R0KY Bypass Right Vertebral Vein to Upper Vein with Nonautologous Tissue Substitute, Open Approach

051R0ZY Bypass Right Vertebral Vein to Upper Vein, Open Approach

051R47Y Bypass Right Vertebral Vein to Upper Vein with Autologous Tissue Substitute, Percutaneous Endoscopic Approach

051R49Y Bypass Right Vertebral Vein to Upper Vein with Autologous Venous Tissue, Percutaneous Endoscopic Approach

051R4AY Bypass Right Vertebral Vein to Upper Vein with Autologous Arterial Tissue, Percutaneous Endoscopic Approach

051R4JY Bypass Right Vertebral Vein to Upper Vein with Synthetic Substitute, Percutaneous Endoscopic Approach

051R4KY Bypass Right Vertebral Vein to Upper Vein with Nonautologous Tissue Substitute, Percutaneous Endoscopic Approach

051R4ZY Bypass Right Vertebral Vein to Upper Vein, Percutaneous Endoscopic Approach

051S07Y Bypass Left Vertebral Vein to Upper Vein with Autologous Tissue Substitute, Open Approach

051S09Y Bypass Left Vertebral Vein to Upper Vein with Autologous Venous Tissue, Open Approach

051S0AY Bypass Left Vertebral Vein to Upper Vein with Autologous Arterial Tissue, Open Approach

051S0JY Bypass Left Vertebral Vein to Upper Vein with Synthetic Substitute, Open Approach

051S0KY Bypass Left Vertebral Vein to Upper Vein with Nonautologous Tissue Substitute, Open Approach

051S0ZY Bypass Left Vertebral Vein to Upper Vein, Open Approach

051S47Y Bypass Left Vertebral Vein to Upper Vein with Autologous Tissue Substitute, Percutaneous Endoscopic Approach

051S49Y Bypass Left Vertebral Vein to Upper Vein with Autologous Venous Tissue, Percutaneous Endoscopic Approach

051S4AY Bypass Left Vertebral Vein to Upper Vein with Autologous Arterial Tissue, Percutaneous Endoscopic Approach

051S4JY Bypass Left Vertebral Vein to Upper Vein with Synthetic Substitute, Percutaneous Endoscopic Approach

051S4KY Bypass Left Vertebral Vein to Upper Vein with Nonautologous Tissue Substitute, Percutaneous Endoscopic Approach

051S4ZY Bypass Left Vertebral Vein to Upper Vein, Percutaneous Endoscopic Approach

051T07Y Bypass Right Face Vein to Upper Vein with Autologous Tissue Substitute, Open Approach

051T09Y Bypass Right Face Vein to Upper Vein with Autologous Venous Tissue, Open Approach

051T0AY Bypass Right Face Vein to Upper Vein with Autologous Arterial Tissue, Open Approach

051T0JY Bypass Right Face Vein to Upper Vein with Synthetic Substitute, Open Approach

051T0KY Bypass Right Face Vein to Upper Vein with Nonautologous Tissue Substitute, Open Approach

051T0ZY Bypass Right Face Vein to Upper Vein, Open Approach

051T47Y Bypass Right Face Vein to Upper Vein with Autologous Tissue Substitute, Percutaneous Endoscopic Approach

051T49Y Bypass Right Face Vein to Upper Vein with Autologous Venous Tissue, Percutaneous Endoscopic Approach

051T4AY Bypass Right Face Vein to Upper Vein with Autologous Arterial Tissue, Percutaneous Endoscopic Approach

051T4JY Bypass Right Face Vein to Upper Vein with Synthetic Substitute, Percutaneous Endoscopic Approach

051T4KY Bypass Right Face Vein to Upper Vein with Nonautologous Tissue Substitute, Percutaneous Endoscopic Approach

051T4ZY Bypass Right Face Vein to Upper Vein, Percutaneous Endoscopic Approach

051V07Y Bypass Left Face Vein to Upper Vein with Autologous Tissue Substitute, Open Approach

051V09Y Bypass Left Face Vein to Upper Vein with Autologous Venous Tissue, Open Approach

051V0AY Bypass Left Face Vein to Upper Vein with Autologous Arterial Tissue, Open Approach

051V0JY Bypass Left Face Vein to Upper Vein with Synthetic Substitute, Open Approach

051V0KY Bypass Left Face Vein to Upper Vein with Nonautologous Tissue Substitute, Open Approach

051V0ZY Bypass Left Face Vein to Upper Vein, Open Approach

051V47Y Bypass Left Face Vein to Upper Vein with Autologous Tissue Substitute, Percutaneous Endoscopic Approach

051V49Y Bypass Left Face Vein to Upper Vein with Autologous Venous Tissue, Percutaneous Endoscopic Approach

051V4AY Bypass Left Face Vein to Upper Vein with Autologous Arterial Tissue, Percutaneous Endoscopic Approach

051V4JY Bypass Left Face Vein to Upper Vein with Synthetic Substitute, Percutaneous Endoscopic Approach

051V4KY Bypass Left Face Vein to Upper Vein with Nonautologous Tissue Substitute, Percutaneous Endoscopic Approach

051V4ZY Bypass Left Face Vein to Upper Vein, Percutaneous Endoscopic Approach

055 – Upper Veins, Destruction

05500ZZ Destruction of Azygos Vein, Open Approach
05503ZZ Destruction of Azygos Vein, Percutaneous Approach
05504ZZ Destruction of Azygos Vein, Percutaneous Endoscopic Approach
05510ZZ Destruction of Hemiazygos Vein, Open Approach
05513ZZ Destruction of Hemiazygos Vein, Percutaneous Approach
05514ZZ Destruction of Hemiazygos Vein, Percutaneous Endoscopic Approach
05530ZZ Destruction of Right Innominate Vein, Open Approach
05533ZZ Destruction of Right Innominate Vein, Percutaneous Approach
05534ZZ Destruction of Right Innominate Vein, Percutaneous Endoscopic Approach
05540ZZ Destruction of Left Innominate Vein, Open Approach
05543ZZ Destruction of Left Innominate Vein, Percutaneous Approach
05544ZZ Destruction of Left Innominate Vein, Percutaneous Endoscopic Approach
05550ZZ Destruction of Right Subclavian Vein, Open Approach
05553ZZ Destruction of Right Subclavian Vein, Percutaneous Approach
05554ZZ Destruction of Right Subclavian Vein, Percutaneous Endoscopic Approach
05560ZZ Destruction of Left Subclavian Vein, Open Approach
05563ZZ Destruction of Left Subclavian Vein, Percutaneous Approach
05564ZZ Destruction of Left Subclavian Vein, Percutaneous Endoscopic Approach
05570ZZ Destruction of Right Axillary Vein, Open Approach
05573ZZ Destruction of Right Axillary Vein, Percutaneous Approach
05574ZZ Destruction of Right Axillary Vein, Percutaneous Endoscopic Approach
05580ZZ Destruction of Left Axillary Vein, Open Approach
05583ZZ Destruction of Left Axillary Vein, Percutaneous Approach
05584ZZ Destruction of Left Axillary Vein, Percutaneous Endoscopic Approach
05590ZZ Destruction of Right Brachial Vein, Open Approach
05593ZZ Destruction of Right Brachial Vein, Percutaneous Approach
05594ZZ Destruction of Right Brachial Vein, Percutaneous Endoscopic Approach
055A0ZZ Destruction of Left Brachial Vein, Open Approach
055A3ZZ Destruction of Left Brachial Vein, Percutaneous Approach
055A4ZZ Destruction of Left Brachial Vein, Percutaneous Endoscopic Approach
055B0ZZ Destruction of Right Basilic Vein, Open Approach
055B3ZZ Destruction of Right Basilic Vein, Percutaneous Approach
055B4ZZ Destruction of Right Basilic Vein, Percutaneous Endoscopic Approach
055C0ZZ Destruction of Left Basilic Vein, Open Approach
055C3ZZ Destruction of Left Basilic Vein, Percutaneous Approach
055C4ZZ Destruction of Left Basilic Vein, Percutaneous Endoscopic Approach
055D0ZZ Destruction of Right Cephalic Vein, Open Approach
055D3ZZ Destruction of Right Cephalic Vein, Percutaneous Approach
055D4ZZ Destruction of Right Cephalic Vein, Percutaneous Endoscopic Approach
055F0ZZ Destruction of Left Cephalic Vein, Open Approach
055F3ZZ Destruction of Left Cephalic Vein, Percutaneous Approach
055F4ZZ Destruction of Left Cephalic Vein, Percutaneous Endoscopic Approach
055G0ZZ Destruction of Right Hand Vein, Open Approach
055G3ZZ Destruction of Right Hand Vein, Percutaneous Approach
055G4ZZ Destruction of Right Hand Vein, Percutaneous Endoscopic Approach
055H0ZZ Destruction of Left Hand Vein, Open Approach
055H3ZZ Destruction of Left Hand Vein, Percutaneous Approach
055H4ZZ Destruction of Left Hand Vein, Percutaneous Endoscopic Approach
055L0ZZ Destruction of Intracranial Vein, Open Approach
055L3ZZ Destruction of Intracranial Vein, Percutaneous Approach
055L4ZZ Destruction of Intracranial Vein, Percutaneous Endoscopic Approach
055M0ZZ Destruction of Right Internal Jugular Vein, Open Approach
055M3ZZ Destruction of Right Internal Jugular Vei Percutaneous Approach
055M4ZZ Destruction of Right Internal Jugular Vei Percutaneous Endoscopic Approach
055N0ZZ Destruction of Left Internal Jugular Vein Open Approach
055N3ZZ Destruction of Left Internal Jugular Vein Percutaneous Approach
055N4ZZ Destruction of Left Internal Jugular Vein Percutaneous Endoscopic Approach
055P0ZZ Destruction of Right External Jugular Vein, Open Approach
055P3ZZ Destruction of Right External Jugular Vein, Percutaneous Approach
055P4ZZ Destruction of Right External Jugular Vein, Percutaneous Endoscopic Approacl
055Q0ZZ Destruction of Left External Jugular Vein Open Approach
055Q3ZZ Destruction of Left External Jugular Vein Percutaneous Approach
055Q4ZZ Destruction of Left External Jugular Vein Percutaneous Endoscopic Approach
055R0ZZ Destruction of Right Vertebral Vein, Ope Approach
055R3ZZ Destruction of Right Vertebral Vein, Percutaneous Approach
055R4ZZ Destruction of Right Vertebral Vein, Percutaneous Endoscopic Approach
055S0ZZ Destruction of Left Vertebral Vein, Open Approach
055S3ZZ Destruction of Left Vertebral Vein, Percutaneous Approach
055S4ZZ Destruction of Left Vertebral Vein, Percutaneous Endoscopic Approach
055T0ZZ Destruction of Right Face Vein, Open Approach
055T3ZZ Destruction of Right Face Vein, Percutaneous Approach
055T4ZZ Destruction of Right Face Vein, Percutaneous Endoscopic Approach
055V0ZZ Destruction of Left Face Vein, Open Approach
055V3ZZ Destruction of Left Face Vein, Percutaneous Approach
055V4ZZ Destruction of Left Face Vein, Percutaneous Endoscopic Approach
055Y0ZZ Destruction of Upper Vein, Open Approach
055Y3ZZ Destruction of Upper Vein, Percutaneous Approach
055Y4ZZ Destruction of Upper Vein, Percutaneous Endoscopic Approach

057 – Upper Veins, Dilation

05700DZ Dilation of Azygos Vein with Intraluminal Device, Open Approach
05700ZZ Dilation of Azygos Vein, Open Approach
05703DZ Dilation of Azygos Vein with Intraluminal Device, Percutaneous Approach
05703ZZ Dilation of Azygos Vein, Percutaneous Approach
05704DZ Dilation of Azygos Vein with Intraluminal Device, Percutaneous Endoscopic Approach
05704ZZ Dilation of Azygos Vein, Percutaneous Endoscopic Approach
05710DZ Dilation of Hemiazygos Vein with Intraluminal Device, Open Approach
05710ZZ Dilation of Hemiazygos Vein, Open Approach
05713DZ Dilation of Hemiazygos Vein with Intraluminal Device, Percutaneous Approach
05713ZZ Dilation of Hemiazygos Vein, Percutaneous Approach
05714DZ Dilation of Hemiazygos Vein with Intraluminal Device, Percutaneous Endoscopic Approach
05714ZZ Dilation of Hemiazygos Vein, Percutaneous Endoscopic Approach
05730DZ Dilation of Right Innominate Vein with Intraluminal Device, Open Approach
05730ZZ Dilation of Right Innominate Vein, Open Approach
05733DZ Dilation of Right Innominate Vein with Intraluminal Device, Percutaneous Approach
05733ZZ Dilation of Right Innominate Vein, Percutaneous Approach
05734DZ Dilation of Right Innominate Vein with Intraluminal Device, Percutaneous Endoscopic Approach
05734ZZ Dilation of Right Innominate Vein, Percutaneous Endoscopic Approach
05740DZ Dilation of Left Innominate Vein with Intraluminal Device, Open Approach
05740ZZ Dilation of Left Innominate Vein, Open Approach
05743DZ Dilation of Left Innominate Vein with Intraluminal Device, Percutaneous Approach
05743ZZ Dilation of Left Innominate Vein, Percutaneous Approach
05744DZ Dilation of Left Innominate Vein with Intraluminal Device, Percutaneous Endoscopic Approach
05744ZZ Dilation of Left Innominate Vein, Percutaneous Endoscopic Approach
05750DZ Dilation of Right Subclavian Vein with Intraluminal Device, Open Approach

5750ZZ Dilation of Right Subclavian Vein, Open Approach
5753DZ Dilation of Right Subclavian Vein with Intraluminal Device, Percutaneous Approach
5753ZZ Dilation of Right Subclavian Vein, Percutaneous Approach
5754DZ Dilation of Right Subclavian Vein with Intraluminal Device, Percutaneous Endoscopic Approach
5754ZZ Dilation of Right Subclavian Vein, Percutaneous Endoscopic Approach
5760DZ Dilation of Left Subclavian Vein with Intraluminal Device, Open Approach
5760ZZ Dilation of Left Subclavian Vein, Open Approach
5763DZ Dilation of Left Subclavian Vein with Intraluminal Device, Percutaneous Approach
5763ZZ Dilation of Left Subclavian Vein, Percutaneous Approach
5764DZ Dilation of Left Subclavian Vein with Intraluminal Device, Percutaneous Endoscopic Approach
5764ZZ Dilation of Left Subclavian Vein, Percutaneous Endoscopic Approach
5770DZ Dilation of Right Axillary Vein with Intraluminal Device, Open Approach
5770ZZ Dilation of Right Axillary Vein, Open Approach
5773DZ Dilation of Right Axillary Vein with Intraluminal Device, Percutaneous Approach
5773ZZ Dilation of Right Axillary Vein, Percutaneous Approach
5774DZ Dilation of Right Axillary Vein with Intraluminal Device, Percutaneous Endoscopic Approach
5774ZZ Dilation of Right Axillary Vein, Percutaneous Endoscopic Approach
5780DZ Dilation of Left Axillary Vein with Intraluminal Device, Open Approach
5780ZZ Dilation of Left Axillary Vein, Open Approach
5783DZ Dilation of Left Axillary Vein with Intraluminal Device, Percutaneous Approach
5783ZZ Dilation of Left Axillary Vein, Percutaneous Approach
5784DZ Dilation of Left Axillary Vein with Intraluminal Device, Percutaneous Endoscopic Approach
5784ZZ Dilation of Left Axillary Vein, Percutaneous Endoscopic Approach
5790DZ Dilation of Right Brachial Vein with Intraluminal Device, Open Approach
05790ZZ Dilation of Right Brachial Vein, Open Approach
05793DZ Dilation of Right Brachial Vein with Intraluminal Device, Percutaneous Approach
05793ZZ Dilation of Right Brachial Vein, Percutaneous Approach
05794DZ Dilation of Right Brachial Vein with Intraluminal Device, Percutaneous Endoscopic Approach
05794ZZ Dilation of Right Brachial Vein, Percutaneous Endoscopic Approach
057A0DZ Dilation of Left Brachial Vein with Intraluminal Device, Open Approach
057A0ZZ Dilation of Left Brachial Vein, Open Approach
057A3DZ Dilation of Left Brachial Vein with Intraluminal Device, Percutaneous Approach
057A3ZZ Dilation of Left Brachial Vein, Percutaneous Approach
057A4DZ Dilation of Left Brachial Vein with Intraluminal Device, Percutaneous Endoscopic Approach
057A4ZZ Dilation of Left Brachial Vein, Percutaneous Endoscopic Approach
057B0DZ Dilation of Right Basilic Vein with Intraluminal Device, Open Approach
057B0ZZ Dilation of Right Basilic Vein, Open Approach
057B3DZ Dilation of Right Basilic Vein with Intraluminal Device, Percutaneous Approach
057B3ZZ Dilation of Right Basilic Vein, Percutaneous Approach
057B4DZ Dilation of Right Basilic Vein with Intraluminal Device, Percutaneous Endoscopic Approach
057B4ZZ Dilation of Right Basilic Vein, Percutaneous Endoscopic Approach
057C0DZ Dilation of Left Basilic Vein with Intraluminal Device, Open Approach
057C0ZZ Dilation of Left Basilic Vein, Open Approach
057C3DZ Dilation of Left Basilic Vein with Intraluminal Device, Percutaneous Approach
057C3ZZ Dilation of Left Basilic Vein, Percutaneous Approach
057C4DZ Dilation of Left Basilic Vein with Intraluminal Device, Percutaneous Endoscopic Approach
057C4ZZ Dilation of Left Basilic Vein, Percutaneous Endoscopic Approach
057D0DZ Dilation of Right Cephalic Vein with Intraluminal Device, Open Approach
057D0ZZ Dilation of Right Cephalic Vein, Open Approach
057D3DZ Dilation of Right Cephalic Vein with Intraluminal Device, Percutaneous Approach
057D3ZZ Dilation of Right Cephalic Vein, Percutaneous Approach
057D4DZ Dilation of Right Cephalic Vein with Intraluminal Device, Percutaneous Endoscopic Approach
057D4ZZ Dilation of Right Cephalic Vein, Percutaneous Endoscopic Approach
057F0DZ Dilation of Left Cephalic Vein with Intraluminal Device, Open Approach
057F0ZZ Dilation of Left Cephalic Vein, Open Approach
057F3DZ Dilation of Left Cephalic Vein with Intraluminal Device, Percutaneous Approach
057F3ZZ Dilation of Left Cephalic Vein, Percutaneous Approach
057F4DZ Dilation of Left Cephalic Vein with Intraluminal Device, Percutaneous Endoscopic Approach
057F4ZZ Dilation of Left Cephalic Vein, Percutaneous Endoscopic Approach
057G0DZ Dilation of Right Hand Vein with Intraluminal Device, Open Approach
057G0ZZ Dilation of Right Hand Vein, Open Approach
057G3DZ Dilation of Right Hand Vein with Intraluminal Device, Percutaneous Approach
057G3ZZ Dilation of Right Hand Vein, Percutaneous Approach
057G4DZ Dilation of Right Hand Vein with Intraluminal Device, Percutaneous Endoscopic Approach
057G4ZZ Dilation of Right Hand Vein, Percutaneous Endoscopic Approach
057H0DZ Dilation of Left Hand Vein with Intraluminal Device, Open Approach
057H0ZZ Dilation of Left Hand Vein, Open Approach
057H3DZ Dilation of Left Hand Vein with Intraluminal Device, Percutaneous Approach
057H3ZZ Dilation of Left Hand Vein, Percutaneous Approach
057H4DZ Dilation of Left Hand Vein with Intraluminal Device, Percutaneous Endoscopic Approach
057H4ZZ Dilation of Left Hand Vein, Percutaneous Endoscopic Approach
057L0DZ Dilation of Intracranial Vein with Intraluminal Device, Open Approach
057L0ZZ Dilation of Intracranial Vein, Open Approach
057L3DZ Dilation of Intracranial Vein with Intraluminal Device, Percutaneous Approach
▲ **057L3ZZ** Dilation of Intracranial Vein, Percutaneous Approach
057L4DZ Dilation of Intracranial Vein with Intraluminal Device, Percutaneous Endoscopic Approach
▲ **057L4ZZ** Dilation of Intracranial Vein, Percutaneous Endoscopic Approach
057M0DZ Dilation of Right Internal Jugular Vein with Intraluminal Device, Open Approach
057M0ZZ Dilation of Right Internal Jugular Vein, Open Approach
057M3DZ Dilation of Right Internal Jugular Vein with Intraluminal Device, Percutaneous Approach
057M3ZZ Dilation of Right Internal Jugular Vein, Percutaneous Approach
057M4DZ Dilation of Right Internal Jugular Vein with Intraluminal Device, Percutaneous Endoscopic Approach
057M4ZZ Dilation of Right Internal Jugular Vein, Percutaneous Endoscopic Approach
057N0DZ Dilation of Left Internal Jugular Vein with Intraluminal Device, Open Approach
057N0ZZ Dilation of Left Internal Jugular Vein, Open Approach
057N3DZ Dilation of Left Internal Jugular Vein with Intraluminal Device, Percutaneous Approach
057N3ZZ Dilation of Left Internal Jugular Vein, Percutaneous Approach
057N4DZ Dilation of Left Internal Jugular Vein with Intraluminal Device, Percutaneous Endoscopic Approach
057N4ZZ Dilation of Left Internal Jugular Vein, Percutaneous Endoscopic Approach
057P0DZ Dilation of Right External Jugular Vein with Intraluminal Device, Open Approach
057P0ZZ Dilation of Right External Jugular Vein, Open Approach
057P3DZ Dilation of Right External Jugular Vein with Intraluminal Device, Percutaneous Approach
057P3ZZ Dilation of Right External Jugular Vein, Percutaneous Approach
057P4DZ Dilation of Right External Jugular Vein with Intraluminal Device, Percutaneous Endoscopic Approach
057P4ZZ Dilation of Right External Jugular Vein, Percutaneous Endoscopic Approach
057Q0DZ Dilation of Left External Jugular Vein with Intraluminal Device, Open Approach
057Q0ZZ Dilation of Left External Jugular Vein, Open Approach
057Q3DZ Dilation of Left External Jugular Vein with Intraluminal Device, Percutaneous Approach
057Q3ZZ Dilation of Left External Jugular Vein, Percutaneous Approach

057Q4DZ Dilation of Left External Jugular Vein with Intraluminal Device, Percutaneous Endoscopic Approach
057Q4ZZ Dilation of Left External Jugular Vein, Percutaneous Endoscopic Approach
057R0DZ Dilation of Right Vertebral Vein with Intraluminal Device, Open Approach
057R0ZZ Dilation of Right Vertebral Vein, Open Approach
057R3DZ Dilation of Right Vertebral Vein with Intraluminal Device, Percutaneous Approach
057R3ZZ Dilation of Right Vertebral Vein, Percutaneous Approach
057R4DZ Dilation of Right Vertebral Vein with Intraluminal Device, Percutaneous Endoscopic Approach
057R4ZZ Dilation of Right Vertebral Vein, Percutaneous Endoscopic Approach
057S0DZ Dilation of Left Vertebral Vein with Intraluminal Device, Open Approach
057S0ZZ Dilation of Left Vertebral Vein, Open Approach
057S3DZ Dilation of Left Vertebral Vein with Intraluminal Device, Percutaneous Approach
057S3ZZ Dilation of Left Vertebral Vein, Percutaneous Approach
057S4DZ Dilation of Left Vertebral Vein with Intraluminal Device, Percutaneous Endoscopic Approach
057S4ZZ Dilation of Left Vertebral Vein, Percutaneous Endoscopic Approach
057T0DZ Dilation of Right Face Vein with Intraluminal Device, Open Approach
057T0ZZ Dilation of Right Face Vein, Open Approach
057T3DZ Dilation of Right Face Vein with Intraluminal Device, Percutaneous Approach
057T3ZZ Dilation of Right Face Vein, Percutaneous Approach
057T4DZ Dilation of Right Face Vein with Intraluminal Device, Percutaneous Endoscopic Approach
057T4ZZ Dilation of Right Face Vein, Percutaneous Endoscopic Approach
057V0DZ Dilation of Left Face Vein with Intraluminal Device, Open Approach
057V0ZZ Dilation of Left Face Vein, Open Approach
057V3DZ Dilation of Left Face Vein with Intraluminal Device, Percutaneous Approach
057V3ZZ Dilation of Left Face Vein, Percutaneous Approach
057V4DZ Dilation of Left Face Vein with Intraluminal Device, Percutaneous Endoscopic Approach
057V4ZZ Dilation of Left Face Vein, Percutaneous Endoscopic Approach
057Y0DZ Dilation of Upper Vein with Intraluminal Device, Open Approach
057Y0ZZ Dilation of Upper Vein, Open Approach
057Y3DZ Dilation of Upper Vein with Intraluminal Device, Percutaneous Approach
057Y3ZZ Dilation of Upper Vein, Percutaneous Approach
057Y4DZ Dilation of Upper Vein with Intraluminal Device, Percutaneous Endoscopic Approach
057Y4ZZ Dilation of Upper Vein, Percutaneous Endoscopic Approach

059 – Upper Veins, Drainage

Review Coding Guidelines B3.4a and B3.4b

Review Coding Guideline B6.2

059000Z Drainage of Azygos Vein with Drainage Device, Open Approach
05900ZX Drainage of Azygos Vein, Open Approach, Diagnostic
05900ZZ Drainage of Azygos Vein, Open Approach
059030Z Drainage of Azygos Vein with Drainage Device, Percutaneous Approach
05903ZX Drainage of Azygos Vein, Percutaneous Approach, Diagnostic
05903ZZ Drainage of Azygos Vein, Percutaneous Approach
059040Z Drainage of Azygos Vein with Drainage Device, Percutaneous Endoscopic Approach
05904ZX Drainage of Azygos Vein, Percutaneous Endoscopic Approach, Diagnostic
05904ZZ Drainage of Azygos Vein, Percutaneous Endoscopic Approach
059100Z Drainage of Hemiazygos Vein with Drainage Device, Open Approach
05910ZX Drainage of Hemiazygos Vein, Open Approach, Diagnostic
05910ZZ Drainage of Hemiazygos Vein, Open Approach
059130Z Drainage of Hemiazygos Vein with Drainage Device, Percutaneous Approach
05913ZX Drainage of Hemiazygos Vein, Percutaneous Approach, Diagnostic
05913ZZ Drainage of Hemiazygos Vein, Percutaneous Approach
059140Z Drainage of Hemiazygos Vein with Drainage Device, Percutaneous Endoscopic Approach
05914ZX Drainage of Hemiazygos Vein, Percutaneous Endoscopic Approach, Diagnostic
05914ZZ Drainage of Hemiazygos Vein, Percutaneous Endoscopic Approach
059300Z Drainage of Right Innominate Vein with Drainage Device, Open Approach
05930ZX Drainage of Right Innominate Vein, Open Approach, Diagnostic
05930ZZ Drainage of Right Innominate Vein, Open Approach
059330Z Drainage of Right Innominate Vein with Drainage Device, Percutaneous Approach
05933ZX Drainage of Right Innominate Vein, Percutaneous Approach, Diagnostic
05933ZZ Drainage of Right Innominate Vein, Percutaneous Approach
059340Z Drainage of Right Innominate Vein with Drainage Device, Percutaneous Endoscopic Approach
05934ZX Drainage of Right Innominate Vein, Percutaneous Endoscopic Approach, Diagnostic
05934ZZ Drainage of Right Innominate Vein, Percutaneous Endoscopic Approach
059400Z Drainage of Left Innominate Vein with Drainage Device, Open Approach
05940ZX Drainage of Left Innominate Vein, Open Approach, Diagnostic
05940ZZ Drainage of Left Innominate Vein, Open Approach
059430Z Drainage of Left Innominate Vein with Drainage Device, Percutaneous Approach
05943ZX Drainage of Left Innominate Vein, Percutaneous Approach, Diagnostic
05943ZZ Drainage of Left Innominate Vein, Percutaneous Approach
059440Z Drainage of Left Innominate Vein with Drainage Device, Percutaneous Endoscopic Approach
05944ZX Drainage of Left Innominate Vein, Percutaneous Endoscopic Approach, Diagnostic
05944ZZ Drainage of Left Innominate Vein, Percutaneous Endoscopic Approach
059500Z Drainage of Right Subclavian Vein with Drainage Device, Open Approach
05950ZX Drainage of Right Subclavian Vein, Open Approach, Diagnostic
05950ZZ Drainage of Right Subclavian Vein, Open Approach
059530Z Drainage of Right Subclavian Vein with Drainage Device, Percutaneous Approach
05953ZX Drainage of Right Subclavian Vein, Percutaneous Approach, Diagnostic
05953ZZ Drainage of Right Subclavian Vein, Percutaneous Approach
059540Z Drainage of Right Subclavian Vein with Drainage Device, Percutaneous Endoscopic Approach
05954ZX Drainage of Right Subclavian Vein, Percutaneous Endoscopic Approach, Diagnostic
05954ZZ Drainage of Right Subclavian Vein, Percutaneous Endoscopic Approach
059600Z Drainage of Left Subclavian Vein with Drainage Device, Open Approach
05960ZX Drainage of Left Subclavian Vein, Open Approach, Diagnostic
05960ZZ Drainage of Left Subclavian Vein, Open Approach
059630Z Drainage of Left Subclavian Vein with Drainage Device, Percutaneous Approach
05963ZX Drainage of Left Subclavian Vein, Percutaneous Approach, Diagnostic
05963ZZ Drainage of Left Subclavian Vein, Percutaneous Approach
059640Z Drainage of Left Subclavian Vein with Drainage Device, Percutaneous Endoscopic Approach
05964ZX Drainage of Left Subclavian Vein, Percutaneous Endoscopic Approach, Diagnostic
05964ZZ Drainage of Left Subclavian Vein, Percutaneous Endoscopic Approach
059700Z Drainage of Right Axillary Vein with Drainage Device, Open Approach
05970ZX Drainage of Right Axillary Vein, Open Approach, Diagnostic
05970ZZ Drainage of Right Axillary Vein, Open Approach
059730Z Drainage of Right Axillary Vein with Drainage Device, Percutaneous Approach
05973ZX Drainage of Right Axillary Vein, Percutaneous Approach, Diagnostic
05973ZZ Drainage of Right Axillary Vein, Percutaneous Approach
059740Z Drainage of Right Axillary Vein with Drainage Device, Percutaneous Endoscopic Approach
05974ZX Drainage of Right Axillary Vein, Percutaneous Endoscopic Approach, Diagnostic

5974ZZ Drainage of Right Axillary Vein, Percutaneous Endoscopic Approach

59800Z Drainage of Left Axillary Vein with Drainage Device, Open Approach

5980ZX Drainage of Left Axillary Vein, Open Approach, Diagnostic

5980ZZ Drainage of Left Axillary Vein, Open Approach

59830Z Drainage of Left Axillary Vein with Drainage Device, Percutaneous Approach

5983ZX Drainage of Left Axillary Vein, Percutaneous Approach, Diagnostic

5983ZZ Drainage of Left Axillary Vein, Percutaneous Approach

59840Z Drainage of Left Axillary Vein with Drainage Device, Percutaneous Endoscopic Approach

5984ZX Drainage of Left Axillary Vein, Percutaneous Endoscopic Approach, Diagnostic

5984ZZ Drainage of Left Axillary Vein, Percutaneous Endoscopic Approach

59900Z Drainage of Right Brachial Vein with Drainage Device, Open Approach

5990ZX Drainage of Right Brachial Vein, Open Approach, Diagnostic

5990ZZ Drainage of Right Brachial Vein, Open Approach

59930Z Drainage of Right Brachial Vein with Drainage Device, Percutaneous Approach

5993ZX Drainage of Right Brachial Vein, Percutaneous Approach, Diagnostic

5993ZZ Drainage of Right Brachial Vein, Percutaneous Approach

59940Z Drainage of Right Brachial Vein with Drainage Device, Percutaneous Endoscopic Approach

5994ZX Drainage of Right Brachial Vein, Percutaneous Endoscopic Approach, Diagnostic

5994ZZ Drainage of Right Brachial Vein, Percutaneous Endoscopic Approach

59A00Z Drainage of Left Brachial Vein with Drainage Device, Open Approach

59A0ZX Drainage of Left Brachial Vein, Open Approach, Diagnostic

59A0ZZ Drainage of Left Brachial Vein, Open Approach

59A30Z Drainage of Left Brachial Vein with Drainage Device, Percutaneous Approach

59A3ZX Drainage of Left Brachial Vein, Percutaneous Approach, Diagnostic

59A3ZZ Drainage of Left Brachial Vein, Percutaneous Approach

59A40Z Drainage of Left Brachial Vein with Drainage Device, Percutaneous Endoscopic Approach

59A4ZX Drainage of Left Brachial Vein, Percutaneous Endoscopic Approach, Diagnostic

59A4ZZ Drainage of Left Brachial Vein, Percutaneous Endoscopic Approach

59B00Z Drainage of Right Basilic Vein with Drainage Device, Open Approach

059B0ZX Drainage of Right Basilic Vein, Open Approach, Diagnostic

059B0ZZ Drainage of Right Basilic Vein, Open Approach

059B30Z Drainage of Right Basilic Vein with Drainage Device, Percutaneous Approach

059B3ZX Drainage of Right Basilic Vein, Percutaneous Approach, Diagnostic

059B3ZZ Drainage of Right Basilic Vein, Percutaneous Approach

059B40Z Drainage of Right Basilic Vein with Drainage Device, Percutaneous Endoscopic Approach

059B4ZX Drainage of Right Basilic Vein, Percutaneous Endoscopic Approach, Diagnostic

059B4ZZ Drainage of Right Basilic Vein, Percutaneous Endoscopic Approach

059C00Z Drainage of Left Basilic Vein with Drainage Device, Open Approach

059C0ZX Drainage of Left Basilic Vein, Open Approach, Diagnostic

059C0ZZ Drainage of Left Basilic Vein, Open Approach

059C30Z Drainage of Left Basilic Vein with Drainage Device, Percutaneous Approach

059C3ZX Drainage of Left Basilic Vein, Percutaneous Approach, Diagnostic

059C3ZZ Drainage of Left Basilic Vein, Percutaneous Approach

059C40Z Drainage of Left Basilic Vein with Drainage Device, Percutaneous Endoscopic Approach

059C4ZX Drainage of Left Basilic Vein, Percutaneous Endoscopic Approach, Diagnostic

059C4ZZ Drainage of Left Basilic Vein, Percutaneous Endoscopic Approach

059D00Z Drainage of Right Cephalic Vein with Drainage Device, Open Approach

059D0ZX Drainage of Right Cephalic Vein, Open Approach, Diagnostic

059D0ZZ Drainage of Right Cephalic Vein, Open Approach

059D30Z Drainage of Right Cephalic Vein with Drainage Device, Percutaneous Approach

059D3ZX Drainage of Right Cephalic Vein, Percutaneous Approach, Diagnostic

059D3ZZ Drainage of Right Cephalic Vein, Percutaneous Approach

059D40Z Drainage of Right Cephalic Vein with Drainage Device, Percutaneous Endoscopic Approach

059D4ZX Drainage of Right Cephalic Vein, Percutaneous Endoscopic Approach, Diagnostic

059D4ZZ Drainage of Right Cephalic Vein, Percutaneous Endoscopic Approach

059F00Z Drainage of Left Cephalic Vein with Drainage Device, Open Approach

059F0ZX Drainage of Left Cephalic Vein, Open Approach, Diagnostic

059F0ZZ Drainage of Left Cephalic Vein, Open Approach

059F30Z Drainage of Left Cephalic Vein with Drainage Device, Percutaneous Approach

059F3ZX Drainage of Left Cephalic Vein, Percutaneous Approach, Diagnostic

059F3ZZ Drainage of Left Cephalic Vein, Percutaneous Approach

059F40Z Drainage of Left Cephalic Vein with Drainage Device, Percutaneous Endoscopic Approach

059F4ZX Drainage of Left Cephalic Vein, Percutaneous Endoscopic Approach, Diagnostic

059F4ZZ Drainage of Left Cephalic Vein, Percutaneous Endoscopic Approach

059G00Z Drainage of Right Hand Vein with Drainage Device, Open Approach

059G0ZX Drainage of Right Hand Vein, Open Approach, Diagnostic

059G0ZZ Drainage of Right Hand Vein, Open Approach

059G30Z Drainage of Right Hand Vein with Drainage Device, Percutaneous Approach

059G3ZX Drainage of Right Hand Vein, Percutaneous Approach, Diagnostic

059G3ZZ Drainage of Right Hand Vein, Percutaneous Approach

059G40Z Drainage of Right Hand Vein with Drainage Device, Percutaneous Endoscopic Approach

059G4ZX Drainage of Right Hand Vein, Percutaneous Endoscopic Approach, Diagnostic

059G4ZZ Drainage of Right Hand Vein, Percutaneous Endoscopic Approach

059H00Z Drainage of Left Hand Vein with Drainage Device, Open Approach

059H0ZX Drainage of Left Hand Vein, Open Approach, Diagnostic

059H0ZZ Drainage of Left Hand Vein, Open Approach

059H30Z Drainage of Left Hand Vein with Drainage Device, Percutaneous Approach

059H3ZX Drainage of Left Hand Vein, Percutaneous Approach, Diagnostic

059H3ZZ Drainage of Left Hand Vein, Percutaneous Approach

059H40Z Drainage of Left Hand Vein with Drainage Device, Percutaneous Endoscopic Approach

059H4ZX Drainage of Left Hand Vein, Percutaneous Endoscopic Approach, Diagnostic

059H4ZZ Drainage of Left Hand Vein, Percutaneous Endoscopic Approach

059L00Z Drainage of Intracranial Vein with Drainage Device, Open Approach

059L0ZX Drainage of Intracranial Vein, Open Approach, Diagnostic

059L0ZZ Drainage of Intracranial Vein, Open Approach

059L30Z Drainage of Intracranial Vein with Drainage Device, Percutaneous Approach

059L3ZX Drainage of Intracranial Vein, Percutaneous Approach, Diagnostic

059L3ZZ Drainage of Intracranial Vein, Percutaneous Approach

059L40Z Drainage of Intracranial Vein with Drainage Device, Percutaneous Endoscopic Approach

059L4ZX Drainage of Intracranial Vein, Percutaneous Endoscopic Approach, Diagnostic

059L4ZZ Drainage of Intracranial Vein, Percutaneous Endoscopic Approach

059M00Z Drainage of Right Internal Jugular Vein with Drainage Device, Open Approach

059M0ZX Drainage of Right Internal Jugular Vein, Open Approach, Diagnostic

059M0ZZ Drainage of Right Internal Jugular Vein, Open Approach

059M30Z Drainage of Right Internal Jugular Vein with Drainage Device, Percutaneous Approach

059M3ZX Drainage of Right Internal Jugular Vein, Percutaneous Approach, Diagnostic

059M3ZZ Drainage of Right Internal Jugular Vein, Percutaneous Approach

059M40Z Drainage of Right Internal Jugular Vein with Drainage Device, Percutaneous Endoscopic Approach

059M4ZX Drainage of Right Internal Jugular Vein, Percutaneous Endoscopic Approach, Diagnostic

059M4ZZ Drainage of Right Internal Jugular Vein, Percutaneous Endoscopic Approach

059N00Z Drainage of Left Internal Jugular Vein with Drainage Device, Open Approach

059N0ZX Drainage of Left Internal Jugular Vein, Open Approach, Diagnostic

059N0ZZ Drainage of Left Internal Jugular Vein, Open Approach

059N30Z Drainage of Left Internal Jugular Vein with Drainage Device, Percutaneous Approach

059N3ZX Drainage of Left Internal Jugular Vein, Percutaneous Approach, Diagnostic

059N3ZZ Drainage of Left Internal Jugular Vein, Percutaneous Approach
059N40Z Drainage of Left Internal Jugular Vein with Drainage Device, Percutaneous Endoscopic Approach
059N4ZX Drainage of Left Internal Jugular Vein, Percutaneous Endoscopic Approach, Diagnostic
059N4ZZ Drainage of Left Internal Jugular Vein, Percutaneous Endoscopic Approach
059P00Z Drainage of Right External Jugular Vein with Drainage Device, Open Approach
059P0ZX Drainage of Right External Jugular Vein, Open Approach, Diagnostic
059P0ZZ Drainage of Right External Jugular Vein, Open Approach
059P30Z Drainage of Right External Jugular Vein with Drainage Device, Percutaneous Approach
059P3ZX Drainage of Right External Jugular Vein, Percutaneous Approach, Diagnostic
059P3ZZ Drainage of Right External Jugular Vein, Percutaneous Approach
059P40Z Drainage of Right External Jugular Vein with Drainage Device, Percutaneous Endoscopic Approach
059P4ZX Drainage of Right External Jugular Vein, Percutaneous Endoscopic Approach, Diagnostic
059P4ZZ Drainage of Right External Jugular Vein, Percutaneous Endoscopic Approach
059Q00Z Drainage of Left External Jugular Vein with Drainage Device, Open Approach
059Q0ZX Drainage of Left External Jugular Vein, Open Approach, Diagnostic
059Q0ZZ Drainage of Left External Jugular Vein, Open Approach
059Q30Z Drainage of Left External Jugular Vein with Drainage Device, Percutaneous Approach
059Q3ZX Drainage of Left External Jugular Vein, Percutaneous Approach, Diagnostic
059Q3ZZ Drainage of Left External Jugular Vein, Percutaneous Approach
059Q40Z Drainage of Left External Jugular Vein with Drainage Device, Percutaneous Endoscopic Approach
059Q4ZX Drainage of Left External Jugular Vein, Percutaneous Endoscopic Approach, Diagnostic
059Q4ZZ Drainage of Left External Jugular Vein, Percutaneous Endoscopic Approach
059R00Z Drainage of Right Vertebral Vein with Drainage Device, Open Approach
059R0ZX Drainage of Right Vertebral Vein, Open Approach, Diagnostic
059R0ZZ Drainage of Right Vertebral Vein, Open Approach
059R30Z Drainage of Right Vertebral Vein with Drainage Device, Percutaneous Approach
059R3ZX Drainage of Right Vertebral Vein, Percutaneous Approach, Diagnostic
059R3ZZ Drainage of Right Vertebral Vein, Percutaneous Approach
059R40Z Drainage of Right Vertebral Vein with Drainage Device, Percutaneous Endoscopic Approach
059R4ZX Drainage of Right Vertebral Vein, Percutaneous Endoscopic Approach, Diagnostic
059R4ZZ Drainage of Right Vertebral Vein, Percutaneous Endoscopic Approach
059S00Z Drainage of Left Vertebral Vein with Drainage Device, Open Approach
059S0ZX Drainage of Left Vertebral Vein, Open Approach, Diagnostic
059S0ZZ Drainage of Left Vertebral Vein, Open Approach
059S30Z Drainage of Left Vertebral Vein with Drainage Device, Percutaneous Approach
059S3ZX Drainage of Left Vertebral Vein, Percutaneous Approach, Diagnostic
059S3ZZ Drainage of Left Vertebral Vein, Percutaneous Approach
059S40Z Drainage of Left Vertebral Vein with Drainage Device, Percutaneous Endoscopic Approach
059S4ZX Drainage of Left Vertebral Vein, Percutaneous Endoscopic Approach, Diagnostic
059S4ZZ Drainage of Left Vertebral Vein, Percutaneous Endoscopic Approach
059T00Z Drainage of Right Face Vein with Drainage Device, Open Approach
059T0ZX Drainage of Right Face Vein, Open Approach, Diagnostic
059T0ZZ Drainage of Right Face Vein, Open Approach
059T30Z Drainage of Right Face Vein with Drainage Device, Percutaneous Approach
059T3ZX Drainage of Right Face Vein, Percutaneous Approach, Diagnostic
059T3ZZ Drainage of Right Face Vein, Percutaneous Approach
059T40Z Drainage of Right Face Vein with Drainage Device, Percutaneous Endoscopic Approach
059T4ZX Drainage of Right Face Vein, Percutaneous Endoscopic Approach, Diagnostic
059T4ZZ Drainage of Right Face Vein, Percutaneous Endoscopic Approach
059V00Z Drainage of Left Face Vein with Drainage Device, Open Approach
059V0ZX Drainage of Left Face Vein, Open Approach, Diagnostic
059V0ZZ Drainage of Left Face Vein, Open Approach
059V30Z Drainage of Left Face Vein with Drainage Device, Percutaneous Approach
059V3ZX Drainage of Left Face Vein, Percutaneous Approach, Diagnostic
059V3ZZ Drainage of Left Face Vein, Percutaneous Approach
059V40Z Drainage of Left Face Vein with Drainage Device, Percutaneous Endoscopic Approach
059V4ZX Drainage of Left Face Vein, Percutaneous Endoscopic Approach, Diagnostic
059V4ZZ Drainage of Left Face Vein, Percutaneous Endoscopic Approach
059Y00Z Drainage of Upper Vein with Drainage Device, Open Approach
059Y0ZX Drainage of Upper Vein, Open Approach, Diagnostic
059Y0ZZ Drainage of Upper Vein, Open Approach
059Y30Z Drainage of Upper Vein with Drainage Device, Percutaneous Approach
059Y3ZX Drainage of Upper Vein, Percutaneous Approach, Diagnostic
059Y3ZZ Drainage of Upper Vein, Percutaneous Approach
059Y40Z Drainage of Upper Vein with Drainage Device, Percutaneous Endoscopic Approach
059Y4ZX Drainage of Upper Vein, Percutaneous Endoscopic Approach, Diagnostic
059Y4ZZ Drainage of Upper Vein, Percutaneous Endoscopic Approach

05B – Upper Veins, Excision

Review Coding Guidelines B3.4a and B3.4b

Review Coding Guideline B3.8

05B00ZX Excision of Azygos Vein, Open Approach, Diagnostic
05B00ZZ Excision of Azygos Vein, Open Approach
05B03ZX Excision of Azygos Vein, Percutaneous Approach, Diagnostic
05B03ZZ Excision of Azygos Vein, Percutaneous Approach
05B04ZX Excision of Azygos Vein, Percutaneous Endoscopic Approach, Diagnostic
05B04ZZ Excision of Azygos Vein, Percutaneous Endoscopic Approach
05B10ZX Excision of Hemiazygos Vein, Open Approach, Diagnostic
05B10ZZ Excision of Hemiazygos Vein, Open Approach
05B13ZX Excision of Hemiazygos Vein, Percutaneous Approach, Diagnostic
05B13ZZ Excision of Hemiazygos Vein, Percutaneous Approach
05B14ZX Excision of Hemiazygos Vein, Percutaneous Endoscopic Approach, Diagnostic
05B14ZZ Excision of Hemiazygos Vein, Percutaneous Endoscopic Approach
05B30ZX Excision of Right Innominate Vein, Open Approach, Diagnostic
05B30ZZ Excision of Right Innominate Vein, Open Approach
05B33ZX Excision of Right Innominate Vein, Percutaneous Approach, Diagnostic
05B33ZZ Excision of Right Innominate Vein, Percutaneous Approach
05B34ZX Excision of Right Innominate Vein, Percutaneous Endoscopic Approach, Diagnostic
05B34ZZ Excision of Right Innominate Vein, Percutaneous Endoscopic Approach
05B40ZX Excision of Left Innominate Vein, Open Approach, Diagnostic
05B40ZZ Excision of Left Innominate Vein, Open Approach
05B43ZX Excision of Left Innominate Vein, Percutaneous Approach, Diagnostic
05B43ZZ Excision of Left Innominate Vein, Percutaneous Approach
05B44ZX Excision of Left Innominate Vein, Percutaneous Endoscopic Approach, Diagnostic
05B44ZZ Excision of Left Innominate Vein, Percutaneous Endoscopic Approach
05B50ZX Excision of Right Subclavian Vein, Open Approach, Diagnostic
05B50ZZ Excision of Right Subclavian Vein, Open Approach
05B53ZX Excision of Right Subclavian Vein, Percutaneous Approach, Diagnostic
05B53ZZ Excision of Right Subclavian Vein, Percutaneous Approach

B54ZX Excision of Right Subclavian Vein, Percutaneous Endoscopic Approach, Diagnostic
B54ZZ Excision of Right Subclavian Vein, Percutaneous Endoscopic Approach
B60ZX Excision of Left Subclavian Vein, Open Approach, Diagnostic
B60ZZ Excision of Left Subclavian Vein, Open Approach
B63ZX Excision of Left Subclavian Vein, Percutaneous Approach, Diagnostic
B63ZZ Excision of Left Subclavian Vein, Percutaneous Approach
B64ZX Excision of Left Subclavian Vein, Percutaneous Endoscopic Approach, Diagnostic
5B64ZZ Excision of Left Subclavian Vein, Percutaneous Endoscopic Approach
5B70ZX Excision of Right Axillary Vein, Open Approach, Diagnostic
5B70ZZ Excision of Right Axillary Vein, Open Approach
5B73ZX Excision of Right Axillary Vein, Percutaneous Approach, Diagnostic
5B73ZZ Excision of Right Axillary Vein, Percutaneous Approach
5B74ZX Excision of Right Axillary Vein, Percutaneous Endoscopic Approach, Diagnostic
5B74ZZ Excision of Right Axillary Vein, Percutaneous Endoscopic Approach
5B80ZX Excision of Left Axillary Vein, Open Approach, Diagnostic
5B80ZZ Excision of Left Axillary Vein, Open Approach
5B83ZX Excision of Left Axillary Vein, Percutaneous Approach, Diagnostic
5B83ZZ Excision of Left Axillary Vein, Percutaneous Approach
5B84ZX Excision of Left Axillary Vein, Percutaneous Endoscopic Approach, Diagnostic
5B84ZZ Excision of Left Axillary Vein, Percutaneous Endoscopic Approach
5B90ZX Excision of Right Brachial Vein, Open Approach, Diagnostic
5B90ZZ Excision of Right Brachial Vein, Open Approach
5B93ZX Excision of Right Brachial Vein, Percutaneous Approach, Diagnostic
5B93ZZ Excision of Right Brachial Vein, Percutaneous Approach
5B94ZX Excision of Right Brachial Vein, Percutaneous Endoscopic Approach, Diagnostic
5B94ZZ Excision of Right Brachial Vein, Percutaneous Endoscopic Approach
5BA0ZX Excision of Left Brachial Vein, Open Approach, Diagnostic
5BA0ZZ Excision of Left Brachial Vein, Open Approach
5BA3ZX Excision of Left Brachial Vein, Percutaneous Approach, Diagnostic
5BA3ZZ Excision of Left Brachial Vein, Percutaneous Approach
5BA4ZX Excision of Left Brachial Vein, Percutaneous Endoscopic Approach, Diagnostic
05BA4ZZ Excision of Left Brachial Vein, Percutaneous Endoscopic Approach
05BB0ZX Excision of Right Basilic Vein, Open Approach, Diagnostic
05BB0ZZ Excision of Right Basilic Vein, Open Approach
05BB3ZX Excision of Right Basilic Vein, Percutaneous Approach, Diagnostic
05BB3ZZ Excision of Right Basilic Vein, Percutaneous Approach
05BB4ZX Excision of Right Basilic Vein, Percutaneous Endoscopic Approach, Diagnostic
05BB4ZZ Excision of Right Basilic Vein, Percutaneous Endoscopic Approach
05BC0ZX Excision of Left Basilic Vein, Open Approach, Diagnostic
05BC0ZZ Excision of Left Basilic Vein, Open Approach
05BC3ZX Excision of Left Basilic Vein, Percutaneous Approach, Diagnostic
05BC3ZZ Excision of Left Basilic Vein, Percutaneous Approach
05BC4ZX Excision of Left Basilic Vein, Percutaneous Endoscopic Approach, Diagnostic
05BC4ZZ Excision of Left Basilic Vein, Percutaneous Endoscopic Approach
05BD0ZX Excision of Right Cephalic Vein, Open Approach, Diagnostic
05BD0ZZ Excision of Right Cephalic Vein, Open Approach
05BD3ZX Excision of Right Cephalic Vein, Percutaneous Approach, Diagnostic
05BD3ZZ Excision of Right Cephalic Vein, Percutaneous Approach
05BD4ZX Excision of Right Cephalic Vein, Percutaneous Endoscopic Approach, Diagnostic
05BD4ZZ Excision of Right Cephalic Vein, Percutaneous Endoscopic Approach
05BF0ZX Excision of Left Cephalic Vein, Open Approach, Diagnostic
05BF0ZZ Excision of Left Cephalic Vein, Open Approach
05BF3ZX Excision of Left Cephalic Vein, Percutaneous Approach, Diagnostic
05BF3ZZ Excision of Left Cephalic Vein, Percutaneous Approach
05BF4ZX Excision of Left Cephalic Vein, Percutaneous Endoscopic Approach, Diagnostic
05BF4ZZ Excision of Left Cephalic Vein, Percutaneous Endoscopic Approach
05BG0ZX Excision of Right Hand Vein, Open Approach, Diagnostic
05BG0ZZ Excision of Right Hand Vein, Open Approach
05BG3ZX Excision of Right Hand Vein, Percutaneous Approach, Diagnostic
05BG3ZZ Excision of Right Hand Vein, Percutaneous Approach
05BG4ZX Excision of Right Hand Vein, Percutaneous Endoscopic Approach, Diagnostic
05BG4ZZ Excision of Right Hand Vein, Percutaneous Endoscopic Approach
05BH0ZX Excision of Left Hand Vein, Open Approach, Diagnostic
05BH0ZZ Excision of Left Hand Vein, Open Approach
05BH3ZX Excision of Left Hand Vein, Percutaneous Approach, Diagnostic
05BH3ZZ Excision of Left Hand Vein, Percutaneous Approach
05BH4ZX Excision of Left Hand Vein, Percutaneous Endoscopic Approach, Diagnostic
05BH4ZZ Excision of Left Hand Vein, Percutaneous Endoscopic Approach
05BL0ZX Excision of Intracranial Vein, Open Approach, Diagnostic
05BL0ZZ Excision of Intracranial Vein, Open Approach
05BL3ZX Excision of Intracranial Vein, Percutaneous Approach, Diagnostic
05BL3ZZ Excision of Intracranial Vein, Percutaneous Approach
05BL4ZX Excision of Intracranial Vein, Percutaneous Endoscopic Approach, Diagnostic
05BL4ZZ Excision of Intracranial Vein, Percutaneous Endoscopic Approach
05BM0ZX Excision of Right Internal Jugular Vein, Open Approach, Diagnostic
05BM0ZZ Excision of Right Internal Jugular Vein, Open Approach
05BM3ZX Excision of Right Internal Jugular Vein, Percutaneous Approach, Diagnostic
05BM3ZZ Excision of Right Internal Jugular Vein, Percutaneous Approach
05BM4ZX Excision of Right Internal Jugular Vein, Percutaneous Endoscopic Approach, Diagnostic
05BM4ZZ Excision of Right Internal Jugular Vein, Percutaneous Endoscopic Approach
05BN0ZX Excision of Left Internal Jugular Vein, Open Approach, Diagnostic
05BN0ZZ Excision of Left Internal Jugular Vein, Open Approach
05BN3ZX Excision of Left Internal Jugular Vein, Percutaneous Approach, Diagnostic
05BN3ZZ Excision of Left Internal Jugular Vein, Percutaneous Approach
05BN4ZX Excision of Left Internal Jugular Vein, Percutaneous Endoscopic Approach, Diagnostic
05BN4ZZ Excision of Left Internal Jugular Vein, Percutaneous Endoscopic Approach
05BP0ZX Excision of Right External Jugular Vein, Open Approach, Diagnostic
05BP0ZZ Excision of Right External Jugular Vein, Open Approach
05BP3ZX Excision of Right External Jugular Vein, Percutaneous Approach, Diagnostic
05BP3ZZ Excision of Right External Jugular Vein, Percutaneous Approach
05BP4ZX Excision of Right External Jugular Vein, Percutaneous Endoscopic Approach, Diagnostic
05BP4ZZ Excision of Right External Jugular Vein, Percutaneous Endoscopic Approach
05BQ0ZX Excision of Left External Jugular Vein, Open Approach, Diagnostic
05BQ0ZZ Excision of Left External Jugular Vein, Open Approach
05BQ3ZX Excision of Left External Jugular Vein, Percutaneous Approach, Diagnostic
05BQ3ZZ Excision of Left External Jugular Vein, Percutaneous Approach
05BQ4ZX Excision of Left External Jugular Vein, Percutaneous Endoscopic Approach, Diagnostic
05BQ4ZZ Excision of Left External Jugular Vein, Percutaneous Endoscopic Approach
05BR0ZX Excision of Right Vertebral Vein, Open Approach, Diagnostic
05BR0ZZ Excision of Right Vertebral Vein, Open Approach
05BR3ZX Excision of Right Vertebral Vein, Percutaneous Approach, Diagnostic
05BR3ZZ Excision of Right Vertebral Vein, Percutaneous Approach
05BR4ZX Excision of Right Vertebral Vein, Percutaneous Endoscopic Approach, Diagnostic
05BR4ZZ Excision of Right Vertebral Vein, Percutaneous Endoscopic Approach
05BS0ZX Excision of Left Vertebral Vein, Open Approach, Diagnostic
05BS0ZZ Excision of Left Vertebral Vein, Open Approach
05BS3ZX Excision of Left Vertebral Vein, Percutaneous Approach, Diagnostic
05BS3ZZ Excision of Left Vertebral Vein, Percutaneous Approach

05BS4ZX Excision of Left Vertebral Vein, Percutaneous Endoscopic Approach, Diagnostic
05BS4ZZ Excision of Left Vertebral Vein, Percutaneous Endoscopic Approach
05BT0ZX Excision of Right Face Vein, Open Approach, Diagnostic
05BT0ZZ Excision of Right Face Vein, Open Approach
05BT3ZX Excision of Right Face Vein, Percutaneous Approach, Diagnostic
05BT3ZZ Excision of Right Face Vein, Percutaneous Approach
05BT4ZX Excision of Right Face Vein, Percutaneous Endoscopic Approach, Diagnostic
05BT4ZZ Excision of Right Face Vein, Percutaneous Endoscopic Approach
05BV0ZX Excision of Left Face Vein, Open Approach, Diagnostic
05BV0ZZ Excision of Left Face Vein, Open Approach
05BV3ZX Excision of Left Face Vein, Percutaneous Approach, Diagnostic
05BV3ZZ Excision of Left Face Vein, Percutaneous Approach
05BV4ZX Excision of Left Face Vein, Percutaneous Endoscopic Approach, Diagnostic
05BV4ZZ Excision of Left Face Vein, Percutaneous Endoscopic Approach
05BY0ZX Excision of Upper Vein, Open Approach, Diagnostic
05BY0ZZ Excision of Upper Vein, Open Approach
05BY3ZX Excision of Upper Vein, Percutaneous Approach, Diagnostic
05BY3ZZ Excision of Upper Vein, Percutaneous Approach
05BY4ZX Excision of Upper Vein, Percutaneous Endoscopic Approach, Diagnostic
05BY4ZZ Excision of Upper Vein, Percutaneous Endoscopic Approach

05C – Upper Veins, Extirpation

05C00ZZ Extirpation of Matter from Azygos Vein, Open Approach
05C03ZZ Extirpation of Matter from Azygos Vein, Percutaneous Approach
05C04ZZ Extirpation of Matter from Azygos Vein, Percutaneous Endoscopic Approach
05C10ZZ Extirpation of Matter from Hemiazygos Vein, Open Approach
05C13ZZ Extirpation of Matter from Hemiazygos Vein, Percutaneous Approach
05C14ZZ Extirpation of Matter from Hemiazygos Vein, Percutaneous Endoscopic Approach
05C30ZZ Extirpation of Matter from Right Innominate Vein, Open Approach
05C33ZZ Extirpation of Matter from Right Innominate Vein, Percutaneous Approach
05C34ZZ Extirpation of Matter from Right Innominate Vein, Percutaneous Endoscopic Approach
05C40ZZ Extirpation of Matter from Left Innominate Vein, Open Approach
05C43ZZ Extirpation of Matter from Left Innominate Vein, Percutaneous Approach
05C44ZZ Extirpation of Matter from Left Innominate Vein, Percutaneous Endoscopic Approach
05C50ZZ Extirpation of Matter from Right Subclavian Vein, Open Approach
05C53ZZ Extirpation of Matter from Right Subclavian Vein, Percutaneous Approach
05C54ZZ Extirpation of Matter from Right Subclavian Vein, Percutaneous Endoscopic Approach
05C60ZZ Extirpation of Matter from Left Subclavian Vein, Open Approach
05C63ZZ Extirpation of Matter from Left Subclavian Vein, Percutaneous Approach
05C64ZZ Extirpation of Matter from Left Subclavian Vein, Percutaneous Endoscopic Approach
05C70ZZ Extirpation of Matter from Right Axillary Vein, Open Approach
05C73ZZ Extirpation of Matter from Right Axillary Vein, Percutaneous Approach
05C74ZZ Extirpation of Matter from Right Axillary Vein, Percutaneous Endoscopic Approach
05C80ZZ Extirpation of Matter from Left Axillary Vein, Open Approach
05C83ZZ Extirpation of Matter from Left Axillary Vein, Percutaneous Approach
05C84ZZ Extirpation of Matter from Left Axillary Vein, Percutaneous Endoscopic Approach
05C90ZZ Extirpation of Matter from Right Brachial Vein, Open Approach
05C93ZZ Extirpation of Matter from Right Brachial Vein, Percutaneous Approach
05C94ZZ Extirpation of Matter from Right Brachial Vein, Percutaneous Endoscopic Approach
05CA0ZZ Extirpation of Matter from Left Brachial Vein, Open Approach
05CA3ZZ Extirpation of Matter from Left Brachial Vein, Percutaneous Approach
05CA4ZZ Extirpation of Matter from Left Brachial Vein, Percutaneous Endoscopic Approach
05CB0ZZ Extirpation of Matter from Right Basilic Vein, Open Approach
05CB3ZZ Extirpation of Matter from Right Basilic Vein, Percutaneous Approach
05CB4ZZ Extirpation of Matter from Right Basilic Vein, Percutaneous Endoscopic Approach
05CC0ZZ Extirpation of Matter from Left Basilic Vein, Open Approach
05CC3ZZ Extirpation of Matter from Left Basilic Vein, Percutaneous Approach
05CC4ZZ Extirpation of Matter from Left Basilic Vein, Percutaneous Endoscopic Approach
05CD0ZZ Extirpation of Matter from Right Cephalic Vein, Open Approach
05CD3ZZ Extirpation of Matter from Right Cephalic Vein, Percutaneous Approach
05CD4ZZ Extirpation of Matter from Right Cephalic Vein, Percutaneous Endoscopic Approach
05CF0ZZ Extirpation of Matter from Left Cephalic Vein, Open Approach
05CF3ZZ Extirpation of Matter from Left Cephalic Vein, Percutaneous Approach
05CF4ZZ Extirpation of Matter from Left Cephalic Vein, Percutaneous Endoscopic Approach
05CG0ZZ Extirpation of Matter from Right Hand Vein, Open Approach
05CG3ZZ Extirpation of Matter from Right Hand Vein, Percutaneous Approach
05CG4ZZ Extirpation of Matter from Right Hand Vein, Percutaneous Endoscopic Approach
05CH0ZZ Extirpation of Matter from Left Hand Vein, Open Approach
05CH3ZZ Extirpation of Matter from Left Hand Vein, Percutaneous Approach
05CH4ZZ Extirpation of Matter from Left Hand Vein, Percutaneous Endoscopic Approach
05CL0ZZ Extirpation of Matter from Intracranial Vein, Open Approach
▲ **05CL3ZZ** Extirpation of Matter from Intracranial Vein, Percutaneous Approach
▲ **05CL4ZZ** Extirpation of Matter from Intracranial Vein, Percutaneous Endoscopic Approach
05CM0ZZ Extirpation of Matter from Right Internal Jugular Vein, Open Approach
05CM3ZZ Extirpation of Matter from Right Internal Jugular Vein, Percutaneous Approach
05CM4ZZ Extirpation of Matter from Right Internal Jugular Vein, Percutaneous Endoscopic Approach
05CN0ZZ Extirpation of Matter from Left Internal Jugular Vein, Open Approach
05CN3ZZ Extirpation of Matter from Left Internal Jugular Vein, Percutaneous Approach
05CN4ZZ Extirpation of Matter from Left Internal Jugular Vein, Percutaneous Endoscopic Approach
05CP0ZZ Extirpation of Matter from Right External Jugular Vein, Open Approach
05CP3ZZ Extirpation of Matter from Right External Jugular Vein, Percutaneous Approach
05CP4ZZ Extirpation of Matter from Right External Jugular Vein, Percutaneous Endoscopic Approach
05CQ0ZZ Extirpation of Matter from Left External Jugular Vein, Open Approach
05CQ3ZZ Extirpation of Matter from Left External Jugular Vein, Percutaneous Approach
05CQ4ZZ Extirpation of Matter from Left External Jugular Vein, Percutaneous Endoscopic Approach
05CR0ZZ Extirpation of Matter from Right Vertebral Vein, Open Approach
05CR3ZZ Extirpation of Matter from Right Vertebral Vein, Percutaneous Approach
05CR4ZZ Extirpation of Matter from Right Vertebral Vein, Percutaneous Endoscopic Approach
05CS0ZZ Extirpation of Matter from Left Vertebral Vein, Open Approach
05CS3ZZ Extirpation of Matter from Left Vertebral Vein, Percutaneous Approach
05CS4ZZ Extirpation of Matter from Left Vertebral Vein, Percutaneous Endoscopic Approach
05CT0ZZ Extirpation of Matter from Right Face Vein, Open Approach
05CT3ZZ Extirpation of Matter from Right Face Vein, Percutaneous Approach
05CT4ZZ Extirpation of Matter from Right Face Vein, Percutaneous Endoscopic Approach
05CV0ZZ Extirpation of Matter from Left Face Vein, Open Approach
05CV3ZZ Extirpation of Matter from Left Face Vein, Percutaneous Approach
05CV4ZZ Extirpation of Matter from Left Face Vein, Percutaneous Endoscopic Approach
05CY0ZZ Extirpation of Matter from Upper Vein, Open Approach
05CY3ZZ Extirpation of Matter from Upper Vein, Percutaneous Approach
05CY4ZZ Extirpation of Matter from Upper Vein, Percutaneous Endoscopic Approach

05D – Upper Veins, Extraction

05D90ZZ Extraction of Right Brachial Vein, Open Approach
05D93ZZ Extraction of Right Brachial Vein, Percutaneous Approach
05DA0ZZ Extraction of Left Brachial Vein, Open Approach

DA3ZZ Extraction of Left Brachial Vein, Percutaneous Approach
DB0ZZ Extraction of Right Basilic Vein, Open Approach
DB3ZZ Extraction of Right Basilic Vein, Percutaneous Approach
DC0ZZ Extraction of Left Basilic Vein, Open Approach
DC3ZZ Extraction of Left Basilic Vein, Percutaneous Approach
05DD0ZZ Extraction of Right Cephalic Vein, Open Approach
05DD3ZZ Extraction of Right Cephalic Vein, Percutaneous Approach
05DF0ZZ Extraction of Left Cephalic Vein, Open Approach
05DF3ZZ Extraction of Left Cephalic Vein, Percutaneous Approach
05DG0ZZ Extraction of Right Hand Vein, Open Approach
05DG3ZZ Extraction of Right Hand Vein, Percutaneous Approach
05DH0ZZ Extraction of Left Hand Vein, Open Approach
05DH3ZZ Extraction of Left Hand Vein, Percutaneous Approach
05DY0ZZ Extraction of Upper Vein, Open Approach
05DY3ZZ Extraction of Upper Vein, Percutaneous Approach

5H – Upper Veins, Insertion

5H003Z Insertion of Infusion Device into Azygos Vein, Open Approach
5H00DZ Insertion of Intraluminal Device into Azygos Vein, Open Approach
5H033Z Insertion of Infusion Device into Azygos Vein, Percutaneous Approach
5H03DZ Insertion of Intraluminal Device into Azygos Vein, Percutaneous Approach
5H043Z Insertion of Infusion Device into Azygos Vein, Percutaneous Endoscopic Approach
5H04DZ Insertion of Intraluminal Device into Azygos Vein, Percutaneous Endoscopic Approach
5H103Z Insertion of Infusion Device into Hemiazygos Vein, Open Approach
5H10DZ Insertion of Intraluminal Device into Hemiazygos Vein, Open Approach
5H133Z Insertion of Infusion Device into Hemiazygos Vein, Percutaneous Approach
5H13DZ Insertion of Intraluminal Device into Hemiazygos Vein, Percutaneous Approach
5H143Z Insertion of Infusion Device into Hemiazygos Vein, Percutaneous Endoscopic Approach
5H14DZ Insertion of Intraluminal Device into Hemiazygos Vein, Percutaneous Endoscopic Approach
5H303Z Insertion of Infusion Device into Right Innominate Vein, Open Approach
5H30DZ Insertion of Intraluminal Device into Right Innominate Vein, Open Approach
5H333Z Insertion of Infusion Device into Right Innominate Vein, Percutaneous Approach
5H33DZ Insertion of Intraluminal Device into Right Innominate Vein, Percutaneous Approach
5H343Z Insertion of Infusion Device into Right Innominate Vein, Percutaneous Endoscopic Approach
5H34DZ Insertion of Intraluminal Device into Right Innominate Vein, Percutaneous Endoscopic Approach
5H403Z Insertion of Infusion Device into Left Innominate Vein, Open Approach
5H40DZ Insertion of Intraluminal Device into Left Innominate Vein, Open Approach
5H433Z Insertion of Infusion Device into Left Innominate Vein, Percutaneous Approach
5H43DZ Insertion of Intraluminal Device into Left Innominate Vein, Percutaneous Approach
5H443Z Insertion of Infusion Device into Left Innominate Vein, Percutaneous Endoscopic Approach
5H44DZ Insertion of Intraluminal Device into Left Innominate Vein, Percutaneous Endoscopic Approach
5H503Z Insertion of Infusion Device into Right Subclavian Vein, Open Approach
5H50DZ Insertion of Intraluminal Device into Right Subclavian Vein, Open Approach
● **05H533Z** Insertion of Infusion Device into Right Subclavian Vein, Percutaneous Approach
05H53DZ Insertion of Intraluminal Device into Right Subclavian Vein, Percutaneous Approach
05H543Z Insertion of Infusion Device into Right Subclavian Vein, Percutaneous Endoscopic Approach
05H54DZ Insertion of Intraluminal Device into Right Subclavian Vein, Percutaneous Endoscopic Approach
05H603Z Insertion of Infusion Device into Left Subclavian Vein, Open Approach
05H60DZ Insertion of Intraluminal Device into Left Subclavian Vein, Open Approach
● **05H633Z** Insertion of Infusion Device into Left Subclavian Vein, Percutaneous Approach
05H63DZ Insertion of Intraluminal Device into Left Subclavian Vein, Percutaneous Approach
05H643Z Insertion of Infusion Device into Left Subclavian Vein, Percutaneous Endoscopic Approach
05H64DZ Insertion of Intraluminal Device into Left Subclavian Vein, Percutaneous Endoscopic Approach
05H703Z Insertion of Infusion Device into Right Axillary Vein, Open Approach
05H70DZ Insertion of Intraluminal Device into Right Axillary Vein, Open Approach
05H733Z Insertion of Infusion Device into Right Axillary Vein, Percutaneous Approach
05H73DZ Insertion of Intraluminal Device into Right Axillary Vein, Percutaneous Approach
05H743Z Insertion of Infusion Device into Right Axillary Vein, Percutaneous Endoscopic Approach
05H74DZ Insertion of Intraluminal Device into Right Axillary Vein, Percutaneous Endoscopic Approach
05H803Z Insertion of Infusion Device into Left Axillary Vein, Open Approach
05H80DZ Insertion of Intraluminal Device into Left Axillary Vein, Open Approach
05H833Z Insertion of Infusion Device into Left Axillary Vein, Percutaneous Approach
05H83DZ Insertion of Intraluminal Device into Left Axillary Vein, Percutaneous Approach
05H843Z Insertion of Infusion Device into Left Axillary Vein, Percutaneous Endoscopic Approach
05H84DZ Insertion of Intraluminal Device into Left Axillary Vein, Percutaneous Endoscopic Approach
05H903Z Insertion of Infusion Device into Right Brachial Vein, Open Approach
05H90DZ Insertion of Intraluminal Device into Right Brachial Vein, Open Approach
05H933Z Insertion of Infusion Device into Right Brachial Vein, Percutaneous Approach
05H93DZ Insertion of Intraluminal Device into Right Brachial Vein, Percutaneous Approach
05H943Z Insertion of Infusion Device into Right Brachial Vein, Percutaneous Endoscopic Approach
05H94DZ Insertion of Intraluminal Device into Right Brachial Vein, Percutaneous Endoscopic Approach
05HA03Z Insertion of Infusion Device into Left Brachial Vein, Open Approach
05HA0DZ Insertion of Intraluminal Device into Left Brachial Vein, Open Approach
05HA33Z Insertion of Infusion Device into Left Brachial Vein, Percutaneous Approach
05HA3DZ Insertion of Intraluminal Device into Left Brachial Vein, Percutaneous Approach
05HA43Z Insertion of Infusion Device into Left Brachial Vein, Percutaneous Endoscopic Approach
05HA4DZ Insertion of Intraluminal Device into Left Brachial Vein, Percutaneous Endoscopic Approach
05HB03Z Insertion of Infusion Device into Right Basilic Vein, Open Approach
05HB0DZ Insertion of Intraluminal Device into Right Basilic Vein, Open Approach
05HB33Z Insertion of Infusion Device into Right Basilic Vein, Percutaneous Approach
05HB3DZ Insertion of Intraluminal Device into Right Basilic Vein, Percutaneous Approach
05HB43Z Insertion of Infusion Device into Right Basilic Vein, Percutaneous Endoscopic Approach
05HB4DZ Insertion of Intraluminal Device into Right Basilic Vein, Percutaneous Endoscopic Approach
05HC03Z Insertion of Infusion Device into Left Basilic Vein, Open Approach
05HC0DZ Insertion of Intraluminal Device into Left Basilic Vein, Open Approach
05HC33Z Insertion of Infusion Device into Left Basilic Vein, Percutaneous Approach
05HC3DZ Insertion of Intraluminal Device into Left Basilic Vein, Percutaneous Approach
05HC43Z Insertion of Infusion Device into Left Basilic Vein, Percutaneous Endoscopic Approach
05HC4DZ Insertion of Intraluminal Device into Left Basilic Vein, Percutaneous Endoscopic Approach
05HD03Z Insertion of Infusion Device into Right Cephalic Vein, Open Approach
05HD0DZ Insertion of Intraluminal Device into Right Cephalic Vein, Open Approach
05HD33Z Insertion of Infusion Device into Right Cephalic Vein, Percutaneous Approach
05HD3DZ Insertion of Intraluminal Device into Right Cephalic Vein, Percutaneous Approach
05HD43Z Insertion of Infusion Device into Right Cephalic Vein, Percutaneous Endoscopic Approach

05HD4DZ Insertion of Intraluminal Device into Right Cephalic Vein, Percutaneous Endoscopic Approach
05HF03Z Insertion of Infusion Device into Left Cephalic Vein, Open Approach
05HF0DZ Insertion of Intraluminal Device into Left Cephalic Vein, Open Approach
05HF33Z Insertion of Infusion Device into Left Cephalic Vein, Percutaneous Approach
05HF3DZ Insertion of Intraluminal Device into Left Cephalic Vein, Percutaneous Approach
05HF43Z Insertion of Infusion Device into Left Cephalic Vein, Percutaneous Endoscopic Approach
05HF4DZ Insertion of Intraluminal Device into Left Cephalic Vein, Percutaneous Endoscopic Approach
05HG03Z Insertion of Infusion Device into Right Hand Vein, Open Approach
05HG0DZ Insertion of Intraluminal Device into Right Hand Vein, Open Approach
05HG33Z Insertion of Infusion Device into Right Hand Vein, Percutaneous Approach
05HG3DZ Insertion of Intraluminal Device into Right Hand Vein, Percutaneous Approach
05HG43Z Insertion of Infusion Device into Right Hand Vein, Percutaneous Endoscopic Approach
05HG4DZ Insertion of Intraluminal Device into Right Hand Vein, Percutaneous Endoscopic Approach
05HH03Z Insertion of Infusion Device into Left Hand Vein, Open Approach
05HH0DZ Insertion of Intraluminal Device into Left Hand Vein, Open Approach
05HH33Z Insertion of Infusion Device into Left Hand Vein, Percutaneous Approach
05HH3DZ Insertion of Intraluminal Device into Left Hand Vein, Percutaneous Approach
05HH43Z Insertion of Infusion Device into Left Hand Vein, Percutaneous Endoscopic Approach
05HH4DZ Insertion of Intraluminal Device into Left Hand Vein, Percutaneous Endoscopic Approach
05HL03Z Insertion of Infusion Device into Intracranial Vein, Open Approach
05HL0DZ Insertion of Intraluminal Device into Intracranial Vein, Open Approach
05HL33Z Insertion of Infusion Device into Intracranial Vein, Percutaneous Approach
05HL3DZ Insertion of Intraluminal Device into Intracranial Vein, Percutaneous Approach
05HL43Z Insertion of Infusion Device into Intracranial Vein, Percutaneous Endoscopic Approach
05HL4DZ Insertion of Intraluminal Device into Intracranial Vein, Percutaneous Endoscopic Approach
05HM03Z Insertion of Infusion Device into Right Internal Jugular Vein, Open Approach
05HM0DZ Insertion of Intraluminal Device into Right Internal Jugular Vein, Open Approach
● **05HM33Z** Insertion of Infusion Device into Right Internal Jugular Vein, Percutaneous Approach
HAC With secondary diagnosis code J95.811
05HM3DZ Insertion of Intraluminal Device into Right Internal Jugular Vein, Percutaneous Approach
05HM43Z Insertion of Infusion Device into Right Internal Jugular Vein, Percutaneous Endoscopic Approach
05HM4DZ Insertion of Intraluminal Device into Right Internal Jugular Vein, Percutaneous Endoscopic Approach
05HN03Z Insertion of Infusion Device into Left Internal Jugular Vein, Open Approach
05HN0DZ Insertion of Intraluminal Device into Left Internal Jugular Vein, Open Approach
● **05HN33Z** Insertion of Infusion Device into Left Internal Jugular Vein, Percutaneous Approach
HAC With secondary diagnosis code J95.811
05HN3DZ Insertion of Intraluminal Device into Left Internal Jugular Vein, Percutaneous Approach
05HN43Z Insertion of Infusion Device into Left Internal Jugular Vein, Percutaneous Endoscopic Approach
05HN4DZ Insertion of Intraluminal Device into Left Internal Jugular Vein, Percutaneous Endoscopic Approach
05HP03Z Insertion of Infusion Device into Right External Jugular Vein, Open Approach
05HP0DZ Insertion of Intraluminal Device into Right External Jugular Vein, Open Approach
● **05HP33Z** Insertion of Infusion Device into Right External Jugular Vein, Percutaneous Approach
HAC With secondary diagnosis code J95.811
05HP3DZ Insertion of Intraluminal Device into Right External Jugular Vein, Percutaneous Approach
05HP43Z Insertion of Infusion Device into Right External Jugular Vein, Percutaneous Endoscopic Approach
05HP4DZ Insertion of Intraluminal Device into Right External Jugular Vein, Percutaneous Endoscopic Approach
05HQ03Z Insertion of Infusion Device into Left External Jugular Vein, Open Approach
05HQ0DZ Insertion of Intraluminal Device into Left External Jugular Vein, Open Approach
● **05HQ33Z** Insertion of Infusion Device into Left External Jugular Vein, Percutaneous Approach
HAC With secondary diagnosis code J95.811
05HQ3DZ Insertion of Intraluminal Device into Left External Jugular Vein, Percutaneous Approach
05HQ43Z Insertion of Infusion Device into Left External Jugular Vein, Percutaneous Endoscopic Approach
05HQ4DZ Insertion of Intraluminal Device into Left External Jugular Vein, Percutaneous Endoscopic Approach
05HR03Z Insertion of Infusion Device into Right Vertebral Vein, Open Approach
05HR0DZ Insertion of Intraluminal Device into Right Vertebral Vein, Open Approach
05HR33Z Insertion of Infusion Device into Right Vertebral Vein, Percutaneous Approach
05HR3DZ Insertion of Intraluminal Device into Right Vertebral Vein, Percutaneous Approach
05HR43Z Insertion of Infusion Device into Right Vertebral Vein, Percutaneous Endoscopic Approach
05HR4DZ Insertion of Intraluminal Device into Rig Vertebral Vein, Percutaneous Endoscopic Approach
05HS03Z Insertion of Infusion Device into Left Vertebral Vein, Open Approach
05HS0DZ Insertion of Intraluminal Device into Left Vertebral Vein, Open Approach
05HS33Z Insertion of Infusion Device into Left Vertebral Vein, Percutaneous Approach
05HS3DZ Insertion of Intraluminal Device into Left Vertebral Vein, Percutaneous Approach
05HS43Z Insertion of Infusion Device into Left Vertebral Vein, Percutaneous Endoscopic Approach
05HS4DZ Insertion of Intraluminal Device into Left Vertebral Vein, Percutaneous Endoscopic Approach
05HT03Z Insertion of Infusion Device into Right Face Vein, Open Approach
05HT0DZ Insertion of Intraluminal Device into Righ Face Vein, Open Approach
05HT33Z Insertion of Infusion Device into Right Face Vein, Percutaneous Approach
05HT3DZ Insertion of Intraluminal Device into Righ Face Vein, Percutaneous Approach
05HT43Z Insertion of Infusion Device into Right Face Vein, Percutaneous Endoscopic Approach
05HT4DZ Insertion of Intraluminal Device into Right Face Vein, Percutaneous Endoscopi Approach
05HV03Z Insertion of Infusion Device into Left Fac Vein, Open Approach
05HV0DZ Insertion of Intraluminal Device into Left Face Vein, Open Approach
05HV33Z Insertion of Infusion Device into Left Fac Vein, Percutaneous Approach
05HV3DZ Insertion of Intraluminal Device into Left Face Vein, Percutaneous Approach
05HV43Z Insertion of Infusion Device into Left Fac Vein, Percutaneous Endoscopic Approach
05HV4DZ Insertion of Intraluminal Device into Left Face Vein, Percutaneous Endoscopic Approach
05HY02Z Insertion of Monitoring Device into Upper Vein, Open Approach
05HY03Z Insertion of Infusion Device into Upper Vein, Open Approach
05HY0DZ Insertion of Intraluminal Device into Upper Vein, Open Approach
05HY32Z Insertion of Monitoring Device into Upper Vein, Percutaneous Approach
05HY33Z Insertion of Infusion Device into Upper Vein, Percutaneous Approach
05HY3DZ Insertion of Intraluminal Device into Upper Vein, Percutaneous Approach
05HY42Z Insertion of Monitoring Device into Upper Vein, Percutaneous Endoscopic Approach
05HY43Z Insertion of Infusion Device into Upper Vein, Percutaneous Endoscopic Approach
05HY4DZ Insertion of Intraluminal Device into Upper Vein, Percutaneous Endoscopic Approach

05J – Upper Veins, Inspection

Review Coding Guidelines B3.11a, B3.11b and B3.11c

05JY0ZZ Inspection of Upper Vein, Open Approach
05JY3ZZ Inspection of Upper Vein, Percutaneous Approach
05JY4ZZ Inspection of Upper Vein, Percutaneous Endoscopic Approach
05JYXZZ Inspection of Upper Vein, External Approach

5L – Upper Veins, Occlusion

eview Coding Guideline B3.12

L00CZ Occlusion of Azygos Vein with Extraluminal Device, Open Approach
L00DZ Occlusion of Azygos Vein with Intraluminal Device, Open Approach
L00ZZ Occlusion of Azygos Vein, Open Approach
L03CZ Occlusion of Azygos Vein with Extraluminal Device, Percutaneous Approach
L03DZ Occlusion of Azygos Vein with Intraluminal Device, Percutaneous Approach
L03ZZ Occlusion of Azygos Vein, Percutaneous Approach
L04CZ Occlusion of Azygos Vein with Extraluminal Device, Percutaneous Endoscopic Approach
L04DZ Occlusion of Azygos Vein with Intraluminal Device, Percutaneous Endoscopic Approach
L04ZZ Occlusion of Azygos Vein, Percutaneous Endoscopic Approach
L10CZ Occlusion of Hemiazygos Vein with Extraluminal Device, Open Approach
5L10DZ Occlusion of Hemiazygos Vein with Intraluminal Device, Open Approach
5L10ZZ Occlusion of Hemiazygos Vein, Open Approach
5L13CZ Occlusion of Hemiazygos Vein with Extraluminal Device, Percutaneous Approach
5L13DZ Occlusion of Hemiazygos Vein with Intraluminal Device, Percutaneous Approach
5L13ZZ Occlusion of Hemiazygos Vein, Percutaneous Approach
5L14CZ Occlusion of Hemiazygos Vein with Extraluminal Device, Percutaneous Endoscopic Approach
5L14DZ Occlusion of Hemiazygos Vein with Intraluminal Device, Percutaneous Endoscopic Approach
5L14ZZ Occlusion of Hemiazygos Vein, Percutaneous Endoscopic Approach
5L30CZ Occlusion of Right Innominate Vein with Extraluminal Device, Open Approach
5L30DZ Occlusion of Right Innominate Vein with Intraluminal Device, Open Approach
5L30ZZ Occlusion of Right Innominate Vein, Open Approach
5L33CZ Occlusion of Right Innominate Vein with Extraluminal Device, Percutaneous Approach
5L33DZ Occlusion of Right Innominate Vein with Intraluminal Device, Percutaneous Approach
5L33ZZ Occlusion of Right Innominate Vein, Percutaneous Approach
5L34CZ Occlusion of Right Innominate Vein with Extraluminal Device, Percutaneous Endoscopic Approach
5L34DZ Occlusion of Right Innominate Vein with Intraluminal Device, Percutaneous Endoscopic Approach
5L34ZZ Occlusion of Right Innominate Vein, Percutaneous Endoscopic Approach
5L40CZ Occlusion of Left Innominate Vein with Extraluminal Device, Open Approach
5L40DZ Occlusion of Left Innominate Vein with Intraluminal Device, Open Approach
5L40ZZ Occlusion of Left Innominate Vein, Open Approach
05L43CZ Occlusion of Left Innominate Vein with Extraluminal Device, Percutaneous Approach
05L43DZ Occlusion of Left Innominate Vein with Intraluminal Device, Percutaneous Approach
05L43ZZ Occlusion of Left Innominate Vein, Percutaneous Approach
05L44CZ Occlusion of Left Innominate Vein with Extraluminal Device, Percutaneous Endoscopic Approach
05L44DZ Occlusion of Left Innominate Vein with Intraluminal Device, Percutaneous Endoscopic Approach
05L44ZZ Occlusion of Left Innominate Vein, Percutaneous Endoscopic Approach
05L50CZ Occlusion of Right Subclavian Vein with Extraluminal Device, Open Approach
05L50DZ Occlusion of Right Subclavian Vein with Intraluminal Device, Open Approach
05L50ZZ Occlusion of Right Subclavian Vein, Open Approach
05L53CZ Occlusion of Right Subclavian Vein with Extraluminal Device, Percutaneous Approach
05L53DZ Occlusion of Right Subclavian Vein with Intraluminal Device, Percutaneous Approach
05L53ZZ Occlusion of Right Subclavian Vein, Percutaneous Approach
05L54CZ Occlusion of Right Subclavian Vein with Extraluminal Device, Percutaneous Endoscopic Approach
05L54DZ Occlusion of Right Subclavian Vein with Intraluminal Device, Percutaneous Endoscopic Approach
05L54ZZ Occlusion of Right Subclavian Vein, Percutaneous Endoscopic Approach
05L60CZ Occlusion of Left Subclavian Vein with Extraluminal Device, Open Approach
05L60DZ Occlusion of Left Subclavian Vein with Intraluminal Device, Open Approach
05L60ZZ Occlusion of Left Subclavian Vein, Open Approach
05L63CZ Occlusion of Left Subclavian Vein with Extraluminal Device, Percutaneous Approach
05L63DZ Occlusion of Left Subclavian Vein with Intraluminal Device, Percutaneous Approach
05L63ZZ Occlusion of Left Subclavian Vein, Percutaneous Approach
05L64CZ Occlusion of Left Subclavian Vein with Extraluminal Device, Percutaneous Endoscopic Approach
05L64DZ Occlusion of Left Subclavian Vein with Intraluminal Device, Percutaneous Endoscopic Approach
05L64ZZ Occlusion of Left Subclavian Vein, Percutaneous Endoscopic Approach
05L70CZ Occlusion of Right Axillary Vein with Extraluminal Device, Open Approach
05L70DZ Occlusion of Right Axillary Vein with Intraluminal Device, Open Approach
05L70ZZ Occlusion of Right Axillary Vein, Open Approach
05L73CZ Occlusion of Right Axillary Vein with Extraluminal Device, Percutaneous Approach
05L73DZ Occlusion of Right Axillary Vein with Intraluminal Device, Percutaneous Approach
05L73ZZ Occlusion of Right Axillary Vein, Percutaneous Approach
05L74CZ Occlusion of Right Axillary Vein with Extraluminal Device, Percutaneous Endoscopic Approach
05L74DZ Occlusion of Right Axillary Vein with Intraluminal Device, Percutaneous Endoscopic Approach
05L74ZZ Occlusion of Right Axillary Vein, Percutaneous Endoscopic Approach
05L80CZ Occlusion of Left Axillary Vein with Extraluminal Device, Open Approach
05L80DZ Occlusion of Left Axillary Vein with Intraluminal Device, Open Approach
05L80ZZ Occlusion of Left Axillary Vein, Open Approach
05L83CZ Occlusion of Left Axillary Vein with Extraluminal Device, Percutaneous Approach
05L83DZ Occlusion of Left Axillary Vein with Intraluminal Device, Percutaneous Approach
05L83ZZ Occlusion of Left Axillary Vein, Percutaneous Approach
05L84CZ Occlusion of Left Axillary Vein with Extraluminal Device, Percutaneous Endoscopic Approach
05L84DZ Occlusion of Left Axillary Vein with Intraluminal Device, Percutaneous Endoscopic Approach
05L84ZZ Occlusion of Left Axillary Vein, Percutaneous Endoscopic Approach
05L90CZ Occlusion of Right Brachial Vein with Extraluminal Device, Open Approach
05L90DZ Occlusion of Right Brachial Vein with Intraluminal Device, Open Approach
05L90ZZ Occlusion of Right Brachial Vein, Open Approach
05L93CZ Occlusion of Right Brachial Vein with Extraluminal Device, Percutaneous Approach
05L93DZ Occlusion of Right Brachial Vein with Intraluminal Device, Percutaneous Approach
05L93ZZ Occlusion of Right Brachial Vein, Percutaneous Approach
05L94CZ Occlusion of Right Brachial Vein with Extraluminal Device, Percutaneous Endoscopic Approach
05L94DZ Occlusion of Right Brachial Vein with Intraluminal Device, Percutaneous Endoscopic Approach
05L94ZZ Occlusion of Right Brachial Vein, Percutaneous Endoscopic Approach
05LA0CZ Occlusion of Left Brachial Vein with Extraluminal Device, Open Approach
05LA0DZ Occlusion of Left Brachial Vein with Intraluminal Device, Open Approach
05LA0ZZ Occlusion of Left Brachial Vein, Open Approach
05LA3CZ Occlusion of Left Brachial Vein with Extraluminal Device, Percutaneous Approach
05LA3DZ Occlusion of Left Brachial Vein with Intraluminal Device, Percutaneous Approach
05LA3ZZ Occlusion of Left Brachial Vein, Percutaneous Approach
05LA4CZ Occlusion of Left Brachial Vein with Extraluminal Device, Percutaneous Endoscopic Approach

05LA4DZ Occlusion of Left Brachial Vein with Intraluminal Device, Percutaneous Endoscopic Approach
05LA4ZZ Occlusion of Left Brachial Vein, Percutaneous Endoscopic Approach
05LB0CZ Occlusion of Right Basilic Vein with Extraluminal Device, Open Approach
05LB0DZ Occlusion of Right Basilic Vein with Intraluminal Device, Open Approach
05LB0ZZ Occlusion of Right Basilic Vein, Open Approach
05LB3CZ Occlusion of Right Basilic Vein with Extraluminal Device, Percutaneous Approach
05LB3DZ Occlusion of Right Basilic Vein with Intraluminal Device, Percutaneous Approach
05LB3ZZ Occlusion of Right Basilic Vein, Percutaneous Approach
05LB4CZ Occlusion of Right Basilic Vein with Extraluminal Device, Percutaneous Endoscopic Approach
05LB4DZ Occlusion of Right Basilic Vein with Intraluminal Device, Percutaneous Endoscopic Approach
05LB4ZZ Occlusion of Right Basilic Vein, Percutaneous Endoscopic Approach
05LC0CZ Occlusion of Left Basilic Vein with Extraluminal Device, Open Approach
05LC0DZ Occlusion of Left Basilic Vein with Intraluminal Device, Open Approach
05LC0ZZ Occlusion of Left Basilic Vein, Open Approach
05LC3CZ Occlusion of Left Basilic Vein with Extraluminal Device, Percutaneous Approach
05LC3DZ Occlusion of Left Basilic Vein with Intraluminal Device, Percutaneous Approach
05LC3ZZ Occlusion of Left Basilic Vein, Percutaneous Approach
05LC4CZ Occlusion of Left Basilic Vein with Extraluminal Device, Percutaneous Endoscopic Approach
05LC4DZ Occlusion of Left Basilic Vein with Intraluminal Device, Percutaneous Endoscopic Approach
05LC4ZZ Occlusion of Left Basilic Vein, Percutaneous Endoscopic Approach
05LD0CZ Occlusion of Right Cephalic Vein with Extraluminal Device, Open Approach
05LD0DZ Occlusion of Right Cephalic Vein with Intraluminal Device, Open Approach
05LD0ZZ Occlusion of Right Cephalic Vein, Open Approach
05LD3CZ Occlusion of Right Cephalic Vein with Extraluminal Device, Percutaneous Approach
05LD3DZ Occlusion of Right Cephalic Vein with Intraluminal Device, Percutaneous Approach
05LD3ZZ Occlusion of Right Cephalic Vein, Percutaneous Approach
05LD4CZ Occlusion of Right Cephalic Vein with Extraluminal Device, Percutaneous Endoscopic Approach
05LD4DZ Occlusion of Right Cephalic Vein with Intraluminal Device, Percutaneous Endoscopic Approach
05LD4ZZ Occlusion of Right Cephalic Vein, Percutaneous Endoscopic Approach
05LF0CZ Occlusion of Left Cephalic Vein with Extraluminal Device, Open Approach
05LF0DZ Occlusion of Left Cephalic Vein with Intraluminal Device, Open Approach
05LF0ZZ Occlusion of Left Cephalic Vein, Open Approach
05LF3CZ Occlusion of Left Cephalic Vein with Extraluminal Device, Percutaneous Approach
05LF3DZ Occlusion of Left Cephalic Vein with Intraluminal Device, Percutaneous Approach
05LF3ZZ Occlusion of Left Cephalic Vein, Percutaneous Approach
05LF4CZ Occlusion of Left Cephalic Vein with Extraluminal Device, Percutaneous Endoscopic Approach
05LF4DZ Occlusion of Left Cephalic Vein with Intraluminal Device, Percutaneous Endoscopic Approach
05LF4ZZ Occlusion of Left Cephalic Vein, Percutaneous Endoscopic Approach
05LG0CZ Occlusion of Right Hand Vein with Extraluminal Device, Open Approach
05LG0DZ Occlusion of Right Hand Vein with Intraluminal Device, Open Approach
05LG0ZZ Occlusion of Right Hand Vein, Open Approach
05LG3CZ Occlusion of Right Hand Vein with Extraluminal Device, Percutaneous Approach
05LG3DZ Occlusion of Right Hand Vein with Intraluminal Device, Percutaneous Approach
05LG3ZZ Occlusion of Right Hand Vein, Percutaneous Approach
05LG4CZ Occlusion of Right Hand Vein with Extraluminal Device, Percutaneous Endoscopic Approach
05LG4DZ Occlusion of Right Hand Vein with Intraluminal Device, Percutaneous Endoscopic Approach
05LG4ZZ Occlusion of Right Hand Vein, Percutaneous Endoscopic Approach
05LH0CZ Occlusion of Left Hand Vein with Extraluminal Device, Open Approach
05LH0DZ Occlusion of Left Hand Vein with Intraluminal Device, Open Approach
05LH0ZZ Occlusion of Left Hand Vein, Open Approach
05LH3CZ Occlusion of Left Hand Vein with Extraluminal Device, Percutaneous Approach
05LH3DZ Occlusion of Left Hand Vein with Intraluminal Device, Percutaneous Approach
05LH3ZZ Occlusion of Left Hand Vein, Percutaneous Approach
05LH4CZ Occlusion of Left Hand Vein with Extraluminal Device, Percutaneous Endoscopic Approach
05LH4DZ Occlusion of Left Hand Vein with Intraluminal Device, Percutaneous Endoscopic Approach
05LH4ZZ Occlusion of Left Hand Vein, Percutaneous Endoscopic Approach
05LL0CZ Occlusion of Intracranial Vein with Extraluminal Device, Open Approach
05LL0DZ Occlusion of Intracranial Vein with Intraluminal Device, Open Approach
05LL0ZZ Occlusion of Intracranial Vein, Open Approach
05LL3CZ Occlusion of Intracranial Vein with Extraluminal Device, Percutaneous Approach
05LL3DZ Occlusion of Intracranial Vein with Intraluminal Device, Percutaneous Approach
05LL3ZZ Occlusion of Intracranial Vein, Percutaneous Approach
05LL4CZ Occlusion of Intracranial Vein with Extraluminal Device, Percutaneous Endoscopic Approach
05LL4DZ Occlusion of Intracranial Vein with Intraluminal Device, Percutaneous Endoscopic Approach
05LL4ZZ Occlusion of Intracranial Vein, Percutaneous Endoscopic Approach
05LM0CZ Occlusion of Right Internal Jugular Vein with Extraluminal Device, Open Approach
05LM0DZ Occlusion of Right Internal Jugular Vein with Intraluminal Device, Open Approach
05LM0ZZ Occlusion of Right Internal Jugular Vein Open Approach
05LM3CZ Occlusion of Right Internal Jugular Vein with Extraluminal Device, Percutaneous Approach
05LM3DZ Occlusion of Right Internal Jugular Vein with Intraluminal Device, Percutaneous Approach
05LM3ZZ Occlusion of Right Internal Jugular Vein, Percutaneous Approach
05LM4CZ Occlusion of Right Internal Jugular Vein with Extraluminal Device, Percutaneous Endoscopic Approach
05LM4DZ Occlusion of Right Internal Jugular Vein with Intraluminal Device, Percutaneous Endoscopic Approach
05LM4ZZ Occlusion of Right Internal Jugular Vein, Percutaneous Endoscopic Approach
05LN0CZ Occlusion of Left Internal Jugular Vein with Extraluminal Device, Open Approach
05LN0DZ Occlusion of Left Internal Jugular Vein with Intraluminal Device, Open Approach
05LN0ZZ Occlusion of Left Internal Jugular Vein, Open Approach
05LN3CZ Occlusion of Left Internal Jugular Vein with Extraluminal Device, Percutaneous Approach
05LN3DZ Occlusion of Left Internal Jugular Vein with Intraluminal Device, Percutaneous Approach
05LN3ZZ Occlusion of Left Internal Jugular Vein, Percutaneous Approach
05LN4CZ Occlusion of Left Internal Jugular Vein with Extraluminal Device, Percutaneous Endoscopic Approach
05LN4DZ Occlusion of Left Internal Jugular Vein with Intraluminal Device, Percutaneous Endoscopic Approach
05LN4ZZ Occlusion of Left Internal Jugular Vein, Percutaneous Endoscopic Approach
05LP0CZ Occlusion of Right External Jugular Vein with Extraluminal Device, Open Approach
05LP0DZ Occlusion of Right External Jugular Vein with Intraluminal Device, Open Approach
05LP0ZZ Occlusion of Right External Jugular Vein, Open Approach
05LP3CZ Occlusion of Right External Jugular Vein with Extraluminal Device, Percutaneous Approach
05LP3DZ Occlusion of Right External Jugular Vein with Intraluminal Device, Percutaneous Approach
05LP3ZZ Occlusion of Right External Jugular Vein, Percutaneous Approach
05LP4CZ Occlusion of Right External Jugular Vein with Extraluminal Device, Percutaneous Endoscopic Approach
05LP4DZ Occlusion of Right External Jugular Vein with Intraluminal Device, Percutaneous Endoscopic Approach
05LP4ZZ Occlusion of Right External Jugular Vein, Percutaneous Endoscopic Approach

LQ0CZ Occlusion of Left External Jugular Vein with Extraluminal Device, Open Approach
LQ0DZ Occlusion of Left External Jugular Vein with Intraluminal Device, Open Approach
LQ0ZZ Occlusion of Left External Jugular Vein, Open Approach
LQ3CZ Occlusion of Left External Jugular Vein with Extraluminal Device, Percutaneous Approach
LQ3DZ Occlusion of Left External Jugular Vein with Intraluminal Device, Percutaneous Approach
LQ3ZZ Occlusion of Left External Jugular Vein, Percutaneous Approach
LQ4CZ Occlusion of Left External Jugular Vein with Extraluminal Device, Percutaneous Endoscopic Approach
LQ4DZ Occlusion of Left External Jugular Vein with Intraluminal Device, Percutaneous Endoscopic Approach
LQ4ZZ Occlusion of Left External Jugular Vein, Percutaneous Endoscopic Approach
LR0CZ Occlusion of Right Vertebral Vein with Extraluminal Device, Open Approach
LR0DZ Occlusion of Right Vertebral Vein with Intraluminal Device, Open Approach
LR0ZZ Occlusion of Right Vertebral Vein, Open Approach
LR3CZ Occlusion of Right Vertebral Vein with Extraluminal Device, Percutaneous Approach
LR3DZ Occlusion of Right Vertebral Vein with Intraluminal Device, Percutaneous Approach
LR3ZZ Occlusion of Right Vertebral Vein, Percutaneous Approach
LR4CZ Occlusion of Right Vertebral Vein with Extraluminal Device, Percutaneous Endoscopic Approach
LR4DZ Occlusion of Right Vertebral Vein with Intraluminal Device, Percutaneous Endoscopic Approach
05LR4ZZ Occlusion of Right Vertebral Vein, Percutaneous Endoscopic Approach
05LS0CZ Occlusion of Left Vertebral Vein with Extraluminal Device, Open Approach
05LS0DZ Occlusion of Left Vertebral Vein with Intraluminal Device, Open Approach
05LS0ZZ Occlusion of Left Vertebral Vein, Open Approach
05LS3CZ Occlusion of Left Vertebral Vein with Extraluminal Device, Percutaneous Approach
05LS3DZ Occlusion of Left Vertebral Vein with Intraluminal Device, Percutaneous Approach
05LS3ZZ Occlusion of Left Vertebral Vein, Percutaneous Approach
05LS4CZ Occlusion of Left Vertebral Vein with Extraluminal Device, Percutaneous Endoscopic Approach
05LS4DZ Occlusion of Left Vertebral Vein with Intraluminal Device, Percutaneous Endoscopic Approach
05LS4ZZ Occlusion of Left Vertebral Vein, Percutaneous Endoscopic Approach
05LT0CZ Occlusion of Right Face Vein with Extraluminal Device, Open Approach
05LT0DZ Occlusion of Right Face Vein with Intraluminal Device, Open Approach
05LT0ZZ Occlusion of Right Face Vein, Open Approach
05LT3CZ Occlusion of Right Face Vein with Extraluminal Device, Percutaneous Approach
05LT3DZ Occlusion of Right Face Vein with Intraluminal Device, Percutaneous Approach
05LT3ZZ Occlusion of Right Face Vein, Percutaneous Approach
05LT4CZ Occlusion of Right Face Vein with Extraluminal Device, Percutaneous Endoscopic Approach
05LT4DZ Occlusion of Right Face Vein with Intraluminal Device, Percutaneous Endoscopic Approach
05LT4ZZ Occlusion of Right Face Vein, Percutaneous Endoscopic Approach
05LV0CZ Occlusion of Left Face Vein with Extraluminal Device, Open Approach
05LV0DZ Occlusion of Left Face Vein with Intraluminal Device, Open Approach
05LV0ZZ Occlusion of Left Face Vein, Open Approach
05LV3CZ Occlusion of Left Face Vein with Extraluminal Device, Percutaneous Approach
05LV3DZ Occlusion of Left Face Vein with Intraluminal Device, Percutaneous Approach
05LV3ZZ Occlusion of Left Face Vein, Percutaneous Approach
05LV4CZ Occlusion of Left Face Vein with Extraluminal Device, Percutaneous Endoscopic Approach
05LV4DZ Occlusion of Left Face Vein with Intraluminal Device, Percutaneous Endoscopic Approach
05LV4ZZ Occlusion of Left Face Vein, Percutaneous Endoscopic Approach
05LY0CZ Occlusion of Upper Vein with Extraluminal Device, Open Approach
05LY0DZ Occlusion of Upper Vein with Intraluminal Device, Open Approach
05LY0ZZ Occlusion of Upper Vein, Open Approach
05LY3CZ Occlusion of Upper Vein with Extraluminal Device, Percutaneous Approach
05LY3DZ Occlusion of Upper Vein with Intraluminal Device, Percutaneous Approach
05LY3ZZ Occlusion of Upper Vein, Percutaneous Approach
05LY4CZ Occlusion of Upper Vein with Extraluminal Device, Percutaneous Endoscopic Approach
05LY4DZ Occlusion of Upper Vein with Intraluminal Device, Percutaneous Endoscopic Approach
05LY4ZZ Occlusion of Upper Vein, Percutaneous Endoscopic Approach

5N – Upper Veins, Release

eview Coding Guidelines B3.13 and B3.14

5N00ZZ Release Azygos Vein, Open Approach
5N03ZZ Release Azygos Vein, Percutaneous Approach
5N04ZZ Release Azygos Vein, Percutaneous Endoscopic Approach
5N10ZZ Release Hemiazygos Vein, Open Approach
5N13ZZ Release Hemiazygos Vein, Percutaneous Approach
5N14ZZ Release Hemiazygos Vein, Percutaneous Endoscopic Approach
5N30ZZ Release Right Innominate Vein, Open Approach
5N33ZZ Release Right Innominate Vein, Percutaneous Approach
5N34ZZ Release Right Innominate Vein, Percutaneous Endoscopic Approach
5N40ZZ Release Left Innominate Vein, Open Approach
5N43ZZ Release Left Innominate Vein, Percutaneous Approach
5N44ZZ Release Left Innominate Vein, Percutaneous Endoscopic Approach
5N50ZZ Release Right Subclavian Vein, Open Approach
5N53ZZ Release Right Subclavian Vein, Percutaneous Approach
05N54ZZ Release Right Subclavian Vein, Percutaneous Endoscopic Approach
05N60ZZ Release Left Subclavian Vein, Open Approach
05N63ZZ Release Left Subclavian Vein, Percutaneous Approach
05N64ZZ Release Left Subclavian Vein, Percutaneous Endoscopic Approach
05N70ZZ Release Right Axillary Vein, Open Approach
05N73ZZ Release Right Axillary Vein, Percutaneous Approach
05N74ZZ Release Right Axillary Vein, Percutaneous Endoscopic Approach
05N80ZZ Release Left Axillary Vein, Open Approach
05N83ZZ Release Left Axillary Vein, Percutaneous Approach
05N84ZZ Release Left Axillary Vein, Percutaneous Endoscopic Approach
05N90ZZ Release Right Brachial Vein, Open Approach
05N93ZZ Release Right Brachial Vein, Percutaneous Approach
05N94ZZ Release Right Brachial Vein, Percutaneous Endoscopic Approach
05NA0ZZ Release Left Brachial Vein, Open Approach
05NA3ZZ Release Left Brachial Vein, Percutaneous Approach
05NA4ZZ Release Left Brachial Vein, Percutaneous Endoscopic Approach
05NB0ZZ Release Right Basilic Vein, Open Approach
05NB3ZZ Release Right Basilic Vein, Percutaneous Approach
05NB4ZZ Release Right Basilic Vein, Percutaneous Endoscopic Approach
05NC0ZZ Release Left Basilic Vein, Open Approach
05NC3ZZ Release Left Basilic Vein, Percutaneous Approach
05NC4ZZ Release Left Basilic Vein, Percutaneous Endoscopic Approach
05ND0ZZ Release Right Cephalic Vein, Open Approach
05ND3ZZ Release Right Cephalic Vein, Percutaneous Approach
05ND4ZZ Release Right Cephalic Vein, Percutaneous Endoscopic Approach
05NF0ZZ Release Left Cephalic Vein, Open Approach
05NF3ZZ Release Left Cephalic Vein, Percutaneous Approach

05NF4ZZ Release Left Cephalic Vein, Percutaneous Endoscopic Approach
05NG0ZZ Release Right Hand Vein, Open Approach
05NG3ZZ Release Right Hand Vein, Percutaneous Approach
05NG4ZZ Release Right Hand Vein, Percutaneous Endoscopic Approach
05NH0ZZ Release Left Hand Vein, Open Approach
05NH3ZZ Release Left Hand Vein, Percutaneous Approach
05NH4ZZ Release Left Hand Vein, Percutaneous Endoscopic Approach
05NL0ZZ Release Intracranial Vein, Open Approach
05NL3ZZ Release Intracranial Vein, Percutaneous Approach
05NL4ZZ Release Intracranial Vein, Percutaneous Endoscopic Approach
05NM0ZZ Release Right Internal Jugular Vein, Open Approach
05NM3ZZ Release Right Internal Jugular Vein, Percutaneous Approach
05NM4ZZ Release Right Internal Jugular Vein, Percutaneous Endoscopic Approach
05NN0ZZ Release Left Internal Jugular Vein, Open Approach
05NN3ZZ Release Left Internal Jugular Vein, Percutaneous Approach
05NN4ZZ Release Left Internal Jugular Vein, Percutaneous Endoscopic Approach
05NP0ZZ Release Right External Jugular Vein, Open Approach
05NP3ZZ Release Right External Jugular Vein, Percutaneous Approach
05NP4ZZ Release Right External Jugular Vein, Percutaneous Endoscopic Approach
05NQ0ZZ Release Left External Jugular Vein, Open Approach
05NQ3ZZ Release Left External Jugular Vein, Percutaneous Approach
05NQ4ZZ Release Left External Jugular Vein, Percutaneous Endoscopic Approach
05NR0ZZ Release Right Vertebral Vein, Open Approach
05NR3ZZ Release Right Vertebral Vein, Percutaneous Approach
05NR4ZZ Release Right Vertebral Vein, Percutaneous Endoscopic Approach
05NS0ZZ Release Left Vertebral Vein, Open Approach
05NS3ZZ Release Left Vertebral Vein, Percutaneous Approach
05NS4ZZ Release Left Vertebral Vein, Percutaneous Endoscopic Approach
05NT0ZZ Release Right Face Vein, Open Approach
05NT3ZZ Release Right Face Vein, Percutaneous Approach
05NT4ZZ Release Right Face Vein, Percutaneous Endoscopic Approach
05NV0ZZ Release Left Face Vein, Open Approach
05NV3ZZ Release Left Face Vein, Percutaneous Approach
05NV4ZZ Release Left Face Vein, Percutaneous Endoscopic Approach
05NY0ZZ Release Upper Vein, Open Approach
05NY3ZZ Release Upper Vein, Percutaneous Approach
05NY4ZZ Release Upper Vein, Percutaneous Endoscopic Approach

05P – Upper Veins, Removal

Review Coding Guideline B6.1c

05PY00Z Removal of Drainage Device from Upper Vein, Open Approach
05PY02Z Removal of Monitoring Device from Upper Vein, Open Approach
05PY03Z Removal of Infusion Device from Upper Vein, Open Approach
05PY07Z Removal of Autologous Tissue Substitute from Upper Vein, Open Approach
05PY0CZ Removal of Extraluminal Device from Upper Vein, Open Approach
05PY0DZ Removal of Intraluminal Device from Upper Vein, Open Approach
05PY0JZ Removal of Synthetic Substitute from Upper Vein, Open Approach
05PY0KZ Removal of Nonautologous Tissue Substitute from Upper Vein, Open Approach
05PY30Z Removal of Drainage Device from Upper Vein, Percutaneous Approach
05PY32Z Removal of Monitoring Device from Upper Vein, Percutaneous Approach
05PY33Z Removal of Infusion Device from Upper Vein, Percutaneous Approach
05PY37Z Removal of Autologous Tissue Substitute from Upper Vein, Percutaneous Approach
05PY3CZ Removal of Extraluminal Device from Upper Vein, Percutaneous Approach
05PY3DZ Removal of Intraluminal Device from Upper Vein, Percutaneous Approach
05PY3JZ Removal of Synthetic Substitute from Upper Vein, Percutaneous Approach
05PY3KZ Removal of Nonautologous Tissue Substitute from Upper Vein, Percutaneous Approach
05PY40Z Removal of Drainage Device from Upper Vein, Percutaneous Endoscopic Approach
05PY42Z Removal of Monitoring Device from Upper Vein, Percutaneous Endoscopic Approach
05PY43Z Removal of Infusion Device from Upper Vein, Percutaneous Endoscopic Approach
05PY47Z Removal of Autologous Tissue Substitute from Upper Vein, Percutaneous Endoscopic Approach
05PY4CZ Removal of Extraluminal Device from Upper Vein, Percutaneous Endoscopic Approach
05PY4DZ Removal of Intraluminal Device from Upper Vein, Percutaneous Endoscopic Approach
05PY4JZ Removal of Synthetic Substitute from Upper Vein, Percutaneous Endoscopic Approach
05PY4KZ Removal of Nonautologous Tissue Substitute from Upper Vein, Percutaneous Endoscopic Approach
05PYX0Z Removal of Drainage Device from Upper Vein, External Approach
05PYX2Z Removal of Monitoring Device from Upper Vein, External Approach
05PYX3Z Removal of Infusion Device from Upper Vein, External Approach
05PYXDZ Removal of Intraluminal Device from Upper Vein, External Approach

05Q – Upper Veins, Repair

05Q00ZZ Repair Azygos Vein, Open Approach
05Q03ZZ Repair Azygos Vein, Percutaneous Approach
05Q04ZZ Repair Azygos Vein, Percutaneous Endoscopic Approach
05Q10ZZ Repair Hemiazygos Vein, Open Approach
05Q13ZZ Repair Hemiazygos Vein, Percutaneous Approach
05Q14ZZ Repair Hemiazygos Vein, Percutaneous Endoscopic Approach
05Q30ZZ Repair Right Innominate Vein, Open Approach
05Q33ZZ Repair Right Innominate Vein, Percutaneous Approach
05Q34ZZ Repair Right Innominate Vein, Percutaneous Endoscopic Approach
05Q40ZZ Repair Left Innominate Vein, Open Approach
05Q43ZZ Repair Left Innominate Vein, Percutaneous Approach
05Q44ZZ Repair Left Innominate Vein, Percutaneous Endoscopic Approach
05Q50ZZ Repair Right Subclavian Vein, Open Approach
05Q53ZZ Repair Right Subclavian Vein, Percutaneous Approach
05Q54ZZ Repair Right Subclavian Vein, Percutaneous Endoscopic Approach
05Q60ZZ Repair Left Subclavian Vein, Open Approach
05Q63ZZ Repair Left Subclavian Vein, Percutaneous Approach
05Q64ZZ Repair Left Subclavian Vein, Percutaneous Endoscopic Approach
05Q70ZZ Repair Right Axillary Vein, Open Approach
05Q73ZZ Repair Right Axillary Vein, Percutaneous Approach
05Q74ZZ Repair Right Axillary Vein, Percutaneous Endoscopic Approach
05Q80ZZ Repair Left Axillary Vein, Open Approach
05Q83ZZ Repair Left Axillary Vein, Percutaneous Approach
05Q84ZZ Repair Left Axillary Vein, Percutaneous Endoscopic Approach
05Q90ZZ Repair Right Brachial Vein, Open Approach
05Q93ZZ Repair Right Brachial Vein, Percutaneous Approach
05Q94ZZ Repair Right Brachial Vein, Percutaneous Endoscopic Approach
05QA0ZZ Repair Left Brachial Vein, Open Approach
05QA3ZZ Repair Left Brachial Vein, Percutaneous Approach
05QA4ZZ Repair Left Brachial Vein, Percutaneous Endoscopic Approach
05QB0ZZ Repair Right Basilic Vein, Open Approach
05QB3ZZ Repair Right Basilic Vein, Percutaneous Approach
05QB4ZZ Repair Right Basilic Vein, Percutaneous Endoscopic Approach
05QC0ZZ Repair Left Basilic Vein, Open Approach
05QC3ZZ Repair Left Basilic Vein, Percutaneous Approach
05QC4ZZ Repair Left Basilic Vein, Percutaneous Endoscopic Approach
05QD0ZZ Repair Right Cephalic Vein, Open Approach
05QD3ZZ Repair Right Cephalic Vein, Percutaneous Approach
05QD4ZZ Repair Right Cephalic Vein, Percutaneous Endoscopic Approach
05QF0ZZ Repair Left Cephalic Vein, Open Approach

QF3ZZ Repair Left Cephalic Vein, Percutaneous Approach
QF4ZZ Repair Left Cephalic Vein, Percutaneous Endoscopic Approach
5QG0ZZ Repair Right Hand Vein, Open Approach
5QG3ZZ Repair Right Hand Vein, Percutaneous Approach
5QG4ZZ Repair Right Hand Vein, Percutaneous Endoscopic Approach
5QH0ZZ Repair Left Hand Vein, Open Approach
5QH3ZZ Repair Left Hand Vein, Percutaneous Approach
5QH4ZZ Repair Left Hand Vein, Percutaneous Endoscopic Approach
5QL0ZZ Repair Intracranial Vein, Open Approach
5QL3ZZ Repair Intracranial Vein, Percutaneous Approach
5QL4ZZ Repair Intracranial Vein, Percutaneous Endoscopic Approach
5QM0ZZ Repair Right Internal Jugular Vein, Open Approach
5QM3ZZ Repair Right Internal Jugular Vein, Percutaneous Approach
05QM4ZZ Repair Right Internal Jugular Vein, Percutaneous Endoscopic Approach
05QN0ZZ Repair Left Internal Jugular Vein, Open Approach
05QN3ZZ Repair Left Internal Jugular Vein, Percutaneous Approach
05QN4ZZ Repair Left Internal Jugular Vein, Percutaneous Endoscopic Approach
05QP0ZZ Repair Right External Jugular Vein, Open Approach
05QP3ZZ Repair Right External Jugular Vein, Percutaneous Approach
05QP4ZZ Repair Right External Jugular Vein, Percutaneous Endoscopic Approach
05QQ0ZZ Repair Left External Jugular Vein, Open Approach
05QQ3ZZ Repair Left External Jugular Vein, Percutaneous Approach
05QQ4ZZ Repair Left External Jugular Vein, Percutaneous Endoscopic Approach
05QR0ZZ Repair Right Vertebral Vein, Open Approach
05QR3ZZ Repair Right Vertebral Vein, Percutaneous Approach
05QR4ZZ Repair Right Vertebral Vein, Percutaneous Endoscopic Approach
05QS0ZZ Repair Left Vertebral Vein, Open Approach
05QS3ZZ Repair Left Vertebral Vein, Percutaneous Approach
05QS4ZZ Repair Left Vertebral Vein, Percutaneous Endoscopic Approach
05QT0ZZ Repair Right Face Vein, Open Approach
05QT3ZZ Repair Right Face Vein, Percutaneous Approach
05QT4ZZ Repair Right Face Vein, Percutaneous Endoscopic Approach
05QV0ZZ Repair Left Face Vein, Open Approach
05QV3ZZ Repair Left Face Vein, Percutaneous Approach
05QV4ZZ Repair Left Face Vein, Percutaneous Endoscopic Approach
05QY0ZZ Repair Upper Vein, Open Approach
05QY3ZZ Repair Upper Vein, Percutaneous Approach
05QY4ZZ Repair Upper Vein, Percutaneous Endoscopic Approach

5R – Upper Veins, Replacement

5R007Z Replacement of Azygos Vein with Autologous Tissue Substitute, Open Approach
5R00JZ Replacement of Azygos Vein with Synthetic Substitute, Open Approach
5R00KZ Replacement of Azygos Vein with Nonautologous Tissue Substitute, Open Approach
5R047Z Replacement of Azygos Vein with Autologous Tissue Substitute, Percutaneous Endoscopic Approach
5R04JZ Replacement of Azygos Vein with Synthetic Substitute, Percutaneous Endoscopic Approach
5R04KZ Replacement of Azygos Vein with Nonautologous Tissue Substitute, Percutaneous Endoscopic Approach
5R107Z Replacement of Hemiazygos Vein with Autologous Tissue Substitute, Open Approach
5R10JZ Replacement of Hemiazygos Vein with Synthetic Substitute, Open Approach
5R10KZ Replacement of Hemiazygos Vein with Nonautologous Tissue Substitute, Open Approach
5R147Z Replacement of Hemiazygos Vein with Autologous Tissue Substitute, Percutaneous Endoscopic Approach
5R14JZ Replacement of Hemiazygos Vein with Synthetic Substitute, Percutaneous Endoscopic Approach
5R14KZ Replacement of Hemiazygos Vein with Nonautologous Tissue Substitute, Percutaneous Endoscopic Approach
5R307Z Replacement of Right Innominate Vein with Autologous Tissue Substitute, Open Approach
5R30JZ Replacement of Right Innominate Vein with Synthetic Substitute, Open Approach
5R30KZ Replacement of Right Innominate Vein with Nonautologous Tissue Substitute, Open Approach
5R347Z Replacement of Right Innominate Vein with Autologous Tissue Substitute, Percutaneous Endoscopic Approach
5R34JZ Replacement of Right Innominate Vein with Synthetic Substitute, Percutaneous Endoscopic Approach
5R34KZ Replacement of Right Innominate Vein with Nonautologous Tissue Substitute, Percutaneous Endoscopic Approach
05R407Z Replacement of Left Innominate Vein with Autologous Tissue Substitute, Open Approach
05R40JZ Replacement of Left Innominate Vein with Synthetic Substitute, Open Approach
05R40KZ Replacement of Left Innominate Vein with Nonautologous Tissue Substitute, Open Approach
05R447Z Replacement of Left Innominate Vein with Autologous Tissue Substitute, Percutaneous Endoscopic Approach
05R44JZ Replacement of Left Innominate Vein with Synthetic Substitute, Percutaneous Endoscopic Approach
05R44KZ Replacement of Left Innominate Vein with Nonautologous Tissue Substitute, Percutaneous Endoscopic Approach
05R507Z Replacement of Right Subclavian Vein with Autologous Tissue Substitute, Open Approach
05R50JZ Replacement of Right Subclavian Vein with Synthetic Substitute, Open Approach
05R50KZ Replacement of Right Subclavian Vein with Nonautologous Tissue Substitute, Open Approach
05R547Z Replacement of Right Subclavian Vein with Autologous Tissue Substitute, Percutaneous Endoscopic Approach
05R54JZ Replacement of Right Subclavian Vein with Synthetic Substitute, Percutaneous Endoscopic Approach
05R54KZ Replacement of Right Subclavian Vein with Nonautologous Tissue Substitute, Percutaneous Endoscopic Approach
05R607Z Replacement of Left Subclavian Vein with Autologous Tissue Substitute, Open Approach
05R60JZ Replacement of Left Subclavian Vein with Synthetic Substitute, Open Approach
05R60KZ Replacement of Left Subclavian Vein with Nonautologous Tissue Substitute, Open Approach
05R647Z Replacement of Left Subclavian Vein with Autologous Tissue Substitute, Percutaneous Endoscopic Approach
05R64JZ Replacement of Left Subclavian Vein with Synthetic Substitute, Percutaneous Endoscopic Approach
05R64KZ Replacement of Left Subclavian Vein with Nonautologous Tissue Substitute, Percutaneous Endoscopic Approach
05R707Z Replacement of Right Axillary Vein with Autologous Tissue Substitute, Open Approach
05R70JZ Replacement of Right Axillary Vein with Synthetic Substitute, Open Approach
05R70KZ Replacement of Right Axillary Vein with Nonautologous Tissue Substitute, Open Approach
05R747Z Replacement of Right Axillary Vein with Autologous Tissue Substitute, Percutaneous Endoscopic Approach
05R74JZ Replacement of Right Axillary Vein with Synthetic Substitute, Percutaneous Endoscopic Approach
05R74KZ Replacement of Right Axillary Vein with Nonautologous Tissue Substitute, Percutaneous Endoscopic Approach
05R807Z Replacement of Left Axillary Vein with Autologous Tissue Substitute, Open Approach
05R80JZ Replacement of Left Axillary Vein with Synthetic Substitute, Open Approach
05R80KZ Replacement of Left Axillary Vein with Nonautologous Tissue Substitute, Open Approach
05R847Z Replacement of Left Axillary Vein with Autologous Tissue Substitute, Percutaneous Endoscopic Approach
05R84JZ Replacement of Left Axillary Vein with Synthetic Substitute, Percutaneous Endoscopic Approach
05R84KZ Replacement of Left Axillary Vein with Nonautologous Tissue Substitute, Percutaneous Endoscopic Approach
05R907Z Replacement of Right Brachial Vein with Autologous Tissue Substitute, Open Approach
05R90JZ Replacement of Right Brachial Vein with Synthetic Substitute, Open Approach
05R90KZ Replacement of Right Brachial Vein with Nonautologous Tissue Substitute, Open Approach
05R947Z Replacement of Right Brachial Vein with Autologous Tissue Substitute, Percutaneous Endoscopic Approach
05R94JZ Replacement of Right Brachial Vein with Synthetic Substitute, Percutaneous Endoscopic Approach
05R94KZ Replacement of Right Brachial Vein with Nonautologous Tissue Substitute, Percutaneous Endoscopic Approach

05RA07Z Replacement of Left Brachial Vein with Autologous Tissue Substitute, Open Approach
05RA0JZ Replacement of Left Brachial Vein with Synthetic Substitute, Open Approach
05RA0KZ Replacement of Left Brachial Vein with Nonautologous Tissue Substitute, Open Approach
05RA47Z Replacement of Left Brachial Vein with Autologous Tissue Substitute, Percutaneous Endoscopic Approach
05RA4JZ Replacement of Left Brachial Vein with Synthetic Substitute, Percutaneous Endoscopic Approach
05RA4KZ Replacement of Left Brachial Vein with Nonautologous Tissue Substitute, Percutaneous Endoscopic Approach
05RB07Z Replacement of Right Basilic Vein with Autologous Tissue Substitute, Open Approach
05RB0JZ Replacement of Right Basilic Vein with Synthetic Substitute, Open Approach
05RB0KZ Replacement of Right Basilic Vein with Nonautologous Tissue Substitute, Open Approach
05RB47Z Replacement of Right Basilic Vein with Autologous Tissue Substitute, Percutaneous Endoscopic Approach
05RB4JZ Replacement of Right Basilic Vein with Synthetic Substitute, Percutaneous Endoscopic Approach
05RB4KZ Replacement of Right Basilic Vein with Nonautologous Tissue Substitute, Percutaneous Endoscopic Approach
05RC07Z Replacement of Left Basilic Vein with Autologous Tissue Substitute, Open Approach
05RC0JZ Replacement of Left Basilic Vein with Synthetic Substitute, Open Approach
05RC0KZ Replacement of Left Basilic Vein with Nonautologous Tissue Substitute, Open Approach
05RC47Z Replacement of Left Basilic Vein with Autologous Tissue Substitute, Percutaneous Endoscopic Approach
05RC4JZ Replacement of Left Basilic Vein with Synthetic Substitute, Percutaneous Endoscopic Approach
05RC4KZ Replacement of Left Basilic Vein with Nonautologous Tissue Substitute, Percutaneous Endoscopic Approach
05RD07Z Replacement of Right Cephalic Vein with Autologous Tissue Substitute, Open Approach
05RD0JZ Replacement of Right Cephalic Vein with Synthetic Substitute, Open Approach
05RD0KZ Replacement of Right Cephalic Vein with Nonautologous Tissue Substitute, Open Approach
05RD47Z Replacement of Right Cephalic Vein with Autologous Tissue Substitute, Percutaneous Endoscopic Approach
05RD4JZ Replacement of Right Cephalic Vein with Synthetic Substitute, Percutaneous Endoscopic Approach
05RD4KZ Replacement of Right Cephalic Vein with Nonautologous Tissue Substitute, Percutaneous Endoscopic Approach
05RF07Z Replacement of Left Cephalic Vein with Autologous Tissue Substitute, Open Approach
05RF0JZ Replacement of Left Cephalic Vein with Synthetic Substitute, Open Approach
05RF0KZ Replacement of Left Cephalic Vein with Nonautologous Tissue Substitute, Open Approach
05RF47Z Replacement of Left Cephalic Vein with Autologous Tissue Substitute, Percutaneous Endoscopic Approach
05RF4JZ Replacement of Left Cephalic Vein with Synthetic Substitute, Percutaneous Endoscopic Approach
05RF4KZ Replacement of Left Cephalic Vein with Nonautologous Tissue Substitute, Percutaneous Endoscopic Approach
05RG07Z Replacement of Right Hand Vein with Autologous Tissue Substitute, Open Approach
05RG0JZ Replacement of Right Hand Vein with Synthetic Substitute, Open Approach
05RG0KZ Replacement of Right Hand Vein with Nonautologous Tissue Substitute, Open Approach
05RG47Z Replacement of Right Hand Vein with Autologous Tissue Substitute, Percutaneous Endoscopic Approach
05RG4JZ Replacement of Right Hand Vein with Synthetic Substitute, Percutaneous Endoscopic Approach
05RG4KZ Replacement of Right Hand Vein with Nonautologous Tissue Substitute, Percutaneous Endoscopic Approach
05RH07Z Replacement of Left Hand Vein with Autologous Tissue Substitute, Open Approach
05RH0JZ Replacement of Left Hand Vein with Synthetic Substitute, Open Approach
05RH0KZ Replacement of Left Hand Vein with Nonautologous Tissue Substitute, Open Approach
05RH47Z Replacement of Left Hand Vein with Autologous Tissue Substitute, Percutaneous Endoscopic Approach
05RH4JZ Replacement of Left Hand Vein with Synthetic Substitute, Percutaneous Endoscopic Approach
05RH4KZ Replacement of Left Hand Vein with Nonautologous Tissue Substitute, Percutaneous Endoscopic Approach
05RL07Z Replacement of Intracranial Vein with Autologous Tissue Substitute, Open Approach
05RL0JZ Replacement of Intracranial Vein with Synthetic Substitute, Open Approach
05RL0KZ Replacement of Intracranial Vein with Nonautologous Tissue Substitute, Open Approach
05RL47Z Replacement of Intracranial Vein with Autologous Tissue Substitute, Percutaneous Endoscopic Approach
05RL4JZ Replacement of Intracranial Vein with Synthetic Substitute, Percutaneous Endoscopic Approach
05RL4KZ Replacement of Intracranial Vein with Nonautologous Tissue Substitute, Percutaneous Endoscopic Approach
05RM07Z Replacement of Right Internal Jugular Vein with Autologous Tissue Substitute, Open Approach
05RM0JZ Replacement of Right Internal Jugular Vein with Synthetic Substitute, Open Approach
05RM0KZ Replacement of Right Internal Jugular Vein with Nonautologous Tissue Substitute, Open Approach
05RM47Z Replacement of Right Internal Jugular Vein with Autologous Tissue Substitute, Percutaneous Endoscopic Approach
05RM4JZ Replacement of Right Internal Jugular Vein with Synthetic Substitute, Percutaneous Endoscopic Approach
05RM4KZ Replacement of Right Internal Jugular Vein with Nonautologous Tissue Substitute, Percutaneous Endoscopic Approach
05RN07Z Replacement of Left Internal Jugular Vein with Autologous Tissue Substitute, Open Approach
05RN0JZ Replacement of Left Internal Jugular Vein with Synthetic Substitute, Open Approach
05RN0KZ Replacement of Left Internal Jugular Vein with Nonautologous Tissue Substitute, Open Approach
05RN47Z Replacement of Left Internal Jugular Vein with Autologous Tissue Substitute, Percutaneous Endoscopic Approach
05RN4JZ Replacement of Left Internal Jugular Vein with Synthetic Substitute, Percutaneous Endoscopic Approach
05RN4KZ Replacement of Left Internal Jugular Vein with Nonautologous Tissue Substitute, Percutaneous Endoscopic Approach
05RP07Z Replacement of Right External Jugular Vein with Autologous Tissue Substitute, Open Approach
05RP0JZ Replacement of Right External Jugular Vein with Synthetic Substitute, Open Approach
05RP0KZ Replacement of Right External Jugular Vein with Nonautologous Tissue Substitute, Open Approach
05RP47Z Replacement of Right External Jugular Vein with Autologous Tissue Substitute, Percutaneous Endoscopic Approach
05RP4JZ Replacement of Right External Jugular Vein with Synthetic Substitute, Percutaneous Endoscopic Approach
05RP4KZ Replacement of Right External Jugular Vein with Nonautologous Tissue Substitute, Percutaneous Endoscopic Approach
05RQ07Z Replacement of Left External Jugular Vein with Autologous Tissue Substitute, Open Approach
05RQ0JZ Replacement of Left External Jugular Vein with Synthetic Substitute, Open Approach
05RQ0KZ Replacement of Left External Jugular Vein with Nonautologous Tissue Substitute, Open Approach
05RQ47Z Replacement of Left External Jugular Vein with Autologous Tissue Substitute, Percutaneous Endoscopic Approach
05RQ4JZ Replacement of Left External Jugular Vein with Synthetic Substitute, Percutaneous Endoscopic Approach
05RQ4KZ Replacement of Left External Jugular Vein with Nonautologous Tissue Substitute, Percutaneous Endoscopic Approach
05RR07Z Replacement of Right Vertebral Vein with Autologous Tissue Substitute, Open Approach
05RR0JZ Replacement of Right Vertebral Vein with Synthetic Substitute, Open Approach
05RR0KZ Replacement of Right Vertebral Vein with Nonautologous Tissue Substitute, Open Approach
05RR47Z Replacement of Right Vertebral Vein with Autologous Tissue Substitute, Percutaneous Endoscopic Approach
05RR4JZ Replacement of Right Vertebral Vein with Synthetic Substitute, Percutaneous Endoscopic Approach
05RR4KZ Replacement of Right Vertebral Vein with Nonautologous Tissue Substitute, Percutaneous Endoscopic Approach
05RS07Z Replacement of Left Vertebral Vein with Autologous Tissue Substitute, Open Approach
05RS0JZ Replacement of Left Vertebral Vein with Synthetic Substitute, Open Approach

5RS0KZ Replacement of Left Vertebral Vein with Nonautologous Tissue Substitute, Open Approach
5RS47Z Replacement of Left Vertebral Vein with Autologous Tissue Substitute, Percutaneous Endoscopic Approach
5RS4JZ Replacement of Left Vertebral Vein with Synthetic Substitute, Percutaneous Endoscopic Approach
5RS4KZ Replacement of Left Vertebral Vein with Nonautologous Tissue Substitute, Percutaneous Endoscopic Approach
5RT07Z Replacement of Right Face Vein with Autologous Tissue Substitute, Open Approach
5RT0JZ Replacement of Right Face Vein with Synthetic Substitute, Open Approach
5RT0KZ Replacement of Right Face Vein with Nonautologous Tissue Substitute, Open Approach
5RT47Z Replacement of Right Face Vein with Autologous Tissue Substitute, Percutaneous Endoscopic Approach
05RT4JZ Replacement of Right Face Vein with Synthetic Substitute, Percutaneous Endoscopic Approach
05RT4KZ Replacement of Right Face Vein with Nonautologous Tissue Substitute, Percutaneous Endoscopic Approach
05RV07Z Replacement of Left Face Vein with Autologous Tissue Substitute, Open Approach
05RV0JZ Replacement of Left Face Vein with Synthetic Substitute, Open Approach
05RV0KZ Replacement of Left Face Vein with Nonautologous Tissue Substitute, Open Approach
05RV47Z Replacement of Left Face Vein with Autologous Tissue Substitute, Percutaneous Endoscopic Approach
05RV4JZ Replacement of Left Face Vein with Synthetic Substitute, Percutaneous Endoscopic Approach
05RV4KZ Replacement of Left Face Vein with Nonautologous Tissue Substitute, Percutaneous Endoscopic Approach
05RY07Z Replacement of Upper Vein with Autologous Tissue Substitute, Open Approach
05RY0JZ Replacement of Upper Vein with Synthetic Substitute, Open Approach
05RY0KZ Replacement of Upper Vein with Nonautologous Tissue Substitute, Open Approach
05RY47Z Replacement of Upper Vein with Autologous Tissue Substitute, Percutaneous Endoscopic Approach
05RY4JZ Replacement of Upper Vein with Synthetic Substitute, Percutaneous Endoscopic Approach
05RY4KZ Replacement of Upper Vein with Nonautologous Tissue Substitute, Percutaneous Endoscopic Approach

5S – *Upper Veins, Reposition*

5S00ZZ Reposition Azygos Vein, Open Approach
5S03ZZ Reposition Azygos Vein, Percutaneous Approach
5S04ZZ Reposition Azygos Vein, Percutaneous Endoscopic Approach
5S10ZZ Reposition Hemiazygos Vein, Open Approach
5S13ZZ Reposition Hemiazygos Vein, Percutaneous Approach
5S14ZZ Reposition Hemiazygos Vein, Percutaneous Endoscopic Approach
5S30ZZ Reposition Right Innominate Vein, Open Approach
5S33ZZ Reposition Right Innominate Vein, Percutaneous Approach
5S34ZZ Reposition Right Innominate Vein, Percutaneous Endoscopic Approach
5S40ZZ Reposition Left Innominate Vein, Open Approach
5S43ZZ Reposition Left Innominate Vein, Percutaneous Approach
5S44ZZ Reposition Left Innominate Vein, Percutaneous Endoscopic Approach
5S50ZZ Reposition Right Subclavian Vein, Open Approach
5S53ZZ Reposition Right Subclavian Vein, Percutaneous Approach
5S54ZZ Reposition Right Subclavian Vein, Percutaneous Endoscopic Approach
5S60ZZ Reposition Left Subclavian Vein, Open Approach
5S63ZZ Reposition Left Subclavian Vein, Percutaneous Approach
5S64ZZ Reposition Left Subclavian Vein, Percutaneous Endoscopic Approach
5S70ZZ Reposition Right Axillary Vein, Open Approach
5S73ZZ Reposition Right Axillary Vein, Percutaneous Approach
5S74ZZ Reposition Right Axillary Vein, Percutaneous Endoscopic Approach
5S80ZZ Reposition Left Axillary Vein, Open Approach
5S83ZZ Reposition Left Axillary Vein, Percutaneous Approach
5S84ZZ Reposition Left Axillary Vein, Percutaneous Endoscopic Approach
5S90ZZ Reposition Right Brachial Vein, Open Approach
5S93ZZ Reposition Right Brachial Vein, Percutaneous Approach
05S94ZZ Reposition Right Brachial Vein, Percutaneous Endoscopic Approach
05SA0ZZ Reposition Left Brachial Vein, Open Approach
05SA3ZZ Reposition Left Brachial Vein, Percutaneous Approach
05SA4ZZ Reposition Left Brachial Vein, Percutaneous Endoscopic Approach
05SB0ZZ Reposition Right Basilic Vein, Open Approach
05SB3ZZ Reposition Right Basilic Vein, Percutaneous Approach
05SB4ZZ Reposition Right Basilic Vein, Percutaneous Endoscopic Approach
05SC0ZZ Reposition Left Basilic Vein, Open Approach
05SC3ZZ Reposition Left Basilic Vein, Percutaneous Approach
05SC4ZZ Reposition Left Basilic Vein, Percutaneous Endoscopic Approach
05SD0ZZ Reposition Right Cephalic Vein, Open Approach
AHA CC: 4Q, 2013, 125-126
05SD3ZZ Reposition Right Cephalic Vein, Percutaneous Approach
05SD4ZZ Reposition Right Cephalic Vein, Percutaneous Endoscopic Approach
05SF0ZZ Reposition Left Cephalic Vein, Open Approach
05SF3ZZ Reposition Left Cephalic Vein, Percutaneous Approach
05SF4ZZ Reposition Left Cephalic Vein, Percutaneous Endoscopic Approach
05SG0ZZ Reposition Right Hand Vein, Open Approach
05SG3ZZ Reposition Right Hand Vein, Percutaneous Approach
05SG4ZZ Reposition Right Hand Vein, Percutaneous Endoscopic Approach
05SH0ZZ Reposition Left Hand Vein, Open Approach
05SH3ZZ Reposition Left Hand Vein, Percutaneous Approach
05SH4ZZ Reposition Left Hand Vein, Percutaneous Endoscopic Approach
05SL0ZZ Reposition Intracranial Vein, Open Approach
05SL3ZZ Reposition Intracranial Vein, Percutaneous Approach
05SL4ZZ Reposition Intracranial Vein, Percutaneous Endoscopic Approach
05SM0ZZ Reposition Right Internal Jugular Vein, Open Approach
05SM3ZZ Reposition Right Internal Jugular Vein, Percutaneous Approach
05SM4ZZ Reposition Right Internal Jugular Vein, Percutaneous Endoscopic Approach
05SN0ZZ Reposition Left Internal Jugular Vein, Open Approach
05SN3ZZ Reposition Left Internal Jugular Vein, Percutaneous Approach
05SN4ZZ Reposition Left Internal Jugular Vein, Percutaneous Endoscopic Approach
05SP0ZZ Reposition Right External Jugular Vein, Open Approach
05SP3ZZ Reposition Right External Jugular Vein, Percutaneous Approach
05SP4ZZ Reposition Right External Jugular Vein, Percutaneous Endoscopic Approach
05SQ0ZZ Reposition Left External Jugular Vein, Open Approach
05SQ3ZZ Reposition Left External Jugular Vein, Percutaneous Approach
05SQ4ZZ Reposition Left External Jugular Vein, Percutaneous Endoscopic Approach
05SR0ZZ Reposition Right Vertebral Vein, Open Approach
05SR3ZZ Reposition Right Vertebral Vein, Percutaneous Approach
05SR4ZZ Reposition Right Vertebral Vein, Percutaneous Endoscopic Approach
05SS0ZZ Reposition Left Vertebral Vein, Open Approach
05SS3ZZ Reposition Left Vertebral Vein, Percutaneous Approach
05SS4ZZ Reposition Left Vertebral Vein, Percutaneous Endoscopic Approach
05ST0ZZ Reposition Right Face Vein, Open Approach
05ST3ZZ Reposition Right Face Vein, Percutaneous Approach
05ST4ZZ Reposition Right Face Vein, Percutaneous Endoscopic Approach
05SV0ZZ Reposition Left Face Vein, Open Approach
05SV3ZZ Reposition Left Face Vein, Percutaneous Approach
05SV4ZZ Reposition Left Face Vein, Percutaneous Endoscopic Approach
05SY0ZZ Reposition Upper Vein, Open Approach
05SY3ZZ Reposition Upper Vein, Percutaneous Approach
05SY4ZZ Reposition Upper Vein, Percutaneous Endoscopic Approach

05U – Upper Veins, Supplement

05U007Z Supplement Azygos Vein with Autologous Tissue Substitute, Open Approach
05U00JZ Supplement Azygos Vein with Synthetic Substitute, Open Approach
05U00KZ Supplement Azygos Vein with Nonautologous Tissue Substitute, Open Approach
05U037Z Supplement Azygos Vein with Autologous Tissue Substitute, Percutaneous Approach
05U03JZ Supplement Azygos Vein with Synthetic Substitute, Percutaneous Approach
05U03KZ Supplement Azygos Vein with Nonautologous Tissue Substitute, Percutaneous Approach
05U047Z Supplement Azygos Vein with Autologous Tissue Substitute, Percutaneous Endoscopic Approach
05U04JZ Supplement Azygos Vein with Synthetic Substitute, Percutaneous Endoscopic Approach
05U04KZ Supplement Azygos Vein with Nonautologous Tissue Substitute, Percutaneous Endoscopic Approach
05U107Z Supplement Hemiazygos Vein with Autologous Tissue Substitute, Open Approach
05U10JZ Supplement Hemiazygos Vein with Synthetic Substitute, Open Approach
05U10KZ Supplement Hemiazygos Vein with Nonautologous Tissue Substitute, Open Approach
05U137Z Supplement Hemiazygos Vein with Autologous Tissue Substitute, Percutaneous Approach
05U13JZ Supplement Hemiazygos Vein with Synthetic Substitute, Percutaneous Approach
05U13KZ Supplement Hemiazygos Vein with Nonautologous Tissue Substitute, Percutaneous Approach
05U147Z Supplement Hemiazygos Vein with Autologous Tissue Substitute, Percutaneous Endoscopic Approach
05U14JZ Supplement Hemiazygos Vein with Synthetic Substitute, Percutaneous Endoscopic Approach
05U14KZ Supplement Hemiazygos Vein with Nonautologous Tissue Substitute, Percutaneous Endoscopic Approach
05U307Z Supplement Right Innominate Vein with Autologous Tissue Substitute, Open Approach
05U30JZ Supplement Right Innominate Vein with Synthetic Substitute, Open Approach
05U30KZ Supplement Right Innominate Vein with Nonautologous Tissue Substitute, Open Approach
05U337Z Supplement Right Innominate Vein with Autologous Tissue Substitute, Percutaneous Approach
05U33JZ Supplement Right Innominate Vein with Synthetic Substitute, Percutaneous Approach
05U33KZ Supplement Right Innominate Vein with Nonautologous Tissue Substitute, Percutaneous Approach
05U347Z Supplement Right Innominate Vein with Autologous Tissue Substitute, Percutaneous Endoscopic Approach
05U34JZ Supplement Right Innominate Vein with Synthetic Substitute, Percutaneous Endoscopic Approach
05U34KZ Supplement Right Innominate Vein with Nonautologous Tissue Substitute, Percutaneous Endoscopic Approach
05U407Z Supplement Left Innominate Vein with Autologous Tissue Substitute, Open Approach
05U40JZ Supplement Left Innominate Vein with Synthetic Substitute, Open Approach
05U40KZ Supplement Left Innominate Vein with Nonautologous Tissue Substitute, Open Approach
05U437Z Supplement Left Innominate Vein with Autologous Tissue Substitute, Percutaneous Approach
05U43JZ Supplement Left Innominate Vein with Synthetic Substitute, Percutaneous Approach
05U43KZ Supplement Left Innominate Vein with Nonautologous Tissue Substitute, Percutaneous Approach
05U447Z Supplement Left Innominate Vein with Autologous Tissue Substitute, Percutaneous Endoscopic Approach
05U44JZ Supplement Left Innominate Vein with Synthetic Substitute, Percutaneous Endoscopic Approach
05U44KZ Supplement Left Innominate Vein with Nonautologous Tissue Substitute, Percutaneous Endoscopic Approach
05U507Z Supplement Right Subclavian Vein with Autologous Tissue Substitute, Open Approach
05U50JZ Supplement Right Subclavian Vein with Synthetic Substitute, Open Approach
05U50KZ Supplement Right Subclavian Vein with Nonautologous Tissue Substitute, Open Approach
05U537Z Supplement Right Subclavian Vein with Autologous Tissue Substitute, Percutaneous Approach
05U53JZ Supplement Right Subclavian Vein with Synthetic Substitute, Percutaneous Approach
05U53KZ Supplement Right Subclavian Vein with Nonautologous Tissue Substitute, Percutaneous Approach
05U547Z Supplement Right Subclavian Vein with Autologous Tissue Substitute, Percutaneous Endoscopic Approach
05U54JZ Supplement Right Subclavian Vein with Synthetic Substitute, Percutaneous Endoscopic Approach
05U54KZ Supplement Right Subclavian Vein with Nonautologous Tissue Substitute, Percutaneous Endoscopic Approach
05U607Z Supplement Left Subclavian Vein with Autologous Tissue Substitute, Open Approach
05U60JZ Supplement Left Subclavian Vein with Synthetic Substitute, Open Approach
05U60KZ Supplement Left Subclavian Vein with Nonautologous Tissue Substitute, Open Approach
05U637Z Supplement Left Subclavian Vein with Autologous Tissue Substitute, Percutaneous Approach
05U63JZ Supplement Left Subclavian Vein with Synthetic Substitute, Percutaneous Approach
05U63KZ Supplement Left Subclavian Vein with Nonautologous Tissue Substitute, Percutaneous Approach
05U647Z Supplement Left Subclavian Vein with Autologous Tissue Substitute, Percutaneous Endoscopic Approach
05U64JZ Supplement Left Subclavian Vein with Synthetic Substitute, Percutaneous Endoscopic Approach
05U64KZ Supplement Left Subclavian Vein with Nonautologous Tissue Substitute, Percutaneous Endoscopic Approach
05U707Z Supplement Right Axillary Vein with Autologous Tissue Substitute, Open Approach
05U70JZ Supplement Right Axillary Vein with Synthetic Substitute, Open Approach
05U70KZ Supplement Right Axillary Vein with Nonautologous Tissue Substitute, Open Approach
05U737Z Supplement Right Axillary Vein with Autologous Tissue Substitute, Percutaneous Approach
05U73JZ Supplement Right Axillary Vein with Synthetic Substitute, Percutaneous Approach
05U73KZ Supplement Right Axillary Vein with Nonautologous Tissue Substitute, Percutaneous Approach
05U747Z Supplement Right Axillary Vein with Autologous Tissue Substitute, Percutaneous Endoscopic Approach
05U74JZ Supplement Right Axillary Vein with Synthetic Substitute, Percutaneous Endoscopic Approach
05U74KZ Supplement Right Axillary Vein with Nonautologous Tissue Substitute, Percutaneous Endoscopic Approach
05U807Z Supplement Left Axillary Vein with Autologous Tissue Substitute, Open Approach
05U80JZ Supplement Left Axillary Vein with Synthetic Substitute, Open Approach
05U80KZ Supplement Left Axillary Vein with Nonautologous Tissue Substitute, Open Approach
05U837Z Supplement Left Axillary Vein with Autologous Tissue Substitute, Percutaneous Approach
05U83JZ Supplement Left Axillary Vein with Synthetic Substitute, Percutaneous Approach
05U83KZ Supplement Left Axillary Vein with Nonautologous Tissue Substitute, Percutaneous Approach
05U847Z Supplement Left Axillary Vein with Autologous Tissue Substitute, Percutaneous Endoscopic Approach
05U84JZ Supplement Left Axillary Vein with Synthetic Substitute, Percutaneous Endoscopic Approach
05U84KZ Supplement Left Axillary Vein with Nonautologous Tissue Substitute, Percutaneous Endoscopic Approach
05U907Z Supplement Right Brachial Vein with Autologous Tissue Substitute, Open Approach
05U90JZ Supplement Right Brachial Vein with Synthetic Substitute, Open Approach
05U90KZ Supplement Right Brachial Vein with Nonautologous Tissue Substitute, Open Approach
05U937Z Supplement Right Brachial Vein with Autologous Tissue Substitute, Percutaneous Approach
05U93JZ Supplement Right Brachial Vein with Synthetic Substitute, Percutaneous Approach
05U93KZ Supplement Right Brachial Vein with Nonautologous Tissue Substitute, Percutaneous Approach
05U947Z Supplement Right Brachial Vein with Autologous Tissue Substitute, Percutaneous Endoscopic Approach
05U94JZ Supplement Right Brachial Vein with Synthetic Substitute, Percutaneous Endoscopic Approach

5U94KZ Supplement Right Brachial Vein with Nonautologous Tissue Substitute, Percutaneous Endoscopic Approach

5UA07Z Supplement Left Brachial Vein with Autologous Tissue Substitute, Open Approach

5UA0JZ Supplement Left Brachial Vein with Synthetic Substitute, Open Approach

5UA0KZ Supplement Left Brachial Vein with Nonautologous Tissue Substitute, Open Approach

5UA37Z Supplement Left Brachial Vein with Autologous Tissue Substitute, Percutaneous Approach

5UA3JZ Supplement Left Brachial Vein with Synthetic Substitute, Percutaneous Approach

5UA3KZ Supplement Left Brachial Vein with Nonautologous Tissue Substitute, Percutaneous Approach

5UA47Z Supplement Left Brachial Vein with Autologous Tissue Substitute, Percutaneous Endoscopic Approach

5UA4JZ Supplement Left Brachial Vein with Synthetic Substitute, Percutaneous Endoscopic Approach

5UA4KZ Supplement Left Brachial Vein with Nonautologous Tissue Substitute, Percutaneous Endoscopic Approach

5UB07Z Supplement Right Basilic Vein with Autologous Tissue Substitute, Open Approach

5UB0JZ Supplement Right Basilic Vein with Synthetic Substitute, Open Approach

5UB0KZ Supplement Right Basilic Vein with Nonautologous Tissue Substitute, Open Approach

5UB37Z Supplement Right Basilic Vein with Autologous Tissue Substitute, Percutaneous Approach

5UB3JZ Supplement Right Basilic Vein with Synthetic Substitute, Percutaneous Approach

5UB3KZ Supplement Right Basilic Vein with Nonautologous Tissue Substitute, Percutaneous Approach

5UB47Z Supplement Right Basilic Vein with Autologous Tissue Substitute, Percutaneous Endoscopic Approach

5UB4JZ Supplement Right Basilic Vein with Synthetic Substitute, Percutaneous Endoscopic Approach

5UB4KZ Supplement Right Basilic Vein with Nonautologous Tissue Substitute, Percutaneous Endoscopic Approach

5UC07Z Supplement Left Basilic Vein with Autologous Tissue Substitute, Open Approach

5UC0JZ Supplement Left Basilic Vein with Synthetic Substitute, Open Approach

5UC0KZ Supplement Left Basilic Vein with Nonautologous Tissue Substitute, Open Approach

5UC37Z Supplement Left Basilic Vein with Autologous Tissue Substitute, Percutaneous Approach

5UC3JZ Supplement Left Basilic Vein with Synthetic Substitute, Percutaneous Approach

5UC3KZ Supplement Left Basilic Vein with Nonautologous Tissue Substitute, Percutaneous Approach

5UC47Z Supplement Left Basilic Vein with Autologous Tissue Substitute, Percutaneous Endoscopic Approach

5UC4JZ Supplement Left Basilic Vein with Synthetic Substitute, Percutaneous Endoscopic Approach

05UC4KZ Supplement Left Basilic Vein with Nonautologous Tissue Substitute, Percutaneous Endoscopic Approach

05UD07Z Supplement Right Cephalic Vein with Autologous Tissue Substitute, Open Approach

05UD0JZ Supplement Right Cephalic Vein with Synthetic Substitute, Open Approach

05UD0KZ Supplement Right Cephalic Vein with Nonautologous Tissue Substitute, Open Approach

05UD37Z Supplement Right Cephalic Vein with Autologous Tissue Substitute, Percutaneous Approach

05UD3JZ Supplement Right Cephalic Vein with Synthetic Substitute, Percutaneous Approach

05UD3KZ Supplement Right Cephalic Vein with Nonautologous Tissue Substitute, Percutaneous Approach

05UD47Z Supplement Right Cephalic Vein with Autologous Tissue Substitute, Percutaneous Endoscopic Approach

05UD4JZ Supplement Right Cephalic Vein with Synthetic Substitute, Percutaneous Endoscopic Approach

05UD4KZ Supplement Right Cephalic Vein with Nonautologous Tissue Substitute, Percutaneous Endoscopic Approach

05UF07Z Supplement Left Cephalic Vein with Autologous Tissue Substitute, Open Approach

05UF0JZ Supplement Left Cephalic Vein with Synthetic Substitute, Open Approach

05UF0KZ Supplement Left Cephalic Vein with Nonautologous Tissue Substitute, Open Approach

05UF37Z Supplement Left Cephalic Vein with Autologous Tissue Substitute, Percutaneous Approach

05UF3JZ Supplement Left Cephalic Vein with Synthetic Substitute, Percutaneous Approach

05UF3KZ Supplement Left Cephalic Vein with Nonautologous Tissue Substitute, Percutaneous Approach

05UF47Z Supplement Left Cephalic Vein with Autologous Tissue Substitute, Percutaneous Endoscopic Approach

05UF4JZ Supplement Left Cephalic Vein with Synthetic Substitute, Percutaneous Endoscopic Approach

05UF4KZ Supplement Left Cephalic Vein with Nonautologous Tissue Substitute, Percutaneous Endoscopic Approach

05UG07Z Supplement Right Hand Vein with Autologous Tissue Substitute, Open Approach

05UG0JZ Supplement Right Hand Vein with Synthetic Substitute, Open Approach

05UG0KZ Supplement Right Hand Vein with Nonautologous Tissue Substitute, Open Approach

05UG37Z Supplement Right Hand Vein with Autologous Tissue Substitute, Percutaneous Approach

05UG3JZ Supplement Right Hand Vein with Synthetic Substitute, Percutaneous Approach

05UG3KZ Supplement Right Hand Vein with Nonautologous Tissue Substitute, Percutaneous Approach

05UG47Z Supplement Right Hand Vein with Autologous Tissue Substitute, Percutaneous Endoscopic Approach

05UG4JZ Supplement Right Hand Vein with Synthetic Substitute, Percutaneous Endoscopic Approach

05UG4KZ Supplement Right Hand Vein with Nonautologous Tissue Substitute, Percutaneous Endoscopic Approach

05UH07Z Supplement Left Hand Vein with Autologous Tissue Substitute, Open Approach

05UH0JZ Supplement Left Hand Vein with Synthetic Substitute, Open Approach

05UH0KZ Supplement Left Hand Vein with Nonautologous Tissue Substitute, Open Approach

05UH37Z Supplement Left Hand Vein with Autologous Tissue Substitute, Percutaneous Approach

05UH3JZ Supplement Left Hand Vein with Synthetic Substitute, Percutaneous Approach

05UH3KZ Supplement Left Hand Vein with Nonautologous Tissue Substitute, Percutaneous Approach

05UH47Z Supplement Left Hand Vein with Autologous Tissue Substitute, Percutaneous Endoscopic Approach

05UH4JZ Supplement Left Hand Vein with Synthetic Substitute, Percutaneous Endoscopic Approach

05UH4KZ Supplement Left Hand Vein with Nonautologous Tissue Substitute, Percutaneous Endoscopic Approach

05UL07Z Supplement Intracranial Vein with Autologous Tissue Substitute, Open Approach

05UL0JZ Supplement Intracranial Vein with Synthetic Substitute, Open Approach

05UL0KZ Supplement Intracranial Vein with Nonautologous Tissue Substitute, Open Approach

05UL37Z Supplement Intracranial Vein with Autologous Tissue Substitute, Percutaneous Approach

05UL3JZ Supplement Intracranial Vein with Synthetic Substitute, Percutaneous Approach

05UL3KZ Supplement Intracranial Vein with Nonautologous Tissue Substitute, Percutaneous Approach

05UL47Z Supplement Intracranial Vein with Autologous Tissue Substitute, Percutaneous Endoscopic Approach

05UL4JZ Supplement Intracranial Vein with Synthetic Substitute, Percutaneous Endoscopic Approach

05UL4KZ Supplement Intracranial Vein with Nonautologous Tissue Substitute, Percutaneous Endoscopic Approach

05UM07Z Supplement Right Internal Jugular Vein with Autologous Tissue Substitute, Open Approach

05UM0JZ Supplement Right Internal Jugular Vein with Synthetic Substitute, Open Approach

05UM0KZ Supplement Right Internal Jugular Vein with Nonautologous Tissue Substitute, Open Approach

05UM37Z Supplement Right Internal Jugular Vein with Autologous Tissue Substitute, Percutaneous Approach

05UM3JZ Supplement Right Internal Jugular Vein with Synthetic Substitute, Percutaneous Approach

05UM3KZ Supplement Right Internal Jugular Vein with Nonautologous Tissue Substitute, Percutaneous Approach

05UM47Z Supplement Right Internal Jugular Vein with Autologous Tissue Substitute, Percutaneous Endoscopic Approach

05UM4JZ Supplement Right Internal Jugular Vein with Synthetic Substitute, Percutaneous Endoscopic Approach

05UM4KZ Supplement Right Internal Jugular Vein with Nonautologous Tissue Substitute, Percutaneous Endoscopic Approach
05UN07Z Supplement Left Internal Jugular Vein with Autologous Tissue Substitute, Open Approach
05UN0JZ Supplement Left Internal Jugular Vein with Synthetic Substitute, Open Approach
05UN0KZ Supplement Left Internal Jugular Vein with Nonautologous Tissue Substitute, Open Approach
05UN37Z Supplement Left Internal Jugular Vein with Autologous Tissue Substitute, Percutaneous Approach
05UN3JZ Supplement Left Internal Jugular Vein with Synthetic Substitute, Percutaneous Approach
05UN3KZ Supplement Left Internal Jugular Vein with Nonautologous Tissue Substitute, Percutaneous Approach
05UN47Z Supplement Left Internal Jugular Vein with Autologous Tissue Substitute, Percutaneous Endoscopic Approach
05UN4JZ Supplement Left Internal Jugular Vein with Synthetic Substitute, Percutaneous Endoscopic Approach
05UN4KZ Supplement Left Internal Jugular Vein with Nonautologous Tissue Substitute, Percutaneous Endoscopic Approach
05UP07Z Supplement Right External Jugular Vein with Autologous Tissue Substitute, Open Approach
05UP0JZ Supplement Right External Jugular Vein with Synthetic Substitute, Open Approach
05UP0KZ Supplement Right External Jugular Vein with Nonautologous Tissue Substitute, Open Approach
05UP37Z Supplement Right External Jugular Vein with Autologous Tissue Substitute, Percutaneous Approach
05UP3JZ Supplement Right External Jugular Vein with Synthetic Substitute, Percutaneous Approach
05UP3KZ Supplement Right External Jugular Vein with Nonautologous Tissue Substitute, Percutaneous Approach
05UP47Z Supplement Right External Jugular Vein with Autologous Tissue Substitute, Percutaneous Endoscopic Approach
05UP4JZ Supplement Right External Jugular Vein with Synthetic Substitute, Percutaneous Endoscopic Approach
05UP4KZ Supplement Right External Jugular Vein with Nonautologous Tissue Substitute, Percutaneous Endoscopic Approach
05UQ07Z Supplement Left External Jugular Vein with Autologous Tissue Substitute, Open Approach
05UQ0JZ Supplement Left External Jugular Vein with Synthetic Substitute, Open Approach
05UQ0KZ Supplement Left External Jugular Vein with Nonautologous Tissue Substitute, Open Approach
05UQ37Z Supplement Left External Jugular Vein with Autologous Tissue Substitute, Percutaneous Approach
05UQ3JZ Supplement Left External Jugular Vein with Synthetic Substitute, Percutaneous Approach
05UQ3KZ Supplement Left External Jugular Vein with Nonautologous Tissue Substitute, Percutaneous Approach
05UQ47Z Supplement Left External Jugular Vein with Autologous Tissue Substitute, Percutaneous Endoscopic Approach
05UQ4JZ Supplement Left External Jugular Vein with Synthetic Substitute, Percutaneous Endoscopic Approach
05UQ4KZ Supplement Left External Jugular Vein with Nonautologous Tissue Substitute, Percutaneous Endoscopic Approach
05UR07Z Supplement Right Vertebral Vein with Autologous Tissue Substitute, Open Approach
05UR0JZ Supplement Right Vertebral Vein with Synthetic Substitute, Open Approach
05UR0KZ Supplement Right Vertebral Vein with Nonautologous Tissue Substitute, Open Approach
05UR37Z Supplement Right Vertebral Vein with Autologous Tissue Substitute, Percutaneous Approach
05UR3JZ Supplement Right Vertebral Vein with Synthetic Substitute, Percutaneous Approach
05UR3KZ Supplement Right Vertebral Vein with Nonautologous Tissue Substitute, Percutaneous Approach
05UR47Z Supplement Right Vertebral Vein with Autologous Tissue Substitute, Percutaneous Endoscopic Approach
05UR4JZ Supplement Right Vertebral Vein with Synthetic Substitute, Percutaneous Endoscopic Approach
05UR4KZ Supplement Right Vertebral Vein with Nonautologous Tissue Substitute, Percutaneous Endoscopic Approach
05US07Z Supplement Left Vertebral Vein with Autologous Tissue Substitute, Open Approach
05US0JZ Supplement Left Vertebral Vein with Synthetic Substitute, Open Approach
05US0KZ Supplement Left Vertebral Vein with Nonautologous Tissue Substitute, Open Approach
05US37Z Supplement Left Vertebral Vein with Autologous Tissue Substitute, Percutaneous Approach
05US3JZ Supplement Left Vertebral Vein with Synthetic Substitute, Percutaneous Approach
05US3KZ Supplement Left Vertebral Vein with Nonautologous Tissue Substitute, Percutaneous Approach
05US47Z Supplement Left Vertebral Vein with Autologous Tissue Substitute, Percutaneous Endoscopic Approach
05US4JZ Supplement Left Vertebral Vein with Synthetic Substitute, Percutaneous Endoscopic Approach
05US4KZ Supplement Left Vertebral Vein with Nonautologous Tissue Substitute, Percutaneous Endoscopic Approach
05UT07Z Supplement Right Face Vein with Autologous Tissue Substitute, Open Approach
05UT0JZ Supplement Right Face Vein with Synthetic Substitute, Open Approach
05UT0KZ Supplement Right Face Vein with Nonautologous Tissue Substitute, Open Approach
05UT37Z Supplement Right Face Vein with Autologous Tissue Substitute, Percutaneous Approach
05UT3JZ Supplement Right Face Vein with Synthet Substitute, Percutaneous Approach
05UT3KZ Supplement Right Face Vein with Nonautologous Tissue Substitute, Percutaneous Approach
05UT47Z Supplement Right Face Vein with Autologous Tissue Substitute, Percutaneous Endoscopic Approach
05UT4JZ Supplement Right Face Vein with Synthetic Substitute, Percutaneous Endoscopic Approach
05UT4KZ Supplement Right Face Vein with Nonautologous Tissue Substitute, Percutaneous Endoscopic Approach
05UV07Z Supplement Left Face Vein with Autologou Tissue Substitute, Open Approach
05UV0JZ Supplement Left Face Vein with Syntheti Substitute, Open Approach
05UV0KZ Supplement Left Face Vein with Nonautologous Tissue Substitute, Open Approach
05UV37Z Supplement Left Face Vein with Autologous Tissue Substitute, Percutaneous Approach
05UV3JZ Supplement Left Face Vein with Syntheti Substitute, Percutaneous Approach
05UV3KZ Supplement Left Face Vein with Nonautologous Tissue Substitute, Percutaneous Approach
05UV47Z Supplement Left Face Vein with Autologous Tissue Substitute, Percutaneous Endoscopic Approach
05UV4JZ Supplement Left Face Vein with Synthetic Substitute, Percutaneous Endoscopic Approach
05UV4KZ Supplement Left Face Vein with Nonautologous Tissue Substitute, Percutaneous Endoscopic Approach
05UY07Z Supplement Upper Vein with Autologous Tissue Substitute, Open Approach
05UY0JZ Supplement Upper Vein with Synthetic Substitute, Open Approach
05UY0KZ Supplement Upper Vein with Nonautologous Tissue Substitute, Open Approach
05UY37Z Supplement Upper Vein with Autologous Tissue Substitute, Percutaneous Approach
05UY3JZ Supplement Upper Vein with Synthetic Substitute, Percutaneous Approach
05UY3KZ Supplement Upper Vein with Nonautologous Tissue Substitute, Percutaneous Approach
05UY47Z Supplement Upper Vein with Autologous Tissue Substitute, Percutaneous Endoscopic Approach
05UY4JZ Supplement Upper Vein with Synthetic Substitute, Percutaneous Endoscopic Approach
05UY4KZ Supplement Upper Vein with Nonautologous Tissue Substitute, Percutaneous Endoscopic Approach

05V – Upper Veins, Restriction

Review Coding Guideline B3.12

05V00CZ Restriction of Azygos Vein with Extraluminal Device, Open Approach
05V00DZ Restriction of Azygos Vein with Intraluminal Device, Open Approach
05V00ZZ Restriction of Azygos Vein, Open Approach
05V03CZ Restriction of Azygos Vein with Extraluminal Device, Percutaneous Approach
05V03DZ Restriction of Azygos Vein with Intraluminal Device, Percutaneous Approach

5V03ZZ Restriction of Azygos Vein, Percutaneous Approach
5V04CZ Restriction of Azygos Vein with Extraluminal Device, Percutaneous Endoscopic Approach
5V04DZ Restriction of Azygos Vein with Intraluminal Device, Percutaneous Endoscopic Approach
5V04ZZ Restriction of Azygos Vein, Percutaneous Endoscopic Approach
5V10CZ Restriction of Hemiazygos Vein with Extraluminal Device, Open Approach
5V10DZ Restriction of Hemiazygos Vein with Intraluminal Device, Open Approach
5V10ZZ Restriction of Hemiazygos Vein, Open Approach
5V13CZ Restriction of Hemiazygos Vein with Extraluminal Device, Percutaneous Approach
5V13DZ Restriction of Hemiazygos Vein with Intraluminal Device, Percutaneous Approach
5V13ZZ Restriction of Hemiazygos Vein, Percutaneous Approach
5V14CZ Restriction of Hemiazygos Vein with Extraluminal Device, Percutaneous Endoscopic Approach
5V14DZ Restriction of Hemiazygos Vein with Intraluminal Device, Percutaneous Endoscopic Approach
5V14ZZ Restriction of Hemiazygos Vein, Percutaneous Endoscopic Approach
5V30CZ Restriction of Right Innominate Vein with Extraluminal Device, Open Approach
5V30DZ Restriction of Right Innominate Vein with Intraluminal Device, Open Approach
5V30ZZ Restriction of Right Innominate Vein, Open Approach
5V33CZ Restriction of Right Innominate Vein with Extraluminal Device, Percutaneous Approach
5V33DZ Restriction of Right Innominate Vein with Intraluminal Device, Percutaneous Approach
5V33ZZ Restriction of Right Innominate Vein, Percutaneous Approach
5V34CZ Restriction of Right Innominate Vein with Extraluminal Device, Percutaneous Endoscopic Approach
5V34DZ Restriction of Right Innominate Vein with Intraluminal Device, Percutaneous Endoscopic Approach
5V34ZZ Restriction of Right Innominate Vein, Percutaneous Endoscopic Approach
5V40CZ Restriction of Left Innominate Vein with Extraluminal Device, Open Approach
5V40DZ Restriction of Left Innominate Vein with Intraluminal Device, Open Approach
5V40ZZ Restriction of Left Innominate Vein, Open Approach
5V43CZ Restriction of Left Innominate Vein with Extraluminal Device, Percutaneous Approach
5V43DZ Restriction of Left Innominate Vein with Intraluminal Device, Percutaneous Approach
5V43ZZ Restriction of Left Innominate Vein, Percutaneous Approach
5V44CZ Restriction of Left Innominate Vein with Extraluminal Device, Percutaneous Endoscopic Approach
05V44DZ Restriction of Left Innominate Vein with Intraluminal Device, Percutaneous Endoscopic Approach
05V44ZZ Restriction of Left Innominate Vein, Percutaneous Endoscopic Approach
05V50CZ Restriction of Right Subclavian Vein with Extraluminal Device, Open Approach
05V50DZ Restriction of Right Subclavian Vein with Intraluminal Device, Open Approach
05V50ZZ Restriction of Right Subclavian Vein, Open Approach
05V53CZ Restriction of Right Subclavian Vein with Extraluminal Device, Percutaneous Approach
05V53DZ Restriction of Right Subclavian Vein with Intraluminal Device, Percutaneous Approach
05V53ZZ Restriction of Right Subclavian Vein, Percutaneous Approach
05V54CZ Restriction of Right Subclavian Vein with Extraluminal Device, Percutaneous Endoscopic Approach
05V54DZ Restriction of Right Subclavian Vein with Intraluminal Device, Percutaneous Endoscopic Approach
05V54ZZ Restriction of Right Subclavian Vein, Percutaneous Endoscopic Approach
05V60CZ Restriction of Left Subclavian Vein with Extraluminal Device, Open Approach
05V60DZ Restriction of Left Subclavian Vein with Intraluminal Device, Open Approach
05V60ZZ Restriction of Left Subclavian Vein, Open Approach
05V63CZ Restriction of Left Subclavian Vein with Extraluminal Device, Percutaneous Approach
05V63DZ Restriction of Left Subclavian Vein with Intraluminal Device, Percutaneous Approach
05V63ZZ Restriction of Left Subclavian Vein, Percutaneous Approach
05V64CZ Restriction of Left Subclavian Vein with Extraluminal Device, Percutaneous Endoscopic Approach
05V64DZ Restriction of Left Subclavian Vein with Intraluminal Device, Percutaneous Endoscopic Approach
05V64ZZ Restriction of Left Subclavian Vein, Percutaneous Endoscopic Approach
05V70CZ Restriction of Right Axillary Vein with Extraluminal Device, Open Approach
05V70DZ Restriction of Right Axillary Vein with Intraluminal Device, Open Approach
05V70ZZ Restriction of Right Axillary Vein, Open Approach
05V73CZ Restriction of Right Axillary Vein with Extraluminal Device, Percutaneous Approach
05V73DZ Restriction of Right Axillary Vein with Intraluminal Device, Percutaneous Approach
05V73ZZ Restriction of Right Axillary Vein, Percutaneous Approach
05V74CZ Restriction of Right Axillary Vein with Extraluminal Device, Percutaneous Endoscopic Approach
05V74DZ Restriction of Right Axillary Vein with Intraluminal Device, Percutaneous Endoscopic Approach
05V74ZZ Restriction of Right Axillary Vein, Percutaneous Endoscopic Approach
05V80CZ Restriction of Left Axillary Vein with Extraluminal Device, Open Approach
05V80DZ Restriction of Left Axillary Vein with Intraluminal Device, Open Approach
05V80ZZ Restriction of Left Axillary Vein, Open Approach
05V83CZ Restriction of Left Axillary Vein with Extraluminal Device, Percutaneous Approach
05V83DZ Restriction of Left Axillary Vein with Intraluminal Device, Percutaneous Approach
05V83ZZ Restriction of Left Axillary Vein, Percutaneous Approach
05V84CZ Restriction of Left Axillary Vein with Extraluminal Device, Percutaneous Endoscopic Approach
05V84DZ Restriction of Left Axillary Vein with Intraluminal Device, Percutaneous Endoscopic Approach
05V84ZZ Restriction of Left Axillary Vein, Percutaneous Endoscopic Approach
05V90CZ Restriction of Right Brachial Vein with Extraluminal Device, Open Approach
05V90DZ Restriction of Right Brachial Vein with Intraluminal Device, Open Approach
05V90ZZ Restriction of Right Brachial Vein, Open Approach
05V93CZ Restriction of Right Brachial Vein with Extraluminal Device, Percutaneous Approach
05V93DZ Restriction of Right Brachial Vein with Intraluminal Device, Percutaneous Approach
05V93ZZ Restriction of Right Brachial Vein, Percutaneous Approach
05V94CZ Restriction of Right Brachial Vein with Extraluminal Device, Percutaneous Endoscopic Approach
05V94DZ Restriction of Right Brachial Vein with Intraluminal Device, Percutaneous Endoscopic Approach
05V94ZZ Restriction of Right Brachial Vein, Percutaneous Endoscopic Approach
05VA0CZ Restriction of Left Brachial Vein with Extraluminal Device, Open Approach
05VA0DZ Restriction of Left Brachial Vein with Intraluminal Device, Open Approach
05VA0ZZ Restriction of Left Brachial Vein, Open Approach
05VA3CZ Restriction of Left Brachial Vein with Extraluminal Device, Percutaneous Approach
05VA3DZ Restriction of Left Brachial Vein with Intraluminal Device, Percutaneous Approach
05VA3ZZ Restriction of Left Brachial Vein, Percutaneous Approach
05VA4CZ Restriction of Left Brachial Vein with Extraluminal Device, Percutaneous Endoscopic Approach
05VA4DZ Restriction of Left Brachial Vein with Intraluminal Device, Percutaneous Endoscopic Approach
05VA4ZZ Restriction of Left Brachial Vein, Percutaneous Endoscopic Approach
05VB0CZ Restriction of Right Basilic Vein with Extraluminal Device, Open Approach
05VB0DZ Restriction of Right Basilic Vein with Intraluminal Device, Open Approach
05VB0ZZ Restriction of Right Basilic Vein, Open Approach
05VB3CZ Restriction of Right Basilic Vein with Extraluminal Device, Percutaneous Approach
05VB3DZ Restriction of Right Basilic Vein with Intraluminal Device, Percutaneous Approach
05VB3ZZ Restriction of Right Basilic Vein, Percutaneous Approach
05VB4CZ Restriction of Right Basilic Vein with Extraluminal Device, Percutaneous Endoscopic Approach
05VB4DZ Restriction of Right Basilic Vein with Intraluminal Device, Percutaneous Endoscopic Approach
05VB4ZZ Restriction of Right Basilic Vein, Percutaneous Endoscopic Approach
05VC0CZ Restriction of Left Basilic Vein with Extraluminal Device, Open Approach

05VC0DZ Restriction of Left Basilic Vein with Intraluminal Device, Open Approach
05VC0ZZ Restriction of Left Basilic Vein, Open Approach
05VC3CZ Restriction of Left Basilic Vein with Extraluminal Device, Percutaneous Approach
05VC3DZ Restriction of Left Basilic Vein with Intraluminal Device, Percutaneous Approach
05VC3ZZ Restriction of Left Basilic Vein, Percutaneous Approach
05VC4CZ Restriction of Left Basilic Vein with Extraluminal Device, Percutaneous Endoscopic Approach
05VC4DZ Restriction of Left Basilic Vein with Intraluminal Device, Percutaneous Endoscopic Approach
05VC4ZZ Restriction of Left Basilic Vein, Percutaneous Endoscopic Approach
05VD0CZ Restriction of Right Cephalic Vein with Extraluminal Device, Open Approach
05VD0DZ Restriction of Right Cephalic Vein with Intraluminal Device, Open Approach
05VD0ZZ Restriction of Right Cephalic Vein, Open Approach
05VD3CZ Restriction of Right Cephalic Vein with Extraluminal Device, Percutaneous Approach
05VD3DZ Restriction of Right Cephalic Vein with Intraluminal Device, Percutaneous Approach
05VD3ZZ Restriction of Right Cephalic Vein, Percutaneous Approach
05VD4CZ Restriction of Right Cephalic Vein with Extraluminal Device, Percutaneous Endoscopic Approach
05VD4DZ Restriction of Right Cephalic Vein with Intraluminal Device, Percutaneous Endoscopic Approach
05VD4ZZ Restriction of Right Cephalic Vein, Percutaneous Endoscopic Approach
05VF0CZ Restriction of Left Cephalic Vein with Extraluminal Device, Open Approach
05VF0DZ Restriction of Left Cephalic Vein with Intraluminal Device, Open Approach
05VF0ZZ Restriction of Left Cephalic Vein, Open Approach
05VF3CZ Restriction of Left Cephalic Vein with Extraluminal Device, Percutaneous Approach
05VF3DZ Restriction of Left Cephalic Vein with Intraluminal Device, Percutaneous Approach
05VF3ZZ Restriction of Left Cephalic Vein, Percutaneous Approach
05VF4CZ Restriction of Left Cephalic Vein with Extraluminal Device, Percutaneous Endoscopic Approach
05VF4DZ Restriction of Left Cephalic Vein with Intraluminal Device, Percutaneous Endoscopic Approach
05VF4ZZ Restriction of Left Cephalic Vein, Percutaneous Endoscopic Approach
05VG0CZ Restriction of Right Hand Vein with Extraluminal Device, Open Approach
05VG0DZ Restriction of Right Hand Vein with Intraluminal Device, Open Approach
05VG0ZZ Restriction of Right Hand Vein, Open Approach
05VG3CZ Restriction of Right Hand Vein with Extraluminal Device, Percutaneous Approach
05VG3DZ Restriction of Right Hand Vein with Intraluminal Device, Percutaneous Approach
05VG3ZZ Restriction of Right Hand Vein, Percutaneous Approach
05VG4CZ Restriction of Right Hand Vein with Extraluminal Device, Percutaneous Endoscopic Approach
05VG4DZ Restriction of Right Hand Vein with Intraluminal Device, Percutaneous Endoscopic Approach
05VG4ZZ Restriction of Right Hand Vein, Percutaneous Endoscopic Approach
05VH0CZ Restriction of Left Hand Vein with Extraluminal Device, Open Approach
05VH0DZ Restriction of Left Hand Vein with Intraluminal Device, Open Approach
05VH0ZZ Restriction of Left Hand Vein, Open Approach
05VH3CZ Restriction of Left Hand Vein with Extraluminal Device, Percutaneous Approach
05VH3DZ Restriction of Left Hand Vein with Intraluminal Device, Percutaneous Approach
05VH3ZZ Restriction of Left Hand Vein, Percutaneous Approach
05VH4CZ Restriction of Left Hand Vein with Extraluminal Device, Percutaneous Endoscopic Approach
05VH4DZ Restriction of Left Hand Vein with Intraluminal Device, Percutaneous Endoscopic Approach
05VH4ZZ Restriction of Left Hand Vein, Percutaneous Endoscopic Approach
05VL0CZ Restriction of Intracranial Vein with Extraluminal Device, Open Approach
05VL0DZ Restriction of Intracranial Vein with Intraluminal Device, Open Approach
05VL0ZZ Restriction of Intracranial Vein, Open Approach
05VL3CZ Restriction of Intracranial Vein with Extraluminal Device, Percutaneous Approach
05VL3DZ Restriction of Intracranial Vein with Intraluminal Device, Percutaneous Approach
05VL3ZZ Restriction of Intracranial Vein, Percutaneous Approach
05VL4CZ Restriction of Intracranial Vein with Extraluminal Device, Percutaneous Endoscopic Approach
05VL4DZ Restriction of Intracranial Vein with Intraluminal Device, Percutaneous Endoscopic Approach
05VL4ZZ Restriction of Intracranial Vein, Percutaneous Endoscopic Approach
05VM0CZ Restriction of Right Internal Jugular Vein with Extraluminal Device, Open Approach
05VM0DZ Restriction of Right Internal Jugular Vein with Intraluminal Device, Open Approach
05VM0ZZ Restriction of Right Internal Jugular Vein, Open Approach
05VM3CZ Restriction of Right Internal Jugular Vein with Extraluminal Device, Percutaneous Approach
05VM3DZ Restriction of Right Internal Jugular Vein with Intraluminal Device, Percutaneous Approach
05VM3ZZ Restriction of Right Internal Jugular Vein, Percutaneous Approach
05VM4CZ Restriction of Right Internal Jugular Vein with Extraluminal Device, Percutaneous Endoscopic Approach
05VM4DZ Restriction of Right Internal Jugular Vein with Intraluminal Device, Percutaneous Endoscopic Approach
05VM4ZZ Restriction of Right Internal Jugular Vein, Percutaneous Endoscopic Approach
05VN0CZ Restriction of Left Internal Jugular Vein with Extraluminal Device, Open Approach
05VN0DZ Restriction of Left Internal Jugular Vein with Intraluminal Device, Open Approach
05VN0ZZ Restriction of Left Internal Jugular Vein, Open Approach
05VN3CZ Restriction of Left Internal Jugular Vein with Extraluminal Device, Percutaneous Approach
05VN3DZ Restriction of Left Internal Jugular Vein with Intraluminal Device, Percutaneous Approach
05VN3ZZ Restriction of Left Internal Jugular Vein, Percutaneous Approach
05VN4CZ Restriction of Left Internal Jugular Vein with Extraluminal Device, Percutaneous Endoscopic Approach
05VN4DZ Restriction of Left Internal Jugular Vein with Intraluminal Device, Percutaneous Endoscopic Approach
05VN4ZZ Restriction of Left Internal Jugular Vein, Percutaneous Endoscopic Approach
05VP0CZ Restriction of Right External Jugular Vein with Extraluminal Device, Open Approach
05VP0DZ Restriction of Right External Jugular Vein with Intraluminal Device, Open Approach
05VP0ZZ Restriction of Right External Jugular Vein, Open Approach
05VP3CZ Restriction of Right External Jugular Vein with Extraluminal Device, Percutaneous Approach
05VP3DZ Restriction of Right External Jugular Vein with Intraluminal Device, Percutaneous Approach
05VP3ZZ Restriction of Right External Jugular Vein Percutaneous Approach
05VP4CZ Restriction of Right External Jugular Vein with Extraluminal Device, Percutaneous Endoscopic Approach
05VP4DZ Restriction of Right External Jugular Vein with Intraluminal Device, Percutaneous Endoscopic Approach
05VP4ZZ Restriction of Right External Jugular Vein Percutaneous Endoscopic Approach
05VQ0CZ Restriction of Left External Jugular Vein with Extraluminal Device, Open Approach
05VQ0DZ Restriction of Left External Jugular Vein with Intraluminal Device, Open Approach
05VQ0ZZ Restriction of Left External Jugular Vein, Open Approach
05VQ3CZ Restriction of Left External Jugular Vein with Extraluminal Device, Percutaneous Approach
05VQ3DZ Restriction of Left External Jugular Vein with Intraluminal Device, Percutaneous Approach
05VQ3ZZ Restriction of Left External Jugular Vein, Percutaneous Approach
05VQ4CZ Restriction of Left External Jugular Vein with Extraluminal Device, Percutaneous Endoscopic Approach
05VQ4DZ Restriction of Left External Jugular Vein with Intraluminal Device, Percutaneous Endoscopic Approach
05VQ4ZZ Restriction of Left External Jugular Vein, Percutaneous Endoscopic Approach
05VR0CZ Restriction of Right Vertebral Vein with Extraluminal Device, Open Approach
05VR0DZ Restriction of Right Vertebral Vein with Intraluminal Device, Open Approach
05VR0ZZ Restriction of Right Vertebral Vein, Open Approach
05VR3CZ Restriction of Right Vertebral Vein with Extraluminal Device, Percutaneous Approach
05VR3DZ Restriction of Right Vertebral Vein with Intraluminal Device, Percutaneous Approach
05VR3ZZ Restriction of Right Vertebral Vein, Percutaneous Approach

5VR4CZ Restriction of Right Vertebral Vein with Extraluminal Device, Percutaneous Endoscopic Approach

5VR4DZ Restriction of Right Vertebral Vein with Intraluminal Device, Percutaneous Endoscopic Approach

5VR4ZZ Restriction of Right Vertebral Vein, Percutaneous Endoscopic Approach

5VS0CZ Restriction of Left Vertebral Vein with Extraluminal Device, Open Approach

5VS0DZ Restriction of Left Vertebral Vein with Intraluminal Device, Open Approach

5VS0ZZ Restriction of Left Vertebral Vein, Open Approach

5VS3CZ Restriction of Left Vertebral Vein with Extraluminal Device, Percutaneous Approach

5VS3DZ Restriction of Left Vertebral Vein with Intraluminal Device, Percutaneous Approach

5VS3ZZ Restriction of Left Vertebral Vein, Percutaneous Approach

5VS4CZ Restriction of Left Vertebral Vein with Extraluminal Device, Percutaneous Endoscopic Approach

5VS4DZ Restriction of Left Vertebral Vein with Intraluminal Device, Percutaneous Endoscopic Approach

5VS4ZZ Restriction of Left Vertebral Vein, Percutaneous Endoscopic Approach

5VT0CZ Restriction of Right Face Vein with Extraluminal Device, Open Approach

05VT0DZ Restriction of Right Face Vein with Intraluminal Device, Open Approach

05VT0ZZ Restriction of Right Face Vein, Open Approach

05VT3CZ Restriction of Right Face Vein with Extraluminal Device, Percutaneous Approach

05VT3DZ Restriction of Right Face Vein with Intraluminal Device, Percutaneous Approach

05VT3ZZ Restriction of Right Face Vein, Percutaneous Approach

05VT4CZ Restriction of Right Face Vein with Extraluminal Device, Percutaneous Endoscopic Approach

05VT4DZ Restriction of Right Face Vein with Intraluminal Device, Percutaneous Endoscopic Approach

05VT4ZZ Restriction of Right Face Vein, Percutaneous Endoscopic Approach

05VV0CZ Restriction of Left Face Vein with Extraluminal Device, Open Approach

05VV0DZ Restriction of Left Face Vein with Intraluminal Device, Open Approach

05VV0ZZ Restriction of Left Face Vein, Open Approach

05VV3CZ Restriction of Left Face Vein with Extraluminal Device, Percutaneous Approach

05VV3DZ Restriction of Left Face Vein with Intraluminal Device, Percutaneous Approach

05VV3ZZ Restriction of Left Face Vein, Percutaneous Approach

05VV4CZ Restriction of Left Face Vein with Extraluminal Device, Percutaneous Endoscopic Approach

05VV4DZ Restriction of Left Face Vein with Intraluminal Device, Percutaneous Endoscopic Approach

05VV4ZZ Restriction of Left Face Vein, Percutaneous Endoscopic Approach

05VY0CZ Restriction of Upper Vein with Extraluminal Device, Open Approach

05VY0DZ Restriction of Upper Vein with Intraluminal Device, Open Approach

05VY0ZZ Restriction of Upper Vein, Open Approach

05VY3CZ Restriction of Upper Vein with Extraluminal Device, Percutaneous Approach

05VY3DZ Restriction of Upper Vein with Intraluminal Device, Percutaneous Approach

05VY3ZZ Restriction of Upper Vein, Percutaneous Approach

05VY4CZ Restriction of Upper Vein with Extraluminal Device, Percutaneous Endoscopic Approach

05VY4DZ Restriction of Upper Vein with Intraluminal Device, Percutaneous Endoscopic Approach

05VY4ZZ Restriction of Upper Vein, Percutaneous Endoscopic Approach

)5W – Upper Veins, Revision

Review Coding Guideline B6.1c

5WY00Z Revision of Drainage Device in Upper Vein, Open Approach

5WY02Z Revision of Monitoring Device in Upper Vein, Open Approach

5WY03Z Revision of Infusion Device in Upper Vein, Open Approach

5WY07Z Revision of Autologous Tissue Substitute in Upper Vein, Open Approach

)5WY0CZ Revision of Extraluminal Device in Upper Vein, Open Approach

05WY0DZ Revision of Intraluminal Device in Upper Vein, Open Approach

05WY0JZ Revision of Synthetic Substitute in Upper Vein, Open Approach

)5WY0KZ Revision of Nonautologous Tissue Substitute in Upper Vein, Open Approach

05WY30Z Revision of Drainage Device in Upper Vein, Percutaneous Approach

05WY32Z Revision of Monitoring Device in Upper Vein, Percutaneous Approach

05WY33Z Revision of Infusion Device in Upper Vein, Percutaneous Approach

05WY37Z Revision of Autologous Tissue Substitute in Upper Vein, Percutaneous Approach

05WY3CZ Revision of Extraluminal Device in Upper Vein, Percutaneous Approach

05WY3DZ Revision of Intraluminal Device in Upper Vein, Percutaneous Approach

05WY3JZ Revision of Synthetic Substitute in Upper Vein, Percutaneous Approach

05WY3KZ Revision of Nonautologous Tissue Substitute in Upper Vein, Percutaneous Approach

05WY40Z Revision of Drainage Device in Upper Vein, Percutaneous Endoscopic Approach

05WY42Z Revision of Monitoring Device in Upper Vein, Percutaneous Endoscopic Approach

05WY43Z Revision of Infusion Device in Upper Vein, Percutaneous Endoscopic Approach

05WY47Z Revision of Autologous Tissue Substitute in Upper Vein, Percutaneous Endoscopic Approach

05WY4CZ Revision of Extraluminal Device in Upper Vein, Percutaneous Endoscopic Approach

05WY4DZ Revision of Intraluminal Device in Upper Vein, Percutaneous Endoscopic Approach

05WY4JZ Revision of Synthetic Substitute in Upper Vein, Percutaneous Endoscopic Approach

05WY4KZ Revision of Nonautologous Tissue Substitute in Upper Vein, Percutaneous Endoscopic Approach

05WYX0Z Revision of Drainage Device in Upper Vein, External Approach

05WYX2Z Revision of Monitoring Device in Upper Vein, External Approach

05WYX3Z Revision of Infusion Device in Upper Vein, External Approach

05WYX7Z Revision of Autologous Tissue Substitute in Upper Vein, External Approach

05WYXCZ Revision of Extraluminal Device in Upper Vein, External Approach

05WYXDZ Revision of Intraluminal Device in Upper Vein, External Approach

05WYXJZ Revision of Synthetic Substitute in Upper Vein, External Approach

05WYXKZ Revision of Nonautologous Tissue Substitute in Upper Vein, External Approach

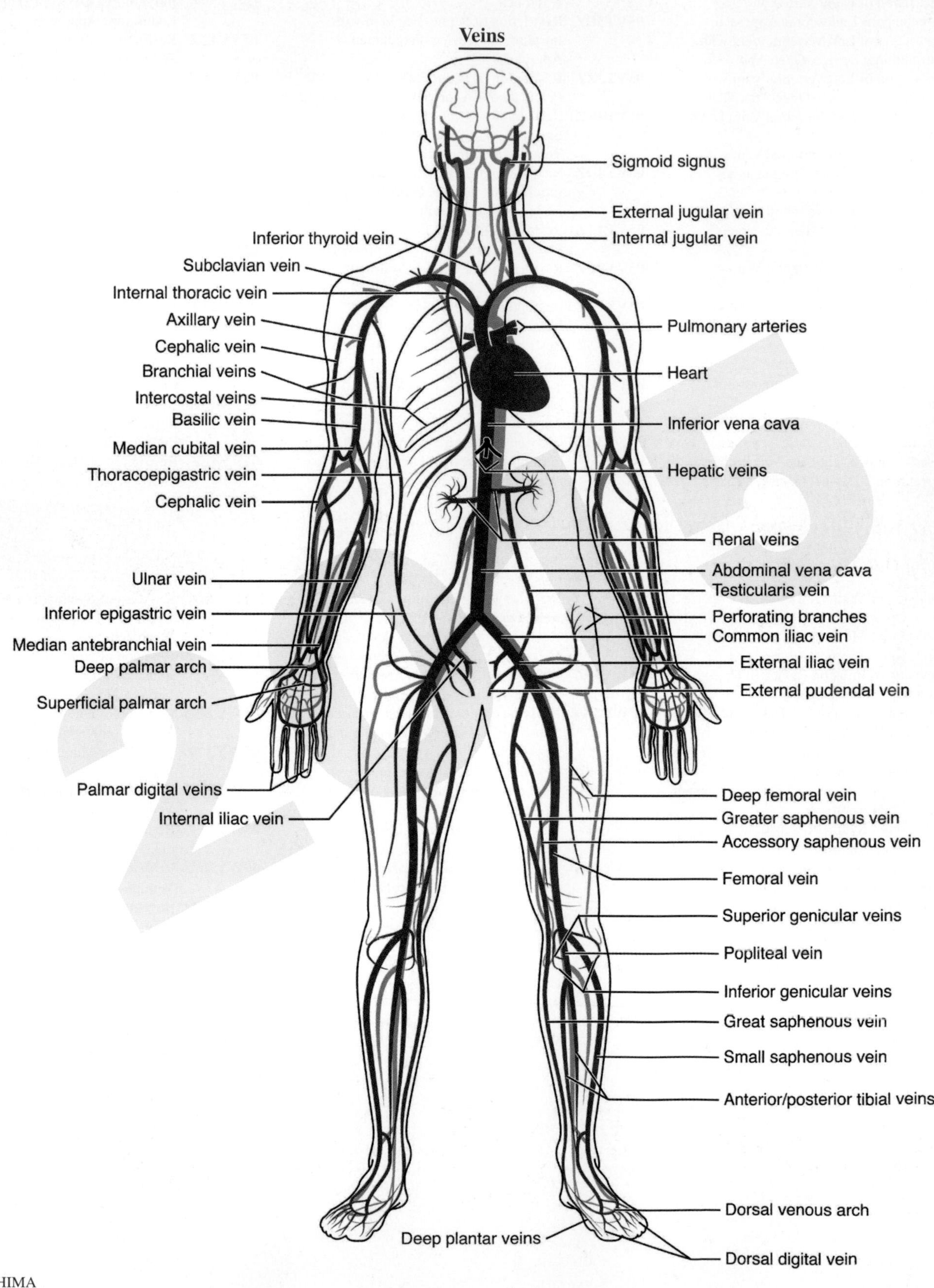
Veins
Sigmoid signus
External jugular vein
Internal jugular vein
Inferior thyroid vein
Subclavian vein
Internal thoracic vein
Axillary vein
Cephalic vein
Branchial veins
Intercostal veins
Basilic vein
Median cubital vein
Thoracoepigastric vein
Cephalic vein
Pulmonary arteries
Heart
Inferior vena cava
Hepatic veins
Renal veins
Abdominal vena cava
Testicularis vein
Ulnar vein
Inferior epigastric vein
Median antebranchial vein
Deep palmar arch
Superficial palmar arch
Perforating branches
Common iliac vein
External iliac vein
External pudendal vein
Palmar digital veins
Internal iliac vein
Deep femoral vein
Greater saphenous vein
Accessory saphenous vein
Femoral vein
Superior genicular veins
Popliteal vein
Inferior genicular veins
Great saphenous vein
Small saphenous vein
Anterior/posterior tibial veins
Dorsal venous arch
Deep plantar veins
Dorsal digital vein

Section 0 **Medical and Surgical**
Body System 6 **Lower Veins**
Operation 1 **Bypass:** Altering the route of passage of the contents of a tubular body part

Body Part (4th)	Approach (5th)	Device (6th)	Qualifier (7th)
0 Inferior Vena Cava	**0** Open **4** Percutaneous Endoscopic	**7** Autologous Tissue Substitute **9** Autologous Venous Tissue **A** Autologous Arterial Tissue **J** Synthetic Substitute **K** Nonautologous Tissue Substitute **Z** No Device	**5** Superior Mesenteric Vein **6** Inferior Mesenteric Vein **Y** Lower Vein
1 Splenic Vein	**0** Open **4** Percutaneous Endoscopic	**7** Autologous Tissue Substitute **9** Autologous Venous Tissue **A** Autologous Arterial Tissue **J** Synthetic Substitute **K** Nonautologous Tissue Substitute **Z** No Device	**9** Renal Vein, Right **B** Renal Vein, Left **Y** Lower Vein
2 Gastric Vein **3** Esophageal Vein **4** Hepatic Vein **5** Superior Mesenteric Vein **6** Inferior Mesenteric Vein **7** Colic Vein **9** Renal Vein, Right **B** Renal Vein, Left **C** Common Iliac Vein, Right **D** Common Iliac Vein, Left **F** External Iliac Vein, Right **G** External Iliac Vein, Left **H** Hypogastric Vein, Right **J** Hypogastric Vein, Left **M** Femoral Vein, Right **N** Femoral Vein, Left **P** Greater Saphenous Vein, Right **Q** Greater Saphenous Vein, Left **R** Lesser Saphenous Vein, Right **S** Lesser Saphenous Vein, Left **T** Foot Vein, Right **V** Foot Vein, Left	**0** Open **4** Percutaneous Endoscopic	**7** Autologous Tissue Substitute **9** Autologous Venous Tissue **A** Autologous Arterial Tissue **J** Synthetic Substitute **K** Nonautologous Tissue Substitute **Z** No Device	**Y** Lower Vein
8 Portal Vein	**0** Open	**7** Autologous Tissue Substitute **9** Autologous Venous Tissue **A** Autologous Arterial Tissue **J** Synthetic Substitute **K** Nonautologous Tissue Substitute **Z** No Device	**9** Renal Vein, Right **B** Renal Vein, Left **Y** Lower Vein
8 Portal Vein	**3** Percutaneous	**D** Intraluminal Device	**Y** Lower Vein
8 Portal Vein	**4** Percutaneous Endoscopic	**7** Autologous Tissue Substitute **9** Autologous Venous Tissue **A** Autologous Arterial Tissue **J** Synthetic Substitute **K** Nonautologous Tissue Substitute **Z** No Device	**9** Renal Vein, Right **B** Renal Vein, Left **Y** Lower Vein
8 Portal Vein	**4** Percutaneous Endoscopic	**D** Intraluminal Device	**Y** Lower Vein

Section 0 **Medical and Surgical**
Body System 6 **Lower Veins**
Operation 5 **Destruction:** Physical eradication of all or a portion of a body part by the direct use of energy, force, or a destructive agent

Body Part (4th)	Approach (5th)	Device (6th)	Qualifier (7th)
0 Inferior Vena Cava **1** Splenic Vein **2** Gastric Vein **3** Esophageal Vein **4** Hepatic Vein **5** Superior Mesenteric Vein **6** Inferior Mesenteric Vein **7** Colic Vein **8** Portal Vein **9** Renal Vein, Right **B** Renal Vein, Left **C** Common Iliac Vein, Right **D** Common Iliac Vein, Left **F** External Iliac Vein, Right **G** External Iliac Vein, Left **H** Hypogastric Vein, Right **J** Hypogastric Vein, Left **M** Femoral Vein, Right **N** Femoral Vein, Left **P** Greater Saphenous Vein, Right **Q** Greater Saphenous Vein, Left **R** Lesser Saphenous Vein, Right **S** Lesser Saphenous Vein, Left **T** Foot Vein, Right **V** Foot Vein, Left	**0** Open **3** Percutaneous **4** Percutaneous Endoscopic	**Z** No Device	**Z** No Qualifier
Y Lower Vein	**0** Open **3** Percutaneous **4** Percutaneous Endoscopic	**Z** No Device	**C** Hemorrhoidal Plexus **Z** No Qualifier

Section 0 **Medical and Surgical**
Body System 6 **Lower Veins**
Operation 7 **Dilation:** Expanding an orifice or the lumen of a tubular body part

Body Part (4th)	Approach (5th)	Device (6th)	Qualifier (7th)
0 Inferior Vena Cava **1** Splenic Vein **2** Gastric Vein **3** Esophageal Vein **4** Hepatic Vein **5** Superior Mesenteric Vein **6** Inferior Mesenteric Vein **7** Colic Vein **8** Portal Vein **9** Renal Vein, Right **B** Renal Vein, Left **C** Common Iliac Vein, Right **D** Common Iliac Vein, Left **F** External Iliac Vein, Right **G** External Iliac Vein, Left **H** Hypogastric Vein, Right **J** Hypogastric Vein, Left **M** Femoral Vein, Right **N** Femoral Vein, Left **P** Greater Saphenous Vein, Right **Q** Greater Saphenous Vein, Left **R** Lesser Saphenous Vein, Right **S** Lesser Saphenous Vein, Left **T** Foot Vein, Right **V** Foot Vein, Left **Y** Lower Vein	**0** Open **3** Percutaneous **4** Percutaneous Endoscopic	**D** Intraluminal Device **Z** No Device	**Z** No Qualifier

ection	**0**	**Medical and Surgical**
ody System	**6**	**Lower Veins**
peration	**9**	**Drainage:** Taking or letting out fluids and/or gases from a body part

Body Part (4th)	Approach (5th)	Device (6th)	Qualifier (7th)
0 Inferior Vena Cava **1** Splenic Vein **2** Gastric Vein **3** Esophageal Vein **4** Hepatic Vein **5** Superior Mesenteric Vein **6** Inferior Mesenteric Vein **7** Colic Vein **8** Portal Vein **9** Renal Vein, Right **B** Renal Vein, Left **C** Common Iliac Vein, Right **D** Common Iliac Vein, Left **F** External Iliac Vein, Right **G** External Iliac Vein, Left **H** Hypogastric Vein, Right **J** Hypogastric Vein, Left **M** Femoral Vein, Right **N** Femoral Vein, Left **P** Greater Saphenous Vein, Right **Q** Greater Saphenous Vein, Left **R** Lesser Saphenous Vein, Right **S** Lesser Saphenous Vein, Left **T** Foot Vein, Right **V** Foot Vein, Left **Y** Lower Vein	**0** Open **3** Percutaneous **4** Percutaneous Endoscopic	**0** Drainage Device	**Z** No Qualifier
0 Inferior Vena Cava **1** Splenic Vein **2** Gastric Vein **3** Esophageal Vein **4** Hepatic Vein **5** Superior Mesenteric Vein **6** Inferior Mesenteric Vein **7** Colic Vein **8** Portal Vein **9** Renal Vein, Right **B** Renal Vein, Left **C** Common Iliac Vein, Right **D** Common Iliac Vein, Left **F** External Iliac Vein, Right **G** External Iliac Vein, Left **H** Hypogastric Vein, Right **J** Hypogastric Vein, Left **M** Femoral Vein, Right **N** Femoral Vein, Left **P** Greater Saphenous Vein, Right **Q** Greater Saphenous Vein, Left **R** Lesser Saphenous Vein, Right **S** Lesser Saphenous Vein, Left **T** Foot Vein, Right **V** Foot Vein, Left **Y** Lower Vein	**0** Open **3** Percutaneous **4** Percutaneous Endoscopic	**Z** No Device	**X** Diagnostic **Z** No Qualifier

Section 0 **Medical and Surgical**
Body System 6 **Lower Veins**
Operation B **Excision:** Cutting out or off, without replacement, a portion of a body part

Body Part (4th)	Approach (5th)	Device (6th)	Qualifier (7th)
0 Inferior Vena Cava **1** Splenic Vein **2** Gastric Vein **3** Esophageal Vein **4** Hepatic Vein **5** Superior Mesenteric Vein **6** Inferior Mesenteric Vein **7** Colic Vein **8** Portal Vein **9** Renal Vein, Right **B** Renal Vein, Left **C** Common Iliac Vein, Right **D** Common Iliac Vein, Left **F** External Iliac Vein, Right **G** External Iliac Vein, Left **H** Hypogastric Vein, Right **J** Hypogastric Vein, Left **M** Femoral Vein, Right **N** Femoral Vein, Left **P** Greater Saphenous Vein, Right **Q** Greater Saphenous Vein, Left **R** Lesser Saphenous Vein, Right **S** Lesser Saphenous Vein, Left **T** Foot Vein, Right **V** Foot Vein, Left	**0** Open **3** Percutaneous **4** Percutaneous Endoscopic	**Z** No Device	**X** Diagnostic **Z** No Qualifier
Y Lower Vein	**0** Open **3** Percutaneous **4** Percutaneous Endoscopic	**Z** No Device	**C** Hemorrhoidal Plexus **X** Diagnostic **Z** No Qualifier

Section 0 **Medical and Surgical**
Body System 6 **Lower Veins**
Operation C **Extirpation:** Taking or cutting out solid matter from a body part

Body Part (4th)	Approach (5th)	Device (6th)	Qualifier (7th)
0 Inferior Vena Cava **1** Splenic Vein **2** Gastric Vein **3** Esophageal Vein **4** Hepatic Vein **5** Superior Mesenteric Vein **6** Inferior Mesenteric Vein **7** Colic Vein **8** Portal Vein **9** Renal Vein, Right **B** Renal Vein, Left **C** Common Iliac Vein, Right **D** Common Iliac Vein, Left **F** External Iliac Vein, Right **G** External Iliac Vein, Left **H** Hypogastric Vein, Right **J** Hypogastric Vein, Left **M** Femoral Vein, Right **N** Femoral Vein, Left **P** Greater Saphenous Vein, Right **Q** Greater Saphenous Vein, Left **R** Lesser Saphenous Vein, Right **S** Lesser Saphenous Vein, Left **T** Foot Vein, Right **V** Foot Vein, Left **Y** Lower Vein	**0** Open **3** Percutaneous **4** Percutaneous Endoscopic	**Z** No Device	**Z** No Qualifier

ection 0 Medical and Surgical
ody System 6 Lower Veins
peration D **Extraction:** Pulling or stripping out or off all or a portion of a body part by the use of force

Body Part (4th)	Approach (5th)	Device (6th)	Qualifier (7th)
M Femoral Vein, Right N Femoral Vein, Left P Greater Saphenous Vein, Right Q Greater Saphenous Vein, Left R Lesser Saphenous Vein, Right S Lesser Saphenous Vein, Left T Foot Vein, Right V Foot Vein, Left Y Lower Vein	0 Open 3 Percutaneous 4 Percutaneous Endoscopic	Z No Device	Z No Qualifier

ection 0 Medical and Surgical
ody System 6 Lower Veins
peration H **Insertion:** Putting in a nonbiological appliance that monitors, assists, performs, or prevents a physiological function but does not physically take the place of a body part

Body Part (4th)	Approach (5th)	Device (6th)	Qualifier (7th)
0 Inferior Vena Cava	0 Open 3 Percutaneous	3 Infusion Device	T Via Umbilical Vein Z No Qualifier
0 Inferior Vena Cava	0 Open 3 Percutaneous	D Intraluminal Device	Z No Qualifier
0 Inferior Vena Cava	4 Percutaneous Endoscopic	3 Infusion Device D Intraluminal Device	Z No Qualifier
1 Splenic Vein 2 Gastric Vein 3 Esophageal Vein 4 Hepatic Vein 5 Superior Mesenteric Vein 6 Inferior Mesenteric Vein 7 Colic Vein 8 Portal Vein 9 Renal Vein, Right B Renal Vein, Left C Common Iliac Vein, Right D Common Iliac Vein, Left F External Iliac Vein, Right G External Iliac Vein, Left H Hypogastric Vein, Right J Hypogastric Vein, Left M Femoral Vein, Right N Femoral Vein, Left P Greater Saphenous Vein, Right Q Greater Saphenous Vein, Left R Lesser Saphenous Vein, Right S Lesser Saphenous Vein, Left T Foot Vein, Right V Foot Vein, Left	0 Open 3 Percutaneous 4 Percutaneous Endoscopic	3 Infusion Device D Intraluminal Device	Z No Qualifier
Y Lower Vein	0 Open 3 Percutaneous 4 Percutaneous Endoscopic	2 Monitoring Device 3 Infusion Device D Intraluminal Device	Z No Qualifier

Section 0 **Medical and Surgical**
Body System 6 **Lower Veins**
Operation J **Inspection:** Visually and/or manually exploring a body part

Body Part (4th)	Approach (5th)	Device (6th)	Qualifier (7th)
Y Lower Vein	**0** Open **3** Percutaneous **4** Percutaneous Endoscopic **X** External	**Z** No Device	**Z** No Qualifier

Section 0 **Medical and Surgical**
Body System 6 **Lower Veins**
Operation L **Occlusion:** Completely closing an orifice or the lumen of a tubular body part

Body Part (4th)	Approach (5th)	Device (6th)	Qualifier (7th)
0 Inferior Vena Cava **1** Splenic Vein **2** Gastric Vein **3** Esophageal Vein **4** Hepatic Vein **5** Superior Mesenteric Vein **6** Inferior Mesenteric Vein **7** Colic Vein **8** Portal Vein **9** Renal Vein, Right **B** Renal Vein, Left **C** Common Iliac Vein, Right **D** Common Iliac Vein, Left **F** External Iliac Vein, Right **G** External Iliac Vein, Left **H** Hypogastric Vein, Right **J** Hypogastric Vein, Left **M** Femoral Vein, Right **N** Femoral Vein, Left **P** Greater Saphenous Vein, Right **Q** Greater Saphenous Vein, Left **R** Lesser Saphenous Vein, Right **S** Lesser Saphenous Vein, Left **T** Foot Vein, Right **V** Foot Vein, Left	**0** Open **3** Percutaneous **4** Percutaneous Endoscopic	**C** Extraluminal Device **D** Intraluminal Device **Z** No Device	**Z** No Qualifier
Y Lower Vein	**0** Open **3** Percutaneous **4** Percutaneous Endoscopic	**C** Extraluminal Device **D** Intraluminal Device **Z** No Device	**C** Hemorrhoidal Plexus **Z** No Qualifier

Section	0	Medical and Surgical
Body System	6	Lower Veins
Operation	N	**Release:** Freeing a body part from an abnormal physical constraint by cutting or by the use of force

Body Part (4th)	Approach (5th)	Device (6th)	Qualifier (7th)
0 Inferior Vena Cava **1** Splenic Vein **2** Gastric Vein **3** Esophageal Vein **4** Hepatic Vein **5** Superior Mesenteric Vein **6** Inferior Mesenteric Vein **7** Colic Vein **8** Portal Vein **9** Renal Vein, Right **B** Renal Vein, Left **C** Common Iliac Vein, Right **D** Common Iliac Vein, Left **F** External Iliac Vein, Right **G** External Iliac Vein, Left **H** Hypogastric Vein, Right **J** Hypogastric Vein, Left **M** Femoral Vein, Right **N** Femoral Vein, Left **P** Greater Saphenous Vein, Right **Q** Greater Saphenous Vein, Left **R** Lesser Saphenous Vein, Right **S** Lesser Saphenous Vein, Left **T** Foot Vein, Right **V** Foot Vein, Left **Y** Lower Vein	**0** Open **3** Percutaneous **4** Percutaneous Endoscopic	**Z** No Device	**Z** No Qualifier

Section	0	Medical and Surgical
Body System	6	Lower Veins
Operation	P	**Removal:** Taking out or off a device from a body part

Body Part (4th)	Approach (5th)	Device (6th)	Qualifier (7th)
Y Lower Vein	**0** Open **3** Percutaneous **4** Percutaneous Endoscopic	**0** Drainage Device **2** Monitoring Device **3** Infusion Device **7** Autologous Tissue Substitute **C** Extraluminal Device **D** Intraluminal Device **J** Synthetic Substitute **K** Nonautologous Tissue Substitute	**Z** No Qualifier
Y Lower Vein	**X** External	**0** Drainage Device **2** Monitoring Device **3** Infusion Device **D** Intraluminal Device	**Z** No Qualifier

Section 0 **Medical and Surgical**
Body System 6 **Lower Veins**
Operation Q **Repair:** Restoring, to the extent possible, a body part to its normal anatomic structure and function

Body Part (4th)	Approach (5th)	Device (6th)	Qualifier (7th)
0 Inferior Vena Cava **1** Splenic Vein **2** Gastric Vein **3** Esophageal Vein **4** Hepatic Vein **5** Superior Mesenteric Vein **6** Inferior Mesenteric Vein **7** Colic Vein **8** Portal Vein **9** Renal Vein, Right **B** Renal Vein, Left **C** Common Iliac Vein, Right **D** Common Iliac Vein, Left **F** External Iliac Vein, Right **G** External Iliac Vein, Left **H** Hypogastric Vein, Right **J** Hypogastric Vein, Left **M** Femoral Vein, Right **N** Femoral Vein, Left **P** Greater Saphenous Vein, Right **Q** Greater Saphenous Vein, Left **R** Lesser Saphenous Vein, Right **S** Lesser Saphenous Vein, Left **T** Foot Vein, Right **V** Foot Vein, Left **Y** Lower Vein	**0** Open **3** Percutaneous **4** Percutaneous Endoscopic	**Z** No Device	**Z** No Qualifier

Section 0 **Medical and Surgical**
Body System 6 **Lower Veins**
Operation R **Replacement:** Putting in or on biological or synthetic material that physically takes the place and/or function of all or a portion of a body part

Body Part (4th)	Approach (5th)	Device (6th)	Qualifier (7th)
0 Inferior Vena Cava **1** Splenic Vein **2** Gastric Vein **3** Esophageal Vein **4** Hepatic Vein **5** Superior Mesenteric Vein **6** Inferior Mesenteric Vein **7** Colic Vein **8** Portal Vein **9** Renal Vein, Right **B** Renal Vein, Left **C** Common Iliac Vein, Right **D** Common Iliac Vein, Left **F** External Iliac Vein, Right **G** External Iliac Vein, Left **H** Hypogastric Vein, Right **J** Hypogastric Vein, Left **M** Femoral Vein, Right **N** Femoral Vein, Left **P** Greater Saphenous Vein, Right **Q** Greater Saphenous Vein, Left **R** Lesser Saphenous Vein, Right **S** Lesser Saphenous Vein, Left **T** Foot Vein, Right **V** Foot Vein, Left **Y** Lower Vein	**0** Open **4** Percutaneous Endoscopic	**7** Autologous Tissue Substitute **J** Synthetic Substitute **K** Nonautologous Tissue Substitute	**Z** No Qualifier

Section 0 **Medical and Surgical**
Body System 6 **Lower Veins**
Operation S **Reposition:** Moving to its normal location, or other suitable location, all or a portion of a body part

Body Part (4th)	Approach (5th)	Device (6th)	Qualifier (7th)
0 Inferior Vena Cava **1** Splenic Vein **2** Gastric Vein **3** Esophageal Vein **4** Hepatic Vein **5** Superior Mesenteric Vein **6** Inferior Mesenteric Vein **7** Colic Vein **8** Portal Vein **9** Renal Vein, Right **B** Renal Vein, Left **C** Common Iliac Vein, Right **D** Common Iliac Vein, Left **F** External Iliac Vein, Right **G** External Iliac Vein, Left **H** Hypogastric Vein, Right **J** Hypogastric Vein, Left **M** Femoral Vein, Right **N** Femoral Vein, Left **P** Greater Saphenous Vein, Right **Q** Greater Saphenous Vein, Left **R** Lesser Saphenous Vein, Right **S** Lesser Saphenous Vein, Left **T** Foot Vein, Right **V** Foot Vein, Left **Y** Lower Vein	**0** Open **3** Percutaneous **4** Percutaneous Endoscopic	**Z** No Device	**Z** No Qualifier

Section 0 **Medical and Surgical**
Body System 6 **Lower Veins**
Operation U **Supplement:** Putting in or on biological or synthetic material that physically reinforces and/or augments the function of a portion of a body part

Body Part (4th)	Approach (5th)	Device (6th)	Qualifier (7th)
0 Inferior Vena Cava **1** Splenic Vein **2** Gastric Vein **3** Esophageal Vein **4** Hepatic Vein **5** Superior Mesenteric Vein **6** Inferior Mesenteric Vein **7** Colic Vein **8** Portal Vein **9** Renal Vein, Right **B** Renal Vein, Left **C** Common Iliac Vein, Right **D** Common Iliac Vein, Left **F** External Iliac Vein, Right **G** External Iliac Vein, Left **H** Hypogastric Vein, Right **J** Hypogastric Vein, Left **M** Femoral Vein, Right **N** Femoral Vein, Left **P** Greater Saphenous Vein, Right **Q** Greater Saphenous Vein, Left **R** Lesser Saphenous Vein, Right **S** Lesser Saphenous Vein, Left **T** Foot Vein, Right **V** Foot Vein, Left **Y** Lower Vein	**0** Open **3** Percutaneous **4** Percutaneous Endoscopic	**7** Autologous Tissue Substitute **J** Synthetic Substitute **K** Nonautologous Tissue Substitute	**Z** No Qualifier

Section 0 **Medical and Surgical**
Body System 6 **Lower Veins**
Operation V **Restriction:** Partially closing an orifice or the lumen of a tubular body part

Body Part (4th)	Approach (5th)	Device (6th)	Qualifier (7th)
0 Inferior Vena Cava **1** Splenic Vein **2** Gastric Vein **3** Esophageal Vein **4** Hepatic Vein **5** Superior Mesenteric Vein **6** Inferior Mesenteric Vein **7** Colic Vein **8** Portal Vein **9** Renal Vein, Right **B** Renal Vein, Left **C** Common Iliac Vein, Right **D** Common Iliac Vein, Left **F** External Iliac Vein, Right **G** External Iliac Vein, Left **H** Hypogastric Vein, Right **J** Hypogastric Vein, Left **M** Femoral Vein, Right **N** Femoral Vein, Left **P** Greater Saphenous Vein, Right **Q** Greater Saphenous Vein, Left **R** Lesser Saphenous Vein, Right **S** Lesser Saphenous Vein, Left **T** Foot Vein, Right **V** Foot Vein, Left **Y** Lower Vein	**0** Open **3** Percutaneous **4** Percutaneous Endoscopic	**C** Extraluminal Device **D** Intraluminal Device **Z** No Device	**Z** No Qualifier

Section 0 **Medical and Surgical**
Body System 6 **Lower Veins**
Operation W **Revision:** Correcting, to the extent possible, a portion of a malfunctioning device or the position of a displaced device

Body Part (4th)	Approach (5th)	Device (6th)	Qualifier (7th)
Y Lower Vein	**0** Open **3** Percutaneous **4** Percutaneous Endoscopic **X** External	**0** Drainage Device **2** Monitoring Device **3** Infusion Device **7** Autologous Tissue Substitute **C** Extraluminal Device **D** Intraluminal Device **J** Synthetic Substitute **K** Nonautologous Tissue Substitute	**Z** No Qualifier

Lower Veins Code Listing 061–06W

061 – Lower Veins, Bypass

Review Coding Guideline B3.6a

0610075 Bypass Inferior Vena Cava to Superior Mesenteric Vein with Autologous Tissue Substitute, Open Approach
0610076 Bypass Inferior Vena Cava to Inferior Mesenteric Vein with Autologous Tissue Substitute, Open Approach
061007Y Bypass Inferior Vena Cava to Lower Vein with Autologous Tissue Substitute, Open Approach
0610095 Bypass Inferior Vena Cava to Superior Mesenteric Vein with Autologous Venous Tissue, Open Approach
0610096 Bypass Inferior Vena Cava to Inferior Mesenteric Vein with Autologous Venous Tissue, Open Approach
061009Y Bypass Inferior Vena Cava to Lower Vein with Autologous Venous Tissue, Open Approach
06100A5 Bypass Inferior Vena Cava to Superior Mesenteric Vein with Autologous Arterial Tissue, Open Approach
06100A6 Bypass Inferior Vena Cava to Inferior Mesenteric Vein with Autologous Arterial Tissue, Open Approach
06100AY Bypass Inferior Vena Cava to Lower Vein with Autologous Arterial Tissue, Open Approach
06100J5 Bypass Inferior Vena Cava to Superior Mesenteric Vein with Synthetic Substitute, Open Approach
06100J6 Bypass Inferior Vena Cava to Inferior Mesenteric Vein with Synthetic Substitute, Open Approach
06100JY Bypass Inferior Vena Cava to Lower Vein with Synthetic Substitute, Open Approach
06100K5 Bypass Inferior Vena Cava to Superior Mesenteric Vein with Nonautologous Tissue Substitute, Open Approach
06100K6 Bypass Inferior Vena Cava to Inferior Mesenteric Vein with Nonautologous Tissue Substitute, Open Approach
06100KY Bypass Inferior Vena Cava to Lower Vein with Nonautologous Tissue Substitute, Open Approach
06100Z5 Bypass Inferior Vena Cava to Superior Mesenteric Vein, Open Approach
06100Z6 Bypass Inferior Vena Cava to Inferior Mesenteric Vein, Open Approach
06100ZY Bypass Inferior Vena Cava to Lower Vein, Open Approach
0610475 Bypass Inferior Vena Cava to Superior Mesenteric Vein with Autologous Tissue

Substitute, Percutaneous Endoscopic Approach

10476 Bypass Inferior Vena Cava to Inferior Mesenteric Vein with Autologous Tissue Substitute, Percutaneous Endoscopic Approach

1047Y Bypass Inferior Vena Cava to Lower Vein with Autologous Tissue Substitute, Percutaneous Endoscopic Approach

10495 Bypass Inferior Vena Cava to Superior Mesenteric Vein with Autologous Venous Tissue, Percutaneous Endoscopic Approach

10496 Bypass Inferior Vena Cava to Inferior Mesenteric Vein with Autologous Venous Tissue, Percutaneous Endoscopic Approach

1049Y Bypass Inferior Vena Cava to Lower Vein with Autologous Venous Tissue, Percutaneous Endoscopic Approach

104A5 Bypass Inferior Vena Cava to Superior Mesenteric Vein with Autologous Arterial Tissue, Percutaneous Endoscopic Approach

104A6 Bypass Inferior Vena Cava to Inferior Mesenteric Vein with Autologous Arterial Tissue, Percutaneous Endoscopic Approach

5104AY Bypass Inferior Vena Cava to Lower Vein with Autologous Arterial Tissue, Percutaneous Endoscopic Approach

5104J5 Bypass Inferior Vena Cava to Superior Mesenteric Vein with Synthetic Substitute, Percutaneous Endoscopic Approach

5104J6 Bypass Inferior Vena Cava to Inferior Mesenteric Vein with Synthetic Substitute, Percutaneous Endoscopic Approach

6104JY Bypass Inferior Vena Cava to Lower Vein with Synthetic Substitute, Percutaneous Endoscopic Approach

6104K5 Bypass Inferior Vena Cava to Superior Mesenteric Vein with Nonautologous Tissue Substitute, Percutaneous Endoscopic Approach

6104K6 Bypass Inferior Vena Cava to Inferior Mesenteric Vein with Nonautologous Tissue Substitute, Percutaneous Endoscopic Approach

6104KY Bypass Inferior Vena Cava to Lower Vein with Nonautologous Tissue Substitute, Percutaneous Endoscopic Approach

6104Z5 Bypass Inferior Vena Cava to Superior Mesenteric Vein, Percutaneous Endoscopic Approach

6104Z6 Bypass Inferior Vena Cava to Inferior Mesenteric Vein, Percutaneous Endoscopic Approach

6104ZY Bypass Inferior Vena Cava to Lower Vein, Percutaneous Endoscopic Approach

611079 Bypass Splenic Vein to Right Renal Vein with Autologous Tissue Substitute, Open Approach

61107B Bypass Splenic Vein to Left Renal Vein with Autologous Tissue Substitute, Open Approach

61107Y Bypass Splenic Vein to Lower Vein with Autologous Tissue Substitute, Open Approach

611099 Bypass Splenic Vein to Right Renal Vein with Autologous Venous Tissue, Open Approach

61109B Bypass Splenic Vein to Left Renal Vein with Autologous Venous Tissue, Open Approach

61109Y Bypass Splenic Vein to Lower Vein with Autologous Venous Tissue, Open Approach

06110A9 Bypass Splenic Vein to Right Renal Vein with Autologous Arterial Tissue, Open Approach

06110AB Bypass Splenic Vein to Left Renal Vein with Autologous Arterial Tissue, Open Approach

06110AY Bypass Splenic Vein to Lower Vein with Autologous Arterial Tissue, Open Approach

06110J9 Bypass Splenic Vein to Right Renal Vein with Synthetic Substitute, Open Approach

06110JB Bypass Splenic Vein to Left Renal Vein with Synthetic Substitute, Open Approach

06110JY Bypass Splenic Vein to Lower Vein with Synthetic Substitute, Open Approach

06110K9 Bypass Splenic Vein to Right Renal Vein with Nonautologous Tissue Substitute, Open Approach

06110KB Bypass Splenic Vein to Left Renal Vein with Nonautologous Tissue Substitute, Open Approach

06110KY Bypass Splenic Vein to Lower Vein with Nonautologous Tissue Substitute, Open Approach

06110Z9 Bypass Splenic Vein to Right Renal Vein, Open Approach

06110ZB Bypass Splenic Vein to Left Renal Vein, Open Approach

06110ZY Bypass Splenic Vein to Lower Vein, Open Approach

0611479 Bypass Splenic Vein to Right Renal Vein with Autologous Tissue Substitute, Percutaneous Endoscopic Approach

061147B Bypass Splenic Vein to Left Renal Vein with Autologous Tissue Substitute, Percutaneous Endoscopic Approach

061147Y Bypass Splenic Vein to Lower Vein with Autologous Tissue Substitute, Percutaneous Endoscopic Approach

0611499 Bypass Splenic Vein to Right Renal Vein with Autologous Venous Tissue, Percutaneous Endoscopic Approach

061149B Bypass Splenic Vein to Left Renal Vein with Autologous Venous Tissue, Percutaneous Endoscopic Approach

061149Y Bypass Splenic Vein to Lower Vein with Autologous Venous Tissue, Percutaneous Endoscopic Approach

06114A9 Bypass Splenic Vein to Right Renal Vein with Autologous Arterial Tissue, Percutaneous Endoscopic Approach

06114AB Bypass Splenic Vein to Left Renal Vein with Autologous Arterial Tissue, Percutaneous Endoscopic Approach

06114AY Bypass Splenic Vein to Lower Vein with Autologous Arterial Tissue, Percutaneous Endoscopic Approach

06114J9 Bypass Splenic Vein to Right Renal Vein with Synthetic Substitute, Percutaneous Endoscopic Approach

06114JB Bypass Splenic Vein to Left Renal Vein with Synthetic Substitute, Percutaneous Endoscopic Approach

06114JY Bypass Splenic Vein to Lower Vein with Synthetic Substitute, Percutaneous Endoscopic Approach

06114K9 Bypass Splenic Vein to Right Renal Vein with Nonautologous Tissue Substitute, Percutaneous Endoscopic Approach

06114KB Bypass Splenic Vein to Left Renal Vein with Nonautologous Tissue Substitute, Percutaneous Endoscopic Approach

06114KY Bypass Splenic Vein to Lower Vein with Nonautologous Tissue Substitute, Percutaneous Endoscopic Approach

06114Z9 Bypass Splenic Vein to Right Renal Vein, Percutaneous Endoscopic Approach

06114ZB Bypass Splenic Vein to Left Renal Vein, Percutaneous Endoscopic Approach

06114ZY Bypass Splenic Vein to Lower Vein, Percutaneous Endoscopic Approach

061207Y Bypass Gastric Vein to Lower Vein with Autologous Tissue Substitute, Open Approach

061209Y Bypass Gastric Vein to Lower Vein with Autologous Venous Tissue, Open Approach

06120AY Bypass Gastric Vein to Lower Vein with Autologous Arterial Tissue, Open Approach

06120JY Bypass Gastric Vein to Lower Vein with Synthetic Substitute, Open Approach

06120KY Bypass Gastric Vein to Lower Vein with Nonautologous Tissue Substitute, Open Approach

06120ZY Bypass Gastric Vein to Lower Vein, Open Approach

061247Y Bypass Gastric Vein to Lower Vein with Autologous Tissue Substitute, Percutaneous Endoscopic Approach

061249Y Bypass Gastric Vein to Lower Vein with Autologous Venous Tissue, Percutaneous Endoscopic Approach

06124AY Bypass Gastric Vein to Lower Vein with Autologous Arterial Tissue, Percutaneous Endoscopic Approach

06124JY Bypass Gastric Vein to Lower Vein with Synthetic Substitute, Percutaneous Endoscopic Approach

06124KY Bypass Gastric Vein to Lower Vein with Nonautologous Tissue Substitute, Percutaneous Endoscopic Approach

06124ZY Bypass Gastric Vein to Lower Vein, Percutaneous Endoscopic Approach

061307Y Bypass Esophageal Vein to Lower Vein with Autologous Tissue Substitute, Open Approach

061309Y Bypass Esophageal Vein to Lower Vein with Autologous Venous Tissue, Open Approach

06130AY Bypass Esophageal Vein to Lower Vein with Autologous Arterial Tissue, Open Approach

06130JY Bypass Esophageal Vein to Lower Vein with Synthetic Substitute, Open Approach

06130KY Bypass Esophageal Vein to Lower Vein with Nonautologous Tissue Substitute, Open Approach

06130ZY Bypass Esophageal Vein to Lower Vein, Open Approach

061347Y Bypass Esophageal Vein to Lower Vein with Autologous Tissue Substitute, Percutaneous Endoscopic Approach

061349Y Bypass Esophageal Vein to Lower Vein with Autologous Venous Tissue, Percutaneous Endoscopic Approach

06134AY Bypass Esophageal Vein to Lower Vein with Autologous Arterial Tissue, Percutaneous Endoscopic Approach

06134JY Bypass Esophageal Vein to Lower Vein with Synthetic Substitute, Percutaneous Endoscopic Approach

06134KY Bypass Esophageal Vein to Lower Vein with Nonautologous Tissue Substitute, Percutaneous Endoscopic Approach

06134ZY Bypass Esophageal Vein to Lower Vein, Percutaneous Endoscopic Approach

061407Y Bypass Hepatic Vein to Lower Vein with Autologous Tissue Substitute, Open Approach

061409Y Bypass Hepatic Vein to Lower Vein with Autologous Venous Tissue, Open Approach

06140AY Bypass Hepatic Vein to Lower Vein with Autologous Arterial Tissue, Open Approach

06140JY Bypass Hepatic Vein to Lower Vein with Synthetic Substitute, Open Approach

06140KY Bypass Hepatic Vein to Lower Vein with Nonautologous Tissue Substitute, Open Approach

06140ZY Bypass Hepatic Vein to Lower Vein, Open Approach

061447Y Bypass Hepatic Vein to Lower Vein with Autologous Tissue Substitute, Percutaneous Endoscopic Approach

061449Y Bypass Hepatic Vein to Lower Vein with Autologous Venous Tissue, Percutaneous Endoscopic Approach

06144AY Bypass Hepatic Vein to Lower Vein with Autologous Arterial Tissue, Percutaneous Endoscopic Approach

06144JY Bypass Hepatic Vein to Lower Vein with Synthetic Substitute, Percutaneous Endoscopic Approach

06144KY Bypass Hepatic Vein to Lower Vein with Nonautologous Tissue Substitute, Percutaneous Endoscopic Approach

06144ZY Bypass Hepatic Vein to Lower Vein, Percutaneous Endoscopic Approach

061507Y Bypass Superior Mesenteric Vein to Lower Vein with Autologous Tissue Substitute, Open Approach

061509Y Bypass Superior Mesenteric Vein to Lower Vein with Autologous Venous Tissue, Open Approach

06150AY Bypass Superior Mesenteric Vein to Lower Vein with Autologous Arterial Tissue, Open Approach

06150JY Bypass Superior Mesenteric Vein to Lower Vein with Synthetic Substitute, Open Approach

06150KY Bypass Superior Mesenteric Vein to Lower Vein with Nonautologous Tissue Substitute, Open Approach

06150ZY Bypass Superior Mesenteric Vein to Lower Vein, Open Approach

061547Y Bypass Superior Mesenteric Vein to Lower Vein with Autologous Tissue Substitute, Percutaneous Endoscopic Approach

061549Y Bypass Superior Mesenteric Vein to Lower Vein with Autologous Venous Tissue, Percutaneous Endoscopic Approach

06154AY Bypass Superior Mesenteric Vein to Lower Vein with Autologous Arterial Tissue, Percutaneous Endoscopic Approach

06154JY Bypass Superior Mesenteric Vein to Lower Vein with Synthetic Substitute, Percutaneous Endoscopic Approach

06154KY Bypass Superior Mesenteric Vein to Lower Vein with Nonautologous Tissue Substitute, Percutaneous Endoscopic Approach

06154ZY Bypass Superior Mesenteric Vein to Lower Vein, Percutaneous Endoscopic Approach

061607Y Bypass Inferior Mesenteric Vein to Lower Vein with Autologous Tissue Substitute, Open Approach

061609Y Bypass Inferior Mesenteric Vein to Lower Vein with Autologous Venous Tissue, Open Approach

06160AY Bypass Inferior Mesenteric Vein to Lower Vein with Autologous Arterial Tissue, Open Approach

06160JY Bypass Inferior Mesenteric Vein to Lower Vein with Synthetic Substitute, Open Approach

06160KY Bypass Inferior Mesenteric Vein to Lower Vein with Nonautologous Tissue Substitute, Open Approach

06160ZY Bypass Inferior Mesenteric Vein to Lower Vein, Open Approach

061647Y Bypass Inferior Mesenteric Vein to Lower Vein with Autologous Tissue Substitute, Percutaneous Endoscopic Approach

061649Y Bypass Inferior Mesenteric Vein to Lower Vein with Autologous Venous Tissue, Percutaneous Endoscopic Approach

06164AY Bypass Inferior Mesenteric Vein to Lower Vein with Autologous Arterial Tissue, Percutaneous Endoscopic Approach

06164JY Bypass Inferior Mesenteric Vein to Lower Vein with Synthetic Substitute, Percutaneous Endoscopic Approach

06164KY Bypass Inferior Mesenteric Vein to Lower Vein with Nonautologous Tissue Substitute, Percutaneous Endoscopic Approach

06164ZY Bypass Inferior Mesenteric Vein to Lower Vein, Percutaneous Endoscopic Approach

061707Y Bypass Colic Vein to Lower Vein with Autologous Tissue Substitute, Open Approach

061709Y Bypass Colic Vein to Lower Vein with Autologous Venous Tissue, Open Approach

06170AY Bypass Colic Vein to Lower Vein with Autologous Arterial Tissue, Open Approach

06170JY Bypass Colic Vein to Lower Vein with Synthetic Substitute, Open Approach

06170KY Bypass Colic Vein to Lower Vein with Nonautologous Tissue Substitute, Open Approach

06170ZY Bypass Colic Vein to Lower Vein, Open Approach

061747Y Bypass Colic Vein to Lower Vein with Autologous Tissue Substitute, Percutaneous Endoscopic Approach

061749Y Bypass Colic Vein to Lower Vein with Autologous Venous Tissue, Percutaneous Endoscopic Approach

06174AY Bypass Colic Vein to Lower Vein with Autologous Arterial Tissue, Percutaneous Endoscopic Approach

06174JY Bypass Colic Vein to Lower Vein with Synthetic Substitute, Percutaneous Endoscopic Approach

06174KY Bypass Colic Vein to Lower Vein with Nonautologous Tissue Substitute, Percutaneous Endoscopic Approach

06174ZY Bypass Colic Vein to Lower Vein, Percutaneous Endoscopic Approach

0618079 Bypass Portal Vein to Right Renal Vein with Autologous Tissue Substitute, Open Approach

061807B Bypass Portal Vein to Left Renal Vein with Autologous Tissue Substitute, Open Approach

061807Y Bypass Portal Vein to Lower Vein with Autologous Tissue Substitute, Open Approach

0618099 Bypass Portal Vein to Right Renal Vein with Autologous Venous Tissue, Open Approach

061809B Bypass Portal Vein to Left Renal Vein with Autologous Venous Tissue, Open Approach

061809Y Bypass Portal Vein to Lower Vein with Autologous Venous Tissue, Open Approach

06180A9 Bypass Portal Vein to Right Renal Vein with Autologous Arterial Tissue, Open Approach

06180AB Bypass Portal Vein to Left Renal Vein with Autologous Arterial Tissue, Open Approach

06180AY Bypass Portal Vein to Lower Vein with Autologous Arterial Tissue, Open Approach

06180J9 Bypass Portal Vein to Right Renal Vein with Synthetic Substitute, Open Approac

06180JB Bypass Portal Vein to Left Renal Vein wi Synthetic Substitute, Open Approach

06180JY Bypass Portal Vein to Lower Vein with Synthetic Substitute, Open Approac

06180K9 Bypass Portal Vein to Right Renal Vein with Nonautologous Tissue Substitute, Open Approach

06180KB Bypass Portal Vein to Left Renal Vein wi Nonautologous Tissue Substitute, Open Approach

06180KY Bypass Portal Vein to Lower Vein with Nonautologous Tissue Substitute, Open Approach

06180Z9 Bypass Portal Vein to Right Renal Vein, Open Approach

06180ZB Bypass Portal Vein to Left Renal Vein, Open Approach

06180ZY Bypass Portal Vein to Lower Vein, Open Approach

06183DY Bypass Portal Vein to Lower Vein with Intraluminal Device, Percutaneous Approach

0618479 Bypass Portal Vein to Right Renal Vein with Autologous Tissue Substitute, Percutaneous Endoscopic Approach

061847B Bypass Portal Vein to Left Renal Vein with Autologous Tissue Substitute, Percutaneous Endoscopic Approach

061847Y Bypass Portal Vein to Lower Vein with Autologous Tissue Substitute, Percutaneous Endoscopic Approach

0618499 Bypass Portal Vein to Right Renal Vein with Autologous Venous Tissue, Percutaneous Endoscopic Approach

061849B Bypass Portal Vein to Left Renal Vein wit Autologous Venous Tissue, Percutaneous Endoscopic Approach

061849Y Bypass Portal Vein to Lower Vein with Autologous Venous Tissue, Percutaneous Endoscopic Approach

06184A9 Bypass Portal Vein to Right Renal Vein with Autologous Arterial Tissue, Percutaneous Endoscopic Approach

06184AB Bypass Portal Vein to Left Renal Vein wit Autologous Arterial Tissue, Percutaneous Endoscopic Approach

06184AY Bypass Portal Vein to Lower Vein with Autologous Arterial Tissue, Percutaneous Endoscopic Approach

06184DY Bypass Portal Vein to Lower Vein with Intraluminal Device, Percutaneous Endoscopic Approach

06184J9 Bypass Portal Vein to Right Renal Vein with Synthetic Substitute, Percutaneous Endoscopic Approach

06184JB Bypass Portal Vein to Left Renal Vein with Synthetic Substitute, Percutaneous Endoscopic Approach

06184JY Bypass Portal Vein to Lower Vein with Synthetic Substitute, Percutaneous Endoscopic Approach

06184K9 Bypass Portal Vein to Right Renal Vein with Nonautologous Tissue Substitute, Percutaneous Endoscopic Approach

06184KB Bypass Portal Vein to Left Renal Vein with Nonautologous Tissue Substitute, Percutaneous Endoscopic Approach

184KY Bypass Portal Vein to Lower Vein with Nonautologous Tissue Substitute, Percutaneous Endoscopic Approach
184Z9 Bypass Portal Vein to Right Renal Vein, Percutaneous Endoscopic Approach
184ZB Bypass Portal Vein to Left Renal Vein, Percutaneous Endoscopic Approach
184ZY Bypass Portal Vein to Lower Vein, Percutaneous Endoscopic Approach
1907Y Bypass Right Renal Vein to Lower Vein with Autologous Tissue Substitute, Open Approach
1909Y Bypass Right Renal Vein to Lower Vein with Autologous Venous Tissue, Open Approach
190AY Bypass Right Renal Vein to Lower Vein with Autologous Arterial Tissue, Open Approach
190JY Bypass Right Renal Vein to Lower Vein with Synthetic Substitute, Open Approach
190KY Bypass Right Renal Vein to Lower Vein with Nonautologous Tissue Substitute, Open Approach
190ZY Bypass Right Renal Vein to Lower Vein, Open Approach
1947Y Bypass Right Renal Vein to Lower Vein with Autologous Tissue Substitute, Percutaneous Endoscopic Approach
1949Y Bypass Right Renal Vein to Lower Vein with Autologous Venous Tissue, Percutaneous Endoscopic Approach
194AY Bypass Right Renal Vein to Lower Vein with Autologous Arterial Tissue, Percutaneous Endoscopic Approach
194JY Bypass Right Renal Vein to Lower Vein with Synthetic Substitute, Percutaneous Endoscopic Approach
194KY Bypass Right Renal Vein to Lower Vein with Nonautologous Tissue Substitute, Percutaneous Endoscopic Approach
194ZY Bypass Right Renal Vein to Lower Vein, Percutaneous Endoscopic Approach
1B07Y Bypass Left Renal Vein to Lower Vein with Autologous Tissue Substitute, Open Approach
1B09Y Bypass Left Renal Vein to Lower Vein with Autologous Venous Tissue, Open Approach
1B0AY Bypass Left Renal Vein to Lower Vein with Autologous Arterial Tissue, Open Approach
1B0JY Bypass Left Renal Vein to Lower Vein with Synthetic Substitute, Open Approach
1B0KY Bypass Left Renal Vein to Lower Vein with Nonautologous Tissue Substitute, Open Approach
61B0ZY Bypass Left Renal Vein to Lower Vein, Open Approach
61B47Y Bypass Left Renal Vein to Lower Vein with Autologous Tissue Substitute, Percutaneous Endoscopic Approach
61B49Y Bypass Left Renal Vein to Lower Vein with Autologous Venous Tissue, Percutaneous Endoscopic Approach
61B4AY Bypass Left Renal Vein to Lower Vein with Autologous Arterial Tissue, Percutaneous Endoscopic Approach
61B4JY Bypass Left Renal Vein to Lower Vein with Synthetic Substitute, Percutaneous Endoscopic Approach
61B4KY Bypass Left Renal Vein to Lower Vein with Nonautologous Tissue Substitute, Percutaneous Endoscopic Approach
61B4ZY Bypass Left Renal Vein to Lower Vein, Percutaneous Endoscopic Approach

061C07Y Bypass Right Common Iliac Vein to Lower Vein with Autologous Tissue Substitute, Open Approach
061C09Y Bypass Right Common Iliac Vein to Lower Vein with Autologous Venous Tissue, Open Approach
061C0AY Bypass Right Common Iliac Vein to Lower Vein with Autologous Arterial Tissue, Open Approach
061C0JY Bypass Right Common Iliac Vein to Lower Vein with Synthetic Substitute, Open Approach
061C0KY Bypass Right Common Iliac Vein to Lower Vein with Nonautologous Tissue Substitute, Open Approach
061C0ZY Bypass Right Common Iliac Vein to Lower Vein, Open Approach
061C47Y Bypass Right Common Iliac Vein to Lower Vein with Autologous Tissue Substitute, Percutaneous Endoscopic Approach
061C49Y Bypass Right Common Iliac Vein to Lower Vein with Autologous Venous Tissue, Percutaneous Endoscopic Approach
061C4AY Bypass Right Common Iliac Vein to Lower Vein with Autologous Arterial Tissue, Percutaneous Endoscopic Approach
061C4JY Bypass Right Common Iliac Vein to Lower Vein with Synthetic Substitute, Percutaneous Endoscopic Approach
061C4KY Bypass Right Common Iliac Vein to Lower Vein with Nonautologous Tissue Substitute, Percutaneous Endoscopic Approach
061C4ZY Bypass Right Common Iliac Vein to Lower Vein, Percutaneous Endoscopic Approach
061D07Y Bypass Left Common Iliac Vein to Lower Vein with Autologous Tissue Substitute, Open Approach
061D09Y Bypass Left Common Iliac Vein to Lower Vein with Autologous Venous Tissue, Open Approach
061D0AY Bypass Left Common Iliac Vein to Lower Vein with Autologous Arterial Tissue, Open Approach
061D0JY Bypass Left Common Iliac Vein to Lower Vein with Synthetic Substitute, Open Approach
061D0KY Bypass Left Common Iliac Vein to Lower Vein with Nonautologous Tissue Substitute, Open Approach
061D0ZY Bypass Left Common Iliac Vein to Lower Vein, Open Approach
061D47Y Bypass Left Common Iliac Vein to Lower Vein with Autologous Tissue Substitute, Percutaneous Endoscopic Approach
061D49Y Bypass Left Common Iliac Vein to Lower Vein with Autologous Venous Tissue, Percutaneous Endoscopic Approach
061D4AY Bypass Left Common Iliac Vein to Lower Vein with Autologous Arterial Tissue, Percutaneous Endoscopic Approach
061D4JY Bypass Left Common Iliac Vein to Lower Vein with Synthetic Substitute, Percutaneous Endoscopic Approach
061D4KY Bypass Left Common Iliac Vein to Lower Vein with Nonautologous Tissue Substitute, Percutaneous Endoscopic Approach
061D4ZY Bypass Left Common Iliac Vein to Lower Vein, Percutaneous Endoscopic Approach
061F07Y Bypass Right External Iliac Vein to Lower Vein with Autologous Tissue Substitute, Open Approach
061F09Y Bypass Right External Iliac Vein to Lower Vein with Autologous Venous Tissue, Open Approach

061F0AY Bypass Right External Iliac Vein to Lower Vein with Autologous Arterial Tissue, Open Approach
061F0JY Bypass Right External Iliac Vein to Lower Vein with Synthetic Substitute, Open Approach
061F0KY Bypass Right External Iliac Vein to Lower Vein with Nonautologous Tissue Substitute, Open Approach
061F0ZY Bypass Right External Iliac Vein to Lower Vein, Open Approach
061F47Y Bypass Right External Iliac Vein to Lower Vein with Autologous Tissue Substitute, Percutaneous Endoscopic Approach
061F49Y Bypass Right External Iliac Vein to Lower Vein with Autologous Venous Tissue, Percutaneous Endoscopic Approach
061F4AY Bypass Right External Iliac Vein to Lower Vein with Autologous Arterial Tissue, Percutaneous Endoscopic Approach
061F4JY Bypass Right External Iliac Vein to Lower Vein with Synthetic Substitute, Percutaneous Endoscopic Approach
061F4KY Bypass Right External Iliac Vein to Lower Vein with Nonautologous Tissue Substitute, Percutaneous Endoscopic Approach
061F4ZY Bypass Right External Iliac Vein to Lower Vein, Percutaneous Endoscopic Approach
061G07Y Bypass Left External Iliac Vein to Lower Vein with Autologous Tissue Substitute, Open Approach
061G09Y Bypass Left External Iliac Vein to Lower Vein with Autologous Venous Tissue, Open Approach
061G0AY Bypass Left External Iliac Vein to Lower Vein with Autologous Arterial Tissue, Open Approach
061G0JY Bypass Left External Iliac Vein to Lower Vein with Synthetic Substitute, Open Approach
061G0KY Bypass Left External Iliac Vein to Lower Vein with Nonautologous Tissue Substitute, Open Approach
061G0ZY Bypass Left External Iliac Vein to Lower Vein, Open Approach
061G47Y Bypass Left External Iliac Vein to Lower Vein with Autologous Tissue Substitute, Percutaneous Endoscopic Approach
061G49Y Bypass Left External Iliac Vein to Lower Vein with Autologous Venous Tissue, Percutaneous Endoscopic Approach
061G4AY Bypass Left External Iliac Vein to Lower Vein with Autologous Arterial Tissue, Percutaneous Endoscopic Approach
061G4JY Bypass Left External Iliac Vein to Lower Vein with Synthetic Substitute, Percutaneous Endoscopic Approach
061G4KY Bypass Left External Iliac Vein to Lower Vein with Nonautologous Tissue Substitute, Percutaneous Endoscopic Approach
061G4ZY Bypass Left External Iliac Vein to Lower Vein, Percutaneous Endoscopic Approach
061H07Y Bypass Right Hypogastric Vein to Lower Vein with Autologous Tissue Substitute, Open Approach
061H09Y Bypass Right Hypogastric Vein to Lower Vein with Autologous Venous Tissue, Open Approach
061H0AY Bypass Right Hypogastric Vein to Lower Vein with Autologous Arterial Tissue, Open Approach
061H0JY Bypass Right Hypogastric Vein to Lower Vein with Synthetic Substitute, Open Approach

061H0KY Bypass Right Hypogastric Vein to Lower Vein with Nonautologous Tissue Substitute, Open Approach
061H0ZY Bypass Right Hypogastric Vein to Lower Vein, Open Approach
061H47Y Bypass Right Hypogastric Vein to Lower Vein with Autologous Tissue Substitute, Percutaneous Endoscopic Approach
061H49Y Bypass Right Hypogastric Vein to Lower Vein with Autologous Venous Tissue, Percutaneous Endoscopic Approach
061H4AY Bypass Right Hypogastric Vein to Lower Vein with Autologous Arterial Tissue, Percutaneous Endoscopic Approach
061H4JY Bypass Right Hypogastric Vein to Lower Vein with Synthetic Substitute, Percutaneous Endoscopic Approach
061H4KY Bypass Right Hypogastric Vein to Lower Vein with Nonautologous Tissue Substitute, Percutaneous Endoscopic Approach
061H4ZY Bypass Right Hypogastric Vein to Lower Vein, Percutaneous Endoscopic Approach
061J07Y Bypass Left Hypogastric Vein to Lower Vein with Autologous Tissue Substitute, Open Approach
061J09Y Bypass Left Hypogastric Vein to Lower Vein with Autologous Venous Tissue, Open Approach
061J0AY Bypass Left Hypogastric Vein to Lower Vein with Autologous Arterial Tissue, Open Approach
061J0JY Bypass Left Hypogastric Vein to Lower Vein with Synthetic Substitute, Open Approach
061J0KY Bypass Left Hypogastric Vein to Lower Vein with Nonautologous Tissue Substitute, Open Approach
061J0ZY Bypass Left Hypogastric Vein to Lower Vein, Open Approach
061J47Y Bypass Left Hypogastric Vein to Lower Vein with Autologous Tissue Substitute, Percutaneous Endoscopic Approach
061J49Y Bypass Left Hypogastric Vein to Lower Vein with Autologous Venous Tissue, Percutaneous Endoscopic Approach
061J4AY Bypass Left Hypogastric Vein to Lower Vein with Autologous Arterial Tissue, Percutaneous Endoscopic Approach
061J4JY Bypass Left Hypogastric Vein to Lower Vein with Synthetic Substitute, Percutaneous Endoscopic Approach
061J4KY Bypass Left Hypogastric Vein to Lower Vein with Nonautologous Tissue Substitute, Percutaneous Endoscopic Approach
061J4ZY Bypass Left Hypogastric Vein to Lower Vein, Percutaneous Endoscopic Approach
061M07Y Bypass Right Femoral Vein to Lower Vein with Autologous Tissue Substitute, Open Approach
061M09Y Bypass Right Femoral Vein to Lower Vein with Autologous Venous Tissue, Open Approach
061M0AY Bypass Right Femoral Vein to Lower Vein with Autologous Arterial Tissue, Open Approach
061M0JY Bypass Right Femoral Vein to Lower Vein with Synthetic Substitute, Open Approach
061M0KY Bypass Right Femoral Vein to Lower Vein with Nonautologous Tissue Substitute, Open Approach
061M0ZY Bypass Right Femoral Vein to Lower Vein, Open Approach
061M47Y Bypass Right Femoral Vein to Lower Vein with Autologous Tissue Substitute, Percutaneous Endoscopic Approach
061M49Y Bypass Right Femoral Vein to Lower Vein with Autologous Venous Tissue, Percutaneous Endoscopic Approach
061M4AY Bypass Right Femoral Vein to Lower Vein with Autologous Arterial Tissue, Percutaneous Endoscopic Approach
061M4JY Bypass Right Femoral Vein to Lower Vein with Synthetic Substitute, Percutaneous Endoscopic Approach
061M4KY Bypass Right Femoral Vein to Lower Vein with Nonautologous Tissue Substitute, Percutaneous Endoscopic Approach
061M4ZY Bypass Right Femoral Vein to Lower Vein, Percutaneous Endoscopic Approach
061N07Y Bypass Left Femoral Vein to Lower Vein with Autologous Tissue Substitute, Open Approach
061N09Y Bypass Left Femoral Vein to Lower Vein with Autologous Venous Tissue, Open Approach
061N0AY Bypass Left Femoral Vein to Lower Vein with Autologous Arterial Tissue, Open Approach
061N0JY Bypass Left Femoral Vein to Lower Vein with Synthetic Substitute, Open Approach
061N0KY Bypass Left Femoral Vein to Lower Vein with Nonautologous Tissue Substitute, Open Approach
061N0ZY Bypass Left Femoral Vein to Lower Vein, Open Approach
061N47Y Bypass Left Femoral Vein to Lower Vein with Autologous Tissue Substitute, Percutaneous Endoscopic Approach
061N49Y Bypass Left Femoral Vein to Lower Vein with Autologous Venous Tissue, Percutaneous Endoscopic Approach
061N4AY Bypass Left Femoral Vein to Lower Vein with Autologous Arterial Tissue, Percutaneous Endoscopic Approach
061N4JY Bypass Left Femoral Vein to Lower Vein with Synthetic Substitute, Percutaneous Endoscopic Approach
061N4KY Bypass Left Femoral Vein to Lower Vein with Nonautologous Tissue Substitute, Percutaneous Endoscopic Approach
061N4ZY Bypass Left Femoral Vein to Lower Vein, Percutaneous Endoscopic Approach
061P07Y Bypass Right Greater Saphenous Vein to Lower Vein with Autologous Tissue Substitute, Open Approach
061P09Y Bypass Right Greater Saphenous Vein to Lower Vein with Autologous Venous Tissue, Open Approach
061P0AY Bypass Right Greater Saphenous Vein to Lower Vein with Autologous Arterial Tissue, Open Approach
061P0JY Bypass Right Greater Saphenous Vein to Lower Vein with Synthetic Substitute, Open Approach
061P0KY Bypass Right Greater Saphenous Vein to Lower Vein with Nonautologous Tissue Substitute, Open Approach
061P0ZY Bypass Right Greater Saphenous Vein to Lower Vein, Open Approach
061P47Y Bypass Right Greater Saphenous Vein to Lower Vein with Autologous Tissue Substitute, Percutaneous Endoscopic Approach
061P49Y Bypass Right Greater Saphenous Vein to Lower Vein with Autologous Venous Tissue, Percutaneous Endoscopic Approach
061P4AY Bypass Right Greater Saphenous Vein to Lower Vein with Autologous Arterial Tissue, Percutaneous Endoscopic Approach
061P4JY Bypass Right Greater Saphenous Vein to Lower Vein with Synthetic Substitute, Percutaneous Endoscopic Approach
061P4KY Bypass Right Greater Saphenous Vein to Lower Vein with Nonautologous Tissue Substitute, Percutaneous Endoscopic Approach
061P4ZY Bypass Right Greater Saphenous Vein to Lower Vein, Percutaneous Endoscopic Approach
061Q07Y Bypass Left Greater Saphenous Vein to Lower Vein with Autologous Tissue Substitute, Open Approach
061Q09Y Bypass Left Greater Saphenous Vein to Lower Vein with Autologous Venous Tissue, Open Approach
061Q0AY Bypass Left Greater Saphenous Vein to Lower Vein with Autologous Arterial Tissue, Open Approach
061Q0JY Bypass Left Greater Saphenous Vein to Lower Vein with Synthetic Substitute, Open Approach
061Q0KY Bypass Left Greater Saphenous Vein to Lower Vein with Nonautologous Tissue Substitute, Open Approach
061Q0ZY Bypass Left Greater Saphenous Vein to Lower Vein, Open Approach
061Q47Y Bypass Left Greater Saphenous Vein to Lower Vein with Autologous Tissue Substitute, Percutaneous Endoscopic Approach
061Q49Y Bypass Left Greater Saphenous Vein to Lower Vein with Autologous Venous Tissue, Percutaneous Endoscopic Approach
061Q4AY Bypass Left Greater Saphenous Vein to Lower Vein with Autologous Arterial Tissue, Percutaneous Endoscopic Approach
061Q4JY Bypass Left Greater Saphenous Vein to Lower Vein with Synthetic Substitute, Percutaneous Endoscopic Approach
061Q4KY Bypass Left Greater Saphenous Vein to Lower Vein with Nonautologous Tissue Substitute, Percutaneous Endoscopic Approach
061Q4ZY Bypass Left Greater Saphenous Vein to Lower Vein, Percutaneous Endoscopic Approach
061R07Y Bypass Right Lesser Saphenous Vein to Lower Vein with Autologous Tissue Substitute, Open Approach
061R09Y Bypass Right Lesser Saphenous Vein to Lower Vein with Autologous Venous Tissue, Open Approach
061R0AY Bypass Right Lesser Saphenous Vein to Lower Vein with Autologous Arterial Tissue, Open Approach
061R0JY Bypass Right Lesser Saphenous Vein to Lower Vein with Synthetic Substitute, Open Approach
061R0KY Bypass Right Lesser Saphenous Vein to Lower Vein with Nonautologous Tissue Substitute, Open Approach
061R0ZY Bypass Right Lesser Saphenous Vein to Lower Vein, Open Approach
061R47Y Bypass Right Lesser Saphenous Vein to Lower Vein with Autologous Tissue Substitute, Percutaneous Endoscopic Approach
061R49Y Bypass Right Lesser Saphenous Vein to Lower Vein with Autologous Venous Tissue, Percutaneous Endoscopic Approach
061R4AY Bypass Right Lesser Saphenous Vein to Lower Vein with Autologous Arterial Tissue, Percutaneous Endoscopic Approach
061R4JY Bypass Right Lesser Saphenous Vein to Lower Vein with Synthetic Substitute, Percutaneous Endoscopic Approach

R4KY Bypass Right Lesser Saphenous Vein to Lower Vein with Nonautologous Tissue Substitute, Percutaneous Endoscopic Approach

R4ZY Bypass Right Lesser Saphenous Vein to Lower Vein, Percutaneous Endoscopic Approach

1S07Y Bypass Left Lesser Saphenous Vein to Lower Vein with Autologous Tissue Substitute, Open Approach

1S09Y Bypass Left Lesser Saphenous Vein to Lower Vein with Autologous Venous Tissue, Open Approach

1S0AY Bypass Left Lesser Saphenous Vein to Lower Vein with Autologous Arterial Tissue, Open Approach

1S0JY Bypass Left Lesser Saphenous Vein to Lower Vein with Synthetic Substitute, Open Approach

1S0KY Bypass Left Lesser Saphenous Vein to Lower Vein with Nonautologous Tissue Substitute, Open Approach

1S0ZY Bypass Left Lesser Saphenous Vein to Lower Vein, Open Approach

1S47Y Bypass Left Lesser Saphenous Vein to Lower Vein with Autologous Tissue Substitute, Percutaneous Endoscopic Approach

1S49Y Bypass Left Lesser Saphenous Vein to Lower Vein with Autologous Venous Tissue, Percutaneous Endoscopic Approach

1S4AY Bypass Left Lesser Saphenous Vein to Lower Vein with Autologous Arterial Tissue, Percutaneous Endoscopic Approach

1S4JY Bypass Left Lesser Saphenous Vein to Lower Vein with Synthetic Substitute, Percutaneous Endoscopic Approach

061S4KY Bypass Left Lesser Saphenous Vein to Lower Vein with Nonautologous Tissue Substitute, Percutaneous Endoscopic Approach

061S4ZY Bypass Left Lesser Saphenous Vein to Lower Vein, Percutaneous Endoscopic Approach

061T07Y Bypass Right Foot Vein to Lower Vein with Autologous Tissue Substitute, Open Approach

061T09Y Bypass Right Foot Vein to Lower Vein with Autologous Venous Tissue, Open Approach

061T0AY Bypass Right Foot Vein to Lower Vein with Autologous Arterial Tissue, Open Approach

061T0JY Bypass Right Foot Vein to Lower Vein with Synthetic Substitute, Open Approach

061T0KY Bypass Right Foot Vein to Lower Vein with Nonautologous Tissue Substitute, Open Approach

061T0ZY Bypass Right Foot Vein to Lower Vein, Open Approach

061T47Y Bypass Right Foot Vein to Lower Vein with Autologous Tissue Substitute, Percutaneous Endoscopic Approach

061T49Y Bypass Right Foot Vein to Lower Vein with Autologous Venous Tissue, Percutaneous Endoscopic Approach

061T4AY Bypass Right Foot Vein to Lower Vein with Autologous Arterial Tissue, Percutaneous Endoscopic Approach

061T4JY Bypass Right Foot Vein to Lower Vein with Synthetic Substitute, Percutaneous Endoscopic Approach

061T4KY Bypass Right Foot Vein to Lower Vein with Nonautologous Tissue Substitute, Percutaneous Endoscopic Approach

061T4ZY Bypass Right Foot Vein to Lower Vein, Percutaneous Endoscopic Approach

061V07Y Bypass Left Foot Vein to Lower Vein with Autologous Tissue Substitute, Open Approach

061V09Y Bypass Left Foot Vein to Lower Vein with Autologous Venous Tissue, Open Approach

061V0AY Bypass Left Foot Vein to Lower Vein with Autologous Arterial Tissue, Open Approach

061V0JY Bypass Left Foot Vein to Lower Vein with Synthetic Substitute, Open Approach

061V0KY Bypass Left Foot Vein to Lower Vein with Nonautologous Tissue Substitute, Open Approach

061V0ZY Bypass Left Foot Vein to Lower Vein, Open Approach

061V47Y Bypass Left Foot Vein to Lower Vein with Autologous Tissue Substitute, Percutaneous Endoscopic Approach

061V49Y Bypass Left Foot Vein to Lower Vein with Autologous Venous Tissue, Percutaneous Endoscopic Approach

061V4AY Bypass Left Foot Vein to Lower Vein with Autologous Arterial Tissue, Percutaneous Endoscopic Approach

061V4JY Bypass Left Foot Vein to Lower Vein with Synthetic Substitute, Percutaneous Endoscopic Approach

061V4KY Bypass Left Foot Vein to Lower Vein with Nonautologous Tissue Substitute, Percutaneous Endoscopic Approach

061V4ZY Bypass Left Foot Vein to Lower Vein, Percutaneous Endoscopic Approach

65 – Lower Veins, Destruction

500ZZ Destruction of Inferior Vena Cava, Open Approach

503ZZ Destruction of Inferior Vena Cava, Percutaneous Approach

504ZZ Destruction of Inferior Vena Cava, Percutaneous Endoscopic Approach

510ZZ Destruction of Splenic Vein, Open Approach

513ZZ Destruction of Splenic Vein, Percutaneous Approach

514ZZ Destruction of Splenic Vein, Percutaneous Endoscopic Approach

520ZZ Destruction of Gastric Vein, Open Approach

523ZZ Destruction of Gastric Vein, Percutaneous Approach

524ZZ Destruction of Gastric Vein, Percutaneous Endoscopic Approach

530ZZ Destruction of Esophageal Vein, Open Approach

6533ZZ Destruction of Esophageal Vein, Percutaneous Approach

6534ZZ Destruction of Esophageal Vein, Percutaneous Endoscopic Approach

6540ZZ Destruction of Hepatic Vein, Open Approach

6543ZZ Destruction of Hepatic Vein, Percutaneous Approach

6544ZZ Destruction of Hepatic Vein, Percutaneous Endoscopic Approach

6550ZZ Destruction of Superior Mesenteric Vein, Open Approach

6553ZZ Destruction of Superior Mesenteric Vein, Percutaneous Approach

6554ZZ Destruction of Superior Mesenteric Vein, Percutaneous Endoscopic Approach

06560ZZ Destruction of Inferior Mesenteric Vein, Open Approach

06563ZZ Destruction of Inferior Mesenteric Vein, Percutaneous Approach

06564ZZ Destruction of Inferior Mesenteric Vein, Percutaneous Endoscopic Approach

06570ZZ Destruction of Colic Vein, Open Approach

06573ZZ Destruction of Colic Vein, Percutaneous Approach

06574ZZ Destruction of Colic Vein, Percutaneous Endoscopic Approach

06580ZZ Destruction of Portal Vein, Open Approach

06583ZZ Destruction of Portal Vein, Percutaneous Approach

06584ZZ Destruction of Portal Vein, Percutaneous Endoscopic Approach

06590ZZ Destruction of Right Renal Vein, Open Approach

06593ZZ Destruction of Right Renal Vein, Percutaneous Approach

06594ZZ Destruction of Right Renal Vein, Percutaneous Endoscopic Approach

065B0ZZ Destruction of Left Renal Vein, Open Approach

065B3ZZ Destruction of Left Renal Vein, Percutaneous Approach

065B4ZZ Destruction of Left Renal Vein, Percutaneous Endoscopic Approach

065C0ZZ Destruction of Right Common Iliac Vein, Open Approach

065C3ZZ Destruction of Right Common Iliac Vein, Percutaneous Approach

065C4ZZ Destruction of Right Common Iliac Vein, Percutaneous Endoscopic Approach

065D0ZZ Destruction of Left Common Iliac Vein, Open Approach

065D3ZZ Destruction of Left Common Iliac Vein, Percutaneous Approach

065D4ZZ Destruction of Left Common Iliac Vein, Percutaneous Endoscopic Approach

065F0ZZ Destruction of Right External Iliac Vein, Open Approach

065F3ZZ Destruction of Right External Iliac Vein, Percutaneous Approach

065F4ZZ Destruction of Right External Iliac Vein, Percutaneous Endoscopic Approach

065G0ZZ Destruction of Left External Iliac Vein, Open Approach

065G3ZZ Destruction of Left External Iliac Vein, Percutaneous Approach

065G4ZZ Destruction of Left External Iliac Vein, Percutaneous Endoscopic Approach

065H0ZZ Destruction of Right Hypogastric Vein, Open Approach

065H3ZZ Destruction of Right Hypogastric Vein, Percutaneous Approach

065H4ZZ Destruction of Right Hypogastric Vein, Percutaneous Endoscopic Approach

065J0ZZ Destruction of Left Hypogastric Vein, Open Approach

065J3ZZ Destruction of Left Hypogastric Vein, Percutaneous Approach

065J4ZZ Destruction of Left Hypogastric Vein, Percutaneous Endoscopic Approach

065M0ZZ Destruction of Right Femoral Vein, Open Approach

065M3ZZ Destruction of Right Femoral Vein, Percutaneous Approach

065M4ZZ Destruction of Right Femoral Vein, Percutaneous Endoscopic Approach

065N0ZZ Destruction of Left Femoral Vein, Open Approach

065N3ZZ Destruction of Left Femoral Vein, Percutaneous Approach
065N4ZZ Destruction of Left Femoral Vein, Percutaneous Endoscopic Approach
065P0ZZ Destruction of Right Greater Saphenous Vein, Open Approach
065P3ZZ Destruction of Right Greater Saphenous Vein, Percutaneous Approach
065P4ZZ Destruction of Right Greater Saphenous Vein, Percutaneous Endoscopic Approach
065Q0ZZ Destruction of Left Greater Saphenous Vein, Open Approach
065Q3ZZ Destruction of Left Greater Saphenous Vein, Percutaneous Approach
065Q4ZZ Destruction of Left Greater Saphenous Vein, Percutaneous Endoscopic Approach
065R0ZZ Destruction of Right Lesser Saphenous Vein, Open Approach
065R3ZZ Destruction of Right Lesser Saphenous Vein, Percutaneous Approach
065R4ZZ Destruction of Right Lesser Saphenous Vein, Percutaneous Endoscopic Approach
065S0ZZ Destruction of Left Lesser Saphenous Vein, Open Approach
065S3ZZ Destruction of Left Lesser Saphenous Vein, Percutaneous Approach
065S4ZZ Destruction of Left Lesser Saphenous Vein, Percutaneous Endoscopic Approach
065T0ZZ Destruction of Right Foot Vein, Open Approach
065T3ZZ Destruction of Right Foot Vein, Percutaneous Approach
065T4ZZ Destruction of Right Foot Vein, Percutaneous Endoscopic Approach
065V0ZZ Destruction of Left Foot Vein, Open Approach
065V3ZZ Destruction of Left Foot Vein, Percutaneous Approach
065V4ZZ Destruction of Left Foot Vein, Percutaneous Endoscopic Approach
065Y0ZC Destruction of Hemorrhoidal Plexus, Op Approach
065Y0ZZ Destruction of Lower Vein, Open Approach
065Y3ZC Destruction of Hemorrhoidal Plexus, Percutaneous Approach
065Y3ZZ Destruction of Lower Vein, Percutaneous Approach
065Y4ZC Destruction of Hemorrhoidal Plexus, Percutaneous Endoscopic Approach
065Y4ZZ Destruction of Lower Vein, Percutaneous Endoscopic Approach

067 – Lower Veins, Dilation

06700DZ Dilation of Inferior Vena Cava with Intraluminal Device, Open Approach
06700ZZ Dilation of Inferior Vena Cava, Open Approach
06703DZ Dilation of Inferior Vena Cava with Intraluminal Device, Percutaneous Approach
06703ZZ Dilation of Inferior Vena Cava, Percutaneous Approach
06704DZ Dilation of Inferior Vena Cava with Intraluminal Device, Percutaneous Endoscopic Approach
06704ZZ Dilation of Inferior Vena Cava, Percutaneous Endoscopic Approach
06710DZ Dilation of Splenic Vein with Intraluminal Device, Open Approach
06710ZZ Dilation of Splenic Vein, Open Approach
06713DZ Dilation of Splenic Vein with Intraluminal Device, Percutaneous Approach
06713ZZ Dilation of Splenic Vein, Percutaneous Approach
06714DZ Dilation of Splenic Vein with Intraluminal Device, Percutaneous Endoscopic Approach
06714ZZ Dilation of Splenic Vein, Percutaneous Endoscopic Approach
06720DZ Dilation of Gastric Vein with Intraluminal Device, Open Approach
06720ZZ Dilation of Gastric Vein, Open Approach
06723DZ Dilation of Gastric Vein with Intraluminal Device, Percutaneous Approach
06723ZZ Dilation of Gastric Vein, Percutaneous Approach
06724DZ Dilation of Gastric Vein with Intraluminal Device, Percutaneous Endoscopic Approach
06724ZZ Dilation of Gastric Vein, Percutaneous Endoscopic Approach
06730DZ Dilation of Esophageal Vein with Intraluminal Device, Open Approach
06730ZZ Dilation of Esophageal Vein, Open Approach
06733DZ Dilation of Esophageal Vein with Intraluminal Device, Percutaneous Approach
06733ZZ Dilation of Esophageal Vein, Percutaneous Approach
06734DZ Dilation of Esophageal Vein with Intraluminal Device, Percutaneous Endoscopic Approach
06734ZZ Dilation of Esophageal Vein, Percutaneous Endoscopic Approach
06740DZ Dilation of Hepatic Vein with Intraluminal Device, Open Approach
06740ZZ Dilation of Hepatic Vein, Open Approach
06743DZ Dilation of Hepatic Vein with Intraluminal Device, Percutaneous Approach
06743ZZ Dilation of Hepatic Vein, Percutaneous Approach
06744DZ Dilation of Hepatic Vein with Intraluminal Device, Percutaneous Endoscopic Approach
06744ZZ Dilation of Hepatic Vein, Percutaneous Endoscopic Approach
06750DZ Dilation of Superior Mesenteric Vein with Intraluminal Device, Open Approach
06750ZZ Dilation of Superior Mesenteric Vein, Open Approach
06753DZ Dilation of Superior Mesenteric Vein with Intraluminal Device, Percutaneous Approach
06753ZZ Dilation of Superior Mesenteric Vein, Percutaneous Approach
06754DZ Dilation of Superior Mesenteric Vein with Intraluminal Device, Percutaneous Endoscopic Approach
06754ZZ Dilation of Superior Mesenteric Vein, Percutaneous Endoscopic Approach
06760DZ Dilation of Inferior Mesenteric Vein with Intraluminal Device, Open Approach
06760ZZ Dilation of Inferior Mesenteric Vein, Open Approach
06763DZ Dilation of Inferior Mesenteric Vein with Intraluminal Device, Percutaneous Approach
06763ZZ Dilation of Inferior Mesenteric Vein, Percutaneous Approach
06764DZ Dilation of Inferior Mesenteric Vein with Intraluminal Device, Percutaneous Endoscopic Approach
06764ZZ Dilation of Inferior Mesenteric Vein, Percutaneous Endoscopic Approach
06770DZ Dilation of Colic Vein with Intraluminal Device, Open Approach
06770ZZ Dilation of Colic Vein, Open Approach
06773DZ Dilation of Colic Vein with Intraluminal Device, Percutaneous Approach
06773ZZ Dilation of Colic Vein, Percutaneous Approach
06774DZ Dilation of Colic Vein with Intraluminal Device, Percutaneous Endoscopic Approach
06774ZZ Dilation of Colic Vein, Percutaneous Endoscopic Approach
06780DZ Dilation of Portal Vein with Intraluminal Device, Open Approach
06780ZZ Dilation of Portal Vein, Open Approach
06783DZ Dilation of Portal Vein with Intraluminal Device, Percutaneous Approach
06783ZZ Dilation of Portal Vein, Percutaneous Approach
06784DZ Dilation of Portal Vein with Intraluminal Device, Percutaneous Endoscopic Approach
06784ZZ Dilation of Portal Vein, Percutaneous Endoscopic Approach
06790DZ Dilation of Right Renal Vein with Intraluminal Device, Open Approach
06790ZZ Dilation of Right Renal Vein, Open Approach
06793DZ Dilation of Right Renal Vein with Intraluminal Device, Percutaneous Approach
06793ZZ Dilation of Right Renal Vein, Percutaneous Approach
06794DZ Dilation of Right Renal Vein with Intraluminal Device, Percutaneous Endoscopic Approach
06794ZZ Dilation of Right Renal Vein, Percutaneous Endoscopic Approach
067B0DZ Dilation of Left Renal Vein with Intraluminal Device, Open Approach
067B0ZZ Dilation of Left Renal Vein, Open Approach
067B3DZ Dilation of Left Renal Vein with Intraluminal Device, Percutaneous Approach
067B3ZZ Dilation of Left Renal Vein, Percutaneous Approach
067B4DZ Dilation of Left Renal Vein with Intraluminal Device, Percutaneous Endoscopic Approach
067B4ZZ Dilation of Left Renal Vein, Percutaneous Endoscopic Approach
067C0DZ Dilation of Right Common Iliac Vein with Intraluminal Device, Open Approach
067C0ZZ Dilation of Right Common Iliac Vein, Open Approach
067C3DZ Dilation of Right Common Iliac Vein with Intraluminal Device, Percutaneous Approach
067C3ZZ Dilation of Right Common Iliac Vein, Percutaneous Approach
067C4DZ Dilation of Right Common Iliac Vein with Intraluminal Device, Percutaneous Endoscopic Approach
067C4ZZ Dilation of Right Common Iliac Vein, Percutaneous Endoscopic Approach
067D0DZ Dilation of Left Common Iliac Vein with Intraluminal Device, Open Approach
067D0ZZ Dilation of Left Common Iliac Vein, Open Approach
067D3DZ Dilation of Left Common Iliac Vein with Intraluminal Device, Percutaneous Approach
067D3ZZ Dilation of Left Common Iliac Vein, Percutaneous Approach

7D4DZ Dilation of Left Common Iliac Vein with Intraluminal Device, Percutaneous Endoscopic Approach
7D4ZZ Dilation of Left Common Iliac Vein, Percutaneous Endoscopic Approach
7F0DZ Dilation of Right External Iliac Vein with Intraluminal Device, Open Approach
7F0ZZ Dilation of Right External Iliac Vein, Open Approach
7F3DZ Dilation of Right External Iliac Vein with Intraluminal Device, Percutaneous Approach
7F3ZZ Dilation of Right External Iliac Vein, Percutaneous Approach
7F4DZ Dilation of Right External Iliac Vein with Intraluminal Device, Percutaneous Endoscopic Approach
7F4ZZ Dilation of Right External Iliac Vein, Percutaneous Endoscopic Approach
7G0DZ Dilation of Left External Iliac Vein with Intraluminal Device, Open Approach
7G0ZZ Dilation of Left External Iliac Vein, Open Approach
7G3DZ Dilation of Left External Iliac Vein with Intraluminal Device, Percutaneous Approach
7G3ZZ Dilation of Left External Iliac Vein, Percutaneous Approach
7G4DZ Dilation of Left External Iliac Vein with Intraluminal Device, Percutaneous Endoscopic Approach
7G4ZZ Dilation of Left External Iliac Vein, Percutaneous Endoscopic Approach
7H0DZ Dilation of Right Hypogastric Vein with Intraluminal Device, Open Approach
7H0ZZ Dilation of Right Hypogastric Vein, Open Approach
7H3DZ Dilation of Right Hypogastric Vein with Intraluminal Device, Percutaneous Approach
7H3ZZ Dilation of Right Hypogastric Vein, Percutaneous Approach
7H4DZ Dilation of Right Hypogastric Vein with Intraluminal Device, Percutaneous Endoscopic Approach
7H4ZZ Dilation of Right Hypogastric Vein, Percutaneous Endoscopic Approach
7J0DZ Dilation of Left Hypogastric Vein with Intraluminal Device, Open Approach
67J0ZZ Dilation of Left Hypogastric Vein, Open Approach
67J3DZ Dilation of Left Hypogastric Vein with Intraluminal Device, Percutaneous Approach
67J3ZZ Dilation of Left Hypogastric Vein, Percutaneous Approach
67J4DZ Dilation of Left Hypogastric Vein with Intraluminal Device, Percutaneous Endoscopic Approach
67J4ZZ Dilation of Left Hypogastric Vein, Percutaneous Endoscopic Approach
67M0DZ Dilation of Right Femoral Vein with Intraluminal Device, Open Approach
067M0ZZ Dilation of Right Femoral Vein, Open Approach
067M3DZ Dilation of Right Femoral Vein with Intraluminal Device, Percutaneous Approach
067M3ZZ Dilation of Right Femoral Vein, Percutaneous Approach
067M4DZ Dilation of Right Femoral Vein with Intraluminal Device, Percutaneous Endoscopic Approach
067M4ZZ Dilation of Right Femoral Vein, Percutaneous Endoscopic Approach
067N0DZ Dilation of Left Femoral Vein with Intraluminal Device, Open Approach
067N0ZZ Dilation of Left Femoral Vein, Open Approach
067N3DZ Dilation of Left Femoral Vein with Intraluminal Device, Percutaneous Approach
067N3ZZ Dilation of Left Femoral Vein, Percutaneous Approach
067N4DZ Dilation of Left Femoral Vein with Intraluminal Device, Percutaneous Endoscopic Approach
067N4ZZ Dilation of Left Femoral Vein, Percutaneous Endoscopic Approach
067P0DZ Dilation of Right Greater Saphenous Vein with Intraluminal Device, Open Approach
067P0ZZ Dilation of Right Greater Saphenous Vein, Open Approach
067P3DZ Dilation of Right Greater Saphenous Vein with Intraluminal Device, Percutaneous Approach
067P3ZZ Dilation of Right Greater Saphenous Vein, Percutaneous Approach
067P4DZ Dilation of Right Greater Saphenous Vein with Intraluminal Device, Percutaneous Endoscopic Approach
067P4ZZ Dilation of Right Greater Saphenous Vein, Percutaneous Endoscopic Approach
067Q0DZ Dilation of Left Greater Saphenous Vein with Intraluminal Device, Open Approach
067Q0ZZ Dilation of Left Greater Saphenous Vein, Open Approach
067Q3DZ Dilation of Left Greater Saphenous Vein with Intraluminal Device, Percutaneous Approach
067Q3ZZ Dilation of Left Greater Saphenous Vein, Percutaneous Approach
067Q4DZ Dilation of Left Greater Saphenous Vein with Intraluminal Device, Percutaneous Endoscopic Approach
067Q4ZZ Dilation of Left Greater Saphenous Vein, Percutaneous Endoscopic Approach
067R0DZ Dilation of Right Lesser Saphenous Vein with Intraluminal Device, Open Approach
067R0ZZ Dilation of Right Lesser Saphenous Vein, Open Approach
067R3DZ Dilation of Right Lesser Saphenous Vein with Intraluminal Device, Percutaneous Approach
067R3ZZ Dilation of Right Lesser Saphenous Vein, Percutaneous Approach
067R4DZ Dilation of Right Lesser Saphenous Vein with Intraluminal Device, Percutaneous Endoscopic Approach
067R4ZZ Dilation of Right Lesser Saphenous Vein, Percutaneous Endoscopic Approach
067S0DZ Dilation of Left Lesser Saphenous Vein with Intraluminal Device, Open Approach
067S0ZZ Dilation of Left Lesser Saphenous Vein, Open Approach
067S3DZ Dilation of Left Lesser Saphenous Vein with Intraluminal Device, Percutaneous Approach
067S3ZZ Dilation of Left Lesser Saphenous Vein, Percutaneous Approach
067S4DZ Dilation of Left Lesser Saphenous Vein with Intraluminal Device, Percutaneous Endoscopic Approach
067S4ZZ Dilation of Left Lesser Saphenous Vein, Percutaneous Endoscopic Approach
067T0DZ Dilation of Right Foot Vein with Intraluminal Device, Open Approach
067T0ZZ Dilation of Right Foot Vein, Open Approach
067T3DZ Dilation of Right Foot Vein with Intraluminal Device, Percutaneous Approach
067T3ZZ Dilation of Right Foot Vein, Percutaneous Approach
067T4DZ Dilation of Right Foot Vein with Intraluminal Device, Percutaneous Endoscopic Approach
067T4ZZ Dilation of Right Foot Vein, Percutaneous Endoscopic Approach
067V0DZ Dilation of Left Foot Vein with Intraluminal Device, Open Approach
067V0ZZ Dilation of Left Foot Vein, Open Approach
067V3DZ Dilation of Left Foot Vein with Intraluminal Device, Percutaneous Approach
067V3ZZ Dilation of Left Foot Vein, Percutaneous Approach
067V4DZ Dilation of Left Foot Vein with Intraluminal Device, Percutaneous Endoscopic Approach
067V4ZZ Dilation of Left Foot Vein, Percutaneous Endoscopic Approach
067Y0DZ Dilation of Lower Vein with Intraluminal Device, Open Approach
067Y0ZZ Dilation of Lower Vein, Open Approach
067Y3DZ Dilation of Lower Vein with Intraluminal Device, Percutaneous Approach
067Y3ZZ Dilation of Lower Vein, Percutaneous Approach
067Y4DZ Dilation of Lower Vein with Intraluminal Device, Percutaneous Endoscopic Approach
067Y4ZZ Dilation of Lower Vein, Percutaneous Endoscopic Approach

69 – Lower Veins, Drainage

eview Coding Guidelines B3.4a and B3.4b

eview Coding Guideline B6.2

69000Z Drainage of Inferior Vena Cava with Drainage Device, Open Approach
6900ZX Drainage of Inferior Vena Cava, Open Approach, Diagnostic
6900ZZ Drainage of Inferior Vena Cava, Open Approach
69030Z Drainage of Inferior Vena Cava with Drainage Device, Percutaneous Approach
06903ZX Drainage of Inferior Vena Cava, Percutaneous Approach, Diagnostic
06903ZZ Drainage of Inferior Vena Cava, Percutaneous Approach
069040Z Drainage of Inferior Vena Cava with Drainage Device, Percutaneous Endoscopic Approach
06904ZX Drainage of Inferior Vena Cava, Percutaneous Endoscopic Approach, Diagnostic
06904ZZ Drainage of Inferior Vena Cava, Percutaneous Endoscopic Approach
069100Z Drainage of Splenic Vein with Drainage Device, Open Approach

06910ZX Drainage of Splenic Vein, Open Approach, Diagnostic
06910ZZ Drainage of Splenic Vein, Open Approach
069130Z Drainage of Splenic Vein with Drainage Device, Percutaneous Approach
06913ZX Drainage of Splenic Vein, Percutaneous Approach, Diagnostic
06913ZZ Drainage of Splenic Vein, Percutaneous Approach
069140Z Drainage of Splenic Vein with Drainage Device, Percutaneous Endoscopic Approach
06914ZX Drainage of Splenic Vein, Percutaneous Endoscopic Approach, Diagnostic
06914ZZ Drainage of Splenic Vein, Percutaneous Endoscopic Approach
069200Z Drainage of Gastric Vein with Drainage Device, Open Approach
06920ZX Drainage of Gastric Vein, Open Approach, Diagnostic
06920ZZ Drainage of Gastric Vein, Open Approach
069230Z Drainage of Gastric Vein with Drainage Device, Percutaneous Approach
06923ZX Drainage of Gastric Vein, Percutaneous Approach, Diagnostic
06923ZZ Drainage of Gastric Vein, Percutaneous Approach
069240Z Drainage of Gastric Vein with Drainage Device, Percutaneous Endoscopic Approach
06924ZX Drainage of Gastric Vein, Percutaneous Endoscopic Approach, Diagnostic
06924ZZ Drainage of Gastric Vein, Percutaneous Endoscopic Approach
069300Z Drainage of Esophageal Vein with Drainage Device, Open Approach
06930ZX Drainage of Esophageal Vein, Open Approach, Diagnostic
06930ZZ Drainage of Esophageal Vein, Open Approach
069330Z Drainage of Esophageal Vein with Drainage Device, Percutaneous Approach
06933ZX Drainage of Esophageal Vein, Percutaneous Approach, Diagnostic
06933ZZ Drainage of Esophageal Vein, Percutaneous Approach
069340Z Drainage of Esophageal Vein with Drainage Device, Percutaneous Endoscopic Approach
06934ZX Drainage of Esophageal Vein, Percutaneous Endoscopic Approach, Diagnostic
06934ZZ Drainage of Esophageal Vein, Percutaneous Endoscopic Approach
069400Z Drainage of Hepatic Vein with Drainage Device, Open Approach
06940ZX Drainage of Hepatic Vein, Open Approach, Diagnostic
06940ZZ Drainage of Hepatic Vein, Open Approach
069430Z Drainage of Hepatic Vein with Drainage Device, Percutaneous Approach
06943ZX Drainage of Hepatic Vein, Percutaneous Approach, Diagnostic
06943ZZ Drainage of Hepatic Vein, Percutaneous Approach
069440Z Drainage of Hepatic Vein with Drainage Device, Percutaneous Endoscopic Approach
06944ZX Drainage of Hepatic Vein, Percutaneous Endoscopic Approach, Diagnostic
06944ZZ Drainage of Hepatic Vein, Percutaneous Endoscopic Approach
069500Z Drainage of Superior Mesenteric Vein with Drainage Device, Open Approach
06950ZX Drainage of Superior Mesenteric Vein, Open Approach, Diagnostic
06950ZZ Drainage of Superior Mesenteric Vein, Open Approach
069530Z Drainage of Superior Mesenteric Vein with Drainage Device, Percutaneous Approach
06953ZX Drainage of Superior Mesenteric Vein, Percutaneous Approach, Diagnostic
06953ZZ Drainage of Superior Mesenteric Vein, Percutaneous Approach
069540Z Drainage of Superior Mesenteric Vein with Drainage Device, Percutaneous Endoscopic Approach
06954ZX Drainage of Superior Mesenteric Vein, Percutaneous Endoscopic Approach, Diagnostic
06954ZZ Drainage of Superior Mesenteric Vein, Percutaneous Endoscopic Approach
069600Z Drainage of Inferior Mesenteric Vein with Drainage Device, Open Approach
06960ZX Drainage of Inferior Mesenteric Vein, Open Approach, Diagnostic
06960ZZ Drainage of Inferior Mesenteric Vein, Open Approach
069630Z Drainage of Inferior Mesenteric Vein with Drainage Device, Percutaneous Approach
06963ZX Drainage of Inferior Mesenteric Vein, Percutaneous Approach, Diagnostic
06963ZZ Drainage of Inferior Mesenteric Vein, Percutaneous Approach
069640Z Drainage of Inferior Mesenteric Vein with Drainage Device, Percutaneous Endoscopic Approach
06964ZX Drainage of Inferior Mesenteric Vein, Percutaneous Endoscopic Approach, Diagnostic
06964ZZ Drainage of Inferior Mesenteric Vein, Percutaneous Endoscopic Approach
069700Z Drainage of Colic Vein with Drainage Device, Open Approach
06970ZX Drainage of Colic Vein, Open Approach, Diagnostic
06970ZZ Drainage of Colic Vein, Open Approach
069730Z Drainage of Colic Vein with Drainage Device, Percutaneous Approach
06973ZX Drainage of Colic Vein, Percutaneous Approach, Diagnostic
06973ZZ Drainage of Colic Vein, Percutaneous Approach
069740Z Drainage of Colic Vein with Drainage Device, Percutaneous Endoscopic Approach
06974ZX Drainage of Colic Vein, Percutaneous Endoscopic Approach, Diagnostic
06974ZZ Drainage of Colic Vein, Percutaneous Endoscopic Approach
069800Z Drainage of Portal Vein with Drainage Device, Open Approach
06980ZX Drainage of Portal Vein, Open Approach, Diagnostic
06980ZZ Drainage of Portal Vein, Open Approach
069830Z Drainage of Portal Vein with Drainage Device, Percutaneous Approach
06983ZX Drainage of Portal Vein, Percutaneous Approach, Diagnostic
06983ZZ Drainage of Portal Vein, Percutaneous Approach
069840Z Drainage of Portal Vein with Drainage Device, Percutaneous Endoscopic Approach
06984ZX Drainage of Portal Vein, Percutaneous Endoscopic Approach, Diagnostic
06984ZZ Drainage of Portal Vein, Percutaneous Endoscopic Approach
069900Z Drainage of Right Renal Vein with Drainage Device, Open Approach
06990ZX Drainage of Right Renal Vein, Open Approach, Diagnostic
06990ZZ Drainage of Right Renal Vein, Open Approach
069930Z Drainage of Right Renal Vein with Drainage Device, Percutaneous Approach
06993ZX Drainage of Right Renal Vein, Percutaneous Approach, Diagnostic
06993ZZ Drainage of Right Renal Vein, Percutaneous Approach
069940Z Drainage of Right Renal Vein with Drainage Device, Percutaneous Endoscopic Approach
06994ZX Drainage of Right Renal Vein, Percutaneous Endoscopic Approach, Diagnostic
06994ZZ Drainage of Right Renal Vein, Percutaneous Endoscopic Approach
069B00Z Drainage of Left Renal Vein with Draina Device, Open Approach
069B0ZX Drainage of Left Renal Vein, Open Approach, Diagnostic
069B0ZZ Drainage of Left Renal Vein, Open Approach
069B30Z Drainage of Left Renal Vein with Draina Device, Percutaneous Approach
069B3ZX Drainage of Left Renal Vein, Percutaneo Approach, Diagnostic
069B3ZZ Drainage of Left Renal Vein, Percutaneo Approach
069B40Z Drainage of Left Renal Vein with Draina Device, Percutaneous Endoscopic Approach
069B4ZX Drainage of Left Renal Vein, Percutaneo Endoscopic Approach, Diagnostic
069B4ZZ Drainage of Left Renal Vein, Percutaneo Endoscopic Approach
069C00Z Drainage of Right Common Iliac Vein with Drainage Device, Open Approach
069C0ZX Drainage of Right Common Iliac Vein, Open Approach, Diagnostic
069C0ZZ Drainage of Right Common Iliac Vein, Open Approach
069C30Z Drainage of Right Common Iliac Vein with Drainage Device, Percutaneous Approach
069C3ZX Drainage of Right Common Iliac Vein, Percutaneous Approach, Diagnostic
069C3ZZ Drainage of Right Common Iliac Vein, Percutaneous Approach
069C40Z Drainage of Right Common Iliac Vein with Drainage Device, Percutaneous Endoscopic Approach
069C4ZX Drainage of Right Common Iliac Vein, Percutaneous Endoscopic Approach, Diagnostic
069C4ZZ Drainage of Right Common Iliac Vein, Percutaneous Endoscopic Approach
069D00Z Drainage of Left Common Iliac Vein with Drainage Device, Open Approach
069D0ZX Drainage of Left Common Iliac Vein, Open Approach, Diagnostic
069D0ZZ Drainage of Left Common Iliac Vein, Open Approach
069D30Z Drainage of Left Common Iliac Vein with Drainage Device, Percutaneous Approach
069D3ZX Drainage of Left Common Iliac Vein, Percutaneous Approach, Diagnostic
069D3ZZ Drainage of Left Common Iliac Vein, Percutaneous Approach
069D40Z Drainage of Left Common Iliac Vein with Drainage Device, Percutaneous Endoscopic Approach
069D4ZX Drainage of Left Common Iliac Vein, Percutaneous Endoscopic Approach, Diagnostic
069D4ZZ Drainage of Left Common Iliac Vein, Percutaneous Endoscopic Approach
069F00Z Drainage of Right External Iliac Vein with Drainage Device, Open Approach
069F0ZX Drainage of Right External Iliac Vein, Open Approach, Diagnostic
069F0ZZ Drainage of Right External Iliac Vein, Open Approach

9F30Z Drainage of Right External Iliac Vein with Drainage Device, Percutaneous Approach

9F3ZX Drainage of Right External Iliac Vein, Percutaneous Approach, Diagnostic

9F3ZZ Drainage of Right External Iliac Vein, Percutaneous Approach

9F40Z Drainage of Right External Iliac Vein with Drainage Device, Percutaneous Endoscopic Approach

9F4ZX Drainage of Right External Iliac Vein, Percutaneous Endoscopic Approach, Diagnostic

9F4ZZ Drainage of Right External Iliac Vein, Percutaneous Endoscopic Approach

9G00Z Drainage of Left External Iliac Vein with Drainage Device, Open Approach

9G0ZX Drainage of Left External Iliac Vein, Open Approach, Diagnostic

9G0ZZ Drainage of Left External Iliac Vein, Open Approach

9G30Z Drainage of Left External Iliac Vein with Drainage Device, Percutaneous Approach

9G3ZX Drainage of Left External Iliac Vein, Percutaneous Approach, Diagnostic

9G3ZZ Drainage of Left External Iliac Vein, Percutaneous Approach

9G40Z Drainage of Left External Iliac Vein with Drainage Device, Percutaneous Endoscopic Approach

9G4ZX Drainage of Left External Iliac Vein, Percutaneous Endoscopic Approach, Diagnostic

9G4ZZ Drainage of Left External Iliac Vein, Percutaneous Endoscopic Approach

9H00Z Drainage of Right Hypogastric Vein with Drainage Device, Open Approach

9H0ZX Drainage of Right Hypogastric Vein, Open Approach, Diagnostic

9H0ZZ Drainage of Right Hypogastric Vein, Open Approach

9H30Z Drainage of Right Hypogastric Vein with Drainage Device, Percutaneous Approach

9H3ZX Drainage of Right Hypogastric Vein, Percutaneous Approach, Diagnostic

9H3ZZ Drainage of Right Hypogastric Vein, Percutaneous Approach

9H40Z Drainage of Right Hypogastric Vein with Drainage Device, Percutaneous Endoscopic Approach

9H4ZX Drainage of Right Hypogastric Vein, Percutaneous Endoscopic Approach, Diagnostic

9H4ZZ Drainage of Right Hypogastric Vein, Percutaneous Endoscopic Approach

69J00Z Drainage of Left Hypogastric Vein with Drainage Device, Open Approach

69J0ZX Drainage of Left Hypogastric Vein, Open Approach, Diagnostic

69J0ZZ Drainage of Left Hypogastric Vein, Open Approach

69J30Z Drainage of Left Hypogastric Vein with Drainage Device, Percutaneous Approach

69J3ZX Drainage of Left Hypogastric Vein, Percutaneous Approach, Diagnostic

69J3ZZ Drainage of Left Hypogastric Vein, Percutaneous Approach

69J40Z Drainage of Left Hypogastric Vein with Drainage Device, Percutaneous Endoscopic Approach

69J4ZX Drainage of Left Hypogastric Vein, Percutaneous Endoscopic Approach, Diagnostic

69J4ZZ Drainage of Left Hypogastric Vein, Percutaneous Endoscopic Approach

69M00Z Drainage of Right Femoral Vein with Drainage Device, Open Approach

69M0ZX Drainage of Right Femoral Vein, Open Approach, Diagnostic

069M0ZZ Drainage of Right Femoral Vein, Open Approach

069M30Z Drainage of Right Femoral Vein with Drainage Device, Percutaneous Approach

069M3ZX Drainage of Right Femoral Vein, Percutaneous Approach, Diagnostic

069M3ZZ Drainage of Right Femoral Vein, Percutaneous Approach

069M40Z Drainage of Right Femoral Vein with Drainage Device, Percutaneous Endoscopic Approach

069M4ZX Drainage of Right Femoral Vein, Percutaneous Endoscopic Approach, Diagnostic

069M4ZZ Drainage of Right Femoral Vein, Percutaneous Endoscopic Approach

069N00Z Drainage of Left Femoral Vein with Drainage Device, Open Approach

069N0ZX Drainage of Left Femoral Vein, Open Approach, Diagnostic

069N0ZZ Drainage of Left Femoral Vein, Open Approach

069N30Z Drainage of Left Femoral Vein with Drainage Device, Percutaneous Approach

069N3ZX Drainage of Left Femoral Vein, Percutaneous Approach, Diagnostic

069N3ZZ Drainage of Left Femoral Vein, Percutaneous Approach

069N40Z Drainage of Left Femoral Vein with Drainage Device, Percutaneous Endoscopic Approach

069N4ZX Drainage of Left Femoral Vein, Percutaneous Endoscopic Approach, Diagnostic

069N4ZZ Drainage of Left Femoral Vein, Percutaneous Endoscopic Approach

069P00Z Drainage of Right Greater Saphenous Vein with Drainage Device, Open Approach

069P0ZX Drainage of Right Greater Saphenous Vein, Open Approach, Diagnostic

069P0ZZ Drainage of Right Greater Saphenous Vein, Open Approach

069P30Z Drainage of Right Greater Saphenous Vein with Drainage Device, Percutaneous Approach

069P3ZX Drainage of Right Greater Saphenous Vein, Percutaneous Approach, Diagnostic

069P3ZZ Drainage of Right Greater Saphenous Vein, Percutaneous Approach

069P40Z Drainage of Right Greater Saphenous Vein with Drainage Device, Percutaneous Endoscopic Approach

069P4ZX Drainage of Right Greater Saphenous Vein, Percutaneous Endoscopic Approach, Diagnostic

069P4ZZ Drainage of Right Greater Saphenous Vein, Percutaneous Endoscopic Approach

069Q00Z Drainage of Left Greater Saphenous Vein with Drainage Device, Open Approach

069Q0ZX Drainage of Left Greater Saphenous Vein, Open Approach, Diagnostic

069Q0ZZ Drainage of Left Greater Saphenous Vein, Open Approach

069Q30Z Drainage of Left Greater Saphenous Vein with Drainage Device, Percutaneous Approach

069Q3ZX Drainage of Left Greater Saphenous Vein, Percutaneous Approach, Diagnostic

069Q3ZZ Drainage of Left Greater Saphenous Vein, Percutaneous Approach

069Q40Z Drainage of Left Greater Saphenous Vein with Drainage Device, Percutaneous Endoscopic Approach

069Q4ZX Drainage of Left Greater Saphenous Vein, Percutaneous Endoscopic Approach, Diagnostic

069Q4ZZ Drainage of Left Greater Saphenous Vein, Percutaneous Endoscopic Approach

069R00Z Drainage of Right Lesser Saphenous Vein with Drainage Device, Open Approach

069R0ZX Drainage of Right Lesser Saphenous Vein, Open Approach, Diagnostic

069R0ZZ Drainage of Right Lesser Saphenous Vein, Open Approach

069R30Z Drainage of Right Lesser Saphenous Vein with Drainage Device, Percutaneous Approach

069R3ZX Drainage of Right Lesser Saphenous Vein, Percutaneous Approach, Diagnostic

069R3ZZ Drainage of Right Lesser Saphenous Vein, Percutaneous Approach

069R40Z Drainage of Right Lesser Saphenous Vein with Drainage Device, Percutaneous Endoscopic Approach

069R4ZX Drainage of Right Lesser Saphenous Vein, Percutaneous Endoscopic Approach, Diagnostic

069R4ZZ Drainage of Right Lesser Saphenous Vein, Percutaneous Endoscopic Approach

069S00Z Drainage of Left Lesser Saphenous Vein with Drainage Device, Open Approach

069S0ZX Drainage of Left Lesser Saphenous Vein, Open Approach, Diagnostic

069S0ZZ Drainage of Left Lesser Saphenous Vein, Open Approach

069S30Z Drainage of Left Lesser Saphenous Vein with Drainage Device, Percutaneous Approach

069S3ZX Drainage of Left Lesser Saphenous Vein, Percutaneous Approach, Diagnostic

069S3ZZ Drainage of Left Lesser Saphenous Vein, Percutaneous Approach

069S40Z Drainage of Left Lesser Saphenous Vein with Drainage Device, Percutaneous Endoscopic Approach

069S4ZX Drainage of Left Lesser Saphenous Vein, Percutaneous Endoscopic Approach, Diagnostic

069S4ZZ Drainage of Left Lesser Saphenous Vein, Percutaneous Endoscopic Approach

069T00Z Drainage of Right Foot Vein with Drainage Device, Open Approach

069T0ZX Drainage of Right Foot Vein, Open Approach, Diagnostic

069T0ZZ Drainage of Right Foot Vein, Open Approach

069T30Z Drainage of Right Foot Vein with Drainage Device, Percutaneous Approach

069T3ZX Drainage of Right Foot Vein, Percutaneous Approach, Diagnostic

069T3ZZ Drainage of Right Foot Vein, Percutaneous Approach

069T40Z Drainage of Right Foot Vein with Drainage Device, Percutaneous Endoscopic Approach

069T4ZX Drainage of Right Foot Vein, Percutaneous Endoscopic Approach, Diagnostic

069T4ZZ Drainage of Right Foot Vein, Percutaneous Endoscopic Approach

069V00Z Drainage of Left Foot Vein with Drainage Device, Open Approach

069V0ZX Drainage of Left Foot Vein, Open Approach, Diagnostic

069V0ZZ Drainage of Left Foot Vein, Open Approach

069V30Z Drainage of Left Foot Vein with Drainage Device, Percutaneous Approach

069V3ZX Drainage of Left Foot Vein, Percutaneous Approach, Diagnostic

069V3ZZ Drainage of Left Foot Vein, Percutaneous Approach

069V40Z Drainage of Left Foot Vein with Drainage Device, Percutaneous Endoscopic Approach

069V4ZX Drainage of Left Foot Vein, Percutaneous Endoscopic Approach, Diagnostic

069V4ZZ Drainage of Left Foot Vein, Percutaneous Endoscopic Approach
069Y00Z Drainage of Lower Vein with Drainage Device, Open Approach
069Y0ZX Drainage of Lower Vein, Open Approach, Diagnostic
069Y0ZZ Drainage of Lower Vein, Open Approach
069Y30Z Drainage of Lower Vein with Drainage Device, Percutaneous Approach
069Y3ZX Drainage of Lower Vein, Percutaneous Approach, Diagnostic
069Y3ZZ Drainage of Lower Vein, Percutaneous Approach
069Y40Z Drainage of Lower Vein with Drainage Device, Percutaneous Endoscopic Approach
069Y4ZX Drainage of Lower Vein, Percutaneous Endoscopic Approach, Diagnostic
069Y4ZZ Drainage of Lower Vein, Percutaneous Endoscopic Approach

06B – Lower Veins, Excision

Review Coding Guidelines B3.4a and B3.4b

Review Coding Guideline B3.8

06B00ZX Excision of Inferior Vena Cava, Open Approach, Diagnostic
06B00ZZ Excision of Inferior Vena Cava, Open Approach
06B03ZX Excision of Inferior Vena Cava, Percutaneous Approach, Diagnostic
06B03ZZ Excision of Inferior Vena Cava, Percutaneous Approach
06B04ZX Excision of Inferior Vena Cava, Percutaneous Endoscopic Approach, Diagnostic
06B04ZZ Excision of Inferior Vena Cava, Percutaneous Endoscopic Approach
06B10ZX Excision of Splenic Vein, Open Approach, Diagnostic
06B10ZZ Excision of Splenic Vein, Open Approach
06B13ZX Excision of Splenic Vein, Percutaneous Approach, Diagnostic
06B13ZZ Excision of Splenic Vein, Percutaneous Approach
06B14ZX Excision of Splenic Vein, Percutaneous Endoscopic Approach, Diagnostic
06B14ZZ Excision of Splenic Vein, Percutaneous Endoscopic Approach
06B20ZX Excision of Gastric Vein, Open Approach, Diagnostic
06B20ZZ Excision of Gastric Vein, Open Approach
06B23ZX Excision of Gastric Vein, Percutaneous Approach, Diagnostic
06B23ZZ Excision of Gastric Vein, Percutaneous Approach
06B24ZX Excision of Gastric Vein, Percutaneous Endoscopic Approach, Diagnostic
06B24ZZ Excision of Gastric Vein, Percutaneous Endoscopic Approach
06B30ZX Excision of Esophageal Vein, Open Approach, Diagnostic
06B30ZZ Excision of Esophageal Vein, Open Approach
06B33ZX Excision of Esophageal Vein, Percutaneous Approach, Diagnostic
06B33ZZ Excision of Esophageal Vein, Percutaneous Approach
06B34ZX Excision of Esophageal Vein, Percutaneous Endoscopic Approach, Diagnostic
06B34ZZ Excision of Esophageal Vein, Percutaneous Endoscopic Approach
06B40ZX Excision of Hepatic Vein, Open Approach, Diagnostic
06B40ZZ Excision of Hepatic Vein, Open Approach
06B43ZX Excision of Hepatic Vein, Percutaneous Approach, Diagnostic
06B43ZZ Excision of Hepatic Vein, Percutaneous Approach
06B44ZX Excision of Hepatic Vein, Percutaneous Endoscopic Approach, Diagnostic
06B44ZZ Excision of Hepatic Vein, Percutaneous Endoscopic Approach
06B50ZX Excision of Superior Mesenteric Vein, Open Approach, Diagnostic
06B50ZZ Excision of Superior Mesenteric Vein, Open Approach
06B53ZX Excision of Superior Mesenteric Vein, Percutaneous Approach, Diagnostic
06B53ZZ Excision of Superior Mesenteric Vein, Percutaneous Approach
06B54ZX Excision of Superior Mesenteric Vein, Percutaneous Endoscopic Approach, Diagnostic
06B54ZZ Excision of Superior Mesenteric Vein, Percutaneous Endoscopic Approach
06B60ZX Excision of Inferior Mesenteric Vein, Open Approach, Diagnostic
06B60ZZ Excision of Inferior Mesenteric Vein, Open Approach
06B63ZX Excision of Inferior Mesenteric Vein, Percutaneous Approach, Diagnostic
06B63ZZ Excision of Inferior Mesenteric Vein, Percutaneous Approach
06B64ZX Excision of Inferior Mesenteric Vein, Percutaneous Endoscopic Approach, Diagnostic
06B64ZZ Excision of Inferior Mesenteric Vein, Percutaneous Endoscopic Approach
06B70ZX Excision of Colic Vein, Open Approach, Diagnostic
06B70ZZ Excision of Colic Vein, Open Approach
06B73ZX Excision of Colic Vein, Percutaneous Approach, Diagnostic
06B73ZZ Excision of Colic Vein, Percutaneous Approach
06B74ZX Excision of Colic Vein, Percutaneous Endoscopic Approach, Diagnostic
06B74ZZ Excision of Colic Vein, Percutaneous Endoscopic Approach
06B80ZX Excision of Portal Vein, Open Approach, Diagnostic
06B80ZZ Excision of Portal Vein, Open Approach
06B83ZX Excision of Portal Vein, Percutaneous Approach, Diagnostic
06B83ZZ Excision of Portal Vein, Percutaneous Approach
06B84ZX Excision of Portal Vein, Percutaneous Endoscopic Approach, Diagnostic
06B84ZZ Excision of Portal Vein, Percutaneous Endoscopic Approach
06B90ZX Excision of Right Renal Vein, Open Approach, Diagnostic
06B90ZZ Excision of Right Renal Vein, Open Approach
06B93ZX Excision of Right Renal Vein, Percutaneous Approach, Diagnostic
06B93ZZ Excision of Right Renal Vein, Percutaneous Approach
06B94ZX Excision of Right Renal Vein, Percutaneous Endoscopic Approach, Diagnostic
06B94ZZ Excision of Right Renal Vein, Percutaneous Endoscopic Approach
06BB0ZX Excision of Left Renal Vein, Open Approach, Diagnostic
06BB0ZZ Excision of Left Renal Vein, Open Approach
06BB3ZX Excision of Left Renal Vein, Percutaneous Approach, Diagnostic
06BB3ZZ Excision of Left Renal Vein, Percutaneous Approach
06BB4ZX Excision of Left Renal Vein, Percutaneous Endoscopic Approach, Diagnostic
06BB4ZZ Excision of Left Renal Vein, Percutaneous Endoscopic Approach
06BC0ZX Excision of Right Common Iliac Vein, Open Approach, Diagnostic
06BC0ZZ Excision of Right Common Iliac Vein, Open Approach
06BC3ZX Excision of Right Common Iliac Vein, Percutaneous Approach, Diagnostic
06BC3ZZ Excision of Right Common Iliac Vein, Percutaneous Approach
06BC4ZX Excision of Right Common Iliac Vein, Percutaneous Endoscopic Approach, Diagnostic
06BC4ZZ Excision of Right Common Iliac Vein, Percutaneous Endoscopic Approach
06BD0ZX Excision of Left Common Iliac Vein, Open Approach, Diagnostic
06BD0ZZ Excision of Left Common Iliac Vein, Open Approach
06BD3ZX Excision of Left Common Iliac Vein, Percutaneous Approach, Diagnostic
06BD3ZZ Excision of Left Common Iliac Vein, Percutaneous Approach
06BD4ZX Excision of Left Common Iliac Vein, Percutaneous Endoscopic Approach, Diagnostic
06BD4ZZ Excision of Left Common Iliac Vein, Percutaneous Endoscopic Approach
06BF0ZX Excision of Right External Iliac Vein, Open Approach, Diagnostic
06BF0ZZ Excision of Right External Iliac Vein, Open Approach
06BF3ZX Excision of Right External Iliac Vein, Percutaneous Approach, Diagnostic
06BF3ZZ Excision of Right External Iliac Vein, Percutaneous Approach
06BF4ZX Excision of Right External Iliac Vein, Percutaneous Endoscopic Approach, Diagnostic
06BF4ZZ Excision of Right External Iliac Vein, Percutaneous Endoscopic Approach
06BG0ZX Excision of Left External Iliac Vein, Open Approach, Diagnostic
06BG0ZZ Excision of Left External Iliac Vein, Open Approach
06BG3ZX Excision of Left External Iliac Vein, Percutaneous Approach, Diagnostic
06BG3ZZ Excision of Left External Iliac Vein, Percutaneous Approach
06BG4ZX Excision of Left External Iliac Vein, Percutaneous Endoscopic Approach, Diagnostic
06BG4ZZ Excision of Left External Iliac Vein, Percutaneous Endoscopic Approach
06BH0ZX Excision of Right Hypogastric Vein, Open Approach, Diagnostic
06BH0ZZ Excision of Right Hypogastric Vein, Open Approach

BH3ZX Excision of Right Hypogastric Vein, Percutaneous Approach, Diagnostic
BH3ZZ Excision of Right Hypogastric Vein, Percutaneous Approach
BH4ZX Excision of Right Hypogastric Vein, Percutaneous Endoscopic Approach, Diagnostic
BH4ZZ Excision of Right Hypogastric Vein, Percutaneous Endoscopic Approach
BJ0ZX Excision of Left Hypogastric Vein, Open Approach, Diagnostic
BJ0ZZ Excision of Left Hypogastric Vein, Open Approach
BJ3ZX Excision of Left Hypogastric Vein, Percutaneous Approach, Diagnostic
BJ3ZZ Excision of Left Hypogastric Vein, Percutaneous Approach
BJ4ZX Excision of Left Hypogastric Vein, Percutaneous Endoscopic Approach, Diagnostic
BJ4ZZ Excision of Left Hypogastric Vein, Percutaneous Endoscopic Approach
BM0ZX Excision of Right Femoral Vein, Open Approach, Diagnostic
BM0ZZ Excision of Right Femoral Vein, Open Approach
BM3ZX Excision of Right Femoral Vein, Percutaneous Approach, Diagnostic
BM3ZZ Excision of Right Femoral Vein, Percutaneous Approach
BM4ZX Excision of Right Femoral Vein, Percutaneous Endoscopic Approach, Diagnostic
BM4ZZ Excision of Right Femoral Vein, Percutaneous Endoscopic Approach
BN0ZX Excision of Left Femoral Vein, Open Approach, Diagnostic
BN0ZZ Excision of Left Femoral Vein, Open Approach
BN3ZX Excision of Left Femoral Vein, Percutaneous Approach, Diagnostic
BN3ZZ Excision of Left Femoral Vein, Percutaneous Approach
BN4ZX Excision of Left Femoral Vein, Percutaneous Endoscopic Approach, Diagnostic
BN4ZZ Excision of Left Femoral Vein, Percutaneous Endoscopic Approach
06BP0ZX Excision of Right Greater Saphenous Vein, Open Approach, Diagnostic
06BP0ZZ Excision of Right Greater Saphenous Vein, Open Approach
AHA CC: 1Q, 2014, 10-11
06BP3ZX Excision of Right Greater Saphenous Vein, Percutaneous Approach, Diagnostic
06BP3ZZ Excision of Right Greater Saphenous Vein, Percutaneous Approach
06BP4ZX Excision of Right Greater Saphenous Vein, Percutaneous Endoscopic Approach, Diagnostic
06BP4ZZ Excision of Right Greater Saphenous Vein, Percutaneous Endoscopic Approach
06BQ0ZX Excision of Left Greater Saphenous Vein, Open Approach, Diagnostic
06BQ0ZZ Excision of Left Greater Saphenous Vein, Open Approach
06BQ3ZX Excision of Left Greater Saphenous Vein, Percutaneous Approach, Diagnostic
06BQ3ZZ Excision of Left Greater Saphenous Vein, Percutaneous Approach
06BQ4ZX Excision of Left Greater Saphenous Vein, Percutaneous Endoscopic Approach, Diagnostic
06BQ4ZZ Excision of Left Greater Saphenous Vein, Percutaneous Endoscopic Approach
06BR0ZX Excision of Right Lesser Saphenous Vein, Open Approach, Diagnostic
06BR0ZZ Excision of Right Lesser Saphenous Vein, Open Approach
06BR3ZX Excision of Right Lesser Saphenous Vein, Percutaneous Approach, Diagnostic
06BR3ZZ Excision of Right Lesser Saphenous Vein, Percutaneous Approach
06BR4ZX Excision of Right Lesser Saphenous Vein, Percutaneous Endoscopic Approach, Diagnostic
06BR4ZZ Excision of Right Lesser Saphenous Vein, Percutaneous Endoscopic Approach
06BS0ZX Excision of Left Lesser Saphenous Vein, Open Approach, Diagnostic
06BS0ZZ Excision of Left Lesser Saphenous Vein, Open Approach
06BS3ZX Excision of Left Lesser Saphenous Vein, Percutaneous Approach, Diagnostic
06BS3ZZ Excision of Left Lesser Saphenous Vein, Percutaneous Approach
06BS4ZX Excision of Left Lesser Saphenous Vein, Percutaneous Endoscopic Approach, Diagnostic
06BS4ZZ Excision of Left Lesser Saphenous Vein, Percutaneous Endoscopic Approach
06BT0ZX Excision of Right Foot Vein, Open Approach, Diagnostic
06BT0ZZ Excision of Right Foot Vein, Open Approach
06BT3ZX Excision of Right Foot Vein, Percutaneous Approach, Diagnostic
06BT3ZZ Excision of Right Foot Vein, Percutaneous Approach
06BT4ZX Excision of Right Foot Vein, Percutaneous Endoscopic Approach, Diagnostic
06BT4ZZ Excision of Right Foot Vein, Percutaneous Endoscopic Approach
06BV0ZX Excision of Left Foot Vein, Open Approach, Diagnostic
06BV0ZZ Excision of Left Foot Vein, Open Approach
06BV3ZX Excision of Left Foot Vein, Percutaneous Approach, Diagnostic
06BV3ZZ Excision of Left Foot Vein, Percutaneous Approach
06BV4ZX Excision of Left Foot Vein, Percutaneous Endoscopic Approach, Diagnostic
06BV4ZZ Excision of Left Foot Vein, Percutaneous Endoscopic Approach
06BY0ZC Excision of Hemorrhoidal Plexus, Open Approach
06BY0ZX Excision of Lower Vein, Open Approach, Diagnostic
06BY0ZZ Excision of Lower Vein, Open Approach
06BY3ZC Excision of Hemorrhoidal Plexus, Percutaneous Approach
06BY3ZX Excision of Lower Vein, Percutaneous Approach, Diagnostic
06BY3ZZ Excision of Lower Vein, Percutaneous Approach
06BY4ZC Excision of Hemorrhoidal Plexus, Percutaneous Endoscopic Approach
06BY4ZX Excision of Lower Vein, Percutaneous Endoscopic Approach, Diagnostic
06BY4ZZ Excision of Lower Vein, Percutaneous Endoscopic Approach

6C – Lower Veins, Extirpation

6C00ZZ Extirpation of Matter from Inferior Vena Cava, Open Approach
6C03ZZ Extirpation of Matter from Inferior Vena Cava, Percutaneous Approach
6C04ZZ Extirpation of Matter from Inferior Vena Cava, Percutaneous Endoscopic Approach
6C10ZZ Extirpation of Matter from Splenic Vein, Open Approach
6C13ZZ Extirpation of Matter from Splenic Vein, Percutaneous Approach
6C14ZZ Extirpation of Matter from Splenic Vein, Percutaneous Endoscopic Approach
6C20ZZ Extirpation of Matter from Gastric Vein, Open Approach
6C23ZZ Extirpation of Matter from Gastric Vein, Percutaneous Approach
6C24ZZ Extirpation of Matter from Gastric Vein, Percutaneous Endoscopic Approach
6C30ZZ Extirpation of Matter from Esophageal Vein, Open Approach
6C33ZZ Extirpation of Matter from Esophageal Vein, Percutaneous Approach
6C34ZZ Extirpation of Matter from Esophageal Vein, Percutaneous Endoscopic Approach
06C40ZZ Extirpation of Matter from Hepatic Vein, Open Approach
06C43ZZ Extirpation of Matter from Hepatic Vein, Percutaneous Approach
06C44ZZ Extirpation of Matter from Hepatic Vein, Percutaneous Endoscopic Approach
06C50ZZ Extirpation of Matter from Superior Mesenteric Vein, Open Approach
06C53ZZ Extirpation of Matter from Superior Mesenteric Vein, Percutaneous Approach
06C54ZZ Extirpation of Matter from Superior Mesenteric Vein, Percutaneous Endoscopic Approach
06C60ZZ Extirpation of Matter from Inferior Mesenteric Vein, Open Approach
06C63ZZ Extirpation of Matter from Inferior Mesenteric Vein, Percutaneous Approach
06C64ZZ Extirpation of Matter from Inferior Mesenteric Vein, Percutaneous Endoscopic Approach
06C70ZZ Extirpation of Matter from Colic Vein, Open Approach
06C73ZZ Extirpation of Matter from Colic Vein, Percutaneous Approach
06C74ZZ Extirpation of Matter from Colic Vein, Percutaneous Endoscopic Approach
06C80ZZ Extirpation of Matter from Portal Vein, Open Approach
06C83ZZ Extirpation of Matter from Portal Vein, Percutaneous Approach
06C84ZZ Extirpation of Matter from Portal Vein, Percutaneous Endoscopic Approach
06C90ZZ Extirpation of Matter from Right Renal Vein, Open Approach
06C93ZZ Extirpation of Matter from Right Renal Vein, Percutaneous Approach
06C94ZZ Extirpation of Matter from Right Renal Vein, Percutaneous Endoscopic Approach
06CB0ZZ Extirpation of Matter from Left Renal Vein, Open Approach
06CB3ZZ Extirpation of Matter from Left Renal Vein, Percutaneous Approach
06CB4ZZ Extirpation of Matter from Left Renal Vein, Percutaneous Endoscopic Approach
06CC0ZZ Extirpation of Matter from Right Common Iliac Vein, Open Approach
06CC3ZZ Extirpation of Matter from Right Common Iliac Vein, Percutaneous Approach
06CC4ZZ Extirpation of Matter from Right Common Iliac Vein, Percutaneous Endoscopic Approach

06CD0ZZ Extirpation of Matter from Left Common Iliac Vein, Open Approach
06CD3ZZ Extirpation of Matter from Left Common Iliac Vein, Percutaneous Approach
06CD4ZZ Extirpation of Matter from Left Common Iliac Vein, Percutaneous Endoscopic Approach
06CF0ZZ Extirpation of Matter from Right External Iliac Vein, Open Approach
06CF3ZZ Extirpation of Matter from Right External Iliac Vein, Percutaneous Approach
06CF4ZZ Extirpation of Matter from Right External Iliac Vein, Percutaneous Endoscopic Approach
06CG0ZZ Extirpation of Matter from Left External Iliac Vein, Open Approach
06CG3ZZ Extirpation of Matter from Left External Iliac Vein, Percutaneous Approach
06CG4ZZ Extirpation of Matter from Left External Iliac Vein, Percutaneous Endoscopic Approach
06CH0ZZ Extirpation of Matter from Right Hypogastric Vein, Open Approach
06CH3ZZ Extirpation of Matter from Right Hypogastric Vein, Percutaneous Approach
06CH4ZZ Extirpation of Matter from Right Hypogastric Vein, Percutaneous Endoscopic Approach
06CJ0ZZ Extirpation of Matter from Left Hypogastric Vein, Open Approach
06CJ3ZZ Extirpation of Matter from Left Hypogastric Vein, Percutaneous Approach
06CJ4ZZ Extirpation of Matter from Left Hypogastric Vein, Percutaneous Endoscopic Approach
06CM0ZZ Extirpation of Matter from Right Femoral Vein, Open Approach
06CM3ZZ Extirpation of Matter from Right Femoral Vein, Percutaneous Approach
06CM4ZZ Extirpation of Matter from Right Femoral Vein, Percutaneous Endoscopic Approach
06CN0ZZ Extirpation of Matter from Left Femoral Vein, Open Approach
06CN3ZZ Extirpation of Matter from Left Femoral Vein, Percutaneous Approach
06CN4ZZ Extirpation of Matter from Left Femoral Vein, Percutaneous Endoscopic Approach
06CP0ZZ Extirpation of Matter from Right Greater Saphenous Vein, Open Approach
06CP3ZZ Extirpation of Matter from Right Greater Saphenous Vein, Percutaneous Approach
06CP4ZZ Extirpation of Matter from Right Greater Saphenous Vein, Percutaneous Endoscopic Approach
06CQ0ZZ Extirpation of Matter from Left Greater Saphenous Vein, Open Approach
06CQ3ZZ Extirpation of Matter from Left Greater Saphenous Vein, Percutaneous Approach
06CQ4ZZ Extirpation of Matter from Left Greater Saphenous Vein, Percutaneous Endoscopic Approach
06CR0ZZ Extirpation of Matter from Right Lesser Saphenous Vein, Open Approach
06CR3ZZ Extirpation of Matter from Right Lesser Saphenous Vein, Percutaneous Approach
06CR4ZZ Extirpation of Matter from Right Lesser Saphenous Vein, Percutaneous Endoscopic Approach
06CS0ZZ Extirpation of Matter from Left Lesser Saphenous Vein, Open Approach
06CS3ZZ Extirpation of Matter from Left Lesser Saphenous Vein, Percutaneous Approach
06CS4ZZ Extirpation of Matter from Left Lesser Saphenous Vein, Percutaneous Endoscopic Approach
06CT0ZZ Extirpation of Matter from Right Foot Vein, Open Approach
06CT3ZZ Extirpation of Matter from Right Foot Vein, Percutaneous Approach
06CT4ZZ Extirpation of Matter from Right Foot Vein, Percutaneous Endoscopic Approach
06CV0ZZ Extirpation of Matter from Left Foot Vein, Open Approach
06CV3ZZ Extirpation of Matter from Left Foot Vein, Percutaneous Approach
06CV4ZZ Extirpation of Matter from Left Foot Vein, Percutaneous Endoscopic Approach
06CY0ZZ Extirpation of Matter from Lower Vein, Open Approach
06CY3ZZ Extirpation of Matter from Lower Vein, Percutaneous Approach
06CY4ZZ Extirpation of Matter from Lower Vein, Percutaneous Endoscopic Approach

06D – Lower Veins, Extraction

06DM0ZZ Extraction of Right Femoral Vein, Open Approach
06DM3ZZ Extraction of Right Femoral Vein, Percutaneous Approach
06DM4ZZ Extraction of Right Femoral Vein, Percutaneous Endoscopic Approach
06DN0ZZ Extraction of Left Femoral Vein, Open Approach
06DN3ZZ Extraction of Left Femoral Vein, Percutaneous Approach
06DN4ZZ Extraction of Left Femoral Vein, Percutaneous Endoscopic Approach
06DP0ZZ Extraction of Right Greater Saphenous Vein, Open Approach
06DP3ZZ Extraction of Right Greater Saphenous Vein, Percutaneous Approach
06DP4ZZ Extraction of Right Greater Saphenous Vein, Percutaneous Endoscopic Approach
06DQ0ZZ Extraction of Left Greater Saphenous Vein, Open Approach
06DQ3ZZ Extraction of Left Greater Saphenous Vein, Percutaneous Approach
06DQ4ZZ Extraction of Left Greater Saphenous Vein, Percutaneous Endoscopic Approach
06DR0ZZ Extraction of Right Lesser Saphenous Vein, Open Approach
06DR3ZZ Extraction of Right Lesser Saphenous Vein, Percutaneous Approach
06DR4ZZ Extraction of Right Lesser Saphenous Vein, Percutaneous Endoscopic Approach
06DS0ZZ Extraction of Left Lesser Saphenous Vein, Open Approach
06DS3ZZ Extraction of Left Lesser Saphenous Vein, Percutaneous Approach
06DS4ZZ Extraction of Left Lesser Saphenous Vein, Percutaneous Endoscopic Approach
06DT0ZZ Extraction of Right Foot Vein, Open Approach
06DT3ZZ Extraction of Right Foot Vein, Percutaneous Approach
06DT4ZZ Extraction of Right Foot Vein, Percutaneous Endoscopic Approach
06DV0ZZ Extraction of Left Foot Vein, Open Approach
06DV3ZZ Extraction of Left Foot Vein, Percutaneous Approach
06DV4ZZ Extraction of Left Foot Vein, Percutaneous Endoscopic Approach
06DY0ZZ Extraction of Lower Vein, Open Approach
06DY3ZZ Extraction of Lower Vein, Percutaneous Approach
06DY4ZZ Extraction of Lower Vein, Percutaneous Endoscopic Approach

06H – Lower Veins, Insertion

06H003T Insertion of Infusion Device, Via Umbilical Vein, into Inferior Vena Cava, Open Approach
06H003Z Insertion of Infusion Device into Inferior Vena Cava, Open Approach
06H00DZ Insertion of Intraluminal Device into Inferior Vena Cava, Open Approach
06H033T Insertion of Infusion Device, Via Umbilical Vein, into Inferior Vena Cava, Percutaneous Approach
06H033Z Insertion of Infusion Device into Inferior Vena Cava, Percutaneous Approach
AHA CC: 3Q, 2013, 18-19
06H03DZ Insertion of Intraluminal Device into Inferior Vena Cava, Percutaneous Approach
06H043Z Insertion of Infusion Device into Inferior Vena Cava, Percutaneous Endoscopic Approach
06H04DZ Insertion of Intraluminal Device into Inferior Vena Cava, Percutaneous Endoscopic Approach
06H103Z Insertion of Infusion Device into Splenic Vein, Open Approach
06H10DZ Insertion of Intraluminal Device into Splenic Vein, Open Approach
06H133Z Insertion of Infusion Device into Splenic Vein, Percutaneous Approach
06H13DZ Insertion of Intraluminal Device into Splenic Vein, Percutaneous Approach
06H143Z Insertion of Infusion Device into Splenic Vein, Percutaneous Endoscopic Approach
06H14DZ Insertion of Intraluminal Device into Splenic Vein, Percutaneous Endoscopic Approach
06H203Z Insertion of Infusion Device into Gastric Vein, Open Approach
06H20DZ Insertion of Intraluminal Device into Gastric Vein, Open Approach
06H233Z Insertion of Infusion Device into Gastric Vein, Percutaneous Approach
06H23DZ Insertion of Intraluminal Device into Gastric Vein, Percutaneous Approach
06H243Z Insertion of Infusion Device into Gastric Vein, Percutaneous Endoscopic Approach
06H24DZ Insertion of Intraluminal Device into Gastric Vein, Percutaneous Endoscopic Approach
06H303Z Insertion of Infusion Device into Esophageal Vein, Open Approach
06H30DZ Insertion of Intraluminal Device into Esophageal Vein, Open Approach
06H333Z Insertion of Infusion Device into Esophageal Vein, Percutaneous Approach
06H33DZ Insertion of Intraluminal Device into Esophageal Vein, Percutaneous Approach
06H343Z Insertion of Infusion Device into Esophageal Vein, Percutaneous Endoscopic Approach
06H34DZ Insertion of Intraluminal Device into Esophageal Vein, Percutaneous Endoscopic Approach
06H403Z Insertion of Infusion Device into Hepatic Vein, Open Approach

H40DZ Insertion of Intraluminal Device into Hepatic Vein, Open Approach

H433Z Insertion of Infusion Device into Hepatic Vein, Percutaneous Approach

H43DZ Insertion of Intraluminal Device into Hepatic Vein, Percutaneous Approach

H443Z Insertion of Infusion Device into Hepatic Vein, Percutaneous Endoscopic Approach

H44DZ Insertion of Intraluminal Device into Hepatic Vein, Percutaneous Endoscopic Approach

H503Z Insertion of Infusion Device into Superior Mesenteric Vein, Open Approach

H50DZ Insertion of Intraluminal Device into Superior Mesenteric Vein, Open Approach

H533Z Insertion of Infusion Device into Superior Mesenteric Vein, Percutaneous Approach

H53DZ Insertion of Intraluminal Device into Superior Mesenteric Vein, Percutaneous Approach

H543Z Insertion of Infusion Device into Superior Mesenteric Vein, Percutaneous Endoscopic Approach

H54DZ Insertion of Intraluminal Device into Superior Mesenteric Vein, Percutaneous Endoscopic Approach

H603Z Insertion of Infusion Device into Inferior Mesenteric Vein, Open Approach

H60DZ Insertion of Intraluminal Device into Inferior Mesenteric Vein, Open Approach

H633Z Insertion of Infusion Device into Inferior Mesenteric Vein, Percutaneous Approach

H63DZ Insertion of Intraluminal Device into Inferior Mesenteric Vein, Percutaneous Approach

H643Z Insertion of Infusion Device into Inferior Mesenteric Vein, Percutaneous Endoscopic Approach

H64DZ Insertion of Intraluminal Device into Inferior Mesenteric Vein, Percutaneous Endoscopic Approach

H703Z Insertion of Infusion Device into Colic Vein, Open Approach

H70DZ Insertion of Intraluminal Device into Colic Vein, Open Approach

H733Z Insertion of Infusion Device into Colic Vein, Percutaneous Approach

H73DZ Insertion of Intraluminal Device into Colic Vein, Percutaneous Approach

H743Z Insertion of Infusion Device into Colic Vein, Percutaneous Endoscopic Approach

H74DZ Insertion of Intraluminal Device into Colic Vein, Percutaneous Endoscopic Approach

6H803Z Insertion of Infusion Device into Portal Vein, Open Approach

6H80DZ Insertion of Intraluminal Device into Portal Vein, Open Approach

6H833Z Insertion of Infusion Device into Portal Vein, Percutaneous Approach

6H83DZ Insertion of Intraluminal Device into Portal Vein, Percutaneous Approach

6H843Z Insertion of Infusion Device into Portal Vein, Percutaneous Endoscopic Approach

6H84DZ Insertion of Intraluminal Device into Portal Vein, Percutaneous Endoscopic Approach

6H903Z Insertion of Infusion Device into Right Renal Vein, Open Approach

6H90DZ Insertion of Intraluminal Device into Right Renal Vein, Open Approach

6H933Z Insertion of Infusion Device into Right Renal Vein, Percutaneous Approach

6H93DZ Insertion of Intraluminal Device into Right Renal Vein, Percutaneous Approach

6H943Z Insertion of Infusion Device into Right Renal Vein, Percutaneous Endoscopic Approach

06H94DZ Insertion of Intraluminal Device into Right Renal Vein, Percutaneous Endoscopic Approach

06HB03Z Insertion of Infusion Device into Left Renal Vein, Open Approach

06HB0DZ Insertion of Intraluminal Device into Left Renal Vein, Open Approach

06HB33Z Insertion of Infusion Device into Left Renal Vein, Percutaneous Approach

06HB3DZ Insertion of Intraluminal Device into Left Renal Vein, Percutaneous Approach

06HB43Z Insertion of Infusion Device into Left Renal Vein, Percutaneous Endoscopic Approach

06HB4DZ Insertion of Intraluminal Device into Left Renal Vein, Percutaneous Endoscopic Approach

06HC03Z Insertion of Infusion Device into Right Common Iliac Vein, Open Approach

06HC0DZ Insertion of Intraluminal Device into Right Common Iliac Vein, Open Approach

06HC33Z Insertion of Infusion Device into Right Common Iliac Vein, Percutaneous Approach

06HC3DZ Insertion of Intraluminal Device into Right Common Iliac Vein, Percutaneous Approach

06HC43Z Insertion of Infusion Device into Right Common Iliac Vein, Percutaneous Endoscopic Approach

06HC4DZ Insertion of Intraluminal Device into Right Common Iliac Vein, Percutaneous Endoscopic Approach

06HD03Z Insertion of Infusion Device into Left Common Iliac Vein, Open Approach

06HD0DZ Insertion of Intraluminal Device into Left Common Iliac Vein, Open Approach

06HD33Z Insertion of Infusion Device into Left Common Iliac Vein, Percutaneous Approach

06HD3DZ Insertion of Intraluminal Device into Left Common Iliac Vein, Percutaneous Approach

06HD43Z Insertion of Infusion Device into Left Common Iliac Vein, Percutaneous Endoscopic Approach

06HD4DZ Insertion of Intraluminal Device into Left Common Iliac Vein, Percutaneous Endoscopic Approach

06HF03Z Insertion of Infusion Device into Right External Iliac Vein, Open Approach

06HF0DZ Insertion of Intraluminal Device into Right External Iliac Vein, Open Approach

06HF33Z Insertion of Infusion Device into Right External Iliac Vein, Percutaneous Approach

06HF3DZ Insertion of Intraluminal Device into Right External Iliac Vein, Percutaneous Approach

06HF43Z Insertion of Infusion Device into Right External Iliac Vein, Percutaneous Endoscopic Approach

06HF4DZ Insertion of Intraluminal Device into Right External Iliac Vein, Percutaneous Endoscopic Approach

06HG03Z Insertion of Infusion Device into Left External Iliac Vein, Open Approach

06HG0DZ Insertion of Intraluminal Device into Left External Iliac Vein, Open Approach

06HG33Z Insertion of Infusion Device into Left External Iliac Vein, Percutaneous Approach

06HG3DZ Insertion of Intraluminal Device into Left External Iliac Vein, Percutaneous Approach

06HG43Z Insertion of Infusion Device into Left External Iliac Vein, Percutaneous Endoscopic Approach

06HG4DZ Insertion of Intraluminal Device into Left External Iliac Vein, Percutaneous Endoscopic Approach

06HH03Z Insertion of Infusion Device into Right Hypogastric Vein, Open Approach

06HH0DZ Insertion of Intraluminal Device into Right Hypogastric Vein, Open Approach

06HH33Z Insertion of Infusion Device into Right Hypogastric Vein, Percutaneous Approach

06HH3DZ Insertion of Intraluminal Device into Right Hypogastric Vein, Percutaneous Approach

06HH43Z Insertion of Infusion Device into Right Hypogastric Vein, Percutaneous Endoscopic Approach

06HH4DZ Insertion of Intraluminal Device into Right Hypogastric Vein, Percutaneous Endoscopic Approach

06HJ03Z Insertion of Infusion Device into Left Hypogastric Vein, Open Approach

06HJ0DZ Insertion of Intraluminal Device into Left Hypogastric Vein, Open Approach

06HJ33Z Insertion of Infusion Device into Left Hypogastric Vein, Percutaneous Approach

06HJ3DZ Insertion of Intraluminal Device into Left Hypogastric Vein, Percutaneous Approach

06HJ43Z Insertion of Infusion Device into Left Hypogastric Vein, Percutaneous Endoscopic Approach

06HJ4DZ Insertion of Intraluminal Device into Left Hypogastric Vein, Percutaneous Endoscopic Approach

06HM03Z Insertion of Infusion Device into Right Femoral Vein, Open Approach

06HM0DZ Insertion of Intraluminal Device into Right Femoral Vein, Open Approach

● **06HM33Z** Insertion of Infusion Device into Right Femoral Vein, Percutaneous Approach

06HM3DZ Insertion of Intraluminal Device into Right Femoral Vein, Percutaneous Approach

06HM43Z Insertion of Infusion Device into Right Femoral Vein, Percutaneous Endoscopic Approach

06HM4DZ Insertion of Intraluminal Device into Right Femoral Vein, Percutaneous Endoscopic Approach

06HN03Z Insertion of Infusion Device into Left Femoral Vein, Open Approach

06HN0DZ Insertion of Intraluminal Device into Left Femoral Vein, Open Approach

● **06HN33Z** Insertion of Infusion Device into Left Femoral Vein, Percutaneous Approach

06HN3DZ Insertion of Intraluminal Device into Left Femoral Vein, Percutaneous Approach

06HN43Z Insertion of Infusion Device into Left Femoral Vein, Percutaneous Endoscopic Approach

06HN4DZ Insertion of Intraluminal Device into Left Femoral Vein, Percutaneous Endoscopic Approach

06HP03Z Insertion of Infusion Device into Right Greater Saphenous Vein, Open Approach

06HP0DZ Insertion of Intraluminal Device into Right Greater Saphenous Vein, Open Approach

06HP33Z Insertion of Infusion Device into Right Greater Saphenous Vein, Percutaneous Approach

06HP3DZ Insertion of Intraluminal Device into Right Greater Saphenous Vein, Percutaneous Approach

06HP43Z Insertion of Infusion Device into Right Greater Saphenous Vein, Percutaneous Endoscopic Approach

06HP4DZ Insertion of Intraluminal Device into Right Greater Saphenous Vein, Percutaneous Endoscopic Approach

06HQ03Z Insertion of Infusion Device into Left Greater Saphenous Vein, Open Approach

06LH3CZ Occlusion of Right Hypogastric Vein with Extraluminal Device, Percutaneous Approach

06LH3DZ Occlusion of Right Hypogastric Vein with Intraluminal Device, Percutaneous Approach

06LH3ZZ Occlusion of Right Hypogastric Vein, Percutaneous Approach

06LH4CZ Occlusion of Right Hypogastric Vein with Extraluminal Device, Percutaneous Endoscopic Approach

06LH4DZ Occlusion of Right Hypogastric Vein with Intraluminal Device, Percutaneous Endoscopic Approach

06LH4ZZ Occlusion of Right Hypogastric Vein, Percutaneous Endoscopic Approach

06LJ0CZ Occlusion of Left Hypogastric Vein with Extraluminal Device, Open Approach

06LJ0DZ Occlusion of Left Hypogastric Vein with Intraluminal Device, Open Approach

06LJ0ZZ Occlusion of Left Hypogastric Vein, Open Approach

06LJ3CZ Occlusion of Left Hypogastric Vein with Extraluminal Device, Percutaneous Approach

06LJ3DZ Occlusion of Left Hypogastric Vein with Intraluminal Device, Percutaneous Approach

06LJ3ZZ Occlusion of Left Hypogastric Vein, Percutaneous Approach

06LJ4CZ Occlusion of Left Hypogastric Vein with Extraluminal Device, Percutaneous Endoscopic Approach

06LJ4DZ Occlusion of Left Hypogastric Vein with Intraluminal Device, Percutaneous Endoscopic Approach

06LJ4ZZ Occlusion of Left Hypogastric Vein, Percutaneous Endoscopic Approach

06LM0CZ Occlusion of Right Femoral Vein with Extraluminal Device, Open Approach

06LM0DZ Occlusion of Right Femoral Vein with Intraluminal Device, Open Approach

06LM0ZZ Occlusion of Right Femoral Vein, Open Approach

06LM3CZ Occlusion of Right Femoral Vein with Extraluminal Device, Percutaneous Approach

06LM3DZ Occlusion of Right Femoral Vein with Intraluminal Device, Percutaneous Approach

06LM3ZZ Occlusion of Right Femoral Vein, Percutaneous Approach

06LM4CZ Occlusion of Right Femoral Vein with Extraluminal Device, Percutaneous Endoscopic Approach

06LM4DZ Occlusion of Right Femoral Vein with Intraluminal Device, Percutaneous Endoscopic Approach

06LM4ZZ Occlusion of Right Femoral Vein, Percutaneous Endoscopic Approach

06LN0CZ Occlusion of Left Femoral Vein with Extraluminal Device, Open Approach

06LN0DZ Occlusion of Left Femoral Vein with Intraluminal Device, Open Approach

06LN0ZZ Occlusion of Left Femoral Vein, Open Approach

06LN3CZ Occlusion of Left Femoral Vein with Extraluminal Device, Percutaneous Approach

06LN3DZ Occlusion of Left Femoral Vein with Intraluminal Device, Percutaneous Approach

06LN3ZZ Occlusion of Left Femoral Vein, Percutaneous Approach

06LN4CZ Occlusion of Left Femoral Vein with Extraluminal Device, Percutaneous Endoscopic Approach

06LN4DZ Occlusion of Left Femoral Vein with Intraluminal Device, Percutaneous Endoscopic Approach

06LN4ZZ Occlusion of Left Femoral Vein, Percutaneous Endoscopic Approach

06LP0CZ Occlusion of Right Greater Saphenous Vein with Extraluminal Device, Open Approach

06LP0DZ Occlusion of Right Greater Saphenous Vein with Intraluminal Device, Open Approach

06LP0ZZ Occlusion of Right Greater Saphenous Vein, Open Approach

06LP3CZ Occlusion of Right Greater Saphenous Vein with Extraluminal Device, Percutaneous Approach

06LP3DZ Occlusion of Right Greater Saphenous Vein with Intraluminal Device, Percutaneous Approach

06LP3ZZ Occlusion of Right Greater Saphenous Vein, Percutaneous Approach

06LP4CZ Occlusion of Right Greater Saphenous Vein with Extraluminal Device, Percutaneous Endoscopic Approach

06LP4DZ Occlusion of Right Greater Saphenous Vein with Intraluminal Device, Percutaneous Endoscopic Approach

06LP4ZZ Occlusion of Right Greater Saphenous Vein, Percutaneous Endoscopic Approach

06LQ0CZ Occlusion of Left Greater Saphenous Vein with Extraluminal Device, Open Approach

06LQ0DZ Occlusion of Left Greater Saphenous Vein with Intraluminal Device, Open Approach

06LQ0ZZ Occlusion of Left Greater Saphenous Vein, Open Approach

06LQ3CZ Occlusion of Left Greater Saphenous Vein with Extraluminal Device, Percutaneous Approach

06LQ3DZ Occlusion of Left Greater Saphenous Vein with Intraluminal Device, Percutaneous Approach

06LQ3ZZ Occlusion of Left Greater Saphenous Vein, Percutaneous Approach

06LQ4CZ Occlusion of Left Greater Saphenous Vein with Extraluminal Device, Percutaneous Endoscopic Approach

06LQ4DZ Occlusion of Left Greater Saphenous Vein with Intraluminal Device, Percutaneous Endoscopic Approach

06LQ4ZZ Occlusion of Left Greater Saphenous Vein, Percutaneous Endoscopic Approach

06LR0CZ Occlusion of Right Lesser Saphenous Vein with Extraluminal Device, Open Approach

06LR0DZ Occlusion of Right Lesser Saphenous Vein with Intraluminal Device, Open Approach

06LR0ZZ Occlusion of Right Lesser Saphenous Vein, Open Approach

06LR3CZ Occlusion of Right Lesser Saphenous Vein with Extraluminal Device, Percutaneous Approach

06LR3DZ Occlusion of Right Lesser Saphenous Vein with Intraluminal Device, Percutaneous Approach

06LR3ZZ Occlusion of Right Lesser Saphenous Vein, Percutaneous Approach

06LR4CZ Occlusion of Right Lesser Saphenous Vein with Extraluminal Device, Percutaneous Endoscopic Approach

06LR4DZ Occlusion of Right Lesser Saphenous Vein with Intraluminal Device, Percutaneous Endoscopic Approach

06LR4ZZ Occlusion of Right Lesser Saphenous Vein, Percutaneous Endoscopic Approach

06LS0CZ Occlusion of Left Lesser Saphenous Vein with Extraluminal Device, Open Approach

06LS0DZ Occlusion of Left Lesser Saphenous Vei with Intraluminal Device, Open Approa

06LS0ZZ Occlusion of Left Lesser Saphenous Vei Open Approach

06LS3CZ Occlusion of Left Lesser Saphenous Vei with Extraluminal Device, Percutaneous Approach

06LS3DZ Occlusion of Left Lesser Saphenous Vei with Intraluminal Device, Percutaneous Endoscopic Approach

06LS3ZZ Occlusion of Left Lesser Saphenous Vei Percutaneous Approach

06LS4CZ Occlusion of Left Lesser Saphenous Vei with Extraluminal Device, Percutaneous Endoscopic Approach

06LS4DZ Occlusion of Left Lesser Saphenous Vei with Intraluminal Device, Percutaneous Endoscopic Approach

06LS4ZZ Occlusion of Left Lesser Saphenous Vei Percutaneous Endoscopic Approach

06LT0CZ Occlusion of Right Foot Vein with Extraluminal Device, Open Approach

06LT0DZ Occlusion of Right Foot Vein with Intraluminal Device, Open Approach

06LT0ZZ Occlusion of Right Foot Vein, Open Approach

06LT3CZ Occlusion of Right Foot Vein with Extraluminal Device, Percutaneous Approach

06LT3DZ Occlusion of Right Foot Vein with Intraluminal Device, Percutaneous Approach

06LT3ZZ Occlusion of Right Foot Vein, Percutaneous Approach

06LT4CZ Occlusion of Right Foot Vein with Extraluminal Device, Percutaneous Endoscopic Approach

06LT4DZ Occlusion of Right Foot Vein with Intraluminal Device, Percutaneous Endoscopic Approach

06LT4ZZ Occlusion of Right Foot Vein, Percutaneous Endoscopic Approach

06LV0CZ Occlusion of Left Foot Vein with Extraluminal Device, Open Approach

06LV0DZ Occlusion of Left Foot Vein with Intraluminal Device, Open Approach

06LV0ZZ Occlusion of Left Foot Vein, Open Approach

06LV3CZ Occlusion of Left Foot Vein with Extraluminal Device, Percutaneous Approach

06LV3DZ Occlusion of Left Foot Vein with Intraluminal Device, Percutaneous Approach

06LV3ZZ Occlusion of Left Foot Vein, Percutaneou Approach

06LV4CZ Occlusion of Left Foot Vein with Extraluminal Device, Percutaneous Endoscopic Approach

06LV4DZ Occlusion of Left Foot Vein with Intraluminal Device, Percutaneous Endoscopic Approach

06LV4ZZ Occlusion of Left Foot Vein, Percutaneou Endoscopic Approach

06LY0CC Occlusion of Hemorrhoidal Plexus with Extraluminal Device, Open Approach

06LY0CZ Occlusion of Lower Vein with Extraluminal Device, Open Approach

06LY0DC Occlusion of Hemorrhoidal Plexus with Intraluminal Device, Open Approach

06LY0DZ Occlusion of Lower Vein with Intralumin Device, Open Approach

06LY0ZC Occlusion of Hemorrhoidal Plexus, Open Approach

06LY0ZZ Occlusion of Lower Vein, Open Approacl

LY3CC Occlusion of Hemorrhoidal Plexus with Extraluminal Device, Percutaneous Approach
LY3CZ Occlusion of Lower Vein with Extraluminal Device, Percutaneous Approach
LY3DC Occlusion of Hemorrhoidal Plexus with Intraluminal Device, Percutaneous Approach
LY3DZ Occlusion of Lower Vein with Intraluminal Device, Percutaneous Approach
06LY3ZC Occlusion of Hemorrhoidal Plexus, Percutaneous Approach
06LY3ZZ Occlusion of Lower Vein, Percutaneous Approach
06LY4CC Occlusion of Hemorrhoidal Plexus with Extraluminal Device, Percutaneous Endoscopic Approach
06LY4CZ Occlusion of Lower Vein with Extraluminal Device, Percutaneous Endoscopic Approach
06LY4DC Occlusion of Hemorrhoidal Plexus with Intraluminal Device, Percutaneous Endoscopic Approach
06LY4DZ Occlusion of Lower Vein with Intraluminal Device, Percutaneous Endoscopic Approach
06LY4ZC Occlusion of Hemorrhoidal Plexus, Percutaneous Endoscopic Approach
06LY4ZZ Occlusion of Lower Vein, Percutaneous Endoscopic Approach

N – Lower Veins, Release

eview Coding Guidelines B3.13 and B3.14

N00ZZ Release Inferior Vena Cava, Open Approach
N03ZZ Release Inferior Vena Cava, Percutaneous Approach
N04ZZ Release Inferior Vena Cava, Percutaneous Endoscopic Approach
N10ZZ Release Splenic Vein, Open Approach
N13ZZ Release Splenic Vein, Percutaneous Approach
N14ZZ Release Splenic Vein, Percutaneous Endoscopic Approach
N20ZZ Release Gastric Vein, Open Approach
N23ZZ Release Gastric Vein, Percutaneous Approach
N24ZZ Release Gastric Vein, Percutaneous Endoscopic Approach
N30ZZ Release Esophageal Vein, Open Approach
N33ZZ Release Esophageal Vein, Percutaneous Approach
N34ZZ Release Esophageal Vein, Percutaneous Endoscopic Approach
N40ZZ Release Hepatic Vein, Open Approach
N43ZZ Release Hepatic Vein, Percutaneous Approach
N44ZZ Release Hepatic Vein, Percutaneous Endoscopic Approach
N50ZZ Release Superior Mesenteric Vein, Open Approach
N53ZZ Release Superior Mesenteric Vein, Percutaneous Approach
N54ZZ Release Superior Mesenteric Vein, Percutaneous Endoscopic Approach
N60ZZ Release Inferior Mesenteric Vein, Open Approach
N63ZZ Release Inferior Mesenteric Vein, Percutaneous Approach
N64ZZ Release Inferior Mesenteric Vein, Percutaneous Endoscopic Approach
N70ZZ Release Colic Vein, Open Approach
N73ZZ Release Colic Vein, Percutaneous Approach
N74ZZ Release Colic Vein, Percutaneous Endoscopic Approach
N80ZZ Release Portal Vein, Open Approach
N83ZZ Release Portal Vein, Percutaneous Approach
N84ZZ Release Portal Vein, Percutaneous Endoscopic Approach
06N90ZZ Release Right Renal Vein, Open Approach
06N93ZZ Release Right Renal Vein, Percutaneous Approach
06N94ZZ Release Right Renal Vein, Percutaneous Endoscopic Approach
06NB0ZZ Release Left Renal Vein, Open Approach
06NB3ZZ Release Left Renal Vein, Percutaneous Approach
06NB4ZZ Release Left Renal Vein, Percutaneous Endoscopic Approach
06NC0ZZ Release Right Common Iliac Vein, Open Approach
06NC3ZZ Release Right Common Iliac Vein, Percutaneous Approach
06NC4ZZ Release Right Common Iliac Vein, Percutaneous Endoscopic Approach
06ND0ZZ Release Left Common Iliac Vein, Open Approach
06ND3ZZ Release Left Common Iliac Vein, Percutaneous Approach
06ND4ZZ Release Left Common Iliac Vein, Percutaneous Endoscopic Approach
06NF0ZZ Release Right External Iliac Vein, Open Approach
06NF3ZZ Release Right External Iliac Vein, Percutaneous Approach
06NF4ZZ Release Right External Iliac Vein, Percutaneous Endoscopic Approach
06NG0ZZ Release Left External Iliac Vein, Open Approach
06NG3ZZ Release Left External Iliac Vein, Percutaneous Approach
06NG4ZZ Release Left External Iliac Vein, Percutaneous Endoscopic Approach
06NH0ZZ Release Right Hypogastric Vein, Open Approach
06NH3ZZ Release Right Hypogastric Vein, Percutaneous Approach
06NH4ZZ Release Right Hypogastric Vein, Percutaneous Endoscopic Approach
06NJ0ZZ Release Left Hypogastric Vein, Open Approach
06NJ3ZZ Release Left Hypogastric Vein, Percutaneous Approach
06NJ4ZZ Release Left Hypogastric Vein, Percutaneous Endoscopic Approach
06NM0ZZ Release Right Femoral Vein, Open Approach
06NM3ZZ Release Right Femoral Vein, Percutaneous Approach
06NM4ZZ Release Right Femoral Vein, Percutaneous Endoscopic Approach
06NN0ZZ Release Left Femoral Vein, Open Approach
06NN3ZZ Release Left Femoral Vein, Percutaneous Approach
06NN4ZZ Release Left Femoral Vein, Percutaneous Endoscopic Approach
06NP0ZZ Release Right Greater Saphenous Vein, Open Approach
06NP3ZZ Release Right Greater Saphenous Vein, Percutaneous Approach
06NP4ZZ Release Right Greater Saphenous Vein, Percutaneous Endoscopic Approach
06NQ0ZZ Release Left Greater Saphenous Vein, Open Approach
06NQ3ZZ Release Left Greater Saphenous Vein, Percutaneous Approach
06NQ4ZZ Release Left Greater Saphenous Vein, Percutaneous Endoscopic Approach
06NR0ZZ Release Right Lesser Saphenous Vein, Open Approach
06NR3ZZ Release Right Lesser Saphenous Vein, Percutaneous Approach
06NR4ZZ Release Right Lesser Saphenous Vein, Percutaneous Endoscopic Approach
06NS0ZZ Release Left Lesser Saphenous Vein, Open Approach
06NS3ZZ Release Left Lesser Saphenous Vein, Percutaneous Approach
06NS4ZZ Release Left Lesser Saphenous Vein, Percutaneous Endoscopic Approach
06NT0ZZ Release Right Foot Vein, Open Approach
06NT3ZZ Release Right Foot Vein, Percutaneous Approach
06NT4ZZ Release Right Foot Vein, Percutaneous Endoscopic Approach
06NV0ZZ Release Left Foot Vein, Open Approach
06NV3ZZ Release Left Foot Vein, Percutaneous Approach
06NV4ZZ Release Left Foot Vein, Percutaneous Endoscopic Approach
06NY0ZZ Release Lower Vein, Open Approach
06NY3ZZ Release Lower Vein, Percutaneous Approach
06NY4ZZ Release Lower Vein, Percutaneous Endoscopic Approach

6P – Lower Veins, Removal

eview Coding Guideline B6.1c

PY00Z Removal of Drainage Device from Lower Vein, Open Approach
PY02Z Removal of Monitoring Device from Lower Vein, Open Approach
PY03Z Removal of Infusion Device from Lower Vein, Open Approach
PY07Z Removal of Autologous Tissue Substitute from Lower Vein, Open Approach
06PY0CZ Removal of Extraluminal Device from Lower Vein, Open Approach
06PY0DZ Removal of Intraluminal Device from Lower Vein, Open Approach
06PY0JZ Removal of Synthetic Substitute from Lower Vein, Open Approach
06PY0KZ Removal of Nonautologous Tissue Substitute from Lower Vein, Open Approach
06PY30Z Removal of Drainage Device from Lower Vein, Percutaneous Approach
06PY32Z Removal of Monitoring Device from Lower Vein, Percutaneous Approach

06PY33Z Removal of Infusion Device from Lower Vein, Percutaneous Approach
06PY37Z Removal of Autologous Tissue Substitute from Lower Vein, Percutaneous Approach
06PY3CZ Removal of Extraluminal Device from Lower Vein, Percutaneous Approach
06PY3DZ Removal of Intraluminal Device from Lower Vein, Percutaneous Approach
06PY3JZ Removal of Synthetic Substitute from Lower Vein, Percutaneous Approach
06PY3KZ Removal of Nonautologous Tissue Substitute from Lower Vein, Percutaneous Approach
06PY40Z Removal of Drainage Device from Lower Vein, Percutaneous Endoscopic Approach
06PY42Z Removal of Monitoring Device from Lower Vein, Percutaneous Endoscopic Approach
06PY43Z Removal of Infusion Device from Lower Vein, Percutaneous Endoscopic Approach
06PY47Z Removal of Autologous Tissue Substitute from Lower Vein, Percutaneous Endoscopic Approach
06PY4CZ Removal of Extraluminal Device from Lower Vein, Percutaneous Endoscopic Approach
06PY4DZ Removal of Intraluminal Device from Lower Vein, Percutaneous Endoscopic Approach
06PY4JZ Removal of Synthetic Substitute from Lower Vein, Percutaneous Endoscopic Approach
06PY4KZ Removal of Nonautologous Tissue Substitute from Lower Vein, Percutaneo Endoscopic Approach
06PYX0Z Removal of Drainage Device from Lowe Vein, External Approach
06PYX2Z Removal of Monitoring Device from Lower Vein, External Approach
06PYX3Z Removal of Infusion Device from Lowe Vein, External Approach
06PYXDZ Removal of Intraluminal Device from Lower Vein, External Approach

06Q – Lower Veins, Repair

06Q00ZZ Repair Inferior Vena Cava, Open Approach
06Q03ZZ Repair Inferior Vena Cava, Percutaneous Approach
06Q04ZZ Repair Inferior Vena Cava, Percutaneous Endoscopic Approach
06Q10ZZ Repair Splenic Vein, Open Approach
06Q13ZZ Repair Splenic Vein, Percutaneous Approach
06Q14ZZ Repair Splenic Vein, Percutaneous Endoscopic Approach
06Q20ZZ Repair Gastric Vein, Open Approach
06Q23ZZ Repair Gastric Vein, Percutaneous Approach
06Q24ZZ Repair Gastric Vein, Percutaneous Endoscopic Approach
06Q30ZZ Repair Esophageal Vein, Open Approach
06Q33ZZ Repair Esophageal Vein, Percutaneous Approach
06Q34ZZ Repair Esophageal Vein, Percutaneous Endoscopic Approach
06Q40ZZ Repair Hepatic Vein, Open Approach
06Q43ZZ Repair Hepatic Vein, Percutaneous Approach
06Q44ZZ Repair Hepatic Vein, Percutaneous Endoscopic Approach
06Q50ZZ Repair Superior Mesenteric Vein, Open Approach
06Q53ZZ Repair Superior Mesenteric Vein, Percutaneous Approach
06Q54ZZ Repair Superior Mesenteric Vein, Percutaneous Endoscopic Approach
06Q60ZZ Repair Inferior Mesenteric Vein, Open Approach
06Q63ZZ Repair Inferior Mesenteric Vein, Percutaneous Approach
06Q64ZZ Repair Inferior Mesenteric Vein, Percutaneous Endoscopic Approach
06Q70ZZ Repair Colic Vein, Open Approach
06Q73ZZ Repair Colic Vein, Percutaneous Approach
06Q74ZZ Repair Colic Vein, Percutaneous Endoscopic Approach
06Q80ZZ Repair Portal Vein, Open Approach
06Q83ZZ Repair Portal Vein, Percutaneous Approach
06Q84ZZ Repair Portal Vein, Percutaneous Endoscopic Approach
06Q90ZZ Repair Right Renal Vein, Open Approach
06Q93ZZ Repair Right Renal Vein, Percutaneous Approach
06Q94ZZ Repair Right Renal Vein, Percutaneous Endoscopic Approach
06QB0ZZ Repair Left Renal Vein, Open Approach
06QB3ZZ Repair Left Renal Vein, Percutaneous Approach
06QB4ZZ Repair Left Renal Vein, Percutaneous Endoscopic Approach
06QC0ZZ Repair Right Common Iliac Vein, Open Approach
06QC3ZZ Repair Right Common Iliac Vein, Percutaneous Approach
06QC4ZZ Repair Right Common Iliac Vein, Percutaneous Endoscopic Approach
06QD0ZZ Repair Left Common Iliac Vein, Open Approach
06QD3ZZ Repair Left Common Iliac Vein, Percutaneous Approach
06QD4ZZ Repair Left Common Iliac Vein, Percutaneous Endoscopic Approach
06QF0ZZ Repair Right External Iliac Vein, Open Approach
06QF3ZZ Repair Right External Iliac Vein, Percutaneous Approach
06QF4ZZ Repair Right External Iliac Vein, Percutaneous Endoscopic Approach
06QG0ZZ Repair Left External Iliac Vein, Open Approach
06QG3ZZ Repair Left External Iliac Vein, Percutaneous Approach
06QG4ZZ Repair Left External Iliac Vein, Percutaneous Endoscopic Approach
06QH0ZZ Repair Right Hypogastric Vein, Open Approach
06QH3ZZ Repair Right Hypogastric Vein, Percutaneous Approach
06QH4ZZ Repair Right Hypogastric Vein, Percutaneous Endoscopic Approach
06QJ0ZZ Repair Left Hypogastric Vein, Open Approach
06QJ3ZZ Repair Left Hypogastric Vein, Percutaneous Approach
06QJ4ZZ Repair Left Hypogastric Vein, Percutaneous Endoscopic Approach
06QM0ZZ Repair Right Femoral Vein, Open Approach
06QM3ZZ Repair Right Femoral Vein, Percutaneou Approach
06QM4ZZ Repair Right Femoral Vein, Percutaneou Endoscopic Approach
06QN0ZZ Repair Left Femoral Vein, Open Approa
06QN3ZZ Repair Left Femoral Vein, Percutaneous Approach
06QN4ZZ Repair Left Femoral Vein, Percutaneous Endoscopic Approach
06QP0ZZ Repair Right Greater Saphenous Vein, Open Approach
06QP3ZZ Repair Right Greater Saphenous Vein, Percutaneous Approach
06QP4ZZ Repair Right Greater Saphenous Vein, Percutaneous Endoscopic Approach
06QQ0ZZ Repair Left Greater Saphenous Vein, Op Approach
06QQ3ZZ Repair Left Greater Saphenous Vein, Percutaneous Approach
06QQ4ZZ Repair Left Greater Saphenous Vein, Percutaneous Endoscopic Approach
06QR0ZZ Repair Right Lesser Saphenous Vein, Open Approach
06QR3ZZ Repair Right Lesser Saphenous Vein, Percutaneous Approach
06QR4ZZ Repair Right Lesser Saphenous Vein, Percutaneous Endoscopic Approach
06QS0ZZ Repair Left Lesser Saphenous Vein, Ope Approach
06QS3ZZ Repair Left Lesser Saphenous Vein, Percutaneous Approach
06QS4ZZ Repair Left Lesser Saphenous Vein, Percutaneous Endoscopic Approach
06QT0ZZ Repair Right Foot Vein, Open Approach
06QT3ZZ Repair Right Foot Vein, Percutaneous Approach
06QT4ZZ Repair Right Foot Vein, Percutaneous Endoscopic Approach
06QV0ZZ Repair Left Foot Vein, Open Approach
06QV3ZZ Repair Left Foot Vein, Percutaneous Approach
06QV4ZZ Repair Left Foot Vein, Percutaneous Endoscopic Approach
06QY0ZZ Repair Lower Vein, Open Approach
06QY3ZZ Repair Lower Vein, Percutaneous Approach
06QY4ZZ Repair Lower Vein, Percutaneous Endoscopic Approach

06R – Lower Veins, Replacement

06R007Z Replacement of Inferior Vena Cava with Autologous Tissue Substitute, Open Approach
06R00JZ Replacement of Inferior Vena Cava with Synthetic Substitute, Open Approach
06R00KZ Replacement of Inferior Vena Cava with Nonautologous Tissue Substitute, Open Approach
06R047Z Replacement of Inferior Vena Cava with Autologous Tissue Substitute, Percutaneous Endoscopic Approach
06R04JZ Replacement of Inferior Vena Cava with Synthetic Substitute, Percutaneous Endoscopic Approach
06R04KZ Replacement of Inferior Vena Cava with Nonautologous Tissue Substitute, Percutaneous Endoscopic Approach
06R107Z Replacement of Splenic Vein with Autologous Tissue Substitute, Open Approach
06R10JZ Replacement of Splenic Vein with Synthetic Substitute, Open Approach
06R10KZ Replacement of Splenic Vein with Nonautologous Tissue Substitute, Open Approach

R147Z Replacement of Splenic Vein with Autologous Tissue Substitute, Percutaneous Endoscopic Approach

R14JZ Replacement of Splenic Vein with Synthetic Substitute, Percutaneous Endoscopic Approach

R14KZ Replacement of Splenic Vein with Nonautologous Tissue Substitute, Percutaneous Endoscopic Approach

R207Z Replacement of Gastric Vein with Autologous Tissue Substitute, Open Approach

R20JZ Replacement of Gastric Vein with Synthetic Substitute, Open Approach

R20KZ Replacement of Gastric Vein with Nonautologous Tissue Substitute, Open Approach

R247Z Replacement of Gastric Vein with Autologous Tissue Substitute, Percutaneous Endoscopic Approach

R24JZ Replacement of Gastric Vein with Synthetic Substitute, Percutaneous Endoscopic Approach

R24KZ Replacement of Gastric Vein with Nonautologous Tissue Substitute, Percutaneous Endoscopic Approach

R307Z Replacement of Esophageal Vein with Autologous Tissue Substitute, Open Approach

R30JZ Replacement of Esophageal Vein with Synthetic Substitute, Open Approach

R30KZ Replacement of Esophageal Vein with Nonautologous Tissue Substitute, Open Approach

R347Z Replacement of Esophageal Vein with Autologous Tissue Substitute, Percutaneous Endoscopic Approach

R34JZ Replacement of Esophageal Vein with Synthetic Substitute, Percutaneous Endoscopic Approach

R34KZ Replacement of Esophageal Vein with Nonautologous Tissue Substitute, Percutaneous Endoscopic Approach

R407Z Replacement of Hepatic Vein with Autologous Tissue Substitute, Open Approach

R40JZ Replacement of Hepatic Vein with Synthetic Substitute, Open Approach

R40KZ Replacement of Hepatic Vein with Nonautologous Tissue Substitute, Open Approach

R447Z Replacement of Hepatic Vein with Autologous Tissue Substitute, Percutaneous Endoscopic Approach

R44JZ Replacement of Hepatic Vein with Synthetic Substitute, Percutaneous Endoscopic Approach

R44KZ Replacement of Hepatic Vein with Nonautologous Tissue Substitute, Percutaneous Endoscopic Approach

R507Z Replacement of Superior Mesenteric Vein with Autologous Tissue Substitute, Open Approach

R50JZ Replacement of Superior Mesenteric Vein with Synthetic Substitute, Open Approach

R50KZ Replacement of Superior Mesenteric Vein with Nonautologous Tissue Substitute, Open Approach

R547Z Replacement of Superior Mesenteric Vein with Autologous Tissue Substitute, Percutaneous Endoscopic Approach

R54JZ Replacement of Superior Mesenteric Vein with Synthetic Substitute, Percutaneous Endoscopic Approach

R54KZ Replacement of Superior Mesenteric Vein with Nonautologous Tissue Substitute, Percutaneous Endoscopic Approach

06R607Z Replacement of Inferior Mesenteric Vein with Autologous Tissue Substitute, Open Approach

06R60JZ Replacement of Inferior Mesenteric Vein with Synthetic Substitute, Open Approach

06R60KZ Replacement of Inferior Mesenteric Vein with Nonautologous Tissue Substitute, Open Approach

06R647Z Replacement of Inferior Mesenteric Vein with Autologous Tissue Substitute, Percutaneous Endoscopic Approach

06R64JZ Replacement of Inferior Mesenteric Vein with Synthetic Substitute, Percutaneous Endoscopic Approach

06R64KZ Replacement of Inferior Mesenteric Vein with Nonautologous Tissue Substitute, Percutaneous Endoscopic Approach

06R707Z Replacement of Colic Vein with Autologous Tissue Substitute, Open Approach

06R70JZ Replacement of Colic Vein with Synthetic Substitute, Open Approach

06R70KZ Replacement of Colic Vein with Nonautologous Tissue Substitute, Open Approach

06R747Z Replacement of Colic Vein with Autologous Tissue Substitute, Percutaneous Endoscopic Approach

06R74JZ Replacement of Colic Vein with Synthetic Substitute, Percutaneous Endoscopic Approach

06R74KZ Replacement of Colic Vein with Nonautologous Tissue Substitute, Percutaneous Endoscopic Approach

06R807Z Replacement of Portal Vein with Autologous Tissue Substitute, Open Approach

06R80JZ Replacement of Portal Vein with Synthetic Substitute, Open Approach

06R80KZ Replacement of Portal Vein with Nonautologous Tissue Substitute, Open Approach

06R847Z Replacement of Portal Vein with Autologous Tissue Substitute, Percutaneous Endoscopic Approach

06R84JZ Replacement of Portal Vein with Synthetic Substitute, Percutaneous Endoscopic Approach

06R84KZ Replacement of Portal Vein with Nonautologous Tissue Substitute, Percutaneous Endoscopic Approach

06R907Z Replacement of Right Renal Vein with Autologous Tissue Substitute, Open Approach

06R90JZ Replacement of Right Renal Vein with Synthetic Substitute, Open Approach

06R90KZ Replacement of Right Renal Vein with Nonautologous Tissue Substitute, Open Approach

06R947Z Replacement of Right Renal Vein with Autologous Tissue Substitute, Percutaneous Endoscopic Approach

06R94JZ Replacement of Right Renal Vein with Synthetic Substitute, Percutaneous Endoscopic Approach

06R94KZ Replacement of Right Renal Vein with Nonautologous Tissue Substitute, Percutaneous Endoscopic Approach

06RB07Z Replacement of Left Renal Vein with Autologous Tissue Substitute, Open Approach

06RB0JZ Replacement of Left Renal Vein with Synthetic Substitute, Open Approach

06RB0KZ Replacement of Left Renal Vein with Nonautologous Tissue Substitute, Open Approach

06RB47Z Replacement of Left Renal Vein with Autologous Tissue Substitute, Percutaneous Endoscopic Approach

06RB4JZ Replacement of Left Renal Vein with Synthetic Substitute, Percutaneous Endoscopic Approach

06RB4KZ Replacement of Left Renal Vein with Nonautologous Tissue Substitute, Percutaneous Endoscopic Approach

06RC07Z Replacement of Right Common Iliac Vein with Autologous Tissue Substitute, Open Approach

06RC0JZ Replacement of Right Common Iliac Vein with Synthetic Substitute, Open Approach

06RC0KZ Replacement of Right Common Iliac Vein with Nonautologous Tissue Substitute, Open Approach

06RC47Z Replacement of Right Common Iliac Vein with Autologous Tissue Substitute, Percutaneous Endoscopic Approach

06RC4JZ Replacement of Right Common Iliac Vein with Synthetic Substitute, Percutaneous Endoscopic Approach

06RC4KZ Replacement of Right Common Iliac Vein with Nonautologous Tissue Substitute, Percutaneous Endoscopic Approach

06RD07Z Replacement of Left Common Iliac Vein with Autologous Tissue Substitute, Open Approach

06RD0JZ Replacement of Left Common Iliac Vein with Synthetic Substitute, Open Approach

06RD0KZ Replacement of Left Common Iliac Vein with Nonautologous Tissue Substitute, Open Approach

06RD47Z Replacement of Left Common Iliac Vein with Autologous Tissue Substitute, Percutaneous Endoscopic Approach

06RD4JZ Replacement of Left Common Iliac Vein with Synthetic Substitute, Percutaneous Endoscopic Approach

06RD4KZ Replacement of Left Common Iliac Vein with Nonautologous Tissue Substitute, Percutaneous Endoscopic Approach

06RF07Z Replacement of Right External Iliac Vein with Autologous Tissue Substitute, Open Approach

06RF0JZ Replacement of Right External Iliac Vein with Synthetic Substitute, Open Approach

06RF0KZ Replacement of Right External Iliac Vein with Nonautologous Tissue Substitute, Open Approach

06RF47Z Replacement of Right External Iliac Vein with Autologous Tissue Substitute, Percutaneous Endoscopic Approach

06RF4JZ Replacement of Right External Iliac Vein with Synthetic Substitute, Percutaneous Endoscopic Approach

06RF4KZ Replacement of Right External Iliac Vein with Nonautologous Tissue Substitute, Percutaneous Endoscopic Approach

06RG07Z Replacement of Left External Iliac Vein with Autologous Tissue Substitute, Open Approach

06RG0JZ Replacement of Left External Iliac Vein with Synthetic Substitute, Open Approach

06RG0KZ Replacement of Left External Iliac Vein with Nonautologous Tissue Substitute, Open Approach

06RG47Z Replacement of Left External Iliac Vein with Autologous Tissue Substitute, Percutaneous Endoscopic Approach

06RG4JZ Replacement of Left External Iliac Vein with Synthetic Substitute, Percutaneous Endoscopic Approach

06RG4KZ Replacement of Left External Iliac Vein with Nonautologous Tissue Substitute, Percutaneous Endoscopic Approach

06RH07Z Replacement of Right Hypogastric Vein with Autologous Tissue Substitute, Open Approach

06RH0JZ Replacement of Right Hypogastric Vein with Synthetic Substitute, Open Approach

06RH0KZ Replacement of Right Hypogastric Vein with Nonautologous Tissue Substitute, Open Approach

06RH47Z Replacement of Right Hypogastric Vein with Autologous Tissue Substitute, Percutaneous Endoscopic Approach

06RH4JZ Replacement of Right Hypogastric Vein with Synthetic Substitute, Percutaneous Endoscopic Approach

06RH4KZ Replacement of Right Hypogastric Vein with Nonautologous Tissue Substitute, Percutaneous Endoscopic Approach

06RJ07Z Replacement of Left Hypogastric Vein with Autologous Tissue Substitute, Open Approach

06RJ0JZ Replacement of Left Hypogastric Vein with Synthetic Substitute, Open Approach

06RJ0KZ Replacement of Left Hypogastric Vein with Nonautologous Tissue Substitute, Open Approach

06RJ47Z Replacement of Left Hypogastric Vein with Autologous Tissue Substitute, Percutaneous Endoscopic Approach

06RJ4JZ Replacement of Left Hypogastric Vein with Synthetic Substitute, Percutaneous Endoscopic Approach

06RJ4KZ Replacement of Left Hypogastric Vein with Nonautologous Tissue Substitute, Percutaneous Endoscopic Approach

06RM07Z Replacement of Right Femoral Vein with Autologous Tissue Substitute, Open Approach

06RM0JZ Replacement of Right Femoral Vein with Synthetic Substitute, Open Approach

06RM0KZ Replacement of Right Femoral Vein with Nonautologous Tissue Substitute, Open Approach

06RM47Z Replacement of Right Femoral Vein with Autologous Tissue Substitute, Percutaneous Endoscopic Approach

06RM4JZ Replacement of Right Femoral Vein with Synthetic Substitute, Percutaneous Endoscopic Approach

06RM4KZ Replacement of Right Femoral Vein with Nonautologous Tissue Substitute, Percutaneous Endoscopic Approach

06RN07Z Replacement of Left Femoral Vein with Autologous Tissue Substitute, Open Approach

06RN0JZ Replacement of Left Femoral Vein with Synthetic Substitute, Open Approach

06RN0KZ Replacement of Left Femoral Vein with Nonautologous Tissue Substitute, Open Approach

06RN47Z Replacement of Left Femoral Vein with Autologous Tissue Substitute, Percutaneous Endoscopic Approach

06RN4JZ Replacement of Left Femoral Vein with Synthetic Substitute, Percutaneous Endoscopic Approach

06RN4KZ Replacement of Left Femoral Vein with Nonautologous Tissue Substitute, Percutaneous Endoscopic Approach

06RP07Z Replacement of Right Greater Saphenous Vein with Autologous Tissue Substitute, Open Approach

06RP0JZ Replacement of Right Greater Saphenous Vein with Synthetic Substitute, Open Approach

06RP0KZ Replacement of Right Greater Saphenous Vein with Nonautologous Tissue Substitute, Open Approach

06RP47Z Replacement of Right Greater Saphenous Vein with Autologous Tissue Substitute, Percutaneous Endoscopic Approach

06RP4JZ Replacement of Right Greater Saphenous Vein with Synthetic Substitute, Percutaneous Endoscopic Approach

06RP4KZ Replacement of Right Greater Saphenous Vein with Nonautologous Tissue Substitute, Percutaneous Endoscopic Approach

06RQ07Z Replacement of Left Greater Saphenous Vein with Autologous Tissue Substitute, Open Approach

06RQ0JZ Replacement of Left Greater Saphenous Vein with Synthetic Substitute, Open Approach

06RQ0KZ Replacement of Left Greater Saphenous Vein with Nonautologous Tissue Substitute, Open Approach

06RQ47Z Replacement of Left Greater Saphenous Vein with Autologous Tissue Substitute, Percutaneous Endoscopic Approach

06RQ4JZ Replacement of Left Greater Saphenous Vein with Synthetic Substitute, Percutaneous Endoscopic Approach

06RQ4KZ Replacement of Left Greater Saphenous Vein with Nonautologous Tissue Substitute, Percutaneous Endoscopic Approach

06RR07Z Replacement of Right Lesser Saphenous Vein with Autologous Tissue Substitute, Open Approach

06RR0JZ Replacement of Right Lesser Saphenous Vein with Synthetic Substitute, Open Approach

06RR0KZ Replacement of Right Lesser Saphenous Vein with Nonautologous Tissue Substitute, Open Approach

06RR47Z Replacement of Right Lesser Saphenous Vein with Autologous Tissue Substitute, Percutaneous Endoscopic Approach

06RR4JZ Replacement of Right Lesser Saphenous Vein with Synthetic Substitute, Percutaneous Endoscopic Approach

06RR4KZ Replacement of Right Lesser Saphenous Vein with Nonautologous Tissue Substitute, Percutaneous Endoscopic Approach

06RS07Z Replacement of Left Lesser Saphenous Vein with Autologous Tissue Substitute, Open Approach

06RS0JZ Replacement of Left Lesser Saphenous Vein with Synthetic Substitute, Open Approach

06RS0KZ Replacement of Left Lesser Saphenous Vein with Nonautologous Tissue Substitute, Open Approach

06RS47Z Replacement of Left Lesser Saphenous Vein with Autologous Tissue Substitute, Percutaneous Endoscopic Approach

06RS4JZ Replacement of Left Lesser Saphenous Vein with Synthetic Substitute, Percutaneous Endoscopic Approach

06RS4KZ Replacement of Left Lesser Saphenous Vein with Nonautologous Tissue Substitute, Percutaneous Endoscopic Approach

06RT07Z Replacement of Right Foot Vein with Autologous Tissue Substitute, Open Approach

06RT0JZ Replacement of Right Foot Vein with Synthetic Substitute, Open Approach

06RT0KZ Replacement of Right Foot Vein with Nonautologous Tissue Substitute, Open Approach

06RT47Z Replacement of Right Foot Vein with Autologous Tissue Substitute, Percutaneous Endoscopic Approach

06RT4JZ Replacement of Right Foot Vein with Synthetic Substitute, Percutaneous Endoscopic Approach

06RT4KZ Replacement of Right Foot Vein with Nonautologous Tissue Substitute, Percutaneous Endoscopic Approach

06RV07Z Replacement of Left Foot Vein with Autologous Tissue Substitute, Open Approach

06RV0JZ Replacement of Left Foot Vein with Synthetic Substitute, Open Approach

06RV0KZ Replacement of Left Foot Vein with Nonautologous Tissue Substitute, Open Approach

06RV47Z Replacement of Left Foot Vein with Autologous Tissue Substitute, Percutaneous Endoscopic Approach

06RV4JZ Replacement of Left Foot Vein with Synthetic Substitute, Percutaneous Endoscopic Approach

06RV4KZ Replacement of Left Foot Vein with Nonautologous Tissue Substitute, Percutaneous Endoscopic Approach

06RY07Z Replacement of Lower Vein with Autologous Tissue Substitute, Open Approach

06RY0JZ Replacement of Lower Vein with Synthe Substitute, Open Approach

06RY0KZ Replacement of Lower Vein with Nonautologous Tissue Substitute, Open Approach

06RY47Z Replacement of Lower Vein with Autologous Tissue Substitute, Percutaneous Endoscopic Approach

06RY4JZ Replacement of Lower Vein with Synthe Substitute, Percutaneous Endoscopic Approach

06RY4KZ Replacement of Lower Vein with Nonautologous Tissue Substitute, Percutaneous Endoscopic Approach

06S – Lower Veins, Reposition

06S00ZZ Reposition Inferior Vena Cava, Open Approach

06S03ZZ Reposition Inferior Vena Cava, Percutaneous Approach

06S04ZZ Reposition Inferior Vena Cava, Percutaneous Endoscopic Approach

06S10ZZ Reposition Splenic Vein, Open Approach

06S13ZZ Reposition Splenic Vein, Percutaneous Approach

06S14ZZ Reposition Splenic Vein, Percutaneous Endoscopic Approach

06S20ZZ Reposition Gastric Vein, Open Approach

06S23ZZ Reposition Gastric Vein, Percutaneous Approach

06S24ZZ Reposition Gastric Vein, Percutaneous Endoscopic Approach

06S30ZZ Reposition Esophageal Vein, Open Approach

06S33ZZ Reposition Esophageal Vein, Percutaneou Approach

06S34ZZ Reposition Esophageal Vein, Percutaneou Endoscopic Approach

40ZZ Reposition Hepatic Vein, Open Approach
43ZZ Reposition Hepatic Vein, Percutaneous Approach
44ZZ Reposition Hepatic Vein, Percutaneous Endoscopic Approach
50ZZ Reposition Superior Mesenteric Vein, Open Approach
S53ZZ Reposition Superior Mesenteric Vein, Percutaneous Approach
S54ZZ Reposition Superior Mesenteric Vein, Percutaneous Endoscopic Approach
S60ZZ Reposition Inferior Mesenteric Vein, Open Approach
S63ZZ Reposition Inferior Mesenteric Vein, Percutaneous Approach
S64ZZ Reposition Inferior Mesenteric Vein, Percutaneous Endoscopic Approach
S70ZZ Reposition Colic Vein, Open Approach
S73ZZ Reposition Colic Vein, Percutaneous Approach
S74ZZ Reposition Colic Vein, Percutaneous Endoscopic Approach
S80ZZ Reposition Portal Vein, Open Approach
S83ZZ Reposition Portal Vein, Percutaneous Approach
S84ZZ Reposition Portal Vein, Percutaneous Endoscopic Approach
S90ZZ Reposition Right Renal Vein, Open Approach
S93ZZ Reposition Right Renal Vein, Percutaneous Approach
S94ZZ Reposition Right Renal Vein, Percutaneous Endoscopic Approach
SB0ZZ Reposition Left Renal Vein, Open Approach
SB3ZZ Reposition Left Renal Vein, Percutaneous Approach
SB4ZZ Reposition Left Renal Vein, Percutaneous Endoscopic Approach
SC0ZZ Reposition Right Common Iliac Vein, Open Approach
SC3ZZ Reposition Right Common Iliac Vein, Percutaneous Approach
06SC4ZZ Reposition Right Common Iliac Vein, Percutaneous Endoscopic Approach
06SD0ZZ Reposition Left Common Iliac Vein, Open Approach
06SD3ZZ Reposition Left Common Iliac Vein, Percutaneous Approach
06SD4ZZ Reposition Left Common Iliac Vein, Percutaneous Endoscopic Approach
06SF0ZZ Reposition Right External Iliac Vein, Open Approach
06SF3ZZ Reposition Right External Iliac Vein, Percutaneous Approach
06SF4ZZ Reposition Right External Iliac Vein, Percutaneous Endoscopic Approach
06SG0ZZ Reposition Left External Iliac Vein, Open Approach
06SG3ZZ Reposition Left External Iliac Vein, Percutaneous Approach
06SG4ZZ Reposition Left External Iliac Vein, Percutaneous Endoscopic Approach
06SH0ZZ Reposition Right Hypogastric Vein, Open Approach
06SH3ZZ Reposition Right Hypogastric Vein, Percutaneous Approach
06SH4ZZ Reposition Right Hypogastric Vein, Percutaneous Endoscopic Approach
06SJ0ZZ Reposition Left Hypogastric Vein, Open Approach
06SJ3ZZ Reposition Left Hypogastric Vein, Percutaneous Approach
06SJ4ZZ Reposition Left Hypogastric Vein, Percutaneous Endoscopic Approach
06SM0ZZ Reposition Right Femoral Vein, Open Approach
06SM3ZZ Reposition Right Femoral Vein, Percutaneous Approach
06SM4ZZ Reposition Right Femoral Vein, Percutaneous Endoscopic Approach
06SN0ZZ Reposition Left Femoral Vein, Open Approach
06SN3ZZ Reposition Left Femoral Vein, Percutaneous Approach
06SN4ZZ Reposition Left Femoral Vein, Percutaneous Endoscopic Approach
06SP0ZZ Reposition Right Greater Saphenous Vein, Open Approach
06SP3ZZ Reposition Right Greater Saphenous Vein, Percutaneous Approach
06SP4ZZ Reposition Right Greater Saphenous Vein, Percutaneous Endoscopic Approach
06SQ0ZZ Reposition Left Greater Saphenous Vein, Open Approach
06SQ3ZZ Reposition Left Greater Saphenous Vein, Percutaneous Approach
06SQ4ZZ Reposition Left Greater Saphenous Vein, Percutaneous Endoscopic Approach
06SR0ZZ Reposition Right Lesser Saphenous Vein, Open Approach
06SR3ZZ Reposition Right Lesser Saphenous Vein, Percutaneous Approach
06SR4ZZ Reposition Right Lesser Saphenous Vein, Percutaneous Endoscopic Approach
06SS0ZZ Reposition Left Lesser Saphenous Vein, Open Approach
06SS3ZZ Reposition Left Lesser Saphenous Vein, Percutaneous Approach
06SS4ZZ Reposition Left Lesser Saphenous Vein, Percutaneous Endoscopic Approach
06ST0ZZ Reposition Right Foot Vein, Open Approach
06ST3ZZ Reposition Right Foot Vein, Percutaneous Approach
06ST4ZZ Reposition Right Foot Vein, Percutaneous Endoscopic Approach
06SV0ZZ Reposition Left Foot Vein, Open Approach
06SV3ZZ Reposition Left Foot Vein, Percutaneous Approach
06SV4ZZ Reposition Left Foot Vein, Percutaneous Endoscopic Approach
06SY0ZZ Reposition Lower Vein, Open Approach
06SY3ZZ Reposition Lower Vein, Percutaneous Approach
06SY4ZZ Reposition Lower Vein, Percutaneous Endoscopic Approach

6U – Lower Veins, Supplement

U007Z Supplement Inferior Vena Cava with Autologous Tissue Substitute, Open Approach
U00JZ Supplement Inferior Vena Cava with Synthetic Substitute, Open Approach
U00KZ Supplement Inferior Vena Cava with Nonautologous Tissue Substitute, Open Approach
U037Z Supplement Inferior Vena Cava with Autologous Tissue Substitute, Percutaneous Approach
U03JZ Supplement Inferior Vena Cava with Synthetic Substitute, Percutaneous Approach
U03KZ Supplement Inferior Vena Cava with Nonautologous Tissue Substitute, Percutaneous Approach
U047Z Supplement Inferior Vena Cava with Autologous Tissue Substitute, Percutaneous Endoscopic Approach
U04JZ Supplement Inferior Vena Cava with Synthetic Substitute, Percutaneous Endoscopic Approach
U04KZ Supplement Inferior Vena Cava with Nonautologous Tissue Substitute, Percutaneous Endoscopic Approach
U107Z Supplement Splenic Vein with Autologous Tissue Substitute, Open Approach
U10JZ Supplement Splenic Vein with Synthetic Substitute, Open Approach
06U10KZ Supplement Splenic Vein with Nonautologous Tissue Substitute, Open Approach
06U137Z Supplement Splenic Vein with Autologous Tissue Substitute, Percutaneous Approach
06U13JZ Supplement Splenic Vein with Synthetic Substitute, Percutaneous Approach
06U13KZ Supplement Splenic Vein with Nonautologous Tissue Substitute, Percutaneous Approach
06U147Z Supplement Splenic Vein with Autologous Tissue Substitute, Percutaneous Endoscopic Approach
06U14JZ Supplement Splenic Vein with Synthetic Substitute, Percutaneous Endoscopic Approach
06U14KZ Supplement Splenic Vein with Nonautologous Tissue Substitute, Percutaneous Endoscopic Approach
06U207Z Supplement Gastric Vein with Autologous Tissue Substitute, Open Approach
06U20JZ Supplement Gastric Vein with Synthetic Substitute, Open Approach
06U20KZ Supplement Gastric Vein with Nonautologous Tissue Substitute, Open Approach
06U237Z Supplement Gastric Vein with Autologous Tissue Substitute, Percutaneous Approach
06U23JZ Supplement Gastric Vein with Synthetic Substitute, Percutaneous Approach
06U23KZ Supplement Gastric Vein with Nonautologous Tissue Substitute, Percutaneous Approach
06U247Z Supplement Gastric Vein with Autologous Tissue Substitute, Percutaneous Endoscopic Approach
06U24JZ Supplement Gastric Vein with Synthetic Substitute, Percutaneous Endoscopic Approach
06U24KZ Supplement Gastric Vein with Nonautologous Tissue Substitute, Percutaneous Endoscopic Approach
06U307Z Supplement Esophageal Vein with Autologous Tissue Substitute, Open Approach
06U30JZ Supplement Esophageal Vein with Synthetic Substitute, Open Approach
06U30KZ Supplement Esophageal Vein with Nonautologous Tissue Substitute, Open Approach
06U337Z Supplement Esophageal Vein with Autologous Tissue Substitute, Percutaneous Approach
06U33JZ Supplement Esophageal Vein with Synthetic Substitute, Percutaneous Approach
06U33KZ Supplement Esophageal Vein with Nonautologous Tissue Substitute, Percutaneous Approach
06U347Z Supplement Esophageal Vein with Autologous Tissue Substitute, Percutaneous Endoscopic Approach

06U34JZ Supplement Esophageal Vein with Synthetic Substitute, Percutaneous Endoscopic Approach
06U34KZ Supplement Esophageal Vein with Nonautologous Tissue Substitute, Percutaneous Endoscopic Approach
06U407Z Supplement Hepatic Vein with Autologous Tissue Substitute, Open Approach
06U40JZ Supplement Hepatic Vein with Synthetic Substitute, Open Approach
06U40KZ Supplement Hepatic Vein with Nonautologous Tissue Substitute, Open Approach
06U437Z Supplement Hepatic Vein with Autologous Tissue Substitute, Percutaneous Approach
06U43JZ Supplement Hepatic Vein with Synthetic Substitute, Percutaneous Approach
06U43KZ Supplement Hepatic Vein with Nonautologous Tissue Substitute, Percutaneous Approach
06U447Z Supplement Hepatic Vein with Autologous Tissue Substitute, Percutaneous Endoscopic Approach
06U44JZ Supplement Hepatic Vein with Synthetic Substitute, Percutaneous Endoscopic Approach
06U44KZ Supplement Hepatic Vein with Nonautologous Tissue Substitute, Percutaneous Endoscopic Approach
06U507Z Supplement Superior Mesenteric Vein with Autologous Tissue Substitute, Open Approach
06U50JZ Supplement Superior Mesenteric Vein with Synthetic Substitute, Open Approach
06U50KZ Supplement Superior Mesenteric Vein with Nonautologous Tissue Substitute, Open Approach
06U537Z Supplement Superior Mesenteric Vein with Autologous Tissue Substitute, Percutaneous Approach
06U53JZ Supplement Superior Mesenteric Vein with Synthetic Substitute, Percutaneous Approach
06U53KZ Supplement Superior Mesenteric Vein with Nonautologous Tissue Substitute, Percutaneous Approach
06U547Z Supplement Superior Mesenteric Vein with Autologous Tissue Substitute, Percutaneous Endoscopic Approach
06U54JZ Supplement Superior Mesenteric Vein with Synthetic Substitute, Percutaneous Endoscopic Approach
06U54KZ Supplement Superior Mesenteric Vein with Nonautologous Tissue Substitute, Percutaneous Endoscopic Approach
06U607Z Supplement Inferior Mesenteric Vein with Autologous Tissue Substitute, Open Approach
06U60JZ Supplement Inferior Mesenteric Vein with Synthetic Substitute, Open Approach
06U60KZ Supplement Inferior Mesenteric Vein with Nonautologous Tissue Substitute, Open Approach
06U637Z Supplement Inferior Mesenteric Vein with Autologous Tissue Substitute, Percutaneous Approach
06U63JZ Supplement Inferior Mesenteric Vein with Synthetic Substitute, Percutaneous Approach
06U63KZ Supplement Inferior Mesenteric Vein with Nonautologous Tissue Substitute, Percutaneous Approach
06U647Z Supplement Inferior Mesenteric Vein with Autologous Tissue Substitute, Percutaneous Endoscopic Approach
06U64JZ Supplement Inferior Mesenteric Vein with Synthetic Substitute, Percutaneous Endoscopic Approach
06U64KZ Supplement Inferior Mesenteric Vein with Nonautologous Tissue Substitute, Percutaneous Endoscopic Approach
06U707Z Supplement Colic Vein with Autologous Tissue Substitute, Open Approach
06U70JZ Supplement Colic Vein with Synthetic Substitute, Open Approach
06U70KZ Supplement Colic Vein with Nonautologous Tissue Substitute, Open Approach
06U737Z Supplement Colic Vein with Autologous Tissue Substitute, Percutaneous Approach
06U73JZ Supplement Colic Vein with Synthetic Substitute, Percutaneous Approach
06U73KZ Supplement Colic Vein with Nonautologous Tissue Substitute, Percutaneous Approach
06U747Z Supplement Colic Vein with Autologous Tissue Substitute, Percutaneous Endoscopic Approach
06U74JZ Supplement Colic Vein with Synthetic Substitute, Percutaneous Endoscopic Approach
06U74KZ Supplement Colic Vein with Nonautologous Tissue Substitute, Percutaneous Endoscopic Approach
06U807Z Supplement Portal Vein with Autologous Tissue Substitute, Open Approach
06U80JZ Supplement Portal Vein with Synthetic Substitute, Open Approach
06U80KZ Supplement Portal Vein with Nonautologous Tissue Substitute, Open Approach
06U837Z Supplement Portal Vein with Autologous Tissue Substitute, Percutaneous Approach
06U83JZ Supplement Portal Vein with Synthetic Substitute, Percutaneous Approach
06U83KZ Supplement Portal Vein with Nonautologous Tissue Substitute, Percutaneous Approach
06U847Z Supplement Portal Vein with Autologous Tissue Substitute, Percutaneous Endoscopic Approach
06U84JZ Supplement Portal Vein with Synthetic Substitute, Percutaneous Endoscopic Approach
06U84KZ Supplement Portal Vein with Nonautologous Tissue Substitute, Percutaneous Endoscopic Approach
06U907Z Supplement Right Renal Vein with Autologous Tissue Substitute, Open Approach
06U90JZ Supplement Right Renal Vein with Synthetic Substitute, Open Approach
06U90KZ Supplement Right Renal Vein with Nonautologous Tissue Substitute, Open Approach
06U937Z Supplement Right Renal Vein with Autologous Tissue Substitute, Percutaneous Approach
06U93JZ Supplement Right Renal Vein with Synthetic Substitute, Percutaneous Approach
06U93KZ Supplement Right Renal Vein with Nonautologous Tissue Substitute, Percutaneous Approach
06U947Z Supplement Right Renal Vein with Autologous Tissue Substitute, Percutaneous Endoscopic Approach
06U94JZ Supplement Right Renal Vein with Synthetic Substitute, Percutaneous Endoscopic Approach
06U94KZ Supplement Right Renal Vein with Nonautologous Tissue Substitute, Percutaneous Endoscopic Approach
06UB07Z Supplement Left Renal Vein with Autologous Tissue Substitute, Open Approach
06UB0JZ Supplement Left Renal Vein with Synthetic Substitute, Open Approach
06UB0KZ Supplement Left Renal Vein with Nonautologous Tissue Substitute, Open Approach
06UB37Z Supplement Left Renal Vein with Autologous Tissue Substitute, Percutaneous Approach
06UB3JZ Supplement Left Renal Vein with Synthetic Substitute, Percutaneous Approach
06UB3KZ Supplement Left Renal Vein with Nonautologous Tissue Substitute, Percutaneous Approach
06UB47Z Supplement Left Renal Vein with Autologous Tissue Substitute, Percutaneous Endoscopic Approach
06UB4JZ Supplement Left Renal Vein with Synthetic Substitute, Percutaneous Endoscopic Approach
06UB4KZ Supplement Left Renal Vein with Nonautologous Tissue Substitute, Percutaneous Endoscopic Approach
06UC07Z Supplement Right Common Iliac Vein with Autologous Tissue Substitute, Open Approach
06UC0JZ Supplement Right Common Iliac Vein with Synthetic Substitute, Open Approach
06UC0KZ Supplement Right Common Iliac Vein with Nonautologous Tissue Substitute, Open Approach
06UC37Z Supplement Right Common Iliac Vein with Autologous Tissue Substitute, Percutaneous Approach
06UC3JZ Supplement Right Common Iliac Vein with Synthetic Substitute, Percutaneous Approach
06UC3KZ Supplement Right Common Iliac Vein with Nonautologous Tissue Substitute, Percutaneous Approach
06UC47Z Supplement Right Common Iliac Vein with Autologous Tissue Substitute, Percutaneous Endoscopic Approach
06UC4JZ Supplement Right Common Iliac Vein with Synthetic Substitute, Percutaneous Endoscopic Approach
06UC4KZ Supplement Right Common Iliac Vein with Nonautologous Tissue Substitute, Percutaneous Endoscopic Approach
06UD07Z Supplement Left Common Iliac Vein with Autologous Tissue Substitute, Open Approach
06UD0JZ Supplement Left Common Iliac Vein with Synthetic Substitute, Open Approach
06UD0KZ Supplement Left Common Iliac Vein with Nonautologous Tissue Substitute, Open Approach
06UD37Z Supplement Left Common Iliac Vein with Autologous Tissue Substitute, Percutaneous Approach
06UD3JZ Supplement Left Common Iliac Vein with Synthetic Substitute, Percutaneous Approach
06UD3KZ Supplement Left Common Iliac Vein with Nonautologous Tissue Substitute, Percutaneous Approach
06UD47Z Supplement Left Common Iliac Vein with Autologous Tissue Substitute, Percutaneous Endoscopic Approach
06UD4JZ Supplement Left Common Iliac Vein with Synthetic Substitute, Percutaneous Endoscopic Approach
06UD4KZ Supplement Left Common Iliac Vein with Nonautologous Tissue Substitute, Percutaneous Endoscopic Approach
06UF07Z Supplement Right External Iliac Vein with Autologous Tissue Substitute, Open Approach

UF0JZ Supplement Right External Iliac Vein with Synthetic Substitute, Open Approach
UF0KZ Supplement Right External Iliac Vein with Nonautologous Tissue Substitute, Open Approach
UF37Z Supplement Right External Iliac Vein with Autologous Tissue Substitute, Percutaneous Approach
UF3JZ Supplement Right External Iliac Vein with Synthetic Substitute, Percutaneous Approach
UF3KZ Supplement Right External Iliac Vein with Nonautologous Tissue Substitute, Percutaneous Approach
UF47Z Supplement Right External Iliac Vein with Autologous Tissue Substitute, Percutaneous Endoscopic Approach
UF4JZ Supplement Right External Iliac Vein with Synthetic Substitute, Percutaneous Endoscopic Approach
UF4KZ Supplement Right External Iliac Vein with Nonautologous Tissue Substitute, Percutaneous Endoscopic Approach
UG07Z Supplement Left External Iliac Vein with Autologous Tissue Substitute, Open Approach
UG0JZ Supplement Left External Iliac Vein with Synthetic Substitute, Open Approach
UG0KZ Supplement Left External Iliac Vein with Nonautologous Tissue Substitute, Open Approach
UG37Z Supplement Left External Iliac Vein with Autologous Tissue Substitute, Percutaneous Approach
UG3JZ Supplement Left External Iliac Vein with Synthetic Substitute, Percutaneous Approach
UG3KZ Supplement Left External Iliac Vein with Nonautologous Tissue Substitute, Percutaneous Approach
UG47Z Supplement Left External Iliac Vein with Autologous Tissue Substitute, Percutaneous Endoscopic Approach
UG4JZ Supplement Left External Iliac Vein with Synthetic Substitute, Percutaneous Endoscopic Approach
UG4KZ Supplement Left External Iliac Vein with Nonautologous Tissue Substitute, Percutaneous Endoscopic Approach
UH07Z Supplement Right Hypogastric Vein with Autologous Tissue Substitute, Open Approach
UH0JZ Supplement Right Hypogastric Vein with Synthetic Substitute, Open Approach
UH0KZ Supplement Right Hypogastric Vein with Nonautologous Tissue Substitute, Open Approach
6UH37Z Supplement Right Hypogastric Vein with Autologous Tissue Substitute, Percutaneous Approach
6UH3JZ Supplement Right Hypogastric Vein with Synthetic Substitute, Percutaneous Approach
6UH3KZ Supplement Right Hypogastric Vein with Nonautologous Tissue Substitute, Percutaneous Approach
6UH47Z Supplement Right Hypogastric Vein with Autologous Tissue Substitute, Percutaneous Endoscopic Approach
6UH4JZ Supplement Right Hypogastric Vein with Synthetic Substitute, Percutaneous Endoscopic Approach
6UH4KZ Supplement Right Hypogastric Vein with Nonautologous Tissue Substitute, Percutaneous Endoscopic Approach
6UJ07Z Supplement Left Hypogastric Vein with Autologous Tissue Substitute, Open Approach

06UJ0JZ Supplement Left Hypogastric Vein with Synthetic Substitute, Open Approach
06UJ0KZ Supplement Left Hypogastric Vein with Nonautologous Tissue Substitute, Open Approach
06UJ37Z Supplement Left Hypogastric Vein with Autologous Tissue Substitute, Percutaneous Approach
06UJ3JZ Supplement Left Hypogastric Vein with Synthetic Substitute, Percutaneous Approach
06UJ3KZ Supplement Left Hypogastric Vein with Nonautologous Tissue Substitute, Percutaneous Approach
06UJ47Z Supplement Left Hypogastric Vein with Autologous Tissue Substitute, Percutaneous Endoscopic Approach
06UJ4JZ Supplement Left Hypogastric Vein with Synthetic Substitute, Percutaneous Endoscopic Approach
06UJ4KZ Supplement Left Hypogastric Vein with Nonautologous Tissue Substitute, Percutaneous Endoscopic Approach
06UM07Z Supplement Right Femoral Vein with Autologous Tissue Substitute, Open Approach
06UM0JZ Supplement Right Femoral Vein with Synthetic Substitute, Open Approach
06UM0KZ Supplement Right Femoral Vein with Nonautologous Tissue Substitute, Open Approach
06UM37Z Supplement Right Femoral Vein with Autologous Tissue Substitute, Percutaneous Approach
06UM3JZ Supplement Right Femoral Vein with Synthetic Substitute, Percutaneous Approach
06UM3KZ Supplement Right Femoral Vein with Nonautologous Tissue Substitute, Percutaneous Approach
06UM47Z Supplement Right Femoral Vein with Autologous Tissue Substitute, Percutaneous Endoscopic Approach
06UM4JZ Supplement Right Femoral Vein with Synthetic Substitute, Percutaneous Endoscopic Approach
06UM4KZ Supplement Right Femoral Vein with Nonautologous Tissue Substitute, Percutaneous Endoscopic Approach
06UN07Z Supplement Left Femoral Vein with Autologous Tissue Substitute, Open Approach
06UN0JZ Supplement Left Femoral Vein with Synthetic Substitute, Open Approach
06UN0KZ Supplement Left Femoral Vein with Nonautologous Tissue Substitute, Open Approach
06UN37Z Supplement Left Femoral Vein with Autologous Tissue Substitute, Percutaneous Approach
06UN3JZ Supplement Left Femoral Vein with Synthetic Substitute, Percutaneous Approach
06UN3KZ Supplement Left Femoral Vein with Nonautologous Tissue Substitute, Percutaneous Approach
06UN47Z Supplement Left Femoral Vein with Autologous Tissue Substitute, Percutaneous Endoscopic Approach
06UN4JZ Supplement Left Femoral Vein with Synthetic Substitute, Percutaneous Endoscopic Approach
06UN4KZ Supplement Left Femoral Vein with Nonautologous Tissue Substitute, Percutaneous Endoscopic Approach
06UP07Z Supplement Right Greater Saphenous Vein with Autologous Tissue Substitute, Open Approach

06UP0JZ Supplement Right Greater Saphenous Vein with Synthetic Substitute, Open Approach
06UP0KZ Supplement Right Greater Saphenous Vein with Nonautologous Tissue Substitute, Open Approach
06UP37Z Supplement Right Greater Saphenous Vein with Autologous Tissue Substitute, Percutaneous Approach
06UP3JZ Supplement Right Greater Saphenous Vein with Synthetic Substitute, Percutaneous Approach
06UP3KZ Supplement Right Greater Saphenous Vein with Nonautologous Tissue Substitute, Percutaneous Approach
06UP47Z Supplement Right Greater Saphenous Vein with Autologous Tissue Substitute, Percutaneous Endoscopic Approach
06UP4JZ Supplement Right Greater Saphenous Vein with Synthetic Substitute, Percutaneous Endoscopic Approach
06UP4KZ Supplement Right Greater Saphenous Vein with Nonautologous Tissue Substitute, Percutaneous Endoscopic Approach
06UQ07Z Supplement Left Greater Saphenous Vein with Autologous Tissue Substitute, Open Approach
06UQ0JZ Supplement Left Greater Saphenous Vein with Synthetic Substitute, Open Approach
06UQ0KZ Supplement Left Greater Saphenous Vein with Nonautologous Tissue Substitute, Open Approach
06UQ37Z Supplement Left Greater Saphenous Vein with Autologous Tissue Substitute, Percutaneous Approach
06UQ3JZ Supplement Left Greater Saphenous Vein with Synthetic Substitute, Percutaneous Approach
06UQ3KZ Supplement Left Greater Saphenous Vein with Nonautologous Tissue Substitute, Percutaneous Approach
06UQ47Z Supplement Left Greater Saphenous Vein with Autologous Tissue Substitute, Percutaneous Endoscopic Approach
06UQ4JZ Supplement Left Greater Saphenous Vein with Synthetic Substitute, Percutaneous Endoscopic Approach
06UQ4KZ Supplement Left Greater Saphenous Vein with Nonautologous Tissue Substitute, Percutaneous Endoscopic Approach
06UR07Z Supplement Right Lesser Saphenous Vein with Autologous Tissue Substitute, Open Approach
06UR0JZ Supplement Right Lesser Saphenous Vein with Synthetic Substitute, Open Approach
06UR0KZ Supplement Right Lesser Saphenous Vein with Nonautologous Tissue Substitute, Open Approach
06UR37Z Supplement Right Lesser Saphenous Vein with Autologous Tissue Substitute, Percutaneous Approach
06UR3JZ Supplement Right Lesser Saphenous Vein with Synthetic Substitute, Percutaneous Approach
06UR3KZ Supplement Right Lesser Saphenous Vein with Nonautologous Tissue Substitute, Percutaneous Approach
06UR47Z Supplement Right Lesser Saphenous Vein with Autologous Tissue Substitute, Percutaneous Endoscopic Approach
06UR4JZ Supplement Right Lesser Saphenous Vein with Synthetic Substitute, Percutaneous Endoscopic Approach
06UR4KZ Supplement Right Lesser Saphenous Vein with Nonautologous Tissue Substitute, Percutaneous Endoscopic Approach

06US07Z Supplement Left Lesser Saphenous Vein with Autologous Tissue Substitute, Open Approach
06US0JZ Supplement Left Lesser Saphenous Vein with Synthetic Substitute, Open Approach
06US0KZ Supplement Left Lesser Saphenous Vein with Nonautologous Tissue Substitute, Open Approach
06US37Z Supplement Left Lesser Saphenous Vein with Autologous Tissue Substitute, Percutaneous Approach
06US3JZ Supplement Left Lesser Saphenous Vein with Synthetic Substitute, Percutaneous Approach
06US3KZ Supplement Left Lesser Saphenous Vein with Nonautologous Tissue Substitute, Percutaneous Approach
06US47Z Supplement Left Lesser Saphenous Vein with Autologous Tissue Substitute, Percutaneous Endoscopic Approach
06US4JZ Supplement Left Lesser Saphenous Vein with Synthetic Substitute, Percutaneous Endoscopic Approach
06US4KZ Supplement Left Lesser Saphenous Vein with Nonautologous Tissue Substitute, Percutaneous Endoscopic Approach
06UT07Z Supplement Right Foot Vein with Autologous Tissue Substitute, Open Approach
06UT0JZ Supplement Right Foot Vein with Synthetic Substitute, Open Approach
06UT0KZ Supplement Right Foot Vein with Nonautologous Tissue Substitute, Open Approach
06UT37Z Supplement Right Foot Vein with Autologous Tissue Substitute, Percutaneous Approach
06UT3JZ Supplement Right Foot Vein with Synthetic Substitute, Percutaneous Approach
06UT3KZ Supplement Right Foot Vein with Nonautologous Tissue Substitute, Percutaneous Approach
06UT47Z Supplement Right Foot Vein with Autologous Tissue Substitute, Percutaneous Endoscopic Approach
06UT4JZ Supplement Right Foot Vein with Synthetic Substitute, Percutaneous Endoscopic Approach
06UT4KZ Supplement Right Foot Vein with Nonautologous Tissue Substitute, Percutaneous Endoscopic Approach
06UV07Z Supplement Left Foot Vein with Autologous Tissue Substitute, Open Approach
06UV0JZ Supplement Left Foot Vein with Synthetic Substitute, Open Approach
06UV0KZ Supplement Left Foot Vein with Nonautologous Tissue Substitute, Open Approach
06UV37Z Supplement Left Foot Vein with Autologous Tissue Substitute, Percutaneous Approach
06UV3JZ Supplement Left Foot Vein with Synthetic Substitute, Percutaneous Approach
06UV3KZ Supplement Left Foot Vein with Nonautologous Tissue Substitute, Percutaneous Approach
06UV47Z Supplement Left Foot Vein with Autologous Tissue Substitute, Percutaneous Endoscopic Approach
06UV4JZ Supplement Left Foot Vein with Synthetic Substitute, Percutaneous Endoscopic Approach
06UV4KZ Supplement Left Foot Vein with Nonautologous Tissue Substitute, Percutaneous Endoscopic Approach
06UY07Z Supplement Lower Vein with Autologous Tissue Substitute, Open Approach
06UY0JZ Supplement Lower Vein with Synthetic Substitute, Open Approach
06UY0KZ Supplement Lower Vein with Nonautologous Tissue Substitute, Open Approach
06UY37Z Supplement Lower Vein with Autologous Tissue Substitute, Percutaneous Approach
06UY3JZ Supplement Lower Vein with Synthetic Substitute, Percutaneous Approach
06UY3KZ Supplement Lower Vein with Nonautologous Tissue Substitute, Percutaneous Approach
06UY47Z Supplement Lower Vein with Autologous Tissue Substitute, Percutaneous Endoscopic Approach
06UY4JZ Supplement Lower Vein with Synthetic Substitute, Percutaneous Endoscopic Approach
06UY4KZ Supplement Lower Vein with Nonautologous Tissue Substitute, Percutaneous Endoscopic Approach

06V – Lower Veins, Restriction

Review Coding Guideline B3.12

06V00CZ Restriction of Inferior Vena Cava with Extraluminal Device, Open Approach
06V00DZ Restriction of Inferior Vena Cava with Intraluminal Device, Open Approach
06V00ZZ Restriction of Inferior Vena Cava, Open Approach
06V03CZ Restriction of Inferior Vena Cava with Extraluminal Device, Percutaneous Approach
06V03DZ Restriction of Inferior Vena Cava with Intraluminal Device, Percutaneous Approach
06V03ZZ Restriction of Inferior Vena Cava, Percutaneous Approach
06V04CZ Restriction of Inferior Vena Cava with Extraluminal Device, Percutaneous Endoscopic Approach
06V04DZ Restriction of Inferior Vena Cava with Intraluminal Device, Percutaneous Endoscopic Approach
06V04ZZ Restriction of Inferior Vena Cava, Percutaneous Endoscopic Approach
06V10CZ Restriction of Splenic Vein with Extraluminal Device, Open Approach
06V10DZ Restriction of Splenic Vein with Intraluminal Device, Open Approach
06V10ZZ Restriction of Splenic Vein, Open Approach
06V13CZ Restriction of Splenic Vein with Extraluminal Device, Percutaneous Approach
06V13DZ Restriction of Splenic Vein with Intraluminal Device, Percutaneous Approach
06V13ZZ Restriction of Splenic Vein, Percutaneous Approach
06V14CZ Restriction of Splenic Vein with Extraluminal Device, Percutaneous Endoscopic Approach
06V14DZ Restriction of Splenic Vein with Intraluminal Device, Percutaneous Endoscopic Approach
06V14ZZ Restriction of Splenic Vein, Percutaneous Endoscopic Approach
06V20CZ Restriction of Gastric Vein with Extraluminal Device, Open Approach
06V20DZ Restriction of Gastric Vein with Intraluminal Device, Open Approach
06V20ZZ Restriction of Gastric Vein, Open Approach
06V23CZ Restriction of Gastric Vein with Extraluminal Device, Percutaneous Approach
06V23DZ Restriction of Gastric Vein with Intraluminal Device, Percutaneous Approach
06V23ZZ Restriction of Gastric Vein, Percutaneous Approach
06V24CZ Restriction of Gastric Vein with Extraluminal Device, Percutaneous Endoscopic Approach
06V24DZ Restriction of Gastric Vein with Intraluminal Device, Percutaneous Endoscopic Approach
06V24ZZ Restriction of Gastric Vein, Percutaneous Endoscopic Approach
06V30CZ Restriction of Esophageal Vein with Extraluminal Device, Open Approach
06V30DZ Restriction of Esophageal Vein with Intraluminal Device, Open Approach
06V30ZZ Restriction of Esophageal Vein, Open Approach
06V33CZ Restriction of Esophageal Vein with Extraluminal Device, Percutaneous Approach
06V33DZ Restriction of Esophageal Vein with Intraluminal Device, Percutaneous Approach
06V33ZZ Restriction of Esophageal Vein, Percutaneous Approach
06V34CZ Restriction of Esophageal Vein with Extraluminal Device, Percutaneous Endoscopic Approach
06V34DZ Restriction of Esophageal Vein with Intraluminal Device, Percutaneous Endoscopic Approach
06V34ZZ Restriction of Esophageal Vein, Percutaneous Endoscopic Approach
06V40CZ Restriction of Hepatic Vein with Extraluminal Device, Open Approach
06V40DZ Restriction of Hepatic Vein with Intraluminal Device, Open Approach
06V40ZZ Restriction of Hepatic Vein, Open Approach
06V43CZ Restriction of Hepatic Vein with Extraluminal Device, Percutaneous Approach
06V43DZ Restriction of Hepatic Vein with Intraluminal Device, Percutaneous Approach
06V43ZZ Restriction of Hepatic Vein, Percutaneous Approach
06V44CZ Restriction of Hepatic Vein with Extraluminal Device, Percutaneous Endoscopic Approach
06V44DZ Restriction of Hepatic Vein with Intraluminal Device, Percutaneous Endoscopic Approach

V44ZZ Restriction of Hepatic Vein, Percutaneous Endoscopic Approach
V50CZ Restriction of Superior Mesenteric Vein with Extraluminal Device, Open Approach
V50DZ Restriction of Superior Mesenteric Vein with Intraluminal Device, Open Approach
V50ZZ Restriction of Superior Mesenteric Vein, Open Approach
V53CZ Restriction of Superior Mesenteric Vein with Extraluminal Device, Percutaneous Approach
V53DZ Restriction of Superior Mesenteric Vein with Intraluminal Device, Percutaneous Approach
V53ZZ Restriction of Superior Mesenteric Vein, Percutaneous Approach
V54CZ Restriction of Superior Mesenteric Vein with Extraluminal Device, Percutaneous Endoscopic Approach
V54DZ Restriction of Superior Mesenteric Vein with Intraluminal Device, Percutaneous Endoscopic Approach
V54ZZ Restriction of Superior Mesenteric Vein, Percutaneous Endoscopic Approach
V60CZ Restriction of Inferior Mesenteric Vein with Extraluminal Device, Open Approach
V60DZ Restriction of Inferior Mesenteric Vein with Intraluminal Device, Open Approach
V60ZZ Restriction of Inferior Mesenteric Vein, Open Approach
V63CZ Restriction of Inferior Mesenteric Vein with Extraluminal Device, Percutaneous Approach
V63DZ Restriction of Inferior Mesenteric Vein with Intraluminal Device, Percutaneous Approach
V63ZZ Restriction of Inferior Mesenteric Vein, Percutaneous Approach
V64CZ Restriction of Inferior Mesenteric Vein with Extraluminal Device, Percutaneous Endoscopic Approach
V64DZ Restriction of Inferior Mesenteric Vein with Intraluminal Device, Percutaneous Endoscopic Approach
V64ZZ Restriction of Inferior Mesenteric Vein, Percutaneous Endoscopic Approach
V70CZ Restriction of Colic Vein with Extraluminal Device, Open Approach
5V70DZ Restriction of Colic Vein with Intraluminal Device, Open Approach
5V70ZZ Restriction of Colic Vein, Open Approach
5V73CZ Restriction of Colic Vein with Extraluminal Device, Percutaneous Approach
5V73DZ Restriction of Colic Vein with Intraluminal Device, Percutaneous Approach
6V73ZZ Restriction of Colic Vein, Percutaneous Approach
6V74CZ Restriction of Colic Vein with Extraluminal Device, Percutaneous Endoscopic Approach
6V74DZ Restriction of Colic Vein with Intraluminal Device, Percutaneous Endoscopic Approach
6V74ZZ Restriction of Colic Vein, Percutaneous Endoscopic Approach
6V80CZ Restriction of Portal Vein with Extraluminal Device, Open Approach
6V80DZ Restriction of Portal Vein with Intraluminal Device, Open Approach
6V80ZZ Restriction of Portal Vein, Open Approach
6V83CZ Restriction of Portal Vein with Extraluminal Device, Percutaneous Approach
6V83DZ Restriction of Portal Vein with Intraluminal Device, Percutaneous Approach
06V83ZZ Restriction of Portal Vein, Percutaneous Approach
06V84CZ Restriction of Portal Vein with Extraluminal Device, Percutaneous Endoscopic Approach
06V84DZ Restriction of Portal Vein with Intraluminal Device, Percutaneous Endoscopic Approach
06V84ZZ Restriction of Portal Vein, Percutaneous Endoscopic Approach
06V90CZ Restriction of Right Renal Vein with Extraluminal Device, Open Approach
06V90DZ Restriction of Right Renal Vein with Intraluminal Device, Open Approach
06V90ZZ Restriction of Right Renal Vein, Open Approach
06V93CZ Restriction of Right Renal Vein with Extraluminal Device, Percutaneous Approach
06V93DZ Restriction of Right Renal Vein with Intraluminal Device, Percutaneous Approach
06V93ZZ Restriction of Right Renal Vein, Percutaneous Approach
06V94CZ Restriction of Right Renal Vein with Extraluminal Device, Percutaneous Endoscopic Approach
06V94DZ Restriction of Right Renal Vein with Intraluminal Device, Percutaneous Endoscopic Approach
06V94ZZ Restriction of Right Renal Vein, Percutaneous Endoscopic Approach
06VB0CZ Restriction of Left Renal Vein with Extraluminal Device, Open Approach
06VB0DZ Restriction of Left Renal Vein with Intraluminal Device, Open Approach
06VB0ZZ Restriction of Left Renal Vein, Open Approach
06VB3CZ Restriction of Left Renal Vein with Extraluminal Device, Percutaneous Approach
06VB3DZ Restriction of Left Renal Vein with Intraluminal Device, Percutaneous Approach
06VB3ZZ Restriction of Left Renal Vein, Percutaneous Approach
06VB4CZ Restriction of Left Renal Vein with Extraluminal Device, Percutaneous Endoscopic Approach
06VB4DZ Restriction of Left Renal Vein with Intraluminal Device, Percutaneous Endoscopic Approach
06VB4ZZ Restriction of Left Renal Vein, Percutaneous Endoscopic Approach
06VC0CZ Restriction of Right Common Iliac Vein with Extraluminal Device, Open Approach
06VC0DZ Restriction of Right Common Iliac Vein with Intraluminal Device, Open Approach
06VC0ZZ Restriction of Right Common Iliac Vein, Open Approach
06VC3CZ Restriction of Right Common Iliac Vein with Extraluminal Device, Percutaneous Approach
06VC3DZ Restriction of Right Common Iliac Vein with Intraluminal Device, Percutaneous Approach
06VC3ZZ Restriction of Right Common Iliac Vein, Percutaneous Approach
06VC4CZ Restriction of Right Common Iliac Vein with Extraluminal Device, Percutaneous Endoscopic Approach
06VC4DZ Restriction of Right Common Iliac Vein with Intraluminal Device, Percutaneous Endoscopic Approach
06VC4ZZ Restriction of Right Common Iliac Vein, Percutaneous Endoscopic Approach
06VD0CZ Restriction of Left Common Iliac Vein with Extraluminal Device, Open Approach
06VD0DZ Restriction of Left Common Iliac Vein with Intraluminal Device, Open Approach
06VD0ZZ Restriction of Left Common Iliac Vein, Open Approach
06VD3CZ Restriction of Left Common Iliac Vein with Extraluminal Device, Percutaneous Approach
06VD3DZ Restriction of Left Common Iliac Vein with Intraluminal Device, Percutaneous Approach
06VD3ZZ Restriction of Left Common Iliac Vein, Percutaneous Approach
06VD4CZ Restriction of Left Common Iliac Vein with Extraluminal Device, Percutaneous Endoscopic Approach
06VD4DZ Restriction of Left Common Iliac Vein with Intraluminal Device, Percutaneous Endoscopic Approach
06VD4ZZ Restriction of Left Common Iliac Vein, Percutaneous Endoscopic Approach
06VF0CZ Restriction of Right External Iliac Vein with Extraluminal Device, Open Approach
06VF0DZ Restriction of Right External Iliac Vein with Intraluminal Device, Open Approach
06VF0ZZ Restriction of Right External Iliac Vein, Open Approach
06VF3CZ Restriction of Right External Iliac Vein with Extraluminal Device, Percutaneous Approach
06VF3DZ Restriction of Right External Iliac Vein with Intraluminal Device, Percutaneous Approach
06VF3ZZ Restriction of Right External Iliac Vein, Percutaneous Approach
06VF4CZ Restriction of Right External Iliac Vein with Extraluminal Device, Percutaneous Endoscopic Approach
06VF4DZ Restriction of Right External Iliac Vein with Intraluminal Device, Percutaneous Endoscopic Approach
06VF4ZZ Restriction of Right External Iliac Vein, Percutaneous Endoscopic Approach
06VG0CZ Restriction of Left External Iliac Vein with Extraluminal Device, Open Approach
06VG0DZ Restriction of Left External Iliac Vein with Intraluminal Device, Open Approach
06VG0ZZ Restriction of Left External Iliac Vein, Open Approach
06VG3CZ Restriction of Left External Iliac Vein with Extraluminal Device, Percutaneous Approach
06VG3DZ Restriction of Left External Iliac Vein with Intraluminal Device, Percutaneous Approach
06VG3ZZ Restriction of Left External Iliac Vein, Percutaneous Approach
06VG4CZ Restriction of Left External Iliac Vein with Extraluminal Device, Percutaneous Endoscopic Approach
06VG4DZ Restriction of Left External Iliac Vein with Intraluminal Device, Percutaneous Endoscopic Approach
06VG4ZZ Restriction of Left External Iliac Vein, Percutaneous Endoscopic Approach
06VH0CZ Restriction of Right Hypogastric Vein with Extraluminal Device, Open Approach
06VH0DZ Restriction of Right Hypogastric Vein with Intraluminal Device, Open Approach
06VH0ZZ Restriction of Right Hypogastric Vein, Open Approach
06VH3CZ Restriction of Right Hypogastric Vein with Extraluminal Device, Percutaneous Approach
06VH3DZ Restriction of Right Hypogastric Vein with Intraluminal Device, Percutaneous Approach
06VH3ZZ Restriction of Right Hypogastric Vein, Percutaneous Approach

06VH4CZ Restriction of Right Hypogastric Vein with Extraluminal Device, Percutaneous Endoscopic Approach
06VH4DZ Restriction of Right Hypogastric Vein with Intraluminal Device, Percutaneous Endoscopic Approach
06VH4ZZ Restriction of Right Hypogastric Vein, Percutaneous Endoscopic Approach
06VJ0CZ Restriction of Left Hypogastric Vein with Extraluminal Device, Open Approach
06VJ0DZ Restriction of Left Hypogastric Vein with Intraluminal Device, Open Approach
06VJ0ZZ Restriction of Left Hypogastric Vein, Open Approach
06VJ3CZ Restriction of Left Hypogastric Vein with Extraluminal Device, Percutaneous Approach
06VJ3DZ Restriction of Left Hypogastric Vein with Intraluminal Device, Percutaneous Approach
06VJ3ZZ Restriction of Left Hypogastric Vein, Percutaneous Approach
06VJ4CZ Restriction of Left Hypogastric Vein with Extraluminal Device, Percutaneous Endoscopic Approach
06VJ4DZ Restriction of Left Hypogastric Vein with Intraluminal Device, Percutaneous Endoscopic Approach
06VJ4ZZ Restriction of Left Hypogastric Vein, Percutaneous Endoscopic Approach
06VM0CZ Restriction of Right Femoral Vein with Extraluminal Device, Open Approach
06VM0DZ Restriction of Right Femoral Vein with Intraluminal Device, Open Approach
06VM0ZZ Restriction of Right Femoral Vein, Open Approach
06VM3CZ Restriction of Right Femoral Vein with Extraluminal Device, Percutaneous Approach
06VM3DZ Restriction of Right Femoral Vein with Intraluminal Device, Percutaneous Approach
06VM3ZZ Restriction of Right Femoral Vein, Percutaneous Approach
06VM4CZ Restriction of Right Femoral Vein with Extraluminal Device, Percutaneous Endoscopic Approach
06VM4DZ Restriction of Right Femoral Vein with Intraluminal Device, Percutaneous Endoscopic Approach
06VM4ZZ Restriction of Right Femoral Vein, Percutaneous Endoscopic Approach
06VN0CZ Restriction of Left Femoral Vein with Extraluminal Device, Open Approach
06VN0DZ Restriction of Left Femoral Vein with Intraluminal Device, Open Approach
06VN0ZZ Restriction of Left Femoral Vein, Open Approach
06VN3CZ Restriction of Left Femoral Vein with Extraluminal Device, Percutaneous Approach
06VN3DZ Restriction of Left Femoral Vein with Intraluminal Device, Percutaneous Approach
06VN3ZZ Restriction of Left Femoral Vein, Percutaneous Approach
06VN4CZ Restriction of Left Femoral Vein with Extraluminal Device, Percutaneous Endoscopic Approach
06VN4DZ Restriction of Left Femoral Vein with Intraluminal Device, Percutaneous Endoscopic Approach
06VN4ZZ Restriction of Left Femoral Vein, Percutaneous Endoscopic Approach
06VP0CZ Restriction of Right Greater Saphenous Vein with Extraluminal Device, Open Approach
06VP0DZ Restriction of Right Greater Saphenous Vein with Intraluminal Device, Open Approach
06VP0ZZ Restriction of Right Greater Saphenous Vein, Open Approach
06VP3CZ Restriction of Right Greater Saphenous Vein with Extraluminal Device, Percutaneous Approach
06VP3DZ Restriction of Right Greater Saphenous Vein with Intraluminal Device, Percutaneous Approach
06VP3ZZ Restriction of Right Greater Saphenous Vein, Percutaneous Approach
06VP4CZ Restriction of Right Greater Saphenous Vein with Extraluminal Device, Percutaneous Endoscopic Approach
06VP4DZ Restriction of Right Greater Saphenous Vein with Intraluminal Device, Percutaneous Endoscopic Approach
06VP4ZZ Restriction of Right Greater Saphenous Vein, Percutaneous Endoscopic Approach
06VQ0CZ Restriction of Left Greater Saphenous Vein with Extraluminal Device, Open Approach
06VQ0DZ Restriction of Left Greater Saphenous Vein with Intraluminal Device, Open Approach
06VQ0ZZ Restriction of Left Greater Saphenous Vein, Open Approach
06VQ3CZ Restriction of Left Greater Saphenous Vein with Extraluminal Device, Percutaneous Approach
06VQ3DZ Restriction of Left Greater Saphenous Vein with Intraluminal Device, Percutaneous Approach
06VQ3ZZ Restriction of Left Greater Saphenous Vein, Percutaneous Approach
06VQ4CZ Restriction of Left Greater Saphenous Vein with Extraluminal Device, Percutaneous Endoscopic Approach
06VQ4DZ Restriction of Left Greater Saphenous Vein with Intraluminal Device, Percutaneous Endoscopic Approach
06VQ4ZZ Restriction of Left Greater Saphenous Vein, Percutaneous Endoscopic Approach
06VR0CZ Restriction of Right Lesser Saphenous Vein with Extraluminal Device, Open Approach
06VR0DZ Restriction of Right Lesser Saphenous Vein with Intraluminal Device, Open Approach
06VR0ZZ Restriction of Right Lesser Saphenous Vein, Open Approach
06VR3CZ Restriction of Right Lesser Saphenous Vein with Extraluminal Device, Percutaneous Approach
06VR3DZ Restriction of Right Lesser Saphenous Vein with Intraluminal Device, Percutaneous Approach
06VR3ZZ Restriction of Right Lesser Saphenous Vein, Percutaneous Approach
06VR4CZ Restriction of Right Lesser Saphenous Vein with Extraluminal Device, Percutaneous Endoscopic Approach
06VR4DZ Restriction of Right Lesser Saphenous Vein with Intraluminal Device, Percutaneous Endoscopic Approach
06VR4ZZ Restriction of Right Lesser Saphenous Vein, Percutaneous Endoscopic Approach
06VS0CZ Restriction of Left Lesser Saphenous Vein with Extraluminal Device, Open Approach
06VS0DZ Restriction of Left Lesser Saphenous Vein with Intraluminal Device, Open Approach
06VS0ZZ Restriction of Left Lesser Saphenous Ve[illegible] Open Approach
06VS3CZ Restriction of Left Lesser Saphenous Ve[illegible] with Extraluminal Device, Percutaneous Approach
06VS3DZ Restriction of Left Lesser Saphenous Ve[illegible] with Intraluminal Device, Percutaneous Approach
06VS3ZZ Restriction of Left Lesser Saphenous Ve[illegible] Percutaneous Approach
06VS4CZ Restriction of Left Lesser Saphenous Ve[illegible] with Extraluminal Device, Percutaneous Endoscopic Approach
06VS4DZ Restriction of Left Lesser Saphenous Ve[illegible] with Intraluminal Device, Percutaneous Endoscopic Approach
06VS4ZZ Restriction of Left Lesser Saphenous Vein, Percutaneous Endoscopic Approach
06VT0CZ Restriction of Right Foot Vein with Extraluminal Device, Open Approach
06VT0DZ Restriction of Right Foot Vein with Intraluminal Device, Open Approach
06VT0ZZ Restriction of Right Foot Vein, Open Approach
06VT3CZ Restriction of Right Foot Vein with Extraluminal Device, Percutaneous Approach
06VT3DZ Restriction of Right Foot Vein with Intraluminal Device, Percutaneous Approach
06VT3ZZ Restriction of Right Foot Vein, Percutaneous Approach
06VT4CZ Restriction of Right Foot Vein with Extraluminal Device, Percutaneous Endoscopic Approach
06VT4DZ Restriction of Right Foot Vein with Intraluminal Device, Percutaneous Endoscopic Approach
06VT4ZZ Restriction of Right Foot Vein, Percutaneous Endoscopic Approach
06VV0CZ Restriction of Left Foot Vein with Extraluminal Device, Open Approach
06VV0DZ Restriction of Left Foot Vein with Intraluminal Device, Open Approach
06VV0ZZ Restriction of Left Foot Vein, Open Approach
06VV3CZ Restriction of Left Foot Vein with Extraluminal Device, Percutaneous Approach
06VV3DZ Restriction of Left Foot Vein with Intraluminal Device, Percutaneous Approach
06VV3ZZ Restriction of Left Foot Vein, Percutaneous Approach
06VV4CZ Restriction of Left Foot Vein with Extraluminal Device, Percutaneous Endoscopic Approach
06VV4DZ Restriction of Left Foot Vein with Intraluminal Device, Percutaneous Endoscopic Approach
06VV4ZZ Restriction of Left Foot Vein, Percutaneous Endoscopic Approach
06VY0CZ Restriction of Lower Vein with Extraluminal Device, Open Approach
06VY0DZ Restriction of Lower Vein with Intraluminal Device, Open Approach
06VY0ZZ Restriction of Lower Vein, Open Approach
06VY3CZ Restriction of Lower Vein with Extraluminal Device, Percutaneous Approach
06VY3DZ Restriction of Lower Vein with Intraluminal Device, Percutaneous Approach
06VY3ZZ Restriction of Lower Vein, Percutaneous Approach

VY4CZ Restriction of Lower Vein with Extraluminal Device, Percutaneous Endoscopic Approach

06VY4DZ Restriction of Lower Vein with Intraluminal Device, Percutaneous Endoscopic Approach

06VY4ZZ Restriction of Lower Vein, Percutaneous Endoscopic Approach

5W – Lower Veins, Revision

eview Coding Guideline B6.1c

WY00Z Revision of Drainage Device in Lower Vein, Open Approach

WY02Z Revision of Monitoring Device in Lower Vein, Open Approach

WY03Z Revision of Infusion Device in Lower Vein, Open Approach

WY07Z Revision of Autologous Tissue Substitute in Lower Vein, Open Approach

WY0CZ Revision of Extraluminal Device in Lower Vein, Open Approach

WY0DZ Revision of Intraluminal Device in Lower Vein, Open Approach

WY0JZ Revision of Synthetic Substitute in Lower Vein, Open Approach

WY0KZ Revision of Nonautologous Tissue Substitute in Lower Vein, Open Approach

WY30Z Revision of Drainage Device in Lower Vein, Percutaneous Approach

WY32Z Revision of Monitoring Device in Lower Vein, Percutaneous Approach

WY33Z Revision of Infusion Device in Lower Vein, Percutaneous Approach

WY37Z Revision of Autologous Tissue Substitute in Lower Vein, Percutaneous Approach

06WY3CZ Revision of Extraluminal Device in Lower Vein, Percutaneous Approach

06WY3DZ Revision of Intraluminal Device in Lower Vein, Percutaneous Approach

06WY3JZ Revision of Synthetic Substitute in Lower Vein, Percutaneous Approach

06WY3KZ Revision of Nonautologous Tissue Substitute in Lower Vein, Percutaneous Approach

06WY40Z Revision of Drainage Device in Lower Vein, Percutaneous Endoscopic Approach

06WY42Z Revision of Monitoring Device in Lower Vein, Percutaneous Endoscopic Approach

06WY43Z Revision of Infusion Device in Lower Vein, Percutaneous Endoscopic Approach

06WY47Z Revision of Autologous Tissue Substitute in Lower Vein, Percutaneous Endoscopic Approach

06WY4CZ Revision of Extraluminal Device in Lower Vein, Percutaneous Endoscopic Approach

06WY4DZ Revision of Intraluminal Device in Lower Vein, Percutaneous Endoscopic Approach

06WY4JZ Revision of Synthetic Substitute in Lower Vein, Percutaneous Endoscopic Approach

06WY4KZ Revision of Nonautologous Tissue Substitute in Lower Vein, Percutaneous Endoscopic Approach

06WYX0Z Revision of Drainage Device in Lower Vein, External Approach

06WYX2Z Revision of Monitoring Device in Lower Vein, External Approach

06WYX3Z Revision of Infusion Device in Lower Vein, External Approach

06WYX7Z Revision of Autologous Tissue Substitute in Lower Vein, External Approach

06WYXCZ Revision of Extraluminal Device in Lower Vein, External Approach

06WYXDZ Revision of Intraluminal Device in Lower Vein, External Approach

06WYXJZ Revision of Synthetic Substitute in Lower Vein, External Approach

06WYXKZ Revision of Nonautologous Tissue Substitute in Lower Vein, External Approach

Lymphatic System

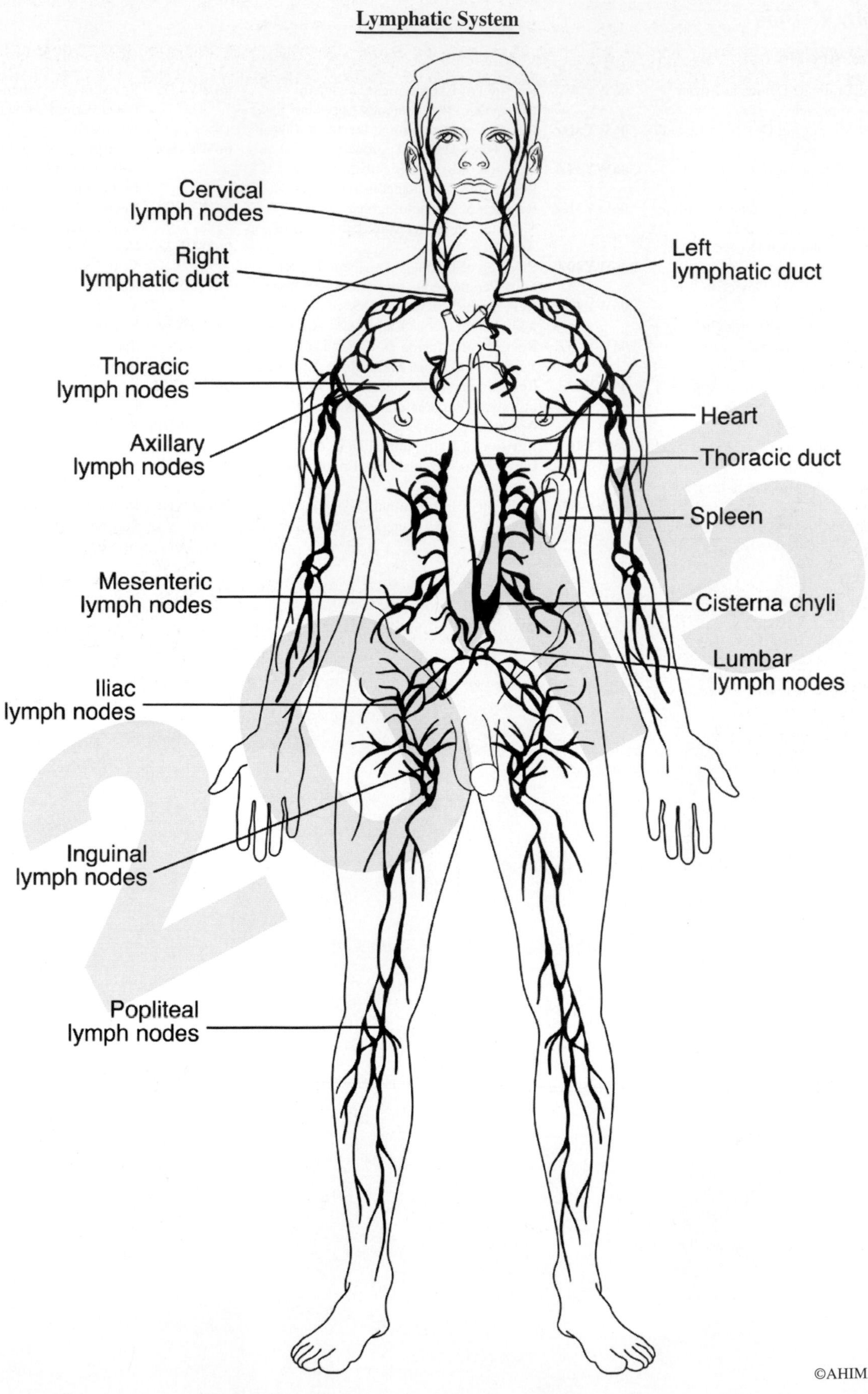
Cervical
lymph nodes
Right
lymphatic duct
Left
lymphatic duct
Thoracic
lymph nodes
Axillary
lymph nodes
Heart
Thoracic duct
Spleen
Mesenteric
lymph nodes
Cisterna chyli
Lumbar
lymph nodes
Iliac
lymph nodes
Inguinal
lymph nodes
Popliteal
lymph nodes
2015
©AHIMA

ction 0 **Medical and Surgical**
ody System 7 **Lymphatic and Hemic Systems**
peration 2 **Change:** Taking out or off a device from a body part and putting back an identical or similar device in or on the same body part without cutting or puncturing the skin or a mucous membrane

Body Part (4th)	Approach (5th)	Device (6th)	Qualifier (7th)
K Thoracic Duct **L** Cisterna Chyli **M** Thymus **N** Lymphatic **P** Spleen **T** Bone Marrow	**X** External	**0** Drainage Device **Y** Other Device	**Z** No Qualifier

ection 0 **Medical and Surgical**
ody System 7 **Lymphatic and Hemic Systems**
peration 5 **Destruction:** Physical eradication of all or a portion of a body part by the direct use of energy, force, or a destructive agent

Body Part (4th)	Approach (5th)	Device (6th)	Qualifier (7th)
0 Lymphatic, Head **1** Lymphatic, Right Neck **2** Lymphatic, Left Neck **3** Lymphatic, Right Upper Extremity **4** Lymphatic, Left Upper Extremity **5** Lymphatic, Right Axillary **6** Lymphatic, Left Axillary **7** Lymphatic, Thorax **8** Lymphatic, Internal Mammary, Right **9** Lymphatic, Internal Mammary, Left **B** Lymphatic, Mesenteric **C** Lymphatic, Pelvis **D** Lymphatic, Aortic **F** Lymphatic, Right Lower Extremity **G** Lymphatic, Left Lower Extremity **H** Lymphatic, Right Inguinal **J** Lymphatic, Left Inguinal **K** Thoracic Duct **L** Cisterna Chyli **M** Thymus **P** Spleen	**0** Open **3** Percutaneous **4** Percutaneous Endoscopic	**Z** No Device	**Z** No Qualifier

Section **0** **Medical and Surgical**
Body System **7** **Lymphatic and Hemic Systems**
Operation **9** **Drainage:** Taking or letting out fluids and/or gases from a body part

Body Part (4th)	Approach (5th)	Device (6th)	Qualifier (7th)
0 Lymphatic, Head **1** Lymphatic, Right Neck **2** Lymphatic, Left Neck **3** Lymphatic, Right Upper Extremity **4** Lymphatic, Left Upper Extremity **5** Lymphatic, Right Axillary **6** Lymphatic, Left Axillary **7** Lymphatic, Thorax **8** Lymphatic, Internal Mammary, Right **9** Lymphatic, Internal Mammary, Left **B** Lymphatic, Mesenteric **C** Lymphatic, Pelvis **D** Lymphatic, Aortic **F** Lymphatic, Right Lower Extremity **G** Lymphatic, Left Lower Extremity **H** Lymphatic, Right Inguinal **J** Lymphatic, Left Inguinal **K** Thoracic Duct **L** Cisterna Chyli **M** Thymus **P** Spleen **T** Bone Marrow	**0** Open **3** Percutaneous **4** Percutaneous Endoscopic	**0** Drainage Device	**Z** No Qualifier
0 Lymphatic, Head **1** Lymphatic, Right Neck **2** Lymphatic, Left Neck **3** Lymphatic, Right Upper Extremity **4** Lymphatic, Left Upper Extremity **5** Lymphatic, Right Axillary **6** Lymphatic, Left Axillary **7** Lymphatic, Thorax **8** Lymphatic, Internal Mammary, Right **9** Lymphatic, Internal Mammary, Left **B** Lymphatic, Mesenteric **C** Lymphatic, Pelvis **D** Lymphatic, Aortic **F** Lymphatic, Right Lower Extremity **G** Lymphatic, Left Lower Extremity **H** Lymphatic, Right Inguinal **J** Lymphatic, Left Inguinal **K** Thoracic Duct **L** Cisterna Chyli **M** Thymus **P** Spleen **T** Bone Marrow	**0** Open **3** Percutaneous **4** Percutaneous Endoscopic	**Z** No Device	**X** Diagnostic **Z** No Qualifier

ection 0 **Medical and Surgical**
dy System 7 **Lymphatic and Hemic Systems**
peration B **Excision:** Cutting out or off, without replacement, a portion of a body part

Body Part (4th)	Approach (5th)	Device (6th)	Qualifier (7th)
0 Lymphatic, Head	0 Open	Z No Device	X Diagnostic
1 Lymphatic, Right Neck	3 Percutaneous		Z No Qualifier
2 Lymphatic, Left Neck	4 Percutaneous Endoscopic		
3 Lymphatic, Right Upper Extremity			
4 Lymphatic, Left Upper Extremity			
5 Lymphatic, Right Axillary			
6 Lymphatic, Left Axillary			
7 Lymphatic, Thorax			
8 Lymphatic, Internal Mammary, Right			
9 Lymphatic, Internal Mammary, Left			
B Lymphatic, Mesenteric			
C Lymphatic, Pelvis			
D Lymphatic, Aortic			
F Lymphatic, Right Lower Extremity			
G Lymphatic, Left Lower Extremity			
H Lymphatic, Right Inguinal			
J Lymphatic, Left Inguinal			
K Thoracic Duct			
L Cisterna Chyli			
M Thymus			
P Spleen			

ection 0 **Medical and Surgical**
ody System 7 **Lymphatic and Hemic Systems**
peration C **Extirpation:** Taking or cutting out solid matter from a body part

Body Part (4th)	Approach (5th)	Device (6th)	Qualifier (7th)
0 Lymphatic, Head	0 Open	Z No Device	Z No Qualifier
1 Lymphatic, Right Neck	3 Percutaneous		
2 Lymphatic, Left Neck	4 Percutaneous Endoscopic		
3 Lymphatic, Right Upper Extremity			
4 Lymphatic, Left Upper Extremity			
5 Lymphatic, Right Axillary			
6 Lymphatic, Left Axillary			
7 Lymphatic, Thorax			
8 Lymphatic, Internal Mammary, Right			
9 Lymphatic, Internal Mammary, Left			
B Lymphatic, Mesenteric			
C Lymphatic, Pelvis			
D Lymphatic, Aortic			
F Lymphatic, Right Lower Extremity			
G Lymphatic, Left Lower Extremity			
H Lymphatic, Right Inguinal			
J Lymphatic, Left Inguinal			
K Thoracic Duct			
L Cisterna Chyli			
M Thymus			
P Spleen			

Section 0 **Medical and Surgical**
Body System 7 **Lymphatic and Hemic Systems**
Operation D **Extraction:** Pulling or stripping out or off all or a portion of a body part by the use of force

Body Part (4th)	Approach (5th)	Device (6th)	Qualifier (7th)
Q Bone Marrow, Sternum	0 Open	Z No Device	X Diagnostic
R Bone Marrow, Iliac	3 Percutaneous		Z No Qualifier
S Bone Marrow, Vertebral			

Section 0 **Medical and Surgical**
Body System 7 **Lymphatic and Hemic Systems**
Operation H **Insertion:** Putting in a nonbiological appliance that monitors, assists, performs, or prevents a physiological function but does not physically take the place of a body part

Body Part (4th)	Approach (5th)	Device (6th)	Qualifier (7th)
K Thoracic Duct **L** Cisterna Chyli **M** Thymus **N** Lymphatic **P** Spleen	**0** Open **3** Percutaneous **4** Percutaneous Endoscopic	**3** Infusion Device	**Z** No Qualifier

Section 0 **Medical and Surgical**
Body System 7 **Lymphatic and Hemic Systems**
Operation J **Inspection:** Visually and/or manually exploring a body part

Body Part (4th)	Approach (5th)	Device (6th)	Qualifier (7th)
K Thoracic Duct **L** Cisterna Chyli **M** Thymus **T** Bone Marrow	**0** Open **3** Percutaneous **4** Percutaneous Endoscopic	**Z** No Device	**Z** No Qualifier
N Lymphatic **P** Spleen	**0** Open **3** Percutaneous **4** Percutaneous Endoscopic **X** External	**Z** No Device	**Z** No Qualifier

Section 0 **Medical and Surgical**
Body System 7 **Lymphatic and Hemic Systems**
Operation L **Occlusion:** Completely closing an orifice or the lumen of a tubular body part

Body Part (4th)	Approach (5th)	Device (6th)	Qualifier (7th)
0 Lymphatic, Head **1** Lymphatic, Right Neck **2** Lymphatic, Left Neck **3** Lymphatic, Right Upper Extremity **4** Lymphatic, Left Upper Extremity **5** Lymphatic, Right Axillary **6** Lymphatic, Left Axillary **7** Lymphatic, Thorax **8** Lymphatic, Internal Mammary, Right **9** Lymphatic, Internal Mammary, Left **B** Lymphatic, Mesenteric **C** Lymphatic, Pelvis **D** Lymphatic, Aortic **F** Lymphatic, Right Lower Extremity **G** Lymphatic, Left Lower Extremity **H** Lymphatic, Right Inguinal **J** Lymphatic, Left Inguinal **K** Thoracic Duct **L** Cisterna Chyli	**0** Open **3** Percutaneous **4** Percutaneous Endoscopic	**C** Extraluminal Device **D** Intraluminal Device **Z** No Device	**Z** No Qualifier

Section 0 Medical and Surgical
Body System 7 Lymphatic and Hemic Systems
Operation N **Release:** Freeing a body part from an abnormal physical constraint by cutting or by the use of force

Body Part (4th)	Approach (5th)	Device (6th)	Qualifier (7th)
0 Lymphatic, Head **1** Lymphatic, Right Neck **2** Lymphatic, Left Neck **3** Lymphatic, Right Upper Extremity **4** Lymphatic, Left Upper Extremity **5** Lymphatic, Right Axillary **6** Lymphatic, Left Axillary **7** Lymphatic, Thorax **8** Lymphatic, Internal Mammary, Right **9** Lymphatic, Internal Mammary, Left **B** Lymphatic, Mesenteric **C** Lymphatic, Pelvis **D** Lymphatic, Aortic **F** Lymphatic, Right Lower Extremity **G** Lymphatic, Left Lower Extremity **H** Lymphatic, Right Inguinal **J** Lymphatic, Left Inguinal **K** Thoracic Duct **L** Cisterna Chyli **M** Thymus **P** Spleen	**0** Open **3** Percutaneous **4** Percutaneous Endoscopic	**Z** No Device	**Z** No Qualifier

Section 0 Medical and Surgical
Body System 7 Lymphatic and Hemic Systems
Operation P **Removal:** Taking out or off a device from a body part

Body Part (4th)	Approach (5th)	Device (6th)	Qualifier (7th)
K Thoracic Duct **L** Cisterna Chyli **N** Lymphatic	**0** Open **3** Percutaneous **4** Percutaneous Endoscopic	**0** Drainage Device **3** Infusion Device **7** Autologous Tissue Substitute **C** Extraluminal Device **D** Intraluminal Device **J** Synthetic Substitute **K** Nonautologous Tissue Substitute	**Z** No Qualifier
K Thoracic Duct **L** Cisterna Chyli **N** Lymphatic	**X** External	**0** Drainage Device **3** Infusion Device **D** Intraluminal Device	**Z** No Qualifier
M Thymus **P** Spleen	**0** Open **3** Percutaneous **4** Percutaneous Endoscopic **X** External	**0** Drainage Device **3** Infusion Device	**Z** No Qualifier
T Bone Marrow	**0** Open **3** Percutaneous **4** Percutaneous Endoscopic **X** External	**0** Drainage Device	**Z** No Qualifier

Section 0 **Medical and Surgical**
Body System 7 **Lymphatic and Hemic Systems**
Operation Q **Repair:** Restoring, to the extent possible, a body part to its normal anatomic structure and function

Body Part (4th)	Approach (5th)	Device (6th)	Qualifier (7th)
0 Lymphatic, Head **1** Lymphatic, Right Neck **2** Lymphatic, Left Neck **3** Lymphatic, Right Upper Extremity **4** Lymphatic, Left Upper Extremity **5** Lymphatic, Right Axillary **6** Lymphatic, Left Axillary **7** Lymphatic, Thorax **8** Lymphatic, Internal Mammary, Right **9** Lymphatic, Internal Mammary, Left **B** Lymphatic, Mesenteric **C** Lymphatic, Pelvis **D** Lymphatic, Aortic **F** Lymphatic, Right Lower Extremity **G** Lymphatic, Left Lower Extremity **H** Lymphatic, Right Inguinal **J** Lymphatic, Left Inguinal **K** Thoracic Duct **L** Cisterna Chyli **M** Thymus **P** Spleen	**0** Open **3** Percutaneous **4** Percutaneous Endoscopic	**Z** No Device	**Z** No Qualifier

Section 0 **Medical and Surgical**
Body System 7 **Lymphatic and Hemic Systems**
Operation S **Reposition:** Moving to its normal location, or other suitable location, all or a portion of a body part

Body Part (4th)	Approach (5th)	Device (6th)	Qualifier (7th)
M Thymus **P** Spleen	**0** Open	**Z** No Device	**Z** No Qualifier

Section 0 **Medical and Surgical**
Body System 7 **Lymphatic and Hemic Systems**
Operation T **Resection:** Cutting out or off, without replacement, all of a body part

Body Part (4th)	Approach (5th)	Device (6th)	Qualifier (7th)
0 Lymphatic, Head **1** Lymphatic, Right Neck **2** Lymphatic, Left Neck **3** Lymphatic, Right Upper Extremity **4** Lymphatic, Left Upper Extremity **5** Lymphatic, Right Axillary **6** Lymphatic, Left Axillary **7** Lymphatic, Thorax **8** Lymphatic, Internal Mammary, Right **9** Lymphatic, Internal Mammary, Left **B** Lymphatic, Mesenteric **C** Lymphatic, Pelvis **D** Lymphatic, Aortic **F** Lymphatic, Right Lower Extremity **G** Lymphatic, Left Lower Extremity **H** Lymphatic, Right Inguinal **J** Lymphatic, Left Inguinal **K** Thoracic Duct **L** Cisterna Chyli **M** Thymus **P** Spleen	**0** Open **4** Percutaneous Endoscopic	**Z** No Device	**Z** No Qualifier

Section 0 **Medical and Surgical**
Body System 7 **Lymphatic and Hemic Systems**
Operation U **Supplement:** Putting in or on biological or synthetic material that physically reinforces and/or augments the function of a portion of a body part

Body Part (4th)	Approach (5th)	Device (6th)	Qualifier (7th)
0 Lymphatic, Head **1** Lymphatic, Right Neck **2** Lymphatic, Left Neck **3** Lymphatic, Right Upper Extremity **4** Lymphatic, Left Upper Extremity **5** Lymphatic, Right Axillary **6** Lymphatic, Left Axillary **7** Lymphatic, Thorax **8** Lymphatic, Internal Mammary, Right **9** Lymphatic, Internal Mammary, Left **B** Lymphatic, Mesenteric **C** Lymphatic, Pelvis **D** Lymphatic, Aortic **F** Lymphatic, Right Lower Extremity **G** Lymphatic, Left Lower Extremity **H** Lymphatic, Right Inguinal **J** Lymphatic, Left Inguinal **K** Thoracic Duct **L** Cisterna Chyli	**0** Open **4** Percutaneous Endoscopic	**7** Autologous Tissue Substitute **J** Synthetic Substitute **K** Nonautologous Tissue Substitute	**Z** No Qualifier

Section 0 **Medical and Surgical**
Body System 7 **Lymphatic and Hemic Systems**
Operation V **Restriction:** Partially closing an orifice or the lumen of a tubular body part

Body Part (4th)	Approach (5th)	Device (6th)	Qualifier (7th)
0 Lymphatic, Head **1** Lymphatic, Right Neck **2** Lymphatic, Left Neck **3** Lymphatic, Right Upper Extremity **4** Lymphatic, Left Upper Extremity **5** Lymphatic, Right Axillary **6** Lymphatic, Left Axillary **7** Lymphatic, Thorax **8** Lymphatic, Internal Mammary, Right **9** Lymphatic, Internal Mammary, Left **B** Lymphatic, Mesenteric **C** Lymphatic, Pelvis **D** Lymphatic, Aortic **F** Lymphatic, Right Lower Extremity **G** Lymphatic, Left Lower Extremity **H** Lymphatic, Right Inguinal **J** Lymphatic, Left Inguinal **K** Thoracic Duct **L** Cisterna Chyli	**0** Open **3** Percutaneous **4** Percutaneous Endoscopic	**C** Extraluminal Device **D** Intraluminal Device **Z** No Device	**Z** No Qualifier

Section 0 **Medical and Surgical**
Body System 7 **Lymphatic and Hemic Systems**
Operation W **Revision:** Correcting, to the extent possible, a portion of a malfunctioning device or the position of a displaced device

Body Part (4th)	Approach (5th)	Device (6th)	Qualifier (7th)
K Thoracic Duct **L** Cisterna Chyli **N** Lymphatic	**0** Open **3** Percutaneous **4** Percutaneous Endoscopic **X** External	**0** Drainage Device **3** Infusion Device **7** Autologous Tissue Substitute **C** Extraluminal Device **D** Intraluminal Device **J** Synthetic Substitute **K** Nonautologous Tissue Substitute	**Z** No Qualifier

Continued →

Section 0 **Medical and Surgical**
Body System 7 **Lymphatic and Hemic Systems**
Operation W **Revision:** Correcting, to the extent possible, a portion of a malfunctioning device or the position of a displaced device

Body Part (4th)	Approach (5th)	Device (6th)	Qualifier (7th)
M Thymus **P** Spleen	**0** Open **3** Percutaneous **4** Percutaneous Endoscopic **X** External	**0** Drainage Device **3** Infusion Device	**Z** No Qualifier
T Bone Marrow	**0** Open **3** Percutaneous **4** Percutaneous Endoscopic **X** External	**0** Drainage Device	**Z** No Qualifier

Section 0 **Medical and Surgical**
Body System 7 **Lymphatic and Hemic Systems**
Operation Y **Transplantation:** Putting in or on all or a portion of a living body part taken from another individual or animal to physically take the place and/or function of all or a portion of a similar body part

Body Part (4th)	Approach (5th)	Device (6th)	Qualifier (7th)
M Thymus **P** Spleen	**0** Open	**Z** No Device	**0** Allogeneic **1** Syngeneic **2** Zooplastic

Lymphatic and Hemic Systems Code Listing 072–07Y

072 – Lymphatic and Hemic Systems, Change

Review Coding Guideline B6.1c

072KX0Z Change Drainage Device in Thoracic Duct, External Approach
072KXYZ Change Other Device in Thoracic Duct, External Approach
072LX0Z Change Drainage Device in Cisterna Chyli, External Approach
072LXYZ Change Other Device in Cisterna Chyli, External Approach
072MX0Z Change Drainage Device in Thymus, External Approach
072MXYZ Change Other Device in Thymus, External Approach
072NX0Z Change Drainage Device in Lymphatic, External Approach
072NXYZ Change Other Device in Lymphatic, External Approach
072PX0Z Change Drainage Device in Spleen, External Approach
072PXYZ Change Other Device in Spleen, External Approach
072TX0Z Change Drainage Device in Bone Marrow, External Approach
072TXYZ Change Other Device in Bone Marrow, External Approach

075 – Lymphatic and Hemic Systems, Destruction

07500ZZ Destruction of Head Lymphatic, Open Approach
07503ZZ Destruction of Head Lymphatic, Percutaneous Approach
07504ZZ Destruction of Head Lymphatic, Percutaneous Endoscopic Approach
07510ZZ Destruction of Right Neck Lymphatic, Open Approach
07513ZZ Destruction of Right Neck Lymphatic, Percutaneous Approach
07514ZZ Destruction of Right Neck Lymphatic, Percutaneous Endoscopic Approach
07520ZZ Destruction of Left Neck Lymphatic, Open Approach
07523ZZ Destruction of Left Neck Lymphatic, Percutaneous Approach
07524ZZ Destruction of Left Neck Lymphatic, Percutaneous Endoscopic Approach
07530ZZ Destruction of Right Upper Extremity Lymphatic, Open Approach
07533ZZ Destruction of Right Upper Extremity Lymphatic, Percutaneous Approach
07534ZZ Destruction of Right Upper Extremity Lymphatic, Percutaneous Endoscopic Approach
07540ZZ Destruction of Left Upper Extremity Lymphatic, Open Approach
07543ZZ Destruction of Left Upper Extremity Lymphatic, Percutaneous Approach
07544ZZ Destruction of Left Upper Extremity Lymphatic, Percutaneous Endoscopic Approach
07550ZZ Destruction of Right Axillary Lymphatic, Open Approach
07553ZZ Destruction of Right Axillary Lymphatic, Percutaneous Approach
07554ZZ Destruction of Right Axillary Lymphatic, Percutaneous Endoscopic Approach
07560ZZ Destruction of Left Axillary Lymphatic, Open Approach
07563ZZ Destruction of Left Axillary Lymphatic, Percutaneous Approach
07564ZZ Destruction of Left Axillary Lymphatic, Percutaneous Endoscopic Approach
07570ZZ Destruction of Thorax Lymphatic, Open Approach
07573ZZ Destruction of Thorax Lymphatic, Percutaneous Approach
07574ZZ Destruction of Thorax Lymphatic, Percutaneous Endoscopic Approach
07580ZZ Destruction of Right Internal Mammary Lymphatic, Open Approach
07583ZZ Destruction of Right Internal Mammary Lymphatic, Percutaneous Approach
07584ZZ Destruction of Right Internal Mammary Lymphatic, Percutaneous Endoscopic Approach
07590ZZ Destruction of Left Internal Mammary Lymphatic, Open Approach
07593ZZ Destruction of Left Internal Mammary Lymphatic, Percutaneous Approach
07594ZZ Destruction of Left Internal Mammary Lymphatic, Percutaneous Endoscopic Approach
075B0ZZ Destruction of Mesenteric Lymphatic, Open Approach
075B3ZZ Destruction of Mesenteric Lymphatic, Percutaneous Approach
075B4ZZ Destruction of Mesenteric Lymphatic, Percutaneous Endoscopic Approach
075C0ZZ Destruction of Pelvis Lymphatic, Open Approach
075C3ZZ Destruction of Pelvis Lymphatic, Percutaneous Approach

5C4ZZ Destruction of Pelvis Lymphatic, Percutaneous Endoscopic Approach
5D0ZZ Destruction of Aortic Lymphatic, Open Approach
5D3ZZ Destruction of Aortic Lymphatic, Percutaneous Approach
5D4ZZ Destruction of Aortic Lymphatic, Percutaneous Endoscopic Approach
5F0ZZ Destruction of Right Lower Extremity Lymphatic, Open Approach
5F3ZZ Destruction of Right Lower Extremity Lymphatic, Percutaneous Approach
5F4ZZ Destruction of Right Lower Extremity Lymphatic, Percutaneous Endoscopic Approach
5G0ZZ Destruction of Left Lower Extremity Lymphatic, Open Approach
5G3ZZ Destruction of Left Lower Extremity Lymphatic, Percutaneous Approach
075G4ZZ Destruction of Left Lower Extremity Lymphatic, Percutaneous Endoscopic Approach
075H0ZZ Destruction of Right Inguinal Lymphatic, Open Approach
075H3ZZ Destruction of Right Inguinal Lymphatic, Percutaneous Approach
075H4ZZ Destruction of Right Inguinal Lymphatic, Percutaneous Endoscopic Approach
075J0ZZ Destruction of Left Inguinal Lymphatic, Open Approach
075J3ZZ Destruction of Left Inguinal Lymphatic, Percutaneous Approach
075J4ZZ Destruction of Left Inguinal Lymphatic, Percutaneous Endoscopic Approach
075K0ZZ Destruction of Thoracic Duct, Open Approach
075K3ZZ Destruction of Thoracic Duct, Percutaneous Approach
075K4ZZ Destruction of Thoracic Duct, Percutaneous Endoscopic Approach
075L0ZZ Destruction of Cisterna Chyli, Open Approach
075L3ZZ Destruction of Cisterna Chyli, Percutaneous Approach
075L4ZZ Destruction of Cisterna Chyli, Percutaneous Endoscopic Approach
075M0ZZ Destruction of Thymus, Open Approach
075M3ZZ Destruction of Thymus, Percutaneous Approach
075M4ZZ Destruction of Thymus, Percutaneous Endoscopic Approach
075P0ZZ Destruction of Spleen, Open Approach
075P3ZZ Destruction of Spleen, Percutaneous Approach
075P4ZZ Destruction of Spleen, Percutaneous Endoscopic Approach

79 – Lymphatic and Hemic Systems, Drainage

eview Coding Guidelines B3.4a and B3.4b

eview Coding Guideline B6.2

79000Z Drainage of Head Lymphatic with Drainage Device, Open Approach
7900ZX Drainage of Head Lymphatic, Open Approach, Diagnostic
7900ZZ Drainage of Head Lymphatic, Open Approach
79030Z Drainage of Head Lymphatic with Drainage Device, Percutaneous Approach
7903ZX Drainage of Head Lymphatic, Percutaneous Approach, Diagnostic
7903ZZ Drainage of Head Lymphatic, Percutaneous Approach
79040Z Drainage of Head Lymphatic with Drainage Device, Percutaneous Endoscopic Approach
7904ZX Drainage of Head Lymphatic, Percutaneous Endoscopic Approach, Diagnostic
7904ZZ Drainage of Head Lymphatic, Percutaneous Endoscopic Approach
79100Z Drainage of Right Neck Lymphatic with Drainage Device, Open Approach
7910ZX Drainage of Right Neck Lymphatic, Open Approach, Diagnostic
7910ZZ Drainage of Right Neck Lymphatic, Open Approach
79130Z Drainage of Right Neck Lymphatic with Drainage Device, Percutaneous Approach
7913ZX Drainage of Right Neck Lymphatic, Percutaneous Approach, Diagnostic
7913ZZ Drainage of Right Neck Lymphatic, Percutaneous Approach
79140Z Drainage of Right Neck Lymphatic with Drainage Device, Percutaneous Endoscopic Approach
7914ZX Drainage of Right Neck Lymphatic, Percutaneous Endoscopic Approach, Diagnostic
07914ZZ Drainage of Right Neck Lymphatic, Percutaneous Endoscopic Approach
079200Z Drainage of Left Neck Lymphatic with Drainage Device, Open Approach
07920ZX Drainage of Left Neck Lymphatic, Open Approach, Diagnostic
07920ZZ Drainage of Left Neck Lymphatic, Open Approach
079230Z Drainage of Left Neck Lymphatic with Drainage Device, Percutaneous Approach
07923ZX Drainage of Left Neck Lymphatic, Percutaneous Approach, Diagnostic
07923ZZ Drainage of Left Neck Lymphatic, Percutaneous Approach
079240Z Drainage of Left Neck Lymphatic with Drainage Device, Percutaneous Endoscopic Approach
07924ZX Drainage of Left Neck Lymphatic, Percutaneous Endoscopic Approach, Diagnostic
07924ZZ Drainage of Left Neck Lymphatic, Percutaneous Endoscopic Approach
079300Z Drainage of Right Upper Extremity Lymphatic with Drainage Device, Open Approach
07930ZX Drainage of Right Upper Extremity Lymphatic, Open Approach, Diagnostic
07930ZZ Drainage of Right Upper Extremity Lymphatic, Open Approach
079330Z Drainage of Right Upper Extremity Lymphatic with Drainage Device, Percutaneous Approach
07933ZX Drainage of Right Upper Extremity Lymphatic, Percutaneous Approach, Diagnostic
07933ZZ Drainage of Right Upper Extremity Lymphatic, Percutaneous Approach
079340Z Drainage of Right Upper Extremity Lymphatic with Drainage Device, Percutaneous Endoscopic Approach
07934ZX Drainage of Right Upper Extremity Lymphatic, Percutaneous Endoscopic Approach, Diagnostic
07934ZZ Drainage of Right Upper Extremity Lymphatic, Percutaneous Endoscopic Approach
079400Z Drainage of Left Upper Extremity Lymphatic with Drainage Device, Open Approach
07940ZX Drainage of Left Upper Extremity Lymphatic, Open Approach, Diagnostic
07940ZZ Drainage of Left Upper Extremity Lymphatic, Open Approach
079430Z Drainage of Left Upper Extremity Lymphatic with Drainage Device, Percutaneous Approach
07943ZX Drainage of Left Upper Extremity Lymphatic, Percutaneous Approach, Diagnostic
07943ZZ Drainage of Left Upper Extremity Lymphatic, Percutaneous Approach
079440Z Drainage of Left Upper Extremity Lymphatic with Drainage Device, Percutaneous Endoscopic Approach
07944ZX Drainage of Left Upper Extremity Lymphatic, Percutaneous Endoscopic Approach, Diagnostic
07944ZZ Drainage of Left Upper Extremity Lymphatic, Percutaneous Endoscopic Approach
079500Z Drainage of Right Axillary Lymphatic with Drainage Device, Open Approach
07950ZX Drainage of Right Axillary Lymphatic, Open Approach, Diagnostic
07950ZZ Drainage of Right Axillary Lymphatic, Open Approach
079530Z Drainage of Right Axillary Lymphatic with Drainage Device, Percutaneous Approach
07953ZX Drainage of Right Axillary Lymphatic, Percutaneous Approach, Diagnostic
07953ZZ Drainage of Right Axillary Lymphatic, Percutaneous Approach
079540Z Drainage of Right Axillary Lymphatic with Drainage Device, Percutaneous Endoscopic Approach
07954ZX Drainage of Right Axillary Lymphatic, Percutaneous Endoscopic Approach, Diagnostic
07954ZZ Drainage of Right Axillary Lymphatic, Percutaneous Endoscopic Approach
079600Z Drainage of Left Axillary Lymphatic with Drainage Device, Open Approach
07960ZX Drainage of Left Axillary Lymphatic, Open Approach, Diagnostic
07960ZZ Drainage of Left Axillary Lymphatic, Open Approach
079630Z Drainage of Left Axillary Lymphatic with Drainage Device, Percutaneous Approach
07963ZX Drainage of Left Axillary Lymphatic, Percutaneous Approach, Diagnostic
07963ZZ Drainage of Left Axillary Lymphatic, Percutaneous Approach
079640Z Drainage of Left Axillary Lymphatic with Drainage Device, Percutaneous Endoscopic Approach
07964ZX Drainage of Left Axillary Lymphatic, Percutaneous Endoscopic Approach, Diagnostic
07964ZZ Drainage of Left Axillary Lymphatic, Percutaneous Endoscopic Approach

079700Z Drainage of Thorax Lymphatic with Drainage Device, Open Approach

07970ZX Drainage of Thorax Lymphatic, Open Approach, Diagnostic

07970ZZ Drainage of Thorax Lymphatic, Open Approach

079730Z Drainage of Thorax Lymphatic with Drainage Device, Percutaneous Approach

07973ZX Drainage of Thorax Lymphatic, Percutaneous Approach, Diagnostic

07973ZZ Drainage of Thorax Lymphatic, Percutaneous Approach

079740Z Drainage of Thorax Lymphatic with Drainage Device, Percutaneous Endoscopic Approach

07974ZX Drainage of Thorax Lymphatic, Percutaneous Endoscopic Approach, Diagnostic

AHA CC: 4Q, 2013, 111-112

07974ZZ Drainage of Thorax Lymphatic, Percutaneous Endoscopic Approach

079800Z Drainage of Right Internal Mammary Lymphatic with Drainage Device, Open Approach

07980ZX Drainage of Right Internal Mammary Lymphatic, Open Approach, Diagnostic

07980ZZ Drainage of Right Internal Mammary Lymphatic, Open Approach

079830Z Drainage of Right Internal Mammary Lymphatic with Drainage Device, Percutaneous Approach

07983ZX Drainage of Right Internal Mammary Lymphatic, Percutaneous Approach, Diagnostic

07983ZZ Drainage of Right Internal Mammary Lymphatic, Percutaneous Approach

079840Z Drainage of Right Internal Mammary Lymphatic with Drainage Device, Percutaneous Endoscopic Approach

07984ZX Drainage of Right Internal Mammary Lymphatic, Percutaneous Endoscopic Approach, Diagnostic

07984ZZ Drainage of Right Internal Mammary Lymphatic, Percutaneous Endoscopic Approach

079900Z Drainage of Left Internal Mammary Lymphatic with Drainage Device, Open Approach

07990ZX Drainage of Left Internal Mammary Lymphatic, Open Approach, Diagnostic

07990ZZ Drainage of Left Internal Mammary Lymphatic, Open Approach

079930Z Drainage of Left Internal Mammary Lymphatic with Drainage Device, Percutaneous Approach

07993ZX Drainage of Left Internal Mammary Lymphatic, Percutaneous Approach, Diagnostic

07993ZZ Drainage of Left Internal Mammary Lymphatic, Percutaneous Approach

079940Z Drainage of Left Internal Mammary Lymphatic with Drainage Device, Percutaneous Endoscopic Approach

07994ZX Drainage of Left Internal Mammary Lymphatic, Percutaneous Endoscopic Approach, Diagnostic

07994ZZ Drainage of Left Internal Mammary Lymphatic, Percutaneous Endoscopic Approach

079B00Z Drainage of Mesenteric Lymphatic with Drainage Device, Open Approach

079B0ZX Drainage of Mesenteric Lymphatic, Open Approach, Diagnostic

079B0ZZ Drainage of Mesenteric Lymphatic, Open Approach

079B30Z Drainage of Mesenteric Lymphatic with Drainage Device, Percutaneous Approach

079B3ZX Drainage of Mesenteric Lymphatic, Percutaneous Approach, Diagnostic

079B3ZZ Drainage of Mesenteric Lymphatic, Percutaneous Approach

079B40Z Drainage of Mesenteric Lymphatic with Drainage Device, Percutaneous Endoscopic Approach

079B4ZX Drainage of Mesenteric Lymphatic, Percutaneous Endoscopic Approach, Diagnostic

079B4ZZ Drainage of Mesenteric Lymphatic, Percutaneous Endoscopic Approach

079C00Z Drainage of Pelvis Lymphatic with Drainage Device, Open Approach

079C0ZX Drainage of Pelvis Lymphatic, Open Approach, Diagnostic

079C0ZZ Drainage of Pelvis Lymphatic, Open Approach

079C30Z Drainage of Pelvis Lymphatic with Drainage Device, Percutaneous Approach

079C3ZX Drainage of Pelvis Lymphatic, Percutaneous Approach, Diagnostic

079C3ZZ Drainage of Pelvis Lymphatic, Percutaneous Approach

079C40Z Drainage of Pelvis Lymphatic with Drainage Device, Percutaneous Endoscopic Approach

079C4ZX Drainage of Pelvis Lymphatic, Percutaneous Endoscopic Approach, Diagnostic

079C4ZZ Drainage of Pelvis Lymphatic, Percutaneous Endoscopic Approach

079D00Z Drainage of Aortic Lymphatic with Drainage Device, Open Approach

079D0ZX Drainage of Aortic Lymphatic, Open Approach, Diagnostic

079D0ZZ Drainage of Aortic Lymphatic, Open Approach

079D30Z Drainage of Aortic Lymphatic with Drainage Device, Percutaneous Approach

079D3ZX Drainage of Aortic Lymphatic, Percutaneous Approach, Diagnostic

079D3ZZ Drainage of Aortic Lymphatic, Percutaneous Approach

079D40Z Drainage of Aortic Lymphatic with Drainage Device, Percutaneous Endoscopic Approach

079D4ZX Drainage of Aortic Lymphatic, Percutaneous Endoscopic Approach, Diagnostic

079D4ZZ Drainage of Aortic Lymphatic, Percutaneous Endoscopic Approach

079F00Z Drainage of Right Lower Extremity Lymphatic with Drainage Device, Open Approach

079F0ZX Drainage of Right Lower Extremity Lymphatic, Open Approach, Diagnostic

079F0ZZ Drainage of Right Lower Extremity Lymphatic, Open Approach

079F30Z Drainage of Right Lower Extremity Lymphatic with Drainage Device, Percutaneous Approach

079F3ZX Drainage of Right Lower Extremity Lymphatic, Percutaneous Approach, Diagnostic

079F3ZZ Drainage of Right Lower Extremity Lymphatic, Percutaneous Approach

079F40Z Drainage of Right Lower Extremity Lymphatic with Drainage Device, Percutaneous Endoscopic Approach

079F4ZX Drainage of Right Lower Extremity Lymphatic, Percutaneous Endoscopic Approach, Diagnostic

079F4ZZ Drainage of Right Lower Extremity Lymphatic, Percutaneous Endoscopic Approach

079G00Z Drainage of Left Lower Extremity Lymphatic with Drainage Device, Open Approach

079G0ZX Drainage of Left Lower Extremity Lymphatic, Open Approach, Diagnostic

079G0ZZ Drainage of Left Lower Extremity Lymphatic, Open Approach

079G30Z Drainage of Left Lower Extremity Lymphatic with Drainage Device, Percutaneous Approach

079G3ZX Drainage of Left Lower Extremity Lymphatic, Percutaneous Approach, Diagnostic

079G3ZZ Drainage of Left Lower Extremity Lymphatic, Percutaneous Approach

079G40Z Drainage of Left Lower Extremity Lymphatic with Drainage Device, Percutaneous Endoscopic Approach

079G4ZX Drainage of Left Lower Extremity Lymphatic, Percutaneous Endoscopic Approach, Diagnostic

079G4ZZ Drainage of Left Lower Extremity Lymphatic, Percutaneous Endoscopic Approach

079H00Z Drainage of Right Inguinal Lymphatic with Drainage Device, Open Approach

079H0ZX Drainage of Right Inguinal Lymphatic, Open Approach, Diagnostic

079H0ZZ Drainage of Right Inguinal Lymphatic, Open Approach

079H30Z Drainage of Right Inguinal Lymphatic with Drainage Device, Percutaneous Approach

079H3ZX Drainage of Right Inguinal Lymphatic, Percutaneous Approach, Diagnostic

079H3ZZ Drainage of Right Inguinal Lymphatic, Percutaneous Approach

079H40Z Drainage of Right Inguinal Lymphatic with Drainage Device, Percutaneous Endoscopic Approach

079H4ZX Drainage of Right Inguinal Lymphatic, Percutaneous Endoscopic Approach, Diagnostic

079H4ZZ Drainage of Right Inguinal Lymphatic, Percutaneous Endoscopic Approach

079J00Z Drainage of Left Inguinal Lymphatic with Drainage Device, Open Approach

079J0ZX Drainage of Left Inguinal Lymphatic, Open Approach, Diagnostic

079J0ZZ Drainage of Left Inguinal Lymphatic, Open Approach

079J30Z Drainage of Left Inguinal Lymphatic with Drainage Device, Percutaneous Approach

079J3ZX Drainage of Left Inguinal Lymphatic, Percutaneous Approach, Diagnostic

079J3ZZ Drainage of Left Inguinal Lymphatic, Percutaneous Approach

079J40Z Drainage of Left Inguinal Lymphatic with Drainage Device, Percutaneous Endoscopic Approach

079J4ZX Drainage of Left Inguinal Lymphatic, Percutaneous Endoscopic Approach, Diagnostic

079J4ZZ Drainage of Left Inguinal Lymphatic, Percutaneous Endoscopic Approach

079K00Z Drainage of Thoracic Duct with Drainage Device, Open Approach

079K0ZX Drainage of Thoracic Duct, Open Approach, Diagnostic

079K0ZZ Drainage of Thoracic Duct, Open Approach

9K30Z Drainage of Thoracic Duct with Drainage Device, Percutaneous Approach
9K3ZX Drainage of Thoracic Duct, Percutaneous Approach, Diagnostic
9K3ZZ Drainage of Thoracic Duct, Percutaneous Approach
9K40Z Drainage of Thoracic Duct with Drainage Device, Percutaneous Endoscopic Approach
9K4ZX Drainage of Thoracic Duct, Percutaneous Endoscopic Approach, Diagnostic
9K4ZZ Drainage of Thoracic Duct, Percutaneous Endoscopic Approach
9L00Z Drainage of Cisterna Chyli with Drainage Device, Open Approach
9L0ZX Drainage of Cisterna Chyli, Open Approach, Diagnostic
9L0ZZ Drainage of Cisterna Chyli, Open Approach
9L30Z Drainage of Cisterna Chyli with Drainage Device, Percutaneous Approach
9L3ZX Drainage of Cisterna Chyli, Percutaneous Approach, Diagnostic
9L3ZZ Drainage of Cisterna Chyli, Percutaneous Approach
9L40Z Drainage of Cisterna Chyli with Drainage Device, Percutaneous Endoscopic Approach
9L4ZX Drainage of Cisterna Chyli, Percutaneous Endoscopic Approach, Diagnostic

079L4ZZ Drainage of Cisterna Chyli, Percutaneous Endoscopic Approach
079M00Z Drainage of Thymus with Drainage Device, Open Approach
079M0ZX Drainage of Thymus, Open Approach, Diagnostic
079M0ZZ Drainage of Thymus, Open Approach
079M30Z Drainage of Thymus with Drainage Device, Percutaneous Approach
079M3ZX Drainage of Thymus, Percutaneous Approach, Diagnostic
079M3ZZ Drainage of Thymus, Percutaneous Approach
079M40Z Drainage of Thymus with Drainage Device, Percutaneous Endoscopic Approach
079M4ZX Drainage of Thymus, Percutaneous Endoscopic Approach, Diagnostic
079M4ZZ Drainage of Thymus, Percutaneous Endoscopic Approach
079P00Z Drainage of Spleen with Drainage Device, Open Approach
079P0ZX Drainage of Spleen, Open Approach, Diagnostic
079P0ZZ Drainage of Spleen, Open Approach
079P30Z Drainage of Spleen with Drainage Device, Percutaneous Approach
079P3ZX Drainage of Spleen, Percutaneous Approach, Diagnostic
079P3ZZ Drainage of Spleen, Percutaneous Approach
079P40Z Drainage of Spleen with Drainage Device, Percutaneous Endoscopic Approach
079P4ZX Drainage of Spleen, Percutaneous Endoscopic Approach, Diagnostic
079P4ZZ Drainage of Spleen, Percutaneous Endoscopic Approach
079T00Z Drainage of Bone Marrow with Drainage Device, Open Approach
079T0ZX Drainage of Bone Marrow, Open Approach, Diagnostic
079T0ZZ Drainage of Bone Marrow, Open Approach
079T30Z Drainage of Bone Marrow with Drainage Device, Percutaneous Approach
079T3ZX Drainage of Bone Marrow, Percutaneous Approach, Diagnostic
079T3ZZ Drainage of Bone Marrow, Percutaneous Approach
079T40Z Drainage of Bone Marrow with Drainage Device, Percutaneous Endoscopic Approach
079T4ZX Drainage of Bone Marrow, Percutaneous Endoscopic Approach, Diagnostic
079T4ZZ Drainage of Bone Marrow, Percutaneous Endoscopic Approach

7B – Lymphatic and Hemic Systems, Excision

eview Coding Guidelines B3.4a and B3.4b

eview Coding Guideline B3.8

7B00ZX Excision of Head Lymphatic, Open Approach, Diagnostic
7B00ZZ Excision of Head Lymphatic, Open Approach
7B03ZX Excision of Head Lymphatic, Percutaneous Approach, Diagnostic
7B03ZZ Excision of Head Lymphatic, Percutaneous Approach
7B04ZX Excision of Head Lymphatic, Percutaneous Endoscopic Approach, Diagnostic
7B04ZZ Excision of Head Lymphatic, Percutaneous Endoscopic Approach
7B10ZX Excision of Right Neck Lymphatic, Open Approach, Diagnostic
7B10ZZ Excision of Right Neck Lymphatic, Open Approach
7B13ZX Excision of Right Neck Lymphatic, Percutaneous Approach, Diagnostic
7B13ZZ Excision of Right Neck Lymphatic, Percutaneous Approach
7B14ZX Excision of Right Neck Lymphatic, Percutaneous Endoscopic Approach, Diagnostic
7B14ZZ Excision of Right Neck Lymphatic, Percutaneous Endoscopic Approach
7B20ZX Excision of Left Neck Lymphatic, Open Approach, Diagnostic
7B20ZZ Excision of Left Neck Lymphatic, Open Approach
7B23ZX Excision of Left Neck Lymphatic, Percutaneous Approach, Diagnostic
)7B23ZZ Excision of Left Neck Lymphatic, Percutaneous Approach
)7B24ZX Excision of Left Neck Lymphatic, Percutaneous Endoscopic Approach, Diagnostic
07B24ZZ Excision of Left Neck Lymphatic, Percutaneous Endoscopic Approach
07B30ZX Excision of Right Upper Extremity Lymphatic, Open Approach, Diagnostic
07B30ZZ Excision of Right Upper Extremity Lymphatic, Open Approach
07B33ZX Excision of Right Upper Extremity Lymphatic, Percutaneous Approach, Diagnostic
07B33ZZ Excision of Right Upper Extremity Lymphatic, Percutaneous Approach
07B34ZX Excision of Right Upper Extremity Lymphatic, Percutaneous Endoscopic Approach, Diagnostic
07B34ZZ Excision of Right Upper Extremity Lymphatic, Percutaneous Endoscopic Approach
07B40ZX Excision of Left Upper Extremity Lymphatic, Open Approach, Diagnostic
07B40ZZ Excision of Left Upper Extremity Lymphatic, Open Approach
07B43ZX Excision of Left Upper Extremity Lymphatic, Percutaneous Approach, Diagnostic
07B43ZZ Excision of Left Upper Extremity Lymphatic, Percutaneous Approach
07B44ZX Excision of Left Upper Extremity Lymphatic, Percutaneous Endoscopic Approach, Diagnostic
07B44ZZ Excision of Left Upper Extremity Lymphatic, Percutaneous Endoscopic Approach
07B50ZX Excision of Right Axillary Lymphatic, Open Approach, Diagnostic
07B50ZZ Excision of Right Axillary Lymphatic, Open Approach
07B53ZX Excision of Right Axillary Lymphatic, Percutaneous Approach, Diagnostic
07B53ZZ Excision of Right Axillary Lymphatic, Percutaneous Approach
07B54ZX Excision of Right Axillary Lymphatic, Percutaneous Endoscopic Approach, Diagnostic
07B54ZZ Excision of Right Axillary Lymphatic, Percutaneous Endoscopic Approach
07B60ZX Excision of Left Axillary Lymphatic, Open Approach, Diagnostic
07B60ZZ Excision of Left Axillary Lymphatic, Open Approach
07B63ZX Excision of Left Axillary Lymphatic, Percutaneous Approach, Diagnostic
07B63ZZ Excision of Left Axillary Lymphatic, Percutaneous Approach
07B64ZX Excision of Left Axillary Lymphatic, Percutaneous Endoscopic Approach, Diagnostic
07B64ZZ Excision of Left Axillary Lymphatic, Percutaneous Endoscopic Approach
07B70ZX Excision of Thorax Lymphatic, Open Approach, Diagnostic
07B70ZZ Excision of Thorax Lymphatic, Open Approach
07B73ZX Excision of Thorax Lymphatic, Percutaneous Approach, Diagnostic
07B73ZZ Excision of Thorax Lymphatic, Percutaneous Approach
07B74ZX Excision of Thorax Lymphatic, Percutaneous Endoscopic Approach, Diagnostic
AHA CC: 1Q, 2014, 20-21, 26
07B74ZZ Excision of Thorax Lymphatic, Percutaneous Endoscopic Approach
07B80ZX Excision of Right Internal Mammary Lymphatic, Open Approach, Diagnostic
07B80ZZ Excision of Right Internal Mammary Lymphatic, Open Approach

07B83ZX Excision of Right Internal Mammary Lymphatic, Percutaneous Approach, Diagnostic

07B83ZZ Excision of Right Internal Mammary Lymphatic, Percutaneous Approach

07B84ZX Excision of Right Internal Mammary Lymphatic, Percutaneous Endoscopic Approach, Diagnostic

07B84ZZ Excision of Right Internal Mammary Lymphatic, Percutaneous Endoscopic Approach

07B90ZX Excision of Left Internal Mammary Lymphatic, Open Approach, Diagnostic

07B90ZZ Excision of Left Internal Mammary Lymphatic, Open Approach

07B93ZX Excision of Left Internal Mammary Lymphatic, Percutaneous Approach, Diagnostic

07B93ZZ Excision of Left Internal Mammary Lymphatic, Percutaneous Approach

07B94ZX Excision of Left Internal Mammary Lymphatic, Percutaneous Endoscopic Approach, Diagnostic

07B94ZZ Excision of Left Internal Mammary Lymphatic, Percutaneous Endoscopic Approach

07BB0ZX Excision of Mesenteric Lymphatic, Open Approach, Diagnostic

07BB0ZZ Excision of Mesenteric Lymphatic, Open Approach

07BB3ZX Excision of Mesenteric Lymphatic, Percutaneous Approach, Diagnostic

07BB3ZZ Excision of Mesenteric Lymphatic, Percutaneous Approach

07BB4ZX Excision of Mesenteric Lymphatic, Percutaneous Endoscopic Approach, Diagnostic

07BB4ZZ Excision of Mesenteric Lymphatic, Percutaneous Endoscopic Approach

07BC0ZX Excision of Pelvis Lymphatic, Open Approach, Diagnostic

07BC0ZZ Excision of Pelvis Lymphatic, Open Approach

07BC3ZX Excision of Pelvis Lymphatic, Percutaneous Approach, Diagnostic

07BC3ZZ Excision of Pelvis Lymphatic, Percutaneous Approach

07BC4ZX Excision of Pelvis Lymphatic, Percutaneous Endoscopic Approach, Diagnostic

07BC4ZZ Excision of Pelvis Lymphatic, Percutaneous Endoscopic Approach

07BD0ZX Excision of Aortic Lymphatic, Open Approach, Diagnostic

07BD0ZZ Excision of Aortic Lymphatic, Open Approach

07BD3ZX Excision of Aortic Lymphatic, Percutaneous Approach, Diagnostic

07BD3ZZ Excision of Aortic Lymphatic, Percutaneous Approach

07BD4ZX Excision of Aortic Lymphatic, Percutaneous Endoscopic Approach, Diagnostic

07BD4ZZ Excision of Aortic Lymphatic, Percutaneous Endoscopic Approach

07BF0ZX Excision of Right Lower Extremity Lymphatic, Open Approach, Diagnostic

07BF0ZZ Excision of Right Lower Extremity Lymphatic, Open Approach

07BF3ZX Excision of Right Lower Extremity Lymphatic, Percutaneous Approach, Diagnostic

07BF3ZZ Excision of Right Lower Extremity Lymphatic, Percutaneous Approach

07BF4ZX Excision of Right Lower Extremity Lymphatic, Percutaneous Endoscopic Approach, Diagnostic

07BF4ZZ Excision of Right Lower Extremity Lymphatic, Percutaneous Endoscopic Approach

07BG0ZX Excision of Left Lower Extremity Lymphatic, Open Approach, Diagnostic

07BG0ZZ Excision of Left Lower Extremity Lymphatic, Open Approach

07BG3ZX Excision of Left Lower Extremity Lymphatic, Percutaneous Approach, Diagnostic

07BG3ZZ Excision of Left Lower Extremity Lymphatic, Percutaneous Approach

07BG4ZX Excision of Left Lower Extremity Lymphatic, Percutaneous Endoscopic Approach, Diagnostic

07BG4ZZ Excision of Left Lower Extremity Lymphatic, Percutaneous Endoscopic Approach

07BH0ZX Excision of Right Inguinal Lymphatic, Open Approach, Diagnostic

07BH0ZZ Excision of Right Inguinal Lymphatic, Open Approach

+ Radical vulvectomy when reported with resection of vulva. *See table 0UT to construct the Resection code.*

07BH3ZX Excision of Right Inguinal Lymphatic, Percutaneous Approach, Diagnostic

07BH3ZZ Excision of Right Inguinal Lymphatic, Percutaneous Approach

07BH4ZX Excision of Right Inguinal Lymphatic, Percutaneous Endoscopic Approach, Diagnostic

07BH4ZZ Excision of Right Inguinal Lymphatic, Percutaneous Endoscopic Approach

+ Radical vulvectomy when reported with resection of vulva. *See table 0UT to construct the Resection code.*

07BJ0ZX Excision of Left Inguinal Lymphatic, Open Approach, Diagnostic

07BJ0ZZ Excision of Left Inguinal Lymphatic, Open Approach

+ Radical vulvectomy when reported with resection of vulva. *See table 0UT to construct the Resection code.*

07BJ3ZX Excision of Left Inguinal Lymphatic, Percutaneous Approach, Diagnostic

07BJ3ZZ Excision of Left Inguinal Lymphatic, Percutaneous Approach

07BJ4ZX Excision of Left Inguinal Lymphatic, Percutaneous Endoscopic Approach, Diagnostic

07BJ4ZZ Excision of Left Inguinal Lymphatic, Percutaneous Endoscopic Approach

+ Radical vulvectomy when reported with resection of vulva. *See table 0UT to construct the Resection code.*

07BK0ZX Excision of Thoracic Duct, Open Approach, Diagnostic

07BK0ZZ Excision of Thoracic Duct, Open Approach

07BK3ZX Excision of Thoracic Duct, Percutaneous Approach, Diagnostic

07BK3ZZ Excision of Thoracic Duct, Percutaneous Approach

07BK4ZX Excision of Thoracic Duct, Percutaneous Endoscopic Approach, Diagnostic

07BK4ZZ Excision of Thoracic Duct, Percutaneous Endoscopic Approach

07BL0ZX Excision of Cisterna Chyli, Open Approach, Diagnostic

07BL0ZZ Excision of Cisterna Chyli, Open Approach

07BL3ZX Excision of Cisterna Chyli, Percutaneous Approach, Diagnostic

07BL3ZZ Excision of Cisterna Chyli, Percutaneous Approach

07BL4ZX Excision of Cisterna Chyli, Percutaneous Endoscopic Approach, Diagnostic

07BL4ZZ Excision of Cisterna Chyli, Percutaneous Endoscopic Approach

07BM0ZX Excision of Thymus, Open Approach, Diagnostic

07BM0ZZ Excision of Thymus, Open Approach

07BM3ZX Excision of Thymus, Percutaneous Approach, Diagnostic

07BM3ZZ Excision of Thymus, Percutaneous Approach

07BM4ZX Excision of Thymus, Percutaneous Endoscopic Approach, Diagnostic

07BM4ZZ Excision of Thymus, Percutaneous Endoscopic Approach

07BP0ZX Excision of Spleen, Open Approach, Diagnostic

07BP0ZZ Excision of Spleen, Open Approach

07BP3ZX Excision of Spleen, Percutaneous Approach, Diagnostic

07BP3ZZ Excision of Spleen, Percutaneous Approach

07BP4ZX Excision of Spleen, Percutaneous Endoscopic Approach, Diagnostic

07BP4ZZ Excision of Spleen, Percutaneous Endoscopic Approach

07C – Lymphatic and Hemic Systems, Extirpation

07C00ZZ Extirpation of Matter from Head Lymphatic, Open Approach

07C03ZZ Extirpation of Matter from Head Lymphatic, Percutaneous Approach

07C04ZZ Extirpation of Matter from Head Lymphatic, Percutaneous Endoscopic Approach

07C10ZZ Extirpation of Matter from Right Neck Lymphatic, Open Approach

07C13ZZ Extirpation of Matter from Right Neck Lymphatic, Percutaneous Approach

07C14ZZ Extirpation of Matter from Right Neck Lymphatic, Percutaneous Endoscopic Approach

07C20ZZ Extirpation of Matter from Left Neck Lymphatic, Open Approach

07C23ZZ Extirpation of Matter from Left Neck Lymphatic, Percutaneous Approach

07C24ZZ Extirpation of Matter from Left Neck Lymphatic, Percutaneous Endoscopic Approach

07C30ZZ Extirpation of Matter from Right Upper Extremity Lymphatic, Open Approach

07C33ZZ Extirpation of Matter from Right Upper Extremity Lymphatic, Percutaneous Approach

07C34ZZ Extirpation of Matter from Right Upper Extremity Lymphatic, Percutaneous Endoscopic Approach

07C40ZZ Extirpation of Matter from Left Upper Extremity Lymphatic, Open Approach

07C43ZZ Extirpation of Matter from Left Upper Extremity Lymphatic, Percutaneous Approach

07C44ZZ Extirpation of Matter from Left Upper Extremity Lymphatic, Percutaneous Endoscopic Approach

07C50ZZ Extirpation of Matter from Right Axillary Lymphatic, Open Approach

07C53ZZ Extirpation of Matter from Right Axillary Lymphatic, Percutaneous Approach

07C54ZZ Extirpation of Matter from Right Axillary Lymphatic, Percutaneous Endoscopic Approach

07C60ZZ Extirpation of Matter from Left Axillary Lymphatic, Open Approach

C63ZZ Extirpation of Matter from Left Axillary Lymphatic, Percutaneous Approach
C64ZZ Extirpation of Matter from Left Axillary Lymphatic, Percutaneous Endoscopic Approach
C70ZZ Extirpation of Matter from Thorax Lymphatic, Open Approach
C73ZZ Extirpation of Matter from Thorax Lymphatic, Percutaneous Approach
C74ZZ Extirpation of Matter from Thorax Lymphatic, Percutaneous Endoscopic Approach
C80ZZ Extirpation of Matter from Right Internal Mammary Lymphatic, Open Approach
C83ZZ Extirpation of Matter from Right Internal Mammary Lymphatic, Percutaneous Approach
C84ZZ Extirpation of Matter from Right Internal Mammary Lymphatic, Percutaneous Endoscopic Approach
C90ZZ Extirpation of Matter from Left Internal Mammary Lymphatic, Open Approach
C93ZZ Extirpation of Matter from Left Internal Mammary Lymphatic, Percutaneous Approach
C94ZZ Extirpation of Matter from Left Internal Mammary Lymphatic, Percutaneous Endoscopic Approach
CB0ZZ Extirpation of Matter from Mesenteric Lymphatic, Open Approach
CB3ZZ Extirpation of Matter from Mesenteric Lymphatic, Percutaneous Approach
CB4ZZ Extirpation of Matter from Mesenteric Lymphatic, Percutaneous Endoscopic Approach
07CC0ZZ Extirpation of Matter from Pelvis Lymphatic, Open Approach
07CC3ZZ Extirpation of Matter from Pelvis Lymphatic, Percutaneous Approach
07CC4ZZ Extirpation of Matter from Pelvis Lymphatic, Percutaneous Endoscopic Approach
07CD0ZZ Extirpation of Matter from Aortic Lymphatic, Open Approach
07CD3ZZ Extirpation of Matter from Aortic Lymphatic, Percutaneous Approach
07CD4ZZ Extirpation of Matter from Aortic Lymphatic, Percutaneous Endoscopic Approach
07CF0ZZ Extirpation of Matter from Right Lower Extremity Lymphatic, Open Approach
07CF3ZZ Extirpation of Matter from Right Lower Extremity Lymphatic, Percutaneous Approach
07CF4ZZ Extirpation of Matter from Right Lower Extremity Lymphatic, Percutaneous Endoscopic Approach
07CG0ZZ Extirpation of Matter from Left Lower Extremity Lymphatic, Open Approach
07CG3ZZ Extirpation of Matter from Left Lower Extremity Lymphatic, Percutaneous Approach
07CG4ZZ Extirpation of Matter from Left Lower Extremity Lymphatic, Percutaneous Endoscopic Approach
07CH0ZZ Extirpation of Matter from Right Inguinal Lymphatic, Open Approach
07CH3ZZ Extirpation of Matter from Right Inguinal Lymphatic, Percutaneous Approach
07CH4ZZ Extirpation of Matter from Right Inguinal Lymphatic, Percutaneous Endoscopic Approach
07CJ0ZZ Extirpation of Matter from Left Inguinal Lymphatic, Open Approach
07CJ3ZZ Extirpation of Matter from Left Inguinal Lymphatic, Percutaneous Approach
07CJ4ZZ Extirpation of Matter from Left Inguinal Lymphatic, Percutaneous Endoscopic Approach
07CK0ZZ Extirpation of Matter from Thoracic Duct, Open Approach
07CK3ZZ Extirpation of Matter from Thoracic Duct, Percutaneous Approach
07CK4ZZ Extirpation of Matter from Thoracic Duct, Percutaneous Endoscopic Approach
07CL0ZZ Extirpation of Matter from Cisterna Chyli, Open Approach
07CL3ZZ Extirpation of Matter from Cisterna Chyli, Percutaneous Approach
07CL4ZZ Extirpation of Matter from Cisterna Chyli, Percutaneous Endoscopic Approach
07CM0ZZ Extirpation of Matter from Thymus, Open Approach
07CM3ZZ Extirpation of Matter from Thymus, Percutaneous Approach
07CM4ZZ Extirpation of Matter from Thymus, Percutaneous Endoscopic Approach
07CP0ZZ Extirpation of Matter from Spleen, Open Approach
07CP3ZZ Extirpation of Matter from Spleen, Percutaneous Approach
07CP4ZZ Extirpation of Matter from Spleen, Percutaneous Endoscopic Approach

7D – Lymphatic and Hemic Systems, Extraction

eview Coding Guidelines B3.4a and B3.4b

7DQ0ZX Extraction of Sternum Bone Marrow, Open Approach, Diagnostic
7DQ0ZZ Extraction of Sternum Bone Marrow, Open Approach
7DQ3ZX Extraction of Sternum Bone Marrow, Percutaneous Approach, Diagnostic
7DQ3ZZ Extraction of Sternum Bone Marrow, Percutaneous Approach
07DR0ZX Extraction of Iliac Bone Marrow, Open Approach, Diagnostic
07DR0ZZ Extraction of Iliac Bone Marrow, Open Approach
07DR3ZX Extraction of Iliac Bone Marrow, Percutaneous Approach, Diagnostic
07DR3ZZ Extraction of Iliac Bone Marrow, Percutaneous Approach
07DS0ZX Extraction of Vertebral Bone Marrow, Open Approach, Diagnostic
07DS0ZZ Extraction of Vertebral Bone Marrow, Open Approach
07DS3ZX Extraction of Vertebral Bone Marrow, Percutaneous Approach, Diagnostic
07DS3ZZ Extraction of Vertebral Bone Marrow, Percutaneous Approach

7H – Lymphatic and Hemic Systems, Insertion

7HK03Z Insertion of Infusion Device into Thoracic Duct, Open Approach
7HK33Z Insertion of Infusion Device into Thoracic Duct, Percutaneous Approach
7HK43Z Insertion of Infusion Device into Thoracic Duct, Percutaneous Endoscopic Approach
7HL03Z Insertion of Infusion Device into Cisterna Chyli, Open Approach
7HL33Z Insertion of Infusion Device into Cisterna Chyli, Percutaneous Approach
07HL43Z Insertion of Infusion Device into Cisterna Chyli, Percutaneous Endoscopic Approach
07HM03Z Insertion of Infusion Device into Thymus, Open Approach
07HM33Z Insertion of Infusion Device into Thymus, Percutaneous Approach
07HM43Z Insertion of Infusion Device into Thymus, Percutaneous Endoscopic Approach
07HN03Z Insertion of Infusion Device into Lymphatic, Open Approach
07HN33Z Insertion of Infusion Device into Lymphatic, Percutaneous Approach
07HN43Z Insertion of Infusion Device into Lymphatic, Percutaneous Endoscopic Approach
07HP03Z Insertion of Infusion Device into Spleen, Open Approach
07HP33Z Insertion of Infusion Device into Spleen, Percutaneous Approach
07HP43Z Insertion of Infusion Device into Spleen, Percutaneous Endoscopic Approach

7J – Lymphatic and Hemic Systems, Inspection

Review Coding Guidelines B3.11a, B3.11b and B3.11c

7JK0ZZ Inspection of Thoracic Duct, Open Approach
7JK3ZZ Inspection of Thoracic Duct, Percutaneous Approach
7JK4ZZ Inspection of Thoracic Duct, Percutaneous Endoscopic Approach
7JL0ZZ Inspection of Cisterna Chyli, Open Approach
07JL3ZZ Inspection of Cisterna Chyli, Percutaneous Approach
07JL4ZZ Inspection of Cisterna Chyli, Percutaneous Endoscopic Approach
07JM0ZZ Inspection of Thymus, Open Approach
07JM3ZZ Inspection of Thymus, Percutaneous Approach
07JM4ZZ Inspection of Thymus, Percutaneous Endoscopic Approach
07JN0ZZ Inspection of Lymphatic, Open Approach
07JN3ZZ Inspection of Lymphatic, Percutaneous Approach
07JN4ZZ Inspection of Lymphatic, Percutaneous Endoscopic Approach
07JNXZZ Inspection of Lymphatic, External Approach
07JP0ZZ Inspection of Spleen, Open Approach

07JP3ZZ Inspection of Spleen, Percutaneous Approach
07JP4ZZ Inspection of Spleen, Percutaneous Endoscopic Approach
07JPXZZ Inspection of Spleen, External Approach
07JT0ZZ Inspection of Bone Marrow, Open Approach
07JT3ZZ Inspection of Bone Marrow, Percutaneous Approach
07JT4ZZ Inspection of Bone Marrow, Percutaneous Endoscopic Approach

07L – Lymphatic and Hemic Systems, Occlusion

07L00CZ Occlusion of Head Lymphatic with Extraluminal Device, Open Approach
07L00DZ Occlusion of Head Lymphatic with Intraluminal Device, Open Approach
07L00ZZ Occlusion of Head Lymphatic, Open Approach
07L03CZ Occlusion of Head Lymphatic with Extraluminal Device, Percutaneous Approach
07L03DZ Occlusion of Head Lymphatic with Intraluminal Device, Percutaneous Approach
07L03ZZ Occlusion of Head Lymphatic, Percutaneous Approach
07L04CZ Occlusion of Head Lymphatic with Extraluminal Device, Percutaneous Endoscopic Approach
07L04DZ Occlusion of Head Lymphatic with Intraluminal Device, Percutaneous Endoscopic Approach
07L04ZZ Occlusion of Head Lymphatic, Percutaneous Endoscopic Approach
07L10CZ Occlusion of Right Neck Lymphatic with Extraluminal Device, Open Approach
07L10DZ Occlusion of Right Neck Lymphatic with Intraluminal Device, Open Approach
07L10ZZ Occlusion of Right Neck Lymphatic, Open Approach
07L13CZ Occlusion of Right Neck Lymphatic with Extraluminal Device, Percutaneous Approach
07L13DZ Occlusion of Right Neck Lymphatic with Intraluminal Device, Percutaneous Approach
07L13ZZ Occlusion of Right Neck Lymphatic, Percutaneous Approach
07L14CZ Occlusion of Right Neck Lymphatic with Extraluminal Device, Percutaneous Endoscopic Approach
07L14DZ Occlusion of Right Neck Lymphatic with Intraluminal Device, Percutaneous Endoscopic Approach
07L14ZZ Occlusion of Right Neck Lymphatic, Percutaneous Endoscopic Approach
07L20CZ Occlusion of Left Neck Lymphatic with Extraluminal Device, Open Approach
07L20DZ Occlusion of Left Neck Lymphatic with Intraluminal Device, Open Approach
07L20ZZ Occlusion of Left Neck Lymphatic, Open Approach
07L23CZ Occlusion of Left Neck Lymphatic with Extraluminal Device, Percutaneous Approach
07L23DZ Occlusion of Left Neck Lymphatic with Intraluminal Device, Percutaneous Approach
07L23ZZ Occlusion of Left Neck Lymphatic, Percutaneous Approach
07L24CZ Occlusion of Left Neck Lymphatic with Extraluminal Device, Percutaneous Endoscopic Approach
07L24DZ Occlusion of Left Neck Lymphatic with Intraluminal Device, Percutaneous Endoscopic Approach
07L24ZZ Occlusion of Left Neck Lymphatic, Percutaneous Endoscopic Approach
07L30CZ Occlusion of Right Upper Extremity Lymphatic with Extraluminal Device, Open Approach
07L30DZ Occlusion of Right Upper Extremity Lymphatic with Intraluminal Device, Open Approach
07L30ZZ Occlusion of Right Upper Extremity Lymphatic, Open Approach
07L33CZ Occlusion of Right Upper Extremity Lymphatic with Extraluminal Device, Percutaneous Approach
07L33DZ Occlusion of Right Upper Extremity Lymphatic with Intraluminal Device, Percutaneous Approach
07L33ZZ Occlusion of Right Upper Extremity Lymphatic, Percutaneous Approach
07L34CZ Occlusion of Right Upper Extremity Lymphatic with Extraluminal Device, Percutaneous Endoscopic Approach
07L34DZ Occlusion of Right Upper Extremity Lymphatic with Intraluminal Device, Percutaneous Endoscopic Approach
07L34ZZ Occlusion of Right Upper Extremity Lymphatic, Percutaneous Endoscopic Approach
07L40CZ Occlusion of Left Upper Extremity Lymphatic with Extraluminal Device, Open Approach
07L40DZ Occlusion of Left Upper Extremity Lymphatic with Intraluminal Device, Open Approach
07L40ZZ Occlusion of Left Upper Extremity Lymphatic, Open Approach
07L43CZ Occlusion of Left Upper Extremity Lymphatic with Extraluminal Device, Percutaneous Approach
07L43DZ Occlusion of Left Upper Extremity Lymphatic with Intraluminal Device, Percutaneous Approach
07L43ZZ Occlusion of Left Upper Extremity Lymphatic, Percutaneous Approach
07L44CZ Occlusion of Left Upper Extremity Lymphatic with Extraluminal Device, Percutaneous Endoscopic Approach
07L44DZ Occlusion of Left Upper Extremity Lymphatic with Intraluminal Device, Percutaneous Endoscopic Approach
07L44ZZ Occlusion of Left Upper Extremity Lymphatic, Percutaneous Endoscopic Approach
07L50CZ Occlusion of Right Axillary Lymphatic with Extraluminal Device, Open Approach
07L50DZ Occlusion of Right Axillary Lymphatic with Intraluminal Device, Open Approach
07L50ZZ Occlusion of Right Axillary Lymphatic, Open Approach
07L53CZ Occlusion of Right Axillary Lymphatic with Extraluminal Device, Percutaneous Approach
07L53DZ Occlusion of Right Axillary Lymphatic with Intraluminal Device, Percutaneous Approach
07L53ZZ Occlusion of Right Axillary Lymphatic, Percutaneous Approach
07L54CZ Occlusion of Right Axillary Lymphatic with Extraluminal Device, Percutaneous Endoscopic Approach
07L54DZ Occlusion of Right Axillary Lymphatic with Intraluminal Device, Percutaneous Endoscopic Approach
07L54ZZ Occlusion of Right Axillary Lymphatic, Percutaneous Endoscopic Approach
07L60CZ Occlusion of Left Axillary Lymphatic with Extraluminal Device, Open Approach
07L60DZ Occlusion of Left Axillary Lymphatic with Intraluminal Device, Open Approach
07L60ZZ Occlusion of Left Axillary Lymphatic, Open Approach
07L63CZ Occlusion of Left Axillary Lymphatic with Extraluminal Device, Percutaneous Approach
07L63DZ Occlusion of Left Axillary Lymphatic with Intraluminal Device, Percutaneous Approach
07L63ZZ Occlusion of Left Axillary Lymphatic, Percutaneous Approach
07L64CZ Occlusion of Left Axillary Lymphatic with Extraluminal Device, Percutaneous Endoscopic Approach
07L64DZ Occlusion of Left Axillary Lymphatic with Intraluminal Device, Percutaneous Endoscopic Approach
07L64ZZ Occlusion of Left Axillary Lymphatic, Percutaneous Endoscopic Approach
07L70CZ Occlusion of Thorax Lymphatic with Extraluminal Device, Open Approach
07L70DZ Occlusion of Thorax Lymphatic with Intraluminal Device, Open Approach
07L70ZZ Occlusion of Thorax Lymphatic, Open Approach
07L73CZ Occlusion of Thorax Lymphatic with Extraluminal Device, Percutaneous Approach
07L73DZ Occlusion of Thorax Lymphatic with Intraluminal Device, Percutaneous Approach
07L73ZZ Occlusion of Thorax Lymphatic, Percutaneous Approach
07L74CZ Occlusion of Thorax Lymphatic with Extraluminal Device, Percutaneous Endoscopic Approach
07L74DZ Occlusion of Thorax Lymphatic with Intraluminal Device, Percutaneous Endoscopic Approach
07L74ZZ Occlusion of Thorax Lymphatic, Percutaneous Endoscopic Approach
07L80CZ Occlusion of Right Internal Mammary Lymphatic with Extraluminal Device, Open Approach
07L80DZ Occlusion of Right Internal Mammary Lymphatic with Intraluminal Device, Open Approach
07L80ZZ Occlusion of Right Internal Mammary Lymphatic, Open Approach
07L83CZ Occlusion of Right Internal Mammary Lymphatic with Extraluminal Device, Percutaneous Approach
07L83DZ Occlusion of Right Internal Mammary Lymphatic with Intraluminal Device, Percutaneous Approach
07L83ZZ Occlusion of Right Internal Mammary Lymphatic, Percutaneous Approach
07L84CZ Occlusion of Right Internal Mammary Lymphatic with Extraluminal Device, Percutaneous Endoscopic Approach
07L84DZ Occlusion of Right Internal Mammary Lymphatic with Intraluminal Device, Percutaneous Endoscopic Approach
07L84ZZ Occlusion of Right Internal Mammary Lymphatic, Percutaneous Endoscopic Approach

.90CZ Occlusion of Left Internal Mammary Lymphatic with Extraluminal Device, Open Approach
L90DZ Occlusion of Left Internal Mammary Lymphatic with Intraluminal Device, Open Approach
L90ZZ Occlusion of Left Internal Mammary Lymphatic, Open Approach
L93CZ Occlusion of Left Internal Mammary Lymphatic with Extraluminal Device, Percutaneous Approach
L93DZ Occlusion of Left Internal Mammary Lymphatic with Intraluminal Device, Percutaneous Approach
L93ZZ Occlusion of Left Internal Mammary Lymphatic, Percutaneous Approach
L94CZ Occlusion of Left Internal Mammary Lymphatic with Extraluminal Device, Percutaneous Endoscopic Approach
L94DZ Occlusion of Left Internal Mammary Lymphatic with Intraluminal Device, Percutaneous Endoscopic Approach
L94ZZ Occlusion of Left Internal Mammary Lymphatic, Percutaneous Endoscopic Approach
LB0CZ Occlusion of Mesenteric Lymphatic with Extraluminal Device, Open Approach
LB0DZ Occlusion of Mesenteric Lymphatic with Intraluminal Device, Open Approach
LB0ZZ Occlusion of Mesenteric Lymphatic, Open Approach
LB3CZ Occlusion of Mesenteric Lymphatic with Extraluminal Device, Percutaneous Approach
LB3DZ Occlusion of Mesenteric Lymphatic with Intraluminal Device, Percutaneous Approach
LB3ZZ Occlusion of Mesenteric Lymphatic, Percutaneous Approach
LB4CZ Occlusion of Mesenteric Lymphatic with Extraluminal Device, Percutaneous Endoscopic Approach
LB4DZ Occlusion of Mesenteric Lymphatic with Intraluminal Device, Percutaneous Endoscopic Approach
LB4ZZ Occlusion of Mesenteric Lymphatic, Percutaneous Endoscopic Approach
LC0CZ Occlusion of Pelvis Lymphatic with Extraluminal Device, Open Approach
7LC0DZ Occlusion of Pelvis Lymphatic with Intraluminal Device, Open Approach
7LC0ZZ Occlusion of Pelvis Lymphatic, Open Approach
7LC3CZ Occlusion of Pelvis Lymphatic with Extraluminal Device, Percutaneous Approach
7LC3DZ Occlusion of Pelvis Lymphatic with Intraluminal Device, Percutaneous Approach
7LC3ZZ Occlusion of Pelvis Lymphatic, Percutaneous Approach
7LC4CZ Occlusion of Pelvis Lymphatic with Extraluminal Device, Percutaneous Endoscopic Approach
7LC4DZ Occlusion of Pelvis Lymphatic with Intraluminal Device, Percutaneous Endoscopic Approach
7LC4ZZ Occlusion of Pelvis Lymphatic, Percutaneous Endoscopic Approach
7LD0CZ Occlusion of Aortic Lymphatic with Extraluminal Device, Open Approach
7LD0DZ Occlusion of Aortic Lymphatic with Intraluminal Device, Open Approach
7LD0ZZ Occlusion of Aortic Lymphatic, Open Approach
7LD3CZ Occlusion of Aortic Lymphatic with Extraluminal Device, Percutaneous Approach
07LD3DZ Occlusion of Aortic Lymphatic with Intraluminal Device, Percutaneous Approach
07LD3ZZ Occlusion of Aortic Lymphatic, Percutaneous Approach
07LD4CZ Occlusion of Aortic Lymphatic with Extraluminal Device, Percutaneous Endoscopic Approach
07LD4DZ Occlusion of Aortic Lymphatic with Intraluminal Device, Percutaneous Endoscopic Approach
07LD4ZZ Occlusion of Aortic Lymphatic, Percutaneous Endoscopic Approach
07LF0CZ Occlusion of Right Lower Extremity Lymphatic with Extraluminal Device, Open Approach
07LF0DZ Occlusion of Right Lower Extremity Lymphatic with Intraluminal Device, Open Approach
07LF0ZZ Occlusion of Right Lower Extremity Lymphatic, Open Approach
07LF3CZ Occlusion of Right Lower Extremity Lymphatic with Extraluminal Device, Percutaneous Approach
07LF3DZ Occlusion of Right Lower Extremity Lymphatic with Intraluminal Device, Percutaneous Approach
07LF3ZZ Occlusion of Right Lower Extremity Lymphatic, Percutaneous Approach
07LF4CZ Occlusion of Right Lower Extremity Lymphatic with Extraluminal Device, Percutaneous Endoscopic Approach
07LF4DZ Occlusion of Right Lower Extremity Lymphatic with Intraluminal Device, Percutaneous Endoscopic Approach
07LF4ZZ Occlusion of Right Lower Extremity Lymphatic, Percutaneous Endoscopic Approach
07LG0CZ Occlusion of Left Lower Extremity Lymphatic with Extraluminal Device, Open Approach
07LG0DZ Occlusion of Left Lower Extremity Lymphatic with Intraluminal Device, Open Approach
07LG0ZZ Occlusion of Left Lower Extremity Lymphatic, Open Approach
07LG3CZ Occlusion of Left Lower Extremity Lymphatic with Extraluminal Device, Percutaneous Approach
07LG3DZ Occlusion of Left Lower Extremity Lymphatic with Intraluminal Device, Percutaneous Approach
07LG3ZZ Occlusion of Left Lower Extremity Lymphatic, Percutaneous Approach
07LG4CZ Occlusion of Left Lower Extremity Lymphatic with Extraluminal Device, Percutaneous Endoscopic Approach
07LG4DZ Occlusion of Left Lower Extremity Lymphatic with Intraluminal Device, Percutaneous Endoscopic Approach
07LG4ZZ Occlusion of Left Lower Extremity Lymphatic, Percutaneous Endoscopic Approach
07LH0CZ Occlusion of Right Inguinal Lymphatic with Extraluminal Device, Open Approach
07LH0DZ Occlusion of Right Inguinal Lymphatic with Intraluminal Device, Open Approach
07LH0ZZ Occlusion of Right Inguinal Lymphatic, Open Approach
07LH3CZ Occlusion of Right Inguinal Lymphatic with Extraluminal Device, Percutaneous Approach
07LH3DZ Occlusion of Right Inguinal Lymphatic with Intraluminal Device, Percutaneous Approach
07LH3ZZ Occlusion of Right Inguinal Lymphatic, Percutaneous Approach
07LH4CZ Occlusion of Right Inguinal Lymphatic with Extraluminal Device, Percutaneous Endoscopic Approach
07LH4DZ Occlusion of Right Inguinal Lymphatic with Intraluminal Device, Percutaneous Endoscopic Approach
07LH4ZZ Occlusion of Right Inguinal Lymphatic, Percutaneous Endoscopic Approach
07LJ0CZ Occlusion of Left Inguinal Lymphatic with Extraluminal Device, Open Approach
07LJ0DZ Occlusion of Left Inguinal Lymphatic with Intraluminal Device, Open Approach
07LJ0ZZ Occlusion of Left Inguinal Lymphatic, Open Approach
07LJ3CZ Occlusion of Left Inguinal Lymphatic with Extraluminal Device, Percutaneous Approach
07LJ3DZ Occlusion of Left Inguinal Lymphatic with Intraluminal Device, Percutaneous Approach
07LJ3ZZ Occlusion of Left Inguinal Lymphatic, Percutaneous Approach
07LJ4CZ Occlusion of Left Inguinal Lymphatic with Extraluminal Device, Percutaneous Endoscopic Approach
07LJ4DZ Occlusion of Left Inguinal Lymphatic with Intraluminal Device, Percutaneous Endoscopic Approach
07LJ4ZZ Occlusion of Left Inguinal Lymphatic, Percutaneous Endoscopic Approach
07LK0CZ Occlusion of Thoracic Duct with Extraluminal Device, Open Approach
07LK0DZ Occlusion of Thoracic Duct with Intraluminal Device, Open Approach
07LK0ZZ Occlusion of Thoracic Duct, Open Approach
07LK3CZ Occlusion of Thoracic Duct with Extraluminal Device, Percutaneous Approach
07LK3DZ Occlusion of Thoracic Duct with Intraluminal Device, Percutaneous Approach
07LK3ZZ Occlusion of Thoracic Duct, Percutaneous Approach
07LK4CZ Occlusion of Thoracic Duct with Extraluminal Device, Percutaneous Endoscopic Approach
07LK4DZ Occlusion of Thoracic Duct with Intraluminal Device, Percutaneous Endoscopic Approach
07LK4ZZ Occlusion of Thoracic Duct, Percutaneous Endoscopic Approach
07LL0CZ Occlusion of Cisterna Chyli with Extraluminal Device, Open Approach
07LL0DZ Occlusion of Cisterna Chyli with Intraluminal Device, Open Approach
07LL0ZZ Occlusion of Cisterna Chyli, Open Approach
07LL3CZ Occlusion of Cisterna Chyli with Extraluminal Device, Percutaneous Approach
07LL3DZ Occlusion of Cisterna Chyli with Intraluminal Device, Percutaneous Approach
07LL3ZZ Occlusion of Cisterna Chyli, Percutaneous Approach
07LL4CZ Occlusion of Cisterna Chyli with Extraluminal Device, Percutaneous Endoscopic Approach
07LL4DZ Occlusion of Cisterna Chyli with Intraluminal Device, Percutaneous Endoscopic Approach
07LL4ZZ Occlusion of Cisterna Chyli, Percutaneous Endoscopic Approach

07N – Lymphatic and Hemic Systems, Release

Review Coding Guidelines B3.13 and B3.14

07N00ZZ Release Head Lymphatic, Open Approach
07N03ZZ Release Head Lymphatic, Percutaneous Approach
07N04ZZ Release Head Lymphatic, Percutaneous Endoscopic Approach
07N10ZZ Release Right Neck Lymphatic, Open Approach
07N13ZZ Release Right Neck Lymphatic, Percutaneous Approach
07N14ZZ Release Right Neck Lymphatic, Percutaneous Endoscopic Approach
07N20ZZ Release Left Neck Lymphatic, Open Approach
07N23ZZ Release Left Neck Lymphatic, Percutaneous Approach
07N24ZZ Release Left Neck Lymphatic, Percutaneous Endoscopic Approach
07N30ZZ Release Right Upper Extremity Lymphatic, Open Approach
07N33ZZ Release Right Upper Extremity Lymphatic, Percutaneous Approach
07N34ZZ Release Right Upper Extremity Lymphatic, Percutaneous Endoscopic Approach
07N40ZZ Release Left Upper Extremity Lymphatic, Open Approach
07N43ZZ Release Left Upper Extremity Lymphatic, Percutaneous Approach
07N44ZZ Release Left Upper Extremity Lymphatic, Percutaneous Endoscopic Approach
07N50ZZ Release Right Axillary Lymphatic, Open Approach
07N53ZZ Release Right Axillary Lymphatic, Percutaneous Approach
07N54ZZ Release Right Axillary Lymphatic, Percutaneous Endoscopic Approach
07N60ZZ Release Left Axillary Lymphatic, Open Approach
07N63ZZ Release Left Axillary Lymphatic, Percutaneous Approach
07N64ZZ Release Left Axillary Lymphatic, Percutaneous Endoscopic Approach
07N70ZZ Release Thorax Lymphatic, Open Approach
07N73ZZ Release Thorax Lymphatic, Percutaneous Approach
07N74ZZ Release Thorax Lymphatic, Percutaneous Endoscopic Approach
07N80ZZ Release Right Internal Mammary Lymphatic, Open Approach
07N83ZZ Release Right Internal Mammary Lymphatic, Percutaneous Approach
07N84ZZ Release Right Internal Mammary Lymphatic, Percutaneous Endoscopic Approach
07N90ZZ Release Left Internal Mammary Lymphatic, Open Approach
07N93ZZ Release Left Internal Mammary Lymphatic, Percutaneous Approach
07N94ZZ Release Left Internal Mammary Lymphatic, Percutaneous Endoscopic Approach
07NB0ZZ Release Mesenteric Lymphatic, Open Approach
07NB3ZZ Release Mesenteric Lymphatic, Percutaneous Approach
07NB4ZZ Release Mesenteric Lymphatic, Percutaneous Endoscopic Approach
07NC0ZZ Release Pelvis Lymphatic, Open Approach
07NC3ZZ Release Pelvis Lymphatic, Percutaneous Approach
07NC4ZZ Release Pelvis Lymphatic, Percutaneous Endoscopic Approach
07ND0ZZ Release Aortic Lymphatic, Open Approach
07ND3ZZ Release Aortic Lymphatic, Percutaneous Approach
07ND4ZZ Release Aortic Lymphatic, Percutaneous Endoscopic Approach
07NF0ZZ Release Right Lower Extremity Lymphatic, Open Approach
07NF3ZZ Release Right Lower Extremity Lymphatic, Percutaneous Approach
07NF4ZZ Release Right Lower Extremity Lymphatic, Percutaneous Endoscopic Approach
07NG0ZZ Release Left Lower Extremity Lymphati Open Approach
07NG3ZZ Release Left Lower Extremity Lymphat Percutaneous Approach
07NG4ZZ Release Left Lower Extremity Lymphati Percutaneous Endoscopic Approach
07NH0ZZ Release Right Inguinal Lymphatic, Ope Approach
07NH3ZZ Release Right Inguinal Lymphatic, Percutaneous Approach
07NH4ZZ Release Right Inguinal Lymphatic, Percutaneous Endoscopic Approach
07NJ0ZZ Release Left Inguinal Lymphatic, Open Approach
07NJ3ZZ Release Left Inguinal Lymphatic, Percutaneous Approach
07NJ4ZZ Release Left Inguinal Lymphatic, Percutaneous Endoscopic Approach
07NK0ZZ Release Thoracic Duct, Open Approach
07NK3ZZ Release Thoracic Duct, Percutaneous Approach
07NK4ZZ Release Thoracic Duct, Percutaneous Endoscopic Approach
07NL0ZZ Release Cisterna Chyli, Open Approach
07NL3ZZ Release Cisterna Chyli, Percutaneous Approach
07NL4ZZ Release Cisterna Chyli, Percutaneous Endoscopic Approach
07NM0ZZ Release Thymus, Open Approach
07NM3ZZ Release Thymus, Percutaneous Approac
07NM4ZZ Release Thymus, Percutaneous Endoscopic Approach
07NP0ZZ Release Spleen, Open Approach
07NP3ZZ Release Spleen, Percutaneous Approach
07NP4ZZ Release Spleen, Percutaneous Endoscopi Approach

07P – Lymphatic and Hemic Systems, Removal

Review Coding Guideline B6.1c

07PK00Z Removal of Drainage Device from Thoracic Duct, Open Approach
07PK03Z Removal of Infusion Device from Thoracic Duct, Open Approach
07PK07Z Removal of Autologous Tissue Substitute from Thoracic Duct, Open Approach
07PK0CZ Removal of Extraluminal Device from Thoracic Duct, Open Approach
07PK0DZ Removal of Intraluminal Device from Thoracic Duct, Open Approach
07PK0JZ Removal of Synthetic Substitute from Thoracic Duct, Open Approach
07PK0KZ Removal of Nonautologous Tissue Substitute from Thoracic Duct, Open Approach
07PK30Z Removal of Drainage Device from Thoracic Duct, Percutaneous Approach
07PK33Z Removal of Infusion Device from Thoracic Duct, Percutaneous Approach
07PK37Z Removal of Autologous Tissue Substitute from Thoracic Duct, Percutaneous Approach
07PK3CZ Removal of Extraluminal Device from Thoracic Duct, Percutaneous Approach
07PK3DZ Removal of Intraluminal Device from Thoracic Duct, Percutaneous Approach
07PK3JZ Removal of Synthetic Substitute from Thoracic Duct, Percutaneous Approach
07PK3KZ Removal of Nonautologous Tissue Substitute from Thoracic Duct, Percutaneous Approach
07PK40Z Removal of Drainage Device from Thoracic Duct, Percutaneous Endoscopic Approach
07PK43Z Removal of Infusion Device from Thoracic Duct, Percutaneous Endoscopic Approach
07PK47Z Removal of Autologous Tissue Substitute from Thoracic Duct, Percutaneous Endoscopic Approach
07PK4CZ Removal of Extraluminal Device from Thoracic Duct, Percutaneous Endoscopic Approach
07PK4DZ Removal of Intraluminal Device from Thoracic Duct, Percutaneous Endoscopic Approach
07PK4JZ Removal of Synthetic Substitute from Thoracic Duct, Percutaneous Endoscopic Approach
07PK4KZ Removal of Nonautologous Tissue Substitute from Thoracic Duct, Percutaneous Endoscopic Approach
07PKX0Z Removal of Drainage Device from Thoracic Duct, External Approach
07PKX3Z Removal of Infusion Device from Thoracic Duct, External Approach
07PKXDZ Removal of Intraluminal Device from Thoracic Duct, External Approach
07PL00Z Removal of Drainage Device from Cisterna Chyli, Open Approach
07PL03Z Removal of Infusion Device from Cistern Chyli, Open Approach
07PL07Z Removal of Autologous Tissue Substitute from Cisterna Chyli, Open Approach
07PL0CZ Removal of Extraluminal Device from Cisterna Chyli, Open Approach
07PL0DZ Removal of Intraluminal Device from Cisterna Chyli, Open Approach
07PL0JZ Removal of Synthetic Substitute from Cisterna Chyli, Open Approach
07PL0KZ Removal of Nonautologous Tissue Substitute from Cisterna Chyli, Open Approach
07PL30Z Removal of Drainage Device from Cisterna Chyli, Percutaneous Approach
07PL33Z Removal of Infusion Device from Cistern Chyli, Percutaneous Approach

L37Z Removal of Autologous Tissue Substitute from Cisterna Chyli, Percutaneous Approach

L3CZ Removal of Extraluminal Device from Cisterna Chyli, Percutaneous Approach

L3DZ Removal of Intraluminal Device from Cisterna Chyli, Percutaneous Approach

PL3JZ Removal of Synthetic Substitute from Cisterna Chyli, Percutaneous Approach

PL3KZ Removal of Nonautologous Tissue Substitute from Cisterna Chyli, Percutaneous Approach

PL40Z Removal of Drainage Device from Cisterna Chyli, Percutaneous Endoscopic Approach

PL43Z Removal of Infusion Device from Cisterna Chyli, Percutaneous Endoscopic Approach

PL47Z Removal of Autologous Tissue Substitute from Cisterna Chyli, Percutaneous Endoscopic Approach

PL4CZ Removal of Extraluminal Device from Cisterna Chyli, Percutaneous Endoscopic Approach

PL4DZ Removal of Intraluminal Device from Cisterna Chyli, Percutaneous Endoscopic Approach

PL4JZ Removal of Synthetic Substitute from Cisterna Chyli, Percutaneous Endoscopic Approach

PL4KZ Removal of Nonautologous Tissue Substitute from Cisterna Chyli, Percutaneous Endoscopic Approach

PLX0Z Removal of Drainage Device from Cisterna Chyli, External Approach

PLX3Z Removal of Infusion Device from Cisterna Chyli, External Approach

PLXDZ Removal of Intraluminal Device from Cisterna Chyli, External Approach

PM00Z Removal of Drainage Device from Thymus, Open Approach

PM03Z Removal of Infusion Device from Thymus, Open Approach

PM30Z Removal of Drainage Device from Thymus, Percutaneous Approach

PM33Z Removal of Infusion Device from Thymus, Percutaneous Approach

07PM40Z Removal of Drainage Device from Thymus, Percutaneous Endoscopic Approach

07PM43Z Removal of Infusion Device from Thymus, Percutaneous Endoscopic Approach

07PMX0Z Removal of Drainage Device from Thymus, External Approach

07PMX3Z Removal of Infusion Device from Thymus, External Approach

07PN00Z Removal of Drainage Device from Lymphatic, Open Approach

07PN03Z Removal of Infusion Device from Lymphatic, Open Approach

07PN07Z Removal of Autologous Tissue Substitute from Lymphatic, Open Approach

07PN0CZ Removal of Extraluminal Device from Lymphatic, Open Approach

07PN0DZ Removal of Intraluminal Device from Lymphatic, Open Approach

07PN0JZ Removal of Synthetic Substitute from Lymphatic, Open Approach

07PN0KZ Removal of Nonautologous Tissue Substitute from Lymphatic, Open Approach

07PN30Z Removal of Drainage Device from Lymphatic, Percutaneous Approach

07PN33Z Removal of Infusion Device from Lymphatic, Percutaneous Approach

07PN37Z Removal of Autologous Tissue Substitute from Lymphatic, Percutaneous Approach

07PN3CZ Removal of Extraluminal Device from Lymphatic, Percutaneous Approach

07PN3DZ Removal of Intraluminal Device from Lymphatic, Percutaneous Approach

07PN3JZ Removal of Synthetic Substitute from Lymphatic, Percutaneous Approach

07PN3KZ Removal of Nonautologous Tissue Substitute from Lymphatic, Percutaneous Approach

07PN40Z Removal of Drainage Device from Lymphatic, Percutaneous Endoscopic Approach

07PN43Z Removal of Infusion Device from Lymphatic, Percutaneous Endoscopic Approach

07PN47Z Removal of Autologous Tissue Substitute from Lymphatic, Percutaneous Endoscopic Approach

07PN4CZ Removal of Extraluminal Device from Lymphatic, Percutaneous Endoscopic Approach

07PN4DZ Removal of Intraluminal Device from Lymphatic, Percutaneous Endoscopic Approach

07PN4JZ Removal of Synthetic Substitute from Lymphatic, Percutaneous Endoscopic Approach

07PN4KZ Removal of Nonautologous Tissue Substitute from Lymphatic, Percutaneous Endoscopic Approach

07PNX0Z Removal of Drainage Device from Lymphatic, External Approach

07PNX3Z Removal of Infusion Device from Lymphatic, External Approach

07PNXDZ Removal of Intraluminal Device from Lymphatic, External Approach

07PP00Z Removal of Drainage Device from Spleen, Open Approach

07PP03Z Removal of Infusion Device from Spleen, Open Approach

07PP30Z Removal of Drainage Device from Spleen, Percutaneous Approach

07PP33Z Removal of Infusion Device from Spleen, Percutaneous Approach

07PP40Z Removal of Drainage Device from Spleen, Percutaneous Endoscopic Approach

07PP43Z Removal of Infusion Device from Spleen, Percutaneous Endoscopic Approach

07PPX0Z Removal of Drainage Device from Spleen, External Approach

07PPX3Z Removal of Infusion Device from Spleen, External Approach

07PT00Z Removal of Drainage Device from Bone Marrow, Open Approach

07PT30Z Removal of Drainage Device from Bone Marrow, Percutaneous Approach

07PT40Z Removal of Drainage Device from Bone Marrow, Percutaneous Endoscopic Approach

07PTX0Z Removal of Drainage Device from Bone Marrow, External Approach

7Q – Lymphatic and Hemic Systems, Repair

Q00ZZ Repair Head Lymphatic, Open Approach

Q03ZZ Repair Head Lymphatic, Percutaneous Approach

Q04ZZ Repair Head Lymphatic, Percutaneous Endoscopic Approach

Q10ZZ Repair Right Neck Lymphatic, Open Approach

7Q13ZZ Repair Right Neck Lymphatic, Percutaneous Approach

Q14ZZ Repair Right Neck Lymphatic, Percutaneous Endoscopic Approach

7Q20ZZ Repair Left Neck Lymphatic, Open Approach

7Q23ZZ Repair Left Neck Lymphatic, Percutaneous Approach

7Q24ZZ Repair Left Neck Lymphatic, Percutaneous Endoscopic Approach

7Q30ZZ Repair Right Upper Extremity Lymphatic, Open Approach

7Q33ZZ Repair Right Upper Extremity Lymphatic, Percutaneous Approach

7Q34ZZ Repair Right Upper Extremity Lymphatic, Percutaneous Endoscopic Approach

7Q40ZZ Repair Left Upper Extremity Lymphatic, Open Approach

07Q43ZZ Repair Left Upper Extremity Lymphatic, Percutaneous Approach

07Q44ZZ Repair Left Upper Extremity Lymphatic, Percutaneous Endoscopic Approach

07Q50ZZ Repair Right Axillary Lymphatic, Open Approach

07Q53ZZ Repair Right Axillary Lymphatic, Percutaneous Approach

07Q54ZZ Repair Right Axillary Lymphatic, Percutaneous Endoscopic Approach

07Q60ZZ Repair Left Axillary Lymphatic, Open Approach

07Q63ZZ Repair Left Axillary Lymphatic, Percutaneous Approach

07Q64ZZ Repair Left Axillary Lymphatic, Percutaneous Endoscopic Approach

07Q70ZZ Repair Thorax Lymphatic, Open Approach

07Q73ZZ Repair Thorax Lymphatic, Percutaneous Approach

07Q74ZZ Repair Thorax Lymphatic, Percutaneous Endoscopic Approach

07Q80ZZ Repair Right Internal Mammary Lymphatic, Open Approach

07Q83ZZ Repair Right Internal Mammary Lymphatic, Percutaneous Approach

07Q84ZZ Repair Right Internal Mammary Lymphatic, Percutaneous Endoscopic Approach

07Q90ZZ Repair Left Internal Mammary Lymphatic, Open Approach

07Q93ZZ Repair Left Internal Mammary Lymphatic, Percutaneous Approach

07Q94ZZ Repair Left Internal Mammary Lymphatic, Percutaneous Endoscopic Approach

07QB0ZZ Repair Mesenteric Lymphatic, Open Approach

07QB3ZZ Repair Mesenteric Lymphatic, Percutaneous Approach

07QB4ZZ Repair Mesenteric Lymphatic, Percutaneous Endoscopic Approach

07QC0ZZ Repair Pelvis Lymphatic, Open Approach

07QC3ZZ Repair Pelvis Lymphatic, Percutaneous Approach

07QC4ZZ Repair Pelvis Lymphatic, Percutaneous Endoscopic Approach

07QD0ZZ Repair Aortic Lymphatic, Open Approach

07QD3ZZ Repair Aortic Lymphatic, Percutaneous Approach

07QD4ZZ Repair Aortic Lymphatic, Percutaneous Endoscopic Approach

07QF0ZZ Repair Right Lower Extremity Lymphatic, Open Approach
07QF3ZZ Repair Right Lower Extremity Lymphatic, Percutaneous Approach
07QF4ZZ Repair Right Lower Extremity Lymphatic, Percutaneous Endoscopic Approach
07QG0ZZ Repair Left Lower Extremity Lymphatic, Open Approach
07QG3ZZ Repair Left Lower Extremity Lymphatic, Percutaneous Approach
07QG4ZZ Repair Left Lower Extremity Lymphatic, Percutaneous Endoscopic Approach
07QH0ZZ Repair Right Inguinal Lymphatic, Open Approach
07QH3ZZ Repair Right Inguinal Lymphatic, Percutaneous Approach
07QH4ZZ Repair Right Inguinal Lymphatic, Percutaneous Endoscopic Approach
07QJ0ZZ Repair Left Inguinal Lymphatic, Open Approach
07QJ3ZZ Repair Left Inguinal Lymphatic, Percutaneous Approach
07QJ4ZZ Repair Left Inguinal Lymphatic, Percutaneous Endoscopic Approach
07QK0ZZ Repair Thoracic Duct, Open Approach
07QK3ZZ Repair Thoracic Duct, Percutaneous Approach
07QK4ZZ Repair Thoracic Duct, Percutaneous Endoscopic Approach
07QL0ZZ Repair Cisterna Chyli, Open Approach
07QL3ZZ Repair Cisterna Chyli, Percutaneous Approach
07QL4ZZ Repair Cisterna Chyli, Percutaneous Endoscopic Approach
07QM0ZZ Repair Thymus, Open Approach
07QM3ZZ Repair Thymus, Percutaneous Approach
07QM4ZZ Repair Thymus, Percutaneous Endoscopic Approach
07QP0ZZ Repair Spleen, Open Approach
07QP3ZZ Repair Spleen, Percutaneous Approach
07QP4ZZ Repair Spleen, Percutaneous Endoscopic Approach

07S – Lymphatic and Hemic Systems, Reposition

07SM0ZZ Reposition Thymus, Open Approach
07SP0ZZ Reposition Spleen, Open Approach

07T – Lymphatic and Hemic Systems, Resection

Review Coding Guideline B3.8

07T00ZZ Resection of Head Lymphatic, Open Approach
07T04ZZ Resection of Head Lymphatic, Percutaneous Endoscopic Approach
07T10ZZ Resection of Right Neck Lymphatic, Open Approach
07T14ZZ Resection of Right Neck Lymphatic, Percutaneous Endoscopic Approach
07T20ZZ Resection of Left Neck Lymphatic, Open Approach
07T24ZZ Resection of Left Neck Lymphatic, Percutaneous Endoscopic Approach
07T30ZZ Resection of Right Upper Extremity Lymphatic, Open Approach
07T34ZZ Resection of Right Upper Extremity Lymphatic, Percutaneous Endoscopic Approach
07T40ZZ Resection of Left Upper Extremity Lymphatic, Open Approach
07T44ZZ Resection of Left Upper Extremity Lymphatic, Percutaneous Endoscopic Approach
07T50ZZ Resection of Right Axillary Lymphatic, Open Approach

+ Mastectomy procedure when reported with resection of breast. *See table 0HT to construct the Resection of breast code. See table 0KT to construct the Resection of thorax muscle code if applicable. See table 07T to report additional lymph node resections.*

07T54ZZ Resection of Right Axillary Lymphatic, Percutaneous Endoscopic Approach
07T60ZZ Resection of Left Axillary Lymphatic, Open Approach

+ Mastectomy procedure when reported with resection of breast. *See table 0HT to construct the Resection of breast code. See table 0KT to construct the Resection of thorax muscle code if applicable. See table 07T to report additional lymph node resections.*

07T64ZZ Resection of Left Axillary Lymphatic, Percutaneous Endoscopic Approach
07T70ZZ Resection of Thorax Lymphatic, Open Approach
07T74ZZ Resection of Thorax Lymphatic, Percutaneous Endoscopic Approach
07T80ZZ Resection of Right Internal Mammary Lymphatic, Open Approach
07T84ZZ Resection of Right Internal Mammary Lymphatic, Percutaneous Endoscopic Approach
07T90ZZ Resection of Left Internal Mammary Lymphatic, Open Approach
07T94ZZ Resection of Left Internal Mammary Lymphatic, Percutaneous Endoscopic Approach
07TB0ZZ Resection of Mesenteric Lymphatic, Open Approach
07TB4ZZ Resection of Mesenteric Lymphatic, Percutaneous Endoscopic Approach
07TC0ZZ Resection of Pelvis Lymphatic, Open Approach
07TC4ZZ Resection of Pelvis Lymphatic, Percutaneous Endoscopic Approach
07TD0ZZ Resection of Aortic Lymphatic, Open Approach
07TD4ZZ Resection of Aortic Lymphatic, Percutaneous Endoscopic Approach
07TF0ZZ Resection of Right Lower Extremity Lymphatic, Open Approach
07TF4ZZ Resection of Right Lower Extremity Lymphatic, Percutaneous Endoscopic Approach
07TG0ZZ Resection of Left Lower Extremity Lymphatic, Open Approach
07TG4ZZ Resection of Left Lower Extremity Lymphatic, Percutaneous Endoscopic Approach
07TH0ZZ Resection of Right Inguinal Lymphatic, Open Approach
07TH4ZZ Resection of Right Inguinal Lymphatic, Percutaneous Endoscopic Approach
07TJ0ZZ Resection of Left Inguinal Lymphatic, Open Approach
07TJ4ZZ Resection of Left Inguinal Lymphatic, Percutaneous Endoscopic Approach
07TK0ZZ Resection of Thoracic Duct, Open Approach
07TK4ZZ Resection of Thoracic Duct, Percutaneous Endoscopic Approach
07TL0ZZ Resection of Cisterna Chyli, Open Approach
07TL4ZZ Resection of Cisterna Chyli, Percutaneous Endoscopic Approach
07TM0ZZ Resection of Thymus, Open Approach
07TM4ZZ Resection of Thymus, Percutaneous Endoscopic Approach
07TP0ZZ Resection of Spleen, Open Approach
07TP4ZZ Resection of Spleen, Percutaneous Endoscopic Approach

07U – Lymphatic and Hemic Systems, Supplement

07U007Z Supplement Head Lymphatic with Autologous Tissue Substitute, Open Approach
07U00JZ Supplement Head Lymphatic with Synthetic Substitute, Open Approach
07U00KZ Supplement Head Lymphatic with Nonautologous Tissue Substitute, Open Approach
07U047Z Supplement Head Lymphatic with Autologous Tissue Substitute, Percutaneous Endoscopic Approach
07U04JZ Supplement Head Lymphatic with Synthetic Substitute, Percutaneous Endoscopic Approach
07U04KZ Supplement Head Lymphatic with Nonautologous Tissue Substitute, Percutaneous Endoscopic Approach
07U107Z Supplement Right Neck Lymphatic with Autologous Tissue Substitute, Open Approach
07U10JZ Supplement Right Neck Lymphatic with Synthetic Substitute, Open Approach
07U10KZ Supplement Right Neck Lymphatic with Nonautologous Tissue Substitute, Open Approach
07U147Z Supplement Right Neck Lymphatic with Autologous Tissue Substitute, Percutaneous Endoscopic Approach
07U14JZ Supplement Right Neck Lymphatic with Synthetic Substitute, Percutaneous Endoscopic Approach
07U14KZ Supplement Right Neck Lymphatic with Nonautologous Tissue Substitute, Percutaneous Endoscopic Approach
07U207Z Supplement Left Neck Lymphatic with Autologous Tissue Substitute, Open Approach
07U20JZ Supplement Left Neck Lymphatic with Synthetic Substitute, Open Approach
07U20KZ Supplement Left Neck Lymphatic with Nonautologous Tissue Substitute, Open Approach
07U247Z Supplement Left Neck Lymphatic with Autologous Tissue Substitute, Percutaneous Endoscopic Approach
07U24JZ Supplement Left Neck Lymphatic with Synthetic Substitute, Percutaneous Endoscopic Approach
07U24KZ Supplement Left Neck Lymphatic with Nonautologous Tissue Substitute, Percutaneous Endoscopic Approach

J307Z Supplement Right Upper Extremity Lymphatic with Autologous Tissue Substitute, Open Approach
J30JZ Supplement Right Upper Extremity Lymphatic with Synthetic Substitute, Open Approach
J30KZ Supplement Right Upper Extremity Lymphatic with Nonautologous Tissue Substitute, Open Approach
J347Z Supplement Right Upper Extremity Lymphatic with Autologous Tissue Substitute, Percutaneous Endoscopic Approach
J34JZ Supplement Right Upper Extremity Lymphatic with Synthetic Substitute, Percutaneous Endoscopic Approach
U34KZ Supplement Right Upper Extremity Lymphatic with Nonautologous Tissue Substitute, Percutaneous Endoscopic Approach
U407Z Supplement Left Upper Extremity Lymphatic with Autologous Tissue Substitute, Open Approach
U40JZ Supplement Left Upper Extremity Lymphatic with Synthetic Substitute, Open Approach
U40KZ Supplement Left Upper Extremity Lymphatic with Nonautologous Tissue Substitute, Open Approach
U447Z Supplement Left Upper Extremity Lymphatic with Autologous Tissue Substitute, Percutaneous Endoscopic Approach
U44JZ Supplement Left Upper Extremity Lymphatic with Synthetic Substitute, Percutaneous Endoscopic Approach
U44KZ Supplement Left Upper Extremity Lymphatic with Nonautologous Tissue Substitute, Percutaneous Endoscopic Approach
U507Z Supplement Right Axillary Lymphatic with Autologous Tissue Substitute, Open Approach
U50JZ Supplement Right Axillary Lymphatic with Synthetic Substitute, Open Approach
U50KZ Supplement Right Axillary Lymphatic with Nonautologous Tissue Substitute, Open Approach
U547Z Supplement Right Axillary Lymphatic with Autologous Tissue Substitute, Percutaneous Endoscopic Approach
U54JZ Supplement Right Axillary Lymphatic with Synthetic Substitute, Percutaneous Endoscopic Approach
U54KZ Supplement Right Axillary Lymphatic with Nonautologous Tissue Substitute, Percutaneous Endoscopic Approach
U607Z Supplement Left Axillary Lymphatic with Autologous Tissue Substitute, Open Approach
U60JZ Supplement Left Axillary Lymphatic with Synthetic Substitute, Open Approach
U60KZ Supplement Left Axillary Lymphatic with Nonautologous Tissue Substitute, Open Approach
U647Z Supplement Left Axillary Lymphatic with Autologous Tissue Substitute, Percutaneous Endoscopic Approach
U64JZ Supplement Left Axillary Lymphatic with Synthetic Substitute, Percutaneous Endoscopic Approach
U64KZ Supplement Left Axillary Lymphatic with Nonautologous Tissue Substitute, Percutaneous Endoscopic Approach
U707Z Supplement Thorax Lymphatic with Autologous Tissue Substitute, Open Approach
U70JZ Supplement Thorax Lymphatic with Synthetic Substitute, Open Approach
07U70KZ Supplement Thorax Lymphatic with Nonautologous Tissue Substitute, Open Approach
07U747Z Supplement Thorax Lymphatic with Autologous Tissue Substitute, Percutaneous Endoscopic Approach
07U74JZ Supplement Thorax Lymphatic with Synthetic Substitute, Percutaneous Endoscopic Approach
07U74KZ Supplement Thorax Lymphatic with Nonautologous Tissue Substitute, Percutaneous Endoscopic Approach
07U807Z Supplement Right Internal Mammary Lymphatic with Autologous Tissue Substitute, Open Approach
07U80JZ Supplement Right Internal Mammary Lymphatic with Synthetic Substitute, Open Approach
07U80KZ Supplement Right Internal Mammary Lymphatic with Nonautologous Tissue Substitute, Open Approach
07U847Z Supplement Right Internal Mammary Lymphatic with Autologous Tissue Substitute, Percutaneous Endoscopic Approach
07U84JZ Supplement Right Internal Mammary Lymphatic with Synthetic Substitute, Percutaneous Endoscopic Approach
07U84KZ Supplement Right Internal Mammary Lymphatic with Nonautologous Tissue Substitute, Percutaneous Endoscopic Approach
07U907Z Supplement Left Internal Mammary Lymphatic with Autologous Tissue Substitute, Open Approach
07U90JZ Supplement Left Internal Mammary Lymphatic with Synthetic Substitute, Open Approach
07U90KZ Supplement Left Internal Mammary Lymphatic with Nonautologous Tissue Substitute, Open Approach
07U947Z Supplement Left Internal Mammary Lymphatic with Autologous Tissue Substitute, Percutaneous Endoscopic Approach
07U94JZ Supplement Left Internal Mammary Lymphatic with Synthetic Substitute, Percutaneous Endoscopic Approach
07U94KZ Supplement Left Internal Mammary Lymphatic with Nonautologous Tissue Substitute, Percutaneous Endoscopic Approach
07UB07Z Supplement Mesenteric Lymphatic with Autologous Tissue Substitute, Open Approach
07UB0JZ Supplement Mesenteric Lymphatic with Synthetic Substitute, Open Approach
07UB0KZ Supplement Mesenteric Lymphatic with Nonautologous Tissue Substitute, Open Approach
07UB47Z Supplement Mesenteric Lymphatic with Autologous Tissue Substitute, Percutaneous Endoscopic Approach
07UB4JZ Supplement Mesenteric Lymphatic with Synthetic Substitute, Percutaneous Endoscopic Approach
07UB4KZ Supplement Mesenteric Lymphatic with Nonautologous Tissue Substitute, Percutaneous Endoscopic Approach
07UC07Z Supplement Pelvis Lymphatic with Autologous Tissue Substitute, Open Approach
07UC0JZ Supplement Pelvis Lymphatic with Synthetic Substitute, Open Approach
07UC0KZ Supplement Pelvis Lymphatic with Nonautologous Tissue Substitute, Open Approach
07UC47Z Supplement Pelvis Lymphatic with Autologous Tissue Substitute, Percutaneous Endoscopic Approach
07UC4JZ Supplement Pelvis Lymphatic with Synthetic Substitute, Percutaneous Endoscopic Approach
07UC4KZ Supplement Pelvis Lymphatic with Nonautologous Tissue Substitute, Percutaneous Endoscopic Approach
07UD07Z Supplement Aortic Lymphatic with Autologous Tissue Substitute, Open Approach
07UD0JZ Supplement Aortic Lymphatic with Synthetic Substitute, Open Approach
07UD0KZ Supplement Aortic Lymphatic with Nonautologous Tissue Substitute, Open Approach
07UD47Z Supplement Aortic Lymphatic with Autologous Tissue Substitute, Percutaneous Endoscopic Approach
07UD4JZ Supplement Aortic Lymphatic with Synthetic Substitute, Percutaneous Endoscopic Approach
07UD4KZ Supplement Aortic Lymphatic with Nonautologous Tissue Substitute, Percutaneous Endoscopic Approach
07UF07Z Supplement Right Lower Extremity Lymphatic with Autologous Tissue Substitute, Open Approach
07UF0JZ Supplement Right Lower Extremity Lymphatic with Synthetic Substitute, Open Approach
07UF0KZ Supplement Right Lower Extremity Lymphatic with Nonautologous Tissue Substitute, Open Approach
07UF47Z Supplement Right Lower Extremity Lymphatic with Autologous Tissue Substitute, Percutaneous Endoscopic Approach
07UF4JZ Supplement Right Lower Extremity Lymphatic with Synthetic Substitute, Percutaneous Endoscopic Approach
07UF4KZ Supplement Right Lower Extremity Lymphatic with Nonautologous Tissue Substitute, Percutaneous Endoscopic Approach
07UG07Z Supplement Left Lower Extremity Lymphatic with Autologous Tissue Substitute, Open Approach
07UG0JZ Supplement Left Lower Extremity Lymphatic with Synthetic Substitute, Open Approach
07UG0KZ Supplement Left Lower Extremity Lymphatic with Nonautologous Tissue Substitute, Open Approach
07UG47Z Supplement Left Lower Extremity Lymphatic with Autologous Tissue Substitute, Percutaneous Endoscopic Approach
07UG4JZ Supplement Left Lower Extremity Lymphatic with Synthetic Substitute, Percutaneous Endoscopic Approach
07UG4KZ Supplement Left Lower Extremity Lymphatic with Nonautologous Tissue Substitute, Percutaneous Endoscopic Approach
07UH07Z Supplement Right Inguinal Lymphatic with Autologous Tissue Substitute, Open Approach
07UH0JZ Supplement Right Inguinal Lymphatic with Synthetic Substitute, Open Approach
07UH0KZ Supplement Right Inguinal Lymphatic with Nonautologous Tissue Substitute, Open Approach
07UH47Z Supplement Right Inguinal Lymphatic with Autologous Tissue Substitute, Percutaneous Endoscopic Approach

07UH4JZ Supplement Right Inguinal Lymphatic with Synthetic Substitute, Percutaneous Endoscopic Approach
07UH4KZ Supplement Right Inguinal Lymphatic with Nonautologous Tissue Substitute, Percutaneous Endoscopic Approach
07UJ07Z Supplement Left Inguinal Lymphatic with Autologous Tissue Substitute, Open Approach
07UJ0JZ Supplement Left Inguinal Lymphatic with Synthetic Substitute, Open Approach
07UJ0KZ Supplement Left Inguinal Lymphatic with Nonautologous Tissue Substitute, Open Approach
07UJ47Z Supplement Left Inguinal Lymphatic with Autologous Tissue Substitute, Percutaneous Endoscopic Approach
07UJ4JZ Supplement Left Inguinal Lymphatic with Synthetic Substitute, Percutaneous Endoscopic Approach
07UJ4KZ Supplement Left Inguinal Lymphatic with Nonautologous Tissue Substitute, Percutaneous Endoscopic Approach
07UK07Z Supplement Thoracic Duct with Autologous Tissue Substitute, Open Approach
07UK0JZ Supplement Thoracic Duct with Synthetic Substitute, Open Approach
07UK0KZ Supplement Thoracic Duct with Nonautologous Tissue Substitute, Open Approach
07UK47Z Supplement Thoracic Duct with Autologous Tissue Substitute, Percutaneous Endoscopic Approach
07UK4JZ Supplement Thoracic Duct with Synthetic Substitute, Percutaneous Endoscopic Approach
07UK4KZ Supplement Thoracic Duct with Nonautologous Tissue Substitute, Percutaneous Endoscopic Approach
07UL07Z Supplement Cisterna Chyli with Autologous Tissue Substitute, Open Approach
07UL0JZ Supplement Cisterna Chyli with Synthetic Substitute, Open Approach
07UL0KZ Supplement Cisterna Chyli with Nonautologous Tissue Substitute, Open Approach
07UL47Z Supplement Cisterna Chyli with Autologous Tissue Substitute, Percutaneous Endoscopic Approach
07UL4JZ Supplement Cisterna Chyli with Synthetic Substitute, Percutaneous Endoscopic Approach
07UL4KZ Supplement Cisterna Chyli with Nonautologous Tissue Substitute, Percutaneous Endoscopic Approach

07V – Lymphatic and Hemic Systems, Restriction

07V00CZ Restriction of Head Lymphatic with Extraluminal Device, Open Approach
07V00DZ Restriction of Head Lymphatic with Intraluminal Device, Open Approach
07V00ZZ Restriction of Head Lymphatic, Open Approach
07V03CZ Restriction of Head Lymphatic with Extraluminal Device, Percutaneous Approach
07V03DZ Restriction of Head Lymphatic with Intraluminal Device, Percutaneous Approach
07V03ZZ Restriction of Head Lymphatic, Percutaneous Approach
07V04CZ Restriction of Head Lymphatic with Extraluminal Device, Percutaneous Endoscopic Approach
07V04DZ Restriction of Head Lymphatic with Intraluminal Device, Percutaneous Endoscopic Approach
07V04ZZ Restriction of Head Lymphatic, Percutaneous Endoscopic Approach
07V10CZ Restriction of Right Neck Lymphatic with Extraluminal Device, Open Approach
07V10DZ Restriction of Right Neck Lymphatic with Intraluminal Device, Open Approach
07V10ZZ Restriction of Right Neck Lymphatic, Open Approach
07V13CZ Restriction of Right Neck Lymphatic with Extraluminal Device, Percutaneous Approach
07V13DZ Restriction of Right Neck Lymphatic with Intraluminal Device, Percutaneous Approach
07V13ZZ Restriction of Right Neck Lymphatic, Percutaneous Approach
07V14CZ Restriction of Right Neck Lymphatic with Extraluminal Device, Percutaneous Endoscopic Approach
07V14DZ Restriction of Right Neck Lymphatic with Intraluminal Device, Percutaneous Endoscopic Approach
07V14ZZ Restriction of Right Neck Lymphatic, Percutaneous Endoscopic Approach
07V20CZ Restriction of Left Neck Lymphatic with Extraluminal Device, Open Approach
07V20DZ Restriction of Left Neck Lymphatic with Intraluminal Device, Open Approach
07V20ZZ Restriction of Left Neck Lymphatic, Open Approach
07V23CZ Restriction of Left Neck Lymphatic with Extraluminal Device, Percutaneous Approach
07V23DZ Restriction of Left Neck Lymphatic with Intraluminal Device, Percutaneous Approach
07V23ZZ Restriction of Left Neck Lymphatic, Percutaneous Approach
07V24CZ Restriction of Left Neck Lymphatic with Extraluminal Device, Percutaneous Endoscopic Approach
07V24DZ Restriction of Left Neck Lymphatic with Intraluminal Device, Percutaneous Endoscopic Approach
07V24ZZ Restriction of Left Neck Lymphatic, Percutaneous Endoscopic Approach
07V30CZ Restriction of Right Upper Extremity Lymphatic with Extraluminal Device, Open Approach
07V30DZ Restriction of Right Upper Extremity Lymphatic with Intraluminal Device, Open Approach
07V30ZZ Restriction of Right Upper Extremity Lymphatic, Open Approach
07V33CZ Restriction of Right Upper Extremity Lymphatic with Extraluminal Device, Percutaneous Approach
07V33DZ Restriction of Right Upper Extremity Lymphatic with Intraluminal Device, Percutaneous Approach
07V33ZZ Restriction of Right Upper Extremity Lymphatic, Percutaneous Approach
07V34CZ Restriction of Right Upper Extremity Lymphatic with Extraluminal Device, Percutaneous Endoscopic Approach
07V34DZ Restriction of Right Upper Extremity Lymphatic with Intraluminal Device, Percutaneous Endoscopic Approach
07V34ZZ Restriction of Right Upper Extremity Lymphatic, Percutaneous Endoscopic Approach
07V40CZ Restriction of Left Upper Extremity Lymphatic with Extraluminal Device, Open Approach
07V40DZ Restriction of Left Upper Extremity Lymphatic with Intraluminal Device, Open Approach
07V40ZZ Restriction of Left Upper Extremity Lymphatic, Open Approach
07V43CZ Restriction of Left Upper Extremity Lymphatic with Extraluminal Device, Percutaneous Approach
07V43DZ Restriction of Left Upper Extremity Lymphatic with Intraluminal Device, Percutaneous Approach
07V43ZZ Restriction of Left Upper Extremity Lymphatic, Percutaneous Approach
07V44CZ Restriction of Left Upper Extremity Lymphatic with Extraluminal Device, Percutaneous Endoscopic Approach
07V44DZ Restriction of Left Upper Extremity Lymphatic with Intraluminal Device, Percutaneous Endoscopic Approach
07V44ZZ Restriction of Left Upper Extremity Lymphatic, Percutaneous Endoscopic Approach
07V50CZ Restriction of Right Axillary Lymphatic with Extraluminal Device, Open Approach
07V50DZ Restriction of Right Axillary Lymphatic with Intraluminal Device, Open Approach
07V50ZZ Restriction of Right Axillary Lymphatic, Open Approach
07V53CZ Restriction of Right Axillary Lymphatic with Extraluminal Device, Percutaneous Approach
07V53DZ Restriction of Right Axillary Lymphatic with Intraluminal Device, Percutaneous Approach
07V53ZZ Restriction of Right Axillary Lymphatic, Percutaneous Approach
07V54CZ Restriction of Right Axillary Lymphatic with Extraluminal Device, Percutaneous Endoscopic Approach
07V54DZ Restriction of Right Axillary Lymphatic with Intraluminal Device, Percutaneous Endoscopic Approach
07V54ZZ Restriction of Right Axillary Lymphatic, Percutaneous Endoscopic Approach
07V60CZ Restriction of Left Axillary Lymphatic with Extraluminal Device, Open Approach
07V60DZ Restriction of Left Axillary Lymphatic with Intraluminal Device, Open Approach
07V60ZZ Restriction of Left Axillary Lymphatic, Open Approach
07V63CZ Restriction of Left Axillary Lymphatic with Extraluminal Device, Percutaneous Approach
07V63DZ Restriction of Left Axillary Lymphatic with Intraluminal Device, Percutaneous Approach
07V63ZZ Restriction of Left Axillary Lymphatic, Percutaneous Approach

V64CZ Restriction of Left Axillary Lymphatic with Extraluminal Device, Percutaneous Endoscopic Approach
V64DZ Restriction of Left Axillary Lymphatic with Intraluminal Device, Percutaneous Endoscopic Approach
V64ZZ Restriction of Left Axillary Lymphatic, Percutaneous Endoscopic Approach
V70CZ Restriction of Thorax Lymphatic with Extraluminal Device, Open Approach
V70DZ Restriction of Thorax Lymphatic with Intraluminal Device, Open Approach
V70ZZ Restriction of Thorax Lymphatic, Open Approach
V73CZ Restriction of Thorax Lymphatic with Extraluminal Device, Percutaneous Approach
V73DZ Restriction of Thorax Lymphatic with Intraluminal Device, Percutaneous Approach
V73ZZ Restriction of Thorax Lymphatic, Percutaneous Approach
V74CZ Restriction of Thorax Lymphatic with Extraluminal Device, Percutaneous Endoscopic Approach
V74DZ Restriction of Thorax Lymphatic with Intraluminal Device, Percutaneous Endoscopic Approach
V74ZZ Restriction of Thorax Lymphatic, Percutaneous Endoscopic Approach
V80CZ Restriction of Right Internal Mammary Lymphatic with Extraluminal Device, Open Approach
V80DZ Restriction of Right Internal Mammary Lymphatic with Intraluminal Device, Open Approach
V80ZZ Restriction of Right Internal Mammary Lymphatic, Open Approach
V83CZ Restriction of Right Internal Mammary Lymphatic with Extraluminal Device, Percutaneous Approach
V83DZ Restriction of Right Internal Mammary Lymphatic with Intraluminal Device, Percutaneous Approach
V83ZZ Restriction of Right Internal Mammary Lymphatic, Percutaneous Approach
V84CZ Restriction of Right Internal Mammary Lymphatic with Extraluminal Device, Percutaneous Endoscopic Approach
V84DZ Restriction of Right Internal Mammary Lymphatic with Intraluminal Device, Percutaneous Endoscopic Approach
V84ZZ Restriction of Right Internal Mammary Lymphatic, Percutaneous Endoscopic Approach
V90CZ Restriction of Left Internal Mammary Lymphatic with Extraluminal Device, Open Approach
7V90DZ Restriction of Left Internal Mammary Lymphatic with Intraluminal Device, Open Approach
7V90ZZ Restriction of Left Internal Mammary Lymphatic, Open Approach
7V93CZ Restriction of Left Internal Mammary Lymphatic with Extraluminal Device, Percutaneous Approach
7V93DZ Restriction of Left Internal Mammary Lymphatic with Intraluminal Device, Percutaneous Approach
7V93ZZ Restriction of Left Internal Mammary Lymphatic, Percutaneous Approach
7V94CZ Restriction of Left Internal Mammary Lymphatic with Extraluminal Device, Percutaneous Endoscopic Approach
7V94DZ Restriction of Left Internal Mammary Lymphatic with Intraluminal Device, Percutaneous Endoscopic Approach

07V94ZZ Restriction of Left Internal Mammary Lymphatic, Percutaneous Endoscopic Approach
07VB0CZ Restriction of Mesenteric Lymphatic with Extraluminal Device, Open Approach
07VB0DZ Restriction of Mesenteric Lymphatic with Intraluminal Device, Open Approach
07VB0ZZ Restriction of Mesenteric Lymphatic, Open Approach
07VB3CZ Restriction of Mesenteric Lymphatic with Extraluminal Device, Percutaneous Approach
07VB3DZ Restriction of Mesenteric Lymphatic with Intraluminal Device, Percutaneous Approach
07VB3ZZ Restriction of Mesenteric Lymphatic, Percutaneous Approach
07VB4CZ Restriction of Mesenteric Lymphatic with Extraluminal Device, Percutaneous Endoscopic Approach
07VB4DZ Restriction of Mesenteric Lymphatic with Intraluminal Device, Percutaneous Endoscopic Approach
07VB4ZZ Restriction of Mesenteric Lymphatic, Percutaneous Endoscopic Approach
07VC0CZ Restriction of Pelvis Lymphatic with Extraluminal Device, Open Approach
07VC0DZ Restriction of Pelvis Lymphatic with Intraluminal Device, Open Approach
07VC0ZZ Restriction of Pelvis Lymphatic, Open Approach
07VC3CZ Restriction of Pelvis Lymphatic with Extraluminal Device, Percutaneous Approach
07VC3DZ Restriction of Pelvis Lymphatic with Intraluminal Device, Percutaneous Approach
07VC3ZZ Restriction of Pelvis Lymphatic, Percutaneous Approach
07VC4CZ Restriction of Pelvis Lymphatic with Extraluminal Device, Percutaneous Endoscopic Approach
07VC4DZ Restriction of Pelvis Lymphatic with Intraluminal Device, Percutaneous Endoscopic Approach
07VC4ZZ Restriction of Pelvis Lymphatic, Percutaneous Endoscopic Approach
07VD0CZ Restriction of Aortic Lymphatic with Extraluminal Device, Open Approach
07VD0DZ Restriction of Aortic Lymphatic with Intraluminal Device, Open Approach
07VD0ZZ Restriction of Aortic Lymphatic, Open Approach
07VD3CZ Restriction of Aortic Lymphatic with Extraluminal Device, Percutaneous Approach
07VD3DZ Restriction of Aortic Lymphatic with Intraluminal Device, Percutaneous Approach
07VD3ZZ Restriction of Aortic Lymphatic, Percutaneous Approach
07VD4CZ Restriction of Aortic Lymphatic with Extraluminal Device, Percutaneous Endoscopic Approach
07VD4DZ Restriction of Aortic Lymphatic with Intraluminal Device, Percutaneous Endoscopic Approach
07VD4ZZ Restriction of Aortic Lymphatic, Percutaneous Endoscopic Approach
07VF0CZ Restriction of Right Lower Extremity Lymphatic with Extraluminal Device, Open Approach
07VF0DZ Restriction of Right Lower Extremity Lymphatic with Intraluminal Device, Open Approach

07VF0ZZ Restriction of Right Lower Extremity Lymphatic, Open Approach
07VF3CZ Restriction of Right Lower Extremity Lymphatic with Extraluminal Device, Percutaneous Approach
07VF3DZ Restriction of Right Lower Extremity Lymphatic with Intraluminal Device, Percutaneous Approach
07VF3ZZ Restriction of Right Lower Extremity Lymphatic, Percutaneous Approach
07VF4CZ Restriction of Right Lower Extremity Lymphatic with Extraluminal Device, Percutaneous Endoscopic Approach
07VF4DZ Restriction of Right Lower Extremity Lymphatic with Intraluminal Device, Percutaneous Endoscopic Approach
07VF4ZZ Restriction of Right Lower Extremity Lymphatic, Percutaneous Endoscopic Approach
07VG0CZ Restriction of Left Lower Extremity Lymphatic with Extraluminal Device, Open Approach
07VG0DZ Restriction of Left Lower Extremity Lymphatic with Intraluminal Device, Open Approach
07VG0ZZ Restriction of Left Lower Extremity Lymphatic, Open Approach
07VG3CZ Restriction of Left Lower Extremity Lymphatic with Extraluminal Device, Percutaneous Approach
07VG3DZ Restriction of Left Lower Extremity Lymphatic with Intraluminal Device, Percutaneous Approach
07VG3ZZ Restriction of Left Lower Extremity Lymphatic, Percutaneous Approach
07VG4CZ Restriction of Left Lower Extremity Lymphatic with Extraluminal Device, Percutaneous Endoscopic Approach
07VG4DZ Restriction of Left Lower Extremity Lymphatic with Intraluminal Device, Percutaneous Endoscopic Approach
07VG4ZZ Restriction of Left Lower Extremity Lymphatic, Percutaneous Endoscopic Approach
07VH0CZ Restriction of Right Inguinal Lymphatic with Extraluminal Device, Open Approach
07VH0DZ Restriction of Right Inguinal Lymphatic with Intraluminal Device, Open Approach
07VH0ZZ Restriction of Right Inguinal Lymphatic, Open Approach
07VH3CZ Restriction of Right Inguinal Lymphatic with Extraluminal Device, Percutaneous Approach
07VH3DZ Restriction of Right Inguinal Lymphatic with Intraluminal Device, Percutaneous Approach
07VH3ZZ Restriction of Right Inguinal Lymphatic, Percutaneous Approach
07VH4CZ Restriction of Right Inguinal Lymphatic with Extraluminal Device, Percutaneous Endoscopic Approach
07VH4DZ Restriction of Right Inguinal Lymphatic with Intraluminal Device, Percutaneous Endoscopic Approach
07VH4ZZ Restriction of Right Inguinal Lymphatic, Percutaneous Endoscopic Approach
07VJ0CZ Restriction of Left Inguinal Lymphatic with Extraluminal Device, Open Approach
07VJ0DZ Restriction of Left Inguinal Lymphatic with Intraluminal Device, Open Approach
07VJ0ZZ Restriction of Left Inguinal Lymphatic, Open Approach
07VJ3CZ Restriction of Left Inguinal Lymphatic with Extraluminal Device, Percutaneous Approach

07VJ3DZ Restriction of Left Inguinal Lymphatic with Intraluminal Device, Percutaneous Approach
07VJ3ZZ Restriction of Left Inguinal Lymphatic, Percutaneous Approach
07VJ4CZ Restriction of Left Inguinal Lymphatic with Extraluminal Device, Percutaneous Endoscopic Approach
07VJ4DZ Restriction of Left Inguinal Lymphatic with Intraluminal Device, Percutaneous Endoscopic Approach
07VJ4ZZ Restriction of Left Inguinal Lymphatic, Percutaneous Endoscopic Approach
07VK0CZ Restriction of Thoracic Duct with Extraluminal Device, Open Approach
07VK0DZ Restriction of Thoracic Duct with Intraluminal Device, Open Approach
07VK0ZZ Restriction of Thoracic Duct, Open Approach
07VK3CZ Restriction of Thoracic Duct with Extraluminal Device, Percutaneous Approach
07VK3DZ Restriction of Thoracic Duct with Intraluminal Device, Percutaneous Approach
07VK3ZZ Restriction of Thoracic Duct, Percutaneous Approach
07VK4CZ Restriction of Thoracic Duct with Extraluminal Device, Percutaneous Endoscopic Approach
07VK4DZ Restriction of Thoracic Duct with Intraluminal Device, Percutaneous Endoscopic Approach
07VK4ZZ Restriction of Thoracic Duct, Percutaneous Endoscopic Approach
07VL0CZ Restriction of Cisterna Chyli with Extraluminal Device, Open Approach
07VL0DZ Restriction of Cisterna Chyli with Intraluminal Device, Open Approach
07VL0ZZ Restriction of Cisterna Chyli, Open Approach
07VL3CZ Restriction of Cisterna Chyli with Extraluminal Device, Percutaneous Approach
07VL3DZ Restriction of Cisterna Chyli with Intraluminal Device, Percutaneous Approach
07VL3ZZ Restriction of Cisterna Chyli, Percutaneous Approach
07VL4CZ Restriction of Cisterna Chyli with Extraluminal Device, Percutaneous Endoscopic Approach
07VL4DZ Restriction of Cisterna Chyli with Intraluminal Device, Percutaneous Endoscopic Approach
07VL4ZZ Restriction of Cisterna Chyli, Percutaneous Endoscopic Approach

07W – Lymphatic and Hemic Systems, Revision

Review Coding Guideline B6.1c

07WK00Z Revision of Drainage Device in Thoracic Duct, Open Approach
07WK03Z Revision of Infusion Device in Thoracic Duct, Open Approach
07WK07Z Revision of Autologous Tissue Substitute in Thoracic Duct, Open Approach
07WK0CZ Revision of Extraluminal Device in Thoracic Duct, Open Approach
07WK0DZ Revision of Intraluminal Device in Thoracic Duct, Open Approach
07WK0JZ Revision of Synthetic Substitute in Thoracic Duct, Open Approach
07WK0KZ Revision of Nonautologous Tissue Substitute in Thoracic Duct, Open Approach
07WK30Z Revision of Drainage Device in Thoracic Duct, Percutaneous Approach
07WK33Z Revision of Infusion Device in Thoracic Duct, Percutaneous Approach
07WK37Z Revision of Autologous Tissue Substitute in Thoracic Duct, Percutaneous Approach
07WK3CZ Revision of Extraluminal Device in Thoracic Duct, Percutaneous Approach
07WK3DZ Revision of Intraluminal Device in Thoracic Duct, Percutaneous Approach
07WK3JZ Revision of Synthetic Substitute in Thoracic Duct, Percutaneous Approach
07WK3KZ Revision of Nonautologous Tissue Substitute in Thoracic Duct, Percutaneous Approach
07WK40Z Revision of Drainage Device in Thoracic Duct, Percutaneous Endoscopic Approach
07WK43Z Revision of Infusion Device in Thoracic Duct, Percutaneous Endoscopic Approach
07WK47Z Revision of Autologous Tissue Substitute in Thoracic Duct, Percutaneous Endoscopic Approach
07WK4CZ Revision of Extraluminal Device in Thoracic Duct, Percutaneous Endoscopic Approach
07WK4DZ Revision of Intraluminal Device in Thoracic Duct, Percutaneous Endoscopic Approach
07WK4JZ Revision of Synthetic Substitute in Thoracic Duct, Percutaneous Endoscopic Approach
07WK4KZ Revision of Nonautologous Tissue Substitute in Thoracic Duct, Percutaneous Endoscopic Approach
07WKX0Z Revision of Drainage Device in Thoracic Duct, External Approach
07WKX3Z Revision of Infusion Device in Thoracic Duct, External Approach
07WKX7Z Revision of Autologous Tissue Substitute in Thoracic Duct, External Approach
07WKXCZ Revision of Extraluminal Device in Thoracic Duct, External Approach
07WKXDZ Revision of Intraluminal Device in Thoracic Duct, External Approach
07WKXJZ Revision of Synthetic Substitute in Thoracic Duct, External Approach
07WKXKZ Revision of Nonautologous Tissue Substitute in Thoracic Duct, External Approach
07WL00Z Revision of Drainage Device in Cisterna Chyli, Open Approach
07WL03Z Revision of Infusion Device in Cisterna Chyli, Open Approach
07WL07Z Revision of Autologous Tissue Substitute in Cisterna Chyli, Open Approach
07WL0CZ Revision of Extraluminal Device in Cisterna Chyli, Open Approach
07WL0DZ Revision of Intraluminal Device in Cisterna Chyli, Open Approach
07WL0JZ Revision of Synthetic Substitute in Cisterna Chyli, Open Approach
07WL0KZ Revision of Nonautologous Tissue Substitute in Cisterna Chyli, Open Approach
07WL30Z Revision of Drainage Device in Cisterna Chyli, Percutaneous Approach
07WL33Z Revision of Infusion Device in Cisterna Chyli, Percutaneous Approach
07WL37Z Revision of Autologous Tissue Substitute in Cisterna Chyli, Percutaneous Approach
07WL3CZ Revision of Extraluminal Device in Cisterna Chyli, Percutaneous Approach
07WL3DZ Revision of Intraluminal Device in Cisterna Chyli, Percutaneous Approach
07WL3JZ Revision of Synthetic Substitute in Cisterna Chyli, Percutaneous Approach
07WL3KZ Revision of Nonautologous Tissue Substitute in Cisterna Chyli, Percutaneous Approach
07WL40Z Revision of Drainage Device in Cisterna Chyli, Percutaneous Endoscopic Approach
07WL43Z Revision of Infusion Device in Cisterna Chyli, Percutaneous Endoscopic Approach
07WL47Z Revision of Autologous Tissue Substitu[te] in Cisterna Chyli, Percutaneous Endoscopic Approach
07WL4CZ Revision of Extraluminal Device in Cisterna Chyli, Percutaneous Endoscop[ic] Approach
07WL4DZ Revision of Intraluminal Device in Cisterna Chyli, Percutaneous Endoscop[ic] Approach
07WL4JZ Revision of Synthetic Substitute in Cisterna Chyli, Percutaneous Endoscop[ic] Approach
07WL4KZ Revision of Nonautologous Tissue Substitute in Cisterna Chyli, Percutaneous Endoscopic Approach
07WLX0Z Revision of Drainage Device in Cistern[a] Chyli, External Approach
07WLX3Z Revision of Infusion Device in Cisterna Chyli, External Approach
07WLX7Z Revision of Autologous Tissue Substitu[te] in Cisterna Chyli, External Approach
07WLXCZ Revision of Extraluminal Device in Cisterna Chyli, External Approach
07WLXDZ Revision of Intraluminal Device in Cisterna Chyli, External Approach
07WLXJZ Revision of Synthetic Substitute in Cisterna Chyli, External Approach
07WLXKZ Revision of Nonautologous Tissue Substitute in Cisterna Chyli, External Approach
07WM00Z Revision of Drainage Device in Thymus[,] Open Approach
07WM03Z Revision of Infusion Device in Thymus, Open Approach
07WM30Z Revision of Drainage Device in Thymus[,] Percutaneous Approach
07WM33Z Revision of Infusion Device in Thymus, Percutaneous Approach
07WM40Z Revision of Drainage Device in Thymus[,] Percutaneous Endoscopic Approach
07WM43Z Revision of Infusion Device in Thymus, Percutaneous Endoscopic Approach
07WMX0Z Revision of Drainage Device in Thymus[,] External Approach
07WMX3Z Revision of Infusion Device in Thymus, External Approach
07WN00Z Revision of Drainage Device in Lymphatic, Open Approach
07WN03Z Revision of Infusion Device in Lymphatic, Open Approach
07WN07Z Revision of Autologous Tissue Substitut[e] in Lymphatic, Open Approach

WN0CZ Revision of Extraluminal Device in Lymphatic, Open Approach
WN0DZ Revision of Intraluminal Device in Lymphatic, Open Approach
WN0JZ Revision of Synthetic Substitute in Lymphatic, Open Approach
WN0KZ Revision of Nonautologous Tissue Substitute in Lymphatic, Open Approach
WN30Z Revision of Drainage Device in Lymphatic, Percutaneous Approach
WN33Z Revision of Infusion Device in Lymphatic, Percutaneous Approach
WN37Z Revision of Autologous Tissue Substitute in Lymphatic, Percutaneous Approach
WN3CZ Revision of Extraluminal Device in Lymphatic, Percutaneous Approach
WN3DZ Revision of Intraluminal Device in Lymphatic, Percutaneous Approach
WN3JZ Revision of Synthetic Substitute in Lymphatic, Percutaneous Approach
WN3KZ Revision of Nonautologous Tissue Substitute in Lymphatic, Percutaneous Approach
WN40Z Revision of Drainage Device in Lymphatic, Percutaneous Endoscopic Approach
WN43Z Revision of Infusion Device in Lymphatic, Percutaneous Endoscopic Approach
07WN47Z Revision of Autologous Tissue Substitute in Lymphatic, Percutaneous Endoscopic Approach
07WN4CZ Revision of Extraluminal Device in Lymphatic, Percutaneous Endoscopic Approach
07WN4DZ Revision of Intraluminal Device in Lymphatic, Percutaneous Endoscopic Approach
07WN4JZ Revision of Synthetic Substitute in Lymphatic, Percutaneous Endoscopic Approach
07WN4KZ Revision of Nonautologous Tissue Substitute in Lymphatic, Percutaneous Endoscopic Approach
07WNX0Z Revision of Drainage Device in Lymphatic, External Approach
07WNX3Z Revision of Infusion Device in Lymphatic, External Approach
07WNX7Z Revision of Autologous Tissue Substitute in Lymphatic, External Approach
07WNXCZ Revision of Extraluminal Device in Lymphatic, External Approach
07WNXDZ Revision of Intraluminal Device in Lymphatic, External Approach
07WNXJZ Revision of Synthetic Substitute in Lymphatic, External Approach
07WNXKZ Revision of Nonautologous Tissue Substitute in Lymphatic, External Approach
07WP00Z Revision of Drainage Device in Spleen, Open Approach
07WP03Z Revision of Infusion Device in Spleen, Open Approach
07WP30Z Revision of Drainage Device in Spleen, Percutaneous Approach
07WP33Z Revision of Infusion Device in Spleen, Percutaneous Approach
07WP40Z Revision of Drainage Device in Spleen, Percutaneous Endoscopic Approach
07WP43Z Revision of Infusion Device in Spleen, Percutaneous Endoscopic Approach
07WPX0Z Revision of Drainage Device in Spleen, External Approach
07WPX3Z Revision of Infusion Device in Spleen, External Approach
07WT00Z Revision of Drainage Device in Bone Marrow, Open Approach
07WT30Z Revision of Drainage Device in Bone Marrow, Percutaneous Approach
07WT40Z Revision of Drainage Device in Bone Marrow, Percutaneous Endoscopic Approach
07WTX0Z Revision of Drainage Device in Bone Marrow, External Approach

7Y – Lymphatic and Hemic Systems, Transplantation

eview Coding Guideline B3.16

'YM0Z0 Transplantation of Thymus, Allogeneic, Open Approach
'YM0Z1 Transplantation of Thymus, Syngeneic, Open Approach
07YM0Z2 Transplantation of Thymus, Zooplastic, Open Approach
07YP0Z0 Transplantation of Spleen, Allogeneic, Open Approach
07YP0Z1 Transplantation of Spleen, Syngeneic, Open Approach
07YP0Z2 Transplantation of Spleen, Zooplastic, Open Approach

Eye

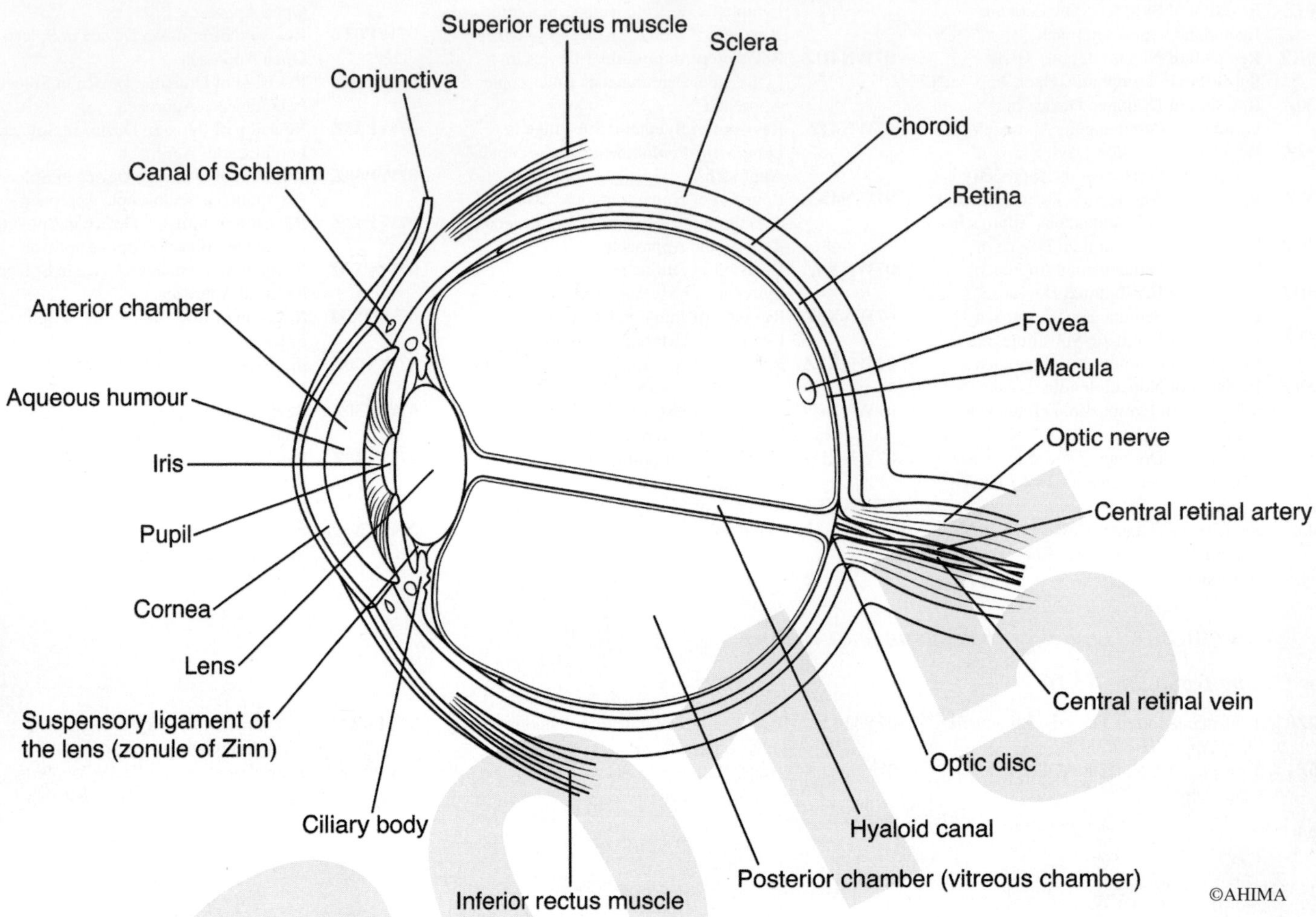

Superior rectus muscle
Sclera
Conjunctiva
Choroid
Canal of Schlemm
Retina
Anterior chamber
Fovea
Macula
Aqueous humour
Optic nerve
Iris
Central retinal artery
Pupil
Cornea
Lens
Central retinal vein
Suspensory ligament of the lens (zonule of Zinn)
Optic disc
Ciliary body
Hyaloid canal
Posterior chamber (vitreous chamber)
Inferior rectus muscle

©AHIMA

Upper eyelid
Lacrimal gland
Superior lacrimal canal
Lacrimal gland ducts
Lacrimal sac
Sclera
Pupil
Lacrimal duct
Iris
Lower eyelid
Inferior lacrimal canal
Lacrimal puncta

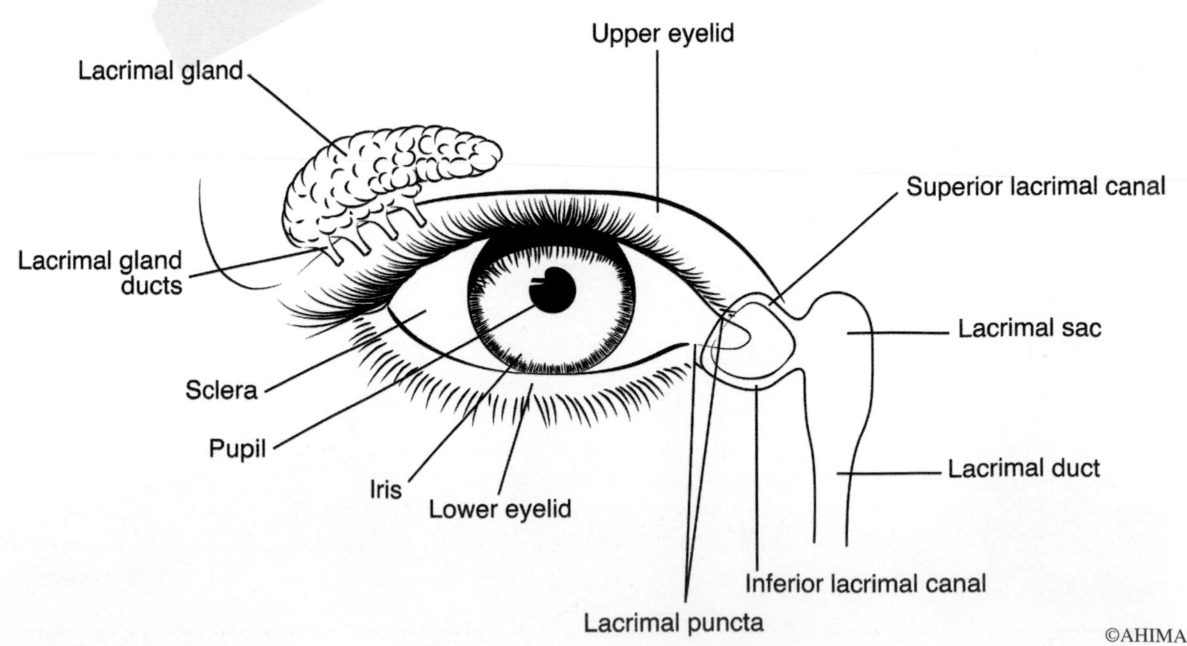

©AHIMA

Eye Muscles

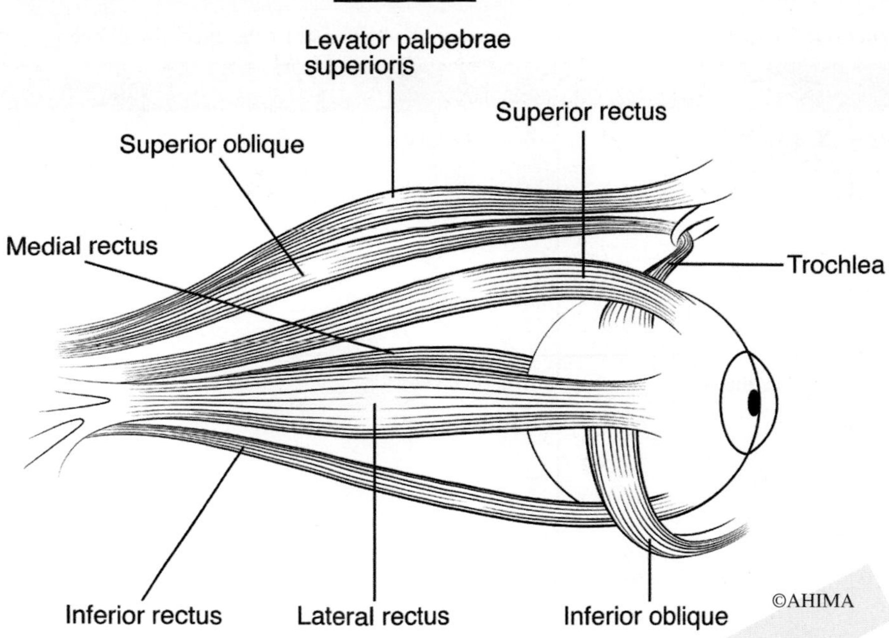

Eye Tables 080–08X

Section 0 **Medical and Surgical**
Body System 8 **Eye**
Operation 0 **Alteration:** Modifying the anatomic structure of a body part without affecting the function of the body part

Body Part (4th)	Approach (5th)	Device (6th)	Qualifier (7th)
N Upper Eyelid, Right **P** Upper Eyelid, Left **Q** Lower Eyelid, Right **R** Lower Eyelid, Left	**0** Open **3** Percutaneous **X** External	**7** Autologous Tissue Substitute **J** Synthetic Substitute **K** Nonautologous Tissue Substitute **Z** No Device	**Z** No Qualifier

Section 0 **Medical and Surgical**
Body System 8 **Eye**
Operation 1 **Bypass:** Altering the route of passage of the contents of a tubular body part

Body Part (4th)	Approach (5th)	Device (6th)	Qualifier (7th)
2 Anterior Chamber, Right **3** Anterior Chamber, Left	**3** Percutaneous	**J** Synthetic Substitute **K** Nonautologous Tissue Substitute **Z** No Device	**4** Sclera
X Lacrimal Duct, Right **Y** Lacrimal Duct, Left	**0** Open **3** Percutaneous	**J** Synthetic Substitute **K** Nonautologous Tissue Substitute **Z** No Device	**3** Nasal Cavity

Section 0 **Medical and Surgical**
Body System 8 **Eye**
Operation 2 **Change:** Taking out or off a device from a body part and putting back an identical or similar device in or on the same body part without cutting or puncturing the skin or a mucous membrane

Body Part (4th)	Approach (5th)	Device (6th)	Qualifier (7th)
0 Eye, Right **1** Eye, Left	**X** External	**0** Drainage Device **Y** Other Device	**Z** No Qualifier

Section 0 **Medical and Surgical**
Body System 8 **Eye**
Operation 5 **Destruction:** Physical eradication of all or a portion of a body part by the direct use of energy, force, or a destructive agent

Body Part (4th)	Approach (5th)	Device (6th)	Qualifier (7th)
0 Eye, Right **1** Eye, Left **6** Sclera, Right **7** Sclera, Left **8** Cornea, Right **9** Cornea, Left **S** Conjunctiva, Right **T** Conjunctiva, Left	**X** External	**Z** No Device	**Z** No Qualifier
2 Anterior Chamber, Right **3** Anterior Chamber, Left **4** Vitreous, Right **5** Vitreous, Left **C** Iris, Right **D** Iris, Left **E** Retina, Right **F** Retina, Left **G** Retinal Vessel, Right **H** Retinal Vessel, Left **J** Lens, Right **K** Lens, Left	**3** Percutaneous	**Z** No Device	**Z** No Qualifier
A Choroid, Right **B** Choroid, Left **L** Extraocular Muscle, Right **M** Extraocular Muscle, Left **V** Lacrimal Gland, Right **W** Lacrimal Gland, Left	**0** Open **3** Percutaneous	**Z** No Device	**Z** No Qualifier
N Upper Eyelid, Right **P** Upper Eyelid, Left **Q** Lower Eyelid, Right **R** Lower Eyelid, Left	**0** Open **3** Percutaneous **X** External	**Z** No Device	**Z** No Qualifier
X Lacrimal Duct, Right **Y** Lacrimal Duct, Left	**0** Open **3** Percutaneous **7** Via Natural or Artificial Opening **8** Via Natural or Artificial Opening Endoscopic	**Z** No Device	**Z** No Qualifier

Section 0 **Medical and Surgical**
Body System 8 **Eye**
Operation 7 **Dilation:** Expanding an orifice or the lumen of a tubular body part

Body Part (4th)	Approach (5th)	Device (6th)	Qualifier (7th)
X Lacrimal Duct, Right **Y** Lacrimal Duct, Left	**0** Open **3** Percutaneous **7** Via Natural or Artificial Opening **8** Via Natural or Artificial Opening Endoscopic	**D** Intraluminal Device **Z** No Device	**Z** No Qualifier

Section 0 **Medical and Surgical**
Body System 8 **Eye**
Operation 9 **Drainage:** Taking or letting out fluids and/or gases from a body part

Body Part (4th)	Approach (5th)	Device (6th)	Qualifier (7th)
0 Eye, Right **1** Eye, Left **6** Sclera, Right **7** Sclera, Left **8** Cornea, Right **9** Cornea, Left **S** Conjunctiva, Right **T** Conjunctiva, Left	**X** External	**0** Drainage Device	**Z** No Qualifier
0 Eye, Right **1** Eye, Left **6** Sclera, Right **7** Sclera, Left **8** Cornea, Right **9** Cornea, Left **S** Conjunctiva, Right **T** Conjunctiva, Left	**X** External	**Z** No Device	**X** Diagnostic **Z** No Qualifier
2 Anterior Chamber, Right **3** Anterior Chamber, Left **4** Vitreous, Right **5** Vitreous, Left **C** Iris, Right **D** Iris, Left **E** Retina, Right **F** Retina, Left **G** Retinal Vessel, Right **H** Retinal Vessel, Left **J** Lens, Right **K** Lens, Left	**3** Percutaneous	**0** Drainage Device	**Z** No Qualifier
2 Anterior Chamber, Right **3** Anterior Chamber, Left **4** Vitreous, Right **5** Vitreous, Left **C** Iris, Right **D** Iris, Left **E** Retina, Right **F** Retina, Left **G** Retinal Vessel, Right **H** Retinal Vessel, Left **J** Lens, Right **K** Lens, Left	**3** Percutaneous	**Z** No Device	**X** Diagnostic **Z** No Qualifier
A Choroid, Right **B** Choroid, Left **L** Extraocular Muscle, Right **M** Extraocular Muscle, Left **V** Lacrimal Gland, Right **W** Lacrimal Gland, Left	**0** Open **3** Percutaneous	**0** Drainage Device	**Z** No Qualifier
A Choroid, Right **B** Choroid, Left **L** Extraocular Muscle, Right **M** Extraocular Muscle, Left **V** Lacrimal Gland, Right **W** Lacrimal Gland, Left	**0** Open **3** Percutaneous	**Z** No Device	**X** Diagnostic **Z** No Qualifier
N Upper Eyelid, Right **P** Upper Eyelid, Left **Q** Lower Eyelid, Right **R** Lower Eyelid, Left	**0** Open **3** Percutaneous **X** External	**0** Drainage Device	**Z** No Qualifier

Continued →

Section 0 **Medical and Surgical**
Body System 8 **Eye**
Operation 9 **Drainage:** Taking or letting out fluids and/or gases from a body part

Body Part (4th)	Approach (5th)	Device (6th)	Qualifier (7th)
N Upper Eyelid, Right **P** Upper Eyelid, Left **Q** Lower Eyelid, Right **R** Lower Eyelid, Left	**0** Open **3** Percutaneous **X** External	**Z** No Device	**X** Diagnostic **Z** No Qualifier
X Lacrimal Duct, Right **Y** Lacrimal Duct, Left	**0** Open **3** Percutaneous **7** Via Natural or Artificial Opening **8** Via Natural or Artificial Opening Endoscopic	**0** Drainage Device	**Z** No Qualifier
X Lacrimal Duct, Right **Y** Lacrimal Duct, Left	**0** Open **3** Percutaneous **7** Via Natural or Artificial Opening **8** Via Natural or Artificial Opening Endoscopic	**Z** No Device	**X** Diagnostic **Z** No Qualifier

Section 0 **Medical and Surgical**
Body System 8 **Eye**
Operation B **Excision:** Cutting out or off, without replacement, a portion of a body part

Body Part (4th)	Approach (5th)	Device (6th)	Qualifier (7th)
0 Eye, Right **1** Eye, Left **N** Upper Eyelid, Right **P** Upper Eyelid, Left **Q** Lower Eyelid, Right **R** Lower Eyelid, Left	**0** Open **3** Percutaneous **X** External	**Z** No Device	**X** Diagnostic **Z** No Qualifier
4 Vitreous, Right **5** Vitreous, Left **C** Iris, Right **D** Iris, Left **E** Retina, Right **F** Retina, Left **J** Lens, Right **K** Lens, Left	**3** Percutaneous	**Z** No Device	**X** Diagnostic **Z** No Qualifier
6 Sclera, Right **7** Sclera, Left **8** Cornea, Right **9** Cornea, Left **S** Conjunctiva, Right **T** Conjunctiva, Left	**X** External	**Z** No Device	**X** Diagnostic **Z** No Qualifier
A Choroid, Right **B** Choroid, Left **L** Extraocular Muscle, Right **M** Extraocular Muscle, Left **V** Lacrimal Gland, Right **W** Lacrimal Gland, Left	**0** Open **3** Percutaneous	**Z** No Device	**X** Diagnostic **Z** No Qualifier
X Lacrimal Duct, Right **Y** Lacrimal Duct, Left	**0** Open **3** Percutaneous **7** Via Natural or Artificial Opening **8** Via Natural or Artificial Opening Endoscopic	**Z** No Device	**X** Diagnostic **Z** No Qualifier

ction	**0**	**Medical and Surgical**
dy System	**8**	**Eye**
eration	**C**	**Extirpation:** Taking or cutting out solid matter from a body part

Body Part (4th)	Approach (5th)	Device (6th)	Qualifier (7th)
0 Eye, Right **1** Eye, Left **6** Sclera, Right **7** Sclera, Left **8** Cornea, Right **9** Cornea, Left **S** Conjunctiva, Right **T** Conjunctiva, Left	**X** External	**Z** No Device	**Z** No Qualifier
2 Anterior Chamber, Right **3** Anterior Chamber, Left **4** Vitreous, Right **5** Vitreous, Left **C** Iris, Right **D** Iris, Left **E** Retina, Right **F** Retina, Left **G** Retinal Vessel, Right	**3** Percutaneous **X** External	**Z** No Device	**Z** No Qualifier
0 Eye, Right **1** Eye, Left **6** Sclera, Right **7** Sclera, Left **8** Cornea, Right **9** Cornea, Left **S** Conjunctiva, Right **T** Conjunctiva, Left	**X** External	**Z** No Device	**Z** No Qualifier
2 Anterior Chamber, Right **3** Anterior Chamber, Left **4** Vitreous, Right **5** Vitreous, Left **C** Iris, Right **D** Iris, Left **E** Retina, Right **F** Retina, Left **G** Retinal Vessel, Right **H** Retinal Vessel, Left **J** Lens, Right **K** Lens, Left	**3** Percutaneous **X** External	**Z** No Device	**Z** No Qualifier
A Choroid, Right **B** Choroid, Left **L** Extraocular Muscle, Right **M** Extraocular Muscle, Left **N** Upper Eyelid, Right **P** Upper Eyelid, Left **Q** Lower Eyelid, Right **R** Lower Eyelid, Left **V** Lacrimal Gland, Right **W** Lacrimal Gland, Left	**0** Open **3** Percutaneous **X** External	**Z** No Device	**Z** No Qualifier
X Lacrimal Duct, Right **Y** Lacrimal Duct, Left	**0** Open **3** Percutaneous **7** Via Natural or Artificial Opening **8** Via Natural or Artificial Opening Endoscopic	**Z** No Device	**Z** No Qualifier

Section 0 Medical and Surgical
Body System 8 Eye
Operation D **Extraction:** Pulling or stripping out or off all or a portion of a body part by the use of force

Body Part (4th)	Approach (5th)	Device (6th)	Qualifier (7th)
8 Cornea, Right 9 Cornea, Left	X External	Z No Device	X Diagnostic Z No Qualifier
J Lens, Right K Lens, Left	3 Percutaneous	Z No Device	Z No Qualifier

Section 0 Medical and Surgical
Body System 8 Eye
Operation F **Fragmentation:** Breaking solid matter in a body part into pieces

Body Part (4th)	Approach (5th)	Device (6th)	Qualifier (7th)
4 Vitreous, Right 5 Vitreous, Left	3 Percutaneous X External	Z No Device	Z No Qualifier

Section 0 Medical and Surgical
Body System 8 Eye
Operation H **Insertion:** Putting in a nonbiological appliance that monitors, assists, performs, or prevents a physiological function but does not physically take the place of a body part

Body Part (4th)	Approach (5th)	Device (6th)	Qualifier (7th)
0 Eye, Right 1 Eye, Left	0 Open	5 Epiretinal Visual Prosthesis	Z No Qualifier
0 Eye, Right 1 Eye, Left	3 Percutaneous X External	1 Radioactive Element 3 Infusion Device	Z No Qualifier

Section 0 Medical and Surgical
Body System 8 Eye
Operation J **Inspection:** Visually and/or manually exploring a body part

Body Part (4th)	Approach (5th)	Device (6th)	Qualifier (7th)
0 Eye, Right 1 Eye, Left J Lens, Right K Lens, Left	X External	Z No Device	Z No Qualifier
L Extraocular Muscle, Right M Extraocular Muscle, Left	0 Open X External	Z No Device	Z No Qualifier

Section 0 Medical and Surgical
Body System 8 Eye
Operation L **Occlusion:** Completely closing an orifice or the lumen of a tubular body part

Body Part (4th)	Approach (5th)	Device (6th)	Qualifier (7th)
X Lacrimal Duct, Right Y Lacrimal Duct, Left	0 Open 3 Percutaneous	C Extraluminal Device D Intraluminal Device Z No Device	Z No Qualifier
X Lacrimal Duct, Right Y Lacrimal Duct, Left	7 Via Natural or Artificial Opening 8 Via Natural or Artificial Opening Endoscopic	D Intraluminal Device Z No Device	Z No Qualifier

ction **0** **Medical and Surgical**
dy System **8** **Eye**
peration **M** **Reattachment:** Putting back in or on all or a portion of a separated body part to its normal location or other suitable location

Body Part (4th)	Approach (5th)	Device (6th)	Qualifier (7th)
N Upper Eyelid, Right **P** Upper Eyelid, Left **Q** Lower Eyelid, Right **R** Lower Eyelid, Left	**X** External	**Z** No Device	**Z** No Qualifier

ction **0** **Medical and Surgical**
dy System **8** **Eye**
peration **N** **Release:** Freeing a body part from an abnormal physical constraint by cutting or by the use of force

Body Part (4th)	Approach (5th)	Device (6th)	Qualifier (7th)
0 Eye, Right **1** Eye, Left **6** Sclera, Right **7** Sclera, Left **8** Cornea, Right **9** Cornea, Left **S** Conjunctiva, Right **T** Conjunctiva, Left	**X** External	**Z** No Device	**Z** No Qualifier
2 Anterior Chamber, Right **3** Anterior Chamber, Left **4** Vitreous, Right **5** Vitreous, Left **C** Iris, Right **D** Iris, Left **E** Retina, Right **F** Retina, Left **G** Retinal Vessel, Right **H** Retinal Vessel, Left **J** Lens, Right **K** Lens, Left	**3** Percutaneous	**Z** No Device	**Z** No Qualifier
A Choroid, Right **B** Choroid, Left **L** Extraocular Muscle, Right **M** Extraocular Muscle, Left **V** Lacrimal Gland, Right **W** Lacrimal Gland, Left	**0** Open **3** Percutaneous	**Z** No Device	**Z** No Qualifier
N Upper Eyelid, Right **P** Upper Eyelid, Left **Q** Lower Eyelid, Right **R** Lower Eyelid, Left	**0** Open **3** Percutaneous **X** External	**Z** No Device	**Z** No Qualifier
X Lacrimal Duct, Right **Y** Lacrimal Duct, Left	**0** Open **3** Percutaneous **7** Via Natural or Artificial Opening **8** Via Natural or Artificial Opening Endoscopic	**Z** No Device	**Z** No Qualifier

Section 0 **Medical and Surgical**
Body System 8 **Eye**
Operation P **Removal:** Taking out or off a device from a body part

Body Part (4th)	Approach (5th)	Device (6th)	Qualifier (7th)
0 Eye, Right **1** Eye, Left	**0** Open **3** Percutaneous **7** Via Natural or Artificial Opening **8** Via Natural or Artificial Opening Endoscopic **X** External	**0** Drainage Device **1** Radioactive Element **3** Infusion Device **7** Autologous Tissue Substitute **C** Extraluminal Device **D** Intraluminal Device **J** Synthetic Substitute **K** Nonautologous Tissue Substitute	**Z** No Qualifier
J Lens, Right **K** Lens, Left	**3** Percutaneous	**J** Synthetic Substitute	**Z** No Qualifier
L Extraocular Muscle, Right **M** Extraocular Muscle, Left	**0** Open **3** Percutaneous	**0** Drainage Device **7** Autologous Tissue Substitute **J** Synthetic Substitute **K** Nonautologous Tissue Substitute	**Z** No Qualifier

Section 0 **Medical and Surgical**
Body System 8 **Eye**
Operation Q **Repair:** Restoring, to the extent possible, a body part to its normal anatomic structure and function

Body Part (4th)	Approach (5th)	Device (6th)	Qualifier (7th)
0 Eye, Right **1** Eye, Left **6** Sclera, Right **7** Sclera, Left **8** Cornea, Right **9** Cornea, Left **S** Conjunctiva, Right **T** Conjunctiva, Left	**X** External	**Z** No Device	**Z** No Qualifier
2 Anterior Chamber, Right **3** Anterior Chamber, Left **4** Vitreous, Right **5** Vitreous, Left **C** Iris, Right **D** Iris, Left **E** Retina, Right **F** Retina, Left **G** Retinal Vessel, Right **H** Retinal Vessel, Left **J** Lens, Right **K** Lens, Left	**3** Percutaneous	**Z** No Device	**Z** No Qualifier
A Choroid, Right **B** Choroid, Left **L** Extraocular Muscle, Right **M** Extraocular Muscle, Left **V** Lacrimal Gland, Right **W** Lacrimal Gland, Left	**0** Open **3** Percutaneous	**Z** No Device	**Z** No Qualifier
N Upper Eyelid, Right **P** Upper Eyelid, Left **Q** Lower Eyelid, Right **R** Lower Eyelid, Left	**0** Open **3** Percutaneous **X** External	**Z** No Device	**Z** No Qualifier
X Lacrimal Duct, Right **Y** Lacrimal Duct, Left	**0** Open **3** Percutaneous **7** Via Natural or Artificial Opening **8** Via Natural or Artificial Opening Endoscopic	**Z** No Device	**Z** No Qualifier

ction **0** **Medical and Surgical**
dy System **8** **Eye**
eration **R** **Replacement:** Putting in or on biological or synthetic material that physically takes the place and/or function of all or a portion of a body part

Body Part (4th)	Approach (5th)	Device (6th)	Qualifier (7th)
0 Eye, Right **1** Eye, Left **A** Choroid, Right **B** Choroid, Left	**0** Open **3** Percutaneous	**7** Autologous Tissue Substitute **J** Synthetic Substitute **K** Nonautologous Tissue Substitute	**Z** No Qualifier
4 Vitreous, Right **5** Vitreous, Left **C** Iris, Right **D** Iris, Left **G** Retinal Vessel, Right **H** Retinal Vessel, Left	**3** Percutaneous	**7** Autologous Tissue Substitute **J** Synthetic Substitute **K** Nonautologous Tissue Substitute	**Z** No Qualifier
0 Eye, Right **1** Eye, Left **A** Choroid, Right **B** Choroid, Left	**0** Open **3** Percutaneous	**7** Autologous Tissue Substitute **J** Synthetic Substitute **K** Nonautologous Tissue Substitute	**Z** No Qualifier
4 Vitreous, Right **5** Vitreous, Left **C** Iris, Right **D** Iris, Left **G** Retinal Vessel, Right **H** Retinal Vessel, Left	**3** Percutaneous	**7** Autologous Tissue Substitute **J** Synthetic Substitute **K** Nonautologous Tissue Substitute	**Z** No Qualifier
6 Sclera, Right **7** Sclera, Left **S** Conjunctiva, Right **T** Conjunctiva, Left	**X** External	**7** Autologous Tissue Substitute **J** Synthetic Substitute **K** Nonautologous Tissue Substitute	**Z** No Qualifier
8 Cornea, Right **9** Cornea, Left	**3** Percutaneous **X** External	**7** Autologous Tissue Substitute **J** Synthetic Substitute **K** Nonautologous Tissue Substitute	**Z** No Qualifier
J Lens, Right **K** Lens, Left	**3** Percutaneous	**0** Synthetic Substitute, Intraocular Telescope **7** Autologous Tissue Substitute **J** Synthetic Substitute **K** Nonautologous Tissue Substitute	**Z** No Qualifier
N Upper Eyelid, Right **P** Upper Eyelid, Left **Q** Lower Eyelid, Right **R** Lower Eyelid, Left	**0** Open **3** Percutaneous **X** External	**7** Autologous Tissue Substitute **J** Synthetic Substitute **K** Nonautologous Tissue Substitute	**Z** No Qualifier
X Lacrimal Duct, Right **Y** Lacrimal Duct, Left	**0** Open **3** Percutaneous **7** Via Natural or Artificial Opening **8** Via Natural or Artificial Opening Endoscopic	**7** Autologous Tissue Substitute **J** Synthetic Substitute **K** Nonautologous Tissue Substitute	**Z** No Qualifier

Section 0 **Medical and Surgical**
Body System 8 **Eye**
Operation S **Reposition:** Moving to its normal location, or other suitable location, all or a portion of a body part

Body Part (4th)	Approach (5th)	Device (6th)	Qualifier (7th)
C Iris, Right **D** Iris, Left **G** Retinal Vessel, Right **H** Retinal Vessel, Left **J** Lens, Right **K** Lens, Left	**3** Percutaneous	**Z** No Device	**Z** No Qualifier
L Extraocular Muscle, Right **M** Extraocular Muscle, Left **V** Lacrimal Gland, Right **W** Lacrimal Gland, Left	**0** Open **3** Percutaneous	**Z** No Device	**Z** No Qualifier
N Upper Eyelid, Right **P** Upper Eyelid, Left **Q** Lower Eyelid, Right **R** Lower Eyelid, Left	**0** Open **3** Percutaneous **X** External	**Z** No Device	**Z** No Qualifier
X Lacrimal Duct, Right **Y** Lacrimal Duct, Left	**0** Open **3** Percutaneous **7** Via Natural or Artificial Opening **8** Via Natural or Artificial Opening Endoscopic	**Z** No Device	**Z** No Qualifier

Section 0 **Medical and Surgical**
Body System 8 **Eye**
Operation T **Resection:** Cutting out or off, without replacement, all of a body part

Body Part (4th)	Approach (5th)	Device (6th)	Qualifier (7th)
0 Eye, Right **1** Eye, Left **8** Cornea, Right **9** Cornea, Left	**X** External	**Z** No Device	**Z** No Qualifier
4 Vitreous, Right **5** Vitreous, Left **C** Iris, Right **D** Iris, Left **J** Lens, Right **K** Lens, Left	**3** Percutaneous	**Z** No Device	**Z** No Qualifier
L Extraocular Muscle, Right **M** Extraocular Muscle, Left **V** Lacrimal Gland, Right **W** Lacrimal Gland, Left	**0** Open **3** Percutaneous	**Z** No Device	**Z** No Qualifier
N Upper Eyelid, Right **P** Upper Eyelid, Left **Q** Lower Eyelid, Right **R** Lower Eyelid, Left	**0** Open **X** External	**Z** No Device	**Z** No Qualifier
X Lacrimal Duct, Right **Y** Lacrimal Duct, Left	**0** Open **3** Percutaneous **7** Via Natural or Artificial Opening **8** Via Natural or Artificial Opening Endoscopic	**Z** No Device	**Z** No Qualifier

Section 0 **Medical and Surgical**
Body System 8 **Eye**
Operation U **Supplement:** Putting in or on biological or synthetic material that physically reinforces and/or augments the function of a portion of a body part

Body Part (4th)	Approach (5th)	Device (6th)	Qualifier (7th)
0 Eye, Right **1** Eye, Left **C** Iris, Right **D** Iris, Left **E** Retina, Right **F** Retina, Left **G** Retinal Vessel, Right **H** Retinal Vessel, Left **L** Extraocular Muscle, Right **M** Extraocular Muscle, Left	**0** Open **3** Percutaneous	**7** Autologous Tissue Substitute **J** Synthetic Substitute **K** Nonautologous Tissue Substitute	**Z** No Qualifier
8 Cornea, Right **9** Cornea, Left **N** Upper Eyelid, Right **P** Upper Eyelid, Left **Q** Lower Eyelid, Right **R** Lower Eyelid, Left	**0** Open **3** Percutaneous **X** External	**7** Autologous Tissue Substitute **J** Synthetic Substitute **K** Nonautologous Tissue Substitute	**Z** No Qualifier
X Lacrimal Duct, Right **Y** Lacrimal Duct, Left	**0** Open **3** Percutaneous **7** Via Natural or Artificial Opening **8** Via Natural or Artificial Opening Endoscopic	**7** Autologous Tissue Substitute **J** Synthetic Substitute **K** Nonautologous Tissue Substitute	**Z** No Qualifier

Section 0 **Medical and Surgical**
Body System 8 **Eye**
Operation V **Restriction:** Partially closing an orifice or the lumen of a tubular body part

Body Part (4th)	Approach (5th)	Device (6th)	Qualifier (7th)
X Lacrimal Duct, Right **Y** Lacrimal Duct, Left	**0** Open **3** Percutaneous	**C** Extraluminal Device **D** Intraluminal Device **Z** No Device	**Z** No Qualifier
X Lacrimal Duct, Right **Y** Lacrimal Duct, Left	**7** Via Natural or Artificial Opening **8** Via Natural or Artificial Opening Endoscopic	**D** Intraluminal Device **Z** No Device	**Z** No Qualifier

Section 0 **Medical and Surgical**
Body System 8 **Eye**
Operation W **Revision:** Correcting, to the extent possible, a portion of a malfunctioning device or the position of a displaced device

Body Part (4th)	Approach (5th)	Device (6th)	Qualifier (7th)
0 Eye, Right **1** Eye, Left	**0** Open **3** Percutaneous **7** Via Natural or Artificial Opening **8** Via Natural or Artificial Opening Endoscopic **X** External	**0** Drainage Device **3** Infusion Device **7** Autologous Tissue Substitute **C** Extraluminal Device **D** Intraluminal Device **J** Synthetic Substitute **K** Nonautologous Tissue Substitute	**Z** No Qualifier
J Lens, Right **K** Lens, Left	**3** Percutaneous **X** External	**J** Synthetic Substitute	**Z** No Qualifier
L Extraocular Muscle, Right **M** Extraocular Muscle, Left	**0** Open **3** Percutaneous	**0** Drainage Device **7** Autologous Tissue Substitute **J** Synthetic Substitute **K** Nonautologous Tissue Substitute	**Z** No Qualifier

Section 0 **Medical and Surgical**
Body System 8 **Eye**
Operation X **Transfer:** Moving, without taking out, all or a portion of a body part to another location to take over the function of all or a portion of a body part

Body Part (4th)	Approach (5th)	Device (6th)	Qualifier (7th)
L Extraocular Muscle, Right **M** Extraocular Muscle, Left	**0** Open **3** Percutaneous	**Z** No Device	**Z** No Qualifier

Eye Code Listing 080–08X

080 – Eye, Alteration

080N07Z Alteration of Right Upper Eyelid with Autologous Tissue Substitute, Open Approach
080N0JZ Alteration of Right Upper Eyelid with Synthetic Substitute, Open Approach
080N0KZ Alteration of Right Upper Eyelid with Nonautologous Tissue Substitute, Open Approach
080N0ZZ Alteration of Right Upper Eyelid, Open Approach
080N37Z Alteration of Right Upper Eyelid with Autologous Tissue Substitute, Percutaneous Approach
080N3JZ Alteration of Right Upper Eyelid with Synthetic Substitute, Percutaneous Approach
080N3KZ Alteration of Right Upper Eyelid with Nonautologous Tissue Substitute, Percutaneous Approach
080N3ZZ Alteration of Right Upper Eyelid, Percutaneous Approach
080NX7Z Alteration of Right Upper Eyelid with Autologous Tissue Substitute, External Approach
080NXJZ Alteration of Right Upper Eyelid with Synthetic Substitute, External Approach
080NXKZ Alteration of Right Upper Eyelid with Nonautologous Tissue Substitute, External Approach
080NXZZ Alteration of Right Upper Eyelid, External Approach
080P07Z Alteration of Left Upper Eyelid with Autologous Tissue Substitute, Open Approach
080P0JZ Alteration of Left Upper Eyelid with Synthetic Substitute, Open Approach
080P0KZ Alteration of Left Upper Eyelid with Nonautologous Tissue Substitute, Open Approach
080P0ZZ Alteration of Left Upper Eyelid, Open Approach
080P37Z Alteration of Left Upper Eyelid with Autologous Tissue Substitute, Percutaneous Approach
080P3JZ Alteration of Left Upper Eyelid with Synthetic Substitute, Percutaneous Approach
080P3KZ Alteration of Left Upper Eyelid with Nonautologous Tissue Substitute, Percutaneous Approach
080P3ZZ Alteration of Left Upper Eyelid, Percutaneous Approach
080PX7Z Alteration of Left Upper Eyelid with Autologous Tissue Substitute, External Approach
080PXJZ Alteration of Left Upper Eyelid with Synthetic Substitute, External Approach
080PXKZ Alteration of Left Upper Eyelid with Nonautologous Tissue Substitute, External Approach
080PXZZ Alteration of Left Upper Eyelid, External Approach
080Q07Z Alteration of Right Lower Eyelid with Autologous Tissue Substitute, Open Approach
080Q0JZ Alteration of Right Lower Eyelid with Synthetic Substitute, Open Approach
080Q0KZ Alteration of Right Lower Eyelid with Nonautologous Tissue Substitute, Open Approach
080Q0ZZ Alteration of Right Lower Eyelid, Open Approach
080Q37Z Alteration of Right Lower Eyelid with Autologous Tissue Substitute, Percutaneous Approach
080Q3JZ Alteration of Right Lower Eyelid with Synthetic Substitute, Percutaneous Approach
080Q3KZ Alteration of Right Lower Eyelid with Nonautologous Tissue Substitute, Percutaneous Approach
080Q3ZZ Alteration of Right Lower Eyelid, Percutaneous Approach
080QX7Z Alteration of Right Lower Eyelid with Autologous Tissue Substitute, External Approach
080QXJZ Alteration of Right Lower Eyelid with Synthetic Substitute, External Approach
080QXKZ Alteration of Right Lower Eyelid with Nonautologous Tissue Substitute, Extern[al] Approach
080QXZZ Alteration of Right Lower Eyelid, Exter[nal] Approach
080R07Z Alteration of Left Lower Eyelid with Autologous Tissue Substitute, Open Approach
080R0JZ Alteration of Left Lower Eyelid with Synthetic Substitute, Open Approach
080R0KZ Alteration of Left Lower Eyelid with Nonautologous Tissue Substitute, Open Approach
080R0ZZ Alteration of Left Lower Eyelid, Open Approach
080R37Z Alteration of Left Lower Eyelid with Autologous Tissue Substitute, Percutaneous Approach
080R3JZ Alteration of Left Lower Eyelid with Synthetic Substitute, Percutaneous Approach
080R3KZ Alteration of Left Lower Eyelid with Nonautologous Tissue Substitute, Percutaneous Approach
080R3ZZ Alteration of Left Lower Eyelid, Percutaneous Approach
080RX7Z Alteration of Left Lower Eyelid with Autologous Tissue Substitute, External Approach
080RXJZ Alteration of Left Lower Eyelid with Synthetic Substitute, External Approach
080RXKZ Alteration of Left Lower Eyelid with Nonautologous Tissue Substitute, Externa[l] Approach
080RXZZ Alteration of Left Lower Eyelid, External Approach

081 – Eye, Bypass

Review Coding Guideline B3.6a

08123J4 Bypass Right Anterior Chamber to Sclera with Synthetic Substitute, Percutaneous Approach
08123K4 Bypass Right Anterior Chamber to Sclera with Nonautologous Tissue Substitute, Percutaneous Approach
08123Z4 Bypass Right Anterior Chamber to Sclera, Percutaneous Approach
08133J4 Bypass Left Anterior Chamber to Sclera with Synthetic Substitute, Percutaneous Approach
08133K4 Bypass Left Anterior Chamber to Sclera with Nonautologous Tissue Substitute, Percutaneous Approach
08133Z4 Bypass Left Anterior Chamber to Sclera, Percutaneous Approach
081X0J3 Bypass Right Lacrimal Duct to Nasal Cavity with Synthetic Substitute, Open Approach
081X0K3 Bypass Right Lacrimal Duct to Nasal Cavity with Nonautologous Tissue Substitute, Open Approach
081X0Z3 Bypass Right Lacrimal Duct to Nasal Cavity, Open Approach
081X3J3 Bypass Right Lacrimal Duct to Nasal Cavity with Synthetic Substitute, Percutaneous Approach
081X3K3 Bypass Right Lacrimal Duct to Nasal Cavity with Nonautologous Tissue Substitute, Percutaneous Approach
081X3Z3 Bypass Right Lacrimal Duct to Nasal Cavity, Percutaneous Approach
081Y0J3 Bypass Left Lacrimal Duct to Nasal Cavity with Synthetic Substitute, Open Approach
081Y0K3 Bypass Left Lacrimal Duct to Nasal Cavity with Nonautologous Tissue Substitute, Open Approach
081Y0Z3 Bypass Left Lacrimal Duct to Nasal Cavity, Open Approach
081Y3J3 Bypass Left Lacrimal Duct to Nasal Cavity with Synthetic Substitute, Percutaneous Approach
081Y3K3 Bypass Left Lacrimal Duct to Nasal Cavity with Nonautologous Tissue Substitute, Percutaneous Approach
081Y3Z3 Bypass Left Lacrimal Duct to Nasal Cavity, Percutaneous Approach

2 – Eye, Change

view Coding Guideline B6.1c

20X0Z Change Drainage Device in Right Eye, External Approach
20XYZ Change Other Device in Right Eye, External Approach
0821X0Z Change Drainage Device in Left Eye, External Approach
0821XYZ Change Other Device in Left Eye, External Approach

5 – Eye, Destruction

50XZZ Destruction of Right Eye, External Approach
51XZZ Destruction of Left Eye, External Approach
523ZZ Destruction of Right Anterior Chamber, Percutaneous Approach
533ZZ Destruction of Left Anterior Chamber, Percutaneous Approach
543ZZ Destruction of Right Vitreous, Percutaneous Approach
553ZZ Destruction of Left Vitreous, Percutaneous Approach
56XZZ Destruction of Right Sclera, External Approach
57XZZ Destruction of Left Sclera, External Approach
58XZZ Destruction of Right Cornea, External Approach
59XZZ Destruction of Left Cornea, External Approach
5A0ZZ Destruction of Right Choroid, Open Approach
5A3ZZ Destruction of Right Choroid, Percutaneous Approach
5B0ZZ Destruction of Left Choroid, Open Approach
5B3ZZ Destruction of Left Choroid, Percutaneous Approach
5C3ZZ Destruction of Right Iris, Percutaneous Approach
5D3ZZ Destruction of Left Iris, Percutaneous Approach
5E3ZZ Destruction of Right Retina, Percutaneous Approach
5F3ZZ Destruction of Left Retina, Percutaneous Approach
085G3ZZ Destruction of Right Retinal Vessel, Percutaneous Approach
085H3ZZ Destruction of Left Retinal Vessel, Percutaneous Approach
085J3ZZ Destruction of Right Lens, Percutaneous Approach
085K3ZZ Destruction of Left Lens, Percutaneous Approach
085L0ZZ Destruction of Right Extraocular Muscle, Open Approach
085L3ZZ Destruction of Right Extraocular Muscle, Percutaneous Approach
085M0ZZ Destruction of Left Extraocular Muscle, Open Approach
085M3ZZ Destruction of Left Extraocular Muscle, Percutaneous Approach
085N0ZZ Destruction of Right Upper Eyelid, Open Approach
085N3ZZ Destruction of Right Upper Eyelid, Percutaneous Approach
085NXZZ Destruction of Right Upper Eyelid, External Approach
085P0ZZ Destruction of Left Upper Eyelid, Open Approach
085P3ZZ Destruction of Left Upper Eyelid, Percutaneous Approach
085PXZZ Destruction of Left Upper Eyelid, External Approach
085Q0ZZ Destruction of Right Lower Eyelid, Open Approach
085Q3ZZ Destruction of Right Lower Eyelid, Percutaneous Approach
085QXZZ Destruction of Right Lower Eyelid, External Approach
085R0ZZ Destruction of Left Lower Eyelid, Open Approach
085R3ZZ Destruction of Left Lower Eyelid, Percutaneous Approach
085RXZZ Destruction of Left Lower Eyelid, External Approach
085SXZZ Destruction of Right Conjunctiva, External Approach
085TXZZ Destruction of Left Conjunctiva, External Approach
085V0ZZ Destruction of Right Lacrimal Gland, Open Approach
085V3ZZ Destruction of Right Lacrimal Gland, Percutaneous Approach
085W0ZZ Destruction of Left Lacrimal Gland, Open Approach
085W3ZZ Destruction of Left Lacrimal Gland, Percutaneous Approach
085X0ZZ Destruction of Right Lacrimal Duct, Open Approach
085X3ZZ Destruction of Right Lacrimal Duct, Percutaneous Approach
085X7ZZ Destruction of Right Lacrimal Duct, Via Natural or Artificial Opening
085X8ZZ Destruction of Right Lacrimal Duct, Via Natural or Artificial Opening Endoscopic
085Y0ZZ Destruction of Left Lacrimal Duct, Open Approach
085Y3ZZ Destruction of Left Lacrimal Duct, Percutaneous Approach
085Y7ZZ Destruction of Left Lacrimal Duct, Via Natural or Artificial Opening
085Y8ZZ Destruction of Left Lacrimal Duct, Via Natural or Artificial Opening Endoscopic

87 – Eye, Dilation

87X0DZ Dilation of Right Lacrimal Duct with Intraluminal Device, Open Approach
87X0ZZ Dilation of Right Lacrimal Duct, Open Approach
87X3DZ Dilation of Right Lacrimal Duct with Intraluminal Device, Percutaneous Approach
87X3ZZ Dilation of Right Lacrimal Duct, Percutaneous Approach
87X7DZ Dilation of Right Lacrimal Duct with Intraluminal Device, Via Natural or Artificial Opening
87X7ZZ Dilation of Right Lacrimal Duct, Via Natural or Artificial Opening
087X8DZ Dilation of Right Lacrimal Duct with Intraluminal Device, Via Natural or Artificial Opening Endoscopic
087X8ZZ Dilation of Right Lacrimal Duct, Via Natural or Artificial Opening Endoscopic
087Y0DZ Dilation of Left Lacrimal Duct with Intraluminal Device, Open Approach
087Y0ZZ Dilation of Left Lacrimal Duct, Open Approach
087Y3DZ Dilation of Left Lacrimal Duct with Intraluminal Device, Percutaneous Approach
087Y3ZZ Dilation of Left Lacrimal Duct, Percutaneous Approach
087Y7DZ Dilation of Left Lacrimal Duct with Intraluminal Device, Via Natural or Artificial Opening
087Y7ZZ Dilation of Left Lacrimal Duct, Via Natural or Artificial Opening
087Y8DZ Dilation of Left Lacrimal Duct with Intraluminal Device, Via Natural or Artificial Opening Endoscopic
087Y8ZZ Dilation of Left Lacrimal Duct, Via Natural or Artificial Opening Endoscopic

89 – Eye, Drainage

Review Coding Guidelines B3.4a and B3.4b

Review Coding Guideline B6.2

890X0Z Drainage of Right Eye with Drainage Device, External Approach
890XZX Drainage of Right Eye, External Approach, Diagnostic
890XZZ Drainage of Right Eye, External Approach
891X0Z Drainage of Left Eye with Drainage Device, External Approach
0891XZX Drainage of Left Eye, External Approach, Diagnostic
0891XZZ Drainage of Left Eye, External Approach
089230Z Drainage of Right Anterior Chamber with Drainage Device, Percutaneous Approach
08923ZX Drainage of Right Anterior Chamber, Percutaneous Approach, Diagnostic
08923ZZ Drainage of Right Anterior Chamber, Percutaneous Approach
089330Z Drainage of Left Anterior Chamber with Drainage Device, Percutaneous Approach
08933ZX Drainage of Left Anterior Chamber, Percutaneous Approach, Diagnostic

08933ZZ Drainage of Left Anterior Chamber, Percutaneous Approach
089430Z Drainage of Right Vitreous with Drainage Device, Percutaneous Approach
08943ZX Drainage of Right Vitreous, Percutaneous Approach, Diagnostic
08943ZZ Drainage of Right Vitreous, Percutaneous Approach
089530Z Drainage of Left Vitreous with Drainage Device, Percutaneous Approach
08953ZX Drainage of Left Vitreous, Percutaneous Approach, Diagnostic
08953ZZ Drainage of Left Vitreous, Percutaneous Approach
0896X0Z Drainage of Right Sclera with Drainage Device, External Approach
0896XZX Drainage of Right Sclera, External Approach, Diagnostic
0896XZZ Drainage of Right Sclera, External Approach
0897X0Z Drainage of Left Sclera with Drainage Device, External Approach
0897XZX Drainage of Left Sclera, External Approach, Diagnostic
0897XZZ Drainage of Left Sclera, External Approach
0898X0Z Drainage of Right Cornea with Drainage Device, External Approach
0898XZX Drainage of Right Cornea, External Approach, Diagnostic
0898XZZ Drainage of Right Cornea, External Approach
0899X0Z Drainage of Left Cornea with Drainage Device, External Approach
0899XZX Drainage of Left Cornea, External Approach, Diagnostic
0899XZZ Drainage of Left Cornea, External Approach
089A00Z Drainage of Right Choroid with Drainage Device, Open Approach
089A0ZX Drainage of Right Choroid, Open Approach, Diagnostic
089A0ZZ Drainage of Right Choroid, Open Approach
089A30Z Drainage of Right Choroid with Drainage Device, Percutaneous Approach
089A3ZX Drainage of Right Choroid, Percutaneous Approach, Diagnostic
089A3ZZ Drainage of Right Choroid, Percutaneous Approach
089B00Z Drainage of Left Choroid with Drainage Device, Open Approach
089B0ZX Drainage of Left Choroid, Open Approach, Diagnostic
089B0ZZ Drainage of Left Choroid, Open Approach
089B30Z Drainage of Left Choroid with Drainage Device, Percutaneous Approach
089B3ZX Drainage of Left Choroid, Percutaneous Approach, Diagnostic
089B3ZZ Drainage of Left Choroid, Percutaneous Approach
089C30Z Drainage of Right Iris with Drainage Device, Percutaneous Approach
089C3ZX Drainage of Right Iris, Percutaneous Approach, Diagnostic
089C3ZZ Drainage of Right Iris, Percutaneous Approach
089D30Z Drainage of Left Iris with Drainage Device, Percutaneous Approach
089D3ZX Drainage of Left Iris, Percutaneous Approach, Diagnostic
089D3ZZ Drainage of Left Iris, Percutaneous Approach
089E30Z Drainage of Right Retina with Drainage Device, Percutaneous Approach
089E3ZX Drainage of Right Retina, Percutaneous Approach, Diagnostic
089E3ZZ Drainage of Right Retina, Percutaneous Approach
089F30Z Drainage of Left Retina with Drainage Device, Percutaneous Approach
089F3ZX Drainage of Left Retina, Percutaneous Approach, Diagnostic
089F3ZZ Drainage of Left Retina, Percutaneous Approach
089G30Z Drainage of Right Retinal Vessel with Drainage Device, Percutaneous Approach
089G3ZX Drainage of Right Retinal Vessel, Percutaneous Approach, Diagnostic
089G3ZZ Drainage of Right Retinal Vessel, Percutaneous Approach
089H30Z Drainage of Left Retinal Vessel with Drainage Device, Percutaneous Approach
089H3ZX Drainage of Left Retinal Vessel, Percutaneous Approach, Diagnostic
089H3ZZ Drainage of Left Retinal Vessel, Percutaneous Approach
089J30Z Drainage of Right Lens with Drainage Device, Percutaneous Approach
089J3ZX Drainage of Right Lens, Percutaneous Approach, Diagnostic
089J3ZZ Drainage of Right Lens, Percutaneous Approach
089K30Z Drainage of Left Lens with Drainage Device, Percutaneous Approach
089K3ZX Drainage of Left Lens, Percutaneous Approach, Diagnostic
089K3ZZ Drainage of Left Lens, Percutaneous Approach
089L00Z Drainage of Right Extraocular Muscle with Drainage Device, Open Approach
089L0ZX Drainage of Right Extraocular Muscle, Open Approach, Diagnostic
089L0ZZ Drainage of Right Extraocular Muscle, Open Approach
089L30Z Drainage of Right Extraocular Muscle with Drainage Device, Percutaneous Approach
089L3ZX Drainage of Right Extraocular Muscle, Percutaneous Approach, Diagnostic
089L3ZZ Drainage of Right Extraocular Muscle, Percutaneous Approach
089M00Z Drainage of Left Extraocular Muscle with Drainage Device, Open Approach
089M0ZX Drainage of Left Extraocular Muscle, Open Approach, Diagnostic
089M0ZZ Drainage of Left Extraocular Muscle, Open Approach
089M30Z Drainage of Left Extraocular Muscle with Drainage Device, Percutaneous Approach
089M3ZX Drainage of Left Extraocular Muscle, Percutaneous Approach, Diagnostic
089M3ZZ Drainage of Left Extraocular Muscle, Percutaneous Approach
089N00Z Drainage of Right Upper Eyelid with Drainage Device, Open Approach
089N0ZX Drainage of Right Upper Eyelid, Open Approach, Diagnostic
089N0ZZ Drainage of Right Upper Eyelid, Open Approach
089N30Z Drainage of Right Upper Eyelid with Drainage Device, Percutaneous Approach
089N3ZX Drainage of Right Upper Eyelid, Percutaneous Approach, Diagnostic
089N3ZZ Drainage of Right Upper Eyelid, Percutaneous Approach
089NX0Z Drainage of Right Upper Eyelid with Drainage Device, External Approach
089NXZX Drainage of Right Upper Eyelid, External Approach, Diagnostic
089NXZZ Drainage of Right Upper Eyelid, External Approach
089P00Z Drainage of Left Upper Eyelid with Drainage Device, Open Approach
089P0ZX Drainage of Left Upper Eyelid, Open Approach, Diagnostic
089P0ZZ Drainage of Left Upper Eyelid, Open Approach
089P30Z Drainage of Left Upper Eyelid with Drainage Device, Percutaneous Approach
089P3ZX Drainage of Left Upper Eyelid, Percutaneous Approach, Diagnostic
089P3ZZ Drainage of Left Upper Eyelid, Percutaneous Approach
089PX0Z Drainage of Left Upper Eyelid with Drainage Device, External Approach
089PXZX Drainage of Left Upper Eyelid, External Approach, Diagnostic
089PXZZ Drainage of Left Upper Eyelid, External Approach
089Q00Z Drainage of Right Lower Eyelid with Drainage Device, Open Approach
089Q0ZX Drainage of Right Lower Eyelid, Open Approach, Diagnostic
089Q0ZZ Drainage of Right Lower Eyelid, Open Approach
089Q30Z Drainage of Right Lower Eyelid with Drainage Device, Percutaneous Approach
089Q3ZX Drainage of Right Lower Eyelid, Percutaneous Approach, Diagnostic
089Q3ZZ Drainage of Right Lower Eyelid, Percutaneous Approach
089QX0Z Drainage of Right Lower Eyelid with Drainage Device, External Approach
089QXZX Drainage of Right Lower Eyelid, External Approach, Diagnostic
089QXZZ Drainage of Right Lower Eyelid, External Approach
089R00Z Drainage of Left Lower Eyelid with Drainage Device, Open Approach
089R0ZX Drainage of Left Lower Eyelid, Open Approach, Diagnostic
089R0ZZ Drainage of Left Lower Eyelid, Open Approach
089R30Z Drainage of Left Lower Eyelid with Drainage Device, Percutaneous Approach
089R3ZX Drainage of Left Lower Eyelid, Percutaneous Approach, Diagnostic
089R3ZZ Drainage of Left Lower Eyelid, Percutaneous Approach
089RX0Z Drainage of Left Lower Eyelid with Drainage Device, External Approach
089RXZX Drainage of Left Lower Eyelid, External Approach, Diagnostic
089RXZZ Drainage of Left Lower Eyelid, External Approach
089SX0Z Drainage of Right Conjunctiva with Drainage Device, External Approach
089SXZX Drainage of Right Conjunctiva, External Approach, Diagnostic
089SXZZ Drainage of Right Conjunctiva, External Approach
089TX0Z Drainage of Left Conjunctiva with Drainage Device, External Approach
089TXZX Drainage of Left Conjunctiva, External Approach, Diagnostic
089TXZZ Drainage of Left Conjunctiva, External Approach
089V00Z Drainage of Right Lacrimal Gland with Drainage Device, Open Approach
089V0ZX Drainage of Right Lacrimal Gland, Open Approach, Diagnostic
089V0ZZ Drainage of Right Lacrimal Gland, Open Approach
089V30Z Drainage of Right Lacrimal Gland with Drainage Device, Percutaneous Approach
089V3ZX Drainage of Right Lacrimal Gland, Percutaneous Approach, Diagnostic
089V3ZZ Drainage of Right Lacrimal Gland, Percutaneous Approach

W00Z Drainage of Left Lacrimal Gland with Drainage Device, Open Approach

W0ZX Drainage of Left Lacrimal Gland, Open Approach, Diagnostic

W0ZZ Drainage of Left Lacrimal Gland, Open Approach

W30Z Drainage of Left Lacrimal Gland with Drainage Device, Percutaneous Approach

W3ZX Drainage of Left Lacrimal Gland, Percutaneous Approach, Diagnostic

W3ZZ Drainage of Left Lacrimal Gland, Percutaneous Approach

X00Z Drainage of Right Lacrimal Duct with Drainage Device, Open Approach

X0ZX Drainage of Right Lacrimal Duct, Open Approach, Diagnostic

X0ZZ Drainage of Right Lacrimal Duct, Open Approach

9X30Z Drainage of Right Lacrimal Duct with Drainage Device, Percutaneous Approach

9X3ZX Drainage of Right Lacrimal Duct, Percutaneous Approach, Diagnostic

089X3ZZ Drainage of Right Lacrimal Duct, Percutaneous Approach

089X70Z Drainage of Right Lacrimal Duct with Drainage Device, Via Natural or Artificial Opening

089X7ZX Drainage of Right Lacrimal Duct, Via Natural or Artificial Opening, Diagnostic

089X7ZZ Drainage of Right Lacrimal Duct, Via Natural or Artificial Opening

089X80Z Drainage of Right Lacrimal Duct with Drainage Device, Via Natural or Artificial Opening Endoscopic

089X8ZX Drainage of Right Lacrimal Duct, Via Natural or Artificial Opening Endoscopic, Diagnostic

089X8ZZ Drainage of Right Lacrimal Duct, Via Natural or Artificial Opening Endoscopic

089Y00Z Drainage of Left Lacrimal Duct with Drainage Device, Open Approach

089Y0ZX Drainage of Left Lacrimal Duct, Open Approach, Diagnostic

089Y0ZZ Drainage of Left Lacrimal Duct, Open Approach

089Y30Z Drainage of Left Lacrimal Duct with Drainage Device, Percutaneous Approach

089Y3ZX Drainage of Left Lacrimal Duct, Percutaneous Approach, Diagnostic

089Y3ZZ Drainage of Left Lacrimal Duct, Percutaneous Approach

089Y70Z Drainage of Left Lacrimal Duct with Drainage Device, Via Natural or Artificial Opening

089Y7ZX Drainage of Left Lacrimal Duct, Via Natural or Artificial Opening, Diagnostic

089Y7ZZ Drainage of Left Lacrimal Duct, Via Natural or Artificial Opening

089Y80Z Drainage of Left Lacrimal Duct with Drainage Device, Via Natural or Artificial Opening Endoscopic

089Y8ZX Drainage of Left Lacrimal Duct, Via Natural or Artificial Opening Endoscopic, Diagnostic

089Y8ZZ Drainage of Left Lacrimal Duct, Via Natural or Artificial Opening Endoscopic

B – Eye, Excision

eview Coding Guidelines B3.4a and B3.4b

eview Coding Guideline B3.8

B00ZX Excision of Right Eye, Open Approach, Diagnostic

B00ZZ Excision of Right Eye, Open Approach

B03ZX Excision of Right Eye, Percutaneous Approach, Diagnostic

B03ZZ Excision of Right Eye, Percutaneous Approach

B0XZX Excision of Right Eye, External Approach, Diagnostic

B0XZZ Excision of Right Eye, External Approach

B10ZX Excision of Left Eye, Open Approach, Diagnostic

B10ZZ Excision of Left Eye, Open Approach

B13ZX Excision of Left Eye, Percutaneous Approach, Diagnostic

B13ZZ Excision of Left Eye, Percutaneous Approach

B1XZX Excision of Left Eye, External Approach, Diagnostic

B1XZZ Excision of Left Eye, External Approach

B43ZX Excision of Right Vitreous, Percutaneous Approach, Diagnostic

B43ZZ Excision of Right Vitreous, Percutaneous Approach

B53ZX Excision of Left Vitreous, Percutaneous Approach, Diagnostic

B53ZZ Excision of Left Vitreous, Percutaneous Approach

B6XZX Excision of Right Sclera, External Approach, Diagnostic

B6XZZ Excision of Right Sclera, External Approach

8B7XZX Excision of Left Sclera, External Approach, Diagnostic

8B7XZZ Excision of Left Sclera, External Approach

B8XZX Excision of Right Cornea, External Approach, Diagnostic

8B8XZZ Excision of Right Cornea, External Approach

8B9XZX Excision of Left Cornea, External Approach, Diagnostic

8B9XZZ Excision of Left Cornea, External Approach

8BA0ZX Excision of Right Choroid, Open Approach, Diagnostic

08BA0ZZ Excision of Right Choroid, Open Approach

08BA3ZX Excision of Right Choroid, Percutaneous Approach, Diagnostic

08BA3ZZ Excision of Right Choroid, Percutaneous Approach

08BB0ZX Excision of Left Choroid, Open Approach, Diagnostic

08BB0ZZ Excision of Left Choroid, Open Approach

08BB3ZX Excision of Left Choroid, Percutaneous Approach, Diagnostic

08BB3ZZ Excision of Left Choroid, Percutaneous Approach

08BC3ZX Excision of Right Iris, Percutaneous Approach, Diagnostic

08BC3ZZ Excision of Right Iris, Percutaneous Approach

08BD3ZX Excision of Left Iris, Percutaneous Approach, Diagnostic

08BD3ZZ Excision of Left Iris, Percutaneous Approach

08BE3ZX Excision of Right Retina, Percutaneous Approach, Diagnostic

08BE3ZZ Excision of Right Retina, Percutaneous Approach

08BF3ZX Excision of Left Retina, Percutaneous Approach, Diagnostic

08BF3ZZ Excision of Left Retina, Percutaneous Approach

08BJ3ZX Excision of Right Lens, Percutaneous Approach, Diagnostic

08BJ3ZZ Excision of Right Lens, Percutaneous Approach

08BK3ZX Excision of Left Lens, Percutaneous Approach, Diagnostic

08BK3ZZ Excision of Left Lens, Percutaneous Approach

08BL0ZX Excision of Right Extraocular Muscle, Open Approach, Diagnostic

08BL0ZZ Excision of Right Extraocular Muscle, Open Approach

08BL3ZX Excision of Right Extraocular Muscle, Percutaneous Approach, Diagnostic

08BL3ZZ Excision of Right Extraocular Muscle, Percutaneous Approach

08BM0ZX Excision of Left Extraocular Muscle, Open Approach, Diagnostic

08BM0ZZ Excision of Left Extraocular Muscle, Open Approach

08BM3ZX Excision of Left Extraocular Muscle, Percutaneous Approach, Diagnostic

08BM3ZZ Excision of Left Extraocular Muscle, Percutaneous Approach

08BN0ZX Excision of Right Upper Eyelid, Open Approach, Diagnostic

08BN0ZZ Excision of Right Upper Eyelid, Open Approach

08BN3ZX Excision of Right Upper Eyelid, Percutaneous Approach, Diagnostic

08BN3ZZ Excision of Right Upper Eyelid, Percutaneous Approach

08BNXZX Excision of Right Upper Eyelid, External Approach, Diagnostic

08BNXZZ Excision of Right Upper Eyelid, External Approach

08BP0ZX Excision of Left Upper Eyelid, Open Approach, Diagnostic

08BP0ZZ Excision of Left Upper Eyelid, Open Approach

08BP3ZX Excision of Left Upper Eyelid, Percutaneous Approach, Diagnostic

08BP3ZZ Excision of Left Upper Eyelid, Percutaneous Approach

08BPXZX Excision of Left Upper Eyelid, External Approach, Diagnostic

08BPXZZ Excision of Left Upper Eyelid, External Approach

08BQ0ZX Excision of Right Lower Eyelid, Open Approach, Diagnostic

08BQ0ZZ Excision of Right Lower Eyelid, Open Approach

08BQ3ZX Excision of Right Lower Eyelid, Percutaneous Approach, Diagnostic

08BQ3ZZ Excision of Right Lower Eyelid, Percutaneous Approach

08BQXZX Excision of Right Lower Eyelid, External Approach, Diagnostic

08BQXZZ Excision of Right Lower Eyelid, External Approach

08BR0ZX Excision of Left Lower Eyelid, Open Approach, Diagnostic

08BR0ZZ Excision of Left Lower Eyelid, Open Approach
08BR3ZX Excision of Left Lower Eyelid, Percutaneous Approach, Diagnostic
08BR3ZZ Excision of Left Lower Eyelid, Percutaneous Approach
08BRXZX Excision of Left Lower Eyelid, External Approach, Diagnostic
08BRXZZ Excision of Left Lower Eyelid, External Approach
08BSXZX Excision of Right Conjunctiva, External Approach, Diagnostic
08BSXZZ Excision of Right Conjunctiva, External Approach
08BTXZX Excision of Left Conjunctiva, External Approach, Diagnostic
08BTXZZ Excision of Left Conjunctiva, External Approach
08BV0ZX Excision of Right Lacrimal Gland, Open Approach, Diagnostic
08BV0ZZ Excision of Right Lacrimal Gland, Open Approach
08BV3ZX Excision of Right Lacrimal Gland, Percutaneous Approach, Diagnostic
08BV3ZZ Excision of Right Lacrimal Gland, Percutaneous Approach
08BW0ZX Excision of Left Lacrimal Gland, Open Approach, Diagnostic
08BW0ZZ Excision of Left Lacrimal Gland, Open Approach
08BW3ZX Excision of Left Lacrimal Gland, Percutaneous Approach, Diagnostic
08BW3ZZ Excision of Left Lacrimal Gland, Percutaneous Approach
08BX0ZX Excision of Right Lacrimal Duct, Open Approach, Diagnostic
08BX0ZZ Excision of Right Lacrimal Duct, Open Approach
08BX3ZX Excision of Right Lacrimal Duct, Percutaneous Approach, Diagnostic
08BX3ZZ Excision of Right Lacrimal Duct, Percutaneous Approach
08BX7ZX Excision of Right Lacrimal Duct, Via Natural or Artificial Opening, Diagnostic
08BX7ZZ Excision of Right Lacrimal Duct, Via Natural or Artificial Opening
08BX8ZX Excision of Right Lacrimal Duct, Via Natural or Artificial Opening Endoscop Diagnostic
08BX8ZZ Excision of Right Lacrimal Duct, Via Natural or Artificial Opening Endoscopi
08BY0ZX Excision of Left Lacrimal Duct, Open Approach, Diagnostic
08BY0ZZ Excision of Left Lacrimal Duct, Open Approach
08BY3ZX Excision of Left Lacrimal Duct, Percutaneous Approach, Diagnostic
08BY3ZZ Excision of Left Lacrimal Duct, Percutaneous Approach
08BY7ZX Excision of Left Lacrimal Duct, Via Natural or Artificial Opening, Diagnosti
08BY7ZZ Excision of Left Lacrimal Duct, Via Natural or Artificial Opening
08BY8ZX Excision of Left Lacrimal Duct, Via Natural or Artificial Opening Endoscopi Diagnostic
08BY8ZZ Excision of Left Lacrimal Duct, Via Natural or Artificial Opening Endoscopi

08C – Eye, Extirpation

08C0XZZ Extirpation of Matter from Right Eye, External Approach
08C1XZZ Extirpation of Matter from Left Eye, External Approach
08C23ZZ Extirpation of Matter from Right Anterior Chamber, Percutaneous Approach
08C2XZZ Extirpation of Matter from Right Anterior Chamber, External Approach
08C33ZZ Extirpation of Matter from Left Anterior Chamber, Percutaneous Approach
08C3XZZ Extirpation of Matter from Left Anterior Chamber, External Approach
08C43ZZ Extirpation of Matter from Right Vitreous, Percutaneous Approach
08C4XZZ Extirpation of Matter from Right Vitreous, External Approach
08C53ZZ Extirpation of Matter from Left Vitreous, Percutaneous Approach
08C5XZZ Extirpation of Matter from Left Vitreous, External Approach
08C6XZZ Extirpation of Matter from Right Sclera, External Approach
08C7XZZ Extirpation of Matter from Left Sclera, External Approach
08C8XZZ Extirpation of Matter from Right Cornea, External Approach
08C9XZZ Extirpation of Matter from Left Cornea, External Approach
08CA0ZZ Extirpation of Matter from Right Choroid, Open Approach
08CA3ZZ Extirpation of Matter from Right Choroid, Percutaneous Approach
08CAXZZ Extirpation of Matter from Right Choroid, External Approach
08CB0ZZ Extirpation of Matter from Left Choroid, Open Approach
08CB3ZZ Extirpation of Matter from Left Choroid, Percutaneous Approach
08CBXZZ Extirpation of Matter from Left Choroid, External Approach
08CC3ZZ Extirpation of Matter from Right Iris, Percutaneous Approach
08CCXZZ Extirpation of Matter from Right Iris, External Approach
08CD3ZZ Extirpation of Matter from Left Iris, Percutaneous Approach
08CDXZZ Extirpation of Matter from Left Iris, External Approach
08CE3ZZ Extirpation of Matter from Right Retina, Percutaneous Approach
08CEXZZ Extirpation of Matter from Right Retina, External Approach
08CF3ZZ Extirpation of Matter from Left Retina, Percutaneous Approach
08CFXZZ Extirpation of Matter from Left Retina, External Approach
08CG3ZZ Extirpation of Matter from Right Retinal Vessel, Percutaneous Approach
08CGXZZ Extirpation of Matter from Right Retinal Vessel, External Approach
08CH3ZZ Extirpation of Matter from Left Retinal Vessel, Percutaneous Approach
08CHXZZ Extirpation of Matter from Left Retinal Vessel, External Approach
08CJ3ZZ Extirpation of Matter from Right Lens, Percutaneous Approach
08CJXZZ Extirpation of Matter from Right Lens, External Approach
08CK3ZZ Extirpation of Matter from Left Lens, Percutaneous Approach
08CKXZZ Extirpation of Matter from Left Lens, External Approach
08CL0ZZ Extirpation of Matter from Right Extraocular Muscle, Open Approach
08CL3ZZ Extirpation of Matter from Right Extraocular Muscle, Percutaneous Approach
08CLXZZ Extirpation of Matter from Right Extraocular Muscle, External Approach
08CM0ZZ Extirpation of Matter from Left Extraocular Muscle, Open Approach
08CM3ZZ Extirpation of Matter from Left Extraocular Muscle, Percutaneous Approach
08CMXZZ Extirpation of Matter from Left Extraocular Muscle, External Approach
08CN0ZZ Extirpation of Matter from Right Upper Eyelid, Open Approach
08CN3ZZ Extirpation of Matter from Right Upper Eyelid, Percutaneous Approach
08CNXZZ Extirpation of Matter from Right Upper Eyelid, External Approach
08CP0ZZ Extirpation of Matter from Left Upper Eyelid, Open Approach
08CP3ZZ Extirpation of Matter from Left Upper Eyelid, Percutaneous Approach
08CPXZZ Extirpation of Matter from Left Upper Eyelid, External Approach
08CQ0ZZ Extirpation of Matter from Right Lower Eyelid, Open Approach
08CQ3ZZ Extirpation of Matter from Right Lower Eyelid, Percutaneous Approach
08CQXZZ Extirpation of Matter from Right Lower Eyelid, External Approach
08CR0ZZ Extirpation of Matter from Left Lower Eyelid, Open Approach
08CR3ZZ Extirpation of Matter from Left Lower Eyelid, Percutaneous Approach
08CRXZZ Extirpation of Matter from Left Lower Eyelid, External Approach
08CSXZZ Extirpation of Matter from Right Conjunctiva, External Approach
08CTXZZ Extirpation of Matter from Left Conjunctiva, External Approach
08CV0ZZ Extirpation of Matter from Right Lacrim Gland, Open Approach
08CV3ZZ Extirpation of Matter from Right Lacrim Gland, Percutaneous Approach
08CVXZZ Extirpation of Matter from Right Lacrim Gland, External Approach
08CW0ZZ Extirpation of Matter from Left Lacrimal Gland, Open Approach
08CW3ZZ Extirpation of Matter from Left Lacrimal Gland, Percutaneous Approach
08CWXZZ Extirpation of Matter from Left Lacrimal Gland, External Approach
08CX0ZZ Extirpation of Matter from Right Lacrima Duct, Open Approach
08CX3ZZ Extirpation of Matter from Right Lacrima Duct, Percutaneous Approach
08CX7ZZ Extirpation of Matter from Right Lacrimal Duct, Via Natural or Artificial Opening
08CX8ZZ Extirpation of Matter from Right Lacrima Duct, Via Natural or Artificial Opening Endoscopic
08CY0ZZ Extirpation of Matter from Left Lacrimal Duct, Open Approach
08CY3ZZ Extirpation of Matter from Left Lacrimal Duct, Percutaneous Approach
08CY7ZZ Extirpation of Matter from Left Lacrimal Duct, Via Natural or Artificial Opening
08CY8ZZ Extirpation of Matter from Left Lacrimal Duct, Via Natural or Artificial Opening Endoscopic

D – Eye, Extraction

view Coding Guidelines B3.4a and B3.4b

- **)8XZX** Extraction of Right Cornea, External Approach, Diagnostic
- **)8XZZ** Extraction of Right Cornea, External Approach
- **08D9XZX** Extraction of Left Cornea, External Approach, Diagnostic
- **08D9XZZ** Extraction of Left Cornea, External Approach
- **08DJ3ZZ** Extraction of Right Lens, Percutaneous Approach
- **08DK3ZZ** Extraction of Left Lens, Percutaneous Approach

F – Eye, Fragmentation

- **F43ZZ** Fragmentation in Right Vitreous, Percutaneous Approach
- **3F4XZZ** Fragmentation in Right Vitreous, External Approach
- **08F53ZZ** Fragmentation in Left Vitreous, Percutaneous Approach
- ▲ **08F5XZZ** Fragmentation in Left Vitreous, External Approach

H – Eye, Insertion

- **H005Z** Insertion of Epiretinal Visual Prosthesis into Right Eye, Open Approach
- **H031Z** Insertion of Radioactive Element into Right Eye, Percutaneous Approach
- **H033Z** Insertion of Infusion Device into Right Eye, Percutaneous Approach
- **H0X1Z** Insertion of Radioactive Element into Right Eye, External Approach
- **08H0X3Z** Insertion of Infusion Device into Right Eye, External Approach
- **08H105Z** Insertion of Epiretinal Visual Prosthesis into Left Eye, Open Approach
- **08H131Z** Insertion of Radioactive Element into Left Eye, Percutaneous Approach
- **08H133Z** Insertion of Infusion Device into Left Eye, Percutaneous Approach
- **08H1X1Z** Insertion of Radioactive Element into Left Eye, External Approach
- **08H1X3Z** Insertion of Infusion Device into Left Eye, External Approach

J – Eye, Inspection

eview Coding Guidelines B3.11a, B3.11b and B3.11c

- **J0XZZ** Inspection of Right Eye, External Approach
- **J1XZZ** Inspection of Left Eye, External Approach
- **JJXZZ** Inspection of Right Lens, External Approach
- **08JKXZZ** Inspection of Left Lens, External Approach
- **08JL0ZZ** Inspection of Right Extraocular Muscle, Open Approach
- **08JLXZZ** Inspection of Right Extraocular Muscle, External Approach
- **08JM0ZZ** Inspection of Left Extraocular Muscle, Open Approach
- **08JMXZZ** Inspection of Left Extraocular Muscle, External Approach

8L – Eye, Occlusion

- **LX0CZ** Occlusion of Right Lacrimal Duct with Extraluminal Device, Open Approach
- **LX0DZ** Occlusion of Right Lacrimal Duct with Intraluminal Device, Open Approach
- **LX0ZZ** Occlusion of Right Lacrimal Duct, Open Approach
- **LX3CZ** Occlusion of Right Lacrimal Duct with Extraluminal Device, Percutaneous Approach
- **LX3DZ** Occlusion of Right Lacrimal Duct with Intraluminal Device, Percutaneous Approach
- **LX3ZZ** Occlusion of Right Lacrimal Duct, Percutaneous Approach
- **LX7DZ** Occlusion of Right Lacrimal Duct with Intraluminal Device, Via Natural or Artificial Opening
- **08LX7ZZ** Occlusion of Right Lacrimal Duct, Via Natural or Artificial Opening
- **08LX8DZ** Occlusion of Right Lacrimal Duct with Intraluminal Device, Via Natural or Artificial Opening Endoscopic
- **08LX8ZZ** Occlusion of Right Lacrimal Duct, Via Natural or Artificial Opening Endoscopic
- **08LY0CZ** Occlusion of Left Lacrimal Duct with Extraluminal Device, Open Approach
- **08LY0DZ** Occlusion of Left Lacrimal Duct with Intraluminal Device, Open Approach
- **08LY0ZZ** Occlusion of Left Lacrimal Duct, Open Approach
- **08LY3CZ** Occlusion of Left Lacrimal Duct with Extraluminal Device, Percutaneous Approach
- **08LY3DZ** Occlusion of Left Lacrimal Duct with Intraluminal Device, Percutaneous Approach
- **08LY3ZZ** Occlusion of Left Lacrimal Duct, Percutaneous Approach
- **08LY7DZ** Occlusion of Left Lacrimal Duct with Intraluminal Device, Via Natural or Artificial Opening
- **08LY7ZZ** Occlusion of Left Lacrimal Duct, Via Natural or Artificial Opening
- **08LY8DZ** Occlusion of Left Lacrimal Duct with Intraluminal Device, Via Natural or Artificial Opening Endoscopic
- **08LY8ZZ** Occlusion of Left Lacrimal Duct, Via Natural or Artificial Opening Endoscopic

8M – Eye, Reattachment

- **8MNXZZ** Reattachment of Right Upper Eyelid, External Approach
- **8MPXZZ** Reattachment of Left Upper Eyelid, External Approach
- **08MQXZZ** Reattachment of Right Lower Eyelid, External Approach
- **08MRXZZ** Reattachment of Left Lower Eyelid, External Approach

8N – Eye, Release

eview Coding Guidelines B3.13 and B3.14

- **8N0XZZ** Release Right Eye, External Approach
- **8N1XZZ** Release Left Eye, External Approach
- **8N23ZZ** Release Right Anterior Chamber, Percutaneous Approach
- **8N33ZZ** Release Left Anterior Chamber, Percutaneous Approach
- **8N43ZZ** Release Right Vitreous, Percutaneous Approach
- **08N53ZZ** Release Left Vitreous, Percutaneous Approach
- **08N6XZZ** Release Right Sclera, External Approach
- **08N7XZZ** Release Left Sclera, External Approach
- **08N8XZZ** Release Right Cornea, External Approach
- **08N9XZZ** Release Left Cornea, External Approach
- **08NA0ZZ** Release Right Choroid, Open Approach
- **08NA3ZZ** Release Right Choroid, Percutaneous Approach
- **08NB0ZZ** Release Left Choroid, Open Approach
- **08NB3ZZ** Release Left Choroid, Percutaneous Approach
- **08NC3ZZ** Release Right Iris, Percutaneous Approach
- **08ND3ZZ** Release Left Iris, Percutaneous Approach

08NE3ZZ Release Right Retina, Percutaneous Approach
08NF3ZZ Release Left Retina, Percutaneous Approach
08NG3ZZ Release Right Retinal Vessel, Percutaneous Approach
08NH3ZZ Release Left Retinal Vessel, Percutaneous Approach
08NJ3ZZ Release Right Lens, Percutaneous Approach
08NK3ZZ Release Left Lens, Percutaneous Approach
08NL0ZZ Release Right Extraocular Muscle, Open Approach
08NL3ZZ Release Right Extraocular Muscle, Percutaneous Approach
08NM0ZZ Release Left Extraocular Muscle, Open Approach
08NM3ZZ Release Left Extraocular Muscle, Percutaneous Approach
08NN0ZZ Release Right Upper Eyelid, Open Approach
08NN3ZZ Release Right Upper Eyelid, Percutaneous Approach
08NNXZZ Release Right Upper Eyelid, External Approach
08NP0ZZ Release Left Upper Eyelid, Open Approach
08NP3ZZ Release Left Upper Eyelid, Percutaneous Approach
08NPXZZ Release Left Upper Eyelid, External Approach
08NQ0ZZ Release Right Lower Eyelid, Open Approach
08NQ3ZZ Release Right Lower Eyelid, Percutaneous Approach
08NQXZZ Release Right Lower Eyelid, External Approach
08NR0ZZ Release Left Lower Eyelid, Open Approach
08NR3ZZ Release Left Lower Eyelid, Percutaneous Approach
08NRXZZ Release Left Lower Eyelid, External Approach
08NSXZZ Release Right Conjunctiva, External Approach
08NTXZZ Release Left Conjunctiva, External Approach
08NV0ZZ Release Right Lacrimal Gland, Open Approach
08NV3ZZ Release Right Lacrimal Gland, Percutaneous Approach
08NW0ZZ Release Left Lacrimal Gland, Open Approach
08NW3ZZ Release Left Lacrimal Gland, Percutaneous Approach
08NX0ZZ Release Right Lacrimal Duct, Open Approach
08NX3ZZ Release Right Lacrimal Duct, Percutaneous Approach
08NX7ZZ Release Right Lacrimal Duct, Via Natur or Artificial Opening
08NX8ZZ Release Right Lacrimal Duct, Via Natur or Artificial Opening Endoscopic
08NY0ZZ Release Left Lacrimal Duct, Open Approach
08NY3ZZ Release Left Lacrimal Duct, Percutaneo Approach
08NY7ZZ Release Left Lacrimal Duct, Via Natural or Artificial Opening
08NY8ZZ Release Left Lacrimal Duct, Via Natural or Artificial Opening Endoscopic

08P – Eye, Removal

Review Coding Guideline B6.1c

08P000Z Removal of Drainage Device from Right Eye, Open Approach
08P001Z Removal of Radioactive Element from Right Eye, Open Approach
08P003Z Removal of Infusion Device from Right Eye, Open Approach
08P007Z Removal of Autologous Tissue Substitute from Right Eye, Open Approach
08P00CZ Removal of Extraluminal Device from Right Eye, Open Approach
08P00DZ Removal of Intraluminal Device from Right Eye, Open Approach
08P00JZ Removal of Synthetic Substitute from Right Eye, Open Approach
08P00KZ Removal of Nonautologous Tissue Substitute from Right Eye, Open Approach
08P030Z Removal of Drainage Device from Right Eye, Percutaneous Approach
08P031Z Removal of Radioactive Element from Right Eye, Percutaneous Approach
08P033Z Removal of Infusion Device from Right Eye, Percutaneous Approach
08P037Z Removal of Autologous Tissue Substitute from Right Eye, Percutaneous Approach
08P03CZ Removal of Extraluminal Device from Right Eye, Percutaneous Approach
08P03DZ Removal of Intraluminal Device from Right Eye, Percutaneous Approach
08P03JZ Removal of Synthetic Substitute from Right Eye, Percutaneous Approach
08P03KZ Removal of Nonautologous Tissue Substitute from Right Eye, Percutaneous Approach
08P070Z Removal of Drainage Device from Right Eye, Via Natural or Artificial Opening
08P071Z Removal of Radioactive Element from Right Eye, Via Natural or Artificial Opening
08P073Z Removal of Infusion Device from Right Eye, Via Natural or Artificial Opening
08P077Z Removal of Autologous Tissue Substitute from Right Eye, Via Natural or Artificial Opening
08P07CZ Removal of Extraluminal Device from Right Eye, Via Natural or Artificial Opening
08P07DZ Removal of Intraluminal Device from Right Eye, Via Natural or Artificial Opening
08P07JZ Removal of Synthetic Substitute from Right Eye, Via Natural or Artificial Opening
08P07KZ Removal of Nonautologous Tissue Substitute from Right Eye, Via Natural or Artificial Opening
08P080Z Removal of Drainage Device from Right Eye, Via Natural or Artificial Opening Endoscopic
08P081Z Removal of Radioactive Element from Right Eye, Via Natural or Artificial Opening Endoscopic
08P083Z Removal of Infusion Device from Right Eye, Via Natural or Artificial Opening Endoscopic
08P087Z Removal of Autologous Tissue Substitute from Right Eye, Via Natural or Artificial Opening Endoscopic
08P08CZ Removal of Extraluminal Device from Right Eye, Via Natural or Artificial Opening Endoscopic
08P08DZ Removal of Intraluminal Device from Right Eye, Via Natural or Artificial Opening Endoscopic
08P08JZ Removal of Synthetic Substitute from Right Eye, Via Natural or Artificial Opening Endoscopic
08P08KZ Removal of Nonautologous Tissue Substitute from Right Eye, Via Natural or Artificial Opening Endoscopic
08P0X0Z Removal of Drainage Device from Right Eye, External Approach
08P0X1Z Removal of Radioactive Element from Right Eye, External Approach
08P0X3Z Removal of Infusion Device from Right Eye, External Approach
08P0X7Z Removal of Autologous Tissue Substitute from Right Eye, External Approach
08P0XCZ Removal of Extraluminal Device from Right Eye, External Approach
08P0XDZ Removal of Intraluminal Device from Right Eye, External Approach
08P0XJZ Removal of Synthetic Substitute from Right Eye, External Approach
08P0XKZ Removal of Nonautologous Tissue Substitute from Right Eye, External Approach
08P100Z Removal of Drainage Device from Left Eye, Open Approach
08P101Z Removal of Radioactive Element from Left Eye, Open Approach
08P103Z Removal of Infusion Device from Left Eye, Open Approach
08P107Z Removal of Autologous Tissue Substitute from Left Eye, Open Approach
08P10CZ Removal of Extraluminal Device from Left Eye, Open Approach
08P10DZ Removal of Intraluminal Device from Le Eye, Open Approach
08P10JZ Removal of Synthetic Substitute from Le Eye, Open Approach
08P10KZ Removal of Nonautologous Tissue Substitute from Left Eye, Open Approac
08P130Z Removal of Drainage Device from Left Eye, Percutaneous Approach
08P131Z Removal of Radioactive Element from Left Eye, Percutaneous Approach
08P133Z Removal of Infusion Device from Left Eye, Percutaneous Approach
08P137Z Removal of Autologous Tissue Substitute from Left Eye, Percutaneous Approach
08P13CZ Removal of Extraluminal Device from Left Eye, Percutaneous Approach
08P13DZ Removal of Intraluminal Device from Le Eye, Percutaneous Approach
08P13JZ Removal of Synthetic Substitute from Le Eye, Percutaneous Approach
08P13KZ Removal of Nonautologous Tissue Substitute from Left Eye, Percutaneous Approach
08P170Z Removal of Drainage Device from Left Eye, Via Natural or Artificial Opening
08P171Z Removal of Radioactive Element from Left Eye, Via Natural or Artificial Openin
08P173Z Removal of Infusion Device from Left Eye, Via Natural or Artificial Openin
08P177Z Removal of Autologous Tissue Substitute from Left Eye, Via Natural or Artificial Opening
08P17CZ Removal of Extraluminal Device from Left Eye, Via Natural or Artificial Openin

P17DZ	Removal of Intraluminal Device from Left Eye, Via Natural or Artificial Opening
P17JZ	Removal of Synthetic Substitute from Left Eye, Via Natural or Artificial Opening
P17KZ	Removal of Nonautologous Tissue Substitute from Left Eye, Via Natural or Artificial Opening
P180Z	Removal of Drainage Device from Left Eye, Via Natural or Artificial Opening Endoscopic
P181Z	Removal of Radioactive Element from Left Eye, Via Natural or Artificial Opening Endoscopic
P183Z	Removal of Infusion Device from Left Eye, Via Natural or Artificial Opening Endoscopic
P187Z	Removal of Autologous Tissue Substitute from Left Eye, Via Natural or Artificial Opening Endoscopic
P18CZ	Removal of Extraluminal Device from Left Eye, Via Natural or Artificial Opening Endoscopic
P18DZ	Removal of Intraluminal Device from Left Eye, Via Natural or Artificial Opening Endoscopic
P18JZ	Removal of Synthetic Substitute from Left Eye, Via Natural or Artificial Opening Endoscopic
P18KZ	Removal of Nonautologous Tissue Substitute from Left Eye, Via Natural or Artificial Opening Endoscopic
P1X0Z	Removal of Drainage Device from Left Eye, External Approach
08P1X1Z	Removal of Radioactive Element from Left Eye, External Approach
08P1X3Z	Removal of Infusion Device from Left Eye, External Approach
08P1X7Z	Removal of Autologous Tissue Substitute from Left Eye, External Approach
08P1XCZ	Removal of Extraluminal Device from Left Eye, External Approach
08P1XDZ	Removal of Intraluminal Device from Left Eye, External Approach
08P1XJZ	Removal of Synthetic Substitute from Left Eye, External Approach
08P1XKZ	Removal of Nonautologous Tissue Substitute from Left Eye, External Approach
08PJ3JZ	Removal of Synthetic Substitute from Right Lens, Percutaneous Approach
08PK3JZ	Removal of Synthetic Substitute from Left Lens, Percutaneous Approach
08PL00Z	Removal of Drainage Device from Right Extraocular Muscle, Open Approach
08PL07Z	Removal of Autologous Tissue Substitute from Right Extraocular Muscle, Open Approach
08PL0JZ	Removal of Synthetic Substitute from Right Extraocular Muscle, Open Approach
08PL0KZ	Removal of Nonautologous Tissue Substitute from Right Extraocular Muscle, Open Approach
08PL30Z	Removal of Drainage Device from Right Extraocular Muscle, Percutaneous Approach
08PL37Z	Removal of Autologous Tissue Substitute from Right Extraocular Muscle, Percutaneous Approach
08PL3JZ	Removal of Synthetic Substitute from Right Extraocular Muscle, Percutaneous Approach
08PL3KZ	Removal of Nonautologous Tissue Substitute from Right Extraocular Muscle, Percutaneous Approach
08PM00Z	Removal of Drainage Device from Left Extraocular Muscle, Open Approach
08PM07Z	Removal of Autologous Tissue Substitute from Left Extraocular Muscle, Open Approach
08PM0JZ	Removal of Synthetic Substitute from Left Extraocular Muscle, Open Approach
08PM0KZ	Removal of Nonautologous Tissue Substitute from Left Extraocular Muscle, Open Approach
08PM30Z	Removal of Drainage Device from Left Extraocular Muscle, Percutaneous Approach
08PM37Z	Removal of Autologous Tissue Substitute from Left Extraocular Muscle, Percutaneous Approach
08PM3JZ	Removal of Synthetic Substitute from Left Extraocular Muscle, Percutaneous Approach
08PM3KZ	Removal of Nonautologous Tissue Substitute from Left Extraocular Muscle, Percutaneous Approach

8Q – Eye, Repair

Q0XZZ	Repair Right Eye, External Approach
Q1XZZ	Repair Left Eye, External Approach
Q23ZZ	Repair Right Anterior Chamber, Percutaneous Approach
Q33ZZ	Repair Left Anterior Chamber, Percutaneous Approach
Q43ZZ	Repair Right Vitreous, Percutaneous Approach
Q53ZZ	Repair Left Vitreous, Percutaneous Approach
Q6XZZ	Repair Right Sclera, External Approach
Q7XZZ	Repair Left Sclera, External Approach
08Q8XZZ	Repair Right Cornea, External Approach
08Q9XZZ	Repair Left Cornea, External Approach
8QA0ZZ	Repair Right Choroid, Open Approach
8QA3ZZ	Repair Right Choroid, Percutaneous Approach
8QB0ZZ	Repair Left Choroid, Open Approach
8QB3ZZ	Repair Left Choroid, Percutaneous Approach
8QC3ZZ	Repair Right Iris, Percutaneous Approach
8QD3ZZ	Repair Left Iris, Percutaneous Approach
8QE3ZZ	Repair Right Retina, Percutaneous Approach
8QF3ZZ	Repair Left Retina, Percutaneous Approach
8QG3ZZ	Repair Right Retinal Vessel, Percutaneous Approach
8QH3ZZ	Repair Left Retinal Vessel, Percutaneous Approach
08QJ3ZZ	Repair Right Lens, Percutaneous Approach
08QK3ZZ	Repair Left Lens, Percutaneous Approach
08QL0ZZ	Repair Right Extraocular Muscle, Open Approach
08QL3ZZ	Repair Right Extraocular Muscle, Percutaneous Approach
08QM0ZZ	Repair Left Extraocular Muscle, Open Approach
08QM3ZZ	Repair Left Extraocular Muscle, Percutaneous Approach
08QN0ZZ	Repair Right Upper Eyelid, Open Approach
08QN3ZZ	Repair Right Upper Eyelid, Percutaneous Approach
08QNXZZ	Repair Right Upper Eyelid, External Approach
08QP0ZZ	Repair Left Upper Eyelid, Open Approach
08QP3ZZ	Repair Left Upper Eyelid, Percutaneous Approach
08QPXZZ	Repair Left Upper Eyelid, External Approach
08QQ0ZZ	Repair Right Lower Eyelid, Open Approach
08QQ3ZZ	Repair Right Lower Eyelid, Percutaneous Approach
08QQXZZ	Repair Right Lower Eyelid, External Approach
08QR0ZZ	Repair Left Lower Eyelid, Open Approach
08QR3ZZ	Repair Left Lower Eyelid, Percutaneous Approach
08QRXZZ	Repair Left Lower Eyelid, External Approach
08QSXZZ	Repair Right Conjunctiva, External Approach
08QTXZZ	Repair Left Conjunctiva, External Approach
08QV0ZZ	Repair Right Lacrimal Gland, Open Approach
08QV3ZZ	Repair Right Lacrimal Gland, Percutaneous Approach
08QW0ZZ	Repair Left Lacrimal Gland, Open Approach
08QW3ZZ	Repair Left Lacrimal Gland, Percutaneous Approach
08QX0ZZ	Repair Right Lacrimal Duct, Open Approach
08QX3ZZ	Repair Right Lacrimal Duct, Percutaneous Approach
08QX7ZZ	Repair Right Lacrimal Duct, Via Natural or Artificial Opening
08QX8ZZ	Repair Right Lacrimal Duct, Via Natural or Artificial Opening Endoscopic
08QY0ZZ	Repair Left Lacrimal Duct, Open Approach
08QY3ZZ	Repair Left Lacrimal Duct, Percutaneous Approach
08QY7ZZ	Repair Left Lacrimal Duct, Via Natural or Artificial Opening
08QY8ZZ	Repair Left Lacrimal Duct, Via Natural or Artificial Opening Endoscopic

8R – Eye, Replacement

8R007Z	Replacement of Right Eye with Autologous Tissue Substitute, Open Approach
8R00JZ	Replacement of Right Eye with Synthetic Substitute, Open Approach
08R00KZ	Replacement of Right Eye with Nonautologous Tissue Substitute, Open Approach
08R037Z	Replacement of Right Eye with Autologous Tissue Substitute, Percutaneous Approach
08R03JZ	Replacement of Right Eye with Synthetic Substitute, Percutaneous Approach
08R03KZ	Replacement of Right Eye with Nonautologous Tissue Substitute, Percutaneous Approach

08R107Z Replacement of Left Eye with Autologous Tissue Substitute, Open Approach
08R10JZ Replacement of Left Eye with Synthetic Substitute, Open Approach
08R10KZ Replacement of Left Eye with Nonautologous Tissue Substitute, Open Approach
08R137Z Replacement of Left Eye with Autologous Tissue Substitute, Percutaneous Approach
08R13JZ Replacement of Left Eye with Synthetic Substitute, Percutaneous Approach
08R13KZ Replacement of Left Eye with Nonautologous Tissue Substitute, Percutaneous Approach
08R437Z Replacement of Right Vitreous with Autologous Tissue Substitute, Percutaneous Approach
08R43JZ Replacement of Right Vitreous with Synthetic Substitute, Percutaneous Approach
08R43KZ Replacement of Right Vitreous with Nonautologous Tissue Substitute, Percutaneous Approach
08R537Z Replacement of Left Vitreous with Autologous Tissue Substitute, Percutaneous Approach
08R53JZ Replacement of Left Vitreous with Synthetic Substitute, Percutaneous Approach
08R53KZ Replacement of Left Vitreous with Nonautologous Tissue Substitute, Percutaneous Approach
08R6X7Z Replacement of Right Sclera with Autologous Tissue Substitute, External Approach
08R6XJZ Replacement of Right Sclera with Synthetic Substitute, External Approach
08R6XKZ Replacement of Right Sclera with Nonautologous Tissue Substitute, External Approach
08R7X7Z Replacement of Left Sclera with Autologous Tissue Substitute, External Approach
08R7XJZ Replacement of Left Sclera with Synthetic Substitute, External Approach
08R7XKZ Replacement of Left Sclera with Nonautologous Tissue Substitute, External Approach
08R837Z Replacement of Right Cornea with Autologous Tissue Substitute, Percutaneous Approach
08R83JZ Replacement of Right Cornea with Synthetic Substitute, Percutaneous Approach
08R83KZ Replacement of Right Cornea with Nonautologous Tissue Substitute, Percutaneous Approach
08R8X7Z Replacement of Right Cornea with Autologous Tissue Substitute, External Approach
08R8XJZ Replacement of Right Cornea with Synthetic Substitute, External Approach
08R8XKZ Replacement of Right Cornea with Nonautologous Tissue Substitute, External Approach
08R937Z Replacement of Left Cornea with Autologous Tissue Substitute, Percutaneous Approach
08R93JZ Replacement of Left Cornea with Synthetic Substitute, Percutaneous Approach
08R93KZ Replacement of Left Cornea with Nonautologous Tissue Substitute, Percutaneous Approach
08R9X7Z Replacement of Left Cornea with Autologous Tissue Substitute, External Approach
08R9XJZ Replacement of Left Cornea with Synthetic Substitute, External Approach
08R9XKZ Replacement of Left Cornea with Nonautologous Tissue Substitute, External Approach
08RA07Z Replacement of Right Choroid with Autologous Tissue Substitute, Open Approach
08RA0JZ Replacement of Right Choroid with Synthetic Substitute, Open Approach
08RA0KZ Replacement of Right Choroid with Nonautologous Tissue Substitute, Open Approach
08RA37Z Replacement of Right Choroid with Autologous Tissue Substitute, Percutaneous Approach
08RA3JZ Replacement of Right Choroid with Synthetic Substitute, Percutaneous Approach
08RA3KZ Replacement of Right Choroid with Nonautologous Tissue Substitute, Percutaneous Approach
08RB07Z Replacement of Left Choroid with Autologous Tissue Substitute, Open Approach
08RB0JZ Replacement of Left Choroid with Synthetic Substitute, Open Approach
08RB0KZ Replacement of Left Choroid with Nonautologous Tissue Substitute, Open Approach
08RB37Z Replacement of Left Choroid with Autologous Tissue Substitute, Percutaneous Approach
08RB3JZ Replacement of Left Choroid with Synthetic Substitute, Percutaneous Approach
08RB3KZ Replacement of Left Choroid with Nonautologous Tissue Substitute, Percutaneous Approach
08RC37Z Replacement of Right Iris with Autologous Tissue Substitute, Percutaneous Approach
08RC3JZ Replacement of Right Iris with Synthetic Substitute, Percutaneous Approach
08RC3KZ Replacement of Right Iris with Nonautologous Tissue Substitute, Percutaneous Approach
08RD37Z Replacement of Left Iris with Autologous Tissue Substitute, Percutaneous Approach
08RD3JZ Replacement of Left Iris with Synthetic Substitute, Percutaneous Approach
08RD3KZ Replacement of Left Iris with Nonautologous Tissue Substitute, Percutaneous Approach
08RG37Z Replacement of Right Retinal Vessel with Autologous Tissue Substitute, Percutaneous Approach
08RG3JZ Replacement of Right Retinal Vessel with Synthetic Substitute, Percutaneous Approach
08RG3KZ Replacement of Right Retinal Vessel with Nonautologous Tissue Substitute, Percutaneous Approach
08RH37Z Replacement of Left Retinal Vessel with Autologous Tissue Substitute, Percutaneous Approach
08RH3JZ Replacement of Left Retinal Vessel with Synthetic Substitute, Percutaneous Approach
08RH3KZ Replacement of Left Retinal Vessel with Nonautologous Tissue Substitute, Percutaneous Approach
08RJ30Z Replacement of Right Lens with Intraocular Telescope, Percutaneous Approach
08RJ37Z Replacement of Right Lens with Autologous Tissue Substitute, Percutaneous Approach
08RJ3JZ Replacement of Right Lens with Synthe Substitute, Percutaneous Approach
08RJ3KZ Replacement of Right Lens with Nonautologous Tissue Substitute, Percutaneous Approach
08RK30Z Replacement of Left Lens with Intraocu Telescope, Percutaneous Approach
08RK37Z Replacement of Left Lens with Autologous Tissue Substitute, Percutaneous Approach
08RK3JZ Replacement of Left Lens with Syntheti Substitute, Percutaneous Approach
08RK3KZ Replacement of Left Lens with Nonautologous Tissue Substitute, Percutaneous Approach
08RN07Z Replacement of Right Upper Eyelid with Autologous Tissue Substitute, Open Approach
08RN0JZ Replacement of Right Upper Eyelid with Synthetic Substitute, Open Approach
08RN0KZ Replacement of Right Upper Eyelid with Nonautologous Tissue Substitute, Open Approach
08RN37Z Replacement of Right Upper Eyelid with Autologous Tissue Substitute, Percutaneous Approach
08RN3JZ Replacement of Right Upper Eyelid with Synthetic Substitute, Percutaneous Approach
08RN3KZ Replacement of Right Upper Eyelid with Nonautologous Tissue Substitute, Percutaneous Approach
08RNX7Z Replacement of Right Upper Eyelid with Autologous Tissue Substitute, External Approach
08RNXJZ Replacement of Right Upper Eyelid with Synthetic Substitute, External Approach
08RNXKZ Replacement of Right Upper Eyelid with Nonautologous Tissue Substitute, Extern Approach
08RP07Z Replacement of Left Upper Eyelid with Autologous Tissue Substitute, Open Approach
08RP0JZ Replacement of Left Upper Eyelid with Synthetic Substitute, Open Approach
08RP0KZ Replacement of Left Upper Eyelid with Nonautologous Tissue Substitute, Open Approach
08RP37Z Replacement of Left Upper Eyelid with Autologous Tissue Substitute, Percutaneous Approach
08RP3JZ Replacement of Left Upper Eyelid with Synthetic Substitute, Percutaneous Approach
08RP3KZ Replacement of Left Upper Eyelid with Nonautologous Tissue Substitute, Percutaneous Approach
08RPX7Z Replacement of Left Upper Eyelid with Autologous Tissue Substitute, External Approach
08RPXJZ Replacement of Left Upper Eyelid with Synthetic Substitute, External Approach
08RPXKZ Replacement of Left Upper Eyelid with Nonautologous Tissue Substitute, External Approach
08RQ07Z Replacement of Right Lower Eyelid with Autologous Tissue Substitute, Open Approach
08RQ0JZ Replacement of Right Lower Eyelid with Synthetic Substitute, Open Approach
08RQ0KZ Replacement of Right Lower Eyelid with Nonautologous Tissue Substitute, Open Approach
08RQ37Z Replacement of Right Lower Eyelid with Autologous Tissue Substitute, Percutaneous Approach

RQ3JZ Replacement of Right Lower Eyelid with Synthetic Substitute, Percutaneous Approach
RQ3KZ Replacement of Right Lower Eyelid with Nonautologous Tissue Substitute, Percutaneous Approach
RQX7Z Replacement of Right Lower Eyelid with Autologous Tissue Substitute, External Approach
RQXJZ Replacement of Right Lower Eyelid with Synthetic Substitute, External Approach
RQXKZ Replacement of Right Lower Eyelid with Nonautologous Tissue Substitute, External Approach
RR07Z Replacement of Left Lower Eyelid with Autologous Tissue Substitute, Open Approach
RR0JZ Replacement of Left Lower Eyelid with Synthetic Substitute, Open Approach
RR0KZ Replacement of Left Lower Eyelid with Nonautologous Tissue Substitute, Open Approach
RR37Z Replacement of Left Lower Eyelid with Autologous Tissue Substitute, Percutaneous Approach
RR3JZ Replacement of Left Lower Eyelid with Synthetic Substitute, Percutaneous Approach
RR3KZ Replacement of Left Lower Eyelid with Nonautologous Tissue Substitute, Percutaneous Approach
RRX7Z Replacement of Left Lower Eyelid with Autologous Tissue Substitute, External Approach
RRXJZ Replacement of Left Lower Eyelid with Synthetic Substitute, External Approach
RRXKZ Replacement of Left Lower Eyelid with Nonautologous Tissue Substitute, External Approach
RSX7Z Replacement of Right Conjunctiva with Autologous Tissue Substitute, External Approach
08RSXJZ Replacement of Right Conjunctiva with Synthetic Substitute, External Approach
08RSXKZ Replacement of Right Conjunctiva with Nonautologous Tissue Substitute, External Approach
08RTX7Z Replacement of Left Conjunctiva with Autologous Tissue Substitute, External Approach
08RTXJZ Replacement of Left Conjunctiva with Synthetic Substitute, External Approach
08RTXKZ Replacement of Left Conjunctiva with Nonautologous Tissue Substitute, External Approach
08RX07Z Replacement of Right Lacrimal Duct with Autologous Tissue Substitute, Open Approach
08RX0JZ Replacement of Right Lacrimal Duct with Synthetic Substitute, Open Approach
08RX0KZ Replacement of Right Lacrimal Duct with Nonautologous Tissue Substitute, Open Approach
08RX37Z Replacement of Right Lacrimal Duct with Autologous Tissue Substitute, Percutaneous Approach
08RX3JZ Replacement of Right Lacrimal Duct with Synthetic Substitute, Percutaneous Approach
08RX3KZ Replacement of Right Lacrimal Duct with Nonautologous Tissue Substitute, Percutaneous Approach
08RX77Z Replacement of Right Lacrimal Duct with Autologous Tissue Substitute, Via Natural or Artificial Opening
08RX7JZ Replacement of Right Lacrimal Duct with Synthetic Substitute, Via Natural or Artificial Opening
08RX7KZ Replacement of Right Lacrimal Duct with Nonautologous Tissue Substitute, Via Natural or Artificial Opening
08RX87Z Replacement of Right Lacrimal Duct with Autologous Tissue Substitute, Via Natural or Artificial Opening Endoscopic
08RX8JZ Replacement of Right Lacrimal Duct with Synthetic Substitute, Via Natural or Artificial Opening Endoscopic
08RX8KZ Replacement of Right Lacrimal Duct with Nonautologous Tissue Substitute, Via Natural or Artificial Opening Endoscopic
08RY07Z Replacement of Left Lacrimal Duct with Autologous Tissue Substitute, Open Approach
08RY0JZ Replacement of Left Lacrimal Duct with Synthetic Substitute, Open Approach
08RY0KZ Replacement of Left Lacrimal Duct with Nonautologous Tissue Substitute, Open Approach
08RY37Z Replacement of Left Lacrimal Duct with Autologous Tissue Substitute, Percutaneous Approach
08RY3JZ Replacement of Left Lacrimal Duct with Synthetic Substitute, Percutaneous Approach
08RY3KZ Replacement of Left Lacrimal Duct with Nonautologous Tissue Substitute, Percutaneous Approach
08RY77Z Replacement of Left Lacrimal Duct with Autologous Tissue Substitute, Via Natural or Artificial Opening
08RY7JZ Replacement of Left Lacrimal Duct with Synthetic Substitute, Via Natural or Artificial Opening
08RY7KZ Replacement of Left Lacrimal Duct with Nonautologous Tissue Substitute, Via Natural or Artificial Opening
08RY87Z Replacement of Left Lacrimal Duct with Autologous Tissue Substitute, Via Natural or Artificial Opening Endoscopic
08RY8JZ Replacement of Left Lacrimal Duct with Synthetic Substitute, Via Natural or Artificial Opening Endoscopic
08RY8KZ Replacement of Left Lacrimal Duct with Nonautologous Tissue Substitute, Via Natural or Artificial Opening Endoscopic

8S – Eye, Reposition

SC3ZZ Reposition Right Iris, Percutaneous Approach
SD3ZZ Reposition Left Iris, Percutaneous Approach
SG3ZZ Reposition Right Retinal Vessel, Percutaneous Approach
SH3ZZ Reposition Left Retinal Vessel, Percutaneous Approach
SJ3ZZ Reposition Right Lens, Percutaneous Approach
SK3ZZ Reposition Left Lens, Percutaneous Approach
SL0ZZ Reposition Right Extraocular Muscle, Open Approach
SL3ZZ Reposition Right Extraocular Muscle, Percutaneous Approach
SM0ZZ Reposition Left Extraocular Muscle, Open Approach
SM3ZZ Reposition Left Extraocular Muscle, Percutaneous Approach
SN0ZZ Reposition Right Upper Eyelid, Open Approach
SN3ZZ Reposition Right Upper Eyelid, Percutaneous Approach
08SNXZZ Reposition Right Upper Eyelid, External Approach
08SP0ZZ Reposition Left Upper Eyelid, Open Approach
08SP3ZZ Reposition Left Upper Eyelid, Percutaneous Approach
08SPXZZ Reposition Left Upper Eyelid, External Approach
08SQ0ZZ Reposition Right Lower Eyelid, Open Approach
08SQ3ZZ Reposition Right Lower Eyelid, Percutaneous Approach
08SQXZZ Reposition Right Lower Eyelid, External Approach
08SR0ZZ Reposition Left Lower Eyelid, Open Approach
08SR3ZZ Reposition Left Lower Eyelid, Percutaneous Approach
08SRXZZ Reposition Left Lower Eyelid, External Approach
08SV0ZZ Reposition Right Lacrimal Gland, Open Approach
08SV3ZZ Reposition Right Lacrimal Gland, Percutaneous Approach
08SW0ZZ Reposition Left Lacrimal Gland, Open Approach
08SW3ZZ Reposition Left Lacrimal Gland, Percutaneous Approach
08SX0ZZ Reposition Right Lacrimal Duct, Open Approach
08SX3ZZ Reposition Right Lacrimal Duct, Percutaneous Approach
08SX7ZZ Reposition Right Lacrimal Duct, Via Natural or Artificial Opening
08SX8ZZ Reposition Right Lacrimal Duct, Via Natural or Artificial Opening Endoscopic
08SY0ZZ Reposition Left Lacrimal Duct, Open Approach
08SY3ZZ Reposition Left Lacrimal Duct, Percutaneous Approach
08SY7ZZ Reposition Left Lacrimal Duct, Via Natural or Artificial Opening
08SY8ZZ Reposition Left Lacrimal Duct, Via Natural or Artificial Opening Endoscopic

8T – Eye, Resection

Review Coding Guideline B3.8

8T0XZZ Resection of Right Eye, External Approach
8T1XZZ Resection of Left Eye, External Approach
08T43ZZ Resection of Right Vitreous, Percutaneous Approach
08T53ZZ Resection of Left Vitreous, Percutaneous Approach

08T8XZZ Resection of Right Cornea, External Approach
08T9XZZ Resection of Left Cornea, External Approach
08TC3ZZ Resection of Right Iris, Percutaneous Approach
08TD3ZZ Resection of Left Iris, Percutaneous Approach
08TJ3ZZ Resection of Right Lens, Percutaneous Approach
08TK3ZZ Resection of Left Lens, Percutaneous Approach
08TL0ZZ Resection of Right Extraocular Muscle, Open Approach
08TL3ZZ Resection of Right Extraocular Muscle, Percutaneous Approach
08TM0ZZ Resection of Left Extraocular Muscle, Open Approach
08TM3ZZ Resection of Left Extraocular Muscle, Percutaneous Approach
08TN0ZZ Resection of Right Upper Eyelid, Open Approach
08TNXZZ Resection of Right Upper Eyelid, External Approach
08TP0ZZ Resection of Left Upper Eyelid, Open Approach
08TPXZZ Resection of Left Upper Eyelid, External Approach
08TQ0ZZ Resection of Right Lower Eyelid, Open Approach
08TQXZZ Resection of Right Lower Eyelid, External Approach
08TR0ZZ Resection of Left Lower Eyelid, Open Approach
08TRXZZ Resection of Left Lower Eyelid, External Approach
08TV0ZZ Resection of Right Lacrimal Gland, Open Approach
08TV3ZZ Resection of Right Lacrimal Gland, Percutaneous Approach
08TW0ZZ Resection of Left Lacrimal Gland, Open Approach
08TW3ZZ Resection of Left Lacrimal Gland, Percutaneous Approach
08TX0ZZ Resection of Right Lacrimal Duct, Open Approach
08TX3ZZ Resection of Right Lacrimal Duct, Percutaneous Approach
08TX7ZZ Resection of Right Lacrimal Duct, Via Natural or Artificial Opening
08TX8ZZ Resection of Right Lacrimal Duct, Via Natural or Artificial Opening Endoscopic
08TY0ZZ Resection of Left Lacrimal Duct, Open Approach
08TY3ZZ Resection of Left Lacrimal Duct, Percutaneous Approach
08TY7ZZ Resection of Left Lacrimal Duct, Via Natural or Artificial Opening
08TY8ZZ Resection of Left Lacrimal Duct, Via Natural or Artificial Opening Endoscopic

08U – Eye, Supplement

08U007Z Supplement of Right Eye with Autologous Tissue Substitute, Open Approach
08U00JZ Supplement of Right Eye with Synthetic Substitute, Open Approach
08U00KZ Supplement of Right Eye with Nonautologous Tissue Substitute, Open Approach
08U037Z Supplement of Right Eye with Autologous Tissue Substitute, Percutaneous Approach
08U03JZ Supplement of Right Eye with Synthetic Substitute, Percutaneous Approach
08U03KZ Supplement of Right Eye with Nonautologous Tissue Substitute, Percutaneous Approach
08U107Z Supplement of Left Eye with Autologous Tissue Substitute, Open Approach
08U10JZ Supplement of Left Eye with Synthetic Substitute, Open Approach
08U10KZ Supplement of Left Eye with Nonautologous Tissue Substitute, Open Approach
08U137Z Supplement of Left Eye with Autologous Tissue Substitute, Percutaneous Approach
08U13JZ Supplement of Left Eye with Synthetic Substitute, Percutaneous Approach
08U13KZ Supplement of Left Eye with Nonautologous Tissue Substitute, Percutaneous Approach
08U807Z Supplement Right Cornea with Autologous Tissue Substitute, Open Approach
08U80JZ Supplement Right Cornea with Synthetic Substitute, Open Approach
▲ **08U80KZ** Supplement Right Cornea with Nonautologous Tissue Substitute, Open Approach
08U837Z Supplement Right Cornea with Autologous Tissue Substitute, Percutaneous Approach
08U83JZ Supplement Right Cornea with Synthetic Substitute, Percutaneous Approach
▲ **08U83KZ** Supplement Right Cornea with Nonautologous Tissue Substitute, Percutaneous Approach
08U8X7Z Supplement Right Cornea with Autologous Tissue Substitute, External Approach
08U8XJZ Supplement Right Cornea with Synthetic Substitute, External Approach
▲ **08U8XKZ** Supplement Right Cornea with Nonautologous Tissue Substitute, External Approach
08U907Z Supplement Left Cornea with Autologous Tissue Substitute, Open Approach
08U90JZ Supplement Left Cornea with Synthetic Substitute, Open Approach
▲ **08U90KZ** Supplement Left Cornea with Nonautologous Tissue Substitute, Open Approach
08U937Z Supplement Left Cornea with Autologous Tissue Substitute, Percutaneous Approach
08U93JZ Supplement Left Cornea with Synthetic Substitute, Percutaneous Approach
▲ **08U93KZ** Supplement Left Cornea with Nonautologous Tissue Substitute, Percutaneous Approach
08U9X7Z Supplement Left Cornea with Autologous Tissue Substitute, External Approach
08U9XJZ Supplement Left Cornea with Synthetic Substitute, External Approach
▲ **08U9XKZ** Supplement Left Cornea with Nonautologous Tissue Substitute, External Approach
08UC07Z Supplement Right Iris with Autologous Tissue Substitute, Open Approach
08UC0JZ Supplement Right Iris with Synthetic Substitute, Open Approach
08UC0KZ Supplement Right Iris with Nonautologous Tissue Substitute, Open Approach
08UC37Z Supplement Right Iris with Autologous Tissue Substitute, Percutaneous Approach
08UC3JZ Supplement Right Iris with Synthetic Substitute, Percutaneous Approach
08UC3KZ Supplement Right Iris with Nonautologous Tissue Substitute, Percutaneous Approach
08UD07Z Supplement Left Iris with Autologous Tissue Substitute, Open Approach
08UD0JZ Supplement Left Iris with Synthetic Substitute, Open Approach
08UD0KZ Supplement Left Iris with Nonautologous Tissue Substitute, Open Approach
08UD37Z Supplement Left Iris with Autologous Tissue Substitute, Percutaneous Approach
08UD3JZ Supplement Left Iris with Synthetic Substitute, Percutaneous Approach
08UD3KZ Supplement Left Iris with Nonautologous Tissue Substitute, Percutaneous Approach
08UE07Z Supplement Right Retina with Autologous Tissue Substitute, Open Approach
08UE0JZ Supplement Right Retina with Synthetic Substitute, Open Approach
08UE0KZ Supplement Right Retina with Nonautologous Tissue Substitute, Open Approach
08UE37Z Supplement Right Retina with Autologous Tissue Substitute, Percutaneous Approach
08UE3JZ Supplement Right Retina with Synthetic Substitute, Percutaneous Approach
08UE3KZ Supplement Right Retina with Nonautologous Tissue Substitute, Percutaneous Approach
08UF07Z Supplement Left Retina with Autologous Tissue Substitute, Open Approach
08UF0JZ Supplement Left Retina with Synthetic Substitute, Open Approach
08UF0KZ Supplement Left Retina with Nonautologous Tissue Substitute, Open Approach
08UF37Z Supplement Left Retina with Autologous Tissue Substitute, Percutaneous Approach
08UF3JZ Supplement Left Retina with Synthetic Substitute, Percutaneous Approach
08UF3KZ Supplement Left Retina with Nonautologous Tissue Substitute, Percutaneous Approach
08UG07Z Supplement Right Retinal Vessel with Autologous Tissue Substitute, Open Approach
08UG0JZ Supplement Right Retinal Vessel with Synthetic Substitute, Open Approach
08UG0KZ Supplement Right Retinal Vessel with Nonautologous Tissue Substitute, Open Approach
08UG37Z Supplement Right Retinal Vessel with Autologous Tissue Substitute, Percutaneous Approach
08UG3JZ Supplement Right Retinal Vessel with Synthetic Substitute, Percutaneous Approach
08UG3KZ Supplement Right Retinal Vessel with Nonautologous Tissue Substitute, Percutaneous Approach
08UH07Z Supplement Left Retinal Vessel with Autologous Tissue Substitute, Open Approach
08UH0JZ Supplement Left Retinal Vessel with Synthetic Substitute, Open Approach
08UH0KZ Supplement Left Retinal Vessel with Nonautologous Tissue Substitute, Open Approach
08UH37Z Supplement Left Retinal Vessel with Autologous Tissue Substitute, Percutaneous Approach
08UH3JZ Supplement Left Retinal Vessel with Synthetic Substitute, Percutaneous Approach
08UH3KZ Supplement Left Retinal Vessel with Nonautologous Tissue Substitute, Percutaneous Approach
08UL07Z Supplement Right Extraocular Muscle with Autologous Tissue Substitute, Open Approach

L0JZ Supplement Right Extraocular Muscle with Synthetic Substitute, Open Approach

L0KZ Supplement Right Extraocular Muscle with Nonautologous Tissue Substitute, Open Approach

JL37Z Supplement Right Extraocular Muscle with Autologous Tissue Substitute, Percutaneous Approach

JL3JZ Supplement Right Extraocular Muscle with Synthetic Substitute, Percutaneous Approach

JL3KZ Supplement Right Extraocular Muscle with Nonautologous Tissue Substitute, Percutaneous Approach

JM07Z Supplement Left Extraocular Muscle with Autologous Tissue Substitute, Open Approach

JM0JZ Supplement Left Extraocular Muscle with Synthetic Substitute, Open Approach

JM0KZ Supplement Left Extraocular Muscle with Nonautologous Tissue Substitute, Open Approach

JM37Z Supplement Left Extraocular Muscle with Autologous Tissue Substitute, Percutaneous Approach

UM3JZ Supplement Left Extraocular Muscle with Synthetic Substitute, Percutaneous Approach

UM3KZ Supplement Left Extraocular Muscle with Nonautologous Tissue Substitute, Percutaneous Approach

UN07Z Supplement Right Upper Eyelid with Autologous Tissue Substitute, Open Approach

UN0JZ Supplement Right Upper Eyelid with Synthetic Substitute, Open Approach

UN0KZ Supplement Right Upper Eyelid with Nonautologous Tissue Substitute, Open Approach

UN37Z Supplement Right Upper Eyelid with Autologous Tissue Substitute, Percutaneous Approach

UN3JZ Supplement Right Upper Eyelid with Synthetic Substitute, Percutaneous Approach

UN3KZ Supplement Right Upper Eyelid with Nonautologous Tissue Substitute, Percutaneous Approach

UNX7Z Supplement Right Upper Eyelid with Autologous Tissue Substitute, External Approach

UNXJZ Supplement Right Upper Eyelid with Synthetic Substitute, External Approach

UNXKZ Supplement Right Upper Eyelid with Nonautologous Tissue Substitute, External Approach

UP07Z Supplement Left Upper Eyelid with Autologous Tissue Substitute, Open Approach

UP0JZ Supplement Left Upper Eyelid with Synthetic Substitute, Open Approach

UP0KZ Supplement Left Upper Eyelid with Nonautologous Tissue Substitute, Open Approach

UP37Z Supplement Left Upper Eyelid with Autologous Tissue Substitute, Percutaneous Approach

08UP3JZ Supplement Left Upper Eyelid with Synthetic Substitute, Percutaneous Approach

08UP3KZ Supplement Left Upper Eyelid with Nonautologous Tissue Substitute, Percutaneous Approach

08UPX7Z Supplement Left Upper Eyelid with Autologous Tissue Substitute, External Approach

08UPXJZ Supplement Left Upper Eyelid with Synthetic Substitute, External Approach

08UPXKZ Supplement Left Upper Eyelid with Nonautologous Tissue Substitute, External Approach

08UQ07Z Supplement Right Lower Eyelid with Autologous Tissue Substitute, Open Approach

08UQ0JZ Supplement Right Lower Eyelid with Synthetic Substitute, Open Approach

08UQ0KZ Supplement Right Lower Eyelid with Nonautologous Tissue Substitute, Open Approach

08UQ37Z Supplement Right Lower Eyelid with Autologous Tissue Substitute, Percutaneous Approach

08UQ3JZ Supplement Right Lower Eyelid with Synthetic Substitute, Percutaneous Approach

08UQ3KZ Supplement Right Lower Eyelid with Nonautologous Tissue Substitute, Percutaneous Approach

08UQX7Z Supplement Right Lower Eyelid with Autologous Tissue Substitute, External Approach

08UQXJZ Supplement Right Lower Eyelid with Synthetic Substitute, External Approach

08UQXKZ Supplement Right Lower Eyelid with Nonautologous Tissue Substitute, External Approach

08UR07Z Supplement Left Lower Eyelid with Autologous Tissue Substitute, Open Approach

08UR0JZ Supplement Left Lower Eyelid with Synthetic Substitute, Open Approach

08UR0KZ Supplement Left Lower Eyelid with Nonautologous Tissue Substitute, Open Approach

08UR37Z Supplement Left Lower Eyelid with Autologous Tissue Substitute, Percutaneous Approach

08UR3JZ Supplement Left Lower Eyelid with Synthetic Substitute, Percutaneous Approach

08UR3KZ Supplement Left Lower Eyelid with Nonautologous Tissue Substitute, Percutaneous Approach

08URX7Z Supplement Left Lower Eyelid with Autologous Tissue Substitute, External Approach

08URXJZ Supplement Left Lower Eyelid with Synthetic Substitute, External Approach

08URXKZ Supplement Left Lower Eyelid with Nonautologous Tissue Substitute, External Approach

08UX07Z Supplement Right Lacrimal Duct with Autologous Tissue Substitute, Open Approach

08UX0JZ Supplement Right Lacrimal Duct with Synthetic Substitute, Open Approach

08UX0KZ Supplement Right Lacrimal Duct with Nonautologous Tissue Substitute, Open Approach

08UX37Z Supplement Right Lacrimal Duct with Autologous Tissue Substitute, Percutaneous Approach

08UX3JZ Supplement Right Lacrimal Duct with Synthetic Substitute, Percutaneous Approach

08UX3KZ Supplement Right Lacrimal Duct with Nonautologous Tissue Substitute, Percutaneous Approach

08UX77Z Supplement Right Lacrimal Duct with Autologous Tissue Substitute, Via Natural or Artificial Opening

08UX7JZ Supplement Right Lacrimal Duct with Synthetic Substitute, Via Natural or Artificial Opening

08UX7KZ Supplement Right Lacrimal Duct with Nonautologous Tissue Substitute, Via Natural or Artificial Opening

08UX87Z Supplement Right Lacrimal Duct with Autologous Tissue Substitute, Via Natural or Artificial Opening Endoscopic

08UX8JZ Supplement Right Lacrimal Duct with Synthetic Substitute, Via Natural or Artificial Opening Endoscopic

08UX8KZ Supplement Right Lacrimal Duct with Nonautologous Tissue Substitute, Via Natural or Artificial Opening Endoscopic

08UY07Z Supplement Left Lacrimal Duct with Autologous Tissue Substitute, Open Approach

08UY0JZ Supplement Left Lacrimal Duct with Synthetic Substitute, Open Approach

08UY0KZ Supplement Left Lacrimal Duct with Nonautologous Tissue Substitute, Open Approach

08UY37Z Supplement Left Lacrimal Duct with Autologous Tissue Substitute, Percutaneous Approach

08UY3JZ Supplement Left Lacrimal Duct with Synthetic Substitute, Percutaneous Approach

08UY3KZ Supplement Left Lacrimal Duct with Nonautologous Tissue Substitute, Percutaneous Approach

08UY77Z Supplement Left Lacrimal Duct with Autologous Tissue Substitute, Via Natural or Artificial Opening

08UY7JZ Supplement Left Lacrimal Duct with Synthetic Substitute, Via Natural or Artificial Opening

08UY7KZ Supplement Left Lacrimal Duct with Nonautologous Tissue Substitute, Via Natural or Artificial Opening

08UY87Z Supplement Left Lacrimal Duct with Autologous Tissue Substitute, Via Natural or Artificial Opening Endoscopic

08UY8JZ Supplement Left Lacrimal Duct with Synthetic Substitute, Via Natural or Artificial Opening Endoscopic

08UY8KZ Supplement Left Lacrimal Duct with Nonautologous Tissue Substitute, Via Natural or Artificial Opening Endoscopic

8V – Eye, Restriction

8VX0CZ Restriction of Right Lacrimal Duct with Extraluminal Device, Open Approach

8VX0DZ Restriction of Right Lacrimal Duct with Intraluminal Device, Open Approach

08VX0ZZ Restriction of Right Lacrimal Duct, Open Approach

08VX3CZ Restriction of Right Lacrimal Duct with Extraluminal Device, Percutaneous Approach

08VX3DZ Restriction of Right Lacrimal Duct with Intraluminal Device, Percutaneous Approach

08VX3ZZ Restriction of Right Lacrimal Duct, Percutaneous Approach

08VX7DZ Restriction of Right Lacrimal Duct with Intraluminal Device, Via Natural or Artificial Opening
08VX7ZZ Restriction of Right Lacrimal Duct, Via Natural or Artificial Opening
08VX8DZ Restriction of Right Lacrimal Duct with Intraluminal Device, Via Natural or Artificial Opening Endoscopic
08VX8ZZ Restriction of Right Lacrimal Duct, Via Natural or Artificial Opening Endoscopic
08VY0CZ Restriction of Left Lacrimal Duct with Extraluminal Device, Open Approach
08VY0DZ Restriction of Left Lacrimal Duct with Intraluminal Device, Open Approach
08VY0ZZ Restriction of Left Lacrimal Duct, Open Approach
08VY3CZ Restriction of Left Lacrimal Duct with Extraluminal Device, Percutaneous Approach
08VY3DZ Restriction of Left Lacrimal Duct with Intraluminal Device, Percutaneous Approach
08VY3ZZ Restriction of Left Lacrimal Duct, Percutaneous Approach
08VY7DZ Restriction of Left Lacrimal Duct with Intraluminal Device, Via Natural or Artificial Opening
08VY7ZZ Restriction of Left Lacrimal Duct, Via Natural or Artificial Opening
08VY8DZ Restriction of Left Lacrimal Duct with Intraluminal Device, Via Natural or Artificial Opening Endoscopic
08VY8ZZ Restriction of Left Lacrimal Duct, Via Natural or Artificial Opening Endoscop

08W – Eye, Revision

Review Coding Guideline B6.1c

08W000Z Revision of Drainage Device in Right Eye, Open Approach
08W003Z Revision of Infusion Device in Right Eye, Open Approach
08W007Z Revision of Autologous Tissue Substitute in Right Eye, Open Approach
08W00CZ Revision of Extraluminal Device in Right Eye, Open Approach
08W00DZ Revision of Intraluminal Device in Right Eye, Open Approach
08W00JZ Revision of Synthetic Substitute in Right Eye, Open Approach
08W00KZ Revision of Nonautologous Tissue Substitute in Right Eye, Open Approach
08W030Z Revision of Drainage Device in Right Eye, Percutaneous Approach
08W033Z Revision of Infusion Device in Right Eye, Percutaneous Approach
08W037Z Revision of Autologous Tissue Substitute in Right Eye, Percutaneous Approach
08W03CZ Revision of Extraluminal Device in Right Eye, Percutaneous Approach
08W03DZ Revision of Intraluminal Device in Right Eye, Percutaneous Approach
08W03JZ Revision of Synthetic Substitute in Right Eye, Percutaneous Approach
08W03KZ Revision of Nonautologous Tissue Substitute in Right Eye, Percutaneous Approach
08W070Z Revision of Drainage Device in Right Eye, Via Natural or Artificial Opening
08W073Z Revision of Infusion Device in Right Eye, Via Natural or Artificial Opening
08W077Z Revision of Autologous Tissue Substitute in Right Eye, Via Natural or Artificial Opening
08W07CZ Revision of Extraluminal Device in Right Eye, Via Natural or Artificial Opening
08W07DZ Revision of Intraluminal Device in Right Eye, Via Natural or Artificial Opening
08W07JZ Revision of Synthetic Substitute in Right Eye, Via Natural or Artificial Opening
08W07KZ Revision of Nonautologous Tissue Substitute in Right Eye, Via Natural or Artificial Opening
08W080Z Revision of Drainage Device in Right Eye, Via Natural or Artificial Opening Endoscopic
08W083Z Revision of Infusion Device in Right Eye, Via Natural or Artificial Opening Endoscopic
08W087Z Revision of Autologous Tissue Substitute in Right Eye, Via Natural or Artificial Opening Endoscopic
08W08CZ Revision of Extraluminal Device in Right Eye, Via Natural or Artificial Opening Endoscopic
08W08DZ Revision of Intraluminal Device in Right Eye, Via Natural or Artificial Opening Endoscopic
08W08JZ Revision of Synthetic Substitute in Right Eye, Via Natural or Artificial Opening Endoscopic
08W08KZ Revision of Nonautologous Tissue Substitute in Right Eye, Via Natural or Artificial Opening Endoscopic
08W0X0Z Revision of Drainage Device in Right Eye, External Approach
08W0X3Z Revision of Infusion Device in Right Eye, External Approach
08W0X7Z Revision of Autologous Tissue Substitute in Right Eye, External Approach
08W0XCZ Revision of Extraluminal Device in Right Eye, External Approach
08W0XDZ Revision of Intraluminal Device in Right Eye, External Approach
08W0XJZ Revision of Synthetic Substitute in Right Eye, External Approach
08W0XKZ Revision of Nonautologous Tissue Substitute in Right Eye, External Approach
08W100Z Revision of Drainage Device in Left Eye, Open Approach
08W103Z Revision of Infusion Device in Left Eye, Open Approach
08W107Z Revision of Autologous Tissue Substitute in Left Eye, Open Approach
08W10CZ Revision of Extraluminal Device in Left Eye, Open Approach
08W10DZ Revision of Intraluminal Device in Left Eye, Open Approach
08W10JZ Revision of Synthetic Substitute in Left Eye, Open Approach
08W10KZ Revision of Nonautologous Tissue Substitute in Left Eye, Open Approach
08W130Z Revision of Drainage Device in Left Eye, Percutaneous Approach
08W133Z Revision of Infusion Device in Left Eye, Percutaneous Approach
08W137Z Revision of Autologous Tissue Substitute in Left Eye, Percutaneous Approach
08W13CZ Revision of Extraluminal Device in Left Eye, Percutaneous Approach
08W13DZ Revision of Intraluminal Device in Left Eye, Percutaneous Approach
08W13JZ Revision of Synthetic Substitute in Left Eye, Percutaneous Approach
08W13KZ Revision of Nonautologous Tissue Substitute in Left Eye, Percutaneous Approach
08W170Z Revision of Drainage Device in Left Eye, Via Natural or Artificial Opening
08W173Z Revision of Infusion Device in Left Eye, Via Natural or Artificial Opening
08W177Z Revision of Autologous Tissue Substitute in Left Eye, Via Natural or Artificial Opening
08W17CZ Revision of Extraluminal Device in Left Eye, Via Natural or Artificial Opening
08W17DZ Revision of Intraluminal Device in Left Eye, Via Natural or Artificial Opening
08W17JZ Revision of Synthetic Substitute in Left Eye, Via Natural or Artificial Opening
08W17KZ Revision of Nonautologous Tissue Substitute in Left Eye, Via Natural or Artificial Opening
08W180Z Revision of Drainage Device in Left Eye, Via Natural or Artificial Opening Endoscopic
08W183Z Revision of Infusion Device in Left Eye, Via Natural or Artificial Opening Endoscopic
08W187Z Revision of Autologous Tissue Substitut in Left Eye, Via Natural or Artificial Opening Endoscopic
08W18CZ Revision of Extraluminal Device in Left Eye, Via Natural or Artificial Opening Endoscopic
08W18DZ Revision of Intraluminal Device in Left Eye, Via Natural or Artificial Opening Endoscopic
08W18JZ Revision of Synthetic Substitute in Left Eye, Via Natural or Artificial Opening Endoscopic
08W18KZ Revision of Nonautologous Tissue Substitute in Left Eye, Via Natural or Artificial Opening Endoscopic
08W1X0Z Revision of Drainage Device in Left Eye External Approach
08W1X3Z Revision of Infusion Device in Left Eye External Approach
08W1X7Z Revision of Autologous Tissue Substitut in Left Eye, External Approach
08W1XCZ Revision of Extraluminal Device in Left Eye, External Approach
08W1XDZ Revision of Intraluminal Device in Left Eye, External Approach
08W1XJZ Revision of Synthetic Substitute in Left Eye, External Approach
08W1XKZ Revision of Nonautologous Tissue Substitute in Left Eye, External Approac
08WJ3JZ Revision of Synthetic Substitute in Righ Lens, Percutaneous Approach
08WJXJZ Revision of Synthetic Substitute in Righ Lens, External Approach
08WK3JZ Revision of Synthetic Substitute in Left Lens, Percutaneous Approach
08WKXJZ Revision of Synthetic Substitute in Left Lens, External Approach
08WL00Z Revision of Drainage Device in Right Extraocular Muscle, Open Approach
08WL07Z Revision of Autologous Tissue Substitute in Right Extraocular Muscle, Open Approach
08WL0JZ Revision of Synthetic Substitute in Right Extraocular Muscle, Open Approach
08WL0KZ Revision of Nonautologous Tissue Substitute in Right Extraocular Muscle, Open Approach

VL30Z Revision of Drainage Device in Right Extraocular Muscle, Percutaneous Approach
VL37Z Revision of Autologous Tissue Substitute in Right Extraocular Muscle, Percutaneous Approach
VL3JZ Revision of Synthetic Substitute in Right Extraocular Muscle, Percutaneous Approach
VL3KZ Revision of Nonautologous Tissue Substitute in Right Extraocular Muscle, Percutaneous Approach
08WM00Z Revision of Drainage Device in Left Extraocular Muscle, Open Approach
08WM07Z Revision of Autologous Tissue Substitute in Left Extraocular Muscle, Open Approach
08WM0JZ Revision of Synthetic Substitute in Left Extraocular Muscle, Open Approach
08WM0KZ Revision of Nonautologous Tissue Substitute in Left Extraocular Muscle, Open Approach
08WM30Z Revision of Drainage Device in Left Extraocular Muscle, Percutaneous Approach
08WM37Z Revision of Autologous Tissue Substitute in Left Extraocular Muscle, Percutaneous Approach
08WM3JZ Revision of Synthetic Substitute in Left Extraocular Muscle, Percutaneous Approach
08WM3KZ Revision of Nonautologous Tissue Substitute in Left Extraocular Muscle, Percutaneous Approach

X – Eye, Transfer

XL0ZZ Transfer Right Extraocular Muscle, Open Approach
XL3ZZ Transfer Right Extraocular Muscle, Percutaneous Approach
08XM0ZZ Transfer Left Extraocular Muscle, Open Approach
08XM3ZZ Transfer Left Extraocular Muscle, Percutaneous Approach

Nose and Sinus

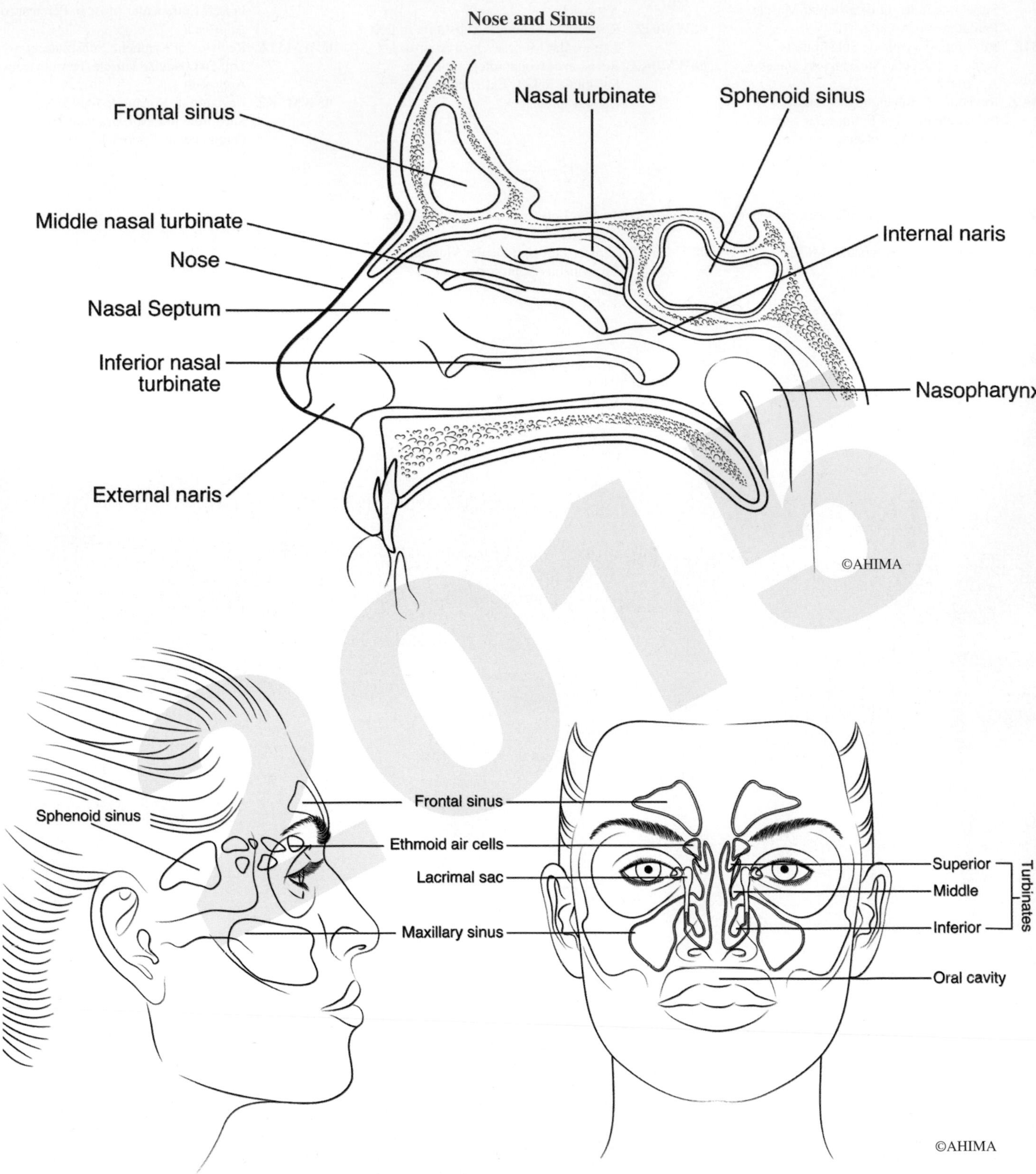
Frontal sinus
Nasal turbinate
Sphenoid sinus
Middle nasal turbinate
Internal naris
Nose
Nasal Septum
Inferior nasal turbinate
Nasopharynx
External naris
©AHIMA
Sphenoid sinus
Frontal sinus
Ethmoid air cells
Lacrimal sac
Maxillary sinus
Superior
Middle
Inferior
Turbinates
Oral cavity
©AHIMA

Ear

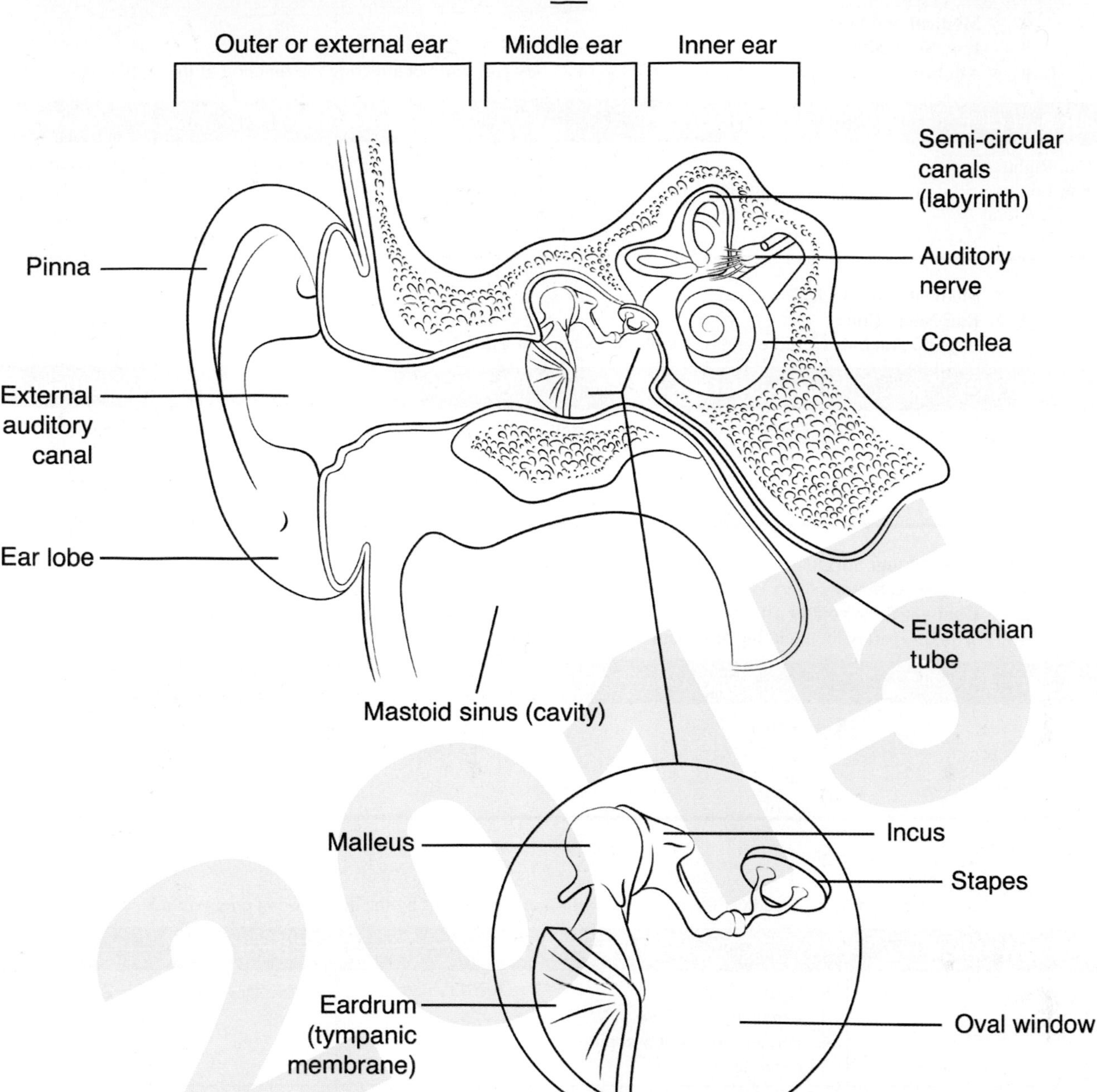

Outer or external ear
Middle ear
Inner ear
Semi-circular canals (labyrinth)
Pinna
Auditory nerve
Cochlea
External auditory canal
Ear lobe
Eustachian tube
Mastoid sinus (cavity)
Malleus
Incus
Stapes
Eardrum (tympanic membrane)
Oval window
Auditory ossicles

Ear, Nose, Sinus Tables 090–09W

Section 0 **Medical and Surgical**
Body System 9 **Ear, Nose, Sinus**
Operation 0 **Alteration:** Modifying the anatomic structure of a body part without affecting the function of the body part

Body Part (4th)	Approach (5th)	Device (6th)	Qualifier (7th)
0 External Ear, Right **1** External Ear, Left **2** External Ear, Bilateral **K** Nose	**0** Open **3** Percutaneous **4** Percutaneous Endoscopic **X** External	**7** Autologous Tissue Substitute **J** Synthetic Substitute **K** Nonautologous Tissue Substitute **Z** No Device	**Z** No Qualifier

Section 0 **Medical and Surgical**
Body System 9 **Ear, Nose, Sinus**
Operation 1 **Bypass:** Altering the route of passage of the contents of a tubular body part

Body Part (4th)	Approach (5th)	Device (6th)	Qualifier (7th)
D Inner Ear, Right **E** Inner Ear, Left	**0** Open	**7** Autologous Tissue Substitute **J** Synthetic Substitute **K** Nonautologous Tissue Substitute **Z** No Device	**0** Endolymphatic

Section 0 **Medical and Surgical**
Body System 9 **Ear, Nose, Sinus**
Operation 2 **Change:** Taking out or off a device from a body part and putting back an identical or similar device in or on the same body part without cutting or puncturing the skin or a mucous membrane

Body Part (4th)	Approach (5th)	Device (6th)	Qualifier (7th)
H Ear, Right **J** Ear, Left **K** Nose **Y** Sinus	**X** External	**0** Drainage Device **Y** Other Device	**Z** No Qualifier

Section 0 **Medical and Surgical**
Body System 9 **Ear, Nose, Sinus**
Operation 5 **Destruction:** Physical eradication of all or a portion of a body part by the direct use of energy, force, or a destructive agent

Body Part (4th)	Approach (5th)	Device (6th)	Qualifier (7th)
0 External Ear, Right **1** External Ear, Left **K** Nose	**0** Open **3** Percutaneous **4** Percutaneous Endoscopic **X** External	**Z** No Device	**Z** No Qualifier
3 External Auditory Canal, Right **4** External Auditory Canal, Left	**0** Open **3** Percutaneous **4** Percutaneous Endoscopic **7** Via Natural or Artificial Opening **8** Via Natural or Artificial Opening Endoscopic **X** External	**Z** No Device	**Z** No Qualifier
5 Middle Ear, Right **6** Middle Ear, Left **9** Auditory Ossicle, Right **A** Auditory Ossicle, Left **D** Inner Ear, Right **E** Inner Ear, Left	**0** Open	**Z** No Device	**Z** No Qualifier
7 Tympanic Membrane, Right **8** Tympanic Membrane, Left **F** Eustachian Tube, Right **G** Eustachian Tube, Left **L** Nasal Turbinate **N** Nasopharynx	**0** Open **3** Percutaneous **4** Percutaneous Endoscopic **7** Via Natural or Artificial Opening **8** Via Natural or Artificial Opening Endoscopic	**Z** No Device	**Z** No Qualifier

Continued →

ction	0	**Medical and Surgical**
dy System	9	**Ear, Nose, Sinus**
eration	5	**Destruction:** Physical eradication of all or a portion of a body part by the direct use of energy, force, or a destructive agent

Body Part (4th)	Approach (5th)	Device (6th)	Qualifier (7th)
Mastoid Sinus, Right Mastoid Sinus, Left I Nasal Septum Accessory Sinus Maxillary Sinus, Right Maxillary Sinus, Left Frontal Sinus, Right Frontal Sinus, Left Ethmoid Sinus, Right Ethmoid Sinus, Left V Sphenoid Sinus, Right Sphenoid Sinus, Left	**0** Open **3** Percutaneous **4** Percutaneous Endoscopic	**Z** No Device	**Z** No Qualifier

ction	0	**Medical and Surgical**
dy System	9	**Ear, Nose, Sinus**
eration	7	**Dilation:** Expanding an orifice or the lumen of a tubular body part

Body Part (4th)	Approach (5th)	Device (6th)	Qualifier (7th)
Eustachian Tube, Right Eustachian Tube, Left	**0** Open **7** Via Natural or Artificial Opening **8** Via Natural or Artificial Opening Endoscopic	**D** Intraluminal Device **Z** No Device	**Z** No Qualifier
Eustachian Tube, Right Eustachian Tube, Left	**3** Percutaneous **4** Percutaneous Endoscopic	**Z** No Device	**Z** No Qualifier

ction	0	**Medical and Surgical**
dy System	9	**Ear, Nose, Sinus**
eration	8	**Division:** Cutting into a body part, without draining fluids and/or gases from the body part, in order to separate or transect a body part

Body Part (4th)	Approach (5th)	Device (6th)	Qualifier (7th)
Nasal Turbinate	**0** Open **3** Percutaneous **4** Percutaneous Endoscopic **7** Via Natural or Artificial Opening **8** Via Natural or Artificial Opening Endoscopic	**Z** No Device	**Z** No Qualifier

ction	0	**Medical and Surgical**
dy System	9	**Ear, Nose, Sinus**
peration	9	**Drainage:** Taking or letting out fluids and/or gases from a body part

Body Part (4th)	Approach (5th)	Device (6th)	Qualifier (7th)
0 External Ear, Right **1** External Ear, Left **K** Nose	**0** Open **3** Percutaneous **4** Percutaneous Endoscopic **X** External	**0** Drainage Device	**Z** No Qualifier
0 External Ear, Right **1** External Ear, Left **K** Nose	**0** Open **3** Percutaneous **4** Percutaneous Endoscopic **X** External	**Z** No Device	**X** Diagnostic **Z** No Qualifier
3 External Auditory Canal, Right **4** External Auditory Canal, Left	**0** Open **3** Percutaneous **4** Percutaneous Endoscopic **7** Via Natural or Artificial Opening **8** Via Natural or Artificial Opening Endoscopic **X** External	**0** Drainage Device	**Z** No Qualifier

Continued →

Section 0 Medical and Surgical
Body System 9 Ear, Nose, Sinus
Operation 9 **Drainage:** Taking or letting out fluids and/or gases from a body part

Body Part (4th)	Approach (5th)	Device (6th)	Qualifier (7th)
3 External Auditory Canal, Right **4** External Auditory Canal, Left	**0** Open **3** Percutaneous **4** Percutaneous Endoscopic **7** Via Natural or Artificial Opening **8** Via Natural or Artificial Opening Endoscopic **X** External	**Z** No Device	**X** Diagnostic **Z** No Qualifier
5 Middle Ear, Right **6** Middle Ear, Left **9** Auditory Ossicle, Right **A** Auditory Ossicle, Left **D** Inner Ear, Right **E** Inner Ear, Left	**0** Open	**0** Drainage Device	**Z** No Qualifier
5 Middle Ear, Right **6** Middle Ear, Left **9** Auditory Ossicle, Right **A** Auditory Ossicle, Left **D** Inner Ear, Right **E** Inner Ear, Left	**0** Open	**Z** No Device	**X** Diagnostic **Z** No Qualifier
7 Tympanic Membrane, Right **8** Tympanic Membrane, Left **F** Eustachian Tube, Right **G** Eustachian Tube, Left **L** Nasal Turbinate **N** Nasopharynx	**0** Open **3** Percutaneous **4** Percutaneous Endoscopic **7** Via Natural or Artificial Opening **8** Via Natural or Artificial Opening Endoscopic	**0** Drainage Device	**Z** No Qualifier
7 Tympanic Membrane, Right **8** Tympanic Membrane, Left **F** Eustachian Tube, Right **G** Eustachian Tube, Left **L** Nasal Turbinate **N** Nasopharynx	**0** Open **3** Percutaneous **4** Percutaneous Endoscopic **7** Via Natural or Artificial Opening **8** Via Natural or Artificial Opening Endoscopic	**Z** No Device	**X** Diagnostic **Z** No Qualifier
B Mastoid Sinus, Right **C** Mastoid Sinus, Left **M** Nasal Septum **P** Accessory Sinus **Q** Maxillary Sinus, Right **R** Maxillary Sinus, Left **S** Frontal Sinus, Right **T** Frontal Sinus, Left **U** Ethmoid Sinus, Right **V** Ethmoid Sinus, Left **W** Sphenoid Sinus, Right **X** Sphenoid Sinus, Left	**0** Open **3** Percutaneous **4** Percutaneous Endoscopic	**0** Drainage Device	**Z** No Qualifier
B Mastoid Sinus, Right **C** Mastoid Sinus, Left **M** Nasal Septum **P** Accessory Sinus **Q** Maxillary Sinus, Right **R** Maxillary Sinus, Left **S** Frontal Sinus, Right **T** Frontal Sinus, Left **U** Ethmoid Sinus, Right **V** Ethmoid Sinus, Left **W** Sphenoid Sinus, Right **X** Sphenoid Sinus, Left	**0** Open **3** Percutaneous **4** Percutaneous Endoscopic	**Z** No Device	**X** Diagnostic **Z** No Qualifier

tion	**0**	**Medical and Surgical**
dy System	**9**	**Ear, Nose, Sinus**
eration	**B**	**Excision:** Cutting out or off, without replacement, a portion of a body part

Body Part (4th)	Approach (5th)	Device (6th)	Qualifier (7th)
External Ear, Right External Ear, Left K Nose	**0** Open **3** Percutaneous **4** Percutaneous Endoscopic **X** External	**Z** No Device	**X** Diagnostic **Z** No Qualifier
External Auditory Canal, Right External Auditory Canal, Left	**0** Open **3** Percutaneous **4** Percutaneous Endoscopic **7** Via Natural or Artificial Opening **8** Via Natural or Artificial Opening Endoscopic **X** External	**Z** No Device	**X** Diagnostic **Z** No Qualifier
Middle Ear, Right Middle Ear, Left Auditory Ossicle, Right A Auditory Ossicle, Left D Inner Ear, Right E Inner Ear, Left	**0** Open	**Z** No Device	**X** Diagnostic **Z** No Qualifier
7 Tympanic Membrane, Right 8 Tympanic Membrane, Left F Eustachian Tube, Right G Eustachian Tube, Left L Nasal Turbinate N Nasopharynx	**0** Open **3** Percutaneous **4** Percutaneous Endoscopic **7** Via Natural or Artificial Opening **8** Via Natural or Artificial Opening Endoscopic	**Z** No Device	**X** Diagnostic **Z** No Qualifier
B Mastoid Sinus, Right **C** Mastoid Sinus, Left **M** Nasal Septum **P** Accessory Sinus **Q** Maxillary Sinus, Right **R** Maxillary Sinus, Left **S** Frontal Sinus, Right **T** Frontal Sinus, Left **U** Ethmoid Sinus, Right **V** Ethmoid Sinus, Left **W** Sphenoid Sinus, Right **X** Sphenoid Sinus, Left	**0** Open **3** Percutaneous **4** Percutaneous Endoscopic	**Z** No Device	**X** Diagnostic **Z** No Qualifier

ection	**0**	**Medical and Surgical**
ody System	**9**	**Ear, Nose, Sinus**
peration	**C**	**Extirpation:** Taking or cutting out solid matter from a body part

Body Part (4th)	Approach (5th)	Device (6th)	Qualifier (7th)
0 External Ear, Right **1** External Ear, Left **K** Nose	**0** Open **3** Percutaneous **4** Percutaneous Endoscopic **X** External	**Z** No Device	**Z** No Qualifier
3 External Auditory Canal, Right **4** External Auditory Canal, Left	**0** Open **3** Percutaneous **4** Percutaneous Endoscopic **7** Via Natural or Artificial Opening **8** Via Natural or Artificial Opening Endoscopic **X** External	**Z** No Device	**Z** No Qualifier

Continued →

Section 0 **Medical and Surgical**
Body System 9 **Ear, Nose, Sinus**
Operation C **Extirpation:** Taking or cutting out solid matter from a body part

Body Part (4th)	Approach (5th)	Device (6th)	Qualifier (7th)
5 Middle Ear, Right **6** Middle Ear, Left **9** Auditory Ossicle, Right **A** Auditory Ossicle, Left **D** Inner Ear, Right **E** Inner Ear, Left	**0** Open	**Z** No Device	**Z** No Qualifier
7 Tympanic Membrane, Right **8** Tympanic Membrane, Left **F** Eustachian Tube, Right **G** Eustachian Tube, Left **L** Nasal Turbinate **N** Nasopharynx	**0** Open **3** Percutaneous **4** Percutaneous Endoscopic **7** Via Natural or Artificial Opening **8** Via Natural or Artificial Opening Endoscopic	**Z** No Device	**Z** No Qualifier
B Mastoid Sinus, Right **C** Mastoid Sinus, Left **M** Nasal Septum **P** Accessory Sinus **Q** Maxillary Sinus, Right **R** Maxillary Sinus, Left **S** Frontal Sinus, Right **T** Frontal Sinus, Left **U** Ethmoid Sinus, Right **V** Ethmoid Sinus, Left **W** Sphenoid Sinus, Right **X** Sphenoid Sinus, Left	**0** Open **3** Percutaneous **4** Percutaneous Endoscopic	**Z** No Device	**Z** No Qualifier

Section 0 **Medical and Surgical**
Body System 9 **Ear, Nose, Sinus**
Operation D **Extraction:** Pulling or stripping out or off all or a portion of a body part by the use of force

Body Part (4th)	Approach (5th)	Device (6th)	Qualifier (7th)
7 Tympanic Membrane, Right **8** Tympanic Membrane, Left **L** Nasal Turbinate	**0** Open **3** Percutaneous **4** Percutaneous Endoscopic **7** Via Natural or Artificial Opening **8** Via Natural or Artificial Opening Endoscopic	**Z** No Device	**Z** No Qualifier
9 Auditory Ossicle, Right **A** Auditory Ossicle, Left	**0** Open	**Z** No Device	**Z** No Qualifier
B Mastoid Sinus, Right **C** Mastoid Sinus, Left **M** Nasal Septum **P** Accessory Sinus **Q** Maxillary Sinus, Right **R** Maxillary Sinus, Left **S** Frontal Sinus, Right **T** Frontal Sinus, Left **U** Ethmoid Sinus, Right **V** Ethmoid Sinus, Left **W** Sphenoid Sinus, Right **X** Sphenoid Sinus, Left	**0** Open **3** Percutaneous **4** Percutaneous Endoscopic	**Z** No Device	**Z** No Qualifier

ction 0 **Medical and Surgical**
dy System 9 **Ear, Nose, Sinus**
eration H **Insertion:** Putting in a nonbiological appliance that monitors, assists, performs, or prevents a physiological function but does not physically take the place of a body part

Body Part (4th)	Approach (5th)	Device (6th)	Qualifier (7th)
D Inner Ear, Right E Inner Ear, Left	**0** Open **3** Percutaneous **4** Percutaneous Endoscopic	**4** Hearing Device, Bone Conduction **5** Hearing Device, Single Channel Cochlear Prosthesis **6** Hearing Device, Multiple Channel Cochlear Prosthesis **S** Hearing Device	**Z** No Qualifier
N Nasopharynx	**7** Via Natural or Artificial Opening **8** Via Natural or Artificial Opening Endoscopic	**B** Intraluminal Device, Airway	**Z** No Qualifier

ction 0 **Medical and Surgical**
dy System 9 **Ear, Nose, Sinus**
peration J **Inspection:** Visually and/or manually exploring a body part

Body Part (4th)	Approach (5th)	Device (6th)	Qualifier (7th)
7 Tympanic Membrane, Right **8** Tympanic Membrane, Left **H** Ear, Right **J** Ear, Left	**0** Open **3** Percutaneous **4** Percutaneous Endoscopic **7** Via Natural or Artificial Opening **8** Via Natural or Artificial Opening Endoscopic **X** External	**Z** No Device	**Z** No Qualifier
D Inner Ear, Right **E** Inner Ear, Left **K** Nose **Y** Sinus	**0** Open **3** Percutaneous **4** Percutaneous Endoscopic **X** External	**Z** No Device	**Z** No Qualifier

ection 0 **Medical and Surgical**
ody System 9 **Ear, Nose, Sinus**
peration M **Reattachment:** Putting back in or on all or a portion of a separated body part to its normal location or other suitable location

Body Part (4th)	Approach (5th)	Device (6th)	Qualifier (7th)
0 External Ear, Right **1** External Ear, Left **K** Nose	**X** External	**Z** No Device	**Z** No Qualifier

ection 0 **Medical and Surgical**
ody System 9 **Ear, Nose, Sinus**
peration N **Release:** Freeing a body part from an abnormal physical constraint by cutting or by the use of force

Body Part (4th)	Approach (5th)	Device (6th)	Qualifier (7th)
0 External Ear, Right **1** External Ear, Left **K** Nose	**0** Open **3** Percutaneous **4** Percutaneous Endoscopic **X** External	**Z** No Device	**Z** No Qualifier
3 External Auditory Canal, Right **4** External Auditory Canal, Left	**0** Open **3** Percutaneous **4** Percutaneous Endoscopic **7** Via Natural or Artificial Opening **8** Via Natural or Artificial Opening Endoscopic **X** External	**Z** No Device	**Z** No Qualifier

Continued →

Section 0 **Medical and Surgical**
Body System 9 **Ear, Nose, Sinus**
Operation N **Release:** Freeing a body part from an abnormal physical constraint by cutting or by the use of force

Body Part (4th)	Approach (5th)	Device (6th)	Qualifier (7th)
5 Middle Ear, Right **6** Middle Ear, Left **9** Auditory Ossicle, Right **A** Auditory Ossicle, Left **D** Inner Ear, Right **E** Inner Ear, Left	**0** Open	**Z** No Device	**Z** No Qualifier
7 Tympanic Membrane, Right **8** Tympanic Membrane, Left **F** Eustachian Tube, Right **G** Eustachian Tube, Left **L** Nasal Turbinate **N** Nasopharynx	**0** Open **3** Percutaneous **4** Percutaneous Endoscopic **7** Via Natural or Artificial Opening **8** Via Natural or Artificial Opening Endoscopic	**Z** No Device	**Z** No Qualifier
B Mastoid Sinus, Right **C** Mastoid Sinus, Left **M** Nasal Septum **P** Accessory Sinus **Q** Maxillary Sinus, Right **R** Maxillary Sinus, Left **S** Frontal Sinus, Right **T** Frontal Sinus, Left **U** Ethmoid Sinus, Right **V** Ethmoid Sinus, Left **W** Sphenoid Sinus, Right **X** Sphenoid Sinus, Left	**0** Open **3** Percutaneous **4** Percutaneous Endoscopic	**Z** No Device	**Z** No Qualifier

Section 0 **Medical and Surgical**
Body System 9 **Ear, Nose, Sinus**
Operation P **Removal:** Taking out or off a device from a body part

Body Part (4th)	Approach (5th)	Device (6th)	Qualifier (7th)
7 Tympanic Membrane, Right **8** Tympanic Membrane, Left	**0** Open **7** Via Natural or Artificial Opening **8** Via Natural or Artificial Opening Endoscopic **X** External	**0** Drainage Device	**Z** No Qualifier
D Inner Ear, Right **E** Inner Ear, Left	**0** Open **7** Via Natural or Artificial Opening **8** Via Natural or Artificial Opening Endoscopic	**S** Hearing Device	**Z** No Qualifier
H Ear, Right **J** Ear, Left **K** Nose	**0** Open **3** Percutaneous **4** Percutaneous Endoscopic **7** Via Natural or Artificial Opening **8** Via Natural or Artificial Opening Endoscopic **X** External	**0** Drainage Device **7** Autologous Tissue Substitute **D** Intraluminal Device **J** Synthetic Substitute **K** Nonautologous Tissue Substitute	**Z** No Qualifier
Y Sinus	**0** Open **3** Percutaneous **4** Percutaneous Endoscopic **X** External	**0** Drainage Device	**Z** No Qualifier

tion 0 **Medical and Surgical**
ly System 9 **Ear, Nose, Sinus**
eration Q **Repair:** Restoring, to the extent possible, a body part to its normal anatomic structure and function

Body Part (4th)	Approach (5th)	Device (6th)	Qualifier (7th)
External Ear, Right External Ear, Left External Ear, Bilateral K Nose	0 Open 3 Percutaneous 4 Percutaneous Endoscopic X External	Z No Device	Z No Qualifier
3 External Auditory Canal, Right External Auditory Canal, Left F Eustachian Tube, Right G Eustachian Tube, Left	0 Open 3 Percutaneous 4 Percutaneous Endoscopic 7 Via Natural or Artificial Opening 8 Via Natural or Artificial Opening Endoscopic X External	Z No Device	Z No Qualifier
5 Middle Ear, Right 6 Middle Ear, Left 9 Auditory Ossicle, Right A Auditory Ossicle, Left D Inner Ear, Right E Inner Ear, Left	0 Open	Z No Device	Z No Qualifier
7 Tympanic Membrane, Right 8 Tympanic Membrane, Left L Nasal Turbinate N Nasopharynx	0 Open 3 Percutaneous 4 Percutaneous Endoscopic 7 Via Natural or Artificial Opening 8 Via Natural or Artificial Opening Endoscopic	Z No Device	Z No Qualifier
B Mastoid Sinus, Right C Mastoid Sinus, Left M Nasal Septum P Accessory Sinus Q Maxillary Sinus, Right R Maxillary Sinus, Left S Frontal Sinus, Right T Frontal Sinus, Left U Ethmoid Sinus, Right V Ethmoid Sinus, Left W Sphenoid Sinus, Right X Sphenoid Sinus, Left	0 Open 3 Percutaneous 4 Percutaneous Endoscopic	Z No Device	Z No Qualifier

ection 0 **Medical and Surgical**
ody System 9 **Ear, Nose, Sinus**
peration R **Replacement:** Putting in or on biological or synthetic material that physically takes the place and/or function of all or a portion of a body part

Body Part (4th)	Approach (5th)	Device (6th)	Qualifier (7th)
0 External Ear, Right 1 External Ear, Left 2 External Ear, Bilateral K Nose	0 Open X External	7 Autologous Tissue Substitute J Synthetic Substitute K Nonautologous Tissue Substitute	Z No Qualifier
5 Middle Ear, Right 6 Middle Ear, Left 9 Auditory Ossicle, Right A Auditory Ossicle, Left D Inner Ear, Right E Inner Ear, Left	0 Open	7 Autologous Tissue Substitute J Synthetic Substitute K Nonautologous Tissue Substitute	Z No Qualifier
7 Tympanic Membrane, Right 8 Tympanic Membrane, Left N Nasopharynx	0 Open 7 Via Natural or Artificial Opening 8 Via Natural or Artificial Opening Endoscopic	7 Autologous Tissue Substitute J Synthetic Substitute K Nonautologous Tissue Substitute	Z No Qualifier

Continued →

Section 0 **Medical and Surgical**
Body System 9 **Ear, Nose, Sinus**
Operation R **Replacement:** Putting in or on biological or synthetic material that physically takes the place and/or function of all or a portion of a body part

Body Part (4th)	Approach (5th)	Device (6th)	Qualifier (7th)
L Nasal Turbinate	**0** Open **3** Percutaneous **4** Percutaneous Endoscopic **7** Via Natural or Artificial Opening **8** Via Natural or Artificial Opening Endoscopic	**7** Autologous Tissue Substitute **J** Synthetic Substitute **K** Nonautologous Tissue Substitute	**Z** No Qualifier
M Nasal Septum	**0** Open **3** Percutaneous **4** Percutaneous Endoscopic	**7** Autologous Tissue Substitute **J** Synthetic Substitute **K** Nonautologous Tissue Substitute	**Z** No Qualifier

Section 0 **Medical and Surgical**
Body System 9 **Ear, Nose, Sinus**
Operation S **Reposition:** Moving to its normal location, or other suitable location, all or a portion of a body part

Body Part (4th)	Approach (5th)	Device (6th)	Qualifier (7th)
0 External Ear, Right **1** External Ear, Left **2** External Ear, Bilateral **K** Nose	**0** Open **4** Percutaneous Endoscopic **X** External	**Z** No Device	**Z** No Qualifier
7 Tympanic Membrane, Right **8** Tympanic Membrane, Left **F** Eustachian Tube, Right **G** Eustachian Tube, Left **L** Nasal Turbinate	**0** Open **4** Percutaneous Endoscopic **7** Via Natural or Artificial Opening **8** Via Natural or Artificial Opening Endoscopic	**Z** No Device	**Z** No Qualifier
9 Auditory Ossicle, Right **A** Auditory Ossicle, Left **M** Nasal Septum	**0** Open **4** Percutaneous Endoscopic	**Z** No Device	**Z** No Qualifier

Section 0 **Medical and Surgical**
Body System 9 **Ear, Nose, Sinus**
Operation T **Resection:** Cutting out or off, without replacement, all of a body part

Body Part (4th)	Approach (5th)	Device (6th)	Qualifier (7th)
0 External Ear, Right **1** External Ear, Left **K** Nose	**0** Open **4** Percutaneous Endoscopic **X** External	**Z** No Device	**Z** No Qualifier
5 Middle Ear, Right **6** Middle Ear, Left **9** Auditory Ossicle, Right **A** Auditory Ossicle, Left **D** Inner Ear, Right **E** Inner Ear, Left	**0** Open	**Z** No Device	**Z** No Qualifier
7 Tympanic Membrane, Right **8** Tympanic Membrane, Left **F** Eustachian Tube, Right **G** Eustachian Tube, Left **L** Nasal Turbinate **N** Nasopharynx	**0** Open **4** Percutaneous Endoscopic **7** Via Natural or Artificial Opening **8** Via Natural or Artificial Opening Endoscopic	**Z** No Device	**Z** No Qualifier

Continued →

09T Continued

ction **0** **Medical and Surgical**
dy System **9** **Ear, Nose, Sinus**
eration **T** **Resection:** Cutting out or off, without replacement, all of a body part

Body Part (4th)	Approach (5th)	Device (6th)	Qualifier (7th)
B Mastoid Sinus, Right **C** Mastoid Sinus, Left **M** Nasal Septum **P** Accessory Sinus **Q** Maxillary Sinus, Right **R** Maxillary Sinus, Left **S** Frontal Sinus, Right **T** Frontal Sinus, Left **U** Ethmoid Sinus, Right **V** Ethmoid Sinus, Left **W** Sphenoid Sinus, Right **X** Sphenoid Sinus, Left	**0** Open **4** Percutaneous Endoscopic	**Z** No Device	**Z** No Qualifier

ction **0** **Medical and Surgical**
dy System **9** **Ear, Nose, Sinus**
peration **U** **Supplement:** Putting in or on biological or synthetic material that physically reinforces and/or augments the function of a portion of a body part

Body Part (4th)	Approach (5th)	Device (6th)	Qualifier (7th)
0 External Ear, Right **1** External Ear, Left **2** External Ear, Bilateral **K** Nose	**0** Open **X** External	**7** Autologous Tissue Substitute **J** Synthetic Substitute **K** Nonautologous Tissue Substitute	**Z** No Qualifier
5 Middle Ear, Right **6** Middle Ear, Left **9** Auditory Ossicle, Right **A** Auditory Ossicle, Left **D** Inner Ear, Right **E** Inner Ear, Left	**0** Open	**7** Autologous Tissue Substitute **J** Synthetic Substitute **K** Nonautologous Tissue Substitute	**Z** No Qualifier
7 Tympanic Membrane, Right **8** Tympanic Membrane, Left **N** Nasopharynx	**0** Open **7** Via Natural or Artificial Opening **8** Via Natural or Artificial Opening Endoscopic	**7** Autologous Tissue Substitute **J** Synthetic Substitute **K** Nonautologous Tissue Substitute	**Z** No Qualifier
L Nasal Turbinate	**0** Open **3** Percutaneous **4** Percutaneous Endoscopic **7** Via Natural or Artificial Opening **8** Via Natural or Artificial Opening Endoscopic	**7** Autologous Tissue Substitute **J** Synthetic Substitute **K** Nonautologous Tissue Substitute	**Z** No Qualifier
M Nasal Septum	**0** Open **3** Percutaneous **4** Percutaneous Endoscopic	**7** Autologous Tissue Substitute **J** Synthetic Substitute **K** Nonautologous Tissue Substitute	**Z** No Qualifier

ection **0** **Medical and Surgical**
ody System **9** **Ear, Nose, Sinus**
peration **W** **Revision:** Correcting, to the extent possible, a portion of a malfunctioning device or the position of a displaced device

Body Part (4th)	Approach (5th)	Device (6th)	Qualifier (7th)
7 Tympanic Membrane, Right **8** Tympanic Membrane, Left **9** Auditory Ossicle, Right **A** Auditory Ossicle, Left	**0** Open **7** Via Natural or Artificial Opening **8** Via Natural or Artificial Opening Endoscopic	**7** Autologous Tissue Substitute **J** Synthetic Substitute **K** Nonautologous Tissue Substitute	**Z** No Qualifier
D Inner Ear, Right **E** Inner Ear, Left	**0** Open **7** Via Natural or Artificial Opening **8** Via Natural or Artificial Opening Endoscopic	**S** Hearing Device	**Z** No Qualifier

Continued →

Section	**0**	**Medical and Surgical**	***09W Continu***
Body System	**9**	**Ear, Nose, Sinus**	
Operation	**W**	**Revision:** Correcting, to the extent possible, a portion of a malfunctioning device or the position of a displaced device	

Body Part (4th)	Approach (5th)	Device (6th)	Qualifier (7th)
H Ear, Right **J** Ear, Left **K** Nose	**0** Open **3** Percutaneous **4** Percutaneous Endoscopic **7** Via Natural or Artificial Opening **8** Via Natural or Artificial Opening Endoscopic **X** External	**0** Drainage Device **7** Autologous Tissue Substitute **D** Intraluminal Device **J** Synthetic Substitute **K** Nonautologous Tissue Substitute	**Z** No Qualifier
Y Sinus	**0** Open **3** Percutaneous **4** Percutaneous Endoscopic **X** External	**0** Drainage Device	**Z** No Qualifier

Ear, Nose, Sinus Coding Listing 090–09W

090 – Ear, Nose, Sinus, Alteration

090007Z Alteration of Right External Ear with Autologous Tissue Substitute, Open Approach
09000JZ Alteration of Right External Ear with Synthetic Substitute, Open Approach
09000KZ Alteration of Right External Ear with Nonautologous Tissue Substitute, Open Approach
09000ZZ Alteration of Right External Ear, Open Approach
090037Z Alteration of Right External Ear with Autologous Tissue Substitute, Percutaneous Approach
09003JZ Alteration of Right External Ear with Synthetic Substitute, Percutaneous Approach
09003KZ Alteration of Right External Ear with Nonautologous Tissue Substitute, Percutaneous Approach
09003ZZ Alteration of Right External Ear, Percutaneous Approach
090047Z Alteration of Right External Ear with Autologous Tissue Substitute, Percutaneous Endoscopic Approach
09004JZ Alteration of Right External Ear with Synthetic Substitute, Percutaneous Endoscopic Approach
09004KZ Alteration of Right External Ear with Nonautologous Tissue Substitute, Percutaneous Endoscopic Approach
09004ZZ Alteration of Right External Ear, Percutaneous Endoscopic Approach
0900X7Z Alteration of Right External Ear with Autologous Tissue Substitute, External Approach
0900XJZ Alteration of Right External Ear with Synthetic Substitute, External Approach
0900XKZ Alteration of Right External Ear with Nonautologous Tissue Substitute, External Approach
0900XZZ Alteration of Right External Ear, External Approach
090107Z Alteration of Left External Ear with Autologous Tissue Substitute, Open Approach
09010JZ Alteration of Left External Ear with Synthetic Substitute, Open Approach
09010KZ Alteration of Left External Ear with Nonautologous Tissue Substitute, Open Approach
09010ZZ Alteration of Left External Ear, Open Approach
090137Z Alteration of Left External Ear with Autologous Tissue Substitute, Percutaneous Approach
09013JZ Alteration of Left External Ear with Synthetic Substitute, Percutaneous Approach
09013KZ Alteration of Left External Ear with Nonautologous Tissue Substitute, Percutaneous Approach
09013ZZ Alteration of Left External Ear, Percutaneous Approach
090147Z Alteration of Left External Ear with Autologous Tissue Substitute, Percutaneous Endoscopic Approach
09014JZ Alteration of Left External Ear with Synthetic Substitute, Percutaneous Endoscopic Approach
09014KZ Alteration of Left External Ear with Nonautologous Tissue Substitute, Percutaneous Endoscopic Approach
09014ZZ Alteration of Left External Ear, Percutaneous Endoscopic Approach
0901X7Z Alteration of Left External Ear with Autologous Tissue Substitute, External Approach
0901XJZ Alteration of Left External Ear with Synthetic Substitute, External Approach
0901XKZ Alteration of Left External Ear with Nonautologous Tissue Substitute, External Approach
0901XZZ Alteration of Left External Ear, External Approach
090207Z Alteration of Bilateral External Ear with Autologous Tissue Substitute, Open Approach
09020JZ Alteration of Bilateral External Ear with Synthetic Substitute, Open Approach
09020KZ Alteration of Bilateral External Ear with Nonautologous Tissue Substitute, Open Approach
09020ZZ Alteration of Bilateral External Ear, Open Approach
090237Z Alteration of Bilateral External Ear with Autologous Tissue Substitute, Percutaneous Approach
09023JZ Alteration of Bilateral External Ear with Synthetic Substitute, Percutaneous Approach
09023KZ Alteration of Bilateral External Ear with Nonautologous Tissue Substitute, Percutaneous Approach
09023ZZ Alteration of Bilateral External Ear, Percutaneous Approach
090247Z Alteration of Bilateral External Ear with Autologous Tissue Substitute, Percutaneous Endoscopic Approach
09024JZ Alteration of Bilateral External Ear with Synthetic Substitute, Percutaneous Endoscopic Approach
09024KZ Alteration of Bilateral External Ear with Nonautologous Tissue Substitute, Percutaneous Endoscopic Approach
09024ZZ Alteration of Bilateral External Ear, Percutaneous Endoscopic Approach
0902X7Z Alteration of Bilateral External Ear with Autologous Tissue Substitute, External Approach
0902XJZ Alteration of Bilateral External Ear with Synthetic Substitute, External Approach
0902XKZ Alteration of Bilateral External Ear with Nonautologous Tissue Substitute, Extern Approach
0902XZZ Alteration of Bilateral External Ear, External Approach
090K07Z Alteration of Nose with Autologous Tissu Substitute, Open Approach
090K0JZ Alteration of Nose with Synthetic Substitute, Open Approach
090K0KZ Alteration of Nose with Nonautologous Tissue Substitute, Open Approach
090K0ZZ Alteration of Nose, Open Approach
090K37Z Alteration of Nose with Autologous Tissu Substitute, Percutaneous Approach
090K3JZ Alteration of Nose with Synthetic Substitute, Percutaneous Approach
090K3KZ Alteration of Nose with Nonautologous Tissue Substitute, Percutaneous Approach
090K3ZZ Alteration of Nose, Percutaneous Approach
090K47Z Alteration of Nose with Autologous Tissu Substitute, Percutaneous Endoscopic Approach
090K4JZ Alteration of Nose with Synthetic Substitute Percutaneous Endoscopic Approach
090K4KZ Alteration of Nose with Nonautologous Tissue Substitute, Percutaneous Endoscopic Approach
090K4ZZ Alteration of Nose, Percutaneous Endoscopic Approach
090KX7Z Alteration of Nose with Autologous Tissu Substitute, External Approach
090KXJZ Alteration of Nose with Synthetic Substitute, External Approach
090KXKZ Alteration of Nose with Nonautologous Tissue Substitute, External Approach
090KXZZ Alteration of Nose, External Approach

1 – Ear, Nose, Sinus, Bypass

view Coding Guideline B3.6a

D070 Bypass Right Inner Ear to Endolymphatic with Autologous Tissue Substitute, Open Approach
D0J0 Bypass Right Inner Ear to Endolymphatic with Synthetic Substitute, Open Approach
D0K0 Bypass Right Inner Ear to Endolymphatic with Nonautologous Tissue Substitute, Open Approach
091D0Z0 Bypass Right Inner Ear to Endolymphatic, Open Approach
091E070 Bypass Left Inner Ear to Endolymphatic with Autologous Tissue Substitute, Open Approach
091E0J0 Bypass Left Inner Ear to Endolymphatic with Synthetic Substitute, Open Approach
091E0K0 Bypass Left Inner Ear to Endolymphatic with Nonautologous Tissue Substitute, Open Approach
091E0Z0 Bypass Left Inner Ear to Endolymphatic, Open Approach

2 – Ear, Nose, Sinus, Change

view Coding Guideline B6.1c

2HX0Z Change Drainage Device in Right Ear, External Approach
2HXYZ Change Other Device in Right Ear, External Approach
2JX0Z Change Drainage Device in Left Ear, External Approach
092JXYZ Change Other Device in Left Ear, External Approach
092KX0Z Change Drainage Device in Nose, External Approach
092KXYZ Change Other Device in Nose, External Approach
092YX0Z Change Drainage Device in Sinus, External Approach
092YXYZ Change Other Device in Sinus, External Approach

5 – Ear, Nose, Sinus, Destruction

500ZZ Destruction of Right External Ear, Open Approach
503ZZ Destruction of Right External Ear, Percutaneous Approach
504ZZ Destruction of Right External Ear, Percutaneous Endoscopic Approach
50XZZ Destruction of Right External Ear, External Approach
510ZZ Destruction of Left External Ear, Open Approach
513ZZ Destruction of Left External Ear, Percutaneous Approach
514ZZ Destruction of Left External Ear, Percutaneous Endoscopic Approach
51XZZ Destruction of Left External Ear, External Approach
530ZZ Destruction of Right External Auditory Canal, Open Approach
533ZZ Destruction of Right External Auditory Canal, Percutaneous Approach
534ZZ Destruction of Right External Auditory Canal, Percutaneous Endoscopic Approach
537ZZ Destruction of Right External Auditory Canal, Via Natural or Artificial Opening
)538ZZ Destruction of Right External Auditory Canal, Via Natural or Artificial Opening Endoscopic
)53XZZ Destruction of Right External Auditory Canal, External Approach
9540ZZ Destruction of Left External Auditory Canal, Open Approach
9543ZZ Destruction of Left External Auditory Canal, Percutaneous Approach
9544ZZ Destruction of Left External Auditory Canal, Percutaneous Endoscopic Approach
9547ZZ Destruction of Left External Auditory Canal, Via Natural or Artificial Opening
9548ZZ Destruction of Left External Auditory Canal, Via Natural or Artificial Opening Endoscopic
954XZZ Destruction of Left External Auditory Canal, External Approach
9550ZZ Destruction of Right Middle Ear, Open Approach
9560ZZ Destruction of Left Middle Ear, Open Approach
9570ZZ Destruction of Right Tympanic Membrane, Open Approach
9573ZZ Destruction of Right Tympanic Membrane, Percutaneous Approach
09574ZZ Destruction of Right Tympanic Membrane, Percutaneous Endoscopic Approach
09577ZZ Destruction of Right Tympanic Membrane, Via Natural or Artificial Opening
09578ZZ Destruction of Right Tympanic Membrane, Via Natural or Artificial Opening Endoscopic
09580ZZ Destruction of Left Tympanic Membrane, Open Approach
09583ZZ Destruction of Left Tympanic Membrane, Percutaneous Approach
09584ZZ Destruction of Left Tympanic Membrane, Percutaneous Endoscopic Approach
09587ZZ Destruction of Left Tympanic Membrane, Via Natural or Artificial Opening
09588ZZ Destruction of Left Tympanic Membrane, Via Natural or Artificial Opening Endoscopic
09590ZZ Destruction of Right Auditory Ossicle, Open Approach
095A0ZZ Destruction of Left Auditory Ossicle, Open Approach
095B0ZZ Destruction of Right Mastoid Sinus, Open Approach
095B3ZZ Destruction of Right Mastoid Sinus, Percutaneous Approach
095B4ZZ Destruction of Right Mastoid Sinus, Percutaneous Endoscopic Approach
095C0ZZ Destruction of Left Mastoid Sinus, Open Approach
095C3ZZ Destruction of Left Mastoid Sinus, Percutaneous Approach
095C4ZZ Destruction of Left Mastoid Sinus, Percutaneous Endoscopic Approach
095D0ZZ Destruction of Right Inner Ear, Open Approach
095E0ZZ Destruction of Left Inner Ear, Open Approach
095F0ZZ Destruction of Right Eustachian Tube, Open Approach
095F3ZZ Destruction of Right Eustachian Tube, Percutaneous Approach
095F4ZZ Destruction of Right Eustachian Tube, Percutaneous Endoscopic Approach
095F7ZZ Destruction of Right Eustachian Tube, Via Natural or Artificial Opening
095F8ZZ Destruction of Right Eustachian Tube, Via Natural or Artificial Opening Endoscopic
095G0ZZ Destruction of Left Eustachian Tube, Open Approach
095G3ZZ Destruction of Left Eustachian Tube, Percutaneous Approach
095G4ZZ Destruction of Left Eustachian Tube, Percutaneous Endoscopic Approach
095G7ZZ Destruction of Left Eustachian Tube, Via Natural or Artificial Opening
095G8ZZ Destruction of Left Eustachian Tube, Via Natural or Artificial Opening Endoscopic
095K0ZZ Destruction of Nose, Open Approach
095K3ZZ Destruction of Nose, Percutaneous Approach
095K4ZZ Destruction of Nose, Percutaneous Endoscopic Approach
095KXZZ Destruction of Nose, External Approach
095L0ZZ Destruction of Nasal Turbinate, Open Approach
095L3ZZ Destruction of Nasal Turbinate, Percutaneous Approach
095L4ZZ Destruction of Nasal Turbinate, Percutaneous Endoscopic Approach
095L7ZZ Destruction of Nasal Turbinate, Via Natural or Artificial Opening
095L8ZZ Destruction of Nasal Turbinate, Via Natural or Artificial Opening Endoscopic
095M0ZZ Destruction of Nasal Septum, Open Approach
095M3ZZ Destruction of Nasal Septum, Percutaneous Approach
095M4ZZ Destruction of Nasal Septum, Percutaneous Endoscopic Approach
095N0ZZ Destruction of Nasopharynx, Open Approach
095N3ZZ Destruction of Nasopharynx, Percutaneous Approach
095N4ZZ Destruction of Nasopharynx, Percutaneous Endoscopic Approach
095N7ZZ Destruction of Nasopharynx, Via Natural or Artificial Opening
095N8ZZ Destruction of Nasopharynx, Via Natural or Artificial Opening Endoscopic
095P0ZZ Destruction of Accessory Sinus, Open Approach
095P3ZZ Destruction of Accessory Sinus, Percutaneous Approach
095P4ZZ Destruction of Accessory Sinus, Percutaneous Endoscopic Approach
095Q0ZZ Destruction of Right Maxillary Sinus, Open Approach
095Q3ZZ Destruction of Right Maxillary Sinus, Percutaneous Approach

095Q4ZZ Destruction of Right Maxillary Sinus, Percutaneous Endoscopic Approach
095R0ZZ Destruction of Left Maxillary Sinus, Open Approach
095R3ZZ Destruction of Left Maxillary Sinus, Percutaneous Approach
095R4ZZ Destruction of Left Maxillary Sinus, Percutaneous Endoscopic Approach
095S0ZZ Destruction of Right Frontal Sinus, Open Approach
095S3ZZ Destruction of Right Frontal Sinus, Percutaneous Approach
095S4ZZ Destruction of Right Frontal Sinus, Percutaneous Endoscopic Approach
095T0ZZ Destruction of Left Frontal Sinus, Open Approach
095T3ZZ Destruction of Left Frontal Sinus, Percutaneous Approach
095T4ZZ Destruction of Left Frontal Sinus, Percutaneous Endoscopic Approach
095U0ZZ Destruction of Right Ethmoid Sinus, Open Approach
095U3ZZ Destruction of Right Ethmoid Sinus, Percutaneous Approach
095U4ZZ Destruction of Right Ethmoid Sinus, Percutaneous Endoscopic Approach
095V0ZZ Destruction of Left Ethmoid Sinus, Open Approach
095V3ZZ Destruction of Left Ethmoid Sinus, Percutaneous Approach
095V4ZZ Destruction of Left Ethmoid Sinus, Percutaneous Endoscopic Approach
095W0ZZ Destruction of Right Sphenoid Sinus, Open Approach
095W3ZZ Destruction of Right Sphenoid Sinus, Percutaneous Approach
095W4ZZ Destruction of Right Sphenoid Sinus, Percutaneous Endoscopic Approach
095X0ZZ Destruction of Left Sphenoid Sinus, Open Approach
095X3ZZ Destruction of Left Sphenoid Sinus, Percutaneous Approach
095X4ZZ Destruction of Left Sphenoid Sinus, Percutaneous Endoscopic Approach

097 – Ear, Nose, Sinus, Dilation

097F0DZ Dilation of Right Eustachian Tube with Intraluminal Device, Open Approach
097F0ZZ Dilation of Right Eustachian Tube, Open Approach
097F3ZZ Dilation of Right Eustachian Tube, Percutaneous Approach
097F4ZZ Dilation of Right Eustachian Tube, Percutaneous Endoscopic Approach
097F7DZ Dilation of Right Eustachian Tube with Intraluminal Device, Via Natural or Artificial Opening
097F7ZZ Dilation of Right Eustachian Tube, Via Natural or Artificial Opening
097F8DZ Dilation of Right Eustachian Tube with Intraluminal Device, Via Natural or Artificial Opening Endoscopic
097F8ZZ Dilation of Right Eustachian Tube, Via Natural or Artificial Opening Endoscopic
097G0DZ Dilation of Left Eustachian Tube with Intraluminal Device, Open Approach
097G0ZZ Dilation of Left Eustachian Tube, Open Approach
097G3ZZ Dilation of Left Eustachian Tube, Percutaneous Approach
097G4ZZ Dilation of Left Eustachian Tube, Percutaneous Endoscopic Approach
097G7DZ Dilation of Left Eustachian Tube with Intraluminal Device, Via Natural or Artificial Opening
097G7ZZ Dilation of Left Eustachian Tube, Via Natural or Artificial Opening
097G8DZ Dilation of Left Eustachian Tube with Intraluminal Device, Via Natural or Artificial Opening Endoscopic
097G8ZZ Dilation of Left Eustachian Tube, Via Natural or Artificial Opening Endoscopic

098 – Ear, Nose, Sinus, Division

098L0ZZ Division of Nasal Turbinate, Open Approach
098L3ZZ Division of Nasal Turbinate, Percutaneous Approach
098L4ZZ Division of Nasal Turbinate, Percutaneous Endoscopic Approach
098L7ZZ Division of Nasal Turbinate, Via Natural or Artificial Opening
098L8ZZ Division of Nasal Turbinate, Via Natural or Artificial Opening Endoscopic

099 – Ear, Nose, Sinus, Drainage

Review Coding Guidelines B3.4a and B3.4b

Review Coding Guideline B6.2

099000Z Drainage of Right External Ear with Drainage Device, Open Approach
09900ZX Drainage of Right External Ear, Open Approach, Diagnostic
09900ZZ Drainage of Right External Ear, Open Approach
099030Z Drainage of Right External Ear with Drainage Device, Percutaneous Approach
09903ZX Drainage of Right External Ear, Percutaneous Approach, Diagnostic
09903ZZ Drainage of Right External Ear, Percutaneous Approach
099040Z Drainage of Right External Ear with Drainage Device, Percutaneous Endoscopic Approach
09904ZX Drainage of Right External Ear, Percutaneous Endoscopic Approach, Diagnostic
09904ZZ Drainage of Right External Ear, Percutaneous Endoscopic Approach
0990X0Z Drainage of Right External Ear with Drainage Device, External Approach
0990XZX Drainage of Right External Ear, External Approach, Diagnostic
0990XZZ Drainage of Right External Ear, External Approach
099100Z Drainage of Left External Ear with Drainage Device, Open Approach
09910ZX Drainage of Left External Ear, Open Approach, Diagnostic
09910ZZ Drainage of Left External Ear, Open Approach
099130Z Drainage of Left External Ear with Drainage Device, Percutaneous Approach
09913ZX Drainage of Left External Ear, Percutaneous Approach, Diagnostic
09913ZZ Drainage of Left External Ear, Percutaneous Approach
099140Z Drainage of Left External Ear with Drainage Device, Percutaneous Endoscopic Approach
09914ZX Drainage of Left External Ear, Percutaneous Endoscopic Approach, Diagnostic
09914ZZ Drainage of Left External Ear, Percutaneous Endoscopic Approach
0991X0Z Drainage of Left External Ear with Drainage Device, External Approach
0991XZX Drainage of Left External Ear, External Approach, Diagnostic
0991XZZ Drainage of Left External Ear, External Approach
099300Z Drainage of Right External Auditory Canal with Drainage Device, Open Approach
09930ZX Drainage of Right External Auditory Canal, Open Approach, Diagnostic
09930ZZ Drainage of Right External Auditory Canal, Open Approach
099330Z Drainage of Right External Auditory Canal with Drainage Device, Percutaneous Approach
09933ZX Drainage of Right External Auditory Canal, Percutaneous Approach, Diagnostic
09933ZZ Drainage of Right External Auditory Canal, Percutaneous Approach
099340Z Drainage of Right External Auditory Canal with Drainage Device, Percutaneous Endoscopic Approach
09934ZX Drainage of Right External Auditory Canal, Percutaneous Endoscopic Approach, Diagnostic
09934ZZ Drainage of Right External Auditory Canal, Percutaneous Endoscopic Approach
099370Z Drainage of Right External Auditory Canal with Drainage Device, Via Natural or Artificial Opening
09937ZX Drainage of Right External Auditory Canal, Via Natural or Artificial Opening, Diagnostic
09937ZZ Drainage of Right External Auditory Canal, Via Natural or Artificial Opening
099380Z Drainage of Right External Auditory Canal with Drainage Device, Via Natural or Artificial Opening Endoscopic
09938ZX Drainage of Right External Auditory Canal, Via Natural or Artificial Opening Endoscopic, Diagnostic
09938ZZ Drainage of Right External Auditory Canal, Via Natural or Artificial Opening Endoscopic

93X0Z Drainage of Right External Auditory Canal with Drainage Device, External Approach

93XZX Drainage of Right External Auditory Canal, External Approach, Diagnostic

93XZZ Drainage of Right External Auditory Canal, External Approach

9400Z Drainage of Left External Auditory Canal with Drainage Device, Open Approach

940ZX Drainage of Left External Auditory Canal, Open Approach, Diagnostic

940ZZ Drainage of Left External Auditory Canal, Open Approach

9430Z Drainage of Left External Auditory Canal with Drainage Device, Percutaneous Approach

943ZX Drainage of Left External Auditory Canal, Percutaneous Approach, Diagnostic

943ZZ Drainage of Left External Auditory Canal, Percutaneous Approach

9440Z Drainage of Left External Auditory Canal with Drainage Device, Percutaneous Endoscopic Approach

944ZX Drainage of Left External Auditory Canal, Percutaneous Endoscopic Approach, Diagnostic

944ZZ Drainage of Left External Auditory Canal, Percutaneous Endoscopic Approach

9470Z Drainage of Left External Auditory Canal with Drainage Device, Via Natural or Artificial Opening

947ZX Drainage of Left External Auditory Canal, Via Natural or Artificial Opening, Diagnostic

947ZZ Drainage of Left External Auditory Canal, Via Natural or Artificial Opening

99480Z Drainage of Left External Auditory Canal with Drainage Device, Via Natural or Artificial Opening Endoscopic

9948ZX Drainage of Left External Auditory Canal, Via Natural or Artificial Opening Endoscopic, Diagnostic

9948ZZ Drainage of Left External Auditory Canal, Via Natural or Artificial Opening Endoscopic

994X0Z Drainage of Left External Auditory Canal with Drainage Device, External Approach

994XZX Drainage of Left External Auditory Canal, External Approach, Diagnostic

994XZZ Drainage of Left External Auditory Canal, External Approach

99500Z Drainage of Right Middle Ear with Drainage Device, Open Approach

9950ZX Drainage of Right Middle Ear, Open Approach, Diagnostic

9950ZZ Drainage of Right Middle Ear, Open Approach

99600Z Drainage of Left Middle Ear with Drainage Device, Open Approach

9960ZX Drainage of Left Middle Ear, Open Approach, Diagnostic

9960ZZ Drainage of Left Middle Ear, Open Approach

99700Z Drainage of Right Tympanic Membrane with Drainage Device, Open Approach

9970ZX Drainage of Right Tympanic Membrane, Open Approach, Diagnostic

9970ZZ Drainage of Right Tympanic Membrane, Open Approach

99730Z Drainage of Right Tympanic Membrane with Drainage Device, Percutaneous Approach

9973ZX Drainage of Right Tympanic Membrane, Percutaneous Approach, Diagnostic

9973ZZ Drainage of Right Tympanic Membrane, Percutaneous Approach

099740Z Drainage of Right Tympanic Membrane with Drainage Device, Percutaneous Endoscopic Approach

09974ZX Drainage of Right Tympanic Membrane, Percutaneous Endoscopic Approach, Diagnostic

09974ZZ Drainage of Right Tympanic Membrane, Percutaneous Endoscopic Approach

099770Z Drainage of Right Tympanic Membrane with Drainage Device, Via Natural or Artificial Opening

09977ZX Drainage of Right Tympanic Membrane, Via Natural or Artificial Opening, Diagnostic

09977ZZ Drainage of Right Tympanic Membrane, Via Natural or Artificial Opening

099780Z Drainage of Right Tympanic Membrane with Drainage Device, Via Natural or Artificial Opening Endoscopic

09978ZX Drainage of Right Tympanic Membrane, Via Natural or Artificial Opening Endoscopic, Diagnostic

09978ZZ Drainage of Right Tympanic Membrane, Via Natural or Artificial Opening Endoscopic

099800Z Drainage of Left Tympanic Membrane with Drainage Device, Open Approach

09980ZX Drainage of Left Tympanic Membrane, Open Approach, Diagnostic

09980ZZ Drainage of Left Tympanic Membrane, Open Approach

099830Z Drainage of Left Tympanic Membrane with Drainage Device, Percutaneous Approach

09983ZX Drainage of Left Tympanic Membrane, Percutaneous Approach, Diagnostic

09983ZZ Drainage of Left Tympanic Membrane, Percutaneous Approach

099840Z Drainage of Left Tympanic Membrane with Drainage Device, Percutaneous Endoscopic Approach

09984ZX Drainage of Left Tympanic Membrane, Percutaneous Endoscopic Approach, Diagnostic

09984ZZ Drainage of Left Tympanic Membrane, Percutaneous Endoscopic Approach

099870Z Drainage of Left Tympanic Membrane with Drainage Device, Via Natural or Artificial Opening

09987ZX Drainage of Left Tympanic Membrane, Via Natural or Artificial Opening, Diagnostic

09987ZZ Drainage of Left Tympanic Membrane, Via Natural or Artificial Opening

099880Z Drainage of Left Tympanic Membrane with Drainage Device, Via Natural or Artificial Opening Endoscopic

09988ZX Drainage of Left Tympanic Membrane, Via Natural or Artificial Opening Endoscopic, Diagnostic

09988ZZ Drainage of Left Tympanic Membrane, Via Natural or Artificial Opening Endoscopic

099900Z Drainage of Right Auditory Ossicle with Drainage Device, Open Approach

09990ZX Drainage of Right Auditory Ossicle, Open Approach, Diagnostic

09990ZZ Drainage of Right Auditory Ossicle, Open Approach

099A00Z Drainage of Left Auditory Ossicle with Drainage Device, Open Approach

099A0ZX Drainage of Left Auditory Ossicle, Open Approach, Diagnostic

099A0ZZ Drainage of Left Auditory Ossicle, Open Approach

099B00Z Drainage of Right Mastoid Sinus with Drainage Device, Open Approach

099B0ZX Drainage of Right Mastoid Sinus, Open Approach, Diagnostic

099B0ZZ Drainage of Right Mastoid Sinus, Open Approach

099B30Z Drainage of Right Mastoid Sinus with Drainage Device, Percutaneous Approach

099B3ZX Drainage of Right Mastoid Sinus, Percutaneous Approach, Diagnostic

099B3ZZ Drainage of Right Mastoid Sinus, Percutaneous Approach

099B40Z Drainage of Right Mastoid Sinus with Drainage Device, Percutaneous Endoscopic Approach

099B4ZX Drainage of Right Mastoid Sinus, Percutaneous Endoscopic Approach, Diagnostic

099B4ZZ Drainage of Right Mastoid Sinus, Percutaneous Endoscopic Approach

099C00Z Drainage of Left Mastoid Sinus with Drainage Device, Open Approach

099C0ZX Drainage of Left Mastoid Sinus, Open Approach, Diagnostic

099C0ZZ Drainage of Left Mastoid Sinus, Open Approach

099C30Z Drainage of Left Mastoid Sinus with Drainage Device, Percutaneous Approach

099C3ZX Drainage of Left Mastoid Sinus, Percutaneous Approach, Diagnostic

099C3ZZ Drainage of Left Mastoid Sinus, Percutaneous Approach

099C40Z Drainage of Left Mastoid Sinus with Drainage Device, Percutaneous Endoscopic Approach

099C4ZX Drainage of Left Mastoid Sinus, Percutaneous Endoscopic Approach, Diagnostic

099C4ZZ Drainage of Left Mastoid Sinus, Percutaneous Endoscopic Approach

099D00Z Drainage of Right Inner Ear with Drainage Device, Open Approach

099D0ZX Drainage of Right Inner Ear, Open Approach, Diagnostic

099D0ZZ Drainage of Right Inner Ear, Open Approach

099E00Z Drainage of Left Inner Ear with Drainage Device, Open Approach

099E0ZX Drainage of Left Inner Ear, Open Approach, Diagnostic

099E0ZZ Drainage of Left Inner Ear, Open Approach

099F00Z Drainage of Right Eustachian Tube with Drainage Device, Open Approach

099F0ZX Drainage of Right Eustachian Tube, Open Approach, Diagnostic

099F0ZZ Drainage of Right Eustachian Tube, Open Approach

099F30Z Drainage of Right Eustachian Tube with Drainage Device, Percutaneous Approach

099F3ZX Drainage of Right Eustachian Tube, Percutaneous Approach, Diagnostic

099F3ZZ Drainage of Right Eustachian Tube, Percutaneous Approach

099F40Z Drainage of Right Eustachian Tube with Drainage Device, Percutaneous Endoscopic Approach

099F4ZX Drainage of Right Eustachian Tube, Percutaneous Endoscopic Approach, Diagnostic

099F4ZZ Drainage of Right Eustachian Tube, Percutaneous Endoscopic Approach

099F70Z Drainage of Right Eustachian Tube with Drainage Device, Via Natural or Artificial Opening

099F7ZX Drainage of Right Eustachian Tube, Via Natural or Artificial Opening, Diagnostic

099F7ZZ Drainage of Right Eustachian Tube, Via Natural or Artificial Opening

099F80Z Drainage of Right Eustachian Tube with Drainage Device, Via Natural or Artificial Opening Endoscopic

099F8ZX Drainage of Right Eustachian Tube, Via Natural or Artificial Opening Endoscopic, Diagnostic

099F8ZZ Drainage of Right Eustachian Tube, Via Natural or Artificial Opening Endoscopic

099G00Z Drainage of Left Eustachian Tube with Drainage Device, Open Approach

099G0ZX Drainage of Left Eustachian Tube, Open Approach, Diagnostic

099G0ZZ Drainage of Left Eustachian Tube, Open Approach

099G30Z Drainage of Left Eustachian Tube with Drainage Device, Percutaneous Approach

099G3ZX Drainage of Left Eustachian Tube, Percutaneous Approach, Diagnostic

099G3ZZ Drainage of Left Eustachian Tube, Percutaneous Approach

099G40Z Drainage of Left Eustachian Tube with Drainage Device, Percutaneous Endoscopic Approach

099G4ZX Drainage of Left Eustachian Tube, Percutaneous Endoscopic Approach, Diagnostic

099G4ZZ Drainage of Left Eustachian Tube, Percutaneous Endoscopic Approach

099G70Z Drainage of Left Eustachian Tube with Drainage Device, Via Natural or Artificial Opening

099G7ZX Drainage of Left Eustachian Tube, Via Natural or Artificial Opening, Diagnostic

099G7ZZ Drainage of Left Eustachian Tube, Via Natural or Artificial Opening

099G80Z Drainage of Left Eustachian Tube with Drainage Device, Via Natural or Artificial Opening Endoscopic

099G8ZX Drainage of Left Eustachian Tube, Via Natural or Artificial Opening Endoscopic, Diagnostic

099G8ZZ Drainage of Left Eustachian Tube, Via Natural or Artificial Opening Endoscopic

099K00Z Drainage of Nose with Drainage Device, Open Approach

099K0ZX Drainage of Nose, Open Approach, Diagnostic

099K0ZZ Drainage of Nose, Open Approach

099K30Z Drainage of Nose with Drainage Device, Percutaneous Approach

099K3ZX Drainage of Nose, Percutaneous Approach, Diagnostic

099K3ZZ Drainage of Nose, Percutaneous Approach

099K40Z Drainage of Nose with Drainage Device, Percutaneous Endoscopic Approach

099K4ZX Drainage of Nose, Percutaneous Endoscopic Approach, Diagnostic

099K4ZZ Drainage of Nose, Percutaneous Endoscopic Approach

099KX0Z Drainage of Nose with Drainage Device, External Approach

099KXZX Drainage of Nose, External Approach, Diagnostic

099KXZZ Drainage of Nose, External Approach

099L00Z Drainage of Nasal Turbinate with Drainage Device, Open Approach

099L0ZX Drainage of Nasal Turbinate, Open Approach, Diagnostic

099L0ZZ Drainage of Nasal Turbinate, Open Approach

099L30Z Drainage of Nasal Turbinate with Drainage Device, Percutaneous Approach

099L3ZX Drainage of Nasal Turbinate, Percutaneous Approach, Diagnostic

099L3ZZ Drainage of Nasal Turbinate, Percutaneous Approach

099L40Z Drainage of Nasal Turbinate with Drainage Device, Percutaneous Endoscopic Approach

099L4ZX Drainage of Nasal Turbinate, Percutaneous Endoscopic Approach, Diagnostic

099L4ZZ Drainage of Nasal Turbinate, Percutaneous Endoscopic Approach

099L70Z Drainage of Nasal Turbinate with Drainage Device, Via Natural or Artificial Opening

099L7ZX Drainage of Nasal Turbinate, Via Natural or Artificial Opening, Diagnostic

099L7ZZ Drainage of Nasal Turbinate, Via Natural or Artificial Opening

099L80Z Drainage of Nasal Turbinate with Drainage Device, Via Natural or Artificial Opening Endoscopic

099L8ZX Drainage of Nasal Turbinate, Via Natural or Artificial Opening Endoscopic, Diagnostic

099L8ZZ Drainage of Nasal Turbinate, Via Natural or Artificial Opening Endoscopic

099M00Z Drainage of Nasal Septum with Drainage Device, Open Approach

099M0ZX Drainage of Nasal Septum, Open Approach, Diagnostic

099M0ZZ Drainage of Nasal Septum, Open Approach

099M30Z Drainage of Nasal Septum with Drainage Device, Percutaneous Approach

099M3ZX Drainage of Nasal Septum, Percutaneous Approach, Diagnostic

099M3ZZ Drainage of Nasal Septum, Percutaneous Approach

099M40Z Drainage of Nasal Septum with Drainage Device, Percutaneous Endoscopic Approach

099M4ZX Drainage of Nasal Septum, Percutaneous Endoscopic Approach, Diagnostic

099M4ZZ Drainage of Nasal Septum, Percutaneous Endoscopic Approach

099N00Z Drainage of Nasopharynx with Drainage Device, Open Approach

099N0ZX Drainage of Nasopharynx, Open Approach, Diagnostic

099N0ZZ Drainage of Nasopharynx, Open Approach

099N30Z Drainage of Nasopharynx with Drainage Device, Percutaneous Approach

099N3ZX Drainage of Nasopharynx, Percutaneous Approach, Diagnostic

099N3ZZ Drainage of Nasopharynx, Percutaneous Approach

099N40Z Drainage of Nasopharynx with Drainage Device, Percutaneous Endoscopic Approach

099N4ZX Drainage of Nasopharynx, Percutaneous Endoscopic Approach, Diagnostic

099N4ZZ Drainage of Nasopharynx, Percutaneous Endoscopic Approach

099N70Z Drainage of Nasopharynx with Drainage Device, Via Natural or Artificial Opening

099N7ZX Drainage of Nasopharynx, Via Natural or Artificial Opening, Diagnostic

099N7ZZ Drainage of Nasopharynx, Via Natural or Artificial Opening

099N80Z Drainage of Nasopharynx with Drainage Device, Via Natural or Artificial Opening Endoscopic

099N8ZX Drainage of Nasopharynx, Via Natural or Artificial Opening Endoscopic, Diagnostic

099N8ZZ Drainage of Nasopharynx, Via Natural or Artificial Opening Endoscopic

099P00Z Drainage of Accessory Sinus with Drainage Device, Open Approach

099P0ZX Drainage of Accessory Sinus, Open Approach, Diagnostic

099P0ZZ Drainage of Accessory Sinus, Open Approach

099P30Z Drainage of Accessory Sinus with Drainage Device, Percutaneous Approac

099P3ZX Drainage of Accessory Sinus, Percutaneous Approach, Diagnostic

099P3ZZ Drainage of Accessory Sinus, Percutaneous Approach

099P40Z Drainage of Accessory Sinus with Drainage Device, Percutaneous Endoscopic Approach

099P4ZX Drainage of Accessory Sinus, Percutaneous Endoscopic Approach, Diagnostic

099P4ZZ Drainage of Accessory Sinus, Percutaneous Endoscopic Approach

099Q00Z Drainage of Right Maxillary Sinus with Drainage Device, Open Approach

099Q0ZX Drainage of Right Maxillary Sinus, Open Approach, Diagnostic

099Q0ZZ Drainage of Right Maxillary Sinus, Open Approach

099Q30Z Drainage of Right Maxillary Sinus with Drainage Device, Percutaneous Approach

099Q3ZX Drainage of Right Maxillary Sinus, Percutaneous Approach, Diagnostic

099Q3ZZ Drainage of Right Maxillary Sinus, Percutaneous Approach

099Q40Z Drainage of Right Maxillary Sinus with Drainage Device, Percutaneous Endoscopic Approach

099Q4ZX Drainage of Right Maxillary Sinus, Percutaneous Endoscopic Approach, Diagnostic

099Q4ZZ Drainage of Right Maxillary Sinus, Percutaneous Endoscopic Approach

099R00Z Drainage of Left Maxillary Sinus with Drainage Device, Open Approach

099R0ZX Drainage of Left Maxillary Sinus, Open Approach, Diagnostic

099R0ZZ Drainage of Left Maxillary Sinus, Open Approach

099R30Z Drainage of Left Maxillary Sinus with Drainage Device, Percutaneous Approach

099R3ZX Drainage of Left Maxillary Sinus, Percutaneous Approach, Diagnostic

099R3ZZ Drainage of Left Maxillary Sinus, Percutaneous Approach

099R40Z Drainage of Left Maxillary Sinus with Drainage Device, Percutaneous Endoscopic Approach

099R4ZX Drainage of Left Maxillary Sinus, Percutaneous Endoscopic Approach, Diagnostic

099R4ZZ Drainage of Left Maxillary Sinus, Percutaneous Endoscopic Approach

099S00Z Drainage of Right Frontal Sinus with Drainage Device, Open Approach

099S0ZX Drainage of Right Frontal Sinus, Open Approach, Diagnostic

099S0ZZ Drainage of Right Frontal Sinus, Open Approach

099S30Z Drainage of Right Frontal Sinus with Drainage Device, Percutaneous Approach

099S3ZX Drainage of Right Frontal Sinus, Percutaneous Approach, Diagnostic

099S3ZZ Drainage of Right Frontal Sinus, Percutaneous Approach

099S40Z Drainage of Right Frontal Sinus with Drainage Device, Percutaneous Endoscopic Approach

099S4ZX Drainage of Right Frontal Sinus, Percutaneous Endoscopic Approach, Diagnostic

099S4ZZ Drainage of Right Frontal Sinus, Percutaneous Endoscopic Approach

9T00Z	Drainage of Left Frontal Sinus with Drainage Device, Open Approach
9T0ZX	Drainage of Left Frontal Sinus, Open Approach, Diagnostic
9T0ZZ	Drainage of Left Frontal Sinus, Open Approach
9T30Z	Drainage of Left Frontal Sinus with Drainage Device, Percutaneous Approach
9T3ZX	Drainage of Left Frontal Sinus, Percutaneous Approach, Diagnostic
9T3ZZ	Drainage of Left Frontal Sinus, Percutaneous Approach
9T40Z	Drainage of Left Frontal Sinus with Drainage Device, Percutaneous Endoscopic Approach
9T4ZX	Drainage of Left Frontal Sinus, Percutaneous Endoscopic Approach, Diagnostic
9T4ZZ	Drainage of Left Frontal Sinus, Percutaneous Endoscopic Approach
9U00Z	Drainage of Right Ethmoid Sinus with Drainage Device, Open Approach
9U0ZX	Drainage of Right Ethmoid Sinus, Open Approach, Diagnostic
9U0ZZ	Drainage of Right Ethmoid Sinus, Open Approach
9U30Z	Drainage of Right Ethmoid Sinus with Drainage Device, Percutaneous Approach
9U3ZX	Drainage of Right Ethmoid Sinus, Percutaneous Approach, Diagnostic
9U3ZZ	Drainage of Right Ethmoid Sinus, Percutaneous Approach
099U40Z	Drainage of Right Ethmoid Sinus with Drainage Device, Percutaneous Endoscopic Approach
099U4ZX	Drainage of Right Ethmoid Sinus, Percutaneous Endoscopic Approach, Diagnostic
099U4ZZ	Drainage of Right Ethmoid Sinus, Percutaneous Endoscopic Approach
099V00Z	Drainage of Left Ethmoid Sinus with Drainage Device, Open Approach
099V0ZX	Drainage of Left Ethmoid Sinus, Open Approach, Diagnostic
099V0ZZ	Drainage of Left Ethmoid Sinus, Open Approach
099V30Z	Drainage of Left Ethmoid Sinus with Drainage Device, Percutaneous Approach
099V3ZX	Drainage of Left Ethmoid Sinus, Percutaneous Approach, Diagnostic
099V3ZZ	Drainage of Left Ethmoid Sinus, Percutaneous Approach
099V40Z	Drainage of Left Ethmoid Sinus with Drainage Device, Percutaneous Endoscopic Approach
099V4ZX	Drainage of Left Ethmoid Sinus, Percutaneous Endoscopic Approach, Diagnostic
099V4ZZ	Drainage of Left Ethmoid Sinus, Percutaneous Endoscopic Approach
099W00Z	Drainage of Right Sphenoid Sinus with Drainage Device, Open Approach
099W0ZX	Drainage of Right Sphenoid Sinus, Open Approach, Diagnostic
099W0ZZ	Drainage of Right Sphenoid Sinus, Open Approach
099W30Z	Drainage of Right Sphenoid Sinus with Drainage Device, Percutaneous Approach
099W3ZX	Drainage of Right Sphenoid Sinus, Percutaneous Approach, Diagnostic
099W3ZZ	Drainage of Right Sphenoid Sinus, Percutaneous Approach
099W40Z	Drainage of Right Sphenoid Sinus with Drainage Device, Percutaneous Endoscopic Approach
099W4ZX	Drainage of Right Sphenoid Sinus, Percutaneous Endoscopic Approach, Diagnostic
099W4ZZ	Drainage of Right Sphenoid Sinus, Percutaneous Endoscopic Approach
099X00Z	Drainage of Left Sphenoid Sinus with Drainage Device, Open Approach
099X0ZX	Drainage of Left Sphenoid Sinus, Open Approach, Diagnostic
099X0ZZ	Drainage of Left Sphenoid Sinus, Open Approach
099X30Z	Drainage of Left Sphenoid Sinus with Drainage Device, Percutaneous Approach
099X3ZX	Drainage of Left Sphenoid Sinus, Percutaneous Approach, Diagnostic
099X3ZZ	Drainage of Left Sphenoid Sinus, Percutaneous Approach
099X40Z	Drainage of Left Sphenoid Sinus with Drainage Device, Percutaneous Endoscopic Approach
099X4ZX	Drainage of Left Sphenoid Sinus, Percutaneous Endoscopic Approach, Diagnostic
099X4ZZ	Drainage of Left Sphenoid Sinus, Percutaneous Endoscopic Approach

9B – Ear, Nose, Sinus, Excision

eview Coding Guidelines B3.4a and B3.4b

eview Coding Guideline B3.8

9B00ZX	Excision of Right External Ear, Open Approach, Diagnostic
9B00ZZ	Excision of Right External Ear, Open Approach
9B03ZX	Excision of Right External Ear, Percutaneous Approach, Diagnostic
9B03ZZ	Excision of Right External Ear, Percutaneous Approach
9B04ZX	Excision of Right External Ear, Percutaneous Endoscopic Approach, Diagnostic
9B04ZZ	Excision of Right External Ear, Percutaneous Endoscopic Approach
9B0XZX	Excision of Right External Ear, External Approach, Diagnostic
9B0XZZ	Excision of Right External Ear, External Approach
9B10ZX	Excision of Left External Ear, Open Approach, Diagnostic
9B10ZZ	Excision of Left External Ear, Open Approach
9B13ZX	Excision of Left External Ear, Percutaneous Approach, Diagnostic
9B13ZZ	Excision of Left External Ear, Percutaneous Approach
9B14ZX	Excision of Left External Ear, Percutaneous Endoscopic Approach, Diagnostic
9B14ZZ	Excision of Left External Ear, Percutaneous Endoscopic Approach
9B1XZX	Excision of Left External Ear, External Approach, Diagnostic
9B1XZZ	Excision of Left External Ear, External Approach
9B30ZX	Excision of Right External Auditory Canal, Open Approach, Diagnostic
09B30ZZ	Excision of Right External Auditory Canal, Open Approach
09B33ZX	Excision of Right External Auditory Canal, Percutaneous Approach, Diagnostic
09B33ZZ	Excision of Right External Auditory Canal, Percutaneous Approach
09B34ZX	Excision of Right External Auditory Canal, Percutaneous Endoscopic Approach, Diagnostic
09B34ZZ	Excision of Right External Auditory Canal, Percutaneous Endoscopic Approach
09B37ZX	Excision of Right External Auditory Canal, Via Natural or Artificial Opening, Diagnostic
09B37ZZ	Excision of Right External Auditory Canal, Via Natural or Artificial Opening
09B38ZX	Excision of Right External Auditory Canal, Via Natural or Artificial Opening Endoscopic, Diagnostic
09B38ZZ	Excision of Right External Auditory Canal, Via Natural or Artificial Opening Endoscopic
09B3XZX	Excision of Right External Auditory Canal, External Approach, Diagnostic
09B3XZZ	Excision of Right External Auditory Canal, External Approach
09B40ZX	Excision of Left External Auditory Canal, Open Approach, Diagnostic
09B40ZZ	Excision of Left External Auditory Canal, Open Approach
09B43ZX	Excision of Left External Auditory Canal, Percutaneous Approach, Diagnostic
09B43ZZ	Excision of Left External Auditory Canal, Percutaneous Approach
09B44ZX	Excision of Left External Auditory Canal, Percutaneous Endoscopic Approach, Diagnostic
09B44ZZ	Excision of Left External Auditory Canal, Percutaneous Endoscopic Approach
09B47ZX	Excision of Left External Auditory Canal, Via Natural or Artificial Opening, Diagnostic
09B47ZZ	Excision of Left External Auditory Canal, Via Natural or Artificial Opening
09B48ZX	Excision of Left External Auditory Canal, Via Natural or Artificial Opening Endoscopic, Diagnostic
09B48ZZ	Excision of Left External Auditory Canal, Via Natural or Artificial Opening Endoscopic
09B4XZX	Excision of Left External Auditory Canal, External Approach, Diagnostic
09B4XZZ	Excision of Left External Auditory Canal, External Approach
09B50ZX	Excision of Right Middle Ear, Open Approach, Diagnostic
09B50ZZ	Excision of Right Middle Ear, Open Approach
09B60ZX	Excision of Left Middle Ear, Open Approach, Diagnostic
09B60ZZ	Excision of Left Middle Ear, Open Approach
09B70ZX	Excision of Right Tympanic Membrane, Open Approach, Diagnostic
09B70ZZ	Excision of Right Tympanic Membrane, Open Approach
09B73ZX	Excision of Right Tympanic Membrane, Percutaneous Approach, Diagnostic
09B73ZZ	Excision of Right Tympanic Membrane, Percutaneous Approach

09B74ZX Excision of Right Tympanic Membrane, Percutaneous Endoscopic Approach, Diagnostic
09B74ZZ Excision of Right Tympanic Membrane, Percutaneous Endoscopic Approach
09B77ZX Excision of Right Tympanic Membrane, Via Natural or Artificial Opening, Diagnostic
09B77ZZ Excision of Right Tympanic Membrane, Via Natural or Artificial Opening
09B78ZX Excision of Right Tympanic Membrane, Via Natural or Artificial Opening Endoscopic, Diagnostic
09B78ZZ Excision of Right Tympanic Membrane, Via Natural or Artificial Opening Endoscopic
09B80ZX Excision of Left Tympanic Membrane, Open Approach, Diagnostic
09B80ZZ Excision of Left Tympanic Membrane, Open Approach
09B83ZX Excision of Left Tympanic Membrane, Percutaneous Approach, Diagnostic
09B83ZZ Excision of Left Tympanic Membrane, Percutaneous Approach
09B84ZX Excision of Left Tympanic Membrane, Percutaneous Endoscopic Approach, Diagnostic
09B84ZZ Excision of Left Tympanic Membrane, Percutaneous Endoscopic Approach
09B87ZX Excision of Left Tympanic Membrane, Via Natural or Artificial Opening, Diagnostic
09B87ZZ Excision of Left Tympanic Membrane, Via Natural or Artificial Opening
09B88ZX Excision of Left Tympanic Membrane, Via Natural or Artificial Opening Endoscopic, Diagnostic
09B88ZZ Excision of Left Tympanic Membrane, Via Natural or Artificial Opening Endoscopic
09B90ZX Excision of Right Auditory Ossicle, Open Approach, Diagnostic
09B90ZZ Excision of Right Auditory Ossicle, Open Approach
09BA0ZX Excision of Left Auditory Ossicle, Open Approach, Diagnostic
09BA0ZZ Excision of Left Auditory Ossicle, Open Approach
09BB0ZX Excision of Right Mastoid Sinus, Open Approach, Diagnostic
09BB0ZZ Excision of Right Mastoid Sinus, Open Approach
09BB3ZX Excision of Right Mastoid Sinus, Percutaneous Approach, Diagnostic
09BB3ZZ Excision of Right Mastoid Sinus, Percutaneous Approach
09BB4ZX Excision of Right Mastoid Sinus, Percutaneous Endoscopic Approach, Diagnostic
09BB4ZZ Excision of Right Mastoid Sinus, Percutaneous Endoscopic Approach
09BC0ZX Excision of Left Mastoid Sinus, Open Approach, Diagnostic
09BC0ZZ Excision of Left Mastoid Sinus, Open Approach
09BC3ZX Excision of Left Mastoid Sinus, Percutaneous Approach, Diagnostic
09BC3ZZ Excision of Left Mastoid Sinus, Percutaneous Approach
09BC4ZX Excision of Left Mastoid Sinus, Percutaneous Endoscopic Approach, Diagnostic
09BC4ZZ Excision of Left Mastoid Sinus, Percutaneous Endoscopic Approach
09BD0ZX Excision of Right Inner Ear, Open Approach, Diagnostic
09BD0ZZ Excision of Right Inner Ear, Open Approach
09BE0ZX Excision of Left Inner Ear, Open Approach, Diagnostic
09BE0ZZ Excision of Left Inner Ear, Open Approach
09BF0ZX Excision of Right Eustachian Tube, Open Approach, Diagnostic
09BF0ZZ Excision of Right Eustachian Tube, Open Approach
09BF3ZX Excision of Right Eustachian Tube, Percutaneous Approach, Diagnostic
09BF3ZZ Excision of Right Eustachian Tube, Percutaneous Approach
09BF4ZX Excision of Right Eustachian Tube, Percutaneous Endoscopic Approach, Diagnostic
09BF4ZZ Excision of Right Eustachian Tube, Percutaneous Endoscopic Approach
09BF7ZX Excision of Right Eustachian Tube, Via Natural or Artificial Opening, Diagnostic
09BF7ZZ Excision of Right Eustachian Tube, Via Natural or Artificial Opening
09BF8ZX Excision of Right Eustachian Tube, Via Natural or Artificial Opening Endoscopic, Diagnostic
09BF8ZZ Excision of Right Eustachian Tube, Via Natural or Artificial Opening Endoscopic
09BG0ZX Excision of Left Eustachian Tube, Open Approach, Diagnostic
09BG0ZZ Excision of Left Eustachian Tube, Open Approach
09BG3ZX Excision of Left Eustachian Tube, Percutaneous Approach, Diagnostic
09BG3ZZ Excision of Left Eustachian Tube, Percutaneous Approach
09BG4ZX Excision of Left Eustachian Tube, Percutaneous Endoscopic Approach, Diagnostic
09BG4ZZ Excision of Left Eustachian Tube, Percutaneous Endoscopic Approach
09BG7ZX Excision of Left Eustachian Tube, Via Natural or Artificial Opening, Diagnostic
09BG7ZZ Excision of Left Eustachian Tube, Via Natural or Artificial Opening
09BG8ZX Excision of Left Eustachian Tube, Via Natural or Artificial Opening Endoscopic, Diagnostic
09BG8ZZ Excision of Left Eustachian Tube, Via Natural or Artificial Opening Endoscopic
09BK0ZX Excision of Nose, Open Approach, Diagnostic
09BK0ZZ Excision of Nose, Open Approach
09BK3ZX Excision of Nose, Percutaneous Approach, Diagnostic
09BK3ZZ Excision of Nose, Percutaneous Approach
09BK4ZX Excision of Nose, Percutaneous Endoscopic Approach, Diagnostic
09BK4ZZ Excision of Nose, Percutaneous Endoscopic Approach
09BKXZX Excision of Nose, External Approach, Diagnostic
09BKXZZ Excision of Nose, External Approach
09BL0ZX Excision of Nasal Turbinate, Open Approach, Diagnostic
09BL0ZZ Excision of Nasal Turbinate, Open Approach
09BL3ZX Excision of Nasal Turbinate, Percutaneous Approach, Diagnostic
09BL3ZZ Excision of Nasal Turbinate, Percutaneous Approach
09BL4ZX Excision of Nasal Turbinate, Percutaneous Endoscopic Approach, Diagnostic
09BL4ZZ Excision of Nasal Turbinate, Percutaneous Endoscopic Approach
09BL7ZX Excision of Nasal Turbinate, Via Natural or Artificial Opening, Diagnostic
09BL7ZZ Excision of Nasal Turbinate, Via Natural or Artificial Opening
09BL8ZX Excision of Nasal Turbinate, Via Natura or Artificial Opening Endoscopic, Diagnostic
09BL8ZZ Excision of Nasal Turbinate, Via Natura or Artificial Opening Endoscopic
09BM0ZX Excision of Nasal Septum, Open Approach, Diagnostic
09BM0ZZ Excision of Nasal Septum, Open Appro
09BM3ZX Excision of Nasal Septum, Percutaneous Approach, Diagnostic
09BM3ZZ Excision of Nasal Septum, Percutaneous Approach
09BM4ZX Excision of Nasal Septum, Percutaneous Endoscopic Approach, Diagnostic
09BM4ZZ Excision of Nasal Septum, Percutaneous Endoscopic Approach
09BN0ZX Excision of Nasopharynx, Open Approa Diagnostic
09BN0ZZ Excision of Nasopharynx, Open Approa
09BN3ZX Excision of Nasopharynx, Percutaneous Approach, Diagnostic
09BN3ZZ Excision of Nasopharynx, Percutaneous Approach
09BN4ZX Excision of Nasopharynx, Percutaneous Endoscopic Approach, Diagnostic
09BN4ZZ Excision of Nasopharynx, Percutaneous Endoscopic Approach
09BN7ZX Excision of Nasopharynx, Via Natural or Artificial Opening, Diagnostic
09BN7ZZ Excision of Nasopharynx, Via Natural or Artificial Opening
09BN8ZX Excision of Nasopharynx, Via Natural or Artificial Opening Endoscopic, Diagnost
09BN8ZZ Excision of Nasopharynx, Via Natural or Artificial Opening Endoscopic
09BP0ZX Excision of Accessory Sinus, Open Approach, Diagnostic
09BP0ZZ Excision of Accessory Sinus, Open Approach
09BP3ZX Excision of Accessory Sinus, Percutaneo Approach, Diagnostic
09BP3ZZ Excision of Accessory Sinus, Percutaneo Approach
09BP4ZX Excision of Accessory Sinus, Percutaneo Endoscopic Approach, Diagnostic
09BP4ZZ Excision of Accessory Sinus, Percutaneo Endoscopic Approach
09BQ0ZX Excision of Right Maxillary Sinus, Open Approach, Diagnostic
09BQ0ZZ Excision of Right Maxillary Sinus, Open Approach
09BQ3ZX Excision of Right Maxillary Sinus, Percutaneous Approach, Diagnostic
09BQ3ZZ Excision of Right Maxillary Sinus, Percutaneous Approach
09BQ4ZX Excision of Right Maxillary Sinus, Percutaneous Endoscopic Approach, Diagnostic
09BQ4ZZ Excision of Right Maxillary Sinus, Percutaneous Endoscopic Approach
09BR0ZX Excision of Left Maxillary Sinus, Open Approach, Diagnostic
09BR0ZZ Excision of Left Maxillary Sinus, Open Approach
09BR3ZX Excision of Left Maxillary Sinus, Percutaneous Approach, Diagnostic
09BR3ZZ Excision of Left Maxillary Sinus, Percutaneous Approach
09BR4ZX Excision of Left Maxillary Sinus, Percutaneous Endoscopic Approach, Diagnostic
09BR4ZZ Excision of Left Maxillary Sinus, Percutaneous Endoscopic Approach
09BS0ZX Excision of Right Frontal Sinus, Open Approach, Diagnostic
09BS0ZZ Excision of Right Frontal Sinus, Open Approach

♀ Female-only ♂ Male-only Limited Coverage ● Non-OR HAC-associated procedure ▲ Non-covered procedures + Combinatio

BS3ZX Excision of Right Frontal Sinus, Percutaneous Approach, Diagnostic
BS3ZZ Excision of Right Frontal Sinus, Percutaneous Approach
BS4ZX Excision of Right Frontal Sinus, Percutaneous Endoscopic Approach, Diagnostic
BS4ZZ Excision of Right Frontal Sinus, Percutaneous Endoscopic Approach
BT0ZX Excision of Left Frontal Sinus, Open Approach, Diagnostic
BT0ZZ Excision of Left Frontal Sinus, Open Approach
BT3ZX Excision of Left Frontal Sinus, Percutaneous Approach, Diagnostic
BT3ZZ Excision of Left Frontal Sinus, Percutaneous Approach
BT4ZX Excision of Left Frontal Sinus, Percutaneous Endoscopic Approach, Diagnostic
BT4ZZ Excision of Left Frontal Sinus, Percutaneous Endoscopic Approach
BU0ZX Excision of Right Ethmoid Sinus, Open Approach, Diagnostic
BU0ZZ Excision of Right Ethmoid Sinus, Open Approach
09BU3ZX Excision of Right Ethmoid Sinus, Percutaneous Approach, Diagnostic
09BU3ZZ Excision of Right Ethmoid Sinus, Percutaneous Approach
09BU4ZX Excision of Right Ethmoid Sinus, Percutaneous Endoscopic Approach, Diagnostic
09BU4ZZ Excision of Right Ethmoid Sinus, Percutaneous Endoscopic Approach
09BV0ZX Excision of Left Ethmoid Sinus, Open Approach, Diagnostic
09BV0ZZ Excision of Left Ethmoid Sinus, Open Approach
09BV3ZX Excision of Left Ethmoid Sinus, Percutaneous Approach, Diagnostic
09BV3ZZ Excision of Left Ethmoid Sinus, Percutaneous Approach
09BV4ZX Excision of Left Ethmoid Sinus, Percutaneous Endoscopic Approach, Diagnostic
09BV4ZZ Excision of Left Ethmoid Sinus, Percutaneous Endoscopic Approach
09BW0ZX Excision of Right Sphenoid Sinus, Open Approach, Diagnostic
09BW0ZZ Excision of Right Sphenoid Sinus, Open Approach
09BW3ZX Excision of Right Sphenoid Sinus, Percutaneous Approach, Diagnostic
09BW3ZZ Excision of Right Sphenoid Sinus, Percutaneous Approach
09BW4ZX Excision of Right Sphenoid Sinus, Percutaneous Endoscopic Approach, Diagnostic
09BW4ZZ Excision of Right Sphenoid Sinus, Percutaneous Endoscopic Approach
09BX0ZX Excision of Left Sphenoid Sinus, Open Approach, Diagnostic
09BX0ZZ Excision of Left Sphenoid Sinus, Open Approach
09BX3ZX Excision of Left Sphenoid Sinus, Percutaneous Approach, Diagnostic
09BX3ZZ Excision of Left Sphenoid Sinus, Percutaneous Approach
09BX4ZX Excision of Left Sphenoid Sinus, Percutaneous Endoscopic Approach, Diagnostic
09BX4ZZ Excision of Left Sphenoid Sinus, Percutaneous Endoscopic Approach

9C – Ear, Nose, Sinus, Extirpation

C00ZZ Extirpation of Matter from Right External Ear, Open Approach
C03ZZ Extirpation of Matter from Right External Ear, Percutaneous Approach
C04ZZ Extirpation of Matter from Right External Ear, Percutaneous Endoscopic Approach
C0XZZ Extirpation of Matter from Right External Ear, External Approach
C10ZZ Extirpation of Matter from Left External Ear, Open Approach
C13ZZ Extirpation of Matter from Left External Ear, Percutaneous Approach
9C14ZZ Extirpation of Matter from Left External Ear, Percutaneous Endoscopic Approach
9C1XZZ Extirpation of Matter from Left External Ear, External Approach
9C30ZZ Extirpation of Matter from Right External Auditory Canal, Open Approach
9C33ZZ Extirpation of Matter from Right External Auditory Canal, Percutaneous Approach
9C34ZZ Extirpation of Matter from Right External Auditory Canal, Percutaneous Endoscopic Approach
9C37ZZ Extirpation of Matter from Right External Auditory Canal, Via Natural or Artificial Opening
9C38ZZ Extirpation of Matter from Right External Auditory Canal, Via Natural or Artificial Opening Endoscopic
9C3XZZ Extirpation of Matter from Right External Auditory Canal, External Approach
9C40ZZ Extirpation of Matter from Left External Auditory Canal, Open Approach
9C43ZZ Extirpation of Matter from Left External Auditory Canal, Percutaneous Approach
9C44ZZ Extirpation of Matter from Left External Auditory Canal, Percutaneous Endoscopic Approach
9C47ZZ Extirpation of Matter from Left External Auditory Canal, Via Natural or Artificial Opening
9C48ZZ Extirpation of Matter from Left External Auditory Canal, Via Natural or Artificial Opening Endoscopic
9C4XZZ Extirpation of Matter from Left External Auditory Canal, External Approach
9C50ZZ Extirpation of Matter from Right Middle Ear, Open Approach
09C60ZZ Extirpation of Matter from Left Middle Ear, Open Approach
09C70ZZ Extirpation of Matter from Right Tympanic Membrane, Open Approach
09C73ZZ Extirpation of Matter from Right Tympanic Membrane, Percutaneous Approach
09C74ZZ Extirpation of Matter from Right Tympanic Membrane, Percutaneous Endoscopic Approach
09C77ZZ Extirpation of Matter from Right Tympanic Membrane, Via Natural or Artificial Opening
09C78ZZ Extirpation of Matter from Right Tympanic Membrane, Via Natural or Artificial Opening Endoscopic
09C80ZZ Extirpation of Matter from Left Tympanic Membrane, Open Approach
09C83ZZ Extirpation of Matter from Left Tympanic Membrane, Percutaneous Approach
09C84ZZ Extirpation of Matter from Left Tympanic Membrane, Percutaneous Endoscopic Approach
09C87ZZ Extirpation of Matter from Left Tympanic Membrane, Via Natural or Artificial Opening
09C88ZZ Extirpation of Matter from Left Tympanic Membrane, Via Natural or Artificial Opening Endoscopic
09C90ZZ Extirpation of Matter from Right Auditory Ossicle, Open Approach
09CA0ZZ Extirpation of Matter from Left Auditory Ossicle, Open Approach
09CB0ZZ Extirpation of Matter from Right Mastoid Sinus, Open Approach
09CB3ZZ Extirpation of Matter from Right Mastoid Sinus, Percutaneous Approach
09CB4ZZ Extirpation of Matter from Right Mastoid Sinus, Percutaneous Endoscopic Approach
09CC0ZZ Extirpation of Matter from Left Mastoid Sinus, Open Approach
09CC3ZZ Extirpation of Matter from Left Mastoid Sinus, Percutaneous Approach
09CC4ZZ Extirpation of Matter from Left Mastoid Sinus, Percutaneous Endoscopic Approach
09CD0ZZ Extirpation of Matter from Right Inner Ear, Open Approach
09CE0ZZ Extirpation of Matter from Left Inner Ear, Open Approach
09CF0ZZ Extirpation of Matter from Right Eustachian Tube, Open Approach
09CF3ZZ Extirpation of Matter from Right Eustachian Tube, Percutaneous Approach
09CF4ZZ Extirpation of Matter from Right Eustachian Tube, Percutaneous Endoscopic Approach
09CF7ZZ Extirpation of Matter from Right Eustachian Tube, Via Natural or Artificial Opening
09CF8ZZ Extirpation of Matter from Right Eustachian Tube, Via Natural or Artificial Opening Endoscopic
09CG0ZZ Extirpation of Matter from Left Eustachian Tube, Open Approach
09CG3ZZ Extirpation of Matter from Left Eustachian Tube, Percutaneous Approach
09CG4ZZ Extirpation of Matter from Left Eustachian Tube, Percutaneous Endoscopic Approach
09CG7ZZ Extirpation of Matter from Left Eustachian Tube, Via Natural or Artificial Opening
09CG8ZZ Extirpation of Matter from Left Eustachian Tube, Via Natural or Artificial Opening Endoscopic
09CK0ZZ Extirpation of Matter from Nose, Open Approach
09CK3ZZ Extirpation of Matter from Nose, Percutaneous Approach
09CK4ZZ Extirpation of Matter from Nose, Percutaneous Endoscopic Approach
09CKXZZ Extirpation of Matter from Nose, External Approach
09CL0ZZ Extirpation of Matter from Nasal Turbinate, Open Approach
09CL3ZZ Extirpation of Matter from Nasal Turbinate, Percutaneous Approach
09CL4ZZ Extirpation of Matter from Nasal Turbinate, Percutaneous Endoscopic Approach
09CL7ZZ Extirpation of Matter from Nasal Turbinate, Via Natural or Artificial Opening
09CL8ZZ Extirpation of Matter from Nasal Turbinate, Via Natural or Artificial Opening Endoscopic

09CM0ZZ Extirpation of Matter from Nasal Septum, Open Approach
09CM3ZZ Extirpation of Matter from Nasal Septum, Percutaneous Approach
09CM4ZZ Extirpation of Matter from Nasal Septum, Percutaneous Endoscopic Approach
09CN0ZZ Extirpation of Matter from Nasopharynx, Open Approach
09CN3ZZ Extirpation of Matter from Nasopharynx, Percutaneous Approach
09CN4ZZ Extirpation of Matter from Nasopharynx, Percutaneous Endoscopic Approach
09CN7ZZ Extirpation of Matter from Nasopharynx, Via Natural or Artificial Opening
09CN8ZZ Extirpation of Matter from Nasopharynx, Via Natural or Artificial Opening Endoscopic
09CP0ZZ Extirpation of Matter from Accessory Sinus, Open Approach
09CP3ZZ Extirpation of Matter from Accessory Sinus, Percutaneous Approach
09CP4ZZ Extirpation of Matter from Accessory Sinus, Percutaneous Endoscopic Approach
09CQ0ZZ Extirpation of Matter from Right Maxillary Sinus, Open Approach
09CQ3ZZ Extirpation of Matter from Right Maxillary Sinus, Percutaneous Approach
09CQ4ZZ Extirpation of Matter from Right Maxillary Sinus, Percutaneous Endoscopic Approach
09CR0ZZ Extirpation of Matter from Left Maxillary Sinus, Open Approach
09CR3ZZ Extirpation of Matter from Left Maxillary Sinus, Percutaneous Approach
09CR4ZZ Extirpation of Matter from Left Maxillary Sinus, Percutaneous Endoscopic Approach
09CS0ZZ Extirpation of Matter from Right Frontal Sinus, Open Approach
09CS3ZZ Extirpation of Matter from Right Frontal Sinus, Percutaneous Approach
09CS4ZZ Extirpation of Matter from Right Frontal Sinus, Percutaneous Endoscopic Approach
09CT0ZZ Extirpation of Matter from Left Frontal Sinus, Open Approach
09CT3ZZ Extirpation of Matter from Left Frontal Sinus, Percutaneous Approach
09CT4ZZ Extirpation of Matter from Left Frontal Sinus, Percutaneous Endoscopic Approach
09CU0ZZ Extirpation of Matter from Right Ethmoid Sinus, Open Approach
09CU3ZZ Extirpation of Matter from Right Ethmo Sinus, Percutaneous Approach
09CU4ZZ Extirpation of Matter from Right Ethmo Sinus, Percutaneous Endoscopic Appro
09CV0ZZ Extirpation of Matter from Left Ethmoi Sinus, Open Approach
09CV3ZZ Extirpation of Matter from Left Ethmoi Sinus, Percutaneous Approach
09CV4ZZ Extirpation of Matter from Left Ethmoi Sinus, Percutaneous Endoscopic Appro
09CW0ZZ Extirpation of Matter from Right Sphen Sinus, Open Approach
09CW3ZZ Extirpation of Matter from Right Sphen Sinus, Percutaneous Approach
09CW4ZZ Extirpation of Matter from Right Sphen Sinus, Percutaneous Endoscopic Appro
09CX0ZZ Extirpation of Matter from Left Sphenoi Sinus, Open Approach
09CX3ZZ Extirpation of Matter from Left Sphenoi Sinus, Percutaneous Approach
09CX4ZZ Extirpation of Matter from Left Sphenoi Sinus, Percutaneous Endoscopic Appro

09D – Ear, Nose, Sinus, Extraction

09D70ZZ Extraction of Right Tympanic Membrane, Open Approach
09D73ZZ Extraction of Right Tympanic Membrane, Percutaneous Approach
09D74ZZ Extraction of Right Tympanic Membrane, Percutaneous Endoscopic Approach
09D77ZZ Extraction of Right Tympanic Membrane, Via Natural or Artificial Opening
09D78ZZ Extraction of Right Tympanic Membrane, Via Natural or Artificial Opening Endoscopic
09D80ZZ Extraction of Left Tympanic Membrane, Open Approach
09D83ZZ Extraction of Left Tympanic Membrane, Percutaneous Approach
09D84ZZ Extraction of Left Tympanic Membrane, Percutaneous Endoscopic Approach
09D87ZZ Extraction of Left Tympanic Membrane, Via Natural or Artificial Opening
09D88ZZ Extraction of Left Tympanic Membrane, Via Natural or Artificial Opening Endoscopic
09D90ZZ Extraction of Right Auditory Ossicle, Open Approach
09DA0ZZ Extraction of Left Auditory Ossicle, Open Approach
09DB0ZZ Extraction of Right Mastoid Sinus, Open Approach
09DB3ZZ Extraction of Right Mastoid Sinus, Percutaneous Approach
09DB4ZZ Extraction of Right Mastoid Sinus, Percutaneous Endoscopic Approach
09DC0ZZ Extraction of Left Mastoid Sinus, Open Approach
09DC3ZZ Extraction of Left Mastoid Sinus, Percutaneous Approach
09DC4ZZ Extraction of Left Mastoid Sinus, Percutaneous Endoscopic Approach
09DL0ZZ Extraction of Nasal Turbinate, Open Approach
09DL3ZZ Extraction of Nasal Turbinate, Percutaneous Approach
09DL4ZZ Extraction of Nasal Turbinate, Percutaneous Endoscopic Approach
09DL7ZZ Extraction of Nasal Turbinate, Via Natural or Artificial Opening
09DL8ZZ Extraction of Nasal Turbinate, Via Natural or Artificial Opening Endoscopic
09DM0ZZ Extraction of Nasal Septum, Open Approach
09DM3ZZ Extraction of Nasal Septum, Percutaneous Approach
09DM4ZZ Extraction of Nasal Septum, Percutaneous Endoscopic Approach
09DP0ZZ Extraction of Accessory Sinus, Open Approach
09DP3ZZ Extraction of Accessory Sinus, Percutaneous Approach
09DP4ZZ Extraction of Accessory Sinus, Percutaneous Endoscopic Approach
09DQ0ZZ Extraction of Right Maxillary Sinus, Open Approach
09DQ3ZZ Extraction of Right Maxillary Sinus, Percutaneous Approach
09DQ4ZZ Extraction of Right Maxillary Sinus, Percutaneous Endoscopic Approach
09DR0ZZ Extraction of Left Maxillary Sinus, Open Approach
09DR3ZZ Extraction of Left Maxillary Sinus, Percutaneous Approach
09DR4ZZ Extraction of Left Maxillary Sinus, Percutaneous Endoscopic Approach
09DS0ZZ Extraction of Right Frontal Sinus, Open Approach
09DS3ZZ Extraction of Right Frontal Sinus, Percutaneous Approach
09DS4ZZ Extraction of Right Frontal Sinus, Percutaneous Endoscopic Approach
09DT0ZZ Extraction of Left Frontal Sinus, Open Approach
09DT3ZZ Extraction of Left Frontal Sinus, Percutaneous Approach
09DT4ZZ Extraction of Left Frontal Sinus, Percutaneous Endoscopic Approach
09DU0ZZ Extraction of Right Ethmoid Sinus, Open Approach
09DU3ZZ Extraction of Right Ethmoid Sinus, Percutaneous Approach
09DU4ZZ Extraction of Right Ethmoid Sinus, Percutaneous Endoscopic Approach
09DV0ZZ Extraction of Left Ethmoid Sinus, Open Approach
09DV3ZZ Extraction of Left Ethmoid Sinus, Percutaneous Approach
09DV4ZZ Extraction of Left Ethmoid Sinus, Percutaneous Endoscopic Approach
09DW0ZZ Extraction of Right Sphenoid Sinus, Open Approach
09DW3ZZ Extraction of Right Sphenoid Sinus, Percutaneous Approach
09DW4ZZ Extraction of Right Sphenoid Sinus, Percutaneous Endoscopic Approach
09DX0ZZ Extraction of Left Sphenoid Sinus, Open Approach
09DX3ZZ Extraction of Left Sphenoid Sinus, Percutaneous Approach
09DX4ZZ Extraction of Left Sphenoid Sinus, Percutaneous Endoscopic Approach

09H – Ear, Nose, Sinus, Insertion

09HD04Z Insertion of Bone Conduction Hearing Device into Right Inner Ear, Open Approach
09HD05Z Insertion of Single Channel Cochlear Prosthesis into Right Inner Ear, Open Approach
09HD06Z Insertion of Multiple Channel Cochlear Prosthesis into Right Inner Ear, Open Approach
09HD0SZ Insertion of Hearing Device into Right Inner Ear, Open Approach
09HD34Z Insertion of Bone Conduction Hearing Device into Right Inner Ear, Percutaneous Approach
09HD35Z Insertion of Single Channel Cochlear Prosthesis into Right Inner Ear, Percutaneous Approach
09HD36Z Insertion of Multiple Channel Cochlear Prosthesis into Right Inner Ear, Percutaneous Approach
09HD3SZ Insertion of Hearing Device into Right Inner Ear, Percutaneous Approach
09HD44Z Insertion of Bone Conduction Hearing Device into Right Inner Ear, Percutaneous Endoscopic Approach
09HD45Z Insertion of Single Channel Cochlear Prosthesis into Right Inner Ear, Percutaneous Endoscopic Approach
09HD46Z Insertion of Multiple Channel Cochlear Prosthesis into Right Inner Ear, Percutaneous Endoscopic Approach

IID4SZ Insertion of Hearing Device into Right Inner Ear, Percutaneous Endoscopic Approach
IE04Z Insertion of Bone Conduction Hearing Device into Left Inner Ear, Open Approach
HE05Z Insertion of Single Channel Cochlear Prosthesis into Left Inner Ear, Open Approach
HE06Z Insertion of Multiple Channel Cochlear Prosthesis into Left Inner Ear, Open Approach
HE0SZ Insertion of Hearing Device into Left Inner Ear, Open Approach
09HE34Z Insertion of Bone Conduction Hearing Device into Left Inner Ear, Percutaneous Approach
09HE35Z Insertion of Single Channel Cochlear Prosthesis into Left Inner Ear, Percutaneous Approach
09HE36Z Insertion of Multiple Channel Cochlear Prosthesis into Left Inner Ear, Percutaneous Approach
09HE3SZ Insertion of Hearing Device into Left Inner Ear, Percutaneous Approach
09HE44Z Insertion of Bone Conduction Hearing Device into Left Inner Ear, Percutaneous Endoscopic Approach
09HE45Z Insertion of Single Channel Cochlear Prosthesis into Left Inner Ear, Percutaneous Endoscopic Approach
09HE46Z Insertion of Multiple Channel Cochlear Prosthesis into Left Inner Ear, Percutaneous Endoscopic Approach
09HE4SZ Insertion of Hearing Device into Left Inner Ear, Percutaneous Endoscopic Approach
09HN7BZ Insertion of Airway into Nasopharynx, Via Natural or Artificial Opening
09HN8BZ Insertion of Airway into Nasopharynx, Via Natural or Artificial Opening Endoscopic

J – Ear, Nose, Sinus, Inspection

view Coding Guidelines B3.11a, B3.11b and B3.11c

J70ZZ Inspection of Right Tympanic Membrane, Open Approach
J73ZZ Inspection of Right Tympanic Membrane, Percutaneous Approach
J74ZZ Inspection of Right Tympanic Membrane, Percutaneous Endoscopic Approach
J77ZZ Inspection of Right Tympanic Membrane, Via Natural or Artificial Opening
J78ZZ Inspection of Right Tympanic Membrane, Via Natural or Artificial Opening Endoscopic
J7XZZ Inspection of Right Tympanic Membrane, External Approach
J80ZZ Inspection of Left Tympanic Membrane, Open Approach
J83ZZ Inspection of Left Tympanic Membrane, Percutaneous Approach
J84ZZ Inspection of Left Tympanic Membrane, Percutaneous Endoscopic Approach
J87ZZ Inspection of Left Tympanic Membrane, Via Natural or Artificial Opening
J88ZZ Inspection of Left Tympanic Membrane, Via Natural or Artificial Opening Endoscopic
J8XZZ Inspection of Left Tympanic Membrane, External Approach
09JD0ZZ Inspection of Right Inner Ear, Open Approach
09JD3ZZ Inspection of Right Inner Ear, Percutaneous Approach
09JD4ZZ Inspection of Right Inner Ear, Percutaneous Endoscopic Approach
09JDXZZ Inspection of Right Inner Ear, External Approach
09JE0ZZ Inspection of Left Inner Ear, Open Approach
09JE3ZZ Inspection of Left Inner Ear, Percutaneous Approach
09JE4ZZ Inspection of Left Inner Ear, Percutaneous Endoscopic Approach
09JEXZZ Inspection of Left Inner Ear, External Approach
09JH0ZZ Inspection of Right Ear, Open Approach
09JH3ZZ Inspection of Right Ear, Percutaneous Approach
09JH4ZZ Inspection of Right Ear, Percutaneous Endoscopic Approach
09JH7ZZ Inspection of Right Ear, Via Natural or Artificial Opening
09JH8ZZ Inspection of Right Ear, Via Natural or Artificial Opening Endoscopic
09JHXZZ Inspection of Right Ear, External Approach
09JJ0ZZ Inspection of Left Ear, Open Approach
09JJ3ZZ Inspection of Left Ear, Percutaneous Approach
09JJ4ZZ Inspection of Left Ear, Percutaneous Endoscopic Approach
09JJ7ZZ Inspection of Left Ear, Via Natural or Artificial Opening
09JJ8ZZ Inspection of Left Ear, Via Natural or Artificial Opening Endoscopic
09JJXZZ Inspection of Left Ear, External Approach
09JK0ZZ Inspection of Nose, Open Approach
09JK3ZZ Inspection of Nose, Percutaneous Approach
09JK4ZZ Inspection of Nose, Percutaneous Endoscopic Approach
09JKXZZ Inspection of Nose, External Approach
09JY0ZZ Inspection of Sinus, Open Approach
09JY3ZZ Inspection of Sinus, Percutaneous Approach
09JY4ZZ Inspection of Sinus, Percutaneous Endoscopic Approach
09JYXZZ Inspection of Sinus, External Approach

9M – Ear, Nose, Sinus, Reattachment

M0XZZ Reattachment of Right External Ear, External Approach
09M1XZZ Reattachment of Left External Ear, External Approach
09MKXZZ Reattachment of Nose, External Approach

9N – Ear, Nose, Sinus, Release

eview Coding Guidelines B3.13 and B3.14

9N00ZZ Release Right External Ear, Open Approach
9N03ZZ Release Right External Ear, Percutaneous Approach
9N04ZZ Release Right External Ear, Percutaneous Endoscopic Approach
9N0XZZ Release Right External Ear, External Approach
9N10ZZ Release Left External Ear, Open Approach
9N13ZZ Release Left External Ear, Percutaneous Approach
9N14ZZ Release Left External Ear, Percutaneous Endoscopic Approach
9N1XZZ Release Left External Ear, External Approach
9N30ZZ Release Right External Auditory Canal, Open Approach
9N33ZZ Release Right External Auditory Canal, Percutaneous Approach
9N34ZZ Release Right External Auditory Canal, Percutaneous Endoscopic Approach
9N37ZZ Release Right External Auditory Canal, Via Natural or Artificial Opening
09N38ZZ Release Right External Auditory Canal, Via Natural or Artificial Opening Endoscopic
09N3XZZ Release Right External Auditory Canal, External Approach
09N40ZZ Release Left External Auditory Canal, Open Approach
09N43ZZ Release Left External Auditory Canal, Percutaneous Approach
09N44ZZ Release Left External Auditory Canal, Percutaneous Endoscopic Approach
09N47ZZ Release Left External Auditory Canal, Via Natural or Artificial Opening
09N48ZZ Release Left External Auditory Canal, Via Natural or Artificial Opening Endoscopic
09N4XZZ Release Left External Auditory Canal, External Approach
09N50ZZ Release Right Middle Ear, Open Approach
09N60ZZ Release Left Middle Ear, Open Approach
09N70ZZ Release Right Tympanic Membrane, Open Approach
09N73ZZ Release Right Tympanic Membrane, Percutaneous Approach
09N74ZZ Release Right Tympanic Membrane, Percutaneous Endoscopic Approach
09N77ZZ Release Right Tympanic Membrane, Via Natural or Artificial Opening
09N78ZZ Release Right Tympanic Membrane, Via Natural or Artificial Opening Endoscopic
09N80ZZ Release Left Tympanic Membrane, Open Approach
09N83ZZ Release Left Tympanic Membrane, Percutaneous Approach
09N84ZZ Release Left Tympanic Membrane, Percutaneous Endoscopic Approach
09N87ZZ Release Left Tympanic Membrane, Via Natural or Artificial Opening
09N88ZZ Release Left Tympanic Membrane, Via Natural or Artificial Opening Endoscopic
09N90ZZ Release Right Auditory Ossicle, Open Approach
09NA0ZZ Release Left Auditory Ossicle, Open Approach

09NB0ZZ Release Right Mastoid Sinus, Open Approach
09NB3ZZ Release Right Mastoid Sinus, Percutaneous Approach
09NB4ZZ Release Right Mastoid Sinus, Percutaneous Endoscopic Approach
09NC0ZZ Release Left Mastoid Sinus, Open Approach
09NC3ZZ Release Left Mastoid Sinus, Percutaneous Approach
09NC4ZZ Release Left Mastoid Sinus, Percutaneous Endoscopic Approach
09ND0ZZ Release Right Inner Ear, Open Approach
09NE0ZZ Release Left Inner Ear, Open Approach
09NF0ZZ Release Right Eustachian Tube, Open Approach
09NF3ZZ Release Right Eustachian Tube, Percutaneous Approach
09NF4ZZ Release Right Eustachian Tube, Percutaneous Endoscopic Approach
09NF7ZZ Release Right Eustachian Tube, Via Natural or Artificial Opening
09NF8ZZ Release Right Eustachian Tube, Via Natural or Artificial Opening Endoscopic
09NG0ZZ Release Left Eustachian Tube, Open Approach
09NG3ZZ Release Left Eustachian Tube, Percutaneous Approach
09NG4ZZ Release Left Eustachian Tube, Percutaneous Endoscopic Approach
09NG7ZZ Release Left Eustachian Tube, Via Natural or Artificial Opening
09NG8ZZ Release Left Eustachian Tube, Via Natural or Artificial Opening Endoscopic
09NK0ZZ Release Nose, Open Approach
09NK3ZZ Release Nose, Percutaneous Approach
09NK4ZZ Release Nose, Percutaneous Endoscopic Approach
09NKXZZ Release Nose, External Approach
09NL0ZZ Release Nasal Turbinate, Open Approach
09NL3ZZ Release Nasal Turbinate, Percutaneous Approach
09NL4ZZ Release Nasal Turbinate, Percutaneous Endoscopic Approach
09NL7ZZ Release Nasal Turbinate, Via Natural or Artificial Opening
09NL8ZZ Release Nasal Turbinate, Via Natural or Artificial Opening Endoscopic
09NM0ZZ Release Nasal Septum, Open Approach
09NM3ZZ Release Nasal Septum, Percutaneous Approach
09NM4ZZ Release Nasal Septum, Percutaneous Endoscopic Approach
09NN0ZZ Release Nasopharynx, Open Approach
09NN3ZZ Release Nasopharynx, Percutaneous Approach
09NN4ZZ Release Nasopharynx, Percutaneous Endoscopic Approach
09NN7ZZ Release Nasopharynx, Via Natural or Artificial Opening
09NN8ZZ Release Nasopharynx, Via Natural or Artificial Opening Endoscopic
09NP0ZZ Release Accessory Sinus, Open Approach
09NP3ZZ Release Accessory Sinus, Percutaneous Approach
09NP4ZZ Release Accessory Sinus, Percutaneous Endoscopic Approach
09NQ0ZZ Release Right Maxillary Sinus, Open Approach
09NQ3ZZ Release Right Maxillary Sinus, Percutaneous Approach
09NQ4ZZ Release Right Maxillary Sinus, Percutaneous Endoscopic Approach
09NR0ZZ Release Left Maxillary Sinus, Open Approach
09NR3ZZ Release Left Maxillary Sinus, Percutaneous Approach
09NR4ZZ Release Left Maxillary Sinus, Percutaneous Endoscopic Approach
09NS0ZZ Release Right Frontal Sinus, Open Approach
09NS3ZZ Release Right Frontal Sinus, Percutane[ous] Approach
09NS4ZZ Release Right Frontal Sinus, Percutane[ous] Endoscopic Approach
09NT0ZZ Release Left Frontal Sinus, Open Approach
09NT3ZZ Release Left Frontal Sinus, Percutaneou[s] Approach
09NT4ZZ Release Left Frontal Sinus, Percutaneou[s] Endoscopic Approach
09NU0ZZ Release Right Ethmoid Sinus, Open Approach
09NU3ZZ Release Right Ethmoid Sinus, Percutaneous Approach
09NU4ZZ Release Right Ethmoid Sinus, Percutaneous Endoscopic Approach
09NV0ZZ Release Left Ethmoid Sinus, Open Approach
09NV3ZZ Release Left Ethmoid Sinus, Percutane[ous] Approach
09NV4ZZ Release Left Ethmoid Sinus, Percutane[ous] Endoscopic Approach
09NW0ZZ Release Right Sphenoid Sinus, Open Approach
09NW3ZZ Release Right Sphenoid Sinus, Percutaneous Approach
09NW4ZZ Release Right Sphenoid Sinus, Percutaneous Endoscopic Approach
09NX0ZZ Release Left Sphenoid Sinus, Open Approach
09NX3ZZ Release Left Sphenoid Sinus, Percutaneous Approach
09NX4ZZ Release Left Sphenoid Sinus, Percutaneous Endoscopic Approach

09P – Ear, Nose, Sinus, Removal

Review Coding Guideline B6.1c

09P700Z Removal of Drainage Device from Right Tympanic Membrane, Open Approach
09P770Z Removal of Drainage Device from Right Tympanic Membrane, Via Natural or Artificial Opening
09P780Z Removal of Drainage Device from Right Tympanic Membrane, Via Natural or Artificial Opening Endoscopic
09P7X0Z Removal of Drainage Device from Right Tympanic Membrane, External Approach
09P800Z Removal of Drainage Device from Left Tympanic Membrane, Open Approach
09P870Z Removal of Drainage Device from Left Tympanic Membrane, Via Natural or Artificial Opening
09P880Z Removal of Drainage Device from Left Tympanic Membrane, Via Natural or Artificial Opening Endoscopic
09P8X0Z Removal of Drainage Device from Left Tympanic Membrane, External Approach
09PD0SZ Removal of Hearing Device from Right Inner Ear, Open Approach
09PD7SZ Removal of Hearing Device from Right Inner Ear, Via Natural or Artificial Opening
09PD8SZ Removal of Hearing Device from Right Inner Ear, Via Natural or Artificial Opening Endoscopic
09PE0SZ Removal of Hearing Device from Left Inner Ear, Open Approach
09PE7SZ Removal of Hearing Device from Left Inner Ear, Via Natural or Artificial Opening
09PE8SZ Removal of Hearing Device from Left Inner Ear, Via Natural or Artificial Opening Endoscopic
09PH00Z Removal of Drainage Device from Right Ear, Open Approach
09PH07Z Removal of Autologous Tissue Substitute from Right Ear, Open Approach
09PH0DZ Removal of Intraluminal Device from Right Ear, Open Approach
09PH0JZ Removal of Synthetic Substitute from Right Ear, Open Approach
09PH0KZ Removal of Nonautologous Tissue Substitute from Right Ear, Open Approach
09PH30Z Removal of Drainage Device from Right Ear, Percutaneous Approach
09PH37Z Removal of Autologous Tissue Substitute from Right Ear, Percutaneous Approach
09PH3DZ Removal of Intraluminal Device from Right Ear, Percutaneous Approach
09PH3JZ Removal of Synthetic Substitute from Right Ear, Percutaneous Approach
09PH3KZ Removal of Nonautologous Tissue Substitute from Right Ear, Percutaneous Approach
09PH40Z Removal of Drainage Device from Right Ear, Percutaneous Endoscopic Approach
09PH47Z Removal of Autologous Tissue Substitute from Right Ear, Percutaneous Endoscopic Approach
09PH4DZ Removal of Intraluminal Device from Right Ear, Percutaneous Endoscopic Approach
09PH4JZ Removal of Synthetic Substitute from Right Ear, Percutaneous Endoscopic Approach
09PH4KZ Removal of Nonautologous Tissue Substitute from Right Ear, Percutaneous Endoscopic Approach
09PH70Z Removal of Drainage Device from Right Ear, Via Natural or Artificial Opening
09PH77Z Removal of Autologous Tissue Substitute from Right Ear, Via Natural or Artificial Opening
09PH7DZ Removal of Intraluminal Device from Right Ear, Via Natural or Artificial Opening
09PH7JZ Removal of Synthetic Substitute from Right Ear, Via Natural or Artificial Opening
09PH7KZ Removal of Nonautologous Tissue Substitute from Right Ear, Via Natural or Artificial Opening
09PH80Z Removal of Drainage Device from Right Ear, Via Natural or Artificial Opening Endoscopic
09PH87Z Removal of Autologous Tissue Substitute from Right Ear, Via Natural or Artificial Opening Endoscopic
09PH8DZ Removal of Intraluminal Device from Right Ear, Via Natural or Artificial Opening Endoscopic

H8JZ Removal of Synthetic Substitute from Right Ear, Via Natural or Artificial Opening Endoscopic
H8KZ Removal of Nonautologous Tissue Substitute from Right Ear, Via Natural or Artificial Opening Endoscopic
HX0Z Removal of Drainage Device from Right Ear, External Approach
HX7Z Removal of Autologous Tissue Substitute from Right Ear, External Approach
HXDZ Removal of Intraluminal Device from Right Ear, External Approach
HXJZ Removal of Synthetic Substitute from Right Ear, External Approach
PHXKZ Removal of Nonautologous Tissue Substitute from Right Ear, External Approach
PJ00Z Removal of Drainage Device from Left Ear, Open Approach
PJ07Z Removal of Autologous Tissue Substitute from Left Ear, Open Approach
PJ0DZ Removal of Intraluminal Device from Left Ear, Open Approach
PJ0JZ Removal of Synthetic Substitute from Left Ear, Open Approach
PJ0KZ Removal of Nonautologous Tissue Substitute from Left Ear, Open Approach
PJ30Z Removal of Drainage Device from Left Ear, Percutaneous Approach
PJ37Z Removal of Autologous Tissue Substitute from Left Ear, Percutaneous Approach
PJ3DZ Removal of Intraluminal Device from Left Ear, Percutaneous Approach
PJ3JZ Removal of Synthetic Substitute from Left Ear, Percutaneous Approach
PJ3KZ Removal of Nonautologous Tissue Substitute from Left Ear, Percutaneous Approach
PJ40Z Removal of Drainage Device from Left Ear, Percutaneous Endoscopic Approach
PJ47Z Removal of Autologous Tissue Substitute from Left Ear, Percutaneous Endoscopic Approach
PJ4DZ Removal of Intraluminal Device from Left Ear, Percutaneous Endoscopic Approach
PJ4JZ Removal of Synthetic Substitute from Left Ear, Percutaneous Endoscopic Approach
PJ4KZ Removal of Nonautologous Tissue Substitute from Left Ear, Percutaneous Endoscopic Approach
PJ70Z Removal of Drainage Device from Left Ear, Via Natural or Artificial Opening
PJ77Z Removal of Autologous Tissue Substitute from Left Ear, Via Natural or Artificial Opening
09PJ7DZ Removal of Intraluminal Device from Left Ear, Via Natural or Artificial Opening
09PJ7JZ Removal of Synthetic Substitute from Left Ear, Via Natural or Artificial Opening
09PJ7KZ Removal of Nonautologous Tissue Substitute from Left Ear, Via Natural or Artificial Opening
09PJ80Z Removal of Drainage Device from Left Ear, Via Natural or Artificial Opening Endoscopic
09PJ87Z Removal of Autologous Tissue Substitute from Left Ear, Via Natural or Artificial Opening Endoscopic
09PJ8DZ Removal of Intraluminal Device from Left Ear, Via Natural or Artificial Opening Endoscopic
09PJ8JZ Removal of Synthetic Substitute from Left Ear, Via Natural or Artificial Opening Endoscopic
09PJ8KZ Removal of Nonautologous Tissue Substitute from Left Ear, Via Natural or Artificial Opening Endoscopic
09PJX0Z Removal of Drainage Device from Left Ear, External Approach
09PJX7Z Removal of Autologous Tissue Substitute from Left Ear, External Approach
09PJXDZ Removal of Intraluminal Device from Left Ear, External Approach
09PJXJZ Removal of Synthetic Substitute from Left Ear, External Approach
09PJXKZ Removal of Nonautologous Tissue Substitute from Left Ear, External Approach
09PK00Z Removal of Drainage Device from Nose, Open Approach
09PK07Z Removal of Autologous Tissue Substitute from Nose, Open Approach
09PK0DZ Removal of Intraluminal Device from Nose, Open Approach
09PK0JZ Removal of Synthetic Substitute from Nose, Open Approach
09PK0KZ Removal of Nonautologous Tissue Substitute from Nose, Open Approach
09PK30Z Removal of Drainage Device from Nose, Percutaneous Approach
09PK37Z Removal of Autologous Tissue Substitute from Nose, Percutaneous Approach
09PK3DZ Removal of Intraluminal Device from Nose, Percutaneous Approach
09PK3JZ Removal of Synthetic Substitute from Nose, Percutaneous Approach
09PK3KZ Removal of Nonautologous Tissue Substitute from Nose, Percutaneous Approach
09PK40Z Removal of Drainage Device from Nose, Percutaneous Endoscopic Approach
09PK47Z Removal of Autologous Tissue Substitute from Nose, Percutaneous Endoscopic Approach
09PK4DZ Removal of Intraluminal Device from Nose, Percutaneous Endoscopic Approach
09PK4JZ Removal of Synthetic Substitute from Nose, Percutaneous Endoscopic Approach
09PK4KZ Removal of Nonautologous Tissue Substitute from Nose, Percutaneous Endoscopic Approach
09PK70Z Removal of Drainage Device from Nose, Via Natural or Artificial Opening
09PK77Z Removal of Autologous Tissue Substitute from Nose, Via Natural or Artificial Opening
09PK7DZ Removal of Intraluminal Device from Nose, Via Natural or Artificial Opening
09PK7JZ Removal of Synthetic Substitute from Nose, Via Natural or Artificial Opening
09PK7KZ Removal of Nonautologous Tissue Substitute from Nose, Via Natural or Artificial Opening
09PK80Z Removal of Drainage Device from Nose, Via Natural or Artificial Opening Endoscopic
09PK87Z Removal of Autologous Tissue Substitute from Nose, Via Natural or Artificial Opening Endoscopic
09PK8DZ Removal of Intraluminal Device from Nose, Via Natural or Artificial Opening Endoscopic
09PK8JZ Removal of Synthetic Substitute from Nose, Via Natural or Artificial Opening Endoscopic
09PK8KZ Removal of Nonautologous Tissue Substitute from Nose, Via Natural or Artificial Opening Endoscopic
09PKX0Z Removal of Drainage Device from Nose, External Approach
09PKX7Z Removal of Autologous Tissue Substitute from Nose, External Approach
09PKXDZ Removal of Intraluminal Device from Nose, External Approach
09PKXJZ Removal of Synthetic Substitute from Nose, External Approach
09PKXKZ Removal of Nonautologous Tissue Substitute from Nose, External Approach
09PY00Z Removal of Drainage Device from Sinus, Open Approach
09PY30Z Removal of Drainage Device from Sinus, Percutaneous Approach
09PY40Z Removal of Drainage Device from Sinus, Percutaneous Endoscopic Approach
09PYX0Z Removal of Drainage Device from Sinus, External Approach

9Q – Ear, Nose, Sinus, Repair

9Q00ZZ Repair Right External Ear, Open Approach
9Q03ZZ Repair Right External Ear, Percutaneous Approach
9Q04ZZ Repair Right External Ear, Percutaneous Endoscopic Approach
9Q0XZZ Repair Right External Ear, External Approach
9Q10ZZ Repair Left External Ear, Open Approach
9Q13ZZ Repair Left External Ear, Percutaneous Approach
9Q14ZZ Repair Left External Ear, Percutaneous Endoscopic Approach
9Q1XZZ Repair Left External Ear, External Approach
9Q20ZZ Repair Bilateral External Ear, Open Approach
9Q23ZZ Repair Bilateral External Ear, Percutaneous Approach
09Q24ZZ Repair Bilateral External Ear, Percutaneous Endoscopic Approach
09Q2XZZ Repair Bilateral External Ear, External Approach
09Q30ZZ Repair Right External Auditory Canal, Open Approach
09Q33ZZ Repair Right External Auditory Canal, Percutaneous Approach
09Q34ZZ Repair Right External Auditory Canal, Percutaneous Endoscopic Approach
09Q37ZZ Repair Right External Auditory Canal, Via Natural or Artificial Opening
09Q38ZZ Repair Right External Auditory Canal, Via Natural or Artificial Opening Endoscopic
09Q3XZZ Repair Right External Auditory Canal, External Approach
09Q40ZZ Repair Left External Auditory Canal, Open Approach
09Q43ZZ Repair Left External Auditory Canal, Percutaneous Approach
09Q44ZZ Repair Left External Auditory Canal, Percutaneous Endoscopic Approach
09Q47ZZ Repair Left External Auditory Canal, Via Natural or Artificial Opening
09Q48ZZ Repair Left External Auditory Canal, Via Natural or Artificial Opening Endoscopic
09Q4XZZ Repair Left External Auditory Canal, External Approach
09Q50ZZ Repair Right Middle Ear, Open Approach
09Q60ZZ Repair Left Middle Ear, Open Approach
09Q70ZZ Repair Right Tympanic Membrane, Open Approach
09Q73ZZ Repair Right Tympanic Membrane, Percutaneous Approach

09Q74ZZ Repair Right Tympanic Membrane, Percutaneous Endoscopic Approach
09Q77ZZ Repair Right Tympanic Membrane, Via Natural or Artificial Opening
09Q78ZZ Repair Right Tympanic Membrane, Via Natural or Artificial Opening Endoscopic
09Q80ZZ Repair Left Tympanic Membrane, Open Approach
09Q83ZZ Repair Left Tympanic Membrane, Percutaneous Approach
09Q84ZZ Repair Left Tympanic Membrane, Percutaneous Endoscopic Approach
09Q87ZZ Repair Left Tympanic Membrane, Via Natural or Artificial Opening
09Q88ZZ Repair Left Tympanic Membrane, Via Natural or Artificial Opening Endoscopic
09Q90ZZ Repair Right Auditory Ossicle, Open Approach
09QA0ZZ Repair Left Auditory Ossicle, Open Approach
09QB0ZZ Repair Right Mastoid Sinus, Open Approach
09QB3ZZ Repair Right Mastoid Sinus, Percutaneous Approach
09QB4ZZ Repair Right Mastoid Sinus, Percutaneous Endoscopic Approach
09QC0ZZ Repair Left Mastoid Sinus, Open Approach
09QC3ZZ Repair Left Mastoid Sinus, Percutaneous Approach
09QC4ZZ Repair Left Mastoid Sinus, Percutaneous Endoscopic Approach
09QD0ZZ Repair Right Inner Ear, Open Approach
09QE0ZZ Repair Left Inner Ear, Open Approach
09QF0ZZ Repair Right Eustachian Tube, Open Approach
09QF3ZZ Repair Right Eustachian Tube, Percutaneous Approach
09QF4ZZ Repair Right Eustachian Tube, Percutaneous Endoscopic Approach
09QF7ZZ Repair Right Eustachian Tube, Via Natural or Artificial Opening
09QF8ZZ Repair Right Eustachian Tube, Via Natural or Artificial Opening Endoscopic
09QFXZZ Repair Right Eustachian Tube, External Approach
09QG0ZZ Repair Left Eustachian Tube, Open Approach
09QG3ZZ Repair Left Eustachian Tube, Percutaneous Approach
09QG4ZZ Repair Left Eustachian Tube, Percutaneous Endoscopic Approach
09QG7ZZ Repair Left Eustachian Tube, Via Natural or Artificial Opening
09QG8ZZ Repair Left Eustachian Tube, Via Natural or Artificial Opening Endoscopic
09QGXZZ Repair Left Eustachian Tube, External Approach
09QK0ZZ Repair Nose, Open Approach
09QK3ZZ Repair Nose, Percutaneous Approach
09QK4ZZ Repair Nose, Percutaneous Endoscopic Approach
09QKXZZ Repair Nose, External Approach
09QL0ZZ Repair Nasal Turbinate, Open Approach
09QL3ZZ Repair Nasal Turbinate, Percutaneous Approach
09QL4ZZ Repair Nasal Turbinate, Percutaneous Endoscopic Approach
09QL7ZZ Repair Nasal Turbinate, Via Natural or Artificial Opening
09QL8ZZ Repair Nasal Turbinate, Via Natural or Artificial Opening Endoscopic
09QM0ZZ Repair Nasal Septum, Open Approach
09QM3ZZ Repair Nasal Septum, Percutaneous Approach
09QM4ZZ Repair Nasal Septum, Percutaneous Endoscopic Approach
09QN0ZZ Repair Nasopharynx, Open Approach
09QN3ZZ Repair Nasopharynx, Percutaneous Approach
09QN4ZZ Repair Nasopharynx, Percutaneous Endoscopic Approach
09QN7ZZ Repair Nasopharynx, Via Natural or Artificial Opening
09QN8ZZ Repair Nasopharynx, Via Natural or Artificial Opening Endoscopic
09QP0ZZ Repair Accessory Sinus, Open Approach
09QP3ZZ Repair Accessory Sinus, Percutaneous Approach
09QP4ZZ Repair Accessory Sinus, Percutaneous Endoscopic Approach
09QQ0ZZ Repair Right Maxillary Sinus, Open Approach
09QQ3ZZ Repair Right Maxillary Sinus, Percutaneous Approach
09QQ4ZZ Repair Right Maxillary Sinus, Percutaneous Endoscopic Approach
09QR0ZZ Repair Left Maxillary Sinus, Open Approach
09QR3ZZ Repair Left Maxillary Sinus, Percutaneous Approach
09QR4ZZ Repair Left Maxillary Sinus, Percutaneous Endoscopic Approach
09QS0ZZ Repair Right Frontal Sinus, Open Approach
09QS3ZZ Repair Right Frontal Sinus, Percutaneous Approach
09QS4ZZ Repair Right Frontal Sinus, Percutaneous Endoscopic Approach
09QT0ZZ Repair Left Frontal Sinus, Open Approach
09QT3ZZ Repair Left Frontal Sinus, Percutaneous Approach
09QT4ZZ Repair Left Frontal Sinus, Percutaneous Endoscopic Approach
AHA CC: 4Q, 2013, 114
09QU0ZZ Repair Right Ethmoid Sinus, Open Approach
09QU3ZZ Repair Right Ethmoid Sinus, Percutaneous Approach
09QU4ZZ Repair Right Ethmoid Sinus, Percutaneous Endoscopic Approach
09QV0ZZ Repair Left Ethmoid Sinus, Open Approach
09QV3ZZ Repair Left Ethmoid Sinus, Percutaneous Approach
09QV4ZZ Repair Left Ethmoid Sinus, Percutaneous Endoscopic Approach
09QW0ZZ Repair Right Sphenoid Sinus, Open Approach
09QW3ZZ Repair Right Sphenoid Sinus, Percutaneous Approach
09QW4ZZ Repair Right Sphenoid Sinus, Percutaneous Endoscopic Approach
09QX0ZZ Repair Left Sphenoid Sinus, Open Approach
09QX3ZZ Repair Left Sphenoid Sinus, Percutaneous Approach
09QX4ZZ Repair Left Sphenoid Sinus, Percutaneous Endoscopic Approach

09R – Ear, Nose, Sinus, Replacement

09R007Z Replacement of Right External Ear with Autologous Tissue Substitute, Open Approach
09R00JZ Replacement of Right External Ear with Synthetic Substitute, Open Approach
09R00KZ Replacement of Right External Ear with Nonautologous Tissue Substitute, Open Approach
09R0X7Z Replacement of Right External Ear with Autologous Tissue Substitute, External Approach
09R0XJZ Replacement of Right External Ear with Synthetic Substitute, External Approach
09R0XKZ Replacement of Right External Ear with Nonautologous Tissue Substitute, External Approach
09R107Z Replacement of Left External Ear with Autologous Tissue Substitute, Open Approach
09R10JZ Replacement of Left External Ear with Synthetic Substitute, Open Approach
09R10KZ Replacement of Left External Ear with Nonautologous Tissue Substitute, Open Approach
09R1X7Z Replacement of Left External Ear with Autologous Tissue Substitute, External Approach
09R1XJZ Replacement of Left External Ear with Synthetic Substitute, External Approach
09R1XKZ Replacement of Left External Ear with Nonautologous Tissue Substitute, External Approach
09R207Z Replacement of Bilateral External Ear with Autologous Tissue Substitute, Open Approach
09R20JZ Replacement of Bilateral External Ear with Synthetic Substitute, Open Approach
09R20KZ Replacement of Bilateral External Ear with Nonautologous Tissue Substitute, Open Approach
09R2X7Z Replacement of Bilateral External Ear with Autologous Tissue Substitute, External Approach
09R2XJZ Replacement of Bilateral External Ear with Synthetic Substitute, External Approach
09R2XKZ Replacement of Bilateral External Ear with Nonautologous Tissue Substitute, External Approach
09R507Z Replacement of Right Middle Ear with Autologous Tissue Substitute, Open Approach
09R50JZ Replacement of Right Middle Ear with Synthetic Substitute, Open Approach
09R50KZ Replacement of Right Middle Ear with Nonautologous Tissue Substitute, Open Approach
09R607Z Replacement of Left Middle Ear with Autologous Tissue Substitute, Open Approach
09R60JZ Replacement of Left Middle Ear with Synthetic Substitute, Open Approach
09R60KZ Replacement of Left Middle Ear with Nonautologous Tissue Substitute, Open Approach
09R707Z Replacement of Right Tympanic Membrane with Autologous Tissue Substitute, Open Approach
09R70JZ Replacement of Right Tympanic Membrane with Synthetic Substitute, Open Approach
09R70KZ Replacement of Right Tympanic Membrane with Nonautologous Tissue Substitute, Open Approach

R777Z Replacement of Right Tympanic Membrane with Autologous Tissue Substitute, Via Natural or Artificial Opening
R77JZ Replacement of Right Tympanic Membrane with Synthetic Substitute, Via Natural or Artificial Opening
R77KZ Replacement of Right Tympanic Membrane with Nonautologous Tissue Substitute, Via Natural or Artificial Opening
R787Z Replacement of Right Tympanic Membrane with Autologous Tissue Substitute, Via Natural or Artificial Opening Endoscopic
R78JZ Replacement of Right Tympanic Membrane with Synthetic Substitute, Via Natural or Artificial Opening Endoscopic
R78KZ Replacement of Right Tympanic Membrane with Nonautologous Tissue Substitute, Via Natural or Artificial Opening Endoscopic
R807Z Replacement of Left Tympanic Membrane with Autologous Tissue Substitute, Open Approach
R80JZ Replacement of Left Tympanic Membrane with Synthetic Substitute, Open Approach
R80KZ Replacement of Left Tympanic Membrane with Nonautologous Tissue Substitute, Open Approach
R877Z Replacement of Left Tympanic Membrane with Autologous Tissue Substitute, Via Natural or Artificial Opening
R87JZ Replacement of Left Tympanic Membrane with Synthetic Substitute, Via Natural or Artificial Opening
R87KZ Replacement of Left Tympanic Membrane with Nonautologous Tissue Substitute, Via Natural or Artificial Opening
R887Z Replacement of Left Tympanic Membrane with Autologous Tissue Substitute, Via Natural or Artificial Opening Endoscopic
R88JZ Replacement of Left Tympanic Membrane with Synthetic Substitute, Via Natural or Artificial Opening Endoscopic
R88KZ Replacement of Left Tympanic Membrane with Nonautologous Tissue Substitute, Via Natural or Artificial Opening Endoscopic
R907Z Replacement of Right Auditory Ossicle with Autologous Tissue Substitute, Open Approach
9R90JZ Replacement of Right Auditory Ossicle with Synthetic Substitute, Open Approach
9R90KZ Replacement of Right Auditory Ossicle with Nonautologous Tissue Substitute, Open Approach
9RA07Z Replacement of Left Auditory Ossicle with Autologous Tissue Substitute, Open Approach
9RA0JZ Replacement of Left Auditory Ossicle with Synthetic Substitute, Open Approach
9RA0KZ Replacement of Left Auditory Ossicle with Nonautologous Tissue Substitute, Open Approach
09RD07Z Replacement of Right Inner Ear with Autologous Tissue Substitute, Open Approach
09RD0JZ Replacement of Right Inner Ear with Synthetic Substitute, Open Approach
09RD0KZ Replacement of Right Inner Ear with Nonautologous Tissue Substitute, Open Approach
09RE07Z Replacement of Left Inner Ear with Autologous Tissue Substitute, Open Approach
09RE0JZ Replacement of Left Inner Ear with Synthetic Substitute, Open Approach
09RE0KZ Replacement of Left Inner Ear with Nonautologous Tissue Substitute, Open Approach
09RK07Z Replacement of Nose with Autologous Tissue Substitute, Open Approach
09RK0JZ Replacement of Nose with Synthetic Substitute, Open Approach
09RK0KZ Replacement of Nose with Nonautologous Tissue Substitute, Open Approach
09RKX7Z Replacement of Nose with Autologous Tissue Substitute, External Approach
09RKXJZ Replacement of Nose with Synthetic Substitute, External Approach
09RKXKZ Replacement of Nose with Nonautologous Tissue Substitute, External Approach
09RL07Z Replacement of Nasal Turbinate with Autologous Tissue Substitute, Open Approach
09RL0JZ Replacement of Nasal Turbinate with Synthetic Substitute, Open Approach
09RL0KZ Replacement of Nasal Turbinate with Nonautologous Tissue Substitute, Open Approach
09RL37Z Replacement of Nasal Turbinate with Autologous Tissue Substitute, Percutaneous Approach
09RL3JZ Replacement of Nasal Turbinate with Synthetic Substitute, Percutaneous Approach
09RL3KZ Replacement of Nasal Turbinate with Nonautologous Tissue Substitute, Percutaneous Approach
09RL47Z Replacement of Nasal Turbinate with Autologous Tissue Substitute, Percutaneous Endoscopic Approach
09RL4JZ Replacement of Nasal Turbinate with Synthetic Substitute, Percutaneous Endoscopic Approach
09RL4KZ Replacement of Nasal Turbinate with Nonautologous Tissue Substitute, Percutaneous Endoscopic Approach
09RL77Z Replacement of Nasal Turbinate with Autologous Tissue Substitute, Via Natural or Artificial Opening
09RL7JZ Replacement of Nasal Turbinate with Synthetic Substitute, Via Natural or Artificial Opening
09RL7KZ Replacement of Nasal Turbinate with Nonautologous Tissue Substitute, Via Natural or Artificial Opening
09RL87Z Replacement of Nasal Turbinate with Autologous Tissue Substitute, Via Natural or Artificial Opening Endoscopic
09RL8JZ Replacement of Nasal Turbinate with Synthetic Substitute, Via Natural or Artificial Opening Endoscopic
09RL8KZ Replacement of Nasal Turbinate with Nonautologous Tissue Substitute, Via Natural or Artificial Opening Endoscopic
09RM07Z Replacement of Nasal Septum with Autologous Tissue Substitute, Open Approach
09RM0JZ Replacement of Nasal Septum with Synthetic Substitute, Open Approach
09RM0KZ Replacement of Nasal Septum with Nonautologous Tissue Substitute, Open Approach
09RM37Z Replacement of Nasal Septum with Autologous Tissue Substitute, Percutaneous Approach
09RM3JZ Replacement of Nasal Septum with Synthetic Substitute, Percutaneous Approach
09RM3KZ Replacement of Nasal Septum with Nonautologous Tissue Substitute, Percutaneous Approach
09RM47Z Replacement of Nasal Septum with Autologous Tissue Substitute, Percutaneous Endoscopic Approach
09RM4JZ Replacement of Nasal Septum with Synthetic Substitute, Percutaneous Endoscopic Approach
09RM4KZ Replacement of Nasal Septum with Nonautologous Tissue Substitute, Percutaneous Endoscopic Approach
09RN07Z Replacement of Nasopharynx with Autologous Tissue Substitute, Open Approach
09RN0JZ Replacement of Nasopharynx with Synthetic Substitute, Open Approach
09RN0KZ Replacement of Nasopharynx with Nonautologous Tissue Substitute, Open Approach
09RN77Z Replacement of Nasopharynx with Autologous Tissue Substitute, Via Natural or Artificial Opening
09RN7JZ Replacement of Nasopharynx with Synthetic Substitute, Via Natural or Artificial Opening
09RN7KZ Replacement of Nasopharynx with Nonautologous Tissue Substitute, Via Natural or Artificial Opening
09RN87Z Replacement of Nasopharynx with Autologous Tissue Substitute, Via Natural or Artificial Opening Endoscopic
09RN8JZ Replacement of Nasopharynx with Synthetic Substitute, Via Natural or Artificial Opening Endoscopic
09RN8KZ Replacement of Nasopharynx with Nonautologous Tissue Substitute, Via Natural or Artificial Opening Endoscopic

9S – Ear, Nose, Sinus, Reposition

9S00ZZ Reposition Right External Ear, Open Approach
9S04ZZ Reposition Right External Ear, Percutaneous Endoscopic Approach
9S0XZZ Reposition Right External Ear, External Approach
9S10ZZ Reposition Left External Ear, Open Approach
9S14ZZ Reposition Left External Ear, Percutaneous Endoscopic Approach
09S1XZZ Reposition Left External Ear, External Approach
09S20ZZ Reposition Bilateral External Ear, Open Approach
09S24ZZ Reposition Bilateral External Ear, Percutaneous Endoscopic Approach
09S2XZZ Reposition Bilateral External Ear, External Approach
09S70ZZ Reposition Right Tympanic Membrane, Open Approach
09S74ZZ Reposition Right Tympanic Membrane, Percutaneous Endoscopic Approach
09S77ZZ Reposition Right Tympanic Membrane, Via Natural or Artificial Opening
09S78ZZ Reposition Right Tympanic Membrane, Via Natural or Artificial Opening Endoscopic
09S80ZZ Reposition Left Tympanic Membrane, Open Approach

09S84ZZ Reposition Left Tympanic Membrane, Percutaneous Endoscopic Approach
09S87ZZ Reposition Left Tympanic Membrane, Via Natural or Artificial Opening
09S88ZZ Reposition Left Tympanic Membrane, Via Natural or Artificial Opening Endoscopic
09S90ZZ Reposition Right Auditory Ossicle, Open Approach
09S94ZZ Reposition Right Auditory Ossicle, Percutaneous Endoscopic Approach
09SA0ZZ Reposition Left Auditory Ossicle, Open Approach
09SA4ZZ Reposition Left Auditory Ossicle, Percutaneous Endoscopic Approach
09SF0ZZ Reposition Right Eustachian Tube, Open Approach
09SF4ZZ Reposition Right Eustachian Tube, Percutaneous Endoscopic Approach
09SF7ZZ Reposition Right Eustachian Tube, Via Natural or Artificial Opening
09SF8ZZ Reposition Right Eustachian Tube, Via Natural or Artificial Opening Endoscopic
09SG0ZZ Reposition Left Eustachian Tube, Open Approach
09SG4ZZ Reposition Left Eustachian Tube, Percutaneous Endoscopic Approach
09SG7ZZ Reposition Left Eustachian Tube, Via Natural or Artificial Opening
09SG8ZZ Reposition Left Eustachian Tube, Via Natural or Artificial Opening Endoscopic
09SK0ZZ Reposition Nose, Open Approach
09SK4ZZ Reposition Nose, Percutaneous Endoscopic Approach
09SKXZZ Reposition Nose, External Approach
09SL0ZZ Reposition Nasal Turbinate, Open Approach
09SL4ZZ Reposition Nasal Turbinate, Percutaneo[us] Endoscopic Approach
09SL7ZZ Reposition Nasal Turbinate, Via Natural [or] Artificial Opening
09SL8ZZ Reposition Nasal Turbinate, Via Natural [or] Artificial Opening Endoscopic
09SM0ZZ Reposition Nasal Septum, Open Approa[ch]
09SM4ZZ Reposition Nasal Septum, Percutaneous Endoscopic Approach

09T – Ear, Nose, Sinus, Resection

Review Coding Guideline B3.8

09T00ZZ Resection of Right External Ear, Open Approach
09T04ZZ Resection of Right External Ear, Percutaneous Endoscopic Approach
09T0XZZ Resection of Right External Ear, External Approach
09T10ZZ Resection of Left External Ear, Open Approach
09T14ZZ Resection of Left External Ear, Percutaneous Endoscopic Approach
09T1XZZ Resection of Left External Ear, External Approach
09T50ZZ Resection of Right Middle Ear, Open Approach
09T60ZZ Resection of Left Middle Ear, Open Approach
09T70ZZ Resection of Right Tympanic Membrane, Open Approach
09T74ZZ Resection of Right Tympanic Membrane, Percutaneous Endoscopic Approach
09T77ZZ Resection of Right Tympanic Membrane, Via Natural or Artificial Opening
09T78ZZ Resection of Right Tympanic Membrane, Via Natural or Artificial Opening Endoscopic
09T80ZZ Resection of Left Tympanic Membrane, Open Approach
09T84ZZ Resection of Left Tympanic Membrane, Percutaneous Endoscopic Approach
09T87ZZ Resection of Left Tympanic Membrane, Via Natural or Artificial Opening
09T88ZZ Resection of Left Tympanic Membrane, Via Natural or Artificial Opening Endoscopic
09T90ZZ Resection of Right Auditory Ossicle, Open Approach
09TA0ZZ Resection of Left Auditory Ossicle, Open Approach
09TB0ZZ Resection of Right Mastoid Sinus, Open Approach
09TB4ZZ Resection of Right Mastoid Sinus, Percutaneous Endoscopic Approach
09TC0ZZ Resection of Left Mastoid Sinus, Open Approach
09TC4ZZ Resection of Left Mastoid Sinus, Percutaneous Endoscopic Approach
09TD0ZZ Resection of Right Inner Ear, Open Approach
09TE0ZZ Resection of Left Inner Ear, Open Approach
09TF0ZZ Resection of Right Eustachian Tube, Open Approach
09TF4ZZ Resection of Right Eustachian Tube, Percutaneous Endoscopic Approach
09TF7ZZ Resection of Right Eustachian Tube, Via Natural or Artificial Opening
09TF8ZZ Resection of Right Eustachian Tube, Via Natural or Artificial Opening Endoscopic
09TG0ZZ Resection of Left Eustachian Tube, Open Approach
09TG4ZZ Resection of Left Eustachian Tube, Percutaneous Endoscopic Approach
09TG7ZZ Resection of Left Eustachian Tube, Via Natural or Artificial Opening
09TG8ZZ Resection of Left Eustachian Tube, Via Natural or Artificial Opening Endoscopic
09TK0ZZ Resection of Nose, Open Approach
09TK4ZZ Resection of Nose, Percutaneous Endoscopic Approach
09TKXZZ Resection of Nose, External Approach
09TL0ZZ Resection of Nasal Turbinate, Open Approach
09TL4ZZ Resection of Nasal Turbinate, Percutaneous Endoscopic Approach
09TL7ZZ Resection of Nasal Turbinate, Via Natural or Artificial Opening
09TL8ZZ Resection of Nasal Turbinate, Via Natural or Artificial Opening Endoscopic
09TM0ZZ Resection of Nasal Septum, Open Approach
09TM4ZZ Resection of Nasal Septum, Percutaneous Endoscopic Approach
09TN0ZZ Resection of Nasopharynx, Open Approach
09TN4ZZ Resection of Nasopharynx, Percutaneous Endoscopic Approach
09TN7ZZ Resection of Nasopharynx, Via Natural o[r] Artificial Opening
09TN8ZZ Resection of Nasopharynx, Via Natural o[r] Artificial Opening Endoscopic
09TP0ZZ Resection of Accessory Sinus, Open Approach
09TP4ZZ Resection of Accessory Sinus, Percutaneous Endoscopic Approach
09TQ0ZZ Resection of Right Maxillary Sinus, Ope[n] Approach
09TQ4ZZ Resection of Right Maxillary Sinus, Percutaneous Endoscopic Approach
09TR0ZZ Resection of Left Maxillary Sinus, Open Approach
09TR4ZZ Resection of Left Maxillary Sinus, Percutaneous Endoscopic Approach
09TS0ZZ Resection of Right Frontal Sinus, Open Approach
09TS4ZZ Resection of Right Frontal Sinus, Percutaneous Endoscopic Approach
09TT0ZZ Resection of Left Frontal Sinus, Open Approach
09TT4ZZ Resection of Left Frontal Sinus, Percutaneous Endoscopic Approach
09TU0ZZ Resection of Right Ethmoid Sinus, Open Approach
09TU4ZZ Resection of Right Ethmoid Sinus, Percutaneous Endoscopic Approach
09TV0ZZ Resection of Left Ethmoid Sinus, Open Approach
09TV4ZZ Resection of Left Ethmoid Sinus, Percutaneous Endoscopic Approach
09TW0ZZ Resection of Right Sphenoid Sinus, Open Approach
09TW4ZZ Resection of Right Sphenoid Sinus, Percutaneous Endoscopic Approach
09TX0ZZ Resection of Left Sphenoid Sinus, Open Approach
09TX4ZZ Resection of Left Sphenoid Sinus, Percutaneous Endoscopic Approach

09U – Ear, Nose, Sinus, Supplement

09U007Z Supplement Right External Ear with Autologous Tissue Substitute, Open Approach
09U00JZ Supplement Right External Ear with Synthetic Substitute, Open Approach
09U00KZ Supplement Right External Ear with Nonautologous Tissue Substitute, Open Approach
09U0X7Z Supplement Right External Ear with Autologous Tissue Substitute, External Approach
09U0XJZ Supplement Right External Ear with Synthetic Substitute, External Approach
09U0XKZ Supplement Right External Ear with Nonautologous Tissue Substitute, External Approach
09U107Z Supplement Left External Ear with Autologous Tissue Substitute, Open Approach
09U10JZ Supplement Left External Ear with Synthetic Substitute, Open Approach
09U10KZ Supplement Left External Ear with Nonautologous Tissue Substitute, Open Approach
09U1X7Z Supplement Left External Ear with Autologous Tissue Substitute, External Approach
09U1XJZ Supplement Left External Ear with Synthetic Substitute, External Approach
09U1XKZ Supplement Left External Ear with Nonautologous Tissue Substitute, External Approach

J207Z Supplement Bilateral External Ear with Autologous Tissue Substitute, Open Approach
J20JZ Supplement Bilateral External Ear with Synthetic Substitute, Open Approach
J20KZ Supplement Bilateral External Ear with Nonautologous Tissue Substitute, Open Approach
J2X7Z Supplement Bilateral External Ear with Autologous Tissue Substitute, External Approach
J2XJZ Supplement Bilateral External Ear with Synthetic Substitute, External Approach
U2XKZ Supplement Bilateral External Ear with Nonautologous Tissue Substitute, External Approach
U507Z Supplement Right Middle Ear with Autologous Tissue Substitute, Open Approach
U50JZ Supplement Right Middle Ear with Synthetic Substitute, Open Approach
U50KZ Supplement Right Middle Ear with Nonautologous Tissue Substitute, Open Approach
U607Z Supplement Left Middle Ear with Autologous Tissue Substitute, Open Approach
U60JZ Supplement Left Middle Ear with Synthetic Substitute, Open Approach
U60KZ Supplement Left Middle Ear with Nonautologous Tissue Substitute, Open Approach
U707Z Supplement Right Tympanic Membrane with Autologous Tissue Substitute, Open Approach
U70JZ Supplement Right Tympanic Membrane with Synthetic Substitute, Open Approach
U70KZ Supplement Right Tympanic Membrane with Nonautologous Tissue Substitute, Open Approach
U777Z Supplement Right Tympanic Membrane with Autologous Tissue Substitute, Via Natural or Artificial Opening
U77JZ Supplement Right Tympanic Membrane with Synthetic Substitute, Via Natural or Artificial Opening
U77KZ Supplement Right Tympanic Membrane with Nonautologous Tissue Substitute, Via Natural or Artificial Opening
U787Z Supplement Right Tympanic Membrane with Autologous Tissue Substitute, Via Natural or Artificial Opening Endoscopic
9U78JZ Supplement Right Tympanic Membrane with Synthetic Substitute, Via Natural or Artificial Opening Endoscopic
9U78KZ Supplement Right Tympanic Membrane with Nonautologous Tissue Substitute, Via Natural or Artificial Opening Endoscopic
9U807Z Supplement Left Tympanic Membrane with Autologous Tissue Substitute, Open Approach
9U80JZ Supplement Left Tympanic Membrane with Synthetic Substitute, Open Approach
9U80KZ Supplement Left Tympanic Membrane with Nonautologous Tissue Substitute, Open Approach
9U877Z Supplement Left Tympanic Membrane with Autologous Tissue Substitute, Via Natural or Artificial Opening
9U87JZ Supplement Left Tympanic Membrane with Synthetic Substitute, Via Natural or Artificial Opening
9U87KZ Supplement Left Tympanic Membrane with Nonautologous Tissue Substitute, Via Natural or Artificial Opening

09U887Z Supplement Left Tympanic Membrane with Autologous Tissue Substitute, Via Natural or Artificial Opening Endoscopic
09U88JZ Supplement Left Tympanic Membrane with Synthetic Substitute, Via Natural or Artificial Opening Endoscopic
09U88KZ Supplement Left Tympanic Membrane with Nonautologous Tissue Substitute, Via Natural or Artificial Opening Endoscopic
09U907Z Supplement Right Auditory Ossicle with Autologous Tissue Substitute, Open Approach
09U90JZ Supplement Right Auditory Ossicle with Synthetic Substitute, Open Approach
09U90KZ Supplement Right Auditory Ossicle with Nonautologous Tissue Substitute, Open Approach
09UA07Z Supplement Left Auditory Ossicle with Autologous Tissue Substitute, Open Approach
09UA0JZ Supplement Left Auditory Ossicle with Synthetic Substitute, Open Approach
09UA0KZ Supplement Left Auditory Ossicle with Nonautologous Tissue Substitute, Open Approach
09UD07Z Supplement Right Inner Ear with Autologous Tissue Substitute, Open Approach
09UD0JZ Supplement Right Inner Ear with Synthetic Substitute, Open Approach
09UD0KZ Supplement Right Inner Ear with Nonautologous Tissue Substitute, Open Approach
09UE07Z Supplement Left Inner Ear with Autologous Tissue Substitute, Open Approach
09UE0JZ Supplement Left Inner Ear with Synthetic Substitute, Open Approach
09UE0KZ Supplement Left Inner Ear with Nonautologous Tissue Substitute, Open Approach
09UK07Z Supplement Nose with Autologous Tissue Substitute, Open Approach
09UK0JZ Supplement Nose with Synthetic Substitute, Open Approach
09UK0KZ Supplement Nose with Nonautologous Tissue Substitute, Open Approach
09UKX7Z Supplement Nose with Autologous Tissue Substitute, External Approach
09UKXJZ Supplement Nose with Synthetic Substitute, External Approach
09UKXKZ Supplement Nose with Nonautologous Tissue Substitute, External Approach
09UL07Z Supplement Nasal Turbinate with Autologous Tissue Substitute, Open Approach
09UL0JZ Supplement Nasal Turbinate with Synthetic Substitute, Open Approach
09UL0KZ Supplement Nasal Turbinate with Nonautologous Tissue Substitute, Open Approach
09UL37Z Supplement Nasal Turbinate with Autologous Tissue Substitute, Percutaneous Approach
09UL3JZ Supplement Nasal Turbinate with Synthetic Substitute, Percutaneous Approach
09UL3KZ Supplement Nasal Turbinate with Nonautologous Tissue Substitute, Percutaneous Approach
09UL47Z Supplement Nasal Turbinate with Autologous Tissue Substitute, Percutaneous Endoscopic Approach
09UL4JZ Supplement Nasal Turbinate with Synthetic Substitute, Percutaneous Endoscopic Approach

09UL4KZ Supplement Nasal Turbinate with Nonautologous Tissue Substitute, Percutaneous Endoscopic Approach
09UL77Z Supplement Nasal Turbinate with Autologous Tissue Substitute, Via Natural or Artificial Opening
09UL7JZ Supplement Nasal Turbinate with Synthetic Substitute, Via Natural or Artificial Opening
09UL7KZ Supplement Nasal Turbinate with Nonautologous Tissue Substitute, Via Natural or Artificial Opening
09UL87Z Supplement Nasal Turbinate with Autologous Tissue Substitute, Via Natural or Artificial Opening Endoscopic
09UL8JZ Supplement Nasal Turbinate with Synthetic Substitute, Via Natural or Artificial Opening Endoscopic
09UL8KZ Supplement Nasal Turbinate with Nonautologous Tissue Substitute, Via Natural or Artificial Opening Endoscopic
09UM07Z Supplement Nasal Septum with Autologous Tissue Substitute, Open Approach
09UM0JZ Supplement Nasal Septum with Synthetic Substitute, Open Approach
09UM0KZ Supplement Nasal Septum with Nonautologous Tissue Substitute, Open Approach
09UM37Z Supplement Nasal Septum with Autologous Tissue Substitute, Percutaneous Approach
09UM3JZ Supplement Nasal Septum with Synthetic Substitute, Percutaneous Approach
09UM3KZ Supplement Nasal Septum with Nonautologous Tissue Substitute, Percutaneous Approach
09UM47Z Supplement Nasal Septum with Autologous Tissue Substitute, Percutaneous Endoscopic Approach
09UM4JZ Supplement Nasal Septum with Synthetic Substitute, Percutaneous Endoscopic Approach
09UM4KZ Supplement Nasal Septum with Nonautologous Tissue Substitute, Percutaneous Endoscopic Approach
09UN07Z Supplement Nasopharynx with Autologous Tissue Substitute, Open Approach
09UN0JZ Supplement Nasopharynx with Synthetic Substitute, Open Approach
09UN0KZ Supplement Nasopharynx with Nonautologous Tissue Substitute, Open Approach
09UN77Z Supplement Nasopharynx with Autologous Tissue Substitute, Via Natural or Artificial Opening
09UN7JZ Supplement Nasopharynx with Synthetic Substitute, Via Natural or Artificial Opening
09UN7KZ Supplement Nasopharynx with Nonautologous Tissue Substitute, Via Natural or Artificial Opening
09UN87Z Supplement Nasopharynx with Autologous Tissue Substitute, Via Natural or Artificial Opening Endoscopic
09UN8JZ Supplement Nasopharynx with Synthetic Substitute, Via Natural or Artificial Opening Endoscopic
09UN8KZ Supplement Nasopharynx with Nonautologous Tissue Substitute, Via Natural or Artificial Opening Endoscopic

09W – Ear, Nose, Sinus, Revision

Review Coding Guideline B6.1c

09W707Z Revision of Autologous Tissue Substitute in Right Tympanic Membrane, Open Approach
09W70JZ Revision of Synthetic Substitute in Right Tympanic Membrane, Open Approach
09W70KZ Revision of Nonautologous Tissue Substitute in Right Tympanic Membrane, Open Approach
09W777Z Revision of Autologous Tissue Substitute in Right Tympanic Membrane, Via Natural or Artificial Opening
09W77JZ Revision of Synthetic Substitute in Right Tympanic Membrane, Via Natural or Artificial Opening
09W77KZ Revision of Nonautologous Tissue Substitute in Right Tympanic Membrane, Via Natural or Artificial Opening
09W787Z Revision of Autologous Tissue Substitute in Right Tympanic Membrane, Via Natural or Artificial Opening Endoscopic
09W78JZ Revision of Synthetic Substitute in Right Tympanic Membrane, Via Natural or Artificial Opening Endoscopic
09W78KZ Revision of Nonautologous Tissue Substitute in Right Tympanic Membrane, Via Natural or Artificial Opening Endoscopic
09W807Z Revision of Autologous Tissue Substitute in Left Tympanic Membrane, Open Approach
09W80JZ Revision of Synthetic Substitute in Left Tympanic Membrane, Open Approach
09W80KZ Revision of Nonautologous Tissue Substitute in Left Tympanic Membrane, Open Approach
09W877Z Revision of Autologous Tissue Substitute in Left Tympanic Membrane, Via Natural or Artificial Opening
09W87JZ Revision of Synthetic Substitute in Left Tympanic Membrane, Via Natural or Artificial Opening
09W87KZ Revision of Nonautologous Tissue Substitute in Left Tympanic Membrane, Via Natural or Artificial Opening
09W887Z Revision of Autologous Tissue Substitute in Left Tympanic Membrane, Via Natural or Artificial Opening Endoscopic
09W88JZ Revision of Synthetic Substitute in Left Tympanic Membrane, Via Natural or Artificial Opening Endoscopic
09W88KZ Revision of Nonautologous Tissue Substitute in Left Tympanic Membrane, Via Natural or Artificial Opening Endoscopic
09W907Z Revision of Autologous Tissue Substitute in Right Auditory Ossicle, Open Approach
09W90JZ Revision of Synthetic Substitute in Right Auditory Ossicle, Open Approach
09W90KZ Revision of Nonautologous Tissue Substitute in Right Auditory Ossicle, Open Approach
09W977Z Revision of Autologous Tissue Substitute in Right Auditory Ossicle, Via Natural or Artificial Opening
09W97JZ Revision of Synthetic Substitute in Right Auditory Ossicle, Via Natural or Artificial Opening
09W97KZ Revision of Nonautologous Tissue Substitute in Right Auditory Ossicle, Via Natural or Artificial Opening
09W987Z Revision of Autologous Tissue Substitute in Right Auditory Ossicle, Via Natural or Artificial Opening Endoscopic
09W98JZ Revision of Synthetic Substitute in Right Auditory Ossicle, Via Natural or Artificial Opening Endoscopic
09W98KZ Revision of Nonautologous Tissue Substitute in Right Auditory Ossicle, Via Natural or Artificial Opening Endoscopic
09WA07Z Revision of Autologous Tissue Substitute in Left Auditory Ossicle, Open Approach
09WA0JZ Revision of Synthetic Substitute in Left Auditory Ossicle, Open Approach
09WA0KZ Revision of Nonautologous Tissue Substitute in Left Auditory Ossicle, Open Approach
09WA77Z Revision of Autologous Tissue Substitute in Left Auditory Ossicle, Via Natural or Artificial Opening
09WA7JZ Revision of Synthetic Substitute in Left Auditory Ossicle, Via Natural or Artificial Opening
09WA7KZ Revision of Nonautologous Tissue Substitute in Left Auditory Ossicle, Via Natural or Artificial Opening
09WA87Z Revision of Autologous Tissue Substitute in Left Auditory Ossicle, Via Natural or Artificial Opening Endoscopic
09WA8JZ Revision of Synthetic Substitute in Left Auditory Ossicle, Via Natural or Artificial Opening Endoscopic
09WA8KZ Revision of Nonautologous Tissue Substitute in Left Auditory Ossicle, Via Natural or Artificial Opening Endoscopic
09WD0SZ Revision of Hearing Device in Right Inner Ear, Open Approach
09WD7SZ Revision of Hearing Device in Right Inner Ear, Via Natural or Artificial Opening
09WD8SZ Revision of Hearing Device in Right Inner Ear, Via Natural or Artificial Opening Endoscopic
09WE0SZ Revision of Hearing Device in Left Inner Ear, Open Approach
09WE7SZ Revision of Hearing Device in Left Inner Ear, Via Natural or Artificial Opening
09WE8SZ Revision of Hearing Device in Left Inner Ear, Via Natural or Artificial Opening Endoscopic
09WH00Z Revision of Drainage Device in Right Ear, Open Approach
09WH07Z Revision of Autologous Tissue Substitute in Right Ear, Open Approach
09WH0DZ Revision of Intraluminal Device in Right Ear, Open Approach
09WH0JZ Revision of Synthetic Substitute in Right Ear, Open Approach
09WH0KZ Revision of Nonautologous Tissue Substitute in Right Ear, Open Approach
09WH30Z Revision of Drainage Device in Right Ear, Percutaneous Approach
09WH37Z Revision of Autologous Tissue Substitute in Right Ear, Percutaneous Approach
09WH3DZ Revision of Intraluminal Device in Right Ear, Percutaneous Approach
09WH3JZ Revision of Synthetic Substitute in Right Ear, Percutaneous Approach
09WH3KZ Revision of Nonautologous Tissue Substitute in Right Ear, Percutaneous Approach
09WH40Z Revision of Drainage Device in Right Ear, Percutaneous Endoscopic Approach
09WH47Z Revision of Autologous Tissue Substitute in Right Ear, Percutaneous Endoscopic Approach
09WH4DZ Revision of Intraluminal Device in Right Ear, Percutaneous Endoscopic Approach
09WH4JZ Revision of Synthetic Substitute in Righ Ear, Percutaneous Endoscopic Approac
09WH4KZ Revision of Nonautologous Tissue Substitute in Right Ear, Percutaneous Endoscopic Approach
09WH70Z Revision of Drainage Device in Right Ear, Via Natural or Artificial Opening
09WH77Z Revision of Autologous Tissue Substitut in Right Ear, Via Natural or Artificial Opening
09WH7DZ Revision of Intraluminal Device in Righ Ear, Via Natural or Artificial Opening
09WH7JZ Revision of Synthetic Substitute in Righ Ear, Via Natural or Artificial Opening
09WH7KZ Revision of Nonautologous Tissue Substitute in Right Ear, Via Natural or Artificial Opening
09WH80Z Revision of Drainage Device in Right Ear, Via Natural or Artificial Opening Endoscopic
09WH87Z Revision of Autologous Tissue Substitut in Right Ear, Via Natural or Artificial Opening Endoscopic
09WH8DZ Revision of Intraluminal Device in Righ Ear, Via Natural or Artificial Opening Endoscopic
09WH8JZ Revision of Synthetic Substitute in Righ Ear, Via Natural or Artificial Opening Endoscopic
09WH8KZ Revision of Nonautologous Tissue Substitute in Right Ear, Via Natural or Artificial Opening Endoscopic
09WHX0Z Revision of Drainage Device in Right Ea External Approach
09WHX7Z Revision of Autologous Tissue Substitu in Right Ear, External Approach
09WHXDZ Revision of Intraluminal Device in Righ Ear, External Approach
09WHXJZ Revision of Synthetic Substitute in Righ Ear, External Approach
09WHXKZ Revision of Nonautologous Tissue Substitute in Right Ear, External Approach
09WJ00Z Revision of Drainage Device in Left Ea Open Approach
09WJ07Z Revision of Autologous Tissue Substitu in Left Ear, Open Approach
09WJ0DZ Revision of Intraluminal Device in Left Ear, Open Approach
09WJ0JZ Revision of Synthetic Substitute in Left Ear, Open Approach
09WJ0KZ Revision of Nonautologous Tissue Substitute in Left Ear, Open Approach
09WJ30Z Revision of Drainage Device in Left Ear Percutaneous Approach
09WJ37Z Revision of Autologous Tissue Substitut in Left Ear, Percutaneous Approach
09WJ3DZ Revision of Intraluminal Device in Left Ear, Percutaneous Approach
09WJ3JZ Revision of Synthetic Substitute in Left Ear, Percutaneous Approach
09WJ3KZ Revision of Nonautologous Tissue Substitute in Left Ear, Percutaneous Approach
09WJ40Z Revision of Drainage Device in Left Ear Percutaneous Endoscopic Approach
09WJ47Z Revision of Autologous Tissue Substitute in Left Ear, Percutaneous Endoscopic Approach
09WJ4DZ Revision of Intraluminal Device in Left Ear, Percutaneous Endoscopic Approach
09WJ4JZ Revision of Synthetic Substitute in Left Ear, Percutaneous Endoscopic Approach

VJ4KZ Revision of Nonautologous Tissue Substitute in Left Ear, Percutaneous Endoscopic Approach
VJ70Z Revision of Drainage Device in Left Ear, Via Natural or Artificial Opening
VJ77Z Revision of Autologous Tissue Substitute in Left Ear, Via Natural or Artificial Opening
VJ7DZ Revision of Intraluminal Device in Left Ear, Via Natural or Artificial Opening
VJ7JZ Revision of Synthetic Substitute in Left Ear, Via Natural or Artificial Opening
VJ7KZ Revision of Nonautologous Tissue Substitute in Left Ear, Via Natural or Artificial Opening
WJ80Z Revision of Drainage Device in Left Ear, Via Natural or Artificial Opening Endoscopic
WJ87Z Revision of Autologous Tissue Substitute in Left Ear, Via Natural or Artificial Opening Endoscopic
WJ8DZ Revision of Intraluminal Device in Left Ear, Via Natural or Artificial Opening Endoscopic
WJ8JZ Revision of Synthetic Substitute in Left Ear, Via Natural or Artificial Opening Endoscopic
WJ8KZ Revision of Nonautologous Tissue Substitute in Left Ear, Via Natural or Artificial Opening Endoscopic
WJX0Z Revision of Drainage Device in Left Ear, External Approach
WJX7Z Revision of Autologous Tissue Substitute in Left Ear, External Approach
WJXDZ Revision of Intraluminal Device in Left Ear, External Approach
WJXJZ Revision of Synthetic Substitute in Left Ear, External Approach
09WJXKZ Revision of Nonautologous Tissue Substitute in Left Ear, External Approach
09WK00Z Revision of Drainage Device in Nose, Open Approach
09WK07Z Revision of Autologous Tissue Substitute in Nose, Open Approach
09WK0DZ Revision of Intraluminal Device in Nose, Open Approach
09WK0JZ Revision of Synthetic Substitute in Nose, Open Approach
09WK0KZ Revision of Nonautologous Tissue Substitute in Nose, Open Approach
09WK30Z Revision of Drainage Device in Nose, Percutaneous Approach
09WK37Z Revision of Autologous Tissue Substitute in Nose, Percutaneous Approach
09WK3DZ Revision of Intraluminal Device in Nose, Percutaneous Approach
09WK3JZ Revision of Synthetic Substitute in Nose, Percutaneous Approach
09WK3KZ Revision of Nonautologous Tissue Substitute in Nose, Percutaneous Approach
09WK40Z Revision of Drainage Device in Nose, Percutaneous Endoscopic Approach
09WK47Z Revision of Autologous Tissue Substitute in Nose, Percutaneous Endoscopic Approach
09WK4DZ Revision of Intraluminal Device in Nose, Percutaneous Endoscopic Approach
09WK4JZ Revision of Synthetic Substitute in Nose, Percutaneous Endoscopic Approach
09WK4KZ Revision of Nonautologous Tissue Substitute in Nose, Percutaneous Endoscopic Approach
09WK70Z Revision of Drainage Device in Nose, Via Natural or Artificial Opening
09WK77Z Revision of Autologous Tissue Substitute in Nose, Via Natural or Artificial Opening
09WK7DZ Revision of Intraluminal Device in Nose, Via Natural or Artificial Opening
09WK7JZ Revision of Synthetic Substitute in Nose, Via Natural or Artificial Opening
09WK7KZ Revision of Nonautologous Tissue Substitute in Nose, Via Natural or Artificial Opening
09WK80Z Revision of Drainage Device in Nose, Via Natural or Artificial Opening Endoscopic
09WK87Z Revision of Autologous Tissue Substitute in Nose, Via Natural or Artificial Opening Endoscopic
09WK8DZ Revision of Intraluminal Device in Nose, Via Natural or Artificial Opening Endoscopic
09WK8JZ Revision of Synthetic Substitute in Nose, Via Natural or Artificial Opening Endoscopic
09WK8KZ Revision of Nonautologous Tissue Substitute in Nose, Via Natural or Artificial Opening Endoscopic
09WKX0Z Revision of Drainage Device in Nose, External Approach
09WKX7Z Revision of Autologous Tissue Substitute in Nose, External Approach
09WKXDZ Revision of Intraluminal Device in Nose, External Approach
09WKXJZ Revision of Synthetic Substitute in Nose, External Approach
09WKXKZ Revision of Nonautologous Tissue Substitute in Nose, External Approach
09WY00Z Revision of Drainage Device in Sinus, Open Approach
09WY30Z Revision of Drainage Device in Sinus, Percutaneous Approach
09WY40Z Revision of Drainage Device in Sinus, Percutaneous Endoscopic Approach
09WYX0Z Revision of Drainage Device in Sinus, External Approach

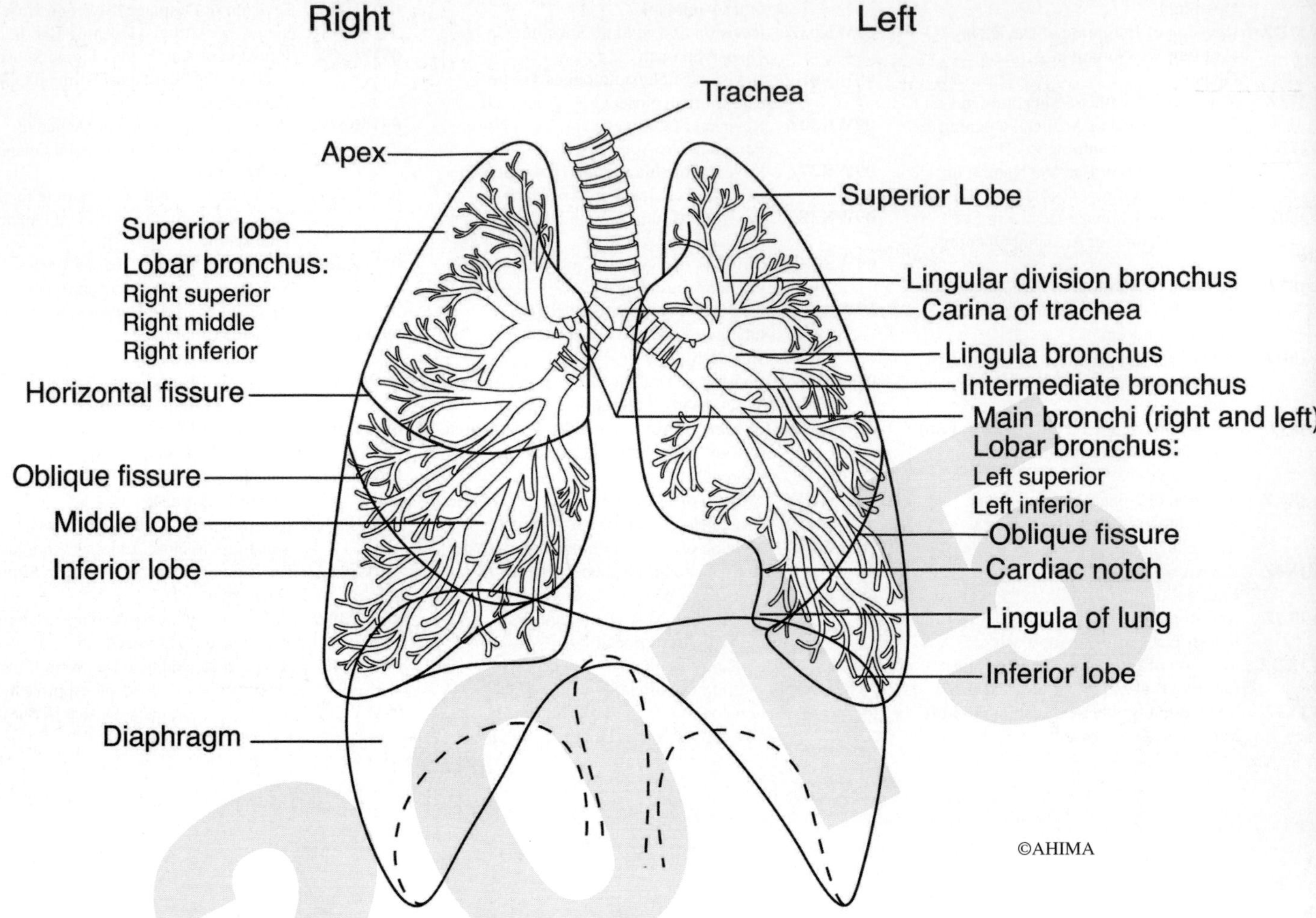
Lungs
Right
Left
Trachea
Apex
Superior Lobe
Superior lobe
Lobar bronchus:
Right superior
Right middle
Right inferior
Lingular division bronchus
Carina of trachea
Lingula bronchus
Intermediate bronchus
Horizontal fissure
Main bronchi (right and left)
Lobar bronchus:
Left superior
Left inferior
Oblique fissure
Middle lobe
Oblique fissure
Inferior lobe
Cardiac notch
Lingula of lung
Inferior lobe
Diaphragm
©AHIMA

tion	**0**	**Medical and Surgical**
ly System	**B**	**Respiratory System**
eration	**1**	**Bypass:** Altering the route of passage of the contents of a tubular body part

Body Part (4th)	Approach (5th)	Device (6th)	Qualifier (7th)
Trachea	**0** Open	**D** Intraluminal Device	**6** Esophagus
Trachea	**0** Open	**F** Tracheostomy Device **Z** No Device	**4** Cutaneous
Trachea	**3** Percutaneous **4** Percutaneous Endoscopic	**F** Tracheostomy Device **Z** No Device	**4** Cutaneous

ction	**0**	**Medical and Surgical**
dy System	**B**	**Respiratory System**
eration	**2**	**Change:** Taking out or off a device from a body part and putting back an identical or similar device in or on the same body part without cutting or puncturing the skin or a mucous membrane

Body Part (4th)	Approach (5th)	Device (6th)	Qualifier (7th)
Tracheobronchial Tree **K** Lung, Right **L** Lung, Left **Q** Pleura **T** Diaphragm	**X** External	**0** Drainage Device **Y** Other Device	**Z** No Qualifier
Trachea	**X** External	**0** Drainage Device **E** Intraluminal Device, Endotracheal Airway **F** Tracheostomy Device **Y** Other Device	**Z** No Qualifier

ction	**0**	**Medical and Surgical**
dy System	**B**	**Respiratory System**
eration	**5**	**Destruction:** Physical eradication of all or a portion of a body part by the direct use of energy, force, or a destructive agent

Body Part (4th)	Approach (5th)	Device (6th)	Qualifier (7th)
1 Trachea **2** Carina **3** Main Bronchus, Right **4** Upper Lobe Bronchus, Right **5** Middle Lobe Bronchus, Right **6** Lower Lobe Bronchus, Right **7** Main Bronchus, Left **8** Upper Lobe Bronchus, Left **9** Lingula Bronchus **B** Lower Lobe Bronchus, Left **C** Upper Lung Lobe, Right **D** Middle Lung Lobe, Right **F** Lower Lung Lobe, Right **G** Upper Lung Lobe, Left **H** Lung Lingula **J** Lower Lung Lobe, Left **K** Lung, Right **L** Lung, Left **M** Lungs, Bilateral	**0** Open **3** Percutaneous **4** Percutaneous Endoscopic **7** Via Natural or Artificial Opening **8** Via Natural or Artificial Opening Endoscopic	**Z** No Device	**Z** No Qualifier
N Pleura, Right **P** Pleura, Left **R** Diaphragm, Right **S** Diaphragm, Left	**0** Open **3** Percutaneous **4** Percutaneous Endoscopic	**Z** No Device	**Z** No Qualifier

Section 0 **Medical and Surgical**
Body System B **Respiratory System**
Operation 7 **Dilation:** Expanding an orifice or the lumen of a tubular body part

Body Part (4th)	Approach (5th)	Device (6th)	Qualifier (7th)
1 Trachea **2** Carina **3** Main Bronchus, Right **4** Upper Lobe Bronchus, Right **5** Middle Lobe Bronchus, Right **6** Lower Lobe Bronchus, Right **7** Main Bronchus, Left **8** Upper Lobe Bronchus, Left **9** Lingula Bronchus **B** Lower Lobe Bronchus, Left	**0** Open **3** Percutaneous **4** Percutaneous Endoscopic **7** Via Natural or Artificial Opening **8** Via Natural or Artificial Opening Endoscopic	**D** Intraluminal Device **Z** No Device	**Z** No Qualifier

Section 0 **Medical and Surgical**
Body System B **Respiratory System**
Operation 9 **Drainage:** Taking or letting out fluids and/or gases from a body part

Body Part (4th)	Approach (5th)	Device (6th)	Qualifier (7th)
1 Trachea **2** Carina **3** Main Bronchus, Right **4** Upper Lobe Bronchus, Right **5** Middle Lobe Bronchus, Right **6** Lower Lobe Bronchus, Right **7** Main Bronchus, Left **8** Upper Lobe Bronchus, Left **9** Lingula Bronchus **B** Lower Lobe Bronchus, Left **C** Upper Lung Lobe, Right **D** Middle Lung Lobe, Right **F** Lower Lung Lobe, Right **G** Upper Lung Lobe, Left **H** Lung Lingula **J** Lower Lung Lobe, Left **K** Lung, Right **L** Lung, Left **M** Lungs, Bilateral	**0** Open **3** Percutaneous **4** Percutaneous Endoscopic **7** Via Natural or Artificial Opening **8** Via Natural or Artificial Opening Endoscopic	**0** Drainage Device	**Z** No Qualifier
1 Trachea **2** Carina **3** Main Bronchus, Right **4** Upper Lobe Bronchus, Right **5** Middle Lobe Bronchus, Right **6** Lower Lobe Bronchus, Right **7** Main Bronchus, Left **8** Upper Lobe Bronchus, Left **9** Lingula Bronchus **B** Lower Lobe Bronchus, Left **C** Upper Lung Lobe, Right **D** Middle Lung Lobe, Right **F** Lower Lung Lobe, Right **G** Upper Lung Lobe, Left **H** Lung Lingula **J** Lower Lung Lobe, Left **K** Lung, Right **L** Lung, Left **M** Lungs, Bilateral	**0** Open **3** Percutaneous **4** Percutaneous Endoscopic **7** Via Natural or Artificial Opening **8** Via Natural or Artificial Opening Endoscopic	**Z** No Device	**X** Diagnostic **Z** No Qualifier
N Pleura, Right **P** Pleura, Left **R** Diaphragm, Right **S** Diaphragm, Left	**0** Open **3** Percutaneous **4** Percutaneous Endoscopic	**0** Drainage Device	**Z** No Qualifier

Continued →

ction 0 Medical and Surgical
dy System B Respiratory System
eration 9 **Drainage:** Taking or letting out fluids and/or gases from a body part

Body Part (4th)	Approach (5th)	Device (6th)	Qualifier (7th)
N Pleura, Right P Pleura, Left R Diaphragm, Right S Diaphragm, Left	0 Open 3 Percutaneous 4 Percutaneous Endoscopic	Z No Device	X Diagnostic Z No Qualifier

ction 0 Medical and Surgical
dy System B Respiratory System
peration B **Excision:** Cutting out or off, without replacement, a portion of a body part

Body Part (4th)	Approach (5th)	Device (6th)	Qualifier (7th)
1 Trachea 2 Carina 3 Main Bronchus, Right 4 Upper Lobe Bronchus, Right 5 Middle Lobe Bronchus, Right 6 Lower Lobe Bronchus, Right 7 Main Bronchus, Left 8 Upper Lobe Bronchus, Left 9 Lingula Bronchus B Lower Lobe Bronchus, Left C Upper Lung Lobe, Right D Middle Lung Lobe, Right F Lower Lung Lobe, Right G Upper Lung Lobe, Left H Lung Lingula J Lower Lung Lobe, Left K Lung, Right L Lung, Left M Lungs, Bilateral	0 Open 3 Percutaneous 4 Percutaneous Endoscopic 7 Via Natural or Artificial Opening 8 Via Natural or Artificial Opening Endoscopic	Z No Device	X Diagnostic Z No Qualifier
N Pleura, Right P Pleura, Left R Diaphragm, Right S Diaphragm, Left	0 Open 3 Percutaneous 4 Percutaneous Endoscopic	Z No Device	X Diagnostic Z No Qualifier

ection 0 Medical and Surgical
ody System B Respiratory System
peration C **Extirpation:** Taking or cutting out solid matter from a body part

Body Part (4th)	Approach (5th)	Device (6th)	Qualifier (7th)
1 Trachea 2 Carina 3 Main Bronchus, Right 4 Upper Lobe Bronchus, Right 5 Middle Lobe Bronchus, Right 6 Lower Lobe Bronchus, Right 7 Main Bronchus, Left 8 Upper Lobe Bronchus, Left 9 Lingula Bronchus B Lower Lobe Bronchus, Left C Upper Lung Lobe, Right D Middle Lung Lobe, Right F Lower Lung Lobe, Right G Upper Lung Lobe, Left H Lung Lingula J Lower Lung Lobe, Left K Lung, Right L Lung, Left M Lungs, Bilateral	0 Open 3 Percutaneous 4 Percutaneous Endoscopic 7 Via Natural or Artificial Opening 8 Via Natural or Artificial Opening Endoscopic	Z No Device	Z No Qualifier

Continued →

0BC Continu

Section 0 **Medical and Surgical**
Body System B **Respiratory System**
Operation C **Extirpation:** Taking or cutting out solid matter from a body part

Body Part (4th)	Approach (5th)	Device (6th)	Qualifier (7th)
N Pleura, Right P Pleura, Left R Diaphragm, Right S Diaphragm, Left	0 Open 3 Percutaneous 4 Percutaneous Endoscopic	Z No Device	Z No Qualifier

Section 0 **Medical and Surgical**
Body System B **Respiratory System**
Operation D **Extraction:** Pulling or stripping out or off all or a portion of a body part by the use of force

Body Part (4th)	Approach (5th)	Device (6th)	Qualifier (7th)
N Pleura, Right P Pleura, Left	0 Open 3 Percutaneous 4 Percutaneous Endoscopic	Z No Device	X Diagnostic Z No Qualifier

Section 0 **Medical and Surgical**
Body System B **Respiratory System**
Operation F **Fragmentation:** Breaking solid matter in a body part into pieces

Body Part (4th)	Approach (5th)	Device (6th)	Qualifier (7th)
1 Trachea 2 Carina 3 Main Bronchus, Right 4 Upper Lobe Bronchus, Right 5 Middle Lobe Bronchus, Right 6 Lower Lobe Bronchus, Right 7 Main Bronchus, Left 8 Upper Lobe Bronchus, Left 9 Lingula Bronchus B Lower Lobe Bronchus, Left	0 Open 3 Percutaneous 4 Percutaneous Endoscopic 7 Via Natural or Artificial Opening 8 Via Natural or Artificial Opening Endoscopic X External	Z No Device	Z No Qualifier

Section 0 **Medical and Surgical**
Body System B **Respiratory System**
Operation H **Insertion:** Putting in a nonbiological appliance that monitors, assists, performs, or prevents a physiological function but does not physically take the place of a body part

Body Part (4th)	Approach (5th)	Device (6th)	Qualifier (7th)
0 Tracheobronchial Tree	0 Open 3 Percutaneous 4 Percutaneous Endoscopic 7 Via Natural or Artificial Opening 8 Via Natural or Artificial Opening Endoscopic	1 Radioactive Element 2 Monitoring Device 3 Infusion Device D Intraluminal Device	Z No Qualifier
1 Trachea	0 Open	2 Monitoring Device D Intraluminal Device	Z No Qualifier
1 Trachea	3 Percutaneous	D Intraluminal Device E Intraluminal Device, Endotracheal Airway	Z No Qualifier
1 Trachea	4 Percutaneous Endoscopic	D Intraluminal Device	Z No Qualifier
1 Trachea	7 Via Natural or Artificial Opening 8 Via Natural or Artificial Opening Endoscopic	2 Monitoring Device D Intraluminal Device E Intraluminal Device, Endotracheal Airway	Z No Qualifier

Continued →

Section 0 **Medical and Surgical**
Body System B **Respiratory System**
Operation H **Insertion:** Putting in a nonbiological appliance that monitors, assists, performs, or prevents a physiological function but does not physically take the place of a body part

Body Part (4th)	Approach (5th)	Device (6th)	Qualifier (7th)
3 Main Bronchus, Right 4 Upper Lobe Bronchus, Right 5 Middle Lobe Bronchus, Right 6 Lower Lobe Bronchus, Right 7 Main Bronchus, Left 8 Upper Lobe Bronchus, Left 9 Lingula Bronchus B Lower Lobe Bronchus, Left	**0** Open **3** Percutaneous **4** Percutaneous Endoscopic **7** Via Natural or Artificial Opening **8** Via Natural or Artificial Opening Endoscopic	**G** Intraluminal Device, Endobronchial Valve	**Z** No Qualifier
K Lung, Right L Lung, Left	**0** Open **3** Percutaneous **4** Percutaneous Endoscopic **7** Via Natural or Artificial Opening **8** Via Natural or Artificial Opening Endoscopic	**1** Radioactive Element **2** Monitoring Device **3** Infusion Device	**Z** No Qualifier
R Diaphragm, Right **S** Diaphragm, Left	**0** Open **3** Percutaneous **4** Percutaneous Endoscopic	**2** Monitoring Device **M** Diaphragmatic Pacemaker Lead	**Z** No Qualifier

Section 0 **Medical and Surgical**
Body System B **Respiratory System**
Operation J **Inspection:** Visually and/or manually exploring a body part

Body Part (4th)	Approach (5th)	Device (6th)	Qualifier (7th)
0 Tracheobronchial Tree **1** Trachea **K** Lung, Right **L** Lung, Left **Q** Pleura **T** Diaphragm	**0** Open **3** Percutaneous **4** Percutaneous Endoscopic **7** Via Natural or Artificial Opening **8** Via Natural or Artificial Opening Endoscopic **X** External	**Z** No Device	**Z** No Qualifier

Section 0 **Medical and Surgical**
Body System B **Respiratory System**
Operation L **Occlusion:** Completely closing an orifice or the lumen of a tubular body part

Body Part (4th)	Approach (5th)	Device (6th)	Qualifier (7th)
1 Trachea **2** Carina **3** Main Bronchus, Right **4** Upper Lobe Bronchus, Right **5** Middle Lobe Bronchus, Right **6** Lower Lobe Bronchus, Right **7** Main Bronchus, Left **8** Upper Lobe Bronchus, Left **9** Lingula Bronchus **B** Lower Lobe Bronchus, Left	**0** Open **3** Percutaneous **4** Percutaneous Endoscopic	**C** Extraluminal Device **D** Intraluminal Device **Z** No Device	**Z** No Qualifier
1 Trachea **2** Carina **3** Main Bronchus, Right **4** Upper Lobe Bronchus, Right **5** Middle Lobe Bronchus, Right **6** Lower Lobe Bronchus, Right **7** Main Bronchus, Left **8** Upper Lobe Bronchus, Left **9** Lingula Bronchus **B** Lower Lobe Bronchus, Left	**7** Via Natural or Artificial Opening **8** Via Natural or Artificial Opening Endoscopic	**D** Intraluminal Device **Z** No Device	**Z** No Qualifier

Section 0 Medical and Surgical
Body System B Respiratory System
Operation M **Reattachment:** Putting back in or on all or a portion of a separated body part to its normal location or other suitable location

Body Part (4th)	Approach (5th)	Device (6th)	Qualifier (7th)
1 Trachea 2 Carina 3 Main Bronchus, Right 4 Upper Lobe Bronchus, Right 5 Middle Lobe Bronchus, Right 6 Lower Lobe Bronchus, Right 7 Main Bronchus, Left 8 Upper Lobe Bronchus, Left 9 Lingula Bronchus B Lower Lobe Bronchus, Left C Upper Lung Lobe, Right D Middle Lung Lobe, Right F Lower Lung Lobe, Right G Upper Lung Lobe, Left H Lung Lingula J Lower Lung Lobe, Left K Lung, Right L Lung, Left R Diaphragm, Right S Diaphragm, Left	0 Open	Z No Device	Z No Qualifier

Section 0 Medical and Surgical
Body System B Respiratory System
Operation N **Release:** Freeing a body part from an abnormal physical constraint by cutting or by the use of force

Body Part (4th)	Approach (5th)	Device (6th)	Qualifier (7th)
1 Trachea 2 Carina 3 Main Bronchus, Right 4 Upper Lobe Bronchus, Right 5 Middle Lobe Bronchus, Right 6 Lower Lobe Bronchus, Right 7 Main Bronchus, Left 8 Upper Lobe Bronchus, Left 9 Lingula Bronchus B Lower Lobe Bronchus, Left C Upper Lung Lobe, Right D Middle Lung Lobe, Right F Lower Lung Lobe, Right G Upper Lung Lobe, Left H Lung Lingula J Lower Lung Lobe, Left K Lung, Right L Lung, Left M Lungs, Bilateral	0 Open 3 Percutaneous 4 Percutaneous Endoscopic 7 Via Natural or Artificial Opening 8 Via Natural or Artificial Opening Endoscopic	Z No Device	Z No Qualifier
N Pleura, Right P Pleura, Left R Diaphragm, Right S Diaphragm, Left	0 Open 3 Percutaneous 4 Percutaneous Endoscopic	Z No Device	Z No Qualifier

ction **0** **Medical and Surgical**
dy System **B** **Respiratory System**
eration **P** **Removal:** Taking out or off a device from a body part

Body Part (4th)	Approach (5th)	Device (6th)	Qualifier (7th)
0 Tracheobronchial Tree	**0** Open **3** Percutaneous **4** Percutaneous Endoscopic **7** Via Natural or Artificial Opening **8** Via Natural or Artificial Opening Endoscopic	**0** Drainage Device **1** Radioactive Element **2** Monitoring Device **3** Infusion Device **7** Autologous Tissue Substitute **C** Extraluminal Device **D** Intraluminal Device **J** Synthetic Substitute **K** Nonautologous Tissue Substitute	**Z** No Qualifier
0 Tracheobronchial Tree	**X** External	**0** Drainage Device **1** Radioactive Element **2** Monitoring Device **3** Infusion Device **D** Intraluminal Device	**Z** No Qualifier
1 Trachea	**0** Open **3** Percutaneous **4** Percutaneous Endoscopic **7** Via Natural or Artificial Opening **8** Via Natural or Artificial Opening Endoscopic	**0** Drainage Device **2** Monitoring Device **7** Autologous Tissue Substitute **C** Extraluminal Device **D** Intraluminal Device **F** Tracheostomy Device **J** Synthetic Substitute **K** Nonautologous Tissue Substitute	**Z** No Qualifier
1 Trachea	**X** External	**0** Drainage Device **2** Monitoring Device **D** Intraluminal Device **F** Tracheostomy Device	**Z** No Qualifier
K Lung, Right **L** Lung, Left	**0** Open **3** Percutaneous **4** Percutaneous Endoscopic **7** Via Natural or Artificial Opening **8** Via Natural or Artificial Opening Endoscopic **X** External	**0** Drainage Device **1** Radioactive Element **2** Monitoring Device **3** Infusion Device	**Z** No Qualifier
Q Pleura	**0** Open **3** Percutaneous **4** Percutaneous Endoscopic **7** Via Natural or Artificial Opening **8** Via Natural or Artificial Opening Endoscopic **X** External	**0** Drainage Device **1** Radioactive Element **2** Monitoring Device	**Z** No Qualifier
T Diaphragm	**0** Open **3** Percutaneous **4** Percutaneous Endoscopic **7** Via Natural or Artificial Opening **8** Via Natural or Artificial Opening Endoscopic	**0** Drainage Device **2** Monitoring Device **7** Autologous Tissue Substitute **J** Synthetic Substitute **K** Nonautologous Tissue Substitute **M** Diaphragmatic Pacemaker Lead	**Z** No Qualifier
T Diaphragm	**X** External	**0** Drainage Device **2** Monitoring Device **M** Diaphragmatic Pacemaker Lead	**Z** No Qualifier

Section 0 **Medical and Surgical**
Body System B **Respiratory System**
Operation Q **Repair:** Restoring, to the extent possible, a body part to its normal anatomic structure and function

Body Part (4th)	Approach (5th)	Device (6th)	Qualifier (7th)
1 Trachea **2** Carina **3** Main Bronchus, Right **4** Upper Lobe Bronchus, Right **5** Middle Lobe Bronchus, Right **6** Lower Lobe Bronchus, Right **7** Main Bronchus, Left **8** Upper Lobe Bronchus, Left **9** Lingula Bronchus **B** Lower Lobe Bronchus, Left **C** Upper Lung Lobe, Right **D** Middle Lung Lobe, Right **F** Lower Lung Lobe, Right **G** Upper Lung Lobe, Left **H** Lung Lingula **J** Lower Lung Lobe, Left **K** Lung, Right **L** Lung, Left **M** Lungs, Bilateral	**0** Open **3** Percutaneous **4** Percutaneous Endoscopic **7** Via Natural or Artificial Opening **8** Via Natural or Artificial Opening Endoscopic	**Z** No Device	**Z** No Qualifier
N Pleura, Right **P** Pleura, Left **R** Diaphragm, Right **S** Diaphragm, Left	**0** Open **3** Percutaneous **4** Percutaneous Endoscopic	**Z** No Device	**Z** No Qualifier

Section 0 **Medical and Surgical**
Body System B **Respiratory System**
Operation S **Reposition:** Moving to its normal location, or other suitable location, all or a portion of a body part

Body Part (4th)	Approach (5th)	Device (6th)	Qualifier (7th)
1 Trachea **2** Carina **3** Main Bronchus, Right **4** Upper Lobe Bronchus, Right **5** Middle Lobe Bronchus, Right **6** Lower Lobe Bronchus, Right **7** Main Bronchus, Left **8** Upper Lobe Bronchus, Left **9** Lingula Bronchus **B** Lower Lobe Bronchus, Left **C** Upper Lung Lobe, Right **D** Middle Lung Lobe, Right **F** Lower Lung Lobe, Right **G** Upper Lung Lobe, Left **H** Lung Lingula **J** Lower Lung Lobe, Left **K** Lung, Right **L** Lung, Left **R** Diaphragm, Right **S** Diaphragm, Left	**0** Open	**Z** No Device	**Z** No Qualifier

Section 0 **Medical and Surgical**
Body System B **Respiratory System**
Operation T **Resection:** Cutting out or off, without replacement, all of a body part

Body Part (4th)	Approach (5th)	Device (6th)	Qualifier (7th)
1 Trachea **2** Carina **3** Main Bronchus, Right **4** Upper Lobe Bronchus, Right **5** Middle Lobe Bronchus, Right **6** Lower Lobe Bronchus, Right **7** Main Bronchus, Left **8** Upper Lobe Bronchus, Left **9** Lingula Bronchus **B** Lower Lobe Bronchus, Left **C** Upper Lung Lobe, Right **D** Middle Lung Lobe, Right **F** Lower Lung Lobe, Right **G** Upper Lung Lobe, Left **H** Lung Lingula **J** Lower Lung Lobe, Left **K** Lung, Right **L** Lung, Left **M** Lungs, Bilateral **R** Diaphragm, Right **S** Diaphragm, Left	**0** Open **4** Percutaneous Endoscopic	**Z** No Device	**Z** No Qualifier

Section 0 **Medical and Surgical**
Body System B **Respiratory System**
Operation U **Supplement:** Putting in or on biological or synthetic material that physically reinforces and/or augments the function of a portion of a body part

Body Part (4th)	Approach (5th)	Device (6th)	Qualifier (7th)
1 Trachea **2** Carina **3** Main Bronchus, Right **4** Upper Lobe Bronchus, Right **5** Middle Lobe Bronchus, Right **6** Lower Lobe Bronchus, Right **7** Main Bronchus, Left **8** Upper Lobe Bronchus, Left **9** Lingula Bronchus **B** Lower Lobe Bronchus, Left **R** Diaphragm, Right **S** Diaphragm, Left	**0** Open **4** Percutaneous Endoscopic	**7** Autologous Tissue Substitute **J** Synthetic Substitute **K** Nonautologous Tissue Substitute	**Z** No Qualifier

Section 0 **Medical and Surgical**
Body System B **Respiratory System**
Operation V **Restriction:** Partially closing an orifice or the lumen of a tubular body part

Body Part (4th)	Approach (5th)	Device (6th)	Qualifier (7th)
1 Trachea **2** Carina **3** Main Bronchus, Right **4** Upper Lobe Bronchus, Right **5** Middle Lobe Bronchus, Right **6** Lower Lobe Bronchus, Right **7** Main Bronchus, Left **8** Upper Lobe Bronchus, Left **9** Lingula Bronchus **B** Lower Lobe Bronchus, Left	**0** Open **3** Percutaneous **4** Percutaneous Endoscopic	**C** Extraluminal Device **D** Intraluminal Device **Z** No Device	**Z** No Qualifier

Continued →

Section 0 **Medical and Surgical**
Body System B **Respiratory System**
Operation V **Restriction:** Partially closing an orifice or the lumen of a tubular body part

Body Part (4th)	Approach (5th)	Device (6th)	Qualifier (7th)
1 Trachea **2** Carina **3** Main Bronchus, Right **4** Upper Lobe Bronchus, Right **5** Middle Lobe Bronchus, Right **6** Lower Lobe Bronchus, Right **7** Main Bronchus, Left **8** Upper Lobe Bronchus, Left **9** Lingula Bronchus **B** Lower Lobe Bronchus, Left	**7** Via Natural or Artificial Opening **8** Via Natural or Artificial Opening Endoscopic	**D** Intraluminal Device **Z** No Device	**Z** No Qualifier

Section 0 **Medical and Surgical**
Body System B **Respiratory System**
Operation W **Revision:** Correcting, to the extent possible, a portion of a malfunctioning device or the position of a displaced device

Body Part (4th)	Approach (5th)	Device (6th)	Qualifier (7th)
0 Tracheobronchial Tree	**0** Open **3** Percutaneous **4** Percutaneous Endoscopic **7** Via Natural or Artificial Opening **8** Via Natural or Artificial Opening Endoscopic **X** External	**0** Drainage Device **2** Monitoring Device **3** Infusion Device **7** Autologous Tissue Substitute **C** Extraluminal Device **D** Intraluminal Device **J** Synthetic Substitute **K** Nonautologous Tissue Substitute	**Z** No Qualifier
1 Trachea	**0** Open **3** Percutaneous **4** Percutaneous Endoscopic **7** Via Natural or Artificial Opening **8** Via Natural or Artificial Opening Endoscopic **X** External	**0** Drainage Device **2** Monitoring Device **7** Autologous Tissue Substitute **C** Extraluminal Device **D** Intraluminal Device **F** Tracheostomy Device **J** Synthetic Substitute **K** Nonautologous Tissue Substitute	**Z** No Qualifier
K Lung, Right **L** Lung, Left	**0** Open **3** Percutaneous **4** Percutaneous Endoscopic **7** Via Natural or Artificial Opening **8** Via Natural or Artificial Opening Endoscopic **X** External	**0** Drainage Device **2** Monitoring Device **3** Infusion Device	**Z** No Qualifier
Q Pleura	**0** Open **3** Percutaneous **4** Percutaneous Endoscopic **7** Via Natural or Artificial Opening **8** Via Natural or Artificial Opening Endoscopic **X** External	**0** Drainage Device **2** Monitoring Device	**Z** No Qualifier
T Diaphragm	**0** Open **3** Percutaneous **4** Percutaneous Endoscopic **7** Via Natural or Artificial Opening **8** Via Natural or Artificial Opening Endoscopic **X** External	**0** Drainage Device **2** Monitoring Device **7** Autologous Tissue Substitute **J** Synthetic Substitute **K** Nonautologous Tissue Substitute **M** Diaphragmatic Pacemaker Lead	**Z** No Qualifier

ction **0** **Medical and Surgical**
dy System **B** **Respiratory System**
eration **Y** **Transplantation:** Putting in or on all or a portion of a living body part taken from another individual or animal to physically take the place and/or function of all or a portion of a similar body part

Body Part (4th)	Approach (5th)	Device (6th)	Qualifier (7th)
C Upper Lung Lobe, Right D Middle Lung Lobe, Right F Lower Lung Lobe, Right G Upper Lung Lobe, Left H Lung Lingula J Lower Lung Lobe, Left K Lung, Right L Lung, Left M Lungs, Bilateral	**0** Open	**Z** No Device	**0** Allogeneic **1** Syngeneic **2** Zooplastic

espiratory System Code Listing 0B1–0BY

B1 – Respiratory System, Bypass

eview Coding Guideline B3.6a

B110D6 Bypass Trachea to Esophagus with Intraluminal Device, Open Approach
B110F4 Bypass Trachea to Cutaneous with Tracheostomy Device, Open Approach
B110Z4 Bypass Trachea to Cutaneous, Open Approach
● **0B113F4** Bypass Trachea to Cutaneous with Tracheostomy Device, Percutaneous Approach
● **0B113Z4** Bypass Trachea to Cutaneous, Percutaneous Approach
0B114F4 Bypass Trachea to Cutaneous with Tracheostomy Device, Percutaneous Endoscopic Approach
0B114Z4 Bypass Trachea to Cutaneous, Percutaneous Endoscopic Approach

B2 – Respiratory System, Change

eview Coding Guideline B6.1c

B20X0Z Change Drainage Device in Tracheobronchial Tree, External Approach
B20XYZ Change Other Device in Tracheobronchial Tree, External Approach
B21X0Z Change Drainage Device in Trachea, External Approach
B21XEZ Change Endotracheal Airway in Trachea, External Approach
B21XFZ Change Tracheostomy Device in Trachea, External Approach
0B21XYZ Change Other Device in Trachea, External Approach
0B2KX0Z Change Drainage Device in Right Lung, External Approach
0B2KXYZ Change Other Device in Right Lung, External Approach
0B2LX0Z Change Drainage Device in Left Lung, External Approach
0B2LXYZ Change Other Device in Left Lung, External Approach
0B2QX0Z Change Drainage Device in Pleura, External Approach
0B2QXYZ Change Other Device in Pleura, External Approach
0B2TX0Z Change Drainage Device in Diaphragm, External Approach
0B2TXYZ Change Other Device in Diaphragm, External Approach

B5 – Respiratory System, Destruction

B510ZZ Destruction of Trachea, Open Approach
B513ZZ Destruction of Trachea, Percutaneous Approach
B514ZZ Destruction of Trachea, Percutaneous Endoscopic Approach
B517ZZ Destruction of Trachea, Via Natural or Artificial Opening
B518ZZ Destruction of Trachea, Via Natural or Artificial Opening Endoscopic
B520ZZ Destruction of Carina, Open Approach
B523ZZ Destruction of Carina, Percutaneous Approach
B524ZZ Destruction of Carina, Percutaneous Endoscopic Approach
B527ZZ Destruction of Carina, Via Natural or Artificial Opening
B528ZZ Destruction of Carina, Via Natural or Artificial Opening Endoscopic
B530ZZ Destruction of Right Main Bronchus, Open Approach
B533ZZ Destruction of Right Main Bronchus, Percutaneous Approach
B534ZZ Destruction of Right Main Bronchus, Percutaneous Endoscopic Approach
B537ZZ Destruction of Right Main Bronchus, Via Natural or Artificial Opening
B538ZZ Destruction of Right Main Bronchus, Via Natural or Artificial Opening Endoscopic
0B540ZZ Destruction of Right Upper Lobe Bronchus, Open Approach
0B543ZZ Destruction of Right Upper Lobe Bronchus, Percutaneous Approach
0B544ZZ Destruction of Right Upper Lobe Bronchus, Percutaneous Endoscopic Approach
0B547ZZ Destruction of Right Upper Lobe Bronchus, Via Natural or Artificial Opening
0B548ZZ Destruction of Right Upper Lobe Bronchus, Via Natural or Artificial Opening Endoscopic
0B550ZZ Destruction of Right Middle Lobe Bronchus, Open Approach
0B553ZZ Destruction of Right Middle Lobe Bronchus, Percutaneous Approach
0B554ZZ Destruction of Right Middle Lobe Bronchus, Percutaneous Endoscopic Approach
0B557ZZ Destruction of Right Middle Lobe Bronchus, Via Natural or Artificial Opening
0B558ZZ Destruction of Right Middle Lobe Bronchus, Via Natural or Artificial Opening Endoscopic
0B560ZZ Destruction of Right Lower Lobe Bronchus, Open Approach
0B563ZZ Destruction of Right Lower Lobe Bronchus, Percutaneous Approach
0B564ZZ Destruction of Right Lower Lobe Bronchus, Percutaneous Endoscopic Approach
0B567ZZ Destruction of Right Lower Lobe Bronchus, Via Natural or Artificial Opening
0B568ZZ Destruction of Right Lower Lobe Bronchus, Via Natural or Artificial Opening Endoscopic
0B570ZZ Destruction of Left Main Bronchus, Open Approach
0B573ZZ Destruction of Left Main Bronchus, Percutaneous Approach
0B574ZZ Destruction of Left Main Bronchus, Percutaneous Endoscopic Approach
0B577ZZ Destruction of Left Main Bronchus, Via Natural or Artificial Opening
0B578ZZ Destruction of Left Main Bronchus, Via Natural or Artificial Opening Endoscopic
0B580ZZ Destruction of Left Upper Lobe Bronchus, Open Approach
0B583ZZ Destruction of Left Upper Lobe Bronchus, Percutaneous Approach
0B584ZZ Destruction of Left Upper Lobe Bronchus, Percutaneous Endoscopic Approach

0B587ZZ Destruction of Left Upper Lobe Bronchus, Via Natural or Artificial Opening
0B588ZZ Destruction of Left Upper Lobe Bronchus, Via Natural or Artificial Opening Endoscopic
0B590ZZ Destruction of Lingula Bronchus, Open Approach
0B593ZZ Destruction of Lingula Bronchus, Percutaneous Approach
0B594ZZ Destruction of Lingula Bronchus, Percutaneous Endoscopic Approach
0B597ZZ Destruction of Lingula Bronchus, Via Natural or Artificial Opening
0B598ZZ Destruction of Lingula Bronchus, Via Natural or Artificial Opening Endoscopic
0B5B0ZZ Destruction of Left Lower Lobe Bronchus, Open Approach
0B5B3ZZ Destruction of Left Lower Lobe Bronchus, Percutaneous Approach
0B5B4ZZ Destruction of Left Lower Lobe Bronchus, Percutaneous Endoscopic Approach
0B5B7ZZ Destruction of Left Lower Lobe Bronchus, Via Natural or Artificial Opening
0B5B8ZZ Destruction of Left Lower Lobe Bronchus, Via Natural or Artificial Opening Endoscopic
0B5C0ZZ Destruction of Right Upper Lung Lobe, Open Approach
0B5C3ZZ Destruction of Right Upper Lung Lobe, Percutaneous Approach
0B5C4ZZ Destruction of Right Upper Lung Lobe, Percutaneous Endoscopic Approach
0B5C7ZZ Destruction of Right Upper Lung Lobe, Via Natural or Artificial Opening
0B5C8ZZ Destruction of Right Upper Lung Lobe, Via Natural or Artificial Opening Endoscopic
0B5D0ZZ Destruction of Right Middle Lung Lobe, Open Approach
0B5D3ZZ Destruction of Right Middle Lung Lobe, Percutaneous Approach
0B5D4ZZ Destruction of Right Middle Lung Lobe, Percutaneous Endoscopic Approach
0B5D7ZZ Destruction of Right Middle Lung Lobe, Via Natural or Artificial Opening
0B5D8ZZ Destruction of Right Middle Lung Lobe, Via Natural or Artificial Opening Endoscopic
0B5F0ZZ Destruction of Right Lower Lung Lobe, Open Approach
0B5F3ZZ Destruction of Right Lower Lung Lobe, Percutaneous Approach
0B5F4ZZ Destruction of Right Lower Lung Lobe, Percutaneous Endoscopic Approach
0B5F7ZZ Destruction of Right Lower Lung Lobe, Via Natural or Artificial Opening
0B5F8ZZ Destruction of Right Lower Lung Lobe, Via Natural or Artificial Opening Endoscopic
0B5G0ZZ Destruction of Left Upper Lung Lobe, Open Approach
0B5G3ZZ Destruction of Left Upper Lung Lobe, Percutaneous Approach
0B5G4ZZ Destruction of Left Upper Lung Lobe, Percutaneous Endoscopic Approach
0B5G7ZZ Destruction of Left Upper Lung Lobe, Via Natural or Artificial Opening
0B5G8ZZ Destruction of Left Upper Lung Lobe, Via Natural or Artificial Opening Endoscopic
0B5H0ZZ Destruction of Lung Lingula, Open Approach
0B5H3ZZ Destruction of Lung Lingula, Percutaneous Approach
0B5H4ZZ Destruction of Lung Lingula, Percutaneous Endoscopic Approach
0B5H7ZZ Destruction of Lung Lingula, Via Natural or Artificial Opening
0B5H8ZZ Destruction of Lung Lingula, Via Natural or Artificial Opening Endoscopic
0B5J0ZZ Destruction of Left Lower Lung Lobe, Open Approach
0B5J3ZZ Destruction of Left Lower Lung Lobe, Percutaneous Approach
0B5J4ZZ Destruction of Left Lower Lung Lobe, Percutaneous Endoscopic Approach
0B5J7ZZ Destruction of Left Lower Lung Lobe, Via Natural or Artificial Opening
0B5J8ZZ Destruction of Left Lower Lung Lobe, Via Natural or Artificial Opening Endoscopic
0B5K0ZZ Destruction of Right Lung, Open Approach
0B5K3ZZ Destruction of Right Lung, Percutaneous Approach
0B5K4ZZ Destruction of Right Lung, Percutaneous Endoscopic Approach
0B5K7ZZ Destruction of Right Lung, Via Natural Artificial Opening
0B5K8ZZ Destruction of Right Lung, Via Natural Artificial Opening Endoscopic
0B5L0ZZ Destruction of Left Lung, Open Approa
0B5L3ZZ Destruction of Left Lung, Percutaneous Approach
0B5L4ZZ Destruction of Left Lung, Percutaneous Endoscopic Approach
0B5L7ZZ Destruction of Left Lung, Via Natural or Artificial Opening
0B5L8ZZ Destruction of Left Lung, Via Natural or Artificial Opening Endoscopic
0B5M0ZZ Destruction of Bilateral Lungs, Open Approach
0B5M3ZZ Destruction of Bilateral Lungs, Percutaneous Approach
0B5M4ZZ Destruction of Bilateral Lungs, Percutaneous Endoscopic Approach
0B5M7ZZ Destruction of Bilateral Lungs, Via Natural or Artificial Opening
0B5M8ZZ Destruction of Bilateral Lungs, Via Natural or Artificial Opening Endoscopic
0B5N0ZZ Destruction of Right Pleura, Open Approach
0B5N3ZZ Destruction of Right Pleura, Percutaneous Approach
0B5N4ZZ Destruction of Right Pleura, Percutaneous Endoscopic Approach
0B5P0ZZ Destruction of Left Pleura, Open Approach
0B5P3ZZ Destruction of Left Pleura, Percutaneous Approach
0B5P4ZZ Destruction of Left Pleura, Percutaneous Endoscopic Approach
0B5R0ZZ Destruction of Right Diaphragm, Open Approach
0B5R3ZZ Destruction of Right Diaphragm, Percutaneous Approach
0B5R4ZZ Destruction of Right Diaphragm, Percutaneous Endoscopic Approach
0B5S0ZZ Destruction of Left Diaphragm, Open Approach
0B5S3ZZ Destruction of Left Diaphragm, Percutaneous Approach
0B5S4ZZ Destruction of Left Diaphragm, Percutaneous Endoscopic Approach

0B7 – Respiratory System, Dilation

0B710DZ Dilation of Trachea with Intraluminal Device, Open Approach
0B710ZZ Dilation of Trachea, Open Approach
0B713DZ Dilation of Trachea with Intraluminal Device, Percutaneous Approach
0B713ZZ Dilation of Trachea, Percutaneous Approach
0B714DZ Dilation of Trachea with Intraluminal Device, Percutaneous Endoscopic Approach
0B714ZZ Dilation of Trachea, Percutaneous Endoscopic Approach
0B717DZ Dilation of Trachea with Intraluminal Device, Via Natural or Artificial Opening
0B717ZZ Dilation of Trachea, Via Natural or Artificial Opening
0B718DZ Dilation of Trachea with Intraluminal Device, Via Natural or Artificial Opening Endoscopic
0B718ZZ Dilation of Trachea, Via Natural or Artificial Opening Endoscopic
0B720DZ Dilation of Carina with Intraluminal Device, Open Approach
0B720ZZ Dilation of Carina, Open Approach
0B723DZ Dilation of Carina with Intraluminal Device, Percutaneous Approach
0B723ZZ Dilation of Carina, Percutaneous Approach
0B724DZ Dilation of Carina with Intraluminal Device, Percutaneous Endoscopic Approach
0B724ZZ Dilation of Carina, Percutaneous Endoscopic Approach
0B727DZ Dilation of Carina with Intraluminal Device, Via Natural or Artificial Opening
0B727ZZ Dilation of Carina, Via Natural or Artificial Opening
0B728DZ Dilation of Carina with Intraluminal Device, Via Natural or Artificial Opening Endoscopic
0B728ZZ Dilation of Carina, Via Natural or Artificial Opening Endoscopic
0B730DZ Dilation of Right Main Bronchus with Intraluminal Device, Open Approach
0B730ZZ Dilation of Right Main Bronchus, Open Approach
0B733DZ Dilation of Right Main Bronchus with Intraluminal Device, Percutaneous Approach
0B733ZZ Dilation of Right Main Bronchus, Percutaneous Approach
0B734DZ Dilation of Right Main Bronchus with Intraluminal Device, Percutaneous Endoscopic Approach
0B734ZZ Dilation of Right Main Bronchus, Percutaneous Endoscopic Approach
0B737DZ Dilation of Right Main Bronchus with Intraluminal Device, Via Natural or Artificial Opening
0B737ZZ Dilation of Right Main Bronchus, Via Natural or Artificial Opening
0B738DZ Dilation of Right Main Bronchus with Intraluminal Device, Via Natural or Artificial Opening Endoscopic
0B738ZZ Dilation of Right Main Bronchus, Via Natural or Artificial Opening Endoscopic
0B740DZ Dilation of Right Upper Lobe Bronchus with Intraluminal Device, Open Approach
0B740ZZ Dilation of Right Upper Lobe Bronchus, Open Approach
0B743DZ Dilation of Right Upper Lobe Bronchus with Intraluminal Device, Percutaneous Approach
0B743ZZ Dilation of Right Upper Lobe Bronchus, Percutaneous Approach
0B744DZ Dilation of Right Upper Lobe Bronchus with Intraluminal Device, Percutaneous Endoscopic Approach
0B744ZZ Dilation of Right Upper Lobe Bronchus, Percutaneous Endoscopic Approach

747DZ Dilation of Right Upper Lobe Bronchus with Intraluminal Device, Via Natural or Artificial Opening
747ZZ Dilation of Right Upper Lobe Bronchus, Via Natural or Artificial Opening
748DZ Dilation of Right Upper Lobe Bronchus with Intraluminal Device, Via Natural or Artificial Opening Endoscopic
748ZZ Dilation of Right Upper Lobe Bronchus, Via Natural or Artificial Opening Endoscopic
750DZ Dilation of Right Middle Lobe Bronchus with Intraluminal Device, Open Approach
750ZZ Dilation of Right Middle Lobe Bronchus, Open Approach
753DZ Dilation of Right Middle Lobe Bronchus with Intraluminal Device, Percutaneous Approach
753ZZ Dilation of Right Middle Lobe Bronchus, Percutaneous Approach
754DZ Dilation of Right Middle Lobe Bronchus with Intraluminal Device, Percutaneous Endoscopic Approach
754ZZ Dilation of Right Middle Lobe Bronchus, Percutaneous Endoscopic Approach
757DZ Dilation of Right Middle Lobe Bronchus with Intraluminal Device, Via Natural or Artificial Opening
B757ZZ Dilation of Right Middle Lobe Bronchus, Via Natural or Artificial Opening
B758DZ Dilation of Right Middle Lobe Bronchus with Intraluminal Device, Via Natural or Artificial Opening Endoscopic
B758ZZ Dilation of Right Middle Lobe Bronchus, Via Natural or Artificial Opening Endoscopic
B760DZ Dilation of Right Lower Lobe Bronchus with Intraluminal Device, Open Approach
B760ZZ Dilation of Right Lower Lobe Bronchus, Open Approach
B763DZ Dilation of Right Lower Lobe Bronchus with Intraluminal Device, Percutaneous Approach
B763ZZ Dilation of Right Lower Lobe Bronchus, Percutaneous Approach
B764DZ Dilation of Right Lower Lobe Bronchus with Intraluminal Device, Percutaneous Endoscopic Approach
B764ZZ Dilation of Right Lower Lobe Bronchus, Percutaneous Endoscopic Approach
B767DZ Dilation of Right Lower Lobe Bronchus with Intraluminal Device, Via Natural or Artificial Opening
B767ZZ Dilation of Right Lower Lobe Bronchus, Via Natural or Artificial Opening
0B768DZ Dilation of Right Lower Lobe Bronchus with Intraluminal Device, Via Natural or Artificial Opening Endoscopic
0B768ZZ Dilation of Right Lower Lobe Bronchus, Via Natural or Artificial Opening Endoscopic
0B770DZ Dilation of Left Main Bronchus with Intraluminal Device, Open Approach
0B770ZZ Dilation of Left Main Bronchus, Open Approach
0B773DZ Dilation of Left Main Bronchus with Intraluminal Device, Percutaneous Approach
0B773ZZ Dilation of Left Main Bronchus, Percutaneous Approach
0B774DZ Dilation of Left Main Bronchus with Intraluminal Device, Percutaneous Endoscopic Approach
0B774ZZ Dilation of Left Main Bronchus, Percutaneous Endoscopic Approach
0B777DZ Dilation of Left Main Bronchus with Intraluminal Device, Via Natural or Artificial Opening
0B777ZZ Dilation of Left Main Bronchus, Via Natural or Artificial Opening
0B778DZ Dilation of Left Main Bronchus with Intraluminal Device, Via Natural or Artificial Opening Endoscopic
0B778ZZ Dilation of Left Main Bronchus, Via Natural or Artificial Opening Endoscopic
0B780DZ Dilation of Left Upper Lobe Bronchus with Intraluminal Device, Open Approach
0B780ZZ Dilation of Left Upper Lobe Bronchus, Open Approach
0B783DZ Dilation of Left Upper Lobe Bronchus with Intraluminal Device, Percutaneous Approach
0B783ZZ Dilation of Left Upper Lobe Bronchus, Percutaneous Approach
0B784DZ Dilation of Left Upper Lobe Bronchus with Intraluminal Device, Percutaneous Endoscopic Approach
0B784ZZ Dilation of Left Upper Lobe Bronchus, Percutaneous Endoscopic Approach
0B787DZ Dilation of Left Upper Lobe Bronchus with Intraluminal Device, Via Natural or Artificial Opening
0B787ZZ Dilation of Left Upper Lobe Bronchus, Via Natural or Artificial Opening
0B788DZ Dilation of Left Upper Lobe Bronchus with Intraluminal Device, Via Natural or Artificial Opening Endoscopic
0B788ZZ Dilation of Left Upper Lobe Bronchus, Via Natural or Artificial Opening Endoscopic
0B790DZ Dilation of Lingula Bronchus with Intraluminal Device, Open Approach
0B790ZZ Dilation of Lingula Bronchus, Open Approach
0B793DZ Dilation of Lingula Bronchus with Intraluminal Device, Percutaneous Approach
0B793ZZ Dilation of Lingula Bronchus, Percutaneous Approach
0B794DZ Dilation of Lingula Bronchus with Intraluminal Device, Percutaneous Endoscopic Approach
0B794ZZ Dilation of Lingula Bronchus, Percutaneous Endoscopic Approach
0B797DZ Dilation of Lingula Bronchus with Intraluminal Device, Via Natural or Artificial Opening
0B797ZZ Dilation of Lingula Bronchus, Via Natural or Artificial Opening
0B798DZ Dilation of Lingula Bronchus with Intraluminal Device, Via Natural or Artificial Opening Endoscopic
0B798ZZ Dilation of Lingula Bronchus, Via Natural or Artificial Opening Endoscopic
0B7B0DZ Dilation of Left Lower Lobe Bronchus with Intraluminal Device, Open Approach
0B7B0ZZ Dilation of Left Lower Lobe Bronchus, Open Approach
0B7B3DZ Dilation of Left Lower Lobe Bronchus with Intraluminal Device, Percutaneous Approach
0B7B3ZZ Dilation of Left Lower Lobe Bronchus, Percutaneous Approach
0B7B4DZ Dilation of Left Lower Lobe Bronchus with Intraluminal Device, Percutaneous Endoscopic Approach
0B7B4ZZ Dilation of Left Lower Lobe Bronchus, Percutaneous Endoscopic Approach
0B7B7DZ Dilation of Left Lower Lobe Bronchus with Intraluminal Device, Via Natural or Artificial Opening
0B7B7ZZ Dilation of Left Lower Lobe Bronchus, Via Natural or Artificial Opening
0B7B8DZ Dilation of Left Lower Lobe Bronchus with Intraluminal Device, Via Natural or Artificial Opening Endoscopic
0B7B8ZZ Dilation of Left Lower Lobe Bronchus, Via Natural or Artificial Opening Endoscopic

B9 – Respiratory System, Drainage

eview Coding Guidelines B3.4a and B3.4b

eview Coding Guideline B6.2

B9100Z Drainage of Trachea with Drainage Device, Open Approach
B910ZX Drainage of Trachea, Open Approach, Diagnostic
0B910ZZ Drainage of Trachea, Open Approach
B9130Z Drainage of Trachea with Drainage Device, Percutaneous Approach
B913ZX Drainage of Trachea, Percutaneous Approach, Diagnostic
0B913ZZ Drainage of Trachea, Percutaneous Approach
0B9140Z Drainage of Trachea with Drainage Device, Percutaneous Endoscopic Approach
0B914ZX Drainage of Trachea, Percutaneous Endoscopic Approach, Diagnostic
0B914ZZ Drainage of Trachea, Percutaneous Endoscopic Approach
0B9170Z Drainage of Trachea with Drainage Device, Via Natural or Artificial Opening
0B917ZX Drainage of Trachea, Via Natural or Artificial Opening, Diagnostic
0B917ZZ Drainage of Trachea, Via Natural or Artificial Opening
0B9180Z Drainage of Trachea with Drainage Device, Via Natural or Artificial Opening Endoscopic
0B918ZX Drainage of Trachea, Via Natural or Artificial Opening Endoscopic, Diagnostic
0B918ZZ Drainage of Trachea, Via Natural or Artificial Opening Endoscopic
0B9200Z Drainage of Carina with Drainage Device, Open Approach
0B920ZX Drainage of Carina, Open Approach, Diagnostic
0B920ZZ Drainage of Carina, Open Approach
0B9230Z Drainage of Carina with Drainage Device, Percutaneous Approach
0B923ZX Drainage of Carina, Percutaneous Approach, Diagnostic
0B923ZZ Drainage of Carina, Percutaneous Approach

0B9240Z Drainage of Carina with Drainage Device, Percutaneous Endoscopic Approach
0B924ZX Drainage of Carina, Percutaneous Endoscopic Approach, Diagnostic
0B924ZZ Drainage of Carina, Percutaneous Endoscopic Approach
0B9270Z Drainage of Carina with Drainage Device, Via Natural or Artificial Opening
0B927ZX Drainage of Carina, Via Natural or Artificial Opening, Diagnostic
0B927ZZ Drainage of Carina, Via Natural or Artificial Opening
0B9280Z Drainage of Carina with Drainage Device, Via Natural or Artificial Opening Endoscopic
0B928ZX Drainage of Carina, Via Natural or Artificial Opening Endoscopic, Diagnostic
0B928ZZ Drainage of Carina, Via Natural or Artificial Opening Endoscopic
0B9300Z Drainage of Right Main Bronchus with Drainage Device, Open Approach
0B930ZX Drainage of Right Main Bronchus, Open Approach, Diagnostic
0B930ZZ Drainage of Right Main Bronchus, Open Approach
0B9330Z Drainage of Right Main Bronchus with Drainage Device, Percutaneous Approach
0B933ZX Drainage of Right Main Bronchus, Percutaneous Approach, Diagnostic
0B933ZZ Drainage of Right Main Bronchus, Percutaneous Approach
0B9340Z Drainage of Right Main Bronchus with Drainage Device, Percutaneous Endoscopic Approach
0B934ZX Drainage of Right Main Bronchus, Percutaneous Endoscopic Approach, Diagnostic
0B934ZZ Drainage of Right Main Bronchus, Percutaneous Endoscopic Approach
0B9370Z Drainage of Right Main Bronchus with Drainage Device, Via Natural or Artificial Opening
0B937ZX Drainage of Right Main Bronchus, Via Natural or Artificial Opening, Diagnostic
0B937ZZ Drainage of Right Main Bronchus, Via Natural or Artificial Opening
0B9380Z Drainage of Right Main Bronchus with Drainage Device, Via Natural or Artificial Opening Endoscopic
0B938ZX Drainage of Right Main Bronchus, Via Natural or Artificial Opening Endoscopic, Diagnostic
0B938ZZ Drainage of Right Main Bronchus, Via Natural or Artificial Opening Endoscopic
0B9400Z Drainage of Right Upper Lobe Bronchus with Drainage Device, Open Approach
0B940ZX Drainage of Right Upper Lobe Bronchus, Open Approach, Diagnostic
0B940ZZ Drainage of Right Upper Lobe Bronchus, Open Approach
0B9430Z Drainage of Right Upper Lobe Bronchus with Drainage Device, Percutaneous Approach
0B943ZX Drainage of Right Upper Lobe Bronchus, Percutaneous Approach, Diagnostic
0B943ZZ Drainage of Right Upper Lobe Bronchus, Percutaneous Approach
0B9440Z Drainage of Right Upper Lobe Bronchus with Drainage Device, Percutaneous Endoscopic Approach
0B944ZX Drainage of Right Upper Lobe Bronchus, Percutaneous Endoscopic Approach, Diagnostic
0B944ZZ Drainage of Right Upper Lobe Bronchus, Percutaneous Endoscopic Approach
0B9470Z Drainage of Right Upper Lobe Bronchus with Drainage Device, Via Natural or Artificial Opening
0B947ZX Drainage of Right Upper Lobe Bronchus, Via Natural or Artificial Opening, Diagnostic
0B947ZZ Drainage of Right Upper Lobe Bronchus, Via Natural or Artificial Opening
0B9480Z Drainage of Right Upper Lobe Bronchus with Drainage Device, Via Natural or Artificial Opening Endoscopic
0B948ZX Drainage of Right Upper Lobe Bronchus, Via Natural or Artificial Opening Endoscopic, Diagnostic
0B948ZZ Drainage of Right Upper Lobe Bronchus, Via Natural or Artificial Opening Endoscopic
0B9500Z Drainage of Right Middle Lobe Bronchus with Drainage Device, Open Approach
0B950ZX Drainage of Right Middle Lobe Bronchus, Open Approach, Diagnostic
0B950ZZ Drainage of Right Middle Lobe Bronchus, Open Approach
0B9530Z Drainage of Right Middle Lobe Bronchus with Drainage Device, Percutaneous Approach
0B953ZX Drainage of Right Middle Lobe Bronchus, Percutaneous Approach, Diagnostic
0B953ZZ Drainage of Right Middle Lobe Bronchus, Percutaneous Approach
0B9540Z Drainage of Right Middle Lobe Bronchus with Drainage Device, Percutaneous Endoscopic Approach
0B954ZX Drainage of Right Middle Lobe Bronchus, Percutaneous Endoscopic Approach, Diagnostic
0B954ZZ Drainage of Right Middle Lobe Bronchus, Percutaneous Endoscopic Approach
0B9570Z Drainage of Right Middle Lobe Bronchus with Drainage Device, Via Natural or Artificial Opening
0B957ZX Drainage of Right Middle Lobe Bronchus, Via Natural or Artificial Opening, Diagnostic
0B957ZZ Drainage of Right Middle Lobe Bronchus, Via Natural or Artificial Opening
0B9580Z Drainage of Right Middle Lobe Bronchus with Drainage Device, Via Natural or Artificial Opening Endoscopic
0B958ZX Drainage of Right Middle Lobe Bronchus, Via Natural or Artificial Opening Endoscopic, Diagnostic
0B958ZZ Drainage of Right Middle Lobe Bronchus, Via Natural or Artificial Opening Endoscopic
0B9600Z Drainage of Right Lower Lobe Bronchus with Drainage Device, Open Approach
0B960ZX Drainage of Right Lower Lobe Bronchus, Open Approach, Diagnostic
0B960ZZ Drainage of Right Lower Lobe Bronchus, Open Approach
0B9630Z Drainage of Right Lower Lobe Bronchus with Drainage Device, Percutaneous Approach
0B963ZX Drainage of Right Lower Lobe Bronchus, Percutaneous Approach, Diagnostic
0B963ZZ Drainage of Right Lower Lobe Bronchus, Percutaneous Approach
0B9640Z Drainage of Right Lower Lobe Bronchus with Drainage Device, Percutaneous Endoscopic Approach
0B964ZX Drainage of Right Lower Lobe Bronchus, Percutaneous Endoscopic Approach, Diagnostic
0B964ZZ Drainage of Right Lower Lobe Bronchus, Percutaneous Endoscopic Approach
0B9670Z Drainage of Right Lower Lobe Bronchu with Drainage Device, Via Natural or Artificial Opening
0B967ZX Drainage of Right Lower Lobe Bronchu Via Natural or Artificial Opening, Diagnostic
0B967ZZ Drainage of Right Lower Lobe Bronchu Via Natural or Artificial Opening
0B9680Z Drainage of Right Lower Lobe Bronchu with Drainage Device, Via Natural or Artificial Opening Endoscopic
0B968ZX Drainage of Right Lower Lobe Bronchus Via Natural or Artificial Opening Endoscopic, Diagnostic
0B968ZZ Drainage of Right Lower Lobe Bronchus Via Natural or Artificial Opening Endoscopic
0B9700Z Drainage of Left Main Bronchus with Drainage Device, Open Approach
0B970ZX Drainage of Left Main Bronchus, Open Approach, Diagnostic
0B970ZZ Drainage of Left Main Bronchus, Open Approach
0B9730Z Drainage of Left Main Bronchus with Drainage Device, Percutaneous Approach
0B973ZX Drainage of Left Main Bronchus, Percutaneous Approach, Diagnostic
0B973ZZ Drainage of Left Main Bronchus, Percutaneous Approach
0B9740Z Drainage of Left Main Bronchus with Drainage Device, Percutaneous Endoscopic Approach
0B974ZX Drainage of Left Main Bronchus, Percutaneous Endoscopic Approach, Diagnostic
0B974ZZ Drainage of Left Main Bronchus, Percutaneous Endoscopic Approach
0B9770Z Drainage of Left Main Bronchus with Drainage Device, Via Natural or Artificial Opening
0B977ZX Drainage of Left Main Bronchus, Via Natural or Artificial Opening, Diagnostic
0B977ZZ Drainage of Left Main Bronchus, Via Natural or Artificial Opening
0B9780Z Drainage of Left Main Bronchus with Drainage Device, Via Natural or Artificial Opening Endoscopic
0B978ZX Drainage of Left Main Bronchus, Via Natural or Artificial Opening Endoscopic, Diagnostic
0B978ZZ Drainage of Left Main Bronchus, Via Natural or Artificial Opening Endoscopic
0B9800Z Drainage of Left Upper Lobe Bronchus with Drainage Device, Open Approach
0B980ZX Drainage of Left Upper Lobe Bronchus, Open Approach, Diagnostic
0B980ZZ Drainage of Left Upper Lobe Bronchus, Open Approach
0B9830Z Drainage of Left Upper Lobe Bronchus with Drainage Device, Percutaneous Approach
0B983ZX Drainage of Left Upper Lobe Bronchus, Percutaneous Approach, Diagnostic
0B983ZZ Drainage of Left Upper Lobe Bronchus, Percutaneous Approach
0B9840Z Drainage of Left Upper Lobe Bronchus with Drainage Device, Percutaneous Endoscopic Approach
0B984ZX Drainage of Left Upper Lobe Bronchus, Percutaneous Endoscopic Approach, Diagnostic
0B984ZZ Drainage of Left Upper Lobe Bronchus, Percutaneous Endoscopic Approach
0B9870Z Drainage of Left Upper Lobe Bronchus with Drainage Device, Via Natural or Artificial Opening

87ZX Drainage of Left Upper Lobe Bronchus, Via Natural or Artificial Opening, Diagnostic

87ZZ Drainage of Left Upper Lobe Bronchus, Via Natural or Artificial Opening

880Z Drainage of Left Upper Lobe Bronchus with Drainage Device, Via Natural or Artificial Opening Endoscopic

88ZX Drainage of Left Upper Lobe Bronchus, Via Natural or Artificial Opening Endoscopic, Diagnostic

88ZZ Drainage of Left Upper Lobe Bronchus, Via Natural or Artificial Opening Endoscopic

9900Z Drainage of Lingula Bronchus with Drainage Device, Open Approach

990ZX Drainage of Lingula Bronchus, Open Approach, Diagnostic

990ZZ Drainage of Lingula Bronchus, Open Approach

9930Z Drainage of Lingula Bronchus with Drainage Device, Percutaneous Approach

993ZX Drainage of Lingula Bronchus, Percutaneous Approach, Diagnostic

993ZZ Drainage of Lingula Bronchus, Percutaneous Approach

9940Z Drainage of Lingula Bronchus with Drainage Device, Percutaneous Endoscopic Approach

994ZX Drainage of Lingula Bronchus, Percutaneous Endoscopic Approach, Diagnostic

994ZZ Drainage of Lingula Bronchus, Percutaneous Endoscopic Approach

9970Z Drainage of Lingula Bronchus with Drainage Device, Via Natural or Artificial Opening

997ZX Drainage of Lingula Bronchus, Via Natural or Artificial Opening, Diagnostic

997ZZ Drainage of Lingula Bronchus, Via Natural or Artificial Opening

9980Z Drainage of Lingula Bronchus with Drainage Device, Via Natural or Artificial Opening Endoscopic

998ZX Drainage of Lingula Bronchus, Via Natural or Artificial Opening Endoscopic, Diagnostic

998ZZ Drainage of Lingula Bronchus, Via Natural or Artificial Opening Endoscopic

39B00Z Drainage of Left Lower Lobe Bronchus with Drainage Device, Open Approach

39B0ZX Drainage of Left Lower Lobe Bronchus, Open Approach, Diagnostic

B9B0ZZ Drainage of Left Lower Lobe Bronchus, Open Approach

B9B30Z Drainage of Left Lower Lobe Bronchus with Drainage Device, Percutaneous Approach

B9B3ZX Drainage of Left Lower Lobe Bronchus, Percutaneous Approach, Diagnostic

B9B3ZZ Drainage of Left Lower Lobe Bronchus, Percutaneous Approach

B9B40Z Drainage of Left Lower Lobe Bronchus with Drainage Device, Percutaneous Endoscopic Approach

B9B4ZX Drainage of Left Lower Lobe Bronchus, Percutaneous Endoscopic Approach, Diagnostic

B9B4ZZ Drainage of Left Lower Lobe Bronchus, Percutaneous Endoscopic Approach

B9B70Z Drainage of Left Lower Lobe Bronchus with Drainage Device, Via Natural or Artificial Opening

B9B7ZX Drainage of Left Lower Lobe Bronchus, Via Natural or Artificial Opening, Diagnostic

0B9B7ZZ Drainage of Left Lower Lobe Bronchus, Via Natural or Artificial Opening

0B9B80Z Drainage of Left Lower Lobe Bronchus with Drainage Device, Via Natural or Artificial Opening Endoscopic

0B9B8ZX Drainage of Left Lower Lobe Bronchus, Via Natural or Artificial Opening Endoscopic, Diagnostic

0B9B8ZZ Drainage of Left Lower Lobe Bronchus, Via Natural or Artificial Opening Endoscopic

0B9C00Z Drainage of Right Upper Lung Lobe with Drainage Device, Open Approach

0B9C0ZX Drainage of Right Upper Lung Lobe, Open Approach, Diagnostic

0B9C0ZZ Drainage of Right Upper Lung Lobe, Open Approach

0B9C30Z Drainage of Right Upper Lung Lobe with Drainage Device, Percutaneous Approach

0B9C3ZX Drainage of Right Upper Lung Lobe, Percutaneous Approach, Diagnostic

0B9C3ZZ Drainage of Right Upper Lung Lobe, Percutaneous Approach

0B9C40Z Drainage of Right Upper Lung Lobe with Drainage Device, Percutaneous Endoscopic Approach

0B9C4ZX Drainage of Right Upper Lung Lobe, Percutaneous Endoscopic Approach, Diagnostic

0B9C4ZZ Drainage of Right Upper Lung Lobe, Percutaneous Endoscopic Approach

0B9C70Z Drainage of Right Upper Lung Lobe with Drainage Device, Via Natural or Artificial Opening

0B9C7ZX Drainage of Right Upper Lung Lobe, Via Natural or Artificial Opening, Diagnostic

0B9C7ZZ Drainage of Right Upper Lung Lobe, Via Natural or Artificial Opening

0B9C80Z Drainage of Right Upper Lung Lobe with Drainage Device, Via Natural or Artificial Opening Endoscopic

0B9C8ZX Drainage of Right Upper Lung Lobe, Via Natural or Artificial Opening Endoscopic, Diagnostic

0B9C8ZZ Drainage of Right Upper Lung Lobe, Via Natural or Artificial Opening Endoscopic

0B9D00Z Drainage of Right Middle Lung Lobe with Drainage Device, Open Approach

0B9D0ZX Drainage of Right Middle Lung Lobe, Open Approach, Diagnostic

0B9D0ZZ Drainage of Right Middle Lung Lobe, Open Approach

0B9D30Z Drainage of Right Middle Lung Lobe with Drainage Device, Percutaneous Approach

0B9D3ZX Drainage of Right Middle Lung Lobe, Percutaneous Approach, Diagnostic

0B9D3ZZ Drainage of Right Middle Lung Lobe, Percutaneous Approach

0B9D40Z Drainage of Right Middle Lung Lobe with Drainage Device, Percutaneous Endoscopic Approach

0B9D4ZX Drainage of Right Middle Lung Lobe, Percutaneous Endoscopic Approach, Diagnostic

0B9D4ZZ Drainage of Right Middle Lung Lobe, Percutaneous Endoscopic Approach

0B9D70Z Drainage of Right Middle Lung Lobe with Drainage Device, Via Natural or Artificial Opening

0B9D7ZX Drainage of Right Middle Lung Lobe, Via Natural or Artificial Opening, Diagnostic

0B9D7ZZ Drainage of Right Middle Lung Lobe, Via Natural or Artificial Opening

0B9D80Z Drainage of Right Middle Lung Lobe with Drainage Device, Via Natural or Artificial Opening Endoscopic

0B9D8ZX Drainage of Right Middle Lung Lobe, Via Natural or Artificial Opening Endoscopic, Diagnostic

0B9D8ZZ Drainage of Right Middle Lung Lobe, Via Natural or Artificial Opening Endoscopic

0B9F00Z Drainage of Right Lower Lung Lobe with Drainage Device, Open Approach

0B9F0ZX Drainage of Right Lower Lung Lobe, Open Approach, Diagnostic

0B9F0ZZ Drainage of Right Lower Lung Lobe, Open Approach

0B9F30Z Drainage of Right Lower Lung Lobe with Drainage Device, Percutaneous Approach

0B9F3ZX Drainage of Right Lower Lung Lobe, Percutaneous Approach, Diagnostic

0B9F3ZZ Drainage of Right Lower Lung Lobe, Percutaneous Approach

0B9F40Z Drainage of Right Lower Lung Lobe with Drainage Device, Percutaneous Endoscopic Approach

0B9F4ZX Drainage of Right Lower Lung Lobe, Percutaneous Endoscopic Approach, Diagnostic

0B9F4ZZ Drainage of Right Lower Lung Lobe, Percutaneous Endoscopic Approach

0B9F70Z Drainage of Right Lower Lung Lobe with Drainage Device, Via Natural or Artificial Opening

0B9F7ZX Drainage of Right Lower Lung Lobe, Via Natural or Artificial Opening, Diagnostic

0B9F7ZZ Drainage of Right Lower Lung Lobe, Via Natural or Artificial Opening

0B9F80Z Drainage of Right Lower Lung Lobe with Drainage Device, Via Natural or Artificial Opening Endoscopic

0B9F8ZX Drainage of Right Lower Lung Lobe, Via Natural or Artificial Opening Endoscopic, Diagnostic

0B9F8ZZ Drainage of Right Lower Lung Lobe, Via Natural or Artificial Opening Endoscopic

0B9G00Z Drainage of Left Upper Lung Lobe with Drainage Device, Open Approach

0B9G0ZX Drainage of Left Upper Lung Lobe, Open Approach, Diagnostic

0B9G0ZZ Drainage of Left Upper Lung Lobe, Open Approach

0B9G30Z Drainage of Left Upper Lung Lobe with Drainage Device, Percutaneous Approach

0B9G3ZX Drainage of Left Upper Lung Lobe, Percutaneous Approach, Diagnostic

0B9G3ZZ Drainage of Left Upper Lung Lobe, Percutaneous Approach

0B9G40Z Drainage of Left Upper Lung Lobe with Drainage Device, Percutaneous Endoscopic Approach

0B9G4ZX Drainage of Left Upper Lung Lobe, Percutaneous Endoscopic Approach, Diagnostic

0B9G4ZZ Drainage of Left Upper Lung Lobe, Percutaneous Endoscopic Approach

0B9G70Z Drainage of Left Upper Lung Lobe with Drainage Device, Via Natural or Artificial Opening

0B9G7ZX Drainage of Left Upper Lung Lobe, Via Natural or Artificial Opening, Diagnostic

0B9G7ZZ Drainage of Left Upper Lung Lobe, Via Natural or Artificial Opening

0B9G80Z Drainage of Left Upper Lung Lobe with Drainage Device, Via Natural or Artificial Opening Endoscopic

0B9G8ZX Drainage of Left Upper Lung Lobe, Via Natural or Artificial Opening Endoscopic, Diagnostic

0B9G8ZZ Drainage of Left Upper Lung Lobe, Via Natural or Artificial Opening Endoscopic

0B9H00Z Drainage of Lung Lingula with Drainage Device, Open Approach

0B9H0ZX Drainage of Lung Lingula, Open Approach, Diagnostic
0B9H0ZZ Drainage of Lung Lingula, Open Approach
0B9H30Z Drainage of Lung Lingula with Drainage Device, Percutaneous Approach
0B9H3ZX Drainage of Lung Lingula, Percutaneous Approach, Diagnostic
0B9H3ZZ Drainage of Lung Lingula, Percutaneous Approach
0B9H40Z Drainage of Lung Lingula with Drainage Device, Percutaneous Endoscopic Approach
0B9H4ZX Drainage of Lung Lingula, Percutaneous Endoscopic Approach, Diagnostic
0B9H4ZZ Drainage of Lung Lingula, Percutaneous Endoscopic Approach
0B9H70Z Drainage of Lung Lingula with Drainage Device, Via Natural or Artificial Opening
0B9H7ZX Drainage of Lung Lingula, Via Natural or Artificial Opening, Diagnostic
0B9H7ZZ Drainage of Lung Lingula, Via Natural or Artificial Opening
0B9H80Z Drainage of Lung Lingula with Drainage Device, Via Natural or Artificial Opening Endoscopic
0B9H8ZX Drainage of Lung Lingula, Via Natural or Artificial Opening Endoscopic, Diagnostic
0B9H8ZZ Drainage of Lung Lingula, Via Natural or Artificial Opening Endoscopic
0B9J00Z Drainage of Left Lower Lung Lobe with Drainage Device, Open Approach
0B9J0ZX Drainage of Left Lower Lung Lobe, Open Approach, Diagnostic
0B9J0ZZ Drainage of Left Lower Lung Lobe, Open Approach
0B9J30Z Drainage of Left Lower Lung Lobe with Drainage Device, Percutaneous Approach
0B9J3ZX Drainage of Left Lower Lung Lobe, Percutaneous Approach, Diagnostic
0B9J3ZZ Drainage of Left Lower Lung Lobe, Percutaneous Approach
0B9J40Z Drainage of Left Lower Lung Lobe with Drainage Device, Percutaneous Endoscopic Approach
0B9J4ZX Drainage of Left Lower Lung Lobe, Percutaneous Endoscopic Approach, Diagnostic
0B9J4ZZ Drainage of Left Lower Lung Lobe, Percutaneous Endoscopic Approach
0B9J70Z Drainage of Left Lower Lung Lobe with Drainage Device, Via Natural or Artificial Opening
0B9J7ZX Drainage of Left Lower Lung Lobe, Via Natural or Artificial Opening, Diagnostic
0B9J7ZZ Drainage of Left Lower Lung Lobe, Via Natural or Artificial Opening
0B9J80Z Drainage of Left Lower Lung Lobe with Drainage Device, Via Natural or Artificial Opening Endoscopic
0B9J8ZX Drainage of Left Lower Lung Lobe, Via Natural or Artificial Opening Endoscopic, Diagnostic
0B9J8ZZ Drainage of Left Lower Lung Lobe, Via Natural or Artificial Opening Endoscopic
0B9K00Z Drainage of Right Lung with Drainage Device, Open Approach
0B9K0ZX Drainage of Right Lung, Open Approach, Diagnostic
0B9K0ZZ Drainage of Right Lung, Open Approach
0B9K30Z Drainage of Right Lung with Drainage Device, Percutaneous Approach
0B9K3ZX Drainage of Right Lung, Percutaneous Approach, Diagnostic
0B9K3ZZ Drainage of Right Lung, Percutaneous Approach
0B9K40Z Drainage of Right Lung with Drainage Device, Percutaneous Endoscopic Approach
0B9K4ZX Drainage of Right Lung, Percutaneous Endoscopic Approach, Diagnostic
0B9K4ZZ Drainage of Right Lung, Percutaneous Endoscopic Approach
0B9K70Z Drainage of Right Lung with Drainage Device, Via Natural or Artificial Opening
0B9K7ZX Drainage of Right Lung, Via Natural or Artificial Opening, Diagnostic
0B9K7ZZ Drainage of Right Lung, Via Natural or Artificial Opening
0B9K80Z Drainage of Right Lung with Drainage Device, Via Natural or Artificial Opening Endoscopic
0B9K8ZX Drainage of Right Lung, Via Natural or Artificial Opening Endoscopic, Diagnostic
0B9K8ZZ Drainage of Right Lung, Via Natural or Artificial Opening Endoscopic
0B9L00Z Drainage of Left Lung with Drainage Device, Open Approach
0B9L0ZX Drainage of Left Lung, Open Approach, Diagnostic
0B9L0ZZ Drainage of Left Lung, Open Approach
0B9L30Z Drainage of Left Lung with Drainage Device, Percutaneous Approach
0B9L3ZX Drainage of Left Lung, Percutaneous Approach, Diagnostic
0B9L3ZZ Drainage of Left Lung, Percutaneous Approach
0B9L40Z Drainage of Left Lung with Drainage Device, Percutaneous Endoscopic Approach
0B9L4ZX Drainage of Left Lung, Percutaneous Endoscopic Approach, Diagnostic
0B9L4ZZ Drainage of Left Lung, Percutaneous Endoscopic Approach
0B9L70Z Drainage of Left Lung with Drainage Device, Via Natural or Artificial Opening
0B9L7ZX Drainage of Left Lung, Via Natural or Artificial Opening, Diagnostic
0B9L7ZZ Drainage of Left Lung, Via Natural or Artificial Opening
0B9L80Z Drainage of Left Lung with Drainage Device, Via Natural or Artificial Opening Endoscopic
0B9L8ZX Drainage of Left Lung, Via Natural or Artificial Opening Endoscopic, Diagnostic
0B9L8ZZ Drainage of Left Lung, Via Natural or Artificial Opening Endoscopic
0B9M00Z Drainage of Bilateral Lungs with Drainage Device, Open Approach
0B9M0ZX Drainage of Bilateral Lungs, Open Approach, Diagnostic
0B9M0ZZ Drainage of Bilateral Lungs, Open Approach
0B9M30Z Drainage of Bilateral Lungs with Drainage Device, Percutaneous Approach
0B9M3ZX Drainage of Bilateral Lungs, Percutaneous Approach, Diagnostic
0B9M3ZZ Drainage of Bilateral Lungs, Percutaneous Approach
0B9M40Z Drainage of Bilateral Lungs with Drainage Device, Percutaneous Endoscopic Approach
0B9M4ZX Drainage of Bilateral Lungs, Percutaneous Endoscopic Approach, Diagnostic
0B9M4ZZ Drainage of Bilateral Lungs, Percutaneous Endoscopic Approach
0B9M70Z Drainage of Bilateral Lungs with Drainage Device, Via Natural or Artificial Opening
0B9M7ZX Drainage of Bilateral Lungs, Via Natural or Artificial Opening, Diagnostic
0B9M7ZZ Drainage of Bilateral Lungs, Via Natural or Artificial Opening
0B9M80Z Drainage of Bilateral Lungs with Drain Device, Via Natural or Artificial Openi Endoscopic
0B9M8ZX Drainage of Bilateral Lungs, Via Natura or Artificial Opening Endoscopic, Diagnostic
0B9M8ZZ Drainage of Bilateral Lungs, Via Natura or Artificial Opening Endoscopic
0B9N00Z Drainage of Right Pleura with Drainage Device, Open Approach
0B9N0ZX Drainage of Right Pleura, Open Approa Diagnostic
0B9N0ZZ Drainage of Right Pleura, Open Approa
0B9N30Z Drainage of Right Pleura with Drainage Device, Percutaneous Approach
0B9N3ZX Drainage of Right Pleura, Percutaneous Approach, Diagnostic
0B9N3ZZ Drainage of Right Pleura, Percutaneous Approach
0B9N40Z Drainage of Right Pleura with Drainage Device, Percutaneous Endoscopic Approach
0B9N4ZX Drainage of Right Pleura, Percutaneous Endoscopic Approach, Diagnostic
0B9N4ZZ Drainage of Right Pleura, Percutaneous Endoscopic Approach
0B9P00Z Drainage of Left Pleura with Drainage Device, Open Approach
0B9P0ZX Drainage of Left Pleura, Open Approach Diagnostic
0B9P0ZZ Drainage of Left Pleura, Open Approach
0B9P30Z Drainage of Left Pleura with Drainage Device, Percutaneous Approach
0B9P3ZX Drainage of Left Pleura, Percutaneous Approach, Diagnostic
0B9P3ZZ Drainage of Left Pleura, Percutaneous Approach
0B9P40Z Drainage of Left Pleura with Drainage Device, Percutaneous Endoscopic Approach
0B9P4ZX Drainage of Left Pleura, Percutaneous Endoscopic Approach, Diagnostic
0B9P4ZZ Drainage of Left Pleura, Percutaneous Endoscopic Approach
0B9R00Z Drainage of Right Diaphragm with Drainage Device, Open Approach
0B9R0ZX Drainage of Right Diaphragm, Open Approach, Diagnostic
0B9R0ZZ Drainage of Right Diaphragm, Open Approach
0B9R30Z Drainage of Right Diaphragm with Drainage Device, Percutaneous Approach
0B9R3ZX Drainage of Right Diaphragm, Percutaneous Approach, Diagnostic
0B9R3ZZ Drainage of Right Diaphragm, Percutaneous Approach
0B9R40Z Drainage of Right Diaphragm with Drainage Device, Percutaneous Endoscopic Approach
0B9R4ZX Drainage of Right Diaphragm, Percutaneous Endoscopic Approach, Diagnostic
0B9R4ZZ Drainage of Right Diaphragm, Percutaneous Endoscopic Approach
0B9S00Z Drainage of Left Diaphragm with Drainage Device, Open Approach
0B9S0ZX Drainage of Left Diaphragm, Open Approach, Diagnostic
0B9S0ZZ Drainage of Left Diaphragm, Open Approach
0B9S30Z Drainage of Left Diaphragm with Drainage Device, Percutaneous Approach
0B9S3ZX Drainage of Left Diaphragm, Percutaneou Approach, Diagnostic
0B9S3ZZ Drainage of Left Diaphragm, Percutaneou Approach

9S40Z Drainage of Left Diaphragm with Drainage Device, Percutaneous Endoscopic Approach

0B9S4ZX Drainage of Left Diaphragm, Percutaneous Endoscopic Approach, Diagnostic

0B9S4ZZ Drainage of Left Diaphragm, Percutaneous Endoscopic Approach

B – Respiratory System, Excision

view Coding Guidelines B3.4a and B3.4b

view Coding Guideline B3.8

B10ZX Excision of Trachea, Open Approach, Diagnostic

B10ZZ Excision of Trachea, Open Approach

B13ZX Excision of Trachea, Percutaneous Approach, Diagnostic

B13ZZ Excision of Trachea, Percutaneous Approach

B14ZX Excision of Trachea, Percutaneous Endoscopic Approach, Diagnostic

B14ZZ Excision of Trachea, Percutaneous Endoscopic Approach

B17ZX Excision of Trachea, Via Natural or Artificial Opening, Diagnostic

B17ZZ Excision of Trachea, Via Natural or Artificial Opening

B18ZX Excision of Trachea, Via Natural or Artificial Opening Endoscopic, Diagnostic

B18ZZ Excision of Trachea, Via Natural or Artificial Opening Endoscopic

B20ZX Excision of Carina, Open Approach, Diagnostic

B20ZZ Excision of Carina, Open Approach

B23ZX Excision of Carina, Percutaneous Approach, Diagnostic

B23ZZ Excision of Carina, Percutaneous Approach

B24ZX Excision of Carina, Percutaneous Endoscopic Approach, Diagnostic

B24ZZ Excision of Carina, Percutaneous Endoscopic Approach

B27ZX Excision of Carina, Via Natural or Artificial Opening, Diagnostic

B27ZZ Excision of Carina, Via Natural or Artificial Opening

B28ZX Excision of Carina, Via Natural or Artificial Opening Endoscopic, Diagnostic

B28ZZ Excision of Carina, Via Natural or Artificial Opening Endoscopic

BB30ZX Excision of Right Main Bronchus, Open Approach, Diagnostic

BB30ZZ Excision of Right Main Bronchus, Open Approach

BB33ZX Excision of Right Main Bronchus, Percutaneous Approach, Diagnostic

BB33ZZ Excision of Right Main Bronchus, Percutaneous Approach

BB34ZX Excision of Right Main Bronchus, Percutaneous Endoscopic Approach, Diagnostic

BB34ZZ Excision of Right Main Bronchus, Percutaneous Endoscopic Approach

BB37ZX Excision of Right Main Bronchus, Via Natural or Artificial Opening, Diagnostic

BB37ZZ Excision of Right Main Bronchus, Via Natural or Artificial Opening

BB38ZX Excision of Right Main Bronchus, Via Natural or Artificial Opening Endoscopic, Diagnostic

BB38ZZ Excision of Right Main Bronchus, Via Natural or Artificial Opening Endoscopic

BB40ZX Excision of Right Upper Lobe Bronchus, Open Approach, Diagnostic

BB40ZZ Excision of Right Upper Lobe Bronchus, Open Approach

BB43ZX Excision of Right Upper Lobe Bronchus, Percutaneous Approach, Diagnostic

0BB43ZZ Excision of Right Upper Lobe Bronchus, Percutaneous Approach

0BB44ZX Excision of Right Upper Lobe Bronchus, Percutaneous Endoscopic Approach, Diagnostic

0BB44ZZ Excision of Right Upper Lobe Bronchus, Percutaneous Endoscopic Approach

0BB47ZX Excision of Right Upper Lobe Bronchus, Via Natural or Artificial Opening, Diagnostic

0BB47ZZ Excision of Right Upper Lobe Bronchus, Via Natural or Artificial Opening

0BB48ZX Excision of Right Upper Lobe Bronchus, Via Natural or Artificial Opening Endoscopic, Diagnostic

0BB48ZZ Excision of Right Upper Lobe Bronchus, Via Natural or Artificial Opening Endoscopic

0BB50ZX Excision of Right Middle Lobe Bronchus, Open Approach, Diagnostic

0BB50ZZ Excision of Right Middle Lobe Bronchus, Open Approach

0BB53ZX Excision of Right Middle Lobe Bronchus, Percutaneous Approach, Diagnostic

0BB53ZZ Excision of Right Middle Lobe Bronchus, Percutaneous Approach

0BB54ZX Excision of Right Middle Lobe Bronchus, Percutaneous Endoscopic Approach, Diagnostic

0BB54ZZ Excision of Right Middle Lobe Bronchus, Percutaneous Endoscopic Approach

0BB57ZX Excision of Right Middle Lobe Bronchus, Via Natural or Artificial Opening, Diagnostic

0BB57ZZ Excision of Right Middle Lobe Bronchus, Via Natural or Artificial Opening

0BB58ZX Excision of Right Middle Lobe Bronchus, Via Natural or Artificial Opening Endoscopic, Diagnostic

0BB58ZZ Excision of Right Middle Lobe Bronchus, Via Natural or Artificial Opening Endoscopic

0BB60ZX Excision of Right Lower Lobe Bronchus, Open Approach, Diagnostic

0BB60ZZ Excision of Right Lower Lobe Bronchus, Open Approach

0BB63ZX Excision of Right Lower Lobe Bronchus, Percutaneous Approach, Diagnostic

0BB63ZZ Excision of Right Lower Lobe Bronchus, Percutaneous Approach

0BB64ZX Excision of Right Lower Lobe Bronchus, Percutaneous Endoscopic Approach, Diagnostic

0BB64ZZ Excision of Right Lower Lobe Bronchus, Percutaneous Endoscopic Approach

0BB67ZX Excision of Right Lower Lobe Bronchus, Via Natural or Artificial Opening, Diagnostic

0BB67ZZ Excision of Right Lower Lobe Bronchus, Via Natural or Artificial Opening

0BB68ZX Excision of Right Lower Lobe Bronchus, Via Natural or Artificial Opening Endoscopic, Diagnostic

0BB68ZZ Excision of Right Lower Lobe Bronchus, Via Natural or Artificial Opening Endoscopic

0BB70ZX Excision of Left Main Bronchus, Open Approach, Diagnostic

0BB70ZZ Excision of Left Main Bronchus, Open Approach

0BB73ZX Excision of Left Main Bronchus, Percutaneous Approach, Diagnostic

0BB73ZZ Excision of Left Main Bronchus, Percutaneous Approach

0BB74ZX Excision of Left Main Bronchus, Percutaneous Endoscopic Approach, Diagnostic

0BB74ZZ Excision of Left Main Bronchus, Percutaneous Endoscopic Approach

0BB77ZX Excision of Left Main Bronchus, Via Natural or Artificial Opening, Diagnostic

0BB77ZZ Excision of Left Main Bronchus, Via Natural or Artificial Opening

0BB78ZX Excision of Left Main Bronchus, Via Natural or Artificial Opening Endoscopic, Diagnostic

0BB78ZZ Excision of Left Main Bronchus, Via Natural or Artificial Opening Endoscopic

0BB80ZX Excision of Left Upper Lobe Bronchus, Open Approach, Diagnostic

0BB80ZZ Excision of Left Upper Lobe Bronchus, Open Approach

0BB83ZX Excision of Left Upper Lobe Bronchus, Percutaneous Approach, Diagnostic

0BB83ZZ Excision of Left Upper Lobe Bronchus, Percutaneous Approach

0BB84ZX Excision of Left Upper Lobe Bronchus, Percutaneous Endoscopic Approach, Diagnostic

0BB84ZZ Excision of Left Upper Lobe Bronchus, Percutaneous Endoscopic Approach

0BB87ZX Excision of Left Upper Lobe Bronchus, Via Natural or Artificial Opening, Diagnostic

0BB87ZZ Excision of Left Upper Lobe Bronchus, Via Natural or Artificial Opening

0BB88ZX Excision of Left Upper Lobe Bronchus, Via Natural or Artificial Opening Endoscopic, Diagnostic

0BB88ZZ Excision of Left Upper Lobe Bronchus, Via Natural or Artificial Opening Endoscopic

0BB90ZX Excision of Lingula Bronchus, Open Approach, Diagnostic

0BB90ZZ Excision of Lingula Bronchus, Open Approach

0BB93ZX Excision of Lingula Bronchus, Percutaneous Approach, Diagnostic

0BB93ZZ Excision of Lingula Bronchus, Percutaneous Approach

0BB94ZX Excision of Lingula Bronchus, Percutaneous Endoscopic Approach, Diagnostic

0BB94ZZ Excision of Lingula Bronchus, Percutaneous Endoscopic Approach

0BB97ZX Excision of Lingula Bronchus, Via Natural or Artificial Opening, Diagnostic

0BB97ZZ Excision of Lingula Bronchus, Via Natural or Artificial Opening

0BB98ZX Excision of Lingula Bronchus, Via Natural or Artificial Opening Endoscopic, Diagnostic

0BB98ZZ Excision of Lingula Bronchus, Via Natural or Artificial Opening Endoscopic
0BBB0ZX Excision of Left Lower Lobe Bronchus, Open Approach, Diagnostic
0BBB0ZZ Excision of Left Lower Lobe Bronchus, Open Approach
0BBB3ZX Excision of Left Lower Lobe Bronchus, Percutaneous Approach, Diagnostic
0BBB3ZZ Excision of Left Lower Lobe Bronchus, Percutaneous Approach
0BBB4ZX Excision of Left Lower Lobe Bronchus, Percutaneous Endoscopic Approach, Diagnostic
0BBB4ZZ Excision of Left Lower Lobe Bronchus, Percutaneous Endoscopic Approach
0BBB7ZX Excision of Left Lower Lobe Bronchus, Via Natural or Artificial Opening, Diagnostic
0BBB7ZZ Excision of Left Lower Lobe Bronchus, Via Natural or Artificial Opening
0BBB8ZX Excision of Left Lower Lobe Bronchus, Via Natural or Artificial Opening Endoscopic, Diagnostic
0BBB8ZZ Excision of Left Lower Lobe Bronchus, Via Natural or Artificial Opening Endoscopic
0BBC0ZX Excision of Right Upper Lung Lobe, Open Approach, Diagnostic
0BBC0ZZ Excision of Right Upper Lung Lobe, Open Approach
0BBC3ZX Excision of Right Upper Lung Lobe, Percutaneous Approach, Diagnostic
0BBC3ZZ Excision of Right Upper Lung Lobe, Percutaneous Approach
0BBC4ZX Excision of Right Upper Lung Lobe, Percutaneous Endoscopic Approach, Diagnostic
0BBC4ZZ Excision of Right Upper Lung Lobe, Percutaneous Endoscopic Approach
0BBC7ZX Excision of Right Upper Lung Lobe, Via Natural or Artificial Opening, Diagnostic
0BBC7ZZ Excision of Right Upper Lung Lobe, Via Natural or Artificial Opening
0BBC8ZX Excision of Right Upper Lung Lobe, Via Natural or Artificial Opening Endoscopic, Diagnostic
0BBC8ZZ Excision of Right Upper Lung Lobe, Via Natural or Artificial Opening Endoscopic
0BBD0ZX Excision of Right Middle Lung Lobe, Open Approach, Diagnostic
0BBD0ZZ Excision of Right Middle Lung Lobe, Open Approach
0BBD3ZX Excision of Right Middle Lung Lobe, Percutaneous Approach, Diagnostic
0BBD3ZZ Excision of Right Middle Lung Lobe, Percutaneous Approach
0BBD4ZX Excision of Right Middle Lung Lobe, Percutaneous Endoscopic Approach, Diagnostic
0BBD4ZZ Excision of Right Middle Lung Lobe, Percutaneous Endoscopic Approach
0BBD7ZX Excision of Right Middle Lung Lobe, Via Natural or Artificial Opening, Diagnostic
0BBD7ZZ Excision of Right Middle Lung Lobe, Via Natural or Artificial Opening
0BBD8ZX Excision of Right Middle Lung Lobe, Via Natural or Artificial Opening Endoscopic, Diagnostic
0BBD8ZZ Excision of Right Middle Lung Lobe, Via Natural or Artificial Opening Endoscopic
0BBF0ZX Excision of Right Lower Lung Lobe, Open Approach, Diagnostic
0BBF0ZZ Excision of Right Lower Lung Lobe, Open Approach
0BBF3ZX Excision of Right Lower Lung Lobe, Percutaneous Approach, Diagnostic
0BBF3ZZ Excision of Right Lower Lung Lobe, Percutaneous Approach
0BBF4ZX Excision of Right Lower Lung Lobe, Percutaneous Endoscopic Approach, Diagnostic
0BBF4ZZ Excision of Right Lower Lung Lobe, Percutaneous Endoscopic Approach
0BBF7ZX Excision of Right Lower Lung Lobe, Via Natural or Artificial Opening, Diagnostic
0BBF7ZZ Excision of Right Lower Lung Lobe, Via Natural or Artificial Opening
0BBF8ZX Excision of Right Lower Lung Lobe, Via Natural or Artificial Opening Endoscopic, Diagnostic
0BBF8ZZ Excision of Right Lower Lung Lobe, Via Natural or Artificial Opening Endoscopic
0BBG0ZX Excision of Left Upper Lung Lobe, Open Approach, Diagnostic
0BBG0ZZ Excision of Left Upper Lung Lobe, Open Approach
0BBG3ZX Excision of Left Upper Lung Lobe, Percutaneous Approach, Diagnostic
0BBG3ZZ Excision of Left Upper Lung Lobe, Percutaneous Approach
0BBG4ZX Excision of Left Upper Lung Lobe, Percutaneous Endoscopic Approach, Diagnostic
0BBG4ZZ Excision of Left Upper Lung Lobe, Percutaneous Endoscopic Approach
0BBG7ZX Excision of Left Upper Lung Lobe, Via Natural or Artificial Opening, Diagnostic
0BBG7ZZ Excision of Left Upper Lung Lobe, Via Natural or Artificial Opening
0BBG8ZX Excision of Left Upper Lung Lobe, Via Natural or Artificial Opening Endoscopic, Diagnostic
0BBG8ZZ Excision of Left Upper Lung Lobe, Via Natural or Artificial Opening Endoscopic
0BBH0ZX Excision of Lung Lingula, Open Approach, Diagnostic
0BBH0ZZ Excision of Lung Lingula, Open Approach
0BBH3ZX Excision of Lung Lingula, Percutaneous Approach, Diagnostic
0BBH3ZZ Excision of Lung Lingula, Percutaneous Approach
0BBH4ZX Excision of Lung Lingula, Percutaneous Endoscopic Approach, Diagnostic
0BBH4ZZ Excision of Lung Lingula, Percutaneous Endoscopic Approach
0BBH7ZX Excision of Lung Lingula, Via Natural or Artificial Opening, Diagnostic
0BBH7ZZ Excision of Lung Lingula, Via Natural or Artificial Opening
0BBH8ZX Excision of Lung Lingula, Via Natural or Artificial Opening Endoscopic, Diagnostic
0BBH8ZZ Excision of Lung Lingula, Via Natural or Artificial Opening Endoscopic
0BBJ0ZX Excision of Left Lower Lung Lobe, Open Approach, Diagnostic
0BBJ0ZZ Excision of Left Lower Lung Lobe, Open Approach
0BBJ3ZX Excision of Left Lower Lung Lobe, Percutaneous Approach, Diagnostic
0BBJ3ZZ Excision of Left Lower Lung Lobe, Percutaneous Approach
0BBJ4ZX Excision of Left Lower Lung Lobe, Percutaneous Endoscopic Approach, Diagnostic
0BBJ4ZZ Excision of Left Lower Lung Lobe, Percutaneous Endoscopic Approach
0BBJ7ZX Excision of Left Lower Lung Lobe, Via Natural or Artificial Opening, Diagnostic
0BBJ7ZZ Excision of Left Lower Lung Lobe, Via Natural or Artificial Opening
0BBJ8ZX Excision of Left Lower Lung Lobe, Via Natural or Artificial Opening Endoscopic, Diagnostic
0BBJ8ZZ Excision of Left Lower Lung Lobe, Via Natural or Artificial Opening Endoscop
0BBK0ZX Excision of Right Lung, Open Approac Diagnostic
0BBK0ZZ Excision of Right Lung, Open Approac
0BBK3ZX Excision of Right Lung, Percutaneous Approach, Diagnostic
0BBK3ZZ Excision of Right Lung, Percutaneous Approach
0BBK4ZX Excision of Right Lung, Percutaneous Endoscopic Approach, Diagnostic
0BBK4ZZ Excision of Right Lung, Percutaneous Endoscopic Approach
0BBK7ZX Excision of Right Lung, Via Natural or Artificial Opening, Diagnostic
0BBK7ZZ Excision of Right Lung, Via Natural or Artificial Opening
0BBK8ZX Excision of Right Lung, Via Natural or Artificial Opening Endoscopic, Diagnos
AHA CC: 1Q, 2014, 20-21
0BBK8ZZ Excision of Right Lung, Via Natural or Artificial Opening Endoscopic
0BBL0ZX Excision of Left Lung, Open Approach, Diagnostic
0BBL0ZZ Excision of Left Lung, Open Approach
0BBL3ZX Excision of Left Lung, Percutaneous Approach, Diagnostic
0BBL3ZZ Excision of Left Lung, Percutaneous Approach
0BBL4ZX Excision of Left Lung, Percutaneous Endoscopic Approach, Diagnostic
0BBL4ZZ Excision of Left Lung, Percutaneous Endoscopic Approach
0BBL7ZX Excision of Left Lung, Via Natural or Artificial Opening, Diagnostic
0BBL7ZZ Excision of Left Lung, Via Natural or Artificial Opening
0BBL8ZX Excision of Left Lung, Via Natural or Artificial Opening Endoscopic, Diagnosti
0BBL8ZZ Excision of Left Lung, Via Natural or Artificial Opening Endoscopic
0BBM0ZX Excision of Bilateral Lungs, Open Approach, Diagnostic
0BBM0ZZ Excision of Bilateral Lungs, Open Approach
0BBM3ZX Excision of Bilateral Lungs, Percutaneou Approach, Diagnostic
0BBM3ZZ Excision of Bilateral Lungs, Percutaneou Approach
0BBM4ZX Excision of Bilateral Lungs, Percutaneou Endoscopic Approach, Diagnostic
0BBM4ZZ Excision of Bilateral Lungs, Percutaneou Endoscopic Approach
0BBM7ZX Excision of Bilateral Lungs, Via Natural c Artificial Opening, Diagnostic
0BBM7ZZ Excision of Bilateral Lungs, Via Natural c Artificial Opening
0BBM8ZX Excision of Bilateral Lungs, Via Natural c Artificial Opening Endoscopic, Diagnostic
0BBM8ZZ Excision of Bilateral Lungs, Via Natural o Artificial Opening Endoscopic
0BBN0ZX Excision of Right Pleura, Open Approach, Diagnostic
0BBN0ZZ Excision of Right Pleura, Open Approach
0BBN3ZX Excision of Right Pleura, Percutaneous Approach, Diagnostic
0BBN3ZZ Excision of Right Pleura, Percutaneous Approach
0BBN4ZX Excision of Right Pleura, Percutaneous Endoscopic Approach, Diagnostic
0BBN4ZZ Excision of Right Pleura, Percutaneous Endoscopic Approach
0BBP0ZX Excision of Left Pleura, Open Approach, Diagnostic
0BBP0ZZ Excision of Left Pleura, Open Approach
0BBP3ZX Excision of Left Pleura, Percutaneous Approach, Diagnostic

P3ZZ Excision of Left Pleura, Percutaneous Approach
P4ZX Excision of Left Pleura, Percutaneous Endoscopic Approach, Diagnostic
P4ZZ Excision of Left Pleura, Percutaneous Endoscopic Approach
R0ZX Excision of Right Diaphragm, Open Approach, Diagnostic
R0ZZ Excision of Right Diaphragm, Open Approach
0BBR3ZX Excision of Right Diaphragm, Percutaneous Approach, Diagnostic
0BBR3ZZ Excision of Right Diaphragm, Percutaneous Approach
0BBR4ZX Excision of Right Diaphragm, Percutaneous Endoscopic Approach, Diagnostic
0BBR4ZZ Excision of Right Diaphragm, Percutaneous Endoscopic Approach
0BBS0ZX Excision of Left Diaphragm, Open Approach, Diagnostic
0BBS0ZZ Excision of Left Diaphragm, Open Approach
0BBS3ZX Excision of Left Diaphragm, Percutaneous Approach, Diagnostic
0BBS3ZZ Excision of Left Diaphragm, Percutaneous Approach
0BBS4ZX Excision of Left Diaphragm, Percutaneous Endoscopic Approach, Diagnostic
0BBS4ZZ Excision of Left Diaphragm, Percutaneous Endoscopic Approach

C – Respiratory System, Extirpation

10ZZ Extirpation of Matter from Trachea, Open Approach
13ZZ Extirpation of Matter from Trachea, Percutaneous Approach
14ZZ Extirpation of Matter from Trachea, Percutaneous Endoscopic Approach
17ZZ Extirpation of Matter from Trachea, Via Natural or Artificial Opening
18ZZ Extirpation of Matter from Trachea, Via Natural or Artificial Opening Endoscopic
20ZZ Extirpation of Matter from Carina, Open Approach
23ZZ Extirpation of Matter from Carina, Percutaneous Approach
24ZZ Extirpation of Matter from Carina, Percutaneous Endoscopic Approach
C27ZZ Extirpation of Matter from Carina, Via Natural or Artificial Opening
C28ZZ Extirpation of Matter from Carina, Via Natural or Artificial Opening Endoscopic
C30ZZ Extirpation of Matter from Right Main Bronchus, Open Approach
C33ZZ Extirpation of Matter from Right Main Bronchus, Percutaneous Approach
C34ZZ Extirpation of Matter from Right Main Bronchus, Percutaneous Endoscopic Approach
C37ZZ Extirpation of Matter from Right Main Bronchus, Via Natural or Artificial Opening
C38ZZ Extirpation of Matter from Right Main Bronchus, Via Natural or Artificial Opening Endoscopic
C40ZZ Extirpation of Matter from Right Upper Lobe Bronchus, Open Approach
C43ZZ Extirpation of Matter from Right Upper Lobe Bronchus, Percutaneous Approach
C44ZZ Extirpation of Matter from Right Upper Lobe Bronchus, Percutaneous Endoscopic Approach
C47ZZ Extirpation of Matter from Right Upper Lobe Bronchus, Via Natural or Artificial Opening
C48ZZ Extirpation of Matter from Right Upper Lobe Bronchus, Via Natural or Artificial Opening Endoscopic
C50ZZ Extirpation of Matter from Right Middle Lobe Bronchus, Open Approach
C53ZZ Extirpation of Matter from Right Middle Lobe Bronchus, Percutaneous Approach
C54ZZ Extirpation of Matter from Right Middle Lobe Bronchus, Percutaneous Endoscopic Approach
BC57ZZ Extirpation of Matter from Right Middle Lobe Bronchus, Via Natural or Artificial Opening
BC58ZZ Extirpation of Matter from Right Middle Lobe Bronchus, Via Natural or Artificial Opening Endoscopic
BC60ZZ Extirpation of Matter from Right Lower Lobe Bronchus, Open Approach
BC63ZZ Extirpation of Matter from Right Lower Lobe Bronchus, Percutaneous Approach
0BC64ZZ Extirpation of Matter from Right Lower Lobe Bronchus, Percutaneous Endoscopic Approach
0BC67ZZ Extirpation of Matter from Right Lower Lobe Bronchus, Via Natural or Artificial Opening
0BC68ZZ Extirpation of Matter from Right Lower Lobe Bronchus, Via Natural or Artificial Opening Endoscopic
0BC70ZZ Extirpation of Matter from Left Main Bronchus, Open Approach
0BC73ZZ Extirpation of Matter from Left Main Bronchus, Percutaneous Approach
0BC74ZZ Extirpation of Matter from Left Main Bronchus, Percutaneous Endoscopic Approach
0BC77ZZ Extirpation of Matter from Left Main Bronchus, Via Natural or Artificial Opening
0BC78ZZ Extirpation of Matter from Left Main Bronchus, Via Natural or Artificial Opening Endoscopic
0BC80ZZ Extirpation of Matter from Left Upper Lobe Bronchus, Open Approach
0BC83ZZ Extirpation of Matter from Left Upper Lobe Bronchus, Percutaneous Approach
0BC84ZZ Extirpation of Matter from Left Upper Lobe Bronchus, Percutaneous Endoscopic Approach
0BC87ZZ Extirpation of Matter from Left Upper Lobe Bronchus, Via Natural or Artificial Opening
0BC88ZZ Extirpation of Matter from Left Upper Lobe Bronchus, Via Natural or Artificial Opening Endoscopic
0BC90ZZ Extirpation of Matter from Lingula Bronchus, Open Approach
0BC93ZZ Extirpation of Matter from Lingula Bronchus, Percutaneous Approach
0BC94ZZ Extirpation of Matter from Lingula Bronchus, Percutaneous Endoscopic Approach
0BC97ZZ Extirpation of Matter from Lingula Bronchus, Via Natural or Artificial Opening
0BC98ZZ Extirpation of Matter from Lingula Bronchus, Via Natural or Artificial Opening Endoscopic
0BCB0ZZ Extirpation of Matter from Left Lower Lobe Bronchus, Open Approach
0BCB3ZZ Extirpation of Matter from Left Lower Lobe Bronchus, Percutaneous Approach
0BCB4ZZ Extirpation of Matter from Left Lower Lobe Bronchus, Percutaneous Endoscopic Approach
0BCB7ZZ Extirpation of Matter from Left Lower Lobe Bronchus, Via Natural or Artificial Opening
0BCB8ZZ Extirpation of Matter from Left Lower Lobe Bronchus, Via Natural or Artificial Opening Endoscopic
0BCC0ZZ Extirpation of Matter from Right Upper Lung Lobe, Open Approach
0BCC3ZZ Extirpation of Matter from Right Upper Lung Lobe, Percutaneous Approach
0BCC4ZZ Extirpation of Matter from Right Upper Lung Lobe, Percutaneous Endoscopic Approach
0BCC7ZZ Extirpation of Matter from Right Upper Lung Lobe, Via Natural or Artificial Opening
0BCC8ZZ Extirpation of Matter from Right Upper Lung Lobe, Via Natural or Artificial Opening Endoscopic
0BCD0ZZ Extirpation of Matter from Right Middle Lung Lobe, Open Approach
0BCD3ZZ Extirpation of Matter from Right Middle Lung Lobe, Percutaneous Approach
0BCD4ZZ Extirpation of Matter from Right Middle Lung Lobe, Percutaneous Endoscopic Approach
0BCD7ZZ Extirpation of Matter from Right Middle Lung Lobe, Via Natural or Artificial Opening
0BCD8ZZ Extirpation of Matter from Right Middle Lung Lobe, Via Natural or Artificial Opening Endoscopic
0BCF0ZZ Extirpation of Matter from Right Lower Lung Lobe, Open Approach
0BCF3ZZ Extirpation of Matter from Right Lower Lung Lobe, Percutaneous Approach
0BCF4ZZ Extirpation of Matter from Right Lower Lung Lobe, Percutaneous Endoscopic Approach
0BCF7ZZ Extirpation of Matter from Right Lower Lung Lobe, Via Natural or Artificial Opening
0BCF8ZZ Extirpation of Matter from Right Lower Lung Lobe, Via Natural or Artificial Opening Endoscopic
0BCG0ZZ Extirpation of Matter from Left Upper Lung Lobe, Open Approach
0BCG3ZZ Extirpation of Matter from Left Upper Lung Lobe, Percutaneous Approach
0BCG4ZZ Extirpation of Matter from Left Upper Lung Lobe, Percutaneous Endoscopic Approach
0BCG7ZZ Extirpation of Matter from Left Upper Lung Lobe, Via Natural or Artificial Opening
0BCG8ZZ Extirpation of Matter from Left Upper Lung Lobe, Via Natural or Artificial Opening Endoscopic
0BCH0ZZ Extirpation of Matter from Lung Lingula, Open Approach
0BCH3ZZ Extirpation of Matter from Lung Lingula, Percutaneous Approach
0BCH4ZZ Extirpation of Matter from Lung Lingula, Percutaneous Endoscopic Approach
0BCH7ZZ Extirpation of Matter from Lung Lingula, Via Natural or Artificial Opening
0BCH8ZZ Extirpation of Matter from Lung Lingula, Via Natural or Artificial Opening Endoscopic
0BCJ0ZZ Extirpation of Matter from Left Lower Lung Lobe, Open Approach

0BCJ3ZZ Extirpation of Matter from Left Lower Lung Lobe, Percutaneous Approach
0BCJ4ZZ Extirpation of Matter from Left Lower Lung Lobe, Percutaneous Endoscopic Approach
0BCJ7ZZ Extirpation of Matter from Left Lower Lung Lobe, Via Natural or Artificial Opening
0BCJ8ZZ Extirpation of Matter from Left Lower Lung Lobe, Via Natural or Artificial Opening Endoscopic
0BCK0ZZ Extirpation of Matter from Right Lung, Open Approach
0BCK3ZZ Extirpation of Matter from Right Lung, Percutaneous Approach
0BCK4ZZ Extirpation of Matter from Right Lung, Percutaneous Endoscopic Approach
0BCK7ZZ Extirpation of Matter from Right Lung, Via Natural or Artificial Opening
0BCK8ZZ Extirpation of Matter from Right Lung, Via Natural or Artificial Opening Endoscopic
0BCL0ZZ Extirpation of Matter from Left Lung, Open Approach
0BCL3ZZ Extirpation of Matter from Left Lung, Percutaneous Approach
0BCL4ZZ Extirpation of Matter from Left Lung, Percutaneous Endoscopic Approach
0BCL7ZZ Extirpation of Matter from Left Lung, Via Natural or Artificial Opening
0BCL8ZZ Extirpation of Matter from Left Lung, Via Natural or Artificial Opening Endoscopic
0BCM0ZZ Extirpation of Matter from Bilateral Lungs, Open Approach
0BCM3ZZ Extirpation of Matter from Bilateral Lungs, Percutaneous Approach
0BCM4ZZ Extirpation of Matter from Bilateral Lungs, Percutaneous Endoscopic Approach
0BCM7ZZ Extirpation of Matter from Bilateral Lungs, Via Natural or Artificial Opening
0BCM8ZZ Extirpation of Matter from Bilateral Lungs, Via Natural or Artificial Opening Endoscopic
0BCN0ZZ Extirpation of Matter from Right Pleura, Open Approach
0BCN3ZZ Extirpation of Matter from Right Pleur Percutaneous Approach
0BCN4ZZ Extirpation of Matter from Right Pleur Percutaneous Endoscopic Approach
0BCP0ZZ Extirpation of Matter from Left Pleura Open Approach
0BCP3ZZ Extirpation of Matter from Left Pleura Percutaneous Approach
0BCP4ZZ Extirpation of Matter from Left Pleura, Percutaneous Endoscopic Approach
0BCR0ZZ Extirpation of Matter from Right Diaphragm, Open Approach
0BCR3ZZ Extirpation of Matter from Right Diaphragm, Percutaneous Approach
0BCR4ZZ Extirpation of Matter from Right Diaphragm, Percutaneous Endoscopic Approach
0BCS0ZZ Extirpation of Matter from Left Diaphragm, Open Approach
0BCS3ZZ Extirpation of Matter from Left Diaphragm, Percutaneous Approach
0BCS4ZZ Extirpation of Matter from Left Diaphragm, Percutaneous Endoscopic Approach

0BD – Respiratory System, Extraction

Review Coding Guidelines B3.4a and B3.4b

0BDN0ZX Extraction of Right Pleura, Open Approach, Diagnostic
0BDN0ZZ Extraction of Right Pleura, Open Approach
0BDN3ZX Extraction of Right Pleura, Percutaneous Approach, Diagnostic
0BDN3ZZ Extraction of Right Pleura, Percutaneous Approach
0BDN4ZX Extraction of Right Pleura, Percutaneous Endoscopic Approach, Diagnostic
0BDN4ZZ Extraction of Right Pleura, Percutaneous Endoscopic Approach
0BDP0ZX Extraction of Left Pleura, Open Approach, Diagnostic
0BDP0ZZ Extraction of Left Pleura, Open Approach
0BDP3ZX Extraction of Left Pleura, Percutaneous Approach, Diagnostic
0BDP3ZZ Extraction of Left Pleura, Percutaneous Approach
0BDP4ZX Extraction of Left Pleura, Percutaneous Endoscopic Approach, Diagnostic
0BDP4ZZ Extraction of Left Pleura, Percutaneous Endoscopic Approach

0BF – Respiratory System, Fragmentation

0BF10ZZ Fragmentation in Trachea, Open Approach
0BF13ZZ Fragmentation in Trachea, Percutaneous Approach
0BF14ZZ Fragmentation in Trachea, Percutaneous Endoscopic Approach
0BF17ZZ Fragmentation in Trachea, Via Natural or Artificial Opening
0BF18ZZ Fragmentation in Trachea, Via Natural or Artificial Opening Endoscopic
▲**0BF1XZZ** Fragmentation in Trachea, External Approach
0BF20ZZ Fragmentation in Carina, Open Approach
0BF23ZZ Fragmentation in Carina, Percutaneous Approach
0BF24ZZ Fragmentation in Carina, Percutaneous Endoscopic Approach
0BF27ZZ Fragmentation in Carina, Via Natural or Artificial Opening
0BF28ZZ Fragmentation in Carina, Via Natural or Artificial Opening Endoscopic
▲**0BF2XZZ** Fragmentation in Carina, External Approach
0BF30ZZ Fragmentation in Right Main Bronchus, Open Approach
0BF33ZZ Fragmentation in Right Main Bronchus, Percutaneous Approach
0BF34ZZ Fragmentation in Right Main Bronchus, Percutaneous Endoscopic Approach
0BF37ZZ Fragmentation in Right Main Bronchus, Via Natural or Artificial Opening
0BF38ZZ Fragmentation in Right Main Bronchus, Via Natural or Artificial Opening Endoscopic
▲**0BF3XZZ** Fragmentation in Right Main Bronchus, External Approach
0BF40ZZ Fragmentation in Right Upper Lobe Bronchus, Open Approach
0BF43ZZ Fragmentation in Right Upper Lobe Bronchus, Percutaneous Approach
0BF44ZZ Fragmentation in Right Upper Lobe Bronchus, Percutaneous Endoscopic Approach
0BF47ZZ Fragmentation in Right Upper Lobe Bronchus, Via Natural or Artificial Opening
0BF48ZZ Fragmentation in Right Upper Lobe Bronchus, Via Natural or Artificial Opening Endoscopic
▲ **0BF4XZZ** Fragmentation in Right Upper Lobe Bronchus, External Approach
0BF50ZZ Fragmentation in Right Middle Lobe Bronchus, Open Approach
0BF53ZZ Fragmentation in Right Middle Lobe Bronchus, Percutaneous Approach
0BF54ZZ Fragmentation in Right Middle Lobe Bronchus, Percutaneous Endoscopic Approach
0BF57ZZ Fragmentation in Right Middle Lobe Bronchus, Via Natural or Artificial Opening
0BF58ZZ Fragmentation in Right Middle Lobe Bronchus, Via Natural or Artificial Opening Endoscopic
▲ **0BF5XZZ** Fragmentation in Right Middle Lobe Bronchus, External Approach
0BF60ZZ Fragmentation in Right Lower Lobe Bronchus, Open Approach
0BF63ZZ Fragmentation in Right Lower Lobe Bronchus, Percutaneous Approach
0BF64ZZ Fragmentation in Right Lower Lobe Bronchus, Percutaneous Endoscopic Approach
0BF67ZZ Fragmentation in Right Lower Lobe Bronchus, Via Natural or Artificial Opening
0BF68ZZ Fragmentation in Right Lower Lobe Bronchus, Via Natural or Artificial Opening Endoscopic
▲ **0BF6XZZ** Fragmentation in Right Lower Lobe Bronchus, External Approach
0BF70ZZ Fragmentation in Left Main Bronchus, Open Approach
0BF73ZZ Fragmentation in Left Main Bronchus, Percutaneous Approach
0BF74ZZ Fragmentation in Left Main Bronchus, Percutaneous Endoscopic Approach
0BF77ZZ Fragmentation in Left Main Bronchus, V Natural or Artificial Opening
0BF78ZZ Fragmentation in Left Main Bronchus, V Natural or Artificial Opening Endoscopic
▲ **0BF7XZZ** Fragmentation in Left Main Bronchus, External Approach
0BF80ZZ Fragmentation in Left Upper Lobe Bronchus, Open Approach
0BF83ZZ Fragmentation in Left Upper Lobe Bronchus, Percutaneous Approach
0BF84ZZ Fragmentation in Left Upper Lobe Bronchus, Percutaneous Endoscopic Approach
0BF87ZZ Fragmentation in Left Upper Lobe Bronchus, Via Natural or Artificial Opening
0BF88ZZ Fragmentation in Left Upper Lobe Bronchus, Via Natural or Artificial Opening Endoscopic
▲ **0BF8XZZ** Fragmentation in Left Upper Lobe Bronchus, External Approach
0BF90ZZ Fragmentation in Lingula Bronchus, Ope Approach

93ZZ Fragmentation in Lingula Bronchus, Percutaneous Approach
94ZZ Fragmentation in Lingula Bronchus, Percutaneous Endoscopic Approach
97ZZ Fragmentation in Lingula Bronchus, Via Natural or Artificial Opening
98ZZ Fragmentation in Lingula Bronchus, Via Natural or Artificial Opening Endoscopic
▲ **0BF9XZZ** Fragmentation in Lingula Bronchus, External Approach
0BFB0ZZ Fragmentation in Left Lower Lobe Bronchus, Open Approach
0BFB3ZZ Fragmentation in Left Lower Lobe Bronchus, Percutaneous Approach
0BFB4ZZ Fragmentation in Left Lower Lobe Bronchus, Percutaneous Endoscopic Approach
0BFB7ZZ Fragmentation in Left Lower Lobe Bronchus, Via Natural or Artificial Opening
0BFB8ZZ Fragmentation in Left Lower Lobe Bronchus, Via Natural or Artificial Opening Endoscopic
▲ **0BFBXZZ** Fragmentation in Left Lower Lobe Bronchus, External Approach

H – Respiratory System, Insertion

H001Z Insertion of Radioactive Element into Tracheobronchial Tree, Open Approach
H002Z Insertion of Monitoring Device into Tracheobronchial Tree, Open Approach
H003Z Insertion of Infusion Device into Tracheobronchial Tree, Open Approach
H00DZ Insertion of Intraluminal Device into Tracheobronchial Tree, Open Approach
H031Z Insertion of Radioactive Element into Tracheobronchial Tree, Percutaneous Approach
H032Z Insertion of Monitoring Device into Tracheobronchial Tree, Percutaneous Approach
H033Z Insertion of Infusion Device into Tracheobronchial Tree, Percutaneous Approach
H03DZ Insertion of Intraluminal Device into Tracheobronchial Tree, Percutaneous Approach
H041Z Insertion of Radioactive Element into Tracheobronchial Tree, Percutaneous Endoscopic Approach
H042Z Insertion of Monitoring Device into Tracheobronchial Tree, Percutaneous Endoscopic Approach
H043Z Insertion of Infusion Device into Tracheobronchial Tree, Percutaneous Endoscopic Approach
H04DZ Insertion of Intraluminal Device into Tracheobronchial Tree, Percutaneous Endoscopic Approach
H071Z Insertion of Radioactive Element into Tracheobronchial Tree, Via Natural or Artificial Opening
H072Z Insertion of Monitoring Device into Tracheobronchial Tree, Via Natural or Artificial Opening
H073Z Insertion of Infusion Device into Tracheobronchial Tree, Via Natural or Artificial Opening
H07DZ Insertion of Intraluminal Device into Tracheobronchial Tree, Via Natural or Artificial Opening
BH081Z Insertion of Radioactive Element into Tracheobronchial Tree, Via Natural or Artificial Opening Endoscopic
BH082Z Insertion of Monitoring Device into Tracheobronchial Tree, Via Natural or Artificial Opening Endoscopic
BH083Z Insertion of Infusion Device into Tracheobronchial Tree, Via Natural or Artificial Opening Endoscopic
BH08DZ Insertion of Intraluminal Device into Tracheobronchial Tree, Via Natural or Artificial Opening Endoscopic
BH102Z Insertion of Monitoring Device into Trachea, Open Approach
BH10DZ Insertion of Intraluminal Device into Trachea, Open Approach
BH13DZ Insertion of Intraluminal Device into Trachea, Percutaneous Approach
BH13EZ Insertion of Endotracheal Airway into Trachea, Percutaneous Approach
0BH14DZ Insertion of Intraluminal Device into Trachea, Percutaneous Endoscopic Approach
0BH172Z Insertion of Monitoring Device into Trachea, Via Natural or Artificial Opening
0BH17DZ Insertion of Intraluminal Device into Trachea, Via Natural or Artificial Opening
0BH17EZ Insertion of Endotracheal Airway into Trachea, Via Natural or Artificial Opening
0BH182Z Insertion of Monitoring Device into Trachea, Via Natural or Artificial Opening Endoscopic
0BH18DZ Insertion of Intraluminal Device into Trachea, Via Natural or Artificial Opening Endoscopic
0BH18EZ Insertion of Endotracheal Airway into Trachea, Via Natural or Artificial Opening Endoscopic
0BH30GZ Insertion of Endobronchial Valve into Right Main Bronchus, Open Approach
0BH33GZ Insertion of Endobronchial Valve into Right Main Bronchus, Percutaneous Approach
0BH34GZ Insertion of Endobronchial Valve into Right Main Bronchus, Percutaneous Endoscopic Approach
0BH37GZ Insertion of Endobronchial Valve into Right Main Bronchus, Via Natural or Artificial Opening
0BH38GZ Insertion of Endobronchial Valve into Right Main Bronchus, Via Natural or Artificial Opening Endoscopic
0BH40GZ Insertion of Endobronchial Valve into Right Upper Lobe Bronchus, Open Approach
0BH43GZ Insertion of Endobronchial Valve into Right Upper Lobe Bronchus, Percutaneous Approach
0BH44GZ Insertion of Endobronchial Valve into Right Upper Lobe Bronchus, Percutaneous Endoscopic Approach
0BH47GZ Insertion of Endobronchial Valve into Right Upper Lobe Bronchus, Via Natural or Artificial Opening
0BH48GZ Insertion of Endobronchial Valve into Right Upper Lobe Bronchus, Via Natural or Artificial Opening Endoscopic
0BH50GZ Insertion of Endobronchial Valve into Right Middle Lobe Bronchus, Open Approach
0BH53GZ Insertion of Endobronchial Valve into Right Middle Lobe Bronchus, Percutaneous Approach
0BH54GZ Insertion of Endobronchial Valve into Right Middle Lobe Bronchus, Percutaneous Endoscopic Approach
0BH57GZ Insertion of Endobronchial Valve into Right Middle Lobe Bronchus, Via Natural or Artificial Opening
0BH58GZ Insertion of Endobronchial Valve into Right Middle Lobe Bronchus, Via Natural or Artificial Opening Endoscopic
0BH60GZ Insertion of Endobronchial Valve into Right Lower Lobe Bronchus, Open Approach
0BH63GZ Insertion of Endobronchial Valve into Right Lower Lobe Bronchus, Percutaneous Approach
0BH64GZ Insertion of Endobronchial Valve into Right Lower Lobe Bronchus, Percutaneous Endoscopic Approach
0BH67GZ Insertion of Endobronchial Valve into Right Lower Lobe Bronchus, Via Natural or Artificial Opening
0BH68GZ Insertion of Endobronchial Valve into Right Lower Lobe Bronchus, Via Natural or Artificial Opening Endoscopic
0BH70GZ Insertion of Endobronchial Valve into Left Main Bronchus, Open Approach
0BH73GZ Insertion of Endobronchial Valve into Left Main Bronchus, Percutaneous Approach
0BH74GZ Insertion of Endobronchial Valve into Left Main Bronchus, Percutaneous Endoscopic Approach
0BH77GZ Insertion of Endobronchial Valve into Left Main Bronchus, Via Natural or Artificial Opening
0BH78GZ Insertion of Endobronchial Valve into Left Main Bronchus, Via Natural or Artificial Opening Endoscopic
0BH80GZ Insertion of Endobronchial Valve into Left Upper Lobe Bronchus, Open Approach
0BH83GZ Insertion of Endobronchial Valve into Left Upper Lobe Bronchus, Percutaneous Approach
0BH84GZ Insertion of Endobronchial Valve into Left Upper Lobe Bronchus, Percutaneous Endoscopic Approach
0BH87GZ Insertion of Endobronchial Valve into Left Upper Lobe Bronchus, Via Natural or Artificial Opening
0BH88GZ Insertion of Endobronchial Valve into Left Upper Lobe Bronchus, Via Natural or Artificial Opening Endoscopic
0BH90GZ Insertion of Endobronchial Valve into Lingula Bronchus, Open Approach
0BH93GZ Insertion of Endobronchial Valve into Lingula Bronchus, Percutaneous Approach
0BH94GZ Insertion of Endobronchial Valve into Lingula Bronchus, Percutaneous Endoscopic Approach
0BH97GZ Insertion of Endobronchial Valve into Lingula Bronchus, Via Natural or Artificial Opening
0BH98GZ Insertion of Endobronchial Valve into Lingula Bronchus, Via Natural or Artificial Opening Endoscopic
0BHB0GZ Insertion of Endobronchial Valve into Left Lower Lobe Bronchus, Open Approach
0BHB3GZ Insertion of Endobronchial Valve into Left Lower Lobe Bronchus, Percutaneous Approach
0BHB4GZ Insertion of Endobronchial Valve into Left Lower Lobe Bronchus, Percutaneous Endoscopic Approach

0BHB7GZ Insertion of Endobronchial Valve into Left Lower Lobe Bronchus, Via Natural or Artificial Opening
0BHB8GZ Insertion of Endobronchial Valve into Left Lower Lobe Bronchus, Via Natural or Artificial Opening Endoscopic
0BHK01Z Insertion of Radioactive Element into Right Lung, Open Approach
0BHK02Z Insertion of Monitoring Device into Right Lung, Open Approach
0BHK03Z Insertion of Infusion Device into Right Lung, Open Approach
0BHK31Z Insertion of Radioactive Element into Right Lung, Percutaneous Approach
0BHK32Z Insertion of Monitoring Device into Right Lung, Percutaneous Approach
0BHK33Z Insertion of Infusion Device into Right Lung, Percutaneous Approach
0BHK41Z Insertion of Radioactive Element into Right Lung, Percutaneous Endoscopic Approach
0BHK42Z Insertion of Monitoring Device into Right Lung, Percutaneous Endoscopic Approach
0BHK43Z Insertion of Infusion Device into Right Lung, Percutaneous Endoscopic Approach
0BHK71Z Insertion of Radioactive Element into Right Lung, Via Natural or Artificial Opening
0BHK72Z Insertion of Monitoring Device into Right Lung, Via Natural or Artificial Opening
0BHK73Z Insertion of Infusion Device into Right Lung, Via Natural or Artificial Opening
0BHK81Z Insertion of Radioactive Element into Right Lung, Via Natural or Artificial Opening Endoscopic
0BHK82Z Insertion of Monitoring Device into Right Lung, Via Natural or Artificial Opening Endoscopic
0BHK83Z Insertion of Infusion Device into Right Lung, Via Natural or Artificial Opening Endoscopic
0BHL01Z Insertion of Radioactive Element into Left Lung, Open Approach
0BHL02Z Insertion of Monitoring Device into Left Lung, Open Approach
0BHL03Z Insertion of Infusion Device into Left Lung, Open Approach
0BHL31Z Insertion of Radioactive Element into Left Lung, Percutaneous Approach
0BHL32Z Insertion of Monitoring Device into Left Lung, Percutaneous Approach
0BHL33Z Insertion of Infusion Device into Left Lung, Percutaneous Approach
0BHL41Z Insertion of Radioactive Element into Left Lung, Percutaneous Endoscopic Approach
0BHL42Z Insertion of Monitoring Device into Left Lung, Percutaneous Endoscopic Approach
0BHL43Z Insertion of Infusion Device into Left Lung, Percutaneous Endoscopic Approach
0BHL71Z Insertion of Radioactive Element into Left Lung, Via Natural or Artificial Opening
0BHL72Z Insertion of Monitoring Device into Left Lung, Via Natural or Artificial Opening
0BHL73Z Insertion of Infusion Device into Left Lung, Via Natural or Artificial Opening
0BHL81Z Insertion of Radioactive Element into Left Lung, Via Natural or Artificial Opening Endoscopic
0BHL82Z Insertion of Monitoring Device into Left Lung, Via Natural or Artificial Opening Endoscopic
0BHL83Z Insertion of Infusion Device into Left Lung, Via Natural or Artificial Openin Endoscopic
0BHR02Z Insertion of Monitoring Device into Right Diaphragm, Open Approach
0BHR0MZ Insertion of Diaphragmatic Pacemaker Lead into Right Diaphragm, Open Approach
0BHR32Z Insertion of Monitoring Device into Ri Diaphragm, Percutaneous Approach
0BHR3MZ Insertion of Diaphragmatic Pacemaker Lead into Right Diaphragm, Percutane Approach
0BHR42Z Insertion of Monitoring Device into Ri Diaphragm, Percutaneous Endoscopic Approach
0BHR4MZ Insertion of Diaphragmatic Pacemaker Lead into Right Diaphragm, Percutane Endoscopic Approach
0BHS02Z Insertion of Monitoring Device into Left Diaphragm, Open Approach
0BHS0MZ Insertion of Diaphragmatic Pacemaker Lead into Left Diaphragm, Open Approach
0BHS32Z Insertion of Monitoring Device into Le Diaphragm, Percutaneous Approach
0BHS3MZ Insertion of Diaphragmatic Pacemaker Lead into Left Diaphragm, Percutaneou Approach
0BHS42Z Insertion of Monitoring Device into Lef Diaphragm, Percutaneous Endoscopic Approach
0BHS4MZ Insertion of Diaphragmatic Pacemaker Lead into Left Diaphragm, Percutaneou Endoscopic Approach

0BJ – Respiratory System, Inspection

Review Coding Guidelines B3.11a, B3.11b and B3.11c

0BJ00ZZ Inspection of Tracheobronchial Tree, Open Approach
0BJ03ZZ Inspection of Tracheobronchial Tree, Percutaneous Approach
0BJ04ZZ Inspection of Tracheobronchial Tree, Percutaneous Endoscopic Approach
0BJ07ZZ Inspection of Tracheobronchial Tree, Via Natural or Artificial Opening
0BJ08ZZ Inspection of Tracheobronchial Tree, Via Natural or Artificial Opening Endoscopic
0BJ0XZZ Inspection of Tracheobronchial Tree, External Approach
0BJ10ZZ Inspection of Trachea, Open Approach
0BJ13ZZ Inspection of Trachea, Percutaneous Approach
0BJ14ZZ Inspection of Trachea, Percutaneous Endoscopic Approach
0BJ17ZZ Inspection of Trachea, Via Natural or Artificial Opening
0BJ18ZZ Inspection of Trachea, Via Natural or Artificial Opening Endoscopic
0BJ1XZZ Inspection of Trachea, External Approach
0BJK0ZZ Inspection of Right Lung, Open Approach
0BJK3ZZ Inspection of Right Lung, Percutaneous Approach
0BJK4ZZ Inspection of Right Lung, Percutaneous Endoscopic Approach
0BJK7ZZ Inspection of Right Lung, Via Natural or Artificial Opening
0BJK8ZZ Inspection of Right Lung, Via Natural or Artificial Opening Endoscopic
0BJKXZZ Inspection of Right Lung, External Approach
0BJL0ZZ Inspection of Left Lung, Open Approach
0BJL3ZZ Inspection of Left Lung, Percutaneous Approach
0BJL4ZZ Inspection of Left Lung, Percutaneous Endoscopic Approach
0BJL7ZZ Inspection of Left Lung, Via Natural or Artificial Opening
0BJL8ZZ Inspection of Left Lung, Via Natural or Artificial Opening Endoscopic
AHA CC: 1Q, 2014, 20
0BJLXZZ Inspection of Left Lung, External Approach
0BJQ0ZZ Inspection of Pleura, Open Approach
0BJQ3ZZ Inspection of Pleura, Percutaneous Approach
0BJQ4ZZ Inspection of Pleura, Percutaneous Endoscopic Approach
0BJQ7ZZ Inspection of Pleura, Via Natural or Artificial Opening
0BJQ8ZZ Inspection of Pleura, Via Natural or Artificial Opening Endoscopic
0BJQXZZ Inspection of Pleura, External Approach
0BJT0ZZ Inspection of Diaphragm, Open Approach
0BJT3ZZ Inspection of Diaphragm, Percutaneous Approach
0BJT4ZZ Inspection of Diaphragm, Percutaneous Endoscopic Approach
0BJT7ZZ Inspection of Diaphragm, Via Natural or Artificial Opening
0BJT8ZZ Inspection of Diaphragm, Via Natural or Artificial Opening Endoscopic
0BJTXZZ Inspection of Diaphragm, External Approach

0BL – Respiratory System, Occlusion

0BL10CZ Occlusion of Trachea with Extraluminal Device, Open Approach
0BL10DZ Occlusion of Trachea with Intraluminal Device, Open Approach
0BL10ZZ Occlusion of Trachea, Open Approach
0BL13CZ Occlusion of Trachea with Extraluminal Device, Percutaneous Approach
0BL13DZ Occlusion of Trachea with Intraluminal Device, Percutaneous Approach
0BL13ZZ Occlusion of Trachea, Percutaneous Approach
0BL14CZ Occlusion of Trachea with Extraluminal Device, Percutaneous Endoscopic Approach
0BL14DZ Occlusion of Trachea with Intraluminal Device, Percutaneous Endoscopic Approach
0BL14ZZ Occlusion of Trachea, Percutaneous Endoscopic Approach
0BL17DZ Occlusion of Trachea with Intraluminal Device, Via Natural or Artificial Opening
0BL17ZZ Occlusion of Trachea, Via Natural or Artificial Opening
0BL18DZ Occlusion of Trachea with Intraluminal Device, Via Natural or Artificial Opening Endoscopic
0BL18ZZ Occlusion of Trachea, Via Natural or Artificial Opening Endoscopic

20CZ Occlusion of Carina with Extraluminal Device, Open Approach
20DZ Occlusion of Carina with Intraluminal Device, Open Approach
20ZZ Occlusion of Carina, Open Approach
23CZ Occlusion of Carina with Extraluminal Device, Percutaneous Approach
23DZ Occlusion of Carina with Intraluminal Device, Percutaneous Approach
23ZZ Occlusion of Carina, Percutaneous Approach
24CZ Occlusion of Carina with Extraluminal Device, Percutaneous Endoscopic Approach
24DZ Occlusion of Carina with Intraluminal Device, Percutaneous Endoscopic Approach
24ZZ Occlusion of Carina, Percutaneous Endoscopic Approach
27DZ Occlusion of Carina with Intraluminal Device, Via Natural or Artificial Opening
27ZZ Occlusion of Carina, Via Natural or Artificial Opening
28DZ Occlusion of Carina with Intraluminal Device, Via Natural or Artificial Opening Endoscopic
28ZZ Occlusion of Carina, Via Natural or Artificial Opening Endoscopic
L30CZ Occlusion of Right Main Bronchus with Extraluminal Device, Open Approach
L30DZ Occlusion of Right Main Bronchus with Intraluminal Device, Open Approach
L30ZZ Occlusion of Right Main Bronchus, Open Approach
L33CZ Occlusion of Right Main Bronchus with Extraluminal Device, Percutaneous Approach
L33DZ Occlusion of Right Main Bronchus with Intraluminal Device, Percutaneous Approach
L33ZZ Occlusion of Right Main Bronchus, Percutaneous Approach
L34CZ Occlusion of Right Main Bronchus with Extraluminal Device, Percutaneous Endoscopic Approach
L34DZ Occlusion of Right Main Bronchus with Intraluminal Device, Percutaneous Endoscopic Approach
BL34ZZ Occlusion of Right Main Bronchus, Percutaneous Endoscopic Approach
BL37DZ Occlusion of Right Main Bronchus with Intraluminal Device, Via Natural or Artificial Opening
BL37ZZ Occlusion of Right Main Bronchus, Via Natural or Artificial Opening
BL38DZ Occlusion of Right Main Bronchus with Intraluminal Device, Via Natural or Artificial Opening Endoscopic
BL38ZZ Occlusion of Right Main Bronchus, Via Natural or Artificial Opening Endoscopic
BL40CZ Occlusion of Right Upper Lobe Bronchus with Extraluminal Device, Open Approach
BL40DZ Occlusion of Right Upper Lobe Bronchus with Intraluminal Device, Open Approach
BL40ZZ Occlusion of Right Upper Lobe Bronchus, Open Approach
BL43CZ Occlusion of Right Upper Lobe Bronchus with Extraluminal Device, Percutaneous Approach
BL43DZ Occlusion of Right Upper Lobe Bronchus with Intraluminal Device, Percutaneous Approach
BL43ZZ Occlusion of Right Upper Lobe Bronchus, Percutaneous Approach
BL44CZ Occlusion of Right Upper Lobe Bronchus with Extraluminal Device, Percutaneous Endoscopic Approach
0BL44DZ Occlusion of Right Upper Lobe Bronchus with Intraluminal Device, Percutaneous Endoscopic Approach
0BL44ZZ Occlusion of Right Upper Lobe Bronchus, Percutaneous Endoscopic Approach
0BL47DZ Occlusion of Right Upper Lobe Bronchus with Intraluminal Device, Via Natural or Artificial Opening
0BL47ZZ Occlusion of Right Upper Lobe Bronchus, Via Natural or Artificial Opening
0BL48DZ Occlusion of Right Upper Lobe Bronchus with Intraluminal Device, Via Natural or Artificial Opening Endoscopic
0BL48ZZ Occlusion of Right Upper Lobe Bronchus, Via Natural or Artificial Opening Endoscopic
0BL50CZ Occlusion of Right Middle Lobe Bronchus with Extraluminal Device, Open Approach
0BL50DZ Occlusion of Right Middle Lobe Bronchus with Intraluminal Device, Open Approach
0BL50ZZ Occlusion of Right Middle Lobe Bronchus, Open Approach
0BL53CZ Occlusion of Right Middle Lobe Bronchus with Extraluminal Device, Percutaneous Approach
0BL53DZ Occlusion of Right Middle Lobe Bronchus with Intraluminal Device, Percutaneous Approach
0BL53ZZ Occlusion of Right Middle Lobe Bronchus, Percutaneous Approach
0BL54CZ Occlusion of Right Middle Lobe Bronchus with Extraluminal Device, Percutaneous Endoscopic Approach
0BL54DZ Occlusion of Right Middle Lobe Bronchus with Intraluminal Device, Percutaneous Endoscopic Approach
0BL54ZZ Occlusion of Right Middle Lobe Bronchus, Percutaneous Endoscopic Approach
0BL57DZ Occlusion of Right Middle Lobe Bronchus with Intraluminal Device, Via Natural or Artificial Opening
0BL57ZZ Occlusion of Right Middle Lobe Bronchus, Via Natural or Artificial Opening
0BL58DZ Occlusion of Right Middle Lobe Bronchus with Intraluminal Device, Via Natural or Artificial Opening Endoscopic
0BL58ZZ Occlusion of Right Middle Lobe Bronchus, Via Natural or Artificial Opening Endoscopic
0BL60CZ Occlusion of Right Lower Lobe Bronchus with Extraluminal Device, Open Approach
0BL60DZ Occlusion of Right Lower Lobe Bronchus with Intraluminal Device, Open Approach
0BL60ZZ Occlusion of Right Lower Lobe Bronchus, Open Approach
0BL63CZ Occlusion of Right Lower Lobe Bronchus with Extraluminal Device, Percutaneous Approach
0BL63DZ Occlusion of Right Lower Lobe Bronchus with Intraluminal Device, Percutaneous Approach
0BL63ZZ Occlusion of Right Lower Lobe Bronchus, Percutaneous Approach
0BL64CZ Occlusion of Right Lower Lobe Bronchus with Extraluminal Device, Percutaneous Endoscopic Approach
0BL64DZ Occlusion of Right Lower Lobe Bronchus with Intraluminal Device, Percutaneous Endoscopic Approach
0BL64ZZ Occlusion of Right Lower Lobe Bronchus, Percutaneous Endoscopic Approach
0BL67DZ Occlusion of Right Lower Lobe Bronchus with Intraluminal Device, Via Natural or Artificial Opening
0BL67ZZ Occlusion of Right Lower Lobe Bronchus, Via Natural or Artificial Opening
0BL68DZ Occlusion of Right Lower Lobe Bronchus with Intraluminal Device, Via Natural or Artificial Opening Endoscopic
0BL68ZZ Occlusion of Right Lower Lobe Bronchus, Via Natural or Artificial Opening Endoscopic
0BL70CZ Occlusion of Left Main Bronchus with Extraluminal Device, Open Approach
0BL70DZ Occlusion of Left Main Bronchus with Intraluminal Device, Open Approach
0BL70ZZ Occlusion of Left Main Bronchus, Open Approach
0BL73CZ Occlusion of Left Main Bronchus with Extraluminal Device, Percutaneous Approach
0BL73DZ Occlusion of Left Main Bronchus with Intraluminal Device, Percutaneous Approach
0BL73ZZ Occlusion of Left Main Bronchus, Percutaneous Approach
0BL74CZ Occlusion of Left Main Bronchus with Extraluminal Device, Percutaneous Endoscopic Approach
0BL74DZ Occlusion of Left Main Bronchus with Intraluminal Device, Percutaneous Endoscopic Approach
0BL74ZZ Occlusion of Left Main Bronchus, Percutaneous Endoscopic Approach
0BL77DZ Occlusion of Left Main Bronchus with Intraluminal Device, Via Natural or Artificial Opening
0BL77ZZ Occlusion of Left Main Bronchus, Via Natural or Artificial Opening
0BL78DZ Occlusion of Left Main Bronchus with Intraluminal Device, Via Natural or Artificial Opening Endoscopic
0BL78ZZ Occlusion of Left Main Bronchus, Via Natural or Artificial Opening Endoscopic
0BL80CZ Occlusion of Left Upper Lobe Bronchus with Extraluminal Device, Open Approach
0BL80DZ Occlusion of Left Upper Lobe Bronchus with Intraluminal Device, Open Approach
0BL80ZZ Occlusion of Left Upper Lobe Bronchus, Open Approach
0BL83CZ Occlusion of Left Upper Lobe Bronchus with Extraluminal Device, Percutaneous Approach
0BL83DZ Occlusion of Left Upper Lobe Bronchus with Intraluminal Device, Percutaneous Approach
0BL83ZZ Occlusion of Left Upper Lobe Bronchus, Percutaneous Approach
0BL84CZ Occlusion of Left Upper Lobe Bronchus with Extraluminal Device, Percutaneous Endoscopic Approach
0BL84DZ Occlusion of Left Upper Lobe Bronchus with Intraluminal Device, Percutaneous Endoscopic Approach
0BL84ZZ Occlusion of Left Upper Lobe Bronchus, Percutaneous Endoscopic Approach
0BL87DZ Occlusion of Left Upper Lobe Bronchus with Intraluminal Device, Via Natural or Artificial Opening
0BL87ZZ Occlusion of Left Upper Lobe Bronchus, Via Natural or Artificial Opening
0BL88DZ Occlusion of Left Upper Lobe Bronchus with Intraluminal Device, Via Natural or Artificial Opening Endoscopic
0BL88ZZ Occlusion of Left Upper Lobe Bronchus, Via Natural or Artificial Opening Endoscopic
0BL90CZ Occlusion of Lingula Bronchus with Extraluminal Device, Open Approach
0BL90DZ Occlusion of Lingula Bronchus with Intraluminal Device, Open Approach

0BL90ZZ Occlusion of Lingula Bronchus, Open Approach
0BL93CZ Occlusion of Lingula Bronchus with Extraluminal Device, Percutaneous Approach
0BL93DZ Occlusion of Lingula Bronchus with Intraluminal Device, Percutaneous Approach
0BL93ZZ Occlusion of Lingula Bronchus, Percutaneous Approach
0BL94CZ Occlusion of Lingula Bronchus with Extraluminal Device, Percutaneous Endoscopic Approach
0BL94DZ Occlusion of Lingula Bronchus with Intraluminal Device, Percutaneous Endoscopic Approach
0BL94ZZ Occlusion of Lingula Bronchus, Percutaneous Endoscopic Approach
0BL97DZ Occlusion of Lingula Bronchus with Intraluminal Device, Via Natural or Artificial Opening
0BL97ZZ Occlusion of Lingula Bronchus, Via Natural or Artificial Opening
0BL98DZ Occlusion of Lingula Bronchus with Intraluminal Device, Via Natural or Artificial Opening Endoscopic
0BL98ZZ Occlusion of Lingula Bronchus, Via Natural or Artificial Opening Endoscopic
0BLB0CZ Occlusion of Left Lower Lobe Bronchus with Extraluminal Device, Open Approach
0BLB0DZ Occlusion of Left Lower Lobe Bronchus with Intraluminal Device, Open Approach
0BLB0ZZ Occlusion of Left Lower Lobe Bronchus, Open Approach
0BLB3CZ Occlusion of Left Lower Lobe Bronchus with Extraluminal Device, Percutaneous Approach
0BLB3DZ Occlusion of Left Lower Lobe Bronchus with Intraluminal Device, Percutaneous Approach
0BLB3ZZ Occlusion of Left Lower Lobe Bronchus, Percutaneous Approach
0BLB4CZ Occlusion of Left Lower Lobe Bronch with Extraluminal Device, Percutaneo Endoscopic Approach
0BLB4DZ Occlusion of Left Lower Lobe Bronch with Intraluminal Device, Percutaneou Endoscopic Approach
0BLB4ZZ Occlusion of Left Lower Lobe Bronch Percutaneous Endoscopic Approach
0BLB7DZ Occlusion of Left Lower Lobe Bronch with Intraluminal Device, Via Natural Artificial Opening
0BLB7ZZ Occlusion of Left Lower Lobe Bronch Via Natural or Artificial Opening
0BLB8DZ Occlusion of Left Lower Lobe Bronch with Intraluminal Device, Via Natural Artificial Opening Endoscopic
0BLB8ZZ Occlusion of Left Lower Lobe Bronch Via Natural or Artificial Opening Endoscopic

0BM – Respiratory System, Reattachment

0BM10ZZ Reattachment of Trachea, Open Approach
0BM20ZZ Reattachment of Carina, Open Approach
0BM30ZZ Reattachment of Right Main Bronchus, Open Approach
0BM40ZZ Reattachment of Right Upper Lobe Bronchus, Open Approach
0BM50ZZ Reattachment of Right Middle Lobe Bronchus, Open Approach
0BM60ZZ Reattachment of Right Lower Lobe Bronchus, Open Approach
0BM70ZZ Reattachment of Left Main Bronchus, Open Approach
0BM80ZZ Reattachment of Left Upper Lobe Bronchus, Open Approach
0BM90ZZ Reattachment of Lingula Bronchus, Open Approach
0BMB0ZZ Reattachment of Left Lower Lobe Bronchus, Open Approach
0BMC0ZZ Reattachment of Right Upper Lung Lobe, Open Approach
0BMD0ZZ Reattachment of Right Middle Lung Lobe, Open Approach
0BMF0ZZ Reattachment of Right Lower Lung Lobe, Open Approach
0BMG0ZZ Reattachment of Left Upper Lung Lobe, Open Approach
0BMH0ZZ Reattachment of Lung Lingula, Open Approach
0BMJ0ZZ Reattachment of Left Lower Lung Lob Open Approach
0BMK0ZZ Reattachment of Right Lung, Open Approach
0BML0ZZ Reattachment of Left Lung, Open Approach
0BMR0ZZ Reattachment of Right Diaphragm, Ope Approach
0BMS0ZZ Reattachment of Left Diaphragm, Open Approach

0BN – Respiratory System, Release

Review Coding Guidelines B3.13 and B3.14

0BN10ZZ Release Trachea, Open Approach
0BN13ZZ Release Trachea, Percutaneous Approach
0BN14ZZ Release Trachea, Percutaneous Endoscopic Approach
0BN17ZZ Release Trachea, Via Natural or Artificial Opening
0BN18ZZ Release Trachea, Via Natural or Artificial Opening Endoscopic
0BN20ZZ Release Carina, Open Approach
0BN23ZZ Release Carina, Percutaneous Approach
0BN24ZZ Release Carina, Percutaneous Endoscopic Approach
0BN27ZZ Release Carina, Via Natural or Artificial Opening
0BN28ZZ Release Carina, Via Natural or Artificial Opening Endoscopic
0BN30ZZ Release Right Main Bronchus, Open Approach
0BN33ZZ Release Right Main Bronchus, Percutaneous Approach
0BN34ZZ Release Right Main Bronchus, Percutaneous Endoscopic Approach
0BN37ZZ Release Right Main Bronchus, Via Natural or Artificial Opening
0BN38ZZ Release Right Main Bronchus, Via Natural or Artificial Opening Endoscopic
0BN40ZZ Release Right Upper Lobe Bronchus, Open Approach
0BN43ZZ Release Right Upper Lobe Bronchus, Percutaneous Approach
0BN44ZZ Release Right Upper Lobe Bronchus, Percutaneous Endoscopic Approach
0BN47ZZ Release Right Upper Lobe Bronchus, Via Natural or Artificial Opening
0BN48ZZ Release Right Upper Lobe Bronchus, Via Natural or Artificial Opening Endoscopic
0BN50ZZ Release Right Middle Lobe Bronchus, Open Approach
0BN53ZZ Release Right Middle Lobe Bronchus, Percutaneous Approach
0BN54ZZ Release Right Middle Lobe Bronchus, Percutaneous Endoscopic Approach
0BN57ZZ Release Right Middle Lobe Bronchus, Via Natural or Artificial Opening
0BN58ZZ Release Right Middle Lobe Bronchus, Via Natural or Artificial Opening Endoscopic
0BN60ZZ Release Right Lower Lobe Bronchus, Open Approach
0BN63ZZ Release Right Lower Lobe Bronchus, Percutaneous Approach
0BN64ZZ Release Right Lower Lobe Bronchus, Percutaneous Endoscopic Approach
0BN67ZZ Release Right Lower Lobe Bronchus, Via Natural or Artificial Opening
0BN68ZZ Release Right Lower Lobe Bronchus, Via Natural or Artificial Opening Endoscopic
0BN70ZZ Release Left Main Bronchus, Open Approach
0BN73ZZ Release Left Main Bronchus, Percutaneous Approach
0BN74ZZ Release Left Main Bronchus, Percutaneous Endoscopic Approach
0BN77ZZ Release Left Main Bronchus, Via Natural or Artificial Opening
0BN78ZZ Release Left Main Bronchus, Via Natural or Artificial Opening Endoscopic
0BN80ZZ Release Left Upper Lobe Bronchus, Open Approach
0BN83ZZ Release Left Upper Lobe Bronchus, Percutaneous Approach
0BN84ZZ Release Left Upper Lobe Bronchus, Percutaneous Endoscopic Approach
0BN87ZZ Release Left Upper Lobe Bronchus, Via Natural or Artificial Opening
0BN88ZZ Release Left Upper Lobe Bronchus, Via Natural or Artificial Opening Endoscopi
0BN90ZZ Release Lingula Bronchus, Open Approach
0BN93ZZ Release Lingula Bronchus, Percutaneou Approach
0BN94ZZ Release Lingula Bronchus, Percutaneou Endoscopic Approach
0BN97ZZ Release Lingula Bronchus, Via Natural Artificial Opening
0BN98ZZ Release Lingula Bronchus, Via Natural Artificial Opening Endoscopic
0BNB0ZZ Release Left Lower Lobe Bronchus, Ope Approach
0BNB3ZZ Release Left Lower Lobe Bronchus, Percutaneous Approach
0BNB4ZZ Release Left Lower Lobe Bronchus, Percutaneous Endoscopic Approach
0BNB7ZZ Release Left Lower Lobe Bronchus, Via Natural or Artificial Opening
0BNB8ZZ Release Left Lower Lobe Bronchus, Via Natural or Artificial Opening Endoscopic
0BNC0ZZ Release Right Upper Lung Lobe, Open Approach
0BNC3ZZ Release Right Upper Lung Lobe, Percutaneous Approach
0BNC4ZZ Release Right Upper Lung Lobe, Percutaneous Endoscopic Approach

C7ZZ Release Right Upper Lung Lobe, Via Natural or Artificial Opening
C8ZZ Release Right Upper Lung Lobe, Via Natural or Artificial Opening Endoscopic
D0ZZ Release Right Middle Lung Lobe, Open Approach
D3ZZ Release Right Middle Lung Lobe, Percutaneous Approach
D4ZZ Release Right Middle Lung Lobe, Percutaneous Endoscopic Approach
D7ZZ Release Right Middle Lung Lobe, Via Natural or Artificial Opening
D8ZZ Release Right Middle Lung Lobe, Via Natural or Artificial Opening Endoscopic
F0ZZ Release Right Lower Lung Lobe, Open Approach
F3ZZ Release Right Lower Lung Lobe, Percutaneous Approach
F4ZZ Release Right Lower Lung Lobe, Percutaneous Endoscopic Approach
F7ZZ Release Right Lower Lung Lobe, Via Natural or Artificial Opening
F8ZZ Release Right Lower Lung Lobe, Via Natural or Artificial Opening Endoscopic
G0ZZ Release Left Upper Lung Lobe, Open Approach
G3ZZ Release Left Upper Lung Lobe, Percutaneous Approach
G4ZZ Release Left Upper Lung Lobe, Percutaneous Endoscopic Approach
G7ZZ Release Left Upper Lung Lobe, Via Natural or Artificial Opening
0BNG8ZZ Release Left Upper Lung Lobe, Via Natural or Artificial Opening Endoscopic
0BNH0ZZ Release Lung Lingula, Open Approach
0BNH3ZZ Release Lung Lingula, Percutaneous Approach
0BNH4ZZ Release Lung Lingula, Percutaneous Endoscopic Approach
0BNH7ZZ Release Lung Lingula, Via Natural or Artificial Opening
0BNH8ZZ Release Lung Lingula, Via Natural or Artificial Opening Endoscopic
0BNJ0ZZ Release Left Lower Lung Lobe, Open Approach
0BNJ3ZZ Release Left Lower Lung Lobe, Percutaneous Approach
0BNJ4ZZ Release Left Lower Lung Lobe, Percutaneous Endoscopic Approach
0BNJ7ZZ Release Left Lower Lung Lobe, Via Natural or Artificial Opening
0BNJ8ZZ Release Left Lower Lung Lobe, Via Natural or Artificial Opening Endoscopic
0BNK0ZZ Release Right Lung, Open Approach
0BNK3ZZ Release Right Lung, Percutaneous Approach
0BNK4ZZ Release Right Lung, Percutaneous Endoscopic Approach
0BNK7ZZ Release Right Lung, Via Natural or Artificial Opening
0BNK8ZZ Release Right Lung, Via Natural or Artificial Opening Endoscopic
0BNL0ZZ Release Left Lung, Open Approach
0BNL3ZZ Release Left Lung, Percutaneous Approach
0BNL4ZZ Release Left Lung, Percutaneous Endoscopic Approach
0BNL7ZZ Release Left Lung, Via Natural or Artificial Opening
0BNL8ZZ Release Left Lung, Via Natural or Artificial Opening Endoscopic
0BNM0ZZ Release Bilateral Lungs, Open Approach
0BNM3ZZ Release Bilateral Lungs, Percutaneous Approach
0BNM4ZZ Release Bilateral Lungs, Percutaneous Endoscopic Approach
0BNM7ZZ Release Bilateral Lungs, Via Natural or Artificial Opening
0BNM8ZZ Release Bilateral Lungs, Via Natural or Artificial Opening Endoscopic
0BNN0ZZ Release Right Pleura, Open Approach
0BNN3ZZ Release Right Pleura, Percutaneous Approach
0BNN4ZZ Release Right Pleura, Percutaneous Endoscopic Approach
0BNP0ZZ Release Left Pleura, Open Approach
0BNP3ZZ Release Left Pleura, Percutaneous Approach
0BNP4ZZ Release Left Pleura, Percutaneous Endoscopic Approach
0BNR0ZZ Release Right Diaphragm, Open Approach
0BNR3ZZ Release Right Diaphragm, Percutaneous Approach
0BNR4ZZ Release Right Diaphragm, Percutaneous Endoscopic Approach
0BNS0ZZ Release Left Diaphragm, Open Approach
0BNS3ZZ Release Left Diaphragm, Percutaneous Approach
0BNS4ZZ Release Left Diaphragm, Percutaneous Endoscopic Approach

P – Respiratory System, Removal

view Coding Guideline B6.1c

P000Z Removal of Drainage Device from Tracheobronchial Tree, Open Approach
P001Z Removal of Radioactive Element from Tracheobronchial Tree, Open Approach
P002Z Removal of Monitoring Device from Tracheobronchial Tree, Open Approach
P003Z Removal of Infusion Device from Tracheobronchial Tree, Open Approach
P007Z Removal of Autologous Tissue Substitute from Tracheobronchial Tree, Open Approach
P00CZ Removal of Extraluminal Device from Tracheobronchial Tree, Open Approach
P00DZ Removal of Intraluminal Device from Tracheobronchial Tree, Open Approach
P00JZ Removal of Synthetic Substitute from Tracheobronchial Tree, Open Approach
P00KZ Removal of Nonautologous Tissue Substitute from Tracheobronchial Tree, Open Approach
P030Z Removal of Drainage Device from Tracheobronchial Tree, Percutaneous Approach
P031Z Removal of Radioactive Element from Tracheobronchial Tree, Percutaneous Approach
P032Z Removal of Monitoring Device from Tracheobronchial Tree, Percutaneous Approach
P033Z Removal of Infusion Device from Tracheobronchial Tree, Percutaneous Approach
BP037Z Removal of Autologous Tissue Substitute from Tracheobronchial Tree, Percutaneous Approach
0BP03CZ Removal of Extraluminal Device from Tracheobronchial Tree, Percutaneous Approach
0BP03DZ Removal of Intraluminal Device from Tracheobronchial Tree, Percutaneous Approach
0BP03JZ Removal of Synthetic Substitute from Tracheobronchial Tree, Percutaneous Approach
0BP03KZ Removal of Nonautologous Tissue Substitute from Tracheobronchial Tree, Percutaneous Approach
0BP040Z Removal of Drainage Device from Tracheobronchial Tree, Percutaneous Endoscopic Approach
0BP041Z Removal of Radioactive Element from Tracheobronchial Tree, Percutaneous Endoscopic Approach
0BP042Z Removal of Monitoring Device from Tracheobronchial Tree, Percutaneous Endoscopic Approach
0BP043Z Removal of Infusion Device from Tracheobronchial Tree, Percutaneous Endoscopic Approach
0BP047Z Removal of Autologous Tissue Substitute from Tracheobronchial Tree, Percutaneous Endoscopic Approach
0BP04CZ Removal of Extraluminal Device from Tracheobronchial Tree, Percutaneous Endoscopic Approach
0BP04DZ Removal of Intraluminal Device from Tracheobronchial Tree, Percutaneous Endoscopic Approach
0BP04JZ Removal of Synthetic Substitute from Tracheobronchial Tree, Percutaneous Endoscopic Approach
0BP04KZ Removal of Nonautologous Tissue Substitute from Tracheobronchial Tree, Percutaneous Endoscopic Approach
0BP070Z Removal of Drainage Device from Tracheobronchial Tree, Via Natural or Artificial Opening
0BP071Z Removal of Radioactive Element from Tracheobronchial Tree, Via Natural or Artificial Opening
0BP072Z Removal of Monitoring Device from Tracheobronchial Tree, Via Natural or Artificial Opening
0BP073Z Removal of Infusion Device from Tracheobronchial Tree, Via Natural or Artificial Opening
0BP077Z Removal of Autologous Tissue Substitute from Tracheobronchial Tree, Via Natural or Artificial Opening
0BP07CZ Removal of Extraluminal Device from Tracheobronchial Tree, Via Natural or Artificial Opening
0BP07DZ Removal of Intraluminal Device from Tracheobronchial Tree, Via Natural or Artificial Opening
0BP07JZ Removal of Synthetic Substitute from Tracheobronchial Tree, Via Natural or Artificial Opening
0BP07KZ Removal of Nonautologous Tissue Substitute from Tracheobronchial Tree, Via Natural or Artificial Opening
0BP080Z Removal of Drainage Device from Tracheobronchial Tree, Via Natural or Artificial Opening Endoscopic
0BP081Z Removal of Radioactive Element from Tracheobronchial Tree, Via Natural or Artificial Opening Endoscopic

0BP082Z Removal of Monitoring Device from Tracheobronchial Tree, Via Natural or Artificial Opening Endoscopic
0BP083Z Removal of Infusion Device from Tracheobronchial Tree, Via Natural or Artificial Opening Endoscopic
0BP087Z Removal of Autologous Tissue Substitute from Tracheobronchial Tree, Via Natural or Artificial Opening Endoscopic
0BP08CZ Removal of Extraluminal Device from Tracheobronchial Tree, Via Natural or Artificial Opening Endoscopic
0BP08DZ Removal of Intraluminal Device from Tracheobronchial Tree, Via Natural or Artificial Opening Endoscopic
0BP08JZ Removal of Synthetic Substitute from Tracheobronchial Tree, Via Natural or Artificial Opening Endoscopic
0BP08KZ Removal of Nonautologous Tissue Substitute from Tracheobronchial Tree, Via Natural or Artificial Opening Endoscopic
0BP0X0Z Removal of Drainage Device from Tracheobronchial Tree, External Approach
0BP0X1Z Removal of Radioactive Element from Tracheobronchial Tree, External Approach
0BP0X2Z Removal of Monitoring Device from Tracheobronchial Tree, External Approach
0BP0X3Z Removal of Infusion Device from Tracheobronchial Tree, External Approach
0BP0XDZ Removal of Intraluminal Device from Tracheobronchial Tree, External Approach
0BP100Z Removal of Drainage Device from Trachea, Open Approach
0BP102Z Removal of Monitoring Device from Trachea, Open Approach
0BP107Z Removal of Autologous Tissue Substitute from Trachea, Open Approach
0BP10CZ Removal of Extraluminal Device from Trachea, Open Approach
0BP10DZ Removal of Intraluminal Device from Trachea, Open Approach
0BP10FZ Removal of Tracheostomy Device from Trachea, Open Approach
0BP10JZ Removal of Synthetic Substitute from Trachea, Open Approach
0BP10KZ Removal of Nonautologous Tissue Substitute from Trachea, Open Approach
0BP130Z Removal of Drainage Device from Trachea, Percutaneous Approach
0BP132Z Removal of Monitoring Device from Trachea, Percutaneous Approach
0BP137Z Removal of Autologous Tissue Substitute from Trachea, Percutaneous Approach
0BP13CZ Removal of Extraluminal Device from Trachea, Percutaneous Approach
0BP13DZ Removal of Intraluminal Device from Trachea, Percutaneous Approach
0BP13FZ Removal of Tracheostomy Device from Trachea, Percutaneous Approach
0BP13JZ Removal of Synthetic Substitute from Trachea, Percutaneous Approach
0BP13KZ Removal of Nonautologous Tissue Substitute from Trachea, Percutaneous Approach
0BP140Z Removal of Drainage Device from Trachea, Percutaneous Endoscopic Approach
0BP142Z Removal of Monitoring Device from Trachea, Percutaneous Endoscopic Approach
0BP147Z Removal of Autologous Tissue Substitute from Trachea, Percutaneous Endoscopic Approach
0BP14CZ Removal of Extraluminal Device from Trachea, Percutaneous Endoscopic Approach
0BP14DZ Removal of Intraluminal Device from Trachea, Percutaneous Endoscopic Approach
0BP14FZ Removal of Tracheostomy Device from Trachea, Percutaneous Endoscopic Approach
0BP14JZ Removal of Synthetic Substitute from Trachea, Percutaneous Endoscopic Approach
0BP14KZ Removal of Nonautologous Tissue Substitute from Trachea, Percutaneous Endoscopic Approach
0BP170Z Removal of Drainage Device from Trachea, Via Natural or Artificial Opening
0BP172Z Removal of Monitoring Device from Trachea, Via Natural or Artificial Opening
0BP177Z Removal of Autologous Tissue Substitute from Trachea, Via Natural or Artificial Opening
0BP17CZ Removal of Extraluminal Device from Trachea, Via Natural or Artificial Opening
0BP17DZ Removal of Intraluminal Device from Trachea, Via Natural or Artificial Opening
0BP17FZ Removal of Tracheostomy Device from Trachea, Via Natural or Artificial Opening
0BP17JZ Removal of Synthetic Substitute from Trachea, Via Natural or Artificial Opening
0BP17KZ Removal of Nonautologous Tissue Substitute from Trachea, Via Natural or Artificial Opening
0BP180Z Removal of Drainage Device from Trachea, Via Natural or Artificial Opening Endoscopic
0BP182Z Removal of Monitoring Device from Trachea, Via Natural or Artificial Opening Endoscopic
0BP187Z Removal of Autologous Tissue Substitute from Trachea, Via Natural or Artificial Opening Endoscopic
0BP18CZ Removal of Extraluminal Device from Trachea, Via Natural or Artificial Opening Endoscopic
0BP18DZ Removal of Intraluminal Device from Trachea, Via Natural or Artificial Opening Endoscopic
0BP18FZ Removal of Tracheostomy Device from Trachea, Via Natural or Artificial Opening Endoscopic
0BP18JZ Removal of Synthetic Substitute from Trachea, Via Natural or Artificial Opening Endoscopic
0BP18KZ Removal of Nonautologous Tissue Substitute from Trachea, Via Natural or Artificial Opening Endoscopic
0BP1X0Z Removal of Drainage Device from Trachea, External Approach
0BP1X2Z Removal of Monitoring Device from Trachea, External Approach
0BP1XDZ Removal of Intraluminal Device from Trachea, External Approach
0BP1XFZ Removal of Tracheostomy Device from Trachea, External Approach
0BPK00Z Removal of Drainage Device from Right Lung, Open Approach
0BPK01Z Removal of Radioactive Element from Right Lung, Open Approach
0BPK02Z Removal of Monitoring Device from Right Lung, Open Approach
0BPK03Z Removal of Infusion Device from Right Lung, Open Approach
0BPK30Z Removal of Drainage Device from Right Lung, Percutaneous Approach
0BPK31Z Removal of Radioactive Element from Right Lung, Percutaneous Approach
0BPK32Z Removal of Monitoring Device from Right Lung, Percutaneous Approach
0BPK33Z Removal of Infusion Device from Righ Lung, Percutaneous Approach
0BPK40Z Removal of Drainage Device from Rig Lung, Percutaneous Endoscopic Appro
0BPK41Z Removal of Radioactive Element from Right Lung, Percutaneous Endoscopic Approach
0BPK42Z Removal of Monitoring Device from R Lung, Percutaneous Endoscopic Appro
0BPK43Z Removal of Infusion Device from Righ Lung, Percutaneous Endoscopic Appro
0BPK70Z Removal of Drainage Device from Rig Lung, Via Natural or Artificial Opening
0BPK71Z Removal of Radioactive Element from Right Lung, Via Natural or Artificial Opening
0BPK72Z Removal of Monitoring Device from R Lung, Via Natural or Artificial Opening
0BPK73Z Removal of Infusion Device from Righ Lung, Via Natural or Artificial Opening
0BPK80Z Removal of Drainage Device from Righ Lung, Via Natural or Artificial Opening Endoscopic
0BPK81Z Removal of Radioactive Element from Right Lung, Via Natural or Artificial Opening Endoscopic
0BPK82Z Removal of Monitoring Device from Ri Lung, Via Natural or Artificial Opening Endoscopic
0BPK83Z Removal of Infusion Device from Right Lung, Via Natural or Artificial Opening Endoscopic
0BPKX0Z Removal of Drainage Device from Righ Lung, External Approach
0BPKX1Z Removal of Radioactive Element from Right Lung, External Approach
0BPKX2Z Removal of Monitoring Device from Ri Lung, External Approach
0BPKX3Z Removal of Infusion Device from Right Lung, External Approach
0BPL00Z Removal of Drainage Device from Left Lung, Open Approach
0BPL01Z Removal of Radioactive Element from Left Lung, Open Approach
0BPL02Z Removal of Monitoring Device from Le Lung, Open Approach
0BPL03Z Removal of Infusion Device from Left Lung, Open Approach
0BPL30Z Removal of Drainage Device from Left Lung, Percutaneous Approach
0BPL31Z Removal of Radioactive Element from Left Lung, Percutaneous Approach
0BPL32Z Removal of Monitoring Device from Le Lung, Percutaneous Approach
0BPL33Z Removal of Infusion Device from Left Lung, Percutaneous Approach
0BPL40Z Removal of Drainage Device from Left Lung, Percutaneous Endoscopic Approac
0BPL41Z Removal of Radioactive Element from Left Lung, Percutaneous Endoscopic Approach
0BPL42Z Removal of Monitoring Device from Lef Lung, Percutaneous Endoscopic Approac
0BPL43Z Removal of Infusion Device from Left Lung, Percutaneous Endoscopic Approac
0BPL70Z Removal of Drainage Device from Left Lung, Via Natural or Artificial Opening
0BPL71Z Removal of Radioactive Element from Left Lung, Via Natural or Artificial Opening
0BPL72Z Removal of Monitoring Device from Left Lung, Via Natural or Artificial Opening
0BPL73Z Removal of Infusion Device from Left Lung, Via Natural or Artificial Opening
0BPL80Z Removal of Drainage Device from Left Lung, Via Natural or Artificial Opening Endoscopic

L81Z Removal of Radioactive Element from Left Lung, Via Natural or Artificial Opening Endoscopic
L82Z Removal of Monitoring Device from Left Lung, Via Natural or Artificial Opening Endoscopic
L83Z Removal of Infusion Device from Left Lung, Via Natural or Artificial Opening Endoscopic
LX0Z Removal of Drainage Device from Left Lung, External Approach
LX1Z Removal of Radioactive Element from Left Lung, External Approach
LX2Z Removal of Monitoring Device from Left Lung, External Approach
LX3Z Removal of Infusion Device from Left Lung, External Approach
Q00Z Removal of Drainage Device from Pleura, Open Approach
Q01Z Removal of Radioactive Element from Pleura, Open Approach
Q02Z Removal of Monitoring Device from Pleura, Open Approach
Q30Z Removal of Drainage Device from Pleura, Percutaneous Approach
Q31Z Removal of Radioactive Element from Pleura, Percutaneous Approach
PQ32Z Removal of Monitoring Device from Pleura, Percutaneous Approach
Q40Z Removal of Drainage Device from Pleura, Percutaneous Endoscopic Approach
PQ41Z Removal of Radioactive Element from Pleura, Percutaneous Endoscopic Approach
PQ42Z Removal of Monitoring Device from Pleura, Percutaneous Endoscopic Approach
PQ70Z Removal of Drainage Device from Pleura, Via Natural or Artificial Opening
PQ71Z Removal of Radioactive Element from Pleura, Via Natural or Artificial Opening
PQ72Z Removal of Monitoring Device from Pleura, Via Natural or Artificial Opening
PQ80Z Removal of Drainage Device from Pleura, Via Natural or Artificial Opening Endoscopic
PQ81Z Removal of Radioactive Element from Pleura, Via Natural or Artificial Opening Endoscopic
0BPQ82Z Removal of Monitoring Device from Pleura, Via Natural or Artificial Opening Endoscopic
0BPQX0Z Removal of Drainage Device from Pleura, External Approach
0BPQX1Z Removal of Radioactive Element from Pleura, External Approach
0BPQX2Z Removal of Monitoring Device from Pleura, External Approach
0BPT00Z Removal of Drainage Device from Diaphragm, Open Approach
0BPT02Z Removal of Monitoring Device from Diaphragm, Open Approach
0BPT07Z Removal of Autologous Tissue Substitute from Diaphragm, Open Approach
0BPT0JZ Removal of Synthetic Substitute from Diaphragm, Open Approach
0BPT0KZ Removal of Nonautologous Tissue Substitute from Diaphragm, Open Approach
0BPT0MZ Removal of Diaphragmatic Pacemaker Lead from Diaphragm, Open Approach
0BPT30Z Removal of Drainage Device from Diaphragm, Percutaneous Approach
0BPT32Z Removal of Monitoring Device from Diaphragm, Percutaneous Approach
0BPT37Z Removal of Autologous Tissue Substitute from Diaphragm, Percutaneous Approach
0BPT3JZ Removal of Synthetic Substitute from Diaphragm, Percutaneous Approach
0BPT3KZ Removal of Nonautologous Tissue Substitute from Diaphragm, Percutaneous Approach
0BPT3MZ Removal of Diaphragmatic Pacemaker Lead from Diaphragm, Percutaneous Approach
0BPT40Z Removal of Drainage Device from Diaphragm, Percutaneous Endoscopic Approach
0BPT42Z Removal of Monitoring Device from Diaphragm, Percutaneous Endoscopic Approach
0BPT47Z Removal of Autologous Tissue Substitute from Diaphragm, Percutaneous Endoscopic Approach
0BPT4JZ Removal of Synthetic Substitute from Diaphragm, Percutaneous Endoscopic Approach
0BPT4KZ Removal of Nonautologous Tissue Substitute from Diaphragm, Percutaneous Endoscopic Approach
0BPT4MZ Removal of Diaphragmatic Pacemaker Lead from Diaphragm, Percutaneous Endoscopic Approach
0BPT70Z Removal of Drainage Device from Diaphragm, Via Natural or Artificial Opening
0BPT72Z Removal of Monitoring Device from Diaphragm, Via Natural or Artificial Opening
0BPT77Z Removal of Autologous Tissue Substitute from Diaphragm, Via Natural or Artificial Opening
0BPT7JZ Removal of Synthetic Substitute from Diaphragm, Via Natural or Artificial Opening
0BPT7KZ Removal of Nonautologous Tissue Substitute from Diaphragm, Via Natural or Artificial Opening
0BPT7MZ Removal of Diaphragmatic Pacemaker Lead from Diaphragm, Via Natural or Artificial Opening
0BPT80Z Removal of Drainage Device from Diaphragm, Via Natural or Artificial Opening Endoscopic
0BPT82Z Removal of Monitoring Device from Diaphragm, Via Natural or Artificial Opening Endoscopic
0BPT87Z Removal of Autologous Tissue Substitute from Diaphragm, Via Natural or Artificial Opening Endoscopic
0BPT8JZ Removal of Synthetic Substitute from Diaphragm, Via Natural or Artificial Opening Endoscopic
0BPT8KZ Removal of Nonautologous Tissue Substitute from Diaphragm, Via Natural or Artificial Opening Endoscopic
0BPT8MZ Removal of Diaphragmatic Pacemaker Lead from Diaphragm, Via Natural or Artificial Opening Endoscopic
0BPTX0Z Removal of Drainage Device from Diaphragm, External Approach
0BPTX2Z Removal of Monitoring Device from Diaphragm, External Approach
0BPTXMZ Removal of Diaphragmatic Pacemaker Lead from Diaphragm, External Approach

3Q – Respiratory System, Repair

Q10ZZ Repair Trachea, Open Approach
Q13ZZ Repair Trachea, Percutaneous Approach
Q14ZZ Repair Trachea, Percutaneous Endoscopic Approach
Q17ZZ Repair Trachea, Via Natural or Artificial Opening
Q18ZZ Repair Trachea, Via Natural or Artificial Opening Endoscopic
Q20ZZ Repair Carina, Open Approach
Q23ZZ Repair Carina, Percutaneous Approach
Q24ZZ Repair Carina, Percutaneous Endoscopic Approach
Q27ZZ Repair Carina, Via Natural or Artificial Opening
Q28ZZ Repair Carina, Via Natural or Artificial Opening Endoscopic
Q30ZZ Repair Right Main Bronchus, Open Approach
Q33ZZ Repair Right Main Bronchus, Percutaneous Approach
Q34ZZ Repair Right Main Bronchus, Percutaneous Endoscopic Approach
Q37ZZ Repair Right Main Bronchus, Via Natural or Artificial Opening
0BQ38ZZ Repair Right Main Bronchus, Via Natural or Artificial Opening Endoscopic
0BQ40ZZ Repair Right Upper Lobe Bronchus, Open Approach
0BQ43ZZ Repair Right Upper Lobe Bronchus, Percutaneous Approach
0BQ44ZZ Repair Right Upper Lobe Bronchus, Percutaneous Endoscopic Approach
0BQ47ZZ Repair Right Upper Lobe Bronchus, Via Natural or Artificial Opening
0BQ48ZZ Repair Right Upper Lobe Bronchus, Via Natural or Artificial Opening Endoscopic
0BQ50ZZ Repair Right Middle Lobe Bronchus, Open Approach
0BQ53ZZ Repair Right Middle Lobe Bronchus, Percutaneous Approach
0BQ54ZZ Repair Right Middle Lobe Bronchus, Percutaneous Endoscopic Approach
0BQ57ZZ Repair Right Middle Lobe Bronchus, Via Natural or Artificial Opening
0BQ58ZZ Repair Right Middle Lobe Bronchus, Via Natural or Artificial Opening Endoscopic
0BQ60ZZ Repair Right Lower Lobe Bronchus, Open Approach
0BQ63ZZ Repair Right Lower Lobe Bronchus, Percutaneous Approach
0BQ64ZZ Repair Right Lower Lobe Bronchus, Percutaneous Endoscopic Approach
0BQ67ZZ Repair Right Lower Lobe Bronchus, Via Natural or Artificial Opening
0BQ68ZZ Repair Right Lower Lobe Bronchus, Via Natural or Artificial Opening Endoscopic
0BQ70ZZ Repair Left Main Bronchus, Open Approach
0BQ73ZZ Repair Left Main Bronchus, Percutaneous Approach
0BQ74ZZ Repair Left Main Bronchus, Percutaneous Endoscopic Approach
0BQ77ZZ Repair Left Main Bronchus, Via Natural or Artificial Opening
0BQ78ZZ Repair Left Main Bronchus, Via Natural or Artificial Opening Endoscopic
0BQ80ZZ Repair Left Upper Lobe Bronchus, Open Approach
0BQ83ZZ Repair Left Upper Lobe Bronchus, Percutaneous Approach

0BQ84ZZ Repair Left Upper Lobe Bronchus, Percutaneous Endoscopic Approach
0BQ87ZZ Repair Left Upper Lobe Bronchus, Via Natural or Artificial Opening
0BQ88ZZ Repair Left Upper Lobe Bronchus, Via Natural or Artificial Opening Endoscopic
0BQ90ZZ Repair Lingula Bronchus, Open Approach
0BQ93ZZ Repair Lingula Bronchus, Percutaneous Approach
0BQ94ZZ Repair Lingula Bronchus, Percutaneous Endoscopic Approach
0BQ97ZZ Repair Lingula Bronchus, Via Natural or Artificial Opening
0BQ98ZZ Repair Lingula Bronchus, Via Natural or Artificial Opening Endoscopic
0BQB0ZZ Repair Left Lower Lobe Bronchus, Open Approach
0BQB3ZZ Repair Left Lower Lobe Bronchus, Percutaneous Approach
0BQB4ZZ Repair Left Lower Lobe Bronchus, Percutaneous Endoscopic Approach
0BQB7ZZ Repair Left Lower Lobe Bronchus, Via Natural or Artificial Opening
0BQB8ZZ Repair Left Lower Lobe Bronchus, Via Natural or Artificial Opening Endoscopic
0BQC0ZZ Repair Right Upper Lung Lobe, Open Approach
0BQC3ZZ Repair Right Upper Lung Lobe, Percutaneous Approach
0BQC4ZZ Repair Right Upper Lung Lobe, Percutaneous Endoscopic Approach
0BQC7ZZ Repair Right Upper Lung Lobe, Via Natural or Artificial Opening
0BQC8ZZ Repair Right Upper Lung Lobe, Via Natural or Artificial Opening Endoscopic
0BQD0ZZ Repair Right Middle Lung Lobe, Open Approach
0BQD3ZZ Repair Right Middle Lung Lobe, Percutaneous Approach
0BQD4ZZ Repair Right Middle Lung Lobe, Percutaneous Endoscopic Approach
0BQD7ZZ Repair Right Middle Lung Lobe, Via Natural or Artificial Opening
0BQD8ZZ Repair Right Middle Lung Lobe, Via Natural or Artificial Opening Endoscopic
0BQF0ZZ Repair Right Lower Lung Lobe, Open Approach
0BQF3ZZ Repair Right Lower Lung Lobe, Percutaneous Approach
0BQF4ZZ Repair Right Lower Lung Lobe, Percutaneous Endoscopic Approach
0BQF7ZZ Repair Right Lower Lung Lobe, Via Natural or Artificial Opening
0BQF8ZZ Repair Right Lower Lung Lobe, Via Natural or Artificial Opening Endoscopic
0BQG0ZZ Repair Left Upper Lung Lobe, Open Approach
0BQG3ZZ Repair Left Upper Lung Lobe, Percutaneous Approach
0BQG4ZZ Repair Left Upper Lung Lobe, Percutaneous Endoscopic Approach
0BQG7ZZ Repair Left Upper Lung Lobe, Via Natural or Artificial Opening
0BQG8ZZ Repair Left Upper Lung Lobe, Via Natural or Artificial Opening Endoscopic
0BQH0ZZ Repair Lung Lingula, Open Approach
0BQH3ZZ Repair Lung Lingula, Percutaneous Approach
0BQH4ZZ Repair Lung Lingula, Percutaneous Endoscopic Approach
0BQH7ZZ Repair Lung Lingula, Via Natural or Artificial Opening
0BQH8ZZ Repair Lung Lingula, Via Natural or Artificial Opening Endoscopic
0BQJ0ZZ Repair Left Lower Lung Lobe, Open Approach
0BQJ3ZZ Repair Left Lower Lung Lobe, Percutaneous Approach
0BQJ4ZZ Repair Left Lower Lung Lobe, Percutaneous Endoscopic Approach
0BQJ7ZZ Repair Left Lower Lung Lobe, Via Natural or Artificial Opening
0BQJ8ZZ Repair Left Lower Lung Lobe, Via Natural or Artificial Opening Endoscopic
0BQK0ZZ Repair Right Lung, Open Approach
0BQK3ZZ Repair Right Lung, Percutaneous Approach
0BQK4ZZ Repair Right Lung, Percutaneous Endoscopic Approach
0BQK7ZZ Repair Right Lung, Via Natural or Artificial Opening
0BQK8ZZ Repair Right Lung, Via Natural or Artificial Opening Endoscopic
0BQL0ZZ Repair Left Lung, Open Approach
0BQL3ZZ Repair Left Lung, Percutaneous Appro
0BQL4ZZ Repair Left Lung, Percutaneous Endoscopic Approach
0BQL7ZZ Repair Left Lung, Via Natural or Artifi Opening
0BQL8ZZ Repair Left Lung, Via Natural or Artifi Opening Endoscopic
0BQM0ZZ Repair Bilateral Lungs, Open Approacl
0BQM3ZZ Repair Bilateral Lungs, Percutaneous Approach
0BQM4ZZ Repair Bilateral Lungs, Percutaneous Endoscopic Approach
0BQM7ZZ Repair Bilateral Lungs, Via Natural or Artificial Opening
0BQM8ZZ Repair Bilateral Lungs, Via Natural or Artificial Opening Endoscopic
0BQN0ZZ Repair Right Pleura, Open Approach
0BQN3ZZ Repair Right Pleura, Percutaneous Approach
0BQN4ZZ Repair Right Pleura, Percutaneous Endoscopic Approach
0BQP0ZZ Repair Left Pleura, Open Approach
0BQP3ZZ Repair Left Pleura, Percutaneous Approach
0BQP4ZZ Repair Left Pleura, Percutaneous Endoscopic Approach
0BQR0ZZ Repair Right Diaphragm, Open Approac
0BQR3ZZ Repair Right Diaphragm, Percutaneous Approach
0BQR4ZZ Repair Right Diaphragm, Percutaneous Endoscopic Approach
0BQS0ZZ Repair Left Diaphragm, Open Approach
0BQS3ZZ Repair Left Diaphragm, Percutaneous Approach
0BQS4ZZ Repair Left Diaphragm, Percutaneous Endoscopic Approach

0BS – Respiratory System, Reposition

0BS10ZZ Reposition Trachea, Open Approach
0BS20ZZ Reposition Carina, Open Approach
0BS30ZZ Reposition Right Main Bronchus, Open Approach
0BS40ZZ Reposition Right Upper Lobe Bronchus, Open Approach
0BS50ZZ Reposition Right Middle Lobe Bronchus, Open Approach
0BS60ZZ Reposition Right Lower Lobe Bronchus, Open Approach
0BS70ZZ Reposition Left Main Bronchus, Open Approach
0BS80ZZ Reposition Left Upper Lobe Bronchus, Open Approach
0BS90ZZ Reposition Lingula Bronchus, Open Approach
0BSB0ZZ Reposition Left Lower Lobe Bronchus, Open Approach
0BSC0ZZ Reposition Right Upper Lung Lobe, Open Approach
0BSD0ZZ Reposition Right Middle Lung Lobe, Open Approach
0BSF0ZZ Reposition Right Lower Lung Lobe, Open Approach
0BSG0ZZ Reposition Left Upper Lung Lobe, Open Approach
0BSH0ZZ Reposition Lung Lingula, Open Approac
0BSJ0ZZ Reposition Left Lower Lung Lobe, Oper Approach
0BSK0ZZ Reposition Right Lung, Open Approach
0BSL0ZZ Reposition Left Lung, Open Approach
0BSR0ZZ Reposition Right Diaphragm, Open Approach
0BSS0ZZ Reposition Left Diaphragm, Open Approach

0BT – Respiratory System, Resection

Review Coding Guideline B3.8

0BT10ZZ Resection of Trachea, Open Approach
0BT14ZZ Resection of Trachea, Percutaneous Endoscopic Approach
0BT20ZZ Resection of Carina, Open Approach
0BT24ZZ Resection of Carina, Percutaneous Endoscopic Approach
0BT30ZZ Resection of Right Main Bronchus, Open Approach
0BT34ZZ Resection of Right Main Bronchus, Percutaneous Endoscopic Approach
0BT40ZZ Resection of Right Upper Lobe Bronchus, Open Approach
0BT44ZZ Resection of Right Upper Lobe Bronchus, Percutaneous Endoscopic Approach
0BT50ZZ Resection of Right Middle Lobe Bronchus, Open Approach
0BT54ZZ Resection of Right Middle Lobe Bronchus, Percutaneous Endoscopic Approach
0BT60ZZ Resection of Right Lower Lobe Bronchus, Open Approach
0BT64ZZ Resection of Right Lower Lobe Bronchus, Percutaneous Endoscopic Approach
0BT70ZZ Resection of Left Main Bronchus, Open Approach
0BT74ZZ Resection of Left Main Bronchus, Percutaneous Endoscopic Approach
0BT80ZZ Resection of Left Upper Lobe Bronchus, Open Approach
0BT84ZZ Resection of Left Upper Lobe Bronchus, Percutaneous Endoscopic Approach
0BT90ZZ Resection of Lingula Bronchus, Open Approach
0BT94ZZ Resection of Lingula Bronchus, Percutaneous Endoscopic Approach

B0ZZ Resection of Left Lower Lobe Bronchus, Open Approach
B4ZZ Resection of Left Lower Lobe Bronchus, Percutaneous Endoscopic Approach
C0ZZ Resection of Right Upper Lung Lobe, Open Approach
C4ZZ Resection of Right Upper Lung Lobe, Percutaneous Endoscopic Approach
D0ZZ Resection of Right Middle Lung Lobe, Open Approach
D4ZZ Resection of Right Middle Lung Lobe, Percutaneous Endoscopic Approach
F0ZZ Resection of Right Lower Lung Lobe, Open Approach
F4ZZ Resection of Right Lower Lung Lobe, Percutaneous Endoscopic Approach
0BTG0ZZ Resection of Left Upper Lung Lobe, Open Approach
0BTG4ZZ Resection of Left Upper Lung Lobe, Percutaneous Endoscopic Approach
0BTH0ZZ Resection of Lung Lingula, Open Approach
0BTH4ZZ Resection of Lung Lingula, Percutaneous Endoscopic Approach
0BTJ0ZZ Resection of Left Lower Lung Lobe, Open Approach
0BTJ4ZZ Resection of Left Lower Lung Lobe, Percutaneous Endoscopic Approach
0BTK0ZZ Resection of Right Lung, Open Approach
0BTK4ZZ Resection of Right Lung, Percutaneous Endoscopic Approach
0BTL0ZZ Resection of Left Lung, Open Approach
0BTL4ZZ Resection of Left Lung, Percutaneous Endoscopic Approach
0BTM0ZZ Resection of Bilateral Lungs, Open Approach
0BTM4ZZ Resection of Bilateral Lungs, Percutaneous Endoscopic Approach
0BTR0ZZ Resection of Right Diaphragm, Open Approach
0BTR4ZZ Resection of Right Diaphragm, Percutaneous Endoscopic Approach
0BTS0ZZ Resection of Left Diaphragm, Open Approach
0BTS4ZZ Resection of Left Diaphragm, Percutaneous Endoscopic Approach

U – Respiratory System, Supplement

J107Z Supplement Trachea with Autologous Tissue Substitute, Open Approach
J10JZ Supplement Trachea with Synthetic Substitute, Open Approach
J10KZ Supplement Trachea with Nonautologous Tissue Substitute, Open Approach
J147Z Supplement Trachea with Autologous Tissue Substitute, Percutaneous Endoscopic Approach
J14JZ Supplement Trachea with Synthetic Substitute, Percutaneous Endoscopic Approach
J14KZ Supplement Trachea with Nonautologous Tissue Substitute, Percutaneous Endoscopic Approach
J207Z Supplement Carina with Autologous Tissue Substitute, Open Approach
J20JZ Supplement Carina with Synthetic Substitute, Open Approach
U20KZ Supplement Carina with Nonautologous Tissue Substitute, Open Approach
U247Z Supplement Carina with Autologous Tissue Substitute, Percutaneous Endoscopic Approach
U24JZ Supplement Carina with Synthetic Substitute, Percutaneous Endoscopic Approach
U24KZ Supplement Carina with Nonautologous Tissue Substitute, Percutaneous Endoscopic Approach
U307Z Supplement Right Main Bronchus with Autologous Tissue Substitute, Open Approach
U30JZ Supplement Right Main Bronchus with Synthetic Substitute, Open Approach
U30KZ Supplement Right Main Bronchus with Nonautologous Tissue Substitute, Open Approach
U347Z Supplement Right Main Bronchus with Autologous Tissue Substitute, Percutaneous Endoscopic Approach
U34JZ Supplement Right Main Bronchus with Synthetic Substitute, Percutaneous Endoscopic Approach
U34KZ Supplement Right Main Bronchus with Nonautologous Tissue Substitute, Percutaneous Endoscopic Approach
U407Z Supplement Right Upper Lobe Bronchus with Autologous Tissue Substitute, Open Approach
U40JZ Supplement Right Upper Lobe Bronchus with Synthetic Substitute, Open Approach
U40KZ Supplement Right Upper Lobe Bronchus with Nonautologous Tissue Substitute, Open Approach
U447Z Supplement Right Upper Lobe Bronchus with Autologous Tissue Substitute, Percutaneous Endoscopic Approach
0BU44JZ Supplement Right Upper Lobe Bronchus with Synthetic Substitute, Percutaneous Endoscopic Approach
0BU44KZ Supplement Right Upper Lobe Bronchus with Nonautologous Tissue Substitute, Percutaneous Endoscopic Approach
0BU507Z Supplement Right Middle Lobe Bronchus with Autologous Tissue Substitute, Open Approach
0BU50JZ Supplement Right Middle Lobe Bronchus with Synthetic Substitute, Open Approach
0BU50KZ Supplement Right Middle Lobe Bronchus with Nonautologous Tissue Substitute, Open Approach
0BU547Z Supplement Right Middle Lobe Bronchus with Autologous Tissue Substitute, Percutaneous Endoscopic Approach
0BU54JZ Supplement Right Middle Lobe Bronchus with Synthetic Substitute, Percutaneous Endoscopic Approach
0BU54KZ Supplement Right Middle Lobe Bronchus with Nonautologous Tissue Substitute, Percutaneous Endoscopic Approach
0BU607Z Supplement Right Lower Lobe Bronchus with Autologous Tissue Substitute, Open Approach
0BU60JZ Supplement Right Lower Lobe Bronchus with Synthetic Substitute, Open Approach
0BU60KZ Supplement Right Lower Lobe Bronchus with Nonautologous Tissue Substitute, Open Approach
0BU647Z Supplement Right Lower Lobe Bronchus with Autologous Tissue Substitute, Percutaneous Endoscopic Approach
0BU64JZ Supplement Right Lower Lobe Bronchus with Synthetic Substitute, Percutaneous Endoscopic Approach
0BU64KZ Supplement Right Lower Lobe Bronchus with Nonautologous Tissue Substitute, Percutaneous Endoscopic Approach
0BU707Z Supplement Left Main Bronchus with Autologous Tissue Substitute, Open Approach
0BU70JZ Supplement Left Main Bronchus with Synthetic Substitute, Open Approach
0BU70KZ Supplement Left Main Bronchus with Nonautologous Tissue Substitute, Open Approach
0BU747Z Supplement Left Main Bronchus with Autologous Tissue Substitute, Percutaneous Endoscopic Approach
0BU74JZ Supplement Left Main Bronchus with Synthetic Substitute, Percutaneous Endoscopic Approach
0BU74KZ Supplement Left Main Bronchus with Nonautologous Tissue Substitute, Percutaneous Endoscopic Approach
0BU807Z Supplement Left Upper Lobe Bronchus with Autologous Tissue Substitute, Open Approach
0BU80JZ Supplement Left Upper Lobe Bronchus with Synthetic Substitute, Open Approach
0BU80KZ Supplement Left Upper Lobe Bronchus with Nonautologous Tissue Substitute, Open Approach
0BU847Z Supplement Left Upper Lobe Bronchus with Autologous Tissue Substitute, Percutaneous Endoscopic Approach
0BU84JZ Supplement Left Upper Lobe Bronchus with Synthetic Substitute, Percutaneous Endoscopic Approach
0BU84KZ Supplement Left Upper Lobe Bronchus with Nonautologous Tissue Substitute, Percutaneous Endoscopic Approach
0BU907Z Supplement Lingula Bronchus with Autologous Tissue Substitute, Open Approach
0BU90JZ Supplement Lingula Bronchus with Synthetic Substitute, Open Approach
0BU90KZ Supplement Lingula Bronchus with Nonautologous Tissue Substitute, Open Approach
0BU947Z Supplement Lingula Bronchus with Autologous Tissue Substitute, Percutaneous Endoscopic Approach
0BU94JZ Supplement Lingula Bronchus with Synthetic Substitute, Percutaneous Endoscopic Approach
0BU94KZ Supplement Lingula Bronchus with Nonautologous Tissue Substitute, Percutaneous Endoscopic Approach
0BUB07Z Supplement Left Lower Lobe Bronchus with Autologous Tissue Substitute, Open Approach
0BUB0JZ Supplement Left Lower Lobe Bronchus with Synthetic Substitute, Open Approach
0BUB0KZ Supplement Left Lower Lobe Bronchus with Nonautologous Tissue Substitute, Open Approach
0BUB47Z Supplement Left Lower Lobe Bronchus with Autologous Tissue Substitute, Percutaneous Endoscopic Approach
0BUB4JZ Supplement Left Lower Lobe Bronchus with Synthetic Substitute, Percutaneous Endoscopic Approach
0BUB4KZ Supplement Left Lower Lobe Bronchus with Nonautologous Tissue Substitute, Percutaneous Endoscopic Approach
0BUR07Z Supplement Right Diaphragm with Autologous Tissue Substitute, Open Approach
0BUR0JZ Supplement Right Diaphragm with Synthetic Substitute, Open Approach

0BUR0KZ Supplement Right Diaphragm with Nonautologous Tissue Substitute, Open Approach
0BUR47Z Supplement Right Diaphragm with Autologous Tissue Substitute, Percutaneous Endoscopic Approach
0BUR4JZ Supplement Right Diaphragm with Synthetic Substitute, Percutaneous Endoscopic Approach
0BUR4KZ Supplement Right Diaphragm with Nonautologous Tissue Substitute, Percutaneous Endoscopic Approach
0BUS07Z Supplement Left Diaphragm with Autologous Tissue Substitute, Open Approach
0BUS0JZ Supplement Left Diaphragm with Synthetic Substitute, Open Approach
0BUS0KZ Supplement Left Diaphragm with Nonautologous Tissue Substitute, Open Approach
0BUS47Z Supplement Left Diaphragm with Autologous Tissue Substitute, Percutaneous Endoscopic Approach
0BUS4JZ Supplement Left Diaphragm with Synthetic Substitute, Percutaneous Endoscopic Approach
0BUS4KZ Supplement Left Diaphragm with Nonautologous Tissue Substitute, Percutaneous Endoscopic Approach

0BV – Respiratory System, Restriction

0BV10CZ Restriction of Trachea with Extraluminal Device, Open Approach
0BV10DZ Restriction of Trachea with Intraluminal Device, Open Approach
0BV10ZZ Restriction of Trachea, Open Approach
0BV13CZ Restriction of Trachea with Extraluminal Device, Percutaneous Approach
0BV13DZ Restriction of Trachea with Intraluminal Device, Percutaneous Approach
0BV13ZZ Restriction of Trachea, Percutaneous Approach
0BV14CZ Restriction of Trachea with Extraluminal Device, Percutaneous Endoscopic Approach
0BV14DZ Restriction of Trachea with Intraluminal Device, Percutaneous Endoscopic Approach
0BV14ZZ Restriction of Trachea, Percutaneous Endoscopic Approach
0BV17DZ Restriction of Trachea with Intraluminal Device, Via Natural or Artificial Opening
0BV17ZZ Restriction of Trachea, Via Natural or Artificial Opening
0BV18DZ Restriction of Trachea with Intraluminal Device, Via Natural or Artificial Opening Endoscopic
0BV18ZZ Restriction of Trachea, Via Natural or Artificial Opening Endoscopic
0BV20CZ Restriction of Carina with Extraluminal Device, Open Approach
0BV20DZ Restriction of Carina with Intraluminal Device, Open Approach
0BV20ZZ Restriction of Carina, Open Approach
0BV23CZ Restriction of Carina with Extraluminal Device, Percutaneous Approach
0BV23DZ Restriction of Carina with Intraluminal Device, Percutaneous Approach
0BV23ZZ Restriction of Carina, Percutaneous Approach
0BV24CZ Restriction of Carina with Extraluminal Device, Percutaneous Endoscopic Approach
0BV24DZ Restriction of Carina with Intraluminal Device, Percutaneous Endoscopic Approach
0BV24ZZ Restriction of Carina, Percutaneous Endoscopic Approach
0BV27DZ Restriction of Carina with Intraluminal Device, Via Natural or Artificial Opening
0BV27ZZ Restriction of Carina, Via Natural or Artificial Opening
0BV28DZ Restriction of Carina with Intraluminal Device, Via Natural or Artificial Opening Endoscopic
0BV28ZZ Restriction of Carina, Via Natural or Artificial Opening Endoscopic
0BV30CZ Restriction of Right Main Bronchus with Extraluminal Device, Open Approach
0BV30DZ Restriction of Right Main Bronchus with Intraluminal Device, Open Approach
0BV30ZZ Restriction of Right Main Bronchus, Open Approach
0BV33CZ Restriction of Right Main Bronchus with Extraluminal Device, Percutaneous Approach
0BV33DZ Restriction of Right Main Bronchus with Intraluminal Device, Percutaneous Approach
0BV33ZZ Restriction of Right Main Bronchus, Percutaneous Approach
0BV34CZ Restriction of Right Main Bronchus with Extraluminal Device, Percutaneous Endoscopic Approach
0BV34DZ Restriction of Right Main Bronchus with Intraluminal Device, Percutaneous Endoscopic Approach
0BV34ZZ Restriction of Right Main Bronchus, Percutaneous Endoscopic Approach
0BV37DZ Restriction of Right Main Bronchus with Intraluminal Device, Via Natural or Artificial Opening
0BV37ZZ Restriction of Right Main Bronchus, Via Natural or Artificial Opening
0BV38DZ Restriction of Right Main Bronchus with Intraluminal Device, Via Natural or Artificial Opening Endoscopic
0BV38ZZ Restriction of Right Main Bronchus, Via Natural or Artificial Opening Endoscopic
0BV40CZ Restriction of Right Upper Lobe Bronchus with Extraluminal Device, Open Approach
0BV40DZ Restriction of Right Upper Lobe Bronchus with Intraluminal Device, Open Approach
0BV40ZZ Restriction of Right Upper Lobe Bronchus, Open Approach
0BV43CZ Restriction of Right Upper Lobe Bronchus with Extraluminal Device, Percutaneous Approach
0BV43DZ Restriction of Right Upper Lobe Bronchus with Intraluminal Device, Percutaneous Approach
0BV43ZZ Restriction of Right Upper Lobe Bronchus, Percutaneous Approach
0BV44CZ Restriction of Right Upper Lobe Bronchus with Extraluminal Device, Percutaneous Endoscopic Approach
0BV44DZ Restriction of Right Upper Lobe Bronchus with Intraluminal Device, Percutaneous Endoscopic Approach
0BV44ZZ Restriction of Right Upper Lobe Bronchus, Percutaneous Endoscopic Approach
0BV47DZ Restriction of Right Upper Lobe Bronchus with Intraluminal Device, Via Natural or Artificial Opening
0BV47ZZ Restriction of Right Upper Lobe Bronchus, Via Natural or Artificial Opening
0BV48DZ Restriction of Right Upper Lobe Bronchus with Intraluminal Device, Via Natural or Artificial Opening Endoscopic
0BV48ZZ Restriction of Right Upper Lobe Bronchus, Via Natural or Artificial Opening Endoscopic
0BV50CZ Restriction of Right Middle Lobe Bronchus with Extraluminal Device, O[pen] Approach
0BV50DZ Restriction of Right Middle Lobe Bronchus with Intraluminal Device, O[pen] Approach
0BV50ZZ Restriction of Right Middle Lobe Bronchus, Open Approach
0BV53CZ Restriction of Right Middle Lobe Bronchus with Extraluminal Device, Percutaneous Approach
0BV53DZ Restriction of Right Middle Lobe Bronchus with Intraluminal Device, Percutaneous Approach
0BV53ZZ Restriction of Right Middle Lobe Bronchus, Percutaneous Approach
0BV54CZ Restriction of Right Middle Lobe Bronchus with Extraluminal Device, Percutaneous Endoscopic Approach
0BV54DZ Restriction of Right Middle Lobe Bronchus with Intraluminal Device, Percutaneous Endoscopic Approach
0BV54ZZ Restriction of Right Middle Lobe Bronchus, Percutaneous Endoscopic Approach
0BV57DZ Restriction of Right Middle Lobe Bronchus with Intraluminal Device, Via Natural or Artificial Openin[g]
0BV57ZZ Restriction of Right Middle Lobe Bronchus, Via Natural or Artificial Opening
0BV58DZ Restriction of Right Middle Lobe Bronchus with Intraluminal Device, Via Natural or Artificial Opening Endoscopi[c]
0BV58ZZ Restriction of Right Middle Lobe Bronchus, Via Natural or Artificial Opening Endoscopic
0BV60CZ Restriction of Right Lower Lobe Bronch[us] with Extraluminal Device, Open Appro[ach]
0BV60DZ Restriction of Right Lower Lobe Bronch[us] with Intraluminal Device, Open Approa[ch]
0BV60ZZ Restriction of Right Lower Lobe Bronchus, Open Approach
0BV63CZ Restriction of Right Lower Lobe Bronch[us] with Extraluminal Device, Percutaneous Approach
0BV63DZ Restriction of Right Lower Lobe Bronch[us] with Intraluminal Device, Percutaneous Approach
0BV63ZZ Restriction of Right Lower Lobe Bronchus, Percutaneous Approach
0BV64CZ Restriction of Right Lower Lobe Bronch[us] with Extraluminal Device, Percutaneous Endoscopic Approach
0BV64DZ Restriction of Right Lower Lobe Bronch[us] with Intraluminal Device, Percutaneous Endoscopic Approach
0BV64ZZ Restriction of Right Lower Lobe Bronchus, Percutaneous Endoscopic Approach

'67DZ Restriction of Right Lower Lobe Bronchus with Intraluminal Device, Via Natural or Artificial Opening
/67ZZ Restriction of Right Lower Lobe Bronchus, Via Natural or Artificial Opening
/68DZ Restriction of Right Lower Lobe Bronchus with Intraluminal Device, Via Natural or Artificial Opening Endoscopic
/68ZZ Restriction of Right Lower Lobe Bronchus, Via Natural or Artificial Opening Endoscopic
V70CZ Restriction of Left Main Bronchus with Extraluminal Device, Open Approach
V70DZ Restriction of Left Main Bronchus with Intraluminal Device, Open Approach
V70ZZ Restriction of Left Main Bronchus, Open Approach
V73CZ Restriction of Left Main Bronchus with Extraluminal Device, Percutaneous Approach
V73DZ Restriction of Left Main Bronchus with Intraluminal Device, Percutaneous Approach
V73ZZ Restriction of Left Main Bronchus, Percutaneous Approach
V74CZ Restriction of Left Main Bronchus with Extraluminal Device, Percutaneous Endoscopic Approach
V74DZ Restriction of Left Main Bronchus with Intraluminal Device, Percutaneous Endoscopic Approach
V74ZZ Restriction of Left Main Bronchus, Percutaneous Endoscopic Approach
V77DZ Restriction of Left Main Bronchus with Intraluminal Device, Via Natural or Artificial Opening
V77ZZ Restriction of Left Main Bronchus, Via Natural or Artificial Opening
V78DZ Restriction of Left Main Bronchus with Intraluminal Device, Via Natural or Artificial Opening Endoscopic
V78ZZ Restriction of Left Main Bronchus, Via Natural or Artificial Opening Endoscopic
V80CZ Restriction of Left Upper Lobe Bronchus with Extraluminal Device, Open Approach
V80DZ Restriction of Left Upper Lobe Bronchus with Intraluminal Device, Open Approach
V80ZZ Restriction of Left Upper Lobe Bronchus, Open Approach
0BV83CZ Restriction of Left Upper Lobe Bronchus with Extraluminal Device, Percutaneous Approach
0BV83DZ Restriction of Left Upper Lobe Bronchus with Intraluminal Device, Percutaneous Approach
0BV83ZZ Restriction of Left Upper Lobe Bronchus, Percutaneous Approach
0BV84CZ Restriction of Left Upper Lobe Bronchus with Extraluminal Device, Percutaneous Endoscopic Approach
0BV84DZ Restriction of Left Upper Lobe Bronchus with Intraluminal Device, Percutaneous Endoscopic Approach
0BV84ZZ Restriction of Left Upper Lobe Bronchus, Percutaneous Endoscopic Approach
0BV87DZ Restriction of Left Upper Lobe Bronchus with Intraluminal Device, Via Natural or Artificial Opening
0BV87ZZ Restriction of Left Upper Lobe Bronchus, Via Natural or Artificial Opening
0BV88DZ Restriction of Left Upper Lobe Bronchus with Intraluminal Device, Via Natural or Artificial Opening Endoscopic
0BV88ZZ Restriction of Left Upper Lobe Bronchus, Via Natural or Artificial Opening Endoscopic
0BV90CZ Restriction of Lingula Bronchus with Extraluminal Device, Open Approach
0BV90DZ Restriction of Lingula Bronchus with Intraluminal Device, Open Approach
0BV90ZZ Restriction of Lingula Bronchus, Open Approach
0BV93CZ Restriction of Lingula Bronchus with Extraluminal Device, Percutaneous Approach
0BV93DZ Restriction of Lingula Bronchus with Intraluminal Device, Percutaneous Approach
0BV93ZZ Restriction of Lingula Bronchus, Percutaneous Approach
0BV94CZ Restriction of Lingula Bronchus with Extraluminal Device, Percutaneous Endoscopic Approach
0BV94DZ Restriction of Lingula Bronchus with Intraluminal Device, Percutaneous Endoscopic Approach
0BV94ZZ Restriction of Lingula Bronchus, Percutaneous Endoscopic Approach
0BV97DZ Restriction of Lingula Bronchus with Intraluminal Device, Via Natural or Artificial Opening
0BV97ZZ Restriction of Lingula Bronchus, Via Natural or Artificial Opening
0BV98DZ Restriction of Lingula Bronchus with Intraluminal Device, Via Natural or Artificial Opening Endoscopic
0BV98ZZ Restriction of Lingula Bronchus, Via Natural or Artificial Opening Endoscopic
0BVB0CZ Restriction of Left Lower Lobe Bronchus with Extraluminal Device, Open Approach
0BVB0DZ Restriction of Left Lower Lobe Bronchus with Intraluminal Device, Open Approach
0BVB0ZZ Restriction of Left Lower Lobe Bronchus, Open Approach
0BVB3CZ Restriction of Left Lower Lobe Bronchus with Extraluminal Device, Percutaneous Approach
0BVB3DZ Restriction of Left Lower Lobe Bronchus with Intraluminal Device, Percutaneous Approach
0BVB3ZZ Restriction of Left Lower Lobe Bronchus, Percutaneous Approach
0BVB4CZ Restriction of Left Lower Lobe Bronchus with Extraluminal Device, Percutaneous Endoscopic Approach
0BVB4DZ Restriction of Left Lower Lobe Bronchus with Intraluminal Device, Percutaneous Endoscopic Approach
0BVB4ZZ Restriction of Left Lower Lobe Bronchus, Percutaneous Endoscopic Approach
0BVB7DZ Restriction of Left Lower Lobe Bronchus with Intraluminal Device, Via Natural or Artificial Opening
0BVB7ZZ Restriction of Left Lower Lobe Bronchus, Via Natural or Artificial Opening
0BVB8DZ Restriction of Left Lower Lobe Bronchus with Intraluminal Device, Via Natural or Artificial Opening Endoscopic
0BVB8ZZ Restriction of Left Lower Lobe Bronchus, Via Natural or Artificial Opening Endoscopic

BW – Respiratory System, Revision

eview Coding Guideline B6.1c

3W000Z Revision of Drainage Device in Tracheobronchial Tree, Open Approach
3W002Z Revision of Monitoring Device in Tracheobronchial Tree, Open Approach
3W003Z Revision of Infusion Device in Tracheobronchial Tree, Open Approach
3W007Z Revision of Autologous Tissue Substitute in Tracheobronchial Tree, Open Approach
BW00CZ Revision of Extraluminal Device in Tracheobronchial Tree, Open Approach
BW00DZ Revision of Intraluminal Device in Tracheobronchial Tree, Open Approach
BW00JZ Revision of Synthetic Substitute in Tracheobronchial Tree, Open Approach
BW00KZ Revision of Nonautologous Tissue Substitute in Tracheobronchial Tree, Open Approach
BW030Z Revision of Drainage Device in Tracheobronchial Tree, Percutaneous Approach
0BW032Z Revision of Monitoring Device in Tracheobronchial Tree, Percutaneous Approach
0BW033Z Revision of Infusion Device in Tracheobronchial Tree, Percutaneous Approach
0BW037Z Revision of Autologous Tissue Substitute in Tracheobronchial Tree, Percutaneous Approach
0BW03CZ Revision of Extraluminal Device in Tracheobronchial Tree, Percutaneous Approach
0BW03DZ Revision of Intraluminal Device in Tracheobronchial Tree, Percutaneous Approach
0BW03JZ Revision of Synthetic Substitute in Tracheobronchial Tree, Percutaneous Approach
0BW03KZ Revision of Nonautologous Tissue Substitute in Tracheobronchial Tree, Percutaneous Approach
0BW040Z Revision of Drainage Device in Tracheobronchial Tree, Percutaneous Endoscopic Approach
0BW042Z Revision of Monitoring Device in Tracheobronchial Tree, Percutaneous Endoscopic Approach
0BW043Z Revision of Infusion Device in Tracheobronchial Tree, Percutaneous Endoscopic Approach
0BW047Z Revision of Autologous Tissue Substitute in Tracheobronchial Tree, Percutaneous Endoscopic Approach
0BW04CZ Revision of Extraluminal Device in Tracheobronchial Tree, Percutaneous Endoscopic Approach
0BW04DZ Revision of Intraluminal Device in Tracheobronchial Tree, Percutaneous Endoscopic Approach
0BW04JZ Revision of Synthetic Substitute in Tracheobronchial Tree, Percutaneous Endoscopic Approach

0BW04KZ Revision of Nonautologous Tissue Substitute in Tracheobronchial Tree, Percutaneous Endoscopic Approach

0BW070Z Revision of Drainage Device in Tracheobronchial Tree, Via Natural or Artificial Opening

0BW072Z Revision of Monitoring Device in Tracheobronchial Tree, Via Natural or Artificial Opening

0BW073Z Revision of Infusion Device in Tracheobronchial Tree, Via Natural or Artificial Opening

0BW077Z Revision of Autologous Tissue Substitute in Tracheobronchial Tree, Via Natural or Artificial Opening

0BW07CZ Revision of Extraluminal Device in Tracheobronchial Tree, Via Natural or Artificial Opening

0BW07DZ Revision of Intraluminal Device in Tracheobronchial Tree, Via Natural or Artificial Opening

0BW07JZ Revision of Synthetic Substitute in Tracheobronchial Tree, Via Natural or Artificial Opening

0BW07KZ Revision of Nonautologous Tissue Substitute in Tracheobronchial Tree, Via Natural or Artificial Opening

0BW080Z Revision of Drainage Device in Tracheobronchial Tree, Via Natural or Artificial Opening Endoscopic

0BW082Z Revision of Monitoring Device in Tracheobronchial Tree, Via Natural or Artificial Opening Endoscopic

0BW083Z Revision of Infusion Device in Tracheobronchial Tree, Via Natural or Artificial Opening Endoscopic

0BW087Z Revision of Autologous Tissue Substitute in Tracheobronchial Tree, Via Natural or Artificial Opening Endoscopic

0BW08CZ Revision of Extraluminal Device in Tracheobronchial Tree, Via Natural or Artificial Opening Endoscopic

0BW08DZ Revision of Intraluminal Device in Tracheobronchial Tree, Via Natural or Artificial Opening Endoscopic

0BW08JZ Revision of Synthetic Substitute in Tracheobronchial Tree, Via Natural or Artificial Opening Endoscopic

0BW08KZ Revision of Nonautologous Tissue Substitute in Tracheobronchial Tree, Via Natural or Artificial Opening Endoscopic

0BW0X0Z Revision of Drainage Device in Tracheobronchial Tree, External Approach

0BW0X2Z Revision of Monitoring Device in Tracheobronchial Tree, External Approach

0BW0X3Z Revision of Infusion Device in Tracheobronchial Tree, External Approach

0BW0X7Z Revision of Autologous Tissue Substitute in Tracheobronchial Tree, External Approach

0BW0XCZ Revision of Extraluminal Device in Tracheobronchial Tree, External Approach

0BW0XDZ Revision of Intraluminal Device in Tracheobronchial Tree, External Approach

0BW0XJZ Revision of Synthetic Substitute in Tracheobronchial Tree, External Approach

0BW0XKZ Revision of Nonautologous Tissue Substitute in Tracheobronchial Tree, External Approach

0BW100Z Revision of Drainage Device in Trachea, Open Approach

0BW102Z Revision of Monitoring Device in Trachea, Open Approach

0BW107Z Revision of Autologous Tissue Substitute in Trachea, Open Approach

0BW10CZ Revision of Extraluminal Device in Trachea, Open Approach

0BW10DZ Revision of Intraluminal Device in Trachea, Open Approach

0BW10FZ Revision of Tracheostomy Device in Trachea, Open Approach

0BW10JZ Revision of Synthetic Substitute in Trachea, Open Approach

0BW10KZ Revision of Nonautologous Tissue Substitute in Trachea, Open Approach

0BW130Z Revision of Drainage Device in Trachea, Percutaneous Approach

0BW132Z Revision of Monitoring Device in Trachea, Percutaneous Approach

0BW137Z Revision of Autologous Tissue Substitute in Trachea, Percutaneous Approach

0BW13CZ Revision of Extraluminal Device in Trachea, Percutaneous Approach

0BW13DZ Revision of Intraluminal Device in Trachea, Percutaneous Approach

0BW13FZ Revision of Tracheostomy Device in Trachea, Percutaneous Approach

0BW13JZ Revision of Synthetic Substitute in Trachea, Percutaneous Approach

0BW13KZ Revision of Nonautologous Tissue Substitute in Trachea, Percutaneous Approach

0BW140Z Revision of Drainage Device in Trachea, Percutaneous Endoscopic Approach

0BW142Z Revision of Monitoring Device in Trachea, Percutaneous Endoscopic Approach

0BW147Z Revision of Autologous Tissue Substitute in Trachea, Percutaneous Endoscopic Approach

0BW14CZ Revision of Extraluminal Device in Trachea, Percutaneous Endoscopic Approach

0BW14DZ Revision of Intraluminal Device in Trachea, Percutaneous Endoscopic Approach

0BW14FZ Revision of Tracheostomy Device in Trachea, Percutaneous Endoscopic Approach

0BW14JZ Revision of Synthetic Substitute in Trachea, Percutaneous Endoscopic Approach

0BW14KZ Revision of Nonautologous Tissue Substitute in Trachea, Percutaneous Endoscopic Approach

0BW170Z Revision of Drainage Device in Trachea, Via Natural or Artificial Opening

0BW172Z Revision of Monitoring Device in Trachea, Via Natural or Artificial Opening

0BW177Z Revision of Autologous Tissue Substitute in Trachea, Via Natural or Artificial Opening

0BW17CZ Revision of Extraluminal Device in Trachea, Via Natural or Artificial Opening

0BW17DZ Revision of Intraluminal Device in Trachea, Via Natural or Artificial Opening

0BW17FZ Revision of Tracheostomy Device in Trachea, Via Natural or Artificial Opening

0BW17JZ Revision of Synthetic Substitute in Trachea, Via Natural or Artificial Opening

0BW17KZ Revision of Nonautologous Tissue Substitute in Trachea, Via Natural or Artificial Opening

0BW180Z Revision of Drainage Device in Trach Via Natural or Artificial Opening Endoscopic

0BW182Z Revision of Monitoring Device in Trachea, Via Natural or Artificial Opening Endoscopic

0BW187Z Revision of Autologous Tissue Substi in Trachea, Via Natural or Artificial Opening Endoscopic

0BW18CZ Revision of Extraluminal Device in Trachea, Via Natural or Artificial Opening Endoscopic

0BW18DZ Revision of Intraluminal Device in Trachea, Via Natural or Artificial Opening Endoscopic

0BW18FZ Revision of Tracheostomy Device in Trachea, Via Natural or Artificial Opening Endoscopic

0BW18JZ Revision of Synthetic Substitute in Trachea, Via Natural or Artificial Opening Endoscopic

0BW18KZ Revision of Nonautologous Tissue Substitute in Trachea, Via Natural or Artificial Opening Endoscopic

0BW1X0Z Revision of Drainage Device in Trache External Approach

0BW1X2Z Revision of Monitoring Device in Trachea, External Approach

0BW1X7Z Revision of Autologous Tissue Substitu in Trachea, External Approach

0BW1XCZ Revision of Extraluminal Device in Trachea, External Approach

0BW1XDZ Revision of Intraluminal Device in Trachea, External Approach

0BW1XFZ Revision of Tracheostomy Device in Trachea, External Approach

0BW1XJZ Revision of Synthetic Substitute in Trachea, External Approach

0BW1XKZ Revision of Nonautologous Tissue Substitute in Trachea, External Approach

0BWK00Z Revision of Drainage Device in Right Lung, Open Approach

0BWK02Z Revision of Monitoring Device in Righ Lung, Open Approach

0BWK03Z Revision of Infusion Device in Right Lung, Open Approach

0BWK30Z Revision of Drainage Device in Right Lung, Percutaneous Approach

0BWK32Z Revision of Monitoring Device in Right Lung, Percutaneous Approach

0BWK33Z Revision of Infusion Device in Right Lung, Percutaneous Approach

0BWK40Z Revision of Drainage Device in Right Lung, Percutaneous Endoscopic Approach

0BWK42Z Revision of Monitoring Device in Right Lung, Percutaneous Endoscopic Approach

0BWK43Z Revision of Infusion Device in Right Lung, Percutaneous Endoscopic Approach

0BWK70Z Revision of Drainage Device in Right Lung, Via Natural or Artificial Opening

0BWK72Z Revision of Monitoring Device in Right Lung, Via Natural or Artificial Opening

0BWK73Z Revision of Infusion Device in Right Lung, Via Natural or Artificial Opening

0BWK80Z Revision of Drainage Device in Right Lung, Via Natural or Artificial Opening Endoscopic

VK82Z Revision of Monitoring Device in Right Lung, Via Natural or Artificial Opening Endoscopic
VK83Z Revision of Infusion Device in Right Lung, Via Natural or Artificial Opening Endoscopic
VKX0Z Revision of Drainage Device in Right Lung, External Approach
VKX2Z Revision of Monitoring Device in Right Lung, External Approach
VKX3Z Revision of Infusion Device in Right Lung, External Approach
VL00Z Revision of Drainage Device in Left Lung, Open Approach
VL02Z Revision of Monitoring Device in Left Lung, Open Approach
VL03Z Revision of Infusion Device in Left Lung, Open Approach
VL30Z Revision of Drainage Device in Left Lung, Percutaneous Approach
VL32Z Revision of Monitoring Device in Left Lung, Percutaneous Approach
WL33Z Revision of Infusion Device in Left Lung, Percutaneous Approach
WL40Z Revision of Drainage Device in Left Lung, Percutaneous Endoscopic Approach
WL42Z Revision of Monitoring Device in Left Lung, Percutaneous Endoscopic Approach
WL43Z Revision of Infusion Device in Left Lung, Percutaneous Endoscopic Approach
WL70Z Revision of Drainage Device in Left Lung, Via Natural or Artificial Opening
WL72Z Revision of Monitoring Device in Left Lung, Via Natural or Artificial Opening
WL73Z Revision of Infusion Device in Left Lung, Via Natural or Artificial Opening
WL80Z Revision of Drainage Device in Left Lung, Via Natural or Artificial Opening Endoscopic
WL82Z Revision of Monitoring Device in Left Lung, Via Natural or Artificial Opening Endoscopic
WL83Z Revision of Infusion Device in Left Lung, Via Natural or Artificial Opening Endoscopic
WLX0Z Revision of Drainage Device in Left Lung, External Approach
WLX2Z Revision of Monitoring Device in Left Lung, External Approach
WLX3Z Revision of Infusion Device in Left Lung, External Approach
WQ00Z Revision of Drainage Device in Pleura, Open Approach
0BWQ02Z Revision of Monitoring Device in Pleura, Open Approach
0BWQ30Z Revision of Drainage Device in Pleura, Percutaneous Approach
0BWQ32Z Revision of Monitoring Device in Pleura, Percutaneous Approach
0BWQ40Z Revision of Drainage Device in Pleura, Percutaneous Endoscopic Approach
0BWQ42Z Revision of Monitoring Device in Pleura, Percutaneous Endoscopic Approach
0BWQ70Z Revision of Drainage Device in Pleura, Via Natural or Artificial Opening
0BWQ72Z Revision of Monitoring Device in Pleura, Via Natural or Artificial Opening
0BWQ80Z Revision of Drainage Device in Pleura, Via Natural or Artificial Opening Endoscopic
0BWQ82Z Revision of Monitoring Device in Pleura, Via Natural or Artificial Opening Endoscopic
0BWQX0Z Revision of Drainage Device in Pleura, External Approach
0BWQX2Z Revision of Monitoring Device in Pleura, External Approach
0BWT00Z Revision of Drainage Device in Diaphragm, Open Approach
0BWT02Z Revision of Monitoring Device in Diaphragm, Open Approach
0BWT07Z Revision of Autologous Tissue Substitute in Diaphragm, Open Approach
0BWT0JZ Revision of Synthetic Substitute in Diaphragm, Open Approach
0BWT0KZ Revision of Nonautologous Tissue Substitute in Diaphragm, Open Approach
0BWT0MZ Revision of Diaphragmatic Pacemaker Lead in Diaphragm, Open Approach
0BWT30Z Revision of Drainage Device in Diaphragm, Percutaneous Approach
0BWT32Z Revision of Monitoring Device in Diaphragm, Percutaneous Approach
0BWT37Z Revision of Autologous Tissue Substitute in Diaphragm, Percutaneous Approach
0BWT3JZ Revision of Synthetic Substitute in Diaphragm, Percutaneous Approach
0BWT3KZ Revision of Nonautologous Tissue Substitute in Diaphragm, Percutaneous Approach
0BWT3MZ Revision of Diaphragmatic Pacemaker Lead in Diaphragm, Percutaneous Approach
0BWT40Z Revision of Drainage Device in Diaphragm, Percutaneous Endoscopic Approach
0BWT42Z Revision of Monitoring Device in Diaphragm, Percutaneous Endoscopic Approach
0BWT47Z Revision of Autologous Tissue Substitute in Diaphragm, Percutaneous Endoscopic Approach
0BWT4JZ Revision of Synthetic Substitute in Diaphragm, Percutaneous Endoscopic Approach
0BWT4KZ Revision of Nonautologous Tissue Substitute in Diaphragm, Percutaneous Endoscopic Approach
0BWT4MZ Revision of Diaphragmatic Pacemaker Lead in Diaphragm, Percutaneous Endoscopic Approach
0BWT70Z Revision of Drainage Device in Diaphragm, Via Natural or Artificial Opening
0BWT72Z Revision of Monitoring Device in Diaphragm, Via Natural or Artificial Opening
0BWT77Z Revision of Autologous Tissue Substitute in Diaphragm, Via Natural or Artificial Opening
0BWT7JZ Revision of Synthetic Substitute in Diaphragm, Via Natural or Artificial Opening
0BWT7KZ Revision of Nonautologous Tissue Substitute in Diaphragm, Via Natural or Artificial Opening
0BWT7MZ Revision of Diaphragmatic Pacemaker Lead in Diaphragm, Via Natural or Artificial Opening
0BWT80Z Revision of Drainage Device in Diaphragm, Via Natural or Artificial Opening Endoscopic
0BWT82Z Revision of Monitoring Device in Diaphragm, Via Natural or Artificial Opening Endoscopic
0BWT87Z Revision of Autologous Tissue Substitute in Diaphragm, Via Natural or Artificial Opening Endoscopic
0BWT8JZ Revision of Synthetic Substitute in Diaphragm, Via Natural or Artificial Opening Endoscopic
0BWT8KZ Revision of Nonautologous Tissue Substitute in Diaphragm, Via Natural or Artificial Opening Endoscopic
0BWT8MZ Revision of Diaphragmatic Pacemaker Lead in Diaphragm, Via Natural or Artificial Opening Endoscopic
0BWTX0Z Revision of Drainage Device in Diaphragm, External Approach
0BWTX2Z Revision of Monitoring Device in Diaphragm, External Approach
0BWTX7Z Revision of Autologous Tissue Substitute in Diaphragm, External Approach
0BWTXJZ Revision of Synthetic Substitute in Diaphragm, External Approach
0BWTXKZ Revision of Nonautologous Tissue Substitute in Diaphragm, External Approach
0BWTXMZ Revision of Diaphragmatic Pacemaker Lead in Diaphragm, External Approach

BY – Respiratory System, Transplantation

eview Coding Guideline B3.16

BYC0Z0 Transplantation of Right Upper Lung Lobe, Allogeneic, Open Approach
BYC0Z1 Transplantation of Right Upper Lung Lobe, Syngeneic, Open Approach
BYC0Z2 Transplantation of Right Upper Lung Lobe, Zooplastic, Open Approach
BYD0Z0 Transplantation of Right Middle Lung Lobe, Allogeneic, Open Approach
BYD0Z1 Transplantation of Right Middle Lung Lobe, Syngeneic, Open Approach
▲ **0BYD0Z2** Transplantation of Right Middle Lung Lobe, Zooplastic, Open Approach
▲ **0BYF0Z0** Transplantation of Right Lower Lung Lobe, Allogeneic, Open Approach
▲ **0BYF0Z1** Transplantation of Right Lower Lung Lobe, Syngeneic, Open Approach
▲ **0BYF0Z2** Transplantation of Right Lower Lung Lobe, Zooplastic, Open Approach
▲ **0BYG0Z0** Transplantation of Left Upper Lung Lobe, Allogeneic, Open Approach
▲ **0BYG0Z1** Transplantation of Left Upper Lung Lobe, Syngeneic, Open Approach
▲ **0BYG0Z2** Transplantation of Left Upper Lung Lobe, Zooplastic, Open Approach
▲ **0BYH0Z0** Transplantation of Lung Lingula, Allogeneic, Open Approach
▲ **0BYH0Z1** Transplantation of Lung Lingula, Syngeneic, Open Approach
▲ **0BYH0Z2** Transplantation of Lung Lingula, Zooplastic, Open Approach

▲ **0BYJ0Z0** Transplantation of Left Lower Lung Lobe, Allogeneic, Open Approach

▲ **0BYJ0Z1** Transplantation of Left Lower Lung Lobe, Syngeneic, Open Approach

▲ **0BYJ0Z2** Transplantation of Left Lower Lung Lobe, Zooplastic, Open Approach

▲ **0BYK0Z0** Transplantation of Right Lung, Allogeneic, Open Approach

▲ **0BYK0Z1** Transplantation of Right Lung, Syngeneic, Open Approach

▲ **0BYK0Z2** Transplantation of Right Lung, Zooplastic, Open Approach

▲ **0BYL0Z0** Transplantation of Left Lung, Allogeneic, Open Approach

▲ **0BYL0Z1** Transplantation of Left Lung, Syngeneic, Open Approach

▲ **0BYL0Z2** Transplantation of Left Lung, Zooplas Open Approach

▲ **0BYM0Z0** Transplantation of Bilateral Lungs, Allogeneic, Open Approach

▲ **0BYM0Z1** Transplantation of Bilateral Lungs, Syngeneic, Open Approach

▲ **0BYM0Z2** Transplantation of Bilateral Lungs, Zooplastic, Open Approach

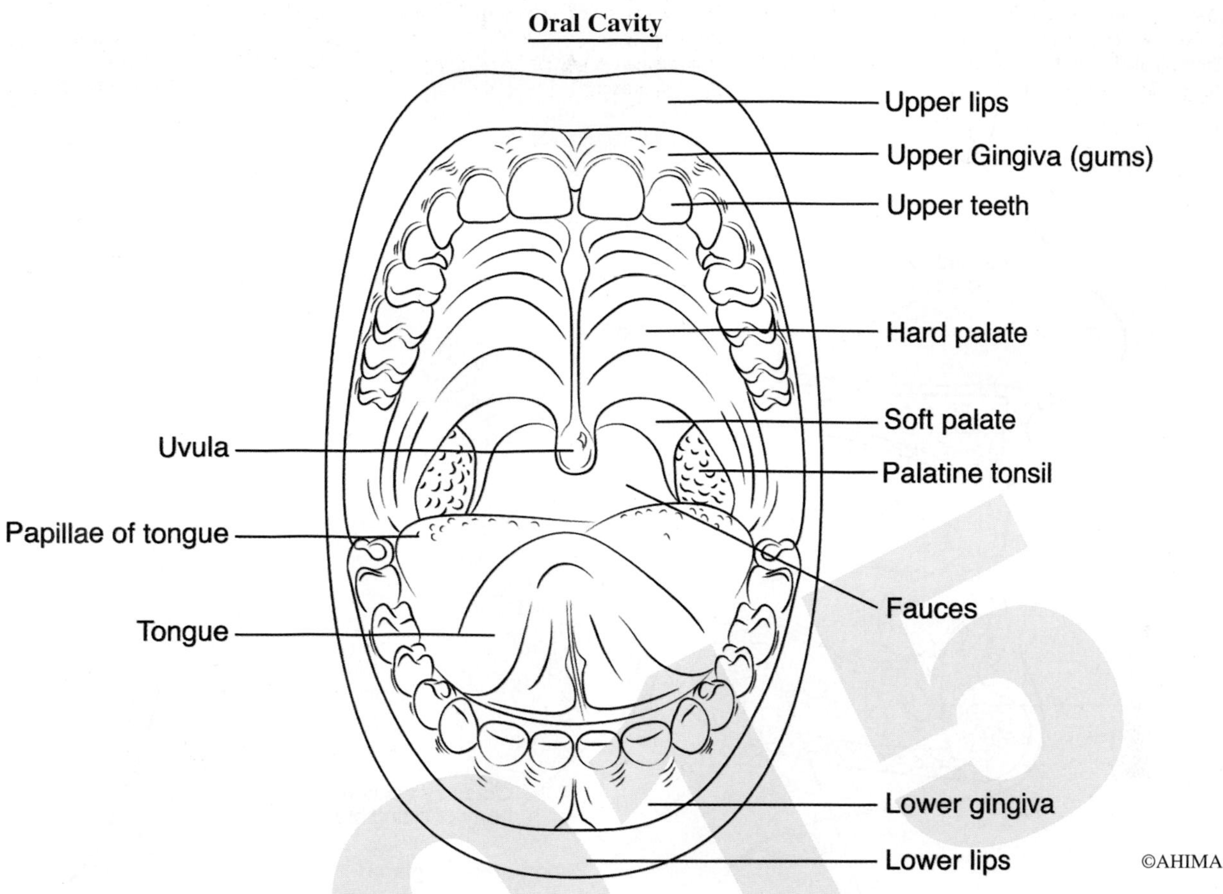
Oral Cavity
Upper lips
Upper Gingiva (gums)
Upper teeth
Hard palate
Soft palate
Uvula
Palatine tonsil
Papillae of tongue
Fauces
Tongue
Lower gingiva
Lower lips
©AHIMA

Glands of the Oral Cavity

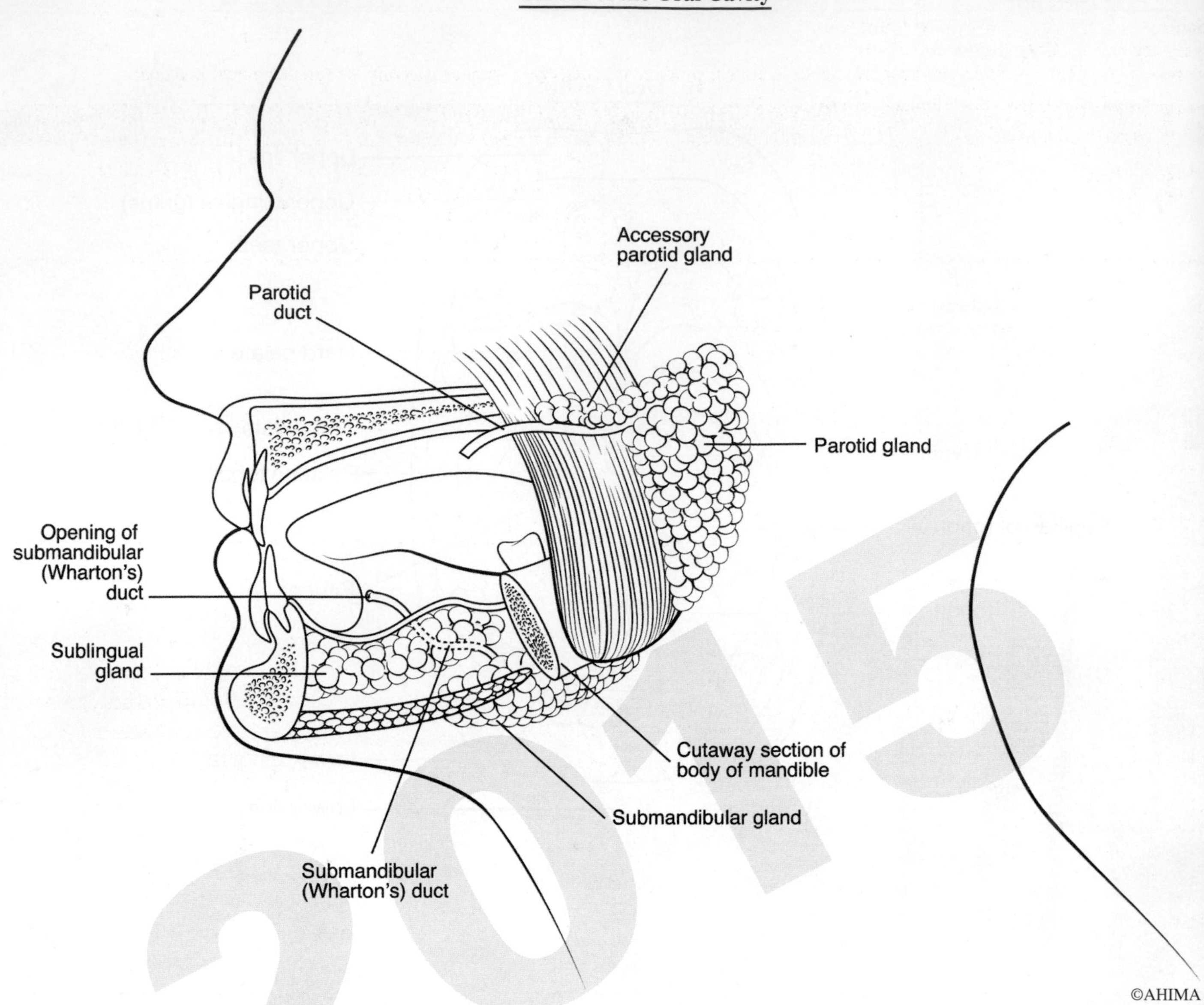

Throat

Tongue

Vocal cord

Epiglottis

Vestibular fold

Pyriform fossa

Esophagus

Trachea

tion 0 **Medical and Surgical**
dy System C **Mouth and Throat**
eration 0 **Alteration:** Modifying the anatomic structure of a body part without affecting the function of the body part

Body Part (4th)	Approach (5th)	Device (6th)	Qualifier (7th)
Upper Lip Lower Lip	**X** External	**7** Autologous Tissue Substitute **J** Synthetic Substitute **K** Nonautologous Tissue Substitute **Z** No Device	**Z** No Qualifier

tion 0 **Medical and Surgical**
dy System C **Mouth and Throat**
eration 2 **Change:** Taking out or off a device from a body part and putting back an identical or similar device in or on the same body part without cutting or puncturing the skin or a mucous membrane

Body Part (4th)	Approach (5th)	Device (6th)	Qualifier (7th)
Salivary Gland Larynx Mouth and Throat	**X** External	**0** Drainage Device **Y** Other Device	**Z** No Qualifier

ction 0 **Medical and Surgical**
dy System C **Mouth and Throat**
eration 5 **Destruction:** Physical eradication of all or a portion of a body part by the direct use of energy, force, or a destructive agent

Body Part (4th)	Approach (5th)	Device (6th)	Qualifier (7th)
Upper Lip Lower Lip Hard Palate Soft Palate Buccal Mucosa Upper Gingiva Lower Gingiva Tongue **N** Uvula **P** Tonsils **Q** Adenoids	**0** Open **3** Percutaneous **X** External	**Z** No Device	**Z** No Qualifier
8 Parotid Gland, Right **9** Parotid Gland, Left **B** Parotid Duct, Right **C** Parotid Duct, Left **D** Sublingual Gland, Right **F** Sublingual Gland, Left **G** Submaxillary Gland, Right **H** Submaxillary Gland, Left **J** Minor Salivary Gland	**0** Open **3** Percutaneous	**Z** No Device	**Z** No Qualifier
M Pharynx **R** Epiglottis **S** Larynx **T** Vocal Cord, Right **V** Vocal Cord, Left	**0** Open **3** Percutaneous **4** Percutaneous Endoscopic **7** Via Natural or Artificial Opening **8** Via Natural or Artificial Opening Endoscopic	**Z** No Device	**Z** No Qualifier
W Upper Tooth **X** Lower Tooth	**0** Open **X** External	**Z** No Device	**0** Single **1** Multiple **2** All

Section 0 **Medical and Surgical**
Body System C **Mouth and Throat**
Operation 7 **Dilation:** Expanding an orifice or the lumen of a tubular body part

Body Part (4th)	Approach (5th)	Device (6th)	Qualifier (7th)
B Parotid Duct, Right **C** Parotid Duct, Left	**0** Open **3** Percutaneous **7** Via Natural or Artificial Opening	**D** Intraluminal Device **Z** No Device	**Z** No Qualifier
M Pharynx	**7** Via Natural or Artificial Opening **8** Via Natural or Artificial Opening Endoscopic	**D** Intraluminal Device **Z** No Device	**Z** No Qualifier
S Larynx	**0** Open **3** Percutaneous **4** Percutaneous Endoscopic **7** Via Natural or Artificial Opening **8** Via Natural or Artificial Opening Endoscopic	**D** Intraluminal Device **Z** No Device	**Z** No Qualifier

Section 0 **Medical and Surgical**
Body System C **Mouth and Throat**
Operation 9 **Drainage:** Taking or letting out fluids and/or gases from a body part

Body Part (4th)	Approach (5th)	Device (6th)	Qualifier (7th)
0 Upper Lip **1** Lower Lip **2** Hard Palate **3** Soft Palate **4** Buccal Mucosa **5** Upper Gingiva **6** Lower Gingiva **7** Tongue **N** Uvula **P** Tonsils **Q** Adenoids	**0** Open **3** Percutaneous **X** External	**0** Drainage Device	**Z** No Qualifier
0 Upper Lip **1** Lower Lip **2** Hard Palate **3** Soft Palate **4** Buccal Mucosa **5** Upper Gingiva **6** Lower Gingiva **7** Tongue **N** Uvula **P** Tonsils **Q** Adenoids	**0** Open **3** Percutaneous **X** External	**Z** No Device	**X** Diagnostic **Z** No Qualifier
8 Parotid Gland, Right **9** Parotid Gland, Left **B** Parotid Duct, Right **C** Parotid Duct, Left **D** Sublingual Gland, Right **F** Sublingual Gland, Left **G** Submaxillary Gland, Right **H** Submaxillary Gland, Left **J** Minor Salivary Gland	**0** Open **3** Percutaneous	**0** Drainage Device	**Z** No Qualifier
8 Parotid Gland, Right **9** Parotid Gland, Left **B** Parotid Duct, Right **C** Parotid Duct, Left	**0** Open **3** Percutaneous	**Z** No Device	**X** Diagnostic **Z** No Qualifier

Continued →

tion	0	**Medical and Surgical**
dy System	C	**Mouth and Throat**
eration	9	**Drainage:** Taking or letting out fluids and/or gases from a body part

Body Part (4th)	Approach (5th)	Device (6th)	Qualifier (7th)
Pharynx Epiglottis Larynx Vocal Cord, Right Vocal Cord, Left	**0** Open **3** Percutaneous **4** Percutaneous Endoscopic **7** Via Natural or Artificial Opening **8** Via Natural or Artificial Opening Endoscopic	**0** Drainage Device	**Z** No Qualifier
Pharynx Epiglottis Larynx Vocal Cord, Right Vocal Cord, Left	**0** Open **3** Percutaneous **4** Percutaneous Endoscopic **7** Via Natural or Artificial Opening **8** Via Natural or Artificial Opening Endoscopic	**Z** No Device	**X** Diagnostic **Z** No Qualifier
Upper Tooth Lower Tooth	**0** Open **X** External	**0** Drainage Device **Z** No Device	**0** Single **1** Multiple **2** All

ction	0	**Medical and Surgical**
dy System	C	**Mouth and Throat**
eration	B	**Excision:** Cutting out or off, without replacement, a portion of a body part

Body Part (4th)	Approach (5th)	Device (6th)	Qualifier (7th)
Upper Lip Lower Lip Hard Palate Soft Palate Buccal Mucosa Upper Gingiva Lower Gingiva Tongue **N** Uvula **P** Tonsils **Q** Adenoids	**0** Open **3** Percutaneous **X** External	**Z** No Device	**X** Diagnostic **Z** No Qualifier
8 Parotid Gland, Right **9** Parotid Gland, Left **B** Parotid Duct, Right **C** Parotid Duct, Left **D** Sublingual Gland, Right **F** Sublingual Gland, Left **G** Submaxillary Gland, Right **H** Submaxillary Gland, Left **J** Minor Salivary Gland	**0** Open **3** Percutaneous	**Z** No Device	**X** Diagnostic **Z** No Qualifier
M Pharynx **R** Epiglottis **S** Larynx **T** Vocal Cord, Right **V** Vocal Cord, Left	**0** Open **3** Percutaneous **4** Percutaneous Endoscopic **7** Via Natural or Artificial Opening **8** Via Natural or Artificial Opening Endoscopic	**Z** No Device	**X** Diagnostic **Z** No Qualifier
W Upper Tooth **X** Lower Tooth	**0** Open **X** External	**Z** No Device	**0** Single **1** Multiple **2** All

Section 0 **Medical and Surgical**
Body System C **Mouth and Throat**
Operation C **Extirpation:** Taking or cutting out solid matter from a body part

Body Part (4th)	Approach (5th)	Device (6th)	Qualifier (7th)
0 Upper Lip **1** Lower Lip **2** Hard Palate **3** Soft Palate **4** Buccal Mucosa **5** Upper Gingiva **6** Lower Gingiva **7** Tongue **N** Uvula **P** Tonsils **Q** Adenoids	**0** Open **3** Percutaneous **X** External	**Z** No Device	**Z** No Qualifier
8 Parotid Gland, Right **9** Parotid Gland, Left **B** Parotid Duct, Right **C** Parotid Duct, Left **D** Sublingual Gland, Right **F** Sublingual Gland, Left **G** Submaxillary Gland, Right **H** Submaxillary Gland, Left **J** Minor Salivary Gland	**0** Open **3** Percutaneous	**Z** No Device	**Z** No Qualifier
M Pharynx **R** Epiglottis **S** Larynx **T** Vocal Cord, Right **V** Vocal Cord, Left	**0** Open **3** Percutaneous **4** Percutaneous Endoscopic **7** Via Natural or Artificial Opening **8** Via Natural or Artificial Opening Endoscopic	**Z** No Device	**Z** No Qualifier
W Upper Tooth **X** Lower Tooth	**0** Open **X** External	**Z** No Device	**0** Single **1** Multiple **2** All

Section 0 **Medical and Surgical**
Body System C **Mouth and Throat**
Operation D **Extraction:** Pulling or stripping out or off all or a portion of a body part by the use of force

Body Part (4th)	Approach (5th)	Device (6th)	Qualifier (7th)
T Vocal Cord, Right **V** Vocal Cord, Left	**0** Open **3** Percutaneous **4** Percutaneous Endoscopic **7** Via Natural or Artificial Opening **8** Via Natural or Artificial Opening Endoscopic	**Z** No Device	**Z** No Qualifier
W Upper Tooth **X** Lower Tooth	**X** External	**Z** No Device	**0** Single **1** Multiple **2** All

Section 0 **Medical and Surgical**
Body System C **Mouth and Throat**
Operation F **Fragmentation:** Breaking solid matter in a body part into pieces

Body Part (4th)	Approach (5th)	Device (6th)	Qualifier (7th)
B Parotid Duct, Right **C** Parotid Duct, Left	**0** Open **3** Percutaneous **7** Via Natural or Artificial Opening **X** External	**Z** No Device	**Z** No Qualifier

tion 0 **Medical and Surgical**
dy System C **Mouth and Throat**
eration H **Insertion:** Putting in a nonbiological appliance that monitors, assists, performs, or prevents a physiological function but does not physically take the place of a body part

Body Part (4th)	Approach (5th)	Device (6th)	Qualifier (7th)
Tongue	**0** Open **3** Percutaneous **X** External	**1** Radioactive Element	**Z** No Qualifier
Mouth and Throat	**7** Via Natural or Artificial Opening **8** Via Natural or Artificial Opening Endoscopic	**B** Intraluminal Device, Airway	**Z** No Qualifier

tion 0 **Medical and Surgical**
dy System C **Mouth and Throat**
eration J **Inspection:** Visually and/or manually exploring a body part

Body Part (4th)	Approach (5th)	Device (6th)	Qualifier (7th)
A SalivaryGland	**0** Open **3** Percutaneous **X** External	**Z** No Device	**Z** No Qualifier
S Larynx Y Mouth and Throat	**0** Open **3** Percutaneous **4** Percutaneous Endoscopic **7** Via Natural or Artificial Opening **8** Via Natural or Artificial Opening Endoscopic **X** External	**Z** No Device	**Z** No Qualifier

ction 0 **Medical and Surgical**
dy System C **Mouth and Throat**
peration L **Occlusion:** Completely closing an orifice or the lumen of a tubular body part

Body Part (4th)	Approach (5th)	Device (6th)	Qualifier (7th)
B Parotid Duct, Right **C** Parotid Duct, Left	**0** Open **3** Percutaneous **4** Percutaneous Endoscopic	**C** Extraluminal Device **D** Intraluminal Device **Z** No Device	**Z** No Qualifier
B Parotid Duct, Right **C** Parotid Duct, Left	**7** Via Natural or Artificial Opening **8** Via Natural or Artificial Opening Endoscopic	**D** Intraluminal Device **Z** No Device	**Z** No Qualifier

ction 0 **Medical and Surgical**
ody System C **Mouth and Throat**
peration M **Reattachment:** Putting back in or on all or a portion of a separated body part to its normal location or other suitable location

Body Part (4th)	Approach (5th)	Device (6th)	Qualifier (7th)
0 Upper Lip **1** Lower Lip **3** Soft Palate **7** Tongue **N** Uvula	**0** Open	**Z** No Device	**Z** No Qualifier
W Upper Tooth **X** Lower Tooth	**0** Open **X** External	**Z** No Device	**0** Single **1** Multiple **2** All

Section 0 **Medical and Surgical**
Body System C **Mouth and Throat**
Operation N **Release:** Freeing a body part from an abnormal physical constraint by cutting or by the use of force

Body Part (4th)	Approach (5th)	Device (6th)	Qualifier (7th)
0 Upper Lip **1** Lower Lip **2** Hard Palate **3** Soft Palate **4** Buccal Mucosa **5** Upper Gingiva **6** Lower Gingiva **7** Tongue **N** Uvula **P** Tonsils **Q** Adenoids	**0** Open **3** Percutaneous **X** External	**Z** No Device	**Z** No Qualifier
8 Parotid Gland, Right **9** Parotid Gland, Left **B** Parotid Duct, Right **C** Parotid Duct, Left **D** Sublingual Gland, Right **F** Sublingual Gland, Left **G** Submaxillary Gland, Right **H** Submaxillary Gland, Left **J** Minor Salivary Gland	**0** Open **3** Percutaneous	**Z** No Device	**Z** No Qualifier
M Pharynx **R** Epiglottis **S** Larynx **T** Vocal Cord, Right **V** Vocal Cord, Left	**0** Open **3** Percutaneous **4** Percutaneous Endoscopic **7** Via Natural or Artificial Opening **8** Via Natural or Artificial Opening Endoscopic	**Z** No Device	**Z** No Qualifier
W Upper Tooth **X** Lower Tooth	**0** Open **X** External	**Z** No Device	**0** Single **1** Multiple **2** All

Section 0 **Medical and Surgical**
Body System C **Mouth and Throat**
Operation P **Removal:** Taking out or off a device from a body part

Body Part (4th)	Approach (5th)	Device (6th)	Qualifier (7th)
A Salivary Gland	**0** Open **3** Percutaneous	**0** Drainage Device **C** Extraluminal Device	**Z** No Qualifier
Y Mouth and Throat	**0** Open **3** Percutaneous **7** Via Natural or Artificial Opening **8** Via Natural or Artificial Opening Endoscopic **X** External	**0** Drainage Device **1** Radioactive Element **7** Autologous Tissue Substitute **D** Intraluminal Device **J** Synthetic Substitute **K** Nonautologous Tissue Substitute	**Z** No Qualifier

tion 0 **Medical and Surgical**
dy System C **Mouth and Throat**
eration Q **Repair:** Restoring, to the extent possible, a body part to its normal anatomic structure and function

Body Part (4th)	Approach (5th)	Device (6th)	Qualifier (7th)
Upper Lip Lower Lip Hard Palate Soft Palate Buccal Mucosa Upper Gingiva Lower Gingiva Tongue N Uvula Tonsils Adenoids	**0** Open **3** Percutaneous **X** External	**Z** No Device	**Z** No Qualifier
Parotid Gland, Right Parotid Gland, Left B Parotid Duct, Right Parotid Duct, Left Sublingual Gland, Right Sublingual Gland, Left G Submaxillary Gland, Right H Submaxillary Gland, Left Minor Salivary Gland	**0** Open **3** Percutaneous	**Z** No Device	**Z** No Qualifier
M Pharynx **R** Epiglottis **S** Larynx **T** Vocal Cord, Right **V** Vocal Cord, Left	**0** Open **3** Percutaneous **4** Percutaneous Endoscopic **7** Via Natural or Artificial Opening **8** Via Natural or Artificial Opening Endoscopic	**Z** No Device	**Z** No Qualifier
W Upper Tooth **X** Lower Tooth	**0** Open **X** External	**Z** No Device	**0** Single **1** Multiple **2** All

ction 0 **Medical and Surgical**
ody System C **Mouth and Throat**
peration R **Replacement:** Putting in or on biological or synthetic material that physically takes the place and/or function of all or a portion of a body part

Body Part (4th)	Approach (5th)	Device (6th)	Qualifier (7th)
0 Upper Lip **1** Lower Lip **2** Hard Palate **3** Soft Palate **4** Buccal Mucosa **5** Upper Gingiva **6** Lower Gingiva **7** Tongue **N** Uvula	**0** Open **3** Percutaneous **X** External	**7** Autologous Tissue Substitute **J** Synthetic Substitute **K** Nonautologous Tissue Substitute	**Z** No Qualifier
B Parotid Duct, Right **C** Parotid Duct, Left	**0** Open **3** Percutaneous	**7** Autologous Tissue Substitute **J** Synthetic Substitute **K** Nonautologous Tissue Substitute	**Z** No Qualifier
M Pharynx **R** Epiglottis **S** Larynx **T** Vocal Cord, Right **V** Vocal Cord, Left	**0** Open **7** Via Natural or Artificial Opening **8** Via Natural or Artificial Opening Endoscopic	**7** Autologous Tissue Substitute **J** Synthetic Substitute **K** Nonautologous Tissue Substitute	**Z** No Qualifier
W Upper Tooth **X** Lower Tooth	**0** Open **X** External	**7** Autologous Tissue Substitute **J** Synthetic Substitute **K** Nonautologous Tissue Substitute	**0** Single **1** Multiple **2** All

Section 0 **Medical and Surgical**
Body System C **Mouth and Throat**
Operation S **Reposition:** Moving to its normal location, or other suitable location, all or a portion of a body part

Body Part (4th)	Approach (5th)	Device (6th)	Qualifier (7th)
0 Upper Lip **1** Lower Lip **2** Hard Palate **3** Soft Palate **7** Tongue **N** Uvula	**0** Open **X** External	**Z** No Device	**Z** No Qualifier
B Parotid Duct, Right **C** Parotid Duct, Left	**0** Open **3** Percutaneous	**Z** No Device	**Z** No Qualifier
R Epiglottis **T** Vocal Cord, Right **V** Vocal Cord, Left	**0** Open **7** Via Natural or Artificial Opening **8** Via Natural or Artificial Opening Endoscopic	**Z** No Device	**Z** No Qualifier
W Upper Tooth **X** Lower Tooth	**0** Open **X** External	**5** External Fixation Device **Z** No Device	**0** Single **1** Multiple **2** All

Section 0 **Medical and Surgical**
Body System C **Mouth and Throat**
Operation T **Resection:** Cutting out or off, without replacement, all of a body part

Body Part (4th)	Approach (5th)	Device (6th)	Qualifier (7th)
0 Upper Lip **1** Lower Lip **2** Hard Palate **3** Soft Palate **7** Tongue **N** Uvula **P** Tonsils **Q** Adenoids	**0** Open **X** External	**Z** No Device	**Z** No Qualifier
8 Parotid Gland, Right **9** Parotid Gland, Left **B** Parotid Duct, Right **C** Parotid Duct, Left **D** Sublingual Gland, Right **F** Sublingual Gland, Left **G** Submaxillary Gland, Right **H** Submaxillary Gland, Left **J** Minor Salivary Gland	**0** Open	**Z** No Device	**Z** No Qualifier
M Pharynx **R** Epiglottis **S** Larynx **T** Vocal Cord, Right **V** Vocal Cord, Left	**0** Open **4** Percutaneous Endoscopic **7** Via Natural or Artificial Opening **8** Via Natural or Artificial Opening Endoscopic	**Z** No Device	**Z** No Qualifier
W Upper Tooth **X** Lower Tooth	**0** Open	**Z** No Device	**0** Single **1** Multiple **2** All

tion	0	**Medical and Surgical**
ly System	C	**Mouth and Throat**
eration	U	**Supplement:** Putting in or on biological or synthetic material that physically reinforces and/or augments the function of a portion of a body part

Body Part (4th)	Approach (5th)	Device (6th)	Qualifier (7th)
Upper Lip Lower Lip Hard Palate Soft Palate Buccal Mucosa Upper Gingiva Lower Gingiva Tongue N Uvula	**0** Open **3** Percutaneous **X** External	**7** Autologous Tissue Substitute **J** Synthetic Substitute **K** Nonautologous Tissue Substitute	**Z** No Qualifier
M Pharynx R Epiglottis S Larynx T Vocal Cord, Right V Vocal Cord, Left	**0** Open **7** Via Natural or Artificial Opening **8** Via Natural or Artificial Opening Endoscopic	**7** Autologous Tissue Substitute **J** Synthetic Substitute **K** Nonautologous Tissue Substitute	**Z** No Qualifier

ction	0	**Medical and Surgical**
dy System	C	**Mouth and Throat**
eration	V	**Restriction:** Partially closing an orifice or the lumen of a tubular body part

Body Part (4th)	Approach (5th)	Device (6th)	Qualifier (7th)
B Parotid Duct, Right C Parotid Duct, Left	**0** Open **3** Percutaneous	**C** Extraluminal Device **D** Intraluminal Device **Z** No Device	**Z** No Qualifier
B Parotid Duct, Right C Parotid Duct, Left	**7** Via Natural or Artificial Opening **8** Via Natural or Artificial Opening Endoscopic	**D** Intraluminal Device **Z** No Device	**Z** No Qualifier

ction	0	**Medical and Surgical**
dy System	C	**Mouth and Throat**
peration	W	**Revision:** Correcting, to the extent possible, a portion of a malfunctioning device or the position of a displaced device

Body Part (4th)	Approach (5th)	Device (6th)	Qualifier (7th)
A Salivary Gland	**0** Open **3** Percutaneous **X** External	**0** Drainage Device **C** Extraluminal Device	**Z** No Qualifier
S Larynx	**0** Open **3** Percutaneous **7** Via Natural or Artificial Opening **8** Via Natural or Artificial Opening Endoscopic **X** External	**0** Drainage Device **7** Autologous Tissue Substitute **D** Intraluminal Device **J** Synthetic Substitute **K** Nonautologous Tissue Substitute	**Z** No Qualifier
Y Mouth and Throat	**0** Open **3** Percutaneous **7** Via Natural or Artificial Opening **8** Via Natural or Artificial Opening Endoscopic **X** External	**0** Drainage Device **1** Radioactive Element **7** Autologous Tissue Substitute **D** Intraluminal Device **J** Synthetic Substitute **K** Nonautologous Tissue Substitute	**Z** No Qualifier

Section 0 **Medical and Surgical**
Body System C **Mouth and Throat**
Operation X **Transfer:** Moving, without taking out, all or a portion of a body part to another location to take over the function of all or a portion of a body part

Body Part (4th)	Approach (5th)	Device (6th)	Qualifier (7th)
0 Upper Lip **1** Lower Lip **3** Soft Palate **4** Buccal Mucosa **5** Upper Gingiva **6** Lower Gingiva **7** Tongue	**0** Open **X** External	**Z** No Device	**Z** No Qualifier

Mouth and Throat Code Listing 0C0–0CX

0C0 – Mouth and Throat, Alteration

0C00X7Z Alteration of Upper Lip with Autologous Tissue Substitute, External Approach
0C00XJZ Alteration of Upper Lip with Synthetic Substitute, External Approach
0C00XKZ Alteration of Upper Lip with Nonautologous Tissue Substitute, External Approach
0C00XZZ Alteration of Upper Lip, External Approach
0C01X7Z Alteration of Lower Lip with Autologous Tissue Substitute, External Approach
0C01XJZ Alteration of Lower Lip with Synthetic Substitute, External Approach
0C01XKZ Alteration of Lower Lip with Nonautologous Tissue Substitute, Exter Approach
0C01XZZ Alteration of Lower Lip, External Approach

0C2 – Mouth and Throat, Change

Review Coding Guideline B6.1c

0C2AX0Z Change Drainage Device in Salivary Gland, External Approach
0C2AXYZ Change Other Device in Salivary Gland, External Approach
0C2SX0Z Change Drainage Device in Larynx, External Approach
0C2SXYZ Change Other Device in Larynx, External Approach
0C2YX0Z Change Drainage Device in Mouth and Throat, External Approach
0C2YXYZ Change Other Device in Mouth and Throat, External Approach

0C5 – Mouth and Throat, Destruction

0C500ZZ Destruction of Upper Lip, Open Approach
0C503ZZ Destruction of Upper Lip, Percutaneous Approach
0C50XZZ Destruction of Upper Lip, External Approach
0C510ZZ Destruction of Lower Lip, Open Approach
0C513ZZ Destruction of Lower Lip, Percutaneous Approach
0C51XZZ Destruction of Lower Lip, External Approach
0C520ZZ Destruction of Hard Palate, Open Approach
0C523ZZ Destruction of Hard Palate, Percutaneous Approach
0C52XZZ Destruction of Hard Palate, External Approach
0C530ZZ Destruction of Soft Palate, Open Approach
0C533ZZ Destruction of Soft Palate, Percutaneous Approach
0C53XZZ Destruction of Soft Palate, External Approach
0C540ZZ Destruction of Buccal Mucosa, Open Approach
0C543ZZ Destruction of Buccal Mucosa, Percutaneous Approach
0C54XZZ Destruction of Buccal Mucosa, External Approach
0C550ZZ Destruction of Upper Gingiva, Open Approach
0C553ZZ Destruction of Upper Gingiva, Percutaneous Approach
0C55XZZ Destruction of Upper Gingiva, External Approach
0C560ZZ Destruction of Lower Gingiva, Open Approach
0C563ZZ Destruction of Lower Gingiva, Percutaneous Approach
0C56XZZ Destruction of Lower Gingiva, External Approach
0C570ZZ Destruction of Tongue, Open Approach
0C573ZZ Destruction of Tongue, Percutaneous Approach
0C57XZZ Destruction of Tongue, External Approach
0C580ZZ Destruction of Right Parotid Gland, Open Approach
0C583ZZ Destruction of Right Parotid Gland, Percutaneous Approach
0C590ZZ Destruction of Left Parotid Gland, Open Approach
0C593ZZ Destruction of Left Parotid Gland, Percutaneous Approach
0C5B0ZZ Destruction of Right Parotid Duct, Open Approach
0C5B3ZZ Destruction of Right Parotid Duct, Percutaneous Approach
0C5C0ZZ Destruction of Left Parotid Duct, Open Approach
0C5C3ZZ Destruction of Left Parotid Duct, Percutaneous Approach
0C5D0ZZ Destruction of Right Sublingual Gland, Open Approach
0C5D3ZZ Destruction of Right Sublingual Gland, Percutaneous Approach
0C5F0ZZ Destruction of Left Sublingual Gland, Open Approach
0C5F3ZZ Destruction of Left Sublingual Gland, Percutaneous Approach
0C5G0ZZ Destruction of Right Submaxillary Gland, Open Approach
0C5G3ZZ Destruction of Right Submaxillary Gland, Percutaneous Approach
0C5H0ZZ Destruction of Left Submaxillary Gland Open Approach
0C5H3ZZ Destruction of Left Submaxillary Gland Percutaneous Approach
0C5J0ZZ Destruction of Minor Salivary Gland, Open Approach
0C5J3ZZ Destruction of Minor Salivary Gland, Percutaneous Approach
0C5M0ZZ Destruction of Pharynx, Open Approach
0C5M3ZZ Destruction of Pharynx, Percutaneous Approach
0C5M4ZZ Destruction of Pharynx, Percutaneous Endoscopic Approach
0C5M7ZZ Destruction of Pharynx, Via Natural or Artificial Opening
0C5M8ZZ Destruction of Pharynx, Via Natural or Artificial Opening Endoscopic
0C5N0ZZ Destruction of Uvula, Open Approach
0C5N3ZZ Destruction of Uvula, Percutaneous Approach
0C5NXZZ Destruction of Uvula, External Approach
0C5P0ZZ Destruction of Tonsils, Open Approach
0C5P3ZZ Destruction of Tonsils, Percutaneous Approach
0C5PXZZ Destruction of Tonsils, External Approach
0C5Q0ZZ Destruction of Adenoids, Open Approach
0C5Q3ZZ Destruction of Adenoids, Percutaneous Approach
0C5QXZZ Destruction of Adenoids, External Approach
0C5R0ZZ Destruction of Epiglottis, Open Approach
0C5R3ZZ Destruction of Epiglottis, Percutaneous Approach
0C5R4ZZ Destruction of Epiglottis, Percutaneous Endoscopic Approach

5R7ZZ Destruction of Epiglottis, Via Natural or Artificial Opening
5R8ZZ Destruction of Epiglottis, Via Natural or Artificial Opening Endoscopic
5S0ZZ Destruction of Larynx, Open Approach
5S3ZZ Destruction of Larynx, Percutaneous Approach
5S4ZZ Destruction of Larynx, Percutaneous Endoscopic Approach
5S7ZZ Destruction of Larynx, Via Natural or Artificial Opening
5S8ZZ Destruction of Larynx, Via Natural or Artificial Opening Endoscopic
5T0ZZ Destruction of Right Vocal Cord, Open Approach
5T3ZZ Destruction of Right Vocal Cord, Percutaneous Approach
5T4ZZ Destruction of Right Vocal Cord, Percutaneous Endoscopic Approach
0C5T7ZZ Destruction of Right Vocal Cord, Via Natural or Artificial Opening
0C5T8ZZ Destruction of Right Vocal Cord, Via Natural or Artificial Opening Endoscopic
0C5V0ZZ Destruction of Left Vocal Cord, Open Approach
0C5V3ZZ Destruction of Left Vocal Cord, Percutaneous Approach
0C5V4ZZ Destruction of Left Vocal Cord, Percutaneous Endoscopic Approach
0C5V7ZZ Destruction of Left Vocal Cord, Via Natural or Artificial Opening
0C5V8ZZ Destruction of Left Vocal Cord, Via Natural or Artificial Opening Endoscopic
0C5W0Z0 Destruction of Upper Tooth, Single, Open Approach
0C5W0Z1 Destruction of Upper Tooth, Multiple, Open Approach
0C5W0Z2 Destruction of Upper Tooth, All, Open Approach
0C5WXZ0 Destruction of Upper Tooth, Single, External Approach
0C5WXZ1 Destruction of Upper Tooth, Multiple, External Approach
0C5WXZ2 Destruction of Upper Tooth, All, External Approach
0C5X0Z0 Destruction of Lower Tooth, Single, Open Approach
0C5X0Z1 Destruction of Lower Tooth, Multiple, Open Approach
0C5X0Z2 Destruction of Lower Tooth, All, Open Approach
0C5XXZ0 Destruction of Lower Tooth, Single, External Approach
0C5XXZ1 Destruction of Lower Tooth, Multiple, External Approach
0C5XXZ2 Destruction of Lower Tooth, All, External Approach

C7 – Mouth and Throat, Dilation

7B0DZ Dilation of Right Parotid Duct with Intraluminal Device, Open Approach
7B0ZZ Dilation of Right Parotid Duct, Open Approach
7B3DZ Dilation of Right Parotid Duct with Intraluminal Device, Percutaneous Approach
7B3ZZ Dilation of Right Parotid Duct, Percutaneous Approach
7B7DZ Dilation of Right Parotid Duct with Intraluminal Device, Via Natural or Artificial Opening
7B7ZZ Dilation of Right Parotid Duct, Via Natural or Artificial Opening
7C0DZ Dilation of Left Parotid Duct with Intraluminal Device, Open Approach
7C0ZZ Dilation of Left Parotid Duct, Open Approach
7C3DZ Dilation of Left Parotid Duct with Intraluminal Device, Percutaneous Approach
0C7C3ZZ Dilation of Left Parotid Duct, Percutaneous Approach
0C7C7DZ Dilation of Left Parotid Duct with Intraluminal Device, Via Natural or Artificial Opening
0C7C7ZZ Dilation of Left Parotid Duct, Via Natural or Artificial Opening
0C7M7DZ Dilation of Pharynx with Intraluminal Device, Via Natural or Artificial Opening
0C7M7ZZ Dilation of Pharynx, Via Natural or Artificial Opening
0C7M8DZ Dilation of Pharynx with Intraluminal Device, Via Natural or Artificial Opening Endoscopic
0C7M8ZZ Dilation of Pharynx, Via Natural or Artificial Opening Endoscopic
0C7S0DZ Dilation of Larynx with Intraluminal Device, Open Approach
0C7S0ZZ Dilation of Larynx, Open Approach
0C7S3DZ Dilation of Larynx with Intraluminal Device, Percutaneous Approach
0C7S3ZZ Dilation of Larynx, Percutaneous Approach
0C7S4DZ Dilation of Larynx with Intraluminal Device, Percutaneous Endoscopic Approach
0C7S4ZZ Dilation of Larynx, Percutaneous Endoscopic Approach
0C7S7DZ Dilation of Larynx with Intraluminal Device, Via Natural or Artificial Opening
0C7S7ZZ Dilation of Larynx, Via Natural or Artificial Opening
0C7S8DZ Dilation of Larynx with Intraluminal Device, Via Natural or Artificial Opening Endoscopic
0C7S8ZZ Dilation of Larynx, Via Natural or Artificial Opening Endoscopic

C9 – Mouth and Throat, Drainage

eview Coding Guidelines B3.4a and B3.4b

eview Coding Guideline B6.2

C9000Z Drainage of Upper Lip with Drainage Device, Open Approach
C900ZX Drainage of Upper Lip, Open Approach, Diagnostic
C900ZZ Drainage of Upper Lip, Open Approach
C9030Z Drainage of Upper Lip with Drainage Device, Percutaneous Approach
C903ZX Drainage of Upper Lip, Percutaneous Approach, Diagnostic
C903ZZ Drainage of Upper Lip, Percutaneous Approach
C90X0Z Drainage of Upper Lip with Drainage Device, External Approach
C90XZX Drainage of Upper Lip, External Approach, Diagnostic
C90XZZ Drainage of Upper Lip, External Approach
C9100Z Drainage of Lower Lip with Drainage Device, Open Approach
C910ZX Drainage of Lower Lip, Open Approach, Diagnostic
C910ZZ Drainage of Lower Lip, Open Approach
C9130Z Drainage of Lower Lip with Drainage Device, Percutaneous Approach
C913ZX Drainage of Lower Lip, Percutaneous Approach, Diagnostic
0C913ZZ Drainage of Lower Lip, Percutaneous Approach
0C91X0Z Drainage of Lower Lip with Drainage Device, External Approach
0C91XZX Drainage of Lower Lip, External Approach, Diagnostic
0C91XZZ Drainage of Lower Lip, External Approach
0C9200Z Drainage of Hard Palate with Drainage Device, Open Approach
0C920ZX Drainage of Hard Palate, Open Approach, Diagnostic
0C920ZZ Drainage of Hard Palate, Open Approach
0C9230Z Drainage of Hard Palate with Drainage Device, Percutaneous Approach
0C923ZX Drainage of Hard Palate, Percutaneous Approach, Diagnostic
0C923ZZ Drainage of Hard Palate, Percutaneous Approach
0C92X0Z Drainage of Hard Palate with Drainage Device, External Approach
0C92XZX Drainage of Hard Palate, External Approach, Diagnostic
0C92XZZ Drainage of Hard Palate, External Approach
0C9300Z Drainage of Soft Palate with Drainage Device, Open Approach
0C930ZX Drainage of Soft Palate, Open Approach, Diagnostic
0C930ZZ Drainage of Soft Palate, Open Approach
0C9330Z Drainage of Soft Palate with Drainage Device, Percutaneous Approach
0C933ZX Drainage of Soft Palate, Percutaneous Approach, Diagnostic
0C933ZZ Drainage of Soft Palate, Percutaneous Approach
0C93X0Z Drainage of Soft Palate with Drainage Device, External Approach
0C93XZX Drainage of Soft Palate, External Approach, Diagnostic
0C93XZZ Drainage of Soft Palate, External Approach
0C9400Z Drainage of Buccal Mucosa with Drainage Device, Open Approach
0C940ZX Drainage of Buccal Mucosa, Open Approach, Diagnostic
0C940ZZ Drainage of Buccal Mucosa, Open Approach
0C9430Z Drainage of Buccal Mucosa with Drainage Device, Percutaneous Approach
0C943ZX Drainage of Buccal Mucosa, Percutaneous Approach, Diagnostic

0C943ZZ Drainage of Buccal Mucosa, Percutaneous Approach
0C94X0Z Drainage of Buccal Mucosa with Drainage Device, External Approach
0C94XZX Drainage of Buccal Mucosa, External Approach, Diagnostic
0C94XZZ Drainage of Buccal Mucosa, External Approach
0C9500Z Drainage of Upper Gingiva with Drainage Device, Open Approach
0C950ZX Drainage of Upper Gingiva, Open Approach, Diagnostic
0C950ZZ Drainage of Upper Gingiva, Open Approach
0C9530Z Drainage of Upper Gingiva with Drainage Device, Percutaneous Approach
0C953ZX Drainage of Upper Gingiva, Percutaneous Approach, Diagnostic
0C953ZZ Drainage of Upper Gingiva, Percutaneous Approach
0C95X0Z Drainage of Upper Gingiva with Drainage Device, External Approach
0C95XZX Drainage of Upper Gingiva, External Approach, Diagnostic
0C95XZZ Drainage of Upper Gingiva, External Approach
0C9600Z Drainage of Lower Gingiva with Drainage Device, Open Approach
0C960ZX Drainage of Lower Gingiva, Open Approach, Diagnostic
0C960ZZ Drainage of Lower Gingiva, Open Approach
0C9630Z Drainage of Lower Gingiva with Drainage Device, Percutaneous Approach
0C963ZX Drainage of Lower Gingiva, Percutaneous Approach, Diagnostic
0C963ZZ Drainage of Lower Gingiva, Percutaneous Approach
0C96X0Z Drainage of Lower Gingiva with Drainage Device, External Approach
0C96XZX Drainage of Lower Gingiva, External Approach, Diagnostic
0C96XZZ Drainage of Lower Gingiva, External Approach
0C9700Z Drainage of Tongue with Drainage Device, Open Approach
0C970ZX Drainage of Tongue, Open Approach, Diagnostic
0C970ZZ Drainage of Tongue, Open Approach
0C9730Z Drainage of Tongue with Drainage Device, Percutaneous Approach
0C973ZX Drainage of Tongue, Percutaneous Approach, Diagnostic
0C973ZZ Drainage of Tongue, Percutaneous Approach
0C97X0Z Drainage of Tongue with Drainage Device, External Approach
0C97XZX Drainage of Tongue, External Approach, Diagnostic
0C97XZZ Drainage of Tongue, External Approach
0C9800Z Drainage of Right Parotid Gland with Drainage Device, Open Approach
0C980ZX Drainage of Right Parotid Gland, Open Approach, Diagnostic
0C980ZZ Drainage of Right Parotid Gland, Open Approach
0C9830Z Drainage of Right Parotid Gland with Drainage Device, Percutaneous Approach
0C983ZX Drainage of Right Parotid Gland, Percutaneous Approach, Diagnostic
0C983ZZ Drainage of Right Parotid Gland, Percutaneous Approach
0C9900Z Drainage of Left Parotid Gland with Drainage Device, Open Approach
0C990ZX Drainage of Left Parotid Gland, Open Approach, Diagnostic
0C990ZZ Drainage of Left Parotid Gland, Open Approach
0C9930Z Drainage of Left Parotid Gland with Drainage Device, Percutaneous Approach
0C993ZX Drainage of Left Parotid Gland, Percutaneous Approach, Diagnostic
0C993ZZ Drainage of Left Parotid Gland, Percutaneous Approach
0C9B00Z Drainage of Right Parotid Duct with Drainage Device, Open Approach
0C9B0ZX Drainage of Right Parotid Duct, Open Approach, Diagnostic
0C9B0ZZ Drainage of Right Parotid Duct, Open Approach
0C9B30Z Drainage of Right Parotid Duct with Drainage Device, Percutaneous Approach
0C9B3ZX Drainage of Right Parotid Duct, Percutaneous Approach, Diagnostic
0C9B3ZZ Drainage of Right Parotid Duct, Percutaneous Approach
0C9C00Z Drainage of Left Parotid Duct with Drainage Device, Open Approach
0C9C0ZX Drainage of Left Parotid Duct, Open Approach, Diagnostic
0C9C0ZZ Drainage of Left Parotid Duct, Open Approach
0C9C30Z Drainage of Left Parotid Duct with Drainage Device, Percutaneous Approach
0C9C3ZX Drainage of Left Parotid Duct, Percutaneous Approach, Diagnostic
0C9C3ZZ Drainage of Left Parotid Duct, Percutaneous Approach
0C9D00Z Drainage of Right Sublingual Gland with Drainage Device, Open Approach
0C9D0ZX Drainage of Right Sublingual Gland, Open Approach, Diagnostic
0C9D0ZZ Drainage of Right Sublingual Gland, Open Approach
0C9D30Z Drainage of Right Sublingual Gland with Drainage Device, Percutaneous Approach
0C9D3ZX Drainage of Right Sublingual Gland, Percutaneous Approach, Diagnostic
0C9D3ZZ Drainage of Right Sublingual Gland, Percutaneous Approach
0C9F00Z Drainage of Left Sublingual Gland with Drainage Device, Open Approach
0C9F0ZX Drainage of Left Sublingual Gland, Open Approach, Diagnostic
0C9F0ZZ Drainage of Left Sublingual Gland, Open Approach
0C9F30Z Drainage of Left Sublingual Gland with Drainage Device, Percutaneous Approach
0C9F3ZX Drainage of Left Sublingual Gland, Percutaneous Approach, Diagnostic
0C9F3ZZ Drainage of Left Sublingual Gland, Percutaneous Approach
0C9G00Z Drainage of Right Submaxillary Gland with Drainage Device, Open Approach
0C9G0ZX Drainage of Right Submaxillary Gland, Open Approach, Diagnostic
0C9G0ZZ Drainage of Right Submaxillary Gland, Open Approach
0C9G30Z Drainage of Right Submaxillary Gland with Drainage Device, Percutaneous Approach
0C9G3ZX Drainage of Right Submaxillary Gland, Percutaneous Approach, Diagnostic
0C9G3ZZ Drainage of Right Submaxillary Gland, Percutaneous Approach
0C9H00Z Drainage of Left Submaxillary Gland with Drainage Device, Open Approach
0C9H0ZX Drainage of Left Submaxillary Gland, Open Approach, Diagnostic
0C9H0ZZ Drainage of Left Submaxillary Gland, Open Approach
0C9H30Z Drainage of Left Submaxillary Gland with Drainage Device, Percutaneous Approach
0C9H3ZX Drainage of Left Submaxillary Gland, Percutaneous Approach, Diagnostic
0C9H3ZZ Drainage of Left Submaxillary Gland, Percutaneous Approach
0C9J00Z Drainage of Minor Salivary Gland with Drainage Device, Open Approach
0C9J0ZX Drainage of Minor Salivary Gland, Ope Approach, Diagnostic
0C9J0ZZ Drainage of Minor Salivary Gland, Ope Approach
0C9J30Z Drainage of Minor Salivary Gland with Drainage Device, Percutaneous Approac
0C9J3ZX Drainage of Minor Salivary Gland, Percutaneous Approach, Diagnostic
0C9J3ZZ Drainage of Minor Salivary Gland, Percutaneous Approach
0C9M00Z Drainage of Pharynx with Drainage Device, Open Approach
0C9M0ZX Drainage of Pharynx, Open Approach, Diagnostic
0C9M0ZZ Drainage of Pharynx, Open Approach
0C9M30Z Drainage of Pharynx with Drainage Device, Percutaneous Approach
0C9M3ZX Drainage of Pharynx, Percutaneous Approach, Diagnostic
0C9M3ZZ Drainage of Pharynx, Percutaneous Approach
0C9M40Z Drainage of Pharynx with Drainage Device, Percutaneous Endoscopic Approach
0C9M4ZX Drainage of Pharynx, Percutaneous Endoscopic Approach, Diagnostic
0C9M4ZZ Drainage of Pharynx, Percutaneous Endoscopic Approach
0C9M70Z Drainage of Pharynx with Drainage Device, Via Natural or Artificial Opening
0C9M7ZX Drainage of Pharynx, Via Natural or Artificial Opening, Diagnostic
0C9M7ZZ Drainage of Pharynx, Via Natural or Artificial Opening
0C9M80Z Drainage of Pharynx with Drainage Device, Via Natural or Artificial Opening Endoscopic
0C9M8ZX Drainage of Pharynx, Via Natural or Artificial Opening Endoscopic, Diagnost
0C9M8ZZ Drainage of Pharynx, Via Natural or Artificial Opening Endoscopic
0C9N00Z Drainage of Uvula with Drainage Device Open Approach
0C9N0ZX Drainage of Uvula, Open Approach, Diagnostic
0C9N0ZZ Drainage of Uvula, Open Approach
0C9N30Z Drainage of Uvula with Drainage Device Percutaneous Approach
0C9N3ZX Drainage of Uvula, Percutaneous Approach, Diagnostic
0C9N3ZZ Drainage of Uvula, Percutaneous Approach
0C9NX0Z Drainage of Uvula with Drainage Device, External Approach
0C9NXZX Drainage of Uvula, External Approach, Diagnostic
0C9NXZZ Drainage of Uvula, External Approach
0C9P00Z Drainage of Tonsils with Drainage Device Open Approach
0C9P0ZX Drainage of Tonsils, Open Approach, Diagnostic
0C9P0ZZ Drainage of Tonsils, Open Approach
0C9P30Z Drainage of Tonsils with Drainage Device Percutaneous Approach
0C9P3ZX Drainage of Tonsils, Percutaneous Approach, Diagnostic
0C9P3ZZ Drainage of Tonsils, Percutaneous Approach
0C9PX0Z Drainage of Tonsils with Drainage Device External Approach
0C9PXZX Drainage of Tonsils, External Approach, Diagnostic

PXZZ Drainage of Tonsils, External Approach
Q00Z Drainage of Adenoids with Drainage Device, Open Approach
Q0ZX Drainage of Adenoids, Open Approach, Diagnostic
Q0ZZ Drainage of Adenoids, Open Approach
Q30Z Drainage of Adenoids with Drainage Device, Percutaneous Approach
Q3ZX Drainage of Adenoids, Percutaneous Approach, Diagnostic
Q3ZZ Drainage of Adenoids, Percutaneous Approach
QX0Z Drainage of Adenoids with Drainage Device, External Approach
9QXZX Drainage of Adenoids, External Approach, Diagnostic
9QXZZ Drainage of Adenoids, External Approach
9R00Z Drainage of Epiglottis with Drainage Device, Open Approach
9R0ZX Drainage of Epiglottis, Open Approach, Diagnostic
9R0ZZ Drainage of Epiglottis, Open Approach
9R30Z Drainage of Epiglottis with Drainage Device, Percutaneous Approach
9R3ZX Drainage of Epiglottis, Percutaneous Approach, Diagnostic
9R3ZZ Drainage of Epiglottis, Percutaneous Approach
9R40Z Drainage of Epiglottis with Drainage Device, Percutaneous Endoscopic Approach
9R4ZX Drainage of Epiglottis, Percutaneous Endoscopic Approach, Diagnostic
9R4ZZ Drainage of Epiglottis, Percutaneous Endoscopic Approach
9R70Z Drainage of Epiglottis with Drainage Device, Via Natural or Artificial Opening
9R7ZX Drainage of Epiglottis, Via Natural or Artificial Opening, Diagnostic
9R7ZZ Drainage of Epiglottis, Via Natural or Artificial Opening
9R80Z Drainage of Epiglottis with Drainage Device, Via Natural or Artificial Opening Endoscopic
C9R8ZX Drainage of Epiglottis, Via Natural or Artificial Opening Endoscopic, Diagnostic
C9R8ZZ Drainage of Epiglottis, Via Natural or Artificial Opening Endoscopic
C9S00Z Drainage of Larynx with Drainage Device, Open Approach
C9S0ZX Drainage of Larynx, Open Approach, Diagnostic
C9S0ZZ Drainage of Larynx, Open Approach
C9S30Z Drainage of Larynx with Drainage Device, Percutaneous Approach
C9S3ZX Drainage of Larynx, Percutaneous Approach, Diagnostic
C9S3ZZ Drainage of Larynx, Percutaneous Approach
C9S40Z Drainage of Larynx with Drainage Device, Percutaneous Endoscopic Approach
C9S4ZX Drainage of Larynx, Percutaneous Endoscopic Approach, Diagnostic
C9S4ZZ Drainage of Larynx, Percutaneous Endoscopic Approach
0C9S70Z Drainage of Larynx with Drainage Device, Via Natural or Artificial Opening
0C9S7ZX Drainage of Larynx, Via Natural or Artificial Opening, Diagnostic
0C9S7ZZ Drainage of Larynx, Via Natural or Artificial Opening
0C9S80Z Drainage of Larynx with Drainage Device, Via Natural or Artificial Opening Endoscopic
0C9S8ZX Drainage of Larynx, Via Natural or Artificial Opening Endoscopic, Diagnostic
0C9S8ZZ Drainage of Larynx, Via Natural or Artificial Opening Endoscopic
0C9T00Z Drainage of Right Vocal Cord with Drainage Device, Open Approach
0C9T0ZX Drainage of Right Vocal Cord, Open Approach, Diagnostic
0C9T0ZZ Drainage of Right Vocal Cord, Open Approach
0C9T30Z Drainage of Right Vocal Cord with Drainage Device, Percutaneous Approach
0C9T3ZX Drainage of Right Vocal Cord, Percutaneous Approach, Diagnostic
0C9T3ZZ Drainage of Right Vocal Cord, Percutaneous Approach
0C9T40Z Drainage of Right Vocal Cord with Drainage Device, Percutaneous Endoscopic Approach
0C9T4ZX Drainage of Right Vocal Cord, Percutaneous Endoscopic Approach, Diagnostic
0C9T4ZZ Drainage of Right Vocal Cord, Percutaneous Endoscopic Approach
0C9T70Z Drainage of Right Vocal Cord with Drainage Device, Via Natural or Artificial Opening
0C9T7ZX Drainage of Right Vocal Cord, Via Natural or Artificial Opening, Diagnostic
0C9T7ZZ Drainage of Right Vocal Cord, Via Natural or Artificial Opening
0C9T80Z Drainage of Right Vocal Cord with Drainage Device, Via Natural or Artificial Opening Endoscopic
0C9T8ZX Drainage of Right Vocal Cord, Via Natural or Artificial Opening Endoscopic, Diagnostic
0C9T8ZZ Drainage of Right Vocal Cord, Via Natural or Artificial Opening Endoscopic
0C9V00Z Drainage of Left Vocal Cord with Drainage Device, Open Approach
0C9V0ZX Drainage of Left Vocal Cord, Open Approach, Diagnostic
0C9V0ZZ Drainage of Left Vocal Cord, Open Approach
0C9V30Z Drainage of Left Vocal Cord with Drainage Device, Percutaneous Approach
0C9V3ZX Drainage of Left Vocal Cord, Percutaneous Approach, Diagnostic
0C9V3ZZ Drainage of Left Vocal Cord, Percutaneous Approach
0C9V40Z Drainage of Left Vocal Cord with Drainage Device, Percutaneous Endoscopic Approach
0C9V4ZX Drainage of Left Vocal Cord, Percutaneous Endoscopic Approach, Diagnostic
0C9V4ZZ Drainage of Left Vocal Cord, Percutaneous Endoscopic Approach
0C9V70Z Drainage of Left Vocal Cord with Drainage Device, Via Natural or Artificial Opening
0C9V7ZX Drainage of Left Vocal Cord, Via Natural or Artificial Opening, Diagnostic
0C9V7ZZ Drainage of Left Vocal Cord, Via Natural or Artificial Opening
0C9V80Z Drainage of Left Vocal Cord with Drainage Device, Via Natural or Artificial Opening Endoscopic
0C9V8ZX Drainage of Left Vocal Cord, Via Natural or Artificial Opening Endoscopic, Diagnostic
0C9V8ZZ Drainage of Left Vocal Cord, Via Natural or Artificial Opening Endoscopic
0C9W000 Drainage of Upper Tooth with Drainage Device, Open Approach, Single
0C9W001 Drainage of Upper Tooth with Drainage Device, Open Approach, Multiple
0C9W002 Drainage of Upper Tooth with Drainage Device, Open Approach, All
0C9W0Z0 Drainage of Upper Tooth, Open Approach, Single
0C9W0Z1 Drainage of Upper Tooth, Open Approach, Multiple
0C9W0Z2 Drainage of Upper Tooth, Open Approach, All
0C9WX00 Drainage of Upper Tooth with Drainage Device, External Approach, Single
0C9WX01 Drainage of Upper Tooth with Drainage Device, External Approach, Multiple
0C9WX02 Drainage of Upper Tooth with Drainage Device, External Approach, All
0C9WXZ0 Drainage of Upper Tooth, External Approach, Single
0C9WXZ1 Drainage of Upper Tooth, External Approach, Multiple
0C9WXZ2 Drainage of Upper Tooth, External Approach, All
0C9X000 Drainage of Lower Tooth with Drainage Device, Open Approach, Single
0C9X001 Drainage of Lower Tooth with Drainage Device, Open Approach, Multiple
0C9X002 Drainage of Lower Tooth with Drainage Device, Open Approach, All
0C9X0Z0 Drainage of Lower Tooth, Open Approach, Single
0C9X0Z1 Drainage of Lower Tooth, Open Approach, Multiple
0C9X0Z2 Drainage of Lower Tooth, Open Approach, All
0C9XX00 Drainage of Lower Tooth with Drainage Device, External Approach, Single
0C9XX01 Drainage of Lower Tooth with Drainage Device, External Approach, Multiple
0C9XX02 Drainage of Lower Tooth with Drainage Device, External Approach, All
0C9XXZ0 Drainage of Lower Tooth, External Approach, Single
0C9XXZ1 Drainage of Lower Tooth, External Approach, Multiple
0C9XXZ2 Drainage of Lower Tooth, External Approach, All

CB – Mouth and Throat, Excision

Review Coding Guidelines B3.4a and B3.4b

Review Coding Guideline B3.8

CB00ZX Excision of Upper Lip, Open Approach, Diagnostic
CB00ZZ Excision of Upper Lip, Open Approach
CB03ZX Excision of Upper Lip, Percutaneous Approach, Diagnostic
0CB03ZZ Excision of Upper Lip, Percutaneous Approach
0CB0XZX Excision of Upper Lip, External Approach, Diagnostic
0CB0XZZ Excision of Upper Lip, External Approach
0CB10ZX Excision of Lower Lip, Open Approach, Diagnostic
0CB10ZZ Excision of Lower Lip, Open Approach
0CB13ZX Excision of Lower Lip, Percutaneous Approach, Diagnostic

0CB13ZZ Excision of Lower Lip, Percutaneous Approach
0CB1XZX Excision of Lower Lip, External Approach, Diagnostic
0CB1XZZ Excision of Lower Lip, External Approach
0CB20ZX Excision of Hard Palate, Open Approach, Diagnostic
0CB20ZZ Excision of Hard Palate, Open Approach
0CB23ZX Excision of Hard Palate, Percutaneous Approach, Diagnostic
0CB23ZZ Excision of Hard Palate, Percutaneous Approach
0CB2XZX Excision of Hard Palate, External Approach, Diagnostic
0CB2XZZ Excision of Hard Palate, External Approach
0CB30ZX Excision of Soft Palate, Open Approach, Diagnostic
0CB30ZZ Excision of Soft Palate, Open Approach
0CB33ZX Excision of Soft Palate, Percutaneous Approach, Diagnostic
0CB33ZZ Excision of Soft Palate, Percutaneous Approach
0CB3XZX Excision of Soft Palate, External Approach, Diagnostic
0CB3XZZ Excision of Soft Palate, External Approach
0CB40ZX Excision of Buccal Mucosa, Open Approach, Diagnostic
0CB40ZZ Excision of Buccal Mucosa, Open Approach
0CB43ZX Excision of Buccal Mucosa, Percutaneous Approach, Diagnostic
0CB43ZZ Excision of Buccal Mucosa, Percutaneous Approach
0CB4XZX Excision of Buccal Mucosa, External Approach, Diagnostic
0CB4XZZ Excision of Buccal Mucosa, External Approach
0CB50ZX Excision of Upper Gingiva, Open Approach, Diagnostic
0CB50ZZ Excision of Upper Gingiva, Open Approach
0CB53ZX Excision of Upper Gingiva, Percutaneous Approach, Diagnostic
0CB53ZZ Excision of Upper Gingiva, Percutaneous Approach
0CB5XZX Excision of Upper Gingiva, External Approach, Diagnostic
0CB5XZZ Excision of Upper Gingiva, External Approach
0CB60ZX Excision of Lower Gingiva, Open Approach, Diagnostic
0CB60ZZ Excision of Lower Gingiva, Open Approach
0CB63ZX Excision of Lower Gingiva, Percutaneous Approach, Diagnostic
0CB63ZZ Excision of Lower Gingiva, Percutaneous Approach
0CB6XZX Excision of Lower Gingiva, External Approach, Diagnostic
0CB6XZZ Excision of Lower Gingiva, External Approach
0CB70ZX Excision of Tongue, Open Approach, Diagnostic
0CB70ZZ Excision of Tongue, Open Approach
0CB73ZX Excision of Tongue, Percutaneous Approach, Diagnostic
0CB73ZZ Excision of Tongue, Percutaneous Approach
0CB7XZX Excision of Tongue, External Approach, Diagnostic
0CB7XZZ Excision of Tongue, External Approach
0CB80ZX Excision of Right Parotid Gland, Open Approach, Diagnostic
0CB80ZZ Excision of Right Parotid Gland, Open Approach
0CB83ZX Excision of Right Parotid Gland, Percutaneous Approach, Diagnostic
0CB83ZZ Excision of Right Parotid Gland, Percutaneous Approach
0CB90ZX Excision of Left Parotid Gland, Open Approach, Diagnostic
0CB90ZZ Excision of Left Parotid Gland, Open Approach
0CB93ZX Excision of Left Parotid Gland, Percutaneous Approach, Diagnostic
0CB93ZZ Excision of Left Parotid Gland, Percutaneous Approach
0CBB0ZX Excision of Right Parotid Duct, Open Approach, Diagnostic
0CBB0ZZ Excision of Right Parotid Duct, Open Approach
0CBB3ZX Excision of Right Parotid Duct, Percutaneous Approach, Diagnostic
0CBB3ZZ Excision of Right Parotid Duct, Percutaneous Approach
0CBC0ZX Excision of Left Parotid Duct, Open Approach, Diagnostic
0CBC0ZZ Excision of Left Parotid Duct, Open Approach
0CBC3ZX Excision of Left Parotid Duct, Percutaneous Approach, Diagnostic
0CBC3ZZ Excision of Left Parotid Duct, Percutaneous Approach
0CBD0ZX Excision of Right Sublingual Gland, Open Approach, Diagnostic
0CBD0ZZ Excision of Right Sublingual Gland, Open Approach
0CBD3ZX Excision of Right Sublingual Gland, Percutaneous Approach, Diagnostic
0CBD3ZZ Excision of Right Sublingual Gland, Percutaneous Approach
0CBF0ZX Excision of Left Sublingual Gland, Open Approach, Diagnostic
0CBF0ZZ Excision of Left Sublingual Gland, Open Approach
0CBF3ZX Excision of Left Sublingual Gland, Percutaneous Approach, Diagnostic
0CBF3ZZ Excision of Left Sublingual Gland, Percutaneous Approach
0CBG0ZX Excision of Right Submaxillary Gland, Open Approach, Diagnostic
0CBG0ZZ Excision of Right Submaxillary Gland, Open Approach
0CBG3ZX Excision of Right Submaxillary Gland, Percutaneous Approach, Diagnostic
0CBG3ZZ Excision of Right Submaxillary Gland, Percutaneous Approach
0CBH0ZX Excision of Left Submaxillary Gland, Open Approach, Diagnostic
0CBH0ZZ Excision of Left Submaxillary Gland, Open Approach
0CBH3ZX Excision of Left Submaxillary Gland, Percutaneous Approach, Diagnostic
0CBH3ZZ Excision of Left Submaxillary Gland, Percutaneous Approach
0CBJ0ZX Excision of Minor Salivary Gland, Open Approach, Diagnostic
0CBJ0ZZ Excision of Minor Salivary Gland, Open Approach
0CBJ3ZX Excision of Minor Salivary Gland, Percutaneous Approach, Diagnostic
0CBJ3ZZ Excision of Minor Salivary Gland, Percutaneous Approach
0CBM0ZX Excision of Pharynx, Open Approach, Diagnostic
0CBM0ZZ Excision of Pharynx, Open Approach
0CBM3ZX Excision of Pharynx, Percutaneous Approach, Diagnostic
0CBM3ZZ Excision of Pharynx, Percutaneous Approach
0CBM4ZX Excision of Pharynx, Percutaneous Endoscopic Approach, Diagnostic
0CBM4ZZ Excision of Pharynx, Percutaneous Endoscopic Approach
0CBM7ZX Excision of Pharynx, Via Natural or Artificial Opening, Diagnostic
0CBM7ZZ Excision of Pharynx, Via Natural or Artificial Opening
0CBM8ZX Excision of Pharynx, Via Natural or Artificial Opening Endoscopic, Diagno
0CBM8ZZ Excision of Pharynx, Via Natural or Artificial Opening Endoscopic
0CBN0ZX Excision of Uvula, Open Approach, Diagnostic
0CBN0ZZ Excision of Uvula, Open Approach
0CBN3ZX Excision of Uvula, Percutaneous Approach, Diagnostic
0CBN3ZZ Excision of Uvula, Percutaneous Appro
0CBNXZX Excision of Uvula, External Approach, Diagnostic
0CBNXZZ Excision of Uvula, External Approach
0CBP0ZX Excision of Tonsils, Open Approach, Diagnostic
0CBP0ZZ Excision of Tonsils, Open Approach
0CBP3ZX Excision of Tonsils, Percutaneous Approach, Diagnostic
0CBP3ZZ Excision of Tonsils, Percutaneous Approach
0CBPXZX Excision of Tonsils, External Approach, Diagnostic
0CBPXZZ Excision of Tonsils, External Approach
0CBQ0ZX Excision of Adenoids, Open Approach, Diagnostic
0CBQ0ZZ Excision of Adenoids, Open Approach
0CBQ3ZX Excision of Adenoids, Percutaneous Approach, Diagnostic
0CBQ3ZZ Excision of Adenoids, Percutaneous Approach
0CBQXZX Excision of Adenoids, External Approac Diagnostic
0CBQXZZ Excision of Adenoids, External Approac
0CBR0ZX Excision of Epiglottis, Open Approach, Diagnostic
0CBR0ZZ Excision of Epiglottis, Open Approach
0CBR3ZX Excision of Epiglottis, Percutaneous Approach, Diagnostic
0CBR3ZZ Excision of Epiglottis, Percutaneous Approach
0CBR4ZX Excision of Epiglottis, Percutaneous Endoscopic Approach, Diagnostic
0CBR4ZZ Excision of Epiglottis, Percutaneous Endoscopic Approach
0CBR7ZX Excision of Epiglottis, Via Natural or Artificial Opening, Diagnostic
0CBR7ZZ Excision of Epiglottis, Via Natural or Artificial Opening
0CBR8ZX Excision of Epiglottis, Via Natural or Artificial Opening Endoscopic, Diagnosti
0CBR8ZZ Excision of Epiglottis, Via Natural or Artificial Opening Endoscopic
0CBS0ZX Excision of Larynx, Open Approach, Diagnostic
0CBS0ZZ Excision of Larynx, Open Approach
0CBS3ZX Excision of Larynx, Percutaneous Approach, Diagnostic
0CBS3ZZ Excision of Larynx, Percutaneous Approach
0CBS4ZX Excision of Larynx, Percutaneous Endoscopic Approach, Diagnostic
0CBS4ZZ Excision of Larynx, Percutaneous Endoscopic Approach
0CBS7ZX Excision of Larynx, Via Natural or Artificial Opening, Diagnostic
0CBS7ZZ Excision of Larynx, Via Natural or Artificial Opening
0CBS8ZX Excision of Larynx, Via Natural or Artificial Opening Endoscopic, Diagnostic
0CBS8ZZ Excision of Larynx, Via Natural or Artificial Opening Endoscopic

BT0ZX Excision of Right Vocal Cord, Open Approach, Diagnostic
BT0ZZ Excision of Right Vocal Cord, Open Approach
BT3ZX Excision of Right Vocal Cord, Percutaneous Approach, Diagnostic
BT3ZZ Excision of Right Vocal Cord, Percutaneous Approach
BT4ZX Excision of Right Vocal Cord, Percutaneous Endoscopic Approach, Diagnostic
BT4ZZ Excision of Right Vocal Cord, Percutaneous Endoscopic Approach
BT7ZX Excision of Right Vocal Cord, Via Natural or Artificial Opening, Diagnostic
BT7ZZ Excision of Right Vocal Cord, Via Natural or Artificial Opening
BT8ZX Excision of Right Vocal Cord, Via Natural or Artificial Opening Endoscopic, Diagnostic
BT8ZZ Excision of Right Vocal Cord, Via Natural or Artificial Opening Endoscopic

0CBV0ZX Excision of Left Vocal Cord, Open Approach, Diagnostic
0CBV0ZZ Excision of Left Vocal Cord, Open Approach
0CBV3ZX Excision of Left Vocal Cord, Percutaneous Approach, Diagnostic
0CBV3ZZ Excision of Left Vocal Cord, Percutaneous Approach
0CBV4ZX Excision of Left Vocal Cord, Percutaneous Endoscopic Approach, Diagnostic
0CBV4ZZ Excision of Left Vocal Cord, Percutaneous Endoscopic Approach
0CBV7ZX Excision of Left Vocal Cord, Via Natural or Artificial Opening, Diagnostic
0CBV7ZZ Excision of Left Vocal Cord, Via Natural or Artificial Opening
0CBV8ZX Excision of Left Vocal Cord, Via Natural or Artificial Opening Endoscopic, Diagnostic
0CBV8ZZ Excision of Left Vocal Cord, Via Natural or Artificial Opening Endoscopic
0CBW0Z0 Excision of Upper Tooth, Open Approach, Single
0CBW0Z1 Excision of Upper Tooth, Open Approach, Multiple
0CBW0Z2 Excision of Upper Tooth, Open Approach, All
0CBWXZ0 Excision of Upper Tooth, External Approach, Single
0CBWXZ1 Excision of Upper Tooth, External Approach, Multiple
0CBWXZ2 Excision of Upper Tooth, External Approach, All
0CBX0Z0 Excision of Lower Tooth, Open Approach, Single
0CBX0Z1 Excision of Lower Tooth, Open Approach, Multiple
0CBX0Z2 Excision of Lower Tooth, Open Approach, All
0CBXXZ0 Excision of Lower Tooth, External Approach, Single
0CBXXZ1 Excision of Lower Tooth, External Approach, Multiple
0CBXXZ2 Excision of Lower Tooth, External Approach, All

CC – Mouth and Throat, Extirpation

CC00ZZ Extirpation of Matter from Upper Lip, Open Approach
CC03ZZ Extirpation of Matter from Upper Lip, Percutaneous Approach
CC0XZZ Extirpation of Matter from Upper Lip, External Approach
CC10ZZ Extirpation of Matter from Lower Lip, Open Approach
CC13ZZ Extirpation of Matter from Lower Lip, Percutaneous Approach
CC1XZZ Extirpation of Matter from Lower Lip, External Approach
CC20ZZ Extirpation of Matter from Hard Palate, Open Approach
CC23ZZ Extirpation of Matter from Hard Palate, Percutaneous Approach
CC2XZZ Extirpation of Matter from Hard Palate, External Approach
CC30ZZ Extirpation of Matter from Soft Palate, Open Approach
CC33ZZ Extirpation of Matter from Soft Palate, Percutaneous Approach
CC3XZZ Extirpation of Matter from Soft Palate, External Approach
CC40ZZ Extirpation of Matter from Buccal Mucosa, Open Approach
CC43ZZ Extirpation of Matter from Buccal Mucosa, Percutaneous Approach
CC4XZZ Extirpation of Matter from Buccal Mucosa, External Approach
CC50ZZ Extirpation of Matter from Upper Gingiva, Open Approach
CC53ZZ Extirpation of Matter from Upper Gingiva, Percutaneous Approach
CC5XZZ Extirpation of Matter from Upper Gingiva, External Approach
CC60ZZ Extirpation of Matter from Lower Gingiva, Open Approach
CC63ZZ Extirpation of Matter from Lower Gingiva, Percutaneous Approach
0CC6XZZ Extirpation of Matter from Lower Gingiva, External Approach
0CC70ZZ Extirpation of Matter from Tongue, Open Approach
0CC73ZZ Extirpation of Matter from Tongue, Percutaneous Approach
0CC7XZZ Extirpation of Matter from Tongue, External Approach
0CC80ZZ Extirpation of Matter from Right Parotid Gland, Open Approach

0CC83ZZ Extirpation of Matter from Right Parotid Gland, Percutaneous Approach
0CC90ZZ Extirpation of Matter from Left Parotid Gland, Open Approach
0CC93ZZ Extirpation of Matter from Left Parotid Gland, Percutaneous Approach
0CCB0ZZ Extirpation of Matter from Right Parotid Duct, Open Approach
0CCB3ZZ Extirpation of Matter from Right Parotid Duct, Percutaneous Approach
0CCC0ZZ Extirpation of Matter from Left Parotid Duct, Open Approach
0CCC3ZZ Extirpation of Matter from Left Parotid Duct, Percutaneous Approach
0CCD0ZZ Extirpation of Matter from Right Sublingual Gland, Open Approach
0CCD3ZZ Extirpation of Matter from Right Sublingual Gland, Percutaneous Approach
0CCF0ZZ Extirpation of Matter from Left Sublingual Gland, Open Approach
0CCF3ZZ Extirpation of Matter from Left Sublingual Gland, Percutaneous Approach
0CCG0ZZ Extirpation of Matter from Right Submaxillary Gland, Open Approach
0CCG3ZZ Extirpation of Matter from Right Submaxillary Gland, Percutaneous Approach
0CCH0ZZ Extirpation of Matter from Left Submaxillary Gland, Open Approach
0CCH3ZZ Extirpation of Matter from Left Submaxillary Gland, Percutaneous Approach
0CCJ0ZZ Extirpation of Matter from Minor Salivary Gland, Open Approach
0CCJ3ZZ Extirpation of Matter from Minor Salivary Gland, Percutaneous Approach
0CCM0ZZ Extirpation of Matter from Pharynx, Open Approach
0CCM3ZZ Extirpation of Matter from Pharynx, Percutaneous Approach
0CCM4ZZ Extirpation of Matter from Pharynx, Percutaneous Endoscopic Approach
0CCM7ZZ Extirpation of Matter from Pharynx, Via Natural or Artificial Opening
0CCM8ZZ Extirpation of Matter from Pharynx, Via Natural or Artificial Opening Endoscopic
0CCN0ZZ Extirpation of Matter from Uvula, Open Approach
0CCN3ZZ Extirpation of Matter from Uvula, Percutaneous Approach
0CCNXZZ Extirpation of Matter from Uvula, External Approach
0CCP0ZZ Extirpation of Matter from Tonsils, Open Approach
0CCP3ZZ Extirpation of Matter from Tonsils, Percutaneous Approach
0CCPXZZ Extirpation of Matter from Tonsils, External Approach
0CCQ0ZZ Extirpation of Matter from Adenoids, Open Approach
0CCQ3ZZ Extirpation of Matter from Adenoids, Percutaneous Approach
0CCQXZZ Extirpation of Matter from Adenoids, External Approach
0CCR0ZZ Extirpation of Matter from Epiglottis, Open Approach
0CCR3ZZ Extirpation of Matter from Epiglottis, Percutaneous Approach
0CCR4ZZ Extirpation of Matter from Epiglottis, Percutaneous Endoscopic Approach
0CCR7ZZ Extirpation of Matter from Epiglottis, Via Natural or Artificial Opening
0CCR8ZZ Extirpation of Matter from Epiglottis, Via Natural or Artificial Opening Endoscopic
0CCS0ZZ Extirpation of Matter from Larynx, Open Approach
0CCS3ZZ Extirpation of Matter from Larynx, Percutaneous Approach
0CCS4ZZ Extirpation of Matter from Larynx, Percutaneous Endoscopic Approach
0CCS7ZZ Extirpation of Matter from Larynx, Via Natural or Artificial Opening
0CCS8ZZ Extirpation of Matter from Larynx, Via Natural or Artificial Opening Endoscopic
0CCT0ZZ Extirpation of Matter from Right Vocal Cord, Open Approach
0CCT3ZZ Extirpation of Matter from Right Vocal Cord, Percutaneous Approach
0CCT4ZZ Extirpation of Matter from Right Vocal Cord, Percutaneous Endoscopic Approach
0CCT7ZZ Extirpation of Matter from Right Vocal Cord, Via Natural or Artificial Opening
0CCT8ZZ Extirpation of Matter from Right Vocal Cord, Via Natural or Artificial Opening Endoscopic
0CCV0ZZ Extirpation of Matter from Left Vocal Cord, Open Approach
0CCV3ZZ Extirpation of Matter from Left Vocal Cord, Percutaneous Approach

0CCV4ZZ Extirpation of Matter from Left Vocal Cord, Percutaneous Endoscopic Approach
0CCV7ZZ Extirpation of Matter from Left Vocal Cord, Via Natural or Artificial Opening
0CCV8ZZ Extirpation of Matter from Left Vocal Cord, Via Natural or Artificial Opening Endoscopic
0CCW0Z0 Extirpation of Matter from Upper Tooth, Single, Open Approach
0CCW0Z1 Extirpation of Matter from Upper Tooth, Multiple, Open Approach
0CCW0Z2 Extirpation of Matter from Upper Tooth, All, Open Approach
0CCWXZ0 Extirpation of Matter from Upper Tooth, Single, External Approach
0CCWXZ1 Extirpation of Matter from Upper Tooth, Multiple, External Approach
0CCWXZ2 Extirpation of Matter from Upper Tooth, All, External Approach
0CCX0Z0 Extirpation of Matter from Lower Tooth, Single, Open Approach
0CCX0Z1 Extirpation of Matter from Lower Tooth, Multiple, Open Approach
0CCX0Z2 Extirpation of Matter from Lower Too All, Open Approach
0CCXXZ0 Extirpation of Matter from Lower Too Single, External Approach
0CCXXZ1 Extirpation of Matter from Lower Too Multiple, External Approach
0CCXXZ2 Extirpation of Matter from Lower Too All, External Approach

0CD – Mouth and Throat, Extraction

0CDT0ZZ Extraction of Right Vocal Cord, Open Approach
0CDT3ZZ Extraction of Right Vocal Cord, Percutaneous Approach
0CDT4ZZ Extraction of Right Vocal Cord, Percutaneous Endoscopic Approach
0CDT7ZZ Extraction of Right Vocal Cord, Via Natural or Artificial Opening
0CDT8ZZ Extraction of Right Vocal Cord, Via Natural or Artificial Opening Endoscopic
0CDV0ZZ Extraction of Left Vocal Cord, Open Approach
0CDV3ZZ Extraction of Left Vocal Cord, Percutaneous Approach
0CDV4ZZ Extraction of Left Vocal Cord, Percutaneous Endoscopic Approach
0CDV7ZZ Extraction of Left Vocal Cord, Via Natural or Artificial Opening
0CDV8ZZ Extraction of Left Vocal Cord, Via Natural or Artificial Opening Endoscopic
0CDWXZ0 Extraction of Upper Tooth, Single, External Approach
0CDWXZ1 Extraction of Upper Tooth, Multiple, External Approach
0CDWXZ2 Extraction of Upper Tooth, All, Extern Approach
0CDXXZ0 Extraction of Lower Tooth, Single, External Approach
0CDXXZ1 Extraction of Lower Tooth, Multiple, External Approach
0CDXXZ2 Extraction of Lower Tooth, All, Extern Approach

0CF – Mouth and Throat, Fragmentation

0CFB0ZZ Fragmentation in Right Parotid Duct, Open Approach
0CFB3ZZ Fragmentation in Right Parotid Duct, Percutaneous Approach
0CFB7ZZ Fragmentation in Right Parotid Duct, Via Natural or Artificial Opening
▲ **0CFBXZZ** Fragmentation in Right Parotid Duct, External Approach
0CFC0ZZ Fragmentation in Left Parotid Duct, Open Approach
0CFC3ZZ Fragmentation in Left Parotid Duct, Percutaneous Approach
0CFC7ZZ Fragmentation in Left Parotid Duct, Via Natural or Artificial Opening
▲ **0CFCXZZ** Fragmentation in Left Parotid Duct, External Approach

0CH – Mouth and Throat, Insertion

0CH701Z Insertion of Radioactive Element into Tongue, Open Approach
0CH731Z Insertion of Radioactive Element into Tongue, Percutaneous Approach
0CH7X1Z Insertion of Radioactive Element into Tongue, External Approach
0CHY7BZ Insertion of Airway into Mouth and Throat, Via Natural or Artificial Opening
0CHY8BZ Insertion of Airway into Mouth and Throat, Via Natural or Artificial Opening Endoscopic

0CJ – Mouth and Throat, Inspection

Review Coding Guidelines B3.11a, B3.11b and B3.11c

0CJA0ZZ Inspection of Salivary Gland, Open Approach
0CJA3ZZ Inspection of Salivary Gland, Percutaneous Approach
0CJAXZZ Inspection of Salivary Gland, External Approach
0CJS0ZZ Inspection of Larynx, Open Approach
0CJS3ZZ Inspection of Larynx, Percutaneous Approach
0CJS4ZZ Inspection of Larynx, Percutaneous Endoscopic Approach
0CJS7ZZ Inspection of Larynx, Via Natural or Artificial Opening
0CJS8ZZ Inspection of Larynx, Via Natural or Artificial Opening Endoscopic
0CJSXZZ Inspection of Larynx, External Approach
0CJY0ZZ Inspection of Mouth and Throat, Open Approach
0CJY3ZZ Inspection of Mouth and Throat, Percutaneous Approach
0CJY4ZZ Inspection of Mouth and Throat, Percutaneous Endoscopic Approach
0CJY7ZZ Inspection of Mouth and Throat, Via Natural or Artificial Opening
0CJY8ZZ Inspection of Mouth and Throat, Via Natural or Artificial Opening Endoscopic
0CJYXZZ Inspection of Mouth and Throat, External Approach

0CL – Mouth and Throat, Occlusion

0CLB0CZ Occlusion of Right Parotid Duct with Extraluminal Device, Open Approach
0CLB0DZ Occlusion of Right Parotid Duct with Intraluminal Device, Open Approach
0CLB0ZZ Occlusion of Right Parotid Duct, Open Approach
0CLB3CZ Occlusion of Right Parotid Duct with Extraluminal Device, Percutaneous Approach
0CLB3DZ Occlusion of Right Parotid Duct with Intraluminal Device, Percutaneous Approach
0CLB3ZZ Occlusion of Right Parotid Duct, Percutaneous Approach
0CLB4CZ Occlusion of Right Parotid Duct with Extraluminal Device, Percutaneous Endoscopic Approach
0CLB4DZ Occlusion of Right Parotid Duct with Intraluminal Device, Percutaneous Endoscopic Approach
0CLB4ZZ Occlusion of Right Parotid Duct, Percutaneous Endoscopic Approach
0CLB7DZ Occlusion of Right Parotid Duct with Intraluminal Device, Via Natural or Artificial Opening
0CLB7ZZ Occlusion of Right Parotid Duct, Via Natural or Artificial Opening
0CLB8DZ Occlusion of Right Parotid Duct with Intraluminal Device, Via Natural or Artificial Opening Endoscopic
0CLB8ZZ Occlusion of Right Parotid Duct, Via Natural or Artificial Opening Endoscopic
0CLC0CZ Occlusion of Left Parotid Duct with Extraluminal Device, Open Approach
0CLC0DZ Occlusion of Left Parotid Duct with Intraluminal Device, Open Approach
0CLC0ZZ Occlusion of Left Parotid Duct, Open Approach
0CLC3CZ Occlusion of Left Parotid Duct with Extraluminal Device, Percutaneous Approach
0CLC3DZ Occlusion of Left Parotid Duct with Intraluminal Device, Percutaneous Approach

.C3ZZ	Occlusion of Left Parotid Duct, Percutaneous Approach
.C4CZ	Occlusion of Left Parotid Duct with Extraluminal Device, Percutaneous Endoscopic Approach
.C4DZ	Occlusion of Left Parotid Duct with Intraluminal Device, Percutaneous Endoscopic Approach
0CLC4ZZ	Occlusion of Left Parotid Duct, Percutaneous Endoscopic Approach
0CLC7DZ	Occlusion of Left Parotid Duct with Intraluminal Device, Via Natural or Artificial Opening
0CLC7ZZ	Occlusion of Left Parotid Duct, Via Natural or Artificial Opening
0CLC8DZ	Occlusion of Left Parotid Duct with Intraluminal Device, Via Natural or Artificial Opening Endoscopic
0CLC8ZZ	Occlusion of Left Parotid Duct, Via Natural or Artificial Opening Endoscopic

:M – Mouth and Throat, Reattachment

M00ZZ	Reattachment of Upper Lip, Open Approach
M10ZZ	Reattachment of Lower Lip, Open Approach
M30ZZ	Reattachment of Soft Palate, Open Approach
M70ZZ	Reattachment of Tongue, Open Approach
MN0ZZ	Reattachment of Uvula, Open Approach
MW0Z0	Reattachment of Upper Tooth, Single, Open Approach
0CMW0Z1	Reattachment of Upper Tooth, Multiple, Open Approach
0CMW0Z2	Reattachment of Upper Tooth, All, Open Approach
0CMWXZ0	Reattachment of Upper Tooth, Single, External Approach
0CMWXZ1	Reattachment of Upper Tooth, Multiple, External Approach
0CMWXZ2	Reattachment of Upper Tooth, All, External Approach
0CMX0Z0	Reattachment of Lower Tooth, Single, Open Approach
0CMX0Z1	Reattachment of Lower Tooth, Multiple, Open Approach
0CMX0Z2	Reattachment of Lower Tooth, All, Open Approach
0CMXXZ0	Reattachment of Lower Tooth, Single, External Approach
0CMXXZ1	Reattachment of Lower Tooth, Multiple, External Approach
0CMXXZ2	Reattachment of Lower Tooth, All, External Approach

:N – Mouth and Throat, Release

ɛview Coding Guidelines B3.13 and B3.14

:N00ZZ	Release Upper Lip, Open Approach
:N03ZZ	Release Upper Lip, Percutaneous Approach
:N0XZZ	Release Upper Lip, External Approach
:N10ZZ	Release Lower Lip, Open Approach
:N13ZZ	Release Lower Lip, Percutaneous Approach
:N1XZZ	Release Lower Lip, External Approach
:N20ZZ	Release Hard Palate, Open Approach
:N23ZZ	Release Hard Palate, Percutaneous Approach
:N2XZZ	Release Hard Palate, External Approach
:N30ZZ	Release Soft Palate, Open Approach
:N33ZZ	Release Soft Palate, Percutaneous Approach
:N3XZZ	Release Soft Palate, External Approach
CN40ZZ	Release Buccal Mucosa, Open Approach
CN43ZZ	Release Buccal Mucosa, Percutaneous Approach
CN4XZZ	Release Buccal Mucosa, External Approach
CN50ZZ	Release Upper Gingiva, Open Approach
CN53ZZ	Release Upper Gingiva, Percutaneous Approach
CN5XZZ	Release Upper Gingiva, External Approach
CN60ZZ	Release Lower Gingiva, Open Approach
CN63ZZ	Release Lower Gingiva, Percutaneous Approach
CN6XZZ	Release Lower Gingiva, External Approach
CN70ZZ	Release Tongue, Open Approach
CN73ZZ	Release Tongue, Percutaneous Approach
CN7XZZ	Release Tongue, External Approach
CN80ZZ	Release Right Parotid Gland, Open Approach
CN83ZZ	Release Right Parotid Gland, Percutaneous Approach
CN90ZZ	Release Left Parotid Gland, Open Approach
CN93ZZ	Release Left Parotid Gland, Percutaneous Approach
CNB0ZZ	Release Right Parotid Duct, Open Approach
CNB3ZZ	Release Right Parotid Duct, Percutaneous Approach
0CNC0ZZ	Release Left Parotid Duct, Open Approach
0CNC3ZZ	Release Left Parotid Duct, Percutaneous Approach
0CND0ZZ	Release Right Sublingual Gland, Open Approach
0CND3ZZ	Release Right Sublingual Gland, Percutaneous Approach
0CNF0ZZ	Release Left Sublingual Gland, Open Approach
0CNF3ZZ	Release Left Sublingual Gland, Percutaneous Approach
0CNG0ZZ	Release Right Submaxillary Gland, Open Approach
0CNG3ZZ	Release Right Submaxillary Gland, Percutaneous Approach
0CNH0ZZ	Release Left Submaxillary Gland, Open Approach
0CNH3ZZ	Release Left Submaxillary Gland, Percutaneous Approach
0CNJ0ZZ	Release Minor Salivary Gland, Open Approach
0CNJ3ZZ	Release Minor Salivary Gland, Percutaneous Approach
0CNM0ZZ	Release Pharynx, Open Approach
0CNM3ZZ	Release Pharynx, Percutaneous Approach
0CNM4ZZ	Release Pharynx, Percutaneous Endoscopic Approach
0CNM7ZZ	Release Pharynx, Via Natural or Artificial Opening
0CNM8ZZ	Release Pharynx, Via Natural or Artificial Opening Endoscopic
0CNN0ZZ	Release Uvula, Open Approach
0CNN3ZZ	Release Uvula, Percutaneous Approach
0CNNXZZ	Release Uvula, External Approach
0CNP0ZZ	Release Tonsils, Open Approach
0CNP3ZZ	Release Tonsils, Percutaneous Approach
0CNPXZZ	Release Tonsils, External Approach
0CNQ0ZZ	Release Adenoids, Open Approach
0CNQ3ZZ	Release Adenoids, Percutaneous Approach
0CNQXZZ	Release Adenoids, External Approach
0CNR0ZZ	Release Epiglottis, Open Approach
0CNR3ZZ	Release Epiglottis, Percutaneous Approach
0CNR4ZZ	Release Epiglottis, Percutaneous Endoscopic Approach
0CNR7ZZ	Release Epiglottis, Via Natural or Artificial Opening
0CNR8ZZ	Release Epiglottis, Via Natural or Artificial Opening Endoscopic
0CNS0ZZ	Release Larynx, Open Approach
0CNS3ZZ	Release Larynx, Percutaneous Approach
0CNS4ZZ	Release Larynx, Percutaneous Endoscopic Approach
0CNS7ZZ	Release Larynx, Via Natural or Artificial Opening
0CNS8ZZ	Release Larynx, Via Natural or Artificial Opening Endoscopic
0CNT0ZZ	Release Right Vocal Cord, Open Approach
0CNT3ZZ	Release Right Vocal Cord, Percutaneous Approach
0CNT4ZZ	Release Right Vocal Cord, Percutaneous Endoscopic Approach
0CNT7ZZ	Release Right Vocal Cord, Via Natural or Artificial Opening
0CNT8ZZ	Release Right Vocal Cord, Via Natural or Artificial Opening Endoscopic
0CNV0ZZ	Release Left Vocal Cord, Open Approach
0CNV3ZZ	Release Left Vocal Cord, Percutaneous Approach
0CNV4ZZ	Release Left Vocal Cord, Percutaneous Endoscopic Approach
0CNV7ZZ	Release Left Vocal Cord, Via Natural or Artificial Opening
0CNV8ZZ	Release Left Vocal Cord, Via Natural or Artificial Opening Endoscopic
0CNW0Z0	Release Upper Tooth, Single, Open Approach
0CNW0Z1	Release Upper Tooth, Multiple, Open Approach
0CNW0Z2	Release Upper Tooth, All, Open Approach
0CNWXZ0	Release Upper Tooth, Single, External Approach
0CNWXZ1	Release Upper Tooth, Multiple, External Approach
0CNWXZ2	Release Upper Tooth, All, External Approach

0CNX0Z0 Release Lower Tooth, Single, Open Approach
0CNX0Z1 Release Lower Tooth, Multiple, Open Approach
0CNX0Z2 Release Lower Tooth, All, Open Approach
0CNXXZ0 Release Lower Tooth, Single, External Approach
0CNXXZ1 Release Lower Tooth, Multiple, Exter Approach
0CNXXZ2 Release Lower Tooth, All, External Approach

0CP – Mouth and Throat, Removal

Review Coding Guideline B6.1c

0CPA00Z Removal of Drainage Device from Salivary Gland, Open Approach
0CPA0CZ Removal of Extraluminal Device from Salivary Gland, Open Approach
0CPA30Z Removal of Drainage Device from Salivary Gland, Percutaneous Approach
0CPA3CZ Removal of Extraluminal Device from Salivary Gland, Percutaneous Approach
0CPS00Z Removal of Drainage Device from Larynx, Open Approach
0CPS07Z Removal of Autologous Tissue Substitute from Larynx, Open Approach
0CPS0DZ Removal of Intraluminal Device from Larynx, Open Approach
0CPS0JZ Removal of Synthetic Substitute from Larynx, Open Approach
0CPS0KZ Removal of Nonautologous Tissue Substitute from Larynx, Open Approach
0CPS30Z Removal of Drainage Device from Larynx, Percutaneous Approach
0CPS37Z Removal of Autologous Tissue Substitute from Larynx, Percutaneous Approach
0CPS3DZ Removal of Intraluminal Device from Larynx, Percutaneous Approach
0CPS3JZ Removal of Synthetic Substitute from Larynx, Percutaneous Approach
0CPS3KZ Removal of Nonautologous Tissue Substitute from Larynx, Percutaneous Approach
0CPS70Z Removal of Drainage Device from Larynx, Via Natural or Artificial Opening
0CPS77Z Removal of Autologous Tissue Substitute from Larynx, Via Natural or Artificial Opening
0CPS7DZ Removal of Intraluminal Device from Larynx, Via Natural or Artificial Opening
0CPS7JZ Removal of Synthetic Substitute from Larynx, Via Natural or Artificial Opening
0CPS7KZ Removal of Nonautologous Tissue Substitute from Larynx, Via Natural or Artificial Opening
0CPS80Z Removal of Drainage Device from Larynx, Via Natural or Artificial Opening Endoscopic
0CPS87Z Removal of Autologous Tissue Substitute from Larynx, Via Natural or Artificial Opening Endoscopic
0CPS8DZ Removal of Intraluminal Device from Larynx, Via Natural or Artificial Opening Endoscopic
0CPS8JZ Removal of Synthetic Substitute from Larynx, Via Natural or Artificial Opening Endoscopic
0CPS8KZ Removal of Nonautologous Tissue Substitute from Larynx, Via Natural or Artificial Opening Endoscopic
0CPSX0Z Removal of Drainage Device from Larynx, External Approach
0CPSX7Z Removal of Autologous Tissue Substitute from Larynx, External Approach
0CPSXDZ Removal of Intraluminal Device from Larynx, External Approach
0CPSXJZ Removal of Synthetic Substitute from Larynx, External Approach
0CPSXKZ Removal of Nonautologous Tissue Substitute from Larynx, External Approach
0CPY00Z Removal of Drainage Device from Mouth and Throat, Open Approach
0CPY01Z Removal of Radioactive Element from Mouth and Throat, Open Approach
0CPY07Z Removal of Autologous Tissue Substitute from Mouth and Throat, Open Approach
0CPY0DZ Removal of Intraluminal Device from Mouth and Throat, Open Approach
0CPY0JZ Removal of Synthetic Substitute from Mouth and Throat, Open Approach
0CPY0KZ Removal of Nonautologous Tissue Substitute from Mouth and Throat, Open Approach
0CPY30Z Removal of Drainage Device from Mouth and Throat, Percutaneous Approach
0CPY31Z Removal of Radioactive Element from Mouth and Throat, Percutaneous Approach
0CPY37Z Removal of Autologous Tissue Substitute from Mouth and Throat, Percutaneous Approach
0CPY3DZ Removal of Intraluminal Device from Mouth and Throat, Percutaneous Approach
0CPY3JZ Removal of Synthetic Substitute from Mouth and Throat, Percutaneous Approach
0CPY3KZ Removal of Nonautologous Tissue Substitute from Mouth and Throat, Percutaneous Approach
0CPY70Z Removal of Drainage Device from Mouth and Throat, Via Natural or Artificial Opening
0CPY71Z Removal of Radioactive Element from Mouth and Throat, Via Natural or Artificial Opening
0CPY77Z Removal of Autologous Tissue Substitu from Mouth and Throat, Via Natural or Artificial Opening
0CPY7DZ Removal of Intraluminal Device from Mouth and Throat, Via Natural or Artificial Opening
0CPY7JZ Removal of Synthetic Substitute from Mouth and Throat, Via Natural or Artificial Opening
0CPY7KZ Removal of Nonautologous Tissue Substitute from Mouth and Throat, Via Natural or Artificial Opening
0CPY80Z Removal of Drainage Device from Mou and Throat, Via Natural or Artificial Opening Endoscopic
0CPY81Z Removal of Radioactive Element from Mouth and Throat, Via Natural or Artificial Opening Endoscopic
0CPY87Z Removal of Autologous Tissue Substitu from Mouth and Throat, Via Natural or Artificial Opening Endoscopic
0CPY8DZ Removal of Intraluminal Device from Mouth and Throat, Via Natural or Artificial Opening Endoscopic
0CPY8JZ Removal of Synthetic Substitute from Mouth and Throat, Via Natural or Artificial Opening Endoscopic
0CPY8KZ Removal of Nonautologous Tissue Substitute from Mouth and Throat, Via Natural or Artificial Opening Endoscopic
0CPYX0Z Removal of Drainage Device from Mou and Throat, External Approach
0CPYX1Z Removal of Radioactive Element from Mouth and Throat, External Approach
0CPYX7Z Removal of Autologous Tissue Substitut from Mouth and Throat, External Approach
0CPYXDZ Removal of Intraluminal Device from Mouth and Throat, External Approach
0CPYXJZ Removal of Synthetic Substitute from Mouth and Throat, External Approach
0CPYXKZ Removal of Nonautologous Tissue Substitute from Mouth and Throat, External Approach

0CQ – Mouth and Throat, Repair

0CQ00ZZ Repair Upper Lip, Open Approach
0CQ03ZZ Repair Upper Lip, Percutaneous Approach
0CQ0XZZ Repair Upper Lip, External Approach
0CQ10ZZ Repair Lower Lip, Open Approach
0CQ13ZZ Repair Lower Lip, Percutaneous Approach
0CQ1XZZ Repair Lower Lip, External Approach
0CQ20ZZ Repair Hard Palate, Open Approach
0CQ23ZZ Repair Hard Palate, Percutaneous Approach
0CQ2XZZ Repair Hard Palate, External Approach
0CQ30ZZ Repair Soft Palate, Open Approach
0CQ33ZZ Repair Soft Palate, Percutaneous Approach
0CQ3XZZ Repair Soft Palate, External Approach
0CQ40ZZ Repair Buccal Mucosa, Open Approach
0CQ43ZZ Repair Buccal Mucosa, Percutaneous Approach
0CQ4XZZ Repair Buccal Mucosa, External Approach
0CQ50ZZ Repair Upper Gingiva, Open Approach
0CQ53ZZ Repair Upper Gingiva, Percutaneous Approach
0CQ5XZZ Repair Upper Gingiva, External Approach
0CQ60ZZ Repair Lower Gingiva, Open Approach
0CQ63ZZ Repair Lower Gingiva, Percutaneous Approach
0CQ6XZZ Repair Lower Gingiva, External Approach
0CQ70ZZ Repair Tongue, Open Approach
0CQ73ZZ Repair Tongue, Percutaneous Approach
0CQ7XZZ Repair Tongue, External Approach
0CQ80ZZ Repair Right Parotid Gland, Open Approach
0CQ83ZZ Repair Right Parotid Gland, Percutaneous Approach
0CQ90ZZ Repair Left Parotid Gland, Open Approach
0CQ93ZZ Repair Left Parotid Gland, Percutaneous Approach
0CQB0ZZ Repair Right Parotid Duct, Open Approach

QB3ZZ Repair Right Parotid Duct, Percutaneous Approach
QC0ZZ Repair Left Parotid Duct, Open Approach
QC3ZZ Repair Left Parotid Duct, Percutaneous Approach
QD0ZZ Repair Right Sublingual Gland, Open Approach
QD3ZZ Repair Right Sublingual Gland, Percutaneous Approach
QF0ZZ Repair Left Sublingual Gland, Open Approach
QF3ZZ Repair Left Sublingual Gland, Percutaneous Approach
QG0ZZ Repair Right Submaxillary Gland, Open Approach
QG3ZZ Repair Right Submaxillary Gland, Percutaneous Approach
QH0ZZ Repair Left Submaxillary Gland, Open Approach
QH3ZZ Repair Left Submaxillary Gland, Percutaneous Approach
QJ0ZZ Repair Minor Salivary Gland, Open Approach
QJ3ZZ Repair Minor Salivary Gland, Percutaneous Approach
CQM0ZZ Repair Pharynx, Open Approach
CQM3ZZ Repair Pharynx, Percutaneous Approach
CQM4ZZ Repair Pharynx, Percutaneous Endoscopic Approach
CQM7ZZ Repair Pharynx, Via Natural or Artificial Opening
CQM8ZZ Repair Pharynx, Via Natural or Artificial Opening Endoscopic
CQN0ZZ Repair Uvula, Open Approach
0CQN3ZZ Repair Uvula, Percutaneous Approach
0CQNXZZ Repair Uvula, External Approach
0CQP0ZZ Repair Tonsils, Open Approach
0CQP3ZZ Repair Tonsils, Percutaneous Approach
0CQPXZZ Repair Tonsils, External Approach
0CQQ0ZZ Repair Adenoids, Open Approach
0CQQ3ZZ Repair Adenoids, Percutaneous Approach
0CQQXZZ Repair Adenoids, External Approach
0CQR0ZZ Repair Epiglottis, Open Approach
0CQR3ZZ Repair Epiglottis, Percutaneous Approach
0CQR4ZZ Repair Epiglottis, Percutaneous Endoscopic Approach
0CQR7ZZ Repair Epiglottis, Via Natural or Artificial Opening
0CQR8ZZ Repair Epiglottis, Via Natural or Artificial Opening Endoscopic
0CQS0ZZ Repair Larynx, Open Approach
0CQS3ZZ Repair Larynx, Percutaneous Approach
0CQS4ZZ Repair Larynx, Percutaneous Endoscopic Approach
0CQS7ZZ Repair Larynx, Via Natural or Artificial Opening
0CQS8ZZ Repair Larynx, Via Natural or Artificial Opening Endoscopic
0CQT0ZZ Repair Right Vocal Cord, Open Approach
0CQT3ZZ Repair Right Vocal Cord, Percutaneous Approach
0CQT4ZZ Repair Right Vocal Cord, Percutaneous Endoscopic Approach
0CQT7ZZ Repair Right Vocal Cord, Via Natural or Artificial Opening
0CQT8ZZ Repair Right Vocal Cord, Via Natural or Artificial Opening Endoscopic
0CQV0ZZ Repair Left Vocal Cord, Open Approach
0CQV3ZZ Repair Left Vocal Cord, Percutaneous Approach
0CQV4ZZ Repair Left Vocal Cord, Percutaneous Endoscopic Approach
0CQV7ZZ Repair Left Vocal Cord, Via Natural or Artificial Opening
0CQV8ZZ Repair Left Vocal Cord, Via Natural or Artificial Opening Endoscopic
0CQW0Z0 Repair of Upper Tooth, Single, Open Approach
0CQW0Z1 Repair of Upper Tooth, Multiple, Open Approach
0CQW0Z2 Repair of Upper Tooth, All, Open Approach
0CQWXZ0 Repair of Upper Tooth, Single, External Approach
0CQWXZ1 Repair of Upper Tooth, Multiple, External Approach
0CQWXZ2 Repair of Upper Tooth, All, External Approach
0CQX0Z0 Repair of Lower Tooth, Single, Open Approach
0CQX0Z1 Repair of Lower Tooth, Multiple, Open Approach
0CQX0Z2 Repair of Lower Tooth, All, Open Approach
0CQXXZ0 Repair of Lower Tooth, Single, External Approach
0CQXXZ1 Repair of Lower Tooth, Multiple, External Approach
0CQXXZ2 Repair of Lower Tooth, All, External Approach

CR – Mouth and Throat, Replacement

CR007Z Replacement of Upper Lip with Autologous Tissue Substitute, Open Approach
CR00JZ Replacement of Upper Lip with Synthetic Substitute, Open Approach
CR00KZ Replacement of Upper Lip with Nonautologous Tissue Substitute, Open Approach
CR037Z Replacement of Upper Lip with Autologous Tissue Substitute, Percutaneous Approach
CR03JZ Replacement of Upper Lip with Synthetic Substitute, Percutaneous Approach
CR03KZ Replacement of Upper Lip with Nonautologous Tissue Substitute, Percutaneous Approach
CR0X7Z Replacement of Upper Lip with Autologous Tissue Substitute, External Approach
CR0XJZ Replacement of Upper Lip with Synthetic Substitute, External Approach
CR0XKZ Replacement of Upper Lip with Nonautologous Tissue Substitute, External Approach
CR107Z Replacement of Lower Lip with Autologous Tissue Substitute, Open Approach
CR10JZ Replacement of Lower Lip with Synthetic Substitute, Open Approach
CR10KZ Replacement of Lower Lip with Nonautologous Tissue Substitute, Open Approach
CR137Z Replacement of Lower Lip with Autologous Tissue Substitute, Percutaneous Approach
CR13JZ Replacement of Lower Lip with Synthetic Substitute, Percutaneous Approach
0CR13KZ Replacement of Lower Lip with Nonautologous Tissue Substitute, Percutaneous Approach
0CR1X7Z Replacement of Lower Lip with Autologous Tissue Substitute, External Approach
0CR1XJZ Replacement of Lower Lip with Synthetic Substitute, External Approach
0CR1XKZ Replacement of Lower Lip with Nonautologous Tissue Substitute, External Approach
0CR207Z Replacement of Hard Palate with Autologous Tissue Substitute, Open Approach
0CR20JZ Replacement of Hard Palate with Synthetic Substitute, Open Approach
0CR20KZ Replacement of Hard Palate with Nonautologous Tissue Substitute, Open Approach
0CR237Z Replacement of Hard Palate with Autologous Tissue Substitute, Percutaneous Approach
0CR23JZ Replacement of Hard Palate with Synthetic Substitute, Percutaneous Approach
0CR23KZ Replacement of Hard Palate with Nonautologous Tissue Substitute, Percutaneous Approach
0CR2X7Z Replacement of Hard Palate with Autologous Tissue Substitute, External Approach
0CR2XJZ Replacement of Hard Palate with Synthetic Substitute, External Approach
0CR2XKZ Replacement of Hard Palate with Nonautologous Tissue Substitute, External Approach
0CR307Z Replacement of Soft Palate with Autologous Tissue Substitute, Open Approach
0CR30JZ Replacement of Soft Palate with Synthetic Substitute, Open Approach
0CR30KZ Replacement of Soft Palate with Nonautologous Tissue Substitute, Open Approach
0CR337Z Replacement of Soft Palate with Autologous Tissue Substitute, Percutaneous Approach
0CR33JZ Replacement of Soft Palate with Synthetic Substitute, Percutaneous Approach
0CR33KZ Replacement of Soft Palate with Nonautologous Tissue Substitute, Percutaneous Approach
0CR3X7Z Replacement of Soft Palate with Autologous Tissue Substitute, External Approach
0CR3XJZ Replacement of Soft Palate with Synthetic Substitute, External Approach
0CR3XKZ Replacement of Soft Palate with Nonautologous Tissue Substitute, External Approach
0CR407Z Replacement of Buccal Mucosa with Autologous Tissue Substitute, Open Approach
0CR40JZ Replacement of Buccal Mucosa with Synthetic Substitute, Open Approach
0CR40KZ Replacement of Buccal Mucosa with Nonautologous Tissue Substitute, Open Approach
0CR437Z Replacement of Buccal Mucosa with Autologous Tissue Substitute, Percutaneous Approach
0CR43JZ Replacement of Buccal Mucosa with Synthetic Substitute, Percutaneous Approach
0CR43KZ Replacement of Buccal Mucosa with Nonautologous Tissue Substitute, Percutaneous Approach

0CR4X7Z Replacement of Buccal Mucosa with Autologous Tissue Substitute, External Approach

0CR4XJZ Replacement of Buccal Mucosa with Synthetic Substitute, External Approach

0CR4XKZ Replacement of Buccal Mucosa with Nonautologous Tissue Substitute, External Approach
AHA CC: 2Q, 2014, 5-6

0CR507Z Replacement of Upper Gingiva with Autologous Tissue Substitute, Open Approach

0CR50JZ Replacement of Upper Gingiva with Synthetic Substitute, Open Approach

0CR50KZ Replacement of Upper Gingiva with Nonautologous Tissue Substitute, Open Approach

0CR537Z Replacement of Upper Gingiva with Autologous Tissue Substitute, Percutaneous Approach

0CR53JZ Replacement of Upper Gingiva with Synthetic Substitute, Percutaneous Approach

0CR53KZ Replacement of Upper Gingiva with Nonautologous Tissue Substitute, Percutaneous Approach

0CR5X7Z Replacement of Upper Gingiva with Autologous Tissue Substitute, External Approach

0CR5XJZ Replacement of Upper Gingiva with Synthetic Substitute, External Approach

0CR5XKZ Replacement of Upper Gingiva with Nonautologous Tissue Substitute, External Approach

0CR607Z Replacement of Lower Gingiva with Autologous Tissue Substitute, Open Approach

0CR60JZ Replacement of Lower Gingiva with Synthetic Substitute, Open Approach

0CR60KZ Replacement of Lower Gingiva with Nonautologous Tissue Substitute, Open Approach

0CR637Z Replacement of Lower Gingiva with Autologous Tissue Substitute, Percutaneous Approach

0CR63JZ Replacement of Lower Gingiva with Synthetic Substitute, Percutaneous Approach

0CR63KZ Replacement of Lower Gingiva with Nonautologous Tissue Substitute, Percutaneous Approach

0CR6X7Z Replacement of Lower Gingiva with Autologous Tissue Substitute, External Approach

0CR6XJZ Replacement of Lower Gingiva with Synthetic Substitute, External Approach

0CR6XKZ Replacement of Lower Gingiva with Nonautologous Tissue Substitute, External Approach

0CR707Z Replacement of Tongue with Autologous Tissue Substitute, Open Approach

0CR70JZ Replacement of Tongue with Synthetic Substitute, Open Approach

0CR70KZ Replacement of Tongue with Nonautologous Tissue Substitute, Open Approach

0CR737Z Replacement of Tongue with Autologous Tissue Substitute, Percutaneous Approach

0CR73JZ Replacement of Tongue with Synthetic Substitute, Percutaneous Approach

0CR73KZ Replacement of Tongue with Nonautologous Tissue Substitute, Percutaneous Approach

0CR7X7Z Replacement of Tongue with Autologous Tissue Substitute, External Approach

0CR7XJZ Replacement of Tongue with Synthetic Substitute, External Approach

0CR7XKZ Replacement of Tongue with Nonautologous Tissue Substitute, External Approach

0CRB07Z Replacement of Right Parotid Duct with Autologous Tissue Substitute, Open Approach

0CRB0JZ Replacement of Right Parotid Duct with Synthetic Substitute, Open Approach

0CRB0KZ Replacement of Right Parotid Duct with Nonautologous Tissue Substitute, Open Approach

0CRB37Z Replacement of Right Parotid Duct with Autologous Tissue Substitute, Percutaneous Approach

0CRB3JZ Replacement of Right Parotid Duct with Synthetic Substitute, Percutaneous Approach

0CRB3KZ Replacement of Right Parotid Duct with Nonautologous Tissue Substitute, Percutaneous Approach

0CRC07Z Replacement of Left Parotid Duct with Autologous Tissue Substitute, Open Approach

0CRC0JZ Replacement of Left Parotid Duct with Synthetic Substitute, Open Approach

0CRC0KZ Replacement of Left Parotid Duct with Nonautologous Tissue Substitute, Open Approach

0CRC37Z Replacement of Left Parotid Duct with Autologous Tissue Substitute, Percutaneous Approach

0CRC3JZ Replacement of Left Parotid Duct with Synthetic Substitute, Percutaneous Approach

0CRC3KZ Replacement of Left Parotid Duct with Nonautologous Tissue Substitute, Percutaneous Approach

0CRM07Z Replacement of Pharynx with Autologous Tissue Substitute, Open Approach

0CRM0JZ Replacement of Pharynx with Synthetic Substitute, Open Approach

0CRM0KZ Replacement of Pharynx with Nonautologous Tissue Substitute, Open Approach

0CRM77Z Replacement of Pharynx with Autologous Tissue Substitute, Via Natural or Artificial Opening

0CRM7JZ Replacement of Pharynx with Synthetic Substitute, Via Natural or Artificial Opening

0CRM7KZ Replacement of Pharynx with Nonautologous Tissue Substitute, Via Natural or Artificial Opening

0CRM87Z Replacement of Pharynx with Autologous Tissue Substitute, Via Natural or Artificial Opening Endoscopic

0CRM8JZ Replacement of Pharynx with Synthetic Substitute, Via Natural or Artificial Opening Endoscopic

0CRM8KZ Replacement of Pharynx with Nonautologous Tissue Substitute, Via Natural or Artificial Opening Endoscopic

0CRN07Z Replacement of Uvula with Autologous Tissue Substitute, Open Approach

0CRN0JZ Replacement of Uvula with Synthetic Substitute, Open Approach

0CRN0KZ Replacement of Uvula with Nonautologous Tissue Substitute, Open Approach

0CRN37Z Replacement of Uvula with Autologous Tissue Substitute, Percutaneous Approach

0CRN3JZ Replacement of Uvula with Synthetic Substitute, Percutaneous Approach

0CRN3KZ Replacement of Uvula with Nonautologous Tissue Substitute, Percutaneous Approach

0CRNX7Z Replacement of Uvula with Autologou Tissue Substitute, External Approach

0CRNXJZ Replacement of Uvula with Synthetic Substitute, External Approach

0CRNXKZ Replacement of Uvula with Nonautologous Tissue Substitute, External Approach

0CRR07Z Replacement of Epiglottis with Autologous Tissue Substitute, Open Approach

0CRR0JZ Replacement of Epiglottis with Synthe Substitute, Open Approach

0CRR0KZ Replacement of Epiglottis with Nonautologous Tissue Substitute, Open Approach

0CRR77Z Replacement of Epiglottis with Autologous Tissue Substitute, Via Natu or Artificial Opening

0CRR7JZ Replacement of Epiglottis with Synthet Substitute, Via Natural or Artificial Opening

0CRR7KZ Replacement of Epiglottis with Nonautologous Tissue Substitute, Via Natural or Artificial Opening

0CRR87Z Replacement of Epiglottis with Autologous Tissue Substitute, Via Natur or Artificial Opening Endoscopic

0CRR8JZ Replacement of Epiglottis with Syntheti Substitute, Via Natural or Artificial Opening Endoscopic

0CRR8KZ Replacement of Epiglottis with Nonautologous Tissue Substitute, Via Natural or Artificial Opening Endoscopic

0CRS07Z Replacement of Larynx with Autologou Tissue Substitute, Open Approach

0CRS0JZ Replacement of Larynx with Synthetic Substitute, Open Approach

0CRS0KZ Replacement of Larynx with Nonautologous Tissue Substitute, Open Approach

0CRS77Z Replacement of Larynx with Autologous Tissue Substitute, Via Natural or Artifici Opening

0CRS7JZ Replacement of Larynx with Synthetic Substitute, Via Natural or Artificial Opening

0CRS7KZ Replacement of Larynx with Nonautologous Tissue Substitute, Via Natural or Artificial Opening

0CRS87Z Replacement of Larynx with Autologous Tissue Substitute, Via Natural or Artificia Opening Endoscopic

0CRS8JZ Replacement of Larynx with Synthetic Substitute, Via Natural or Artificial Opening Endoscopic

0CRS8KZ Replacement of Larynx with Nonautologous Tissue Substitute, Via Natural or Artificial Opening Endoscopic

0CRT07Z Replacement of Right Vocal Cord with Autologous Tissue Substitute, Open Approach

0CRT0JZ Replacement of Right Vocal Cord with Synthetic Substitute, Open Approach

0CRT0KZ Replacement of Right Vocal Cord with Nonautologous Tissue Substitute, Open Approach

0CRT77Z Replacement of Right Vocal Cord with Autologous Tissue Substitute, Via Natura or Artificial Opening

RT7JZ Replacement of Right Vocal Cord with Synthetic Substitute, Via Natural or Artificial Opening

RT7KZ Replacement of Right Vocal Cord with Nonautologous Tissue Substitute, Via Natural or Artificial Opening

RT87Z Replacement of Right Vocal Cord with Autologous Tissue Substitute, Via Natural or Artificial Opening Endoscopic

RT8JZ Replacement of Right Vocal Cord with Synthetic Substitute, Via Natural or Artificial Opening Endoscopic

RT8KZ Replacement of Right Vocal Cord with Nonautologous Tissue Substitute, Via Natural or Artificial Opening Endoscopic

RV07Z Replacement of Left Vocal Cord with Autologous Tissue Substitute, Open Approach

RV0JZ Replacement of Left Vocal Cord with Synthetic Substitute, Open Approach

RV0KZ Replacement of Left Vocal Cord with Nonautologous Tissue Substitute, Open Approach

RV77Z Replacement of Left Vocal Cord with Autologous Tissue Substitute, Via Natural or Artificial Opening

RV7JZ Replacement of Left Vocal Cord with Synthetic Substitute, Via Natural or Artificial Opening

RV7KZ Replacement of Left Vocal Cord with Nonautologous Tissue Substitute, Via Natural or Artificial Opening

RV87Z Replacement of Left Vocal Cord with Autologous Tissue Substitute, Via Natural or Artificial Opening Endoscopic

RV8JZ Replacement of Left Vocal Cord with Synthetic Substitute, Via Natural or Artificial Opening Endoscopic

RV8KZ Replacement of Left Vocal Cord with Nonautologous Tissue Substitute, Via Natural or Artificial Opening Endoscopic

RW070 Replacement of Upper Tooth, Single, with Autologous Tissue Substitute, Open Approach

RW071 Replacement of Upper Tooth, Multiple, with Autologous Tissue Substitute, Open Approach

0CRW072 Replacement of Upper Tooth, All, with Autologous Tissue Substitute, Open Approach

0CRW0J0 Replacement of Upper Tooth, Single, with Synthetic Substitute, Open Approach

0CRW0J1 Replacement of Upper Tooth, Multiple, with Synthetic Substitute, Open Approach

0CRW0J2 Replacement of Upper Tooth, All, with Synthetic Substitute, Open Approach

0CRW0K0 Replacement of Upper Tooth, Single, with Nonautologous Tissue Substitute, Open Approach

0CRW0K1 Replacement of Upper Tooth, Multiple, with Nonautologous Tissue Substitute, Open Approach

0CRW0K2 Replacement of Upper Tooth, All, with Nonautologous Tissue Substitute, Open Approach

0CRWX70 Replacement of Upper Tooth, Single, with Autologous Tissue Substitute, External Approach

0CRWX71 Replacement of Upper Tooth, Multiple, with Autologous Tissue Substitute, External Approach

0CRWX72 Replacement of Upper Tooth, All, with Autologous Tissue Substitute, External Approach

0CRWXJ0 Replacement of Upper Tooth, Single, with Synthetic Substitute, External Approach

0CRWXJ1 Replacement of Upper Tooth, Multiple, with Synthetic Substitute, External Approach

0CRWXJ2 Replacement of Upper Tooth, All, with Synthetic Substitute, External Approach

0CRWXK0 Replacement of Upper Tooth, Single, with Nonautologous Tissue Substitute, External Approach

0CRWXK1 Replacement of Upper Tooth, Multiple, with Nonautologous Tissue Substitute, External Approach

0CRWXK2 Replacement of Upper Tooth, All, with Nonautologous Tissue Substitute, External Approach

0CRX070 Replacement of Lower Tooth, Single, with Autologous Tissue Substitute, Open Approach

0CRX071 Replacement of Lower Tooth, Multiple, with Autologous Tissue Substitute, Open Approach

0CRX072 Replacement of Lower Tooth, All, with Autologous Tissue Substitute, Open Approach

0CRX0J0 Replacement of Lower Tooth, Single, with Synthetic Substitute, Open Approach

0CRX0J1 Replacement of Lower Tooth, Multiple, with Synthetic Substitute, Open Approach

0CRX0J2 Replacement of Lower Tooth, All, with Synthetic Substitute, Open Approach

0CRX0K0 Replacement of Lower Tooth, Single, with Nonautologous Tissue Substitute, Open Approach

0CRX0K1 Replacement of Lower Tooth, Multiple, with Nonautologous Tissue Substitute, Open Approach

0CRX0K2 Replacement of Lower Tooth, All, with Nonautologous Tissue Substitute, Open Approach

0CRXX70 Replacement of Lower Tooth, Single, with Autologous Tissue Substitute, External Approach

0CRXX71 Replacement of Lower Tooth, Multiple, with Autologous Tissue Substitute, External Approach

0CRXX72 Replacement of Lower Tooth, All, with Autologous Tissue Substitute, External Approach

0CRXXJ0 Replacement of Lower Tooth, Single, with Synthetic Substitute, External Approach

0CRXXJ1 Replacement of Lower Tooth, Multiple, with Synthetic Substitute, External Approach

0CRXXJ2 Replacement of Lower Tooth, All, with Synthetic Substitute, External Approach

0CRXXK0 Replacement of Lower Tooth, Single, with Nonautologous Tissue Substitute, External Approach

0CRXXK1 Replacement of Lower Tooth, Multiple, with Nonautologous Tissue Substitute, External Approach

0CRXXK2 Replacement of Lower Tooth, All, with Nonautologous Tissue Substitute, External Approach

CS – Mouth and Throat, Reposition

CS00ZZ Reposition Upper Lip, Open Approach

CS0XZZ Reposition Upper Lip, External Approach

CS10ZZ Reposition Lower Lip, Open Approach

CS1XZZ Reposition Lower Lip, External Approach

CS20ZZ Reposition Hard Palate, Open Approach

CS2XZZ Reposition Hard Palate, External Approach

CS30ZZ Reposition Soft Palate, Open Approach

CS3XZZ Reposition Soft Palate, External Approach

CS70ZZ Reposition Tongue, Open Approach

CS7XZZ Reposition Tongue, External Approach

CSB0ZZ Reposition Right Parotid Duct, Open Approach

CSB3ZZ Reposition Right Parotid Duct, Percutaneous Approach

CSC0ZZ Reposition Left Parotid Duct, Open Approach

CSC3ZZ Reposition Left Parotid Duct, Percutaneous Approach

CSN0ZZ Reposition Uvula, Open Approach

CSNXZZ Reposition Uvula, External Approach

CSR0ZZ Reposition Epiglottis, Open Approach

0CSR7ZZ Reposition Epiglottis, Via Natural or Artificial Opening

0CSR8ZZ Reposition Epiglottis, Via Natural or Artificial Opening Endoscopic

0CST0ZZ Reposition Right Vocal Cord, Open Approach

0CST7ZZ Reposition Right Vocal Cord, Via Natural or Artificial Opening

0CST8ZZ Reposition Right Vocal Cord, Via Natural or Artificial Opening Endoscopic

0CSV0ZZ Reposition Left Vocal Cord, Open Approach

0CSV7ZZ Reposition Left Vocal Cord, Via Natural or Artificial Opening

0CSV8ZZ Reposition Left Vocal Cord, Via Natural or Artificial Opening Endoscopic

0CSW050 Reposition Upper Tooth with External Fixation Device, Single, Open Approach

0CSW051 Reposition Upper Tooth with External Fixation Device, Multiple, Open Approach

0CSW052 Reposition Upper Tooth with External Fixation Device, All, Open Approach

0CSW0Z0 Reposition Upper Tooth, Single, Open Approach

0CSW0Z1 Reposition Upper Tooth, Multiple, Open Approach

0CSW0Z2 Reposition Upper Tooth, All, Open Approach

0CSWX50 Reposition Upper Tooth, Single, with External Fixation Device, External Approach

0CSWX51 Reposition Upper Tooth, Multiple, with External Fixation Device, External Approach

0CSWX52 Reposition Upper Tooth, All, with External Fixation Device, External Approach

0CSWXZ0 Reposition Upper Tooth, Single, External Approach

0CSWXZ1 Reposition Upper Tooth, Multiple, External Approach

0CSWXZ2 Reposition Upper Tooth, All, External Approach

0CSX050 Reposition Lower Tooth with External Fixation Device, Single, Open Approach

0CSX051 Reposition Lower Tooth with External Fixation Device, Multiple, Open Approach
0CSX052 Reposition Lower Tooth with External Fixation Device, All, Open Approach
0CSX0Z0 Reposition Lower Tooth, Single, Open Approach
0CSX0Z1 Reposition Lower Tooth, Multiple, Open Approach
0CSX0Z2 Reposition Lower Tooth, All, Open Approach
0CSXX50 Reposition Lower Tooth, Single, with External Fixation Device, External Approach
0CSXX51 Reposition Lower Tooth, Multiple, with External Fixation Device, External Approach
0CSXX52 Reposition Lower Tooth, All, with External Fixation Device, External Approach
0CSXXZ0 Reposition Lower Tooth, Single, Exte[rnal] Approach
0CSXXZ1 Reposition Lower Tooth, Multiple, External Approach
0CSXXZ2 Reposition Lower Tooth, All, External Approach

0CT – Mouth and Throat, Resection

Review Coding Guideline B3.8

0CT00ZZ Resection of Upper Lip, Open Approach
0CT0XZZ Resection of Upper Lip, External Approach
0CT10ZZ Resection of Lower Lip, Open Approach
0CT1XZZ Resection of Lower Lip, External Approach
0CT20ZZ Resection of Hard Palate, Open Approach
0CT2XZZ Resection of Hard Palate, External Approach
0CT30ZZ Resection of Soft Palate, Open Approach
0CT3XZZ Resection of Soft Palate, External Approach
0CT70ZZ Resection of Tongue, Open Approach
0CT7XZZ Resection of Tongue, External Approach
0CT80ZZ Resection of Right Parotid Gland, Open Approach
0CT90ZZ Resection of Left Parotid Gland, Open Approach
0CTB0ZZ Resection of Right Parotid Duct, Open Approach
0CTC0ZZ Resection of Left Parotid Duct, Open Approach
0CTD0ZZ Resection of Right Sublingual Gland, Open Approach
0CTF0ZZ Resection of Left Sublingual Gland, Open Approach
0CTG0ZZ Resection of Right Submaxillary Gland, Open Approach
0CTH0ZZ Resection of Left Submaxillary Gland, Open Approach
0CTJ0ZZ Resection of Minor Salivary Gland, Open Approach
0CTM0ZZ Resection of Pharynx, Open Approach
0CTM4ZZ Resection of Pharynx, Percutaneous Endoscopic Approach
0CTM7ZZ Resection of Pharynx, Via Natural or Artificial Opening
0CTM8ZZ Resection of Pharynx, Via Natural or Artificial Opening Endoscopic
0CTN0ZZ Resection of Uvula, Open Approach
0CTNXZZ Resection of Uvula, External Approach
0CTP0ZZ Resection of Tonsils, Open Approach
0CTPXZZ Resection of Tonsils, External Approach
0CTQ0ZZ Resection of Adenoids, Open Approach
0CTQXZZ Resection of Adenoids, External Approach
0CTR0ZZ Resection of Epiglottis, Open Approach
0CTR4ZZ Resection of Epiglottis, Percutaneous Endoscopic Approach
0CTR7ZZ Resection of Epiglottis, Via Natural or Artificial Opening
0CTR8ZZ Resection of Epiglottis, Via Natural or Artificial Opening Endoscopic
0CTS0ZZ Resection of Larynx, Open Approach
0CTS4ZZ Resection of Larynx, Percutaneous Endoscopic Approach
0CTS7ZZ Resection of Larynx, Via Natural or Artificial Opening
0CTS8ZZ Resection of Larynx, Via Natural or Artificial Opening Endoscopic
0CTT0ZZ Resection of Right Vocal Cord, Open Approach
0CTT4ZZ Resection of Right Vocal Cord, Percutaneous Endoscopic Approach
0CTT7ZZ Resection of Right Vocal Cord, Via Natural or Artificial Opening
0CTT8ZZ Resection of Right Vocal Cord, Via Natural or Artificial Opening Endoscop[ic]
0CTV0ZZ Resection of Left Vocal Cord, Open Approach
0CTV4ZZ Resection of Left Vocal Cord, Percutaneous Endoscopic Approach
0CTV7ZZ Resection of Left Vocal Cord, Via Natu[ral] or Artificial Opening
0CTV8ZZ Resection of Left Vocal Cord, Via Natu[ral] or Artificial Opening Endoscopic
0CTW0Z0 Resection of Upper Tooth, Single, Ope[n] Approach
0CTW0Z1 Resection of Upper Tooth, Multiple, Open Approach
0CTW0Z2 Resection of Upper Tooth, All, Open Approach
0CTX0Z0 Resection of Lower Tooth, Single, Ope[n] Approach
0CTX0Z1 Resection of Lower Tooth, Multiple, Open Approach
0CTX0Z2 Resection of Lower Tooth, All, Open Approach

0CU – Mouth and Throat, Supplement

0CU007Z Supplement Upper Lip with Autologous Tissue Substitute, Open Approach
0CU00JZ Supplement Upper Lip with Synthetic Substitute, Open Approach
0CU00KZ Supplement Upper Lip with Nonautologous Tissue Substitute, Open Approach
0CU037Z Supplement Upper Lip with Autologous Tissue Substitute, Percutaneous Approach
0CU03JZ Supplement Upper Lip with Synthetic Substitute, Percutaneous Approach
0CU03KZ Supplement Upper Lip with Nonautologous Tissue Substitute, Percutaneous Approach
0CU0X7Z Supplement Upper Lip with Autologous Tissue Substitute, External Approach
0CU0XJZ Supplement Upper Lip with Synthetic Substitute, External Approach
0CU0XKZ Supplement Upper Lip with Nonautologous Tissue Substitute, External Approach
0CU107Z Supplement Lower Lip with Autologous Tissue Substitute, Open Approach
0CU10JZ Supplement Lower Lip with Synthetic Substitute, Open Approach
0CU10KZ Supplement Lower Lip with Nonautologous Tissue Substitute, Open Approach
0CU137Z Supplement Lower Lip with Autologous Tissue Substitute, Percutaneous Approach
0CU13JZ Supplement Lower Lip with Synthetic Substitute, Percutaneous Approach
0CU13KZ Supplement Lower Lip with Nonautologous Tissue Substitute, Percutaneous Approach
0CU1X7Z Supplement Lower Lip with Autologous Tissue Substitute, External Approach
0CU1XJZ Supplement Lower Lip with Synthetic Substitute, External Approach
0CU1XKZ Supplement Lower Lip with Nonautologous Tissue Substitute, External Approach
0CU207Z Supplement Hard Palate with Autologous Tissue Substitute, Open Approach
0CU20JZ Supplement Hard Palate with Synthetic Substitute, Open Approach
0CU20KZ Supplement Hard Palate with Nonautologous Tissue Substitute, Open Approach
0CU237Z Supplement Hard Palate with Autologous Tissue Substitute, Percutaneous Approach
0CU23JZ Supplement Hard Palate with Synthetic Substitute, Percutaneous Approach
0CU23KZ Supplement Hard Palate with Nonautologous Tissue Substitute, Percutaneous Approach
0CU2X7Z Supplement Hard Palate with Autologou[s] Tissue Substitute, External Approach
0CU2XJZ Supplement Hard Palate with Synthetic Substitute, External Approach
0CU2XKZ Supplement Hard Palate with Nonautologous Tissue Substitute, External Approach
0CU307Z Supplement Soft Palate with Autologous Tissue Substitute, Open Approach
0CU30JZ Supplement Soft Palate with Synthetic Substitute, Open Approach
0CU30KZ Supplement Soft Palate with Nonautologous Tissue Substitute, Open Approach
0CU337Z Supplement Soft Palate with Autologous Tissue Substitute, Percutaneous Approach
0CU33JZ Supplement Soft Palate with Synthetic Substitute, Percutaneous Approach
0CU33KZ Supplement Soft Palate with Nonautologous Tissue Substitute, Percutaneous Approach
0CU3X7Z Supplement Soft Palate with Autologous Tissue Substitute, External Approach
0CU3XJZ Supplement Soft Palate with Synthetic Substitute, External Approach

J3XKZ Supplement Soft Palate with Nonautologous Tissue Substitute, External Approach
J407Z Supplement Buccal Mucosa with Autologous Tissue Substitute, Open Approach
J40JZ Supplement Buccal Mucosa with Synthetic Substitute, Open Approach
J40KZ Supplement Buccal Mucosa with Nonautologous Tissue Substitute, Open Approach
J437Z Supplement Buccal Mucosa with Autologous Tissue Substitute, Percutaneous Approach
J43JZ Supplement Buccal Mucosa with Synthetic Substitute, Percutaneous Approach
J43KZ Supplement Buccal Mucosa with Nonautologous Tissue Substitute, Percutaneous Approach
U4X7Z Supplement Buccal Mucosa with Autologous Tissue Substitute, External Approach
U4XJZ Supplement Buccal Mucosa with Synthetic Substitute, External Approach
U4XKZ Supplement Buccal Mucosa with Nonautologous Tissue Substitute, External Approach
U507Z Supplement Upper Gingiva with Autologous Tissue Substitute, Open Approach
U50JZ Supplement Upper Gingiva with Synthetic Substitute, Open Approach
U50KZ Supplement Upper Gingiva with Nonautologous Tissue Substitute, Open Approach
U537Z Supplement Upper Gingiva with Autologous Tissue Substitute, Percutaneous Approach
U53JZ Supplement Upper Gingiva with Synthetic Substitute, Percutaneous Approach
U53KZ Supplement Upper Gingiva with Nonautologous Tissue Substitute, Percutaneous Approach
U5X7Z Supplement Upper Gingiva with Autologous Tissue Substitute, External Approach
U5XJZ Supplement Upper Gingiva with Synthetic Substitute, External Approach
U5XKZ Supplement Upper Gingiva with Nonautologous Tissue Substitute, External Approach
CU607Z Supplement Lower Gingiva with Autologous Tissue Substitute, Open Approach
CU60JZ Supplement Lower Gingiva with Synthetic Substitute, Open Approach
CU60KZ Supplement Lower Gingiva with Nonautologous Tissue Substitute, Open Approach
CU637Z Supplement Lower Gingiva with Autologous Tissue Substitute, Percutaneous Approach
CU63JZ Supplement Lower Gingiva with Synthetic Substitute, Percutaneous Approach
CU63KZ Supplement Lower Gingiva with Nonautologous Tissue Substitute, Percutaneous Approach
CU6X7Z Supplement Lower Gingiva with Autologous Tissue Substitute, External Approach
CU6XJZ Supplement Lower Gingiva with Synthetic Substitute, External Approach
0CU6XKZ Supplement Lower Gingiva with Nonautologous Tissue Substitute, External Approach
0CU707Z Supplement Tongue with Autologous Tissue Substitute, Open Approach
0CU70JZ Supplement Tongue with Synthetic Substitute, Open Approach
0CU70KZ Supplement Tongue with Nonautologous Tissue Substitute, Open Approach
0CU737Z Supplement Tongue with Autologous Tissue Substitute, Percutaneous Approach
0CU73JZ Supplement Tongue with Synthetic Substitute, Percutaneous Approach
0CU73KZ Supplement Tongue with Nonautologous Tissue Substitute, Percutaneous Approach
0CU7X7Z Supplement Tongue with Autologous Tissue Substitute, External Approach
0CU7XJZ Supplement Tongue with Synthetic Substitute, External Approach
0CU7XKZ Supplement Tongue with Nonautologous Tissue Substitute, External Approach
0CUM07Z Supplement Pharynx with Autologous Tissue Substitute, Open Approach
0CUM0JZ Supplement Pharynx with Synthetic Substitute, Open Approach
0CUM0KZ Supplement Pharynx with Nonautologous Tissue Substitute, Open Approach
0CUM77Z Supplement Pharynx with Autologous Tissue Substitute, Via Natural or Artificial Opening
0CUM7JZ Supplement Pharynx with Synthetic Substitute, Via Natural or Artificial Opening
0CUM7KZ Supplement Pharynx with Nonautologous Tissue Substitute, Via Natural or Artificial Opening
0CUM87Z Supplement Pharynx with Autologous Tissue Substitute, Via Natural or Artificial Opening Endoscopic
0CUM8JZ Supplement Pharynx with Synthetic Substitute, Via Natural or Artificial Opening Endoscopic
0CUM8KZ Supplement Pharynx with Nonautologous Tissue Substitute, Via Natural or Artificial Opening Endoscopic
0CUN07Z Supplement Uvula with Autologous Tissue Substitute, Open Approach
0CUN0JZ Supplement Uvula with Synthetic Substitute, Open Approach
0CUN0KZ Supplement Uvula with Nonautologous Tissue Substitute, Open Approach
0CUN37Z Supplement Uvula with Autologous Tissue Substitute, Percutaneous Approach
0CUN3JZ Supplement Uvula with Synthetic Substitute, Percutaneous Approach
0CUN3KZ Supplement Uvula with Nonautologous Tissue Substitute, Percutaneous Approach
0CUNX7Z Supplement Uvula with Autologous Tissue Substitute, External Approach
0CUNXJZ Supplement Uvula with Synthetic Substitute, External Approach
0CUNXKZ Supplement Uvula with Nonautologous Tissue Substitute, External Approach
0CUR07Z Supplement Epiglottis with Autologous Tissue Substitute, Open Approach
0CUR0JZ Supplement Epiglottis with Synthetic Substitute, Open Approach
0CUR0KZ Supplement Epiglottis with Nonautologous Tissue Substitute, Open Approach
0CUR77Z Supplement Epiglottis with Autologous Tissue Substitute, Via Natural or Artificial Opening
0CUR7JZ Supplement Epiglottis with Synthetic Substitute, Via Natural or Artificial Opening
0CUR7KZ Supplement Epiglottis with Nonautologous Tissue Substitute, Via Natural or Artificial Opening
0CUR87Z Supplement Epiglottis with Autologous Tissue Substitute, Via Natural or Artificial Opening Endoscopic
0CUR8JZ Supplement Epiglottis with Synthetic Substitute, Via Natural or Artificial Opening Endoscopic
0CUR8KZ Supplement Epiglottis with Nonautologous Tissue Substitute, Via Natural or Artificial Opening Endoscopic
0CUS07Z Supplement Larynx with Autologous Tissue Substitute, Open Approach
0CUS0JZ Supplement Larynx with Synthetic Substitute, Open Approach
0CUS0KZ Supplement Larynx with Nonautologous Tissue Substitute, Open Approach
0CUS77Z Supplement Larynx with Autologous Tissue Substitute, Via Natural or Artificial Opening
0CUS7JZ Supplement Larynx with Synthetic Substitute, Via Natural or Artificial Opening
0CUS7KZ Supplement Larynx with Nonautologous Tissue Substitute, Via Natural or Artificial Opening
0CUS87Z Supplement Larynx with Autologous Tissue Substitute, Via Natural or Artificial Opening Endoscopic
0CUS8JZ Supplement Larynx with Synthetic Substitute, Via Natural or Artificial Opening Endoscopic
0CUS8KZ Supplement Larynx with Nonautologous Tissue Substitute, Via Natural or Artificial Opening Endoscopic
0CUT07Z Supplement Right Vocal Cord with Autologous Tissue Substitute, Open Approach
0CUT0JZ Supplement Right Vocal Cord with Synthetic Substitute, Open Approach
0CUT0KZ Supplement Right Vocal Cord with Nonautologous Tissue Substitute, Open Approach
0CUT77Z Supplement Right Vocal Cord with Autologous Tissue Substitute, Via Natural or Artificial Opening
0CUT7JZ Supplement Right Vocal Cord with Synthetic Substitute, Via Natural or Artificial Opening
0CUT7KZ Supplement Right Vocal Cord with Nonautologous Tissue Substitute, Via Natural or Artificial Opening
0CUT87Z Supplement Right Vocal Cord with Autologous Tissue Substitute, Via Natural or Artificial Opening Endoscopic
0CUT8JZ Supplement Right Vocal Cord with Synthetic Substitute, Via Natural or Artificial Opening Endoscopic
0CUT8KZ Supplement Right Vocal Cord with Nonautologous Tissue Substitute, Via Natural or Artificial Opening Endoscopic
0CUV07Z Supplement Left Vocal Cord with Autologous Tissue Substitute, Open Approach
0CUV0JZ Supplement Left Vocal Cord with Synthetic Substitute, Open Approach
0CUV0KZ Supplement Left Vocal Cord with Nonautologous Tissue Substitute, Open Approach
0CUV77Z Supplement Left Vocal Cord with Autologous Tissue Substitute, Via Natural or Artificial Opening

0CUV7JZ Supplement Left Vocal Cord with Synthetic Substitute, Via Natural or Artificial Opening
0CUV7KZ Supplement Left Vocal Cord with Nonautologous Tissue Substitute, Via Natural or Artificial Opening
0CUV87Z Supplement Left Vocal Cord with Autologous Tissue Substitute, Via Natural or Artificial Opening Endoscopic
0CUV8JZ Supplement Left Vocal Cord with Synthetic Substitute, Via Natural or Artificial Opening Endoscopic
0CUV8KZ Supplement Left Vocal Cord with Nonautologous Tissue Substitute, Via Natural or Artificial Opening Endosco

0CV – Mouth and Throat, Restriction

0CVB0CZ Restriction of Right Parotid Duct with Extraluminal Device, Open Approach
0CVB0DZ Restriction of Right Parotid Duct with Intraluminal Device, Open Approach
0CVB0ZZ Restriction of Right Parotid Duct, Open Approach
0CVB3CZ Restriction of Right Parotid Duct with Extraluminal Device, Percutaneous Approach
0CVB3DZ Restriction of Right Parotid Duct with Intraluminal Device, Percutaneous Approach
0CVB3ZZ Restriction of Right Parotid Duct, Percutaneous Approach
0CVB7DZ Restriction of Right Parotid Duct with Intraluminal Device, Via Natural or Artificial Opening
0CVB7ZZ Restriction of Right Parotid Duct, Via Natural or Artificial Opening
0CVB8DZ Restriction of Right Parotid Duct with Intraluminal Device, Via Natural or Artificial Opening Endoscopic
0CVB8ZZ Restriction of Right Parotid Duct, Via Natural or Artificial Opening Endoscopic
0CVC0CZ Restriction of Left Parotid Duct with Extraluminal Device, Open Approach
0CVC0DZ Restriction of Left Parotid Duct with Intraluminal Device, Open Approach
0CVC0ZZ Restriction of Left Parotid Duct, Open Approach
0CVC3CZ Restriction of Left Parotid Duct with Extraluminal Device, Percutaneous Approach
0CVC3DZ Restriction of Left Parotid Duct with Intraluminal Device, Percutaneous Approach
0CVC3ZZ Restriction of Left Parotid Duct, Percutaneous Approach
0CVC7DZ Restriction of Left Parotid Duct with Intraluminal Device, Via Natural or Artificial Opening
0CVC7ZZ Restriction of Left Parotid Duct, Via Natural or Artificial Opening
0CVC8DZ Restriction of Left Parotid Duct with Intraluminal Device, Via Natural or Artificial Opening Endoscopic
0CVC8ZZ Restriction of Left Parotid Duct, Via Natural or Artificial Opening Endoscop

0CW – Mouth and Throat, Revision

Review Coding Guideline B6.1c

0CWA00Z Revision of Drainage Device in Salivary Gland, Open Approach
0CWA0CZ Revision of Extraluminal Device in Salivary Gland, Open Approach
0CWA30Z Revision of Drainage Device in Salivary Gland, Percutaneous Approach
0CWA3CZ Revision of Extraluminal Device in Salivary Gland, Percutaneous Approach
0CWAX0Z Revision of Drainage Device in Salivary Gland, External Approach
0CWAXCZ Revision of Extraluminal Device in Salivary Gland, External Approach
0CWS00Z Revision of Drainage Device in Larynx, Open Approach
0CWS07Z Revision of Autologous Tissue Substitute in Larynx, Open Approach
0CWS0DZ Revision of Intraluminal Device in Larynx, Open Approach
0CWS0JZ Revision of Synthetic Substitute in Larynx, Open Approach
0CWS0KZ Revision of Nonautologous Tissue Substitute in Larynx, Open Approach
0CWS30Z Revision of Drainage Device in Larynx, Percutaneous Approach
0CWS37Z Revision of Autologous Tissue Substitute in Larynx, Percutaneous Approach
0CWS3DZ Revision of Intraluminal Device in Larynx, Percutaneous Approach
0CWS3JZ Revision of Synthetic Substitute in Larynx, Percutaneous Approach
0CWS3KZ Revision of Nonautologous Tissue Substitute in Larynx, Percutaneous Approach
0CWS70Z Revision of Drainage Device in Larynx, Via Natural or Artificial Opening
0CWS77Z Revision of Autologous Tissue Substitute in Larynx, Via Natural or Artificial Opening
0CWS7DZ Revision of Intraluminal Device in Larynx, Via Natural or Artificial Opening
0CWS7JZ Revision of Synthetic Substitute in Larynx, Via Natural or Artificial Opening
0CWS7KZ Revision of Nonautologous Tissue Substitute in Larynx, Via Natural or Artificial Opening
0CWS80Z Revision of Drainage Device in Larynx, Via Natural or Artificial Opening Endoscopic
0CWS87Z Revision of Autologous Tissue Substitute in Larynx, Via Natural or Artificial Opening Endoscopic
0CWS8DZ Revision of Intraluminal Device in Larynx, Via Natural or Artificial Opening Endoscopic
0CWS8JZ Revision of Synthetic Substitute in Larynx, Via Natural or Artificial Opening Endoscopic
0CWS8KZ Revision of Nonautologous Tissue Substitute in Larynx, Via Natural or Artificial Opening Endoscopic
0CWSX0Z Revision of Drainage Device in Larynx, External Approach
0CWSX7Z Revision of Autologous Tissue Substitute in Larynx, External Approach
0CWSXDZ Revision of Intraluminal Device in Larynx, External Approach
0CWSXJZ Revision of Synthetic Substitute in Larynx, External Approach
0CWSXKZ Revision of Nonautologous Tissue Substitute in Larynx, External Approach
0CWY00Z Revision of Drainage Device in Mouth and Throat, Open Approach
0CWY01Z Revision of Radioactive Element in Mouth and Throat, Open Approach
0CWY07Z Revision of Autologous Tissue Substitute in Mouth and Throat, Open Approach
0CWY0DZ Revision of Intraluminal Device in Mouth and Throat, Open Approach
0CWY0JZ Revision of Synthetic Substitute in Mouth and Throat, Open Approach
0CWY0KZ Revision of Nonautologous Tissue Substitute in Mouth and Throat, Open Approach
0CWY30Z Revision of Drainage Device in Mouth and Throat, Percutaneous Approach
0CWY31Z Revision of Radioactive Element in Mouth and Throat, Percutaneous Approach
0CWY37Z Revision of Autologous Tissue Substitute in Mouth and Throat, Percutaneous Approach
0CWY3DZ Revision of Intraluminal Device in Mouth and Throat, Percutaneous Approach
0CWY3JZ Revision of Synthetic Substitute in Mouth and Throat, Percutaneous Approach
0CWY3KZ Revision of Nonautologous Tissue Substitute in Mouth and Throat, Percutaneous Approach
0CWY70Z Revision of Drainage Device in Mouth and Throat, Via Natural or Artificial Opening
0CWY71Z Revision of Radioactive Element in Mouth and Throat, Via Natural or Artificial Opening
0CWY77Z Revision of Autologous Tissue Substitute in Mouth and Throat, Via Natural or Artificial Opening
0CWY7DZ Revision of Intraluminal Device in Mouth and Throat, Via Natural or Artificial Opening
0CWY7JZ Revision of Synthetic Substitute in Mouth and Throat, Via Natural or Artificial Opening
0CWY7KZ Revision of Nonautologous Tissue Substitute in Mouth and Throat, Via Natural or Artificial Opening
0CWY80Z Revision of Drainage Device in Mouth and Throat, Via Natural or Artificial Opening Endoscopic
0CWY81Z Revision of Radioactive Element in Mouth and Throat, Via Natural or Artificial Opening Endoscopic
0CWY87Z Revision of Autologous Tissue Substitute in Mouth and Throat, Via Natural or Artificial Opening Endoscopic
0CWY8DZ Revision of Intraluminal Device in Mouth and Throat, Via Natural or Artificial Opening Endoscopic

WY8JZ Revision of Synthetic Substitute in Mouth and Throat, Via Natural or Artificial Opening Endoscopic
WY8KZ Revision of Nonautologous Tissue Substitute in Mouth and Throat, Via Natural or Artificial Opening Endoscopic
0CWYX0Z Revision of Drainage Device in Mouth and Throat, External Approach
0CWYX1Z Revision of Radioactive Element in Mouth and Throat, External Approach
0CWYX7Z Revision of Autologous Tissue Substitute in Mouth and Throat, External Approach
0CWYXDZ Revision of Intraluminal Device in Mouth and Throat, External Approach
0CWYXJZ Revision of Synthetic Substitute in Mouth and Throat, External Approach
0CWYXKZ Revision of Nonautologous Tissue Substitute in Mouth and Throat, External Approach

X – Mouth and Throat, Transfer

X00ZZ Transfer Upper Lip, Open Approach
X0XZZ Transfer Upper Lip, External Approach
X10ZZ Transfer Lower Lip, Open Approach
X1XZZ Transfer Lower Lip, External Approach
X30ZZ Transfer Soft Palate, Open Approach
X3XZZ Transfer Soft Palate, External Approach
0CX40ZZ Transfer Buccal Mucosa, Open Approach
0CX4XZZ Transfer Buccal Mucosa, External Approach
0CX50ZZ Transfer Upper Gingiva, Open Approach
0CX5XZZ Transfer Upper Gingiva, External Approach
0CX60ZZ Transfer Lower Gingiva, Open Approach
0CX6XZZ Transfer Lower Gingiva, External Approach
0CX70ZZ Transfer Tongue, Open Approach
0CX7XZZ Transfer Tongue, External Approach

Upper Gastrointestinal System

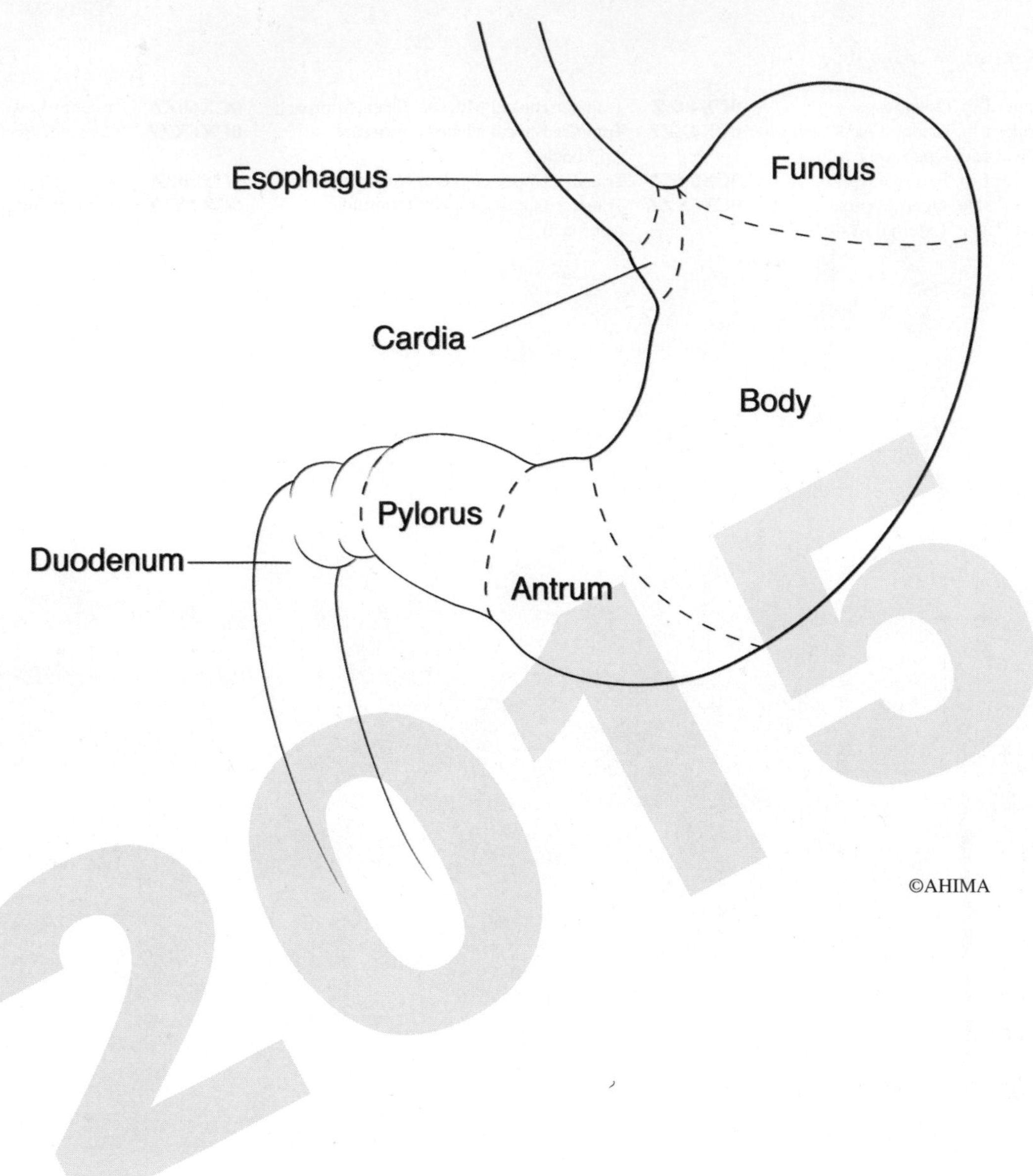

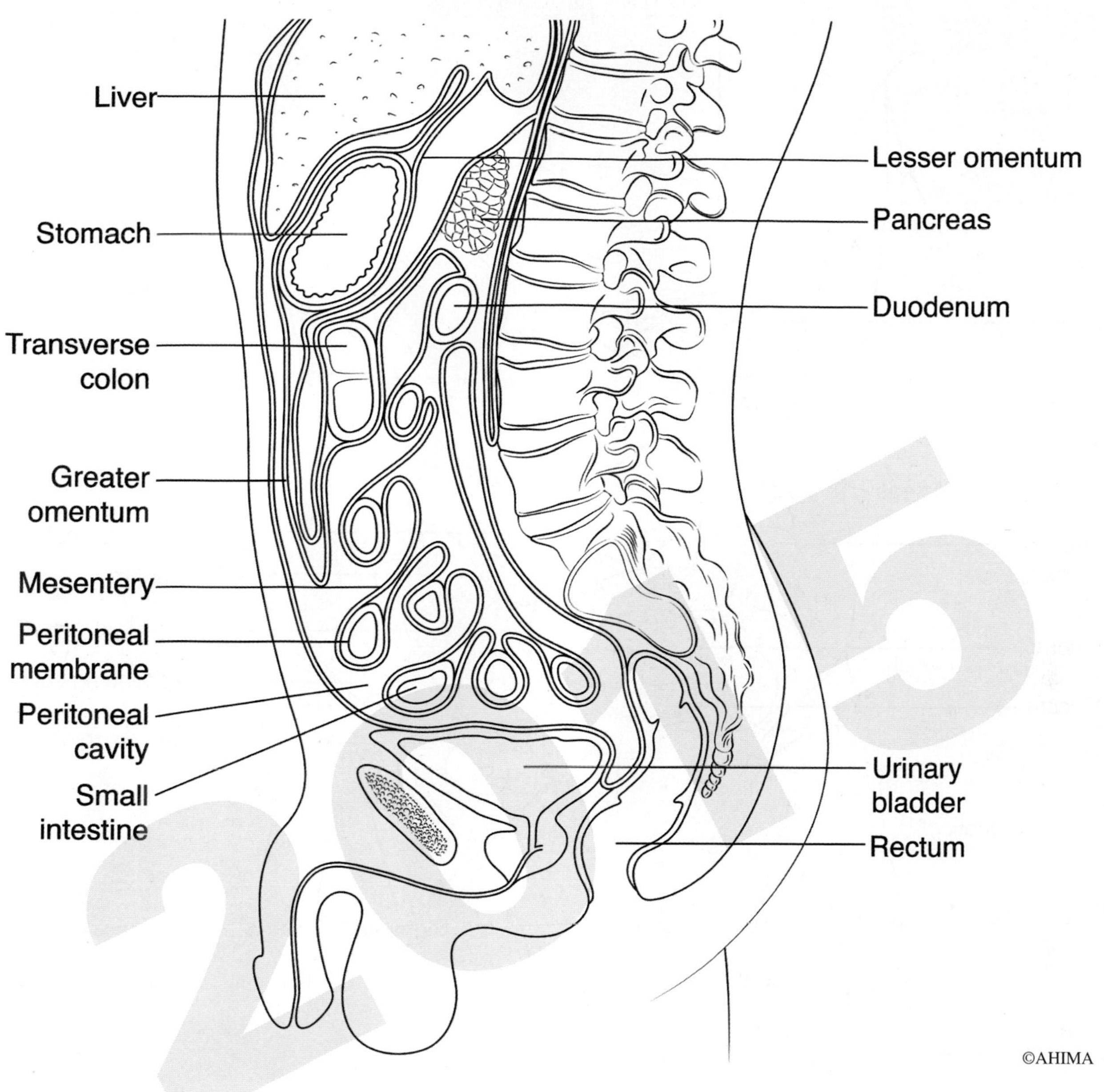
Liver
Stomach
Transverse colon
Greater omentum
Mesentery
Peritoneal membrane
Peritoneal cavity
Small intestine
Lesser omentum
Pancreas
Duodenum
Urinary bladder
Rectum
©AHIMA

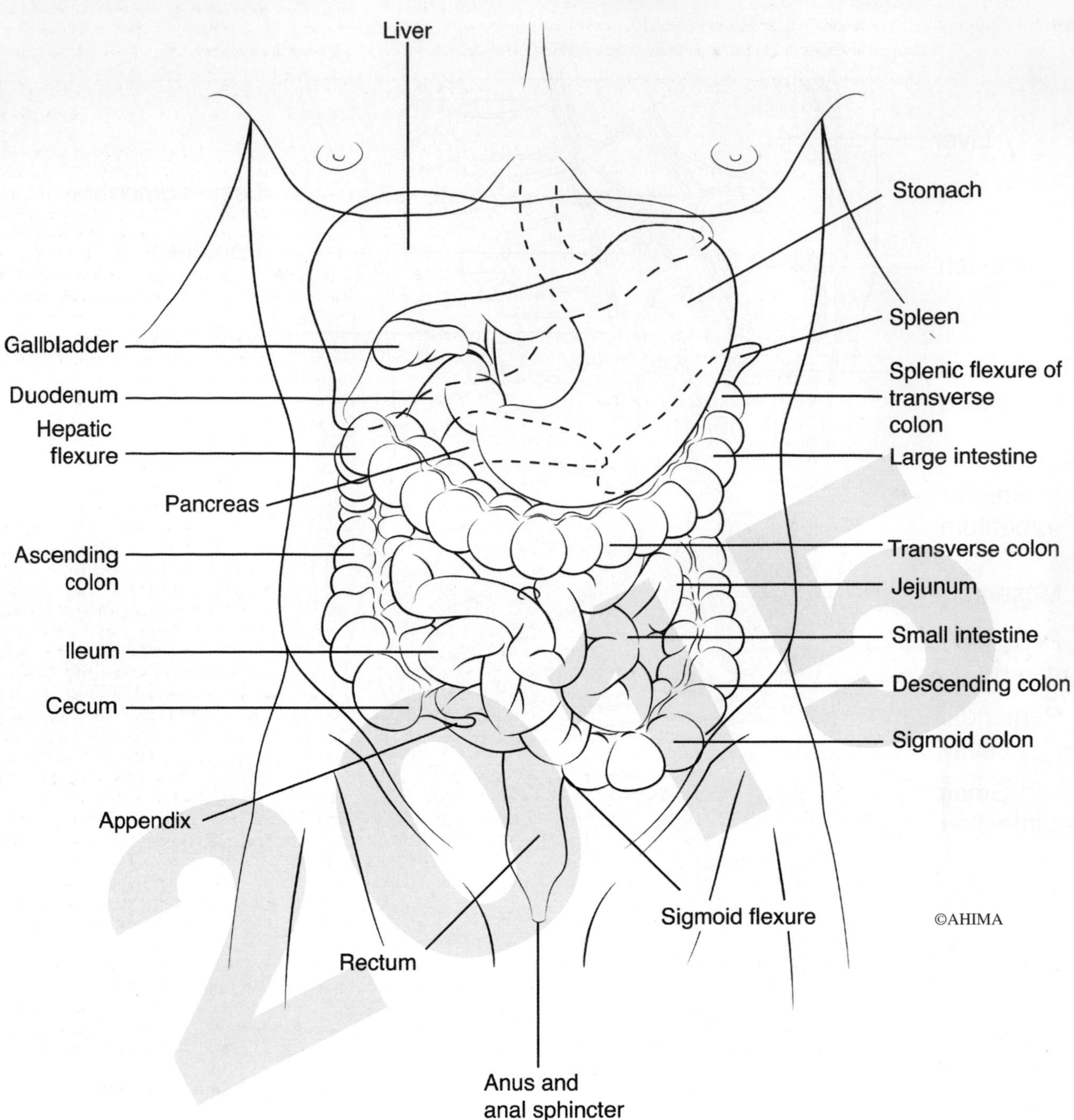
Liver
Stomach
Spleen
Gallbladder
Duodenum
Splenic flexure of transverse colon
Hepatic flexure
Large intestine
Pancreas
Ascending colon
Transverse colon
Jejunum
Small intestine
Ileum
Descending colon
Cecum
Sigmoid colon
Appendix
Sigmoid flexure
©AHIMA
Rectum
Anus and anal sphincter

strointestinal System Tables 0D1–0DY

tion	0	**Medical and Surgical**
dy System	D	**Gastrointestinal System**
eration	1	**Bypass:** Altering the route of passage of the contents of a tubular body part

Body Part (4th)	Approach (5th)	Device (6th)	Qualifier (7th)
Esophagus, Upper Esophagus, Middle Esophagus, Lower Esophagus	**0** Open **4** Percutaneous Endoscopic **8** Via Natural or Artificial Opening Endoscopic	**7** Autologous Tissue Substitute **J** Synthetic Substitute **K** Nonautologous Tissue Substitute **Z** No Device	**4** Cutaneous **6** Stomach **9** Duodenum **A** Jejunum **B** Ileum
Esophagus, Upper Esophagus, Middle Esophagus, Lower Esophagus	**3** Percutaneous	**J** Synthetic Substitute	**4** Cutaneous
Stomach Duodenum	**0** Open **4** Percutaneous Endoscopic **8** Via Natural or Artificial Opening Endoscopic	**7** Autologous Tissue Substitute **J** Synthetic Substitute **K** Nonautologous Tissue Substitute **Z** No Device	**4** Cutaneous **9** Duodenum **A** Jejunum **B** Ileum **L** Transverse Colon
Stomach Duodenum	**3** Percutaneous	**J** Synthetic Substitute	**4** Cutaneous
A Jejunum	**0** Open **4** Percutaneous Endoscopic **8** Via Natural or Artificial Opening Endoscopic	**7** Autologous Tissue Substitute **J** Synthetic Substitute **K** Nonautologous Tissue Substitute **Z** No Device	**4** Cutaneous **A** Jejunum **B** Ileum **H** Cecum **K** Ascending Colon **L** Transverse Colon **M** Descending Colon **N** Sigmoid Colon **P** Rectum **Q** Anus
A Jejunum	**3** Percutaneous	**J** Synthetic Substitute	**4** Cutaneous
B Ileum	**0** Open **4** Percutaneous Endoscopic **8** Via Natural or Artificial Opening Endoscopic	**7** Autologous Tissue Substitute **J** Synthetic Substitute **K** Nonautologous Tissue Substitute **Z** No Device	**4** Cutaneous **B** Ileum **H** Cecum **K** Ascending Colon **L** Transverse Colon **M** Descending Colon **N** Sigmoid Colon **P** Rectum **Q** Anus
B Ileum	**3** Percutaneous	**J** Synthetic Substitute	**4** Cutaneous
H Cecum	**0** Open **4** Percutaneous Endoscopic **8** Via Natural or Artificial Opening Endoscopic	**7** Autologous Tissue Substitute **J** Synthetic Substitute **K** Nonautologous Tissue Substitute **Z** No Device	**4** Cutaneous **H** Cecum **K** Ascending Colon **L** Transverse Colon **M** Descending Colon **N** Sigmoid Colon **P** Rectum
H Cecum	**3** Percutaneous	**J** Synthetic Substitute	**4** Cutaneous
K Ascending Colon	**0** Open **4** Percutaneous Endoscopic **8** Via Natural or Artificial Opening Endoscopic	**7** Autologous Tissue Substitute **J** Synthetic Substitute **K** Nonautologous Tissue Substitute **Z** No Device	**4** Cutaneous **K** Ascending Colon **L** Transverse Colon **M** Descending Colon **N** Sigmoid Colon **P** Rectum
K Ascending Colon	**3** Percutaneous	**J** Synthetic Substitute	**4** Cutaneous

Continued →

0D1 Contin

Section 0 **Medical and Surgical**
Body System D **Gastrointestinal System**
Operation 1 **Bypass:** Altering the route of passage of the contents of a tubular body part

Body Part (4th)	Approach (5th)	Device (6th)	Qualifier (7th)
L Transverse Colon	**0** Open **4** Percutaneous Endoscopic **8** Via Natural or Artificial Opening Endoscopic	**7** Autologous Tissue Substitute **J** Synthetic Substitute **K** Nonautologous Tissue Substitute **Z** No Device	**4** Cutaneous **L** Transverse Colon **M** escending Colon **N** Sigmoid Colon **P** Rectum
L Transverse Colon	**3** Percutaneous	**J** Synthetic Substitute	**4** Cutaneous
M Descending Colon	**0** Open **4** Percutaneous Endoscopic **8** Via Natural or Artificial Opening Endoscopic	**7** Autologous Tissue Substitute **J** Synthetic Substitute **K** Nonautologous Tissue Substitute **Z** No Device	**4** Cutaneous **M** Descending Colon **N** Sigmoid Colon **P** Rectum
M Descending Colon	**3** Percutaneous	**J** Synthetic Substitute	**4** Cutaneous
N Sigmoid Colon	**0** Open **4** Percutaneous Endoscopic **8** Via Natural or Artificial Opening Endoscopic	**7** Autologous Tissue Substitute **J** Synthetic Substitute **K** Nonautologous Tissue Substitute **Z** No Device	**4** Cutaneous **N** Sigmoid Colon **P** Rectum
N Sigmoid Colon	**3** Percutaneous	**J** Synthetic Substitute	**4** Cutaneous

Section 0 **Medical and Surgical**
Body System D **Gastrointestinal System**
Operation 2 **Change:** Taking out or off a device from a body part and putting back an identical or similar device in or on the same body part without cutting or puncturing the skin or a mucous membrane

Body Part (4th)	Approach (5th)	Device (6th)	Qualifier (7th)
0 Upper Intestinal Tract **D** Lower Intestinal Tract	**X** External	**0** Drainage Device **U** Feeding Device **Y** Other Device	**Z** No Qualifier
U Omentum **V** Mesentery **W** Peritoneum	**X** External	**0** Drainage Device **Y** Other Device	**Z** No Qualifier

tion	0	**Medical and Surgical**
dy System	D	**Gastrointestinal System**
eration	5	**Destruction:** Physical eradication of all or a portion of a body part by the direct use of energy, force, or a destructive agent

Body Part (4th)	Approach (5th)	Device (6th)	Qualifier (7th)
Esophagus, Upper Esophagus, Middle Esophagus, Lower Esophagogastric Junction Esophagus Stomach Stomach, Pylorus Small Intestine Duodenum A Jejunum B Ileum C Ileocecal Valve E Large Intestine F Large Intestine, Right G Large Intestine, Left H Cecum J Appendix K Ascending Colon L Transverse Colon M Descending Colon N Sigmoid Colon P Rectum	0 Open 3 Percutaneous 4 Percutaneous Endoscopic 7 Via Natural or Artificial Opening 8 Via Natural or Artificial Opening Endoscopic	Z No Device	Z No Qualifier
Q Anus	0 Open 3 Percutaneous 4 Percutaneous Endoscopic 7 Via Natural or Artificial Opening 8 Via Natural or Artificial Opening Endoscopic X External	Z No Device	Z No Qualifier
R Anal Sphincter S Greater Omentum T Lesser Omentum V Mesentery W Peritoneum	0 Open 3 Percutaneous 4 Percutaneous Endoscopic	Z No Device	Z No Qualifier

ction	0	**Medical and Surgical**
dy System	D	**Gastrointestinal System**
peration	7	**Dilation:** Expanding an orifice or the lumen of a tubular body part

Body Part (4th)	Approach (5th)	Device (6th)	Qualifier (7th)
1 Esophagus, Upper 2 Esophagus, Middle 3 Esophagus, Lower 4 Esophagogastric Junction 5 Esophagus 6 Stomach 7 Stomach, Pylorus 8 Small Intestine 9 Duodenum A Jejunum B Ileum C Ileocecal Valve E Large Intestine F Large Intestine, Right G Large Intestine, Left H Cecum K Ascending Colon L Transverse Colon M Descending Colon N Sigmoid Colon P Rectum Q Anus	0 Open 3 Percutaneous 4 Percutaneous Endoscopic 7 Via Natural or Artificial Opening 8 Via Natural or Artificial Opening Endoscopic	D Intraluminal Device Z No Device	Z No Qualifier

Section 0 **Medical and Surgical**
Body System D **Gastrointestinal System**
Operation 8 **Division:** Cutting into a body part, without draining fluids and/or gases from the body part, in order to separate or transect a body part

Body Part (4th)	Approach (5th)	Device (6th)	Qualifier (7th)
4 Esophagogastric Junction **7** Stomach, Pylorus	**0** Open **3** Percutaneous **4** Percutaneous Endoscopic **7** Via Natural or Artificial Opening **8** Via Natural or Artificial Opening Endoscopic	**Z** No Device	**Z** No Qualifier
R Anal Sphincter	**0** Open **3** Percutaneous	**Z** No Device	**Z** No Qualifier

Section 0 **Medical and Surgical**
Body System D **Gastrointestinal System**
Operation 9 **Drainage:** Taking or letting out fluids and/or gases from a body part

Body Part (4th)	Approach (5th)	Device (6th)	Qualifier (7th)
1 Esophagus, Upper **2** Esophagus, Middle **3** Esophagus, Lower **4** Esophagogastric Junction **5** Esophagus **6** Stomach **7** Stomach, Pylorus **8** Small Intestine **9** Duodenum **A** Jejunum **B** Ileum **C** Ileocecal Valve **E** Large Intestine **F** Large Intestine, Right **G** Large Intestine, Left **H** Cecum **J** Appendix **K** Ascending Colon **L** Transverse Colon **M** Descending Colon **N** Sigmoid Colon **P** Rectum	**0** Open **3** Percutaneous **4** Percutaneous Endoscopic **7** Via Natural or Artificial Opening **8** Via Natural or Artificial Opening Endoscopic	**0** Drainage Device	**Z** No Qualifier
1 Esophagus, Upper **2** Esophagus, Middle **3** Esophagus, Lower **4** Esophagogastric Junction **5** Esophagus **6** Stomach **7** Stomach, Pylorus **8** Small Intestine **9** Duodenum **A** Jejunum **B** Ileum **C** Ileocecal Valve **E** Large Intestine **F** Large Intestine, Right **G** Large Intestine, Left **H** Cecum **J** Appendix **K** Ascending Colon **L** Transverse Colon **M** Descending Colon **N** Sigmoid Colon **P** Rectum	**0** Open **3** Percutaneous **4** Percutaneous Endoscopic **7** Via Natural or Artificial Opening **8** Via Natural or Artificial Opening Endoscopic	**Z** No Device	**X** Diagnostic **Z** No Qualifier

Continued →

Section 0 Medical and Surgical
Body System D Gastrointestinal System
Operation 9 Drainage: Taking or letting out fluids and/or gases from a body part

Body Part (4th)	Approach (5th)	Device (6th)	Qualifier (7th)
Q Anus	0 Open 3 Percutaneous 4 Percutaneous Endoscopic 7 Via Natural or Artificial Opening 8 Via Natural or Artificial Opening Endoscopic X External	0 Drainage Device	Z No Qualifier
Q Anus	0 Open 3 Percutaneous 4 Percutaneous Endoscopic 7 Via Natural or Artificial Opening 8 Via Natural or Artificial Opening Endoscopic X External	Z No Device	X Diagnostic Z No Qualifier
R Anal Sphincter S Greater Omentum T Lesser Omentum V Mesentery W Peritoneum	0 Open 3 Percutaneous 4 Percutaneous Endoscopic	0 Drainage Device	Z No Qualifier
R Anal Sphincter S Greater Omentum T Lesser Omentum V Mesentery W Peritoneum	0 Open 3 Percutaneous 4 Percutaneous Endoscopic	Z No Device	X Diagnostic Z No Qualifier

Section 0 Medical and Surgical
Body System D Gastrointestinal System
Operation B Excision: Cutting out or off, without replacement, a portion of a body part

Body Part (4th)	Approach (5th)	Device (6th)	Qualifier (7th)
1 Esophagus, Upper 2 Esophagus, Middle 3 Esophagus, Lower 4 Esophagogastric Junction 5 Esophagus 7 Stomach, Pylorus 8 Small Intestine 9 Duodenum A Jejunum B Ileum C Ileocecal Valve E Large Intestine F Large Intestine, Right G Large Intestine, Left H Cecum J Appendix K Ascending Colon L Transverse Colon M Descending Colon N Sigmoid Colon P Rectum	0 Open 3 Percutaneous 4 Percutaneous Endoscopic 7 Via Natural or Artificial Opening 8 Via Natural or Artificial Opening Endoscopic	Z No Device	X Diagnostic Z No Qualifier
6 Stomach	0 Open 3 Percutaneous 4 Percutaneous Endoscopic 7 Via Natural or Artificial Opening 8 Via Natural or Artificial Opening Endoscopic	Z No Device	3 Vertical X Diagnostic Z No Qualifier

Continued →

Section 0 **Medical and Surgical**
Body System D **Gastrointestinal System**
Operation B **Excision:** Cutting out or off, without replacement, a portion of a body part

Body Part (4th)	Approach (5th)	Device (6th)	Qualifier (7th)
Q Anus	**0** Open **3** Percutaneous **4** Percutaneous Endoscopic **7** Via Natural or Artificial Opening **8** Via Natural or Artificial Opening Endoscopic **X** External	**Z** No Device	**X** Diagnostic **Z** No Qualifier
R Anal Sphincter **S** Greater Omentum **T** Lesser Omentum **V** Mesentery **W** Peritoneum	**0** Open **3** Percutaneous **4** Percutaneous Endoscopic	**Z** No Device	**X** Diagnostic **Z** No Qualifier

Section 0 **Medical and Surgical**
Body System D **Gastrointestinal System**
Operation C **Extirpation:** Taking or cutting out solid matter from a body part

Body Part (4th)	Approach (5th)	Device (6th)	Qualifier (7th)
1 Esophagus, Upper **2** Esophagus, Middle **3** Esophagus, Lower **4** Esophagogastric Junction **5** Esophagus **6** Stomach **7** Stomach, Pylorus **8** Small Intestine **9** Duodenum **A** Jejunum **B** Ileum **C** Ileocecal Valve **E** Large Intestine **F** Large Intestine, Right **G** Large Intestine, Left **H** Cecum **J** Appendix **K** Ascending Colon **L** Transverse Colon **M** Descending Colon **N** Sigmoid Colon **P** Rectum	**0** Open **3** Percutaneous **4** Percutaneous Endoscopic **7** Via Natural or Artificial Opening **8** Via Natural or Artificial Opening Endoscopic	**Z** No Device	**Z** No Qualifier
Q Anus	**0** Open **3** Percutaneous **4** Percutaneous Endoscopic **7** Via Natural or Artificial Opening **8** Via Natural or Artificial Opening Endoscopic **X** External	**Z** No Device	**Z** No Qualifier
R Anal Sphincter **S** Greater Omentum **T** Lesser Omentum **V** Mesentery **W** Peritoneum	**0** Open **3** Percutaneous **4** Percutaneous Endoscopic	**Z** No Device	**Z** No Qualifier

tion 0 **Medical and Surgical**
ly System D **Gastrointestinal System**
eration F **Fragmentation:** Breaking solid matter in a body part into pieces

Body Part (4th)	Approach (5th)	Device (6th)	Qualifier (7th)
Esophagus Stomach Small Intestine Duodenum Jejunum Ileum Large Intestine Large Intestine, Right Large Intestine, Left Cecum Appendix Ascending Colon Transverse Colon Descending Colon Sigmoid Colon Rectum Anus	**0** Open **3** Percutaneous **4** Percutaneous Endoscopic **7** Via Natural or Artificial Opening **8** Via Natural or Artificial Opening Endoscopic **X** External	**Z** No Device	**Z** No Qualifier

ction 0 **Medical and Surgical**
dy System D **Gastrointestinal System**
eration H **Insertion:** Putting in a nonbiological appliance that monitors, assists, performs, or prevents a physiological function but does not physically take the place of a body part

Body Part (4th)	Approach (5th)	Device (6th)	Qualifier (7th)
5 Esophagus	**0** Open **3** Percutaneous **4** Percutaneous Endoscopic	**1** Radioactive Element **2** Monitoring Device **3** Infusion Device **D** Intraluminal Device **U** Feeding Device	**Z** No Qualifier
5 Esophagus	**7** Via Natural or Artificial Opening **8** Via Natural or Artificial Opening Endoscopic	**1** Radioactive Element **2** Monitoring Device **3** Infusion Device **B** Intraluminal Device, Airway **D** Intraluminal Device **U** Feeding Device	**Z** No Qualifier
6 Stomach	**0** Open **3** Percutaneous **4** Percutaneous Endoscopic	**2** Monitoring Device **3** Infusion Device **D** Intraluminal Device **M** Stimulator Lead **U** Feeding Device	**Z** No Qualifier
6 Stomach	**7** Via Natural or Artificial Opening **8** Via Natural or Artificial Opening Endoscopic	**2** Monitoring Device **3** Infusion Device **D** Intraluminal Device **U** Feeding Device	**Z** No Qualifier
8 Small Intestine **9** Duodenum **A** Jejunum **B** Ileum	**0** Open **3** Percutaneous **4** Percutaneous Endoscopic **7** Via Natural or Artificial Opening **8** Via Natural or Artificial Opening Endoscopic	**2** Monitoring Device **3** Infusion Device **D** Intraluminal Device **U** Feeding Device	**Z** No Qualifier
E Large Intestine	**0** Open **3** Percutaneous **4** Percutaneous Endoscopic **7** Via Natural or Artificial Opening **8** Via Natural or Artificial Opening Endoscopic	**D** Intraluminal Device	**Z** No Qualifier

Continued →

0DH Continu

Section 0 **Medical and Surgical**
Body System D **Gastrointestinal System**
Operation H **Insertion:** Putting in a nonbiological appliance that monitors, assists, performs, or prevents a physiological function but doe not physically take the place of a body part

Body Part (4th)	Approach (5th)	Device (6th)	Qualifier (7th)
P Rectum	**0** Open **3** Percutaneous **4** Percutaneous Endoscopic **7** Via Natural or Artificial Opening **8** Via Natural or Artificial Opening Endoscopic	**1** Radioactive Element **D** Intraluminal Device	**Z** No Qualifier
Q Anus	**0** Open **3** Percutaneous **4** Percutaneous Endoscopic	**D** Intraluminal Device **L** Artificial Sphincter	**Z** No Qualifier
Q Anus	**7** Via Natural or Artificial Opening **8** Via Natural or Artificial Opening Endoscopic	**D** Intraluminal Device	**Z** No Qualifier
R Anal Sphincter	**0** Open **3** Percutaneous **4** Percutaneous Endoscopic	**M** Stimulator Lead	**Z** No Qualifier

Section 0 **Medical and Surgical**
Body System D **Gastrointestinal System**
Operation J **Inspection:** Visually and/or manually exploring a body part

Body Part (4th)	Approach (5th)	Device (6th)	Qualifier (7th)
0 Upper Intestinal Tract **6** Stomach **D** Lower Intestinal Tract	**0** Open **3** Percutaneous **4** Percutaneous Endoscopic **7** Via Natural or Artificial Opening **8** Via Natural or Artificial Opening Endoscopic **X** External	**Z** No Device	**Z** No Qualifier
U Omentum **V** Mesentery **W** Peritoneum	**0** Open **3** Percutaneous **4** Percutaneous Endoscopic **X** External	**Z** No Device	**Z** No Qualifier

Section 0 **Medical and Surgical**
Body System D **Gastrointestinal System**
Operation L **Occlusion:** Completely closing an orifice or the lumen of a tubular body part

Body Part (4th)	Approach (5th)	Device (6th)	Qualifier (7th)
1 Esophagus, Upper **2** Esophagus, Middle **3** Esophagus, Lower **4** Esophagogastric Junction **5** Esophagus **6** Stomach **7** Stomach, Pylorus **8** Small Intestine **9** Duodenum **A** Jejunum **B** Ileum **C** Ileocecal Valve **E** Large Intestine **F** Large Intestine, Right **G** Large Intestine, Left **H** Cecum **K** Ascending Colon **L** Transverse Colon **M** Descending Colon **N** Sigmoid Colon **P** Rectum	**0** Open **3** Percutaneous **4** Percutaneous Endoscopic	**C** Extraluminal Device **D** Intraluminal Device **Z** No Device	**Z** No Qualifier

Continued →

Section 0 **Medical and Surgical**
Body System D **Gastrointestinal System**
Operation L **Occlusion:** Completely closing an orifice or the lumen of a tubular body part

Body Part (4th)	Approach (5th)	Device (6th)	Qualifier (7th)
Esophagus, Upper **2** Esophagus, Middle **3** Esophagus, Lower **4** Esophagogastric Junction **5** Esophagus **6** Stomach **7** Stomach, Pylorus **8** Small Intestine **9** Duodenum **A** Jejunum **B** Ileum **C** Ileocecal Valve **E** Large Intestine **F** Large Intestine, Right **G** Large Intestine, Left **H** Cecum **K** Ascending Colon **L** Transverse Colon **M** Descending Colon **N** Sigmoid Colon **P** Rectum	**7** Via Natural or Artificial Opening **8** Via Natural or Artificial Opening Endoscopic	**D** Intraluminal Device **Z** No Device	**Z** No Qualifier
Q Anus	**0** Open **3** Percutaneous **4** Percutaneous Endoscopic **X** External	**C** Extraluminal Device **D** Intraluminal Device **Z** No Device	**Z** No Qualifier
Q Anus	**7** Via Natural or Artificial Opening **8** Via Natural or Artificial Opening Endoscopic	**D** Intraluminal Device **Z** No Device	**Z** No Qualifier

Section 0 **Medical and Surgical**
Body System D **Gastrointestinal System**
Operation M **Reattachment:** Putting back in or on all or a portion of a separated body part to its normal location or other suitable location

Body Part (4th)	Approach (5th)	Device (6th)	Qualifier (7th)
5 Esophagus **6** Stomach **8** Small Intestine **9** Duodenum **A** Jejunum **B** Ileum **E** Large Intestine **F** Large Intestine, Right **G** Large Intestine, Left **H** Cecum **K** Ascending Colon **L** Transverse Colon **M** Descending Colon **N** Sigmoid Colon **P** Rectum	**0** Open **4** Percutaneous Endoscopic	**Z** No Device	**Z** No Qualifier

Section 0 **Medical and Surgical**
Body System D **Gastrointestinal System**
Operation N **Release:** Freeing a body part from an abnormal physical constraint by cutting or by the use of force

Body Part (4th)	Approach (5th)	Device (6th)	Qualifier (7th)
1 Esophagus, Upper **2** Esophagus, Middle **3** Esophagus, Lower **4** Esophagogastric Junction **5** Esophagus **6** Stomach **7** Stomach, Pylorus **8** Small Intestine **9** Duodenum **A** Jejunum **B** Ileum **C** Ileocecal Valve **E** Large Intestine **F** Large Intestine, Right **G** Large Intestine, Left **H** Cecum **J** Appendix **K** Ascending Colon **L** Transverse Colon **M** Descending Colon **N** Sigmoid Colon **P** Rectum	**0** Open **3** Percutaneous **4** Percutaneous Endoscopic **7** Via Natural or Artificial Opening **8** Via Natural or Artificial Opening Endoscopic	**Z** No Device	**Z** No Qualifier
Q Anus	**0** Open **3** Percutaneous **4** Percutaneous Endoscopic **7** Via Natural or Artificial Opening **8** Via Natural or Artificial Opening Endoscopic **X** External	**Z** No Device	**Z** No Qualifier
R Anal Sphincter **S** Greater Omentum **T** Lesser Omentum **V** Mesentery **W** Peritoneum	**0** Open **3** Percutaneous **4** Percutaneous Endoscopic	**Z** No Device	**Z** No Qualifier

Section 0 **Medical and Surgical**
Body System D **Gastrointestinal System**
Operation P **Removal:** Taking out or off a device from a body part

Body Part (4th)	Approach (5th)	Device (6th)	Qualifier (7th)
0 Upper Intestinal Tract **D** Lower Intestinal Tract	**0** Open **3** Percutaneous **4** Percutaneous Endoscopic **7** Via Natural or Artificial Opening **8** Via Natural or Artificial Opening Endoscopic	**0** Drainage Device **2** Monitoring Device **3** Infusion Device **7** Autologous Tissue Substitute **C** Extraluminal Device **D** Intraluminal Device **J** Synthetic Substitute **K** Nonautologous Tissue Substitute **U** Feeding Device	**Z** No Qualifier
0 Upper Intestinal Tract **D** Lower Intestinal Tract	**X** External	**0** Drainage Device **2** Monitoring Device **3** Infusion Device **D** Intraluminal Device **U** Feeding Device	**Z** No Qualifier
5 Esophagus	**0** Open **3** Percutaneous **4** Percutaneous Endoscopic	**1** Radioactive Element **2** Monitoring Device **3** Infusion Device **U** Feeding Device	**Z** No Qualifier

Continued →

ction	**0**	**Medical and Surgical**
dy System	**D**	**Gastrointestinal System**
eration	**P**	**Removal:** Taking out or off a device from a body part

Body Part (4th)	Approach (5th)	Device (6th)	Qualifier (7th)
5 Esophagus	**7** Via Natural or Artificial Opening **8** Via Natural or Artificial Opening Endoscopic	**1** Radioactive Element **D** Intraluminal Device	**Z** No Qualifier
5 Esophagus	**X** External	**1** Radioactive Element **2** Monitoring Device **3** Infusion Device **D** Intraluminal Device **U** Feeding Device	**Z** No Qualifier
6 Stomach	**0** Open **3** Percutaneous **4** Percutaneous Endoscopic	**0** Drainage Device **2** Monitoring Device **3** Infusion Device **7** Autologous Tissue Substitute **C** Extraluminal Device **D** Intraluminal Device **J** Synthetic Substitute **K** Nonautologous Tissue Substitute **M** Stimulator Lead **U** Feeding Device	**Z** No Qualifier
6 Stomach	**7** Via Natural or Artificial Opening **8** Via Natural or Artificial Opening Endoscopic	**0** Drainage Device **2** Monitoring Device **3** Infusion Device **7** Autologous Tissue Substitute **C** Extraluminal Device **D** Intraluminal Device **J** Synthetic Substitute **K** Nonautologous Tissue Substitute **U** Feeding Device	**Z** No Qualifier
6 Stomach	**X** External	**0** Drainage Device **2** Monitoring Device **3** Infusion Device **D** Intraluminal Device **U** Feeding Device	**Z** No Qualifier
P Rectum	**0** Open **3** Percutaneous **4** Percutaneous Endoscopic **7** Via Natural or Artificial Opening **8** Via Natural or Artificial Opening Endoscopic **X** External	**1** Radioactive Element	**Z** No Qualifier
Q Anus	**0** Open **3** Percutaneous **4** Percutaneous Endoscopic **7** Via Natural or Artificial Opening **8** Via Natural or Artificial Opening Endoscopic	**L** Artificial Sphincter	**Z** No Qualifier
R Anal Sphincter	**0** Open **3** Percutaneous **4** Percutaneous Endoscopic	**M** Stimulator Lead	**Z** No Qualifier
U Omentum **V** Mesentery **W** Peritoneum	**0** Open **3** Percutaneous **4** Percutaneous Endoscopic	**0** Drainage Device **1** Radioactive Element **7** Autologous Tissue Substitute **J** Synthetic Substitute **K** Nonautologous Tissue Substitute	**Z** No Qualifier

Section 0 **Medical and Surgical**
Body System D **Gastrointestinal System**
Operation Q **Repair:** Restoring, to the extent possible, a body part to its normal anatomic structure and function

Body Part (4th)	Approach (5th)	Device (6th)	Qualifier (7th)
1 Esophagus, Upper **2** Esophagus, Middle **3** Esophagus, Lower **4** Esophagogastric Junction **5** Esophagus **6** Stomach **7** Stomach, Pylorus **8** Small Intestine **9** Duodenum **A** Jejunum **B** Ileum **C** Ileocecal Valve **E** Large Intestine **F** Large Intestine, Right **G** Large Intestine, Left **H** Cecum **J** Appendix **K** Ascending Colon **L** Transverse Colon **M** Descending Colon **N** Sigmoid Colon **P** Rectum	**0** Open **3** Percutaneous **4** Percutaneous Endoscopic **7** Via Natural or Artificial Opening **8** Via Natural or Artificial Opening Endoscopic	**Z** No Device	**Z** No Qualifier
Q Anus	**0** Open **3** Percutaneous **4** Percutaneous Endoscopic **7** Via Natural or Artificial Opening **8** Via Natural or Artificial Opening Endoscopic **X** External	**Z** No Device	**Z** No Qualifier
R Anal Sphincter **S** Greater Omentum **T** Lesser Omentum **V** Mesentery **W** Peritoneum	**0** Open **3** Percutaneous **4** Percutaneous Endoscopic	**Z** No Device	**Z** No Qualifier

Section 0 **Medical and Surgical**
Body System D **Gastrointestinal System**
Operation R **Replacement:** Putting in or on biological or synthetic material that physically takes the place and/or function of all or a portion of a body part

Body Part (4th)	Approach (5th)	Device (6th)	Qualifier (7th)
5 Esophagus	**0** Open **4** Percutaneous Endoscopic **7** Via Natural or Artificial Opening **8** Via Natural or Artificial Opening Endoscopic	**7** Autologous Tissue Substitute **J** Synthetic Substitute **K** Nonautologous Tissue Substitute	**Z** No Qualifier
R Anal Sphincter **S** Greater Omentum **T** Lesser Omentum **V** Mesentery **W** Peritoneum	**0** Open **4** Percutaneous Endoscopic	**7** Autologous Tissue Substitute **J** Synthetic Substitute **K** Nonautologous Tissue Substitute	**Z** No Qualifier

tion	0	**Medical and Surgical**
dy System	D	**Gastrointestinal System**
eration	S	**Reposition:** Moving to its normal location, or other suitable location, all or a portion of a body part

Body Part (4th)	Approach (5th)	Device (6th)	Qualifier (7th)
Esophagus Stomach Duodenum A Jejunum B Ileum H Cecum K Ascending Colon L Transverse Colon M Descending Colon N Sigmoid Colon P Rectum Q Anus	**0** Open **4** Percutaneous Endoscopic **7** Via Natural or Artificial Opening **8** Via Natural or Artificial Opening Endoscopic **X** External	**Z** No Device	**Z** No Qualifier

ction	0	**Medical and Surgical**
dy System	D	**Gastrointestinal System**
peration	T	**Resection:** Cutting out or off, without replacement, all of a body part

Body Part (4th)	Approach (5th)	Device (6th)	Qualifier (7th)
1 Esophagus, Upper **2** Esophagus, Middle **3** Esophagus, Lower **4** Esophagogastric Junction **5** Esophagus **6** Stomach **7** Stomach, Pylorus **8** Small Intestine **9** Duodenum **A** Jejunum **B** Ileum **C** Ileocecal Valve **E** Large Intestine **F** Large Intestine, Right **G** Large Intestine, Left **H** Cecum **J** Appendix **K** Ascending Colon **L** Transverse Colon **M** Descending Colon **N** Sigmoid Colon **P** Rectum **Q** Anus	**0** Open **4** Percutaneous Endoscopic **7** Via Natural or Artificial Opening **8** Via Natural or Artificial Opening Endoscopic	**Z** No Device	**Z** No Qualifier
R Anal Sphincter **S** Greater Omentum **T** Lesser Omentum	**0** Open **4** Percutaneous Endoscopic	**Z** No Device	**Z** No Qualifier

Section 0 **Medical and Surgical**
Body System D **Gastrointestinal System**
Operation U **Supplement:** Putting in or on biological or synthetic material that physically reinforces and/or augments the function of a portion of a body part

Body Part (4th)	Approach (5th)	Device (6th)	Qualifier (7th)
1 Esophagus, Upper **2** Esophagus, Middle **3** Esophagus, Lower **4** Esophagogastric Junction **5** Esophagus **6** Stomach **7** Stomach, Pylorus **8** Small Intestine **9** Duodenum **A** Jejunum **B** Ileum **C** Ileocecal Valve **E** Large Intestine **F** Large Intestine, Right **G** Large Intestine, Left **H** Cecum **K** Ascending Colon **L** Transverse Colon **M** Descending Colon **N** Sigmoid Colon **P** Rectum	**0** Open **4** Percutaneous Endoscopic **7** Via Natural or Artificial Opening **8** Via Natural or Artificial Opening Endoscopic	**7** Autologous Tissue Substitute **J** Synthetic Substitute **K** Nonautologous Tissue Substitute	**Z** No Qualifier
Q Anus	**0** Open **4** Percutaneous Endoscopic **7** Via Natural or Artificial Opening **8** Via Natural or Artificial Opening Endoscopic **X** External	**7** Autologous Tissue Substitute **J** Synthetic Substitute **K** Nonautologous Tissue Substitute	**Z** No Qualifier
R Anal Sphincter **S** Greater Omentum **T** Lesser Omentum **V** Mesentery **W** Peritoneum	**0** Open **4** Percutaneous Endoscopic	**7** Autologous Tissue Substitute **J** Synthetic Substitute **K** Nonautologous Tissue Substitute	**Z** No Qualifier

Section 0 **Medical and Surgical**
Body System D **Gastrointestinal System**
Operation V **Restriction:** Partially closing an orifice or the lumen of a tubular body part

Body Part (4th)	Approach (5th)	Device (6th)	Qualifier (7th)
1 Esophagus, Upper **2** Esophagus, Middle **3** Esophagus, Lower **4** Esophagogastric Junction **5** Esophagus **6** Stomach **7** Stomach, Pylorus **8** Small Intestine **9** Duodenum **A** Jejunum **B** Ileum **C** Ileocecal Valve **E** Large Intestine **F** Large Intestine, Right **G** Large Intestine, Left **H** Cecum **K** Ascending Colon **L** Transverse Colon **M** Descending Colon **N** Sigmoid Colon **P** Rectum	**0** Open **3** Percutaneous **4** Percutaneous Endoscopic	**C** Extraluminal Device **D** Intraluminal Device **Z** No Device	**Z** No Qualifier

Continued →

Section 0 **Medical and Surgical**
Body System D **Gastrointestinal System**
Operation V **Restriction:** Partially closing an orifice or the lumen of a tubular body part

Body Part (4th)	Approach (5th)	Device (6th)	Qualifier (7th)
Esophagus, Upper Esophagus, Middle 3 Esophagus, Lower 4 Esophagogastric Junction 5 Esophagus 6 Stomach 7 Stomach, Pylorus 8 Small Intestine 9 Duodenum A Jejunum B Ileum C Ileocecal Valve E Large Intestine F Large Intestine, Right G Large Intestine, Left H Cecum K Ascending Colon L Transverse Colon M Descending Colon N Sigmoid Colon P Rectum	**7** Via Natural or Artificial Opening **8** Via Natural or Artificial Opening Endoscopic	**D** Intraluminal Device **Z** No Device	**Z** No Qualifier
Q Anus	**0** Open **3** Percutaneous **4** Percutaneous Endoscopic **X** External	**C** Extraluminal Device **D** Intraluminal Device **Z** No Device	**Z** No Qualifier
Q Anus	**7** Via Natural or Artificial Opening **8** Via Natural or Artificial Opening Endoscopic	**D** Intraluminal Device **Z** No Device	**Z** No Qualifier

Section 0 **Medical and Surgical**
Body System D **Gastrointestinal System**
Operation W **Revision:** Correcting, to the extent possible, a portion of a malfunctioning device or the position of a displaced device

Body Part (4th)	Approach (5th)	Device (6th)	Qualifier (7th)
0 Upper Intestinal Tract **D** Lower Intestinal Tract	**0** Open **3** Percutaneous **4** Percutaneous Endoscopic **7** Via Natural or Artificial Opening **8** Via Natural or Artificial Opening Endoscopic **X** External	**0** Drainage Device **2** Monitoring Device **3** Infusion Device **7** Autologous Tissue Substitute **C** Extraluminal Device **D** Intraluminal Device **J** Synthetic Substitute **K** Nonautologous Tissue Substitute **U** Feeding Device	**Z** No Qualifier
5 Esophagus	**7** Via Natural or Artificial Opening **8** Via Natural or Artificial Opening Endoscopic **X** External	**D** Intraluminal Device	**Z** No Qualifier
6 Stomach	**0** Open **3** Percutaneous **4** Percutaneous Endoscopic	**0** Drainage Device **2** Monitoring Device **3** Infusion Device **7** Autologous Tissue Substitute **C** Extraluminal Device **D** Intraluminal Device **J** Synthetic Substitute **K** Nonautologous Tissue Substitute **M** Stimulator Lead **U** Feeding Device	**Z** No Qualifier

Continued →

Section 0 **Medical and Surgical**
Body System D **Gastrointestinal System**
Operation W **Revision:** Correcting, to the extent possible, a portion of a malfunctioning device or the position of a displaced device

Body Part (4th)	Approach (5th)	Device (6th)	Qualifier (7th)
6 Stomach	**7** Via Natural or Artificial Opening **8** Via Natural or Artificial Opening Endoscopic **X** External	**0** Drainage Device **2** Monitoring Device **3** Infusion Device **7** Autologous Tissue Substitute **C** Extraluminal Device **D** Intraluminal Device **J** Synthetic Substitute **K** Nonautologous Tissue Substitute **U** Feeding Device	**Z** No Qualifier
8 Small Intestine **E** Large Intestine	**0** Open **4** Percutaneous Endoscopic **7** Via Natural or Artificial Opening **8** Via Natural or Artificial Opening Endoscopic	**7** Autologous Tissue Substitute **J** Synthetic Substitute **K** Nonautologous Tissue Substitute	**Z** No Qualifier
Q Anus	**0** Open **3** Percutaneous **4** Percutaneous Endoscopic **7** Via Natural or Artificial Opening **8** Via Natural or Artificial Opening Endoscopic	**L** Artificial Sphincter	**Z** No Qualifier
R Anal Sphincter	**0** Open **3** Percutaneous **4** Percutaneous Endoscopic	**M** Stimulator Lead	**Z** No Qualifier
U Omentum **V** Mesentery **W** Peritoneum	**0** Open **3** Percutaneous **4** Percutaneous Endoscopic	**0** Drainage Device **7** Autologous Tissue Substitute **J** Synthetic Substitute **K** Nonautologous Tissue Substitute	**Z** No Qualifier

Section 0 **Medical and Surgical**
Body System D **Gastrointestinal System**
Operation X **Transfer:** Moving, without taking out, all or a portion of a body part to another location to take over the function of all or a portion of a body part

Body Part (4th)	Approach (5th)	Device (6th)	Qualifier (7th)
6 Stomach **8** Small Intestine **E** Large Intestine	**0** Open **4** Percutaneous Endoscopic	**Z** No Device	**5** Esophagus

Section 0 **Medical and Surgical**
Body System D **Gastrointestinal System**
Operation Y **Transplantation:** Putting in or on all or a portion of a living body part taken from another individual or animal to physically take the place and/or function of all or a portion of a similar body part

Body Part (4th)	Approach (5th)	Device (6th)	Qualifier (7th)
5 Esophagus **6** Stomach **8** Small Intestine **E** Large Intestine	**0** Open	**Z** No Device	**0** Allogeneic **1** Syngeneic **2** Zooplastic

strointestinal System Code Listing 0D1–0DY

view Coding Guideline B4.8

1 – Gastrointestinal System, Bypass

view Coding Guideline B3.6a

11074 Bypass Upper Esophagus to Cutaneous with Autologous Tissue Substitute, Open Approach

11076 Bypass Upper Esophagus to Stomach with Autologous Tissue Substitute, Open Approach

11079 Bypass Upper Esophagus to Duodenum with Autologous Tissue Substitute, Open Approach

1107A Bypass Upper Esophagus to Jejunum with Autologous Tissue Substitute, Open Approach

1107B Bypass Upper Esophagus to Ileum with Autologous Tissue Substitute, Open Approach

110J4 Bypass Upper Esophagus to Cutaneous with Synthetic Substitute, Open Approach

110J6 Bypass Upper Esophagus to Stomach with Synthetic Substitute, Open Approach

110J9 Bypass Upper Esophagus to Duodenum with Synthetic Substitute, Open Approach

110JA Bypass Upper Esophagus to Jejunum with Synthetic Substitute, Open Approach

110JB Bypass Upper Esophagus to Ileum with Synthetic Substitute, Open Approach

110K4 Bypass Upper Esophagus to Cutaneous with Nonautologous Tissue Substitute, Open Approach

110K6 Bypass Upper Esophagus to Stomach with Nonautologous Tissue Substitute, Open Approach

110K9 Bypass Upper Esophagus to Duodenum with Nonautologous Tissue Substitute, Open Approach

110KA Bypass Upper Esophagus to Jejunum with Nonautologous Tissue Substitute, Open Approach

110KB Bypass Upper Esophagus to Ileum with Nonautologous Tissue Substitute, Open Approach

110Z4 Bypass Upper Esophagus to Cutaneous, Open Approach

110Z6 Bypass Upper Esophagus to Stomach, Open Approach

110Z9 Bypass Upper Esophagus to Duodenum, Open Approach

110ZA Bypass Upper Esophagus to Jejunum, Open Approach

D110ZB Bypass Upper Esophagus to Ileum, Open Approach

D113J4 Bypass Upper Esophagus to Cutaneous with Synthetic Substitute, Percutaneous Approach

D11474 Bypass Upper Esophagus to Cutaneous with Autologous Tissue Substitute, Percutaneous Endoscopic Approach

D11476 Bypass Upper Esophagus to Stomach with Autologous Tissue Substitute, Percutaneous Endoscopic Approach

D11479 Bypass Upper Esophagus to Duodenum with Autologous Tissue Substitute, Percutaneous Endoscopic Approach

D1147A Bypass Upper Esophagus to Jejunum with Autologous Tissue Substitute, Percutaneous Endoscopic Approach

D1147B Bypass Upper Esophagus to Ileum with Autologous Tissue Substitute, Percutaneous Endoscopic Approach

0D114J4 Bypass Upper Esophagus to Cutaneous with Synthetic Substitute, Percutaneous Endoscopic Approach

0D114J6 Bypass Upper Esophagus to Stomach with Synthetic Substitute, Percutaneous Endoscopic Approach

0D114J9 Bypass Upper Esophagus to Duodenum with Synthetic Substitute, Percutaneous Endoscopic Approach

0D114JA Bypass Upper Esophagus to Jejunum with Synthetic Substitute, Percutaneous Endoscopic Approach

0D114JB Bypass Upper Esophagus to Ileum with Synthetic Substitute, Percutaneous Endoscopic Approach

0D114K4 Bypass Upper Esophagus to Cutaneous with Nonautologous Tissue Substitute, Percutaneous Endoscopic Approach

0D114K6 Bypass Upper Esophagus to Stomach with Nonautologous Tissue Substitute, Percutaneous Endoscopic Approach

0D114K9 Bypass Upper Esophagus to Duodenum with Nonautologous Tissue Substitute, Percutaneous Endoscopic Approach

0D114KA Bypass Upper Esophagus to Jejunum with Nonautologous Tissue Substitute, Percutaneous Endoscopic Approach

0D114KB Bypass Upper Esophagus to Ileum with Nonautologous Tissue Substitute, Percutaneous Endoscopic Approach

0D114Z4 Bypass Upper Esophagus to Cutaneous, Percutaneous Endoscopic Approach

0D114Z6 Bypass Upper Esophagus to Stomach, Percutaneous Endoscopic Approach

0D114Z9 Bypass Upper Esophagus to Duodenum, Percutaneous Endoscopic Approach

0D114ZA Bypass Upper Esophagus to Jejunum, Percutaneous Endoscopic Approach

0D114ZB Bypass Upper Esophagus to Ileum, Percutaneous Endoscopic Approach

0D11874 Bypass Upper Esophagus to Cutaneous with Autologous Tissue Substitute, Via Natural or Artificial Opening Endoscopic

0D11876 Bypass Upper Esophagus to Stomach with Autologous Tissue Substitute, Via Natural or Artificial Opening Endoscopic

0D11879 Bypass Upper Esophagus to Duodenum with Autologous Tissue Substitute, Via Natural or Artificial Opening Endoscopic

0D1187A Bypass Upper Esophagus to Jejunum with Autologous Tissue Substitute, Via Natural or Artificial Opening Endoscopic

0D1187B Bypass Upper Esophagus to Ileum with Autologous Tissue Substitute, Via Natural or Artificial Opening Endoscopic

0D118J4 Bypass Upper Esophagus to Cutaneous with Synthetic Substitute, Via Natural or Artificial Opening Endoscopic

0D118J6 Bypass Upper Esophagus to Stomach with Synthetic Substitute, Via Natural or Artificial Opening Endoscopic

0D118J9 Bypass Upper Esophagus to Duodenum with Synthetic Substitute, Via Natural or Artificial Opening Endoscopic

0D118JA Bypass Upper Esophagus to Jejunum with Synthetic Substitute, Via Natural or Artificial Opening Endoscopic

0D118JB Bypass Upper Esophagus to Ileum with Synthetic Substitute, Via Natural or Artificial Opening Endoscopic

0D118K4 Bypass Upper Esophagus to Cutaneous with Nonautologous Tissue Substitute, Via Natural or Artificial Opening Endoscopic

0D118K6 Bypass Upper Esophagus to Stomach with Nonautologous Tissue Substitute, Via Natural or Artificial Opening Endoscopic

0D118K9 Bypass Upper Esophagus to Duodenum with Nonautologous Tissue Substitute, Via Natural or Artificial Opening Endoscopic

0D118KA Bypass Upper Esophagus to Jejunum with Nonautologous Tissue Substitute, Via Natural or Artificial Opening Endoscopic

0D118KB Bypass Upper Esophagus to Ileum with Nonautologous Tissue Substitute, Via Natural or Artificial Opening Endoscopic

0D118Z4 Bypass Upper Esophagus to Cutaneous, Via Natural or Artificial Opening Endoscopic

0D118Z6 Bypass Upper Esophagus to Stomach, Via Natural or Artificial Opening Endoscopic

0D118Z9 Bypass Upper Esophagus to Duodenum, Via Natural or Artificial Opening Endoscopic

0D118ZA Bypass Upper Esophagus to Jejunum, Via Natural or Artificial Opening Endoscopic

0D118ZB Bypass Upper Esophagus to Ileum, Via Natural or Artificial Opening Endoscopic

0D12074 Bypass Middle Esophagus to Cutaneous with Autologous Tissue Substitute, Open Approach

0D12076 Bypass Middle Esophagus to Stomach with Autologous Tissue Substitute, Open Approach

0D12079 Bypass Middle Esophagus to Duodenum with Autologous Tissue Substitute, Open Approach

0D1207A Bypass Middle Esophagus to Jejunum with Autologous Tissue Substitute, Open Approach

0D1207B Bypass Middle Esophagus to Ileum with Autologous Tissue Substitute, Open Approach

0D120J4 Bypass Middle Esophagus to Cutaneous with Synthetic Substitute, Open Approach

0D120J6 Bypass Middle Esophagus to Stomach with Synthetic Substitute, Open Approach

0D120J9 Bypass Middle Esophagus to Duodenum with Synthetic Substitute, Open Approach

0D120JA Bypass Middle Esophagus to Jejunum with Synthetic Substitute, Open Approach

0D120JB Bypass Middle Esophagus to Ileum with Synthetic Substitute, Open Approach

0D120K4 Bypass Middle Esophagus to Cutaneous with Nonautologous Tissue Substitute, Open Approach

0D120K6 Bypass Middle Esophagus to Stomach with Nonautologous Tissue Substitute, Open Approach

0D120K9 Bypass Middle Esophagus to Duodenum with Nonautologous Tissue Substitute, Open Approach

0D120KA Bypass Middle Esophagus to Jejunum with Nonautologous Tissue Substitute, Open Approach

0D120KB Bypass Middle Esophagus to Ileum with Nonautologous Tissue Substitute, Open Approach

0D120Z4 Bypass Middle Esophagus to Cutaneous, Open Approach

0D120Z6 Bypass Middle Esophagus to Stomach, Open Approach
0D120Z9 Bypass Middle Esophagus to Duodenum, Open Approach
0D120ZA Bypass Middle Esophagus to Jejunum, Open Approach
0D120ZB Bypass Middle Esophagus to Ileum, Open Approach
0D123J4 Bypass Middle Esophagus to Cutaneous with Synthetic Substitute, Percutaneous Approach
0D12474 Bypass Middle Esophagus to Cutaneous with Autologous Tissue Substitute, Percutaneous Endoscopic Approach
0D12476 Bypass Middle Esophagus to Stomach with Autologous Tissue Substitute, Percutaneous Endoscopic Approach
0D12479 Bypass Middle Esophagus to Duodenum with Autologous Tissue Substitute, Percutaneous Endoscopic Approach
0D1247A Bypass Middle Esophagus to Jejunum with Autologous Tissue Substitute, Percutaneous Endoscopic Approach
0D1247B Bypass Middle Esophagus to Ileum with Autologous Tissue Substitute, Percutaneous Endoscopic Approach
0D124J4 Bypass Middle Esophagus to Cutaneous with Synthetic Substitute, Percutaneous Endoscopic Approach
0D124J6 Bypass Middle Esophagus to Stomach with Synthetic Substitute, Percutaneous Endoscopic Approach
0D124J9 Bypass Middle Esophagus to Duodenum with Synthetic Substitute, Percutaneous Endoscopic Approach
0D124JA Bypass Middle Esophagus to Jejunum with Synthetic Substitute, Percutaneous Endoscopic Approach
0D124JB Bypass Middle Esophagus to Ileum with Synthetic Substitute, Percutaneous Endoscopic Approach
0D124K4 Bypass Middle Esophagus to Cutaneous with Nonautologous Tissue Substitute, Percutaneous Endoscopic Approach
0D124K6 Bypass Middle Esophagus to Stomach with Nonautologous Tissue Substitute, Percutaneous Endoscopic Approach
0D124K9 Bypass Middle Esophagus to Duodenum with Nonautologous Tissue Substitute, Percutaneous Endoscopic Approach
0D124KA Bypass Middle Esophagus to Jejunum with Nonautologous Tissue Substitute, Percutaneous Endoscopic Approach
0D124KB Bypass Middle Esophagus to Ileum with Nonautologous Tissue Substitute, Percutaneous Endoscopic Approach
0D124Z4 Bypass Middle Esophagus to Cutaneous, Percutaneous Endoscopic Approach
0D124Z6 Bypass Middle Esophagus to Stomach, Percutaneous Endoscopic Approach
0D124Z9 Bypass Middle Esophagus to Duodenum, Percutaneous Endoscopic Approach
0D124ZA Bypass Middle Esophagus to Jejunum, Percutaneous Endoscopic Approach
0D124ZB Bypass Middle Esophagus to Ileum, Percutaneous Endoscopic Approach
0D12874 Bypass Middle Esophagus to Cutaneous with Autologous Tissue Substitute, Via Natural or Artificial Opening Endoscopic
0D12876 Bypass Middle Esophagus to Stomach with Autologous Tissue Substitute, Via Natural or Artificial Opening Endoscopic
0D12879 Bypass Middle Esophagus to Duodenum with Autologous Tissue Substitute, Via Natural or Artificial Opening Endoscopic
0D1287A Bypass Middle Esophagus to Jejunum with Autologous Tissue Substitute, Via Natural or Artificial Opening Endoscopic
0D1287B Bypass Middle Esophagus to Ileum with Autologous Tissue Substitute, Via Natural or Artificial Opening Endoscopic
0D128J4 Bypass Middle Esophagus to Cutaneous with Synthetic Substitute, Via Natural or Artificial Opening Endoscopic
0D128J6 Bypass Middle Esophagus to Stomach with Synthetic Substitute, Via Natural or Artificial Opening Endoscopic
0D128J9 Bypass Middle Esophagus to Duodenum with Synthetic Substitute, Via Natural or Artificial Opening Endoscopic
0D128JA Bypass Middle Esophagus to Jejunum with Synthetic Substitute, Via Natural or Artificial Opening Endoscopic
0D128JB Bypass Middle Esophagus to Ileum with Synthetic Substitute, Via Natural or Artificial Opening Endoscopic
0D128K4 Bypass Middle Esophagus to Cutaneous with Nonautologous Tissue Substitute, Via Natural or Artificial Opening Endoscopic
0D128K6 Bypass Middle Esophagus to Stomach with Nonautologous Tissue Substitute, Via Natural or Artificial Opening Endoscopic
0D128K9 Bypass Middle Esophagus to Duodenum with Nonautologous Tissue Substitute, Via Natural or Artificial Opening Endoscopic
0D128KA Bypass Middle Esophagus to Jejunum with Nonautologous Tissue Substitute, Via Natural or Artificial Opening Endoscopic
0D128KB Bypass Middle Esophagus to Ileum with Nonautologous Tissue Substitute, Via Natural or Artificial Opening Endoscopic
0D128Z4 Bypass Middle Esophagus to Cutaneous, Via Natural or Artificial Opening Endoscopic
0D128Z6 Bypass Middle Esophagus to Stomach, Via Natural or Artificial Opening Endoscopic
0D128Z9 Bypass Middle Esophagus to Duodenum, Via Natural or Artificial Opening Endoscopic
0D128ZA Bypass Middle Esophagus to Jejunum, Via Natural or Artificial Opening Endoscopic
0D128ZB Bypass Middle Esophagus to Ileum, Via Natural or Artificial Opening Endoscopic
0D13074 Bypass Lower Esophagus to Cutaneous with Autologous Tissue Substitute, Open Approach
0D13076 Bypass Lower Esophagus to Stomach with Autologous Tissue Substitute, Open Approach
0D13079 Bypass Lower Esophagus to Duodenum with Autologous Tissue Substitute, Open Approach
0D1307A Bypass Lower Esophagus to Jejunum with Autologous Tissue Substitute, Open Approach
0D1307B Bypass Lower Esophagus to Ileum with Autologous Tissue Substitute, Open Approach
0D130J4 Bypass Lower Esophagus to Cutaneous with Synthetic Substitute, Open Approach
0D130J6 Bypass Lower Esophagus to Stomach with Synthetic Substitute, Open Approach
0D130J9 Bypass Lower Esophagus to Duodenum with Synthetic Substitute, Open Approach
0D130JA Bypass Lower Esophagus to Jejunum with Synthetic Substitute, Open Approach
0D130JB Bypass Lower Esophagus to Ileum with Synthetic Substitute, Open Approach
0D130K4 Bypass Lower Esophagus to Cutaneous with Nonautologous Tissue Substitute, Open Approach
0D130K6 Bypass Lower Esophagus to Stomach with Nonautologous Tissue Substitute, Open Approach
0D130K9 Bypass Lower Esophagus to Duodenum with Nonautologous Tissue Substitute, Open Approach
0D130KA Bypass Lower Esophagus to Jejunum w Nonautologous Tissue Substitute, Oper Approach
0D130KB Bypass Lower Esophagus to Ileum wit Nonautologous Tissue Substitute, Open Approach
0D130Z4 Bypass Lower Esophagus to Cutaneous Open Approach
0D130Z6 Bypass Lower Esophagus to Stomach, Open Approach
0D130Z9 Bypass Lower Esophagus to Duodenum Open Approach
0D130ZA Bypass Lower Esophagus to Jejunum, Open Approach
0D130ZB Bypass Lower Esophagus to Ileum, Op Approach
0D133J4 Bypass Lower Esophagus to Cutaneous with Synthetic Substitute, Percutaneous Approach
0D13474 Bypass Lower Esophagus to Cutaneous with Autologous Tissue Substitute, Percutaneous Endoscopic Approach
0D13476 Bypass Lower Esophagus to Stomach with Autologous Tissue Substitute, Percutaneous Endoscopic Approach
0D13479 Bypass Lower Esophagus to Duodenum with Autologous Tissue Substitute, Percutaneous Endoscopic Approach
0D1347A Bypass Lower Esophagus to Jejunum with Autologous Tissue Substitute, Percutaneous Endoscopic Approach
0D1347B Bypass Lower Esophagus to Ileum with Autologous Tissue Substitute, Percutaneous Endoscopic Approach
0D134J4 Bypass Lower Esophagus to Cutaneous with Synthetic Substitute, Percutaneous Endoscopic Approach
0D134J6 Bypass Lower Esophagus to Stomach with Synthetic Substitute, Percutaneous Endoscopic Approach
0D134J9 Bypass Lower Esophagus to Duodenum with Synthetic Substitute, Percutaneous Endoscopic Approach
0D134JA Bypass Lower Esophagus to Jejunum with Synthetic Substitute, Percutaneous Endoscopic Approach
0D134JB Bypass Lower Esophagus to Ileum with Synthetic Substitute, Percutaneous Endoscopic Approach
0D134K4 Bypass Lower Esophagus to Cutaneous with Nonautologous Tissue Substitute, Percutaneous Endoscopic Approach
0D134K6 Bypass Lower Esophagus to Stomach with Nonautologous Tissue Substitute, Percutaneous Endoscopic Approach
0D134K9 Bypass Lower Esophagus to Duodenum with Nonautologous Tissue Substitute, Percutaneous Endoscopic Approach
0D134KA Bypass Lower Esophagus to Jejunum with Nonautologous Tissue Substitute, Percutaneous Endoscopic Approach
0D134KB Bypass Lower Esophagus to Ileum with Nonautologous Tissue Substitute, Percutaneous Endoscopic Approach
0D134Z4 Bypass Lower Esophagus to Cutaneous, Percutaneous Endoscopic Approach
0D134Z6 Bypass Lower Esophagus to Stomach, Percutaneous Endoscopic Approach
0D134Z9 Bypass Lower Esophagus to Duodenum, Percutaneous Endoscopic Approach
0D134ZA Bypass Lower Esophagus to Jejunum, Percutaneous Endoscopic Approach
0D134ZB Bypass Lower Esophagus to Ileum, Percutaneous Endoscopic Approach

3874 Bypass Lower Esophagus to Cutaneous with Autologous Tissue Substitute, Via Natural or Artificial Opening Endoscopic
3876 Bypass Lower Esophagus to Stomach with Autologous Tissue Substitute, Via Natural or Artificial Opening Endoscopic
13879 Bypass Lower Esophagus to Duodenum with Autologous Tissue Substitute, Via Natural or Artificial Opening Endoscopic
1387A Bypass Lower Esophagus to Jejunum with Autologous Tissue Substitute, Via Natural or Artificial Opening Endoscopic
1387B Bypass Lower Esophagus to Ileum with Autologous Tissue Substitute, Via Natural or Artificial Opening Endoscopic
138J4 Bypass Lower Esophagus to Cutaneous with Synthetic Substitute, Via Natural or Artificial Opening Endoscopic
138J6 Bypass Lower Esophagus to Stomach with Synthetic Substitute, Via Natural or Artificial Opening Endoscopic
138J9 Bypass Lower Esophagus to Duodenum with Synthetic Substitute, Via Natural or Artificial Opening Endoscopic
138JA Bypass Lower Esophagus to Jejunum with Synthetic Substitute, Via Natural or Artificial Opening Endoscopic
138JB Bypass Lower Esophagus to Ileum with Synthetic Substitute, Via Natural or Artificial Opening Endoscopic
138K4 Bypass Lower Esophagus to Cutaneous with Nonautologous Tissue Substitute, Via Natural or Artificial Opening Endoscopic
138K6 Bypass Lower Esophagus to Stomach with Nonautologous Tissue Substitute, Via Natural or Artificial Opening Endoscopic
138K9 Bypass Lower Esophagus to Duodenum with Nonautologous Tissue Substitute, Via Natural or Artificial Opening Endoscopic
138KA Bypass Lower Esophagus to Jejunum with Nonautologous Tissue Substitute, Via Natural or Artificial Opening Endoscopic
138KB Bypass Lower Esophagus to Ileum with Nonautologous Tissue Substitute, Via Natural or Artificial Opening Endoscopic
)138Z4 Bypass Lower Esophagus to Cutaneous, Via Natural or Artificial Opening Endoscopic
)138Z6 Bypass Lower Esophagus to Stomach, Via Natural or Artificial Opening Endoscopic
)138Z9 Bypass Lower Esophagus to Duodenum, Via Natural or Artificial Opening Endoscopic
)138ZA Bypass Lower Esophagus to Jejunum, Via Natural or Artificial Opening Endoscopic
)138ZB Bypass Lower Esophagus to Ileum, Via Natural or Artificial Opening Endoscopic
)15074 Bypass Esophagus to Cutaneous with Autologous Tissue Substitute, Open Approach
D15076 Bypass Esophagus to Stomach with Autologous Tissue Substitute, Open Approach
D15079 Bypass Esophagus to Duodenum with Autologous Tissue Substitute, Open Approach
D1507A Bypass Esophagus to Jejunum with Autologous Tissue Substitute, Open Approach
D1507B Bypass Esophagus to Ileum with Autologous Tissue Substitute, Open Approach
D150J4 Bypass Esophagus to Cutaneous with Synthetic Substitute, Open Approach
D150J6 Bypass Esophagus to Stomach with Synthetic Substitute, Open Approach

0D150J9 Bypass Esophagus to Duodenum with Synthetic Substitute, Open Approach
0D150JA Bypass Esophagus to Jejunum with Synthetic Substitute, Open Approach
0D150JB Bypass Esophagus to Ileum with Synthetic Substitute, Open Approach
0D150K4 Bypass Esophagus to Cutaneous with Nonautologous Tissue Substitute, Open Approach
0D150K6 Bypass Esophagus to Stomach with Nonautologous Tissue Substitute, Open Approach
0D150K9 Bypass Esophagus to Duodenum with Nonautologous Tissue Substitute, Open Approach
0D150KA Bypass Esophagus to Jejunum with Nonautologous Tissue Substitute, Open Approach
0D150KB Bypass Esophagus to Ileum with Nonautologous Tissue Substitute, Open Approach
0D150Z4 Bypass Esophagus to Cutaneous, Open Approach
0D150Z6 Bypass Esophagus to Stomach, Open Approach
0D150Z9 Bypass Esophagus to Duodenum, Open Approach
0D150ZA Bypass Esophagus to Jejunum, Open Approach
0D150ZB Bypass Esophagus to Ileum, Open Approach
0D153J4 Bypass Esophagus to Cutaneous with Synthetic Substitute, Percutaneous Approach
0D15474 Bypass Esophagus to Cutaneous with Autologous Tissue Substitute, Percutaneous Endoscopic Approach
0D15476 Bypass Esophagus to Stomach with Autologous Tissue Substitute, Percutaneous Endoscopic Approach
0D15479 Bypass Esophagus to Duodenum with Autologous Tissue Substitute, Percutaneous Endoscopic Approach
0D1547A Bypass Esophagus to Jejunum with Autologous Tissue Substitute, Percutaneous Endoscopic Approach
0D1547B Bypass Esophagus to Ileum with Autologous Tissue Substitute, Percutaneous Endoscopic Approach
0D154J4 Bypass Esophagus to Cutaneous with Synthetic Substitute, Percutaneous Endoscopic Approach
0D154J6 Bypass Esophagus to Stomach with Synthetic Substitute, Percutaneous Endoscopic Approach
0D154J9 Bypass Esophagus to Duodenum with Synthetic Substitute, Percutaneous Endoscopic Approach
0D154JA Bypass Esophagus to Jejunum with Synthetic Substitute, Percutaneous Endoscopic Approach
0D154JB Bypass Esophagus to Ileum with Synthetic Substitute, Percutaneous Endoscopic Approach
0D154K4 Bypass Esophagus to Cutaneous with Nonautologous Tissue Substitute, Percutaneous Endoscopic Approach
0D154K6 Bypass Esophagus to Stomach with Nonautologous Tissue Substitute, Percutaneous Endoscopic Approach
0D154K9 Bypass Esophagus to Duodenum with Nonautologous Tissue Substitute, Percutaneous Endoscopic Approach
0D154KA Bypass Esophagus to Jejunum with Nonautologous Tissue Substitute, Percutaneous Endoscopic Approach

0D154KB Bypass Esophagus to Ileum with Nonautologous Tissue Substitute, Percutaneous Endoscopic Approach
0D154Z4 Bypass Esophagus to Cutaneous, Percutaneous Endoscopic Approach
0D154Z6 Bypass Esophagus to Stomach, Percutaneous Endoscopic Approach
0D154Z9 Bypass Esophagus to Duodenum, Percutaneous Endoscopic Approach
0D154ZA Bypass Esophagus to Jejunum, Percutaneous Endoscopic Approach
0D154ZB Bypass Esophagus to Ileum, Percutaneous Endoscopic Approach
0D15874 Bypass Esophagus to Cutaneous with Autologous Tissue Substitute, Via Natural or Artificial Opening Endoscopic
0D15876 Bypass Esophagus to Stomach with Autologous Tissue Substitute, Via Natural or Artificial Opening Endoscopic
0D15879 Bypass Esophagus to Duodenum with Autologous Tissue Substitute, Via Natural or Artificial Opening Endoscopic
0D1587A Bypass Esophagus to Jejunum with Autologous Tissue Substitute, Via Natural or Artificial Opening Endoscopic
0D1587B Bypass Esophagus to Ileum with Autologous Tissue Substitute, Via Natural or Artificial Opening Endoscopic
0D158J4 Bypass Esophagus to Cutaneous with Synthetic Substitute, Via Natural or Artificial Opening Endoscopic
0D158J6 Bypass Esophagus to Stomach with Synthetic Substitute, Via Natural or Artificial Opening Endoscopic
0D158J9 Bypass Esophagus to Duodenum with Synthetic Substitute, Via Natural or Artificial Opening Endoscopic
0D158JA Bypass Esophagus to Jejunum with Synthetic Substitute, Via Natural or Artificial Opening Endoscopic
0D158JB Bypass Esophagus to Ileum with Synthetic Substitute, Via Natural or Artificial Opening Endoscopic
0D158K4 Bypass Esophagus to Cutaneous with Nonautologous Tissue Substitute, Via Natural or Artificial Opening Endoscopic
0D158K6 Bypass Esophagus to Stomach with Nonautologous Tissue Substitute, Via Natural or Artificial Opening Endoscopic
0D158K9 Bypass Esophagus to Duodenum with Nonautologous Tissue Substitute, Via Natural or Artificial Opening Endoscopic
0D158KA Bypass Esophagus to Jejunum with Nonautologous Tissue Substitute, Via Natural or Artificial Opening Endoscopic
0D158KB Bypass Esophagus to Ileum with Nonautologous Tissue Substitute, Via Natural or Artificial Opening Endoscopic
0D158Z4 Bypass Esophagus to Cutaneous, Via Natural or Artificial Opening Endoscopic
0D158Z6 Bypass Esophagus to Stomach, Via Natural or Artificial Opening Endoscopic
0D158Z9 Bypass Esophagus to Duodenum, Via Natural or Artificial Opening Endoscopic
0D158ZA Bypass Esophagus to Jejunum, Via Natural or Artificial Opening Endoscopic
0D158ZB Bypass Esophagus to Ileum, Via Natural or Artificial Opening Endoscopic
0D16074 Bypass Stomach to Cutaneous with Autologous Tissue Substitute, Open Approach
0D16079 Bypass Stomach to Duodenum with Autologous Tissue Substitute, Open Approach

HAC When reported with principal diagnosis code K66.01 and secondary diagnosis code K68.11, K95.01, K95.81 or T81.4XXA

0D1607A Bypass Stomach to Jejunum with Autologous Tissue Substitute, Open Approach

0D1607B Bypass Stomach to Ileum with Autologous Tissue Substitute, Open Approach
HAC When reported with principal diagnosis code K66.01 and secondary diagnosis code K68.11, K95.01, K95.81 or T81.4XXA

0D1607L Bypass Stomach to Transverse Colon with Autologous Tissue Substitute, Open Approach
HAC When reported with principal diagnosis code K66.01 and secondary diagnosis code K68.11, K95.01, K95.81 or T81.4XXA

0D160J4 Bypass Stomach to Cutaneous with Synthetic Substitute, Open Approach

0D160J9 Bypass Stomach to Duodenum with Synthetic Substitute, Open Approach
HAC When reported with principal diagnosis code K66.01 and secondary diagnosis code K68.11, K95.01, K95.81 or T81.4XXA

0D160JA Bypass Stomach to Jejunum with Synthetic Substitute, Open Approach
HAC When reported with principal diagnosis code K66.01 and secondary diagnosis code K68.11, K95.01, K95.81 or T81.4XXA

0D160JB Bypass Stomach to Ileum with Synthetic Substitute, Open Approach
HAC When reported with principal diagnosis code K66.01 and secondary diagnosis code K68.11, K95.01, K95.81 or T81.4XXA

0D160JL Bypass Stomach to Transverse Colon with Synthetic Substitute, Open Approach
HAC When reported with principal diagnosis code K66.01 and secondary diagnosis code K68.11, K95.01, K95.81 or T81.4XXA

0D160K4 Bypass Stomach to Cutaneous with Nonautologous Tissue Substitute, Open Approach

0D160K9 Bypass Stomach to Duodenum with Nonautologous Tissue Substitute, Open Approach
HAC When reported with principal diagnosis code K66.01 and secondary diagnosis code K68.11, K95.01, K95.81 or T81.4XXA

0D160KA Bypass Stomach to Jejunum with Nonautologous Tissue Substitute, Open Approach
HAC When reported with principal diagnosis code K66.01 and secondary diagnosis code K68.11, K95.01, K95.81 or T81.4XXA

0D160KB Bypass Stomach to Ileum with Nonautologous Tissue Substitute, Open Approach
HAC When reported with principal diagnosis code K66.01 and secondary diagnosis code K68.11, K95.01, K95.81 or T81.4XXA

0D160KL Bypass Stomach to Transverse Colon with Nonautologous Tissue Substitute, Open Approach
HAC When reported with principal diagnosis code K66.01 and secondary diagnosis code K68.11, K95.01, K95.81 or T81.4XXA

0D160Z4 Bypass Stomach to Cutaneous, Open Approach

0D160Z9 Bypass Stomach to Duodenum, Open Approach
HAC When reported with principal diagnosis code K66.01 and secondary diagnosis code K68.11, K95.01, K95.81 or T81.4XXA

0D160ZA Bypass Stomach to Jejunum, Open Approach
HAC When reported with principal diagnosis code K66.01 and secondary diagnosis code K68.11, K95.01, K95.81 or T81.4XXA

0D160ZB Bypass Stomach to Ileum, Open Approach
HAC When reported with principal diagnosis code K66.01 and secondary diagnosis code K68.11, K95.01, K95.81 or T81.4XXA

0D160ZL Bypass Stomach to Transverse Colon, Open Approach
HAC When reported with principal diagnosis code K66.01 and secondary diagnosis code K68.11, K95.01, K95.81 or T81.4XXA

0D163J4 Bypass Stomach to Cutaneous with Synthetic Substitute, Percutaneous Approach

0D16474 Bypass Stomach to Cutaneous with Autologous Tissue Substitute, Percutaneous Endoscopic Approach

0D16479 Bypass Stomach to Duodenum with Autologous Tissue Substitute, Percutaneous Endoscopic Approach
HAC When reported with principal diagnosis code K66.01 and secondary diagnosis code K68.11, K95.01, K95.81 or T81.4XXA

0D1647A Bypass Stomach to Jejunum with Autologous Tissue Substitute, Percutaneous Endoscopic Approach
HAC When reported with principal diagnosis code K66.01 and secondary diagnosis code K68.11, K95.01, K95.81 or T81.4XXA

0D1647B Bypass Stomach to Ileum with Autologous Tissue Substitute, Percutaneous Endoscopic Approach
HAC When reported with principal diagnosis code K66.01 and secondary diagnosis code K68.11, K95.01, K95.81 or T81.4XXA

0D1647L Bypass Stomach to Transverse Colon with Autologous Tissue Substitute, Percutaneous Endoscopic Approach
HAC When reported with principal diagnosis code K66.01 and secondary diagnosis code K68.11, K95.01, K95.81 or T81.4XXA

0D164J4 Bypass Stomach to Cutaneous with Synthetic Substitute, Percutaneous Endoscopic Approach

0D164J9 Bypass Stomach to Duodenum with Synthetic Substitute, Percutaneous Endoscopic Approach
HAC When reported with principal diagnosis code K66.01 and secondary diagnosis code K68.11, K95.01, K95.81 or T81.4XXA

0D164JA Bypass Stomach to Jejunum with Synthetic Substitute, Percutaneous Endoscopic Approach
HAC When reported with principal diagnosis code K66.01 and secondary diagnosis code K68.11, K95.01, K95.81 or T81.4XXA

0D164JB Bypass Stomach to Ileum with Synthetic Substitute, Percutaneous Endoscopic Approach
HAC When reported with principal diagnosis code K66.01 and secondary diagnosis code K68.11, K95.01, K95.81 or T81.4XXA

0D164JL Bypass Stomach to Transverse Colon with Synthetic Substitute, Percutaneous Endoscopic Approach
HAC When reported with principal diagnosis code K66.01 and secondary diagnosis code K68.11, K95.01, K95.81 or T81.4XXA

0D164K4 Bypass Stomach to Cutaneous with Nonautologous Tissue Substitute, Percutaneous Endoscopic Approach

0D164K9 Bypass Stomach to Duodenum with Nonautologous Tissue Substitute, Percutaneous Endoscopic Approach
HAC When reported with principal diagnosis code K66.01 and secondary diagnosis code K68.11, K95.01, K95.81 or T81.4XXA

0D164KA Bypass Stomach to Jejunum with Nonautologous Tissue Substitute, Percutaneous Endoscopic Approach
HAC When reported with principal diagnosis code K66.01 and secondary diagnosis code K68.11, K95.01, K95.81 or T81.4XXA

0D164KB Bypass Stomach to Ileum with Nonautologous Tissue Substitute, Percutaneous Endoscopic Approach
HAC When reported with principal diagnosis code K66.01 and secondary diagnosis code K68.11, K95.01, K95.81 or T81.4XXA

0D164KL Bypass Stomach to Transverse Colon with Nonautologous Tissue Substitute, Percutaneous Endoscopic Approach
HAC When reported with principal diagnosis code K66.01 and secondary diagnosis code K68.11, K95.01, K95.81 or T81.4XXA

0D164Z4 Bypass Stomach to Cutaneous, Percutaneous Endoscopic Approach

0D164Z9 Bypass Stomach to Duodenum, Percutaneous Endoscopic Approach
HAC When reported with principal diagnosis code K66.01 and secondary diagnosis code K68.11, K95.01, K95.81 or T81.4XXA

0D164ZA Bypass Stomach to Jejunum, Percutaneous Endoscopic Approach
HAC When reported with principal diagnosis code K66.01 and secondary diagnosis code K68.11, K95.01, K95.81 or T81.4XXA

0D164ZB Bypass Stomach to Ileum, Percutaneous Endoscopic Approach
HAC When reported with principal diagnosis code K66.01 and secondary diagnosis code K68.11, K95.01, K95.81 or T81.4XXA

0D164ZL Bypass Stomach to Transverse Colon, Percutaneous Endoscopic Approach

0D16874 Bypass Stomach to Cutaneous with Autologous Tissue Substitute, Via Natural or Artificial Opening Endoscopic

0D16879 Bypass Stomach to Duodenum with Autologous Tissue Substitute, Via Natural or Artificial Opening Endoscopic
HAC When reported with principal diagnosis code K66.01 and secondary diagnosis code K68.11, K95.01, K95.81 or T81.4XXA

687A Bypass Stomach to Jejunum with Autologous Tissue Substitute, Via Natural or Artificial Opening Endoscopic
HAC When reported with principal diagnosis code K66.01 and secondary diagnosis code K68.11, K95.01, K95.81 or T81.4XXA

687B Bypass Stomach to Ileum with Autologous Tissue Substitute, Via Natural or Artificial Opening Endoscopic
HAC When reported with principal diagnosis code K66.01 and secondary diagnosis code K68.11, K95.01, K95.81 or T81.4XXA

687L Bypass Stomach to Transverse Colon with Autologous Tissue Substitute, Via Natural or Artificial Opening Endoscopic
HAC When reported with principal diagnosis code K66.01 and secondary diagnosis code K68.11, K95.01, K95.81 or T81.4XXA

168J4 Bypass Stomach to Cutaneous with Synthetic Substitute, Via Natural or Artificial Opening Endoscopic

168J9 Bypass Stomach to Duodenum with Synthetic Substitute, Via Natural or Artificial Opening Endoscopic
HAC When reported with principal diagnosis code K66.01 and secondary diagnosis code K68.11, K95.01, K95.81 or T81.4XXA

168JA Bypass Stomach to Jejunum with Synthetic Substitute, Via Natural or Artificial Opening Endoscopic
HAC When reported with principal diagnosis code K66.01 and secondary diagnosis code K68.11, K95.01, K95.81 or T81.4XXA

168JB Bypass Stomach to Ileum with Synthetic Substitute, Via Natural or Artificial Opening Endoscopic
HAC When reported with principal diagnosis code K66.01 and secondary diagnosis code K68.11, K95.01, K95.81 or T81.4XXA

168JL Bypass Stomach to Transverse Colon with Synthetic Substitute, Via Natural or Artificial Opening Endoscopic
HAC When reported with principal diagnosis code K66.01 and secondary diagnosis code K68.11, K95.01, K95.81 or T81.4XXA

168K4 Bypass Stomach to Cutaneous with Nonautologous Tissue Substitute, Via Natural or Artificial Opening Endoscopic

168K9 Bypass Stomach to Duodenum with Nonautologous Tissue Substitute, Via Natural or Artificial Opening Endoscopic
HAC When reported with principal diagnosis code K66.01 and secondary diagnosis code K68.11, K95.01, K95.81 or T81.4XXA

168KA Bypass Stomach to Jejunum with Nonautologous Tissue Substitute, Via Natural or Artificial Opening Endoscopic
HAC When reported with principal diagnosis code K66.01 and secondary diagnosis code K68.11, K95.01, K95.81 or T81.4XXA

168KB Bypass Stomach to Ileum with Nonautologous Tissue Substitute, Via Natural or Artificial Opening Endoscopic

168KL Bypass Stomach to Transverse Colon with Nonautologous Tissue Substitute, Via Natural or Artificial Opening Endoscopic
HAC When reported with principal diagnosis code K66.01 and secondary diagnosis code K68.11, K95.01, K95.81 or T81.4XXA

0D168Z4 Bypass Stomach to Cutaneous, Via Natural or Artificial Opening Endoscopic

0D168Z9 Bypass Stomach to Duodenum, Via Natural or Artificial Opening Endoscopic
HAC When reported with principal diagnosis code K66.01 and secondary diagnosis code K68.11, K95.01, K95.81 or T81.4XXA

0D168ZA Bypass Stomach to Jejunum, Via Natural or Artificial Opening Endoscopic
HAC When reported with principal diagnosis code K66.01 and secondary diagnosis code K68.11, K95.01, K95.81 or T81.4XXA

0D168ZB Bypass Stomach to Ileum, Via Natural or Artificial Opening Endoscopic
HAC When reported with principal diagnosis code K66.01 and secondary diagnosis code K68.11, K95.01, K95.81 or T81.4XXA

0D168ZL Bypass Stomach to Transverse Colon, Via Natural or Artificial Opening Endoscopic
HAC When reported with principal diagnosis code K66.01 and secondary diagnosis code K68.11, K95.01, K95.81 or T81.4XXA

0D19074 Bypass Duodenum to Cutaneous with Autologous Tissue Substitute, Open Approach

0D19079 Bypass Duodenum to Duodenum with Autologous Tissue Substitute, Open Approach

0D1907A Bypass Duodenum to Jejunum with Autologous Tissue Substitute, Open Approach

0D1907B Bypass Duodenum to Ileum with Autologous Tissue Substitute, Open Approach

0D1907L Bypass Duodenum to Transverse Colon with Autologous Tissue Substitute, Open Approach

0D190J4 Bypass Duodenum to Cutaneous with Synthetic Substitute, Open Approach

0D190J9 Bypass Duodenum to Duodenum with Synthetic Substitute, Open Approach

0D190JA Bypass Duodenum to Jejunum with Synthetic Substitute, Open Approach

0D190JB Bypass Duodenum to Ileum with Synthetic Substitute, Open Approach

0D190JL Bypass Duodenum to Transverse Colon with Synthetic Substitute, Open Approach

0D190K4 Bypass Duodenum to Cutaneous with Nonautologous Tissue Substitute, Open Approach

0D190K9 Bypass Duodenum to Duodenum with Nonautologous Tissue Substitute, Open Approach

0D190KA Bypass Duodenum to Jejunum with Nonautologous Tissue Substitute, Open Approach

0D190KB Bypass Duodenum to Ileum with Nonautologous Tissue Substitute, Open Approach

0D190KL Bypass Duodenum to Transverse Colon with Nonautologous Tissue Substitute, Open Approach

0D190Z4 Bypass Duodenum to Cutaneous, Open Approach

0D190Z9 Bypass Duodenum to Duodenum, Open Approach

0D190ZA Bypass Duodenum to Jejunum, Open Approach

0D190ZB Bypass Duodenum to Ileum, Open Approach

0D190ZL Bypass Duodenum to Transverse Colon, Open Approach

0D193J4 Bypass Duodenum to Cutaneous with Synthetic Substitute, Percutaneous Approach

0D19474 Bypass Duodenum to Cutaneous with Autologous Tissue Substitute, Percutaneous Endoscopic Approach

0D19479 Bypass Duodenum to Duodenum with Autologous Tissue Substitute, Percutaneous Endoscopic Approach

0D1947A Bypass Duodenum to Jejunum with Autologous Tissue Substitute, Percutaneous Endoscopic Approach

0D1947B Bypass Duodenum to Ileum with Autologous Tissue Substitute, Percutaneous Endoscopic Approach

0D1947L Bypass Duodenum to Transverse Colon with Autologous Tissue Substitute, Percutaneous Endoscopic Approach

0D194J4 Bypass Duodenum to Cutaneous with Synthetic Substitute, Percutaneous Endoscopic Approach

0D194J9 Bypass Duodenum to Duodenum with Synthetic Substitute, Percutaneous Endoscopic Approach

0D194JA Bypass Duodenum to Jejunum with Synthetic Substitute, Percutaneous Endoscopic Approach

0D194JB Bypass Duodenum to Ileum with Synthetic Substitute, Percutaneous Endoscopic Approach

0D194JL Bypass Duodenum to Transverse Colon with Synthetic Substitute, Percutaneous Endoscopic Approach

0D194K4 Bypass Duodenum to Cutaneous with Nonautologous Tissue Substitute, Percutaneous Endoscopic Approach

0D194K9 Bypass Duodenum to Duodenum with Nonautologous Tissue Substitute, Percutaneous Endoscopic Approach

0D194KA Bypass Duodenum to Jejunum with Nonautologous Tissue Substitute, Percutaneous Endoscopic Approach

0D194KB Bypass Duodenum to Ileum with Nonautologous Tissue Substitute, Percutaneous Endoscopic Approach

0D194KL Bypass Duodenum to Transverse Colon with Nonautologous Tissue Substitute, Percutaneous Endoscopic Approach

0D194Z4 Bypass Duodenum to Cutaneous, Percutaneous Endoscopic Approach

0D194Z9 Bypass Duodenum to Duodenum, Percutaneous Endoscopic Approach

0D194ZA Bypass Duodenum to Jejunum, Percutaneous Endoscopic Approach

0D194ZB Bypass Duodenum to Ileum, Percutaneous Endoscopic Approach

0D194ZL Bypass Duodenum to Transverse Colon, Percutaneous Endoscopic Approach

0D19874 Bypass Duodenum to Cutaneous with Autologous Tissue Substitute, Via Natural or Artificial Opening Endoscopic

0D19879 Bypass Duodenum to Duodenum with Autologous Tissue Substitute, Via Natural or Artificial Opening Endoscopic

0D1987A Bypass Duodenum to Jejunum with Autologous Tissue Substitute, Via Natural or Artificial Opening Endoscopic

0D1987B Bypass Duodenum to Ileum with Autologous Tissue Substitute, Via Natural or Artificial Opening Endoscopic

0D1987L Bypass Duodenum to Transverse Colon with Autologous Tissue Substitute, Via Natural or Artificial Opening Endoscopic

0D198J4 Bypass Duodenum to Cutaneous with Synthetic Substitute, Via Natural or Artificial Opening Endoscopic

0D198J9 Bypass Duodenum to Duodenum with Synthetic Substitute, Via Natural or Artificial Opening Endoscopic
0D198JA Bypass Duodenum to Jejunum with Synthetic Substitute, Via Natural or Artificial Opening Endoscopic
0D198JB Bypass Duodenum to Ileum with Synthetic Substitute, Via Natural or Artificial Opening Endoscopic
0D198JL Bypass Duodenum to Transverse Colon with Synthetic Substitute, Via Natural or Artificial Opening Endoscopic
0D198K4 Bypass Duodenum to Cutaneous with Nonautologous Tissue Substitute, Via Natural or Artificial Opening Endoscopic
0D198K9 Bypass Duodenum to Duodenum with Nonautologous Tissue Substitute, Via Natural or Artificial Opening Endoscopic
0D198KA Bypass Duodenum to Jejunum with Nonautologous Tissue Substitute, Via Natural or Artificial Opening Endoscopic
0D198KB Bypass Duodenum to Ileum with Nonautologous Tissue Substitute, Via Natural or Artificial Opening Endoscopic
0D198KL Bypass Duodenum to Transverse Colon with Nonautologous Tissue Substitute, Via Natural or Artificial Opening Endoscopic
0D198Z4 Bypass Duodenum to Cutaneous, Via Natural or Artificial Opening Endoscopic
0D198Z9 Bypass Duodenum to Duodenum, Via Natural or Artificial Opening Endoscopic
0D198ZA Bypass Duodenum to Jejunum, Via Natural or Artificial Opening Endoscopic
0D198ZB Bypass Duodenum to Ileum, Via Natural or Artificial Opening Endoscopic
0D198ZL Bypass Duodenum to Transverse Colon, Via Natural or Artificial Opening Endoscopic
0D1A074 Bypass Jejunum to Cutaneous with Autologous Tissue Substitute, Open Approach
0D1A07A Bypass Jejunum to Jejunum with Autologous Tissue Substitute, Open Approach
0D1A07B Bypass Jejunum to Ileum with Autologous Tissue Substitute, Open Approach
0D1A07H Bypass Jejunum to Cecum with Autologous Tissue Substitute, Open Approach
0D1A07K Bypass Jejunum to Ascending Colon with Autologous Tissue Substitute, Open Approach
0D1A07L Bypass Jejunum to Transverse Colon with Autologous Tissue Substitute, Open Approach
0D1A07M Bypass Jejunum to Descending Colon with Autologous Tissue Substitute, Open Approach
0D1A07N Bypass Jejunum to Sigmoid Colon with Autologous Tissue Substitute, Open Approach
0D1A07P Bypass Jejunum to Rectum with Autologous Tissue Substitute, Open Approach
0D1A07Q Bypass Jejunum to Anus with Autologous Tissue Substitute, Open Approach
0D1A0J4 Bypass Jejunum to Cutaneous with Synthetic Substitute, Open Approach
0D1A0JA Bypass Jejunum to Jejunum with Synthetic Substitute, Open Approach
0D1A0JB Bypass Jejunum to Ileum with Synthetic Substitute, Open Approach
0D1A0JH Bypass Jejunum to Cecum with Synthetic Substitute, Open Approach
0D1A0JK Bypass Jejunum to Ascending Colon with Synthetic Substitute, Open Approach
0D1A0JL Bypass Jejunum to Transverse Colon with Synthetic Substitute, Open Approach
0D1A0JM Bypass Jejunum to Descending Colon with Synthetic Substitute, Open Approach
0D1A0JN Bypass Jejunum to Sigmoid Colon with Synthetic Substitute, Open Approach
0D1A0JP Bypass Jejunum to Rectum with Synthetic Substitute, Open Approach
0D1A0JQ Bypass Jejunum to Anus with Synthetic Substitute, Open Approach
0D1A0K4 Bypass Jejunum to Cutaneous with Nonautologous Tissue Substitute, Open Approach
0D1A0KA Bypass Jejunum to Jejunum with Nonautologous Tissue Substitute, Open Approach
0D1A0KB Bypass Jejunum to Ileum with Nonautologous Tissue Substitute, Open Approach
0D1A0KH Bypass Jejunum to Cecum with Nonautologous Tissue Substitute, Open Approach
0D1A0KK Bypass Jejunum to Ascending Colon with Nonautologous Tissue Substitute, Open Approach
0D1A0KL Bypass Jejunum to Transverse Colon with Nonautologous Tissue Substitute, Open Approach
0D1A0KM Bypass Jejunum to Descending Colon with Nonautologous Tissue Substitute, Open Approach
0D1A0KN Bypass Jejunum to Sigmoid Colon with Nonautologous Tissue Substitute, Open Approach
0D1A0KP Bypass Jejunum to Rectum with Nonautologous Tissue Substitute, Open Approach
0D1A0KQ Bypass Jejunum to Anus with Nonautologous Tissue Substitute, Open Approach
0D1A0Z4 Bypass Jejunum to Cutaneous, Open Approach
0D1A0ZA Bypass Jejunum to Jejunum, Open Approach
0D1A0ZB Bypass Jejunum to Ileum, Open Approach
0D1A0ZH Bypass Jejunum to Cecum, Open Approach
0D1A0ZK Bypass Jejunum to Ascending Colon, Open Approach
0D1A0ZL Bypass Jejunum to Transverse Colon, Open Approach
0D1A0ZM Bypass Jejunum to Descending Colon, Open Approach
0D1A0ZN Bypass Jejunum to Sigmoid Colon, Open Approach
0D1A0ZP Bypass Jejunum to Rectum, Open Approach
0D1A0ZQ Bypass Jejunum to Anus, Open Approach
0D1A3J4 Bypass Jejunum to Cutaneous with Synthetic Substitute, Percutaneous Approach
0D1A474 Bypass Jejunum to Cutaneous with Autologous Tissue Substitute, Percutaneous Endoscopic Approach
0D1A47A Bypass Jejunum to Jejunum with Autologous Tissue Substitute, Percutaneous Endoscopic Approach
0D1A47B Bypass Jejunum to Ileum with Autologous Tissue Substitute, Percutaneous Endoscopic Approach
0D1A47H Bypass Jejunum to Cecum with Autologous Tissue Substitute, Percutaneous Endoscopic Approach
0D1A47K Bypass Jejunum to Ascending Colon with Autologous Tissue Substitute, Percutaneous Endoscopic Approach
0D1A47L Bypass Jejunum to Transverse Colon with Autologous Tissue Substitute, Percutaneous Endoscopic Approach
0D1A47M Bypass Jejunum to Descending Colon with Autologous Tissue Substitute, Percutaneous Endoscopic Approach
0D1A47N Bypass Jejunum to Sigmoid Colon with Autologous Tissue Substitute, Percutaneous Endoscopic Approach
0D1A47P Bypass Jejunum to Rectum with Autologous Tissue Substitute, Percutaneous Endoscopic Approach
0D1A47Q Bypass Jejunum to Anus with Autologo[us] Tissue Substitute, Percutaneous Endoscopic Approach
0D1A4J4 Bypass Jejunum to Cutaneous with Synthetic Substitute, Percutaneous Endoscopic Approach
0D1A4JA Bypass Jejunum to Jejunum with Synth[etic] Substitute, Percutaneous Endoscopic Approach
0D1A4JB Bypass Jejunum to Ileum with Syntheti[c] Substitute, Percutaneous Endoscopic Approach
0D1A4JH Bypass Jejunum to Cecum with Synthe[tic] Substitute, Percutaneous Endoscopic Approach
0D1A4JK Bypass Jejunum to Ascending Colon with Synthetic Substitute, Percutaneous Endoscopic Approach
0D1A4JL Bypass Jejunum to Transverse Colon with Synthetic Substitute, Percutaneous Endoscopic Approach
0D1A4JM Bypass Jejunum to Descending Colon with Synthetic Substitute, Percutaneous Endoscopic Approach
0D1A4JN Bypass Jejunum to Sigmoid Colon with Synthetic Substitute, Percutaneous Endoscopic Approach
0D1A4JP Bypass Jejunum to Rectum with Synthe[tic] Substitute, Percutaneous Endoscopic Approach
0D1A4JQ Bypass Jejunum to Anus with Synthetic Substitute, Percutaneous Endoscopic Approach
0D1A4K4 Bypass Jejunum to Cutaneous with Nonautologous Tissue Substitute, Percutaneous Endoscopic Approach
0D1A4KA Bypass Jejunum to Jejunum with Nonautologous Tissue Substitute, Percutaneous Endoscopic Approach
0D1A4KB Bypass Jejunum to Ileum with Nonautologous Tissue Substitute, Percutaneous Endoscopic Approach
0D1A4KH Bypass Jejunum to Cecum with Nonautologous Tissue Substitute, Percutaneous Endoscopic Approach
0D1A4KK Bypass Jejunum to Ascending Colon with Nonautologous Tissue Substitute, Percutaneous Endoscopic Approach
0D1A4KL Bypass Jejunum to Transverse Colon with Nonautologous Tissue Substitute, Percutaneous Endoscopic Approach
0D1A4KM Bypass Jejunum to Descending Colon with Nonautologous Tissue Substitute, Percutaneous Endoscopic Approach
0D1A4KN Bypass Jejunum to Sigmoid Colon with Nonautologous Tissue Substitute, Percutaneous Endoscopic Approach
0D1A4KP Bypass Jejunum to Rectum with Nonautologous Tissue Substitute, Percutaneous Endoscopic Approach

A4KQ Bypass Jejunum to Anus with Nonautologous Tissue Substitute, Percutaneous Endoscopic Approach
A4Z4 Bypass Jejunum to Cutaneous, Percutaneous Endoscopic Approach
A4ZA Bypass Jejunum to Jejunum, Percutaneous Endoscopic Approach
A4ZB Bypass Jejunum to Ileum, Percutaneous Endoscopic Approach
A4ZH Bypass Jejunum to Cecum, Percutaneous Endoscopic Approach
A4ZK Bypass Jejunum to Ascending Colon, Percutaneous Endoscopic Approach
A4ZL Bypass Jejunum to Transverse Colon, Percutaneous Endoscopic Approach
A4ZM Bypass Jejunum to Descending Colon, Percutaneous Endoscopic Approach
A4ZN Bypass Jejunum to Sigmoid Colon, Percutaneous Endoscopic Approach
1A4ZP Bypass Jejunum to Rectum, Percutaneous Endoscopic Approach
1A4ZQ Bypass Jejunum to Anus, Percutaneous Endoscopic Approach
1A874 Bypass Jejunum to Cutaneous with Autologous Tissue Substitute, Via Natural or Artificial Opening Endoscopic
1A87A Bypass Jejunum to Jejunum with Autologous Tissue Substitute, Via Natural or Artificial Opening Endoscopic
1A87B Bypass Jejunum to Ileum with Autologous Tissue Substitute, Via Natural or Artificial Opening Endoscopic
1A87H Bypass Jejunum to Cecum with Autologous Tissue Substitute, Via Natural or Artificial Opening Endoscopic
1A87K Bypass Jejunum to Ascending Colon with Autologous Tissue Substitute, Via Natural or Artificial Opening Endoscopic
1A87L Bypass Jejunum to Transverse Colon with Autologous Tissue Substitute, Via Natural or Artificial Opening Endoscopic
1A87M Bypass Jejunum to Descending Colon with Autologous Tissue Substitute, Via Natural or Artificial Opening Endoscopic
1A87N Bypass Jejunum to Sigmoid Colon with Autologous Tissue Substitute, Via Natural or Artificial Opening Endoscopic
1A87P Bypass Jejunum to Rectum with Autologous Tissue Substitute, Via Natural or Artificial Opening Endoscopic
1A87Q Bypass Jejunum to Anus with Autologous Tissue Substitute, Via Natural or Artificial Opening Endoscopic
1A8J4 Bypass Jejunum to Cutaneous with Synthetic Substitute, Via Natural or Artificial Opening Endoscopic
1A8JA Bypass Jejunum to Jejunum with Synthetic Substitute, Via Natural or Artificial Opening Endoscopic
1A8JB Bypass Jejunum to Ileum with Synthetic Substitute, Via Natural or Artificial Opening Endoscopic
D1A8JH Bypass Jejunum to Cecum with Synthetic Substitute, Via Natural or Artificial Opening Endoscopic
D1A8JK Bypass Jejunum to Ascending Colon with Synthetic Substitute, Via Natural or Artificial Opening Endoscopic
D1A8JL Bypass Jejunum to Transverse Colon with Synthetic Substitute, Via Natural or Artificial Opening Endoscopic
D1A8JM Bypass Jejunum to Descending Colon with Synthetic Substitute, Via Natural or Artificial Opening Endoscopic
0D1A8JN Bypass Jejunum to Sigmoid Colon with Synthetic Substitute, Via Natural or Artificial Opening Endoscopic
0D1A8JP Bypass Jejunum to Rectum with Synthetic Substitute, Via Natural or Artificial Opening Endoscopic
0D1A8JQ Bypass Jejunum to Anus with Synthetic Substitute, Via Natural or Artificial Opening Endoscopic
0D1A8K4 Bypass Jejunum to Cutaneous with Nonautologous Tissue Substitute, Via Natural or Artificial Opening Endoscopic
0D1A8KA Bypass Jejunum to Jejunum with Nonautologous Tissue Substitute, Via Natural or Artificial Opening Endoscopic
0D1A8KB Bypass Jejunum to Ileum with Nonautologous Tissue Substitute, Via Natural or Artificial Opening Endoscopic
0D1A8KH Bypass Jejunum to Cecum with Nonautologous Tissue Substitute, Via Natural or Artificial Opening Endoscopic
0D1A8KK Bypass Jejunum to Ascending Colon with Nonautologous Tissue Substitute, Via Natural or Artificial Opening Endoscopic
0D1A8KL Bypass Jejunum to Transverse Colon with Nonautologous Tissue Substitute, Via Natural or Artificial Opening Endoscopic
0D1A8KM Bypass Jejunum to Descending Colon with Nonautologous Tissue Substitute, Via Natural or Artificial Opening Endoscopic
0D1A8KN Bypass Jejunum to Sigmoid Colon with Nonautologous Tissue Substitute, Via Natural or Artificial Opening Endoscopic
0D1A8KP Bypass Jejunum to Rectum with Nonautologous Tissue Substitute, Via Natural or Artificial Opening Endoscopic
0D1A8KQ Bypass Jejunum to Anus with Nonautologous Tissue Substitute, Via Natural or Artificial Opening Endoscopic
0D1A8Z4 Bypass Jejunum to Cutaneous, Via Natural or Artificial Opening Endoscopic
0D1A8ZA Bypass Jejunum to Jejunum, Via Natural or Artificial Opening Endoscopic
0D1A8ZB Bypass Jejunum to Ileum, Via Natural or Artificial Opening Endoscopic
0D1A8ZH Bypass Jejunum to Cecum, Via Natural or Artificial Opening Endoscopic
0D1A8ZK Bypass Jejunum to Ascending Colon, Via Natural or Artificial Opening Endoscopic
0D1A8ZL Bypass Jejunum to Transverse Colon, Via Natural or Artificial Opening Endoscopic
0D1A8ZM Bypass Jejunum to Descending Colon, Via Natural or Artificial Opening Endoscopic
0D1A8ZN Bypass Jejunum to Sigmoid Colon, Via Natural or Artificial Opening Endoscopic
0D1A8ZP Bypass Jejunum to Rectum, Via Natural or Artificial Opening Endoscopic
0D1A8ZQ Bypass Jejunum to Anus, Via Natural or Artificial Opening Endoscopic
0D1B074 Bypass Ileum to Cutaneous with Autologous Tissue Substitute, Open Approach
0D1B07B Bypass Ileum to Ileum with Autologous Tissue Substitute, Open Approach
0D1B07H Bypass Ileum to Cecum with Autologous Tissue Substitute, Open Approach
0D1B07K Bypass Ileum to Ascending Colon with Autologous Tissue Substitute, Open Approach
0D1B07L Bypass Ileum to Transverse Colon with Autologous Tissue Substitute, Open Approach
0D1B07M Bypass Ileum to Descending Colon with Autologous Tissue Substitute, Open Approach
0D1B07N Bypass Ileum to Sigmoid Colon with Autologous Tissue Substitute, Open Approach
0D1B07P Bypass Ileum to Rectum with Autologous Tissue Substitute, Open Approach
0D1B07Q Bypass Ileum to Anus with Autologous Tissue Substitute, Open Approach
0D1B0J4 Bypass Ileum to Cutaneous with Synthetic Substitute, Open Approach
0D1B0JB Bypass Ileum to Ileum with Synthetic Substitute, Open Approach
0D1B0JH Bypass Ileum to Cecum with Synthetic Substitute, Open Approach
0D1B0JK Bypass Ileum to Ascending Colon with Synthetic Substitute, Open Approach
0D1B0JL Bypass Ileum to Transverse Colon with Synthetic Substitute, Open Approach
0D1B0JM Bypass Ileum to Descending Colon with Synthetic Substitute, Open Approach
0D1B0JN Bypass Ileum to Sigmoid Colon with Synthetic Substitute, Open Approach
0D1B0JP Bypass Ileum to Rectum with Synthetic Substitute, Open Approach
0D1B0JQ Bypass Ileum to Anus with Synthetic Substitute, Open Approach
0D1B0K4 Bypass Ileum to Cutaneous with Nonautologous Tissue Substitute, Open Approach
0D1B0KB Bypass Ileum to Ileum with Nonautologous Tissue Substitute, Open Approach
0D1B0KH Bypass Ileum to Cecum with Nonautologous Tissue Substitute, Open Approach
0D1B0KK Bypass Ileum to Ascending Colon with Nonautologous Tissue Substitute, Open Approach
0D1B0KL Bypass Ileum to Transverse Colon with Nonautologous Tissue Substitute, Open Approach
0D1B0KM Bypass Ileum to Descending Colon with Nonautologous Tissue Substitute, Open Approach
0D1B0KN Bypass Ileum to Sigmoid Colon with Nonautologous Tissue Substitute, Open Approach
0D1B0KP Bypass Ileum to Rectum with Nonautologous Tissue Substitute, Open Approach
0D1B0KQ Bypass Ileum to Anus with Nonautologous Tissue Substitute, Open Approach
0D1B0Z4 Bypass Ileum to Cutaneous, Open Approach
0D1B0ZB Bypass Ileum to Ileum, Open Approach
0D1B0ZH Bypass Ileum to Cecum, Open Approach
0D1B0ZK Bypass Ileum to Ascending Colon, Open Approach
0D1B0ZL Bypass Ileum to Transverse Colon, Open Approach
0D1B0ZM Bypass Ileum to Descending Colon, Open Approach
0D1B0ZN Bypass Ileum to Sigmoid Colon, Open Approach
0D1B0ZP Bypass Ileum to Rectum, Open Approach
0D1B0ZQ Bypass Ileum to Anus, Open Approach
0D1B3J4 Bypass Ileum to Cutaneous with Synthetic Substitute, Percutaneous Approach
0D1B474 Bypass Ileum to Cutaneous with Autologous Tissue Substitute, Percutaneous Endoscopic Approach
0D1B47B Bypass Ileum to Ileum with Autologous Tissue Substitute, Percutaneous Endoscopic Approach

0D1B47H Bypass Ileum to Cecum with Autologous Tissue Substitute, Percutaneous Endoscopic Approach

0D1B47K Bypass Ileum to Ascending Colon with Autologous Tissue Substitute, Percutaneous Endoscopic Approach

0D1B47L Bypass Ileum to Transverse Colon with Autologous Tissue Substitute, Percutaneous Endoscopic Approach

0D1B47M Bypass Ileum to Descending Colon with Autologous Tissue Substitute, Percutaneous Endoscopic Approach

0D1B47N Bypass Ileum to Sigmoid Colon with Autologous Tissue Substitute, Percutaneous Endoscopic Approach

0D1B47P Bypass Ileum to Rectum with Autologous Tissue Substitute, Percutaneous Endoscopic Approach

0D1B47Q Bypass Ileum to Anus with Autologous Tissue Substitute, Percutaneous Endoscopic Approach

0D1B4J4 Bypass Ileum to Cutaneous with Synthetic Substitute, Percutaneous Endoscopic Approach

0D1B4JB Bypass Ileum to Ileum with Synthetic Substitute, Percutaneous Endoscopic Approach

0D1B4JH Bypass Ileum to Cecum with Synthetic Substitute, Percutaneous Endoscopic Approach

0D1B4JK Bypass Ileum to Ascending Colon with Synthetic Substitute, Percutaneous Endoscopic Approach

0D1B4JL Bypass Ileum to Transverse Colon with Synthetic Substitute, Percutaneous Endoscopic Approach

0D1B4JM Bypass Ileum to Descending Colon with Synthetic Substitute, Percutaneous Endoscopic Approach

0D1B4JN Bypass Ileum to Sigmoid Colon with Synthetic Substitute, Percutaneous Endoscopic Approach

0D1B4JP Bypass Ileum to Rectum with Synthetic Substitute, Percutaneous Endoscopic Approach

0D1B4JQ Bypass Ileum to Anus with Synthetic Substitute, Percutaneous Endoscopic Approach

0D1B4K4 Bypass Ileum to Cutaneous with Nonautologous Tissue Substitute, Percutaneous Endoscopic Approach

0D1B4KB Bypass Ileum to Ileum with Nonautologous Tissue Substitute, Percutaneous Endoscopic Approach

0D1B4KH Bypass Ileum to Cecum with Nonautologous Tissue Substitute, Percutaneous Endoscopic Approach

0D1B4KK Bypass Ileum to Ascending Colon with Nonautologous Tissue Substitute, Percutaneous Endoscopic Approach

0D1B4KL Bypass Ileum to Transverse Colon with Nonautologous Tissue Substitute, Percutaneous Endoscopic Approach

0D1B4KM Bypass Ileum to Descending Colon with Nonautologous Tissue Substitute, Percutaneous Endoscopic Approach

0D1B4KN Bypass Ileum to Sigmoid Colon with Nonautologous Tissue Substitute, Percutaneous Endoscopic Approach

0D1B4KP Bypass Ileum to Rectum with Nonautologous Tissue Substitute, Percutaneous Endoscopic Approach

0D1B4KQ Bypass Ileum to Anus with Nonautologous Tissue Substitute, Percutaneous Endoscopic Approach

0D1B4Z4 Bypass Ileum to Cutaneous, Percutaneous Endoscopic Approach

0D1B4ZB Bypass Ileum to Ileum, Percutaneous Endoscopic Approach

0D1B4ZH Bypass Ileum to Cecum, Percutaneous Endoscopic Approach

0D1B4ZK Bypass Ileum to Ascending Colon, Percutaneous Endoscopic Approach

0D1B4ZL Bypass Ileum to Transverse Colon, Percutaneous Endoscopic Approach

0D1B4ZM Bypass Ileum to Descending Colon, Percutaneous Endoscopic Approach

0D1B4ZN Bypass Ileum to Sigmoid Colon, Percutaneous Endoscopic Approach

0D1B4ZP Bypass Ileum to Rectum, Percutaneous Endoscopic Approach

0D1B4ZQ Bypass Ileum to Anus, Percutaneous Endoscopic Approach

0D1B874 Bypass Ileum to Cutaneous with Autologous Tissue Substitute, Via Natural or Artificial Opening Endoscopic

0D1B87B Bypass Ileum to Ileum with Autologous Tissue Substitute, Via Natural or Artificial Opening Endoscopic

0D1B87H Bypass Ileum to Cecum with Autologous Tissue Substitute, Via Natural or Artificial Opening Endoscopic

0D1B87K Bypass Ileum to Ascending Colon with Autologous Tissue Substitute, Via Natural or Artificial Opening Endoscopic

0D1B87L Bypass Ileum to Transverse Colon with Autologous Tissue Substitute, Via Natural or Artificial Opening Endoscopic

0D1B87M Bypass Ileum to Descending Colon with Autologous Tissue Substitute, Via Natural or Artificial Opening Endoscopic

0D1B87N Bypass Ileum to Sigmoid Colon with Autologous Tissue Substitute, Via Natural or Artificial Opening Endoscopic

0D1B87P Bypass Ileum to Rectum with Autologous Tissue Substitute, Via Natural or Artificial Opening Endoscopic

0D1B87Q Bypass Ileum to Anus with Autologous Tissue Substitute, Via Natural or Artificial Opening Endoscopic

0D1B8J4 Bypass Ileum to Cutaneous with Synthetic Substitute, Via Natural or Artificial Opening Endoscopic

0D1B8JB Bypass Ileum to Ileum with Synthetic Substitute, Via Natural or Artificial Opening Endoscopic

0D1B8JH Bypass Ileum to Cecum with Synthetic Substitute, Via Natural or Artificial Opening Endoscopic

0D1B8JK Bypass Ileum to Ascending Colon with Synthetic Substitute, Via Natural or Artificial Opening Endoscopic

0D1B8JL Bypass Ileum to Transverse Colon with Synthetic Substitute, Via Natural or Artificial Opening Endoscopic

0D1B8JM Bypass Ileum to Descending Colon with Synthetic Substitute, Via Natural or Artificial Opening Endoscopic

0D1B8JN Bypass Ileum to Sigmoid Colon with Synthetic Substitute, Via Natural or Artificial Opening Endoscopic

0D1B8JP Bypass Ileum to Rectum with Synthetic Substitute, Via Natural or Artificial Opening Endoscopic

0D1B8JQ Bypass Ileum to Anus with Synthetic Substitute, Via Natural or Artificial Opening Endoscopic

0D1B8K4 Bypass Ileum to Cutaneous with Nonautologous Tissue Substitute, Via Natural or Artificial Opening Endoscopic

0D1B8KB Bypass Ileum to Ileum with Nonautologous Tissue Substitute, Via Natural or Artificial Opening Endoscopic

0D1B8KH Bypass Ileum to Cecum with Nonautologous Tissue Substitute, Via Natural or Artificial Opening Endosco

0D1B8KK Bypass Ileum to Ascending Colon wit Nonautologous Tissue Substitute, Via Natural or Artificial Opening Endosco

0D1B8KL Bypass Ileum to Transverse Colon wi Nonautologous Tissue Substitute, Via Natural or Artificial Opening Endosco

0D1B8KM Bypass Ileum to Descending Colon wi Nonautologous Tissue Substitute, Via Natural or Artificial Opening Endosco

0D1B8KN Bypass Ileum to Sigmoid Colon with Nonautologous Tissue Substitute, Via Natural or Artificial Opening Endosco

0D1B8KP Bypass Ileum to Rectum with Nonautologous Tissue Substitute, Via Natural or Artificial Opening Endosco

0D1B8KQ Bypass Ileum to Anus with Nonautologous Tissue Substitute, Via Natural or Artificial Opening Endosco

0D1B8Z4 Bypass Ileum to Cutaneous, Via Natur or Artificial Opening Endoscopic

0D1B8ZB Bypass Ileum to Ileum, Via Natural or Artificial Opening Endoscopic

0D1B8ZH Bypass Ileum to Cecum, Via Natural or Artificial Opening Endoscopic

0D1B8ZK Bypass Ileum to Ascending Colon, Via Natural or Artificial Opening Endoscop

0D1B8ZL Bypass Ileum to Transverse Colon, Via Natural or Artificial Opening Endoscop

0D1B8ZM Bypass Ileum to Descending Colon, Vi Natural or Artificial Opening Endoscop

0D1B8ZN Bypass Ileum to Sigmoid Colon, Via Natural or Artificial Opening Endoscop

0D1B8ZP Bypass Ileum to Rectum, Via Natural o Artificial Opening Endoscopic

0D1B8ZQ Bypass Ileum to Anus, Via Natural or Artificial Opening Endoscopic

0D1H074 Bypass Cecum to Cutaneous with Autologous Tissue Substitute, Open Approach

0D1H07H Bypass Cecum to Cecum with Autolog Tissue Substitute, Open Approach

0D1H07K Bypass Cecum to Ascending Colon wit Autologous Tissue Substitute, Open Approach

0D1H07L Bypass Cecum to Transverse Colon wit Autologous Tissue Substitute, Open Approach

0D1H07M Bypass Cecum to Descending Colon with Autologous Tissue Substitute, Ope Approach

0D1H07N Bypass Cecum to Sigmoid Colon with Autologous Tissue Substitute, Open Approach

0D1H07P Bypass Cecum to Rectum with Autologo Tissue Substitute, Open Approach

0D1H0J4 Bypass Cecum to Cutaneous with Synthetic Substitute, Open Approach

0D1H0JH Bypass Cecum to Cecum with Synthetic Substitute, Open Approach

0D1H0JK Bypass Cecum to Ascending Colon with Synthetic Substitute, Open Approach

0D1H0JL Bypass Cecum to Transverse Colon wit Synthetic Substitute, Open Approach

0D1H0JM Bypass Cecum to Descending Colon wit Synthetic Substitute, Open Approach

0D1H0JN Bypass Cecum to Sigmoid Colon with Synthetic Substitute, Open Approach

0D1H0JP Bypass Cecum to Rectum with Syntheti Substitute, Open Approach

0D1H0K4 Bypass Cecum to Cutaneous with Nonautologous Tissue Substitute, Open Approach

0D1H0KH Bypass Cecum to Cecum with Nonautologous Tissue Substitute, Open Approach

H0KK Bypass Cecum to Ascending Colon with Nonautologous Tissue Substitute, Open Approach

H0KL Bypass Cecum to Transverse Colon with Nonautologous Tissue Substitute, Open Approach

H0KM Bypass Cecum to Descending Colon with Nonautologous Tissue Substitute, Open Approach

H0KN Bypass Cecum to Sigmoid Colon with Nonautologous Tissue Substitute, Open Approach

H0KP Bypass Cecum to Rectum with Nonautologous Tissue Substitute, Open Approach

H0Z4 Bypass Cecum to Cutaneous, Open Approach

H0ZH Bypass Cecum to Cecum, Open Approach

H0ZK Bypass Cecum to Ascending Colon, Open Approach

H0ZL Bypass Cecum to Transverse Colon, Open Approach

H0ZM Bypass Cecum to Descending Colon, Open Approach

H0ZN Bypass Cecum to Sigmoid Colon, Open Approach

H0ZP Bypass Cecum to Rectum, Open Approach

H3J4 Bypass Cecum to Cutaneous with Synthetic Substitute, Percutaneous Approach

1H474 Bypass Cecum to Cutaneous with Autologous Tissue Substitute, Percutaneous Endoscopic Approach

1H47H Bypass Cecum to Cecum with Autologous Tissue Substitute, Percutaneous Endoscopic Approach

1H47K Bypass Cecum to Ascending Colon with Autologous Tissue Substitute, Percutaneous Endoscopic Approach

1H47L Bypass Cecum to Transverse Colon with Autologous Tissue Substitute, Percutaneous Endoscopic Approach

1H47M Bypass Cecum to Descending Colon with Autologous Tissue Substitute, Percutaneous Endoscopic Approach

1H47N Bypass Cecum to Sigmoid Colon with Autologous Tissue Substitute, Percutaneous Endoscopic Approach

1H47P Bypass Cecum to Rectum with Autologous Tissue Substitute, Percutaneous Endoscopic Approach

1H4J4 Bypass Cecum to Cutaneous with Synthetic Substitute, Percutaneous Endoscopic Approach

1H4JH Bypass Cecum to Cecum with Synthetic Substitute, Percutaneous Endoscopic Approach

1H4JK Bypass Cecum to Ascending Colon with Synthetic Substitute, Percutaneous Endoscopic Approach

1H4JL Bypass Cecum to Transverse Colon with Synthetic Substitute, Percutaneous Endoscopic Approach

1H4JM Bypass Cecum to Descending Colon with Synthetic Substitute, Percutaneous Endoscopic Approach

1H4JN Bypass Cecum to Sigmoid Colon with Synthetic Substitute, Percutaneous Endoscopic Approach

D1H4JP Bypass Cecum to Rectum with Synthetic Substitute, Percutaneous Endoscopic Approach

D1H4K4 Bypass Cecum to Cutaneous with Nonautologous Tissue Substitute, Percutaneous Endoscopic Approach

D1H4KH Bypass Cecum to Cecum with Nonautologous Tissue Substitute, Percutaneous Endoscopic Approach

0D1H4KK Bypass Cecum to Ascending Colon with Nonautologous Tissue Substitute, Percutaneous Endoscopic Approach

0D1H4KL Bypass Cecum to Transverse Colon with Nonautologous Tissue Substitute, Percutaneous Endoscopic Approach

0D1H4KM Bypass Cecum to Descending Colon with Nonautologous Tissue Substitute, Percutaneous Endoscopic Approach

0D1H4KN Bypass Cecum to Sigmoid Colon with Nonautologous Tissue Substitute, Percutaneous Endoscopic Approach

0D1H4KP Bypass Cecum to Rectum with Nonautologous Tissue Substitute, Percutaneous Endoscopic Approach

0D1H4Z4 Bypass Cecum to Cutaneous, Percutaneous Endoscopic Approach

0D1H4ZH Bypass Cecum to Cecum, Percutaneous Endoscopic Approach

0D1H4ZK Bypass Cecum to Ascending Colon, Percutaneous Endoscopic Approach

0D1H4ZL Bypass Cecum to Transverse Colon, Percutaneous Endoscopic Approach

0D1H4ZM Bypass Cecum to Descending Colon, Percutaneous Endoscopic Approach

0D1H4ZN Bypass Cecum to Sigmoid Colon, Percutaneous Endoscopic Approach

0D1H4ZP Bypass Cecum to Rectum, Percutaneous Endoscopic Approach

0D1H874 Bypass Cecum to Cutaneous with Autologous Tissue Substitute, Via Natural or Artificial Opening Endoscopic

0D1H87H Bypass Cecum to Cecum with Autologous Tissue Substitute, Via Natural or Artificial Opening Endoscopic

0D1H87K Bypass Cecum to Ascending Colon with Autologous Tissue Substitute, Via Natural or Artificial Opening Endoscopic

0D1H87L Bypass Cecum to Transverse Colon with Autologous Tissue Substitute, Via Natural or Artificial Opening Endoscopic

0D1H87M Bypass Cecum to Descending Colon with Autologous Tissue Substitute, Via Natural or Artificial Opening Endoscopic

0D1H87N Bypass Cecum to Sigmoid Colon with Autologous Tissue Substitute, Via Natural or Artificial Opening Endoscopic

0D1H87P Bypass Cecum to Rectum with Autologous Tissue Substitute, Via Natural or Artificial Opening Endoscopic

0D1H8J4 Bypass Cecum to Cutaneous with Synthetic Substitute, Via Natural or Artificial Opening Endoscopic

0D1H8JH Bypass Cecum to Cecum with Synthetic Substitute, Via Natural or Artificial Opening Endoscopic

0D1H8JK Bypass Cecum to Ascending Colon with Synthetic Substitute, Via Natural or Artificial Opening Endoscopic

0D1H8JL Bypass Cecum to Transverse Colon with Synthetic Substitute, Via Natural or Artificial Opening Endoscopic

0D1H8JM Bypass Cecum to Descending Colon with Synthetic Substitute, Via Natural or Artificial Opening Endoscopic

0D1H8JN Bypass Cecum to Sigmoid Colon with Synthetic Substitute, Via Natural or Artificial Opening Endoscopic

0D1H8JP Bypass Cecum to Rectum with Synthetic Substitute, Via Natural or Artificial Opening Endoscopic

0D1H8K4 Bypass Cecum to Cutaneous with Nonautologous Tissue Substitute, Via Natural or Artificial Opening Endoscopic

0D1H8KH Bypass Cecum to Cecum with Nonautologous Tissue Substitute, Via Natural or Artificial Opening Endoscopic

0D1H8KK Bypass Cecum to Ascending Colon with Nonautologous Tissue Substitute, Via Natural or Artificial Opening Endoscopic

0D1H8KL Bypass Cecum to Transverse Colon with Nonautologous Tissue Substitute, Via Natural or Artificial Opening Endoscopic

0D1H8KM Bypass Cecum to Descending Colon with Nonautologous Tissue Substitute, Via Natural or Artificial Opening Endoscopic

0D1H8KN Bypass Cecum to Sigmoid Colon with Nonautologous Tissue Substitute, Via Natural or Artificial Opening Endoscopic

0D1H8KP Bypass Cecum to Rectum with Nonautologous Tissue Substitute, Via Natural or Artificial Opening Endoscopic

0D1H8Z4 Bypass Cecum to Cutaneous, Via Natural or Artificial Opening Endoscopic

0D1H8ZH Bypass Cecum to Cecum, Via Natural or Artificial Opening Endoscopic

0D1H8ZK Bypass Cecum to Ascending Colon, Via Natural or Artificial Opening Endoscopic

0D1H8ZL Bypass Cecum to Transverse Colon, Via Natural or Artificial Opening Endoscopic

0D1H8ZM Bypass Cecum to Descending Colon, Via Natural or Artificial Opening Endoscopic

0D1H8ZN Bypass Cecum to Sigmoid Colon, Via Natural or Artificial Opening Endoscopic

0D1H8ZP Bypass Cecum to Rectum, Via Natural or Artificial Opening Endoscopic

0D1K074 Bypass Ascending Colon to Cutaneous with Autologous Tissue Substitute, Open Approach

0D1K07K Bypass Ascending Colon to Ascending Colon with Autologous Tissue Substitute, Open Approach

0D1K07L Bypass Ascending Colon to Transverse Colon with Autologous Tissue Substitute, Open Approach

0D1K07M Bypass Ascending Colon to Descending Colon with Autologous Tissue Substitute, Open Approach

0D1K07N Bypass Ascending Colon to Sigmoid Colon with Autologous Tissue Substitute, Open Approach

0D1K07P Bypass Ascending Colon to Rectum with Autologous Tissue Substitute, Open Approach

0D1K0J4 Bypass Ascending Colon to Cutaneous with Synthetic Substitute, Open Approach

0D1K0JK Bypass Ascending Colon to Ascending Colon with Synthetic Substitute, Open Approach

0D1K0JL Bypass Ascending Colon to Transverse Colon with Synthetic Substitute, Open Approach

0D1K0JM Bypass Ascending Colon to Descending Colon with Synthetic Substitute, Open Approach

0D1K0JN Bypass Ascending Colon to Sigmoid Colon with Synthetic Substitute, Open Approach

0D1K0JP Bypass Ascending Colon to Rectum with Synthetic Substitute, Open Approach

0D1K0K4 Bypass Ascending Colon to Cutaneous with Nonautologous Tissue Substitute, Open Approach

0D1K0KK Bypass Ascending Colon to Ascending Colon with Nonautologous Tissue Substitute, Open Approach

0D1K0KL Bypass Ascending Colon to Transverse Colon with Nonautologous Tissue Substitute, Open Approach

0D1K0KM Bypass Ascending Colon to Descending Colon with Nonautologous Tissue Substitute, Open Approach

0D1K0KN Bypass Ascending Colon to Sigmoid Colon with Nonautologous Tissue Substitute, Open Approach

0D1K0KP Bypass Ascending Colon to Rectum with Nonautologous Tissue Substitute, Open Approach
0D1K0Z4 Bypass Ascending Colon to Cutaneous, Open Approach
0D1K0ZK Bypass Ascending Colon to Ascending Colon, Open Approach
0D1K0ZL Bypass Ascending Colon to Transverse Colon, Open Approach
0D1K0ZM Bypass Ascending Colon to Descending Colon, Open Approach
0D1K0ZN Bypass Ascending Colon to Sigmoid Colon, Open Approach
0D1K0ZP Bypass Ascending Colon to Rectum, Open Approach
0D1K3J4 Bypass Ascending Colon to Cutaneous with Synthetic Substitute, Percutaneous Approach
0D1K474 Bypass Ascending Colon to Cutaneous with Autologous Tissue Substitute, Percutaneous Endoscopic Approach
0D1K47K Bypass Ascending Colon to Ascending Colon with Autologous Tissue Substitute, Percutaneous Endoscopic Approach
0D1K47L Bypass Ascending Colon to Transverse Colon with Autologous Tissue Substitute, Percutaneous Endoscopic Approach
0D1K47M Bypass Ascending Colon to Descending Colon with Autologous Tissue Substitute, Percutaneous Endoscopic Approach
0D1K47N Bypass Ascending Colon to Sigmoid Colon with Autologous Tissue Substitute, Percutaneous Endoscopic Approach
0D1K47P Bypass Ascending Colon to Rectum with Autologous Tissue Substitute, Percutaneous Endoscopic Approach
0D1K4J4 Bypass Ascending Colon to Cutaneous with Synthetic Substitute, Percutaneous Endoscopic Approach
0D1K4JK Bypass Ascending Colon to Ascending Colon with Synthetic Substitute, Percutaneous Endoscopic Approach
0D1K4JL Bypass Ascending Colon to Transverse Colon with Synthetic Substitute, Percutaneous Endoscopic Approach
0D1K4JM Bypass Ascending Colon to Descending Colon with Synthetic Substitute, Percutaneous Endoscopic Approach
0D1K4JN Bypass Ascending Colon to Sigmoid Colon with Synthetic Substitute, Percutaneous Endoscopic Approach
0D1K4JP Bypass Ascending Colon to Rectum with Synthetic Substitute, Percutaneous Endoscopic Approach
0D1K4K4 Bypass Ascending Colon to Cutaneous with Nonautologous Tissue Substitute, Percutaneous Endoscopic Approach
0D1K4KK Bypass Ascending Colon to Ascending Colon with Nonautologous Tissue Substitute, Percutaneous Endoscopic Approach
0D1K4KL Bypass Ascending Colon to Transverse Colon with Nonautologous Tissue Substitute, Percutaneous Endoscopic Approach
0D1K4KM Bypass Ascending Colon to Descending Colon with Nonautologous Tissue Substitute, Percutaneous Endoscopic Approach
0D1K4KN Bypass Ascending Colon to Sigmoid Colon with Nonautologous Tissue Substitute, Percutaneous Endoscopic Approach
0D1K4KP Bypass Ascending Colon to Rectum with Nonautologous Tissue Substitute, Percutaneous Endoscopic Approach
0D1K4Z4 Bypass Ascending Colon to Cutaneous, Percutaneous Endoscopic Approach
0D1K4ZK Bypass Ascending Colon to Ascending Colon, Percutaneous Endoscopic Approach
0D1K4ZL Bypass Ascending Colon to Transverse Colon, Percutaneous Endoscopic Approach
0D1K4ZM Bypass Ascending Colon to Descending Colon, Percutaneous Endoscopic Approach
0D1K4ZN Bypass Ascending Colon to Sigmoid Colon, Percutaneous Endoscopic Approach
0D1K4ZP Bypass Ascending Colon to Rectum, Percutaneous Endoscopic Approach
0D1K874 Bypass Ascending Colon to Cutaneous with Autologous Tissue Substitute, Via Natural or Artificial Opening Endoscopic
0D1K87K Bypass Ascending Colon to Ascending Colon with Autologous Tissue Substitute, Via Natural or Artificial Opening Endoscopic
0D1K87L Bypass Ascending Colon to Transverse Colon with Autologous Tissue Substitute, Via Natural or Artificial Opening Endoscopic
0D1K87M Bypass Ascending Colon to Descending Colon with Autologous Tissue Substitute, Via Natural or Artificial Opening Endoscopic
0D1K87N Bypass Ascending Colon to Sigmoid Colon with Autologous Tissue Substitute, Via Natural or Artificial Opening Endoscopic
0D1K87P Bypass Ascending Colon to Rectum with Autologous Tissue Substitute, Via Natural or Artificial Opening Endoscopic
0D1K8J4 Bypass Ascending Colon to Cutaneous with Synthetic Substitute, Via Natural or Artificial Opening Endoscopic
0D1K8JK Bypass Ascending Colon to Ascending Colon with Synthetic Substitute, Via Natural or Artificial Opening Endoscopic
0D1K8JL Bypass Ascending Colon to Transverse Colon with Synthetic Substitute, Via Natural or Artificial Opening Endoscopic
0D1K8JM Bypass Ascending Colon to Descending Colon with Synthetic Substitute, Via Natural or Artificial Opening Endoscopic
0D1K8JN Bypass Ascending Colon to Sigmoid Colon with Synthetic Substitute, Via Natural or Artificial Opening Endoscopic
0D1K8JP Bypass Ascending Colon to Rectum with Synthetic Substitute, Via Natural or Artificial Opening Endoscopic
0D1K8K4 Bypass Ascending Colon to Cutaneous with Nonautologous Tissue Substitute, Via Natural or Artificial Opening Endoscopic
0D1K8KK Bypass Ascending Colon to Ascending Colon with Nonautologous Tissue Substitute, Via Natural or Artificial Opening Endoscopic
0D1K8KL Bypass Ascending Colon to Transverse Colon with Nonautologous Tissue Substitute, Via Natural or Artificial Opening Endoscopic
0D1K8KM Bypass Ascending Colon to Descending Colon with Nonautologous Tissue Substitute, Via Natural or Artificial Opening Endoscopic
0D1K8KN Bypass Ascending Colon to Sigmoid Colon with Nonautologous Tissue Substitute, Via Natural or Artificial Opening Endoscopic
0D1K8KP Bypass Ascending Colon to Rectum with Nonautologous Tissue Substitute, Via Natural or Artificial Opening Endoscopic
0D1K8Z4 Bypass Ascending Colon to Cutaneous, Via Natural or Artificial Opening Endoscopic
0D1K8ZK Bypass Ascending Colon to Ascending Colon, Via Natural or Artificial Opening Endoscopic
0D1K8ZL Bypass Ascending Colon to Transverse Colon, Via Natural or Artificial Opening Endoscopic
0D1K8ZM Bypass Ascending Colon to Descending Colon, Via Natural or Artificial Opening Endoscopic
0D1K8ZN Bypass Ascending Colon to Sigmoid Colon, Via Natural or Artificial Opening Endoscopic
0D1K8ZP Bypass Ascending Colon to Rectum, Via Natural or Artificial Opening Endoscopic
0D1L074 Bypass Transverse Colon to Cutaneous with Autologous Tissue Substitute, Open Approach
0D1L07L Bypass Transverse Colon to Transverse Colon with Autologous Tissue Substitute, Open Approach
0D1L07M Bypass Transverse Colon to Descending Colon with Autologous Tissue Substitute, Open Approach
0D1L07N Bypass Transverse Colon to Sigmoid Colon with Autologous Tissue Substitute, Open Approach
0D1L07P Bypass Transverse Colon to Rectum with Autologous Tissue Substitute, Open Approach
0D1L0J4 Bypass Transverse Colon to Cutaneous with Synthetic Substitute, Open Approach
0D1L0JL Bypass Transverse Colon to Transverse Colon with Synthetic Substitute, Open Approach
0D1L0JM Bypass Transverse Colon to Descending Colon with Synthetic Substitute, Open Approach
0D1L0JN Bypass Transverse Colon to Sigmoid Colon with Synthetic Substitute, Open Approach
0D1L0JP Bypass Transverse Colon to Rectum with Synthetic Substitute, Open Approach
0D1L0K4 Bypass Transverse Colon to Cutaneous with Nonautologous Tissue Substitute, Open Approach
0D1L0KL Bypass Transverse Colon to Transverse Colon with Nonautologous Tissue Substitute, Open Approach
0D1L0KM Bypass Transverse Colon to Descending Colon with Nonautologous Tissue Substitute, Open Approach
0D1L0KN Bypass Transverse Colon to Sigmoid Colon with Nonautologous Tissue Substitute, Open Approach
0D1L0KP Bypass Transverse Colon to Rectum with Nonautologous Tissue Substitute, Open Approach
0D1L0Z4 Bypass Transverse Colon to Cutaneous, Open Approach
0D1L0ZL Bypass Transverse Colon to Transverse Colon, Open Approach
0D1L0ZM Bypass Transverse Colon to Descending Colon, Open Approach
0D1L0ZN Bypass Transverse Colon to Sigmoid Colon, Open Approach
0D1L0ZP Bypass Transverse Colon to Rectum, Open Approach
0D1L3J4 Bypass Transverse Colon to Cutaneous with Synthetic Substitute, Percutaneous Approach
0D1L474 Bypass Transverse Colon to Cutaneous with Autologous Tissue Substitute, Percutaneous Endoscopic Approach

L47L Bypass Transverse Colon to Transverse Colon with Autologous Tissue Substitute, Percutaneous Endoscopic Approach
L47M Bypass Transverse Colon to Descending Colon with Autologous Tissue Substitute, Percutaneous Endoscopic Approach
L47N Bypass Transverse Colon to Sigmoid Colon with Autologous Tissue Substitute, Percutaneous Endoscopic Approach
L47P Bypass Transverse Colon to Rectum with Autologous Tissue Substitute, Percutaneous Endoscopic Approach
L4J4 Bypass Transverse Colon to Cutaneous with Synthetic Substitute, Percutaneous Endoscopic Approach
L4JL Bypass Transverse Colon to Transverse Colon with Synthetic Substitute, Percutaneous Endoscopic Approach
L4JM Bypass Transverse Colon to Descending Colon with Synthetic Substitute, Percutaneous Endoscopic Approach
L4JN Bypass Transverse Colon to Sigmoid Colon with Synthetic Substitute, Percutaneous Endoscopic Approach
L4JP Bypass Transverse Colon to Rectum with Synthetic Substitute, Percutaneous Endoscopic Approach
L4K4 Bypass Transverse Colon to Cutaneous with Nonautologous Tissue Substitute, Percutaneous Endoscopic Approach
L4KL Bypass Transverse Colon to Transverse Colon with Nonautologous Tissue Substitute, Percutaneous Endoscopic Approach
L4KM Bypass Transverse Colon to Descending Colon with Nonautologous Tissue Substitute, Percutaneous Endoscopic Approach
L4KN Bypass Transverse Colon to Sigmoid Colon with Nonautologous Tissue Substitute, Percutaneous Endoscopic Approach
1L4KP Bypass Transverse Colon to Rectum with Nonautologous Tissue Substitute, Percutaneous Endoscopic Approach
1L4Z4 Bypass Transverse Colon to Cutaneous, Percutaneous Endoscopic Approach
1L4ZL Bypass Transverse Colon to Transverse Colon, Percutaneous Endoscopic Approach
1L4ZM Bypass Transverse Colon to Descending Colon, Percutaneous Endoscopic Approach
1L4ZN Bypass Transverse Colon to Sigmoid Colon, Percutaneous Endoscopic Approach
1L4ZP Bypass Transverse Colon to Rectum, Percutaneous Endoscopic Approach
1L874 Bypass Transverse Colon to Cutaneous with Autologous Tissue Substitute, Via Natural or Artificial Opening Endoscopic
1L87L Bypass Transverse Colon to Transverse Colon with Autologous Tissue Substitute, Via Natural or Artificial Opening Endoscopic
1L87M Bypass Transverse Colon to Descending Colon with Autologous Tissue Substitute, Via Natural or Artificial Opening Endoscopic
)1L87N Bypass Transverse Colon to Sigmoid Colon with Autologous Tissue Substitute, Via Natural or Artificial Opening Endoscopic
)1L87P Bypass Transverse Colon to Rectum with Autologous Tissue Substitute, Via Natural or Artificial Opening Endoscopic

0D1L8J4 Bypass Transverse Colon to Cutaneous with Synthetic Substitute, Via Natural or Artificial Opening Endoscopic
0D1L8JL Bypass Transverse Colon to Transverse Colon with Synthetic Substitute, Via Natural or Artificial Opening Endoscopic
0D1L8JM Bypass Transverse Colon to Descending Colon with Synthetic Substitute, Via Natural or Artificial Opening Endoscopic
0D1L8JN Bypass Transverse Colon to Sigmoid Colon with Synthetic Substitute, Via Natural or Artificial Opening Endoscopic
0D1L8JP Bypass Transverse Colon to Rectum with Synthetic Substitute, Via Natural or Artificial Opening Endoscopic
0D1L8K4 Bypass Transverse Colon to Cutaneous with Nonautologous Tissue Substitute, Via Natural or Artificial Opening Endoscopic
0D1L8KL Bypass Transverse Colon to Transverse Colon with Nonautologous Tissue Substitute, Via Natural or Artificial Opening Endoscopic
0D1L8KM Bypass Transverse Colon to Descending Colon with Nonautologous Tissue Substitute, Via Natural or Artificial Opening Endoscopic
0D1L8KN Bypass Transverse Colon to Sigmoid Colon with Nonautologous Tissue Substitute, Via Natural or Artificial Opening Endoscopic
0D1L8KP Bypass Transverse Colon to Rectum with Nonautologous Tissue Substitute, Via Natural or Artificial Opening Endoscopic
0D1L8Z4 Bypass Transverse Colon to Cutaneous, Via Natural or Artificial Opening Endoscopic
0D1L8ZL Bypass Transverse Colon to Transverse Colon, Via Natural or Artificial Opening Endoscopic
0D1L8ZM Bypass Transverse Colon to Descending Colon, Via Natural or Artificial Opening Endoscopic
0D1L8ZN Bypass Transverse Colon to Sigmoid Colon, Via Natural or Artificial Opening Endoscopic
0D1L8ZP Bypass Transverse Colon to Rectum, Via Natural or Artificial Opening Endoscopic
0D1M074 Bypass Descending Colon to Cutaneous with Autologous Tissue Substitute, Open Approach
0D1M07M Bypass Descending Colon to Descending Colon with Autologous Tissue Substitute, Open Approach
0D1M07N Bypass Descending Colon to Sigmoid Colon with Autologous Tissue Substitute, Open Approach
0D1M07P Bypass Descending Colon to Rectum with Autologous Tissue Substitute, Open Approach
0D1M0J4 Bypass Descending Colon to Cutaneous with Synthetic Substitute, Open Approach
0D1M0JM Bypass Descending Colon to Descending Colon with Synthetic Substitute, Open Approach
0D1M0JN Bypass Descending Colon to Sigmoid Colon with Synthetic Substitute, Open Approach
0D1M0JP Bypass Descending Colon to Rectum with Synthetic Substitute, Open Approach
0D1M0K4 Bypass Descending Colon to Cutaneous with Nonautologous Tissue Substitute, Open Approach
0D1M0KM Bypass Descending Colon to Descending Colon with Nonautologous Tissue Substitute, Open Approach

0D1M0KN Bypass Descending Colon to Sigmoid Colon with Nonautologous Tissue Substitute, Open Approach
0D1M0KP Bypass Descending Colon to Rectum with Nonautologous Tissue Substitute, Open Approach
0D1M0Z4 Bypass Descending Colon to Cutaneous, Open Approach
0D1M0ZM Bypass Descending Colon to Descending Colon, Open Approach
0D1M0ZN Bypass Descending Colon to Sigmoid Colon, Open Approach
0D1M0ZP Bypass Descending Colon to Rectum, Open Approach
0D1M3J4 Bypass Descending Colon to Cutaneous with Synthetic Substitute, Percutaneous Approach
0D1M474 Bypass Descending Colon to Cutaneous with Autologous Tissue Substitute, Percutaneous Endoscopic Approach
0D1M47M Bypass Descending Colon to Descending Colon with Autologous Tissue Substitute, Percutaneous Endoscopic Approach
0D1M47N Bypass Descending Colon to Sigmoid Colon with Autologous Tissue Substitute, Percutaneous Endoscopic Approach
0D1M47P Bypass Descending Colon to Rectum with Autologous Tissue Substitute, Percutaneous Endoscopic Approach
0D1M4J4 Bypass Descending Colon to Cutaneous with Synthetic Substitute, Percutaneous Endoscopic Approach
0D1M4JM Bypass Descending Colon to Descending Colon with Synthetic Substitute, Percutaneous Endoscopic Approach
0D1M4JN Bypass Descending Colon to Sigmoid Colon with Synthetic Substitute, Percutaneous Endoscopic Approach
0D1M4JP Bypass Descending Colon to Rectum with Synthetic Substitute, Percutaneous Endoscopic Approach
0D1M4K4 Bypass Descending Colon to Cutaneous with Nonautologous Tissue Substitute, Percutaneous Endoscopic Approach
0D1M4KM Bypass Descending Colon to Descending Colon with Nonautologous Tissue Substitute, Percutaneous Endoscopic Approach
0D1M4KN Bypass Descending Colon to Sigmoid Colon with Nonautologous Tissue Substitute, Percutaneous Endoscopic Approach
0D1M4KP Bypass Descending Colon to Rectum with Nonautologous Tissue Substitute, Percutaneous Endoscopic Approach
0D1M4Z4 Bypass Descending Colon to Cutaneous, Percutaneous Endoscopic Approach
0D1M4ZM Bypass Descending Colon to Descending Colon, Percutaneous Endoscopic Approach
0D1M4ZN Bypass Descending Colon to Sigmoid Colon, Percutaneous Endoscopic Approach
0D1M4ZP Bypass Descending Colon to Rectum, Percutaneous Endoscopic Approach
0D1M874 Bypass Descending Colon to Cutaneous with Autologous Tissue Substitute, Via Natural or Artificial Opening Endoscopic
0D1M87M Bypass Descending Colon to Descending Colon with Autologous Tissue Substitute, Via Natural or Artificial Opening Endoscopic
0D1M87N Bypass Descending Colon to Sigmoid Colon with Autologous Tissue Substitute, Via Natural or Artificial Opening Endoscopic

0D1M87P Bypass Descending Colon to Rectum with Autologous Tissue Substitute, Via Natural or Artificial Opening Endoscopic

0D1M8J4 Bypass Descending Colon to Cutaneous with Synthetic Substitute, Via Natural or Artificial Opening Endoscopic

0D1M8JM Bypass Descending Colon to Descending Colon with Synthetic Substitute, Via Natural or Artificial Opening Endoscopic

0D1M8JN Bypass Descending Colon to Sigmoid Colon with Synthetic Substitute, Via Natural or Artificial Opening Endoscopic

0D1M8JP Bypass Descending Colon to Rectum with Synthetic Substitute, Via Natural or Artificial Opening Endoscopic

0D1M8K4 Bypass Descending Colon to Cutaneous with Nonautologous Tissue Substitute, Via Natural or Artificial Opening Endoscopic

0D1M8KM Bypass Descending Colon to Descending Colon with Nonautologous Tissue Substitute, Via Natural or Artificial Opening Endoscopic

0D1M8KN Bypass Descending Colon to Sigmoid Colon with Nonautologous Tissue Substitute, Via Natural or Artificial Opening Endoscopic

0D1M8KP Bypass Descending Colon to Rectum with Nonautologous Tissue Substitute, Via Natural or Artificial Opening Endoscopic

0D1M8Z4 Bypass Descending Colon to Cutaneous, Via Natural or Artificial Opening Endoscopic

0D1M8ZM Bypass Descending Colon to Descending Colon, Via Natural or Artificial Opening Endoscopic

0D1M8ZN Bypass Descending Colon to Sigmoid Colon, Via Natural or Artificial Opening Endoscopic

0D1M8ZP Bypass Descending Colon to Rectum, Via Natural or Artificial Opening Endoscopic

0D1N074 Bypass Sigmoid Colon to Cutaneous with Autologous Tissue Substitute, Open Approach

0D1N07N Bypass Sigmoid Colon to Sigmoid Colon with Autologous Tissue Substitute, Open Approach

0D1N07P Bypass Sigmoid Colon to Rectum with Autologous Tissue Substitute, Open Approach

0D1N0J4 Bypass Sigmoid Colon to Cutaneous with Synthetic Substitute, Open Approach

0D1N0JN Bypass Sigmoid Colon to Sigmoid Colon with Synthetic Substitute, Open Approach

0D1N0JP Bypass Sigmoid Colon to Rectum with Synthetic Substitute, Open Approach

0D1N0K4 Bypass Sigmoid Colon to Cutaneous with Nonautologous Tissue Substitute, Open Approach

0D1N0KN Bypass Sigmoid Colon to Sigmoid Colon with Nonautologous Tissue Substitute, Open Approach

0D1N0KP Bypass Sigmoid Colon to Rectum with Nonautologous Tissue Substitute, Open Approach

0D1N0Z4 Bypass Sigmoid Colon to Cutaneous, Open Approach

0D1N0ZN Bypass Sigmoid Colon to Sigmoid Colon, Open Approach

0D1N0ZP Bypass Sigmoid Colon to Rectum, Open Approach

0D1N3J4 Bypass Sigmoid Colon to Cutaneous with Synthetic Substitute, Percutaneous Approach

0D1N474 Bypass Sigmoid Colon to Cutaneous with Autologous Tissue Substitute, Percutaneous Endoscopic Approach

0D1N47N Bypass Sigmoid Colon to Sigmoid Colon with Autologous Tissue Substitute, Percutaneous Endoscopic Approach

0D1N47P Bypass Sigmoid Colon to Rectum with Autologous Tissue Substitute, Percutaneous Endoscopic Approach

0D1N4J4 Bypass Sigmoid Colon to Cutaneous with Synthetic Substitute, Percutaneous Endoscopic Approach

0D1N4JN Bypass Sigmoid Colon to Sigmoid Colon with Synthetic Substitute, Percutaneous Endoscopic Approach

0D1N4JP Bypass Sigmoid Colon to Rectum with Synthetic Substitute, Percutaneous Endoscopic Approach

0D1N4K4 Bypass Sigmoid Colon to Cutaneous with Nonautologous Tissue Substitute, Percutaneous Endoscopic Approach

0D1N4KN Bypass Sigmoid Colon to Sigmoid C with Nonautologous Tissue Substitut Percutaneous Endoscopic Approach

0D1N4KP Bypass Sigmoid Colon to Rectum with Nonautologous Tissue Substitut Percutaneous Endoscopic Approach

0D1N4Z4 Bypass Sigmoid Colon to Cutaneous, Percutaneous Endoscopic Approach

0D1N4ZN Bypass Sigmoid Colon to Sigmoid Colon, Percutaneous Endoscopic Approach

0D1N4ZP Bypass Sigmoid Colon to Rectum, Percutaneous Endoscopic Approach

0D1N874 Bypass Sigmoid Colon to Cutaneous with Autologous Tissue Substitute, Vi Natural or Artificial Opening Endosc

0D1N87N Bypass Sigmoid Colon to Sigmoid Co with Autologous Tissue Substitute, Vi Natural or Artificial Opening Endosc

0D1N87P Bypass Sigmoid Colon to Rectum with Autologous Tissue Substitute, Vi Natural or Artificial Opening Endosc

0D1N8J4 Bypass Sigmoid Colon to Cutaneous with Synthetic Substitute, Via Natural Artificial Opening Endoscopic

0D1N8JN Bypass Sigmoid Colon to Sigmoid Co with Synthetic Substitute, Via Natural Artificial Opening Endoscopic

0D1N8JP Bypass Sigmoid Colon to Rectum with Synthetic Substitute, Via Natural or Artificial Opening Endoscopic

0D1N8K4 Bypass Sigmoid Colon to Cutaneous w Nonautologous Tissue Substitute, Via Natural or Artificial Opening Endosco

0D1N8KN Bypass Sigmoid Colon to Sigmoid Co with Nonautologous Tissue Substitute, Via Natural or Artificial Opening Endoscopic

0D1N8KP Bypass Sigmoid Colon to Rectum with Nonautologous Tissue Substitute, Via Natural or Artificial Opening Endosco

0D1N8Z4 Bypass Sigmoid Colon to Cutaneous, Natural or Artificial Opening Endosco

0D1N8ZN Bypass Sigmoid Colon to Sigmoid Colon, Via Natural or Artificial Openin Endoscopic

0D1N8ZP Bypass Sigmoid Colon to Rectum, Via Natural or Artificial Opening Endosco

0D2 – Gastrointestinal System, Change

Review Coding Guideline B6.1c

0D20X0Z Change Drainage Device in Upper Intestinal Tract, External Approach

0D20XUZ Change Feeding Device in Upper Intestinal Tract, External Approach

0D20XYZ Change Other Device in Upper Intestinal Tract, External Approach

0D2DX0Z Change Drainage Device in Lower Intestinal Tract, External Approach

0D2DXUZ Change Feeding Device in Lower Intestinal Tract, External Approach

0D2DXYZ Change Other Device in Lower Intestinal Tract, External Approach

0D2UX0Z Change Drainage Device in Omentum, External Approach

0D2UXYZ Change Other Device in Omentum, External Approach

0D2VX0Z Change Drainage Device in Mesentery, External Approach

0D2VXYZ Change Other Device in Mesentery, External Approach

0D2WX0Z Change Drainage Device in Peritoneum External Approach

0D2WXYZ Change Other Device in Peritoneum, External Approach

0D5 – Gastrointestinal System, Destruction

0D510ZZ Destruction of Upper Esophagus, Open Approach

0D513ZZ Destruction of Upper Esophagus, Percutaneous Approach

0D514ZZ Destruction of Upper Esophagus, Percutaneous Endoscopic Approach

0D517ZZ Destruction of Upper Esophagus, Via Natural or Artificial Opening

0D518ZZ Destruction of Upper Esophagus, Via Natural or Artificial Opening Endoscopic

0D520ZZ Destruction of Middle Esophagus, Open Approach

0D523ZZ Destruction of Middle Esophagus, Percutaneous Approach

0D524ZZ Destruction of Middle Esophagus, Percutaneous Endoscopic Approach

0D527ZZ Destruction of Middle Esophagus, Via Natural or Artificial Opening

0D528ZZ Destruction of Middle Esophagus, Via Natural or Artificial Opening Endoscopic

0D530ZZ Destruction of Lower Esophagus, Open Approach

0D533ZZ Destruction of Lower Esophagus, Percutaneous Approach

0D534ZZ Destruction of Lower Esophagus, Percutaneous Endoscopic Approach

0D537ZZ Destruction of Lower Esophagus, Via Natural or Artificial Opening

0D538ZZ Destruction of Lower Esophagus, Via Natural or Artificial Opening Endoscopic

40ZZ Destruction of Esophagogastric Junction, Open Approach
43ZZ Destruction of Esophagogastric Junction, Percutaneous Approach
44ZZ Destruction of Esophagogastric Junction, Percutaneous Endoscopic Approach
47ZZ Destruction of Esophagogastric Junction, Via Natural or Artificial Opening
48ZZ Destruction of Esophagogastric Junction, Via Natural or Artificial Opening Endoscopic
50ZZ Destruction of Esophagus, Open Approach
53ZZ Destruction of Esophagus, Percutaneous Approach
54ZZ Destruction of Esophagus, Percutaneous Endoscopic Approach
57ZZ Destruction of Esophagus, Via Natural or Artificial Opening
58ZZ Destruction of Esophagus, Via Natural or Artificial Opening Endoscopic
560ZZ Destruction of Stomach, Open Approach
563ZZ Destruction of Stomach, Percutaneous Approach
564ZZ Destruction of Stomach, Percutaneous Endoscopic Approach
567ZZ Destruction of Stomach, Via Natural or Artificial Opening
568ZZ Destruction of Stomach, Via Natural or Artificial Opening Endoscopic
570ZZ Destruction of Stomach, Pylorus, Open Approach
573ZZ Destruction of Stomach, Pylorus, Percutaneous Approach
574ZZ Destruction of Stomach, Pylorus, Percutaneous Endoscopic Approach
577ZZ Destruction of Stomach, Pylorus, Via Natural or Artificial Opening
578ZZ Destruction of Stomach, Pylorus, Via Natural or Artificial Opening Endoscopic
580ZZ Destruction of Small Intestine, Open Approach
583ZZ Destruction of Small Intestine, Percutaneous Approach
584ZZ Destruction of Small Intestine, Percutaneous Endoscopic Approach
587ZZ Destruction of Small Intestine, Via Natural or Artificial Opening
588ZZ Destruction of Small Intestine, Via Natural or Artificial Opening Endoscopic
590ZZ Destruction of Duodenum, Open Approach
593ZZ Destruction of Duodenum, Percutaneous Approach
594ZZ Destruction of Duodenum, Percutaneous Endoscopic Approach
597ZZ Destruction of Duodenum, Via Natural or Artificial Opening
598ZZ Destruction of Duodenum, Via Natural or Artificial Opening Endoscopic
5A0ZZ Destruction of Jejunum, Open Approach
5A3ZZ Destruction of Jejunum, Percutaneous Approach
5A4ZZ Destruction of Jejunum, Percutaneous Endoscopic Approach
5A7ZZ Destruction of Jejunum, Via Natural or Artificial Opening
5A8ZZ Destruction of Jejunum, Via Natural or Artificial Opening Endoscopic
5B0ZZ Destruction of Ileum, Open Approach
D5B3ZZ Destruction of Ileum, Percutaneous Approach
D5B4ZZ Destruction of Ileum, Percutaneous Endoscopic Approach
D5B7ZZ Destruction of Ileum, Via Natural or Artificial Opening
0D5B8ZZ Destruction of Ileum, Via Natural or Artificial Opening Endoscopic
0D5C0ZZ Destruction of Ileocecal Valve, Open Approach
0D5C3ZZ Destruction of Ileocecal Valve, Percutaneous Approach
0D5C4ZZ Destruction of Ileocecal Valve, Percutaneous Endoscopic Approach
0D5C7ZZ Destruction of Ileocecal Valve, Via Natural or Artificial Opening
0D5C8ZZ Destruction of Ileocecal Valve, Via Natural or Artificial Opening Endoscopic
0D5E0ZZ Destruction of Large Intestine, Open Approach
0D5E3ZZ Destruction of Large Intestine, Percutaneous Approach
0D5E4ZZ Destruction of Large Intestine, Percutaneous Endoscopic Approach
0D5E7ZZ Destruction of Large Intestine, Via Natural or Artificial Opening
0D5E8ZZ Destruction of Large Intestine, Via Natural or Artificial Opening Endoscopic
0D5F0ZZ Destruction of Right Large Intestine, Open Approach
0D5F3ZZ Destruction of Right Large Intestine, Percutaneous Approach
0D5F4ZZ Destruction of Right Large Intestine, Percutaneous Endoscopic Approach
0D5F7ZZ Destruction of Right Large Intestine, Via Natural or Artificial Opening
0D5F8ZZ Destruction of Right Large Intestine, Via Natural or Artificial Opening Endoscopic
0D5G0ZZ Destruction of Left Large Intestine, Open Approach
0D5G3ZZ Destruction of Left Large Intestine, Percutaneous Approach
0D5G4ZZ Destruction of Left Large Intestine, Percutaneous Endoscopic Approach
0D5G7ZZ Destruction of Left Large Intestine, Via Natural or Artificial Opening
0D5G8ZZ Destruction of Left Large Intestine, Via Natural or Artificial Opening Endoscopic
0D5H0ZZ Destruction of Cecum, Open Approach
0D5H3ZZ Destruction of Cecum, Percutaneous Approach
0D5H4ZZ Destruction of Cecum, Percutaneous Endoscopic Approach
0D5H7ZZ Destruction of Cecum, Via Natural or Artificial Opening
0D5H8ZZ Destruction of Cecum, Via Natural or Artificial Opening Endoscopic
0D5J0ZZ Destruction of Appendix, Open Approach
0D5J3ZZ Destruction of Appendix, Percutaneous Approach
0D5J4ZZ Destruction of Appendix, Percutaneous Endoscopic Approach
0D5J7ZZ Destruction of Appendix, Via Natural or Artificial Opening
0D5J8ZZ Destruction of Appendix, Via Natural or Artificial Opening Endoscopic
0D5K0ZZ Destruction of Ascending Colon, Open Approach
0D5K3ZZ Destruction of Ascending Colon, Percutaneous Approach
0D5K4ZZ Destruction of Ascending Colon, Percutaneous Endoscopic Approach
0D5K7ZZ Destruction of Ascending Colon, Via Natural or Artificial Opening
0D5K8ZZ Destruction of Ascending Colon, Via Natural or Artificial Opening Endoscopic
0D5L0ZZ Destruction of Transverse Colon, Open Approach
0D5L3ZZ Destruction of Transverse Colon, Percutaneous Approach
0D5L4ZZ Destruction of Transverse Colon, Percutaneous Endoscopic Approach
0D5L7ZZ Destruction of Transverse Colon, Via Natural or Artificial Opening
0D5L8ZZ Destruction of Transverse Colon, Via Natural or Artificial Opening Endoscopic
0D5M0ZZ Destruction of Descending Colon, Open Approach
0D5M3ZZ Destruction of Descending Colon, Percutaneous Approach
0D5M4ZZ Destruction of Descending Colon, Percutaneous Endoscopic Approach
0D5M7ZZ Destruction of Descending Colon, Via Natural or Artificial Opening
0D5M8ZZ Destruction of Descending Colon, Via Natural or Artificial Opening Endoscopic
0D5N0ZZ Destruction of Sigmoid Colon, Open Approach
0D5N3ZZ Destruction of Sigmoid Colon, Percutaneous Approach
0D5N4ZZ Destruction of Sigmoid Colon, Percutaneous Endoscopic Approach
0D5N7ZZ Destruction of Sigmoid Colon, Via Natural or Artificial Opening
0D5N8ZZ Destruction of Sigmoid Colon, Via Natural or Artificial Opening Endoscopic
0D5P0ZZ Destruction of Rectum, Open Approach
0D5P3ZZ Destruction of Rectum, Percutaneous Approach
0D5P4ZZ Destruction of Rectum, Percutaneous Endoscopic Approach
0D5P7ZZ Destruction of Rectum, Via Natural or Artificial Opening
0D5P8ZZ Destruction of Rectum, Via Natural or Artificial Opening Endoscopic
0D5Q0ZZ Destruction of Anus, Open Approach
0D5Q3ZZ Destruction of Anus, Percutaneous Approach
0D5Q4ZZ Destruction of Anus, Percutaneous Endoscopic Approach
0D5Q7ZZ Destruction of Anus, Via Natural or Artificial Opening
0D5Q8ZZ Destruction of Anus, Via Natural or Artificial Opening Endoscopic
0D5QXZZ Destruction of Anus, External Approach
0D5R0ZZ Destruction of Anal Sphincter, Open Approach
0D5R3ZZ Destruction of Anal Sphincter, Percutaneous Approach
0D5R4ZZ Destruction of Anal Sphincter, Percutaneous Endoscopic Approach
0D5S0ZZ Destruction of Greater Omentum, Open Approach
0D5S3ZZ Destruction of Greater Omentum, Percutaneous Approach
0D5S4ZZ Destruction of Greater Omentum, Percutaneous Endoscopic Approach
0D5T0ZZ Destruction of Lesser Omentum, Open Approach
0D5T3ZZ Destruction of Lesser Omentum, Percutaneous Approach
0D5T4ZZ Destruction of Lesser Omentum, Percutaneous Endoscopic Approach
0D5V0ZZ Destruction of Mesentery, Open Approach
0D5V3ZZ Destruction of Mesentery, Percutaneous Approach
0D5V4ZZ Destruction of Mesentery, Percutaneous Endoscopic Approach
0D5W0ZZ Destruction of Peritoneum, Open Approach
0D5W3ZZ Destruction of Peritoneum, Percutaneous Approach
0D5W4ZZ Destruction of Peritoneum, Percutaneous Endoscopic Approach

0D7 – Gastrointestinal System, Dilation

0D710DZ Dilation of Upper Esophagus with Intraluminal Device, Open Approach
0D710ZZ Dilation of Upper Esophagus, Open Approach
0D713DZ Dilation of Upper Esophagus with Intraluminal Device, Percutaneous Approach
0D713ZZ Dilation of Upper Esophagus, Percutaneous Approach
0D714DZ Dilation of Upper Esophagus with Intraluminal Device, Percutaneous Endoscopic Approach
0D714ZZ Dilation of Upper Esophagus, Percutaneous Endoscopic Approach
0D717DZ Dilation of Upper Esophagus with Intraluminal Device, Via Natural or Artificial Opening
0D717ZZ Dilation of Upper Esophagus, Via Natural or Artificial Opening
0D718DZ Dilation of Upper Esophagus with Intraluminal Device, Via Natural or Artificial Opening Endoscopic
0D718ZZ Dilation of Upper Esophagus, Via Natural or Artificial Opening Endoscopic
0D720DZ Dilation of Middle Esophagus with Intraluminal Device, Open Approach
0D720ZZ Dilation of Middle Esophagus, Open Approach
0D723DZ Dilation of Middle Esophagus with Intraluminal Device, Percutaneous Approach
0D723ZZ Dilation of Middle Esophagus, Percutaneous Approach
0D724DZ Dilation of Middle Esophagus with Intraluminal Device, Percutaneous Endoscopic Approach
0D724ZZ Dilation of Middle Esophagus, Percutaneous Endoscopic Approach
0D727DZ Dilation of Middle Esophagus with Intraluminal Device, Via Natural or Artificial Opening
0D727ZZ Dilation of Middle Esophagus, Via Natural or Artificial Opening
0D728DZ Dilation of Middle Esophagus with Intraluminal Device, Via Natural or Artificial Opening Endoscopic
0D728ZZ Dilation of Middle Esophagus, Via Natural or Artificial Opening Endoscopic
0D730DZ Dilation of Lower Esophagus with Intraluminal Device, Open Approach
0D730ZZ Dilation of Lower Esophagus, Open Approach
0D733DZ Dilation of Lower Esophagus with Intraluminal Device, Percutaneous Approach
0D733ZZ Dilation of Lower Esophagus, Percutaneous Approach
0D734DZ Dilation of Lower Esophagus with Intraluminal Device, Percutaneous Endoscopic Approach
0D734ZZ Dilation of Lower Esophagus, Percutaneous Endoscopic Approach
0D737DZ Dilation of Lower Esophagus with Intraluminal Device, Via Natural or Artificial Opening
0D737ZZ Dilation of Lower Esophagus, Via Natural or Artificial Opening
0D738DZ Dilation of Lower Esophagus with Intraluminal Device, Via Natural or Artificial Opening Endoscopic
0D738ZZ Dilation of Lower Esophagus, Via Natural or Artificial Opening Endoscopic
0D740DZ Dilation of Esophagogastric Junction with Intraluminal Device, Open Approach
0D740ZZ Dilation of Esophagogastric Junction, Open Approach
0D743DZ Dilation of Esophagogastric Junction with Intraluminal Device, Percutaneous Approach
0D743ZZ Dilation of Esophagogastric Junction, Percutaneous Approach
0D744DZ Dilation of Esophagogastric Junction with Intraluminal Device, Percutaneous Endoscopic Approach
0D744ZZ Dilation of Esophagogastric Junction, Percutaneous Endoscopic Approach
0D747DZ Dilation of Esophagogastric Junction with Intraluminal Device, Via Natural or Artificial Opening
0D747ZZ Dilation of Esophagogastric Junction, Via Natural or Artificial Opening
0D748DZ Dilation of Esophagogastric Junction with Intraluminal Device, Via Natural or Artificial Opening Endoscopic
0D748ZZ Dilation of Esophagogastric Junction, Via Natural or Artificial Opening Endoscopic
0D750DZ Dilation of Esophagus with Intraluminal Device, Open Approach
0D750ZZ Dilation of Esophagus, Open Approach
0D753DZ Dilation of Esophagus with Intraluminal Device, Percutaneous Approach
0D753ZZ Dilation of Esophagus, Percutaneous Approach
0D754DZ Dilation of Esophagus with Intraluminal Device, Percutaneous Endoscopic Approach
0D754ZZ Dilation of Esophagus, Percutaneous Endoscopic Approach
0D757DZ Dilation of Esophagus with Intraluminal Device, Via Natural or Artificial Opening
0D757ZZ Dilation of Esophagus, Via Natural or Artificial Opening
0D758DZ Dilation of Esophagus with Intraluminal Device, Via Natural or Artificial Opening Endoscopic
0D758ZZ Dilation of Esophagus, Via Natural or Artificial Opening Endoscopic
0D760DZ Dilation of Stomach with Intraluminal Device, Open Approach
0D760ZZ Dilation of Stomach, Open Approach
0D763DZ Dilation of Stomach with Intraluminal Device, Percutaneous Approach
0D763ZZ Dilation of Stomach, Percutaneous Approach
0D764DZ Dilation of Stomach with Intraluminal Device, Percutaneous Endoscopic Approach
0D764ZZ Dilation of Stomach, Percutaneous Endoscopic Approach
0D767DZ Dilation of Stomach with Intraluminal Device, Via Natural or Artificial Opening
0D767ZZ Dilation of Stomach, Via Natural or Artificial Opening
0D768DZ Dilation of Stomach with Intraluminal Device, Via Natural or Artificial Opening Endoscopic
0D768ZZ Dilation of Stomach, Via Natural or Artificial Opening Endoscopic
0D770DZ Dilation of Stomach, Pylorus with Intraluminal Device, Open Approach
0D770ZZ Dilation of Stomach, Pylorus, Open Approach
0D773DZ Dilation of Stomach, Pylorus with Intraluminal Device, Percutaneous Approach
0D773ZZ Dilation of Stomach, Pylorus, Percutaneous Approach
0D774DZ Dilation of Stomach, Pylorus with Intraluminal Device, Percutaneous Endoscopic Approach
0D774ZZ Dilation of Stomach, Pylorus, Percutaneous Endoscopic Approach
0D777DZ Dilation of Stomach, Pylorus with Intraluminal Device, Via Natural or Artificial Opening
0D777ZZ Dilation of Stomach, Pylorus, Via Natu or Artificial Opening
0D778DZ Dilation of Stomach, Pylorus with Intraluminal Device, Via Natural or Artificial Opening Endoscopic
● **0D778ZZ** Dilation of Stomach, Pylorus, Via Natu or Artificial Opening Endoscopic
0D780DZ Dilation of Small Intestine with Intraluminal Device, Open Approach
0D780ZZ Dilation of Small Intestine, Open Approach
0D783DZ Dilation of Small Intestine with Intraluminal Device, Percutaneous Approach
0D783ZZ Dilation of Small Intestine, Percutaneou Approach
0D784DZ Dilation of Small Intestine with Intraluminal Device, Percutaneous Endoscopic Approach
0D784ZZ Dilation of Small Intestine, Percutaneou Endoscopic Approach
0D787DZ Dilation of Small Intestine with Intraluminal Device, Via Natural or Artificial Opening
0D787ZZ Dilation of Small Intestine, Via Natural Artificial Opening
0D788DZ Dilation of Small Intestine with Intraluminal Device, Via Natural or Artificial Opening Endoscopic
0D788ZZ Dilation of Small Intestine, Via Natural Artificial Opening Endoscopic
0D790DZ Dilation of Duodenum with Intralumina Device, Open Approach
0D790ZZ Dilation of Duodenum, Open Approach
0D793DZ Dilation of Duodenum with Intralumina Device, Percutaneous Approach
0D793ZZ Dilation of Duodenum, Percutaneous Approach
0D794DZ Dilation of Duodenum with Intraluminal Device, Percutaneous Endoscopic Approach
0D794ZZ Dilation of Duodenum, Percutaneous Endoscopic Approach
0D797DZ Dilation of Duodenum with Intraluminal Device, Via Natural or Artificial Opening
0D797ZZ Dilation of Duodenum, Via Natural or Artificial Opening
0D798DZ Dilation of Duodenum with Intraluminal Device, Via Natural or Artificial Opening Endoscopic
0D798ZZ Dilation of Duodenum, Via Natural or Artificial Opening Endoscopic
0D7A0DZ Dilation of Jejunum with Intraluminal Device, Open Approach
0D7A0ZZ Dilation of Jejunum, Open Approach
0D7A3DZ Dilation of Jejunum with Intraluminal Device, Percutaneous Approach
0D7A3ZZ Dilation of Jejunum, Percutaneous Approach
0D7A4DZ Dilation of Jejunum with Intraluminal Device, Percutaneous Endoscopic Approach
0D7A4ZZ Dilation of Jejunum, Percutaneous Endoscopic Approach
0D7A7DZ Dilation of Jejunum with Intraluminal Device, Via Natural or Artificial Opening
0D7A7ZZ Dilation of Jejunum, Via Natural or Artificial Opening
0D7A8DZ Dilation of Jejunum with Intraluminal Device, Via Natural or Artificial Opening Endoscopic

A8ZZ Dilation of Jejunum, Via Natural or Artificial Opening Endoscopic
B0DZ Dilation of Ileum with Intraluminal Device, Open Approach
B0ZZ Dilation of Ileum, Open Approach
B3DZ Dilation of Ileum with Intraluminal Device, Percutaneous Approach
B3ZZ Dilation of Ileum, Percutaneous Approach
B4DZ Dilation of Ileum with Intraluminal Device, Percutaneous Endoscopic Approach
B4ZZ Dilation of Ileum, Percutaneous Endoscopic Approach
B7DZ Dilation of Ileum with Intraluminal Device, Via Natural or Artificial Opening
B7ZZ Dilation of Ileum, Via Natural or Artificial Opening
B8DZ Dilation of Ileum with Intraluminal Device, Via Natural or Artificial Opening Endoscopic
B8ZZ Dilation of Ileum, Via Natural or Artificial Opening Endoscopic
7C0DZ Dilation of Ileocecal Valve with Intraluminal Device, Open Approach
7C0ZZ Dilation of Ileocecal Valve, Open Approach
7C3DZ Dilation of Ileocecal Valve with Intraluminal Device, Percutaneous Approach
7C3ZZ Dilation of Ileocecal Valve, Percutaneous Approach
7C4DZ Dilation of Ileocecal Valve with Intraluminal Device, Percutaneous Endoscopic Approach
7C4ZZ Dilation of Ileocecal Valve, Percutaneous Endoscopic Approach
7C7DZ Dilation of Ileocecal Valve with Intraluminal Device, Via Natural or Artificial Opening
7C7ZZ Dilation of Ileocecal Valve, Via Natural or Artificial Opening
7C8DZ Dilation of Ileocecal Valve with Intraluminal Device, Via Natural or Artificial Opening Endoscopic
7C8ZZ Dilation of Ileocecal Valve, Via Natural or Artificial Opening Endoscopic
7E0DZ Dilation of Large Intestine with Intraluminal Device, Open Approach
7E0ZZ Dilation of Large Intestine, Open Approach
7E3DZ Dilation of Large Intestine with Intraluminal Device, Percutaneous Approach
7E3ZZ Dilation of Large Intestine, Percutaneous Approach
7E4DZ Dilation of Large Intestine with Intraluminal Device, Percutaneous Endoscopic Approach
7E4ZZ Dilation of Large Intestine, Percutaneous Endoscopic Approach
7E7DZ Dilation of Large Intestine with Intraluminal Device, Via Natural or Artificial Opening
7E7ZZ Dilation of Large Intestine, Via Natural or Artificial Opening
7E8DZ Dilation of Large Intestine with Intraluminal Device, Via Natural or Artificial Opening Endoscopic
7E8ZZ Dilation of Large Intestine, Via Natural or Artificial Opening Endoscopic
7F0DZ Dilation of Right Large Intestine with Intraluminal Device, Open Approach
7F0ZZ Dilation of Right Large Intestine, Open Approach
D7F3DZ Dilation of Right Large Intestine with Intraluminal Device, Percutaneous Approach
0D7F3ZZ Dilation of Right Large Intestine, Percutaneous Approach
0D7F4DZ Dilation of Right Large Intestine with Intraluminal Device, Percutaneous Endoscopic Approach
0D7F4ZZ Dilation of Right Large Intestine, Percutaneous Endoscopic Approach
0D7F7DZ Dilation of Right Large Intestine with Intraluminal Device, Via Natural or Artificial Opening
0D7F7ZZ Dilation of Right Large Intestine, Via Natural or Artificial Opening
0D7F8DZ Dilation of Right Large Intestine with Intraluminal Device, Via Natural or Artificial Opening Endoscopic
0D7F8ZZ Dilation of Right Large Intestine, Via Natural or Artificial Opening Endoscopic
0D7G0DZ Dilation of Left Large Intestine with Intraluminal Device, Open Approach
0D7G0ZZ Dilation of Left Large Intestine, Open Approach
0D7G3DZ Dilation of Left Large Intestine with Intraluminal Device, Percutaneous Approach
0D7G3ZZ Dilation of Left Large Intestine, Percutaneous Approach
0D7G4DZ Dilation of Left Large Intestine with Intraluminal Device, Percutaneous Endoscopic Approach
0D7G4ZZ Dilation of Left Large Intestine, Percutaneous Endoscopic Approach
0D7G7DZ Dilation of Left Large Intestine with Intraluminal Device, Via Natural or Artificial Opening
0D7G7ZZ Dilation of Left Large Intestine, Via Natural or Artificial Opening
0D7G8DZ Dilation of Left Large Intestine with Intraluminal Device, Via Natural or Artificial Opening Endoscopic
0D7G8ZZ Dilation of Left Large Intestine, Via Natural or Artificial Opening Endoscopic
0D7H0DZ Dilation of Cecum with Intraluminal Device, Open Approach
0D7H0ZZ Dilation of Cecum, Open Approach
0D7H3DZ Dilation of Cecum with Intraluminal Device, Percutaneous Approach
0D7H3ZZ Dilation of Cecum, Percutaneous Approach
0D7H4DZ Dilation of Cecum with Intraluminal Device, Percutaneous Endoscopic Approach
0D7H4ZZ Dilation of Cecum, Percutaneous Endoscopic Approach
0D7H7DZ Dilation of Cecum with Intraluminal Device, Via Natural or Artificial Opening
0D7H7ZZ Dilation of Cecum, Via Natural or Artificial Opening
0D7H8DZ Dilation of Cecum with Intraluminal Device, Via Natural or Artificial Opening Endoscopic
0D7H8ZZ Dilation of Cecum, Via Natural or Artificial Opening Endoscopic
0D7K0DZ Dilation of Ascending Colon with Intraluminal Device, Open Approach
0D7K0ZZ Dilation of Ascending Colon, Open Approach
0D7K3DZ Dilation of Ascending Colon with Intraluminal Device, Percutaneous Approach
0D7K3ZZ Dilation of Ascending Colon, Percutaneous Approach
0D7K4DZ Dilation of Ascending Colon with Intraluminal Device, Percutaneous Endoscopic Approach
0D7K4ZZ Dilation of Ascending Colon, Percutaneous Endoscopic Approach
0D7K7DZ Dilation of Ascending Colon with Intraluminal Device, Via Natural or Artificial Opening
0D7K7ZZ Dilation of Ascending Colon, Via Natural or Artificial Opening
0D7K8DZ Dilation of Ascending Colon with Intraluminal Device, Via Natural or Artificial Opening Endoscopic
0D7K8ZZ Dilation of Ascending Colon, Via Natural or Artificial Opening Endoscopic
0D7L0DZ Dilation of Transverse Colon with Intraluminal Device, Open Approach
0D7L0ZZ Dilation of Transverse Colon, Open Approach
0D7L3DZ Dilation of Transverse Colon with Intraluminal Device, Percutaneous Approach
0D7L3ZZ Dilation of Transverse Colon, Percutaneous Approach
0D7L4DZ Dilation of Transverse Colon with Intraluminal Device, Percutaneous Endoscopic Approach
0D7L4ZZ Dilation of Transverse Colon, Percutaneous Endoscopic Approach
0D7L7DZ Dilation of Transverse Colon with Intraluminal Device, Via Natural or Artificial Opening
0D7L7ZZ Dilation of Transverse Colon, Via Natural or Artificial Opening
0D7L8DZ Dilation of Transverse Colon with Intraluminal Device, Via Natural or Artificial Opening Endoscopic
0D7L8ZZ Dilation of Transverse Colon, Via Natural or Artificial Opening Endoscopic
0D7M0DZ Dilation of Descending Colon with Intraluminal Device, Open Approach
0D7M0ZZ Dilation of Descending Colon, Open Approach
0D7M3DZ Dilation of Descending Colon with Intraluminal Device, Percutaneous Approach
0D7M3ZZ Dilation of Descending Colon, Percutaneous Approach
0D7M4DZ Dilation of Descending Colon with Intraluminal Device, Percutaneous Endoscopic Approach
0D7M4ZZ Dilation of Descending Colon, Percutaneous Endoscopic Approach
0D7M7DZ Dilation of Descending Colon with Intraluminal Device, Via Natural or Artificial Opening
0D7M7ZZ Dilation of Descending Colon, Via Natural or Artificial Opening
0D7M8DZ Dilation of Descending Colon with Intraluminal Device, Via Natural or Artificial Opening Endoscopic
0D7M8ZZ Dilation of Descending Colon, Via Natural or Artificial Opening Endoscopic
0D7N0DZ Dilation of Sigmoid Colon with Intraluminal Device, Open Approach
0D7N0ZZ Dilation of Sigmoid Colon, Open Approach
0D7N3DZ Dilation of Sigmoid Colon with Intraluminal Device, Percutaneous Approach
0D7N3ZZ Dilation of Sigmoid Colon, Percutaneous Approach
0D7N4DZ Dilation of Sigmoid Colon with Intraluminal Device, Percutaneous Endoscopic Approach
0D7N4ZZ Dilation of Sigmoid Colon, Percutaneous Endoscopic Approach

0D7N7DZ Dilation of Sigmoid Colon with Intraluminal Device, Via Natural or Artificial Opening
0D7N7ZZ Dilation of Sigmoid Colon, Via Natural or Artificial Opening
0D7N8DZ Dilation of Sigmoid Colon with Intraluminal Device, Via Natural or Artificial Opening Endoscopic
0D7N8ZZ Dilation of Sigmoid Colon, Via Natural or Artificial Opening Endoscopic
0D7P0DZ Dilation of Rectum with Intraluminal Device, Open Approach
0D7P0ZZ Dilation of Rectum, Open Approach
0D7P3DZ Dilation of Rectum with Intraluminal Device, Percutaneous Approach
0D7P3ZZ Dilation of Rectum, Percutaneous Approach
0D7P4DZ Dilation of Rectum with Intraluminal Device, Percutaneous Endoscopic Approach
0D7P4ZZ Dilation of Rectum, Percutaneous Endoscopic Approach
0D7P7DZ Dilation of Rectum with Intraluminal Device, Via Natural or Artificial Opening
0D7P7ZZ Dilation of Rectum, Via Natural or Artificial Opening
0D7P8DZ Dilation of Rectum with Intraluminal Device, Via Natural or Artificial Opening Endoscopic
0D7P8ZZ Dilation of Rectum, Via Natural or Artificial Opening Endoscopic
0D7Q0DZ Dilation of Anus with Intraluminal Device, Open Approach
0D7Q0ZZ Dilation of Anus, Open Approach
0D7Q3DZ Dilation of Anus with Intraluminal Device, Percutaneous Approach
0D7Q3ZZ Dilation of Anus, Percutaneous Appro
0D7Q4DZ Dilation of Anus with Intraluminal Device, Percutaneous Endoscopic Approach
0D7Q4ZZ Dilation of Anus, Percutaneous Endoscopic Approach
0D7Q7DZ Dilation of Anus with Intraluminal Device, Via Natural or Artificial Open
0D7Q7ZZ Dilation of Anus, Via Natural or Artifi Opening
0D7Q8DZ Dilation of Anus with Intraluminal Device, Via Natural or Artificial Openi Endoscopic
0D7Q8ZZ Dilation of Anus, Via Natural or Artifi Opening Endoscopic

0D8 – Gastrointestinal System, Division

Review Coding Guideline B3.14

0D840ZZ Division of Esophagogastric Junction, Open Approach
0D843ZZ Division of Esophagogastric Junction, Percutaneous Approach
0D844ZZ Division of Esophagogastric Junction, Percutaneous Endoscopic Approach
0D847ZZ Division of Esophagogastric Junction, Via Natural or Artificial Opening
0D848ZZ Division of Esophagogastric Junction, Via Natural or Artificial Opening Endoscopic
0D870ZZ Division of Stomach, Pylorus, Open Approach
0D873ZZ Division of Stomach, Pylorus, Percutaneous Approach
0D874ZZ Division of Stomach, Pylorus, Percutaneous Endoscopic Approach
0D877ZZ Division of Stomach, Pylorus, Via Natu or Artificial Opening
0D878ZZ Division of Stomach, Pylorus, Via Natu or Artificial Opening Endoscopic
0D8R0ZZ Division of Anal Sphincter, Open Approach
0D8R3ZZ Division of Anal Sphincter, Percutaneou Approach

0D9 – Gastrointestinal System, Drainage

Review Coding Guidelines B3.4a and B3.4b

Review Coding Guideline B6.2

0D9100Z Drainage of Upper Esophagus with Drainage Device, Open Approach
0D910ZX Drainage of Upper Esophagus, Open Approach, Diagnostic
0D910ZZ Drainage of Upper Esophagus, Open Approach
0D9130Z Drainage of Upper Esophagus with Drainage Device, Percutaneous Approach
0D913ZX Drainage of Upper Esophagus, Percutaneous Approach, Diagnostic
0D913ZZ Drainage of Upper Esophagus, Percutaneous Approach
0D9140Z Drainage of Upper Esophagus with Drainage Device, Percutaneous Endoscopic Approach
0D914ZX Drainage of Upper Esophagus, Percutaneous Endoscopic Approach, Diagnostic
0D914ZZ Drainage of Upper Esophagus, Percutaneous Endoscopic Approach
0D9170Z Drainage of Upper Esophagus with Drainage Device, Via Natural or Artificial Opening
0D917ZX Drainage of Upper Esophagus, Via Natural or Artificial Opening, Diagnostic
0D917ZZ Drainage of Upper Esophagus, Via Natural or Artificial Opening
0D9180Z Drainage of Upper Esophagus with Drainage Device, Via Natural or Artificial Opening Endoscopic
0D918ZX Drainage of Upper Esophagus, Via Natural or Artificial Opening Endoscopic, Diagnostic
0D918ZZ Drainage of Upper Esophagus, Via Natural or Artificial Opening Endoscopic
0D9200Z Drainage of Middle Esophagus with Drainage Device, Open Approach
0D920ZX Drainage of Middle Esophagus, Open Approach, Diagnostic
0D920ZZ Drainage of Middle Esophagus, Open Approach
0D9230Z Drainage of Middle Esophagus with Drainage Device, Percutaneous Approach
0D923ZX Drainage of Middle Esophagus, Percutaneous Approach, Diagnostic
0D923ZZ Drainage of Middle Esophagus, Percutaneous Approach
0D9240Z Drainage of Middle Esophagus with Drainage Device, Percutaneous Endoscopic Approach
0D924ZX Drainage of Middle Esophagus, Percutaneous Endoscopic Approach, Diagnostic
0D924ZZ Drainage of Middle Esophagus, Percutaneous Endoscopic Approach
0D9270Z Drainage of Middle Esophagus with Drainage Device, Via Natural or Artificial Opening
0D927ZX Drainage of Middle Esophagus, Via Natural or Artificial Opening, Diagnostic
0D927ZZ Drainage of Middle Esophagus, Via Natural or Artificial Opening
0D9280Z Drainage of Middle Esophagus with Drainage Device, Via Natural or Artificial Opening Endoscopic
0D928ZX Drainage of Middle Esophagus, Via Natural or Artificial Opening Endoscopic, Diagnostic
0D928ZZ Drainage of Middle Esophagus, Via Natural or Artificial Opening Endoscopic
0D9300Z Drainage of Lower Esophagus with Drainage Device, Open Approach
0D930ZX Drainage of Lower Esophagus, Open Approach, Diagnostic
0D930ZZ Drainage of Lower Esophagus, Open Approach
0D9330Z Drainage of Lower Esophagus with Drainage Device, Percutaneous Approac
0D933ZX Drainage of Lower Esophagus, Percutaneous Approach, Diagnostic
0D933ZZ Drainage of Lower Esophagus, Percutaneous Approach
0D9340Z Drainage of Lower Esophagus with Drainage Device, Percutaneous Endoscopic Approach
0D934ZX Drainage of Lower Esophagus, Percutaneous Endoscopic Approach, Diagnostic
0D934ZZ Drainage of Lower Esophagus, Percutaneous Endoscopic Approach
0D9370Z Drainage of Lower Esophagus with Drainage Device, Via Natural or Artifici Opening
0D937ZX Drainage of Lower Esophagus, Via Natural or Artificial Opening, Diagnostic
0D937ZZ Drainage of Lower Esophagus, Via Natural or Artificial Opening
0D9380Z Drainage of Lower Esophagus with Drainage Device, Via Natural or Artifici Opening Endoscopic
0D938ZX Drainage of Lower Esophagus, Via Natural or Artificial Opening Endoscopic Diagnostic
0D938ZZ Drainage of Lower Esophagus, Via Natural or Artificial Opening Endoscopic
0D9400Z Drainage of Esophagogastric Junction with Drainage Device, Open Approach
0D940ZX Drainage of Esophagogastric Junction, Open Approach, Diagnostic
0D940ZZ Drainage of Esophagogastric Junction, Open Approach
0D9430Z Drainage of Esophagogastric Junction with Drainage Device, Percutaneous Approach

43ZX Drainage of Esophagogastric Junction, Percutaneous Approach, Diagnostic

43ZZ Drainage of Esophagogastric Junction, Percutaneous Approach

440Z Drainage of Esophagogastric Junction with Drainage Device, Percutaneous Endoscopic Approach

44ZX Drainage of Esophagogastric Junction, Percutaneous Endoscopic Approach, Diagnostic

44ZZ Drainage of Esophagogastric Junction, Percutaneous Endoscopic Approach

470Z Drainage of Esophagogastric Junction with Drainage Device, Via Natural or Artificial Opening

)47ZX Drainage of Esophagogastric Junction, Via Natural or Artificial Opening, Diagnostic

47ZZ Drainage of Esophagogastric Junction, Via Natural or Artificial Opening

)480Z Drainage of Esophagogastric Junction with Drainage Device, Via Natural or Artificial Opening Endoscopic

)48ZX Drainage of Esophagogastric Junction, Via Natural or Artificial Opening Endoscopic, Diagnostic

948ZZ Drainage of Esophagogastric Junction, Via Natural or Artificial Opening Endoscopic

9500Z Drainage of Esophagus with Drainage Device, Open Approach

950ZX Drainage of Esophagus, Open Approach, Diagnostic

950ZZ Drainage of Esophagus, Open Approach

9530Z Drainage of Esophagus with Drainage Device, Percutaneous Approach

953ZX Drainage of Esophagus, Percutaneous Approach, Diagnostic

953ZZ Drainage of Esophagus, Percutaneous Approach

9540Z Drainage of Esophagus with Drainage Device, Percutaneous Endoscopic Approach

954ZX Drainage of Esophagus, Percutaneous Endoscopic Approach, Diagnostic

954ZZ Drainage of Esophagus, Percutaneous Endoscopic Approach

9570Z Drainage of Esophagus with Drainage Device, Via Natural or Artificial Opening

957ZX Drainage of Esophagus, Via Natural or Artificial Opening, Diagnostic

957ZZ Drainage of Esophagus, Via Natural or Artificial Opening

9580Z Drainage of Esophagus with Drainage Device, Via Natural or Artificial Opening Endoscopic

)958ZX Drainage of Esophagus, Via Natural or Artificial Opening Endoscopic, Diagnostic

)958ZZ Drainage of Esophagus, Via Natural or Artificial Opening Endoscopic

)9600Z Drainage of Stomach with Drainage Device, Open Approach

)960ZX Drainage of Stomach, Open Approach, Diagnostic

)960ZZ Drainage of Stomach, Open Approach

)9630Z Drainage of Stomach with Drainage Device, Percutaneous Approach

)963ZX Drainage of Stomach, Percutaneous Approach, Diagnostic

)963ZZ Drainage of Stomach, Percutaneous Approach

)9640Z Drainage of Stomach with Drainage Device, Percutaneous Endoscopic Approach

D964ZX Drainage of Stomach, Percutaneous Endoscopic Approach, Diagnostic

0D964ZZ Drainage of Stomach, Percutaneous Endoscopic Approach

0D9670Z Drainage of Stomach with Drainage Device, Via Natural or Artificial Opening

0D967ZX Drainage of Stomach, Via Natural or Artificial Opening, Diagnostic

0D967ZZ Drainage of Stomach, Via Natural or Artificial Opening

0D9680Z Drainage of Stomach with Drainage Device, Via Natural or Artificial Opening Endoscopic

0D968ZX Drainage of Stomach, Via Natural or Artificial Opening Endoscopic, Diagnostic

0D968ZZ Drainage of Stomach, Via Natural or Artificial Opening Endoscopic

0D9700Z Drainage of Stomach, Pylorus with Drainage Device, Open Approach

0D970ZX Drainage of Stomach, Pylorus, Open Approach, Diagnostic

0D970ZZ Drainage of Stomach, Pylorus, Open Approach

0D9730Z Drainage of Stomach, Pylorus with Drainage Device, Percutaneous Approach

0D973ZX Drainage of Stomach, Pylorus, Percutaneous Approach, Diagnostic

0D973ZZ Drainage of Stomach, Pylorus, Percutaneous Approach

0D9740Z Drainage of Stomach, Pylorus with Drainage Device, Percutaneous Endoscopic Approach

0D974ZX Drainage of Stomach, Pylorus, Percutaneous Endoscopic Approach, Diagnostic

0D974ZZ Drainage of Stomach, Pylorus, Percutaneous Endoscopic Approach

0D9770Z Drainage of Stomach, Pylorus with Drainage Device, Via Natural or Artificial Opening

0D977ZX Drainage of Stomach, Pylorus, Via Natural or Artificial Opening, Diagnostic

0D977ZZ Drainage of Stomach, Pylorus, Via Natural or Artificial Opening

0D9780Z Drainage of Stomach, Pylorus with Drainage Device, Via Natural or Artificial Opening Endoscopic

0D978ZX Drainage of Stomach, Pylorus, Via Natural or Artificial Opening Endoscopic, Diagnostic

0D978ZZ Drainage of Stomach, Pylorus, Via Natural or Artificial Opening Endoscopic

0D9800Z Drainage of Small Intestine with Drainage Device, Open Approach

0D980ZX Drainage of Small Intestine, Open Approach, Diagnostic

0D980ZZ Drainage of Small Intestine, Open Approach

0D9830Z Drainage of Small Intestine with Drainage Device, Percutaneous Approach

0D983ZX Drainage of Small Intestine, Percutaneous Approach, Diagnostic

0D983ZZ Drainage of Small Intestine, Percutaneous Approach

0D9840Z Drainage of Small Intestine with Drainage Device, Percutaneous Endoscopic Approach

0D984ZX Drainage of Small Intestine, Percutaneous Endoscopic Approach, Diagnostic

0D984ZZ Drainage of Small Intestine, Percutaneous Endoscopic Approach

0D9870Z Drainage of Small Intestine with Drainage Device, Via Natural or Artificial Opening

0D987ZX Drainage of Small Intestine, Via Natural or Artificial Opening, Diagnostic

0D987ZZ Drainage of Small Intestine, Via Natural or Artificial Opening

0D9880Z Drainage of Small Intestine with Drainage Device, Via Natural or Artificial Opening Endoscopic

0D988ZX Drainage of Small Intestine, Via Natural or Artificial Opening Endoscopic, Diagnostic

0D988ZZ Drainage of Small Intestine, Via Natural or Artificial Opening Endoscopic

0D9900Z Drainage of Duodenum with Drainage Device, Open Approach

0D990ZX Drainage of Duodenum, Open Approach, Diagnostic

0D990ZZ Drainage of Duodenum, Open Approach

0D9930Z Drainage of Duodenum with Drainage Device, Percutaneous Approach

0D993ZX Drainage of Duodenum, Percutaneous Approach, Diagnostic

0D993ZZ Drainage of Duodenum, Percutaneous Approach

0D9940Z Drainage of Duodenum with Drainage Device, Percutaneous Endoscopic Approach

0D994ZX Drainage of Duodenum, Percutaneous Endoscopic Approach, Diagnostic

0D994ZZ Drainage of Duodenum, Percutaneous Endoscopic Approach

0D9970Z Drainage of Duodenum with Drainage Device, Via Natural or Artificial Opening

0D997ZX Drainage of Duodenum, Via Natural or Artificial Opening, Diagnostic

0D997ZZ Drainage of Duodenum, Via Natural or Artificial Opening

0D9980Z Drainage of Duodenum with Drainage Device, Via Natural or Artificial Opening Endoscopic

0D998ZX Drainage of Duodenum, Via Natural or Artificial Opening Endoscopic, Diagnostic

0D998ZZ Drainage of Duodenum, Via Natural or Artificial Opening Endoscopic

0D9A00Z Drainage of Jejunum with Drainage Device, Open Approach

0D9A0ZX Drainage of Jejunum, Open Approach, Diagnostic

0D9A0ZZ Drainage of Jejunum, Open Approach

0D9A30Z Drainage of Jejunum with Drainage Device, Percutaneous Approach

0D9A3ZX Drainage of Jejunum, Percutaneous Approach, Diagnostic

0D9A3ZZ Drainage of Jejunum, Percutaneous Approach

0D9A40Z Drainage of Jejunum with Drainage Device, Percutaneous Endoscopic Approach

0D9A4ZX Drainage of Jejunum, Percutaneous Endoscopic Approach, Diagnostic

0D9A4ZZ Drainage of Jejunum, Percutaneous Endoscopic Approach

0D9A70Z Drainage of Jejunum with Drainage Device, Via Natural or Artificial Opening

0D9A7ZX Drainage of Jejunum, Via Natural or Artificial Opening, Diagnostic

0D9A7ZZ Drainage of Jejunum, Via Natural or Artificial Opening

0D9A80Z Drainage of Jejunum with Drainage Device, Via Natural or Artificial Opening Endoscopic

0D9A8ZX Drainage of Jejunum, Via Natural or Artificial Opening Endoscopic, Diagnostic

0D9A8ZZ Drainage of Jejunum, Via Natural or Artificial Opening Endoscopic

0D9B00Z Drainage of Ileum with Drainage Device, Open Approach

0D9B0ZX Drainage of Ileum, Open Approach, Diagnostic

0D9B0ZZ Drainage of Ileum, Open Approach

0D9B30Z Drainage of Ileum with Drainage Device, Percutaneous Approach

0D9B3ZX Drainage of Ileum, Percutaneous Approach, Diagnostic
0D9B3ZZ Drainage of Ileum, Percutaneous Approach
0D9B40Z Drainage of Ileum with Drainage Device, Percutaneous Endoscopic Approach
0D9B4ZX Drainage of Ileum, Percutaneous Endoscopic Approach, Diagnostic
0D9B4ZZ Drainage of Ileum, Percutaneous Endoscopic Approach
0D9B70Z Drainage of Ileum with Drainage Device, Via Natural or Artificial Opening
0D9B7ZX Drainage of Ileum, Via Natural or Artificial Opening, Diagnostic
0D9B7ZZ Drainage of Ileum, Via Natural or Artificial Opening
0D9B80Z Drainage of Ileum with Drainage Device, Via Natural or Artificial Opening Endoscopic
0D9B8ZX Drainage of Ileum, Via Natural or Artificial Opening Endoscopic, Diagnostic
0D9B8ZZ Drainage of Ileum, Via Natural or Artificial Opening Endoscopic
0D9C00Z Drainage of Ileocecal Valve with Drainage Device, Open Approach
0D9C0ZX Drainage of Ileocecal Valve, Open Approach, Diagnostic
0D9C0ZZ Drainage of Ileocecal Valve, Open Approach
0D9C30Z Drainage of Ileocecal Valve with Drainage Device, Percutaneous Approach
0D9C3ZX Drainage of Ileocecal Valve, Percutaneous Approach, Diagnostic
0D9C3ZZ Drainage of Ileocecal Valve, Percutaneous Approach
0D9C40Z Drainage of Ileocecal Valve with Drainage Device, Percutaneous Endoscopic Approach
0D9C4ZX Drainage of Ileocecal Valve, Percutaneous Endoscopic Approach, Diagnostic
0D9C4ZZ Drainage of Ileocecal Valve, Percutaneous Endoscopic Approach
0D9C70Z Drainage of Ileocecal Valve with Drainage Device, Via Natural or Artificial Opening
0D9C7ZX Drainage of Ileocecal Valve, Via Natural or Artificial Opening, Diagnostic
0D9C7ZZ Drainage of Ileocecal Valve, Via Natural or Artificial Opening
0D9C80Z Drainage of Ileocecal Valve with Drainage Device, Via Natural or Artificial Opening Endoscopic
0D9C8ZX Drainage of Ileocecal Valve, Via Natural or Artificial Opening Endoscopic, Diagnostic
0D9C8ZZ Drainage of Ileocecal Valve, Via Natural or Artificial Opening Endoscopic
0D9E00Z Drainage of Large Intestine with Drainage Device, Open Approach
0D9E0ZX Drainage of Large Intestine, Open Approach, Diagnostic
0D9E0ZZ Drainage of Large Intestine, Open Approach
0D9E30Z Drainage of Large Intestine with Drainage Device, Percutaneous Approach
0D9E3ZX Drainage of Large Intestine, Percutaneous Approach, Diagnostic
0D9E3ZZ Drainage of Large Intestine, Percutaneous Approach
0D9E40Z Drainage of Large Intestine with Drainage Device, Percutaneous Endoscopic Approach
0D9E4ZX Drainage of Large Intestine, Percutaneous Endoscopic Approach, Diagnostic
0D9E4ZZ Drainage of Large Intestine, Percutaneous Endoscopic Approach
0D9E70Z Drainage of Large Intestine with Drainage Device, Via Natural or Artificial Opening
0D9E7ZX Drainage of Large Intestine, Via Natural or Artificial Opening, Diagnostic
0D9E7ZZ Drainage of Large Intestine, Via Natural or Artificial Opening
0D9E80Z Drainage of Large Intestine with Drainage Device, Via Natural or Artificial Opening Endoscopic
0D9E8ZX Drainage of Large Intestine, Via Natural or Artificial Opening Endoscopic, Diagnostic
0D9E8ZZ Drainage of Large Intestine, Via Natural or Artificial Opening Endoscopic
0D9F00Z Drainage of Right Large Intestine with Drainage Device, Open Approach
0D9F0ZX Drainage of Right Large Intestine, Open Approach, Diagnostic
0D9F0ZZ Drainage of Right Large Intestine, Open Approach
0D9F30Z Drainage of Right Large Intestine with Drainage Device, Percutaneous Approach
0D9F3ZX Drainage of Right Large Intestine, Percutaneous Approach, Diagnostic
0D9F3ZZ Drainage of Right Large Intestine, Percutaneous Approach
0D9F40Z Drainage of Right Large Intestine with Drainage Device, Percutaneous Endoscopic Approach
0D9F4ZX Drainage of Right Large Intestine, Percutaneous Endoscopic Approach, Diagnostic
0D9F4ZZ Drainage of Right Large Intestine, Percutaneous Endoscopic Approach
0D9F70Z Drainage of Right Large Intestine with Drainage Device, Via Natural or Artificial Opening
0D9F7ZX Drainage of Right Large Intestine, Via Natural or Artificial Opening, Diagnostic
0D9F7ZZ Drainage of Right Large Intestine, Via Natural or Artificial Opening
0D9F80Z Drainage of Right Large Intestine with Drainage Device, Via Natural or Artificial Opening Endoscopic
0D9F8ZX Drainage of Right Large Intestine, Via Natural or Artificial Opening Endoscopic, Diagnostic
0D9F8ZZ Drainage of Right Large Intestine, Via Natural or Artificial Opening Endoscopic
0D9G00Z Drainage of Left Large Intestine with Drainage Device, Open Approach
0D9G0ZX Drainage of Left Large Intestine, Open Approach, Diagnostic
0D9G0ZZ Drainage of Left Large Intestine, Open Approach
0D9G30Z Drainage of Left Large Intestine with Drainage Device, Percutaneous Approach
0D9G3ZX Drainage of Left Large Intestine, Percutaneous Approach, Diagnostic
0D9G3ZZ Drainage of Left Large Intestine, Percutaneous Approach
0D9G40Z Drainage of Left Large Intestine with Drainage Device, Percutaneous Endoscopic Approach
0D9G4ZX Drainage of Left Large Intestine, Percutaneous Endoscopic Approach, Diagnostic
0D9G4ZZ Drainage of Left Large Intestine, Percutaneous Endoscopic Approach
0D9G70Z Drainage of Left Large Intestine with Drainage Device, Via Natural or Artificial Opening
0D9G7ZX Drainage of Left Large Intestine, Via Natural or Artificial Opening, Diagnostic
0D9G7ZZ Drainage of Left Large Intestine, Via Natural or Artificial Opening
0D9G80Z Drainage of Left Large Intestine with Drainage Device, Via Natural or Artificial Opening Endoscopic
0D9G8ZX Drainage of Left Large Intestine, Via Natural or Artificial Opening Endoscop Diagnostic
0D9G8ZZ Drainage of Left Large Intestine, Via Natural or Artificial Opening Endoscopic
0D9H00Z Drainage of Cecum with Drainage Dev Open Approach
0D9H0ZX Drainage of Cecum, Open Approach, Diagnostic
0D9H0ZZ Drainage of Cecum, Open Approach
0D9H30Z Drainage of Cecum with Drainage Dev Percutaneous Approach
0D9H3ZX Drainage of Cecum, Percutaneous Approach, Diagnostic
0D9H3ZZ Drainage of Cecum, Percutaneous Approach
0D9H40Z Drainage of Cecum with Drainage Dev Percutaneous Endoscopic Approach
0D9H4ZX Drainage of Cecum, Percutaneous Endoscopic Approach, Diagnostic
0D9H4ZZ Drainage of Cecum, Percutaneous Endoscopic Approach
0D9H70Z Drainage of Cecum with Drainage Devi Via Natural or Artificial Opening
0D9H7ZX Drainage of Cecum, Via Natural or Artificial Opening, Diagnostic
0D9H7ZZ Drainage of Cecum, Via Natural or Artificial Opening
0D9H80Z Drainage of Cecum with Drainage Device, Via Natural or Artificial Openin Endoscopic
0D9H8ZX Drainage of Cecum, Via Natural or Artificial Opening Endoscopic, Diagnos
0D9H8ZZ Drainage of Cecum, Via Natural or Artificial Opening Endoscopic
0D9J00Z Drainage of Appendix with Drainage Device, Open Approach
0D9J0ZX Drainage of Appendix, Open Approach, Diagnostic
0D9J0ZZ Drainage of Appendix, Open Approach
0D9J30Z Drainage of Appendix with Drainage Device, Percutaneous Approach
0D9J3ZX Drainage of Appendix, Percutaneous Approach, Diagnostic
0D9J3ZZ Drainage of Appendix, Percutaneous Approach
0D9J40Z Drainage of Appendix with Drainage Device, Percutaneous Endoscopic Approach
0D9J4ZX Drainage of Appendix, Percutaneous Endoscopic Approach, Diagnostic
0D9J4ZZ Drainage of Appendix, Percutaneous Endoscopic Approach
0D9J70Z Drainage of Appendix with Drainage Device, Via Natural or Artificial Opening
0D9J7ZX Drainage of Appendix, Via Natural or Artificial Opening, Diagnostic
0D9J7ZZ Drainage of Appendix, Via Natural or Artificial Opening
0D9J80Z Drainage of Appendix with Drainage Device, Via Natural or Artificial Opening Endoscopic
0D9J8ZX Drainage of Appendix, Via Natural or Artificial Opening Endoscopic, Diagnost
0D9J8ZZ Drainage of Appendix, Via Natural or Artificial Opening Endoscopic
0D9K00Z Drainage of Ascending Colon with Drainage Device, Open Approach
0D9K0ZX Drainage of Ascending Colon, Open Approach, Diagnostic
0D9K0ZZ Drainage of Ascending Colon, Open Approach
0D9K30Z Drainage of Ascending Colon with Drainage Device, Percutaneous Approach
0D9K3ZX Drainage of Ascending Colon, Percutaneous Approach, Diagnostic

0D9K3ZZ Drainage of Ascending Colon, Percutaneous Approach
0D9K40Z Drainage of Ascending Colon with Drainage Device, Percutaneous Endoscopic Approach
0D9K4ZX Drainage of Ascending Colon, Percutaneous Endoscopic Approach, Diagnostic
0D9K4ZZ Drainage of Ascending Colon, Percutaneous Endoscopic Approach
0D9K70Z Drainage of Ascending Colon with Drainage Device, Via Natural or Artificial Opening
0D9K7ZX Drainage of Ascending Colon, Via Natural or Artificial Opening, Diagnostic
0D9K7ZZ Drainage of Ascending Colon, Via Natural or Artificial Opening
0D9K80Z Drainage of Ascending Colon with Drainage Device, Via Natural or Artificial Opening Endoscopic
0D9K8ZX Drainage of Ascending Colon, Via Natural or Artificial Opening Endoscopic, Diagnostic
0D9K8ZZ Drainage of Ascending Colon, Via Natural or Artificial Opening Endoscopic
0D9L00Z Drainage of Transverse Colon with Drainage Device, Open Approach
0D9L0ZX Drainage of Transverse Colon, Open Approach, Diagnostic
0D9L0ZZ Drainage of Transverse Colon, Open Approach
0D9L30Z Drainage of Transverse Colon with Drainage Device, Percutaneous Approach
0D9L3ZX Drainage of Transverse Colon, Percutaneous Approach, Diagnostic
0D9L3ZZ Drainage of Transverse Colon, Percutaneous Approach
0D9L40Z Drainage of Transverse Colon with Drainage Device, Percutaneous Endoscopic Approach
0D9L4ZX Drainage of Transverse Colon, Percutaneous Endoscopic Approach, Diagnostic
0D9L4ZZ Drainage of Transverse Colon, Percutaneous Endoscopic Approach
0D9L70Z Drainage of Transverse Colon with Drainage Device, Via Natural or Artificial Opening
0D9L7ZX Drainage of Transverse Colon, Via Natural or Artificial Opening, Diagnostic
0D9L7ZZ Drainage of Transverse Colon, Via Natural or Artificial Opening
0D9L80Z Drainage of Transverse Colon with Drainage Device, Via Natural or Artificial Opening Endoscopic
0D9L8ZX Drainage of Transverse Colon, Via Natural or Artificial Opening Endoscopic, Diagnostic
0D9L8ZZ Drainage of Transverse Colon, Via Natural or Artificial Opening Endoscopic
0D9M00Z Drainage of Descending Colon with Drainage Device, Open Approach
0D9M0ZX Drainage of Descending Colon, Open Approach, Diagnostic
0D9M0ZZ Drainage of Descending Colon, Open Approach
0D9M30Z Drainage of Descending Colon with Drainage Device, Percutaneous Approach
0D9M3ZX Drainage of Descending Colon, Percutaneous Approach, Diagnostic
0D9M3ZZ Drainage of Descending Colon, Percutaneous Approach
0D9M40Z Drainage of Descending Colon with Drainage Device, Percutaneous Endoscopic Approach
0D9M4ZX Drainage of Descending Colon, Percutaneous Endoscopic Approach, Diagnostic
0D9M4ZZ Drainage of Descending Colon, Percutaneous Endoscopic Approach
0D9M70Z Drainage of Descending Colon with Drainage Device, Via Natural or Artificial Opening
0D9M7ZX Drainage of Descending Colon, Via Natural or Artificial Opening, Diagnostic
0D9M7ZZ Drainage of Descending Colon, Via Natural or Artificial Opening
0D9M80Z Drainage of Descending Colon with Drainage Device, Via Natural or Artificial Opening Endoscopic
0D9M8ZX Drainage of Descending Colon, Via Natural or Artificial Opening Endoscopic, Diagnostic
0D9M8ZZ Drainage of Descending Colon, Via Natural or Artificial Opening Endoscopic
0D9N00Z Drainage of Sigmoid Colon with Drainage Device, Open Approach
0D9N0ZX Drainage of Sigmoid Colon, Open Approach, Diagnostic
0D9N0ZZ Drainage of Sigmoid Colon, Open Approach
0D9N30Z Drainage of Sigmoid Colon with Drainage Device, Percutaneous Approach
0D9N3ZX Drainage of Sigmoid Colon, Percutaneous Approach, Diagnostic
0D9N3ZZ Drainage of Sigmoid Colon, Percutaneous Approach
0D9N40Z Drainage of Sigmoid Colon with Drainage Device, Percutaneous Endoscopic Approach
0D9N4ZX Drainage of Sigmoid Colon, Percutaneous Endoscopic Approach, Diagnostic
0D9N4ZZ Drainage of Sigmoid Colon, Percutaneous Endoscopic Approach
0D9N70Z Drainage of Sigmoid Colon with Drainage Device, Via Natural or Artificial Opening
0D9N7ZX Drainage of Sigmoid Colon, Via Natural or Artificial Opening, Diagnostic
0D9N7ZZ Drainage of Sigmoid Colon, Via Natural or Artificial Opening
0D9N80Z Drainage of Sigmoid Colon with Drainage Device, Via Natural or Artificial Opening Endoscopic
0D9N8ZX Drainage of Sigmoid Colon, Via Natural or Artificial Opening Endoscopic, Diagnostic
0D9N8ZZ Drainage of Sigmoid Colon, Via Natural or Artificial Opening Endoscopic
0D9P00Z Drainage of Rectum with Drainage Device, Open Approach
0D9P0ZX Drainage of Rectum, Open Approach, Diagnostic
0D9P0ZZ Drainage of Rectum, Open Approach
0D9P30Z Drainage of Rectum with Drainage Device, Percutaneous Approach
0D9P3ZX Drainage of Rectum, Percutaneous Approach, Diagnostic
0D9P3ZZ Drainage of Rectum, Percutaneous Approach
0D9P40Z Drainage of Rectum with Drainage Device, Percutaneous Endoscopic Approach
0D9P4ZX Drainage of Rectum, Percutaneous Endoscopic Approach, Diagnostic
0D9P4ZZ Drainage of Rectum, Percutaneous Endoscopic Approach
0D9P70Z Drainage of Rectum with Drainage Device, Via Natural or Artificial Opening
0D9P7ZX Drainage of Rectum, Via Natural or Artificial Opening, Diagnostic
0D9P7ZZ Drainage of Rectum, Via Natural or Artificial Opening
0D9P80Z Drainage of Rectum with Drainage Device, Via Natural or Artificial Opening Endoscopic
0D9P8ZX Drainage of Rectum, Via Natural or Artificial Opening Endoscopic, Diagnostic
0D9P8ZZ Drainage of Rectum, Via Natural or Artificial Opening Endoscopic
0D9Q00Z Drainage of Anus with Drainage Device, Open Approach
0D9Q0ZX Drainage of Anus, Open Approach, Diagnostic
0D9Q0ZZ Drainage of Anus, Open Approach
0D9Q30Z Drainage of Anus with Drainage Device, Percutaneous Approach
0D9Q3ZX Drainage of Anus, Percutaneous Approach, Diagnostic
0D9Q3ZZ Drainage of Anus, Percutaneous Approach
0D9Q40Z Drainage of Anus with Drainage Device, Percutaneous Endoscopic Approach
0D9Q4ZX Drainage of Anus, Percutaneous Endoscopic Approach, Diagnostic
0D9Q4ZZ Drainage of Anus, Percutaneous Endoscopic Approach
0D9Q70Z Drainage of Anus with Drainage Device, Via Natural or Artificial Opening
0D9Q7ZX Drainage of Anus, Via Natural or Artificial Opening, Diagnostic
0D9Q7ZZ Drainage of Anus, Via Natural or Artificial Opening
0D9Q80Z Drainage of Anus with Drainage Device, Via Natural or Artificial Opening Endoscopic
0D9Q8ZX Drainage of Anus, Via Natural or Artificial Opening Endoscopic, Diagnostic
0D9Q8ZZ Drainage of Anus, Via Natural or Artificial Opening Endoscopic
0D9QX0Z Drainage of Anus with Drainage Device, External Approach
0D9QXZX Drainage of Anus, External Approach, Diagnostic
0D9QXZZ Drainage of Anus, External Approach
0D9R00Z Drainage of Anal Sphincter with Drainage Device, Open Approach
0D9R0ZX Drainage of Anal Sphincter, Open Approach, Diagnostic
0D9R0ZZ Drainage of Anal Sphincter, Open Approach
0D9R30Z Drainage of Anal Sphincter with Drainage Device, Percutaneous Approach
0D9R3ZX Drainage of Anal Sphincter, Percutaneous Approach, Diagnostic
0D9R3ZZ Drainage of Anal Sphincter, Percutaneous Approach
0D9R40Z Drainage of Anal Sphincter with Drainage Device, Percutaneous Endoscopic Approach
0D9R4ZX Drainage of Anal Sphincter, Percutaneous Endoscopic Approach, Diagnostic
0D9R4ZZ Drainage of Anal Sphincter, Percutaneous Endoscopic Approach
0D9S00Z Drainage of Greater Omentum with Drainage Device, Open Approach
0D9S0ZX Drainage of Greater Omentum, Open Approach, Diagnostic
0D9S0ZZ Drainage of Greater Omentum, Open Approach
0D9S30Z Drainage of Greater Omentum with Drainage Device, Percutaneous Approach
0D9S3ZX Drainage of Greater Omentum, Percutaneous Approach, Diagnostic
0D9S3ZZ Drainage of Greater Omentum, Percutaneous Approach
0D9S40Z Drainage of Greater Omentum with Drainage Device, Percutaneous Endoscopic Approach

0D9S4ZX Drainage of Greater Omentum, Percutaneous Endoscopic Approach, Diagnostic
0D9S4ZZ Drainage of Greater Omentum, Percutaneous Endoscopic Approach
0D9T00Z Drainage of Lesser Omentum with Drainage Device, Open Approach
0D9T0ZX Drainage of Lesser Omentum, Open Approach, Diagnostic
0D9T0ZZ Drainage of Lesser Omentum, Open Approach
0D9T30Z Drainage of Lesser Omentum with Drainage Device, Percutaneous Approach
0D9T3ZX Drainage of Lesser Omentum, Percutaneous Approach, Diagnostic
0D9T3ZZ Drainage of Lesser Omentum, Percutaneous Approach
0D9T40Z Drainage of Lesser Omentum with Drainage Device, Percutaneous Endoscopic Approach
0D9T4ZX Drainage of Lesser Omentum, Percutaneous Endoscopic Approach, Diagnostic
0D9T4ZZ Drainage of Lesser Omentum, Percutaneous Endoscopic Approach
0D9V00Z Drainage of Mesentery with Drainage Device, Open Approach
0D9V0ZX Drainage of Mesentery, Open Approach, Diagnostic
0D9V0ZZ Drainage of Mesentery, Open Approach
0D9V30Z Drainage of Mesentery with Drainage Device, Percutaneous Approach
0D9V3ZX Drainage of Mesentery, Percutaneous Approach, Diagnostic
0D9V3ZZ Drainage of Mesentery, Percutaneous Approach
0D9V40Z Drainage of Mesentery with Drainage Device, Percutaneous Endoscopic Approach
0D9V4ZX Drainage of Mesentery, Percutaneous Endoscopic Approach, Diagnostic
0D9V4ZZ Drainage of Mesentery, Percutaneous Endoscopic Approach
0D9W00Z Drainage of Peritoneum with Drainage Device, Open Approach
0D9W0ZX Drainage of Peritoneum, Open Approac Diagnostic
0D9W0ZZ Drainage of Peritoneum, Open Approac
0D9W30Z Drainage of Peritoneum with Drainage Device, Percutaneous Approach
0D9W3ZX Drainage of Peritoneum, Percutaneous Approach, Diagnostic
0D9W3ZZ Drainage of Peritoneum, Percutaneous Approach
0D9W40Z Drainage of Peritoneum with Drainage Device, Percutaneous Endoscopic Approach
0D9W4ZX Drainage of Peritoneum, Percutaneous Endoscopic Approach, Diagnostic
0D9W4ZZ Drainage of Peritoneum, Percutaneous Endoscopic Approach

0DB – Gastrointestinal System, Excision

Review Coding Guidelines B3.4a and B3.4b

Review Coding Guideline B3.8

0DB10ZX Excision of Upper Esophagus, Open Approach, Diagnostic
0DB10ZZ Excision of Upper Esophagus, Open Approach
0DB13ZX Excision of Upper Esophagus, Percutaneous Approach, Diagnostic
0DB13ZZ Excision of Upper Esophagus, Percutaneous Approach
0DB14ZX Excision of Upper Esophagus, Percutaneous Endoscopic Approach, Diagnostic
0DB14ZZ Excision of Upper Esophagus, Percutaneous Endoscopic Approach
0DB17ZX Excision of Upper Esophagus, Via Natural or Artificial Opening, Diagnostic
0DB17ZZ Excision of Upper Esophagus, Via Natural or Artificial Opening
0DB18ZX Excision of Upper Esophagus, Via Natural or Artificial Opening Endoscopic, Diagnostic
0DB18ZZ Excision of Upper Esophagus, Via Natural or Artificial Opening Endoscopic
0DB20ZX Excision of Middle Esophagus, Open Approach, Diagnostic
0DB20ZZ Excision of Middle Esophagus, Open Approach
0DB23ZX Excision of Middle Esophagus, Percutaneous Approach, Diagnostic
0DB23ZZ Excision of Middle Esophagus, Percutaneous Approach
0DB24ZX Excision of Middle Esophagus, Percutaneous Endoscopic Approach, Diagnostic
0DB24ZZ Excision of Middle Esophagus, Percutaneous Endoscopic Approach
0DB27ZX Excision of Middle Esophagus, Via Natural or Artificial Opening, Diagnostic
0DB27ZZ Excision of Middle Esophagus, Via Natural or Artificial Opening
0DB28ZX Excision of Middle Esophagus, Via Natural or Artificial Opening Endoscopic, Diagnostic
0DB28ZZ Excision of Middle Esophagus, Via Natural or Artificial Opening Endoscopic
0DB30ZX Excision of Lower Esophagus, Open Approach, Diagnostic
0DB30ZZ Excision of Lower Esophagus, Open Approach
0DB33ZX Excision of Lower Esophagus, Percutaneous Approach, Diagnostic
0DB33ZZ Excision of Lower Esophagus, Percutaneous Approach
0DB34ZX Excision of Lower Esophagus, Percutaneous Endoscopic Approach, Diagnostic
0DB34ZZ Excision of Lower Esophagus, Percutaneous Endoscopic Approach
0DB37ZX Excision of Lower Esophagus, Via Natural or Artificial Opening, Diagnostic
0DB37ZZ Excision of Lower Esophagus, Via Natural or Artificial Opening
0DB38ZX Excision of Lower Esophagus, Via Natural or Artificial Opening Endoscopic, Diagnostic
0DB38ZZ Excision of Lower Esophagus, Via Natural or Artificial Opening Endoscopic
0DB40ZX Excision of Esophagogastric Junction, Open Approach, Diagnostic
0DB40ZZ Excision of Esophagogastric Junction, Open Approach
0DB43ZX Excision of Esophagogastric Junction, Percutaneous Approach, Diagnostic
0DB43ZZ Excision of Esophagogastric Junction, Percutaneous Approach
0DB44ZX Excision of Esophagogastric Junction, Percutaneous Endoscopic Approach, Diagnostic
0DB44ZZ Excision of Esophagogastric Junction, Percutaneous Endoscopic Approach
0DB47ZX Excision of Esophagogastric Junction, Via Natural or Artificial Opening, Diagnostic
0DB47ZZ Excision of Esophagogastric Junction, Via Natural or Artificial Opening
0DB48ZX Excision of Esophagogastric Junction, Via Natural or Artificial Opening Endoscopic, Diagnostic
0DB48ZZ Excision of Esophagogastric Junction, Via Natural or Artificial Opening Endoscopic
0DB50ZX Excision of Esophagus, Open Approach, Diagnostic
0DB50ZZ Excision of Esophagus, Open Approach
0DB53ZX Excision of Esophagus, Percutaneous Approach, Diagnostic
0DB53ZZ Excision of Esophagus, Percutaneous Approach
0DB54ZX Excision of Esophagus, Percutaneous Endoscopic Approach, Diagnostic
0DB54ZZ Excision of Esophagus, Percutaneous Endoscopic Approach
0DB57ZX Excision of Esophagus, Via Natural or Artificial Opening, Diagnostic
0DB57ZZ Excision of Esophagus, Via Natural or Artificial Opening
0DB58ZX Excision of Esophagus, Via Natural or Artificial Opening Endoscopic, Diagnost
0DB58ZZ Excision of Esophagus, Via Natural or Artificial Opening Endoscopic
0DB60Z3 Excision of Stomach, Open Approach, Vertical
0DB60ZX Excision of Stomach, Open Approach, Diagnostic
0DB60ZZ Excision of Stomach, Open Approach
0DB63Z3 Excision of Stomach, Percutaneous Approach, Vertical
0DB63ZX Excision of Stomach, Percutaneous Approach, Diagnostic
0DB63ZZ Excision of Stomach, Percutaneous Approach
0DB64Z3 Excision of Stomach, Percutaneous Endoscopic Approach, Vertical
0DB64ZX Excision of Stomach, Percutaneous Endoscopic Approach, Diagnostic
0DB64ZZ Excision of Stomach, Percutaneous Endoscopic Approach
0DB67Z3 Excision of Stomach, Via Natural or Artificial Opening, Vertical
0DB67ZX Excision of Stomach, Via Natural or Artificial Opening, Diagnostic
0DB67ZZ Excision of Stomach, Via Natural or Artificial Opening
0DB68Z3 Excision of Stomach, Via Natural or Artificial Opening Endoscopic, Vertical
0DB68ZX Excision of Stomach, Via Natural or Artificial Opening Endoscopic, Diagnosti
0DB68ZZ Excision of Stomach, Via Natural or Artificial Opening Endoscopic
0DB70ZX Excision of Stomach, Pylorus, Open Approach, Diagnostic
0DB70ZZ Excision of Stomach, Pylorus, Open Approach
0DB73ZX Excision of Stomach, Pylorus, Percutaneous Approach, Diagnostic
0DB73ZZ Excision of Stomach, Pylorus, Percutaneous Approach

B74ZX Excision of Stomach, Pylorus, Percutaneous Endoscopic Approach, Diagnostic
B74ZZ Excision of Stomach, Pylorus, Percutaneous Endoscopic Approach
B77ZX Excision of Stomach, Pylorus, Via Natural or Artificial Opening, Diagnostic
B77ZZ Excision of Stomach, Pylorus, Via Natural or Artificial Opening
B78ZX Excision of Stomach, Pylorus, Via Natural or Artificial Opening Endoscopic, Diagnostic
B78ZZ Excision of Stomach, Pylorus, Via Natural or Artificial Opening Endoscopic
B80ZX Excision of Small Intestine, Open Approach, Diagnostic
B80ZZ Excision of Small Intestine, Open Approach
B83ZX Excision of Small Intestine, Percutaneous Approach, Diagnostic
B83ZZ Excision of Small Intestine, Percutaneous Approach
B84ZX Excision of Small Intestine, Percutaneous Endoscopic Approach, Diagnostic
B84ZZ Excision of Small Intestine, Percutaneous Endoscopic Approach
B87ZX Excision of Small Intestine, Via Natural or Artificial Opening, Diagnostic
B87ZZ Excision of Small Intestine, Via Natural or Artificial Opening
B88ZX Excision of Small Intestine, Via Natural or Artificial Opening Endoscopic, Diagnostic
B88ZZ Excision of Small Intestine, Via Natural or Artificial Opening Endoscopic
B90ZX Excision of Duodenum, Open Approach, Diagnostic
B90ZZ Excision of Duodenum, Open Approach
B93ZX Excision of Duodenum, Percutaneous Approach, Diagnostic
B93ZZ Excision of Duodenum, Percutaneous Approach
B94ZX Excision of Duodenum, Percutaneous Endoscopic Approach, Diagnostic
B94ZZ Excision of Duodenum, Percutaneous Endoscopic Approach
B97ZX Excision of Duodenum, Via Natural or Artificial Opening, Diagnostic
B97ZZ Excision of Duodenum, Via Natural or Artificial Opening
B98ZX Excision of Duodenum, Via Natural or Artificial Opening Endoscopic, Diagnostic
B98ZZ Excision of Duodenum, Via Natural or Artificial Opening Endoscopic
BA0ZX Excision of Jejunum, Open Approach, Diagnostic
BA0ZZ Excision of Jejunum, Open Approach
DBA3ZX Excision of Jejunum, Percutaneous Approach, Diagnostic
DBA3ZZ Excision of Jejunum, Percutaneous Approach
DBA4ZX Excision of Jejunum, Percutaneous Endoscopic Approach, Diagnostic
DBA4ZZ Excision of Jejunum, Percutaneous Endoscopic Approach
DBA7ZX Excision of Jejunum, Via Natural or Artificial Opening, Diagnostic
DBA7ZZ Excision of Jejunum, Via Natural or Artificial Opening
DBA8ZX Excision of Jejunum, Via Natural or Artificial Opening Endoscopic, Diagnostic
DBA8ZZ Excision of Jejunum, Via Natural or Artificial Opening Endoscopic
DBB0ZX Excision of Ileum, Open Approach, Diagnostic
DBB0ZZ Excision of Ileum, Open Approach
0DBB3ZX Excision of Ileum, Percutaneous Approach, Diagnostic
0DBB3ZZ Excision of Ileum, Percutaneous Approach
0DBB4ZX Excision of Ileum, Percutaneous Endoscopic Approach, Diagnostic
0DBB4ZZ Excision of Ileum, Percutaneous Endoscopic Approach
0DBB7ZX Excision of Ileum, Via Natural or Artificial Opening, Diagnostic
0DBB7ZZ Excision of Ileum, Via Natural or Artificial Opening
0DBB8ZX Excision of Ileum, Via Natural or Artificial Opening Endoscopic, Diagnostic
0DBB8ZZ Excision of Ileum, Via Natural or Artificial Opening Endoscopic
0DBC0ZX Excision of Ileocecal Valve, Open Approach, Diagnostic
0DBC0ZZ Excision of Ileocecal Valve, Open Approach
0DBC3ZX Excision of Ileocecal Valve, Percutaneous Approach, Diagnostic
0DBC3ZZ Excision of Ileocecal Valve, Percutaneous Approach
0DBC4ZX Excision of Ileocecal Valve, Percutaneous Endoscopic Approach, Diagnostic
0DBC4ZZ Excision of Ileocecal Valve, Percutaneous Endoscopic Approach
0DBC7ZX Excision of Ileocecal Valve, Via Natural or Artificial Opening, Diagnostic
0DBC7ZZ Excision of Ileocecal Valve, Via Natural or Artificial Opening
0DBC8ZX Excision of Ileocecal Valve, Via Natural or Artificial Opening Endoscopic, Diagnostic
0DBC8ZZ Excision of Ileocecal Valve, Via Natural or Artificial Opening Endoscopic
0DBE0ZX Excision of Large Intestine, Open Approach, Diagnostic
0DBE0ZZ Excision of Large Intestine, Open Approach
0DBE3ZX Excision of Large Intestine, Percutaneous Approach, Diagnostic
0DBE3ZZ Excision of Large Intestine, Percutaneous Approach
0DBE4ZX Excision of Large Intestine, Percutaneous Endoscopic Approach, Diagnostic
0DBE4ZZ Excision of Large Intestine, Percutaneous Endoscopic Approach
0DBE7ZX Excision of Large Intestine, Via Natural or Artificial Opening, Diagnostic
0DBE7ZZ Excision of Large Intestine, Via Natural or Artificial Opening
0DBE8ZX Excision of Large Intestine, Via Natural or Artificial Opening Endoscopic, Diagnostic
0DBE8ZZ Excision of Large Intestine, Via Natural or Artificial Opening Endoscopic
0DBF0ZX Excision of Right Large Intestine, Open Approach, Diagnostic
0DBF0ZZ Excision of Right Large Intestine, Open Approach
0DBF3ZX Excision of Right Large Intestine, Percutaneous Approach, Diagnostic
0DBF3ZZ Excision of Right Large Intestine, Percutaneous Approach
0DBF4ZX Excision of Right Large Intestine, Percutaneous Endoscopic Approach, Diagnostic
0DBF4ZZ Excision of Right Large Intestine, Percutaneous Endoscopic Approach
0DBF7ZX Excision of Right Large Intestine, Via Natural or Artificial Opening, Diagnostic
0DBF7ZZ Excision of Right Large Intestine, Via Natural or Artificial Opening
0DBF8ZX Excision of Right Large Intestine, Via Natural or Artificial Opening Endoscopic, Diagnostic
0DBF8ZZ Excision of Right Large Intestine, Via Natural or Artificial Opening Endoscopic
0DBG0ZX Excision of Left Large Intestine, Open Approach, Diagnostic
0DBG0ZZ Excision of Left Large Intestine, Open Approach
0DBG3ZX Excision of Left Large Intestine, Percutaneous Approach, Diagnostic
0DBG3ZZ Excision of Left Large Intestine, Percutaneous Approach
0DBG4ZX Excision of Left Large Intestine, Percutaneous Endoscopic Approach, Diagnostic
0DBG4ZZ Excision of Left Large Intestine, Percutaneous Endoscopic Approach
0DBG7ZX Excision of Left Large Intestine, Via Natural or Artificial Opening, Diagnostic
0DBG7ZZ Excision of Left Large Intestine, Via Natural or Artificial Opening
0DBG8ZX Excision of Left Large Intestine, Via Natural or Artificial Opening Endoscopic, Diagnostic
0DBG8ZZ Excision of Left Large Intestine, Via Natural or Artificial Opening Endoscopic
0DBH0ZX Excision of Cecum, Open Approach, Diagnostic
0DBH0ZZ Excision of Cecum, Open Approach
0DBH3ZX Excision of Cecum, Percutaneous Approach, Diagnostic
0DBH3ZZ Excision of Cecum, Percutaneous Approach
0DBH4ZX Excision of Cecum, Percutaneous Endoscopic Approach, Diagnostic
0DBH4ZZ Excision of Cecum, Percutaneous Endoscopic Approach
0DBH7ZX Excision of Cecum, Via Natural or Artificial Opening, Diagnostic
0DBH7ZZ Excision of Cecum, Via Natural or Artificial Opening
0DBH8ZX Excision of Cecum, Via Natural or Artificial Opening Endoscopic, Diagnostic
0DBH8ZZ Excision of Cecum, Via Natural or Artificial Opening Endoscopic
0DBJ0ZX Excision of Appendix, Open Approach, Diagnostic
0DBJ0ZZ Excision of Appendix, Open Approach
0DBJ3ZX Excision of Appendix, Percutaneous Approach, Diagnostic
0DBJ3ZZ Excision of Appendix, Percutaneous Approach
0DBJ4ZX Excision of Appendix, Percutaneous Endoscopic Approach, Diagnostic
0DBJ4ZZ Excision of Appendix, Percutaneous Endoscopic Approach
0DBJ7ZX Excision of Appendix, Via Natural or Artificial Opening, Diagnostic
0DBJ7ZZ Excision of Appendix, Via Natural or Artificial Opening
0DBJ8ZX Excision of Appendix, Via Natural or Artificial Opening Endoscopic, Diagnostic
0DBJ8ZZ Excision of Appendix, Via Natural or Artificial Opening Endoscopic
0DBK0ZX Excision of Ascending Colon, Open Approach, Diagnostic
0DBK0ZZ Excision of Ascending Colon, Open Approach
0DBK3ZX Excision of Ascending Colon, Percutaneous Approach, Diagnostic
0DBK3ZZ Excision of Ascending Colon, Percutaneous Approach
0DBK4ZX Excision of Ascending Colon, Percutaneous Endoscopic Approach, Diagnostic

0DBK4ZZ Excision of Ascending Colon, Percutaneous Endoscopic Approach
0DBK7ZX Excision of Ascending Colon, Via Natural or Artificial Opening, Diagnostic
0DBK7ZZ Excision of Ascending Colon, Via Natural or Artificial Opening
0DBK8ZX Excision of Ascending Colon, Via Natural or Artificial Opening Endoscopic, Diagnostic
0DBK8ZZ Excision of Ascending Colon, Via Natural or Artificial Opening Endoscopic
0DBL0ZX Excision of Transverse Colon, Open Approach, Diagnostic
0DBL0ZZ Excision of Transverse Colon, Open Approach
0DBL3ZX Excision of Transverse Colon, Percutaneous Approach, Diagnostic
0DBL3ZZ Excision of Transverse Colon, Percutaneous Approach
0DBL4ZX Excision of Transverse Colon, Percutaneous Endoscopic Approach, Diagnostic
0DBL4ZZ Excision of Transverse Colon, Percutaneous Endoscopic Approach
0DBL7ZX Excision of Transverse Colon, Via Natural or Artificial Opening, Diagnostic
0DBL7ZZ Excision of Transverse Colon, Via Natural or Artificial Opening
0DBL8ZX Excision of Transverse Colon, Via Natural or Artificial Opening Endoscopic, Diagnostic
0DBL8ZZ Excision of Transverse Colon, Via Natural or Artificial Opening Endoscopic
0DBM0ZX Excision of Descending Colon, Open Approach, Diagnostic
0DBM0ZZ Excision of Descending Colon, Open Approach
0DBM3ZX Excision of Descending Colon, Percutaneous Approach, Diagnostic
0DBM3ZZ Excision of Descending Colon, Percutaneous Approach
0DBM4ZX Excision of Descending Colon, Percutaneous Endoscopic Approach, Diagnostic
0DBM4ZZ Excision of Descending Colon, Percutaneous Endoscopic Approach
0DBM7ZX Excision of Descending Colon, Via Natural or Artificial Opening, Diagnostic
0DBM7ZZ Excision of Descending Colon, Via Natural or Artificial Opening
0DBM8ZX Excision of Descending Colon, Via Natural or Artificial Opening Endoscopic, Diagnostic
0DBM8ZZ Excision of Descending Colon, Via Natural or Artificial Opening Endoscopic
0DBN0ZX Excision of Sigmoid Colon, Open Approach, Diagnostic
0DBN0ZZ Excision of Sigmoid Colon, Open Approach
0DBN3ZX Excision of Sigmoid Colon, Percutaneous Approach, Diagnostic
0DBN3ZZ Excision of Sigmoid Colon, Percutaneous Approach
0DBN4ZX Excision of Sigmoid Colon, Percutaneous Endoscopic Approach, Diagnostic
0DBN4ZZ Excision of Sigmoid Colon, Percutaneous Endoscopic Approach
0DBN7ZX Excision of Sigmoid Colon, Via Natural or Artificial Opening, Diagnostic
0DBN7ZZ Excision of Sigmoid Colon, Via Natural or Artificial Opening
0DBN8ZX Excision of Sigmoid Colon, Via Natural or Artificial Opening Endoscopic, Diagnostic
0DBN8ZZ Excision of Sigmoid Colon, Via Natural or Artificial Opening Endoscopic
0DBP0ZX Excision of Rectum, Open Approach, Diagnostic
0DBP0ZZ Excision of Rectum, Open Approach
0DBP3ZX Excision of Rectum, Percutaneous Approach, Diagnostic
0DBP3ZZ Excision of Rectum, Percutaneous Approach
0DBP4ZX Excision of Rectum, Percutaneous Endoscopic Approach, Diagnostic
0DBP4ZZ Excision of Rectum, Percutaneous Endoscopic Approach
0DBP7ZX Excision of Rectum, Via Natural or Artificial Opening, Diagnostic
0DBP7ZZ Excision of Rectum, Via Natural or Artificial Opening
0DBP8ZX Excision of Rectum, Via Natural or Artificial Opening Endoscopic, Diagnostic
0DBP8ZZ Excision of Rectum, Via Natural or Artificial Opening Endoscopic
0DBQ0ZX Excision of Anus, Open Approach, Diagnostic
0DBQ0ZZ Excision of Anus, Open Approach
0DBQ3ZX Excision of Anus, Percutaneous Approach, Diagnostic
0DBQ3ZZ Excision of Anus, Percutaneous Approach
0DBQ4ZX Excision of Anus, Percutaneous Endoscopic Approach, Diagnostic
0DBQ4ZZ Excision of Anus, Percutaneous Endoscopic Approach
0DBQ7ZX Excision of Anus, Via Natural or Artificial Opening, Diagnostic
0DBQ7ZZ Excision of Anus, Via Natural or Artificial Opening
0DBQ8ZX Excision of Anus, Via Natural or Artificial Opening Endoscopic, Diagnostic
0DBQ8ZZ Excision of Anus, Via Natural or Artificial Opening Endoscopic
0DBQXZX Excision of Anus, External Approach, Diagnostic
0DBQXZZ Excision of Anus, External Approach
0DBR0ZX Excision of Anal Sphincter, Open Approach, Diagnostic
0DBR0ZZ Excision of Anal Sphincter, Open Approach
0DBR3ZX Excision of Anal Sphincter, Percutaneous Approach, Diagnostic
0DBR3ZZ Excision of Anal Sphincter, Percutaneous Approach
0DBR4ZX Excision of Anal Sphincter, Percutaneous Endoscopic Approach, Diagnostic
0DBR4ZZ Excision of Anal Sphincter, Percutaneous Endoscopic Approach
0DBS0ZX Excision of Greater Omentum, Open Approach, Diagnostic
0DBS0ZZ Excision of Greater Omentum, Open Approach
0DBS3ZX Excision of Greater Omentum, Percutaneous Approach, Diagnostic
0DBS3ZZ Excision of Greater Omentum, Percutaneous Approach
0DBS4ZX Excision of Greater Omentum, Percutaneous Endoscopic Approach, Diagnostic
0DBS4ZZ Excision of Greater Omentum, Percutaneous Endoscopic Approach
0DBT0ZX Excision of Lesser Omentum, Open Approach, Diagnostic
0DBT0ZZ Excision of Lesser Omentum, Open Approach
0DBT3ZX Excision of Lesser Omentum, Percutaneous Approach, Diagnostic
0DBT3ZZ Excision of Lesser Omentum, Percutaneous Approach
0DBT4ZX Excision of Lesser Omentum, Percutaneous Endoscopic Approach, Diagnostic
0DBT4ZZ Excision of Lesser Omentum, Percutaneous Endoscopic Approach
0DBV0ZX Excision of Mesentery, Open Approach, Diagnostic
0DBV0ZZ Excision of Mesentery, Open Approach
0DBV3ZX Excision of Mesentery, Percutaneous Approach, Diagnostic
0DBV3ZZ Excision of Mesentery, Percutaneous Approach
0DBV4ZX Excision of Mesentery, Percutaneous Endoscopic Approach, Diagnostic
0DBV4ZZ Excision of Mesentery, Percutaneous Endoscopic Approach
0DBW0ZX Excision of Peritoneum, Open Approach, Diagnostic
0DBW0ZZ Excision of Peritoneum, Open Approach
0DBW3ZX Excision of Peritoneum, Percutaneous Approach, Diagnostic
0DBW3ZZ Excision of Peritoneum, Percutaneous Approach
0DBW4ZX Excision of Peritoneum, Percutaneous Endoscopic Approach, Diagnostic
0DBW4ZZ Excision of Peritoneum, Percutaneous Endoscopic Approach

0DC – Gastrointestinal System, Extirpation

0DC10ZZ Extirpation of Matter from Upper Esophagus, Open Approach
0DC13ZZ Extirpation of Matter from Upper Esophagus, Percutaneous Approach
0DC14ZZ Extirpation of Matter from Upper Esophagus, Percutaneous Endoscopic Approach
0DC17ZZ Extirpation of Matter from Upper Esophagus, Via Natural or Artificial Opening
0DC18ZZ Extirpation of Matter from Upper Esophagus, Via Natural or Artificial Opening Endoscopic
0DC20ZZ Extirpation of Matter from Middle Esophagus, Open Approach
0DC23ZZ Extirpation of Matter from Middle Esophagus, Percutaneous Approach
0DC24ZZ Extirpation of Matter from Middle Esophagus, Percutaneous Endoscopic Approach
0DC27ZZ Extirpation of Matter from Middle Esophagus, Via Natural or Artificial Opening
0DC28ZZ Extirpation of Matter from Middle Esophagus, Via Natural or Artificial Opening Endoscopic
0DC30ZZ Extirpation of Matter from Lower Esophagus, Open Approach
0DC33ZZ Extirpation of Matter from Lower Esophagus, Percutaneous Approach
0DC34ZZ Extirpation of Matter from Lower Esophagus, Percutaneous Endoscopic Approach
0DC37ZZ Extirpation of Matter from Lower Esophagus, Via Natural or Artificial Opening
0DC38ZZ Extirpation of Matter from Lower Esophagus, Via Natural or Artificial Opening Endoscopic

C40ZZ Extirpation of Matter from Esophagogastric Junction, Open Approach
C43ZZ Extirpation of Matter from Esophagogastric Junction, Percutaneous Approach
C44ZZ Extirpation of Matter from Esophagogastric Junction, Percutaneous Endoscopic Approach
C47ZZ Extirpation of Matter from Esophagogastric Junction, Via Natural or Artificial Opening
C48ZZ Extirpation of Matter from Esophagogastric Junction, Via Natural or Artificial Opening Endoscopic
C50ZZ Extirpation of Matter from Esophagus, Open Approach
C53ZZ Extirpation of Matter from Esophagus, Percutaneous Approach
C54ZZ Extirpation of Matter from Esophagus, Percutaneous Endoscopic Approach
C57ZZ Extirpation of Matter from Esophagus, Via Natural or Artificial Opening
C58ZZ Extirpation of Matter from Esophagus, Via Natural or Artificial Opening Endoscopic
C60ZZ Extirpation of Matter from Stomach, Open Approach
C63ZZ Extirpation of Matter from Stomach, Percutaneous Approach
C64ZZ Extirpation of Matter from Stomach, Percutaneous Endoscopic Approach
C67ZZ Extirpation of Matter from Stomach, Via Natural or Artificial Opening
C68ZZ Extirpation of Matter from Stomach, Via Natural or Artificial Opening Endoscopic
C70ZZ Extirpation of Matter from Stomach, Pylorus, Open Approach
C73ZZ Extirpation of Matter from Stomach, Pylorus, Percutaneous Approach
C74ZZ Extirpation of Matter from Stomach, Pylorus, Percutaneous Endoscopic Approach
C77ZZ Extirpation of Matter from Stomach, Pylorus, Via Natural or Artificial Opening
C78ZZ Extirpation of Matter from Stomach, Pylorus, Via Natural or Artificial Opening Endoscopic
C80ZZ Extirpation of Matter from Small Intestine, Open Approach
C83ZZ Extirpation of Matter from Small Intestine, Percutaneous Approach
C84ZZ Extirpation of Matter from Small Intestine, Percutaneous Endoscopic Approach
C87ZZ Extirpation of Matter from Small Intestine, Via Natural or Artificial Opening
C88ZZ Extirpation of Matter from Small Intestine, Via Natural or Artificial Opening Endoscopic
C90ZZ Extirpation of Matter from Duodenum, Open Approach
DC93ZZ Extirpation of Matter from Duodenum, Percutaneous Approach
DC94ZZ Extirpation of Matter from Duodenum, Percutaneous Endoscopic Approach
DC97ZZ Extirpation of Matter from Duodenum, Via Natural or Artificial Opening
DC98ZZ Extirpation of Matter from Duodenum, Via Natural or Artificial Opening Endoscopic
DCA0ZZ Extirpation of Matter from Jejunum, Open Approach
DCA3ZZ Extirpation of Matter from Jejunum, Percutaneous Approach
0DCA4ZZ Extirpation of Matter from Jejunum, Percutaneous Endoscopic Approach
0DCA7ZZ Extirpation of Matter from Jejunum, Via Natural or Artificial Opening
0DCA8ZZ Extirpation of Matter from Jejunum, Via Natural or Artificial Opening Endoscopic
0DCB0ZZ Extirpation of Matter from Ileum, Open Approach
0DCB3ZZ Extirpation of Matter from Ileum, Percutaneous Approach
0DCB4ZZ Extirpation of Matter from Ileum, Percutaneous Endoscopic Approach
0DCB7ZZ Extirpation of Matter from Ileum, Via Natural or Artificial Opening
0DCB8ZZ Extirpation of Matter from Ileum, Via Natural or Artificial Opening Endoscopic
0DCC0ZZ Extirpation of Matter from Ileocecal Valve, Open Approach
0DCC3ZZ Extirpation of Matter from Ileocecal Valve, Percutaneous Approach
0DCC4ZZ Extirpation of Matter from Ileocecal Valve, Percutaneous Endoscopic Approach
0DCC7ZZ Extirpation of Matter from Ileocecal Valve, Via Natural or Artificial Opening
0DCC8ZZ Extirpation of Matter from Ileocecal Valve, Via Natural or Artificial Opening Endoscopic
0DCE0ZZ Extirpation of Matter from Large Intestine, Open Approach
0DCE3ZZ Extirpation of Matter from Large Intestine, Percutaneous Approach
0DCE4ZZ Extirpation of Matter from Large Intestine, Percutaneous Endoscopic Approach
0DCE7ZZ Extirpation of Matter from Large Intestine, Via Natural or Artificial Opening
0DCE8ZZ Extirpation of Matter from Large Intestine, Via Natural or Artificial Opening Endoscopic
0DCF0ZZ Extirpation of Matter from Right Large Intestine, Open Approach
0DCF3ZZ Extirpation of Matter from Right Large Intestine, Percutaneous Approach
0DCF4ZZ Extirpation of Matter from Right Large Intestine, Percutaneous Endoscopic Approach
0DCF7ZZ Extirpation of Matter from Right Large Intestine, Via Natural or Artificial Opening
0DCF8ZZ Extirpation of Matter from Right Large Intestine, Via Natural or Artificial Opening Endoscopic
0DCG0ZZ Extirpation of Matter from Left Large Intestine, Open Approach
0DCG3ZZ Extirpation of Matter from Left Large Intestine, Percutaneous Approach
0DCG4ZZ Extirpation of Matter from Left Large Intestine, Percutaneous Endoscopic Approach
0DCG7ZZ Extirpation of Matter from Left Large Intestine, Via Natural or Artificial Opening
0DCG8ZZ Extirpation of Matter from Left Large Intestine, Via Natural or Artificial Opening Endoscopic
0DCH0ZZ Extirpation of Matter from Cecum, Open Approach
0DCH3ZZ Extirpation of Matter from Cecum, Percutaneous Approach
0DCH4ZZ Extirpation of Matter from Cecum, Percutaneous Endoscopic Approach
0DCH7ZZ Extirpation of Matter from Cecum, Via Natural or Artificial Opening
0DCH8ZZ Extirpation of Matter from Cecum, Via Natural or Artificial Opening Endoscopic
0DCJ0ZZ Extirpation of Matter from Appendix, Open Approach
0DCJ3ZZ Extirpation of Matter from Appendix, Percutaneous Approach
0DCJ4ZZ Extirpation of Matter from Appendix, Percutaneous Endoscopic Approach
0DCJ7ZZ Extirpation of Matter from Appendix, Via Natural or Artificial Opening
0DCJ8ZZ Extirpation of Matter from Appendix, Via Natural or Artificial Opening Endoscopic
0DCK0ZZ Extirpation of Matter from Ascending Colon, Open Approach
0DCK3ZZ Extirpation of Matter from Ascending Colon, Percutaneous Approach
0DCK4ZZ Extirpation of Matter from Ascending Colon, Percutaneous Endoscopic Approach
0DCK7ZZ Extirpation of Matter from Ascending Colon, Via Natural or Artificial Opening
0DCK8ZZ Extirpation of Matter from Ascending Colon, Via Natural or Artificial Opening Endoscopic
0DCL0ZZ Extirpation of Matter from Transverse Colon, Open Approach
0DCL3ZZ Extirpation of Matter from Transverse Colon, Percutaneous Approach
0DCL4ZZ Extirpation of Matter from Transverse Colon, Percutaneous Endoscopic Approach
0DCL7ZZ Extirpation of Matter from Transverse Colon, Via Natural or Artificial Opening
0DCL8ZZ Extirpation of Matter from Transverse Colon, Via Natural or Artificial Opening Endoscopic
0DCM0ZZ Extirpation of Matter from Descending Colon, Open Approach
0DCM3ZZ Extirpation of Matter from Descending Colon, Percutaneous Approach
0DCM4ZZ Extirpation of Matter from Descending Colon, Percutaneous Endoscopic Approach
0DCM7ZZ Extirpation of Matter from Descending Colon, Via Natural or Artificial Opening
0DCM8ZZ Extirpation of Matter from Descending Colon, Via Natural or Artificial Opening Endoscopic
0DCN0ZZ Extirpation of Matter from Sigmoid Colon, Open Approach
0DCN3ZZ Extirpation of Matter from Sigmoid Colon, Percutaneous Approach
0DCN4ZZ Extirpation of Matter from Sigmoid Colon, Percutaneous Endoscopic Approach
0DCN7ZZ Extirpation of Matter from Sigmoid Colon, Via Natural or Artificial Opening
0DCN8ZZ Extirpation of Matter from Sigmoid Colon, Via Natural or Artificial Opening Endoscopic
0DCP0ZZ Extirpation of Matter from Rectum, Open Approach
0DCP3ZZ Extirpation of Matter from Rectum, Percutaneous Approach
0DCP4ZZ Extirpation of Matter from Rectum, Percutaneous Endoscopic Approach
0DCP7ZZ Extirpation of Matter from Rectum, Via Natural or Artificial Opening
0DCP8ZZ Extirpation of Matter from Rectum, Via Natural or Artificial Opening Endoscopic
0DCQ0ZZ Extirpation of Matter from Anus, Open Approach
0DCQ3ZZ Extirpation of Matter from Anus, Percutaneous Approach
0DCQ4ZZ Extirpation of Matter from Anus, Percutaneous Endoscopic Approach

0DCQ7ZZ Extirpation of Matter from Anus, Via Natural or Artificial Opening
0DCQ8ZZ Extirpation of Matter from Anus, Via Natural or Artificial Opening Endoscopic
0DCQXZZ Extirpation of Matter from Anus, External Approach
0DCR0ZZ Extirpation of Matter from Anal Sphincter, Open Approach
0DCR3ZZ Extirpation of Matter from Anal Sphincter, Percutaneous Approach
0DCR4ZZ Extirpation of Matter from Anal Sphincter, Percutaneous Endoscopic Approach
0DCS0ZZ Extirpation of Matter from Greater Omentum, Open Approach
0DCS3ZZ Extirpation of Matter from Greater Omentum, Percutaneous Approach
0DCS4ZZ Extirpation of Matter from Greater Omentum, Percutaneous Endoscopic Approach
0DCT0ZZ Extirpation of Matter from Lesser Omentum, Open Approach
0DCT3ZZ Extirpation of Matter from Lesser Omentum, Percutaneous Approach
0DCT4ZZ Extirpation of Matter from Lesser Omentum, Percutaneous Endoscopic Approach
0DCV0ZZ Extirpation of Matter from Mesentery, Open Approach
0DCV3ZZ Extirpation of Matter from Mesentery, Percutaneous Approach
0DCV4ZZ Extirpation of Matter from Mesentery, Percutaneous Endoscopic Approach
0DCW0ZZ Extirpation of Matter from Peritoneum, Open Approach
0DCW3ZZ Extirpation of Matter from Peritoneum, Percutaneous Approach
0DCW4ZZ Extirpation of Matter from Peritoneum, Percutaneous Endoscopic Approach

0DF – Gastrointestinal System, Fragmentation

0DF50ZZ Fragmentation in Esophagus, Open Approach
0DF53ZZ Fragmentation in Esophagus, Percutaneous Approach
0DF54ZZ Fragmentation in Esophagus, Percutaneous Endoscopic Approach
0DF57ZZ Fragmentation in Esophagus, Via Natural or Artificial Opening
0DF58ZZ Fragmentation in Esophagus, Via Natural or Artificial Opening Endoscopic
▲ **0DF5XZZ** Fragmentation in Esophagus, External Approach
0DF60ZZ Fragmentation in Stomach, Open Approach
0DF63ZZ Fragmentation in Stomach, Percutaneous Approach
0DF64ZZ Fragmentation in Stomach, Percutaneous Endoscopic Approach
0DF67ZZ Fragmentation in Stomach, Via Natural or Artificial Opening
0DF68ZZ Fragmentation in Stomach, Via Natural or Artificial Opening Endoscopic
▲ **0DF6XZZ** Fragmentation in Stomach, External Approach
0DF80ZZ Fragmentation in Small Intestine, Open Approach
0DF83ZZ Fragmentation in Small Intestine, Percutaneous Approach
0DF84ZZ Fragmentation in Small Intestine, Percutaneous Endoscopic Approach
0DF87ZZ Fragmentation in Small Intestine, Via Natural or Artificial Opening
0DF88ZZ Fragmentation in Small Intestine, Via Natural or Artificial Opening Endoscopic
▲ **0DF8XZZ** Fragmentation in Small Intestine, External Approach
0DF90ZZ Fragmentation in Duodenum, Open Approach
0DF93ZZ Fragmentation in Duodenum, Percutaneous Approach
0DF94ZZ Fragmentation in Duodenum, Percutaneous Endoscopic Approach
0DF97ZZ Fragmentation in Duodenum, Via Natural or Artificial Opening
0DF98ZZ Fragmentation in Duodenum, Via Natural or Artificial Opening Endoscopic
▲ **0DF9XZZ** Fragmentation in Duodenum, External Approach
0DFA0ZZ Fragmentation in Jejunum, Open Approach
0DFA3ZZ Fragmentation in Jejunum, Percutaneous Approach
0DFA4ZZ Fragmentation in Jejunum, Percutaneous Endoscopic Approach
0DFA7ZZ Fragmentation in Jejunum, Via Natural or Artificial Opening
0DFA8ZZ Fragmentation in Jejunum, Via Natural or Artificial Opening Endoscopic
▲ **0DFAXZZ** Fragmentation in Jejunum, External Approach
0DFB0ZZ Fragmentation in Ileum, Open Approach
0DFB3ZZ Fragmentation in Ileum, Percutaneous Approach
0DFB4ZZ Fragmentation in Ileum, Percutaneous Endoscopic Approach
0DFB7ZZ Fragmentation in Ileum, Via Natural or Artificial Opening
0DFB8ZZ Fragmentation in Ileum, Via Natural or Artificial Opening Endoscopic
▲ **0DFBXZZ** Fragmentation in Ileum, External Approach
0DFE0ZZ Fragmentation in Large Intestine, Open Approach
0DFE3ZZ Fragmentation in Large Intestine, Percutaneous Approach
0DFE4ZZ Fragmentation in Large Intestine, Percutaneous Endoscopic Approach
0DFE7ZZ Fragmentation in Large Intestine, Via Natural or Artificial Opening
0DFE8ZZ Fragmentation in Large Intestine, Via Natural or Artificial Opening Endoscopic
▲ **0DFEXZZ** Fragmentation in Large Intestine, External Approach
0DFF0ZZ Fragmentation in Right Large Intestine, Open Approach
0DFF3ZZ Fragmentation in Right Large Intestine, Percutaneous Approach
0DFF4ZZ Fragmentation in Right Large Intestine, Percutaneous Endoscopic Approach
0DFF7ZZ Fragmentation in Right Large Intestine, Via Natural or Artificial Opening
0DFF8ZZ Fragmentation in Right Large Intestine, Via Natural or Artificial Opening Endoscopic
▲ **0DFFXZZ** Fragmentation in Right Large Intestine, External Approach
0DFG0ZZ Fragmentation in Left Large Intestine, Open Approach
0DFG3ZZ Fragmentation in Left Large Intestine, Percutaneous Approach
0DFG4ZZ Fragmentation in Left Large Intestine, Percutaneous Endoscopic Approach
0DFG7ZZ Fragmentation in Left Large Intestine, Via Natural or Artificial Opening
0DFG8ZZ Fragmentation in Left Large Intestine, Via Natural or Artificial Opening Endoscopic
▲ **0DFGXZZ** Fragmentation in Left Large Intestine, External Approach
0DFH0ZZ Fragmentation in Cecum, Open Approach
0DFH3ZZ Fragmentation in Cecum, Percutaneous Approach
0DFH4ZZ Fragmentation in Cecum, Percutaneous Endoscopic Approach
0DFH7ZZ Fragmentation in Cecum, Via Natural or Artificial Opening
0DFH8ZZ Fragmentation in Cecum, Via Natural or Artificial Opening Endoscopic
▲ **0DFHXZZ** Fragmentation in Cecum, External Approach
0DFJ0ZZ Fragmentation in Appendix, Open Approach
0DFJ3ZZ Fragmentation in Appendix, Percutaneous Approach
0DFJ4ZZ Fragmentation in Appendix, Percutaneous Endoscopic Approach
0DFJ7ZZ Fragmentation in Appendix, Via Natural or Artificial Opening
0DFJ8ZZ Fragmentation in Appendix, Via Natural or Artificial Opening Endoscopic
▲ **0DFJXZZ** Fragmentation in Appendix, External Approach
0DFK0ZZ Fragmentation in Ascending Colon, Open Approach
0DFK3ZZ Fragmentation in Ascending Colon, Percutaneous Approach
0DFK4ZZ Fragmentation in Ascending Colon, Percutaneous Endoscopic Approach
0DFK7ZZ Fragmentation in Ascending Colon, Via Natural or Artificial Opening
0DFK8ZZ Fragmentation in Ascending Colon, Via Natural or Artificial Opening Endoscopic
▲ **0DFKXZZ** Fragmentation in Ascending Colon, External Approach
0DFL0ZZ Fragmentation in Transverse Colon, Open Approach
0DFL3ZZ Fragmentation in Transverse Colon, Percutaneous Approach
0DFL4ZZ Fragmentation in Transverse Colon, Percutaneous Endoscopic Approach
0DFL7ZZ Fragmentation in Transverse Colon, Via Natural or Artificial Opening
0DFL8ZZ Fragmentation in Transverse Colon, Via Natural or Artificial Opening Endoscopic
▲ **0DFLXZZ** Fragmentation in Transverse Colon, External Approach
0DFM0ZZ Fragmentation in Descending Colon, Open Approach
0DFM3ZZ Fragmentation in Descending Colon, Percutaneous Approach
0DFM4ZZ Fragmentation in Descending Colon, Percutaneous Endoscopic Approach
0DFM7ZZ Fragmentation in Descending Colon, Via Natural or Artificial Opening
0DFM8ZZ Fragmentation in Descending Colon, Via Natural or Artificial Opening Endoscopic
▲ **0DFMXZZ** Fragmentation in Descending Colon, External Approach
0DFN0ZZ Fragmentation in Sigmoid Colon, Open Approach
0DFN3ZZ Fragmentation in Sigmoid Colon, Percutaneous Approach
0DFN4ZZ Fragmentation in Sigmoid Colon, Percutaneous Endoscopic Approach
0DFN7ZZ Fragmentation in Sigmoid Colon, Via Natural or Artificial Opening
0DFN8ZZ Fragmentation in Sigmoid Colon, Via Natural or Artificial Opening Endoscopic
▲ **0DFNXZZ** Fragmentation in Sigmoid Colon, External Approach

FP0ZZ Fragmentation in Rectum, Open Approach
FP3ZZ Fragmentation in Rectum, Percutaneous Approach
FP4ZZ Fragmentation in Rectum, Percutaneous Endoscopic Approach
FP7ZZ Fragmentation in Rectum, Via Natural or Artificial Opening
0DFP8ZZ Fragmentation in Rectum, Via Natural or Artificial Opening Endoscopic
▲ **0DFPXZZ** Fragmentation in Rectum, External Approach
0DFQ0ZZ Fragmentation in Anus, Open Approach
0DFQ3ZZ Fragmentation in Anus, Percutaneous Approach
0DFQ4ZZ Fragmentation in Anus, Percutaneous Endoscopic Approach
0DFQ7ZZ Fragmentation in Anus, Via Natural or Artificial Opening
0DFQ8ZZ Fragmentation in Anus, Via Natural or Artificial Opening Endoscopic
▲ **0DFQXZZ** Fragmentation in Anus, External Approach

)H – Gastrointestinal System, Insertion

H501Z Insertion of Radioactive Element into Esophagus, Open Approach
H502Z Insertion of Monitoring Device into Esophagus, Open Approach
H503Z Insertion of Infusion Device into Esophagus, Open Approach
H50DZ Insertion of Intraluminal Device into Esophagus, Open Approach
H50UZ Insertion of Feeding Device into Esophagus, Open Approach
H531Z Insertion of Radioactive Element into Esophagus, Percutaneous Approach
H532Z Insertion of Monitoring Device into Esophagus, Percutaneous Approach
H533Z Insertion of Infusion Device into Esophagus, Percutaneous Approach
H53DZ Insertion of Intraluminal Device into Esophagus, Percutaneous Approach
H53UZ Insertion of Feeding Device into Esophagus, Percutaneous Approach
)H541Z Insertion of Radioactive Element into Esophagus, Percutaneous Endoscopic Approach
)H542Z Insertion of Monitoring Device into Esophagus, Percutaneous Endoscopic Approach
)H543Z Insertion of Infusion Device into Esophagus, Percutaneous Endoscopic Approach
)H54DZ Insertion of Intraluminal Device into Esophagus, Percutaneous Endoscopic Approach
)H54UZ Insertion of Feeding Device into Esophagus, Percutaneous Endoscopic Approach
)H571Z Insertion of Radioactive Element into Esophagus, Via Natural or Artificial Opening
DH572Z Insertion of Monitoring Device into Esophagus, Via Natural or Artificial Opening
DH573Z Insertion of Infusion Device into Esophagus, Via Natural or Artificial Opening
DH57BZ Insertion of Airway into Esophagus, Via Natural or Artificial Opening
DH57DZ Insertion of Intraluminal Device into Esophagus, Via Natural or Artificial Opening
DH57UZ Insertion of Feeding Device into Esophagus, Via Natural or Artificial Opening
DH581Z Insertion of Radioactive Element into Esophagus, Via Natural or Artificial Opening Endoscopic
DH582Z Insertion of Monitoring Device into Esophagus, Via Natural or Artificial Opening Endoscopic
DH583Z Insertion of Infusion Device into Esophagus, Via Natural or Artificial Opening Endoscopic
DH58BZ Insertion of Airway into Esophagus, Via Natural or Artificial Opening Endoscopic
DH58DZ Insertion of Intraluminal Device into Esophagus, Via Natural or Artificial Opening Endoscopic
0DH58UZ Insertion of Feeding Device into Esophagus, Via Natural or Artificial Opening Endoscopic
0DH602Z Insertion of Monitoring Device into Stomach, Open Approach
0DH603Z Insertion of Infusion Device into Stomach, Open Approach
0DH60DZ Insertion of Intraluminal Device into Stomach, Open Approach
0DH60MZ Insertion of Stimulator Lead into Stomach, Open Approach
0DH60UZ Insertion of Feeding Device into Stomach, Open Approach
0DH632Z Insertion of Monitoring Device into Stomach, Percutaneous Approach
0DH633Z Insertion of Infusion Device into Stomach, Percutaneous Approach
0DH63DZ Insertion of Intraluminal Device into Stomach, Percutaneous Approach
0DH63MZ Insertion of Stimulator Lead into Stomach, Percutaneous Approach
0DH63UZ Insertion of Feeding Device into Stomach, Percutaneous Approach
AHA CC: 4Q, 2013, 117
0DH642Z Insertion of Monitoring Device into Stomach, Percutaneous Endoscopic Approach
0DH643Z Insertion of Infusion Device into Stomach, Percutaneous Endoscopic Approach
0DH64DZ Insertion of Intraluminal Device into Stomach, Percutaneous Endoscopic Approach
0DH64MZ Insertion of Stimulator Lead into Stomach, Percutaneous Endoscopic Approach
0DH64UZ Insertion of Feeding Device into Stomach, Percutaneous Endoscopic Approach
0DH672Z Insertion of Monitoring Device into Stomach, Via Natural or Artificial Opening
0DH673Z Insertion of Infusion Device into Stomach, Via Natural or Artificial Opening
0DH67DZ Insertion of Intraluminal Device into Stomach, Via Natural or Artificial Opening
● **0DH67UZ** Insertion of Feeding Device into Stomach, Via Natural or Artificial Opening
0DH682Z Insertion of Monitoring Device into Stomach, Via Natural or Artificial Opening Endoscopic
0DH683Z Insertion of Infusion Device into Stomach, Via Natural or Artificial Opening Endoscopic
0DH68DZ Insertion of Intraluminal Device into Stomach, Via Natural or Artificial Opening Endoscopic
● **0DH68UZ** Insertion of Feeding Device into Stomach, Via Natural or Artificial Opening Endoscopic
0DH802Z Insertion of Monitoring Device into Small Intestine, Open Approach
0DH803Z Insertion of Infusion Device into Small Intestine, Open Approach
0DH80DZ Insertion of Intraluminal Device into Small Intestine, Open Approach
0DH80UZ Insertion of Feeding Device into Small Intestine, Open Approach
0DH832Z Insertion of Monitoring Device into Small Intestine, Percutaneous Approach
0DH833Z Insertion of Infusion Device into Small Intestine, Percutaneous Approach
0DH83DZ Insertion of Intraluminal Device into Small Intestine, Percutaneous Approach
0DH83UZ Insertion of Feeding Device into Small Intestine, Percutaneous Approach
0DH842Z Insertion of Monitoring Device into Small Intestine, Percutaneous Endoscopic Approach
0DH843Z Insertion of Infusion Device into Small Intestine, Percutaneous Endoscopic Approach
0DH84DZ Insertion of Intraluminal Device into Small Intestine, Percutaneous Endoscopic Approach
0DH84UZ Insertion of Feeding Device into Small Intestine, Percutaneous Endoscopic Approach
0DH872Z Insertion of Monitoring Device into Small Intestine, Via Natural or Artificial Opening
0DH873Z Insertion of Infusion Device into Small Intestine, Via Natural or Artificial Opening
0DH87DZ Insertion of Intraluminal Device into Small Intestine, Via Natural or Artificial Opening
0DH87UZ Insertion of Feeding Device into Small Intestine, Via Natural or Artificial Opening
0DH882Z Insertion of Monitoring Device into Small Intestine, Via Natural or Artificial Opening Endoscopic
0DH883Z Insertion of Infusion Device into Small Intestine, Via Natural or Artificial Opening Endoscopic
0DH88DZ Insertion of Intraluminal Device into Small Intestine, Via Natural or Artificial Opening Endoscopic
0DH88UZ Insertion of Feeding Device into Small Intestine, Via Natural or Artificial Opening Endoscopic
0DH902Z Insertion of Monitoring Device into Duodenum, Open Approach
0DH903Z Insertion of Infusion Device into Duodenum, Open Approach
0DH90DZ Insertion of Intraluminal Device into Duodenum, Open Approach
0DH90UZ Insertion of Feeding Device into Duodenum, Open Approach
0DH932Z Insertion of Monitoring Device into Duodenum, Percutaneous Approach
0DH933Z Insertion of Infusion Device into Duodenum, Percutaneous Approach
0DH93DZ Insertion of Intraluminal Device into Duodenum, Percutaneous Approach

0DH93UZ Insertion of Feeding Device into Duodenum, Percutaneous Approach
0DH942Z Insertion of Monitoring Device into Duodenum, Percutaneous Endoscopic Approach
0DH943Z Insertion of Infusion Device into Duodenum, Percutaneous Endoscopic Approach
0DH94DZ Insertion of Intraluminal Device into Duodenum, Percutaneous Endoscopic Approach
0DH94UZ Insertion of Feeding Device into Duodenum, Percutaneous Endoscopic Approach
0DH972Z Insertion of Monitoring Device into Duodenum, Via Natural or Artificial Opening
0DH973Z Insertion of Infusion Device into Duodenum, Via Natural or Artificial Opening
0DH97DZ Insertion of Intraluminal Device into Duodenum, Via Natural or Artificial Opening
0DH97UZ Insertion of Feeding Device into Duodenum, Via Natural or Artificial Opening
0DH982Z Insertion of Monitoring Device into Duodenum, Via Natural or Artificial Opening Endoscopic
0DH983Z Insertion of Infusion Device into Duodenum, Via Natural or Artificial Opening Endoscopic
0DH98DZ Insertion of Intraluminal Device into Duodenum, Via Natural or Artificial Opening Endoscopic
0DH98UZ Insertion of Feeding Device into Duodenum, Via Natural or Artificial Opening Endoscopic
0DHA02Z Insertion of Monitoring Device into Jejunum, Open Approach
0DHA03Z Insertion of Infusion Device into Jejunum, Open Approach
0DHA0DZ Insertion of Intraluminal Device into Jejunum, Open Approach
0DHA0UZ Insertion of Feeding Device into Jejunum, Open Approach
0DHA32Z Insertion of Monitoring Device into Jejunum, Percutaneous Approach
0DHA33Z Insertion of Infusion Device into Jejunum, Percutaneous Approach
0DHA3DZ Insertion of Intraluminal Device into Jejunum, Percutaneous Approach
0DHA3UZ Insertion of Feeding Device into Jejunum, Percutaneous Approach
0DHA42Z Insertion of Monitoring Device into Jejunum, Percutaneous Endoscopic Approach
0DHA43Z Insertion of Infusion Device into Jejunum, Percutaneous Endoscopic Approach
0DHA4DZ Insertion of Intraluminal Device into Jejunum, Percutaneous Endoscopic Approach
0DHA4UZ Insertion of Feeding Device into Jejunum, Percutaneous Endoscopic Approach
0DHA72Z Insertion of Monitoring Device into Jejunum, Via Natural or Artificial Opening
0DHA73Z Insertion of Infusion Device into Jejunum, Via Natural or Artificial Opening
0DHA7DZ Insertion of Intraluminal Device into Jejunum, Via Natural or Artificial Opening
0DHA7UZ Insertion of Feeding Device into Jejunum, Via Natural or Artificial Opening
0DHA82Z Insertion of Monitoring Device into Jejunum, Via Natural or Artificial Opening Endoscopic
0DHA83Z Insertion of Infusion Device into Jejunum, Via Natural or Artificial Opening Endoscopic
0DHA8DZ Insertion of Intraluminal Device into Jejunum, Via Natural or Artificial Opening Endoscopic
0DHA8UZ Insertion of Feeding Device into Jejunum, Via Natural or Artificial Opening Endoscopic
0DHB02Z Insertion of Monitoring Device into Ileum, Open Approach
0DHB03Z Insertion of Infusion Device into Ileum, Open Approach
0DHB0DZ Insertion of Intraluminal Device into Ileum, Open Approach
0DHB0UZ Insertion of Feeding Device into Ileum, Open Approach
0DHB32Z Insertion of Monitoring Device into Ileum, Percutaneous Approach
0DHB33Z Insertion of Infusion Device into Ileum, Percutaneous Approach
0DHB3DZ Insertion of Intraluminal Device into Ileum, Percutaneous Approach
0DHB3UZ Insertion of Feeding Device into Ileum, Percutaneous Approach
0DHB42Z Insertion of Monitoring Device into Ileum, Percutaneous Endoscopic Approach
0DHB43Z Insertion of Infusion Device into Ileum, Percutaneous Endoscopic Approach
0DHB4DZ Insertion of Intraluminal Device into Ileum, Percutaneous Endoscopic Approach
0DHB4UZ Insertion of Feeding Device into Ileum, Percutaneous Endoscopic Approach
0DHB72Z Insertion of Monitoring Device into Ileum, Via Natural or Artificial Opening
0DHB73Z Insertion of Infusion Device into Ileum, Via Natural or Artificial Opening
0DHB7DZ Insertion of Intraluminal Device into Ileum, Via Natural or Artificial Opening
0DHB7UZ Insertion of Feeding Device into Ileum, Via Natural or Artificial Opening
0DHB82Z Insertion of Monitoring Device into Ileum, Via Natural or Artificial Opening Endoscopic
0DHB83Z Insertion of Infusion Device into Ileum, Via Natural or Artificial Opening Endoscopic
0DHB8DZ Insertion of Intraluminal Device into Ileum, Via Natural or Artificial Opening Endoscopic
0DHB8UZ Insertion of Feeding Device into Ileum, Via Natural or Artificial Opening Endoscopic
0DHE0DZ Insertion of Intraluminal Device into Large Intestine, Open Approach
0DHE3DZ Insertion of Intraluminal Device into Large Intestine, Percutaneous Approach
0DHE4DZ Insertion of Intraluminal Device into Large Intestine, Percutaneous Endoscopic Approach
0DHE7DZ Insertion of Intraluminal Device into Large Intestine, Via Natural or Artificial Opening
0DHE8DZ Insertion of Intraluminal Device into Large Intestine, Via Natural or Artificial Opening Endoscopic
0DHP01Z Insertion of Radioactive Element into Rectum, Open Approach
0DHP0DZ Insertion of Intraluminal Device into Rectum, Open Approach
0DHP31Z Insertion of Radioactive Element into Rectum, Percutaneous Approach
0DHP3DZ Insertion of Intraluminal Device into Rectum, Percutaneous Approach
0DHP41Z Insertion of Radioactive Element into Rectum, Percutaneous Endoscopic Approach
0DHP4DZ Insertion of Intraluminal Device into Rectum, Percutaneous Endoscopic Approach
0DHP71Z Insertion of Radioactive Element into Rectum, Via Natural or Artificial Opening
0DHP7DZ Insertion of Intraluminal Device into Rectum, Via Natural or Artificial Opening
0DHP81Z Insertion of Radioactive Element into Rectum, Via Natural or Artificial Opening Endoscopic
0DHP8DZ Insertion of Intraluminal Device into Rectum, Via Natural or Artificial Opening Endoscopic
0DHQ0DZ Insertion of Intraluminal Device into Anus, Open Approach
0DHQ0LZ Insertion of Artificial Sphincter into Anus, Open Approach
0DHQ3DZ Insertion of Intraluminal Device into Anus, Percutaneous Approach
0DHQ3LZ Insertion of Artificial Sphincter into Anus, Percutaneous Approach
0DHQ4DZ Insertion of Intraluminal Device into Anus, Percutaneous Endoscopic Approach
0DHQ4LZ Insertion of Artificial Sphincter into Anus, Percutaneous Endoscopic Approach
0DHQ7DZ Insertion of Intraluminal Device into Anus, Via Natural or Artificial Opening
0DHQ8DZ Insertion of Intraluminal Device into Anus, Via Natural or Artificial Opening Endoscopic
0DHR0MZ Insertion of Stimulator Lead into Anal Sphincter, Open Approach
0DHR3MZ Insertion of Stimulator Lead into Anal Sphincter, Percutaneous Approach
0DHR4MZ Insertion of Stimulator Lead into Anal Sphincter, Percutaneous Endoscopic Approach

0DJ – Gastrointestinal System, Inspection

Review Coding Guidelines B3.11a, B3.11b and B3.11c

0DJ00ZZ Inspection of Upper Intestinal Tract, Open Approach
0DJ03ZZ Inspection of Upper Intestinal Tract, Percutaneous Approach
0DJ04ZZ Inspection of Upper Intestinal Tract, Percutaneous Endoscopic Approach
0DJ07ZZ Inspection of Upper Intestinal Tract, Via Natural or Artificial Opening
0DJ08ZZ Inspection of Upper Intestinal Tract, Via Natural or Artificial Opening Endoscopic
0DJ0XZZ Inspection of Upper Intestinal Tract, External Approach

J60ZZ Inspection of Stomach, Open Approach
J63ZZ Inspection of Stomach, Percutaneous Approach
J64ZZ Inspection of Stomach, Percutaneous Endoscopic Approach
J67ZZ Inspection of Stomach, Via Natural or Artificial Opening
J68ZZ Inspection of Stomach, Via Natural or Artificial Opening Endoscopic
J6XZZ Inspection of Stomach, External Approach
JD0ZZ Inspection of Lower Intestinal Tract, Open Approach
JD3ZZ Inspection of Lower Intestinal Tract, Percutaneous Approach
0DJD4ZZ Inspection of Lower Intestinal Tract, Percutaneous Endoscopic Approach
0DJD7ZZ Inspection of Lower Intestinal Tract, Via Natural or Artificial Opening
0DJD8ZZ Inspection of Lower Intestinal Tract, Via Natural or Artificial Opening Endoscopic
0DJDXZZ Inspection of Lower Intestinal Tract, External Approach
0DJU0ZZ Inspection of Omentum, Open Approach
0DJU3ZZ Inspection of Omentum, Percutaneous Approach
0DJU4ZZ Inspection of Omentum, Percutaneous Endoscopic Approach
0DJUXZZ Inspection of Omentum, External Approach
0DJV0ZZ Inspection of Mesentery, Open Approach
0DJV3ZZ Inspection of Mesentery, Percutaneous Approach
0DJV4ZZ Inspection of Mesentery, Percutaneous Endoscopic Approach
0DJVXZZ Inspection of Mesentery, External Approach
0DJW0ZZ Inspection of Peritoneum, Open Approach
0DJW3ZZ Inspection of Peritoneum, Percutaneous Approach
0DJW4ZZ Inspection of Peritoneum, Percutaneous Endoscopic Approach
0DJWXZZ Inspection of Peritoneum, External Approach

)L – Gastrointestinal System, Occlusion

L10CZ Occlusion of Upper Esophagus with Extraluminal Device, Open Approach
L10DZ Occlusion of Upper Esophagus with Intraluminal Device, Open Approach
L10ZZ Occlusion of Upper Esophagus, Open Approach
L13CZ Occlusion of Upper Esophagus with Extraluminal Device, Percutaneous Approach
)L13DZ Occlusion of Upper Esophagus with Intraluminal Device, Percutaneous Approach
)L13ZZ Occlusion of Upper Esophagus, Percutaneous Approach
L14CZ Occlusion of Upper Esophagus with Extraluminal Device, Percutaneous Endoscopic Approach
)L14DZ Occlusion of Upper Esophagus with Intraluminal Device, Percutaneous Endoscopic Approach
)L14ZZ Occlusion of Upper Esophagus, Percutaneous Endoscopic Approach
DL17DZ Occlusion of Upper Esophagus with Intraluminal Device, Via Natural or Artificial Opening
DL17ZZ Occlusion of Upper Esophagus, Via Natural or Artificial Opening
DL18DZ Occlusion of Upper Esophagus with Intraluminal Device, Via Natural or Artificial Opening Endoscopic
DL18ZZ Occlusion of Upper Esophagus, Via Natural or Artificial Opening Endoscopic
DL20CZ Occlusion of Middle Esophagus with Extraluminal Device, Open Approach
DL20DZ Occlusion of Middle Esophagus with Intraluminal Device, Open Approach
DL20ZZ Occlusion of Middle Esophagus, Open Approach
DL23CZ Occlusion of Middle Esophagus with Extraluminal Device, Percutaneous Approach
DL23DZ Occlusion of Middle Esophagus with Intraluminal Device, Percutaneous Approach
DL23ZZ Occlusion of Middle Esophagus, Percutaneous Approach
DL24CZ Occlusion of Middle Esophagus with Extraluminal Device, Percutaneous Endoscopic Approach
DL24DZ Occlusion of Middle Esophagus with Intraluminal Device, Percutaneous Endoscopic Approach
DL24ZZ Occlusion of Middle Esophagus, Percutaneous Endoscopic Approach
)DL27DZ Occlusion of Middle Esophagus with Intraluminal Device, Via Natural or Artificial Opening
0DL27ZZ Occlusion of Middle Esophagus, Via Natural or Artificial Opening
0DL28DZ Occlusion of Middle Esophagus with Intraluminal Device, Via Natural or Artificial Opening Endoscopic
0DL28ZZ Occlusion of Middle Esophagus, Via Natural or Artificial Opening Endoscopic
0DL30CZ Occlusion of Lower Esophagus with Extraluminal Device, Open Approach
0DL30DZ Occlusion of Lower Esophagus with Intraluminal Device, Open Approach
0DL30ZZ Occlusion of Lower Esophagus, Open Approach
0DL33CZ Occlusion of Lower Esophagus with Extraluminal Device, Percutaneous Approach
0DL33DZ Occlusion of Lower Esophagus with Intraluminal Device, Percutaneous Approach
0DL33ZZ Occlusion of Lower Esophagus, Percutaneous Approach
0DL34CZ Occlusion of Lower Esophagus with Extraluminal Device, Percutaneous Endoscopic Approach
0DL34DZ Occlusion of Lower Esophagus with Intraluminal Device, Percutaneous Endoscopic Approach
0DL34ZZ Occlusion of Lower Esophagus, Percutaneous Endoscopic Approach
0DL37DZ Occlusion of Lower Esophagus with Intraluminal Device, Via Natural or Artificial Opening
0DL37ZZ Occlusion of Lower Esophagus, Via Natural or Artificial Opening
0DL38DZ Occlusion of Lower Esophagus with Intraluminal Device, Via Natural or Artificial Opening Endoscopic
0DL38ZZ Occlusion of Lower Esophagus, Via Natural or Artificial Opening Endoscopic
0DL40CZ Occlusion of Esophagogastric Junction with Extraluminal Device, Open Approach
0DL40DZ Occlusion of Esophagogastric Junction with Intraluminal Device, Open Approach
0DL40ZZ Occlusion of Esophagogastric Junction, Open Approach
0DL43CZ Occlusion of Esophagogastric Junction with Extraluminal Device, Percutaneous Approach
0DL43DZ Occlusion of Esophagogastric Junction with Intraluminal Device, Percutaneous Approach
0DL43ZZ Occlusion of Esophagogastric Junction, Percutaneous Approach
0DL44CZ Occlusion of Esophagogastric Junction with Extraluminal Device, Percutaneous Endoscopic Approach
0DL44DZ Occlusion of Esophagogastric Junction with Intraluminal Device, Percutaneous Endoscopic Approach
0DL44ZZ Occlusion of Esophagogastric Junction, Percutaneous Endoscopic Approach
0DL47DZ Occlusion of Esophagogastric Junction with Intraluminal Device, Via Natural or Artificial Opening
0DL47ZZ Occlusion of Esophagogastric Junction, Via Natural or Artificial Opening
0DL48DZ Occlusion of Esophagogastric Junction with Intraluminal Device, Via Natural or Artificial Opening Endoscopic
0DL48ZZ Occlusion of Esophagogastric Junction, Via Natural or Artificial Opening Endoscopic
0DL50CZ Occlusion of Esophagus with Extraluminal Device, Open Approach
0DL50DZ Occlusion of Esophagus with Intraluminal Device, Open Approach
0DL50ZZ Occlusion of Esophagus, Open Approach
0DL53CZ Occlusion of Esophagus with Extraluminal Device, Percutaneous Approach
0DL53DZ Occlusion of Esophagus with Intraluminal Device, Percutaneous Approach
0DL53ZZ Occlusion of Esophagus, Percutaneous Approach
0DL54CZ Occlusion of Esophagus with Extraluminal Device, Percutaneous Endoscopic Approach
0DL54DZ Occlusion of Esophagus with Intraluminal Device, Percutaneous Endoscopic Approach
0DL54ZZ Occlusion of Esophagus, Percutaneous Endoscopic Approach
0DL57DZ Occlusion of Esophagus with Intraluminal Device, Via Natural or Artificial Opening
0DL57ZZ Occlusion of Esophagus, Via Natural or Artificial Opening
0DL58DZ Occlusion of Esophagus with Intraluminal Device, Via Natural or Artificial Opening Endoscopic
0DL58ZZ Occlusion of Esophagus, Via Natural or Artificial Opening Endoscopic
0DL60CZ Occlusion of Stomach with Extraluminal Device, Open Approach
0DL60DZ Occlusion of Stomach with Intraluminal Device, Open Approach
0DL60ZZ Occlusion of Stomach, Open Approach
0DL63CZ Occlusion of Stomach with Extraluminal Device, Percutaneous Approach

0DL63DZ Occlusion of Stomach with Intraluminal Device, Percutaneous Approach
0DL63ZZ Occlusion of Stomach, Percutaneous Approach
0DL64CZ Occlusion of Stomach with Extraluminal Device, Percutaneous Endoscopic Approach
0DL64DZ Occlusion of Stomach with Intraluminal Device, Percutaneous Endoscopic Approach
0DL64ZZ Occlusion of Stomach, Percutaneous Endoscopic Approach
0DL67DZ Occlusion of Stomach with Intraluminal Device, Via Natural or Artificial Opening
0DL67ZZ Occlusion of Stomach, Via Natural or Artificial Opening
0DL68DZ Occlusion of Stomach with Intraluminal Device, Via Natural or Artificial Opening Endoscopic
0DL68ZZ Occlusion of Stomach, Via Natural or Artificial Opening Endoscopic
0DL70CZ Occlusion of Stomach, Pylorus with Extraluminal Device, Open Approach
0DL70DZ Occlusion of Stomach, Pylorus with Intraluminal Device, Open Approach
0DL70ZZ Occlusion of Stomach, Pylorus, Open Approach
0DL73CZ Occlusion of Stomach, Pylorus with Extraluminal Device, Percutaneous Approach
0DL73DZ Occlusion of Stomach, Pylorus with Intraluminal Device, Percutaneous Approach
0DL73ZZ Occlusion of Stomach, Pylorus, Percutaneous Approach
0DL74CZ Occlusion of Stomach, Pylorus with Extraluminal Device, Percutaneous Endoscopic Approach
0DL74DZ Occlusion of Stomach, Pylorus with Intraluminal Device, Percutaneous Endoscopic Approach
0DL74ZZ Occlusion of Stomach, Pylorus, Percutaneous Endoscopic Approach
0DL77DZ Occlusion of Stomach, Pylorus with Intraluminal Device, Via Natural or Artificial Opening
0DL77ZZ Occlusion of Stomach, Pylorus, Via Natural or Artificial Opening
0DL78DZ Occlusion of Stomach, Pylorus with Intraluminal Device, Via Natural or Artificial Opening Endoscopic
0DL78ZZ Occlusion of Stomach, Pylorus, Via Natural or Artificial Opening Endoscopic
0DL80CZ Occlusion of Small Intestine with Extraluminal Device, Open Approach
0DL80DZ Occlusion of Small Intestine with Intraluminal Device, Open Approach
0DL80ZZ Occlusion of Small Intestine, Open Approach
0DL83CZ Occlusion of Small Intestine with Extraluminal Device, Percutaneous Approach
0DL83DZ Occlusion of Small Intestine with Intraluminal Device, Percutaneous Approach
0DL83ZZ Occlusion of Small Intestine, Percutaneous Approach
0DL84CZ Occlusion of Small Intestine with Extraluminal Device, Percutaneous Endoscopic Approach
0DL84DZ Occlusion of Small Intestine with Intraluminal Device, Percutaneous Endoscopic Approach
0DL84ZZ Occlusion of Small Intestine, Percutaneous Endoscopic Approach
0DL87DZ Occlusion of Small Intestine with Intraluminal Device, Via Natural or Artificial Opening
0DL87ZZ Occlusion of Small Intestine, Via Natural or Artificial Opening
0DL88DZ Occlusion of Small Intestine with Intraluminal Device, Via Natural or Artificial Opening Endoscopic
0DL88ZZ Occlusion of Small Intestine, Via Natural or Artificial Opening Endoscopic
0DL90CZ Occlusion of Duodenum with Extraluminal Device, Open Approach
0DL90DZ Occlusion of Duodenum with Intraluminal Device, Open Approach
0DL90ZZ Occlusion of Duodenum, Open Approach
0DL93CZ Occlusion of Duodenum with Extraluminal Device, Percutaneous Approach
0DL93DZ Occlusion of Duodenum with Intraluminal Device, Percutaneous Approach
0DL93ZZ Occlusion of Duodenum, Percutaneous Approach
0DL94CZ Occlusion of Duodenum with Extraluminal Device, Percutaneous Endoscopic Approach
0DL94DZ Occlusion of Duodenum with Intraluminal Device, Percutaneous Endoscopic Approach
0DL94ZZ Occlusion of Duodenum, Percutaneous Endoscopic Approach
0DL97DZ Occlusion of Duodenum with Intraluminal Device, Via Natural or Artificial Opening
0DL97ZZ Occlusion of Duodenum, Via Natural or Artificial Opening
0DL98DZ Occlusion of Duodenum with Intraluminal Device, Via Natural or Artificial Opening Endoscopic
0DL98ZZ Occlusion of Duodenum, Via Natural or Artificial Opening Endoscopic
0DLA0CZ Occlusion of Jejunum with Extraluminal Device, Open Approach
0DLA0DZ Occlusion of Jejunum with Intraluminal Device, Open Approach
0DLA0ZZ Occlusion of Jejunum, Open Approach
0DLA3CZ Occlusion of Jejunum with Extraluminal Device, Percutaneous Approach
0DLA3DZ Occlusion of Jejunum with Intraluminal Device, Percutaneous Approach
0DLA3ZZ Occlusion of Jejunum, Percutaneous Approach
0DLA4CZ Occlusion of Jejunum with Extraluminal Device, Percutaneous Endoscopic Approach
0DLA4DZ Occlusion of Jejunum with Intraluminal Device, Percutaneous Endoscopic Approach
0DLA4ZZ Occlusion of Jejunum, Percutaneous Endoscopic Approach
0DLA7DZ Occlusion of Jejunum with Intraluminal Device, Via Natural or Artificial Opening
0DLA7ZZ Occlusion of Jejunum, Via Natural or Artificial Opening
0DLA8DZ Occlusion of Jejunum with Intraluminal Device, Via Natural or Artificial Opening Endoscopic
0DLA8ZZ Occlusion of Jejunum, Via Natural or Artificial Opening Endoscopic
0DLB0CZ Occlusion of Ileum with Extraluminal Device, Open Approach
0DLB0DZ Occlusion of Ileum with Intraluminal Device, Open Approach
0DLB0ZZ Occlusion of Ileum, Open Approach
0DLB3CZ Occlusion of Ileum with Extraluminal Device, Percutaneous Approach
0DLB3DZ Occlusion of Ileum with Intraluminal Device, Percutaneous Approach
0DLB3ZZ Occlusion of Ileum, Percutaneous Approach
0DLB4CZ Occlusion of Ileum with Extraluminal Device, Percutaneous Endoscopic Approach
0DLB4DZ Occlusion of Ileum with Intraluminal Device, Percutaneous Endoscopic Approach
0DLB4ZZ Occlusion of Ileum, Percutaneous Endoscopic Approach
0DLB7DZ Occlusion of Ileum with Intraluminal Device, Via Natural or Artificial Openi
0DLB7ZZ Occlusion of Ileum, Via Natural or Artificial Opening
0DLB8DZ Occlusion of Ileum with Intraluminal Device, Via Natural or Artificial Openi Endoscopic
0DLB8ZZ Occlusion of Ileum, Via Natural or Artificial Opening Endoscopic
0DLC0CZ Occlusion of Ileocecal Valve with Extraluminal Device, Open Approach
0DLC0DZ Occlusion of Ileocecal Valve with Intraluminal Device, Open Approach
0DLC0ZZ Occlusion of Ileocecal Valve, Open Approach
0DLC3CZ Occlusion of Ileocecal Valve with Extraluminal Device, Percutaneous Approach
0DLC3DZ Occlusion of Ileocecal Valve with Intraluminal Device, Percutaneous Approach
0DLC3ZZ Occlusion of Ileocecal Valve, Percutaneous Approach
0DLC4CZ Occlusion of Ileocecal Valve with Extraluminal Device, Percutaneous Endoscopic Approach
0DLC4DZ Occlusion of Ileocecal Valve with Intraluminal Device, Percutaneous Endoscopic Approach
0DLC4ZZ Occlusion of Ileocecal Valve, Percutaneous Endoscopic Approach
0DLC7DZ Occlusion of Ileocecal Valve with Intraluminal Device, Via Natural or Artificial Opening
0DLC7ZZ Occlusion of Ileocecal Valve, Via Natura or Artificial Opening
0DLC8DZ Occlusion of Ileocecal Valve with Intraluminal Device, Via Natural or Artificial Opening Endoscopic
0DLC8ZZ Occlusion of Ileocecal Valve, Via Natura or Artificial Opening Endoscopic
0DLE0CZ Occlusion of Large Intestine with Extraluminal Device, Open Approach
0DLE0DZ Occlusion of Large Intestine with Intraluminal Device, Open Approach
0DLE0ZZ Occlusion of Large Intestine, Open Approach
0DLE3CZ Occlusion of Large Intestine with Extraluminal Device, Percutaneous Approach
0DLE3DZ Occlusion of Large Intestine with Intraluminal Device, Percutaneous Approach
0DLE3ZZ Occlusion of Large Intestine, Percutaneous Approach
0DLE4CZ Occlusion of Large Intestine with Extraluminal Device, Percutaneous Endoscopic Approach
0DLE4DZ Occlusion of Large Intestine with Intraluminal Device, Percutaneous Endoscopic Approach
0DLE4ZZ Occlusion of Large Intestine, Percutaneous Endoscopic Approach

LE7DZ Occlusion of Large Intestine with Intraluminal Device, Via Natural or Artificial Opening
LE7ZZ Occlusion of Large Intestine, Via Natural or Artificial Opening
LE8DZ Occlusion of Large Intestine with Intraluminal Device, Via Natural or Artificial Opening Endoscopic
LE8ZZ Occlusion of Large Intestine, Via Natural or Artificial Opening Endoscopic
LF0CZ Occlusion of Right Large Intestine with Extraluminal Device, Open Approach
LF0DZ Occlusion of Right Large Intestine with Intraluminal Device, Open Approach
LF0ZZ Occlusion of Right Large Intestine, Open Approach
LF3CZ Occlusion of Right Large Intestine with Extraluminal Device, Percutaneous Approach
LF3DZ Occlusion of Right Large Intestine with Intraluminal Device, Percutaneous Approach
LF3ZZ Occlusion of Right Large Intestine, Percutaneous Approach
)LF4CZ Occlusion of Right Large Intestine with Extraluminal Device, Percutaneous Endoscopic Approach
)LF4DZ Occlusion of Right Large Intestine with Intraluminal Device, Percutaneous Endoscopic Approach
)LF4ZZ Occlusion of Right Large Intestine, Percutaneous Endoscopic Approach
)LF7DZ Occlusion of Right Large Intestine with Intraluminal Device, Via Natural or Artificial Opening
)LF7ZZ Occlusion of Right Large Intestine, Via Natural or Artificial Opening
)LF8DZ Occlusion of Right Large Intestine with Intraluminal Device, Via Natural or Artificial Opening Endoscopic
DLF8ZZ Occlusion of Right Large Intestine, Via Natural or Artificial Opening Endoscopic
DLG0CZ Occlusion of Left Large Intestine with Extraluminal Device, Open Approach
DLG0DZ Occlusion of Left Large Intestine with Intraluminal Device, Open Approach
DLG0ZZ Occlusion of Left Large Intestine, Open Approach
DLG3CZ Occlusion of Left Large Intestine with Extraluminal Device, Percutaneous Approach
DLG3DZ Occlusion of Left Large Intestine with Intraluminal Device, Percutaneous Approach
DLG3ZZ Occlusion of Left Large Intestine, Percutaneous Approach
DLG4CZ Occlusion of Left Large Intestine with Extraluminal Device, Percutaneous Endoscopic Approach
DLG4DZ Occlusion of Left Large Intestine with Intraluminal Device, Percutaneous Endoscopic Approach
DLG4ZZ Occlusion of Left Large Intestine, Percutaneous Endoscopic Approach
DLG7DZ Occlusion of Left Large Intestine with Intraluminal Device, Via Natural or Artificial Opening
DLG7ZZ Occlusion of Left Large Intestine, Via Natural or Artificial Opening
DLG8DZ Occlusion of Left Large Intestine with Intraluminal Device, Via Natural or Artificial Opening Endoscopic
)DLG8ZZ Occlusion of Left Large Intestine, Via Natural or Artificial Opening Endoscopic
)DLH0CZ Occlusion of Cecum with Extraluminal Device, Open Approach
0DLH0DZ Occlusion of Cecum with Intraluminal Device, Open Approach
0DLH0ZZ Occlusion of Cecum, Open Approach
0DLH3CZ Occlusion of Cecum with Extraluminal Device, Percutaneous Approach
0DLH3DZ Occlusion of Cecum with Intraluminal Device, Percutaneous Approach
0DLH3ZZ Occlusion of Cecum, Percutaneous Approach
0DLH4CZ Occlusion of Cecum with Extraluminal Device, Percutaneous Endoscopic Approach
0DLH4DZ Occlusion of Cecum with Intraluminal Device, Percutaneous Endoscopic Approach
0DLH4ZZ Occlusion of Cecum, Percutaneous Endoscopic Approach
0DLH7DZ Occlusion of Cecum with Intraluminal Device, Via Natural or Artificial Opening
0DLH7ZZ Occlusion of Cecum, Via Natural or Artificial Opening
0DLH8DZ Occlusion of Cecum with Intraluminal Device, Via Natural or Artificial Opening Endoscopic
0DLH8ZZ Occlusion of Cecum, Via Natural or Artificial Opening Endoscopic
0DLK0CZ Occlusion of Ascending Colon with Extraluminal Device, Open Approach
0DLK0DZ Occlusion of Ascending Colon with Intraluminal Device, Open Approach
0DLK0ZZ Occlusion of Ascending Colon, Open Approach
0DLK3CZ Occlusion of Ascending Colon with Extraluminal Device, Percutaneous Approach
0DLK3DZ Occlusion of Ascending Colon with Intraluminal Device, Percutaneous Approach
0DLK3ZZ Occlusion of Ascending Colon, Percutaneous Approach
0DLK4CZ Occlusion of Ascending Colon with Extraluminal Device, Percutaneous Endoscopic Approach
0DLK4DZ Occlusion of Ascending Colon with Intraluminal Device, Percutaneous Endoscopic Approach
0DLK4ZZ Occlusion of Ascending Colon, Percutaneous Endoscopic Approach
0DLK7DZ Occlusion of Ascending Colon with Intraluminal Device, Via Natural or Artificial Opening
0DLK7ZZ Occlusion of Ascending Colon, Via Natural or Artificial Opening
0DLK8DZ Occlusion of Ascending Colon with Intraluminal Device, Via Natural or Artificial Opening Endoscopic
0DLK8ZZ Occlusion of Ascending Colon, Via Natural or Artificial Opening Endoscopic
0DLL0CZ Occlusion of Transverse Colon with Extraluminal Device, Open Approach
0DLL0DZ Occlusion of Transverse Colon with Intraluminal Device, Open Approach
0DLL0ZZ Occlusion of Transverse Colon, Open Approach
0DLL3CZ Occlusion of Transverse Colon with Extraluminal Device, Percutaneous Approach
0DLL3DZ Occlusion of Transverse Colon with Intraluminal Device, Percutaneous Approach
0DLL3ZZ Occlusion of Transverse Colon, Percutaneous Approach
0DLL4CZ Occlusion of Transverse Colon with Extraluminal Device, Percutaneous Endoscopic Approach
0DLL4DZ Occlusion of Transverse Colon with Intraluminal Device, Percutaneous Endoscopic Approach
0DLL4ZZ Occlusion of Transverse Colon, Percutaneous Endoscopic Approach
0DLL7DZ Occlusion of Transverse Colon with Intraluminal Device, Via Natural or Artificial Opening
0DLL7ZZ Occlusion of Transverse Colon, Via Natural or Artificial Opening
0DLL8DZ Occlusion of Transverse Colon with Intraluminal Device, Via Natural or Artificial Opening Endoscopic
0DLL8ZZ Occlusion of Transverse Colon, Via Natural or Artificial Opening Endoscopic
0DLM0CZ Occlusion of Descending Colon with Extraluminal Device, Open Approach
0DLM0DZ Occlusion of Descending Colon with Intraluminal Device, Open Approach
0DLM0ZZ Occlusion of Descending Colon, Open Approach
0DLM3CZ Occlusion of Descending Colon with Extraluminal Device, Percutaneous Approach
0DLM3DZ Occlusion of Descending Colon with Intraluminal Device, Percutaneous Approach
0DLM3ZZ Occlusion of Descending Colon, Percutaneous Approach
0DLM4CZ Occlusion of Descending Colon with Extraluminal Device, Percutaneous Endoscopic Approach
0DLM4DZ Occlusion of Descending Colon with Intraluminal Device, Percutaneous Endoscopic Approach
0DLM4ZZ Occlusion of Descending Colon, Percutaneous Endoscopic Approach
0DLM7DZ Occlusion of Descending Colon with Intraluminal Device, Via Natural or Artificial Opening
0DLM7ZZ Occlusion of Descending Colon, Via Natural or Artificial Opening
0DLM8DZ Occlusion of Descending Colon with Intraluminal Device, Via Natural or Artificial Opening Endoscopic
0DLM8ZZ Occlusion of Descending Colon, Via Natural or Artificial Opening Endoscopic
0DLN0CZ Occlusion of Sigmoid Colon with Extraluminal Device, Open Approach
0DLN0DZ Occlusion of Sigmoid Colon with Intraluminal Device, Open Approach
0DLN0ZZ Occlusion of Sigmoid Colon, Open Approach
0DLN3CZ Occlusion of Sigmoid Colon with Extraluminal Device, Percutaneous Approach
0DLN3DZ Occlusion of Sigmoid Colon with Intraluminal Device, Percutaneous Approach
0DLN3ZZ Occlusion of Sigmoid Colon, Percutaneous Approach
0DLN4CZ Occlusion of Sigmoid Colon with Extraluminal Device, Percutaneous Endoscopic Approach
0DLN4DZ Occlusion of Sigmoid Colon with Intraluminal Device, Percutaneous Endoscopic Approach
0DLN4ZZ Occlusion of Sigmoid Colon, Percutaneous Endoscopic Approach
0DLN7DZ Occlusion of Sigmoid Colon with Intraluminal Device, Via Natural or Artificial Opening
0DLN7ZZ Occlusion of Sigmoid Colon, Via Natural or Artificial Opening
0DLN8DZ Occlusion of Sigmoid Colon with Intraluminal Device, Via Natural or Artificial Opening Endoscopic

0DLN8ZZ Occlusion of Sigmoid Colon, Via Natural or Artificial Opening Endoscopic
0DLP0CZ Occlusion of Rectum with Extraluminal Device, Open Approach
0DLP0DZ Occlusion of Rectum with Intraluminal Device, Open Approach
0DLP0ZZ Occlusion of Rectum, Open Approach
0DLP3CZ Occlusion of Rectum with Extraluminal Device, Percutaneous Approach
0DLP3DZ Occlusion of Rectum with Intraluminal Device, Percutaneous Approach
0DLP3ZZ Occlusion of Rectum, Percutaneous Approach
0DLP4CZ Occlusion of Rectum with Extraluminal Device, Percutaneous Endoscopic Approach
0DLP4DZ Occlusion of Rectum with Intraluminal Device, Percutaneous Endoscopic Approach
0DLP4ZZ Occlusion of Rectum, Percutaneous Endoscopic Approach
0DLP7DZ Occlusion of Rectum with Intraluminal Device, Via Natural or Artificial Opening
0DLP7ZZ Occlusion of Rectum, Via Natural or Artificial Opening
0DLP8DZ Occlusion of Rectum with Intraluminal Device, Via Natural or Artificial Opening Endoscopic
0DLP8ZZ Occlusion of Rectum, Via Natural or Artificial Opening Endoscopic
0DLQ0CZ Occlusion of Anus with Extraluminal Device, Open Approach
0DLQ0DZ Occlusion of Anus with Intraluminal Device, Open Approach
0DLQ0ZZ Occlusion of Anus, Open Approach
0DLQ3CZ Occlusion of Anus with Extraluminal Device, Percutaneous Approach
0DLQ3DZ Occlusion of Anus with Intraluminal Device, Percutaneous Approach
0DLQ3ZZ Occlusion of Anus, Percutaneous Approach
0DLQ4CZ Occlusion of Anus with Extraluminal Device, Percutaneous Endoscopic Approach
0DLQ4DZ Occlusion of Anus with Intraluminal Device, Percutaneous Endoscopic Approach
0DLQ4ZZ Occlusion of Anus, Percutaneous Endoscopic Approach
0DLQ7DZ Occlusion of Anus with Intraluminal Device, Via Natural or Artificial Openi
0DLQ7ZZ Occlusion of Anus, Via Natural or Artificial Opening
0DLQ8DZ Occlusion of Anus with Intraluminal Device, Via Natural or Artificial Openi Endoscopic
0DLQ8ZZ Occlusion of Anus, Via Natural or Artificial Opening Endoscopic
0DLQXCZ Occlusion of Anus with Extraluminal Device, External Approach
0DLQXDZ Occlusion of Anus with Intraluminal Device, External Approach
0DLQXZZ Occlusion of Anus, External Approach

0DM – Gastrointestinal System, Reattachment

0DM50ZZ Reattachment of Esophagus, Open Approach
0DM54ZZ Reattachment of Esophagus, Percutaneous Endoscopic Approach
0DM60ZZ Reattachment of Stomach, Open Approach
0DM64ZZ Reattachment of Stomach, Percutaneous Endoscopic Approach
0DM80ZZ Reattachment of Small Intestine, Open Approach
0DM84ZZ Reattachment of Small Intestine, Percutaneous Endoscopic Approach
0DM90ZZ Reattachment of Duodenum, Open Approach
0DM94ZZ Reattachment of Duodenum, Percutaneous Endoscopic Approach
0DMA0ZZ Reattachment of Jejunum, Open Approach
0DMA4ZZ Reattachment of Jejunum, Percutaneous Endoscopic Approach
0DMB0ZZ Reattachment of Ileum, Open Approach
0DMB4ZZ Reattachment of Ileum, Percutaneous Endoscopic Approach
0DME0ZZ Reattachment of Large Intestine, Open Approach
0DME4ZZ Reattachment of Large Intestine, Percutaneous Endoscopic Approach
0DMF0ZZ Reattachment of Right Large Intestine, Open Approach
0DMF4ZZ Reattachment of Right Large Intestine, Percutaneous Endoscopic Approach
0DMG0ZZ Reattachment of Left Large Intestine, Open Approach
0DMG4ZZ Reattachment of Left Large Intestine, Percutaneous Endoscopic Approach
0DMH0ZZ Reattachment of Cecum, Open Approach
0DMH4ZZ Reattachment of Cecum, Percutaneous Endoscopic Approach
0DMK0ZZ Reattachment of Ascending Colon, Open Approach
0DMK4ZZ Reattachment of Ascending Colon, Percutaneous Endoscopic Approach
0DML0ZZ Reattachment of Transverse Colon, Ope Approach
0DML4ZZ Reattachment of Transverse Colon, Percutaneous Endoscopic Approach
0DMM0ZZ Reattachment of Descending Colon, Open Approach
0DMM4ZZ Reattachment of Descending Colon, Percutaneous Endoscopic Approach
0DMN0ZZ Reattachment of Sigmoid Colon, Open Approach
0DMN4ZZ Reattachment of Sigmoid Colon, Percutaneous Endoscopic Approach
0DMP0ZZ Reattachment of Rectum, Open Approa
0DMP4ZZ Reattachment of Rectum, Percutaneous Endoscopic Approach

0DN – Gastrointestinal System, Release

Review Coding Guideline B3.13

Review Coding Guideline B3.14

0DN10ZZ Release Upper Esophagus, Open Approach
0DN13ZZ Release Upper Esophagus, Percutaneous Approach
0DN14ZZ Release Upper Esophagus, Percutaneous Endoscopic Approach
0DN17ZZ Release Upper Esophagus, Via Natural or Artificial Opening
0DN18ZZ Release Upper Esophagus, Via Natural or Artificial Opening Endoscopic
0DN20ZZ Release Middle Esophagus, Open Approach
0DN23ZZ Release Middle Esophagus, Percutaneous Approach
0DN24ZZ Release Middle Esophagus, Percutaneous Endoscopic Approach
0DN27ZZ Release Middle Esophagus, Via Natural or Artificial Opening
0DN28ZZ Release Middle Esophagus, Via Natural or Artificial Opening Endoscopic
0DN30ZZ Release Lower Esophagus, Open Approach
0DN33ZZ Release Lower Esophagus, Percutaneous Approach
0DN34ZZ Release Lower Esophagus, Percutaneous Endoscopic Approach
0DN37ZZ Release Lower Esophagus, Via Natural or Artificial Opening
0DN38ZZ Release Lower Esophagus, Via Natural or Artificial Opening Endoscopic
0DN40ZZ Release Esophagogastric Junction, Open Approach
0DN43ZZ Release Esophagogastric Junction, Percutaneous Approach
0DN44ZZ Release Esophagogastric Junction, Percutaneous Endoscopic Approach
0DN47ZZ Release Esophagogastric Junction, Via Natural or Artificial Opening
0DN48ZZ Release Esophagogastric Junction, Via Natural or Artificial Opening Endoscopic
0DN50ZZ Release Esophagus, Open Approach
0DN53ZZ Release Esophagus, Percutaneous Approach
0DN54ZZ Release Esophagus, Percutaneous Endoscopic Approach
0DN57ZZ Release Esophagus, Via Natural or Artificial Opening
0DN58ZZ Release Esophagus, Via Natural or Artificial Opening Endoscopic
0DN60ZZ Release Stomach, Open Approach
0DN63ZZ Release Stomach, Percutaneous Approac
0DN64ZZ Release Stomach, Percutaneous Endoscopic Approach
0DN67ZZ Release Stomach, Via Natural or Artificia Opening
0DN68ZZ Release Stomach, Via Natural or Artificia Opening Endoscopic
0DN70ZZ Release Stomach, Pylorus, Open Approach
0DN73ZZ Release Stomach, Pylorus, Percutaneous Approach
0DN74ZZ Release Stomach, Pylorus, Percutaneous Endoscopic Approach
0DN77ZZ Release Stomach, Pylorus, Via Natural or Artificial Opening
0DN78ZZ Release Stomach, Pylorus, Via Natural or Artificial Opening Endoscopic
0DN80ZZ Release Small Intestine, Open Approach
0DN83ZZ Release Small Intestine, Percutaneous Approach
0DN84ZZ Release Small Intestine, Percutaneous Endoscopic Approach

N87ZZ	Release Small Intestine, Via Natural or Artificial Opening
N88ZZ	Release Small Intestine, Via Natural or Artificial Opening Endoscopic
N90ZZ	Release Duodenum, Open Approach
N93ZZ	Release Duodenum, Percutaneous Approach
N94ZZ	Release Duodenum, Percutaneous Endoscopic Approach
N97ZZ	Release Duodenum, Via Natural or Artificial Opening
N98ZZ	Release Duodenum, Via Natural or Artificial Opening Endoscopic
NA0ZZ	Release Jejunum, Open Approach
NA3ZZ	Release Jejunum, Percutaneous Approach
NA4ZZ	Release Jejunum, Percutaneous Endoscopic Approach
NA7ZZ	Release Jejunum, Via Natural or Artificial Opening
NA8ZZ	Release Jejunum, Via Natural or Artificial Opening Endoscopic
NB0ZZ	Release Ileum, Open Approach
NB3ZZ	Release Ileum, Percutaneous Approach
NB4ZZ	Release Ileum, Percutaneous Endoscopic Approach
NB7ZZ	Release Ileum, Via Natural or Artificial Opening
NB8ZZ	Release Ileum, Via Natural or Artificial Opening Endoscopic
NC0ZZ	Release Ileocecal Valve, Open Approach
NC3ZZ	Release Ileocecal Valve, Percutaneous Approach
NC4ZZ	Release Ileocecal Valve, Percutaneous Endoscopic Approach
NC7ZZ	Release Ileocecal Valve, Via Natural or Artificial Opening
NC8ZZ	Release Ileocecal Valve, Via Natural or Artificial Opening Endoscopic
NE0ZZ	Release Large Intestine, Open Approach
NE3ZZ	Release Large Intestine, Percutaneous Approach
NE4ZZ	Release Large Intestine, Percutaneous Endoscopic Approach
NE7ZZ	Release Large Intestine, Via Natural or Artificial Opening
NE8ZZ	Release Large Intestine, Via Natural or Artificial Opening Endoscopic
NF0ZZ	Release Right Large Intestine, Open Approach
NF3ZZ	Release Right Large Intestine, Percutaneous Approach
NF4ZZ	Release Right Large Intestine, Percutaneous Endoscopic Approach
NF7ZZ	Release Right Large Intestine, Via Natural or Artificial Opening
NF8ZZ	Release Right Large Intestine, Via Natural or Artificial Opening Endoscopic
0DNG0ZZ	Release Left Large Intestine, Open Approach
0DNG3ZZ	Release Left Large Intestine, Percutaneous Approach
0DNG4ZZ	Release Left Large Intestine, Percutaneous Endoscopic Approach
0DNG7ZZ	Release Left Large Intestine, Via Natural or Artificial Opening
0DNG8ZZ	Release Left Large Intestine, Via Natural or Artificial Opening Endoscopic
0DNH0ZZ	Release Cecum, Open Approach
0DNH3ZZ	Release Cecum, Percutaneous Approach
0DNH4ZZ	Release Cecum, Percutaneous Endoscopic Approach
0DNH7ZZ	Release Cecum, Via Natural or Artificial Opening
0DNH8ZZ	Release Cecum, Via Natural or Artificial Opening Endoscopic
0DNJ0ZZ	Release Appendix, Open Approach
0DNJ3ZZ	Release Appendix, Percutaneous Approach
0DNJ4ZZ	Release Appendix, Percutaneous Endoscopic Approach
0DNJ7ZZ	Release Appendix, Via Natural or Artificial Opening
0DNJ8ZZ	Release Appendix, Via Natural or Artificial Opening Endoscopic
0DNK0ZZ	Release Ascending Colon, Open Approach
0DNK3ZZ	Release Ascending Colon, Percutaneous Approach
0DNK4ZZ	Release Ascending Colon, Percutaneous Endoscopic Approach
0DNK7ZZ	Release Ascending Colon, Via Natural or Artificial Opening
0DNK8ZZ	Release Ascending Colon, Via Natural or Artificial Opening Endoscopic
0DNL0ZZ	Release Transverse Colon, Open Approach
0DNL3ZZ	Release Transverse Colon, Percutaneous Approach
0DNL4ZZ	Release Transverse Colon, Percutaneous Endoscopic Approach
0DNL7ZZ	Release Transverse Colon, Via Natural or Artificial Opening
0DNL8ZZ	Release Transverse Colon, Via Natural or Artificial Opening Endoscopic
0DNM0ZZ	Release Descending Colon, Open Approach
0DNM3ZZ	Release Descending Colon, Percutaneous Approach
0DNM4ZZ	Release Descending Colon, Percutaneous Endoscopic Approach
0DNM7ZZ	Release Descending Colon, Via Natural or Artificial Opening
0DNM8ZZ	Release Descending Colon, Via Natural or Artificial Opening Endoscopic
0DNN0ZZ	Release Sigmoid Colon, Open Approach
0DNN3ZZ	Release Sigmoid Colon, Percutaneous Approach
0DNN4ZZ	Release Sigmoid Colon, Percutaneous Endoscopic Approach
0DNN7ZZ	Release Sigmoid Colon, Via Natural or Artificial Opening
0DNN8ZZ	Release Sigmoid Colon, Via Natural or Artificial Opening Endoscopic
0DNP0ZZ	Release Rectum, Open Approach
0DNP3ZZ	Release Rectum, Percutaneous Approach
0DNP4ZZ	Release Rectum, Percutaneous Endoscopic Approach
0DNP7ZZ	Release Rectum, Via Natural or Artificial Opening
0DNP8ZZ	Release Rectum, Via Natural or Artificial Opening Endoscopic
0DNQ0ZZ	Release Anus, Open Approach
0DNQ3ZZ	Release Anus, Percutaneous Approach
0DNQ4ZZ	Release Anus, Percutaneous Endoscopic Approach
0DNQ7ZZ	Release Anus, Via Natural or Artificial Opening
0DNQ8ZZ	Release Anus, Via Natural or Artificial Opening Endoscopic
0DNQXZZ	Release Anus, External Approach
0DNR0ZZ	Release Anal Sphincter, Open Approach
0DNR3ZZ	Release Anal Sphincter, Percutaneous Approach
0DNR4ZZ	Release Anal Sphincter, Percutaneous Endoscopic Approach
0DNS0ZZ	Release Greater Omentum, Open Approach
0DNS3ZZ	Release Greater Omentum, Percutaneous Approach
0DNS4ZZ	Release Greater Omentum, Percutaneous Endoscopic Approach
0DNT0ZZ	Release Lesser Omentum, Open Approach
0DNT3ZZ	Release Lesser Omentum, Percutaneous Approach
0DNT4ZZ	Release Lesser Omentum, Percutaneous Endoscopic Approach
0DNV0ZZ	Release Mesentery, Open Approach
0DNV3ZZ	Release Mesentery, Percutaneous Approach
0DNV4ZZ	Release Mesentery, Percutaneous Endoscopic Approach
0DNW0ZZ	Release Peritoneum, Open Approach
0DNW3ZZ	Release Peritoneum, Percutaneous Approach
0DNW4ZZ	Release Peritoneum, Percutaneous Endoscopic Approach

DP – Gastrointestinal System, Removal

eview Coding Guideline B6.1c

DP000Z	Removal of Drainage Device from Upper Intestinal Tract, Open Approach
DP002Z	Removal of Monitoring Device from Upper Intestinal Tract, Open Approach
DP003Z	Removal of Infusion Device from Upper Intestinal Tract, Open Approach
DP007Z	Removal of Autologous Tissue Substitute from Upper Intestinal Tract, Open Approach
DP00CZ	Removal of Extraluminal Device from Upper Intestinal Tract, Open Approach
DP00DZ	Removal of Intraluminal Device from Upper Intestinal Tract, Open Approach
DP00JZ	Removal of Synthetic Substitute from Upper Intestinal Tract, Open Approach
0DP00KZ	Removal of Nonautologous Tissue Substitute from Upper Intestinal Tract, Open Approach
0DP00UZ	Removal of Feeding Device from Upper Intestinal Tract, Open Approach
0DP030Z	Removal of Drainage Device from Upper Intestinal Tract, Percutaneous Approach
0DP032Z	Removal of Monitoring Device from Upper Intestinal Tract, Percutaneous Approach
0DP033Z	Removal of Infusion Device from Upper Intestinal Tract, Percutaneous Approach
0DP037Z	Removal of Autologous Tissue Substitute from Upper Intestinal Tract, Percutaneous Approach
0DP03CZ	Removal of Extraluminal Device from Upper Intestinal Tract, Percutaneous Approach
0DP03DZ	Removal of Intraluminal Device from Upper Intestinal Tract, Percutaneous Approach
0DP03JZ	Removal of Synthetic Substitute from Upper Intestinal Tract, Percutaneous Approach
0DP03KZ	Removal of Nonautologous Tissue Substitute from Upper Intestinal Tract, Percutaneous Approach
0DP03UZ	Removal of Feeding Device from Upper Intestinal Tract, Percutaneous Approach

0DP040Z Removal of Drainage Device from Upper Intestinal Tract, Percutaneous Endoscopic Approach
0DP042Z Removal of Monitoring Device from Upper Intestinal Tract, Percutaneous Endoscopic Approach
0DP043Z Removal of Infusion Device from Upper Intestinal Tract, Percutaneous Endoscopic Approach
0DP047Z Removal of Autologous Tissue Substitute from Upper Intestinal Tract, Percutaneous Endoscopic Approach
0DP04CZ Removal of Extraluminal Device from Upper Intestinal Tract, Percutaneous Endoscopic Approach
0DP04DZ Removal of Intraluminal Device from Upper Intestinal Tract, Percutaneous Endoscopic Approach
0DP04JZ Removal of Synthetic Substitute from Upper Intestinal Tract, Percutaneous Endoscopic Approach
0DP04KZ Removal of Nonautologous Tissue Substitute from Upper Intestinal Tract, Percutaneous Endoscopic Approach
0DP04UZ Removal of Feeding Device from Upper Intestinal Tract, Percutaneous Endoscopic Approach
0DP070Z Removal of Drainage Device from Upper Intestinal Tract, Via Natural or Artificial Opening
0DP072Z Removal of Monitoring Device from Upper Intestinal Tract, Via Natural or Artificial Opening
0DP073Z Removal of Infusion Device from Upper Intestinal Tract, Via Natural or Artificial Opening
0DP077Z Removal of Autologous Tissue Substitute from Upper Intestinal Tract, Via Natural or Artificial Opening
0DP07CZ Removal of Extraluminal Device from Upper Intestinal Tract, Via Natural or Artificial Opening
0DP07DZ Removal of Intraluminal Device from Upper Intestinal Tract, Via Natural or Artificial Opening
0DP07JZ Removal of Synthetic Substitute from Upper Intestinal Tract, Via Natural or Artificial Opening
0DP07KZ Removal of Nonautologous Tissue Substitute from Upper Intestinal Tract, Via Natural or Artificial Opening
0DP07UZ Removal of Feeding Device from Upper Intestinal Tract, Via Natural or Artificial Opening
0DP080Z Removal of Drainage Device from Upper Intestinal Tract, Via Natural or Artificial Opening Endoscopic
0DP082Z Removal of Monitoring Device from Upper Intestinal Tract, Via Natural or Artificial Opening Endoscopic
0DP083Z Removal of Infusion Device from Upper Intestinal Tract, Via Natural or Artificial Opening Endoscopic
0DP087Z Removal of Autologous Tissue Substitute from Upper Intestinal Tract, Via Natural or Artificial Opening Endoscopic
0DP08CZ Removal of Extraluminal Device from Upper Intestinal Tract, Via Natural or Artificial Opening Endoscopic
0DP08DZ Removal of Intraluminal Device from Upper Intestinal Tract, Via Natural or Artificial Opening Endoscopic
0DP08JZ Removal of Synthetic Substitute from Upper Intestinal Tract, Via Natural or Artificial Opening Endoscopic
0DP08KZ Removal of Nonautologous Tissue Substitute from Upper Intestinal Tract, Via Natural or Artificial Opening Endoscopic
0DP08UZ Removal of Feeding Device from Upper Intestinal Tract, Via Natural or Artificial Opening Endoscopic
0DP0X0Z Removal of Drainage Device from Upper Intestinal Tract, External Approach
0DP0X2Z Removal of Monitoring Device from Upper Intestinal Tract, External Approach
0DP0X3Z Removal of Infusion Device from Upper Intestinal Tract, External Approach
0DP0XDZ Removal of Intraluminal Device from Upper Intestinal Tract, External Approach
0DP0XUZ Removal of Feeding Device from Upper Intestinal Tract, External Approach
0DP501Z Removal of Radioactive Element from Esophagus, Open Approach
0DP502Z Removal of Monitoring Device from Esophagus, Open Approach
0DP503Z Removal of Infusion Device from Esophagus, Open Approach
0DP50UZ Removal of Feeding Device from Esophagus, Open Approach
0DP531Z Removal of Radioactive Element from Esophagus, Percutaneous Approach
0DP532Z Removal of Monitoring Device from Esophagus, Percutaneous Approach
0DP533Z Removal of Infusion Device from Esophagus, Percutaneous Approach
0DP53UZ Removal of Feeding Device from Esophagus, Percutaneous Approach
0DP541Z Removal of Radioactive Element from Esophagus, Percutaneous Endoscopic Approach
0DP542Z Removal of Monitoring Device from Esophagus, Percutaneous Endoscopic Approach
0DP543Z Removal of Infusion Device from Esophagus, Percutaneous Endoscopic Approach
0DP54UZ Removal of Feeding Device from Esophagus, Percutaneous Endoscopic Approach
0DP571Z Removal of Radioactive Element from Esophagus, Via Natural or Artificial Opening
0DP57DZ Removal of Intraluminal Device from Esophagus, Via Natural or Artificial Opening
0DP581Z Removal of Radioactive Element from Esophagus, Via Natural or Artificial Opening Endoscopic
0DP58DZ Removal of Intraluminal Device from Esophagus, Via Natural or Artificial Opening Endoscopic
0DP5X1Z Removal of Radioactive Element from Esophagus, External Approach
0DP5X2Z Removal of Monitoring Device from Esophagus, External Approach
0DP5X3Z Removal of Infusion Device from Esophagus, External Approach
0DP5XDZ Removal of Intraluminal Device from Esophagus, External Approach
0DP5XUZ Removal of Feeding Device from Esophagus, External Approach
0DP600Z Removal of Drainage Device from Stomach, Open Approach
0DP602Z Removal of Monitoring Device from Stomach, Open Approach
0DP603Z Removal of Infusion Device from Stomach, Open Approach
0DP607Z Removal of Autologous Tissue Substitute from Stomach, Open Approach
0DP60CZ Removal of Extraluminal Device from Stomach, Open Approach
0DP60DZ Removal of Intraluminal Device from Stomach, Open Approach
0DP60JZ Removal of Synthetic Substitute from Stomach, Open Approach
0DP60KZ Removal of Nonautologous Tissue Substitute from Stomach, Open Approa
0DP60MZ Removal of Stimulator Lead from Stomach, Open Approach
0DP60UZ Removal of Feeding Device from Stomach, Open Approach
0DP630Z Removal of Drainage Device from Stomach, Percutaneous Approach
0DP632Z Removal of Monitoring Device from Stomach, Percutaneous Approach
0DP633Z Removal of Infusion Device from Stomach, Percutaneous Approach
0DP637Z Removal of Autologous Tissue Substitu from Stomach, Percutaneous Approach
0DP63CZ Removal of Extraluminal Device from Stomach, Percutaneous Approach
0DP63DZ Removal of Intraluminal Device from Stomach, Percutaneous Approach
0DP63JZ Removal of Synthetic Substitute from Stomach, Percutaneous Approach
0DP63KZ Removal of Nonautologous Tissue Substitute from Stomach, Percutaneous Approach
0DP63MZ Removal of Stimulator Lead from Stomach, Percutaneous Approach
0DP63UZ Removal of Feeding Device from Stomach, Percutaneous Approach
0DP640Z Removal of Drainage Device from Stomach, Percutaneous Endoscopic Approach
0DP642Z Removal of Monitoring Device from Stomach, Percutaneous Endoscopic Approach
0DP643Z Removal of Infusion Device from Stomach, Percutaneous Endoscopic Approach
0DP647Z Removal of Autologous Tissue Substitute from Stomach, Percutaneous Endoscopic Approach
0DP64CZ Removal of Extraluminal Device from Stomach, Percutaneous Endoscopic Approach
0DP64DZ Removal of Intraluminal Device from Stomach, Percutaneous Endoscopic Approach
0DP64JZ Removal of Synthetic Substitute from Stomach, Percutaneous Endoscopic Approach
0DP64KZ Removal of Nonautologous Tissue Substitute from Stomach, Percutaneous Endoscopic Approach
0DP64MZ Removal of Stimulator Lead from Stomach, Percutaneous Endoscopic Approach
0DP64UZ Removal of Feeding Device from Stomach, Percutaneous Endoscopic Approach
0DP670Z Removal of Drainage Device from Stomach, Via Natural or Artificial Opening
0DP672Z Removal of Monitoring Device from Stomach, Via Natural or Artificial Opening
0DP673Z Removal of Infusion Device from Stomach, Via Natural or Artificial Opening
0DP677Z Removal of Autologous Tissue Substitute from Stomach, Via Natural or Artificial Opening
0DP67CZ Removal of Extraluminal Device from Stomach, Via Natural or Artificial Opening
0DP67DZ Removal of Intraluminal Device from Stomach, Via Natural or Artificial Opening

•67JZ Removal of Synthetic Substitute from Stomach, Via Natural or Artificial Opening

•67KZ Removal of Nonautologous Tissue Substitute from Stomach, Via Natural or Artificial Opening

•67UZ Removal of Feeding Device from Stomach, Via Natural or Artificial Opening

•P680Z Removal of Drainage Device from Stomach, Via Natural or Artificial Opening Endoscopic

•P682Z Removal of Monitoring Device from Stomach, Via Natural or Artificial Opening Endoscopic

•P683Z Removal of Infusion Device from Stomach, Via Natural or Artificial Opening Endoscopic

•P687Z Removal of Autologous Tissue Substitute from Stomach, Via Natural or Artificial Opening Endoscopic

•P68CZ Removal of Extraluminal Device from Stomach, Via Natural or Artificial Opening Endoscopic

•P68DZ Removal of Intraluminal Device from Stomach, Via Natural or Artificial Opening Endoscopic

•P68JZ Removal of Synthetic Substitute from Stomach, Via Natural or Artificial Opening Endoscopic

•P68KZ Removal of Nonautologous Tissue Substitute from Stomach, Via Natural or Artificial Opening Endoscopic

•P68UZ Removal of Feeding Device from Stomach, Via Natural or Artificial Opening Endoscopic

•P6X0Z Removal of Drainage Device from Stomach, External Approach

•P6X2Z Removal of Monitoring Device from Stomach, External Approach

•P6X3Z Removal of Infusion Device from Stomach, External Approach

•P6XDZ Removal of Intraluminal Device from Stomach, External Approach

•P6XUZ Removal of Feeding Device from Stomach, External Approach

•PD00Z Removal of Drainage Device from Lower Intestinal Tract, Open Approach

•PD02Z Removal of Monitoring Device from Lower Intestinal Tract, Open Approach

•DPD03Z Removal of Infusion Device from Lower Intestinal Tract, Open Approach

•DPD07Z Removal of Autologous Tissue Substitute from Lower Intestinal Tract, Open Approach

•DPD0CZ Removal of Extraluminal Device from Lower Intestinal Tract, Open Approach

•DPD0DZ Removal of Intraluminal Device from Lower Intestinal Tract, Open Approach

•DPD0JZ Removal of Synthetic Substitute from Lower Intestinal Tract, Open Approach

•DPD0KZ Removal of Nonautologous Tissue Substitute from Lower Intestinal Tract, Open Approach

DPD0UZ Removal of Feeding Device from Lower Intestinal Tract, Open Approach

DPD30Z Removal of Drainage Device from Lower Intestinal Tract, Percutaneous Approach

•DPD32Z Removal of Monitoring Device from Lower Intestinal Tract, Percutaneous Approach

•DPD33Z Removal of Infusion Device from Lower Intestinal Tract, Percutaneous Approach

•DPD37Z Removal of Autologous Tissue Substitute from Lower Intestinal Tract, Percutaneous Approach

•DPD3CZ Removal of Extraluminal Device from Lower Intestinal Tract, Percutaneous Approach

0DPD3DZ Removal of Intraluminal Device from Lower Intestinal Tract, Percutaneous Approach

0DPD3JZ Removal of Synthetic Substitute from Lower Intestinal Tract, Percutaneous Approach

0DPD3KZ Removal of Nonautologous Tissue Substitute from Lower Intestinal Tract, Percutaneous Approach

0DPD3UZ Removal of Feeding Device from Lower Intestinal Tract, Percutaneous Approach

0DPD40Z Removal of Drainage Device from Lower Intestinal Tract, Percutaneous Endoscopic Approach

0DPD42Z Removal of Monitoring Device from Lower Intestinal Tract, Percutaneous Endoscopic Approach

0DPD43Z Removal of Infusion Device from Lower Intestinal Tract, Percutaneous Endoscopic Approach

0DPD47Z Removal of Autologous Tissue Substitute from Lower Intestinal Tract, Percutaneous Endoscopic Approach

0DPD4CZ Removal of Extraluminal Device from Lower Intestinal Tract, Percutaneous Endoscopic Approach

0DPD4DZ Removal of Intraluminal Device from Lower Intestinal Tract, Percutaneous Endoscopic Approach

0DPD4JZ Removal of Synthetic Substitute from Lower Intestinal Tract, Percutaneous Endoscopic Approach

0DPD4KZ Removal of Nonautologous Tissue Substitute from Lower Intestinal Tract, Percutaneous Endoscopic Approach

0DPD4UZ Removal of Feeding Device from Lower Intestinal Tract, Percutaneous Endoscopic Approach

0DPD70Z Removal of Drainage Device from Lower Intestinal Tract, Via Natural or Artificial Opening

0DPD72Z Removal of Monitoring Device from Lower Intestinal Tract, Via Natural or Artificial Opening

0DPD73Z Removal of Infusion Device from Lower Intestinal Tract, Via Natural or Artificial Opening

0DPD77Z Removal of Autologous Tissue Substitute from Lower Intestinal Tract, Via Natural or Artificial Opening

0DPD7CZ Removal of Extraluminal Device from Lower Intestinal Tract, Via Natural or Artificial Opening

0DPD7DZ Removal of Intraluminal Device from Lower Intestinal Tract, Via Natural or Artificial Opening

0DPD7JZ Removal of Synthetic Substitute from Lower Intestinal Tract, Via Natural or Artificial Opening

0DPD7KZ Removal of Nonautologous Tissue Substitute from Lower Intestinal Tract, Via Natural or Artificial Opening

0DPD7UZ Removal of Feeding Device from Lower Intestinal Tract, Via Natural or Artificial Opening

0DPD80Z Removal of Drainage Device from Lower Intestinal Tract, Via Natural or Artificial Opening Endoscopic

0DPD82Z Removal of Monitoring Device from Lower Intestinal Tract, Via Natural or Artificial Opening Endoscopic

0DPD83Z Removal of Infusion Device from Lower Intestinal Tract, Via Natural or Artificial Opening Endoscopic

0DPD87Z Removal of Autologous Tissue Substitute from Lower Intestinal Tract, Via Natural or Artificial Opening Endoscopic

0DPD8CZ Removal of Extraluminal Device from Lower Intestinal Tract, Via Natural or Artificial Opening Endoscopic

0DPD8DZ Removal of Intraluminal Device from Lower Intestinal Tract, Via Natural or Artificial Opening Endoscopic

0DPD8JZ Removal of Synthetic Substitute from Lower Intestinal Tract, Via Natural or Artificial Opening Endoscopic

0DPD8KZ Removal of Nonautologous Tissue Substitute from Lower Intestinal Tract, Via Natural or Artificial Opening Endoscopic

0DPD8UZ Removal of Feeding Device from Lower Intestinal Tract, Via Natural or Artificial Opening Endoscopic

0DPDX0Z Removal of Drainage Device from Lower Intestinal Tract, External Approach

0DPDX2Z Removal of Monitoring Device from Lower Intestinal Tract, External Approach

0DPDX3Z Removal of Infusion Device from Lower Intestinal Tract, External Approach

0DPDXDZ Removal of Intraluminal Device from Lower Intestinal Tract, External Approach

0DPDXUZ Removal of Feeding Device from Lower Intestinal Tract, External Approach

0DPP01Z Removal of Radioactive Element from Rectum, Open Approach

0DPP31Z Removal of Radioactive Element from Rectum, Percutaneous Approach

0DPP41Z Removal of Radioactive Element from Rectum, Percutaneous Endoscopic Approach

0DPP71Z Removal of Radioactive Element from Rectum, Via Natural or Artificial Opening

0DPP81Z Removal of Radioactive Element from Rectum, Via Natural or Artificial Opening Endoscopic

0DPPX1Z Removal of Radioactive Element from Rectum, External Approach

0DPQ0LZ Removal of Artificial Sphincter from Anus, Open Approach

0DPQ3LZ Removal of Artificial Sphincter from Anus, Percutaneous Approach

0DPQ4LZ Removal of Artificial Sphincter from Anus, Percutaneous Endoscopic Approach

0DPQ7LZ Removal of Artificial Sphincter from Anus, Via Natural or Artificial Opening

0DPQ8LZ Removal of Artificial Sphincter from Anus, Via Natural or Artificial Opening Endoscopic

0DPR0MZ Removal of Stimulator Lead from Anal Sphincter, Open Approach

0DPR3MZ Removal of Stimulator Lead from Anal Sphincter, Percutaneous Approach

0DPR4MZ Removal of Stimulator Lead from Anal Sphincter, Percutaneous Endoscopic Approach

0DPU00Z Removal of Drainage Device from Omentum, Open Approach

0DPU01Z Removal of Radioactive Element from Omentum, Open Approach

0DPU07Z Removal of Autologous Tissue Substitute from Omentum, Open Approach

0DPU0JZ Removal of Synthetic Substitute from Omentum, Open Approach

0DPU0KZ Removal of Nonautologous Tissue Substitute from Omentum, Open Approach

0DPU30Z Removal of Drainage Device from Omentum, Percutaneous Approach

0DPU31Z Removal of Radioactive Element from Omentum, Percutaneous Approach

0DPU37Z Removal of Autologous Tissue Substitute from Omentum, Percutaneous Approach

0DPU3JZ Removal of Synthetic Substitute from Omentum, Percutaneous Approach

0DPU3KZ Removal of Nonautologous Tissue Substitute from Omentum, Percutaneous Approach
0DPU40Z Removal of Drainage Device from Omentum, Percutaneous Endoscopic Approach
0DPU41Z Removal of Radioactive Element from Omentum, Percutaneous Endoscopic Approach
0DPU47Z Removal of Autologous Tissue Substitute from Omentum, Percutaneous Endoscopic Approach
0DPU4JZ Removal of Synthetic Substitute from Omentum, Percutaneous Endoscopic Approach
0DPU4KZ Removal of Nonautologous Tissue Substitute from Omentum, Percutaneous Endoscopic Approach
0DPV00Z Removal of Drainage Device from Mesentery, Open Approach
0DPV01Z Removal of Radioactive Element from Mesentery, Open Approach
0DPV07Z Removal of Autologous Tissue Substitute from Mesentery, Open Approach
0DPV0JZ Removal of Synthetic Substitute from Mesentery, Open Approach
0DPV0KZ Removal of Nonautologous Tissue Substitute from Mesentery, Open Approach
0DPV30Z Removal of Drainage Device from Mesentery, Percutaneous Approach
0DPV31Z Removal of Radioactive Element from Mesentery, Percutaneous Approach
0DPV37Z Removal of Autologous Tissue Substitute from Mesentery, Percutaneous Approach
0DPV3JZ Removal of Synthetic Substitute from Mesentery, Percutaneous Approach
0DPV3KZ Removal of Nonautologous Tissue Substitute from Mesentery, Percutaneous Approach
0DPV40Z Removal of Drainage Device from Mesentery, Percutaneous Endoscopic Approach
0DPV41Z Removal of Radioactive Element from Mesentery, Percutaneous Endoscopic Approach
0DPV47Z Removal of Autologous Tissue Substitute from Mesentery, Percutaneous Endoscopic Approach
0DPV4JZ Removal of Synthetic Substitute from Mesentery, Percutaneous Endoscopic Approach
0DPV4KZ Removal of Nonautologous Tissue Substitute from Mesentery, Percutaneous Endoscopic Approach
0DPW00Z Removal of Drainage Device from Peritoneum, Open Approach
0DPW01Z Removal of Radioactive Element from Peritoneum, Open Approach
0DPW07Z Removal of Autologous Tissue Substitute from Peritoneum, Open Approach
0DPW0JZ Removal of Synthetic Substitute from Peritoneum, Open Approach
0DPW0KZ Removal of Nonautologous Tissue Substitute from Peritoneum, Open Approach
0DPW30Z Removal of Drainage Device from Peritoneum, Percutaneous Appro
0DPW31Z Removal of Radioactive Element from Peritoneum, Percutaneous Approach
0DPW37Z Removal of Autologous Tissue Substit from Peritoneum, Percutaneous Appro
0DPW3JZ Removal of Synthetic Substitute from Peritoneum, Percutaneous Appro
0DPW3KZ Removal of Nonautologous Tissue Substitute from Peritoneum, Percutane Approach
0DPW40Z Removal of Drainage Device from Peritoneum, Percutaneous Endoscopic Approach
0DPW41Z Removal of Radioactive Element from Peritoneum, Percutaneous Endoscopic Approach
0DPW47Z Removal of Autologous Tissue Substitu from Peritoneum, Percutaneous Endoscopic Approach
0DPW4JZ Removal of Synthetic Substitute from Peritoneum, Percutaneous Endoscopic Approach
0DPW4KZ Removal of Nonautologous Tissue Substitute from Peritoneum, Percutanec Endoscopic Approach

0DQ – Gastrointestinal System, Repair

0DQ10ZZ Repair Upper Esophagus, Open Approach
0DQ13ZZ Repair Upper Esophagus, Percutaneous Approach
0DQ14ZZ Repair Upper Esophagus, Percutaneous Endoscopic Approach
0DQ17ZZ Repair Upper Esophagus, Via Natural or Artificial Opening
0DQ18ZZ Repair Upper Esophagus, Via Natural or Artificial Opening Endoscopic
0DQ20ZZ Repair Middle Esophagus, Open Approach
0DQ23ZZ Repair Middle Esophagus, Percutaneous Approach
0DQ24ZZ Repair Middle Esophagus, Percutaneous Endoscopic Approach
0DQ27ZZ Repair Middle Esophagus, Via Natural or Artificial Opening
0DQ28ZZ Repair Middle Esophagus, Via Natural or Artificial Opening Endoscopic
0DQ30ZZ Repair Lower Esophagus, Open Approach
0DQ33ZZ Repair Lower Esophagus, Percutaneous Approach
0DQ34ZZ Repair Lower Esophagus, Percutaneous Endoscopic Approach
0DQ37ZZ Repair Lower Esophagus, Via Natural or Artificial Opening
0DQ38ZZ Repair Lower Esophagus, Via Natural or Artificial Opening Endoscopic
0DQ40ZZ Repair Esophagogastric Junction, Open Approach
0DQ43ZZ Repair Esophagogastric Junction, Percutaneous Approach
0DQ44ZZ Repair Esophagogastric Junction, Percutaneous Endoscopic Approach
0DQ47ZZ Repair Esophagogastric Junction, Via Natural or Artificial Opening
0DQ48ZZ Repair Esophagogastric Junction, Via Natural or Artificial Opening Endoscopic
0DQ50ZZ Repair Esophagus, Open Approach
0DQ53ZZ Repair Esophagus, Percutaneous Approach
0DQ54ZZ Repair Esophagus, Percutaneous Endoscopic Approach
0DQ57ZZ Repair Esophagus, Via Natural or Artificial Opening
0DQ58ZZ Repair Esophagus, Via Natural or Artificial Opening Endoscopic
0DQ60ZZ Repair Stomach, Open Approach
0DQ63ZZ Repair Stomach, Percutaneous Approach
0DQ64ZZ Repair Stomach, Percutaneous Endoscopic Approach
0DQ67ZZ Repair Stomach, Via Natural or Artificial Opening
0DQ68ZZ Repair Stomach, Via Natural or Artificial Opening Endoscopic
0DQ70ZZ Repair Stomach, Pylorus, Open Approach
0DQ73ZZ Repair Stomach, Pylorus, Percutaneous Approach
0DQ74ZZ Repair Stomach, Pylorus, Percutaneous Endoscopic Approach
0DQ77ZZ Repair Stomach, Pylorus, Via Natural or Artificial Opening
0DQ78ZZ Repair Stomach, Pylorus, Via Natural or Artificial Opening Endoscopic
0DQ80ZZ Repair Small Intestine, Open Approach
+ Ileostomy takedown when performed with code 0WQFXZ2, Repair of abdominal wall, stoma, external approach.
0DQ83ZZ Repair Small Intestine, Percutaneous Approach
0DQ84ZZ Repair Small Intestine, Percutaneous Endoscopic Approach
0DQ87ZZ Repair Small Intestine, Via Natural or Artificial Opening
0DQ88ZZ Repair Small Intestine, Via Natural or Artificial Opening Endoscopic
0DQ90ZZ Repair Duodenum, Open Approach
+ Duodenostomy takedown when performed with code 0WQFXZ2, Repair of abdominal wall, stoma, external approach.
0DQ93ZZ Repair Duodenum, Percutaneous Approach
0DQ94ZZ Repair Duodenum, Percutaneous Endoscopic Approach
0DQ97ZZ Repair Duodenum, Via Natural or Artificial Opening
0DQ98ZZ Repair Duodenum, Via Natural or Artificial Opening Endoscopic
0DQA0ZZ Repair Jejunum, Open Approach
+ Jejunostomy takedown when performec with code 0WQFXZ2, Repair of abdominal wall, stoma, external approach.
0DQA3ZZ Repair Jejunum, Percutaneous Approac
0DQA4ZZ Repair Jejunum, Percutaneous Endoscopic Approach
0DQA7ZZ Repair Jejunum, Via Natural or Artificia Opening
0DQA8ZZ Repair Jejunum, Via Natural or Artificia Opening Endoscopic
0DQB0ZZ Repair Ileum, Open Approach
+ Ileostomy takedown when performed with code 0WQFXZ2, Repair of abdominal wall, stoma, external approach.
0DQB3ZZ Repair Ileum, Percutaneous Approach
0DQB4ZZ Repair Ileum, Percutaneous Endoscopic Approach
0DQB7ZZ Repair Ileum, Via Natural or Artificial Opening
0DQB8ZZ Repair Ileum, Via Natural or Artificial Opening Endoscopic
0DQC0ZZ Repair Ileocecal Valve, Open Approach
0DQC3ZZ Repair Ileocecal Valve, Percutaneous Approach
0DQC4ZZ Repair Ileocecal Valve, Percutaneous Endoscopic Approach
0DQC7ZZ Repair Ileocecal Valve, Via Natural or Artificial Opening
0DQC8ZZ Repair Ileocecal Valve, Via Natural or Artificial Opening Endoscopic
0DQE0ZZ Repair Large Intestine, Open Approach
+ Colostomy takedown when performed with code 0WQFXZ2, Repair of abdominal wall, stoma, external approach.
0DQE3ZZ Repair Large Intestine, Percutaneous Approach
0DQE4ZZ Repair Large Intestine, Percutaneous Endoscopic Approach
0DQE7ZZ Repair Large Intestine, Via Natural or Artificial Opening

E8ZZ Repair Large Intestine, Via Natural or Artificial Opening Endoscopic
F0ZZ Repair Right Large Intestine, Open Approach
+ Colostomy takedown when performed with code 0WQFXZ2, Repair of abdominal wall, stoma, external approach.
QF3ZZ Repair Right Large Intestine, Percutaneous Approach
QF4ZZ Repair Right Large Intestine, Percutaneous Endoscopic Approach
QF7ZZ Repair Right Large Intestine, Via Natural or Artificial Opening
QF8ZZ Repair Right Large Intestine, Via Natural or Artificial Opening Endoscopic
QG0ZZ Repair Left Large Intestine, Open Approach
+ Colostomy takedown when performed with code 0WQFXZ2, Repair of abdominal wall, stoma, external approach.
QG3ZZ Repair Left Large Intestine, Percutaneous Approach
QG4ZZ Repair Left Large Intestine, Percutaneous Endoscopic Approach
QG7ZZ Repair Left Large Intestine, Via Natural or Artificial Opening
QG8ZZ Repair Left Large Intestine, Via Natural or Artificial Opening Endoscopic
QH0ZZ Repair Cecum, Open Approach
+ Cecostomy takedown when performed with code 0WQFXZ2, Repair of abdominal wall, stoma, external approach.
QH3ZZ Repair Cecum, Percutaneous Approach
QH4ZZ Repair Cecum, Percutaneous Endoscopic Approach
QH7ZZ Repair Cecum, Via Natural or Artificial Opening
QH8ZZ Repair Cecum, Via Natural or Artificial Opening Endoscopic
QJ0ZZ Repair Appendix, Open Approach
QJ3ZZ Repair Appendix, Percutaneous Approach
QJ4ZZ Repair Appendix, Percutaneous Endoscopic Approach
QJ7ZZ Repair Appendix, Via Natural or Artificial Opening
QJ8ZZ Repair Appendix, Via Natural or Artificial Opening Endoscopic
QK0ZZ Repair Ascending Colon, Open Approach
+ Colostomy takedown when performed with code 0WQFXZ2, Repair of abdominal wall, stoma, external approach.
0DQK3ZZ Repair Ascending Colon, Percutaneous Approach
0DQK4ZZ Repair Ascending Colon, Percutaneous Endoscopic Approach
0DQK7ZZ Repair Ascending Colon, Via Natural or Artificial Opening
0DQK8ZZ Repair Ascending Colon, Via Natural or Artificial Opening Endoscopic
0DQL0ZZ Repair Transverse Colon, Open Approach
+ Colostomy takedown when performed with code 0WQFXZ2, Repair of abdominal wall, stoma, external approach.
0DQL3ZZ Repair Transverse Colon, Percutaneous Approach
0DQL4ZZ Repair Transverse Colon, Percutaneous Endoscopic Approach
0DQL7ZZ Repair Transverse Colon, Via Natural or Artificial Opening
0DQL8ZZ Repair Transverse Colon, Via Natural or Artificial Opening Endoscopic
0DQM0ZZ Repair Descending Colon, Open Approach
+ Colostomy takedown when performed with code 0WQFXZ2, Repair of abdominal wall, stoma, external approach.
0DQM3ZZ Repair Descending Colon, Percutaneous Approach
0DQM4ZZ Repair Descending Colon, Percutaneous Endoscopic Approach
0DQM7ZZ Repair Descending Colon, Via Natural or Artificial Opening
0DQM8ZZ Repair Descending Colon, Via Natural or Artificial Opening Endoscopic
0DQN0ZZ Repair Sigmoid Colon, Open Approach
+ Colostomy takedown when performed with code 0WQFXZ2, Repair of abdominal wall, stoma, external approach.
0DQN3ZZ Repair Sigmoid Colon, Percutaneous Approach
0DQN4ZZ Repair Sigmoid Colon, Percutaneous Endoscopic Approach
0DQN7ZZ Repair Sigmoid Colon, Via Natural or Artificial Opening
0DQN8ZZ Repair Sigmoid Colon, Via Natural or Artificial Opening Endoscopic
0DQP0ZZ Repair Rectum, Open Approach
0DQP3ZZ Repair Rectum, Percutaneous Approach
0DQP4ZZ Repair Rectum, Percutaneous Endoscopic Approach
0DQP7ZZ Repair Rectum, Via Natural or Artificial Opening
0DQP8ZZ Repair Rectum, Via Natural or Artificial Opening Endoscopic
0DQQ0ZZ Repair Anus, Open Approach
0DQQ3ZZ Repair Anus, Percutaneous Approach
0DQQ4ZZ Repair Anus, Percutaneous Endoscopic Approach
0DQQ7ZZ Repair Anus, Via Natural or Artificial Opening
0DQQ8ZZ Repair Anus, Via Natural or Artificial Opening Endoscopic
0DQQXZZ Repair Anus, External Approach
0DQR0ZZ Repair Anal Sphincter, Open Approach
0DQR3ZZ Repair Anal Sphincter, Percutaneous Approach
0DQR4ZZ Repair Anal Sphincter, Percutaneous Endoscopic Approach
0DQS0ZZ Repair Greater Omentum, Open Approach
0DQS3ZZ Repair Greater Omentum, Percutaneous Approach
0DQS4ZZ Repair Greater Omentum, Percutaneous Endoscopic Approach
0DQT0ZZ Repair Lesser Omentum, Open Approach
0DQT3ZZ Repair Lesser Omentum, Percutaneous Approach
0DQT4ZZ Repair Lesser Omentum, Percutaneous Endoscopic Approach
0DQV0ZZ Repair Mesentery, Open Approach
0DQV3ZZ Repair Mesentery, Percutaneous Approach
0DQV4ZZ Repair Mesentery, Percutaneous Endoscopic Approach
0DQW0ZZ Repair Peritoneum, Open Approach
0DQW3ZZ Repair Peritoneum, Percutaneous Approach
0DQW4ZZ Repair Peritoneum, Percutaneous Endoscopic Approach

DR – *Gastrointestinal System, Replacement*

DR507Z Replacement of Esophagus with Autologous Tissue Substitute, Open Approach
DR50JZ Replacement of Esophagus with Synthetic Substitute, Open Approach
DR50KZ Replacement of Esophagus with Nonautologous Tissue Substitute, Open Approach
DR547Z Replacement of Esophagus with Autologous Tissue Substitute, Percutaneous Endoscopic Approach
DR54JZ Replacement of Esophagus with Synthetic Substitute, Percutaneous Endoscopic Approach
DR54KZ Replacement of Esophagus with Nonautologous Tissue Substitute, Percutaneous Endoscopic Approach
DR577Z Replacement of Esophagus with Autologous Tissue Substitute, Via Natural or Artificial Opening
DR57JZ Replacement of Esophagus with Synthetic Substitute, Via Natural or Artificial Opening
DR57KZ Replacement of Esophagus with Nonautologous Tissue Substitute, Via Natural or Artificial Opening
0DR587Z Replacement of Esophagus with Autologous Tissue Substitute, Via Natural or Artificial Opening Endoscopic
0DR58JZ Replacement of Esophagus with Synthetic Substitute, Via Natural or Artificial Opening Endoscopic
0DR58KZ Replacement of Esophagus with Nonautologous Tissue Substitute, Via Natural or Artificial Opening Endoscopic
0DRR07Z Replacement of Anal Sphincter with Autologous Tissue Substitute, Open Approach
0DRR0JZ Replacement of Anal Sphincter with Synthetic Substitute, Open Approach
0DRR0KZ Replacement of Anal Sphincter with Nonautologous Tissue Substitute, Open Approach
0DRR47Z Replacement of Anal Sphincter with Autologous Tissue Substitute, Percutaneous Endoscopic Approach
0DRR4JZ Replacement of Anal Sphincter with Synthetic Substitute, Percutaneous Endoscopic Approach
0DRR4KZ Replacement of Anal Sphincter with Nonautologous Tissue Substitute, Percutaneous Endoscopic Approach
0DRS07Z Replacement of Greater Omentum with Autologous Tissue Substitute, Open Approach
0DRS0JZ Replacement of Greater Omentum with Synthetic Substitute, Open Approach
0DRS0KZ Replacement of Greater Omentum with Nonautologous Tissue Substitute, Open Approach
0DRS47Z Replacement of Greater Omentum with Autologous Tissue Substitute, Percutaneous Endoscopic Approach
0DRS4JZ Replacement of Greater Omentum with Synthetic Substitute, Percutaneous Endoscopic Approach
0DRS4KZ Replacement of Greater Omentum with Nonautologous Tissue Substitute, Percutaneous Endoscopic Approach
0DRT07Z Replacement of Lesser Omentum with Autologous Tissue Substitute, Open Approach
0DRT0JZ Replacement of Lesser Omentum with Synthetic Substitute, Open Approach

0DRT0KZ Replacement of Lesser Omentum with Nonautologous Tissue Substitute, Open Approach
0DRT47Z Replacement of Lesser Omentum with Autologous Tissue Substitute, Percutaneous Endoscopic Approach
0DRT4JZ Replacement of Lesser Omentum with Synthetic Substitute, Percutaneous Endoscopic Approach
0DRT4KZ Replacement of Lesser Omentum with Nonautologous Tissue Substitute, Percutaneous Endoscopic Approach
0DRV07Z Replacement of Mesentery with Autologous Tissue Substitute, Open Approach
0DRV0JZ Replacement of Mesentery with Synthetic Substitute, Open Approach
0DRV0KZ Replacement of Mesentery with Nonautologous Tissue Substitute, Open Approach
0DRV47Z Replacement of Mesentery with Autologous Tissue Substitute, Percutaneous Endoscopic Approach
0DRV4JZ Replacement of Mesentery with Synthetic Substitute, Percutaneous Endoscopic Approach
0DRV4KZ Replacement of Mesentery with Nonautologous Tissue Substitute, Percutaneous Endoscopic Approach
0DRW07Z Replacement of Peritoneum with Autologous Tissue Substitute, Open Approach
0DRW0JZ Replacement of Peritoneum with Synthetic Substitute, Open Approach
0DRW0KZ Replacement of Peritoneum with Nonautologous Tissue Substitute, Op[en] Approach
0DRW47Z Replacement of Peritoneum with Autologous Tissue Substitute, Percutaneous Endoscopic Approach
0DRW4JZ Replacement of Peritoneum with Synthetic Substitute, Percutaneous Endoscopic Approach
0DRW4KZ Replacement of Peritoneum with Nonautologous Tissue Substitute, Percutaneous Endoscopic Approach

0DS – Gastrointestinal System, Reposition

0DS50ZZ Reposition Esophagus, Open Approach
0DS54ZZ Reposition Esophagus, Percutaneous Endoscopic Approach
0DS57ZZ Reposition Esophagus, Via Natural or Artificial Opening
0DS58ZZ Reposition Esophagus, Via Natural or Artificial Opening Endoscopic
0DS5XZZ Reposition Esophagus, External Approach
0DS60ZZ Reposition Stomach, Open Approach
0DS64ZZ Reposition Stomach, Percutaneous Endoscopic Approach
0DS67ZZ Reposition Stomach, Via Natural or Artificial Opening
0DS68ZZ Reposition Stomach, Via Natural or Artificial Opening Endoscopic
● 0DS6XZZ Reposition Stomach, External Approach
0DS90ZZ Reposition Duodenum, Open Approach
0DS94ZZ Reposition Duodenum, Percutaneous Endoscopic Approach
0DS97ZZ Reposition Duodenum, Via Natural or Artificial Opening
0DS98ZZ Reposition Duodenum, Via Natural or Artificial Opening Endoscopic
0DS9XZZ Reposition Duodenum, External Approach
0DSA0ZZ Reposition Jejunum, Open Approach
0DSA4ZZ Reposition Jejunum, Percutaneous Endoscopic Approach
0DSA7ZZ Reposition Jejunum, Via Natural or Artificial Opening
0DSA8ZZ Reposition Jejunum, Via Natural or Artificial Opening Endoscopic
0DSAXZZ Reposition Jejunum, External Approach
0DSB0ZZ Reposition Ileum, Open Approach
0DSB4ZZ Reposition Ileum, Percutaneous Endoscopic Approach
0DSB7ZZ Reposition Ileum, Via Natural or Artificial Opening
0DSB8ZZ Reposition Ileum, Via Natural or Artificial Opening Endoscopic
0DSBXZZ Reposition Ileum, External Approach
0DSH0ZZ Reposition Cecum, Open Approach
0DSH4ZZ Reposition Cecum, Percutaneous Endoscopic Approach
0DSH7ZZ Reposition Cecum, Via Natural or Artificial Opening
0DSH8ZZ Reposition Cecum, Via Natural or Artificial Opening Endoscopic
0DSHXZZ Reposition Cecum, External Approach
0DSK0ZZ Reposition Ascending Colon, Open Approach
0DSK4ZZ Reposition Ascending Colon, Percutaneous Endoscopic Approach
0DSK7ZZ Reposition Ascending Colon, Via Natural or Artificial Opening
0DSK8ZZ Reposition Ascending Colon, Via Natural or Artificial Opening Endoscopic
0DSKXZZ Reposition Ascending Colon, External Approach
0DSL0ZZ Reposition Transverse Colon, Open Approach
0DSL4ZZ Reposition Transverse Colon, Percutaneous Endoscopic Approach
0DSL7ZZ Reposition Transverse Colon, Via Natural or Artificial Opening
0DSL8ZZ Reposition Transverse Colon, Via Natural or Artificial Opening Endoscopic
0DSLXZZ Reposition Transverse Colon, External Approach
0DSM0ZZ Reposition Descending Colon, Open Approach
0DSM4ZZ Reposition Descending Colon, Percutaneous Endoscopic Approach
0DSM7ZZ Reposition Descending Colon, Via Natural or Artificial Opening
0DSM8ZZ Reposition Descending Colon, Via Natural or Artificial Opening Endoscop[ic]
0DSMXZZ Reposition Descending Colon, Externa[l] Approach
0DSN0ZZ Reposition Sigmoid Colon, Open Approach
0DSN4ZZ Reposition Sigmoid Colon, Percutaneo[us] Endoscopic Approach
0DSN7ZZ Reposition Sigmoid Colon, Via Natural [or] Artificial Opening
0DSN8ZZ Reposition Sigmoid Colon, Via Natural [or] Artificial Opening Endoscopic
0DSNXZZ Reposition Sigmoid Colon, External Approach
0DSP0ZZ Reposition Rectum, Open Approach
0DSP4ZZ Reposition Rectum, Percutaneous Endoscopic Approach
0DSP7ZZ Reposition Rectum, Via Natural or Artificial Opening
0DSP8ZZ Reposition Rectum, Via Natural or Artificial Opening Endoscopic
0DSPXZZ Reposition Rectum, External Approach
0DSQ0ZZ Reposition Anus, Open Approach
0DSQ4ZZ Reposition Anus, Percutaneous Endoscopic Approach
0DSQ7ZZ Reposition Anus, Via Natural or Artifici[al] Opening
0DSQ8ZZ Reposition Anus, Via Natural or Artifici[al] Opening Endoscopic
0DSQXZZ Reposition Anus, External Approach

0DT – Gastrointestinal System, Resection

Review Coding Guideline B3.8

0DT10ZZ Resection of Upper Esophagus, Open Approach
0DT14ZZ Resection of Upper Esophagus, Percutaneous Endoscopic Approach
0DT17ZZ Resection of Upper Esophagus, Via Natural or Artificial Opening
0DT18ZZ Resection of Upper Esophagus, Via Natural or Artificial Opening Endoscopic
0DT20ZZ Resection of Middle Esophagus, Open Approach
0DT24ZZ Resection of Middle Esophagus, Percutaneous Endoscopic Approach
0DT27ZZ Resection of Middle Esophagus, Via Natural or Artificial Opening
0DT28ZZ Resection of Middle Esophagus, Via Natural or Artificial Opening Endoscopic
0DT30ZZ Resection of Lower Esophagus, Open Approach
0DT34ZZ Resection of Lower Esophagus, Percutaneous Endoscopic Approach
0DT37ZZ Resection of Lower Esophagus, Via Natural or Artificial Opening
0DT38ZZ Resection of Lower Esophagus, Via Natural or Artificial Opening Endoscopic
0DT40ZZ Resection of Esophagogastric Junction, Open Approach
0DT44ZZ Resection of Esophagogastric Junction, Percutaneous Endoscopic Approach
0DT47ZZ Resection of Esophagogastric Junction, Via Natural or Artificial Opening
0DT48ZZ Resection of Esophagogastric Junction, Via Natural or Artificial Opening Endoscopic
0DT50ZZ Resection of Esophagus, Open Approach
0DT54ZZ Resection of Esophagus, Percutaneous Endoscopic Approach
0DT57ZZ Resection of Esophagus, Via Natural or Artificial Opening
0DT58ZZ Resection of Esophagus, Via Natural or Artificial Opening Endoscopic
0DT60ZZ Resection of Stomach, Open Approach

64ZZ Resection of Stomach, Percutaneous Endoscopic Approach
67ZZ Resection of Stomach, Via Natural or Artificial Opening
68ZZ Resection of Stomach, Via Natural or Artificial Opening Endoscopic
70ZZ Resection of Stomach, Pylorus, Open Approach
74ZZ Resection of Stomach, Pylorus, Percutaneous Endoscopic Approach
77ZZ Resection of Stomach, Pylorus, Via Natural or Artificial Opening
78ZZ Resection of Stomach, Pylorus, Via Natural or Artificial Opening Endoscopic
T80ZZ Resection of Small Intestine, Open Approach
T84ZZ Resection of Small Intestine, Percutaneous Endoscopic Approach
T87ZZ Resection of Small Intestine, Via Natural or Artificial Opening
T88ZZ Resection of Small Intestine, Via Natural or Artificial Opening Endoscopic
T90ZZ Resection of Duodenum, Open Approach
+ Pancreaticododenectomy when reported with Resection of the pancreas. *See table 0FT to construct the Resection code.*
T94ZZ Resection of Duodenum, Percutaneous Endoscopic Approach
T97ZZ Resection of Duodenum, Via Natural or Artificial Opening
T98ZZ Resection of Duodenum, Via Natural or Artificial Opening Endoscopic
TA0ZZ Resection of Jejunum, Open Approach
TA4ZZ Resection of Jejunum, Percutaneous Endoscopic Approach
TA7ZZ Resection of Jejunum, Via Natural or Artificial Opening
TA8ZZ Resection of Jejunum, Via Natural or Artificial Opening Endoscopic
TB0ZZ Resection of Ileum, Open Approach
TB4ZZ Resection of Ileum, Percutaneous Endoscopic Approach
TB7ZZ Resection of Ileum, Via Natural or Artificial Opening
TB8ZZ Resection of Ileum, Via Natural or Artificial Opening Endoscopic
TC0ZZ Resection of Ileocecal Valve, Open Approach
TC4ZZ Resection of Ileocecal Valve, Percutaneous Endoscopic Approach
0DTC7ZZ Resection of Ileocecal Valve, Via Natural or Artificial Opening
0DTC8ZZ Resection of Ileocecal Valve, Via Natural or Artificial Opening Endoscopic
0DTE0ZZ Resection of Large Intestine, Open Approach
0DTE4ZZ Resection of Large Intestine, Percutaneous Endoscopic Approach
0DTE7ZZ Resection of Large Intestine, Via Natural or Artificial Opening
0DTE8ZZ Resection of Large Intestine, Via Natural or Artificial Opening Endoscopic
0DTF0ZZ Resection of Right Large Intestine, Open Approach
0DTF4ZZ Resection of Right Large Intestine, Percutaneous Endoscopic Approach
0DTF7ZZ Resection of Right Large Intestine, Via Natural or Artificial Opening
0DTF8ZZ Resection of Right Large Intestine, Via Natural or Artificial Opening Endoscopic
0DTG0ZZ Resection of Left Large Intestine, Open Approach
0DTG4ZZ Resection of Left Large Intestine, Percutaneous Endoscopic Approach
0DTG7ZZ Resection of Left Large Intestine, Via Natural or Artificial Opening
0DTG8ZZ Resection of Left Large Intestine, Via Natural or Artificial Opening Endoscopic
0DTH0ZZ Resection of Cecum, Open Approach
0DTH4ZZ Resection of Cecum, Percutaneous Endoscopic Approach
0DTH7ZZ Resection of Cecum, Via Natural or Artificial Opening
0DTH8ZZ Resection of Cecum, Via Natural or Artificial Opening Endoscopic
0DTJ0ZZ Resection of Appendix, Open Approach
0DTJ4ZZ Resection of Appendix, Percutaneous Endoscopic Approach
0DTJ7ZZ Resection of Appendix, Via Natural or Artificial Opening
0DTJ8ZZ Resection of Appendix, Via Natural or Artificial Opening Endoscopic
0DTK0ZZ Resection of Ascending Colon, Open Approach
0DTK4ZZ Resection of Ascending Colon, Percutaneous Endoscopic Approach
0DTK7ZZ Resection of Ascending Colon, Via Natural or Artificial Opening
0DTK8ZZ Resection of Ascending Colon, Via Natural or Artificial Opening Endoscopic
0DTL0ZZ Resection of Transverse Colon, Open Approach
0DTL4ZZ Resection of Transverse Colon, Percutaneous Endoscopic Approach
0DTL7ZZ Resection of Transverse Colon, Via Natural or Artificial Opening
0DTL8ZZ Resection of Transverse Colon, Via Natural or Artificial Opening Endoscopic
0DTM0ZZ Resection of Descending Colon, Open Approach
0DTM4ZZ Resection of Descending Colon, Percutaneous Endoscopic Approach
0DTM7ZZ Resection of Descending Colon, Via Natural or Artificial Opening
0DTM8ZZ Resection of Descending Colon, Via Natural or Artificial Opening Endoscopic
0DTN0ZZ Resection of Sigmoid Colon, Open Approach
0DTN4ZZ Resection of Sigmoid Colon, Percutaneous Endoscopic Approach
0DTN7ZZ Resection of Sigmoid Colon, Via Natural or Artificial Opening
0DTN8ZZ Resection of Sigmoid Colon, Via Natural or Artificial Opening Endoscopic
0DTP0ZZ Resection of Rectum, Open Approach
0DTP4ZZ Resection of Rectum, Percutaneous Endoscopic Approach
0DTP7ZZ Resection of Rectum, Via Natural or Artificial Opening
0DTP8ZZ Resection of Rectum, Via Natural or Artificial Opening Endoscopic
0DTQ0ZZ Resection of Anus, Open Approach
0DTQ4ZZ Resection of Anus, Percutaneous Endoscopic Approach
0DTQ7ZZ Resection of Anus, Via Natural or Artificial Opening
0DTQ8ZZ Resection of Anus, Via Natural or Artificial Opening Endoscopic
0DTR0ZZ Resection of Anal Sphincter, Open Approach
0DTR4ZZ Resection of Anal Sphincter, Percutaneous Endoscopic Approach
0DTS0ZZ Resection of Greater Omentum, Open Approach
0DTS4ZZ Resection of Greater Omentum, Percutaneous Endoscopic Approach
0DTT0ZZ Resection of Lesser Omentum, Open Approach
0DTT4ZZ Resection of Lesser Omentum, Percutaneous Endoscopic Approach

DU – Gastrointestinal System, Supplement

U107Z Supplement Upper Esophagus with Autologous Tissue Substitute, Open Approach
U10JZ Supplement Upper Esophagus with Synthetic Substitute, Open Approach
U10KZ Supplement Upper Esophagus with Nonautologous Tissue Substitute, Open Approach
U147Z Supplement Upper Esophagus with Autologous Tissue Substitute, Percutaneous Endoscopic Approach
DU14JZ Supplement Upper Esophagus with Synthetic Substitute, Percutaneous Endoscopic Approach
DU14KZ Supplement Upper Esophagus with Nonautologous Tissue Substitute, Percutaneous Endoscopic Approach
DU177Z Supplement Upper Esophagus with Autologous Tissue Substitute, Via Natural or Artificial Opening
DU17JZ Supplement Upper Esophagus with Synthetic Substitute, Via Natural or Artificial Opening
0DU17KZ Supplement Upper Esophagus with Nonautologous Tissue Substitute, Via Natural or Artificial Opening
0DU187Z Supplement Upper Esophagus with Autologous Tissue Substitute, Via Natural or Artificial Opening Endoscopic
0DU18JZ Supplement Upper Esophagus with Synthetic Substitute, Via Natural or Artificial Opening Endoscopic
0DU18KZ Supplement Upper Esophagus with Nonautologous Tissue Substitute, Via Natural or Artificial Opening Endoscopic
0DU207Z Supplement Middle Esophagus with Autologous Tissue Substitute, Open Approach
0DU20JZ Supplement Middle Esophagus with Synthetic Substitute, Open Approach
0DU20KZ Supplement Middle Esophagus with Nonautologous Tissue Substitute, Open Approach
0DU247Z Supplement Middle Esophagus with Autologous Tissue Substitute, Percutaneous Endoscopic Approach
0DU24JZ Supplement Middle Esophagus with Synthetic Substitute, Percutaneous Endoscopic Approach
0DU24KZ Supplement Middle Esophagus with Nonautologous Tissue Substitute, Percutaneous Endoscopic Approach
0DU277Z Supplement Middle Esophagus with Autologous Tissue Substitute, Via Natural or Artificial Opening
0DU27JZ Supplement Middle Esophagus with Synthetic Substitute, Via Natural or Artificial Opening
0DU27KZ Supplement Middle Esophagus with Nonautologous Tissue Substitute, Via Natural or Artificial Opening
0DU287Z Supplement Middle Esophagus with Autologous Tissue Substitute, Via Natural or Artificial Opening Endoscopic
0DU28JZ Supplement Middle Esophagus with Synthetic Substitute, Via Natural or Artificial Opening Endoscopic
0DU28KZ Supplement Middle Esophagus with Nonautologous Tissue Substitute, Via Natural or Artificial Opening Endoscopic

0DU307Z Supplement Lower Esophagus with Autologous Tissue Substitute, Open Approach

0DU30JZ Supplement Lower Esophagus with Synthetic Substitute, Open Approach

0DU30KZ Supplement Lower Esophagus with Nonautologous Tissue Substitute, Open Approach

0DU347Z Supplement Lower Esophagus with Autologous Tissue Substitute, Percutaneous Endoscopic Approach

0DU34JZ Supplement Lower Esophagus with Synthetic Substitute, Percutaneous Endoscopic Approach

0DU34KZ Supplement Lower Esophagus with Nonautologous Tissue Substitute, Percutaneous Endoscopic Approach

0DU377Z Supplement Lower Esophagus with Autologous Tissue Substitute, Via Natural or Artificial Opening

0DU37JZ Supplement Lower Esophagus with Synthetic Substitute, Via Natural or Artificial Opening

0DU37KZ Supplement Lower Esophagus with Nonautologous Tissue Substitute, Via Natural or Artificial Opening

0DU387Z Supplement Lower Esophagus with Autologous Tissue Substitute, Via Natural or Artificial Opening Endoscopic

0DU38JZ Supplement Lower Esophagus with Synthetic Substitute, Via Natural or Artificial Opening Endoscopic

0DU38KZ Supplement Lower Esophagus with Nonautologous Tissue Substitute, Via Natural or Artificial Opening Endoscopic

0DU407Z Supplement Esophagogastric Junction with Autologous Tissue Substitute, Open Approach

0DU40JZ Supplement Esophagogastric Junction with Synthetic Substitute, Open Approach

0DU40KZ Supplement Esophagogastric Junction with Nonautologous Tissue Substitute, Open Approach

0DU447Z Supplement Esophagogastric Junction with Autologous Tissue Substitute, Percutaneous Endoscopic Approach

0DU44JZ Supplement Esophagogastric Junction with Synthetic Substitute, Percutaneous Endoscopic Approach

0DU44KZ Supplement Esophagogastric Junction with Nonautologous Tissue Substitute, Percutaneous Endoscopic Approach

0DU477Z Supplement Esophagogastric Junction with Autologous Tissue Substitute, Via Natural or Artificial Opening

0DU47JZ Supplement Esophagogastric Junction with Synthetic Substitute, Via Natural or Artificial Opening

0DU47KZ Supplement Esophagogastric Junction with Nonautologous Tissue Substitute, Via Natural or Artificial Opening

0DU487Z Supplement Esophagogastric Junction with Autologous Tissue Substitute, Via Natural or Artificial Opening Endoscopic

0DU48JZ Supplement Esophagogastric Junction with Synthetic Substitute, Via Natural or Artificial Opening Endoscopic

0DU48KZ Supplement Esophagogastric Junction with Nonautologous Tissue Substitute, Via Natural or Artificial Opening Endoscopic

0DU507Z Supplement Esophagus with Autologous Tissue Substitute, Open Approach

0DU50JZ Supplement Esophagus with Synthetic Substitute, Open Approach

0DU50KZ Supplement Esophagus with Nonautologous Tissue Substitute, Open Approach

0DU547Z Supplement Esophagus with Autologous Tissue Substitute, Percutaneous Endoscopic Approach

0DU54JZ Supplement Esophagus with Synthetic Substitute, Percutaneous Endoscopic Approach

0DU54KZ Supplement Esophagus with Nonautologous Tissue Substitute, Percutaneous Endoscopic Approach

0DU577Z Supplement Esophagus with Autologous Tissue Substitute, Via Natural or Artificial Opening

0DU57JZ Supplement Esophagus with Synthetic Substitute, Via Natural or Artificial Opening

0DU57KZ Supplement Esophagus with Nonautologous Tissue Substitute, Via Natural or Artificial Opening

0DU587Z Supplement Esophagus with Autologous Tissue Substitute, Via Natural or Artificial Opening Endoscopic

0DU58JZ Supplement Esophagus with Synthetic Substitute, Via Natural or Artificial Opening Endoscopic

0DU58KZ Supplement Esophagus with Nonautologous Tissue Substitute, Via Natural or Artificial Opening Endoscopic

0DU607Z Supplement Stomach with Autologous Tissue Substitute, Open Approach

0DU60JZ Supplement Stomach with Synthetic Substitute, Open Approach

0DU60KZ Supplement Stomach with Nonautologous Tissue Substitute, Open Approach

0DU647Z Supplement Stomach with Autologous Tissue Substitute, Percutaneous Endoscopic Approach

0DU64JZ Supplement Stomach with Synthetic Substitute, Percutaneous Endoscopic Approach

0DU64KZ Supplement Stomach with Nonautologous Tissue Substitute, Percutaneous Endoscopic Approach

0DU677Z Supplement Stomach with Autologous Tissue Substitute, Via Natural or Artificial Opening

0DU67JZ Supplement Stomach with Synthetic Substitute, Via Natural or Artificial Opening

0DU67KZ Supplement Stomach with Nonautologous Tissue Substitute, Via Natural or Artificial Opening

0DU687Z Supplement Stomach with Autologous Tissue Substitute, Via Natural or Artificial Opening Endoscopic

0DU68JZ Supplement Stomach with Synthetic Substitute, Via Natural or Artificial Opening Endoscopic

0DU68KZ Supplement Stomach with Nonautologous Tissue Substitute, Via Natural or Artificial Opening Endoscopic

0DU707Z Supplement Stomach, Pylorus with Autologous Tissue Substitute, Open Approach

0DU70JZ Supplement Stomach, Pylorus with Synthetic Substitute, Open Approach

0DU70KZ Supplement Stomach, Pylorus with Nonautologous Tissue Substitute, Open Approach

0DU747Z Supplement Stomach, Pylorus with Autologous Tissue Substitute, Percutaneous Endoscopic Approach

0DU74JZ Supplement Stomach, Pylorus with Synthetic Substitute, Percutaneous Endoscopic Approach

0DU74KZ Supplement Stomach, Pylorus with Nonautologous Tissue Substitute, Percutaneous Endoscopic Approach

0DU777Z Supplement Stomach, Pylorus with Autologous Tissue Substitute, Via Nat or Artificial Opening

0DU77JZ Supplement Stomach, Pylorus with Synthetic Substitute, Via Natural or Artificial Opening

0DU77KZ Supplement Stomach, Pylorus with Nonautologous Tissue Substitute, Via Natural or Artificial Opening

0DU787Z Supplement Stomach, Pylorus with Autologous Tissue Substitute, Via Nat or Artificial Opening Endoscopic

0DU78JZ Supplement Stomach, Pylorus with Synthetic Substitute, Via Natural or Artificial Opening Endoscopic

0DU78KZ Supplement Stomach, Pylorus with Nonautologous Tissue Substitute, Via Natural or Artificial Opening Endoscopic

0DU807Z Supplement Small Intestine with Autologous Tissue Substitute, Open Approach

0DU80JZ Supplement Small Intestine with Synthetic Substitute, Open Approach

0DU80KZ Supplement Small Intestine with Nonautologous Tissue Substitute, Open Approach

0DU847Z Supplement Small Intestine with Autologous Tissue Substitute, Percutaneous Endoscopic Approach

0DU84JZ Supplement Small Intestine with Synthetic Substitute, Percutaneous Endoscopic Approach

0DU84KZ Supplement Small Intestine with Nonautologous Tissue Substitute, Percutaneous Endoscopic Approach

0DU877Z Supplement Small Intestine with Autologous Tissue Substitute, Via Natu or Artificial Opening

0DU87JZ Supplement Small Intestine with Synthetic Substitute, Via Natural or Artificial Opening

0DU87KZ Supplement Small Intestine with Nonautologous Tissue Substitute, Via Natural or Artificial Opening

0DU887Z Supplement Small Intestine with Autologous Tissue Substitute, Via Natu or Artificial Opening Endoscopic

0DU88JZ Supplement Small Intestine with Synthetic Substitute, Via Natural or Artificial Opening Endoscopic

0DU88KZ Supplement Small Intestine with Nonautologous Tissue Substitute, Via Natural or Artificial Opening Endoscopi

0DU907Z Supplement Duodenum with Autologous Tissue Substitute, Open Approach

0DU90JZ Supplement Duodenum with Synthetic Substitute, Open Approach

0DU90KZ Supplement Duodenum with Nonautologous Tissue Substitute, Open Approach

0DU947Z Supplement Duodenum with Autologous Tissue Substitute, Percutaneous Endoscopic Approach

0DU94JZ Supplement Duodenum with Synthetic Substitute, Percutaneous Endoscopic Approach

0DU94KZ Supplement Duodenum with Nonautologous Tissue Substitute, Percutaneous Endoscopic Approach

J977Z Supplement Duodenum with Autologous Tissue Substitute, Via Natural or Artificial Opening

J97JZ Supplement Duodenum with Synthetic Substitute, Via Natural or Artificial Opening

J97KZ Supplement Duodenum with Nonautologous Tissue Substitute, Via Natural or Artificial Opening

J987Z Supplement Duodenum with Autologous Tissue Substitute, Via Natural or Artificial Opening Endoscopic

J98JZ Supplement Duodenum with Synthetic Substitute, Via Natural or Artificial Opening Endoscopic

U98KZ Supplement Duodenum with Nonautologous Tissue Substitute, Via Natural or Artificial Opening Endoscopic

UA07Z Supplement Jejunum with Autologous Tissue Substitute, Open Approach

UA0JZ Supplement Jejunum with Synthetic Substitute, Open Approach

UA0KZ Supplement Jejunum with Nonautologous Tissue Substitute, Open Approach

UA47Z Supplement Jejunum with Autologous Tissue Substitute, Percutaneous Endoscopic Approach

UA4JZ Supplement Jejunum with Synthetic Substitute, Percutaneous Endoscopic Approach

UA4KZ Supplement Jejunum with Nonautologous Tissue Substitute, Percutaneous Endoscopic Approach

UA77Z Supplement Jejunum with Autologous Tissue Substitute, Via Natural or Artificial Opening

UA7JZ Supplement Jejunum with Synthetic Substitute, Via Natural or Artificial Opening

UA7KZ Supplement Jejunum with Nonautologous Tissue Substitute, Via Natural or Artificial Opening

UA87Z Supplement Jejunum with Autologous Tissue Substitute, Via Natural or Artificial Opening Endoscopic

UA8JZ Supplement Jejunum with Synthetic Substitute, Via Natural or Artificial Opening Endoscopic

UA8KZ Supplement Jejunum with Nonautologous Tissue Substitute, Via Natural or Artificial Opening Endoscopic

UB07Z Supplement Ileum with Autologous Tissue Substitute, Open Approach

UB0JZ Supplement Ileum with Synthetic Substitute, Open Approach

UB0KZ Supplement Ileum with Nonautologous Tissue Substitute, Open Approach

UB47Z Supplement Ileum with Autologous Tissue Substitute, Percutaneous Endoscopic Approach

DUB4JZ Supplement Ileum with Synthetic Substitute, Percutaneous Endoscopic Approach

DUB4KZ Supplement Ileum with Nonautologous Tissue Substitute, Percutaneous Endoscopic Approach

DUB77Z Supplement Ileum with Autologous Tissue Substitute, Via Natural or Artificial Opening

DUB7JZ Supplement Ileum with Synthetic Substitute, Via Natural or Artificial Opening

DUB7KZ Supplement Ileum with Nonautologous Tissue Substitute, Via Natural or Artificial Opening

0DUB87Z Supplement Ileum with Autologous Tissue Substitute, Via Natural or Artificial Opening Endoscopic

0DUB8JZ Supplement Ileum with Synthetic Substitute, Via Natural or Artificial Opening Endoscopic

0DUB8KZ Supplement Ileum with Nonautologous Tissue Substitute, Via Natural or Artificial Opening Endoscopic

0DUC07Z Supplement Ileocecal Valve with Autologous Tissue Substitute, Open Approach

0DUC0JZ Supplement Ileocecal Valve with Synthetic Substitute, Open Approach

0DUC0KZ Supplement Ileocecal Valve with Nonautologous Tissue Substitute, Open Approach

0DUC47Z Supplement Ileocecal Valve with Autologous Tissue Substitute, Percutaneous Endoscopic Approach

0DUC4JZ Supplement Ileocecal Valve with Synthetic Substitute, Percutaneous Endoscopic Approach

0DUC4KZ Supplement Ileocecal Valve with Nonautologous Tissue Substitute, Percutaneous Endoscopic Approach

0DUC77Z Supplement Ileocecal Valve with Autologous Tissue Substitute, Via Natural or Artificial Opening

0DUC7JZ Supplement Ileocecal Valve with Synthetic Substitute, Via Natural or Artificial Opening

0DUC7KZ Supplement Ileocecal Valve with Nonautologous Tissue Substitute, Via Natural or Artificial Opening

0DUC87Z Supplement Ileocecal Valve with Autologous Tissue Substitute, Via Natural or Artificial Opening Endoscopic

0DUC8JZ Supplement Ileocecal Valve with Synthetic Substitute, Via Natural or Artificial Opening Endoscopic

0DUC8KZ Supplement Ileocecal Valve with Nonautologous Tissue Substitute, Via Natural or Artificial Opening Endoscopic

0DUE07Z Supplement Large Intestine with Autologous Tissue Substitute, Open Approach

0DUE0JZ Supplement Large Intestine with Synthetic Substitute, Open Approach

0DUE0KZ Supplement Large Intestine with Nonautologous Tissue Substitute, Open Approach

0DUE47Z Supplement Large Intestine with Autologous Tissue Substitute, Percutaneous Endoscopic Approach

0DUE4JZ Supplement Large Intestine with Synthetic Substitute, Percutaneous Endoscopic Approach

0DUE4KZ Supplement Large Intestine with Nonautologous Tissue Substitute, Percutaneous Endoscopic Approach

0DUE77Z Supplement Large Intestine with Autologous Tissue Substitute, Via Natural or Artificial Opening

0DUE7JZ Supplement Large Intestine with Synthetic Substitute, Via Natural or Artificial Opening

0DUE7KZ Supplement Large Intestine with Nonautologous Tissue Substitute, Via Natural or Artificial Opening

0DUE87Z Supplement Large Intestine with Autologous Tissue Substitute, Via Natural or Artificial Opening Endoscopic

0DUE8JZ Supplement Large Intestine with Synthetic Substitute, Via Natural or Artificial Opening Endoscopic

0DUE8KZ Supplement Large Intestine with Nonautologous Tissue Substitute, Via Natural or Artificial Opening Endoscopic

0DUF07Z Supplement Right Large Intestine with Autologous Tissue Substitute, Open Approach

0DUF0JZ Supplement Right Large Intestine with Synthetic Substitute, Open Approach

0DUF0KZ Supplement Right Large Intestine with Nonautologous Tissue Substitute, Open Approach

0DUF47Z Supplement Right Large Intestine with Autologous Tissue Substitute, Percutaneous Endoscopic Approach

0DUF4JZ Supplement Right Large Intestine with Synthetic Substitute, Percutaneous Endoscopic Approach

0DUF4KZ Supplement Right Large Intestine with Nonautologous Tissue Substitute, Percutaneous Endoscopic Approach

0DUF77Z Supplement Right Large Intestine with Autologous Tissue Substitute, Via Natural or Artificial Opening

0DUF7JZ Supplement Right Large Intestine with Synthetic Substitute, Via Natural or Artificial Opening

0DUF7KZ Supplement Right Large Intestine with Nonautologous Tissue Substitute, Via Natural or Artificial Opening

0DUF87Z Supplement Right Large Intestine with Autologous Tissue Substitute, Via Natural or Artificial Opening Endoscopic

0DUF8JZ Supplement Right Large Intestine with Synthetic Substitute, Via Natural or Artificial Opening Endoscopic

0DUF8KZ Supplement Right Large Intestine with Nonautologous Tissue Substitute, Via Natural or Artificial Opening Endoscopic

0DUG07Z Supplement Left Large Intestine with Autologous Tissue Substitute, Open Approach

0DUG0JZ Supplement Left Large Intestine with Synthetic Substitute, Open Approach

0DUG0KZ Supplement Left Large Intestine with Nonautologous Tissue Substitute, Open Approach

0DUG47Z Supplement Left Large Intestine with Autologous Tissue Substitute, Percutaneous Endoscopic Approach

0DUG4JZ Supplement Left Large Intestine with Synthetic Substitute, Percutaneous Endoscopic Approach

0DUG4KZ Supplement Left Large Intestine with Nonautologous Tissue Substitute, Percutaneous Endoscopic Approach

0DUG77Z Supplement Left Large Intestine with Autologous Tissue Substitute, Via Natural or Artificial Opening

0DUG7JZ Supplement Left Large Intestine with Synthetic Substitute, Via Natural or Artificial Opening

0DUG7KZ Supplement Left Large Intestine with Nonautologous Tissue Substitute, Via Natural or Artificial Opening

0DUG87Z Supplement Left Large Intestine with Autologous Tissue Substitute, Via Natural or Artificial Opening Endoscopic

0DUG8JZ Supplement Left Large Intestine with Synthetic Substitute, Via Natural or Artificial Opening Endoscopic

0DUG8KZ Supplement Left Large Intestine with Nonautologous Tissue Substitute, Via Natural or Artificial Opening Endoscopic

0DUH07Z Supplement Cecum with Autologous Tissue Substitute, Open Approach

0DUH0JZ Supplement Cecum with Synthetic Substitute, Open Approach

0DUH0KZ Supplement Cecum with Nonautologous Tissue Substitute, Open Approach

0DUH47Z Supplement Cecum with Autologous Tissue Substitute, Percutaneous Endoscopic Approach

0DUH4JZ Supplement Cecum with Synthetic Substitute, Percutaneous Endoscopic Approach

0DUH4KZ Supplement Cecum with Nonautologous Tissue Substitute, Percutaneous Endoscopic Approach

0DUH77Z Supplement Cecum with Autologous Tissue Substitute, Via Natural or Artificial Opening

0DUH7JZ Supplement Cecum with Synthetic Substitute, Via Natural or Artificial Opening

0DUH7KZ Supplement Cecum with Nonautologous Tissue Substitute, Via Natural or Artificial Opening

0DUH87Z Supplement Cecum with Autologous Tissue Substitute, Via Natural or Artificial Opening Endoscopic

0DUH8JZ Supplement Cecum with Synthetic Substitute, Via Natural or Artificial Opening Endoscopic

0DUH8KZ Supplement Cecum with Nonautologous Tissue Substitute, Via Natural or Artificial Opening Endoscopic

0DUK07Z Supplement Ascending Colon with Autologous Tissue Substitute, Open Approach

0DUK0JZ Supplement Ascending Colon with Synthetic Substitute, Open Approach

0DUK0KZ Supplement Ascending Colon with Nonautologous Tissue Substitute, Open Approach

0DUK47Z Supplement Ascending Colon with Autologous Tissue Substitute, Percutaneous Endoscopic Approach

0DUK4JZ Supplement Ascending Colon with Synthetic Substitute, Percutaneous Endoscopic Approach

0DUK4KZ Supplement Ascending Colon with Nonautologous Tissue Substitute, Percutaneous Endoscopic Approach

0DUK77Z Supplement Ascending Colon with Autologous Tissue Substitute, Via Natural or Artificial Opening

0DUK7JZ Supplement Ascending Colon with Synthetic Substitute, Via Natural or Artificial Opening

0DUK7KZ Supplement Ascending Colon with Nonautologous Tissue Substitute, Via Natural or Artificial Opening

0DUK87Z Supplement Ascending Colon with Autologous Tissue Substitute, Via Natural or Artificial Opening Endoscopic

0DUK8JZ Supplement Ascending Colon with Synthetic Substitute, Via Natural or Artificial Opening Endoscopic

0DUK8KZ Supplement Ascending Colon with Nonautologous Tissue Substitute, Via Natural or Artificial Opening Endoscopic

0DUL07Z Supplement Transverse Colon with Autologous Tissue Substitute, Open Approach

0DUL0JZ Supplement Transverse Colon with Synthetic Substitute, Open Approach

0DUL0KZ Supplement Transverse Colon with Nonautologous Tissue Substitute, Open Approach

0DUL47Z Supplement Transverse Colon with Autologous Tissue Substitute, Percutaneous Endoscopic Approach

0DUL4JZ Supplement Transverse Colon with Synthetic Substitute, Percutaneous Endoscopic Approach

0DUL4KZ Supplement Transverse Colon with Nonautologous Tissue Substitute, Percutaneous Endoscopic Approach

0DUL77Z Supplement Transverse Colon with Autologous Tissue Substitute, Via Natural or Artificial Opening

0DUL7JZ Supplement Transverse Colon with Synthetic Substitute, Via Natural or Artificial Opening

0DUL7KZ Supplement Transverse Colon with Nonautologous Tissue Substitute, Via Natural or Artificial Opening

0DUL87Z Supplement Transverse Colon with Autologous Tissue Substitute, Via Natural or Artificial Opening Endoscopic

0DUL8JZ Supplement Transverse Colon with Synthetic Substitute, Via Natural or Artificial Opening Endoscopic

0DUL8KZ Supplement Transverse Colon with Nonautologous Tissue Substitute, Via Natural or Artificial Opening Endoscopic

0DUM07Z Supplement Descending Colon with Autologous Tissue Substitute, Open Approach

0DUM0JZ Supplement Descending Colon with Synthetic Substitute, Open Approach

0DUM0KZ Supplement Descending Colon with Nonautologous Tissue Substitute, Open Approach

0DUM47Z Supplement Descending Colon with Autologous Tissue Substitute, Percutaneous Endoscopic Approach

0DUM4JZ Supplement Descending Colon with Synthetic Substitute, Percutaneous Endoscopic Approach

0DUM4KZ Supplement Descending Colon with Nonautologous Tissue Substitute, Percutaneous Endoscopic Approach

0DUM77Z Supplement Descending Colon with Autologous Tissue Substitute, Via Natural or Artificial Opening

0DUM7JZ Supplement Descending Colon with Synthetic Substitute, Via Natural or Artificial Opening

0DUM7KZ Supplement Descending Colon with Nonautologous Tissue Substitute, Via Natural or Artificial Opening

0DUM87Z Supplement Descending Colon with Autologous Tissue Substitute, Via Natural or Artificial Opening Endoscopic

0DUM8JZ Supplement Descending Colon with Synthetic Substitute, Via Natural or Artificial Opening Endoscopic

0DUM8KZ Supplement Descending Colon with Nonautologous Tissue Substitute, Via Natural or Artificial Opening Endoscopic

0DUN07Z Supplement Sigmoid Colon with Autologous Tissue Substitute, Open Approach

0DUN0JZ Supplement Sigmoid Colon with Synthetic Substitute, Open Approach

0DUN0KZ Supplement Sigmoid Colon with Nonautologous Tissue Substitute, Open Approach

0DUN47Z Supplement Sigmoid Colon with Autologous Tissue Substitute, Percutaneous Endoscopic Approach

0DUN4JZ Supplement Sigmoid Colon with Synthetic Substitute, Percutaneous Endoscopic Approach

0DUN4KZ Supplement Sigmoid Colon with Nonautologous Tissue Substitute, Percutaneous Endoscopic Approach

0DUN77Z Supplement Sigmoid Colon with Autologous Tissue Substitute, Via Nat or Artificial Opening

0DUN7JZ Supplement Sigmoid Colon with Synthetic Substitute, Via Natural or Artificial Opening

0DUN7KZ Supplement Sigmoid Colon with Nonautologous Tissue Substitute, Via Natural or Artificial Opening

0DUN87Z Supplement Sigmoid Colon with Autologous Tissue Substitute, Via Nat or Artificial Opening Endoscopic

0DUN8JZ Supplement Sigmoid Colon with Synthetic Substitute, Via Natural or Artificial Opening Endoscopic

0DUN8KZ Supplement Sigmoid Colon with Nonautologous Tissue Substitute, Via Natural or Artificial Opening Endoscopic

0DUP07Z Supplement Rectum with Autologous Tissue Substitute, Open Approach

0DUP0JZ Supplement Rectum with Synthetic Substitute, Open Approach

0DUP0KZ Supplement Rectum with Nonautologo Tissue Substitute, Open Approach

0DUP47Z Supplement Rectum with Autologous Tissue Substitute, Percutaneous Endoscopic Approach

0DUP4JZ Supplement Rectum with Synthetic Substitute, Percutaneous Endoscopic Approach

0DUP4KZ Supplement Rectum with Nonautologo Tissue Substitute, Percutaneous Endoscopic Approach

0DUP77Z Supplement Rectum with Autologous Tissue Substitute, Via Natural or Artific Opening

0DUP7JZ Supplement Rectum with Synthetic Substitute, Via Natural or Artificial Opening

0DUP7KZ Supplement Rectum with Nonautologo Tissue Substitute, Via Natural or Artific Opening

0DUP87Z Supplement Rectum with Autologous Tissue Substitute, Via Natural or Artific Opening Endoscopic

0DUP8JZ Supplement Rectum with Synthetic Substitute, Via Natural or Artificial Opening Endoscopic

0DUP8KZ Supplement Rectum with Nonautologou Tissue Substitute, Via Natural or Artifici Opening Endoscopic

0DUQ07Z Supplement Anus with Autologous Tissu Substitute, Open Approach

0DUQ0JZ Supplement Anus with Synthetic Substitute, Open Approach

0DUQ0KZ Supplement Anus with Nonautologous Tissue Substitute, Open Approach

0DUQ47Z Supplement Anus with Autologous Tissu Substitute, Percutaneous Endoscopic Approach

0DUQ4JZ Supplement Anus with Synthetic Substitute, Percutaneous Endoscopic Approach

0DUQ4KZ Supplement Anus with Nonautologous Tissue Substitute, Percutaneous Endoscopic Approach

0DUQ77Z Supplement Anus with Autologous Tissue Substitute, Via Natural or Artifici Opening

0DUQ7JZ Supplement Anus with Synthetic Substitute, Via Natural or Artificial Opening

0DUQ7KZ Supplement Anus with Nonautologous Tissue Substitute, Via Natural or Artifici Opening

[cut off]Q87Z Supplement Anus with Autologous Tissue Substitute, Via Natural or Artificial Opening Endoscopic
[cut off]Q8JZ Supplement Anus with Synthetic Substitute, Via Natural or Artificial Opening Endoscopic
[cut off]JQ8KZ Supplement Anus with Nonautologous Tissue Substitute, Via Natural or Artificial Opening Endoscopic
[cut off]JQX7Z Supplement Anus with Autologous Tissue Substitute, External Approach
[cut off]JQXJZ Supplement Anus with Synthetic Substitute, External Approach
[cut off]JQXKZ Supplement Anus with Nonautologous Tissue Substitute, External Approach
[cut off]JR07Z Supplement Anal Sphincter with Autologous Tissue Substitute, Open Approach
[cut off]JR0JZ Supplement Anal Sphincter with Synthetic Substitute, Open Approach
[cut off]UR0KZ Supplement Anal Sphincter with Nonautologous Tissue Substitute, Open Approach
[cut off]UR47Z Supplement Anal Sphincter with Autologous Tissue Substitute, Percutaneous Endoscopic Approach
[cut off]UR4JZ Supplement Anal Sphincter with Synthetic Substitute, Percutaneous Endoscopic Approach
[cut off]UR4KZ Supplement Anal Sphincter with Nonautologous Tissue Substitute, Percutaneous Endoscopic Approach
[cut off]US07Z Supplement Greater Omentum with Autologous Tissue Substitute, Open Approach
0DUS0JZ Supplement Greater Omentum with Synthetic Substitute, Open Approach
0DUS0KZ Supplement Greater Omentum with Nonautologous Tissue Substitute, Open Approach
0DUS47Z Supplement Greater Omentum with Autologous Tissue Substitute, Percutaneous Endoscopic Approach
0DUS4JZ Supplement Greater Omentum with Synthetic Substitute, Percutaneous Endoscopic Approach
0DUS4KZ Supplement Greater Omentum with Nonautologous Tissue Substitute, Percutaneous Endoscopic Approach
0DUT07Z Supplement Lesser Omentum with Autologous Tissue Substitute, Open Approach
0DUT0JZ Supplement Lesser Omentum with Synthetic Substitute, Open Approach
0DUT0KZ Supplement Lesser Omentum with Nonautologous Tissue Substitute, Open Approach
0DUT47Z Supplement Lesser Omentum with Autologous Tissue Substitute, Percutaneous Endoscopic Approach
0DUT4JZ Supplement Lesser Omentum with Synthetic Substitute, Percutaneous Endoscopic Approach
0DUT4KZ Supplement Lesser Omentum with Nonautologous Tissue Substitute, Percutaneous Endoscopic Approach
0DUV07Z Supplement Mesentery with Autologous Tissue Substitute, Open Approach
0DUV0JZ Supplement Mesentery with Synthetic Substitute, Open Approach
0DUV0KZ Supplement Mesentery with Nonautologous Tissue Substitute, Open Approach
0DUV47Z Supplement Mesentery with Autologous Tissue Substitute, Percutaneous Endoscopic Approach
0DUV4JZ Supplement Mesentery with Synthetic Substitute, Percutaneous Endoscopic Approach
0DUV4KZ Supplement Mesentery with Nonautologous Tissue Substitute, Percutaneous Endoscopic Approach
0DUW07Z Supplement Peritoneum with Autologous Tissue Substitute, Open Approach
0DUW0JZ Supplement Peritoneum with Synthetic Substitute, Open Approach
0DUW0KZ Supplement Peritoneum with Nonautologous Tissue Substitute, Open Approach
0DUW47Z Supplement Peritoneum with Autologous Tissue Substitute, Percutaneous Endoscopic Approach
0DUW4JZ Supplement Peritoneum with Synthetic Substitute, Percutaneous Endoscopic Approach
0DUW4KZ Supplement Peritoneum with Nonautologous Tissue Substitute, Percutaneous Endoscopic Approach

[cut off]V – Gastrointestinal System, Restriction

[cut off]V10CZ Restriction of Upper Esophagus with Extraluminal Device, Open Approach
[cut off]V10DZ Restriction of Upper Esophagus with Intraluminal Device, Open Approach
[cut off]V10ZZ Restriction of Upper Esophagus, Open Approach
[cut off]V13CZ Restriction of Upper Esophagus with Extraluminal Device, Percutaneous Approach
[cut off]V13DZ Restriction of Upper Esophagus with Intraluminal Device, Percutaneous Approach
[cut off]V13ZZ Restriction of Upper Esophagus, Percutaneous Approach
[cut off]V14CZ Restriction of Upper Esophagus with Extraluminal Device, Percutaneous Endoscopic Approach
[cut off]V14DZ Restriction of Upper Esophagus with Intraluminal Device, Percutaneous Endoscopic Approach
[cut off]V14ZZ Restriction of Upper Esophagus, Percutaneous Endoscopic Approach
[cut off]V17DZ Restriction of Upper Esophagus with Intraluminal Device, Via Natural or Artificial Opening
[cut off]DV17ZZ Restriction of Upper Esophagus, Via Natural or Artificial Opening
[cut off]DV18DZ Restriction of Upper Esophagus with Intraluminal Device, Via Natural or Artificial Opening Endoscopic
[cut off]DV18ZZ Restriction of Upper Esophagus, Via Natural or Artificial Opening Endoscopic
[cut off]DV20CZ Restriction of Middle Esophagus with Extraluminal Device, Open Approach
[cut off]DV20DZ Restriction of Middle Esophagus with Intraluminal Device, Open Approach
0DV20ZZ Restriction of Middle Esophagus, Open Approach
0DV23CZ Restriction of Middle Esophagus with Extraluminal Device, Percutaneous Approach
0DV23DZ Restriction of Middle Esophagus with Intraluminal Device, Percutaneous Approach
0DV23ZZ Restriction of Middle Esophagus, Percutaneous Approach
0DV24CZ Restriction of Middle Esophagus with Extraluminal Device, Percutaneous Endoscopic Approach
0DV24DZ Restriction of Middle Esophagus with Intraluminal Device, Percutaneous Endoscopic Approach
0DV24ZZ Restriction of Middle Esophagus, Percutaneous Endoscopic Approach
0DV27DZ Restriction of Middle Esophagus with Intraluminal Device, Via Natural or Artificial Opening
0DV27ZZ Restriction of Middle Esophagus, Via Natural or Artificial Opening
0DV28DZ Restriction of Middle Esophagus with Intraluminal Device, Via Natural or Artificial Opening Endoscopic
0DV28ZZ Restriction of Middle Esophagus, Via Natural or Artificial Opening Endoscopic
0DV30CZ Restriction of Lower Esophagus with Extraluminal Device, Open Approach
0DV30DZ Restriction of Lower Esophagus with Intraluminal Device, Open Approach
0DV30ZZ Restriction of Lower Esophagus, Open Approach
0DV33CZ Restriction of Lower Esophagus with Extraluminal Device, Percutaneous Approach
0DV33DZ Restriction of Lower Esophagus with Intraluminal Device, Percutaneous Approach
0DV33ZZ Restriction of Lower Esophagus, Percutaneous Approach
0DV34CZ Restriction of Lower Esophagus with Extraluminal Device, Percutaneous Endoscopic Approach
0DV34DZ Restriction of Lower Esophagus with Intraluminal Device, Percutaneous Endoscopic Approach
0DV34ZZ Restriction of Lower Esophagus, Percutaneous Endoscopic Approach
0DV37DZ Restriction of Lower Esophagus with Intraluminal Device, Via Natural or Artificial Opening
0DV37ZZ Restriction of Lower Esophagus, Via Natural or Artificial Opening
0DV38DZ Restriction of Lower Esophagus with Intraluminal Device, Via Natural or Artificial Opening Endoscopic
0DV38ZZ Restriction of Lower Esophagus, Via Natural or Artificial Opening Endoscopic
0DV40CZ Restriction of Esophagogastric Junction with Extraluminal Device, Open Approach
0DV40DZ Restriction of Esophagogastric Junction with Intraluminal Device, Open Approach
0DV40ZZ Restriction of Esophagogastric Junction, Open Approach
0DV43CZ Restriction of Esophagogastric Junction with Extraluminal Device, Percutaneous Approach
0DV43DZ Restriction of Esophagogastric Junction with Intraluminal Device, Percutaneous Approach

0DV43ZZ Restriction of Esophagogastric Junction, Percutaneous Approach

0DV44CZ Restriction of Esophagogastric Junction with Extraluminal Device, Percutaneous Endoscopic Approach

0DV44DZ Restriction of Esophagogastric Junction with Intraluminal Device, Percutaneous Endoscopic Approach

0DV44ZZ Restriction of Esophagogastric Junction, Percutaneous Endoscopic Approach

0DV47DZ Restriction of Esophagogastric Junction with Intraluminal Device, Via Natural or Artificial Opening

0DV47ZZ Restriction of Esophagogastric Junction, Via Natural or Artificial Opening

0DV48DZ Restriction of Esophagogastric Junction with Intraluminal Device, Via Natural or Artificial Opening Endoscopic

0DV48ZZ Restriction of Esophagogastric Junction, Via Natural or Artificial Opening Endoscopic

0DV50CZ Restriction of Esophagus with Extraluminal Device, Open Approach

0DV50DZ Restriction of Esophagus with Intraluminal Device, Open Approach

0DV50ZZ Restriction of Esophagus, Open Approach

0DV53CZ Restriction of Esophagus with Extraluminal Device, Percutaneous Approach

0DV53DZ Restriction of Esophagus with Intraluminal Device, Percutaneous Approach

0DV53ZZ Restriction of Esophagus, Percutaneous Approach

0DV54CZ Restriction of Esophagus with Extraluminal Device, Percutaneous Endoscopic Approach

0DV54DZ Restriction of Esophagus with Intraluminal Device, Percutaneous Endoscopic Approach

0DV54ZZ Restriction of Esophagus, Percutaneous Endoscopic Approach

0DV57DZ Restriction of Esophagus with Intraluminal Device, Via Natural or Artificial Opening

0DV57ZZ Restriction of Esophagus, Via Natural or Artificial Opening

0DV58DZ Restriction of Esophagus with Intraluminal Device, Via Natural or Artificial Opening Endoscopic

0DV58ZZ Restriction of Esophagus, Via Natural or Artificial Opening Endoscopic

0DV60CZ Restriction of Stomach with Extraluminal Device, Open Approach

0DV60DZ Restriction of Stomach with Intraluminal Device, Open Approach

0DV60ZZ Restriction of Stomach, Open Approach

0DV63CZ Restriction of Stomach with Extraluminal Device, Percutaneous Approach

0DV63DZ Restriction of Stomach with Intraluminal Device, Percutaneous Approach

0DV63ZZ Restriction of Stomach, Percutaneous Approach

0DV64CZ Restriction of Stomach with Extraluminal Device, Percutaneous Endoscopic Approach

HAC When reported with principal diagnosis code K66.01 and secondary diagnosis code K68.11, K95.01, K95.81 or T81.4XXA

0DV64DZ Restriction of Stomach with Intraluminal Device, Percutaneous Endoscopic Approach

0DV64ZZ Restriction of Stomach, Percutaneous Endoscopic Approach

▲ **0DV67DZ** Restriction of Stomach with Intraluminal Device, Via Natural or Artificial Opening

0DV67ZZ Restriction of Stomach, Via Natural or Artificial Opening

▲ **0DV68DZ** Restriction of Stomach with Intraluminal Device, Via Natural or Artificial Opening Endoscopic

0DV68ZZ Restriction of Stomach, Via Natural or Artificial Opening Endoscopic

0DV70CZ Restriction of Stomach, Pylorus with Extraluminal Device, Open Approach

0DV70DZ Restriction of Stomach, Pylorus with Intraluminal Device, Open Approach

0DV70ZZ Restriction of Stomach, Pylorus, Open Approach

0DV73CZ Restriction of Stomach, Pylorus with Extraluminal Device, Percutaneous Approach

0DV73DZ Restriction of Stomach, Pylorus with Intraluminal Device, Percutaneous Approach

0DV73ZZ Restriction of Stomach, Pylorus, Percutaneous Approach

0DV74CZ Restriction of Stomach, Pylorus with Extraluminal Device, Percutaneous Endoscopic Approach

0DV74DZ Restriction of Stomach, Pylorus with Intraluminal Device, Percutaneous Endoscopic Approach

0DV74ZZ Restriction of Stomach, Pylorus, Percutaneous Endoscopic Approach

0DV77DZ Restriction of Stomach, Pylorus with Intraluminal Device, Via Natural or Artificial Opening

0DV77ZZ Restriction of Stomach, Pylorus, Via Natural or Artificial Opening

0DV78DZ Restriction of Stomach, Pylorus with Intraluminal Device, Via Natural or Artificial Opening Endoscopic

0DV78ZZ Restriction of Stomach, Pylorus, Via Natural or Artificial Opening Endoscopic

0DV80CZ Restriction of Small Intestine with Extraluminal Device, Open Approach

0DV80DZ Restriction of Small Intestine with Intraluminal Device, Open Approach

0DV80ZZ Restriction of Small Intestine, Open Approach

0DV83CZ Restriction of Small Intestine with Extraluminal Device, Percutaneous Approach

0DV83DZ Restriction of Small Intestine with Intraluminal Device, Percutaneous Approach

0DV83ZZ Restriction of Small Intestine, Percutaneous Approach

0DV84CZ Restriction of Small Intestine with Extraluminal Device, Percutaneous Endoscopic Approach

0DV84DZ Restriction of Small Intestine with Intraluminal Device, Percutaneous Endoscopic Approach

0DV84ZZ Restriction of Small Intestine, Percutaneous Endoscopic Approach

0DV87DZ Restriction of Small Intestine with Intraluminal Device, Via Natural or Artificial Opening

0DV87ZZ Restriction of Small Intestine, Via Natural or Artificial Opening

0DV88DZ Restriction of Small Intestine with Intraluminal Device, Via Natural or Artificial Opening Endoscopic

0DV88ZZ Restriction of Small Intestine, Via Natural or Artificial Opening Endoscopic

0DV90CZ Restriction of Duodenum with Extraluminal Device, Open Approach

0DV90DZ Restriction of Duodenum with Intraluminal Device, Open Approach

0DV90ZZ Restriction of Duodenum, Open Appr

0DV93CZ Restriction of Duodenum with Extraluminal Device, Percutaneous Approach

0DV93DZ Restriction of Duodenum with Intraluminal Device, Percutaneous Approach

0DV93ZZ Restriction of Duodenum, Percutaneou Approach

0DV94CZ Restriction of Duodenum with Extraluminal Device, Percutaneous Endoscopic Approach

0DV94DZ Restriction of Duodenum with Intraluminal Device, Percutaneous Endoscopic Approach

0DV94ZZ Restriction of Duodenum, Percutaneou Endoscopic Approach

0DV97DZ Restriction of Duodenum with Intraluminal Device, Via Natural or Artificial Opening

0DV97ZZ Restriction of Duodenum, Via Natural Artificial Opening

0DV98DZ Restriction of Duodenum with Intraluminal Device, Via Natural or Artificial Opening Endoscopic

0DV98ZZ Restriction of Duodenum, Via Natural Artificial Opening Endoscopic

0DVA0CZ Restriction of Jejunum with Extralumin Device, Open Approach

0DVA0DZ Restriction of Jejunum with Intralumin Device, Open Approach

0DVA0ZZ Restriction of Jejunum, Open Approach

0DVA3CZ Restriction of Jejunum with Extraluminal Device, Percutaneous Approach

0DVA3DZ Restriction of Jejunum with Intralumina Device, Percutaneous Approach

0DVA3ZZ Restriction of Jejunum, Percutaneous Approach

0DVA4CZ Restriction of Jejunum with Extralumin Device, Percutaneous Endoscopic Approach

0DVA4DZ Restriction of Jejunum with Intralumina Device, Percutaneous Endoscopic Approach

0DVA4ZZ Restriction of Jejunum, Percutaneous Endoscopic Approach

0DVA7DZ Restriction of Jejunum with Intraluminal Device, Via Natural or Artificial Opening

0DVA7ZZ Restriction of Jejunum, Via Natural or Artificial Opening

0DVA8DZ Restriction of Jejunum with Intraluminal Device, Via Natural or Artificial Opening Endoscopic

0DVA8ZZ Restriction of Jejunum, Via Natural or Artificial Opening Endoscopic

0DVB0CZ Restriction of Ileum with Extraluminal Device, Open Approach

0DVB0DZ Restriction of Ileum with Intraluminal Device, Open Approach

0DVB0ZZ Restriction of Ileum, Open Approach

0DVB3CZ Restriction of Ileum with Extraluminal Device, Percutaneous Approach

0DVB3DZ Restriction of Ileum with Intraluminal Device, Percutaneous Approach

0DVB3ZZ Restriction of Ileum, Percutaneous Approach

0DVB4CZ Restriction of Ileum with Extraluminal Device, Percutaneous Endoscopic Approach

0DVB4DZ Restriction of Ileum with Intraluminal Device, Percutaneous Endoscopic Approach

B4ZZ Restriction of Ileum, Percutaneous Endoscopic Approach
B7DZ Restriction of Ileum with Intraluminal Device, Via Natural or Artificial Opening
B7ZZ Restriction of Ileum, Via Natural or Artificial Opening
B8DZ Restriction of Ileum with Intraluminal Device, Via Natural or Artificial Opening Endoscopic
B8ZZ Restriction of Ileum, Via Natural or Artificial Opening Endoscopic
C0CZ Restriction of Ileocecal Valve with Extraluminal Device, Open Approach
C0DZ Restriction of Ileocecal Valve with Intraluminal Device, Open Approach
C0ZZ Restriction of Ileocecal Valve, Open Approach
C3CZ Restriction of Ileocecal Valve with Extraluminal Device, Percutaneous Approach
C3DZ Restriction of Ileocecal Valve with Intraluminal Device, Percutaneous Approach
VC3ZZ Restriction of Ileocecal Valve, Percutaneous Approach
C4CZ Restriction of Ileocecal Valve with Extraluminal Device, Percutaneous Endoscopic Approach
VC4DZ Restriction of Ileocecal Valve with Intraluminal Device, Percutaneous Endoscopic Approach
VC4ZZ Restriction of Ileocecal Valve, Percutaneous Endoscopic Approach
VC7DZ Restriction of Ileocecal Valve with Intraluminal Device, Via Natural or Artificial Opening
VC7ZZ Restriction of Ileocecal Valve, Via Natural or Artificial Opening
VC8DZ Restriction of Ileocecal Valve with Intraluminal Device, Via Natural or Artificial Opening Endoscopic
VC8ZZ Restriction of Ileocecal Valve, Via Natural or Artificial Opening Endoscopic
VE0CZ Restriction of Large Intestine with Extraluminal Device, Open Approach
VE0DZ Restriction of Large Intestine with Intraluminal Device, Open Approach
VE0ZZ Restriction of Large Intestine, Open Approach
VE3CZ Restriction of Large Intestine with Extraluminal Device, Percutaneous Approach
VE3DZ Restriction of Large Intestine with Intraluminal Device, Percutaneous Approach
VE3ZZ Restriction of Large Intestine, Percutaneous Approach
VE4CZ Restriction of Large Intestine with Extraluminal Device, Percutaneous Endoscopic Approach
VE4DZ Restriction of Large Intestine with Intraluminal Device, Percutaneous Endoscopic Approach
VE4ZZ Restriction of Large Intestine, Percutaneous Endoscopic Approach
VE7DZ Restriction of Large Intestine with Intraluminal Device, Via Natural or Artificial Opening
DVE7ZZ Restriction of Large Intestine, Via Natural or Artificial Opening
DVE8DZ Restriction of Large Intestine with Intraluminal Device, Via Natural or Artificial Opening Endoscopic
DVE8ZZ Restriction of Large Intestine, Via Natural or Artificial Opening Endoscopic
0DVF0CZ Restriction of Right Large Intestine with Extraluminal Device, Open Approach
0DVF0DZ Restriction of Right Large Intestine with Intraluminal Device, Open Approach
0DVF0ZZ Restriction of Right Large Intestine, Open Approach
0DVF3CZ Restriction of Right Large Intestine with Extraluminal Device, Percutaneous Approach
0DVF3DZ Restriction of Right Large Intestine with Intraluminal Device, Percutaneous Approach
0DVF3ZZ Restriction of Right Large Intestine, Percutaneous Approach
0DVF4CZ Restriction of Right Large Intestine with Extraluminal Device, Percutaneous Endoscopic Approach
0DVF4DZ Restriction of Right Large Intestine with Intraluminal Device, Percutaneous Endoscopic Approach
0DVF4ZZ Restriction of Right Large Intestine, Percutaneous Endoscopic Approach
0DVF7DZ Restriction of Right Large Intestine with Intraluminal Device, Via Natural or Artificial Opening
0DVF7ZZ Restriction of Right Large Intestine, Via Natural or Artificial Opening
0DVF8DZ Restriction of Right Large Intestine with Intraluminal Device, Via Natural or Artificial Opening Endoscopic
0DVF8ZZ Restriction of Right Large Intestine, Via Natural or Artificial Opening Endoscopic
0DVG0CZ Restriction of Left Large Intestine with Extraluminal Device, Open Approach
0DVG0DZ Restriction of Left Large Intestine with Intraluminal Device, Open Approach
0DVG0ZZ Restriction of Left Large Intestine, Open Approach
0DVG3CZ Restriction of Left Large Intestine with Extraluminal Device, Percutaneous Approach
0DVG3DZ Restriction of Left Large Intestine with Intraluminal Device, Percutaneous Approach
0DVG3ZZ Restriction of Left Large Intestine, Percutaneous Approach
0DVG4CZ Restriction of Left Large Intestine with Extraluminal Device, Percutaneous Endoscopic Approach
0DVG4DZ Restriction of Left Large Intestine with Intraluminal Device, Percutaneous Endoscopic Approach
0DVG4ZZ Restriction of Left Large Intestine, Percutaneous Endoscopic Approach
0DVG7DZ Restriction of Left Large Intestine with Intraluminal Device, Via Natural or Artificial Opening
0DVG7ZZ Restriction of Left Large Intestine, Via Natural or Artificial Opening
0DVG8DZ Restriction of Left Large Intestine with Intraluminal Device, Via Natural or Artificial Opening Endoscopic
0DVG8ZZ Restriction of Left Large Intestine, Via Natural or Artificial Opening Endoscopic
0DVH0CZ Restriction of Cecum with Extraluminal Device, Open Approach
0DVH0DZ Restriction of Cecum with Intraluminal Device, Open Approach
0DVH0ZZ Restriction of Cecum, Open Approach
0DVH3CZ Restriction of Cecum with Extraluminal Device, Percutaneous Approach
0DVH3DZ Restriction of Cecum with Intraluminal Device, Percutaneous Approach
0DVH3ZZ Restriction of Cecum, Percutaneous Approach
0DVH4CZ Restriction of Cecum with Extraluminal Device, Percutaneous Endoscopic Approach
0DVH4DZ Restriction of Cecum with Intraluminal Device, Percutaneous Endoscopic Approach
0DVH4ZZ Restriction of Cecum, Percutaneous Endoscopic Approach
0DVH7DZ Restriction of Cecum with Intraluminal Device, Via Natural or Artificial Opening
0DVH7ZZ Restriction of Cecum, Via Natural or Artificial Opening
0DVH8DZ Restriction of Cecum with Intraluminal Device, Via Natural or Artificial Opening Endoscopic
0DVH8ZZ Restriction of Cecum, Via Natural or Artificial Opening Endoscopic
0DVK0CZ Restriction of Ascending Colon with Extraluminal Device, Open Approach
0DVK0DZ Restriction of Ascending Colon with Intraluminal Device, Open Approach
0DVK0ZZ Restriction of Ascending Colon, Open Approach
0DVK3CZ Restriction of Ascending Colon with Extraluminal Device, Percutaneous Approach
0DVK3DZ Restriction of Ascending Colon with Intraluminal Device, Percutaneous Approach
0DVK3ZZ Restriction of Ascending Colon, Percutaneous Approach
0DVK4CZ Restriction of Ascending Colon with Extraluminal Device, Percutaneous Endoscopic Approach
0DVK4DZ Restriction of Ascending Colon with Intraluminal Device, Percutaneous Endoscopic Approach
0DVK4ZZ Restriction of Ascending Colon, Percutaneous Endoscopic Approach
0DVK7DZ Restriction of Ascending Colon with Intraluminal Device, Via Natural or Artificial Opening
0DVK7ZZ Restriction of Ascending Colon, Via Natural or Artificial Opening
0DVK8DZ Restriction of Ascending Colon with Intraluminal Device, Via Natural or Artificial Opening Endoscopic
0DVK8ZZ Restriction of Ascending Colon, Via Natural or Artificial Opening Endoscopic
0DVL0CZ Restriction of Transverse Colon with Extraluminal Device, Open Approach
0DVL0DZ Restriction of Transverse Colon with Intraluminal Device, Open Approach
0DVL0ZZ Restriction of Transverse Colon, Open Approach
0DVL3CZ Restriction of Transverse Colon with Extraluminal Device, Percutaneous Approach
0DVL3DZ Restriction of Transverse Colon with Intraluminal Device, Percutaneous Approach
0DVL3ZZ Restriction of Transverse Colon, Percutaneous Approach
0DVL4CZ Restriction of Transverse Colon with Extraluminal Device, Percutaneous Endoscopic Approach
0DVL4DZ Restriction of Transverse Colon with Intraluminal Device, Percutaneous Endoscopic Approach
0DVL4ZZ Restriction of Transverse Colon, Percutaneous Endoscopic Approach
0DVL7DZ Restriction of Transverse Colon with Intraluminal Device, Via Natural or Artificial Opening

0DVL7ZZ Restriction of Transverse Colon, Via Natural or Artificial Opening
0DVL8DZ Restriction of Transverse Colon with Intraluminal Device, Via Natural or Artificial Opening Endoscopic
0DVL8ZZ Restriction of Transverse Colon, Via Natural or Artificial Opening Endoscopic
0DVM0CZ Restriction of Descending Colon with Extraluminal Device, Open Approach
0DVM0DZ Restriction of Descending Colon with Intraluminal Device, Open Approach
0DVM0ZZ Restriction of Descending Colon, Open Approach
0DVM3CZ Restriction of Descending Colon with Extraluminal Device, Percutaneous Approach
0DVM3DZ Restriction of Descending Colon with Intraluminal Device, Percutaneous Approach
0DVM3ZZ Restriction of Descending Colon, Percutaneous Approach
0DVM4CZ Restriction of Descending Colon with Extraluminal Device, Percutaneous Endoscopic Approach
0DVM4DZ Restriction of Descending Colon with Intraluminal Device, Percutaneous Endoscopic Approach
0DVM4ZZ Restriction of Descending Colon, Percutaneous Endoscopic Approach
0DVM7DZ Restriction of Descending Colon with Intraluminal Device, Via Natural or Artificial Opening
0DVM7ZZ Restriction of Descending Colon, Via Natural or Artificial Opening
0DVM8DZ Restriction of Descending Colon with Intraluminal Device, Via Natural or Artificial Opening Endoscopic
0DVM8ZZ Restriction of Descending Colon, Via Natural or Artificial Opening Endoscopic
0DVN0CZ Restriction of Sigmoid Colon with Extraluminal Device, Open Approach
0DVN0DZ Restriction of Sigmoid Colon with Intraluminal Device, Open Approach
0DVN0ZZ Restriction of Sigmoid Colon, Open Approach
0DVN3CZ Restriction of Sigmoid Colon with Extraluminal Device, Percutaneous Approach
0DVN3DZ Restriction of Sigmoid Colon with Intraluminal Device, Percutaneous Approach
0DVN3ZZ Restriction of Sigmoid Colon, Percutaneous Approach
0DVN4CZ Restriction of Sigmoid Colon with Extraluminal Device, Percutaneous Endoscopic Approach
0DVN4DZ Restriction of Sigmoid Colon with Intraluminal Device, Percutaneous Endoscopic Approach
0DVN4ZZ Restriction of Sigmoid Colon, Percutaneous Endoscopic Approach
0DVN7DZ Restriction of Sigmoid Colon with Intraluminal Device, Via Natural or Artificial Opening
0DVN7ZZ Restriction of Sigmoid Colon, Via Natural or Artificial Opening
0DVN8DZ Restriction of Sigmoid Colon with Intraluminal Device, Via Natural or Artificial Opening Endoscopic
0DVN8ZZ Restriction of Sigmoid Colon, Via Natural or Artificial Opening Endoscopic
0DVP0CZ Restriction of Rectum with Extraluminal Device, Open Approach
0DVP0DZ Restriction of Rectum with Intraluminal Device, Open Approach
0DVP0ZZ Restriction of Rectum, Open Approach
0DVP3CZ Restriction of Rectum with Extraluminal Device, Percutaneous Approach
0DVP3DZ Restriction of Rectum with Intraluminal Device, Percutaneous Approach
0DVP3ZZ Restriction of Rectum, Percutaneous Approach
0DVP4CZ Restriction of Rectum with Extraluminal Device, Percutaneous Endoscopic Approach
0DVP4DZ Restriction of Rectum with Intraluminal Device, Percutaneous Endoscopic Approach
0DVP4ZZ Restriction of Rectum, Percutaneous Endoscopic Approach
0DVP7DZ Restriction of Rectum with Intralumi Device, Via Natural or Artificial Opening
0DVP7ZZ Restriction of Rectum, Via Natural or Artificial Opening
0DVP8DZ Restriction of Rectum with Intralumir Device, Via Natural or Artificial Open Endoscopic
0DVP8ZZ Restriction of Rectum, Via Natural or Artificial Opening Endoscopic
0DVQ0CZ Restriction of Anus with Extraluminal Device, Open Approach
0DVQ0DZ Restriction of Anus with Intraluminal Device, Open Approach
0DVQ0ZZ Restriction of Anus, Open Approach
0DVQ3CZ Restriction of Anus with Extraluminal Device, Percutaneous Approach
0DVQ3DZ Restriction of Anus with Intraluminal Device, Percutaneous Approach
0DVQ3ZZ Restriction of Anus, Percutaneous Approach
0DVQ4CZ Restriction of Anus with Extraluminal Device, Percutaneous Endoscopic Approach
0DVQ4DZ Restriction of Anus with Intraluminal Device, Percutaneous Endoscopic Approach
0DVQ4ZZ Restriction of Anus, Percutaneous Endoscopic Approach
0DVQ7DZ Restriction of Anus with Intraluminal Device, Via Natural or Artificial Opening
0DVQ7ZZ Restriction of Anus, Via Natural or Artificial Opening
0DVQ8DZ Restriction of Anus with Intraluminal Device, Via Natural or Artificial Openi Endoscopic
0DVQ8ZZ Restriction of Anus, Via Natural or Artificial Opening Endoscopic
0DVQXCZ Restriction of Anus with Extraluminal Device, External Approach
0DVQXDZ Restriction of Anus with Intraluminal Device, External Approach
0DVQXZZ Restriction of Anus, External Approach

0DW – Gastrointestinal System, Revision

Review Coding Guideline B6.1c

0DW000Z Revision of Drainage Device in Upper Intestinal Tract, Open Approach
0DW002Z Revision of Monitoring Device in Upper Intestinal Tract, Open Approach
0DW003Z Revision of Infusion Device in Upper Intestinal Tract, Open Approach
0DW007Z Revision of Autologous Tissue Substitute in Upper Intestinal Tract, Open Approach
0DW00CZ Revision of Extraluminal Device in Upper Intestinal Tract, Open Approach
0DW00DZ Revision of Intraluminal Device in Upper Intestinal Tract, Open Approach
0DW00JZ Revision of Synthetic Substitute in Upper Intestinal Tract, Open Approach
0DW00KZ Revision of Nonautologous Tissue Substitute in Upper Intestinal Tract, Open Approach
0DW00UZ Revision of Feeding Device in Upper Intestinal Tract, Open Approach
0DW030Z Revision of Drainage Device in Upper Intestinal Tract, Percutaneous Approach
0DW032Z Revision of Monitoring Device in Upper Intestinal Tract, Percutaneous Approach
0DW033Z Revision of Infusion Device in Upper Intestinal Tract, Percutaneous Approach
0DW037Z Revision of Autologous Tissue Substitute in Upper Intestinal Tract, Percutaneous Approach
0DW03CZ Revision of Extraluminal Device in Upper Intestinal Tract, Percutaneous Approach
0DW03DZ Revision of Intraluminal Device in Upper Intestinal Tract, Percutaneous Approach
0DW03JZ Revision of Synthetic Substitute in Upper Intestinal Tract, Percutaneous Approach
0DW03KZ Revision of Nonautologous Tissue Substitute in Upper Intestinal Tract, Percutaneous Approach
0DW03UZ Revision of Feeding Device in Upper Intestinal Tract, Percutaneous Approach
0DW040Z Revision of Drainage Device in Upper Intestinal Tract, Percutaneous Endoscopic Approach
0DW042Z Revision of Monitoring Device in Upper Intestinal Tract, Percutaneous Endoscopic Approach
0DW043Z Revision of Infusion Device in Upper Intestinal Tract, Percutaneous Endoscopic Approach
0DW047Z Revision of Autologous Tissue Substitute in Upper Intestinal Tract, Percutaneous Endoscopic Approach
0DW04CZ Revision of Extraluminal Device in Upper Intestinal Tract, Percutaneous Endoscopic Approach
0DW04DZ Revision of Intraluminal Device in Upper Intestinal Tract, Percutaneous Endoscopic Approach
0DW04JZ Revision of Synthetic Substitute in Upper Intestinal Tract, Percutaneous Endoscopic Approach
0DW04KZ Revision of Nonautologous Tissue Substitute in Upper Intestinal Tract, Percutaneous Endoscopic Approach
0DW04UZ Revision of Feeding Device in Upper Intestinal Tract, Percutaneous Endoscopic Approach
0DW070Z Revision of Drainage Device in Upper Intestinal Tract, Via Natural or Artificial Opening

/072Z Revision of Monitoring Device in Upper Intestinal Tract, Via Natural or Artificial Opening
/073Z Revision of Infusion Device in Upper Intestinal Tract, Via Natural or Artificial Opening
/077Z Revision of Autologous Tissue Substitute in Upper Intestinal Tract, Via Natural or Artificial Opening
V07CZ Revision of Extraluminal Device in Upper Intestinal Tract, Via Natural or Artificial Opening
V07DZ Revision of Intraluminal Device in Upper Intestinal Tract, Via Natural or Artificial Opening
V07JZ Revision of Synthetic Substitute in Upper Intestinal Tract, Via Natural or Artificial Opening
V07KZ Revision of Nonautologous Tissue Substitute in Upper Intestinal Tract, Via Natural or Artificial Opening
V07UZ Revision of Feeding Device in Upper Intestinal Tract, Via Natural or Artificial Opening
V080Z Revision of Drainage Device in Upper Intestinal Tract, Via Natural or Artificial Opening Endoscopic
V082Z Revision of Monitoring Device in Upper Intestinal Tract, Via Natural or Artificial Opening Endoscopic
W083Z Revision of Infusion Device in Upper Intestinal Tract, Via Natural or Artificial Opening Endoscopic
W087Z Revision of Autologous Tissue Substitute in Upper Intestinal Tract, Via Natural or Artificial Opening Endoscopic
W08CZ Revision of Extraluminal Device in Upper Intestinal Tract, Via Natural or Artificial Opening Endoscopic
W08DZ Revision of Intraluminal Device in Upper Intestinal Tract, Via Natural or Artificial Opening Endoscopic
W08JZ Revision of Synthetic Substitute in Upper Intestinal Tract, Via Natural or Artificial Opening Endoscopic
W08KZ Revision of Nonautologous Tissue Substitute in Upper Intestinal Tract, Via Natural or Artificial Opening Endoscopic
W08UZ Revision of Feeding Device in Upper Intestinal Tract, Via Natural or Artificial Opening Endoscopic
W0X0Z Revision of Drainage Device in Upper Intestinal Tract, External Approach
W0X2Z Revision of Monitoring Device in Upper Intestinal Tract, External Approach
W0X3Z Revision of Infusion Device in Upper Intestinal Tract, External Approach
W0X7Z Revision of Autologous Tissue Substitute in Upper Intestinal Tract, External Approach
DW0XCZ Revision of Extraluminal Device in Upper Intestinal Tract, External Approach
DW0XDZ Revision of Intraluminal Device in Upper Intestinal Tract, External Approach
DW0XJZ Revision of Synthetic Substitute in Upper Intestinal Tract, External Approach
DW0XKZ Revision of Nonautologous Tissue Substitute in Upper Intestinal Tract, External Approach
DW0XUZ Revision of Feeding Device in Upper Intestinal Tract, External Approach
DW57DZ Revision of Intraluminal Device in Esophagus, Via Natural or Artificial Opening
0DW58DZ Revision of Intraluminal Device in Esophagus, Via Natural or Artificial Opening Endoscopic
0DW5XDZ Revision of Intraluminal Device in Esophagus, External Approach
0DW600Z Revision of Drainage Device in Stomach, Open Approach
0DW602Z Revision of Monitoring Device in Stomach, Open Approach
0DW603Z Revision of Infusion Device in Stomach, Open Approach
0DW607Z Revision of Autologous Tissue Substitute in Stomach, Open Approach
0DW60CZ Revision of Extraluminal Device in Stomach, Open Approach
0DW60DZ Revision of Intraluminal Device in Stomach, Open Approach
0DW60JZ Revision of Synthetic Substitute in Stomach, Open Approach
0DW60KZ Revision of Nonautologous Tissue Substitute in Stomach, Open Approach
0DW60MZ Revision of Stimulator Lead in Stomach, Open Approach
0DW60UZ Revision of Feeding Device in Stomach, Open Approach
0DW630Z Revision of Drainage Device in Stomach, Percutaneous Approach
0DW632Z Revision of Monitoring Device in Stomach, Percutaneous Approach
0DW633Z Revision of Infusion Device in Stomach, Percutaneous Approach
0DW637Z Revision of Autologous Tissue Substitute in Stomach, Percutaneous Approach
0DW63CZ Revision of Extraluminal Device in Stomach, Percutaneous Approach
0DW63DZ Revision of Intraluminal Device in Stomach, Percutaneous Approach
0DW63JZ Revision of Synthetic Substitute in Stomach, Percutaneous Approach
0DW63KZ Revision of Nonautologous Tissue Substitute in Stomach, Percutaneous Approach
0DW63MZ Revision of Stimulator Lead in Stomach, Percutaneous Approach
0DW63UZ Revision of Feeding Device in Stomach, Percutaneous Approach
0DW640Z Revision of Drainage Device in Stomach, Percutaneous Endoscopic Approach
0DW642Z Revision of Monitoring Device in Stomach, Percutaneous Endoscopic Approach
0DW643Z Revision of Infusion Device in Stomach, Percutaneous Endoscopic Approach
0DW647Z Revision of Autologous Tissue Substitute in Stomach, Percutaneous Endoscopic Approach
0DW64CZ Revision of Extraluminal Device in Stomach, Percutaneous Endoscopic Approach
0DW64DZ Revision of Intraluminal Device in Stomach, Percutaneous Endoscopic Approach
0DW64JZ Revision of Synthetic Substitute in Stomach, Percutaneous Endoscopic Approach
0DW64KZ Revision of Nonautologous Tissue Substitute in Stomach, Percutaneous Endoscopic Approach
0DW64MZ Revision of Stimulator Lead in Stomach, Percutaneous Endoscopic Approach
0DW64UZ Revision of Feeding Device in Stomach, Percutaneous Endoscopic Approach
0DW670Z Revision of Drainage Device in Stomach, Via Natural or Artificial Opening
0DW672Z Revision of Monitoring Device in Stomach, Via Natural or Artificial Opening
0DW673Z Revision of Infusion Device in Stomach, Via Natural or Artificial Opening
0DW677Z Revision of Autologous Tissue Substitute in Stomach, Via Natural or Artificial Opening
0DW67CZ Revision of Extraluminal Device in Stomach, Via Natural or Artificial Opening
0DW67DZ Revision of Intraluminal Device in Stomach, Via Natural or Artificial Opening
0DW67JZ Revision of Synthetic Substitute in Stomach, Via Natural or Artificial Opening
0DW67KZ Revision of Nonautologous Tissue Substitute in Stomach, Via Natural or Artificial Opening
0DW67UZ Revision of Feeding Device in Stomach, Via Natural or Artificial Opening
0DW680Z Revision of Drainage Device in Stomach, Via Natural or Artificial Opening Endoscopic
0DW682Z Revision of Monitoring Device in Stomach, Via Natural or Artificial Opening Endoscopic
0DW683Z Revision of Infusion Device in Stomach, Via Natural or Artificial Opening Endoscopic
0DW687Z Revision of Autologous Tissue Substitute in Stomach, Via Natural or Artificial Opening Endoscopic
0DW68CZ Revision of Extraluminal Device in Stomach, Via Natural or Artificial Opening Endoscopic
0DW68DZ Revision of Intraluminal Device in Stomach, Via Natural or Artificial Opening Endoscopic
0DW68JZ Revision of Synthetic Substitute in Stomach, Via Natural or Artificial Opening Endoscopic
0DW68KZ Revision of Nonautologous Tissue Substitute in Stomach, Via Natural or Artificial Opening Endoscopic
0DW68UZ Revision of Feeding Device in Stomach, Via Natural or Artificial Opening Endoscopic
0DW6X0Z Revision of Drainage Device in Stomach, External Approach
0DW6X2Z Revision of Monitoring Device in Stomach, External Approach
0DW6X3Z Revision of Infusion Device in Stomach, External Approach
0DW6X7Z Revision of Autologous Tissue Substitute in Stomach, External Approach
0DW6XCZ Revision of Extraluminal Device in Stomach, External Approach
0DW6XDZ Revision of Intraluminal Device in Stomach, External Approach
0DW6XJZ Revision of Synthetic Substitute in Stomach, External Approach
0DW6XKZ Revision of Nonautologous Tissue Substitute in Stomach, External Approach
0DW6XUZ Revision of Feeding Device in Stomach, External Approach
0DW807Z Revision of Autologous Tissue Substitute in Small Intestine, Open Approach
0DW80JZ Revision of Synthetic Substitute in Small Intestine, Open Approach
0DW80KZ Revision of Nonautologous Tissue Substitute in Small Intestine, Open Approach
0DW847Z Revision of Autologous Tissue Substitute in Small Intestine, Percutaneous Endoscopic Approach

0DW84JZ Revision of Synthetic Substitute in Small Intestine, Percutaneous Endoscopic Approach

0DW84KZ Revision of Nonautologous Tissue Substitute in Small Intestine, Percutaneous Endoscopic Approach

0DW877Z Revision of Autologous Tissue Substitute in Small Intestine, Via Natural or Artificial Opening

0DW87JZ Revision of Synthetic Substitute in Small Intestine, Via Natural or Artificial Opening

0DW87KZ Revision of Nonautologous Tissue Substitute in Small Intestine, Via Natural or Artificial Opening

0DW887Z Revision of Autologous Tissue Substitute in Small Intestine, Via Natural or Artificial Opening Endoscopic

0DW88JZ Revision of Synthetic Substitute in Small Intestine, Via Natural or Artificial Opening Endoscopic

0DW88KZ Revision of Nonautologous Tissue Substitute in Small Intestine, Via Natural or Artificial Opening Endoscopic

0DWD00Z Revision of Drainage Device in Lower Intestinal Tract, Open Approach

0DWD02Z Revision of Monitoring Device in Lower Intestinal Tract, Open Approach

0DWD03Z Revision of Infusion Device in Lower Intestinal Tract, Open Approach

0DWD07Z Revision of Autologous Tissue Substitute in Lower Intestinal Tract, Open Approach

0DWD0CZ Revision of Extraluminal Device in Lower Intestinal Tract, Open Approach

0DWD0DZ Revision of Intraluminal Device in Lower Intestinal Tract, Open Approach

0DWD0JZ Revision of Synthetic Substitute in Lower Intestinal Tract, Open Approach

0DWD0KZ Revision of Nonautologous Tissue Substitute in Lower Intestinal Tract, Open Approach

0DWD0UZ Revision of Feeding Device in Lower Intestinal Tract, Open Approach

0DWD30Z Revision of Drainage Device in Lower Intestinal Tract, Percutaneous Approach

0DWD32Z Revision of Monitoring Device in Lower Intestinal Tract, Percutaneous Approach

0DWD33Z Revision of Infusion Device in Lower Intestinal Tract, Percutaneous Approach

0DWD37Z Revision of Autologous Tissue Substitute in Lower Intestinal Tract, Percutaneous Approach

0DWD3CZ Revision of Extraluminal Device in Lower Intestinal Tract, Percutaneous Approach

0DWD3DZ Revision of Intraluminal Device in Lower Intestinal Tract, Percutaneous Approach

0DWD3JZ Revision of Synthetic Substitute in Lower Intestinal Tract, Percutaneous Approach

0DWD3KZ Revision of Nonautologous Tissue Substitute in Lower Intestinal Tract, Percutaneous Approach

0DWD3UZ Revision of Feeding Device in Lower Intestinal Tract, Percutaneous Approach

0DWD40Z Revision of Drainage Device in Lower Intestinal Tract, Percutaneous Endoscopic Approach

0DWD42Z Revision of Monitoring Device in Lower Intestinal Tract, Percutaneous Endoscopic Approach

0DWD43Z Revision of Infusion Device in Lower Intestinal Tract, Percutaneous Endoscopic Approach

0DWD47Z Revision of Autologous Tissue Substitute in Lower Intestinal Tract, Percutaneous Endoscopic Approach

0DWD4CZ Revision of Extraluminal Device in Lower Intestinal Tract, Percutaneous Endoscopic Approach

0DWD4DZ Revision of Intraluminal Device in Lower Intestinal Tract, Percutaneous Endoscopic Approach

0DWD4JZ Revision of Synthetic Substitute in Lower Intestinal Tract, Percutaneous Endoscopic Approach

0DWD4KZ Revision of Nonautologous Tissue Substitute in Lower Intestinal Tract, Percutaneous Endoscopic Approach

0DWD4UZ Revision of Feeding Device in Lower Intestinal Tract, Percutaneous Endoscopic Approach

0DWD70Z Revision of Drainage Device in Lower Intestinal Tract, Via Natural or Artificial Opening

0DWD72Z Revision of Monitoring Device in Lower Intestinal Tract, Via Natural or Artificial Opening

0DWD73Z Revision of Infusion Device in Lower Intestinal Tract, Via Natural or Artificial Opening

0DWD77Z Revision of Autologous Tissue Substitute in Lower Intestinal Tract, Via Natural or Artificial Opening

0DWD7CZ Revision of Extraluminal Device in Lower Intestinal Tract, Via Natural or Artificial Opening

0DWD7DZ Revision of Intraluminal Device in Lower Intestinal Tract, Via Natural or Artificial Opening

0DWD7JZ Revision of Synthetic Substitute in Lower Intestinal Tract, Via Natural or Artificial Opening

0DWD7KZ Revision of Nonautologous Tissue Substitute in Lower Intestinal Tract, Via Natural or Artificial Opening

0DWD7UZ Revision of Feeding Device in Lower Intestinal Tract, Via Natural or Artificial Opening

0DWD80Z Revision of Drainage Device in Lower Intestinal Tract, Via Natural or Artificial Opening Endoscopic

0DWD82Z Revision of Monitoring Device in Lower Intestinal Tract, Via Natural or Artificial Opening Endoscopic

0DWD83Z Revision of Infusion Device in Lower Intestinal Tract, Via Natural or Artificial Opening Endoscopic

0DWD87Z Revision of Autologous Tissue Substitute in Lower Intestinal Tract, Via Natural or Artificial Opening Endoscopic

0DWD8CZ Revision of Extraluminal Device in Lower Intestinal Tract, Via Natural or Artificial Opening Endoscopic

0DWD8DZ Revision of Intraluminal Device in Lower Intestinal Tract, Via Natural or Artificial Opening Endoscopic

0DWD8JZ Revision of Synthetic Substitute in Lower Intestinal Tract, Via Natural or Artificial Opening Endoscopic

0DWD8KZ Revision of Nonautologous Tissue Substitute in Lower Intestinal Tract, Via Natural or Artificial Opening Endoscopic

0DWD8UZ Revision of Feeding Device in Lower Intestinal Tract, Via Natural or Artificial Opening Endoscopic

0DWDX0Z Revision of Drainage Device in Lower Intestinal Tract, External Approach

0DWDX2Z Revision of Monitoring Device in Lower Intestinal Tract, External Approach

0DWDX3Z Revision of Infusion Device in Lowe Intestinal Tract, External Approach

0DWDX7Z Revision of Autologous Tissue Substitute in Lower Intestinal Tract, External Approach

0DWDXCZ Revision of Extraluminal Device in Lower Intestinal Tract, External Approach

0DWDXDZ Revision of Intraluminal Device in Lower Intestinal Tract, External Approach

0DWDXJZ Revision of Synthetic Substitute in Lc Intestinal Tract, External Approach

0DWDXKZ Revision of Nonautologous Tissue Substitute in Lower Intestinal Tract, External Approach

0DWDXUZ Revision of Feeding Device in Lower Intestinal Tract, External Approach

0DWE07Z Revision of Autologous Tissue Substi in Large Intestine, Open Approach

0DWE0JZ Revision of Synthetic Substitute in La Intestine, Open Approach

0DWE0KZ Revision of Nonautologous Tissue Substitute in Large Intestine, Open Approach

0DWE47Z Revision of Autologous Tissue Substit in Large Intestine, Percutaneous Endoscopic Approach

0DWE4JZ Revision of Synthetic Substitute in La Intestine, Percutaneous Endoscopic Approach

0DWE4KZ Revision of Nonautologous Tissue Substitute in Large Intestine, Percutaneous Endoscopic Approach

0DWE77Z Revision of Autologous Tissue Substit in Large Intestine, Via Natural or Artificial Opening

0DWE7JZ Revision of Synthetic Substitute in Large Intestine, Via Natural or Artificia Opening

0DWE7KZ Revision of Nonautologous Tissue Substitute in Large Intestine, Via Natur or Artificial Opening

0DWE87Z Revision of Autologous Tissue Substitu in Large Intestine, Via Natural or Artificial Opening Endoscopic

0DWE8JZ Revision of Synthetic Substitute in Large Intestine, Via Natural or Artificia Opening Endoscopic

0DWE8KZ Revision of Nonautologous Tissue Substitute in Large Intestine, Via Natur or Artificial Opening Endoscopic

0DWQ0LZ Revision of Artificial Sphincter in Anus Open Approach

0DWQ3LZ Revision of Artificial Sphincter in Anus Percutaneous Approach

0DWQ4LZ Revision of Artificial Sphincter in Anus Percutaneous Endoscopic Approach

0DWQ7LZ Revision of Artificial Sphincter in Anus Via Natural or Artificial Opening

0DWQ8LZ Revision of Artificial Sphincter in Anus, Via Natural or Artificial Opening Endoscopic

0DWR0MZ Revision of Stimulator Lead in Anal Sphincter, Open Approach

0DWR3MZ Revision of Stimulator Lead in Anal Sphincter, Percutaneous Approach

0DWR4MZ Revision of Stimulator Lead in Anal Sphincter, Percutaneous Endoscopic Approach

0DWU00Z Revision of Drainage Device in Omentum, Open Approach

0DWU07Z Revision of Autologous Tissue Substitut in Omentum, Open Approach

VU0JZ Revision of Synthetic Substitute in Omentum, Open Approach
VU0KZ Revision of Nonautologous Tissue Substitute in Omentum, Open Approach
VU30Z Revision of Drainage Device in Omentum, Percutaneous Approach
VU37Z Revision of Autologous Tissue Substitute in Omentum, Percutaneous Approach
VU3JZ Revision of Synthetic Substitute in Omentum, Percutaneous Approach
VU3KZ Revision of Nonautologous Tissue Substitute in Omentum, Percutaneous Approach
VU40Z Revision of Drainage Device in Omentum, Percutaneous Endoscopic Approach
VU47Z Revision of Autologous Tissue Substitute in Omentum, Percutaneous Endoscopic Approach
WU4JZ Revision of Synthetic Substitute in Omentum, Percutaneous Endoscopic Approach
WU4KZ Revision of Nonautologous Tissue Substitute in Omentum, Percutaneous Endoscopic Approach
WV00Z Revision of Drainage Device in Mesentery, Open Approach
WV07Z Revision of Autologous Tissue Substitute in Mesentery, Open Approach
0DWV0JZ Revision of Synthetic Substitute in Mesentery, Open Approach
0DWV0KZ Revision of Nonautologous Tissue Substitute in Mesentery, Open Approach
0DWV30Z Revision of Drainage Device in Mesentery, Percutaneous Approach
0DWV37Z Revision of Autologous Tissue Substitute in Mesentery, Percutaneous Approach
0DWV3JZ Revision of Synthetic Substitute in Mesentery, Percutaneous Approach
0DWV3KZ Revision of Nonautologous Tissue Substitute in Mesentery, Percutaneous Approach
0DWV40Z Revision of Drainage Device in Mesentery, Percutaneous Endoscopic Approach
0DWV47Z Revision of Autologous Tissue Substitute in Mesentery, Percutaneous Endoscopic Approach
0DWV4JZ Revision of Synthetic Substitute in Mesentery, Percutaneous Endoscopic Approach
0DWV4KZ Revision of Nonautologous Tissue Substitute in Mesentery, Percutaneous Endoscopic Approach
0DWW00Z Revision of Drainage Device in Peritoneum, Open Approach
0DWW07Z Revision of Autologous Tissue Substitute in Peritoneum, Open Approach
0DWW0JZ Revision of Synthetic Substitute in Peritoneum, Open Approach
0DWW0KZ Revision of Nonautologous Tissue Substitute in Peritoneum, Open Approach
0DWW30Z Revision of Drainage Device in Peritoneum, Percutaneous Approach
0DWW37Z Revision of Autologous Tissue Substitute in Peritoneum, Percutaneous Approach
0DWW3JZ Revision of Synthetic Substitute in Peritoneum, Percutaneous Approach
0DWW3KZ Revision of Nonautologous Tissue Substitute in Peritoneum, Percutaneous Approach
0DWW40Z Revision of Drainage Device in Peritoneum, Percutaneous Endoscopic Approach
0DWW47Z Revision of Autologous Tissue Substitute in Peritoneum, Percutaneous Endoscopic Approach
0DWW4JZ Revision of Synthetic Substitute in Peritoneum, Percutaneous Endoscopic Approach
0DWW4KZ Revision of Nonautologous Tissue Substitute in Peritoneum, Percutaneous Endoscopic Approach

)X – Gastrointestinal System, Transfer

X60Z5 Transfer Stomach to Esophagus, Open Approach
X64Z5 Transfer Stomach to Esophagus, Percutaneous Endoscopic Approach
0DX80Z5 Transfer Small Intestine to Esophagus, Open Approach
0DX84Z5 Transfer Small Intestine to Esophagus, Percutaneous Endoscopic Approach
0DXE0Z5 Transfer Large Intestine to Esophagus, Open Approach
0DXE4Z5 Transfer Large Intestine to Esophagus, Percutaneous Endoscopic Approach

)Y – Gastrointestinal System, Transplantation

view Coding Guideline B3.16

Y50Z0 Transplantation of Esophagus, Allogeneic, Open Approach
Y50Z1 Transplantation of Esophagus, Syngeneic, Open Approach
Y50Z2 Transplantation of Esophagus, Zooplastic, Open Approach
Y60Z0 Transplantation of Stomach, Allogeneic, Open Approach
0DY60Z1 Transplantation of Stomach, Syngeneic, Open Approach
0DY60Z2 Transplantation of Stomach, Zooplastic, Open Approach
0DY80Z0 Transplantation of Small Intestine, Allogeneic, Open Approach
0DY80Z1 Transplantation of Small Intestine, Syngeneic, Open Approach
0DY80Z2 Transplantation of Small Intestine, Zooplastic, Open Approach
0DYE0Z0 Transplantation of Large Intestine, Allogeneic, Open Approach
0DYE0Z1 Transplantation of Large Intestine, Syngeneic, Open Approach`
0DYE0Z2 Transplantation of Large Intestine, Zooplastic, Open Approach

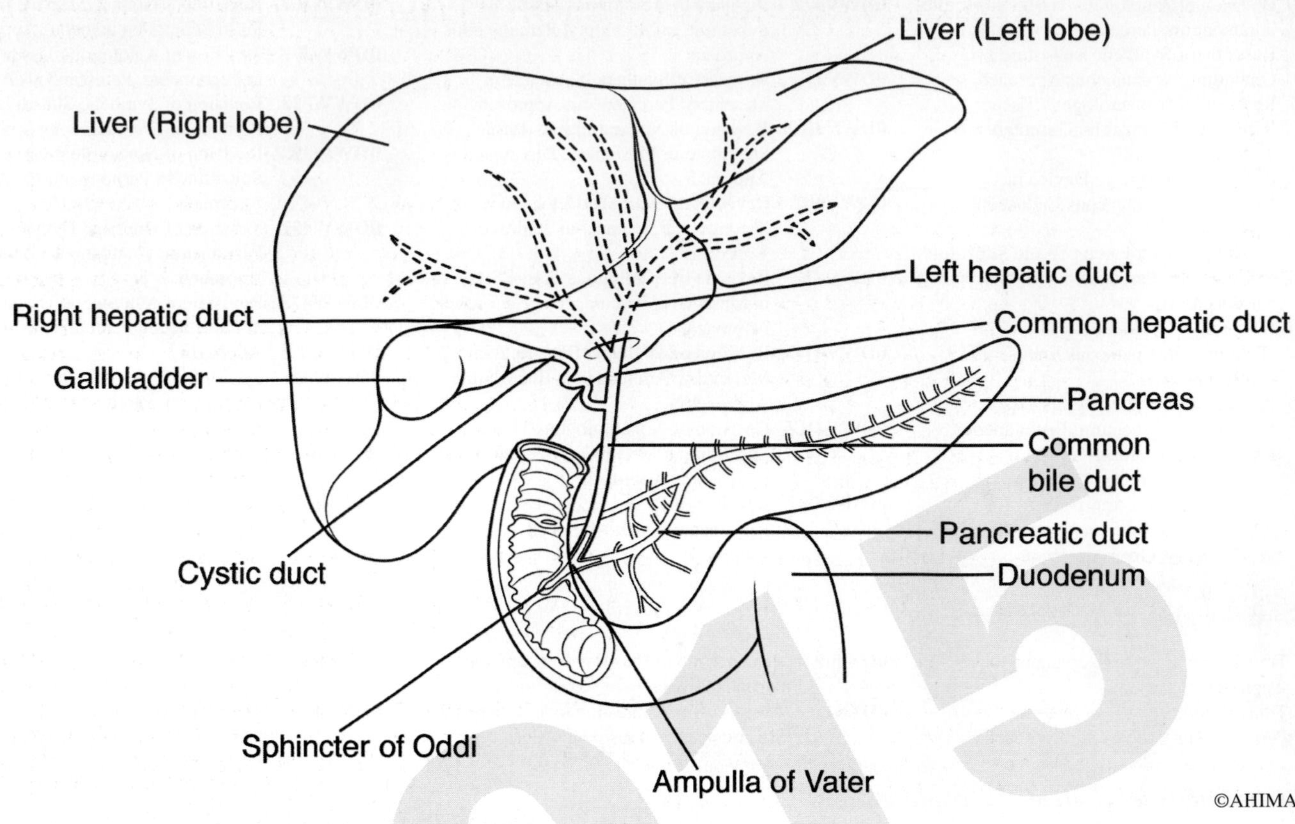
Hepatobiliary System and Pancreas
Liver (Left lobe)
Liver (Right lobe)
Left hepatic duct
Right hepatic duct
Common hepatic duct
Gallbladder
Pancreas
Common
bile duct
Pancreatic duct
Cystic duct
Duodenum
Sphincter of Oddi
Ampulla of Vater
©AHIMA

tion	**0**	**Medical and Surgical**
y System	**F**	**Hepatobiliary System and Pancreas**
ration	**1**	**Bypass:** Altering the route of passage of the contents of a tubular body part

Body Part (4th)	Approach (5th)	Device (6th)	Qualifier (7th)
Gallbladder Hepatic Duct, Right Hepatic Duct, Left Cystic Duct Common Bile Duct	**0** Open **4** Percutaneous Endoscopic	**D** Intraluminal Device **Z** No Device	**3** Duodenum **4** Stomach **5** Hepatic Duct, Right **6** Hepatic Duct, Left **7** Hepatic Duct, Caudate **8** Cystic Duct **9** Common Bile Duct **B** Small Intestine
Pancreatic Duct Pancreatic Duct, Accessory Pancreas	**0** Open **4** Percutaneous Endoscopic	**D** Intraluminal Device **Z** No Device	**3** Duodenum **B** Small Intestine **C** Large Intestine

tion	**0**	**Medical and Surgical**
dy System	**F**	**Hepatobiliary System and Pancreas**
eration	**2**	**Change:** Taking out or off a device from a body part and putting back an identical or similar device in or on the same body part without cutting or puncturing the skin or a mucous membrane

Body Part (4th)	Approach (5th)	Device (6th)	Qualifier (7th)
Liver Gallbladder **B** Hepatobiliary Duct **D** Pancreatic Duct **G** Pancreas	**X** External	**0** Drainage Device **Y** Other Device	**Z** No Qualifier

ction	**0**	**Medical and Surgical**
dy System	**F**	**Hepatobiliary System and Pancreas**
eration	**5**	**Destruction:** Physical eradication of all or a portion of a body part by the direct use of energy, force, or a destructive agent

Body Part (4th)	Approach (5th)	Device (6th)	Qualifier (7th)
0 Liver **1** Liver, Right Lobe **2** Liver, Left Lobe **4** Gallbladder **G** Pancreas	**0** Open **3** Percutaneous **4** Percutaneous Endoscopic	**Z** No Device	**Z** No Qualifier
5 Hepatic Duct, Right **6** Hepatic Duct, Left **8** Cystic Duct **9** Common Bile Duct **C** Ampulla of Vater **D** Pancreatic Duct **F** Pancreatic Duct, Accessory	**0** Open **3** Percutaneous **4** Percutaneous Endoscopic **7** Via Natural or Artificial Opening **8** Via Natural or Artificial Opening Endoscopic	**Z** No Device	**Z** No Qualifier

ction	**0**	**Medical and Surgical**
dy System	**F**	**Hepatobiliary System and Pancreas**
peration	**7**	**Dilation:** Expanding an orifice or the lumen of a tubular body part

Body Part (4th)	Approach (5th)	Device (6th)	Qualifier (7th)
5 Hepatic Duct, Right **6** Hepatic Duct, Left **8** Cystic Duct **9** Common Bile Duct **C** Ampulla of Vater **D** Pancreatic Duct **F** Pancreatic Duct, Accessory	**0** Open **3** Percutaneous **4** Percutaneous Endoscopic **7** Via Natural or Artificial Opening **8** Via Natural or Artificial Opening Endoscopic	**D** Intraluminal Device **Z** No Device	**Z** No Qualifier

Section 0 **Medical and Surgical**
Body System F **Hepatobiliary System and Pancreas**
Operation 8 **Division:** Cutting into a body part, without draining fluids and/or gases from the body part, in order to separate or transect a body part

Body Part (4th)	Approach (5th)	Device (6th)	Qualifier (7th)
G Pancreas	0 Open 3 Percutaneous 4 Percutaneous Endoscopic	Z No Device	Z No Qualifier

Section 0 **Medical and Surgical**
Body System F **Hepatobiliary System and Pancreas**
Operation 9 **Drainage:** Taking or letting out fluids and/or gases from a body part

Body Part (4th)	Approach (5th)	Device (6th)	Qualifier (7th)
0 Liver 1 Liver, Right Lobe 2 Liver, Left Lobe 4 Gallbladder G Pancreas	0 Open 3 Percutaneous 4 Percutaneous Endoscopic	0 Drainage Device	Z No Qualifier
0 Liver 1 Liver, Right Lobe 2 Liver, Left Lobe 4 Gallbladder G Pancreas	0 Open 3 Percutaneous 4 Percutaneous Endoscopic	Z No Device	X Diagnostic Z No Qualifier
5 Hepatic Duct, Right 6 Hepatic Duct, Left 8 Cystic Duct 9 Common Bile Duct C Ampulla of Vater D Pancreatic Duct F Pancreatic Duct, Accessory	0 Open 3 Percutaneous 4 Percutaneous Endoscopic 7 Via Natural or Artificial Opening 8 Via Natural or Artificial Opening Endoscopic	0 Drainage Device	Z No Qualifier
5 Hepatic Duct, Right 6 Hepatic Duct, Left 8 Cystic Duct 9 Common Bile Duct C Ampulla of Vater D Pancreatic Duct F Pancreatic Duct, Accessory	0 Open 3 Percutaneous 4 Percutaneous Endoscopic 7 Via Natural or Artificial Opening 8 Via Natural or Artificial Opening Endoscopic	Z No Device	X Diagnostic Z No Qualifier

Section 0 **Medical and Surgical**
Body System F **Hepatobiliary System and Pancreas**
Operation B **Excision:** Cutting out or off, without replacement, a portion of a body part

Body Part (4th)	Approach (5th)	Device (6th)	Qualifier (7th)
0 Liver 1 Liver, Right Lobe 2 Liver, Left Lobe 4 Gallbladder G Pancreas	0 Open 3 Percutaneous 4 Percutaneous Endoscopic	Z No Device	X Diagnostic Z No Qualifier
5 Hepatic Duct, Right 6 Hepatic Duct, Left 8 Cystic Duct 9 Common Bile Duct C Ampulla of Vater D Pancreatic Duct F Pancreatic Duct, Accessory	0 Open 3 Percutaneous 4 Percutaneous Endoscopic 7 Via Natural or Artificial Opening 8 Via Natural or Artificial Opening Endoscopic	Z No Device	X Diagnostic Z No Qualifier

tion 0 **Medical and Surgical**
ly System F **Hepatobiliary System and Pancreas**
eration C **Extirpation:** Taking or cutting out solid matter from a body part

Body Part (4th)	Approach (5th)	Device (6th)	Qualifier (7th)
Liver Liver, Right Lobe Liver, Left Lobe Gallbladder Pancreas	**0** Open **3** Percutaneous **4** Percutaneous Endoscopic	**Z** No Device	**Z** No Qualifier
Hepatic Duct, Right Hepatic Duct, Left Cystic Duct Common Bile Duct Ampulla of Vater Pancreatic Duct Pancreatic Duct, Accessory	**0** Open **3** Percutaneous **4** Percutaneous Endoscopic **7** Via Natural or Artificial Opening **8** Via Natural or Artificial Opening Endoscopic	**Z** No Device	**Z** No Qualifier

ction 0 **Medical and Surgical**
dy System F **Hepatobiliary System and Pancreas**
eration F **Fragmentation:** Breaking solid matter in a body part into pieces

Body Part (4th)	Approach (5th)	Device (6th)	Qualifier (7th)
4 Gallbladder **5** Hepatic Duct, Right **6** Hepatic Duct, Left **8** Cystic Duct **9** Common Bile Duct **C** Ampulla of Vater **D** Pancreatic Duct **F** Pancreatic Duct, Accessory	**0** Open **3** Percutaneous **4** Percutaneous Endoscopic **7** Via Natural or Artificial Opening **8** Via Natural or Artificial Opening Endoscopic **X** External	**Z** No Device	**Z** No Qualifier

ction 0 **Medical and Surgical**
ody System F **Hepatobiliary System and Pancreas**
peration H **Insertion:** Putting in a nonbiological appliance that monitors, assists, performs, or prevents a physiological function but does not physically take the place of a body part

Body Part (4th)	Approach (5th)	Device (6th)	Qualifier (7th)
0 Liver **1** Liver, Right Lobe **2** Liver, Left Lobe **4** Gallbladder **G** Pancreas	**0** Open **3** Percutaneous **4** Percutaneous Endoscopic	**2** Monitoring Device **3** Infusion Device	**Z** No Qualifier
B Hepatobiliary Duct **D** Pancreatic Duct	**0** Open **3** Percutaneous **4** Percutaneous Endoscopic **7** Via Natural or Artificial Opening **8** Via Natural or Artificial Opening Endoscopic	**1** Radioactive Element **2** Monitoring Device **3** Infusion Device **D** Intraluminal Device	**Z** No Qualifier

ection 0 **Medical and Surgical**
ody System F **Hepatobiliary System and Pancreas**
peration J **Inspection:** Visually and/or manually exploring a body part

Body Part (4th)	Approach (5th)	Device (6th)	Qualifier (7th)
0 Liver **4** Gallbladder **G** Pancreas	**0** Open **3** Percutaneous **4** Percutaneous Endoscopic **X** External	**Z** No Device	**Z** No Qualifier

Continued →

Section 0 **Medical and Surgical**
Body System F **Hepatobiliary System and Pancreas**
Operation J **Inspection:** Visually and/or manually exploring a body part

Body Part (4th)	Approach (5th)	Device (6th)	Qualifier (7th)
B Hepatobiliary Duct **D** Pancreatic Duct	**0** Open **3** Percutaneous **4** Percutaneous Endoscopic **7** Via Natural or Artificial Opening **8** Via Natural or Artificial Opening Endoscopic	**Z** No Device	**Z** No Qualifier

Section 0 **Medical and Surgical**
Body System F **Hepatobiliary System and Pancreas**
Operation L **Occlusion:** Completely closing an orifice or the lumen of a tubular body part

Body Part (4th)	Approach (5th)	Device (6th)	Qualifier (7th)
5 Hepatic Duct, Right **6** Hepatic Duct, Left **8** Cystic Duct **9** Common Bile Duct **C** Ampulla of Vater **D** Pancreatic Duct **F** Pancreatic Duct, Accessory	**0** Open **3** Percutaneous **4** Percutaneous Endoscopic	**C** Extraluminal Device **D** Intraluminal Device **Z** No Device	**Z** No Qualifier
5 Hepatic Duct, Right **6** Hepatic Duct, Left **8** Cystic Duct **9** Common Bile Duct **C** Ampulla of Vater **D** Pancreatic Duct **F** Pancreatic Duct, Accessory	**7** Via Natural or Artificial Opening **8** Via Natural or Artificial Opening Endoscopic	**D** Intraluminal Device **Z** No Device	**Z** No Qualifier

Section 0 **Medical and Surgical**
Body System F **Hepatobiliary System and Pancreas**
Operation M **Reattachment:** Putting back in or on all or a portion of a separated body part to its normal location or other suitable location

Body Part (4th)	Approach (5th)	Device (6th)	Qualifier (7th)
0 Liver **1** Liver, Right Lobe **2** Liver, Left Lobe **4** Gallbladder **5** Hepatic Duct, Right **6** Hepatic Duct, Left **8** Cystic Duct **9** Common Bile Duct **C** Ampulla of Vater **D** Pancreatic Duct **F** Pancreatic Duct, Accessory **G** Pancreas	**0** Open **4** Percutaneous Endoscopic	**Z** No Device	**Z** No Qualifier

Section 0 **Medical and Surgical**
Body System F **Hepatobiliary System and Pancreas**
Operation N **Release:** Freeing a body part from an abnormal physical constraint by cutting or by the use of force

Body Part (4th)	Approach (5th)	Device (6th)	Qualifier (7th)
0 Liver **1** Liver, Right Lobe **2** Liver, Left Lobe **4** Gallbladder **G** Pancreas	**0** Open **3** Percutaneous **4** Percutaneous Endoscopic	**Z** No Device	**Z** No Qualifier

Continued →

tion	0	**Medical and Surgical**
dy System	F	**Hepatobiliary System and Pancreas**
eration	N	**Release:** Freeing a body part from an abnormal physical constraint by cutting or by the use of force

Body Part (4th)	Approach (5th)	Device (6th)	Qualifier (7th)
Hepatic Duct, Right Hepatic Duct, Left Cystic Duct Common Bile Duct Ampulla of Vater Pancreatic Duct Pancreatic Duct, Accessory	**0** Open **3** Percutaneous **4** Percutaneous Endoscopic **7** Via Natural or Artificial Opening **8** Via Natural or Artificial Opening Endoscopic	**Z** No Device	**Z** No Qualifier

tion	0	**Medical and Surgical**
dy System	F	**Hepatobiliary System and Pancreas**
eration	P	**Removal:** Taking out or off a device from a body part

Body Part (4th)	Approach (5th)	Device (6th)	Qualifier (7th)
Liver	**0** Open **3** Percutaneous **4** Percutaneous Endoscopic **X** External	**0** Drainage Device **2** Monitoring Device **3** Infusion Device	**Z** No Qualifier
Gallbladder Pancreas	**0** Open **3** Percutaneous **4** Percutaneous Endoscopic **X** External	**0** Drainage Device **2** Monitoring Device **3** Infusion Device **D** Intraluminal Device	**Z** No Qualifier
B Hepatobiliary Duct **D** Pancreatic Duct	**0** Open **3** Percutaneous **4** Percutaneous Endoscopic **7** Via Natural or Artificial Opening **8** Via Natural or Artificial Opening Endoscopic	**0** Drainage Device **1** Radioactive Element **2** Monitoring Device **3** Infusion Device **7** Autologous Tissue Substitute **C** Extraluminal Device **D** Intraluminal Device **J** Synthetic Substitute **K** Nonautologous Tissue Substitute	**Z** No Qualifier
B Hepatobiliary Duct **D** Pancreatic Duct	**X** External	**0** Drainage Device **1** Radioactive Element **2** Monitoring Device **3** Infusion Device **D** Intraluminal Device	**Z** No Qualifier

ction	0	**Medical and Surgical**
ody System	F	**Hepatobiliary System and Pancreas**
peration	Q	**Repair:** Restoring, to the extent possible, a body part to its normal anatomic structure and function

Body Part (4th)	Approach (5th)	Device (6th)	Qualifier (7th)
0 Liver **1** Liver, Right Lobe **2** Liver, Left Lobe **4** Gallbladder **G** Pancreas	**0** Open **3** Percutaneous **4** Percutaneous Endoscopic	**Z** No Device	**Z** No Qualifier
5 Hepatic Duct, Right **6** Hepatic Duct, Left **8** Cystic Duct **9** Common Bile Duct **C** Ampulla of Vater **D** Pancreatic Duct **F** Pancreatic Duct, Accessory	**0** Open **3** Percutaneous **4** Percutaneous Endoscopic **7** Via Natural or Artificial Opening **8** Via Natural or Artificial Opening Endoscopic	**Z** No Device	**Z** No Qualifier

Section 0 **Medical and Surgical**
Body System F **Hepatobiliary System and Pancreas**
Operation R **Replacement:** Putting in or on biological or synthetic material that physically takes the place and/or function of all or a portion of a body part

Body Part (4th)	Approach (5th)	Device (6th)	Qualifier (7th)
5 Hepatic Duct, Right 6 Hepatic Duct, Left 8 Cystic Duct 9 Common Bile Duct C Ampulla of Vater D Pancreatic Duct F Pancreatic Duct, Accessory	0 Open 4 Percutaneous Endoscopic	7 Autologous Tissue Substitute J Synthetic Substitute K Nonautologous Tissue Substitute	Z No Qualifier

Section 0 **Medical and Surgical**
Body System F **Hepatobiliary System and Pancreas**
Operation S **Reposition:** Moving to its normal location, or other suitable location, all or a portion of a body part

Body Part (4th)	Approach (5th)	Device (6th)	Qualifier (7th)
0 Liver 4 Gallbladder 5 Hepatic Duct, Right 6 Hepatic Duct, Left 8 Cystic Duct 9 Common Bile Duct C Ampulla of Vater D Pancreatic Duct F Pancreatic Duct, Accessory G Pancreas	0 Open 4 Percutaneous Endoscopic	Z No Device	Z No Qualifier

Section 0 **Medical and Surgical**
Body System F **Hepatobiliary System and Pancreas**
Operation T **Resection:** Cutting out or off, without replacement, all of a body part

Body Part (4th)	Approach (5th)	Device (6th)	Qualifier (7th)
0 Liver 1 Liver, Right Lobe 2 Liver, Left Lobe 4 Gallbladder G Pancreas	0 Open 4 Percutaneous Endoscopic	Z No Device	Z No Qualifier
5 Hepatic Duct, Right 6 Hepatic Duct, Left 8 Cystic Duct 9 Common Bile Duct C Ampulla of Vater D Pancreatic Duct F Pancreatic Duct, Accessory	0 Open 4 Percutaneous Endoscopic 7 Via Natural or Artificial Opening 8 Via Natural or Artificial Opening Endoscopic	Z No Device	Z No Qualifier

Section 0 **Medical and Surgical**
Body System F **Hepatobiliary System and Pancreas**
Operation U **Supplement:** Putting in or on biological or synthetic material that physically reinforces and/or augments the function of a portion of a body part

Body Part (4th)	Approach (5th)	Device (6th)	Qualifier (7th)
5 Hepatic Duct, Right 6 Hepatic Duct, Left 8 Cystic Duct 9 Common Bile Duct C Ampulla of Vater D Pancreatic Duct F Pancreatic Duct, Accessory	0 Open 3 Percutaneous 4 Percutaneous Endoscopic	7 Autologous Tissue Substitute J Synthetic Substitute K Nonautologous Tissue Substitute	Z No Qualifier

tion	0	**Medical and Surgical**
ly System	F	**Hepatobiliary System and Pancreas**
eration	V	**Restriction:** Partially closing an orifice or the lumen of a tubular body part

Body Part (4th)	Approach (5th)	Device (6th)	Qualifier (7th)
Hepatic Duct, Right Hepatic Duct, Left Cystic Duct Common Bile Duct Ampulla of Vater Pancreatic Duct Pancreatic Duct, Accessory	**0** Open **3** Percutaneous **4** Percutaneous Endoscopic	**C** Extraluminal Device **D** Intraluminal Device **Z** No Device	**Z** No Qualifier
Hepatic Duct, Right Hepatic Duct, Left Cystic Duct Common Bile Duct C Ampulla of Vater D Pancreatic Duct Pancreatic Duct, Accessory	**7** Via Natural or Artificial Opening **8** Via Natural or Artificial Opening Endoscopic	**D** Intraluminal Device **Z** No Device	**Z** No Qualifier

ction	0	**Medical and Surgical**
dy System	F	**Hepatobiliary System and Pancreas**
eration	W	**Revision:** Correcting, to the extent possible, a portion of a malfunctioning device or the position of a displaced device

Body Part (4th)	Approach (5th)	Device (6th)	Qualifier (7th)
Liver	**0** Open **3** Percutaneous **4** Percutaneous Endoscopic **X** External	**0** Drainage Device **2** Monitoring Device **3** Infusion Device	**Z** No Qualifier
4 Gallbladder G Pancreas	**0** Open **3** Percutaneous **4** Percutaneous Endoscopic **X** External	**0** Drainage Device **2** Monitoring Device **3** Infusion Device **D** Intraluminal Device	**Z** No Qualifier
B Hepatobiliary Duct D Pancreatic Duct	**0** Open **3** Percutaneous **4** Percutaneous Endoscopic **7** Via Natural or Artificial Opening **8** Via Natural or Artificial Opening Endoscopic **X** External	**0** Drainage Device **2** Monitoring Device **3** Infusion Device **7** Autologous Tissue Substitute **C** Extraluminal Device **D** Intraluminal Device **J** Synthetic Substitute **K** Nonautologous Tissue Substitute	**Z** No Qualifier

ction	0	**Medical and Surgical**
ody System	F	**Hepatobiliary System and Pancreas**
peration	Y	**Transplantation:** Putting in or on all or a portion of a living body part taken from another individual or animal to physically take the place and/or function of all or a portion of a similar body part

Body Part (4th)	Approach (5th)	Device (6th)	Qualifier (7th)
0 Liver **G** Pancreas	**0** Open	**Z** No Device	**0** Allogeneic **1** Syngeneic **2** Zooplastic

lepatobiliary System and Pancreas Code Listing 0F1–0FY

F1 – Hepatobiliary System and Pancreas, Bypass

eview Coding Guideline B3.6a

F140D3 Bypass Gallbladder to Duodenum with Intraluminal Device, Open Approach
F140D4 Bypass Gallbladder to Stomach with Intraluminal Device, Open Approach
F140D5 Bypass Gallbladder to Right Hepatic Duct with Intraluminal Device, Open Approach
0F140D6 Bypass Gallbladder to Left Hepatic Duct with Intraluminal Device, Open Approach
0F140D7 Bypass Gallbladder to Caudate Hepatic Duct with Intraluminal Device, Open Approach
0F140D8 Bypass Gallbladder to Cystic Duct with Intraluminal Device, Open Approach
0F140D9 Bypass Gallbladder to Common Bile Duct with Intraluminal Device, Open Approach
0F140DB Bypass Gallbladder to Small Intestine with Intraluminal Device, Open Approach
0F140Z3 Bypass Gallbladder to Duodenum, Open Approach

0F140Z4 Bypass Gallbladder to Stomach, Open Approach
0F140Z5 Bypass Gallbladder to Right Hepatic Duct, Open Approach
0F140Z6 Bypass Gallbladder to Left Hepatic Duct, Open Approach
0F140Z7 Bypass Gallbladder to Caudate Hepatic Duct, Open Approach
0F140Z8 Bypass Gallbladder to Cystic Duct, Open Approach
0F140Z9 Bypass Gallbladder to Common Bile Duct, Open Approach
0F140ZB Bypass Gallbladder to Small Intestine, Open Approach
0F144D3 Bypass Gallbladder to Duodenum with Intraluminal Device, Percutaneous Endoscopic Approach
0F144D4 Bypass Gallbladder to Stomach with Intraluminal Device, Percutaneous Endoscopic Approach
0F144D5 Bypass Gallbladder to Right Hepatic Duct with Intraluminal Device, Percutaneous Endoscopic Approach
0F144D6 Bypass Gallbladder to Left Hepatic Duct with Intraluminal Device, Percutaneous Endoscopic Approach
0F144D7 Bypass Gallbladder to Caudate Hepatic Duct with Intraluminal Device, Percutaneous Endoscopic Approach
0F144D8 Bypass Gallbladder to Cystic Duct with Intraluminal Device, Percutaneous Endoscopic Approach
0F144D9 Bypass Gallbladder to Common Bile Duct with Intraluminal Device, Percutaneous Endoscopic Approach
0F144DB Bypass Gallbladder to Small Intestine with Intraluminal Device, Percutaneous Endoscopic Approach
0F144Z3 Bypass Gallbladder to Duodenum, Percutaneous Endoscopic Approach
0F144Z4 Bypass Gallbladder to Stomach, Percutaneous Endoscopic Approach
0F144Z5 Bypass Gallbladder to Right Hepatic Duct, Percutaneous Endoscopic Approach
0F144Z6 Bypass Gallbladder to Left Hepatic Duct, Percutaneous Endoscopic Approach
0F144Z7 Bypass Gallbladder to Caudate Hepatic Duct, Percutaneous Endoscopic Approach
0F144Z8 Bypass Gallbladder to Cystic Duct, Percutaneous Endoscopic Approach
0F144Z9 Bypass Gallbladder to Common Bile Duct, Percutaneous Endoscopic Approach
0F144ZB Bypass Gallbladder to Small Intestine, Percutaneous Endoscopic Approach
0F150D3 Bypass Right Hepatic Duct to Duodenum with Intraluminal Device, Open Approach
0F150D4 Bypass Right Hepatic Duct to Stomach with Intraluminal Device, Open Approach
0F150D5 Bypass Right Hepatic Duct to Right Hepatic Duct with Intraluminal Device, Open Approach
0F150D6 Bypass Right Hepatic Duct to Left Hepatic Duct with Intraluminal Device, Open Approach
0F150D7 Bypass Right Hepatic Duct to Caudate Hepatic Duct with Intraluminal Device, Open Approach
0F150D8 Bypass Right Hepatic Duct to Cystic Duct with Intraluminal Device, Open Approach
0F150D9 Bypass Right Hepatic Duct to Common Bile Duct with Intraluminal Device, Open Approach
0F150DB Bypass Right Hepatic Duct to Small Intestine with Intraluminal Device, Open Approach
0F150Z3 Bypass Right Hepatic Duct to Duodenum, Open Approach
0F150Z4 Bypass Right Hepatic Duct to Stomach, Open Approach
0F150Z5 Bypass Right Hepatic Duct to Right Hepatic Duct, Open Approach
0F150Z6 Bypass Right Hepatic Duct to Left Hepatic Duct, Open Approach
0F150Z7 Bypass Right Hepatic Duct to Caudate Hepatic Duct, Open Approach
0F150Z8 Bypass Right Hepatic Duct to Cystic Duct, Open Approach
0F150Z9 Bypass Right Hepatic Duct to Common Bile Duct, Open Approach
0F150ZB Bypass Right Hepatic Duct to Small Intestine, Open Approach
0F154D3 Bypass Right Hepatic Duct to Duodenum with Intraluminal Device, Percutaneous Endoscopic Approach
0F154D4 Bypass Right Hepatic Duct to Stomach with Intraluminal Device, Percutaneous Endoscopic Approach
0F154D5 Bypass Right Hepatic Duct to Right Hepatic Duct with Intraluminal Device, Percutaneous Endoscopic Approach
0F154D6 Bypass Right Hepatic Duct to Left Hepatic Duct with Intraluminal Device, Percutaneous Endoscopic Approach
0F154D7 Bypass Right Hepatic Duct to Caudate Hepatic Duct with Intraluminal Device, Percutaneous Endoscopic Approach
0F154D8 Bypass Right Hepatic Duct to Cystic Duct with Intraluminal Device, Percutaneous Endoscopic Approach
0F154D9 Bypass Right Hepatic Duct to Common Bile Duct with Intraluminal Device, Percutaneous Endoscopic Approach
0F154DB Bypass Right Hepatic Duct to Small Intestine with Intraluminal Device, Percutaneous Endoscopic Approach
0F154Z3 Bypass Right Hepatic Duct to Duodenum, Percutaneous Endoscopic Approach
0F154Z4 Bypass Right Hepatic Duct to Stomach, Percutaneous Endoscopic Approach
0F154Z5 Bypass Right Hepatic Duct to Right Hepatic Duct, Percutaneous Endoscopic Approach
0F154Z6 Bypass Right Hepatic Duct to Left Hepatic Duct, Percutaneous Endoscopic Approach
0F154Z7 Bypass Right Hepatic Duct to Caudate Hepatic Duct, Percutaneous Endoscopic Approach
0F154Z8 Bypass Right Hepatic Duct to Cystic Duct, Percutaneous Endoscopic Approach
0F154Z9 Bypass Right Hepatic Duct to Common Bile Duct, Percutaneous Endoscopic Approach
0F154ZB Bypass Right Hepatic Duct to Small Intestine, Percutaneous Endoscopic Approach
0F160D3 Bypass Left Hepatic Duct to Duodenum with Intraluminal Device, Open Approach
0F160D4 Bypass Left Hepatic Duct to Stomach with Intraluminal Device, Open Approach
0F160D5 Bypass Left Hepatic Duct to Right Hepatic Duct with Intraluminal Device, Open Approach
0F160D6 Bypass Left Hepatic Duct to Left Hepatic Duct with Intraluminal Device, Open Approach
0F160D7 Bypass Left Hepatic Duct to Caudate Hepatic Duct with Intraluminal Device, Open Approach
0F160D8 Bypass Left Hepatic Duct to Cystic Duct with Intraluminal Device, Open Approach
0F160D9 Bypass Left Hepatic Duct to Common Bile Duct with Intraluminal Device, Op Approach
0F160DB Bypass Left Hepatic Duct to Small Intestine with Intraluminal Device, Ope Approach
0F160Z3 Bypass Left Hepatic Duct to Duodenum Open Approach
0F160Z4 Bypass Left Hepatic Duct to Stomach, Open Approach
0F160Z5 Bypass Left Hepatic Duct to Right Hep Duct, Open Approach
0F160Z6 Bypass Left Hepatic Duct to Left Hepa Duct, Open Approach
0F160Z7 Bypass Left Hepatic Duct to Caudate Hepatic Duct, Open Approach
0F160Z8 Bypass Left Hepatic Duct to Cystic Duc Open Approach
0F160Z9 Bypass Left Hepatic Duct to Common Bile Duct, Open Approach
0F160ZB Bypass Left Hepatic Duct to Small Intestine, Open Approach
0F164D3 Bypass Left Hepatic Duct to Duodenum with Intraluminal Device, Percutaneous Endoscopic Approach
0F164D4 Bypass Left Hepatic Duct to Stomach with Intraluminal Device, Percutaneous Endoscopic Approach
0F164D5 Bypass Left Hepatic Duct to Right Hepatic Duct with Intraluminal Device, Percutaneous Endoscopic Approach
0F164D6 Bypass Left Hepatic Duct to Left Hepatic Duct with Intraluminal Device, Percutaneous Endoscopic Approach
0F164D7 Bypass Left Hepatic Duct to Caudate Hepatic Duct with Intraluminal Device, Percutaneous Endoscopic Approach
0F164D8 Bypass Left Hepatic Duct to Cystic Duc with Intraluminal Device, Percutaneous Endoscopic Approach
0F164D9 Bypass Left Hepatic Duct to Common Bile Duct with Intraluminal Device, Percutaneous Endoscopic Approach
0F164DB Bypass Left Hepatic Duct to Small Intestine with Intraluminal Device, Percutaneous Endoscopic Approach
0F164Z3 Bypass Left Hepatic Duct to Duodenum, Percutaneous Endoscopic Approach
0F164Z4 Bypass Left Hepatic Duct to Stomach, Percutaneous Endoscopic Approach
0F164Z5 Bypass Left Hepatic Duct to Right Hepatic Duct, Percutaneous Endoscopic Approach
0F164Z6 Bypass Left Hepatic Duct to Left Hepatic Duct, Percutaneous Endoscopic Approac
0F164Z7 Bypass Left Hepatic Duct to Caudate Hepatic Duct, Percutaneous Endoscopic Approach
0F164Z8 Bypass Left Hepatic Duct to Cystic Duct, Percutaneous Endoscopic Approach
0F164Z9 Bypass Left Hepatic Duct to Common Bile Duct, Percutaneous Endoscopic Approach
0F164ZB Bypass Left Hepatic Duct to Small Intestine, Percutaneous Endoscopic Approach
0F180D3 Bypass Cystic Duct to Duodenum with Intraluminal Device, Open Approach
0F180D4 Bypass Cystic Duct to Stomach with Intraluminal Device, Open Approach
0F180D5 Bypass Cystic Duct to Right Hepatic Duc with Intraluminal Device, Open Approach
0F180D6 Bypass Cystic Duct to Left Hepatic Duct with Intraluminal Device, Open Approach
0F180D7 Bypass Cystic Duct to Caudate Hepatic Duct with Intraluminal Device, Open Approach

80D8 Bypass Cystic Duct to Cystic Duct with Intraluminal Device, Open Approach
80D9 Bypass Cystic Duct to Common Bile Duct with Intraluminal Device, Open Approach
80DB Bypass Cystic Duct to Small Intestine with Intraluminal Device, Open Approach
80Z3 Bypass Cystic Duct to Duodenum, Open Approach
80Z4 Bypass Cystic Duct to Stomach, Open Approach
80Z5 Bypass Cystic Duct to Right Hepatic Duct, Open Approach
180Z6 Bypass Cystic Duct to Left Hepatic Duct, Open Approach
180Z7 Bypass Cystic Duct to Caudate Hepatic Duct, Open Approach
180Z8 Bypass Cystic Duct to Cystic Duct, Open Approach
180Z9 Bypass Cystic Duct to Common Bile Duct, Open Approach
180ZB Bypass Cystic Duct to Small Intestine, Open Approach
184D3 Bypass Cystic Duct to Duodenum with Intraluminal Device, Percutaneous Endoscopic Approach
184D4 Bypass Cystic Duct to Stomach with Intraluminal Device, Percutaneous Endoscopic Approach
184D5 Bypass Cystic Duct to Right Hepatic Duct with Intraluminal Device, Percutaneous Endoscopic Approach
184D6 Bypass Cystic Duct to Left Hepatic Duct with Intraluminal Device, Percutaneous Endoscopic Approach
184D7 Bypass Cystic Duct to Caudate Hepatic Duct with Intraluminal Device, Percutaneous Endoscopic Approach
184D8 Bypass Cystic Duct to Cystic Duct with Intraluminal Device, Percutaneous Endoscopic Approach
184D9 Bypass Cystic Duct to Common Bile Duct with Intraluminal Device, Percutaneous Endoscopic Approach
184DB Bypass Cystic Duct to Small Intestine with Intraluminal Device, Percutaneous Endoscopic Approach
184Z3 Bypass Cystic Duct to Duodenum, Percutaneous Endoscopic Approach
184Z4 Bypass Cystic Duct to Stomach, Percutaneous Endoscopic Approach
184Z5 Bypass Cystic Duct to Right Hepatic Duct, Percutaneous Endoscopic Approach
184Z6 Bypass Cystic Duct to Left Hepatic Duct, Percutaneous Endoscopic Approach
184Z7 Bypass Cystic Duct to Caudate Hepatic Duct, Percutaneous Endoscopic Approach
F184Z8 Bypass Cystic Duct to Cystic Duct, Percutaneous Endoscopic Approach
F184Z9 Bypass Cystic Duct to Common Bile Duct, Percutaneous Endoscopic Approach
F184ZB Bypass Cystic Duct to Small Intestine, Percutaneous Endoscopic Approach
F190D3 Bypass Common Bile Duct to Duodenum with Intraluminal Device, Open Approach
F190D4 Bypass Common Bile Duct to Stomach with Intraluminal Device, Open Approach
F190D5 Bypass Common Bile Duct to Right Hepatic Duct with Intraluminal Device, Open Approach
F190D6 Bypass Common Bile Duct to Left Hepatic Duct with Intraluminal Device, Open Approach
F190D7 Bypass Common Bile Duct to Caudate Hepatic Duct with Intraluminal Device, Open Approach
F190D8 Bypass Common Bile Duct to Cystic Duct with Intraluminal Device, Open Approach
0F190D9 Bypass Common Bile Duct to Common Bile Duct with Intraluminal Device, Open Approach
0F190DB Bypass Common Bile Duct to Small Intestine with Intraluminal Device, Open Approach
0F190Z3 Bypass Common Bile Duct to Duodenum, Open Approach
0F190Z4 Bypass Common Bile Duct to Stomach, Open Approach
0F190Z5 Bypass Common Bile Duct to Right Hepatic Duct, Open Approach
0F190Z6 Bypass Common Bile Duct to Left Hepatic Duct, Open Approach
0F190Z7 Bypass Common Bile Duct to Caudate Hepatic Duct, Open Approach
0F190Z8 Bypass Common Bile Duct to Cystic Duct, Open Approach
0F190Z9 Bypass Common Bile Duct to Common Bile Duct, Open Approach
0F190ZB Bypass Common Bile Duct to Small Intestine, Open Approach
0F194D3 Bypass Common Bile Duct to Duodenum with Intraluminal Device, Percutaneous Endoscopic Approach
0F194D4 Bypass Common Bile Duct to Stomach with Intraluminal Device, Percutaneous Endoscopic Approach
0F194D5 Bypass Common Bile Duct to Right Hepatic Duct with Intraluminal Device, Percutaneous Endoscopic Approach
0F194D6 Bypass Common Bile Duct to Left Hepatic Duct with Intraluminal Device, Percutaneous Endoscopic Approach
0F194D7 Bypass Common Bile Duct to Caudate Hepatic Duct with Intraluminal Device, Percutaneous Endoscopic Approach
0F194D8 Bypass Common Bile Duct to Cystic Duct with Intraluminal Device, Percutaneous Endoscopic Approach
0F194D9 Bypass Common Bile Duct to Common Bile Duct with Intraluminal Device, Percutaneous Endoscopic Approach
0F194DB Bypass Common Bile Duct to Small Intestine with Intraluminal Device, Percutaneous Endoscopic Approach
0F194Z3 Bypass Common Bile Duct to Duodenum, Percutaneous Endoscopic Approach
0F194Z4 Bypass Common Bile Duct to Stomach, Percutaneous Endoscopic Approach
0F194Z5 Bypass Common Bile Duct to Right Hepatic Duct, Percutaneous Endoscopic Approach
0F194Z6 Bypass Common Bile Duct to Left Hepatic Duct, Percutaneous Endoscopic Approach
0F194Z7 Bypass Common Bile Duct to Caudate Hepatic Duct, Percutaneous Endoscopic Approach
0F194Z8 Bypass Common Bile Duct to Cystic Duct, Percutaneous Endoscopic Approach
0F194Z9 Bypass Common Bile Duct to Common Bile Duct, Percutaneous Endoscopic Approach
0F194ZB Bypass Common Bile Duct to Small Intestine, Percutaneous Endoscopic Approach
0F1D0D3 Bypass Pancreatic Duct to Duodenum with Intraluminal Device, Open Approach
0F1D0DB Bypass Pancreatic Duct to Small Intestine with Intraluminal Device, Open Approach
0F1D0DC Bypass Pancreatic Duct to Large Intestine with Intraluminal Device, Open Approach
0F1D0Z3 Bypass Pancreatic Duct to Duodenum, Open Approach
0F1D0ZB Bypass Pancreatic Duct to Small Intestine, Open Approach
0F1D0ZC Bypass Pancreatic Duct to Large Intestine, Open Approach
0F1D4D3 Bypass Pancreatic Duct to Duodenum with Intraluminal Device, Percutaneous Endoscopic Approach
0F1D4DB Bypass Pancreatic Duct to Small Intestine with Intraluminal Device, Percutaneous Endoscopic Approach
0F1D4DC Bypass Pancreatic Duct to Large Intestine with Intraluminal Device, Percutaneous Endoscopic Approach
0F1D4Z3 Bypass Pancreatic Duct to Duodenum, Percutaneous Endoscopic Approach
0F1D4ZB Bypass Pancreatic Duct to Small Intestine, Percutaneous Endoscopic Approach
0F1D4ZC Bypass Pancreatic Duct to Large Intestine, Percutaneous Endoscopic Approach
0F1F0D3 Bypass Accessory Pancreatic Duct to Duodenum with Intraluminal Device, Open Approach
0F1F0DB Bypass Accessory Pancreatic Duct to Small Intestine with Intraluminal Device, Open Approach
0F1F0DC Bypass Accessory Pancreatic Duct to Large Intestine with Intraluminal Device, Open Approach
0F1F0Z3 Bypass Accessory Pancreatic Duct to Duodenum, Open Approach
0F1F0ZB Bypass Accessory Pancreatic Duct to Small Intestine, Open Approach
0F1F0ZC Bypass Accessory Pancreatic Duct to Large Intestine, Open Approach
0F1F4D3 Bypass Accessory Pancreatic Duct to Duodenum with Intraluminal Device, Percutaneous Endoscopic Approach
0F1F4DB Bypass Accessory Pancreatic Duct to Small Intestine with Intraluminal Device, Percutaneous Endoscopic Approach
0F1F4DC Bypass Accessory Pancreatic Duct to Large Intestine with Intraluminal Device, Percutaneous Endoscopic Approach
0F1F4Z3 Bypass Accessory Pancreatic Duct to Duodenum, Percutaneous Endoscopic Approach
0F1F4ZB Bypass Accessory Pancreatic Duct to Small Intestine, Percutaneous Endoscopic Approach
0F1F4ZC Bypass Accessory Pancreatic Duct to Large Intestine, Percutaneous Endoscopic Approach
0F1G0D3 Bypass Pancreas to Duodenum with Intraluminal Device, Open Approach
0F1G0DB Bypass Pancreas to Small Intestine with Intraluminal Device, Open Approach
0F1G0DC Bypass Pancreas to Large Intestine with Intraluminal Device, Open Approach
0F1G0Z3 Bypass Pancreas to Duodenum, Open Approach
0F1G0ZB Bypass Pancreas to Small Intestine, Open Approach
0F1G0ZC Bypass Pancreas to Large Intestine, Open Approach
0F1G4D3 Bypass Pancreas to Duodenum with Intraluminal Device, Percutaneous Endoscopic Approach
0F1G4DB Bypass Pancreas to Small Intestine with Intraluminal Device, Percutaneous Endoscopic Approach
0F1G4DC Bypass Pancreas to Large Intestine with Intraluminal Device, Percutaneous Endoscopic Approach
0F1G4Z3 Bypass Pancreas to Duodenum, Percutaneous Endoscopic Approach
0F1G4ZB Bypass Pancreas to Small Intestine, Percutaneous Endoscopic Approach
0F1G4ZC Bypass Pancreas to Large Intestine, Percutaneous Endoscopic Approach

0F2 – Hepatobiliary System and Pancreas, Change

Review Coding Guideline B6.1c

0F20X0Z Change Drainage Device in Liver, External Approach
0F20XYZ Change Other Device in Liver, External Approach
0F24X0Z Change Drainage Device in Gallbladder, External Approach
0F24XYZ Change Other Device in Gallbladder, External Approach
0F2BX0Z Change Drainage Device in Hepatobiliary Duct, External Approach
0F2BXYZ Change Other Device in Hepatobiliary Duct, External Approach
0F2DX0Z Change Drainage Device in Pancreatic Duct, External Approach
0F2DXYZ Change Other Device in Pancreatic Duct, External Approach
0F2GX0Z Change Drainage Device in Pancreas, External Approach
0F2GXYZ Change Other Device in Pancreas, External Approach

0F5 – Hepatobiliary System and Pancreas, Destruction

0F500ZZ Destruction of Liver, Open Approach
0F503ZZ Destruction of Liver, Percutaneous Approach
0F504ZZ Destruction of Liver, Percutaneous Endoscopic Approach
0F510ZZ Destruction of Right Lobe Liver, Open Approach
0F513ZZ Destruction of Right Lobe Liver, Percutaneous Approach
0F514ZZ Destruction of Right Lobe Liver, Percutaneous Endoscopic Approach
0F520ZZ Destruction of Left Lobe Liver, Open Approach
0F523ZZ Destruction of Left Lobe Liver, Percutaneous Approach
0F524ZZ Destruction of Left Lobe Liver, Percutaneous Endoscopic Approach
0F540ZZ Destruction of Gallbladder, Open Approach
0F543ZZ Destruction of Gallbladder, Percutaneous Approach
0F544ZZ Destruction of Gallbladder, Percutaneous Endoscopic Approach
0F550ZZ Destruction of Right Hepatic Duct, Open Approach
0F553ZZ Destruction of Right Hepatic Duct, Percutaneous Approach
0F554ZZ Destruction of Right Hepatic Duct, Percutaneous Endoscopic Approach
0F557ZZ Destruction of Right Hepatic Duct, Via Natural or Artificial Opening
0F558ZZ Destruction of Right Hepatic Duct, Via Natural or Artificial Opening Endoscopic
0F560ZZ Destruction of Left Hepatic Duct, Open Approach
0F563ZZ Destruction of Left Hepatic Duct, Percutaneous Approach
0F564ZZ Destruction of Left Hepatic Duct, Percutaneous Endoscopic Approach
0F567ZZ Destruction of Left Hepatic Duct, Via Natural or Artificial Opening
0F568ZZ Destruction of Left Hepatic Duct, Via Natural or Artificial Opening Endoscopic
0F580ZZ Destruction of Cystic Duct, Open Approach
0F583ZZ Destruction of Cystic Duct, Percutaneous Approach
0F584ZZ Destruction of Cystic Duct, Percutaneous Endoscopic Approach
0F587ZZ Destruction of Cystic Duct, Via Natural or Artificial Opening
0F588ZZ Destruction of Cystic Duct, Via Natural or Artificial Opening Endoscopic
0F590ZZ Destruction of Common Bile Duct, Open Approach
0F593ZZ Destruction of Common Bile Duct, Percutaneous Approach
0F594ZZ Destruction of Common Bile Duct, Percutaneous Endoscopic Approach
0F597ZZ Destruction of Common Bile Duct, Via Natural or Artificial Opening
0F598ZZ Destruction of Common Bile Duct, Via Natural or Artificial Opening Endoscopic
0F5C0ZZ Destruction of Ampulla of Vater, Open Approach
0F5C3ZZ Destruction of Ampulla of Vater, Percutaneous Approach
0F5C4ZZ Destruction of Ampulla of Vater, Percutaneous Endoscopic Approach
0F5C7ZZ Destruction of Ampulla of Vater, Via Natural or Artificial Opening
0F5C8ZZ Destruction of Ampulla of Vater, Via Natural or Artificial Opening Endoscop
0F5D0ZZ Destruction of Pancreatic Duct, Open Approach
0F5D3ZZ Destruction of Pancreatic Duct, Percutaneous Approach
0F5D4ZZ Destruction of Pancreatic Duct, Percutaneous Endoscopic Approach
0F5D7ZZ Destruction of Pancreatic Duct, Via Natural or Artificial Opening
0F5D8ZZ Destruction of Pancreatic Duct, Via Natural or Artificial Opening Endoscopi
0F5F0ZZ Destruction of Accessory Pancreatic Du Open Approach
0F5F3ZZ Destruction of Accessory Pancreatic Du Percutaneous Approach
0F5F4ZZ Destruction of Accessory Pancreatic Du Percutaneous Endoscopic Approach
0F5F7ZZ Destruction of Accessory Pancreatic Du Via Natural or Artificial Opening
0F5F8ZZ Destruction of Accessory Pancreatic Duct, Via Natural or Artificial Opening Endoscopic
0F5G0ZZ Destruction of Pancreas, Open Approach
0F5G3ZZ Destruction of Pancreas, Percutaneous Approach
0F5G4ZZ Destruction of Pancreas, Percutaneous Endoscopic Approach

0F7 – Hepatobiliary System and Pancreas, Dilation

0F750DZ Dilation of Right Hepatic Duct with Intraluminal Device, Open Approach
0F750ZZ Dilation of Right Hepatic Duct, Open Approach
0F753DZ Dilation of Right Hepatic Duct with Intraluminal Device, Percutaneous Approach
0F753ZZ Dilation of Right Hepatic Duct, Percutaneous Approach
0F754DZ Dilation of Right Hepatic Duct with Intraluminal Device, Percutaneous Endoscopic Approach
0F754ZZ Dilation of Right Hepatic Duct, Percutaneous Endoscopic Approach
● **0F757DZ** Dilation of Right Hepatic Duct with Intraluminal Device, Via Natural or Artificial Opening
0F757ZZ Dilation of Right Hepatic Duct, Via Natural or Artificial Opening
● **0F758DZ** Dilation of Right Hepatic Duct with Intraluminal Device, Via Natural or Artificial Opening Endoscopic
0F758ZZ Dilation of Right Hepatic Duct, Via Natural or Artificial Opening Endoscopic
0F760DZ Dilation of Left Hepatic Duct with Intraluminal Device, Open Approach
0F760ZZ Dilation of Left Hepatic Duct, Open Approach
0F763DZ Dilation of Left Hepatic Duct with Intraluminal Device, Percutaneous Approach
0F763ZZ Dilation of Left Hepatic Duct, Percutaneous Approach
0F764DZ Dilation of Left Hepatic Duct with Intraluminal Device, Percutaneous Endoscopic Approach
0F764ZZ Dilation of Left Hepatic Duct, Percutaneous Endoscopic Approach
● **0F767DZ** Dilation of Left Hepatic Duct with Intraluminal Device, Via Natural or Artificial Opening
0F767ZZ Dilation of Left Hepatic Duct, Via Natural or Artificial Opening
● **0F768DZ** Dilation of Left Hepatic Duct with Intraluminal Device, Via Natural or Artificial Opening Endoscopic
0F768ZZ Dilation of Left Hepatic Duct, Via Natural or Artificial Opening Endoscopic
0F780DZ Dilation of Cystic Duct with Intraluminal Device, Open Approach
0F780ZZ Dilation of Cystic Duct, Open Approach
0F783DZ Dilation of Cystic Duct with Intralumina Device, Percutaneous Approach
0F783ZZ Dilation of Cystic Duct, Percutaneous Approach
0F784DZ Dilation of Cystic Duct with Intralumina Device, Percutaneous Endoscopic Approach
0F784ZZ Dilation of Cystic Duct, Percutaneous Endoscopic Approach
● **0F787DZ** Dilation of Cystic Duct with Intraluminal Device, Via Natural or Artificial Opening
0F787ZZ Dilation of Cystic Duct, Via Natural or Artificial Opening
● **0F788DZ** Dilation of Cystic Duct with Intraluminal Device, Via Natural or Artificial Opening Endoscopic
0F788ZZ Dilation of Cystic Duct, Via Natural or Artificial Opening Endoscopic
0F790DZ Dilation of Common Bile Duct with Intraluminal Device, Open Approach
0F790ZZ Dilation of Common Bile Duct, Open Approach
0F793DZ Dilation of Common Bile Duct with Intraluminal Device, Percutaneous Approach

93ZZ	Dilation of Common Bile Duct, Percutaneous Approach
94DZ	Dilation of Common Bile Duct with Intraluminal Device, Percutaneous Endoscopic Approach
94ZZ	Dilation of Common Bile Duct, Percutaneous Endoscopic Approach
797DZ	Dilation of Common Bile Duct with Intraluminal Device, Via Natural or Artificial Opening
97ZZ	Dilation of Common Bile Duct, Via Natural or Artificial Opening
F798DZ	Dilation of Common Bile Duct with Intraluminal Device, Via Natural or Artificial Opening Endoscopic
798ZZ	Dilation of Common Bile Duct, Via Natural or Artificial Opening Endoscopic
7C0DZ	Dilation of Ampulla of Vater with Intraluminal Device, Open Approach
7C0ZZ	Dilation of Ampulla of Vater, Open Approach
7C3DZ	Dilation of Ampulla of Vater with Intraluminal Device, Percutaneous Approach
7C3ZZ	Dilation of Ampulla of Vater, Percutaneous Approach
7C4DZ	Dilation of Ampulla of Vater with Intraluminal Device, Percutaneous Endoscopic Approach
7C4ZZ	Dilation of Ampulla of Vater, Percutaneous Endoscopic Approach
0F7C7DZ	Dilation of Ampulla of Vater with Intraluminal Device, Via Natural or Artificial Opening
0F7C7ZZ	Dilation of Ampulla of Vater, Via Natural or Artificial Opening
0F7C8DZ	Dilation of Ampulla of Vater with Intraluminal Device, Via Natural or Artificial Opening Endoscopic
0F7C8ZZ	Dilation of Ampulla of Vater, Via Natural or Artificial Opening Endoscopic
0F7D0DZ	Dilation of Pancreatic Duct with Intraluminal Device, Open Approach
0F7D0ZZ	Dilation of Pancreatic Duct, Open Approach
0F7D3DZ	Dilation of Pancreatic Duct with Intraluminal Device, Percutaneous Approach
0F7D3ZZ	Dilation of Pancreatic Duct, Percutaneous Approach
0F7D4DZ	Dilation of Pancreatic Duct with Intraluminal Device, Percutaneous Endoscopic Approach
0F7D4ZZ	Dilation of Pancreatic Duct, Percutaneous Endoscopic Approach
● 0F7D7DZ	Dilation of Pancreatic Duct with Intraluminal Device, Via Natural or Artificial Opening
0F7D7ZZ	Dilation of Pancreatic Duct, Via Natural or Artificial Opening
● 0F7D8DZ	Dilation of Pancreatic Duct with Intraluminal Device, Via Natural or Artificial Opening Endoscopic
0F7D8ZZ	Dilation of Pancreatic Duct, Via Natural or Artificial Opening Endoscopic
0F7F0DZ	Dilation of Accessory Pancreatic Duct with Intraluminal Device, Open Approach
0F7F0ZZ	Dilation of Accessory Pancreatic Duct, Open Approach
0F7F3DZ	Dilation of Accessory Pancreatic Duct with Intraluminal Device, Percutaneous Approach
0F7F3ZZ	Dilation of Accessory Pancreatic Duct, Percutaneous Approach
0F7F4DZ	Dilation of Accessory Pancreatic Duct with Intraluminal Device, Percutaneous Endoscopic Approach
0F7F4ZZ	Dilation of Accessory Pancreatic Duct, Percutaneous Endoscopic Approach
0F7F7DZ	Dilation of Accessory Pancreatic Duct with Intraluminal Device, Via Natural or Artificial Opening
0F7F7ZZ	Dilation of Accessory Pancreatic Duct, Via Natural or Artificial Opening
0F7F8DZ	Dilation of Accessory Pancreatic Duct with Intraluminal Device, Via Natural or Artificial Opening Endoscopic
0F7F8ZZ	Dilation of Accessory Pancreatic Duct, Via Natural or Artificial Opening Endoscopic

F8 – Hepatobiliary System and Pancreas, Division

eview Coding Guideline B3.14

8G0ZZ	Division of Pancreas, Open Approach
0F8G3ZZ	Division of Pancreas, Percutaneous Approach
0F8G4ZZ	Division of Pancreas, Percutaneous Endoscopic Approach

F9 – Hepatobiliary System and Pancreas, Drainage

eview Coding Guidelines B3.4a and B3.4b

eview Coding Guideline B6.2

F9000Z	Drainage of Liver with Drainage Device, Open Approach
F900ZX	Drainage of Liver, Open Approach, Diagnostic
F900ZZ	Drainage of Liver, Open Approach
F9030Z	Drainage of Liver with Drainage Device, Percutaneous Approach
F903ZX	Drainage of Liver, Percutaneous Approach, Diagnostic
F903ZZ	Drainage of Liver, Percutaneous Approach
F9040Z	Drainage of Liver with Drainage Device, Percutaneous Endoscopic Approach
F904ZX	Drainage of Liver, Percutaneous Endoscopic Approach, Diagnostic
F904ZZ	Drainage of Liver, Percutaneous Endoscopic Approach
F9100Z	Drainage of Right Lobe Liver with Drainage Device, Open Approach
F910ZX	Drainage of Right Lobe Liver, Open Approach, Diagnostic
F910ZZ	Drainage of Right Lobe Liver, Open Approach
F9130Z	Drainage of Right Lobe Liver with Drainage Device, Percutaneous Approach
F913ZX	Drainage of Right Lobe Liver, Percutaneous Approach, Diagnostic
F913ZZ	Drainage of Right Lobe Liver, Percutaneous Approach
F9140Z	Drainage of Right Lobe Liver with Drainage Device, Percutaneous Endoscopic Approach
0F914ZX	Drainage of Right Lobe Liver, Percutaneous Endoscopic Approach, Diagnostic
0F914ZZ	Drainage of Right Lobe Liver, Percutaneous Endoscopic Approach
0F9200Z	Drainage of Left Lobe Liver with Drainage Device, Open Approach
0F920ZX	Drainage of Left Lobe Liver, Open Approach, Diagnostic
0F920ZZ	Drainage of Left Lobe Liver, Open Approach
0F9230Z	Drainage of Left Lobe Liver with Drainage Device, Percutaneous Approach
0F923ZX	Drainage of Left Lobe Liver, Percutaneous Approach, Diagnostic
0F923ZZ	Drainage of Left Lobe Liver, Percutaneous Approach
0F9240Z	Drainage of Left Lobe Liver with Drainage Device, Percutaneous Endoscopic Approach
0F924ZX	Drainage of Left Lobe Liver, Percutaneous Endoscopic Approach, Diagnostic
0F924ZZ	Drainage of Left Lobe Liver, Percutaneous Endoscopic Approach
0F9400Z	Drainage of Gallbladder with Drainage Device, Open Approach
0F940ZX	Drainage of Gallbladder, Open Approach, Diagnostic
0F940ZZ	Drainage of Gallbladder, Open Approach
0F9430Z	Drainage of Gallbladder with Drainage Device, Percutaneous Approach
0F943ZX	Drainage of Gallbladder, Percutaneous Approach, Diagnostic
0F943ZZ	Drainage of Gallbladder, Percutaneous Approach
0F9440Z	Drainage of Gallbladder with Drainage Device, Percutaneous Endoscopic Approach
0F944ZX	Drainage of Gallbladder, Percutaneous Endoscopic Approach, Diagnostic
0F944ZZ	Drainage of Gallbladder, Percutaneous Endoscopic Approach
0F9500Z	Drainage of Right Hepatic Duct with Drainage Device, Open Approach
0F950ZX	Drainage of Right Hepatic Duct, Open Approach, Diagnostic
0F950ZZ	Drainage of Right Hepatic Duct, Open Approach
0F9530Z	Drainage of Right Hepatic Duct with Drainage Device, Percutaneous Approach
0F953ZX	Drainage of Right Hepatic Duct, Percutaneous Approach, Diagnostic
0F953ZZ	Drainage of Right Hepatic Duct, Percutaneous Approach
0F9540Z	Drainage of Right Hepatic Duct with Drainage Device, Percutaneous Endoscopic Approach
0F954ZX	Drainage of Right Hepatic Duct, Percutaneous Endoscopic Approach, Diagnostic
0F954ZZ	Drainage of Right Hepatic Duct, Percutaneous Endoscopic Approach
0F9570Z	Drainage of Right Hepatic Duct with Drainage Device, Via Natural or Artificial Opening
0F957ZX	Drainage of Right Hepatic Duct, Via Natural or Artificial Opening, Diagnostic

0F957ZZ Drainage of Right Hepatic Duct, Via Natural or Artificial Opening

0F9580Z Drainage of Right Hepatic Duct with Drainage Device, Via Natural or Artificial Opening Endoscopic

0F958ZX Drainage of Right Hepatic Duct, Via Natural or Artificial Opening Endoscopic, Diagnostic

0F958ZZ Drainage of Right Hepatic Duct, Via Natural or Artificial Opening Endoscopic

0F9600Z Drainage of Left Hepatic Duct with Drainage Device, Open Approach

0F960ZX Drainage of Left Hepatic Duct, Open Approach, Diagnostic

0F960ZZ Drainage of Left Hepatic Duct, Open Approach

0F9630Z Drainage of Left Hepatic Duct with Drainage Device, Percutaneous Approach

0F963ZX Drainage of Left Hepatic Duct, Percutaneous Approach, Diagnostic

0F963ZZ Drainage of Left Hepatic Duct, Percutaneous Approach

0F9640Z Drainage of Left Hepatic Duct with Drainage Device, Percutaneous Endoscopic Approach

0F964ZX Drainage of Left Hepatic Duct, Percutaneous Endoscopic Approach, Diagnostic

0F964ZZ Drainage of Left Hepatic Duct, Percutaneous Endoscopic Approach

0F9670Z Drainage of Left Hepatic Duct with Drainage Device, Via Natural or Artificial Opening

0F967ZX Drainage of Left Hepatic Duct, Via Natural or Artificial Opening, Diagnostic

0F967ZZ Drainage of Left Hepatic Duct, Via Natural or Artificial Opening

0F9680Z Drainage of Left Hepatic Duct with Drainage Device, Via Natural or Artificial Opening Endoscopic

0F968ZX Drainage of Left Hepatic Duct, Via Natural or Artificial Opening Endoscopic, Diagnostic

0F968ZZ Drainage of Left Hepatic Duct, Via Natural or Artificial Opening Endoscopic

0F9800Z Drainage of Cystic Duct with Drainage Device, Open Approach

0F980ZX Drainage of Cystic Duct, Open Approach, Diagnostic

0F980ZZ Drainage of Cystic Duct, Open Approach

0F9830Z Drainage of Cystic Duct with Drainage Device, Percutaneous Approach

0F983ZX Drainage of Cystic Duct, Percutaneous Approach, Diagnostic

0F983ZZ Drainage of Cystic Duct, Percutaneous Approach

0F9840Z Drainage of Cystic Duct with Drainage Device, Percutaneous Endoscopic Approach

0F984ZX Drainage of Cystic Duct, Percutaneous Endoscopic Approach, Diagnostic

0F984ZZ Drainage of Cystic Duct, Percutaneous Endoscopic Approach

0F9870Z Drainage of Cystic Duct with Drainage Device, Via Natural or Artificial Opening

0F987ZX Drainage of Cystic Duct, Via Natural or Artificial Opening, Diagnostic

0F987ZZ Drainage of Cystic Duct, Via Natural or Artificial Opening

0F9880Z Drainage of Cystic Duct with Drainage Device, Via Natural or Artificial Opening Endoscopic

0F988ZX Drainage of Cystic Duct, Via Natural or Artificial Opening Endoscopic, Diagnostic

0F988ZZ Drainage of Cystic Duct, Via Natural or Artificial Opening Endoscopic

0F9900Z Drainage of Common Bile Duct with Drainage Device, Open Approach

0F990ZX Drainage of Common Bile Duct, Open Approach, Diagnostic

0F990ZZ Drainage of Common Bile Duct, Open Approach

0F9930Z Drainage of Common Bile Duct with Drainage Device, Percutaneous Approach

0F993ZX Drainage of Common Bile Duct, Percutaneous Approach, Diagnostic

0F993ZZ Drainage of Common Bile Duct, Percutaneous Approach

0F9940Z Drainage of Common Bile Duct with Drainage Device, Percutaneous Endoscopic Approach

0F994ZX Drainage of Common Bile Duct, Percutaneous Endoscopic Approach, Diagnostic

0F994ZZ Drainage of Common Bile Duct, Percutaneous Endoscopic Approach

0F9970Z Drainage of Common Bile Duct with Drainage Device, Via Natural or Artificial Opening

0F997ZX Drainage of Common Bile Duct, Via Natural or Artificial Opening, Diagnostic

0F997ZZ Drainage of Common Bile Duct, Via Natural or Artificial Opening

0F9980Z Drainage of Common Bile Duct with Drainage Device, Via Natural or Artificial Opening Endoscopic

0F998ZX Drainage of Common Bile Duct, Via Natural or Artificial Opening Endoscopic, Diagnostic

0F998ZZ Drainage of Common Bile Duct, Via Natural or Artificial Opening Endoscopic

0F9C00Z Drainage of Ampulla of Vater with Drainage Device, Open Approach

0F9C0ZX Drainage of Ampulla of Vater, Open Approach, Diagnostic

0F9C0ZZ Drainage of Ampulla of Vater, Open Approach

0F9C30Z Drainage of Ampulla of Vater with Drainage Device, Percutaneous Approach

0F9C3ZX Drainage of Ampulla of Vater, Percutaneous Approach, Diagnostic

0F9C3ZZ Drainage of Ampulla of Vater, Percutaneous Approach

0F9C40Z Drainage of Ampulla of Vater with Drainage Device, Percutaneous Endoscopic Approach

0F9C4ZX Drainage of Ampulla of Vater, Percutaneous Endoscopic Approach, Diagnostic

0F9C4ZZ Drainage of Ampulla of Vater, Percutaneous Endoscopic Approach

0F9C70Z Drainage of Ampulla of Vater with Drainage Device, Via Natural or Artificial Opening

0F9C7ZX Drainage of Ampulla of Vater, Via Natural or Artificial Opening, Diagnostic

0F9C7ZZ Drainage of Ampulla of Vater, Via Natural or Artificial Opening

0F9C80Z Drainage of Ampulla of Vater with Drainage Device, Via Natural or Artificial Opening Endoscopic

0F9C8ZX Drainage of Ampulla of Vater, Via Natural or Artificial Opening Endoscopic, Diagnostic

0F9C8ZZ Drainage of Ampulla of Vater, Via Natural or Artificial Opening Endoscopic

0F9D00Z Drainage of Pancreatic Duct with Drainage Device, Open Approach

0F9D0ZX Drainage of Pancreatic Duct, Open Approach, Diagnostic

0F9D0ZZ Drainage of Pancreatic Duct, Open Approach

0F9D30Z Drainage of Pancreatic Duct with Drainage Device, Percutaneous Approach

0F9D3ZX Drainage of Pancreatic Duct, Percutaneous Approach, Diagnostic

0F9D3ZZ Drainage of Pancreatic Duct, Percutane Approach

0F9D40Z Drainage of Pancreatic Duct with Drainage Device, Percutaneous Endoscopic Approach

0F9D4ZX Drainage of Pancreatic Duct, Percutane Endoscopic Approach, Diagnostic

0F9D4ZZ Drainage of Pancreatic Duct, Percutane Endoscopic Approach

0F9D70Z Drainage of Pancreatic Duct with Drain Device, Via Natural or Artificial Openir

0F9D7ZX Drainage of Pancreatic Duct, Via Natur or Artificial Opening, Diagnostic

0F9D7ZZ Drainage of Pancreatic Duct, Via Natur or Artificial Opening

0F9D80Z Drainage of Pancreatic Duct with Drainage Device, Via Natural or Artifici Opening Endoscopic

0F9D8ZX Drainage of Pancreatic Duct, Via Natura Artificial Opening Endoscopic, Diagnos

0F9D8ZZ Drainage of Pancreatic Duct, Via Natura or Artificial Opening Endoscopic

0F9F00Z Drainage of Accessory Pancreatic Duct with Drainage Device, Open Approach

0F9F0ZX Drainage of Accessory Pancreatic Duct, Open Approach, Diagnostic

0F9F0ZZ Drainage of Accessory Pancreatic Duct, Open Approach

0F9F30Z Drainage of Accessory Pancreatic Duct with Drainage Device, Percutaneous Approach

0F9F3ZX Drainage of Accessory Pancreatic Duct, Percutaneous Approach, Diagnostic

0F9F3ZZ Drainage of Accessory Pancreatic Duct, Percutaneous Approach

0F9F40Z Drainage of Accessory Pancreatic Duct with Drainage Device, Percutaneous Endoscopic Approach

0F9F4ZX Drainage of Accessory Pancreatic Duct, Percutaneous Endoscopic Approach, Diagnostic

0F9F4ZZ Drainage of Accessory Pancreatic Duct, Percutaneous Endoscopic Approach

0F9F70Z Drainage of Accessory Pancreatic Duct with Drainage Device, Via Natural or Artificial Opening

0F9F7ZX Drainage of Accessory Pancreatic Duct, Via Natural or Artificial Opening, Diagnostic

0F9F7ZZ Drainage of Accessory Pancreatic Duct, Via Natural or Artificial Opening

0F9F80Z Drainage of Accessory Pancreatic Duct with Drainage Device, Via Natural or Artificial Opening Endoscopic

0F9F8ZX Drainage of Accessory Pancreatic Duct, Via Natural or Artificial Opening Endoscopic, Diagnostic

0F9F8ZZ Drainage of Accessory Pancreatic Duct, Via Natural or Artificial Opening Endoscopic

0F9G00Z Drainage of Pancreas with Drainage Device, Open Approach

0F9G0ZX Drainage of Pancreas, Open Approach, Diagnostic

0F9G0ZZ Drainage of Pancreas, Open Approach

0F9G30Z Drainage of Pancreas with Drainage Device, Percutaneous Approach

0F9G3ZX Drainage of Pancreas, Percutaneous Approach, Diagnostic

0F9G3ZZ Drainage of Pancreas, Percutaneous Approach

0F9G40Z Drainage of Pancreas with Drainage Device, Percutaneous Endoscopic Approach

0F9G4ZX Drainage of Pancreas, Percutaneous Endoscopic Approach, Diagnostic

0F9G4ZZ Drainage of Pancreas, Percutaneous Endoscopic Approach

B – Hepatobiliary System and Pancreas, Excision

view Coding Guidelines B3.4a and B3.4b

view Coding Guideline B3.8

B00ZX Excision of Liver, Open Approach, Diagnostic
B00ZZ Excision of Liver, Open Approach
B03ZX Excision of Liver, Percutaneous Approach, Diagnostic
B03ZZ Excision of Liver, Percutaneous Approach
B04ZX Excision of Liver, Percutaneous Endoscopic Approach, Diagnostic
B04ZZ Excision of Liver, Percutaneous Endoscopic Approach
B10ZX Excision of Right Lobe Liver, Open Approach, Diagnostic
B10ZZ Excision of Right Lobe Liver, Open Approach
B13ZX Excision of Right Lobe Liver, Percutaneous Approach, Diagnostic
B13ZZ Excision of Right Lobe Liver, Percutaneous Approach
B14ZX Excision of Right Lobe Liver, Percutaneous Endoscopic Approach, Diagnostic
B14ZZ Excision of Right Lobe Liver, Percutaneous Endoscopic Approach
B20ZX Excision of Left Lobe Liver, Open Approach, Diagnostic
B20ZZ Excision of Left Lobe Liver, Open Approach
B23ZX Excision of Left Lobe Liver, Percutaneous Approach, Diagnostic
B23ZZ Excision of Left Lobe Liver, Percutaneous Approach
B24ZX Excision of Left Lobe Liver, Percutaneous Endoscopic Approach, Diagnostic
B24ZZ Excision of Left Lobe Liver, Percutaneous Endoscopic Approach
FB40ZX Excision of Gallbladder, Open Approach, Diagnostic
B40ZZ Excision of Gallbladder, Open Approach
FB43ZX Excision of Gallbladder, Percutaneous Approach, Diagnostic
FB43ZZ Excision of Gallbladder, Percutaneous Approach
FB44ZX Excision of Gallbladder, Percutaneous Endoscopic Approach, Diagnostic
FB44ZZ Excision of Gallbladder, Percutaneous Endoscopic Approach
FB50ZX Excision of Right Hepatic Duct, Open Approach, Diagnostic
FB50ZZ Excision of Right Hepatic Duct, Open Approach
FB53ZX Excision of Right Hepatic Duct, Percutaneous Approach, Diagnostic
FB53ZZ Excision of Right Hepatic Duct, Percutaneous Approach
FB54ZX Excision of Right Hepatic Duct, Percutaneous Endoscopic Approach, Diagnostic
FB54ZZ Excision of Right Hepatic Duct, Percutaneous Endoscopic Approach
FB57ZX Excision of Right Hepatic Duct, Via Natural or Artificial Opening, Diagnostic
FB57ZZ Excision of Right Hepatic Duct, Via Natural or Artificial Opening
FB58ZX Excision of Right Hepatic Duct, Via Natural or Artificial Opening Endoscopic, Diagnostic
FB58ZZ Excision of Right Hepatic Duct, Via Natural or Artificial Opening Endoscopic
FB60ZX Excision of Left Hepatic Duct, Open Approach, Diagnostic
0FB60ZZ Excision of Left Hepatic Duct, Open Approach
0FB63ZX Excision of Left Hepatic Duct, Percutaneous Approach, Diagnostic
0FB63ZZ Excision of Left Hepatic Duct, Percutaneous Approach
0FB64ZX Excision of Left Hepatic Duct, Percutaneous Endoscopic Approach, Diagnostic
0FB64ZZ Excision of Left Hepatic Duct, Percutaneous Endoscopic Approach
0FB67ZX Excision of Left Hepatic Duct, Via Natural or Artificial Opening, Diagnostic
0FB67ZZ Excision of Left Hepatic Duct, Via Natural or Artificial Opening
0FB68ZX Excision of Left Hepatic Duct, Via Natural or Artificial Opening Endoscopic, Diagnostic
0FB68ZZ Excision of Left Hepatic Duct, Via Natural or Artificial Opening Endoscopic
0FB80ZX Excision of Cystic Duct, Open Approach, Diagnostic
0FB80ZZ Excision of Cystic Duct, Open Approach
0FB83ZX Excision of Cystic Duct, Percutaneous Approach, Diagnostic
0FB83ZZ Excision of Cystic Duct, Percutaneous Approach
0FB84ZX Excision of Cystic Duct, Percutaneous Endoscopic Approach, Diagnostic
0FB84ZZ Excision of Cystic Duct, Percutaneous Endoscopic Approach
0FB87ZX Excision of Cystic Duct, Via Natural or Artificial Opening, Diagnostic
0FB87ZZ Excision of Cystic Duct, Via Natural or Artificial Opening
0FB88ZX Excision of Cystic Duct, Via Natural or Artificial Opening Endoscopic, Diagnostic
0FB88ZZ Excision of Cystic Duct, Via Natural or Artificial Opening Endoscopic
0FB90ZX Excision of Common Bile Duct, Open Approach, Diagnostic
0FB90ZZ Excision of Common Bile Duct, Open Approach
0FB93ZX Excision of Common Bile Duct, Percutaneous Approach, Diagnostic
0FB93ZZ Excision of Common Bile Duct, Percutaneous Approach
0FB94ZX Excision of Common Bile Duct, Percutaneous Endoscopic Approach, Diagnostic
0FB94ZZ Excision of Common Bile Duct, Percutaneous Endoscopic Approach
0FB97ZX Excision of Common Bile Duct, Via Natural or Artificial Opening, Diagnostic
0FB97ZZ Excision of Common Bile Duct, Via Natural or Artificial Opening
0FB98ZX Excision of Common Bile Duct, Via Natural or Artificial Opening Endoscopic, Diagnostic
0FB98ZZ Excision of Common Bile Duct, Via Natural or Artificial Opening Endoscopic
0FBC0ZX Excision of Ampulla of Vater, Open Approach, Diagnostic
0FBC0ZZ Excision of Ampulla of Vater, Open Approach
0FBC3ZX Excision of Ampulla of Vater, Percutaneous Approach, Diagnostic
0FBC3ZZ Excision of Ampulla of Vater, Percutaneous Approach
0FBC4ZX Excision of Ampulla of Vater, Percutaneous Endoscopic Approach, Diagnostic
0FBC4ZZ Excision of Ampulla of Vater, Percutaneous Endoscopic Approach
0FBC7ZX Excision of Ampulla of Vater, Via Natural or Artificial Opening, Diagnostic
0FBC7ZZ Excision of Ampulla of Vater, Via Natural or Artificial Opening
0FBC8ZX Excision of Ampulla of Vater, Via Natural or Artificial Opening Endoscopic, Diagnostic
0FBC8ZZ Excision of Ampulla of Vater, Via Natural or Artificial Opening Endoscopic
0FBD0ZX Excision of Pancreatic Duct, Open Approach, Diagnostic
0FBD0ZZ Excision of Pancreatic Duct, Open Approach
0FBD3ZX Excision of Pancreatic Duct, Percutaneous Approach, Diagnostic
0FBD3ZZ Excision of Pancreatic Duct, Percutaneous Approach
0FBD4ZX Excision of Pancreatic Duct, Percutaneous Endoscopic Approach, Diagnostic
0FBD4ZZ Excision of Pancreatic Duct, Percutaneous Endoscopic Approach
0FBD7ZX Excision of Pancreatic Duct, Via Natural or Artificial Opening, Diagnostic
0FBD7ZZ Excision of Pancreatic Duct, Via Natural or Artificial Opening
0FBD8ZX Excision of Pancreatic Duct, Via Natural or Artificial Opening Endoscopic, Diagnostic
0FBD8ZZ Excision of Pancreatic Duct, Via Natural or Artificial Opening Endoscopic
0FBF0ZX Excision of Accessory Pancreatic Duct, Open Approach, Diagnostic
0FBF0ZZ Excision of Accessory Pancreatic Duct, Open Approach
0FBF3ZX Excision of Accessory Pancreatic Duct, Percutaneous Approach, Diagnostic
0FBF3ZZ Excision of Accessory Pancreatic Duct, Percutaneous Approach
0FBF4ZX Excision of Accessory Pancreatic Duct, Percutaneous Endoscopic Approach, Diagnostic
0FBF4ZZ Excision of Accessory Pancreatic Duct, Percutaneous Endoscopic Approach
0FBF7ZX Excision of Accessory Pancreatic Duct, Via Natural or Artificial Opening, Diagnostic
0FBF7ZZ Excision of Accessory Pancreatic Duct, Via Natural or Artificial Opening
0FBF8ZX Excision of Accessory Pancreatic Duct, Via Natural or Artificial Opening Endoscopic, Diagnostic
0FBF8ZZ Excision of Accessory Pancreatic Duct, Via Natural or Artificial Opening Endoscopic
0FBG0ZX Excision of Pancreas, Open Approach, Diagnostic
0FBG0ZZ Excision of Pancreas, Open Approach
0FBG3ZX Excision of Pancreas, Percutaneous Approach, Diagnostic
0FBG3ZZ Excision of Pancreas, Percutaneous Approach
0FBG4ZX Excision of Pancreas, Percutaneous Endoscopic Approach, Diagnostic
0FBG4ZZ Excision of Pancreas, Percutaneous Endoscopic Approach

0FC – Hepatobiliary System and Pancreas, Extirpation

0FC00ZZ Extirpation of Matter from Liver, Open Approach
0FC03ZZ Extirpation of Matter from Liver, Percutaneous Approach
0FC04ZZ Extirpation of Matter from Liver, Percutaneous Endoscopic Approach
0FC10ZZ Extirpation of Matter from Right Lobe Liver, Open Approach
0FC13ZZ Extirpation of Matter from Right Lobe Liver, Percutaneous Approach
0FC14ZZ Extirpation of Matter from Right Lobe Liver, Percutaneous Endoscopic Approach
0FC20ZZ Extirpation of Matter from Left Lobe Liver, Open Approach
0FC23ZZ Extirpation of Matter from Left Lobe Liver, Percutaneous Approach
0FC24ZZ Extirpation of Matter from Left Lobe Liver, Percutaneous Endoscopic Approach
0FC40ZZ Extirpation of Matter from Gallbladder, Open Approach
0FC43ZZ Extirpation of Matter from Gallbladder, Percutaneous Approach
0FC44ZZ Extirpation of Matter from Gallbladder, Percutaneous Endoscopic Approach
0FC50ZZ Extirpation of Matter from Right Hepatic Duct, Open Approach
0FC53ZZ Extirpation of Matter from Right Hepatic Duct, Percutaneous Approach
0FC54ZZ Extirpation of Matter from Right Hepatic Duct, Percutaneous Endoscopic Approach
0FC57ZZ Extirpation of Matter from Right Hepatic Duct, Via Natural or Artificial Opening
0FC58ZZ Extirpation of Matter from Right Hepatic Duct, Via Natural or Artificial Opening Endoscopic
0FC60ZZ Extirpation of Matter from Left Hepatic Duct, Open Approach
0FC63ZZ Extirpation of Matter from Left Hepatic Duct, Percutaneous Approach
0FC64ZZ Extirpation of Matter from Left Hepatic Duct, Percutaneous Endoscopic Approach
0FC67ZZ Extirpation of Matter from Left Hepatic Duct, Via Natural or Artificial Opening
0FC68ZZ Extirpation of Matter from Left Hepatic Duct, Via Natural or Artificial Opening Endoscopic
0FC80ZZ Extirpation of Matter from Cystic Duct, Open Approach
0FC83ZZ Extirpation of Matter from Cystic Duct, Percutaneous Approach
0FC84ZZ Extirpation of Matter from Cystic Duct, Percutaneous Endoscopic Approach
0FC87ZZ Extirpation of Matter from Cystic Duct, Via Natural or Artificial Opening
0FC88ZZ Extirpation of Matter from Cystic Duct, Via Natural or Artificial Opening Endoscopic
0FC90ZZ Extirpation of Matter from Common Bile Duct, Open Approach
0FC93ZZ Extirpation of Matter from Common Bile Duct, Percutaneous Approach
0FC94ZZ Extirpation of Matter from Common Bile Duct, Percutaneous Endoscopic Approach
0FC97ZZ Extirpation of Matter from Common Bile Duct, Via Natural or Artificial Opening
0FC98ZZ Extirpation of Matter from Common Bile Duct, Via Natural or Artificial Opening Endoscopic
0FCC0ZZ Extirpation of Matter from Ampulla of Vater, Open Approach
0FCC3ZZ Extirpation of Matter from Ampulla of Vater, Percutaneous Approach
0FCC4ZZ Extirpation of Matter from Ampulla of Vater, Percutaneous Endoscopic Approach
0FCC7ZZ Extirpation of Matter from Ampulla of Vater, Via Natural or Artificial Opening
0FCC8ZZ Extirpation of Matter from Ampulla of Vater, Via Natural or Artificial Opening Endoscopic
0FCD0ZZ Extirpation of Matter from Pancreatic Duct, Open Approach
0FCD3ZZ Extirpation of Matter from Pancreatic Duct, Percutaneous Approach
0FCD4ZZ Extirpation of Matter from Pancreatic Duct, Percutaneous Endoscopic Approach
0FCD7ZZ Extirpation of Matter from Pancreatic Duct, Via Natural or Artificial Opening
0FCD8ZZ Extirpation of Matter from Pancreatic Duct, Via Natural or Artificial Opening Endoscopic
0FCF0ZZ Extirpation of Matter from Accessory Pancreatic Duct, Open Approach
0FCF3ZZ Extirpation of Matter from Accessory Pancreatic Duct, Percutaneous Approach
0FCF4ZZ Extirpation of Matter from Accessory Pancreatic Duct, Percutaneous Endoscopic Approach
0FCF7ZZ Extirpation of Matter from Accessory Pancreatic Duct, Via Natural or Artificial Opening
0FCF8ZZ Extirpation of Matter from Accessory Pancreatic Duct, Via Natural or Artificial Opening Endoscopic
0FCG0ZZ Extirpation of Matter from Pancreas, Open Approach
0FCG3ZZ Extirpation of Matter from Pancreas, Percutaneous Approach
0FCG4ZZ Extirpation of Matter from Pancreas, Percutaneous Endoscopic Approach

0FF – Hepatobiliary System and Pancreas, Fragmentation

0FF40ZZ Fragmentation in Gallbladder, Open Approach
0FF43ZZ Fragmentation in Gallbladder, Percutaneous Approach
0FF44ZZ Fragmentation in Gallbladder, Percutaneous Endoscopic Approach
0FF47ZZ Fragmentation in Gallbladder, Via Natural or Artificial Opening
0FF48ZZ Fragmentation in Gallbladder, Via Natural or Artificial Opening Endoscopic
▲ **0FF4XZZ** Fragmentation in Gallbladder, External Approach
0FF50ZZ Fragmentation in Right Hepatic Duct, Open Approach
0FF53ZZ Fragmentation in Right Hepatic Duct, Percutaneous Approach
0FF54ZZ Fragmentation in Right Hepatic Duct, Percutaneous Endoscopic Approach
0FF57ZZ Fragmentation in Right Hepatic Duct, Via Natural or Artificial Opening
0FF58ZZ Fragmentation in Right Hepatic Duct, Via Natural or Artificial Opening Endoscopic
▲ **0FF5XZZ** Fragmentation in Right Hepatic Duct, External Approach
0FF60ZZ Fragmentation in Left Hepatic Duct, Open Approach
0FF63ZZ Fragmentation in Left Hepatic Duct, Percutaneous Approach
0FF64ZZ Fragmentation in Left Hepatic Duct, Percutaneous Endoscopic Approach
0FF67ZZ Fragmentation in Left Hepatic Duct, Via Natural or Artificial Opening
0FF68ZZ Fragmentation in Left Hepatic Duct, Via Natural or Artificial Opening Endoscopic
▲ **0FF6XZZ** Fragmentation in Left Hepatic Duct, External Approach
0FF80ZZ Fragmentation in Cystic Duct, Open Approach
0FF83ZZ Fragmentation in Cystic Duct, Percutaneous Approach
0FF84ZZ Fragmentation in Cystic Duct, Percutaneous Endoscopic Approach
0FF87ZZ Fragmentation in Cystic Duct, Via Natural or Artificial Opening
0FF88ZZ Fragmentation in Cystic Duct, Via Natural or Artificial Opening Endoscopic
▲ **0FF8XZZ** Fragmentation in Cystic Duct, External Approach
0FF90ZZ Fragmentation in Common Bile Duct, Open Approach
0FF93ZZ Fragmentation in Common Bile Duct, Percutaneous Approach
0FF94ZZ Fragmentation in Common Bile Duct, Percutaneous Endoscopic Approach
0FF97ZZ Fragmentation in Common Bile Duct, Via Natural or Artificial Opening
0FF98ZZ Fragmentation in Common Bile Duct, Via Natural or Artificial Opening Endoscopic
▲ **0FF9XZZ** Fragmentation in Common Bile Duct, External Approach
0FFC0ZZ Fragmentation in Ampulla of Vater, Open Approach
0FFC3ZZ Fragmentation in Ampulla of Vater, Percutaneous Approach
0FFC4ZZ Fragmentation in Ampulla of Vater, Percutaneous Endoscopic Approach
0FFC7ZZ Fragmentation in Ampulla of Vater, Via Natural or Artificial Opening
0FFC8ZZ Fragmentation in Ampulla of Vater, Via Natural or Artificial Opening Endoscopic
▲ **0FFCXZZ** Fragmentation in Ampulla of Vater, External Approach
0FFD0ZZ Fragmentation in Pancreatic Duct, Open Approach
0FFD3ZZ Fragmentation in Pancreatic Duct, Percutaneous Approach
0FFD4ZZ Fragmentation in Pancreatic Duct, Percutaneous Endoscopic Approach
0FFD7ZZ Fragmentation in Pancreatic Duct, Via Natural or Artificial Opening
0FFD8ZZ Fragmentation in Pancreatic Duct, Via Natural or Artificial Opening Endoscopic
▲ **0FFDXZZ** Fragmentation in Pancreatic Duct, External Approach
0FFF0ZZ Fragmentation in Accessory Pancreatic Duct, Open Approach
0FFF3ZZ Fragmentation in Accessory Pancreatic Duct, Percutaneous Approach
0FFF4ZZ Fragmentation in Accessory Pancreatic Duct, Percutaneous Endoscopic Approach
0FFF7ZZ Fragmentation in Accessory Pancreatic Duct, Via Natural or Artificial Opening
0FFF8ZZ Fragmentation in Accessory Pancreatic Duct, Via Natural or Artificial Opening Endoscopic
▲ **0FFFXZZ** Fragmentation in Accessory Pancreatic Duct, External Approach

H – Hepatobiliary System and Pancreas, Insertion

I002Z Insertion of Monitoring Device into Liver, Open Approach
I003Z Insertion of Infusion Device into Liver, Open Approach
I032Z Insertion of Monitoring Device into Liver, Percutaneous Approach
I033Z Insertion of Infusion Device into Liver, Percutaneous Approach
I042Z Insertion of Monitoring Device into Liver, Percutaneous Endoscopic Approach
I043Z Insertion of Infusion Device into Liver, Percutaneous Endoscopic Approach
H102Z Insertion of Monitoring Device into Right Lobe Liver, Open Approach
H103Z Insertion of Infusion Device into Right Lobe Liver, Open Approach
H132Z Insertion of Monitoring Device into Right Lobe Liver, Percutaneous Approach
H133Z Insertion of Infusion Device into Right Lobe Liver, Percutaneous Approach
H142Z Insertion of Monitoring Device into Right Lobe Liver, Percutaneous Endoscopic Approach
H143Z Insertion of Infusion Device into Right Lobe Liver, Percutaneous Endoscopic Approach
H202Z Insertion of Monitoring Device into Left Lobe Liver, Open Approach
H203Z Insertion of Infusion Device into Left Lobe Liver, Open Approach
H232Z Insertion of Monitoring Device into Left Lobe Liver, Percutaneous Approach
H233Z Insertion of Infusion Device into Left Lobe Liver, Percutaneous Approach
H242Z Insertion of Monitoring Device into Left Lobe Liver, Percutaneous Endoscopic Approach
H243Z Insertion of Infusion Device into Left Lobe Liver, Percutaneous Endoscopic Approach
H402Z Insertion of Monitoring Device into Gallbladder, Open Approach
H403Z Insertion of Infusion Device into Gallbladder, Open Approach
H432Z Insertion of Monitoring Device into Gallbladder, Percutaneous Approach
H433Z Insertion of Infusion Device into Gallbladder, Percutaneous Approach
H442Z Insertion of Monitoring Device into Gallbladder, Percutaneous Endoscopic Approach
FH443Z Insertion of Infusion Device into Gallbladder, Percutaneous Endoscopic Approach
FHB01Z Insertion of Radioactive Element into Hepatobiliary Duct, Open Approach
FHB02Z Insertion of Monitoring Device into Hepatobiliary Duct, Open Approach
0FHB03Z Insertion of Infusion Device into Hepatobiliary Duct, Open Approach
0FHB0DZ Insertion of Intraluminal Device into Hepatobiliary Duct, Open Approach
0FHB31Z Insertion of Radioactive Element into Hepatobiliary Duct, Percutaneous Approach
0FHB32Z Insertion of Monitoring Device into Hepatobiliary Duct, Percutaneous Approach
0FHB33Z Insertion of Infusion Device into Hepatobiliary Duct, Percutaneous Approach
0FHB3DZ Insertion of Intraluminal Device into Hepatobiliary Duct, Percutaneous Approach
0FHB41Z Insertion of Radioactive Element into Hepatobiliary Duct, Percutaneous Endoscopic Approach
0FHB42Z Insertion of Monitoring Device into Hepatobiliary Duct, Percutaneous Endoscopic Approach
0FHB43Z Insertion of Infusion Device into Hepatobiliary Duct, Percutaneous Endoscopic Approach
0FHB4DZ Insertion of Intraluminal Device into Hepatobiliary Duct, Percutaneous Endoscopic Approach
0FHB71Z Insertion of Radioactive Element into Hepatobiliary Duct, Via Natural or Artificial Opening
0FHB72Z Insertion of Monitoring Device into Hepatobiliary Duct, Via Natural or Artificial Opening
0FHB73Z Insertion of Infusion Device into Hepatobiliary Duct, Via Natural or Artificial Opening
0FHB7DZ Insertion of Intraluminal Device into Hepatobiliary Duct, Via Natural or Artificial Opening
0FHB81Z Insertion of Radioactive Element into Hepatobiliary Duct, Via Natural or Artificial Opening Endoscopic
0FHB82Z Insertion of Monitoring Device into Hepatobiliary Duct, Via Natural or Artificial Opening Endoscopic
0FHB83Z Insertion of Infusion Device into Hepatobiliary Duct, Via Natural or Artificial Opening Endoscopic
● **0FHB8DZ** Insertion of Intraluminal Device into Hepatobiliary Duct, Via Natural or Artificial Opening Endoscopic
0FHD01Z Insertion of Radioactive Element into Pancreatic Duct, Open Approach
0FHD02Z Insertion of Monitoring Device into Pancreatic Duct, Open Approach
0FHD03Z Insertion of Infusion Device into Pancreatic Duct, Open Approach
0FHD0DZ Insertion of Intraluminal Device into Pancreatic Duct, Open Approach
0FHD31Z Insertion of Radioactive Element into Pancreatic Duct, Percutaneous Approach
0FHD32Z Insertion of Monitoring Device into Pancreatic Duct, Percutaneous Approach
0FHD33Z Insertion of Infusion Device into Pancreatic Duct, Percutaneous Approach
0FHD3DZ Insertion of Intraluminal Device into Pancreatic Duct, Percutaneous Approach
0FHD41Z Insertion of Radioactive Element into Pancreatic Duct, Percutaneous Endoscopic Approach
0FHD42Z Insertion of Monitoring Device into Pancreatic Duct, Percutaneous Endoscopic Approach
0FHD43Z Insertion of Infusion Device into Pancreatic Duct, Percutaneous Endoscopic Approach
0FHD4DZ Insertion of Intraluminal Device into Pancreatic Duct, Percutaneous Endoscopic Approach
0FHD71Z Insertion of Radioactive Element into Pancreatic Duct, Via Natural or Artificial Opening
0FHD72Z Insertion of Monitoring Device into Pancreatic Duct, Via Natural or Artificial Opening
0FHD73Z Insertion of Infusion Device into Pancreatic Duct, Via Natural or Artificial Opening
0FHD7DZ Insertion of Intraluminal Device into Pancreatic Duct, Via Natural or Artificial Opening
0FHD81Z Insertion of Radioactive Element into Pancreatic Duct, Via Natural or Artificial Opening Endoscopic
0FHD82Z Insertion of Monitoring Device into Pancreatic Duct, Via Natural or Artificial Opening Endoscopic
0FHD83Z Insertion of Infusion Device into Pancreatic Duct, Via Natural or Artificial Opening Endoscopic
0FHD8DZ Insertion of Intraluminal Device into Pancreatic Duct, Via Natural or Artificial Opening Endoscopic
0FHG02Z Insertion of Monitoring Device into Pancreas, Open Approach
0FHG03Z Insertion of Infusion Device into Pancreas, Open Approach
0FHG32Z Insertion of Monitoring Device into Pancreas, Percutaneous Approach
0FHG33Z Insertion of Infusion Device into Pancreas, Percutaneous Approach
0FHG42Z Insertion of Monitoring Device into Pancreas, Percutaneous Endoscopic Approach
0FHG43Z Insertion of Infusion Device into Pancreas, Percutaneous Endoscopic Approach

FJ – Hepatobiliary System and Pancreas, Inspection

eview Coding Guidelines B3.11a, B3.11b and B3.11c

FJ00ZZ Inspection of Liver, Open Approach
FJ03ZZ Inspection of Liver, Percutaneous Approach
FJ04ZZ Inspection of Liver, Percutaneous Endoscopic Approach
FJ0XZZ Inspection of Liver, External Approach
FJ40ZZ Inspection of Gallbladder, Open Approach
FJ43ZZ Inspection of Gallbladder, Percutaneous Approach
FJ44ZZ Inspection of Gallbladder, Percutaneous Endoscopic Approach
FJ4XZZ Inspection of Gallbladder, External Approach
0FJB0ZZ Inspection of Hepatobiliary Duct, Open Approach
0FJB3ZZ Inspection of Hepatobiliary Duct, Percutaneous Approach
0FJB4ZZ Inspection of Hepatobiliary Duct, Percutaneous Endoscopic Approach
0FJB7ZZ Inspection of Hepatobiliary Duct, Via Natural or Artificial Opening
0FJB8ZZ Inspection of Hepatobiliary Duct, Via Natural or Artificial Opening Endoscopic
0FJD0ZZ Inspection of Pancreatic Duct, Open Approach
0FJD3ZZ Inspection of Pancreatic Duct, Percutaneous Approach
0FJD4ZZ Inspection of Pancreatic Duct, Percutaneous Endoscopic Approach
0FJD7ZZ Inspection of Pancreatic Duct, Via Natural or Artificial Opening
0FJD8ZZ Inspection of Pancreatic Duct, Via Natural or Artificial Opening Endoscopic
0FJG0ZZ Inspection of Pancreas, Open Approach
0FJG3ZZ Inspection of Pancreas, Percutaneous Approach
0FJG4ZZ Inspection of Pancreas, Percutaneous Endoscopic Approach
0FJGXZZ Inspection of Pancreas, External Approach

0FL50CZ Occlusion of Right Hepatic Duct with Extraluminal Device, Open Approach
0FL50DZ Occlusion of Right Hepatic Duct with Intraluminal Device, Open Approach
0FL50ZZ Occlusion of Right Hepatic Duct, Open Approach
0FL53CZ Occlusion of Right Hepatic Duct with Extraluminal Device, Percutaneous Approach
0FL53DZ Occlusion of Right Hepatic Duct with Intraluminal Device, Percutaneous Approach
0FL53ZZ Occlusion of Right Hepatic Duct, Percutaneous Approach
0FL54CZ Occlusion of Right Hepatic Duct with Extraluminal Device, Percutaneous Endoscopic Approach
0FL54DZ Occlusion of Right Hepatic Duct with Intraluminal Device, Percutaneous Endoscopic Approach
0FL54ZZ Occlusion of Right Hepatic Duct, Percutaneous Endoscopic Approach
0FL57DZ Occlusion of Right Hepatic Duct with Intraluminal Device, Via Natural or Artificial Opening
0FL57ZZ Occlusion of Right Hepatic Duct, Via Natural or Artificial Opening
0FL58DZ Occlusion of Right Hepatic Duct with Intraluminal Device, Via Natural or Artificial Opening Endoscopic
0FL58ZZ Occlusion of Right Hepatic Duct, Via Natural or Artificial Opening Endoscopic
0FL60CZ Occlusion of Left Hepatic Duct with Extraluminal Device, Open Approach
0FL60DZ Occlusion of Left Hepatic Duct with Intraluminal Device, Open Approach
0FL60ZZ Occlusion of Left Hepatic Duct, Open Approach
0FL63CZ Occlusion of Left Hepatic Duct with Extraluminal Device, Percutaneous Approach
0FL63DZ Occlusion of Left Hepatic Duct with Intraluminal Device, Percutaneous Approach
0FL63ZZ Occlusion of Left Hepatic Duct, Percutaneous Approach
0FL64CZ Occlusion of Left Hepatic Duct with Extraluminal Device, Percutaneous Endoscopic Approach
0FL64DZ Occlusion of Left Hepatic Duct with Intraluminal Device, Percutaneous Endoscopic Approach
0FL64ZZ Occlusion of Left Hepatic Duct, Percutaneous Endoscopic Approach
0FL67DZ Occlusion of Left Hepatic Duct with Intraluminal Device, Via Natural or Artificial Opening
0FL67ZZ Occlusion of Left Hepatic Duct, Via Natural or Artificial Opening
0FL68DZ Occlusion of Left Hepatic Duct with Intraluminal Device, Via Natural or Artificial Opening Endoscopic
0FL68ZZ Occlusion of Left Hepatic Duct, Via Natural or Artificial Opening Endoscopic
0FL80CZ Occlusion of Cystic Duct with Extraluminal Device, Open Approach
0FL80DZ Occlusion of Cystic Duct with Intraluminal Device, Open Approach
0FL80ZZ Occlusion of Cystic Duct, Open Approach
0FL83CZ Occlusion of Cystic Duct with Extraluminal Device, Percutaneous Approach
0FL83DZ Occlusion of Cystic Duct with Intraluminal Device, Percutaneous Approach
0FL83ZZ Occlusion of Cystic Duct, Percutaneous Approach
0FL84CZ Occlusion of Cystic Duct with Extraluminal Device, Percutaneous Endoscopic Approach
0FL84DZ Occlusion of Cystic Duct with Intraluminal Device, Percutaneous Endoscopic Approach
0FL84ZZ Occlusion of Cystic Duct, Percutaneous Endoscopic Approach
0FL87DZ Occlusion of Cystic Duct with Intraluminal Device, Via Natural or Artificial Opening
0FL87ZZ Occlusion of Cystic Duct, Via Natural or Artificial Opening
0FL88DZ Occlusion of Cystic Duct with Intraluminal Device, Via Natural or Artificial Opening Endoscopic
0FL88ZZ Occlusion of Cystic Duct, Via Natural or Artificial Opening Endoscopic
0FL90CZ Occlusion of Common Bile Duct with Extraluminal Device, Open Approach
0FL90DZ Occlusion of Common Bile Duct with Intraluminal Device, Open Approach
0FL90ZZ Occlusion of Common Bile Duct, Open Approach
0FL93CZ Occlusion of Common Bile Duct with Extraluminal Device, Percutaneous Approach
0FL93DZ Occlusion of Common Bile Duct with Intraluminal Device, Percutaneous Approach
0FL93ZZ Occlusion of Common Bile Duct, Percutaneous Approach
0FL94CZ Occlusion of Common Bile Duct with Extraluminal Device, Percutaneous Endoscopic Approach
0FL94DZ Occlusion of Common Bile Duct with Intraluminal Device, Percutaneous Endoscopic Approach
0FL94ZZ Occlusion of Common Bile Duct, Percutaneous Endoscopic Approach
0FL97DZ Occlusion of Common Bile Duct with Intraluminal Device, Via Natural or Artificial Opening
0FL97ZZ Occlusion of Common Bile Duct, Via Natural or Artificial Opening
0FL98DZ Occlusion of Common Bile Duct with Intraluminal Device, Via Natural or Artificial Opening Endoscopic
0FL98ZZ Occlusion of Common Bile Duct, Via Natural or Artificial Opening Endoscopic
0FLC0CZ Occlusion of Ampulla of Vater with Extraluminal Device, Open Approach
0FLC0DZ Occlusion of Ampulla of Vater with Intraluminal Device, Open Approach
0FLC0ZZ Occlusion of Ampulla of Vater, Open Approach
0FLC3CZ Occlusion of Ampulla of Vater with Extraluminal Device, Percutaneous Approach
0FLC3DZ Occlusion of Ampulla of Vater with Intraluminal Device, Percutaneous Approach
0FLC3ZZ Occlusion of Ampulla of Vater, Percutaneous Approach
0FLC4CZ Occlusion of Ampulla of Vater with Extraluminal Device, Percutaneous Endoscopic Approach
0FLC4DZ Occlusion of Ampulla of Vater with Intraluminal Device, Percutaneous Endoscopic Approach
0FLC4ZZ Occlusion of Ampulla of Vater, Percutaneous Endoscopic Approach
0FLC7DZ Occlusion of Ampulla of Vater with Intraluminal Device, Via Natural or Artificial Opening
0FLC7ZZ Occlusion of Ampulla of Vater, Via Natural or Artificial Opening
0FLC8DZ Occlusion of Ampulla of Vater with Intraluminal Device, Via Natural or Artificial Opening Endoscopic
0FLC8ZZ Occlusion of Ampulla of Vater, Via Natural or Artificial Opening Endoscop
0FLD0CZ Occlusion of Pancreatic Duct with Extraluminal Device, Open Approach
0FLD0DZ Occlusion of Pancreatic Duct with Intraluminal Device, Open Approach
0FLD0ZZ Occlusion of Pancreatic Duct, Open Approach
0FLD3CZ Occlusion of Pancreatic Duct with Extraluminal Device, Percutaneous Approach
0FLD3DZ Occlusion of Pancreatic Duct with Intraluminal Device, Percutaneous Approach
0FLD3ZZ Occlusion of Pancreatic Duct, Percutaneous Approach
0FLD4CZ Occlusion of Pancreatic Duct with Extraluminal Device, Percutaneous Endoscopic Approach
0FLD4DZ Occlusion of Pancreatic Duct with Intraluminal Device, Percutaneous Endoscopic Approach
0FLD4ZZ Occlusion of Pancreatic Duct, Percutaneous Endoscopic Approach
0FLD7DZ Occlusion of Pancreatic Duct with Intraluminal Device, Via Natural or Artificial Opening
0FLD7ZZ Occlusion of Pancreatic Duct, Via Natur or Artificial Opening
0FLD8DZ Occlusion of Pancreatic Duct with Intraluminal Device, Via Natural or Artificial Opening Endoscopic
0FLD8ZZ Occlusion of Pancreatic Duct, Via Natur or Artificial Opening Endoscopic
0FLF0CZ Occlusion of Accessory Pancreatic Duct with Extraluminal Device, Open Approach
0FLF0DZ Occlusion of Accessory Pancreatic Duct with Intraluminal Device, Open Approac
0FLF0ZZ Occlusion of Accessory Pancreatic Duct, Open Approach
0FLF3CZ Occlusion of Accessory Pancreatic Duct with Extraluminal Device, Percutaneous Approach
0FLF3DZ Occlusion of Accessory Pancreatic Duct with Intraluminal Device, Percutaneous Approach
0FLF3ZZ Occlusion of Accessory Pancreatic Duct, Percutaneous Approach
0FLF4CZ Occlusion of Accessory Pancreatic Duct with Extraluminal Device, Percutaneous Endoscopic Approach
0FLF4DZ Occlusion of Accessory Pancreatic Duct with Intraluminal Device, Percutaneous Endoscopic Approach
0FLF4ZZ Occlusion of Accessory Pancreatic Duct, Percutaneous Endoscopic Approach
0FLF7DZ Occlusion of Accessory Pancreatic Duct with Intraluminal Device, Via Natural or Artificial Opening
0FLF7ZZ Occlusion of Accessory Pancreatic Duct, Via Natural or Artificial Opening
0FLF8DZ Occlusion of Accessory Pancreatic Duct with Intraluminal Device, Via Natural or Artificial Opening Endoscopic
0FLF8ZZ Occlusion of Accessory Pancreatic Duct, Via Natural or Artificial Opening Endoscopic

M – Hepatobiliary System and Pancreas, Reattachment

M00ZZ Reattachment of Liver, Open Approach
M04ZZ Reattachment of Liver, Percutaneous Endoscopic Approach
M10ZZ Reattachment of Right Lobe Liver, Open Approach
M14ZZ Reattachment of Right Lobe Liver, Percutaneous Endoscopic Approach
M20ZZ Reattachment of Left Lobe Liver, Open Approach
M24ZZ Reattachment of Left Lobe Liver, Percutaneous Endoscopic Approach
M40ZZ Reattachment of Gallbladder, Open Approach
M44ZZ Reattachment of Gallbladder, Percutaneous Endoscopic Approach
0FM50ZZ Reattachment of Right Hepatic Duct, Open Approach
0FM54ZZ Reattachment of Right Hepatic Duct, Percutaneous Endoscopic Approach
0FM60ZZ Reattachment of Left Hepatic Duct, Open Approach
0FM64ZZ Reattachment of Left Hepatic Duct, Percutaneous Endoscopic Approach
0FM80ZZ Reattachment of Cystic Duct, Open Approach
0FM84ZZ Reattachment of Cystic Duct, Percutaneous Endoscopic Approach
0FM90ZZ Reattachment of Common Bile Duct, Open Approach
0FM94ZZ Reattachment of Common Bile Duct, Percutaneous Endoscopic Approach
0FMC0ZZ Reattachment of Ampulla of Vater, Open Approach
0FMC4ZZ Reattachment of Ampulla of Vater, Percutaneous Endoscopic Approach
0FMD0ZZ Reattachment of Pancreatic Duct, Open Approach
0FMD4ZZ Reattachment of Pancreatic Duct, Percutaneous Endoscopic Approach
0FMF0ZZ Reattachment of Accessory Pancreatic Duct, Open Approach
0FMF4ZZ Reattachment of Accessory Pancreatic Duct, Percutaneous Endoscopic Approach
0FMG0ZZ Reattachment of Pancreas, Open Approach
0FMG4ZZ Reattachment of Pancreas, Percutaneous Endoscopic Approach

N – Hepatobiliary System and Pancreas, Release

eview Coding Guideline B3.13

eview Coding Guideline B3.14

N00ZZ Release Liver, Open Approach
N03ZZ Release Liver, Percutaneous Approach
N04ZZ Release Liver, Percutaneous Endoscopic Approach
N10ZZ Release Right Lobe Liver, Open Approach
N13ZZ Release Right Lobe Liver, Percutaneous Approach
N14ZZ Release Right Lobe Liver, Percutaneous Endoscopic Approach
N20ZZ Release Left Lobe Liver, Open Approach
N23ZZ Release Left Lobe Liver, Percutaneous Approach
N24ZZ Release Left Lobe Liver, Percutaneous Endoscopic Approach
N40ZZ Release Gallbladder, Open Approach
N43ZZ Release Gallbladder, Percutaneous Approach
FN44ZZ Release Gallbladder, Percutaneous Endoscopic Approach
FN50ZZ Release Right Hepatic Duct, Open Approach
FN53ZZ Release Right Hepatic Duct, Percutaneous Approach
FN54ZZ Release Right Hepatic Duct, Percutaneous Endoscopic Approach
FN57ZZ Release Right Hepatic Duct, Via Natural or Artificial Opening
FN58ZZ Release Right Hepatic Duct, Via Natural or Artificial Opening Endoscopic
FN60ZZ Release Left Hepatic Duct, Open Approach
0FN63ZZ Release Left Hepatic Duct, Percutaneous Approach
0FN64ZZ Release Left Hepatic Duct, Percutaneous Endoscopic Approach
0FN67ZZ Release Left Hepatic Duct, Via Natural or Artificial Opening
0FN68ZZ Release Left Hepatic Duct, Via Natural or Artificial Opening Endoscopic
0FN80ZZ Release Cystic Duct, Open Approach
0FN83ZZ Release Cystic Duct, Percutaneous Approach
0FN84ZZ Release Cystic Duct, Percutaneous Endoscopic Approach
0FN87ZZ Release Cystic Duct, Via Natural or Artificial Opening
0FN88ZZ Release Cystic Duct, Via Natural or Artificial Opening Endoscopic
0FN90ZZ Release Common Bile Duct, Open Approach
0FN93ZZ Release Common Bile Duct, Percutaneous Approach
0FN94ZZ Release Common Bile Duct, Percutaneous Endoscopic Approach
0FN97ZZ Release Common Bile Duct, Via Natural or Artificial Opening
0FN98ZZ Release Common Bile Duct, Via Natural or Artificial Opening Endoscopic
0FNC0ZZ Release Ampulla of Vater, Open Approach
0FNC3ZZ Release Ampulla of Vater, Percutaneous Approach
0FNC4ZZ Release Ampulla of Vater, Percutaneous Endoscopic Approach
0FNC7ZZ Release Ampulla of Vater, Via Natural or Artificial Opening
0FNC8ZZ Release Ampulla of Vater, Via Natural or Artificial Opening Endoscopic
0FND0ZZ Release Pancreatic Duct, Open Approach
0FND3ZZ Release Pancreatic Duct, Percutaneous Approach
0FND4ZZ Release Pancreatic Duct, Percutaneous Endoscopic Approach
0FND7ZZ Release Pancreatic Duct, Via Natural or Artificial Opening
0FND8ZZ Release Pancreatic Duct, Via Natural or Artificial Opening Endoscopic
0FNF0ZZ Release Accessory Pancreatic Duct, Open Approach
0FNF3ZZ Release Accessory Pancreatic Duct, Percutaneous Approach
0FNF4ZZ Release Accessory Pancreatic Duct, Percutaneous Endoscopic Approach
0FNF7ZZ Release Accessory Pancreatic Duct, Via Natural or Artificial Opening
0FNF8ZZ Release Accessory Pancreatic Duct, Via Natural or Artificial Opening Endoscopic
0FNG0ZZ Release Pancreas, Open Approach
0FNG3ZZ Release Pancreas, Percutaneous Approach
0FNG4ZZ Release Pancreas, Percutaneous Endoscopic Approach

FP – Hepatobiliary System and Pancreas, Removal

Review Coding Guideline B6.1c

FP000Z Removal of Drainage Device from Liver, Open Approach
FP002Z Removal of Monitoring Device from Liver, Open Approach
FP003Z Removal of Infusion Device from Liver, Open Approach
FP030Z Removal of Drainage Device from Liver, Percutaneous Approach
FP032Z Removal of Monitoring Device from Liver, Percutaneous Approach
FP033Z Removal of Infusion Device from Liver, Percutaneous Approach
FP040Z Removal of Drainage Device from Liver, Percutaneous Endoscopic Approach
FP042Z Removal of Monitoring Device from Liver, Percutaneous Endoscopic Approach
0FP043Z Removal of Infusion Device from Liver, Percutaneous Endoscopic Approach
0FP0X0Z Removal of Drainage Device from Liver, External Approach
0FP0X2Z Removal of Monitoring Device from Liver, External Approach
0FP0X3Z Removal of Infusion Device from Liver, External Approach
0FP400Z Removal of Drainage Device from Gallbladder, Open Approach
0FP402Z Removal of Monitoring Device from Gallbladder, Open Approach
0FP403Z Removal of Infusion Device from Gallbladder, Open Approach
0FP40DZ Removal of Intraluminal Device from Gallbladder, Open Approach
0FP430Z Removal of Drainage Device from Gallbladder, Percutaneous Approach
0FP432Z Removal of Monitoring Device from Gallbladder, Percutaneous Approach
0FP433Z Removal of Infusion Device from Gallbladder, Percutaneous Approach
0FP43DZ Removal of Intraluminal Device from Gallbladder, Percutaneous Approach
0FP440Z Removal of Drainage Device from Gallbladder, Percutaneous Endoscopic Approach
0FP442Z Removal of Monitoring Device from Gallbladder, Percutaneous Endoscopic Approach
0FP443Z Removal of Infusion Device from Gallbladder, Percutaneous Endoscopic Approach

0FP44DZ Removal of Intraluminal Device from Gallbladder, Percutaneous Endoscopic Approach
0FP4X0Z Removal of Drainage Device from Gallbladder, External Approach
0FP4X2Z Removal of Monitoring Device from Gallbladder, External Approach
0FP4X3Z Removal of Infusion Device from Gallbladder, External Approach
0FP4XDZ Removal of Intraluminal Device from Gallbladder, External Approach
0FPB00Z Removal of Drainage Device from Hepatobiliary Duct, Open Approach
0FPB01Z Removal of Radioactive Element from Hepatobiliary Duct, Open Approach
0FPB02Z Removal of Monitoring Device from Hepatobiliary Duct, Open Approach
0FPB03Z Removal of Infusion Device from Hepatobiliary Duct, Open Approach
0FPB07Z Removal of Autologous Tissue Substitute from Hepatobiliary Duct, Open Approach
0FPB0CZ Removal of Extraluminal Device from Hepatobiliary Duct, Open Approach
0FPB0DZ Removal of Intraluminal Device from Hepatobiliary Duct, Open Approach
0FPB0JZ Removal of Synthetic Substitute from Hepatobiliary Duct, Open Approach
0FPB0KZ Removal of Nonautologous Tissue Substitute from Hepatobiliary Duct, Open Approach
0FPB30Z Removal of Drainage Device from Hepatobiliary Duct, Percutaneous Approach
0FPB31Z Removal of Radioactive Element from Hepatobiliary Duct, Percutaneous Approach
0FPB32Z Removal of Monitoring Device from Hepatobiliary Duct, Percutaneous Approach
0FPB33Z Removal of Infusion Device from Hepatobiliary Duct, Percutaneous Approach
0FPB37Z Removal of Autologous Tissue Substitute from Hepatobiliary Duct, Percutaneous Approach
0FPB3CZ Removal of Extraluminal Device from Hepatobiliary Duct, Percutaneous Approach
0FPB3DZ Removal of Intraluminal Device from Hepatobiliary Duct, Percutaneous Approach
0FPB3JZ Removal of Synthetic Substitute from Hepatobiliary Duct, Percutaneous Approach
0FPB3KZ Removal of Nonautologous Tissue Substitute from Hepatobiliary Duct, Percutaneous Approach
0FPB40Z Removal of Drainage Device from Hepatobiliary Duct, Percutaneous Endoscopic Approach
0FPB41Z Removal of Radioactive Element from Hepatobiliary Duct, Percutaneous Endoscopic Approach
0FPB42Z Removal of Monitoring Device from Hepatobiliary Duct, Percutaneous Endoscopic Approach
0FPB43Z Removal of Infusion Device from Hepatobiliary Duct, Percutaneous Endoscopic Approach
0FPB47Z Removal of Autologous Tissue Substitute from Hepatobiliary Duct, Percutaneous Endoscopic Approach
0FPB4CZ Removal of Extraluminal Device from Hepatobiliary Duct, Percutaneous Endoscopic Approach
0FPB4DZ Removal of Intraluminal Device from Hepatobiliary Duct, Percutaneous Endoscopic Approach
0FPB4JZ Removal of Synthetic Substitute from Hepatobiliary Duct, Percutaneous Endoscopic Approach
0FPB4KZ Removal of Nonautologous Tissue Substitute from Hepatobiliary Duct, Percutaneous Endoscopic Approach
0FPB70Z Removal of Drainage Device from Hepatobiliary Duct, Via Natural or Artificial Opening
0FPB71Z Removal of Radioactive Element from Hepatobiliary Duct, Via Natural or Artificial Opening
0FPB72Z Removal of Monitoring Device from Hepatobiliary Duct, Via Natural or Artificial Opening
0FPB73Z Removal of Infusion Device from Hepatobiliary Duct, Via Natural or Artificial Opening
0FPB77Z Removal of Autologous Tissue Substitute from Hepatobiliary Duct, Via Natural or Artificial Opening
0FPB7CZ Removal of Extraluminal Device from Hepatobiliary Duct, Via Natural or Artificial Opening
0FPB7DZ Removal of Intraluminal Device from Hepatobiliary Duct, Via Natural or Artificial Opening
0FPB7JZ Removal of Synthetic Substitute from Hepatobiliary Duct, Via Natural or Artificial Opening
0FPB7KZ Removal of Nonautologous Tissue Substitute from Hepatobiliary Duct, Via Natural or Artificial Opening
0FPB80Z Removal of Drainage Device from Hepatobiliary Duct, Via Natural or Artificial Opening Endoscopic
0FPB81Z Removal of Radioactive Element from Hepatobiliary Duct, Via Natural or Artificial Opening Endoscopic
0FPB82Z Removal of Monitoring Device from Hepatobiliary Duct, Via Natural or Artificial Opening Endoscopic
0FPB83Z Removal of Infusion Device from Hepatobiliary Duct, Via Natural or Artificial Opening Endoscopic
0FPB87Z Removal of Autologous Tissue Substitute from Hepatobiliary Duct, Via Natural or Artificial Opening Endoscopic
0FPB8CZ Removal of Extraluminal Device from Hepatobiliary Duct, Via Natural or Artificial Opening Endoscopic
0FPB8DZ Removal of Intraluminal Device from Hepatobiliary Duct, Via Natural or Artificial Opening Endoscopic
0FPB8JZ Removal of Synthetic Substitute from Hepatobiliary Duct, Via Natural or Artificial Opening Endoscopic
0FPB8KZ Removal of Nonautologous Tissue Substitute from Hepatobiliary Duct, Via Natural or Artificial Opening Endoscopic
0FPBX0Z Removal of Drainage Device from Hepatobiliary Duct, External Approach
0FPBX1Z Removal of Radioactive Element from Hepatobiliary Duct, External Approach
0FPBX2Z Removal of Monitoring Device from Hepatobiliary Duct, External Approach
0FPBX3Z Removal of Infusion Device from Hepatobiliary Duct, External Approach
● **0FPBXDZ** Removal of Intraluminal Device from Hepatobiliary Duct, External Approach
0FPD00Z Removal of Drainage Device from Pancreatic Duct, Open Approach
0FPD01Z Removal of Radioactive Element from Pancreatic Duct, Open Approach
0FPD02Z Removal of Monitoring Device from Pancreatic Duct, Open Approach
0FPD03Z Removal of Infusion Device from Pancreatic Duct, Open Approach
0FPD07Z Removal of Autologous Tissue Substitu from Pancreatic Duct, Open Approach
0FPD0CZ Removal of Extraluminal Device from Pancreatic Duct, Open Approach
0FPD0DZ Removal of Intraluminal Device from Pancreatic Duct, Open Approach
0FPD0JZ Removal of Synthetic Substitute from Pancreatic Duct, Open Approach
0FPD0KZ Removal of Nonautologous Tissue Substitute from Pancreatic Duct, Open Approach
0FPD30Z Removal of Drainage Device from Pancreatic Duct, Percutaneous Approach
0FPD31Z Removal of Radioactive Element from Pancreatic Duct, Percutaneous Approach
0FPD32Z Removal of Monitoring Device from Pancreatic Duct, Percutaneous Approac
0FPD33Z Removal of Infusion Device from Pancreatic Duct, Percutaneous Approac
0FPD37Z Removal of Autologous Tissue Substitu from Pancreatic Duct, Percutaneous Approach
0FPD3CZ Removal of Extraluminal Device from Pancreatic Duct, Percutaneous Approach
0FPD3DZ Removal of Intraluminal Device from Pancreatic Duct, Percutaneous Approach
0FPD3JZ Removal of Synthetic Substitute from Pancreatic Duct, Percutaneous Approach
0FPD3KZ Removal of Nonautologous Tissue Substitute from Pancreatic Duct, Percutaneous Approach
0FPD40Z Removal of Drainage Device from Pancreatic Duct, Percutaneous Endoscop Approach
0FPD41Z Removal of Radioactive Element from Pancreatic Duct, Percutaneous Endoscop Approach
0FPD42Z Removal of Monitoring Device from Pancreatic Duct, Percutaneous Endoscop Approach
0FPD43Z Removal of Infusion Device from Pancreatic Duct, Percutaneous Endoscopi Approach
0FPD47Z Removal of Autologous Tissue Substitute from Pancreatic Duct, Percutaneous Endoscopic Approach
0FPD4CZ Removal of Extraluminal Device from Pancreatic Duct, Percutaneous Endoscopi Approach
0FPD4DZ Removal of Intraluminal Device from Pancreatic Duct, Percutaneous Endoscopi Approach
0FPD4JZ Removal of Synthetic Substitute from Pancreatic Duct, Percutaneous Endoscopi Approach
0FPD4KZ Removal of Nonautologous Tissue Substitute from Pancreatic Duct, Percutaneous Endoscopic Approach
0FPD70Z Removal of Drainage Device from Pancreatic Duct, Via Natural or Artificial Opening
0FPD71Z Removal of Radioactive Element from Pancreatic Duct, Via Natural or Artificial Opening
0FPD72Z Removal of Monitoring Device from Pancreatic Duct, Via Natural or Artificial Opening
0FPD73Z Removal of Infusion Device from Pancreatic Duct, Via Natural or Artificial Opening
0FPD77Z Removal of Autologous Tissue Substitute from Pancreatic Duct, Via Natural or Artificial Opening
0FPD7CZ Removal of Extraluminal Device from Pancreatic Duct, Via Natural or Artificial Opening

D7DZ Removal of Intraluminal Device from Pancreatic Duct, Via Natural or Artificial Opening
D7JZ Removal of Synthetic Substitute from Pancreatic Duct, Via Natural or Artificial Opening
D7KZ Removal of Nonautologous Tissue Substitute from Pancreatic Duct, Via Natural or Artificial Opening
D80Z Removal of Drainage Device from Pancreatic Duct, Via Natural or Artificial Opening Endoscopic
D81Z Removal of Radioactive Element from Pancreatic Duct, Via Natural or Artificial Opening Endoscopic
D82Z Removal of Monitoring Device from Pancreatic Duct, Via Natural or Artificial Opening Endoscopic
D83Z Removal of Infusion Device from Pancreatic Duct, Via Natural or Artificial Opening Endoscopic
D87Z Removal of Autologous Tissue Substitute from Pancreatic Duct, Via Natural or Artificial Opening Endoscopic
D8CZ Removal of Extraluminal Device from Pancreatic Duct, Via Natural or Artificial Opening Endoscopic
0FPD8DZ Removal of Intraluminal Device from Pancreatic Duct, Via Natural or Artificial Opening Endoscopic
0FPD8JZ Removal of Synthetic Substitute from Pancreatic Duct, Via Natural or Artificial Opening Endoscopic
0FPD8KZ Removal of Nonautologous Tissue Substitute from Pancreatic Duct, Via Natural or Artificial Opening Endoscopic
0FPDX0Z Removal of Drainage Device from Pancreatic Duct, External Approach
0FPDX1Z Removal of Radioactive Element from Pancreatic Duct, External Approach
0FPDX2Z Removal of Monitoring Device from Pancreatic Duct, External Approach
0FPDX3Z Removal of Infusion Device from Pancreatic Duct, External Approach
● 0FPDXDZ Removal of Intraluminal Device from Pancreatic Duct, External Approach
0FPG00Z Removal of Drainage Device from Pancreas, Open Approach
0FPG02Z Removal of Monitoring Device from Pancreas, Open Approach
0FPG03Z Removal of Infusion Device from Pancreas, Open Approach
0FPG0DZ Removal of Intraluminal Device from Pancreas, Open Approach
0FPG30Z Removal of Drainage Device from Pancreas, Percutaneous Approach
0FPG32Z Removal of Monitoring Device from Pancreas, Percutaneous Approach
0FPG33Z Removal of Infusion Device from Pancreas, Percutaneous Approach
0FPG3DZ Removal of Intraluminal Device from Pancreas, Percutaneous Approach
0FPG40Z Removal of Drainage Device from Pancreas, Percutaneous Endoscopic Approach
0FPG42Z Removal of Monitoring Device from Pancreas, Percutaneous Endoscopic Approach
0FPG43Z Removal of Infusion Device from Pancreas, Percutaneous Endoscopic Approach
0FPG4DZ Removal of Intraluminal Device from Pancreas, Percutaneous Endoscopic Approach
0FPGX0Z Removal of Drainage Device from Pancreas, External Approach
0FPGX2Z Removal of Monitoring Device from Pancreas, External Approach
0FPGX3Z Removal of Infusion Device from Pancreas, External Approach
0FPGXDZ Removal of Intraluminal Device from Pancreas, External Approach

FQ – Hepatobiliary System and Pancreas, Repair

Q00ZZ Repair Liver, Open Approach
AHA CC: 4Q, 2013, 109-111
Q03ZZ Repair Liver, Percutaneous Approach
Q04ZZ Repair Liver, Percutaneous Endoscopic Approach
Q10ZZ Repair Right Lobe Liver, Open Approach
Q13ZZ Repair Right Lobe Liver, Percutaneous Approach
Q14ZZ Repair Right Lobe Liver, Percutaneous Endoscopic Approach
Q20ZZ Repair Left Lobe Liver, Open Approach
Q23ZZ Repair Left Lobe Liver, Percutaneous Approach
Q24ZZ Repair Left Lobe Liver, Percutaneous Endoscopic Approach
Q40ZZ Repair Gallbladder, Open Approach
Q43ZZ Repair Gallbladder, Percutaneous Approach
Q44ZZ Repair Gallbladder, Percutaneous Endoscopic Approach
FQ50ZZ Repair Right Hepatic Duct, Open Approach
FQ53ZZ Repair Right Hepatic Duct, Percutaneous Approach
FQ54ZZ Repair Right Hepatic Duct, Percutaneous Endoscopic Approach
FQ57ZZ Repair Right Hepatic Duct, Via Natural or Artificial Opening
FQ58ZZ Repair Right Hepatic Duct, Via Natural or Artificial Opening Endoscopic
FQ60ZZ Repair Left Hepatic Duct, Open Approach
0FQ63ZZ Repair Left Hepatic Duct, Percutaneous Approach
0FQ64ZZ Repair Left Hepatic Duct, Percutaneous Endoscopic Approach
0FQ67ZZ Repair Left Hepatic Duct, Via Natural or Artificial Opening
0FQ68ZZ Repair Left Hepatic Duct, Via Natural or Artificial Opening Endoscopic
0FQ80ZZ Repair Cystic Duct, Open Approach
0FQ83ZZ Repair Cystic Duct, Percutaneous Approach
0FQ84ZZ Repair Cystic Duct, Percutaneous Endoscopic Approach
0FQ87ZZ Repair Cystic Duct, Via Natural or Artificial Opening
0FQ88ZZ Repair Cystic Duct, Via Natural or Artificial Opening Endoscopic
0FQ90ZZ Repair Common Bile Duct, Open Approach
0FQ93ZZ Repair Common Bile Duct, Percutaneous Approach
0FQ94ZZ Repair Common Bile Duct, Percutaneous Endoscopic Approach
0FQ97ZZ Repair Common Bile Duct, Via Natural or Artificial Opening
0FQ98ZZ Repair Common Bile Duct, Via Natural or Artificial Opening Endoscopic
0FQC0ZZ Repair Ampulla of Vater, Open Approach
0FQC3ZZ Repair Ampulla of Vater, Percutaneous Approach
0FQC4ZZ Repair Ampulla of Vater, Percutaneous Endoscopic Approach
0FQC7ZZ Repair Ampulla of Vater, Via Natural or Artificial Opening
0FQC8ZZ Repair Ampulla of Vater, Via Natural or Artificial Opening Endoscopic
0FQD0ZZ Repair Pancreatic Duct, Open Approach
0FQD3ZZ Repair Pancreatic Duct, Percutaneous Approach
0FQD4ZZ Repair Pancreatic Duct, Percutaneous Endoscopic Approach
0FQD7ZZ Repair Pancreatic Duct, Via Natural or Artificial Opening
0FQD8ZZ Repair Pancreatic Duct, Via Natural or Artificial Opening Endoscopic
0FQF0ZZ Repair Accessory Pancreatic Duct, Open Approach
0FQF3ZZ Repair Accessory Pancreatic Duct, Percutaneous Approach
0FQF4ZZ Repair Accessory Pancreatic Duct, Percutaneous Endoscopic Approach
0FQF7ZZ Repair Accessory Pancreatic Duct, Via Natural or Artificial Opening
0FQF8ZZ Repair Accessory Pancreatic Duct, Via Natural or Artificial Opening Endoscopic
0FQG0ZZ Repair Pancreas, Open Approach
0FQG3ZZ Repair Pancreas, Percutaneous Approach
0FQG4ZZ Repair Pancreas, Percutaneous Endoscopic Approach

FR – Hepatobiliary System and Pancreas, Replacement

FR507Z Replacement of Right Hepatic Duct with Autologous Tissue Substitute, Open Approach
FR50JZ Replacement of Right Hepatic Duct with Synthetic Substitute, Open Approach
FR50KZ Replacement of Right Hepatic Duct with Nonautologous Tissue Substitute, Open Approach
FR547Z Replacement of Right Hepatic Duct with Autologous Tissue Substitute, Percutaneous Endoscopic Approach
0FR54JZ Replacement of Right Hepatic Duct with Synthetic Substitute, Percutaneous Endoscopic Approach
0FR54KZ Replacement of Right Hepatic Duct with Nonautologous Tissue Substitute, Percutaneous Endoscopic Approach
0FR607Z Replacement of Left Hepatic Duct with Autologous Tissue Substitute, Open Approach
0FR60JZ Replacement of Left Hepatic Duct with Synthetic Substitute, Open Approach
0FR60KZ Replacement of Left Hepatic Duct with Nonautologous Tissue Substitute, Open Approach
0FR647Z Replacement of Left Hepatic Duct with Autologous Tissue Substitute, Percutaneous Endoscopic Approach
0FR64JZ Replacement of Left Hepatic Duct with Synthetic Substitute, Percutaneous Endoscopic Approach
0FR64KZ Replacement of Left Hepatic Duct with Nonautologous Tissue Substitute, Percutaneous Endoscopic Approach

0FR807Z Replacement of Cystic Duct with Autologous Tissue Substitute, Open Approach
0FR80JZ Replacement of Cystic Duct with Synthetic Substitute, Open Approach
0FR80KZ Replacement of Cystic Duct with Nonautologous Tissue Substitute, Open Approach
0FR847Z Replacement of Cystic Duct with Autologous Tissue Substitute, Percutaneous Endoscopic Approach
0FR84JZ Replacement of Cystic Duct with Synthetic Substitute, Percutaneous Endoscopic Approach
0FR84KZ Replacement of Cystic Duct with Nonautologous Tissue Substitute, Percutaneous Endoscopic Approach
0FR907Z Replacement of Common Bile Duct with Autologous Tissue Substitute, Open Approach
0FR90JZ Replacement of Common Bile Duct with Synthetic Substitute, Open Approach
0FR90KZ Replacement of Common Bile Duct with Nonautologous Tissue Substitute, Open Approach
0FR947Z Replacement of Common Bile Duct with Autologous Tissue Substitute, Percutaneous Endoscopic Approach
0FR94JZ Replacement of Common Bile Duct with Synthetic Substitute, Percutaneous Endoscopic Approach
0FR94KZ Replacement of Common Bile Duct with Nonautologous Tissue Substitute, Percutaneous Endoscopic Approach
0FRC07Z Replacement of Ampulla of Vater with Autologous Tissue Substitute, Open Approach
0FRC0JZ Replacement of Ampulla of Vater with Synthetic Substitute, Open Approach
0FRC0KZ Replacement of Ampulla of Vater with Nonautologous Tissue Substitute, Open Approach
0FRC47Z Replacement of Ampulla of Vater with Autologous Tissue Substitute, Percutaneous Endoscopic Approach
0FRC4JZ Replacement of Ampulla of Vater with Synthetic Substitute, Percutaneous Endoscopic Approach
0FRC4KZ Replacement of Ampulla of Vater with Nonautologous Tissue Substitute, Percutaneous Endoscopic Approach
0FRD07Z Replacement of Pancreatic Duct with Autologous Tissue Substitute, Open Approach
0FRD0JZ Replacement of Pancreatic Duct with Synthetic Substitute, Open Approach
0FRD0KZ Replacement of Pancreatic Duct with Nonautologous Tissue Substitute, Ope Approach
0FRD47Z Replacement of Pancreatic Duct with Autologous Tissue Substitute, Percutaneous Endoscopic Approach
0FRD4JZ Replacement of Pancreatic Duct with Synthetic Substitute, Percutaneous Endoscopic Approach
0FRD4KZ Replacement of Pancreatic Duct with Nonautologous Tissue Substitute, Percutaneous Endoscopic Approach
0FRF07Z Replacement of Accessory Pancreatic Duct with Autologous Tissue Substitut Open Approach
0FRF0JZ Replacement of Accessory Pancreatic D with Synthetic Substitute, Open Approa
0FRF0KZ Replacement of Accessory Pancreatic Duct with Nonautologous Tissue Substitute, Open Approach
0FRF47Z Replacement of Accessory Pancreatic Duct with Autologous Tissue Substitute, Percutaneous Endoscopic Approach
0FRF4JZ Replacement of Accessory Pancreatic D with Synthetic Substitute, Percutaneous Endoscopic Approach
0FRF4KZ Replacement of Accessory Pancreatic D with Nonautologous Tissue Substitute, Percutaneous Endoscopic Approach

0FS – Hepatobiliary System and Pancreas, Reposition

0FS00ZZ Reposition Liver, Open Approach
0FS04ZZ Reposition Liver, Percutaneous Endoscopic Approach
0FS40ZZ Reposition Gallbladder, Open Approach
0FS44ZZ Reposition Gallbladder, Percutaneous Endoscopic Approach
0FS50ZZ Reposition Right Hepatic Duct, Open Approach
0FS54ZZ Reposition Right Hepatic Duct, Percutaneous Endoscopic Approach
0FS60ZZ Reposition Left Hepatic Duct, Open Approach
0FS64ZZ Reposition Left Hepatic Duct, Percutaneous Endoscopic Approach
0FS80ZZ Reposition Cystic Duct, Open Approach
0FS84ZZ Reposition Cystic Duct, Percutaneous Endoscopic Approach
0FS90ZZ Reposition Common Bile Duct, Open Approach
0FS94ZZ Reposition Common Bile Duct, Percutaneous Endoscopic Approach
0FSC0ZZ Reposition Ampulla of Vater, Open Approach
0FSC4ZZ Reposition Ampulla of Vater, Percutaneous Endoscopic Approach
0FSD0ZZ Reposition Pancreatic Duct, Open Approach
0FSD4ZZ Reposition Pancreatic Duct, Percutaneo Endoscopic Approach
0FSF0ZZ Reposition Accessory Pancreatic Duct, Open Approach
0FSF4ZZ Reposition Accessory Pancreatic Duct, Percutaneous Endoscopic Approach
0FSG0ZZ Reposition Pancreas, Open Approach
0FSG4ZZ Reposition Pancreas, Percutaneous Endoscopic Approach

0FT – Hepatobiliary System and Pancreas, Resection

Review Coding Guideline B3.8

0FT00ZZ Resection of Liver, Open Approach
AHA CC: 4Q, 2012, 99-101
0FT04ZZ Resection of Liver, Percutaneous Endoscopic Approach
0FT10ZZ Resection of Right Lobe Liver, Open Approach
0FT14ZZ Resection of Right Lobe Liver, Percutaneous Endoscopic Approach
0FT20ZZ Resection of Left Lobe Liver, Open Approach
0FT24ZZ Resection of Left Lobe Liver, Percutaneous Endoscopic Approach
0FT40ZZ Resection of Gallbladder, Open Approach
0FT44ZZ Resection of Gallbladder, Percutaneous Endoscopic Approach
0FT50ZZ Resection of Right Hepatic Duct, Open Approach
0FT54ZZ Resection of Right Hepatic Duct, Percutaneous Endoscopic Approach
0FT57ZZ Resection of Right Hepatic Duct, Via Natural or Artificial Opening
0FT58ZZ Resection of Right Hepatic Duct, Via Natural or Artificial Opening Endoscopic
0FT60ZZ Resection of Left Hepatic Duct, Open Approach
0FT64ZZ Resection of Left Hepatic Duct, Percutaneous Endoscopic Approach
0FT67ZZ Resection of Left Hepatic Duct, Via Natural or Artificial Opening
0FT68ZZ Resection of Left Hepatic Duct, Via Natural or Artificial Opening Endoscopic
0FT80ZZ Resection of Cystic Duct, Open Approach
0FT84ZZ Resection of Cystic Duct, Percutaneous Endoscopic Approach
0FT87ZZ Resection of Cystic Duct, Via Natural or Artificial Opening
0FT88ZZ Resection of Cystic Duct, Via Natural or Artificial Opening Endoscopic
0FT90ZZ Resection of Common Bile Duct, Open Approach
0FT94ZZ Resection of Common Bile Duct, Percutaneous Endoscopic Approach
0FT97ZZ Resection of Common Bile Duct, Via Natural or Artificial Opening
0FT98ZZ Resection of Common Bile Duct, Via Natural or Artificial Opening Endoscopic
0FTC0ZZ Resection of Ampulla of Vater, Open Approach
0FTC4ZZ Resection of Ampulla of Vater, Percutaneous Endoscopic Approach
0FTC7ZZ Resection of Ampulla of Vater, Via Natu or Artificial Opening
0FTC8ZZ Resection of Ampulla of Vater, Via Natur or Artificial Opening Endoscopic
0FTD0ZZ Resection of Pancreatic Duct, Open Approach
0FTD4ZZ Resection of Pancreatic Duct, Percutaneous Endoscopic Approach
0FTD7ZZ Resection of Pancreatic Duct, Via Natura or Artificial Opening
0FTD8ZZ Resection of Pancreatic Duct, Via Natura or Artificial Opening Endoscopic
0FTF0ZZ Resection of Accessory Pancreatic Duct, Open Approach
0FTF4ZZ Resection of Accessory Pancreatic Duct, Percutaneous Endoscopic Approach
0FTF7ZZ Resection of Accessory Pancreatic Duct, Via Natural or Artificial Opening
0FTF8ZZ Resection of Accessory Pancreatic Duct, Via Natural or Artificial Opening Endoscopic
0FTG0ZZ Resection of Pancreas, Open Approach
0FTG4ZZ Resection of Pancreas, Percutaneous Endoscopic Approach

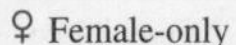
♀ Female-only ♂ Male-only Limited Coverage ● Non-OR HAC-associated procedure ▲ Non-covered procedures + Combinatio

U – Hepatobiliary System and Pancreas, Supplement

507Z Supplement Right Hepatic Duct with Autologous Tissue Substitute, Open Approach
J50JZ Supplement Right Hepatic Duct with Synthetic Substitute, Open Approach
J50KZ Supplement Right Hepatic Duct with Nonautologous Tissue Substitute, Open Approach
J537Z Supplement Right Hepatic Duct with Autologous Tissue Substitute, Percutaneous Approach
J53JZ Supplement Right Hepatic Duct with Synthetic Substitute, Percutaneous Approach
U53KZ Supplement Right Hepatic Duct with Nonautologous Tissue Substitute, Percutaneous Approach
U547Z Supplement Right Hepatic Duct with Autologous Tissue Substitute, Percutaneous Endoscopic Approach
U54JZ Supplement Right Hepatic Duct with Synthetic Substitute, Percutaneous Endoscopic Approach
U54KZ Supplement Right Hepatic Duct with Nonautologous Tissue Substitute, Percutaneous Endoscopic Approach
U607Z Supplement Left Hepatic Duct with Autologous Tissue Substitute, Open Approach
U60JZ Supplement Left Hepatic Duct with Synthetic Substitute, Open Approach
U60KZ Supplement Left Hepatic Duct with Nonautologous Tissue Substitute, Open Approach
U637Z Supplement Left Hepatic Duct with Autologous Tissue Substitute, Percutaneous Approach
U63JZ Supplement Left Hepatic Duct with Synthetic Substitute, Percutaneous Approach
U63KZ Supplement Left Hepatic Duct with Nonautologous Tissue Substitute, Percutaneous Approach
U647Z Supplement Left Hepatic Duct with Autologous Tissue Substitute, Percutaneous Endoscopic Approach
U64JZ Supplement Left Hepatic Duct with Synthetic Substitute, Percutaneous Endoscopic Approach
FU64KZ Supplement Left Hepatic Duct with Nonautologous Tissue Substitute, Percutaneous Endoscopic Approach
FU807Z Supplement Cystic Duct with Autologous Tissue Substitute, Open Approach
FU80JZ Supplement Cystic Duct with Synthetic Substitute, Open Approach
FU80KZ Supplement Cystic Duct with Nonautologous Tissue Substitute, Open Approach
0FU837Z Supplement Cystic Duct with Autologous Tissue Substitute, Percutaneous Approach
0FU83JZ Supplement Cystic Duct with Synthetic Substitute, Percutaneous Approach
0FU83KZ Supplement Cystic Duct with Nonautologous Tissue Substitute, Percutaneous Approach
0FU847Z Supplement Cystic Duct with Autologous Tissue Substitute, Percutaneous Endoscopic Approach
0FU84JZ Supplement Cystic Duct with Synthetic Substitute, Percutaneous Endoscopic Approach
0FU84KZ Supplement Cystic Duct with Nonautologous Tissue Substitute, Percutaneous Endoscopic Approach
0FU907Z Supplement Common Bile Duct with Autologous Tissue Substitute, Open Approach
0FU90JZ Supplement Common Bile Duct with Synthetic Substitute, Open Approach
0FU90KZ Supplement Common Bile Duct with Nonautologous Tissue Substitute, Open Approach
0FU937Z Supplement Common Bile Duct with Autologous Tissue Substitute, Percutaneous Approach
0FU93JZ Supplement Common Bile Duct with Synthetic Substitute, Percutaneous Approach
0FU93KZ Supplement Common Bile Duct with Nonautologous Tissue Substitute, Percutaneous Approach
0FU947Z Supplement Common Bile Duct with Autologous Tissue Substitute, Percutaneous Endoscopic Approach
0FU94JZ Supplement Common Bile Duct with Synthetic Substitute, Percutaneous Endoscopic Approach
0FU94KZ Supplement Common Bile Duct with Nonautologous Tissue Substitute, Percutaneous Endoscopic Approach
0FUC07Z Supplement Ampulla of Vater with Autologous Tissue Substitute, Open Approach
0FUC0JZ Supplement Ampulla of Vater with Synthetic Substitute, Open Approach
0FUC0KZ Supplement Ampulla of Vater with Nonautologous Tissue Substitute, Open Approach
0FUC37Z Supplement Ampulla of Vater with Autologous Tissue Substitute, Percutaneous Approach
0FUC3JZ Supplement Ampulla of Vater with Synthetic Substitute, Percutaneous Approach
0FUC3KZ Supplement Ampulla of Vater with Nonautologous Tissue Substitute, Percutaneous Approach
0FUC47Z Supplement Ampulla of Vater with Autologous Tissue Substitute, Percutaneous Endoscopic Approach
0FUC4JZ Supplement Ampulla of Vater with Synthetic Substitute, Percutaneous Endoscopic Approach
0FUC4KZ Supplement Ampulla of Vater with Nonautologous Tissue Substitute, Percutaneous Endoscopic Approach
0FUD07Z Supplement Pancreatic Duct with Autologous Tissue Substitute, Open Approach
0FUD0JZ Supplement Pancreatic Duct with Synthetic Substitute, Open Approach
0FUD0KZ Supplement Pancreatic Duct with Nonautologous Tissue Substitute, Open Approach
0FUD37Z Supplement Pancreatic Duct with Autologous Tissue Substitute, Percutaneous Approach
0FUD3JZ Supplement Pancreatic Duct with Synthetic Substitute, Percutaneous Approach
0FUD3KZ Supplement Pancreatic Duct with Nonautologous Tissue Substitute, Percutaneous Approach
0FUD47Z Supplement Pancreatic Duct with Autologous Tissue Substitute, Percutaneous Endoscopic Approach
0FUD4JZ Supplement Pancreatic Duct with Synthetic Substitute, Percutaneous Endoscopic Approach
0FUD4KZ Supplement Pancreatic Duct with Nonautologous Tissue Substitute, Percutaneous Endoscopic Approach
0FUF07Z Supplement Accessory Pancreatic Duct with Autologous Tissue Substitute, Open Approach
0FUF0JZ Supplement Accessory Pancreatic Duct with Synthetic Substitute, Open Approach
0FUF0KZ Supplement Accessory Pancreatic Duct with Nonautologous Tissue Substitute, Open Approach
0FUF37Z Supplement Accessory Pancreatic Duct with Autologous Tissue Substitute, Percutaneous Approach
0FUF3JZ Supplement Accessory Pancreatic Duct with Synthetic Substitute, Percutaneous Approach
0FUF3KZ Supplement Accessory Pancreatic Duct with Nonautologous Tissue Substitute, Percutaneous Approach
0FUF47Z Supplement Accessory Pancreatic Duct with Autologous Tissue Substitute, Percutaneous Endoscopic Approach
0FUF4JZ Supplement Accessory Pancreatic Duct with Synthetic Substitute, Percutaneous Endoscopic Approach
0FUF4KZ Supplement Accessory Pancreatic Duct with Nonautologous Tissue Substitute, Percutaneous Endoscopic Approach

FV – Hepatobiliary System and Pancreas, Restriction

FV50CZ Restriction of Right Hepatic Duct with Extraluminal Device, Open Approach
FV50DZ Restriction of Right Hepatic Duct with Intraluminal Device, Open Approach
FV50ZZ Restriction of Right Hepatic Duct, Open Approach
FV53CZ Restriction of Right Hepatic Duct with Extraluminal Device, Percutaneous Approach
FV53DZ Restriction of Right Hepatic Duct with Intraluminal Device, Percutaneous Approach
0FV53ZZ Restriction of Right Hepatic Duct, Percutaneous Approach
0FV54CZ Restriction of Right Hepatic Duct with Extraluminal Device, Percutaneous Endoscopic Approach
0FV54DZ Restriction of Right Hepatic Duct with Intraluminal Device, Percutaneous Endoscopic Approach
0FV54ZZ Restriction of Right Hepatic Duct, Percutaneous Endoscopic Approach
0FV57DZ Restriction of Right Hepatic Duct with Intraluminal Device, Via Natural or Artificial Opening
0FV57ZZ Restriction of Right Hepatic Duct, Via Natural or Artificial Opening
0FV58DZ Restriction of Right Hepatic Duct with Intraluminal Device, Via Natural or Artificial Opening Endoscopic
0FV58ZZ Restriction of Right Hepatic Duct, Via Natural or Artificial Opening Endoscopic
0FV60CZ Restriction of Left Hepatic Duct with Extraluminal Device, Open Approach

0FV60DZ Restriction of Left Hepatic Duct with Intraluminal Device, Open Approach
0FV60ZZ Restriction of Left Hepatic Duct, Open Approach
0FV63CZ Restriction of Left Hepatic Duct with Extraluminal Device, Percutaneous Approach
0FV63DZ Restriction of Left Hepatic Duct with Intraluminal Device, Percutaneous Approach
0FV63ZZ Restriction of Left Hepatic Duct, Percutaneous Approach
0FV64CZ Restriction of Left Hepatic Duct with Extraluminal Device, Percutaneous Endoscopic Approach
0FV64DZ Restriction of Left Hepatic Duct with Intraluminal Device, Percutaneous Endoscopic Approach
0FV64ZZ Restriction of Left Hepatic Duct, Percutaneous Endoscopic Approach
0FV67DZ Restriction of Left Hepatic Duct with Intraluminal Device, Via Natural or Artificial Opening
0FV67ZZ Restriction of Left Hepatic Duct, Via Natural or Artificial Opening
0FV68DZ Restriction of Left Hepatic Duct with Intraluminal Device, Via Natural or Artificial Opening Endoscopic
0FV68ZZ Restriction of Left Hepatic Duct, Via Natural or Artificial Opening Endoscopic
0FV80CZ Restriction of Cystic Duct with Extraluminal Device, Open Approach
0FV80DZ Restriction of Cystic Duct with Intraluminal Device, Open Approach
0FV80ZZ Restriction of Cystic Duct, Open Approach
0FV83CZ Restriction of Cystic Duct with Extraluminal Device, Percutaneous Approach
0FV83DZ Restriction of Cystic Duct with Intraluminal Device, Percutaneous Approach
0FV83ZZ Restriction of Cystic Duct, Percutaneous Approach
0FV84CZ Restriction of Cystic Duct with Extraluminal Device, Percutaneous Endoscopic Approach
0FV84DZ Restriction of Cystic Duct with Intraluminal Device, Percutaneous Endoscopic Approach
0FV84ZZ Restriction of Cystic Duct, Percutaneous Endoscopic Approach
0FV87DZ Restriction of Cystic Duct with Intraluminal Device, Via Natural or Artificial Opening
0FV87ZZ Restriction of Cystic Duct, Via Natural or Artificial Opening
0FV88DZ Restriction of Cystic Duct with Intraluminal Device, Via Natural or Artificial Opening Endoscopic
0FV88ZZ Restriction of Cystic Duct, Via Natural or Artificial Opening Endoscopic
0FV90CZ Restriction of Common Bile Duct with Extraluminal Device, Open Approach
0FV90DZ Restriction of Common Bile Duct with Intraluminal Device, Open Approach
0FV90ZZ Restriction of Common Bile Duct, Open Approach
0FV93CZ Restriction of Common Bile Duct with Extraluminal Device, Percutaneous Approach
0FV93DZ Restriction of Common Bile Duct with Intraluminal Device, Percutaneous Approach
0FV93ZZ Restriction of Common Bile Duct, Percutaneous Approach
0FV94CZ Restriction of Common Bile Duct with Extraluminal Device, Percutaneous Endoscopic Approach
0FV94DZ Restriction of Common Bile Duct with Intraluminal Device, Percutaneous Endoscopic Approach
0FV94ZZ Restriction of Common Bile Duct, Percutaneous Endoscopic Approach
0FV97DZ Restriction of Common Bile Duct with Intraluminal Device, Via Natural or Artificial Opening
0FV97ZZ Restriction of Common Bile Duct, Via Natural or Artificial Opening
0FV98DZ Restriction of Common Bile Duct with Intraluminal Device, Via Natural or Artificial Opening Endoscopic
0FV98ZZ Restriction of Common Bile Duct, Via Natural or Artificial Opening Endoscopic
0FVC0CZ Restriction of Ampulla of Vater with Extraluminal Device, Open Approach
0FVC0DZ Restriction of Ampulla of Vater with Intraluminal Device, Open Approach
0FVC0ZZ Restriction of Ampulla of Vater, Open Approach
0FVC3CZ Restriction of Ampulla of Vater with Extraluminal Device, Percutaneous Approach
0FVC3DZ Restriction of Ampulla of Vater with Intraluminal Device, Percutaneous Approach
0FVC3ZZ Restriction of Ampulla of Vater, Percutaneous Approach
0FVC4CZ Restriction of Ampulla of Vater with Extraluminal Device, Percutaneous Endoscopic Approach
0FVC4DZ Restriction of Ampulla of Vater with Intraluminal Device, Percutaneous Endoscopic Approach
0FVC4ZZ Restriction of Ampulla of Vater, Percutaneous Endoscopic Approach
0FVC7DZ Restriction of Ampulla of Vater with Intraluminal Device, Via Natural or Artificial Opening
0FVC7ZZ Restriction of Ampulla of Vater, Via Natural or Artificial Opening
0FVC8DZ Restriction of Ampulla of Vater with Intraluminal Device, Via Natural or Artificial Opening Endoscopic
0FVC8ZZ Restriction of Ampulla of Vater, Via Natural or Artificial Opening Endoscopic
0FVD0CZ Restriction of Pancreatic Duct with Extraluminal Device, Open Approach
0FVD0DZ Restriction of Pancreatic Duct with Intraluminal Device, Open Approach
0FVD0ZZ Restriction of Pancreatic Duct, Open Approach
0FVD3CZ Restriction of Pancreatic Duct with Extraluminal Device, Percutaneous Approach
0FVD3DZ Restriction of Pancreatic Duct with Intraluminal Device, Percutaneous Approach
0FVD3ZZ Restriction of Pancreatic Duct, Percutaneous Approach
0FVD4CZ Restriction of Pancreatic Duct with Extraluminal Device, Percutaneous Endoscopic Approach
0FVD4DZ Restriction of Pancreatic Duct with Intraluminal Device, Percutaneous Endoscopic Approach
0FVD4ZZ Restriction of Pancreatic Duct, Percutaneous Endoscopic Approach
0FVD7DZ Restriction of Pancreatic Duct with Intraluminal Device, Via Natural or Artificial Opening
0FVD7ZZ Restriction of Pancreatic Duct, Via Natu or Artificial Opening
0FVD8DZ Restriction of Pancreatic Duct with Intraluminal Device, Via Natural or Artificial Opening Endoscopic
0FVD8ZZ Restriction of Pancreatic Duct, Via Natu or Artificial Opening Endoscopic
0FVF0CZ Restriction of Accessory Pancreatic Duc with Extraluminal Device, Open Approa
0FVF0DZ Restriction of Accessory Pancreatic Duc with Intraluminal Device, Open Approa
0FVF0ZZ Restriction of Accessory Pancreatic Duc Open Approach
0FVF3CZ Restriction of Accessory Pancreatic Duc with Extraluminal Device, Percutaneous Approach
0FVF3DZ Restriction of Accessory Pancreatic Duc with Intraluminal Device, Percutaneous Approach
0FVF3ZZ Restriction of Accessory Pancreatic Duc Percutaneous Approach
0FVF4CZ Restriction of Accessory Pancreatic Duc with Extraluminal Device, Percutaneous Endoscopic Approach
0FVF4DZ Restriction of Accessory Pancreatic Duc with Intraluminal Device, Percutaneous Endoscopic Approach
0FVF4ZZ Restriction of Accessory Pancreatic Duct Percutaneous Endoscopic Approach
0FVF7DZ Restriction of Accessory Pancreatic Duct with Intraluminal Device, Via Natural or Artificial Opening
0FVF7ZZ Restriction of Accessory Pancreatic Duct Via Natural or Artificial Opening
0FVF8DZ Restriction of Accessory Pancreatic Duct with Intraluminal Device, Via Natural or Artificial Opening Endoscopic
0FVF8ZZ Restriction of Accessory Pancreatic Duct, Via Natural or Artificial Opening Endoscopic

0FW – Hepatobiliary System and Pancreas, Revision

Review Coding Guideline B6.1c

0FW000Z Revision of Drainage Device in Liver, Open Approach
0FW002Z Revision of Monitoring Device in Liver, Open Approach
0FW003Z Revision of Infusion Device in Liver, Open Approach
0FW030Z Revision of Drainage Device in Liver, Percutaneous Approach
0FW032Z Revision of Monitoring Device in Liver, Percutaneous Approach
0FW033Z Revision of Infusion Device in Liver, Percutaneous Approach
0FW040Z Revision of Drainage Device in Liver, Percutaneous Endoscopic Approach
0FW042Z Revision of Monitoring Device in Liver, Percutaneous Endoscopic Approach
0FW043Z Revision of Infusion Device in Liver, Percutaneous Endoscopic Approach
0FW0X0Z Revision of Drainage Device in Liver, External Approach
0FW0X2Z Revision of Monitoring Device in Liver, External Approach
0FW0X3Z Revision of Infusion Device in Liver, External Approach

V400Z Revision of Drainage Device in Gallbladder, Open Approach
V402Z Revision of Monitoring Device in Gallbladder, Open Approach
V403Z Revision of Infusion Device in Gallbladder, Open Approach
V40DZ Revision of Intraluminal Device in Gallbladder, Open Approach
V430Z Revision of Drainage Device in Gallbladder, Percutaneous Approach
V432Z Revision of Monitoring Device in Gallbladder, Percutaneous Approach
V433Z Revision of Infusion Device in Gallbladder, Percutaneous Approach
V43DZ Revision of Intraluminal Device in Gallbladder, Percutaneous Approach
V440Z Revision of Drainage Device in Gallbladder, Percutaneous Endoscopic Approach
W442Z Revision of Monitoring Device in Gallbladder, Percutaneous Endoscopic Approach
W443Z Revision of Infusion Device in Gallbladder, Percutaneous Endoscopic Approach
W44DZ Revision of Intraluminal Device in Gallbladder, Percutaneous Endoscopic Approach
W4X0Z Revision of Drainage Device in Gallbladder, External Approach
W4X2Z Revision of Monitoring Device in Gallbladder, External Approach
W4X3Z Revision of Infusion Device in Gallbladder, External Approach
W4XDZ Revision of Intraluminal Device in Gallbladder, External Approach
WB00Z Revision of Drainage Device in Hepatobiliary Duct, Open Approach
WB02Z Revision of Monitoring Device in Hepatobiliary Duct, Open Approach
WB03Z Revision of Infusion Device in Hepatobiliary Duct, Open Approach
WB07Z Revision of Autologous Tissue Substitute in Hepatobiliary Duct, Open Approach
WB0CZ Revision of Extraluminal Device in Hepatobiliary Duct, Open Approach
WB0DZ Revision of Intraluminal Device in Hepatobiliary Duct, Open Approach
WB0JZ Revision of Synthetic Substitute in Hepatobiliary Duct, Open Approach
WB0KZ Revision of Nonautologous Tissue Substitute in Hepatobiliary Duct, Open Approach
FWB30Z Revision of Drainage Device in Hepatobiliary Duct, Percutaneous Approach
FWB32Z Revision of Monitoring Device in Hepatobiliary Duct, Percutaneous Approach
FWB33Z Revision of Infusion Device in Hepatobiliary Duct, Percutaneous Approach
FWB37Z Revision of Autologous Tissue Substitute in Hepatobiliary Duct, Percutaneous Approach
FWB3CZ Revision of Extraluminal Device in Hepatobiliary Duct, Percutaneous Approach
FWB3DZ Revision of Intraluminal Device in Hepatobiliary Duct, Percutaneous Approach
FWB3JZ Revision of Synthetic Substitute in Hepatobiliary Duct, Percutaneous Approach
FWB3KZ Revision of Nonautologous Tissue Substitute in Hepatobiliary Duct, Percutaneous Approach

0FWB40Z Revision of Drainage Device in Hepatobiliary Duct, Percutaneous Endoscopic Approach
0FWB42Z Revision of Monitoring Device in Hepatobiliary Duct, Percutaneous Endoscopic Approach
0FWB43Z Revision of Infusion Device in Hepatobiliary Duct, Percutaneous Endoscopic Approach
0FWB47Z Revision of Autologous Tissue Substitute in Hepatobiliary Duct, Percutaneous Endoscopic Approach
0FWB4CZ Revision of Extraluminal Device in Hepatobiliary Duct, Percutaneous Endoscopic Approach
0FWB4DZ Revision of Intraluminal Device in Hepatobiliary Duct, Percutaneous Endoscopic Approach
0FWB4JZ Revision of Synthetic Substitute in Hepatobiliary Duct, Percutaneous Endoscopic Approach
0FWB4KZ Revision of Nonautologous Tissue Substitute in Hepatobiliary Duct, Percutaneous Endoscopic Approach
0FWB70Z Revision of Drainage Device in Hepatobiliary Duct, Via Natural or Artificial Opening
0FWB72Z Revision of Monitoring Device in Hepatobiliary Duct, Via Natural or Artificial Opening
0FWB73Z Revision of Infusion Device in Hepatobiliary Duct, Via Natural or Artificial Opening
0FWB77Z Revision of Autologous Tissue Substitute in Hepatobiliary Duct, Via Natural or Artificial Opening
0FWB7CZ Revision of Extraluminal Device in Hepatobiliary Duct, Via Natural or Artificial Opening
0FWB7DZ Revision of Intraluminal Device in Hepatobiliary Duct, Via Natural or Artificial Opening
0FWB7JZ Revision of Synthetic Substitute in Hepatobiliary Duct, Via Natural or Artificial Opening
0FWB7KZ Revision of Nonautologous Tissue Substitute in Hepatobiliary Duct, Via Natural or Artificial Opening
0FWB80Z Revision of Drainage Device in Hepatobiliary Duct, Via Natural or Artificial Opening Endoscopic
0FWB82Z Revision of Monitoring Device in Hepatobiliary Duct, Via Natural or Artificial Opening Endoscopic
0FWB83Z Revision of Infusion Device in Hepatobiliary Duct, Via Natural or Artificial Opening Endoscopic
0FWB87Z Revision of Autologous Tissue Substitute in Hepatobiliary Duct, Via Natural or Artificial Opening Endoscopic
0FWB8CZ Revision of Extraluminal Device in Hepatobiliary Duct, Via Natural or Artificial Opening Endoscopic
0FWB8DZ Revision of Intraluminal Device in Hepatobiliary Duct, Via Natural or Artificial Opening Endoscopic
0FWB8JZ Revision of Synthetic Substitute in Hepatobiliary Duct, Via Natural or Artificial Opening Endoscopic
0FWB8KZ Revision of Nonautologous Tissue Substitute in Hepatobiliary Duct, Via Natural or Artificial Opening Endoscopic
0FWBX0Z Revision of Drainage Device in Hepatobiliary Duct, External Approach
0FWBX2Z Revision of Monitoring Device in Hepatobiliary Duct, External Approach
0FWBX3Z Revision of Infusion Device in Hepatobiliary Duct, External Approach

0FWBX7Z Revision of Autologous Tissue Substitute in Hepatobiliary Duct, External Approach
0FWBXCZ Revision of Extraluminal Device in Hepatobiliary Duct, External Approach
0FWBXDZ Revision of Intraluminal Device in Hepatobiliary Duct, External Approach
0FWBXJZ Revision of Synthetic Substitute in Hepatobiliary Duct, External Approach
0FWBXKZ Revision of Nonautologous Tissue Substitute in Hepatobiliary Duct, External Approach
0FWD00Z Revision of Drainage Device in Pancreatic Duct, Open Approach
0FWD02Z Revision of Monitoring Device in Pancreatic Duct, Open Approach
0FWD03Z Revision of Infusion Device in Pancreatic Duct, Open Approach
0FWD07Z Revision of Autologous Tissue Substitute in Pancreatic Duct, Open Approach
0FWD0CZ Revision of Extraluminal Device in Pancreatic Duct, Open Approach
0FWD0DZ Revision of Intraluminal Device in Pancreatic Duct, Open Approach
0FWD0JZ Revision of Synthetic Substitute in Pancreatic Duct, Open Approach
0FWD0KZ Revision of Nonautologous Tissue Substitute in Pancreatic Duct, Open Approach
0FWD30Z Revision of Drainage Device in Pancreatic Duct, Percutaneous Approach
0FWD32Z Revision of Monitoring Device in Pancreatic Duct, Percutaneous Approach
0FWD33Z Revision of Infusion Device in Pancreatic Duct, Percutaneous Approach
0FWD37Z Revision of Autologous Tissue Substitute in Pancreatic Duct, Percutaneous Approach
0FWD3CZ Revision of Extraluminal Device in Pancreatic Duct, Percutaneous Approach
0FWD3DZ Revision of Intraluminal Device in Pancreatic Duct, Percutaneous Approach
0FWD3JZ Revision of Synthetic Substitute in Pancreatic Duct, Percutaneous Approach
0FWD3KZ Revision of Nonautologous Tissue Substitute in Pancreatic Duct, Percutaneous Approach
0FWD40Z Revision of Drainage Device in Pancreatic Duct, Percutaneous Endoscopic Approach
0FWD42Z Revision of Monitoring Device in Pancreatic Duct, Percutaneous Endoscopic Approach
0FWD43Z Revision of Infusion Device in Pancreatic Duct, Percutaneous Endoscopic Approach
0FWD47Z Revision of Autologous Tissue Substitute in Pancreatic Duct, Percutaneous Endoscopic Approach
0FWD4CZ Revision of Extraluminal Device in Pancreatic Duct, Percutaneous Endoscopic Approach
0FWD4DZ Revision of Intraluminal Device in Pancreatic Duct, Percutaneous Endoscopic Approach
0FWD4JZ Revision of Synthetic Substitute in Pancreatic Duct, Percutaneous Endoscopic Approach
0FWD4KZ Revision of Nonautologous Tissue Substitute in Pancreatic Duct, Percutaneous Endoscopic Approach
0FWD70Z Revision of Drainage Device in Pancreatic Duct, Via Natural or Artificial Opening
0FWD72Z Revision of Monitoring Device in Pancreatic Duct, Via Natural or Artificial Opening
0FWD73Z Revision of Infusion Device in Pancreatic Duct, Via Natural or Artificial Opening

0FWD77Z Revision of Autologous Tissue Substitute in Pancreatic Duct, Via Natural or Artificial Opening
0FWD7CZ Revision of Extraluminal Device in Pancreatic Duct, Via Natural or Artificial Opening
0FWD7DZ Revision of Intraluminal Device in Pancreatic Duct, Via Natural or Artificial Opening
0FWD7JZ Revision of Synthetic Substitute in Pancreatic Duct, Via Natural or Artificial Opening
0FWD7KZ Revision of Nonautologous Tissue Substitute in Pancreatic Duct, Via Natural or Artificial Opening
0FWD80Z Revision of Drainage Device in Pancreatic Duct, Via Natural or Artificial Opening Endoscopic
0FWD82Z Revision of Monitoring Device in Pancreatic Duct, Via Natural or Artificial Opening Endoscopic
0FWD83Z Revision of Infusion Device in Pancreatic Duct, Via Natural or Artificial Opening Endoscopic
0FWD87Z Revision of Autologous Tissue Substitute in Pancreatic Duct, Via Natural or Artificial Opening Endoscopic
0FWD8CZ Revision of Extraluminal Device in Pancreatic Duct, Via Natural or Artificial Opening Endoscopic
0FWD8DZ Revision of Intraluminal Device in Pancreatic Duct, Via Natural or Artificial Opening Endoscopic
0FWD8JZ Revision of Synthetic Substitute in Pancreatic Duct, Via Natural or Artificial Opening Endoscopic
0FWD8KZ Revision of Nonautologous Tissue Substitute in Pancreatic Duct, Via Natural or Artificial Opening Endoscopic
0FWDX0Z Revision of Drainage Device in Pancreatic Duct, External Approach
0FWDX2Z Revision of Monitoring Device in Pancreatic Duct, External Approach
0FWDX3Z Revision of Infusion Device in Pancreatic Duct, External Approach
0FWDX7Z Revision of Autologous Tissue Substitute in Pancreatic Duct, External Approach
0FWDXCZ Revision of Extraluminal Device in Pancreatic Duct, External Approach
0FWDXDZ Revision of Intraluminal Device in Pancreatic Duct, External Approach
0FWDXJZ Revision of Synthetic Substitute in Pancreatic Duct, External Approach
0FWDXKZ Revision of Nonautologous Tissue Substitute in Pancreatic Duct, External Approach
0FWG00Z Revision of Drainage Device in Pancreas, Open Approach
0FWG02Z Revision of Monitoring Device in Pancreas, Open Approach
0FWG03Z Revision of Infusion Device in Pancre[illegible] Open Approach
0FWG0DZ Revision of Intraluminal Device in Pancreas, Open Approach
0FWG30Z Revision of Drainage Device in Panc[illegible] Percutaneous Approach
0FWG32Z Revision of Monitoring Device in Pancreas, Percutaneous Approach
0FWG33Z Revision of Infusion Device in Pancre[illegible] Percutaneous Approach
0FWG3DZ Revision of Intraluminal Device in Pancreas, Percutaneous Approach
0FWG40Z Revision of Drainage Device in Pancr[illegible] Percutaneous Endoscopic Approach
0FWG42Z Revision of Monitoring Device in Pancreas, Percutaneous Endoscopic Approach
0FWG43Z Revision of Infusion Device in Pancre[illegible] Percutaneous Endoscopic Approach
0FWG4DZ Revision of Intraluminal Device in Pancreas, Percutaneous Endoscopic Approach
0FWGX0Z Revision of Drainage Device in Pancre[illegible] External Approach
0FWGX2Z Revision of Monitoring Device in Pancreas, External Approach
0FWGX3Z Revision of Infusion Device in Pancre[illegible] External Approach
0FWGXDZ Revision of Intraluminal Device in Pancreas, External Approach

0FY – Hepatobiliary System and Pancreas, Transplantation

Review Coding Guideline B3.16

0FY00Z0 Transplantation of Liver, Allogeneic, Open Approach
AHA CC: 4Q, 2012, 99-101
0FY00Z1 Transplantation of Liver, Syngeneic, Open Approach
0FY00Z2 Transplantation of Liver, Zooplastic, Open Approach
0FYG0Z0 Transplantation of Pancreas, Allogeneic, Open Approach
▲ *When reported without an associated kidney transplant code (0TY00Z0, 0TY00Z1, 0TY00Z2, 0TY10Z0, 0TY10Z1 or 0TY10Z2) and without one of the following diagnosis codes E10.10-E10.9, E89.1*
0FYG0Z1 Transplantation of Pancreas, Syngeneic, Open Approah
▲ *When reported without an associated kidney transplant code (0TY00Z0, 0TY00Z1, 0TY00Z2, 0TY10Z0, 0TY10Z1 or 0TY10Z2) and without one of the following diagnosis codes E10.10-E10.9, E89.1*
▲ **0FYG0Z2** Transplantation of Pancreas, Zooplastic, Open Approach

Endocrine System

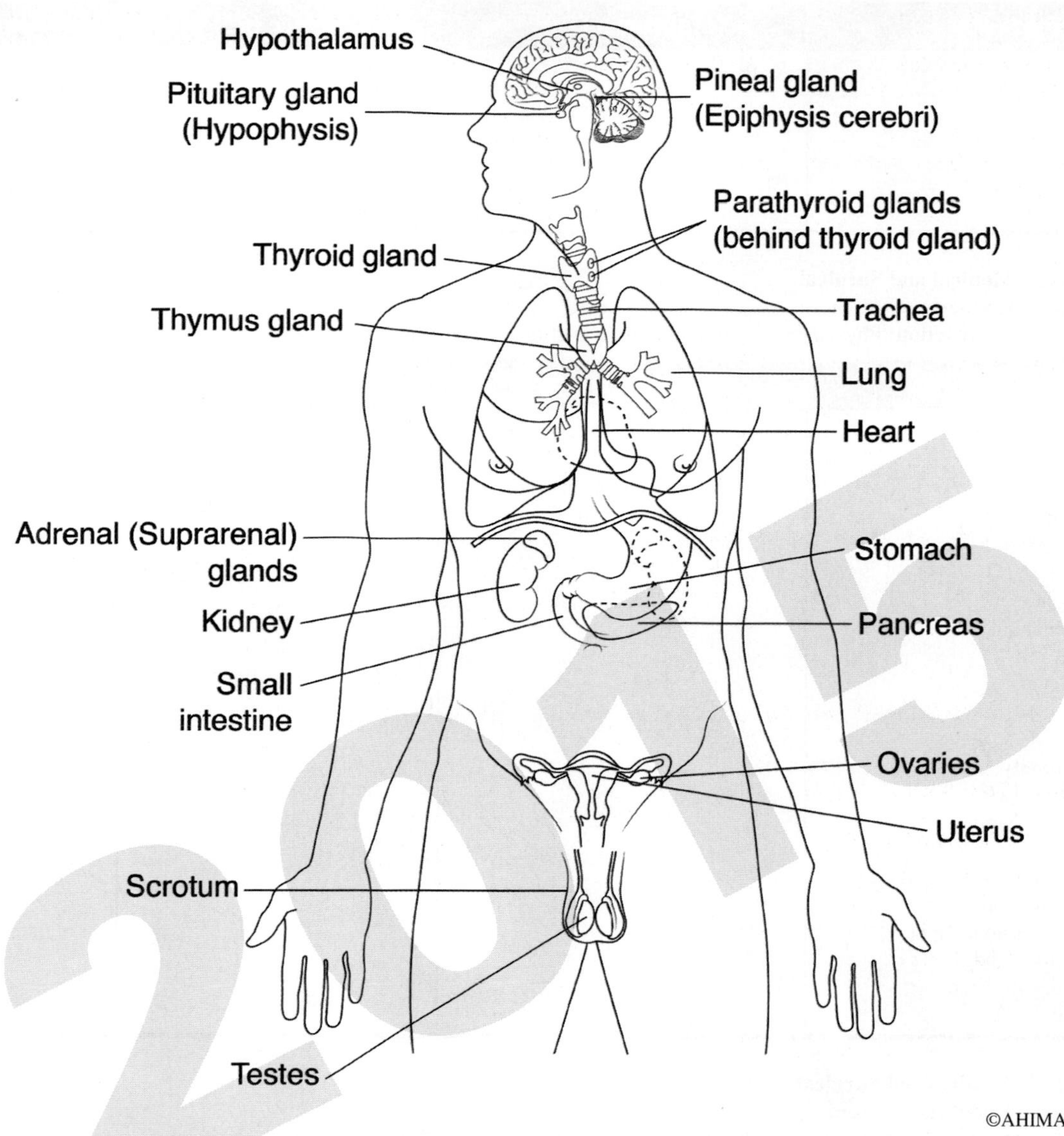
Hypothalamus
Pituitary gland
(Hypophysis)
Pineal gland
(Epiphysis cerebri)
Parathyroid glands
(behind thyroid gland)
Thyroid gland
Thymus gland
Trachea
Lung
Heart
Adrenal (Suprarenal)
glands
Stomach
Kidney
Pancreas
Small
intestine
Ovaries
Uterus
Scrotum
Testes
2015

Endocrine System Tables 0G2–0GW

Section 0 **Medical and Surgical**
Body System G **Endocrine System**
Operation 2 **Change:** Taking out or off a device from a body part and putting back an identical or similar device in or on the same body part without cutting or puncturing the skin or a mucous membrane

Body Part (4th)	Approach (5th)	Device (6th)	Qualifier (7th)
0 Pituitary Gland **1** Pineal Body **5** Adrenal Gland **K** Thyroid Gland **R** Parathyroid Gland **S** Endocrine Gland	**X** External	**0** Drainage Device **Y** Other Device	**Z** No Qualifier

Section 0 **Medical and Surgical**
Body System G **Endocrine System**
Operation 5 **Destruction:** Physical eradication of all or a portion of a body part by the direct use of energy, force, or a destructive agent

Body Part (4th)	Approach (5th)	Device (6th)	Qualifier (7th)
0 Pituitary Gland **1** Pineal Body **2** Adrenal Gland, Left **3** Adrenal Gland, Right **4** Adrenal Glands, Bilateral **6** Carotid Body, Left **7** Carotid Body, Right **8** Carotid Bodies, Bilateral **9** Para-aortic Body **B** Coccygeal Glomus **C** Glomus Jugulare **D** Aortic Body **F** Paraganglion Extremity **G** Thyroid Gland Lobe, Left **H** Thyroid Gland Lobe, Right **K** Thyroid Gland **L** Superior Parathyroid Gland, Right **M** Superior Parathyroid Gland, Left **N** Inferior Parathyroid Gland, Right **P** Inferior Parathyroid Gland, Left **Q** Parathyroid Glands, Multiple **R** Parathyroid Gland	**0** Open **3** Percutaneous **4** Percutaneous Endoscopic	**Z** No Device	**Z** No Qualifier

Section 0 **Medical and Surgical**
Body System G **Endocrine System**
Operation 8 **Division:** Cutting into a body part, without draining fluids and/or gases from the body part, in order to separate or transect a body part

Body Part (4th)	Approach (5th)	Device (6th)	Qualifier (7th)
0 Pituitary Gland **J** Thyroid Gland Isthmus	**0** Open **3** Percutaneous **4** Percutaneous Endoscopic	**Z** No Device	**Z** No Qualifier

tion 0 Medical and Surgical
y System G Endocrine System
ration 9 Drainage: Taking or letting out fluids and/or gases from a body part

Body Part (4th)	Approach (5th)	Device (6th)	Qualifier (7th)
Pituitary Gland	**0** Open	**0** Drainage Device	**Z** No Qualifier
Pineal Body	**3** Percutaneous		
Adrenal Gland, Left	**4** Percutaneous Endoscopic		
Adrenal Gland, Right			
Adrenal Glands, Bilateral			
Carotid Body, Left			
Carotid Body, Right			
Carotid Bodies, Bilateral			
Para-aortic Body			
Coccygeal Glomus			
C Glomus Jugulare			
D Aortic Body			
Paraganglion Extremity			
G Thyroid Gland Lobe, Left			
H Thyroid Gland Lobe, Right			
K Thyroid Gland			
L Superior Parathyroid Gland, Right			
M Superior Parathyroid Gland, Left			
N Inferior Parathyroid Gland, Right			
P Inferior Parathyroid Gland, Left			
Q Parathyroid Glands, Multiple			
R Parathyroid Gland			
0 Pituitary Gland	**0** Open	**Z** No Device	**X** Diagnostic
Pineal Body	**3** Percutaneous		**Z** No Qualifier
2 Adrenal Gland, Left	**4** Percutaneous Endoscopic		
3 Adrenal Gland, Right			
4 Adrenal Glands, Bilateral			
6 Carotid Body, Left			
7 Carotid Body, Right			
8 Carotid Bodies, Bilateral			
9 Para-aortic Body			
B Coccygeal Glomus			
C Glomus Jugulare			
D Aortic Body			
F Paraganglion Extremity			
G Thyroid Gland Lobe, Left			
H Thyroid Gland Lobe, Right			
K Thyroid Gland			
L Superior Parathyroid Gland, Right			
M Superior Parathyroid Gland, Left			
N Inferior Parathyroid Gland, Right			
P Inferior Parathyroid Gland, Left			
Q Parathyroid Glands, Multiple			
R Parathyroid Gland			

Section 0 **Medical and Surgical**
Body System G **Endocrine System**
Operation B **Excision:** Cutting out or off, without replacement, a portion of a body part

Body Part (4th)	Approach (5th)	Device (6th)	Qualifier (7th)
0 Pituitary Gland **1** Pineal Body **2** Adrenal Gland, Left **3** Adrenal Gland, Right **4** Adrenal Glands, Bilateral **6** Carotid Body, Left **7** Carotid Body, Right **8** Carotid Bodies, Bilateral **9** Para-aortic Body **B** Coccygeal Glomus **C** Glomus Jugulare **D** Aortic Body **F** Paraganglion Extremity **G** Thyroid Gland Lobe, Left **H** Thyroid Gland Lobe, Right **L** Superior Parathyroid Gland, Right **M** Superior Parathyroid Gland, Left **N** Inferior Parathyroid Gland, Right **P** Inferior Parathyroid Gland, Left **Q** Parathyroid Glands, Multiple **R** Parathyroid Gland	**0** Open **3** Percutaneous **4** Percutaneous Endoscopic	**Z** No Device	**X** Diagnostic **Z** No Qualifier

Section 0 **Medical and Surgical**
Body System G **Endocrine System**
Operation C **Extirpation:** Taking or cutting out solid matter from a body part

Body Part (4th)	Approach (5th)	Device (6th)	Qualifier (7th)
0 Pituitary Gland **1** Pineal Body **2** Adrenal Gland, Left **3** Adrenal Gland, Right **4** Adrenal Glands, Bilateral **6** Carotid Body, Left **7** Carotid Body, Right **8** Carotid Bodies, Bilateral **9** Para-aortic Body **B** Coccygeal Glomus **C** Glomus Jugulare **D** Aortic Body **F** Paraganglion Extremity **G** Thyroid Gland Lobe, Left **H** Thyroid Gland Lobe, Right **K** Thyroid Gland **L** Superior Parathyroid Gland, Right **M** Superior Parathyroid Gland, Left **N** Inferior Parathyroid Gland, Right **P** Inferior Parathyroid Gland, Left **Q** Parathyroid Glands, Multiple **R** Parathyroid Gland	**0** Open **3** Percutaneous **4** Percutaneous Endoscopic	**Z** No Device	**Z** No Qualifier

Section 0 **Medical and Surgical**
Body System G **Endocrine System**
Operation H **Insertion:** Putting in a nonbiological appliance that monitors, assists, performs, or prevents a physiological function but does not physically take the place of a body part

Body Part (4th)	Approach (5th)	Device (6th)	Qualifier (7th)
S Endocrine Gland	**0** Open **3** Percutaneous **4** Percutaneous Endoscopic	**2** Monitoring Device **3** Infusion Device	**Z** No Qualifier

ion	0	**Medical and Surgical**
y System	G	**Endocrine System**
eration	J	**Inspection:** Visually and/or manually exploring a body part

Body Part (4th)	Approach (5th)	Device (6th)	Qualifier (7th)
Pituitary Gland Pineal Body Adrenal Gland Thyroid Gland Parathyroid Gland Endocrine Gland	**0** Open **3** Percutaneous **4** Percutaneous Endoscopic	**Z** No Device	**Z** No Qualifier

tion	0	**Medical and Surgical**
dy System	G	**Endocrine System**
eration	M	**Reattachment:** Putting back in or on all or a portion of a separated body part to its normal location or other suitable location

Body Part (4th)	Approach (5th)	Device (6th)	Qualifier (7th)
Adrenal Gland, Left Adrenal Gland, Right Thyroid Gland Lobe, Left Thyroid Gland Lobe, Right Superior Parathyroid Gland, Right Superior Parathyroid Gland, Left Inferior Parathyroid Gland, Right Inferior Parathyroid Gland, Left Parathyroid Glands, Multiple Parathyroid Gland	**0** Open **4** Percutaneous Endoscopic	**Z** No Device	**Z** No Qualifier

tion	0	**Medical and Surgical**
dy System	G	**Endocrine System**
eration	N	**Release:** Freeing a body part from an abnormal physical constraint by cutting or by the use of force

Body Part (4th)	Approach (5th)	Device (6th)	Qualifier (7th)
Pituitary Gland Pineal Body Adrenal Gland, Left Adrenal Gland, Right Adrenal Glands, Bilateral Carotid Body, Left Carotid Body, Right Carotid Bodies, Bilateral Para-aortic Body **B** Coccygeal Glomus **C** Glomus Jugulare **D** Aortic Body **F** Paraganglion Extremity **G** Thyroid Gland Lobe, Left **H** Thyroid Gland Lobe, Right **K** Thyroid Gland **L** Superior Parathyroid Gland, Right **M** Superior Parathyroid Gland, Left **N** Inferior Parathyroid Gland, Right **P** Inferior Parathyroid Gland, Left **Q** Parathyroid Glands, Multiple **R** Parathyroid Gland	**0** Open **3** Percutaneous **4** Percutaneous Endoscopic	**Z** No Device	**Z** No Qualifier

Section 0 **Medical and Surgical**
Body System G **Endocrine System**
Operation P **Removal:** Taking out or off a device from a body part

Body Part (4th)	Approach (5th)	Device (6th)	Qualifier (7th)
0 Pituitary Gland **1** Pineal Body **5** Adrenal Gland **K** Thyroid Gland **R** Parathyroid Gland	**0** Open **3** Percutaneous **4** Percutaneous Endoscopic **X** External	**0** Drainage Device	**Z** No Qualifier
S Endocrine Gland	**0** Open **3** Percutaneous **4** Percutaneous Endoscopic **X** External	**0** Drainage Device **2** Monitoring Device **3** Infusion Device	**Z** No Qualifier

Section 0 **Medical and Surgical**
Body System G **Endocrine System**
Operation Q **Repair:** Restoring, to the extent possible, a body part to its normal anatomic structure and function

Body Part (4th)	Approach (5th)	Device (6th)	Qualifier (7th)
0 Pituitary Gland **1** Pineal Body **2** Adrenal Gland, Left **3** Adrenal Gland, Right **4** Adrenal Glands, Bilateral **6** Carotid Body, Left **7** Carotid Body, Right **8** Carotid Bodies, Bilateral **9** Para-aortic Body **B** Coccygeal Glomus **C** Glomus Jugulare **D** Aortic Body **F** Paraganglion Extremity **G** Thyroid Gland Lobe, Left **H** Thyroid Gland Lobe, Right **J** Thyroid Gland Isthmus **K** Thyroid Gland **L** Superior Parathyroid Gland, Right **M** Superior Parathyroid Gland, Left **N** Inferior Parathyroid Gland, Right **P** Inferior Parathyroid Gland, Left **Q** Parathyroid Glands, Multiple **R** Parathyroid Gland	**0** Open **3** Percutaneous **4** Percutaneous Endoscopic	**Z** No Device	**Z** No Qualifier

Section 0 **Medical and Surgical**
Body System G **Endocrine System**
Operation S **Reposition:** Moving to its normal location, or other suitable location, all or a portion of a body part

Body Part (4th)	Approach (5th)	Device (6th)	Qualifier (7th)
2 Adrenal Gland, Left **3** Adrenal Gland, Right **G** Thyroid Gland Lobe, Left **H** Thyroid Gland Lobe, Right **L** Superior Parathyroid Gland, Right **M** Superior Parathyroid Gland, Left **N** Inferior Parathyroid Gland, Right **P** Inferior Parathyroid Gland, Left **Q** Parathyroid Glands, Multiple **R** Parathyroid Gland	**0** Open **4** Percutaneous Endoscopic	**Z** No Device	**Z** No Qualifier

tion	0	Medical and Surgical
dy System	G	Endocrine System
eration	T	**Resection:** Cutting out or off, without replacement, all of a body part

Body Part (4th)	Approach (5th)	Device (6th)	Qualifier (7th)
Pituitary Gland Pineal Body Adrenal Gland, Left Adrenal Gland, Right Adrenal Glands, Bilateral Carotid Body, Left Carotid Body, Right Carotid Bodies, Bilateral Para-aortic Body Coccygeal Glomus Glomus Jugulare Aortic Body Paraganglion Extremity Thyroid Gland Lobe, Left Thyroid Gland Lobe, Right Thyroid Gland Superior Parathyroid Gland, Right Superior Parathyroid Gland, Left Inferior Parathyroid Gland, Right Inferior Parathyroid Gland, Left Parathyroid Glands, Multiple Parathyroid Gland	**0** Open **4** Percutaneous Endoscopic	**Z** No Device	**Z** No Qualifier

ction	0	Medical and Surgical
dy System	G	Endocrine System
eration	W	**Revision:** Correcting, to the extent possible, a portion of a malfunctioning device or the position of a displaced device

Body Part (4th)	Approach (5th)	Device (6th)	Qualifier (7th)
Pituitary Gland Pineal Body 5 Adrenal Gland K Thyroid Gland R Parathyroid Gland	**0** Open **3** Percutaneous **4** Percutaneous Endoscopic **X** External	**0** Drainage Device	**Z** No Qualifier
S Endocrine Gland	**0** Open **3** Percutaneous **4** Percutaneous Endoscopic **X** External	**0** Drainage Device **2** Monitoring Device **3** Infusion Device	**Z** No Qualifier

ndocrine System Code Listing 0G2–0GW

G2 – Endocrine System, Change

eview Coding Guideline B6.1c

20X0Z Change Drainage Device in Pituitary Gland, External Approach
20XYZ Change Other Device in Pituitary Gland, External Approach
21X0Z Change Drainage Device in Pineal Body, External Approach
21XYZ Change Other Device in Pineal Body, External Approach
0G25X0Z Change Drainage Device in Adrenal Gland, External Approach
0G25XYZ Change Other Device in Adrenal Gland, External Approach
0G2KX0Z Change Drainage Device in Thyroid Gland, External Approach
0G2KXYZ Change Other Device in Thyroid Gland, External Approach
0G2RX0Z Change Drainage Device in Parathyroid Gland, External Approach
0G2RXYZ Change Other Device in Parathyroid Gland, External Approach
0G2SX0Z Change Drainage Device in Endocrine Gland, External Approach
0G2SXYZ Change Other Device in Endocrine Gland, External Approach

G5 – Endocrine System, Destruction

G500ZZ Destruction of Pituitary Gland, Open Approach
G503ZZ Destruction of Pituitary Gland, Percutaneous Approach
G504ZZ Destruction of Pituitary Gland, Percutaneous Endoscopic Approach
G510ZZ Destruction of Pineal Body, Open Approach
0G513ZZ Destruction of Pineal Body, Percutaneous Approach
0G514ZZ Destruction of Pineal Body, Percutaneous Endoscopic Approach
0G520ZZ Destruction of Left Adrenal Gland, Open Approach
0G523ZZ Destruction of Left Adrenal Gland, Percutaneous Approach
0G524ZZ Destruction of Left Adrenal Gland, Percutaneous Endoscopic Approach
0G530ZZ Destruction of Right Adrenal Gland, Open Approach
0G533ZZ Destruction of Right Adrenal Gland, Percutaneous Approach
0G534ZZ Destruction of Right Adrenal Gland, Percutaneous Endoscopic Approach

0G540ZZ Destruction of Bilateral Adrenal Glands, Open Approach
0G543ZZ Destruction of Bilateral Adrenal Glands, Percutaneous Approach
0G544ZZ Destruction of Bilateral Adrenal Glands, Percutaneous Endoscopic Approach
0G560ZZ Destruction of Left Carotid Body, Open Approach
0G563ZZ Destruction of Left Carotid Body, Percutaneous Approach
0G564ZZ Destruction of Left Carotid Body, Percutaneous Endoscopic Approach
0G570ZZ Destruction of Right Carotid Body, Open Approach
0G573ZZ Destruction of Right Carotid Body, Percutaneous Approach
0G574ZZ Destruction of Right Carotid Body, Percutaneous Endoscopic Approach
0G580ZZ Destruction of Bilateral Carotid Bodies, Open Approach
0G583ZZ Destruction of Bilateral Carotid Bodies, Percutaneous Approach
0G584ZZ Destruction of Bilateral Carotid Bodies, Percutaneous Endoscopic Approach
0G590ZZ Destruction of Para-aortic Body, Open Approach
0G593ZZ Destruction of Para-aortic Body, Percutaneous Approach
0G594ZZ Destruction of Para-aortic Body, Percutaneous Endoscopic Approach
0G5B0ZZ Destruction of Coccygeal Glomus, Open Approach
0G5B3ZZ Destruction of Coccygeal Glomus, Percutaneous Approach
0G5B4ZZ Destruction of Coccygeal Glomus, Percutaneous Endoscopic Approach
0G5C0ZZ Destruction of Glomus Jugulare, Open Approach
0G5C3ZZ Destruction of Glomus Jugulare, Percutaneous Approach
0G5C4ZZ Destruction of Glomus Jugulare, Percutaneous Endoscopic Approach
0G5D0ZZ Destruction of Aortic Body, Open Approach
0G5D3ZZ Destruction of Aortic Body, Percutaneous Approach
0G5D4ZZ Destruction of Aortic Body, Percutaneous Endoscopic Approach
0G5F0ZZ Destruction of Paraganglion Extremity, Open Approach
0G5F3ZZ Destruction of Paraganglion Extremity, Percutaneous Approach
0G5F4ZZ Destruction of Paraganglion Extremity, Percutaneous Endoscopic Approach
0G5G0ZZ Destruction of Left Thyroid Gland Lobe, Open Approach
0G5G3ZZ Destruction of Left Thyroid Gland Lobe, Percutaneous Approach
0G5G4ZZ Destruction of Left Thyroid Gland Lobe, Percutaneous Endoscopic Approach
0G5H0ZZ Destruction of Right Thyroid Gland Lobe, Open Approach
0G5H3ZZ Destruction of Right Thyroid Gland Lobe, Percutaneous Approach
0G5H4ZZ Destruction of Right Thyroid Gland Lobe, Percutaneous Endoscopic Approach
0G5K0ZZ Destruction of Thyroid Gland, Open Approach
0G5K3ZZ Destruction of Thyroid Gland, Percutaneous Approach
0G5K4ZZ Destruction of Thyroid Gland, Percutaneous Endoscopic Approach
0G5L0ZZ Destruction of Right Superior Parathyroid Gland, Open Approach
0G5L3ZZ Destruction of Right Superior Parathyroid Gland, Percutaneous Approach
0G5L4ZZ Destruction of Right Superior Parathyr Gland, Percutaneous Endoscopic Approach
0G5M0ZZ Destruction of Left Superior Parathyro Gland, Open Approach
0G5M3ZZ Destruction of Left Superior Parathyroi Gland, Percutaneous Approach
0G5M4ZZ Destruction of Left Superior Parathyroi Gland, Percutaneous Endoscopic Approach
0G5N0ZZ Destruction of Right Inferior Parathyro Gland, Open Approach
0G5N3ZZ Destruction of Right Inferior Parathyro Gland, Percutaneous Approach
0G5N4ZZ Destruction of Right Inferior Parathyro Gland, Percutaneous Endoscopic Approach
0G5P0ZZ Destruction of Left Inferior Parathyroid Gland, Open Approach
0G5P3ZZ Destruction of Left Inferior Parathyroid Gland, Percutaneous Approach
0G5P4ZZ Destruction of Left Inferior Parathyroid Gland, Percutaneous Endoscopic Approach
0G5Q0ZZ Destruction of Multiple Parathyroid Glands, Open Approach
0G5Q3ZZ Destruction of Multiple Parathyroid Glands, Percutaneous Approach
0G5Q4ZZ Destruction of Multiple Parathyroid Glands, Percutaneous Endoscopic Approach
0G5R0ZZ Destruction of Parathyroid Gland, Open Approach
0G5R3ZZ Destruction of Parathyroid Gland, Percutaneous Approach
0G5R4ZZ Destruction of Parathyroid Gland, Percutaneous Endoscopic Approach

0G8 – Endocrine System, Division

Review Coding Guideline B3.14

0G800ZZ Division of Pituitary Gland, Open Approach
0G803ZZ Division of Pituitary Gland, Percutaneous Approach
0G804ZZ Division of Pituitary Gland, Percutaneous Endoscopic Approach
0G8J0ZZ Division of Thyroid Gland Isthmus, Open Approach
0G8J3ZZ Division of Thyroid Gland Isthmus, Percutaneous Approach
0G8J4ZZ Division of Thyroid Gland Isthmus, Percutaneous Endoscopic Approach

0G9 – Endocrine System, Drainage

Review Coding Guidelines B3.4a and B3.4b

Review Coding Guideline B6.2

0G9000Z Drainage of Pituitary Gland with Drainage Device, Open Approach
0G900ZX Drainage of Pituitary Gland, Open Approach, Diagnostic
0G900ZZ Drainage of Pituitary Gland, Open Approach
0G9030Z Drainage of Pituitary Gland with Drainage Device, Percutaneous Approach
0G903ZX Drainage of Pituitary Gland, Percutaneous Approach, Diagnostic
0G903ZZ Drainage of Pituitary Gland, Percutaneous Approach
0G9040Z Drainage of Pituitary Gland with Drainage Device, Percutaneous Endoscopic Approach
0G904ZX Drainage of Pituitary Gland, Percutaneous Endoscopic Approach, Diagnostic
0G904ZZ Drainage of Pituitary Gland, Percutaneous Endoscopic Approach
0G9100Z Drainage of Pineal Body with Drainage Device, Open Approach
0G910ZX Drainage of Pineal Body, Open Approach, Diagnostic
0G910ZZ Drainage of Pineal Body, Open Approach
0G9130Z Drainage of Pineal Body with Drainage Device, Percutaneous Approach
0G913ZX Drainage of Pineal Body, Percutaneous Approach, Diagnostic
0G913ZZ Drainage of Pineal Body, Percutaneous Approach
0G9140Z Drainage of Pineal Body with Drainage Device, Percutaneous Endoscopic Approach
0G914ZX Drainage of Pineal Body, Percutaneous Endoscopic Approach, Diagnostic
0G914ZZ Drainage of Pineal Body, Percutaneous Endoscopic Approach
0G9200Z Drainage of Left Adrenal Gland with Drainage Device, Open Approach
0G920ZX Drainage of Left Adrenal Gland, Open Approach, Diagnostic
0G920ZZ Drainage of Left Adrenal Gland, Open Approach
0G9230Z Drainage of Left Adrenal Gland with Drainage Device, Percutaneous Approach
0G923ZX Drainage of Left Adrenal Gland, Percutaneous Approach, Diagnostic
0G923ZZ Drainage of Left Adrenal Gland, Percutaneous Approach
0G9240Z Drainage of Left Adrenal Gland with Drainage Device, Percutaneous Endoscopic Approach
0G924ZX Drainage of Left Adrenal Gland, Percutaneous Endoscopic Approach, Diagnostic
0G924ZZ Drainage of Left Adrenal Gland, Percutaneous Endoscopic Approach
0G9300Z Drainage of Right Adrenal Gland with Drainage Device, Open Approach
0G930ZX Drainage of Right Adrenal Gland, Open Approach, Diagnostic
0G930ZZ Drainage of Right Adrenal Gland, Open Approach
0G9330Z Drainage of Right Adrenal Gland with Drainage Device, Percutaneous Approach
0G933ZX Drainage of Right Adrenal Gland, Percutaneous Approach, Diagnostic
0G933ZZ Drainage of Right Adrenal Gland, Percutaneous Approach

340Z Drainage of Right Adrenal Gland with Drainage Device, Percutaneous Endoscopic Approach
34ZX Drainage of Right Adrenal Gland, Percutaneous Endoscopic Approach, Diagnostic
34ZZ Drainage of Right Adrenal Gland, Percutaneous Endoscopic Approach
400Z Drainage of Bilateral Adrenal Glands with Drainage Device, Open Approach
40ZX Drainage of Bilateral Adrenal Glands, Open Approach, Diagnostic
40ZZ Drainage of Bilateral Adrenal Glands, Open Approach
430Z Drainage of Bilateral Adrenal Glands with Drainage Device, Percutaneous Approach
43ZX Drainage of Bilateral Adrenal Glands, Percutaneous Approach, Diagnostic
43ZZ Drainage of Bilateral Adrenal Glands, Percutaneous Approach
440Z Drainage of Bilateral Adrenal Glands with Drainage Device, Percutaneous Endoscopic Approach
944ZX Drainage of Bilateral Adrenal Glands, Percutaneous Endoscopic Approach, Diagnostic
944ZZ Drainage of Bilateral Adrenal Glands, Percutaneous Endoscopic Approach
9600Z Drainage of Left Carotid Body with Drainage Device, Open Approach
960ZX Drainage of Left Carotid Body, Open Approach, Diagnostic
960ZZ Drainage of Left Carotid Body, Open Approach
9630Z Drainage of Left Carotid Body with Drainage Device, Percutaneous Approach
963ZX Drainage of Left Carotid Body, Percutaneous Approach, Diagnostic
963ZZ Drainage of Left Carotid Body, Percutaneous Approach
9640Z Drainage of Left Carotid Body with Drainage Device, Percutaneous Endoscopic Approach
964ZX Drainage of Left Carotid Body, Percutaneous Endoscopic Approach, Diagnostic
964ZZ Drainage of Left Carotid Body, Percutaneous Endoscopic Approach
9700Z Drainage of Right Carotid Body with Drainage Device, Open Approach
970ZX Drainage of Right Carotid Body, Open Approach, Diagnostic
970ZZ Drainage of Right Carotid Body, Open Approach
9730Z Drainage of Right Carotid Body with Drainage Device, Percutaneous Approach
973ZX Drainage of Right Carotid Body, Percutaneous Approach, Diagnostic
973ZZ Drainage of Right Carotid Body, Percutaneous Approach
9740Z Drainage of Right Carotid Body with Drainage Device, Percutaneous Endoscopic Approach
974ZX Drainage of Right Carotid Body, Percutaneous Endoscopic Approach, Diagnostic
974ZZ Drainage of Right Carotid Body, Percutaneous Endoscopic Approach
G9800Z Drainage of Bilateral Carotid Bodies with Drainage Device, Open Approach
G980ZX Drainage of Bilateral Carotid Bodies, Open Approach, Diagnostic
G980ZZ Drainage of Bilateral Carotid Bodies, Open Approach
G9830Z Drainage of Bilateral Carotid Bodies with Drainage Device, Percutaneous Approach
0G983ZX Drainage of Bilateral Carotid Bodies, Percutaneous Approach, Diagnostic
0G983ZZ Drainage of Bilateral Carotid Bodies, Percutaneous Approach
0G9840Z Drainage of Bilateral Carotid Bodies with Drainage Device, Percutaneous Endoscopic Approach
0G984ZX Drainage of Bilateral Carotid Bodies, Percutaneous Endoscopic Approach, Diagnostic
0G984ZZ Drainage of Bilateral Carotid Bodies, Percutaneous Endoscopic Approach
0G9900Z Drainage of Para-aortic Body with Drainage Device, Open Approach
0G990ZX Drainage of Para-aortic Body, Open Approach, Diagnostic
0G990ZZ Drainage of Para-aortic Body, Open Approach
0G9930Z Drainage of Para-aortic Body with Drainage Device, Percutaneous Approach
0G993ZX Drainage of Para-aortic Body, Percutaneous Approach, Diagnostic
0G993ZZ Drainage of Para-aortic Body, Percutaneous Approach
0G9940Z Drainage of Para-aortic Body with Drainage Device, Percutaneous Endoscopic Approach
0G994ZX Drainage of Para-aortic Body, Percutaneous Endoscopic Approach, Diagnostic
0G994ZZ Drainage of Para-aortic Body, Percutaneous Endoscopic Approach
0G9B00Z Drainage of Coccygeal Glomus with Drainage Device, Open Approach
0G9B0ZX Drainage of Coccygeal Glomus, Open Approach, Diagnostic
0G9B0ZZ Drainage of Coccygeal Glomus, Open Approach
0G9B30Z Drainage of Coccygeal Glomus with Drainage Device, Percutaneous Approach
0G9B3ZX Drainage of Coccygeal Glomus, Percutaneous Approach, Diagnostic
0G9B3ZZ Drainage of Coccygeal Glomus, Percutaneous Approach
0G9B40Z Drainage of Coccygeal Glomus with Drainage Device, Percutaneous Endoscopic Approach
0G9B4ZX Drainage of Coccygeal Glomus, Percutaneous Endoscopic Approach, Diagnostic
0G9B4ZZ Drainage of Coccygeal Glomus, Percutaneous Endoscopic Approach
0G9C00Z Drainage of Glomus Jugulare with Drainage Device, Open Approach
0G9C0ZX Drainage of Glomus Jugulare, Open Approach, Diagnostic
0G9C0ZZ Drainage of Glomus Jugulare, Open Approach
0G9C30Z Drainage of Glomus Jugulare with Drainage Device, Percutaneous Approach
0G9C3ZX Drainage of Glomus Jugulare, Percutaneous Approach, Diagnostic
0G9C3ZZ Drainage of Glomus Jugulare, Percutaneous Approach
0G9C40Z Drainage of Glomus Jugulare with Drainage Device, Percutaneous Endoscopic Approach
0G9C4ZX Drainage of Glomus Jugulare, Percutaneous Endoscopic Approach, Diagnostic
0G9C4ZZ Drainage of Glomus Jugulare, Percutaneous Endoscopic Approach
0G9D00Z Drainage of Aortic Body with Drainage Device, Open Approach
0G9D0ZX Drainage of Aortic Body, Open Approach, Diagnostic
0G9D0ZZ Drainage of Aortic Body, Open Approach
0G9D30Z Drainage of Aortic Body with Drainage Device, Percutaneous Approach
0G9D3ZX Drainage of Aortic Body, Percutaneous Approach, Diagnostic
0G9D3ZZ Drainage of Aortic Body, Percutaneous Approach
0G9D40Z Drainage of Aortic Body with Drainage Device, Percutaneous Endoscopic Approach
0G9D4ZX Drainage of Aortic Body, Percutaneous Endoscopic Approach, Diagnostic
0G9D4ZZ Drainage of Aortic Body, Percutaneous Endoscopic Approach
0G9F00Z Drainage of Paraganglion Extremity with Drainage Device, Open Approach
0G9F0ZX Drainage of Paraganglion Extremity, Open Approach, Diagnostic
0G9F0ZZ Drainage of Paraganglion Extremity, Open Approach
0G9F30Z Drainage of Paraganglion Extremity with Drainage Device, Percutaneous Approach
0G9F3ZX Drainage of Paraganglion Extremity, Percutaneous Approach, Diagnostic
0G9F3ZZ Drainage of Paraganglion Extremity, Percutaneous Approach
0G9F40Z Drainage of Paraganglion Extremity with Drainage Device, Percutaneous Endoscopic Approach
0G9F4ZX Drainage of Paraganglion Extremity, Percutaneous Endoscopic Approach, Diagnostic
0G9F4ZZ Drainage of Paraganglion Extremity, Percutaneous Endoscopic Approach
0G9G00Z Drainage of Left Thyroid Gland Lobe with Drainage Device, Open Approach
0G9G0ZX Drainage of Left Thyroid Gland Lobe, Open Approach, Diagnostic
0G9G0ZZ Drainage of Left Thyroid Gland Lobe, Open Approach
0G9G30Z Drainage of Left Thyroid Gland Lobe with Drainage Device, Percutaneous Approach
0G9G3ZX Drainage of Left Thyroid Gland Lobe, Percutaneous Approach, Diagnostic
0G9G3ZZ Drainage of Left Thyroid Gland Lobe, Percutaneous Approach
0G9G40Z Drainage of Left Thyroid Gland Lobe with Drainage Device, Percutaneous Endoscopic Approach
0G9G4ZX Drainage of Left Thyroid Gland Lobe, Percutaneous Endoscopic Approach, Diagnostic
0G9G4ZZ Drainage of Left Thyroid Gland Lobe, Percutaneous Endoscopic Approach
0G9H00Z Drainage of Right Thyroid Gland Lobe with Drainage Device, Open Approach
0G9H0ZX Drainage of Right Thyroid Gland Lobe, Open Approach, Diagnostic
0G9H0ZZ Drainage of Right Thyroid Gland Lobe, Open Approach
0G9H30Z Drainage of Right Thyroid Gland Lobe with Drainage Device, Percutaneous Approach
0G9H3ZX Drainage of Right Thyroid Gland Lobe, Percutaneous Approach, Diagnostic
0G9H3ZZ Drainage of Right Thyroid Gland Lobe, Percutaneous Approach
0G9H40Z Drainage of Right Thyroid Gland Lobe with Drainage Device, Percutaneous Endoscopic Approach
0G9H4ZX Drainage of Right Thyroid Gland Lobe, Percutaneous Endoscopic Approach, Diagnostic
0G9H4ZZ Drainage of Right Thyroid Gland Lobe, Percutaneous Endoscopic Approach
0G9K00Z Drainage of Thyroid Gland with Drainage Device, Open Approach

0G9K0ZX Drainage of Thyroid Gland, Open Approach, Diagnostic
0G9K0ZZ Drainage of Thyroid Gland, Open Approach
0G9K30Z Drainage of Thyroid Gland with Drainage Device, Percutaneous Approach
0G9K3ZX Drainage of Thyroid Gland, Percutaneous Approach, Diagnostic
0G9K3ZZ Drainage of Thyroid Gland, Percutaneous Approach
0G9K40Z Drainage of Thyroid Gland with Drainage Device, Percutaneous Endoscopic Approach
0G9K4ZX Drainage of Thyroid Gland, Percutaneous Endoscopic Approach, Diagnostic
0G9K4ZZ Drainage of Thyroid Gland, Percutaneous Endoscopic Approach
0G9L00Z Drainage of Right Superior Parathyroid Gland with Drainage Device, Open Approach
0G9L0ZX Drainage of Right Superior Parathyroid Gland, Open Approach, Diagnostic
0G9L0ZZ Drainage of Right Superior Parathyroid Gland, Open Approach
0G9L30Z Drainage of Right Superior Parathyroid Gland with Drainage Device, Percutaneous Approach
0G9L3ZX Drainage of Right Superior Parathyroid Gland, Percutaneous Approach, Diagnostic
0G9L3ZZ Drainage of Right Superior Parathyroid Gland, Percutaneous Approach
0G9L40Z Drainage of Right Superior Parathyroid Gland with Drainage Device, Percutaneous Endoscopic Approach
0G9L4ZX Drainage of Right Superior Parathyroid Gland, Percutaneous Endoscopic Approach, Diagnostic
0G9L4ZZ Drainage of Right Superior Parathyroid Gland, Percutaneous Endoscopic Approach
0G9M00Z Drainage of Left Superior Parathyroid Gland with Drainage Device, Open Approach
0G9M0ZX Drainage of Left Superior Parathyroid Gland, Open Approach, Diagnostic
0G9M0ZZ Drainage of Left Superior Parathyroid Gland, Open Approach
0G9M30Z Drainage of Left Superior Parathyroid Gland with Drainage Device, Percutaneous Approach
0G9M3ZX Drainage of Left Superior Parathyroid Gland, Percutaneous Approach, Diagnostic
0G9M3ZZ Drainage of Left Superior Parathyroid Gland, Percutaneous Approach
0G9M40Z Drainage of Left Superior Parathyroid Gland with Drainage Device, Percutaneous Endoscopic Approach
0G9M4ZX Drainage of Left Superior Parathyroid Gland, Percutaneous Endoscopic Approach, Diagnostic
0G9M4ZZ Drainage of Left Superior Parathyroid Gland, Percutaneous Endoscopic Approach
0G9N00Z Drainage of Right Inferior Parathyroid Gland with Drainage Device, Open Approach
0G9N0ZX Drainage of Right Inferior Parathyroid Gland, Open Approach, Diagnostic
0G9N0ZZ Drainage of Right Inferior Parathyroid Gland, Open Approach
0G9N30Z Drainage of Right Inferior Parathyroid Gland with Drainage Device, Percutaneous Approach
0G9N3ZX Drainage of Right Inferior Parathyroid Gland, Percutaneous Approach, Diagnostic
0G9N3ZZ Drainage of Right Inferior Parathyroid Gland, Percutaneous Approach
0G9N40Z Drainage of Right Inferior Parathyroid Gland with Drainage Device, Percutaneous Endoscopic Approach
0G9N4ZX Drainage of Right Inferior Parathyroid Gland, Percutaneous Endoscopic Approach, Diagnostic
0G9N4ZZ Drainage of Right Inferior Parathyroid Gland, Percutaneous Endoscopic Approach
0G9P00Z Drainage of Left Inferior Parathyroid Gland with Drainage Device, Open Approach
0G9P0ZX Drainage of Left Inferior Parathyroid Gland, Open Approach, Diagnostic
0G9P0ZZ Drainage of Left Inferior Parathyroid Gland, Open Approach
0G9P30Z Drainage of Left Inferior Parathyroid Gland with Drainage Device, Percutaneous Approach
0G9P3ZX Drainage of Left Inferior Parathyroid Gland, Percutaneous Approach, Diagnostic
0G9P3ZZ Drainage of Left Inferior Parathyroid Gland, Percutaneous Approach
0G9P40Z Drainage of Left Inferior Parathyroid Gland with Drainage Device, Percutaneous Endoscopic Approach
0G9P4ZX Drainage of Left Inferior Parathyroid Gland, Percutaneous Endoscopic Approach, Diagnostic
0G9P4ZZ Drainage of Left Inferior Parathyroid Gland, Percutaneous Endoscopic Approach
0G9Q00Z Drainage of Multiple Parathyroid Glands with Drainage Device, Open Approach
0G9Q0ZX Drainage of Multiple Parathyroid Glan[ds,] Open Approach, Diagnostic
0G9Q0ZZ Drainage of Multiple Parathyroid Glan[ds,] Open Approach
0G9Q30Z Drainage of Multiple Parathyroid Glan[ds] with Drainage Device, Percutaneous Approach
0G9Q3ZX Drainage of Multiple Parathyroid Glan[ds,] Percutaneous Approach, Diagnostic
0G9Q3ZZ Drainage of Multiple Parathyroid Gland[s,] Percutaneous Approach
0G9Q4ZX Drainage of Multiple Parathyroid Gland[s,] Percutaneous Endoscopic Approach, Diagnostic
0G9Q4ZZ Drainage of Multiple Parathyroid Gland[s,] Percutaneous Endoscopic Approach
0G9R00Z Drainage of Parathyroid Gland with Drainage Device, Open Approach
0G9R0ZX Drainage of Parathyroid Gland, Open Approach, Diagnostic
0G9R0ZZ Drainage of Parathyroid Gland, Open Approach
0G9R30Z Drainage of Parathyroid Gland with Drainage Device, Percutaneous Approach
0G9R3ZX Drainage of Parathyroid Gland, Percutaneous Approach, Diagnostic
0G9R3ZZ Drainage of Parathyroid Gland, Percutaneous Approach
0G9R40Z Drainage of Parathyroid Gland with Drainage Device, Percutaneous Endoscopic Approach
0G9R4ZX Drainage of Parathyroid Gland, Percutaneous Endoscopic Approach, Diagnostic
0G9R4ZZ Drainage of Parathyroid Gland, Percutaneous Endoscopic Approach

0GB – Endocrine System, Excision

Review Coding Guidelines B3.4a and B3.4b

Review Coding Guideline B3.8

0GB00ZX Excision of Pituitary Gland, Open Approach, Diagnostic
0GB00ZZ Excision of Pituitary Gland, Open Approach
0GB03ZX Excision of Pituitary Gland, Percutaneous Approach, Diagnostic
0GB03ZZ Excision of Pituitary Gland, Percutaneous Approach
0GB04ZX Excision of Pituitary Gland, Percutaneous Endoscopic Approach, Diagnostic
0GB04ZZ Excision of Pituitary Gland, Percutaneous Endoscopic Approach
0GB10ZX Excision of Pineal Body, Open Approach, Diagnostic
0GB10ZZ Excision of Pineal Body, Open Approach
0GB13ZX Excision of Pineal Body, Percutaneous Approach, Diagnostic
0GB13ZZ Excision of Pineal Body, Percutaneous Approach
0GB14ZX Excision of Pineal Body, Percutaneous Endoscopic Approach, Diagnostic
0GB14ZZ Excision of Pineal Body, Percutaneous Endoscopic Approach
0GB20ZX Excision of Left Adrenal Gland, Open Approach, Diagnostic
0GB20ZZ Excision of Left Adrenal Gland, Open Approach
0GB23ZX Excision of Left Adrenal Gland, Percutaneous Approach, Diagnostic
0GB23ZZ Excision of Left Adrenal Gland, Percutaneous Approach
0GB24ZX Excision of Left Adrenal Gland, Percutaneous Endoscopic Approach, Diagnostic
0GB24ZZ Excision of Left Adrenal Gland, Percutaneous Endoscopic Approach
0GB30ZX Excision of Right Adrenal Gland, Open Approach, Diagnostic
0GB30ZZ Excision of Right Adrenal Gland, Open Approach
0GB33ZX Excision of Right Adrenal Gland, Percutaneous Approach, Diagnostic
0GB33ZZ Excision of Right Adrenal Gland, Percutaneous Approach
0GB34ZX Excision of Right Adrenal Gland, Percutaneous Endoscopic Approach, Diagnostic
0GB34ZZ Excision of Right Adrenal Gland, Percutaneous Endoscopic Approach
0GB40ZX Excision of Bilateral Adrenal Glands, Open Approach, Diagnostic
0GB40ZZ Excision of Bilateral Adrenal Glands, Open Approach
0GB43ZX Excision of Bilateral Adrenal Glands, Percutaneous Approach, Diagnostic
0GB43ZZ Excision of Bilateral Adrenal Glands, Percutaneous Approach
0GB44ZX Excision of Bilateral Adrenal Glands, Percutaneous Endoscopic Approach, Diagnostic
0GB44ZZ Excision of Bilateral Adrenal Glands, Percutaneous Endoscopic Approach

B60ZX Excision of Left Carotid Body, Open Approach, Diagnostic
B60ZZ Excision of Left Carotid Body, Open Approach
B63ZX Excision of Left Carotid Body, Percutaneous Approach, Diagnostic
B63ZZ Excision of Left Carotid Body, Percutaneous Approach
B64ZX Excision of Left Carotid Body, Percutaneous Endoscopic Approach, Diagnostic
B64ZZ Excision of Left Carotid Body, Percutaneous Endoscopic Approach
B70ZX Excision of Right Carotid Body, Open Approach, Diagnostic
B70ZZ Excision of Right Carotid Body, Open Approach
B73ZX Excision of Right Carotid Body, Percutaneous Approach, Diagnostic
B73ZZ Excision of Right Carotid Body, Percutaneous Approach
B74ZX Excision of Right Carotid Body, Percutaneous Endoscopic Approach, Diagnostic
B74ZZ Excision of Right Carotid Body, Percutaneous Endoscopic Approach
B80ZX Excision of Bilateral Carotid Bodies, Open Approach, Diagnostic
B80ZZ Excision of Bilateral Carotid Bodies, Open Approach
B83ZX Excision of Bilateral Carotid Bodies, Percutaneous Approach, Diagnostic
B83ZZ Excision of Bilateral Carotid Bodies, Percutaneous Approach
B84ZX Excision of Bilateral Carotid Bodies, Percutaneous Endoscopic Approach, Diagnostic
B84ZZ Excision of Bilateral Carotid Bodies, Percutaneous Endoscopic Approach
B90ZX Excision of Para-aortic Body, Open Approach, Diagnostic
B90ZZ Excision of Para-aortic Body, Open Approach
B93ZX Excision of Para-aortic Body, Percutaneous Approach, Diagnostic
B93ZZ Excision of Para-aortic Body, Percutaneous Approach
B94ZX Excision of Para-aortic Body, Percutaneous Endoscopic Approach, Diagnostic
B94ZZ Excision of Para-aortic Body, Percutaneous Endoscopic Approach
BB0ZX Excision of Coccygeal Glomus, Open Approach, Diagnostic
BB0ZZ Excision of Coccygeal Glomus, Open Approach
BB3ZX Excision of Coccygeal Glomus, Percutaneous Approach, Diagnostic
BB3ZZ Excision of Coccygeal Glomus, Percutaneous Approach
BB4ZX Excision of Coccygeal Glomus, Percutaneous Endoscopic Approach, Diagnostic
GBB4ZZ Excision of Coccygeal Glomus, Percutaneous Endoscopic Approach
GBC0ZX Excision of Glomus Jugulare, Open Approach, Diagnostic
GBC0ZZ Excision of Glomus Jugulare, Open Approach
GBC3ZX Excision of Glomus Jugulare, Percutaneous Approach, Diagnostic
0GBC3ZZ Excision of Glomus Jugulare, Percutaneous Approach
0GBC4ZX Excision of Glomus Jugulare, Percutaneous Endoscopic Approach, Diagnostic
0GBC4ZZ Excision of Glomus Jugulare, Percutaneous Endoscopic Approach
0GBD0ZX Excision of Aortic Body, Open Approach, Diagnostic
0GBD0ZZ Excision of Aortic Body, Open Approach
0GBD3ZX Excision of Aortic Body, Percutaneous Approach, Diagnostic
0GBD3ZZ Excision of Aortic Body, Percutaneous Approach
0GBD4ZX Excision of Aortic Body, Percutaneous Endoscopic Approach, Diagnostic
0GBD4ZZ Excision of Aortic Body, Percutaneous Endoscopic Approach
0GBF0ZX Excision of Paraganglion Extremity, Open Approach, Diagnostic
0GBF0ZZ Excision of Paraganglion Extremity, Open Approach
0GBF3ZX Excision of Paraganglion Extremity, Percutaneous Approach, Diagnostic
0GBF3ZZ Excision of Paraganglion Extremity, Percutaneous Approach
0GBF4ZX Excision of Paraganglion Extremity, Percutaneous Endoscopic Approach, Diagnostic
0GBF4ZZ Excision of Paraganglion Extremity, Percutaneous Endoscopic Approach
0GBG0ZX Excision of Left Thyroid Gland Lobe, Open Approach, Diagnostic
0GBG0ZZ Excision of Left Thyroid Gland Lobe, Open Approach
0GBG3ZX Excision of Left Thyroid Gland Lobe, Percutaneous Approach, Diagnostic
0GBG3ZZ Excision of Left Thyroid Gland Lobe, Percutaneous Approach
0GBG4ZX Excision of Left Thyroid Gland Lobe, Percutaneous Endoscopic Approach, Diagnostic
0GBG4ZZ Excision of Left Thyroid Gland Lobe, Percutaneous Endoscopic Approach
0GBH0ZX Excision of Right Thyroid Gland Lobe, Open Approach, Diagnostic
0GBH0ZZ Excision of Right Thyroid Gland Lobe, Open Approach
0GBH3ZX Excision of Right Thyroid Gland Lobe, Percutaneous Approach, Diagnostic
0GBH3ZZ Excision of Right Thyroid Gland Lobe, Percutaneous Approach
0GBH4ZX Excision of Right Thyroid Gland Lobe, Percutaneous Endoscopic Approach, Diagnostic
0GBH4ZZ Excision of Right Thyroid Gland Lobe, Percutaneous Endoscopic Approach
0GBL0ZX Excision of Right Superior Parathyroid Gland, Open Approach, Diagnostic
0GBL0ZZ Excision of Right Superior Parathyroid Gland, Open Approach
0GBL3ZX Excision of Right Superior Parathyroid Gland, Percutaneous Approach, Diagnostic
0GBL3ZZ Excision of Right Superior Parathyroid Gland, Percutaneous Approach
0GBL4ZX Excision of Right Superior Parathyroid Gland, Percutaneous Endoscopic Approach, Diagnostic
0GBL4ZZ Excision of Right Superior Parathyroid Gland, Percutaneous Endoscopic Approach
0GBM0ZX Excision of Left Superior Parathyroid Gland, Open Approach, Diagnostic
0GBM0ZZ Excision of Left Superior Parathyroid Gland, Open Approach
0GBM3ZX Excision of Left Superior Parathyroid Gland, Percutaneous Approach, Diagnostic
0GBM3ZZ Excision of Left Superior Parathyroid Gland, Percutaneous Approach
0GBM4ZX Excision of Left Superior Parathyroid Gland, Percutaneous Endoscopic Approach, Diagnostic
0GBM4ZZ Excision of Left Superior Parathyroid Gland, Percutaneous Endoscopic Approach
0GBN0ZX Excision of Right Inferior Parathyroid Gland, Open Approach, Diagnostic
0GBN0ZZ Excision of Right Inferior Parathyroid Gland, Open Approach
0GBN3ZX Excision of Right Inferior Parathyroid Gland, Percutaneous Approach, Diagnostic
0GBN3ZZ Excision of Right Inferior Parathyroid Gland, Percutaneous Approach
0GBN4ZX Excision of Right Inferior Parathyroid Gland, Percutaneous Endoscopic Approach, Diagnostic
0GBN4ZZ Excision of Right Inferior Parathyroid Gland, Percutaneous Endoscopic Approach
0GBP0ZX Excision of Left Inferior Parathyroid Gland, Open Approach, Diagnostic
0GBP0ZZ Excision of Left Inferior Parathyroid Gland, Open Approach
0GBP3ZX Excision of Left Inferior Parathyroid Gland, Percutaneous Approach, Diagnostic
0GBP3ZZ Excision of Left Inferior Parathyroid Gland, Percutaneous Approach
0GBP4ZX Excision of Left Inferior Parathyroid Gland, Percutaneous Endoscopic Approach, Diagnostic
0GBP4ZZ Excision of Left Inferior Parathyroid Gland, Percutaneous Endoscopic Approach
0GBQ0ZX Excision of Multiple Parathyroid Glands, Open Approach, Diagnostic
0GBQ0ZZ Excision of Multiple Parathyroid Glands, Open Approach
0GBQ3ZX Excision of Multiple Parathyroid Glands, Percutaneous Approach, Diagnostic
0GBQ3ZZ Excision of Multiple Parathyroid Glands, Percutaneous Approach
0GBQ4ZX Excision of Multiple Parathyroid Glands, Percutaneous Endoscopic Approach, Diagnostic
0GBQ4ZZ Excision of Multiple Parathyroid Glands, Percutaneous Endoscopic Approach
0GBR0ZX Excision of Parathyroid Gland, Open Approach, Diagnostic
0GBR0ZZ Excision of Parathyroid Gland, Open Approach
0GBR3ZX Excision of Parathyroid Gland, Percutaneous Approach, Diagnostic
0GBR3ZZ Excision of Parathyroid Gland, Percutaneous Approach
0GBR4ZX Excision of Parathyroid Gland, Percutaneous Endoscopic Approach, Diagnostic
0GBR4ZZ Excision of Parathyroid Gland, Percutaneous Endoscopic Approach

GC – Endocrine System, Extirpation

GC00ZZ Extirpation of Matter from Pituitary Gland, Open Approach
GC03ZZ Extirpation of Matter from Pituitary Gland, Percutaneous Approach
0GC04ZZ Extirpation of Matter from Pituitary Gland, Percutaneous Endoscopic Approach
0GC10ZZ Extirpation of Matter from Pineal Body, Open Approach
0GC13ZZ Extirpation of Matter from Pineal Body, Percutaneous Approach

0GC14ZZ Extirpation of Matter from Pineal Body, Percutaneous Endoscopic Approach
0GC20ZZ Extirpation of Matter from Left Adrenal Gland, Open Approach
0GC23ZZ Extirpation of Matter from Left Adrenal Gland, Percutaneous Approach
0GC24ZZ Extirpation of Matter from Left Adrenal Gland, Percutaneous Endoscopic Approach
0GC30ZZ Extirpation of Matter from Right Adrenal Gland, Open Approach
0GC33ZZ Extirpation of Matter from Right Adrenal Gland, Percutaneous Approach
0GC34ZZ Extirpation of Matter from Right Adrenal Gland, Percutaneous Endoscopic Approach
0GC40ZZ Extirpation of Matter from Bilateral Adrenal Glands, Open Approach
0GC43ZZ Extirpation of Matter from Bilateral Adrenal Glands, Percutaneous Approach
0GC44ZZ Extirpation of Matter from Bilateral Adrenal Glands, Percutaneous Endoscopic Approach
0GC60ZZ Extirpation of Matter from Left Carotid Body, Open Approach
0GC63ZZ Extirpation of Matter from Left Carotid Body, Percutaneous Approach
0GC64ZZ Extirpation of Matter from Left Carotid Body, Percutaneous Endoscopic Approach
0GC70ZZ Extirpation of Matter from Right Carotid Body, Open Approach
0GC73ZZ Extirpation of Matter from Right Carotid Body, Percutaneous Approach
0GC74ZZ Extirpation of Matter from Right Carotid Body, Percutaneous Endoscopic Approach
0GC80ZZ Extirpation of Matter from Bilateral Carotid Bodies, Open Approach
0GC83ZZ Extirpation of Matter from Bilateral Carotid Bodies, Percutaneous Approach
0GC84ZZ Extirpation of Matter from Bilateral Carotid Bodies, Percutaneous Endoscopic Approach
0GC90ZZ Extirpation of Matter from Para-aortic Body, Open Approach
0GC93ZZ Extirpation of Matter from Para-aortic Body, Percutaneous Approach
0GC94ZZ Extirpation of Matter from Para-aortic Body, Percutaneous Endoscopic Approach
0GCB0ZZ Extirpation of Matter from Coccygeal Glomus, Open Approach
0GCB3ZZ Extirpation of Matter from Coccygeal Glomus, Percutaneous Approach
0GCB4ZZ Extirpation of Matter from Coccygeal Glomus, Percutaneous Endoscopic Approach
0GCC0ZZ Extirpation of Matter from Glomus Jugulare, Open Approach
0GCC3ZZ Extirpation of Matter from Glomus Jugulare, Percutaneous Approach
0GCC4ZZ Extirpation of Matter from Glomus Jugulare, Percutaneous Endoscopic Approach
0GCD0ZZ Extirpation of Matter from Aortic Body, Open Approach
0GCD3ZZ Extirpation of Matter from Aortic Body, Percutaneous Approach
0GCD4ZZ Extirpation of Matter from Aortic Body, Percutaneous Endoscopic Approach
0GCF0ZZ Extirpation of Matter from Paraganglion Extremity, Open Approach
0GCF3ZZ Extirpation of Matter from Paraganglion Extremity, Percutaneous Approach
0GCF4ZZ Extirpation of Matter from Paraganglion Extremity, Percutaneous Endoscopic Approach
0GCG0ZZ Extirpation of Matter from Left Thyroid Gland Lobe, Open Approach
0GCG3ZZ Extirpation of Matter from Left Thyroid Gland Lobe, Percutaneous Approach
0GCG4ZZ Extirpation of Matter from Left Thyroid Gland Lobe, Percutaneous Endoscopic Approach
0GCH0ZZ Extirpation of Matter from Right Thyroid Gland Lobe, Open Approach
0GCH3ZZ Extirpation of Matter from Right Thyroid Gland Lobe, Percutaneous Approach
0GCH4ZZ Extirpation of Matter from Right Thyroid Gland Lobe, Percutaneous Endoscopic Approach
0GCK0ZZ Extirpation of Matter from Thyroid Gland, Open Approach
0GCK3ZZ Extirpation of Matter from Thyroid Gland, Percutaneous Approach
0GCK4ZZ Extirpation of Matter from Thyroid Gland, Percutaneous Endoscopic Approach
0GCL0ZZ Extirpation of Matter from Right Super Parathyroid Gland, Open Approach
0GCL3ZZ Extirpation of Matter from Right Super Parathyroid Gland, Percutaneous Approach
0GCL4ZZ Extirpation of Matter from Right Super Parathyroid Gland, Percutaneous Endoscopic Approach
0GCM0ZZ Extirpation of Matter from Left Superic Parathyroid Gland, Open Approach
0GCM3ZZ Extirpation of Matter from Left Superic Parathyroid Gland, Percutaneous Approach
0GCM4ZZ Extirpation of Matter from Left Superic Parathyroid Gland, Percutaneous Endoscopic Approach
0GCN0ZZ Extirpation of Matter from Right Inferic Parathyroid Gland, Open Approach
0GCN3ZZ Extirpation of Matter from Right Inferi Parathyroid Gland, Percutaneous Approach
0GCN4ZZ Extirpation of Matter from Right Inferic Parathyroid Gland, Percutaneous Endoscopic Approach
0GCP0ZZ Extirpation of Matter from Left Inferior Parathyroid Gland, Open Approach
0GCP3ZZ Extirpation of Matter from Left Inferior Parathyroid Gland, Percutaneous Approach
0GCP4ZZ Extirpation of Matter from Left Inferior Parathyroid Gland, Percutaneous Endoscopic Approach
0GCQ0ZZ Extirpation of Matter from Multiple Parathyroid Glands, Open Approach
0GCQ3ZZ Extirpation of Matter from Multiple Parathyroid Glands, Percutaneous Approach
0GCQ4ZZ Extirpation of Matter from Multiple Parathyroid Glands, Percutaneous Endoscopic Approach
0GCR0ZZ Extirpation of Matter from Parathyroid Gland, Open Approach
0GCR3ZZ Extirpation of Matter from Parathyroid Gland, Percutaneous Approach
0GCR4ZZ Extirpation of Matter from Parathyroid Gland, Percutaneous Endoscopic Approach

0GH – Endocrine System, Insertion

0GHS02Z Insertion of Monitoring Device into Endocrine Gland, Open Approach
0GHS03Z Insertion of Infusion Device into Endocrine Gland, Open Approach
0GHS32Z Insertion of Monitoring Device into Endocrine Gland, Percutaneous Approach
0GHS33Z Insertion of Infusion Device into Endocrine Gland, Percutaneous Approach
0GHS42Z Insertion of Monitoring Device into Endocrine Gland, Percutaneous Endoscopic Approach
0GHS43Z Insertion of Infusion Device into Endocrine Gland, Percutaneous Endoscopic Approach

0GJ – Endocrine System, Inspection

Review Coding Guidelines B3.11a, B3.11b and B3.11c

0GJ00ZZ Inspection of Pituitary Gland, Open Approach
0GJ03ZZ Inspection of Pituitary Gland, Percutaneous Approach
0GJ04ZZ Inspection of Pituitary Gland, Percutaneous Endoscopic Approach
0GJ10ZZ Inspection of Pineal Body, Open Approach
0GJ13ZZ Inspection of Pineal Body, Percutaneous Approach
0GJ14ZZ Inspection of Pineal Body, Percutaneous Endoscopic Approach
0GJ50ZZ Inspection of Adrenal Gland, Open Approach
0GJ53ZZ Inspection of Adrenal Gland, Percutaneous Approach
0GJ54ZZ Inspection of Adrenal Gland, Percutaneous Endoscopic Approach
0GJK0ZZ Inspection of Thyroid Gland, Open Approach
0GJK3ZZ Inspection of Thyroid Gland, Percutaneous Approach
0GJK4ZZ Inspection of Thyroid Gland, Percutaneous Endoscopic Approach
0GJR0ZZ Inspection of Parathyroid Gland, Open Approach
0GJR3ZZ Inspection of Parathyroid Gland, Percutaneous Approach
0GJR4ZZ Inspection of Parathyroid Gland, Percutaneous Endoscopic Approach
0GJS0ZZ Inspection of Endocrine Gland, Open Approach
0GJS3ZZ Inspection of Endocrine Gland, Percutaneous Approach
0GJS4ZZ Inspection of Endocrine Gland, Percutaneous Endoscopic Approach

M – Endocrine System, Reattachment

M20ZZ Reattachment of Left Adrenal Gland, Open Approach
M24ZZ Reattachment of Left Adrenal Gland, Percutaneous Endoscopic Approach
M30ZZ Reattachment of Right Adrenal Gland, Open Approach
M34ZZ Reattachment of Right Adrenal Gland, Percutaneous Endoscopic Approach
MG0ZZ Reattachment of Left Thyroid Gland Lobe, Open Approach
MG4ZZ Reattachment of Left Thyroid Gland Lobe, Percutaneous Endoscopic Approach
MH0ZZ Reattachment of Right Thyroid Gland Lobe, Open Approach
0GMH4ZZ Reattachment of Right Thyroid Gland Lobe, Percutaneous Endoscopic Approach
0GML0ZZ Reattachment of Right Superior Parathyroid Gland, Open Approach
0GML4ZZ Reattachment of Right Superior Parathyroid Gland, Percutaneous Endoscopic Approach
0GMM0ZZ Reattachment of Left Superior Parathyroid Gland, Open Approach
0GMM4ZZ Reattachment of Left Superior Parathyroid Gland, Percutaneous Endoscopic Approach
0GMN0ZZ Reattachment of Right Inferior Parathyroid Gland, Open Approach
0GMN4ZZ Reattachment of Right Inferior Parathyroid Gland, Percutaneous Endoscopic Approach
0GMP0ZZ Reattachment of Left Inferior Parathyroid Gland, Open Approach
0GMP4ZZ Reattachment of Left Inferior Parathyroid Gland, Percutaneous Endoscopic Approach
0GMQ0ZZ Reattachment of Multiple Parathyroid Glands, Open Approach
0GMQ4ZZ Reattachment of Multiple Parathyroid Glands, Percutaneous Endoscopic Approach
0GMR0ZZ Reattachment of Parathyroid Gland, Open Approach
0GMR4ZZ Reattachment of Parathyroid Gland, Percutaneous Endoscopic Approach

N – Endocrine System, Release

view Coding Guideline B3.13

view Coding Guideline B3.14

N00ZZ Release Pituitary Gland, Open Approach
N03ZZ Release Pituitary Gland, Percutaneous Approach
N04ZZ Release Pituitary Gland, Percutaneous Endoscopic Approach
N10ZZ Release Pineal Body, Open Approach
N13ZZ Release Pineal Body, Percutaneous Approach
N14ZZ Release Pineal Body, Percutaneous Endoscopic Approach
N20ZZ Release Left Adrenal Gland, Open Approach
N23ZZ Release Left Adrenal Gland, Percutaneous Approach
N24ZZ Release Left Adrenal Gland, Percutaneous Endoscopic Approach
N30ZZ Release Right Adrenal Gland, Open Approach
N33ZZ Release Right Adrenal Gland, Percutaneous Approach
N34ZZ Release Right Adrenal Gland, Percutaneous Endoscopic Approach
N40ZZ Release Bilateral Adrenal Glands, Open Approach
N43ZZ Release Bilateral Adrenal Glands, Percutaneous Approach
N44ZZ Release Bilateral Adrenal Glands, Percutaneous Endoscopic Approach
N60ZZ Release Left Carotid Body, Open Approach
N63ZZ Release Left Carotid Body, Percutaneous Approach
N64ZZ Release Left Carotid Body, Percutaneous Endoscopic Approach
N70ZZ Release Right Carotid Body, Open Approach
GN73ZZ Release Right Carotid Body, Percutaneous Approach
GN74ZZ Release Right Carotid Body, Percutaneous Endoscopic Approach
0GN80ZZ Release Bilateral Carotid Bodies, Open Approach
0GN83ZZ Release Bilateral Carotid Bodies, Percutaneous Approach
0GN84ZZ Release Bilateral Carotid Bodies, Percutaneous Endoscopic Approach
0GN90ZZ Release Para-aortic Body, Open Approach
0GN93ZZ Release Para-aortic Body, Percutaneous Approach
0GN94ZZ Release Para-aortic Body, Percutaneous Endoscopic Approach
0GNB0ZZ Release Coccygeal Glomus, Open Approach
0GNB3ZZ Release Coccygeal Glomus, Percutaneous Approach
0GNB4ZZ Release Coccygeal Glomus, Percutaneous Endoscopic Approach
0GNC0ZZ Release Glomus Jugulare, Open Approach
0GNC3ZZ Release Glomus Jugulare, Percutaneous Approach
0GNC4ZZ Release Glomus Jugulare, Percutaneous Endoscopic Approach
0GND0ZZ Release Aortic Body, Open Approach
0GND3ZZ Release Aortic Body, Percutaneous Approach
0GND4ZZ Release Aortic Body, Percutaneous Endoscopic Approach
0GNF0ZZ Release Paraganglion Extremity, Open Approach
0GNF3ZZ Release Paraganglion Extremity, Percutaneous Approach
0GNF4ZZ Release Paraganglion Extremity, Percutaneous Endoscopic Approach
0GNG0ZZ Release Left Thyroid Gland Lobe, Open Approach
0GNG3ZZ Release Left Thyroid Gland Lobe, Percutaneous Approach
0GNG4ZZ Release Left Thyroid Gland Lobe, Percutaneous Endoscopic Approach
0GNH0ZZ Release Right Thyroid Gland Lobe, Open Approach
0GNH3ZZ Release Right Thyroid Gland Lobe, Percutaneous Approach
0GNH4ZZ Release Right Thyroid Gland Lobe, Percutaneous Endoscopic Approach
0GNK0ZZ Release Thyroid Gland, Open Approach
0GNK3ZZ Release Thyroid Gland, Percutaneous Approach
0GNK4ZZ Release Thyroid Gland, Percutaneous Endoscopic Approach
0GNL0ZZ Release Right Superior Parathyroid Gland, Open Approach
0GNL3ZZ Release Right Superior Parathyroid Gland, Percutaneous Approach
0GNL4ZZ Release Right Superior Parathyroid Gland, Percutaneous Endoscopic Approach
0GNM0ZZ Release Left Superior Parathyroid Gland, Open Approach
0GNM3ZZ Release Left Superior Parathyroid Gland, Percutaneous Approach
0GNM4ZZ Release Left Superior Parathyroid Gland, Percutaneous Endoscopic Approach
0GNN0ZZ Release Right Inferior Parathyroid Gland, Open Approach
0GNN3ZZ Release Right Inferior Parathyroid Gland, Percutaneous Approach
0GNN4ZZ Release Right Inferior Parathyroid Gland, Percutaneous Endoscopic Approach
0GNP0ZZ Release Left Inferior Parathyroid Gland, Open Approach
0GNP3ZZ Release Left Inferior Parathyroid Gland, Percutaneous Approach
0GNP4ZZ Release Left Inferior Parathyroid Gland, Percutaneous Endoscopic Approach
0GNQ0ZZ Release Multiple Parathyroid Glands, Open Approach
0GNQ3ZZ Release Multiple Parathyroid Glands, Percutaneous Approach
0GNQ4ZZ Release Multiple Parathyroid Glands, Percutaneous Endoscopic Approach
0GNR0ZZ Release Parathyroid Gland, Open Approach
0GNR3ZZ Release Parathyroid Gland, Percutaneous Approach
0GNR4ZZ Release Parathyroid Gland, Percutaneous Endoscopic Approach

GP – Endocrine System, Removal

eview Coding Guideline B6.1c

GP000Z Removal of Drainage Device from Pituitary Gland, Open Approach
GP030Z Removal of Drainage Device from Pituitary Gland, Percutaneous Approach
0GP040Z Removal of Drainage Device from Pituitary Gland, Percutaneous Endoscopic Approach
0GP0X0Z Removal of Drainage Device from Pituitary Gland, External Approach
0GP100Z Removal of Drainage Device from Pineal Body, Open Approach

0GP130Z Removal of Drainage Device from Pineal Body, Percutaneous Approach
0GP140Z Removal of Drainage Device from Pineal Body, Percutaneous Endoscopic Approach
0GP1X0Z Removal of Drainage Device from Pineal Body, External Approach
0GP500Z Removal of Drainage Device from Adrenal Gland, Open Approach
0GP530Z Removal of Drainage Device from Adrenal Gland, Percutaneous Approach
0GP540Z Removal of Drainage Device from Adrenal Gland, Percutaneous Endoscopic Approach
0GP5X0Z Removal of Drainage Device from Adrenal Gland, External Approach
0GPK00Z Removal of Drainage Device from Thyroid Gland, Open Approach
0GPK30Z Removal of Drainage Device from Thyroid Gland, Percutaneous Approach
0GPK40Z Removal of Drainage Device from Thyroid Gland, Percutaneous Endoscopic Approach
0GPKX0Z Removal of Drainage Device from Thyroid Gland, External Approach
0GPR00Z Removal of Drainage Device from Parathyroid Gland, Open Approach
0GPR30Z Removal of Drainage Device from Parathyroid Gland, Percutaneous Approach
0GPR40Z Removal of Drainage Device from Parathyroid Gland, Percutaneous Endoscopic Approach
0GPRX0Z Removal of Drainage Device from Parathyroid Gland, External Approach
0GPS00Z Removal of Drainage Device from Endocrine Gland, Open Approach
0GPS02Z Removal of Monitoring Device from Endocrine Gland, Open Approach
0GPS03Z Removal of Infusion Device from Endocrine Gland, Open Approach
0GPS30Z Removal of Drainage Device from Endocrine Gland, Percutaneous Appro
0GPS32Z Removal of Monitoring Device from Endocrine Gland, Percutaneous Appro
0GPS33Z Removal of Infusion Device from Endocrine Gland, Percutaneous Appro
0GPS40Z Removal of Drainage Device from Endocrine Gland, Percutaneous Endoscopic Approach
0GPS42Z Removal of Monitoring Device from Endocrine Gland, Percutaneous Endoscopic Approach
0GPS43Z Removal of Infusion Device from Endocrine Gland, Percutaneous Endoscopic Approach
0GPSX0Z Removal of Drainage Device from Endocrine Gland, External Approach
0GPSX2Z Removal of Monitoring Device from Endocrine Gland, External Approach
0GPSX3Z Removal of Infusion Device from Endocrine Gland, External Approach

0GQ – Endocrine System, Repair

0GQ00ZZ Repair Pituitary Gland, Open Approach
0GQ03ZZ Repair Pituitary Gland, Percutaneous Approach
0GQ04ZZ Repair Pituitary Gland, Percutaneous Endoscopic Approach
0GQ10ZZ Repair Pineal Body, Open Approach
0GQ13ZZ Repair Pineal Body, Percutaneous Approach
0GQ14ZZ Repair Pineal Body, Percutaneous Endoscopic Approach
0GQ20ZZ Repair Left Adrenal Gland, Open Approach
0GQ23ZZ Repair Left Adrenal Gland, Percutaneous Approach
0GQ24ZZ Repair Left Adrenal Gland, Percutaneous Endoscopic Approach
0GQ30ZZ Repair Right Adrenal Gland, Open Approach
0GQ33ZZ Repair Right Adrenal Gland, Percutaneous Approach
0GQ34ZZ Repair Right Adrenal Gland, Percutaneous Endoscopic Approach
0GQ40ZZ Repair Bilateral Adrenal Glands, Open Approach
0GQ43ZZ Repair Bilateral Adrenal Glands, Percutaneous Approach
0GQ44ZZ Repair Bilateral Adrenal Glands, Percutaneous Endoscopic Approach
0GQ60ZZ Repair Left Carotid Body, Open Approach
0GQ63ZZ Repair Left Carotid Body, Percutaneous Approach
0GQ64ZZ Repair Left Carotid Body, Percutaneous Endoscopic Approach
0GQ70ZZ Repair Right Carotid Body, Open Approach
0GQ73ZZ Repair Right Carotid Body, Percutaneous Approach
0GQ74ZZ Repair Right Carotid Body, Percutaneous Endoscopic Approach
0GQ80ZZ Repair Bilateral Carotid Bodies, Open Approach
0GQ83ZZ Repair Bilateral Carotid Bodies, Percutaneous Approach
0GQ84ZZ Repair Bilateral Carotid Bodies, Percutaneous Endoscopic Approach
0GQ90ZZ Repair Para-aortic Body, Open Approach
0GQ93ZZ Repair Para-aortic Body, Percutaneous Approach
0GQ94ZZ Repair Para-aortic Body, Percutaneous Endoscopic Approach
0GQB0ZZ Repair Coccygeal Glomus, Open Approach
0GQB3ZZ Repair Coccygeal Glomus, Percutaneous Approach
0GQB4ZZ Repair Coccygeal Glomus, Percutaneous Endoscopic Approach
0GQC0ZZ Repair Glomus Jugulare, Open Approach
0GQC3ZZ Repair Glomus Jugulare, Percutaneous Approach
0GQC4ZZ Repair Glomus Jugulare, Percutaneous Endoscopic Approach
0GQD0ZZ Repair Aortic Body, Open Approach
0GQD3ZZ Repair Aortic Body, Percutaneous Approach
0GQD4ZZ Repair Aortic Body, Percutaneous Endoscopic Approach
0GQF0ZZ Repair Paraganglion Extremity, Open Approach
0GQF3ZZ Repair Paraganglion Extremity, Percutaneous Approach
0GQF4ZZ Repair Paraganglion Extremity, Percutaneous Endoscopic Approach
0GQG0ZZ Repair Left Thyroid Gland Lobe, Open Approach
0GQG3ZZ Repair Left Thyroid Gland Lobe, Percutaneous Approach
0GQG4ZZ Repair Left Thyroid Gland Lobe, Percutaneous Endoscopic Approach
0GQH0ZZ Repair Right Thyroid Gland Lobe, Open Approach
0GQH3ZZ Repair Right Thyroid Gland Lobe, Percutaneous Approach
0GQH4ZZ Repair Right Thyroid Gland Lobe, Percutaneous Endoscopic Approach
0GQJ0ZZ Repair Thyroid Gland Isthmus, Open Approach
0GQJ3ZZ Repair Thyroid Gland Isthmus, Percutaneous Approach
0GQJ4ZZ Repair Thyroid Gland Isthmus, Percutaneous Endoscopic Approach
0GQK0ZZ Repair Thyroid Gland, Open Approach
0GQK3ZZ Repair Thyroid Gland, Percutaneous Approach
0GQK4ZZ Repair Thyroid Gland, Percutaneous Endoscopic Approach
0GQL0ZZ Repair Right Superior Parathyroid Glan Open Approach
0GQL3ZZ Repair Right Superior Parathyroid Glan Percutaneous Approach
0GQL4ZZ Repair Right Superior Parathyroid Glan Percutaneous Endoscopic Approach
0GQM0ZZ Repair Left Superior Parathyroid Gland, Open Approach
0GQM3ZZ Repair Left Superior Parathyroid Gland, Percutaneous Approach
0GQM4ZZ Repair Left Superior Parathyroid Gland, Percutaneous Endoscopic Approach
0GQN0ZZ Repair Right Inferior Parathyroid Gland, Open Approach
0GQN3ZZ Repair Right Inferior Parathyroid Gland, Percutaneous Approach
0GQN4ZZ Repair Right Inferior Parathyroid Gland, Percutaneous Endoscopic Approach
0GQP0ZZ Repair Left Inferior Parathyroid Gland, Open Approach
0GQP3ZZ Repair Left Inferior Parathyroid Gland, Percutaneous Approach
0GQP4ZZ Repair Left Inferior Parathyroid Gland, Percutaneous Endoscopic Approach
0GQQ0ZZ Repair Multiple Parathyroid Glands, Ope Approach
0GQQ3ZZ Repair Multiple Parathyroid Glands, Percutaneous Approach
0GQQ4ZZ Repair Multiple Parathyroid Glands, Percutaneous Endoscopic Approach
0GQR0ZZ Repair Parathyroid Gland, Open Approac
0GQR3ZZ Repair Parathyroid Gland, Percutaneous Approach
0GQR4ZZ Repair Parathyroid Gland, Percutaneous Endoscopic Approach

0GS – Endocrine System, Reposition

0GS20ZZ Reposition Left Adrenal Gland, Open Approach
0GS24ZZ Reposition Left Adrenal Gland, Percutaneous Endoscopic Approach
0GS30ZZ Reposition Right Adrenal Gland, Open Approach
0GS34ZZ Reposition Right Adrenal Gland, Percutaneous Endoscopic Approach
0GSG0ZZ Reposition Left Thyroid Gland Lobe, Open Approach
0GSG4ZZ Reposition Left Thyroid Gland Lobe, Percutaneous Endoscopic Approach
0GSH0ZZ Reposition Right Thyroid Gland Lobe, Open Approach
0GSH4ZZ Reposition Right Thyroid Gland Lobe, Percutaneous Endoscopic Approach
0GSL0ZZ Reposition Right Superior Parathyroid Gland, Open Approach

L4ZZ Reposition Right Superior Parathyroid Gland, Percutaneous Endoscopic Approach
M0ZZ Reposition Left Superior Parathyroid Gland, Open Approach
M4ZZ Reposition Left Superior Parathyroid Gland, Percutaneous Endoscopic Approach
N0ZZ Reposition Right Inferior Parathyroid Gland, Open Approach
0GSN4ZZ Reposition Right Inferior Parathyroid Gland, Percutaneous Endoscopic Approach
0GSP0ZZ Reposition Left Inferior Parathyroid Gland, Open Approach
0GSP4ZZ Reposition Left Inferior Parathyroid Gland, Percutaneous Endoscopic Approach
0GSQ0ZZ Reposition Multiple Parathyroid Glands, Open Approach
0GSQ4ZZ Reposition Multiple Parathyroid Glands, Percutaneous Endoscopic Approach
0GSR0ZZ Reposition Parathyroid Gland, Open Approach
0GSR4ZZ Reposition Parathyroid Gland, Percutaneous Endoscopic Approach

T – Endocrine System, Resection

view Coding Guideline B3.8

T00ZZ Resection of Pituitary Gland, Open Approach
T04ZZ Resection of Pituitary Gland, Percutaneous Endoscopic Approach
T10ZZ Resection of Pineal Body, Open Approach
T14ZZ Resection of Pineal Body, Percutaneous Endoscopic Approach
T20ZZ Resection of Left Adrenal Gland, Open Approach
T24ZZ Resection of Left Adrenal Gland, Percutaneous Endoscopic Approach
T30ZZ Resection of Right Adrenal Gland, Open Approach
T34ZZ Resection of Right Adrenal Gland, Percutaneous Endoscopic Approach
T40ZZ Resection of Bilateral Adrenal Glands, Open Approach
T44ZZ Resection of Bilateral Adrenal Glands, Percutaneous Endoscopic Approach
T60ZZ Resection of Left Carotid Body, Open Approach
T64ZZ Resection of Left Carotid Body, Percutaneous Endoscopic Approach
T70ZZ Resection of Right Carotid Body, Open Approach
T74ZZ Resection of Right Carotid Body, Percutaneous Endoscopic Approach
T80ZZ Resection of Bilateral Carotid Bodies, Open Approach
T84ZZ Resection of Bilateral Carotid Bodies, Percutaneous Endoscopic Approach
0GT90ZZ Resection of Para-aortic Body, Open Approach
0GT94ZZ Resection of Para-aortic Body, Percutaneous Endoscopic Approach
0GTB0ZZ Resection of Coccygeal Glomus, Open Approach
0GTB4ZZ Resection of Coccygeal Glomus, Percutaneous Endoscopic Approach
0GTC0ZZ Resection of Glomus Jugulare, Open Approach
0GTC4ZZ Resection of Glomus Jugulare, Percutaneous Endoscopic Approach
0GTD0ZZ Resection of Aortic Body, Open Approach
0GTD4ZZ Resection of Aortic Body, Percutaneous Endoscopic Approach
0GTF0ZZ Resection of Paraganglion Extremity, Open Approach
0GTF4ZZ Resection of Paraganglion Extremity, Percutaneous Endoscopic Approach
0GTG0ZZ Resection of Left Thyroid Gland Lobe, Open Approach
0GTG4ZZ Resection of Left Thyroid Gland Lobe, Percutaneous Endoscopic Approach
0GTH0ZZ Resection of Right Thyroid Gland Lobe, Open Approach
0GTH4ZZ Resection of Right Thyroid Gland Lobe, Percutaneous Endoscopic Approach
0GTK0ZZ Resection of Thyroid Gland, Open Approach
0GTK4ZZ Resection of Thyroid Gland, Percutaneous Endoscopic Approach
0GTL0ZZ Resection of Right Superior Parathyroid Gland, Open Approach
0GTL4ZZ Resection of Right Superior Parathyroid Gland, Percutaneous Endoscopic Approach
0GTM0ZZ Resection of Left Superior Parathyroid Gland, Open Approach
0GTM4ZZ Resection of Left Superior Parathyroid Gland, Percutaneous Endoscopic Approach
0GTN0ZZ Resection of Right Inferior Parathyroid Gland, Open Approach
0GTN4ZZ Resection of Right Inferior Parathyroid Gland, Percutaneous Endoscopic Approach
0GTP0ZZ Resection of Left Inferior Parathyroid Gland, Open Approach
0GTP4ZZ Resection of Left Inferior Parathyroid Gland, Percutaneous Endoscopic Approach
0GTQ0ZZ Resection of Multiple Parathyroid Glands, Open Approach
0GTQ4ZZ Resection of Multiple Parathyroid Glands, Percutaneous Endoscopic Approach
0GTR0ZZ Resection of Parathyroid Gland, Open Approach
0GTR4ZZ Resection of Parathyroid Gland, Percutaneous Endoscopic Approach

GW – Endocrine System, Revision

eview Coding Guideline B6.1c

W000Z Revision of Drainage Device in Pituitary Gland, Open Approach
W030Z Revision of Drainage Device in Pituitary Gland, Percutaneous Approach
W040Z Revision of Drainage Device in Pituitary Gland, Percutaneous Endoscopic Approach
W0X0Z Revision of Drainage Device in Pituitary Gland, External Approach
W100Z Revision of Drainage Device in Pineal Body, Open Approach
W130Z Revision of Drainage Device in Pineal Body, Percutaneous Approach
W140Z Revision of Drainage Device in Pineal Body, Percutaneous Endoscopic Approach
W1X0Z Revision of Drainage Device in Pineal Body, External Approach
W500Z Revision of Drainage Device in Adrenal Gland, Open Approach
GW530Z Revision of Drainage Device in Adrenal Gland, Percutaneous Approach
GW540Z Revision of Drainage Device in Adrenal Gland, Percutaneous Endoscopic Approach
0GW5X0Z Revision of Drainage Device in Adrenal Gland, External Approach
0GWK00Z Revision of Drainage Device in Thyroid Gland, Open Approach
0GWK30Z Revision of Drainage Device in Thyroid Gland, Percutaneous Approach
0GWK40Z Revision of Drainage Device in Thyroid Gland, Percutaneous Endoscopic Approach
0GWKX0Z Revision of Drainage Device in Thyroid Gland, External Approach
0GWR00Z Revision of Drainage Device in Parathyroid Gland, Open Approach
0GWR30Z Revision of Drainage Device in Parathyroid Gland, Percutaneous Approach
0GWR40Z Revision of Drainage Device in Parathyroid Gland, Percutaneous Endoscopic Approach
0GWRX0Z Revision of Drainage Device in Parathyroid Gland, External Approach
0GWS00Z Revision of Drainage Device in Endocrine Gland, Open Approach
0GWS02Z Revision of Monitoring Device in Endocrine Gland, Open Approach
0GWS03Z Revision of Infusion Device in Endocrine Gland, Open Approach
0GWS30Z Revision of Drainage Device in Endocrine Gland, Percutaneous Approach
0GWS32Z Revision of Monitoring Device in Endocrine Gland, Percutaneous Approach
0GWS33Z Revision of Infusion Device in Endocrine Gland, Percutaneous Approach
0GWS40Z Revision of Drainage Device in Endocrine Gland, Percutaneous Endoscopic Approach
0GWS42Z Revision of Monitoring Device in Endocrine Gland, Percutaneous Endoscopic Approach
0GWS43Z Revision of Infusion Device in Endocrine Gland, Percutaneous Endoscopic Approach
0GWSX0Z Revision of Drainage Device in Endocrine Gland, External Approach
0GWSX2Z Revision of Monitoring Device in Endocrine Gland, External Approach
0GWSX3Z Revision of Infusion Device in Endocrine Gland, External Approach

Skin and Subcutaneous Tissue

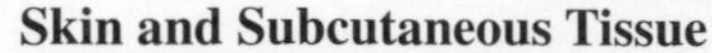

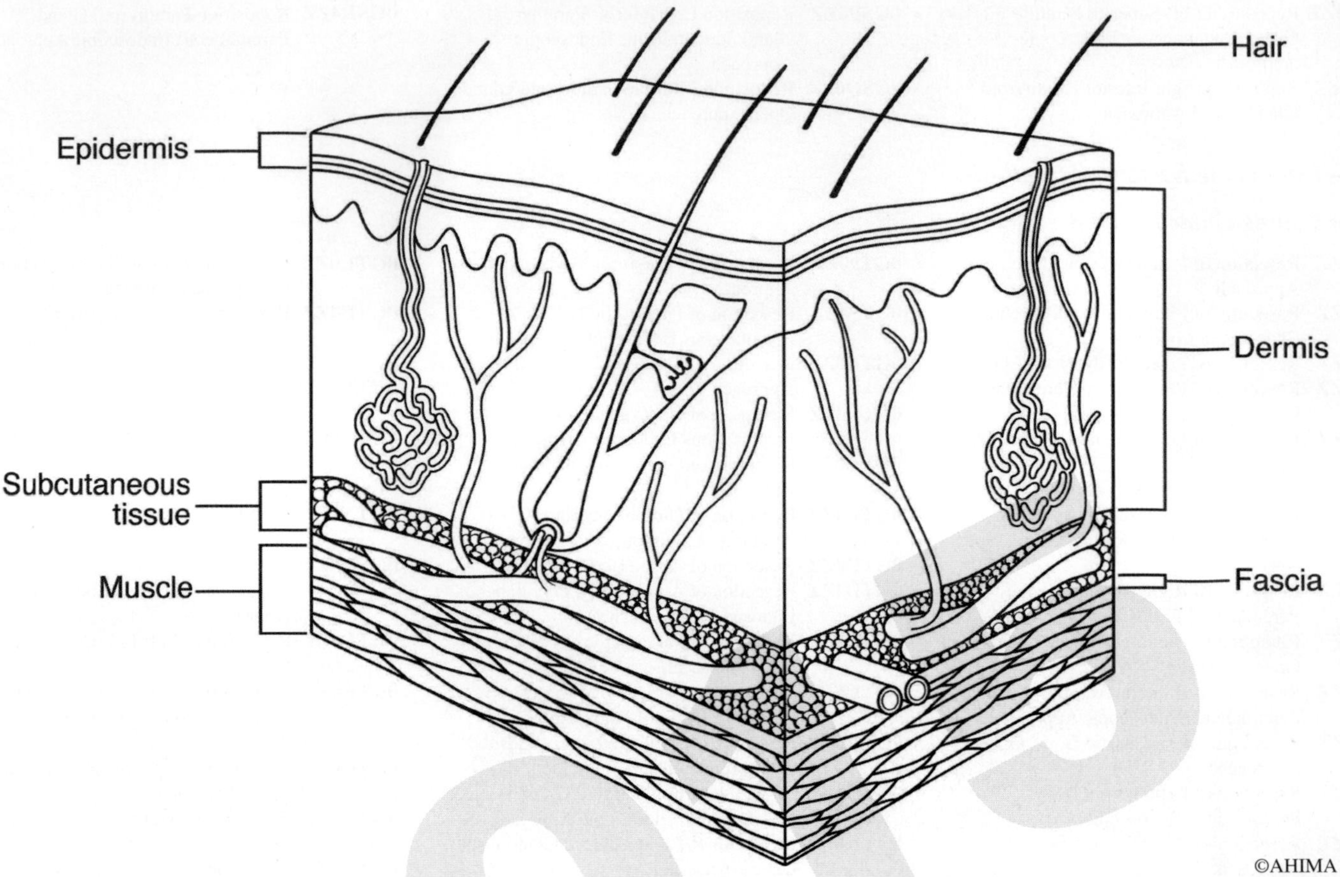

Breast

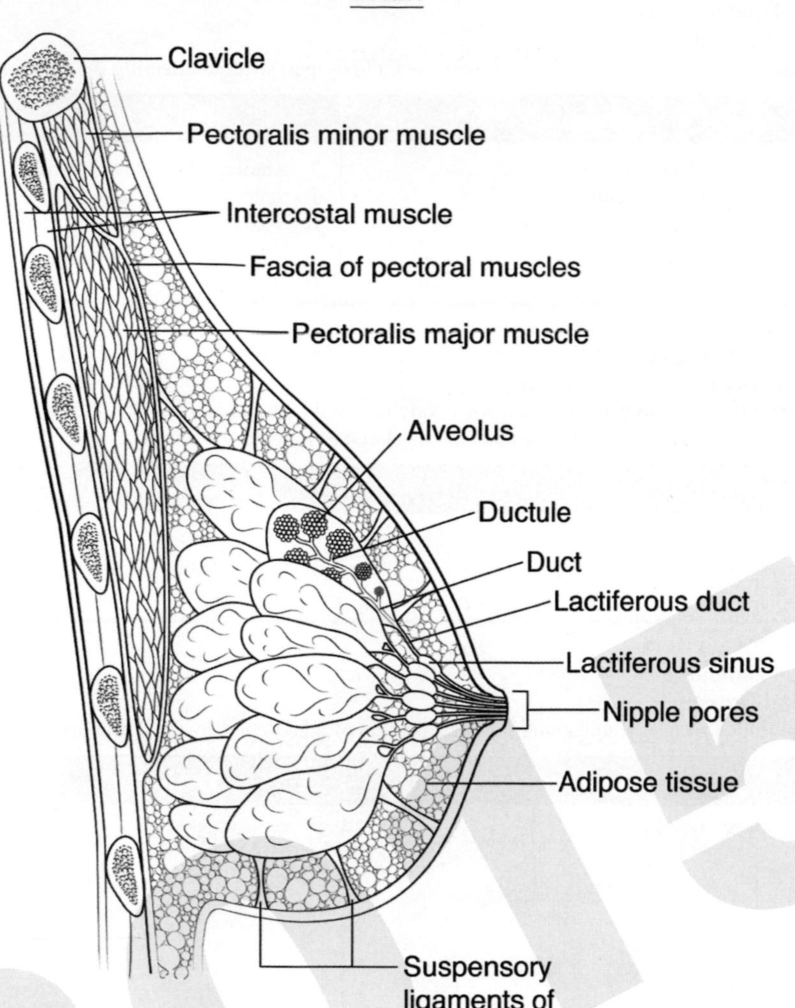
Clavicle
Pectoralis minor muscle
Intercostal muscle
Fascia of pectoral muscles
Pectoralis major muscle
Alveolus
Ductule
Duct
Lactiferous duct
Lactiferous sinus
Nipple pores
Adipose tissue
Suspensory ligaments of Cooper
©AHIMA

Nail Bed

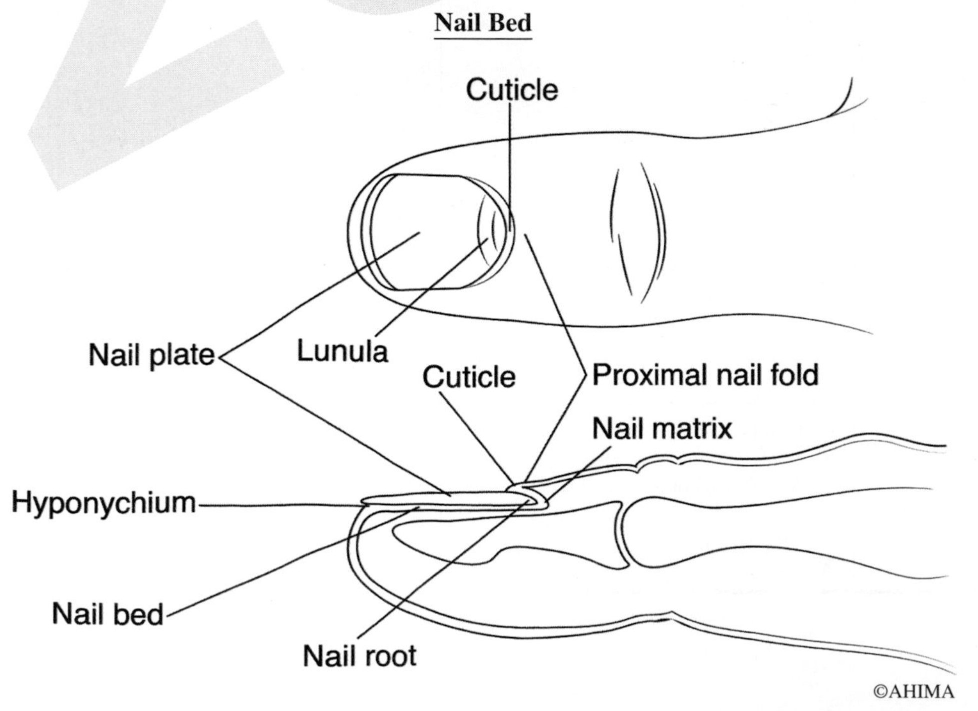
Cuticle
Nail plate
Lunula
Cuticle
Proximal nail fold
Nail matrix
Hyponychium
Nail bed
Nail root
©AHIMA

Skin and Breast Tables 0H0–0HX

Section 0 **Medical and Surgical**
Body System H **Skin and Breast**
Operation 0 **Alteration:** Modifying the anatomic structure of a body part without affecting the function of the body part

Body Part (4th)	Approach (5th)	Device (6th)	Qualifier (7th)
T Breast, Right **U** Breast, Left **V** Breast, Bilateral	**0** Open **3** Percutaneous **X** External	**7** Autologous Tissue Substitute **J** Synthetic Substitute **K** Nonautologous Tissue Substitute **Z** No Device	**Z** No Qualifier

Section 0 **Medical and Surgical**
Body System H **Skin and Breast**
Operation 2 **Change:** Taking out or off a device from a body part and putting back an identical or similar device in or on the same body part without cutting or puncturing the skin or a mucous membrane

Body Part (4th)	Approach (5th)	Device (6th)	Qualifier (7th)
P Skin **T** Breast, Right **U** Breast, Left	**X** External	**0** Drainage Device **Y** Other Device	**Z** No Qualifier

Section 0 **Medical and Surgical**
Body System H **Skin and Breast**
Operation 5 **Destruction:** Physical eradication of all or a portion of a body part by the direct use of energy, force, or a destructive agent

Body Part (4th)	Approach (5th)	Device (6th)	Qualifier (7th)
0 Skin, Scalp **1** Skin, Face **2** Skin, Right Ear **3** Skin, Left Ear **4** Skin, Neck **5** Skin, Chest **6** Skin, Back **7** Skin, Abdomen **8** Skin, Buttock **9** Skin, Perineum **A** Skin, Genitalia **B** Skin, Right Upper Arm **C** Skin, Left Upper Arm **D** Skin, Right Lower Arm **E** Skin, Left Lower Arm **F** Skin, Right Hand **G** Skin, Left Hand **H** Skin, Right Upper Leg **J** Skin, Left Upper Leg **K** Skin, Right Lower Leg **L** Skin, Left Lower Leg **M** Skin, Right Foot **N** Skin, Left Foot	**X** External	**Z** No Device	**D** Multiple **Z** No Qualifier
Q Finger Nail **R** Toe Nail	**X** External	**Z** No Device	**Z** No Qualifier
T Breast, Right **U** Breast, Left **V** Breast, Bilateral **W** Nipple, Right **X** Nipple, Left	**0** Open **3** Percutaneous **7** Via Natural or Artificial Opening **8** Via Natural or Artificial Opening Endoscopic **X** External	**Z** No Device	**Z** No Qualifier

tion 0 **Medical and Surgical**
dy System H **Skin and Breast**
eration 8 **Division:** Cutting into a body part, without draining fluids and/or gases from the body part, in order to separate or transect a body part

Body Part (4th)	Approach (5th)	Device (6th)	Qualifier (7th)
Skin, Scalp	**X** External	**Z** No Device	**Z** No Qualifier
Skin, Face			
Skin, Right Ear			
Skin, Left Ear			
4 Skin, Neck			
5 Skin, Chest			
6 Skin, Back			
7 Skin, Abdomen			
8 Skin, Buttock			
9 Skin, Perineum			
A Skin, Genitalia			
B Skin, Right Upper Arm			
C Skin, Left Upper Arm			
D Skin, Right Lower Arm			
E Skin, Left Lower Arm			
F Skin, Right Hand			
G Skin, Left Hand			
H Skin, Right Upper Leg			
J Skin, Left Upper Leg			
K Skin, Right Lower Leg			
L Skin, Left Lower Leg			
M Skin, Right Foot			
N Skin, Left Foot			

ction 0 **Medical and Surgical**
dy System H **Skin and Breast**
peration 9 **Drainage:** Taking or letting out fluids and/or gases from a body part

Body Part (4th)	Approach (5th)	Device (6th)	Qualifier (7th)
0 Skin, Scalp	**X** External	**0** Drainage Device	**Z** No Qualifier
1 Skin, Face			
2 Skin, Right Ear			
3 Skin, Left Ear			
4 Skin, Neck			
5 Skin, Chest			
6 Skin, Back			
7 Skin, Abdomen			
8 Skin, Buttock			
9 Skin, Perineum			
A Skin, Genitalia			
B Skin, Right Upper Arm			
C Skin, Left Upper Arm			
D Skin, Right Lower Arm			
E Skin, Left Lower Arm			
F Skin, Right Hand			
G Skin, Left Hand			
H Skin, Right Upper Leg			
J Skin, Left Upper Leg			
K Skin, Right Lower Leg			
L Skin, Left Lower Leg			
M Skin, Right Foot			
N Skin, Left Foot			
Q Finger Nail			
R Toe Nail			

Continued →

Section 0 **Medical and Surgical**
Body System H **Skin and Breast**
Operation 9 **Drainage:** Taking or letting out fluids and/or gases from a body part

0H9 Contin

Body Part (4th)	Approach (5th)	Device (6th)	Qualifier (7th)
0 Skin, Scalp **1** Skin, Face **2** Skin, Right Ear **3** Skin, Left Ear **4** Skin, Neck **5** Skin, Chest **6** Skin, Back **7** Skin, Abdomen **8** Skin, Buttock **9** Skin, Perineum **A** Skin, Genitalia **B** Skin, Right Upper Arm **C** Skin, Left Upper Arm **D** Skin, Right Lower Arm **E** Skin, Left Lower Arm **F** Skin, Right Hand **G** Skin, Left Hand **H** Skin, Right Upper Leg **J** Skin, Left Upper Leg **K** Skin, Right Lower Leg **L** Skin, Left Lower Leg **M** Skin, Right Foot **N** Skin, Left Foot **Q** Finger Nail **R** Toe Nail	**X** External	**Z** No Device	**X** Diagnostic **Z** No Qualifier
T Breast, Right **U** Breast, Left **V** Breast, Bilateral **W** Nipple, Right **X** Nipple, Left	**0** Open **3** Percutaneous **7** Via Natural or Artificial Opening **8** Via Natural or Artificial Opening Endoscopic **X** External	**0** Drainage Device	**Z** No Qualifier
T Breast, Right **U** Breast, Left **V** Breast, Bilateral **W** Nipple, Right **X** Nipple, Left	**0** Open **3** Percutaneous **7** Via Natural or Artificial Opening **8** Via Natural or Artificial Opening Endoscopic **X** External	**Z** No Device	**X** Diagnostic **Z** No Qualifier

Section	**0**	**Medical and Surgical**
Body System	**H**	**Skin and Breast**
Operation	**B**	**Excision:** Cutting out or off, without replacement, a portion of a body part

Body Part (4th)	Approach (5th)	Device (6th)	Qualifier (7th)
0 Skin, Scalp Skin, Face **2** Skin, Right Ear **3** Skin, Left Ear **4** Skin, Neck **5** Skin, Chest **6** Skin, Back **7** Skin, Abdomen **8** Skin, Buttock **9** Skin, Perineum **A** Skin, Genitalia **B** Skin, Right Upper Arm **C** Skin, Left Upper Arm **D** Skin, Right Lower Arm **E** Skin, Left Lower Arm **F** Skin, Right Hand **G** Skin, Left Hand **H** Skin, Right Upper Leg **J** Skin, Left Upper Leg **K** Skin, Right Lower Leg **L** Skin, Left Lower Leg **M** Skin, Right Foot **N** Skin, Left Foot **Q** Finger Nail **R** Toe Nail	**X** External	**Z** No Device	**X** Diagnostic **Z** No Qualifier
T Breast, Right **U** Breast, Left **V** Breast, Bilateral **W** Nipple, Right **X** Nipple, Left **Y** Supernumerary Breast	**0** Open **3** Percutaneous **7** Via Natural or Artificial Opening **8** Via Natural or Artificial Opening Endoscopic **X** External	**Z** No Device	**X** Diagnostic **Z** No Qualifier

Section 0 **Medical and Surgical**
Body System H **Skin and Breast**
Operation C **Extirpation:** Taking or cutting out solid matter from a body part

Body Part (4th)	Approach (5th)	Device (6th)	Qualifier (7th)
0 Skin, Scalp **1** Skin, Face **2** Skin, Right Ear **3** Skin, Left Ear **4** Skin, Neck **5** Skin, Chest **6** Skin, Back **7** Skin, Abdomen **8** Skin, Buttock **9** Skin, Perineum **A** Skin, Genitalia **B** Skin, Right Upper Arm **C** Skin, Left Upper Arm **D** Skin, Right Lower Arm **E** Skin, Left Lower Arm **F** Skin, Right Hand **G** Skin, Left Hand **H** Skin, Right Upper Leg **J** Skin, Left Upper Leg **K** Skin, Right Lower Leg **L** Skin, Left Lower Leg **M** Skin, Right Foot **N** Skin, Left Foot **Q** Finger Nail **R** Toe Nail	**X** External	**Z** No Device	**Z** No Qualifier
T Breast, Right **U** Breast, Left **V** Breast, Bilateral **W** Nipple, Right **X** Nipple, Left	**0** Open **3** Percutaneous **7** Via Natural or Artificial Opening **8** Via Natural or Artificial Opening Endoscopic **X** External	**Z** No Device	**Z** No Qualifier

tion **0** **Medical and Surgical**
dy System **H** **Skin and Breast**
eration **D** **Extraction:** Pulling or stripping out or off all or a portion of a body part by the use of force

Body Part (4th)	Approach (5th)	Device (6th)	Qualifier (7th)
Skin, Scalp Skin, Face Skin, Right Ear Skin, Left Ear Skin, Neck Skin, Chest Skin, Back Skin, Abdomen Skin, Buttock Skin, Perineum **A** Skin, Genitalia **B** Skin, Right Upper Arm **C** Skin, Left Upper Arm **D** Skin, Right Lower Arm **E** Skin, Left Lower Arm **F** Skin, Right Hand **G** Skin, Left Hand **H** Skin, Right Upper Leg **J** Skin, Left Upper Leg **K** Skin, Right Lower Leg **L** Skin, Left Lower Leg **M** Skin, Right Foot **N** Skin, Left Foot **Q** Finger Nail **R** Toe Nail **S** Hair	**X** External	**Z** No Device	**Z** No Qualifier

ection **0** **Medical and Surgical**
ody System **H** **Skin and Breast**
peration **H** **Insertion:** Putting in a nonbiological appliance that monitors, assists, performs, or prevents a physiological function but does not physically take the place of a body part

Body Part (4th)	Approach (5th)	Device (6th)	Qualifier (7th)
T Breast, Right **U** Breast, Left **V** Breast, Bilateral **W** Nipple, Right **X** Nipple, Left	**0** Open **3** Percutaneous **7** Via Natural or Artificial Opening **8** Via Natural or Artificial Opening Endoscopic	**1** Radioactive Element **N** Tissue Expander	**Z** No Qualifier
T Breast, Right **U** Breast, Left **V** Breast, Bilateral **W** Nipple, Right **X** Nipple, Left	**X** External	**1** Radioactive Element	**Z** No Qualifier

ection **0** **Medical and Surgical**
ody System **H** **Skin and Breast**
peration **J** **Inspection:** Visually and/or manually exploring a body part

Body Part (4th)	Approach (5th)	Device (6th)	Qualifier (7th)
P Skin **Q** Finger Nail **R** Toe Nail	**X** External	**Z** No Device	**Z** No Qualifier
T Breast, Right **U** Breast, Left	**0** Open **3** Percutaneous **7** Via Natural or Artificial Opening **8** Via Natural or Artificial Opening Endoscopic **X** External	**Z** No Device	**Z** No Qualifier

Section 0 **Medical and Surgical**
Body System H **Skin and Breast**
Operation M **Reattachment:** Putting back in or on all or a portion of a separated body part to its normal location or other suitable locatio

Body Part (4th)	Approach (5th)	Device (6th)	Qualifier (7th)
0 Skin, Scalp **1** Skin, Face **2** Skin, Right Ear **3** Skin, Left Ear **4** Skin, Neck **5** Skin, Chest **6** Skin, Back **7** Skin, Abdomen **8** Skin, Buttock **9** Skin, Perineum **A** Skin, Genitalia **B** Skin, Right Upper Arm **C** Skin, Left Upper Arm **D** Skin, Right Lower Arm **E** Skin, Left Lower Arm **F** Skin, Right Hand **G** Skin, Left Hand **H** Skin, Right Upper Leg **J** Skin, Left Upper Leg **K** Skin, Right Lower Leg **L** Skin, Left Lower Leg **M** Skin, Right Foot **N** Skin, Left Foot **T** Breast, Right **U** Breast, Left **V** Breast, Bilateral **W** Nipple, Right **X** Nipple, Left	**X** External	**Z** No Device	**Z** No Qualifier

Section 0 **Medical and Surgical**
Body System H **Skin and Breast**
Operation N **Release:** Freeing a body part from an abnormal physical constraint by cutting or by the use of force

Body Part (4th)	Approach (5th)	Device (6th)	Qualifier (7th)
0 Skin, Scalp **1** Skin, Face **2** Skin, Right Ear **3** Skin, Left Ear **4** Skin, Neck **5** Skin, Chest **6** Skin, Back **7** Skin, Abdomen **8** Skin, Buttock **9** Skin, Perineum **A** Skin, Genitalia **B** Skin, Right Upper Arm **C** Skin, Left Upper Arm **D** Skin, Right Lower Arm **E** Skin, Left Lower Arm **F** Skin, Right Hand **G** Skin, Left Hand **H** Skin, Right Upper Leg **J** Skin, Left Upper Leg	**X** External	**Z** No Device	**Z** No Qualifier

Continued →

tion	0	**Medical and Surgical**
ly System	H	**Skin and Breast**
eration	N	**Release:** Freeing a body part from an abnormal physical constraint by cutting or by the use of force

Body Part (4th)	Approach (5th)	Device (6th)	Qualifier (7th)
K Skin, Right Lower Leg L Skin, Left Lower Leg M Skin, Right Foot N Skin, Left Foot Q Finger Nail R Toe Nail T Breast, Right U Breast, Left V Breast, Bilateral W Nipple, Right X Nipple, Left	**0** Open **3** Percutaneous **7** Via Natural or Artificial Opening **8** Via Natural or Artificial Opening Endoscopic **X** External	**Z** No Device	**Z** No Qualifier

ction	0	**Medical and Surgical**
dy System	H	**Skin and Breast**
eration	P	**Removal:** Taking out or off a device from a body part

Body Part (4th)	Approach (5th)	Device (6th)	Qualifier (7th)
P Skin **Q** Finger Nail **R** Toe Nail	**X** External	**0** Drainage Device **7** Autologous Tissue Substitute **J** Synthetic Substitute **K** Nonautologous Tissue Substitute	**Z** No Qualifier
S Hair	**X** External	**7** Autologous Tissue Substitute **J** Synthetic Substitute **K** Nonautologous Tissue Substitute	**Z** No Qualifier
T Breast, Right **U** Breast, Left	**0** Open **3** Percutaneous **7** Via Natural or Artificial Opening **8** Via Natural or Artificial Opening Endoscopic	**0** Drainage Device **1** Radioactive Element **7** Autologous Tissue Substitute **J** Synthetic Substitute **K** Nonautologous Tissue Substitute **N** Tissue Expander	**Z** No Qualifier
T Breast, Right **U** Breast, Left	**X** External	**0** Drainage Device **1** Radioactive Element **7** Autologous Tissue Substitute **J** Synthetic Substitute **K** Nonautologous Tissue Substitute	**Z** No Qualifier

Section 0 **Medical and Surgical**
Body System H **Skin and Breast**
Operation Q **Repair:** Restoring, to the extent possible, a body part to its normal anatomic structure and function

Body Part (4th)	Approach (5th)	Device (6th)	Qualifier (7th)
0 Skin, Scalp **1** Skin, Face **2** Skin, Right Ear **3** Skin, Left Ear **4** Skin, Neck **5** Skin, Chest **6** Skin, Back **7** Skin, Abdomen **8** Skin, Buttock **9** Skin, Perineum **A** Skin, Genitalia **B** Skin, Right Upper Arm **C** Skin, Left Upper Arm **D** Skin, Right Lower Arm **E** Skin, Left Lower Arm **F** Skin, Right Hand **G** Skin, Left Hand **H** Skin, Right Upper Leg **J** Skin, Left Upper Leg **K** Skin, Right Lower Leg **L** Skin, Left Lower Leg **M** Skin, Right Foot **N** Skin, Left Foot **Q** Finger Nail **R** Toe Nail	**X** External	**Z** No Device	**Z** No Qualifier
T Breast, Right **U** Breast, Left **V** Breast, Bilateral **W** Nipple, Right **X** Nipple, Left **Y** Supernumerary Breast	**0** Open **3** Percutaneous **7** Via Natural or Artificial Opening **8** Via Natural or Artificial Opening Endoscopic **X** External	**Z** No Device	**Z** No Qualifier

Section 0 **Medical and Surgical**
Body System H **Skin and Breast**
Operation R **Replacement:** Putting in or on biological or synthetic material that physically takes the place and/or function of all or a portion of a body part

Body Part (4th)	Approach (5th)	Device (6th)	Qualifier (7th)
0 Skin, Scalp **1** Skin, Face **2** Skin, Right Ear **3** Skin, Left Ear **4** Skin, Neck **5** Skin, Chest **6** Skin, Back **7** Skin, Abdomen **8** Skin, Buttock **9** Skin, Perineum **A** Skin, Genitalia **B** Skin, Right Upper Arm **C** Skin, Left Upper Arm **D** Skin, Right Lower Arm **E** Skin, Left Lower Arm **F** Skin, Right Hand **G** Skin, Left Hand **H** Skin, Right Upper Leg **J** Skin, Left Upper Leg **K** Skin, Right Lower Leg **L** Skin, Left Lower Leg **M** Skin, Right Foot **N** Skin, Left Foot	**X** External	**7** Autologous Tissue Substitute **K** Nonautologous Tissue Substitute	**3** Full Thickness **4** Partial Thickness

Continued →

Section 0 **Medical and Surgical**
Body System H **Skin and Breast**
Operation R **Replacement:** Putting in or on biological or synthetic material that physically takes the place and/or function of all or a portion of a body part

Body Part (4th)	Approach (5th)	Device (6th)	Qualifier (7th)
Skin, Scalp Skin, Face Skin, Right Ear Skin, Left Ear Skin, Neck Skin, Chest Skin, Back Skin, Abdomen Skin, Buttock Skin, Perineum **A** Skin, Genitalia **B** Skin, Right Upper Arm **C** Skin, Left Upper Arm **D** Skin, Right Lower Arm **E** Skin, Left Lower Arm **F** Skin, Right Hand **G** Skin, Left Hand **H** Skin, Right Upper Leg **J** Skin, Left Upper Leg **K** Skin, Right Lower Leg **L** Skin, Left Lower Leg **M** Skin, Right Foot **N** Skin, Left Foot	**X** External	**J** Synthetic Substitute	**3** Full Thickness **4** Partial Thickness **Z** No Qualifier
Q Finger Nail **R** Toe Nail **S** Hair	**X** External	**7** Autologous Tissue Substitute **J** Synthetic Substitute **K** Nonautologous Tissue Substitute	**Z** No Qualifier
T Breast, Right **U** Breast, Left **V** Breast, Bilateral	**0** Open	**7** Autologous Tissue Substitute	**5** Latissimus Dorsi Myocutaneous Flap **6** Transverse Rectus Abdominis Myocutaneous Flap **7** Deep Inferior Epigastric Artery Perforator Flap **8** Superficial Inferior Epigastric Artery Flap **9** Gluteal Artery Perforator Flap **Z** No Qualifier
T Breast, Right **U** Breast, Left **V** Breast, Bilateral	**0** Open	**J** Synthetic Substitute **K** Nonautologous Tissue Substitute	**Z** No Qualifier
T Breast, Right **U** Breast, Left **V** Breast, Bilateral	**3** Percutaneous **X** External	**7** Autologous Tissue Substitute **J** Synthetic Substitute **K** Nonautologous Tissue Substitute	**Z** No Qualifier
W Nipple, Right **X** Nipple, Left	**0** Open **3** Percutaneous **X** External	**7** Autologous Tissue Substitute **J** Synthetic Substitute **K** Nonautologous Tissue Substitute	**Z** No Qualifier

Section 0 **Medical and Surgical**
Body System H **Skin and Breast**
Operation S **Reposition:** Moving to its normal location, or other suitable location, all or a portion of a body part

Body Part (4th)	Approach (5th)	Device (6th)	Qualifier (7th)
S Hair **W** Nipple, Right **X** Nipple, Left	**X** External	**Z** No Device	**Z** No Qualifier
T Breast, Right **U** Breast, Left **V** Breast, Bilateral	**0** Open	**Z** No Device	**Z** No Qualifier

Section 0 **Medical and Surgical**
Body System H **Skin and Breast**
Operation T **Resection:** Cutting out or off, without replacement, all of a body part

Body Part (4th)	Approach (5th)	Device (6th)	Qualifier (7th)
Q Finger Nail **R** Toe Nail **W** Nipple, Right **X** Nipple, Left	**X** External	**Z** No Device	**Z** No Qualifier
T Breast, Right **U** Breast, Left **V** Breast, Bilateral **Y** Supernumerary Breast	**0** Open	**Z** No Device	**Z** No Qualifier

Section 0 **Medical and Surgical**
Body System H **Skin and Breast**
Operation U **Supplement:** Putting in or on biological or synthetic material that physically reinforces and/or augments the function of a portion of a body part

Body Part (4th)	Approach (5th)	Device (6th)	Qualifier (7th)
T Breast, Right **U** Breast, Left **V** Breast, Bilateral **W** Nipple, Right **X** Nipple, Left	**0** Open **3** Percutaneous **7** Via Natural or Artificial Opening **8** Via Natural or Artificial Opening Endoscopic **X** External	**7** Autologous Tissue Substitute **J** Synthetic Substitute **K** Nonautologous Tissue Substitute	**Z** No Qualifier

Section 0 **Medical and Surgical**
Body System H **Skin and Breast**
Operation W **Revision:** Correcting, to the extent possible, a portion of a malfunctioning device or the position of a displaced device

Body Part (4th)	Approach (5th)	Device (6th)	Qualifier (7th)
P Skin **Q** Finger Nail **R** Toe Nail	**X** External	**0** Drainage Device **7** Autologous Tissue Substitute **J** Synthetic Substitute **K** Nonautologous Tissue Substitute	**Z** No Qualifier
S Hair	**X** External	**7** Autologous Tissue Substitute **J** Synthetic Substitute **K** Nonautologous Tissue Substitute	**Z** No Qualifier
T Breast, Right **U** Breast, Left	**0** Open **3** Percutaneous **7** Via Natural or Artificial Opening **8** Via Natural or Artificial Opening Endoscopic	**0** Drainage Device **7** Autologous Tissue Substitute **J** Synthetic Substitute **K** Nonautologous Tissue Substitute **N** Tissue Expander	**Z** No Qualifier
T Breast, Right **U** Breast, Left	**X** External	**0** Drainage Device **7** Autologous Tissue Substitute **J** Synthetic Substitute **K** Nonautologous Tissue Substitute	**Z** No Qualifier

Section **0** **Medical and Surgical**
Body System **H** **Skin and Breast**
Operation **X** **Transfer:** Moving, without taking out, all or a portion of a body part to another location to take over the function of all or a portion of a body part

Body Part (4th)	Approach (5th)	Device (6th)	Qualifier (7th)
Skin, Scalp Skin, Face Skin, Right Ear Skin, Left Ear Skin, Neck Skin, Chest Skin, Back Skin, Abdomen Skin, Buttock Skin, Perineum Skin, Genitalia B Skin, Right Upper Arm C Skin, Left Upper Arm D Skin, Right Lower Arm E Skin, Left Lower Arm F Skin, Right Hand G Skin, Left Hand H Skin, Right Upper Leg J Skin, Left Upper Leg K Skin, Right Lower Leg L Skin, Left Lower Leg M Skin, Right Foot N Skin, Left Foot	X External	Z No Device	Z No Qualifier

Skin and Breast Code Listing 0H0–0HX

0H0 – Skin and Breast, Alteration

0H0T07Z Alteration of Right Breast with Autologous Tissue Substitute, Open Approach
0H0T0JZ Alteration of Right Breast with Synthetic Substitute, Open Approach
0H0T0KZ Alteration of Right Breast with Nonautologous Tissue Substitute, Open Approach
0H0T0ZZ Alteration of Right Breast, Open Approach
0H0T37Z Alteration of Right Breast with Autologous Tissue Substitute, Percutaneous Approach
0H0T3JZ Alteration of Right Breast with Synthetic Substitute, Percutaneous Approach
0H0T3KZ Alteration of Right Breast with Nonautologous Tissue Substitute, Percutaneous Approach
0H0T3ZZ Alteration of Right Breast, Percutaneous Approach
0H0TX7Z Alteration of Right Breast with Autologous Tissue Substitute, External Approach
0H0TXJZ Alteration of Right Breast with Synthetic Substitute, External Approach
0H0TXKZ Alteration of Right Breast with Nonautologous Tissue Substitute, External Approach
0H0TXZZ Alteration of Right Breast, External Approach
0H0U07Z Alteration of Left Breast with Autologous Tissue Substitute, Open Approach
0H0U0JZ Alteration of Left Breast with Synthetic Substitute, Open Approach
0H0U0KZ Alteration of Left Breast with Nonautologous Tissue Substitute, Open Approach
0H0U0ZZ Alteration of Left Breast, Open Approach
0H0U37Z Alteration of Left Breast with Autologous Tissue Substitute, Percutaneous Approach
0H0U3JZ Alteration of Left Breast with Synthetic Substitute, Percutaneous Approach
0H0U3KZ Alteration of Left Breast with Nonautologous Tissue Substitute, Percutaneous Approach
0H0U3ZZ Alteration of Left Breast, Percutaneous Approach
0H0UX7Z Alteration of Left Breast with Autologous Tissue Substitute, External Approach
0H0UXJZ Alteration of Left Breast with Synthetic Substitute, External Approach
0H0UXKZ Alteration of Left Breast with Nonautologous Tissue Substitute, External Approach
0H0UXZZ Alteration of Left Breast, External Approach
0H0V07Z Alteration of Bilateral Breast with Autologous Tissue Substitute, Open Approach
0H0V0JZ Alteration of Bilateral Breast with Synthetic Substitute, Open Approach
0H0V0KZ Alteration of Bilateral Breast with Nonautologous Tissue Substitute, Open Approach
0H0V0ZZ Alteration of Bilateral Breast, Open Approach
0H0V37Z Alteration of Bilateral Breast with Autologous Tissue Substitute, Percutaneous Approach
0H0V3JZ Alteration of Bilateral Breast with Synthetic Substitute, Percutaneous Approach
0H0V3KZ Alteration of Bilateral Breast with Nonautologous Tissue Substitute, Percutaneous Approach
0H0V3ZZ Alteration of Bilateral Breast, Percutaneous Approach
0H0VX7Z Alteration of Bilateral Breast with Autologous Tissue Substitute, External Approach
0H0VXJZ Alteration of Bilateral Breast with Synthetic Substitute, External Approach
0H0VXKZ Alteration of Bilateral Breast with Nonautologous Tissue Substitute, External Approach
0H0VXZZ Alteration of Bilateral Breast, External Approach

0H2 – Skin and Breast, Change

Review Coding Guideline B6.1c

0H2PX0Z Change Drainage Device in Skin, External Approach
0H2PXYZ Change Other Device in Skin, External Approach
0H2TX0Z Change Drainage Device in Right Breast, External Approach
0H2TXYZ Change Other Device in Right Breast, External Approach
0H2UX0Z Change Drainage Device in Left Breast, External Approach
0H2UXYZ Change Other Device in Left Breast, External Approach

0H5 – Skin and Breast, Destruction

● **0H50XZD** Destruction of Scalp Skin, Multiple, External Approach
● **0H50XZZ** Destruction of Scalp Skin, External Approach
● **0H51XZD** Destruction of Face Skin, Multiple, External Approach
● **0H51XZZ** Destruction of Face Skin, External Approach
0H52XZD Destruction of Right Ear Skin, Multiple, External Approach
0H52XZZ Destruction of Right Ear Skin, External Approach
0H53XZD Destruction of Left Ear Skin, Multiple, External Approach
0H53XZZ Destruction of Left Ear Skin, External Approach
● **0H54XZD** Destruction of Neck Skin, Multiple, External Approach
● **0H54XZZ** Destruction of Neck Skin, External Approach
● **0H55XZD** Destruction of Chest Skin, Multiple, External Approach
● **0H55XZZ** Destruction of Chest Skin, External Approach
● **0H56XZD** Destruction of Back Skin, Multiple, External Approach
● **0H56XZZ** Destruction of Back Skin, External Approach
● **0H57XZD** Destruction of Abdomen Skin, Multiple, External Approach
● **0H57XZZ** Destruction of Abdomen Skin, External Approach
● **0H58XZD** Destruction of Buttock Skin, Multiple, External Approach
● **0H58XZZ** Destruction of Buttock Skin, External Approach
● **0H59XZD** Destruction of Perineum Skin, Multiple, External Approach
● **0H59XZZ** Destruction of Perineum Skin, External Approach
● **0H5AXZD** Destruction of Genitalia Skin, Multiple, External Approach
● **0H5AXZZ** Destruction of Genitalia Skin, External Approach
● **0H5BXZD** Destruction of Right Upper Arm Skin, Multiple, External Approach
● **0H5BXZZ** Destruction of Right Upper Arm Skin, External Approach
● **0H5CXZD** Destruction of Left Upper Arm Skin, Multiple, External Approach
● **0H5CXZZ** Destruction of Left Upper Arm Skin, External Approach
● **0H5DXZD** Destruction of Right Lower Arm Skin, Multiple, External Approach
● **0H5DXZZ** Destruction of Right Lower Arm Skin, External Approach
● **0H5EXZD** Destruction of Left Lower Arm Skin, Multiple, External Approach
● **0H5EXZZ** Destruction of Left Lower Arm Skin, External Approach
● **0H5FXZD** Destruction of Right Hand Skin, Multiple, External Approach
● **0H5FXZZ** Destruction of Right Hand Skin, External Approach
● **0H5GXZD** Destruction of Left Hand Skin, Multiple, External Approach
● **0H5GXZZ** Destruction of Left Hand Skin, External Approach
● **0H5HXZD** Destruction of Right Upper Leg Skin, Multiple, External Approach
● **0H5HXZZ** Destruction of Right Upper Leg Skin, External Approach
● **0H5JXZD** Destruction of Left Upper Leg Skin, Multiple, External Approach
● **0H5JXZZ** Destruction of Left Upper Leg Skin, External Approach
● **0H5KXZD** Destruction of Right Lower Leg Skin, Multiple, External Approach
● **0H5KXZZ** Destruction of Right Lower Leg Skin, External Approach
● **0H5LXZD** Destruction of Left Lower Leg Skin, Multiple, External Approach
● **0H5LXZZ** Destruction of Left Lower Leg Skin, External Approach
● **0H5MXZD** Destruction of Right Foot Skin, Multiple, External Approach
● **0H5MXZZ** Destruction of Right Foot Skin, External Approach
● **0H5NXZD** Destruction of Left Foot Skin, Multiple, External Approach
● **0H5NXZZ** Destruction of Left Foot Skin, External Approach
● **0H5QXZZ** Destruction of Finger Nail, External Approach
● **0H5RXZZ** Destruction of Toe Nail, External Approach
0H5T0ZZ Destruction of Right Breast, Open Approach
0H5T3ZZ Destruction of Right Breast, Percutaneous Approach
0H5T7ZZ Destruction of Right Breast, Via Natur or Artificial Opening
0H5T8ZZ Destruction of Right Breast, Via Natural or Artificial Opening Endoscopic
0H5TXZZ Destruction of Right Breast, External Approach
0H5U0ZZ Destruction of Left Breast, Open Approach
0H5U3ZZ Destruction of Left Breast, Percutaneo Approach
0H5U7ZZ Destruction of Left Breast, Via Natural Artificial Opening
0H5U8ZZ Destruction of Left Breast, Via Natural Artificial Opening Endoscopic
0H5UXZZ Destruction of Left Breast, External Approach
0H5V0ZZ Destruction of Bilateral Breast, Open Approach
0H5V3ZZ Destruction of Bilateral Breast, Percutaneous Approach
0H5V7ZZ Destruction of Bilateral Breast, Via Natural or Artificial Opening
0H5V8ZZ Destruction of Bilateral Breast, Via Natural or Artificial Opening Endoscopic
0H5VXZZ Destruction of Bilateral Breast, Externa Approach
0H5W0ZZ Destruction of Right Nipple, Open Approach
0H5W3ZZ Destruction of Right Nipple, Percutaneous Approach
0H5W7ZZ Destruction of Right Nipple, Via Natura or Artificial Opening
0H5W8ZZ Destruction of Right Nipple, Via Natura or Artificial Opening Endoscopic
0H5WXZZ Destruction of Right Nipple, External Approach
0H5X0ZZ Destruction of Left Nipple, Open Approach
0H5X3ZZ Destruction of Left Nipple, Percutaneou Approach
0H5X7ZZ Destruction of Left Nipple, Via Natural Artificial Opening
0H5X8ZZ Destruction of Left Nipple, Via Natural Artificial Opening Endoscopic
0H5XXZZ Destruction of Left Nipple, External Approach

0H8 – Skin and Breast, Division

Review Coding Guideline B3.14

0H80XZZ Division of Scalp Skin, External Approach
0H81XZZ Division of Face Skin, External Approach
0H82XZZ Division of Right Ear Skin, External Approach
0H83XZZ Division of Left Ear Skin, External Approach
0H84XZZ Division of Neck Skin, External Approach
0H85XZZ Division of Chest Skin, External Approach
0H86XZZ Division of Back Skin, External Approach
0H87XZZ Division of Abdomen Skin, External Approach
0H88XZZ Division of Buttock Skin, External Approach
0H89XZZ Division of Perineum Skin, External Approach
0H8AXZZ Division of Genitalia Skin, External Approach
0H8BXZZ Division of Right Upper Arm Skin, External Approach
0H8CXZZ Division of Left Upper Arm Skin, External Approach
0H8DXZZ Division of Right Lower Arm Skin, External Approach
0H8EXZZ Division of Left Lower Arm Skin, External Approach
0H8FXZZ Division of Right Hand Skin, External Approach
0H8GXZZ Division of Left Hand Skin, External Approach
0H8HXZZ Division of Right Upper Leg Skin, External Approach
0H8JXZZ Division of Left Upper Leg Skin, Extern Approach
0H8KXZZ Division of Right Lower Leg Skin, External Approach
0H8LXZZ Division of Left Lower Leg Skin, External Approach
0H8MXZZ Division of Right Foot Skin, External Approach
0H8NXZZ Division of Left Foot Skin, External Approach

9 – Skin and Breast, Drainage

view Coding Guidelines B3.4a and B3.4b

view Coding Guideline B6.2

0X0Z Drainage of Scalp Skin with Drainage Device, External Approach
90XZX Drainage of Scalp Skin, External Approach, Diagnostic
90XZZ Drainage of Scalp Skin, External Approach
91X0Z Drainage of Face Skin with Drainage Device, External Approach
91XZX Drainage of Face Skin, External Approach, Diagnostic
91XZZ Drainage of Face Skin, External Approach
92X0Z Drainage of Right Ear Skin with Drainage Device, External Approach
92XZX Drainage of Right Ear Skin, External Approach, Diagnostic
92XZZ Drainage of Right Ear Skin, External Approach
93X0Z Drainage of Left Ear Skin with Drainage Device, External Approach
93XZX Drainage of Left Ear Skin, External Approach, Diagnostic
93XZZ Drainage of Left Ear Skin, External Approach
94X0Z Drainage of Neck Skin with Drainage Device, External Approach
94XZX Drainage of Neck Skin, External Approach, Diagnostic
94XZZ Drainage of Neck Skin, External Approach
95X0Z Drainage of Chest Skin with Drainage Device, External Approach
95XZX Drainage of Chest Skin, External Approach, Diagnostic
95XZZ Drainage of Chest Skin, External Approach
96X0Z Drainage of Back Skin with Drainage Device, External Approach
96XZX Drainage of Back Skin, External Approach, Diagnostic
96XZZ Drainage of Back Skin, External Approach
97X0Z Drainage of Abdomen Skin with Drainage Device, External Approach
97XZX Drainage of Abdomen Skin, External Approach, Diagnostic
97XZZ Drainage of Abdomen Skin, External Approach
H98X0Z Drainage of Buttock Skin with Drainage Device, External Approach
H98XZX Drainage of Buttock Skin, External Approach, Diagnostic
H98XZZ Drainage of Buttock Skin, External Approach
H99X0Z Drainage of Perineum Skin with Drainage Device, External Approach
H99XZX Drainage of Perineum Skin, External Approach, Diagnostic
H99XZZ Drainage of Perineum Skin, External Approach
H9AX0Z Drainage of Genitalia Skin with Drainage Device, External Approach
H9AXZX Drainage of Genitalia Skin, External Approach, Diagnostic
H9AXZZ Drainage of Genitalia Skin, External Approach
H9BX0Z Drainage of Right Upper Arm Skin with Drainage Device, External Approach
H9BXZX Drainage of Right Upper Arm Skin, External Approach, Diagnostic
H9BXZZ Drainage of Right Upper Arm Skin, External Approach
0H9CX0Z Drainage of Left Upper Arm Skin with Drainage Device, External Approach
0H9CXZX Drainage of Left Upper Arm Skin, External Approach, Diagnostic
0H9CXZZ Drainage of Left Upper Arm Skin, External Approach
0H9DX0Z Drainage of Right Lower Arm Skin with Drainage Device, External Approach
0H9DXZX Drainage of Right Lower Arm Skin, External Approach, Diagnostic
0H9DXZZ Drainage of Right Lower Arm Skin, External Approach
0H9EX0Z Drainage of Left Lower Arm Skin with Drainage Device, External Approach
0H9EXZX Drainage of Left Lower Arm Skin, External Approach, Diagnostic
0H9EXZZ Drainage of Left Lower Arm Skin, External Approach
0H9FX0Z Drainage of Right Hand Skin with Drainage Device, External Approach
0H9FXZX Drainage of Right Hand Skin, External Approach, Diagnostic
0H9FXZZ Drainage of Right Hand Skin, External Approach
0H9GX0Z Drainage of Left Hand Skin with Drainage Device, External Approach
0H9GXZX Drainage of Left Hand Skin, External Approach, Diagnostic
0H9GXZZ Drainage of Left Hand Skin, External Approach
0H9HX0Z Drainage of Right Upper Leg Skin with Drainage Device, External Approach
0H9HXZX Drainage of Right Upper Leg Skin, External Approach, Diagnostic
0H9HXZZ Drainage of Right Upper Leg Skin, External Approach
0H9JX0Z Drainage of Left Upper Leg Skin with Drainage Device, External Approach
0H9JXZX Drainage of Left Upper Leg Skin, External Approach, Diagnostic
0H9JXZZ Drainage of Left Upper Leg Skin, External Approach
0H9KX0Z Drainage of Right Lower Leg Skin with Drainage Device, External Approach
0H9KXZX Drainage of Right Lower Leg Skin, External Approach, Diagnostic
0H9KXZZ Drainage of Right Lower Leg Skin, External Approach
0H9LX0Z Drainage of Left Lower Leg Skin with Drainage Device, External Approach
0H9LXZX Drainage of Left Lower Leg Skin, External Approach, Diagnostic
0H9LXZZ Drainage of Left Lower Leg Skin, External Approach
0H9MX0Z Drainage of Right Foot Skin with Drainage Device, External Approach
0H9MXZX Drainage of Right Foot Skin, External Approach, Diagnostic
0H9MXZZ Drainage of Right Foot Skin, External Approach
0H9NX0Z Drainage of Left Foot Skin with Drainage Device, External Approach
0H9NXZX Drainage of Left Foot Skin, External Approach, Diagnostic
0H9NXZZ Drainage of Left Foot Skin, External Approach
0H9QX0Z Drainage of Finger Nail with Drainage Device, External Approach
0H9QXZX Drainage of Finger Nail, External Approach, Diagnostic
0H9QXZZ Drainage of Finger Nail, External Approach
0H9RX0Z Drainage of Toe Nail with Drainage Device, External Approach
0H9RXZX Drainage of Toe Nail, External Approach, Diagnostic
0H9RXZZ Drainage of Toe Nail, External Approach
0H9T00Z Drainage of Right Breast with Drainage Device, Open Approach
0H9T0ZX Drainage of Right Breast, Open Approach, Diagnostic
0H9T0ZZ Drainage of Right Breast, Open Approach
0H9T30Z Drainage of Right Breast with Drainage Device, Percutaneous Approach
0H9T3ZX Drainage of Right Breast, Percutaneous Approach, Diagnostic
0H9T3ZZ Drainage of Right Breast, Percutaneous Approach
0H9T70Z Drainage of Right Breast with Drainage Device, Via Natural or Artificial Opening
0H9T7ZX Drainage of Right Breast, Via Natural or Artificial Opening, Diagnostic
0H9T7ZZ Drainage of Right Breast, Via Natural or Artificial Opening
0H9T80Z Drainage of Right Breast with Drainage Device, Via Natural or Artificial Opening Endoscopic
0H9T8ZX Drainage of Right Breast, Via Natural or Artificial Opening Endoscopic, Diagnostic
0H9T8ZZ Drainage of Right Breast, Via Natural or Artificial Opening Endoscopic
0H9TX0Z Drainage of Right Breast with Drainage Device, External Approach
0H9TXZX Drainage of Right Breast, External Approach, Diagnostic
0H9TXZZ Drainage of Right Breast, External Approach
0H9U00Z Drainage of Left Breast with Drainage Device, Open Approach
0H9U0ZX Drainage of Left Breast, Open Approach, Diagnostic
0H9U0ZZ Drainage of Left Breast, Open Approach
0H9U30Z Drainage of Left Breast with Drainage Device, Percutaneous Approach
0H9U3ZX Drainage of Left Breast, Percutaneous Approach, Diagnostic
0H9U3ZZ Drainage of Left Breast, Percutaneous Approach
0H9U70Z Drainage of Left Breast with Drainage Device, Via Natural or Artificial Opening
0H9U7ZX Drainage of Left Breast, Via Natural or Artificial Opening, Diagnostic
0H9U7ZZ Drainage of Left Breast, Via Natural or Artificial Opening
0H9U80Z Drainage of Left Breast with Drainage Device, Via Natural or Artificial Opening Endoscopic
0H9U8ZX Drainage of Left Breast, Via Natural or Artificial Opening Endoscopic, Diagnostic
0H9U8ZZ Drainage of Left Breast, Via Natural or Artificial Opening Endoscopic
0H9UX0Z Drainage of Left Breast with Drainage Device, External Approach
0H9UXZX Drainage of Left Breast, External Approach, Diagnostic
0H9UXZZ Drainage of Left Breast, External Approach
0H9V00Z Drainage of Bilateral Breast with Drainage Device, Open Approach
0H9V0ZX Drainage of Bilateral Breast, Open Approach, Diagnostic

0H9V0ZZ Drainage of Bilateral Breast, Open Approach
0H9V30Z Drainage of Bilateral Breast with Drainage Device, Percutaneous Approach
0H9V3ZX Drainage of Bilateral Breast, Percutaneous Approach, Diagnostic
0H9V3ZZ Drainage of Bilateral Breast, Percutaneous Approach
0H9V70Z Drainage of Bilateral Breast with Drainage Device, Via Natural or Artificial Opening
0H9V7ZX Drainage of Bilateral Breast, Via Natural or Artificial Opening, Diagnostic
0H9V7ZZ Drainage of Bilateral Breast, Via Natural or Artificial Opening
0H9V80Z Drainage of Bilateral Breast with Drainage Device, Via Natural or Artificial Opening Endoscopic
0H9V8ZX Drainage of Bilateral Breast, Via Natural or Artificial Opening Endoscopic, Diagnostic
0H9V8ZZ Drainage of Bilateral Breast, Via Natural or Artificial Opening Endoscopic
0H9VX0Z Drainage of Bilateral Breast with Drainage Device, External Approach
0H9VXZX Drainage of Bilateral Breast, External Approach, Diagnostic
0H9VXZZ Drainage of Bilateral Breast, External Approach
0H9W00Z Drainage of Right Nipple with Drainage Device, Open Approach
0H9W0ZX Drainage of Right Nipple, Open Approach, Diagnostic
0H9W0ZZ Drainage of Right Nipple, Open Approach
0H9W30Z Drainage of Right Nipple with Drainage Device, Percutaneous Approach
0H9W3ZX Drainage of Right Nipple, Percutaneous Approach, Diagnostic
0H9W3ZZ Drainage of Right Nipple, Percutaneous Approach
0H9W70Z Drainage of Right Nipple with Drainage Device, Via Natural or Artificial Opening
0H9W7ZX Drainage of Right Nipple, Via Natural or Artificial Opening, Diagnostic
0H9W7ZZ Drainage of Right Nipple, Via Natural or Artificial Opening
0H9W80Z Drainage of Right Nipple with Drainage Device, Via Natural or Artificial Opening Endoscopic
0H9W8ZX Drainage of Right Nipple, Via Natural or Artificial Opening Endoscopic, Diagnostic
0H9W8ZZ Drainage of Right Nipple, Via Natural or Artificial Opening Endoscopic
0H9WX0Z Drainage of Right Nipple with Drainage Device, External Approach
0H9WXZX Drainage of Right Nipple, External Approach, Diagnostic
0H9WXZZ Drainage of Right Nipple, External Approach
0H9X00Z Drainage of Left Nipple with Drainage Device, Open Approach
0H9X0ZX Drainage of Left Nipple, Open Approach, Diagnostic
0H9X0ZZ Drainage of Left Nipple, Open Approach
0H9X30Z Drainage of Left Nipple with Drainage Device, Percutaneous Approach
0H9X3ZX Drainage of Left Nipple, Percutaneous Approach, Diagnostic
0H9X3ZZ Drainage of Left Nipple, Percutaneous Approach
0H9X70Z Drainage of Left Nipple with Drainage Device, Via Natural or Artificial Opening
0H9X7ZX Drainage of Left Nipple, Via Natural or Artificial Opening, Diagnostic
0H9X7ZZ Drainage of Left Nipple, Via Natural or Artificial Opening
0H9X80Z Drainage of Left Nipple with Drainage Device, Via Natural or Artificial Opening Endoscopic
0H9X8ZX Drainage of Left Nipple, Via Natural or Artificial Opening Endoscopic, Diagnostic
0H9X8ZZ Drainage of Left Nipple, Via Natural or Artificial Opening Endoscopic
0H9XX0Z Drainage of Left Nipple with Drainage Device, External Approach
0H9XXZX Drainage of Left Nipple, External Approach, Diagnostic
0H9XXZZ Drainage of Left Nipple, External Approach

0HB – Skin and Breast, Excision

Review Coding Guidelines 3B.4a and 3B.4b

Review Coding Guideline B3.5

Review Coding Guideline B3.8

0HB0XZX Excision of Scalp Skin, External Approach, Diagnostic
0HB0XZZ Excision of Scalp Skin, External Approach
0HB1XZX Excision of Face Skin, External Approach, Diagnostic
0HB1XZZ Excision of Face Skin, External Approach
0HB2XZX Excision of Right Ear Skin, External Approach, Diagnostic
0HB2XZZ Excision of Right Ear Skin, External Approach
0HB3XZX Excision of Left Ear Skin, External Approach, Diagnostic
0HB3XZZ Excision of Left Ear Skin, External Approach
0HB4XZX Excision of Neck Skin, External Approach, Diagnostic
0HB4XZZ Excision of Neck Skin, External Approach
0HB5XZX Excision of Chest Skin, External Approach, Diagnostic
0HB5XZZ Excision of Chest Skin, External Approach
0HB6XZX Excision of Back Skin, External Approach, Diagnostic
0HB6XZZ Excision of Back Skin, External Approach
0HB7XZX Excision of Abdomen Skin, External Approach, Diagnostic
0HB7XZZ Excision of Abdomen Skin, External Approach
0HB8XZX Excision of Buttock Skin, External Approach, Diagnostic
0HB8XZZ Excision of Buttock Skin, External Approach
0HB9XZX Excision of Perineum Skin, External Approach, Diagnostic
● **0HB9XZZ** Excision of Perineum Skin, External Approach
0HBAXZX Excision of Genitalia Skin, External Approach, Diagnostic
0HBAXZZ Excision of Genitalia Skin, External Approach
0HBBXZX Excision of Right Upper Arm Skin, External Approach, Diagnostic
0HBBXZZ Excision of Right Upper Arm Skin, External Approach
0HBCXZX Excision of Left Upper Arm Skin, External Approach, Diagnostic
0HBCXZZ Excision of Left Upper Arm Skin, External Approach
0HBDXZX Excision of Right Lower Arm Skin, External Approach, Diagnostic
0HBDXZZ Excision of Right Lower Arm Skin, External Approach
0HBEXZX Excision of Left Lower Arm Skin, External Approach, Diagnostic
0HBEXZZ Excision of Left Lower Arm Skin, External Approach
0HBFXZX Excision of Right Hand Skin, External Approach, Diagnostic
0HBFXZZ Excision of Right Hand Skin, External Approach
0HBGXZX Excision of Left Hand Skin, External Approach, Diagnostic
0HBGXZZ Excision of Left Hand Skin, External Approach
0HBHXZX Excision of Right Upper Leg Skin, External Approach, Diagnostic
0HBHXZZ Excision of Right Upper Leg Skin, External Approach
0HBJXZX Excision of Left Upper Leg Skin, External Approach, Diagnostic
0HBJXZZ Excision of Left Upper Leg Skin, External Approach
0HBKXZX Excision of Right Lower Leg Skin, External Approach, Diagnostic
0HBKXZZ Excision of Right Lower Leg Skin, External Approach
0HBLXZX Excision of Left Lower Leg Skin, External Approach, Diagnostic
0HBLXZZ Excision of Left Lower Leg Skin, External Approach
0HBMXZX Excision of Right Foot Skin, External Approach, Diagnostic
0HBMXZZ Excision of Right Foot Skin, External Approach
0HBNXZX Excision of Left Foot Skin, External Approach, Diagnostic
0HBNXZZ Excision of Left Foot Skin, External Approach
0HBQXZX Excision of Finger Nail, External Approach, Diagnostic
0HBQXZZ Excision of Finger Nail, External Approach
0HBRXZX Excision of Toe Nail, External Approach, Diagnostic
0HBRXZZ Excision of Toe Nail, External Approach
0HBT0ZX Excision of Right Breast, Open Approach, Diagnostic
0HBT0ZZ Excision of Right Breast, Open Approach
0HBT3ZX Excision of Right Breast, Percutaneous Approach, Diagnostic
0HBT3ZZ Excision of Right Breast, Percutaneous Approach
0HBT7ZX Excision of Right Breast, Via Natural or Artificial Opening, Diagnostic
0HBT7ZZ Excision of Right Breast, Via Natural or Artificial Opening
0HBT8ZX Excision of Right Breast, Via Natural or Artificial Opening Endoscopic, Diagnostic

3T8ZZ Excision of Right Breast, Via Natural or Artificial Opening Endoscopic
3TXZX Excision of Right Breast, External Approach, Diagnostic
3TXZZ Excision of Right Breast, External Approach
3U0ZX Excision of Left Breast, Open Approach, Diagnostic
BU0ZZ Excision of Left Breast, Open Approach
BU3ZX Excision of Left Breast, Percutaneous Approach, Diagnostic
BU3ZZ Excision of Left Breast, Percutaneous Approach
BU7ZX Excision of Left Breast, Via Natural or Artificial Opening, Diagnostic
BU7ZZ Excision of Left Breast, Via Natural or Artificial Opening
BU8ZX Excision of Left Breast, Via Natural or Artificial Opening Endoscopic, Diagnostic
BU8ZZ Excision of Left Breast, Via Natural or Artificial Opening Endoscopic
BUXZX Excision of Left Breast, External Approach, Diagnostic
BUXZZ Excision of Left Breast, External Approach
IBV0ZX Excision of Bilateral Breast, Open Approach, Diagnostic
IBV0ZZ Excision of Bilateral Breast, Open Approach
IBV3ZX Excision of Bilateral Breast, Percutaneous Approach, Diagnostic
IBV3ZZ Excision of Bilateral Breast, Percutaneous Approach
IBV7ZX Excision of Bilateral Breast, Via Natural or Artificial Opening, Diagnostic
0HBV7ZZ Excision of Bilateral Breast, Via Natural or Artificial Opening
0HBV8ZX Excision of Bilateral Breast, Via Natural or Artificial Opening Endoscopic, Diagnostic
0HBV8ZZ Excision of Bilateral Breast, Via Natural or Artificial Opening Endoscopic
0HBVXZX Excision of Bilateral Breast, External Approach, Diagnostic
0HBVXZZ Excision of Bilateral Breast, External Approach
0HBW0ZX Excision of Right Nipple, Open Approach, Diagnostic
0HBW0ZZ Excision of Right Nipple, Open Approach
0HBW3ZX Excision of Right Nipple, Percutaneous Approach, Diagnostic
0HBW3ZZ Excision of Right Nipple, Percutaneous Approach
0HBW7ZX Excision of Right Nipple, Via Natural or Artificial Opening, Diagnostic
0HBW7ZZ Excision of Right Nipple, Via Natural or Artificial Opening
0HBW8ZX Excision of Right Nipple, Via Natural or Artificial Opening Endoscopic, Diagnostic
0HBW8ZZ Excision of Right Nipple, Via Natural or Artificial Opening Endoscopic
0HBWXZX Excision of Right Nipple, External Approach, Diagnostic
0HBWXZZ Excision of Right Nipple, External Approach
0HBX0ZX Excision of Left Nipple, Open Approach, Diagnostic
0HBX0ZZ Excision of Left Nipple, Open Approach
0HBX3ZX Excision of Left Nipple, Percutaneous Approach, Diagnostic
0HBX3ZZ Excision of Left Nipple, Percutaneous Approach
0HBX7ZX Excision of Left Nipple, Via Natural or Artificial Opening, Diagnostic
0HBX7ZZ Excision of Left Nipple, Via Natural or Artificial Opening
0HBX8ZX Excision of Left Nipple, Via Natural or Artificial Opening Endoscopic, Diagnostic
0HBX8ZZ Excision of Left Nipple, Via Natural or Artificial Opening Endoscopic
0HBXXZX Excision of Left Nipple, External Approach, Diagnostic
0HBXXZZ Excision of Left Nipple, External Approach
0HBY0ZX Excision of Supernumerary Breast, Open Approach, Diagnostic
0HBY0ZZ Excision of Supernumerary Breast, Open Approach
0HBY3ZX Excision of Supernumerary Breast, Percutaneous Approach, Diagnostic
0HBY3ZZ Excision of Supernumerary Breast, Percutaneous Approach
0HBY7ZX Excision of Supernumerary Breast, Via Natural or Artificial Opening, Diagnostic
0HBY7ZZ Excision of Supernumerary Breast, Via Natural or Artificial Opening
0HBY8ZX Excision of Supernumerary Breast, Via Natural or Artificial Opening Endoscopic, Diagnostic
0HBY8ZZ Excision of Supernumerary Breast, Via Natural or Artificial Opening Endoscopic
0HBYXZX Excision of Supernumerary Breast, External Approach, Diagnostic
0HBYXZZ Excision of Supernumerary Breast, External Approach

HC – Skin and Breast, Extirpation

IC0XZZ Extirpation of Matter from Scalp Skin, External Approach
IC1XZZ Extirpation of Matter from Face Skin, External Approach
IC2XZZ Extirpation of Matter from Right Ear Skin, External Approach
IC3XZZ Extirpation of Matter from Left Ear Skin, External Approach
IC4XZZ Extirpation of Matter from Neck Skin, External Approach
IC5XZZ Extirpation of Matter from Chest Skin, External Approach
HC6XZZ Extirpation of Matter from Back Skin, External Approach
HC7XZZ Extirpation of Matter from Abdomen Skin, External Approach
HC8XZZ Extirpation of Matter from Buttock Skin, External Approach
HC9XZZ Extirpation of Matter from Perineum Skin, External Approach
HCAXZZ Extirpation of Matter from Genitalia Skin, External Approach
HCBXZZ Extirpation of Matter from Right Upper Arm Skin, External Approach
HCCXZZ Extirpation of Matter from Left Upper Arm Skin, External Approach
HCDXZZ Extirpation of Matter from Right Lower Arm Skin, External Approach
HCEXZZ Extirpation of Matter from Left Lower Arm Skin, External Approach
HCFXZZ Extirpation of Matter from Right Hand Skin, External Approach
HCGXZZ Extirpation of Matter from Left Hand Skin, External Approach
HCHXZZ Extirpation of Matter from Right Upper Leg Skin, External Approach
0HCJXZZ Extirpation of Matter from Left Upper Leg Skin, External Approach
0HCKXZZ Extirpation of Matter from Right Lower Leg Skin, External Approach
0HCLXZZ Extirpation of Matter from Left Lower Leg Skin, External Approach
0HCMXZZ Extirpation of Matter from Right Foot Skin, External Approach
0HCNXZZ Extirpation of Matter from Left Foot Skin, External Approach
0HCQXZZ Extirpation of Matter from Finger Nail, External Approach
0HCRXZZ Extirpation of Matter from Toe Nail, External Approach
0HCT0ZZ Extirpation of Matter from Right Breast, Open Approach
0HCT3ZZ Extirpation of Matter from Right Breast, Percutaneous Approach
0HCT7ZZ Extirpation of Matter from Right Breast, Via Natural or Artificial Opening
0HCT8ZZ Extirpation of Matter from Right Breast, Via Natural or Artificial Opening Endoscopic
0HCTXZZ Extirpation of Matter from Right Breast, External Approach
0HCU0ZZ Extirpation of Matter from Left Breast, Open Approach
0HCU3ZZ Extirpation of Matter from Left Breast, Percutaneous Approach
0HCU7ZZ Extirpation of Matter from Left Breast, Via Natural or Artificial Opening
0HCU8ZZ Extirpation of Matter from Left Breast, Via Natural or Artificial Opening Endoscopic
0HCUXZZ Extirpation of Matter from Left Breast, External Approach
0HCV0ZZ Extirpation of Matter from Bilateral Breast, Open Approach
0HCV3ZZ Extirpation of Matter from Bilateral Breast, Percutaneous Approach
0HCV7ZZ Extirpation of Matter from Bilateral Breast, Via Natural or Artificial Opening
0HCV8ZZ Extirpation of Matter from Bilateral Breast, Via Natural or Artificial Opening Endoscopic
0HCVXZZ Extirpation of Matter from Bilateral Breast, External Approach
0HCW0ZZ Extirpation of Matter from Right Nipple, Open Approach
0HCW3ZZ Extirpation of Matter from Right Nipple, Percutaneous Approach
0HCW7ZZ Extirpation of Matter from Right Nipple, Via Natural or Artificial Opening
0HCW8ZZ Extirpation of Matter from Right Nipple, Via Natural or Artificial Opening Endoscopic
0HCWXZZ Extirpation of Matter from Right Nipple, External Approach
0HCX0ZZ Extirpation of Matter from Left Nipple, Open Approach
0HCX3ZZ Extirpation of Matter from Left Nipple, Percutaneous Approach
0HCX7ZZ Extirpation of Matter from Left Nipple, Via Natural or Artificial Opening
0HCX8ZZ Extirpation of Matter from Left Nipple, Via Natural or Artificial Opening Endoscopic
0HCXXZZ Extirpation of Matter from Left Nipple, External Approach

0HD – Skin and Breast, Extraction

0HD0XZZ Extraction of Scalp Skin, External Approach
0HD1XZZ Extraction of Face Skin, External Approach
0HD2XZZ Extraction of Right Ear Skin, External Approach
0HD3XZZ Extraction of Left Ear Skin, External Approach
0HD4XZZ Extraction of Neck Skin, External Approach
0HD5XZZ Extraction of Chest Skin, External Approach
0HD6XZZ Extraction of Back Skin, External Approach
0HD7XZZ Extraction of Abdomen Skin, External Approach
0HD8XZZ Extraction of Buttock Skin, External Approach
0HD9XZZ Extraction of Perineum Skin, External Approach
0HDAXZZ Extraction of Genitalia Skin, External Approach
0HDBXZZ Extraction of Right Upper Arm Skin, External Approach
0HDCXZZ Extraction of Left Upper Arm Skin, External Approach
0HDDXZZ Extraction of Right Lower Arm Skin, External Approach
0HDEXZZ Extraction of Left Lower Arm Skin, External Approach
0HDFXZZ Extraction of Right Hand Skin, External Approach
0HDGXZZ Extraction of Left Hand Skin, External Approach
0HDHXZZ Extraction of Right Upper Leg Skin, External Approach
0HDJXZZ Extraction of Left Upper Leg Skin, External Approach
0HDKXZZ Extraction of Right Lower Leg Skin, External Approach
0HDLXZZ Extraction of Left Lower Leg Skin, External Approach
0HDMXZZ Extraction of Right Foot Skin, External Approach
0HDNXZZ Extraction of Left Foot Skin, External Approach
0HDQXZZ Extraction of Finger Nail, External Approach
0HDRXZZ Extraction of Toe Nail, External Approach
0HDSXZZ Extraction of Hair, External Approach

0HH – Skin and Breast, Insertion

0HHT01Z Insertion of Radioactive Element into Right Breast, Open Approach
0HHT0NZ Insertion of Tissue Expander into Right Breast, Open Approach
0HHT31Z Insertion of Radioactive Element into Right Breast, Percutaneous Approach
0HHT3NZ Insertion of Tissue Expander into Right Breast, Percutaneous Approach
0HHT71Z Insertion of Radioactive Element into Right Breast, Via Natural or Artificial Opening
0HHT7NZ Insertion of Tissue Expander into Right Breast, Via Natural or Artificial Opening
0HHT81Z Insertion of Radioactive Element into Right Breast, Via Natural or Artificial Opening Endoscopic
0HHT8NZ Insertion of Tissue Expander into Right Breast, Via Natural or Artificial Opening Endoscopic
0HHTX1Z Insertion of Radioactive Element into Right Breast, External Approach
0HHU01Z Insertion of Radioactive Element into Left Breast, Open Approach
0HHU0NZ Insertion of Tissue Expander into Left Breast, Open Approach
AHA CC: 4Q, 2013, 107
0HHU31Z Insertion of Radioactive Element into Left Breast, Percutaneous Approach
0HHU3NZ Insertion of Tissue Expander into Left Breast, Percutaneous Approach
0HHU71Z Insertion of Radioactive Element into Left Breast, Via Natural or Artificial Opening
0HHU7NZ Insertion of Tissue Expander into Left Breast, Via Natural or Artificial Opening
0HHU81Z Insertion of Radioactive Element into Left Breast, Via Natural or Artificial Opening Endoscopic
0HHU8NZ Insertion of Tissue Expander into Left Breast, Via Natural or Artificial Opening Endoscopic
0HHUX1Z Insertion of Radioactive Element into Left Breast, External Approach
0HHV01Z Insertion of Radioactive Element into Bilateral Breast, Open Approach
0HHV0NZ Insertion of Tissue Expander into Bilateral Breast, Open Approach
0HHV31Z Insertion of Radioactive Element into Bilateral Breast, Percutaneous Approach
0HHV3NZ Insertion of Tissue Expander into Bilateral Breast, Percutaneous Approach
0HHV71Z Insertion of Radioactive Element into Bilateral Breast, Via Natural or Artificial Opening
0HHV7NZ Insertion of Tissue Expander into Bilateral Breast, Via Natural or Artificial Opening
0HHV81Z Insertion of Radioactive Element into Bilateral Breast, Via Natural or Artificial Opening Endoscopic
0HHV8NZ Insertion of Tissue Expander into Bilateral Breast, Via Natural or Artificial Opening Endoscopic
0HHVX1Z Insertion of Radioactive Element into Bilateral Breast, External Approach
0HHW01Z Insertion of Radioactive Element into Right Nipple, Open Approach
0HHW0NZ Insertion of Tissue Expander into Right Nipple, Open Approach
0HHW31Z Insertion of Radioactive Element into Right Nipple, Percutaneous Approach
0HHW3NZ Insertion of Tissue Expander into Right Nipple, Percutaneous Approach
0HHW71Z Insertion of Radioactive Element into Right Nipple, Via Natural or Artificial Opening
0HHW7NZ Insertion of Tissue Expander into Right Nipple, Via Natural or Artificial Opening
0HHW81Z Insertion of Radioactive Element into Right Nipple, Via Natural or Artificial Opening Endoscopic
0HHW8NZ Insertion of Tissue Expander into Right Nipple, Via Natural or Artificial Opening Endoscopic
0HHWX1Z Insertion of Radioactive Element into Right Nipple, External Approach
0HHX01Z Insertion of Radioactive Element into Left Nipple, Open Approach
0HHX0NZ Insertion of Tissue Expander into Left Nipple, Open Approach
0HHX31Z Insertion of Radioactive Element into Left Nipple, Percutaneous Approach
0HHX3NZ Insertion of Tissue Expander into Left Nipple, Percutaneous Approach
0HHX71Z Insertion of Radioactive Element into Left Nipple, Via Natural or Artificial Opening
0HHX7NZ Insertion of Tissue Expander into Left Nipple, Via Natural or Artificial Opening
0HHX81Z Insertion of Radioactive Element into Left Nipple, Via Natural or Artificial Opening Endoscopic
0HHX8NZ Insertion of Tissue Expander into Left Nipple, Via Natural or Artificial Opening Endoscopic
0HHXX1Z Insertion of Radioactive Element into Left Nipple, External Approach

0HJ – Skin and Breast, Inspection

Review Coding Guideline B3.5

Review Coding Guidelines B3.11a, B3.11b and B3.11c

0HJPXZZ Inspection of Skin, External Approach
0HJQXZZ Inspection of Finger Nail, External Approach
0HJRXZZ Inspection of Toe Nail, External Approach
0HJT0ZZ Inspection of Right Breast, Open Approach
0HJT3ZZ Inspection of Right Breast, Percutaneous Approach
0HJT7ZZ Inspection of Right Breast, Via Natural or Artificial Opening
0HJT8ZZ Inspection of Right Breast, Via Natural or Artificial Opening Endoscopic
0HJTXZZ Inspection of Right Breast, External Approach
0HJU0ZZ Inspection of Left Breast, Open Approach
0HJU3ZZ Inspection of Left Breast, Percutaneous Approach
0HJU7ZZ Inspection of Left Breast, Via Natural or Artificial Opening
0HJU8ZZ Inspection of Left Breast, Via Natural or Artificial Opening Endoscopic
0HJUXZZ Inspection of Left Breast, External Approach

M – Skin and Breast, Reattachment

10XZZ	Reattachment of Scalp Skin, External Approach
11XZZ	Reattachment of Face Skin, External Approach
12XZZ	Reattachment of Right Ear Skin, External Approach
13XZZ	Reattachment of Left Ear Skin, External Approach
14XZZ	Reattachment of Neck Skin, External Approach
15XZZ	Reattachment of Chest Skin, External Approach
16XZZ	Reattachment of Back Skin, External Approach
17XZZ	Reattachment of Abdomen Skin, External Approach
18XZZ	Reattachment of Buttock Skin, External Approach
19XZZ	Reattachment of Perineum Skin, External Approach
0HMAXZZ	Reattachment of Genitalia Skin, External Approach
0HMBXZZ	Reattachment of Right Upper Arm Skin, External Approach
0HMCXZZ	Reattachment of Left Upper Arm Skin, External Approach
0HMDXZZ	Reattachment of Right Lower Arm Skin, External Approach
0HMEXZZ	Reattachment of Left Lower Arm Skin, External Approach
0HMFXZZ	Reattachment of Right Hand Skin, External Approach
0HMGXZZ	Reattachment of Left Hand Skin, External Approach
0HMHXZZ	Reattachment of Right Upper Leg Skin, External Approach
0HMJXZZ	Reattachment of Left Upper Leg Skin, External Approach
0HMKXZZ	Reattachment of Right Lower Leg Skin, External Approach
0HMLXZZ	Reattachment of Left Lower Leg Skin, External Approach
0HMMXZZ	Reattachment of Right Foot Skin, External Approach
0HMNXZZ	Reattachment of Left Foot Skin, External Approach
0HMTXZZ	Reattachment of Right Breast, External Approach
0HMUXZZ	Reattachment of Left Breast, External Approach
0HMVXZZ	Reattachment of Bilateral Breast, External Approach
0HMWXZZ	Reattachment of Right Nipple, External Approach
0HMXXZZ	Reattachment of Left Nipple, External Approach

N – Skin and Breast, Release

view Coding Guideline B3.13

view Coding Guideline B3.14

N0XZZ	Release Scalp Skin, External Approach
N1XZZ	Release Face Skin, External Approach
N2XZZ	Release Right Ear Skin, External Approach
N3XZZ	Release Left Ear Skin, External Approach
N4XZZ	Release Neck Skin, External Approach
N5XZZ	Release Chest Skin, External Approach
N6XZZ	Release Back Skin, External Approach
N7XZZ	Release Abdomen Skin, External Approach
N8XZZ	Release Buttock Skin, External Approach
N9XZZ	Release Perineum Skin, External Approach
NAXZZ	Release Genitalia Skin, External Approach
NBXZZ	Release Right Upper Arm Skin, External Approach
NCXZZ	Release Left Upper Arm Skin, External Approach
NDXZZ	Release Right Lower Arm Skin, External Approach
NEXZZ	Release Left Lower Arm Skin, External Approach
NFXZZ	Release Right Hand Skin, External Approach
NGXZZ	Release Left Hand Skin, External Approach
0HNHXZZ	Release Right Upper Leg Skin, External Approach
0HNJXZZ	Release Left Upper Leg Skin, External Approach
0HNKXZZ	Release Right Lower Leg Skin, External Approach
0HNLXZZ	Release Left Lower Leg Skin, External Approach
0HNMXZZ	Release Right Foot Skin, External Approach
0HNNXZZ	Release Left Foot Skin, External Approach
0HNQXZZ	Release Finger Nail, External Approach
0HNRXZZ	Release Toe Nail, External Approach
0HNT0ZZ	Release Right Breast, Open Approach
0HNT3ZZ	Release Right Breast, Percutaneous Approach
0HNT7ZZ	Release Right Breast, Via Natural or Artificial Opening
0HNT8ZZ	Release Right Breast, Via Natural or Artificial Opening Endoscopic
0HNTXZZ	Release Right Breast, External Approach
0HNU0ZZ	Release Left Breast, Open Approach
0HNU3ZZ	Release Left Breast, Percutaneous Approach
0HNU7ZZ	Release Left Breast, Via Natural or Artificial Opening
0HNU8ZZ	Release Left Breast, Via Natural or Artificial Opening Endoscopic
0HNUXZZ	Release Left Breast, External Approach
0HNV0ZZ	Release Bilateral Breast, Open Approach
0HNV3ZZ	Release Bilateral Breast, Percutaneous Approach
0HNV7ZZ	Release Bilateral Breast, Via Natural or Artificial Opening
0HNV8ZZ	Release Bilateral Breast, Via Natural or Artificial Opening Endoscopic
0HNVXZZ	Release Bilateral Breast, External Approach
0HNW0ZZ	Release Right Nipple, Open Approach
0HNW3ZZ	Release Right Nipple, Percutaneous Approach
0HNW7ZZ	Release Right Nipple, Via Natural or Artificial Opening
0HNW8ZZ	Release Right Nipple, Via Natural or Artificial Opening Endoscopic
0HNWXZZ	Release Right Nipple, External Approach
0HNX0ZZ	Release Left Nipple, Open Approach
0HNX3ZZ	Release Left Nipple, Percutaneous Approach
0HNX7ZZ	Release Left Nipple, Via Natural or Artificial Opening
0HNX8ZZ	Release Left Nipple, Via Natural or Artificial Opening Endoscopic
0HNXXZZ	Release Left Nipple, External Approach

HP – Skin and Breast, Removal

eview Coding Guideline B6.1c

HPPX0Z	Removal of Drainage Device from Skin, External Approach
HPPX7Z	Removal of Autologous Tissue Substitute from Skin, External Approach
HPPXJZ	Removal of Synthetic Substitute from Skin, External Approach
HPPXKZ	Removal of Nonautologous Tissue Substitute from Skin, External Approach
HPQX0Z	Removal of Drainage Device from Finger Nail, External Approach
HPQX7Z	Removal of Autologous Tissue Substitute from Finger Nail, External Approach
HPQXJZ	Removal of Synthetic Substitute from Finger Nail, External Approach
0HPQXKZ	Removal of Nonautologous Tissue Substitute from Finger Nail, External Approach
0HPRX0Z	Removal of Drainage Device from Toe Nail, External Approach
0HPRX7Z	Removal of Autologous Tissue Substitute from Toe Nail, External Approach
0HPRXJZ	Removal of Synthetic Substitute from Toe Nail, External Approach
0HPRXKZ	Removal of Nonautologous Tissue Substitute from Toe Nail, External Approach
0HPSX7Z	Removal of Autologous Tissue Substitute from Hair, External Approach
0HPSXJZ	Removal of Synthetic Substitute from Hair, External Approach
0HPSXKZ	Removal of Nonautologous Tissue Substitute from Hair, External Approach
0HPT00Z	Removal of Drainage Device from Right Breast, Open Approach
0HPT01Z	Removal of Radioactive Element from Right Breast, Open Approach
0HPT07Z	Removal of Autologous Tissue Substitute from Right Breast, Open Approach
0HPT0JZ	Removal of Synthetic Substitute from Right Breast, Open Approach
0HPT0KZ	Removal of Nonautologous Tissue Substitute from Right Breast, Open Approach

0HPT0NZ Removal of Tissue Expander from Right Breast, Open Approach
0HPT30Z Removal of Drainage Device from Right Breast, Percutaneous Approach
0HPT31Z Removal of Radioactive Element from Right Breast, Percutaneous Approach
0HPT37Z Removal of Autologous Tissue Substitute from Right Breast, Percutaneous Approach
0HPT3JZ Removal of Synthetic Substitute from Right Breast, Percutaneous Approach
0HPT3KZ Removal of Nonautologous Tissue Substitute from Right Breast, Percutaneous Approach
0HPT3NZ Removal of Tissue Expander from Right Breast, Percutaneous Approach
0HPT70Z Removal of Drainage Device from Right Breast, Via Natural or Artificial Opening
0HPT71Z Removal of Radioactive Element from Right Breast, Via Natural or Artificial Opening
0HPT77Z Removal of Autologous Tissue Substitute from Right Breast, Via Natural or Artificial Opening
0HPT7JZ Removal of Synthetic Substitute from Right Breast, Via Natural or Artificial Opening
0HPT7KZ Removal of Nonautologous Tissue Substitute from Right Breast, Via Natural or Artificial Opening
0HPT7NZ Removal of Tissue Expander from Right Breast, Via Natural or Artificial Opening
0HPT80Z Removal of Drainage Device from Right Breast, Via Natural or Artificial Opening Endoscopic
0HPT81Z Removal of Radioactive Element from Right Breast, Via Natural or Artificial Opening Endoscopic
0HPT87Z Removal of Autologous Tissue Substitute from Right Breast, Via Natural or Artificial Opening Endoscopic
0HPT8JZ Removal of Synthetic Substitute from Right Breast, Via Natural or Artificial Opening Endoscopic
0HPT8KZ Removal of Nonautologous Tissue Substitute from Right Breast, Via Natural or Artificial Opening Endoscopic
0HPT8NZ Removal of Tissue Expander from Right Breast, Via Natural or Artificial Opening Endoscopic
0HPTX0Z Removal of Drainage Device from Right Breast, External Approach
0HPTX1Z Removal of Radioactive Element from Right Breast, External Approach
0HPTX7Z Removal of Autologous Tissue Substitute from Right Breast, External Approach
0HPTXJZ Removal of Synthetic Substitute from Right Breast, External Approach
0HPTXKZ Removal of Nonautologous Tissue Substitute from Right Breast, External Approach
0HPU00Z Removal of Drainage Device from Left Breast, Open Approach
0HPU01Z Removal of Radioactive Element from Left Breast, Open Approach
0HPU07Z Removal of Autologous Tissue Substitute from Left Breast, Open Approach
0HPU0JZ Removal of Synthetic Substitute from Left Breast, Open Approach
0HPU0KZ Removal of Nonautologous Tissue Substitute from Left Breast, Open Approach
0HPU0NZ Removal of Tissue Expander from Left Breast, Open Approach
0HPU30Z Removal of Drainage Device from Left Breast, Percutaneous Approach
0HPU31Z Removal of Radioactive Element from Left Breast, Percutaneous Approach
0HPU37Z Removal of Autologous Tissue Substitute from Left Breast, Percutaneous Approach
0HPU3JZ Removal of Synthetic Substitute from Left Breast, Percutaneous Approach
0HPU3KZ Removal of Nonautologous Tissue Substitute from Left Breast, Percutaneous Approach
0HPU3NZ Removal of Tissue Expander from Left Breast, Percutaneous Approach
0HPU70Z Removal of Drainage Device from Left Breast, Via Natural or Artificial Opening
0HPU71Z Removal of Radioactive Element fror Left Breast, Via Natural or Artificial Opening
0HPU77Z Removal of Autologous Tissue Substit from Left Breast, Via Natural or Artifi Opening
0HPU7JZ Removal of Synthetic Substitute from Left Breast, Via Natural or Artificial Opening
0HPU7KZ Removal of Nonautologous Tissue Substitute from Left Breast, Via Natur or Artificial Opening
0HPU7NZ Removal of Tissue Expander from Left Breast, Via Natural or Artificial Opening
0HPU80Z Removal of Drainage Device from Lef Breast, Via Natural or Artificial Openir Endoscopic
0HPU81Z Removal of Radioactive Element from Left Breast, Via Natural or Artificial Opening Endoscopic
0HPU87Z Removal of Autologous Tissue Substitute from Left Breast, Via Natural or Artificia Opening Endoscopic
0HPU8JZ Removal of Synthetic Substitute from Left Breast, Via Natural or Artific Opening Endoscopic
0HPU8KZ Removal of Nonautologous Tissue Substitute from Left Breast, Via Natural Artificial Opening Endoscopic
0HPU8NZ Removal of Tissue Expander from Left Breast, Via Natural or Artificial Openin Endoscopic
0HPUX0Z Removal of Drainage Device from Left Breast, External Approach
0HPUX1Z Removal of Radioactive Element from L Breast, External Approach
0HPUX7Z Removal of Autologous Tissue Substitu from Left Breast, External Approach
0HPUXJZ Removal of Synthetic Substitute from Le Breast, External Approach
0HPUXKZ Removal of Nonautologous Tissue Substitute from Left Breast, External Approach

0HQ – Skin and Breast, Repair

Review Coding Guideline B3.5

0HQ0XZZ Repair Scalp Skin, External Approach
0HQ1XZZ Repair Face Skin, External Approach
0HQ2XZZ Repair Right Ear Skin, External Approach
0HQ3XZZ Repair Left Ear Skin, External Approach
0HQ4XZZ Repair Neck Skin, External Approach
0HQ5XZZ Repair Chest Skin, External Approach
0HQ6XZZ Repair Back Skin, External Approach
0HQ7XZZ Repair Abdomen Skin, External Approach
0HQ8XZZ Repair Buttock Skin, External Approach
● **0HQ9XZZ** Repair Perineum Skin, External Approach
0HQAXZZ Repair Genitalia Skin, External Approach
0HQBXZZ Repair Right Upper Arm Skin, External Approach
0HQCXZZ Repair Left Upper Arm Skin, External Approach
0HQDXZZ Repair Right Lower Arm Skin, External Approach
0HQEXZZ Repair Left Lower Arm Skin, External Approach
0HQFXZZ Repair Right Hand Skin, External Approach
0HQGXZZ Repair Left Hand Skin, External Approach
0HQHXZZ Repair Right Upper Leg Skin, External Approach
0HQJXZZ Repair Left Upper Leg Skin, External Approach
0HQKXZZ Repair Right Lower Leg Skin, External Approach
0HQLXZZ Repair Left Lower Leg Skin, External Approach
0HQMXZZ Repair Right Foot Skin, External Approach
0HQNXZZ Repair Left Foot Skin, External Approach
0HQQXZZ Repair Finger Nail, External Approach
0HQRXZZ Repair Toe Nail, External Approach
0HQT0ZZ Repair Right Breast, Open Approach
0HQT3ZZ Repair Right Breast, Percutaneous Approach
0HQT7ZZ Repair Right Breast, Via Natural or Artificial Opening
0HQT8ZZ Repair Right Breast, Via Natural or Artificial Opening Endoscopic
0HQTXZZ Repair Right Breast, External Approach
0HQU0ZZ Repair Left Breast, Open Approach
0HQU3ZZ Repair Left Breast, Percutaneous Approach
0HQU7ZZ Repair Left Breast, Via Natural or Artificial Opening
0HQU8ZZ Repair Left Breast, Via Natural or Artificial Opening Endoscopic
0HQUXZZ Repair Left Breast, External Approach
0HQV0ZZ Repair Bilateral Breast, Open Approach
0HQV3ZZ Repair Bilateral Breast, Percutaneous Approach
0HQV7ZZ Repair Bilateral Breast, Via Natural or Artificial Opening
0HQV8ZZ Repair Bilateral Breast, Via Natural or Artificial Opening Endoscopic
0HQVXZZ Repair Bilateral Breast, External Approach
0HQW0ZZ Repair Right Nipple, Open Approach
0HQW3ZZ Repair Right Nipple, Percutaneous Approach
0HQW7ZZ Repair Right Nipple, Via Natural or Artificial Opening
0HQW8ZZ Repair Right Nipple, Via Natural or Artificial Opening Endoscopic
0HQWXZZ Repair Right Nipple, External Approach
0HQX0ZZ Repair Left Nipple, Open Approach
0HQX3ZZ Repair Left Nipple, Percutaneous Approach
0HQX7ZZ Repair Left Nipple, Via Natural or Artificial Opening
0HQX8ZZ Repair Left Nipple, Via Natural or Artificial Opening Endoscopic

XXZZ Repair Left Nipple, External Approach
Y0ZZ Repair Supernumerary Breast, Open Approach
0HQY3ZZ Repair Supernumerary Breast, Percutaneous Approach
0HQY7ZZ Repair Supernumerary Breast, Via Natural or Artificial Opening
0HQY8ZZ Repair Supernumerary Breast, Via Natural or Artificial Opening Endoscopic
0HQYXZZ Repair Supernumerary Breast, External Approach

R – Skin and Breast, Replacement

R0X73 Replacement of Scalp Skin with Autologous Tissue Substitute, Full Thickness, External Approach
R0X74 Replacement of Scalp Skin with Autologous Tissue Substitute, Partial Thickness, External Approach
R0XJ3 Replacement of Scalp Skin with Synthetic Substitute, Full Thickness, External Approach
R0XJ4 Replacement of Scalp Skin with Synthetic Substitute, Partial Thickness, External Approach
R0XJZ Replacement of Scalp Skin with Synthetic Substitute, External Approach
R0XK3 Replacement of Scalp Skin with Nonautologous Tissue Substitute, Full Thickness, External Approach
R0XK4 Replacement of Scalp Skin with Nonautologous Tissue Substitute, Partial Thickness, External Approach
R1X73 Replacement of Face Skin with Autologous Tissue Substitute, Full Thickness, External Approach
R1X74 Replacement of Face Skin with Autologous Tissue Substitute, Partial Thickness, External Approach
R1XJ3 Replacement of Face Skin with Synthetic Substitute, Full Thickness, External Approach
R1XJ4 Replacement of Face Skin with Synthetic Substitute, Partial Thickness, External Approach
R1XJZ Replacement of Face Skin with Synthetic Substitute, External Approach
R1XK3 Replacement of Face Skin with Nonautologous Tissue Substitute, Full Thickness, External Approach
R1XK4 Replacement of Face Skin with Nonautologous Tissue Substitute, Partial Thickness, External Approach
R2X73 Replacement of Right Ear Skin with Autologous Tissue Substitute, Full Thickness, External Approach
R2X74 Replacement of Right Ear Skin with Autologous Tissue Substitute, Partial Thickness, External Approach
R2XJ3 Replacement of Right Ear Skin with Synthetic Substitute, Full Thickness, External Approach
R2XJ4 Replacement of Right Ear Skin with Synthetic Substitute, Partial Thickness, External Approach
R2XJZ Replacement of Right Ear Skin with Synthetic Substitute, External Approach
R2XK3 Replacement of Right Ear Skin with Nonautologous Tissue Substitute, Full Thickness, External Approach
R2XK4 Replacement of Right Ear Skin with Nonautologous Tissue Substitute, Partial Thickness, External Approach
HR3X73 Replacement of Left Ear Skin with Autologous Tissue Substitute, Full Thickness, External Approach
HR3X74 Replacement of Left Ear Skin with Autologous Tissue Substitute, Partial Thickness, External Approach
HR3XJ3 Replacement of Left Ear Skin with Synthetic Substitute, Full Thickness, External Approach
0HR3XJ4 Replacement of Left Ear Skin with Synthetic Substitute, Partial Thickness, External Approach
0HR3XJZ Replacement of Left Ear Skin with Synthetic Substitute, External Approach
0HR3XK3 Replacement of Left Ear Skin with Nonautologous Tissue Substitute, Full Thickness, External Approach
0HR3XK4 Replacement of Left Ear Skin with Nonautologous Tissue Substitute, Partial Thickness, External Approach
0HR4X73 Replacement of Neck Skin with Autologous Tissue Substitute, Full Thickness, External Approach
0HR4X74 Replacement of Neck Skin with Autologous Tissue Substitute, Partial Thickness, External Approach
0HR4XJ3 Replacement of Neck Skin with Synthetic Substitute, Full Thickness, External Approach
0HR4XJ4 Replacement of Neck Skin with Synthetic Substitute, Partial Thickness, External Approach
0HR4XJZ Replacement of Neck Skin with Synthetic Substitute, External Approach
0HR4XK3 Replacement of Neck Skin with Nonautologous Tissue Substitute, Full Thickness, External Approach
0HR4XK4 Replacement of Neck Skin with Nonautologous Tissue Substitute, Partial Thickness, External Approach
0HR5X73 Replacement of Chest Skin with Autologous Tissue Substitute, Full Thickness, External Approach
0HR5X74 Replacement of Chest Skin with Autologous Tissue Substitute, Partial Thickness, External Approach
0HR5XJ3 Replacement of Chest Skin with Synthetic Substitute, Full Thickness, External Approach
0HR5XJ4 Replacement of Chest Skin with Synthetic Substitute, Partial Thickness, External Approach
0HR5XJZ Replacement of Chest Skin with Synthetic Substitute, External Approach
0HR5XK3 Replacement of Chest Skin with Nonautologous Tissue Substitute, Full Thickness, External Approach
0HR5XK4 Replacement of Chest Skin with Nonautologous Tissue Substitute, Partial Thickness, External Approach
0HR6X73 Replacement of Back Skin with Autologous Tissue Substitute, Full Thickness, External Approach
0HR6X74 Replacement of Back Skin with Autologous Tissue Substitute, Partial Thickness, External Approach
0HR6XJ3 Replacement of Back Skin with Synthetic Substitute, Full Thickness, External Approach
0HR6XJ4 Replacement of Back Skin with Synthetic Substitute, Partial Thickness, External Approach
0HR6XJZ Replacement of Back Skin with Synthetic Substitute, External Approach
0HR6XK3 Replacement of Back Skin with Nonautologous Tissue Substitute, Full Thickness, External Approach
0HR6XK4 Replacement of Back Skin with Nonautologous Tissue Substitute, Partial Thickness, External Approach
0HR7X73 Replacement of Abdomen Skin with Autologous Tissue Substitute, Full Thickness, External Approach
0HR7X74 Replacement of Abdomen Skin with Autologous Tissue Substitute, Partial Thickness, External Approach
0HR7XJ3 Replacement of Abdomen Skin with Synthetic Substitute, Full Thickness, External Approach
0HR7XJ4 Replacement of Abdomen Skin with Synthetic Substitute, Partial Thickness, External Approach
0HR7XJZ Replacement of Abdomen Skin with Synthetic Substitute, External Approach
0HR7XK3 Replacement of Abdomen Skin with Nonautologous Tissue Substitute, Full Thickness, External Approach
0HR7XK4 Replacement of Abdomen Skin with Nonautologous Tissue Substitute, Partial Thickness, External Approach
0HR8X73 Replacement of Buttock Skin with Autologous Tissue Substitute, Full Thickness, External Approach
0HR8X74 Replacement of Buttock Skin with Autologous Tissue Substitute, Partial Thickness, External Approach
0HR8XJ3 Replacement of Buttock Skin with Synthetic Substitute, Full Thickness, External Approach
0HR8XJ4 Replacement of Buttock Skin with Synthetic Substitute, Partial Thickness, External Approach
0HR8XJZ Replacement of Buttock Skin with Synthetic Substitute, External Approach
0HR8XK3 Replacement of Buttock Skin with Nonautologous Tissue Substitute, Full Thickness, External Approach
0HR8XK4 Replacement of Buttock Skin with Nonautologous Tissue Substitute, Partial Thickness, External Approach
0HR9X73 Replacement of Perineum Skin with Autologous Tissue Substitute, Full Thickness, External Approach
0HR9X74 Replacement of Perineum Skin with Autologous Tissue Substitute, Partial Thickness, External Approach
0HR9XJ3 Replacement of Perineum Skin with Synthetic Substitute, Full Thickness, External Approach
0HR9XJ4 Replacement of Perineum Skin with Synthetic Substitute, Partial Thickness, External Approach
0HR9XJZ Replacement of Perineum Skin with Synthetic Substitute, External Approach
0HR9XK3 Replacement of Perineum Skin with Nonautologous Tissue Substitute, Full Thickness, External Approach
0HR9XK4 Replacement of Perineum Skin with Nonautologous Tissue Substitute, Partial Thickness, External Approach
0HRAX73 Replacement of Genitalia Skin with Autologous Tissue Substitute, Full Thickness, External Approach
0HRAX74 Replacement of Genitalia Skin with Autologous Tissue Substitute, Partial Thickness, External Approach
0HRAXJ3 Replacement of Genitalia Skin with Synthetic Substitute, Full Thickness, External Approach

0HRAXJ4 Replacement of Genitalia Skin with Synthetic Substitute, Partial Thickness, External Approach

0HRAXJZ Replacement of Genitalia Skin with Synthetic Substitute, External Approach

0HRAXK3 Replacement of Genitalia Skin with Nonautologous Tissue Substitute, Full Thickness, External Approach

0HRAXK4 Replacement of Genitalia Skin with Nonautologous Tissue Substitute, Partial Thickness, External Approach

0HRBX73 Replacement of Right Upper Arm Skin with Autologous Tissue Substitute, Full Thickness, External Approach

0HRBX74 Replacement of Right Upper Arm Skin with Autologous Tissue Substitute, Partial Thickness, External Approach

0HRBXJ3 Replacement of Right Upper Arm Skin with Synthetic Substitute, Full Thickness, External Approach

0HRBXJ4 Replacement of Right Upper Arm Skin with Synthetic Substitute, Partial Thickness, External Approach

0HRBXJZ Replacement of Right Upper Arm Skin with Synthetic Substitute, External Approach

0HRBXK3 Replacement of Right Upper Arm Skin with Nonautologous Tissue Substitute, Full Thickness, External Approach

0HRBXK4 Replacement of Right Upper Arm Skin with Nonautologous Tissue Substitute, Partial Thickness, External Approach

0HRCX73 Replacement of Left Upper Arm Skin with Autologous Tissue Substitute, Full Thickness, External Approach

0HRCX74 Replacement of Left Upper Arm Skin with Autologous Tissue Substitute, Partial Thickness, External Approach

0HRCXJ3 Replacement of Left Upper Arm Skin with Synthetic Substitute, Full Thickness, External Approach

0HRCXJ4 Replacement of Left Upper Arm Skin with Synthetic Substitute, Partial Thickness, External Approach

0HRCXJZ Replacement of Left Upper Arm Skin with Synthetic Substitute, External Approach

0HRCXK3 Replacement of Left Upper Arm Skin with Nonautologous Tissue Substitute, Full Thickness, External Approach

0HRCXK4 Replacement of Left Upper Arm Skin with Nonautologous Tissue Substitute, Partial Thickness, External Approach

0HRDX73 Replacement of Right Lower Arm Skin with Autologous Tissue Substitute, Full Thickness, External Approach

0HRDX74 Replacement of Right Lower Arm Skin with Autologous Tissue Substitute, Partial Thickness, External Approach

0HRDXJ3 Replacement of Right Lower Arm Skin with Synthetic Substitute, Full Thickness, External Approach

0HRDXJ4 Replacement of Right Lower Arm Skin with Synthetic Substitute, Partial Thickness, External Approach

0HRDXJZ Replacement of Right Lower Arm Skin with Synthetic Substitute, External Approach

0HRDXK3 Replacement of Right Lower Arm Skin with Nonautologous Tissue Substitute, Full Thickness, External Approach

0HRDXK4 Replacement of Right Lower Arm Skin with Nonautologous Tissue Substitute, Partial Thickness, External Approach

0HREX73 Replacement of Left Lower Arm Skin with Autologous Tissue Substitute, Full Thickness, External Approach

0HREX74 Replacement of Left Lower Arm Skin with Autologous Tissue Substitute, Partial Thickness, External Approach

0HREXJ3 Replacement of Left Lower Arm Skin with Synthetic Substitute, Full Thickness, External Approach

0HREXJ4 Replacement of Left Lower Arm Skin with Synthetic Substitute, Partial Thickness, External Approach

0HREXJZ Replacement of Left Lower Arm Skin with Synthetic Substitute, External Approach

0HREXK3 Replacement of Left Lower Arm Skin with Nonautologous Tissue Substitute, Full Thickness, External Approach

0HREXK4 Replacement of Left Lower Arm Skin with Nonautologous Tissue Substitute, Partial Thickness, External Approach

0HRFX73 Replacement of Right Hand Skin with Autologous Tissue Substitute, Full Thickness, External Approach

0HRFX74 Replacement of Right Hand Skin with Autologous Tissue Substitute, Partial Thickness, External Approach

0HRFXJ3 Replacement of Right Hand Skin with Synthetic Substitute, Full Thickness, External Approach

0HRFXJ4 Replacement of Right Hand Skin with Synthetic Substitute, Partial Thickness, External Approach

0HRFXJZ Replacement of Right Hand Skin with Synthetic Substitute, External Approach

0HRFXK3 Replacement of Right Hand Skin with Nonautologous Tissue Substitute, Full Thickness, External Approach

0HRFXK4 Replacement of Right Hand Skin with Nonautologous Tissue Substitute, Partial Thickness, External Approach

0HRGX73 Replacement of Left Hand Skin with Autologous Tissue Substitute, Full Thickness, External Approach

0HRGX74 Replacement of Left Hand Skin with Autologous Tissue Substitute, Partial Thickness, External Approach

0HRGXJ3 Replacement of Left Hand Skin with Synthetic Substitute, Full Thickness, External Approach

0HRGXJ4 Replacement of Left Hand Skin with Synthetic Substitute, Partial Thickness, External Approach

0HRGXJZ Replacement of Left Hand Skin with Synthetic Substitute, External Approach

0HRGXK3 Replacement of Left Hand Skin with Nonautologous Tissue Substitute, Full Thickness, External Approach

0HRGXK4 Replacement of Left Hand Skin with Nonautologous Tissue Substitute, Partial Thickness, External Approach

0HRHX73 Replacement of Right Upper Leg Skin with Autologous Tissue Substitute, Full Thickness, External Approach

0HRHX74 Replacement of Right Upper Leg Skin with Autologous Tissue Substitute, Partial Thickness, External Approach

0HRHXJ3 Replacement of Right Upper Leg Skin with Synthetic Substitute, Full Thickness, External Approach

0HRHXJ4 Replacement of Right Upper Leg Skin with Synthetic Substitute, Partial Thickness, External Approach

0HRHXJZ Replacement of Right Upper Leg Skin with Synthetic Substitute, External Approach

0HRHXK3 Replacement of Right Upper Leg Ski with Nonautologous Tissue Substitute Full Thickness, External Approach

0HRHXK4 Replacement of Right Upper Leg Ski with Nonautologous Tissue Substitute Partial Thickness, External Approach

0HRJX73 Replacement of Left Upper Leg Skin with Autologous Tissue Substitute, Fu Thickness, External Approach

0HRJX74 Replacement of Left Upper Leg Skin with Autologous Tissue Substitute, Partial Thickness, External Approach

0HRJXJ3 Replacement of Left Upper Leg Skin with Synthetic Substitute, Full Thickn External Approach

0HRJXJ4 Replacement of Left Upper Leg Skin with Synthetic Substitute, Partial Thickness, External Approach

0HRJXJZ Replacement of Left Upper Leg Skin with Synthetic Substitute, External Approach

0HRJXK3 Replacement of Left Upper Leg Skin with Nonautologous Tissue Substitute Full Thickness, External Approach

0HRJXK4 Replacement of Left Upper Leg Skin with Nonautologous Tissue Substitute, Partial Thickness, External Approach

0HRKX73 Replacement of Right Lower Leg Skin with Autologous Tissue Substitute, Fu Thickness, External Approach

0HRKX74 Replacement of Right Lower Leg Skin with Autologous Tissue Substitute, Partial Thickness, External Approach

0HRKXJ3 Replacement of Right Lower Leg Skin with Synthetic Substitute, Full Thickne External Approach

0HRKXJ4 Replacement of Right Lower Leg Skin with Synthetic Substitute, Partial Thickness, External Approach

0HRKXJZ Replacement of Right Lower Leg Skin with Synthetic Substitute, External Approach

0HRKXK3 Replacement of Right Lower Leg Skin with Nonautologous Tissue Substitute, Full Thickness, External Approach

0HRKXK4 Replacement of Right Lower Leg Skin with Nonautologous Tissue Substitute, Partial Thickness, External Approach

0HRLX73 Replacement of Left Lower Leg Skin with Autologous Tissue Substitute, Full Thickness, External Approach

0HRLX74 Replacement of Left Lower Leg Skin with Autologous Tissue Substitute, Partial Thickness, External Approach

0HRLXJ3 Replacement of Left Lower Leg Skin with Synthetic Substitute, Full Thickne External Approach

0HRLXJ4 Replacement of Left Lower Leg Skin with Synthetic Substitute, Partial Thickness, External Approach

0HRLXJZ Replacement of Left Lower Leg Skin with Synthetic Substitute, External Approach

0HRLXK3 Replacement of Left Lower Leg Skin with Nonautologous Tissue Substitute, Full Thickness, External Approach

0HRLXK4 Replacement of Left Lower Leg Skin with Nonautologous Tissue Substitute, Partial Thickness, External Approach

0HRMX73 Replacement of Right Foot Skin with Autologous Tissue Substitute, Full Thickness, External Approach

0HRMX74 Replacement of Right Foot Skin with Autologous Tissue Substitute, Partial Thickness, External Approach

0HRMXJ3 Replacement of Right Foot Skin with Synthetic Substitute, Full Thickness, External Approach

RMXJ4 Replacement of Right Foot Skin with Synthetic Substitute, Partial Thickness, External Approach

RMXJZ Replacement of Right Foot Skin with Synthetic Substitute, External Approach

RMXK3 Replacement of Right Foot Skin with Nonautologous Tissue Substitute, Full Thickness, External Approach

RMXK4 Replacement of Right Foot Skin with Nonautologous Tissue Substitute, Partial Thickness, External Approach

RNX73 Replacement of Left Foot Skin with Autologous Tissue Substitute, Full Thickness, External Approach

RNX74 Replacement of Left Foot Skin with Autologous Tissue Substitute, Partial Thickness, External Approach

RNXJ3 Replacement of Left Foot Skin with Synthetic Substitute, Full Thickness, External Approach

RNXJ4 Replacement of Left Foot Skin with Synthetic Substitute, Partial Thickness, External Approach

RNXJZ Replacement of Left Foot Skin with Synthetic Substitute, External Approach

RNXK3 Replacement of Left Foot Skin with Nonautologous Tissue Substitute, Full Thickness, External Approach

RNXK4 Replacement of Left Foot Skin with Nonautologous Tissue Substitute, Partial Thickness, External Approach

RQX7Z Replacement of Finger Nail with Autologous Tissue Substitute, External Approach

RQXJZ Replacement of Finger Nail with Synthetic Substitute, External Approach

RQXKZ Replacement of Finger Nail with Nonautologous Tissue Substitute, External Approach

RRX7Z Replacement of Toe Nail with Autologous Tissue Substitute, External Approach

RRXJZ Replacement of Toe Nail with Synthetic Substitute, External Approach

RRXKZ Replacement of Toe Nail with Nonautologous Tissue Substitute, External Approach

RSX7Z Replacement of Hair with Autologous Tissue Substitute, External Approach

RSXJZ Replacement of Hair with Synthetic Substitute, External Approach

RSXKZ Replacement of Hair with Nonautologous Tissue Substitute, External Approach

HRT075 Replacement of Right Breast using Latissimus Dorsi Myocutaneous Flap, Open Approach

HRT076 Replacement of Right Breast using Transverse Rectus Abdominis Myocutaneous Flap, Open Approach

HRT077 Replacement of Right Breast using Deep Inferior Epigastric Artery Perforator Flap, Open Approach

HRT078 Replacement of Right Breast using Superficial Inferior Epigastric Artery Flap, Open Approach

HRT079 Replacement of Right Breast using Gluteal Artery Perforator Flap, Open Approach

HRT07Z Replacement of Right Breast with Autologous Tissue Substitute, Open Approach

HRT0JZ Replacement of Right Breast with Synthetic Substitute, Open Approach

HRT0KZ Replacement of Right Breast with Nonautologous Tissue Substitute, Open Approach

HRT37Z Replacement of Right Breast with Autologous Tissue Substitute, Percutaneous Approach

+ Breast replacement when reported with Extraction of subcutaneous tissue and fascia (4th characters 6,7,8,9,L or M). *See table 0JD to construct the Extraction code.*

0HRT3JZ Replacement of Right Breast with Synthetic Substitute, Percutaneous Approach

0HRT3KZ Replacement of Right Breast with Nonautologous Tissue Substitute, Percutaneous Approach

0HRTX7Z Replacement of Right Breast with Autologous Tissue Substitute, External Approach

0HRTXJZ Replacement of Right Breast with Synthetic Substitute, External Approach

0HRTXKZ Replacement of Right Breast with Nonautologous Tissue Substitute, External Approach

0HRU075 Replacement of Left Breast using Latissimus Dorsi Myocutaneous Flap, Open Approach

0HRU076 Replacement of Left Breast using Transverse Rectus Abdominis Myocutaneous Flap, Open Approach

0HRU077 Replacement of Left Breast using Deep Inferior Epigastric Artery Perforator Flap, Open Approach

0HRU078 Replacement of Left Breast using Superficial Inferior Epigastric Artery Flap, Open Approach

0HRU079 Replacement of Left Breast using Gluteal Artery Perforator Flap, Open Approach

0HRU07Z Replacement of Left Breast with Autologous Tissue Substitute, Open Approach

0HRU0JZ Replacement of Left Breast with Synthetic Substitute, Open Approach

0HRU0KZ Replacement of Left Breast with Nonautologous Tissue Substitute, Open Approach

0HRU37Z Replacement of Left Breast with Autologous Tissue Substitute, Percutaneous Approach

0HRU3JZ Replacement of Left Breast with Synthetic Substitute, Percutaneous Approach

+ Breast replacement when reported with Extraction of subcutaneous tissue and fascia (4th characters 6,7,8,9,L or M). *See table 0JD to construct the Extraction code.*

0HRU3KZ Replacement of Left Breast with Nonautologous Tissue Substitute, Percutaneous Approach

0HRUX7Z Replacement of Left Breast with Autologous Tissue Substitute, External Approach

0HRUXJZ Replacement of Left Breast with Synthetic Substitute, External Approach

0HRUXKZ Replacement of Left Breast with Nonautologous Tissue Substitute, External Approach

0HRV075 Replacement of Bilateral Breast using Latissimus Dorsi Myocutaneous Flap, Open Approach

0HRV076 Replacement of Bilateral Breast using Transverse Rectus Abdominis Myocutaneous Flap, Open Approach

0HRV077 Replacement of Bilateral Breast using Deep Inferior Epigastric Artery Perforator Flap, Open Approach

0HRV078 Replacement of Bilateral Breast using Superficial Inferior Epigastric Artery Flap, Open Approach

0HRV079 Replacement of Bilateral Breast using Gluteal Artery Perforator Flap, Open Approach

0HRV07Z Replacement of Bilateral Breast with Autologous Tissue Substitute, Open Approach

0HRV0JZ Replacement of Bilateral Breast with Synthetic Substitute, Open Approach

0HRV0KZ Replacement of Bilateral Breast with Nonautologous Tissue Substitute, Open Approach

0HRV37Z Replacement of Bilateral Breast with Autologous Tissue Substitute, Percutaneous Approach

+ Breast replacement when reported with Extraction of subcutaneous tissue and fascia (4th characters 6,7,8,9,L or M). *See table 0JD to construct the Extraction code.*

0HRV3JZ Replacement of Bilateral Breast with Synthetic Substitute, Percutaneous Approach

0HRV3KZ Replacement of Bilateral Breast with Nonautologous Tissue Substitute, Percutaneous Approach

0HRVX7Z Replacement of Bilateral Breast with Autologous Tissue Substitute, External Approach

0HRVXJZ Replacement of Bilateral Breast with Synthetic Substitute, External Approach

0HRVXKZ Replacement of Bilateral Breast with Nonautologous Tissue Substitute, External Approach

0HRW07Z Replacement of Right Nipple with Autologous Tissue Substitute, Open Approach

0HRW0JZ Replacement of Right Nipple with Synthetic Substitute, Open Approach

0HRW0KZ Replacement of Right Nipple with Nonautologous Tissue Substitute, Open Approach

0HRW37Z Replacement of Right Nipple with Autologous Tissue Substitute, Percutaneous Approach

0HRW3JZ Replacement of Right Nipple with Synthetic Substitute, Percutaneous Approach

0HRW3KZ Replacement of Right Nipple with Nonautologous Tissue Substitute, Percutaneous Approach

0HRWX7Z Replacement of Right Nipple with Autologous Tissue Substitute, External Approach

0HRWXJZ Replacement of Right Nipple with Synthetic Substitute, External Approach

0HRWXKZ Replacement of Right Nipple with Nonautologous Tissue Substitute, External Approach

0HRX07Z Replacement of Left Nipple with Autologous Tissue Substitute, Open Approach

0HRX0JZ Replacement of Left Nipple with Synthetic Substitute, Open Approach

0HRX0KZ Replacement of Left Nipple with Nonautologous Tissue Substitute, Open Approach

0HRX37Z Replacement of Left Nipple with Autologous Tissue Substitute, Percutaneous Approach

0HRX3JZ Replacement of Left Nipple with Synthetic Substitute, Percutaneous Approach

0HRX3KZ Replacement of Left Nipple with Nonautologous Tissue Substitute, Percutaneous Approach

0HRXX7Z Replacement of Left Nipple with Autologous Tissue Substitute, External Approach

0HRXXJZ Replacement of Left Nipple with Synthetic Substitute, External Approach

0HRXXKZ Replacement of Left Nipple with Nonautologous Tissue Substitute, External Approach

0HS – Skin and Breast, Reposition

0HSSXZZ Reposition Hair, External Approach
0HST0ZZ Reposition Right Breast, Open Approach
0HSU0ZZ Reposition Left Breast, Open Approach
0HSV0ZZ Reposition Bilateral Breast, Open Approach
0HSWXZZ Reposition Right Nipple, External Approach
0HSXXZZ Reposition Left Nipple, External Approach

0HT – Skin and Breast, Resection

Review Coding Guideline B3.8

0HTQXZZ Resection of Finger Nail, External Approach
0HTRXZZ Resection of Toe Nail, External Approach
0HTT0ZZ Resection of Right Breast, Open Approach
0HTU0ZZ Resection of Left Breast, Open Approach
0HTV0ZZ Resection of Bilateral Breast, Open Approach
0HTWXZZ Resection of Right Nipple, External Approach
0HTXXZZ Resection of Left Nipple, External Approach
0HTY0ZZ Resection of Supernumerary Breast, Open Approach

0HU – Skin and Breast, Supplement

0HUT07Z Supplement Right Breast with Autologous Tissue Substitute, Open Approach
0HUT0JZ Supplement Right Breast with Synthetic Substitute, Open Approach
0HUT0KZ Supplement Right Breast with Nonautologous Tissue Substitute, Open Approach
0HUT37Z Supplement Right Breast with Autologous Tissue Substitute, Percutaneous Approach
0HUT3JZ Supplement Right Breast with Synthetic Substitute, Percutaneous Approach
0HUT3KZ Supplement Right Breast with Nonautologous Tissue Substitute, Percutaneous Approach
0HUT77Z Supplement Right Breast with Autologous Tissue Substitute, Via Natural or Artificial Opening
0HUT7JZ Supplement Right Breast with Synthetic Substitute, Via Natural or Artificial Opening
0HUT7KZ Supplement Right Breast with Nonautologous Tissue Substitute, Via Natural or Artificial Opening
0HUT87Z Supplement Right Breast with Autologous Tissue Substitute, Via Natural or Artificial Opening Endoscopic
0HUT8JZ Supplement Right Breast with Synthetic Substitute, Via Natural or Artificial Opening Endoscopic
0HUT8KZ Supplement Right Breast with Nonautologous Tissue Substitute, Via Natural or Artificial Opening Endoscopic
0HUTX7Z Supplement Right Breast with Autologous Tissue Substitute, External Approach
0HUTXJZ Supplement Right Breast with Synthetic Substitute, External Approach
0HUTXKZ Supplement Right Breast with Nonautologous Tissue Substitute, External Approach
0HUU07Z Supplement Left Breast with Autologous Tissue Substitute, Open Approach
0HUU0JZ Supplement Left Breast with Synthetic Substitute, Open Approach
0HUU0KZ Supplement Left Breast with Nonautologous Tissue Substitute, Open Approach
0HUU37Z Supplement Left Breast with Autologous Tissue Substitute, Percutaneous Approach
0HUU3JZ Supplement Left Breast with Synthetic Substitute, Percutaneous Approach
0HUU3KZ Supplement Left Breast with Nonautologous Tissue Substitute, Percutaneous Approach
0HUU77Z Supplement Left Breast with Autologous Tissue Substitute, Via Natural or Artificial Opening
0HUU7JZ Supplement Left Breast with Synthetic Substitute, Via Natural or Artificial Opening
0HUU7KZ Supplement Left Breast with Nonautologous Tissue Substitute, Via Natural or Artificial Opening
0HUU87Z Supplement Left Breast with Autologous Tissue Substitute, Via Natural or Artificial Opening Endoscopic
0HUU8JZ Supplement Left Breast with Synthetic Substitute, Via Natural or Artificial Opening Endoscopic
0HUU8KZ Supplement Left Breast with Nonautologous Tissue Substitute, Via Natural or Artificial Opening Endoscopic
0HUUX7Z Supplement Left Breast with Autologous Tissue Substitute, External Approach
0HUUXJZ Supplement Left Breast with Synthetic Substitute, External Approach
0HUUXKZ Supplement Left Breast with Nonautologous Tissue Substitute, External Approach
0HUV07Z Supplement Bilateral Breast with Autologous Tissue Substitute, Open Approach
0HUV0JZ Supplement Bilateral Breast with Synthetic Substitute, Open Approach
0HUV0KZ Supplement Bilateral Breast with Nonautologous Tissue Substitute, Open Approach
0HUV37Z Supplement Bilateral Breast with Autologous Tissue Substitute, Percutaneous Approach
0HUV3JZ Supplement Bilateral Breast with Synthetic Substitute, Percutaneous Approach
0HUV3KZ Supplement Bilateral Breast with Nonautologous Tissue Substitute, Percutaneous Approach
0HUV77Z Supplement Bilateral Breast with Autologous Tissue Substitute, Via Natural or Artificial Opening
0HUV7JZ Supplement Bilateral Breast with Synthetic Substitute, Via Natural or Artificial Opening
0HUV7KZ Supplement Bilateral Breast with Nonautologous Tissue Substitute, Via Natural or Artificial Opening
0HUV87Z Supplement Bilateral Breast with Autologous Tissue Substitute, Via Natural or Artificial Opening Endoscopic
0HUV8JZ Supplement Bilateral Breast with Synthetic Substitute, Via Natural or Artificial Opening Endoscopic
0HUV8KZ Supplement Bilateral Breast with Nonautologous Tissue Substitute, Via Natural or Artificial Opening Endoscc
0HUVX7Z Supplement Bilateral Breast with Autologous Tissue Substitute, Externa Approach
0HUVXJZ Supplement Bilateral Breast with Synthetic Substitute, External Approa
0HUVXKZ Supplement Bilateral Breast with Nonautologous Tissue Substitute, External Approach
0HUW07Z Supplement Right Nipple with Autologous Tissue Substitute, Open Approach
0HUW0JZ Supplement Right Nipple with Synthe Substitute, Open Approach
0HUW0KZ Supplement Right Nipple with Nonautologous Tissue Substitute, Ope Approach
0HUW37Z Supplement Right Nipple with Autologous Tissue Substitute, Percutaneous Approach
0HUW3JZ Supplement Right Nipple with Synthe Substitute, Percutaneous Approach
0HUW3KZ Supplement Right Nipple with Nonautologous Tissue Substitute, Percutaneous Approach
0HUW77Z Supplement Right Nipple with Autologous Tissue Substitute, Via Natural or Artificial Opening
0HUW7JZ Supplement Right Nipple with Synthet Substitute, Via Natural or Artificial Opening
0HUW7KZ Supplement Right Nipple with Nonautologous Tissue Substitute, Via Natural or Artificial Opening
0HUW87Z Supplement Right Nipple with Autologous Tissue Substitute, Via Natural or Artificial Opening Endoscop
0HUW8JZ Supplement Right Nipple with Synthet Substitute, Via Natural or Artificial Opening Endoscopic
0HUW8KZ Supplement Right Nipple with Nonautologous Tissue Substitute, Via Natural or Artificial Opening Endoscop
0HUWX7Z Supplement Right Nipple with Autologous Tissue Substitute, External Approach
0HUWXJZ Supplement Right Nipple with Syntheti Substitute, External Approach
0HUWXKZ Supplement Right Nipple with Nonautologous Tissue Substitute, External Approach
0HUX07Z Supplement Left Nipple with Autologous Tissue Substitute, Open Approach
0HUX0JZ Supplement Left Nipple with Synthetic Substitute, Open Approach

JX0KZ Supplement Left Nipple with Nonautologous Tissue Substitute, Open Approach
JX37Z Supplement Left Nipple with Autologous Tissue Substitute, Percutaneous Approach
JX3JZ Supplement Left Nipple with Synthetic Substitute, Percutaneous Approach
JX3KZ Supplement Left Nipple with Nonautologous Tissue Substitute, Percutaneous Approach
JX77Z Supplement Left Nipple with Autologous Tissue Substitute, Via Natural or Artificial Opening
0HUX7JZ Supplement Left Nipple with Synthetic Substitute, Via Natural or Artificial Opening
0HUX7KZ Supplement Left Nipple with Nonautologous Tissue Substitute, Via Natural or Artificial Opening
0HUX87Z Supplement Left Nipple with Autologous Tissue Substitute, Via Natural or Artificial Opening Endoscopic
0HUX8JZ Supplement Left Nipple with Synthetic Substitute, Via Natural or Artificial Opening Endoscopic
0HUX8KZ Supplement Left Nipple with Nonautologous Tissue Substitute, Via Natural or Artificial Opening Endoscopic
0HUXX7Z Supplement Left Nipple with Autologous Tissue Substitute, External Approach
0HUXXJZ Supplement Left Nipple with Synthetic Substitute, External Approach
0HUXXKZ Supplement Left Nipple with Nonautologous Tissue Substitute, External Approach

W – Skin and Breast, Revision

view Coding Guideline B6.1c

WPX0Z Revision of Drainage Device in Skin, External Approach
WPX7Z Revision of Autologous Tissue Substitute in Skin, External Approach
WPXJZ Revision of Synthetic Substitute in Skin, External Approach
WPXKZ Revision of Nonautologous Tissue Substitute in Skin, External Approach
WQX0Z Revision of Drainage Device in Finger Nail, External Approach
WQX7Z Revision of Autologous Tissue Substitute in Finger Nail, External Approach
WQXJZ Revision of Synthetic Substitute in Finger Nail, External Approach
WQXKZ Revision of Nonautologous Tissue Substitute in Finger Nail, External Approach
WRX0Z Revision of Drainage Device in Toe Nail, External Approach
WRX7Z Revision of Autologous Tissue Substitute in Toe Nail, External Approach
WRXJZ Revision of Synthetic Substitute in Toe Nail, External Approach
WRXKZ Revision of Nonautologous Tissue Substitute in Toe Nail, External Approach
WSX7Z Revision of Autologous Tissue Substitute in Hair, External Approach
WSXJZ Revision of Synthetic Substitute in Hair, External Approach
WSXKZ Revision of Nonautologous Tissue Substitute in Hair, External Approach
WT00Z Revision of Drainage Device in Right Breast, Open Approach
WT07Z Revision of Autologous Tissue Substitute in Right Breast, Open Approach
WT0JZ Revision of Synthetic Substitute in Right Breast, Open Approach
WT0KZ Revision of Nonautologous Tissue Substitute in Right Breast, Open Approach
WT0NZ Revision of Tissue Expander in Right Breast, Open Approach
WT30Z Revision of Drainage Device in Right Breast, Percutaneous Approach
WT37Z Revision of Autologous Tissue Substitute in Right Breast, Percutaneous Approach
HWT3JZ Revision of Synthetic Substitute in Right Breast, Percutaneous Approach
0HWT3KZ Revision of Nonautologous Tissue Substitute in Right Breast, Percutaneous Approach
0HWT3NZ Revision of Tissue Expander in Right Breast, Percutaneous Approach
0HWT70Z Revision of Drainage Device in Right Breast, Via Natural or Artificial Opening
0HWT77Z Revision of Autologous Tissue Substitute in Right Breast, Via Natural or Artificial Opening
0HWT7JZ Revision of Synthetic Substitute in Right Breast, Via Natural or Artificial Opening
0HWT7KZ Revision of Nonautologous Tissue Substitute in Right Breast, Via Natural or Artificial Opening
0HWT7NZ Revision of Tissue Expander in Right Breast, Via Natural or Artificial Opening
0HWT80Z Revision of Drainage Device in Right Breast, Via Natural or Artificial Opening Endoscopic
0HWT87Z Revision of Autologous Tissue Substitute in Right Breast, Via Natural or Artificial Opening Endoscopic
0HWT8JZ Revision of Synthetic Substitute in Right Breast, Via Natural or Artificial Opening Endoscopic
0HWT8KZ Revision of Nonautologous Tissue Substitute in Right Breast, Via Natural or Artificial Opening Endoscopic
0HWT8NZ Revision of Tissue Expander in Right Breast, Via Natural or Artificial Opening Endoscopic
0HWTX0Z Revision of Drainage Device in Right Breast, External Approach
0HWTX7Z Revision of Autologous Tissue Substitute in Right Breast, External Approach
0HWTXJZ Revision of Synthetic Substitute in Right Breast, External Approach
0HWTXKZ Revision of Nonautologous Tissue Substitute in Right Breast, External Approach
0HWU00Z Revision of Drainage Device in Left Breast, Open Approach
0HWU07Z Revision of Autologous Tissue Substitute in Left Breast, Open Approach
0HWU0JZ Revision of Synthetic Substitute in Left Breast, Open Approach
0HWU0KZ Revision of Nonautologous Tissue Substitute in Left Breast, Open Approach
0HWU0NZ Revision of Tissue Expander in Left Breast, Open Approach
0HWU30Z Revision of Drainage Device in Left Breast, Percutaneous Approach
0HWU37Z Revision of Autologous Tissue Substitute in Left Breast, Percutaneous Approach
0HWU3JZ Revision of Synthetic Substitute in Left Breast, Percutaneous Approach
0HWU3KZ Revision of Nonautologous Tissue Substitute in Left Breast, Percutaneous Approach
0HWU3NZ Revision of Tissue Expander in Left Breast, Percutaneous Approach
0HWU70Z Revision of Drainage Device in Left Breast, Via Natural or Artificial Opening
0HWU77Z Revision of Autologous Tissue Substitute in Left Breast, Via Natural or Artificial Opening
0HWU7JZ Revision of Synthetic Substitute in Left Breast, Via Natural or Artificial Opening
0HWU7KZ Revision of Nonautologous Tissue Substitute in Left Breast, Via Natural or Artificial Opening
0HWU7NZ Revision of Tissue Expander in Left Breast, Via Natural or Artificial Opening
0HWU80Z Revision of Drainage Device in Left Breast, Via Natural or Artificial Opening Endoscopic
0HWU87Z Revision of Autologous Tissue Substitute in Left Breast, Via Natural or Artificial Opening Endoscopic
0HWU8JZ Revision of Synthetic Substitute in Left Breast, Via Natural or Artificial Opening Endoscopic
0HWU8KZ Revision of Nonautologous Tissue Substitute in Left Breast, Via Natural or Artificial Opening Endoscopic
0HWU8NZ Revision of Tissue Expander in Left Breast, Via Natural or Artificial Opening Endoscopic
0HWUX0Z Revision of Drainage Device in Left Breast, External Approach
0HWUX7Z Revision of Autologous Tissue Substitute in Left Breast, External Approach
0HWUXJZ Revision of Synthetic Substitute in Left Breast, External Approach
0HWUXKZ Revision of Nonautologous Tissue Substitute in Left Breast, External Approach

HX – Skin and Breast, Transfer

HX0XZZ Transfer Scalp Skin, External Approach
HX1XZZ Transfer Face Skin, External Approach
0HX2XZZ Transfer Right Ear Skin, External Approach
0HX3XZZ Transfer Left Ear Skin, External Approach

0HX4XZZ Transfer Neck Skin, External Approach
0HX5XZZ Transfer Chest Skin, External Approach
0HX6XZZ Transfer Back Skin, External Approach
0HX7XZZ Transfer Abdomen Skin, External Approach
0HX8XZZ Transfer Buttock Skin, External Approach
0HX9XZZ Transfer Perineum Skin, External Approach
0HXAXZZ Transfer Genitalia Skin, External Approach
0HXBXZZ Transfer Right Upper Arm Skin, External Approach
0HXCXZZ Transfer Left Upper Arm Skin, External Approach
0HXDXZZ Transfer Right Lower Arm Skin, External Approach
0HXEXZZ Transfer Left Lower Arm Skin, External Approach
0HXFXZZ Transfer Right Hand Skin, External Approach
0HXGXZZ Transfer Left Hand Skin, External Approach
0HXHXZZ Transfer Right Upper Leg Skin, External Approach
0HXJXZZ Transfer Left Upper Leg Skin, Externa Approach
0HXKXZZ Transfer Right Lower Leg Skin, Exter Approach
0HXLXZZ Transfer Left Lower Leg Skin, Externa Approach
0HXMXZZ Transfer Right Foot Skin, External Approach
0HXNXZZ Transfer Left Foot Skin, External Approach

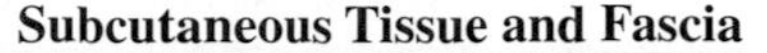

Subcutaneous Tissue and Fascia

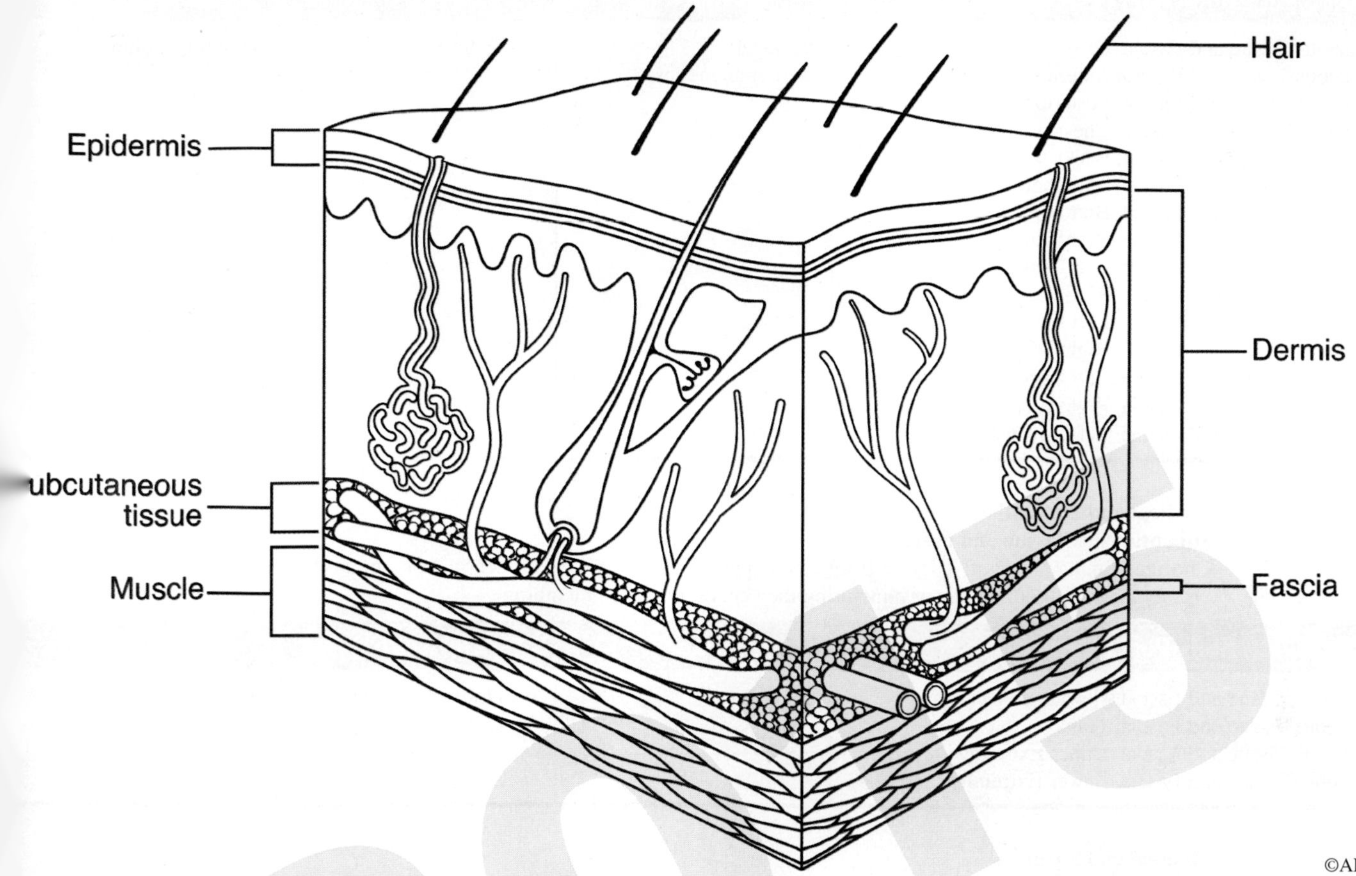

©AHIMA

Subcutaneous Tissue and Fascia Tables 0J0–0JX

Section 0 **Medical and Surgical**
Body System J **Subcutaneous Tissue and Fascia**
Operation 0 **Alteration:** Modifying the anatomic structure of a body part without affecting the function of the body part

Body Part (4th)	Approach (5th)	Device (6th)	Qualifier (7th)
1 Subcutaneous Tissue and Fascia, Face **4** Subcutaneous Tissue and Fascia, Anterior Neck **5** Subcutaneous Tissue and Fascia, Posterior Neck **6** Subcutaneous Tissue and Fascia, Chest **7** Subcutaneous Tissue and Fascia, Back **8** Subcutaneous Tissue and Fascia, Abdomen **9** Subcutaneous Tissue and Fascia, Buttock **D** Subcutaneous Tissue and Fascia, Right Upper Arm **F** Subcutaneous Tissue and Fascia, Left Upper Arm **G** Subcutaneous Tissue and Fascia, Right Lower Arm **H** Subcutaneous Tissue and Fascia, Left Lower Arm **L** Subcutaneous Tissue and Fascia, Right Upper Leg **M** Subcutaneous Tissue and Fascia, Left Upper Leg **N** Subcutaneous Tissue and Fascia, Right Lower Leg **P** Subcutaneous Tissue and Fascia, Left Lower Leg	**0** Open **3** Percutaneous	**Z** No Device	**Z** No Qualifier

Section 0 **Medical and Surgical**
Body System J **Subcutaneous Tissue and Fascia**
Operation 2 **Change:** Taking out or off a device from a body part and putting back an identical or similar device in or on the same body part without cutting or puncturing the skin or a mucous membrane

Body Part (4th)	Approach (5th)	Device (6th)	Qualifier (7th)
S Subcutaneous Tissue and Fascia, Head and Neck **T** Subcutaneous Tissue and Fascia, Trunk **V** Subcutaneous Tissue and Fascia, Upper Extremity **W** Subcutaneous Tissue and Fascia, Lower Extremity	**X** External	**0** Drainage Device **Y** Other Device	**Z** No Qualifier

Section 0 **Medical and Surgical**
Body System J **Subcutaneous Tissue and Fascia**
Operation 5 **Destruction:** Physical eradication of all or a portion of a body part by the direct use of energy, force, or a destructive agent

Body Part (4th)	Approach (5th)	Device (6th)	Qualifier (7th)
0 Subcutaneous Tissue and Fascia, Scalp **1** Subcutaneous Tissue and Fascia, Face **4** Subcutaneous Tissue and Fascia, Anterior Neck **5** Subcutaneous Tissue and Fascia, Posterior Neck **6** Subcutaneous Tissue and Fascia, Chest **7** Subcutaneous Tissue and Fascia, Back **8** Subcutaneous Tissue and Fascia, Abdomen **9** Subcutaneous Tissue and Fascia, Buttock **B** Subcutaneous Tissue and Fascia, Perineum **C** Subcutaneous Tissue and Fascia, Pelvic Region **D** Subcutaneous Tissue and Fascia, Right Upper Arm **F** Subcutaneous Tissue and Fascia, Left Upper Arm **G** Subcutaneous Tissue and Fascia, Right Lower Arm **H** Subcutaneous Tissue and Fascia, Left Lower Arm **J** Subcutaneous Tissue and Fascia, Right Hand **K** Subcutaneous Tissue and Fascia, Left Hand **L** Subcutaneous Tissue and Fascia, Right Upper Leg **M** Subcutaneous Tissue and Fascia, Left Upper Leg **N** Subcutaneous Tissue and Fascia, Right Lower Leg **P** Subcutaneous Tissue and Fascia, Left Lower Leg **Q** Subcutaneous Tissue and Fascia, Right Foot **R** Subcutaneous Tissue and Fascia, Left Foot	**0** Open **3** Percutaneous	**Z** No Device	**Z** No Qualifier

tion	0	**Medical and Surgical**
ly System	J	**Subcutaneous Tissue and Fascia**
eration	8	**Division:** Cutting into a body part, without draining fluids and/or gases from the body part, in order to separate or transect a body part

Body Part (4th)	Approach (5th)	Device (6th)	Qualifier (7th)
Subcutaneous Tissue and Fascia, Scalp	**0** Open	**Z** No Device	**Z** No Qualifier
Subcutaneous Tissue and Fascia, Face	**3** Percutaneous		
Subcutaneous Tissue and Fascia, Anterior Neck			
Subcutaneous Tissue and Fascia, Posterior Neck			
Subcutaneous Tissue and Fascia, Chest			
Subcutaneous Tissue and Fascia, Back			
Subcutaneous Tissue and Fascia, Abdomen			
Subcutaneous Tissue and Fascia, Buttock			
B Subcutaneous Tissue and Fascia, Perineum			
C Subcutaneous Tissue and Fascia, Pelvic Region			
D Subcutaneous Tissue and Fascia, Right Upper Arm			
F Subcutaneous Tissue and Fascia, Left Upper Arm			
G Subcutaneous Tissue and Fascia, Right Lower Arm			
H Subcutaneous Tissue and Fascia, Left Lower Arm			
J Subcutaneous Tissue and Fascia, Right Hand			
K Subcutaneous Tissue and Fascia, Left Hand			
L Subcutaneous Tissue and Fascia, Right Upper Leg			
M Subcutaneous Tissue and Fascia, Left Upper Leg			
N Subcutaneous Tissue and Fascia, Right Lower Leg			
P Subcutaneous Tissue and Fascia, Left Lower Leg			
Q Subcutaneous Tissue and Fascia, Right Foot			
R Subcutaneous Tissue and Fascia, Left Foot			
S Subcutaneous Tissue and Fascia, Head and Neck			
T Subcutaneous Tissue and Fascia, Trunk			
V Subcutaneous Tissue and Fascia, Upper Extremity			
W Subcutaneous Tissue and Fascia, Lower Extremity			

ction	0	**Medical and Surgical**
dy System	J	**Subcutaneous Tissue and Fascia**
peration	9	**Drainage:** Taking or letting out fluids and/or gases from a body part

Body Part (4th)	Approach (5th)	Device (6th)	Qualifier (7th)
0 Subcutaneous Tissue and Fascia, Scalp	**0** Open	**0** Drainage Device	**Z** No Qualifier
1 Subcutaneous Tissue and Fascia, Face	**3** Percutaneous		
4 Subcutaneous Tissue and Fascia, Anterior Neck			
5 Subcutaneous Tissue and Fascia, Posterior Neck			
6 Subcutaneous Tissue and Fascia, Chest			
7 Subcutaneous Tissue and Fascia, Back			
8 Subcutaneous Tissue and Fascia, Abdomen			
9 Subcutaneous Tissue and Fascia, Buttock			
B Subcutaneous Tissue and Fascia, Perineum			
C Subcutaneous Tissue and Fascia, Pelvic Region			
D Subcutaneous Tissue and Fascia, Right Upper Arm			
F Subcutaneous Tissue and Fascia, Left Upper Arm			
G Subcutaneous Tissue and Fascia, Right Lower Arm			
H Subcutaneous Tissue and Fascia, Left Lower Arm			
J Subcutaneous Tissue and Fascia, Right Hand			
K Subcutaneous Tissue and Fascia, Left Hand			
L Subcutaneous Tissue and Fascia, Right Upper Leg			
M Subcutaneous Tissue and Fascia, Left Upper Leg			
N Subcutaneous Tissue and Fascia, Right Lower Leg			
P Subcutaneous Tissue and Fascia, Left Lower Leg			
Q Subcutaneous Tissue and Fascia, Right Foot			
R Subcutaneous Tissue and Fascia, Left Foot			

Continued →

Section 0 **Medical and Surgical**
Body System J **Subcutaneous Tissue and Fascia**
Operation 9 **Drainage:** Taking or letting out fluids and/or gases from a body part

Body Part (4th)	Approach (5th)	Device (6th)	Qualifier (7th)
0 Subcutaneous Tissue and Fascia, Scalp	**0** Open	**Z** No Device	**X** Diagnostic
1 Subcutaneous Tissue and Fascia, Face	**3** Percutaneous		**Z** No Qualifier
4 Subcutaneous Tissue and Fascia, Anterior Neck			
5 Subcutaneous Tissue and Fascia, Posterior Neck			
6 Subcutaneous Tissue and Fascia, Chest			
7 Subcutaneous Tissue and Fascia, Back			
8 Subcutaneous Tissue and Fascia, Abdomen			
9 Subcutaneous Tissue and Fascia, Buttock			
B Subcutaneous Tissue and Fascia, Perineum			
C Subcutaneous Tissue and Fascia, Pelvic Region			
D Subcutaneous Tissue and Fascia, Right Upper Arm			
F Subcutaneous Tissue and Fascia, Left Upper Arm			
G Subcutaneous Tissue and Fascia, Right Lower Arm			
H Subcutaneous Tissue and Fascia, Left Lower Arm			
J Subcutaneous Tissue and Fascia, Right Hand			
K Subcutaneous Tissue and Fascia, Left Hand			
L Subcutaneous Tissue and Fascia, Right Upper Leg			
M Subcutaneous Tissue and Fascia, Left Upper Leg			
N Subcutaneous Tissue and Fascia, Right Lower Leg			
P Subcutaneous Tissue and Fascia, Left Lower Leg			
Q Subcutaneous Tissue and Fascia, Right Foot			
R Subcutaneous Tissue and Fascia, Left Foot			

Section 0 **Medical and Surgical**
Body System J **Subcutaneous Tissue and Fascia**
Operation B **Excision:** Cutting out or off, without replacement, a portion of a body part

Body Part (4th)	Approach (5th)	Device (6th)	Qualifier (7th)
0 Subcutaneous Tissue and Fascia, Scalp	**0** Open	**Z** No Device	**X** Diagnostic
1 Subcutaneous Tissue and Fascia, Face	**3** Percutaneous		**Z** No Qualifier
4 Subcutaneous Tissue and Fascia, Anterior Neck			
5 Subcutaneous Tissue and Fascia, Posterior Neck			
6 Subcutaneous Tissue and Fascia, Chest			
7 Subcutaneous Tissue and Fascia, Back			
8 Subcutaneous Tissue and Fascia, Abdomen			
9 Subcutaneous Tissue and Fascia, Buttock			
B Subcutaneous Tissue and Fascia, Perineum			
C Subcutaneous Tissue and Fascia, Pelvic Region			
D Subcutaneous Tissue and Fascia, Right Upper Arm			
F Subcutaneous Tissue and Fascia, Left Upper Arm			
G Subcutaneous Tissue and Fascia, Right Lower Arm			
H Subcutaneous Tissue and Fascia, Left Lower Arm			
J Subcutaneous Tissue and Fascia, Right Hand			
K Subcutaneous Tissue and Fascia, Left Hand			
L Subcutaneous Tissue and Fascia, Right Upper Leg			
M Subcutaneous Tissue and Fascia, Left Upper Leg			
N Subcutaneous Tissue and Fascia, Right Lower Leg			
P Subcutaneous Tissue and Fascia, Left Lower Leg			
Q Subcutaneous Tissue and Fascia, Right Foot			
R Subcutaneous Tissue and Fascia, Left Foot			

tion	0	**Medical and Surgical**
ly System	J	**Subcutaneous Tissue and Fascia**
eration	C	**Extirpation:** Taking or cutting out solid matter from a body part

Body Part (4th)	Approach (5th)	Device (6th)	Qualifier (7th)
Subcutaneous Tissue and Fascia, Scalp	**0** Open	**Z** No Device	**Z** No Qualifier
Subcutaneous Tissue and Fascia, Face	**3** Percutaneous		
Subcutaneous Tissue and Fascia, Anterior Neck			
Subcutaneous Tissue and Fascia, Posterior Neck			
Subcutaneous Tissue and Fascia, Chest			
Subcutaneous Tissue and Fascia, Back			
Subcutaneous Tissue and Fascia, Abdomen			
Subcutaneous Tissue and Fascia, Buttock			
Subcutaneous Tissue and Fascia, Perineum			
Subcutaneous Tissue and Fascia, Pelvic Region			
Subcutaneous Tissue and Fascia, Right Upper Arm			
Subcutaneous Tissue and Fascia, Left Upper Arm			
Subcutaneous Tissue and Fascia, Right Lower Arm			
Subcutaneous Tissue and Fascia, Left Lower Arm			
Subcutaneous Tissue and Fascia, Right Hand			
Subcutaneous Tissue and Fascia, Left Hand			
Subcutaneous Tissue and Fascia, Right Upper Leg			
M Subcutaneous Tissue and Fascia, Left Upper Leg			
Subcutaneous Tissue and Fascia, Right Lower Leg			
Subcutaneous Tissue and Fascia, Left Lower Leg			
Subcutaneous Tissue and Fascia, Right Foot			
R Subcutaneous Tissue and Fascia, Left Foot			

ction	0	**Medical and Surgical**
dy System	J	**Subcutaneous Tissue and Fascia**
eration	D	**Extraction:** Pulling or stripping out or off all or a portion of a body part by the use of force

Body Part (4th)	Approach (5th)	Device (6th)	Qualifier (7th)
Subcutaneous Tissue and Fascia, Scalp	**0** Open	**Z** No Device	**Z** No Qualifier
Subcutaneous Tissue and Fascia, Face	**3** Percutaneous		
Subcutaneous Tissue and Fascia, Anterior Neck			
5 Subcutaneous Tissue and Fascia, Posterior Neck			
Subcutaneous Tissue and Fascia, Chest			
7 Subcutaneous Tissue and Fascia, Back			
8 Subcutaneous Tissue and Fascia, Abdomen			
9 Subcutaneous Tissue and Fascia, Buttock			
B Subcutaneous Tissue and Fascia, Perineum			
C Subcutaneous Tissue and Fascia, Pelvic Region			
D Subcutaneous Tissue and Fascia, Right Upper Arm			
F Subcutaneous Tissue and Fascia, Left Upper Arm			
G Subcutaneous Tissue and Fascia, Right Lower Arm			
H Subcutaneous Tissue and Fascia, Left Lower Arm			
J Subcutaneous Tissue and Fascia, Right Hand			
K Subcutaneous Tissue and Fascia, Left Hand			
L Subcutaneous Tissue and Fascia, Right Upper Leg			
M Subcutaneous Tissue and Fascia, Left Upper Leg			
N Subcutaneous Tissue and Fascia, Right Lower Leg			
P Subcutaneous Tissue and Fascia, Left Lower Leg			
Q Subcutaneous Tissue and Fascia, Right Foot			
R Subcutaneous Tissue and Fascia, Left Foot			

Section	**0**	**Medical and Surgical**
Body System	**J**	**Subcutaneous Tissue and Fascia**
Operation	**H**	**Insertion:** Putting in a nonbiological appliance that monitors, assists, performs, or prevents a physiological function but do not physically take the place of a body part

Body Part (4th)	Approach (5th)	Device (6th)	Qualifier (7th
0 Subcutaneous Tissue and Fascia, Scalp **1** Subcutaneous Tissue and Fascia, Face **4** Subcutaneous Tissue and Fascia, Anterior Neck **5** Subcutaneous Tissue and Fascia, Posterior Neck **9** Subcutaneous Tissue and Fascia, Buttock **B** Subcutaneous Tissue and Fascia, Perineum **C** Subcutaneous Tissue and Fascia, Pelvic Region **J** Subcutaneous Tissue and Fascia, Right Hand **K** Subcutaneous Tissue and Fascia, Left Hand **Q** Subcutaneous Tissue and Fascia, Right Foot **R** Subcutaneous Tissue and Fascia, Left Foot	**0** Open **3** Percutaneous	**N** Tissue Expander	**Z** No Qualifier
6 Subcutaneous Tissue and Fascia, Chest **8** Subcutaneous Tissue and Fascia, Abdomen	**0** Open **3** Percutaneous	**0** Monitoring Device, Hemodynamic **2** Monitoring Device **4** Pacemaker, Single Chamber **5** Pacemaker, Single Chamber Rate Responsive **6** Pacemaker, Dual Chamber **7** Cardiac Resynchronization Pacemaker Pulse Generator **8** Defibrillator Generator **9** Cardiac Resynchronization Defibrillator Pulse Generator **A** Contractility Modulation Device **B** Stimulator Generator, Single Array **C** Stimulator Generator, Single Array Rechargeable **D** Stimulator Generator, Multiple Array **E** Stimulator Generator, Multiple Array Rechargeable **H** Contraceptive Device **M** Stimulator Generator **N** Tissue Expander **P** Cardiac Rhythm Related Device **V** Infusion Device, Pump **W** Vascular Access Device, Reservoir **X** Vascular Access Device	**Z** No Qualifier
7 Subcutaneous Tissue and Fascia, Back	**0** Open **3** Percutaneous	**B** Stimulator Generator, Single Array **C** Stimulator Generator, Single Array Rechargeable **D** Stimulator Generator, Multiple Array **E** Stimulator Generator, Multiple Array Rechargeable **M** Stimulator Generator **N** Tissue Expander **V** Infusion Device, Pump	**Z** No Qualifier
D Subcutaneous Tissue and Fascia, Right Upper Arm **F** Subcutaneous Tissue and Fascia, Left Upper Arm **G** Subcutaneous Tissue and Fascia, Right Lower Arm **H** Subcutaneous Tissue and Fascia, Left Lower Arm **L** Subcutaneous Tissue and Fascia, Right Upper Leg **M** Subcutaneous Tissue and Fascia, Left Upper Leg **N** Subcutaneous Tissue and Fascia, Right Lower Leg **P** Subcutaneous Tissue and Fascia, Left Lower Leg	**0** Open **3** Percutaneous	**H** Contraceptive Device **N** Tissue Expander **V** Infusion Device, Pump **W** Vascular Access Device, Reservoir **X** Vascular Access Device	**Z** No Qualifier
S Subcutaneous Tissue and Fascia, Head and Neck **V** Subcutaneous Tissue and Fascia, Upper Extremity **W** Subcutaneous Tissue and Fascia, Lower Extremity	**0** Open **3** Percutaneous	**1** Radioactive Element **3** Infusion Device	**Z** No Qualifier
T Subcutaneous Tissue and Fascia, Trunk	**0** Open **3** Percutaneous	**1** Radioactive Element **3** Infusion Device **V** Infusion Device, Pump	**Z** No Qualifier

Section 0 **Medical and Surgical**
Body System J **Subcutaneous Tissue and Fascia**
Operation J **Inspection:** Visually and/or manually exploring a body part

Body Part (4th)	Approach (5th)	Device (6th)	Qualifier (7th)
Subcutaneous Tissue and Fascia, Head and Neck Subcutaneous Tissue and Fascia, Trunk Subcutaneous Tissue and Fascia, Upper Extremity **W** Subcutaneous Tissue and Fascia, Lower Extremity	**0** Open **3** Percutaneous **X** External	**Z** No Device	**Z** No Qualifier

Section 0 **Medical and Surgical**
Body System J **Subcutaneous Tissue and Fascia**
Operation N **Release:** Freeing a body part from an abnormal physical constraint by cutting or by the use of force

Body Part (4th)	Approach (5th)	Device (6th)	Qualifier (7th)
Subcutaneous Tissue and Fascia, Scalp Subcutaneous Tissue and Fascia, Face Subcutaneous Tissue and Fascia, Anterior Neck **5** Subcutaneous Tissue and Fascia, Posterior Neck **6** Subcutaneous Tissue and Fascia, Chest **7** Subcutaneous Tissue and Fascia, Back **8** Subcutaneous Tissue and Fascia, Abdomen **9** Subcutaneous Tissue and Fascia, Buttock **B** Subcutaneous Tissue and Fascia, Perineum **C** Subcutaneous Tissue and Fascia, Pelvic Region **D** Subcutaneous Tissue and Fascia, Right Upper Arm **F** Subcutaneous Tissue and Fascia, Left Upper Arm **G** Subcutaneous Tissue and Fascia, Right Lower Arm **H** Subcutaneous Tissue and Fascia, Left Lower Arm **J** Subcutaneous Tissue and Fascia, Right Hand **K** Subcutaneous Tissue and Fascia, Left Hand **L** Subcutaneous Tissue and Fascia, Right Upper Leg **M** Subcutaneous Tissue and Fascia, Left Upper Leg **N** Subcutaneous Tissue and Fascia, Right Lower Leg **P** Subcutaneous Tissue and Fascia, Left Lower Leg **Q** Subcutaneous Tissue and Fascia, Right Foot **R** Subcutaneous Tissue and Fascia, Left Foot	**0** Open **3** Percutaneous **X** External	**Z** No Device	**Z** No Qualifier

Section 0 **Medical and Surgical**
Body System J **Subcutaneous Tissue and Fascia**
Operation P **Removal:** Taking out or off a device from a body part

Body Part (4th)	Approach (5th)	Device (6th)	Qualifier (7th)
S Subcutaneous Tissue and Fascia, Head and Neck	**0** Open **3** Percutaneous	**0** Drainage Device **1** Radioactive Element **3** Infusion Device **7** Autologous Tissue Substitute **J** Synthetic Substitute **K** Nonautologous Tissue Substitute **N** Tissue Expander	**Z** No Qualifier
S Subcutaneous Tissue and Fascia, Head and Neck	**X** External	**0** Drainage Device **1** Radioactive Element **3** Infusion Device	**Z** No Qualifier

Continued →

Section 0 **Medical and Surgical**
Body System J **Subcutaneous Tissue and Fascia**
Operation P **Removal:** Taking out or off a device from a body part

0JP Contin

Body Part (4th)	Approach (5th)	Device (6th)	Qualifier (7th)
T Subcutaneous Tissue and Fascia, Trunk	**0** Open **3** Percutaneous	**0** Drainage Device **1** Radioactive Element **2** Monitoring Device **3** Infusion Device **7** Autologous Tissue Substitute **H** Contraceptive Device **J** Synthetic Substitute **K** Nonautologous Tissue Substitute **M** Stimulator Generator **N** Tissue Expander **P** Cardiac Rhythm Related Device **V** Infusion Device, Pump **W** Vascular Access Device, Reservoir **X** Vascular Access Device	**Z** No Qualifier
T Subcutaneous Tissue and Fascia, Trunk	**X** External	**0** Drainage Device **1** Radioactive Element **2** Monitoring Device **3** Infusion Device **H** Contraceptive Device **V** Infusion Device, Pump **X** Vascular Access Device	**Z** No Qualifier
V Subcutaneous Tissue and Fascia, Upper Extremity **W** Subcutaneous Tissue and Fascia, Lower Extremity	**0** Open **3** Percutaneous	**0** Drainage Device **1** Radioactive Element **3** Infusion Device **7** Autologous Tissue Substitute **H** Contraceptive Device **J** Synthetic Substitute **K** Nonautologous Tissue Substitute **N** Tissue Expander **V** Infusion Device, Pump **W** Vascular Access Device, Reservoir **X** Vascular Access Device	**Z** No Qualifier
V Subcutaneous Tissue and Fascia, Upper Extremity **W** Subcutaneous Tissue and Fascia, Lower Extremity	**X** External	**0** Drainage Device **1** Radioactive Element **3** Infusion Device **H** Contraceptive Device **V** Infusion Device, Pump **X** Vascular Access Device	**Z** No Qualifier

Section 0 **Medical and Surgical**
Body System J **Subcutaneous Tissue and Fascia**
Operation Q **Repair:** Restoring, to the extent possible, a body part to its normal anatomic structure and function

Body Part (4th)	Approach (5th)	Device (6th)	Qualifier (7th)
0 Subcutaneous Tissue and Fascia, Scalp	**0** Open	**Z** No Device	**Z** No Qualifier
1 Subcutaneous Tissue and Fascia, Face	**3** Percutaneous		
4 Subcutaneous Tissue and Fascia, Anterior Neck			
5 Subcutaneous Tissue and Fascia, Posterior Neck			
6 Subcutaneous Tissue and Fascia, Chest			
7 Subcutaneous Tissue and Fascia, Back			
8 Subcutaneous Tissue and Fascia, Abdomen			
9 Subcutaneous Tissue and Fascia, Buttock			
B Subcutaneous Tissue and Fascia, Perineum			
C Subcutaneous Tissue and Fascia, Pelvic Region			
D Subcutaneous Tissue and Fascia, Right Upper Arm			
F Subcutaneous Tissue and Fascia, Left Upper Arm			
G Subcutaneous Tissue and Fascia, Right Lower Arm			
H Subcutaneous Tissue and Fascia, Left Lower Arm			
J Subcutaneous Tissue and Fascia, Right Hand			
K Subcutaneous Tissue and Fascia, Left Hand			
L Subcutaneous Tissue and Fascia, Right Upper Leg			
M Subcutaneous Tissue and Fascia, Left Upper Leg			
N Subcutaneous Tissue and Fascia, Right Lower Leg			
P Subcutaneous Tissue and Fascia, Left Lower Leg			
Q Subcutaneous Tissue and Fascia, Right Foot			
R Subcutaneous Tissue and Fascia, Left Foot			

Section 0 **Medical and Surgical**
Body System J **Subcutaneous Tissue and Fascia**
Operation R **Replacement:** Putting in or on biological or synthetic material that physically takes the place and/or function of all or a portion of a body part

Body Part (4th)	Approach (5th)	Device (6th)	Qualifier (7th)
0 Subcutaneous Tissue and Fascia, Scalp	**0** Open	**7** Autologous Tissue Substitute	**Z** No Qualifier
1 Subcutaneous Tissue and Fascia, Face	**3** Percutaneous	**J** Synthetic Substitute	
4 Subcutaneous Tissue and Fascia, Anterior Neck		**K** Nonautologous Tissue Substitute	
5 Subcutaneous Tissue and Fascia, Posterior Neck			
6 Subcutaneous Tissue and Fascia, Chest			
7 Subcutaneous Tissue and Fascia, Back			
8 Subcutaneous Tissue and Fascia, Abdomen			
9 Subcutaneous Tissue and Fascia, Buttock			
B Subcutaneous Tissue and Fascia, Perineum			
C Subcutaneous Tissue and Fascia, Pelvic Region			
D Subcutaneous Tissue and Fascia, Right Upper Arm			
F Subcutaneous Tissue and Fascia, Left Upper Arm			
G Subcutaneous Tissue and Fascia, Right Lower Arm			
H Subcutaneous Tissue and Fascia, Left Lower Arm			
J Subcutaneous Tissue and Fascia, Right Hand			
K Subcutaneous Tissue and Fascia, Left Hand			
L Subcutaneous Tissue and Fascia, Right Upper Leg			
M Subcutaneous Tissue and Fascia, Left Upper Leg			
N Subcutaneous Tissue and Fascia, Right Lower Leg			
P Subcutaneous Tissue and Fascia, Left Lower Leg			
Q Subcutaneous Tissue and Fascia, Right Foot			
R Subcutaneous Tissue and Fascia, Left Foot			

Section 0 **Medical and Surgical**
Body System J **Subcutaneous Tissue and Fascia**
Operation U **Supplement:** Putting in or on biological or synthetic material that physically reinforces and/or augments the function of a portion of a body part

Body Part (4th)	Approach (5th)	Device (6th)	Qualifier (7th)
0 Subcutaneous Tissue and Fascia, Scalp **1** Subcutaneous Tissue and Fascia, Face **4** Subcutaneous Tissue and Fascia, Anterior Neck **5** Subcutaneous Tissue and Fascia, Posterior Neck **6** Subcutaneous Tissue and Fascia, Chest **7** Subcutaneous Tissue and Fascia, Back **8** Subcutaneous Tissue and Fascia, Abdomen **9** Subcutaneous Tissue and Fascia, Buttock **B** Subcutaneous Tissue and Fascia, Perineum **C** Subcutaneous Tissue and Fascia, Pelvic Region **D** Subcutaneous Tissue and Fascia, Right Upper Arm **F** Subcutaneous Tissue and Fascia, Left Upper Arm **G** Subcutaneous Tissue and Fascia, Right Lower Arm **H** Subcutaneous Tissue and Fascia, Left Lower Arm **J** Subcutaneous Tissue and Fascia, Right Hand **K** Subcutaneous Tissue and Fascia, Left Hand **L** Subcutaneous Tissue and Fascia, Right Upper Leg **M** Subcutaneous Tissue and Fascia, Left Upper Leg **N** Subcutaneous Tissue and Fascia, Right Lower Leg **P** Subcutaneous Tissue and Fascia, Left Lower Leg **Q** Subcutaneous Tissue and Fascia, Right Foot **R** Subcutaneous Tissue and Fascia, Left Foot	**0** Open **3** Percutaneous	**7** Autologous Tissue Substitute **J** Synthetic Substitute **K** Nonautologous Tissue Substitute	**Z** No Qualifier

Section 0 **Medical and Surgical**
Body System J **Subcutaneous Tissue and Fascia**
Operation W **Revision:** Correcting, to the extent possible, a portion of a malfunctioning device or the position of a displaced device

Body Part (4th)	Approach (5th)	Device (6th)	Qualifier (7th)
S Subcutaneous Tissue and Fascia, Head and Neck	**0** Open **3** Percutaneous **X** External	**0** Drainage Device **3** Infusion Device **7** Autologous Tissue Substitute **J** Synthetic Substitute **K** Nonautologous Tissue Substitute **N** Tissue Expander	**Z** No Qualifier
T Subcutaneous Tissue and Fascia, Trunk	**0** Open **3** Percutaneous **X** External	**0** Drainage Device **2** Monitoring Device **3** Infusion Device **7** Autologous Tissue Substitute **H** Contraceptive Device **J** Synthetic Substitute **K** Nonautologous Tissue Substitute **M** Stimulator Generator **N** Tissue Expander **P** Cardiac Rhythm Related Device **V** Infusion Device, Pump **W** Vascular Access Device, Reservoir **X** Vascular Access Device	**Z** No Qualifier
V Subcutaneous Tissue and Fascia, Upper Extremity **W** Subcutaneous Tissue and Fascia, Lower Extremity	**0** Open **3** Percutaneous **X** External	**0** Drainage Device **3** Infusion Device **7** Autologous Tissue Substitute **H** Contraceptive Device **J** Synthetic Substitute **K** Nonautologous Tissue Substitute **N** Tissue Expander **V** Infusion Device, Pump **W** Vascular Access Device, Reservoir **X** Vascular Access Device	**Z** No Qualifier

ction 0 **Medical and Surgical**
dy System J **Subcutaneous Tissue and Fascia**
eration X **Transfer:** Moving, without taking out, all or a portion of a body part to another location to take over the function of all or a portion of a body part

Body Part (4th)	Approach (5th)	Device (6th)	Qualifier (7th)
0 Subcutaneous Tissue and Fascia, Scalp 1 Subcutaneous Tissue and Fascia, Face 4 Subcutaneous Tissue and Fascia, Anterior Neck 5 Subcutaneous Tissue and Fascia, Posterior Neck 6 Subcutaneous Tissue and Fascia, Chest 7 Subcutaneous Tissue and Fascia, Back 8 Subcutaneous Tissue and Fascia, Abdomen 9 Subcutaneous Tissue and Fascia, Buttock B Subcutaneous Tissue and Fascia, Perineum C Subcutaneous Tissue and Fascia, Pelvic Region D Subcutaneous Tissue and Fascia, Right Upper Arm F Subcutaneous Tissue and Fascia, Left Upper Arm G Subcutaneous Tissue and Fascia, Right Lower Arm H Subcutaneous Tissue and Fascia, Left Lower Arm J Subcutaneous Tissue and Fascia, Right Hand K Subcutaneous Tissue and Fascia, Left Hand L Subcutaneous Tissue and Fascia, Right Upper Leg M Subcutaneous Tissue and Fascia, Left Upper Leg N Subcutaneous Tissue and Fascia, Right Lower Leg P Subcutaneous Tissue and Fascia, Left Lower Leg Q Subcutaneous Tissue and Fascia, Right Foot R Subcutaneous Tissue and Fascia, Left Foot	0 Open 3 Percutaneous	Z No Device	B Skin and Subcutaneous Tissue C Skin, Subcutaneous Tissue and Fascia Z No Qualifier

ubcutaneous Tissue and Fascia Code Listing 0J0–0JX

eview Coding Guideline B4.5

eview Coding Guideline B4.6

J0 – Subcutaneous Tissue and Fascia, Alteration

J010ZZ Alteration of Face Subcutaneous Tissue and Fascia, Open Approach
J013ZZ Alteration of Face Subcutaneous Tissue and Fascia, Percutaneous Approach
J040ZZ Alteration of Anterior Neck Subcutaneous Tissue and Fascia, Open Approach
J043ZZ Alteration of Anterior Neck Subcutaneous Tissue and Fascia, Percutaneous Approach
J050ZZ Alteration of Posterior Neck Subcutaneous Tissue and Fascia, Open Approach
J053ZZ Alteration of Posterior Neck Subcutaneous Tissue and Fascia, Percutaneous Approach
J060ZZ Alteration of Chest Subcutaneous Tissue and Fascia, Open Approach
J063ZZ Alteration of Chest Subcutaneous Tissue and Fascia, Percutaneous Approach
J070ZZ Alteration of Back Subcutaneous Tissue and Fascia, Open Approach
J073ZZ Alteration of Back Subcutaneous Tissue and Fascia, Percutaneous Approach
J080ZZ Alteration of Abdomen Subcutaneous Tissue and Fascia, Open Approach
J083ZZ Alteration of Abdomen Subcutaneous Tissue and Fascia, Percutaneous Approach
J090ZZ Alteration of Buttock Subcutaneous Tissue and Fascia, Open Approach
0J093ZZ Alteration of Buttock Subcutaneous Tissue and Fascia, Percutaneous Approach
0J0D0ZZ Alteration of Right Upper Arm Subcutaneous Tissue and Fascia, Open Approach
0J0D3ZZ Alteration of Right Upper Arm Subcutaneous Tissue and Fascia, Percutaneous Approach
0J0F0ZZ Alteration of Left Upper Arm Subcutaneous Tissue and Fascia, Open Approach
0J0F3ZZ Alteration of Left Upper Arm Subcutaneous Tissue and Fascia, Percutaneous Approach
0J0G0ZZ Alteration of Right Lower Arm Subcutaneous Tissue and Fascia, Open Approach
0J0G3ZZ Alteration of Right Lower Arm Subcutaneous Tissue and Fascia, Percutaneous Approach
0J0H0ZZ Alteration of Left Lower Arm Subcutaneous Tissue and Fascia, Open Approach
0J0H3ZZ Alteration of Left Lower Arm Subcutaneous Tissue and Fascia, Percutaneous Approach
0J0L0ZZ Alteration of Right Upper Leg Subcutaneous Tissue and Fascia, Open Approach
0J0L3ZZ Alteration of Right Upper Leg Subcutaneous Tissue and Fascia, Percutaneous Approach
0J0M0ZZ Alteration of Left Upper Leg Subcutaneous Tissue and Fascia, Open Approach
0J0M3ZZ Alteration of Left Upper Leg Subcutaneous Tissue and Fascia, Percutaneous Approach
0J0N0ZZ Alteration of Right Lower Leg Subcutaneous Tissue and Fascia, Open Approach
0J0N3ZZ Alteration of Right Lower Leg Subcutaneous Tissue and Fascia, Percutaneous Approach
0J0P0ZZ Alteration of Left Lower Leg Subcutaneous Tissue and Fascia, Open Approach
0J0P3ZZ Alteration of Left Lower Leg Subcutaneous Tissue and Fascia, Percutaneous Approach

J2 – Subcutaneous Tissue and Fascia, Change

Review Coding Guideline B6.1c

J2SX0Z Change Drainage Device in Head and Neck Subcutaneous Tissue and Fascia, External Approach
J2SXYZ Change Other Device in Head and Neck Subcutaneous Tissue and Fascia, External Approach
0J2TX0Z Change Drainage Device in Trunk Subcutaneous Tissue and Fascia, External Approach
0J2TXYZ Change Other Device in Trunk Subcutaneous Tissue and Fascia, External Approach
0J2VX0Z Change Drainage Device in Upper Extremity Subcutaneous Tissue and Fascia, External Approach
0J2VXYZ Change Other Device in Upper Extremity Subcutaneous Tissue and Fascia, External Approach

0J2WX0Z Change Drainage Device in Lower Extremity Subcutaneous Tissue and Fascia, External Approach

0J2WXYZ Change Other Device in Lower Extremity Subcutaneous Tissue and Fascia, External Approach

0J5 – Subcutaneous Tissue and Fascia, Destruction

● **0J500ZZ** Destruction of Scalp Subcutaneous Tissue and Fascia, Open Approach

● **0J503ZZ** Destruction of Scalp Subcutaneous Tissue and Fascia, Percutaneous Approach

● **0J510ZZ** Destruction of Face Subcutaneous Tissue and Fascia, Open Approach

● **0J513ZZ** Destruction of Face Subcutaneous Tissue and Fascia, Percutaneous Approach

● **0J540ZZ** Destruction of Anterior Neck Subcutaneous Tissue and Fascia, Open Approach

● **0J543ZZ** Destruction of Anterior Neck Subcutaneous Tissue and Fascia, Percutaneous Approach

● **0J550ZZ** Destruction of Posterior Neck Subcutaneous Tissue and Fascia, Open Approach

● **0J553ZZ** Destruction of Posterior Neck Subcutaneous Tissue and Fascia, Percutaneous Approach

● **0J560ZZ** Destruction of Chest Subcutaneous Tissue and Fascia, Open Approach

● **0J563ZZ** Destruction of Chest Subcutaneous Tissue and Fascia, Percutaneous Approach

● **0J570ZZ** Destruction of Back Subcutaneous Tissue and Fascia, Open Approach

● **0J573ZZ** Destruction of Back Subcutaneous Tissue and Fascia, Percutaneous Approach

● **0J580ZZ** Destruction of Abdomen Subcutaneous Tissue and Fascia, Open Approach

● **0J583ZZ** Destruction of Abdomen Subcutaneous Tissue and Fascia, Percutaneous Approach

● **0J590ZZ** Destruction of Buttock Subcutaneous Tissue and Fascia, Open Approach

● **0J593ZZ** Destruction of Buttock Subcutaneous Tissue and Fascia, Percutaneous Approach

● **0J5B0ZZ** Destruction of Perineum Subcutaneous Tissue and Fascia, Open Approach

● **0J5B3ZZ** Destruction of Perineum Subcutaneous Tissue and Fascia, Percutaneous Approach

● **0J5C0ZZ** Destruction of Pelvic Region Subcutaneous Tissue and Fascia, Open Approach

● **0J5C3ZZ** Destruction of Pelvic Region Subcutaneous Tissue and Fascia, Percutaneous Approach

● **0J5D0ZZ** Destruction of Right Upper Arm Subcutaneous Tissue and Fascia, Open Approach

● **0J5D3ZZ** Destruction of Right Upper Arm Subcutaneous Tissue and Fascia, Percutaneous Approach

● **0J5F0ZZ** Destruction of Left Upper Arm Subcutaneous Tissue and Fascia, Open Approach

● **0J5F3ZZ** Destruction of Left Upper Arm Subcutaneous Tissue and Fascia, Percutaneous Approach

● **0J5G0ZZ** Destruction of Right Lower Arm Subcutaneous Tissue and Fascia, Open Approach

● **0J5G3ZZ** Destruction of Right Lower Arm Subcutaneous Tissue and Fascia, Percutaneous Approach

● **0J5H0ZZ** Destruction of Left Lower Arm Subcutaneous Tissue and Fascia, Open Approach

● **0J5H3ZZ** Destruction of Left Lower Arm Subcutaneous Tissue and Fascia, Percutaneous Approach

● **0J5J0ZZ** Destruction of Right Hand Subcutaneous Tissue and Fascia, Open Approach

● **0J5J3ZZ** Destruction of Right Hand Subcutaneous Tissue and Fascia, Percutaneous Approach

● **0J5K0ZZ** Destruction of Left Hand Subcutaneous Tissue and Fascia, Open Approach

● **0J5K3ZZ** Destruction of Left Hand Subcutaneous Tissue and Fascia, Percutaneous Approa

● **0J5L0ZZ** Destruction of Right Upper Leg Subcutaneous Tissue and Fascia, Open Approach

● **0J5L3ZZ** Destruction of Right Upper Leg Subcutaneous Tissue and Fascia, Percutaneous Approach

● **0J5M0ZZ** Destruction of Left Upper Leg Subcutaneous Tissue and Fascia, Open Approach

● **0J5M3ZZ** Destruction of Left Upper Leg Subcutaneous Tissue and Fascia, Percutaneous Approach

● **0J5N0ZZ** Destruction of Right Lower Leg Subcutaneous Tissue and Fascia, Open Approach

● **0J5N3ZZ** Destruction of Right Lower Leg Subcutaneous Tissue and Fascia, Percutaneous Approach

● **0J5P0ZZ** Destruction of Left Lower Leg Subcutaneous Tissue and Fascia, Open Approach

● **0J5P3ZZ** Destruction of Left Lower Leg Subcutaneous Tissue and Fascia, Percutaneous Approach

● **0J5Q0ZZ** Destruction of Right Foot Subcutaneous Tissue and Fascia, Open Approach

● **0J5Q3ZZ** Destruction of Right Foot Subcutaneous Tissue and Fascia, Percutaneous Approac

● **0J5R0ZZ** Destruction of Left Foot Subcutaneous Tissue and Fascia, Open Approach

● **0J5R3ZZ** Destruction of Left Foot Subcutaneous Tissue and Fascia, Percutaneous Approac

0J8 – Subcutaneous Tissue and Fascia, Division

Review Coding Guideline B3.14

0J800ZZ Division of Scalp Subcutaneous Tissue and Fascia, Open Approach

0J803ZZ Division of Scalp Subcutaneous Tissue and Fascia, Percutaneous Approach

0J810ZZ Division of Face Subcutaneous Tissue and Fascia, Open Approach

0J813ZZ Division of Face Subcutaneous Tissue and Fascia, Percutaneous Approach

0J840ZZ Division of Anterior Neck Subcutaneous Tissue and Fascia, Open Approach

0J843ZZ Division of Anterior Neck Subcutaneous Tissue and Fascia, Percutaneous Approach

0J850ZZ Division of Posterior Neck Subcutaneous Tissue and Fascia, Open Approach

0J853ZZ Division of Posterior Neck Subcutaneous Tissue and Fascia, Percutaneous Approach

0J860ZZ Division of Chest Subcutaneous Tissue and Fascia, Open Approach

0J863ZZ Division of Chest Subcutaneous Tissue and Fascia, Percutaneous Approach

0J870ZZ Division of Back Subcutaneous Tissue and Fascia, Open Approach

0J873ZZ Division of Back Subcutaneous Tissue and Fascia, Percutaneous Approach

0J880ZZ Division of Abdomen Subcutaneous Tissue and Fascia, Open Approach

0J883ZZ Division of Abdomen Subcutaneous Tissue and Fascia, Percutaneous Approach

0J890ZZ Division of Buttock Subcutaneous Tissue and Fascia, Open Approach

0J893ZZ Division of Buttock Subcutaneous Tissue and Fascia, Percutaneous Approach

0J8B0ZZ Division of Perineum Subcutaneous Tissue and Fascia, Open Approach

0J8B3ZZ Division of Perineum Subcutaneous Tissue and Fascia, Percutaneous Approach

0J8C0ZZ Division of Pelvic Region Subcutaneous Tissue and Fascia, Open Approach

0J8C3ZZ Division of Pelvic Region Subcutaneous Tissue and Fascia, Percutaneous Approach

0J8D0ZZ Division of Right Upper Arm Subcutaneous Tissue and Fascia, Open Approach

0J8D3ZZ Division of Right Upper Arm Subcutaneous Tissue and Fascia, Percutaneous Approach

0J8F0ZZ Division of Left Upper Arm Subcutaneous Tissue and Fascia, Open Approach

0J8F3ZZ Division of Left Upper Arm Subcutaneous Tissue and Fascia, Percutaneous Approach

0J8G0ZZ Division of Right Lower Arm Subcutaneous Tissue and Fascia, Open Approach

0J8G3ZZ Division of Right Lower Arm Subcutaneous Tissue and Fascia, Percutaneous Approach

0J8H0ZZ Division of Left Lower Arm Subcutaneou Tissue and Fascia, Open Approach

0J8H3ZZ Division of Left Lower Arm Subcutaneou Tissue and Fascia, Percutaneous Approac

0J8J0ZZ Division of Right Hand Subcutaneous Tissue and Fascia, Open Approach

0J8J3ZZ Division of Right Hand Subcutaneous Tissue and Fascia, Percutaneous Approac

0J8K0ZZ Division of Left Hand Subcutaneous Tissue and Fascia, Open Approach

0J8K3ZZ Division of Left Hand Subcutaneous Tissue and Fascia, Percutaneous Approac

0J8L0ZZ Division of Right Upper Leg Subcutaneous Tissue and Fascia, Open Approach

0J8L3ZZ Division of Right Upper Leg Subcutaneous Tissue and Fascia, Percutaneous Approach

0J8M0ZZ Division of Left Upper Leg Subcutaneous Tissue and Fascia, Open Approach

0J8M3ZZ Division of Left Upper Leg Subcutaneous Tissue and Fascia, Percutaneous Approach

0J8N0ZZ Division of Right Lower Leg Subcutaneous Tissue and Fascia, Open Approach

0J8N3ZZ Division of Right Lower Leg Subcutaneous Tissue and Fascia, Percutaneous Approach

·P0ZZ	Division of Left Lower Leg Subcutaneous Tissue and Fascia, Open Approach
·P3ZZ	Division of Left Lower Leg Subcutaneous Tissue and Fascia, Percutaneous Approach
·Q0ZZ	Division of Right Foot Subcutaneous Tissue and Fascia, Open Approach
·Q3ZZ	Division of Right Foot Subcutaneous Tissue and Fascia, Percutaneous Approach
·R0ZZ	Division of Left Foot Subcutaneous Tissue and Fascia, Open Approach
0J8R3ZZ	Division of Left Foot Subcutaneous Tissue and Fascia, Percutaneous Approach
0J8S0ZZ	Division of Head and Neck Subcutaneous Tissue and Fascia, Open Approach
0J8S3ZZ	Division of Head and Neck Subcutaneous Tissue and Fascia, Percutaneous Approach
0J8T0ZZ	Division of Trunk Subcutaneous Tissue and Fascia, Open Approach
0J8T3ZZ	Division of Trunk Subcutaneous Tissue and Fascia, Percutaneous Approach
0J8V0ZZ	Division of Upper Extremity Subcutaneous Tissue and Fascia, Open Approach
0J8V3ZZ	Division of Upper Extremity Subcutaneous Tissue and Fascia, Percutaneous Approach
0J8W0ZZ	Division of Lower Extremity Subcutaneous Tissue and Fascia, Open Approach
0J8W3ZZ	Division of Lower Extremity Subcutaneous Tissue and Fascia, Percutaneous Approach

9 – Subcutaneous Tissue and Fascia, Drainage

·view Coding Guidelines B3.4a and B3.4b

·view Coding Guideline B6.2

9000Z	Drainage of Scalp Subcutaneous Tissue and Fascia with Drainage Device, Open Approach
900ZX	Drainage of Scalp Subcutaneous Tissue and Fascia, Open Approach, Diagnostic
900ZZ	Drainage of Scalp Subcutaneous Tissue and Fascia, Open Approach
9030Z	Drainage of Scalp Subcutaneous Tissue and Fascia with Drainage Device, Percutaneous Approach
903ZX	Drainage of Scalp Subcutaneous Tissue and Fascia, Percutaneous Approach, Diagnostic
903ZZ	Drainage of Scalp Subcutaneous Tissue and Fascia, Percutaneous Approach
9100Z	Drainage of Face Subcutaneous Tissue and Fascia with Drainage Device, Open Approach
910ZX	Drainage of Face Subcutaneous Tissue and Fascia, Open Approach, Diagnostic
910ZZ	Drainage of Face Subcutaneous Tissue and Fascia, Open Approach
9130Z	Drainage of Face Subcutaneous Tissue and Fascia with Drainage Device, Percutaneous Approach
913ZX	Drainage of Face Subcutaneous Tissue and Fascia, Percutaneous Approach, Diagnostic
913ZZ	Drainage of Face Subcutaneous Tissue and Fascia, Percutaneous Approach
9400Z	Drainage of Anterior Neck Subcutaneous Tissue and Fascia with Drainage Device, Open Approach
J940ZX	Drainage of Anterior Neck Subcutaneous Tissue and Fascia, Open Approach, Diagnostic
J940ZZ	Drainage of Anterior Neck Subcutaneous Tissue and Fascia, Open Approach
J9430Z	Drainage of Anterior Neck Subcutaneous Tissue and Fascia with Drainage Device, Percutaneous Approach
J943ZX	Drainage of Anterior Neck Subcutaneous Tissue and Fascia, Percutaneous Approach, Diagnostic
J943ZZ	Drainage of Anterior Neck Subcutaneous Tissue and Fascia, Percutaneous Approach
·J9500Z	Drainage of Posterior Neck Subcutaneous Tissue and Fascia with Drainage Device, Open Approach
·J950ZX	Drainage of Posterior Neck Subcutaneous Tissue and Fascia, Open Approach, Diagnostic
·J950ZZ	Drainage of Posterior Neck Subcutaneous Tissue and Fascia, Open Approach
·J9530Z	Drainage of Posterior Neck Subcutaneous Tissue and Fascia with Drainage Device, Percutaneous Approach
·J953ZX	Drainage of Posterior Neck Subcutaneous Tissue and Fascia, Percutaneous Approach, Diagnostic
)J953ZZ	Drainage of Posterior Neck Subcutaneous Tissue and Fascia, Percutaneous Approach
0J9600Z	Drainage of Chest Subcutaneous Tissue and Fascia with Drainage Device, Open Approach
0J960ZX	Drainage of Chest Subcutaneous Tissue and Fascia, Open Approach, Diagnostic
0J960ZZ	Drainage of Chest Subcutaneous Tissue and Fascia, Open Approach
0J9630Z	Drainage of Chest Subcutaneous Tissue and Fascia with Drainage Device, Percutaneous Approach
0J963ZX	Drainage of Chest Subcutaneous Tissue and Fascia, Percutaneous Approach, Diagnostic
0J963ZZ	Drainage of Chest Subcutaneous Tissue and Fascia, Percutaneous Approach
0J9700Z	Drainage of Back Subcutaneous Tissue and Fascia with Drainage Device, Open Approach
0J970ZX	Drainage of Back Subcutaneous Tissue and Fascia, Open Approach, Diagnostic
0J970ZZ	Drainage of Back Subcutaneous Tissue and Fascia, Open Approach
0J9730Z	Drainage of Back Subcutaneous Tissue and Fascia with Drainage Device, Percutaneous Approach
0J973ZX	Drainage of Back Subcutaneous Tissue and Fascia, Percutaneous Approach, Diagnostic
0J973ZZ	Drainage of Back Subcutaneous Tissue and Fascia, Percutaneous Approach
0J9800Z	Drainage of Abdomen Subcutaneous Tissue and Fascia with Drainage Device, Open Approach
0J980ZX	Drainage of Abdomen Subcutaneous Tissue and Fascia, Open Approach, Diagnostic
0J980ZZ	Drainage of Abdomen Subcutaneous Tissue and Fascia, Open Approach
0J9830Z	Drainage of Abdomen Subcutaneous Tissue and Fascia with Drainage Device, Percutaneous Approach
0J983ZX	Drainage of Abdomen Subcutaneous Tissue and Fascia, Percutaneous Approach, Diagnostic
0J983ZZ	Drainage of Abdomen Subcutaneous Tissue and Fascia, Percutaneous Approach
0J9900Z	Drainage of Buttock Subcutaneous Tissue and Fascia with Drainage Device, Open Approach
0J990ZX	Drainage of Buttock Subcutaneous Tissue and Fascia, Open Approach, Diagnostic
0J990ZZ	Drainage of Buttock Subcutaneous Tissue and Fascia, Open Approach
0J9930Z	Drainage of Buttock Subcutaneous Tissue and Fascia with Drainage Device, Percutaneous Approach
0J993ZX	Drainage of Buttock Subcutaneous Tissue and Fascia, Percutaneous Approach, Diagnostic
0J993ZZ	Drainage of Buttock Subcutaneous Tissue and Fascia, Percutaneous Approach
0J9B00Z	Drainage of Perineum Subcutaneous Tissue and Fascia with Drainage Device, Open Approach
0J9B0ZX	Drainage of Perineum Subcutaneous Tissue and Fascia, Open Approach, Diagnostic
0J9B0ZZ	Drainage of Perineum Subcutaneous Tissue and Fascia, Open Approach
0J9B30Z	Drainage of Perineum Subcutaneous Tissue and Fascia with Drainage Device, Percutaneous Approach
0J9B3ZX	Drainage of Perineum Subcutaneous Tissue and Fascia, Percutaneous Approach, Diagnostic
0J9B3ZZ	Drainage of Perineum Subcutaneous Tissue and Fascia, Percutaneous Approach
0J9C00Z	Drainage of Pelvic Region Subcutaneous Tissue and Fascia with Drainage Device, Open Approach
0J9C0ZX	Drainage of Pelvic Region Subcutaneous Tissue and Fascia, Open Approach, Diagnostic
0J9C0ZZ	Drainage of Pelvic Region Subcutaneous Tissue and Fascia, Open Approach
0J9C30Z	Drainage of Pelvic Region Subcutaneous Tissue and Fascia with Drainage Device, Percutaneous Approach
0J9C3ZX	Drainage of Pelvic Region Subcutaneous Tissue and Fascia, Percutaneous Approach, Diagnostic
0J9C3ZZ	Drainage of Pelvic Region Subcutaneous Tissue and Fascia, Percutaneous Approach
0J9D00Z	Drainage of Right Upper Arm Subcutaneous Tissue and Fascia with Drainage Device, Open Approach
0J9D0ZX	Drainage of Right Upper Arm Subcutaneous Tissue and Fascia, Open Approach, Diagnostic
0J9D0ZZ	Drainage of Right Upper Arm Subcutaneous Tissue and Fascia, Open Approach
0J9D30Z	Drainage of Right Upper Arm Subcutaneous Tissue and Fascia with Drainage Device, Percutaneous Approach
0J9D3ZX	Drainage of Right Upper Arm Subcutaneous Tissue and Fascia, Percutaneous Approach, Diagnostic
0J9D3ZZ	Drainage of Right Upper Arm Subcutaneous Tissue and Fascia, Percutaneous Approach
0J9F00Z	Drainage of Left Upper Arm Subcutaneous Tissue and Fascia with Drainage Device, Open Approach
0J9F0ZX	Drainage of Left Upper Arm Subcutaneous Tissue and Fascia, Open Approach, Diagnostic
0J9F0ZZ	Drainage of Left Upper Arm Subcutaneous Tissue and Fascia, Open Approach
0J9F30Z	Drainage of Left Upper Arm Subcutaneous Tissue and Fascia with Drainage Device, Percutaneous Approach

0J9F3ZX Drainage of Left Upper Arm Subcutaneous Tissue and Fascia, Percutaneous Approach, Diagnostic
0J9F3ZZ Drainage of Left Upper Arm Subcutaneous Tissue and Fascia, Percutaneous Approach
0J9G00Z Drainage of Right Lower Arm Subcutaneous Tissue and Fascia with Drainage Device, Open Approach
0J9G0ZX Drainage of Right Lower Arm Subcutaneous Tissue and Fascia, Open Approach, Diagnostic
0J9G0ZZ Drainage of Right Lower Arm Subcutaneous Tissue and Fascia, Open Approach
0J9G30Z Drainage of Right Lower Arm Subcutaneous Tissue and Fascia with Drainage Device, Percutaneous Approach
0J9G3ZX Drainage of Right Lower Arm Subcutaneous Tissue and Fascia, Percutaneous Approach, Diagnostic
0J9G3ZZ Drainage of Right Lower Arm Subcutaneous Tissue and Fascia, Percutaneous Approach
0J9H00Z Drainage of Left Lower Arm Subcutaneous Tissue and Fascia with Drainage Device, Open Approach
0J9H0ZX Drainage of Left Lower Arm Subcutaneous Tissue and Fascia, Open Approach, Diagnostic
0J9H0ZZ Drainage of Left Lower Arm Subcutaneous Tissue and Fascia, Open Approach
0J9H30Z Drainage of Left Lower Arm Subcutaneous Tissue and Fascia with Drainage Device, Percutaneous Approach
0J9H3ZX Drainage of Left Lower Arm Subcutaneous Tissue and Fascia, Percutaneous Approach, Diagnostic
0J9H3ZZ Drainage of Left Lower Arm Subcutaneous Tissue and Fascia, Percutaneous Approach
0J9J00Z Drainage of Right Hand Subcutaneous Tissue and Fascia with Drainage Device, Open Approach
0J9J0ZX Drainage of Right Hand Subcutaneous Tissue and Fascia, Open Approach, Diagnostic
0J9J0ZZ Drainage of Right Hand Subcutaneous Tissue and Fascia, Open Approach
0J9J30Z Drainage of Right Hand Subcutaneous Tissue and Fascia with Drainage Device, Percutaneous Approach
0J9J3ZX Drainage of Right Hand Subcutaneous Tissue and Fascia, Percutaneous Approach, Diagnostic
● **0J9J3ZZ** Drainage of Right Hand Subcutaneous Tissue and Fascia, Percutaneous Approach
0J9K00Z Drainage of Left Hand Subcutaneous Tissue and Fascia with Drainage Device, Open Approach
0J9K0ZX Drainage of Left Hand Subcutaneous Tissue and Fascia, Open Approach, Diagnostic
0J9K0ZZ Drainage of Left Hand Subcutaneous Tissue and Fascia, Open Approach
0J9K30Z Drainage of Left Hand Subcutaneous Tissue and Fascia with Drainage Device, Percutaneous Approach
0J9K3ZX Drainage of Left Hand Subcutaneous Tissue and Fascia, Percutaneous Approach, Diagnostic
● **0J9K3ZZ** Drainage of Left Hand Subcutaneous Tissue and Fascia, Percutaneous Approach
0J9L00Z Drainage of Right Upper Leg Subcutaneous Tissue and Fascia with Drainage Device, Open Approach
0J9L0ZX Drainage of Right Upper Leg Subcutaneous Tissue and Fascia, Open Approach, Diagnostic
0J9L0ZZ Drainage of Right Upper Leg Subcutaneous Tissue and Fascia, Open Approach
0J9L30Z Drainage of Right Upper Leg Subcutaneous Tissue and Fascia with Drainage Device, Percutaneous Approach
0J9L3ZX Drainage of Right Upper Leg Subcutaneous Tissue and Fascia, Percutaneous Approach, Diagnostic
0J9L3ZZ Drainage of Right Upper Leg Subcutaneous Tissue and Fascia, Percutaneous Approach
0J9M00Z Drainage of Left Upper Leg Subcutaneous Tissue and Fascia with Drainage Device, Open Approach
0J9M0ZX Drainage of Left Upper Leg Subcutaneous Tissue and Fascia, Open Approach, Diagnostic
0J9M0ZZ Drainage of Left Upper Leg Subcutaneous Tissue and Fascia, Open Approach
0J9M30Z Drainage of Left Upper Leg Subcutaneous Tissue and Fascia with Drainage Device, Percutaneous Approach
0J9M3ZX Drainage of Left Upper Leg Subcutaneous Tissue and Fascia, Percutaneous Approach, Diagnostic
0J9M3ZZ Drainage of Left Upper Leg Subcutaneous Tissue and Fascia, Percutaneous Approach
0J9N00Z Drainage of Right Lower Leg Subcutaneous Tissue and Fascia with Drainage Device, Open Approach
0J9N0ZX Drainage of Right Lower Leg Subcutaneous Tissue and Fascia, Open Approach, Diagnostic
0J9N0ZZ Drainage of Right Lower Leg Subcutaneous Tissue and Fascia, Open Approach
0J9N30Z Drainage of Right Lower Leg Subcutaneous Tissue and Fascia with Drainage Device, Percutaneous Approa
0J9N3ZX Drainage of Right Lower Leg Subcutaneous Tissue and Fascia, Percutaneous Approach, Diagnostic
0J9N3ZZ Drainage of Right Lower Leg Subcutaneous Tissue and Fascia, Percutaneous Approach
0J9P00Z Drainage of Left Lower Leg Subcutane Tissue and Fascia with Drainage Device Open Approach
0J9P0ZX Drainage of Left Lower Leg Subcutane Tissue and Fascia, Open Approach, Diagnostic
0J9P0ZZ Drainage of Left Lower Leg Subcutane Tissue and Fascia, Open Approach
0J9P30Z Drainage of Left Lower Leg Subcutane Tissue and Fascia with Drainage Device Percutaneous Approach
0J9P3ZX Drainage of Left Lower Leg Subcutane Tissue and Fascia, Percutaneous Approach, Diagnostic
0J9P3ZZ Drainage of Left Lower Leg Subcutane Tissue and Fascia, Percutaneous Approa
0J9Q00Z Drainage of Right Foot Subcutaneous Tissue and Fascia with Drainage Device Open Approach
0J9Q0ZX Drainage of Right Foot Subcutaneous Tissue and Fascia, Open Approach, Diagnostic
0J9Q0ZZ Drainage of Right Foot Subcutaneous Tissue and Fascia, Open Approach
0J9Q30Z Drainage of Right Foot Subcutaneous Tissue and Fascia with Drainage Device, Percutaneous Approach
0J9Q3ZX Drainage of Right Foot Subcutaneous Tissue and Fascia, Percutaneous Approach, Diagnostic
0J9Q3ZZ Drainage of Right Foot Subcutaneous Tissue and Fascia, Percutaneous Approac
0J9R00Z Drainage of Left Foot Subcutaneous Tissue and Fascia with Drainage Device, Open Approach
0J9R0ZX Drainage of Left Foot Subcutaneous Tissue and Fascia, Open Approach, Diagnostic
0J9R0ZZ Drainage of Left Foot Subcutaneous Tissue and Fascia, Open Approach
0J9R30Z Drainage of Left Foot Subcutaneous Tissue and Fascia with Drainage Device, Percutaneous Approach
0J9R3ZX Drainage of Left Foot Subcutaneous Tissue and Fascia, Percutaneous Approach, Diagnostic
0J9R3ZZ Drainage of Left Foot Subcutaneous Tissue and Fascia, Percutaneous Approac

0JB – Subcutaneous Tissue and Fascia, Excision

Review Coding Guidelines B3.4a and B3.4b

Review Coding Guideline B3.5

Review Coding Guideline B3.8

0JB00ZX Excision of Scalp Subcutaneous Tissue and Fascia, Open Approach, Diagnostic
0JB00ZZ Excision of Scalp Subcutaneous Tissue and Fascia, Open Approach
0JB03ZX Excision of Scalp Subcutaneous Tissue and Fascia, Percutaneous Approach, Diagnostic
0JB03ZZ Excision of Scalp Subcutaneous Tissue and Fascia, Percutaneous Approach
0JB10ZX Excision of Face Subcutaneous Tissue and Fascia, Open Approach, Diagnostic
0JB10ZZ Excision of Face Subcutaneous Tissue and Fascia, Open Approach
0JB13ZX Excision of Face Subcutaneous Tissue and Fascia, Percutaneous Approach, Diagnostic
0JB13ZZ Excision of Face Subcutaneous Tissue and Fascia, Percutaneous Approach
0JB40ZX Excision of Anterior Neck Subcutaneous Tissue and Fascia, Open Approach, Diagnostic
0JB40ZZ Excision of Anterior Neck Subcutaneous Tissue and Fascia, Open Approach
0JB43ZX Excision of Anterior Neck Subcutaneous Tissue and Fascia, Percutaneous Approach, Diagnostic
0JB43ZZ Excision of Anterior Neck Subcutaneous Tissue and Fascia, Percutaneous Approach
0JB50ZX Excision of Posterior Neck Subcutaneous Tissue and Fascia, Open Approach, Diagnostic
0JB50ZZ Excision of Posterior Neck Subcutaneous Tissue and Fascia, Open Approach

53ZX Excision of Posterior Neck Subcutaneous Tissue and Fascia, Percutaneous Approach, Diagnostic
53ZZ Excision of Posterior Neck Subcutaneous Tissue and Fascia, Percutaneous Approach
60ZX Excision of Chest Subcutaneous Tissue and Fascia, Open Approach, Diagnostic
60ZZ Excision of Chest Subcutaneous Tissue and Fascia, Open Approach
63ZX Excision of Chest Subcutaneous Tissue and Fascia, Percutaneous Approach, Diagnostic
63ZZ Excision of Chest Subcutaneous Tissue and Fascia, Percutaneous Approach
B70ZX Excision of Back Subcutaneous Tissue and Fascia, Open Approach, Diagnostic
B70ZZ Excision of Back Subcutaneous Tissue and Fascia, Open Approach
B73ZX Excision of Back Subcutaneous Tissue and Fascia, Percutaneous Approach, Diagnostic
B73ZZ Excision of Back Subcutaneous Tissue and Fascia, Percutaneous Approach
B80ZX Excision of Abdomen Subcutaneous Tissue and Fascia, Open Approach, Diagnostic
B80ZZ Excision of Abdomen Subcutaneous Tissue and Fascia, Open Approach
B83ZX Excision of Abdomen Subcutaneous Tissue and Fascia, Percutaneous Approach, Diagnostic
B83ZZ Excision of Abdomen Subcutaneous Tissue and Fascia, Percutaneous Approach
B90ZX Excision of Buttock Subcutaneous Tissue and Fascia, Open Approach, Diagnostic
B90ZZ Excision of Buttock Subcutaneous Tissue and Fascia, Open Approach
B93ZX Excision of Buttock Subcutaneous Tissue and Fascia, Percutaneous Approach, Diagnostic
B93ZZ Excision of Buttock Subcutaneous Tissue and Fascia, Percutaneous Approach
BB0ZX Excision of Perineum Subcutaneous Tissue and Fascia, Open Approach, Diagnostic
JBB0ZZ Excision of Perineum Subcutaneous Tissue and Fascia, Open Approach
JBB3ZX Excision of Perineum Subcutaneous Tissue and Fascia, Percutaneous Approach, Diagnostic
JBB3ZZ Excision of Perineum Subcutaneous Tissue and Fascia, Percutaneous Approach
JBC0ZX Excision of Pelvic Region Subcutaneous Tissue and Fascia, Open Approach, Diagnostic
JBC0ZZ Excision of Pelvic Region Subcutaneous Tissue and Fascia, Open Approach
JBC3ZX Excision of Pelvic Region Subcutaneous Tissue and Fascia, Percutaneous Approach, Diagnostic
JBC3ZZ Excision of Pelvic Region Subcutaneous Tissue and Fascia, Percutaneous Approach
JBD0ZX Excision of Right Upper Arm Subcutaneous Tissue and Fascia, Open Approach, Diagnostic
0JBD0ZZ Excision of Right Upper Arm Subcutaneous Tissue and Fascia, Open Approach
0JBD3ZX Excision of Right Upper Arm Subcutaneous Tissue and Fascia, Percutaneous Approach, Diagnostic
0JBD3ZZ Excision of Right Upper Arm Subcutaneous Tissue and Fascia, Percutaneous Approach
0JBF0ZX Excision of Left Upper Arm Subcutaneous Tissue and Fascia, Open Approach, Diagnostic
0JBF0ZZ Excision of Left Upper Arm Subcutaneous Tissue and Fascia, Open Approach
0JBF3ZX Excision of Left Upper Arm Subcutaneous Tissue and Fascia, Percutaneous Approach, Diagnostic
0JBF3ZZ Excision of Left Upper Arm Subcutaneous Tissue and Fascia, Percutaneous Approach
0JBG0ZX Excision of Right Lower Arm Subcutaneous Tissue and Fascia, Open Approach, Diagnostic
0JBG0ZZ Excision of Right Lower Arm Subcutaneous Tissue and Fascia, Open Approach
0JBG3ZX Excision of Right Lower Arm Subcutaneous Tissue and Fascia, Percutaneous Approach, Diagnostic
0JBG3ZZ Excision of Right Lower Arm Subcutaneous Tissue and Fascia, Percutaneous Approach
0JBH0ZX Excision of Left Lower Arm Subcutaneous Tissue and Fascia, Open Approach, Diagnostic
0JBH0ZZ Excision of Left Lower Arm Subcutaneous Tissue and Fascia, Open Approach
0JBH3ZX Excision of Left Lower Arm Subcutaneous Tissue and Fascia, Percutaneous Approach, Diagnostic
0JBH3ZZ Excision of Left Lower Arm Subcutaneous Tissue and Fascia, Percutaneous Approach
0JBJ0ZX Excision of Right Hand Subcutaneous Tissue and Fascia, Open Approach, Diagnostic
0JBJ0ZZ Excision of Right Hand Subcutaneous Tissue and Fascia, Open Approach
0JBJ3ZX Excision of Right Hand Subcutaneous Tissue and Fascia, Percutaneous Approach, Diagnostic
0JBJ3ZZ Excision of Right Hand Subcutaneous Tissue and Fascia, Percutaneous Approach
0JBK0ZX Excision of Left Hand Subcutaneous Tissue and Fascia, Open Approach, Diagnostic
0JBK0ZZ Excision of Left Hand Subcutaneous Tissue and Fascia, Open Approach
0JBK3ZX Excision of Left Hand Subcutaneous Tissue and Fascia, Percutaneous Approach, Diagnostic
0JBK3ZZ Excision of Left Hand Subcutaneous Tissue and Fascia, Percutaneous Approach
0JBL0ZX Excision of Right Upper Leg Subcutaneous Tissue and Fascia, Open Approach, Diagnostic
0JBL0ZZ Excision of Right Upper Leg Subcutaneous Tissue and Fascia, Open Approach
0JBL3ZX Excision of Right Upper Leg Subcutaneous Tissue and Fascia, Percutaneous Approach, Diagnostic
0JBL3ZZ Excision of Right Upper Leg Subcutaneous Tissue and Fascia, Percutaneous Approach
0JBM0ZX Excision of Left Upper Leg Subcutaneous Tissue and Fascia, Open Approach, Diagnostic
0JBM0ZZ Excision of Left Upper Leg Subcutaneous Tissue and Fascia, Open Approach
0JBM3ZX Excision of Left Upper Leg Subcutaneous Tissue and Fascia, Percutaneous Approach, Diagnostic
0JBM3ZZ Excision of Left Upper Leg Subcutaneous Tissue and Fascia, Percutaneous Approach
0JBN0ZX Excision of Right Lower Leg Subcutaneous Tissue and Fascia, Open Approach, Diagnostic
0JBN0ZZ Excision of Right Lower Leg Subcutaneous Tissue and Fascia, Open Approach
0JBN3ZX Excision of Right Lower Leg Subcutaneous Tissue and Fascia, Percutaneous Approach, Diagnostic
0JBN3ZZ Excision of Right Lower Leg Subcutaneous Tissue and Fascia, Percutaneous Approach
0JBP0ZX Excision of Left Lower Leg Subcutaneous Tissue and Fascia, Open Approach, Diagnostic
0JBP0ZZ Excision of Left Lower Leg Subcutaneous Tissue and Fascia, Open Approach
0JBP3ZX Excision of Left Lower Leg Subcutaneous Tissue and Fascia, Percutaneous Approach, Diagnostic
0JBP3ZZ Excision of Left Lower Leg Subcutaneous Tissue and Fascia, Percutaneous Approach
0JBQ0ZX Excision of Right Foot Subcutaneous Tissue and Fascia, Open Approach, Diagnostic
0JBQ0ZZ Excision of Right Foot Subcutaneous Tissue and Fascia, Open Approach
0JBQ3ZX Excision of Right Foot Subcutaneous Tissue and Fascia, Percutaneous Approach, Diagnostic
0JBQ3ZZ Excision of Right Foot Subcutaneous Tissue and Fascia, Percutaneous Approach
0JBR0ZX Excision of Left Foot Subcutaneous Tissue and Fascia, Open Approach, Diagnostic
0JBR0ZZ Excision of Left Foot Subcutaneous Tissue and Fascia, Open Approach
0JBR3ZX Excision of Left Foot Subcutaneous Tissue and Fascia, Percutaneous Approach, Diagnostic
0JBR3ZZ Excision of Left Foot Subcutaneous Tissue and Fascia, Percutaneous Approach

JC – *Subcutaneous Tissue and Fascia, Extirpation*

JC00ZZ Extirpation of Matter from Scalp Subcutaneous Tissue and Fascia, Open Approach
JC03ZZ Extirpation of Matter from Scalp Subcutaneous Tissue and Fascia, Percutaneous Approach
0JC10ZZ Extirpation of Matter from Face Subcutaneous Tissue and Fascia, Open Approach
0JC13ZZ Extirpation of Matter from Face Subcutaneous Tissue and Fascia, Percutaneous Approach
0JC40ZZ Extirpation of Matter from Anterior Neck Subcutaneous Tissue and Fascia, Open Approach
0JC43ZZ Extirpation of Matter from Anterior Neck Subcutaneous Tissue and Fascia, Percutaneous Approach
0JC50ZZ Extirpation of Matter from Posterior Neck Subcutaneous Tissue and Fascia, Open Approach
0JC53ZZ Extirpation of Matter from Posterior Neck Subcutaneous Tissue and Fascia, Percutaneous Approach
0JC60ZZ Extirpation of Matter from Chest Subcutaneous Tissue and Fascia, Open Approach

0JC63ZZ Extirpation of Matter from Chest Subcutaneous Tissue and Fascia, Percutaneous Approach
0JC70ZZ Extirpation of Matter from Back Subcutaneous Tissue and Fascia, Open Approach
0JC73ZZ Extirpation of Matter from Back Subcutaneous Tissue and Fascia, Percutaneous Approach
0JC80ZZ Extirpation of Matter from Abdomen Subcutaneous Tissue and Fascia, Open Approach
0JC83ZZ Extirpation of Matter from Abdomen Subcutaneous Tissue and Fascia, Percutaneous Approach
0JC90ZZ Extirpation of Matter from Buttock Subcutaneous Tissue and Fascia, Open Approach
0JC93ZZ Extirpation of Matter from Buttock Subcutaneous Tissue and Fascia, Percutaneous Approach
0JCB0ZZ Extirpation of Matter from Perineum Subcutaneous Tissue and Fascia, Open Approach
0JCB3ZZ Extirpation of Matter from Perineum Subcutaneous Tissue and Fascia, Percutaneous Approach
0JCC0ZZ Extirpation of Matter from Pelvic Region Subcutaneous Tissue and Fascia, Open Approach
0JCC3ZZ Extirpation of Matter from Pelvic Region Subcutaneous Tissue and Fascia, Percutaneous Approach
0JCD0ZZ Extirpation of Matter from Right Upper Arm Subcutaneous Tissue and Fascia, Open Approach
0JCD3ZZ Extirpation of Matter from Right Upper Arm Subcutaneous Tissue and Fascia, Percutaneous Approach
0JCF0ZZ Extirpation of Matter from Left Upper Arm Subcutaneous Tissue and Fascia, Open Approach
0JCF3ZZ Extirpation of Matter from Left Upper Arm Subcutaneous Tissue and Fascia, Percutaneous Approach
0JCG0ZZ Extirpation of Matter from Right Lower Arm Subcutaneous Tissue and Fascia, Open Approach
0JCG3ZZ Extirpation of Matter from Right Lower Arm Subcutaneous Tissue and Fascia, Percutaneous Approach
0JCH0ZZ Extirpation of Matter from Left Lower Arm Subcutaneous Tissue and Fascia, Open Approach
0JCH3ZZ Extirpation of Matter from Left Lower Arm Subcutaneous Tissue and Fascia, Percutaneous Approach
0JCJ0ZZ Extirpation of Matter from Right Hand Subcutaneous Tissue and Fascia, Open Approach
0JCJ3ZZ Extirpation of Matter from Right Hand Subcutaneous Tissue and Fascia, Percutaneous Approach
0JCK0ZZ Extirpation of Matter from Left Hand Subcutaneous Tissue and Fascia, Open Approach
0JCK3ZZ Extirpation of Matter from Left Hand Subcutaneous Tissue and Fascia, Percutaneous Approach
0JCL0ZZ Extirpation of Matter from Right Upper Leg Subcutaneous Tissue and Fascia, Open Approach
0JCL3ZZ Extirpation of Matter from Right Uppe Leg Subcutaneous Tissue and Fascia, Percutaneous Approach
0JCM0ZZ Extirpation of Matter from Left Upper Leg Subcutaneous Tissue and Fascia, Open Approach
0JCM3ZZ Extirpation of Matter from Left Upper Leg Subcutaneous Tissue and Fascia, Percutaneous Approach
0JCN0ZZ Extirpation of Matter from Right Lowe Leg Subcutaneous Tissue and Fascia, Open Approach
0JCN3ZZ Extirpation of Matter from Right Lowe Leg Subcutaneous Tissue and Fascia, Percutaneous Approach
0JCP0ZZ Extirpation of Matter from Left Lower Leg Subcutaneous Tissue and Fascia, Open Approach
0JCP3ZZ Extirpation of Matter from Left Lower Leg Subcutaneous Tissue and Fascia, Percutaneous Approach
0JCQ0ZZ Extirpation of Matter from Right Foot Subcutaneous Tissue and Fascia, Open Approach
0JCQ3ZZ Extirpation of Matter from Right Foot Subcutaneous Tissue and Fascia, Percutaneous Approach
0JCR0ZZ Extirpation of Matter from Left Foot Subcutaneous Tissue and Fascia, Open Approach
0JCR3ZZ Extirpation of Matter from Left Foot Subcutaneous Tissue and Fascia, Percutaneous Approach

0JD – Subcutaneous Tissue and Fascia, Extraction

0JD00ZZ Extraction of Scalp Subcutaneous Tissue and Fascia, Open Approach
0JD03ZZ Extraction of Scalp Subcutaneous Tissue and Fascia, Percutaneous Approach
0JD10ZZ Extraction of Face Subcutaneous Tissue and Fascia, Open Approach
0JD13ZZ Extraction of Face Subcutaneous Tissue and Fascia, Percutaneous Approach
0JD40ZZ Extraction of Anterior Neck Subcutaneous Tissue and Fascia, Open Approach
0JD43ZZ Extraction of Anterior Neck Subcutaneous Tissue and Fascia, Percutaneous Approach
0JD50ZZ Extraction of Posterior Neck Subcutaneous Tissue and Fascia, Open Approach
0JD53ZZ Extraction of Posterior Neck Subcutaneous Tissue and Fascia, Percutaneous Approach
0JD60ZZ Extraction of Chest Subcutaneous Tissue and Fascia, Open Approach
0JD63ZZ Extraction of Chest Subcutaneous Tissue and Fascia, Percutaneous Approach
0JD70ZZ Extraction of Back Subcutaneous Tissue and Fascia, Open Approach
0JD73ZZ Extraction of Back Subcutaneous Tissue and Fascia, Percutaneous Approach
0JD80ZZ Extraction of Abdomen Subcutaneous Tissue and Fascia, Open Approach
0JD83ZZ Extraction of Abdomen Subcutaneous Tissue and Fascia, Percutaneous Approach
0JD90ZZ Extraction of Buttock Subcutaneous Tissue and Fascia, Open Approach
0JD93ZZ Extraction of Buttock Subcutaneous Tissue and Fascia, Percutaneous Approach
0JDB0ZZ Extraction of Perineum Subcutaneous Tissue and Fascia, Open Approach
0JDB3ZZ Extraction of Perineum Subcutaneous Tissue and Fascia, Percutaneous Approach
0JDC0ZZ Extraction of Pelvic Region Subcutaneous Tissue and Fascia, Open Approach
0JDC3ZZ Extraction of Pelvic Region Subcutaneous Tissue and Fascia, Percutaneous Approach
0JDD0ZZ Extraction of Right Upper Arm Subcutaneous Tissue and Fascia, Open Approach
0JDD3ZZ Extraction of Right Upper Arm Subcutaneous Tissue and Fascia, Percutaneous Approach
0JDF0ZZ Extraction of Left Upper Arm Subcutaneous Tissue and Fascia, Open Approach
0JDF3ZZ Extraction of Left Upper Arm Subcutaneous Tissue and Fascia, Percutaneous Approach
0JDG0ZZ Extraction of Right Lower Arm Subcutaneous Tissue and Fascia, Open Approach
0JDG3ZZ Extraction of Right Lower Arm Subcutaneous Tissue and Fascia, Percutaneous Approach
0JDH0ZZ Extraction of Left Lower Arm Subcutaneous Tissue and Fascia, Open Approach
0JDH3ZZ Extraction of Left Lower Arm Subcutaneous Tissue and Fascia, Percutaneous Approach
0JDJ0ZZ Extraction of Right Hand Subcutaneous Tissue and Fascia, Open Approach
0JDJ3ZZ Extraction of Right Hand Subcutaneous Tissue and Fascia, Percutaneous Approach
0JDK0ZZ Extraction of Left Hand Subcutaneous Tissue and Fascia, Open Approach
0JDK3ZZ Extraction of Left Hand Subcutaneous Tissue and Fascia, Percutaneous Approach
0JDL0ZZ Extraction of Right Upper Leg Subcutaneous Tissue and Fascia, Open Approach
0JDL3ZZ Extraction of Right Upper Leg Subcutaneous Tissue and Fascia, Percutaneous Approach
0JDM0ZZ Extraction of Left Upper Leg Subcutaneous Tissue and Fascia, Open Approach
0JDM3ZZ Extraction of Left Upper Leg Subcutaneous Tissue and Fascia, Percutaneous Approach
0JDN0ZZ Extraction of Right Lower Leg Subcutaneous Tissue and Fascia, Open Approach
0JDN3ZZ Extraction of Right Lower Leg Subcutaneous Tissue and Fascia, Percutaneous Approach
0JDP0ZZ Extraction of Left Lower Leg Subcutaneous Tissue and Fascia, Open Approach
0JDP3ZZ Extraction of Left Lower Leg Subcutaneous Tissue and Fascia, Percutaneous Approach
0JDQ0ZZ Extraction of Right Foot Subcutaneous Tissue and Fascia, Open Approach
0JDQ3ZZ Extraction of Right Foot Subcutaneous Tissue and Fascia, Percutaneous Approach
0JDR0ZZ Extraction of Left Foot Subcutaneous Tissue and Fascia, Open Approach
0JDR3ZZ Extraction of Left Foot Subcutaneous Tissue and Fascia, Percutaneous Approach

00NZ Insertion of Tissue Expander into Scalp Subcutaneous Tissue and Fascia, Open Approach

03NZ Insertion of Tissue Expander into Scalp Subcutaneous Tissue and Fascia, Percutaneous Approach

10NZ Insertion of Tissue Expander into Face Subcutaneous Tissue and Fascia, Open Approach

13NZ Insertion of Tissue Expander into Face Subcutaneous Tissue and Fascia, Percutaneous Approach

40NZ Insertion of Tissue Expander into Anterior Neck Subcutaneous Tissue and Fascia, Open Approach

43NZ Insertion of Tissue Expander into Anterior Neck Subcutaneous Tissue and Fascia, Percutaneous Approach

50NZ Insertion of Tissue Expander into Posterior Neck Subcutaneous Tissue and Fascia, Open Approach

H53NZ Insertion of Tissue Expander into Posterior Neck Subcutaneous Tissue and Fascia, Percutaneous Approach

H600Z Insertion of Hemodynamic Monitoring Device into Chest Subcutaneous Tissue and Fascia, Open Approach

JH602Z Insertion of Monitoring Device into Chest Subcutaneous Tissue and Fascia, Open Approach

JH604Z Insertion of Pacemaker, Single Chamber into Chest Subcutaneous Tissue and Fascia, Open Approach

HAC With a secondary diagnosis code of K68.11, T81.4XXA, T82.6XXA, T82.7XXA

\+ Pacemaker device when reported with an Insertion of a cardiac lead (6th character J or M) into the coronary vein, atrium, ventricle or pericardium (4th characters 4, 6, 7, K, L and N). *See table 02H to construct the Insertion code.* When a device is replaced, also report the Removal of the cardiac rhythm device (6th character P) from the trunk subcutaneous tissue and fascia. *See table 0JP to construct the Removal code.* When a cardiac lead is replaced, also report the Removal of the cardiac lead (6th character M) from the heart. *See table 02P to construct the Removal code.*

JH605Z Insertion of Pacemaker, Single Chamber Rate Responsive into Chest Subcutaneous Tissue and Fascia, Open Approach

HAC With a secondary diagnosis code of K68.11, T81.4XXA, T82.6XXA, T82.7XXA

\+ Pacemaker device when reported with an Insertion of a cardiac lead (6th character J or M) into the coronary vein, atrium, ventricle or pericardium (4th characters 4, 6, 7, K, L and N). *See table 02H to construct the Insertion code.* When a device is replaced, also report the Removal of the cardiac rhythm device (6th character P) from the trunk subcutaneous tissue and fascia. *See table 0JP to construct the Removal code.* When a cardiac lead is replaced, also report the Removal of the cardiac lead (6th character M) from the heart. *See table 02P to construct the Removal code.*

0JH606Z Insertion of Pacemaker, Dual Chamber into Chest Subcutaneous Tissue and Fascia, Open Approach

HAC With a secondary diagnosis code of K68.11, T81.4XXA, T82.6XXA, T82.7XXA

\+ Pacemaker device when reported with an Insertion of a cardiac lead (6th character J or M) into the coronary vein, atrium, ventricle or pericardium (4th characters 4, 6, 7, K, L and N). *See table 02H to construct the Insertion code.* When a device is replaced, also report the Removal of the cardiac rhythm device (6th character P) from the trunk subcutaneous tissue and fascia. *See table 0JP to construct the Removal code.* When a cardiac lead is replaced, also report the Removal of the cardiac lead (6th character M) from the heart. *See table 02P to construct the Removal code.*

0JH607Z Insertion of Cardiac Resynchronization Pacemaker Pulse Generator into Chest Subcutaneous Tissue and Fascia, Open Approach

HAC With a secondary diagnosis code of K68.11, T81.4XXA, T82.6XXA, T82.7XXA

\+ Pacemaker device when reported with an Insertion of a cardiac lead (6th character J or M) into the coronary vein, atrium, ventricle or pericardium (4th characters 4, 6, 7, K, L and N). *See table 02H to construct the Insertion code.* When a cardiac lead is replaced, also report the Removal of the cardiac lead (6th character M) from the heart. *See table 02P to construct the Removal code.*

0JH608Z Insertion of Defibrillator Generator into Chest Subcutaneous Tissue and Fascia, Open Approach

AHA CC: 4Q, 2012, 104-106

HAC With a secondary diagnosis code of K68.11, T81.4XXA, T82.6XXA, T82.7XXA

\+ Cardioverter-Defibrillator lead(s)/generator when reported with Insertion of a defibrillator cardiac lead (6th character K) into the coronary vein, atrium, or ventricle. Also applicable with Insertion of pacemaker cardiac lead, defibrillator cardiac lead or cardiac lead (6th characters J, K, M) into the pericardium. *See table 02H to construct the Insertion code.*

0JH609Z Insertion of Cardiac Resynchronization Defibrillator
Pulse Generator into Chest Subcutaneous Tissue and Fascia, Open Approach

HAC With a secondary diagnosis code of K68.11, T81.4XXA, T82.6XXA, T82.7XXA

\+ Cardioverter-Defibrillator lead(s)/generator when reported with Insertion of a defibrillator cardiac lead (6th character K) into the atrium, or ventricle. Also applicable with Insertion of pacemaker cardiac lead, defibrillator cardiac lead or cardiac lead (6th characters J, K, M) into the coronary vein or pericardium. *See table 02H to construct the Insertion code.*

0JH60AZ Insertion of Contractility Modulation Device into Chest Subcutaneous Tissue and Fascia, Open Approach

\+ Cardioverter-Defibrillator lead(s)/generator when reported with Insertion of a cardiac lead (6th character M) into the left ventricle. *See table 02H to construct the Insertion code.*

0JH60BZ Insertion of Single Array Stimulator Generator into Chest Subcutaneous Tissue and Fascia, Open Approach

\+ Neurotransmitter/Neurostimulator when reported with an Insertion of a neurostimulator lead (6th character M) into the cranial nerve, spinal canal or spinal cord. *See table 00H to construct the Insertion code.* Also applicable when reported with Insertion of neurostimulator lead (6th character M) into the peripheral nerve. *See table 01H to construct the Insertion code.* Also applicable when reported with Insertion of a stimulator lead (6th character M) into the stomach. *See table 0DH to construct the Insertion code.*

0JH60CZ Insertion of Single Array Rechargeable Stimulator Generator into Chest Subcutaneous Tissue and Fascia, Open Approach

\+ Neurotransmitter/Neurostimulator when reported with an Insertion of a neurostimulator lead (6th character M) into the cranial nerve, spinal canal or spinal cord. *See table 00H to construct the Insertion code.* Also applicable when reported with Insertion of neurostimulator lead (6th character M) into the peripheral nerve. *See table 01H to construct the Insertion code.* Also applicable when reported with Insertion of a stimulator lead (6th character M) into the stomach. *See table 0DH to construct the Insertion code.*

0JH60DZ Insertion of Multiple Array Stimulator Generator into Chest Subcutaneous Tissue and Fascia, Open Approach

\+ Major brain device implant when reported with an Insertion of a neurostimulator lead (6th character M) into the brain or cerebral ventricle. *See table 00H to construct the Insertion code.*

\+ Neurotransmitter/Neurostimulator when reported with an Insertion of a neurostimulator lead (6th character M) into the cranial nerve, spinal canal or spinal cord. *See table 00H to construct the Insertion code.* Also applicable when reported with Insertion of neurostimulator lead (6th character M) into the peripheral nerve. *See table 01H to construct the Insertion code.* Also applicable when reported with Insertion of a stimulator lead (6th character M) into the stomach. *See table 0DH to construct the Insertion code.*

0JH60EZ Insertion of Multiple Array Rechargeable Stimulator Generator into Chest Subcutaneous Tissue and Fascia, Open Approach

\+ Major brain device implant when reported with an Insertion of a neurostimulator lead (6th character M) into the brain or cerebral ventricle. *See table 00H to construct the Insertion code.*

\+ Neurotransmitter/Neurostimulator when reported with an Insertion of a neurostimulator lead (6th character M) into the cranial nerve, spinal canal or spinal cord. *See table 00H to construct the Insertion code.* Also applicable when reported with Insertion of neurostimulator lead (6th character M) into the peripheral nerve. *See table 01H to construct the Insertion code.* Also applicable when reported with Insertion of a stimulator lead (6th character M) into the stomach. *See table 0DH to construct the Insertion code.*

● **0JH60HZ** Insertion of Contraceptive Device into Chest Subcutaneous Tissue and Fascia, Open Approach

0JH60MZ Insertion of Stimulator Generator into Chest Subcutaneous Tissue and Fascia, Open Approach

0JH60NZ Insertion of Tissue Expander into Chest Subcutaneous Tissue and Fascia, Open Approach

0JH60PZ Insertion of Cardiac Rhythm Related Device into Chest Subcutaneous Tissue and Fascia, Open Approach

AHA CC: 4Q, 2012, 104-106

HAC With a secondary diagnosis code of K68.11, T81.4XXA, T82.6XXA, T82.7XXA

\+ Pacemaker device when reported with an Insertion of a cardiac lead (6th character J or M) into the coronary vein, atrium, ventricle or pericardium (4th characters 4, 6, 7, K, L and N). *See table 02H to construct the Insertion code.* When a cardiac lead is replaced, also report the Removal of the cardiac lead (6th character M) from the heart. *See table 02P to construct the Removal code.*

0JH60VZ Insertion of Infusion Pump into Chest Subcutaneous Tissue and Fascia, Open Approach

● **0JH60WZ** Insertion of Reservoir into Chest Subcutaneous Tissue and Fascia, Open Approach

● **0JH60XZ** Insertion of Vascular Access Device into Chest Subcutaneous Tissue and Fascia, Open Approach

0JH630Z Insertion of Hemodynamic Monitoring Device into Chest Subcutaneous Tissue and Fascia, Percutaneous Approach

● **0JH632Z** Insertion of Monitoring Device into Chest Subcutaneous Tissue and Fascia, Percutaneous Approach

● **0JH634Z** Insertion of Pacemaker, Single Chamber into Chest Subcutaneous Tissue and Fascia, Percutaneous Approach

HAC With a secondary diagnosis code of K68.11, T81.4XXA, T82.6XXA, T82.7XXA

\+ Pacemaker device when reported with an Insertion of a cardiac lead (6th character J or M) into the coronary vein, atrium, ventricle or pericardium (4th characters 4, 6, 7, K, L and N). *See table 02H to construct the Insertion code.* When a device is replaced, also report the Removal of the cardiac rhythm device (6th character P) from the trunk subcutaneous tissue and fascia. *See table 0JP to construct the Removal code.* When a cardiac lead is replaced, also report the Removal of the cardiac lead (6th character M) from the heart. *See table 02P to construct the Removal code.*

● **0JH635Z** Insertion of Pacemaker, Single Chamber Rate Responsive into Chest Subcutaneous Tissue and Fascia, Percutaneous Approach

HAC With a secondary diagnosis code of K68.11, T81.4XXA, T82.6XXA, T82.7XXA

\+ Pacemaker device when reported with an Insertion of a cardiac lead (6th character J or M) into the coronary vein, atrium, ventricle or pericardium (4th characters 4, 6, 7, K, L and N). *See table 02H to construct the Insertion code.* When a device is replaced, also report the Removal of the cardiac rhythm device (6th character P) from the trunk subcutaneous tissue and fascia. *See table 0JP to construct the Removal code.* When a cardiac lead is replaced, also report the Removal of the cardiac lead (6th character M) from the heart. *See table 02P to construct the Removal code.*

● **0JH636Z** Insertion of Pacemaker, Dual Chamber into Chest Subcutaneous Tissue and Fascia, Percutaneous Approach

HAC With a secondary diagnosis code of K68.11, T81.4XXA, T82.6XXA, T82.7XXA

\+ Pacemaker device when reported with an Insertion of a cardiac lead (6th character J or M) into the coronary vein, atrium, ventricle or pericardium (4th characters 4, 6, 7, K, L and N). *See table 02H to construct the Insertion code.* When a device is replaced, also report the Removal of the cardiac rhythm device (6th character P) from the trunk subcutaneous tissue and fascia. *See table 0JP to construct the Removal code.* When a cardiac lead is replaced, also report the Removal of the cardiac lead (6th character M) from the heart. *See table 02P to construct the Removal code.*

0JH637Z Insertion of Cardiac Resynchronization Pacemaker Pulse Generator into Chest Subcutaneous Tissue and Fascia, Percutaneous Approach

HAC With a secondary diagnosis code of K68.11, T81.4XXA, T82.6XXA, T82.7XXA

\+ Pacemaker device when reported with an Insertion of a cardiac lead (6th character J or M) into the coronary vein, atrium, ventricle or pericardium (4th characters 4, 6, 7, K, L and N). *See table 02H to construct the Insertion code.* When a cardiac lead is replaced, also report the Removal of the cardiac lead (6th character M) from the heart. *See table 02P to construct the Removal code.*

0JH638Z Insertion of Defibrillator Generator into Chest Subcutaneous Tissue and Fascia, Percutaneous Approach

HAC With a secondary diagnosis code of K68.11, T81.4XXA, T82.6XXA, T82.7XXA

\+ Cardioverter-Defibrillator lead(s)/generator when reported with Insertion of a defibrillator cardiac lead (6th character K) into the coronary vein, atrium, or ventricle. Also applicable with Insertion of pacemaker cardiac lead, defibrillator cardiac lead or cardiac lead (6th characters J, K, M) into the pericardium. *See table 02H to construct the Insertion code.*

0JH639Z Insertion of Cardiac Resynchronization Defibrillator Pulse Generator into Chest Subcutaneous Tissue and Fascia, Percutaneous Approach

HAC With a secondary diagnosis code of K68.11, T81.4XXA, T82.6XXA, T82.7XXA

\+ Cardioverter-Defibrillator lead(s)/generator when reported with Insertion of a defibrillator cardiac lead (6th character K) into the atrium, or ventricle. Also applicable with Insertion of pacemaker cardiac lead, defibrillator cardiac lead or cardiac lead (6th characters J, K, M) into the coronary vein or pericardium. *See table 02H to construct the Insertion code.*

0JH63AZ Insertion of Contractility Modulation Device into Chest Subcutaneous Tissue and Fascia, Percutaneous Approach

\+ Cardioverter-Defibrillator lead(s)/generator when reported with Insertion of a cardiac lead (6th character M) into the left ventricle. *See table 02H to constru the Insertion code.*

0JH63BZ Insertion of Single Array Stimulator Generator into Chest Subcutaneous Tis and Fascia, Percutaneous Approach

\+ Neurotransmitter/Neurostimulator when reported with an Insertion of a neurostimulator lead (6th character M) into the cranial nerve, spinal canal or spinal cord. *See table 00H to construct the Insertion code.* Also applicable whe reported with Insertion of neurostimula lead (6th character M) into the peripher nerve. *See table 01H to construct the Insertion code.* Also applicable when reported with Insertion of a stimulator l (6th character M) into the stomach. *See table 0DH to construct the Insertion co*

0JH63CZ Insertion of Single Array Rechargeable Stimulator Generator into Chest Subcutaneous Tissue and Fascia, Percutaneous Approach

\+ Neurotransmitter/Neurostimulator when reported with an Insertion of a neurostimulator lead (6th character M) into the cranial nerve, spinal canal or spinal cord. *See table 00H to construct the Insertion code.* Also applicable whe reported with Insertion of neurostimulat lead (6th character M) into the periphera nerve. *See table 01H to construct the Insertion code.* Also applicable when reported with Insertion of a stimulator le (6th character M) into the stomach. *See table 0DH to construct the Insertion co*

0JH63DZ Insertion of Multiple Array Stimulator Generator into Chest Subcutaneous Tiss and Fascia, Percutaneous Approach

\+ Major brain device implant when reporte with an Insertion of a neurostimulator le (6th character M) into the brain or cereb ventricle. *See table 00H to construct the Insertion code.*

\+ Neurotransmitter/Neurostimulator when reported with an Insertion of a neurostimulator lead (6th character M) into the cranial nerve, spinal canal or spinal cord. *See table 00H to construct the Insertion code.* Also applicable when reported with Insertion of neurostimulato lead (6th character M) into the periphera nerve. *See table 01H to construct the Insertion code.* Also applicable when reported with Insertion of a stimulator le (6th character M) into the stomach. *See table 0DH to construct the Insertion code*

0JH63EZ Insertion of Multiple Array Rechargeable Stimulator Generator into Chest Subcutaneous Tissue and Fascia, Percutaneous Approach

\+ Major brain device implant when reporte with an Insertion of a neurostimulator lea (6th character M) into the brain or cerebr ventricle. *See table 00H to construct the Insertion code.*

\+ Neurotransmitter/Neurostimulator when reported with an Insertion of a neurostimulator lead (6th character M) into the cranial nerve, spinal canal or spinal cord. *See table 00H to construct the Insertion code.* Also applicable when reported with Insertion of neurostimulator lead (6th character M) into the peripheral nerve. *See table 01H to construct the Insertion code.* Also applicable when reported with Insertion of a stimulator lea (6th character M) into the stomach. *See table 0DH to construct the Insertion code*

H63HZ Insertion of Contraceptive Device into Chest Subcutaneous Tissue and Fascia, Percutaneous Approach

63MZ Insertion of Stimulator Generator into Chest Subcutaneous Tissue and Fascia, Percutaneous Approach

63NZ Insertion of Tissue Expander into Chest Subcutaneous Tissue and Fascia, Percutaneous Approach

63PZ Insertion of Cardiac Rhythm Related Device into Chest Subcutaneous Tissue and Fascia, Percutaneous Approach

HAC With a secondary diagnosis code of K68.11, T81.4XXA, T82.6XXA, T82.7XXA

+ Pacemaker device when reported with an Insertion of a cardiac lead (6th character J or M) into the coronary vein, atrium, ventricle or pericardium (4th characters 4, 6, 7, K, L and N). *See table 02H to construct the Insertion code.* When a cardiac lead is replaced, also report the Removal of the cardiac lead (6th character M) from the heart. *See table 02P to construct the Removal code.*

H63VZ Insertion of Infusion Pump into Chest Subcutaneous Tissue and Fascia, Percutaneous Approach

JH63WZ Insertion of Reservoir into Chest Subcutaneous Tissue and Fascia, Percutaneous Approach

JH63XZ Insertion of Vascular Access Device into Chest Subcutaneous Tissue and Fascia, Percutaneous Approach

AHA CC: 4Q, 2013, 116-117

HAC With secondary diagnosis code J95.811

H70BZ Insertion of Single Array Stimulator Generator into Back Subcutaneous Tissue and Fascia, Open Approach

+ Neurotransmitter/Neurostimulator when reported with an Insertion of a neurostimulator lead (6th character M) into the cranial nerve, spinal canal or spinal cord. *See table 00H to construct the Insertion code.* Also applicable when reported with Insertion of neurostimulator lead (6th character M) into the peripheral nerve. *See table 01H to construct the Insertion code.* Also applicable when reported with Insertion of a stimulator lead (6th character M) into the stomach. *See table 0DH to construct the Insertion code.*

H70CZ Insertion of Single Array Rechargeable Stimulator Generator into Back Subcutaneous Tissue and Fascia, Open Approach

+ Neurotransmitter/Neurostimulator when reported with an Insertion of a neurostimulator lead (6th character M) into the cranial nerve, spinal canal or spinal cord. *See table 00H to construct the Insertion code.* Also applicable when reported with Insertion of neurostimulator lead (6th character M) into the peripheral nerve. *See table 01H to construct the Insertion code.* Also applicable when reported with Insertion of a stimulator lead (6th character M) into the stomach. *See table 0DH to construct the Insertion code.*

JH70DZ Insertion of Multiple Array Stimulator Generator into Back Subcutaneous Tissue and Fascia, Open Approach

+ Major brain device implant when reported with an Insertion of a neurostimulator lead (6th character M) into the brain or cerebral ventricle. *See table 00H to construct the Insertion code.*

+ Neurotransmitter/Neurostimulator when reported with an Insertion of a neurostimulator lead (6th character M) into the cranial nerve, spinal canal or spinal cord. *See table 00H to construct the Insertion code.* Also applicable when reported with Insertion of neurostimulator lead (6th character M) into the peripheral nerve. *See table 01H to construct the Insertion code.* Also applicable when reported with Insertion of a stimulator lead (6th character M) into the stomach. *See table 0DH to construct the Insertion code.*

0JH70EZ Insertion of Multiple Array Rechargeable Stimulator Generator into Back Subcutaneous Tissue and Fascia, Open Approach

+ Major brain device implant when reported with an Insertion of a neurostimulator lead (6th character M) into the brain or cerebral ventricle. *See table 00H to construct the Insertion code.*

+ Neurotransmitter/Neurostimulator when reported with an Insertion of a neurostimulator lead (6th character M) into the cranial nerve, spinal canal or spinal cord. *See table 00H to construct the Insertion code.* Also applicable when reported with Insertion of neurostimulator lead (6th character M) into the peripheral nerve. *See table 01H to construct the Insertion code.* Also applicable when reported with Insertion of a stimulator lead (6th character M) into the stomach. *See table 0DH to construct the Insertion code.*

▲ **0JH70MZ** Insertion of Stimulator Generator into Back Subcutaneous Tissue and Fascia, Open Approach

0JH70NZ Insertion of Tissue Expander into Back Subcutaneous Tissue and Fascia, Open Approach

0JH70VZ Insertion of Infusion Pump into Back Subcutaneous Tissue and Fascia, Open Approach

0JH73BZ Insertion of Single Array Stimulator Generator into Back Subcutaneous Tissue and Fascia, Percutaneous Approach

+ Neurotransmitter/Neurostimulator when reported with an Insertion of a neurostimulator lead (6th character M) into the cranial nerve, spinal canal or spinal cord. *See table 00H to construct the Insertion code.* Also applicable when reported with Insertion of neurostimulator lead (6th character M) into the peripheral nerve. *See table 01H to construct the Insertion code.* Also applicable when reported with Insertion of a stimulator lead (6th character M) into the stomach. *See table 0DH to construct the Insertion code.*

0JH73CZ Insertion of Single Array Rechargeable Stimulator Generator into Back Subcutaneous Tissue and Fascia, Percutaneous Approach

+ Neurotransmitter/Neurostimulator when reported with an Insertion of a neurostimulator lead (6th character M) into the cranial nerve, spinal canal or spinal cord. *See table 00H to construct the Insertion code.* Also applicable when reported with Insertion of neurostimulator lead (6th character M) into the peripheral nerve. *See table 01H to construct the Insertion code.* Also applicable when reported with Insertion of a stimulator lead (6th character M) into the stomach. *See table 0DH to construct the Insertion code.*

0JH73DZ Insertion of Multiple Array Stimulator Generator into Back Subcutaneous Tissue and Fascia, Percutaneous Approach

+ Major brain device implant when reported with an Insertion of a neurostimulator lead (6th character M) into the brain or cerebral ventricle. *See table 00H to construct the Insertion code.*

+ Neurotransmitter/Neurostimulator when reported with an Insertion of a neurostimulator lead (6th character M) into the cranial nerve, spinal canal or spinal cord. *See table 00H to construct the Insertion code.* Also applicable when reported with Insertion of neurostimulator lead (6th character M) into the peripheral nerve. *See table 01H to construct the Insertion code.* Also applicable when reported with Insertion of a stimulator lead (6th character M) into the stomach. *See table 0DH to construct the Insertion code.*

0JH73EZ Insertion of Multiple Array Rechargeable Stimulator Generator into Back Subcutaneous Tissue and Fascia, Percutaneous Approach

+ Major brain device implant when reported with an Insertion of a neurostimulator lead (6th character M) into the brain or cerebral ventricle. *See table 00H to construct the Insertion code.*

+ Neurotransmitter/Neurostimulator when reported with an Insertion of a neurostimulator lead (6th character M) into the cranial nerve, spinal canal or spinal cord. *See table 00H to construct the Insertion code.* Also applicable when reported with Insertion of neurostimulator lead (6th character M) into the peripheral nerve. *See table 01H to construct the Insertion code.* Also applicable when reported with Insertion of a stimulator lead (6th character M) into the stomach. *See table 0DH to construct the Insertion code.*

▲ **0JH73MZ** Insertion of Stimulator Generator into Back Subcutaneous Tissue and Fascia, Percutaneous Approach

0JH73NZ Insertion of Tissue Expander into Back Subcutaneous Tissue and Fascia, Percutaneous Approach

0JH73VZ Insertion of Infusion Pump into Back Subcutaneous Tissue and Fascia, Percutaneous Approach

0JH800Z Insertion of Hemodynamic Monitoring Device into Abdomen Subcutaneous Tissue and Fascia, Open Approach

● **0JH802Z** Insertion of Monitoring Device into Abdomen Subcutaneous Tissue and Fascia, Open Approach

● **0JH804Z** Insertion of Pacemaker, Single Chamber into Abdomen Subcutaneous Tissue and Fascia, Open Approach

HAC With a secondary diagnosis code of K68.11, T81.4XXA, T82.6XXA, T82.7XXA

+ Pacemaker device when reported with an Insertion of a cardiac lead (6th character J or M) into the coronary vein, atrium, ventricle or pericardium (4th characters 4, 6, 7, K, L and N). *See table 02H to construct the Insertion code.* When a device is replaced, also report the

Note continued

Continued note

Removal of the cardiac rhythm device (6th character P) from the trunk subcutaneous tissue and fascia. *See table 0JP to construct the Removal code.* When a cardiac lead is replaced, also report the Removal of the cardiac lead (6th character M) from the heart. *See table 02P to construct the Removal code.*

● **0JH805Z** Insertion of Pacemaker, Single Chamber Rate Responsive into Abdomen Subcutaneous Tissue and Fascia, Open Approach

HAC With a secondary diagnosis code of K68.11, T81.4XXA, T82.6XXA, T82.7XXA

+ Pacemaker device when reported with an Insertion of a cardiac lead (6th character J or M) into the coronary vein, atrium, ventricle or pericardium (4th characters 4, 6, 7, K, L and N). *See table 02H to construct the Insertion code.* When a device is replaced, also report the Removal of the cardiac rhythm device (6th character P) from the trunk subcutaneous tissue and fascia. *See table 0JP to construct the Removal code.* When a cardiac lead is replaced, also report the Removal of the cardiac lead (6th character M) from the heart. *See table 02P to construct the Removal code.*

● **0JH806Z** Insertion of Pacemaker, Dual Chamber into Abdomen Subcutaneous Tissue and Fascia, Open Approach

HAC With a secondary diagnosis code of K68.11, T81.4XXA, T82.6XXA, T82.7XXA

+ Pacemaker device when reported with an Insertion of a cardiac lead (6th character J or M) into the coronary vein, atrium, ventricle or pericardium (4th characters 4, 6, 7, K, L and N). *See table 02H to construct the Insertion code.* When a device is replaced, also report the Removal of the cardiac rhythm device (6th character P) from the trunk subcutaneous tissue and fascia. *See table 0JP to construct the Removal code.* When a cardiac lead is replaced, also report the Removal of the cardiac lead (6th character M) from the heart. *See table 02P to construct the Removal code.*

0JH807Z Insertion of Cardiac Resynchronization Pacemaker Pulse Generator into Abdomen Subcutaneous Tissue and Fascia, Open Approach

HAC With a secondary diagnosis code of K68.11, T81.4XXA, T82.6XXA, T82.7XXA

+ Pacemaker device when reported with an Insertion of a cardiac lead (6th character J or M) into the coronary vein, atrium, ventricle or pericardium (4th characters 4, 6, 7, K, L and N). *See table 02H to construct the Insertion code.* When a cardiac lead is replaced, also report the Removal of the cardiac lead (6th character M) from the heart. *See table 02P to construct the Removal code.*

0JH808Z Insertion of Defibrillator Generator into Abdomen Subcutaneous Tissue and Fascia, Open Approach

HAC With a secondary diagnosis code of K68.11, T81.4XXA, T82.6XXA, T82.7XXA

+ Cardioverter-Defibrillator lead(s)/generator when reported with Insertion of a defibrillator cardiac lead (6th character K) into the coronary vein, atrium, or ventricle. Also applicable with Insertion of pacemaker cardiac lead, defibrillator cardiac lead or cardiac lead (6th characters J, K, M) into the pericardium. *See table 02H to construct the Insertion code.*

0JH809Z Insertion of Cardiac Resynchronization Defibrillator Pulse Generator into Abdomen Subcutaneous Tissue and Fascia, Open Approach

HAC With a secondary diagnosis code of K68.11, T81.4XXA, T82.6XXA, T82.7XXA

+ Cardioverter-Defibrillator lead(s)/generator when reported with Insertion of a defibrillator cardiac lead (6th character K) into the atrium, or ventricle. Also applicable with Insertion of pacemaker cardiac lead, defibrillator cardiac lead or cardiac lead (6th characters J, K, M) into the coronary vein or pericardium. *See table 02H to construct the Insertion code.*

0JH80AZ Insertion of Contractility Modulation Device into Abdomen Subcutaneous Tissue and Fascia, Open Approach

+ Cardioverter-Defibrillator lead(s)/generator when reported with Insertion of a cardiac lead (6th character M) into the left ventricle. *See table 02H to construct the Insertion code.*

0JH80BZ Insertion of Single Array Stimulator Generator into Abdomen Subcutaneous Tissue and Fascia, Open Approach

+ Neurotransmitter/Neurostimulator when reported with an Insertion of a neurostimulator lead (6th character M) into the cranial nerve, spinal canal or spinal cord. *See table 00H to construct the Insertion code.* Also applicable when reported with Insertion of neurostimulator lead (6th character M) into the peripheral nerve. *See table 01H to construct the Insertion code.* Also applicable when reported with Insertion of a stimulator lead (6th character M) into the stomach. *See table 0DH to construct the Insertion code.*

0JH80CZ Insertion of Single Array Rechargeable Stimulator Generator into Abdomen Subcutaneous Tissue and Fascia, Open Approach

+ Neurotransmitter/Neurostimulator when reported with an Insertion of a neurostimulator lead (6th character M) into the cranial nerve, spinal canal or spinal cord. *See table 00H to construct the Insertion code.* Also applicable when reported with Insertion of neurostimulator lead (6th character M) into the peripheral nerve. *See table 01H to construct the Insertion code.* Also applicable when reported with Insertion of a stimulator lead (6th character M) into the stomach. *See table 0DH to construct the Insertion code.*

0JH80DZ Insertion of Multiple Array Stimulator Generator into Abdomen Subcutaneous Tissue and Fascia, Open Approach

+ Major brain device implant when reported with an Insertion of a neurostimulator lead (6th character M) into the brain or cerebral ventricle. *See table 00H to construct the Insertion code.*

+ Neurotransmitter/Neurostimulator when reported with an Insertion of a neurostimulator lead (6th character M) into the cranial nerve, spinal canal or spinal cord. *See table 00H to construct the Insertion code.* Also applicable when reported with Insertion of neurostimulator lead (6th character M) into the peripheral nerve. *See table 01H to construct the Insertion code.* Also applicable when reported with Insertion of a stimulator lead (6th character M) into the stomach. *See table 0DH to construct the Insertion code.*

0JH80EZ Insertion of Multiple Array Rechargeable Stimulator Generator into Abdomen Subcutaneous Tissue and Fascia, Open Approach

+ Major brain device implant when reported with an Insertion of a neurostimulator lead (6th character M) into the brain or cerebral ventricle. *See table 00H to construct the Insertion code.*

+ Neurotransmitter/Neurostimulator when reported with an Insertion of a neurostimulator lead (6th character M) into the cranial nerve, spinal canal or spinal cord. *See table 00H to construct the Insertion code.* Also applicable when reported with Insertion of neurostimulator lead (6th character M) into the peripheral nerve. *See table 01H to construct the Insertion code.* Also applicable when reported with Insertion of a stimulator lead (6th character M) into the stomach. *See table 0DH to construct the Insertion code.*

● **0JH80HZ** Insertion of Contraceptive Device into Abdomen Subcutaneous Tissue and Fascia, Open Approach

▲ **0JH80MZ** Insertion of Stimulator Generator into Abdomen Subcutaneous Tissue and Fascia, Open Approach

0JH80NZ Insertion of Tissue Expander into Abdomen Subcutaneous Tissue and Fascia, Open Approach

0JH80PZ Insertion of Cardiac Rhythm Related Device into Abdomen Subcutaneous Tissue and Fascia, Open Approach

HAC With a secondary diagnosis code of K68.11, T81.4XXA, T82.6XXA, T82.7XXA

+ Pacemaker device when reported with an Insertion of a cardiac lead (6th character J or M) into the coronary vein, atrium, ventricle or pericardium (4th characters 4, 6, 7, K, L and N). *See table 02H to construct the Insertion code.* When a cardiac lead is replaced, also report the Removal of the cardiac lead (6th character M) from the heart. *See table 02P to construct the Removal code.*

0JH80VZ Insertion of Infusion Pump into Abdomen Subcutaneous Tissue and Fascia, Open Approach

● **0JH80WZ** Insertion of Reservoir into Abdomen Subcutaneous Tissue and Fascia, Open Approach

● **0JH80XZ** Insertion of Vascular Access Device into Abdomen Subcutaneous Tissue and Fascia, Open Approach

0JH830Z Insertion of Hemodynamic Monitoring Device into Abdomen Subcutaneous Tissue and Fascia, Percutaneous Approach

● **0JH832Z** Insertion of Monitoring Device into Abdomen Subcutaneous Tissue and Fascia, Percutaneous Approach

H834Z Insertion of Pacemaker, Single Chamber into Abdomen Subcutaneous Tissue and Fascia, Percutaneous Approach

HAC With a secondary diagnosis code of K68.11, T81.4XXA, T82.6XXA, T82.7XXA

+ Pacemaker device when reported with an Insertion of a cardiac lead (6th character J or M) into the coronary vein, atrium, ventricle or pericardium (4th characters 4, 6, 7, K, L and N). *See table 02H to construct the Insertion code.* When a device is replaced, also report the Removal of the cardiac rhythm device (6th character P) from the trunk subcutaneous tissue and fascia. *See table 0JP to construct the Removal code.* When a cardiac lead is replaced, also report the Removal of the cardiac lead (6th character M) from the heart. *See table 02P to construct the Removal code.*

JH835Z Insertion of Pacemaker, Single Chamber Rate Responsive into Abdomen Subcutaneous Tissue and Fascia, Percutaneous Approach

HAC With a secondary diagnosis code of K68.11, T81.4XXA, T82.6XXA, T82.7XXA

+ Pacemaker device when reported with an Insertion of a cardiac lead (6th character J or M) into the coronary vein, atrium, ventricle or pericardium (4th characters 4, 6, 7, K, L and N). *See table 02H to construct the Insertion code.* When a device is replaced, also report the Removal of the cardiac rhythm device (6th character P) from the trunk subcutaneous tissue and fascia. *See table 0JP to construct the Removal code.* When a cardiac lead is replaced, also report the Removal of the cardiac lead (6th character M) from the heart. *See table 02P to construct the Removal code.*

JH836Z Insertion of Pacemaker, Dual Chamber into Abdomen Subcutaneous Tissue and Fascia, Percutaneous Approach

HAC With a secondary diagnosis code of K68.11, T81.4XXA, T82.6XXA, T82.7XXA

+ Pacemaker device when reported with an Insertion of a cardiac lead (6th character J or M) into the coronary vein, atrium, ventricle or pericardium (4th characters 4, 6, 7, K, L and N). *See table 02H to construct the Insertion code.* When a device is replaced, also report the Removal of the cardiac rhythm device (6th character P) from the trunk subcutaneous tissue and fascia. *See table 0JP to construct the Removal code.* When a cardiac lead is replaced, also report the Removal of the cardiac lead (6th character M) from the heart. *See table 02P to construct the Removal code.*

JH837Z Insertion of Cardiac Resynchronization Pacemaker Pulse Generator into Abdomen Subcutaneous Tissue and Fascia, Percutaneous Approach

HAC With a secondary diagnosis code of K68.11, T81.4XXA, T82.6XXA, T82.7XXA

+ Pacemaker device when reported with an Insertion of a cardiac lead (6th character J or M) into the coronary vein, atrium, ventricle or pericardium (4th characters 4, 6, 7, K, L and N). *See table 02H to construct the Insertion code.* When a cardiac lead is replaced, also report the Removal of the cardiac lead (6th character M) from the heart. *See table 02P to construct the Removal code.*

0JH838Z Insertion of Defibrillator Generator into Abdomen Subcutaneous Tissue and Fascia, Percutaneous Approach

HAC With a secondary diagnosis code of K68.11, T81.4XXA, T82.6XXA, T82.7XXA

+ Cardioverter-Defibrillator lead(s)/generator when reported with Insertion of a defibrillator cardiac lead (6th character K) into the coronary vein, atrium, or ventricle. Also applicable with Insertion of pacemaker cardiac lead, defibrillator cardiac lead or cardiac lead (6th characters J, K, M) into the pericardium. *See table 02H to construct the Insertion code.*

0JH839Z Insertion of Cardiac Resynchronization Defibrillator Pulse Generator into Abdomen Subcutaneous Tissue and Fascia, Percutaneous Approach

HAC With a secondary diagnosis code of K68.11, T81.4XXA, T82.6XXA, T82.7XXA

+ Cardioverter-Defibrillator lead(s)/generator when reported with Insertion of a defibrillator cardiac lead (6th character K) into the atrium, or ventricle. Also applicable with Insertion of pacemaker cardiac lead, defibrillator cardiac lead or cardiac lead (6th characters J, K, M) into the coronary vein or pericardium. *See table 02H to construct the Insertion code.*

0JH83AZ Insertion of Contractility Modulation Device into Abdomen Subcutaneous Tissue and Fascia, Percutaneous Approach

+ Cardioverter-Defibrillator lead(s)/generator when reported with Insertion of a cardiac lead (6th character M) into the left ventricle. *See table 02H to construct the Insertion code.*

0JH83BZ Insertion of Single Array Stimulator Generator into Abdomen Subcutaneous Tissue and Fascia, Percutaneous Approach

+ Neurotransmitter/Neurostimulator when reported with an Insertion of a neurostimulator lead (6th character M) into the cranial nerve, spinal canal or spinal cord. *See table 00H to construct the Insertion code.* Also applicable when reported with Insertion of neurostimulator lead (6th character M) into the peripheral nerve. *See table 01H to construct the Insertion code.* Also applicable when reported with Insertion of a stimulator lead (6th character M) into the stomach. *See table 0DH to construct the Insertion code.*

0JH83CZ Insertion of Single Array Rechargeable Stimulator Generator into Abdomen Subcutaneous Tissue and Fascia, Percutaneous Approach

+ Neurotransmitter/Neurostimulator when reported with an Insertion of a neurostimulator lead (6th character M) into the cranial nerve, spinal canal or spinal cord. *See table 00H to construct the Insertion code.* Also applicable when reported with Insertion of neurostimulator lead (6th character M) into the peripheral nerve. *See table 01H to construct the Insertion code.* Also applicable when reported with Insertion of a stimulator lead (6th character M) into the stomach. *See table 0DH to construct the Insertion code.*

0JH83DZ Insertion of Multiple Array Stimulator Generator into Abdomen Subcutaneous Tissue and Fascia, Percutaneous Approach

+ Major brain device implant when reported with an Insertion of a neurostimulator lead (6th character M) into the brain or cerebral ventricle. *See table 00H to construct the Insertion code.*

+ Neurotransmitter/Neurostimulator when reported with an Insertion of a neurostimulator lead (6th character M) into the cranial nerve, spinal canal or spinal cord. *See table 00H to construct the Insertion code.* Also applicable when reported with Insertion of neurostimulator lead (6th character M) into the peripheral nerve. *See table 01H to construct the Insertion code.* Also applicable when reported with Insertion of a stimulator lead (6th character M) into the stomach. *See table 0DH to construct the Insertion code.*

0JH83EZ Insertion of Multiple Array Rechargeable Stimulator Generator into Abdomen Subcutaneous Tissue and Fascia, Percutaneous Approach

+ Major brain device implant when reported with an Insertion of a neurostimulator lead (6th character M) into the brain or cerebral ventricle. *See table 00H to construct the Insertion code.*

+ Neurotransmitter/Neurostimulator when reported with an Insertion of a neurostimulator lead (6th character M) into the cranial nerve, spinal canal or spinal cord. *See table 00H to construct the Insertion code.* Also applicable when reported with Insertion of neurostimulator lead (6th character M) into the peripheral nerve. *See table 01H to construct the Insertion code.* Also applicable when reported with Insertion of a stimulator lead (6th character M) into the stomach. *See table 0DH to construct the Insertion code.*

● **0JH83HZ** Insertion of Contraceptive Device into Abdomen Subcutaneous Tissue and Fascia, Percutaneous Approach

▲ **0JH83MZ** Insertion of Stimulator Generator into Abdomen Subcutaneous Tissue and Fascia, Percutaneous Approach

0JH83NZ Insertion of Tissue Expander into Abdomen Subcutaneous Tissue and Fascia, Percutaneous Approach

0JH83PZ Insertion of Cardiac Rhythm Related Device into Abdomen Subcutaneous Tissue and Fascia, Percutaneous Approach

HAC With a secondary diagnosis code of K68.11, T81.4XXA, T82.6XXA, T82.7XXA

+ Pacemaker device when reported with an Insertion of a cardiac lead (6th character J or M) into the coronary vein, atrium, ventricle or pericardium (4th characters 4, 6, 7, K, L and N). *See table 02H to construct the Insertion code.* When a cardiac lead is replaced, also report the Removal of the cardiac lead (6th character M) from the heart. *See table 02P to construct the Removal code.*

0JH83VZ Insertion of Infusion Pump into Abdomen Subcutaneous Tissue and Fascia, Percutaneous Approach

● **0JH83WZ** Insertion of Reservoir into Abdomen Subcutaneous Tissue and Fascia, Percutaneous Approach

● **0JH83XZ** Insertion of Vascular Access Device into Abdomen Subcutaneous Tissue and Fascia, Percutaneous Approach

0JH90NZ Insertion of Tissue Expander into Buttock Subcutaneous Tissue and Fascia, Open Approach

0JH93NZ Insertion of Tissue Expander into Buttock Subcutaneous Tissue and Fascia, Percutaneous Approach

0JHB0NZ Insertion of Tissue Expander into Perineum Subcutaneous Tissue and Fascia, Open Approach

0JHB3NZ Insertion of Tissue Expander into Perineum Subcutaneous Tissue and Fascia, Percutaneous Approach

0JHC0NZ Insertion of Tissue Expander into Pelvic Region Subcutaneous Tissue and Fascia, Open Approach

0JHC3NZ Insertion of Tissue Expander into Pelvic Region Subcutaneous Tissue and Fascia, Percutaneous Approach

0JHD0HZ Insertion of Contraceptive Device into Right Upper Arm Subcutaneous Tissue and Fascia, Open Approach

0JHD0NZ Insertion of Tissue Expander into Right Upper Arm Subcutaneous Tissue and Fascia, Open Approach

0JHD0VZ Insertion of Infusion Pump into Right Upper Arm Subcutaneous Tissue and Fascia, Open Approach

● **0JHD0WZ** Insertion of Reservoir into Right Upper Arm Subcutaneous Tissue and Fascia, Open Approach

● **0JHD0XZ** Insertion of Vascular Access Device into Right Upper Arm Subcutaneous Tissue and Fascia, Open Approach

0JHD3HZ Insertion of Contraceptive Device into Right Upper Arm Subcutaneous Tissue and Fascia, Percutaneous Approach

0JHD3NZ Insertion of Tissue Expander into Right Upper Arm Subcutaneous Tissue and Fascia, Percutaneous Approach

0JHD3VZ Insertion of Infusion Pump into Right Upper Arm Subcutaneous Tissue and Fascia, Percutaneous Approach

● **0JHD3WZ** Insertion of Reservoir into Right Upper Arm Subcutaneous Tissue and Fascia, Percutaneous Approach

● **0JHD3XZ** Insertion of Vascular Access Device into Right Upper Arm Subcutaneous Tissue and Fascia, Percutaneous Approach

0JHF0HZ Insertion of Contraceptive Device into Left Upper Arm Subcutaneous Tissue and Fascia, Open Approach

0JHF0NZ Insertion of Tissue Expander into Left Upper Arm Subcutaneous Tissue and Fascia, Open Approach

0JHF0VZ Insertion of Infusion Pump into Left Upper Arm Subcutaneous Tissue and Fascia, Open Approach

● **0JHF0WZ** Insertion of Reservoir into Left Upper Arm Subcutaneous Tissue and Fascia, Open Approach

● **0JHF0XZ** Insertion of Vascular Access Device into Left Upper Arm Subcutaneous Tissue and Fascia, Open Approach

0JHF3HZ Insertion of Contraceptive Device into Left Upper Arm Subcutaneous Tissue and Fascia, Percutaneous Approach

0JHF3NZ Insertion of Tissue Expander into Left Upper Arm Subcutaneous Tissue and Fascia, Percutaneous Approach

0JHF3VZ Insertion of Infusion Pump into Left Upper Arm Subcutaneous Tissue and Fascia, Percutaneous Approach

● **0JHF3WZ** Insertion of Reservoir into Left Upper Arm Subcutaneous Tissue and Fascia, Percutaneous Approach

● **0JHF3XZ** Insertion of Vascular Access Device into Left Upper Arm Subcutaneous Tissue and Fascia, Percutaneous Approach

0JHG0HZ Insertion of Contraceptive Device into Right Lower Arm Subcutaneous Tissue and Fascia, Open Approach

0JHG0NZ Insertion of Tissue Expander into Right Lower Arm Subcutaneous Tissue and Fascia, Open Approach

0JHG0VZ Insertion of Infusion Pump into Right Lower Arm Subcutaneous Tissue and Fascia, Open Approach

● **0JHG0WZ** Insertion of Reservoir into Right Lower Arm Subcutaneous Tissue and Fascia, Open Approach

● **0JHG0XZ** Insertion of Vascular Access Device into Right Lower Arm Subcutaneous Tissue and Fascia, Open Approach

0JHG3HZ Insertion of Contraceptive Device into Right Lower Arm Subcutaneous Tissue and Fascia, Percutaneous Approach

0JHG3NZ Insertion of Tissue Expander into Right Lower Arm Subcutaneous Tissue and Fascia, Percutaneous Approach

0JHG3VZ Insertion of Infusion Pump into Right Lower Arm Subcutaneous Tissue and Fascia, Percutaneous Approach

● **0JHG3WZ** Insertion of Reservoir into Right Lower Arm Subcutaneous Tissue and Fascia, Percutaneous Approach

● **0JHG3XZ** Insertion of Vascular Access Device into Right Lower Arm Subcutaneous Tissue and Fascia, Percutaneous Approach

0JHH0HZ Insertion of Contraceptive Device into Left Lower Arm Subcutaneous Tissue and Fascia, Open Approach

0JHH0NZ Insertion of Tissue Expander into Left Lower Arm Subcutaneous Tissue and Fascia, Open Approach

0JHH0VZ Insertion of Infusion Pump into Left Lower Arm Subcutaneous Tissue and Fascia, Open Approach

● **0JHH0WZ** Insertion of Reservoir into Left Lower Arm Subcutaneous Tissue and Fascia, Open Approach

● **0JHH0XZ** Insertion of Vascular Access Device into Left Lower Arm Subcutaneous Tissue and Fascia, Open Approach

0JHH3HZ Insertion of Contraceptive Device into Left Lower Arm Subcutaneous Tissue and Fascia, Percutaneous Approach

0JHH3NZ Insertion of Tissue Expander into Left Lower Arm Subcutaneous Tissue and Fascia, Percutaneous Approach

0JHH3VZ Insertion of Infusion Pump into Left Lower Arm Subcutaneous Tissue and Fascia, Percutaneous Approach

● **0JHH3WZ** Insertion of Reservoir into Left Lower Arm Subcutaneous Tissue and Fascia, Percutaneous Approach

● **0JHH3XZ** Insertion of Vascular Access Device into Left Lower Arm Subcutaneous Tissue and Fascia, Percutaneous Approach

0JHJ0NZ Insertion of Tissue Expander into Right Hand Subcutaneous Tissue and Fascia, Open Approach

0JHJ3NZ Insertion of Tissue Expander into Right Hand Subcutaneous Tissue and Fascia, Percutaneous Approach

0JHK0NZ Insertion of Tissue Expander into Left Hand Subcutaneous Tissue and Fascia, Open Approach

0JHK3NZ Insertion of Tissue Expander into Left Hand Subcutaneous Tissue and Fascia, Percutaneous Approach

0JHL0HZ Insertion of Contraceptive Device into Right Upper Leg Subcutaneous Tissue and Fascia, Open Approach

0JHL0NZ Insertion of Tissue Expander into Right Upper Leg Subcutaneous Tissue and Fascia, Open Approach

0JHL0VZ Insertion of Infusion Pump into Right Upper Leg Subcutaneous Tissue and Fascia, Open Approach

● **0JHL0WZ** Insertion of Reservoir into Right Uppe Leg Subcutaneous Tissue and Fascia, Open Approach

● **0JHL0XZ** Insertion of Vascular Access Device in Right Upper Leg Subcutaneous Tissue and Fascia, Open Approach

0JHL3HZ Insertion of Contraceptive Device into Right Upper Leg Subcutaneous Tissue and Fascia, Percutaneous Approach

0JHL3NZ Insertion of Tissue Expander into Right Upper Leg Subcutaneous Tissue and Fascia, Percutaneous Approach

0JHL3VZ Insertion of Infusion Pump into Right Upper Leg Subcutaneous Tissue and Fascia, Percutaneous Approach

● **0JHL3WZ** Insertion of Reservoir into Right Upper Leg Subcutaneous Tissue and Fascia, Percutaneous Approach

● **0JHL3XZ** Insertion of Vascular Access Device int Right Upper Leg Subcutaneous Tissue and Fascia, Percutaneous Approach

0JHM0HZ Insertion of Contraceptive Device into Left Upper Leg Subcutaneous Tissue ar Fascia, Open Approach

0JHM0NZ Insertion of Tissue Expander into Left Upper Leg Subcutaneous Tissue and Fascia, Open Approach

0JHM0VZ Insertion of Infusion Pump into Left Upper Leg Subcutaneous Tissue and Fascia, Open Approach

● **0JHM0WZ** Insertion of Reservoir into Left Upper Leg Subcutaneous Tissue and Fascia, Open Approach

● **0JHM0XZ** Insertion of Vascular Access Device into Left Upper Leg Subcutaneous Tissue an Fascia, Open Approach

0JHM3HZ Insertion of Contraceptive Device into Left Upper Leg Subcutaneous Tissue an Fascia, Percutaneous Approach

0JHM3NZ Insertion of Tissue Expander into Left Upper Leg Subcutaneous Tissue and Fascia, Percutaneous Approach

0JHM3VZ Insertion of Infusion Pump into Left Upper Leg Subcutaneous Tissue and Fascia, Percutaneous Approach

● **0JHM3WZ** Insertion of Reservoir into Left Upper Leg Subcutaneous Tissue and Fascia, Percutaneous Approach

● **0JHM3XZ** Insertion of Vascular Access Device into Left Upper Leg Subcutaneous Tissue an Fascia, Percutaneous Approach

0JHN0HZ Insertion of Contraceptive Device into Right Lower Leg Subcutaneous Tissue and Fascia, Open Approach

0JHN0NZ Insertion of Tissue Expander into Right Lower Leg Subcutaneous Tissue and Fascia, Open Approach

0JHN0VZ Insertion of Infusion Pump into Right Lower Leg Subcutaneous Tissue and Fascia, Open Approach

● **0JHN0WZ** Insertion of Reservoir into Right Lower Leg Subcutaneous Tissue and Fascia, Open Approach

● **0JHN0XZ** Insertion of Vascular Access Device into Right Lower Leg Subcutaneous Tissue and Fascia, Open Approach

● **0JHN3HZ** Insertion of Contraceptive Device into Right Lower Leg Subcutaneous Tissue and Fascia, Percutaneous Approach

0JHN3NZ Insertion of Tissue Expander into Right Lower Leg Subcutaneous Tissue and Fascia, Percutaneous Approach

0JHN3VZ Insertion of Infusion Pump into Right Lower Leg Subcutaneous Tissue and Fascia, Percutaneous Approach

● **0JHN3WZ** Insertion of Reservoir into Right Lower Leg Subcutaneous Tissue and Fascia, Percutaneous Approach

HN3XZ Insertion of Vascular Access Device into Right Lower Leg Subcutaneous Tissue and Fascia, Percutaneous Approach
HP0HZ Insertion of Contraceptive Device into Left Lower Leg Subcutaneous Tissue and Fascia, Open Approach
IP0NZ Insertion of Tissue Expander into Left Lower Leg Subcutaneous Tissue and Fascia, Open Approach
IP0VZ Insertion of Infusion Pump into Left Lower Leg Subcutaneous Tissue and Fascia, Open Approach
JHP0WZ Insertion of Reservoir into Left Lower Leg Subcutaneous Tissue and Fascia, Open Approach
JHP0XZ Insertion of Vascular Access Device into Left Lower Leg Subcutaneous Tissue and Fascia, Open Approach
JHP3HZ Insertion of Contraceptive Device into Left Lower Leg Subcutaneous Tissue and Fascia, Percutaneous Approach
HP3NZ Insertion of Tissue Expander into Left Lower Leg Subcutaneous Tissue and Fascia, Percutaneous Approach
HP3VZ Insertion of Infusion Pump into Left Lower Leg Subcutaneous Tissue and Fascia, Percutaneous Approach
JHP3WZ Insertion of Reservoir into Left Lower Leg Subcutaneous Tissue and Fascia, Percutaneous Approach
JHP3XZ Insertion of Vascular Access Device into Left Lower Leg Subcutaneous Tissue and Fascia, Percutaneous Approach
0JHQ0NZ Insertion of Tissue Expander into Right Foot Subcutaneous Tissue and Fascia, Open Approach
0JHQ3NZ Insertion of Tissue Expander into Right Foot Subcutaneous Tissue and Fascia, Percutaneous Approach
0JHR0NZ Insertion of Tissue Expander into Left Foot Subcutaneous Tissue and Fascia, Open Approach
0JHR3NZ Insertion of Tissue Expander into Left Foot Subcutaneous Tissue and Fascia, Percutaneous Approach
0JHS01Z Insertion of Radioactive Element into Head and Neck Subcutaneous Tissue and Fascia, Open Approach
0JHS03Z Insertion of Infusion Device into Head and Neck Subcutaneous Tissue and Fascia, Open Approach
0JHS31Z Insertion of Radioactive Element into Head and Neck Subcutaneous Tissue and Fascia, Percutaneous Approach
0JHS33Z Insertion of Infusion Device into Head and Neck Subcutaneous Tissue and Fascia, Percutaneous Approach
0JHT01Z Insertion of Radioactive Element into Trunk Subcutaneous Tissue and Fascia, Open Approach
0JHT03Z Insertion of Infusion Device into Trunk Subcutaneous Tissue and Fascia, Open Approach
0JHT0VZ Insertion of Infusion Pump into Trunk Subcutaneous Tissue and Fascia, Open Approach
0JHT31Z Insertion of Radioactive Element into Trunk Subcutaneous Tissue and Fascia, Percutaneous Approach
0JHT33Z Insertion of Infusion Device into Trunk Subcutaneous Tissue and Fascia, Percutaneous Approach
0JHT3VZ Insertion of Infusion Pump into Trunk Subcutaneous Tissue and Fascia, Percutaneous Approach
0JHV01Z Insertion of Radioactive Element into Upper Extremity Subcutaneous Tissue and Fascia, Open Approach
0JHV03Z Insertion of Infusion Device into Upper Extremity Subcutaneous Tissue and Fascia, Open Approach
0JHV31Z Insertion of Radioactive Element into Upper Extremity Subcutaneous Tissue and Fascia, Percutaneous Approach
0JHV33Z Insertion of Infusion Device into Upper Extremity Subcutaneous Tissue and Fascia, Percutaneous Approach
0JHW01Z Insertion of Radioactive Element into Lower Extremity Subcutaneous Tissue and Fascia, Open Approach
0JHW03Z Insertion of Infusion Device into Lower Extremity Subcutaneous Tissue and Fascia, Open Approach
0JHW31Z Insertion of Radioactive Element into Lower Extremity Subcutaneous Tissue and Fascia, Percutaneous Approach
0JHW33Z Insertion of Infusion Device into Lower Extremity Subcutaneous Tissue and Fascia, Percutaneous Approach

JJ – Subcutaneous Tissue and Fascia, Inspection

eview Coding Guideline B3.5

eview Coding Guidelines B3.11a, B3.11b and B3.11c

JS0ZZ Inspection of Head and Neck Subcutaneous Tissue and Fascia, Open Approach
JS3ZZ Inspection of Head and Neck Subcutaneous Tissue and Fascia, Percutaneous Approach
JSXZZ Inspection of Head and Neck Subcutaneous Tissue and Fascia, External Approach
JJT0ZZ Inspection of Trunk Subcutaneous Tissue and Fascia, Open Approach
0JJT3ZZ Inspection of Trunk Subcutaneous Tissue and Fascia, Percutaneous Approach
0JJTXZZ Inspection of Trunk Subcutaneous Tissue and Fascia, External Approach
0JJV0ZZ Inspection of Upper Extremity Subcutaneous Tissue and Fascia, Open Approach
0JJV3ZZ Inspection of Upper Extremity Subcutaneous Tissue and Fascia, Percutaneous Approach
0JJVXZZ Inspection of Upper Extremity Subcutaneous Tissue and Fascia, External Approach
0JJW0ZZ Inspection of Lower Extremity Subcutaneous Tissue and Fascia, Open Approach
0JJW3ZZ Inspection of Lower Extremity Subcutaneous Tissue and Fascia, Percutaneous Approach
0JJWXZZ Inspection of Lower Extremity Subcutaneous Tissue and Fascia, External Approach

JN – Subcutaneous Tissue and Fascia, Release

eview Coding Guideline B3.13

eview Coding Guideline B3.14

JN00ZZ Release Scalp Subcutaneous Tissue and Fascia, Open Approach
JN03ZZ Release Scalp Subcutaneous Tissue and Fascia, Percutaneous Approach
JN0XZZ Release Scalp Subcutaneous Tissue and Fascia, External Approach
JN10ZZ Release Face Subcutaneous Tissue and Fascia, Open Approach
JN13ZZ Release Face Subcutaneous Tissue and Fascia, Percutaneous Approach
JN1XZZ Release Face Subcutaneous Tissue and Fascia, External Approach
JN40ZZ Release Anterior Neck Subcutaneous Tissue and Fascia, Open Approach
JN43ZZ Release Anterior Neck Subcutaneous Tissue and Fascia, Percutaneous Approach
JN4XZZ Release Anterior Neck Subcutaneous Tissue and Fascia, External Approach
0JN50ZZ Release Posterior Neck Subcutaneous Tissue and Fascia, Open Approach
0JN53ZZ Release Posterior Neck Subcutaneous Tissue and Fascia, Percutaneous Approach
0JN5XZZ Release Posterior Neck Subcutaneous Tissue and Fascia, External Approach
0JN60ZZ Release Chest Subcutaneous Tissue and Fascia, Open Approach
0JN63ZZ Release Chest Subcutaneous Tissue and Fascia, Percutaneous Approach
0JN6XZZ Release Chest Subcutaneous Tissue and Fascia, External Approach
0JN70ZZ Release Back Subcutaneous Tissue and Fascia, Open Approach
0JN73ZZ Release Back Subcutaneous Tissue and Fascia, Percutaneous Approach
0JN7XZZ Release Back Subcutaneous Tissue and Fascia, External Approach
0JN80ZZ Release Abdomen Subcutaneous Tissue and Fascia, Open Approach
0JN83ZZ Release Abdomen Subcutaneous Tissue and Fascia, Percutaneous Approach
0JN8XZZ Release Abdomen Subcutaneous Tissue and Fascia, External Approach
0JN90ZZ Release Buttock Subcutaneous Tissue and Fascia, Open Approach
0JN93ZZ Release Buttock Subcutaneous Tissue and Fascia, Percutaneous Approach
0JN9XZZ Release Buttock Subcutaneous Tissue and Fascia, External Approach
0JNB0ZZ Release Perineum Subcutaneous Tissue and Fascia, Open Approach
0JNB3ZZ Release Perineum Subcutaneous Tissue and Fascia, Percutaneous Approach
0JNBXZZ Release Perineum Subcutaneous Tissue and Fascia, External Approach

0JNC0ZZ Release Pelvic Region Subcutaneous Tissue and Fascia, Open Approach
0JNC3ZZ Release Pelvic Region Subcutaneous Tissue and Fascia, Percutaneous Approach
0JNCXZZ Release Pelvic Region Subcutaneous Tissue and Fascia, External Approach
0JND0ZZ Release Right Upper Arm Subcutaneous Tissue and Fascia, Open Approach
0JND3ZZ Release Right Upper Arm Subcutaneous Tissue and Fascia, Percutaneous Approach
0JNDXZZ Release Right Upper Arm Subcutaneous Tissue and Fascia, External Approach
0JNF0ZZ Release Left Upper Arm Subcutaneous Tissue and Fascia, Open Approach
0JNF3ZZ Release Left Upper Arm Subcutaneous Tissue and Fascia, Percutaneous Approach
0JNFXZZ Release Left Upper Arm Subcutaneous Tissue and Fascia, External Approach
0JNG0ZZ Release Right Lower Arm Subcutaneous Tissue and Fascia, Open Approach
0JNG3ZZ Release Right Lower Arm Subcutaneous Tissue and Fascia, Percutaneous Approach
0JNGXZZ Release Right Lower Arm Subcutaneous Tissue and Fascia, External Approach
0JNH0ZZ Release Left Lower Arm Subcutaneous Tissue and Fascia, Open Approach
0JNH3ZZ Release Left Lower Arm Subcutaneous Tissue and Fascia, Percutaneous Approach
0JNHXZZ Release Left Lower Arm Subcutaneous Tissue and Fascia, External Approach
0JNJ0ZZ Release Right Hand Subcutaneous Tissue and Fascia, Open Approach
0JNJ3ZZ Release Right Hand Subcutaneous Tissue and Fascia, Percutaneous Approach
0JNJXZZ Release Right Hand Subcutaneous Tissue and Fascia, External Approach
0JNK0ZZ Release Left Hand Subcutaneous Tissue and Fascia, Open Approach
0JNK3ZZ Release Left Hand Subcutaneous Tissue and Fascia, Percutaneous Approach
0JNKXZZ Release Left Hand Subcutaneous Tissue and Fascia, External Approach
0JNL0ZZ Release Right Upper Leg Subcutaneous Tissue and Fascia, Open Approach
0JNL3ZZ Release Right Upper Leg Subcutaneous Tissue and Fascia, Percutaneous Approach
0JNLXZZ Release Right Upper Leg Subcutaneous Tissue and Fascia, External Approach
0JNM0ZZ Release Left Upper Leg Subcutaneous Tissue and Fascia, Open Approach
0JNM3ZZ Release Left Upper Leg Subcutaneous Tissue and Fascia, Percutaneous Approach
0JNMXZZ Release Left Upper Leg Subcutaneous Tissue and Fascia, External Approach
0JNN0ZZ Release Right Lower Leg Subcutaneous Tissue and Fascia, Open Approach
0JNN3ZZ Release Right Lower Leg Subcutaneous Tissue and Fascia, Percutaneous Approach
0JNNXZZ Release Right Lower Leg Subcutaneous Tissue and Fascia, External Approach
0JNP0ZZ Release Left Lower Leg Subcutaneous Tissue and Fascia, Open Approach
0JNP3ZZ Release Left Lower Leg Subcutaneous Tissue and Fascia, Percutaneous Approach
0JNPXZZ Release Left Lower Leg Subcutaneous Tissue and Fascia, External Approach
0JNQ0ZZ Release Right Foot Subcutaneous Tissue and Fascia, Open Approach
0JNQ3ZZ Release Right Foot Subcutaneous Tissue and Fascia, Percutaneous Approach
0JNQXZZ Release Right Foot Subcutaneous Tissue and Fascia, External Approach
0JNR0ZZ Release Left Foot Subcutaneous Tissue and Fascia, Open Approach
0JNR3ZZ Release Left Foot Subcutaneous Tissue and Fascia, Percutaneous Approach
0JNRXZZ Release Left Foot Subcutaneous Tissue and Fascia, External Approach

0JP – Subcutaneous Tissue and Fascia, Removal

Review Coding Guideline B6.1c

0JPS00Z Removal of Drainage Device from Head and Neck Subcutaneous Tissue and Fascia, Open Approach
0JPS01Z Removal of Radioactive Element from Head and Neck Subcutaneous Tissue and Fascia, Open Approach
0JPS03Z Removal of Infusion Device from Head and Neck Subcutaneous Tissue and Fascia, Open Approach
0JPS07Z Removal of Autologous Tissue Substitute from Head and Neck Subcutaneous Tissue and Fascia, Open Approach
0JPS0JZ Removal of Synthetic Substitute from Head and Neck Subcutaneous Tissue and Fascia, Open Approach
0JPS0KZ Removal of Nonautologous Tissue Substitute from Head and Neck Subcutaneous Tissue and Fascia, Open Approach
0JPS0NZ Removal of Tissue Expander from Head and Neck Subcutaneous Tissue and Fascia, Open Approach
0JPS30Z Removal of Drainage Device from Head and Neck Subcutaneous Tissue and Fascia, Percutaneous Approach
0JPS31Z Removal of Radioactive Element from Head and Neck Subcutaneous Tissue and Fascia, Percutaneous Approach
0JPS33Z Removal of Infusion Device from Head and Neck Subcutaneous Tissue and Fascia, Percutaneous Approach
0JPS37Z Removal of Autologous Tissue Substitute from Head and Neck Subcutaneous Tissue and Fascia, Percutaneous Approach
0JPS3JZ Removal of Synthetic Substitute from Head and Neck Subcutaneous Tissue and Fascia, Percutaneous Approach
0JPS3KZ Removal of Nonautologous Tissue Substitute from Head and Neck Subcutaneous Tissue and Fascia, Percutaneous Approach
0JPS3NZ Removal of Tissue Expander from Head and Neck Subcutaneous Tissue and Fascia, Percutaneous Approach
0JPSX0Z Removal of Drainage Device from Head and Neck Subcutaneous Tissue and Fascia, External Approach
0JPSX1Z Removal of Radioactive Element from Head and Neck Subcutaneous Tissue and Fascia, External Approach
0JPSX3Z Removal of Infusion Device from Head and Neck Subcutaneous Tissue and Fascia, External Approach
0JPT00Z Removal of Drainage Device from Trunk Subcutaneous Tissue and Fascia, Open Approach
0JPT01Z Removal of Radioactive Element from Trunk Subcutaneous Tissue and Fascia, Open Approach
0JPT02Z Removal of Monitoring Device from Trunk Subcutaneous Tissue and Fascia, Open Approach
0JPT03Z Removal of Infusion Device from Trunk Subcutaneous Tissue and Fascia, Open Approach
0JPT07Z Removal of Autologous Tissue Substitute from Trunk Subcutaneous Tissue and Fascia, Open Approach
0JPT0HZ Removal of Contraceptive Device from Trunk Subcutaneous Tissue and Fascia, Open Approach
0JPT0JZ Removal of Synthetic Substitute from Trunk Subcutaneous Tissue and Fascia, Open Approach
0JPT0KZ Removal of Nonautologous Tissue Substitute from Trunk Subcutaneous Tissue and Fascia, Open Approach
0JPT0MZ Removal of Stimulator Generator from Trunk Subcutaneous Tissue and Fascia, Open Approach
0JPT0NZ Removal of Tissue Expander from Trunk Subcutaneous Tissue and Fascia, Open Approach
AHA CC: 4Q, 2013, 109-111
0JPT0PZ Removal of Cardiac Rhythm Related Device from Trunk Subcutaneous Tissue and Fascia, Open Approach
AHA CC: 4Q, 2012, 104-106
HAC With a secondary diagnosis code of K68.11, T81.4XXA, T82.6XXA, T82.7XXA
0JPT0VZ Removal of Infusion Pump from Trunk Subcutaneous Tissue and Fascia, Open Approach
0JPT0WZ Removal of Reservoir from Trunk Subcutaneous Tissue and Fascia, Open Approach
0JPT0XZ Removal of Vascular Access Device from Trunk Subcutaneous Tissue and Fascia, Open Approach
0JPT30Z Removal of Drainage Device from Trunk Subcutaneous Tissue and Fascia, Percutaneous Approach
0JPT31Z Removal of Radioactive Element from Trunk Subcutaneous Tissue and Fascia, Percutaneous Approach
0JPT32Z Removal of Monitoring Device from Trunk Subcutaneous Tissue and Fascia, Percutaneous Approach
0JPT33Z Removal of Infusion Device from Trunk Subcutaneous Tissue and Fascia, Percutaneous Approach
0JPT37Z Removal of Autologous Tissue Substitute from Trunk Subcutaneous Tissue and Fascia, Percutaneous Approach
0JPT3HZ Removal of Contraceptive Device from Trunk Subcutaneous Tissue and Fascia, Percutaneous Approach
0JPT3JZ Removal of Synthetic Substitute from Trunk Subcutaneous Tissue and Fascia, Percutaneous Approach
0JPT3KZ Removal of Nonautologous Tissue Substitute from Trunk Subcutaneous Tissue and Fascia, Percutaneous Approach
0JPT3MZ Removal of Stimulator Generator from Trunk Subcutaneous Tissue and Fascia, Percutaneous Approach
0JPT3NZ Removal of Tissue Expander from Trunk Subcutaneous Tissue and Fascia, Percutaneous Approach
0JPT3PZ Removal of Cardiac Rhythm Related Device from Trunk Subcutaneous Tissue and Fascia, Percutaneous Approach
HAC With a secondary diagnosis code of K68.11, T81.4XXA, T82.6XXA, T82.7XXA
0JPT3VZ Removal of Infusion Pump from Trunk Subcutaneous Tissue and Fascia, Percutaneous Approach
0JPT3WZ Removal of Reservoir from Trunk Subcutaneous Tissue and Fascia, Percutaneous Approach

T3XZ Removal of Vascular Access Device from Trunk Subcutaneous Tissue and Fascia, Percutaneous Approach
TX0Z Removal of Drainage Device from Trunk Subcutaneous Tissue and Fascia, External Approach
TX1Z Removal of Radioactive Element from Trunk Subcutaneous Tissue and Fascia, External Approach
TX2Z Removal of Monitoring Device from Trunk Subcutaneous Tissue and Fascia, External Approach
TX3Z Removal of Infusion Device from Trunk Subcutaneous Tissue and Fascia, External Approach
TXHZ Removal of Contraceptive Device from Trunk Subcutaneous Tissue and Fascia, External Approach
TXVZ Removal of Infusion Pump from Trunk Subcutaneous Tissue and Fascia, External Approach
TXXZ Removal of Vascular Access Device from Trunk Subcutaneous Tissue and Fascia, External Approach
V00Z Removal of Drainage Device from Upper Extremity Subcutaneous Tissue and Fascia, Open Approach
V01Z Removal of Radioactive Element from Upper Extremity Subcutaneous Tissue and Fascia, Open Approach
PV03Z Removal of Infusion Device from Upper Extremity Subcutaneous Tissue and Fascia, Open Approach
PV07Z Removal of Autologous Tissue Substitute from Upper Extremity Subcutaneous Tissue and Fascia, Open Approach
PV0HZ Removal of Contraceptive Device from Upper Extremity Subcutaneous Tissue and Fascia, Open Approach
PV0JZ Removal of Synthetic Substitute from Upper Extremity Subcutaneous Tissue and Fascia, Open Approach
PV0KZ Removal of Nonautologous Tissue Substitute from Upper Extremity Subcutaneous Tissue and Fascia, Open Approach
PV0NZ Removal of Tissue Expander from Upper Extremity Subcutaneous Tissue and Fascia, Open Approach
PV0VZ Removal of Infusion Pump from Upper Extremity Subcutaneous Tissue and Fascia, Open Approach
PV0WZ Removal of Reservoir from Upper Extremity Subcutaneous Tissue and Fascia, Open Approach
PV0XZ Removal of Vascular Access Device from Upper Extremity Subcutaneous Tissue and Fascia, Open Approach
PV30Z Removal of Drainage Device from Upper Extremity Subcutaneous Tissue and Fascia, Percutaneous Approach
PV31Z Removal of Radioactive Element from Upper Extremity Subcutaneous Tissue and Fascia, Percutaneous Approach
JPV33Z Removal of Infusion Device from Upper Extremity Subcutaneous Tissue and Fascia, Percutaneous Approach
0JPV37Z Removal of Autologous Tissue Substitute from Upper Extremity Subcutaneous Tissue and Fascia, Percutaneous Approach
0JPV3HZ Removal of Contraceptive Device from Upper Extremity Subcutaneous Tissue and Fascia, Percutaneous Approach
0JPV3JZ Removal of Synthetic Substitute from Upper Extremity Subcutaneous Tissue and Fascia, Percutaneous Approach
0JPV3KZ Removal of Nonautologous Tissue Substitute from Upper Extremity Subcutaneous Tissue and Fascia, Percutaneous Approach
0JPV3NZ Removal of Tissue Expander from Upper Extremity Subcutaneous Tissue and Fascia, Percutaneous Approach
0JPV3VZ Removal of Infusion Pump from Upper Extremity Subcutaneous Tissue and Fascia, Percutaneous Approach
0JPV3WZ Removal of Reservoir from Upper Extremity Subcutaneous Tissue and Fascia, Percutaneous Approach
0JPV3XZ Removal of Vascular Access Device from Upper Extremity Subcutaneous Tissue and Fascia, Percutaneous Approach
0JPVX0Z Removal of Drainage Device from Upper Extremity Subcutaneous Tissue and Fascia, External Approach
0JPVX1Z Removal of Radioactive Element from Upper Extremity Subcutaneous Tissue and Fascia, External Approach
0JPVX3Z Removal of Infusion Device from Upper Extremity Subcutaneous Tissue and Fascia, External Approach
0JPVXHZ Removal of Contraceptive Device from Upper Extremity Subcutaneous Tissue and Fascia, External Approach
0JPVXVZ Removal of Infusion Pump from Upper Extremity Subcutaneous Tissue and Fascia, External Approach
0JPVXXZ Removal of Vascular Access Device from Upper Extremity Subcutaneous Tissue and Fascia, External Approach
0JPW00Z Removal of Drainage Device from Lower Extremity Subcutaneous Tissue and Fascia, Open Approach
0JPW01Z Removal of Radioactive Element from Lower Extremity Subcutaneous Tissue and Fascia, Open Approach
0JPW03Z Removal of Infusion Device from Lower Extremity Subcutaneous Tissue and Fascia, Open Approach
0JPW07Z Removal of Autologous Tissue Substitute from Lower Extremity Subcutaneous Tissue and Fascia, Open Approach
0JPW0HZ Removal of Contraceptive Device from Lower Extremity Subcutaneous Tissue and Fascia, Open Approach
0JPW0JZ Removal of Synthetic Substitute from Lower Extremity Subcutaneous Tissue and Fascia, Open Approach
0JPW0KZ Removal of Nonautologous Tissue Substitute from Lower Extremity Subcutaneous Tissue and Fascia, Open Approach
0JPW0NZ Removal of Tissue Expander from Lower Extremity Subcutaneous Tissue and Fascia, Open Approach
0JPW0VZ Removal of Infusion Pump from Lower Extremity Subcutaneous Tissue and Fascia, Open Approach
0JPW0WZ Removal of Reservoir from Lower Extremity Subcutaneous Tissue and Fascia, Open Approach
0JPW0XZ Removal of Vascular Access Device from Lower Extremity Subcutaneous Tissue and Fascia, Open Approach
0JPW30Z Removal of Drainage Device from Lower Extremity Subcutaneous Tissue and Fascia, Percutaneous Approach
0JPW31Z Removal of Radioactive Element from Lower Extremity Subcutaneous Tissue and Fascia, Percutaneous Approach
0JPW33Z Removal of Infusion Device from Lower Extremity Subcutaneous Tissue and Fascia, Percutaneous Approach
0JPW37Z Removal of Autologous Tissue Substitute from Lower Extremity Subcutaneous Tissue and Fascia, Percutaneous Approach
0JPW3HZ Removal of Contraceptive Device from Lower Extremity Subcutaneous Tissue and Fascia, Percutaneous Approach
0JPW3JZ Removal of Synthetic Substitute from Lower Extremity Subcutaneous Tissue and Fascia, Percutaneous Approach
0JPW3KZ Removal of Nonautologous Tissue Substitute from Lower Extremity Subcutaneous Tissue and Fascia, Percutaneous Approach
0JPW3NZ Removal of Tissue Expander from Lower Extremity Subcutaneous Tissue and Fascia, Percutaneous Approach
0JPW3VZ Removal of Infusion Pump from Lower Extremity Subcutaneous Tissue and Fascia, Percutaneous Approach
0JPW3WZ Removal of Reservoir from Lower Extremity Subcutaneous Tissue and Fascia, Percutaneous Approach
0JPW3XZ Removal of Vascular Access Device from Lower Extremity Subcutaneous Tissue and Fascia, Percutaneous Approach
0JPWX0Z Removal of Drainage Device from Lower Extremity Subcutaneous Tissue and Fascia, External Approach
0JPWX1Z Removal of Radioactive Element from Lower Extremity Subcutaneous Tissue and Fascia, External Approach
0JPWX3Z Removal of Infusion Device from Lower Extremity Subcutaneous Tissue and Fascia, External Approach
0JPWXHZ Removal of Contraceptive Device from Lower Extremity Subcutaneous Tissue and Fascia, External Approach
0JPWXVZ Removal of Infusion Pump from Lower Extremity Subcutaneous Tissue and Fascia, External Approach
0JPWXXZ Removal of Vascular Access Device from Lower Extremity Subcutaneous Tissue and Fascia, External Approach

JQ – Subcutaneous Tissue and Fascia, Repair

eview Coding Guideline B3.5

JQ00ZZ Repair Scalp Subcutaneous Tissue and Fascia, Open Approach
JQ03ZZ Repair Scalp Subcutaneous Tissue and Fascia, Percutaneous Approach
JQ10ZZ Repair Face Subcutaneous Tissue and Fascia, Open Approach
0JQ13ZZ Repair Face Subcutaneous Tissue and Fascia, Percutaneous Approach
0JQ40ZZ Repair Anterior Neck Subcutaneous Tissue and Fascia, Open Approach
0JQ43ZZ Repair Anterior Neck Subcutaneous Tissue and Fascia, Percutaneous Approach
0JQ50ZZ Repair Posterior Neck Subcutaneous Tissue and Fascia, Open Approach
0JQ53ZZ Repair Posterior Neck Subcutaneous Tissue and Fascia, Percutaneous Approach
0JQ60ZZ Repair Chest Subcutaneous Tissue and Fascia, Open Approach

0JQ63ZZ Repair Chest Subcutaneous Tissue and Fascia, Percutaneous Approach
0JQ70ZZ Repair Back Subcutaneous Tissue and Fascia, Open Approach
0JQ73ZZ Repair Back Subcutaneous Tissue and Fascia, Percutaneous Approach
0JQ80ZZ Repair Abdomen Subcutaneous Tissue and Fascia, Open Approach
0JQ83ZZ Repair Abdomen Subcutaneous Tissue and Fascia, Percutaneous Approach
0JQ90ZZ Repair Buttock Subcutaneous Tissue and Fascia, Open Approach
0JQ93ZZ Repair Buttock Subcutaneous Tissue and Fascia, Percutaneous Approach
0JQB0ZZ Repair Perineum Subcutaneous Tissue and Fascia, Open Approach
0JQB3ZZ Repair Perineum Subcutaneous Tissue and Fascia, Percutaneous Approach
0JQC0ZZ Repair Pelvic Region Subcutaneous Tissue and Fascia, Open Approach
0JQC3ZZ Repair Pelvic Region Subcutaneous Tissue and Fascia, Percutaneous Approach
0JQD0ZZ Repair Right Upper Arm Subcutaneous Tissue and Fascia, Open Approach
0JQD3ZZ Repair Right Upper Arm Subcutaneous Tissue and Fascia, Percutaneous Approach
0JQF0ZZ Repair Left Upper Arm Subcutaneous Tissue and Fascia, Open Approach
0JQF3ZZ Repair Left Upper Arm Subcutaneous Tissue and Fascia, Percutaneous Approach
0JQG0ZZ Repair Right Lower Arm Subcutaneous Tissue and Fascia, Open Approach
0JQG3ZZ Repair Right Lower Arm Subcutaneous Tissue and Fascia, Percutaneous Approach
0JQH0ZZ Repair Left Lower Arm Subcutaneous Tissue and Fascia, Open Approach
0JQH3ZZ Repair Left Lower Arm Subcutaneous Tissue and Fascia, Percutaneous Approach
0JQJ0ZZ Repair Right Hand Subcutaneous Tissue and Fascia, Open Approach
0JQJ3ZZ Repair Right Hand Subcutaneous Tissue and Fascia, Percutaneous Approach
0JQK0ZZ Repair Left Hand Subcutaneous Tissue and Fascia, Open Approach
0JQK3ZZ Repair Left Hand Subcutaneous Tissue and Fascia, Percutaneous Approach
0JQL0ZZ Repair Right Upper Leg Subcutaneous Tissue and Fascia, Open Approach
0JQL3ZZ Repair Right Upper Leg Subcutaneous Tissue and Fascia, Percutaneous Appro
0JQM0ZZ Repair Left Upper Leg Subcutaneous Tissue and Fascia, Open Approach
0JQM3ZZ Repair Left Upper Leg Subcutaneous Tissue and Fascia, Percutaneous Appro
0JQN0ZZ Repair Right Lower Leg Subcutaneous Tissue and Fascia, Open Approach
0JQN3ZZ Repair Right Lower Leg Subcutaneous Tissue and Fascia, Percutaneous Appro
0JQP0ZZ Repair Left Lower Leg Subcutaneous Tissue and Fascia, Open Approach
0JQP3ZZ Repair Left Lower Leg Subcutaneous Tissue and Fascia, Percutaneous Appro
0JQQ0ZZ Repair Right Foot Subcutaneous Tissue and Fascia, Open Approach
0JQQ3ZZ Repair Right Foot Subcutaneous Tissue and Fascia, Percutaneous Approach
0JQR0ZZ Repair Left Foot Subcutaneous Tissue a Fascia, Open Approach
0JQR3ZZ Repair Left Foot Subcutaneous Tissue a Fascia, Percutaneous Approach

0JR – Subcutaneous Tissue and Fascia, Replacement

0JR007Z Replacement of Scalp Subcutaneous Tissue and Fascia with Autologous Tissue Substitute, Open Approach
0JR00JZ Replacement of Scalp Subcutaneous Tissue and Fascia with Synthetic Substitute, Open Approach
0JR00KZ Replacement of Scalp Subcutaneous Tissue and Fascia with Nonautologous Tissue Substitute, Open Approach
0JR037Z Replacement of Scalp Subcutaneous Tissue and Fascia with Autologous Tissue Substitute, Percutaneous Approach
0JR03JZ Replacement of Scalp Subcutaneous Tissue and Fascia with Synthetic Substitute, Percutaneous Approach
0JR03KZ Replacement of Scalp Subcutaneous Tissue and Fascia with Nonautologous Tissue Substitute, Percutaneous Approach
0JR107Z Replacement of Face Subcutaneous Tissue and Fascia with Autologous Tissue Substitute, Open Approach
0JR10JZ Replacement of Face Subcutaneous Tissue and Fascia with Synthetic Substitute, Open Approach
0JR10KZ Replacement of Face Subcutaneous Tissue and Fascia with Nonautologous Tissue Substitute, Open Approach
0JR137Z Replacement of Face Subcutaneous Tissue and Fascia with Autologous Tissue Substitute, Percutaneous Approach
0JR13JZ Replacement of Face Subcutaneous Tissue and Fascia with Synthetic Substitute, Percutaneous Approach
0JR13KZ Replacement of Face Subcutaneous Tissue and Fascia with Nonautologous Tissue Substitute, Percutaneous Approach
0JR407Z Replacement of Anterior Neck Subcutaneous Tissue and Fascia with Autologous Tissue Substitute, Open Approach
0JR40JZ Replacement of Anterior Neck Subcutaneous Tissue and Fascia with Synthetic Substitute, Open Approach
0JR40KZ Replacement of Anterior Neck Subcutaneous Tissue and Fascia with Nonautologous Tissue Substitute, Open Approach
0JR437Z Replacement of Anterior Neck Subcutaneous Tissue and Fascia with Autologous Tissue Substitute, Percutaneous Approach
0JR43JZ Replacement of Anterior Neck Subcutaneous Tissue and Fascia with Synthetic Substitute, Percutaneous Approach
0JR43KZ Replacement of Anterior Neck Subcutaneous Tissue and Fascia with Nonautologous Tissue Substitute, Percutaneous Approach
0JR507Z Replacement of Posterior Neck Subcutaneous Tissue and Fascia with Autologous Tissue Substitute, Open Approach
0JR50JZ Replacement of Posterior Neck Subcutaneous Tissue and Fascia with Synthetic Substitute, Open Approach
0JR50KZ Replacement of Posterior Neck Subcutaneous Tissue and Fascia with Nonautologous Tissue Substitute, Open Approach
0JR537Z Replacement of Posterior Neck Subcutaneous Tissue and Fascia with Autologous Tissue Substitute, Percutaneous Approach
0JR53JZ Replacement of Posterior Neck Subcutaneous Tissue and Fascia with Synthetic Substitute, Percutaneous Approach
0JR53KZ Replacement of Posterior Neck Subcutaneous Tissue and Fascia with Nonautologous Tissue Substitute, Percutaneous Approach
0JR607Z Replacement of Chest Subcutaneous Tissue and Fascia with Autologous Tissue Substitute, Open Approach
0JR60JZ Replacement of Chest Subcutaneous Tissue and Fascia with Synthetic Substitute, Open Approach
0JR60KZ Replacement of Chest Subcutaneous Tissue and Fascia with Nonautologous Tissue Substitute, Open Approach
0JR637Z Replacement of Chest Subcutaneous Tissue and Fascia with Autologous Tissue Substitute, Percutaneous Approach
0JR63JZ Replacement of Chest Subcutaneous Tissue and Fascia with Synthetic Substitute, Percutaneous Approach
0JR63KZ Replacement of Chest Subcutaneous Tissue and Fascia with Nonautologous Tissue Substitute, Percutaneous Approach
0JR707Z Replacement of Back Subcutaneous Tissue and Fascia with Autologous Tiss Substitute, Open Approach
0JR70JZ Replacement of Back Subcutaneous Tis and Fascia with Synthetic Substitute, O Approach
0JR70KZ Replacement of Back Subcutaneous Tis and Fascia with Nonautologous Tissue Substitute, Open Approach
0JR737Z Replacement of Back Subcutaneous Tissue and Fascia with Autologous Tissu Substitute, Percutaneous Approach
0JR73JZ Replacement of Back Subcutaneous Tis and Fascia with Synthetic Substitute, Percutaneous Approach
0JR73KZ Replacement of Back Subcutaneous Tis and Fascia with Nonautologous Tissue Substitute, Percutaneous Approach
0JR807Z Replacement of Abdomen Subcutaneous Tissue and Fascia with Autologous Tissu Substitute, Open Approach
0JR80JZ Replacement of Abdomen Subcutaneous Tissue and Fascia with Synthetic Substitute, Open Approach
0JR80KZ Replacement of Abdomen Subcutaneous Tissue and Fascia with Nonautologous Tissue Substitute, Open Approach
0JR837Z Replacement of Abdomen Subcutaneous Tissue and Fascia with Autologous Tissu Substitute, Percutaneous Approach
0JR83JZ Replacement of Abdomen Subcutaneous Tissue and Fascia with Synthetic Substitute, Percutaneous Approach
0JR83KZ Replacement of Abdomen Subcutaneous Tissue and Fascia with Nonautologous Tissue Substitute, Percutaneous Approac
0JR907Z Replacement of Buttock Subcutaneous Tissue and Fascia with Autologous Tissue Substitute, Open Approach
0JR90JZ Replacement of Buttock Subcutaneous Tissue and Fascia with Synthetic Substitute, Open Approach
0JR90KZ Replacement of Buttock Subcutaneous Tissue and Fascia with Nonautologous Tissue Substitute, Open Approach
0JR937Z Replacement of Buttock Subcutaneous Tissue and Fascia with Autologous Tissue Substitute, Percutaneous Approach
0JR93JZ Replacement of Buttock Subcutaneous Tissue and Fascia with Synthetic Substitute, Percutaneous Approach

93KZ Replacement of Buttock Subcutaneous Tissue and Fascia with Nonautologous Tissue Substitute, Percutaneous Approach

B07Z Replacement of Perineum Subcutaneous Tissue and Fascia with Autologous Tissue Substitute, Open Approach

B0JZ Replacement of Perineum Subcutaneous Tissue and Fascia with Synthetic Substitute, Open Approach

B0KZ Replacement of Perineum Subcutaneous Tissue and Fascia with Nonautologous Tissue Substitute, Open Approach

B37Z Replacement of Perineum Subcutaneous Tissue and Fascia with Autologous Tissue Substitute, Percutaneous Approach

B3JZ Replacement of Perineum Subcutaneous Tissue and Fascia with Synthetic Substitute, Percutaneous Approach

B3KZ Replacement of Perineum Subcutaneous Tissue and Fascia with Nonautologous Tissue Substitute, Percutaneous Approach

RC07Z Replacement of Pelvic Region Subcutaneous Tissue and Fascia with Autologous Tissue Substitute, Open Approach

RC0JZ Replacement of Pelvic Region Subcutaneous Tissue and Fascia with Synthetic Substitute, Open Approach

RC0KZ Replacement of Pelvic Region Subcutaneous Tissue and Fascia with Nonautologous Tissue Substitute, Open Approach

RC37Z Replacement of Pelvic Region Subcutaneous Tissue and Fascia with Autologous Tissue Substitute, Percutaneous Approach

RC3JZ Replacement of Pelvic Region Subcutaneous Tissue and Fascia with Synthetic Substitute, Percutaneous Approach

RC3KZ Replacement of Pelvic Region Subcutaneous Tissue and Fascia with Nonautologous Tissue Substitute, Percutaneous Approach

RD07Z Replacement of Right Upper Arm Subcutaneous Tissue and Fascia with Autologous Tissue Substitute, Open Approach

RD0JZ Replacement of Right Upper Arm Subcutaneous Tissue and Fascia with Synthetic Substitute, Open Approach

RD0KZ Replacement of Right Upper Arm Subcutaneous Tissue and Fascia with Nonautologous Tissue Substitute, Open Approach

RD37Z Replacement of Right Upper Arm Subcutaneous Tissue and Fascia with Autologous Tissue Substitute, Percutaneous Approach

RD3JZ Replacement of Right Upper Arm Subcutaneous Tissue and Fascia with Synthetic Substitute, Percutaneous Approach

RD3KZ Replacement of Right Upper Arm Subcutaneous Tissue and Fascia with Nonautologous Tissue Substitute, Percutaneous Approach

JRF07Z Replacement of Left Upper Arm Subcutaneous Tissue and Fascia with Autologous Tissue Substitute, Open Approach

JRF0JZ Replacement of Left Upper Arm Subcutaneous Tissue and Fascia with Synthetic Substitute, Open Approach

JRF0KZ Replacement of Left Upper Arm Subcutaneous Tissue and Fascia with Nonautologous Tissue Substitute, Open Approach

0JRF37Z Replacement of Left Upper Arm Subcutaneous Tissue and Fascia with Autologous Tissue Substitute, Percutaneous Approach

0JRF3JZ Replacement of Left Upper Arm Subcutaneous Tissue and Fascia with Synthetic Substitute, Percutaneous Approach

0JRF3KZ Replacement of Left Upper Arm Subcutaneous Tissue and Fascia with Nonautologous Tissue Substitute, Percutaneous Approach

0JRG07Z Replacement of Right Lower Arm Subcutaneous Tissue and Fascia with Autologous Tissue Substitute, Open Approach

0JRG0JZ Replacement of Right Lower Arm Subcutaneous Tissue and Fascia with Synthetic Substitute, Open Approach

0JRG0KZ Replacement of Right Lower Arm Subcutaneous Tissue and Fascia with Nonautologous Tissue Substitute, Open Approach

0JRG37Z Replacement of Right Lower Arm Subcutaneous Tissue and Fascia with Autologous Tissue Substitute, Percutaneous Approach

0JRG3JZ Replacement of Right Lower Arm Subcutaneous Tissue and Fascia with Synthetic Substitute, Percutaneous Approach

0JRG3KZ Replacement of Right Lower Arm Subcutaneous Tissue and Fascia with Nonautologous Tissue Substitute, Percutaneous Approach

0JRH07Z Replacement of Left Lower Arm Subcutaneous Tissue and Fascia with Autologous Tissue Substitute, Open Approach

0JRH0JZ Replacement of Left Lower Arm Subcutaneous Tissue and Fascia with Synthetic Substitute, Open Approach

0JRH0KZ Replacement of Left Lower Arm Subcutaneous Tissue and Fascia with Nonautologous Tissue Substitute, Open Approach

0JRH37Z Replacement of Left Lower Arm Subcutaneous Tissue and Fascia with Autologous Tissue Substitute, Percutaneous Approach

0JRH3JZ Replacement of Left Lower Arm Subcutaneous Tissue and Fascia with Synthetic Substitute, Percutaneous Approach

0JRH3KZ Replacement of Left Lower Arm Subcutaneous Tissue and Fascia with Nonautologous Tissue Substitute, Percutaneous Approach

0JRJ07Z Replacement of Right Hand Subcutaneous Tissue and Fascia with Autologous Tissue Substitute, Open Approach

0JRJ0JZ Replacement of Right Hand Subcutaneous Tissue and Fascia with Synthetic Substitute, Open Approach

0JRJ0KZ Replacement of Right Hand Subcutaneous Tissue and Fascia with Nonautologous Tissue Substitute, Open Approach

0JRJ37Z Replacement of Right Hand Subcutaneous Tissue and Fascia with Autologous Tissue Substitute, Percutaneous Approach

0JRJ3JZ Replacement of Right Hand Subcutaneous Tissue and Fascia with Synthetic Substitute, Percutaneous Approach

0JRJ3KZ Replacement of Right Hand Subcutaneous Tissue and Fascia with Nonautologous Tissue Substitute, Percutaneous Approach

0JRK07Z Replacement of Left Hand Subcutaneous Tissue and Fascia with Autologous Tissue Substitute, Open Approach

0JRK0JZ Replacement of Left Hand Subcutaneous Tissue and Fascia with Synthetic Substitute, Open Approach

0JRK0KZ Replacement of Left Hand Subcutaneous Tissue and Fascia with Nonautologous Tissue Substitute, Open Approach

0JRK37Z Replacement of Left Hand Subcutaneous Tissue and Fascia with Autologous Tissue Substitute, Percutaneous Approach

0JRK3JZ Replacement of Left Hand Subcutaneous Tissue and Fascia with Synthetic Substitute, Percutaneous Approach

0JRK3KZ Replacement of Left Hand Subcutaneous Tissue and Fascia with Nonautologous Tissue Substitute, Percutaneous Approach

0JRL07Z Replacement of Right Upper Leg Subcutaneous Tissue and Fascia with Autologous Tissue Substitute, Open Approach

0JRL0JZ Replacement of Right Upper Leg Subcutaneous Tissue and Fascia with Synthetic Substitute, Open Approach

0JRL0KZ Replacement of Right Upper Leg Subcutaneous Tissue and Fascia with Nonautologous Tissue Substitute, Open Approach

0JRL37Z Replacement of Right Upper Leg Subcutaneous Tissue and Fascia with Autologous Tissue Substitute, Percutaneous Approach

0JRL3JZ Replacement of Right Upper Leg Subcutaneous Tissue and Fascia with Synthetic Substitute, Percutaneous Approach

0JRL3KZ Replacement of Right Upper Leg Subcutaneous Tissue and Fascia with Nonautologous Tissue Substitute, Percutaneous Approach

0JRM07Z Replacement of Left Upper Leg Subcutaneous Tissue and Fascia with Autologous Tissue Substitute, Open Approach

0JRM0JZ Replacement of Left Upper Leg Subcutaneous Tissue and Fascia with Synthetic Substitute, Open Approach

0JRM0KZ Replacement of Left Upper Leg Subcutaneous Tissue and Fascia with Nonautologous Tissue Substitute, Open Approach

0JRM37Z Replacement of Left Upper Leg Subcutaneous Tissue and Fascia with Autologous Tissue Substitute, Percutaneous Approach

0JRM3JZ Replacement of Left Upper Leg Subcutaneous Tissue and Fascia with Synthetic Substitute, Percutaneous Approach

0JRM3KZ Replacement of Left Upper Leg Subcutaneous Tissue and Fascia with Nonautologous Tissue Substitute, Percutaneous Approach

0JRN07Z Replacement of Right Lower Leg Subcutaneous Tissue and Fascia with Autologous Tissue Substitute, Open Approach

0JRN0JZ Replacement of Right Lower Leg Subcutaneous Tissue and Fascia with Synthetic Substitute, Open Approach

0JRN0KZ Replacement of Right Lower Leg Subcutaneous Tissue and Fascia with Nonautologous Tissue Substitute, Open Approach

0JRN37Z Replacement of Right Lower Leg Subcutaneous Tissue and Fascia with Autologous Tissue Substitute, Percutaneous Approach
0JRN3JZ Replacement of Right Lower Leg Subcutaneous Tissue and Fascia with Synthetic Substitute, Percutaneous Approach
0JRN3KZ Replacement of Right Lower Leg Subcutaneous Tissue and Fascia with Nonautologous Tissue Substitute, Percutaneous Approach
0JRP07Z Replacement of Left Lower Leg Subcutaneous Tissue and Fascia with Autologous Tissue Substitute, Open Approach
0JRP0JZ Replacement of Left Lower Leg Subcutaneous Tissue and Fascia with Synthetic Substitute, Open Approach
0JRP0KZ Replacement of Left Lower Leg Subcutaneous Tissue and Fascia with Nonautologous Tissue Substitute, Open Approach
0JRP37Z Replacement of Left Lower Leg Subcutaneous Tissue and Fascia with Autologous Tissue Substitute, Percutaneous Approach
0JRP3JZ Replacement of Left Lower Leg Subcutaneous Tissue and Fascia with Synthetic Substitute, Percutaneous Approach
0JRP3KZ Replacement of Left Lower Leg Subcutaneous Tissue and Fascia with Nonautologous Tissue Substitute, Percutaneous Approach
0JRQ07Z Replacement of Right Foot Subcutaneous Tissue and Fascia with Autologous Tissue Substitute, Open Approach
0JRQ0JZ Replacement of Right Foot Subcutaneous Tissue and Fascia with Synthetic Substitute, Open Approach
0JRQ0KZ Replacement of Right Foot Subcutaneous Tissue and Fascia with Nonautologous Tissue Substitute, Open Approach
0JRQ37Z Replacement of Right Foot Subcutaneous Tissue and Fascia with Autologous Tissue Substitute, Percutaneous Approach
0JRQ3JZ Replacement of Right Foot Subcutane Tissue and Fascia with Synthetic Substitute, Percutaneous Approach
0JRQ3KZ Replacement of Right Foot Subcutane Tissue and Fascia with Nonautologous Tissue Substitute, Percutaneous Appro
0JRR07Z Replacement of Left Foot Subcutaneou Tissue and Fascia with Autologous Tis Substitute, Open Approach
0JRR0JZ Replacement of Left Foot Subcutaneou Tissue and Fascia with Synthetic Substitute, Open Approach
0JRR0KZ Replacement of Left Foot Subcutaneou Tissue and Fascia with Nonautologous Tissue Substitute, Open Approach
0JRR37Z Replacement of Left Foot Subcutaneou Tissue and Fascia with Autologous Tiss Substitute, Percutaneous Approach
0JRR3JZ Replacement of Left Foot Subcutaneou Tissue and Fascia with Synthetic Substitute, Percutaneous Approach
0JRR3KZ Replacement of Left Foot Subcutaneou Tissue and Fascia with Nonautologous Tissue Substitute, Percutaneous Appro

0JU – Subcutaneous Tissue and Fascia, Supplement

0JU007Z Supplement of Scalp Subcutaneous Tissue and Fascia with Autologous Tissue Substitute, Open Approach
0JU00JZ Supplement of Scalp Subcutaneous Tissue and Fascia with Synthetic Substitute, Open Approach
0JU00KZ Supplement of Scalp Subcutaneous Tissue and Fascia with Nonautologous Tissue Substitute, Open Approach
0JU037Z Supplement of Scalp Subcutaneous Tissue and Fascia with Autologous Tissue Substitute, Percutaneous Approach
0JU03JZ Supplement of Scalp Subcutaneous Tissue and Fascia with Synthetic Substitute, Percutaneous Approach
0JU03KZ Supplement of Scalp Subcutaneous Tissue and Fascia with Nonautologous Tissue Substitute, Percutaneous Approach
0JU107Z Supplement of Face Subcutaneous Tissue and Fascia with Autologous Tissue Substitute, Open Approach
0JU10JZ Supplement of Face Subcutaneous Tissue and Fascia with Synthetic Substitute, Open Approach
0JU10KZ Supplement of Face Subcutaneous Tissue and Fascia with Nonautologous Tissue Substitute, Open Approach
0JU137Z Supplement of Face Subcutaneous Tissue and Fascia with Autologous Tissue Substitute, Percutaneous Approach
0JU13JZ Supplement of Face Subcutaneous Tissue and Fascia with Synthetic Substitute, Percutaneous Approach
0JU13KZ Supplement of Face Subcutaneous Tissue and Fascia with Nonautologous Tissue Substitute, Percutaneous Approach
0JU407Z Supplement of Anterior Neck Subcutaneous Tissue and Fascia with Autologous Tissue Substitute, Open Approach
0JU40JZ Supplement of Anterior Neck Subcutaneous Tissue and Fascia with Synthetic Substitute, Open Approach
0JU40KZ Supplement of Anterior Neck Subcutaneous Tissue and Fascia with Nonautologous Tissue Substitute, Open Approach
0JU437Z Supplement of Anterior Neck Subcutaneous Tissue and Fascia with Autologous Tissue Substitute, Percutaneous Approach
0JU43JZ Supplement of Anterior Neck Subcutaneous Tissue and Fascia with Synthetic Substitute, Percutaneous Approach
0JU43KZ Supplement of Anterior Neck Subcutaneous Tissue and Fascia with Nonautologous Tissue Substitute, Percutaneous Approach
0JU507Z Supplement of Posterior Neck Subcutaneous Tissue and Fascia with Autologous Tissue Substitute, Open Approach
0JU50JZ Supplement of Posterior Neck Subcutaneous Tissue and Fascia with Synthetic Substitute, Open Approach
0JU50KZ Supplement of Posterior Neck Subcutaneous Tissue and Fascia with Nonautologous Tissue Substitute, Open Approach
0JU537Z Supplement of Posterior Neck Subcutaneous Tissue and Fascia with Autologous Tissue Substitute, Percutaneous Approach
0JU53JZ Supplement of Posterior Neck Subcutaneous Tissue and Fascia with Synthetic Substitute, Percutaneous Approach
0JU53KZ Supplement of Posterior Neck Subcutaneous Tissue and Fascia with Nonautologous Tissue Substitute, Percutaneous Approach
0JU607Z Supplement of Chest Subcutaneous Tissue and Fascia with Autologous Tissue Substitute, Open Approach
0JU60JZ Supplement of Chest Subcutaneous Tissue and Fascia with Synthetic Substitute, Open Approach
0JU60KZ Supplement of Chest Subcutaneous Tissue and Fascia with Nonautologous Tissue Substitute, Open Approach
0JU637Z Supplement of Chest Subcutaneous Tissue and Fascia with Autologous Tissue Substitute, Percutaneous Approach
0JU63JZ Supplement of Chest Subcutaneous Tissue and Fascia with Synthetic Substitute, Percutaneous Approach
0JU63KZ Supplement of Chest Subcutaneous Tissue and Fascia with Nonautologous Tissue Substitute, Percutaneous Approach
0JU707Z Supplement of Back Subcutaneous Tissue and Fascia with Autologous Tissue Substitute, Open Approach
0JU70JZ Supplement of Back Subcutaneous Tiss and Fascia with Synthetic Substitute, O Approach
0JU70KZ Supplement of Back Subcutaneous Tiss and Fascia with Nonautologous Tissue Substitute, Open Approach
0JU737Z Supplement of Back Subcutaneous Tissue and Fascia with Autologous Tiss Substitute, Percutaneous Approach
0JU73JZ Supplement of Back Subcutaneous Tiss and Fascia with Synthetic Substitute, Percutaneous Approach
0JU73KZ Supplement of Back Subcutaneous Tissu and Fascia with Nonautologous Tissue Substitute, Percutaneous Approach
0JU807Z Supplement of Abdomen Subcutaneous Tissue and Fascia with Autologous Tissu Substitute, Open Approach
0JU80JZ Supplement of Abdomen Subcutaneous Tissue and Fascia with Synthetic Substitute, Open Approach
0JU80KZ Supplement of Abdomen Subcutaneous Tissue and Fascia with Nonautologous Tissue Substitute, Open Approach
0JU837Z Supplement of Abdomen Subcutaneous Tissue and Fascia with Autologous Tissu Substitute, Percutaneous Approach
0JU83JZ Supplement of Abdomen Subcutaneous Tissue and Fascia with Synthetic Substitute, Percutaneous Approach
0JU83KZ Supplement of Abdomen Subcutaneous Tissue and Fascia with Nonautologous Tissue Substitute, Percutaneous Approac
0JU907Z Supplement of Buttock Subcutaneous Tissue and Fascia with Autologous Tissu Substitute, Open Approach
0JU90JZ Supplement of Buttock Subcutaneous Tissue and Fascia with Synthetic Substitute, Open Approach
0JU90KZ Supplement of Buttock Subcutaneous Tissue and Fascia with Nonautologous Tissue Substitute, Open Approach
0JU937Z Supplement of Buttock Subcutaneous Tissue and Fascia with Autologous Tissue Substitute, Percutaneous Approach
0JU93JZ Supplement of Buttock Subcutaneous Tissue and Fascia with Synthetic Substitute, Percutaneous Approach
0JU93KZ Supplement of Buttock Subcutaneous Tissue and Fascia with Nonautologous Tissue Substitute, Percutaneous Approach

B07Z Supplement of Perineum Subcutaneous Tissue and Fascia with Autologous Tissue Substitute, Open Approach

B0JZ Supplement of Perineum Subcutaneous Tissue and Fascia with Synthetic Substitute, Open Approach

B0KZ Supplement of Perineum Subcutaneous Tissue and Fascia with Nonautologous Tissue Substitute, Open Approach

B37Z Supplement of Perineum Subcutaneous Tissue and Fascia with Autologous Tissue Substitute, Percutaneous Approach

B3JZ Supplement of Perineum Subcutaneous Tissue and Fascia with Synthetic Substitute, Percutaneous Approach

JB3KZ Supplement of Perineum Subcutaneous Tissue and Fascia with Nonautologous Tissue Substitute, Percutaneous Approach

JC07Z Supplement of Pelvic Region Subcutaneous Tissue and Fascia with Autologous Tissue Substitute, Open Approach

JC0JZ Supplement of Pelvic Region Subcutaneous Tissue and Fascia with Synthetic Substitute, Open Approach

JC0KZ Supplement of Pelvic Region Subcutaneous Tissue and Fascia with Nonautologous Tissue Substitute, Open Approach

JC37Z Supplement of Pelvic Region Subcutaneous Tissue and Fascia with Autologous Tissue Substitute, Percutaneous Approach

UC3JZ Supplement of Pelvic Region Subcutaneous Tissue and Fascia with Synthetic Substitute, Percutaneous Approach

UC3KZ Supplement of Pelvic Region Subcutaneous Tissue and Fascia with Nonautologous Tissue Substitute, Percutaneous Approach

UD07Z Supplement of Right Upper Arm Subcutaneous Tissue and Fascia with Autologous Tissue Substitute, Open Approach

UD0JZ Supplement of Right Upper Arm Subcutaneous Tissue and Fascia with Synthetic Substitute, Open Approach

UD0KZ Supplement of Right Upper Arm Subcutaneous Tissue and Fascia with Nonautologous Tissue Substitute, Open Approach

UD37Z Supplement of Right Upper Arm Subcutaneous Tissue and Fascia with Autologous Tissue Substitute, Percutaneous Approach

UD3JZ Supplement of Right Upper Arm Subcutaneous Tissue and Fascia with Synthetic Substitute, Percutaneous Approach

UD3KZ Supplement of Right Upper Arm Subcutaneous Tissue and Fascia with Nonautologous Tissue Substitute, Percutaneous Approach

UF07Z Supplement of Left Upper Arm Subcutaneous Tissue and Fascia with Autologous Tissue Substitute, Open Approach

JUF0JZ Supplement of Left Upper Arm Subcutaneous Tissue and Fascia with Synthetic Substitute, Open Approach

JUF0KZ Supplement of Left Upper Arm Subcutaneous Tissue and Fascia with Nonautologous Tissue Substitute, Open Approach

JUF37Z Supplement of Left Upper Arm Subcutaneous Tissue and Fascia with Autologous Tissue Substitute, Percutaneous Approach

0JUF3JZ Supplement of Left Upper Arm Subcutaneous Tissue and Fascia with Synthetic Substitute, Percutaneous Approach

0JUF3KZ Supplement of Left Upper Arm Subcutaneous Tissue and Fascia with Nonautologous Tissue Substitute, Percutaneous Approach

0JUG07Z Supplement of Right Lower Arm Subcutaneous Tissue and Fascia with Autologous Tissue Substitute, Open Approach

0JUG0JZ Supplement of Right Lower Arm Subcutaneous Tissue and Fascia with Synthetic Substitute, Open Approach

0JUG0KZ Supplement of Right Lower Arm Subcutaneous Tissue and Fascia with Nonautologous Tissue Substitute, Open Approach

0JUG37Z Supplement of Right Lower Arm Subcutaneous Tissue and Fascia with Autologous Tissue Substitute, Percutaneous Approach

0JUG3JZ Supplement of Right Lower Arm Subcutaneous Tissue and Fascia with Synthetic Substitute, Percutaneous Approach

0JUG3KZ Supplement of Right Lower Arm Subcutaneous Tissue and Fascia with Nonautologous Tissue Substitute, Percutaneous Approach

0JUH07Z Supplement of Left Lower Arm Subcutaneous Tissue and Fascia with Autologous Tissue Substitute, Open Approach

0JUH0JZ Supplement of Left Lower Arm Subcutaneous Tissue and Fascia with Synthetic Substitute, Open Approach

0JUH0KZ Supplement of Left Lower Arm Subcutaneous Tissue and Fascia with Nonautologous Tissue Substitute, Open Approach

0JUH37Z Supplement of Left Lower Arm Subcutaneous Tissue and Fascia with Autologous Tissue Substitute, Percutaneous Approach

0JUH3JZ Supplement of Left Lower Arm Subcutaneous Tissue and Fascia with Synthetic Substitute, Percutaneous Approach

0JUH3KZ Supplement of Left Lower Arm Subcutaneous Tissue and Fascia with Nonautologous Tissue Substitute, Percutaneous Approach

0JUJ07Z Supplement of Right Hand Subcutaneous Tissue and Fascia with Autologous Tissue Substitute, Open Approach

0JUJ0JZ Supplement of Right Hand Subcutaneous Tissue and Fascia with Synthetic Substitute, Open Approach

0JUJ0KZ Supplement of Right Hand Subcutaneous Tissue and Fascia with Nonautologous Tissue Substitute, Open Approach

0JUJ37Z Supplement of Right Hand Subcutaneous Tissue and Fascia with Autologous Tissue Substitute, Percutaneous Approach

0JUJ3JZ Supplement of Right Hand Subcutaneous Tissue and Fascia with Synthetic Substitute, Percutaneous Approach

0JUJ3KZ Supplement of Right Hand Subcutaneous Tissue and Fascia with Nonautologous Tissue Substitute, Percutaneous Approach

0JUK07Z Supplement of Left Hand Subcutaneous Tissue and Fascia with Autologous Tissue Substitute, Open Approach

0JUK0JZ Supplement of Left Hand Subcutaneous Tissue and Fascia with Synthetic Substitute, Open Approach

0JUK0KZ Supplement of Left Hand Subcutaneous Tissue and Fascia with Nonautologous Tissue Substitute, Open Approach

0JUK37Z Supplement of Left Hand Subcutaneous Tissue and Fascia with Autologous Tissue Substitute, Percutaneous Approach

0JUK3JZ Supplement of Left Hand Subcutaneous Tissue and Fascia with Synthetic Substitute, Percutaneous Approach

0JUK3KZ Supplement of Left Hand Subcutaneous Tissue and Fascia with Nonautologous Tissue Substitute, Percutaneous Approach

0JUL07Z Supplement of Right Upper Leg Subcutaneous Tissue and Fascia with Autologous Tissue Substitute, Open Approach

0JUL0JZ Supplement of Right Upper Leg Subcutaneous Tissue and Fascia with Synthetic Substitute, Open Approach

0JUL0KZ Supplement of Right Upper Leg Subcutaneous Tissue and Fascia with Nonautologous Tissue Substitute, Open Approach

0JUL37Z Supplement of Right Upper Leg Subcutaneous Tissue and Fascia with Autologous Tissue Substitute, Percutaneous Approach

0JUL3JZ Supplement of Right Upper Leg Subcutaneous Tissue and Fascia with Synthetic Substitute, Percutaneous Approach

0JUL3KZ Supplement of Right Upper Leg Subcutaneous Tissue and Fascia with Nonautologous Tissue Substitute, Percutaneous Approach

0JUM07Z Supplement of Left Upper Leg Subcutaneous Tissue and Fascia with Autologous Tissue Substitute, Open Approach

0JUM0JZ Supplement of Left Upper Leg Subcutaneous Tissue and Fascia with Synthetic Substitute, Open Approach

0JUM0KZ Supplement of Left Upper Leg Subcutaneous Tissue and Fascia with Nonautologous Tissue Substitute, Open Approach

0JUM37Z Supplement of Left Upper Leg Subcutaneous Tissue and Fascia with Autologous Tissue Substitute, Percutaneous Approach

0JUM3JZ Supplement of Left Upper Leg Subcutaneous Tissue and Fascia with Synthetic Substitute, Percutaneous Approach

0JUM3KZ Supplement of Left Upper Leg Subcutaneous Tissue and Fascia with Nonautologous Tissue Substitute, Percutaneous Approach

0JUN07Z Supplement of Right Lower Leg Subcutaneous Tissue and Fascia with Autologous Tissue Substitute, Open Approach

0JUN0JZ Supplement of Right Lower Leg Subcutaneous Tissue and Fascia with Synthetic Substitute, Open Approach

0JUN0KZ Supplement of Right Lower Leg Subcutaneous Tissue and Fascia with Nonautologous Tissue Substitute, Open Approach

0JUN37Z Supplement of Right Lower Leg Subcutaneous Tissue and Fascia with Autologous Tissue Substitute, Percutaneous Approach

0JUN3JZ Supplement of Right Lower Leg Subcutaneous Tissue and Fascia with Synthetic Substitute, Percutaneous Approach

0JUN3KZ Supplement of Right Lower Leg Subcutaneous Tissue and Fascia with Nonautologous Tissue Substitute, Percutaneous Approach

0JUP07Z Supplement of Left Lower Leg Subcutaneous Tissue and Fascia with Autologous Tissue Substitute, Open Approach

0JUP0JZ Supplement of Left Lower Leg Subcutaneous Tissue and Fascia with Synthetic Substitute, Open Approach

0JUP0KZ Supplement of Left Lower Leg Subcutaneous Tissue and Fascia with Nonautologous Tissue Substitute, Open Approach

0JUP37Z Supplement of Left Lower Leg Subcutaneous Tissue and Fascia with Autologous Tissue Substitute, Percutaneous Approach

0JUP3JZ Supplement of Left Lower Leg Subcutaneous Tissue and Fascia with Synthetic Substitute, Percutaneous Approach

0JUP3KZ Supplement of Left Lower Leg Subcutaneous Tissue and Fascia with Nonautologous Tissue Substitute, Percutaneous Approach

0JUQ07Z Supplement of Right Foot Subcutaneous Tissue and Fascia with Autologous Tissue Substitute, Open Approach

0JUQ0JZ Supplement of Right Foot Subcutaneous Tissue and Fascia with Synthetic Substitute, Open Approach

0JUQ0KZ Supplement of Right Foot Subcutaneous Tissue and Fascia with Nonautologous Tissue Substitute, Open Approach

0JUQ37Z Supplement of Right Foot Subcutaneous Tissue and Fascia with Autologous Tissue Substitute, Percutaneous Approach

0JUQ3JZ Supplement of Right Foot Subcutaneous Tissue and Fascia with Synthetic Substitute, Percutaneous Approach

0JUQ3KZ Supplement of Right Foot Subcutaneou[s] Tissue and Fascia with Nonautologous Tissue Substitute, Percutaneous Approach

0JUR07Z Supplement of Left Foot Subcutaneous Tissue and Fascia with Autologous Tiss[ue] Substitute, Open Approach

0JUR0JZ Supplement of Left Foot Subcutaneous Tissue and Fascia with Synthetic Substitute, Open Approach

0JUR0KZ Supplement of Left Foot Subcutaneous Tissue and Fascia with Nonautologous Tissue Substitute, Open Approach

0JUR37Z Supplement of Left Foot Subcutaneous Tissue and Fascia with Autologous Tissue Substitute, Percutaneous Approach

0JUR3JZ Supplement of Left Foot Subcutaneous Tissue and Fascia with Synthetic Substitute, Percutaneous Approach

0JUR3KZ Supplement of Left Foot Subcutaneous Tissue and Fascia with Nonautologous Tissue Substitute, Percutaneous Approach

0JW – Subcutaneous Tissue and Fascia, Revision

Review Coding Guideline B6.1c

● **0JWS00Z** Revision of Drainage Device in Head and Neck Subcutaneous Tissue and Fascia, Open Approach

● **0JWS03Z** Revision of Infusion Device in Head and Neck Subcutaneous Tissue and Fascia, Open Approach

● **0JWS07Z** Revision of Autologous Tissue Substitute in Head and Neck Subcutaneous Tissue and Fascia, Open Approach

● **0JWS0JZ** Revision of Synthetic Substitute in Head and Neck Subcutaneous Tissue and Fascia, Open Approach

● **0JWS0KZ** Revision of Nonautologous Tissue Substitute in Head and Neck Subcutaneous Tissue and Fascia, Open Approach

● **0JWS0NZ** Revision of Tissue Expander in Head and Neck Subcutaneous Tissue and Fascia, Open Approach

● **0JWS30Z** Revision of Drainage Device in Head and Neck Subcutaneous Tissue and Fascia, Percutaneous Approach

● **0JWS33Z** Revision of Infusion Device in Head and Neck Subcutaneous Tissue and Fascia, Percutaneous Approach

● **0JWS37Z** Revision of Autologous Tissue Substitute in Head and Neck Subcutaneous Tissue and Fascia, Percutaneous Approach

● **0JWS3JZ** Revision of Synthetic Substitute in Head and Neck Subcutaneous Tissue and Fascia, Percutaneous Approach

● **0JWS3KZ** Revision of Nonautologous Tissue Substitute in Head and Neck Subcutaneous Tissue and Fascia, Percutaneous Approach

● **0JWS3NZ** Revision of Tissue Expander in Head and Neck Subcutaneous Tissue and Fascia, Percutaneous Approach

0JWSX0Z Revision of Drainage Device in Head and Neck Subcutaneous Tissue and Fascia, External Approach

0JWSX3Z Revision of Infusion Device in Head and Neck Subcutaneous Tissue and Fascia, External Approach

0JWSX7Z Revision of Autologous Tissue Substitute in Head and Neck Subcutaneous Tissue and Fascia, External Approach

0JWSXJZ Revision of Synthetic Substitute in Head and Neck Subcutaneous Tissue and Fascia, External Approach

0JWSXKZ Revision of Nonautologous Tissue Substitute in Head and Neck Subcutaneous Tissue and Fascia, External Approach

0JWSXNZ Revision of Tissue Expander in Head and Neck Subcutaneous Tissue and Fascia, External Approach

● **0JWT00Z** Revision of Drainage Device in Trunk Subcutaneous Tissue and Fascia, Open Approach

● **0JWT02Z** Revision of Monitoring Device in Trunk Subcutaneous Tissue and Fascia, Open Approach

● **0JWT03Z** Revision of Infusion Device in Trunk Subcutaneous Tissue and Fascia, Open Approach

● **0JWT07Z** Revision of Autologous Tissue Substitute in Trunk Subcutaneous Tissue and Fascia, Open Approach

● **0JWT0HZ** Revision of Contraceptive Device in Trunk Subcutaneous Tissue and Fascia, Open Approach

● **0JWT0JZ** Revision of Synthetic Substitute in Trunk Subcutaneous Tissue and Fascia, Open Approach

● **0JWT0KZ** Revision of Nonautologous Tissue Substitute in Trunk Subcutaneous Tissue and Fascia, Open Approach

0JWT0MZ Revision of Stimulator Generator in Trunk Subcutaneous Tissue and Fascia, Open Approach

● **0JWT0NZ** Revision of Tissue Expander in Trunk Subcutaneous Tissue and Fascia, Open Approach

0JWT0PZ Revision of Cardiac Rhythm Related Device in Trunk Subcutaneous Tissue and Fascia, Open Approach

AHA CC: 4Q, 2012, 104-106

HAC With a secondary diagnosis code of K68.11, T81.4XXA, T82.6XXA, T82.7XXA

● **0JWT0VZ** Revision of Infusion Pump in Trunk Subcutaneous Tissue and Fascia, Open Approach

● **0JWT0WZ** Revision of Reservoir in Trunk Subcutaneous Tissue and Fascia, Open Approach

● **0JWT0XZ** Revision of Vascular Access Device in Trunk Subcutaneous Tissue and Fascia, Open Approach

● **0JWT30Z** Revision of Drainage Device in Trunk Subcutaneous Tissue and Fascia, Percutaneous Approach

● **0JWT32Z** Revision of Monitoring Device in Trunk Subcutaneous Tissue and Fascia, Percutaneous Approach

● **0JWT33Z** Revision of Infusion Device in Trunk Subcutaneous Tissue and Fascia, Percutaneous Approach

● **0JWT37Z** Revision of Autologous Tissue Substitute in Trunk Subcutaneous Tissue and Fascia, Percutaneous Approach

● **0JWT3HZ** Revision of Contraceptive Device in Trunk Subcutaneous Tissue and Fascia, Percutaneous Approach

● **0JWT3JZ** Revision of Synthetic Substitute in Trunk Subcutaneous Tissue and Fascia, Percutaneous Approach

● **0JWT3KZ** Revision of Nonautologous Tissue Substitute in Trunk Subcutaneous Tissue and Fascia, Percutaneous Approach

0JWT3MZ Revision of Stimulator Generator in Trunk Subcutaneous Tissue and Fascia, Percutaneous Approach

● **0JWT3NZ** Revision of Tissue Expander in Trunk Subcutaneous Tissue and Fascia, Percutaneous Approach

0JWT3PZ Revision of Cardiac Rhythm Related Device in Trunk Subcutaneous Tissue and Fascia, Percutaneous Approach

HAC With a secondary diagnosis code of K68.11, T81.4XXA, T82.6XXA, T82.7XXA

● **0JWT3VZ** Revision of Infusion Pump in Trunk Subcutaneous Tissue and Fascia, Percutaneous Approach

● **0JWT3WZ** Revision of Reservoir in Trunk Subcutaneous Tissue and Fascia, Percutaneous Approach

WT3XZ Revision of Vascular Access Device in Trunk Subcutaneous Tissue and Fascia, Percutaneous Approach

TX0Z Revision of Drainage Device in Trunk Subcutaneous Tissue and Fascia, External Approach

TX2Z Revision of Monitoring Device in Trunk Subcutaneous Tissue and Fascia, External Approach

VTX3Z Revision of Infusion Device in Trunk Subcutaneous Tissue and Fascia, External Approach

VTX7Z Revision of Autologous Tissue Substitute in Trunk Subcutaneous Tissue and Fascia, External Approach

VTXHZ Revision of Contraceptive Device in Trunk Subcutaneous Tissue and Fascia, External Approach

VTXJZ Revision of Synthetic Substitute in Trunk Subcutaneous Tissue and Fascia, External Approach

VTXKZ Revision of Nonautologous Tissue Substitute in Trunk Subcutaneous Tissue and Fascia, External Approach

VTXMZ Revision of Stimulator Generator in Trunk Subcutaneous Tissue and Fascia, External Approach

VTXNZ Revision of Tissue Expander in Trunk Subcutaneous Tissue and Fascia, External Approach

WTXPZ Revision of Cardiac Rhythm Related Device in Trunk Subcutaneous Tissue and Fascia, External Approach

WTXVZ Revision of Infusion Pump in Trunk Subcutaneous Tissue and Fascia, External Approach

WTXWZ Revision of Reservoir in Trunk Subcutaneous Tissue and Fascia, External Approach

WTXXZ Revision of Vascular Access Device in Trunk Subcutaneous Tissue and Fascia, External Approach

JWV00Z Revision of Drainage Device in Upper Extremity Subcutaneous Tissue and Fascia, Open Approach

JWV03Z Revision of Infusion Device in Upper Extremity Subcutaneous Tissue and Fascia, Open Approach

JWV07Z Revision of Autologous Tissue Substitute in Upper Extremity Subcutaneous Tissue and Fascia, Open Approach

JWV0HZ Revision of Contraceptive Device in Upper Extremity Subcutaneous Tissue and Fascia, Open Approach

JWV0JZ Revision of Synthetic Substitute in Upper Extremity Subcutaneous Tissue and Fascia, Open Approach

JWV0KZ Revision of Nonautologous Tissue Substitute in Upper Extremity Subcutaneous Tissue and Fascia, Open Approach

JWV0NZ Revision of Tissue Expander in Upper Extremity Subcutaneous Tissue and Fascia, Open Approach

JWV0VZ Revision of Infusion Pump in Upper Extremity Subcutaneous Tissue and Fascia, Open Approach

JWV0WZ Revision of Reservoir in Upper Extremity Subcutaneous Tissue and Fascia, Open Approach

JWV0XZ Revision of Vascular Access Device in Upper Extremity Subcutaneous Tissue and Fascia, Open Approach

JWV30Z Revision of Drainage Device in Upper Extremity Subcutaneous Tissue and Fascia, Percutaneous Approach

● 0JWV33Z Revision of Infusion Device in Upper Extremity Subcutaneous Tissue and Fascia, Percutaneous Approach

● 0JWV37Z Revision of Autologous Tissue Substitute in Upper Extremity Subcutaneous Tissue and Fascia, Percutaneous Approach

● 0JWV3HZ Revision of Contraceptive Device in Upper Extremity Subcutaneous Tissue and Fascia, Percutaneous Approach

● 0JWV3JZ Revision of Synthetic Substitute in Upper Extremity Subcutaneous Tissue and Fascia, Percutaneous Approach

● 0JWV3KZ Revision of Nonautologous Tissue Substitute in Upper Extremity Subcutaneous Tissue and Fascia, Percutaneous Approach

● 0JWV3NZ Revision of Tissue Expander in Upper Extremity Subcutaneous Tissue and Fascia, Percutaneous Approach

● 0JWV3VZ Revision of Infusion Pump in Upper Extremity Subcutaneous Tissue and Fascia, Percutaneous Approach

● 0JWV3WZ Revision of Reservoir in Upper Extremity Subcutaneous Tissue and Fascia, Percutaneous Approach

● 0JWV3XZ Revision of Vascular Access Device in Upper Extremity Subcutaneous Tissue and Fascia, Percutaneous Approach

0JWVX0Z Revision of Drainage Device in Upper Extremity Subcutaneous Tissue and Fascia, External Approach

0JWVX3Z Revision of Infusion Device in Upper Extremity Subcutaneous Tissue and Fascia, External Approach

0JWVX7Z Revision of Autologous Tissue Substitute in Upper Extremity Subcutaneous Tissue and Fascia, External Approach

0JWVXHZ Revision of Contraceptive Device in Upper Extremity Subcutaneous Tissue and Fascia, External Approach

0JWVXJZ Revision of Synthetic Substitute in Upper Extremity Subcutaneous Tissue and Fascia, External Approach

0JWVXKZ Revision of Nonautologous Tissue Substitute in Upper Extremity Subcutaneous Tissue and Fascia, External Approach

0JWVXNZ Revision of Tissue Expander in Upper Extremity Subcutaneous Tissue and Fascia, External Approach

0JWVXVZ Revision of Infusion Pump in Upper Extremity Subcutaneous Tissue and Fascia, External Approach

0JWVXWZ Revision of Reservoir in Upper Extremity Subcutaneous Tissue and Fascia, External Approach

0JWVXXZ Revision of Vascular Access Device in Upper Extremity Subcutaneous Tissue and Fascia, External Approach

● 0JWW00Z Revision of Drainage Device in Lower Extremity Subcutaneous Tissue and Fascia, Open Approach

● 0JWW03Z Revision of Infusion Device in Lower Extremity Subcutaneous Tissue and Fascia, Open Approach

● 0JWW07Z Revision of Autologous Tissue Substitute in Lower Extremity Subcutaneous Tissue and Fascia, Open Approach

● 0JWW0HZ Revision of Contraceptive Device in Lower Extremity Subcutaneous Tissue and Fascia, Open Approach

● 0JWW0JZ Revision of Synthetic Substitute in Lower Extremity Subcutaneous Tissue and Fascia, Open Approach

● 0JWW0KZ Revision of Nonautologous Tissue Substitute in Lower Extremity Subcutaneous Tissue and Fascia, Open Approach

● 0JWW0NZ Revision of Tissue Expander in Lower Extremity Subcutaneous Tissue and Fascia, Open Approach

● 0JWW0VZ Revision of Infusion Pump in Lower Extremity Subcutaneous Tissue and Fascia, Open Approach

● 0JWW0WZ Revision of Reservoir in Lower Extremity Subcutaneous Tissue and Fascia, Open Approach

● 0JWW0XZ Revision of Vascular Access Device in Lower Extremity Subcutaneous Tissue and Fascia, Open Approach

● 0JWW30Z Revision of Drainage Device in Lower Extremity Subcutaneous Tissue and Fascia, Percutaneous Approach

● 0JWW33Z Revision of Infusion Device in Lower Extremity Subcutaneous Tissue and Fascia, Percutaneous Approach

● 0JWW37Z Revision of Autologous Tissue Substitute in Lower Extremity Subcutaneous Tissue and Fascia, Percutaneous Approach

● 0JWW3HZ Revision of Contraceptive Device in Lower Extremity Subcutaneous Tissue and Fascia, Percutaneous Approach

● 0JWW3JZ Revision of Synthetic Substitute in Lower Extremity Subcutaneous Tissue and Fascia, Percutaneous Approach

● 0JWW3KZ Revision of Nonautologous Tissue Substitute in Lower Extremity Subcutaneous Tissue and Fascia, Percutaneous Approach

● 0JWW3NZ Revision of Tissue Expander in Lower Extremity Subcutaneous Tissue and Fascia, Percutaneous Approach

● 0JWW3VZ Revision of Infusion Pump in Lower Extremity Subcutaneous Tissue and Fascia, Percutaneous Approach

● 0JWW3WZ Revision of Reservoir in Lower Extremity Subcutaneous Tissue and Fascia, Percutaneous Approach

● 0JWW3XZ Revision of Vascular Access Device in Lower Extremity Subcutaneous Tissue and Fascia, Percutaneous Approach

0JWWX0Z Revision of Drainage Device in Lower Extremity Subcutaneous Tissue and Fascia, External Approach

0JWWX3Z Revision of Infusion Device in Lower Extremity Subcutaneous Tissue and Fascia, External Approach

0JWWX7Z Revision of Autologous Tissue Substitute in Lower Extremity Subcutaneous Tissue and Fascia, External Approach

0JWWXHZ Revision of Contraceptive Device in Lower Extremity Subcutaneous Tissue and Fascia, External Approach

0JWWXJZ Revision of Synthetic Substitute in Lower Extremity Subcutaneous Tissue and Fascia, External Approach

0JWWXKZ Revision of Nonautologous Tissue Substitute in Lower Extremity Subcutaneous Tissue and Fascia, External Approach

0JWWXNZ Revision of Tissue Expander in Lower Extremity Subcutaneous Tissue and Fascia, External Approach

0JWWXVZ Revision of Infusion Pump in Lower Extremity Subcutaneous Tissue and Fascia, External Approach

0JWWXWZ Revision of Reservoir in Lower Extremity Subcutaneous Tissue and Fascia, External Approach

0JWWXXZ Revision of Vascular Access Device in Lower Extremity Subcutaneous Tissue and Fascia, External Approach

0JX – Subcutaneous Tissue and Fascia, Transfer

0JX00ZB Transfer Scalp Subcutaneous Tissue and Fascia with Skin and Subcutaneous Tissue, Open Approach

0JX00ZC Transfer Scalp Subcutaneous Tissue and Fascia with Skin, Subcutaneous Tissue and Fascia, Open Approach

0JX00ZZ Transfer Scalp Subcutaneous Tissue and Fascia, Open Approach

0JX03ZB Transfer Scalp Subcutaneous Tissue and Fascia with Skin and Subcutaneous Tissue, Percutaneous Approach

0JX03ZC Transfer Scalp Subcutaneous Tissue and Fascia with Skin, Subcutaneous Tissue and Fascia, Percutaneous Approach

0JX03ZZ Transfer Scalp Subcutaneous Tissue and Fascia, Percutaneous Approach

0JX10ZB Transfer Face Subcutaneous Tissue and Fascia with Skin and Subcutaneous Tissue, Open Approach

0JX10ZC Transfer Face Subcutaneous Tissue and Fascia with Skin, Subcutaneous Tissue and Fascia, Open Approach

0JX10ZZ Transfer Face Subcutaneous Tissue and Fascia, Open Approach

0JX13ZB Transfer Face Subcutaneous Tissue and Fascia with Skin and Subcutaneous Tissue, Percutaneous Approach

0JX13ZC Transfer Face Subcutaneous Tissue and Fascia with Skin, Subcutaneous Tissue and Fascia, Percutaneous Approach

0JX13ZZ Transfer Face Subcutaneous Tissue and Fascia, Percutaneous Approach

0JX40ZB Transfer Anterior Neck Subcutaneous Tissue and Fascia with Skin and Subcutaneous Tissue, Open Approach

0JX40ZC Transfer Anterior Neck Subcutaneous Tissue and Fascia with Skin, Subcutaneous Tissue and Fascia, Open Approach

0JX40ZZ Transfer Anterior Neck Subcutaneous Tissue and Fascia, Open Approach

0JX43ZB Transfer Anterior Neck Subcutaneous Tissue and Fascia with Skin and Subcutaneous Tissue, Percutaneous Approach

0JX43ZC Transfer Anterior Neck Subcutaneous Tissue and Fascia with Skin, Subcutaneous Tissue and Fascia, Percutaneous Approach

0JX43ZZ Transfer Anterior Neck Subcutaneous Tissue and Fascia, Percutaneous Approach

0JX50ZB Transfer Posterior Neck Subcutaneous Tissue and Fascia with Skin and Subcutaneous Tissue, Open Approach

0JX50ZC Transfer Posterior Neck Subcutaneous Tissue and Fascia with Skin, Subcutaneous Tissue and Fascia, Open Approach

0JX50ZZ Transfer Posterior Neck Subcutaneous Tissue and Fascia, Open Approach

0JX53ZB Transfer Posterior Neck Subcutaneous Tissue and Fascia with Skin and Subcutaneous Tissue, Percutaneous Approach

0JX53ZC Transfer Posterior Neck Subcutaneous Tissue and Fascia with Skin, Subcutaneous Tissue and Fascia, Percutaneous Approach

0JX53ZZ Transfer Posterior Neck Subcutaneous Tissue and Fascia, Percutaneous Approach

0JX60ZB Transfer Chest Subcutaneous Tissue and Fascia with Skin and Subcutaneous Tissue, Open Approach
AHA CC: 4Q, 2013, 109-111

0JX60ZC Transfer Chest Subcutaneous Tissue and Fascia with Skin, Subcutaneous Tissue and Fascia, Open Approach

0JX60ZZ Transfer Chest Subcutaneous Tissue and Fascia, Open Approach

0JX63ZB Transfer Chest Subcutaneous Tissue and Fascia with Skin and Subcutaneous Tissue, Percutaneous Approach

0JX63ZC Transfer Chest Subcutaneous Tissue and Fascia with Skin, Subcutaneous Tissue and Fascia, Percutaneous Approach

0JX63ZZ Transfer Chest Subcutaneous Tissue and Fascia, Percutaneous Approach

0JX70ZB Transfer Back Subcutaneous Tissue and Fascia with Skin and Subcutaneous Tissue, Open Approach

0JX70ZC Transfer Back Subcutaneous Tissue and Fascia with Skin, Subcutaneous Tissue and Fascia, Open Approach

0JX70ZZ Transfer Back Subcutaneous Tissue and Fascia, Open Approach

0JX73ZB Transfer Back Subcutaneous Tissue and Fascia with Skin and Subcutaneous Tissue, Percutaneous Approach

0JX73ZC Transfer Back Subcutaneous Tissue and Fascia with Skin, Subcutaneous Tissue and Fascia, Percutaneous Approach

0JX73ZZ Transfer Back Subcutaneous Tissue and Fascia, Percutaneous Approach

0JX80ZB Transfer Abdomen Subcutaneous Tissue and Fascia with Skin and Subcutaneous Tissue, Open Approach
AHA CC: 4Q, 2013, 109-111

0JX80ZC Transfer Abdomen Subcutaneous Tissue and Fascia with Skin, Subcutaneous Tissue and Fascia, Open Approach

0JX80ZZ Transfer Abdomen Subcutaneous Tissue and Fascia, Open Approach

0JX83ZB Transfer Abdomen Subcutaneous Tissue and Fascia with Skin and Subcutaneous Tissue, Percutaneous Approach

0JX83ZC Transfer Abdomen Subcutaneous Tissue and Fascia with Skin, Subcutaneous Tissue and Fascia, Percutaneous Approach

0JX83ZZ Transfer Abdomen Subcutaneous Tissue and Fascia, Percutaneous Approach

0JX90ZB Transfer Buttock Subcutaneous Tissue and Fascia with Skin and Subcutaneous Tissue, Open Approach

0JX90ZC Transfer Buttock Subcutaneous Tissue and Fascia with Skin, Subcutaneous Tissue and Fascia, Open Approach

0JX90ZZ Transfer Buttock Subcutaneous Tissue and Fascia, Open Approach

0JX93ZB Transfer Buttock Subcutaneous Tissue and Fascia with Skin and Subcutaneous Tissue, Percutaneous Approach

0JX93ZC Transfer Buttock Subcutaneous Tissue and Fascia with Skin, Subcutaneous Tissue and Fascia, Percutaneous Approach

0JX93ZZ Transfer Buttock Subcutaneous Tissue and Fascia, Percutaneous Approach

0JXB0ZB Transfer Perineum Subcutaneous Tissue and Fascia with Skin and Subcutaneous Tissue, Open Approach

0JXB0ZC Transfer Perineum Subcutaneous Tissue and Fascia with Skin, Subcutaneous Tissue and Fascia, Open Approach

0JXB0ZZ Transfer Perineum Subcutaneous Tissue and Fascia, Open Approach

0JXB3ZB Transfer Perineum Subcutaneous Tissue and Fascia with Skin and Subcutaneous Tissue, Percutaneous Approach

0JXB3ZC Transfer Perineum Subcutaneous Tissue and Fascia with Skin, Subcutaneous Tissue and Fascia, Percutaneous Approach

0JXB3ZZ Transfer Perineum Subcutaneous Tissue and Fascia, Percutaneous Approach

0JXC0ZB Transfer Pelvic Region Subcutaneous Tissue and Fascia with Skin and Subcutaneous Tissue, Open Approach

0JXC0ZC Transfer Pelvic Region Subcutaneous Tissue and Fascia with Skin, Subcutane Tissue and Fascia, Open Approach

0JXC0ZZ Transfer Pelvic Region Subcutaneous Tissue and Fascia, Open Approach

0JXC3ZB Transfer Pelvic Region Subcutaneous Tissue and Fascia with Skin and Subcutaneous Tissue, Percutaneous Approach

0JXC3ZC Transfer Pelvic Region Subcutaneous Tissue and Fascia with Skin, Subcutane Tissue and Fascia, Percutaneous Appro

0JXC3ZZ Transfer Pelvic Region Subcutaneous Tissue and Fascia, Percutaneous Appro

0JXD0ZB Transfer Right Upper Arm Subcutaneo Tissue and Fascia with Skin and Subcutaneous Tissue, Open Approach

0JXD0ZC Transfer Right Upper Arm Subcutaneou Tissue and Fascia with Skin, Subcutane Tissue and Fascia, Open Approach

0JXD0ZZ Transfer Right Upper Arm Subcutaneou Tissue and Fascia, Open Approach

0JXD3ZB Transfer Right Upper Arm Subcutaneou Tissue and Fascia with Skin and Subcutaneous Tissue, Percutaneous Approach

0JXD3ZC Transfer Right Upper Arm Subcutaneou Tissue and Fascia with Skin, Subcutane Tissue and Fascia, Percutaneous Approa

0JXD3ZZ Transfer Right Upper Arm Subcutaneou Tissue and Fascia, Percutaneous Approa

0JXF0ZB Transfer Left Upper Arm Subcutaneous Tissue and Fascia with Skin and Subcutaneous Tissue, Open Approach

0JXF0ZC Transfer Left Upper Arm Subcutaneous Tissue and Fascia with Skin, Subcutane Tissue and Fascia, Open Approach

0JXF0ZZ Transfer Left Upper Arm Subcutaneous Tissue and Fascia, Open Approach

0JXF3ZB Transfer Left Upper Arm Subcutaneous Tissue and Fascia with Skin and Subcutaneous Tissue, Percutaneous Approach

0JXF3ZC Transfer Left Upper Arm Subcutaneous Tissue and Fascia with Skin, Subcutaneo Tissue and Fascia, Percutaneous Approa

0JXF3ZZ Transfer Left Upper Arm Subcutaneous Tissue and Fascia, Percutaneous Approac

0JXG0ZB Transfer Right Lower Arm Subcutaneous Tissue and Fascia with Skin and Subcutaneous Tissue, Open Approach

0JXG0ZC Transfer Right Lower Arm Subcutaneous Tissue and Fascia with Skin, Subcutaneo Tissue and Fascia, Open Approach

0JXG0ZZ Transfer Right Lower Arm Subcutaneous Tissue and Fascia, Open Approach

0JXG3ZB Transfer Right Lower Arm Subcutaneous Tissue and Fascia with Skin and Subcutaneous Tissue, Percutaneous Approach

0JXG3ZC Transfer Right Lower Arm Subcutaneous Tissue and Fascia with Skin, Subcutaneo Tissue and Fascia, Percutaneous Approac

0JXG3ZZ Transfer Right Lower Arm Subcutaneous Tissue and Fascia, Percutaneous Approac

0JXH0ZB Transfer Left Lower Arm Subcutaneous Tissue and Fascia with Skin and Subcutaneous Tissue, Open Approach

0JXH0ZC Transfer Left Lower Arm Subcutaneous Tissue and Fascia with Skin, Subcutaneou Tissue and Fascia, Open Approach

0JXH0ZZ Transfer Left Lower Arm Subcutaneous Tissue and Fascia, Open Approach

H3ZB Transfer Left Lower Arm Subcutaneous Tissue and Fascia with Skin and Subcutaneous Tissue, Percutaneous Approach

H3ZC Transfer Left Lower Arm Subcutaneous Tissue and Fascia with Skin, Subcutaneous Tissue and Fascia, Percutaneous Approach

H3ZZ Transfer Left Lower Arm Subcutaneous Tissue and Fascia, Percutaneous Approach

J0ZB Transfer Right Hand Subcutaneous Tissue and Fascia with Skin and Subcutaneous Tissue, Open Approach

J0ZC Transfer Right Hand Subcutaneous Tissue and Fascia with Skin, Subcutaneous Tissue and Fascia, Open Approach

J0ZZ Transfer Right Hand Subcutaneous Tissue and Fascia, Open Approach

J3ZB Transfer Right Hand Subcutaneous Tissue and Fascia with Skin and Subcutaneous Tissue, Percutaneous Approach

J3ZC Transfer Right Hand Subcutaneous Tissue and Fascia with Skin, Subcutaneous Tissue and Fascia, Percutaneous Approach

XJ3ZZ Transfer Right Hand Subcutaneous Tissue and Fascia, Percutaneous Approach

XK0ZB Transfer Left Hand Subcutaneous Tissue and Fascia with Skin and Subcutaneous Tissue, Open Approach

XK0ZC Transfer Left Hand Subcutaneous Tissue and Fascia with Skin, Subcutaneous Tissue and Fascia, Open Approach

XK0ZZ Transfer Left Hand Subcutaneous Tissue and Fascia, Open Approach

XK3ZB Transfer Left Hand Subcutaneous Tissue and Fascia with Skin and Subcutaneous Tissue, Percutaneous Approach

XK3ZC Transfer Left Hand Subcutaneous Tissue and Fascia with Skin, Subcutaneous Tissue and Fascia, Percutaneous Approach

XK3ZZ Transfer Left Hand Subcutaneous Tissue and Fascia, Percutaneous Approach

XL0ZB Transfer Right Upper Leg Subcutaneous Tissue and Fascia with Skin and Subcutaneous Tissue, Open Approach

XL0ZC Transfer Right Upper Leg Subcutaneous Tissue and Fascia with Skin, Subcutaneous Tissue and Fascia, Open Approach

XL0ZZ Transfer Right Upper Leg Subcutaneous Tissue and Fascia, Open Approach

0JXL3ZB Transfer Right Upper Leg Subcutaneous Tissue and Fascia with Skin and Subcutaneous Tissue, Percutaneous Approach

0JXL3ZC Transfer Right Upper Leg Subcutaneous Tissue and Fascia with Skin, Subcutaneous Tissue and Fascia, Percutaneous Approach

0JXL3ZZ Transfer Right Upper Leg Subcutaneous Tissue and Fascia, Percutaneous Approach

0JXM0ZB Transfer Left Upper Leg Subcutaneous Tissue and Fascia with Skin and Subcutaneous Tissue, Open Approach

0JXM0ZC Transfer Left Upper Leg Subcutaneous Tissue and Fascia with Skin, Subcutaneous Tissue and Fascia, Open Approach

0JXM0ZZ Transfer Left Upper Leg Subcutaneous Tissue and Fascia, Open Approach

0JXM3ZB Transfer Left Upper Leg Subcutaneous Tissue and Fascia with Skin and Subcutaneous Tissue, Percutaneous Approach

0JXM3ZC Transfer Left Upper Leg Subcutaneous Tissue and Fascia with Skin, Subcutaneous Tissue and Fascia, Percutaneous Approach

0JXM3ZZ Transfer Left Upper Leg Subcutaneous Tissue and Fascia, Percutaneous Approach

0JXN0ZB Transfer Right Lower Leg Subcutaneous Tissue and Fascia with Skin and Subcutaneous Tissue, Open Approach

0JXN0ZC Transfer Right Lower Leg Subcutaneous Tissue and Fascia with Skin, Subcutaneous Tissue and Fascia, Open Approach

0JXN0ZZ Transfer Right Lower Leg Subcutaneous Tissue and Fascia, Open Approach

0JXN3ZB Transfer Right Lower Leg Subcutaneous Tissue and Fascia with Skin and Subcutaneous Tissue, Percutaneous Approach

0JXN3ZC Transfer Right Lower Leg Subcutaneous Tissue and Fascia with Skin, Subcutaneous Tissue and Fascia, Percutaneous Approach

0JXN3ZZ Transfer Right Lower Leg Subcutaneous Tissue and Fascia, Percutaneous Approach

0JXP0ZB Transfer Left Lower Leg Subcutaneous Tissue and Fascia with Skin and Subcutaneous Tissue, Open Approach

0JXP0ZC Transfer Left Lower Leg Subcutaneous Tissue and Fascia with Skin, Subcutaneous Tissue and Fascia, Open Approach

0JXP0ZZ Transfer Left Lower Leg Subcutaneous Tissue and Fascia, Open Approach

0JXP3ZB Transfer Left Lower Leg Subcutaneous Tissue and Fascia with Skin and Subcutaneous Tissue, Percutaneous Approach

0JXP3ZC Transfer Left Lower Leg Subcutaneous Tissue and Fascia with Skin, Subcutaneous Tissue and Fascia, Percutaneous Approach

0JXP3ZZ Transfer Left Lower Leg Subcutaneous Tissue and Fascia, Percutaneous Approach

0JXQ0ZB Transfer Right Foot Subcutaneous Tissue and Fascia with Skin and Subcutaneous Tissue, Open Approach

0JXQ0ZC Transfer Right Foot Subcutaneous Tissue and Fascia with Skin, Subcutaneous Tissue and Fascia, Open Approach

0JXQ0ZZ Transfer Right Foot Subcutaneous Tissue and Fascia, Open Approach

0JXQ3ZB Transfer Right Foot Subcutaneous Tissue and Fascia with Skin and Subcutaneous Tissue, Percutaneous Approach

0JXQ3ZC Transfer Right Foot Subcutaneous Tissue and Fascia with Skin, Subcutaneous Tissue and Fascia, Percutaneous Approach

0JXQ3ZZ Transfer Right Foot Subcutaneous Tissue and Fascia, Percutaneous Approach

0JXR0ZB Transfer Left Foot Subcutaneous Tissue and Fascia with Skin and Subcutaneous Tissue, Open Approach

0JXR0ZC Transfer Left Foot Subcutaneous Tissue and Fascia with Skin, Subcutaneous Tissue and Fascia, Open Approach

0JXR0ZZ Transfer Left Foot Subcutaneous Tissue and Fascia, Open Approach

0JXR3ZB Transfer Left Foot Subcutaneous Tissue and Fascia with Skin and Subcutaneous Tissue, Percutaneous Approach

0JXR3ZC Transfer Left Foot Subcutaneous Tissue and Fascia with Skin, Subcutaneous Tissue and Fascia, Percutaneous Approach

0JXR3ZZ Transfer Left Foot Subcutaneous Tissue and Fascia, Percutaneous Approach

Muscles

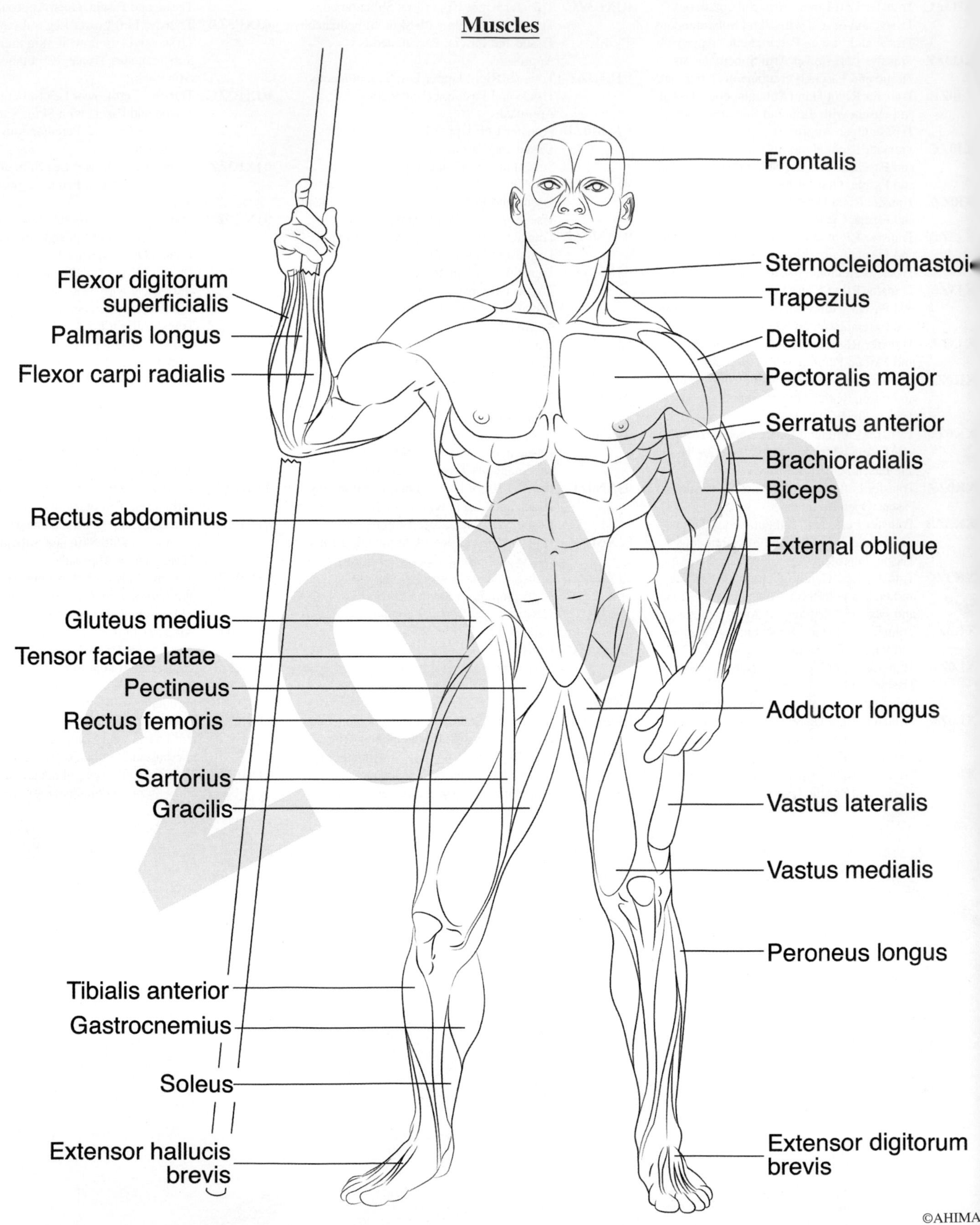
Frontalis
Flexor digitorum superficialis
Sternocleidomastoi
Trapezius
Palmaris longus
Deltoid
Flexor carpi radialis
Pectoralis major
Serratus anterior
Brachioradialis
Biceps
Rectus abdominus
External oblique
Gluteus medius
Tensor faciae latae
Pectineus
Adductor longus
Rectus femoris
Sartorius
Vastus lateralis
Gracilis
Vastus medialis
Peroneus longus
Tibialis anterior
Gastrocnemius
Soleus
Extensor hallucis brevis
Extensor digitorum brevis
2015

Muscles of the Hand

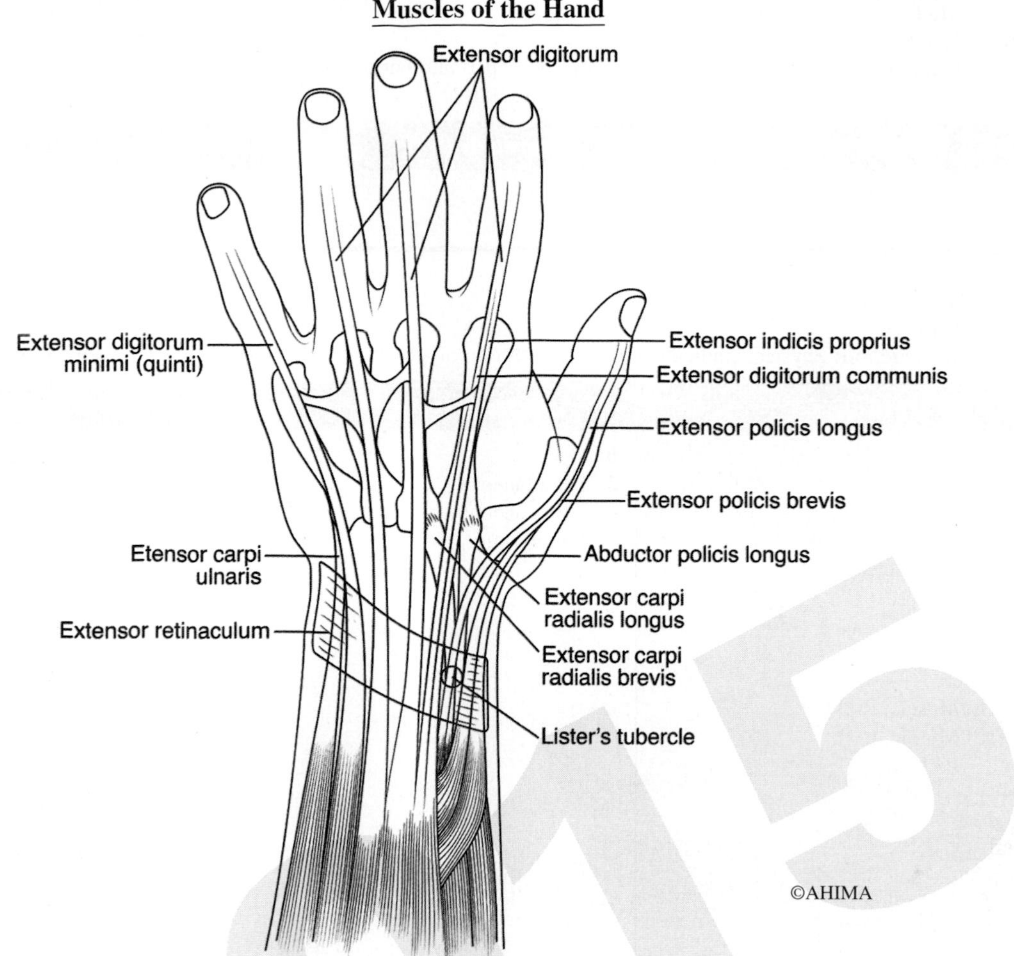

Extensor digitorum
Extensor digitorum minimi (quinti)
Extensor indicis proprius
Extensor digitorum communis
Extensor policis longus
Extensor policis brevis
Etensor carpi ulnaris
Abductor policis longus
Extensor carpi radialis longus
Extensor retinaculum
Extensor carpi radialis brevis
Lister's tubercle
©AHIMA

Muscles of the Foot

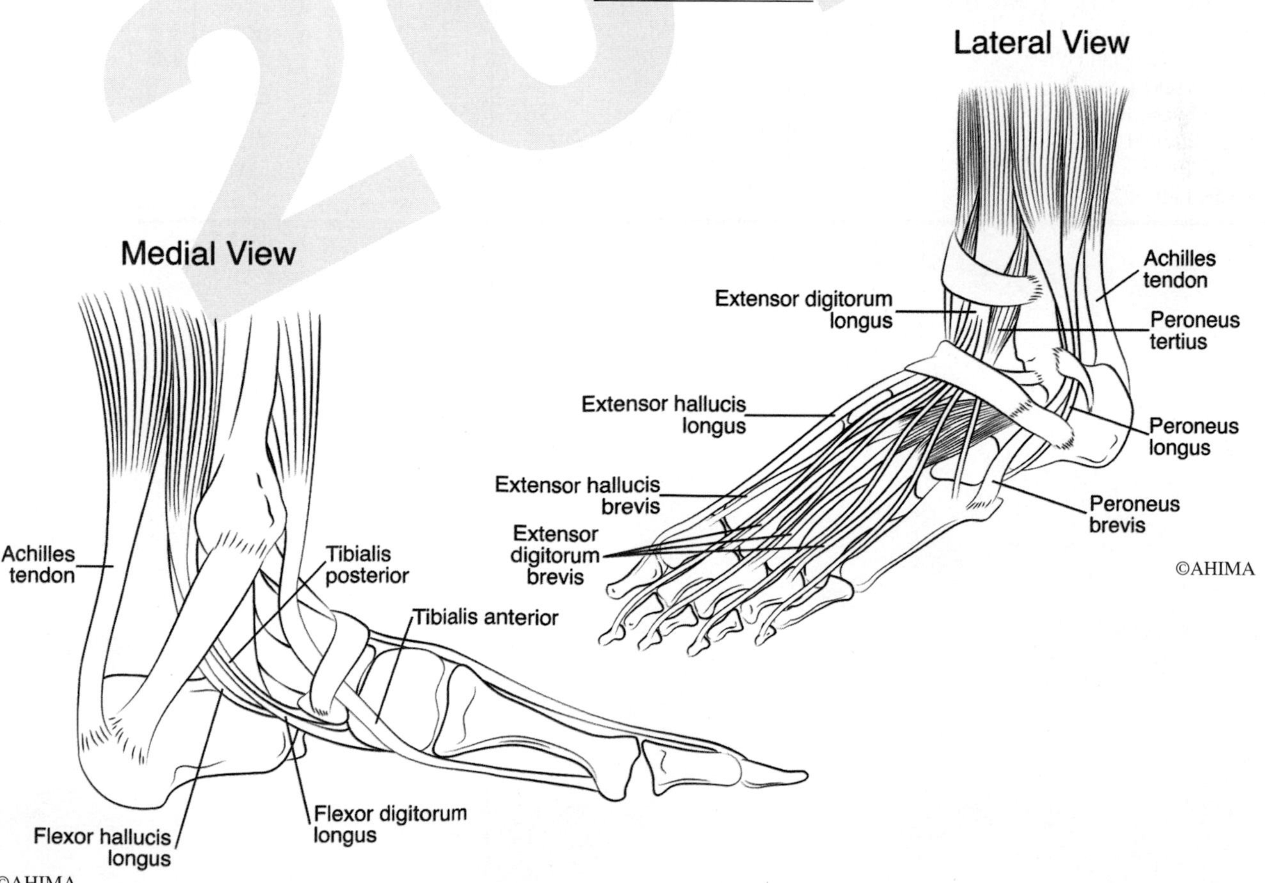

Lateral View
Achilles tendon
Extensor digitorum longus
Peroneus tertius
Extensor hallucis longus
Peroneus longus
Extensor hallucis brevis
Peroneus brevis
Extensor digitorum brevis
©AHIMA
Medial View
Achilles tendon
Tibialis posterior
Tibialis anterior
Flexor digitorum longus
Flexor hallucis longus
©AHIMA

Muscles Tables 0K2–0KX

Section 0 **Medical and Surgical**
Body System K **Muscles**
Operation 2 **Change:** Taking out or off a device from a body part and putting back an identical or similar device in or on the same body part without cutting or puncturing the skin or a mucous membrane

Body Part (4th)	Approach (5th)	Device (6th)	Qualifier (7th)
X Upper Muscle **Y** Lower Muscle	**X** External	**0** Drainage Device **Y** Other Device	**Z** No Qualifier

Section 0 **Medical and Surgical**
Body System K **Muscles**
Operation 5 **Destruction:** Physical eradication of all or a portion of a body part by the direct use of energy, force, or a destructive agent

Body Part (4th)	Approach (5th)	Device (6th)	Qualifier (7th)
0 Head Muscle **1** Facial Muscle **2** Neck Muscle, Right **3** Neck Muscle, Left **4** Tongue, Palate, Pharynx Muscle **5** Shoulder Muscle, Right **6** Shoulder Muscle, Left **7** Upper Arm Muscle, Right **8** Upper Arm Muscle, Left **9** Lower Arm and Wrist Muscle, Right **B** Lower Arm and Wrist Muscle, Left **C** Hand Muscle, Right **D** Hand Muscle, Left **F** Trunk Muscle, Right **G** Trunk Muscle, Left **H** Thorax Muscle, Right **J** Thorax Muscle, Left **K** Abdomen Muscle, Right **L** Abdomen Muscle, Left **M** Perineum Muscle **N** Hip Muscle, Right **P** Hip Muscle, Left **Q** Upper Leg Muscle, Right **R** Upper Leg Muscle, Left **S** Lower Leg Muscle, Right **T** Lower Leg Muscle, Left **V** Foot Muscle, Right **W** Foot Muscle, Left	**0** Open **3** Percutaneous **4** Percutaneous Endoscopic	**Z** No Device	**Z** No Qualifier

tion **0** **Medical and Surgical**
ly System **K** **Muscles**
eration **8** **Division:** Cutting into a body part, without draining fluids and/or gases from the body part, in order to separate or transect a body part

Body Part (4th)	Approach (5th)	Device (6th)	Qualifier (7th)
Head Muscle Facial Muscle Neck Muscle, Right Neck Muscle, Left Tongue, Palate, Pharynx Muscle Shoulder Muscle, Right Shoulder Muscle, Left Upper Arm Muscle, Right Upper Arm Muscle, Left Lower Arm and Wrist Muscle, Right Lower Arm and Wrist Muscle, Left Hand Muscle, Right Hand Muscle, Left Trunk Muscle, Right Trunk Muscle, Left Thorax Muscle, Right Thorax Muscle, Left K Abdomen Muscle, Right Abdomen Muscle, Left M Perineum Muscle N Hip Muscle, Right P Hip Muscle, Left Q Upper Leg Muscle, Right R Upper Leg Muscle, Left S Lower Leg Muscle, Right T Lower Leg Muscle, Left V Foot Muscle, Right W Foot Muscle, Left	**0** Open **3** Percutaneous **4** Percutaneous Endoscopic	**Z** No Device	**Z** No Qualifier

Section 0 **Medical and Surgical**
Body System K **Muscles**
Operation 9 **Drainage:** Taking or letting out fluids and/or gases from a body part

Body Part (4th)	Approach (5th)	Device (6th)	Qualifier (7th)
0 Head Muscle **1** Facial Muscle **2** Neck Muscle, Right **3** Neck Muscle, Left **4** Tongue, Palate, Pharynx Muscle **5** Shoulder Muscle, Right **6** Shoulder Muscle, Left **7** Upper Arm Muscle, Right **8** Upper Arm Muscle, Left **9** Lower Arm and Wrist Muscle, Right **B** Lower Arm and Wrist Muscle, Left **C** Hand Muscle, Right **D** Hand Muscle, Left **F** Trunk Muscle, Right **G** Trunk Muscle, Left **H** Thorax Muscle, Right **J** Thorax Muscle, Left **K** Abdomen Muscle, Right **L** Abdomen Muscle, Left **M** Perineum Muscle **N** Hip Muscle, Right **P** Hip Muscle, Left **Q** Upper Leg Muscle, Right **R** Upper Leg Muscle, Left **S** Lower Leg Muscle, Right **T** Lower Leg Muscle, Left **V** Foot Muscle, Right **W** Foot Muscle, Left	**0** Open **3** Percutaneous **4** Percutaneous Endoscopic	**0** Drainage Device	**Z** No Qualifier
0 Head Muscle **1** Facial Muscle **2** Neck Muscle, Right **3** Neck Muscle, Left **4** Tongue, Palate, Pharynx Muscle **5** Shoulder Muscle, Right **6** Shoulder Muscle, Left **7** Upper Arm Muscle, Right **8** Upper Arm Muscle, Left **9** Lower Arm and Wrist Muscle, Right **B** Lower Arm and Wrist Muscle, Left **C** Hand Muscle, Right **D** Hand Muscle, Left **F** Trunk Muscle, Right **G** Trunk Muscle, Left **H** Thorax Muscle, Right **J** Thorax Muscle, Left **K** Abdomen Muscle, Right **L** Abdomen Muscle, Left **M** Perineum Muscle **N** Hip Muscle, Right **P** Hip Muscle, Left **Q** Upper Leg Muscle, Right **R** Upper Leg Muscle, Left **S** Lower Leg Muscle, Right **T** Lower Leg Muscle, Left **V** Foot Muscle, Right **W** Foot Muscle, Left	**0** Open **3** Percutaneous **4** Percutaneous Endoscopic	**Z** No Device	**X** Diagnostic **Z** No Qualifier

tion	**0**	**Medical and Surgical**
dy System	**K**	**Muscles**
eration	**B**	**Excision:** Cutting out or off, without replacement, a portion of a body part

Body Part (4th)	Approach (5th)	Device (6th)	Qualifier (7th)
Head Muscle	**0** Open	**Z** No Device	**X** Diagnostic
Facial Muscle	**3** Percutaneous		**Z** No Qualifier
Neck Muscle, Right	**4** Percutaneous Endoscopic		
Neck Muscle, Left			
Tongue, Palate, Pharynx Muscle			
Shoulder Muscle, Right			
Shoulder Muscle, Left			
Upper Arm Muscle, Right			
Upper Arm Muscle, Left			
Lower Arm and Wrist Muscle, Right			
Lower Arm and Wrist Muscle, Left			
Hand Muscle, Right			
Hand Muscle, Left			
Trunk Muscle, Right			
Trunk Muscle, Left			
H Thorax Muscle, Right			
J Thorax Muscle, Left			
K Abdomen Muscle, Right			
L Abdomen Muscle, Left			
M Perineum Muscle			
N Hip Muscle, Right			
P Hip Muscle, Left			
Q Upper Leg Muscle, Right			
R Upper Leg Muscle, Left			
S Lower Leg Muscle, Right			
T Lower Leg Muscle, Left			
V Foot Muscle, Right			
W Foot Muscle, Left			

ection	**0**	**Medical and Surgical**
ody System	**K**	**Muscles**
peration	**C**	**Extirpation:** Taking or cutting out solid matter from a body part

Body Part (4th)	Approach (5th)	Device (6th)	Qualifier (7th)
0 Head Muscle	**0** Open	**Z** No Device	**Z** No Qualifier
1 Facial Muscle	**3** Percutaneous		
2 Neck Muscle, Right	**4** Percutaneous Endoscopic		
3 Neck Muscle, Left			
4 Tongue, Palate, Pharynx Muscle			
5 Shoulder Muscle, Right			
6 Shoulder Muscle, Left			
7 Upper Arm Muscle, Right			
8 Upper Arm Muscle, Left			
9 Lower Arm and Wrist Muscle, Right			
B Lower Arm and Wrist Muscle, Left			
C Hand Muscle, Right			
D Hand Muscle, Left			
F Trunk Muscle, Right			
G Trunk Muscle, Left			
H Thorax Muscle, Right			
J Thorax Muscle, Left			
K Abdomen Muscle, Right			
L Abdomen Muscle, Left			
M Perineum Muscle			
N Hip Muscle, Right			
P Hip Muscle, Left			
Q Upper Leg Muscle, Right			
R Upper Leg Muscle, Left			
S Lower Leg Muscle, Right			
T Lower Leg Muscle, Left			
V Foot Muscle, Right			
W Foot Muscle, Left			

Section 0 **Medical and Surgical**
Body System K **Muscles**
Operation H **Insertion:** Putting in a nonbiological appliance that monitors, assists, performs, or prevents a physiological function but do[es] not physically take the place of a body part

Body Part (4th)	Approach (5th)	Device (6th)	Qualifier (7th)
X Upper Muscle **Y** Lower Muscle	**0** Open **3** Percutaneous **4** Percutaneous Endoscopic	**M** Stimulator Lead	**Z** No Qualifier

Section 0 **Medical and Surgical**
Body System K **Muscles**
Operation J **Inspection:** Visually and/or manually exploring a body part

Body Part (4th)	Approach (5th)	Device (6th)	Qualifier (7th)
X Upper Muscle **Y** Lower Muscle	**0** Open **3** Percutaneous **4** Percutaneous Endoscopic **X** External	**Z** No Device	**Z** No Qualifier

Section 0 **Medical and Surgical**
Body System K **Muscles**
Operation M **Reattachment:** Putting back in or on all or a portion of a separated body part to its normal location or other suitable locatio[n]

Body Part (4th)	Approach (5th)	Device (6th)	Qualifier (7th)
0 Head Muscle **1** Facial Muscle **2** Neck Muscle, Right **3** Neck Muscle, Left **4** Tongue, Palate, Pharynx Muscle **5** Shoulder Muscle, Right **6** Shoulder Muscle, Left **7** Upper Arm Muscle, Right **8** Upper Arm Muscle, Left **9** Lower Arm and Wrist Muscle, Right **B** Lower Arm and Wrist Muscle, Left **C** Hand Muscle, Right **D** Hand Muscle, Left **F** Trunk Muscle, Right **G** Trunk Muscle, Left **H** Thorax Muscle, Right **J** Thorax Muscle, Left **K** Abdomen Muscle, Right **L** Abdomen Muscle, Left **M** Perineum Muscle **N** Hip Muscle, Right **P** Hip Muscle, Left **Q** Upper Leg Muscle, Right **R** Upper Leg Muscle, Left **S** Lower Leg Muscle, Right **T** Lower Leg Muscle, Left **V** Foot Muscle, Right **W** Foot Muscle, Left	**0** Open **4** Percutaneous Endoscopic	**Z** No Device	**Z** No Qualifier

Section 0 **Medical and Surgical**
Body System K **Muscles**
Operation N **Release:** Freeing a body part from an abnormal physical constraint by cutting or by the use of force

Body Part (4th)	Approach (5th)	Device (6th)	Qualifier (7th)
0 Head Muscle Facial Muscle 2 Neck Muscle, Right 3 Neck Muscle, Left 4 Tongue, Palate, Pharynx Muscle 5 Shoulder Muscle, Right 6 Shoulder Muscle, Left 7 Upper Arm Muscle, Right 8 Upper Arm Muscle, Left 9 Lower Arm and Wrist Muscle, Right B Lower Arm and Wrist Muscle, Left C Hand Muscle, Right D Hand Muscle, Left F Trunk Muscle, Right G Trunk Muscle, Left H Thorax Muscle, Right J Thorax Muscle, Left K Abdomen Muscle, Right L Abdomen Muscle, Left M Perineum Muscle N Hip Muscle, Right P Hip Muscle, Left Q Upper Leg Muscle, Right R Upper Leg Muscle, Left S Lower Leg Muscle, Right T Lower Leg Muscle, Left V Foot Muscle, Right W Foot Muscle, Left	0 Open 3 Percutaneous 4 Percutaneous Endoscopic X External	Z No Device	Z No Qualifier

Section 0 **Medical and Surgical**
Body System K **Muscles**
Operation P **Removal:** Taking out or off a device from a body part

Body Part (4th)	Approach (5th)	Device (6th)	Qualifier (7th)
X Upper Muscle Y Lower Muscle	0 Open 3 Percutaneous 4 Percutaneous Endoscopic	0 Drainage Device 7 Autologous Tissue Substitute J Synthetic Substitute K Nonautologous Tissue Substitute M Stimulator Lead	Z No Qualifier
X Upper Muscle Y Lower Muscle	X External	0 Drainage Device M Stimulator Lead	Z No Qualifier

Section 0 **Medical and Surgical**
Body System K **Muscles**
Operation Q **Repair:** Restoring, to the extent possible, a body part to its normal anatomic structure and function

Body Part (4th)	Approach (5th)	Device (6th)	Qualifier (7th)
0 Head Muscle	**0** Open	**Z** No Device	**Z** No Qualifier
1 Facial Muscle	**3** Percutaneous		
2 Neck Muscle, Right	**4** Percutaneous Endoscopic		
3 Neck Muscle, Left			
4 Tongue, Palate, Pharynx Muscle			
5 Shoulder Muscle, Right			
6 Shoulder Muscle, Left			
7 Upper Arm Muscle, Right			
8 Upper Arm Muscle, Left			
9 Lower Arm and Wrist Muscle, Right			
B Lower Arm and Wrist Muscle, Left			
C Hand Muscle, Right			
D Hand Muscle, Left			
F Trunk Muscle, Right			
G Trunk Muscle, Left			
H Thorax Muscle, Right			
J Thorax Muscle, Left			
K Abdomen Muscle, Right			
L Abdomen Muscle, Left			
M Perineum Muscle			
N Hip Muscle, Right			
P Hip Muscle, Left			
Q Upper Leg Muscle, Right			
R Upper Leg Muscle, Left			
S Lower Leg Muscle, Right			
T Lower Leg Muscle, Left			
V Foot Muscle, Right			
W Foot Muscle, Left			

Section 0 **Medical and Surgical**
Body System K **Muscles**
Operation S **Reposition:** Moving to its normal location, or other suitable location, all or a portion of a body part

Body Part (4th)	Approach (5th)	Device (6th)	Qualifier (7th)
0 Head Muscle	**0** Open	**Z** No Device	**Z** No Qualifier
1 Facial Muscle	**4** Percutaneous Endoscopic		
2 Neck Muscle, Right			
3 Neck Muscle, Left			
4 Tongue, Palate, Pharynx Muscle			
5 Shoulder Muscle, Right			
6 Shoulder Muscle, Left			
7 Upper Arm Muscle, Right			
8 Upper Arm Muscle, Left			
9 Lower Arm and Wrist Muscle, Right			
B Lower Arm and Wrist Muscle, Left			
C Hand Muscle, Right			
D Hand Muscle, Left			
F Trunk Muscle, Right			
G Trunk Muscle, Left			
H Thorax Muscle, Right			
J Thorax Muscle, Left			
K Abdomen Muscle, Right			
L Abdomen Muscle, Left			
M Perineum Muscle			
N Hip Muscle, Right			
P Hip Muscle, Left			
Q Upper Leg Muscle, Right			
R Upper Leg Muscle, Left			
S Lower Leg Muscle, Right			
T Lower Leg Muscle, Left			
V Foot Muscle, Right			
W Foot Muscle, Left			

Section 0 **Medical and Surgical**
Body System K **Muscles**
Operation T **Resection:** Cutting out or off, without replacement, all of a body part

Body Part (4th)	Approach (5th)	Device (6th)	Qualifier (7th)
0 Head Muscle 1 Facial Muscle 2 Neck Muscle, Right 3 Neck Muscle, Left 4 Tongue, Palate, Pharynx Muscle 5 Shoulder Muscle, Right 6 Shoulder Muscle, Left 7 Upper Arm Muscle, Right 8 Upper Arm Muscle, Left 9 Lower Arm and Wrist Muscle, Right B Lower Arm and Wrist Muscle, Left C Hand Muscle, Right D Hand Muscle, Left F Trunk Muscle, Right G Trunk Muscle, Left H Thorax Muscle, Right J Thorax Muscle, Left K Abdomen Muscle, Right L Abdomen Muscle, Left M Perineum Muscle N Hip Muscle, Right P Hip Muscle, Left Q Upper Leg Muscle, Right R Upper Leg Muscle, Left S Lower Leg Muscle, Right T Lower Leg Muscle, Left V Foot Muscle, Right W Foot Muscle, Left	0 Open 4 Percutaneous Endoscopic	Z No Device	Z No Qualifier

Section 0 **Medical and Surgical**
Body System K **Muscles**
Operation U **Supplement:** Putting in or on biological or synthetic material that physically reinforces and/or augments the function of a portion of a body part

Body Part (4th)	Approach (5th)	Device (6th)	Qualifier (7th)
0 Head Muscle 1 Facial Muscle 2 Neck Muscle, Right 3 Neck Muscle, Left 4 Tongue, Palate, Pharynx Muscle 5 Shoulder Muscle, Right 6 Shoulder Muscle, Left 7 Upper Arm Muscle, Right 8 Upper Arm Muscle, Left 9 Lower Arm and Wrist Muscle, Right B Lower Arm and Wrist Muscle, Left C Hand Muscle, Right D Hand Muscle, Left F Trunk Muscle, Right G Trunk Muscle, Left H Thorax Muscle, Right J Thorax Muscle, Left K Abdomen Muscle, Right L Abdomen Muscle, Left M Perineum Muscle N Hip Muscle, Right P Hip Muscle, Left Q Upper Leg Muscle, Right R Upper Leg Muscle, Left S Lower Leg Muscle, Right T Lower Leg Muscle, Left V Foot Muscle, Right W Foot Muscle, Left	0 Open 4 Percutaneous Endoscopic	7 Autologous Tissue Substitute J Synthetic Substitute K Nonautologous Tissue Substitute	Z No Qualifier

Section 0 **Medical and Surgical**
Body System K **Muscles**
Operation W **Revision:** Correcting, to the extent possible, a portion of a malfunctioning device or the position of a displaced device

Body Part (4th)	Approach (5th)	Device (6th)	Qualifier (7th)
X Upper Muscle **Y** Lower Muscle	**0** Open **3** Percutaneous **4** Percutaneous Endoscopic **X** External	**0** Drainage Device **7** Autologous Tissue Substitute **J** Synthetic Substitute **K** Nonautologous Tissue Substitute **M** Stimulator Lead	**Z** No Qualifier

Section 0 **Medical and Surgical**
Body System K **Muscles**
Operation X **Transfer:** Moving, without taking out, all or a portion of a body part to another location to take over the function of all or a portion of a body part

Body Part (4th)	Approach (5th)	Device (6th)	Qualifier (7th)
0 Head Muscle **1** Facial Muscle **2** Neck Muscle, Right **3** Neck Muscle, Left **4** Tongue, Palate, Pharynx Muscle **5** Shoulder Muscle, Right **6** Shoulder Muscle, Left **7** Upper Arm Muscle, Right **8** Upper Arm Muscle, Left **9** Lower Arm and Wrist Muscle, Right **B** Lower Arm and Wrist Muscle, Left **C** Hand Muscle, Right **D** Hand Muscle, Left **F** Trunk Muscle, Right **G** Trunk Muscle, Left **H** Thorax Muscle, Right **J** Thorax Muscle, Left **M** Perineum Muscle **N** Hip Muscle, Right **P** Hip Muscle, Left **Q** Upper Leg Muscle, Right **R** Upper Leg Muscle, Left **S** Lower Leg Muscle, Right **T** Lower Leg Muscle, Left **V** Foot Muscle, Right **W** Foot Muscle, Left	**0** Open **4** Percutaneous Endoscopic	**Z** No Device	**0** Skin **1** Subcutaneous Tissue **2** Skin and Subcutaneous Tissue **Z** No Qualifier
K Abdomen Muscle, Right **L** Abdomen Muscle, Left	**0** Open **4** Percutaneous Endoscopic	**Z** No Device	**0** Skin **1** Subcutaneous Tissue **2** Skin and Subcutaneous Tissue **6** Transverse Rectus Abdominis Myocutaneous Flap **Z** No Qualifier

Muscles Code Listing 0K2–0KX

0K2 – Muscles, Change

Review Coding Guideline B6.1c

0K2XX0Z Change Drainage Device in Upper Muscle, External Approach
0K2XXYZ Change Other Device in Upper Muscle, External Approach
0K2YX0Z Change Drainage Device in Lower Muscle, External Approach
0K2YXYZ Change Other Device in Lower Muscle, External Approach

0K5 – Muscles, Destruction

0K500ZZ Destruction of Head Muscle, Open Approach
0K503ZZ Destruction of Head Muscle, Percutaneous Approach
0K504ZZ Destruction of Head Muscle, Percutaneous Endoscopic Approach
0K510ZZ Destruction of Facial Muscle, Open Approach
0K513ZZ Destruction of Facial Muscle, Percutaneous Approach
0K514ZZ Destruction of Facial Muscle, Percutaneous Endoscopic Approach

520ZZ Destruction of Right Neck Muscle, Open Approach
523ZZ Destruction of Right Neck Muscle, Percutaneous Approach
524ZZ Destruction of Right Neck Muscle, Percutaneous Endoscopic Approach
530ZZ Destruction of Left Neck Muscle, Open Approach
533ZZ Destruction of Left Neck Muscle, Percutaneous Approach
534ZZ Destruction of Left Neck Muscle, Percutaneous Endoscopic Approach
540ZZ Destruction of Tongue, Palate, Pharynx Muscle, Open Approach
543ZZ Destruction of Tongue, Palate, Pharynx Muscle, Percutaneous Approach
544ZZ Destruction of Tongue, Palate, Pharynx Muscle, Percutaneous Endoscopic Approach
550ZZ Destruction of Right Shoulder Muscle, Open Approach
553ZZ Destruction of Right Shoulder Muscle, Percutaneous Approach
554ZZ Destruction of Right Shoulder Muscle, Percutaneous Endoscopic Approach
560ZZ Destruction of Left Shoulder Muscle, Open Approach
563ZZ Destruction of Left Shoulder Muscle, Percutaneous Approach
564ZZ Destruction of Left Shoulder Muscle, Percutaneous Endoscopic Approach
570ZZ Destruction of Right Upper Arm Muscle, Open Approach
573ZZ Destruction of Right Upper Arm Muscle, Percutaneous Approach
574ZZ Destruction of Right Upper Arm Muscle, Percutaneous Endoscopic Approach
580ZZ Destruction of Left Upper Arm Muscle, Open Approach
583ZZ Destruction of Left Upper Arm Muscle, Percutaneous Approach
K584ZZ Destruction of Left Upper Arm Muscle, Percutaneous Endoscopic Approach
K590ZZ Destruction of Right Lower Arm and Wrist Muscle, Open Approach
K593ZZ Destruction of Right Lower Arm and Wrist Muscle, Percutaneous Approach
K594ZZ Destruction of Right Lower Arm and Wrist Muscle, Percutaneous Endoscopic Approach
K5B0ZZ Destruction of Left Lower Arm and Wrist Muscle, Open Approach
0K5B3ZZ Destruction of Left Lower Arm and Wrist Muscle, Percutaneous Approach
0K5B4ZZ Destruction of Left Lower Arm and Wrist Muscle, Percutaneous Endoscopic Approach
0K5C0ZZ Destruction of Right Hand Muscle, Open Approach
0K5C3ZZ Destruction of Right Hand Muscle, Percutaneous Approach
0K5C4ZZ Destruction of Right Hand Muscle, Percutaneous Endoscopic Approach
0K5D0ZZ Destruction of Left Hand Muscle, Open Approach
0K5D3ZZ Destruction of Left Hand Muscle, Percutaneous Approach
0K5D4ZZ Destruction of Left Hand Muscle, Percutaneous Endoscopic Approach
0K5F0ZZ Destruction of Right Trunk Muscle, Open Approach
0K5F3ZZ Destruction of Right Trunk Muscle, Percutaneous Approach
0K5F4ZZ Destruction of Right Trunk Muscle, Percutaneous Endoscopic Approach
0K5G0ZZ Destruction of Left Trunk Muscle, Open Approach
0K5G3ZZ Destruction of Left Trunk Muscle, Percutaneous Approach
0K5G4ZZ Destruction of Left Trunk Muscle, Percutaneous Endoscopic Approach
0K5H0ZZ Destruction of Right Thorax Muscle, Open Approach
0K5H3ZZ Destruction of Right Thorax Muscle, Percutaneous Approach
0K5H4ZZ Destruction of Right Thorax Muscle, Percutaneous Endoscopic Approach
0K5J0ZZ Destruction of Left Thorax Muscle, Open Approach
0K5J3ZZ Destruction of Left Thorax Muscle, Percutaneous Approach
0K5J4ZZ Destruction of Left Thorax Muscle, Percutaneous Endoscopic Approach
0K5K0ZZ Destruction of Right Abdomen Muscle, Open Approach
0K5K3ZZ Destruction of Right Abdomen Muscle, Percutaneous Approach
0K5K4ZZ Destruction of Right Abdomen Muscle, Percutaneous Endoscopic Approach
0K5L0ZZ Destruction of Left Abdomen Muscle, Open Approach
0K5L3ZZ Destruction of Left Abdomen Muscle, Percutaneous Approach
0K5L4ZZ Destruction of Left Abdomen Muscle, Percutaneous Endoscopic Approach
0K5M0ZZ Destruction of Perineum Muscle, Open Approach
0K5M3ZZ Destruction of Perineum Muscle, Percutaneous Approach
0K5M4ZZ Destruction of Perineum Muscle, Percutaneous Endoscopic Approach
0K5N0ZZ Destruction of Right Hip Muscle, Open Approach
0K5N3ZZ Destruction of Right Hip Muscle, Percutaneous Approach
0K5N4ZZ Destruction of Right Hip Muscle, Percutaneous Endoscopic Approach
0K5P0ZZ Destruction of Left Hip Muscle, Open Approach
0K5P3ZZ Destruction of Left Hip Muscle, Percutaneous Approach
0K5P4ZZ Destruction of Left Hip Muscle, Percutaneous Endoscopic Approach
0K5Q0ZZ Destruction of Right Upper Leg Muscle, Open Approach
0K5Q3ZZ Destruction of Right Upper Leg Muscle, Percutaneous Approach
0K5Q4ZZ Destruction of Right Upper Leg Muscle, Percutaneous Endoscopic Approach
0K5R0ZZ Destruction of Left Upper Leg Muscle, Open Approach
0K5R3ZZ Destruction of Left Upper Leg Muscle, Percutaneous Approach
0K5R4ZZ Destruction of Left Upper Leg Muscle, Percutaneous Endoscopic Approach
0K5S0ZZ Destruction of Right Lower Leg Muscle, Open Approach
0K5S3ZZ Destruction of Right Lower Leg Muscle, Percutaneous Approach
0K5S4ZZ Destruction of Right Lower Leg Muscle, Percutaneous Endoscopic Approach
0K5T0ZZ Destruction of Left Lower Leg Muscle, Open Approach
0K5T3ZZ Destruction of Left Lower Leg Muscle, Percutaneous Approach
0K5T4ZZ Destruction of Left Lower Leg Muscle, Percutaneous Endoscopic Approach
0K5V0ZZ Destruction of Right Foot Muscle, Open Approach
0K5V3ZZ Destruction of Right Foot Muscle, Percutaneous Approach
0K5V4ZZ Destruction of Right Foot Muscle, Percutaneous Endoscopic Approach
0K5W0ZZ Destruction of Left Foot Muscle, Open Approach
0K5W3ZZ Destruction of Left Foot Muscle, Percutaneous Approach
0K5W4ZZ Destruction of Left Foot Muscle, Percutaneous Endoscopic Approach

K8 – Muscles, Division

eview Coding Guideline B3.14

K800ZZ Division of Head Muscle, Open Approach
K803ZZ Division of Head Muscle, Percutaneous Approach
K804ZZ Division of Head Muscle, Percutaneous Endoscopic Approach
K810ZZ Division of Facial Muscle, Open Approach
K813ZZ Division of Facial Muscle, Percutaneous Approach
K814ZZ Division of Facial Muscle, Percutaneous Endoscopic Approach
K820ZZ Division of Right Neck Muscle, Open Approach
K823ZZ Division of Right Neck Muscle, Percutaneous Approach
K824ZZ Division of Right Neck Muscle, Percutaneous Endoscopic Approach
0K830ZZ Division of Left Neck Muscle, Open Approach
0K833ZZ Division of Left Neck Muscle, Percutaneous Approach
0K834ZZ Division of Left Neck Muscle, Percutaneous Endoscopic Approach
0K840ZZ Division of Tongue, Palate, Pharynx Muscle, Open Approach
0K843ZZ Division of Tongue, Palate, Pharynx Muscle, Percutaneous Approach
0K844ZZ Division of Tongue, Palate, Pharynx Muscle, Percutaneous Endoscopic Approach
0K850ZZ Division of Right Shoulder Muscle, Open Approach
0K853ZZ Division of Right Shoulder Muscle, Percutaneous Approach
0K854ZZ Division of Right Shoulder Muscle, Percutaneous Endoscopic Approach
0K860ZZ Division of Left Shoulder Muscle, Open Approach
0K863ZZ Division of Left Shoulder Muscle, Percutaneous Approach
0K864ZZ Division of Left Shoulder Muscle, Percutaneous Endoscopic Approach
0K870ZZ Division of Right Upper Arm Muscle, Open Approach
0K873ZZ Division of Right Upper Arm Muscle, Percutaneous Approach
0K874ZZ Division of Right Upper Arm Muscle, Percutaneous Endoscopic Approach
0K880ZZ Division of Left Upper Arm Muscle, Open Approach

0K883ZZ Division of Left Upper Arm Muscle, Percutaneous Approach
0K884ZZ Division of Left Upper Arm Muscle, Percutaneous Endoscopic Approach
0K890ZZ Division of Right Lower Arm and Wrist Muscle, Open Approach
0K893ZZ Division of Right Lower Arm and Wrist Muscle, Percutaneous Approach
0K894ZZ Division of Right Lower Arm and Wrist Muscle, Percutaneous Endoscopic Approach
0K8B0ZZ Division of Left Lower Arm and Wrist Muscle, Open Approach
0K8B3ZZ Division of Left Lower Arm and Wrist Muscle, Percutaneous Approach
0K8B4ZZ Division of Left Lower Arm and Wrist Muscle, Percutaneous Endoscopic Approach
0K8C0ZZ Division of Right Hand Muscle, Open Approach
0K8C3ZZ Division of Right Hand Muscle, Percutaneous Approach
0K8C4ZZ Division of Right Hand Muscle, Percutaneous Endoscopic Approach
0K8D0ZZ Division of Left Hand Muscle, Open Approach
0K8D3ZZ Division of Left Hand Muscle, Percutaneous Approach
0K8D4ZZ Division of Left Hand Muscle, Percutaneous Endoscopic Approach
0K8F0ZZ Division of Right Trunk Muscle, Open Approach
0K8F3ZZ Division of Right Trunk Muscle, Percutaneous Approach
0K8F4ZZ Division of Right Trunk Muscle, Percutaneous Endoscopic Approach
0K8G0ZZ Division of Left Trunk Muscle, Open Approach
0K8G3ZZ Division of Left Trunk Muscle, Percutaneous Approach
0K8G4ZZ Division of Left Trunk Muscle, Percutaneous Endoscopic Approach
0K8H0ZZ Division of Right Thorax Muscle, Open Approach
0K8H3ZZ Division of Right Thorax Muscle, Percutaneous Approach
0K8H4ZZ Division of Right Thorax Muscle, Percutaneous Endoscopic Approach
0K8J0ZZ Division of Left Thorax Muscle, Open Approach
0K8J3ZZ Division of Left Thorax Muscle, Percutaneous Approach
0K8J4ZZ Division of Left Thorax Muscle, Percutaneous Endoscopic Approach
0K8K0ZZ Division of Right Abdomen Muscle, Open Approach
0K8K3ZZ Division of Right Abdomen Muscle, Percutaneous Approach
0K8K4ZZ Division of Right Abdomen Muscle, Percutaneous Endoscopic Approach
0K8L0ZZ Division of Left Abdomen Muscle, Open Approach
0K8L3ZZ Division of Left Abdomen Muscle, Percutaneous Approach
0K8L4ZZ Division of Left Abdomen Muscle, Percutaneous Endoscopic Approach
0K8M0ZZ Division of Perineum Muscle, Open Approach
0K8M3ZZ Division of Perineum Muscle, Percutaneous Approach
0K8M4ZZ Division of Perineum Muscle, Percutaneous Endoscopic Approach
0K8N0ZZ Division of Right Hip Muscle, Open Approach
0K8N3ZZ Division of Right Hip Muscle, Percutaneous Approach
0K8N4ZZ Division of Right Hip Muscle, Percutaneous Endoscopic Approach
0K8P0ZZ Division of Left Hip Muscle, Open Approach
0K8P3ZZ Division of Left Hip Muscle, Percutane[ous] Approach
0K8P4ZZ Division of Left Hip Muscle, Percutane[ous] Endoscopic Approach
0K8Q0ZZ Division of Right Upper Leg Muscle, Open Approach
0K8Q3ZZ Division of Right Upper Leg Muscle, Percutaneous Approach
0K8Q4ZZ Division of Right Upper Leg Muscle, Percutaneous Endoscopic Approach
0K8R0ZZ Division of Left Upper Leg Muscle, Op[en] Approach
0K8R3ZZ Division of Left Upper Leg Muscle, Percutaneous Approach
0K8R4ZZ Division of Left Upper Leg Muscle, Percutaneous Endoscopic Approach
0K8S0ZZ Division of Right Lower Leg Muscle, Open Approach
0K8S3ZZ Division of Right Lower Leg Muscle, Percutaneous Approach
0K8S4ZZ Division of Right Lower Leg Muscle, Percutaneous Endoscopic Approach
0K8T0ZZ Division of Left Lower Leg Muscle, Op[en] Approach
0K8T3ZZ Division of Left Lower Leg Muscle, Percutaneous Approach
0K8T4ZZ Division of Left Lower Leg Muscle, Percutaneous Endoscopic Approach
0K8V0ZZ Division of Right Foot Muscle, Open Approach
0K8V3ZZ Division of Right Foot Muscle, Percutaneous Approach
0K8V4ZZ Division of Right Foot Muscle, Percutaneous Endoscopic Approach
0K8W0ZZ Division of Left Foot Muscle, Open Approach
0K8W3ZZ Division of Left Foot Muscle, Percutaneous Approach
0K8W4ZZ Division of Left Foot Muscle, Percutaneous Endoscopic Approach

0K9 – Muscles, Drainage

Review Coding Guidelines B3.4a and B3.4b

Review Coding Guideline B6.2

0K9000Z Drainage of Head Muscle with Drainage Device, Open Approach
0K900ZX Drainage of Head Muscle, Open Approach, Diagnostic
0K900ZZ Drainage of Head Muscle, Open Approach
0K9030Z Drainage of Head Muscle with Drainage Device, Percutaneous Approach
0K903ZX Drainage of Head Muscle, Percutaneous Approach, Diagnostic
0K903ZZ Drainage of Head Muscle, Percutaneous Approach
0K9040Z Drainage of Head Muscle with Drainage Device, Percutaneous Endoscopic Approach
0K904ZX Drainage of Head Muscle, Percutaneous Endoscopic Approach, Diagnostic
0K904ZZ Drainage of Head Muscle, Percutaneous Endoscopic Approach
0K9100Z Drainage of Facial Muscle with Drainage Device, Open Approach
0K910ZX Drainage of Facial Muscle, Open Approach, Diagnostic
0K910ZZ Drainage of Facial Muscle, Open Approach
0K9130Z Drainage of Facial Muscle with Drainage Device, Percutaneous Approach
0K913ZX Drainage of Facial Muscle, Percutaneous Approach, Diagnostic
0K913ZZ Drainage of Facial Muscle, Percutaneous Approach
0K9140Z Drainage of Facial Muscle with Drainage Device, Percutaneous Endoscopic Approach
0K914ZX Drainage of Facial Muscle, Percutaneous Endoscopic Approach, Diagnostic
0K914ZZ Drainage of Facial Muscle, Percutaneous Endoscopic Approach
0K9200Z Drainage of Right Neck Muscle with Drainage Device, Open Approach
0K920ZX Drainage of Right Neck Muscle, Open Approach, Diagnostic
0K920ZZ Drainage of Right Neck Muscle, Open Approach
0K9230Z Drainage of Right Neck Muscle with Drainage Device, Percutaneous Approach
0K923ZX Drainage of Right Neck Muscle, Percutaneous Approach, Diagnostic
0K923ZZ Drainage of Right Neck Muscle, Percutaneous Approach
0K9240Z Drainage of Right Neck Muscle with Drainage Device, Percutaneous Endoscopic Approach
0K924ZX Drainage of Right Neck Muscle, Percutaneous Endoscopic Approach, Diagnostic
0K924ZZ Drainage of Right Neck Muscle, Percutaneous Endoscopic Approach
0K9300Z Drainage of Left Neck Muscle with Drainage Device, Open Approach
0K930ZX Drainage of Left Neck Muscle, Open Approach, Diagnostic
0K930ZZ Drainage of Left Neck Muscle, Open Approach
0K9330Z Drainage of Left Neck Muscle with Drainage Device, Percutaneous Approach
0K933ZX Drainage of Left Neck Muscle, Percutaneous Approach, Diagnostic
0K933ZZ Drainage of Left Neck Muscle, Percutaneous Approach
0K9340Z Drainage of Left Neck Muscle with Drainage Device, Percutaneous Endoscopic Approach
0K934ZX Drainage of Left Neck Muscle, Percutaneous Endoscopic Approach, Diagnostic
0K934ZZ Drainage of Left Neck Muscle, Percutaneous Endoscopic Approach
0K9400Z Drainage of Tongue, Palate, Pharynx Muscle with Drainage Device, Open Approach
0K940ZX Drainage of Tongue, Palate, Pharynx Muscle, Open Approach, Diagnostic

940ZZ Drainage of Tongue, Palate, Pharynx Muscle, Open Approach
9430Z Drainage of Tongue, Palate, Pharynx Muscle with Drainage Device, Percutaneous Approach
943ZX Drainage of Tongue, Palate, Pharynx Muscle, Percutaneous Approach, Diagnostic
943ZZ Drainage of Tongue, Palate, Pharynx Muscle, Percutaneous Approach
9440Z Drainage of Tongue, Palate, Pharynx Muscle with Drainage Device, Percutaneous Endoscopic Approach
944ZX Drainage of Tongue, Palate, Pharynx Muscle, Percutaneous Endoscopic Approach, Diagnostic
944ZZ Drainage of Tongue, Palate, Pharynx Muscle, Percutaneous Endoscopic Approach
9500Z Drainage of Right Shoulder Muscle with Drainage Device, Open Approach
950ZX Drainage of Right Shoulder Muscle, Open Approach, Diagnostic
950ZZ Drainage of Right Shoulder Muscle, Open Approach
9530Z Drainage of Right Shoulder Muscle with Drainage Device, Percutaneous Approach
953ZX Drainage of Right Shoulder Muscle, Percutaneous Approach, Diagnostic
953ZZ Drainage of Right Shoulder Muscle, Percutaneous Approach
9540Z Drainage of Right Shoulder Muscle with Drainage Device, Percutaneous Endoscopic Approach
K954ZX Drainage of Right Shoulder Muscle, Percutaneous Endoscopic Approach, Diagnostic
K954ZZ Drainage of Right Shoulder Muscle, Percutaneous Endoscopic Approach
K9600Z Drainage of Left Shoulder Muscle with Drainage Device, Open Approach
K960ZX Drainage of Left Shoulder Muscle, Open Approach, Diagnostic
K960ZZ Drainage of Left Shoulder Muscle, Open Approach
K9630Z Drainage of Left Shoulder Muscle with Drainage Device, Percutaneous Approach
K963ZX Drainage of Left Shoulder Muscle, Percutaneous Approach, Diagnostic
K963ZZ Drainage of Left Shoulder Muscle, Percutaneous Approach
K9640Z Drainage of Left Shoulder Muscle with Drainage Device, Percutaneous Endoscopic Approach
K964ZX Drainage of Left Shoulder Muscle, Percutaneous Endoscopic Approach, Diagnostic
K964ZZ Drainage of Left Shoulder Muscle, Percutaneous Endoscopic Approach
K9700Z Drainage of Right Upper Arm Muscle with Drainage Device, Open Approach
K970ZX Drainage of Right Upper Arm Muscle, Open Approach, Diagnostic
K970ZZ Drainage of Right Upper Arm Muscle, Open Approach
K9730Z Drainage of Right Upper Arm Muscle with Drainage Device, Percutaneous Approach
0K973ZX Drainage of Right Upper Arm Muscle, Percutaneous Approach, Diagnostic
0K973ZZ Drainage of Right Upper Arm Muscle, Percutaneous Approach
0K9740Z Drainage of Right Upper Arm Muscle with Drainage Device, Percutaneous Endoscopic Approach
0K974ZX Drainage of Right Upper Arm Muscle, Percutaneous Endoscopic Approach, Diagnostic
0K974ZZ Drainage of Right Upper Arm Muscle, Percutaneous Endoscopic Approach
0K9800Z Drainage of Left Upper Arm Muscle with Drainage Device, Open Approach
0K980ZX Drainage of Left Upper Arm Muscle, Open Approach, Diagnostic
0K980ZZ Drainage of Left Upper Arm Muscle, Open Approach
0K9830Z Drainage of Left Upper Arm Muscle with Drainage Device, Percutaneous Approach
0K983ZX Drainage of Left Upper Arm Muscle, Percutaneous Approach, Diagnostic
0K983ZZ Drainage of Left Upper Arm Muscle, Percutaneous Approach
0K9840Z Drainage of Left Upper Arm Muscle with Drainage Device, Percutaneous Endoscopic Approach
0K984ZX Drainage of Left Upper Arm Muscle, Percutaneous Endoscopic Approach, Diagnostic
0K984ZZ Drainage of Left Upper Arm Muscle, Percutaneous Endoscopic Approach
0K9900Z Drainage of Right Lower Arm and Wrist Muscle with Drainage Device, Open Approach
0K990ZX Drainage of Right Lower Arm and Wrist Muscle, Open Approach, Diagnostic
0K990ZZ Drainage of Right Lower Arm and Wrist Muscle, Open Approach
0K9930Z Drainage of Right Lower Arm and Wrist Muscle with Drainage Device, Percutaneous Approach
0K993ZX Drainage of Right Lower Arm and Wrist Muscle, Percutaneous Approach, Diagnostic
0K993ZZ Drainage of Right Lower Arm and Wrist Muscle, Percutaneous Approach
0K9940Z Drainage of Right Lower Arm and Wrist Muscle with Drainage Device, Percutaneous Endoscopic Approach
0K994ZX Drainage of Right Lower Arm and Wrist Muscle, Percutaneous Endoscopic Approach, Diagnostic
0K994ZZ Drainage of Right Lower Arm and Wrist Muscle, Percutaneous Endoscopic Approach
0K9B00Z Drainage of Left Lower Arm and Wrist Muscle with Drainage Device, Open Approach
0K9B0ZX Drainage of Left Lower Arm and Wrist Muscle, Open Approach, Diagnostic
0K9B0ZZ Drainage of Left Lower Arm and Wrist Muscle, Open Approach
0K9B30Z Drainage of Left Lower Arm and Wrist Muscle with Drainage Device, Percutaneous Approach
0K9B3ZX Drainage of Left Lower Arm and Wrist Muscle, Percutaneous Approach, Diagnostic
0K9B3ZZ Drainage of Left Lower Arm and Wrist Muscle, Percutaneous Approach
0K9B40Z Drainage of Left Lower Arm and Wrist Muscle with Drainage Device, Percutaneous Endoscopic Approach
0K9B4ZX Drainage of Left Lower Arm and Wrist Muscle, Percutaneous Endoscopic Approach, Diagnostic
0K9B4ZZ Drainage of Left Lower Arm and Wrist Muscle, Percutaneous Endoscopic Approach
0K9C00Z Drainage of Right Hand Muscle with Drainage Device, Open Approach
0K9C0ZX Drainage of Right Hand Muscle, Open Approach, Diagnostic
0K9C0ZZ Drainage of Right Hand Muscle, Open Approach
0K9C30Z Drainage of Right Hand Muscle with Drainage Device, Percutaneous Approach
0K9C3ZX Drainage of Right Hand Muscle, Percutaneous Approach, Diagnostic
0K9C3ZZ Drainage of Right Hand Muscle, Percutaneous Approach
0K9C40Z Drainage of Right Hand Muscle with Drainage Device, Percutaneous Endoscopic Approach
0K9C4ZX Drainage of Right Hand Muscle, Percutaneous Endoscopic Approach, Diagnostic
0K9C4ZZ Drainage of Right Hand Muscle, Percutaneous Endoscopic Approach
0K9D00Z Drainage of Left Hand Muscle with Drainage Device, Open Approach
0K9D0ZX Drainage of Left Hand Muscle, Open Approach, Diagnostic
0K9D0ZZ Drainage of Left Hand Muscle, Open Approach
0K9D30Z Drainage of Left Hand Muscle with Drainage Device, Percutaneous Approach
0K9D3ZX Drainage of Left Hand Muscle, Percutaneous Approach, Diagnostic
0K9D3ZZ Drainage of Left Hand Muscle, Percutaneous Approach
0K9D40Z Drainage of Left Hand Muscle with Drainage Device, Percutaneous Endoscopic Approach
0K9D4ZX Drainage of Left Hand Muscle, Percutaneous Endoscopic Approach, Diagnostic
0K9D4ZZ Drainage of Left Hand Muscle, Percutaneous Endoscopic Approach
0K9F00Z Drainage of Right Trunk Muscle with Drainage Device, Open Approach
0K9F0ZX Drainage of Right Trunk Muscle, Open Approach, Diagnostic
0K9F0ZZ Drainage of Right Trunk Muscle, Open Approach
0K9F30Z Drainage of Right Trunk Muscle with Drainage Device, Percutaneous Approach
0K9F3ZX Drainage of Right Trunk Muscle, Percutaneous Approach, Diagnostic
0K9F3ZZ Drainage of Right Trunk Muscle, Percutaneous Approach
0K9F40Z Drainage of Right Trunk Muscle with Drainage Device, Percutaneous Endoscopic Approach
0K9F4ZX Drainage of Right Trunk Muscle, Percutaneous Endoscopic Approach, Diagnostic
0K9F4ZZ Drainage of Right Trunk Muscle, Percutaneous Endoscopic Approach
0K9G00Z Drainage of Left Trunk Muscle with Drainage Device, Open Approach
0K9G0ZX Drainage of Left Trunk Muscle, Open Approach, Diagnostic
0K9G0ZZ Drainage of Left Trunk Muscle, Open Approach
0K9G30Z Drainage of Left Trunk Muscle with Drainage Device, Percutaneous Approach
0K9G3ZX Drainage of Left Trunk Muscle, Percutaneous Approach, Diagnostic
0K9G3ZZ Drainage of Left Trunk Muscle, Percutaneous Approach
0K9G40Z Drainage of Left Trunk Muscle with Drainage Device, Percutaneous Endoscopic Approach
0K9G4ZX Drainage of Left Trunk Muscle, Percutaneous Endoscopic Approach, Diagnostic

0K9G4ZZ Drainage of Left Trunk Muscle, Percutaneous Endoscopic Approach
0K9H00Z Drainage of Right Thorax Muscle with Drainage Device, Open Approach
0K9H0ZX Drainage of Right Thorax Muscle, Open Approach, Diagnostic
0K9H0ZZ Drainage of Right Thorax Muscle, Open Approach
0K9H30Z Drainage of Right Thorax Muscle with Drainage Device, Percutaneous Approach
0K9H3ZX Drainage of Right Thorax Muscle, Percutaneous Approach, Diagnostic
0K9H3ZZ Drainage of Right Thorax Muscle, Percutaneous Approach
0K9H40Z Drainage of Right Thorax Muscle with Drainage Device, Percutaneous Endoscopic Approach
0K9H4ZX Drainage of Right Thorax Muscle, Percutaneous Endoscopic Approach, Diagnostic
0K9H4ZZ Drainage of Right Thorax Muscle, Percutaneous Endoscopic Approach
0K9J00Z Drainage of Left Thorax Muscle with Drainage Device, Open Approach
0K9J0ZX Drainage of Left Thorax Muscle, Open Approach, Diagnostic
0K9J0ZZ Drainage of Left Thorax Muscle, Open Approach
0K9J30Z Drainage of Left Thorax Muscle with Drainage Device, Percutaneous Approach
0K9J3ZX Drainage of Left Thorax Muscle, Percutaneous Approach, Diagnostic
0K9J3ZZ Drainage of Left Thorax Muscle, Percutaneous Approach
0K9J40Z Drainage of Left Thorax Muscle with Drainage Device, Percutaneous Endoscopic Approach
0K9J4ZX Drainage of Left Thorax Muscle, Percutaneous Endoscopic Approach, Diagnostic
0K9J4ZZ Drainage of Left Thorax Muscle, Percutaneous Endoscopic Approach
0K9K00Z Drainage of Right Abdomen Muscle with Drainage Device, Open Approach
0K9K0ZX Drainage of Right Abdomen Muscle, Open Approach, Diagnostic
0K9K0ZZ Drainage of Right Abdomen Muscle, Open Approach
0K9K30Z Drainage of Right Abdomen Muscle with Drainage Device, Percutaneous Approach
0K9K3ZX Drainage of Right Abdomen Muscle, Percutaneous Approach, Diagnostic
0K9K3ZZ Drainage of Right Abdomen Muscle, Percutaneous Approach
0K9K40Z Drainage of Right Abdomen Muscle with Drainage Device, Percutaneous Endoscopic Approach
0K9K4ZX Drainage of Right Abdomen Muscle, Percutaneous Endoscopic Approach, Diagnostic
0K9K4ZZ Drainage of Right Abdomen Muscle, Percutaneous Endoscopic Approach
0K9L00Z Drainage of Left Abdomen Muscle with Drainage Device, Open Approach
0K9L0ZX Drainage of Left Abdomen Muscle, Open Approach, Diagnostic
0K9L0ZZ Drainage of Left Abdomen Muscle, Open Approach
0K9L30Z Drainage of Left Abdomen Muscle with Drainage Device, Percutaneous Approach
0K9L3ZX Drainage of Left Abdomen Muscle, Percutaneous Approach, Diagnostic
0K9L3ZZ Drainage of Left Abdomen Muscle, Percutaneous Approach
0K9L40Z Drainage of Left Abdomen Muscle with Drainage Device, Percutaneous Endoscopic Approach
0K9L4ZX Drainage of Left Abdomen Muscle, Percutaneous Endoscopic Approach, Diagnostic
0K9L4ZZ Drainage of Left Abdomen Muscle, Percutaneous Endoscopic Approach
0K9M00Z Drainage of Perineum Muscle with Drainage Device, Open Approach
0K9M0ZX Drainage of Perineum Muscle, Open Approach, Diagnostic
0K9M0ZZ Drainage of Perineum Muscle, Open Approach
0K9M30Z Drainage of Perineum Muscle with Drainage Device, Percutaneous Approach
0K9M3ZX Drainage of Perineum Muscle, Percutaneous Approach, Diagnostic
0K9M3ZZ Drainage of Perineum Muscle, Percutaneous Approach
0K9M40Z Drainage of Perineum Muscle with Drainage Device, Percutaneous Endoscopic Approach
0K9M4ZX Drainage of Perineum Muscle, Percutaneous Endoscopic Approach, Diagnostic
0K9M4ZZ Drainage of Perineum Muscle, Percutaneous Endoscopic Approach
0K9N00Z Drainage of Right Hip Muscle with Drainage Device, Open Approach
0K9N0ZX Drainage of Right Hip Muscle, Open Approach, Diagnostic
0K9N0ZZ Drainage of Right Hip Muscle, Open Approach
0K9N30Z Drainage of Right Hip Muscle with Drainage Device, Percutaneous Approach
0K9N3ZX Drainage of Right Hip Muscle, Percutaneous Approach, Diagnostic
0K9N3ZZ Drainage of Right Hip Muscle, Percutaneous Approach
0K9N40Z Drainage of Right Hip Muscle with Drainage Device, Percutaneous Endoscopic Approach
0K9N4ZX Drainage of Right Hip Muscle, Percutaneous Endoscopic Approach, Diagnostic
0K9N4ZZ Drainage of Right Hip Muscle, Percutaneous Endoscopic Approach
0K9P00Z Drainage of Left Hip Muscle with Drainage Device, Open Approach
0K9P0ZX Drainage of Left Hip Muscle, Open Approach, Diagnostic
0K9P0ZZ Drainage of Left Hip Muscle, Open Approach
0K9P30Z Drainage of Left Hip Muscle with Drainage Device, Percutaneous Approach
0K9P3ZX Drainage of Left Hip Muscle, Percutaneous Approach, Diagnostic
0K9P3ZZ Drainage of Left Hip Muscle, Percutaneous Approach
0K9P40Z Drainage of Left Hip Muscle with Drainage Device, Percutaneous Endoscopic Approach
0K9P4ZX Drainage of Left Hip Muscle, Percutaneous Endoscopic Approach, Diagnostic
0K9P4ZZ Drainage of Left Hip Muscle, Percutaneous Endoscopic Approach
0K9Q00Z Drainage of Right Upper Leg Muscle with Drainage Device, Open Approach
0K9Q0ZX Drainage of Right Upper Leg Muscle, Open Approach, Diagnostic
0K9Q0ZZ Drainage of Right Upper Leg Muscle, Open Approach
0K9Q30Z Drainage of Right Upper Leg Muscle with Drainage Device, Percutaneous Approach
0K9Q3ZX Drainage of Right Upper Leg Muscle, Percutaneous Approach, Diagnostic
0K9Q3ZZ Drainage of Right Upper Leg Muscle, Percutaneous Approach
0K9Q40Z Drainage of Right Upper Leg Muscle with Drainage Device, Percutaneous Endoscopic Approach
0K9Q4ZX Drainage of Right Upper Leg Muscle, Percutaneous Endoscopic Approach, Diagnostic
0K9Q4ZZ Drainage of Right Upper Leg Muscle, Percutaneous Endoscopic Approach
0K9R00Z Drainage of Left Upper Leg Muscle with Drainage Device, Open Approach
0K9R0ZX Drainage of Left Upper Leg Muscle, Open Approach, Diagnostic
0K9R0ZZ Drainage of Left Upper Leg Muscle, Open Approach
0K9R30Z Drainage of Left Upper Leg Muscle with Drainage Device, Percutaneous Approach
0K9R3ZX Drainage of Left Upper Leg Muscle, Percutaneous Approach, Diagnostic
0K9R3ZZ Drainage of Left Upper Leg Muscle, Percutaneous Approach
0K9R40Z Drainage of Left Upper Leg Muscle with Drainage Device, Percutaneous Endoscopic Approach
0K9R4ZX Drainage of Left Upper Leg Muscle, Percutaneous Endoscopic Approach, Diagnostic
0K9R4ZZ Drainage of Left Upper Leg Muscle, Percutaneous Endoscopic Approach
0K9S00Z Drainage of Right Lower Leg Muscle with Drainage Device, Open Approach
0K9S0ZX Drainage of Right Lower Leg Muscle, Open Approach, Diagnostic
0K9S0ZZ Drainage of Right Lower Leg Muscle, Open Approach
0K9S30Z Drainage of Right Lower Leg Muscle with Drainage Device, Percutaneous Approach
0K9S3ZX Drainage of Right Lower Leg Muscle, Percutaneous Approach, Diagnostic
0K9S3ZZ Drainage of Right Lower Leg Muscle, Percutaneous Approach
0K9S40Z Drainage of Right Lower Leg Muscle with Drainage Device, Percutaneous Endoscopic Approach
0K9S4ZX Drainage of Right Lower Leg Muscle, Percutaneous Endoscopic Approach, Diagnostic
0K9S4ZZ Drainage of Right Lower Leg Muscle, Percutaneous Endoscopic Approach
0K9T00Z Drainage of Left Lower Leg Muscle with Drainage Device, Open Approach
0K9T0ZX Drainage of Left Lower Leg Muscle, Open Approach, Diagnostic
0K9T0ZZ Drainage of Left Lower Leg Muscle, Open Approach
0K9T30Z Drainage of Left Lower Leg Muscle with Drainage Device, Percutaneous Approach
0K9T3ZX Drainage of Left Lower Leg Muscle, Percutaneous Approach, Diagnostic
0K9T3ZZ Drainage of Left Lower Leg Muscle, Percutaneous Approach
0K9T40Z Drainage of Left Lower Leg Muscle with Drainage Device, Percutaneous Endoscopic Approach
0K9T4ZX Drainage of Left Lower Leg Muscle, Percutaneous Endoscopic Approach, Diagnostic

9T4ZZ Drainage of Left Lower Leg Muscle, Percutaneous Endoscopic Approach
9V00Z Drainage of Right Foot Muscle with Drainage Device, Open Approach
9V0ZX Drainage of Right Foot Muscle, Open Approach, Diagnostic
9V0ZZ Drainage of Right Foot Muscle, Open Approach
9V30Z Drainage of Right Foot Muscle with Drainage Device, Percutaneous Approach
9V3ZX Drainage of Right Foot Muscle, Percutaneous Approach, Diagnostic
9V3ZZ Drainage of Right Foot Muscle, Percutaneous Approach
0K9V40Z Drainage of Right Foot Muscle with Drainage Device, Percutaneous Endoscopic Approach
0K9V4ZX Drainage of Right Foot Muscle, Percutaneous Endoscopic Approach, Diagnostic
0K9V4ZZ Drainage of Right Foot Muscle, Percutaneous Endoscopic Approach
0K9W00Z Drainage of Left Foot Muscle with Drainage Device, Open Approach
0K9W0ZX Drainage of Left Foot Muscle, Open Approach, Diagnostic
0K9W0ZZ Drainage of Left Foot Muscle, Open Approach
0K9W30Z Drainage of Left Foot Muscle with Drainage Device, Percutaneous Approach
0K9W3ZX Drainage of Left Foot Muscle, Percutaneous Approach, Diagnostic
0K9W3ZZ Drainage of Left Foot Muscle, Percutaneous Approach
0K9W40Z Drainage of Left Foot Muscle with Drainage Device, Percutaneous Endoscopic Approach
0K9W4ZX Drainage of Left Foot Muscle, Percutaneous Endoscopic Approach, Diagnostic
0K9W4ZZ Drainage of Left Foot Muscle, Percutaneous Endoscopic Approach

KB – Muscles, Excision

view Coding Guidelines B3.4a and B3.4b

view Coding Guideline B3.5

view Coding Guideline B3.8

B00ZX Excision of Head Muscle, Open Approach, Diagnostic
B00ZZ Excision of Head Muscle, Open Approach
B03ZX Excision of Head Muscle, Percutaneous Approach, Diagnostic
B03ZZ Excision of Head Muscle, Percutaneous Approach
KB04ZX Excision of Head Muscle, Percutaneous Endoscopic Approach, Diagnostic
KB04ZZ Excision of Head Muscle, Percutaneous Endoscopic Approach
KB10ZX Excision of Facial Muscle, Open Approach, Diagnostic
KB10ZZ Excision of Facial Muscle, Open Approach
KB13ZX Excision of Facial Muscle, Percutaneous Approach, Diagnostic
KB13ZZ Excision of Facial Muscle, Percutaneous Approach
KB14ZX Excision of Facial Muscle, Percutaneous Endoscopic Approach, Diagnostic
KB14ZZ Excision of Facial Muscle, Percutaneous Endoscopic Approach
KB20ZX Excision of Right Neck Muscle, Open Approach, Diagnostic
KB20ZZ Excision of Right Neck Muscle, Open Approach
KB23ZX Excision of Right Neck Muscle, Percutaneous Approach, Diagnostic
KB23ZZ Excision of Right Neck Muscle, Percutaneous Approach
KB24ZX Excision of Right Neck Muscle, Percutaneous Endoscopic Approach, Diagnostic
KB24ZZ Excision of Right Neck Muscle, Percutaneous Endoscopic Approach
KB30ZX Excision of Left Neck Muscle, Open Approach, Diagnostic
KB30ZZ Excision of Left Neck Muscle, Open Approach
KB33ZX Excision of Left Neck Muscle, Percutaneous Approach, Diagnostic
KB33ZZ Excision of Left Neck Muscle, Percutaneous Approach
KB34ZX Excision of Left Neck Muscle, Percutaneous Endoscopic Approach, Diagnostic
KB34ZZ Excision of Left Neck Muscle, Percutaneous Endoscopic Approach
KB40ZX Excision of Tongue, Palate, Pharynx Muscle, Open Approach, Diagnostic
0KB40ZZ Excision of Tongue, Palate, Pharynx Muscle, Open Approach
0KB43ZX Excision of Tongue, Palate, Pharynx Muscle, Percutaneous Approach, Diagnostic
0KB43ZZ Excision of Tongue, Palate, Pharynx Muscle, Percutaneous Approach
0KB44ZX Excision of Tongue, Palate, Pharynx Muscle, Percutaneous Endoscopic Approach, Diagnostic
0KB44ZZ Excision of Tongue, Palate, Pharynx Muscle, Percutaneous Endoscopic Approach
0KB50ZX Excision of Right Shoulder Muscle, Open Approach, Diagnostic
0KB50ZZ Excision of Right Shoulder Muscle, Open Approach
0KB53ZX Excision of Right Shoulder Muscle, Percutaneous Approach, Diagnostic
0KB53ZZ Excision of Right Shoulder Muscle, Percutaneous Approach
0KB54ZX Excision of Right Shoulder Muscle, Percutaneous Endoscopic Approach, Diagnostic
0KB54ZZ Excision of Right Shoulder Muscle, Percutaneous Endoscopic Approach
0KB60ZX Excision of Left Shoulder Muscle, Open Approach, Diagnostic
0KB60ZZ Excision of Left Shoulder Muscle, Open Approach
0KB63ZX Excision of Left Shoulder Muscle, Percutaneous Approach, Diagnostic
0KB63ZZ Excision of Left Shoulder Muscle, Percutaneous Approach
0KB64ZX Excision of Left Shoulder Muscle, Percutaneous Endoscopic Approach, Diagnostic
0KB64ZZ Excision of Left Shoulder Muscle, Percutaneous Endoscopic Approach
0KB70ZX Excision of Right Upper Arm Muscle, Open Approach, Diagnostic
0KB70ZZ Excision of Right Upper Arm Muscle, Open Approach
0KB73ZX Excision of Right Upper Arm Muscle, Percutaneous Approach, Diagnostic
0KB73ZZ Excision of Right Upper Arm Muscle, Percutaneous Approach
0KB74ZX Excision of Right Upper Arm Muscle, Percutaneous Endoscopic Approach, Diagnostic
0KB74ZZ Excision of Right Upper Arm Muscle, Percutaneous Endoscopic Approach
0KB80ZX Excision of Left Upper Arm Muscle, Open Approach, Diagnostic
0KB80ZZ Excision of Left Upper Arm Muscle, Open Approach
0KB83ZX Excision of Left Upper Arm Muscle, Percutaneous Approach, Diagnostic
0KB83ZZ Excision of Left Upper Arm Muscle, Percutaneous Approach
0KB84ZX Excision of Left Upper Arm Muscle, Percutaneous Endoscopic Approach, Diagnostic
0KB84ZZ Excision of Left Upper Arm Muscle, Percutaneous Endoscopic Approach
0KB90ZX Excision of Right Lower Arm and Wrist Muscle, Open Approach, Diagnostic
0KB90ZZ Excision of Right Lower Arm and Wrist Muscle, Open Approach
0KB93ZX Excision of Right Lower Arm and Wrist Muscle, Percutaneous Approach, Diagnostic
0KB93ZZ Excision of Right Lower Arm and Wrist Muscle, Percutaneous Approach
0KB94ZX Excision of Right Lower Arm and Wrist Muscle, Percutaneous Endoscopic Approach, Diagnostic
0KB94ZZ Excision of Right Lower Arm and Wrist Muscle, Percutaneous Endoscopic Approach
0KBB0ZX Excision of Left Lower Arm and Wrist Muscle, Open Approach, Diagnostic
0KBB0ZZ Excision of Left Lower Arm and Wrist Muscle, Open Approach
0KBB3ZX Excision of Left Lower Arm and Wrist Muscle, Percutaneous Approach, Diagnostic
0KBB3ZZ Excision of Left Lower Arm and Wrist Muscle, Percutaneous Approach
0KBB4ZX Excision of Left Lower Arm and Wrist Muscle, Percutaneous Endoscopic Approach, Diagnostic
0KBB4ZZ Excision of Left Lower Arm and Wrist Muscle, Percutaneous Endoscopic Approach
0KBC0ZX Excision of Right Hand Muscle, Open Approach, Diagnostic
0KBC0ZZ Excision of Right Hand Muscle, Open Approach
0KBC3ZX Excision of Right Hand Muscle, Percutaneous Approach, Diagnostic
0KBC3ZZ Excision of Right Hand Muscle, Percutaneous Approach

0KBC4ZX Excision of Right Hand Muscle, Percutaneous Endoscopic Approach, Diagnostic
0KBC4ZZ Excision of Right Hand Muscle, Percutaneous Endoscopic Approach
0KBD0ZX Excision of Left Hand Muscle, Open Approach, Diagnostic
0KBD0ZZ Excision of Left Hand Muscle, Open Approach
0KBD3ZX Excision of Left Hand Muscle, Percutaneous Approach, Diagnostic
0KBD3ZZ Excision of Left Hand Muscle, Percutaneous Approach
0KBD4ZX Excision of Left Hand Muscle, Percutaneous Endoscopic Approach, Diagnostic
0KBD4ZZ Excision of Left Hand Muscle, Percutaneous Endoscopic Approach
0KBF0ZX Excision of Right Trunk Muscle, Open Approach, Diagnostic
0KBF0ZZ Excision of Right Trunk Muscle, Open Approach
0KBF3ZX Excision of Right Trunk Muscle, Percutaneous Approach, Diagnostic
0KBF3ZZ Excision of Right Trunk Muscle, Percutaneous Approach
0KBF4ZX Excision of Right Trunk Muscle, Percutaneous Endoscopic Approach, Diagnostic
0KBF4ZZ Excision of Right Trunk Muscle, Percutaneous Endoscopic Approach
0KBG0ZX Excision of Left Trunk Muscle, Open Approach, Diagnostic
0KBG0ZZ Excision of Left Trunk Muscle, Open Approach
0KBG3ZX Excision of Left Trunk Muscle, Percutaneous Approach, Diagnostic
0KBG3ZZ Excision of Left Trunk Muscle, Percutaneous Approach
0KBG4ZX Excision of Left Trunk Muscle, Percutaneous Endoscopic Approach, Diagnostic
0KBG4ZZ Excision of Left Trunk Muscle, Percutaneous Endoscopic Approach
0KBH0ZX Excision of Right Thorax Muscle, Open Approach, Diagnostic
0KBH0ZZ Excision of Right Thorax Muscle, Open Approach
0KBH3ZX Excision of Right Thorax Muscle, Percutaneous Approach, Diagnostic
0KBH3ZZ Excision of Right Thorax Muscle, Percutaneous Approach
0KBH4ZX Excision of Right Thorax Muscle, Percutaneous Endoscopic Approach, Diagnostic
0KBH4ZZ Excision of Right Thorax Muscle, Percutaneous Endoscopic Approach
0KBJ0ZX Excision of Left Thorax Muscle, Open Approach, Diagnostic
0KBJ0ZZ Excision of Left Thorax Muscle, Open Approach
0KBJ3ZX Excision of Left Thorax Muscle, Percutaneous Approach, Diagnostic
0KBJ3ZZ Excision of Left Thorax Muscle, Percutaneous Approach
0KBJ4ZX Excision of Left Thorax Muscle, Percutaneous Endoscopic Approach, Diagnostic
0KBJ4ZZ Excision of Left Thorax Muscle, Percutaneous Endoscopic Approach
0KBK0ZX Excision of Right Abdomen Muscle, Open Approach, Diagnostic
0KBK0ZZ Excision of Right Abdomen Muscle, Open Approach
0KBK3ZX Excision of Right Abdomen Muscle, Percutaneous Approach, Diagnostic
0KBK3ZZ Excision of Right Abdomen Muscle, Percutaneous Approach
0KBK4ZX Excision of Right Abdomen Muscle, Percutaneous Endoscopic Approach, Diagnostic
0KBK4ZZ Excision of Right Abdomen Muscle, Percutaneous Endoscopic Approach
0KBL0ZX Excision of Left Abdomen Muscle, Open Approach, Diagnostic
0KBL0ZZ Excision of Left Abdomen Muscle, Open Approach
0KBL3ZX Excision of Left Abdomen Muscle, Percutaneous Approach, Diagnostic
0KBL3ZZ Excision of Left Abdomen Muscle, Percutaneous Approach
0KBL4ZX Excision of Left Abdomen Muscle, Percutaneous Endoscopic Approach, Diagnostic
0KBL4ZZ Excision of Left Abdomen Muscle, Percutaneous Endoscopic Approach
0KBM0ZX Excision of Perineum Muscle, Open Approach, Diagnostic
0KBM0ZZ Excision of Perineum Muscle, Open Approach
0KBM3ZX Excision of Perineum Muscle, Percutaneous Approach, Diagnostic
0KBM3ZZ Excision of Perineum Muscle, Percutaneous Approach
0KBM4ZX Excision of Perineum Muscle, Percutaneous Endoscopic Approach, Diagnostic
0KBM4ZZ Excision of Perineum Muscle, Percutaneous Endoscopic Approach
0KBN0ZX Excision of Right Hip Muscle, Open Approach, Diagnostic
0KBN0ZZ Excision of Right Hip Muscle, Open Approach
0KBN3ZX Excision of Right Hip Muscle, Percutaneous Approach, Diagnostic
0KBN3ZZ Excision of Right Hip Muscle, Percutaneous Approach
0KBN4ZX Excision of Right Hip Muscle, Percutaneous Endoscopic Approach, Diagnostic
0KBN4ZZ Excision of Right Hip Muscle, Percutaneous Endoscopic Approach
0KBP0ZX Excision of Left Hip Muscle, Open Approach, Diagnostic
0KBP0ZZ Excision of Left Hip Muscle, Open Approach
0KBP3ZX Excision of Left Hip Muscle, Percutaneous Approach, Diagnostic
0KBP3ZZ Excision of Left Hip Muscle, Percutaneous Approach
0KBP4ZX Excision of Left Hip Muscle, Percutaneous Endoscopic Approach, Diagnostic
0KBP4ZZ Excision of Left Hip Muscle, Percutaneous Endoscopic Approach
0KBQ0ZX Excision of Right Upper Leg Muscle, Open Approach, Diagnostic
0KBQ0ZZ Excision of Right Upper Leg Muscle, Open Approach
0KBQ3ZX Excision of Right Upper Leg Muscle, Percutaneous Approach, Diagnostic
0KBQ3ZZ Excision of Right Upper Leg Muscle, Percutaneous Approach
0KBQ4ZX Excision of Right Upper Leg Muscle, Percutaneous Endoscopic Approach, Diagnostic
0KBQ4ZZ Excision of Right Upper Leg Muscle, Percutaneous Endoscopic Approach
0KBR0ZX Excision of Left Upper Leg Muscle, O Approach, Diagnostic
0KBR0ZZ Excision of Left Upper Leg Muscle, O Approach
0KBR3ZX Excision of Left Upper Leg Muscle, Percutaneous Approach, Diagnostic
0KBR3ZZ Excision of Left Upper Leg Muscle, Percutaneous Approach
0KBR4ZX Excision of Left Upper Leg Muscle, Percutaneous Endoscopic Approach, Diagnostic
0KBR4ZZ Excision of Left Upper Leg Muscle, Percutaneous Endoscopic Approach
0KBS0ZX Excision of Right Lower Leg Muscle, Open Approach, Diagnostic
0KBS0ZZ Excision of Right Lower Leg Muscle, Open Approach
0KBS3ZX Excision of Right Lower Leg Muscle, Percutaneous Approach, Diagnostic
0KBS3ZZ Excision of Right Lower Leg Muscle, Percutaneous Approach
0KBS4ZX Excision of Right Lower Leg Muscle, Percutaneous Endoscopic Approach, Diagnostic
0KBS4ZZ Excision of Right Lower Leg Muscle, Percutaneous Endoscopic Approach
0KBT0ZX Excision of Left Lower Leg Muscle, Op Approach, Diagnostic
0KBT0ZZ Excision of Left Lower Leg Muscle, Op Approach
0KBT3ZX Excision of Left Lower Leg Muscle, Percutaneous Approach, Diagnostic
0KBT3ZZ Excision of Left Lower Leg Muscle, Percutaneous Approach
0KBT4ZX Excision of Left Lower Leg Muscle, Percutaneous Endoscopic Approach, Diagnostic
0KBT4ZZ Excision of Left Lower Leg Muscle, Percutaneous Endoscopic Approach
0KBV0ZX Excision of Right Foot Muscle, Open Approach, Diagnostic
0KBV0ZZ Excision of Right Foot Muscle, Open Approach
0KBV3ZX Excision of Right Foot Muscle, Percutaneous Approach, Diagnostic
0KBV3ZZ Excision of Right Foot Muscle, Percutaneous Approach
0KBV4ZX Excision of Right Foot Muscle, Percutaneous Endoscopic Approach, Diagnostic
0KBV4ZZ Excision of Right Foot Muscle, Percutaneous Endoscopic Approach
0KBW0ZX Excision of Left Foot Muscle, Open Approach, Diagnostic
0KBW0ZZ Excision of Left Foot Muscle, Open Approach
0KBW3ZX Excision of Left Foot Muscle, Percutaneous Approach, Diagnostic
0KBW3ZZ Excision of Left Foot Muscle, Percutaneous Approach
0KBW4ZX Excision of Left Foot Muscle, Percutaneous Endoscopic Approach, Diagnostic
0KBW4ZZ Excision of Left Foot Muscle, Percutaneous Endoscopic Approach

0KC – Muscles, Extirpation

0KC00ZZ Extirpation of Matter from Head Muscle, Open Approach
0KC03ZZ Extirpation of Matter from Head Muscle, Percutaneous Approach
0KC04ZZ Extirpation of Matter from Head Muscle, Percutaneous Endoscopic Approach

C10ZZ Extirpation of Matter from Facial Muscle, Open Approach

C13ZZ Extirpation of Matter from Facial Muscle, Percutaneous Approach

C14ZZ Extirpation of Matter from Facial Muscle, Percutaneous Endoscopic Approach

C20ZZ Extirpation of Matter from Right Neck Muscle, Open Approach

C23ZZ Extirpation of Matter from Right Neck Muscle, Percutaneous Approach

C24ZZ Extirpation of Matter from Right Neck Muscle, Percutaneous Endoscopic Approach

C30ZZ Extirpation of Matter from Left Neck Muscle, Open Approach

C33ZZ Extirpation of Matter from Left Neck Muscle, Percutaneous Approach

C34ZZ Extirpation of Matter from Left Neck Muscle, Percutaneous Endoscopic Approach

C40ZZ Extirpation of Matter from Tongue, Palate, Pharynx Muscle, Open Approach

C43ZZ Extirpation of Matter from Tongue, Palate, Pharynx Muscle, Percutaneous Approach

C44ZZ Extirpation of Matter from Tongue, Palate, Pharynx Muscle, Percutaneous Endoscopic Approach

C50ZZ Extirpation of Matter from Right Shoulder Muscle, Open Approach

C53ZZ Extirpation of Matter from Right Shoulder Muscle, Percutaneous Approach

C54ZZ Extirpation of Matter from Right Shoulder Muscle, Percutaneous Endoscopic Approach

C60ZZ Extirpation of Matter from Left Shoulder Muscle, Open Approach

C63ZZ Extirpation of Matter from Left Shoulder Muscle, Percutaneous Approach

C64ZZ Extirpation of Matter from Left Shoulder Muscle, Percutaneous Endoscopic Approach

C70ZZ Extirpation of Matter from Right Upper Arm Muscle, Open Approach

C73ZZ Extirpation of Matter from Right Upper Arm Muscle, Percutaneous Approach

KC74ZZ Extirpation of Matter from Right Upper Arm Muscle, Percutaneous Endoscopic Approach

KC80ZZ Extirpation of Matter from Left Upper Arm Muscle, Open Approach

KC83ZZ Extirpation of Matter from Left Upper Arm Muscle, Percutaneous Approach

KC84ZZ Extirpation of Matter from Left Upper Arm Muscle, Percutaneous Endoscopic Approach

KC90ZZ Extirpation of Matter from Right Lower Arm and Wrist Muscle, Open Approach

KC93ZZ Extirpation of Matter from Right Lower Arm and Wrist Muscle, Percutaneous Approach

0KC94ZZ Extirpation of Matter from Right Lower Arm and Wrist Muscle, Percutaneous Endoscopic Approach

0KCB0ZZ Extirpation of Matter from Left Lower Arm and Wrist Muscle, Open Approach

0KCB3ZZ Extirpation of Matter from Left Lower Arm and Wrist Muscle, Percutaneous Approach

0KCB4ZZ Extirpation of Matter from Left Lower Arm and Wrist Muscle, Percutaneous Endoscopic Approach

0KCC0ZZ Extirpation of Matter from Right Hand Muscle, Open Approach

0KCC3ZZ Extirpation of Matter from Right Hand Muscle, Percutaneous Approach

0KCC4ZZ Extirpation of Matter from Right Hand Muscle, Percutaneous Endoscopic Approach

0KCD0ZZ Extirpation of Matter from Left Hand Muscle, Open Approach

0KCD3ZZ Extirpation of Matter from Left Hand Muscle, Percutaneous Approach

0KCD4ZZ Extirpation of Matter from Left Hand Muscle, Percutaneous Endoscopic Approach

0KCF0ZZ Extirpation of Matter from Right Trunk Muscle, Open Approach

0KCF3ZZ Extirpation of Matter from Right Trunk Muscle, Percutaneous Approach

0KCF4ZZ Extirpation of Matter from Right Trunk Muscle, Percutaneous Endoscopic Approach

0KCG0ZZ Extirpation of Matter from Left Trunk Muscle, Open Approach

0KCG3ZZ Extirpation of Matter from Left Trunk Muscle, Percutaneous Approach

0KCG4ZZ Extirpation of Matter from Left Trunk Muscle, Percutaneous Endoscopic Approach

0KCH0ZZ Extirpation of Matter from Right Thorax Muscle, Open Approach

0KCH3ZZ Extirpation of Matter from Right Thorax Muscle, Percutaneous Approach

0KCH4ZZ Extirpation of Matter from Right Thorax Muscle, Percutaneous Endoscopic Approach

0KCJ0ZZ Extirpation of Matter from Left Thorax Muscle, Open Approach

0KCJ3ZZ Extirpation of Matter from Left Thorax Muscle, Percutaneous Approach

0KCJ4ZZ Extirpation of Matter from Left Thorax Muscle, Percutaneous Endoscopic Approach

0KCK0ZZ Extirpation of Matter from Right Abdomen Muscle, Open Approach

0KCK3ZZ Extirpation of Matter from Right Abdomen Muscle, Percutaneous Approach

0KCK4ZZ Extirpation of Matter from Right Abdomen Muscle, Percutaneous Endoscopic Approach

0KCL0ZZ Extirpation of Matter from Left Abdomen Muscle, Open Approach

0KCL3ZZ Extirpation of Matter from Left Abdomen Muscle, Percutaneous Approach

0KCL4ZZ Extirpation of Matter from Left Abdomen Muscle, Percutaneous Endoscopic Approach

0KCM0ZZ Extirpation of Matter from Perineum Muscle, Open Approach

0KCM3ZZ Extirpation of Matter from Perineum Muscle, Percutaneous Approach

0KCM4ZZ Extirpation of Matter from Perineum Muscle, Percutaneous Endoscopic Approach

0KCN0ZZ Extirpation of Matter from Right Hip Muscle, Open Approach

0KCN3ZZ Extirpation of Matter from Right Hip Muscle, Percutaneous Approach

0KCN4ZZ Extirpation of Matter from Right Hip Muscle, Percutaneous Endoscopic Approach

0KCP0ZZ Extirpation of Matter from Left Hip Muscle, Open Approach

0KCP3ZZ Extirpation of Matter from Left Hip Muscle, Percutaneous Approach

0KCP4ZZ Extirpation of Matter from Left Hip Muscle, Percutaneous Endoscopic Approach

0KCQ0ZZ Extirpation of Matter from Right Upper Leg Muscle, Open Approach

0KCQ3ZZ Extirpation of Matter from Right Upper Leg Muscle, Percutaneous Approach

0KCQ4ZZ Extirpation of Matter from Right Upper Leg Muscle, Percutaneous Endoscopic Approach

0KCR0ZZ Extirpation of Matter from Left Upper Leg Muscle, Open Approach

0KCR3ZZ Extirpation of Matter from Left Upper Leg Muscle, Percutaneous Approach

0KCR4ZZ Extirpation of Matter from Left Upper Leg Muscle, Percutaneous Endoscopic Approach

0KCS0ZZ Extirpation of Matter from Right Lower Leg Muscle, Open Approach

0KCS3ZZ Extirpation of Matter from Right Lower Leg Muscle, Percutaneous Approach

0KCS4ZZ Extirpation of Matter from Right Lower Leg Muscle, Percutaneous Endoscopic Approach

0KCT0ZZ Extirpation of Matter from Left Lower Leg Muscle, Open Approach

0KCT3ZZ Extirpation of Matter from Left Lower Leg Muscle, Percutaneous Approach

0KCT4ZZ Extirpation of Matter from Left Lower Leg Muscle, Percutaneous Endoscopic Approach

0KCV0ZZ Extirpation of Matter from Right Foot Muscle, Open Approach

0KCV3ZZ Extirpation of Matter from Right Foot Muscle, Percutaneous Approach

0KCV4ZZ Extirpation of Matter from Right Foot Muscle, Percutaneous Endoscopic Approach

0KCW0ZZ Extirpation of Matter from Left Foot Muscle, Open Approach

0KCW3ZZ Extirpation of Matter from Left Foot Muscle, Percutaneous Approach

0KCW4ZZ Extirpation of Matter from Left Foot Muscle, Percutaneous Endoscopic Approach

KH – Muscles, Insertion

KHX0MZ Insertion of Stimulator Lead into Upper Muscle, Open Approach

KHX3MZ Insertion of Stimulator Lead into Upper Muscle, Percutaneous Approach

0KHX4MZ Insertion of Stimulator Lead into Upper Muscle, Percutaneous Endoscopic Approach

0KHY0MZ Insertion of Stimulator Lead into Lower Muscle, Open Approach

0KHY3MZ Insertion of Stimulator Lead into Lower Muscle, Percutaneous Approach

0KHY4MZ Insertion of Stimulator Lead into Lower Muscle, Percutaneous Endoscopic Approach

0KJ – Muscles, Inspection

Review Coding Guideline B3.5

Review Coding Guidelines B3.11a, B3.11b and B3.11c

0KJX0ZZ Inspection of Upper Muscle, Open Approach
0KJX3ZZ Inspection of Upper Muscle, Percutaneous Approach
0KJX4ZZ Inspection of Upper Muscle, Percutaneous Endoscopic Approach
0KJXXZZ Inspection of Upper Muscle, External Approach
0KJY0ZZ Inspection of Lower Muscle, Open Approach
0KJY3ZZ Inspection of Lower Muscle, Percutaneous Approach
0KJY4ZZ Inspection of Lower Muscle, Percutane Endoscopic Approach
0KJYXZZ Inspection of Lower Muscle, External Approach

0KM – Muscles, Reattachment

0KM00ZZ Reattachment of Head Muscle, Open Approach
0KM04ZZ Reattachment of Head Muscle, Percutaneous Endoscopic Approach
0KM10ZZ Reattachment of Facial Muscle, Open Approach
0KM14ZZ Reattachment of Facial Muscle, Percutaneous Endoscopic Approach
0KM20ZZ Reattachment of Right Neck Muscle, Open Approach
0KM24ZZ Reattachment of Right Neck Muscle, Percutaneous Endoscopic Approach
0KM30ZZ Reattachment of Left Neck Muscle, Open Approach
0KM34ZZ Reattachment of Left Neck Muscle, Percutaneous Endoscopic Approach
0KM40ZZ Reattachment of Tongue, Palate, Pharynx Muscle, Open Approach
0KM44ZZ Reattachment of Tongue, Palate, Pharynx Muscle, Percutaneous Endoscopic Approach
0KM50ZZ Reattachment of Right Shoulder Muscle, Open Approach
0KM54ZZ Reattachment of Right Shoulder Muscle, Percutaneous Endoscopic Approach
0KM60ZZ Reattachment of Left Shoulder Muscle, Open Approach
0KM64ZZ Reattachment of Left Shoulder Muscle, Percutaneous Endoscopic Approach
0KM70ZZ Reattachment of Right Upper Arm Muscle, Open Approach
0KM74ZZ Reattachment of Right Upper Arm Muscle, Percutaneous Endoscopic Approach
0KM80ZZ Reattachment of Left Upper Arm Muscle, Open Approach
0KM84ZZ Reattachment of Left Upper Arm Muscle, Percutaneous Endoscopic Approach
0KM90ZZ Reattachment of Right Lower Arm and Wrist Muscle, Open Approach
0KM94ZZ Reattachment of Right Lower Arm and Wrist Muscle, Percutaneous Endoscopic Approach
0KMB0ZZ Reattachment of Left Lower Arm and Wrist Muscle, Open Approach
0KMB4ZZ Reattachment of Left Lower Arm and Wrist Muscle, Percutaneous Endoscopic Approach
0KMC0ZZ Reattachment of Right Hand Muscle, Open Approach
0KMC4ZZ Reattachment of Right Hand Muscle, Percutaneous Endoscopic Approach
0KMD0ZZ Reattachment of Left Hand Muscle, Open Approach
0KMD4ZZ Reattachment of Left Hand Muscle, Percutaneous Endoscopic Approach
0KMF0ZZ Reattachment of Right Trunk Muscle, Open Approach
0KMF4ZZ Reattachment of Right Trunk Muscle, Percutaneous Endoscopic Approach
0KMG0ZZ Reattachment of Left Trunk Muscle, Open Approach
0KMG4ZZ Reattachment of Left Trunk Muscle, Percutaneous Endoscopic Approach
0KMH0ZZ Reattachment of Right Thorax Muscle, Open Approach
0KMH4ZZ Reattachment of Right Thorax Muscle, Percutaneous Endoscopic Approach
0KMJ0ZZ Reattachment of Left Thorax Muscle, Open Approach
0KMJ4ZZ Reattachment of Left Thorax Muscle, Percutaneous Endoscopic Approach
0KMK0ZZ Reattachment of Right Abdomen Muscle, Open Approach
0KMK4ZZ Reattachment of Right Abdomen Muscle, Percutaneous Endoscopic Approach
0KML0ZZ Reattachment of Left Abdomen Muscle, Open Approach
0KML4ZZ Reattachment of Left Abdomen Muscle, Percutaneous Endoscopic Approach
0KMM0ZZ Reattachment of Perineum Muscle, Op Approach
0KMM4ZZ Reattachment of Perineum Muscle, Percutaneous Endoscopic Approach
0KMN0ZZ Reattachment of Right Hip Muscle, O Approach
0KMN4ZZ Reattachment of Right Hip Muscle, Percutaneous Endoscopic Approach
0KMP0ZZ Reattachment of Left Hip Muscle, Ope Approach
0KMP4ZZ Reattachment of Left Hip Muscle, Percutaneous Endoscopic Approach
0KMQ0ZZ Reattachment of Right Upper Leg Muscle, Open Approach
0KMQ4ZZ Reattachment of Right Upper Leg Muscle, Percutaneous Endoscopic Approach
0KMR0ZZ Reattachment of Left Upper Leg Muscl Open Approach
0KMR4ZZ Reattachment of Left Upper Leg Muscl Percutaneous Endoscopic Approach
0KMS0ZZ Reattachment of Right Lower Leg Muscle, Open Approach
0KMS4ZZ Reattachment of Right Lower Leg Muscle, Percutaneous Endoscopic Approach
0KMT0ZZ Reattachment of Left Lower Leg Muscl Open Approach
0KMT4ZZ Reattachment of Left Lower Leg Musc Percutaneous Endoscopic Approach
0KMV0ZZ Reattachment of Right Foot Muscle, Open Approach
0KMV4ZZ Reattachment of Right Foot Muscle, Percutaneous Endoscopic Approach
0KMW0ZZ Reattachment of Left Foot Muscle, Ope Approach
0KMW4ZZ Reattachment of Left Foot Muscle, Percutaneous Endoscopic Approach

0KN – Muscles, Release

Review Coding Guideline B3.13

Review Coding Guideline B3.14

0KN00ZZ Release Head Muscle, Open Approach
0KN03ZZ Release Head Muscle, Percutaneous Approach
0KN04ZZ Release Head Muscle, Percutaneous Endoscopic Approach
0KN0XZZ Release Head Muscle, External Approach
0KN10ZZ Release Facial Muscle, Open Approach
0KN13ZZ Release Facial Muscle, Percutaneous Approach
0KN14ZZ Release Facial Muscle, Percutaneous Endoscopic Approach
0KN1XZZ Release Facial Muscle, External Approach
0KN20ZZ Release Right Neck Muscle, Open Approach
0KN23ZZ Release Right Neck Muscle, Percutaneous Approach
0KN24ZZ Release Right Neck Muscle, Percutaneous Endoscopic Approach
0KN2XZZ Release Right Neck Muscle, External Approach
0KN30ZZ Release Left Neck Muscle, Open Approach
0KN33ZZ Release Left Neck Muscle, Percutaneous Approach
0KN34ZZ Release Left Neck Muscle, Percutaneous Endoscopic Approach
0KN3XZZ Release Left Neck Muscle, External Approach
0KN40ZZ Release Tongue, Palate, Pharynx Muscle, Open Approach
0KN43ZZ Release Tongue, Palate, Pharynx Muscle, Percutaneous Approach
0KN44ZZ Release Tongue, Palate, Pharynx Muscle, Percutaneous Endoscopic Approach
0KN4XZZ Release Tongue, Palate, Pharynx Muscle, External Approach
0KN50ZZ Release Right Shoulder Muscle, Open Approach
0KN53ZZ Release Right Shoulder Muscle, Percutaneous Approach
0KN54ZZ Release Right Shoulder Muscle, Percutaneous Endoscopic Approach
0KN5XZZ Release Right Shoulder Muscle, External Approach

N60ZZ Release Left Shoulder Muscle, Open Approach
N63ZZ Release Left Shoulder Muscle, Percutaneous Approach
N64ZZ Release Left Shoulder Muscle, Percutaneous Endoscopic Approach
N6XZZ Release Left Shoulder Muscle, External Approach
N70ZZ Release Right Upper Arm Muscle, Open Approach
N73ZZ Release Right Upper Arm Muscle, Percutaneous Approach
N74ZZ Release Right Upper Arm Muscle, Percutaneous Endoscopic Approach
N7XZZ Release Right Upper Arm Muscle, External Approach
N80ZZ Release Left Upper Arm Muscle, Open Approach
N83ZZ Release Left Upper Arm Muscle, Percutaneous Approach
N84ZZ Release Left Upper Arm Muscle, Percutaneous Endoscopic Approach
N8XZZ Release Left Upper Arm Muscle, External Approach
N90ZZ Release Right Lower Arm and Wrist Muscle, Open Approach
N93ZZ Release Right Lower Arm and Wrist Muscle, Percutaneous Approach
N94ZZ Release Right Lower Arm and Wrist Muscle, Percutaneous Endoscopic Approach
KN9XZZ Release Right Lower Arm and Wrist Muscle, External Approach
KNB0ZZ Release Left Lower Arm and Wrist Muscle, Open Approach
KNB3ZZ Release Left Lower Arm and Wrist Muscle, Percutaneous Approach
KNB4ZZ Release Left Lower Arm and Wrist Muscle, Percutaneous Endoscopic Approach
KNBXZZ Release Left Lower Arm and Wrist Muscle, External Approach
KNC0ZZ Release Right Hand Muscle, Open Approach
KNC3ZZ Release Right Hand Muscle, Percutaneous Approach
KNC4ZZ Release Right Hand Muscle, Percutaneous Endoscopic Approach
KNCXZZ Release Right Hand Muscle, External Approach
KND0ZZ Release Left Hand Muscle, Open Approach
KND3ZZ Release Left Hand Muscle, Percutaneous Approach
KND4ZZ Release Left Hand Muscle, Percutaneous Endoscopic Approach
KNDXZZ Release Left Hand Muscle, External Approach
KNF0ZZ Release Right Trunk Muscle, Open Approach
0KNF3ZZ Release Right Trunk Muscle, Percutaneous Approach
0KNF4ZZ Release Right Trunk Muscle, Percutaneous Endoscopic Approach
0KNFXZZ Release Right Trunk Muscle, External Approach
0KNG0ZZ Release Left Trunk Muscle, Open Approach
0KNG3ZZ Release Left Trunk Muscle, Percutaneous Approach
0KNG4ZZ Release Left Trunk Muscle, Percutaneous Endoscopic Approach
0KNGXZZ Release Left Trunk Muscle, External Approach
0KNH0ZZ Release Right Thorax Muscle, Open Approach
0KNH3ZZ Release Right Thorax Muscle, Percutaneous Approach
0KNH4ZZ Release Right Thorax Muscle, Percutaneous Endoscopic Approach
0KNHXZZ Release Right Thorax Muscle, External Approach
0KNJ0ZZ Release Left Thorax Muscle, Open Approach
0KNJ3ZZ Release Left Thorax Muscle, Percutaneous Approach
0KNJ4ZZ Release Left Thorax Muscle, Percutaneous Endoscopic Approach
0KNJXZZ Release Left Thorax Muscle, External Approach
0KNK0ZZ Release Right Abdomen Muscle, Open Approach
0KNK3ZZ Release Right Abdomen Muscle, Percutaneous Approach
0KNK4ZZ Release Right Abdomen Muscle, Percutaneous Endoscopic Approach
0KNKXZZ Release Right Abdomen Muscle, External Approach
0KNL0ZZ Release Left Abdomen Muscle, Open Approach
0KNL3ZZ Release Left Abdomen Muscle, Percutaneous Approach
0KNL4ZZ Release Left Abdomen Muscle, Percutaneous Endoscopic Approach
0KNLXZZ Release Left Abdomen Muscle, External Approach
0KNM0ZZ Release Perineum Muscle, Open Approach
0KNM3ZZ Release Perineum Muscle, Percutaneous Approach
0KNM4ZZ Release Perineum Muscle, Percutaneous Endoscopic Approach
0KNMXZZ Release Perineum Muscle, External Approach
0KNN0ZZ Release Right Hip Muscle, Open Approach
0KNN3ZZ Release Right Hip Muscle, Percutaneous Approach
0KNN4ZZ Release Right Hip Muscle, Percutaneous Endoscopic Approach
0KNNXZZ Release Right Hip Muscle, External Approach
0KNP0ZZ Release Left Hip Muscle, Open Approach
0KNP3ZZ Release Left Hip Muscle, Percutaneous Approach
0KNP4ZZ Release Left Hip Muscle, Percutaneous Endoscopic Approach
0KNPXZZ Release Left Hip Muscle, External Approach
0KNQ0ZZ Release Right Upper Leg Muscle, Open Approach
0KNQ3ZZ Release Right Upper Leg Muscle, Percutaneous Approach
0KNQ4ZZ Release Right Upper Leg Muscle, Percutaneous Endoscopic Approach
0KNQXZZ Release Right Upper Leg Muscle, External Approach
0KNR0ZZ Release Left Upper Leg Muscle, Open Approach
0KNR3ZZ Release Left Upper Leg Muscle, Percutaneous Approach
0KNR4ZZ Release Left Upper Leg Muscle, Percutaneous Endoscopic Approach
0KNRXZZ Release Left Upper Leg Muscle, External Approach
0KNS0ZZ Release Right Lower Leg Muscle, Open Approach
0KNS3ZZ Release Right Lower Leg Muscle, Percutaneous Approach
0KNS4ZZ Release Right Lower Leg Muscle, Percutaneous Endoscopic Approach
0KNSXZZ Release Right Lower Leg Muscle, External Approach
0KNT0ZZ Release Left Lower Leg Muscle, Open Approach
0KNT3ZZ Release Left Lower Leg Muscle, Percutaneous Approach
0KNT4ZZ Release Left Lower Leg Muscle, Percutaneous Endoscopic Approach
0KNTXZZ Release Left Lower Leg Muscle, External Approach
0KNV0ZZ Release Right Foot Muscle, Open Approach
0KNV3ZZ Release Right Foot Muscle, Percutaneous Approach
0KNV4ZZ Release Right Foot Muscle, Percutaneous Endoscopic Approach
0KNVXZZ Release Right Foot Muscle, External Approach
0KNW0ZZ Release Left Foot Muscle, Open Approach
0KNW3ZZ Release Left Foot Muscle, Percutaneous Approach
0KNW4ZZ Release Left Foot Muscle, Percutaneous Endoscopic Approach
0KNWXZZ Release Left Foot Muscle, External Approach

KP – Muscles, Removal

eview Coding Guideline B6.1c

KPX00Z Removal of Drainage Device from Upper Muscle, Open Approach
KPX07Z Removal of Autologous Tissue Substitute from Upper Muscle, Open Approach
KPX0JZ Removal of Synthetic Substitute from Upper Muscle, Open Approach
KPX0KZ Removal of Nonautologous Tissue Substitute from Upper Muscle, Open Approach
KPX0MZ Removal of Stimulator Lead from Upper Muscle, Open Approach
0KPX30Z Removal of Drainage Device from Upper Muscle, Percutaneous Approach
0KPX37Z Removal of Autologous Tissue Substitute from Upper Muscle, Percutaneous Approach
0KPX3JZ Removal of Synthetic Substitute from Upper Muscle, Percutaneous Approach
0KPX3KZ Removal of Nonautologous Tissue Substitute from Upper Muscle, Percutaneous Approach
0KPX3MZ Removal of Stimulator Lead from Upper Muscle, Percutaneous Approach
0KPX40Z Removal of Drainage Device from Upper Muscle, Percutaneous Endoscopic Approach
0KPX47Z Removal of Autologous Tissue Substitute from Upper Muscle, Percutaneous Endoscopic Approach
0KPX4JZ Removal of Synthetic Substitute from Upper Muscle, Percutaneous Endoscopic Approach
0KPX4KZ Removal of Nonautologous Tissue Substitute from Upper Muscle, Percutaneous Endoscopic Approach

0KPX4MZ Removal of Stimulator Lead from Upper Muscle, Percutaneous Endoscopic Approach
0KPXX0Z Removal of Drainage Device from Upper Muscle, External Approach
0KPXXMZ Removal of Stimulator Lead from Upper Muscle, External Approach
0KPY00Z Removal of Drainage Device from Lower Muscle, Open Approach
0KPY07Z Removal of Autologous Tissue Substitute from Lower Muscle, Open Approach
0KPY0JZ Removal of Synthetic Substitute from Lower Muscle, Open Approach
0KPY0KZ Removal of Nonautologous Tissue Substitute from Lower Muscle, Open Approach
0KPY0MZ Removal of Stimulator Lead from Lower Muscle, Open Approach
0KPY30Z Removal of Drainage Device from Lower Muscle, Percutaneous Approach
0KPY37Z Removal of Autologous Tissue Substitute from Lower Muscle, Percutaneous Approach
0KPY3JZ Removal of Synthetic Substitute from Lower Muscle, Percutaneous Approach
0KPY3KZ Removal of Nonautologous Tissue Substitute from Lower Muscle, Percutaneous Approach
0KPY3MZ Removal of Stimulator Lead from Lower Muscle, Percutaneous Approach
0KPY40Z Removal of Drainage Device from Lower Muscle, Percutaneous Endoscopic Approach
0KPY47Z Removal of Autologous Tissue Substitute from Lower Muscle, Percutaneous Endoscopic Approach
0KPY4JZ Removal of Synthetic Substitute from Lower Muscle, Percutaneous Endoscopic Approach
0KPY4KZ Removal of Nonautologous Tissue Substitute from Lower Muscle, Percutaneous Endoscopic Approach
0KPY4MZ Removal of Stimulator Lead from Lower Muscle, Percutaneous Endoscopic Approach
0KPYX0Z Removal of Drainage Device from Lower Muscle, External Approach
0KPYXMZ Removal of Stimulator Lead from Lower Muscle, External Approach

0KQ – Muscles, Repair

Review Coding Guideline B3.5

0KQ00ZZ Repair Head Muscle, Open Approach
0KQ03ZZ Repair Head Muscle, Percutaneous Approach
0KQ04ZZ Repair Head Muscle, Percutaneous Endoscopic Approach
0KQ10ZZ Repair Facial Muscle, Open Approach
0KQ13ZZ Repair Facial Muscle, Percutaneous Approach
0KQ14ZZ Repair Facial Muscle, Percutaneous Endoscopic Approach
0KQ20ZZ Repair Right Neck Muscle, Open Approach
0KQ23ZZ Repair Right Neck Muscle, Percutaneous Approach
0KQ24ZZ Repair Right Neck Muscle, Percutaneous Endoscopic Approach
0KQ30ZZ Repair Left Neck Muscle, Open Approach
0KQ33ZZ Repair Left Neck Muscle, Percutaneous Approach
0KQ34ZZ Repair Left Neck Muscle, Percutaneous Endoscopic Approach
0KQ40ZZ Repair Tongue, Palate, Pharynx Muscle, Open Approach
0KQ43ZZ Repair Tongue, Palate, Pharynx Muscle, Percutaneous Approach
0KQ44ZZ Repair Tongue, Palate, Pharynx Muscle, Percutaneous Endoscopic Approach
0KQ50ZZ Repair Right Shoulder Muscle, Open Approach
0KQ53ZZ Repair Right Shoulder Muscle, Percutaneous Approach
0KQ54ZZ Repair Right Shoulder Muscle, Percutaneous Endoscopic Approach
0KQ60ZZ Repair Left Shoulder Muscle, Open Approach
0KQ63ZZ Repair Left Shoulder Muscle, Percutaneous Approach
0KQ64ZZ Repair Left Shoulder Muscle, Percutaneous Endoscopic Approach
0KQ70ZZ Repair Right Upper Arm Muscle, Open Approach
0KQ73ZZ Repair Right Upper Arm Muscle, Percutaneous Approach
0KQ74ZZ Repair Right Upper Arm Muscle, Percutaneous Endoscopic Approach
0KQ80ZZ Repair Left Upper Arm Muscle, Open Approach
0KQ83ZZ Repair Left Upper Arm Muscle, Percutaneous Approach
0KQ84ZZ Repair Left Upper Arm Muscle, Percutaneous Endoscopic Approach
0KQ90ZZ Repair Right Lower Arm and Wrist Muscle, Open Approach
0KQ93ZZ Repair Right Lower Arm and Wrist Muscle, Percutaneous Approach
0KQ94ZZ Repair Right Lower Arm and Wrist Muscle, Percutaneous Endoscopic Approach
0KQB0ZZ Repair Left Lower Arm and Wrist Muscle, Open Approach
0KQB3ZZ Repair Left Lower Arm and Wrist Muscle, Percutaneous Approach
0KQB4ZZ Repair Left Lower Arm and Wrist Muscle, Percutaneous Endoscopic Approach
0KQC0ZZ Repair Right Hand Muscle, Open Approach
0KQC3ZZ Repair Right Hand Muscle, Percutaneous Approach
0KQC4ZZ Repair Right Hand Muscle, Percutaneous Endoscopic Approach
0KQD0ZZ Repair Left Hand Muscle, Open Approach
0KQD3ZZ Repair Left Hand Muscle, Percutaneous Approach
0KQD4ZZ Repair Left Hand Muscle, Percutaneous Endoscopic Approach
0KQF0ZZ Repair Right Trunk Muscle, Open Approach
0KQF3ZZ Repair Right Trunk Muscle, Percutaneous Approach
0KQF4ZZ Repair Right Trunk Muscle, Percutaneous Endoscopic Approach
0KQG0ZZ Repair Left Trunk Muscle, Open Approach
0KQG3ZZ Repair Left Trunk Muscle, Percutaneous Approach
0KQG4ZZ Repair Left Trunk Muscle, Percutaneous Endoscopic Approach
0KQH0ZZ Repair Right Thorax Muscle, Open Approach
0KQH3ZZ Repair Right Thorax Muscle, Percutaneous Approach
0KQH4ZZ Repair Right Thorax Muscle, Percutaneous Endoscopic Approach
0KQJ0ZZ Repair Left Thorax Muscle, Open Approach
0KQJ3ZZ Repair Left Thorax Muscle, Percutaneous Approach
0KQJ4ZZ Repair Left Thorax Muscle, Percutaneous Endoscopic Approach
0KQK0ZZ Repair Right Abdomen Muscle, Open Approach
0KQK3ZZ Repair Right Abdomen Muscle, Percutaneous Approach
0KQK4ZZ Repair Right Abdomen Muscle, Percutaneous Endoscopic Approach
0KQL0ZZ Repair Left Abdomen Muscle, Open Approach
0KQL3ZZ Repair Left Abdomen Muscle, Percutaneous Approach
0KQL4ZZ Repair Left Abdomen Muscle, Percutaneous Endoscopic Approach
0KQM0ZZ Repair Perineum Muscle, Open Approach
AHA CC: 4Q, 2013, 120
0KQM3ZZ Repair Perineum Muscle, Percutaneous Approach
0KQM4ZZ Repair Perineum Muscle, Percutaneous Endoscopic Approach
0KQN0ZZ Repair Right Hip Muscle, Open Approach
0KQN3ZZ Repair Right Hip Muscle, Percutaneous Approach
0KQN4ZZ Repair Right Hip Muscle, Percutaneous Endoscopic Approach
0KQP0ZZ Repair Left Hip Muscle, Open Approach
0KQP3ZZ Repair Left Hip Muscle, Percutaneous Approach
0KQP4ZZ Repair Left Hip Muscle, Percutaneous Endoscopic Approach
0KQQ0ZZ Repair Right Upper Leg Muscle, Open Approach
0KQQ3ZZ Repair Right Upper Leg Muscle, Percutaneous Approach
0KQQ4ZZ Repair Right Upper Leg Muscle, Percutaneous Endoscopic Approach
0KQR0ZZ Repair Left Upper Leg Muscle, Open Approach
0KQR3ZZ Repair Left Upper Leg Muscle, Percutaneous Approach
0KQR4ZZ Repair Left Upper Leg Muscle, Percutaneous Endoscopic Approach
0KQS0ZZ Repair Right Lower Leg Muscle, Open Approach
0KQS3ZZ Repair Right Lower Leg Muscle, Percutaneous Approach
0KQS4ZZ Repair Right Lower Leg Muscle, Percutaneous Endoscopic Approach
0KQT0ZZ Repair Left Lower Leg Muscle, Open Approach
0KQT3ZZ Repair Left Lower Leg Muscle, Percutaneous Approach
0KQT4ZZ Repair Left Lower Leg Muscle, Percutaneous Endoscopic Approach
0KQV0ZZ Repair Right Foot Muscle, Open Approach
0KQV3ZZ Repair Right Foot Muscle, Percutaneous Approach
0KQV4ZZ Repair Right Foot Muscle, Percutaneous Endoscopic Approach
0KQW0ZZ Repair Left Foot Muscle, Open Approach
0KQW3ZZ Repair Left Foot Muscle, Percutaneous Approach
0KQW4ZZ Repair Left Foot Muscle, Percutaneous Endoscopic Approach

S – Muscles, Reposition

S00ZZ Reposition Head Muscle, Open Approach
S04ZZ Reposition Head Muscle, Percutaneous Endoscopic Approach
S10ZZ Reposition Facial Muscle, Open Approach
S14ZZ Reposition Facial Muscle, Percutaneous Endoscopic Approach
S20ZZ Reposition Right Neck Muscle, Open Approach
S24ZZ Reposition Right Neck Muscle, Percutaneous Endoscopic Approach
S30ZZ Reposition Left Neck Muscle, Open Approach
S34ZZ Reposition Left Neck Muscle, Percutaneous Endoscopic Approach
S40ZZ Reposition Tongue, Palate, Pharynx Muscle, Open Approach
S44ZZ Reposition Tongue, Palate, Pharynx Muscle, Percutaneous Endoscopic Approach
S50ZZ Reposition Right Shoulder Muscle, Open Approach
S54ZZ Reposition Right Shoulder Muscle, Percutaneous Endoscopic Approach
S60ZZ Reposition Left Shoulder Muscle, Open Approach
S64ZZ Reposition Left Shoulder Muscle, Percutaneous Endoscopic Approach
S70ZZ Reposition Right Upper Arm Muscle, Open Approach
S74ZZ Reposition Right Upper Arm Muscle, Percutaneous Endoscopic Approach
S80ZZ Reposition Left Upper Arm Muscle, Open Approach
S84ZZ Reposition Left Upper Arm Muscle, Percutaneous Endoscopic Approach
S90ZZ Reposition Right Lower Arm and Wrist Muscle, Open Approach
0KS94ZZ Reposition Right Lower Arm and Wrist Muscle, Percutaneous Endoscopic Approach
0KSB0ZZ Reposition Left Lower Arm and Wrist Muscle, Open Approach
0KSB4ZZ Reposition Left Lower Arm and Wrist Muscle, Percutaneous Endoscopic Approach
0KSC0ZZ Reposition Right Hand Muscle, Open Approach
0KSC4ZZ Reposition Right Hand Muscle, Percutaneous Endoscopic Approach
0KSD0ZZ Reposition Left Hand Muscle, Open Approach
0KSD4ZZ Reposition Left Hand Muscle, Percutaneous Endoscopic Approach
0KSF0ZZ Reposition Right Trunk Muscle, Open Approach
0KSF4ZZ Reposition Right Trunk Muscle, Percutaneous Endoscopic Approach
0KSG0ZZ Reposition Left Trunk Muscle, Open Approach
0KSG4ZZ Reposition Left Trunk Muscle, Percutaneous Endoscopic Approach
0KSH0ZZ Reposition Right Thorax Muscle, Open Approach
0KSH4ZZ Reposition Right Thorax Muscle, Percutaneous Endoscopic Approach
0KSJ0ZZ Reposition Left Thorax Muscle, Open Approach
0KSJ4ZZ Reposition Left Thorax Muscle, Percutaneous Endoscopic Approach
0KSK0ZZ Reposition Right Abdomen Muscle, Open Approach
0KSK4ZZ Reposition Right Abdomen Muscle, Percutaneous Endoscopic Approach
0KSL0ZZ Reposition Left Abdomen Muscle, Open Approach
0KSL4ZZ Reposition Left Abdomen Muscle, Percutaneous Endoscopic Approach
0KSM0ZZ Reposition Perineum Muscle, Open Approach
0KSM4ZZ Reposition Perineum Muscle, Percutaneous Endoscopic Approach
0KSN0ZZ Reposition Right Hip Muscle, Open Approach
0KSN4ZZ Reposition Right Hip Muscle, Percutaneous Endoscopic Approach
0KSP0ZZ Reposition Left Hip Muscle, Open Approach
0KSP4ZZ Reposition Left Hip Muscle, Percutaneous Endoscopic Approach
0KSQ0ZZ Reposition Right Upper Leg Muscle, Open Approach
0KSQ4ZZ Reposition Right Upper Leg Muscle, Percutaneous Endoscopic Approach
0KSR0ZZ Reposition Left Upper Leg Muscle, Open Approach
0KSR4ZZ Reposition Left Upper Leg Muscle, Percutaneous Endoscopic Approach
0KSS0ZZ Reposition Right Lower Leg Muscle, Open Approach
0KSS4ZZ Reposition Right Lower Leg Muscle, Percutaneous Endoscopic Approach
0KST0ZZ Reposition Left Lower Leg Muscle, Open Approach
0KST4ZZ Reposition Left Lower Leg Muscle, Percutaneous Endoscopic Approach
0KSV0ZZ Reposition Right Foot Muscle, Open Approach
0KSV4ZZ Reposition Right Foot Muscle, Percutaneous Endoscopic Approach
0KSW0ZZ Reposition Left Foot Muscle, Open Approach
0KSW4ZZ Reposition Left Foot Muscle, Percutaneous Endoscopic Approach

KT – Muscles, Resection

eview Coding Guideline B3.8

KT00ZZ Resection of Head Muscle, Open Approach
KT04ZZ Resection of Head Muscle, Percutaneous Endoscopic Approach
KT10ZZ Resection of Facial Muscle, Open Approach
KT14ZZ Resection of Facial Muscle, Percutaneous Endoscopic Approach
KT20ZZ Resection of Right Neck Muscle, Open Approach
KT24ZZ Resection of Right Neck Muscle, Percutaneous Endoscopic Approach
KT30ZZ Resection of Left Neck Muscle, Open Approach
KT34ZZ Resection of Left Neck Muscle, Percutaneous Endoscopic Approach
KT40ZZ Resection of Tongue, Palate, Pharynx Muscle, Open Approach
KT44ZZ Resection of Tongue, Palate, Pharynx Muscle, Percutaneous Endoscopic Approach
KT50ZZ Resection of Right Shoulder Muscle, Open Approach
KT54ZZ Resection of Right Shoulder Muscle, Percutaneous Endoscopic Approach
KT60ZZ Resection of Left Shoulder Muscle, Open Approach
KT64ZZ Resection of Left Shoulder Muscle, Percutaneous Endoscopic Approach
KT70ZZ Resection of Right Upper Arm Muscle, Open Approach
0KT74ZZ Resection of Right Upper Arm Muscle, Percutaneous Endoscopic Approach
0KT80ZZ Resection of Left Upper Arm Muscle, Open Approach
0KT84ZZ Resection of Left Upper Arm Muscle, Percutaneous Endoscopic Approach
0KT90ZZ Resection of Right Lower Arm and Wrist Muscle, Open Approach
0KT94ZZ Resection of Right Lower Arm and Wrist Muscle, Percutaneous Endoscopic Approach
0KTB0ZZ Resection of Left Lower Arm and Wrist Muscle, Open Approach
0KTB4ZZ Resection of Left Lower Arm and Wrist Muscle, Percutaneous Endoscopic Approach
0KTC0ZZ Resection of Right Hand Muscle, Open Approach
0KTC4ZZ Resection of Right Hand Muscle, Percutaneous Endoscopic Approach
0KTD0ZZ Resection of Left Hand Muscle, Open Approach
0KTD4ZZ Resection of Left Hand Muscle, Percutaneous Endoscopic Approach
0KTF0ZZ Resection of Right Trunk Muscle, Open Approach
0KTF4ZZ Resection of Right Trunk Muscle, Percutaneous Endoscopic Approach
0KTG0ZZ Resection of Left Trunk Muscle, Open Approach
0KTG4ZZ Resection of Left Trunk Muscle, Percutaneous Endoscopic Approach
0KTH0ZZ Resection of Right Thorax Muscle, Open Approach
0KTH4ZZ Resection of Right Thorax Muscle, Percutaneous Endoscopic Approach
0KTJ0ZZ Resection of Left Thorax Muscle, Open Approach
0KTJ4ZZ Resection of Left Thorax Muscle, Percutaneous Endoscopic Approach
0KTK0ZZ Resection of Right Abdomen Muscle, Open Approach
0KTK4ZZ Resection of Right Abdomen Muscle, Percutaneous Endoscopic Approach
0KTL0ZZ Resection of Left Abdomen Muscle, Open Approach
0KTL4ZZ Resection of Left Abdomen Muscle, Percutaneous Endoscopic Approach
0KTM0ZZ Resection of Perineum Muscle, Open Approach
0KTM4ZZ Resection of Perineum Muscle, Percutaneous Endoscopic Approach
0KTN0ZZ Resection of Right Hip Muscle, Open Approach
0KTN4ZZ Resection of Right Hip Muscle, Percutaneous Endoscopic Approach
0KTP0ZZ Resection of Left Hip Muscle, Open Approach
0KTP4ZZ Resection of Left Hip Muscle, Percutaneous Endoscopic Approach
0KTQ0ZZ Resection of Right Upper Leg Muscle, Open Approach

0KTQ4ZZ Resection of Right Upper Leg Muscle, Percutaneous Endoscopic Approach
0KTR0ZZ Resection of Left Upper Leg Muscle, Open Approach
0KTR4ZZ Resection of Left Upper Leg Muscle, Percutaneous Endoscopic Approach
0KTS0ZZ Resection of Right Lower Leg Muscle, Open Approach
0KTS4ZZ Resection of Right Lower Leg Muscle, Percutaneous Endoscopic Approach
0KTT0ZZ Resection of Left Lower Leg Muscle, Open Approach
0KTT4ZZ Resection of Left Lower Leg Muscle, Percutaneous Endoscopic Approach
0KTV0ZZ Resection of Right Foot Muscle, Open Approach
0KTV4ZZ Resection of Right Foot Muscle, Percutaneous Endoscopic Approach
0KTW0ZZ Resection of Left Foot Muscle, Open Approach
0KTW4ZZ Resection of Left Foot Muscle, Percutaneous Endoscopic Approach

0KU – Muscles, Supplement

0KU007Z Supplement Head Muscle with Autologous Tissue Substitute, Open Approach
0KU00JZ Supplement Head Muscle with Synthetic Substitute, Open Approach
0KU00KZ Supplement Head Muscle with Nonautologous Tissue Substitute, Open Approach
0KU047Z Supplement Head Muscle with Autologous Tissue Substitute, Percutaneous Endoscopic Approach
0KU04JZ Supplement Head Muscle with Synthetic Substitute, Percutaneous Endoscopic Approach
0KU04KZ Supplement Head Muscle with Nonautologous Tissue Substitute, Percutaneous Endoscopic Approach
0KU107Z Supplement Facial Muscle with Autologous Tissue Substitute, Open Approach
0KU10JZ Supplement Facial Muscle with Synthetic Substitute, Open Approach
0KU10KZ Supplement Facial Muscle with Nonautologous Tissue Substitute, Open Approach
0KU147Z Supplement Facial Muscle with Autologous Tissue Substitute, Percutaneous Endoscopic Approach
0KU14JZ Supplement Facial Muscle with Synthetic Substitute, Percutaneous Endoscopic Approach
0KU14KZ Supplement Facial Muscle with Nonautologous Tissue Substitute, Percutaneous Endoscopic Approach
0KU207Z Supplement Right Neck Muscle with Autologous Tissue Substitute, Open Approach
0KU20JZ Supplement Right Neck Muscle with Synthetic Substitute, Open Approach
0KU20KZ Supplement Right Neck Muscle with Nonautologous Tissue Substitute, Open Approach
0KU247Z Supplement Right Neck Muscle with Autologous Tissue Substitute, Percutaneous Endoscopic Approach
0KU24JZ Supplement Right Neck Muscle with Synthetic Substitute, Percutaneous Endoscopic Approach
0KU24KZ Supplement Right Neck Muscle with Nonautologous Tissue Substitute, Percutaneous Endoscopic Approach
0KU307Z Supplement Left Neck Muscle with Autologous Tissue Substitute, Open Approach
0KU30JZ Supplement Left Neck Muscle with Synthetic Substitute, Open Approach
0KU30KZ Supplement Left Neck Muscle with Nonautologous Tissue Substitute, Open Approach
0KU347Z Supplement Left Neck Muscle with Autologous Tissue Substitute, Percutaneous Endoscopic Approach
0KU34JZ Supplement Left Neck Muscle with Synthetic Substitute, Percutaneous Endoscopic Approach
0KU34KZ Supplement Left Neck Muscle with Nonautologous Tissue Substitute, Percutaneous Endoscopic Approach
0KU407Z Supplement Tongue, Palate, Pharynx Muscle with Autologous Tissue Substitute, Open Approach
0KU40JZ Supplement Tongue, Palate, Pharynx Muscle with Synthetic Substitute, Open Approach
0KU40KZ Supplement Tongue, Palate, Pharynx Muscle with Nonautologous Tissue Substitute, Open Approach
0KU447Z Supplement Tongue, Palate, Pharynx Muscle with Autologous Tissue Substitute, Percutaneous Endoscopic Approach
0KU44JZ Supplement Tongue, Palate, Pharynx Muscle with Synthetic Substitute, Percutaneous Endoscopic Approach
0KU44KZ Supplement Tongue, Palate, Pharynx Muscle with Nonautologous Tissue Substitute, Percutaneous Endoscopic Approach
0KU507Z Supplement Right Shoulder Muscle with Autologous Tissue Substitute, Open Approach
0KU50JZ Supplement Right Shoulder Muscle with Synthetic Substitute, Open Approach
0KU50KZ Supplement Right Shoulder Muscle with Nonautologous Tissue Substitute, Open Approach
0KU547Z Supplement Right Shoulder Muscle with Autologous Tissue Substitute, Percutaneous Endoscopic Approach
0KU54JZ Supplement Right Shoulder Muscle with Synthetic Substitute, Percutaneous Endoscopic Approach
0KU54KZ Supplement Right Shoulder Muscle with Nonautologous Tissue Substitute, Percutaneous Endoscopic Approach
0KU607Z Supplement Left Shoulder Muscle with Autologous Tissue Substitute, Open Approach
0KU60JZ Supplement Left Shoulder Muscle with Synthetic Substitute, Open Approach
0KU60KZ Supplement Left Shoulder Muscle with Nonautologous Tissue Substitute, Open Approach
0KU647Z Supplement Left Shoulder Muscle with Autologous Tissue Substitute, Percutaneous Endoscopic Approach
0KU64JZ Supplement Left Shoulder Muscle with Synthetic Substitute, Percutaneous Endoscopic Approach
0KU64KZ Supplement Left Shoulder Muscle with Nonautologous Tissue Substitute, Percutaneous Endoscopic Approach
0KU707Z Supplement Right Upper Arm Muscle with Autologous Tissue Substitute, Open Approach
0KU70JZ Supplement Right Upper Arm Muscle with Synthetic Substitute, Open Approach
0KU70KZ Supplement Right Upper Arm Muscle with Nonautologous Tissue Substitute, Open Approach
0KU747Z Supplement Right Upper Arm Muscle with Autologous Tissue Substitute, Percutaneous Endoscopic Approach
0KU74JZ Supplement Right Upper Arm Muscle with Synthetic Substitute, Percutaneou Endoscopic Approach
0KU74KZ Supplement Right Upper Arm Muscle with Nonautologous Tissue Substitute, Percutaneous Endoscopic Approach
0KU807Z Supplement Left Upper Arm Muscle with Autologous Tissue Substitute, Op Approach
0KU80JZ Supplement Left Upper Arm Muscle w Synthetic Substitute, Open Approach
0KU80KZ Supplement Left Upper Arm Muscle w Nonautologous Tissue Substitute, Open Approach
0KU847Z Supplement Left Upper Arm Muscle with Autologous Tissue Substitute, Percutaneous Endoscopic Approach
0KU84JZ Supplement Left Upper Arm Muscle with Synthetic Substitute, Percutaneous Endoscopic Approach
0KU84KZ Supplement Left Upper Arm Muscle with Nonautologous Tissue Substitute, Percutaneous Endoscopic Approach
0KU907Z Supplement Right Lower Arm and Wrist Muscle with Autologous Tissue Substitute, Open Approach
0KU90JZ Supplement Right Lower Arm and Wris Muscle with Synthetic Substitute, Open Approach
0KU90KZ Supplement Right Lower Arm and Wris Muscle with Nonautologous Tissue Substitute, Open Approach
0KU947Z Supplement Right Lower Arm and Wrist Muscle with Autologous Tissue Substitute, Percutaneous Endoscopic Approach
0KU94JZ Supplement Right Lower Arm and Wrist Muscle with Synthetic Substitute, Percutaneous Endoscopic Approach
0KU94KZ Supplement Right Lower Arm and Wrist Muscle with Nonautologous Tissue Substitute, Percutaneous Endoscopic Approach
0KUB07Z Supplement Left Lower Arm and Wrist Muscle with Autologous Tissue Substitute, Open Approach
0KUB0JZ Supplement Left Lower Arm and Wrist Muscle with Synthetic Substitute, Open Approach
0KUB0KZ Supplement Left Lower Arm and Wrist Muscle with Nonautologous Tissue Substitute, Open Approach
0KUB47Z Supplement Left Lower Arm and Wrist Muscle with Autologous Tissue Substitute, Percutaneous Endoscopic Approach
0KUB4JZ Supplement Left Lower Arm and Wrist Muscle with Synthetic Substitute, Percutaneous Endoscopic Approach
0KUB4KZ Supplement Left Lower Arm and Wrist Muscle with Nonautologous Tissue Substitute, Percutaneous Endoscopic Approach

JC07Z Supplement Right Hand Muscle with Autologous Tissue Substitute, Open Approach

JC0JZ Supplement Right Hand Muscle with Synthetic Substitute, Open Approach

JC0KZ Supplement Right Hand Muscle with Nonautologous Tissue Substitute, Open Approach

JC47Z Supplement Right Hand Muscle with Autologous Tissue Substitute, Percutaneous Endoscopic Approach

UC4JZ Supplement Right Hand Muscle with Synthetic Substitute, Percutaneous Endoscopic Approach

UC4KZ Supplement Right Hand Muscle with Nonautologous Tissue Substitute, Percutaneous Endoscopic Approach

UD07Z Supplement Left Hand Muscle with Autologous Tissue Substitute, Open Approach

UD0JZ Supplement Left Hand Muscle with Synthetic Substitute, Open Approach

UD0KZ Supplement Left Hand Muscle with Nonautologous Tissue Substitute, Open Approach

UD47Z Supplement Left Hand Muscle with Autologous Tissue Substitute, Percutaneous Endoscopic Approach

UD4JZ Supplement Left Hand Muscle with Synthetic Substitute, Percutaneous Endoscopic Approach

UD4KZ Supplement Left Hand Muscle with Nonautologous Tissue Substitute, Percutaneous Endoscopic Approach

UF07Z Supplement Right Trunk Muscle with Autologous Tissue Substitute, Open Approach

UF0JZ Supplement Right Trunk Muscle with Synthetic Substitute, Open Approach

UF0KZ Supplement Right Trunk Muscle with Nonautologous Tissue Substitute, Open Approach

UF47Z Supplement Right Trunk Muscle with Autologous Tissue Substitute, Percutaneous Endoscopic Approach

UF4JZ Supplement Right Trunk Muscle with Synthetic Substitute, Percutaneous Endoscopic Approach

UF4KZ Supplement Right Trunk Muscle with Nonautologous Tissue Substitute, Percutaneous Endoscopic Approach

UG07Z Supplement Left Trunk Muscle with Autologous Tissue Substitute, Open Approach

UG0JZ Supplement Left Trunk Muscle with Synthetic Substitute, Open Approach

KUG0KZ Supplement Left Trunk Muscle with Nonautologous Tissue Substitute, Open Approach

KUG47Z Supplement Left Trunk Muscle with Autologous Tissue Substitute, Percutaneous Endoscopic Approach

KUG4JZ Supplement Left Trunk Muscle with Synthetic Substitute, Percutaneous Endoscopic Approach

KUG4KZ Supplement Left Trunk Muscle with Nonautologous Tissue Substitute, Percutaneous Endoscopic Approach

KUH07Z Supplement Right Thorax Muscle with Autologous Tissue Substitute, Open Approach

KUH0JZ Supplement Right Thorax Muscle with Synthetic Substitute, Open Approach

0KUH0KZ Supplement Right Thorax Muscle with Nonautologous Tissue Substitute, Open Approach

0KUH47Z Supplement Right Thorax Muscle with Autologous Tissue Substitute, Percutaneous Endoscopic Approach

0KUH4JZ Supplement Right Thorax Muscle with Synthetic Substitute, Percutaneous Endoscopic Approach

0KUH4KZ Supplement Right Thorax Muscle with Nonautologous Tissue Substitute, Percutaneous Endoscopic Approach

0KUJ07Z Supplement Left Thorax Muscle with Autologous Tissue Substitute, Open Approach

0KUJ0JZ Supplement Left Thorax Muscle with Synthetic Substitute, Open Approach

0KUJ0KZ Supplement Left Thorax Muscle with Nonautologous Tissue Substitute, Open Approach

0KUJ47Z Supplement Left Thorax Muscle with Autologous Tissue Substitute, Percutaneous Endoscopic Approach

0KUJ4JZ Supplement Left Thorax Muscle with Synthetic Substitute, Percutaneous Endoscopic Approach

0KUJ4KZ Supplement Left Thorax Muscle with Nonautologous Tissue Substitute, Percutaneous Endoscopic Approach

0KUK07Z Supplement Right Abdomen Muscle with Autologous Tissue Substitute, Open Approach

0KUK0JZ Supplement Right Abdomen Muscle with Synthetic Substitute, Open Approach

0KUK0KZ Supplement Right Abdomen Muscle with Nonautologous Tissue Substitute, Open Approach

0KUK47Z Supplement Right Abdomen Muscle with Autologous Tissue Substitute, Percutaneous Endoscopic Approach

0KUK4JZ Supplement Right Abdomen Muscle with Synthetic Substitute, Percutaneous Endoscopic Approach

0KUK4KZ Supplement Right Abdomen Muscle with Nonautologous Tissue Substitute, Percutaneous Endoscopic Approach

0KUL07Z Supplement Left Abdomen Muscle with Autologous Tissue Substitute, Open Approach

0KUL0JZ Supplement Left Abdomen Muscle with Synthetic Substitute, Open Approach

0KUL0KZ Supplement Left Abdomen Muscle with Nonautologous Tissue Substitute, Open Approach

0KUL47Z Supplement Left Abdomen Muscle with Autologous Tissue Substitute, Percutaneous Endoscopic Approach

0KUL4JZ Supplement Left Abdomen Muscle with Synthetic Substitute, Percutaneous Endoscopic Approach

0KUL4KZ Supplement Left Abdomen Muscle with Nonautologous Tissue Substitute, Percutaneous Endoscopic Approach

0KUM07Z Supplement Perineum Muscle with Autologous Tissue Substitute, Open Approach

0KUM0JZ Supplement Perineum Muscle with Synthetic Substitute, Open Approach

0KUM0KZ Supplement Perineum Muscle with Nonautologous Tissue Substitute, Open Approach

0KUM47Z Supplement Perineum Muscle with Autologous Tissue Substitute, Percutaneous Endoscopic Approach

0KUM4JZ Supplement Perineum Muscle with Synthetic Substitute, Percutaneous Endoscopic Approach

0KUM4KZ Supplement Perineum Muscle with Nonautologous Tissue Substitute, Percutaneous Endoscopic Approach

0KUN07Z Supplement Right Hip Muscle with Autologous Tissue Substitute, Open Approach

0KUN0JZ Supplement Right Hip Muscle with Synthetic Substitute, Open Approach

0KUN0KZ Supplement Right Hip Muscle with Nonautologous Tissue Substitute, Open Approach

0KUN47Z Supplement Right Hip Muscle with Autologous Tissue Substitute, Percutaneous Endoscopic Approach

0KUN4JZ Supplement Right Hip Muscle with Synthetic Substitute, Percutaneous Endoscopic Approach

0KUN4KZ Supplement Right Hip Muscle with Nonautologous Tissue Substitute, Percutaneous Endoscopic Approach

0KUP07Z Supplement Left Hip Muscle with Autologous Tissue Substitute, Open Approach

0KUP0JZ Supplement Left Hip Muscle with Synthetic Substitute, Open Approach

0KUP0KZ Supplement Left Hip Muscle with Nonautologous Tissue Substitute, Open Approach

0KUP47Z Supplement Left Hip Muscle with Autologous Tissue Substitute, Percutaneous Endoscopic Approach

0KUP4JZ Supplement Left Hip Muscle with Synthetic Substitute, Percutaneous Endoscopic Approach

0KUP4KZ Supplement Left Hip Muscle with Nonautologous Tissue Substitute, Percutaneous Endoscopic Approach

0KUQ07Z Supplement Right Upper Leg Muscle with Autologous Tissue Substitute, Open Approach

0KUQ0JZ Supplement Right Upper Leg Muscle with Synthetic Substitute, Open Approach

0KUQ0KZ Supplement Right Upper Leg Muscle with Nonautologous Tissue Substitute, Open Approach

0KUQ47Z Supplement Right Upper Leg Muscle with Autologous Tissue Substitute, Percutaneous Endoscopic Approach

0KUQ4JZ Supplement Right Upper Leg Muscle with Synthetic Substitute, Percutaneous Endoscopic Approach

0KUQ4KZ Supplement Right Upper Leg Muscle with Nonautologous Tissue Substitute, Percutaneous Endoscopic Approach

0KUR07Z Supplement Left Upper Leg Muscle with Autologous Tissue Substitute, Open Approach

0KUR0JZ Supplement Left Upper Leg Muscle with Synthetic Substitute, Open Approach

0KUR0KZ Supplement Left Upper Leg Muscle with Nonautologous Tissue Substitute, Open Approach

0KUR47Z Supplement Left Upper Leg Muscle with Autologous Tissue Substitute, Percutaneous Endoscopic Approach

0KUR4JZ Supplement Left Upper Leg Muscle with Synthetic Substitute, Percutaneous Endoscopic Approach

0KUR4KZ Supplement Left Upper Leg Muscle with Nonautologous Tissue Substitute, Percutaneous Endoscopic Approach

0KUS07Z Supplement Right Lower Leg Muscle with Autologous Tissue Substitute, Open Approach

0KUS0JZ Supplement Right Lower Leg Muscle with Synthetic Substitute, Open Approach
0KUS0KZ Supplement Right Lower Leg Muscle with Nonautologous Tissue Substitute, Open Approach
0KUS47Z Supplement Right Lower Leg Muscle with Autologous Tissue Substitute, Percutaneous Endoscopic Approach
0KUS4JZ Supplement Right Lower Leg Muscle with Synthetic Substitute, Percutaneous Endoscopic Approach
0KUS4KZ Supplement Right Lower Leg Muscle with Nonautologous Tissue Substitute, Percutaneous Endoscopic Approach
0KUT07Z Supplement Left Lower Leg Muscle with Autologous Tissue Substitute, Open Approach
0KUT0JZ Supplement Left Lower Leg Muscle with Synthetic Substitute, Open Approach
0KUT0KZ Supplement Left Lower Leg Muscle with Nonautologous Tissue Substitute, Open Approach
0KUT47Z Supplement Left Lower Leg Muscle with Autologous Tissue Substitute, Percutaneous Endoscopic Approach
0KUT4JZ Supplement Left Lower Leg Muscle with Synthetic Substitute, Percutaneous Endoscopic Approach
0KUT4KZ Supplement Left Lower Leg Muscle with Nonautologous Tissue Substitute, Percutaneous Endoscopic Approach
0KUV07Z Supplement Right Foot Muscle with Autologous Tissue Substitute, Open Approach
0KUV0JZ Supplement Right Foot Muscle with Synthetic Substitute, Open Approach
0KUV0KZ Supplement Right Foot Muscle with Nonautologous Tissue Substitute, Open Approach
0KUV47Z Supplement Right Foot Muscle with Autologous Tissue Substitute, Percutaneous Endoscopic Approach
0KUV4JZ Supplement Right Foot Muscle with Synthetic Substitute, Percutaneous Endoscopic Approach
0KUV4KZ Supplement Right Foot Muscle with Nonautologous Tissue Substitute, Percutaneous Endoscopic Approach
0KUW07Z Supplement Left Foot Muscle with Autologous Tissue Substitute, Open Approach
0KUW0JZ Supplement Left Foot Muscle with Synthetic Substitute, Open Approach
0KUW0KZ Supplement Left Foot Muscle with Nonautologous Tissue Substitute, Ope Approach
0KUW47Z Supplement Left Foot Muscle with Autologous Tissue Substitute, Percutaneous Endoscopic Approach
0KUW4JZ Supplement Left Foot Muscle with Synthetic Substitute, Percutaneous Endoscopic Approach
0KUW4KZ Supplement Left Foot Muscle with Nonautologous Tissue Substitute, Percutaneous Endoscopic Approach

0KW – Muscles, Revision

Review Coding Guideline B6.1c

0KWX00Z Revision of Drainage Device in Upper Muscle, Open Approach
0KWX07Z Revision of Autologous Tissue Substitute in Upper Muscle, Open Approach
0KWX0JZ Revision of Synthetic Substitute in Upper Muscle, Open Approach
0KWX0KZ Revision of Nonautologous Tissue Substitute in Upper Muscle, Open Approach
0KWX0MZ Revision of Stimulator Lead in Upper Muscle, Open Approach
0KWX30Z Revision of Drainage Device in Upper Muscle, Percutaneous Approach
0KWX37Z Revision of Autologous Tissue Substitute in Upper Muscle, Percutaneous Approach
0KWX3JZ Revision of Synthetic Substitute in Upper Muscle, Percutaneous Approach
0KWX3KZ Revision of Nonautologous Tissue Substitute in Upper Muscle, Percutaneous Approach
0KWX3MZ Revision of Stimulator Lead in Upper Muscle, Percutaneous Approach
0KWX40Z Revision of Drainage Device in Upper Muscle, Percutaneous Endoscopic Approach
0KWX47Z Revision of Autologous Tissue Substitute in Upper Muscle, Percutaneous Endoscopic Approach
0KWX4JZ Revision of Synthetic Substitute in Upper Muscle, Percutaneous Endoscopic Approach
0KWX4KZ Revision of Nonautologous Tissue Substitute in Upper Muscle, Percutaneous Endoscopic Approach
0KWX4MZ Revision of Stimulator Lead in Upper Muscle, Percutaneous Endoscopic Approach
0KWXX0Z Revision of Drainage Device in Upper Muscle, External Approach
0KWXX7Z Revision of Autologous Tissue Substitute in Upper Muscle, External Approach
0KWXXJZ Revision of Synthetic Substitute in Upper Muscle, External Approach
0KWXXKZ Revision of Nonautologous Tissue Substitute in Upper Muscle, External Approach
0KWXXMZ Revision of Stimulator Lead in Upper Muscle, External Approach
0KWY00Z Revision of Drainage Device in Lower Muscle, Open Approach
0KWY07Z Revision of Autologous Tissue Substitute in Lower Muscle, Open Approach
0KWY0JZ Revision of Synthetic Substitute in Lower Muscle, Open Approach
0KWY0KZ Revision of Nonautologous Tissue Substitute in Lower Muscle, Open Approach
0KWY0MZ Revision of Stimulator Lead in Lower Muscle, Open Approach
0KWY30Z Revision of Drainage Device in Lower Muscle, Percutaneous Approach
0KWY37Z Revision of Autologous Tissue Substitute in Lower Muscle, Percutaneous Approach
0KWY3JZ Revision of Synthetic Substitute in Lower Muscle, Percutaneous Approac
0KWY3KZ Revision of Nonautologous Tissue Substitute in Lower Muscle, Percutaneous Approach
0KWY3MZ Revision of Stimulator Lead in Lower Muscle, Percutaneous Approach
0KWY40Z Revision of Drainage Device in Lower Muscle, Percutaneous Endoscopic Approach
0KWY47Z Revision of Autologous Tissue Substitute in Lower Muscle, Percutaneous Endoscopic Approach
0KWY4JZ Revision of Synthetic Substitute in Lower Muscle, Percutaneous Endoscopic Approach
0KWY4KZ Revision of Nonautologous Tissue Substitute in Lower Muscle, Percutaneous Endoscopic Approach
0KWY4MZ Revision of Stimulator Lead in Lower Muscle, Percutaneous Endoscopic Approach
0KWYX0Z Revision of Drainage Device in Lower Muscle, External Approach
0KWYX7Z Revision of Autologous Tissue Substitute in Lower Muscle, External Approach
0KWYXJZ Revision of Synthetic Substitute in Lower Muscle, External Approach
0KWYXKZ Revision of Nonautologous Tissue Substitute in Lower Muscle, External Approach
0KWYXMZ Revision of Stimulator Lead in Lower Muscle, External Approach

0KX – Muscles, Transfer

0KX00Z0 Transfer Head Muscle with Skin, Open Approach
0KX00Z1 Transfer Head Muscle with Subcutaneous Tissue, Open Approach
0KX00Z2 Transfer Head Muscle with Skin and Subcutaneous Tissue, Open Approach
0KX00ZZ Transfer Head Muscle, Open Approach
0KX04Z0 Transfer Head Muscle with Skin, Percutaneous Endoscopic Approach
0KX04Z1 Transfer Head Muscle with Subcutaneous Tissue, Percutaneous Endoscopic Approach
0KX04Z2 Transfer Head Muscle with Skin and Subcutaneous Tissue, Percutaneous Endoscopic Approach
0KX04ZZ Transfer Head Muscle, Percutaneous Endoscopic Approach
0KX10Z0 Transfer Facial Muscle with Skin, Open Approach
0KX10Z1 Transfer Facial Muscle with Subcutaneous Tissue, Open Approach
0KX10Z2 Transfer Facial Muscle with Skin and Subcutaneous Tissue, Open Approach
0KX10ZZ Transfer Facial Muscle, Open Approach
0KX14Z0 Transfer Facial Muscle with Skin, Percutaneous Endoscopic Approach
0KX14Z1 Transfer Facial Muscle with Subcutaneou Tissue, Percutaneous Endoscopic Approach
0KX14Z2 Transfer Facial Muscle with Skin and Subcutaneous Tissue, Percutaneous Endoscopic Approach
0KX14ZZ Transfer Facial Muscle, Percutaneous Endoscopic Approach
0KX20Z0 Transfer Right Neck Muscle with Skin, Open Approach

K20Z1 Transfer Right Neck Muscle with Subcutaneous Tissue, Open Approach
K20Z2 Transfer Right Neck Muscle with Skin and Subcutaneous Tissue, Open Approach
K20ZZ Transfer Right Neck Muscle, Open Approach
K24Z0 Transfer Right Neck Muscle with Skin, Percutaneous Endoscopic Approach
K24Z1 Transfer Right Neck Muscle with Subcutaneous Tissue, Percutaneous Endoscopic Approach
K24Z2 Transfer Right Neck Muscle with Skin and Subcutaneous Tissue, Percutaneous Endoscopic Approach
K24ZZ Transfer Right Neck Muscle, Percutaneous Endoscopic Approach
X30Z0 Transfer Left Neck Muscle with Skin, Open Approach
X30Z1 Transfer Left Neck Muscle with Subcutaneous Tissue, Open Approach
X30Z2 Transfer Left Neck Muscle with Skin and Subcutaneous Tissue, Open Approach
X30ZZ Transfer Left Neck Muscle, Open Approach
X34Z0 Transfer Left Neck Muscle with Skin, Percutaneous Endoscopic Approach
X34Z1 Transfer Left Neck Muscle with Subcutaneous Tissue, Percutaneous Endoscopic Approach
X34Z2 Transfer Left Neck Muscle with Skin and Subcutaneous Tissue, Percutaneous Endoscopic Approach
X34ZZ Transfer Left Neck Muscle, Percutaneous Endoscopic Approach
X40Z0 Transfer Tongue, Palate, Pharynx Muscle with Skin, Open Approach
X40Z1 Transfer Tongue, Palate, Pharynx Muscle with Subcutaneous Tissue, Open Approach
X40Z2 Transfer Tongue, Palate, Pharynx Muscle with Skin and Subcutaneous Tissue, Open Approach
X40ZZ Transfer Tongue, Palate, Pharynx Muscle, Open Approach
X44Z0 Transfer Tongue, Palate, Pharynx Muscle with Skin, Percutaneous Endoscopic Approach
X44Z1 Transfer Tongue, Palate, Pharynx Muscle with Subcutaneous Tissue, Percutaneous Endoscopic Approach
KX44Z2 Transfer Tongue, Palate, Pharynx Muscle with Skin and Subcutaneous Tissue, Percutaneous Endoscopic Approach
KX44ZZ Transfer Tongue, Palate, Pharynx Muscle, Percutaneous Endoscopic Approach
KX50Z0 Transfer Right Shoulder Muscle with Skin, Open Approach
KX50Z1 Transfer Right Shoulder Muscle with Subcutaneous Tissue, Open Approach
KX50Z2 Transfer Right Shoulder Muscle with Skin and Subcutaneous Tissue, Open Approach
KX50ZZ Transfer Right Shoulder Muscle, Open Approach
KX54Z0 Transfer Right Shoulder Muscle with Skin, Percutaneous Endoscopic Approach
KX54Z1 Transfer Right Shoulder Muscle with Subcutaneous Tissue, Percutaneous Endoscopic Approach
KX54Z2 Transfer Right Shoulder Muscle with Skin and Subcutaneous Tissue, Percutaneous Endoscopic Approach
KX54ZZ Transfer Right Shoulder Muscle, Percutaneous Endoscopic Approach
KX60Z0 Transfer Left Shoulder Muscle with Skin, Open Approach
KX60Z1 Transfer Left Shoulder Muscle with Subcutaneous Tissue, Open Approach
0KX60Z2 Transfer Left Shoulder Muscle with Skin and Subcutaneous Tissue, Open Approach
0KX60ZZ Transfer Left Shoulder Muscle, Open Approach
0KX64Z0 Transfer Left Shoulder Muscle with Skin, Percutaneous Endoscopic Approach
0KX64Z1 Transfer Left Shoulder Muscle with Subcutaneous Tissue, Percutaneous Endoscopic Approach
0KX64Z2 Transfer Left Shoulder Muscle with Skin and Subcutaneous Tissue, Percutaneous Endoscopic Approach
0KX64ZZ Transfer Left Shoulder Muscle, Percutaneous Endoscopic Approach
0KX70Z0 Transfer Right Upper Arm Muscle with Skin, Open Approach
0KX70Z1 Transfer Right Upper Arm Muscle with Subcutaneous Tissue, Open Approach
0KX70Z2 Transfer Right Upper Arm Muscle with Skin and Subcutaneous Tissue, Open Approach
0KX70ZZ Transfer Right Upper Arm Muscle, Open Approach
0KX74Z0 Transfer Right Upper Arm Muscle with Skin, Percutaneous Endoscopic Approach
0KX74Z1 Transfer Right Upper Arm Muscle with Subcutaneous Tissue, Percutaneous Endoscopic Approach
0KX74Z2 Transfer Right Upper Arm Muscle with Skin and Subcutaneous Tissue, Percutaneous Endoscopic Approach
0KX74ZZ Transfer Right Upper Arm Muscle, Percutaneous Endoscopic Approach
0KX80Z0 Transfer Left Upper Arm Muscle with Skin, Open Approach
0KX80Z1 Transfer Left Upper Arm Muscle with Subcutaneous Tissue, Open Approach
0KX80Z2 Transfer Left Upper Arm Muscle with Skin and Subcutaneous Tissue, Open Approach
0KX80ZZ Transfer Left Upper Arm Muscle, Open Approach
0KX84Z0 Transfer Left Upper Arm Muscle with Skin, Percutaneous Endoscopic Approach
0KX84Z1 Transfer Left Upper Arm Muscle with Subcutaneous Tissue, Percutaneous Endoscopic Approach
0KX84Z2 Transfer Left Upper Arm Muscle with Skin and Subcutaneous Tissue, Percutaneous Endoscopic Approach
0KX84ZZ Transfer Left Upper Arm Muscle, Percutaneous Endoscopic Approach
0KX90Z0 Transfer Right Lower Arm and Wrist Muscle with Skin, Open Approach
0KX90Z1 Transfer Right Lower Arm and Wrist Muscle with Subcutaneous Tissue, Open Approach
0KX90Z2 Transfer Right Lower Arm and Wrist Muscle with Skin and Subcutaneous Tissue, Open Approach
0KX90ZZ Transfer Right Lower Arm and Wrist Muscle, Open Approach
0KX94Z0 Transfer Right Lower Arm and Wrist Muscle with Skin, Percutaneous Endoscopic Approach
0KX94Z1 Transfer Right Lower Arm and Wrist Muscle with Subcutaneous Tissue, Percutaneous Endoscopic Approach
0KX94Z2 Transfer Right Lower Arm and Wrist Muscle with Skin and Subcutaneous Tissue, Percutaneous Endoscopic Approach
0KX94ZZ Transfer Right Lower Arm and Wrist Muscle, Percutaneous Endoscopic Approach
0KXB0Z0 Transfer Left Lower Arm and Wrist Muscle with Skin, Open Approach
0KXB0Z1 Transfer Left Lower Arm and Wrist Muscle with Subcutaneous Tissue, Open Approach
0KXB0Z2 Transfer Left Lower Arm and Wrist Muscle with Skin and Subcutaneous Tissue, Open Approach
0KXB0ZZ Transfer Left Lower Arm and Wrist Muscle, Open Approach
0KXB4Z0 Transfer Left Lower Arm and Wrist Muscle with Skin, Percutaneous Endoscopic Approach
0KXB4Z1 Transfer Left Lower Arm and Wrist Muscle with Subcutaneous Tissue, Percutaneous Endoscopic Approach
0KXB4Z2 Transfer Left Lower Arm and Wrist Muscle with Skin and Subcutaneous Tissue, Percutaneous Endoscopic Approach
0KXB4ZZ Transfer Left Lower Arm and Wrist Muscle, Percutaneous Endoscopic Approach
0KXC0Z0 Transfer Right Hand Muscle with Skin, Open Approach
0KXC0Z1 Transfer Right Hand Muscle with Subcutaneous Tissue, Open Approach
0KXC0Z2 Transfer Right Hand Muscle with Skin and Subcutaneous Tissue, Open Approach
0KXC0ZZ Transfer Right Hand Muscle, Open Approach
0KXC4Z0 Transfer Right Hand Muscle with Skin, Percutaneous Endoscopic Approach
0KXC4Z1 Transfer Right Hand Muscle with Subcutaneous Tissue, Percutaneous Endoscopic Approach
0KXC4Z2 Transfer Right Hand Muscle with Skin and Subcutaneous Tissue, Percutaneous Endoscopic Approach
0KXC4ZZ Transfer Right Hand Muscle, Percutaneous Endoscopic Approach
0KXD0Z0 Transfer Left Hand Muscle with Skin, Open Approach
0KXD0Z1 Transfer Left Hand Muscle with Subcutaneous Tissue, Open Approach
0KXD0Z2 Transfer Left Hand Muscle with Skin and Subcutaneous Tissue, Open Approach
0KXD0ZZ Transfer Left Hand Muscle, Open Approach
0KXD4Z0 Transfer Left Hand Muscle with Skin, Percutaneous Endoscopic Approach
0KXD4Z1 Transfer Left Hand Muscle with Subcutaneous Tissue, Percutaneous Endoscopic Approach
0KXD4Z2 Transfer Left Hand Muscle with Skin and Subcutaneous Tissue, Percutaneous Endoscopic Approach
0KXD4ZZ Transfer Left Hand Muscle, Percutaneous Endoscopic Approach
0KXF0Z0 Transfer Right Trunk Muscle with Skin, Open Approach
0KXF0Z1 Transfer Right Trunk Muscle with Subcutaneous Tissue, Open Approach
0KXF0Z2 Transfer Right Trunk Muscle with Skin and Subcutaneous Tissue, Open Approach
0KXF0ZZ Transfer Right Trunk Muscle, Open Approach
0KXF4Z0 Transfer Right Trunk Muscle with Skin, Percutaneous Endoscopic Approach
0KXF4Z1 Transfer Right Trunk Muscle with Subcutaneous Tissue, Percutaneous Endoscopic Approach
0KXF4Z2 Transfer Right Trunk Muscle with Skin and Subcutaneous Tissue, Percutaneous Endoscopic Approach

0KXF4ZZ Transfer Right Trunk Muscle, Percutaneous Endoscopic Approach
0KXG0Z0 Transfer Left Trunk Muscle with Skin, Open Approach
0KXG0Z1 Transfer Left Trunk Muscle with Subcutaneous Tissue, Open Approach
0KXG0Z2 Transfer Left Trunk Muscle with Skin and Subcutaneous Tissue, Open Approach
0KXG0ZZ Transfer Left Trunk Muscle, Open Approach
0KXG4Z0 Transfer Left Trunk Muscle with Skin, Percutaneous Endoscopic Approach
0KXG4Z1 Transfer Left Trunk Muscle with Subcutaneous Tissue, Percutaneous Endoscopic Approach
0KXG4Z2 Transfer Left Trunk Muscle with Skin and Subcutaneous Tissue, Percutaneous Endoscopic Approach
0KXG4ZZ Transfer Left Trunk Muscle, Percutaneous Endoscopic Approach
0KXH0Z0 Transfer Right Thorax Muscle with Skin, Open Approach
0KXH0Z1 Transfer Right Thorax Muscle with Subcutaneous Tissue, Open Approach
0KXH0Z2 Transfer Right Thorax Muscle with Skin and Subcutaneous Tissue, Open Approach
0KXH0ZZ Transfer Right Thorax Muscle, Open Approach
0KXH4Z0 Transfer Right Thorax Muscle with Skin, Percutaneous Endoscopic Approach
0KXH4Z1 Transfer Right Thorax Muscle with Subcutaneous Tissue, Percutaneous Endoscopic Approach
0KXH4Z2 Transfer Right Thorax Muscle with Skin and Subcutaneous Tissue, Percutaneous Endoscopic Approach
0KXH4ZZ Transfer Right Thorax Muscle, Percutaneous Endoscopic Approach
0KXJ0Z0 Transfer Left Thorax Muscle with Skin, Open Approach
0KXJ0Z1 Transfer Left Thorax Muscle with Subcutaneous Tissue, Open Approach
0KXJ0Z2 Transfer Left Thorax Muscle with Skin and Subcutaneous Tissue, Open Approach
0KXJ0ZZ Transfer Left Thorax Muscle, Open Approach
0KXJ4Z0 Transfer Left Thorax Muscle with Skin, Percutaneous Endoscopic Approach
0KXJ4Z1 Transfer Left Thorax Muscle with Subcutaneous Tissue, Percutaneous Endoscopic Approach
0KXJ4Z2 Transfer Left Thorax Muscle with Skin and Subcutaneous Tissue, Percutaneous Endoscopic Approach
0KXJ4ZZ Transfer Left Thorax Muscle, Percutaneous Endoscopic Approach
0KXK0Z0 Transfer Right Abdomen Muscle with Skin, Open Approach
0KXK0Z1 Transfer Right Abdomen Muscle with Subcutaneous Tissue, Open Approach
0KXK0Z2 Transfer Right Abdomen Muscle with Skin and Subcutaneous Tissue, Open Approach
0KXK0Z6 Transfer Right Abdomen Muscle, Transverse Rectus Abdominis Myocutaneous Flap, Open Approach
0KXK0ZZ Transfer Right Abdomen Muscle, Open Approach
0KXK4Z0 Transfer Right Abdomen Muscle with Skin, Percutaneous Endoscopic Approach
0KXK4Z1 Transfer Right Abdomen Muscle with Subcutaneous Tissue, Percutaneous Endoscopic Approach
0KXK4Z2 Transfer Right Abdomen Muscle with Skin and Subcutaneous Tissue, Percutaneous Endoscopic Approach
0KXK4Z6 Transfer Right Abdomen Muscle, Transverse Rectus Abdominis Myocutaneous Flap, Percutaneous Endoscopic Approach
0KXK4ZZ Transfer Right Abdomen Muscle, Percutaneous Endoscopic Approach
0KXL0Z0 Transfer Left Abdomen Muscle with Skin, Open Approach
0KXL0Z1 Transfer Left Abdomen Muscle with Subcutaneous Tissue, Open Approach
0KXL0Z2 Transfer Left Abdomen Muscle with Skin and Subcutaneous Tissue, Open Approach
0KXL0Z6 Transfer Left Abdomen Muscle, Transverse Rectus Abdominis Myocutaneous Flap, Open Approach
AHA CC: 2Q, 2014, 10-11
0KXL0ZZ Transfer Left Abdomen Muscle, Open Approach
0KXL4Z0 Transfer Left Abdomen Muscle with Skin, Percutaneous Endoscopic Approach
0KXL4Z1 Transfer Left Abdomen Muscle with Subcutaneous Tissue, Percutaneous Endoscopic Approach
0KXL4Z2 Transfer Left Abdomen Muscle with Skin and Subcutaneous Tissue, Percutaneous Endoscopic Approach
0KXL4Z6 Transfer Left Abdomen Muscle, Transverse Rectus Abdominis Myocutaneous Flap, Percutaneous Endoscopic Approach
0KXL4ZZ Transfer Left Abdomen Muscle, Percutaneous Endoscopic Approach
0KXM0Z0 Transfer Perineum Muscle with Skin, Open Approach
0KXM0Z1 Transfer Perineum Muscle with Subcutaneous Tissue, Open Approach
0KXM0Z2 Transfer Perineum Muscle with Skin and Subcutaneous Tissue, Open Approach
0KXM0ZZ Transfer Perineum Muscle, Open Approach
0KXM4Z0 Transfer Perineum Muscle with Skin, Percutaneous Endoscopic Approach
0KXM4Z1 Transfer Perineum Muscle with Subcutaneous Tissue, Percutaneous Endoscopic Approach
0KXM4Z2 Transfer Perineum Muscle with Skin and Subcutaneous Tissue, Percutaneous Endoscopic Approach
0KXM4ZZ Transfer Perineum Muscle, Percutaneous Endoscopic Approach
0KXN0Z0 Transfer Right Hip Muscle with Skin, Open Approach
0KXN0Z1 Transfer Right Hip Muscle with Subcutaneous Tissue, Open Approach
0KXN0Z2 Transfer Right Hip Muscle with Skin and Subcutaneous Tissue, Open Approach
0KXN0ZZ Transfer Right Hip Muscle, Open Approach
0KXN4Z0 Transfer Right Hip Muscle with Skin, Percutaneous Endoscopic Approach
0KXN4Z1 Transfer Right Hip Muscle with Subcutaneous Tissue, Percutaneous Endoscopic Approach
0KXN4Z2 Transfer Right Hip Muscle with Skin and Subcutaneous Tissue, Percutaneous Endoscopic Approach
0KXN4ZZ Transfer Right Hip Muscle, Percutaneous Endoscopic Approach
0KXP0Z0 Transfer Left Hip Muscle with Skin, Open Approach
0KXP0Z1 Transfer Left Hip Muscle with Subcutaneous Tissue, Open Approach
0KXP0Z2 Transfer Left Hip Muscle with Skin an[d] Subcutaneous Tissue, Open Approach
0KXP0ZZ Transfer Left Hip Muscle, Open Approach
0KXP4Z0 Transfer Left Hip Muscle with Skin, Percutaneous Endoscopic Approach
0KXP4Z1 Transfer Left Hip Muscle with Subcutaneous Tissue, Percutaneous Endoscopic Approach
0KXP4Z2 Transfer Left Hip Muscle with Skin and Subcutaneous Tissue, Percutaneou[s] Endoscopic Approach
0KXP4ZZ Transfer Left Hip Muscle, Percutaneou[s] Endoscopic Approach
0KXQ0Z0 Transfer Right Upper Leg Muscle with Skin, Open Approach
0KXQ0Z1 Transfer Right Upper Leg Muscle with Subcutaneous Tissue, Open Approach
0KXQ0Z2 Transfer Right Upper Leg Muscle with Skin and Subcutaneous Tissue, Open Approach
0KXQ0ZZ Transfer Right Upper Leg Muscle, Ope[n] Approach
0KXQ4Z0 Transfer Right Upper Leg Muscle with Skin, Percutaneous Endoscopic Approach
0KXQ4Z1 Transfer Right Upper Leg Muscle with Subcutaneous Tissue, Percutaneous Endoscopic Approach
0KXQ4Z2 Transfer Right Upper Leg Muscle with Skin and Subcutaneous Tissue, Percutaneous Endoscopic Approach
0KXQ4ZZ Transfer Right Upper Leg Muscle, Percutaneous Endoscopic Approach
0KXR0Z0 Transfer Left Upper Leg Muscle with Skin, Open Approach
0KXR0Z1 Transfer Left Upper Leg Muscle with Subcutaneous Tissue, Open Approach
0KXR0Z2 Transfer Left Upper Leg Muscle with Skin and Subcutaneous Tissue, Open Approach
0KXR0ZZ Transfer Left Upper Leg Muscle, Open Approach
0KXR4Z0 Transfer Left Upper Leg Muscle with Skin, Percutaneous Endoscopic Approach
0KXR4Z1 Transfer Left Upper Leg Muscle with Subcutaneous Tissue, Percutaneous Endoscopic Approach
0KXR4Z2 Transfer Left Upper Leg Muscle with Skin and Subcutaneous Tissue, Percutaneous Endoscopic Approach
0KXR4ZZ Transfer Left Upper Leg Muscle, Percutaneous Endoscopic Approach
0KXS0Z0 Transfer Right Lower Leg Muscle with Skin, Open Approach
0KXS0Z1 Transfer Right Lower Leg Muscle with Subcutaneous Tissue, Open Approach
0KXS0Z2 Transfer Right Lower Leg Muscle with Skin and Subcutaneous Tissue, Open Approach
0KXS0ZZ Transfer Right Lower Leg Muscle, Open Approach
0KXS4Z0 Transfer Right Lower Leg Muscle with Skin, Percutaneous Endoscopic Approac[h]
0KXS4Z1 Transfer Right Lower Leg Muscle with Subcutaneous Tissue, Percutaneous Endoscopic Approach
0KXS4Z2 Transfer Right Lower Leg Muscle with Skin and Subcutaneous Tissue, Percutaneous Endoscopic Approach
0KXS4ZZ Transfer Right Lower Leg Muscle, Percutaneous Endoscopic Approach
0KXT0Z0 Transfer Left Lower Leg Muscle with Skin, Open Approach
0KXT0Z1 Transfer Left Lower Leg Muscle with Subcutaneous Tissue, Open Approach

XT0Z2 Transfer Left Lower Leg Muscle with Skin and Subcutaneous Tissue, Open Approach

XT0ZZ Transfer Left Lower Leg Muscle, Open Approach

XT4Z0 Transfer Left Lower Leg Muscle with Skin, Percutaneous Endoscopic Approach

XT4Z1 Transfer Left Lower Leg Muscle with Subcutaneous Tissue, Percutaneous Endoscopic Approach

XT4Z2 Transfer Left Lower Leg Muscle with Skin and Subcutaneous Tissue, Percutaneous Endoscopic Approach

XT4ZZ Transfer Left Lower Leg Muscle, Percutaneous Endoscopic Approach

XV0Z0 Transfer Right Foot Muscle with Skin, Open Approach

0KXV0Z1 Transfer Right Foot Muscle with Subcutaneous Tissue, Open Approach

0KXV0Z2 Transfer Right Foot Muscle with Skin and Subcutaneous Tissue, Open Approach

0KXV0ZZ Transfer Right Foot Muscle, Open Approach

0KXV4Z0 Transfer Right Foot Muscle with Skin, Percutaneous Endoscopic Approach

0KXV4Z1 Transfer Right Foot Muscle with Subcutaneous Tissue, Percutaneous Endoscopic Approach

0KXV4Z2 Transfer Right Foot Muscle with Skin and Subcutaneous Tissue, Percutaneous Endoscopic Approach

0KXV4ZZ Transfer Right Foot Muscle, Percutaneous Endoscopic Approach

0KXW0Z0 Transfer Left Foot Muscle with Skin, Open Approach

0KXW0Z1 Transfer Left Foot Muscle with Subcutaneous Tissue, Open Approach

0KXW0Z2 Transfer Left Foot Muscle with Skin and Subcutaneous Tissue, Open Approach

0KXW0ZZ Transfer Left Foot Muscle, Open Approach

0KXW4Z0 Transfer Left Foot Muscle with Skin, Percutaneous Endoscopic Approach

0KXW4Z1 Transfer Left Foot Muscle with Subcutaneous Tissue, Percutaneous Endoscopic Approach

0KXW4Z2 Transfer Left Foot Muscle with Skin and Subcutaneous Tissue, Percutaneous Endoscopic Approach

0KXW4ZZ Transfer Left Foot Muscle, Percutaneous Endoscopic Approach

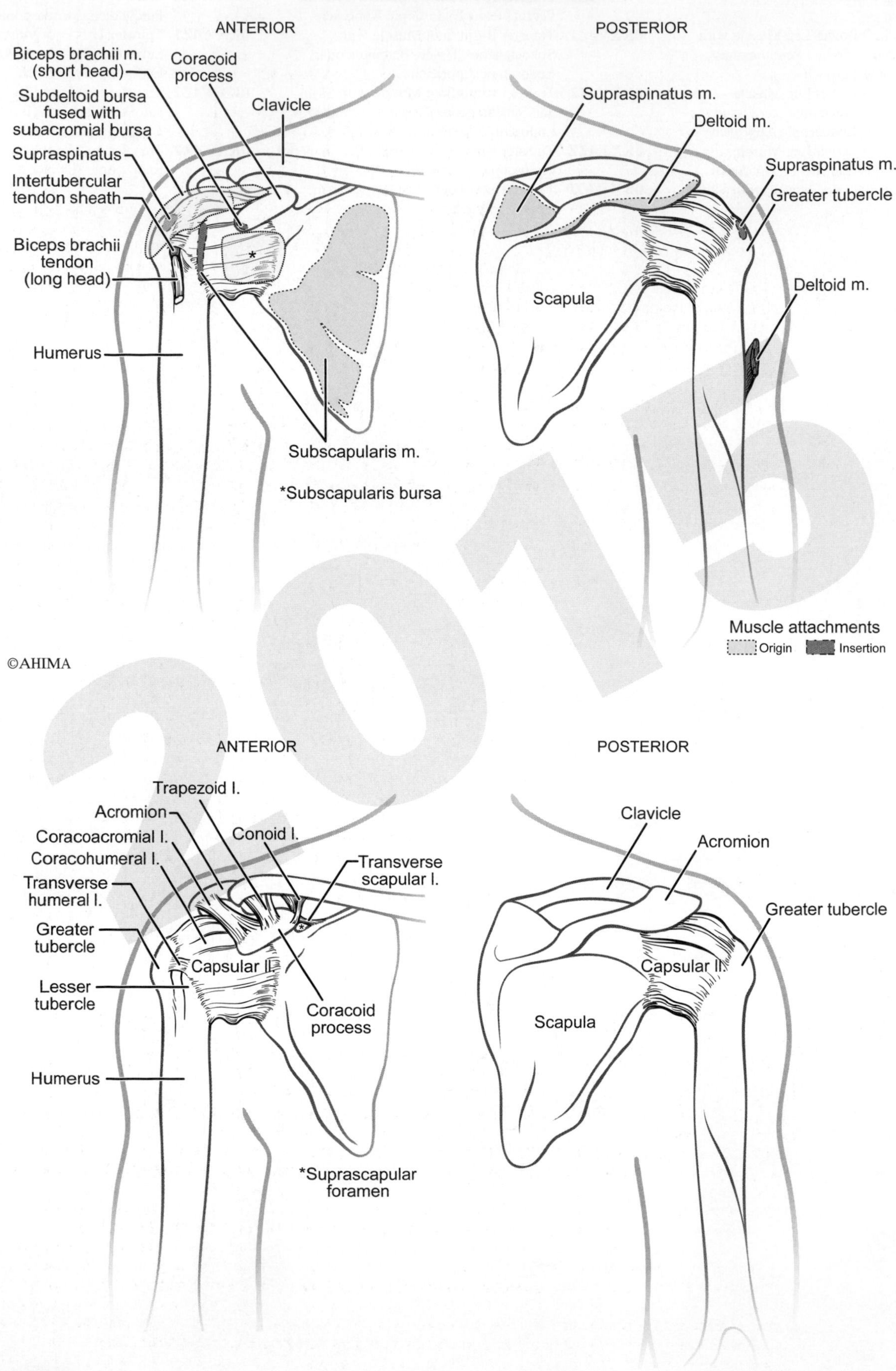
Shoulder Tendons and Ligaments
ANTERIOR
POSTERIOR
Biceps brachii m. (short head)
Coracoid process
Subdeltoid bursa fused with subacromial bursa
Clavicle
Supraspinatus
Intertubercular tendon sheath
Biceps brachii tendon (long head)
Humerus
Subscapularis m.
*Subscapularis bursa
Supraspinatus m.
Deltoid m.
Supraspinatus m.
Greater tubercle
Scapula
Deltoid m.
Muscle attachments
Origin
Insertion
©AHIMA
ANTERIOR
POSTERIOR
Trapezoid l.
Acromion
Coracoacromial l.
Conoid l.
Coracohumeral l.
Transverse scapular l.
Transverse humeral l.
Greater tubercle
Capsular ll.
Lesser tubercle
Coracoid process
Humerus
*Suprascapular foramen
Clavicle
Acromion
Greater tubercle
Capsular ll.
Scapula
©AHIMA

Hip Tendons and Ligaments

ANTERIOR

Anterior sacroiliac l.
Iliopectinea bursa
Pubofemoral l.
Iliofemoral l.
Greater trochanter
Lesser trochanter
Intertrochanteric line

POSTERIOR

Posterior sacroiliac ll.
**Sacrospinous l.
Iliotibial band
Acetabular labrum
Iliofemoral l.
Ischiofemoral l.
Greater trochanter
Zona orbicularis
Protrusion of synovial membrane
Lesser trochanter
*Sacrotuberous l.

Knee Tendons and Ligaments

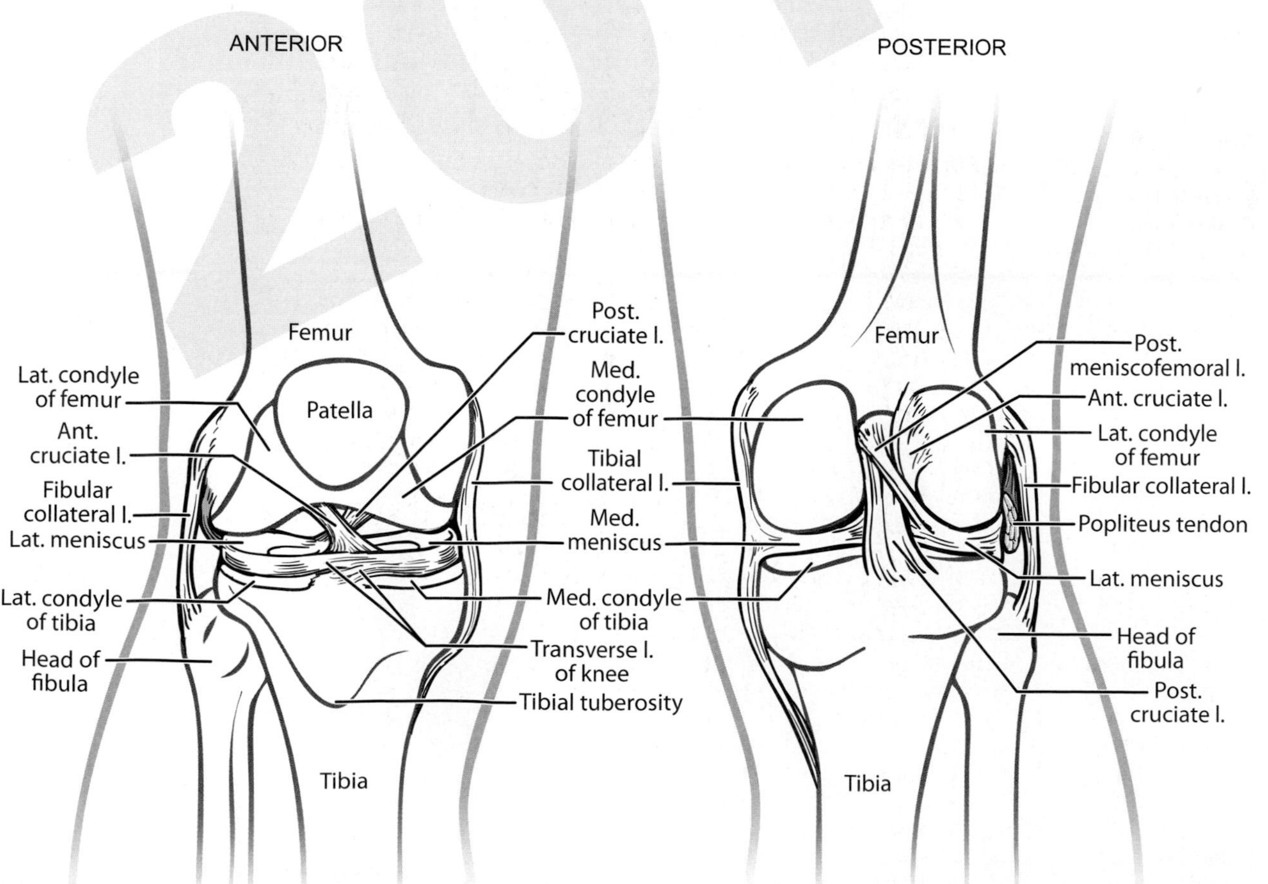

Tendons Tables 0L2–0LX

Section 0 **Medical and Surgical**
Body System L **Tendons**
Operation 2 **Change:** Taking out or off a device from a body part and putting back an identical or similar device in or on the same body part without cutting or puncturing the skin or a mucous membrane

Body Part (4th)	Approach (5th)	Device (6th)	Qualifier (7th)
X Upper Tendon **Y** Lower Tendon	**X** External	**0** Drainage Device **Y** Other Device	**Z** No Qualifier

Section 0 **Medical and Surgical**
Body System L **Tendons**
Operation 5 **Destruction:** Physical eradication of all or a portion of a body part by the direct use of energy, force, or a destructive agent

Body Part (4th)	Approach (5th)	Device (6th)	Qualifier (7th)
0 Head and Neck Tendon **1** Shoulder Tendon, Right **2** Shoulder Tendon, Left **3** Upper Arm Tendon, Right **4** Upper Arm Tendon, Left **5** Lower Arm and Wrist Tendon, Right **6** Lower Arm and Wrist Tendon, Left **7** Hand Tendon, Right **8** Hand Tendon, Left **9** Trunk Tendon, Right **B** Trunk Tendon, Left **C** Thorax Tendon, Right **D** Thorax Tendon, Left **F** Abdomen Tendon, Right **G** Abdomen Tendon, Left **H** Perineum Tendon **J** Hip Tendon, Right **K** Hip Tendon, Left **L** Upper Leg Tendon, Right **M** Upper Leg Tendon, Left **N** Lower Leg Tendon, Right **P** Lower Leg Tendon, Left **Q** Knee Tendon, Right **R** Knee Tendon, Left **S** Ankle Tendon, Right **T** Ankle Tendon, Left **V** Foot Tendon, Right **W** Foot Tendon, Left	**0** Open **3** Percutaneous **4** Percutaneous Endoscopic	**Z** No Device	**Z** No Qualifier

tion	0	**Medical and Surgical**
dy System	L	**Tendons**
eration	8	**Division:** Cutting into a body part, without draining fluids and/or gases from the body part, in order to separate or transect a body part

Body Part (4th)	Approach (5th)	Device (6th)	Qualifier (7th)
Head and Neck Tendon Shoulder Tendon, Right Shoulder Tendon, Left Upper Arm Tendon, Right Upper Arm Tendon, Left Lower Arm and Wrist Tendon, Right Lower Arm and Wrist Tendon, Left Hand Tendon, Right Hand Tendon, Left Trunk Tendon, Right Trunk Tendon, Left Thorax Tendon, Right Thorax Tendon, Left Abdomen Tendon, Right Abdomen Tendon, Left H Perineum Tendon J Hip Tendon, Right K Hip Tendon, Left L Upper Leg Tendon, Right M Upper Leg Tendon, Left N Lower Leg Tendon, Right P Lower Leg Tendon, Left Q Knee Tendon, Right R Knee Tendon, Left S Ankle Tendon, Right T Ankle Tendon, Left V Foot Tendon, Right W Foot Tendon, Left	0 Open 3 Percutaneous 4 Percutaneous Endoscopic	Z No Device	Z No Qualifier

ction	0	**Medical and Surgical**
dy System	L	**Tendons**
peration	9	**Drainage:** Taking or letting out fluids and/or gases from a body part

Body Part (4th)	Approach (5th)	Device (6th)	Qualifier (7th)
0 Head and Neck Tendon 1 Shoulder Tendon, Right 2 Shoulder Tendon, Left 3 Upper Arm Tendon, Right 4 Upper Arm Tendon, Left 5 Lower Arm and Wrist Tendon, Right 6 Lower Arm and Wrist Tendon, Left 7 Hand Tendon, Right 8 Hand Tendon, Left 9 Trunk Tendon, Right B Trunk Tendon, Left C Thorax Tendon, Right D Thorax Tendon, Left F Abdomen Tendon, Right G Abdomen Tendon, Left H Perineum Tendon J Hip Tendon, Right K Hip Tendon, Left L Upper Leg Tendon, Right M Upper Leg Tendon, Left N Lower Leg Tendon, Right P Lower Leg Tendon, Left Q Knee Tendon, Right R Knee Tendon, Left S Ankle Tendon, Right T Ankle Tendon, Left V Foot Tendon, Right W Foot Tendon, Left	0 Open 3 Percutaneous 4 Percutaneous Endoscopic	0 Drainage Device	Z No Qualifier

Continued →

Section 0 **Medical and Surgical**
Body System L **Tendons**
Operation 9 **Drainage:** Taking or letting out fluids and/or gases from a body part

Body Part (4th)	Approach (5th)	Device (6th)	Qualifier (7th)
0 Head and Neck Tendon **1** Shoulder Tendon, Right **2** Shoulder Tendon, Left **3** Upper Arm Tendon, Right **4** Upper Arm Tendon, Left **5** Lower Arm and Wrist Tendon, Right **6** Lower Arm and Wrist Tendon, Left **7** Hand Tendon, Right **8** Hand Tendon, Left **9** Trunk Tendon, Right **B** Trunk Tendon, Left **C** Thorax Tendon, Right **D** Thorax Tendon, Left **F** Abdomen Tendon, Right **G** Abdomen Tendon, Left **H** Perineum Tendon **J** Hip Tendon, Right **K** Hip Tendon, Left **L** Upper Leg Tendon, Right **M** Upper Leg Tendon, Left **N** Lower Leg Tendon, Right **P** Lower Leg Tendon, Left **Q** Knee Tendon, Right **R** Knee Tendon, Left **S** Ankle Tendon, Right **T** Ankle Tendon, Left **V** Foot Tendon, Right **W** Foot Tendon, Left	**0** Open **3** Percutaneous **4** Percutaneous Endoscopic	**Z** No Device	**X** Diagnostic **Z** No Qualifier

Section 0 **Medical and Surgical**
Body System L **Tendons**
Operation B **Excision:** Cutting out or off, without replacement, a portion of a body part

Body Part (4th)	Approach (5th)	Device (6th)	Qualifier (7th)
0 Head and Neck Tendon **1** Shoulder Tendon, Right **2** Shoulder Tendon, Left **3** Upper Arm Tendon, Right **4** Upper Arm Tendon, Left **5** Lower Arm and Wrist Tendon, Right **6** Lower Arm and Wrist Tendon, Left **7** Hand Tendon, Right **8** Hand Tendon, Left **9** Trunk Tendon, Right **B** Trunk Tendon, Left **C** Thorax Tendon, Right **D** Thorax Tendon, Left **F** Abdomen Tendon, Right **G** Abdomen Tendon, Left **H** Perineum Tendon **J** Hip Tendon, Right **K** Hip Tendon, Left **L** Upper Leg Tendon, Right **M** Upper Leg Tendon, Left **N** Lower Leg Tendon, Right **P** Lower Leg Tendon, Left **Q** Knee Tendon, Right **R** Knee Tendon, Left **S** Ankle Tendon, Right **T** Ankle Tendon, Left **V** Foot Tendon, Right **W** Foot Tendon, Left	**0** Open **3** Percutaneous **4** Percutaneous Endoscopic	**Z** No Device	**X** Diagnostic **Z** No Qualifier

Section 0 **Medical and Surgical**
Body System L **Tendons**
Operation C **Extirpation:** Taking or cutting out solid matter from a body part

Body Part (4th)	Approach (5th)	Device (6th)	Qualifier (7th)
0 Head and Neck Tendon **1** Shoulder Tendon, Right **2** Shoulder Tendon, Left **3** Upper Arm Tendon, Right **4** Upper Arm Tendon, Left **5** Lower Arm and Wrist Tendon, Right **6** Lower Arm and Wrist Tendon, Left **7** Hand Tendon, Right **8** Hand Tendon, Left **9** Trunk Tendon, Right **B** Trunk Tendon, Left **C** Thorax Tendon, Right **D** Thorax Tendon, Left **F** Abdomen Tendon, Right **G** Abdomen Tendon, Left **H** Perineum Tendon **J** Hip Tendon, Right **K** Hip Tendon, Left **L** Upper Leg Tendon, Right **M** Upper Leg Tendon, Left **N** Lower Leg Tendon, Right **P** Lower Leg Tendon, Left **Q** Knee Tendon, Right **R** Knee Tendon, Left **S** Ankle Tendon, Right **T** Ankle Tendon, Left **V** Foot Tendon, Right **W** Foot Tendon, Left	**0** Open **3** Percutaneous **4** Percutaneous Endoscopic	**Z** No Device	**Z** No Qualifier

Section 0 **Medical and Surgical**
Body System L **Tendons**
Operation J **Inspection:** Visually and/or manually exploring a body part

Body Part (4th)	Approach (5th)	Device (6th)	Qualifier (7th)
X Upper Tendon **Y** Lower Tendon	**0** Open **3** Percutaneous **4** Percutaneous Endoscopic **X** External	**Z** No Device	**Z** No Qualifier

Section 0 **Medical and Surgical**
Body System L **Tendons**
Operation M **Reattachment:** Putting back in or on all or a portion of a separated body part to its normal location or other suitable location

Body Part (4th)	Approach (5th)	Device (6th)	Qualifier (7th)
0 Head and Neck Tendon **1** Shoulder Tendon, Right **2** Shoulder Tendon, Left **3** Upper Arm Tendon, Right **4** Upper Arm Tendon, Left **5** Lower Arm and Wrist Tendon, Right **6** Lower Arm and Wrist Tendon, Left **7** Hand Tendon, Right **8** Hand Tendon, Left **9** Trunk Tendon, Right **B** Trunk Tendon, Left **C** Thorax Tendon, Right **D** Thorax Tendon, Left **F** Abdomen Tendon, Right **G** Abdomen Tendon, Left **H** Perineum Tendon **J** Hip Tendon, Right **K** Hip Tendon, Left **L** Upper Leg Tendon, Right **M** Upper Leg Tendon, Left **N** Lower Leg Tendon, Right **P** Lower Leg Tendon, Left **Q** Knee Tendon, Right **R** Knee Tendon, Left **S** Ankle Tendon, Right **T** Ankle Tendon, Left **V** Foot Tendon, Right **W** Foot Tendon, Left	**0** Open **4** Percutaneous Endoscopic	**Z** No Device	**Z** No Qualifier

Section 0 **Medical and Surgical**
Body System L **Tendons**
Operation N **Release:** Freeing a body part from an abnormal physical constraint by cutting or by the use of force

Body Part (4th)	Approach (5th)	Device (6th)	Qualifier (7th)
0 Head and Neck Tendon **1** Shoulder Tendon, Right **2** Shoulder Tendon, Left **3** Upper Arm Tendon, Right **4** Upper Arm Tendon, Left **5** Lower Arm and Wrist Tendon, Right **6** Lower Arm and Wrist Tendon, Left **7** Hand Tendon, Right **8** Hand Tendon, Left **9** Trunk Tendon, Right **B** Trunk Tendon, Left **C** Thorax Tendon, Right **D** Thorax Tendon, Left **F** Abdomen Tendon, Right **G** Abdomen Tendon, Left **H** Perineum Tendon **J** Hip Tendon, Right **K** Hip Tendon, Left **L** Upper Leg Tendon, Right **M** Upper Leg Tendon, Left **N** Lower Leg Tendon, Right **P** Lower Leg Tendon, Left **Q** Knee Tendon, Right **R** Knee Tendon, Left **S** Ankle Tendon, Right **T** Ankle Tendon, Left **V** Foot Tendon, Right **W** Foot Tendon, Left	**0** Open **3** Percutaneous **4** Percutaneous Endoscopic **X** External	**Z** No Device	**Z** No Qualifier

tion	0	**Medical and Surgical**
dy System	L	**Tendons**
eration	P	**Removal:** Taking out or off a device from a body part

Body Part (4th)	Approach (5th)	Device (6th)	Qualifier (7th)
X Upper Tendon **Y** Lower Tendon	**0** Open **3** Percutaneous **4** Percutaneous Endoscopic	**0** Drainage Device **7** Autologous Tissue Substitute **J** Synthetic Substitute **K** Nonautologous Tissue Substitute	**Z** No Qualifier
X Upper Tendon **Y** Lower Tendon	**X** External	**0** Drainage Device	**Z** No Qualifier

tion	0	**Medical and Surgical**
dy System	L	**Tendons**
eration	Q	**Repair:** Restoring, to the extent possible, a body part to its normal anatomic structure and function

Body Part (4th)	Approach (5th)	Device (6th)	Qualifier (7th)
0 Head and Neck Tendon **1** Shoulder Tendon, Right **2** Shoulder Tendon, Left **3** Upper Arm Tendon, Right **4** Upper Arm Tendon, Left **5** Lower Arm and Wrist Tendon, Right **6** Lower Arm and Wrist Tendon, Left **7** Hand Tendon, Right **8** Hand Tendon, Left **9** Trunk Tendon, Right **B** Trunk Tendon, Left **C** Thorax Tendon, Right **D** Thorax Tendon, Left **F** Abdomen Tendon, Right **G** Abdomen Tendon, Left **H** Perineum Tendon **J** Hip Tendon, Right **K** Hip Tendon, Left **L** Upper Leg Tendon, Right **M** Upper Leg Tendon, Left **N** Lower Leg Tendon, Right **P** Lower Leg Tendon, Left **Q** Knee Tendon, Right **R** Knee Tendon, Left **S** Ankle Tendon, Right **T** Ankle Tendon, Left **V** Foot Tendon, Right **W** Foot Tendon, Left	**0** Open **3** Percutaneous **4** Percutaneous Endoscopic	**Z** No Device	**Z** No Qualifier

Section 0 **Medical and Surgical**
Body System L **Tendons**
Operation R **Replacement:** Putting in or on biological or synthetic material that physically takes the place and/or function of all or a portion of a body part

Body Part (4th)	Approach (5th)	Device (6th)	Qualifier (7th)
0 Head and Neck Tendon **1** Shoulder Tendon, Right **2** Shoulder Tendon, Left **3** Upper Arm Tendon, Right **4** Upper Arm Tendon, Left **5** Lower Arm and Wrist Tendon, Right **6** Lower Arm and Wrist Tendon, Left **7** Hand Tendon, Right **8** Hand Tendon, Left **9** Trunk Tendon, Right **B** Trunk Tendon, Left **C** Thorax Tendon, Right **D** Thorax Tendon, Left **F** Abdomen Tendon, Right **G** Abdomen Tendon, Left **H** Perineum Tendon **J** Hip Tendon, Right **K** Hip Tendon, Left **L** Upper Leg Tendon, Right **M** Upper Leg Tendon, Left **N** Lower Leg Tendon, Right **P** Lower Leg Tendon, Left **Q** Knee Tendon, Right **R** Knee Tendon, Left **S** Ankle Tendon, Right **T** Ankle Tendon, Left **V** Foot Tendon, Right **W** Foot Tendon, Left	**0** Open **4** Percutaneous Endoscopic	**7** Autologous Tissue Substitute **J** Synthetic Substitute **K** Nonautologous Tissue Substitute	**Z** No Qualifier

Section 0 **Medical and Surgical**
Body System L **Tendons**
Operation S **Reposition:** Moving to its normal location, or other suitable location, all or a portion of a body part

Body Part (4th)	Approach (5th)	Device (6th)	Qualifier (7th)
0 Head and Neck Tendon **1** Shoulder Tendon, Right **2** Shoulder Tendon, Left **3** Upper Arm Tendon, Right **4** Upper Arm Tendon, Left **5** Lower Arm and Wrist Tendon, Right **6** Lower Arm and Wrist Tendon, Left **7** Hand Tendon, Right **8** Hand Tendon, Left **9** Trunk Tendon, Right **B** Trunk Tendon, Left **C** Thorax Tendon, Right **D** Thorax Tendon, Left **F** Abdomen Tendon, Right **G** Abdomen Tendon, Left **H** Perineum Tendon **J** Hip Tendon, Right **K** Hip Tendon, Left **L** Upper Leg Tendon, Right **M** Upper Leg Tendon, Left **N** Lower Leg Tendon, Right **P** Lower Leg Tendon, Left **Q** Knee Tendon, Right **R** Knee Tendon, Left **S** Ankle Tendon, Right **T** Ankle Tendon, Left **V** Foot Tendon, Right **W** Foot Tendon, Left	**0** Open **4** Percutaneous Endoscopic	**Z** No Device	**Z** No Qualifier

tion **0** **Medical and Surgical**
dy System **L** **Tendons**
eration **T** **Resection:** Cutting out or off, without replacement, all of a body part

Body Part (4th)	Approach (5th)	Device (6th)	Qualifier (7th)
Head and Neck Tendon	**0** Open	**Z** No Device	**Z** No Qualifier
Shoulder Tendon, Right	**4** Percutaneous Endoscopic		
Shoulder Tendon, Left			
Upper Arm Tendon, Right			
Upper Arm Tendon, Left			
Lower Arm and Wrist Tendon, Right			
Lower Arm and Wrist Tendon, Left			
Hand Tendon, Right			
Hand Tendon, Left			
Trunk Tendon, Right			
Trunk Tendon, Left			
Thorax Tendon, Right			
Thorax Tendon, Left			
Abdomen Tendon, Right			
Abdomen Tendon, Left			
Perineum Tendon			
Hip Tendon, Right			
K Hip Tendon, Left			
Upper Leg Tendon, Right			
M Upper Leg Tendon, Left			
N Lower Leg Tendon, Right			
P Lower Leg Tendon, Left			
Q Knee Tendon, Right			
R Knee Tendon, Left			
S Ankle Tendon, Right			
T Ankle Tendon, Left			
V Foot Tendon, Right			
W Foot Tendon, Left			

ction **0** **Medical and Surgical**
ody System **L** **Tendons**
peration **U** **Supplement:** Putting in or on biological or synthetic material that physically reinforces and/or augments the function of a portion of a body part

Body Part (4th)	Approach (5th)	Device (6th)	Qualifier (7th)
0 Head and Neck Tendon	**0** Open	**7** Autologous Tissue Substitute	**Z** No Qualifier
1 Shoulder Tendon, Right	**4** Percutaneous Endoscopic	**J** Synthetic Substitute	
2 Shoulder Tendon, Left		**K** Nonautologous Tissue Substitute	
3 Upper Arm Tendon, Right			
4 Upper Arm Tendon, Left			
5 Lower Arm and Wrist Tendon, Right			
6 Lower Arm and Wrist Tendon, Left			
7 Hand Tendon, Right			
8 Hand Tendon, Left			
9 Trunk Tendon, Right			
B Trunk Tendon, Left			
C Thorax Tendon, Right			
D Thorax Tendon, Left			
F Abdomen Tendon, Right			
G Abdomen Tendon, Left			
H Perineum Tendon			
J Hip Tendon, Right			
K Hip Tendon, Left			
L Upper Leg Tendon, Right			
M Upper Leg Tendon, Left			
N Lower Leg Tendon, Right			
P Lower Leg Tendon, Left			
Q Knee Tendon, Right			
R Knee Tendon, Left			
S Ankle Tendon, Right			
T Ankle Tendon, Left			
V Foot Tendon, Right			
W Foot Tendon, Left			

Section 0 Medical and Surgical
Body System L Tendons
Operation W **Revision:** Correcting, to the extent possible, a portion of a malfunctioning device or the position of a displaced device

Body Part (4th)	Approach (5th)	Device (6th)	Qualifier (7th)
X Upper Tendon **Y** Lower Tendon	**0** Open **3** Percutaneous **4** Percutaneous Endoscopic **X** External	**0** Drainage Device **7** Autologous Tissue Substitute **J** Synthetic Substitute **K** Nonautologous Tissue Substitute	**Z** No Qualifier

Section 0 Medical and Surgical
Body System L Tendons
Operation X **Transfer:** Moving, without taking out, all or a portion of a body part to another location to take over the function of all or a portion of a body part

Body Part (4th)	Approach (5th)	Device (6th)	Qualifier (7th)
0 Head and Neck Tendon **1** Shoulder Tendon, Right **2** Shoulder Tendon, Left **3** Upper Arm Tendon, Right **4** Upper Arm Tendon, Left **5** Lower Arm and Wrist Tendon, Right **6** Lower Arm and Wrist Tendon, Left **7** Hand Tendon, Right **8** Hand Tendon, Left **9** Trunk Tendon, Right **B** Trunk Tendon, Left **C** Thorax Tendon, Right **D** Thorax Tendon, Left **F** Abdomen Tendon, Right **G** Abdomen Tendon, Left **H** Perineum Tendon **J** Hip Tendon, Right **K** Hip Tendon, Left **L** Upper Leg Tendon, Right **M** Upper Leg Tendon, Left **N** Lower Leg Tendon, Right **P** Lower Leg Tendon, Left **Q** Knee Tendon, Right **R** Knee Tendon, Left **S** Ankle Tendon, Right **T** Ankle Tendon, Left **V** Foot Tendon, Right **W** Foot Tendon, Left	**0** Open **4** Percutaneous Endoscopic	**Z** No Device	**Z** No Qualifier

Tendons Code Listing 0L2–0LX

Review Coding Guideline B4.5

0L2 – Tendons, Change

Review Coding Guideline B6.1c

0L2XX0Z Change Drainage Device in Upper Tendon, External Approach
0L2XXYZ Change Other Device in Upper Tendon, External Approach
0L2YX0Z Change Drainage Device in Lower Tendon, External Approach
0L2YXYZ Change Other Device in Lower Tendon, External Approach

0L5 – Tendons, Destruction

0L500ZZ Destruction of Head and Neck Tendon, Open Approach
0L503ZZ Destruction of Head and Neck Tendon, Percutaneous Approach
0L504ZZ Destruction of Head and Neck Tendon, Percutaneous Endoscopic Approach
0L510ZZ Destruction of Right Shoulder Tendon, Open Approach
0L513ZZ Destruction of Right Shoulder Tendon, Percutaneous Approach
0L514ZZ Destruction of Right Shoulder Tendon, Percutaneous Endoscopic Approach
0L520ZZ Destruction of Left Shoulder Tendon, Open Approach
0L523ZZ Destruction of Left Shoulder Tendon, Percutaneous Approach
0L524ZZ Destruction of Left Shoulder Tendon, Percutaneous Endoscopic Approach
0L530ZZ Destruction of Right Upper Arm Tendon, Open Approach
0L533ZZ Destruction of Right Upper Arm Tendon, Percutaneous Approach
0L534ZZ Destruction of Right Upper Arm Tendon, Percutaneous Endoscopic Approach
0L540ZZ Destruction of Left Upper Arm Tendon, Open Approach
0L543ZZ Destruction of Left Upper Arm Tendon, Percutaneous Approach

544ZZ Destruction of Left Upper Arm Tendon, Percutaneous Endoscopic Approach
550ZZ Destruction of Right Lower Arm and Wrist Tendon, Open Approach
553ZZ Destruction of Right Lower Arm and Wrist Tendon, Percutaneous Approach
554ZZ Destruction of Right Lower Arm and Wrist Tendon, Percutaneous Endoscopic Approach
560ZZ Destruction of Left Lower Arm and Wrist Tendon, Open Approach
563ZZ Destruction of Left Lower Arm and Wrist Tendon, Percutaneous Approach
564ZZ Destruction of Left Lower Arm and Wrist Tendon, Percutaneous Endoscopic Approach
570ZZ Destruction of Right Hand Tendon, Open Approach
573ZZ Destruction of Right Hand Tendon, Percutaneous Approach
574ZZ Destruction of Right Hand Tendon, Percutaneous Endoscopic Approach
580ZZ Destruction of Left Hand Tendon, Open Approach
583ZZ Destruction of Left Hand Tendon, Percutaneous Approach
L584ZZ Destruction of Left Hand Tendon, Percutaneous Endoscopic Approach
L590ZZ Destruction of Right Trunk Tendon, Open Approach
L593ZZ Destruction of Right Trunk Tendon, Percutaneous Approach
L594ZZ Destruction of Right Trunk Tendon, Percutaneous Endoscopic Approach
L5B0ZZ Destruction of Left Trunk Tendon, Open Approach
L5B3ZZ Destruction of Left Trunk Tendon, Percutaneous Approach
L5B4ZZ Destruction of Left Trunk Tendon, Percutaneous Endoscopic Approach
L5C0ZZ Destruction of Right Thorax Tendon, Open Approach
L5C3ZZ Destruction of Right Thorax Tendon, Percutaneous Approach
L5C4ZZ Destruction of Right Thorax Tendon, Percutaneous Endoscopic Approach
L5D0ZZ Destruction of Left Thorax Tendon, Open Approach
0L5D3ZZ Destruction of Left Thorax Tendon, Percutaneous Approach
0L5D4ZZ Destruction of Left Thorax Tendon, Percutaneous Endoscopic Approach
0L5F0ZZ Destruction of Right Abdomen Tendon, Open Approach
0L5F3ZZ Destruction of Right Abdomen Tendon, Percutaneous Approach
0L5F4ZZ Destruction of Right Abdomen Tendon, Percutaneous Endoscopic Approach
0L5G0ZZ Destruction of Left Abdomen Tendon, Open Approach
0L5G3ZZ Destruction of Left Abdomen Tendon, Percutaneous Approach
0L5G4ZZ Destruction of Left Abdomen Tendon, Percutaneous Endoscopic Approach
0L5H0ZZ Destruction of Perineum Tendon, Open Approach
0L5H3ZZ Destruction of Perineum Tendon, Percutaneous Approach
0L5H4ZZ Destruction of Perineum Tendon, Percutaneous Endoscopic Approach
0L5J0ZZ Destruction of Right Hip Tendon, Open Approach
0L5J3ZZ Destruction of Right Hip Tendon, Percutaneous Approach
0L5J4ZZ Destruction of Right Hip Tendon, Percutaneous Endoscopic Approach
0L5K0ZZ Destruction of Left Hip Tendon, Open Approach
0L5K3ZZ Destruction of Left Hip Tendon, Percutaneous Approach
0L5K4ZZ Destruction of Left Hip Tendon, Percutaneous Endoscopic Approach
0L5L0ZZ Destruction of Right Upper Leg Tendon, Open Approach
0L5L3ZZ Destruction of Right Upper Leg Tendon, Percutaneous Approach
0L5L4ZZ Destruction of Right Upper Leg Tendon, Percutaneous Endoscopic Approach
0L5M0ZZ Destruction of Left Upper Leg Tendon, Open Approach
0L5M3ZZ Destruction of Left Upper Leg Tendon, Percutaneous Approach
0L5M4ZZ Destruction of Left Upper Leg Tendon, Percutaneous Endoscopic Approach
0L5N0ZZ Destruction of Right Lower Leg Tendon, Open Approach
0L5N3ZZ Destruction of Right Lower Leg Tendon, Percutaneous Approach
0L5N4ZZ Destruction of Right Lower Leg Tendon, Percutaneous Endoscopic Approach
0L5P0ZZ Destruction of Left Lower Leg Tendon, Open Approach
0L5P3ZZ Destruction of Left Lower Leg Tendon, Percutaneous Approach
0L5P4ZZ Destruction of Left Lower Leg Tendon, Percutaneous Endoscopic Approach
0L5Q0ZZ Destruction of Right Knee Tendon, Open Approach
0L5Q3ZZ Destruction of Right Knee Tendon, Percutaneous Approach
0L5Q4ZZ Destruction of Right Knee Tendon, Percutaneous Endoscopic Approach
0L5R0ZZ Destruction of Left Knee Tendon, Open Approach
0L5R3ZZ Destruction of Left Knee Tendon, Percutaneous Approach
0L5R4ZZ Destruction of Left Knee Tendon, Percutaneous Endoscopic Approach
0L5S0ZZ Destruction of Right Ankle Tendon, Open Approach
0L5S3ZZ Destruction of Right Ankle Tendon, Percutaneous Approach
0L5S4ZZ Destruction of Right Ankle Tendon, Percutaneous Endoscopic Approach
0L5T0ZZ Destruction of Left Ankle Tendon, Open Approach
0L5T3ZZ Destruction of Left Ankle Tendon, Percutaneous Approach
0L5T4ZZ Destruction of Left Ankle Tendon, Percutaneous Endoscopic Approach
0L5V0ZZ Destruction of Right Foot Tendon, Open Approach
0L5V3ZZ Destruction of Right Foot Tendon, Percutaneous Approach
0L5V4ZZ Destruction of Right Foot Tendon, Percutaneous Endoscopic Approach
0L5W0ZZ Destruction of Left Foot Tendon, Open Approach
0L5W3ZZ Destruction of Left Foot Tendon, Percutaneous Approach
0L5W4ZZ Destruction of Left Foot Tendon, Percutaneous Endoscopic Approach

)L8 – Tendons, Division

Review Coding Guideline B3.14

L800ZZ Division of Head and Neck Tendon, Open Approach
L803ZZ Division of Head and Neck Tendon, Percutaneous Approach
L804ZZ Division of Head and Neck Tendon, Percutaneous Endoscopic Approach
L810ZZ Division of Right Shoulder Tendon, Open Approach
)L813ZZ Division of Right Shoulder Tendon, Percutaneous Approach
L814ZZ Division of Right Shoulder Tendon, Percutaneous Endoscopic Approach
)L820ZZ Division of Left Shoulder Tendon, Open Approach
0L823ZZ Division of Left Shoulder Tendon, Percutaneous Approach
0L824ZZ Division of Left Shoulder Tendon, Percutaneous Endoscopic Approach
0L830ZZ Division of Right Upper Arm Tendon, Open Approach
0L833ZZ Division of Right Upper Arm Tendon, Percutaneous Approach
0L834ZZ Division of Right Upper Arm Tendon, Percutaneous Endoscopic Approach
0L840ZZ Division of Left Upper Arm Tendon, Open Approach
0L843ZZ Division of Left Upper Arm Tendon, Percutaneous Approach
0L844ZZ Division of Left Upper Arm Tendon, Percutaneous Endoscopic Approach
0L850ZZ Division of Right Lower Arm and Wrist Tendon, Open Approach
0L853ZZ Division of Right Lower Arm and Wrist Tendon, Percutaneous Approach
0L854ZZ Division of Right Lower Arm and Wrist Tendon, Percutaneous Endoscopic Approach
0L860ZZ Division of Left Lower Arm and Wrist Tendon, Open Approach
0L863ZZ Division of Left Lower Arm and Wrist Tendon, Percutaneous Approach
0L864ZZ Division of Left Lower Arm and Wrist Tendon, Percutaneous Endoscopic Approach
0L870ZZ Division of Right Hand Tendon, Open Approach
0L873ZZ Division of Right Hand Tendon, Percutaneous Approach
0L874ZZ Division of Right Hand Tendon, Percutaneous Endoscopic Approach
0L880ZZ Division of Left Hand Tendon, Open Approach
0L883ZZ Division of Left Hand Tendon, Percutaneous Approach
0L884ZZ Division of Left Hand Tendon, Percutaneous Endoscopic Approach
0L890ZZ Division of Right Trunk Tendon, Open Approach
0L893ZZ Division of Right Trunk Tendon, Percutaneous Approach
0L894ZZ Division of Right Trunk Tendon, Percutaneous Endoscopic Approach
0L8B0ZZ Division of Left Trunk Tendon, Open Approach
0L8B3ZZ Division of Left Trunk Tendon, Percutaneous Approach

0L8B4ZZ Division of Left Trunk Tendon, Percutaneous Endoscopic Approach
0L8C0ZZ Division of Right Thorax Tendon, Open Approach
0L8C3ZZ Division of Right Thorax Tendon, Percutaneous Approach
0L8C4ZZ Division of Right Thorax Tendon, Percutaneous Endoscopic Approach
0L8D0ZZ Division of Left Thorax Tendon, Open Approach
0L8D3ZZ Division of Left Thorax Tendon, Percutaneous Approach
0L8D4ZZ Division of Left Thorax Tendon, Percutaneous Endoscopic Approach
0L8F0ZZ Division of Right Abdomen Tendon, Open Approach
0L8F3ZZ Division of Right Abdomen Tendon, Percutaneous Approach
0L8F4ZZ Division of Right Abdomen Tendon, Percutaneous Endoscopic Approach
0L8G0ZZ Division of Left Abdomen Tendon, Open Approach
0L8G3ZZ Division of Left Abdomen Tendon, Percutaneous Approach
0L8G4ZZ Division of Left Abdomen Tendon, Percutaneous Endoscopic Approach
0L8H0ZZ Division of Perineum Tendon, Open Approach
0L8H3ZZ Division of Perineum Tendon, Percutaneous Approach
0L8H4ZZ Division of Perineum Tendon, Percutaneous Endoscopic Approach
0L8J0ZZ Division of Right Hip Tendon, Open Approach
0L8J3ZZ Division of Right Hip Tendon, Percutaneous Approach
0L8J4ZZ Division of Right Hip Tendon, Percutaneous Endoscopic Approach
0L8K0ZZ Division of Left Hip Tendon, Open Approach
0L8K3ZZ Division of Left Hip Tendon, Percutaneous Approach
0L8K4ZZ Division of Left Hip Tendon, Percutaneous Endoscopic Approach
0L8L0ZZ Division of Right Upper Leg Tendon, Open Approach
0L8L3ZZ Division of Right Upper Leg Tendon, Percutaneous Approach
0L8L4ZZ Division of Right Upper Leg Tendon, Percutaneous Endoscopic Approach
0L8M0ZZ Division of Left Upper Leg Tendon, Open Approach
0L8M3ZZ Division of Left Upper Leg Tendon, Percutaneous Approach
0L8M4ZZ Division of Left Upper Leg Tendon, Percutaneous Endoscopic Approach
0L8N0ZZ Division of Right Lower Leg Tendon, Open Approach
0L8N3ZZ Division of Right Lower Leg Tendon, Percutaneous Approach
0L8N4ZZ Division of Right Lower Leg Tendon, Percutaneous Endoscopic Approach
0L8P0ZZ Division of Left Lower Leg Tendon, Open Approach
0L8P3ZZ Division of Left Lower Leg Tendon, Percutaneous Approach
0L8P4ZZ Division of Left Lower Leg Tendon, Percutaneous Endoscopic Approach
0L8Q0ZZ Division of Right Knee Tendon, Open Approach
0L8Q3ZZ Division of Right Knee Tendon, Percutaneous Approach
0L8Q4ZZ Division of Right Knee Tendon, Percutaneous Endoscopic Approach
0L8R0ZZ Division of Left Knee Tendon, Open Approach
0L8R3ZZ Division of Left Knee Tendon, Percutaneous Approach
0L8R4ZZ Division of Left Knee Tendon, Percutaneous Endoscopic Approach
0L8S0ZZ Division of Right Ankle Tendon, Open Approach
0L8S3ZZ Division of Right Ankle Tendon, Percutaneous Approach
0L8S4ZZ Division of Right Ankle Tendon, Percutaneous Endoscopic Approach
0L8T0ZZ Division of Left Ankle Tendon, Open Approach
0L8T3ZZ Division of Left Ankle Tendon, Percutaneous Approach
0L8T4ZZ Division of Left Ankle Tendon, Percutaneous Endoscopic Approach
0L8V0ZZ Division of Right Foot Tendon, Open Approach
0L8V3ZZ Division of Right Foot Tendon, Percutaneous Approach
0L8V4ZZ Division of Right Foot Tendon, Percutaneous Endoscopic Approach
0L8W0ZZ Division of Left Foot Tendon, Open Approach
0L8W3ZZ Division of Left Foot Tendon, Percutaneous Approach
0L8W4ZZ Division of Left Foot Tendon, Percutaneous Endoscopic Approach

0L9 – Tendons, Drainage

Review Coding Guidelines B3.4a and B3.4b

Review Coding Guideline B6.2

0L9000Z Drainage of Head and Neck Tendon with Drainage Device, Open Approach
0L900ZX Drainage of Head and Neck Tendon, Open Approach, Diagnostic
0L900ZZ Drainage of Head and Neck Tendon, Open Approach
0L9030Z Drainage of Head and Neck Tendon with Drainage Device, Percutaneous Approach
0L903ZX Drainage of Head and Neck Tendon, Percutaneous Approach, Diagnostic
0L903ZZ Drainage of Head and Neck Tendon, Percutaneous Approach
0L9040Z Drainage of Head and Neck Tendon with Drainage Device, Percutaneous Endoscopic Approach
0L904ZX Drainage of Head and Neck Tendon, Percutaneous Endoscopic Approach, Diagnostic
0L904ZZ Drainage of Head and Neck Tendon, Percutaneous Endoscopic Approach
0L9100Z Drainage of Right Shoulder Tendon with Drainage Device, Open Approach
0L910ZX Drainage of Right Shoulder Tendon, Open Approach, Diagnostic
0L910ZZ Drainage of Right Shoulder Tendon, Open Approach
0L9130Z Drainage of Right Shoulder Tendon with Drainage Device, Percutaneous Approach
0L913ZX Drainage of Right Shoulder Tendon, Percutaneous Approach, Diagnostic
0L913ZZ Drainage of Right Shoulder Tendon, Percutaneous Approach
0L9140Z Drainage of Right Shoulder Tendon with Drainage Device, Percutaneous Endoscopic Approach
0L914ZX Drainage of Right Shoulder Tendon, Percutaneous Endoscopic Approach, Diagnostic
0L914ZZ Drainage of Right Shoulder Tendon, Percutaneous Endoscopic Approach
0L9200Z Drainage of Left Shoulder Tendon with Drainage Device, Open Approach
0L920ZX Drainage of Left Shoulder Tendon, Open Approach, Diagnostic
0L920ZZ Drainage of Left Shoulder Tendon, Open Approach
0L9230Z Drainage of Left Shoulder Tendon with Drainage Device, Percutaneous Approach
0L923ZX Drainage of Left Shoulder Tendon, Percutaneous Approach, Diagnostic
0L923ZZ Drainage of Left Shoulder Tendon, Percutaneous Approach
0L9240Z Drainage of Left Shoulder Tendon with Drainage Device, Percutaneous Endoscopic Approach
0L924ZX Drainage of Left Shoulder Tendon, Percutaneous Endoscopic Approach, Diagnostic
0L924ZZ Drainage of Left Shoulder Tendon, Percutaneous Endoscopic Approach
0L9300Z Drainage of Right Upper Arm Tendon with Drainage Device, Open Approach
0L930ZX Drainage of Right Upper Arm Tendon, Open Approach, Diagnostic
0L930ZZ Drainage of Right Upper Arm Tendon, Open Approach
0L9330Z Drainage of Right Upper Arm Tendon with Drainage Device, Percutaneous Approach
0L933ZX Drainage of Right Upper Arm Tendon, Percutaneous Approach, Diagnostic
0L933ZZ Drainage of Right Upper Arm Tendon, Percutaneous Approach
0L9340Z Drainage of Right Upper Arm Tendon with Drainage Device, Percutaneous Endoscopic Approach
0L934ZX Drainage of Right Upper Arm Tendon, Percutaneous Endoscopic Approach, Diagnostic
0L934ZZ Drainage of Right Upper Arm Tendon, Percutaneous Endoscopic Approach
0L9400Z Drainage of Left Upper Arm Tendon with Drainage Device, Open Approach
0L940ZX Drainage of Left Upper Arm Tendon, Open Approach, Diagnostic
0L940ZZ Drainage of Left Upper Arm Tendon, Open Approach
0L9430Z Drainage of Left Upper Arm Tendon with Drainage Device, Percutaneous Approach
0L943ZX Drainage of Left Upper Arm Tendon, Percutaneous Approach, Diagnostic
0L943ZZ Drainage of Left Upper Arm Tendon, Percutaneous Approach
0L9440Z Drainage of Left Upper Arm Tendon with Drainage Device, Percutaneous Endoscopic Approach
0L944ZX Drainage of Left Upper Arm Tendon, Percutaneous Endoscopic Approach, Diagnostic
0L944ZZ Drainage of Left Upper Arm Tendon, Percutaneous Endoscopic Approach

9500Z Drainage of Right Lower Arm and Wrist Tendon with Drainage Device, Open Approach
950ZX Drainage of Right Lower Arm and Wrist Tendon, Open Approach, Diagnostic
950ZZ Drainage of Right Lower Arm and Wrist Tendon, Open Approach
9530Z Drainage of Right Lower Arm and Wrist Tendon with Drainage Device, Percutaneous Approach
953ZX Drainage of Right Lower Arm and Wrist Tendon, Percutaneous Approach, Diagnostic
953ZZ Drainage of Right Lower Arm and Wrist Tendon, Percutaneous Approach
9540Z Drainage of Right Lower Arm and Wrist Tendon with Drainage Device, Percutaneous Endoscopic Approach
954ZX Drainage of Right Lower Arm and Wrist Tendon, Percutaneous Endoscopic Approach, Diagnostic
954ZZ Drainage of Right Lower Arm and Wrist Tendon, Percutaneous Endoscopic Approach
9600Z Drainage of Left Lower Arm and Wrist Tendon with Drainage Device, Open Approach
960ZX Drainage of Left Lower Arm and Wrist Tendon, Open Approach, Diagnostic
960ZZ Drainage of Left Lower Arm and Wrist Tendon, Open Approach
9630Z Drainage of Left Lower Arm and Wrist Tendon with Drainage Device, Percutaneous Approach
963ZX Drainage of Left Lower Arm and Wrist Tendon, Percutaneous Approach, Diagnostic
963ZZ Drainage of Left Lower Arm and Wrist Tendon, Percutaneous Approach
9640Z Drainage of Left Lower Arm and Wrist Tendon with Drainage Device, Percutaneous Endoscopic Approach
L964ZX Drainage of Left Lower Arm and Wrist Tendon, Percutaneous Endoscopic Approach, Diagnostic
L964ZZ Drainage of Left Lower Arm and Wrist Tendon, Percutaneous Endoscopic Approach
L9700Z Drainage of Right Hand Tendon with Drainage Device, Open Approach
L970ZX Drainage of Right Hand Tendon, Open Approach, Diagnostic
L970ZZ Drainage of Right Hand Tendon, Open Approach
L9730Z Drainage of Right Hand Tendon with Drainage Device, Percutaneous Approach
L973ZX Drainage of Right Hand Tendon, Percutaneous Approach, Diagnostic
L973ZZ Drainage of Right Hand Tendon, Percutaneous Approach
L9740Z Drainage of Right Hand Tendon with Drainage Device, Percutaneous Endoscopic Approach
L974ZX Drainage of Right Hand Tendon, Percutaneous Endoscopic Approach, Diagnostic
L974ZZ Drainage of Right Hand Tendon, Percutaneous Endoscopic Approach
L9800Z Drainage of Left Hand Tendon with Drainage Device, Open Approach
L980ZX Drainage of Left Hand Tendon, Open Approach, Diagnostic
L980ZZ Drainage of Left Hand Tendon, Open Approach
L9830Z Drainage of Left Hand Tendon with Drainage Device, Percutaneous Approach
0L983ZX Drainage of Left Hand Tendon, Percutaneous Approach, Diagnostic
0L983ZZ Drainage of Left Hand Tendon, Percutaneous Approach
0L9840Z Drainage of Left Hand Tendon with Drainage Device, Percutaneous Endoscopic Approach
0L984ZX Drainage of Left Hand Tendon, Percutaneous Endoscopic Approach, Diagnostic
0L984ZZ Drainage of Left Hand Tendon, Percutaneous Endoscopic Approach
0L9900Z Drainage of Right Trunk Tendon with Drainage Device, Open Approach
0L990ZX Drainage of Right Trunk Tendon, Open Approach, Diagnostic
0L990ZZ Drainage of Right Trunk Tendon, Open Approach
0L9930Z Drainage of Right Trunk Tendon with Drainage Device, Percutaneous Approach
0L993ZX Drainage of Right Trunk Tendon, Percutaneous Approach, Diagnostic
0L993ZZ Drainage of Right Trunk Tendon, Percutaneous Approach
0L9940Z Drainage of Right Trunk Tendon with Drainage Device, Percutaneous Endoscopic Approach
0L994ZX Drainage of Right Trunk Tendon, Percutaneous Endoscopic Approach, Diagnostic
0L994ZZ Drainage of Right Trunk Tendon, Percutaneous Endoscopic Approach
0L9B00Z Drainage of Left Trunk Tendon with Drainage Device, Open Approach
0L9B0ZX Drainage of Left Trunk Tendon, Open Approach, Diagnostic
0L9B0ZZ Drainage of Left Trunk Tendon, Open Approach
0L9B30Z Drainage of Left Trunk Tendon with Drainage Device, Percutaneous Approach
0L9B3ZX Drainage of Left Trunk Tendon, Percutaneous Approach, Diagnostic
0L9B3ZZ Drainage of Left Trunk Tendon, Percutaneous Approach
0L9B40Z Drainage of Left Trunk Tendon with Drainage Device, Percutaneous Endoscopic Approach
0L9B4ZX Drainage of Left Trunk Tendon, Percutaneous Endoscopic Approach, Diagnostic
0L9B4ZZ Drainage of Left Trunk Tendon, Percutaneous Endoscopic Approach
0L9C00Z Drainage of Right Thorax Tendon with Drainage Device, Open Approach
0L9C0ZX Drainage of Right Thorax Tendon, Open Approach, Diagnostic
0L9C0ZZ Drainage of Right Thorax Tendon, Open Approach
0L9C30Z Drainage of Right Thorax Tendon with Drainage Device, Percutaneous Approach
0L9C3ZX Drainage of Right Thorax Tendon, Percutaneous Approach, Diagnostic
0L9C3ZZ Drainage of Right Thorax Tendon, Percutaneous Approach
0L9C40Z Drainage of Right Thorax Tendon with Drainage Device, Percutaneous Endoscopic Approach
0L9C4ZX Drainage of Right Thorax Tendon, Percutaneous Endoscopic Approach, Diagnostic
0L9C4ZZ Drainage of Right Thorax Tendon, Percutaneous Endoscopic Approach
0L9D00Z Drainage of Left Thorax Tendon with Drainage Device, Open Approach
0L9D0ZX Drainage of Left Thorax Tendon, Open Approach, Diagnostic
0L9D0ZZ Drainage of Left Thorax Tendon, Open Approach
0L9D30Z Drainage of Left Thorax Tendon with Drainage Device, Percutaneous Approach
0L9D3ZX Drainage of Left Thorax Tendon, Percutaneous Approach, Diagnostic
0L9D3ZZ Drainage of Left Thorax Tendon, Percutaneous Approach
0L9D40Z Drainage of Left Thorax Tendon with Drainage Device, Percutaneous Endoscopic Approach
0L9D4ZX Drainage of Left Thorax Tendon, Percutaneous Endoscopic Approach, Diagnostic
0L9D4ZZ Drainage of Left Thorax Tendon, Percutaneous Endoscopic Approach
0L9F00Z Drainage of Right Abdomen Tendon with Drainage Device, Open Approach
0L9F0ZX Drainage of Right Abdomen Tendon, Open Approach, Diagnostic
0L9F0ZZ Drainage of Right Abdomen Tendon, Open Approach
0L9F30Z Drainage of Right Abdomen Tendon with Drainage Device, Percutaneous Approach
0L9F3ZX Drainage of Right Abdomen Tendon, Percutaneous Approach, Diagnostic
0L9F3ZZ Drainage of Right Abdomen Tendon, Percutaneous Approach
0L9F40Z Drainage of Right Abdomen Tendon with Drainage Device, Percutaneous Endoscopic Approach
0L9F4ZX Drainage of Right Abdomen Tendon, Percutaneous Endoscopic Approach, Diagnostic
0L9F4ZZ Drainage of Right Abdomen Tendon, Percutaneous Endoscopic Approach
0L9G00Z Drainage of Left Abdomen Tendon with Drainage Device, Open Approach
0L9G0ZX Drainage of Left Abdomen Tendon, Open Approach, Diagnostic
0L9G0ZZ Drainage of Left Abdomen Tendon, Open Approach
0L9G30Z Drainage of Left Abdomen Tendon with Drainage Device, Percutaneous Approach
0L9G3ZX Drainage of Left Abdomen Tendon, Percutaneous Approach, Diagnostic
0L9G3ZZ Drainage of Left Abdomen Tendon, Percutaneous Approach
0L9G40Z Drainage of Left Abdomen Tendon with Drainage Device, Percutaneous Endoscopic Approach
0L9G4ZX Drainage of Left Abdomen Tendon, Percutaneous Endoscopic Approach, Diagnostic
0L9G4ZZ Drainage of Left Abdomen Tendon, Percutaneous Endoscopic Approach
0L9H00Z Drainage of Perineum Tendon with Drainage Device, Open Approach
0L9H0ZX Drainage of Perineum Tendon, Open Approach, Diagnostic
0L9H0ZZ Drainage of Perineum Tendon, Open Approach
0L9H30Z Drainage of Perineum Tendon with Drainage Device, Percutaneous Approach
0L9H3ZX Drainage of Perineum Tendon, Percutaneous Approach, Diagnostic
0L9H3ZZ Drainage of Perineum Tendon, Percutaneous Approach
0L9H40Z Drainage of Perineum Tendon with Drainage Device, Percutaneous Endoscopic Approach
0L9H4ZX Drainage of Perineum Tendon, Percutaneous Endoscopic Approach, Diagnostic
0L9H4ZZ Drainage of Perineum Tendon, Percutaneous Endoscopic Approach

0L9J00Z Drainage of Right Hip Tendon with Drainage Device, Open Approach
0L9J0ZX Drainage of Right Hip Tendon, Open Approach, Diagnostic
0L9J0ZZ Drainage of Right Hip Tendon, Open Approach
0L9J30Z Drainage of Right Hip Tendon with Drainage Device, Percutaneous Approach
0L9J3ZX Drainage of Right Hip Tendon, Percutaneous Approach, Diagnostic
0L9J3ZZ Drainage of Right Hip Tendon, Percutaneous Approach
0L9J40Z Drainage of Right Hip Tendon with Drainage Device, Percutaneous Endoscopic Approach
0L9J4ZX Drainage of Right Hip Tendon, Percutaneous Endoscopic Approach, Diagnostic
0L9J4ZZ Drainage of Right Hip Tendon, Percutaneous Endoscopic Approach
0L9K00Z Drainage of Left Hip Tendon with Drainage Device, Open Approach
0L9K0ZX Drainage of Left Hip Tendon, Open Approach, Diagnostic
0L9K0ZZ Drainage of Left Hip Tendon, Open Approach
0L9K30Z Drainage of Left Hip Tendon with Drainage Device, Percutaneous Approach
0L9K3ZX Drainage of Left Hip Tendon, Percutaneous Approach, Diagnostic
0L9K3ZZ Drainage of Left Hip Tendon, Percutaneous Approach
0L9K40Z Drainage of Left Hip Tendon with Drainage Device, Percutaneous Endoscopic Approach
0L9K4ZX Drainage of Left Hip Tendon, Percutaneous Endoscopic Approach, Diagnostic
0L9K4ZZ Drainage of Left Hip Tendon, Percutaneous Endoscopic Approach
0L9L00Z Drainage of Right Upper Leg Tendon with Drainage Device, Open Approach
0L9L0ZX Drainage of Right Upper Leg Tendon, Open Approach, Diagnostic
0L9L0ZZ Drainage of Right Upper Leg Tendon, Open Approach
0L9L30Z Drainage of Right Upper Leg Tendon with Drainage Device, Percutaneous Approach
0L9L3ZX Drainage of Right Upper Leg Tendon, Percutaneous Approach, Diagnostic
0L9L3ZZ Drainage of Right Upper Leg Tendon, Percutaneous Approach
0L9L40Z Drainage of Right Upper Leg Tendon with Drainage Device, Percutaneous Endoscopic Approach
0L9L4ZX Drainage of Right Upper Leg Tendon, Percutaneous Endoscopic Approach, Diagnostic
0L9L4ZZ Drainage of Right Upper Leg Tendon, Percutaneous Endoscopic Approach
0L9M00Z Drainage of Left Upper Leg Tendon with Drainage Device, Open Approach
0L9M0ZX Drainage of Left Upper Leg Tendon, Open Approach, Diagnostic
0L9M0ZZ Drainage of Left Upper Leg Tendon, Open Approach
0L9M30Z Drainage of Left Upper Leg Tendon with Drainage Device, Percutaneous Approach
0L9M3ZX Drainage of Left Upper Leg Tendon, Percutaneous Approach, Diagnostic
0L9M3ZZ Drainage of Left Upper Leg Tendon, Percutaneous Approach
0L9M40Z Drainage of Left Upper Leg Tendon with Drainage Device, Percutaneous Endoscopic Approach
0L9M4ZX Drainage of Left Upper Leg Tendon, Percutaneous Endoscopic Approach, Diagnostic
0L9M4ZZ Drainage of Left Upper Leg Tendon, Percutaneous Endoscopic Approach
0L9N00Z Drainage of Right Lower Leg Tendon with Drainage Device, Open Approach
0L9N0ZX Drainage of Right Lower Leg Tendon, Open Approach, Diagnostic
0L9N0ZZ Drainage of Right Lower Leg Tendon, Open Approach
0L9N30Z Drainage of Right Lower Leg Tendon with Drainage Device, Percutaneous Approach
0L9N3ZX Drainage of Right Lower Leg Tendon, Percutaneous Approach, Diagnostic
0L9N3ZZ Drainage of Right Lower Leg Tendon, Percutaneous Approach
0L9N40Z Drainage of Right Lower Leg Tendon with Drainage Device, Percutaneous Endoscopic Approach
0L9N4ZX Drainage of Right Lower Leg Tendon, Percutaneous Endoscopic Approach, Diagnostic
0L9N4ZZ Drainage of Right Lower Leg Tendon, Percutaneous Endoscopic Approach
0L9P00Z Drainage of Left Lower Leg Tendon with Drainage Device, Open Approach
0L9P0ZX Drainage of Left Lower Leg Tendon, Open Approach, Diagnostic
0L9P0ZZ Drainage of Left Lower Leg Tendon, Open Approach
0L9P30Z Drainage of Left Lower Leg Tendon with Drainage Device, Percutaneous Approach
0L9P3ZX Drainage of Left Lower Leg Tendon, Percutaneous Approach, Diagnostic
0L9P3ZZ Drainage of Left Lower Leg Tendon, Percutaneous Approach
0L9P40Z Drainage of Left Lower Leg Tendon with Drainage Device, Percutaneous Endoscopic Approach
0L9P4ZX Drainage of Left Lower Leg Tendon, Percutaneous Endoscopic Approach, Diagnostic
0L9P4ZZ Drainage of Left Lower Leg Tendon, Percutaneous Endoscopic Approach
0L9Q00Z Drainage of Right Knee Tendon with Drainage Device, Open Approach
0L9Q0ZX Drainage of Right Knee Tendon, Open Approach, Diagnostic
0L9Q0ZZ Drainage of Right Knee Tendon, Open Approach
0L9Q30Z Drainage of Right Knee Tendon with Drainage Device, Percutaneous Approach
0L9Q3ZX Drainage of Right Knee Tendon, Percutaneous Approach, Diagnostic
0L9Q3ZZ Drainage of Right Knee Tendon, Percutaneous Approach
0L9Q40Z Drainage of Right Knee Tendon with Drainage Device, Percutaneous Endoscopic Approach
0L9Q4ZX Drainage of Right Knee Tendon, Percutaneous Endoscopic Approach, Diagnostic
0L9Q4ZZ Drainage of Right Knee Tendon, Percutaneous Endoscopic Approach
0L9R00Z Drainage of Left Knee Tendon with Drainage Device, Open Approach
0L9R0ZX Drainage of Left Knee Tendon, Open Approach, Diagnostic
0L9R0ZZ Drainage of Left Knee Tendon, Open Approach
0L9R30Z Drainage of Left Knee Tendon with Drainage Device, Percutaneous Approach
0L9R3ZX Drainage of Left Knee Tendon, Percutaneous Approach, Diagnostic
0L9R3ZZ Drainage of Left Knee Tendon, Percutaneous Approach
0L9R40Z Drainage of Left Knee Tendon with Drainage Device, Percutaneous Endoscopic Approach
0L9R4ZX Drainage of Left Knee Tendon, Percutaneous Endoscopic Approach, Diagnostic
0L9R4ZZ Drainage of Left Knee Tendon, Percutaneous Endoscopic Approach
0L9S00Z Drainage of Right Ankle Tendon with Drainage Device, Open Approach
0L9S0ZX Drainage of Right Ankle Tendon, Open Approach, Diagnostic
0L9S0ZZ Drainage of Right Ankle Tendon, Open Approach
0L9S30Z Drainage of Right Ankle Tendon with Drainage Device, Percutaneous Approach
0L9S3ZX Drainage of Right Ankle Tendon, Percutaneous Approach, Diagnostic
0L9S3ZZ Drainage of Right Ankle Tendon, Percutaneous Approach
0L9S40Z Drainage of Right Ankle Tendon with Drainage Device, Percutaneous Endoscopic Approach
0L9S4ZX Drainage of Right Ankle Tendon, Percutaneous Endoscopic Approach, Diagnostic
0L9S4ZZ Drainage of Right Ankle Tendon, Percutaneous Endoscopic Approach
0L9T00Z Drainage of Left Ankle Tendon with Drainage Device, Open Approach
0L9T0ZX Drainage of Left Ankle Tendon, Open Approach, Diagnostic
0L9T0ZZ Drainage of Left Ankle Tendon, Open Approach
0L9T30Z Drainage of Left Ankle Tendon with Drainage Device, Percutaneous Approach
0L9T3ZX Drainage of Left Ankle Tendon, Percutaneous Approach, Diagnostic
0L9T3ZZ Drainage of Left Ankle Tendon, Percutaneous Approach
0L9T40Z Drainage of Left Ankle Tendon with Drainage Device, Percutaneous Endoscopic Approach
0L9T4ZX Drainage of Left Ankle Tendon, Percutaneous Endoscopic Approach, Diagnostic
0L9T4ZZ Drainage of Left Ankle Tendon, Percutaneous Endoscopic Approach
0L9V00Z Drainage of Right Foot Tendon with Drainage Device, Open Approach
0L9V0ZX Drainage of Right Foot Tendon, Open Approach, Diagnostic
0L9V0ZZ Drainage of Right Foot Tendon, Open Approach
0L9V30Z Drainage of Right Foot Tendon with Drainage Device, Percutaneous Approach
0L9V3ZX Drainage of Right Foot Tendon, Percutaneous Approach, Diagnostic
0L9V3ZZ Drainage of Right Foot Tendon, Percutaneous Approach
0L9V40Z Drainage of Right Foot Tendon with Drainage Device, Percutaneous Endoscopic Approach
0L9V4ZX Drainage of Right Foot Tendon, Percutaneous Endoscopic Approach, Diagnostic
0L9V4ZZ Drainage of Right Foot Tendon, Percutaneous Endoscopic Approach
0L9W00Z Drainage of Left Foot Tendon with Drainage Device, Open Approach
0L9W0ZX Drainage of Left Foot Tendon, Open Approach, Diagnostic
0L9W0ZZ Drainage of Left Foot Tendon, Open Approach
0L9W30Z Drainage of Left Foot Tendon with Drainage Device, Percutaneous Approach

W3ZX Drainage of Left Foot Tendon, Percutaneous Approach, Diagnostic
W3ZZ Drainage of Left Foot Tendon, Percutaneous Approach
0L9W40Z Drainage of Left Foot Tendon with Drainage Device, Percutaneous Endoscopic Approach
0L9W4ZX Drainage of Left Foot Tendon, Percutaneous Endoscopic Approach, Diagnostic
0L9W4ZZ Drainage of Left Foot Tendon, Percutaneous Endoscopic Approach

B – Tendons, Excision

view Coding Guidelines B3.4a and B3.4b

view Coding Guideline B3.5

view Coding Guideline B3.8

B00ZX Excision of Head and Neck Tendon, Open Approach, Diagnostic
B00ZZ Excision of Head and Neck Tendon, Open Approach
B03ZX Excision of Head and Neck Tendon, Percutaneous Approach, Diagnostic
B03ZZ Excision of Head and Neck Tendon, Percutaneous Approach
B04ZX Excision of Head and Neck Tendon, Percutaneous Endoscopic Approach, Diagnostic
B04ZZ Excision of Head and Neck Tendon, Percutaneous Endoscopic Approach
B10ZX Excision of Right Shoulder Tendon, Open Approach, Diagnostic
B10ZZ Excision of Right Shoulder Tendon, Open Approach
B13ZX Excision of Right Shoulder Tendon, Percutaneous Approach, Diagnostic
B13ZZ Excision of Right Shoulder Tendon, Percutaneous Approach
B14ZX Excision of Right Shoulder Tendon, Percutaneous Endoscopic Approach, Diagnostic
B14ZZ Excision of Right Shoulder Tendon, Percutaneous Endoscopic Approach
B20ZX Excision of Left Shoulder Tendon, Open Approach, Diagnostic
LB20ZZ Excision of Left Shoulder Tendon, Open Approach
LB23ZX Excision of Left Shoulder Tendon, Percutaneous Approach, Diagnostic
LB23ZZ Excision of Left Shoulder Tendon, Percutaneous Approach
LB24ZX Excision of Left Shoulder Tendon, Percutaneous Endoscopic Approach, Diagnostic
LB24ZZ Excision of Left Shoulder Tendon, Percutaneous Endoscopic Approach
LB30ZX Excision of Right Upper Arm Tendon, Open Approach, Diagnostic
LB30ZZ Excision of Right Upper Arm Tendon, Open Approach
LB33ZX Excision of Right Upper Arm Tendon, Percutaneous Approach, Diagnostic
LB33ZZ Excision of Right Upper Arm Tendon, Percutaneous Approach
LB34ZX Excision of Right Upper Arm Tendon, Percutaneous Endoscopic Approach, Diagnostic
LB34ZZ Excision of Right Upper Arm Tendon, Percutaneous Endoscopic Approach
LB40ZX Excision of Left Upper Arm Tendon, Open Approach, Diagnostic
LB40ZZ Excision of Left Upper Arm Tendon, Open Approach
LB43ZX Excision of Left Upper Arm Tendon, Percutaneous Approach, Diagnostic
LB43ZZ Excision of Left Upper Arm Tendon, Percutaneous Approach
0LB44ZX Excision of Left Upper Arm Tendon, Percutaneous Endoscopic Approach, Diagnostic
0LB44ZZ Excision of Left Upper Arm Tendon, Percutaneous Endoscopic Approach
0LB50ZX Excision of Right Lower Arm and Wrist Tendon, Open Approach, Diagnostic
0LB50ZZ Excision of Right Lower Arm and Wrist Tendon, Open Approach
0LB53ZX Excision of Right Lower Arm and Wrist Tendon, Percutaneous Approach, Diagnostic
0LB53ZZ Excision of Right Lower Arm and Wrist Tendon, Percutaneous Approach
0LB54ZX Excision of Right Lower Arm and Wrist Tendon, Percutaneous Endoscopic Approach, Diagnostic
0LB54ZZ Excision of Right Lower Arm and Wrist Tendon, Percutaneous Endoscopic Approach
0LB60ZX Excision of Left Lower Arm and Wrist Tendon, Open Approach, Diagnostic
0LB60ZZ Excision of Left Lower Arm and Wrist Tendon, Open Approach
0LB63ZX Excision of Left Lower Arm and Wrist Tendon, Percutaneous Approach, Diagnostic
0LB63ZZ Excision of Left Lower Arm and Wrist Tendon, Percutaneous Approach
0LB64ZX Excision of Left Lower Arm and Wrist Tendon, Percutaneous Endoscopic Approach, Diagnostic
0LB64ZZ Excision of Left Lower Arm and Wrist Tendon, Percutaneous Endoscopic Approach
0LB70ZX Excision of Right Hand Tendon, Open Approach, Diagnostic
0LB70ZZ Excision of Right Hand Tendon, Open Approach
0LB73ZX Excision of Right Hand Tendon, Percutaneous Approach, Diagnostic
0LB73ZZ Excision of Right Hand Tendon, Percutaneous Approach
0LB74ZX Excision of Right Hand Tendon, Percutaneous Endoscopic Approach, Diagnostic
0LB74ZZ Excision of Right Hand Tendon, Percutaneous Endoscopic Approach
0LB80ZX Excision of Left Hand Tendon, Open Approach, Diagnostic
0LB80ZZ Excision of Left Hand Tendon, Open Approach
0LB83ZX Excision of Left Hand Tendon, Percutaneous Approach, Diagnostic
0LB83ZZ Excision of Left Hand Tendon, Percutaneous Approach
0LB84ZX Excision of Left Hand Tendon, Percutaneous Endoscopic Approach, Diagnostic
0LB84ZZ Excision of Left Hand Tendon, Percutaneous Endoscopic Approach
0LB90ZX Excision of Right Trunk Tendon, Open Approach, Diagnostic
0LB90ZZ Excision of Right Trunk Tendon, Open Approach
0LB93ZX Excision of Right Trunk Tendon, Percutaneous Approach, Diagnostic
0LB93ZZ Excision of Right Trunk Tendon, Percutaneous Approach
0LB94ZX Excision of Right Trunk Tendon, Percutaneous Endoscopic Approach, Diagnostic
0LB94ZZ Excision of Right Trunk Tendon, Percutaneous Endoscopic Approach
0LBB0ZX Excision of Left Trunk Tendon, Open Approach, Diagnostic
0LBB0ZZ Excision of Left Trunk Tendon, Open Approach
0LBB3ZX Excision of Left Trunk Tendon, Percutaneous Approach, Diagnostic
0LBB3ZZ Excision of Left Trunk Tendon, Percutaneous Approach
0LBB4ZX Excision of Left Trunk Tendon, Percutaneous Endoscopic Approach, Diagnostic
0LBB4ZZ Excision of Left Trunk Tendon, Percutaneous Endoscopic Approach
0LBC0ZX Excision of Right Thorax Tendon, Open Approach, Diagnostic
0LBC0ZZ Excision of Right Thorax Tendon, Open Approach
0LBC3ZX Excision of Right Thorax Tendon, Percutaneous Approach, Diagnostic
0LBC3ZZ Excision of Right Thorax Tendon, Percutaneous Approach
0LBC4ZX Excision of Right Thorax Tendon, Percutaneous Endoscopic Approach, Diagnostic
0LBC4ZZ Excision of Right Thorax Tendon, Percutaneous Endoscopic Approach
0LBD0ZX Excision of Left Thorax Tendon, Open Approach, Diagnostic
0LBD0ZZ Excision of Left Thorax Tendon, Open Approach
0LBD3ZX Excision of Left Thorax Tendon, Percutaneous Approach, Diagnostic
0LBD3ZZ Excision of Left Thorax Tendon, Percutaneous Approach
0LBD4ZX Excision of Left Thorax Tendon, Percutaneous Endoscopic Approach, Diagnostic
0LBD4ZZ Excision of Left Thorax Tendon, Percutaneous Endoscopic Approach
0LBF0ZX Excision of Right Abdomen Tendon, Open Approach, Diagnostic
0LBF0ZZ Excision of Right Abdomen Tendon, Open Approach
0LBF3ZX Excision of Right Abdomen Tendon, Percutaneous Approach, Diagnostic
0LBF3ZZ Excision of Right Abdomen Tendon, Percutaneous Approach
0LBF4ZX Excision of Right Abdomen Tendon, Percutaneous Endoscopic Approach, Diagnostic
0LBF4ZZ Excision of Right Abdomen Tendon, Percutaneous Endoscopic Approach

0LBG0ZX Excision of Left Abdomen Tendon, Open Approach, Diagnostic
0LBG0ZZ Excision of Left Abdomen Tendon, Open Approach
0LBG3ZX Excision of Left Abdomen Tendon, Percutaneous Approach, Diagnostic
0LBG3ZZ Excision of Left Abdomen Tendon, Percutaneous Approach
0LBG4ZX Excision of Left Abdomen Tendon, Percutaneous Endoscopic Approach, Diagnostic
0LBG4ZZ Excision of Left Abdomen Tendon, Percutaneous Endoscopic Approach
0LBH0ZX Excision of Perineum Tendon, Open Approach, Diagnostic
0LBH0ZZ Excision of Perineum Tendon, Open Approach
0LBH3ZX Excision of Perineum Tendon, Percutaneous Approach, Diagnostic
0LBH3ZZ Excision of Perineum Tendon, Percutaneous Approach
0LBH4ZX Excision of Perineum Tendon, Percutaneous Endoscopic Approach, Diagnostic
0LBH4ZZ Excision of Perineum Tendon, Percutaneous Endoscopic Approach
0LBJ0ZX Excision of Right Hip Tendon, Open Approach, Diagnostic
0LBJ0ZZ Excision of Right Hip Tendon, Open Approach
0LBJ3ZX Excision of Right Hip Tendon, Percutaneous Approach, Diagnostic
0LBJ3ZZ Excision of Right Hip Tendon, Percutaneous Approach
0LBJ4ZX Excision of Right Hip Tendon, Percutaneous Endoscopic Approach, Diagnostic
0LBJ4ZZ Excision of Right Hip Tendon, Percutaneous Endoscopic Approach
0LBK0ZX Excision of Left Hip Tendon, Open Approach, Diagnostic
0LBK0ZZ Excision of Left Hip Tendon, Open Approach
0LBK3ZX Excision of Left Hip Tendon, Percutaneous Approach, Diagnostic
0LBK3ZZ Excision of Left Hip Tendon, Percutaneous Approach
0LBK4ZX Excision of Left Hip Tendon, Percutaneous Endoscopic Approach, Diagnostic
0LBK4ZZ Excision of Left Hip Tendon, Percutaneous Endoscopic Approach
0LBL0ZX Excision of Right Upper Leg Tendon, Open Approach, Diagnostic
0LBL0ZZ Excision of Right Upper Leg Tendon, Open Approach
0LBL3ZX Excision of Right Upper Leg Tendon, Percutaneous Approach, Diagnostic
0LBL3ZZ Excision of Right Upper Leg Tendon, Percutaneous Approach
0LBL4ZX Excision of Right Upper Leg Tendon, Percutaneous Endoscopic Approach, Diagnostic
0LBL4ZZ Excision of Right Upper Leg Tendon, Percutaneous Endoscopic Approach
0LBM0ZX Excision of Left Upper Leg Tendon, Open Approach, Diagnostic
0LBM0ZZ Excision of Left Upper Leg Tendon, Open Approach
0LBM3ZX Excision of Left Upper Leg Tendon, Percutaneous Approach, Diagnostic
0LBM3ZZ Excision of Left Upper Leg Tendon, Percutaneous Approach
0LBM4ZX Excision of Left Upper Leg Tendon, Percutaneous Endoscopic Approach, Diagnostic
0LBM4ZZ Excision of Left Upper Leg Tendon, Percutaneous Endoscopic Approach
0LBN0ZX Excision of Right Lower Leg Tendon, Open Approach, Diagnostic
0LBN0ZZ Excision of Right Lower Leg Tendon, Open Approach
0LBN3ZX Excision of Right Lower Leg Tendon, Percutaneous Approach, Diagnostic
0LBN3ZZ Excision of Right Lower Leg Tendon, Percutaneous Approach
0LBN4ZX Excision of Right Lower Leg Tendon, Percutaneous Endoscopic Approach, Diagnostic
0LBN4ZZ Excision of Right Lower Leg Tendon, Percutaneous Endoscopic Approach
0LBP0ZX Excision of Left Lower Leg Tendon, Open Approach, Diagnostic
0LBP0ZZ Excision of Left Lower Leg Tendon, Open Approach
0LBP3ZX Excision of Left Lower Leg Tendon, Percutaneous Approach, Diagnostic
0LBP3ZZ Excision of Left Lower Leg Tendon, Percutaneous Approach
0LBP4ZX Excision of Left Lower Leg Tendon, Percutaneous Endoscopic Approach, Diagnostic
0LBP4ZZ Excision of Left Lower Leg Tendon, Percutaneous Endoscopic Approach
0LBQ0ZX Excision of Right Knee Tendon, Open Approach, Diagnostic
0LBQ0ZZ Excision of Right Knee Tendon, Open Approach
0LBQ3ZX Excision of Right Knee Tendon, Percutaneous Approach, Diagnostic
0LBQ3ZZ Excision of Right Knee Tendon, Percutaneous Approach
0LBQ4ZX Excision of Right Knee Tendon, Percutaneous Endoscopic Approach, Diagnostic
0LBQ4ZZ Excision of Right Knee Tendon, Percutaneous Endoscopic Approach
0LBR0ZX Excision of Left Knee Tendon, Open Approach, Diagnostic
0LBR0ZZ Excision of Left Knee Tendon, Open Approach
0LBR3ZX Excision of Left Knee Tendon, Percutaneous Approach, Diagnostic
0LBR3ZZ Excision of Left Knee Tendon, Percutaneous Approach
0LBR4ZX Excision of Left Knee Tendon, Percutaneous Endoscopic Approach, Diagnostic
0LBR4ZZ Excision of Left Knee Tendon, Percutaneous Endoscopic Approach
0LBS0ZX Excision of Right Ankle Tendon, Open Approach, Diagnostic
0LBS0ZZ Excision of Right Ankle Tendon, Open Approach
0LBS3ZX Excision of Right Ankle Tendon, Percutaneous Approach, Diagnostic
0LBS3ZZ Excision of Right Ankle Tendon, Percutaneous Approach
0LBS4ZX Excision of Right Ankle Tendon, Percutaneous Endoscopic Approach, Diagnostic
0LBS4ZZ Excision of Right Ankle Tendon, Percutaneous Endoscopic Approach
0LBT0ZX Excision of Left Ankle Tendon, Open Approach, Diagnostic
0LBT0ZZ Excision of Left Ankle Tendon, Open Approach
0LBT3ZX Excision of Left Ankle Tendon, Percutaneous Approach, Diagnostic
0LBT3ZZ Excision of Left Ankle Tendon, Percutaneous Approach
0LBT4ZX Excision of Left Ankle Tendon, Percutaneous Endoscopic Approach, Diagnostic
0LBT4ZZ Excision of Left Ankle Tendon, Percutaneous Endoscopic Approach
0LBV0ZX Excision of Right Foot Tendon, Open Approach, Diagnostic
0LBV0ZZ Excision of Right Foot Tendon, Open Approach
0LBV3ZX Excision of Right Foot Tendon, Percutaneous Approach, Diagnostic
0LBV3ZZ Excision of Right Foot Tendon, Percutaneous Approach
0LBV4ZX Excision of Right Foot Tendon, Percutaneous Endoscopic Approach, Diagnostic
0LBV4ZZ Excision of Right Foot Tendon, Percutaneous Endoscopic Approach
0LBW0ZX Excision of Left Foot Tendon, Open Approach, Diagnostic
0LBW0ZZ Excision of Left Foot Tendon, Open Approach
0LBW3ZX Excision of Left Foot Tendon, Percutaneous Approach, Diagnostic
0LBW3ZZ Excision of Left Foot Tendon, Percutaneous Approach
0LBW4ZX Excision of Left Foot Tendon, Percutaneous Endoscopic Approach, Diagnostic
0LBW4ZZ Excision of Left Foot Tendon, Percutaneous Endoscopic Approach

0LC – Tendons, Extirpation

0LC00ZZ Extirpation of Matter from Head and Neck Tendon, Open Approach
0LC03ZZ Extirpation of Matter from Head and Neck Tendon, Percutaneous Approach
0LC04ZZ Extirpation of Matter from Head and Neck Tendon, Percutaneous Endoscopic Approach
0LC10ZZ Extirpation of Matter from Right Shoulder Tendon, Open Approach
0LC13ZZ Extirpation of Matter from Right Shoulder Tendon, Percutaneous Approach
0LC14ZZ Extirpation of Matter from Right Shoulder Tendon, Percutaneous Endoscopic Approach
0LC20ZZ Extirpation of Matter from Left Shoulder Tendon, Open Approach
0LC23ZZ Extirpation of Matter from Left Shoulder Tendon, Percutaneous Approach
0LC24ZZ Extirpation of Matter from Left Shoulder Tendon, Percutaneous Endoscopic Approach
0LC30ZZ Extirpation of Matter from Right Upper Arm Tendon, Open Approach
0LC33ZZ Extirpation of Matter from Right Upper Arm Tendon, Percutaneous Approach
0LC34ZZ Extirpation of Matter from Right Upper Arm Tendon, Percutaneous Endoscopic Approach
0LC40ZZ Extirpation of Matter from Left Upper Arm Tendon, Open Approach
0LC43ZZ Extirpation of Matter from Left Upper Arm Tendon, Percutaneous Approach

C44ZZ Extirpation of Matter from Left Upper Arm Tendon, Percutaneous Endoscopic Approach

C50ZZ Extirpation of Matter from Right Lower Arm and Wrist Tendon, Open Approach

C53ZZ Extirpation of Matter from Right Lower Arm and Wrist Tendon, Percutaneous Approach

C54ZZ Extirpation of Matter from Right Lower Arm and Wrist Tendon, Percutaneous Endoscopic Approach

C60ZZ Extirpation of Matter from Left Lower Arm and Wrist Tendon, Open Approach

C63ZZ Extirpation of Matter from Left Lower Arm and Wrist Tendon, Percutaneous Approach

C64ZZ Extirpation of Matter from Left Lower Arm and Wrist Tendon, Percutaneous Endoscopic Approach

C70ZZ Extirpation of Matter from Right Hand Tendon, Open Approach

C73ZZ Extirpation of Matter from Right Hand Tendon, Percutaneous Approach

C74ZZ Extirpation of Matter from Right Hand Tendon, Percutaneous Endoscopic Approach

C80ZZ Extirpation of Matter from Left Hand Tendon, Open Approach

C83ZZ Extirpation of Matter from Left Hand Tendon, Percutaneous Approach

C84ZZ Extirpation of Matter from Left Hand Tendon, Percutaneous Endoscopic Approach

LC90ZZ Extirpation of Matter from Right Trunk Tendon, Open Approach

LC93ZZ Extirpation of Matter from Right Trunk Tendon, Percutaneous Approach

LC94ZZ Extirpation of Matter from Right Trunk Tendon, Percutaneous Endoscopic Approach

LCB0ZZ Extirpation of Matter from Left Trunk Tendon, Open Approach

LCB3ZZ Extirpation of Matter from Left Trunk Tendon, Percutaneous Approach

LCB4ZZ Extirpation of Matter from Left Trunk Tendon, Percutaneous Endoscopic Approach

LCC0ZZ Extirpation of Matter from Right Thorax Tendon, Open Approach

LCC3ZZ Extirpation of Matter from Right Thorax Tendon, Percutaneous Approach

LCC4ZZ Extirpation of Matter from Right Thorax Tendon, Percutaneous Endoscopic Approach

LCD0ZZ Extirpation of Matter from Left Thorax Tendon, Open Approach

0LCD3ZZ Extirpation of Matter from Left Thorax Tendon, Percutaneous Approach

0LCD4ZZ Extirpation of Matter from Left Thorax Tendon, Percutaneous Endoscopic Approach

0LCF0ZZ Extirpation of Matter from Right Abdomen Tendon, Open Approach

0LCF3ZZ Extirpation of Matter from Right Abdomen Tendon, Percutaneous Approach

0LCF4ZZ Extirpation of Matter from Right Abdomen Tendon, Percutaneous Endoscopic Approach

0LCG0ZZ Extirpation of Matter from Left Abdomen Tendon, Open Approach

0LCG3ZZ Extirpation of Matter from Left Abdomen Tendon, Percutaneous Approach

0LCG4ZZ Extirpation of Matter from Left Abdomen Tendon, Percutaneous Endoscopic Approach

0LCH0ZZ Extirpation of Matter from Perineum Tendon, Open Approach

0LCH3ZZ Extirpation of Matter from Perineum Tendon, Percutaneous Approach

0LCH4ZZ Extirpation of Matter from Perineum Tendon, Percutaneous Endoscopic Approach

0LCJ0ZZ Extirpation of Matter from Right Hip Tendon, Open Approach

0LCJ3ZZ Extirpation of Matter from Right Hip Tendon, Percutaneous Approach

0LCJ4ZZ Extirpation of Matter from Right Hip Tendon, Percutaneous Endoscopic Approach

0LCK0ZZ Extirpation of Matter from Left Hip Tendon, Open Approach

0LCK3ZZ Extirpation of Matter from Left Hip Tendon, Percutaneous Approach

0LCK4ZZ Extirpation of Matter from Left Hip Tendon, Percutaneous Endoscopic Approach

0LCL0ZZ Extirpation of Matter from Right Upper Leg Tendon, Open Approach

0LCL3ZZ Extirpation of Matter from Right Upper Leg Tendon, Percutaneous Approach

0LCL4ZZ Extirpation of Matter from Right Upper Leg Tendon, Percutaneous Endoscopic Approach

0LCM0ZZ Extirpation of Matter from Left Upper Leg Tendon, Open Approach

0LCM3ZZ Extirpation of Matter from Left Upper Leg Tendon, Percutaneous Approach

0LCM4ZZ Extirpation of Matter from Left Upper Leg Tendon, Percutaneous Endoscopic Approach

0LCN0ZZ Extirpation of Matter from Right Lower Leg Tendon, Open Approach

0LCN3ZZ Extirpation of Matter from Right Lower Leg Tendon, Percutaneous Approach

0LCN4ZZ Extirpation of Matter from Right Lower Leg Tendon, Percutaneous Endoscopic Approach

0LCP0ZZ Extirpation of Matter from Left Lower Leg Tendon, Open Approach

0LCP3ZZ Extirpation of Matter from Left Lower Leg Tendon, Percutaneous Approach

0LCP4ZZ Extirpation of Matter from Left Lower Leg Tendon, Percutaneous Endoscopic Approach

0LCQ0ZZ Extirpation of Matter from Right Knee Tendon, Open Approach

0LCQ3ZZ Extirpation of Matter from Right Knee Tendon, Percutaneous Approach

0LCQ4ZZ Extirpation of Matter from Right Knee Tendon, Percutaneous Endoscopic Approach

0LCR0ZZ Extirpation of Matter from Left Knee Tendon, Open Approach

0LCR3ZZ Extirpation of Matter from Left Knee Tendon, Percutaneous Approach

0LCR4ZZ Extirpation of Matter from Left Knee Tendon, Percutaneous Endoscopic Approach

0LCS0ZZ Extirpation of Matter from Right Ankle Tendon, Open Approach

0LCS3ZZ Extirpation of Matter from Right Ankle Tendon, Percutaneous Approach

0LCS4ZZ Extirpation of Matter from Right Ankle Tendon, Percutaneous Endoscopic Approach

0LCT0ZZ Extirpation of Matter from Left Ankle Tendon, Open Approach

0LCT3ZZ Extirpation of Matter from Left Ankle Tendon, Percutaneous Approach

0LCT4ZZ Extirpation of Matter from Left Ankle Tendon, Percutaneous Endoscopic Approach

0LCV0ZZ Extirpation of Matter from Right Foot Tendon, Open Approach

0LCV3ZZ Extirpation of Matter from Right Foot Tendon, Percutaneous Approach

0LCV4ZZ Extirpation of Matter from Right Foot Tendon, Percutaneous Endoscopic Approach

0LCW0ZZ Extirpation of Matter from Left Foot Tendon, Open Approach

0LCW3ZZ Extirpation of Matter from Left Foot Tendon, Percutaneous Approach

0LCW4ZZ Extirpation of Matter from Left Foot Tendon, Percutaneous Endoscopic Approach

0LJ – Tendons, Inspection

Review Coding Guidelines B3.5

Review Coding Guidelines B3.11a, B3.11b and B3.11c

LJX0ZZ Inspection of Upper Tendon, Open Approach

LJX3ZZ Inspection of Upper Tendon, Percutaneous Approach

0LJX4ZZ Inspection of Upper Tendon, Percutaneous Endoscopic Approach

0LJXXZZ Inspection of Upper Tendon, External Approach

0LJY0ZZ Inspection of Lower Tendon, Open Approach

0LJY3ZZ Inspection of Lower Tendon, Percutaneous Approach

0LJY4ZZ Inspection of Lower Tendon, Percutaneous Endoscopic Approach

0LJYXZZ Inspection of Lower Tendon, External Approach

0LM – Tendons, Reattachment

0LM00ZZ Reattachment of Head and Neck Tendon, Open Approach

0LM04ZZ Reattachment of Head and Neck Tendon, Percutaneous Endoscopic Approach

0LM10ZZ Reattachment of Right Shoulder Tendon, Open Approach

0LM14ZZ Reattachment of Right Shoulder Tendon, Percutaneous Endoscopic Approach

0LM20ZZ Reattachment of Left Shoulder Tendon, Open Approach

0LM24ZZ Reattachment of Left Shoulder Tendon, Percutaneous Endoscopic Approach

0LM30ZZ Reattachment of Right Upper Arm Tendon, Open Approach
0LM34ZZ Reattachment of Right Upper Arm Tendon, Percutaneous Endoscopic Approach
0LM40ZZ Reattachment of Left Upper Arm Tendon, Open Approach
0LM44ZZ Reattachment of Left Upper Arm Tendon, Percutaneous Endoscopic Approach
0LM50ZZ Reattachment of Right Lower Arm and Wrist Tendon, Open Approach
0LM54ZZ Reattachment of Right Lower Arm and Wrist Tendon, Percutaneous Endoscopic Approach
0LM60ZZ Reattachment of Left Lower Arm and Wrist Tendon, Open Approach
0LM64ZZ Reattachment of Left Lower Arm and Wrist Tendon, Percutaneous Endoscopic Approach
0LM70ZZ Reattachment of Right Hand Tendon, Open Approach
0LM74ZZ Reattachment of Right Hand Tendon, Percutaneous Endoscopic Approach
0LM80ZZ Reattachment of Left Hand Tendon, Open Approach
0LM84ZZ Reattachment of Left Hand Tendon, Percutaneous Endoscopic Approach
0LM90ZZ Reattachment of Right Trunk Tendon, Open Approach
0LM94ZZ Reattachment of Right Trunk Tendon, Percutaneous Endoscopic Approach
0LMB0ZZ Reattachment of Left Trunk Tendon, Open Approach
0LMB4ZZ Reattachment of Left Trunk Tendon, Percutaneous Endoscopic Approach
0LMC0ZZ Reattachment of Right Thorax Tendon, Open Approach
0LMC4ZZ Reattachment of Right Thorax Tendon, Percutaneous Endoscopic Approach
0LMD0ZZ Reattachment of Left Thorax Tendon, Open Approach
0LMD4ZZ Reattachment of Left Thorax Tendon, Percutaneous Endoscopic Approach
0LMF0ZZ Reattachment of Right Abdomen Tendon, Open Approach
0LMF4ZZ Reattachment of Right Abdomen Tendon, Percutaneous Endoscopic Approach
0LMG0ZZ Reattachment of Left Abdomen Tendon, Open Approach
0LMG4ZZ Reattachment of Left Abdomen Tendon, Percutaneous Endoscopic Approach
0LMH0ZZ Reattachment of Perineum Tendon, Open Approach
0LMH4ZZ Reattachment of Perineum Tendon, Percutaneous Endoscopic Approach
0LMJ0ZZ Reattachment of Right Hip Tendon, Open Approach
0LMJ4ZZ Reattachment of Right Hip Tendon, Percutaneous Endoscopic Approach
0LMK0ZZ Reattachment of Left Hip Tendon, Open Approach
0LMK4ZZ Reattachment of Left Hip Tendon, Percutaneous Endoscopic Approach
0LML0ZZ Reattachment of Right Upper Leg Tendon, Open Approach
0LML4ZZ Reattachment of Right Upper Leg Tendon, Percutaneous Endoscopic Approach
0LMM0ZZ Reattachment of Left Upper Leg Tendon, Open Approach
0LMM4ZZ Reattachment of Left Upper Leg Tend Percutaneous Endoscopic Approach
0LMN0ZZ Reattachment of Right Lower Leg Tendon, Open Approach
0LMN4ZZ Reattachment of Right Lower Leg Tendon, Percutaneous Endoscopic Approach
0LMP0ZZ Reattachment of Left Lower Leg Tend Open Approach
0LMP4ZZ Reattachment of Left Lower Leg Tend Percutaneous Endoscopic Approach
0LMQ0ZZ Reattachment of Right Knee Tendon, Open Approach
0LMQ4ZZ Reattachment of Right Knee Tendon, Percutaneous Endoscopic Approach
0LMR0ZZ Reattachment of Left Knee Tendon, Open Approach
0LMR4ZZ Reattachment of Left Knee Tendon, Percutaneous Endoscopic Approach
0LMS0ZZ Reattachment of Right Ankle Tendon, Open Approach
0LMS4ZZ Reattachment of Right Ankle Tendon, Percutaneous Endoscopic Approach
0LMT0ZZ Reattachment of Left Ankle Tendon, Open Approach
0LMT4ZZ Reattachment of Left Ankle Tendon, Percutaneous Endoscopic Approach
0LMV0ZZ Reattachment of Right Foot Tendon, Open Approach
0LMV4ZZ Reattachment of Right Foot Tendon, Percutaneous Endoscopic Approach
0LMW0ZZ Reattachment of Left Foot Tendon, Op Approach
0LMW4ZZ Reattachment of Left Foot Tendon, Percutaneous Endoscopic Approach

0LN – Tendons, Release

Review Coding Guideline B3.13

Review Coding Guideline B3.14

0LN00ZZ Release Head and Neck Tendon, Open Approach
0LN03ZZ Release Head and Neck Tendon, Percutaneous Approach
0LN04ZZ Release Head and Neck Tendon, Percutaneous Endoscopic Approach
0LN0XZZ Release Head and Neck Tendon, External Approach
0LN10ZZ Release Right Shoulder Tendon, Open Approach
0LN13ZZ Release Right Shoulder Tendon, Percutaneous Approach
0LN14ZZ Release Right Shoulder Tendon, Percutaneous Endoscopic Approach
0LN1XZZ Release Right Shoulder Tendon, External Approach
0LN20ZZ Release Left Shoulder Tendon, Open Approach
0LN23ZZ Release Left Shoulder Tendon, Percutaneous Approach
0LN24ZZ Release Left Shoulder Tendon, Percutaneous Endoscopic Approach
0LN2XZZ Release Left Shoulder Tendon, External Approach
0LN30ZZ Release Right Upper Arm Tendon, Open Approach
0LN33ZZ Release Right Upper Arm Tendon, Percutaneous Approach
0LN34ZZ Release Right Upper Arm Tendon, Percutaneous Endoscopic Approach
0LN3XZZ Release Right Upper Arm Tendon, External Approach
0LN40ZZ Release Left Upper Arm Tendon, Open Approach
0LN43ZZ Release Left Upper Arm Tendon, Percutaneous Approach
0LN44ZZ Release Left Upper Arm Tendon, Percutaneous Endoscopic Approach
0LN4XZZ Release Left Upper Arm Tendon, External Approach
0LN50ZZ Release Right Lower Arm and Wrist Tendon, Open Approach
0LN53ZZ Release Right Lower Arm and Wrist Tendon, Percutaneous Approach
0LN54ZZ Release Right Lower Arm and Wrist Tendon, Percutaneous Endoscopic Approach
0LN5XZZ Release Right Lower Arm and Wrist Tendon, External Approach
0LN60ZZ Release Left Lower Arm and Wrist Tendon, Open Approach
0LN63ZZ Release Left Lower Arm and Wrist Tendon, Percutaneous Approach
0LN64ZZ Release Left Lower Arm and Wrist Tendon, Percutaneous Endoscopic Approach
0LN6XZZ Release Left Lower Arm and Wrist Tendon, External Approach
0LN70ZZ Release Right Hand Tendon, Open Approach
0LN73ZZ Release Right Hand Tendon, Percutaneous Approach
0LN74ZZ Release Right Hand Tendon, Percutaneous Endoscopic Approach
0LN7XZZ Release Right Hand Tendon, External Approach
0LN80ZZ Release Left Hand Tendon, Open Approach
0LN83ZZ Release Left Hand Tendon, Percutaneous Approach
0LN84ZZ Release Left Hand Tendon, Percutaneous Endoscopic Approach
0LN8XZZ Release Left Hand Tendon, External Approach
0LN90ZZ Release Right Trunk Tendon, Open Approach
0LN93ZZ Release Right Trunk Tendon, Percutaneous Approach
0LN94ZZ Release Right Trunk Tendon, Percutaneous Endoscopic Approach
0LN9XZZ Release Right Trunk Tendon, External Approach
0LNB0ZZ Release Left Trunk Tendon, Open Approach
0LNB3ZZ Release Left Trunk Tendon, Percutaneous Approach
0LNB4ZZ Release Left Trunk Tendon, Percutaneous Endoscopic Approach
0LNBXZZ Release Left Trunk Tendon, External Approach

NC0ZZ Release Right Thorax Tendon, Open Approach
NC3ZZ Release Right Thorax Tendon, Percutaneous Approach
NC4ZZ Release Right Thorax Tendon, Percutaneous Endoscopic Approach
NCXZZ Release Right Thorax Tendon, External Approach
ND0ZZ Release Left Thorax Tendon, Open Approach
ND3ZZ Release Left Thorax Tendon, Percutaneous Approach
ND4ZZ Release Left Thorax Tendon, Percutaneous Endoscopic Approach
NDXZZ Release Left Thorax Tendon, External Approach
NF0ZZ Release Right Abdomen Tendon, Open Approach
NF3ZZ Release Right Abdomen Tendon, Percutaneous Approach
NF4ZZ Release Right Abdomen Tendon, Percutaneous Endoscopic Approach
NFXZZ Release Right Abdomen Tendon, External Approach
NG0ZZ Release Left Abdomen Tendon, Open Approach
NG3ZZ Release Left Abdomen Tendon, Percutaneous Approach
NG4ZZ Release Left Abdomen Tendon, Percutaneous Endoscopic Approach
NGXZZ Release Left Abdomen Tendon, External Approach
NH0ZZ Release Perineum Tendon, Open Approach
NH3ZZ Release Perineum Tendon, Percutaneous Approach
NH4ZZ Release Perineum Tendon, Percutaneous Endoscopic Approach
NHXZZ Release Perineum Tendon, External Approach
NJ0ZZ Release Right Hip Tendon, Open Approach
NJ3ZZ Release Right Hip Tendon, Percutaneous Approach
0LNJ4ZZ Release Right Hip Tendon, Percutaneous Endoscopic Approach
0LNJXZZ Release Right Hip Tendon, External Approach
0LNK0ZZ Release Left Hip Tendon, Open Approach
0LNK3ZZ Release Left Hip Tendon, Percutaneous Approach
0LNK4ZZ Release Left Hip Tendon, Percutaneous Endoscopic Approach
0LNKXZZ Release Left Hip Tendon, External Approach
0LNL0ZZ Release Right Upper Leg Tendon, Open Approach
0LNL3ZZ Release Right Upper Leg Tendon, Percutaneous Approach
0LNL4ZZ Release Right Upper Leg Tendon, Percutaneous Endoscopic Approach
0LNLXZZ Release Right Upper Leg Tendon, External Approach
0LNM0ZZ Release Left Upper Leg Tendon, Open Approach
0LNM3ZZ Release Left Upper Leg Tendon, Percutaneous Approach
0LNM4ZZ Release Left Upper Leg Tendon, Percutaneous Endoscopic Approach
0LNMXZZ Release Left Upper Leg Tendon, External Approach
0LNN0ZZ Release Right Lower Leg Tendon, Open Approach
0LNN3ZZ Release Right Lower Leg Tendon, Percutaneous Approach
0LNN4ZZ Release Right Lower Leg Tendon, Percutaneous Endoscopic Approach
0LNNXZZ Release Right Lower Leg Tendon, External Approach
0LNP0ZZ Release Left Lower Leg Tendon, Open Approach
0LNP3ZZ Release Left Lower Leg Tendon, Percutaneous Approach
0LNP4ZZ Release Left Lower Leg Tendon, Percutaneous Endoscopic Approach
0LNPXZZ Release Left Lower Leg Tendon, External Approach
0LNQ0ZZ Release Right Knee Tendon, Open Approach
0LNQ3ZZ Release Right Knee Tendon, Percutaneous Approach
0LNQ4ZZ Release Right Knee Tendon, Percutaneous Endoscopic Approach
0LNQXZZ Release Right Knee Tendon, External Approach
0LNR0ZZ Release Left Knee Tendon, Open Approach
0LNR3ZZ Release Left Knee Tendon, Percutaneous Approach
0LNR4ZZ Release Left Knee Tendon, Percutaneous Endoscopic Approach
0LNRXZZ Release Left Knee Tendon, External Approach
0LNS0ZZ Release Right Ankle Tendon, Open Approach
0LNS3ZZ Release Right Ankle Tendon, Percutaneous Approach
0LNS4ZZ Release Right Ankle Tendon, Percutaneous Endoscopic Approach
0LNSXZZ Release Right Ankle Tendon, External Approach
0LNT0ZZ Release Left Ankle Tendon, Open Approach
0LNT3ZZ Release Left Ankle Tendon, Percutaneous Approach
0LNT4ZZ Release Left Ankle Tendon, Percutaneous Endoscopic Approach
0LNTXZZ Release Left Ankle Tendon, External Approach
0LNV0ZZ Release Right Foot Tendon, Open Approach
0LNV3ZZ Release Right Foot Tendon, Percutaneous Approach
0LNV4ZZ Release Right Foot Tendon, Percutaneous Endoscopic Approach
0LNVXZZ Release Right Foot Tendon, External Approach
0LNW0ZZ Release Left Foot Tendon, Open Approach
0LNW3ZZ Release Left Foot Tendon, Percutaneous Approach
0LNW4ZZ Release Left Foot Tendon, Percutaneous Endoscopic Approach
0LNWXZZ Release Left Foot Tendon, External Approach

LP – Tendons, Removal

eview Coding Guideline B6.1c

LPX00Z Removal of Drainage Device from Upper Tendon, Open Approach
LPX07Z Removal of Autologous Tissue Substitute from Upper Tendon, Open Approach
LPX0JZ Removal of Synthetic Substitute from Upper Tendon, Open Approach
LPX0KZ Removal of Nonautologous Tissue Substitute from Upper Tendon, Open Approach
LPX30Z Removal of Drainage Device from Upper Tendon, Percutaneous Approach
LPX37Z Removal of Autologous Tissue Substitute from Upper Tendon, Percutaneous Approach
LPX3JZ Removal of Synthetic Substitute from Upper Tendon, Percutaneous Approach
LPX3KZ Removal of Nonautologous Tissue Substitute from Upper Tendon, Percutaneous Approach
LPX40Z Removal of Drainage Device from Upper Tendon, Percutaneous Endoscopic Approach
0LPX47Z Removal of Autologous Tissue Substitute from Upper Tendon, Percutaneous Endoscopic Approach
0LPX4JZ Removal of Synthetic Substitute from Upper Tendon, Percutaneous Endoscopic Approach
0LPX4KZ Removal of Nonautologous Tissue Substitute from Upper Tendon, Percutaneous Endoscopic Approach
0LPXX0Z Removal of Drainage Device from Upper Tendon, External Approach
0LPY00Z Removal of Drainage Device from Lower Tendon, Open Approach
0LPY07Z Removal of Autologous Tissue Substitute from Lower Tendon, Open Approach
0LPY0JZ Removal of Synthetic Substitute from Lower Tendon, Open Approach
0LPY0KZ Removal of Nonautologous Tissue Substitute from Lower Tendon, Open Approach
0LPY30Z Removal of Drainage Device from Lower Tendon, Percutaneous Approach
0LPY37Z Removal of Autologous Tissue Substitute from Lower Tendon, Percutaneous Approach
0LPY3JZ Removal of Synthetic Substitute from Lower Tendon, Percutaneous Approach
0LPY3KZ Removal of Nonautologous Tissue Substitute from Lower Tendon, Percutaneous Approach
0LPY40Z Removal of Drainage Device from Lower Tendon, Percutaneous Endoscopic Approach
0LPY47Z Removal of Autologous Tissue Substitute from Lower Tendon, Percutaneous Endoscopic Approach
0LPY4JZ Removal of Synthetic Substitute from Lower Tendon, Percutaneous Endoscopic Approach
0LPY4KZ Removal of Nonautologous Tissue Substitute from Lower Tendon, Percutaneous Endoscopic Approach
0LPYX0Z Removal of Drainage Device from Lower Tendon, External Approach

0LQ – Tendons, Repair

Review Coding Guideline B3.5

0LQ00ZZ Repair Head and Neck Tendon, Open Approach
0LQ03ZZ Repair Head and Neck Tendon, Percutaneous Approach
0LQ04ZZ Repair Head and Neck Tendon, Percutaneous Endoscopic Approach
0LQ10ZZ Repair Right Shoulder Tendon, Open Approach
0LQ13ZZ Repair Right Shoulder Tendon, Percutaneous Approach
0LQ14ZZ Repair Right Shoulder Tendon, Percutaneous Endoscopic Approach
AHA CC: 3Q, 2013, 20-22
0LQ20ZZ Repair Left Shoulder Tendon, Open Approach
0LQ23ZZ Repair Left Shoulder Tendon, Percutaneous Approach
0LQ24ZZ Repair Left Shoulder Tendon, Percutaneous Endoscopic Approach
0LQ30ZZ Repair Right Upper Arm Tendon, Open Approach
0LQ33ZZ Repair Right Upper Arm Tendon, Percutaneous Approach
0LQ34ZZ Repair Right Upper Arm Tendon, Percutaneous Endoscopic Approach
0LQ40ZZ Repair Left Upper Arm Tendon, Open Approach
0LQ43ZZ Repair Left Upper Arm Tendon, Percutaneous Approach
0LQ44ZZ Repair Left Upper Arm Tendon, Percutaneous Endoscopic Approach
0LQ50ZZ Repair Right Lower Arm and Wrist Tendon, Open Approach
0LQ53ZZ Repair Right Lower Arm and Wrist Tendon, Percutaneous Approach
0LQ54ZZ Repair Right Lower Arm and Wrist Tendon, Percutaneous Endoscopic Approach
0LQ60ZZ Repair Left Lower Arm and Wrist Tendon, Open Approach
0LQ63ZZ Repair Left Lower Arm and Wrist Tendon, Percutaneous Approach
0LQ64ZZ Repair Left Lower Arm and Wrist Tendon, Percutaneous Endoscopic Approach
0LQ70ZZ Repair Right Hand Tendon, Open Approach
0LQ73ZZ Repair Right Hand Tendon, Percutaneous Approach
0LQ74ZZ Repair Right Hand Tendon, Percutaneous Endoscopic Approach
0LQ80ZZ Repair Left Hand Tendon, Open Approach
0LQ83ZZ Repair Left Hand Tendon, Percutaneous Approach
0LQ84ZZ Repair Left Hand Tendon, Percutaneous Endoscopic Approach
0LQ90ZZ Repair Right Trunk Tendon, Open Approach
0LQ93ZZ Repair Right Trunk Tendon, Percutaneous Approach
0LQ94ZZ Repair Right Trunk Tendon, Percutaneous Endoscopic Approach
0LQB0ZZ Repair Left Trunk Tendon, Open Approach
0LQB3ZZ Repair Left Trunk Tendon, Percutaneous Approach
0LQB4ZZ Repair Left Trunk Tendon, Percutaneous Endoscopic Approach
0LQC0ZZ Repair Right Thorax Tendon, Open Approach
0LQC3ZZ Repair Right Thorax Tendon, Percutaneous Approach
0LQC4ZZ Repair Right Thorax Tendon, Percutaneous Endoscopic Approach
0LQD0ZZ Repair Left Thorax Tendon, Open Approach
0LQD3ZZ Repair Left Thorax Tendon, Percutaneous Approach
0LQD4ZZ Repair Left Thorax Tendon, Percutaneous Endoscopic Approach
0LQF0ZZ Repair Right Abdomen Tendon, Open Approach
0LQF3ZZ Repair Right Abdomen Tendon, Percutaneous Approach
0LQF4ZZ Repair Right Abdomen Tendon, Percutaneous Endoscopic Approach
0LQG0ZZ Repair Left Abdomen Tendon, Open Approach
0LQG3ZZ Repair Left Abdomen Tendon, Percutaneous Approach
0LQG4ZZ Repair Left Abdomen Tendon, Percutaneous Endoscopic Approach
0LQH0ZZ Repair Perineum Tendon, Open Approach
0LQH3ZZ Repair Perineum Tendon, Percutaneous Approach
0LQH4ZZ Repair Perineum Tendon, Percutaneous Endoscopic Approach
0LQJ0ZZ Repair Right Hip Tendon, Open Approach
0LQJ3ZZ Repair Right Hip Tendon, Percutaneous Approach
0LQJ4ZZ Repair Right Hip Tendon, Percutaneous Endoscopic Approach
0LQK0ZZ Repair Left Hip Tendon, Open Approach
0LQK3ZZ Repair Left Hip Tendon, Percutaneous Approach
0LQK4ZZ Repair Left Hip Tendon, Percutaneous Endoscopic Approach
0LQL0ZZ Repair Right Upper Leg Tendon, Open Approach
0LQL3ZZ Repair Right Upper Leg Tendon, Percutaneous Approach
0LQL4ZZ Repair Right Upper Leg Tendon, Percutaneous Endoscopic Approach
0LQM0ZZ Repair Left Upper Leg Tendon, Open Approach
0LQM3ZZ Repair Left Upper Leg Tendon, Percutaneous Approach
0LQM4ZZ Repair Left Upper Leg Tendon, Percutaneous Endoscopic Approach
0LQN0ZZ Repair Right Lower Leg Tendon, Oper Approach
0LQN3ZZ Repair Right Lower Leg Tendon, Percutaneous Approach
0LQN4ZZ Repair Right Lower Leg Tendon, Percutaneous Endoscopic Approach
0LQP0ZZ Repair Left Lower Leg Tendon, Open Approach
0LQP3ZZ Repair Left Lower Leg Tendon, Percutaneous Approach
0LQP4ZZ Repair Left Lower Leg Tendon, Percutaneous Endoscopic Approach
0LQQ0ZZ Repair Right Knee Tendon, Open Approach
0LQQ3ZZ Repair Right Knee Tendon, Percutaneo Approach
0LQQ4ZZ Repair Right Knee Tendon, Percutaneo Endoscopic Approach
0LQR0ZZ Repair Left Knee Tendon, Open Approach
0LQR3ZZ Repair Left Knee Tendon, Percutaneous Approach
0LQR4ZZ Repair Left Knee Tendon, Percutaneous Endoscopic Approach
0LQS0ZZ Repair Right Ankle Tendon, Open Approach
0LQS3ZZ Repair Right Ankle Tendon, Percutaneous Approach
0LQS4ZZ Repair Right Ankle Tendon, Percutaneous Endoscopic Approach
0LQT0ZZ Repair Left Ankle Tendon, Open Approach
0LQT3ZZ Repair Left Ankle Tendon, Percutaneou Approach
0LQT4ZZ Repair Left Ankle Tendon, Percutaneou Endoscopic Approach
0LQV0ZZ Repair Right Foot Tendon, Open Approach
0LQV3ZZ Repair Right Foot Tendon, Percutaneous Approach
0LQV4ZZ Repair Right Foot Tendon, Percutaneous Endoscopic Approach
0LQW0ZZ Repair Left Foot Tendon, Open Approac
0LQW3ZZ Repair Left Foot Tendon, Percutaneous Approach
0LQW4ZZ Repair Left Foot Tendon, Percutaneous Endoscopic Approach

0LR – Tendons, Replacement

0LR007Z Replacement of Head and Neck Tendon with Autologous Tissue Substitute, Open Approach
0LR00JZ Replacement of Head and Neck Tendon with Synthetic Substitute, Open Approach
0LR00KZ Replacement of Head and Neck Tendon with Nonautologous Tissue Substitute, Open Approach
0LR047Z Replacement of Head and Neck Tendon with Autologous Tissue Substitute, Percutaneous Endoscopic Approach
0LR04JZ Replacement of Head and Neck Tendon with Synthetic Substitute, Percutaneous Endoscopic Approach
0LR04KZ Replacement of Head and Neck Tendon with Nonautologous Tissue Substitute, Percutaneous Endoscopic Approach
0LR107Z Replacement of Right Shoulder Tendon with Autologous Tissue Substitute, Open Approach
0LR10JZ Replacement of Right Shoulder Tendon with Synthetic Substitute, Open Approach
0LR10KZ Replacement of Right Shoulder Tendon with Nonautologous Tissue Substitute, Open Approach
0LR147Z Replacement of Right Shoulder Tendon with Autologous Tissue Substitute, Percutaneous Endoscopic Approach
0LR14JZ Replacement of Right Shoulder Tendon with Synthetic Substitute, Percutaneous Endoscopic Approach
0LR14KZ Replacement of Right Shoulder Tendon with Nonautologous Tissue Substitute, Percutaneous Endoscopic Approach

R207Z Replacement of Left Shoulder Tendon with Autologous Tissue Substitute, Open Approach

R20JZ Replacement of Left Shoulder Tendon with Synthetic Substitute, Open Approach

R20KZ Replacement of Left Shoulder Tendon with Nonautologous Tissue Substitute, Open Approach

R247Z Replacement of Left Shoulder Tendon with Autologous Tissue Substitute, Percutaneous Endoscopic Approach

R24JZ Replacement of Left Shoulder Tendon with Synthetic Substitute, Percutaneous Endoscopic Approach

R24KZ Replacement of Left Shoulder Tendon with Nonautologous Tissue Substitute, Percutaneous Endoscopic Approach

R307Z Replacement of Right Upper Arm Tendon with Autologous Tissue Substitute, Open Approach

R30JZ Replacement of Right Upper Arm Tendon with Synthetic Substitute, Open Approach

R30KZ Replacement of Right Upper Arm Tendon with Nonautologous Tissue Substitute, Open Approach

R347Z Replacement of Right Upper Arm Tendon with Autologous Tissue Substitute, Percutaneous Endoscopic Approach

R34JZ Replacement of Right Upper Arm Tendon with Synthetic Substitute, Percutaneous Endoscopic Approach

R34KZ Replacement of Right Upper Arm Tendon with Nonautologous Tissue Substitute, Percutaneous Endoscopic Approach

R407Z Replacement of Left Upper Arm Tendon with Autologous Tissue Substitute, Open Approach

R40JZ Replacement of Left Upper Arm Tendon with Synthetic Substitute, Open Approach

R40KZ Replacement of Left Upper Arm Tendon with Nonautologous Tissue Substitute, Open Approach

R447Z Replacement of Left Upper Arm Tendon with Autologous Tissue Substitute, Percutaneous Endoscopic Approach

R44JZ Replacement of Left Upper Arm Tendon with Synthetic Substitute, Percutaneous Endoscopic Approach

R44KZ Replacement of Left Upper Arm Tendon with Nonautologous Tissue Substitute, Percutaneous Endoscopic Approach

R507Z Replacement of Right Lower Arm and Wrist Tendon with Autologous Tissue Substitute, Open Approach

R50JZ Replacement of Right Lower Arm and Wrist Tendon with Synthetic Substitute, Open Approach

LR50KZ Replacement of Right Lower Arm and Wrist Tendon with Nonautologous Tissue Substitute, Open Approach

LR547Z Replacement of Right Lower Arm and Wrist Tendon with Autologous Tissue Substitute, Percutaneous Endoscopic Approach

LR54JZ Replacement of Right Lower Arm and Wrist Tendon with Synthetic Substitute, Percutaneous Endoscopic Approach

LR54KZ Replacement of Right Lower Arm and Wrist Tendon with Nonautologous Tissue Substitute, Percutaneous Endoscopic Approach

LR607Z Replacement of Left Lower Arm and Wrist Tendon with Autologous Tissue Substitute, Open Approach

LR60JZ Replacement of Left Lower Arm and Wrist Tendon with Synthetic Substitute, Open Approach

0LR60KZ Replacement of Left Lower Arm and Wrist Tendon with Nonautologous Tissue Substitute, Open Approach

0LR647Z Replacement of Left Lower Arm and Wrist Tendon with Autologous Tissue Substitute, Percutaneous Endoscopic Approach

0LR64JZ Replacement of Left Lower Arm and Wrist Tendon with Synthetic Substitute, Percutaneous Endoscopic Approach

0LR64KZ Replacement of Left Lower Arm and Wrist Tendon with Nonautologous Tissue Substitute, Percutaneous Endoscopic Approach

0LR707Z Replacement of Right Hand Tendon with Autologous Tissue Substitute, Open Approach

0LR70JZ Replacement of Right Hand Tendon with Synthetic Substitute, Open Approach

0LR70KZ Replacement of Right Hand Tendon with Nonautologous Tissue Substitute, Open Approach

0LR747Z Replacement of Right Hand Tendon with Autologous Tissue Substitute, Percutaneous Endoscopic Approach

0LR74JZ Replacement of Right Hand Tendon with Synthetic Substitute, Percutaneous Endoscopic Approach

0LR74KZ Replacement of Right Hand Tendon with Nonautologous Tissue Substitute, Percutaneous Endoscopic Approach

0LR807Z Replacement of Left Hand Tendon with Autologous Tissue Substitute, Open Approach

0LR80JZ Replacement of Left Hand Tendon with Synthetic Substitute, Open Approach

0LR80KZ Replacement of Left Hand Tendon with Nonautologous Tissue Substitute, Open Approach

0LR847Z Replacement of Left Hand Tendon with Autologous Tissue Substitute, Percutaneous Endoscopic Approach

0LR84JZ Replacement of Left Hand Tendon with Synthetic Substitute, Percutaneous Endoscopic Approach

0LR84KZ Replacement of Left Hand Tendon with Nonautologous Tissue Substitute, Percutaneous Endoscopic Approach

0LR907Z Replacement of Right Trunk Tendon with Autologous Tissue Substitute, Open Approach

0LR90JZ Replacement of Right Trunk Tendon with Synthetic Substitute, Open Approach

0LR90KZ Replacement of Right Trunk Tendon with Nonautologous Tissue Substitute, Open Approach

0LR947Z Replacement of Right Trunk Tendon with Autologous Tissue Substitute, Percutaneous Endoscopic Approach

0LR94JZ Replacement of Right Trunk Tendon with Synthetic Substitute, Percutaneous Endoscopic Approach

0LR94KZ Replacement of Right Trunk Tendon with Nonautologous Tissue Substitute, Percutaneous Endoscopic Approach

0LRB07Z Replacement of Left Trunk Tendon with Autologous Tissue Substitute, Open Approach

0LRB0JZ Replacement of Left Trunk Tendon with Synthetic Substitute, Open Approach

0LRB0KZ Replacement of Left Trunk Tendon with Nonautologous Tissue Substitute, Open Approach

0LRB47Z Replacement of Left Trunk Tendon with Autologous Tissue Substitute, Percutaneous Endoscopic Approach

0LRB4JZ Replacement of Left Trunk Tendon with Synthetic Substitute, Percutaneous Endoscopic Approach

0LRB4KZ Replacement of Left Trunk Tendon with Nonautologous Tissue Substitute, Percutaneous Endoscopic Approach

0LRC07Z Replacement of Right Thorax Tendon with Autologous Tissue Substitute, Open Approach

0LRC0JZ Replacement of Right Thorax Tendon with Synthetic Substitute, Open Approach

0LRC0KZ Replacement of Right Thorax Tendon with Nonautologous Tissue Substitute, Open Approach

0LRC47Z Replacement of Right Thorax Tendon with Autologous Tissue Substitute, Percutaneous Endoscopic Approach

0LRC4JZ Replacement of Right Thorax Tendon with Synthetic Substitute, Percutaneous Endoscopic Approach

0LRC4KZ Replacement of Right Thorax Tendon with Nonautologous Tissue Substitute, Percutaneous Endoscopic Approach

0LRD07Z Replacement of Left Thorax Tendon with Autologous Tissue Substitute, Open Approach

0LRD0JZ Replacement of Left Thorax Tendon with Synthetic Substitute, Open Approach

0LRD0KZ Replacement of Left Thorax Tendon with Nonautologous Tissue Substitute, Open Approach

0LRD47Z Replacement of Left Thorax Tendon with Autologous Tissue Substitute, Percutaneous Endoscopic Approach

0LRD4JZ Replacement of Left Thorax Tendon with Synthetic Substitute, Percutaneous Endoscopic Approach

0LRD4KZ Replacement of Left Thorax Tendon with Nonautologous Tissue Substitute, Percutaneous Endoscopic Approach

0LRF07Z Replacement of Right Abdomen Tendon with Autologous Tissue Substitute, Open Approach

0LRF0JZ Replacement of Right Abdomen Tendon with Synthetic Substitute, Open Approach

0LRF0KZ Replacement of Right Abdomen Tendon with Nonautologous Tissue Substitute, Open Approach

0LRF47Z Replacement of Right Abdomen Tendon with Autologous Tissue Substitute, Percutaneous Endoscopic Approach

0LRF4JZ Replacement of Right Abdomen Tendon with Synthetic Substitute, Percutaneous Endoscopic Approach

0LRF4KZ Replacement of Right Abdomen Tendon with Nonautologous Tissue Substitute, Percutaneous Endoscopic Approach

0LRG07Z Replacement of Left Abdomen Tendon with Autologous Tissue Substitute, Open Approach

0LRG0JZ Replacement of Left Abdomen Tendon with Synthetic Substitute, Open Approach

0LRG0KZ Replacement of Left Abdomen Tendon with Nonautologous Tissue Substitute, Open Approach

0LRG47Z Replacement of Left Abdomen Tendon with Autologous Tissue Substitute, Percutaneous Endoscopic Approach

0LRG4JZ Replacement of Left Abdomen Tendon with Synthetic Substitute, Percutaneous Endoscopic Approach

0LRG4KZ Replacement of Left Abdomen Tendon with Nonautologous Tissue Substitute, Percutaneous Endoscopic Approach

0LRH07Z Replacement of Perineum Tendon with Autologous Tissue Substitute, Open Approach
0LRH0JZ Replacement of Perineum Tendon with Synthetic Substitute, Open Approach
0LRH0KZ Replacement of Perineum Tendon with Nonautologous Tissue Substitute, Open Approach
0LRH47Z Replacement of Perineum Tendon with Autologous Tissue Substitute, Percutaneous Endoscopic Approach
0LRH4JZ Replacement of Perineum Tendon with Synthetic Substitute, Percutaneous Endoscopic Approach
0LRH4KZ Replacement of Perineum Tendon with Nonautologous Tissue Substitute, Percutaneous Endoscopic Approach
0LRJ07Z Replacement of Right Hip Tendon with Autologous Tissue Substitute, Open Approach
0LRJ0JZ Replacement of Right Hip Tendon with Synthetic Substitute, Open Approach
0LRJ0KZ Replacement of Right Hip Tendon with Nonautologous Tissue Substitute, Open Approach
0LRJ47Z Replacement of Right Hip Tendon with Autologous Tissue Substitute, Percutaneous Endoscopic Approach
0LRJ4JZ Replacement of Right Hip Tendon with Synthetic Substitute, Percutaneous Endoscopic Approach
0LRJ4KZ Replacement of Right Hip Tendon with Nonautologous Tissue Substitute, Percutaneous Endoscopic Approach
0LRK07Z Replacement of Left Hip Tendon with Autologous Tissue Substitute, Open Approach
0LRK0JZ Replacement of Left Hip Tendon with Synthetic Substitute, Open Approach
0LRK0KZ Replacement of Left Hip Tendon with Nonautologous Tissue Substitute, Open Approach
0LRK47Z Replacement of Left Hip Tendon with Autologous Tissue Substitute, Percutaneous Endoscopic Approach
0LRK4JZ Replacement of Left Hip Tendon with Synthetic Substitute, Percutaneous Endoscopic Approach
0LRK4KZ Replacement of Left Hip Tendon with Nonautologous Tissue Substitute, Percutaneous Endoscopic Approach
0LRL07Z Replacement of Right Upper Leg Tendon with Autologous Tissue Substitute, Open Approach
0LRL0JZ Replacement of Right Upper Leg Tendon with Synthetic Substitute, Open Approach
0LRL0KZ Replacement of Right Upper Leg Tendon with Nonautologous Tissue Substitute, Open Approach
0LRL47Z Replacement of Right Upper Leg Tendon with Autologous Tissue Substitute, Percutaneous Endoscopic Approach
0LRL4JZ Replacement of Right Upper Leg Tendon with Synthetic Substitute, Percutaneous Endoscopic Approach
0LRL4KZ Replacement of Right Upper Leg Tendon with Nonautologous Tissue Substitute, Percutaneous Endoscopic Approach
0LRM07Z Replacement of Left Upper Leg Tendon with Autologous Tissue Substitute, Open Approach
0LRM0JZ Replacement of Left Upper Leg Tendon with Synthetic Substitute, Open Approach
0LRM0KZ Replacement of Left Upper Leg Tendon with Nonautologous Tissue Substitute, Open Approach
0LRM47Z Replacement of Left Upper Leg Tendon with Autologous Tissue Substitute, Percutaneous Endoscopic Approach
0LRM4JZ Replacement of Left Upper Leg Tendon with Synthetic Substitute, Percutaneous Endoscopic Approach
0LRM4KZ Replacement of Left Upper Leg Tendon with Nonautologous Tissue Substitute, Percutaneous Endoscopic Approach
0LRN07Z Replacement of Right Lower Leg Tendon with Autologous Tissue Substitute, Open Approach
0LRN0JZ Replacement of Right Lower Leg Tendon with Synthetic Substitute, Open Approach
0LRN0KZ Replacement of Right Lower Leg Tendon with Nonautologous Tissue Substitute, Open Approach
0LRN47Z Replacement of Right Lower Leg Tendon with Autologous Tissue Substitute, Percutaneous Endoscopic Approach
0LRN4JZ Replacement of Right Lower Leg Tendon with Synthetic Substitute, Percutaneous Endoscopic Approach
0LRN4KZ Replacement of Right Lower Leg Tendon with Nonautologous Tissue Substitute, Percutaneous Endoscopic Approach
0LRP07Z Replacement of Left Lower Leg Tendon with Autologous Tissue Substitute, Open Approach
0LRP0JZ Replacement of Left Lower Leg Tendon with Synthetic Substitute, Open Approach
0LRP0KZ Replacement of Left Lower Leg Tendon with Nonautologous Tissue Substitute, Open Approach
0LRP47Z Replacement of Left Lower Leg Tendon with Autologous Tissue Substitute, Percutaneous Endoscopic Approach
0LRP4JZ Replacement of Left Lower Leg Tendon with Synthetic Substitute, Percutaneous Endoscopic Approach
0LRP4KZ Replacement of Left Lower Leg Tendon with Nonautologous Tissue Substitute, Percutaneous Endoscopic Approach
0LRQ07Z Replacement of Right Knee Tendon with Autologous Tissue Substitute, Open Approach
0LRQ0JZ Replacement of Right Knee Tendon with Synthetic Substitute, Open Approach
0LRQ0KZ Replacement of Right Knee Tendon with Nonautologous Tissue Substitute, Open Approach
0LRQ47Z Replacement of Right Knee Tendon with Autologous Tissue Substitute, Percutaneous Endoscopic Approach
0LRQ4JZ Replacement of Right Knee Tendon with Synthetic Substitute, Percutaneous Endoscopic Approach
0LRQ4KZ Replacement of Right Knee Tendon with Nonautologous Tissue Substitute, Percutaneous Endoscopic Approach
0LRR07Z Replacement of Left Knee Tendon with Autologous Tissue Substitute, Open Approach
0LRR0JZ Replacement of Left Knee Tendon with Synthetic Substitute, Open Approach
0LRR0KZ Replacement of Left Knee Tendon with Nonautologous Tissue Substitute, Open Approach
0LRR47Z Replacement of Left Knee Tendon with Autologous Tissue Substitute, Percutaneous Endoscopic Approach
0LRR4JZ Replacement of Left Knee Tendon with Synthetic Substitute, Percutaneous Endoscopic Approach
0LRR4KZ Replacement of Left Knee Tendon with Nonautologous Tissue Substitute Percutaneous Endoscopic Approach
0LRS07Z Replacement of Right Ankle Tendon with Autologous Tissue Substitute, Op Approach
0LRS0JZ Replacement of Right Ankle Tendon with Synthetic Substitute, Open Approach
0LRS0KZ Replacement of Right Ankle Tendon w Nonautologous Tissue Substitute, Ope Approach
0LRS47Z Replacement of Right Ankle Tendon with Autologous Tissue Substitute, Percutaneous Endoscopic Approach
0LRS4JZ Replacement of Right Ankle Tendon with Synthetic Substitute, Percutaneou Endoscopic Approach
0LRS4KZ Replacement of Right Ankle Tendon with Nonautologous Tissue Substitute, Percutaneous Endoscopic Approach
0LRT07Z Replacement of Left Ankle Tendon wi Autologous Tissue Substitute, Open Approach
0LRT0JZ Replacement of Left Ankle Tendon with Synthetic Substitute, Open Approach
0LRT0KZ Replacement of Left Ankle Tendon wit Nonautologous Tissue Substitute, Oper Approach
0LRT47Z Replacement of Left Ankle Tendon with Autologous Tissue Substitute, Percutaneous Endoscopic Approach
0LRT4JZ Replacement of Left Ankle Tendon with Synthetic Substitute, Percutaneous Endoscopic Approach
0LRT4KZ Replacement of Left Ankle Tendon with Nonautologous Tissue Substitute, Percutaneous Endoscopic Approach
0LRV07Z Replacement of Right Foot Tendon wit Autologous Tissue Substitute, Open Approach
0LRV0JZ Replacement of Right Foot Tendon with Synthetic Substitute, Open Approach
0LRV0KZ Replacement of Right Foot Tendon with Nonautologous Tissue Substitute, Open Approach
0LRV47Z Replacement of Right Foot Tendon with Autologous Tissue Substitute, Percutaneous Endoscopic Approach
0LRV4JZ Replacement of Right Foot Tendon with Synthetic Substitute, Percutaneous Endoscopic Approach
0LRV4KZ Replacement of Right Foot Tendon with Nonautologous Tissue Substitute, Percutaneous Endoscopic Approach
0LRW07Z Replacement of Left Foot Tendon with Autologous Tissue Substitute, Open Approach
0LRW0JZ Replacement of Left Foot Tendon with Synthetic Substitute, Open Approach
0LRW0KZ Replacement of Left Foot Tendon with Nonautologous Tissue Substitute, Open Approach
0LRW47Z Replacement of Left Foot Tendon with Autologous Tissue Substitute, Percutaneous Endoscopic Approach
0LRW4JZ Replacement of Left Foot Tendon with Synthetic Substitute, Percutaneous Endoscopic Approach
0LRW4KZ Replacement of Left Foot Tendon with Nonautologous Tissue Substitute, Percutaneous Endoscopic Approach

S – Tendons, Reposition

S00ZZ Reposition Head and Neck Tendon, Open Approach
S04ZZ Reposition Head and Neck Tendon, Percutaneous Endoscopic Approach
S10ZZ Reposition Right Shoulder Tendon, Open Approach
S14ZZ Reposition Right Shoulder Tendon, Percutaneous Endoscopic Approach
S20ZZ Reposition Left Shoulder Tendon, Open Approach
S24ZZ Reposition Left Shoulder Tendon, Percutaneous Endoscopic Approach
S30ZZ Reposition Right Upper Arm Tendon, Open Approach
S34ZZ Reposition Right Upper Arm Tendon, Percutaneous Endoscopic Approach
S40ZZ Reposition Left Upper Arm Tendon, Open Approach
.S44ZZ Reposition Left Upper Arm Tendon, Percutaneous Endoscopic Approach
.S50ZZ Reposition Right Lower Arm and Wrist Tendon, Open Approach
.S54ZZ Reposition Right Lower Arm and Wrist Tendon, Percutaneous Endoscopic Approach
.S60ZZ Reposition Left Lower Arm and Wrist Tendon, Open Approach
.S64ZZ Reposition Left Lower Arm and Wrist Tendon, Percutaneous Endoscopic Approach
.S70ZZ Reposition Right Hand Tendon, Open Approach
.S74ZZ Reposition Right Hand Tendon, Percutaneous Endoscopic Approach
.S80ZZ Reposition Left Hand Tendon, Open Approach
.S84ZZ Reposition Left Hand Tendon, Percutaneous Endoscopic Approach
0LS90ZZ Reposition Right Trunk Tendon, Open Approach
0LS94ZZ Reposition Right Trunk Tendon, Percutaneous Endoscopic Approach
0LSB0ZZ Reposition Left Trunk Tendon, Open Approach
0LSB4ZZ Reposition Left Trunk Tendon, Percutaneous Endoscopic Approach
0LSC0ZZ Reposition Right Thorax Tendon, Open Approach
0LSC4ZZ Reposition Right Thorax Tendon, Percutaneous Endoscopic Approach
0LSD0ZZ Reposition Left Thorax Tendon, Open Approach
0LSD4ZZ Reposition Left Thorax Tendon, Percutaneous Endoscopic Approach
0LSF0ZZ Reposition Right Abdomen Tendon, Open Approach
0LSF4ZZ Reposition Right Abdomen Tendon, Percutaneous Endoscopic Approach
0LSG0ZZ Reposition Left Abdomen Tendon, Open Approach
0LSG4ZZ Reposition Left Abdomen Tendon, Percutaneous Endoscopic Approach
0LSH0ZZ Reposition Perineum Tendon, Open Approach
0LSH4ZZ Reposition Perineum Tendon, Percutaneous Endoscopic Approach
0LSJ0ZZ Reposition Right Hip Tendon, Open Approach
0LSJ4ZZ Reposition Right Hip Tendon, Percutaneous Endoscopic Approach
0LSK0ZZ Reposition Left Hip Tendon, Open Approach
0LSK4ZZ Reposition Left Hip Tendon, Percutaneous Endoscopic Approach
0LSL0ZZ Reposition Right Upper Leg Tendon, Open Approach
0LSL4ZZ Reposition Right Upper Leg Tendon, Percutaneous Endoscopic Approach
0LSM0ZZ Reposition Left Upper Leg Tendon, Open Approach
0LSM4ZZ Reposition Left Upper Leg Tendon, Percutaneous Endoscopic Approach
0LSN0ZZ Reposition Right Lower Leg Tendon, Open Approach
0LSN4ZZ Reposition Right Lower Leg Tendon, Percutaneous Endoscopic Approach
0LSP0ZZ Reposition Left Lower Leg Tendon, Open Approach
0LSP4ZZ Reposition Left Lower Leg Tendon, Percutaneous Endoscopic Approach
0LSQ0ZZ Reposition Right Knee Tendon, Open Approach
0LSQ4ZZ Reposition Right Knee Tendon, Percutaneous Endoscopic Approach
0LSR0ZZ Reposition Left Knee Tendon, Open Approach
0LSR4ZZ Reposition Left Knee Tendon, Percutaneous Endoscopic Approach
0LSS0ZZ Reposition Right Ankle Tendon, Open Approach
0LSS4ZZ Reposition Right Ankle Tendon, Percutaneous Endoscopic Approach
0LST0ZZ Reposition Left Ankle Tendon, Open Approach
0LST4ZZ Reposition Left Ankle Tendon, Percutaneous Endoscopic Approach
0LSV0ZZ Reposition Right Foot Tendon, Open Approach
0LSV4ZZ Reposition Right Foot Tendon, Percutaneous Endoscopic Approach
0LSW0ZZ Reposition Left Foot Tendon, Open Approach
0LSW4ZZ Reposition Left Foot Tendon, Percutaneous Endoscopic Approach

LT – Tendons, Resection

eview Coding Guideline B3.8

LT00ZZ Resection of Head and Neck Tendon, Open Approach
LT04ZZ Resection of Head and Neck Tendon, Percutaneous Endoscopic Approach
LT10ZZ Resection of Right Shoulder Tendon, Open Approach
LT14ZZ Resection of Right Shoulder Tendon, Percutaneous Endoscopic Approach
LT20ZZ Resection of Left Shoulder Tendon, Open Approach
LT24ZZ Resection of Left Shoulder Tendon, Percutaneous Endoscopic Approach
LT30ZZ Resection of Right Upper Arm Tendon, Open Approach
LT34ZZ Resection of Right Upper Arm Tendon, Percutaneous Endoscopic Approach
LT40ZZ Resection of Left Upper Arm Tendon, Open Approach
LT44ZZ Resection of Left Upper Arm Tendon, Percutaneous Endoscopic Approach
)LT50ZZ Resection of Right Lower Arm and Wrist Tendon, Open Approach
LT54ZZ Resection of Right Lower Arm and Wrist Tendon, Percutaneous Endoscopic Approach
)LT60ZZ Resection of Left Lower Arm and Wrist Tendon, Open Approach
)LT64ZZ Resection of Left Lower Arm and Wrist Tendon, Percutaneous Endoscopic Approach
0LT70ZZ Resection of Right Hand Tendon, Open Approach
0LT74ZZ Resection of Right Hand Tendon, Percutaneous Endoscopic Approach
0LT80ZZ Resection of Left Hand Tendon, Open Approach
0LT84ZZ Resection of Left Hand Tendon, Percutaneous Endoscopic Approach
0LT90ZZ Resection of Right Trunk Tendon, Open Approach
0LT94ZZ Resection of Right Trunk Tendon, Percutaneous Endoscopic Approach
0LTB0ZZ Resection of Left Trunk Tendon, Open Approach
0LTB4ZZ Resection of Left Trunk Tendon, Percutaneous Endoscopic Approach
0LTC0ZZ Resection of Right Thorax Tendon, Open Approach
0LTC4ZZ Resection of Right Thorax Tendon, Percutaneous Endoscopic Approach
0LTD0ZZ Resection of Left Thorax Tendon, Open Approach
0LTD4ZZ Resection of Left Thorax Tendon, Percutaneous Endoscopic Approach
0LTF0ZZ Resection of Right Abdomen Tendon, Open Approach
0LTF4ZZ Resection of Right Abdomen Tendon, Percutaneous Endoscopic Approach
0LTG0ZZ Resection of Left Abdomen Tendon, Open Approach
0LTG4ZZ Resection of Left Abdomen Tendon, Percutaneous Endoscopic Approach
0LTH0ZZ Resection of Perineum Tendon, Open Approach
0LTH4ZZ Resection of Perineum Tendon, Percutaneous Endoscopic Approach
0LTJ0ZZ Resection of Right Hip Tendon, Open Approach
0LTJ4ZZ Resection of Right Hip Tendon, Percutaneous Endoscopic Approach
0LTK0ZZ Resection of Left Hip Tendon, Open Approach
0LTK4ZZ Resection of Left Hip Tendon, Percutaneous Endoscopic Approach
0LTL0ZZ Resection of Right Upper Leg Tendon, Open Approach
0LTL4ZZ Resection of Right Upper Leg Tendon, Percutaneous Endoscopic Approach
0LTM0ZZ Resection of Left Upper Leg Tendon, Open Approach
0LTM4ZZ Resection of Left Upper Leg Tendon, Percutaneous Endoscopic Approach
0LTN0ZZ Resection of Right Lower Leg Tendon, Open Approach
0LTN4ZZ Resection of Right Lower Leg Tendon, Percutaneous Endoscopic Approach
0LTP0ZZ Resection of Left Lower Leg Tendon, Open Approach
0LTP4ZZ Resection of Left Lower Leg Tendon, Percutaneous Endoscopic Approach
0LTQ0ZZ Resection of Right Knee Tendon, Open Approach
0LTQ4ZZ Resection of Right Knee Tendon, Percutaneous Endoscopic Approach

0LTR0ZZ Resection of Left Knee Tendon, Open Approach
0LTR4ZZ Resection of Left Knee Tendon, Percutaneous Endoscopic Approach
0LTS0ZZ Resection of Right Ankle Tendon, Open Approach
0LTS4ZZ Resection of Right Ankle Tendon, Percutaneous Endoscopic Approach
0LTT0ZZ Resection of Left Ankle Tendon, Open Approach
0LTT4ZZ Resection of Left Ankle Tendon, Percutaneous Endoscopic Approach
0LTV0ZZ Resection of Right Foot Tendon, Open Approach
0LTV4ZZ Resection of Right Foot Tendon, Percutaneous Endoscopic Approach
0LTW0ZZ Resection of Left Foot Tendon, Open Approach
0LTW4ZZ Resection of Left Foot Tendon, Percutaneous Endoscopic Approach

0LU – Tendons, Supplement

0LU007Z Supplement Head and Neck Tendon with Autologous Tissue Substitute, Open Approach
0LU00JZ Supplement Head and Neck Tendon with Synthetic Substitute, Open Approach
0LU00KZ Supplement Head and Neck Tendon with Nonautologous Tissue Substitute, Open Approach
0LU047Z Supplement Head and Neck Tendon with Autologous Tissue Substitute, Percutaneous Endoscopic Approach
0LU04JZ Supplement Head and Neck Tendon with Synthetic Substitute, Percutaneous Endoscopic Approach
0LU04KZ Supplement Head and Neck Tendon with Nonautologous Tissue Substitute, Percutaneous Endoscopic Approach
0LU107Z Supplement Right Shoulder Tendon with Autologous Tissue Substitute, Open Approach
0LU10JZ Supplement Right Shoulder Tendon with Synthetic Substitute, Open Approach
0LU10KZ Supplement Right Shoulder Tendon with Nonautologous Tissue Substitute, Open Approach
0LU147Z Supplement Right Shoulder Tendon with Autologous Tissue Substitute, Percutaneous Endoscopic Approach
0LU14JZ Supplement Right Shoulder Tendon with Synthetic Substitute, Percutaneous Endoscopic Approach
0LU14KZ Supplement Right Shoulder Tendon with Nonautologous Tissue Substitute, Percutaneous Endoscopic Approach
0LU207Z Supplement Left Shoulder Tendon with Autologous Tissue Substitute, Open Approach
0LU20JZ Supplement Left Shoulder Tendon with Synthetic Substitute, Open Approach
0LU20KZ Supplement Left Shoulder Tendon with Nonautologous Tissue Substitute, Open Approach
0LU247Z Supplement Left Shoulder Tendon with Autologous Tissue Substitute, Percutaneous Endoscopic Approach
0LU24JZ Supplement Left Shoulder Tendon with Synthetic Substitute, Percutaneous Endoscopic Approach
0LU24KZ Supplement Left Shoulder Tendon with Nonautologous Tissue Substitute, Percutaneous Endoscopic Approach
0LU307Z Supplement Right Upper Arm Tendon with Autologous Tissue Substitute, Open Approach
0LU30JZ Supplement Right Upper Arm Tendon with Synthetic Substitute, Open Approach
0LU30KZ Supplement Right Upper Arm Tendon with Nonautologous Tissue Substitute, Open Approach
0LU347Z Supplement Right Upper Arm Tendon with Autologous Tissue Substitute, Percutaneous Endoscopic Approach
0LU34JZ Supplement Right Upper Arm Tendon with Synthetic Substitute, Percutaneous Endoscopic Approach
0LU34KZ Supplement Right Upper Arm Tendon with Nonautologous Tissue Substitute, Percutaneous Endoscopic Approach
0LU407Z Supplement Left Upper Arm Tendon with Autologous Tissue Substitute, Open Approach
0LU40JZ Supplement Left Upper Arm Tendon with Synthetic Substitute, Open Approach
0LU40KZ Supplement Left Upper Arm Tendon with Nonautologous Tissue Substitute, Open Approach
0LU447Z Supplement Left Upper Arm Tendon with Autologous Tissue Substitute, Percutaneous Endoscopic Approach
0LU44JZ Supplement Left Upper Arm Tendon with Synthetic Substitute, Percutaneous Endoscopic Approach
0LU44KZ Supplement Left Upper Arm Tendon with Nonautologous Tissue Substitute, Percutaneous Endoscopic Approach
0LU507Z Supplement Right Lower Arm and Wrist Tendon with Autologous Tissue Substitute, Open Approach
0LU50JZ Supplement Right Lower Arm and Wrist Tendon with Synthetic Substitute, Open Approach
0LU50KZ Supplement Right Lower Arm and Wrist Tendon with Nonautologous Tissue Substitute, Open Approach
0LU547Z Supplement Right Lower Arm and Wrist Tendon with Autologous Tissue Substitute, Percutaneous Endoscopic Approach
0LU54JZ Supplement Right Lower Arm and Wrist Tendon with Synthetic Substitute, Percutaneous Endoscopic Approach
0LU54KZ Supplement Right Lower Arm and Wrist Tendon with Nonautologous Tissue Substitute, Percutaneous Endoscopic Approach
0LU607Z Supplement Left Lower Arm and Wrist Tendon with Autologous Tissue Substitute, Open Approach
0LU60JZ Supplement Left Lower Arm and Wrist Tendon with Synthetic Substitute, Open Approach
0LU60KZ Supplement Left Lower Arm and Wrist Tendon with Nonautologous Tissue Substitute, Open Approach
0LU647Z Supplement Left Lower Arm and Wrist Tendon with Autologous Tissue Substitute, Percutaneous Endoscopic Approach
0LU64JZ Supplement Left Lower Arm and Wrist Tendon with Synthetic Substitute, Percutaneous Endoscopic Approach
0LU64KZ Supplement Left Lower Arm and Wrist Tendon with Nonautologous Tissue Substitute, Percutaneous Endoscopic Approach
0LU707Z Supplement Right Hand Tendon with Autologous Tissue Substitute, Open Approach
0LU70JZ Supplement Right Hand Tendon with Synthetic Substitute, Open Approach
0LU70KZ Supplement Right Hand Tendon with Nonautologous Tissue Substitute, Open Approach
0LU747Z Supplement Right Hand Tendon with Autologous Tissue Substitute, Percutaneous Endoscopic Approach
0LU74JZ Supplement Right Hand Tendon with Synthetic Substitute, Percutaneous Endoscopic Approach
0LU74KZ Supplement Right Hand Tendon with Nonautologous Tissue Substitute, Percutaneous Endoscopic Approach
0LU807Z Supplement Left Hand Tendon with Autologous Tissue Substitute, Open Approach
0LU80JZ Supplement Left Hand Tendon with Synthetic Substitute, Open Approac
0LU80KZ Supplement Left Hand Tendon with Nonautologous Tissue Substitute, Open Approach
0LU847Z Supplement Left Hand Tendon with Autologous Tissue Substitute, Percutaneous Endoscopic Approach
0LU84JZ Supplement Left Hand Tendon with Synthetic Substitute, Percutaneous Endoscopic Approach
0LU84KZ Supplement Left Hand Tendon with Nonautologous Tissue Substitute, Percutaneous Endoscopic Approach
0LU907Z Supplement Right Trunk Tendon with Autologous Tissue Substitute, Open Approach
0LU90JZ Supplement Right Trunk Tendon with Synthetic Substitute, Open Approach
0LU90KZ Supplement Right Trunk Tendon with Nonautologous Tissue Substitute, Open Approach
0LU947Z Supplement Right Trunk Tendon with Autologous Tissue Substitute, Percutaneous Endoscopic Approach
0LU94JZ Supplement Right Trunk Tendon with Synthetic Substitute, Percutaneous Endoscopic Approach
0LU94KZ Supplement Right Trunk Tendon with Nonautologous Tissue Substitute, Percutaneous Endoscopic Approach
0LUB07Z Supplement Left Trunk Tendon with Autologous Tissue Substitute, Open Approach
0LUB0JZ Supplement Left Trunk Tendon with Synthetic Substitute, Open Approach
0LUB0KZ Supplement Left Trunk Tendon with Nonautologous Tissue Substitute, Open Approach
0LUB47Z Supplement Left Trunk Tendon with Autologous Tissue Substitute, Percutaneous Endoscopic Approach
0LUB4JZ Supplement Left Trunk Tendon with Synthetic Substitute, Percutaneous Endoscopic Approach
0LUB4KZ Supplement Left Trunk Tendon with Nonautologous Tissue Substitute, Percutaneous Endoscopic Approach
0LUC07Z Supplement Right Thorax Tendon with Autologous Tissue Substitute, Open Approach

JC0JZ Supplement Right Thorax Tendon with Synthetic Substitute, Open Approach

JC0KZ Supplement Right Thorax Tendon with Nonautologous Tissue Substitute, Open Approach

UC47Z Supplement Right Thorax Tendon with Autologous Tissue Substitute, Percutaneous Endoscopic Approach

UC4JZ Supplement Right Thorax Tendon with Synthetic Substitute, Percutaneous Endoscopic Approach

UC4KZ Supplement Right Thorax Tendon with Nonautologous Tissue Substitute, Percutaneous Endoscopic Approach

UD07Z Supplement Left Thorax Tendon with Autologous Tissue Substitute, Open Approach

UD0JZ Supplement Left Thorax Tendon with Synthetic Substitute, Open Approach

UD0KZ Supplement Left Thorax Tendon with Nonautologous Tissue Substitute, Open Approach

UD47Z Supplement Left Thorax Tendon with Autologous Tissue Substitute, Percutaneous Endoscopic Approach

UD4JZ Supplement Left Thorax Tendon with Synthetic Substitute, Percutaneous Endoscopic Approach

UD4KZ Supplement Left Thorax Tendon with Nonautologous Tissue Substitute, Percutaneous Endoscopic Approach

UF07Z Supplement Right Abdomen Tendon with Autologous Tissue Substitute, Open Approach

UF0JZ Supplement Right Abdomen Tendon with Synthetic Substitute, Open Approach

UF0KZ Supplement Right Abdomen Tendon with Nonautologous Tissue Substitute, Open Approach

UF47Z Supplement Right Abdomen Tendon with Autologous Tissue Substitute, Percutaneous Endoscopic Approach

UF4JZ Supplement Right Abdomen Tendon with Synthetic Substitute, Percutaneous Endoscopic Approach

UF4KZ Supplement Right Abdomen Tendon with Nonautologous Tissue Substitute, Percutaneous Endoscopic Approach

UG07Z Supplement Left Abdomen Tendon with Autologous Tissue Substitute, Open Approach

LUG0JZ Supplement Left Abdomen Tendon with Synthetic Substitute, Open Approach

LUG0KZ Supplement Left Abdomen Tendon with Nonautologous Tissue Substitute, Open Approach

LUG47Z Supplement Left Abdomen Tendon with Autologous Tissue Substitute, Percutaneous Endoscopic Approach

LUG4JZ Supplement Left Abdomen Tendon with Synthetic Substitute, Percutaneous Endoscopic Approach

LUG4KZ Supplement Left Abdomen Tendon with Nonautologous Tissue Substitute, Percutaneous Endoscopic Approach

LUH07Z Supplement Perineum Tendon with Autologous Tissue Substitute, Open Approach

LUH0JZ Supplement Perineum Tendon with Synthetic Substitute, Open Approach

LUH0KZ Supplement Perineum Tendon with Nonautologous Tissue Substitute, Open Approach

LUH47Z Supplement Perineum Tendon with Autologous Tissue Substitute, Percutaneous Endoscopic Approach

0LUH4JZ Supplement Perineum Tendon with Synthetic Substitute, Percutaneous Endoscopic Approach

0LUH4KZ Supplement Perineum Tendon with Nonautologous Tissue Substitute, Percutaneous Endoscopic Approach

0LUJ07Z Supplement Right Hip Tendon with Autologous Tissue Substitute, Open Approach

0LUJ0JZ Supplement Right Hip Tendon with Synthetic Substitute, Open Approach

0LUJ0KZ Supplement Right Hip Tendon with Nonautologous Tissue Substitute, Open Approach

0LUJ47Z Supplement Right Hip Tendon with Autologous Tissue Substitute, Percutaneous Endoscopic Approach

0LUJ4JZ Supplement Right Hip Tendon with Synthetic Substitute, Percutaneous Endoscopic Approach

0LUJ4KZ Supplement Right Hip Tendon with Nonautologous Tissue Substitute, Percutaneous Endoscopic Approach

0LUK07Z Supplement Left Hip Tendon with Autologous Tissue Substitute, Open Approach

0LUK0JZ Supplement Left Hip Tendon with Synthetic Substitute, Open Approach

0LUK0KZ Supplement Left Hip Tendon with Nonautologous Tissue Substitute, Open Approach

0LUK47Z Supplement Left Hip Tendon with Autologous Tissue Substitute, Percutaneous Endoscopic Approach

0LUK4JZ Supplement Left Hip Tendon with Synthetic Substitute, Percutaneous Endoscopic Approach

0LUK4KZ Supplement Left Hip Tendon with Nonautologous Tissue Substitute, Percutaneous Endoscopic Approach

0LUL07Z Supplement Right Upper Leg Tendon with Autologous Tissue Substitute, Open Approach

0LUL0JZ Supplement Right Upper Leg Tendon with Synthetic Substitute, Open Approach

0LUL0KZ Supplement Right Upper Leg Tendon with Nonautologous Tissue Substitute, Open Approach

0LUL47Z Supplement Right Upper Leg Tendon with Autologous Tissue Substitute, Percutaneous Endoscopic Approach

0LUL4JZ Supplement Right Upper Leg Tendon with Synthetic Substitute, Percutaneous Endoscopic Approach

0LUL4KZ Supplement Right Upper Leg Tendon with Nonautologous Tissue Substitute, Percutaneous Endoscopic Approach

0LUM07Z Supplement Left Upper Leg Tendon with Autologous Tissue Substitute, Open Approach

0LUM0JZ Supplement Left Upper Leg Tendon with Synthetic Substitute, Open Approach

0LUM0KZ Supplement Left Upper Leg Tendon with Nonautologous Tissue Substitute, Open Approach

0LUM47Z Supplement Left Upper Leg Tendon with Autologous Tissue Substitute, Percutaneous Endoscopic Approach

0LUM4JZ Supplement Left Upper Leg Tendon with Synthetic Substitute, Percutaneous Endoscopic Approach

0LUM4KZ Supplement Left Upper Leg Tendon with Nonautologous Tissue Substitute, Percutaneous Endoscopic Approach

0LUN07Z Supplement Right Lower Leg Tendon with Autologous Tissue Substitute, Open Approach

0LUN0JZ Supplement Right Lower Leg Tendon with Synthetic Substitute, Open Approach

0LUN0KZ Supplement Right Lower Leg Tendon with Nonautologous Tissue Substitute, Open Approach

0LUN47Z Supplement Right Lower Leg Tendon with Autologous Tissue Substitute, Percutaneous Endoscopic Approach

0LUN4JZ Supplement Right Lower Leg Tendon with Synthetic Substitute, Percutaneous Endoscopic Approach

0LUN4KZ Supplement Right Lower Leg Tendon with Nonautologous Tissue Substitute, Percutaneous Endoscopic Approach

0LUP07Z Supplement Left Lower Leg Tendon with Autologous Tissue Substitute, Open Approach

0LUP0JZ Supplement Left Lower Leg Tendon with Synthetic Substitute, Open Approach

0LUP0KZ Supplement Left Lower Leg Tendon with Nonautologous Tissue Substitute, Open Approach

0LUP47Z Supplement Left Lower Leg Tendon with Autologous Tissue Substitute, Percutaneous Endoscopic Approach

0LUP4JZ Supplement Left Lower Leg Tendon with Synthetic Substitute, Percutaneous Endoscopic Approach

0LUP4KZ Supplement Left Lower Leg Tendon with Nonautologous Tissue Substitute, Percutaneous Endoscopic Approach

0LUQ07Z Supplement Right Knee Tendon with Autologous Tissue Substitute, Open Approach

0LUQ0JZ Supplement Right Knee Tendon with Synthetic Substitute, Open Approach

0LUQ0KZ Supplement Right Knee Tendon with Nonautologous Tissue Substitute, Open Approach

0LUQ47Z Supplement Right Knee Tendon with Autologous Tissue Substitute, Percutaneous Endoscopic Approach

0LUQ4JZ Supplement Right Knee Tendon with Synthetic Substitute, Percutaneous Endoscopic Approach

0LUQ4KZ Supplement Right Knee Tendon with Nonautologous Tissue Substitute, Percutaneous Endoscopic Approach

0LUR07Z Supplement Left Knee Tendon with Autologous Tissue Substitute, Open Approach

0LUR0JZ Supplement Left Knee Tendon with Synthetic Substitute, Open Approach

0LUR0KZ Supplement Left Knee Tendon with Nonautologous Tissue Substitute, Open Approach

0LUR47Z Supplement Left Knee Tendon with Autologous Tissue Substitute, Percutaneous Endoscopic Approach

0LUR4JZ Supplement Left Knee Tendon with Synthetic Substitute, Percutaneous Endoscopic Approach

0LUR4KZ Supplement Left Knee Tendon with Nonautologous Tissue Substitute, Percutaneous Endoscopic Approach

0LUS07Z Supplement Right Ankle Tendon with Autologous Tissue Substitute, Open Approach

0LUS0JZ Supplement Right Ankle Tendon with Synthetic Substitute, Open Approach

0LUS0KZ Supplement Right Ankle Tendon with Nonautologous Tissue Substitute, Open Approach

0LUS47Z Supplement Right Ankle Tendon with Autologous Tissue Substitute, Percutaneous Endoscopic Approach

0LUS4JZ Supplement Right Ankle Tendon with Synthetic Substitute, Percutaneous Endoscopic Approach
0LUS4KZ Supplement Right Ankle Tendon with Nonautologous Tissue Substitute, Percutaneous Endoscopic Approach
0LUT07Z Supplement Left Ankle Tendon with Autologous Tissue Substitute, Open Approach
0LUT0JZ Supplement Left Ankle Tendon with Synthetic Substitute, Open Approach
0LUT0KZ Supplement Left Ankle Tendon with Nonautologous Tissue Substitute, Open Approach
0LUT47Z Supplement Left Ankle Tendon with Autologous Tissue Substitute, Percutaneous Endoscopic Approach
0LUT4JZ Supplement Left Ankle Tendon with Synthetic Substitute, Percutaneous Endoscopic Approach
0LUT4KZ Supplement Left Ankle Tendon with Nonautologous Tissue Substitute, Percutaneous Endoscopic Approach
0LUV07Z Supplement Right Foot Tendon with Autologous Tissue Substitute, Open Approach
0LUV0JZ Supplement Right Foot Tendon with Synthetic Substitute, Open Approach
0LUV0KZ Supplement Right Foot Tendon with Nonautologous Tissue Substitute, Open Approach
0LUV47Z Supplement Right Foot Tendon with Autologous Tissue Substitute, Percutaneous Endoscopic Approach
0LUV4JZ Supplement Right Foot Tendon with Synthetic Substitute, Percutaneous Endoscopic Approach
0LUV4KZ Supplement Right Foot Tendon with Nonautologous Tissue Substitute, Percutaneous Endoscopic Approach
0LUW07Z Supplement Left Foot Tendon with Autologous Tissue Substitute, Open Approach
0LUW0JZ Supplement Left Foot Tendon with Synthetic Substitute, Open Approach
0LUW0KZ Supplement Left Foot Tendon with Nonautologous Tissue Substitute, Ope Approach
0LUW47Z Supplement Left Foot Tendon with Autologous Tissue Substitute, Percutaneous Endoscopic Approach
0LUW4JZ Supplement Left Foot Tendon with Synthetic Substitute, Percutaneous Endoscopic Approach
0LUW4KZ Supplement Left Foot Tendon with Nonautologous Tissue Substitute, Percutaneous Endoscopic Approach

0LW – Tendons, Revision

Review Coding Guideline B6.1c

0LWX00Z Revision of Drainage Device in Upper Tendon, Open Approach
0LWX07Z Revision of Autologous Tissue Substitute in Upper Tendon, Open Approach
0LWX0JZ Revision of Synthetic Substitute in Upper Tendon, Open Approach
0LWX0KZ Revision of Nonautologous Tissue Substitute in Upper Tendon, Open Approach
0LWX30Z Revision of Drainage Device in Upper Tendon, Percutaneous Approach
0LWX37Z Revision of Autologous Tissue Substitute in Upper Tendon, Percutaneous Approach
0LWX3JZ Revision of Synthetic Substitute in Upper Tendon, Percutaneous Approach
0LWX3KZ Revision of Nonautologous Tissue Substitute in Upper Tendon, Percutaneous Approach
0LWX40Z Revision of Drainage Device in Upper Tendon, Percutaneous Endoscopic Approach
0LWX47Z Revision of Autologous Tissue Substitute in Upper Tendon, Percutaneous Endoscopic Approach
0LWX4JZ Revision of Synthetic Substitute in Upper Tendon, Percutaneous Endoscopic Approach
0LWX4KZ Revision of Nonautologous Tissue Substitute in Upper Tendon, Percutaneous Endoscopic Approach
0LWXX0Z Revision of Drainage Device in Upper Tendon, External Approach
0LWXX7Z Revision of Autologous Tissue Substitute in Upper Tendon, External Approach
0LWXXJZ Revision of Synthetic Substitute in Upper Tendon, External Approach
0LWXXKZ Revision of Nonautologous Tissue Substitute in Upper Tendon, External Approach
0LWY00Z Revision of Drainage Device in Lower Tendon, Open Approach
0LWY07Z Revision of Autologous Tissue Substitute in Lower Tendon, Open Approach
0LWY0JZ Revision of Synthetic Substitute in Lower Tendon, Open Approach
0LWY0KZ Revision of Nonautologous Tissue Substitute in Lower Tendon, Open Approach
0LWY30Z Revision of Drainage Device in Lower Tendon, Percutaneous Approach
0LWY37Z Revision of Autologous Tissue Substitute in Lower Tendon, Percutaneous Approach
0LWY3JZ Revision of Synthetic Substitute in Lower Tendon, Percutaneous Approach
0LWY3KZ Revision of Nonautologous Tissue Substitute in Lower Tendon, Percutaneous Approach
0LWY40Z Revision of Drainage Device in Lower Tendon, Percutaneous Endoscopic Approach
0LWY47Z Revision of Autologous Tissue Substitu in Lower Tendon, Percutaneous Endoscopic Approach
0LWY4JZ Revision of Synthetic Substitute in Lower Tendon, Percutaneous Endoscop Approach
0LWY4KZ Revision of Nonautologous Tissue Substitute in Lower Tendon, Percutaneous Endoscopic Approach
0LWYX0Z Revision of Drainage Device in Lower Tendon, External Approach
0LWYX7Z Revision of Autologous Tissue Substitu in Lower Tendon, External Approach
0LWYXJZ Revision of Synthetic Substitute in Lower Tendon, External Approach
0LWYXKZ Revision of Nonautologous Tissue Substitute in Lower Tendon, External Approach

0LX – Tendons, Transfer

0LX00ZZ Transfer Head and Neck Tendon, Open Approach
0LX04ZZ Transfer Head and Neck Tendon, Percutaneous Endoscopic Approach
0LX10ZZ Transfer Right Shoulder Tendon, Open Approach
0LX14ZZ Transfer Right Shoulder Tendon, Percutaneous Endoscopic Approach
0LX20ZZ Transfer Left Shoulder Tendon, Open Approach
0LX24ZZ Transfer Left Shoulder Tendon, Percutaneous Endoscopic Approach
0LX30ZZ Transfer Right Upper Arm Tendon, Open Approach
0LX34ZZ Transfer Right Upper Arm Tendon, Percutaneous Endoscopic Approach
0LX40ZZ Transfer Left Upper Arm Tendon, Open Approach
0LX44ZZ Transfer Left Upper Arm Tendon, Percutaneous Endoscopic Approach
0LX50ZZ Transfer Right Lower Arm and Wrist Tendon, Open Approach
0LX54ZZ Transfer Right Lower Arm and Wrist Tendon, Percutaneous Endoscopic Approach
0LX60ZZ Transfer Left Lower Arm and Wrist Tendon, Open Approach
0LX64ZZ Transfer Left Lower Arm and Wrist Tendon, Percutaneous Endoscopic Approach
0LX70ZZ Transfer Right Hand Tendon, Open Approach
0LX74ZZ Transfer Right Hand Tendon, Percutaneous Endoscopic Approach
0LX80ZZ Transfer Left Hand Tendon, Open Approach
0LX84ZZ Transfer Left Hand Tendon, Percutaneous Endoscopic Approach
0LX90ZZ Transfer Right Trunk Tendon, Open Approach
0LX94ZZ Transfer Right Trunk Tendon, Percutaneous Endoscopic Approach
0LXB0ZZ Transfer Left Trunk Tendon, Open Approach
0LXB4ZZ Transfer Left Trunk Tendon, Percutaneou Endoscopic Approach
0LXC0ZZ Transfer Right Thorax Tendon, Open Approach
0LXC4ZZ Transfer Right Thorax Tendon, Percutaneous Endoscopic Approach
0LXD0ZZ Transfer Left Thorax Tendon, Open Approach
0LXD4ZZ Transfer Left Thorax Tendon, Percutaneous Endoscopic Approach
0LXF0ZZ Transfer Right Abdomen Tendon, Open Approach
0LXF4ZZ Transfer Right Abdomen Tendon, Percutaneous Endoscopic Approach
0LXG0ZZ Transfer Left Abdomen Tendon, Open Approach
0LXG4ZZ Transfer Left Abdomen Tendon, Percutaneous Endoscopic Approach
0LXH0ZZ Transfer Perineum Tendon, Open Approach
0LXH4ZZ Transfer Perineum Tendon, Percutaneous Endoscopic Approach

J0ZZ Transfer Right Hip Tendon, Open Approach
J4ZZ Transfer Right Hip Tendon, Percutaneous Endoscopic Approach
K0ZZ Transfer Left Hip Tendon, Open Approach
K4ZZ Transfer Left Hip Tendon, Percutaneous Endoscopic Approach
L0ZZ Transfer Right Upper Leg Tendon, Open Approach
L4ZZ Transfer Right Upper Leg Tendon, Percutaneous Endoscopic Approach
M0ZZ Transfer Left Upper Leg Tendon, Open Approach
M4ZZ Transfer Left Upper Leg Tendon, Percutaneous Endoscopic Approach

0LXN0ZZ Transfer Right Lower Leg Tendon, Open Approach
0LXN4ZZ Transfer Right Lower Leg Tendon, Percutaneous Endoscopic Approach
0LXP0ZZ Transfer Left Lower Leg Tendon, Open Approach
0LXP4ZZ Transfer Left Lower Leg Tendon, Percutaneous Endoscopic Approach
0LXQ0ZZ Transfer Right Knee Tendon, Open Approach
0LXQ4ZZ Transfer Right Knee Tendon, Percutaneous Endoscopic Approach
0LXR0ZZ Transfer Left Knee Tendon, Open Approach
0LXR4ZZ Transfer Left Knee Tendon, Percutaneous Endoscopic Approach
0LXS0ZZ Transfer Right Ankle Tendon, Open Approach
0LXS4ZZ Transfer Right Ankle Tendon, Percutaneous Endoscopic Approach
0LXT0ZZ Transfer Left Ankle Tendon, Open Approach
0LXT4ZZ Transfer Left Ankle Tendon, Percutaneous Endoscopic Approach
0LXV0ZZ Transfer Right Foot Tendon, Open Approach
0LXV4ZZ Transfer Right Foot Tendon, Percutaneous Endoscopic Approach
0LXW0ZZ Transfer Left Foot Tendon, Open Approach
0LXW4ZZ Transfer Left Foot Tendon, Percutaneous Endoscopic Approach

Bursa of the Knee

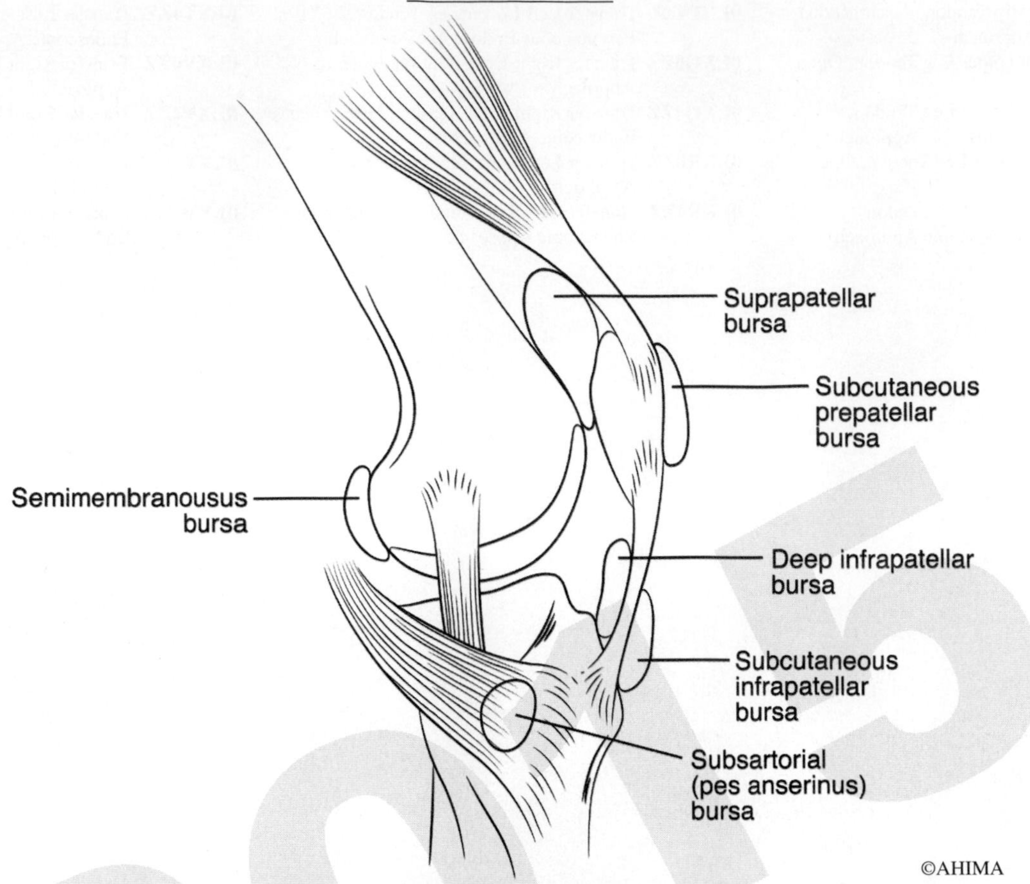
Suprapatellar bursa
Subcutaneous prepatellar bursa
Semimembranousus bursa
Deep infrapatellar bursa
Subcutaneous infrapatellar bursa
Subsartorial (pes anserinus) bursa
©AHIMA

Ligaments of the Knee

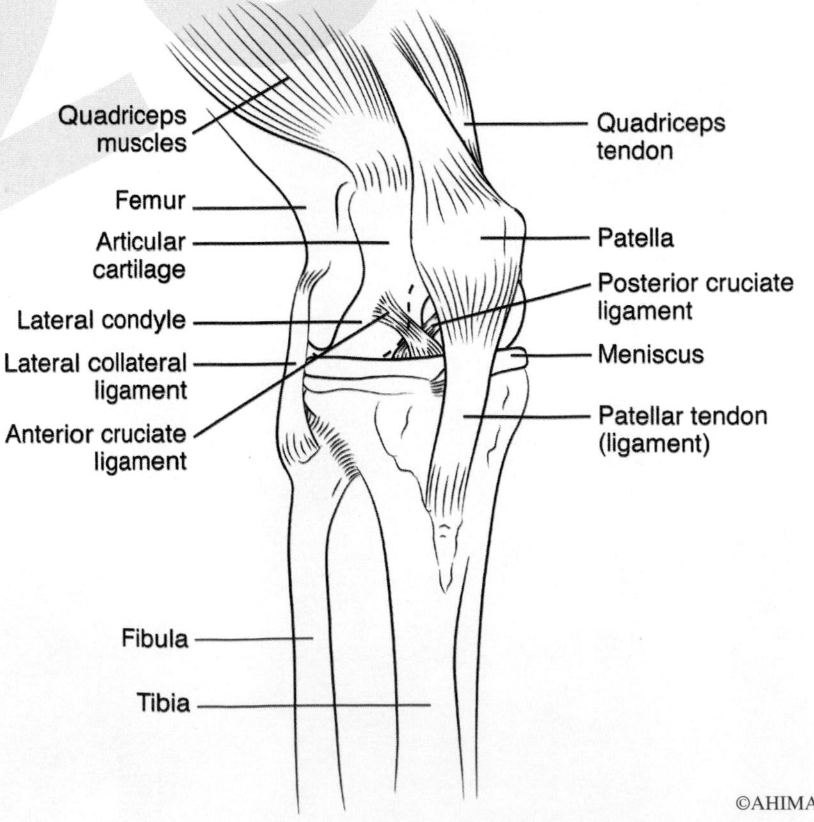
Quadriceps muscles
Quadriceps tendon
Femur
Articular cartilage
Patella
Posterior cruciate ligament
Lateral condyle
Meniscus
Lateral collateral ligament
Anterior cruciate ligament
Patellar tendon (ligament)
Fibula
Tibia
©AHIMA

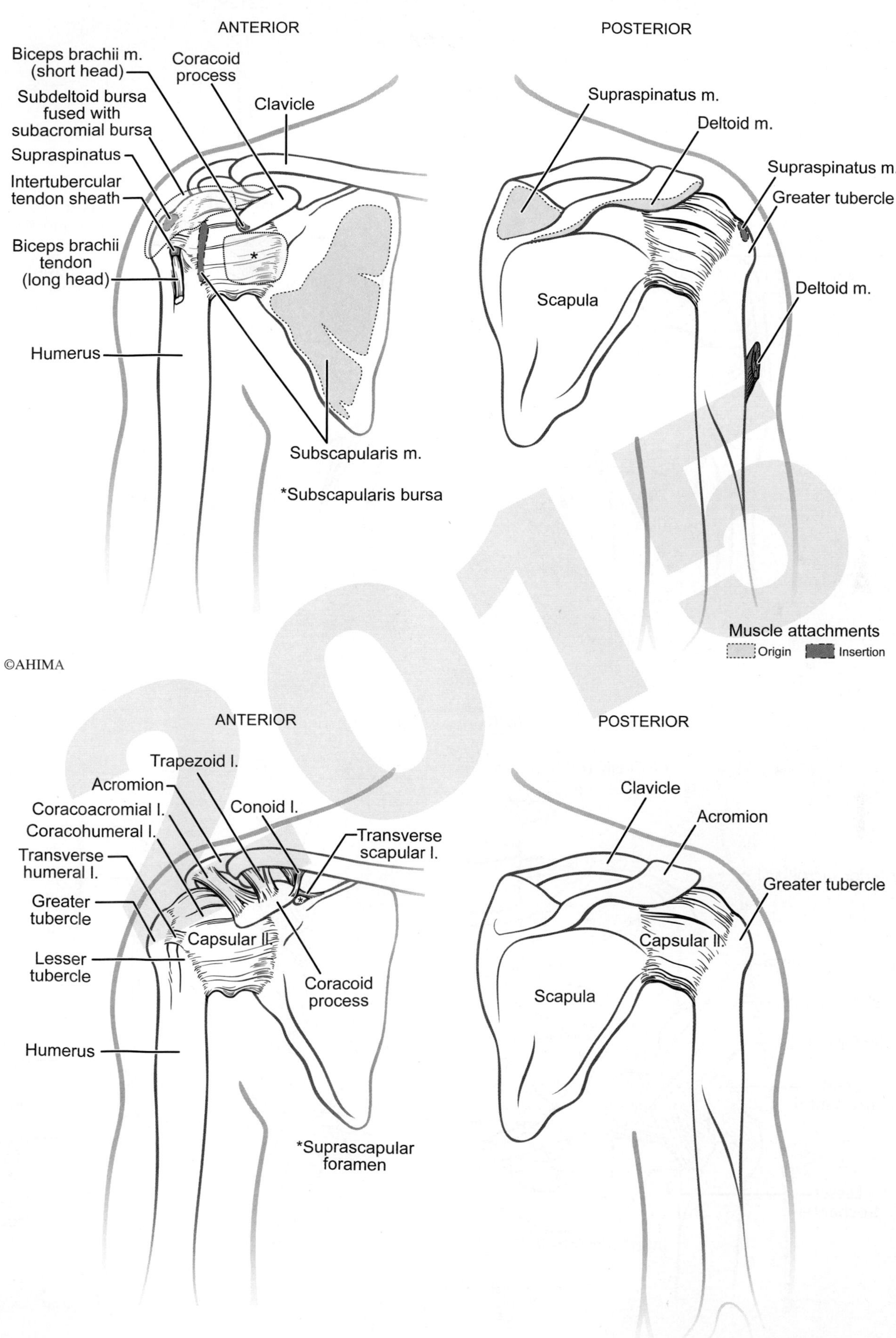
ANTERIOR
POSTERIOR
Biceps brachii m. (short head)
Coracoid process
Clavicle
Subdeltoid bursa fused with subacromial bursa
Supraspinatus
Intertubercular tendon sheath
Biceps brachii tendon (long head)
Humerus
Subscapularis m.
*Subscapularis bursa
Supraspinatus m.
Deltoid m.
Supraspinatus m.
Greater tubercle
Deltoid m.
Scapula
Muscle attachments
Origin
Insertion
©AHIMA
ANTERIOR
POSTERIOR
Trapezoid l.
Acromion
Coracoacromial l.
Conoid l.
Coracohumeral l.
Transverse scapular l.
Transverse humeral l.
Greater tubercle
Capsular ll.
Lesser tubercle
Coracoid process
Humerus
*Suprascapular foramen
Clavicle
Acromion
Greater tubercle
Capsular ll.
Scapula
©AHIMA

Knee Tendons and Ligaments

ANTERIOR
POSTERIOR
Femur
Patella
Lat. condyle of femur
Ant. cruciate l.
Fibular collateral l.
Lat. meniscus
Lat. condyle of tibia
Head of fibula
Post. cruciate l.
Med. condyle of femur
Tibial collateral l.
Med. meniscus
Med. condyle of tibia
Transverse l. of knee
Tibial tuberosity
Tibia
Femur
Post. meniscofemoral l.
Ant. cruciate l.
Lat. condyle of femur
Fibular collateral l.
Popliteus tendon
Lat. meniscus
Head of fibula
Post. cruciate l.
Tibia

Hip Tendons and Ligaments

ANTERIOR
POSTERIOR
Anterior sacroiliac l.
Iliopectinea bursa
Pubofemoral l.
Iliofemoral l.
Greater trochanter
Lesser trochanter
Intertrochanteric line
*
**
*
Posterior sacroiliac ll.
**Sacrospinous l.
Iliotibial band
Acetabular labrum
Iliofemoral l.
Ischiofemoral l.
Greater trochanter
Zona orbicularis
Protrusion of synovial membrane
Lesser trochanter
*Sacrotuberous l.

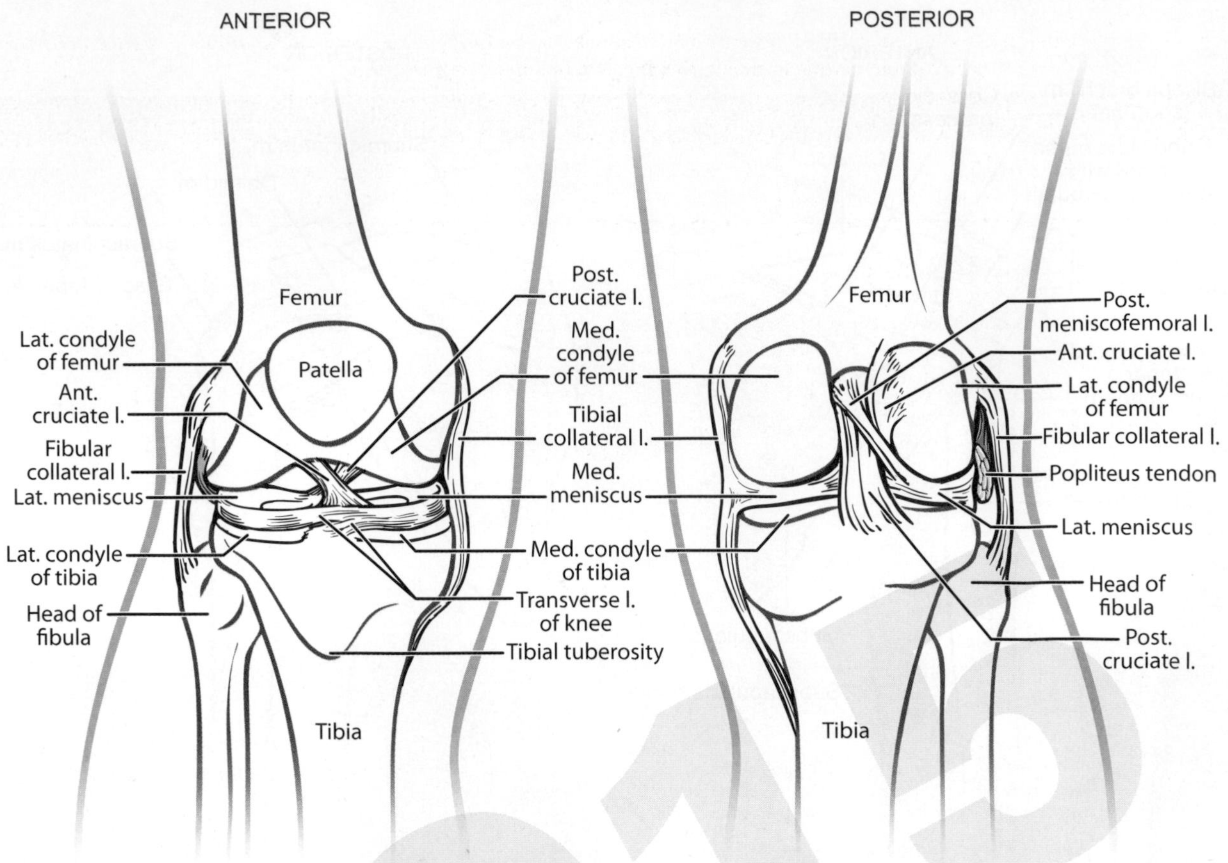

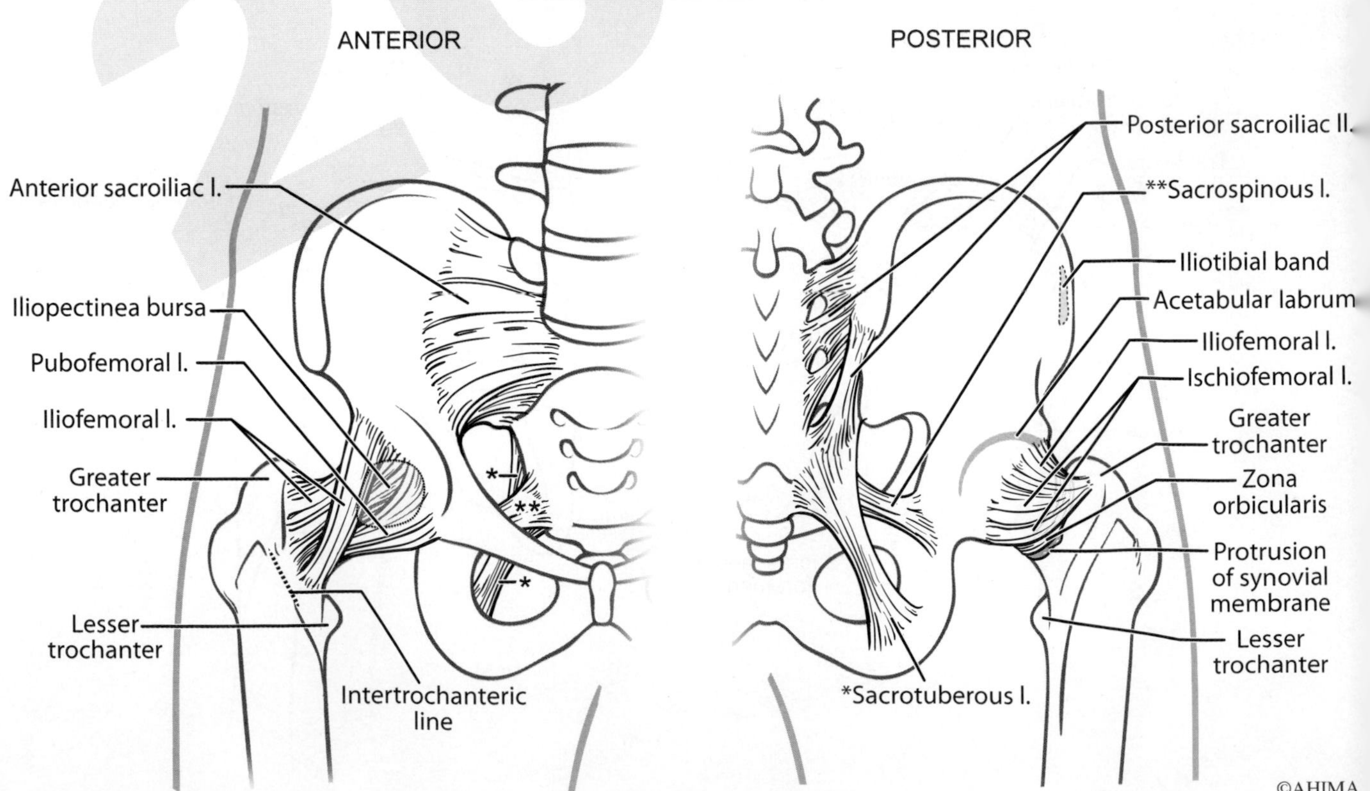

tion 0 **Medical and Surgical**
dy System M **Bursae and Ligaments**
eration 2 **Change:** Taking out or off a device from a body part and putting back an identical or similar device in or on the same body part without cutting or puncturing the skin or a mucous membrane

Body Part (4th)	Approach (5th)	Device (6th)	Qualifier (7th)
X Upper Bursa and Ligament Y Lower Bursa and Ligament	**X** External	**0** Drainage Device **Y** Other Device	**Z** No Qualifier

ction 0 **Medical and Surgical**
dy System M **Bursae and Ligaments**
eration 5 **Destruction:** Physical eradication of all or a portion of a body part by the direct use of energy, force, or a destructive agent

Body Part (4th)	Approach (5th)	Device (6th)	Qualifier (7th)
0 Head and Neck Bursa and Ligament 1 Shoulder Bursa and Ligament, Right 2 Shoulder Bursa and Ligament, Left 3 Elbow Bursa and Ligament, Right 4 Elbow Bursa and Ligament, Left 5 Wrist Bursa and Ligament, Right 6 Wrist Bursa and Ligament, Left 7 Hand Bursa and Ligament, Right 8 Hand Bursa and Ligament, Left 9 Upper Extremity Bursa and Ligament, Right **B** Upper Extremity Bursa and Ligament, Left **C** Trunk Bursa and Ligament, Right **D** Trunk Bursa and Ligament, Left **F** Thorax Bursa and Ligament, Right **G** Thorax Bursa and Ligament, Left **H** Abdomen Bursa and Ligament, Right **J** Abdomen Bursa and Ligament, Left **K** Perineum Bursa and Ligament **L** Hip Bursa and Ligament, Right **M** Hip Bursa and Ligament, Left **N** Knee Bursa and Ligament, Right **P** Knee Bursa and Ligament, Left **Q** Ankle Bursa and Ligament, Right **R** Ankle Bursa and Ligament, Left **S** Foot Bursa and Ligament, Right **T** Foot Bursa and Ligament, Left **V** Lower Extremity Bursa and Ligament, Right **W** Lower Extremity Bursa and Ligament, Left	**0** Open **3** Percutaneous **4** Percutaneous Endoscopic	**Z** No Device	**Z** No Qualifier

Section 0 **Medical and Surgical**
Body System M **Bursae and Ligaments**
Operation 8 **Division:** Cutting into a body part, without draining fluids and/or gases from the body part, in order to separate or transect a body part

Body Part (4th)	Approach (5th)	Device (6th)	Qualifier (7th)
0 Head and Neck Bursa and Ligament 1 Shoulder Bursa and Ligament, Right 2 Shoulder Bursa and Ligament, Left 3 Elbow Bursa and Ligament, Right 4 Elbow Bursa and Ligament, Left 5 Wrist Bursa and Ligament, Right 6 Wrist Bursa and Ligament, Left 7 Hand Bursa and Ligament, Right 8 Hand Bursa and Ligament, Left 9 Upper Extremity Bursa and Ligament, Right B Upper Extremity Bursa and Ligament, Left C Trunk Bursa and Ligament, Right D Trunk Bursa and Ligament, Left F Thorax Bursa and Ligament, Right G Thorax Bursa and Ligament, Left H Abdomen Bursa and Ligament, Right J Abdomen Bursa and Ligament, Left K Perineum Bursa and Ligament L Hip Bursa and Ligament, Right M Hip Bursa and Ligament, Left N Knee Bursa and Ligament, Right P Knee Bursa and Ligament, Left Q Ankle Bursa and Ligament, Right R Ankle Bursa and Ligament, Left S Foot Bursa and Ligament, Right T Foot Bursa and Ligament, Left V Lower Extremity Bursa and Ligament, Right W Lower Extremity Bursa and Ligament, Left	0 Open 3 Percutaneous 4 Percutaneous Endoscopic	Z No Device	Z No Qualifier

Section 0 **Medical and Surgical**
Body System M **Bursae and Ligaments**
Operation 9 **Drainage:** Taking or letting out fluids and/or gases from a body part

Body Part (4th)	Approach (5th)	Device (6th)	Qualifier (7th)
0 Head and Neck Bursa and Ligament 1 Shoulder Bursa and Ligament, Right 2 Shoulder Bursa and Ligament, Left 3 Elbow Bursa and Ligament, Right 4 Elbow Bursa and Ligament, Left 5 Wrist Bursa and Ligament, Right 6 Wrist Bursa and Ligament, Left 7 Hand Bursa and Ligament, Right 8 Hand Bursa and Ligament, Left 9 Upper Extremity Bursa and Ligament, Right B Upper Extremity Bursa and Ligament, Left C Trunk Bursa and Ligament, Right D Trunk Bursa and Ligament, Left F Thorax Bursa and Ligament, Right G Thorax Bursa and Ligament, Left H Abdomen Bursa and Ligament, Right J Abdomen Bursa and Ligament, Left K Perineum Bursa and Ligament L Hip Bursa and Ligament, Right M Hip Bursa and Ligament, Left N Knee Bursa and Ligament, Right P Knee Bursa and Ligament, Left Q Ankle Bursa and Ligament, Right R Ankle Bursa and Ligament, Left S Foot Bursa and Ligament, Right T Foot Bursa and Ligament, Left V Lower Extremity Bursa and Ligament, Right W Lower Extremity Bursa and Ligament, Left	0 Open 3 Percutaneous 4 Percutaneous Endoscopic	0 Drainage Device	Z No Qualifier

Continued →

tion 0 **Medical and Surgical**
ly System M **Bursae and Ligaments**
eration 9 **Drainage:** Taking or letting out fluids and/or gases from a body part

Body Part (4th)	Approach (5th)	Device (6th)	Qualifier (7th)
Head and Neck Bursa and Ligament	**0** Open	**Z** No Device	**X** Diagnostic
Shoulder Bursa and Ligament, Right	**3** Percutaneous		**Z** No Qualifier
Shoulder Bursa and Ligament, Left	**4** Percutaneous Endoscopic		
Elbow Bursa and Ligament, Right			
Elbow Bursa and Ligament, Left			
Wrist Bursa and Ligament, Right			
Wrist Bursa and Ligament, Left			
Hand Bursa and Ligament, Right			
Hand Bursa and Ligament, Left			
Upper Extremity Bursa and Ligament, Right			
Upper Extremity Bursa and Ligament, Left			
Trunk Bursa and Ligament, Right			
Trunk Bursa and Ligament, Left			
Thorax Bursa and Ligament, Right			
Thorax Bursa and Ligament, Left			
Abdomen Bursa and Ligament, Right			
Abdomen Bursa and Ligament, Left			
Perineum Bursa and Ligament			
Hip Bursa and Ligament, Right			
M Hip Bursa and Ligament, Left			
N Knee Bursa and Ligament, Right			
Knee Bursa and Ligament, Left			
Q Ankle Bursa and Ligament, Right			
R Ankle Bursa and Ligament, Left			
Foot Bursa and Ligament, Right			
T Foot Bursa and Ligament, Left			
V Lower Extremity Bursa and Ligament, Right			
W Lower Extremity Bursa and Ligament, Left			

ction 0 **Medical and Surgical**
dy System M **Bursae and Ligaments**
peration B **Excision:** Cutting out or off, without replacement, a portion of a body part

Body Part (4th)	Approach (5th)	Device (6th)	Qualifier (7th)
0 Head and Neck Bursa and Ligament	**0** Open	**Z** No Device	**X** Diagnostic
1 Shoulder Bursa and Ligament, Right	**3** Percutaneous		**Z** No Qualifier
2 Shoulder Bursa and Ligament, Left	**4** Percutaneous Endoscopic		
3 Elbow Bursa and Ligament, Right			
4 Elbow Bursa and Ligament, Left			
5 Wrist Bursa and Ligament, Right			
6 Wrist Bursa and Ligament, Left			
7 Hand Bursa and Ligament, Right			
8 Hand Bursa and Ligament, Left			
9 Upper Extremity Bursa and Ligament, Right			
B Upper Extremity Bursa and Ligament, Left			
C Trunk Bursa and Ligament, Right			
D Trunk Bursa and Ligament, Left			
F Thorax Bursa and Ligament, Right			
G Thorax Bursa and Ligament, Left			
H Abdomen Bursa and Ligament, Right			
J Abdomen Bursa and Ligament, Left			
K Perineum Bursa and Ligament			
L Hip Bursa and Ligament, Right			
M Hip Bursa and Ligament, Left			
N Knee Bursa and Ligament, Right			
P Knee Bursa and Ligament, Left			
Q Ankle Bursa and Ligament, Right			
R Ankle Bursa and Ligament, Left			
S Foot Bursa and Ligament, Right			
T Foot Bursa and Ligament, Left			
V Lower Extremity Bursa and Ligament, Right			
W Lower Extremity Bursa and Ligament, Left			

Section 0 **Medical and Surgical**
Body System M **Bursae and Ligaments**
Operation C **Extirpation:** Taking or cutting out solid matter from a body part

Body Part (4th)	Approach (5th)	Device (6th)	Qualifier (7th)
0 Head and Neck Bursa and Ligament **1** Shoulder Bursa and Ligament, Right **2** Shoulder Bursa and Ligament, Left **3** Elbow Bursa and Ligament, Right **4** Elbow Bursa and Ligament, Left **5** Wrist Bursa and Ligament, Right **6** Wrist Bursa and Ligament, Left **7** Hand Bursa and Ligament, Right **8** Hand Bursa and Ligament, Left **9** Upper Extremity Bursa and Ligament, Right **B** Upper Extremity Bursa and Ligament, Left **C** Trunk Bursa and Ligament, Right **D** Trunk Bursa and Ligament, Left **F** Thorax Bursa and Ligament, Right **G** Thorax Bursa and Ligament, Left **H** Abdomen Bursa and Ligament, Right **J** Abdomen Bursa and Ligament, Left **K** Perineum Bursa and Ligament **L** Hip Bursa and Ligament, Right **M** Hip Bursa and Ligament, Left **N** Knee Bursa and Ligament, Right **P** Knee Bursa and Ligament, Left **Q** Ankle Bursa and Ligament, Right **R** Ankle Bursa and Ligament, Left **S** Foot Bursa and Ligament, Right **T** Foot Bursa and Ligament, Left **V** Lower Extremity Bursa and Ligament, Right **W** Lower Extremity Bursa and Ligament, Left	**0** Open **3** Percutaneous **4** Percutaneous Endoscopic	**Z** No Device	**Z** No Qualifier

Section 0 **Medical and Surgical**
Body System M **Bursae and Ligaments**
Operation D **Extraction:** Pulling or stripping out or off all or a portion of a body part by the use of force

Body Part (4th)	Approach (5th)	Device (6th)	Qualifier (7th)
0 Head and Neck Bursa and Ligament **1** Shoulder Bursa and Ligament, Right **2** Shoulder Bursa and Ligament, Left **3** Elbow Bursa and Ligament, Right **4** Elbow Bursa and Ligament, Left **5** Wrist Bursa and Ligament, Right **6** Wrist Bursa and Ligament, Left **7** Hand Bursa and Ligament, Right **8** Hand Bursa and Ligament, Left **9** Upper Extremity Bursa and Ligament, Right **B** Upper Extremity Bursa and Ligament, Left **C** Trunk Bursa and Ligament, Right **D** Trunk Bursa and Ligament, Left **F** Thorax Bursa and Ligament, Right **G** Thorax Bursa and Ligament, Left **H** Abdomen Bursa and Ligament, Right **J** Abdomen Bursa and Ligament, Left **K** Perineum Bursa and Ligament **L** Hip Bursa and Ligament, Right **M** Hip Bursa and Ligament, Left **N** Knee Bursa and Ligament, Right **P** Knee Bursa and Ligament, Left **Q** Ankle Bursa and Ligament, Right **R** Ankle Bursa and Ligament, Left **S** Foot Bursa and Ligament, Right **T** Foot Bursa and Ligament, Left **V** Lower Extremity Bursa and Ligament, Right **W** Lower Extremity Bursa and Ligament, Left	**0** Open **3** Percutaneous **4** Percutaneous Endoscopic	**Z** No Device	**Z** No Qualifier

Section	**0**	**Medical and Surgical**
Body System	**M**	**Bursae and Ligaments**
Operation	**J**	**Inspection:** Visually and/or manually exploring a body part

Body Part (4th)	Approach (5th)	Device (6th)	Qualifier (7th)
X Upper Bursa and Ligament **Y** Lower Bursa and Ligament	**0** Open **3** Percutaneous **4** Percutaneous Endoscopic **X** External	**Z** No Device	**Z** No Qualifier

Section	**0**	**Medical and Surgical**
Body System	**M**	**Bursae and Ligaments**
Operation	**M**	**Reattachment:** Putting back in or on all or a portion of a separated body part to its normal location or other suitable location

Body Part (4th)	Approach (5th)	Device (6th)	Qualifier (7th)
0 Head and Neck Bursa and Ligament **1** Shoulder Bursa and Ligament, Right **2** Shoulder Bursa and Ligament, Left **3** Elbow Bursa and Ligament, Right **4** Elbow Bursa and Ligament, Left **5** Wrist Bursa and Ligament, Right **6** Wrist Bursa and Ligament, Left **7** Hand Bursa and Ligament, Right **8** Hand Bursa and Ligament, Left **9** Upper Extremity Bursa and Ligament, Right **B** Upper Extremity Bursa and Ligament, Left **C** Trunk Bursa and Ligament, Right **D** Trunk Bursa and Ligament, Left **F** Thorax Bursa and Ligament, Right **G** Thorax Bursa and Ligament, Left **H** Abdomen Bursa and Ligament, Right **J** Abdomen Bursa and Ligament, Left **K** Perineum Bursa and Ligament **L** Hip Bursa and Ligament, Right **M** Hip Bursa and Ligament, Left **N** Knee Bursa and Ligament, Right **P** Knee Bursa and Ligament, Left **Q** Ankle Bursa and Ligament, Right **R** Ankle Bursa and Ligament, Left **S** Foot Bursa and Ligament, Right **T** Foot Bursa and Ligament, Left **V** Lower Extremity Bursa and Ligament, Right **W** Lower Extremity Bursa and Ligament, Left	**0** Open **4** Percutaneous Endoscopic	**Z** No Device	**Z** No Qualifier

Section 0 **Medical and Surgical**
Body System M **Bursae and Ligaments**
Operation N **Release:** Freeing a body part from an abnormal physical constraint by cutting or by the use of force

Body Part (4th)	Approach (5th)	Device (6th)	Qualifier (7th)
0 Head and Neck Bursa and Ligament **1** Shoulder Bursa and Ligament, Right **2** Shoulder Bursa and Ligament, Left **3** Elbow Bursa and Ligament, Right **4** Elbow Bursa and Ligament, Left **5** Wrist Bursa and Ligament, Right **6** Wrist Bursa and Ligament, Left **7** Hand Bursa and Ligament, Right **8** Hand Bursa and Ligament, Left **9** Upper Extremity Bursa and Ligament, Right **B** Upper Extremity Bursa and Ligament, Left **C** Trunk Bursa and Ligament, Right **D** Trunk Bursa and Ligament, Left **F** Thorax Bursa and Ligament, Right **G** Thorax Bursa and Ligament, Left **H** Abdomen Bursa and Ligament, Right **J** Abdomen Bursa and Ligament, Left **K** Perineum Bursa and Ligament **L** Hip Bursa and Ligament, Right **M** Hip Bursa and Ligament, Left **N** Knee Bursa and Ligament, Right **P** Knee Bursa and Ligament, Left **Q** Ankle Bursa and Ligament, Right **R** Ankle Bursa and Ligament, Left **S** Foot Bursa and Ligament, Right **T** Foot Bursa and Ligament, Left **V** Lower Extremity Bursa and Ligament, Right **W** Lower Extremity Bursa and Ligament, Left	**0** Open **3** Percutaneous **4** Percutaneous Endoscopic **X** External	**Z** No Device	**Z** No Qualifier

Section 0 **Medical and Surgical**
Body System M **Bursae and Ligaments**
Operation P **Removal:** Taking out or off a device from a body part

Body Part (4th)	Approach (5th)	Device (6th)	Qualifier (7th)
X Upper Bursa and Ligament **Y** Lower Bursa and Ligament	**0** Open **3** Percutaneous **4** Percutaneous Endoscopic	**0** Drainage Device **7** Autologous Tissue Substitute **J** Synthetic Substitute **K** Nonautologous Tissue Substitute	**Z** No Qualifier
X Upper Bursa and Ligament **Y** Lower Bursa and Ligament	**X** External	**0** Drainage Device	**Z** No Qualifier

Section 0 **Medical and Surgical**
Body System M **Bursae and Ligaments**
Operation Q **Repair:** Restoring, to the extent possible, a body part to its normal anatomic structure and function

Body Part (4th)	Approach (5th)	Device (6th)	Qualifier (7th)
0 Head and Neck Bursa and Ligament **1** Shoulder Bursa and Ligament, Right **2** Shoulder Bursa and Ligament, Left **3** Elbow Bursa and Ligament, Right **4** Elbow Bursa and Ligament, Left **5** Wrist Bursa and Ligament, Right **6** Wrist Bursa and Ligament, Left **7** Hand Bursa and Ligament, Right **8** Hand Bursa and Ligament, Left **9** Upper Extremity Bursa and Ligament, Right **B** Upper Extremity Bursa and Ligament, Left **C** Trunk Bursa and Ligament, Right **D** Trunk Bursa and Ligament, Left **F** Thorax Bursa and Ligament, Right **G** Thorax Bursa and Ligament, Left **H** Abdomen Bursa and Ligament, Right **J** Abdomen Bursa and Ligament, Left **K** Perineum Bursa and Ligament **L** Hip Bursa and Ligament, Right **M** Hip Bursa and Ligament, Left **N** Knee Bursa and Ligaxment, Right **P** Knee Bursa and Ligament, Left **Q** Ankle Bursa and Ligament, Right **R** Ankle Bursa and Ligament, Left **S** Foot Bursa and Ligament, Right **T** Foot Bursa and Ligament, Left **V** Lower Extremity Bursa and Ligament, Right **W** Lower Extremity Bursa and Ligament, Left	**0** Open **3** Percutaneous **4** Percutaneous Endoscopic	**Z** No Device	**Z** No Qualifier

Section 0 **Medical and Surgical**
Body System M **Bursae and Ligaments**
Operation S **Reposition:** Moving to its normal location, or other suitable location, all or a portion of a body part

Body Part (4th)	Approach (5th)	Device (6th)	Qualifier (7th)
0 Head and Neck Bursa and Ligament **1** Shoulder Bursa and Ligament, Right **2** Shoulder Bursa and Ligament, Left **3** Elbow Bursa and Ligament, Right **4** Elbow Bursa and Ligament, Left **5** Wrist Bursa and Ligament, Right **6** Wrist Bursa and Ligament, Left **7** Hand Bursa and Ligament, Right **8** Hand Bursa and Ligament, Left **9** Upper Extremity Bursa and Ligament, Right **B** Upper Extremity Bursa and Ligament, Left **C** Trunk Bursa and Ligament, Right **D** Trunk Bursa and Ligament, Left **F** Thorax Bursa and Ligament, Right **G** Thorax Bursa and Ligament, Left **H** Abdomen Bursa and Ligament, Right **J** Abdomen Bursa and Ligament, Left **K** Perineum Bursa and Ligament **L** Hip Bursa and Ligament, Right **M** Hip Bursa and Ligament, Left **N** Knee Bursa and Ligament, Right **P** Knee Bursa and Ligament, Left **Q** Ankle Bursa and Ligament, Right **R** Ankle Bursa and Ligament, Left **S** Foot Bursa and Ligament, Right **T** Foot Bursa and Ligament, Left **V** Lower Extremity Bursa and Ligament, Right **W** Lower Extremity Bursa and Ligament, Left	**0** Open **4** Percutaneous Endoscopic	**Z** No Device	**Z** No Qualifier

Section 0 **Medical and Surgical**
Body System M **Bursae and Ligaments**
Operation T **Resection:** Cutting out or off, without replacement, all of a body part

Body Part (4th)	Approach (5th)	Device (6th)	Qualifier (7th)
0 Head and Neck Bursa and Ligament **1** Shoulder Bursa and Ligament, Right **2** Shoulder Bursa and Ligament, Left **3** Elbow Bursa and Ligament, Right **4** Elbow Bursa and Ligament, Left **5** Wrist Bursa and Ligament, Right **6** Wrist Bursa and Ligament, Left **7** Hand Bursa and Ligament, Right **8** Hand Bursa and Ligament, Left **9** Upper Extremity Bursa and Ligament, Right **B** Upper Extremity Bursa and Ligament, Left **C** Trunk Bursa and Ligament, Right **D** Trunk Bursa and Ligament, Left **F** Thorax Bursa and Ligament, Right **G** Thorax Bursa and Ligament, Left **H** Abdomen Bursa and Ligament, Right **J** Abdomen Bursa and Ligament, Left **K** Perineum Bursa and Ligament **L** Hip Bursa and Ligament, Right **M** Hip Bursa and Ligament, Left **N** Knee Bursa and Ligament, Right **P** Knee Bursa and Ligament, Left **Q** Ankle Bursa and Ligament, Right **R** Ankle Bursa and Ligament, Left **S** Foot Bursa and Ligament, Right **T** Foot Bursa and Ligament, Left **V** Lower Extremity Bursa and Ligament, Right **W** Lower Extremity Bursa and Ligament, Left	**0** Open **4** Percutaneous Endoscopic	**Z** No Device	**Z** No Qualifier

Section 0 **Medical and Surgical**
Body System M **Bursae and Ligaments**
Operation U **Supplement:** Putting in or on biological or synthetic material that physically reinforces and/or augments the function of a portion of a body part

Body Part (4th)	Approach (5th)	Device (6th)	Qualifier (7th)
0 Head and Neck Bursa and Ligament **1** Shoulder Bursa and Ligament, Right **2** Shoulder Bursa and Ligament, Left **3** Elbow Bursa and Ligament, Right **4** Elbow Bursa and Ligament, Left **5** Wrist Bursa and Ligament, Right **6** Wrist Bursa and Ligament, Left **7** Hand Bursa and Ligament, Right **8** Hand Bursa and Ligament, Left **9** Upper Extremity Bursa and Ligament, Right **B** Upper Extremity Bursa and Ligament, Left **C** Trunk Bursa and Ligament, Right **D** Trunk Bursa and Ligament, Left **F** Thorax Bursa and Ligament, Right **G** Thorax Bursa and Ligament, Left **H** Abdomen Bursa and Ligament, Right **J** Abdomen Bursa and Ligament, Left **K** Perineum Bursa and Ligament **L** Hip Bursa and Ligament, Right **M** Hip Bursa and Ligament, Left **N** Knee Bursa and Ligament, Right **P** Knee Bursa and Ligament, Left **Q** Ankle Bursa and Ligament, Right **R** Ankle Bursa and Ligament, Left **S** Foot Bursa and Ligament, Right **T** Foot Bursa and Ligament, Left **V** Lower Extremity Bursa and Ligament, Right **W** Lower Extremity Bursa and Ligament, Left	**0** Open **4** Percutaneous Endoscopic	**7** Autologous Tissue Substitute **J** Synthetic Substitute **K** Nonautologous Tissue Substitute	**Z** No Qualifier

-tion	**0**	**Medical and Surgical**
-ly System	**M**	**Bursae and Ligaments**
-eration	**W**	**Revision:** Correcting, to the extent possible, a portion of a malfunctioning device or the position of a displaced device

Body Part (4th)	Approach (5th)	Device (6th)	Qualifier (7th)
Upper Bursa and Ligament Lower Bursa and Ligament	**0** Open **3** Percutaneous **4** Percutaneous Endoscopic **X** External	**0** Drainage Device **7** Autologous Tissue Substitute **J** Synthetic Substitute **K** Nonautologous Tissue Substitute	**Z** No Qualifier

-tion	**0**	**Medical and Surgical**
-ly System	**M**	**Bursae and Ligaments**
-eration	**X**	**Transfer:** Moving, without taking out, all or a portion of a body part to another location to take over the function of all or a portion of a body part

Body Part (4th)	Approach (5th)	Device (6th)	Qualifier (7th)
Head and Neck Bursa and Ligament Shoulder Bursa and Ligament, Right Shoulder Bursa and Ligament, Left Elbow Bursa and Ligament, Right Elbow Bursa and Ligament, Left Wrist Bursa and Ligament, Right Wrist Bursa and Ligament, Left Hand Bursa and Ligament, Right Hand Bursa and Ligament, Left Upper Extremity Bursa and Ligament, Right Upper Extremity Bursa and Ligament, Left Trunk Bursa and Ligament, Right Trunk Bursa and Ligament, Left Thorax Bursa and Ligament, Right Thorax Bursa and Ligament, Left I Abdomen Bursa and Ligament, Right Abdomen Bursa and Ligament, Left Perineum Bursa and Ligament Hip Bursa and Ligament, Right M Hip Bursa and Ligament, Left N Knee Bursa and Ligament, Right P Knee Bursa and Ligament, Left Q Ankle Bursa and Ligament, Right R Ankle Bursa and Ligament, Left Foot Bursa and Ligament, Right T Foot Bursa and Ligament, Left V Lower Extremity Bursa and Ligament, Right W Lower Extremity Bursa and Ligament, Left	**0** Open **4** Percutaneous Endoscopic	**Z** No Device	**Z** No Qualifier

-ursae and Ligaments Code Listing 0M2–0MX

-eview Coding Guideline B4.5

-M2 – Bursae and Ligaments, Change

-M2XX0Z Change Drainage Device in Upper Bursa and Ligament, External Approach

-M2XXYZ Change Other Device in Upper Bursa and Ligament, External Approach

0M2YX0Z Change Drainage Device in Lower Bursa and Ligament, External Approach

0M2YXYZ Change Other Device in Lower Bursa and Ligament, External Approach

-M5 – Bursae and Ligaments, Destruction

-eview Coding Guideline B6.1c

-M500ZZ Destruction of Head and Neck Bursa and Ligament, Open Approach

-M503ZZ Destruction of Head and Neck Bursa and Ligament, Percutaneous Approach

0M504ZZ Destruction of Head and Neck Bursa and Ligament, Percutaneous Endoscopic Approach

0M510ZZ Destruction of Right Shoulder Bursa and Ligament, Open Approach

0M513ZZ Destruction of Right Shoulder Bursa and Ligament, Percutaneous Approach

0M514ZZ Destruction of Right Shoulder Bursa and Ligament, Percutaneous Endoscopic Approach

0M520ZZ Destruction of Left Shoulder Bursa and Ligament, Open Approach
0M523ZZ Destruction of Left Shoulder Bursa and Ligament, Percutaneous Approach
0M524ZZ Destruction of Left Shoulder Bursa and Ligament, Percutaneous Endoscopic Approach
0M530ZZ Destruction of Right Elbow Bursa and Ligament, Open Approach
0M533ZZ Destruction of Right Elbow Bursa and Ligament, Percutaneous Approach
0M534ZZ Destruction of Right Elbow Bursa and Ligament, Percutaneous Endoscopic Approach
0M540ZZ Destruction of Left Elbow Bursa and Ligament, Open Approach
0M543ZZ Destruction of Left Elbow Bursa and Ligament, Percutaneous Approach
0M544ZZ Destruction of Left Elbow Bursa and Ligament, Percutaneous Endoscopic Approach
0M550ZZ Destruction of Right Wrist Bursa and Ligament, Open Approach
0M553ZZ Destruction of Right Wrist Bursa and Ligament, Percutaneous Approach
0M554ZZ Destruction of Right Wrist Bursa and Ligament, Percutaneous Endoscopic Approach
0M560ZZ Destruction of Left Wrist Bursa and Ligament, Open Approach
0M563ZZ Destruction of Left Wrist Bursa and Ligament, Percutaneous Approach
0M564ZZ Destruction of Left Wrist Bursa and Ligament, Percutaneous Endoscopic Approach
0M570ZZ Destruction of Right Hand Bursa and Ligament, Open Approach
0M573ZZ Destruction of Right Hand Bursa and Ligament, Percutaneous Approach
0M574ZZ Destruction of Right Hand Bursa and Ligament, Percutaneous Endoscopic Approach
0M580ZZ Destruction of Left Hand Bursa and Ligament, Open Approach
0M583ZZ Destruction of Left Hand Bursa and Ligament, Percutaneous Approach
0M584ZZ Destruction of Left Hand Bursa and Ligament, Percutaneous Endoscopic Approach
0M590ZZ Destruction of Right Upper Extremity Bursa and Ligament, Open Approach
0M593ZZ Destruction of Right Upper Extremity Bursa and Ligament, Percutaneous Approach
0M594ZZ Destruction of Right Upper Extremity Bursa and Ligament, Percutaneous Endoscopic Approach
0M5B0ZZ Destruction of Left Upper Extremity Bursa and Ligament, Open Approach
0M5B3ZZ Destruction of Left Upper Extremity Bursa and Ligament, Percutaneous Approach
0M5B4ZZ Destruction of Left Upper Extremity Bursa and Ligament, Percutaneous Endoscopic Approach
0M5C0ZZ Destruction of Right Trunk Bursa and Ligament, Open Approach
0M5C3ZZ Destruction of Right Trunk Bursa and Ligament, Percutaneous Approach
0M5C4ZZ Destruction of Right Trunk Bursa and Ligament, Percutaneous Endoscopic Approach
0M5D0ZZ Destruction of Left Trunk Bursa and Ligament, Open Approach
0M5D3ZZ Destruction of Left Trunk Bursa and Ligament, Percutaneous Approach
0M5D4ZZ Destruction of Left Trunk Bursa and Ligament, Percutaneous Endoscopic Approach
0M5F0ZZ Destruction of Right Thorax Bursa and Ligament, Open Approach
0M5F3ZZ Destruction of Right Thorax Bursa and Ligament, Percutaneous Approach
0M5F4ZZ Destruction of Right Thorax Bursa and Ligament, Percutaneous Endoscopic Approach
0M5G0ZZ Destruction of Left Thorax Bursa and Ligament, Open Approach
0M5G3ZZ Destruction of Left Thorax Bursa and Ligament, Percutaneous Approach
0M5G4ZZ Destruction of Left Thorax Bursa and Ligament, Percutaneous Endoscopic Approach
0M5H0ZZ Destruction of Right Abdomen Bursa and Ligament, Open Approach
0M5H3ZZ Destruction of Right Abdomen Bursa and Ligament, Percutaneous Approach
0M5H4ZZ Destruction of Right Abdomen Bursa and Ligament, Percutaneous Endoscopic Approach
0M5J0ZZ Destruction of Left Abdomen Bursa and Ligament, Open Approach
0M5J3ZZ Destruction of Left Abdomen Bursa and Ligament, Percutaneous Approach
0M5J4ZZ Destruction of Left Abdomen Bursa and Ligament, Percutaneous Endoscopic Approach
0M5K0ZZ Destruction of Perineum Bursa and Ligament, Open Approach
0M5K3ZZ Destruction of Perineum Bursa and Ligament, Percutaneous Approach
0M5K4ZZ Destruction of Perineum Bursa and Ligament, Percutaneous Endoscopic Approach
0M5L0ZZ Destruction of Right Hip Bursa and Ligament, Open Approach
0M5L3ZZ Destruction of Right Hip Bursa and Ligament, Percutaneous Approach
0M5L4ZZ Destruction of Right Hip Bursa and Ligament, Percutaneous Endoscopic Approach
0M5M0ZZ Destruction of Left Hip Bursa and Ligament, Open Approach
0M5M3ZZ Destruction of Left Hip Bursa and Ligament, Percutaneous Approach
0M5M4ZZ Destruction of Left Hip Bursa and Ligament, Percutaneous Endoscopic Approach
0M5N0ZZ Destruction of Right Knee Bursa and Ligament, Open Approach
0M5N3ZZ Destruction of Right Knee Bursa and Ligament, Percutaneous Approach
0M5N4ZZ Destruction of Right Knee Bursa and Ligament, Percutaneous Endoscopic Approach
0M5P0ZZ Destruction of Left Knee Bursa and Ligament, Open Approach
0M5P3ZZ Destruction of Left Knee Bursa and Ligament, Percutaneous Approach
0M5P4ZZ Destruction of Left Knee Bursa and Ligament, Percutaneous Endoscopic Approach
0M5Q0ZZ Destruction of Right Ankle Bursa and Ligament, Open Approach
0M5Q3ZZ Destruction of Right Ankle Bursa and Ligament, Percutaneous Approach
0M5Q4ZZ Destruction of Right Ankle Bursa and Ligament, Percutaneous Endoscopic Approach
0M5R0ZZ Destruction of Left Ankle Bursa and Ligament, Open Approach
0M5R3ZZ Destruction of Left Ankle Bursa and Ligament, Percutaneous Approach
0M5R4ZZ Destruction of Left Ankle Bursa and Ligament, Percutaneous Endoscopic Approach
0M5S0ZZ Destruction of Right Foot Bursa and Ligament, Open Approach
0M5S3ZZ Destruction of Right Foot Bursa and Ligament, Percutaneous Approach
0M5S4ZZ Destruction of Right Foot Bursa and Ligament, Percutaneous Endoscopic Approach
0M5T0ZZ Destruction of Left Foot Bursa and Ligament, Open Approach
0M5T3ZZ Destruction of Left Foot Bursa and Ligament, Percutaneous Approach
0M5T4ZZ Destruction of Left Foot Bursa and Ligament, Percutaneous Endoscopic Approach
0M5V0ZZ Destruction of Right Lower Extremity Bursa and Ligament, Open Approach
0M5V3ZZ Destruction of Right Lower Extremity Bursa and Ligament, Percutaneous Approach
0M5V4ZZ Destruction of Right Lower Extremity Bursa and Ligament, Percutaneous Endoscopic Approach
0M5W0ZZ Destruction of Left Lower Extremity Bursa and Ligament, Open Approach
0M5W3ZZ Destruction of Left Lower Extremity Bursa and Ligament, Percutaneous Approach
0M5W4ZZ Destruction of Left Lower Extremity Bursa and Ligament, Percutaneous Endoscopic Approach

0M8 – Bursae and Ligaments, Division

Review Coding Guideline B3.14

0M800ZZ Division of Head and Neck Bursa and Ligament, Open Approach
0M803ZZ Division of Head and Neck Bursa and Ligament, Percutaneous Approach
0M804ZZ Division of Head and Neck Bursa and Ligament, Percutaneous Endoscopic Approach
0M810ZZ Division of Right Shoulder Bursa and Ligament, Open Approach
0M813ZZ Division of Right Shoulder Bursa and Ligament, Percutaneous Approach
0M814ZZ Division of Right Shoulder Bursa and Ligament, Percutaneous Endoscopic Approach
0M820ZZ Division of Left Shoulder Bursa and Ligament, Open Approach
0M823ZZ Division of Left Shoulder Bursa and Ligament, Percutaneous Approach
0M824ZZ Division of Left Shoulder Bursa and Ligament, Percutaneous Endoscopic Approach

830ZZ	Division of Right Elbow Bursa and Ligament, Open Approach
833ZZ	Division of Right Elbow Bursa and Ligament, Percutaneous Approach
834ZZ	Division of Right Elbow Bursa and Ligament, Percutaneous Endoscopic Approach
840ZZ	Division of Left Elbow Bursa and Ligament, Open Approach
843ZZ	Division of Left Elbow Bursa and Ligament, Percutaneous Approach
844ZZ	Division of Left Elbow Bursa and Ligament, Percutaneous Endoscopic Approach
850ZZ	Division of Right Wrist Bursa and Ligament, Open Approach
853ZZ	Division of Right Wrist Bursa and Ligament, Percutaneous Approach
854ZZ	Division of Right Wrist Bursa and Ligament, Percutaneous Endoscopic Approach
860ZZ	Division of Left Wrist Bursa and Ligament, Open Approach
863ZZ	Division of Left Wrist Bursa and Ligament, Percutaneous Approach
864ZZ	Division of Left Wrist Bursa and Ligament, Percutaneous Endoscopic Approach
870ZZ	Division of Right Hand Bursa and Ligament, Open Approach
873ZZ	Division of Right Hand Bursa and Ligament, Percutaneous Approach
874ZZ	Division of Right Hand Bursa and Ligament, Percutaneous Endoscopic Approach
880ZZ	Division of Left Hand Bursa and Ligament, Open Approach
883ZZ	Division of Left Hand Bursa and Ligament, Percutaneous Approach
884ZZ	Division of Left Hand Bursa and Ligament, Percutaneous Endoscopic Approach
890ZZ	Division of Right Upper Extremity Bursa and Ligament, Open Approach
893ZZ	Division of Right Upper Extremity Bursa and Ligament, Percutaneous Approach
894ZZ	Division of Right Upper Extremity Bursa and Ligament, Percutaneous Endoscopic Approach
18B0ZZ	Division of Left Upper Extremity Bursa and Ligament, Open Approach
18B3ZZ	Division of Left Upper Extremity Bursa and Ligament, Percutaneous Approach
18B4ZZ	Division of Left Upper Extremity Bursa and Ligament, Percutaneous Endoscopic Approach
M8C0ZZ	Division of Right Trunk Bursa and Ligament, Open Approach
0M8C3ZZ	Division of Right Trunk Bursa and Ligament, Percutaneous Approach
0M8C4ZZ	Division of Right Trunk Bursa and Ligament, Percutaneous Endoscopic Approach
0M8D0ZZ	Division of Left Trunk Bursa and Ligament, Open Approach
0M8D3ZZ	Division of Left Trunk Bursa and Ligament, Percutaneous Approach
0M8D4ZZ	Division of Left Trunk Bursa and Ligament, Percutaneous Endoscopic Approach
0M8F0ZZ	Division of Right Thorax Bursa and Ligament, Open Approach
0M8F3ZZ	Division of Right Thorax Bursa and Ligament, Percutaneous Approach
0M8F4ZZ	Division of Right Thorax Bursa and Ligament, Percutaneous Endoscopic Approach
0M8G0ZZ	Division of Left Thorax Bursa and Ligament, Open Approach
0M8G3ZZ	Division of Left Thorax Bursa and Ligament, Percutaneous Approach
0M8G4ZZ	Division of Left Thorax Bursa and Ligament, Percutaneous Endoscopic Approach
0M8H0ZZ	Division of Right Abdomen Bursa and Ligament, Open Approach
0M8H3ZZ	Division of Right Abdomen Bursa and Ligament, Percutaneous Approach
0M8H4ZZ	Division of Right Abdomen Bursa and Ligament, Percutaneous Endoscopic Approach
0M8J0ZZ	Division of Left Abdomen Bursa and Ligament, Open Approach
0M8J3ZZ	Division of Left Abdomen Bursa and Ligament, Percutaneous Approach
0M8J4ZZ	Division of Left Abdomen Bursa and Ligament, Percutaneous Endoscopic Approach
0M8K0ZZ	Division of Perineum Bursa and Ligament, Open Approach
0M8K3ZZ	Division of Perineum Bursa and Ligament, Percutaneous Approach
0M8K4ZZ	Division of Perineum Bursa and Ligament, Percutaneous Endoscopic Approach
0M8L0ZZ	Division of Right Hip Bursa and Ligament, Open Approach
0M8L3ZZ	Division of Right Hip Bursa and Ligament, Percutaneous Approach
0M8L4ZZ	Division of Right Hip Bursa and Ligament, Percutaneous Endoscopic Approach
0M8M0ZZ	Division of Left Hip Bursa and Ligament, Open Approach
0M8M3ZZ	Division of Left Hip Bursa and Ligament, Percutaneous Approach
0M8M4ZZ	Division of Left Hip Bursa and Ligament, Percutaneous Endoscopic Approach
0M8N0ZZ	Division of Right Knee Bursa and Ligament, Open Approach
0M8N3ZZ	Division of Right Knee Bursa and Ligament, Percutaneous Approach
0M8N4ZZ	Division of Right Knee Bursa and Ligament, Percutaneous Endoscopic Approach
0M8P0ZZ	Division of Left Knee Bursa and Ligament, Open Approach
0M8P3ZZ	Division of Left Knee Bursa and Ligament, Percutaneous Approach
0M8P4ZZ	Division of Left Knee Bursa and Ligament, Percutaneous Endoscopic Approach
0M8Q0ZZ	Division of Right Ankle Bursa and Ligament, Open Approach
0M8Q3ZZ	Division of Right Ankle Bursa and Ligament, Percutaneous Approach
0M8Q4ZZ	Division of Right Ankle Bursa and Ligament, Percutaneous Endoscopic Approach
0M8R0ZZ	Division of Left Ankle Bursa and Ligament, Open Approach
0M8R3ZZ	Division of Left Ankle Bursa and Ligament, Percutaneous Approach
0M8R4ZZ	Division of Left Ankle Bursa and Ligament, Percutaneous Endoscopic Approach
0M8S0ZZ	Division of Right Foot Bursa and Ligament, Open Approach
0M8S3ZZ	Division of Right Foot Bursa and Ligament, Percutaneous Approach
0M8S4ZZ	Division of Right Foot Bursa and Ligament, Percutaneous Endoscopic Approach
0M8T0ZZ	Division of Left Foot Bursa and Ligament, Open Approach
0M8T3ZZ	Division of Left Foot Bursa and Ligament, Percutaneous Approach
0M8T4ZZ	Division of Left Foot Bursa and Ligament, Percutaneous Endoscopic Approach
0M8V0ZZ	Division of Right Lower Extremity Bursa and Ligament, Open Approach
0M8V3ZZ	Division of Right Lower Extremity Bursa and Ligament, Percutaneous Approach
0M8V4ZZ	Division of Right Lower Extremity Bursa and Ligament, Percutaneous Endoscopic Approach
0M8W0ZZ	Division of Left Lower Extremity Bursa and Ligament, Open Approach
0M8W3ZZ	Division of Left Lower Extremity Bursa and Ligament, Percutaneous Approach
0M8W4ZZ	Division of Left Lower Extremity Bursa and Ligament, Percutaneous Endoscopic Approach

M9 – Bursae and Ligaments, Drainage

?eview Coding Guidelines B3.4a and B3.4b

?eview Coding Guideline B6.2

M9000Z	Drainage of Head and Neck Bursa and Ligament with Drainage Device, Open Approach
M900ZX	Drainage of Head and Neck Bursa and Ligament, Open Approach, Diagnostic
M900ZZ	Drainage of Head and Neck Bursa and Ligament, Open Approach
0M9030Z	Drainage of Head and Neck Bursa and Ligament with Drainage Device, Percutaneous Approach
0M903ZX	Drainage of Head and Neck Bursa and Ligament, Percutaneous Approach, Diagnostic
0M903ZZ	Drainage of Head and Neck Bursa and Ligament, Percutaneous Approach
0M9040Z	Drainage of Head and Neck Bursa and Ligament with Drainage Device, Percutaneous Endoscopic Approach
0M904ZX	Drainage of Head and Neck Bursa and Ligament, Percutaneous Endoscopic Approach, Diagnostic
0M904ZZ	Drainage of Head and Neck Bursa and Ligament, Percutaneous Endoscopic Approach

0M9100Z Drainage of Right Shoulder Bursa and Ligament with Drainage Device, Open Approach

0M910ZX Drainage of Right Shoulder Bursa and Ligament, Open Approach, Diagnostic

0M910ZZ Drainage of Right Shoulder Bursa and Ligament, Open Approach

0M9130Z Drainage of Right Shoulder Bursa and Ligament with Drainage Device, Percutaneous Approach

0M913ZX Drainage of Right Shoulder Bursa and Ligament, Percutaneous Approach, Diagnostic

0M913ZZ Drainage of Right Shoulder Bursa and Ligament, Percutaneous Approach

0M9140Z Drainage of Right Shoulder Bursa and Ligament with Drainage Device, Percutaneous Endoscopic Approach

0M914ZX Drainage of Right Shoulder Bursa and Ligament, Percutaneous Endoscopic Approach, Diagnostic

0M914ZZ Drainage of Right Shoulder Bursa and Ligament, Percutaneous Endoscopic Approach

0M9200Z Drainage of Left Shoulder Bursa and Ligament with Drainage Device, Open Approach

0M920ZX Drainage of Left Shoulder Bursa and Ligament, Open Approach, Diagnostic

0M920ZZ Drainage of Left Shoulder Bursa and Ligament, Open Approach

0M9230Z Drainage of Left Shoulder Bursa and Ligament with Drainage Device, Percutaneous Approach

0M923ZX Drainage of Left Shoulder Bursa and Ligament, Percutaneous Approach, Diagnostic

0M923ZZ Drainage of Left Shoulder Bursa and Ligament, Percutaneous Approach

0M9240Z Drainage of Left Shoulder Bursa and Ligament with Drainage Device, Percutaneous Endoscopic Approach

0M924ZX Drainage of Left Shoulder Bursa and Ligament, Percutaneous Endoscopic Approach, Diagnostic

0M924ZZ Drainage of Left Shoulder Bursa and Ligament, Percutaneous Endoscopic Approach

0M9300Z Drainage of Right Elbow Bursa and Ligament with Drainage Device, Open Approach

0M930ZX Drainage of Right Elbow Bursa and Ligament, Open Approach, Diagnostic

0M930ZZ Drainage of Right Elbow Bursa and Ligament, Open Approach

0M9330Z Drainage of Right Elbow Bursa and Ligament with Drainage Device, Percutaneous Approach

0M933ZX Drainage of Right Elbow Bursa and Ligament, Percutaneous Approach, Diagnostic

0M933ZZ Drainage of Right Elbow Bursa and Ligament, Percutaneous Approach

0M9340Z Drainage of Right Elbow Bursa and Ligament with Drainage Device, Percutaneous Endoscopic Approach

0M934ZX Drainage of Right Elbow Bursa and Ligament, Percutaneous Endoscopic Approach, Diagnostic

0M934ZZ Drainage of Right Elbow Bursa and Ligament, Percutaneous Endoscopic Approach

0M9400Z Drainage of Left Elbow Bursa and Ligament with Drainage Device, Open Approach

0M940ZX Drainage of Left Elbow Bursa and Ligament, Open Approach, Diagnostic

0M940ZZ Drainage of Left Elbow Bursa and Ligament, Open Approach

0M9430Z Drainage of Left Elbow Bursa and Ligament with Drainage Device, Percutaneous Approach

0M943ZX Drainage of Left Elbow Bursa and Ligament, Percutaneous Approach, Diagnostic

0M943ZZ Drainage of Left Elbow Bursa and Ligament, Percutaneous Approach

0M9440Z Drainage of Left Elbow Bursa and Ligament with Drainage Device, Percutaneous Endoscopic Approach

0M944ZX Drainage of Left Elbow Bursa and Ligament, Percutaneous Endoscopic Approach, Diagnostic

0M944ZZ Drainage of Left Elbow Bursa and Ligament, Percutaneous Endoscopic Approach

0M9500Z Drainage of Right Wrist Bursa and Ligament with Drainage Device, Open Approach

0M950ZX Drainage of Right Wrist Bursa and Ligament, Open Approach, Diagnostic

0M950ZZ Drainage of Right Wrist Bursa and Ligament, Open Approach

0M9530Z Drainage of Right Wrist Bursa and Ligament with Drainage Device, Percutaneous Approach

0M953ZX Drainage of Right Wrist Bursa and Ligament, Percutaneous Approach, Diagnostic

0M953ZZ Drainage of Right Wrist Bursa and Ligament, Percutaneous Approach

0M9540Z Drainage of Right Wrist Bursa and Ligament with Drainage Device, Percutaneous Endoscopic Approach

0M954ZX Drainage of Right Wrist Bursa and Ligament, Percutaneous Endoscopic Approach, Diagnostic

0M954ZZ Drainage of Right Wrist Bursa and Ligament, Percutaneous Endoscopic Approach

0M9600Z Drainage of Left Wrist Bursa and Ligament with Drainage Device, Open Approach

0M960ZX Drainage of Left Wrist Bursa and Ligament, Open Approach, Diagnostic

0M960ZZ Drainage of Left Wrist Bursa and Ligament, Open Approach

0M9630Z Drainage of Left Wrist Bursa and Ligament with Drainage Device, Percutaneous Approach

0M963ZX Drainage of Left Wrist Bursa and Ligament, Percutaneous Approach, Diagnostic

0M963ZZ Drainage of Left Wrist Bursa and Ligament, Percutaneous Approach

0M9640Z Drainage of Left Wrist Bursa and Ligament with Drainage Device, Percutaneous Endoscopic Approach

0M964ZX Drainage of Left Wrist Bursa and Ligament, Percutaneous Endoscopic Approach, Diagnostic

0M964ZZ Drainage of Left Wrist Bursa and Ligament, Percutaneous Endoscopic Approach

0M9700Z Drainage of Right Hand Bursa and Ligament with Drainage Device, Open Approach

0M970ZX Drainage of Right Hand Bursa and Ligament, Open Approach, Diagnostic

0M970ZZ Drainage of Right Hand Bursa and Ligament, Open Approach

0M9730Z Drainage of Right Hand Bursa and Ligament with Drainage Device, Percutaneous Approach

0M973ZX Drainage of Right Hand Bursa and Ligament, Percutaneous Approach, Diagnostic

0M973ZZ Drainage of Right Hand Bursa and Ligament, Percutaneous Approach

0M9740Z Drainage of Right Hand Bursa and Ligament with Drainage Device, Percutaneous Endoscopic Approach

0M974ZX Drainage of Right Hand Bursa and Ligament, Percutaneous Endoscopic Approach, Diagnostic

0M974ZZ Drainage of Right Hand Bursa and Ligament, Percutaneous Endoscopic Approach

0M9800Z Drainage of Left Hand Bursa and Ligament with Drainage Device, Open Approach

0M980ZX Drainage of Left Hand Bursa and Ligament, Open Approach, Diagnostic

0M980ZZ Drainage of Left Hand Bursa and Ligament, Open Approach

0M9830Z Drainage of Left Hand Bursa and Ligament with Drainage Device, Percutaneous Approach

0M983ZX Drainage of Left Hand Bursa and Ligament, Percutaneous Approach, Diagnostic

0M983ZZ Drainage of Left Hand Bursa and Ligament, Percutaneous Approach

0M9840Z Drainage of Left Hand Bursa and Ligament with Drainage Device, Percutaneous Endoscopic Approach

0M984ZX Drainage of Left Hand Bursa and Ligament, Percutaneous Endoscopic Approach, Diagnostic

0M984ZZ Drainage of Left Hand Bursa and Ligament, Percutaneous Endoscopic Approach

0M9900Z Drainage of Right Upper Extremity Burs and Ligament with Drainage Device, Op Approach

0M990ZX Drainage of Right Upper Extremity Bursa and Ligament, Open Approach, Diagnostic

0M990ZZ Drainage of Right Upper Extremity Burs and Ligament, Open Approach

0M9930Z Drainage of Right Upper Extremity Burs and Ligament with Drainage Device, Percutaneous Approach

0M993ZX Drainage of Right Upper Extremity Burs and Ligament, Percutaneous Approach, Diagnostic

0M993ZZ Drainage of Right Upper Extremity Burs and Ligament, Percutaneous Approach

0M9940Z Drainage of Right Upper Extremity Burs and Ligament with Drainage Device, Percutaneous Endoscopic Approach

0M994ZX Drainage of Right Upper Extremity Burs and Ligament, Percutaneous Endoscopic Approach, Diagnostic

0M994ZZ Drainage of Right Upper Extremity Burs and Ligament, Percutaneous Endoscopic Approach

0M9B00Z Drainage of Left Upper Extremity Bursa and Ligament with Drainage Device, Ope Approach

0M9B0ZX Drainage of Left Upper Extremity Bursa and Ligament, Open Approach, Diagnosti

0M9B0ZZ Drainage of Left Upper Extremity Bursa and Ligament, Open Approach

0M9B30Z Drainage of Left Upper Extremity Bursa and Ligament with Drainage Device, Percutaneous Approach

M9B3ZX Drainage of Left Upper Extremity Bursa and Ligament, Percutaneous Approach, Diagnostic

M9B3ZZ Drainage of Left Upper Extremity Bursa and Ligament, Percutaneous Approach

M9B40Z Drainage of Left Upper Extremity Bursa and Ligament with Drainage Device, Percutaneous Endoscopic Approach

M9B4ZX Drainage of Left Upper Extremity Bursa and Ligament, Percutaneous Endoscopic Approach, Diagnostic

M9B4ZZ Drainage of Left Upper Extremity Bursa and Ligament, Percutaneous Endoscopic Approach

M9C00Z Drainage of Right Trunk Bursa and Ligament with Drainage Device, Open Approach

M9C0ZX Drainage of Right Trunk Bursa and Ligament, Open Approach, Diagnostic

M9C0ZZ Drainage of Right Trunk Bursa and Ligament, Open Approach

M9C30Z Drainage of Right Trunk Bursa and Ligament with Drainage Device, Percutaneous Approach

M9C3ZX Drainage of Right Trunk Bursa and Ligament, Percutaneous Approach, Diagnostic

M9C3ZZ Drainage of Right Trunk Bursa and Ligament, Percutaneous Approach

M9C40Z Drainage of Right Trunk Bursa and Ligament with Drainage Device, Percutaneous Endoscopic Approach

M9C4ZX Drainage of Right Trunk Bursa and Ligament, Percutaneous Endoscopic Approach, Diagnostic

M9C4ZZ Drainage of Right Trunk Bursa and Ligament, Percutaneous Endoscopic Approach

M9D00Z Drainage of Left Trunk Bursa and Ligament with Drainage Device, Open Approach

M9D0ZX Drainage of Left Trunk Bursa and Ligament, Open Approach, Diagnostic

M9D0ZZ Drainage of Left Trunk Bursa and Ligament, Open Approach

M9D30Z Drainage of Left Trunk Bursa and Ligament with Drainage Device, Percutaneous Approach

M9D3ZX Drainage of Left Trunk Bursa and Ligament, Percutaneous Approach, Diagnostic

M9D3ZZ Drainage of Left Trunk Bursa and Ligament, Percutaneous Approach

0M9D40Z Drainage of Left Trunk Bursa and Ligament with Drainage Device, Percutaneous Endoscopic Approach

0M9D4ZX Drainage of Left Trunk Bursa and Ligament, Percutaneous Endoscopic Approach, Diagnostic

0M9D4ZZ Drainage of Left Trunk Bursa and Ligament, Percutaneous Endoscopic Approach

0M9F00Z Drainage of Right Thorax Bursa and Ligament with Drainage Device, Open Approach

0M9F0ZX Drainage of Right Thorax Bursa and Ligament, Open Approach, Diagnostic

0M9F0ZZ Drainage of Right Thorax Bursa and Ligament, Open Approach

0M9F30Z Drainage of Right Thorax Bursa and Ligament with Drainage Device, Percutaneous Approach

0M9F3ZX Drainage of Right Thorax Bursa and Ligament, Percutaneous Approach, Diagnostic

0M9F3ZZ Drainage of Right Thorax Bursa and Ligament, Percutaneous Approach

0M9F40Z Drainage of Right Thorax Bursa and Ligament with Drainage Device, Percutaneous Endoscopic Approach

0M9F4ZX Drainage of Right Thorax Bursa and Ligament, Percutaneous Endoscopic Approach, Diagnostic

0M9F4ZZ Drainage of Right Thorax Bursa and Ligament, Percutaneous Endoscopic Approach

0M9G00Z Drainage of Left Thorax Bursa and Ligament with Drainage Device, Open Approach

0M9G0ZX Drainage of Left Thorax Bursa and Ligament, Open Approach, Diagnostic

0M9G0ZZ Drainage of Left Thorax Bursa and Ligament, Open Approach

0M9G30Z Drainage of Left Thorax Bursa and Ligament with Drainage Device, Percutaneous Approach

0M9G3ZX Drainage of Left Thorax Bursa and Ligament, Percutaneous Approach, Diagnostic

0M9G3ZZ Drainage of Left Thorax Bursa and Ligament, Percutaneous Approach

0M9G40Z Drainage of Left Thorax Bursa and Ligament with Drainage Device, Percutaneous Endoscopic Approach

0M9G4ZX Drainage of Left Thorax Bursa and Ligament, Percutaneous Endoscopic Approach, Diagnostic

0M9G4ZZ Drainage of Left Thorax Bursa and Ligament, Percutaneous Endoscopic Approach

0M9H00Z Drainage of Right Abdomen Bursa and Ligament with Drainage Device, Open Approach

0M9H0ZX Drainage of Right Abdomen Bursa and Ligament, Open Approach, Diagnostic

0M9H0ZZ Drainage of Right Abdomen Bursa and Ligament, Open Approach

0M9H30Z Drainage of Right Abdomen Bursa and Ligament with Drainage Device, Percutaneous Approach

0M9H3ZX Drainage of Right Abdomen Bursa and Ligament, Percutaneous Approach, Diagnostic

0M9H3ZZ Drainage of Right Abdomen Bursa and Ligament, Percutaneous Approach

0M9H40Z Drainage of Right Abdomen Bursa and Ligament with Drainage Device, Percutaneous Endoscopic Approach

0M9H4ZX Drainage of Right Abdomen Bursa and Ligament, Percutaneous Endoscopic Approach, Diagnostic

0M9H4ZZ Drainage of Right Abdomen Bursa and Ligament, Percutaneous Endoscopic Approach

0M9J00Z Drainage of Left Abdomen Bursa and Ligament with Drainage Device, Open Approach

0M9J0ZX Drainage of Left Abdomen Bursa and Ligament, Open Approach, Diagnostic

0M9J0ZZ Drainage of Left Abdomen Bursa and Ligament, Open Approach

0M9J30Z Drainage of Left Abdomen Bursa and Ligament with Drainage Device, Percutaneous Approach

0M9J3ZX Drainage of Left Abdomen Bursa and Ligament, Percutaneous Approach, Diagnostic

0M9J3ZZ Drainage of Left Abdomen Bursa and Ligament, Percutaneous Approach

0M9J40Z Drainage of Left Abdomen Bursa and Ligament with Drainage Device, Percutaneous Endoscopic Approach

0M9J4ZX Drainage of Left Abdomen Bursa and Ligament, Percutaneous Endoscopic Approach, Diagnostic

0M9J4ZZ Drainage of Left Abdomen Bursa and Ligament, Percutaneous Endoscopic Approach

0M9K00Z Drainage of Perineum Bursa and Ligament with Drainage Device, Open Approach

0M9K0ZX Drainage of Perineum Bursa and Ligament, Open Approach, Diagnostic

0M9K0ZZ Drainage of Perineum Bursa and Ligament, Open Approach

0M9K30Z Drainage of Perineum Bursa and Ligament with Drainage Device, Percutaneous Approach

0M9K3ZX Drainage of Perineum Bursa and Ligament, Percutaneous Approach, Diagnostic

0M9K3ZZ Drainage of Perineum Bursa and Ligament, Percutaneous Approach

0M9K40Z Drainage of Perineum Bursa and Ligament with Drainage Device, Percutaneous Endoscopic Approach

0M9K4ZX Drainage of Perineum Bursa and Ligament, Percutaneous Endoscopic Approach, Diagnostic

0M9K4ZZ Drainage of Perineum Bursa and Ligament, Percutaneous Endoscopic Approach

0M9L00Z Drainage of Right Hip Bursa and Ligament with Drainage Device, Open Approach

0M9L0ZX Drainage of Right Hip Bursa and Ligament, Open Approach, Diagnostic

0M9L0ZZ Drainage of Right Hip Bursa and Ligament, Open Approach

0M9L30Z Drainage of Right Hip Bursa and Ligament with Drainage Device, Percutaneous Approach

0M9L3ZX Drainage of Right Hip Bursa and Ligament, Percutaneous Approach, Diagnostic

0M9L3ZZ Drainage of Right Hip Bursa and Ligament, Percutaneous Approach

0M9L40Z Drainage of Right Hip Bursa and Ligament with Drainage Device, Percutaneous Endoscopic Approach

0M9L4ZX Drainage of Right Hip Bursa and Ligament, Percutaneous Endoscopic Approach, Diagnostic

0M9L4ZZ Drainage of Right Hip Bursa and Ligament, Percutaneous Endoscopic Approach

0M9M00Z Drainage of Left Hip Bursa and Ligament with Drainage Device, Open Approach

0M9M0ZX Drainage of Left Hip Bursa and Ligament, Open Approach, Diagnostic

0M9M0ZZ Drainage of Left Hip Bursa and Ligament, Open Approach

0M9M30Z Drainage of Left Hip Bursa and Ligament with Drainage Device, Percutaneous Approach

0M9M3ZX Drainage of Left Hip Bursa and Ligament, Percutaneous Approach, Diagnostic

0M9M3ZZ Drainage of Left Hip Bursa and Ligament, Percutaneous Approach

0M9M40Z Drainage of Left Hip Bursa and Ligament with Drainage Device, Percutaneous Endoscopic Approach

0M9M4ZX Drainage of Left Hip Bursa and Ligament, Percutaneous Endoscopic Approach, Diagnostic

0M9M4ZZ Drainage of Left Hip Bursa and Ligament, Percutaneous Endoscopic Approach

0M9N00Z Drainage of Right Knee Bursa and Ligament with Drainage Device, Open Approach

0M9N0ZX Drainage of Right Knee Bursa and Ligament, Open Approach, Diagnostic

0M9N0ZZ Drainage of Right Knee Bursa and Ligament, Open Approach

0M9N30Z Drainage of Right Knee Bursa and Ligament with Drainage Device, Percutaneous Approach

0M9N3ZX Drainage of Right Knee Bursa and Ligament, Percutaneous Approach, Diagnostic

0M9N3ZZ Drainage of Right Knee Bursa and Ligament, Percutaneous Approach

0M9N40Z Drainage of Right Knee Bursa and Ligament with Drainage Device, Percutaneous Endoscopic Approach

0M9N4ZX Drainage of Right Knee Bursa and Ligament, Percutaneous Endoscopic Approach, Diagnostic

0M9N4ZZ Drainage of Right Knee Bursa and Ligament, Percutaneous Endoscopic Approach

0M9P00Z Drainage of Left Knee Bursa and Ligament with Drainage Device, Open Approach

0M9P0ZX Drainage of Left Knee Bursa and Ligament, Open Approach, Diagnostic

0M9P0ZZ Drainage of Left Knee Bursa and Ligament, Open Approach

0M9P30Z Drainage of Left Knee Bursa and Ligament with Drainage Device, Percutaneous Approach

0M9P3ZX Drainage of Left Knee Bursa and Ligament, Percutaneous Approach, Diagnostic

0M9P3ZZ Drainage of Left Knee Bursa and Ligament, Percutaneous Approach

0M9P40Z Drainage of Left Knee Bursa and Ligament with Drainage Device, Percutaneous Endoscopic Approach

0M9P4ZX Drainage of Left Knee Bursa and Ligament, Percutaneous Endoscopic Approach, Diagnostic

0M9P4ZZ Drainage of Left Knee Bursa and Ligament, Percutaneous Endoscopic Approach

0M9Q00Z Drainage of Right Ankle Bursa and Ligament with Drainage Device, Open Approach

0M9Q0ZX Drainage of Right Ankle Bursa and Ligament, Open Approach, Diagnostic

0M9Q0ZZ Drainage of Right Ankle Bursa and Ligament, Open Approach

0M9Q30Z Drainage of Right Ankle Bursa and Ligament with Drainage Device, Percutaneous Approach

0M9Q3ZX Drainage of Right Ankle Bursa and Ligament, Percutaneous Approach, Diagnostic

0M9Q3ZZ Drainage of Right Ankle Bursa and Ligament, Percutaneous Approach

0M9Q40Z Drainage of Right Ankle Bursa and Ligament with Drainage Device, Percutaneous Endoscopic Approach

0M9Q4ZX Drainage of Right Ankle Bursa and Ligament, Percutaneous Endoscopic Approach, Diagnostic

0M9Q4ZZ Drainage of Right Ankle Bursa and Ligament, Percutaneous Endoscopic Approach

0M9R00Z Drainage of Left Ankle Bursa and Ligament with Drainage Device, Open Approach

0M9R0ZX Drainage of Left Ankle Bursa and Ligament, Open Approach, Diagnostic

0M9R0ZZ Drainage of Left Ankle Bursa and Ligament, Open Approach

0M9R30Z Drainage of Left Ankle Bursa and Ligament with Drainage Device, Percutaneous Approach

0M9R3ZX Drainage of Left Ankle Bursa and Ligament, Percutaneous Approach, Diagnostic

0M9R3ZZ Drainage of Left Ankle Bursa and Ligament, Percutaneous Approach

0M9R40Z Drainage of Left Ankle Bursa and Ligament with Drainage Device, Percutaneous Endoscopic Approach

0M9R4ZX Drainage of Left Ankle Bursa and Ligament, Percutaneous Endoscopic Approach, Diagnostic

0M9R4ZZ Drainage of Left Ankle Bursa and Ligament, Percutaneous Endoscopic Approach

0M9S00Z Drainage of Right Foot Bursa and Ligament with Drainage Device, Open Approach

0M9S0ZX Drainage of Right Foot Bursa and Ligament, Open Approach, Diagnostic

0M9S0ZZ Drainage of Right Foot Bursa and Ligament, Open Approach

0M9S30Z Drainage of Right Foot Bursa and Ligament with Drainage Device, Percutaneous Approach

0M9S3ZX Drainage of Right Foot Bursa and Ligament, Percutaneous Approach, Diagnostic

0M9S3ZZ Drainage of Right Foot Bursa and Ligament, Percutaneous Approach

0M9S40Z Drainage of Right Foot Bursa and Ligament with Drainage Device, Percutaneous Endoscopic Approach

0M9S4ZX Drainage of Right Foot Bursa and Ligament, Percutaneous Endoscopic Approach, Diagnostic

0M9S4ZZ Drainage of Right Foot Bursa and Ligament, Percutaneous Endoscopic Approach

0M9T00Z Drainage of Left Foot Bursa and Ligament with Drainage Device, Open Approach

0M9T0ZX Drainage of Left Foot Bursa and Ligament, Open Approach, Diagnostic

0M9T0ZZ Drainage of Left Foot Bursa and Ligament, Open Approach

0M9T30Z Drainage of Left Foot Bursa and Ligament with Drainage Device, Percutaneous Approach

0M9T3ZX Drainage of Left Foot Bursa and Ligament, Percutaneous Approach, Diagnostic

0M9T3ZZ Drainage of Left Foot Bursa and Ligament, Percutaneous Approach

0M9T40Z Drainage of Left Foot Bursa and Ligament with Drainage Device, Percutaneous Endoscopic Approach

0M9T4ZX Drainage of Left Foot Bursa and Ligament, Percutaneous Endoscopic Approach, Diagnostic

0M9T4ZZ Drainage of Left Foot Bursa and Ligament, Percutaneous Endoscopic Approach

0M9V00Z Drainage of Right Lower Extremity Bursa and Ligament with Drainage Device, Open Approach

0M9V0ZX Drainage of Right Lower Extremity Bursa and Ligament, Open Approach, Diagnostic

0M9V0ZZ Drainage of Right Lower Extremity Bursa and Ligament, Open Approach

0M9V30Z Drainage of Right Lower Extremity Bursa and Ligament with Drainage Device, Percutaneous Approach

0M9V3ZX Drainage of Right Lower Extremity Bursa and Ligament, Percutaneous Approach, Diagnostic

0M9V3ZZ Drainage of Right Lower Extremity Bursa and Ligament, Percutaneous Approach

0M9V40Z Drainage of Right Lower Extremity Bursa and Ligament with Drainage Device, Percutaneous Endoscopic Approach

0M9V4ZX Drainage of Right Lower Extremity Bursa and Ligament, Percutaneous Endoscopic Approach, Diagnostic

0M9V4ZZ Drainage of Right Lower Extremity Bursa and Ligament, Percutaneous Endoscopic Approach

0M9W00Z Drainage of Left Lower Extremity Bursa and Ligament with Drainage Device, Open Approach

0M9W0ZX Drainage of Left Lower Extremity Bursa and Ligament, Open Approach, Diagnostic

0M9W0ZZ Drainage of Left Lower Extremity Bursa and Ligament, Open Approach

0M9W30Z Drainage of Left Lower Extremity Bursa and Ligament with Drainage Device, Percutaneous Approach

0M9W3ZX Drainage of Left Lower Extremity Bursa and Ligament, Percutaneous Approach, Diagnostic

0M9W3ZZ Drainage of Left Lower Extremity Bursa and Ligament, Percutaneous Approach

0M9W40Z Drainage of Left Lower Extremity Bursa and Ligament with Drainage Device, Percutaneous Endoscopic Approach

0M9W4ZX Drainage of Left Lower Extremity Bursa and Ligament, Percutaneous Endoscopic Approach, Diagnostic

0M9W4ZZ Drainage of Left Lower Extremity Bursa and Ligament, Percutaneous Endoscopic Approach

0MB – Bursae and Ligaments, Excision

Review Coding Guidelines B3.4a and B3.4b

Review Coding Guideline B3.5

Review Coding Guideline B3.8

0MB00ZX Excision of Head and Neck Bursa and Ligament, Open Approach, Diagnostic

0MB00ZZ Excision of Head and Neck Bursa and Ligament, Open Approach

0MB03ZX Excision of Head and Neck Bursa and Ligament, Percutaneous Approach, Diagnostic

IB03ZZ Excision of Head and Neck Bursa and Ligament, Percutaneous Approach
IB04ZX Excision of Head and Neck Bursa and Ligament, Percutaneous Endoscopic Approach, Diagnostic
IB04ZZ Excision of Head and Neck Bursa and Ligament, Percutaneous Endoscopic Approach
IB10ZX Excision of Right Shoulder Bursa and Ligament, Open Approach, Diagnostic
IB10ZZ Excision of Right Shoulder Bursa and Ligament, Open Approach
IB13ZX Excision of Right Shoulder Bursa and Ligament, Percutaneous Approach, Diagnostic
IB13ZZ Excision of Right Shoulder Bursa and Ligament, Percutaneous Approach
IB14ZX Excision of Right Shoulder Bursa and Ligament, Percutaneous Endoscopic Approach, Diagnostic
IB14ZZ Excision of Right Shoulder Bursa and Ligament, Percutaneous Endoscopic Approach
MB20ZX Excision of Left Shoulder Bursa and Ligament, Open Approach, Diagnostic
MB20ZZ Excision of Left Shoulder Bursa and Ligament, Open Approach
MB23ZX Excision of Left Shoulder Bursa and Ligament, Percutaneous Approach, Diagnostic
MB23ZZ Excision of Left Shoulder Bursa and Ligament, Percutaneous Approach
MB24ZX Excision of Left Shoulder Bursa and Ligament, Percutaneous Endoscopic Approach, Diagnostic
MB24ZZ Excision of Left Shoulder Bursa and Ligament, Percutaneous Endoscopic Approach
MB30ZX Excision of Right Elbow Bursa and Ligament, Open Approach, Diagnostic
MB30ZZ Excision of Right Elbow Bursa and Ligament, Open Approach
MB33ZX Excision of Right Elbow Bursa and Ligament, Percutaneous Approach, Diagnostic
MB33ZZ Excision of Right Elbow Bursa and Ligament, Percutaneous Approach
MB34ZX Excision of Right Elbow Bursa and Ligament, Percutaneous Endoscopic Approach, Diagnostic
MB34ZZ Excision of Right Elbow Bursa and Ligament, Percutaneous Endoscopic Approach
MB40ZX Excision of Left Elbow Bursa and Ligament, Open Approach, Diagnostic
MB40ZZ Excision of Left Elbow Bursa and Ligament, Open Approach
MB43ZX Excision of Left Elbow Bursa and Ligament, Percutaneous Approach, Diagnostic
MB43ZZ Excision of Left Elbow Bursa and Ligament, Percutaneous Approach
MB44ZX Excision of Left Elbow Bursa and Ligament, Percutaneous Endoscopic Approach, Diagnostic
0MB44ZZ Excision of Left Elbow Bursa and Ligament, Percutaneous Endoscopic Approach
0MB50ZX Excision of Right Wrist Bursa and Ligament, Open Approach, Diagnostic
0MB50ZZ Excision of Right Wrist Bursa and Ligament, Open Approach
0MB53ZX Excision of Right Wrist Bursa and Ligament, Percutaneous Approach, Diagnostic
0MB53ZZ Excision of Right Wrist Bursa and Ligament, Percutaneous Approach
0MB54ZX Excision of Right Wrist Bursa and Ligament, Percutaneous Endoscopic Approach, Diagnostic
0MB54ZZ Excision of Right Wrist Bursa and Ligament, Percutaneous Endoscopic Approach
0MB60ZX Excision of Left Wrist Bursa and Ligament, Open Approach, Diagnostic
0MB60ZZ Excision of Left Wrist Bursa and Ligament, Open Approach
0MB63ZX Excision of Left Wrist Bursa and Ligament, Percutaneous Approach, Diagnostic
0MB63ZZ Excision of Left Wrist Bursa and Ligament, Percutaneous Approach
0MB64ZX Excision of Left Wrist Bursa and Ligament, Percutaneous Endoscopic Approach, Diagnostic
0MB64ZZ Excision of Left Wrist Bursa and Ligament, Percutaneous Endoscopic Approach
0MB70ZX Excision of Right Hand Bursa and Ligament, Open Approach, Diagnostic
0MB70ZZ Excision of Right Hand Bursa and Ligament, Open Approach
0MB73ZX Excision of Right Hand Bursa and Ligament, Percutaneous Approach, Diagnostic
0MB73ZZ Excision of Right Hand Bursa and Ligament, Percutaneous Approach
0MB74ZX Excision of Right Hand Bursa and Ligament, Percutaneous Endoscopic Approach, Diagnostic
0MB74ZZ Excision of Right Hand Bursa and Ligament, Percutaneous Endoscopic Approach
0MB80ZX Excision of Left Hand Bursa and Ligament, Open Approach, Diagnostic
0MB80ZZ Excision of Left Hand Bursa and Ligament, Open Approach
0MB83ZX Excision of Left Hand Bursa and Ligament, Percutaneous Approach, Diagnostic
0MB83ZZ Excision of Left Hand Bursa and Ligament, Percutaneous Approach
0MB84ZX Excision of Left Hand Bursa and Ligament, Percutaneous Endoscopic Approach, Diagnostic
0MB84ZZ Excision of Left Hand Bursa and Ligament, Percutaneous Endoscopic Approach
0MB90ZX Excision of Right Upper Extremity Bursa and Ligament, Open Approach, Diagnostic
0MB90ZZ Excision of Right Upper Extremity Bursa and Ligament, Open Approach
0MB93ZX Excision of Right Upper Extremity Bursa and Ligament, Percutaneous Approach, Diagnostic
0MB93ZZ Excision of Right Upper Extremity Bursa and Ligament, Percutaneous Approach
0MB94ZX Excision of Right Upper Extremity Bursa and Ligament, Percutaneous Endoscopic Approach, Diagnostic
0MB94ZZ Excision of Right Upper Extremity Bursa and Ligament, Percutaneous Endoscopic Approach
0MBB0ZX Excision of Left Upper Extremity Bursa and Ligament, Open Approach, Diagnostic
0MBB0ZZ Excision of Left Upper Extremity Bursa and Ligament, Open Approach
0MBB3ZX Excision of Left Upper Extremity Bursa and Ligament, Percutaneous Approach, Diagnostic
0MBB3ZZ Excision of Left Upper Extremity Bursa and Ligament, Percutaneous Approach
0MBB4ZX Excision of Left Upper Extremity Bursa and Ligament, Percutaneous Endoscopic Approach, Diagnostic
0MBB4ZZ Excision of Left Upper Extremity Bursa and Ligament, Percutaneous Endoscopic Approach
0MBC0ZX Excision of Right Trunk Bursa and Ligament, Open Approach, Diagnostic
0MBC0ZZ Excision of Right Trunk Bursa and Ligament, Open Approach
0MBC3ZX Excision of Right Trunk Bursa and Ligament, Percutaneous Approach, Diagnostic
0MBC3ZZ Excision of Right Trunk Bursa and Ligament, Percutaneous Approach
0MBC4ZX Excision of Right Trunk Bursa and Ligament, Percutaneous Endoscopic Approach, Diagnostic
0MBC4ZZ Excision of Right Trunk Bursa and Ligament, Percutaneous Endoscopic Approach
0MBD0ZX Excision of Left Trunk Bursa and Ligament, Open Approach, Diagnostic
0MBD0ZZ Excision of Left Trunk Bursa and Ligament, Open Approach
0MBD3ZX Excision of Left Trunk Bursa and Ligament, Percutaneous Approach, Diagnostic
0MBD3ZZ Excision of Left Trunk Bursa and Ligament, Percutaneous Approach
0MBD4ZX Excision of Left Trunk Bursa and Ligament, Percutaneous Endoscopic Approach, Diagnostic
0MBD4ZZ Excision of Left Trunk Bursa and Ligament, Percutaneous Endoscopic Approach
0MBF0ZX Excision of Right Thorax Bursa and Ligament, Open Approach, Diagnostic
0MBF0ZZ Excision of Right Thorax Bursa and Ligament, Open Approach
0MBF3ZX Excision of Right Thorax Bursa and Ligament, Percutaneous Approach, Diagnostic
0MBF3ZZ Excision of Right Thorax Bursa and Ligament, Percutaneous Approach
0MBF4ZX Excision of Right Thorax Bursa and Ligament, Percutaneous Endoscopic Approach, Diagnostic
0MBF4ZZ Excision of Right Thorax Bursa and Ligament, Percutaneous Endoscopic Approach
0MBG0ZX Excision of Left Thorax Bursa and Ligament, Open Approach, Diagnostic
0MBG0ZZ Excision of Left Thorax Bursa and Ligament, Open Approach
0MBG3ZX Excision of Left Thorax Bursa and Ligament, Percutaneous Approach, Diagnostic
0MBG3ZZ Excision of Left Thorax Bursa and Ligament, Percutaneous Approach
0MBG4ZX Excision of Left Thorax Bursa and Ligament, Percutaneous Endoscopic Approach, Diagnostic
0MBG4ZZ Excision of Left Thorax Bursa and Ligament, Percutaneous Endoscopic Approach
0MBH0ZX Excision of Right Abdomen Bursa and Ligament, Open Approach, Diagnostic
0MBH0ZZ Excision of Right Abdomen Bursa and Ligament, Open Approach
0MBH3ZX Excision of Right Abdomen Bursa and Ligament, Percutaneous Approach, Diagnostic
0MBH3ZZ Excision of Right Abdomen Bursa and Ligament, Percutaneous Approach

0MBH4ZX Excision of Right Abdomen Bursa and Ligament, Percutaneous Endoscopic Approach, Diagnostic
0MBH4ZZ Excision of Right Abdomen Bursa and Ligament, Percutaneous Endoscopic Approach
0MBJ0ZX Excision of Left Abdomen Bursa and Ligament, Open Approach, Diagnostic
0MBJ0ZZ Excision of Left Abdomen Bursa and Ligament, Open Approach
0MBJ3ZX Excision of Left Abdomen Bursa and Ligament, Percutaneous Approach, Diagnostic
0MBJ3ZZ Excision of Left Abdomen Bursa and Ligament, Percutaneous Approach
0MBJ4ZX Excision of Left Abdomen Bursa and Ligament, Percutaneous Endoscopic Approach, Diagnostic
0MBJ4ZZ Excision of Left Abdomen Bursa and Ligament, Percutaneous Endoscopic Approach
0MBK0ZX Excision of Perineum Bursa and Ligament, Open Approach, Diagnostic
0MBK0ZZ Excision of Perineum Bursa and Ligament, Open Approach
0MBK3ZX Excision of Perineum Bursa and Ligament, Percutaneous Approach, Diagnostic
0MBK3ZZ Excision of Perineum Bursa and Ligament, Percutaneous Approach
0MBK4ZX Excision of Perineum Bursa and Ligament, Percutaneous Endoscopic Approach, Diagnostic
0MBK4ZZ Excision of Perineum Bursa and Ligament, Percutaneous Endoscopic Approach
0MBL0ZX Excision of Right Hip Bursa and Ligament, Open Approach, Diagnostic
0MBL0ZZ Excision of Right Hip Bursa and Ligament, Open Approach
0MBL3ZX Excision of Right Hip Bursa and Ligament, Percutaneous Approach, Diagnostic
0MBL3ZZ Excision of Right Hip Bursa and Ligament, Percutaneous Approach
0MBL4ZX Excision of Right Hip Bursa and Ligament, Percutaneous Endoscopic Approach, Diagnostic
0MBL4ZZ Excision of Right Hip Bursa and Ligament, Percutaneous Endoscopic Approach
0MBM0ZX Excision of Left Hip Bursa and Ligament, Open Approach, Diagnostic
0MBM0ZZ Excision of Left Hip Bursa and Ligament, Open Approach
0MBM3ZX Excision of Left Hip Bursa and Ligament, Percutaneous Approach, Diagnostic
0MBM3ZZ Excision of Left Hip Bursa and Ligament, Percutaneous Approach
0MBM4ZX Excision of Left Hip Bursa and Ligament, Percutaneous Endoscopic Approach, Diagnostic
0MBM4ZZ Excision of Left Hip Bursa and Ligament, Percutaneous Endoscopic Approach
0MBN0ZX Excision of Right Knee Bursa and Ligament, Open Approach, Diagnostic
0MBN0ZZ Excision of Right Knee Bursa and Ligament, Open Approach
0MBN3ZX Excision of Right Knee Bursa and Ligament, Percutaneous Approach, Diagnostic
0MBN3ZZ Excision of Right Knee Bursa and Ligament, Percutaneous Approach
0MBN4ZX Excision of Right Knee Bursa and Ligament, Percutaneous Endoscopic Approach, Diagnostic
0MBN4ZZ Excision of Right Knee Bursa and Ligament, Percutaneous Endoscopic Approach
0MBP0ZX Excision of Left Knee Bursa and Ligament, Open Approach, Diagnostic
0MBP0ZZ Excision of Left Knee Bursa and Ligament, Open Approach
0MBP3ZX Excision of Left Knee Bursa and Ligament, Percutaneous Approach, Diagnostic
0MBP3ZZ Excision of Left Knee Bursa and Ligament, Percutaneous Approach
0MBP4ZX Excision of Left Knee Bursa and Ligament, Percutaneous Endoscopic Approach, Diagnostic
0MBP4ZZ Excision of Left Knee Bursa and Ligament, Percutaneous Endoscopic Approach
0MBQ0ZX Excision of Right Ankle Bursa and Ligament, Open Approach, Diagnostic
0MBQ0ZZ Excision of Right Ankle Bursa and Ligament, Open Approach
0MBQ3ZX Excision of Right Ankle Bursa and Ligament, Percutaneous Approach, Diagnostic
0MBQ3ZZ Excision of Right Ankle Bursa and Ligament, Percutaneous Approach
0MBQ4ZX Excision of Right Ankle Bursa and Ligament, Percutaneous Endoscopic Approach, Diagnostic
0MBQ4ZZ Excision of Right Ankle Bursa and Ligament, Percutaneous Endoscopic Approach
0MBR0ZX Excision of Left Ankle Bursa and Ligament, Open Approach, Diagnostic
0MBR0ZZ Excision of Left Ankle Bursa and Ligament, Open Approach
0MBR3ZX Excision of Left Ankle Bursa and Ligament, Percutaneous Approach, Diagnostic
0MBR3ZZ Excision of Left Ankle Bursa and Ligament, Percutaneous Approach
0MBR4ZX Excision of Left Ankle Bursa and Ligament, Percutaneous Endoscopic Approach, Diagnostic
0MBR4ZZ Excision of Left Ankle Bursa and Ligament, Percutaneous Endoscopic Approach
0MBS0ZX Excision of Right Foot Bursa and Ligament, Open Approach, Diagnostic
0MBS0ZZ Excision of Right Foot Bursa and Ligament, Open Approach
0MBS3ZX Excision of Right Foot Bursa and Ligament, Percutaneous Approach, Diagnostic
0MBS3ZZ Excision of Right Foot Bursa and Ligament, Percutaneous Approach
0MBS4ZX Excision of Right Foot Bursa and Ligament, Percutaneous Endoscopic Approach, Diagnostic
0MBS4ZZ Excision of Right Foot Bursa and Ligament, Percutaneous Endoscopic Approach
0MBT0ZX Excision of Left Foot Bursa and Ligament, Open Approach, Diagnostic
0MBT0ZZ Excision of Left Foot Bursa and Ligament, Open Approach
0MBT3ZX Excision of Left Foot Bursa and Ligament, Percutaneous Approach, Diagnostic
0MBT3ZZ Excision of Left Foot Bursa and Ligament, Percutaneous Approach
0MBT4ZX Excision of Left Foot Bursa and Ligament, Percutaneous Endoscopic Approach, Diagnostic
0MBT4ZZ Excision of Left Foot Bursa and Ligament, Percutaneous Endoscopic Approach
0MBV0ZX Excision of Right Lower Extremity Bursa and Ligament, Open Approach, Diagnostic
0MBV0ZZ Excision of Right Lower Extremity Burs and Ligament, Open Approach
0MBV3ZX Excision of Right Lower Extremity Burs and Ligament, Percutaneous Approach, Diagnostic
0MBV3ZZ Excision of Right Lower Extremity Burs and Ligament, Percutaneous Approach
0MBV4ZX Excision of Right Lower Extremity Burs and Ligament, Percutaneous Endoscopic Approach, Diagnostic
0MBV4ZZ Excision of Right Lower Extremity Burs and Ligament, Percutaneous Endoscopic Approach
0MBW0ZX Excision of Left Lower Extremity Bursa and Ligament, Open Approach, Diagnostic
0MBW0ZZ Excision of Left Lower Extremity Bursa and Ligament, Open Approach
0MBW3ZX Excision of Left Lower Extremity Bursa and Ligament, Percutaneous Approach, Diagnostic
0MBW3ZZ Excision of Left Lower Extremity Bursa and Ligament, Percutaneous Approach
0MBW4ZX Excision of Left Lower Extremity Bursa and Ligament, Percutaneous Endoscopic Approach, Diagnostic
0MBW4ZZ Excision of Left Lower Extremity Bursa and Ligament, Percutaneous Endoscopic Approach

0MC – Bursae and Ligaments, Extirpation

0MC00ZZ Extirpation of Matter from Head and Neck Bursa and Ligament, Open Approach
0MC03ZZ Extirpation of Matter from Head and Neck Bursa and Ligament, Percutaneous Approach
0MC04ZZ Extirpation of Matter from Head and Neck Bursa and Ligament, Percutaneous Endoscopic Approach
0MC10ZZ Extirpation of Matter from Right Shoulder Bursa and Ligament, Open Approach
0MC13ZZ Extirpation of Matter from Right Shoulder Bursa and Ligament, Percutaneous Approach
0MC14ZZ Extirpation of Matter from Right Shoulder Bursa and Ligament, Percutaneous Endoscopic Approach
0MC20ZZ Extirpation of Matter from Left Shoulder Bursa and Ligament, Open Approach
0MC23ZZ Extirpation of Matter from Left Shoulder Bursa and Ligament, Percutaneous Approach
0MC24ZZ Extirpation of Matter from Left Shoulder Bursa and Ligament, Percutaneous Endoscopic Approach
0MC30ZZ Extirpation of Matter from Right Elbow Bursa and Ligament, Open Approach
0MC33ZZ Extirpation of Matter from Right Elbow Bursa and Ligament, Percutaneous Approach
0MC34ZZ Extirpation of Matter from Right Elbow Bursa and Ligament, Percutaneous Endoscopic Approach

C40ZZ Extirpation of Matter from Left Elbow Bursa and Ligament, Open Approach
C43ZZ Extirpation of Matter from Left Elbow Bursa and Ligament, Percutaneous Approach
C44ZZ Extirpation of Matter from Left Elbow Bursa and Ligament, Percutaneous Endoscopic Approach
IC50ZZ Extirpation of Matter from Right Wrist Bursa and Ligament, Open Approach
IC53ZZ Extirpation of Matter from Right Wrist Bursa and Ligament, Percutaneous Approach
IC54ZZ Extirpation of Matter from Right Wrist Bursa and Ligament, Percutaneous Endoscopic Approach
IC60ZZ Extirpation of Matter from Left Wrist Bursa and Ligament, Open Approach
IC63ZZ Extirpation of Matter from Left Wrist Bursa and Ligament, Percutaneous Approach
IC64ZZ Extirpation of Matter from Left Wrist Bursa and Ligament, Percutaneous Endoscopic Approach
MC70ZZ Extirpation of Matter from Right Hand Bursa and Ligament, Open Approach
MC73ZZ Extirpation of Matter from Right Hand Bursa and Ligament, Percutaneous Approach
MC74ZZ Extirpation of Matter from Right Hand Bursa and Ligament, Percutaneous Endoscopic Approach
MC80ZZ Extirpation of Matter from Left Hand Bursa and Ligament, Open Approach
MC83ZZ Extirpation of Matter from Left Hand Bursa and Ligament, Percutaneous Approach
MC84ZZ Extirpation of Matter from Left Hand Bursa and Ligament, Percutaneous Endoscopic Approach
MC90ZZ Extirpation of Matter from Right Upper Extremity Bursa and Ligament, Open Approach
MC93ZZ Extirpation of Matter from Right Upper Extremity Bursa and Ligament, Percutaneous Approach
MC94ZZ Extirpation of Matter from Right Upper Extremity Bursa and Ligament, Percutaneous Endoscopic Approach
MCB0ZZ Extirpation of Matter from Left Upper Extremity Bursa and Ligament, Open Approach
MCB3ZZ Extirpation of Matter from Left Upper Extremity Bursa and Ligament, Percutaneous Approach
MCB4ZZ Extirpation of Matter from Left Upper Extremity Bursa and Ligament, Percutaneous Endoscopic Approach
MCC0ZZ Extirpation of Matter from Right Trunk Bursa and Ligament, Open Approach
MCC3ZZ Extirpation of Matter from Right Trunk Bursa and Ligament, Percutaneous Approach
MCC4ZZ Extirpation of Matter from Right Trunk Bursa and Ligament, Percutaneous Endoscopic Approach
0MCD0ZZ Extirpation of Matter from Left Trunk Bursa and Ligament, Open Approach
0MCD3ZZ Extirpation of Matter from Left Trunk Bursa and Ligament, Percutaneous Approach
0MCD4ZZ Extirpation of Matter from Left Trunk Bursa and Ligament, Percutaneous Endoscopic Approach
0MCF0ZZ Extirpation of Matter from Right Thorax Bursa and Ligament, Open Approach
0MCF3ZZ Extirpation of Matter from Right Thorax Bursa and Ligament, Percutaneous Approach
0MCF4ZZ Extirpation of Matter from Right Thorax Bursa and Ligament, Percutaneous Endoscopic Approach
0MCG0ZZ Extirpation of Matter from Left Thorax Bursa and Ligament, Open Approach
0MCG3ZZ Extirpation of Matter from Left Thorax Bursa and Ligament, Percutaneous Approach
0MCG4ZZ Extirpation of Matter from Left Thorax Bursa and Ligament, Percutaneous Endoscopic Approach
0MCH0ZZ Extirpation of Matter from Right Abdomen Bursa and Ligament, Open Approach
0MCH3ZZ Extirpation of Matter from Right Abdomen Bursa and Ligament, Percutaneous Approach
0MCH4ZZ Extirpation of Matter from Right Abdomen Bursa and Ligament, Percutaneous Endoscopic Approach
0MCJ0ZZ Extirpation of Matter from Left Abdomen Bursa and Ligament, Open Approach
0MCJ3ZZ Extirpation of Matter from Left Abdomen Bursa and Ligament, Percutaneous Approach
0MCJ4ZZ Extirpation of Matter from Left Abdomen Bursa and Ligament, Percutaneous Endoscopic Approach
0MCK0ZZ Extirpation of Matter from Perineum Bursa and Ligament, Open Approach
0MCK3ZZ Extirpation of Matter from Perineum Bursa and Ligament, Percutaneous Approach
0MCK4ZZ Extirpation of Matter from Perineum Bursa and Ligament, Percutaneous Endoscopic Approach
0MCL0ZZ Extirpation of Matter from Right Hip Bursa and Ligament, Open Approach
0MCL3ZZ Extirpation of Matter from Right Hip Bursa and Ligament, Percutaneous Approach
0MCL4ZZ Extirpation of Matter from Right Hip Bursa and Ligament, Percutaneous Endoscopic Approach
0MCM0ZZ Extirpation of Matter from Left Hip Bursa and Ligament, Open Approach
0MCM3ZZ Extirpation of Matter from Left Hip Bursa and Ligament, Percutaneous Approach
0MCM4ZZ Extirpation of Matter from Left Hip Bursa and Ligament, Percutaneous Endoscopic Approach
0MCN0ZZ Extirpation of Matter from Right Knee Bursa and Ligament, Open Approach
0MCN3ZZ Extirpation of Matter from Right Knee Bursa and Ligament, Percutaneous Approach
0MCN4ZZ Extirpation of Matter from Right Knee Bursa and Ligament, Percutaneous Endoscopic Approach
0MCP0ZZ Extirpation of Matter from Left Knee Bursa and Ligament, Open Approach
0MCP3ZZ Extirpation of Matter from Left Knee Bursa and Ligament, Percutaneous Approach
0MCP4ZZ Extirpation of Matter from Left Knee Bursa and Ligament, Percutaneous Endoscopic Approach
0MCQ0ZZ Extirpation of Matter from Right Ankle Bursa and Ligament, Open Approach
0MCQ3ZZ Extirpation of Matter from Right Ankle Bursa and Ligament, Percutaneous Approach
0MCQ4ZZ Extirpation of Matter from Right Ankle Bursa and Ligament, Percutaneous Endoscopic Approach
0MCR0ZZ Extirpation of Matter from Left Ankle Bursa and Ligament, Open Approach
0MCR3ZZ Extirpation of Matter from Left Ankle Bursa and Ligament, Percutaneous Approach
0MCR4ZZ Extirpation of Matter from Left Ankle Bursa and Ligament, Percutaneous Endoscopic Approach
0MCS0ZZ Extirpation of Matter from Right Foot Bursa and Ligament, Open Approach
0MCS3ZZ Extirpation of Matter from Right Foot Bursa and Ligament, Percutaneous Approach
0MCS4ZZ Extirpation of Matter from Right Foot Bursa and Ligament, Percutaneous Endoscopic Approach
0MCT0ZZ Extirpation of Matter from Left Foot Bursa and Ligament, Open Approach
0MCT3ZZ Extirpation of Matter from Left Foot Bursa and Ligament, Percutaneous Approach
0MCT4ZZ Extirpation of Matter from Left Foot Bursa and Ligament, Percutaneous Endoscopic Approach
0MCV0ZZ Extirpation of Matter from Right Lower Extremity Bursa and Ligament, Open Approach
0MCV3ZZ Extirpation of Matter from Right Lower Extremity Bursa and Ligament, Percutaneous Approach
0MCV4ZZ Extirpation of Matter from Right Lower Extremity Bursa and Ligament, Percutaneous Endoscopic Approach
0MCW0ZZ Extirpation of Matter from Left Lower Extremity Bursa and Ligament, Open Approach
0MCW3ZZ Extirpation of Matter from Left Lower Extremity Bursa and Ligament, Percutaneous Approach
0MCW4ZZ Extirpation of Matter from Left Lower Extremity Bursa and Ligament, Percutaneous Endoscopic Approach

0MD – Bursae and Ligaments, Extraction

0MD00ZZ Extraction of Head and Neck Bursa and Ligament, Open Approach
0MD03ZZ Extraction of Head and Neck Bursa and Ligament, Percutaneous Approach
0MD04ZZ Extraction of Head and Neck Bursa and Ligament, Percutaneous Endoscopic Approach
0MD10ZZ Extraction of Right Shoulder Bursa and Ligament, Open Approach
0MD13ZZ Extraction of Right Shoulder Bursa and Ligament, Percutaneous Approach
0MD14ZZ Extraction of Right Shoulder Bursa and Ligament, Percutaneous Endoscopic Approach
0MD20ZZ Extraction of Left Shoulder Bursa and Ligament, Open Approach
0MD23ZZ Extraction of Left Shoulder Bursa and Ligament, Percutaneous Approach
0MD24ZZ Extraction of Left Shoulder Bursa and Ligament, Percutaneous Endoscopic Approach

0MD30ZZ Extraction of Right Elbow Bursa and Ligament, Open Approach
0MD33ZZ Extraction of Right Elbow Bursa and Ligament, Percutaneous Approach
0MD34ZZ Extraction of Right Elbow Bursa and Ligament, Percutaneous Endoscopic Approach
0MD40ZZ Extraction of Left Elbow Bursa and Ligament, Open Approach
0MD43ZZ Extraction of Left Elbow Bursa and Ligament, Percutaneous Approach
0MD44ZZ Extraction of Left Elbow Bursa and Ligament, Percutaneous Endoscopic Approach
0MD50ZZ Extraction of Right Wrist Bursa and Ligament, Open Approach
0MD53ZZ Extraction of Right Wrist Bursa and Ligament, Percutaneous Approach
0MD54ZZ Extraction of Right Wrist Bursa and Ligament, Percutaneous Endoscopic Approach
0MD60ZZ Extraction of Left Wrist Bursa and Ligament, Open Approach
0MD63ZZ Extraction of Left Wrist Bursa and Ligament, Percutaneous Approach
0MD64ZZ Extraction of Left Wrist Bursa and Ligament, Percutaneous Endoscopic Approach
0MD70ZZ Extraction of Right Hand Bursa and Ligament, Open Approach
0MD73ZZ Extraction of Right Hand Bursa and Ligament, Percutaneous Approach
0MD74ZZ Extraction of Right Hand Bursa and Ligament, Percutaneous Endoscopic Approach
0MD80ZZ Extraction of Left Hand Bursa and Ligament, Open Approach
0MD83ZZ Extraction of Left Hand Bursa and Ligament, Percutaneous Approach
0MD84ZZ Extraction of Left Hand Bursa and Ligament, Percutaneous Endoscopic Approach
0MD90ZZ Extraction of Right Upper Extremity Bursa and Ligament, Open Approach
0MD93ZZ Extraction of Right Upper Extremity Bursa and Ligament, Percutaneous Approach
0MD94ZZ Extraction of Right Upper Extremity Bursa and Ligament, Percutaneous Endoscopic Approach
0MDB0ZZ Extraction of Left Upper Extremity Bursa and Ligament, Open Approach
0MDB3ZZ Extraction of Left Upper Extremity Bursa and Ligament, Percutaneous Approach
0MDB4ZZ Extraction of Left Upper Extremity Bursa and Ligament, Percutaneous Endoscopic Approach
0MDC0ZZ Extraction of Right Trunk Bursa and Ligament, Open Approach
0MDC3ZZ Extraction of Right Trunk Bursa and Ligament, Percutaneous Approach
0MDC4ZZ Extraction of Right Trunk Bursa and Ligament, Percutaneous Endoscopic Approach
0MDD0ZZ Extraction of Left Trunk Bursa and Ligament, Open Approach
0MDD3ZZ Extraction of Left Trunk Bursa and Ligament, Percutaneous Approach
0MDD4ZZ Extraction of Left Trunk Bursa and Ligament, Percutaneous Endoscopic Approach
0MDF0ZZ Extraction of Right Thorax Bursa and Ligament, Open Approach
0MDF3ZZ Extraction of Right Thorax Bursa and Ligament, Percutaneous Approach
0MDF4ZZ Extraction of Right Thorax Bursa and Ligament, Percutaneous Endoscopic Approach
0MDG0ZZ Extraction of Left Thorax Bursa and Ligament, Open Approach
0MDG3ZZ Extraction of Left Thorax Bursa and Ligament, Percutaneous Approach
0MDG4ZZ Extraction of Left Thorax Bursa and Ligament, Percutaneous Endoscopic Approach
0MDH0ZZ Extraction of Right Abdomen Bursa and Ligament, Open Approach
0MDH3ZZ Extraction of Right Abdomen Bursa and Ligament, Percutaneous Approach
0MDH4ZZ Extraction of Right Abdomen Bursa and Ligament, Percutaneous Endoscopic Approach
0MDJ0ZZ Extraction of Left Abdomen Bursa and Ligament, Open Approach
0MDJ3ZZ Extraction of Left Abdomen Bursa and Ligament, Percutaneous Approach
0MDJ4ZZ Extraction of Left Abdomen Bursa and Ligament, Percutaneous Endoscopic Approach
0MDK0ZZ Extraction of Perineum Bursa and Ligament, Open Approach
0MDK3ZZ Extraction of Perineum Bursa and Ligament, Percutaneous Approach
0MDK4ZZ Extraction of Perineum Bursa and Ligament, Percutaneous Endoscopic Approach
0MDL0ZZ Extraction of Right Hip Bursa and Ligament, Open Approach
0MDL3ZZ Extraction of Right Hip Bursa and Ligament, Percutaneous Approach
0MDL4ZZ Extraction of Right Hip Bursa and Ligament, Percutaneous Endoscopic Approach
0MDM0ZZ Extraction of Left Hip Bursa and Ligament, Open Approach
0MDM3ZZ Extraction of Left Hip Bursa and Ligament, Percutaneous Approach
0MDM4ZZ Extraction of Left Hip Bursa and Ligament, Percutaneous Endoscopic Approach
0MDN0ZZ Extraction of Right Knee Bursa and Ligament, Open Approach
0MDN3ZZ Extraction of Right Knee Bursa and Ligament, Percutaneous Approach
0MDN4ZZ Extraction of Right Knee Bursa and Ligament, Percutaneous Endoscopic Approach
0MDP0ZZ Extraction of Left Knee Bursa and Ligament, Open Approach
0MDP3ZZ Extraction of Left Knee Bursa and Ligament, Percutaneous Approach
0MDP4ZZ Extraction of Left Knee Bursa and Ligament, Percutaneous Endoscopic Approach
0MDQ0ZZ Extraction of Right Ankle Bursa and Ligament, Open Approach
0MDQ3ZZ Extraction of Right Ankle Bursa and Ligament, Percutaneous Approach
0MDQ4ZZ Extraction of Right Ankle Bursa and Ligament, Percutaneous Endoscopic Approach
0MDR0ZZ Extraction of Left Ankle Bursa and Ligament, Open Approach
0MDR3ZZ Extraction of Left Ankle Bursa and Ligament, Percutaneous Approach
0MDR4ZZ Extraction of Left Ankle Bursa and Ligament, Percutaneous Endoscopic Approach
0MDS0ZZ Extraction of Right Foot Bursa and Ligament, Open Approach
0MDS3ZZ Extraction of Right Foot Bursa and Ligament, Percutaneous Approach
0MDS4ZZ Extraction of Right Foot Bursa and Ligament, Percutaneous Endoscopic Approach
0MDT0ZZ Extraction of Left Foot Bursa and Ligament, Open Approach
0MDT3ZZ Extraction of Left Foot Bursa and Ligament, Percutaneous Approach
0MDT4ZZ Extraction of Left Foot Bursa and Ligament, Percutaneous Endoscopic Approach
0MDV0ZZ Extraction of Right Lower Extremity Bursa and Ligament, Open Approach
0MDV3ZZ Extraction of Right Lower Extremity Bursa and Ligament, Percutaneous Approach
0MDV4ZZ Extraction of Right Lower Extremity Bursa and Ligament, Percutaneous Endoscopic Approach
0MDW0ZZ Extraction of Left Lower Extremity Bursa and Ligament, Open Approach
0MDW3ZZ Extraction of Left Lower Extremity Bursa and Ligament, Percutaneous Approach
0MDW4ZZ Extraction of Left Lower Extremity Bursa and Ligament, Percutaneous Endoscopic Approach

0MJ – Bursae and Ligaments, Inspection

Review Coding Guideline B3.5

Review Coding Guidelines B3.11a, B3.11b and B3.11c

0MJX0ZZ Inspection of Upper Bursa and Ligament, Open Approach
0MJX3ZZ Inspection of Upper Bursa and Ligament, Percutaneous Approach
0MJX4ZZ Inspection of Upper Bursa and Ligament, Percutaneous Endoscopic Approach
0MJXXZZ Inspection of Upper Bursa and Ligament, External Approach
0MJY0ZZ Inspection of Lower Bursa and Ligament, Open Approach
0MJY3ZZ Inspection of Lower Bursa and Ligament, Percutaneous Approach
0MJY4ZZ Inspection of Lower Bursa and Ligament, Percutaneous Endoscopic Approach
0MJYXZZ Inspection of Lower Bursa and Ligament, External Approach

1M – Bursae and Ligaments, Reattachment

1M00ZZ Reattachment of Head and Neck Bursa and Ligament, Open Approach
1M04ZZ Reattachment of Head and Neck Bursa and Ligament, Percutaneous Endoscopic Approach
1M10ZZ Reattachment of Right Shoulder Bursa and Ligament, Open Approach
1M14ZZ Reattachment of Right Shoulder Bursa and Ligament, Percutaneous Endoscopic Approach
AHA CC: 3Q, 2013, 20-22
1M20ZZ Reattachment of Left Shoulder Bursa and Ligament, Open Approach
1M24ZZ Reattachment of Left Shoulder Bursa and Ligament, Percutaneous Endoscopic Approach
1M30ZZ Reattachment of Right Elbow Bursa and Ligament, Open Approach
1M34ZZ Reattachment of Right Elbow Bursa and Ligament, Percutaneous Endoscopic Approach
1M40ZZ Reattachment of Left Elbow Bursa and Ligament, Open Approach
1M44ZZ Reattachment of Left Elbow Bursa and Ligament, Percutaneous Endoscopic Approach
MM50ZZ Reattachment of Right Wrist Bursa and Ligament, Open Approach
MM54ZZ Reattachment of Right Wrist Bursa and Ligament, Percutaneous Endoscopic Approach
MM60ZZ Reattachment of Left Wrist Bursa and Ligament, Open Approach
MM64ZZ Reattachment of Left Wrist Bursa and Ligament, Percutaneous Endoscopic Approach
MM70ZZ Reattachment of Right Hand Bursa and Ligament, Open Approach
MM74ZZ Reattachment of Right Hand Bursa and Ligament, Percutaneous Endoscopic Approach
MM80ZZ Reattachment of Left Hand Bursa and Ligament, Open Approach
MM84ZZ Reattachment of Left Hand Bursa and Ligament, Percutaneous Endoscopic Approach
MM90ZZ Reattachment of Right Upper Extremity Bursa and Ligament, Open Approach
0MM94ZZ Reattachment of Right Upper Extremity Bursa and Ligament, Percutaneous Endoscopic Approach
0MMB0ZZ Reattachment of Left Upper Extremity Bursa and Ligament, Open Approach
0MMB4ZZ Reattachment of Left Upper Extremity Bursa and Ligament, Percutaneous Endoscopic Approach
0MMC0ZZ Reattachment of Right Trunk Bursa and Ligament, Open Approach
0MMC4ZZ Reattachment of Right Trunk Bursa and Ligament, Percutaneous Endoscopic Approach
0MMD0ZZ Reattachment of Left Trunk Bursa and Ligament, Open Approach
0MMD4ZZ Reattachment of Left Trunk Bursa and Ligament, Percutaneous Endoscopic Approach
0MMF0ZZ Reattachment of Right Thorax Bursa and Ligament, Open Approach
0MMF4ZZ Reattachment of Right Thorax Bursa and Ligament, Percutaneous Endoscopic Approach
0MMG0ZZ Reattachment of Left Thorax Bursa and Ligament, Open Approach
0MMG4ZZ Reattachment of Left Thorax Bursa and Ligament, Percutaneous Endoscopic Approach
0MMH0ZZ Reattachment of Right Abdomen Bursa and Ligament, Open Approach
0MMH4ZZ Reattachment of Right Abdomen Bursa and Ligament, Percutaneous Endoscopic Approach
0MMJ0ZZ Reattachment of Left Abdomen Bursa and Ligament, Open Approach
0MMJ4ZZ Reattachment of Left Abdomen Bursa and Ligament, Percutaneous Endoscopic Approach
0MMK0ZZ Reattachment of Perineum Bursa and Ligament, Open Approach
0MMK4ZZ Reattachment of Perineum Bursa and Ligament, Percutaneous Endoscopic Approach
0MML0ZZ Reattachment of Right Hip Bursa and Ligament, Open Approach
0MML4ZZ Reattachment of Right Hip Bursa and Ligament, Percutaneous Endoscopic Approach
0MMM0ZZ Reattachment of Left Hip Bursa and Ligament, Open Approach
0MMM4ZZ Reattachment of Left Hip Bursa and Ligament, Percutaneous Endoscopic Approach
0MMN0ZZ Reattachment of Right Knee Bursa and Ligament, Open Approach
0MMN4ZZ Reattachment of Right Knee Bursa and Ligament, Percutaneous Endoscopic Approach
0MMP0ZZ Reattachment of Left Knee Bursa and Ligament, Open Approach
0MMP4ZZ Reattachment of Left Knee Bursa and Ligament, Percutaneous Endoscopic Approach
0MMQ0ZZ Reattachment of Right Ankle Bursa and Ligament, Open Approach
0MMQ4ZZ Reattachment of Right Ankle Bursa and Ligament, Percutaneous Endoscopic Approach
0MMR0ZZ Reattachment of Left Ankle Bursa and Ligament, Open Approach
0MMR4ZZ Reattachment of Left Ankle Bursa and Ligament, Percutaneous Endoscopic Approach
0MMS0ZZ Reattachment of Right Foot Bursa and Ligament, Open Approach
0MMS4ZZ Reattachment of Right Foot Bursa and Ligament, Percutaneous Endoscopic Approach
0MMT0ZZ Reattachment of Left Foot Bursa and Ligament, Open Approach
0MMT4ZZ Reattachment of Left Foot Bursa and Ligament, Percutaneous Endoscopic Approach
0MMV0ZZ Reattachment of Right Lower Extremity Bursa and Ligament, Open Approach
0MMV4ZZ Reattachment of Right Lower Extremity Bursa and Ligament, Percutaneous Endoscopic Approach
0MMW0ZZ Reattachment of Left Lower Extremity Bursa and Ligament, Open Approach
0MMW4ZZ Reattachment of Left Lower Extremity Bursa and Ligament, Percutaneous Endoscopic Approach

0MN – Bursae and Ligaments, Release

Review Coding Guideline B3.13

Review Coding Guideline B3.14

0MN00ZZ Release Head and Neck Bursa and Ligament, Open Approach
0MN03ZZ Release Head and Neck Bursa and Ligament, Percutaneous Approach
0MN04ZZ Release Head and Neck Bursa and Ligament, Percutaneous Endoscopic Approach
0MN0XZZ Release Head and Neck Bursa and Ligament, External Approach
0MN10ZZ Release Right Shoulder Bursa and Ligament, Open Approach
0MN13ZZ Release Right Shoulder Bursa and Ligament, Percutaneous Approach
0MN14ZZ Release Right Shoulder Bursa and Ligament, Percutaneous Endoscopic Approach
0MN1XZZ Release Right Shoulder Bursa and Ligament, External Approach
0MN20ZZ Release Left Shoulder Bursa and Ligament, Open Approach
0MN23ZZ Release Left Shoulder Bursa and Ligament, Percutaneous Approach
0MN24ZZ Release Left Shoulder Bursa and Ligament, Percutaneous Endoscopic Approach
0MN2XZZ Release Left Shoulder Bursa and Ligament, External Approach
0MN30ZZ Release Right Elbow Bursa and Ligament, Open Approach
0MN33ZZ Release Right Elbow Bursa and Ligament, Percutaneous Approach
0MN34ZZ Release Right Elbow Bursa and Ligament, Percutaneous Endoscopic Approach
0MN3XZZ Release Right Elbow Bursa and Ligament, External Approach
0MN40ZZ Release Left Elbow Bursa and Ligament, Open Approach
0MN43ZZ Release Left Elbow Bursa and Ligament, Percutaneous Approach
0MN44ZZ Release Left Elbow Bursa and Ligament, Percutaneous Endoscopic Approach
0MN4XZZ Release Left Elbow Bursa and Ligament, External Approach
0MN50ZZ Release Right Wrist Bursa and Ligament, Open Approach
0MN53ZZ Release Right Wrist Bursa and Ligament, Percutaneous Approach
0MN54ZZ Release Right Wrist Bursa and Ligament, Percutaneous Endoscopic Approach
0MN5XZZ Release Right Wrist Bursa and Ligament, External Approach
0MN60ZZ Release Left Wrist Bursa and Ligament, Open Approach

0MN63ZZ Release Left Wrist Bursa and Ligament, Percutaneous Approach
0MN64ZZ Release Left Wrist Bursa and Ligament, Percutaneous Endoscopic Approach
0MN6XZZ Release Left Wrist Bursa and Ligament, External Approach
0MN70ZZ Release Right Hand Bursa and Ligament, Open Approach
0MN73ZZ Release Right Hand Bursa and Ligament, Percutaneous Approach
0MN74ZZ Release Right Hand Bursa and Ligament, Percutaneous Endoscopic Approach
0MN7XZZ Release Right Hand Bursa and Ligament, External Approach
0MN80ZZ Release Left Hand Bursa and Ligament, Open Approach
0MN83ZZ Release Left Hand Bursa and Ligament, Percutaneous Approach
0MN84ZZ Release Left Hand Bursa and Ligament, Percutaneous Endoscopic Approach
0MN8XZZ Release Left Hand Bursa and Ligament, External Approach
0MN90ZZ Release Right Upper Extremity Bursa and Ligament, Open Approach
0MN93ZZ Release Right Upper Extremity Bursa and Ligament, Percutaneous Approach
0MN94ZZ Release Right Upper Extremity Bursa and Ligament, Percutaneous Endoscopic Approach
0MN9XZZ Release Right Upper Extremity Bursa and Ligament, External Approach
0MNB0ZZ Release Left Upper Extremity Bursa and Ligament, Open Approach
0MNB3ZZ Release Left Upper Extremity Bursa and Ligament, Percutaneous Approach
0MNB4ZZ Release Left Upper Extremity Bursa and Ligament, Percutaneous Endoscopic Approach
0MNBXZZ Release Left Upper Extremity Bursa and Ligament, External Approach
0MNC0ZZ Release Right Trunk Bursa and Ligament, Open Approach
0MNC3ZZ Release Right Trunk Bursa and Ligament, Percutaneous Approach
0MNC4ZZ Release Right Trunk Bursa and Ligament, Percutaneous Endoscopic Approach
0MNCXZZ Release Right Trunk Bursa and Ligament, External Approach
0MND0ZZ Release Left Trunk Bursa and Ligament, Open Approach
0MND3ZZ Release Left Trunk Bursa and Ligament, Percutaneous Approach
0MND4ZZ Release Left Trunk Bursa and Ligament, Percutaneous Endoscopic Approach
0MNDXZZ Release Left Trunk Bursa and Ligament, External Approach
0MNF0ZZ Release Right Thorax Bursa and Ligament, Open Approach
0MNF3ZZ Release Right Thorax Bursa and Ligament, Percutaneous Approach
0MNF4ZZ Release Right Thorax Bursa and Ligament, Percutaneous Endoscopic Approach
0MNFXZZ Release Right Thorax Bursa and Ligament, External Approach
0MNG0ZZ Release Left Thorax Bursa and Ligament, Open Approach
0MNG3ZZ Release Left Thorax Bursa and Ligament, Percutaneous Approach
0MNG4ZZ Release Left Thorax Bursa and Ligament, Percutaneous Endoscopic Approach
0MNGXZZ Release Left Thorax Bursa and Ligament, External Approach
0MNH0ZZ Release Right Abdomen Bursa and Ligament, Open Approach
0MNH3ZZ Release Right Abdomen Bursa and Ligament, Percutaneous Approach
0MNH4ZZ Release Right Abdomen Bursa and Ligament, Percutaneous Endoscopic Approach
0MNHXZZ Release Right Abdomen Bursa and Ligament, External Approach
0MNJ0ZZ Release Left Abdomen Bursa and Ligament, Open Approach
0MNJ3ZZ Release Left Abdomen Bursa and Ligament, Percutaneous Approach
0MNJ4ZZ Release Left Abdomen Bursa and Ligament, Percutaneous Endoscopic Approach
0MNJXZZ Release Left Abdomen Bursa and Ligament, External Approach
0MNK0ZZ Release Perineum Bursa and Ligament, Open Approach
0MNK3ZZ Release Perineum Bursa and Ligament, Percutaneous Approach
0MNK4ZZ Release Perineum Bursa and Ligament, Percutaneous Endoscopic Approach
0MNKXZZ Release Perineum Bursa and Ligament, External Approach
0MNL0ZZ Release Right Hip Bursa and Ligament, Open Approach
0MNL3ZZ Release Right Hip Bursa and Ligament, Percutaneous Approach
0MNL4ZZ Release Right Hip Bursa and Ligament, Percutaneous Endoscopic Approach
0MNLXZZ Release Right Hip Bursa and Ligament, External Approach
0MNM0ZZ Release Left Hip Bursa and Ligament, Open Approach
0MNM3ZZ Release Left Hip Bursa and Ligament, Percutaneous Approach
0MNM4ZZ Release Left Hip Bursa and Ligament, Percutaneous Endoscopic Approach
0MNMXZZ Release Left Hip Bursa and Ligament, External Approach
0MNN0ZZ Release Right Knee Bursa and Ligament, Open Approach
0MNN3ZZ Release Right Knee Bursa and Ligament, Percutaneous Approach
0MNN4ZZ Release Right Knee Bursa and Ligament, Percutaneous Endoscopic Approach
0MNNXZZ Release Right Knee Bursa and Ligament, External Approach
0MNP0ZZ Release Left Knee Bursa and Ligament, Open Approach
0MNP3ZZ Release Left Knee Bursa and Ligament, Percutaneous Approach
0MNP4ZZ Release Left Knee Bursa and Ligament, Percutaneous Endoscopic Approach
0MNPXZZ Release Left Knee Bursa and Ligament, External Approach
0MNQ0ZZ Release Right Ankle Bursa and Ligament, Open Approach
0MNQ3ZZ Release Right Ankle Bursa and Ligament, Percutaneous Approach
0MNQ4ZZ Release Right Ankle Bursa and Ligament, Percutaneous Endoscopic Approach
0MNQXZZ Release Right Ankle Bursa and Ligament, External Approach
0MNR0ZZ Release Left Ankle Bursa and Ligament, Open Approach
0MNR3ZZ Release Left Ankle Bursa and Ligament, Percutaneous Approach
0MNR4ZZ Release Left Ankle Bursa and Ligament, Percutaneous Endoscopic Approach
0MNRXZZ Release Left Ankle Bursa and Ligament, External Approach
0MNS0ZZ Release Right Foot Bursa and Ligament, Open Approach
0MNS3ZZ Release Right Foot Bursa and Ligament, Percutaneous Approach
0MNS4ZZ Release Right Foot Bursa and Ligament, Percutaneous Endoscopic Approach
0MNSXZZ Release Right Foot Bursa and Ligament, External Approach
0MNT0ZZ Release Left Foot Bursa and Ligament, Open Approach
0MNT3ZZ Release Left Foot Bursa and Ligament, Percutaneous Approach
0MNT4ZZ Release Left Foot Bursa and Ligament, Percutaneous Endoscopic Approach
0MNTXZZ Release Left Foot Bursa and Ligament, External Approach
0MNV0ZZ Release Right Lower Extremity Bursa and Ligament, Open Approach
0MNV3ZZ Release Right Lower Extremity Bursa and Ligament, Percutaneous Approach
0MNV4ZZ Release Right Lower Extremity Bursa and Ligament, Percutaneous Endoscopic Approach
0MNVXZZ Release Right Lower Extremity Bursa and Ligament, External Approach
0MNW0ZZ Release Left Lower Extremity Bursa and Ligament, Open Approach
0MNW3ZZ Release Left Lower Extremity Bursa and Ligament, Percutaneous Approach
0MNW4ZZ Release Left Lower Extremity Bursa and Ligament, Percutaneous Endoscopic Approach
0MNWXZZ Release Left Lower Extremity Bursa and Ligament, External Approach

0MP – Bursae and Ligaments, Removal

Review Coding Guideline B6.1c

0MPX00Z Removal of Drainage Device from Upper Bursa and Ligament, Open Approach
0MPX07Z Removal of Autologous Tissue Substitute from Upper Bursa and Ligament, Open Approach
0MPX0JZ Removal of Synthetic Substitute from Upper Bursa and Ligament, Open Approach
0MPX0KZ Removal of Nonautologous Tissue Substitute from Upper Bursa and Ligament, Open Approach
0MPX30Z Removal of Drainage Device from Upper Bursa and Ligament, Percutaneous Approach
0MPX37Z Removal of Autologous Tissue Substitute from Upper Bursa and Ligament, Percutaneous Approach
0MPX3JZ Removal of Synthetic Substitute from Upper Bursa and Ligament, Percutaneous Approach
0MPX3KZ Removal of Nonautologous Tissue Substitute from Upper Bursa and Ligament, Percutaneous Approach
0MPX40Z Removal of Drainage Device from Upper Bursa and Ligament, Percutaneous Endoscopic Approach

PX47Z Removal of Autologous Tissue Substitute from Upper Bursa and Ligament, Percutaneous Endoscopic Approach
PX4JZ Removal of Synthetic Substitute from Upper Bursa and Ligament, Percutaneous Endoscopic Approach
PX4KZ Removal of Nonautologous Tissue Substitute from Upper Bursa and Ligament, Percutaneous Endoscopic Approach
IPXX0Z Removal of Drainage Device from Upper Bursa and Ligament, External Approach
IPY00Z Removal of Drainage Device from Lower Bursa and Ligament, Open Approach
IPY07Z Removal of Autologous Tissue Substitute from Lower Bursa and Ligament, Open Approach
0MPY0JZ Removal of Synthetic Substitute from Lower Bursa and Ligament, Open Approach
0MPY0KZ Removal of Nonautologous Tissue Substitute from Lower Bursa and Ligament, Open Approach
0MPY30Z Removal of Drainage Device from Lower Bursa and Ligament, Percutaneous Approach
0MPY37Z Removal of Autologous Tissue Substitute from Lower Bursa and Ligament, Percutaneous Approach
0MPY3JZ Removal of Synthetic Substitute from Lower Bursa and Ligament, Percutaneous Approach
0MPY3KZ Removal of Nonautologous Tissue Substitute from Lower Bursa and Ligament, Percutaneous Approach
0MPY40Z Removal of Drainage Device from Lower Bursa and Ligament, Percutaneous Endoscopic Approach
0MPY47Z Removal of Autologous Tissue Substitute from Lower Bursa and Ligament, Percutaneous Endoscopic Approach
0MPY4JZ Removal of Synthetic Substitute from Lower Bursa and Ligament, Percutaneous Endoscopic Approach
0MPY4KZ Removal of Nonautologous Tissue Substitute from Lower Bursa and Ligament, Percutaneous Endoscopic Approach
0MPYX0Z Removal of Drainage Device from Lower Bursa and Ligament, External Approach

MQ – Bursae and Ligaments, Repair

eview Coding Guideline B3.5

IQ00ZZ Repair Head and Neck Bursa and Ligament, Open Approach
IQ03ZZ Repair Head and Neck Bursa and Ligament, Percutaneous Approach
IQ04ZZ Repair Head and Neck Bursa and Ligament, Percutaneous Endoscopic Approach
IQ10ZZ Repair Right Shoulder Bursa and Ligament, Open Approach
IQ13ZZ Repair Right Shoulder Bursa and Ligament, Percutaneous Approach
IQ14ZZ Repair Right Shoulder Bursa and Ligament, Percutaneous Endoscopic Approach
MQ20ZZ Repair Left Shoulder Bursa and Ligament, Open Approach
MQ23ZZ Repair Left Shoulder Bursa and Ligament, Percutaneous Approach
MQ24ZZ Repair Left Shoulder Bursa and Ligament, Percutaneous Endoscopic Approach
MQ30ZZ Repair Right Elbow Bursa and Ligament, Open Approach
MQ33ZZ Repair Right Elbow Bursa and Ligament, Percutaneous Approach
MQ34ZZ Repair Right Elbow Bursa and Ligament, Percutaneous Endoscopic Approach
MQ40ZZ Repair Left Elbow Bursa and Ligament, Open Approach
MQ43ZZ Repair Left Elbow Bursa and Ligament, Percutaneous Approach
MQ44ZZ Repair Left Elbow Bursa and Ligament, Percutaneous Endoscopic Approach
MQ50ZZ Repair Right Wrist Bursa and Ligament, Open Approach
MQ53ZZ Repair Right Wrist Bursa and Ligament, Percutaneous Approach
MQ54ZZ Repair Right Wrist Bursa and Ligament, Percutaneous Endoscopic Approach
MQ60ZZ Repair Left Wrist Bursa and Ligament, Open Approach
MQ63ZZ Repair Left Wrist Bursa and Ligament, Percutaneous Approach
MQ64ZZ Repair Left Wrist Bursa and Ligament, Percutaneous Endoscopic Approach
MQ70ZZ Repair Right Hand Bursa and Ligament, Open Approach
MQ73ZZ Repair Right Hand Bursa and Ligament, Percutaneous Approach
MQ74ZZ Repair Right Hand Bursa and Ligament, Percutaneous Endoscopic Approach
0MQ80ZZ Repair Left Hand Bursa and Ligament, Open Approach
0MQ83ZZ Repair Left Hand Bursa and Ligament, Percutaneous Approach
0MQ84ZZ Repair Left Hand Bursa and Ligament, Percutaneous Endoscopic Approach
0MQ90ZZ Repair Right Upper Extremity Bursa and Ligament, Open Approach
0MQ93ZZ Repair Right Upper Extremity Bursa and Ligament, Percutaneous Approach
0MQ94ZZ Repair Right Upper Extremity Bursa and Ligament, Percutaneous Endoscopic Approach
0MQB0ZZ Repair Left Upper Extremity Bursa and Ligament, Open Approach
0MQB3ZZ Repair Left Upper Extremity Bursa and Ligament, Percutaneous Approach
0MQB4ZZ Repair Left Upper Extremity Bursa and Ligament, Percutaneous Endoscopic Approach
0MQC0ZZ Repair Right Trunk Bursa and Ligament, Open Approach
0MQC3ZZ Repair Right Trunk Bursa and Ligament, Percutaneous Approach
0MQC4ZZ Repair Right Trunk Bursa and Ligament, Percutaneous Endoscopic Approach
0MQD0ZZ Repair Left Trunk Bursa and Ligament, Open Approach
0MQD3ZZ Repair Left Trunk Bursa and Ligament, Percutaneous Approach
0MQD4ZZ Repair Left Trunk Bursa and Ligament, Percutaneous Endoscopic Approach
0MQF0ZZ Repair Right Thorax Bursa and Ligament, Open Approach
0MQF3ZZ Repair Right Thorax Bursa and Ligament, Percutaneous Approach
0MQF4ZZ Repair Right Thorax Bursa and Ligament, Percutaneous Endoscopic Approach
0MQG0ZZ Repair Left Thorax Bursa and Ligament, Open Approach
0MQG3ZZ Repair Left Thorax Bursa and Ligament, Percutaneous Approach
0MQG4ZZ Repair Left Thorax Bursa and Ligament, Percutaneous Endoscopic Approach
0MQH0ZZ Repair Right Abdomen Bursa and Ligament, Open Approach
0MQH3ZZ Repair Right Abdomen Bursa and Ligament, Percutaneous Approach
0MQH4ZZ Repair Right Abdomen Bursa and Ligament, Percutaneous Endoscopic Approach
0MQJ0ZZ Repair Left Abdomen Bursa and Ligament, Open Approach
0MQJ3ZZ Repair Left Abdomen Bursa and Ligament, Percutaneous Approach
0MQJ4ZZ Repair Left Abdomen Bursa and Ligament, Percutaneous Endoscopic Approach
0MQK0ZZ Repair Perineum Bursa and Ligament, Open Approach
0MQK3ZZ Repair Perineum Bursa and Ligament, Percutaneous Approach
0MQK4ZZ Repair Perineum Bursa and Ligament, Percutaneous Endoscopic Approach
0MQL0ZZ Repair Right Hip Bursa and Ligament, Open Approach
0MQL3ZZ Repair Right Hip Bursa and Ligament, Percutaneous Approach
0MQL4ZZ Repair Right Hip Bursa and Ligament, Percutaneous Endoscopic Approach
0MQM0ZZ Repair Left Hip Bursa and Ligament, Open Approach
0MQM3ZZ Repair Left Hip Bursa and Ligament, Percutaneous Approach
0MQM4ZZ Repair Left Hip Bursa and Ligament, Percutaneous Endoscopic Approach
0MQN0ZZ Repair Right Knee Bursa and Ligament, Open Approach
0MQN3ZZ Repair Right Knee Bursa and Ligament, Percutaneous Approach
0MQN4ZZ Repair Right Knee Bursa and Ligament, Percutaneous Endoscopic Approach
0MQP0ZZ Repair Left Knee Bursa and Ligament, Open Approach
0MQP3ZZ Repair Left Knee Bursa and Ligament, Percutaneous Approach
0MQP4ZZ Repair Left Knee Bursa and Ligament, Percutaneous Endoscopic Approach
0MQQ0ZZ Repair Right Ankle Bursa and Ligament, Open Approach
0MQQ3ZZ Repair Right Ankle Bursa and Ligament, Percutaneous Approach
0MQQ4ZZ Repair Right Ankle Bursa and Ligament, Percutaneous Endoscopic Approach
0MQR0ZZ Repair Left Ankle Bursa and Ligament, Open Approach
0MQR3ZZ Repair Left Ankle Bursa and Ligament, Percutaneous Approach
0MQR4ZZ Repair Left Ankle Bursa and Ligament, Percutaneous Endoscopic Approach
0MQS0ZZ Repair Right Foot Bursa and Ligament, Open Approach

0MQS3ZZ Repair Right Foot Bursa and Ligament, Percutaneous Approach
0MQS4ZZ Repair Right Foot Bursa and Ligament, Percutaneous Endoscopic Approach
0MQT0ZZ Repair Left Foot Bursa and Ligament, Open Approach
0MQT3ZZ Repair Left Foot Bursa and Ligament, Percutaneous Approach
0MQT4ZZ Repair Left Foot Bursa and Ligament, Percutaneous Endoscopic Approach
0MQV0ZZ Repair Right Lower Extremity Bursa and Ligament, Open Approach
0MQV3ZZ Repair Right Lower Extremity Bursa and Ligament, Percutaneous Approach
0MQV4ZZ Repair Right Lower Extremity Bursa and Ligament, Percutaneous Endoscopic Approach
0MQW0ZZ Repair Left Lower Extremity Bursa a Ligament, Open Approach
0MQW3ZZ Repair Left Lower Extremity Bursa a Ligament, Percutaneous Approach
0MQW4ZZ Repair Left Lower Extremity Bursa a Ligament, Percutaneous Endoscopic Approach

0MS – Bursae and Ligaments, Reposition

0MS00ZZ Reposition Head and Neck Bursa and Ligament, Open Approach
0MS04ZZ Reposition Head and Neck Bursa and Ligament, Percutaneous Endoscopic Approach
0MS10ZZ Reposition Right Shoulder Bursa and Ligament, Open Approach
0MS14ZZ Reposition Right Shoulder Bursa and Ligament, Percutaneous Endoscopic Approach
0MS20ZZ Reposition Left Shoulder Bursa and Ligament, Open Approach
0MS24ZZ Reposition Left Shoulder Bursa and Ligament, Percutaneous Endoscopic Approach
0MS30ZZ Reposition Right Elbow Bursa and Ligament, Open Approach
0MS34ZZ Reposition Right Elbow Bursa and Ligament, Percutaneous Endoscopic Approach
0MS40ZZ Reposition Left Elbow Bursa and Ligament, Open Approach
0MS44ZZ Reposition Left Elbow Bursa and Ligament, Percutaneous Endoscopic Approach
0MS50ZZ Reposition Right Wrist Bursa and Ligament, Open Approach
0MS54ZZ Reposition Right Wrist Bursa and Ligament, Percutaneous Endoscopic Approach
0MS60ZZ Reposition Left Wrist Bursa and Ligament, Open Approach
0MS64ZZ Reposition Left Wrist Bursa and Ligament, Percutaneous Endoscopic Approach
0MS70ZZ Reposition Right Hand Bursa and Ligament, Open Approach
0MS74ZZ Reposition Right Hand Bursa and Ligament, Percutaneous Endoscopic Approach
0MS80ZZ Reposition Left Hand Bursa and Ligament, Open Approach
0MS84ZZ Reposition Left Hand Bursa and Ligament, Percutaneous Endoscopic Approach
0MS90ZZ Reposition Right Upper Extremity Bursa and Ligament, Open Approach
0MS94ZZ Reposition Right Upper Extremity Bursa and Ligament, Percutaneous Endoscopic Approach
0MSB0ZZ Reposition Left Upper Extremity Bursa and Ligament, Open Approach
0MSB4ZZ Reposition Left Upper Extremity Bursa and Ligament, Percutaneous Endoscopic Approach
0MSC0ZZ Reposition Right Trunk Bursa and Ligament, Open Approach
0MSC4ZZ Reposition Right Trunk Bursa and Ligament, Percutaneous Endoscopic Approach
0MSD0ZZ Reposition Left Trunk Bursa and Ligament, Open Approach
0MSD4ZZ Reposition Left Trunk Bursa and Ligament, Percutaneous Endoscopic Approach
0MSF0ZZ Reposition Right Thorax Bursa and Ligament, Open Approach
0MSF4ZZ Reposition Right Thorax Bursa and Ligament, Percutaneous Endoscopic Approach
0MSG0ZZ Reposition Left Thorax Bursa and Ligament, Open Approach
0MSG4ZZ Reposition Left Thorax Bursa and Ligament, Percutaneous Endoscopic Approach
0MSH0ZZ Reposition Right Abdomen Bursa and Ligament, Open Approach
0MSH4ZZ Reposition Right Abdomen Bursa and Ligament, Percutaneous Endoscopic Approach
0MSJ0ZZ Reposition Left Abdomen Bursa and Ligament, Open Approach
0MSJ4ZZ Reposition Left Abdomen Bursa and Ligament, Percutaneous Endoscopic Approach
0MSK0ZZ Reposition Perineum Bursa and Ligament, Open Approach
0MSK4ZZ Reposition Perineum Bursa and Ligament, Percutaneous Endoscopic Approach
0MSL0ZZ Reposition Right Hip Bursa and Ligament, Open Approach
0MSL4ZZ Reposition Right Hip Bursa and Ligament, Percutaneous Endoscopic Approach
0MSM0ZZ Reposition Left Hip Bursa and Ligame Open Approach
0MSM4ZZ Reposition Left Hip Bursa and Ligame Percutaneous Endoscopic Approach
0MSN0ZZ Reposition Right Knee Bursa and Ligament, Open Approach
0MSN4ZZ Reposition Right Knee Bursa and Ligament, Percutaneous Endoscopic Approach
0MSP0ZZ Reposition Left Knee Bursa and Ligament, Open Approach
0MSP4ZZ Reposition Left Knee Bursa and Ligament, Percutaneous Endoscopic Approach
0MSQ0ZZ Reposition Right Ankle Bursa and Ligament, Open Approach
0MSQ4ZZ Reposition Right Ankle Bursa and Ligament, Percutaneous Endoscopic Approach
0MSR0ZZ Reposition Left Ankle Bursa and Ligament, Open Approach
0MSR4ZZ Reposition Left Ankle Bursa and Ligament, Percutaneous Endoscopic Approach
0MSS0ZZ Reposition Right Foot Bursa and Ligament, Open Approach
0MSS4ZZ Reposition Right Foot Bursa and Ligament, Percutaneous Endoscopic Approach
0MST0ZZ Reposition Left Foot Bursa and Ligament, Open Approach
0MST4ZZ Reposition Left Foot Bursa and Ligament, Percutaneous Endoscopic Approach
0MSV0ZZ Reposition Right Lower Extremity Burs and Ligament, Open Approach
0MSV4ZZ Reposition Right Lower Extremity Burs and Ligament, Percutaneous Endoscopic Approach
0MSW0ZZ Reposition Left Lower Extremity Bursa and Ligament, Open Approach
0MSW4ZZ Reposition Left Lower Extremity Bursa and Ligament, Percutaneous Endoscopic Approach

0MT – Bursae and Ligaments, Resection

Review Coding Guideline B3.8

0MT00ZZ Resection of Head and Neck Bursa and Ligament, Open Approach
0MT04ZZ Resection of Head and Neck Bursa and Ligament, Percutaneous Endoscopic Approach
0MT10ZZ Resection of Right Shoulder Bursa and Ligament, Open Approach
0MT14ZZ Resection of Right Shoulder Bursa and Ligament, Percutaneous Endoscopic Approach
0MT20ZZ Resection of Left Shoulder Bursa and Ligament, Open Approach
0MT24ZZ Resection of Left Shoulder Bursa and Ligament, Percutaneous Endoscopic Approach
0MT30ZZ Resection of Right Elbow Bursa and Ligament, Open Approach
0MT34ZZ Resection of Right Elbow Bursa and Ligament, Percutaneous Endoscopic Approach
0MT40ZZ Resection of Left Elbow Bursa and Ligament, Open Approach
0MT44ZZ Resection of Left Elbow Bursa and Ligament, Percutaneous Endoscopic Approach
0MT50ZZ Resection of Right Wrist Bursa and Ligament, Open Approach
0MT54ZZ Resection of Right Wrist Bursa and Ligament, Percutaneous Endoscopic Approach
0MT60ZZ Resection of Left Wrist Bursa and Ligament, Open Approach
0MT64ZZ Resection of Left Wrist Bursa and Ligament, Percutaneous Endoscopic Approach
0MT70ZZ Resection of Right Hand Bursa and Ligament, Open Approach

T74ZZ	Resection of Right Hand Bursa and Ligament, Percutaneous Endoscopic Approach
T80ZZ	Resection of Left Hand Bursa and Ligament, Open Approach
T84ZZ	Resection of Left Hand Bursa and Ligament, Percutaneous Endoscopic Approach
T90ZZ	Resection of Right Upper Extremity Bursa and Ligament, Open Approach
T94ZZ	Resection of Right Upper Extremity Bursa and Ligament, Percutaneous Endoscopic Approach
TB0ZZ	Resection of Left Upper Extremity Bursa and Ligament, Open Approach
TB4ZZ	Resection of Left Upper Extremity Bursa and Ligament, Percutaneous Endoscopic Approach
TC0ZZ	Resection of Right Trunk Bursa and Ligament, Open Approach
TC4ZZ	Resection of Right Trunk Bursa and Ligament, Percutaneous Endoscopic Approach
TD0ZZ	Resection of Left Trunk Bursa and Ligament, Open Approach
TD4ZZ	Resection of Left Trunk Bursa and Ligament, Percutaneous Endoscopic Approach
TF0ZZ	Resection of Right Thorax Bursa and Ligament, Open Approach
TF4ZZ	Resection of Right Thorax Bursa and Ligament, Percutaneous Endoscopic Approach
TG0ZZ	Resection of Left Thorax Bursa and Ligament, Open Approach
0MTG4ZZ	Resection of Left Thorax Bursa and Ligament, Percutaneous Endoscopic Approach
0MTH0ZZ	Resection of Right Abdomen Bursa and Ligament, Open Approach
0MTH4ZZ	Resection of Right Abdomen Bursa and Ligament, Percutaneous Endoscopic Approach
0MTJ0ZZ	Resection of Left Abdomen Bursa and Ligament, Open Approach
0MTJ4ZZ	Resection of Left Abdomen Bursa and Ligament, Percutaneous Endoscopic Approach
0MTK0ZZ	Resection of Perineum Bursa and Ligament, Open Approach
0MTK4ZZ	Resection of Perineum Bursa and Ligament, Percutaneous Endoscopic Approach
0MTL0ZZ	Resection of Right Hip Bursa and Ligament, Open Approach
0MTL4ZZ	Resection of Right Hip Bursa and Ligament, Percutaneous Endoscopic Approach
0MTM0ZZ	Resection of Left Hip Bursa and Ligament, Open Approach
0MTM4ZZ	Resection of Left Hip Bursa and Ligament, Percutaneous Endoscopic Approach
0MTN0ZZ	Resection of Right Knee Bursa and Ligament, Open Approach
0MTN4ZZ	Resection of Right Knee Bursa and Ligament, Percutaneous Endoscopic Approach
0MTP0ZZ	Resection of Left Knee Bursa and Ligament, Open Approach
0MTP4ZZ	Resection of Left Knee Bursa and Ligament, Percutaneous Endoscopic Approach
0MTQ0ZZ	Resection of Right Ankle Bursa and Ligament, Open Approach
0MTQ4ZZ	Resection of Right Ankle Bursa and Ligament, Percutaneous Endoscopic Approach
0MTR0ZZ	Resection of Left Ankle Bursa and Ligament, Open Approach
0MTR4ZZ	Resection of Left Ankle Bursa and Ligament, Percutaneous Endoscopic Approach
0MTS0ZZ	Resection of Right Foot Bursa and Ligament, Open Approach
0MTS4ZZ	Resection of Right Foot Bursa and Ligament, Percutaneous Endoscopic Approach
0MTT0ZZ	Resection of Left Foot Bursa and Ligament, Open Approach
0MTT4ZZ	Resection of Left Foot Bursa and Ligament, Percutaneous Endoscopic Approach
0MTV0ZZ	Resection of Right Lower Extremity Bursa and Ligament, Open Approach
0MTV4ZZ	Resection of Right Lower Extremity Bursa and Ligament, Percutaneous Endoscopic Approach
0MTW0ZZ	Resection of Left Lower Extremity Bursa and Ligament, Open Approach
0MTW4ZZ	Resection of Left Lower Extremity Bursa and Ligament, Percutaneous Endoscopic Approach

MU – Bursae and Ligaments, Supplement

IU007Z	Supplement Head and Neck Bursa and Ligament with Autologous Tissue Substitute, Open Approach
IU00JZ	Supplement Head and Neck Bursa and Ligament with Synthetic Substitute, Open Approach
IU00KZ	Supplement Head and Neck Bursa and Ligament with Nonautologous Tissue Substitute, Open Approach
IU047Z	Supplement Head and Neck Bursa and Ligament with Autologous Tissue Substitute, Percutaneous Endoscopic Approach
IU04JZ	Supplement Head and Neck Bursa and Ligament with Synthetic Substitute, Percutaneous Endoscopic Approach
MU04KZ	Supplement Head and Neck Bursa and Ligament with Nonautologous Tissue Substitute, Percutaneous Endoscopic Approach
MU107Z	Supplement Right Shoulder Bursa and Ligament with Autologous Tissue Substitute, Open Approach
MU10JZ	Supplement Right Shoulder Bursa and Ligament with Synthetic Substitute, Open Approach
MU10KZ	Supplement Right Shoulder Bursa and Ligament with Nonautologous Tissue Substitute, Open Approach
MU147Z	Supplement Right Shoulder Bursa and Ligament with Autologous Tissue Substitute, Percutaneous Endoscopic Approach
MU14JZ	Supplement Right Shoulder Bursa and Ligament with Synthetic Substitute, Percutaneous Endoscopic Approach
MU14KZ	Supplement Right Shoulder Bursa and Ligament with Nonautologous Tissue Substitute, Percutaneous Endoscopic Approach
0MU207Z	Supplement Left Shoulder Bursa and Ligament with Autologous Tissue Substitute, Open Approach
0MU20JZ	Supplement Left Shoulder Bursa and Ligament with Synthetic Substitute, Open Approach
0MU20KZ	Supplement Left Shoulder Bursa and Ligament with Nonautologous Tissue Substitute, Open Approach
0MU247Z	Supplement Left Shoulder Bursa and Ligament with Autologous Tissue Substitute, Percutaneous Endoscopic Approach
0MU24JZ	Supplement Left Shoulder Bursa and Ligament with Synthetic Substitute, Percutaneous Endoscopic Approach
0MU24KZ	Supplement Left Shoulder Bursa and Ligament with Nonautologous Tissue Substitute, Percutaneous Endoscopic Approach
0MU307Z	Supplement Right Elbow Bursa and Ligament with Autologous Tissue Substitute, Open Approach
0MU30JZ	Supplement Right Elbow Bursa and Ligament with Synthetic Substitute, Open Approach
0MU30KZ	Supplement Right Elbow Bursa and Ligament with Nonautologous Tissue Substitute, Open Approach
0MU347Z	Supplement Right Elbow Bursa and Ligament with Autologous Tissue Substitute, Percutaneous Endoscopic Approach
0MU34JZ	Supplement Right Elbow Bursa and Ligament with Synthetic Substitute, Percutaneous Endoscopic Approach
0MU34KZ	Supplement Right Elbow Bursa and Ligament with Nonautologous Tissue Substitute, Percutaneous Endoscopic Approach
0MU407Z	Supplement Left Elbow Bursa and Ligament with Autologous Tissue Substitute, Open Approach
0MU40JZ	Supplement Left Elbow Bursa and Ligament with Synthetic Substitute, Open Approach
0MU40KZ	Supplement Left Elbow Bursa and Ligament with Nonautologous Tissue Substitute, Open Approach
0MU447Z	Supplement Left Elbow Bursa and Ligament with Autologous Tissue Substitute, Percutaneous Endoscopic Approach
0MU44JZ	Supplement Left Elbow Bursa and Ligament with Synthetic Substitute, Percutaneous Endoscopic Approach
0MU44KZ	Supplement Left Elbow Bursa and Ligament with Nonautologous Tissue Substitute, Percutaneous Endoscopic Approach
0MU507Z	Supplement Right Wrist Bursa and Ligament with Autologous Tissue Substitute, Open Approach
0MU50JZ	Supplement Right Wrist Bursa and Ligament with Synthetic Substitute, Open Approach
0MU50KZ	Supplement Right Wrist Bursa and Ligament with Nonautologous Tissue Substitute, Open Approach
0MU547Z	Supplement Right Wrist Bursa and Ligament with Autologous Tissue Substitute, Percutaneous Endoscopic Approach

0MU54JZ Supplement Right Wrist Bursa and Ligament with Synthetic Substitute, Percutaneous Endoscopic Approach
0MU54KZ Supplement Right Wrist Bursa and Ligament with Nonautologous Tissue Substitute, Percutaneous Endoscopic Approach
0MU607Z Supplement Left Wrist Bursa and Ligament with Autologous Tissue Substitute, Open Approach
0MU60JZ Supplement Left Wrist Bursa and Ligament with Synthetic Substitute, Open Approach
0MU60KZ Supplement Left Wrist Bursa and Ligament with Nonautologous Tissue Substitute, Open Approach
0MU647Z Supplement Left Wrist Bursa and Ligament with Autologous Tissue Substitute, Percutaneous Endoscopic Approach
0MU64JZ Supplement Left Wrist Bursa and Ligament with Synthetic Substitute, Percutaneous Endoscopic Approach
0MU64KZ Supplement Left Wrist Bursa and Ligament with Nonautologous Tissue Substitute, Percutaneous Endoscopic Approach
0MU707Z Supplement Right Hand Bursa and Ligament with Autologous Tissue Substitute, Open Approach
0MU70JZ Supplement Right Hand Bursa and Ligament with Synthetic Substitute, Open Approach
0MU70KZ Supplement Right Hand Bursa and Ligament with Nonautologous Tissue Substitute, Open Approach
0MU747Z Supplement Right Hand Bursa and Ligament with Autologous Tissue Substitute, Percutaneous Endoscopic Approach
0MU74JZ Supplement Right Hand Bursa and Ligament with Synthetic Substitute, Percutaneous Endoscopic Approach
0MU74KZ Supplement Right Hand Bursa and Ligament with Nonautologous Tissue Substitute, Percutaneous Endoscopic Approach
0MU807Z Supplement Left Hand Bursa and Ligament with Autologous Tissue Substitute, Open Approach
0MU80JZ Supplement Left Hand Bursa and Ligament with Synthetic Substitute, Open Approach
0MU80KZ Supplement Left Hand Bursa and Ligament with Nonautologous Tissue Substitute, Open Approach
0MU847Z Supplement Left Hand Bursa and Ligament with Autologous Tissue Substitute, Percutaneous Endoscopic Approach
0MU84JZ Supplement Left Hand Bursa and Ligament with Synthetic Substitute, Percutaneous Endoscopic Approach
0MU84KZ Supplement Left Hand Bursa and Ligament with Nonautologous Tissue Substitute, Percutaneous Endoscopic Approach
0MU907Z Supplement Right Upper Extremity Bursa and Ligament with Autologous Tissue Substitute, Open Approach
0MU90JZ Supplement Right Upper Extremity Bursa and Ligament with Synthetic Substitute, Open Approach
0MU90KZ Supplement Right Upper Extremity Bursa and Ligament with Nonautologous Tissue Substitute, Open Approach
0MU947Z Supplement Right Upper Extremity Bursa and Ligament with Autologous Tissue Substitute, Percutaneous Endoscopic Approach
0MU94JZ Supplement Right Upper Extremity Bursa and Ligament with Synthetic Substitute, Percutaneous Endoscopic Approach
0MU94KZ Supplement Right Upper Extremity Bursa and Ligament with Nonautologous Tissue Substitute, Percutaneous Endoscopic Approach
0MUB07Z Supplement Left Upper Extremity Bursa and Ligament with Autologous Tissue Substitute, Open Approach
0MUB0JZ Supplement Left Upper Extremity Bursa and Ligament with Synthetic Substitute, Open Approach
0MUB0KZ Supplement Left Upper Extremity Bursa and Ligament with Nonautologous Tissue Substitute, Open Approach
0MUB47Z Supplement Left Upper Extremity Bursa and Ligament with Autologous Tissue Substitute, Percutaneous Endoscopic Approach
0MUB4JZ Supplement Left Upper Extremity Bursa and Ligament with Synthetic Substitute, Percutaneous Endoscopic Approach
0MUB4KZ Supplement Left Upper Extremity Bursa and Ligament with Nonautologous Tissue Substitute, Percutaneous Endoscopic Approach
0MUC07Z Supplement Right Trunk Bursa and Ligament with Autologous Tissue Substitute, Open Approach
0MUC0JZ Supplement Right Trunk Bursa and Ligament with Synthetic Substitute, Open Approach
0MUC0KZ Supplement Right Trunk Bursa and Ligament with Nonautologous Tissue Substitute, Open Approach
0MUC47Z Supplement Right Trunk Bursa and Ligament with Autologous Tissue Substitute, Percutaneous Endoscopic Approach
0MUC4JZ Supplement Right Trunk Bursa and Ligament with Synthetic Substitute, Percutaneous Endoscopic Approach
0MUC4KZ Supplement Right Trunk Bursa and Ligament with Nonautologous Tissue Substitute, Percutaneous Endoscopic Approach
0MUD07Z Supplement Left Trunk Bursa and Ligament with Autologous Tissue Substitute, Open Approach
0MUD0JZ Supplement Left Trunk Bursa and Ligament with Synthetic Substitute, Open Approach
0MUD0KZ Supplement Left Trunk Bursa and Ligament with Nonautologous Tissue Substitute, Open Approach
0MUD47Z Supplement Left Trunk Bursa and Ligament with Autologous Tissue Substitute, Percutaneous Endoscopic Approach
0MUD4JZ Supplement Left Trunk Bursa and Ligament with Synthetic Substitute, Percutaneous Endoscopic Approach
0MUD4KZ Supplement Left Trunk Bursa and Ligament with Nonautologous Tissue Substitute, Percutaneous Endoscopic Approach
0MUF07Z Supplement Right Thorax Bursa and Ligament with Autologous Tissue Substitute, Open Approach
0MUF0JZ Supplement Right Thorax Bursa and Ligament with Synthetic Substitute, Open Approach
0MUF0KZ Supplement Right Thorax Bursa and Ligament with Nonautologous Tissue Substitute, Open Approach
0MUF47Z Supplement Right Thorax Bursa and Ligament with Autologous Tissue Substitute, Percutaneous Endoscopic Approach
0MUF4JZ Supplement Right Thorax Bursa and Ligament with Synthetic Substitute, Percutaneous Endoscopic Approach
0MUF4KZ Supplement Right Thorax Bursa and Ligament with Nonautologous Tissue Substitute, Percutaneous Endoscopic Approach
0MUG07Z Supplement Left Thorax Bursa and Ligament with Autologous Tissue Substitute, Open Approach
0MUG0JZ Supplement Left Thorax Bursa and Ligament with Synthetic Substitute, Open Approach
0MUG0KZ Supplement Left Thorax Bursa and Ligament with Nonautologous Tissue Substitute, Open Approach
0MUG47Z Supplement Left Thorax Bursa and Ligament with Autologous Tissue Substitute, Percutaneous Endoscopic Approach
0MUG4JZ Supplement Left Thorax Bursa and Ligament with Synthetic Substitute, Percutaneous Endoscopic Approach
0MUG4KZ Supplement Left Thorax Bursa and Ligament with Nonautologous Tissue Substitute, Percutaneous Endoscopic Approach
0MUH07Z Supplement Right Abdomen Bursa and Ligament with Autologous Tissue Substitute, Open Approach
0MUH0JZ Supplement Right Abdomen Bursa and Ligament with Synthetic Substitute, Open Approach
0MUH0KZ Supplement Right Abdomen Bursa and Ligament with Nonautologous Tissue Substitute, Open Approach
0MUH47Z Supplement Right Abdomen Bursa and Ligament with Autologous Tissue Substitute, Percutaneous Endoscopic Approach
0MUH4JZ Supplement Right Abdomen Bursa and Ligament with Synthetic Substitute, Percutaneous Endoscopic Approach
0MUH4KZ Supplement Right Abdomen Bursa and Ligament with Nonautologous Tissue Substitute, Percutaneous Endoscopic Approach
0MUJ07Z Supplement Left Abdomen Bursa and Ligament with Autologous Tissue Substitute, Open Approach
0MUJ0JZ Supplement Left Abdomen Bursa and Ligament with Synthetic Substitute, Open Approach
0MUJ0KZ Supplement Left Abdomen Bursa and Ligament with Nonautologous Tissue Substitute, Open Approach
0MUJ47Z Supplement Left Abdomen Bursa and Ligament with Autologous Tissue Substitute, Percutaneous Endoscopic Approach
0MUJ4JZ Supplement Left Abdomen Bursa and Ligament with Synthetic Substitute, Percutaneous Endoscopic Approach
0MUJ4KZ Supplement Left Abdomen Bursa and Ligament with Nonautologous Tissue Substitute, Percutaneous Endoscopic Approach

1UK07Z Supplement Perineum Bursa and Ligament with Autologous Tissue Substitute, Open Approach

1UK0JZ Supplement Perineum Bursa and Ligament with Synthetic Substitute, Open Approach

1UK0KZ Supplement Perineum Bursa and Ligament with Nonautologous Tissue Substitute, Open Approach

MUK47Z Supplement Perineum Bursa and Ligament with Autologous Tissue Substitute, Percutaneous Endoscopic Approach

MUK4JZ Supplement Perineum Bursa and Ligament with Synthetic Substitute, Percutaneous Endoscopic Approach

MUK4KZ Supplement Perineum Bursa and Ligament with Nonautologous Tissue Substitute, Percutaneous Endoscopic Approach

MUL07Z Supplement Right Hip Bursa and Ligament with Autologous Tissue Substitute, Open Approach

MUL0JZ Supplement Right Hip Bursa and Ligament with Synthetic Substitute, Open Approach

MUL0KZ Supplement Right Hip Bursa and Ligament with Nonautologous Tissue Substitute, Open Approach

MUL47Z Supplement Right Hip Bursa and Ligament with Autologous Tissue Substitute, Percutaneous Endoscopic Approach

MUL4JZ Supplement Right Hip Bursa and Ligament with Synthetic Substitute, Percutaneous Endoscopic Approach

MUL4KZ Supplement Right Hip Bursa and Ligament with Nonautologous Tissue Substitute, Percutaneous Endoscopic Approach

MUM07Z Supplement Left Hip Bursa and Ligament with Autologous Tissue Substitute, Open Approach

MUM0JZ Supplement Left Hip Bursa and Ligament with Synthetic Substitute, Open Approach

MUM0KZ Supplement Left Hip Bursa and Ligament with Nonautologous Tissue Substitute, Open Approach

MUM47Z Supplement Left Hip Bursa and Ligament with Autologous Tissue Substitute, Percutaneous Endoscopic Approach

MUM4JZ Supplement Left Hip Bursa and Ligament with Synthetic Substitute, Percutaneous Endoscopic Approach

MUM4KZ Supplement Left Hip Bursa and Ligament with Nonautologous Tissue Substitute, Percutaneous Endoscopic Approach

0MUN07Z Supplement Right Knee Bursa and Ligament with Autologous Tissue Substitute, Open Approach

0MUN0JZ Supplement Right Knee Bursa and Ligament with Synthetic Substitute, Open Approach

0MUN0KZ Supplement Right Knee Bursa and Ligament with Nonautologous Tissue Substitute, Open Approach

0MUN47Z Supplement Right Knee Bursa and Ligament with Autologous Tissue Substitute, Percutaneous Endoscopic Approach

0MUN4JZ Supplement Right Knee Bursa and Ligament with Synthetic Substitute, Percutaneous Endoscopic Approach

0MUN4KZ Supplement Right Knee Bursa and Ligament with Nonautologous Tissue Substitute, Percutaneous Endoscopic Approach

0MUP07Z Supplement Left Knee Bursa and Ligament with Autologous Tissue Substitute, Open Approach

0MUP0JZ Supplement Left Knee Bursa and Ligament with Synthetic Substitute, Open Approach

0MUP0KZ Supplement Left Knee Bursa and Ligament with Nonautologous Tissue Substitute, Open Approach

0MUP47Z Supplement Left Knee Bursa and Ligament with Autologous Tissue Substitute, Percutaneous Endoscopic Approach

0MUP4JZ Supplement Left Knee Bursa and Ligament with Synthetic Substitute, Percutaneous Endoscopic Approach

0MUP4KZ Supplement Left Knee Bursa and Ligament with Nonautologous Tissue Substitute, Percutaneous Endoscopic Approach

0MUQ07Z Supplement Right Ankle Bursa and Ligament with Autologous Tissue Substitute, Open Approach

0MUQ0JZ Supplement Right Ankle Bursa and Ligament with Synthetic Substitute, Open Approach

0MUQ0KZ Supplement Right Ankle Bursa and Ligament with Nonautologous Tissue Substitute, Open Approach

0MUQ47Z Supplement Right Ankle Bursa and Ligament with Autologous Tissue Substitute, Percutaneous Endoscopic Approach

0MUQ4JZ Supplement Right Ankle Bursa and Ligament with Synthetic Substitute, Percutaneous Endoscopic Approach

0MUQ4KZ Supplement Right Ankle Bursa and Ligament with Nonautologous Tissue Substitute, Percutaneous Endoscopic Approach

0MUR07Z Supplement Left Ankle Bursa and Ligament with Autologous Tissue Substitute, Open Approach

0MUR0JZ Supplement Left Ankle Bursa and Ligament with Synthetic Substitute, Open Approach

0MUR0KZ Supplement Left Ankle Bursa and Ligament with Nonautologous Tissue Substitute, Open Approach

0MUR47Z Supplement Left Ankle Bursa and Ligament with Autologous Tissue Substitute, Percutaneous Endoscopic Approach

0MUR4JZ Supplement Left Ankle Bursa and Ligament with Synthetic Substitute, Percutaneous Endoscopic Approach

0MUR4KZ Supplement Left Ankle Bursa and Ligament with Nonautologous Tissue Substitute, Percutaneous Endoscopic Approach

0MUS07Z Supplement Right Foot Bursa and Ligament with Autologous Tissue Substitute, Open Approach

0MUS0JZ Supplement Right Foot Bursa and Ligament with Synthetic Substitute, Open Approach

0MUS0KZ Supplement Right Foot Bursa and Ligament with Nonautologous Tissue Substitute, Open Approach

0MUS47Z Supplement Right Foot Bursa and Ligament with Autologous Tissue Substitute, Percutaneous Endoscopic Approach

0MUS4JZ Supplement Right Foot Bursa and Ligament with Synthetic Substitute, Percutaneous Endoscopic Approach

0MUS4KZ Supplement Right Foot Bursa and Ligament with Nonautologous Tissue Substitute, Percutaneous Endoscopic Approach

0MUT07Z Supplement Left Foot Bursa and Ligament with Autologous Tissue Substitute, Open Approach

0MUT0JZ Supplement Left Foot Bursa and Ligament with Synthetic Substitute, Open Approach

0MUT0KZ Supplement Left Foot Bursa and Ligament with Nonautologous Tissue Substitute, Open Approach

0MUT47Z Supplement Left Foot Bursa and Ligament with Autologous Tissue Substitute, Percutaneous Endoscopic Approach

0MUT4JZ Supplement Left Foot Bursa and Ligament with Synthetic Substitute, Percutaneous Endoscopic Approach

0MUT4KZ Supplement Left Foot Bursa and Ligament with Nonautologous Tissue Substitute, Percutaneous Endoscopic Approach

0MUV07Z Supplement Right Lower Extremity Bursa and Ligament with Autologous Tissue Substitute, Open Approach

0MUV0JZ Supplement Right Lower Extremity Bursa and Ligament with Synthetic Substitute, Open Approach

0MUV0KZ Supplement Right Lower Extremity Bursa and Ligament with Nonautologous Tissue Substitute, Open Approach

0MUV47Z Supplement Right Lower Extremity Bursa and Ligament with Autologous Tissue Substitute, Percutaneous Endoscopic Approach

0MUV4JZ Supplement Right Lower Extremity Bursa and Ligament with Synthetic Substitute, Percutaneous Endoscopic Approach

0MUV4KZ Supplement Right Lower Extremity Bursa and Ligament with Nonautologous Tissue Substitute, Percutaneous Endoscopic Approach

0MUW07Z Supplement Left Lower Extremity Bursa and Ligament with Autologous Tissue Substitute, Open Approach

0MUW0JZ Supplement Left Lower Extremity Bursa and Ligament with Synthetic Substitute, Open Approach

0MUW0KZ Supplement Left Lower Extremity Bursa and Ligament with Nonautologous Tissue Substitute, Open Approach

0MUW47Z Supplement Left Lower Extremity Bursa and Ligament with Autologous Tissue Substitute, Percutaneous Endoscopic Approach

0MUW4JZ Supplement Left Lower Extremity Bursa and Ligament with Synthetic Substitute, Percutaneous Endoscopic Approach

0MUW4KZ Supplement Left Lower Extremity Bursa and Ligament with Nonautologous Tissue Substitute, Percutaneous Endoscopic Approach

0MW – Bursae and Ligaments, Revision

Review Coding Guideline B6.1c

0MWX00Z Revision of Drainage Device in Upper Bursa and Ligament, Open Approach
0MWX07Z Revision of Autologous Tissue Substitute in Upper Bursa and Ligament, Open Approach
0MWX0JZ Revision of Synthetic Substitute in Upper Bursa and Ligament, Open Approach
0MWX0KZ Revision of Nonautologous Tissue Substitute in Upper Bursa and Ligament, Open Approach
0MWX30Z Revision of Drainage Device in Upper Bursa and Ligament, Percutaneous Approach
0MWX37Z Revision of Autologous Tissue Substitute in Upper Bursa and Ligament, Percutaneous Approach
0MWX3JZ Revision of Synthetic Substitute in Upper Bursa and Ligament, Percutaneous Approach
0MWX3KZ Revision of Nonautologous Tissue Substitute in Upper Bursa and Ligament, Percutaneous Approach
0MWX40Z Revision of Drainage Device in Upper Bursa and Ligament, Percutaneous Endoscopic Approach
0MWX47Z Revision of Autologous Tissue Substitute in Upper Bursa and Ligament, Percutaneous Endoscopic Approach
0MWX4JZ Revision of Synthetic Substitute in Upper Bursa and Ligament, Percutaneous Endoscopic Approach
0MWX4KZ Revision of Nonautologous Tissue Substitute in Upper Bursa and Ligament, Percutaneous Endoscopic Approach
0MWXX0Z Revision of Drainage Device in Upper Bursa and Ligament, External Approach
0MWXX7Z Revision of Autologous Tissue Substitute in Upper Bursa and Ligament, External Approach
0MWXXJZ Revision of Synthetic Substitute in Upper Bursa and Ligament, External Approach
0MWXXKZ Revision of Nonautologous Tissue Substitute in Upper Bursa and Ligament, External Approach
0MWY00Z Revision of Drainage Device in Lower Bursa and Ligament, Open Approach
0MWY07Z Revision of Autologous Tissue Substitute in Lower Bursa and Ligament, Open Approach
0MWY0JZ Revision of Synthetic Substitute in Lower Bursa and Ligament, Open Approach
0MWY0KZ Revision of Nonautologous Tissue Substitute in Lower Bursa and Ligament, Open Approach
0MWY30Z Revision of Drainage Device in Lower Bursa and Ligament, Percutaneous Approach
0MWY37Z Revision of Autologous Tissue Substitute in Lower Bursa and Ligament, Percutaneous Approach
0MWY3JZ Revision of Synthetic Substitute in Lower Bursa and Ligament, Percutaneous Approach
0MWY3KZ Revision of Nonautologous Tissue Substitute in Lower Bursa and Ligament, Percutaneous Approach
0MWY40Z Revision of Drainage Device in Lower Bursa and Ligament, Percutaneous Endoscopic Approach
0MWY47Z Revision of Autologous Tissue Substitute in Lower Bursa and Ligament, Percutaneous Endoscopic Approach
0MWY4JZ Revision of Synthetic Substitute in Lower Bursa and Ligament, Percutaneous Endoscopic Approach
0MWY4KZ Revision of Nonautologous Tissue Substitute in Lower Bursa and Ligament, Percutaneous Endoscopic Approach
0MWYX0Z Revision of Drainage Device in Lower Bursa and Ligament, External Approach
0MWYX7Z Revision of Autologous Tissue Substitute in Lower Bursa and Ligament, External Approach
0MWYXJZ Revision of Synthetic Substitute in Lower Bursa and Ligament, External Approach
0MWYXKZ Revision of Nonautologous Tissue Substitute in Lower Bursa and Ligament, External Approach

0MX – Bursae and Ligaments, Transfer

0MX00ZZ Transfer Head and Neck Bursa and Ligament, Open Approach
0MX04ZZ Transfer Head and Neck Bursa and Ligament, Percutaneous Endoscopic Approach
0MX10ZZ Transfer Right Shoulder Bursa and Ligament, Open Approach
0MX14ZZ Transfer Right Shoulder Bursa and Ligament, Percutaneous Endoscopic Approach
0MX20ZZ Transfer Left Shoulder Bursa and Ligament, Open Approach
0MX24ZZ Transfer Left Shoulder Bursa and Ligament, Percutaneous Endoscopic Approach
0MX30ZZ Transfer Right Elbow Bursa and Ligament, Open Approach
0MX34ZZ Transfer Right Elbow Bursa and Ligament, Percutaneous Endoscopic Approach
0MX40ZZ Transfer Left Elbow Bursa and Ligament, Open Approach
0MX44ZZ Transfer Left Elbow Bursa and Ligament, Percutaneous Endoscopic Approach
0MX50ZZ Transfer Right Wrist Bursa and Ligament, Open Approach
0MX54ZZ Transfer Right Wrist Bursa and Ligament, Percutaneous Endoscopic Approach
0MX60ZZ Transfer Left Wrist Bursa and Ligament, Open Approach
0MX64ZZ Transfer Left Wrist Bursa and Ligament, Percutaneous Endoscopic Approach
0MX70ZZ Transfer Right Hand Bursa and Ligament, Open Approach
0MX74ZZ Transfer Right Hand Bursa and Ligament, Percutaneous Endoscopic Approach
0MX80ZZ Transfer Left Hand Bursa and Ligament, Open Approach
0MX84ZZ Transfer Left Hand Bursa and Ligament, Percutaneous Endoscopic Approach
0MX90ZZ Transfer Right Upper Extremity Bursa and Ligament, Open Approach
0MX94ZZ Transfer Right Upper Extremity Bursa and Ligament, Percutaneous Endoscopic Approach
0MXB0ZZ Transfer Left Upper Extremity Bursa and Ligament, Open Approach
0MXB4ZZ Transfer Left Upper Extremity Bursa and Ligament, Percutaneous Endoscopic Approach
0MXC0ZZ Transfer Right Trunk Bursa and Ligament, Open Approach
0MXC4ZZ Transfer Right Trunk Bursa and Ligament, Percutaneous Endoscopic Approach
0MXD0ZZ Transfer Left Trunk Bursa and Ligament, Open Approach
0MXD4ZZ Transfer Left Trunk Bursa and Ligament, Percutaneous Endoscopic Approach
0MXF0ZZ Transfer Right Thorax Bursa and Ligament, Open Approach
0MXF4ZZ Transfer Right Thorax Bursa and Ligament, Percutaneous Endoscopic Approach
0MXG0ZZ Transfer Left Thorax Bursa and Ligament, Open Approach
0MXG4ZZ Transfer Left Thorax Bursa and Ligament, Percutaneous Endoscopic Approach
0MXH0ZZ Transfer Right Abdomen Bursa and Ligament, Open Approach
0MXH4ZZ Transfer Right Abdomen Bursa and Ligament, Percutaneous Endoscopic Approach
0MXJ0ZZ Transfer Left Abdomen Bursa and Ligament, Open Approach
0MXJ4ZZ Transfer Left Abdomen Bursa and Ligament, Percutaneous Endoscopic Approach
0MXK0ZZ Transfer Perineum Bursa and Ligament, Open Approach
0MXK4ZZ Transfer Perineum Bursa and Ligament, Percutaneous Endoscopic Approach
0MXL0ZZ Transfer Right Hip Bursa and Ligament, Open Approach
0MXL4ZZ Transfer Right Hip Bursa and Ligament, Percutaneous Endoscopic Approach
0MXM0ZZ Transfer Left Hip Bursa and Ligament, Open Approach
0MXM4ZZ Transfer Left Hip Bursa and Ligament, Percutaneous Endoscopic Approach
0MXN0ZZ Transfer Right Knee Bursa and Ligament, Open Approach
0MXN4ZZ Transfer Right Knee Bursa and Ligament, Percutaneous Endoscopic Approach
0MXP0ZZ Transfer Left Knee Bursa and Ligament, Open Approach
0MXP4ZZ Transfer Left Knee Bursa and Ligament, Percutaneous Endoscopic Approach
0MXQ0ZZ Transfer Right Ankle Bursa and Ligament, Open Approach
0MXQ4ZZ Transfer Right Ankle Bursa and Ligament, Percutaneous Endoscopic Approach
0MXR0ZZ Transfer Left Ankle Bursa and Ligament, Open Approach
0MXR4ZZ Transfer Left Ankle Bursa and Ligament, Percutaneous Endoscopic Approach

0MXS0ZZ Transfer Right Foot Bursa and Ligament, Open Approach
0MXS4ZZ Transfer Right Foot Bursa and Ligament, Percutaneous Endoscopic Approach
0MXT0ZZ Transfer Left Foot Bursa and Ligament, Open Approach
0MXT4ZZ Transfer Left Foot Bursa and Ligament, Percutaneous Endoscopic Approach
0MXV0ZZ Transfer Right Lower Extremity Bursa and Ligament, Open Approach
0MXV4ZZ Transfer Right Lower Extremity Bursa and Ligament, Percutaneous Endoscopic Approach
0MXW0ZZ Transfer Left Lower Extremity Bursa and Ligament, Open Approach
0MXW4ZZ Transfer Left Lower Extremity Bursa and Ligament, Percutaneous Endoscopic Approach

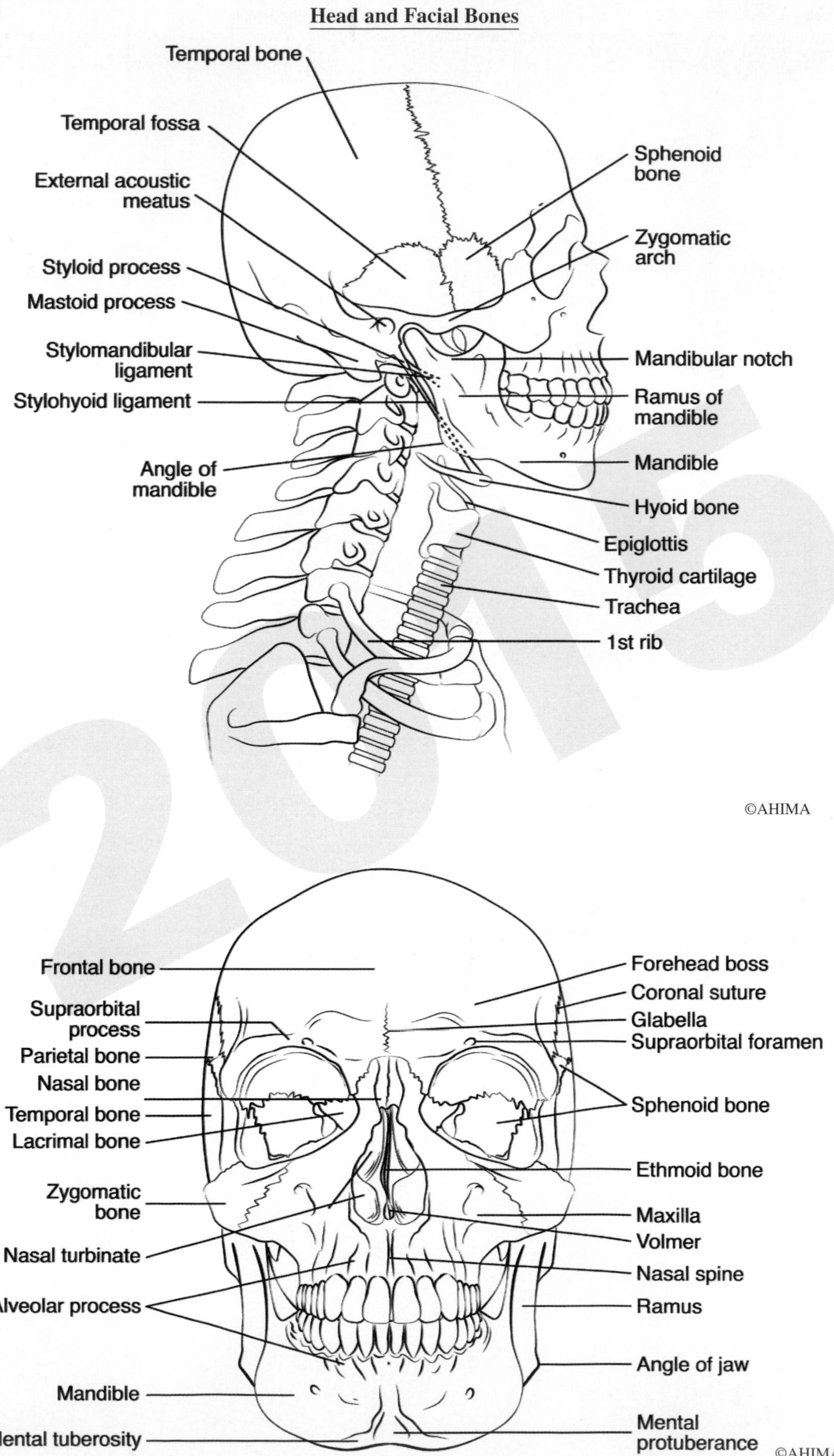
Head and Facial Bones
Temporal bone
Temporal fossa
External acoustic meatus
Styloid process
Mastoid process
Stylomandibular ligament
Stylohyoid ligament
Angle of mandible
Sphenoid bone
Zygomatic arch
Mandibular notch
Ramus of mandible
Mandible
Hyoid bone
Epiglottis
Thyroid cartilage
Trachea
1st rib
©AHIMA
Frontal bone
Supraorbital process
Parietal bone
Nasal bone
Temporal bone
Lacrimal bone
Zygomatic bone
Nasal turbinate
Alveolar process
Mandible
Mental tuberosity
Forehead boss
Coronal suture
Glabella
Supraorbital foramen
Sphenoid bone
Ethmoid bone
Maxilla
Volmer
Nasal spine
Ramus
Angle of jaw
Mental protuberance
©AHIMA

ad and Facial Bones Tables 0N2–0NW

tion 0 **Medical and Surgical**
dy System N **Head and Facial Bones**
eration 2 **Change:** Taking out or off a device from a body part and putting back an identical or similar device in or on the same body part without cutting or puncturing the skin or a mucous membrane

Body Part (4th)	Approach (5th)	Device (6th)	Qualifier (7th)
Skull Nasal Bone Facial Bone	**X** External	**0** Drainage Device **Y** Other Device	**Z** No Qualifier

tion 0 **Medical and Surgical**
dy System N **Head and Facial Bones**
eration 5 **Destruction:** Physical eradication of all or a portion of a body part by the direct use of energy, force, or a destructive agent

Body Part (4th)	Approach (5th)	Device (6th)	Qualifier (7th)
Skull Frontal Bone, Right Frontal Bone, Left Parietal Bone, Right Parietal Bone, Left Temporal Bone, Right Temporal Bone, Left Occipital Bone, Right Occipital Bone, Left Nasal Bone Sphenoid Bone, Right Sphenoid Bone, Left Ethmoid Bone, Right Ethmoid Bone, Left Lacrimal Bone, Right Lacrimal Bone, Left **K** Palatine Bone, Right **L** Palatine Bone, Left **M** Zygomatic Bone, Right **N** Zygomatic Bone, Left **P** Orbit, Right **Q** Orbit, Left **R** Maxilla, Right **S** Maxilla, Left **T** Mandible, Right **V** Mandible, Left **X** Hyoid Bone	**0** Open **3** Percutaneous **4** Percutaneous Endoscopic	**Z** No Device	**Z** No Qualifier

Section 0 **Medical and Surgical**
Body System N **Head and Facial Bones**
Operation 8 **Division:** Cutting into a body part, without draining fluids and/or gases from the body part, in order to separate or transect a body part

Body Part (4th)	Approach (5th)	Device (6th)	Qualifier (7th)
0 Skull **1** Frontal Bone, Right **2** Frontal Bone, Left **3** Parietal Bone, Right **4** Parietal Bone, Left **5** Temporal Bone, Right **6** Temporal Bone, Left **7** Occipital Bone, Right **8** Occipital Bone, Left **B** Nasal Bone **C** Sphenoid Bone, Right **D** Sphenoid Bone, Left **F** Ethmoid Bone, Right **G** Ethmoid Bone, Left **H** Lacrimal Bone, Right **J** Lacrimal Bone, Left **K** Palatine Bone, Right **L** Palatine Bone, Left **M** Zygomatic Bone, Right **N** Zygomatic Bone, Left **P** Orbit, Right **Q** Orbit, Left **R** Maxilla, Right **S** Maxilla, Left **T** Mandible, Right **V** Mandible, Left **X** Hyoid Bone	**0** Open **3** Percutaneous **4** Percutaneous Endoscopic	**Z** No Device	**Z** No Qualifier

Section 0 **Medical and Surgical**
Body System N **Head and Facial Bones**
Operation 9 **Drainage:** Taking or letting out fluids and/or gases from a body part

Body Part (4th)	Approach (5th)	Device (6th)	Qualifier (7th)
0 Skull **1** Frontal Bone, Right **2** Frontal Bone, Left **3** Parietal Bone, Right **4** Parietal Bone, Left **5** Temporal Bone, Right **6** Temporal Bone, Left **7** Occipital Bone, Right **8** Occipital Bone, Left **B** Nasal Bone **C** Sphenoid Bone, Right **D** Sphenoid Bone, Left **F** Ethmoid Bone, Right **G** Ethmoid Bone, Left **H** Lacrimal Bone, Right **J** Lacrimal Bone, Left **K** Palatine Bone, Right **L** Palatine Bone, Left **M** Zygomatic Bone, Right **N** Zygomatic Bone, Left **P** Orbit, Right **Q** Orbit, Left **R** Maxilla, Right **S** Maxilla, Left **T** Mandible, Right **V** Mandible, Left **X** Hyoid Bone	**0** Open **3** Percutaneous **4** Percutaneous Endoscopic	**0** Drainage Device	**Z** No Qualifier

Continued →

tion	0	**Medical and Surgical**
ly System	N	**Head and Facial Bones**
eration	9	**Drainage:** Taking or letting out fluids and/or gases from a body part

Body Part (4th)	Approach (5th)	Device (6th)	Qualifier (7th)
Skull Frontal Bone, Right Frontal Bone, Left Parietal Bone, Right Parietal Bone, Left Temporal Bone, Right Temporal Bone, Left Occipital Bone, Right Occipital Bone, Left Nasal Bone Sphenoid Bone, Right Sphenoid Bone, Left Ethmoid Bone, Right Ethmoid Bone, Left Lacrimal Bone, Right Lacrimal Bone, Left Palatine Bone, Right Palatine Bone, Left Zygomatic Bone, Right Zygomatic Bone, Left P Orbit, Right Orbit, Left R Maxilla, Right Maxilla, Left T Mandible, Right V Mandible, Left X Hyoid Bone	**0** Open **3** Percutaneous **4** Percutaneous Endoscopic	**Z** No Device	**X** Diagnostic **Z** No Qualifier

ction	0	**Medical and Surgical**
dy System	N	**Head and Facial Bones**
peration	B	**Excision:** Cutting out or off, without replacement, a portion of a body part

Body Part (4th)	Approach (5th)	Device (6th)	Qualifier (7th)
0 Skull **1** Frontal Bone, Right **2** Frontal Bone, Left **3** Parietal Bone, Right **4** Parietal Bone, Left **5** Temporal Bone, Right **6** Temporal Bone, Left **7** Occipital Bone, Right **8** Occipital Bone, Left **B** Nasal Bone **C** Sphenoid Bone, Right **D** Sphenoid Bone, Left **F** Ethmoid Bone, Right **G** Ethmoid Bone, Left **H** Lacrimal Bone, Right **J** Lacrimal Bone, Left **K** Palatine Bone, Right **L** Palatine Bone, Left **M** Zygomatic Bone, Right **N** Zygomatic Bone, Left **P** Orbit, Right **Q** Orbit, Left **R** Maxilla, Right **S** Maxilla, Left **T** Mandible, Right **V** Mandible, Left **X** Hyoid Bone	**0** Open **3** Percutaneous **4** Percutaneous Endoscopic	**Z** No Device	**X** Diagnostic **Z** No Qualifier

Section 0 **Medical and Surgical**
Body System N **Head and Facial Bones**
Operation C **Extirpation: Taking or cutting out solid matter from a body part**

Body Part (4th)	Approach (5th)	Device (6th)	Qualifier (7th)
1 Frontal Bone, Right **2** Frontal Bone, Left **3** Parietal Bone, Right **4** Parietal Bone, Left **5** Temporal Bone, Right **6** Temporal Bone, Left **7** Occipital Bone, Right **8** Occipital Bone, Left **B** Nasal Bone **C** Sphenoid Bone, Right **D** Sphenoid Bone, Left **F** Ethmoid Bone, Right **G** Ethmoid Bone, Left **H** Lacrimal Bone, Right **J** Lacrimal Bone, Left **K** Palatine Bone, Right **L** Palatine Bone, Left **M** Zygomatic Bone, Right **N** Zygomatic Bone, Left **P** Orbit, Right **Q** Orbit, Left **R** Maxilla, Right **S** Maxilla, Left **T** Mandible, Right **V** Mandible, Left **X** Hyoid Bone	**0** Open **3** Percutaneous **4** Percutaneous Endoscopic	**Z** No Device	**Z** No Qualifier

Section 0 **Medical and Surgical**
Body System N **Head and Facial Bones**
Operation H **Insertion:** Putting in a nonbiological appliance that monitors, assists, performs, or prevents a physiological function but does not physically take the place of a body part

Body Part (4th)	Approach (5th)	Device (6th)	Qualifier (7th)
0 Skull	**0** Open	**4** Internal Fixation Device **5** External Fixation Device **M** Bone Growth Stimulator **N** Neurostimulator Generator	**Z** No Qualifier
0 Skull	**3** Percutaneous **4** Percutaneous Endoscopic	**4** Internal Fixation Device **5** External Fixation Device **M** Bone Growth Stimulator	**Z** No Qualifier
1 Frontal Bone, Right **2** Frontal Bone, Left **3** Parietal Bone, Right **4** Parietal Bone, Left **7** Occipital Bone, Right **8** Occipital Bone, Left **C** Sphenoid Bone, Right **D** Sphenoid Bone, Left **F** Ethmoid Bone, Right **G** Ethmoid Bone, Left **H** Lacrimal Bone, Right **J** Lacrimal Bone, Left **K** Palatine Bone, Right **L** Palatine Bone, Left **M** Zygomatic Bone, Right **N** Zygomatic Bone, Left **P** Orbit, Right **Q** Orbit, Left **X** Hyoid Bone	**0** Open **3** Percutaneous **4** Percutaneous Endoscopic	**4** Internal Fixation Device	**Z** No Qualifier

Continued →

tion	**0**	**Medical and Surgical**
dy System	**N**	**Head and Facial Bones**
eration	**H**	**Insertion:** Putting in a nonbiological appliance that monitors, assists, performs, or prevents a physiological function but does not physically take the place of a body part

Body Part (4th)	Approach (5th)	Device (6th)	Qualifier (7th)
Temporal Bone, Right Temporal Bone, Left	**0** Open **3** Percutaneous **4** Percutaneous Endoscopic	**4** Internal Fixation Device **S** Hearing Device	**Z** No Qualifier
B Nasal Bone	**0** Open **3** Percutaneous **4** Percutaneous Endoscopic	**4** Internal Fixation Device **M** Bone Growth Stimulator	**Z** No Qualifier
R Maxilla, Right **S** Maxilla, Left **T** Mandible, Right **V** Mandible, Left	**0** Open **3** Percutaneous **4** Percutaneous Endoscopic	**4** Internal Fixation Device **5** External Fixation Device	**Z** No Qualifier
W Facial Bone	**0** Open **3** Percutaneous **4** Percutaneous Endoscopic	**M** Bone Growth Stimulator	**Z** No Qualifier

ction	**0**	**Medical and Surgical**
dy System	**N**	**Head and Facial Bones**
peration	**J**	**Inspection:** Visually and/or manually exploring a body part

Body Part (4th)	Approach (5th)	Device (6th)	Qualifier (7th)
0 Skull **B** Nasal Bone **W** Facial Bone	**0** Open **3** Percutaneous **4** Percutaneous Endoscopic **X** External	**Z** No Device	**Z** No Qualifier

ction	**0**	**Medical and Surgical**
ody System	**N**	**Head and Facial Bones**
peration	**N**	**Release:** Freeing a body part from an abnormal physical constraint by cutting or by the use of force

Body Part (4th)	Approach (5th)	Device (6th)	Qualifier (7th)
1 Frontal Bone, Right **2** Frontal Bone, Left **3** Parietal Bone, Right **4** Parietal Bone, Left **5** Temporal Bone, Right **6** Temporal Bone, Left **7** Occipital Bone, Right **8** Occipital Bone, Left **B** Nasal Bone **C** Sphenoid Bone, Right **D** Sphenoid Bone, Left **F** Ethmoid Bone, Right **G** Ethmoid Bone, Left **H** Lacrimal Bone, Right **J** Lacrimal Bone, Left **K** Palatine Bone, Right **L** Palatine Bone, Left **M** Zygomatic Bone, Right **N** Zygomatic Bone, Left **P** Orbit, Right **Q** Orbit, Left **R** Maxilla, Right **S** Maxilla, Left **T** Mandible, Right **V** Mandible, Left **X** Hyoid Bone	**0** Open **3** Percutaneous **4** Percutaneous Endoscopic	**Z** No Device	**Z** No Qualifier

Section 0 **Medical and Surgical**
Body System N **Head and Facial Bones**
Operation P **Removal:** Taking out or off a device from a body part

Body Part (4th)	Approach (5th)	Device (6th)	Qualifier (7th)
0 Skull	**0** Open	**0** Drainage Device **4** Internal Fixation Device **5** External Fixation Device **7** Autologous Tissue Substitute **J** Synthetic Substitute **K** Nonautologous Tissue Substitute **M** Bone Growth Stimulator **N** Neurostimulator Generator **S** Hearing Device	**Z** No Qualifier
0 Skull	**3** Percutaneous **4** Percutaneous Endoscopic	**0** Drainage Device **4** Internal Fixation Device **5** External Fixation Device **7** Autologous Tissue Substitute **J** Synthetic Substitute **K** Nonautologous Tissue Substitute **M** Bone Growth Stimulator **S** Hearing Device	**Z** No Qualifier
0 Skull	**X** External	**0** Drainage Device **4** Internal Fixation Device **5** External Fixation Device **M** Bone Growth Stimulator **S** Hearing Device	**Z** No Qualifier
B Nasal Bone **W** Facial Bone	**0** Open **3** Percutaneous **4** Percutaneous Endoscopic	**0** Drainage Device **4** Internal Fixation Device **7** Autologous Tissue Substitute **J** Synthetic Substitute **K** Nonautologous Tissue Substitute **M** Bone Growth Stimulator	**Z** No Qualifier
B Nasal Bone **W** Facial Bone	**X** External	**0** Drainage Device **4** Internal Fixation Device **M** Bone Growth Stimulator	**Z** No Qualifier

tion	**0**	**Medical and Surgical**
dy System	**N**	**Head and Facial Bones**
eration	**Q**	**Repair:** Restoring, to the extent possible, a body part to its normal anatomic structure and function

Body Part (4th)	Approach (5th)	Device (6th)	Qualifier (7th)
Skull Frontal Bone, Right Frontal Bone, Left Parietal Bone, Right Parietal Bone, Left 5 Temporal Bone, Right 6 Temporal Bone, Left 7 Occipital Bone, Right 8 Occipital Bone, Left B Nasal Bone C Sphenoid Bone, Right D Sphenoid Bone, Left F Ethmoid Bone, Right G Ethmoid Bone, Left H Lacrimal Bone, Right J Lacrimal Bone, Left K Palatine Bone, Right L Palatine Bone, Left M Zygomatic Bone, Right N Zygomatic Bone, Left P Orbit, Right Q Orbit, Left R Maxilla, Right S Maxilla, Left T Mandible, Right V Mandible, Left X Hyoid Bone	**0** Open **3** Percutaneous **4** Percutaneous Endoscopic **X** External	**Z** No Device	**Z** No Qualifier

ction	**0**	**Medical and Surgical**
dy System	**N**	**Head and Facial Bones**
peration	**R**	**Replacement:** Putting in or on biological or synthetic material that physically takes the place and/or function of all or a portion of a body part

Body Part (4th)	Approach (5th)	Device (6th)	Qualifier (7th)
0 Skull **1** Frontal Bone, Right **2** Frontal Bone, Left **3** Parietal Bone, Right **4** Parietal Bone, Left **5** Temporal Bone, Right **6** Temporal Bone, Left **7** Occipital Bone, Right **8** Occipital Bone, Left **B** Nasal Bone **C** Sphenoid Bone, Right **D** Sphenoid Bone, Left **F** Ethmoid Bone, Right **G** Ethmoid Bone, Left **H** Lacrimal Bone, Right **J** Lacrimal Bone, Left **K** Palatine Bone, Right **L** Palatine Bone, Left **M** Zygomatic Bone, Right **N** Zygomatic Bone, Left **P** Orbit, Right **Q** Orbit, Left **R** Maxilla, Right **S** Maxilla, Left **T** Mandible, Right **V** Mandible, Left **X** Hyoid Bone	**0** Open **3** Percutaneous **4** Percutaneous Endoscopic	**7** Autologous Tissue Substitute **J** Synthetic Substitute **K** Nonautologous Tissue Substitute	**Z** No Qualifier

Section 0 **Medical and Surgical**
Body System N **Head and Facial Bones**
Operation S **Reposition:** Moving to its normal location, or other suitable location, all or a portion of a body part

Body Part (4th)	Approach (5th)	Device (6th)	Qualifier (7th)
0 Skull **R** Maxilla, Right **S** Maxilla, Left **T** Mandible, Right **V** Mandible, Left	**0** Open **3** Percutaneous **4** Percutaneous Endoscopic	**4** Internal Fixation Device **5** External Fixation Device **Z** No Device	**Z** No Qualifier
0 Skull **R** Maxilla, Right **S** Maxilla, Left **T** Mandible, Right **V** Mandible, Left	**X** External	**Z** No Device	**Z** No Qualifier
1 Frontal Bone, Right **2** Frontal Bone, Left **3** Parietal Bone, Right **4** Parietal Bone, Left **5** Temporal Bone, Right **6** Temporal Bone, Left **7** Occipital Bone, Right **8** Occipital Bone, Left **B** Nasal Bone **C** Sphenoid Bone, Right **D** Sphenoid Bone, Left **F** Ethmoid Bone, Right **G** Ethmoid Bone, Left **H** Lacrimal Bone, Right **J** Lacrimal Bone, Left **K** Palatine Bone, Right **L** Palatine Bone, Left **M** Zygomatic Bone, Right **N** Zygomatic Bone, Left **P** Orbit, Right **Q** Orbit, Left **X** Hyoid Bone	**0** Open **3** Percutaneous **4** Percutaneous Endoscopic	**4** Internal Fixation Device **Z** No Device	**Z** No Qualifier
1 Frontal Bone, Right **2** Frontal Bone, Left **3** Parietal Bone, Right **4** Parietal Bone, Left **5** Temporal Bone, Right **6** Temporal Bone, Left **7** Occipital Bone, Right **8** Occipital Bone, Left **B** Nasal Bone **C** Sphenoid Bone, Right **D** Sphenoid Bone, Left **F** Ethmoid Bone, Right **G** Ethmoid Bone, Left **H** Lacrimal Bone, Right **J** Lacrimal Bone, Left **K** Palatine Bone, Right **L** Palatine Bone, Left **M** Zygomatic Bone, Right **N** Zygomatic Bone, Left **P** Orbit, Right **Q** Orbit, Left **X** Hyoid Bone	**X** External	**Z** No Device	**Z** No Qualifier

ction 0 **Medical and Surgical**
dy System N **Head and Facial Bones**
eration T **Resection:** Cutting out or off, without replacement, all of a body part

Body Part (4th)	Approach (5th)	Device (6th)	Qualifier (7th)
Frontal Bone, Right 2 Frontal Bone, Left 3 Parietal Bone, Right 4 Parietal Bone, Left 5 Temporal Bone, Right 6 Temporal Bone, Left 7 Occipital Bone, Right 8 Occipital Bone, Left B Nasal Bone C Sphenoid Bone, Right D Sphenoid Bone, Left F Ethmoid Bone, Right G Ethmoid Bone, Left H Lacrimal Bone, Right J Lacrimal Bone, Left K Palatine Bone, Right L Palatine Bone, Left M Zygomatic Bone, Right N Zygomatic Bone, Left P Orbit, Right Q Orbit, Left R Maxilla, Right S Maxilla, Left T Mandible, Right V Mandible, Left X Hyoid Bone	**0** Open	**Z** No Device	**Z** No Qualifier

ction 0 **Medical and Surgical**
ody System N **Head and Facial Bones**
peration U **Supplement:** Putting in or on biological or synthetic material that physically reinforces and/or augments the function of a portion of a body part

Body Part (4th)	Approach (5th)	Device (6th)	Qualifier (7th)
0 Skull **1** Frontal Bone, Right **2** Frontal Bone, Left **3** Parietal Bone, Right **4** Parietal Bone, Left **5** Temporal Bone, Right **6** Temporal Bone, Left **7** Occipital Bone, Right **8** Occipital Bone, Left **B** Nasal Bone **C** Sphenoid Bone, Right **D** Sphenoid Bone, Left **F** Ethmoid Bone, Right **G** Ethmoid Bone, Left **H** Lacrimal Bone, Right **J** Lacrimal Bone, Left **K** Palatine Bone, Right **L** Palatine Bone, Left **M** Zygomatic Bone, Right **N** Zygomatic Bone, Left **P** Orbit, Right **Q** Orbit, Left **R** Maxilla, Right **S** Maxilla, Left **T** Mandible, Right **V** Mandible, Left **X** Hyoid Bone	**0** Open **3** Percutaneous **4** Percutaneous Endoscopic	**7** Autologous Tissue Substitute **J** Synthetic Substitute **K** Nonautologous Tissue Substitute	**Z** No Qualifier

Section 0 **Medical and Surgical**
Body System N **Head and Facial Bones**
Operation W **Revision:** Correcting, to the extent possible, a portion of a malfunctioning device or the position of a displaced device

Body Part (4th)	Approach (5th)	Device (6th)	Qualifier (7th)
0 Skull	**0** Open	**0** Drainage Device **4** Internal Fixation Device **5** External Fixation Device **7** Autologous Tissue Substitute **J** Synthetic Substitute **K** Nonautologous Tissue Substitute **M** Bone Growth Stimulator **N** Neurostimulator Generator **S** Hearing Device	**Z** No Qualifier
0 Skull	**3** Percutaneous **4** Percutaneous Endoscopic **X** External	**0** Drainage Device **4** Internal Fixation Device **5** External Fixation Device **7** Autologous Tissue Substitute **J** Synthetic Substitute **K** Nonautologous Tissue Substitute **M** Bone Growth Stimulator **S** Hearing Device	**Z** No Qualifier
B Nasal Bone **W** Facial Bone	**0** Open **3** Percutaneous **4** Percutaneous Endoscopic **X** External	**0** Drainage Device **4** Internal Fixation Device **7** Autologous Tissue Substitute **J** Synthetic Substitute **K** Nonautologous Tissue Substitute **M** Bone Growth Stimulator	**Z** No Qualifier

Head and Facial Bones Code Listing 0N2–0NW

0N2 – Head and Facial Bones, Change

Review Coding Guideline B6.1c

0N20X0Z Change Drainage Device in Skull, External Approach
0N20XYZ Change Other Device in Skull, External Approach
0N2BX0Z Change Drainage Device in Nasal Bone, External Approach
0N2BXYZ Change Other Device in Nasal Bone, External Approach
0N2WX0Z Change Drainage Device in Facial Bone External Approach
0N2WXYZ Change Other Device in Facial Bone, External Approach

0N5 – Head and Facial Bones, Destruction

0N500ZZ Destruction of Skull, Open Approach
0N503ZZ Destruction of Skull, Percutaneous Approach
0N504ZZ Destruction of Skull, Percutaneous Endoscopic Approach
0N510ZZ Destruction of Right Frontal Bone, Open Approach
0N513ZZ Destruction of Right Frontal Bone, Percutaneous Approach
0N514ZZ Destruction of Right Frontal Bone, Percutaneous Endoscopic Approach
0N520ZZ Destruction of Left Frontal Bone, Open Approach
0N523ZZ Destruction of Left Frontal Bone, Percutaneous Approach
0N524ZZ Destruction of Left Frontal Bone, Percutaneous Endoscopic Approach
0N530ZZ Destruction of Right Parietal Bone, Open Approach
0N533ZZ Destruction of Right Parietal Bone, Percutaneous Approach
0N534ZZ Destruction of Right Parietal Bone, Percutaneous Endoscopic Approach
0N540ZZ Destruction of Left Parietal Bone, Open Approach
0N543ZZ Destruction of Left Parietal Bone, Percutaneous Approach
0N544ZZ Destruction of Left Parietal Bone, Percutaneous Endoscopic Approach
0N550ZZ Destruction of Right Temporal Bone, Open Approach
0N553ZZ Destruction of Right Temporal Bone, Percutaneous Approach
0N554ZZ Destruction of Right Temporal Bone, Percutaneous Endoscopic Approach
0N560ZZ Destruction of Left Temporal Bone, Open Approach
0N563ZZ Destruction of Left Temporal Bone, Percutaneous Approach
0N564ZZ Destruction of Left Temporal Bone, Percutaneous Endoscopic Approach
0N570ZZ Destruction of Right Occipital Bone, Open Approach
0N573ZZ Destruction of Right Occipital Bone, Percutaneous Approach
0N574ZZ Destruction of Right Occipital Bone, Percutaneous Endoscopic Approach
0N580ZZ Destruction of Left Occipital Bone, Open Approach
0N583ZZ Destruction of Left Occipital Bone, Percutaneous Approach
0N584ZZ Destruction of Left Occipital Bone, Percutaneous Endoscopic Approach
0N5B0ZZ Destruction of Nasal Bone, Open Approach
0N5B3ZZ Destruction of Nasal Bone, Percutaneous Approach
0N5B4ZZ Destruction of Nasal Bone, Percutaneous Endoscopic Approach
0N5C0ZZ Destruction of Right Sphenoid Bone, Open Approach
0N5C3ZZ Destruction of Right Sphenoid Bone, Percutaneous Approach
0N5C4ZZ Destruction of Right Sphenoid Bone, Percutaneous Endoscopic Approach
0N5D0ZZ Destruction of Left Sphenoid Bone, Open Approach
0N5D3ZZ Destruction of Left Sphenoid Bone, Percutaneous Approach
0N5D4ZZ Destruction of Left Sphenoid Bone, Percutaneous Endoscopic Approach
0N5F0ZZ Destruction of Right Ethmoid Bone, Open Approach
0N5F3ZZ Destruction of Right Ethmoid Bone, Percutaneous Approach
0N5F4ZZ Destruction of Right Ethmoid Bone, Percutaneous Endoscopic Approach
0N5G0ZZ Destruction of Left Ethmoid Bone, Open Approach
0N5G3ZZ Destruction of Left Ethmoid Bone, Percutaneous Approach
0N5G4ZZ Destruction of Left Ethmoid Bone, Percutaneous Endoscopic Approach

5H0ZZ Destruction of Right Lacrimal Bone, Open Approach
5H3ZZ Destruction of Right Lacrimal Bone, Percutaneous Approach
5H4ZZ Destruction of Right Lacrimal Bone, Percutaneous Endoscopic Approach
5J0ZZ Destruction of Left Lacrimal Bone, Open Approach
5J3ZZ Destruction of Left Lacrimal Bone, Percutaneous Approach
5J4ZZ Destruction of Left Lacrimal Bone, Percutaneous Endoscopic Approach
5K0ZZ Destruction of Right Palatine Bone, Open Approach
5K3ZZ Destruction of Right Palatine Bone, Percutaneous Approach
5K4ZZ Destruction of Right Palatine Bone, Percutaneous Endoscopic Approach
5L0ZZ Destruction of Left Palatine Bone, Open Approach
5L3ZZ Destruction of Left Palatine Bone, Percutaneous Approach
5L4ZZ Destruction of Left Palatine Bone, Percutaneous Endoscopic Approach
5M0ZZ Destruction of Right Zygomatic Bone, Open Approach
0N5M3ZZ Destruction of Right Zygomatic Bone, Percutaneous Approach
0N5M4ZZ Destruction of Right Zygomatic Bone, Percutaneous Endoscopic Approach
0N5N0ZZ Destruction of Left Zygomatic Bone, Open Approach
0N5N3ZZ Destruction of Left Zygomatic Bone, Percutaneous Approach
0N5N4ZZ Destruction of Left Zygomatic Bone, Percutaneous Endoscopic Approach
0N5P0ZZ Destruction of Right Orbit, Open Approach
0N5P3ZZ Destruction of Right Orbit, Percutaneous Approach
0N5P4ZZ Destruction of Right Orbit, Percutaneous Endoscopic Approach
0N5Q0ZZ Destruction of Left Orbit, Open Approach
0N5Q3ZZ Destruction of Left Orbit, Percutaneous Approach
0N5Q4ZZ Destruction of Left Orbit, Percutaneous Endoscopic Approach
0N5R0ZZ Destruction of Right Maxilla, Open Approach
0N5R3ZZ Destruction of Right Maxilla, Percutaneous Approach
0N5R4ZZ Destruction of Right Maxilla, Percutaneous Endoscopic Approach
0N5S0ZZ Destruction of Left Maxilla, Open Approach
0N5S3ZZ Destruction of Left Maxilla, Percutaneous Approach
0N5S4ZZ Destruction of Left Maxilla, Percutaneous Endoscopic Approach
0N5T0ZZ Destruction of Right Mandible, Open Approach
0N5T3ZZ Destruction of Right Mandible, Percutaneous Approach
0N5T4ZZ Destruction of Right Mandible, Percutaneous Endoscopic Approach
0N5V0ZZ Destruction of Left Mandible, Open Approach
0N5V3ZZ Destruction of Left Mandible, Percutaneous Approach
0N5V4ZZ Destruction of Left Mandible, Percutaneous Endoscopic Approach
0N5X0ZZ Destruction of Hyoid Bone, Open Approach
0N5X3ZZ Destruction of Hyoid Bone, Percutaneous Approach
0N5X4ZZ Destruction of Hyoid Bone, Percutaneous Endoscopic Approach

N8 – Head and Facial Bones, Division

eview Coding Guideline B3.14

N800ZZ Division of Skull, Open Approach
N803ZZ Division of Skull, Percutaneous Approach
N804ZZ Division of Skull, Percutaneous Endoscopic Approach
N810ZZ Division of Right Frontal Bone, Open Approach
N813ZZ Division of Right Frontal Bone, Percutaneous Approach
N814ZZ Division of Right Frontal Bone, Percutaneous Endoscopic Approach
N820ZZ Division of Left Frontal Bone, Open Approach
N823ZZ Division of Left Frontal Bone, Percutaneous Approach
N824ZZ Division of Left Frontal Bone, Percutaneous Endoscopic Approach
N830ZZ Division of Right Parietal Bone, Open Approach
N833ZZ Division of Right Parietal Bone, Percutaneous Approach
N834ZZ Division of Right Parietal Bone, Percutaneous Endoscopic Approach
N840ZZ Division of Left Parietal Bone, Open Approach
N843ZZ Division of Left Parietal Bone, Percutaneous Approach
N844ZZ Division of Left Parietal Bone, Percutaneous Endoscopic Approach
N850ZZ Division of Right Temporal Bone, Open Approach
N853ZZ Division of Right Temporal Bone, Percutaneous Approach
N854ZZ Division of Right Temporal Bone, Percutaneous Endoscopic Approach
N860ZZ Division of Left Temporal Bone, Open Approach
N863ZZ Division of Left Temporal Bone, Percutaneous Approach
N864ZZ Division of Left Temporal Bone, Percutaneous Endoscopic Approach
N870ZZ Division of Right Occipital Bone, Open Approach
N873ZZ Division of Right Occipital Bone, Percutaneous Approach
N874ZZ Division of Right Occipital Bone, Percutaneous Endoscopic Approach
0N880ZZ Division of Left Occipital Bone, Open Approach
0N883ZZ Division of Left Occipital Bone, Percutaneous Approach
0N884ZZ Division of Left Occipital Bone, Percutaneous Endoscopic Approach
0N8B0ZZ Division of Nasal Bone, Open Approach
0N8B3ZZ Division of Nasal Bone, Percutaneous Approach
0N8B4ZZ Division of Nasal Bone, Percutaneous Endoscopic Approach
0N8C0ZZ Division of Right Sphenoid Bone, Open Approach
0N8C3ZZ Division of Right Sphenoid Bone, Percutaneous Approach
0N8C4ZZ Division of Right Sphenoid Bone, Percutaneous Endoscopic Approach
0N8D0ZZ Division of Left Sphenoid Bone, Open Approach
0N8D3ZZ Division of Left Sphenoid Bone, Percutaneous Approach
0N8D4ZZ Division of Left Sphenoid Bone, Percutaneous Endoscopic Approach
0N8F0ZZ Division of Right Ethmoid Bone, Open Approach
0N8F3ZZ Division of Right Ethmoid Bone, Percutaneous Approach
0N8F4ZZ Division of Right Ethmoid Bone, Percutaneous Endoscopic Approach
0N8G0ZZ Division of Left Ethmoid Bone, Open Approach
0N8G3ZZ Division of Left Ethmoid Bone, Percutaneous Approach
0N8G4ZZ Division of Left Ethmoid Bone, Percutaneous Endoscopic Approach
0N8H0ZZ Division of Right Lacrimal Bone, Open Approach
0N8H3ZZ Division of Right Lacrimal Bone, Percutaneous Approach
0N8H4ZZ Division of Right Lacrimal Bone, Percutaneous Endoscopic Approach
0N8J0ZZ Division of Left Lacrimal Bone, Open Approach
0N8J3ZZ Division of Left Lacrimal Bone, Percutaneous Approach
0N8J4ZZ Division of Left Lacrimal Bone, Percutaneous Endoscopic Approach
0N8K0ZZ Division of Right Palatine Bone, Open Approach
0N8K3ZZ Division of Right Palatine Bone, Percutaneous Approach
0N8K4ZZ Division of Right Palatine Bone, Percutaneous Endoscopic Approach
0N8L0ZZ Division of Left Palatine Bone, Open Approach
0N8L3ZZ Division of Left Palatine Bone, Percutaneous Approach
0N8L4ZZ Division of Left Palatine Bone, Percutaneous Endoscopic Approach
0N8M0ZZ Division of Right Zygomatic Bone, Open Approach
0N8M3ZZ Division of Right Zygomatic Bone, Percutaneous Approach
0N8M4ZZ Division of Right Zygomatic Bone, Percutaneous Endoscopic Approach
0N8N0ZZ Division of Left Zygomatic Bone, Open Approach
0N8N3ZZ Division of Left Zygomatic Bone, Percutaneous Approach
0N8N4ZZ Division of Left Zygomatic Bone, Percutaneous Endoscopic Approach
0N8P0ZZ Division of Right Orbit, Open Approach
0N8P3ZZ Division of Right Orbit, Percutaneous Approach
0N8P4ZZ Division of Right Orbit, Percutaneous Endoscopic Approach
0N8Q0ZZ Division of Left Orbit, Open Approach
0N8Q3ZZ Division of Left Orbit, Percutaneous Approach
0N8Q4ZZ Division of Left Orbit, Percutaneous Endoscopic Approach
0N8R0ZZ Division of Right Maxilla, Open Approach
0N8R3ZZ Division of Right Maxilla, Percutaneous Approach
0N8R4ZZ Division of Right Maxilla, Percutaneous Endoscopic Approach
0N8S0ZZ Division of Left Maxilla, Open Approach
0N8S3ZZ Division of Left Maxilla, Percutaneous Approach
0N8S4ZZ Division of Left Maxilla, Percutaneous Endoscopic Approach

0N8T0ZZ Division of Right Mandible, Open Approach
0N8T3ZZ Division of Right Mandible, Percutaneous Approach
0N8T4ZZ Division of Right Mandible, Percutaneous Endoscopic Approach
0N8V0ZZ Division of Left Mandible, Open Approach
0N8V3ZZ Division of Left Mandible, Percutaneous Approach
0N8V4ZZ Division of Left Mandible, Percutaneous Endoscopic Approach
0N8X0ZZ Division of Hyoid Bone, Open Approach
0N8X3ZZ Division of Hyoid Bone, Percutaneous Approach
0N8X4ZZ Division of Hyoid Bone, Percutaneous Endoscopic Approach

0N9 – Head and Facial Bones, Drainage

Review Coding Guidelines B3.4a and B3.4b

Review Coding Guideline B6.2

0N9000Z Drainage of Skull with Drainage Device, Open Approach
0N900ZX Drainage of Skull, Open Approach, Diagnostic
0N900ZZ Drainage of Skull, Open Approach
0N9030Z Drainage of Skull with Drainage Device, Percutaneous Approach
0N903ZX Drainage of Skull, Percutaneous Approach, Diagnostic
0N903ZZ Drainage of Skull, Percutaneous Approach
0N9040Z Drainage of Skull with Drainage Device, Percutaneous Endoscopic Approach
0N904ZX Drainage of Skull, Percutaneous Endoscopic Approach, Diagnostic
0N904ZZ Drainage of Skull, Percutaneous Endoscopic Approach
0N9100Z Drainage of Right Frontal Bone with Drainage Device, Open Approach
0N910ZX Drainage of Right Frontal Bone, Open Approach, Diagnostic
0N910ZZ Drainage of Right Frontal Bone, Open Approach
0N9130Z Drainage of Right Frontal Bone with Drainage Device, Percutaneous Approach
0N913ZX Drainage of Right Frontal Bone, Percutaneous Approach, Diagnostic
0N913ZZ Drainage of Right Frontal Bone, Percutaneous Approach
0N9140Z Drainage of Right Frontal Bone with Drainage Device, Percutaneous Endoscopic Approach
0N914ZX Drainage of Right Frontal Bone, Percutaneous Endoscopic Approach, Diagnostic
0N914ZZ Drainage of Right Frontal Bone, Percutaneous Endoscopic Approach
0N9200Z Drainage of Left Frontal Bone with Drainage Device, Open Approach
0N920ZX Drainage of Left Frontal Bone, Open Approach, Diagnostic
0N920ZZ Drainage of Left Frontal Bone, Open Approach
0N9230Z Drainage of Left Frontal Bone with Drainage Device, Percutaneous Approach
0N923ZX Drainage of Left Frontal Bone, Percutaneous Approach, Diagnostic
0N923ZZ Drainage of Left Frontal Bone, Percutaneous Approach
0N9240Z Drainage of Left Frontal Bone with Drainage Device, Percutaneous Endoscopic Approach
0N924ZX Drainage of Left Frontal Bone, Percutaneous Endoscopic Approach, Diagnostic
0N924ZZ Drainage of Left Frontal Bone, Percutaneous Endoscopic Approach
0N9300Z Drainage of Right Parietal Bone with Drainage Device, Open Approach
0N930ZX Drainage of Right Parietal Bone, Open Approach, Diagnostic
0N930ZZ Drainage of Right Parietal Bone, Open Approach
0N9330Z Drainage of Right Parietal Bone with Drainage Device, Percutaneous Approach
0N933ZX Drainage of Right Parietal Bone, Percutaneous Approach, Diagnostic
0N933ZZ Drainage of Right Parietal Bone, Percutaneous Approach
0N9340Z Drainage of Right Parietal Bone with Drainage Device, Percutaneous Endoscopic Approach
0N934ZX Drainage of Right Parietal Bone, Percutaneous Endoscopic Approach, Diagnostic
0N934ZZ Drainage of Right Parietal Bone, Percutaneous Endoscopic Approach
0N9400Z Drainage of Left Parietal Bone with Drainage Device, Open Approach
0N940ZX Drainage of Left Parietal Bone, Open Approach, Diagnostic
0N940ZZ Drainage of Left Parietal Bone, Open Approach
0N9430Z Drainage of Left Parietal Bone with Drainage Device, Percutaneous Approach
0N943ZX Drainage of Left Parietal Bone, Percutaneous Approach, Diagnostic
0N943ZZ Drainage of Left Parietal Bone, Percutaneous Approach
0N9440Z Drainage of Left Parietal Bone with Drainage Device, Percutaneous Endoscopic Approach
0N944ZX Drainage of Left Parietal Bone, Percutaneous Endoscopic Approach, Diagnostic
0N944ZZ Drainage of Left Parietal Bone, Percutaneous Endoscopic Approach
0N9500Z Drainage of Right Temporal Bone with Drainage Device, Open Approach
0N950ZX Drainage of Right Temporal Bone, Open Approach, Diagnostic
0N950ZZ Drainage of Right Temporal Bone, Open Approach
0N9530Z Drainage of Right Temporal Bone with Drainage Device, Percutaneous Approach
0N953ZX Drainage of Right Temporal Bone, Percutaneous Approach, Diagnostic
0N953ZZ Drainage of Right Temporal Bone, Percutaneous Approach
0N9540Z Drainage of Right Temporal Bone with Drainage Device, Percutaneous Endoscopic Approach
0N954ZX Drainage of Right Temporal Bone, Percutaneous Endoscopic Approach, Diagnostic
0N954ZZ Drainage of Right Temporal Bone, Percutaneous Endoscopic Approach
0N9600Z Drainage of Left Temporal Bone with Drainage Device, Open Approach
0N960ZX Drainage of Left Temporal Bone, Open Approach, Diagnostic
0N960ZZ Drainage of Left Temporal Bone, Open Approach
0N9630Z Drainage of Left Temporal Bone with Drainage Device, Percutaneous Approach
0N963ZX Drainage of Left Temporal Bone, Percutaneous Approach, Diagnostic
0N963ZZ Drainage of Left Temporal Bone, Percutaneous Approach
0N9640Z Drainage of Left Temporal Bone with Drainage Device, Percutaneous Endoscopic Approach
0N964ZX Drainage of Left Temporal Bone, Percutaneous Endoscopic Approach, Diagnostic
0N964ZZ Drainage of Left Temporal Bone, Percutaneous Endoscopic Approach
0N9700Z Drainage of Right Occipital Bone with Drainage Device, Open Approach
0N970ZX Drainage of Right Occipital Bone, Open Approach, Diagnostic
0N970ZZ Drainage of Right Occipital Bone, Open Approach
0N9730Z Drainage of Right Occipital Bone with Drainage Device, Percutaneous Approach
0N973ZX Drainage of Right Occipital Bone, Percutaneous Approach, Diagnostic
0N973ZZ Drainage of Right Occipital Bone, Percutaneous Approach
0N9740Z Drainage of Right Occipital Bone with Drainage Device, Percutaneous Endoscopic Approach
0N974ZX Drainage of Right Occipital Bone, Percutaneous Endoscopic Approach, Diagnostic
0N974ZZ Drainage of Right Occipital Bone, Percutaneous Endoscopic Approach
0N9800Z Drainage of Left Occipital Bone with Drainage Device, Open Approach
0N980ZX Drainage of Left Occipital Bone, Open Approach, Diagnostic
0N980ZZ Drainage of Left Occipital Bone, Open Approach
0N9830Z Drainage of Left Occipital Bone with Drainage Device, Percutaneous Approach
0N983ZX Drainage of Left Occipital Bone, Percutaneous Approach, Diagnostic
0N983ZZ Drainage of Left Occipital Bone, Percutaneous Approach
0N9840Z Drainage of Left Occipital Bone with Drainage Device, Percutaneous Endoscopic Approach
0N984ZX Drainage of Left Occipital Bone, Percutaneous Endoscopic Approach, Diagnostic
0N984ZZ Drainage of Left Occipital Bone, Percutaneous Endoscopic Approach
0N9B00Z Drainage of Nasal Bone with Drainage Device, Open Approach
0N9B0ZX Drainage of Nasal Bone, Open Approach, Diagnostic
0N9B0ZZ Drainage of Nasal Bone, Open Approach
0N9B30Z Drainage of Nasal Bone with Drainage Device, Percutaneous Approach
0N9B3ZX Drainage of Nasal Bone, Percutaneous Approach, Diagnostic
0N9B3ZZ Drainage of Nasal Bone, Percutaneous Approach
0N9B40Z Drainage of Nasal Bone with Drainage Device, Percutaneous Endoscopic Approach

B4ZX Drainage of Nasal Bone, Percutaneous Endoscopic Approach, Diagnostic

B4ZZ Drainage of Nasal Bone, Percutaneous Endoscopic Approach

C00Z Drainage of Right Sphenoid Bone with Drainage Device, Open Approach

C0ZX Drainage of Right Sphenoid Bone, Open Approach, Diagnostic

C0ZZ Drainage of Right Sphenoid Bone, Open Approach

C30Z Drainage of Right Sphenoid Bone with Drainage Device, Percutaneous Approach

C3ZX Drainage of Right Sphenoid Bone, Percutaneous Approach, Diagnostic

9C3ZZ Drainage of Right Sphenoid Bone, Percutaneous Approach

9C40Z Drainage of Right Sphenoid Bone with Drainage Device, Percutaneous Endoscopic Approach

9C4ZX Drainage of Right Sphenoid Bone, Percutaneous Endoscopic Approach, Diagnostic

9C4ZZ Drainage of Right Sphenoid Bone, Percutaneous Endoscopic Approach

9D00Z Drainage of Left Sphenoid Bone with Drainage Device, Open Approach

9D0ZX Drainage of Left Sphenoid Bone, Open Approach, Diagnostic

9D0ZZ Drainage of Left Sphenoid Bone, Open Approach

9D30Z Drainage of Left Sphenoid Bone with Drainage Device, Percutaneous Approach

9D3ZX Drainage of Left Sphenoid Bone, Percutaneous Approach, Diagnostic

9D3ZZ Drainage of Left Sphenoid Bone, Percutaneous Approach

9D40Z Drainage of Left Sphenoid Bone with Drainage Device, Percutaneous Endoscopic Approach

9D4ZX Drainage of Left Sphenoid Bone, Percutaneous Endoscopic Approach, Diagnostic

9D4ZZ Drainage of Left Sphenoid Bone, Percutaneous Endoscopic Approach

N9F00Z Drainage of Right Ethmoid Bone with Drainage Device, Open Approach

N9F0ZX Drainage of Right Ethmoid Bone, Open Approach, Diagnostic

N9F0ZZ Drainage of Right Ethmoid Bone, Open Approach

N9F30Z Drainage of Right Ethmoid Bone with Drainage Device, Percutaneous Approach

N9F3ZX Drainage of Right Ethmoid Bone, Percutaneous Approach, Diagnostic

N9F3ZZ Drainage of Right Ethmoid Bone, Percutaneous Approach

N9F40Z Drainage of Right Ethmoid Bone with Drainage Device, Percutaneous Endoscopic Approach

N9F4ZX Drainage of Right Ethmoid Bone, Percutaneous Endoscopic Approach, Diagnostic

N9F4ZZ Drainage of Right Ethmoid Bone, Percutaneous Endoscopic Approach

N9G00Z Drainage of Left Ethmoid Bone with Drainage Device, Open Approach

N9G0ZX Drainage of Left Ethmoid Bone, Open Approach, Diagnostic

N9G0ZZ Drainage of Left Ethmoid Bone, Open Approach

N9G30Z Drainage of Left Ethmoid Bone with Drainage Device, Percutaneous Approach

N9G3ZX Drainage of Left Ethmoid Bone, Percutaneous Approach, Diagnostic

N9G3ZZ Drainage of Left Ethmoid Bone, Percutaneous Approach

0N9G40Z Drainage of Left Ethmoid Bone with Drainage Device, Percutaneous Endoscopic Approach

0N9G4ZX Drainage of Left Ethmoid Bone, Percutaneous Endoscopic Approach, Diagnostic

0N9G4ZZ Drainage of Left Ethmoid Bone, Percutaneous Endoscopic Approach

0N9H00Z Drainage of Right Lacrimal Bone with Drainage Device, Open Approach

0N9H0ZX Drainage of Right Lacrimal Bone, Open Approach, Diagnostic

0N9H0ZZ Drainage of Right Lacrimal Bone, Open Approach

0N9H30Z Drainage of Right Lacrimal Bone with Drainage Device, Percutaneous Approach

0N9H3ZX Drainage of Right Lacrimal Bone, Percutaneous Approach, Diagnostic

0N9H3ZZ Drainage of Right Lacrimal Bone, Percutaneous Approach

0N9H40Z Drainage of Right Lacrimal Bone with Drainage Device, Percutaneous Endoscopic Approach

0N9H4ZX Drainage of Right Lacrimal Bone, Percutaneous Endoscopic Approach, Diagnostic

0N9H4ZZ Drainage of Right Lacrimal Bone, Percutaneous Endoscopic Approach

0N9J00Z Drainage of Left Lacrimal Bone with Drainage Device, Open Approach

0N9J0ZX Drainage of Left Lacrimal Bone, Open Approach, Diagnostic

0N9J0ZZ Drainage of Left Lacrimal Bone, Open Approach

0N9J30Z Drainage of Left Lacrimal Bone with Drainage Device, Percutaneous Approach

0N9J3ZX Drainage of Left Lacrimal Bone, Percutaneous Approach, Diagnostic

0N9J3ZZ Drainage of Left Lacrimal Bone, Percutaneous Approach

0N9J40Z Drainage of Left Lacrimal Bone with Drainage Device, Percutaneous Endoscopic Approach

0N9J4ZX Drainage of Left Lacrimal Bone, Percutaneous Endoscopic Approach, Diagnostic

0N9J4ZZ Drainage of Left Lacrimal Bone, Percutaneous Endoscopic Approach

0N9K00Z Drainage of Right Palatine Bone with Drainage Device, Open Approach

0N9K0ZX Drainage of Right Palatine Bone, Open Approach, Diagnostic

0N9K0ZZ Drainage of Right Palatine Bone, Open Approach

0N9K30Z Drainage of Right Palatine Bone with Drainage Device, Percutaneous Approach

0N9K3ZX Drainage of Right Palatine Bone, Percutaneous Approach, Diagnostic

0N9K3ZZ Drainage of Right Palatine Bone, Percutaneous Approach

0N9K40Z Drainage of Right Palatine Bone with Drainage Device, Percutaneous Endoscopic Approach

0N9K4ZX Drainage of Right Palatine Bone, Percutaneous Endoscopic Approach, Diagnostic

0N9K4ZZ Drainage of Right Palatine Bone, Percutaneous Endoscopic Approach

0N9L00Z Drainage of Left Palatine Bone with Drainage Device, Open Approach

0N9L0ZX Drainage of Left Palatine Bone, Open Approach, Diagnostic

0N9L0ZZ Drainage of Left Palatine Bone, Open Approach

0N9L30Z Drainage of Left Palatine Bone with Drainage Device, Percutaneous Approach

0N9L3ZX Drainage of Left Palatine Bone, Percutaneous Approach, Diagnostic

0N9L3ZZ Drainage of Left Palatine Bone, Percutaneous Approach

0N9L40Z Drainage of Left Palatine Bone with Drainage Device, Percutaneous Endoscopic Approach

0N9L4ZX Drainage of Left Palatine Bone, Percutaneous Endoscopic Approach, Diagnostic

0N9L4ZZ Drainage of Left Palatine Bone, Percutaneous Endoscopic Approach

0N9M00Z Drainage of Right Zygomatic Bone with Drainage Device, Open Approach

0N9M0ZX Drainage of Right Zygomatic Bone, Open Approach, Diagnostic

0N9M0ZZ Drainage of Right Zygomatic Bone, Open Approach

0N9M30Z Drainage of Right Zygomatic Bone with Drainage Device, Percutaneous Approach

0N9M3ZX Drainage of Right Zygomatic Bone, Percutaneous Approach, Diagnostic

0N9M3ZZ Drainage of Right Zygomatic Bone, Percutaneous Approach

0N9M40Z Drainage of Right Zygomatic Bone with Drainage Device, Percutaneous Endoscopic Approach

0N9M4ZX Drainage of Right Zygomatic Bone, Percutaneous Endoscopic Approach, Diagnostic

0N9M4ZZ Drainage of Right Zygomatic Bone, Percutaneous Endoscopic Approach

0N9N00Z Drainage of Left Zygomatic Bone with Drainage Device, Open Approach

0N9N0ZX Drainage of Left Zygomatic Bone, Open Approach, Diagnostic

0N9N0ZZ Drainage of Left Zygomatic Bone, Open Approach

0N9N30Z Drainage of Left Zygomatic Bone with Drainage Device, Percutaneous Approach

0N9N3ZX Drainage of Left Zygomatic Bone, Percutaneous Approach, Diagnostic

0N9N3ZZ Drainage of Left Zygomatic Bone, Percutaneous Approach

0N9N40Z Drainage of Left Zygomatic Bone with Drainage Device, Percutaneous Endoscopic Approach

0N9N4ZX Drainage of Left Zygomatic Bone, Percutaneous Endoscopic Approach, Diagnostic

0N9N4ZZ Drainage of Left Zygomatic Bone, Percutaneous Endoscopic Approach

0N9P00Z Drainage of Right Orbit with Drainage Device, Open Approach

0N9P0ZX Drainage of Right Orbit, Open Approach, Diagnostic

0N9P0ZZ Drainage of Right Orbit, Open Approach

0N9P30Z Drainage of Right Orbit with Drainage Device, Percutaneous Approach

0N9P3ZX Drainage of Right Orbit, Percutaneous Approach, Diagnostic

0N9P3ZZ Drainage of Right Orbit, Percutaneous Approach

0N9P40Z Drainage of Right Orbit with Drainage Device, Percutaneous Endoscopic Approach

0N9P4ZX Drainage of Right Orbit, Percutaneous Endoscopic Approach, Diagnostic

0N9P4ZZ Drainage of Right Orbit, Percutaneous Endoscopic Approach

0N9Q00Z Drainage of Left Orbit with Drainage Device, Open Approach

0N9Q0ZX Drainage of Left Orbit, Open Approach, Diagnostic

0N9Q0ZZ Drainage of Left Orbit, Open Approach

0N9Q30Z Drainage of Left Orbit with Drainage Device, Percutaneous Approach

0N9Q3ZX Drainage of Left Orbit, Percutaneous Approach, Diagnostic
0N9Q3ZZ Drainage of Left Orbit, Percutaneous Approach
0N9Q40Z Drainage of Left Orbit with Drainage Device, Percutaneous Endoscopic Approach
0N9Q4ZX Drainage of Left Orbit, Percutaneous Endoscopic Approach, Diagnostic
0N9Q4ZZ Drainage of Left Orbit, Percutaneous Endoscopic Approach
0N9R00Z Drainage of Right Maxilla with Drainage Device, Open Approach
0N9R0ZX Drainage of Right Maxilla, Open Approach, Diagnostic
0N9R0ZZ Drainage of Right Maxilla, Open Approach
0N9R30Z Drainage of Right Maxilla with Drainage Device, Percutaneous Approach
0N9R3ZX Drainage of Right Maxilla, Percutaneous Approach, Diagnostic
0N9R3ZZ Drainage of Right Maxilla, Percutaneous Approach
0N9R40Z Drainage of Right Maxilla with Drainage Device, Percutaneous Endoscopic Approach
0N9R4ZX Drainage of Right Maxilla, Percutaneous Endoscopic Approach, Diagnostic
0N9R4ZZ Drainage of Right Maxilla, Percutaneous Endoscopic Approach
0N9S00Z Drainage of Left Maxilla with Drainage Device, Open Approach
0N9S0ZX Drainage of Left Maxilla, Open Approach, Diagnostic
0N9S0ZZ Drainage of Left Maxilla, Open Approach
0N9S30Z Drainage of Left Maxilla with Drainage Device, Percutaneous Approach
0N9S3ZX Drainage of Left Maxilla, Percutaneous Approach, Diagnostic
0N9S3ZZ Drainage of Left Maxilla, Percutaneous Approach
0N9S40Z Drainage of Left Maxilla with Drainage Device, Percutaneous Endoscopic Approach
0N9S4ZX Drainage of Left Maxilla, Percutaneous Endoscopic Approach, Diagnostic
0N9S4ZZ Drainage of Left Maxilla, Percutaneous Endoscopic Approach
0N9T00Z Drainage of Right Mandible with Drainage Device, Open Approach
0N9T0ZX Drainage of Right Mandible, Open Approach, Diagnostic
0N9T0ZZ Drainage of Right Mandible, Open Approach
0N9T30Z Drainage of Right Mandible with Drainage Device, Percutaneous Approach
0N9T3ZX Drainage of Right Mandible, Percutaneous Approach, Diagnostic
0N9T3ZZ Drainage of Right Mandible, Percutaneous Approach
0N9T40Z Drainage of Right Mandible with Drainage Device, Percutaneous Endoscopic Approach
0N9T4ZX Drainage of Right Mandible, Percutaneous Endoscopic Approach, Diagnostic
0N9T4ZZ Drainage of Right Mandible, Percutaneous Endoscopic Approach
0N9V00Z Drainage of Left Mandible with Drainage Device, Open Approach
0N9V0ZX Drainage of Left Mandible, Open Approach, Diagnostic
0N9V0ZZ Drainage of Left Mandible, Open Approach
0N9V30Z Drainage of Left Mandible with Draina Device, Percutaneous Approach
0N9V3ZX Drainage of Left Mandible, Percutaneo Approach, Diagnostic
0N9V3ZZ Drainage of Left Mandible, Percutaneo Approach
0N9V40Z Drainage of Left Mandible with Draina Device, Percutaneous Endoscopic Approach
0N9V4ZX Drainage of Left Mandible, Percutaneo Endoscopic Approach, Diagnostic
0N9V4ZZ Drainage of Left Mandible, Percutaneou Endoscopic Approach
0N9X00Z Drainage of Hyoid Bone with Drainage Device, Open Approach
0N9X0ZX Drainage of Hyoid Bone, Open Approac Diagnostic
0N9X0ZZ Drainage of Hyoid Bone, Open Approac
0N9X30Z Drainage of Hyoid Bone with Drainage Device, Percutaneous Approach
0N9X3ZX Drainage of Hyoid Bone, Percutaneous Approach, Diagnostic
0N9X3ZZ Drainage of Hyoid Bone, Percutaneous Approach
0N9X40Z Drainage of Hyoid Bone with Drainage Device, Percutaneous Endoscopic Approach
0N9X4ZX Drainage of Hyoid Bone, Percutaneous Endoscopic Approach, Diagnostic
0N9X4ZZ Drainage of Hyoid Bone, Percutaneous Endoscopic Approach

0NB – Head and Facial Bones, Excision

Review Coding Guidelines B3.4a and B3.4b

Review Coding Guideline B3.5

Review Coding Guideline B3.8

0NB00ZX Excision of Skull, Open Approach, Diagnostic
0NB00ZZ Excision of Skull, Open Approach
0NB03ZX Excision of Skull, Percutaneous Approach, Diagnostic
0NB03ZZ Excision of Skull, Percutaneous Approach
0NB04ZX Excision of Skull, Percutaneous Endoscopic Approach, Diagnostic
0NB04ZZ Excision of Skull, Percutaneous Endoscopic Approach
0NB10ZX Excision of Right Frontal Bone, Open Approach, Diagnostic
0NB10ZZ Excision of Right Frontal Bone, Open Approach
0NB13ZX Excision of Right Frontal Bone, Percutaneous Approach, Diagnostic
0NB13ZZ Excision of Right Frontal Bone, Percutaneous Approach
0NB14ZX Excision of Right Frontal Bone, Percutaneous Endoscopic Approach, Diagnostic
0NB14ZZ Excision of Right Frontal Bone, Percutaneous Endoscopic Approach
0NB20ZX Excision of Left Frontal Bone, Open Approach, Diagnostic
0NB20ZZ Excision of Left Frontal Bone, Open Approach
0NB23ZX Excision of Left Frontal Bone, Percutaneous Approach, Diagnostic
0NB23ZZ Excision of Left Frontal Bone, Percutaneous Approach
0NB24ZX Excision of Left Frontal Bone, Percutaneous Endoscopic Approach, Diagnostic
0NB24ZZ Excision of Left Frontal Bone, Percutaneous Endoscopic Approach
0NB30ZX Excision of Right Parietal Bone, Open Approach, Diagnostic
0NB30ZZ Excision of Right Parietal Bone, Open Approach
0NB33ZX Excision of Right Parietal Bone, Percutaneous Approach, Diagnostic
0NB33ZZ Excision of Right Parietal Bone, Percutaneous Approach
0NB34ZX Excision of Right Parietal Bone, Percutaneous Endoscopic Approach, Diagnostic
0NB34ZZ Excision of Right Parietal Bone, Percutaneous Endoscopic Approach
0NB40ZX Excision of Left Parietal Bone, Open Approach, Diagnostic
0NB40ZZ Excision of Left Parietal Bone, Open Approach
0NB43ZX Excision of Left Parietal Bone, Percutaneous Approach, Diagnostic
0NB43ZZ Excision of Left Parietal Bone, Percutaneous Approach
0NB44ZX Excision of Left Parietal Bone, Percutaneous Endoscopic Approach, Diagnostic
0NB44ZZ Excision of Left Parietal Bone, Percutaneous Endoscopic Approach
0NB50ZX Excision of Right Temporal Bone, Open Approach, Diagnostic
0NB50ZZ Excision of Right Temporal Bone, Open Approach
0NB53ZX Excision of Right Temporal Bone, Percutaneous Approach, Diagnostic
0NB53ZZ Excision of Right Temporal Bone, Percutaneous Approach
0NB54ZX Excision of Right Temporal Bone, Percutaneous Endoscopic Approach, Diagnostic
0NB54ZZ Excision of Right Temporal Bone, Percutaneous Endoscopic Approach
0NB60ZX Excision of Left Temporal Bone, Open Approach, Diagnostic
0NB60ZZ Excision of Left Temporal Bone, Open Approach
0NB63ZX Excision of Left Temporal Bone, Percutaneous Approach, Diagnostic
0NB63ZZ Excision of Left Temporal Bone, Percutaneous Approach
0NB64ZX Excision of Left Temporal Bone, Percutaneous Endoscopic Approach, Diagnostic
0NB64ZZ Excision of Left Temporal Bone, Percutaneous Endoscopic Approach
0NB70ZX Excision of Right Occipital Bone, Open Approach, Diagnostic
0NB70ZZ Excision of Right Occipital Bone, Open Approach
0NB73ZX Excision of Right Occipital Bone, Percutaneous Approach, Diagnostic
0NB73ZZ Excision of Right Occipital Bone, Percutaneous Approach
0NB74ZX Excision of Right Occipital Bone, Percutaneous Endoscopic Approach, Diagnostic
0NB74ZZ Excision of Right Occipital Bone, Percutaneous Endoscopic Approach

B80ZX Excision of Left Occipital Bone, Open Approach, Diagnostic
B80ZZ Excision of Left Occipital Bone, Open Approach
B83ZX Excision of Left Occipital Bone, Percutaneous Approach, Diagnostic
B83ZZ Excision of Left Occipital Bone, Percutaneous Approach
B84ZX Excision of Left Occipital Bone, Percutaneous Endoscopic Approach, Diagnostic
B84ZZ Excision of Left Occipital Bone, Percutaneous Endoscopic Approach
BB0ZX Excision of Nasal Bone, Open Approach, Diagnostic
BB0ZZ Excision of Nasal Bone, Open Approach
BB3ZX Excision of Nasal Bone, Percutaneous Approach, Diagnostic
BB3ZZ Excision of Nasal Bone, Percutaneous Approach
BB4ZX Excision of Nasal Bone, Percutaneous Endoscopic Approach, Diagnostic
BB4ZZ Excision of Nasal Bone, Percutaneous Endoscopic Approach
BC0ZX Excision of Right Sphenoid Bone, Open Approach, Diagnostic
BC0ZZ Excision of Right Sphenoid Bone, Open Approach
BC3ZX Excision of Right Sphenoid Bone, Percutaneous Approach, Diagnostic
BC3ZZ Excision of Right Sphenoid Bone, Percutaneous Approach
BC4ZX Excision of Right Sphenoid Bone, Percutaneous Endoscopic Approach, Diagnostic
BC4ZZ Excision of Right Sphenoid Bone, Percutaneous Endoscopic Approach
BD0ZX Excision of Left Sphenoid Bone, Open Approach, Diagnostic
BD0ZZ Excision of Left Sphenoid Bone, Open Approach
BD3ZX Excision of Left Sphenoid Bone, Percutaneous Approach, Diagnostic
BD3ZZ Excision of Left Sphenoid Bone, Percutaneous Approach
BD4ZX Excision of Left Sphenoid Bone, Percutaneous Endoscopic Approach, Diagnostic
BD4ZZ Excision of Left Sphenoid Bone, Percutaneous Endoscopic Approach
NBF0ZX Excision of Right Ethmoid Bone, Open Approach, Diagnostic
NBF0ZZ Excision of Right Ethmoid Bone, Open Approach
NBF3ZX Excision of Right Ethmoid Bone, Percutaneous Approach, Diagnostic
NBF3ZZ Excision of Right Ethmoid Bone, Percutaneous Approach
NBF4ZX Excision of Right Ethmoid Bone, Percutaneous Endoscopic Approach, Diagnostic
NBF4ZZ Excision of Right Ethmoid Bone, Percutaneous Endoscopic Approach
NBG0ZX Excision of Left Ethmoid Bone, Open Approach, Diagnostic
NBG0ZZ Excision of Left Ethmoid Bone, Open Approach
NBG3ZX Excision of Left Ethmoid Bone, Percutaneous Approach, Diagnostic
NBG3ZZ Excision of Left Ethmoid Bone, Percutaneous Approach
NBG4ZX Excision of Left Ethmoid Bone, Percutaneous Endoscopic Approach, Diagnostic
NBG4ZZ Excision of Left Ethmoid Bone, Percutaneous Endoscopic Approach
NBH0ZX Excision of Right Lacrimal Bone, Open Approach, Diagnostic
0NBH0ZZ Excision of Right Lacrimal Bone, Open Approach
0NBH3ZX Excision of Right Lacrimal Bone, Percutaneous Approach, Diagnostic
0NBH3ZZ Excision of Right Lacrimal Bone, Percutaneous Approach
0NBH4ZX Excision of Right Lacrimal Bone, Percutaneous Endoscopic Approach, Diagnostic
0NBH4ZZ Excision of Right Lacrimal Bone, Percutaneous Endoscopic Approach
0NBJ0ZX Excision of Left Lacrimal Bone, Open Approach, Diagnostic
0NBJ0ZZ Excision of Left Lacrimal Bone, Open Approach
0NBJ3ZX Excision of Left Lacrimal Bone, Percutaneous Approach, Diagnostic
0NBJ3ZZ Excision of Left Lacrimal Bone, Percutaneous Approach
0NBJ4ZX Excision of Left Lacrimal Bone, Percutaneous Endoscopic Approach, Diagnostic
0NBJ4ZZ Excision of Left Lacrimal Bone, Percutaneous Endoscopic Approach
0NBK0ZX Excision of Right Palatine Bone, Open Approach, Diagnostic
0NBK0ZZ Excision of Right Palatine Bone, Open Approach
0NBK3ZX Excision of Right Palatine Bone, Percutaneous Approach, Diagnostic
0NBK3ZZ Excision of Right Palatine Bone, Percutaneous Approach
0NBK4ZX Excision of Right Palatine Bone, Percutaneous Endoscopic Approach, Diagnostic
0NBK4ZZ Excision of Right Palatine Bone, Percutaneous Endoscopic Approach
0NBL0ZX Excision of Left Palatine Bone, Open Approach, Diagnostic
0NBL0ZZ Excision of Left Palatine Bone, Open Approach
0NBL3ZX Excision of Left Palatine Bone, Percutaneous Approach, Diagnostic
0NBL3ZZ Excision of Left Palatine Bone, Percutaneous Approach
0NBL4ZX Excision of Left Palatine Bone, Percutaneous Endoscopic Approach, Diagnostic
0NBL4ZZ Excision of Left Palatine Bone, Percutaneous Endoscopic Approach
0NBM0ZX Excision of Right Zygomatic Bone, Open Approach, Diagnostic
0NBM0ZZ Excision of Right Zygomatic Bone, Open Approach
0NBM3ZX Excision of Right Zygomatic Bone, Percutaneous Approach, Diagnostic
0NBM3ZZ Excision of Right Zygomatic Bone, Percutaneous Approach
0NBM4ZX Excision of Right Zygomatic Bone, Percutaneous Endoscopic Approach, Diagnostic
0NBM4ZZ Excision of Right Zygomatic Bone, Percutaneous Endoscopic Approach
0NBN0ZX Excision of Left Zygomatic Bone, Open Approach, Diagnostic
0NBN0ZZ Excision of Left Zygomatic Bone, Open Approach
0NBN3ZX Excision of Left Zygomatic Bone, Percutaneous Approach, Diagnostic
0NBN3ZZ Excision of Left Zygomatic Bone, Percutaneous Approach
0NBN4ZX Excision of Left Zygomatic Bone, Percutaneous Endoscopic Approach, Diagnostic
0NBN4ZZ Excision of Left Zygomatic Bone, Percutaneous Endoscopic Approach
0NBP0ZX Excision of Right Orbit, Open Approach, Diagnostic
0NBP0ZZ Excision of Right Orbit, Open Approach
0NBP3ZX Excision of Right Orbit, Percutaneous Approach, Diagnostic
0NBP3ZZ Excision of Right Orbit, Percutaneous Approach
0NBP4ZX Excision of Right Orbit, Percutaneous Endoscopic Approach, Diagnostic
0NBP4ZZ Excision of Right Orbit, Percutaneous Endoscopic Approach
0NBQ0ZX Excision of Left Orbit, Open Approach, Diagnostic
0NBQ0ZZ Excision of Left Orbit, Open Approach
0NBQ3ZX Excision of Left Orbit, Percutaneous Approach, Diagnostic
0NBQ3ZZ Excision of Left Orbit, Percutaneous Approach
0NBQ4ZX Excision of Left Orbit, Percutaneous Endoscopic Approach, Diagnostic
0NBQ4ZZ Excision of Left Orbit, Percutaneous Endoscopic Approach
0NBR0ZX Excision of Right Maxilla, Open Approach, Diagnostic
0NBR0ZZ Excision of Right Maxilla, Open Approach
0NBR3ZX Excision of Right Maxilla, Percutaneous Approach, Diagnostic
0NBR3ZZ Excision of Right Maxilla, Percutaneous Approach
0NBR4ZX Excision of Right Maxilla, Percutaneous Endoscopic Approach, Diagnostic
0NBR4ZZ Excision of Right Maxilla, Percutaneous Endoscopic Approach
0NBS0ZX Excision of Left Maxilla, Open Approach, Diagnostic
0NBS0ZZ Excision of Left Maxilla, Open Approach
0NBS3ZX Excision of Left Maxilla, Percutaneous Approach, Diagnostic
0NBS3ZZ Excision of Left Maxilla, Percutaneous Approach
0NBS4ZX Excision of Left Maxilla, Percutaneous Endoscopic Approach, Diagnostic
0NBS4ZZ Excision of Left Maxilla, Percutaneous Endoscopic Approach
0NBT0ZX Excision of Right Mandible, Open Approach, Diagnostic
0NBT0ZZ Excision of Right Mandible, Open Approach
0NBT3ZX Excision of Right Mandible, Percutaneous Approach, Diagnostic
0NBT3ZZ Excision of Right Mandible, Percutaneous Approach
0NBT4ZX Excision of Right Mandible, Percutaneous Endoscopic Approach, Diagnostic
0NBT4ZZ Excision of Right Mandible, Percutaneous Endoscopic Approach
0NBV0ZX Excision of Left Mandible, Open Approach, Diagnostic
0NBV0ZZ Excision of Left Mandible, Open Approach
0NBV3ZX Excision of Left Mandible, Percutaneous Approach, Diagnostic
0NBV3ZZ Excision of Left Mandible, Percutaneous Approach
0NBV4ZX Excision of Left Mandible, Percutaneous Endoscopic Approach, Diagnostic
0NBV4ZZ Excision of Left Mandible, Percutaneous Endoscopic Approach
0NBX0ZX Excision of Hyoid Bone, Open Approach, Diagnostic
0NBX0ZZ Excision of Hyoid Bone, Open Approach
0NBX3ZX Excision of Hyoid Bone, Percutaneous Approach, Diagnostic
0NBX3ZZ Excision of Hyoid Bone, Percutaneous Approach
0NBX4ZX Excision of Hyoid Bone, Percutaneous Endoscopic Approach, Diagnostic
0NBX4ZZ Excision of Hyoid Bone, Percutaneous Endoscopic Approach

0NC – Head and Facial Bones, Extirpation

0NC10ZZ Extirpation of Matter from Right Frontal Bone, Open Approach
0NC13ZZ Extirpation of Matter from Right Frontal Bone, Percutaneous Approach
0NC14ZZ Extirpation of Matter from Right Frontal Bone, Percutaneous Endoscopic Approach
0NC20ZZ Extirpation of Matter from Left Frontal Bone, Open Approach
0NC23ZZ Extirpation of Matter from Left Frontal Bone, Percutaneous Approach
0NC24ZZ Extirpation of Matter from Left Frontal Bone, Percutaneous Endoscopic Approach
0NC30ZZ Extirpation of Matter from Right Parietal Bone, Open Approach
0NC33ZZ Extirpation of Matter from Right Parietal Bone, Percutaneous Approach
0NC34ZZ Extirpation of Matter from Right Parietal Bone, Percutaneous Endoscopic Approach
0NC40ZZ Extirpation of Matter from Left Parietal Bone, Open Approach
0NC43ZZ Extirpation of Matter from Left Parietal Bone, Percutaneous Approach
0NC44ZZ Extirpation of Matter from Left Parietal Bone, Percutaneous Endoscopic Approach
0NC50ZZ Extirpation of Matter from Right Temporal Bone, Open Approach
0NC53ZZ Extirpation of Matter from Right Temporal Bone, Percutaneous Approach
0NC54ZZ Extirpation of Matter from Right Temporal Bone, Percutaneous Endoscopic Approach
0NC60ZZ Extirpation of Matter from Left Temporal Bone, Open Approach
0NC63ZZ Extirpation of Matter from Left Temporal Bone, Percutaneous Approach
0NC64ZZ Extirpation of Matter from Left Temporal Bone, Percutaneous Endoscopic Approach
0NC70ZZ Extirpation of Matter from Right Occipital Bone, Open Approach
0NC73ZZ Extirpation of Matter from Right Occipital Bone, Percutaneous Approach
0NC74ZZ Extirpation of Matter from Right Occipital Bone, Percutaneous Endoscopic Approach
0NC80ZZ Extirpation of Matter from Left Occipital Bone, Open Approach
0NC83ZZ Extirpation of Matter from Left Occipital Bone, Percutaneous Approach
0NC84ZZ Extirpation of Matter from Left Occipital Bone, Percutaneous Endoscopic Approach
0NCB0ZZ Extirpation of Matter from Nasal Bone, Open Approach
0NCB3ZZ Extirpation of Matter from Nasal Bone, Percutaneous Approach
0NCB4ZZ Extirpation of Matter from Nasal Bone, Percutaneous Endoscopic Approach
0NCC0ZZ Extirpation of Matter from Right Sphenoid Bone, Open Approach
0NCC3ZZ Extirpation of Matter from Right Sphenoid Bone, Percutaneous Approach
0NCC4ZZ Extirpation of Matter from Right Sphenoid Bone, Percutaneous Endoscopic Approach
0NCD0ZZ Extirpation of Matter from Left Sphenoid Bone, Open Approach
0NCD3ZZ Extirpation of Matter from Left Sphenoid Bone, Percutaneous Approach
0NCD4ZZ Extirpation of Matter from Left Sphenoid Bone, Percutaneous Endoscopic Approach
0NCF0ZZ Extirpation of Matter from Right Ethmoid Bone, Open Approach
0NCF3ZZ Extirpation of Matter from Right Ethmoid Bone, Percutaneous Approach
0NCF4ZZ Extirpation of Matter from Right Ethmoid Bone, Percutaneous Endoscopic Approach
0NCG0ZZ Extirpation of Matter from Left Ethmoid Bone, Open Approach
0NCG3ZZ Extirpation of Matter from Left Ethmoid Bone, Percutaneous Approach
0NCG4ZZ Extirpation of Matter from Left Ethmoid Bone, Percutaneous Endoscopic Approach
0NCH0ZZ Extirpation of Matter from Right Lacrimal Bone, Open Approach
0NCH3ZZ Extirpation of Matter from Right Lacrimal Bone, Percutaneous Approach
0NCH4ZZ Extirpation of Matter from Right Lacrimal Bone, Percutaneous Endoscopic Approach
0NCJ0ZZ Extirpation of Matter from Left Lacrimal Bone, Open Approach
0NCJ3ZZ Extirpation of Matter from Left Lacrimal Bone, Percutaneous Approach
0NCJ4ZZ Extirpation of Matter from Left Lacrimal Bone, Percutaneous Endoscopic Approach
0NCK0ZZ Extirpation of Matter from Right Palatine Bone, Open Approach
0NCK3ZZ Extirpation of Matter from Right Palatine Bone, Percutaneous Approach
0NCK4ZZ Extirpation of Matter from Right Palatine Bone, Percutaneous Endoscopic Approach
0NCL0ZZ Extirpation of Matter from Left Palatine Bone, Open Approach
0NCL3ZZ Extirpation of Matter from Left Palatine Bone, Percutaneous Approach
0NCL4ZZ Extirpation of Matter from Left Palatine Bone, Percutaneous Endoscopic Approach
0NCM0ZZ Extirpation of Matter from Right Zygomatic Bone, Open Approach
0NCM3ZZ Extirpation of Matter from Right Zygomatic Bone, Percutaneous Appro
0NCM4ZZ Extirpation of Matter from Right Zygomatic Bone, Percutaneous Endoscopic Approach
0NCN0ZZ Extirpation of Matter from Left Zygomatic Bone, Open Approach
0NCN3ZZ Extirpation of Matter from Left Zygomatic Bone, Percutaneous Approa
0NCN4ZZ Extirpation of Matter from Left Zygomatic Bone, Percutaneous Endoscopic Approach
0NCP0ZZ Extirpation of Matter from Right Orbit, Open Approach
0NCP3ZZ Extirpation of Matter from Right Orbit, Percutaneous Approach
0NCP4ZZ Extirpation of Matter from Right Orbit, Percutaneous Endoscopic Approach
0NCQ0ZZ Extirpation of Matter from Left Orbit, Open Approach
0NCQ3ZZ Extirpation of Matter from Left Orbit, Percutaneous Approach
0NCQ4ZZ Extirpation of Matter from Left Orbit, Percutaneous Endoscopic Approa
0NCR0ZZ Extirpation of Matter from Right Maxil Open Approach
0NCR3ZZ Extirpation of Matter from Right Maxil Percutaneous Approach
0NCR4ZZ Extirpation of Matter from Right Maxil Percutaneous Endoscopic Approach
0NCS0ZZ Extirpation of Matter from Left Maxilla Open Approach
0NCS3ZZ Extirpation of Matter from Left Maxilla Percutaneous Approach
0NCS4ZZ Extirpation of Matter from Left Maxilla Percutaneous Endoscopic Approach
0NCT0ZZ Extirpation of Matter from Right Mandible, Open Approach
0NCT3ZZ Extirpation of Matter from Right Mandible, Percutaneous Approach
0NCT4ZZ Extirpation of Matter from Right Mandib Percutaneous Endoscopic Approach
0NCV0ZZ Extirpation of Matter from Left Mandib Open Approach
0NCV3ZZ Extirpation of Matter from Left Mandib Percutaneous Approach
0NCV4ZZ Extirpation of Matter from Left Mandib Percutaneous Endoscopic Approach
0NCX0ZZ Extirpation of Matter from Hyoid Bone, Open Approach
0NCX3ZZ Extirpation of Matter from Hyoid Bone, Percutaneous Approach
0NCX4ZZ Extirpation of Matter from Hyoid Bone, Percutaneous Endoscopic Approach

0NH – Head and Facial Bones, Insertion

0NH004Z Insertion of Internal Fixation Device into Skull, Open Approach
0NH005Z Insertion of External Fixation Device into Skull, Open Approach
0NH00MZ Insertion of Bone Growth Stimulator into Skull, Open Approach
0NH00NZ Insertion of Neurostimulator Generator into Skull, Open Approach
+ Major brain device implant when reported with an Insertion of a neurostimulator lead (6th character M) into the brain or cerebral ventricle. See table 00H to construct the Insertion code.
0NH034Z Insertion of Internal Fixation Device into Skull, Percutaneous Approach
0NH035Z Insertion of External Fixation Device into Skull, Percutaneous Approach
0NH03MZ Insertion of Bone Growth Stimulator into Skull, Percutaneous Approach
0NH044Z Insertion of Internal Fixation Device into Skull, Percutaneous Endoscopic Approach
0NH045Z Insertion of External Fixation Device into Skull, Percutaneous Endoscopic Approach
0NH04MZ Insertion of Bone Growth Stimulator into Skull, Percutaneous Endoscopic Approach
0NH104Z Insertion of Internal Fixation Device into Right Frontal Bone, Open Approach
0NH134Z Insertion of Internal Fixation Device into Right Frontal Bone, Percutaneous Approach
0NH144Z Insertion of Internal Fixation Device into Right Frontal Bone, Percutaneous Endoscopic Approach
0NH204Z Insertion of Internal Fixation Device into Left Frontal Bone, Open Approach
0NH234Z Insertion of Internal Fixation Device into Left Frontal Bone, Percutaneous Approach
0NH244Z Insertion of Internal Fixation Device into Left Frontal Bone, Percutaneous Endoscopic Approach
0NH304Z Insertion of Internal Fixation Device into Right Parietal Bone, Open Approach
0NH334Z Insertion of Internal Fixation Device into Right Parietal Bone, Percutaneous Approach
0NH344Z Insertion of Internal Fixation Device into Right Parietal Bone, Percutaneous Endoscopic Approach
0NH404Z Insertion of Internal Fixation Device into Left Parietal Bone, Open Approach
0NH434Z Insertion of Internal Fixation Device into Left Parietal Bone, Percutaneous Approach

H444Z Insertion of Internal Fixation Device into Left Parietal Bone, Percutaneous Endoscopic Approach

H504Z Insertion of Internal Fixation Device into Right Temporal Bone, Open Approach

H50SZ Insertion of Hearing Device into Right Temporal Bone, Open Approach

H534Z Insertion of Internal Fixation Device into Right Temporal Bone, Percutaneous Approach

H53SZ Insertion of Hearing Device into Right Temporal Bone, Percutaneous Approach

H544Z Insertion of Internal Fixation Device into Right Temporal Bone, Percutaneous Endoscopic Approach

H54SZ Insertion of Hearing Device into Right Temporal Bone, Percutaneous Endoscopic Approach

NH604Z Insertion of Internal Fixation Device into Left Temporal Bone, Open Approach

NH60SZ Insertion of Hearing Device into Left Temporal Bone, Open Approach

NH634Z Insertion of Internal Fixation Device into Left Temporal Bone, Percutaneous Approach

NH63SZ Insertion of Hearing Device into Left Temporal Bone, Percutaneous Approach

NH644Z Insertion of Internal Fixation Device into Left Temporal Bone, Percutaneous Endoscopic Approach

NH64SZ Insertion of Hearing Device into Left Temporal Bone, Percutaneous Endoscopic Approach

NH704Z Insertion of Internal Fixation Device into Right Occipital Bone, Open Approach

NH734Z Insertion of Internal Fixation Device into Right Occipital Bone, Percutaneous Approach

NH744Z Insertion of Internal Fixation Device into Right Occipital Bone, Percutaneous Endoscopic Approach

NH804Z Insertion of Internal Fixation Device into Left Occipital Bone, Open Approach

NH834Z Insertion of Internal Fixation Device into Left Occipital Bone, Percutaneous Approach

NH844Z Insertion of Internal Fixation Device into Left Occipital Bone, Percutaneous Endoscopic Approach

NHB04Z Insertion of Internal Fixation Device into Nasal Bone, Open Approach

NHB0MZ Insertion of Bone Growth Stimulator into Nasal Bone, Open Approach

NHB34Z Insertion of Internal Fixation Device into Nasal Bone, Percutaneous Approach

NHB3MZ Insertion of Bone Growth Stimulator into Nasal Bone, Percutaneous Approach

NHB44Z Insertion of Internal Fixation Device into Nasal Bone, Percutaneous Endoscopic Approach

0NHB4MZ Insertion of Bone Growth Stimulator into Nasal Bone, Percutaneous Endoscopic Approach

0NHC04Z Insertion of Internal Fixation Device into Right Sphenoid Bone, Open Approach

0NHC34Z Insertion of Internal Fixation Device into Right Sphenoid Bone, Percutaneous Approach

0NHC44Z Insertion of Internal Fixation Device into Right Sphenoid Bone, Percutaneous Endoscopic Approach

0NHD04Z Insertion of Internal Fixation Device into Left Sphenoid Bone, Open Approach

0NHD34Z Insertion of Internal Fixation Device into Left Sphenoid Bone, Percutaneous Approach

0NHD44Z Insertion of Internal Fixation Device into Left Sphenoid Bone, Percutaneous Endoscopic Approach

0NHF04Z Insertion of Internal Fixation Device into Right Ethmoid Bone, Open Approach

0NHF34Z Insertion of Internal Fixation Device into Right Ethmoid Bone, Percutaneous Approach

0NHF44Z Insertion of Internal Fixation Device into Right Ethmoid Bone, Percutaneous Endoscopic Approach

0NHG04Z Insertion of Internal Fixation Device into Left Ethmoid Bone, Open Approach

0NHG34Z Insertion of Internal Fixation Device into Left Ethmoid Bone, Percutaneous Approach

0NHG44Z Insertion of Internal Fixation Device into Left Ethmoid Bone, Percutaneous Endoscopic Approach

0NHH04Z Insertion of Internal Fixation Device into Right Lacrimal Bone, Open Approach

0NHH34Z Insertion of Internal Fixation Device into Right Lacrimal Bone, Percutaneous Approach

0NHH44Z Insertion of Internal Fixation Device into Right Lacrimal Bone, Percutaneous Endoscopic Approach

0NHJ04Z Insertion of Internal Fixation Device into Left Lacrimal Bone, Open Approach

0NHJ34Z Insertion of Internal Fixation Device into Left Lacrimal Bone, Percutaneous Approach

0NHJ44Z Insertion of Internal Fixation Device into Left Lacrimal Bone, Percutaneous Endoscopic Approach

0NHK04Z Insertion of Internal Fixation Device into Right Palatine Bone, Open Approach

0NHK34Z Insertion of Internal Fixation Device into Right Palatine Bone, Percutaneous Approach

0NHK44Z Insertion of Internal Fixation Device into Right Palatine Bone, Percutaneous Endoscopic Approach

0NHL04Z Insertion of Internal Fixation Device into Left Palatine Bone, Open Approach

0NHL34Z Insertion of Internal Fixation Device into Left Palatine Bone, Percutaneous Approach

0NHL44Z Insertion of Internal Fixation Device into Left Palatine Bone, Percutaneous Endoscopic Approach

0NHM04Z Insertion of Internal Fixation Device into Right Zygomatic Bone, Open Approach

0NHM34Z Insertion of Internal Fixation Device into Right Zygomatic Bone, Percutaneous Approach

0NHM44Z Insertion of Internal Fixation Device into Right Zygomatic Bone, Percutaneous Endoscopic Approach

0NHN04Z Insertion of Internal Fixation Device into Left Zygomatic Bone, Open Approach

0NHN34Z Insertion of Internal Fixation Device into Left Zygomatic Bone, Percutaneous Approach

0NHN44Z Insertion of Internal Fixation Device into Left Zygomatic Bone, Percutaneous Endoscopic Approach

0NHP04Z Insertion of Internal Fixation Device into Right Orbit, Open Approach

0NHP34Z Insertion of Internal Fixation Device into Right Orbit, Percutaneous Approach

0NHP44Z Insertion of Internal Fixation Device into Right Orbit, Percutaneous Endoscopic Approach

0NHQ04Z Insertion of Internal Fixation Device into Left Orbit, Open Approach

0NHQ34Z Insertion of Internal Fixation Device into Left Orbit, Percutaneous Approach

0NHQ44Z Insertion of Internal Fixation Device into Left Orbit, Percutaneous Endoscopic Approach

0NHR04Z Insertion of Internal Fixation Device into Right Maxilla, Open Approach

0NHR05Z Insertion of External Fixation Device into Right Maxilla, Open Approach

0NHR34Z Insertion of Internal Fixation Device into Right Maxilla, Percutaneous Approach

0NHR35Z Insertion of External Fixation Device into Right Maxilla, Percutaneous Approach

0NHR44Z Insertion of Internal Fixation Device into Right Maxilla, Percutaneous Endoscopic Approach

0NHR45Z Insertion of External Fixation Device into Right Maxilla, Percutaneous Endoscopic Approach

0NHS04Z Insertion of Internal Fixation Device into Left Maxilla, Open Approach

0NHS05Z Insertion of External Fixation Device into Left Maxilla, Open Approach

0NHS34Z Insertion of Internal Fixation Device into Left Maxilla, Percutaneous Approach

0NHS35Z Insertion of External Fixation Device into Left Maxilla, Percutaneous Approach

0NHS44Z Insertion of Internal Fixation Device into Left Maxilla, Percutaneous Endoscopic Approach

0NHS45Z Insertion of External Fixation Device into Left Maxilla, Percutaneous Endoscopic Approach

0NHT04Z Insertion of Internal Fixation Device into Right Mandible, Open Approach

0NHT05Z Insertion of External Fixation Device into Right Mandible, Open Approach

0NHT34Z Insertion of Internal Fixation Device into Right Mandible, Percutaneous Approach

0NHT35Z Insertion of External Fixation Device into Right Mandible, Percutaneous Approach

0NHT44Z Insertion of Internal Fixation Device into Right Mandible, Percutaneous Endoscopic Approach

0NHT45Z Insertion of External Fixation Device into Right Mandible, Percutaneous Endoscopic Approach

0NHV04Z Insertion of Internal Fixation Device into Left Mandible, Open Approach

0NHV05Z Insertion of External Fixation Device into Left Mandible, Open Approach

0NHV34Z Insertion of Internal Fixation Device into Left Mandible, Percutaneous Approach

0NHV35Z Insertion of External Fixation Device into Left Mandible, Percutaneous Approach

0NHV44Z Insertion of Internal Fixation Device into Left Mandible, Percutaneous Endoscopic Approach

0NHV45Z Insertion of External Fixation Device into Left Mandible, Percutaneous Endoscopic Approach

0NHW0MZ Insertion of Bone Growth Stimulator into Facial Bone, Open Approach

0NHW3MZ Insertion of Bone Growth Stimulator into Facial Bone, Percutaneous Approach

0NHW4MZ Insertion of Bone Growth Stimulator into Facial Bone, Percutaneous Endoscopic Approach

0NHX04Z Insertion of Internal Fixation Device into Hyoid Bone, Open Approach

0NHX34Z Insertion of Internal Fixation Device into Hyoid Bone, Percutaneous Approach

0NHX44Z Insertion of Internal Fixation Device into Hyoid Bone, Percutaneous Endoscopic Approach

0NJ – Head and Facial Bones, Inspection

Review Coding Guideline B3.5

Review Coding Guidelines B3.11a, B3.11b and B3.11c

0NJ00ZZ Inspection of Skull, Open Approach
0NJ03ZZ Inspection of Skull, Percutaneous Approach
0NJ04ZZ Inspection of Skull, Percutaneous Endoscopic Approach
0NJ0XZZ Inspection of Skull, External Approach
0NJB0ZZ Inspection of Nasal Bone, Open Approach
0NJB3ZZ Inspection of Nasal Bone, Percutaneous Approach
0NJB4ZZ Inspection of Nasal Bone, Percutaneous Endoscopic Approach
0NJBXZZ Inspection of Nasal Bone, External Approach
0NJW0ZZ Inspection of Facial Bone, Open Approach
0NJW3ZZ Inspection of Facial Bone, Percutaneous Approach
0NJW4ZZ Inspection of Facial Bone, Percutaneous Endoscopic Approach
0NJWXZZ Inspection of Facial Bone, External Approach

0NN – Head and Facial Bones, Release

Review Coding Guideline B3.13

Review Coding Guideline B3.14

0NN10ZZ Release Right Frontal Bone, Open Approach
0NN13ZZ Release Right Frontal Bone, Percutaneous Approach
0NN14ZZ Release Right Frontal Bone, Percutaneous Endoscopic Approach
0NN20ZZ Release Left Frontal Bone, Open Approach
0NN23ZZ Release Left Frontal Bone, Percutaneous Approach
0NN24ZZ Release Left Frontal Bone, Percutaneous Endoscopic Approach
0NN30ZZ Release Right Parietal Bone, Open Approach
0NN33ZZ Release Right Parietal Bone, Percutaneous Approach
0NN34ZZ Release Right Parietal Bone, Percutaneous Endoscopic Approach
0NN40ZZ Release Left Parietal Bone, Open Approach
0NN43ZZ Release Left Parietal Bone, Percutaneous Approach
0NN44ZZ Release Left Parietal Bone, Percutaneous Endoscopic Approach
0NN50ZZ Release Right Temporal Bone, Open Approach
0NN53ZZ Release Right Temporal Bone, Percutaneous Approach
0NN54ZZ Release Right Temporal Bone, Percutaneous Endoscopic Approach
0NN60ZZ Release Left Temporal Bone, Open Approach
0NN63ZZ Release Left Temporal Bone, Percutaneous Approach
0NN64ZZ Release Left Temporal Bone, Percutaneous Endoscopic Approach
0NN70ZZ Release Right Occipital Bone, Open Approach
0NN73ZZ Release Right Occipital Bone, Percutaneous Approach
0NN74ZZ Release Right Occipital Bone, Percutaneous Endoscopic Approach
0NN80ZZ Release Left Occipital Bone, Open Approach
0NN83ZZ Release Left Occipital Bone, Percutaneous Approach
0NN84ZZ Release Left Occipital Bone, Percutaneous Endoscopic Approach
0NNB0ZZ Release Nasal Bone, Open Approach
0NNB3ZZ Release Nasal Bone, Percutaneous Approach
0NNB4ZZ Release Nasal Bone, Percutaneous Endoscopic Approach
0NNC0ZZ Release Right Sphenoid Bone, Open Approach
0NNC3ZZ Release Right Sphenoid Bone, Percutaneous Approach
0NNC4ZZ Release Right Sphenoid Bone, Percutaneous Endoscopic Approach
0NND0ZZ Release Left Sphenoid Bone, Open Approach
0NND3ZZ Release Left Sphenoid Bone, Percutaneous Approach
0NND4ZZ Release Left Sphenoid Bone, Percutaneous Endoscopic Approach
0NNF0ZZ Release Right Ethmoid Bone, Open Approach
0NNF3ZZ Release Right Ethmoid Bone, Percutaneous Approach
0NNF4ZZ Release Right Ethmoid Bone, Percutaneous Endoscopic Approach
0NNG0ZZ Release Left Ethmoid Bone, Open Approach
0NNG3ZZ Release Left Ethmoid Bone, Percutaneous Approach
0NNG4ZZ Release Left Ethmoid Bone, Percutaneous Endoscopic Approach
0NNH0ZZ Release Right Lacrimal Bone, Open Approach
0NNH3ZZ Release Right Lacrimal Bone, Percutaneous Approach
0NNH4ZZ Release Right Lacrimal Bone, Percutaneous Endoscopic Approach
0NNJ0ZZ Release Left Lacrimal Bone, Open Approach
0NNJ3ZZ Release Left Lacrimal Bone, Percutaneous Approach
0NNJ4ZZ Release Left Lacrimal Bone, Percutaneous Endoscopic Approach
0NNK0ZZ Release Right Palatine Bone, Open Approach
0NNK3ZZ Release Right Palatine Bone, Percutaneous Approach
0NNK4ZZ Release Right Palatine Bone, Percutaneous Endoscopic Approach
0NNL0ZZ Release Left Palatine Bone, Open Approach
0NNL3ZZ Release Left Palatine Bone, Percutaneous Approach
0NNL4ZZ Release Left Palatine Bone, Percutaneous Endoscopic Approach
0NNM0ZZ Release Right Zygomatic Bone, Open Approach
0NNM3ZZ Release Right Zygomatic Bone, Percutaneous Approach
0NNM4ZZ Release Right Zygomatic Bone, Percutaneous Endoscopic Approach
0NNN0ZZ Release Left Zygomatic Bone, Open Approach
0NNN3ZZ Release Left Zygomatic Bone, Percutaneous Approach
0NNN4ZZ Release Left Zygomatic Bone, Percutaneous Endoscopic Approach
0NNP0ZZ Release Right Orbit, Open Approach
0NNP3ZZ Release Right Orbit, Percutaneous Approach
0NNP4ZZ Release Right Orbit, Percutaneous Endoscopic Approach
0NNQ0ZZ Release Left Orbit, Open Approach
0NNQ3ZZ Release Left Orbit, Percutaneous Approach
0NNQ4ZZ Release Left Orbit, Percutaneous Endoscopic Approach
0NNR0ZZ Release Right Maxilla, Open Approach
0NNR3ZZ Release Right Maxilla, Percutaneous Approach
0NNR4ZZ Release Right Maxilla, Percutaneous Endoscopic Approach
0NNS0ZZ Release Left Maxilla, Open Approach
0NNS3ZZ Release Left Maxilla, Percutaneous Approach
0NNS4ZZ Release Left Maxilla, Percutaneous Endoscopic Approach
0NNT0ZZ Release Right Mandible, Open Approach
0NNT3ZZ Release Right Mandible, Percutaneous Approach
0NNT4ZZ Release Right Mandible, Percutaneous Endoscopic Approach
0NNV0ZZ Release Left Mandible, Open Approach
0NNV3ZZ Release Left Mandible, Percutaneous Approach
0NNV4ZZ Release Left Mandible, Percutaneous Endoscopic Approach
0NNX0ZZ Release Hyoid Bone, Open Approach
0NNX3ZZ Release Hyoid Bone, Percutaneous Approach
0NNX4ZZ Release Hyoid Bone, Percutaneous Endoscopic Approach

0NP – Head and Facial Bones, Removal

Review Coding Guideline B6.1c

0NP000Z Removal of Drainage Device from Skull, Open Approach
0NP004Z Removal of Internal Fixation Device from Skull, Open Approach
0NP005Z Removal of External Fixation Device from Skull, Open Approach

P007Z Removal of Autologous Tissue Substitute from Skull, Open Approach
P00JZ Removal of Synthetic Substitute from Skull, Open Approach
P00KZ Removal of Nonautologous Tissue Substitute from Skull, Open Approach
P00MZ Removal of Bone Growth Stimulator from Skull, Open Approach
P00NZ Removal of Neurostimulator Generator from Skull, Open Approach
P00SZ Removal of Hearing Device from Skull, Open Approach
P030Z Removal of Drainage Device from Skull, Percutaneous Approach
P034Z Removal of Internal Fixation Device from Skull, Percutaneous Approach
P035Z Removal of External Fixation Device from Skull, Percutaneous Approach
NP037Z Removal of Autologous Tissue Substitute from Skull, Percutaneous Approach
NP03JZ Removal of Synthetic Substitute from Skull, Percutaneous Approach
NP03KZ Removal of Nonautologous Tissue Substitute from Skull, Percutaneous Approach
NP03MZ Removal of Bone Growth Stimulator from Skull, Percutaneous Approach
NP03SZ Removal of Hearing Device from Skull, Percutaneous Approach
NP040Z Removal of Drainage Device from Skull, Percutaneous Endoscopic Approach
NP044Z Removal of Internal Fixation Device from Skull, Percutaneous Endoscopic Approach
NP045Z Removal of External Fixation Device from Skull, Percutaneous Endoscopic Approach
NP047Z Removal of Autologous Tissue Substitute from Skull, Percutaneous Endoscopic Approach
NP04JZ Removal of Synthetic Substitute from Skull, Percutaneous Endoscopic Approach
NP04KZ Removal of Nonautologous Tissue Substitute from Skull, Percutaneous Endoscopic Approach
NP04MZ Removal of Bone Growth Stimulator from Skull, Percutaneous Endoscopic Approach
NP04SZ Removal of Hearing Device from Skull, Percutaneous Endoscopic Approach
NP0X0Z Removal of Drainage Device from Skull, External Approach
0NP0X4Z Removal of Internal Fixation Device from Skull, External Approach
0NP0X5Z Removal of External Fixation Device from Skull, External Approach
0NP0XMZ Removal of Bone Growth Stimulator from Skull, External Approach
0NP0XSZ Removal of Hearing Device from Skull, External Approach
0NPB00Z Removal of Drainage Device from Nasal Bone, Open Approach
0NPB04Z Removal of Internal Fixation Device from Nasal Bone, Open Approach
0NPB07Z Removal of Autologous Tissue Substitute from Nasal Bone, Open Approach
0NPB0JZ Removal of Synthetic Substitute from Nasal Bone, Open Approach
0NPB0KZ Removal of Nonautologous Tissue Substitute from Nasal Bone, Open Approach
0NPB0MZ Removal of Bone Growth Stimulator from Nasal Bone, Open Approach
0NPB30Z Removal of Drainage Device from Nasal Bone, Percutaneous Approach
0NPB34Z Removal of Internal Fixation Device from Nasal Bone, Percutaneous Approach
0NPB37Z Removal of Autologous Tissue Substitute from Nasal Bone, Percutaneous Approach
0NPB3JZ Removal of Synthetic Substitute from Nasal Bone, Percutaneous Approach
0NPB3KZ Removal of Nonautologous Tissue Substitute from Nasal Bone, Percutaneous Approach
0NPB3MZ Removal of Bone Growth Stimulator from Nasal Bone, Percutaneous Approach
0NPB40Z Removal of Drainage Device from Nasal Bone, Percutaneous Endoscopic Approach
0NPB44Z Removal of Internal Fixation Device from Nasal Bone, Percutaneous Endoscopic Approach
0NPB47Z Removal of Autologous Tissue Substitute from Nasal Bone, Percutaneous Endoscopic Approach
0NPB4JZ Removal of Synthetic Substitute from Nasal Bone, Percutaneous Endoscopic Approach
0NPB4KZ Removal of Nonautologous Tissue Substitute from Nasal Bone, Percutaneous Endoscopic Approach
0NPB4MZ Removal of Bone Growth Stimulator from Nasal Bone, Percutaneous Endoscopic Approach
0NPBX0Z Removal of Drainage Device from Nasal Bone, External Approach
0NPBX4Z Removal of Internal Fixation Device from Nasal Bone, External Approach
0NPBXMZ Removal of Bone Growth Stimulator from Nasal Bone, External Approach
0NPW00Z Removal of Drainage Device from Facial Bone, Open Approach
0NPW04Z Removal of Internal Fixation Device from Facial Bone, Open Approach
0NPW07Z Removal of Autologous Tissue Substitute from Facial Bone, Open Approach
0NPW0JZ Removal of Synthetic Substitute from Facial Bone, Open Approach
0NPW0KZ Removal of Nonautologous Tissue Substitute from Facial Bone, Open Approach
0NPW0MZ Removal of Bone Growth Stimulator from Facial Bone, Open Approach
0NPW30Z Removal of Drainage Device from Facial Bone, Percutaneous Approach
0NPW34Z Removal of Internal Fixation Device from Facial Bone, Percutaneous Approach
0NPW37Z Removal of Autologous Tissue Substitute from Facial Bone, Percutaneous Approach
0NPW3JZ Removal of Synthetic Substitute from Facial Bone, Percutaneous Approach
0NPW3KZ Removal of Nonautologous Tissue Substitute from Facial Bone, Percutaneous Approach
0NPW3MZ Removal of Bone Growth Stimulator from Facial Bone, Percutaneous Approach
0NPW40Z Removal of Drainage Device from Facial Bone, Percutaneous Endoscopic Approach
0NPW44Z Removal of Internal Fixation Device from Facial Bone, Percutaneous Endoscopic Approach
0NPW47Z Removal of Autologous Tissue Substitute from Facial Bone, Percutaneous Endoscopic Approach
0NPW4JZ Removal of Synthetic Substitute from Facial Bone, Percutaneous Endoscopic Approach
0NPW4KZ Removal of Nonautologous Tissue Substitute from Facial Bone, Percutaneous Endoscopic Approach
0NPW4MZ Removal of Bone Growth Stimulator from Facial Bone, Percutaneous Endoscopic Approach
0NPWX0Z Removal of Drainage Device from Facial Bone, External Approach
0NPWX4Z Removal of Internal Fixation Device from Facial Bone, External Approach
0NPWXMZ Removal of Bone Growth Stimulator from Facial Bone, External Approach

0NQ – Head and Facial Bones, Repair

Review Coding Guideline B3.5

0NQ00ZZ Repair Skull, Open Approach
0NQ03ZZ Repair Skull, Percutaneous Approach
0NQ04ZZ Repair Skull, Percutaneous Endoscopic Approach
0NQ0XZZ Repair Skull, External Approach
0NQ10ZZ Repair Right Frontal Bone, Open Approach
0NQ13ZZ Repair Right Frontal Bone, Percutaneous Approach
0NQ14ZZ Repair Right Frontal Bone, Percutaneous Endoscopic Approach
0NQ1XZZ Repair Right Frontal Bone, External Approach
0NQ20ZZ Repair Left Frontal Bone, Open Approach
0NQ23ZZ Repair Left Frontal Bone, Percutaneous Approach
0NQ24ZZ Repair Left Frontal Bone, Percutaneous Endoscopic Approach
0NQ2XZZ Repair Left Frontal Bone, External Approach
0NQ30ZZ Repair Right Parietal Bone, Open Approach
0NQ33ZZ Repair Right Parietal Bone, Percutaneous Approach
0NQ34ZZ Repair Right Parietal Bone, Percutaneous Endoscopic Approach
0NQ3XZZ Repair Right Parietal Bone, External Approach
0NQ40ZZ Repair Left Parietal Bone, Open Approach
0NQ43ZZ Repair Left Parietal Bone, Percutaneous Approach
0NQ44ZZ Repair Left Parietal Bone, Percutaneous Endoscopic Approach
0NQ4XZZ Repair Left Parietal Bone, External Approach
0NQ50ZZ Repair Right Temporal Bone, Open Approach
0NQ53ZZ Repair Right Temporal Bone, Percutaneous Approach
0NQ54ZZ Repair Right Temporal Bone, Percutaneous Endoscopic Approach
0NQ5XZZ Repair Right Temporal Bone, External Approach
0NQ60ZZ Repair Left Temporal Bone, Open Approach

0NQ63ZZ Repair Left Temporal Bone, Percutaneous Approach
0NQ64ZZ Repair Left Temporal Bone, Percutaneous Endoscopic Approach
0NQ6XZZ Repair Left Temporal Bone, External Approach
0NQ70ZZ Repair Right Occipital Bone, Open Approach
0NQ73ZZ Repair Right Occipital Bone, Percutaneous Approach
0NQ74ZZ Repair Right Occipital Bone, Percutaneous Endoscopic Approach
0NQ7XZZ Repair Right Occipital Bone, External Approach
0NQ80ZZ Repair Left Occipital Bone, Open Approach
0NQ83ZZ Repair Left Occipital Bone, Percutaneous Approach
0NQ84ZZ Repair Left Occipital Bone, Percutaneous Endoscopic Approach
0NQ8XZZ Repair Left Occipital Bone, External Approach
0NQB0ZZ Repair Nasal Bone, Open Approach
0NQB3ZZ Repair Nasal Bone, Percutaneous Approach
0NQB4ZZ Repair Nasal Bone, Percutaneous Endoscopic Approach
0NQBXZZ Repair Nasal Bone, External Approach
0NQC0ZZ Repair Right Sphenoid Bone, Open Approach
0NQC3ZZ Repair Right Sphenoid Bone, Percutaneous Approach
0NQC4ZZ Repair Right Sphenoid Bone, Percutaneous Endoscopic Approach
0NQCXZZ Repair Right Sphenoid Bone, External Approach
0NQD0ZZ Repair Left Sphenoid Bone, Open Approach
0NQD3ZZ Repair Left Sphenoid Bone, Percutaneous Approach
0NQD4ZZ Repair Left Sphenoid Bone, Percutaneous Endoscopic Approach
0NQDXZZ Repair Left Sphenoid Bone, External Approach
0NQF0ZZ Repair Right Ethmoid Bone, Open Approach
0NQF3ZZ Repair Right Ethmoid Bone, Percutaneous Approach
0NQF4ZZ Repair Right Ethmoid Bone, Percutaneous Endoscopic Approach
0NQFXZZ Repair Right Ethmoid Bone, External Approach
0NQG0ZZ Repair Left Ethmoid Bone, Open Approach
0NQG3ZZ Repair Left Ethmoid Bone, Percutaneous Approach
0NQG4ZZ Repair Left Ethmoid Bone, Percutaneous Endoscopic Approach
0NQGXZZ Repair Left Ethmoid Bone, External Approach
0NQH0ZZ Repair Right Lacrimal Bone, Open Approach
0NQH3ZZ Repair Right Lacrimal Bone, Percutaneous Approach
0NQH4ZZ Repair Right Lacrimal Bone, Percutaneous Endoscopic Approach
0NQHXZZ Repair Right Lacrimal Bone, External Approach
0NQJ0ZZ Repair Left Lacrimal Bone, Open Approach
0NQJ3ZZ Repair Left Lacrimal Bone, Percutaneous Approach
0NQJ4ZZ Repair Left Lacrimal Bone, Percutaneous Endoscopic Approach
0NQJXZZ Repair Left Lacrimal Bone, External Approach
0NQK0ZZ Repair Right Palatine Bone, Open Approach
0NQK3ZZ Repair Right Palatine Bone, Percutaneous Approach
0NQK4ZZ Repair Right Palatine Bone, Percutaneous Endoscopic Approach
0NQKXZZ Repair Right Palatine Bone, External Approach
0NQL0ZZ Repair Left Palatine Bone, Open Approach
0NQL3ZZ Repair Left Palatine Bone, Percutaneous Approach
0NQL4ZZ Repair Left Palatine Bone, Percutaneous Endoscopic Approach
0NQLXZZ Repair Left Palatine Bone, External Approach
0NQM0ZZ Repair Right Zygomatic Bone, Open Approach
0NQM3ZZ Repair Right Zygomatic Bone, Percutaneous Approach
0NQM4ZZ Repair Right Zygomatic Bone, Percutaneous Endoscopic Approach
0NQMXZZ Repair Right Zygomatic Bone, External Approach
0NQN0ZZ Repair Left Zygomatic Bone, Open Approach
0NQN3ZZ Repair Left Zygomatic Bone, Percutaneous Approach
0NQN4ZZ Repair Left Zygomatic Bone, Percutaneous Endoscopic Approach
0NQNXZZ Repair Left Zygomatic Bone, External Approach
0NQP0ZZ Repair Right Orbit, Open Approach
0NQP3ZZ Repair Right Orbit, Percutaneous Approach
0NQP4ZZ Repair Right Orbit, Percutaneous Endoscopic Approach
0NQPXZZ Repair Right Orbit, External Approach
0NQQ0ZZ Repair Left Orbit, Open Approach
0NQQ3ZZ Repair Left Orbit, Percutaneous Approach
0NQQ4ZZ Repair Left Orbit, Percutaneous Endoscopic Approach
0NQQXZZ Repair Left Orbit, External Approach
0NQR0ZZ Repair Right Maxilla, Open Approach
0NQR3ZZ Repair Right Maxilla, Percutaneous Approach
0NQR4ZZ Repair Right Maxilla, Percutaneous Endoscopic Approach
0NQRXZZ Repair Right Maxilla, External Approac
0NQS0ZZ Repair Left Maxilla, Open Approach
0NQS3ZZ Repair Left Maxilla, Percutaneous Approach
0NQS4ZZ Repair Left Maxilla, Percutaneous Endoscopic Approach
0NQSXZZ Repair Left Maxilla, External Approach
0NQT0ZZ Repair Right Mandible, Open Approach
0NQT3ZZ Repair Right Mandible, Percutaneous Approach
0NQT4ZZ Repair Right Mandible, Percutaneous Endoscopic Approach
0NQTXZZ Repair Right Mandible, External Approach
0NQV0ZZ Repair Left Mandible, Open Approach
0NQV3ZZ Repair Left Mandible, Percutaneous Approach
0NQV4ZZ Repair Left Mandible, Percutaneous Endoscopic Approach
0NQVXZZ Repair Left Mandible, External Approac
0NQX0ZZ Repair Hyoid Bone, Open Approach
0NQX3ZZ Repair Hyoid Bone, Percutaneous Approach
0NQX4ZZ Repair Hyoid Bone, Percutaneous Endoscopic Approach
0NQXXZZ Repair Hyoid Bone, External Approach

*0N*R – *Head and Facial Bones, Replacement*

0NR007Z Replacement of Skull with Autologous Tissue Substitute, Open Approach
0NR00JZ Replacement of Skull with Synthetic Substitute, Open Approach
0NR00KZ Replacement of Skull with Nonautologous Tissue Substitute, Open Approach
0NR037Z Replacement of Skull with Autologous Tissue Substitute, Percutaneous Approach
0NR03JZ Replacement of Skull with Synthetic Substitute, Percutaneous Approach
0NR03KZ Replacement of Skull with Nonautologous Tissue Substitute, Percutaneous Approach
0NR047Z Replacement of Skull with Autologous Tissue Substitute, Percutaneous Endoscopic Approach
0NR04JZ Replacement of Skull with Synthetic Substitute, Percutaneous Endoscopic Approach
0NR04KZ Replacement of Skull with Nonautologous Tissue Substitute, Percutaneous Endoscopic Approach
0NR107Z Replacement of Right Frontal Bone with Autologous Tissue Substitute, Open Approach
0NR10JZ Replacement of Right Frontal Bone with Synthetic Substitute, Open Approach
0NR10KZ Replacement of Right Frontal Bone with Nonautologous Tissue Substitute, Open Approach
0NR137Z Replacement of Right Frontal Bone with Autologous Tissue Substitute, Percutaneous Approach
0NR13JZ Replacement of Right Frontal Bone with Synthetic Substitute, Percutaneous Approach
0NR13KZ Replacement of Right Frontal Bone with Nonautologous Tissue Substitute, Percutaneous Approach
0NR147Z Replacement of Right Frontal Bone with Autologous Tissue Substitute, Percutaneous Endoscopic Approach
0NR14JZ Replacement of Right Frontal Bone with Synthetic Substitute, Percutaneous Endoscopic Approach
0NR14KZ Replacement of Right Frontal Bone with Nonautologous Tissue Substitute, Percutaneous Endoscopic Approach
0NR207Z Replacement of Left Frontal Bone with Autologous Tissue Substitute, Open Approach
0NR20JZ Replacement of Left Frontal Bone with Synthetic Substitute, Open Approach
0NR20KZ Replacement of Left Frontal Bone with Nonautologous Tissue Substitute, Open Approach
0NR237Z Replacement of Left Frontal Bone with Autologous Tissue Substitute, Percutaneous Approach
0NR23JZ Replacement of Left Frontal Bone with Synthetic Substitute, Percutaneous Approach
0NR23KZ Replacement of Left Frontal Bone with Nonautologous Tissue Substitute, Percutaneous Approach
0NR247Z Replacement of Left Frontal Bone with Autologous Tissue Substitute, Percutaneous Endoscopic Approach

R24JZ Replacement of Left Frontal Bone with Synthetic Substitute, Percutaneous Endoscopic Approach
R24KZ Replacement of Left Frontal Bone with Nonautologous Tissue Substitute, Percutaneous Endoscopic Approach
R307Z Replacement of Right Parietal Bone with Autologous Tissue Substitute, Open Approach
R30JZ Replacement of Right Parietal Bone with Synthetic Substitute, Open Approach
R30KZ Replacement of Right Parietal Bone with Nonautologous Tissue Substitute, Open Approach
R337Z Replacement of Right Parietal Bone with Autologous Tissue Substitute, Percutaneous Approach
R33JZ Replacement of Right Parietal Bone with Synthetic Substitute, Percutaneous Approach
R33KZ Replacement of Right Parietal Bone with Nonautologous Tissue Substitute, Percutaneous Approach
NR347Z Replacement of Right Parietal Bone with Autologous Tissue Substitute, Percutaneous Endoscopic Approach
NR34JZ Replacement of Right Parietal Bone with Synthetic Substitute, Percutaneous Endoscopic Approach
NR34KZ Replacement of Right Parietal Bone with Nonautologous Tissue Substitute, Percutaneous Endoscopic Approach
NR407Z Replacement of Left Parietal Bone with Autologous Tissue Substitute, Open Approach
NR40JZ Replacement of Left Parietal Bone with Synthetic Substitute, Open Approach
NR40KZ Replacement of Left Parietal Bone with Nonautologous Tissue Substitute, Open Approach
NR437Z Replacement of Left Parietal Bone with Autologous Tissue Substitute, Percutaneous Approach
NR43JZ Replacement of Left Parietal Bone with Synthetic Substitute, Percutaneous Approach
NR43KZ Replacement of Left Parietal Bone with Nonautologous Tissue Substitute, Percutaneous Approach
NR447Z Replacement of Left Parietal Bone with Autologous Tissue Substitute, Percutaneous Endoscopic Approach
NR44JZ Replacement of Left Parietal Bone with Synthetic Substitute, Percutaneous Endoscopic Approach
NR44KZ Replacement of Left Parietal Bone with Nonautologous Tissue Substitute, Percutaneous Endoscopic Approach
NR507Z Replacement of Right Temporal Bone with Autologous Tissue Substitute, Open Approach
NR50JZ Replacement of Right Temporal Bone with Synthetic Substitute, Open Approach
0NR50KZ Replacement of Right Temporal Bone with Nonautologous Tissue Substitute, Open Approach
0NR537Z Replacement of Right Temporal Bone with Autologous Tissue Substitute, Percutaneous Approach
0NR53JZ Replacement of Right Temporal Bone with Synthetic Substitute, Percutaneous Approach
0NR53KZ Replacement of Right Temporal Bone with Nonautologous Tissue Substitute, Percutaneous Approach
0NR547Z Replacement of Right Temporal Bone with Autologous Tissue Substitute, Percutaneous Endoscopic Approach
0NR54JZ Replacement of Right Temporal Bone with Synthetic Substitute, Percutaneous Endoscopic Approach
0NR54KZ Replacement of Right Temporal Bone with Nonautologous Tissue Substitute, Percutaneous Endoscopic Approach
0NR607Z Replacement of Left Temporal Bone with Autologous Tissue Substitute, Open Approach
0NR60JZ Replacement of Left Temporal Bone with Synthetic Substitute, Open Approach
0NR60KZ Replacement of Left Temporal Bone with Nonautologous Tissue Substitute, Open Approach
0NR637Z Replacement of Left Temporal Bone with Autologous Tissue Substitute, Percutaneous Approach
0NR63JZ Replacement of Left Temporal Bone with Synthetic Substitute, Percutaneous Approach
0NR63KZ Replacement of Left Temporal Bone with Nonautologous Tissue Substitute, Percutaneous Approach
0NR647Z Replacement of Left Temporal Bone with Autologous Tissue Substitute, Percutaneous Endoscopic Approach
0NR64JZ Replacement of Left Temporal Bone with Synthetic Substitute, Percutaneous Endoscopic Approach
0NR64KZ Replacement of Left Temporal Bone with Nonautologous Tissue Substitute, Percutaneous Endoscopic Approach
0NR707Z Replacement of Right Occipital Bone with Autologous Tissue Substitute, Open Approach
0NR70JZ Replacement of Right Occipital Bone with Synthetic Substitute, Open Approach
0NR70KZ Replacement of Right Occipital Bone with Nonautologous Tissue Substitute, Open Approach
0NR737Z Replacement of Right Occipital Bone with Autologous Tissue Substitute, Percutaneous Approach
0NR73JZ Replacement of Right Occipital Bone with Synthetic Substitute, Percutaneous Approach
0NR73KZ Replacement of Right Occipital Bone with Nonautologous Tissue Substitute, Percutaneous Approach
0NR747Z Replacement of Right Occipital Bone with Autologous Tissue Substitute, Percutaneous Endoscopic Approach
0NR74JZ Replacement of Right Occipital Bone with Synthetic Substitute, Percutaneous Endoscopic Approach
0NR74KZ Replacement of Right Occipital Bone with Nonautologous Tissue Substitute, Percutaneous Endoscopic Approach
0NR807Z Replacement of Left Occipital Bone with Autologous Tissue Substitute, Open Approach
0NR80JZ Replacement of Left Occipital Bone with Synthetic Substitute, Open Approach
0NR80KZ Replacement of Left Occipital Bone with Nonautologous Tissue Substitute, Open Approach
0NR837Z Replacement of Left Occipital Bone with Autologous Tissue Substitute, Percutaneous Approach
0NR83JZ Replacement of Left Occipital Bone with Synthetic Substitute, Percutaneous Approach
0NR83KZ Replacement of Left Occipital Bone with Nonautologous Tissue Substitute, Percutaneous Approach
0NR847Z Replacement of Left Occipital Bone with Autologous Tissue Substitute, Percutaneous Endoscopic Approach
0NR84JZ Replacement of Left Occipital Bone with Synthetic Substitute, Percutaneous Endoscopic Approach
0NR84KZ Replacement of Left Occipital Bone with Nonautologous Tissue Substitute, Percutaneous Endoscopic Approach
0NRB07Z Replacement of Nasal Bone with Autologous Tissue Substitute, Open Approach
0NRB0JZ Replacement of Nasal Bone with Synthetic Substitute, Open Approach
0NRB0KZ Replacement of Nasal Bone with Nonautologous Tissue Substitute, Open Approach
0NRB37Z Replacement of Nasal Bone with Autologous Tissue Substitute, Percutaneous Approach
0NRB3JZ Replacement of Nasal Bone with Synthetic Substitute, Percutaneous Approach
0NRB3KZ Replacement of Nasal Bone with Nonautologous Tissue Substitute, Percutaneous Approach
0NRB47Z Replacement of Nasal Bone with Autologous Tissue Substitute, Percutaneous Endoscopic Approach
0NRB4JZ Replacement of Nasal Bone with Synthetic Substitute, Percutaneous Endoscopic Approach
0NRB4KZ Replacement of Nasal Bone with Nonautologous Tissue Substitute, Percutaneous Endoscopic Approach
0NRC07Z Replacement of Right Sphenoid Bone with Autologous Tissue Substitute, Open Approach
0NRC0JZ Replacement of Right Sphenoid Bone with Synthetic Substitute, Open Approach
0NRC0KZ Replacement of Right Sphenoid Bone with Nonautologous Tissue Substitute, Open Approach
0NRC37Z Replacement of Right Sphenoid Bone with Autologous Tissue Substitute, Percutaneous Approach
0NRC3JZ Replacement of Right Sphenoid Bone with Synthetic Substitute, Percutaneous Approach
0NRC3KZ Replacement of Right Sphenoid Bone with Nonautologous Tissue Substitute, Percutaneous Approach
0NRC47Z Replacement of Right Sphenoid Bone with Autologous Tissue Substitute, Percutaneous Endoscopic Approach
0NRC4JZ Replacement of Right Sphenoid Bone with Synthetic Substitute, Percutaneous Endoscopic Approach
0NRC4KZ Replacement of Right Sphenoid Bone with Nonautologous Tissue Substitute, Percutaneous Endoscopic Approach
0NRD07Z Replacement of Left Sphenoid Bone with Autologous Tissue Substitute, Open Approach
0NRD0JZ Replacement of Left Sphenoid Bone with Synthetic Substitute, Open Approach
0NRD0KZ Replacement of Left Sphenoid Bone with Nonautologous Tissue Substitute, Open Approach
0NRD37Z Replacement of Left Sphenoid Bone with Autologous Tissue Substitute, Percutaneous Approach
0NRD3JZ Replacement of Left Sphenoid Bone with Synthetic Substitute, Percutaneous Approach
0NRD3KZ Replacement of Left Sphenoid Bone with Nonautologous Tissue Substitute, Percutaneous Approach
0NRD47Z Replacement of Left Sphenoid Bone with Autologous Tissue Substitute, Percutaneous Endoscopic Approach

0NRD4JZ Replacement of Left Sphenoid Bone with Synthetic Substitute, Percutaneous Endoscopic Approach
0NRD4KZ Replacement of Left Sphenoid Bone with Nonautologous Tissue Substitute, Percutaneous Endoscopic Approach
0NRF07Z Replacement of Right Ethmoid Bone with Autologous Tissue Substitute, Open Approach
0NRF0JZ Replacement of Right Ethmoid Bone with Synthetic Substitute, Open Approach
0NRF0KZ Replacement of Right Ethmoid Bone with Nonautologous Tissue Substitute, Open Approach
0NRF37Z Replacement of Right Ethmoid Bone with Autologous Tissue Substitute, Percutaneous Approach
0NRF3JZ Replacement of Right Ethmoid Bone with Synthetic Substitute, Percutaneous Approach
0NRF3KZ Replacement of Right Ethmoid Bone with Nonautologous Tissue Substitute, Percutaneous Approach
0NRF47Z Replacement of Right Ethmoid Bone with Autologous Tissue Substitute, Percutaneous Endoscopic Approach
0NRF4JZ Replacement of Right Ethmoid Bone with Synthetic Substitute, Percutaneous Endoscopic Approach
0NRF4KZ Replacement of Right Ethmoid Bone with Nonautologous Tissue Substitute, Percutaneous Endoscopic Approach
0NRG07Z Replacement of Left Ethmoid Bone with Autologous Tissue Substitute, Open Approach
0NRG0JZ Replacement of Left Ethmoid Bone with Synthetic Substitute, Open Approach
0NRG0KZ Replacement of Left Ethmoid Bone with Nonautologous Tissue Substitute, Open Approach
0NRG37Z Replacement of Left Ethmoid Bone with Autologous Tissue Substitute, Percutaneous Approach
0NRG3JZ Replacement of Left Ethmoid Bone with Synthetic Substitute, Percutaneous Approach
0NRG3KZ Replacement of Left Ethmoid Bone with Nonautologous Tissue Substitute, Percutaneous Approach
0NRG47Z Replacement of Left Ethmoid Bone with Autologous Tissue Substitute, Percutaneous Endoscopic Approach
0NRG4JZ Replacement of Left Ethmoid Bone with Synthetic Substitute, Percutaneous Endoscopic Approach
0NRG4KZ Replacement of Left Ethmoid Bone with Nonautologous Tissue Substitute, Percutaneous Endoscopic Approach
0NRH07Z Replacement of Right Lacrimal Bone with Autologous Tissue Substitute, Open Approach
0NRH0JZ Replacement of Right Lacrimal Bone with Synthetic Substitute, Open Approach
0NRH0KZ Replacement of Right Lacrimal Bone with Nonautologous Tissue Substitute, Open Approach
0NRH37Z Replacement of Right Lacrimal Bone with Autologous Tissue Substitute, Percutaneous Approach
0NRH3JZ Replacement of Right Lacrimal Bone with Synthetic Substitute, Percutaneous Approach
0NRH3KZ Replacement of Right Lacrimal Bone with Nonautologous Tissue Substitute, Percutaneous Approach
0NRH47Z Replacement of Right Lacrimal Bone with Autologous Tissue Substitute, Percutaneous Endoscopic Approach
0NRH4JZ Replacement of Right Lacrimal Bone with Synthetic Substitute, Percutaneous Endoscopic Approach
0NRH4KZ Replacement of Right Lacrimal Bone with Nonautologous Tissue Substitute, Percutaneous Endoscopic Approach
0NRJ07Z Replacement of Left Lacrimal Bone with Autologous Tissue Substitute, Open Approach
0NRJ0JZ Replacement of Left Lacrimal Bone with Synthetic Substitute, Open Approach
0NRJ0KZ Replacement of Left Lacrimal Bone with Nonautologous Tissue Substitute, Open Approach
0NRJ37Z Replacement of Left Lacrimal Bone with Autologous Tissue Substitute, Percutaneous Approach
0NRJ3JZ Replacement of Left Lacrimal Bone with Synthetic Substitute, Percutaneous Approach
0NRJ3KZ Replacement of Left Lacrimal Bone with Nonautologous Tissue Substitute, Percutaneous Approach
0NRJ47Z Replacement of Left Lacrimal Bone with Autologous Tissue Substitute, Percutaneous Endoscopic Approach
0NRJ4JZ Replacement of Left Lacrimal Bone with Synthetic Substitute, Percutaneous Endoscopic Approach
0NRJ4KZ Replacement of Left Lacrimal Bone with Nonautologous Tissue Substitute, Percutaneous Endoscopic Approach
0NRK07Z Replacement of Right Palatine Bone with Autologous Tissue Substitute, Open Approach
0NRK0JZ Replacement of Right Palatine Bone with Synthetic Substitute, Open Approach
0NRK0KZ Replacement of Right Palatine Bone with Nonautologous Tissue Substitute, Open Approach
0NRK37Z Replacement of Right Palatine Bone with Autologous Tissue Substitute, Percutaneous Approach
0NRK3JZ Replacement of Right Palatine Bone with Synthetic Substitute, Percutaneous Approach
0NRK3KZ Replacement of Right Palatine Bone with Nonautologous Tissue Substitute, Percutaneous Approach
0NRK47Z Replacement of Right Palatine Bone with Autologous Tissue Substitute, Percutaneous Endoscopic Approach
0NRK4JZ Replacement of Right Palatine Bone with Synthetic Substitute, Percutaneous Endoscopic Approach
0NRK4KZ Replacement of Right Palatine Bone with Nonautologous Tissue Substitute, Percutaneous Endoscopic Approach
0NRL07Z Replacement of Left Palatine Bone with Autologous Tissue Substitute, Open Approach
0NRL0JZ Replacement of Left Palatine Bone with Synthetic Substitute, Open Approach
0NRL0KZ Replacement of Left Palatine Bone with Nonautologous Tissue Substitute, Open Approach
0NRL37Z Replacement of Left Palatine Bone with Autologous Tissue Substitute, Percutaneous Approach
0NRL3JZ Replacement of Left Palatine Bone with Synthetic Substitute, Percutaneous Approach
0NRL3KZ Replacement of Left Palatine Bone with Nonautologous Tissue Substitute, Percutaneous Approach
0NRL47Z Replacement of Left Palatine Bone with Autologous Tissue Substitute, Percutaneous Endoscopic Approach
0NRL4JZ Replacement of Left Palatine Bone with Synthetic Substitute, Percutaneous Endoscopic Approach
0NRL4KZ Replacement of Left Palatine Bone with Nonautologous Tissue Substitute, Percutaneous Endoscopic Approach
0NRM07Z Replacement of Right Zygomatic Bone with Autologous Tissue Substitute, Open Approach
0NRM0JZ Replacement of Right Zygomatic Bone with Synthetic Substitute, Open Approach
0NRM0KZ Replacement of Right Zygomatic Bone with Nonautologous Tissue Substitute, Open Approach
0NRM37Z Replacement of Right Zygomatic Bone with Autologous Tissue Substitute, Percutaneous Approach
0NRM3JZ Replacement of Right Zygomatic Bone with Synthetic Substitute, Percutaneous Approach
0NRM3KZ Replacement of Right Zygomatic Bone with Nonautologous Tissue Substitute, Percutaneous Approach
0NRM47Z Replacement of Right Zygomatic Bone with Autologous Tissue Substitute, Percutaneous Endoscopic Approach
0NRM4JZ Replacement of Right Zygomatic Bone with Synthetic Substitute, Percutaneous Endoscopic Approach
0NRM4KZ Replacement of Right Zygomatic Bone with Nonautologous Tissue Substitute, Percutaneous Endoscopic Approach
0NRN07Z Replacement of Left Zygomatic Bone with Autologous Tissue Substitute, Open Approach
0NRN0JZ Replacement of Left Zygomatic Bone with Synthetic Substitute, Open Approach
0NRN0KZ Replacement of Left Zygomatic Bone with Nonautologous Tissue Substitute, Open Approach
0NRN37Z Replacement of Left Zygomatic Bone with Autologous Tissue Substitute, Percutaneous Approach
0NRN3JZ Replacement of Left Zygomatic Bone with Synthetic Substitute, Percutaneous Approach
0NRN3KZ Replacement of Left Zygomatic Bone with Nonautologous Tissue Substitute, Percutaneous Approach
0NRN47Z Replacement of Left Zygomatic Bone with Autologous Tissue Substitute, Percutaneous Endoscopic Approach
0NRN4JZ Replacement of Left Zygomatic Bone with Synthetic Substitute, Percutaneous Endoscopic Approach
0NRN4KZ Replacement of Left Zygomatic Bone with Nonautologous Tissue Substitute, Percutaneous Endoscopic Approach
0NRP07Z Replacement of Right Orbit with Autologous Tissue Substitute, Open Approach
0NRP0JZ Replacement of Right Orbit with Synthetic Substitute, Open Approach
0NRP0KZ Replacement of Right Orbit with Nonautologous Tissue Substitute, Open Approach
0NRP37Z Replacement of Right Orbit with Autologous Tissue Substitute, Percutaneous Approach
0NRP3JZ Replacement of Right Orbit with Synthetic Substitute, Percutaneous Approach
0NRP3KZ Replacement of Right Orbit with Nonautologous Tissue Substitute, Percutaneous Approach

RP47Z Replacement of Right Orbit with Autologous Tissue Substitute, Percutaneous Endoscopic Approach

RP4JZ Replacement of Right Orbit with Synthetic Substitute, Percutaneous Endoscopic Approach

RP4KZ Replacement of Right Orbit with Nonautologous Tissue Substitute, Percutaneous Endoscopic Approach

RQ07Z Replacement of Left Orbit with Autologous Tissue Substitute, Open Approach

NRQ0JZ Replacement of Left Orbit with Synthetic Substitute, Open Approach

NRQ0KZ Replacement of Left Orbit with Nonautologous Tissue Substitute, Open Approach

NRQ37Z Replacement of Left Orbit with Autologous Tissue Substitute, Percutaneous Approach

NRQ3JZ Replacement of Left Orbit with Synthetic Substitute, Percutaneous Approach

NRQ3KZ Replacement of Left Orbit with Nonautologous Tissue Substitute, Percutaneous Approach

NRQ47Z Replacement of Left Orbit with Autologous Tissue Substitute, Percutaneous Endoscopic Approach

NRQ4JZ Replacement of Left Orbit with Synthetic Substitute, Percutaneous Endoscopic Approach

NRQ4KZ Replacement of Left Orbit with Nonautologous Tissue Substitute, Percutaneous Endoscopic Approach

NRR07Z Replacement of Right Maxilla with Autologous Tissue Substitute, Open Approach

NRR0JZ Replacement of Right Maxilla with Synthetic Substitute, Open Approach

NRR0KZ Replacement of Right Maxilla with Nonautologous Tissue Substitute, Open Approach

NRR37Z Replacement of Right Maxilla with Autologous Tissue Substitute, Percutaneous Approach

NRR3JZ Replacement of Right Maxilla with Synthetic Substitute, Percutaneous Approach

NRR3KZ Replacement of Right Maxilla with Nonautologous Tissue Substitute, Percutaneous Approach

NRR47Z Replacement of Right Maxilla with Autologous Tissue Substitute, Percutaneous Endoscopic Approach

0NRR4JZ Replacement of Right Maxilla with Synthetic Substitute, Percutaneous Endoscopic Approach

0NRR4KZ Replacement of Right Maxilla with Nonautologous Tissue Substitute, Percutaneous Endoscopic Approach

0NRS07Z Replacement of Left Maxilla with Autologous Tissue Substitute, Open Approach

0NRS0JZ Replacement of Left Maxilla with Synthetic Substitute, Open Approach

0NRS0KZ Replacement of Left Maxilla with Nonautologous Tissue Substitute, Open Approach

0NRS37Z Replacement of Left Maxilla with Autologous Tissue Substitute, Percutaneous Approach

0NRS3JZ Replacement of Left Maxilla with Synthetic Substitute, Percutaneous Approach

0NRS3KZ Replacement of Left Maxilla with Nonautologous Tissue Substitute, Percutaneous Approach

0NRS47Z Replacement of Left Maxilla with Autologous Tissue Substitute, Percutaneous Endoscopic Approach

0NRS4JZ Replacement of Left Maxilla with Synthetic Substitute, Percutaneous Endoscopic Approach

0NRS4KZ Replacement of Left Maxilla with Nonautologous Tissue Substitute, Percutaneous Endoscopic Approach

0NRT07Z Replacement of Right Mandible with Autologous Tissue Substitute, Open Approach

0NRT0JZ Replacement of Right Mandible with Synthetic Substitute, Open Approach

0NRT0KZ Replacement of Right Mandible with Nonautologous Tissue Substitute, Open Approach

0NRT37Z Replacement of Right Mandible with Autologous Tissue Substitute, Percutaneous Approach

0NRT3JZ Replacement of Right Mandible with Synthetic Substitute, Percutaneous Approach

0NRT3KZ Replacement of Right Mandible with Nonautologous Tissue Substitute, Percutaneous Approach

0NRT47Z Replacement of Right Mandible with Autologous Tissue Substitute, Percutaneous Endoscopic Approach

0NRT4JZ Replacement of Right Mandible with Synthetic Substitute, Percutaneous Endoscopic Approach

0NRT4KZ Replacement of Right Mandible with Nonautologous Tissue Substitute, Percutaneous Endoscopic Approach

0NRV07Z Replacement of Left Mandible with Autologous Tissue Substitute, Open Approach

0NRV0JZ Replacement of Left Mandible with Synthetic Substitute, Open Approach

0NRV0KZ Replacement of Left Mandible with Nonautologous Tissue Substitute, Open Approach

0NRV37Z Replacement of Left Mandible with Autologous Tissue Substitute, Percutaneous Approach

0NRV3JZ Replacement of Left Mandible with Synthetic Substitute, Percutaneous Approach

0NRV3KZ Replacement of Left Mandible with Nonautologous Tissue Substitute, Percutaneous Approach

0NRV47Z Replacement of Left Mandible with Autologous Tissue Substitute, Percutaneous Endoscopic Approach

0NRV4JZ Replacement of Left Mandible with Synthetic Substitute, Percutaneous Endoscopic Approach

0NRV4KZ Replacement of Left Mandible with Nonautologous Tissue Substitute, Percutaneous Endoscopic Approach

0NRX07Z Replacement of Hyoid Bone with Autologous Tissue Substitute, Open Approach

0NRX0JZ Replacement of Hyoid Bone with Synthetic Substitute, Open Approach

0NRX0KZ Replacement of Hyoid Bone with Nonautologous Tissue Substitute, Open Approach

0NRX37Z Replacement of Hyoid Bone with Autologous Tissue Substitute, Percutaneous Approach

0NRX3JZ Replacement of Hyoid Bone with Synthetic Substitute, Percutaneous Approach

0NRX3KZ Replacement of Hyoid Bone with Nonautologous Tissue Substitute, Percutaneous Approach

0NRX47Z Replacement of Hyoid Bone with Autologous Tissue Substitute, Percutaneous Endoscopic Approach

0NRX4JZ Replacement of Hyoid Bone with Synthetic Substitute, Percutaneous Endoscopic Approach

0NRX4KZ Replacement of Hyoid Bone with Nonautologous Tissue Substitute, Percutaneous Endoscopic Approach

NS – Head and Facial Bones, Reposition

Review Coding Guideline B3.15

NS004Z Reposition Skull with Internal Fixation Device, Open Approach

NS005Z Reposition Skull with External Fixation Device, Open Approach
AHA CC: 3Q, 2013, 24-25

0NS00ZZ Reposition Skull, Open Approach

0NS034Z Reposition Skull with Internal Fixation Device, Percutaneous Approach

0NS035Z Reposition Skull with External Fixation Device, Percutaneous Approach

0NS03ZZ Reposition Skull, Percutaneous Approach

0NS044Z Reposition Skull with Internal Fixation Device, Percutaneous Endoscopic Approach

0NS045Z Reposition Skull with External Fixation Device, Percutaneous Endoscopic Approach

0NS04ZZ Reposition Skull, Percutaneous Endoscopic Approach

0NS0XZZ Reposition Skull, External Approach

0NS104Z Reposition Right Frontal Bone with Internal Fixation Device, Open Approach
AHA CC: 3Q, 2013, 25

0NS10ZZ Reposition Right Frontal Bone, Open Approach

0NS134Z Reposition Right Frontal Bone with Internal Fixation Device, Percutaneous Approach

0NS13ZZ Reposition Right Frontal Bone, Percutaneous Approach

0NS144Z Reposition Right Frontal Bone with Internal Fixation Device, Percutaneous Endoscopic Approach

0NS14ZZ Reposition Right Frontal Bone, Percutaneous Endoscopic Approach

0NS1XZZ Reposition Right Frontal Bone, External Approach

0NS204Z Reposition Left Frontal Bone with Internal Fixation Device, Open Approach

0NS20ZZ Reposition Left Frontal Bone, Open Approach

0NS234Z Reposition Left Frontal Bone with Internal Fixation Device, Percutaneous Approach

0NS23ZZ Reposition Left Frontal Bone, Percutaneous Approach

0NS244Z Reposition Left Frontal Bone with Internal Fixation Device, Percutaneous Endoscopic Approach

0NS24ZZ Reposition Left Frontal Bone, Percutaneous Endoscopic Approach

0NS2XZZ Reposition Left Frontal Bone, External Approach
0NS304Z Reposition Right Parietal Bone with Internal Fixation Device, Open Approach
0NS30ZZ Reposition Right Parietal Bone, Open Approach
0NS334Z Reposition Right Parietal Bone with Internal Fixation Device, Percutaneous Approach
0NS33ZZ Reposition Right Parietal Bone, Percutaneous Approach
0NS344Z Reposition Right Parietal Bone with Internal Fixation Device, Percutaneous Endoscopic Approach
0NS34ZZ Reposition Right Parietal Bone, Percutaneous Endoscopic Approach
0NS3XZZ Reposition Right Parietal Bone, External Approach
0NS404Z Reposition Left Parietal Bone with Internal Fixation Device, Open Approach
0NS40ZZ Reposition Left Parietal Bone, Open Approach
0NS434Z Reposition Left Parietal Bone with Internal Fixation Device, Percutaneous Approach
0NS43ZZ Reposition Left Parietal Bone, Percutaneous Approach
0NS444Z Reposition Left Parietal Bone with Internal Fixation Device, Percutaneous Endoscopic Approach
0NS44ZZ Reposition Left Parietal Bone, Percutaneous Endoscopic Approach
0NS4XZZ Reposition Left Parietal Bone, External Approach
0NS504Z Reposition Right Temporal Bone with Internal Fixation Device, Open Approach
0NS50ZZ Reposition Right Temporal Bone, Open Approach
0NS534Z Reposition Right Temporal Bone with Internal Fixation Device, Percutaneous Approach
0NS53ZZ Reposition Right Temporal Bone, Percutaneous Approach
0NS544Z Reposition Right Temporal Bone with Internal Fixation Device, Percutaneous Endoscopic Approach
0NS54ZZ Reposition Right Temporal Bone, Percutaneous Endoscopic Approach
0NS5XZZ Reposition Right Temporal Bone, External Approach
0NS604Z Reposition Left Temporal Bone with Internal Fixation Device, Open Approach
0NS60ZZ Reposition Left Temporal Bone, Open Approach
0NS634Z Reposition Left Temporal Bone with Internal Fixation Device, Percutaneous Approach
0NS63ZZ Reposition Left Temporal Bone, Percutaneous Approach
0NS644Z Reposition Left Temporal Bone with Internal Fixation Device, Percutaneous Endoscopic Approach
0NS64ZZ Reposition Left Temporal Bone, Percutaneous Endoscopic Approach
0NS6XZZ Reposition Left Temporal Bone, External Approach
0NS704Z Reposition Right Occipital Bone with Internal Fixation Device, Open Approach
0NS70ZZ Reposition Right Occipital Bone, Open Approach
0NS734Z Reposition Right Occipital Bone with Internal Fixation Device, Percutaneous Approach
0NS73ZZ Reposition Right Occipital Bone, Percutaneous Approach
0NS744Z Reposition Right Occipital Bone with Internal Fixation Device, Percutaneous Endoscopic Approach
0NS74ZZ Reposition Right Occipital Bone, Percutaneous Endoscopic Approach
0NS7XZZ Reposition Right Occipital Bone, External Approach
0NS804Z Reposition Left Occipital Bone with Internal Fixation Device, Open Approach
0NS80ZZ Reposition Left Occipital Bone, Open Approach
0NS834Z Reposition Left Occipital Bone with Internal Fixation Device, Percutaneous Approach
0NS83ZZ Reposition Left Occipital Bone, Percutaneous Approach
0NS844Z Reposition Left Occipital Bone with Internal Fixation Device, Percutaneous Endoscopic Approach
0NS84ZZ Reposition Left Occipital Bone, Percutaneous Endoscopic Approach
0NS8XZZ Reposition Left Occipital Bone, External Approach
0NSB04Z Reposition Nasal Bone with Internal Fixation Device, Open Approach
0NSB0ZZ Reposition Nasal Bone, Open Approach
0NSB34Z Reposition Nasal Bone with Internal Fixation Device, Percutaneous Approach
0NSB3ZZ Reposition Nasal Bone, Percutaneous Approach
0NSB44Z Reposition Nasal Bone with Internal Fixation Device, Percutaneous Endoscopic Approach
0NSB4ZZ Reposition Nasal Bone, Percutaneous Endoscopic Approach
0NSBXZZ Reposition Nasal Bone, External Approach
0NSC04Z Reposition Right Sphenoid Bone with Internal Fixation Device, Open Approach
0NSC0ZZ Reposition Right Sphenoid Bone, Open Approach
0NSC34Z Reposition Right Sphenoid Bone with Internal Fixation Device, Percutaneous Approach
0NSC3ZZ Reposition Right Sphenoid Bone, Percutaneous Approach
0NSC44Z Reposition Right Sphenoid Bone with Internal Fixation Device, Percutaneous Endoscopic Approach
0NSC4ZZ Reposition Right Sphenoid Bone, Percutaneous Endoscopic Approach
0NSCXZZ Reposition Right Sphenoid Bone, External Approach
0NSD04Z Reposition Left Sphenoid Bone with Internal Fixation Device, Open Approach
0NSD0ZZ Reposition Left Sphenoid Bone, Open Approach
0NSD34Z Reposition Left Sphenoid Bone with Internal Fixation Device, Percutaneous Approach
0NSD3ZZ Reposition Left Sphenoid Bone, Percutaneous Approach
0NSD44Z Reposition Left Sphenoid Bone with Internal Fixation Device, Percutaneous Endoscopic Approach
0NSD4ZZ Reposition Left Sphenoid Bone, Percutaneous Endoscopic Approach
0NSDXZZ Reposition Left Sphenoid Bone, External Approach
0NSF04Z Reposition Right Ethmoid Bone with Internal Fixation Device, Open Approach
0NSF0ZZ Reposition Right Ethmoid Bone, Open Approach
0NSF34Z Reposition Right Ethmoid Bone with Internal Fixation Device, Percutaneous Approach
0NSF3ZZ Reposition Right Ethmoid Bone, Percutaneous Approach
0NSF44Z Reposition Right Ethmoid Bone with Internal Fixation Device, Percutaneous Endoscopic Approach
0NSF4ZZ Reposition Right Ethmoid Bone, Percutaneous Endoscopic Approach
0NSFXZZ Reposition Right Ethmoid Bone, Extern Approach
0NSG04Z Reposition Left Ethmoid Bone with Internal Fixation Device, Open Approach
0NSG0ZZ Reposition Left Ethmoid Bone, Open Approach
0NSG34Z Reposition Left Ethmoid Bone with Internal Fixation Device, Percutaneous Approach
0NSG3ZZ Reposition Left Ethmoid Bone, Percutaneous Approach
0NSG44Z Reposition Left Ethmoid Bone with Internal Fixation Device, Percutaneous Endoscopic Approach
0NSG4ZZ Reposition Left Ethmoid Bone, Percutaneous Endoscopic Approach
0NSGXZZ Reposition Left Ethmoid Bone, External Approach
0NSH04Z Reposition Right Lacrimal Bone with Internal Fixation Device, Open Approach
0NSH0ZZ Reposition Right Lacrimal Bone, Open Approach
0NSH34Z Reposition Right Lacrimal Bone with Internal Fixation Device, Percutaneous Approach
0NSH3ZZ Reposition Right Lacrimal Bone, Percutaneous Approach
0NSH44Z Reposition Right Lacrimal Bone with Internal Fixation Device, Percutaneous Endoscopic Approach
0NSH4ZZ Reposition Right Lacrimal Bone, Percutaneous Endoscopic Approach
0NSHXZZ Reposition Right Lacrimal Bone, Externa Approach
0NSJ04Z Reposition Left Lacrimal Bone with Internal Fixation Device, Open Approach
0NSJ0ZZ Reposition Left Lacrimal Bone, Open Approach
0NSJ34Z Reposition Left Lacrimal Bone with Internal Fixation Device, Percutaneous Approach
0NSJ3ZZ Reposition Left Lacrimal Bone, Percutaneous Approach
0NSJ44Z Reposition Left Lacrimal Bone with Internal Fixation Device, Percutaneous Endoscopic Approach
0NSJ4ZZ Reposition Left Lacrimal Bone, Percutaneous Endoscopic Approach
0NSJXZZ Reposition Left Lacrimal Bone, External Approach
0NSK04Z Reposition Right Palatine Bone with Internal Fixation Device, Open Approach
0NSK0ZZ Reposition Right Palatine Bone, Open Approach
0NSK34Z Reposition Right Palatine Bone with Internal Fixation Device, Percutaneous Approach
0NSK3ZZ Reposition Right Palatine Bone, Percutaneous Approach
0NSK44Z Reposition Right Palatine Bone with Internal Fixation Device, Percutaneous Endoscopic Approach

SK4ZZ Reposition Right Palatine Bone, Percutaneous Endoscopic Approach
SKXZZ Reposition Right Palatine Bone, External Approach
SL04Z Reposition Left Palatine Bone with Internal Fixation Device, Open Approach
SL0ZZ Reposition Left Palatine Bone, Open Approach
SL34Z Reposition Left Palatine Bone with Internal Fixation Device, Percutaneous Approach
SL3ZZ Reposition Left Palatine Bone, Percutaneous Approach
SL44Z Reposition Left Palatine Bone with Internal Fixation Device, Percutaneous Endoscopic Approach
SL4ZZ Reposition Left Palatine Bone, Percutaneous Endoscopic Approach
SLXZZ Reposition Left Palatine Bone, External Approach
SM04Z Reposition Right Zygomatic Bone with Internal Fixation Device, Open Approach
SM0ZZ Reposition Right Zygomatic Bone, Open Approach
SM34Z Reposition Right Zygomatic Bone with Internal Fixation Device, Percutaneous Approach
SM3ZZ Reposition Right Zygomatic Bone, Percutaneous Approach
SM44Z Reposition Right Zygomatic Bone with Internal Fixation Device, Percutaneous Endoscopic Approach
SM4ZZ Reposition Right Zygomatic Bone, Percutaneous Endoscopic Approach
SMXZZ Reposition Right Zygomatic Bone, External Approach
SN04Z Reposition Left Zygomatic Bone with Internal Fixation Device, Open Approach
SN0ZZ Reposition Left Zygomatic Bone, Open Approach
SN34Z Reposition Left Zygomatic Bone with Internal Fixation Device, Percutaneous Approach
SN3ZZ Reposition Left Zygomatic Bone, Percutaneous Approach
SN44Z Reposition Left Zygomatic Bone with Internal Fixation Device, Percutaneous Endoscopic Approach
SN4ZZ Reposition Left Zygomatic Bone, Percutaneous Endoscopic Approach
SNXZZ Reposition Left Zygomatic Bone, External Approach
NSP04Z Reposition Right Orbit with Internal Fixation Device, Open Approach
NSP0ZZ Reposition Right Orbit, Open Approach
NSP34Z Reposition Right Orbit with Internal Fixation Device, Percutaneous Approach
NSP3ZZ Reposition Right Orbit, Percutaneous Approach
0NSP44Z Reposition Right Orbit with Internal Fixation Device, Percutaneous Endoscopic Approach
0NSP4ZZ Reposition Right Orbit, Percutaneous Endoscopic Approach
0NSPXZZ Reposition Right Orbit, External Approach
0NSQ04Z Reposition Left Orbit with Internal Fixation Device, Open Approach
0NSQ0ZZ Reposition Left Orbit, Open Approach
0NSQ34Z Reposition Left Orbit with Internal Fixation Device, Percutaneous Approach
0NSQ3ZZ Reposition Left Orbit, Percutaneous Approach
0NSQ44Z Reposition Left Orbit with Internal Fixation Device, Percutaneous Endoscopic Approach
0NSQ4ZZ Reposition Left Orbit, Percutaneous Endoscopic Approach
0NSQXZZ Reposition Left Orbit, External Approach
0NSR04Z Reposition Right Maxilla with Internal Fixation Device, Open Approach
0NSR05Z Reposition Right Maxilla with External Fixation Device, Open Approach
0NSR0ZZ Reposition Right Maxilla, Open Approach
0NSR34Z Reposition Right Maxilla with Internal Fixation Device, Percutaneous Approach
0NSR35Z Reposition Right Maxilla with External Fixation Device, Percutaneous Approach
0NSR3ZZ Reposition Right Maxilla, Percutaneous Approach
0NSR44Z Reposition Right Maxilla with Internal Fixation Device, Percutaneous Endoscopic Approach
0NSR45Z Reposition Right Maxilla with External Fixation Device, Percutaneous Endoscopic Approach
0NSR4ZZ Reposition Right Maxilla, Percutaneous Endoscopic Approach
0NSRXZZ Reposition Right Maxilla, External Approach
0NSS04Z Reposition Left Maxilla with Internal Fixation Device, Open Approach
0NSS05Z Reposition Left Maxilla with External Fixation Device, Open Approach
0NSS0ZZ Reposition Left Maxilla, Open Approach
0NSS34Z Reposition Left Maxilla with Internal Fixation Device, Percutaneous Approach
0NSS35Z Reposition Left Maxilla with External Fixation Device, Percutaneous Approach
0NSS3ZZ Reposition Left Maxilla, Percutaneous Approach
0NSS44Z Reposition Left Maxilla with Internal Fixation Device, Percutaneous Endoscopic Approach
0NSS45Z Reposition Left Maxilla with External Fixation Device, Percutaneous Endoscopic Approach
0NSS4ZZ Reposition Left Maxilla, Percutaneous Endoscopic Approach
0NSSXZZ Reposition Left Maxilla, External Approach
0NST04Z Reposition Right Mandible with Internal Fixation Device, Open Approach
0NST05Z Reposition Right Mandible with External Fixation Device, Open Approach
0NST0ZZ Reposition Right Mandible, Open Approach
0NST34Z Reposition Right Mandible with Internal Fixation Device, Percutaneous Approach
0NST35Z Reposition Right Mandible with External Fixation Device, Percutaneous Approach
0NST3ZZ Reposition Right Mandible, Percutaneous Approach
0NST44Z Reposition Right Mandible with Internal Fixation Device, Percutaneous Endoscopic Approach
0NST45Z Reposition Right Mandible with External Fixation Device, Percutaneous Endoscopic Approach
0NST4ZZ Reposition Right Mandible, Percutaneous Endoscopic Approach
0NSTXZZ Reposition Right Mandible, External Approach
0NSV04Z Reposition Left Mandible with Internal Fixation Device, Open Approach
0NSV05Z Reposition Left Mandible with External Fixation Device, Open Approach
0NSV0ZZ Reposition Left Mandible, Open Approach
0NSV34Z Reposition Left Mandible with Internal Fixation Device, Percutaneous Approach
0NSV35Z Reposition Left Mandible with External Fixation Device, Percutaneous Approach
0NSV3ZZ Reposition Left Mandible, Percutaneous Approach
0NSV44Z Reposition Left Mandible with Internal Fixation Device, Percutaneous Endoscopic Approach
0NSV45Z Reposition Left Mandible with External Fixation Device, Percutaneous Endoscopic Approach
0NSV4ZZ Reposition Left Mandible, Percutaneous Endoscopic Approach
0NSVXZZ Reposition Left Mandible, External Approach
0NSX04Z Reposition Hyoid Bone with Internal Fixation Device, Open Approach
0NSX0ZZ Reposition Hyoid Bone, Open Approach
0NSX34Z Reposition Hyoid Bone with Internal Fixation Device, Percutaneous Approach
0NSX3ZZ Reposition Hyoid Bone, Percutaneous Approach
0NSX44Z Reposition Hyoid Bone with Internal Fixation Device, Percutaneous Endoscopic Approach
0NSX4ZZ Reposition Hyoid Bone, Percutaneous Endoscopic Approach
0NSXXZZ Reposition Hyoid Bone, External Approach

NT – Head and Facial Bones, Resection

Review Coding Guideline B3.8

NT10ZZ Resection of Right Frontal Bone, Open Approach
NT20ZZ Resection of Left Frontal Bone, Open Approach
NT30ZZ Resection of Right Parietal Bone, Open Approach
NT40ZZ Resection of Left Parietal Bone, Open Approach
NT50ZZ Resection of Right Temporal Bone, Open Approach
0NT60ZZ Resection of Left Temporal Bone, Open Approach
0NT70ZZ Resection of Right Occipital Bone, Open Approach
0NT80ZZ Resection of Left Occipital Bone, Open Approach
0NTB0ZZ Resection of Nasal Bone, Open Approach
0NTC0ZZ Resection of Right Sphenoid Bone, Open Approach
0NTD0ZZ Resection of Left Sphenoid Bone, Open Approach
0NTF0ZZ Resection of Right Ethmoid Bone, Open Approach
0NTG0ZZ Resection of Left Ethmoid Bone, Open Approach
0NTH0ZZ Resection of Right Lacrimal Bone, Open Approach
0NTJ0ZZ Resection of Left Lacrimal Bone, Open Approach
0NTK0ZZ Resection of Right Palatine Bone, Open Approach
0NTL0ZZ Resection of Left Palatine Bone, Open Approach
0NTM0ZZ Resection of Right Zygomatic Bone, Open Approach

0NTN0ZZ Resection of Left Zygomatic Bone, Open Approach
0NTP0ZZ Resection of Right Orbit, Open Approach
0NTQ0ZZ Resection of Left Orbit, Open Approach
0NTR0ZZ Resection of Right Maxilla, Open Approach
0NTS0ZZ Resection of Left Maxilla, Open Approach
0NTT0ZZ Resection of Right Mandible, Open Approach
0NTV0ZZ Resection of Left Mandible, Open Approach
0NTX0ZZ Resection of Hyoid Bone, Open Appro...

0NU – Head and Facial Bones, Supplement

0NU007Z Supplement Skull with Autologous Tissue Substitute, Open Approach
0NU00JZ Supplement Skull with Synthetic Substitute, Open Approach
AHA CC: 3Q, 2013, 24-25
0NU00KZ Supplement Skull with Nonautologous Tissue Substitute, Open Approach
0NU037Z Supplement Skull with Autologous Tissue Substitute, Percutaneous Approach
0NU03JZ Supplement Skull with Synthetic Substitute, Percutaneous Approach
0NU03KZ Supplement Skull with Nonautologous Tissue Substitute, Percutaneous Approach
0NU047Z Supplement Skull with Autologous Tissue Substitute, Percutaneous Endoscopic Approach
0NU04JZ Supplement Skull with Synthetic Substitute, Percutaneous Endoscopic Approach
0NU04KZ Supplement Skull with Nonautologous Tissue Substitute, Percutaneous Endoscopic Approach
0NU107Z Supplement Right Frontal Bone with Autologous Tissue Substitute, Open Approach
0NU10JZ Supplement Right Frontal Bone with Synthetic Substitute, Open Approach
0NU10KZ Supplement Right Frontal Bone with Nonautologous Tissue Substitute, Open Approach
0NU137Z Supplement Right Frontal Bone with Autologous Tissue Substitute, Percutaneous Approach
0NU13JZ Supplement Right Frontal Bone with Synthetic Substitute, Percutaneous Approach
0NU13KZ Supplement Right Frontal Bone with Nonautologous Tissue Substitute, Percutaneous Approach
0NU147Z Supplement Right Frontal Bone with Autologous Tissue Substitute, Percutaneous Endoscopic Approach
0NU14JZ Supplement Right Frontal Bone with Synthetic Substitute, Percutaneous Endoscopic Approach
0NU14KZ Supplement Right Frontal Bone with Nonautologous Tissue Substitute, Percutaneous Endoscopic Approach
0NU207Z Supplement Left Frontal Bone with Autologous Tissue Substitute, Open Approach
0NU20JZ Supplement Left Frontal Bone with Synthetic Substitute, Open Approach
0NU20KZ Supplement Left Frontal Bone with Nonautologous Tissue Substitute, Open Approach
0NU237Z Supplement Left Frontal Bone with Autologous Tissue Substitute, Percutaneous Approach
0NU23JZ Supplement Left Frontal Bone with Synthetic Substitute, Percutaneous Approach
0NU23KZ Supplement Left Frontal Bone with Nonautologous Tissue Substitute, Percutaneous Approach
0NU247Z Supplement Left Frontal Bone with Autologous Tissue Substitute, Percutaneous Endoscopic Approach
0NU24JZ Supplement Left Frontal Bone with Synthetic Substitute, Percutaneous Endoscopic Approach
0NU24KZ Supplement Left Frontal Bone with Nonautologous Tissue Substitute, Percutaneous Endoscopic Approach
0NU307Z Supplement Right Parietal Bone with Autologous Tissue Substitute, Open Approach
0NU30JZ Supplement Right Parietal Bone with Synthetic Substitute, Open Approach
0NU30KZ Supplement Right Parietal Bone with Nonautologous Tissue Substitute, Open Approach
0NU337Z Supplement Right Parietal Bone with Autologous Tissue Substitute, Percutaneous Approach
0NU33JZ Supplement Right Parietal Bone with Synthetic Substitute, Percutaneous Approach
0NU33KZ Supplement Right Parietal Bone with Nonautologous Tissue Substitute, Percutaneous Approach
0NU347Z Supplement Right Parietal Bone with Autologous Tissue Substitute, Percutaneous Endoscopic Approach
0NU34JZ Supplement Right Parietal Bone with Synthetic Substitute, Percutaneous Endoscopic Approach
0NU34KZ Supplement Right Parietal Bone with Nonautologous Tissue Substitute, Percutaneous Endoscopic Approach
0NU407Z Supplement Left Parietal Bone with Autologous Tissue Substitute, Open Approach
0NU40JZ Supplement Left Parietal Bone with Synthetic Substitute, Open Approach
0NU40KZ Supplement Left Parietal Bone with Nonautologous Tissue Substitute, Open Approach
0NU437Z Supplement Left Parietal Bone with Autologous Tissue Substitute, Percutaneous Approach
0NU43JZ Supplement Left Parietal Bone with Synthetic Substitute, Percutaneous Approach
0NU43KZ Supplement Left Parietal Bone with Nonautologous Tissue Substitute, Percutaneous Approach
0NU447Z Supplement Left Parietal Bone with Autologous Tissue Substitute, Percutaneous Endoscopic Approach
0NU44JZ Supplement Left Parietal Bone with Synthetic Substitute, Percutaneous Endoscopic Approach
0NU44KZ Supplement Left Parietal Bone with Nonautologous Tissue Substitute, Percutaneous Endoscopic Approach
0NU507Z Supplement Right Temporal Bone with Autologous Tissue Substitute, Open Approach
0NU50JZ Supplement Right Temporal Bone with Synthetic Substitute, Open Approach
0NU50KZ Supplement Right Temporal Bone with Nonautologous Tissue Substitute, Open Approach
0NU537Z Supplement Right Temporal Bone with Autologous Tissue Substitute, Percutaneous Approach
0NU53JZ Supplement Right Temporal Bone with Synthetic Substitute, Percutaneous Approach
0NU53KZ Supplement Right Temporal Bone with Nonautologous Tissue Substitute, Percutaneous Approach
0NU547Z Supplement Right Temporal Bone with Autologous Tissue Substitute, Percutaneous Endoscopic Approach
0NU54JZ Supplement Right Temporal Bone with Synthetic Substitute, Percutaneous Endoscopic Approach
0NU54KZ Supplement Right Temporal Bone with Nonautologous Tissue Substitute, Percutaneous Endoscopic Approach
0NU607Z Supplement Left Temporal Bone with Autologous Tissue Substitute, Open Approach
0NU60JZ Supplement Left Temporal Bone with Synthetic Substitute, Open Approach
0NU60KZ Supplement Left Temporal Bone with Nonautologous Tissue Substitute, Open Approach
0NU637Z Supplement Left Temporal Bone with Autologous Tissue Substitute, Percutaneous Approach
0NU63JZ Supplement Left Temporal Bone with Synthetic Substitute, Percutaneous Approach
0NU63KZ Supplement Left Temporal Bone with Nonautologous Tissue Substitute, Percutaneous Approach
0NU647Z Supplement Left Temporal Bone with Autologous Tissue Substitute, Percutaneous Endoscopic Approach
0NU64JZ Supplement Left Temporal Bone with Synthetic Substitute, Percutaneous Endoscopic Approach
0NU64KZ Supplement Left Temporal Bone with Nonautologous Tissue Substitute, Percutaneous Endoscopic Approach
0NU707Z Supplement Right Occipital Bone with Autologous Tissue Substitute, Open Approach
0NU70JZ Supplement Right Occipital Bone with Synthetic Substitute, Open Approach
0NU70KZ Supplement Right Occipital Bone with Nonautologous Tissue Substitute, Open Approach
0NU737Z Supplement Right Occipital Bone with Autologous Tissue Substitute, Percutaneous Approach
0NU73JZ Supplement Right Occipital Bone with Synthetic Substitute, Percutaneous Approach
0NU73KZ Supplement Right Occipital Bone with Nonautologous Tissue Substitute, Percutaneous Approach
0NU747Z Supplement Right Occipital Bone with Autologous Tissue Substitute, Percutaneous Endoscopic Approach
0NU74JZ Supplement Right Occipital Bone with Synthetic Substitute, Percutaneous Endoscopic Approach
0NU74KZ Supplement Right Occipital Bone with Nonautologous Tissue Substitute, Percutaneous Endoscopic Approach

U807Z Supplement Left Occipital Bone with Autologous Tissue Substitute, Open Approach

U80JZ Supplement Left Occipital Bone with Synthetic Substitute, Open Approach

U80KZ Supplement Left Occipital Bone with Nonautologous Tissue Substitute, Open Approach

U837Z Supplement Left Occipital Bone with Autologous Tissue Substitute, Percutaneous Approach

U83JZ Supplement Left Occipital Bone with Synthetic Substitute, Percutaneous Approach

U83KZ Supplement Left Occipital Bone with Nonautologous Tissue Substitute, Percutaneous Approach

U847Z Supplement Left Occipital Bone with Autologous Tissue Substitute, Percutaneous Endoscopic Approach

U84JZ Supplement Left Occipital Bone with Synthetic Substitute, Percutaneous Endoscopic Approach

U84KZ Supplement Left Occipital Bone with Nonautologous Tissue Substitute, Percutaneous Endoscopic Approach

UB07Z Supplement Nasal Bone with Autologous Tissue Substitute, Open Approach

UB0JZ Supplement Nasal Bone with Synthetic Substitute, Open Approach

UB0KZ Supplement Nasal Bone with Nonautologous Tissue Substitute, Open Approach

UB37Z Supplement Nasal Bone with Autologous Tissue Substitute, Percutaneous Approach

NUB3JZ Supplement Nasal Bone with Synthetic Substitute, Percutaneous Approach

NUB3KZ Supplement Nasal Bone with Nonautologous Tissue Substitute, Percutaneous Approach

NUB47Z Supplement Nasal Bone with Autologous Tissue Substitute, Percutaneous Endoscopic Approach

NUB4JZ Supplement Nasal Bone with Synthetic Substitute, Percutaneous Endoscopic Approach

NUB4KZ Supplement Nasal Bone with Nonautologous Tissue Substitute, Percutaneous Endoscopic Approach

NUC07Z Supplement Right Sphenoid Bone with Autologous Tissue Substitute, Open Approach

NUC0JZ Supplement Right Sphenoid Bone with Synthetic Substitute, Open Approach

NUC0KZ Supplement Right Sphenoid Bone with Nonautologous Tissue Substitute, Open Approach

NUC37Z Supplement Right Sphenoid Bone with Autologous Tissue Substitute, Percutaneous Approach

NUC3JZ Supplement Right Sphenoid Bone with Synthetic Substitute, Percutaneous Approach

NUC3KZ Supplement Right Sphenoid Bone with Nonautologous Tissue Substitute, Percutaneous Approach

NUC47Z Supplement Right Sphenoid Bone with Autologous Tissue Substitute, Percutaneous Endoscopic Approach

NUC4JZ Supplement Right Sphenoid Bone with Synthetic Substitute, Percutaneous Endoscopic Approach

NUC4KZ Supplement Right Sphenoid Bone with Nonautologous Tissue Substitute, Percutaneous Endoscopic Approach

0NUD07Z Supplement Left Sphenoid Bone with Autologous Tissue Substitute, Open Approach

0NUD0JZ Supplement Left Sphenoid Bone with Synthetic Substitute, Open Approach

0NUD0KZ Supplement Left Sphenoid Bone with Nonautologous Tissue Substitute, Open Approach

0NUD37Z Supplement Left Sphenoid Bone with Autologous Tissue Substitute, Percutaneous Approach

0NUD3JZ Supplement Left Sphenoid Bone with Synthetic Substitute, Percutaneous Approach

0NUD3KZ Supplement Left Sphenoid Bone with Nonautologous Tissue Substitute, Percutaneous Approach

0NUD47Z Supplement Left Sphenoid Bone with Autologous Tissue Substitute, Percutaneous Endoscopic Approach

0NUD4JZ Supplement Left Sphenoid Bone with Synthetic Substitute, Percutaneous Endoscopic Approach

0NUD4KZ Supplement Left Sphenoid Bone with Nonautologous Tissue Substitute, Percutaneous Endoscopic Approach

0NUF07Z Supplement Right Ethmoid Bone with Autologous Tissue Substitute, Open Approach

0NUF0JZ Supplement Right Ethmoid Bone with Synthetic Substitute, Open Approach

0NUF0KZ Supplement Right Ethmoid Bone with Nonautologous Tissue Substitute, Open Approach

0NUF37Z Supplement Right Ethmoid Bone with Autologous Tissue Substitute, Percutaneous Approach

0NUF3JZ Supplement Right Ethmoid Bone with Synthetic Substitute, Percutaneous Approach

0NUF3KZ Supplement Right Ethmoid Bone with Nonautologous Tissue Substitute, Percutaneous Approach

0NUF47Z Supplement Right Ethmoid Bone with Autologous Tissue Substitute, Percutaneous Endoscopic Approach

0NUF4JZ Supplement Right Ethmoid Bone with Synthetic Substitute, Percutaneous Endoscopic Approach

0NUF4KZ Supplement Right Ethmoid Bone with Nonautologous Tissue Substitute, Percutaneous Endoscopic Approach

0NUG07Z Supplement Left Ethmoid Bone with Autologous Tissue Substitute, Open Approach

0NUG0JZ Supplement Left Ethmoid Bone with Synthetic Substitute, Open Approach

0NUG0KZ Supplement Left Ethmoid Bone with Nonautologous Tissue Substitute, Open Approach

0NUG37Z Supplement Left Ethmoid Bone with Autologous Tissue Substitute, Percutaneous Approach

0NUG3JZ Supplement Left Ethmoid Bone with Synthetic Substitute, Percutaneous Approach

0NUG3KZ Supplement Left Ethmoid Bone with Nonautologous Tissue Substitute, Percutaneous Approach

0NUG47Z Supplement Left Ethmoid Bone with Autologous Tissue Substitute, Percutaneous Endoscopic Approach

0NUG4JZ Supplement Left Ethmoid Bone with Synthetic Substitute, Percutaneous Endoscopic Approach

0NUG4KZ Supplement Left Ethmoid Bone with Nonautologous Tissue Substitute, Percutaneous Endoscopic Approach

0NUH07Z Supplement Right Lacrimal Bone with Autologous Tissue Substitute, Open Approach

0NUH0JZ Supplement Right Lacrimal Bone with Synthetic Substitute, Open Approach

0NUH0KZ Supplement Right Lacrimal Bone with Nonautologous Tissue Substitute, Open Approach

0NUH37Z Supplement Right Lacrimal Bone with Autologous Tissue Substitute, Percutaneous Approach

0NUH3JZ Supplement Right Lacrimal Bone with Synthetic Substitute, Percutaneous Approach

0NUH3KZ Supplement Right Lacrimal Bone with Nonautologous Tissue Substitute, Percutaneous Approach

0NUH47Z Supplement Right Lacrimal Bone with Autologous Tissue Substitute, Percutaneous Endoscopic Approach

0NUH4JZ Supplement Right Lacrimal Bone with Synthetic Substitute, Percutaneous Endoscopic Approach

0NUH4KZ Supplement Right Lacrimal Bone with Nonautologous Tissue Substitute, Percutaneous Endoscopic Approach

0NUJ07Z Supplement Left Lacrimal Bone with Autologous Tissue Substitute, Open Approach

0NUJ0JZ Supplement Left Lacrimal Bone with Synthetic Substitute, Open Approach

0NUJ0KZ Supplement Left Lacrimal Bone with Nonautologous Tissue Substitute, Open Approach

0NUJ37Z Supplement Left Lacrimal Bone with Autologous Tissue Substitute, Percutaneous Approach

0NUJ3JZ Supplement Left Lacrimal Bone with Synthetic Substitute, Percutaneous Approach

0NUJ3KZ Supplement Left Lacrimal Bone with Nonautologous Tissue Substitute, Percutaneous Approach

0NUJ47Z Supplement Left Lacrimal Bone with Autologous Tissue Substitute, Percutaneous Endoscopic Approach

0NUJ4JZ Supplement Left Lacrimal Bone with Synthetic Substitute, Percutaneous Endoscopic Approach

0NUJ4KZ Supplement Left Lacrimal Bone with Nonautologous Tissue Substitute, Percutaneous Endoscopic Approach

0NUK07Z Supplement Right Palatine Bone with Autologous Tissue Substitute, Open Approach

0NUK0JZ Supplement Right Palatine Bone with Synthetic Substitute, Open Approach

0NUK0KZ Supplement Right Palatine Bone with Nonautologous Tissue Substitute, Open Approach

0NUK37Z Supplement Right Palatine Bone with Autologous Tissue Substitute, Percutaneous Approach

0NUK3JZ Supplement Right Palatine Bone with Synthetic Substitute, Percutaneous Approach

0NUK3KZ Supplement Right Palatine Bone with Nonautologous Tissue Substitute, Percutaneous Approach

0NUK47Z Supplement Right Palatine Bone with Autologous Tissue Substitute, Percutaneous Endoscopic Approach

0NUK4JZ Supplement Right Palatine Bone with Synthetic Substitute, Percutaneous Endoscopic Approach

0NUK4KZ Supplement Right Palatine Bone with Nonautologous Tissue Substitute, Percutaneous Endoscopic Approach

0NUL07Z Supplement Left Palatine Bone with Autologous Tissue Substitute, Open Approach

0NUL0JZ Supplement Left Palatine Bone with Synthetic Substitute, Open Approach

0NUL0KZ Supplement Left Palatine Bone with Nonautologous Tissue Substitute, Open Approach

0NUL37Z Supplement Left Palatine Bone with Autologous Tissue Substitute, Percutaneous Approach

0NUL3JZ Supplement Left Palatine Bone with Synthetic Substitute, Percutaneous Approach

0NUL3KZ Supplement Left Palatine Bone with Nonautologous Tissue Substitute, Percutaneous Approach

0NUL47Z Supplement Left Palatine Bone with Autologous Tissue Substitute, Percutaneous Endoscopic Approach

0NUL4JZ Supplement Left Palatine Bone with Synthetic Substitute, Percutaneous Endoscopic Approach

0NUL4KZ Supplement Left Palatine Bone with Nonautologous Tissue Substitute, Percutaneous Endoscopic Approach

0NUM07Z Supplement Right Zygomatic Bone with Autologous Tissue Substitute, Open Approach

0NUM0JZ Supplement Right Zygomatic Bone with Synthetic Substitute, Open Approach

0NUM0KZ Supplement Right Zygomatic Bone with Nonautologous Tissue Substitute, Open Approach

0NUM37Z Supplement Right Zygomatic Bone with Autologous Tissue Substitute, Percutaneous Approach

0NUM3JZ Supplement Right Zygomatic Bone with Synthetic Substitute, Percutaneous Approach

0NUM3KZ Supplement Right Zygomatic Bone with Nonautologous Tissue Substitute, Percutaneous Approach

0NUM47Z Supplement Right Zygomatic Bone with Autologous Tissue Substitute, Percutaneous Endoscopic Approach

0NUM4JZ Supplement Right Zygomatic Bone with Synthetic Substitute, Percutaneous Endoscopic Approach

0NUM4KZ Supplement Right Zygomatic Bone with Nonautologous Tissue Substitute, Percutaneous Endoscopic Approach

0NUN07Z Supplement Left Zygomatic Bone with Autologous Tissue Substitute, Open Approach

0NUN0JZ Supplement Left Zygomatic Bone with Synthetic Substitute, Open Approach

0NUN0KZ Supplement Left Zygomatic Bone with Nonautologous Tissue Substitute, Open Approach

0NUN37Z Supplement Left Zygomatic Bone with Autologous Tissue Substitute, Percutaneous Approach

0NUN3JZ Supplement Left Zygomatic Bone with Synthetic Substitute, Percutaneous Approach

0NUN3KZ Supplement Left Zygomatic Bone with Nonautologous Tissue Substitute, Percutaneous Approach

0NUN47Z Supplement Left Zygomatic Bone with Autologous Tissue Substitute, Percutaneous Endoscopic Approach

0NUN4JZ Supplement Left Zygomatic Bone with Synthetic Substitute, Percutaneous Endoscopic Approach

0NUN4KZ Supplement Left Zygomatic Bone with Nonautologous Tissue Substitute, Percutaneous Endoscopic Approach

0NUP07Z Supplement Right Orbit with Autologous Tissue Substitute, Open Approach

0NUP0JZ Supplement Right Orbit with Synthetic Substitute, Open Approach

0NUP0KZ Supplement Right Orbit with Nonautologous Tissue Substitute, Open Approach

0NUP37Z Supplement Right Orbit with Autologous Tissue Substitute, Percutaneous Approach

0NUP3JZ Supplement Right Orbit with Synthetic Substitute, Percutaneous Approach

0NUP3KZ Supplement Right Orbit with Nonautologous Tissue Substitute, Percutaneous Approach

0NUP47Z Supplement Right Orbit with Autologous Tissue Substitute, Percutaneous Endoscopic Approach

0NUP4JZ Supplement Right Orbit with Synthetic Substitute, Percutaneous Endoscopic Approach

0NUP4KZ Supplement Right Orbit with Nonautologous Tissue Substitute, Percutaneous Endoscopic Approach

0NUQ07Z Supplement Left Orbit with Autologous Tissue Substitute, Open Approach

0NUQ0JZ Supplement Left Orbit with Synthetic Substitute, Open Approach

0NUQ0KZ Supplement Left Orbit with Nonautologous Tissue Substitute, Open Approach

0NUQ37Z Supplement Left Orbit with Autologous Tissue Substitute, Percutaneous Approach

0NUQ3JZ Supplement Left Orbit with Synthetic Substitute, Percutaneous Approach

0NUQ3KZ Supplement Left Orbit with Nonautologous Tissue Substitute, Percutaneous Approach

0NUQ47Z Supplement Left Orbit with Autologous Tissue Substitute, Percutaneous Endoscopic Approach

0NUQ4JZ Supplement Left Orbit with Synthetic Substitute, Percutaneous Endoscopic Approach

0NUQ4KZ Supplement Left Orbit with Nonautologous Tissue Substitute, Percutaneous Endoscopic Approach

0NUR07Z Supplement Right Maxilla with Autologous Tissue Substitute, Open Approach

0NUR0JZ Supplement Right Maxilla with Synthetic Substitute, Open Approach

0NUR0KZ Supplement Right Maxilla with Nonautologous Tissue Substitute, Open Approach

0NUR37Z Supplement Right Maxilla with Autologous Tissue Substitute, Percutaneous Approach

0NUR3JZ Supplement Right Maxilla with Synthetic Substitute, Percutaneous Approach

0NUR3KZ Supplement Right Maxilla with Nonautologous Tissue Substitute, Percutaneous Approach

0NUR47Z Supplement Right Maxilla with Autologous Tissue Substitute, Percutaneous Endoscopic Approach

0NUR4JZ Supplement Right Maxilla with Synthetic Substitute, Percutaneous Endoscopic Approach

0NUR4KZ Supplement Right Maxilla with Nonautologous Tissue Substitute, Percutaneous Endoscopic Approach

0NUS07Z Supplement Left Maxilla with Autolog Tissue Substitute, Open Approach

0NUS0JZ Supplement Left Maxilla with Synthet Substitute, Open Approach

0NUS0KZ Supplement Left Maxilla with Nonautologous Tissue Substitute, Oper Approach

0NUS37Z Supplement Left Maxilla with Autologous Tissue Substitute, Percutaneous Approach

0NUS3JZ Supplement Left Maxilla with Syntheti Substitute, Percutaneous Approach

0NUS3KZ Supplement Left Maxilla with Nonautologous Tissue Substitute, Percutaneous Approach

0NUS47Z Supplement Left Maxilla with Autolog Tissue Substitute, Percutaneous Endoscopic Approach

0NUS4JZ Supplement Left Maxilla with Syntheti Substitute, Percutaneous Endoscopic Approach

0NUS4KZ Supplement Left Maxilla with Nonautologous Tissue Substitute, Percutaneous Endoscopic Approach

0NUT07Z Supplement Right Mandible with Autologous Tissue Substitute, Open Approach

0NUT0JZ Supplement Right Mandible with Synthetic Substitute, Open Approach

0NUT0KZ Supplement Right Mandible with Nonautologous Tissue Substitute, Open Approach

0NUT37Z Supplement Right Mandible with Autologous Tissue Substitute, Percutaneous Approach

0NUT3JZ Supplement Right Mandible with Synthetic Substitute, Percutaneous Approach

0NUT3KZ Supplement Right Mandible with Nonautologous Tissue Substitute, Percutaneous Approach

0NUT47Z Supplement Right Mandible with Autologous Tissue Substitute, Percutaneous Endoscopic Approach

0NUT4JZ Supplement Right Mandible with Synthetic Substitute, Percutaneous Endoscopic Approach

0NUT4KZ Supplement Right Mandible with Nonautologous Tissue Substitute, Percutaneous Endoscopic Approach

0NUV07Z Supplement Left Mandible with Autologous Tissue Substitute, Open Approach

0NUV0JZ Supplement Left Mandible with Syntheti Substitute, Open Approach

0NUV0KZ Supplement Left Mandible with Nonautologous Tissue Substitute, Open Approach

0NUV37Z Supplement Left Mandible with Autologous Tissue Substitute, Percutaneous Approach

0NUV3JZ Supplement Left Mandible with Syntheti Substitute, Percutaneous Approach

0NUV3KZ Supplement Left Mandible with Nonautologous Tissue Substitute, Percutaneous Approach

0NUV47Z Supplement Left Mandible with Autologous Tissue Substitute, Percutaneous Endoscopic Approach

0NUV4JZ Supplement Left Mandible with Syntheti Substitute, Percutaneous Endoscopic Approach

0NUV4KZ Supplement Left Mandible with Nonautologous Tissue Substitute, Percutaneous Endoscopic Approach

0NUX07Z Supplement Hyoid Bone with Autologous Tissue Substitute, Open Approach

UX0JZ Supplement Hyoid Bone with Synthetic Substitute, Open Approach

UX0KZ Supplement Hyoid Bone with Nonautologous Tissue Substitute, Open Approach

UX37Z Supplement Hyoid Bone with Autologous Tissue Substitute, Percutaneous Approach

0NUX3JZ Supplement Hyoid Bone with Synthetic Substitute, Percutaneous Approach

0NUX3KZ Supplement Hyoid Bone with Nonautologous Tissue Substitute, Percutaneous Approach

0NUX47Z Supplement Hyoid Bone with Autologous Tissue Substitute, Percutaneous Endoscopic Approach

0NUX4JZ Supplement Hyoid Bone with Synthetic Substitute, Percutaneous Endoscopic Approach

0NUX4KZ Supplement Hyoid Bone with Nonautologous Tissue Substitute, Percutaneous Endoscopic Approach

NW – Head and Facial Bones, Revision

eview Coding Guideline B6.1c

W000Z Revision of Drainage Device in Skull, Open Approach

W004Z Revision of Internal Fixation Device in Skull, Open Approach

W005Z Revision of External Fixation Device in Skull, Open Approach

W007Z Revision of Autologous Tissue Substitute in Skull, Open Approach

W00JZ Revision of Synthetic Substitute in Skull, Open Approach

NW00KZ Revision of Nonautologous Tissue Substitute in Skull, Open Approach

NW00MZ Revision of Bone Growth Stimulator in Skull, Open Approach

NW00NZ Revision of Neurostimulator Generator in Skull, Open Approach

NW00SZ Revision of Hearing Device in Skull, Open Approach

NW030Z Revision of Drainage Device in Skull, Percutaneous Approach

NW034Z Revision of Internal Fixation Device in Skull, Percutaneous Approach

NW035Z Revision of External Fixation Device in Skull, Percutaneous Approach

NW037Z Revision of Autologous Tissue Substitute in Skull, Percutaneous Approach

NW03JZ Revision of Synthetic Substitute in Skull, Percutaneous Approach

NW03KZ Revision of Nonautologous Tissue Substitute in Skull, Percutaneous Approach

NW03MZ Revision of Bone Growth Stimulator in Skull, Percutaneous Approach

NW03SZ Revision of Hearing Device in Skull, Percutaneous Approach

NW040Z Revision of Drainage Device in Skull, Percutaneous Endoscopic Approach

NW044Z Revision of Internal Fixation Device in Skull, Percutaneous Endoscopic Approach

NW045Z Revision of External Fixation Device in Skull, Percutaneous Endoscopic Approach

NW047Z Revision of Autologous Tissue Substitute in Skull, Percutaneous Endoscopic Approach

NW04JZ Revision of Synthetic Substitute in Skull, Percutaneous Endoscopic Approach

NW04KZ Revision of Nonautologous Tissue Substitute in Skull, Percutaneous Endoscopic Approach

NW04MZ Revision of Bone Growth Stimulator in Skull, Percutaneous Endoscopic Approach

0NW04SZ Revision of Hearing Device in Skull, Percutaneous Endoscopic Approach

0NW0X0Z Revision of Drainage Device in Skull, External Approach

0NW0X4Z Revision of Internal Fixation Device in Skull, External Approach

0NW0X5Z Revision of External Fixation Device in Skull, External Approach

0NW0X7Z Revision of Autologous Tissue Substitute in Skull, External Approach

0NW0XJZ Revision of Synthetic Substitute in Skull, External Approach

0NW0XKZ Revision of Nonautologous Tissue Substitute in Skull, External Approach

0NW0XMZ Revision of Bone Growth Stimulator in Skull, External Approach

0NW0XSZ Revision of Hearing Device in Skull, External Approach

0NWB00Z Revision of Drainage Device in Nasal Bone, Open Approach

0NWB04Z Revision of Internal Fixation Device in Nasal Bone, Open Approach

0NWB07Z Revision of Autologous Tissue Substitute in Nasal Bone, Open Approach

0NWB0JZ Revision of Synthetic Substitute in Nasal Bone, Open Approach

0NWB0KZ Revision of Nonautologous Tissue Substitute in Nasal Bone, Open Approach

0NWB0MZ Revision of Bone Growth Stimulator in Nasal Bone, Open Approach

0NWB30Z Revision of Drainage Device in Nasal Bone, Percutaneous Approach

0NWB34Z Revision of Internal Fixation Device in Nasal Bone, Percutaneous Approach

0NWB37Z Revision of Autologous Tissue Substitute in Nasal Bone, Percutaneous Approach

0NWB3JZ Revision of Synthetic Substitute in Nasal Bone, Percutaneous Approach

0NWB3KZ Revision of Nonautologous Tissue Substitute in Nasal Bone, Percutaneous Approach

0NWB3MZ Revision of Bone Growth Stimulator in Nasal Bone, Percutaneous Approach

0NWB40Z Revision of Drainage Device in Nasal Bone, Percutaneous Endoscopic Approach

0NWB44Z Revision of Internal Fixation Device in Nasal Bone, Percutaneous Endoscopic Approach

0NWB47Z Revision of Autologous Tissue Substitute in Nasal Bone, Percutaneous Endoscopic Approach

0NWB4JZ Revision of Synthetic Substitute in Nasal Bone, Percutaneous Endoscopic Approach

0NWB4KZ Revision of Nonautologous Tissue Substitute in Nasal Bone, Percutaneous Endoscopic Approach

0NWB4MZ Revision of Bone Growth Stimulator in Nasal Bone, Percutaneous Endoscopic Approach

0NWBX0Z Revision of Drainage Device in Nasal Bone, External Approach

0NWBX4Z Revision of Internal Fixation Device in Nasal Bone, External Approach

0NWBX7Z Revision of Autologous Tissue Substitute in Nasal Bone, External Approach

0NWBXJZ Revision of Synthetic Substitute in Nasal Bone, External Approach

0NWBXKZ Revision of Nonautologous Tissue Substitute in Nasal Bone, External Approach

0NWBXMZ Revision of Bone Growth Stimulator in Nasal Bone, External Approach

0NWW00Z Revision of Drainage Device in Facial Bone, Open Approach

0NWW04Z Revision of Internal Fixation Device in Facial Bone, Open Approach

0NWW07Z Revision of Autologous Tissue Substitute in Facial Bone, Open Approach

0NWW0JZ Revision of Synthetic Substitute in Facial Bone, Open Approach

0NWW0KZ Revision of Nonautologous Tissue Substitute in Facial Bone, Open Approach

0NWW0MZ Revision of Bone Growth Stimulator in Facial Bone, Open Approach

0NWW30Z Revision of Drainage Device in Facial Bone, Percutaneous Approach

0NWW34Z Revision of Internal Fixation Device in Facial Bone, Percutaneous Approach

0NWW37Z Revision of Autologous Tissue Substitute in Facial Bone, Percutaneous Approach

0NWW3JZ Revision of Synthetic Substitute in Facial Bone, Percutaneous Approach

0NWW3KZ Revision of Nonautologous Tissue Substitute in Facial Bone, Percutaneous Approach

0NWW3MZ Revision of Bone Growth Stimulator in Facial Bone, Percutaneous Approach

0NWW40Z Revision of Drainage Device in Facial Bone, Percutaneous Endoscopic Approach

0NWW44Z Revision of Internal Fixation Device in Facial Bone, Percutaneous Endoscopic Approach

0NWW47Z Revision of Autologous Tissue Substitute in Facial Bone, Percutaneous Endoscopic Approach

0NWW4JZ Revision of Synthetic Substitute in Facial Bone, Percutaneous Endoscopic Approach

0NWW4KZ Revision of Nonautologous Tissue Substitute in Facial Bone, Percutaneous Endoscopic Approach

0NWW4MZ Revision of Bone Growth Stimulator in Facial Bone, Percutaneous Endoscopic Approach

0NWWX0Z Revision of Drainage Device in Facial Bone, External Approach

0NWWX4Z Revision of Internal Fixation Device in Facial Bone, External Approach

0NWWX7Z Revision of Autologous Tissue Substitute in Facial Bone, External Approach

0NWWXJZ Revision of Synthetic Substitute in Facial Bone, External Approach

0NWWXKZ Revision of Nonautologous Tissue Substitute in Facial Bone, External Approach

0NWWXMZ Revision of Bone Growth Stimulator in Facial Bone, External Approach

Bones - Front and Back Views

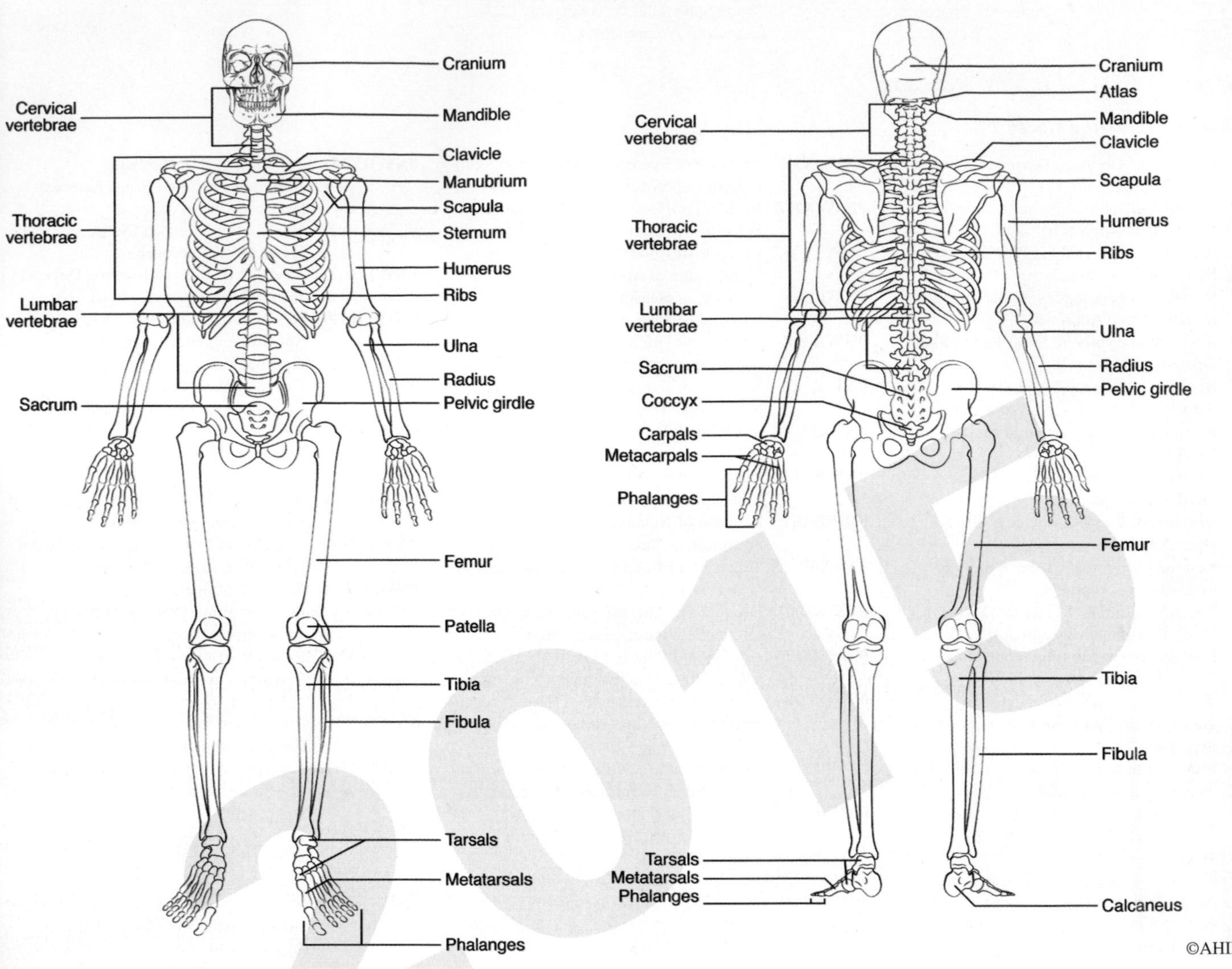

Vertebrae

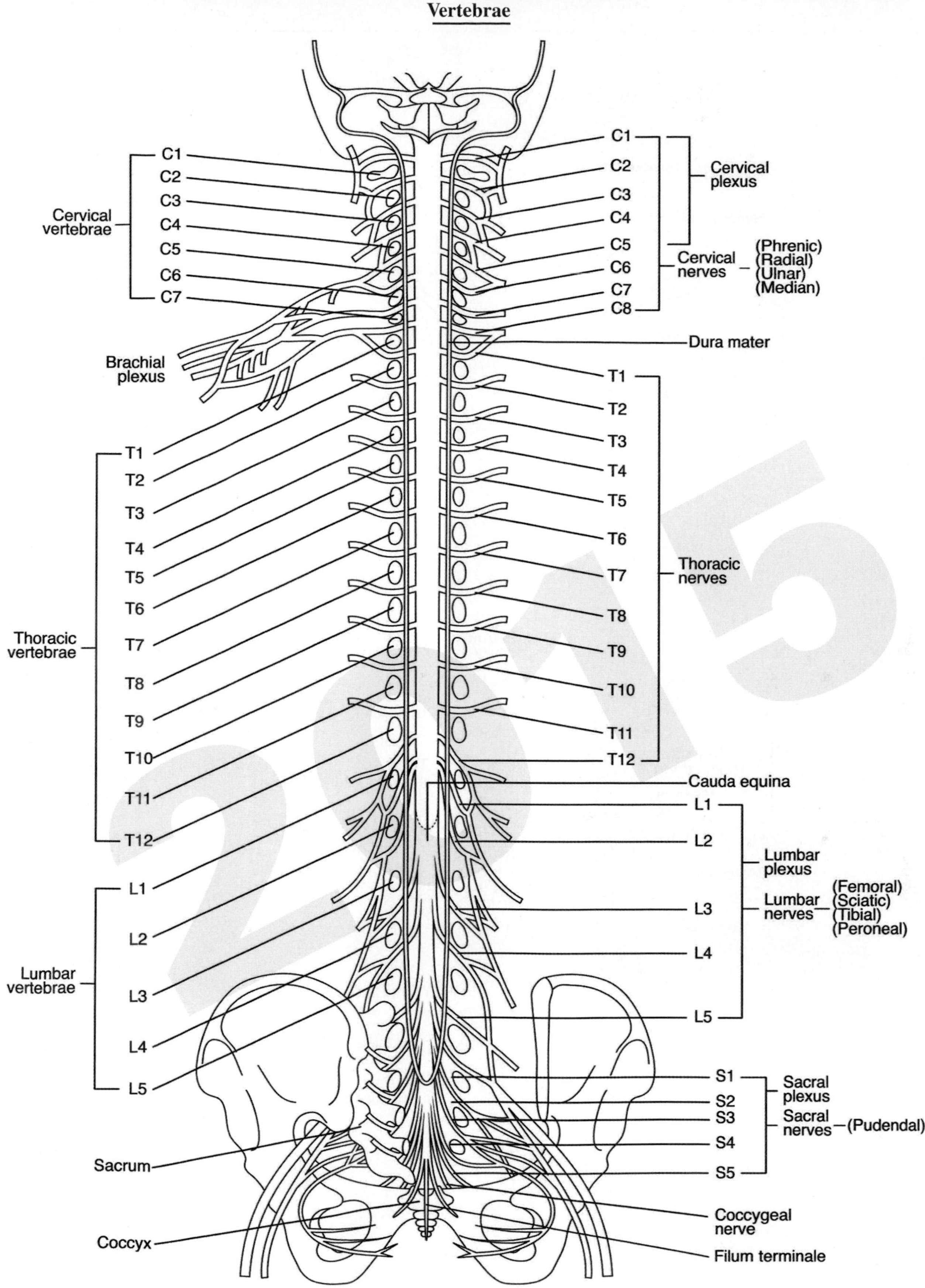

C1
C2
C3
C4
C5
C6
C7
Cervical vertebrae
Brachial plexus
T1
T2
T3
T4
T5
T6
T7
T8
T9
T10
T11
T12
Thoracic vertebrae
L1
L2
L3
L4
L5
Lumbar vertebrae
Sacrum
Coccyx
C1
C2
C3
C4
C5
C6
C7
C8
Cervical plexus
Cervical nerves
(Phrenic)
(Radial)
(Ulnar)
(Median)
Dura mater
T1
T2
T3
T4
T5
T6
T7
T8
T9
T10
T11
T12
Thoracic nerves
Cauda equina
L1
L2
L3
L4
L5
Lumbar plexus
Lumbar nerves
(Femoral)
(Sciatic)
(Tibial)
(Peroneal)
S1
S2
S3
S4
S5
Sacral plexus
Sacral nerves
(Pudendal)
Coccygeal nerve
Filum terminale
2015

Cross-section Spine

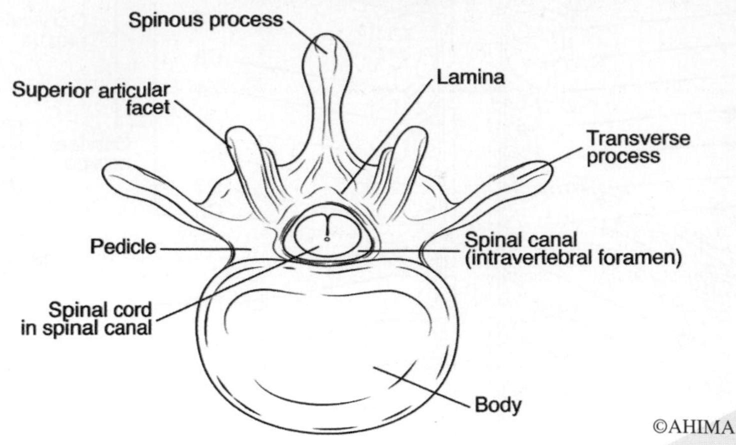
Spinous process
Lamina
Superior articular facet
Transverse process
Pedicle
Spinal canal (intravertebral foramen)
Spinal cord in spinal canal
Body

Hand Bones

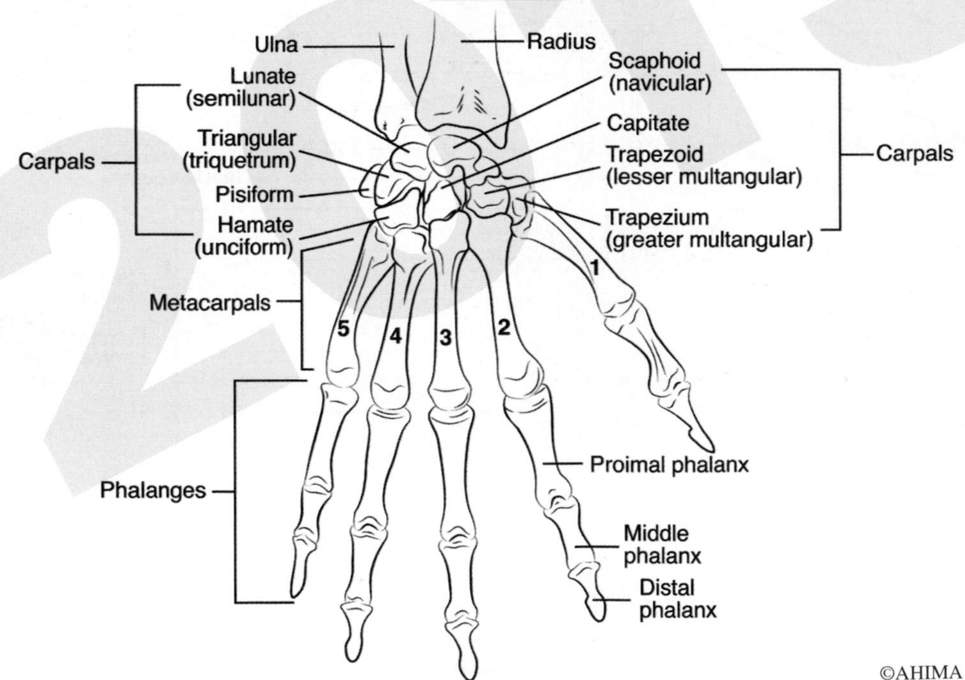
Ulna
Radius
Lunate (semilunar)
Scaphoid (navicular)
Carpals
Triangular (triquetrum)
Capitate
Trapezoid (lesser multangular)
Carpals
Pisiform
Hamate (unciform)
Trapezium (greater multangular)
1
Metacarpals
5
4
3
2
Phalanges
Proimal phalanx
Middle phalanx
Distal phalanx

Section	**0**	**Medical and Surgical**
Body System	**P**	**Upper Bones**
Operation	**2**	**Change:** Taking out or off a device from a body part and putting back an identical or similar device in or on the same body part without cutting or puncturing the skin or a mucous membrane

Body Part (4th)	Approach (5th)	Device (6th)	Qualifier (7th)
Y Upper Bone	**X** External	**0** Drainage Device **Y** Other Device	**Z** No Qualifier

Section	**0**	**Medical and Surgical**
Body System	**P**	**Upper Bones**
Operation	**5**	**Destruction:** Physical eradication of all or a portion of a body part by the direct use of energy, force, or a destructive agent

Body Part (4th)	Approach (5th)	Device (6th)	Qualifier (7th)
0 Sternum **1** Rib, Right **2** Rib, Left **3** Cervical Vertebra **4** Thoracic Vertebra **5** Scapula, Right **6** Scapula, Left **7** Glenoid Cavity, Right **8** Glenoid Cavity, Left **9** Clavicle, Right **B** Clavicle, Left **C** Humeral Head, Right **D** Humeral Head, Left **F** Humeral Shaft, Right **G** Humeral Shaft, Left **H** Radius, Right **J** Radius, Left **K** Ulna, Right **L** Ulna, Left **M** Carpal, Right **N** Carpal, Left **P** Metacarpal, Right **Q** Metacarpal, Left **R** Thumb Phalanx, Right **S** Thumb Phalanx, Left **T** Finger Phalanx, Right **V** Finger Phalanx, Left	**0** Open **3** Percutaneous **4** Percutaneous Endoscopic	**Z** No Device	**Z** No Qualifier

Section 0 **Medical and Surgical**
Body System P **Upper Bones**
Operation 8 **Division:** Cutting into a body part, without draining fluids and/or gases from the body part, in order to separate or transect a body part

Body Part (4th)	Approach (5th)	Device (6th)	Qualifier (7th)
0 Sternum **1** Rib, Right **2** Rib, Left **3** Cervical Vertebra **4** Thoracic Vertebra **5** Scapula, Right **6** Scapula, Left **7** Glenoid Cavity, Right **8** Glenoid Cavity, Left **9** Clavicle, Right **B** Clavicle, Left **C** Humeral Head, Right **D** Humeral Head, Left **F** Humeral Shaft, Right **G** Humeral Shaft, Left **H** Radius, Right **J** Radius, Left **K** Ulna, Right **L** Ulna, Left **M** Carpal, Right **N** Carpal, Left **P** Metacarpal, Right **Q** Metacarpal, Left **R** Thumb Phalanx, Right **S** Thumb Phalanx, Left **T** Finger Phalanx, Right **V** Finger Phalanx, Left	**0** Open **3** Percutaneous **4** Percutaneous Endoscopic	**Z** No Device	**Z** No Qualifier

Section 0 **Medical and Surgical**
Body System P **Upper Bones**
Operation 9 **Drainage:** Taking or letting out fluids and/or gases from a body part

Body Part (4th)	Approach (5th)	Device (6th)	Qualifier (7th)
0 Sternum **1** Rib, Right **2** Rib, Left **3** Cervical Vertebra **4** Thoracic Vertebra **5** Scapula, Right **6** Scapula, Left **7** Glenoid Cavity, Right **8** Glenoid Cavity, Left **9** Clavicle, Right **B** Clavicle, Left **C** Humeral Head, Right **D** Humeral Head, Left **F** Humeral Shaft, Right **G** Humeral Shaft, Left **H** Radius, Right **J** Radius, Left **K** Ulna, Right **L** Ulna, Left **M** Carpal, Right **N** Carpal, Left **P** Metacarpal, Right **Q** Metacarpal, Left **R** Thumb Phalanx, Right **S** Thumb Phalanx, Left **T** Finger Phalanx, Right **V** Finger Phalanx, Left	**0** Open **3** Percutaneous **4** Percutaneous Endoscopic	**0** Drainage Device	**Z** No Qualifier

Continued →

tion	0	**Medical and Surgical**
dy System	P	**Upper Bones**
eration	9	**Drainage:** Taking or letting out fluids and/or gases from a body part

Body Part (4th)	Approach (5th)	Device (6th)	Qualifier (7th)
Sternum Rib, Right Rib, Left Cervical Vertebra Thoracic Vertebra Scapula, Right Scapula, Left Glenoid Cavity, Right Glenoid Cavity, Left Clavicle, Right Clavicle, Left Humeral Head, Right Humeral Head, Left Humeral Shaft, Right Humeral Shaft, Left H Radius, Right Radius, Left K Ulna, Right L Ulna, Left M Carpal, Right N Carpal, Left P Metacarpal, Right Q Metacarpal, Left R Thumb Phalanx, Right S Thumb Phalanx, Left T Finger Phalanx, Right V Finger Phalanx, Left	0 Open 3 Percutaneous 4 Percutaneous Endoscopic	Z No Device	X Diagnostic Z No Qualifier

ction	0	**Medical and Surgical**
dy System	P	**Upper Bones**
peration	B	**Excision:** Cutting out or off, without replacement, a portion of a body part

Body Part (4th)	Approach (5th)	Device (6th)	Qualifier (7th)
0 Sternum 1 Rib, Right 2 Rib, Left 3 Cervical Vertebra 4 Thoracic Vertebra 5 Scapula, Right 6 Scapula, Left 7 Glenoid Cavity, Right 8 Glenoid Cavity, Left 9 Clavicle, Right B Clavicle, Left C Humeral Head, Right D Humeral Head, Left F Humeral Shaft, Right G Humeral Shaft, Left H Radius, Right J Radius, Left K Ulna, Right L Ulna, Left M Carpal, Right N Carpal, Left P Metacarpal, Right Q Metacarpal, Left R Thumb Phalanx, Right S Thumb Phalanx, Left T Finger Phalanx, Right V Finger Phalanx, Left	0 Open 3 Percutaneous 4 Percutaneous Endoscopic	Z No Device	X Diagnostic Z No Qualifier

Section 0 **Medical and Surgical**
Body System P **Upper Bones**
Operation C **Extirpation:** Taking or cutting out solid matter from a body part

Body Part (4th)	Approach (5th)	Device (6th)	Qualifier (7th)
0 Sternum **1** Rib, Right **2** Rib, Left **3** Cervical Vertebra **4** Thoracic Vertebra **5** Scapula, Right **6** Scapula, Left **7** Glenoid Cavity, Right **8** Glenoid Cavity, Left **9** Clavicle, Right **B** Clavicle, Left **C** Humeral Head, Right **D** Humeral Head, Left **F** Humeral Shaft, Right **G** Humeral Shaft, Left **H** Radius, Right **J** Radius, Left **K** Ulna, Right **L** Ulna, Left **M** Carpal, Right **N** Carpal, Left **P** Metacarpal, Right **Q** Metacarpal, Left **R** Thumb Phalanx, Right **S** Thumb Phalanx, Left **T** Finger Phalanx, Right **V** Finger Phalanx, Left	**0** Open **3** Percutaneous **4** Percutaneous Endoscopic	**Z** No Device	**Z** No Qualifier

Section 0 **Medical and Surgical**
Body System P **Upper Bones**
Operation H **Insertion:** Putting in a nonbiological appliance that monitors, assists, performs, or prevents a physiological function but does not physically take the place of a body part

Body Part (4th)	Approach (5th)	Device (6th)	Qualifier (7th)
0 Sternum	**0** Open **3** Percutaneous **4** Percutaneous Endoscopic	**0** Internal Fixation Device, Rigid Plate **4** Internal Fixation Device	**Z** No Qualifier
1 Rib, Right **2** Rib, Left **3** Cervical Vertebra **4** Thoracic Vertebra **5** Scapula, Right **6** Scapula, Left **7** Glenoid Cavity, Right **8** Glenoid Cavity, Left **9** Clavicle, Right **B** Clavicle, Left	**0** Open **3** Percutaneous **4** Percutaneous Endoscopic	**4** Internal Fixation Device	**Z** No Qualifier
C Humeral Head, Right **D** Humeral Head, Left **F** Humeral Shaft, Right **G** Humeral Shaft, Left **H** Radius, Right **J** Radius, Left **K** Ulna, Right **L** Ulna, Left	**0** Open **3** Percutaneous **4** Percutaneous Endoscopic	**4** Internal Fixation Device **5** External Fixation Device **6** Internal Fixation Device, Intramedullary **8** External Fixation Device, Limb Lengthening **B** External Fixation Device, Monoplanar **C** External Fixation Device, Ring **D** External Fixation Device, Hybrid	**Z** No Qualifier

Continued →

Section 0 **Medical and Surgical**
Body System P **Upper Bones**
Operation H **Insertion:** Putting in a nonbiological appliance that monitors, assists, performs, or prevents a physiological function but does not physically take the place of a body part

Body Part (4th)	Approach (5th)	Device (6th)	Qualifier (7th)
M Carpal, Right **N** Carpal, Left **P** Metacarpal, Right **Q** Metacarpal, Left **R** Thumb Phalanx, Right **S** Thumb Phalanx, Left **T** Finger Phalanx, Right **V** Finger Phalanx, Left	**0** Open **3** Percutaneous **4** Percutaneous Endoscopic	**4** Internal Fixation Device **5** External Fixation Device	**Z** No Qualifier
Y Upper Bone	**0** Open **3** Percutaneous **4** Percutaneous Endoscopic	**M** Bone Growth Stimulator	**Z** No Qualifier

Section 0 **Medical and Surgical**
Body System P **Upper Bones**
Operation J **Inspection:** Visually and/or manually exploring a body part

Body Part (4th)	Approach (5th)	Device (6th)	Qualifier (7th)
Y Upper Bone	**0** Open **3** Percutaneous **4** Percutaneous Endoscopic **X** External	**Z** No Device	**Z** No Qualifier

Section 0 **Medical and Surgical**
Body System P **Upper Bones**
Operation N **Release:** Freeing a body part from an abnormal physical constraint by cutting or by the use of force

Body Part (4th)	Approach (5th)	Device (6th)	Qualifier (7th)
0 Sternum **1** Rib, Right **2** Rib, Left **3** Cervical Vertebra **4** Thoracic Vertebra **5** Scapula, Right **6** Scapula, Left **7** Glenoid Cavity, Right **8** Glenoid Cavity, Left **9** Clavicle, Right **B** Clavicle, Left **C** Humeral Head, Right **D** Humeral Head, Left **F** Humeral Shaft, Right **G** Humeral Shaft, Left **H** Radius, Right **J** Radius, Left **K** Ulna, Right **L** Ulna, Left **M** Carpal, Right **N** Carpal, Left **P** Metacarpal, Right **Q** Metacarpal, Left **R** Thumb Phalanx, Right **S** Thumb Phalanx, Left **T** Finger Phalanx, Right **V** Finger Phalanx, Left	**0** Open **3** Percutaneous **4** Percutaneous Endoscopic	**Z** No Device	**Z** No Qualifier

Section **0** **Medical and Surgical**
Body System **P** **Upper Bones**
Operation **P** **Removal:** Taking out or off a device from a body part

Body Part (4th)	Approach (5th)	Device (6th)	Qualifier (7th)
0 Sternum **1** Rib, Right **2** Rib, Left **3** Cervical Vertebra **4** Thoracic Vertebra **5** Scapula, Right **6** Scapula, Left **7** Glenoid Cavity, Right **8** Glenoid Cavity, Left **9** Clavicle, Right **B** Clavicle, Left	**0** Open **3** Percutaneous **4** Percutaneous Endoscopic	**4** Internal Fixation Device **7** Autologous Tissue Substitute **J** Synthetic Substitute **K** Nonautologous Tissue Substitute	**Z** No Qualifier
0 Sternum **1** Rib, Right **2** Rib, Left **3** Cervical Vertebra **4** Thoracic Vertebra **5** Scapula, Right **6** Scapula, Left **7** Glenoid Cavity, Right **8** Glenoid Cavity, Left **9** Clavicle, Right **B** Clavicle, Left	**X** External	**4** Internal Fixation Device	**Z** No Qualifier
C Humeral Head, Right **D** Humeral Head, Left **F** Humeral Shaft, Right **G** Humeral Shaft, Left **H** Radius, Right **J** Radius, Left **K** Ulna, Right **L** Ulna, Left **M** Carpal, Right **N** Carpal, Left **P** Metacarpal, Right **Q** Metacarpal, Left **R** Thumb Phalanx, Right **S** Thumb Phalanx, Left **T** Finger Phalanx, Right **V** Finger Phalanx, Left	**0** Open **3** Percutaneous **4** Percutaneous Endoscopic	**4** Internal Fixation Device **5** External Fixation Device **7** Autologous Tissue Substitute **J** Synthetic Substitute **K** Nonautologous Tissue Substitute	**Z** No Qualifier
C Humeral Head, Right **D** Humeral Head, Left **F** Humeral Shaft, Right **G** Humeral Shaft, Left **H** Radius, Right **J** Radius, Left **K** Ulna, Right **L** Ulna, Left **M** Carpal, Right **N** Carpal, Left **P** Metacarpal, Right **Q** Metacarpal, Left **R** Thumb Phalanx, Right **S** Thumb Phalanx, Left **T** Finger Phalanx, Right **V** Finger Phalanx, Left	**X** External	**4** Internal Fixation Device **5** External Fixation Device	**Z** No Qualifier
Y Upper Bone	**0** Open **3** Percutaneous **4** Percutaneous Endoscopic **X** External	**0** Drainage Device **M** Bone Growth Stimulator	**Z** No Qualifier

ction **0** **Medical and Surgical**
dy System **P** **Upper Bones**
eration **Q** **Repair:** Restoring, to the extent possible, a body part to its normal anatomic structure and function

Body Part (4th)	Approach (5th)	Device (6th)	Qualifier (7th)
0 Sternum **1** Rib, Right **2** Rib, Left **3** Cervical Vertebra **4** Thoracic Vertebra **5** Scapula, Right **6** Scapula, Left **7** Glenoid Cavity, Right **8** Glenoid Cavity, Left **9** Clavicle, Right **B** Clavicle, Left **C** Humeral Head, Right **D** Humeral Head, Left **F** Humeral Shaft, Right **G** Humeral Shaft, Left **H** Radius, Right **J** Radius, Left **K** Ulna, Right **L** Ulna, Left **M** Carpal, Right **N** Carpal, Left **P** Metacarpal, Right **Q** Metacarpal, Left **R** Thumb Phalanx, Right **S** Thumb Phalanx, Left **T** Finger Phalanx, Right **V** Finger Phalanx, Left	**0** Open **3** Percutaneous **4** Percutaneous Endoscopic **X** External	**Z** No Device	**Z** No Qualifier

ction **0** **Medical and Surgical**
ody System **P** **Upper Bones**
peration **R** **Replacement:** Putting in or on biological or synthetic material that physically takes the place and/or function of all or a portion of a body part

Body Part (4th)	Approach (5th)	Device (6th)	Qualifier (7th)
0 Sternum **1** Rib, Right **2** Rib, Left **3** Cervical Vertebra **4** Thoracic Vertebra **5** Scapula, Right **6** Scapula, Left **7** Glenoid Cavity, Right **8** Glenoid Cavity, Left **9** Clavicle, Right **B** Clavicle, Left **C** Humeral Head, Right **D** Humeral Head, Left **F** Humeral Shaft, Right **G** Humeral Shaft, Left **H** Radius, Right **J** Radius, Left **K** Ulna, Right **L** Ulna, Left **M** Carpal, Right **N** Carpal, Left **P** Metacarpal, Right **Q** Metacarpal, Left **R** Thumb Phalanx, Right **S** Thumb Phalanx, Left **T** Finger Phalanx, Right **V** Finger Phalanx, Left	**0** Open **3** Percutaneous **4** Percutaneous Endoscopic	**7** Autologous Tissue Substitute **J** Synthetic Substitute **K** Nonautologous Tissue Substitute	**Z** No Qualifier

Section 0 **Medical and Surgical**
Body System P **Upper Bones**
Operation S **Reposition:** Moving to its normal location, or other suitable location, all or a portion of a body part

Body Part (4th)	Approach (5th)	Device (6th)	Qualifier (7th)
0 Sternum	**0** Open **3** Percutaneous **4** Percutaneous Endoscopic	**0** Internal Fixation Device, Rigid Plate **4** Internal Fixation Device **Z** No Device	**Z** No Qualifier
0 Sternum	**X** External	**Z** No Device	**Z** No Qualifier
1 Rib, Right **2** Rib, Left **3** Cervical Vertebra **4** Thoracic Vertebra **5** Scapula, Right **6** Scapula, Left **7** Glenoid Cavity, Right **8** Glenoid Cavity, Left **9** Clavicle, Right **B** Clavicle, Left	**0** Open **3** Percutaneous **4** Percutaneous Endoscopic	**4** Internal Fixation Device **Z** No Device	**Z** No Qualifier
1 Rib, Right **2** Rib, Left **3** Cervical Vertebra **4** Thoracic Vertebra **5** Scapula, Right **6** Scapula, Left **7** Glenoid Cavity, Right **8** Glenoid Cavity, Left **9** Clavicle, Right **B** Clavicle, Left	**X** External	**Z** No Device	**Z** No Qualifier
C Humeral Head, Right **D** Humeral Head, Left **F** Humeral Shaft, Right **G** Humeral Shaft, Left **H** Radius, Right **J** Radius, Left **K** Ulna, Right **L** Ulna, Left	**0** Open **3** Percutaneous **4** Percutaneous Endoscopic	**4** Internal Fixation Device **5** External Fixation Device **6** Internal Fixation Device, Intramedullary **B** External Fixation Device, Monoplanar **C** External Fixation Device, Ring **D** External Fixation Device, Hybrid **Z** No Device	**Z** No Qualifier
C Humeral Head, Right **D** Humeral Head, Left **F** Humeral Shaft, Right **G** Humeral Shaft, Left **H** Radius, Right **J** Radius, Left **K** Ulna, Right **L** Ulna, Left	**X** External	**Z** No Device	**Z** No Qualifier
M Carpal, Right **N** Carpal, Left **P** Metacarpal, Right **Q** Metacarpal, Left **R** Thumb Phalanx, Right **S** Thumb Phalanx, Left **T** Finger Phalanx, Right **V** Finger Phalanx, Left	**0** Open **3** Percutaneous **4** Percutaneous Endoscopic	**4** Internal Fixation Device **5** External Fixation Device **Z** No Device	**Z** No Qualifier
M Carpal, Right **N** Carpal, Left **P** Metacarpal, Right **Q** Metacarpal, Left **R** Thumb Phalanx, Right **S** Thumb Phalanx, Left **T** Finger Phalanx, Right **V** Finger Phalanx, Left	**X** External	**Z** No Device	**Z** No Qualifier

ection **0** **Medical and Surgical**
ody System **P** **Upper Bones**
peration **T** **Resection:** Cutting out or off, without replacement, all of a body part

Body Part (4th)	Approach (5th)	Device (6th)	Qualifier (7th)
0 Sternum	**0** Open	**Z** No Device	**Z** No Qualifier
1 Rib, Right			
2 Rib, Left			
5 Scapula, Right			
6 Scapula, Left			
7 Glenoid Cavity, Right			
8 Glenoid Cavity, Left			
9 Clavicle, Right			
B Clavicle, Left			
C Humeral Head, Right			
D Humeral Head, Left			
F Humeral Shaft, Right			
G Humeral Shaft, Left			
H Radius, Right			
J Radius, Left			
K Ulna, Right			
L Ulna, Left			
M Carpal, Right			
N Carpal, Left			
P Metacarpal, Right			
Q Metacarpal, Left			
R Thumb Phalanx, Right			
S Thumb Phalanx, Left			
T Finger Phalanx, Right			
V Finger Phalanx, Left			

ection **0** **Medical and Surgical**
ody System **P** **Upper Bones**
peration **U** **Supplement:** Putting in or on biological or synthetic material that physically reinforces and/or augments the function of a portion of a body part

Body Part (4th)	Approach (5th)	Device (6th)	Qualifier (7th)
0 Sternum	**0** Open	**7** Autologous Tissue Substitute	**Z** No Qualifier
1 Rib, Right	**3** Percutaneous	**J** Synthetic Substitute	
2 Rib, Left	**4** Percutaneous Endoscopic	**K** Nonautologous Tissue Substitute	
3 Cervical Vertebra			
4 Thoracic Vertebra			
5 Scapula, Right			
6 Scapula, Left			
7 Glenoid Cavity, Right			
8 Glenoid Cavity, Left			
9 Clavicle, Right			
B Clavicle, Left			
C Humeral Head, Right			
D Humeral Head, Left			
F Humeral Shaft, Right			
G Humeral Shaft, Left			
H Radius, Right			
J Radius, Left			
K Ulna, Right			
L Ulna, Left			
M Carpal, Right			
N Carpal, Left			
P Metacarpal, Right			
Q Metacarpal, Left			
R Thumb Phalanx, Right			
S Thumb Phalanx, Left			
T Finger Phalanx, Right			
V Finger Phalanx, Left			

Section 0 **Medical and Surgical**
Body System P **Upper Bones**
Operation W **Revision:** Correcting, to the extent possible, a portion of a malfunctioning device or the position of a displaced device

Body Part (4th)	Approach (5th)	Device (6th)	Qualifier (7th)
0 Sternum **1** Rib, Right **2** Rib, Left **3** Cervical Vertebra **4** Thoracic Vertebra **5** Scapula, Right **6** Scapula, Left **7** Glenoid Cavity, Right **8** Glenoid Cavity, Left **9** Clavicle, Right **B** Clavicle, Left	**0** Open **3** Percutaneous **4** Percutaneous Endoscopic **X** External	**4** Internal Fixation Device **7** Autologous Tissue Substitute **J** Synthetic Substitute **K** Nonautologous Tissue Substitute	**Z** No Qualifier
C Humeral Head, Right **D** Humeral Head, Left **F** Humeral Shaft, Right **G** Humeral Shaft, Left **H** Radius, Right **J** Radius, Left **K** Ulna, Right **L** Ulna, Left **M** Carpal, Right **N** Carpal, Left **P** Metacarpal, Right **Q** Metacarpal, Left **R** Thumb Phalanx, Right **S** Thumb Phalanx, Left **T** Finger Phalanx, Right **V** Finger Phalanx, Left	**0** Open **3** Percutaneous **4** Percutaneous Endoscopic **X** External	**4** Internal Fixation Device **5** External Fixation Device **7** Autologous Tissue Substitute **J** Synthetic Substitute **K** Nonautologous Tissue Substitute	**Z** No Qualifier
Y Upper Bone	**0** Open **3** Percutaneous **4** Percutaneous Endoscopic **X** External	**0** Drainage Device **M** Bone Growth Stimulator	**Z** No Qualifier

Upper Bones Code Listing 0P2–0PW

0P2 – Upper Bones, Change

Review Coding Guideline B6.1c

0P2YX0Z Change Drainage Device in Upper Bone, External Approach

0P2YXYZ Change Other Device in Upper Bone, External Approach

0P5 – Upper Bones, Destruction

0P500ZZ Destruction of Sternum, Open Approach
0P503ZZ Destruction of Sternum, Percutaneous Approach
0P504ZZ Destruction of Sternum, Percutaneous Endoscopic Approach
0P510ZZ Destruction of Right Rib, Open Approach
0P513ZZ Destruction of Right Rib, Percutaneous Approach
0P514ZZ Destruction of Right Rib, Percutaneous Endoscopic Approach
0P520ZZ Destruction of Left Rib, Open Approach
0P523ZZ Destruction of Left Rib, Percutaneous Approach
0P524ZZ Destruction of Left Rib, Percutaneous Endoscopic Approach
0P530ZZ Destruction of Cervical Vertebra, Open Approach
0P533ZZ Destruction of Cervical Vertebra, Percutaneous Approach
0P534ZZ Destruction of Cervical Vertebra, Percutaneous Endoscopic Approach
0P540ZZ Destruction of Thoracic Vertebra, Open Approach
0P543ZZ Destruction of Thoracic Vertebra, Percutaneous Approach
0P544ZZ Destruction of Thoracic Vertebra, Percutaneous Endoscopic Approach
0P550ZZ Destruction of Right Scapula, Open Approach
0P553ZZ Destruction of Right Scapula, Percutaneous Approach
0P554ZZ Destruction of Right Scapula, Percutaneous Endoscopic Approach
0P560ZZ Destruction of Left Scapula, Open Approach
0P563ZZ Destruction of Left Scapula, Percutaneous Approach
0P564ZZ Destruction of Left Scapula, Percutaneous Endoscopic Approach
0P570ZZ Destruction of Right Glenoid Cavity, Open Approach
0P573ZZ Destruction of Right Glenoid Cavity, Percutaneous Approach
0P574ZZ Destruction of Right Glenoid Cavity, Percutaneous Endoscopic Approach
0P580ZZ Destruction of Left Glenoid Cavity, Open Approach
0P583ZZ Destruction of Left Glenoid Cavity, Percutaneous Approach
0P584ZZ Destruction of Left Glenoid Cavity, Percutaneous Endoscopic Approach
0P590ZZ Destruction of Right Clavicle, Open Approach
0P593ZZ Destruction of Right Clavicle, Percutaneous Approach

594ZZ Destruction of Right Clavicle, Percutaneous Endoscopic Approach
5B0ZZ Destruction of Left Clavicle, Open Approach
5B3ZZ Destruction of Left Clavicle, Percutaneous Approach
5B4ZZ Destruction of Left Clavicle, Percutaneous Endoscopic Approach
5C0ZZ Destruction of Right Humeral Head, Open Approach
5C3ZZ Destruction of Right Humeral Head, Percutaneous Approach
5C4ZZ Destruction of Right Humeral Head, Percutaneous Endoscopic Approach
P5D0ZZ Destruction of Left Humeral Head, Open Approach
P5D3ZZ Destruction of Left Humeral Head, Percutaneous Approach
P5D4ZZ Destruction of Left Humeral Head, Percutaneous Endoscopic Approach
P5F0ZZ Destruction of Right Humeral Shaft, Open Approach
P5F3ZZ Destruction of Right Humeral Shaft, Percutaneous Approach
P5F4ZZ Destruction of Right Humeral Shaft, Percutaneous Endoscopic Approach
P5G0ZZ Destruction of Left Humeral Shaft, Open Approach
P5G3ZZ Destruction of Left Humeral Shaft, Percutaneous Approach
P5G4ZZ Destruction of Left Humeral Shaft, Percutaneous Endoscopic Approach
P5H0ZZ Destruction of Right Radius, Open Approach
0P5H3ZZ Destruction of Right Radius, Percutaneous Approach
0P5H4ZZ Destruction of Right Radius, Percutaneous Endoscopic Approach
0P5J0ZZ Destruction of Left Radius, Open Approach
0P5J3ZZ Destruction of Left Radius, Percutaneous Approach
0P5J4ZZ Destruction of Left Radius, Percutaneous Endoscopic Approach
0P5K0ZZ Destruction of Right Ulna, Open Approach
0P5K3ZZ Destruction of Right Ulna, Percutaneous Approach
0P5K4ZZ Destruction of Right Ulna, Percutaneous Endoscopic Approach
0P5L0ZZ Destruction of Left Ulna, Open Approach
0P5L3ZZ Destruction of Left Ulna, Percutaneous Approach
0P5L4ZZ Destruction of Left Ulna, Percutaneous Endoscopic Approach
0P5M0ZZ Destruction of Right Carpal, Open Approach
0P5M3ZZ Destruction of Right Carpal, Percutaneous Approach
0P5M4ZZ Destruction of Right Carpal, Percutaneous Endoscopic Approach
0P5N0ZZ Destruction of Left Carpal, Open Approach
0P5N3ZZ Destruction of Left Carpal, Percutaneous Approach
0P5N4ZZ Destruction of Left Carpal, Percutaneous Endoscopic Approach
0P5P0ZZ Destruction of Right Metacarpal, Open Approach
0P5P3ZZ Destruction of Right Metacarpal, Percutaneous Approach
0P5P4ZZ Destruction of Right Metacarpal, Percutaneous Endoscopic Approach
0P5Q0ZZ Destruction of Left Metacarpal, Open Approach
0P5Q3ZZ Destruction of Left Metacarpal, Percutaneous Approach
0P5Q4ZZ Destruction of Left Metacarpal, Percutaneous Endoscopic Approach
0P5R0ZZ Destruction of Right Thumb Phalanx, Open Approach
0P5R3ZZ Destruction of Right Thumb Phalanx, Percutaneous Approach
0P5R4ZZ Destruction of Right Thumb Phalanx, Percutaneous Endoscopic Approach
0P5S0ZZ Destruction of Left Thumb Phalanx, Open Approach
0P5S3ZZ Destruction of Left Thumb Phalanx, Percutaneous Approach
0P5S4ZZ Destruction of Left Thumb Phalanx, Percutaneous Endoscopic Approach
0P5T0ZZ Destruction of Right Finger Phalanx, Open Approach
0P5T3ZZ Destruction of Right Finger Phalanx, Percutaneous Approach
0P5T4ZZ Destruction of Right Finger Phalanx, Percutaneous Endoscopic Approach
0P5V0ZZ Destruction of Left Finger Phalanx, Open Approach
0P5V3ZZ Destruction of Left Finger Phalanx, Percutaneous Approach
0P5V4ZZ Destruction of Left Finger Phalanx, Percutaneous Endoscopic Approach

P8 – Upper Bones, Division

eview Coding Guideline B3.14

P800ZZ Division of Sternum, Open Approach
P803ZZ Division of Sternum, Percutaneous Approach
P804ZZ Division of Sternum, Percutaneous Endoscopic Approach
P810ZZ Division of Right Rib, Open Approach
P813ZZ Division of Right Rib, Percutaneous Approach
P814ZZ Division of Right Rib, Percutaneous Endoscopic Approach
P820ZZ Division of Left Rib, Open Approach
P823ZZ Division of Left Rib, Percutaneous Approach
P824ZZ Division of Left Rib, Percutaneous Endoscopic Approach
P830ZZ Division of Cervical Vertebra, Open Approach
P833ZZ Division of Cervical Vertebra, Percutaneous Approach
P834ZZ Division of Cervical Vertebra, Percutaneous Endoscopic Approach
P840ZZ Division of Thoracic Vertebra, Open Approach
P843ZZ Division of Thoracic Vertebra, Percutaneous Approach
P844ZZ Division of Thoracic Vertebra, Percutaneous Endoscopic Approach
P850ZZ Division of Right Scapula, Open Approach
P853ZZ Division of Right Scapula, Percutaneous Approach
P854ZZ Division of Right Scapula, Percutaneous Endoscopic Approach
P860ZZ Division of Left Scapula, Open Approach
0P863ZZ Division of Left Scapula, Percutaneous Approach
0P864ZZ Division of Left Scapula, Percutaneous Endoscopic Approach
P870ZZ Division of Right Glenoid Cavity, Open Approach
0P873ZZ Division of Right Glenoid Cavity, Percutaneous Approach
0P874ZZ Division of Right Glenoid Cavity, Percutaneous Endoscopic Approach
0P880ZZ Division of Left Glenoid Cavity, Open Approach
0P883ZZ Division of Left Glenoid Cavity, Percutaneous Approach
0P884ZZ Division of Left Glenoid Cavity, Percutaneous Endoscopic Approach
0P890ZZ Division of Right Clavicle, Open Approach
0P893ZZ Division of Right Clavicle, Percutaneous Approach
0P894ZZ Division of Right Clavicle, Percutaneous Endoscopic Approach
0P8B0ZZ Division of Left Clavicle, Open Approach
0P8B3ZZ Division of Left Clavicle, Percutaneous Approach
0P8B4ZZ Division of Left Clavicle, Percutaneous Endoscopic Approach
0P8C0ZZ Division of Right Humeral Head, Open Approach
0P8C3ZZ Division of Right Humeral Head, Percutaneous Approach
0P8C4ZZ Division of Right Humeral Head, Percutaneous Endoscopic Approach
0P8D0ZZ Division of Left Humeral Head, Open Approach
0P8D3ZZ Division of Left Humeral Head, Percutaneous Approach
0P8D4ZZ Division of Left Humeral Head, Percutaneous Endoscopic Approach
0P8F0ZZ Division of Right Humeral Shaft, Open Approach
0P8F3ZZ Division of Right Humeral Shaft, Percutaneous Approach
0P8F4ZZ Division of Right Humeral Shaft, Percutaneous Endoscopic Approach
0P8G0ZZ Division of Left Humeral Shaft, Open Approach
0P8G3ZZ Division of Left Humeral Shaft, Percutaneous Approach
0P8G4ZZ Division of Left Humeral Shaft, Percutaneous Endoscopic Approach
0P8H0ZZ Division of Right Radius, Open Approach
0P8H3ZZ Division of Right Radius, Percutaneous Approach
0P8H4ZZ Division of Right Radius, Percutaneous Endoscopic Approach
0P8J0ZZ Division of Left Radius, Open Approach
0P8J3ZZ Division of Left Radius, Percutaneous Approach
0P8J4ZZ Division of Left Radius, Percutaneous Endoscopic Approach
0P8K0ZZ Division of Right Ulna, Open Approach
0P8K3ZZ Division of Right Ulna, Percutaneous Approach
0P8K4ZZ Division of Right Ulna, Percutaneous Endoscopic Approach
0P8L0ZZ Division of Left Ulna, Open Approach
0P8L3ZZ Division of Left Ulna, Percutaneous Approach
0P8L4ZZ Division of Left Ulna, Percutaneous Endoscopic Approach
0P8M0ZZ Division of Right Carpal, Open Approach
0P8M3ZZ Division of Right Carpal, Percutaneous Approach
0P8M4ZZ Division of Right Carpal, Percutaneous Endoscopic Approach
0P8N0ZZ Division of Left Carpal, Open Approach
0P8N3ZZ Division of Left Carpal, Percutaneous Approach
0P8N4ZZ Division of Left Carpal, Percutaneous Endoscopic Approach

0P8P0ZZ Division of Right Metacarpal, Open Approach
0P8P3ZZ Division of Right Metacarpal, Percutaneous Approach
0P8P4ZZ Division of Right Metacarpal, Percutaneous Endoscopic Approach
0P8Q0ZZ Division of Left Metacarpal, Open Approach
0P8Q3ZZ Division of Left Metacarpal, Percutaneous Approach
0P8Q4ZZ Division of Left Metacarpal, Percutaneous Endoscopic Approach
0P8R0ZZ Division of Right Thumb Phalanx, Open Approach
0P8R3ZZ Division of Right Thumb Phalanx, Percutaneous Approach
0P8R4ZZ Division of Right Thumb Phalanx, Percutaneous Endoscopic Approach
0P8S0ZZ Division of Left Thumb Phalanx, Open Approach
0P8S3ZZ Division of Left Thumb Phalanx, Percutaneous Approach
0P8S4ZZ Division of Left Thumb Phalanx, Percutaneous Endoscopic Approach
0P8T0ZZ Division of Right Finger Phalanx, Open Approach
0P8T3ZZ Division of Right Finger Phalanx, Percutaneous Approach
0P8T4ZZ Division of Right Finger Phalanx, Percutaneous Endoscopic Approach
0P8V0ZZ Division of Left Finger Phalanx, Open Approach
0P8V3ZZ Division of Left Finger Phalanx, Percutaneous Approach
0P8V4ZZ Division of Left Finger Phalanx, Percutaneous Endoscopic Approach

0P9 – Upper Bones, Drainage

Review Coding Guidelines B3.4a and B3.4b

Review Coding Guideline B6.2

0P9000Z Drainage of Sternum with Drainage Device, Open Approach
0P900ZX Drainage of Sternum, Open Approach, Diagnostic
0P900ZZ Drainage of Sternum, Open Approach
0P9030Z Drainage of Sternum with Drainage Device, Percutaneous Approach
0P903ZX Drainage of Sternum, Percutaneous Approach, Diagnostic
0P903ZZ Drainage of Sternum, Percutaneous Approach
0P9040Z Drainage of Sternum with Drainage Device, Percutaneous Endoscopic Approach
0P904ZX Drainage of Sternum, Percutaneous Endoscopic Approach, Diagnostic
0P904ZZ Drainage of Sternum, Percutaneous Endoscopic Approach
0P9100Z Drainage of Right Rib with Drainage Device, Open Approach
0P910ZX Drainage of Right Rib, Open Approach, Diagnostic
0P910ZZ Drainage of Right Rib, Open Approach
0P9130Z Drainage of Right Rib with Drainage Device, Percutaneous Approach
0P913ZX Drainage of Right Rib, Percutaneous Approach, Diagnostic
0P913ZZ Drainage of Right Rib, Percutaneous Approach
0P9140Z Drainage of Right Rib with Drainage Device, Percutaneous Endoscopic Approach
0P914ZX Drainage of Right Rib, Percutaneous Endoscopic Approach, Diagnostic
0P914ZZ Drainage of Right Rib, Percutaneous Endoscopic Approach
0P9200Z Drainage of Left Rib with Drainage Device, Open Approach
0P920ZX Drainage of Left Rib, Open Approach, Diagnostic
0P920ZZ Drainage of Left Rib, Open Approach
0P9230Z Drainage of Left Rib with Drainage Device, Percutaneous Approach
0P923ZX Drainage of Left Rib, Percutaneous Approach, Diagnostic
0P923ZZ Drainage of Left Rib, Percutaneous Approach
0P9240Z Drainage of Left Rib with Drainage Device, Percutaneous Endoscopic Approach
0P924ZX Drainage of Left Rib, Percutaneous Endoscopic Approach, Diagnostic
0P924ZZ Drainage of Left Rib, Percutaneous Endoscopic Approach
0P9300Z Drainage of Cervical Vertebra with Drainage Device, Open Approach
0P930ZX Drainage of Cervical Vertebra, Open Approach, Diagnostic
0P930ZZ Drainage of Cervical Vertebra, Open Approach
0P9330Z Drainage of Cervical Vertebra with Drainage Device, Percutaneous Approach
0P933ZX Drainage of Cervical Vertebra, Percutaneous Approach, Diagnostic
0P933ZZ Drainage of Cervical Vertebra, Percutaneous Approach
0P9340Z Drainage of Cervical Vertebra with Drainage Device, Percutaneous Endoscopic Approach
0P934ZX Drainage of Cervical Vertebra, Percutaneous Endoscopic Approach, Diagnostic
0P934ZZ Drainage of Cervical Vertebra, Percutaneous Endoscopic Approach
0P9400Z Drainage of Thoracic Vertebra with Drainage Device, Open Approach
0P940ZX Drainage of Thoracic Vertebra, Open Approach, Diagnostic
0P940ZZ Drainage of Thoracic Vertebra, Open Approach
0P9430Z Drainage of Thoracic Vertebra with Drainage Device, Percutaneous Approach
0P943ZX Drainage of Thoracic Vertebra, Percutaneous Approach, Diagnostic
0P943ZZ Drainage of Thoracic Vertebra, Percutaneous Approach
0P9440Z Drainage of Thoracic Vertebra with Drainage Device, Percutaneous Endoscopic Approach
0P944ZX Drainage of Thoracic Vertebra, Percutaneous Endoscopic Approach, Diagnostic
0P944ZZ Drainage of Thoracic Vertebra, Percutaneous Endoscopic Approach
0P9500Z Drainage of Right Scapula with Drainage Device, Open Approach
0P950ZX Drainage of Right Scapula, Open Approach, Diagnostic
0P950ZZ Drainage of Right Scapula, Open Approach
0P9530Z Drainage of Right Scapula with Drainage Device, Percutaneous Approach
0P953ZX Drainage of Right Scapula, Percutaneous Approach, Diagnostic
0P953ZZ Drainage of Right Scapula, Percutaneous Approach
0P9540Z Drainage of Right Scapula with Drainage Device, Percutaneous Endoscopic Approach
0P954ZX Drainage of Right Scapula, Percutaneous Endoscopic Approach, Diagnostic
0P954ZZ Drainage of Right Scapula, Percutaneous Endoscopic Approach
0P9600Z Drainage of Left Scapula with Drainage Device, Open Approach
0P960ZX Drainage of Left Scapula, Open Approach, Diagnostic
0P960ZZ Drainage of Left Scapula, Open Approach
0P9630Z Drainage of Left Scapula with Drainage Device, Percutaneous Approach
0P963ZX Drainage of Left Scapula, Percutaneous Approach, Diagnostic
0P963ZZ Drainage of Left Scapula, Percutaneous Approach
0P9640Z Drainage of Left Scapula with Drainage Device, Percutaneous Endoscopic Approach
0P964ZX Drainage of Left Scapula, Percutaneous Endoscopic Approach, Diagnostic
0P964ZZ Drainage of Left Scapula, Percutaneous Endoscopic Approach
0P9700Z Drainage of Right Glenoid Cavity with Drainage Device, Open Approach
0P970ZX Drainage of Right Glenoid Cavity, Open Approach, Diagnostic
0P970ZZ Drainage of Right Glenoid Cavity, Open Approach
0P9730Z Drainage of Right Glenoid Cavity with Drainage Device, Percutaneous Approach
0P973ZX Drainage of Right Glenoid Cavity, Percutaneous Approach, Diagnostic
0P973ZZ Drainage of Right Glenoid Cavity, Percutaneous Approach
0P9740Z Drainage of Right Glenoid Cavity with Drainage Device, Percutaneous Endoscopic Approach
0P974ZX Drainage of Right Glenoid Cavity, Percutaneous Endoscopic Approach, Diagnostic
0P974ZZ Drainage of Right Glenoid Cavity, Percutaneous Endoscopic Approach
0P9800Z Drainage of Left Glenoid Cavity with Drainage Device, Open Approach
0P980ZX Drainage of Left Glenoid Cavity, Open Approach, Diagnostic
0P980ZZ Drainage of Left Glenoid Cavity, Open Approach
0P9830Z Drainage of Left Glenoid Cavity with Drainage Device, Percutaneous Approach
0P983ZX Drainage of Left Glenoid Cavity, Percutaneous Approach, Diagnostic
0P983ZZ Drainage of Left Glenoid Cavity, Percutaneous Approach
0P9840Z Drainage of Left Glenoid Cavity with Drainage Device, Percutaneous Endoscopic Approach
0P984ZX Drainage of Left Glenoid Cavity, Percutaneous Endoscopic Approach, Diagnostic
0P984ZZ Drainage of Left Glenoid Cavity, Percutaneous Endoscopic Approach
0P9900Z Drainage of Right Clavicle with Drainage Device, Open Approach

990ZX Drainage of Right Clavicle, Open Approach, Diagnostic
990ZZ Drainage of Right Clavicle, Open Approach
9930Z Drainage of Right Clavicle with Drainage Device, Percutaneous Approach
993ZX Drainage of Right Clavicle, Percutaneous Approach, Diagnostic
993ZZ Drainage of Right Clavicle, Percutaneous Approach
9940Z Drainage of Right Clavicle with Drainage Device, Percutaneous Endoscopic Approach
994ZX Drainage of Right Clavicle, Percutaneous Endoscopic Approach, Diagnostic
994ZZ Drainage of Right Clavicle, Percutaneous Endoscopic Approach
9B00Z Drainage of Left Clavicle with Drainage Device, Open Approach
9B0ZX Drainage of Left Clavicle, Open Approach, Diagnostic
9B0ZZ Drainage of Left Clavicle, Open Approach
9B30Z Drainage of Left Clavicle with Drainage Device, Percutaneous Approach
9B3ZX Drainage of Left Clavicle, Percutaneous Approach, Diagnostic
9B3ZZ Drainage of Left Clavicle, Percutaneous Approach
9B40Z Drainage of Left Clavicle with Drainage Device, Percutaneous Endoscopic Approach
9B4ZX Drainage of Left Clavicle, Percutaneous Endoscopic Approach, Diagnostic
9B4ZZ Drainage of Left Clavicle, Percutaneous Endoscopic Approach
9C00Z Drainage of Right Humeral Head with Drainage Device, Open Approach
9C0ZX Drainage of Right Humeral Head, Open Approach, Diagnostic
9C0ZZ Drainage of Right Humeral Head, Open Approach
9C30Z Drainage of Right Humeral Head with Drainage Device, Percutaneous Approach
9C3ZX Drainage of Right Humeral Head, Percutaneous Approach, Diagnostic
9C3ZZ Drainage of Right Humeral Head, Percutaneous Approach
9C40Z Drainage of Right Humeral Head with Drainage Device, Percutaneous Endoscopic Approach
9C4ZX Drainage of Right Humeral Head, Percutaneous Endoscopic Approach, Diagnostic
P9C4ZZ Drainage of Right Humeral Head, Percutaneous Endoscopic Approach
P9D00Z Drainage of Left Humeral Head with Drainage Device, Open Approach
P9D0ZX Drainage of Left Humeral Head, Open Approach, Diagnostic
P9D0ZZ Drainage of Left Humeral Head, Open Approach
P9D30Z Drainage of Left Humeral Head with Drainage Device, Percutaneous Approach
P9D3ZX Drainage of Left Humeral Head, Percutaneous Approach, Diagnostic
P9D3ZZ Drainage of Left Humeral Head, Percutaneous Approach
P9D40Z Drainage of Left Humeral Head with Drainage Device, Percutaneous Endoscopic Approach
P9D4ZX Drainage of Left Humeral Head, Percutaneous Endoscopic Approach, Diagnostic
P9D4ZZ Drainage of Left Humeral Head, Percutaneous Endoscopic Approach
P9F00Z Drainage of Right Humeral Shaft with Drainage Device, Open Approach

0P9F0ZX Drainage of Right Humeral Shaft, Open Approach, Diagnostic
0P9F0ZZ Drainage of Right Humeral Shaft, Open Approach
0P9F30Z Drainage of Right Humeral Shaft with Drainage Device, Percutaneous Approach
0P9F3ZX Drainage of Right Humeral Shaft, Percutaneous Approach, Diagnostic
0P9F3ZZ Drainage of Right Humeral Shaft, Percutaneous Approach
0P9F40Z Drainage of Right Humeral Shaft with Drainage Device, Percutaneous Endoscopic Approach
0P9F4ZX Drainage of Right Humeral Shaft, Percutaneous Endoscopic Approach, Diagnostic
0P9F4ZZ Drainage of Right Humeral Shaft, Percutaneous Endoscopic Approach
0P9G00Z Drainage of Left Humeral Shaft with Drainage Device, Open Approach
0P9G0ZX Drainage of Left Humeral Shaft, Open Approach, Diagnostic
0P9G0ZZ Drainage of Left Humeral Shaft, Open Approach
0P9G30Z Drainage of Left Humeral Shaft with Drainage Device, Percutaneous Approach
0P9G3ZX Drainage of Left Humeral Shaft, Percutaneous Approach, Diagnostic
0P9G3ZZ Drainage of Left Humeral Shaft, Percutaneous Approach
0P9G40Z Drainage of Left Humeral Shaft with Drainage Device, Percutaneous Endoscopic Approach
0P9G4ZX Drainage of Left Humeral Shaft, Percutaneous Endoscopic Approach, Diagnostic
0P9G4ZZ Drainage of Left Humeral Shaft, Percutaneous Endoscopic Approach
0P9H00Z Drainage of Right Radius with Drainage Device, Open Approach
0P9H0ZX Drainage of Right Radius, Open Approach, Diagnostic
0P9H0ZZ Drainage of Right Radius, Open Approach
0P9H30Z Drainage of Right Radius with Drainage Device, Percutaneous Approach
0P9H3ZX Drainage of Right Radius, Percutaneous Approach, Diagnostic
0P9H3ZZ Drainage of Right Radius, Percutaneous Approach
0P9H40Z Drainage of Right Radius with Drainage Device, Percutaneous Endoscopic Approach
0P9H4ZX Drainage of Right Radius, Percutaneous Endoscopic Approach, Diagnostic
0P9H4ZZ Drainage of Right Radius, Percutaneous Endoscopic Approach
0P9J00Z Drainage of Left Radius with Drainage Device, Open Approach
0P9J0ZX Drainage of Left Radius, Open Approach, Diagnostic
0P9J0ZZ Drainage of Left Radius, Open Approach
0P9J30Z Drainage of Left Radius with Drainage Device, Percutaneous Approach
0P9J3ZX Drainage of Left Radius, Percutaneous Approach, Diagnostic
0P9J3ZZ Drainage of Left Radius, Percutaneous Approach
0P9J40Z Drainage of Left Radius with Drainage Device, Percutaneous Endoscopic Approach
0P9J4ZX Drainage of Left Radius, Percutaneous Endoscopic Approach, Diagnostic
0P9J4ZZ Drainage of Left Radius, Percutaneous Endoscopic Approach
0P9K00Z Drainage of Right Ulna with Drainage Device, Open Approach

0P9K0ZX Drainage of Right Ulna, Open Approach, Diagnostic
0P9K0ZZ Drainage of Right Ulna, Open Approach
0P9K30Z Drainage of Right Ulna with Drainage Device, Percutaneous Approach
0P9K3ZX Drainage of Right Ulna, Percutaneous Approach, Diagnostic
0P9K3ZZ Drainage of Right Ulna, Percutaneous Approach
0P9K40Z Drainage of Right Ulna with Drainage Device, Percutaneous Endoscopic Approach
0P9K4ZX Drainage of Right Ulna, Percutaneous Endoscopic Approach, Diagnostic
0P9K4ZZ Drainage of Right Ulna, Percutaneous Endoscopic Approach
0P9L00Z Drainage of Left Ulna with Drainage Device, Open Approach
0P9L0ZX Drainage of Left Ulna, Open Approach, Diagnostic
0P9L0ZZ Drainage of Left Ulna, Open Approach
0P9L30Z Drainage of Left Ulna with Drainage Device, Percutaneous Approach
0P9L3ZX Drainage of Left Ulna, Percutaneous Approach, Diagnostic
0P9L3ZZ Drainage of Left Ulna, Percutaneous Approach
0P9L40Z Drainage of Left Ulna with Drainage Device, Percutaneous Endoscopic Approach
0P9L4ZX Drainage of Left Ulna, Percutaneous Endoscopic Approach, Diagnostic
0P9L4ZZ Drainage of Left Ulna, Percutaneous Endoscopic Approach
0P9M00Z Drainage of Right Carpal with Drainage Device, Open Approach
0P9M0ZX Drainage of Right Carpal, Open Approach, Diagnostic
0P9M0ZZ Drainage of Right Carpal, Open Approach
0P9M30Z Drainage of Right Carpal with Drainage Device, Percutaneous Approach
0P9M3ZX Drainage of Right Carpal, Percutaneous Approach, Diagnostic
0P9M3ZZ Drainage of Right Carpal, Percutaneous Approach
0P9M40Z Drainage of Right Carpal with Drainage Device, Percutaneous Endoscopic Approach
0P9M4ZX Drainage of Right Carpal, Percutaneous Endoscopic Approach, Diagnostic
0P9M4ZZ Drainage of Right Carpal, Percutaneous Endoscopic Approach
0P9N00Z Drainage of Left Carpal with Drainage Device, Open Approach
0P9N0ZX Drainage of Left Carpal, Open Approach, Diagnostic
0P9N0ZZ Drainage of Left Carpal, Open Approach
0P9N30Z Drainage of Left Carpal with Drainage Device, Percutaneous Approach
0P9N3ZX Drainage of Left Carpal, Percutaneous Approach, Diagnostic
0P9N3ZZ Drainage of Left Carpal, Percutaneous Approach
0P9N40Z Drainage of Left Carpal with Drainage Device, Percutaneous Endoscopic Approach
0P9N4ZX Drainage of Left Carpal, Percutaneous Endoscopic Approach, Diagnostic
0P9N4ZZ Drainage of Left Carpal, Percutaneous Endoscopic Approach
0P9P00Z Drainage of Right Metacarpal with Drainage Device, Open Approach
0P9P0ZX Drainage of Right Metacarpal, Open Approach, Diagnostic
0P9P0ZZ Drainage of Right Metacarpal, Open Approach

0P9P30Z Drainage of Right Metacarpal with Drainage Device, Percutaneous Approach

0P9P3ZX Drainage of Right Metacarpal, Percutaneous Approach, Diagnostic

0P9P3ZZ Drainage of Right Metacarpal, Percutaneous Approach

0P9P40Z Drainage of Right Metacarpal with Drainage Device, Percutaneous Endoscopic Approach

0P9P4ZX Drainage of Right Metacarpal, Percutaneous Endoscopic Approach, Diagnostic

0P9P4ZZ Drainage of Right Metacarpal, Percutaneous Endoscopic Approach

0P9Q00Z Drainage of Left Metacarpal with Drainage Device, Open Approach

0P9Q0ZX Drainage of Left Metacarpal, Open Approach, Diagnostic

0P9Q0ZZ Drainage of Left Metacarpal, Open Approach

0P9Q30Z Drainage of Left Metacarpal with Drainage Device, Percutaneous Approach

0P9Q3ZX Drainage of Left Metacarpal, Percutaneous Approach, Diagnostic

0P9Q3ZZ Drainage of Left Metacarpal, Percutaneous Approach

0P9Q40Z Drainage of Left Metacarpal with Drainage Device, Percutaneous Endoscopic Approach

0P9Q4ZX Drainage of Left Metacarpal, Percutaneous Endoscopic Approach, Diagnostic

0P9Q4ZZ Drainage of Left Metacarpal, Percutaneous Endoscopic Approach

0P9R00Z Drainage of Right Thumb Phalanx with Drainage Device, Open Approach

0P9R0ZX Drainage of Right Thumb Phalanx, Open Approach, Diagnostic

0P9R0ZZ Drainage of Right Thumb Phalanx, Open Approach

0P9R30Z Drainage of Right Thumb Phalanx with Drainage Device, Percutaneous Approach

0P9R3ZX Drainage of Right Thumb Phalanx, Percutaneous Approach, Diagnostic

0P9R3ZZ Drainage of Right Thumb Phalanx, Percutaneous Approach

0P9R40Z Drainage of Right Thumb Phalanx with Drainage Device, Percutaneous Endoscopic Approach

0P9R4ZX Drainage of Right Thumb Phalanx, Percutaneous Endoscopic Approach, Diagnostic

0P9R4ZZ Drainage of Right Thumb Phalanx, Percutaneous Endoscopic Approach

0P9S00Z Drainage of Left Thumb Phalanx with Drainage Device, Open Approach

0P9S0ZX Drainage of Left Thumb Phalanx, Open Approach, Diagnostic

0P9S0ZZ Drainage of Left Thumb Phalanx, Open Approach

0P9S30Z Drainage of Left Thumb Phalanx with Drainage Device, Percutaneous Approach

0P9S3ZX Drainage of Left Thumb Phalanx, Percutaneous Approach, Diagnostic

0P9S3ZZ Drainage of Left Thumb Phalanx, Percutaneous Approach

0P9S40Z Drainage of Left Thumb Phalanx with Drainage Device, Percutaneous Endoscopic Approach

0P9S4ZX Drainage of Left Thumb Phalanx, Percutaneous Endoscopic Approach, Diagnostic

0P9S4ZZ Drainage of Left Thumb Phalanx, Percutaneous Endoscopic Approach

0P9T00Z Drainage of Right Finger Phalanx with Drainage Device, Open Approach

0P9T0ZX Drainage of Right Finger Phalanx, Open Approach, Diagnostic

0P9T0ZZ Drainage of Right Finger Phalanx, Open Approach

0P9T30Z Drainage of Right Finger Phalanx with Drainage Device, Percutaneous Approach

0P9T3ZX Drainage of Right Finger Phalanx, Percutaneous Approach, Diagnostic

0P9T3ZZ Drainage of Right Finger Phalanx, Percutaneous Approach

0P9T40Z Drainage of Right Finger Phalanx with Drainage Device, Percutaneous Endoscopic Approach

0P9T4ZX Drainage of Right Finger Phalanx, Percutaneous Endoscopic Approach, Diagnostic

0P9T4ZZ Drainage of Right Finger Phalanx, Percutaneous Endoscopic Approach

0P9V00Z Drainage of Left Finger Phalanx with Drainage Device, Open Approach

0P9V0ZX Drainage of Left Finger Phalanx, Open Approach, Diagnostic

0P9V0ZZ Drainage of Left Finger Phalanx, Open Approach

0P9V30Z Drainage of Left Finger Phalanx with Drainage Device, Percutaneous Approach

0P9V3ZX Drainage of Left Finger Phalanx, Percutaneous Approach, Diagnostic

0P9V3ZZ Drainage of Left Finger Phalanx, Percutaneous Approach

0P9V40Z Drainage of Left Finger Phalanx with Drainage Device, Percutaneous Endoscopic Approach

0P9V4ZX Drainage of Left Finger Phalanx, Percutaneous Endoscopic Approach, Diagnostic

0P9V4ZZ Drainage of Left Finger Phalanx, Percutaneous Endoscopic Approach

0PB – Upper Bones, Excision

Review Coding Guideline B3.5

Review Coding Guidelines B3.4a and B3.4b

Review Coding Guideline B3.8

0PB00ZX Excision of Sternum, Open Approach, Diagnostic

0PB00ZZ Excision of Sternum, Open Approach

0PB03ZX Excision of Sternum, Percutaneous Approach, Diagnostic

0PB03ZZ Excision of Sternum, Percutaneous Approach

0PB04ZX Excision of Sternum, Percutaneous Endoscopic Approach, Diagnostic

0PB04ZZ Excision of Sternum, Percutaneous Endoscopic Approach

0PB10ZX Excision of Right Rib, Open Approach, Diagnostic

0PB10ZZ Excision of Right Rib, Open Approach
AHA CC: 4Q, 2012, 101-102; 4Q, 2013, 109-111

0PB13ZX Excision of Right Rib, Percutaneous Approach, Diagnostic

0PB13ZZ Excision of Right Rib, Percutaneous Approach

0PB14ZX Excision of Right Rib, Percutaneous Endoscopic Approach, Diagnostic

0PB14ZZ Excision of Right Rib, Percutaneous Endoscopic Approach

0PB20ZX Excision of Left Rib, Open Approach, Diagnostic

0PB20ZZ Excision of Left Rib, Open Approach
AHA CC: 4Q, 2013, 109-111

0PB23ZX Excision of Left Rib, Percutaneous Approach, Diagnostic

0PB23ZZ Excision of Left Rib, Percutaneous Approach

0PB24ZX Excision of Left Rib, Percutaneous Endoscopic Approach, Diagnostic

0PB24ZZ Excision of Left Rib, Percutaneous Endoscopic Approach

0PB30ZX Excision of Cervical Vertebra, Open Approach, Diagnostic

0PB30ZZ Excision of Cervical Vertebra, Open Approach

0PB33ZX Excision of Cervical Vertebra, Percutaneous Approach, Diagnostic

0PB33ZZ Excision of Cervical Vertebra, Percutaneous Approach

0PB34ZX Excision of Cervical Vertebra, Percutaneous Endoscopic Approach, Diagnostic

0PB34ZZ Excision of Cervical Vertebra, Percutaneous Endoscopic Approach

0PB40ZX Excision of Thoracic Vertebra, Open Approach, Diagnostic

0PB40ZZ Excision of Thoracic Vertebra, Open Approach

0PB43ZX Excision of Thoracic Vertebra, Percutaneous Approach, Diagnostic

0PB43ZZ Excision of Thoracic Vertebra, Percutaneous Approach

0PB44ZX Excision of Thoracic Vertebra, Percutaneous Endoscopic Approach, Diagnostic

0PB44ZZ Excision of Thoracic Vertebra, Percutaneous Endoscopic Approach

0PB50ZX Excision of Right Scapula, Open Approach, Diagnostic

0PB50ZZ Excision of Right Scapula, Open Approach

0PB53ZX Excision of Right Scapula, Percutaneous Approach, Diagnostic

0PB53ZZ Excision of Right Scapula, Percutaneous Approach

0PB54ZX Excision of Right Scapula, Percutaneous Endoscopic Approach, Diagnostic

0PB54ZZ Excision of Right Scapula, Percutaneous Endoscopic Approach
AHA CC: 3Q, 2013, 20-22

0PB60ZX Excision of Left Scapula, Open Approach, Diagnostic

0PB60ZZ Excision of Left Scapula, Open Approach

0PB63ZX Excision of Left Scapula, Percutaneous Approach, Diagnostic

0PB63ZZ Excision of Left Scapula, Percutaneous Approach

0PB64ZX Excision of Left Scapula, Percutaneous Endoscopic Approach, Diagnostic

0PB64ZZ Excision of Left Scapula, Percutaneous Endoscopic Approach

0PB70ZX Excision of Right Glenoid Cavity, Open Approach, Diagnostic

0PB70ZZ Excision of Right Glenoid Cavity, Open Approach

0PB73ZX Excision of Right Glenoid Cavity, Percutaneous Approach, Diagnostic

B73ZZ Excision of Right Glenoid Cavity, Percutaneous Approach

B74ZX Excision of Right Glenoid Cavity, Percutaneous Endoscopic Approach, Diagnostic

B74ZZ Excision of Right Glenoid Cavity, Percutaneous Endoscopic Approach

B80ZX Excision of Left Glenoid Cavity, Open Approach, Diagnostic

B80ZZ Excision of Left Glenoid Cavity, Open Approach

B83ZX Excision of Left Glenoid Cavity, Percutaneous Approach, Diagnostic

B83ZZ Excision of Left Glenoid Cavity, Percutaneous Approach

B84ZX Excision of Left Glenoid Cavity, Percutaneous Endoscopic Approach, Diagnostic

B84ZZ Excision of Left Glenoid Cavity, Percutaneous Endoscopic Approach

B90ZX Excision of Right Clavicle, Open Approach, Diagnostic

B90ZZ Excision of Right Clavicle, Open Approach

B93ZX Excision of Right Clavicle, Percutaneous Approach, Diagnostic

B93ZZ Excision of Right Clavicle, Percutaneous Approach

B94ZX Excision of Right Clavicle, Percutaneous Endoscopic Approach, Diagnostic

B94ZZ Excision of Right Clavicle, Percutaneous Endoscopic Approach

BB0ZX Excision of Left Clavicle, Open Approach, Diagnostic

BB0ZZ Excision of Left Clavicle, Open Approach

PBB3ZX Excision of Left Clavicle, Percutaneous Approach, Diagnostic

PBB3ZZ Excision of Left Clavicle, Percutaneous Approach

PBB4ZX Excision of Left Clavicle, Percutaneous Endoscopic Approach, Diagnostic

PBB4ZZ Excision of Left Clavicle, Percutaneous Endoscopic Approach

PBC0ZX Excision of Right Humeral Head, Open Approach, Diagnostic

PBC0ZZ Excision of Right Humeral Head, Open Approach

PBC3ZX Excision of Right Humeral Head, Percutaneous Approach, Diagnostic

PBC3ZZ Excision of Right Humeral Head, Percutaneous Approach

PBC4ZX Excision of Right Humeral Head, Percutaneous Endoscopic Approach, Diagnostic

PBC4ZZ Excision of Right Humeral Head, Percutaneous Endoscopic Approach

PBD0ZX Excision of Left Humeral Head, Open Approach, Diagnostic

PBD0ZZ Excision of Left Humeral Head, Open Approach

PBD3ZX Excision of Left Humeral Head, Percutaneous Approach, Diagnostic

PBD3ZZ Excision of Left Humeral Head, Percutaneous Approach

PBD4ZX Excision of Left Humeral Head, Percutaneous Endoscopic Approach, Diagnostic

PBD4ZZ Excision of Left Humeral Head, Percutaneous Endoscopic Approach

PBF0ZX Excision of Right Humeral Shaft, Open Approach, Diagnostic

PBF0ZZ Excision of Right Humeral Shaft, Open Approach

PBF3ZX Excision of Right Humeral Shaft, Percutaneous Approach, Diagnostic

PBF3ZZ Excision of Right Humeral Shaft, Percutaneous Approach

0PBF4ZX Excision of Right Humeral Shaft, Percutaneous Endoscopic Approach, Diagnostic

0PBF4ZZ Excision of Right Humeral Shaft, Percutaneous Endoscopic Approach

0PBG0ZX Excision of Left Humeral Shaft, Open Approach, Diagnostic

0PBG0ZZ Excision of Left Humeral Shaft, Open Approach

0PBG3ZX Excision of Left Humeral Shaft, Percutaneous Approach, Diagnostic

0PBG3ZZ Excision of Left Humeral Shaft, Percutaneous Approach

0PBG4ZX Excision of Left Humeral Shaft, Percutaneous Endoscopic Approach, Diagnostic

0PBG4ZZ Excision of Left Humeral Shaft, Percutaneous Endoscopic Approach

0PBH0ZX Excision of Right Radius, Open Approach, Diagnostic

0PBH0ZZ Excision of Right Radius, Open Approach

0PBH3ZX Excision of Right Radius, Percutaneous Approach, Diagnostic

0PBH3ZZ Excision of Right Radius, Percutaneous Approach

0PBH4ZX Excision of Right Radius, Percutaneous Endoscopic Approach, Diagnostic

0PBH4ZZ Excision of Right Radius, Percutaneous Endoscopic Approach

0PBJ0ZX Excision of Left Radius, Open Approach, Diagnostic

0PBJ0ZZ Excision of Left Radius, Open Approach

0PBJ3ZX Excision of Left Radius, Percutaneous Approach, Diagnostic

0PBJ3ZZ Excision of Left Radius, Percutaneous Approach

0PBJ4ZX Excision of Left Radius, Percutaneous Endoscopic Approach, Diagnostic

0PBJ4ZZ Excision of Left Radius, Percutaneous Endoscopic Approach

0PBK0ZX Excision of Right Ulna, Open Approach, Diagnostic

0PBK0ZZ Excision of Right Ulna, Open Approach

0PBK3ZX Excision of Right Ulna, Percutaneous Approach, Diagnostic

0PBK3ZZ Excision of Right Ulna, Percutaneous Approach

0PBK4ZX Excision of Right Ulna, Percutaneous Endoscopic Approach, Diagnostic

0PBK4ZZ Excision of Right Ulna, Percutaneous Endoscopic Approach

0PBL0ZX Excision of Left Ulna, Open Approach, Diagnostic

0PBL0ZZ Excision of Left Ulna, Open Approach

0PBL3ZX Excision of Left Ulna, Percutaneous Approach, Diagnostic

0PBL3ZZ Excision of Left Ulna, Percutaneous Approach

0PBL4ZX Excision of Left Ulna, Percutaneous Endoscopic Approach, Diagnostic

0PBL4ZZ Excision of Left Ulna, Percutaneous Endoscopic Approach

0PBM0ZX Excision of Right Carpal, Open Approach, Diagnostic

0PBM0ZZ Excision of Right Carpal, Open Approach

0PBM3ZX Excision of Right Carpal, Percutaneous Approach, Diagnostic

0PBM3ZZ Excision of Right Carpal, Percutaneous Approach

0PBM4ZX Excision of Right Carpal, Percutaneous Endoscopic Approach, Diagnostic

0PBM4ZZ Excision of Right Carpal, Percutaneous Endoscopic Approach

0PBN0ZX Excision of Left Carpal, Open Approach, Diagnostic

0PBN0ZZ Excision of Left Carpal, Open Approach

0PBN3ZX Excision of Left Carpal, Percutaneous Approach, Diagnostic

0PBN3ZZ Excision of Left Carpal, Percutaneous Approach

0PBN4ZX Excision of Left Carpal, Percutaneous Endoscopic Approach, Diagnostic

0PBN4ZZ Excision of Left Carpal, Percutaneous Endoscopic Approach

0PBP0ZX Excision of Right Metacarpal, Open Approach, Diagnostic

0PBP0ZZ Excision of Right Metacarpal, Open Approach

0PBP3ZX Excision of Right Metacarpal, Percutaneous Approach, Diagnostic

0PBP3ZZ Excision of Right Metacarpal, Percutaneous Approach

0PBP4ZX Excision of Right Metacarpal, Percutaneous Endoscopic Approach, Diagnostic

0PBP4ZZ Excision of Right Metacarpal, Percutaneous Endoscopic Approach

0PBQ0ZX Excision of Left Metacarpal, Open Approach, Diagnostic

0PBQ0ZZ Excision of Left Metacarpal, Open Approach

0PBQ3ZX Excision of Left Metacarpal, Percutaneous Approach, Diagnostic

0PBQ3ZZ Excision of Left Metacarpal, Percutaneous Approach

0PBQ4ZX Excision of Left Metacarpal, Percutaneous Endoscopic Approach, Diagnostic

0PBQ4ZZ Excision of Left Metacarpal, Percutaneous Endoscopic Approach

0PBR0ZX Excision of Right Thumb Phalanx, Open Approach, Diagnostic

0PBR0ZZ Excision of Right Thumb Phalanx, Open Approach

0PBR3ZX Excision of Right Thumb Phalanx, Percutaneous Approach, Diagnostic

0PBR3ZZ Excision of Right Thumb Phalanx, Percutaneous Approach

0PBR4ZX Excision of Right Thumb Phalanx, Percutaneous Endoscopic Approach, Diagnostic

0PBR4ZZ Excision of Right Thumb Phalanx, Percutaneous Endoscopic Approach

0PBS0ZX Excision of Left Thumb Phalanx, Open Approach, Diagnostic

0PBS0ZZ Excision of Left Thumb Phalanx, Open Approach

0PBS3ZX Excision of Left Thumb Phalanx, Percutaneous Approach, Diagnostic

0PBS3ZZ Excision of Left Thumb Phalanx, Percutaneous Approach

0PBS4ZX Excision of Left Thumb Phalanx, Percutaneous Endoscopic Approach, Diagnostic

0PBS4ZZ Excision of Left Thumb Phalanx, Percutaneous Endoscopic Approach

0PBT0ZX Excision of Right Finger Phalanx, Open Approach, Diagnostic

0PBT0ZZ Excision of Right Finger Phalanx, Open Approach

0PBT3ZX Excision of Right Finger Phalanx, Percutaneous Approach, Diagnostic

0PBT3ZZ Excision of Right Finger Phalanx, Percutaneous Approach

0PBT4ZX Excision of Right Finger Phalanx, Percutaneous Endoscopic Approach, Diagnostic

0PBT4ZZ Excision of Right Finger Phalanx, Percutaneous Endoscopic Approach

0PBV0ZX Excision of Left Finger Phalanx, Open Approach, Diagnostic

0PBV0ZZ Excision of Left Finger Phalanx, Open Approach

0PBV3ZX Excision of Left Finger Phalanx, Percutaneous Approach, Diagnostic

0PBV3ZZ Excision of Left Finger Phalanx, Percutaneous Approach

0PBV4ZX Excision of Left Finger Phalanx, Percutaneous Endoscopic Approach, Diagnostic

0PBV4ZZ Excision of Left Finger Phalanx, Percutaneous Endoscopic Approach

0PC – Upper Bones, Extirpation

0PC00ZZ Extirpation of Matter from Sternum, Open Approach

0PC03ZZ Extirpation of Matter from Sternum, Percutaneous Approach

0PC04ZZ Extirpation of Matter from Sternum, Percutaneous Endoscopic Approach

0PC10ZZ Extirpation of Matter from Right Rib, Open Approach

0PC13ZZ Extirpation of Matter from Right Rib, Percutaneous Approach

0PC14ZZ Extirpation of Matter from Right Rib, Percutaneous Endoscopic Approach

0PC20ZZ Extirpation of Matter from Left Rib, Open Approach

0PC23ZZ Extirpation of Matter from Left Rib, Percutaneous Approach

0PC24ZZ Extirpation of Matter from Left Rib, Percutaneous Endoscopic Approach

0PC30ZZ Extirpation of Matter from Cervical Vertebra, Open Approach

0PC33ZZ Extirpation of Matter from Cervical Vertebra, Percutaneous Approach

0PC34ZZ Extirpation of Matter from Cervical Vertebra, Percutaneous Endoscopic Approach

0PC40ZZ Extirpation of Matter from Thoracic Vertebra, Open Approach

0PC43ZZ Extirpation of Matter from Thoracic Vertebra, Percutaneous Approach

0PC44ZZ Extirpation of Matter from Thoracic Vertebra, Percutaneous Endoscopic Approach

0PC50ZZ Extirpation of Matter from Right Scapula, Open Approach

0PC53ZZ Extirpation of Matter from Right Scapula, Percutaneous Approach

0PC54ZZ Extirpation of Matter from Right Scapula, Percutaneous Endoscopic Approach

0PC60ZZ Extirpation of Matter from Left Scapula, Open Approach

0PC63ZZ Extirpation of Matter from Left Scapula, Percutaneous Approach

0PC64ZZ Extirpation of Matter from Left Scapula, Percutaneous Endoscopic Approach

0PC70ZZ Extirpation of Matter from Right Glenoid Cavity, Open Approach

0PC73ZZ Extirpation of Matter from Right Glenoid Cavity, Percutaneous Approach

0PC74ZZ Extirpation of Matter from Right Glenoid Cavity, Percutaneous Endoscopic Approach

0PC80ZZ Extirpation of Matter from Left Glenoid Cavity, Open Approach

0PC83ZZ Extirpation of Matter from Left Glenoid Cavity, Percutaneous Approach

0PC84ZZ Extirpation of Matter from Left Glenoid Cavity, Percutaneous Endoscopic Approach

0PC90ZZ Extirpation of Matter from Right Clavicle, Open Approach

0PC93ZZ Extirpation of Matter from Right Clavicle, Percutaneous Approach

0PC94ZZ Extirpation of Matter from Right Clavicle, Percutaneous Endoscopic Approach

0PCB0ZZ Extirpation of Matter from Left Clavicle, Open Approach

0PCB3ZZ Extirpation of Matter from Left Clavicle, Percutaneous Approach

0PCB4ZZ Extirpation of Matter from Left Clavicle, Percutaneous Endoscopic Approach

0PCC0ZZ Extirpation of Matter from Right Humeral Head, Open Approach

0PCC3ZZ Extirpation of Matter from Right Humeral Head, Percutaneous Approach

0PCC4ZZ Extirpation of Matter from Right Humeral Head, Percutaneous Endoscopic Approach

0PCD0ZZ Extirpation of Matter from Left Humeral Head, Open Approach

0PCD3ZZ Extirpation of Matter from Left Humeral Head, Percutaneous Approach

0PCD4ZZ Extirpation of Matter from Left Humeral Head, Percutaneous Endoscopic Approach

0PCF0ZZ Extirpation of Matter from Right Humeral Shaft, Open Approach

0PCF3ZZ Extirpation of Matter from Right Humeral Shaft, Percutaneous Approach

0PCF4ZZ Extirpation of Matter from Right Humeral Shaft, Percutaneous Endoscopic Approach

0PCG0ZZ Extirpation of Matter from Left Humeral Shaft, Open Approach

0PCG3ZZ Extirpation of Matter from Left Humeral Shaft, Percutaneous Approach

0PCG4ZZ Extirpation of Matter from Left Humeral Shaft, Percutaneous Endoscopic Approach

0PCH0ZZ Extirpation of Matter from Right Radius, Open Approach

0PCH3ZZ Extirpation of Matter from Right Radius, Percutaneous Approach

0PCH4ZZ Extirpation of Matter from Right Radius, Percutaneous Endoscopic Approach

0PCJ0ZZ Extirpation of Matter from Left Radius, Open Approach

0PCJ3ZZ Extirpation of Matter from Left Radius, Percutaneous Approach

0PCJ4ZZ Extirpation of Matter from Left Radius, Percutaneous Endoscopic Approach

0PCK0ZZ Extirpation of Matter from Right Ulna, Open Approach

0PCK3ZZ Extirpation of Matter from Right Ulna, Percutaneous Approach

0PCK4ZZ Extirpation of Matter from Right Ulna, Percutaneous Endoscopic Approach

0PCL0ZZ Extirpation of Matter from Left Ulna, Open Approach

0PCL3ZZ Extirpation of Matter from Left Ulna, Percutaneous Approach

0PCL4ZZ Extirpation of Matter from Left Ulna, Percutaneous Endoscopic Approach

0PCM0ZZ Extirpation of Matter from Right Carpal, Open Approach

0PCM3ZZ Extirpation of Matter from Right Carpal, Percutaneous Approach

0PCM4ZZ Extirpation of Matter from Right Carpal, Percutaneous Endoscopic Approach

0PCN0ZZ Extirpation of Matter from Left Carpal, Open Approach

0PCN3ZZ Extirpation of Matter from Left Carpal, Percutaneous Approach

0PCN4ZZ Extirpation of Matter from Left Carpal, Percutaneous Endoscopic Approach

0PCP0ZZ Extirpation of Matter from Right Metacarpal, Open Approach

0PCP3ZZ Extirpation of Matter from Right Metacarpal, Percutaneous Approach

0PCP4ZZ Extirpation of Matter from Right Metacarpal, Percutaneous Endoscopic Approach

0PCQ0ZZ Extirpation of Matter from Left Metacarpal, Open Approach

0PCQ3ZZ Extirpation of Matter from Left Metacarpal, Percutaneous Approach

0PCQ4ZZ Extirpation of Matter from Left Metacarpal, Percutaneous Endoscopic Approach

0PCR0ZZ Extirpation of Matter from Right Thumb Phalanx, Open Approach

0PCR3ZZ Extirpation of Matter from Right Thumb Phalanx, Percutaneous Approach

0PCR4ZZ Extirpation of Matter from Right Thumb Phalanx, Percutaneous Endoscopic Approach

0PCS0ZZ Extirpation of Matter from Left Thumb Phalanx, Open Approach

0PCS3ZZ Extirpation of Matter from Left Thumb Phalanx, Percutaneous Approach

0PCS4ZZ Extirpation of Matter from Left Thumb Phalanx, Percutaneous Endoscopic Approach

0PCT0ZZ Extirpation of Matter from Right Finger Phalanx, Open Approach

0PCT3ZZ Extirpation of Matter from Right Finger Phalanx, Percutaneous Approach

0PCT4ZZ Extirpation of Matter from Right Finger Phalanx, Percutaneous Endoscopic Approach

0PCV0ZZ Extirpation of Matter from Left Finger Phalanx, Open Approach

0PCV3ZZ Extirpation of Matter from Left Finger Phalanx, Percutaneous Approach

0PCV4ZZ Extirpation of Matter from Left Finger Phalanx, Percutaneous Endoscopic Approach

0PH – Upper Bones, Insertion

0PH000Z Insertion of Rigid Plate Internal Fixation Device into Sternum, Open Approach

0PH004Z Insertion of Internal Fixation Device into Sternum, Open Approach

0PH030Z Insertion of Rigid Plate Internal Fixation Device into Sternum, Percutaneous Approach

0PH034Z Insertion of Internal Fixation Device into Sternum, Percutaneous Approach

0PH040Z Insertion of Rigid Plate Internal Fixation Device into Sternum, Percutaneous Endoscopic Approach

0PH044Z Insertion of Internal Fixation Device into Sternum, Percutaneous Endoscopic Approach

0PH104Z Insertion of Internal Fixation Device into Right Rib, Open Approach

0PH134Z Insertion of Internal Fixation Device into Right Rib, Percutaneous Approach

0PH144Z Insertion of Internal Fixation Device into Right Rib, Percutaneous Endoscopic Approach

0PH204Z Insertion of Internal Fixation Device into Left Rib, Open Approach

0PH234Z Insertion of Internal Fixation Device into Left Rib, Percutaneous Approach

0PH244Z Insertion of Internal Fixation Device into Left Rib, Percutaneous Endoscopic Approach
0PH304Z Insertion of Internal Fixation Device into Cervical Vertebra, Open Approach
0PH334Z Insertion of Internal Fixation Device into Cervical Vertebra, Percutaneous Approach
0PH344Z Insertion of Internal Fixation Device into Cervical Vertebra, Percutaneous Endoscopic Approach
0PH404Z Insertion of Internal Fixation Device into Thoracic Vertebra, Open Approach
0PH434Z Insertion of Internal Fixation Device into Thoracic Vertebra, Percutaneous Approach
0PH444Z Insertion of Internal Fixation Device into Thoracic Vertebra, Percutaneous Endoscopic Approach
0PH504Z Insertion of Internal Fixation Device into Right Scapula, Open Approach
0PH534Z Insertion of Internal Fixation Device into Right Scapula, Percutaneous Approach
0PH544Z Insertion of Internal Fixation Device into Right Scapula, Percutaneous Endoscopic Approach
0PH604Z Insertion of Internal Fixation Device into Left Scapula, Open Approach
0PH634Z Insertion of Internal Fixation Device into Left Scapula, Percutaneous Approach
0PH644Z Insertion of Internal Fixation Device into Left Scapula, Percutaneous Endoscopic Approach
0PH704Z Insertion of Internal Fixation Device into Right Glenoid Cavity, Open Approach
0PH734Z Insertion of Internal Fixation Device into Right Glenoid Cavity, Percutaneous Approach
0PH744Z Insertion of Internal Fixation Device into Right Glenoid Cavity, Percutaneous Endoscopic Approach
0PH804Z Insertion of Internal Fixation Device into Left Glenoid Cavity, Open Approach
0PH834Z Insertion of Internal Fixation Device into Left Glenoid Cavity, Percutaneous Approach
0PH844Z Insertion of Internal Fixation Device into Left Glenoid Cavity, Percutaneous Endoscopic Approach
0PH904Z Insertion of Internal Fixation Device into Right Clavicle, Open Approach
0PH934Z Insertion of Internal Fixation Device into Right Clavicle, Percutaneous Approach
0PH944Z Insertion of Internal Fixation Device into Right Clavicle, Percutaneous Endoscopic Approach
0PHB04Z Insertion of Internal Fixation Device into Left Clavicle, Open Approach
0PHB34Z Insertion of Internal Fixation Device into Left Clavicle, Percutaneous Approach
0PHB44Z Insertion of Internal Fixation Device into Left Clavicle, Percutaneous Endoscopic Approach
0PHC04Z Insertion of Internal Fixation Device into Right Humeral Head, Open Approach
0PHC05Z Insertion of External Fixation Device into Right Humeral Head, Open Approach
0PHC06Z Insertion of Intramedullary Internal Fixation Device into Right Humeral Head, Open Approach
0PHC08Z Insertion of Limb Lengthening External Fixation Device into Right Humeral Head, Open Approach
0PHC0BZ Insertion of Monoplanar External Fixation Device into Right Humeral Head, Open Approach
0PHC0CZ Insertion of Ring External Fixation Device into Right Humeral Head, Open Approach
0PHC0DZ Insertion of Hybrid External Fixation Device into Right Humeral Head, Open Approach
0PHC34Z Insertion of Internal Fixation Device into Right Humeral Head, Percutaneous Approach
0PHC35Z Insertion of External Fixation Device into Right Humeral Head, Percutaneous Approach
0PHC36Z Insertion of Intramedullary Internal Fixation Device into Right Humeral Head, Percutaneous Approach
0PHC38Z Insertion of Limb Lengthening External Fixation Device into Right Humeral Head, Percutaneous Approach
0PHC3BZ Insertion of Monoplanar External Fixation Device into Right Humeral Head, Percutaneous Approach
0PHC3CZ Insertion of Ring External Fixation Device into Right Humeral Head, Percutaneous Approach
0PHC3DZ Insertion of Hybrid External Fixation Device into Right Humeral Head, Percutaneous Approach
0PHC44Z Insertion of Internal Fixation Device into Right Humeral Head, Percutaneous Endoscopic Approach
0PHC45Z Insertion of External Fixation Device into Right Humeral Head, Percutaneous Endoscopic Approach
0PHC46Z Insertion of Intramedullary Internal Fixation Device into Right Humeral Head, Percutaneous Endoscopic Approach
0PHC48Z Insertion of Limb Lengthening External Fixation Device into Right Humeral Head, Percutaneous Endoscopic Approach
0PHC4BZ Insertion of Monoplanar External Fixation Device into Right Humeral Head, Percutaneous Endoscopic Approach
0PHC4CZ Insertion of Ring External Fixation Device into Right Humeral Head, Percutaneous Endoscopic Approach
0PHC4DZ Insertion of Hybrid External Fixation Device into Right Humeral Head, Percutaneous Endoscopic Approach
0PHD04Z Insertion of Internal Fixation Device into Left Humeral Head, Open Approach
0PHD05Z Insertion of External Fixation Device into Left Humeral Head, Open Approach
0PHD06Z Insertion of Intramedullary Internal Fixation Device into Left Humeral Head, Open Approach
0PHD08Z Insertion of Limb Lengthening External Fixation Device into Left Humeral Head, Open Approach
0PHD0BZ Insertion of Monoplanar External Fixation Device into Left Humeral Head, Open Approach
0PHD0CZ Insertion of Ring External Fixation Device into Left Humeral Head, Open Approach
0PHD0DZ Insertion of Hybrid External Fixation Device into Left Humeral Head, Open Approach
0PHD34Z Insertion of Internal Fixation Device into Left Humeral Head, Percutaneous Approach
0PHD35Z Insertion of External Fixation Device into Left Humeral Head, Percutaneous Approach
0PHD36Z Insertion of Intramedullary Internal Fixation Device into Left Humeral Head, Percutaneous Approach
0PHD38Z Insertion of Limb Lengthening External Fixation Device into Left Humeral Head, Percutaneous Approach
0PHD3BZ Insertion of Monoplanar External Fixation Device into Left Humeral Head, Percutaneous Approach
0PHD3CZ Insertion of Ring External Fixation Device into Left Humeral Head, Percutaneous Approach
0PHD3DZ Insertion of Hybrid External Fixation Device into Left Humeral Head, Percutaneous Approach
0PHD44Z Insertion of Internal Fixation Device into Left Humeral Head, Percutaneous Endoscopic Approach
0PHD45Z Insertion of External Fixation Device into Left Humeral Head, Percutaneous Endoscopic Approach
0PHD46Z Insertion of Intramedullary Internal Fixation Device into Left Humeral Head, Percutaneous Endoscopic Approach
0PHD48Z Insertion of Limb Lengthening External Fixation Device into Left Humeral Head, Percutaneous Endoscopic Approach
0PHD4BZ Insertion of Monoplanar External Fixation Device into Left Humeral Head, Percutaneous Endoscopic Approach
0PHD4CZ Insertion of Ring External Fixation Device into Left Humeral Head, Percutaneous Endoscopic Approach
0PHD4DZ Insertion of Hybrid External Fixation Device into Left Humeral Head, Percutaneous Endoscopic Approach
0PHF04Z Insertion of Internal Fixation Device into Right Humeral Shaft, Open Approach
0PHF05Z Insertion of External Fixation Device into Right Humeral Shaft, Open Approach
0PHF06Z Insertion of Intramedullary Internal Fixation Device into Right Humeral Shaft, Open Approach
0PHF08Z Insertion of Limb Lengthening External Fixation Device into Right Humeral Shaft, Open Approach
0PHF0BZ Insertion of Monoplanar External Fixation Device into Right Humeral Shaft, Open Approach
0PHF0CZ Insertion of Ring External Fixation Device into Right Humeral Shaft, Open Approach
0PHF0DZ Insertion of Hybrid External Fixation Device into Right Humeral Shaft, Open Approach
0PHF34Z Insertion of Internal Fixation Device into Right Humeral Shaft, Percutaneous Approach
0PHF35Z Insertion of External Fixation Device into Right Humeral Shaft, Percutaneous Approach
0PHF36Z Insertion of Intramedullary Internal Fixation Device into Right Humeral Shaft, Percutaneous Approach
0PHF38Z Insertion of Limb Lengthening External Fixation Device into Right Humeral Shaft, Percutaneous Approach
0PHF3BZ Insertion of Monoplanar External Fixation Device into Right Humeral Shaft, Percutaneous Approach
0PHF3CZ Insertion of Ring External Fixation Device into Right Humeral Shaft, Percutaneous Approach
0PHF3DZ Insertion of Hybrid External Fixation Device into Right Humeral Shaft, Percutaneous Approach
0PHF44Z Insertion of Internal Fixation Device into Right Humeral Shaft, Percutaneous Endoscopic Approach
0PHF45Z Insertion of External Fixation Device into Right Humeral Shaft, Percutaneous Endoscopic Approach

0PHF46Z Insertion of Intramedullary Internal Fixation Device into Right Humeral Shaft, Percutaneous Endoscopic Approach
0PHF48Z Insertion of Limb Lengthening External Fixation Device into Right Humeral Shaft, Percutaneous Endoscopic Approach
0PHF4BZ Insertion of Monoplanar External Fixation Device into Right Humeral Shaft, Percutaneous Endoscopic Approach
0PHF4CZ Insertion of Ring External Fixation Device into Right Humeral Shaft, Percutaneous Endoscopic Approach
0PHF4DZ Insertion of Hybrid External Fixation Device into Right Humeral Shaft, Percutaneous Endoscopic Approach
0PHG04Z Insertion of Internal Fixation Device into Left Humeral Shaft, Open Approach
0PHG05Z Insertion of External Fixation Device into Left Humeral Shaft, Open Approach
0PHG06Z Insertion of Intramedullary Internal Fixation Device into Left Humeral Shaft, Open Approach
0PHG08Z Insertion of Limb Lengthening External Fixation Device into Left Humeral Shaft, Open Approach
0PHG0BZ Insertion of Monoplanar External Fixation Device into Left Humeral Shaft, Open Approach
0PHG0CZ Insertion of Ring External Fixation Device into Left Humeral Shaft, Open Approach
0PHG0DZ Insertion of Hybrid External Fixation Device into Left Humeral Shaft, Open Approach
0PHG34Z Insertion of Internal Fixation Device into Left Humeral Shaft, Percutaneous Approach
0PHG35Z Insertion of External Fixation Device into Left Humeral Shaft, Percutaneous Approach
0PHG36Z Insertion of Intramedullary Internal Fixation Device into Left Humeral Shaft, Percutaneous Approach
0PHG38Z Insertion of Limb Lengthening External Fixation Device into Left Humeral Shaft, Percutaneous Approach
0PHG3BZ Insertion of Monoplanar External Fixation Device into Left Humeral Shaft, Percutaneous Approach
0PHG3CZ Insertion of Ring External Fixation Device into Left Humeral Shaft, Percutaneous Approach
0PHG3DZ Insertion of Hybrid External Fixation Device into Left Humeral Shaft, Percutaneous Approach
0PHG44Z Insertion of Internal Fixation Device into Left Humeral Shaft, Percutaneous Endoscopic Approach
0PHG45Z Insertion of External Fixation Device into Left Humeral Shaft, Percutaneous Endoscopic Approach
0PHG46Z Insertion of Intramedullary Internal Fixation Device into Left Humeral Shaft, Percutaneous Endoscopic Approach
0PHG48Z Insertion of Limb Lengthening External Fixation Device into Left Humeral Shaft, Percutaneous Endoscopic Approach
0PHG4BZ Insertion of Monoplanar External Fixation Device into Left Humeral Shaft, Percutaneous Endoscopic Approach
0PHG4CZ Insertion of Ring External Fixation Device into Left Humeral Shaft, Percutaneous Endoscopic Approach
0PHG4DZ Insertion of Hybrid External Fixation Device into Left Humeral Shaft, Percutaneous Endoscopic Approach
0PHH04Z Insertion of Internal Fixation Device into Right Radius, Open Approach
0PHH05Z Insertion of External Fixation Device into Right Radius, Open Approach
0PHH06Z Insertion of Intramedullary Internal Fixation Device into Right Radius, Open Approach
0PHH08Z Insertion of Limb Lengthening External Fixation Device into Right Radius, Open Approach
0PHH0BZ Insertion of Monoplanar External Fixation Device into Right Radius, Open Approach
0PHH0CZ Insertion of Ring External Fixation Device into Right Radius, Open Approach
0PHH0DZ Insertion of Hybrid External Fixation Device into Right Radius, Open Approach
0PHH34Z Insertion of Internal Fixation Device into Right Radius, Percutaneous Approach
0PHH35Z Insertion of External Fixation Device into Right Radius, Percutaneous Approach
0PHH36Z Insertion of Intramedullary Internal Fixation Device into Right Radius, Percutaneous Approach
0PHH38Z Insertion of Limb Lengthening External Fixation Device into Right Radius, Percutaneous Approach
0PHH3BZ Insertion of Monoplanar External Fixation Device into Right Radius, Percutaneous Approach
0PHH3CZ Insertion of Ring External Fixation Device into Right Radius, Percutaneous Approach
0PHH3DZ Insertion of Hybrid External Fixation Device into Right Radius, Percutaneous Approach
0PHH44Z Insertion of Internal Fixation Device into Right Radius, Percutaneous Endoscopic Approach
0PHH45Z Insertion of External Fixation Device into Right Radius, Percutaneous Endoscopic Approach
0PHH46Z Insertion of Intramedullary Internal Fixation Device into Right Radius, Percutaneous Endoscopic Approach
0PHH48Z Insertion of Limb Lengthening External Fixation Device into Right Radius, Percutaneous Endoscopic Approach
0PHH4BZ Insertion of Monoplanar External Fixation Device into Right Radius, Percutaneous Endoscopic Approach
0PHH4CZ Insertion of Ring External Fixation Device into Right Radius, Percutaneous Endoscopic Approach
0PHH4DZ Insertion of Hybrid External Fixation Device into Right Radius, Percutaneous Endoscopic Approach
0PHJ04Z Insertion of Internal Fixation Device into Left Radius, Open Approach
0PHJ05Z Insertion of External Fixation Device into Left Radius, Open Approach
0PHJ06Z Insertion of Intramedullary Internal Fixation Device into Left Radius, Open Approach
0PHJ08Z Insertion of Limb Lengthening External Fixation Device into Left Radius, Open Approach
0PHJ0BZ Insertion of Monoplanar External Fixation Device into Left Radius, Open Approach
0PHJ0CZ Insertion of Ring External Fixation Device into Left Radius, Open Approach
0PHJ0DZ Insertion of Hybrid External Fixation Device into Left Radius, Open Approach
0PHJ34Z Insertion of Internal Fixation Device into Left Radius, Percutaneous Approach
0PHJ35Z Insertion of External Fixation Device into Left Radius, Percutaneous Approach
0PHJ36Z Insertion of Intramedullary Internal Fixation Device into Left Radius, Percutaneous Approach
0PHJ38Z Insertion of Limb Lengthening External Fixation Device into Left Radius, Percutaneous Approach
0PHJ3BZ Insertion of Monoplanar External Fixatio Device into Left Radius, Percutaneous Approach
0PHJ3CZ Insertion of Ring External Fixation Device into Left Radius, Percutaneous Approach
0PHJ3DZ Insertion of Hybrid External Fixation Device into Left Radius, Percutaneous Approach
0PHJ44Z Insertion of Internal Fixation Device into Left Radius, Percutaneous Endoscopic Approach
0PHJ45Z Insertion of External Fixation Device intc Left Radius, Percutaneous Endoscopic Approach
0PHJ46Z Insertion of Intramedullary Internal Fixation Device into Left Radius, Percutaneous Endoscopic Approach
0PHJ48Z Insertion of Limb Lengthening External Fixation Device into Left Radius, Percutaneous Endoscopic Approach
0PHJ4BZ Insertion of Monoplanar External Fixatio Device into Left Radius, Percutaneous Endoscopic Approach
0PHJ4CZ Insertion of Ring External Fixation Devic into Left Radius, Percutaneous Endoscopi Approach
0PHJ4DZ Insertion of Hybrid External Fixation Device into Left Radius, Percutaneous Endoscopic Approach
0PHK04Z Insertion of Internal Fixation Device into Right Ulna, Open Approach
0PHK05Z Insertion of External Fixation Device into Right Ulna, Open Approach
0PHK06Z Insertion of Intramedullary Internal Fixation Device into Right Ulna, Open Approach
0PHK08Z Insertion of Limb Lengthening External Fixation Device into Right Ulna, Open Approach
0PHK0BZ Insertion of Monoplanar External Fixation Device into Right Ulna, Open Approach
0PHK0CZ Insertion of Ring External Fixation Device into Right Ulna, Open Approach
0PHK0DZ Insertion of Hybrid External Fixation Device into Right Ulna, Open Approach
0PHK34Z Insertion of Internal Fixation Device into Right Ulna, Percutaneous Approach
0PHK35Z Insertion of External Fixation Device into Right Ulna, Percutaneous Approach
0PHK36Z Insertion of Intramedullary Internal Fixation Device into Right Ulna, Percutaneous Approach
0PHK38Z Insertion of Limb Lengthening External Fixation Device into Right Ulna, Percutaneous Approach
0PHK3BZ Insertion of Monoplanar External Fixation Device into Right Ulna, Percutaneous Approach
0PHK3CZ Insertion of Ring External Fixation Device into Right Ulna, Percutaneous Approach
0PHK3DZ Insertion of Hybrid External Fixation Device into Right Ulna, Percutaneous Approach
0PHK44Z Insertion of Internal Fixation Device into Right Ulna, Percutaneous Endoscopic Approach
0PHK45Z Insertion of External Fixation Device into Right Ulna, Percutaneous Endoscopic Approach
0PHK46Z Insertion of Intramedullary Internal Fixation Device into Right Ulna, Percutaneous Endoscopic Approach

HK48Z Insertion of Limb Lengthening External Fixation Device into Right Ulna, Percutaneous Endoscopic Approach
HK4BZ Insertion of Monoplanar External Fixation Device into Right Ulna, Percutaneous Endoscopic Approach
HK4CZ Insertion of Ring External Fixation Device into Right Ulna, Percutaneous Endoscopic Approach
HK4DZ Insertion of Hybrid External Fixation Device into Right Ulna, Percutaneous Endoscopic Approach
PHL04Z Insertion of Internal Fixation Device into Left Ulna, Open Approach
PHL05Z Insertion of External Fixation Device into Left Ulna, Open Approach
PHL06Z Insertion of Intramedullary Internal Fixation Device into Left Ulna, Open Approach
PHL08Z Insertion of Limb Lengthening External Fixation Device into Left Ulna, Open Approach
PHL0BZ Insertion of Monoplanar External Fixation Device into Left Ulna, Open Approach
PHL0CZ Insertion of Ring External Fixation Device into Left Ulna, Open Approach
PHL0DZ Insertion of Hybrid External Fixation Device into Left Ulna, Open Approach
PHL34Z Insertion of Internal Fixation Device into Left Ulna, Percutaneous Approach
PHL35Z Insertion of External Fixation Device into Left Ulna, Percutaneous Approach
PHL36Z Insertion of Intramedullary Internal Fixation Device into Left Ulna, Percutaneous Approach
PHL38Z Insertion of Limb Lengthening External Fixation Device into Left Ulna, Percutaneous Approach
PHL3BZ Insertion of Monoplanar External Fixation Device into Left Ulna, Percutaneous Approach
PHL3CZ Insertion of Ring External Fixation Device into Left Ulna, Percutaneous Approach
PHL3DZ Insertion of Hybrid External Fixation Device into Left Ulna, Percutaneous Approach
PHL44Z Insertion of Internal Fixation Device into Left Ulna, Percutaneous Endoscopic Approach
PHL45Z Insertion of External Fixation Device into Left Ulna, Percutaneous Endoscopic Approach
PHL46Z Insertion of Intramedullary Internal Fixation Device into Left Ulna, Percutaneous Endoscopic Approach
PHL48Z Insertion of Limb Lengthening External Fixation Device into Left Ulna, Percutaneous Endoscopic Approach
0PHL4BZ Insertion of Monoplanar External Fixation Device into Left Ulna, Percutaneous Endoscopic Approach
0PHL4CZ Insertion of Ring External Fixation Device into Left Ulna, Percutaneous Endoscopic Approach
0PHL4DZ Insertion of Hybrid External Fixation Device into Left Ulna, Percutaneous Endoscopic Approach
0PHM04Z Insertion of Internal Fixation Device into Right Carpal, Open Approach
0PHM05Z Insertion of External Fixation Device into Right Carpal, Open Approach
0PHM34Z Insertion of Internal Fixation Device into Right Carpal, Percutaneous Approach
0PHM35Z Insertion of External Fixation Device into Right Carpal, Percutaneous Approach
0PHM44Z Insertion of Internal Fixation Device into Right Carpal, Percutaneous Endoscopic Approach
0PHM45Z Insertion of External Fixation Device into Right Carpal, Percutaneous Endoscopic Approach
0PHN04Z Insertion of Internal Fixation Device into Left Carpal, Open Approach
0PHN05Z Insertion of External Fixation Device into Left Carpal, Open Approach
0PHN34Z Insertion of Internal Fixation Device into Left Carpal, Percutaneous Approach
0PHN35Z Insertion of External Fixation Device into Left Carpal, Percutaneous Approach
0PHN44Z Insertion of Internal Fixation Device into Left Carpal, Percutaneous Endoscopic Approach
0PHN45Z Insertion of External Fixation Device into Left Carpal, Percutaneous Endoscopic Approach
0PHP04Z Insertion of Internal Fixation Device into Right Metacarpal, Open Approach
0PHP05Z Insertion of External Fixation Device into Right Metacarpal, Open Approach
0PHP34Z Insertion of Internal Fixation Device into Right Metacarpal, Percutaneous Approach
0PHP35Z Insertion of External Fixation Device into Right Metacarpal, Percutaneous Approach
0PHP44Z Insertion of Internal Fixation Device into Right Metacarpal, Percutaneous Endoscopic Approach
0PHP45Z Insertion of External Fixation Device into Right Metacarpal, Percutaneous Endoscopic Approach
0PHQ04Z Insertion of Internal Fixation Device into Left Metacarpal, Open Approach
0PHQ05Z Insertion of External Fixation Device into Left Metacarpal, Open Approach
0PHQ34Z Insertion of Internal Fixation Device into Left Metacarpal, Percutaneous Approach
0PHQ35Z Insertion of External Fixation Device into Left Metacarpal, Percutaneous Approach
0PHQ44Z Insertion of Internal Fixation Device into Left Metacarpal, Percutaneous Endoscopic Approach
0PHQ45Z Insertion of External Fixation Device into Left Metacarpal, Percutaneous Endoscopic Approach
0PHR04Z Insertion of Internal Fixation Device into Right Thumb Phalanx, Open Approach
0PHR05Z Insertion of External Fixation Device into Right Thumb Phalanx, Open Approach
0PHR34Z Insertion of Internal Fixation Device into Right Thumb Phalanx, Percutaneous Approach
0PHR35Z Insertion of External Fixation Device into Right Thumb Phalanx, Percutaneous Approach
0PHR44Z Insertion of Internal Fixation Device into Right Thumb Phalanx, Percutaneous Endoscopic Approach
0PHR45Z Insertion of External Fixation Device into Right Thumb Phalanx, Percutaneous Endoscopic Approach
0PHS04Z Insertion of Internal Fixation Device into Left Thumb Phalanx, Open Approach
0PHS05Z Insertion of External Fixation Device into Left Thumb Phalanx, Open Approach
0PHS34Z Insertion of Internal Fixation Device into Left Thumb Phalanx, Percutaneous Approach
0PHS35Z Insertion of External Fixation Device into Left Thumb Phalanx, Percutaneous Approach
0PHS44Z Insertion of Internal Fixation Device into Left Thumb Phalanx, Percutaneous Endoscopic Approach
0PHS45Z Insertion of External Fixation Device into Left Thumb Phalanx, Percutaneous Endoscopic Approach
0PHT04Z Insertion of Internal Fixation Device into Right Finger Phalanx, Open Approach
0PHT05Z Insertion of External Fixation Device into Right Finger Phalanx, Open Approach
0PHT34Z Insertion of Internal Fixation Device into Right Finger Phalanx, Percutaneous Approach
0PHT35Z Insertion of External Fixation Device into Right Finger Phalanx, Percutaneous Approach
0PHT44Z Insertion of Internal Fixation Device into Right Finger Phalanx, Percutaneous Endoscopic Approach
0PHT45Z Insertion of External Fixation Device into Right Finger Phalanx, Percutaneous Endoscopic Approach
0PHV04Z Insertion of Internal Fixation Device into Left Finger Phalanx, Open Approach
0PHV05Z Insertion of External Fixation Device into Left Finger Phalanx, Open Approach
0PHV34Z Insertion of Internal Fixation Device into Left Finger Phalanx, Percutaneous Approach
0PHV35Z Insertion of External Fixation Device into Left Finger Phalanx, Percutaneous Approach
0PHV44Z Insertion of Internal Fixation Device into Left Finger Phalanx, Percutaneous Endoscopic Approach
0PHV45Z Insertion of External Fixation Device into Left Finger Phalanx, Percutaneous Endoscopic Approach
0PHY0MZ Insertion of Bone Growth Stimulator into Upper Bone, Open Approach
0PHY3MZ Insertion of Bone Growth Stimulator into Upper Bone, Percutaneous Approach
0PHY4MZ Insertion of Bone Growth Stimulator into Upper Bone, Percutaneous Endoscopic Approach

0PJ – Upper Bones, Inspection

Review Coding Guideline B3.5

Review Coding Guidelines B3.11a, B3.11b and B3.11c

0PJY0ZZ Inspection of Upper Bone, Open Approach
0PJY3ZZ Inspection of Upper Bone, Percutaneous Approach
0PJY4ZZ Inspection of Upper Bone, Percutaneous Endoscopic Approach
0PJYXZZ Inspection of Upper Bone, External Approach

0PN – Upper Bones, Release

Review Coding Guideline B3.13

Review Coding Guideline B3.14

0PN00ZZ Release Sternum, Open Approach
0PN03ZZ Release Sternum, Percutaneous Approach
0PN04ZZ Release Sternum, Percutaneous Endoscopic Approach
0PN10ZZ Release Right Rib, Open Approach
0PN13ZZ Release Right Rib, Percutaneous Approach
0PN14ZZ Release Right Rib, Percutaneous Endoscopic Approach
0PN20ZZ Release Left Rib, Open Approach
0PN23ZZ Release Left Rib, Percutaneous Approach
0PN24ZZ Release Left Rib, Percutaneous Endoscopic Approach
0PN30ZZ Release Cervical Vertebra, Open Approach
0PN33ZZ Release Cervical Vertebra, Percutaneous Approach
0PN34ZZ Release Cervical Vertebra, Percutaneous Endoscopic Approach
0PN40ZZ Release Thoracic Vertebra, Open Approach
0PN43ZZ Release Thoracic Vertebra, Percutaneous Approach
0PN44ZZ Release Thoracic Vertebra, Percutaneous Endoscopic Approach
0PN50ZZ Release Right Scapula, Open Approach
0PN53ZZ Release Right Scapula, Percutaneous Approach
0PN54ZZ Release Right Scapula, Percutaneous Endoscopic Approach
0PN60ZZ Release Left Scapula, Open Approach
0PN63ZZ Release Left Scapula, Percutaneous Approach
0PN64ZZ Release Left Scapula, Percutaneous Endoscopic Approach
0PN70ZZ Release Right Glenoid Cavity, Open Approach
0PN73ZZ Release Right Glenoid Cavity, Percutaneous Approach
0PN74ZZ Release Right Glenoid Cavity, Percutaneous Endoscopic Approach
0PN80ZZ Release Left Glenoid Cavity, Open Approach
0PN83ZZ Release Left Glenoid Cavity, Percutaneous Approach
0PN84ZZ Release Left Glenoid Cavity, Percutaneous Endoscopic Approach
0PN90ZZ Release Right Clavicle, Open Approach
0PN93ZZ Release Right Clavicle, Percutaneous Approach
0PN94ZZ Release Right Clavicle, Percutaneous Endoscopic Approach
0PNB0ZZ Release Left Clavicle, Open Approach
0PNB3ZZ Release Left Clavicle, Percutaneous Approach
0PNB4ZZ Release Left Clavicle, Percutaneous Endoscopic Approach
0PNC0ZZ Release Right Humeral Head, Open Approach
0PNC3ZZ Release Right Humeral Head, Percutaneous Approach
0PNC4ZZ Release Right Humeral Head, Percutaneous Endoscopic Approach
0PND0ZZ Release Left Humeral Head, Open Approach
0PND3ZZ Release Left Humeral Head, Percutaneous Approach
0PND4ZZ Release Left Humeral Head, Percutaneous Endoscopic Approach
0PNF0ZZ Release Right Humeral Shaft, Open Approach
0PNF3ZZ Release Right Humeral Shaft, Percutaneous Approach
0PNF4ZZ Release Right Humeral Shaft, Percutaneous Endoscopic Approach
0PNG0ZZ Release Left Humeral Shaft, Open Approach
0PNG3ZZ Release Left Humeral Shaft, Percutaneous Approach
0PNG4ZZ Release Left Humeral Shaft, Percutaneous Endoscopic Approach
0PNH0ZZ Release Right Radius, Open Approach
0PNH3ZZ Release Right Radius, Percutaneous Approach
0PNH4ZZ Release Right Radius, Percutaneous Endoscopic Approach
0PNJ0ZZ Release Left Radius, Open Approach
0PNJ3ZZ Release Left Radius, Percutaneous Approach
0PNJ4ZZ Release Left Radius, Percutaneous Endoscopic Approach
0PNK0ZZ Release Right Ulna, Open Approach
0PNK3ZZ Release Right Ulna, Percutaneous Approach
0PNK4ZZ Release Right Ulna, Percutaneous Endoscopic Approach
0PNL0ZZ Release Left Ulna, Open Approach
0PNL3ZZ Release Left Ulna, Percutaneous Approa
0PNL4ZZ Release Left Ulna, Percutaneous Endoscopic Approach
0PNM0ZZ Release Right Carpal, Open Approach
0PNM3ZZ Release Right Carpal, Percutaneous Approach
0PNM4ZZ Release Right Carpal, Percutaneous Endoscopic Approach
0PNN0ZZ Release Left Carpal, Open Approach
0PNN3ZZ Release Left Carpal, Percutaneous Approach
0PNN4ZZ Release Left Carpal, Percutaneous Endoscopic Approach
0PNP0ZZ Release Right Metacarpal, Open Approac
0PNP3ZZ Release Right Metacarpal, Percutaneous Approach
0PNP4ZZ Release Right Metacarpal, Percutaneous Endoscopic Approach
0PNQ0ZZ Release Left Metacarpal, Open Approach
0PNQ3ZZ Release Left Metacarpal, Percutaneous Approach
0PNQ4ZZ Release Left Metacarpal, Percutaneous Endoscopic Approach
0PNR0ZZ Release Right Thumb Phalanx, Open Approach
0PNR3ZZ Release Right Thumb Phalanx, Percutaneous Approach
0PNR4ZZ Release Right Thumb Phalanx, Percutaneous Endoscopic Approach
0PNS0ZZ Release Left Thumb Phalanx, Open Approach
0PNS3ZZ Release Left Thumb Phalanx, Percutaneous Approach
0PNS4ZZ Release Left Thumb Phalanx, Percutaneous Endoscopic Approach
0PNT0ZZ Release Right Finger Phalanx, Open Approach
0PNT3ZZ Release Right Finger Phalanx, Percutaneous Approach
0PNT4ZZ Release Right Finger Phalanx, Percutaneous Endoscopic Approach
0PNV0ZZ Release Left Finger Phalanx, Open Approach
0PNV3ZZ Release Left Finger Phalanx, Percutaneou Approach
0PNV4ZZ Release Left Finger Phalanx, Percutaneou Endoscopic Approach

0PP – Upper Bones, Removal

Review Coding Guideline B6.1c

0PP004Z Removal of Internal Fixation Device from Sternum, Open Approach
0PP007Z Removal of Autologous Tissue Substitute from Sternum, Open Approach
0PP00JZ Removal of Synthetic Substitute from Sternum, Open Approach
0PP00KZ Removal of Nonautologous Tissue Substitute from Sternum, Open Approach
0PP034Z Removal of Internal Fixation Device from Sternum, Percutaneous Approach
0PP037Z Removal of Autologous Tissue Substitute from Sternum, Percutaneous Approach
0PP03JZ Removal of Synthetic Substitute from Sternum, Percutaneous Approach
0PP03KZ Removal of Nonautologous Tissue Substitute from Sternum, Percutaneous Approach
0PP044Z Removal of Internal Fixation Device from Sternum, Percutaneous Endoscopic Approach
0PP047Z Removal of Autologous Tissue Substitute from Sternum, Percutaneous Endoscopic Approach
0PP04JZ Removal of Synthetic Substitute from Sternum, Percutaneous Endoscopic Approach
0PP04KZ Removal of Nonautologous Tissue Substitute from Sternum, Percutaneous Endoscopic Approach
0PP0X4Z Removal of Internal Fixation Device from Sternum, External Approach
0PP104Z Removal of Internal Fixation Device from Right Rib, Open Approach
0PP107Z Removal of Autologous Tissue Substitute from Right Rib, Open Approach
0PP10JZ Removal of Synthetic Substitute from Right Rib, Open Approach
0PP10KZ Removal of Nonautologous Tissue Substitute from Right Rib, Open Approach
0PP134Z Removal of Internal Fixation Device from Right Rib, Percutaneous Approach
0PP137Z Removal of Autologous Tissue Substitute from Right Rib, Percutaneous Approach
0PP13JZ Removal of Synthetic Substitute from Right Rib, Percutaneous Approach
0PP13KZ Removal of Nonautologous Tissue Substitute from Right Rib, Percutaneous Approach
0PP144Z Removal of Internal Fixation Device from Right Rib, Percutaneous Endoscopic Approach
0PP147Z Removal of Autologous Tissue Substitute from Right Rib, Percutaneous Endoscopic Approach

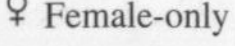
♀ Female-only ♂ Male-only Limited Coverage ● Non-OR HAC-associated procedure ▲ Non-covered procedures Combination

P14JZ Removal of Synthetic Substitute from Right Rib, Percutaneous Endoscopic Approach

P14KZ Removal of Nonautologous Tissue Substitute from Right Rib, Percutaneous Endoscopic Approach

P1X4Z Removal of Internal Fixation Device from Right Rib, External Approach

P204Z Removal of Internal Fixation Device from Left Rib, Open Approach

P207Z Removal of Autologous Tissue Substitute from Left Rib, Open Approach

P20JZ Removal of Synthetic Substitute from Left Rib, Open Approach

PP20KZ Removal of Nonautologous Tissue Substitute from Left Rib, Open Approach

PP234Z Removal of Internal Fixation Device from Left Rib, Percutaneous Approach

PP237Z Removal of Autologous Tissue Substitute from Left Rib, Percutaneous Approach

PP23JZ Removal of Synthetic Substitute from Left Rib, Percutaneous Approach

PP23KZ Removal of Nonautologous Tissue Substitute from Left Rib, Percutaneous Approach

PP244Z Removal of Internal Fixation Device from Left Rib, Percutaneous Endoscopic Approach

PP247Z Removal of Autologous Tissue Substitute from Left Rib, Percutaneous Endoscopic Approach

PP24JZ Removal of Synthetic Substitute from Left Rib, Percutaneous Endoscopic Approach

PP24KZ Removal of Nonautologous Tissue Substitute from Left Rib, Percutaneous Endoscopic Approach

PP2X4Z Removal of Internal Fixation Device from Left Rib, External Approach

PP304Z Removal of Internal Fixation Device from Cervical Vertebra, Open Approach

PP307Z Removal of Autologous Tissue Substitute from Cervical Vertebra, Open Approach

PP30JZ Removal of Synthetic Substitute from Cervical Vertebra, Open Approach

PP30KZ Removal of Nonautologous Tissue Substitute from Cervical Vertebra, Open Approach

PP334Z Removal of Internal Fixation Device from Cervical Vertebra, Percutaneous Approach

PP337Z Removal of Autologous Tissue Substitute from Cervical Vertebra, Percutaneous Approach

PP33JZ Removal of Synthetic Substitute from Cervical Vertebra, Percutaneous Approach

PP33KZ Removal of Nonautologous Tissue Substitute from Cervical Vertebra, Percutaneous Approach

PP344Z Removal of Internal Fixation Device from Cervical Vertebra, Percutaneous Endoscopic Approach

PP347Z Removal of Autologous Tissue Substitute from Cervical Vertebra, Percutaneous Endoscopic Approach

PP34JZ Removal of Synthetic Substitute from Cervical Vertebra, Percutaneous Endoscopic Approach

PP34KZ Removal of Nonautologous Tissue Substitute from Cervical Vertebra, Percutaneous Endoscopic Approach

0PP3X4Z Removal of Internal Fixation Device from Cervical Vertebra, External Approach

0PP404Z Removal of Internal Fixation Device from Thoracic Vertebra, Open Approach

0PP407Z Removal of Autologous Tissue Substitute from Thoracic Vertebra, Open Approach

0PP40JZ Removal of Synthetic Substitute from Thoracic Vertebra, Open Approach

0PP40KZ Removal of Nonautologous Tissue Substitute from Thoracic Vertebra, Open Approach

0PP434Z Removal of Internal Fixation Device from Thoracic Vertebra, Percutaneous Approach

0PP437Z Removal of Autologous Tissue Substitute from Thoracic Vertebra, Percutaneous Approach

0PP43JZ Removal of Synthetic Substitute from Thoracic Vertebra, Percutaneous Approach

0PP43KZ Removal of Nonautologous Tissue Substitute from Thoracic Vertebra, Percutaneous Approach

0PP444Z Removal of Internal Fixation Device from Thoracic Vertebra, Percutaneous Endoscopic Approach

0PP447Z Removal of Autologous Tissue Substitute from Thoracic Vertebra, Percutaneous Endoscopic Approach

0PP44JZ Removal of Synthetic Substitute from Thoracic Vertebra, Percutaneous Endoscopic Approach

0PP44KZ Removal of Nonautologous Tissue Substitute from Thoracic Vertebra, Percutaneous Endoscopic Approach

0PP4X4Z Removal of Internal Fixation Device from Thoracic Vertebra, External Approach

0PP504Z Removal of Internal Fixation Device from Right Scapula, Open Approach

0PP507Z Removal of Autologous Tissue Substitute from Right Scapula, Open Approach

0PP50JZ Removal of Synthetic Substitute from Right Scapula, Open Approach

0PP50KZ Removal of Nonautologous Tissue Substitute from Right Scapula, Open Approach

0PP534Z Removal of Internal Fixation Device from Right Scapula, Percutaneous Approach

0PP537Z Removal of Autologous Tissue Substitute from Right Scapula, Percutaneous Approach

0PP53JZ Removal of Synthetic Substitute from Right Scapula, Percutaneous Approach

0PP53KZ Removal of Nonautologous Tissue Substitute from Right Scapula, Percutaneous Approach

0PP544Z Removal of Internal Fixation Device from Right Scapula, Percutaneous Endoscopic Approach

0PP547Z Removal of Autologous Tissue Substitute from Right Scapula, Percutaneous Endoscopic Approach

0PP54JZ Removal of Synthetic Substitute from Right Scapula, Percutaneous Endoscopic Approach

0PP54KZ Removal of Nonautologous Tissue Substitute from Right Scapula, Percutaneous Endoscopic Approach

0PP5X4Z Removal of Internal Fixation Device from Right Scapula, External Approach

0PP604Z Removal of Internal Fixation Device from Left Scapula, Open Approach

0PP607Z Removal of Autologous Tissue Substitute from Left Scapula, Open Approach

0PP60JZ Removal of Synthetic Substitute from Left Scapula, Open Approach

0PP60KZ Removal of Nonautologous Tissue Substitute from Left Scapula, Open Approach

0PP634Z Removal of Internal Fixation Device from Left Scapula, Percutaneous Approach

0PP637Z Removal of Autologous Tissue Substitute from Left Scapula, Percutaneous Approach

0PP63JZ Removal of Synthetic Substitute from Left Scapula, Percutaneous Approach

0PP63KZ Removal of Nonautologous Tissue Substitute from Left Scapula, Percutaneous Approach

0PP644Z Removal of Internal Fixation Device from Left Scapula, Percutaneous Endoscopic Approach

0PP647Z Removal of Autologous Tissue Substitute from Left Scapula, Percutaneous Endoscopic Approach

0PP64JZ Removal of Synthetic Substitute from Left Scapula, Percutaneous Endoscopic Approach

0PP64KZ Removal of Nonautologous Tissue Substitute from Left Scapula, Percutaneous Endoscopic Approach

0PP6X4Z Removal of Internal Fixation Device from Left Scapula, External Approach

0PP704Z Removal of Internal Fixation Device from Right Glenoid Cavity, Open Approach

0PP707Z Removal of Autologous Tissue Substitute from Right Glenoid Cavity, Open Approach

0PP70JZ Removal of Synthetic Substitute from Right Glenoid Cavity, Open Approach

0PP70KZ Removal of Nonautologous Tissue Substitute from Right Glenoid Cavity, Open Approach

0PP734Z Removal of Internal Fixation Device from Right Glenoid Cavity, Percutaneous Approach

0PP737Z Removal of Autologous Tissue Substitute from Right Glenoid Cavity, Percutaneous Approach

0PP73JZ Removal of Synthetic Substitute from Right Glenoid Cavity, Percutaneous Approach

0PP73KZ Removal of Nonautologous Tissue Substitute from Right Glenoid Cavity, Percutaneous Approach

0PP744Z Removal of Internal Fixation Device from Right Glenoid Cavity, Percutaneous Endoscopic Approach

0PP747Z Removal of Autologous Tissue Substitute from Right Glenoid Cavity, Percutaneous Endoscopic Approach

0PP74JZ Removal of Synthetic Substitute from Right Glenoid Cavity, Percutaneous Endoscopic Approach

0PP74KZ Removal of Nonautologous Tissue Substitute from Right Glenoid Cavity, Percutaneous Endoscopic Approach

0PP7X4Z Removal of Internal Fixation Device from Right Glenoid Cavity, External Approach

0PP804Z Removal of Internal Fixation Device from Left Glenoid Cavity, Open Approach

0PP807Z Removal of Autologous Tissue Substitute from Left Glenoid Cavity, Open Approach

0PP80JZ Removal of Synthetic Substitute from Left Glenoid Cavity, Open Approach

0PP80KZ Removal of Nonautologous Tissue Substitute from Left Glenoid Cavity, Open Approach

0PP834Z Removal of Internal Fixation Device from Left Glenoid Cavity, Percutaneous Approach

0PP837Z Removal of Autologous Tissue Substitute from Left Glenoid Cavity, Percutaneous Approach

0PP83JZ Removal of Synthetic Substitute from Left Glenoid Cavity, Percutaneous Approach

0PP83KZ Removal of Nonautologous Tissue Substitute from Left Glenoid Cavity, Percutaneous Approach

0PP844Z Removal of Internal Fixation Device from Left Glenoid Cavity, Percutaneous Endoscopic Approach

0PP847Z Removal of Autologous Tissue Substitute from Left Glenoid Cavity, Percutaneous Endoscopic Approach
0PP84JZ Removal of Synthetic Substitute from Left Glenoid Cavity, Percutaneous Endoscopic Approach
0PP84KZ Removal of Nonautologous Tissue Substitute from Left Glenoid Cavity, Percutaneous Endoscopic Approach
0PP8X4Z Removal of Internal Fixation Device from Left Glenoid Cavity, External Approach
0PP904Z Removal of Internal Fixation Device from Right Clavicle, Open Approach
0PP907Z Removal of Autologous Tissue Substitute from Right Clavicle, Open Approach
0PP90JZ Removal of Synthetic Substitute from Right Clavicle, Open Approach
0PP90KZ Removal of Nonautologous Tissue Substitute from Right Clavicle, Open Approach
0PP934Z Removal of Internal Fixation Device from Right Clavicle, Percutaneous Approach
0PP937Z Removal of Autologous Tissue Substitute from Right Clavicle, Percutaneous Approach
0PP93JZ Removal of Synthetic Substitute from Right Clavicle, Percutaneous Approach
0PP93KZ Removal of Nonautologous Tissue Substitute from Right Clavicle, Percutaneous Approach
0PP944Z Removal of Internal Fixation Device from Right Clavicle, Percutaneous Endoscopic Approach
0PP947Z Removal of Autologous Tissue Substitute from Right Clavicle, Percutaneous Endoscopic Approach
0PP94JZ Removal of Synthetic Substitute from Right Clavicle, Percutaneous Endoscopic Approach
0PP94KZ Removal of Nonautologous Tissue Substitute from Right Clavicle, Percutaneous Endoscopic Approach
0PP9X4Z Removal of Internal Fixation Device from Right Clavicle, External Approach
0PPB04Z Removal of Internal Fixation Device from Left Clavicle, Open Approach
0PPB07Z Removal of Autologous Tissue Substitute from Left Clavicle, Open Approach
0PPB0JZ Removal of Synthetic Substitute from Left Clavicle, Open Approach
0PPB0KZ Removal of Nonautologous Tissue Substitute from Left Clavicle, Open Approach
0PPB34Z Removal of Internal Fixation Device from Left Clavicle, Percutaneous Approach
0PPB37Z Removal of Autologous Tissue Substitute from Left Clavicle, Percutaneous Approach
0PPB3JZ Removal of Synthetic Substitute from Left Clavicle, Percutaneous Approach
0PPB3KZ Removal of Nonautologous Tissue Substitute from Left Clavicle, Percutaneous Approach
0PPB44Z Removal of Internal Fixation Device from Left Clavicle, Percutaneous Endoscopic Approach
0PPB47Z Removal of Autologous Tissue Substitute from Left Clavicle, Percutaneous Endoscopic Approach
0PPB4JZ Removal of Synthetic Substitute from Left Clavicle, Percutaneous Endoscopic Approach
0PPB4KZ Removal of Nonautologous Tissue Substitute from Left Clavicle, Percutaneous Endoscopic Approach
0PPBX4Z Removal of Internal Fixation Device from Left Clavicle, External Approach
0PPC04Z Removal of Internal Fixation Device from Right Humeral Head, Open Approach
0PPC05Z Removal of External Fixation Device from Right Humeral Head, Open Approach
0PPC07Z Removal of Autologous Tissue Substitute from Right Humeral Head, Open Approach
0PPC0JZ Removal of Synthetic Substitute from Right Humeral Head, Open Approach
0PPC0KZ Removal of Nonautologous Tissue Substitute from Right Humeral Head, Open Approach
0PPC34Z Removal of Internal Fixation Device from Right Humeral Head, Percutaneous Approach
0PPC35Z Removal of External Fixation Device from Right Humeral Head, Percutaneous Approach
0PPC37Z Removal of Autologous Tissue Substitute from Right Humeral Head, Percutaneous Approach
0PPC3JZ Removal of Synthetic Substitute from Right Humeral Head, Percutaneous Approach
0PPC3KZ Removal of Nonautologous Tissue Substitute from Right Humeral Head, Percutaneous Approach
0PPC44Z Removal of Internal Fixation Device from Right Humeral Head, Percutaneous Endoscopic Approach
0PPC45Z Removal of External Fixation Device from Right Humeral Head, Percutaneous Endoscopic Approach
0PPC47Z Removal of Autologous Tissue Substitute from Right Humeral Head, Percutaneous Endoscopic Approach
0PPC4JZ Removal of Synthetic Substitute from Right Humeral Head, Percutaneous Endoscopic Approach
0PPC4KZ Removal of Nonautologous Tissue Substitute from Right Humeral Head, Percutaneous Endoscopic Approach
0PPCX4Z Removal of Internal Fixation Device from Right Humeral Head, External Approach
0PPCX5Z Removal of External Fixation Device from Right Humeral Head, External Approach
0PPD04Z Removal of Internal Fixation Device from Left Humeral Head, Open Approach
0PPD05Z Removal of External Fixation Device from Left Humeral Head, Open Approach
0PPD07Z Removal of Autologous Tissue Substitute from Left Humeral Head, Open Approach
0PPD0JZ Removal of Synthetic Substitute from Left Humeral Head, Open Approach
0PPD0KZ Removal of Nonautologous Tissue Substitute from Left Humeral Head, Open Approach
0PPD34Z Removal of Internal Fixation Device from Left Humeral Head, Percutaneous Approach
0PPD35Z Removal of External Fixation Device from Left Humeral Head, Percutaneous Approach
0PPD37Z Removal of Autologous Tissue Substitute from Left Humeral Head, Percutaneous Approach
0PPD3JZ Removal of Synthetic Substitute from Left Humeral Head, Percutaneous Approach
0PPD3KZ Removal of Nonautologous Tissue Substitute from Left Humeral Head, Percutaneous Approach
0PPD44Z Removal of Internal Fixation Device from Left Humeral Head, Percutaneous Endoscopic Approach
0PPD45Z Removal of External Fixation Device from Left Humeral Head, Percutaneous Endoscopic Approach
0PPD47Z Removal of Autologous Tissue Substitute from Left Humeral Head, Percutaneous Endoscopic Approach
0PPD4JZ Removal of Synthetic Substitute from Left Humeral Head, Percutaneous Endoscopic Approach
0PPD4KZ Removal of Nonautologous Tissue Substitute from Left Humeral Head, Percutaneous Endoscopic Approach
0PPDX4Z Removal of Internal Fixation Device from Left Humeral Head, External Approach
0PPDX5Z Removal of External Fixation Device from Left Humeral Head, External Approach
0PPF04Z Removal of Internal Fixation Device from Right Humeral Shaft, Open Approach
0PPF05Z Removal of External Fixation Device from Right Humeral Shaft, Open Approach
0PPF07Z Removal of Autologous Tissue Substitute from Right Humeral Shaft, Open Approach
0PPF0JZ Removal of Synthetic Substitute from Right Humeral Shaft, Open Approach
0PPF0KZ Removal of Nonautologous Tissue Substitute from Right Humeral Shaft, Open Approach
0PPF34Z Removal of Internal Fixation Device from Right Humeral Shaft, Percutaneous Approach
0PPF35Z Removal of External Fixation Device from Right Humeral Shaft, Percutaneous Approach
0PPF37Z Removal of Autologous Tissue Substitute from Right Humeral Shaft, Percutaneous Approach
0PPF3JZ Removal of Synthetic Substitute from Right Humeral Shaft, Percutaneous Approach
0PPF3KZ Removal of Nonautologous Tissue Substitute from Right Humeral Shaft, Percutaneous Approach
0PPF44Z Removal of Internal Fixation Device from Right Humeral Shaft, Percutaneous Endoscopic Approach
0PPF45Z Removal of External Fixation Device from Right Humeral Shaft, Percutaneous Endoscopic Approach
0PPF47Z Removal of Autologous Tissue Substitute from Right Humeral Shaft, Percutaneous Endoscopic Approach
0PPF4JZ Removal of Synthetic Substitute from Right Humeral Shaft, Percutaneous Endoscopic Approach
0PPF4KZ Removal of Nonautologous Tissue Substitute from Right Humeral Shaft, Percutaneous Endoscopic Approach
0PPFX4Z Removal of Internal Fixation Device from Right Humeral Shaft, External Approach
0PPFX5Z Removal of External Fixation Device from Right Humeral Shaft, External Approach
0PPG04Z Removal of Internal Fixation Device from Left Humeral Shaft, Open Approach
0PPG05Z Removal of External Fixation Device from Left Humeral Shaft, Open Approach
0PPG07Z Removal of Autologous Tissue Substitute from Left Humeral Shaft, Open Approach
0PPG0JZ Removal of Synthetic Substitute from Left Humeral Shaft, Open Approach
0PPG0KZ Removal of Nonautologous Tissue Substitute from Left Humeral Shaft, Open Approach
0PPG34Z Removal of Internal Fixation Device from Left Humeral Shaft, Percutaneous Approach

PG35Z Removal of External Fixation Device from Left Humeral Shaft, Percutaneous Approach
PG37Z Removal of Autologous Tissue Substitute from Left Humeral Shaft, Percutaneous Approach
PG3JZ Removal of Synthetic Substitute from Left Humeral Shaft, Percutaneous Approach
PG3KZ Removal of Nonautologous Tissue Substitute from Left Humeral Shaft, Percutaneous Approach
PG44Z Removal of Internal Fixation Device from Left Humeral Shaft, Percutaneous Endoscopic Approach
PG45Z Removal of External Fixation Device from Left Humeral Shaft, Percutaneous Endoscopic Approach
PG47Z Removal of Autologous Tissue Substitute from Left Humeral Shaft, Percutaneous Endoscopic Approach
PG4JZ Removal of Synthetic Substitute from Left Humeral Shaft, Percutaneous Endoscopic Approach
PG4KZ Removal of Nonautologous Tissue Substitute from Left Humeral Shaft, Percutaneous Endoscopic Approach
PGX4Z Removal of Internal Fixation Device from Left Humeral Shaft, External Approach
PGX5Z Removal of External Fixation Device from Left Humeral Shaft, External Approach
PPH04Z Removal of Internal Fixation Device from Right Radius, Open Approach
PPH05Z Removal of External Fixation Device from Right Radius, Open Approach
PPH07Z Removal of Autologous Tissue Substitute from Right Radius, Open Approach
PPH0JZ Removal of Synthetic Substitute from Right Radius, Open Approach
PPH0KZ Removal of Nonautologous Tissue Substitute from Right Radius, Open Approach
PPH34Z Removal of Internal Fixation Device from Right Radius, Percutaneous Approach
PPH35Z Removal of External Fixation Device from Right Radius, Percutaneous Approach
PPH37Z Removal of Autologous Tissue Substitute from Right Radius, Percutaneous Approach
PPH3JZ Removal of Synthetic Substitute from Right Radius, Percutaneous Approach
PPH3KZ Removal of Nonautologous Tissue Substitute from Right Radius, Percutaneous Approach
PPH44Z Removal of Internal Fixation Device from Right Radius, Percutaneous Endoscopic Approach
PPH45Z Removal of External Fixation Device from Right Radius, Percutaneous Endoscopic Approach
0PPH47Z Removal of Autologous Tissue Substitute from Right Radius, Percutaneous Endoscopic Approach
0PPH4JZ Removal of Synthetic Substitute from Right Radius, Percutaneous Endoscopic Approach
0PPH4KZ Removal of Nonautologous Tissue Substitute from Right Radius, Percutaneous Endoscopic Approach
0PPHX4Z Removal of Internal Fixation Device from Right Radius, External Approach
0PPHX5Z Removal of External Fixation Device from Right Radius, External Approach
0PPJ04Z Removal of Internal Fixation Device from Left Radius, Open Approach
0PPJ05Z Removal of External Fixation Device from Left Radius, Open Approach
0PPJ07Z Removal of Autologous Tissue Substitute from Left Radius, Open Approach
0PPJ0JZ Removal of Synthetic Substitute from Left Radius, Open Approach
0PPJ0KZ Removal of Nonautologous Tissue Substitute from Left Radius, Open Approach
0PPJ34Z Removal of Internal Fixation Device from Left Radius, Percutaneous Approach
0PPJ35Z Removal of External Fixation Device from Left Radius, Percutaneous Approach
0PPJ37Z Removal of Autologous Tissue Substitute from Left Radius, Percutaneous Approach
0PPJ3JZ Removal of Synthetic Substitute from Left Radius, Percutaneous Approach
0PPJ3KZ Removal of Nonautologous Tissue Substitute from Left Radius, Percutaneous Approach
0PPJ44Z Removal of Internal Fixation Device from Left Radius, Percutaneous Endoscopic Approach
0PPJ45Z Removal of External Fixation Device from Left Radius, Percutaneous Endoscopic Approach
0PPJ47Z Removal of Autologous Tissue Substitute from Left Radius, Percutaneous Endoscopic Approach
0PPJ4JZ Removal of Synthetic Substitute from Left Radius, Percutaneous Endoscopic Approach
0PPJ4KZ Removal of Nonautologous Tissue Substitute from Left Radius, Percutaneous Endoscopic Approach
0PPJX4Z Removal of Internal Fixation Device from Left Radius, External Approach
0PPJX5Z Removal of External Fixation Device from Left Radius, External Approach
0PPK04Z Removal of Internal Fixation Device from Right Ulna, Open Approach
0PPK05Z Removal of External Fixation Device from Right Ulna, Open Approach
0PPK07Z Removal of Autologous Tissue Substitute from Right Ulna, Open Approach
0PPK0JZ Removal of Synthetic Substitute from Right Ulna, Open Approach
0PPK0KZ Removal of Nonautologous Tissue Substitute from Right Ulna, Open Approach
0PPK34Z Removal of Internal Fixation Device from Right Ulna, Percutaneous Approach
0PPK35Z Removal of External Fixation Device from Right Ulna, Percutaneous Approach
0PPK37Z Removal of Autologous Tissue Substitute from Right Ulna, Percutaneous Approach
0PPK3JZ Removal of Synthetic Substitute from Right Ulna, Percutaneous Approach
0PPK3KZ Removal of Nonautologous Tissue Substitute from Right Ulna, Percutaneous Approach
0PPK44Z Removal of Internal Fixation Device from Right Ulna, Percutaneous Endoscopic Approach
0PPK45Z Removal of External Fixation Device from Right Ulna, Percutaneous Endoscopic Approach
0PPK47Z Removal of Autologous Tissue Substitute from Right Ulna, Percutaneous Endoscopic Approach
0PPK4JZ Removal of Synthetic Substitute from Right Ulna, Percutaneous Endoscopic Approach
0PPK4KZ Removal of Nonautologous Tissue Substitute from Right Ulna, Percutaneous Endoscopic Approach
0PPKX4Z Removal of Internal Fixation Device from Right Ulna, External Approach
0PPKX5Z Removal of External Fixation Device from Right Ulna, External Approach
0PPL04Z Removal of Internal Fixation Device from Left Ulna, Open Approach
0PPL05Z Removal of External Fixation Device from Left Ulna, Open Approach
0PPL07Z Removal of Autologous Tissue Substitute from Left Ulna, Open Approach
0PPL0JZ Removal of Synthetic Substitute from Left Ulna, Open Approach
0PPL0KZ Removal of Nonautologous Tissue Substitute from Left Ulna, Open Approach
0PPL34Z Removal of Internal Fixation Device from Left Ulna, Percutaneous Approach
0PPL35Z Removal of External Fixation Device from Left Ulna, Percutaneous Approach
0PPL37Z Removal of Autologous Tissue Substitute from Left Ulna, Percutaneous Approach
0PPL3JZ Removal of Synthetic Substitute from Left Ulna, Percutaneous Approach
0PPL3KZ Removal of Nonautologous Tissue Substitute from Left Ulna, Percutaneous Approach
0PPL44Z Removal of Internal Fixation Device from Left Ulna, Percutaneous Endoscopic Approach
0PPL45Z Removal of External Fixation Device from Left Ulna, Percutaneous Endoscopic Approach
0PPL47Z Removal of Autologous Tissue Substitute from Left Ulna, Percutaneous Endoscopic Approach
0PPL4JZ Removal of Synthetic Substitute from Left Ulna, Percutaneous Endoscopic Approach
0PPL4KZ Removal of Nonautologous Tissue Substitute from Left Ulna, Percutaneous Endoscopic Approach
0PPLX4Z Removal of Internal Fixation Device from Left Ulna, External Approach
0PPLX5Z Removal of External Fixation Device from Left Ulna, External Approach
0PPM04Z Removal of Internal Fixation Device from Right Carpal, Open Approach
0PPM05Z Removal of External Fixation Device from Right Carpal, Open Approach
0PPM07Z Removal of Autologous Tissue Substitute from Right Carpal, Open Approach
0PPM0JZ Removal of Synthetic Substitute from Right Carpal, Open Approach
0PPM0KZ Removal of Nonautologous Tissue Substitute from Right Carpal, Open Approach
0PPM34Z Removal of Internal Fixation Device from Right Carpal, Percutaneous Approach
0PPM35Z Removal of External Fixation Device from Right Carpal, Percutaneous Approach
0PPM37Z Removal of Autologous Tissue Substitute from Right Carpal, Percutaneous Approach
0PPM3JZ Removal of Synthetic Substitute from Right Carpal, Percutaneous Approach
0PPM3KZ Removal of Nonautologous Tissue Substitute from Right Carpal, Percutaneous Approach
0PPM44Z Removal of Internal Fixation Device from Right Carpal, Percutaneous Endoscopic Approach
0PPM45Z Removal of External Fixation Device from Right Carpal, Percutaneous Endoscopic Approach
0PPM47Z Removal of Autologous Tissue Substitute from Right Carpal, Percutaneous Endoscopic Approach
0PPM4JZ Removal of Synthetic Substitute from Right Carpal, Percutaneous Endoscopic Approach

0PPM4KZ Removal of Nonautologous Tissue Substitute from Right Carpal, Percutaneous Endoscopic Approach
0PPMX4Z Removal of Internal Fixation Device from Right Carpal, External Approach
0PPMX5Z Removal of External Fixation Device from Right Carpal, External Approach
0PPN04Z Removal of Internal Fixation Device from Left Carpal, Open Approach
0PPN05Z Removal of External Fixation Device from Left Carpal, Open Approach
0PPN07Z Removal of Autologous Tissue Substitute from Left Carpal, Open Approach
0PPN0JZ Removal of Synthetic Substitute from Left Carpal, Open Approach
0PPN0KZ Removal of Nonautologous Tissue Substitute from Left Carpal, Open Approach
0PPN34Z Removal of Internal Fixation Device from Left Carpal, Percutaneous Approach
0PPN35Z Removal of External Fixation Device from Left Carpal, Percutaneous Approach
0PPN37Z Removal of Autologous Tissue Substitute from Left Carpal, Percutaneous Approach
0PPN3JZ Removal of Synthetic Substitute from Left Carpal, Percutaneous Approach
0PPN3KZ Removal of Nonautologous Tissue Substitute from Left Carpal, Percutaneous Approach
0PPN44Z Removal of Internal Fixation Device from Left Carpal, Percutaneous Endoscopic Approach
0PPN45Z Removal of External Fixation Device from Left Carpal, Percutaneous Endoscopic Approach
0PPN47Z Removal of Autologous Tissue Substitute from Left Carpal, Percutaneous Endoscopic Approach
0PPN4JZ Removal of Synthetic Substitute from Left Carpal, Percutaneous Endoscopic Approach
0PPN4KZ Removal of Nonautologous Tissue Substitute from Left Carpal, Percutaneous Endoscopic Approach
0PPNX4Z Removal of Internal Fixation Device from Left Carpal, External Approach
0PPNX5Z Removal of External Fixation Device from Left Carpal, External Approach
0PPP04Z Removal of Internal Fixation Device from Right Metacarpal, Open Approach
0PPP05Z Removal of External Fixation Device from Right Metacarpal, Open Approach
0PPP07Z Removal of Autologous Tissue Substitute from Right Metacarpal, Open Approach
0PPP0JZ Removal of Synthetic Substitute from Right Metacarpal, Open Approach
0PPP0KZ Removal of Nonautologous Tissue Substitute from Right Metacarpal, Open Approach
0PPP34Z Removal of Internal Fixation Device from Right Metacarpal, Percutaneous Approach
0PPP35Z Removal of External Fixation Device from Right Metacarpal, Percutaneous Approach
0PPP37Z Removal of Autologous Tissue Substitute from Right Metacarpal, Percutaneous Approach
0PPP3JZ Removal of Synthetic Substitute from Right Metacarpal, Percutaneous Approach
0PPP3KZ Removal of Nonautologous Tissue Substitute from Right Metacarpal, Percutaneous Approach
0PPP44Z Removal of Internal Fixation Device from Right Metacarpal, Percutaneous Endoscopic Approach
0PPP45Z Removal of External Fixation Device from Right Metacarpal, Percutaneous Endoscopic Approach
0PPP47Z Removal of Autologous Tissue Substitute from Right Metacarpal, Percutaneous Endoscopic Approach
0PPP4JZ Removal of Synthetic Substitute from Right Metacarpal, Percutaneous Endoscopic Approach
0PPP4KZ Removal of Nonautologous Tissue Substitute from Right Metacarpal, Percutaneous Endoscopic Approach
0PPPX4Z Removal of Internal Fixation Device from Right Metacarpal, External Approach
0PPPX5Z Removal of External Fixation Device from Right Metacarpal, External Approach
0PPQ04Z Removal of Internal Fixation Device from Left Metacarpal, Open Approach
0PPQ05Z Removal of External Fixation Device from Left Metacarpal, Open Approach
0PPQ07Z Removal of Autologous Tissue Substitute from Left Metacarpal, Open Approach
0PPQ0JZ Removal of Synthetic Substitute from Left Metacarpal, Open Approach
0PPQ0KZ Removal of Nonautologous Tissue Substitute from Left Metacarpal, Open Approach
0PPQ34Z Removal of Internal Fixation Device from Left Metacarpal, Percutaneous Approach
0PPQ35Z Removal of External Fixation Device from Left Metacarpal, Percutaneous Approach
0PPQ37Z Removal of Autologous Tissue Substitute from Left Metacarpal, Percutaneous Approach
0PPQ3JZ Removal of Synthetic Substitute from Left Metacarpal, Percutaneous Approach
0PPQ3KZ Removal of Nonautologous Tissue Substitute from Left Metacarpal, Percutaneous Approach
0PPQ44Z Removal of Internal Fixation Device from Left Metacarpal, Percutaneous Endoscopic Approach
0PPQ45Z Removal of External Fixation Device from Left Metacarpal, Percutaneous Endoscopic Approach
0PPQ47Z Removal of Autologous Tissue Substitute from Left Metacarpal, Percutaneous Endoscopic Approach
0PPQ4JZ Removal of Synthetic Substitute from Left Metacarpal, Percutaneous Endoscopic Approach
0PPQ4KZ Removal of Nonautologous Tissue Substitute from Left Metacarpal, Percutaneous Endoscopic Approach
0PPQX4Z Removal of Internal Fixation Device from Left Metacarpal, External Approach
0PPQX5Z Removal of External Fixation Device from Left Metacarpal, External Approach
0PPR04Z Removal of Internal Fixation Device from Right Thumb Phalanx, Open Approach
0PPR05Z Removal of External Fixation Device from Right Thumb Phalanx, Open Approach
0PPR07Z Removal of Autologous Tissue Substitute from Right Thumb Phalanx, Open Approach
0PPR0JZ Removal of Synthetic Substitute from Right Thumb Phalanx, Open Approach
0PPR0KZ Removal of Nonautologous Tissue Substitute from Right Thumb Phalanx, Open Approach
0PPR34Z Removal of Internal Fixation Device from Right Thumb Phalanx, Percutaneous Approach
0PPR35Z Removal of External Fixation Device from Right Thumb Phalanx, Percutaneous Approach
0PPR37Z Removal of Autologous Tissue Substitute from Right Thumb Phalanx, Percutaneous Approach
0PPR3JZ Removal of Synthetic Substitute from Right Thumb Phalanx, Percutaneous Approach
0PPR3KZ Removal of Nonautologous Tissue Substitute from Right Thumb Phalanx, Percutaneous Approach
0PPR44Z Removal of Internal Fixation Device from Right Thumb Phalanx, Percutaneous Endoscopic Approach
0PPR45Z Removal of External Fixation Device from Right Thumb Phalanx, Percutaneous Endoscopic Approach
0PPR47Z Removal of Autologous Tissue Substitute from Right Thumb Phalanx, Percutaneous Endoscopic Approach
0PPR4JZ Removal of Synthetic Substitute from Right Thumb Phalanx, Percutaneous Endoscopic Approach
0PPR4KZ Removal of Nonautologous Tissue Substitute from Right Thumb Phalanx, Percutaneous Endoscopic Approach
0PPRX4Z Removal of Internal Fixation Device from Right Thumb Phalanx, External Approach
0PPRX5Z Removal of External Fixation Device from Right Thumb Phalanx, External Approach
0PPS04Z Removal of Internal Fixation Device from Left Thumb Phalanx, Open Approach
0PPS05Z Removal of External Fixation Device from Left Thumb Phalanx, Open Approach
0PPS07Z Removal of Autologous Tissue Substitute from Left Thumb Phalanx, Open Approach
0PPS0JZ Removal of Synthetic Substitute from Left Thumb Phalanx, Open Approach
0PPS0KZ Removal of Nonautologous Tissue Substitute from Left Thumb Phalanx, Open Approach
0PPS34Z Removal of Internal Fixation Device from Left Thumb Phalanx, Percutaneous Approach
0PPS35Z Removal of External Fixation Device from Left Thumb Phalanx, Percutaneous Approach
0PPS37Z Removal of Autologous Tissue Substitute from Left Thumb Phalanx, Percutaneous Approach
0PPS3JZ Removal of Synthetic Substitute from Left Thumb Phalanx, Percutaneous Approach
0PPS3KZ Removal of Nonautologous Tissue Substitute from Left Thumb Phalanx, Percutaneous Approach
0PPS44Z Removal of Internal Fixation Device from Left Thumb Phalanx, Percutaneous Endoscopic Approach
0PPS45Z Removal of External Fixation Device from Left Thumb Phalanx, Percutaneous Endoscopic Approach
0PPS47Z Removal of Autologous Tissue Substitute from Left Thumb Phalanx, Percutaneous Endoscopic Approach
0PPS4JZ Removal of Synthetic Substitute from Left Thumb Phalanx, Percutaneous Endoscopic Approach
0PPS4KZ Removal of Nonautologous Tissue Substitute from Left Thumb Phalanx, Percutaneous Endoscopic Approach
0PPSX4Z Removal of Internal Fixation Device from Left Thumb Phalanx, External Approach
0PPSX5Z Removal of External Fixation Device from Left Thumb Phalanx, External Approach
0PPT04Z Removal of Internal Fixation Device from Right Finger Phalanx, Open Approach

PT05Z Removal of External Fixation Device from Right Finger Phalanx, Open Approach
PT07Z Removal of Autologous Tissue Substitute from Right Finger Phalanx, Open Approach
PT0JZ Removal of Synthetic Substitute from Right Finger Phalanx, Open Approach
PT0KZ Removal of Nonautologous Tissue Substitute from Right Finger Phalanx, Open Approach
PT34Z Removal of Internal Fixation Device from Right Finger Phalanx, Percutaneous Approach
PT35Z Removal of External Fixation Device from Right Finger Phalanx, Percutaneous Approach
PT37Z Removal of Autologous Tissue Substitute from Right Finger Phalanx, Percutaneous Approach
PT3JZ Removal of Synthetic Substitute from Right Finger Phalanx, Percutaneous Approach
PT3KZ Removal of Nonautologous Tissue Substitute from Right Finger Phalanx, Percutaneous Approach
PT44Z Removal of Internal Fixation Device from Right Finger Phalanx, Percutaneous Endoscopic Approach
PT45Z Removal of External Fixation Device from Right Finger Phalanx, Percutaneous Endoscopic Approach
PPT47Z Removal of Autologous Tissue Substitute from Right Finger Phalanx, Percutaneous Endoscopic Approach
PPT4JZ Removal of Synthetic Substitute from Right Finger Phalanx, Percutaneous Endoscopic Approach
0PPT4KZ Removal of Nonautologous Tissue Substitute from Right Finger Phalanx, Percutaneous Endoscopic Approach
0PPTX4Z Removal of Internal Fixation Device from Right Finger Phalanx, External Approach
0PPTX5Z Removal of External Fixation Device from Right Finger Phalanx, External Approach
0PPV04Z Removal of Internal Fixation Device from Left Finger Phalanx, Open Approach
0PPV05Z Removal of External Fixation Device from Left Finger Phalanx, Open Approach
0PPV07Z Removal of Autologous Tissue Substitute from Left Finger Phalanx, Open Approach
0PPV0JZ Removal of Synthetic Substitute from Left Finger Phalanx, Open Approach
0PPV0KZ Removal of Nonautologous Tissue Substitute from Left Finger Phalanx, Open Approach
0PPV34Z Removal of Internal Fixation Device from Left Finger Phalanx, Percutaneous Approach
0PPV35Z Removal of External Fixation Device from Left Finger Phalanx, Percutaneous Approach
0PPV37Z Removal of Autologous Tissue Substitute from Left Finger Phalanx, Percutaneous Approach
0PPV3JZ Removal of Synthetic Substitute from Left Finger Phalanx, Percutaneous Approach
0PPV3KZ Removal of Nonautologous Tissue Substitute from Left Finger Phalanx, Percutaneous Approach
0PPV44Z Removal of Internal Fixation Device from Left Finger Phalanx, Percutaneous Endoscopic Approach
0PPV45Z Removal of External Fixation Device from Left Finger Phalanx, Percutaneous Endoscopic Approach
0PPV47Z Removal of Autologous Tissue Substitute from Left Finger Phalanx, Percutaneous Endoscopic Approach
0PPV4JZ Removal of Synthetic Substitute from Left Finger Phalanx, Percutaneous Endoscopic Approach
0PPV4KZ Removal of Nonautologous Tissue Substitute from Left Finger Phalanx, Percutaneous Endoscopic Approach
0PPVX4Z Removal of Internal Fixation Device from Left Finger Phalanx, External Approach
0PPVX5Z Removal of External Fixation Device from Left Finger Phalanx, External Approach
0PPY00Z Removal of Drainage Device from Upper Bone, Open Approach
0PPY0MZ Removal of Bone Growth Stimulator from Upper Bone, Open Approach
0PPY30Z Removal of Drainage Device from Upper Bone, Percutaneous Approach
0PPY3MZ Removal of Bone Growth Stimulator from Upper Bone, Percutaneous Approach
0PPY40Z Removal of Drainage Device from Upper Bone, Percutaneous Endoscopic Approach
0PPY4MZ Removal of Bone Growth Stimulator from Upper Bone, Percutaneous Endoscopic Approach
0PPYX0Z Removal of Drainage Device from Upper Bone, External Approach
0PPYXMZ Removal of Bone Growth Stimulator from Upper Bone, External Approach

PQ – Upper Bones, Repair

eview Coding Guideline B3.5

PQ00ZZ Repair Sternum, Open Approach
PQ03ZZ Repair Sternum, Percutaneous Approach
PQ04ZZ Repair Sternum, Percutaneous Endoscopic Approach
PQ0XZZ Repair Sternum, External Approach
PQ10ZZ Repair Right Rib, Open Approach
PQ13ZZ Repair Right Rib, Percutaneous Approach
PQ14ZZ Repair Right Rib, Percutaneous Endoscopic Approach
PQ1XZZ Repair Right Rib, External Approach
PQ20ZZ Repair Left Rib, Open Approach
PQ23ZZ Repair Left Rib, Percutaneous Approach
PQ24ZZ Repair Left Rib, Percutaneous Endoscopic Approach
PQ2XZZ Repair Left Rib, External Approach
PQ30ZZ Repair Cervical Vertebra, Open Approach
PQ33ZZ Repair Cervical Vertebra, Percutaneous Approach
PQ34ZZ Repair Cervical Vertebra, Percutaneous Endoscopic Approach
PQ3XZZ Repair Cervical Vertebra, External Approach
0PQ40ZZ Repair Thoracic Vertebra, Open Approach
0PQ43ZZ Repair Thoracic Vertebra, Percutaneous Approach
0PQ44ZZ Repair Thoracic Vertebra, Percutaneous Endoscopic Approach
0PQ4XZZ Repair Thoracic Vertebra, External Approach
0PQ50ZZ Repair Right Scapula, Open Approach
0PQ53ZZ Repair Right Scapula, Percutaneous Approach
0PQ54ZZ Repair Right Scapula, Percutaneous Endoscopic Approach
0PQ5XZZ Repair Right Scapula, External Approach
0PQ60ZZ Repair Left Scapula, Open Approach
0PQ63ZZ Repair Left Scapula, Percutaneous Approach
0PQ64ZZ Repair Left Scapula, Percutaneous Endoscopic Approach
0PQ6XZZ Repair Left Scapula, External Approach
0PQ70ZZ Repair Right Glenoid Cavity, Open Approach
0PQ73ZZ Repair Right Glenoid Cavity, Percutaneous Approach
0PQ74ZZ Repair Right Glenoid Cavity, Percutaneous Endoscopic Approach
0PQ7XZZ Repair Right Glenoid Cavity, External Approach
0PQ80ZZ Repair Left Glenoid Cavity, Open Approach
0PQ83ZZ Repair Left Glenoid Cavity, Percutaneous Approach
0PQ84ZZ Repair Left Glenoid Cavity, Percutaneous Endoscopic Approach
0PQ8XZZ Repair Left Glenoid Cavity, External Approach
0PQ90ZZ Repair Right Clavicle, Open Approach
0PQ93ZZ Repair Right Clavicle, Percutaneous Approach
0PQ94ZZ Repair Right Clavicle, Percutaneous Endoscopic Approach
0PQ9XZZ Repair Right Clavicle, External Approach
0PQB0ZZ Repair Left Clavicle, Open Approach
0PQB3ZZ Repair Left Clavicle, Percutaneous Approach
0PQB4ZZ Repair Left Clavicle, Percutaneous Endoscopic Approach
0PQBXZZ Repair Left Clavicle, External Approach
0PQC0ZZ Repair Right Humeral Head, Open Approach
0PQC3ZZ Repair Right Humeral Head, Percutaneous Approach
0PQC4ZZ Repair Right Humeral Head, Percutaneous Endoscopic Approach
0PQCXZZ Repair Right Humeral Head, External Approach
0PQD0ZZ Repair Left Humeral Head, Open Approach
0PQD3ZZ Repair Left Humeral Head, Percutaneous Approach
0PQD4ZZ Repair Left Humeral Head, Percutaneous Endoscopic Approach
0PQDXZZ Repair Left Humeral Head, External Approach
0PQF0ZZ Repair Right Humeral Shaft, Open Approach
0PQF3ZZ Repair Right Humeral Shaft, Percutaneous Approach
0PQF4ZZ Repair Right Humeral Shaft, Percutaneous Endoscopic Approach
0PQFXZZ Repair Right Humeral Shaft, External Approach
0PQG0ZZ Repair Left Humeral Shaft, Open Approach
0PQG3ZZ Repair Left Humeral Shaft, Percutaneous Approach
0PQG4ZZ Repair Left Humeral Shaft, Percutaneous Endoscopic Approach
0PQGXZZ Repair Left Humeral Shaft, External Approach
0PQH0ZZ Repair Right Radius, Open Approach
0PQH3ZZ Repair Right Radius, Percutaneous Approach

0PQH4ZZ Repair Right Radius, Percutaneous Endoscopic Approach
0PQHXZZ Repair Right Radius, External Approach
0PQJ0ZZ Repair Left Radius, Open Approach
0PQJ3ZZ Repair Left Radius, Percutaneous Approach
0PQJ4ZZ Repair Left Radius, Percutaneous Endoscopic Approach
0PQJXZZ Repair Left Radius, External Approach
0PQK0ZZ Repair Right Ulna, Open Approach
0PQK3ZZ Repair Right Ulna, Percutaneous Approach
0PQK4ZZ Repair Right Ulna, Percutaneous Endoscopic Approach
0PQKXZZ Repair Right Ulna, External Approach
0PQL0ZZ Repair Left Ulna, Open Approach
0PQL3ZZ Repair Left Ulna, Percutaneous Approach
0PQL4ZZ Repair Left Ulna, Percutaneous Endoscopic Approach
0PQLXZZ Repair Left Ulna, External Approach
0PQM0ZZ Repair Right Carpal, Open Approach
0PQM3ZZ Repair Right Carpal, Percutaneous Approach
0PQM4ZZ Repair Right Carpal, Percutaneous Endoscopic Approach
0PQMXZZ Repair Right Carpal, External Approach
0PQN0ZZ Repair Left Carpal, Open Approach
0PQN3ZZ Repair Left Carpal, Percutaneous Approach
0PQN4ZZ Repair Left Carpal, Percutaneous Endoscopic Approach
0PQNXZZ Repair Left Carpal, External Approach
0PQP0ZZ Repair Right Metacarpal, Open Approach
0PQP3ZZ Repair Right Metacarpal, Percutaneous Approach
0PQP4ZZ Repair Right Metacarpal, Percutaneous Endoscopic Approach
0PQPXZZ Repair Right Metacarpal, External Approach
0PQQ0ZZ Repair Left Metacarpal, Open Approach
0PQQ3ZZ Repair Left Metacarpal, Percutaneous Approach
0PQQ4ZZ Repair Left Metacarpal, Percutaneous Endoscopic Approach
0PQQXZZ Repair Left Metacarpal, External Approach
0PQR0ZZ Repair Right Thumb Phalanx, Open Approach
0PQR3ZZ Repair Right Thumb Phalanx, Percutaneous Approach
0PQR4ZZ Repair Right Thumb Phalanx, Percutaneous Endoscopic Approach
0PQRXZZ Repair Right Thumb Phalanx, External Approach
0PQS0ZZ Repair Left Thumb Phalanx, Open Approach
0PQS3ZZ Repair Left Thumb Phalanx, Percutaneous Approach
0PQS4ZZ Repair Left Thumb Phalanx, Percutaneous Endoscopic Approach
0PQSXZZ Repair Left Thumb Phalanx, External Approach
0PQT0ZZ Repair Right Finger Phalanx, Open Approach
0PQT3ZZ Repair Right Finger Phalanx, Percutaneous Approach
0PQT4ZZ Repair Right Finger Phalanx, Percutaneous Endoscopic Approach
0PQTXZZ Repair Right Finger Phalanx, External Approach
0PQV0ZZ Repair Left Finger Phalanx, Open Approach
0PQV3ZZ Repair Left Finger Phalanx, Percutaneous Approach
0PQV4ZZ Repair Left Finger Phalanx, Percutaneous Endoscopic Approach
0PQVXZZ Repair Left Finger Phalanx, External Approach

0PR – Upper Bones, Replacement

0PR007Z Replacement of Sternum with Autologous Tissue Substitute, Open Approach
0PR00JZ Replacement of Sternum with Synthetic Substitute, Open Approach
0PR00KZ Replacement of Sternum with Nonautologous Tissue Substitute, Open Approach
0PR037Z Replacement of Sternum with Autologous Tissue Substitute, Percutaneous Approach
0PR03JZ Replacement of Sternum with Synthetic Substitute, Percutaneous Approach
0PR03KZ Replacement of Sternum with Nonautologous Tissue Substitute, Percutaneous Approach
0PR047Z Replacement of Sternum with Autologous Tissue Substitute, Percutaneous Endoscopic Approach
0PR04JZ Replacement of Sternum with Synthetic Substitute, Percutaneous Endoscopic Approach
0PR04KZ Replacement of Sternum with Nonautologous Tissue Substitute, Percutaneous Endoscopic Approach
0PR107Z Replacement of Right Rib with Autologous Tissue Substitute, Open Approach
0PR10JZ Replacement of Right Rib with Synthetic Substitute, Open Approach
0PR10KZ Replacement of Right Rib with Nonautologous Tissue Substitute, Open Approach
0PR137Z Replacement of Right Rib with Autologous Tissue Substitute, Percutaneous Approach
0PR13JZ Replacement of Right Rib with Synthetic Substitute, Percutaneous Approach
0PR13KZ Replacement of Right Rib with Nonautologous Tissue Substitute, Percutaneous Approach
0PR147Z Replacement of Right Rib with Autologous Tissue Substitute, Percutaneous Endoscopic Approach
0PR14JZ Replacement of Right Rib with Synthetic Substitute, Percutaneous Endoscopic Approach
0PR14KZ Replacement of Right Rib with Nonautologous Tissue Substitute, Percutaneous Endoscopic Approach
0PR207Z Replacement of Left Rib with Autologous Tissue Substitute, Open Approach
0PR20JZ Replacement of Left Rib with Synthetic Substitute, Open Approach
0PR20KZ Replacement of Left Rib with Nonautologous Tissue Substitute, Open Approach
0PR237Z Replacement of Left Rib with Autologous Tissue Substitute, Percutaneous Approach
0PR23JZ Replacement of Left Rib with Synthetic Substitute, Percutaneous Approach
0PR23KZ Replacement of Left Rib with Nonautologous Tissue Substitute, Percutaneous Approach
0PR247Z Replacement of Left Rib with Autologous Tissue Substitute, Percutaneous Endoscopic Approach
0PR24JZ Replacement of Left Rib with Synthetic Substitute, Percutaneous Endoscopic Approach
0PR24KZ Replacement of Left Rib with Nonautologous Tissue Substitute, Percutaneous Endoscopic Approach
0PR307Z Replacement of Cervical Vertebra with Autologous Tissue Substitute, Open Approach
0PR30JZ Replacement of Cervical Vertebra with Synthetic Substitute, Open Approach
0PR30KZ Replacement of Cervical Vertebra with Nonautologous Tissue Substitute, Open Approach
0PR337Z Replacement of Cervical Vertebra with Autologous Tissue Substitute, Percutaneous Approach
0PR33JZ Replacement of Cervical Vertebra with Synthetic Substitute, Percutaneous Approach
0PR33KZ Replacement of Cervical Vertebra with Nonautologous Tissue Substitute, Percutaneous Approach
0PR347Z Replacement of Cervical Vertebra with Autologous Tissue Substitute, Percutaneous Endoscopic Approach
0PR34JZ Replacement of Cervical Vertebra with Synthetic Substitute, Percutaneous Endoscopic Approach
0PR34KZ Replacement of Cervical Vertebra with Nonautologous Tissue Substitute, Percutaneous Endoscopic Approach
0PR407Z Replacement of Thoracic Vertebra with Autologous Tissue Substitute, Open Approach
0PR40JZ Replacement of Thoracic Vertebra with Synthetic Substitute, Open Approach
0PR40KZ Replacement of Thoracic Vertebra with Nonautologous Tissue Substitute, Open Approach
0PR437Z Replacement of Thoracic Vertebra with Autologous Tissue Substitute, Percutaneous Approach
0PR43JZ Replacement of Thoracic Vertebra with Synthetic Substitute, Percutaneous Approach
0PR43KZ Replacement of Thoracic Vertebra with Nonautologous Tissue Substitute, Percutaneous Approach
0PR447Z Replacement of Thoracic Vertebra with Autologous Tissue Substitute, Percutaneous Endoscopic Approach
0PR44JZ Replacement of Thoracic Vertebra with Synthetic Substitute, Percutaneous Endoscopic Approach
0PR44KZ Replacement of Thoracic Vertebra with Nonautologous Tissue Substitute, Percutaneous Endoscopic Approach
0PR507Z Replacement of Right Scapula with Autologous Tissue Substitute, Open Approach
0PR50JZ Replacement of Right Scapula with Synthetic Substitute, Open Approach
0PR50KZ Replacement of Right Scapula with Nonautologous Tissue Substitute, Open Approach
0PR537Z Replacement of Right Scapula with Autologous Tissue Substitute, Percutaneous Approach
0PR53JZ Replacement of Right Scapula with Synthetic Substitute, Percutaneous Approach
0PR53KZ Replacement of Right Scapula with Nonautologous Tissue Substitute, Percutaneous Approach
0PR547Z Replacement of Right Scapula with Autologous Tissue Substitute, Percutaneous Endoscopic Approach
0PR54JZ Replacement of Right Scapula with Synthetic Substitute, Percutaneous Endoscopic Approach

R54KZ Replacement of Right Scapula with Nonautologous Tissue Substitute, Percutaneous Endoscopic Approach
R607Z Replacement of Left Scapula with Autologous Tissue Substitute, Open Approach
R60JZ Replacement of Left Scapula with Synthetic Substitute, Open Approach
R60KZ Replacement of Left Scapula with Nonautologous Tissue Substitute, Open Approach
R637Z Replacement of Left Scapula with Autologous Tissue Substitute, Percutaneous Approach
R63JZ Replacement of Left Scapula with Synthetic Substitute, Percutaneous Approach
R63KZ Replacement of Left Scapula with Nonautologous Tissue Substitute, Percutaneous Approach
R647Z Replacement of Left Scapula with Autologous Tissue Substitute, Percutaneous Endoscopic Approach
R64JZ Replacement of Left Scapula with Synthetic Substitute, Percutaneous Endoscopic Approach
R64KZ Replacement of Left Scapula with Nonautologous Tissue Substitute, Percutaneous Endoscopic Approach
R707Z Replacement of Right Glenoid Cavity with Autologous Tissue Substitute, Open Approach
R70JZ Replacement of Right Glenoid Cavity with Synthetic Substitute, Open Approach
R70KZ Replacement of Right Glenoid Cavity with Nonautologous Tissue Substitute, Open Approach
R737Z Replacement of Right Glenoid Cavity with Autologous Tissue Substitute, Percutaneous Approach
R73JZ Replacement of Right Glenoid Cavity with Synthetic Substitute, Percutaneous Approach
PR73KZ Replacement of Right Glenoid Cavity with Nonautologous Tissue Substitute, Percutaneous Approach
PR747Z Replacement of Right Glenoid Cavity with Autologous Tissue Substitute, Percutaneous Endoscopic Approach
PR74JZ Replacement of Right Glenoid Cavity with Synthetic Substitute, Percutaneous Endoscopic Approach
PR74KZ Replacement of Right Glenoid Cavity with Nonautologous Tissue Substitute, Percutaneous Endoscopic Approach
PR807Z Replacement of Left Glenoid Cavity with Autologous Tissue Substitute, Open Approach
PR80JZ Replacement of Left Glenoid Cavity with Synthetic Substitute, Open Approach
PR80KZ Replacement of Left Glenoid Cavity with Nonautologous Tissue Substitute, Open Approach
PR837Z Replacement of Left Glenoid Cavity with Autologous Tissue Substitute, Percutaneous Approach
PR83JZ Replacement of Left Glenoid Cavity with Synthetic Substitute, Percutaneous Approach
PR83KZ Replacement of Left Glenoid Cavity with Nonautologous Tissue Substitute, Percutaneous Approach
PR847Z Replacement of Left Glenoid Cavity with Autologous Tissue Substitute, Percutaneous Endoscopic Approach
0PR84JZ Replacement of Left Glenoid Cavity with Synthetic Substitute, Percutaneous Endoscopic Approach
0PR84KZ Replacement of Left Glenoid Cavity with Nonautologous Tissue Substitute, Percutaneous Endoscopic Approach
0PR907Z Replacement of Right Clavicle with Autologous Tissue Substitute, Open Approach
0PR90JZ Replacement of Right Clavicle with Synthetic Substitute, Open Approach
0PR90KZ Replacement of Right Clavicle with Nonautologous Tissue Substitute, Open Approach
0PR937Z Replacement of Right Clavicle with Autologous Tissue Substitute, Percutaneous Approach
0PR93JZ Replacement of Right Clavicle with Synthetic Substitute, Percutaneous Approach
0PR93KZ Replacement of Right Clavicle with Nonautologous Tissue Substitute, Percutaneous Approach
0PR947Z Replacement of Right Clavicle with Autologous Tissue Substitute, Percutaneous Endoscopic Approach
0PR94JZ Replacement of Right Clavicle with Synthetic Substitute, Percutaneous Endoscopic Approach
0PR94KZ Replacement of Right Clavicle with Nonautologous Tissue Substitute, Percutaneous Endoscopic Approach
0PRB07Z Replacement of Left Clavicle with Autologous Tissue Substitute, Open Approach
0PRB0JZ Replacement of Left Clavicle with Synthetic Substitute, Open Approach
0PRB0KZ Replacement of Left Clavicle with Nonautologous Tissue Substitute, Open Approach
0PRB37Z Replacement of Left Clavicle with Autologous Tissue Substitute, Percutaneous Approach
0PRB3JZ Replacement of Left Clavicle with Synthetic Substitute, Percutaneous Approach
0PRB3KZ Replacement of Left Clavicle with Nonautologous Tissue Substitute, Percutaneous Approach
0PRB47Z Replacement of Left Clavicle with Autologous Tissue Substitute, Percutaneous Endoscopic Approach
0PRB4JZ Replacement of Left Clavicle with Synthetic Substitute, Percutaneous Endoscopic Approach
0PRB4KZ Replacement of Left Clavicle with Nonautologous Tissue Substitute, Percutaneous Endoscopic Approach
0PRC07Z Replacement of Right Humeral Head with Autologous Tissue Substitute, Open Approach
0PRC0JZ Replacement of Right Humeral Head with Synthetic Substitute, Open Approach
0PRC0KZ Replacement of Right Humeral Head with Nonautologous Tissue Substitute, Open Approach
0PRC37Z Replacement of Right Humeral Head with Autologous Tissue Substitute, Percutaneous Approach
0PRC3JZ Replacement of Right Humeral Head with Synthetic Substitute, Percutaneous Approach
0PRC3KZ Replacement of Right Humeral Head with Nonautologous Tissue Substitute, Percutaneous Approach
0PRC47Z Replacement of Right Humeral Head with Autologous Tissue Substitute, Percutaneous Endoscopic Approach
0PRC4JZ Replacement of Right Humeral Head with Synthetic Substitute, Percutaneous Endoscopic Approach
0PRC4KZ Replacement of Right Humeral Head with Nonautologous Tissue Substitute, Percutaneous Endoscopic Approach
0PRD07Z Replacement of Left Humeral Head with Autologous Tissue Substitute, Open Approach
0PRD0JZ Replacement of Left Humeral Head with Synthetic Substitute, Open Approach
0PRD0KZ Replacement of Left Humeral Head with Nonautologous Tissue Substitute, Open Approach
0PRD37Z Replacement of Left Humeral Head with Autologous Tissue Substitute, Percutaneous Approach
0PRD3JZ Replacement of Left Humeral Head with Synthetic Substitute, Percutaneous Approach
0PRD3KZ Replacement of Left Humeral Head with Nonautologous Tissue Substitute, Percutaneous Approach
0PRD47Z Replacement of Left Humeral Head with Autologous Tissue Substitute, Percutaneous Endoscopic Approach
0PRD4JZ Replacement of Left Humeral Head with Synthetic Substitute, Percutaneous Endoscopic Approach
0PRD4KZ Replacement of Left Humeral Head with Nonautologous Tissue Substitute, Percutaneous Endoscopic Approach
0PRF07Z Replacement of Right Humeral Shaft with Autologous Tissue Substitute, Open Approach
0PRF0JZ Replacement of Right Humeral Shaft with Synthetic Substitute, Open Approach
0PRF0KZ Replacement of Right Humeral Shaft with Nonautologous Tissue Substitute, Open Approach
0PRF37Z Replacement of Right Humeral Shaft with Autologous Tissue Substitute, Percutaneous Approach
0PRF3JZ Replacement of Right Humeral Shaft with Synthetic Substitute, Percutaneous Approach
0PRF3KZ Replacement of Right Humeral Shaft with Nonautologous Tissue Substitute, Percutaneous Approach
0PRF47Z Replacement of Right Humeral Shaft with Autologous Tissue Substitute, Percutaneous Endoscopic Approach
0PRF4JZ Replacement of Right Humeral Shaft with Synthetic Substitute, Percutaneous Endoscopic Approach
0PRF4KZ Replacement of Right Humeral Shaft with Nonautologous Tissue Substitute, Percutaneous Endoscopic Approach
0PRG07Z Replacement of Left Humeral Shaft with Autologous Tissue Substitute, Open Approach
0PRG0JZ Replacement of Left Humeral Shaft with Synthetic Substitute, Open Approach
0PRG0KZ Replacement of Left Humeral Shaft with Nonautologous Tissue Substitute, Open Approach
0PRG37Z Replacement of Left Humeral Shaft with Autologous Tissue Substitute, Percutaneous Approach
0PRG3JZ Replacement of Left Humeral Shaft with Synthetic Substitute, Percutaneous Approach

0PRG3KZ Replacement of Left Humeral Shaft with Nonautologous Tissue Substitute, Percutaneous Approach
0PRG47Z Replacement of Left Humeral Shaft with Autologous Tissue Substitute, Percutaneous Endoscopic Approach
0PRG4JZ Replacement of Left Humeral Shaft with Synthetic Substitute, Percutaneous Endoscopic Approach
0PRG4KZ Replacement of Left Humeral Shaft with Nonautologous Tissue Substitute, Percutaneous Endoscopic Approach
0PRH07Z Replacement of Right Radius with Autologous Tissue Substitute, Open Approach
0PRH0JZ Replacement of Right Radius with Synthetic Substitute, Open Approach
0PRH0KZ Replacement of Right Radius with Nonautologous Tissue Substitute, Open Approach
0PRH37Z Replacement of Right Radius with Autologous Tissue Substitute, Percutaneous Approach
0PRH3JZ Replacement of Right Radius with Synthetic Substitute, Percutaneous Approach
0PRH3KZ Replacement of Right Radius with Nonautologous Tissue Substitute, Percutaneous Approach
0PRH47Z Replacement of Right Radius with Autologous Tissue Substitute, Percutaneous Endoscopic Approach
0PRH4JZ Replacement of Right Radius with Synthetic Substitute, Percutaneous Endoscopic Approach
0PRH4KZ Replacement of Right Radius with Nonautologous Tissue Substitute, Percutaneous Endoscopic Approach
0PRJ07Z Replacement of Left Radius with Autologous Tissue Substitute, Open Approach
0PRJ0JZ Replacement of Left Radius with Synthetic Substitute, Open Approach
0PRJ0KZ Replacement of Left Radius with Nonautologous Tissue Substitute, Open Approach
0PRJ37Z Replacement of Left Radius with Autologous Tissue Substitute, Percutaneous Approach
0PRJ3JZ Replacement of Left Radius with Synthetic Substitute, Percutaneous Approach
0PRJ3KZ Replacement of Left Radius with Nonautologous Tissue Substitute, Percutaneous Approach
0PRJ47Z Replacement of Left Radius with Autologous Tissue Substitute, Percutaneous Endoscopic Approach
0PRJ4JZ Replacement of Left Radius with Synthetic Substitute, Percutaneous Endoscopic Approach
0PRJ4KZ Replacement of Left Radius with Nonautologous Tissue Substitute, Percutaneous Endoscopic Approach
0PRK07Z Replacement of Right Ulna with Autologous Tissue Substitute, Open Approach
0PRK0JZ Replacement of Right Ulna with Synthetic Substitute, Open Approach
0PRK0KZ Replacement of Right Ulna with Nonautologous Tissue Substitute, Open Approach
0PRK37Z Replacement of Right Ulna with Autologous Tissue Substitute, Percutaneous Approach
0PRK3JZ Replacement of Right Ulna with Synthetic Substitute, Percutaneous Approach
0PRK3KZ Replacement of Right Ulna with Nonautologous Tissue Substitute, Percutaneous Approach
0PRK47Z Replacement of Right Ulna with Autologous Tissue Substitute, Percutaneous Endoscopic Approach
0PRK4JZ Replacement of Right Ulna with Synthetic Substitute, Percutaneous Endoscopic Approach
0PRK4KZ Replacement of Right Ulna with Nonautologous Tissue Substitute, Percutaneous Endoscopic Approach
0PRL07Z Replacement of Left Ulna with Autologous Tissue Substitute, Open Approach
0PRL0JZ Replacement of Left Ulna with Synthetic Substitute, Open Approach
0PRL0KZ Replacement of Left Ulna with Nonautologous Tissue Substitute, Open Approach
0PRL37Z Replacement of Left Ulna with Autologous Tissue Substitute, Percutaneous Approach
0PRL3JZ Replacement of Left Ulna with Synthetic Substitute, Percutaneous Approach
0PRL3KZ Replacement of Left Ulna with Nonautologous Tissue Substitute, Percutaneous Approach
0PRL47Z Replacement of Left Ulna with Autologous Tissue Substitute, Percutaneous Endoscopic Approach
0PRL4JZ Replacement of Left Ulna with Synthetic Substitute, Percutaneous Endoscopic Approach
0PRL4KZ Replacement of Left Ulna with Nonautologous Tissue Substitute, Percutaneous Endoscopic Approach
0PRM07Z Replacement of Right Carpal with Autologous Tissue Substitute, Open Approach
0PRM0JZ Replacement of Right Carpal with Synthetic Substitute, Open Approach
0PRM0KZ Replacement of Right Carpal with Nonautologous Tissue Substitute, Open Approach
0PRM37Z Replacement of Right Carpal with Autologous Tissue Substitute, Percutaneous Approach
0PRM3JZ Replacement of Right Carpal with Synthetic Substitute, Percutaneous Approach
0PRM3KZ Replacement of Right Carpal with Nonautologous Tissue Substitute, Percutaneous Approach
0PRM47Z Replacement of Right Carpal with Autologous Tissue Substitute, Percutaneous Endoscopic Approach
0PRM4JZ Replacement of Right Carpal with Synthetic Substitute, Percutaneous Endoscopic Approach
0PRM4KZ Replacement of Right Carpal with Nonautologous Tissue Substitute, Percutaneous Endoscopic Approach
0PRN07Z Replacement of Left Carpal with Autologous Tissue Substitute, Open Approach
0PRN0JZ Replacement of Left Carpal with Synthetic Substitute, Open Approach
0PRN0KZ Replacement of Left Carpal with Nonautologous Tissue Substitute, Open Approach
0PRN37Z Replacement of Left Carpal with Autologous Tissue Substitute, Percutaneous Approach
0PRN3JZ Replacement of Left Carpal with Synthetic Substitute, Percutaneous Approach
0PRN3KZ Replacement of Left Carpal with Nonautologous Tissue Substitute, Percutaneous Approach
0PRN47Z Replacement of Left Carpal with Autologous Tissue Substitute, Percutaneous Endoscopic Approach
0PRN4JZ Replacement of Left Carpal with Synthetic Substitute, Percutaneous Endoscopic Approach
0PRN4KZ Replacement of Left Carpal with Nonautologous Tissue Substitute, Percutaneous Endoscopic Approach
0PRP07Z Replacement of Right Metacarpal with Autologous Tissue Substitute, Open Approach
0PRP0JZ Replacement of Right Metacarpal with Synthetic Substitute, Open Approach
0PRP0KZ Replacement of Right Metacarpal with Nonautologous Tissue Substitute, Open Approach
0PRP37Z Replacement of Right Metacarpal with Autologous Tissue Substitute, Percutaneous Approach
0PRP3JZ Replacement of Right Metacarpal with Synthetic Substitute, Percutaneous Approach
0PRP3KZ Replacement of Right Metacarpal with Nonautologous Tissue Substitute, Percutaneous Approach
0PRP47Z Replacement of Right Metacarpal with Autologous Tissue Substitute, Percutaneous Endoscopic Approach
0PRP4JZ Replacement of Right Metacarpal with Synthetic Substitute, Percutaneous Endoscopic Approach
0PRP4KZ Replacement of Right Metacarpal with Nonautologous Tissue Substitute, Percutaneous Endoscopic Approach
0PRQ07Z Replacement of Left Metacarpal with Autologous Tissue Substitute, Open Approach
0PRQ0JZ Replacement of Left Metacarpal with Synthetic Substitute, Open Approach
0PRQ0KZ Replacement of Left Metacarpal with Nonautologous Tissue Substitute, Open Approach
0PRQ37Z Replacement of Left Metacarpal with Autologous Tissue Substitute, Percutaneous Approach
0PRQ3JZ Replacement of Left Metacarpal with Synthetic Substitute, Percutaneous Approach
0PRQ3KZ Replacement of Left Metacarpal with Nonautologous Tissue Substitute, Percutaneous Approach
0PRQ47Z Replacement of Left Metacarpal with Autologous Tissue Substitute, Percutaneous Endoscopic Approach
0PRQ4JZ Replacement of Left Metacarpal with Synthetic Substitute, Percutaneous Endoscopic Approach
0PRQ4KZ Replacement of Left Metacarpal with Nonautologous Tissue Substitute, Percutaneous Endoscopic Approach
0PRR07Z Replacement of Right Thumb Phalanx with Autologous Tissue Substitute, Open Approach
0PRR0JZ Replacement of Right Thumb Phalanx with Synthetic Substitute, Open Approach
0PRR0KZ Replacement of Right Thumb Phalanx with Nonautologous Tissue Substitute, Open Approach
0PRR37Z Replacement of Right Thumb Phalanx with Autologous Tissue Substitute, Percutaneous Approach

0PRR3JZ Replacement of Right Thumb Phalanx with Synthetic Substitute, Percutaneous Approach
0PRR3KZ Replacement of Right Thumb Phalanx with Nonautologous Tissue Substitute, Percutaneous Approach
0PRR47Z Replacement of Right Thumb Phalanx with Autologous Tissue Substitute, Percutaneous Endoscopic Approach
0PRR4JZ Replacement of Right Thumb Phalanx with Synthetic Substitute, Percutaneous Endoscopic Approach
0PRR4KZ Replacement of Right Thumb Phalanx with Nonautologous Tissue Substitute, Percutaneous Endoscopic Approach
0PRS07Z Replacement of Left Thumb Phalanx with Autologous Tissue Substitute, Open Approach
0PRS0JZ Replacement of Left Thumb Phalanx with Synthetic Substitute, Open Approach
0PRS0KZ Replacement of Left Thumb Phalanx with Nonautologous Tissue Substitute, Open Approach
0PRS37Z Replacement of Left Thumb Phalanx with Autologous Tissue Substitute, Percutaneous Approach
0PRS3JZ Replacement of Left Thumb Phalanx with Synthetic Substitute, Percutaneous Approach
0PRS3KZ Replacement of Left Thumb Phalanx with Nonautologous Tissue Substitute, Percutaneous Approach
0PRS47Z Replacement of Left Thumb Phalanx with Autologous Tissue Substitute, Percutaneous Endoscopic Approach
0PRS4JZ Replacement of Left Thumb Phalanx with Synthetic Substitute, Percutaneous Endoscopic Approach
0PRS4KZ Replacement of Left Thumb Phalanx with Nonautologous Tissue Substitute, Percutaneous Endoscopic Approach
0PRT07Z Replacement of Right Finger Phalanx with Autologous Tissue Substitute, Open Approach
0PRT0JZ Replacement of Right Finger Phalanx with Synthetic Substitute, Open Approach
0PRT0KZ Replacement of Right Finger Phalanx with Nonautologous Tissue Substitute, Open Approach
0PRT37Z Replacement of Right Finger Phalanx with Autologous Tissue Substitute, Percutaneous Approach
0PRT3JZ Replacement of Right Finger Phalanx with Synthetic Substitute, Percutaneous Approach
0PRT3KZ Replacement of Right Finger Phalanx with Nonautologous Tissue Substitute, Percutaneous Approach
0PRT47Z Replacement of Right Finger Phalanx with Autologous Tissue Substitute, Percutaneous Endoscopic Approach
0PRT4JZ Replacement of Right Finger Phalanx with Synthetic Substitute, Percutaneous Endoscopic Approach
0PRT4KZ Replacement of Right Finger Phalanx with Nonautologous Tissue Substitute, Percutaneous Endoscopic Approach
0PRV07Z Replacement of Left Finger Phalanx with Autologous Tissue Substitute, Open Approach
0PRV0JZ Replacement of Left Finger Phalanx with Synthetic Substitute, Open Approach
0PRV0KZ Replacement of Left Finger Phalanx with Nonautologous Tissue Substitute, Open Approach
0PRV37Z Replacement of Left Finger Phalanx with Autologous Tissue Substitute, Percutaneous Approach
0PRV3JZ Replacement of Left Finger Phalanx with Synthetic Substitute, Percutaneous Approach
0PRV3KZ Replacement of Left Finger Phalanx with Nonautologous Tissue Substitute, Percutaneous Approach
0PRV47Z Replacement of Left Finger Phalanx with Autologous Tissue Substitute, Percutaneous Endoscopic Approach
0PRV4JZ Replacement of Left Finger Phalanx with Synthetic Substitute, Percutaneous Endoscopic Approach
0PRV4KZ Replacement of Left Finger Phalanx with Nonautologous Tissue Substitute, Percutaneous Endoscopic Approach

0PS – Upper Bones, Reposition

Review Coding Guideline B3.15

0PS000Z Reposition Sternum with Rigid Plate Internal Fixation Device, Open Approach
0PS004Z Reposition Sternum with Internal Fixation Device, Open Approach
0PS00ZZ Reposition Sternum, Open Approach
0PS030Z Reposition Sternum with Rigid Plate Internal Fixation Device, Percutaneous Approach
0PS034Z Reposition Sternum with Internal Fixation Device, Percutaneous Approach
0PS03ZZ Reposition Sternum, Percutaneous Approach
0PS040Z Reposition Sternum with Rigid Plate Internal Fixation Device, Percutaneous Endoscopic Approach
0PS044Z Reposition Sternum with Internal Fixation Device, Percutaneous Endoscopic Approach
0PS04ZZ Reposition Sternum, Percutaneous Endoscopic Approach
0PS0XZZ Reposition Sternum, External Approach
0PS104Z Reposition Right Rib with Internal Fixation Device, Open Approach
0PS10ZZ Reposition Right Rib, Open Approach
0PS134Z Reposition Right Rib with Internal Fixation Device, Percutaneous Approach
0PS13ZZ Reposition Right Rib, Percutaneous Approach
0PS144Z Reposition Right Rib with Internal Fixation Device, Percutaneous Endoscopic Approach
0PS14ZZ Reposition Right Rib, Percutaneous Endoscopic Approach
0PS1XZZ Reposition Right Rib, External Approach
0PS204Z Reposition Left Rib with Internal Fixation Device, Open Approach
0PS20ZZ Reposition Left Rib, Open Approach
0PS234Z Reposition Left Rib with Internal Fixation Device, Percutaneous Approach
0PS23ZZ Reposition Left Rib, Percutaneous Approach
0PS244Z Reposition Left Rib with Internal Fixation Device, Percutaneous Endoscopic Approach
0PS24ZZ Reposition Left Rib, Percutaneous Endoscopic Approach
0PS2XZZ Reposition Left Rib, External Approach
0PS304Z Reposition Cervical Vertebra with Internal Fixation Device, Open Approach
0PS30ZZ Reposition Cervical Vertebra, Open Approach
0PS334Z Reposition Cervical Vertebra with Internal Fixation Device, Percutaneous Approach
0PS33ZZ Reposition Cervical Vertebra, Percutaneous Approach
+ *See table 0PU to construct a code for Supplement with synthetic substitute.*
0PS344Z Reposition Cervical Vertebra with Internal Fixation Device, Percutaneous Endoscopic Approach
0PS34ZZ Reposition Cervical Vertebra, Percutaneous Endoscopic Approach
0PS3XZZ Reposition Cervical Vertebra, External Approach
0PS404Z Reposition Thoracic Vertebra with Internal Fixation Device, Open Approach
0PS40ZZ Reposition Thoracic Vertebra, Open Approach
0PS434Z Reposition Thoracic Vertebra with Internal Fixation Device, Percutaneous Approach
0PS43ZZ Reposition Thoracic Vertebra, Percutaneous Approach
+ *See table 0PU to construct a code for Supplement with synthetic substitute.*
0PS444Z Reposition Thoracic Vertebra with Internal Fixation Device, Percutaneous Endoscopic Approach
0PS44ZZ Reposition Thoracic Vertebra, Percutaneous Endoscopic Approach
0PS4XZZ Reposition Thoracic Vertebra, External Approach
0PS504Z Reposition Right Scapula with Internal Fixation Device, Open Approach
0PS50ZZ Reposition Right Scapula, Open Approach
0PS534Z Reposition Right Scapula with Internal Fixation Device, Percutaneous Approach
0PS53ZZ Reposition Right Scapula, Percutaneous Approach
0PS544Z Reposition Right Scapula with Internal Fixation Device, Percutaneous Endoscopic Approach
0PS54ZZ Reposition Right Scapula, Percutaneous Endoscopic Approach
0PS5XZZ Reposition Right Scapula, External Approach
0PS604Z Reposition Left Scapula with Internal Fixation Device, Open Approach
0PS60ZZ Reposition Left Scapula, Open Approach
0PS634Z Reposition Left Scapula with Internal Fixation Device, Percutaneous Approach
0PS63ZZ Reposition Left Scapula, Percutaneous Approach
0PS644Z Reposition Left Scapula with Internal Fixation Device, Percutaneous Endoscopic Approach
0PS64ZZ Reposition Left Scapula, Percutaneous Endoscopic Approach
0PS6XZZ Reposition Left Scapula, External Approach
0PS704Z Reposition Right Glenoid Cavity with Internal Fixation Device, Open Approach
0PS70ZZ Reposition Right Glenoid Cavity, Open Approach
0PS734Z Reposition Right Glenoid Cavity with Internal Fixation Device, Percutaneous Approach
0PS73ZZ Reposition Right Glenoid Cavity, Percutaneous Approach
0PS744Z Reposition Right Glenoid Cavity with Internal Fixation Device, Percutaneous Endoscopic Approach

0PS74ZZ Reposition Right Glenoid Cavity, Percutaneous Endoscopic Approach
0PS7XZZ Reposition Right Glenoid Cavity, External Approach
0PS804Z Reposition Left Glenoid Cavity with Internal Fixation Device, Open Approach
0PS80ZZ Reposition Left Glenoid Cavity, Open Approach
0PS834Z Reposition Left Glenoid Cavity with Internal Fixation Device, Percutaneous Approach
0PS83ZZ Reposition Left Glenoid Cavity, Percutaneous Approach
0PS844Z Reposition Left Glenoid Cavity with Internal Fixation Device, Percutaneous Endoscopic Approach
0PS84ZZ Reposition Left Glenoid Cavity, Percutaneous Endoscopic Approach
0PS8XZZ Reposition Left Glenoid Cavity, External Approach
0PS904Z Reposition Right Clavicle with Internal Fixation Device, Open Approach
0PS90ZZ Reposition Right Clavicle, Open Approach
0PS934Z Reposition Right Clavicle with Internal Fixation Device, Percutaneous Approach
0PS93ZZ Reposition Right Clavicle, Percutaneous Approach
0PS944Z Reposition Right Clavicle with Internal Fixation Device, Percutaneous Endoscopic Approach
0PS94ZZ Reposition Right Clavicle, Percutaneous Endoscopic Approach
0PS9XZZ Reposition Right Clavicle, External Approach
0PSB04Z Reposition Left Clavicle with Internal Fixation Device, Open Approach
0PSB0ZZ Reposition Left Clavicle, Open Approach
0PSB34Z Reposition Left Clavicle with Internal Fixation Device, Percutaneous Approach
0PSB3ZZ Reposition Left Clavicle, Percutaneous Approach
0PSB44Z Reposition Left Clavicle with Internal Fixation Device, Percutaneous Endoscopic Approach
0PSB4ZZ Reposition Left Clavicle, Percutaneous Endoscopic Approach
0PSBXZZ Reposition Left Clavicle, External Approach
0PSC04Z Reposition Right Humeral Head with Internal Fixation Device, Open Approach
0PSC05Z Reposition Right Humeral Head with External Fixation Device, Open Approach
0PSC06Z Reposition Right Humeral Head with Intramedullary Internal Fixation Device, Open Approach
0PSC0BZ Reposition Right Humeral Head with Monoplanar External Fixation Device, Open Approach
0PSC0CZ Reposition Right Humeral Head with Ring External Fixation Device, Open Approach
0PSC0DZ Reposition Right Humeral Head with Hybrid External Fixation Device, Open Approach
0PSC0ZZ Reposition Right Humeral Head, Open Approach
0PSC34Z Reposition Right Humeral Head with Internal Fixation Device, Percutaneous Approach
0PSC35Z Reposition Right Humeral Head with External Fixation Device, Percutaneous Approach
0PSC36Z Reposition Right Humeral Head with Intramedullary Internal Fixation Device, Percutaneous Approach
0PSC3BZ Reposition Right Humeral Head with Monoplanar External Fixation Device, Percutaneous Approach
0PSC3CZ Reposition Right Humeral Head with Ring External Fixation Device, Percutaneous Approach
0PSC3DZ Reposition Right Humeral Head with Hybrid External Fixation Device, Percutaneous Approach
0PSC3ZZ Reposition Right Humeral Head, Percutaneous Approach
0PSC44Z Reposition Right Humeral Head with Internal Fixation Device, Percutaneous Endoscopic Approach
0PSC45Z Reposition Right Humeral Head with External Fixation Device, Percutaneous Endoscopic Approach
0PSC46Z Reposition Right Humeral Head with Intramedullary Internal Fixation Device, Percutaneous Endoscopic Approach
0PSC4BZ Reposition Right Humeral Head with Monoplanar External Fixation Device, Percutaneous Endoscopic Approach
0PSC4CZ Reposition Right Humeral Head with Ring External Fixation Device, Percutaneous Endoscopic Approach
0PSC4DZ Reposition Right Humeral Head with Hybrid External Fixation Device, Percutaneous Endoscopic Approach
0PSC4ZZ Reposition Right Humeral Head, Percutaneous Endoscopic Approach
0PSCXZZ Reposition Right Humeral Head, External Approach
0PSD04Z Reposition Left Humeral Head with Internal Fixation Device, Open Approach
0PSD05Z Reposition Left Humeral Head with External Fixation Device, Open Approach
0PSD06Z Reposition Left Humeral Head with Intramedullary Internal Fixation Device, Open Approach
0PSD0BZ Reposition Left Humeral Head with Monoplanar External Fixation Device, Open Approach
0PSD0CZ Reposition Left Humeral Head with Ring External Fixation Device, Open Approach
0PSD0DZ Reposition Left Humeral Head with Hybrid External Fixation Device, Open Approach
0PSD0ZZ Reposition Left Humeral Head, Open Approach
0PSD34Z Reposition Left Humeral Head with Internal Fixation Device, Percutaneous Approach
0PSD35Z Reposition Left Humeral Head with External Fixation Device, Percutaneous Approach
0PSD36Z Reposition Left Humeral Head with Intramedullary Internal Fixation Device, Percutaneous Approach
0PSD3BZ Reposition Left Humeral Head with Monoplanar External Fixation Device, Percutaneous Approach
0PSD3CZ Reposition Left Humeral Head with Ring External Fixation Device, Percutaneous Approach
0PSD3DZ Reposition Left Humeral Head with Hybrid External Fixation Device, Percutaneous Approach
0PSD3ZZ Reposition Left Humeral Head, Percutaneous Approach
0PSD44Z Reposition Left Humeral Head with Internal Fixation Device, Percutaneous Endoscopic Approach
0PSD45Z Reposition Left Humeral Head with External Fixation Device, Percutaneous Endoscopic Approach
0PSD46Z Reposition Left Humeral Head with Intramedullary Internal Fixation Device, Percutaneous Endoscopic Approach
0PSD4BZ Reposition Left Humeral Head with Monoplanar External Fixation Device, Percutaneous Endoscopic Approach
0PSD4CZ Reposition Left Humeral Head with Ring External Fixation Device, Percutaneous Endoscopic Approach
0PSD4DZ Reposition Left Humeral Head with Hybrid External Fixation Device, Percutaneous Endoscopic Approach
0PSD4ZZ Reposition Left Humeral Head, Percutaneous Endoscopic Approach
0PSDXZZ Reposition Left Humeral Head, External Approach
0PSF04Z Reposition Right Humeral Shaft with Internal Fixation Device, Open Approach
0PSF05Z Reposition Right Humeral Shaft with External Fixation Device, Open Approach
0PSF06Z Reposition Right Humeral Shaft with Intramedullary Internal Fixation Device, Open Approach
0PSF0BZ Reposition Right Humeral Shaft with Monoplanar External Fixation Device, Open Approach
0PSF0CZ Reposition Right Humeral Shaft with Ring External Fixation Device, Open Approach
0PSF0DZ Reposition Right Humeral Shaft with Hybrid External Fixation Device, Open Approach
0PSF0ZZ Reposition Right Humeral Shaft, Open Approach
0PSF34Z Reposition Right Humeral Shaft with Internal Fixation Device, Percutaneous Approach
0PSF35Z Reposition Right Humeral Shaft with External Fixation Device, Percutaneous Approach
0PSF36Z Reposition Right Humeral Shaft with Intramedullary Internal Fixation Device, Percutaneous Approach
0PSF3BZ Reposition Right Humeral Shaft with Monoplanar External Fixation Device, Percutaneous Approach
0PSF3CZ Reposition Right Humeral Shaft with Ring External Fixation Device, Percutaneous Approach
0PSF3DZ Reposition Right Humeral Shaft with Hybrid External Fixation Device, Percutaneous Approach
0PSF3ZZ Reposition Right Humeral Shaft, Percutaneous Approach
0PSF44Z Reposition Right Humeral Shaft with Internal Fixation Device, Percutaneous Endoscopic Approach
0PSF45Z Reposition Right Humeral Shaft with External Fixation Device, Percutaneous Endoscopic Approach
0PSF46Z Reposition Right Humeral Shaft with Intramedullary Internal Fixation Device, Percutaneous Endoscopic Approach
0PSF4BZ Reposition Right Humeral Shaft with Monoplanar External Fixation Device, Percutaneous Endoscopic Approach
0PSF4CZ Reposition Right Humeral Shaft with Ring External Fixation Device, Percutaneous Endoscopic Approach
0PSF4DZ Reposition Right Humeral Shaft with Hybrid External Fixation Device, Percutaneous Endoscopic Approach
0PSF4ZZ Reposition Right Humeral Shaft, Percutaneous Endoscopic Approach
0PSFXZZ Reposition Right Humeral Shaft, External Approach
0PSG04Z Reposition Left Humeral Shaft with Internal Fixation Device, Open Approach
0PSG05Z Reposition Left Humeral Shaft with External Fixation Device, Open Approach

SG06Z Reposition Left Humeral Shaft with Intramedullary Internal Fixation Device, Open Approach
SG0BZ Reposition Left Humeral Shaft with Monoplanar External Fixation Device, Open Approach
SG0CZ Reposition Left Humeral Shaft with Ring External Fixation Device, Open Approach
SG0DZ Reposition Left Humeral Shaft with Hybrid External Fixation Device, Open Approach
SG0ZZ Reposition Left Humeral Shaft, Open Approach
SG34Z Reposition Left Humeral Shaft with Internal Fixation Device, Percutaneous Approach
SG35Z Reposition Left Humeral Shaft with External Fixation Device, Percutaneous Approach
PSG36Z Reposition Left Humeral Shaft with Intramedullary Internal Fixation Device, Percutaneous Approach
PSG3BZ Reposition Left Humeral Shaft with Monoplanar External Fixation Device, Percutaneous Approach
PSG3CZ Reposition Left Humeral Shaft with Ring External Fixation Device, Percutaneous Approach
PSG3DZ Reposition Left Humeral Shaft with Hybrid External Fixation Device, Percutaneous Approach
PSG3ZZ Reposition Left Humeral Shaft, Percutaneous Approach
PSG44Z Reposition Left Humeral Shaft with Internal Fixation Device, Percutaneous Endoscopic Approach
PSG45Z Reposition Left Humeral Shaft with External Fixation Device, Percutaneous Endoscopic Approach
PSG46Z Reposition Left Humeral Shaft with Intramedullary Internal Fixation Device, Percutaneous Endoscopic Approach
PSG4BZ Reposition Left Humeral Shaft with Monoplanar External Fixation Device, Percutaneous Endoscopic Approach
PSG4CZ Reposition Left Humeral Shaft with Ring External Fixation Device, Percutaneous Endoscopic Approach
PSG4DZ Reposition Left Humeral Shaft with Hybrid External Fixation Device, Percutaneous Endoscopic Approach
PSG4ZZ Reposition Left Humeral Shaft, Percutaneous Endoscopic Approach
)PSGXZZ Reposition Left Humeral Shaft, External Approach
)PSH04Z Reposition Right Radius with Internal Fixation Device, Open Approach
0PSH05Z Reposition Right Radius with External Fixation Device, Open Approach
0PSH06Z Reposition Right Radius with Intramedullary Internal Fixation Device, Open Approach
0PSH0BZ Reposition Right Radius with Monoplanar External Fixation Device, Open Approach
0PSH0CZ Reposition Right Radius with Ring External Fixation Device, Open Approach
0PSH0DZ Reposition Right Radius with Hybrid External Fixation Device, Open Approach
0PSH0ZZ Reposition Right Radius, Open Approach
0PSH34Z Reposition Right Radius with Internal Fixation Device, Percutaneous Approach
0PSH35Z Reposition Right Radius with External Fixation Device, Percutaneous Approach
0PSH36Z Reposition Right Radius with Intramedullary Internal Fixation Device, Percutaneous Approach
0PSH3BZ Reposition Right Radius with Monoplanar External Fixation Device, Percutaneous Approach
0PSH3CZ Reposition Right Radius with Ring External Fixation Device, Percutaneous Approach
0PSH3DZ Reposition Right Radius with Hybrid External Fixation Device, Percutaneous Approach
0PSH3ZZ Reposition Right Radius, Percutaneous Approach
0PSH44Z Reposition Right Radius with Internal Fixation Device, Percutaneous Endoscopic Approach
0PSH45Z Reposition Right Radius with External Fixation Device, Percutaneous Endoscopic Approach
0PSH46Z Reposition Right Radius with Intramedullary Internal Fixation Device, Percutaneous Endoscopic Approach
0PSH4BZ Reposition Right Radius with Monoplanar External Fixation Device, Percutaneous Endoscopic Approach
0PSH4CZ Reposition Right Radius with Ring External Fixation Device, Percutaneous Endoscopic Approach
0PSH4DZ Reposition Right Radius with Hybrid External Fixation Device, Percutaneous Endoscopic Approach
0PSH4ZZ Reposition Right Radius, Percutaneous Endoscopic Approach
0PSHXZZ Reposition Right Radius, External Approach
0PSJ04Z Reposition Left Radius with Internal Fixation Device, Open Approach
0PSJ05Z Reposition Left Radius with External Fixation Device, Open Approach
0PSJ06Z Reposition Left Radius with Intramedullary Internal Fixation Device, Open Approach
0PSJ0BZ Reposition Left Radius with Monoplanar External Fixation Device, Open Approach
0PSJ0CZ Reposition Left Radius with Ring External Fixation Device, Open Approach
0PSJ0DZ Reposition Left Radius with Hybrid External Fixation Device, Open Approach
0PSJ0ZZ Reposition Left Radius, Open Approach
0PSJ34Z Reposition Left Radius with Internal Fixation Device, Percutaneous Approach
0PSJ35Z Reposition Left Radius with External Fixation Device, Percutaneous Approach
0PSJ36Z Reposition Left Radius with Intramedullary Internal Fixation Device, Percutaneous Approach
0PSJ3BZ Reposition Left Radius with Monoplanar External Fixation Device, Percutaneous Approach
0PSJ3CZ Reposition Left Radius with Ring External Fixation Device, Percutaneous Approach
0PSJ3DZ Reposition Left Radius with Hybrid External Fixation Device, Percutaneous Approach
0PSJ3ZZ Reposition Left Radius, Percutaneous Approach
0PSJ44Z Reposition Left Radius with Internal Fixation Device, Percutaneous Endoscopic Approach
0PSJ45Z Reposition Left Radius with External Fixation Device, Percutaneous Endoscopic Approach
0PSJ46Z Reposition Left Radius with Intramedullary Internal Fixation Device, Percutaneous Endoscopic Approach
0PSJ4BZ Reposition Left Radius with Monoplanar External Fixation Device, Percutaneous Endoscopic Approach
0PSJ4CZ Reposition Left Radius with Ring External Fixation Device, Percutaneous Endoscopic Approach
0PSJ4DZ Reposition Left Radius with Hybrid External Fixation Device, Percutaneous Endoscopic Approach
0PSJ4ZZ Reposition Left Radius, Percutaneous Endoscopic Approach
0PSJXZZ Reposition Left Radius, External Approach
0PSK04Z Reposition Right Ulna with Internal Fixation Device, Open Approach
0PSK05Z Reposition Right Ulna with External Fixation Device, Open Approach
0PSK06Z Reposition Right Ulna with Intramedullary Internal Fixation Device, Open Approach
0PSK0BZ Reposition Right Ulna with Monoplanar External Fixation Device, Open Approach
0PSK0CZ Reposition Right Ulna with Ring External Fixation Device, Open Approach
0PSK0DZ Reposition Right Ulna with Hybrid External Fixation Device, Open Approach
0PSK0ZZ Reposition Right Ulna, Open Approach
0PSK34Z Reposition Right Ulna with Internal Fixation Device, Percutaneous Approach
0PSK35Z Reposition Right Ulna with External Fixation Device, Percutaneous Approach
0PSK36Z Reposition Right Ulna with Intramedullary Internal Fixation Device, Percutaneous Approach
0PSK3BZ Reposition Right Ulna with Monoplanar External Fixation Device, Percutaneous Approach
0PSK3CZ Reposition Right Ulna with Ring External Fixation Device, Percutaneous Approach
0PSK3DZ Reposition Right Ulna with Hybrid External Fixation Device, Percutaneous Approach
0PSK3ZZ Reposition Right Ulna, Percutaneous Approach
0PSK44Z Reposition Right Ulna with Internal Fixation Device, Percutaneous Endoscopic Approach
0PSK45Z Reposition Right Ulna with External Fixation Device, Percutaneous Endoscopic Approach
0PSK46Z Reposition Right Ulna with Intramedullary Internal Fixation Device, Percutaneous Endoscopic Approach
0PSK4BZ Reposition Right Ulna with Monoplanar External Fixation Device, Percutaneous Endoscopic Approach
0PSK4CZ Reposition Right Ulna with Ring External Fixation Device, Percutaneous Endoscopic Approach
0PSK4DZ Reposition Right Ulna with Hybrid External Fixation Device, Percutaneous Endoscopic Approach
0PSK4ZZ Reposition Right Ulna, Percutaneous Endoscopic Approach
0PSKXZZ Reposition Right Ulna, External Approach
0PSL04Z Reposition Left Ulna with Internal Fixation Device, Open Approach
0PSL05Z Reposition Left Ulna with External Fixation Device, Open Approach

0PSL06Z Reposition Left Ulna with Intramedullary Internal Fixation Device, Open Approach
0PSL0BZ Reposition Left Ulna with Monoplanar External Fixation Device, Open Approach
0PSL0CZ Reposition Left Ulna with Ring External Fixation Device, Open Approach
0PSL0DZ Reposition Left Ulna with Hybrid External Fixation Device, Open Approach
0PSL0ZZ Reposition Left Ulna, Open Approach
0PSL34Z Reposition Left Ulna with Internal Fixation Device, Percutaneous Approach
0PSL35Z Reposition Left Ulna with External Fixation Device, Percutaneous Approach
0PSL36Z Reposition Left Ulna with Intramedullary Internal Fixation Device, Percutaneous Approach
0PSL3BZ Reposition Left Ulna with Monoplanar External Fixation Device, Percutaneous Approach
0PSL3CZ Reposition Left Ulna with Ring External Fixation Device, Percutaneous Approach
0PSL3DZ Reposition Left Ulna with Hybrid External Fixation Device, Percutaneous Approach
0PSL3ZZ Reposition Left Ulna, Percutaneous Approach
0PSL44Z Reposition Left Ulna with Internal Fixation Device, Percutaneous Endoscopic Approach
0PSL45Z Reposition Left Ulna with External Fixation Device, Percutaneous Endoscopic Approach
0PSL46Z Reposition Left Ulna with Intramedullary Internal Fixation Device, Percutaneous Endoscopic Approach
0PSL4BZ Reposition Left Ulna with Monoplanar External Fixation Device, Percutaneous Endoscopic Approach
0PSL4CZ Reposition Left Ulna with Ring External Fixation Device, Percutaneous Endoscopic Approach
0PSL4DZ Reposition Left Ulna with Hybrid External Fixation Device, Percutaneous Endoscopic Approach
0PSL4ZZ Reposition Left Ulna, Percutaneous Endoscopic Approach
0PSLXZZ Reposition Left Ulna, External Approach
0PSM04Z Reposition Right Carpal with Internal Fixation Device, Open Approach
0PSM05Z Reposition Right Carpal with External Fixation Device, Open Approach
0PSM0ZZ Reposition Right Carpal, Open Approach
0PSM34Z Reposition Right Carpal with Internal Fixation Device, Percutaneous Approach
0PSM35Z Reposition Right Carpal with External Fixation Device, Percutaneous Approach
0PSM3ZZ Reposition Right Carpal, Percutaneous Approach
0PSM44Z Reposition Right Carpal with Internal Fixation Device, Percutaneous Endoscopic Approach
0PSM45Z Reposition Right Carpal with External Fixation Device, Percutaneous Endoscopic Approach
0PSM4ZZ Reposition Right Carpal, Percutaneous Endoscopic Approach
0PSMXZZ Reposition Right Carpal, External Approach
0PSN04Z Reposition Left Carpal with Internal Fixation Device, Open Approach
0PSN05Z Reposition Left Carpal with External Fixation Device, Open Approach
0PSN0ZZ Reposition Left Carpal, Open Approach
0PSN34Z Reposition Left Carpal with Internal Fixation Device, Percutaneous Approach
0PSN35Z Reposition Left Carpal with External Fixation Device, Percutaneous Approach
0PSN3ZZ Reposition Left Carpal, Percutaneous Approach
0PSN44Z Reposition Left Carpal with Internal Fixation Device, Percutaneous Endoscopic Approach
0PSN45Z Reposition Left Carpal with External Fixation Device, Percutaneous Endoscopic Approach
0PSN4ZZ Reposition Left Carpal, Percutaneous Endoscopic Approach
0PSNXZZ Reposition Left Carpal, External Approach
0PSP04Z Reposition Right Metacarpal with Internal Fixation Device, Open Approach
0PSP05Z Reposition Right Metacarpal with External Fixation Device, Open Approach
0PSP0ZZ Reposition Right Metacarpal, Open Approach
0PSP34Z Reposition Right Metacarpal with Internal Fixation Device, Percutaneous Approach
0PSP35Z Reposition Right Metacarpal with External Fixation Device, Percutaneous Approach
0PSP3ZZ Reposition Right Metacarpal, Percutaneous Approach
0PSP44Z Reposition Right Metacarpal with Internal Fixation Device, Percutaneous Endoscopic Approach
0PSP45Z Reposition Right Metacarpal with External Fixation Device, Percutaneous Endoscopic Approach
0PSP4ZZ Reposition Right Metacarpal, Percutaneous Endoscopic Approach
0PSPXZZ Reposition Right Metacarpal, External Approach
0PSQ04Z Reposition Left Metacarpal with Internal Fixation Device, Open Approach
0PSQ05Z Reposition Left Metacarpal with External Fixation Device, Open Approach
0PSQ0ZZ Reposition Left Metacarpal, Open Approach
0PSQ34Z Reposition Left Metacarpal with Internal Fixation Device, Percutaneous Approach
0PSQ35Z Reposition Left Metacarpal with External Fixation Device, Percutaneous Approach
0PSQ3ZZ Reposition Left Metacarpal, Percutaneous Approach
0PSQ44Z Reposition Left Metacarpal with Internal Fixation Device, Percutaneous Endoscopic Approach
0PSQ45Z Reposition Left Metacarpal with External Fixation Device, Percutaneous Endoscopic Approach
0PSQ4ZZ Reposition Left Metacarpal, Percutaneous Endoscopic Approach
0PSQXZZ Reposition Left Metacarpal, External Approach
0PSR04Z Reposition Right Thumb Phalanx with Internal Fixation Device, Open Approach
0PSR05Z Reposition Right Thumb Phalanx with External Fixation Device, Open Approach
0PSR0ZZ Reposition Right Thumb Phalanx, Open Approach
0PSR34Z Reposition Right Thumb Phalanx with Internal Fixation Device, Percutaneous Approach
0PSR35Z Reposition Right Thumb Phalanx with External Fixation Device, Percutaneous Approach
0PSR3ZZ Reposition Right Thumb Phalanx, Percutaneous Approach
0PSR44Z Reposition Right Thumb Phalanx with Internal Fixation Device, Percutaneous Endoscopic Approach
0PSR45Z Reposition Right Thumb Phalanx with External Fixation Device, Percutaneous Endoscopic Approach
0PSR4ZZ Reposition Right Thumb Phalanx, Percutaneous Endoscopic Approach
0PSRXZZ Reposition Right Thumb Phalanx, External Approach
0PSS04Z Reposition Left Thumb Phalanx with Internal Fixation Device, Open Approach
0PSS05Z Reposition Left Thumb Phalanx with External Fixation Device, Open Approach
0PSS0ZZ Reposition Left Thumb Phalanx, Open Approach
0PSS34Z Reposition Left Thumb Phalanx with Internal Fixation Device, Percutaneous Approach
0PSS35Z Reposition Left Thumb Phalanx with External Fixation Device, Percutaneous Approach
0PSS3ZZ Reposition Left Thumb Phalanx, Percutaneous Approach
0PSS44Z Reposition Left Thumb Phalanx with Internal Fixation Device, Percutaneous Endoscopic Approach
0PSS45Z Reposition Left Thumb Phalanx with External Fixation Device, Percutaneous Endoscopic Approach
0PSS4ZZ Reposition Left Thumb Phalanx, Percutaneous Endoscopic Approach
0PSSXZZ Reposition Left Thumb Phalanx, External Approach
0PST04Z Reposition Right Finger Phalanx with Internal Fixation Device, Open Approach
0PST05Z Reposition Right Finger Phalanx with External Fixation Device, Open Approach
0PST0ZZ Reposition Right Finger Phalanx, Open Approach
0PST34Z Reposition Right Finger Phalanx with Internal Fixation Device, Percutaneous Approach
0PST35Z Reposition Right Finger Phalanx with External Fixation Device, Percutaneous Approach
0PST3ZZ Reposition Right Finger Phalanx, Percutaneous Approach
0PST44Z Reposition Right Finger Phalanx with Internal Fixation Device, Percutaneous Endoscopic Approach
0PST45Z Reposition Right Finger Phalanx with External Fixation Device, Percutaneous Endoscopic Approach
0PST4ZZ Reposition Right Finger Phalanx, Percutaneous Endoscopic Approach
0PSTXZZ Reposition Right Finger Phalanx, External Approach
0PSV04Z Reposition Left Finger Phalanx with Internal Fixation Device, Open Approach
0PSV05Z Reposition Left Finger Phalanx with External Fixation Device, Open Approach
0PSV0ZZ Reposition Left Finger Phalanx, Open Approach
0PSV34Z Reposition Left Finger Phalanx with Internal Fixation Device, Percutaneous Approach
0PSV35Z Reposition Left Finger Phalanx with External Fixation Device, Percutaneous Approach
0PSV3ZZ Reposition Left Finger Phalanx, Percutaneous Approach
0PSV44Z Reposition Left Finger Phalanx with Internal Fixation Device, Percutaneous Endoscopic Approach
0PSV45Z Reposition Left Finger Phalanx with External Fixation Device, Percutaneous Endoscopic Approach
0PSV4ZZ Reposition Left Finger Phalanx, Percutaneous Endoscopic Approach
0PSVXZZ Reposition Left Finger Phalanx, External Approach

T – Upper Bones, Resection

view Coding Guideline B3.8

T00ZZ Resection of Sternum, Open Approach
T10ZZ Resection of Right Rib, Open Approach
T20ZZ Resection of Left Rib, Open Approach
T50ZZ Resection of Right Scapula, Open Approach
T60ZZ Resection of Left Scapula, Open Approach
T70ZZ Resection of Right Glenoid Cavity, Open Approach
T80ZZ Resection of Left Glenoid Cavity, Open Approach
T90ZZ Resection of Right Clavicle, Open Approach
TB0ZZ Resection of Left Clavicle, Open Approach
0PTC0ZZ Resection of Right Humeral Head, Open Approach
0PTD0ZZ Resection of Left Humeral Head, Open Approach
0PTF0ZZ Resection of Right Humeral Shaft, Open Approach
0PTG0ZZ Resection of Left Humeral Shaft, Open Approach
0PTH0ZZ Resection of Right Radius, Open Approach
0PTJ0ZZ Resection of Left Radius, Open Approach
0PTK0ZZ Resection of Right Ulna, Open Approach
0PTL0ZZ Resection of Left Ulna, Open Approach
0PTM0ZZ Resection of Right Carpal, Open Approach
0PTN0ZZ Resection of Left Carpal, Open Approach
0PTP0ZZ Resection of Right Metacarpal, Open Approach
0PTQ0ZZ Resection of Left Metacarpal, Open Approach
0PTR0ZZ Resection of Right Thumb Phalanx, Open Approach
0PTS0ZZ Resection of Left Thumb Phalanx, Open Approach
0PTT0ZZ Resection of Right Finger Phalanx, Open Approach
0PTV0ZZ Resection of Left Finger Phalanx, Open Approach

U – Upper Bones, Supplement

U007Z Supplement Sternum with Autologous Tissue Substitute, Open Approach
U00JZ Supplement Sternum with Synthetic Substitute, Open Approach
AHA CC: 4Q, 2013, 109-111
U00KZ Supplement Sternum with Nonautologous Tissue Substitute, Open Approach
U037Z Supplement Sternum with Autologous Tissue Substitute, Percutaneous Approach
U03JZ Supplement Sternum with Synthetic Substitute, Percutaneous Approach
U03KZ Supplement Sternum with Nonautologous Tissue Substitute, Percutaneous Approach
U047Z Supplement Sternum with Autologous Tissue Substitute, Percutaneous Endoscopic Approach
U04JZ Supplement Sternum with Synthetic Substitute, Percutaneous Endoscopic Approach
U04KZ Supplement Sternum with Nonautologous Tissue Substitute, Percutaneous Endoscopic Approach
PU107Z Supplement Right Rib with Autologous Tissue Substitute, Open Approach
U10JZ Supplement Right Rib with Synthetic Substitute, Open Approach
U10KZ Supplement Right Rib with Nonautologous Tissue Substitute, Open Approach
PU137Z Supplement Right Rib with Autologous Tissue Substitute, Percutaneous Approach
PU13JZ Supplement Right Rib with Synthetic Substitute, Percutaneous Approach
PU13KZ Supplement Right Rib with Nonautologous Tissue Substitute, Percutaneous Approach
PU147Z Supplement Right Rib with Autologous Tissue Substitute, Percutaneous Endoscopic Approach
PU14JZ Supplement Right Rib with Synthetic Substitute, Percutaneous Endoscopic Approach
PU14KZ Supplement Right Rib with Nonautologous Tissue Substitute, Percutaneous Endoscopic Approach
PU207Z Supplement Left Rib with Autologous Tissue Substitute, Open Approach
PU20JZ Supplement Left Rib with Synthetic Substitute, Open Approach
PU20KZ Supplement Left Rib with Nonautologous Tissue Substitute, Open Approach
PU237Z Supplement Left Rib with Autologous Tissue Substitute, Percutaneous Approach
PU23JZ Supplement Left Rib with Synthetic Substitute, Percutaneous Approach
0PU23KZ Supplement Left Rib with Nonautologous Tissue Substitute, Percutaneous Approach
0PU247Z Supplement Left Rib with Autologous Tissue Substitute, Percutaneous Endoscopic Approach
0PU24JZ Supplement Left Rib with Synthetic Substitute, Percutaneous Endoscopic Approach
0PU24KZ Supplement Left Rib with Nonautologous Tissue Substitute, Percutaneous Endoscopic Approach
0PU307Z Supplement Cervical Vertebra with Autologous Tissue Substitute, Open Approach
0PU30JZ Supplement Cervical Vertebra with Synthetic Substitute, Open Approach
0PU30KZ Supplement Cervical Vertebra with Nonautologous Tissue Substitute, Open Approach
0PU337Z Supplement Cervical Vertebra with Autologous Tissue Substitute, Percutaneous Approach
0PU33JZ Supplement Cervical Vertebra with Synthetic Substitute, Percutaneous Approach
0PU33KZ Supplement Cervical Vertebra with Nonautologous Tissue Substitute, Percutaneous Approach
0PU347Z Supplement Cervical Vertebra with Autologous Tissue Substitute, Percutaneous Endoscopic Approach
0PU34JZ Supplement Cervical Vertebra with Synthetic Substitute, Percutaneous Endoscopic Approach
0PU34KZ Supplement Cervical Vertebra with Nonautologous Tissue Substitute, Percutaneous Endoscopic Approach
0PU407Z Supplement Thoracic Vertebra with Autologous Tissue Substitute, Open Approach
0PU40JZ Supplement Thoracic Vertebra with Synthetic Substitute, Open Approach
0PU40KZ Supplement Thoracic Vertebra with Nonautologous Tissue Substitute, Open Approach
0PU437Z Supplement Thoracic Vertebra with Autologous Tissue Substitute, Percutaneous Approach
0PU43JZ Supplement Thoracic Vertebra with Synthetic Substitute, Percutaneous Approach
0PU43KZ Supplement Thoracic Vertebra with Nonautologous Tissue Substitute, Percutaneous Approach
0PU447Z Supplement Thoracic Vertebra with Autologous Tissue Substitute, Percutaneous Endoscopic Approach
0PU44JZ Supplement Thoracic Vertebra with Synthetic Substitute, Percutaneous Endoscopic Approach
0PU44KZ Supplement Thoracic Vertebra with Nonautologous Tissue Substitute, Percutaneous Endoscopic Approach
0PU507Z Supplement Right Scapula with Autologous Tissue Substitute, Open Approach
0PU50JZ Supplement Right Scapula with Synthetic Substitute, Open Approach
0PU50KZ Supplement Right Scapula with Nonautologous Tissue Substitute, Open Approach
0PU537Z Supplement Right Scapula with Autologous Tissue Substitute, Percutaneous Approach
0PU53JZ Supplement Right Scapula with Synthetic Substitute, Percutaneous Approach
0PU53KZ Supplement Right Scapula with Nonautologous Tissue Substitute, Percutaneous Approach
0PU547Z Supplement Right Scapula with Autologous Tissue Substitute, Percutaneous Endoscopic Approach
0PU54JZ Supplement Right Scapula with Synthetic Substitute, Percutaneous Endoscopic Approach
0PU54KZ Supplement Right Scapula with Nonautologous Tissue Substitute, Percutaneous Endoscopic Approach
0PU607Z Supplement Left Scapula with Autologous Tissue Substitute, Open Approach
0PU60JZ Supplement Left Scapula with Synthetic Substitute, Open Approach
0PU60KZ Supplement Left Scapula with Nonautologous Tissue Substitute, Open Approach
0PU637Z Supplement Left Scapula with Autologous Tissue Substitute, Percutaneous Approach
0PU63JZ Supplement Left Scapula with Synthetic Substitute, Percutaneous Approach
0PU63KZ Supplement Left Scapula with Nonautologous Tissue Substitute, Percutaneous Approach
0PU647Z Supplement Left Scapula with Autologous Tissue Substitute, Percutaneous Endoscopic Approach
0PU64JZ Supplement Left Scapula with Synthetic Substitute, Percutaneous Endoscopic Approach

0PU64KZ Supplement Left Scapula with Nonautologous Tissue Substitute, Percutaneous Endoscopic Approach
0PU707Z Supplement Right Glenoid Cavity with Autologous Tissue Substitute, Open Approach
0PU70JZ Supplement Right Glenoid Cavity with Synthetic Substitute, Open Approach
0PU70KZ Supplement Right Glenoid Cavity with Nonautologous Tissue Substitute, Open Approach
0PU737Z Supplement Right Glenoid Cavity with Autologous Tissue Substitute, Percutaneous Approach
0PU73JZ Supplement Right Glenoid Cavity with Synthetic Substitute, Percutaneous Approach
0PU73KZ Supplement Right Glenoid Cavity with Nonautologous Tissue Substitute, Percutaneous Approach
0PU747Z Supplement Right Glenoid Cavity with Autologous Tissue Substitute, Percutaneous Endoscopic Approach
0PU74JZ Supplement Right Glenoid Cavity with Synthetic Substitute, Percutaneous Endoscopic Approach
0PU74KZ Supplement Right Glenoid Cavity with Nonautologous Tissue Substitute, Percutaneous Endoscopic Approach
0PU807Z Supplement Left Glenoid Cavity with Autologous Tissue Substitute, Open Approach
0PU80JZ Supplement Left Glenoid Cavity with Synthetic Substitute, Open Approach
0PU80KZ Supplement Left Glenoid Cavity with Nonautologous Tissue Substitute, Open Approach
0PU837Z Supplement Left Glenoid Cavity with Autologous Tissue Substitute, Percutaneous Approach
0PU83JZ Supplement Left Glenoid Cavity with Synthetic Substitute, Percutaneous Approach
0PU83KZ Supplement Left Glenoid Cavity with Nonautologous Tissue Substitute, Percutaneous Approach
0PU847Z Supplement Left Glenoid Cavity with Autologous Tissue Substitute, Percutaneous Endoscopic Approach
0PU84JZ Supplement Left Glenoid Cavity with Synthetic Substitute, Percutaneous Endoscopic Approach
0PU84KZ Supplement Left Glenoid Cavity with Nonautologous Tissue Substitute, Percutaneous Endoscopic Approach
0PU907Z Supplement Right Clavicle with Autologous Tissue Substitute, Open Approach
0PU90JZ Supplement Right Clavicle with Synthetic Substitute, Open Approach
0PU90KZ Supplement Right Clavicle with Nonautologous Tissue Substitute, Open Approach
0PU937Z Supplement Right Clavicle with Autologous Tissue Substitute, Percutaneous Approach
0PU93JZ Supplement Right Clavicle with Synthetic Substitute, Percutaneous Approach
0PU93KZ Supplement Right Clavicle with Nonautologous Tissue Substitute, Percutaneous Approach
0PU947Z Supplement Right Clavicle with Autologous Tissue Substitute, Percutaneous Endoscopic Approach
0PU94JZ Supplement Right Clavicle with Synthetic Substitute, Percutaneous Endoscopic Approach
0PU94KZ Supplement Right Clavicle with Nonautologous Tissue Substitute, Percutaneous Endoscopic Approach
0PUB07Z Supplement Left Clavicle with Autologous Tissue Substitute, Open Approach
0PUB0JZ Supplement Left Clavicle with Synthetic Substitute, Open Approach
0PUB0KZ Supplement Left Clavicle with Nonautologous Tissue Substitute, Open Approach
0PUB37Z Supplement Left Clavicle with Autologous Tissue Substitute, Percutaneous Approach
0PUB3JZ Supplement Left Clavicle with Synthetic Substitute, Percutaneous Approach
0PUB3KZ Supplement Left Clavicle with Nonautologous Tissue Substitute, Percutaneous Approach
0PUB47Z Supplement Left Clavicle with Autologous Tissue Substitute, Percutaneous Endoscopic Approach
0PUB4JZ Supplement Left Clavicle with Synthetic Substitute, Percutaneous Endoscopic Approach
0PUB4KZ Supplement Left Clavicle with Nonautologous Tissue Substitute, Percutaneous Endoscopic Approach
0PUC07Z Supplement Right Humeral Head with Autologous Tissue Substitute, Open Approach
0PUC0JZ Supplement Right Humeral Head with Synthetic Substitute, Open Approach
0PUC0KZ Supplement Right Humeral Head with Nonautologous Tissue Substitute, Open Approach
0PUC37Z Supplement Right Humeral Head with Autologous Tissue Substitute, Percutaneous Approach
0PUC3JZ Supplement Right Humeral Head with Synthetic Substitute, Percutaneous Approach
0PUC3KZ Supplement Right Humeral Head with Nonautologous Tissue Substitute, Percutaneous Approach
0PUC47Z Supplement Right Humeral Head with Autologous Tissue Substitute, Percutaneous Endoscopic Approach
0PUC4JZ Supplement Right Humeral Head with Synthetic Substitute, Percutaneous Endoscopic Approach
0PUC4KZ Supplement Right Humeral Head with Nonautologous Tissue Substitute, Percutaneous Endoscopic Approach
0PUD07Z Supplement Left Humeral Head with Autologous Tissue Substitute, Open Approach
0PUD0JZ Supplement Left Humeral Head with Synthetic Substitute, Open Approach
0PUD0KZ Supplement Left Humeral Head with Nonautologous Tissue Substitute, Open Approach
0PUD37Z Supplement Left Humeral Head with Autologous Tissue Substitute, Percutaneous Approach
0PUD3JZ Supplement Left Humeral Head with Synthetic Substitute, Percutaneous Approach
0PUD3KZ Supplement Left Humeral Head with Nonautologous Tissue Substitute, Percutaneous Approach
0PUD47Z Supplement Left Humeral Head with Autologous Tissue Substitute, Percutaneous Endoscopic Approach
0PUD4JZ Supplement Left Humeral Head with Synthetic Substitute, Percutaneous Endoscopic Approach
0PUD4KZ Supplement Left Humeral Head with Nonautologous Tissue Substitute, Percutaneous Endoscopic Approach
0PUF07Z Supplement Right Humeral Shaft with Autologous Tissue Substitute, Open Approach
0PUF0JZ Supplement Right Humeral Shaft with Synthetic Substitute, Open Approach
0PUF0KZ Supplement Right Humeral Shaft with Nonautologous Tissue Substitute, Open Approach
0PUF37Z Supplement Right Humeral Shaft with Autologous Tissue Substitute, Percutaneous Approach
0PUF3JZ Supplement Right Humeral Shaft with Synthetic Substitute, Percutaneous Approach
0PUF3KZ Supplement Right Humeral Shaft with Nonautologous Tissue Substitute, Percutaneous Approach
0PUF47Z Supplement Right Humeral Shaft with Autologous Tissue Substitute, Percutaneous Endoscopic Approach
0PUF4JZ Supplement Right Humeral Shaft with Synthetic Substitute, Percutaneous Endoscopic Approach
0PUF4KZ Supplement Right Humeral Shaft with Nonautologous Tissue Substitute, Percutaneous Endoscopic Approach
0PUG07Z Supplement Left Humeral Shaft with Autologous Tissue Substitute, Open Approach
0PUG0JZ Supplement Left Humeral Shaft with Synthetic Substitute, Open Approach
0PUG0KZ Supplement Left Humeral Shaft with Nonautologous Tissue Substitute, Open Approach
0PUG37Z Supplement Left Humeral Shaft with Autologous Tissue Substitute, Percutaneous Approach
0PUG3JZ Supplement Left Humeral Shaft with Synthetic Substitute, Percutaneous Approach
0PUG3KZ Supplement Left Humeral Shaft with Nonautologous Tissue Substitute, Percutaneous Approach
0PUG47Z Supplement Left Humeral Shaft with Autologous Tissue Substitute, Percutaneous Endoscopic Approach
0PUG4JZ Supplement Left Humeral Shaft with Synthetic Substitute, Percutaneous Endoscopic Approach
0PUG4KZ Supplement Left Humeral Shaft with Nonautologous Tissue Substitute, Percutaneous Endoscopic Approach
0PUH07Z Supplement Right Radius with Autologous Tissue Substitute, Open Approach
0PUH0JZ Supplement Right Radius with Synthetic Substitute, Open Approach
0PUH0KZ Supplement Right Radius with Nonautologous Tissue Substitute, Open Approach
0PUH37Z Supplement Right Radius with Autologous Tissue Substitute, Percutaneous Approach
0PUH3JZ Supplement Right Radius with Synthetic Substitute, Percutaneous Approach
0PUH3KZ Supplement Right Radius with Nonautologous Tissue Substitute, Percutaneous Approach
0PUH47Z Supplement Right Radius with Autologous Tissue Substitute, Percutaneous Endoscopic Approach
0PUH4JZ Supplement Right Radius with Synthetic Substitute, Percutaneous Endoscopic Approach

UH4KZ Supplement Right Radius with Nonautologous Tissue Substitute, Percutaneous Endoscopic Approach

UJ07Z Supplement Left Radius with Autologous Tissue Substitute, Open Approach

UJ0JZ Supplement Left Radius with Synthetic Substitute, Open Approach

UJ0KZ Supplement Left Radius with Nonautologous Tissue Substitute, Open Approach

UJ37Z Supplement Left Radius with Autologous Tissue Substitute, Percutaneous Approach

UJ3JZ Supplement Left Radius with Synthetic Substitute, Percutaneous Approach

UJ3KZ Supplement Left Radius with Nonautologous Tissue Substitute, Percutaneous Approach

UJ47Z Supplement Left Radius with Autologous Tissue Substitute, Percutaneous Endoscopic Approach

UJ4JZ Supplement Left Radius with Synthetic Substitute, Percutaneous Endoscopic Approach

UJ4KZ Supplement Left Radius with Nonautologous Tissue Substitute, Percutaneous Endoscopic Approach

UK07Z Supplement Right Ulna with Autologous Tissue Substitute, Open Approach

UK0JZ Supplement Right Ulna with Synthetic Substitute, Open Approach

UK0KZ Supplement Right Ulna with Nonautologous Tissue Substitute, Open Approach

UK37Z Supplement Right Ulna with Autologous Tissue Substitute, Percutaneous Approach

UK3JZ Supplement Right Ulna with Synthetic Substitute, Percutaneous Approach

UK3KZ Supplement Right Ulna with Nonautologous Tissue Substitute, Percutaneous Approach

PUK47Z Supplement Right Ulna with Autologous Tissue Substitute, Percutaneous Endoscopic Approach

PUK4JZ Supplement Right Ulna with Synthetic Substitute, Percutaneous Endoscopic Approach

PUK4KZ Supplement Right Ulna with Nonautologous Tissue Substitute, Percutaneous Endoscopic Approach

PUL07Z Supplement Left Ulna with Autologous Tissue Substitute, Open Approach

PUL0JZ Supplement Left Ulna with Synthetic Substitute, Open Approach

PUL0KZ Supplement Left Ulna with Nonautologous Tissue Substitute, Open Approach

PUL37Z Supplement Left Ulna with Autologous Tissue Substitute, Percutaneous Approach

PUL3JZ Supplement Left Ulna with Synthetic Substitute, Percutaneous Approach

PUL3KZ Supplement Left Ulna with Nonautologous Tissue Substitute, Percutaneous Approach

PUL47Z Supplement Left Ulna with Autologous Tissue Substitute, Percutaneous Endoscopic Approach

PUL4JZ Supplement Left Ulna with Synthetic Substitute, Percutaneous Endoscopic Approach

PUL4KZ Supplement Left Ulna with Nonautologous Tissue Substitute, Percutaneous Endoscopic Approach

PUM07Z Supplement Right Carpal with Autologous Tissue Substitute, Open Approach

0PUM0JZ Supplement Right Carpal with Synthetic Substitute, Open Approach

0PUM0KZ Supplement Right Carpal with Nonautologous Tissue Substitute, Open Approach

0PUM37Z Supplement Right Carpal with Autologous Tissue Substitute, Percutaneous Approach

0PUM3JZ Supplement Right Carpal with Synthetic Substitute, Percutaneous Approach

0PUM3KZ Supplement Right Carpal with Nonautologous Tissue Substitute, Percutaneous Approach

0PUM47Z Supplement Right Carpal with Autologous Tissue Substitute, Percutaneous Endoscopic Approach

0PUM4JZ Supplement Right Carpal with Synthetic Substitute, Percutaneous Endoscopic Approach

0PUM4KZ Supplement Right Carpal with Nonautologous Tissue Substitute, Percutaneous Endoscopic Approach

0PUN07Z Supplement Left Carpal with Autologous Tissue Substitute, Open Approach

0PUN0JZ Supplement Left Carpal with Synthetic Substitute, Open Approach

0PUN0KZ Supplement Left Carpal with Nonautologous Tissue Substitute, Open Approach

0PUN37Z Supplement Left Carpal with Autologous Tissue Substitute, Percutaneous Approach

0PUN3JZ Supplement Left Carpal with Synthetic Substitute, Percutaneous Approach

0PUN3KZ Supplement Left Carpal with Nonautologous Tissue Substitute, Percutaneous Approach

0PUN47Z Supplement Left Carpal with Autologous Tissue Substitute, Percutaneous Endoscopic Approach

0PUN4JZ Supplement Left Carpal with Synthetic Substitute, Percutaneous Endoscopic Approach

0PUN4KZ Supplement Left Carpal with Nonautologous Tissue Substitute, Percutaneous Endoscopic Approach

0PUP07Z Supplement Right Metacarpal with Autologous Tissue Substitute, Open Approach

0PUP0JZ Supplement Right Metacarpal with Synthetic Substitute, Open Approach

0PUP0KZ Supplement Right Metacarpal with Nonautologous Tissue Substitute, Open Approach

0PUP37Z Supplement Right Metacarpal with Autologous Tissue Substitute, Percutaneous Approach

0PUP3JZ Supplement Right Metacarpal with Synthetic Substitute, Percutaneous Approach

0PUP3KZ Supplement Right Metacarpal with Nonautologous Tissue Substitute, Percutaneous Approach

0PUP47Z Supplement Right Metacarpal with Autologous Tissue Substitute, Percutaneous Endoscopic Approach

0PUP4JZ Supplement Right Metacarpal with Synthetic Substitute, Percutaneous Endoscopic Approach

0PUP4KZ Supplement Right Metacarpal with Nonautologous Tissue Substitute, Percutaneous Endoscopic Approach

0PUQ07Z Supplement Left Metacarpal with Autologous Tissue Substitute, Open Approach

0PUQ0JZ Supplement Left Metacarpal with Synthetic Substitute, Open Approach

0PUQ0KZ Supplement Left Metacarpal with Nonautologous Tissue Substitute, Open Approach

0PUQ37Z Supplement Left Metacarpal with Autologous Tissue Substitute, Percutaneous Approach

0PUQ3JZ Supplement Left Metacarpal with Synthetic Substitute, Percutaneous Approach

0PUQ3KZ Supplement Left Metacarpal with Nonautologous Tissue Substitute, Percutaneous Approach

0PUQ47Z Supplement Left Metacarpal with Autologous Tissue Substitute, Percutaneous Endoscopic Approach

0PUQ4JZ Supplement Left Metacarpal with Synthetic Substitute, Percutaneous Endoscopic Approach

0PUQ4KZ Supplement Left Metacarpal with Nonautologous Tissue Substitute, Percutaneous Endoscopic Approach

0PUR07Z Supplement Right Thumb Phalanx with Autologous Tissue Substitute, Open Approach

0PUR0JZ Supplement Right Thumb Phalanx with Synthetic Substitute, Open Approach

0PUR0KZ Supplement Right Thumb Phalanx with Nonautologous Tissue Substitute, Open Approach

0PUR37Z Supplement Right Thumb Phalanx with Autologous Tissue Substitute, Percutaneous Approach

0PUR3JZ Supplement Right Thumb Phalanx with Synthetic Substitute, Percutaneous Approach

0PUR3KZ Supplement Right Thumb Phalanx with Nonautologous Tissue Substitute, Percutaneous Approach

0PUR47Z Supplement Right Thumb Phalanx with Autologous Tissue Substitute, Percutaneous Endoscopic Approach

0PUR4JZ Supplement Right Thumb Phalanx with Synthetic Substitute, Percutaneous Endoscopic Approach

0PUR4KZ Supplement Right Thumb Phalanx with Nonautologous Tissue Substitute, Percutaneous Endoscopic Approach

0PUS07Z Supplement Left Thumb Phalanx with Autologous Tissue Substitute, Open Approach

0PUS0JZ Supplement Left Thumb Phalanx with Synthetic Substitute, Open Approach

0PUS0KZ Supplement Left Thumb Phalanx with Nonautologous Tissue Substitute, Open Approach

0PUS37Z Supplement Left Thumb Phalanx with Autologous Tissue Substitute, Percutaneous Approach

0PUS3JZ Supplement Left Thumb Phalanx with Synthetic Substitute, Percutaneous Approach

0PUS3KZ Supplement Left Thumb Phalanx with Nonautologous Tissue Substitute, Percutaneous Approach

0PUS47Z Supplement Left Thumb Phalanx with Autologous Tissue Substitute, Percutaneous Endoscopic Approach

0PUS4JZ Supplement Left Thumb Phalanx with Synthetic Substitute, Percutaneous Endoscopic Approach

0PUS4KZ Supplement Left Thumb Phalanx with Nonautologous Tissue Substitute, Percutaneous Endoscopic Approach

0PUT07Z Supplement Right Finger Phalanx with Autologous Tissue Substitute, Open Approach

0PUT0JZ Supplement Right Finger Phalanx with Synthetic Substitute, Open Approach
0PUT0KZ Supplement Right Finger Phalanx with Nonautologous Tissue Substitute, Open Approach
0PUT37Z Supplement Right Finger Phalanx with Autologous Tissue Substitute, Percutaneous Approach
0PUT3JZ Supplement Right Finger Phalanx with Synthetic Substitute, Percutaneous Approach
0PUT3KZ Supplement Right Finger Phalanx with Nonautologous Tissue Substitute, Percutaneous Approach
0PUT47Z Supplement Right Finger Phalanx with Autologous Tissue Substitute, Percutaneous Endoscopic Approach
0PUT4JZ Supplement Right Finger Phalanx with Synthetic Substitute, Percutaneous Endoscopic Approach
0PUT4KZ Supplement Right Finger Phalanx with Nonautologous Tissue Substitute, Percutaneous Endoscopic Approach
0PUV07Z Supplement Left Finger Phalanx with Autologous Tissue Substitute, Open Approach
0PUV0JZ Supplement Left Finger Phalanx with Synthetic Substitute, Open Approach
0PUV0KZ Supplement Left Finger Phalanx with Nonautologous Tissue Substitute, Open Approach
0PUV37Z Supplement Left Finger Phalanx with Autologous Tissue Substitute, Percutaneous Approach
0PUV3JZ Supplement Left Finger Phalanx with Synthetic Substitute, Percutaneous Approach
0PUV3KZ Supplement Left Finger Phalanx with Nonautologous Tissue Substitute, Percutaneous Approach
0PUV47Z Supplement Left Finger Phalanx with Autologous Tissue Substitute, Percutaneous Endoscopic Approach
0PUV4JZ Supplement Left Finger Phalanx with Synthetic Substitute, Percutaneous Endoscopic Approach
0PUV4KZ Supplement Left Finger Phalanx with Nonautologous Tissue Substitute, Percutaneous Endoscopic Approach

0PW – Upper Bones, Revision

Review Coding Guideline B6.1c

0PW004Z Revision of Internal Fixation Device in Sternum, Open Approach
0PW007Z Revision of Autologous Tissue Substitute in Sternum, Open Approach
0PW00JZ Revision of Synthetic Substitute in Sternum, Open Approach
0PW00KZ Revision of Nonautologous Tissue Substitute in Sternum, Open Approach
0PW034Z Revision of Internal Fixation Device in Sternum, Percutaneous Approach
0PW037Z Revision of Autologous Tissue Substitute in Sternum, Percutaneous Approach
0PW03JZ Revision of Synthetic Substitute in Sternum, Percutaneous Approach
0PW03KZ Revision of Nonautologous Tissue Substitute in Sternum, Percutaneous Approach
0PW044Z Revision of Internal Fixation Device in Sternum, Percutaneous Endoscopic Approach
0PW047Z Revision of Autologous Tissue Substitute in Sternum, Percutaneous Endoscopic Approach
0PW04JZ Revision of Synthetic Substitute in Sternum, Percutaneous Endoscopic Approach
0PW04KZ Revision of Nonautologous Tissue Substitute in Sternum, Percutaneous Endoscopic Approach
0PW0X4Z Revision of Internal Fixation Device in Sternum, External Approach
0PW0X7Z Revision of Autologous Tissue Substitute in Sternum, External Approach
0PW0XJZ Revision of Synthetic Substitute in Sternum, External Approach
0PW0XKZ Revision of Nonautologous Tissue Substitute in Sternum, External Approach
0PW104Z Revision of Internal Fixation Device in Right Rib, Open Approach
0PW107Z Revision of Autologous Tissue Substitute in Right Rib, Open Approach
0PW10JZ Revision of Synthetic Substitute in Right Rib, Open Approach
0PW10KZ Revision of Nonautologous Tissue Substitute in Right Rib, Open Approach
0PW134Z Revision of Internal Fixation Device in Right Rib, Percutaneous Approach
0PW137Z Revision of Autologous Tissue Substitute in Right Rib, Percutaneous Approach
0PW13JZ Revision of Synthetic Substitute in Right Rib, Percutaneous Approach
0PW13KZ Revision of Nonautologous Tissue Substitute in Right Rib, Percutaneous Approach
0PW144Z Revision of Internal Fixation Device in Right Rib, Percutaneous Endoscopic Approach
0PW147Z Revision of Autologous Tissue Substitute in Right Rib, Percutaneous Endoscopic Approach
0PW14JZ Revision of Synthetic Substitute in Right Rib, Percutaneous Endoscopic Approach
0PW14KZ Revision of Nonautologous Tissue Substitute in Right Rib, Percutaneous Endoscopic Approach
0PW1X4Z Revision of Internal Fixation Device in Right Rib, External Approach
0PW1X7Z Revision of Autologous Tissue Substitute in Right Rib, External Approach
0PW1XJZ Revision of Synthetic Substitute in Right Rib, External Approach
0PW1XKZ Revision of Nonautologous Tissue Substitute in Right Rib, External Approach
0PW204Z Revision of Internal Fixation Device in Left Rib, Open Approach
0PW207Z Revision of Autologous Tissue Substitute in Left Rib, Open Approach
0PW20JZ Revision of Synthetic Substitute in Left Rib, Open Approach
0PW20KZ Revision of Nonautologous Tissue Substitute in Left Rib, Open Approach
0PW234Z Revision of Internal Fixation Device in Left Rib, Percutaneous Approach
0PW237Z Revision of Autologous Tissue Substitute in Left Rib, Percutaneous Approach
0PW23JZ Revision of Synthetic Substitute in Left Rib, Percutaneous Approach
0PW23KZ Revision of Nonautologous Tissue Substitute in Left Rib, Percutaneous Approach
0PW244Z Revision of Internal Fixation Device in Left Rib, Percutaneous Endoscopic Approach
0PW247Z Revision of Autologous Tissue Substitute in Left Rib, Percutaneous Endoscopic Approach
0PW24JZ Revision of Synthetic Substitute in Left Rib, Percutaneous Endoscopic Approach
0PW24KZ Revision of Nonautologous Tissue Substitute in Left Rib, Percutaneous Endoscopic Approach
0PW2X4Z Revision of Internal Fixation Device in Left Rib, External Approach
0PW2X7Z Revision of Autologous Tissue Substitute in Left Rib, External Approach
0PW2XJZ Revision of Synthetic Substitute in Left Rib, External Approach
0PW2XKZ Revision of Nonautologous Tissue Substitute in Left Rib, External Approac
0PW304Z Revision of Internal Fixation Device in Cervical Vertebra, Open Approach
0PW307Z Revision of Autologous Tissue Substitut in Cervical Vertebra, Open Approach
0PW30JZ Revision of Synthetic Substitute in Cervical Vertebra, Open Approach
0PW30KZ Revision of Nonautologous Tissue Substitute in Cervical Vertebra, Open Approach
0PW334Z Revision of Internal Fixation Device in Cervical Vertebra, Percutaneous Approa
0PW337Z Revision of Autologous Tissue Substitut in Cervical Vertebra, Percutaneous Approach
0PW33JZ Revision of Synthetic Substitute in Cervical Vertebra, Percutaneous Approac
0PW33KZ Revision of Nonautologous Tissue Substitute in Cervical Vertebra, Percutaneous Approach
0PW344Z Revision of Internal Fixation Device in Cervical Vertebra, Percutaneous Endoscopic Approach
0PW347Z Revision of Autologous Tissue Substitute in Cervical Vertebra, Percutaneous Endoscopic Approach
0PW34JZ Revision of Synthetic Substitute in Cervical Vertebra, Percutaneous Endoscopic Approach
0PW34KZ Revision of Nonautologous Tissue Substitute in Cervical Vertebra, Percutaneous Endoscopic Approach
0PW3X4Z Revision of Internal Fixation Device in Cervical Vertebra, External Approach
0PW3X7Z Revision of Autologous Tissue Substitute in Cervical Vertebra, External Approach
0PW3XJZ Revision of Synthetic Substitute in Cervical Vertebra, External Approach
0PW3XKZ Revision of Nonautologous Tissue Substitute in Cervical Vertebra, External Approach
0PW404Z Revision of Internal Fixation Device in Thoracic Vertebra, Open Approach
0PW407Z Revision of Autologous Tissue Substitute in Thoracic Vertebra, Open Approach
0PW40JZ Revision of Synthetic Substitute in Thoracic Vertebra, Open Approach
0PW40KZ Revision of Nonautologous Tissue Substitute in Thoracic Vertebra, Open Approach
0PW434Z Revision of Internal Fixation Device in Thoracic Vertebra, Percutaneous Approach

W437Z Revision of Autologous Tissue Substitute in Thoracic Vertebra, Percutaneous Approach
W43JZ Revision of Synthetic Substitute in Thoracic Vertebra, Percutaneous Approach
W43KZ Revision of Nonautologous Tissue Substitute in Thoracic Vertebra, Percutaneous Approach
W444Z Revision of Internal Fixation Device in Thoracic Vertebra, Percutaneous Endoscopic Approach
W447Z Revision of Autologous Tissue Substitute in Thoracic Vertebra, Percutaneous Endoscopic Approach
W44JZ Revision of Synthetic Substitute in Thoracic Vertebra, Percutaneous Endoscopic Approach
W44KZ Revision of Nonautologous Tissue Substitute in Thoracic Vertebra, Percutaneous Endoscopic Approach
W4X4Z Revision of Internal Fixation Device in Thoracic Vertebra, External Approach
W4X7Z Revision of Autologous Tissue Substitute in Thoracic Vertebra, External Approach
W4XJZ Revision of Synthetic Substitute in Thoracic Vertebra, External Approach
W4XKZ Revision of Nonautologous Tissue Substitute in Thoracic Vertebra, External Approach
W504Z Revision of Internal Fixation Device in Right Scapula, Open Approach
W507Z Revision of Autologous Tissue Substitute in Right Scapula, Open Approach
PW50JZ Revision of Synthetic Substitute in Right Scapula, Open Approach
PW50KZ Revision of Nonautologous Tissue Substitute in Right Scapula, Open Approach
PW534Z Revision of Internal Fixation Device in Right Scapula, Percutaneous Approach
PW537Z Revision of Autologous Tissue Substitute in Right Scapula, Percutaneous Approach
PW53JZ Revision of Synthetic Substitute in Right Scapula, Percutaneous Approach
PW53KZ Revision of Nonautologous Tissue Substitute in Right Scapula, Percutaneous Approach
PW544Z Revision of Internal Fixation Device in Right Scapula, Percutaneous Endoscopic Approach
PW547Z Revision of Autologous Tissue Substitute in Right Scapula, Percutaneous Endoscopic Approach
PW54JZ Revision of Synthetic Substitute in Right Scapula, Percutaneous Endoscopic Approach
PW54KZ Revision of Nonautologous Tissue Substitute in Right Scapula, Percutaneous Endoscopic Approach
PW5X4Z Revision of Internal Fixation Device in Right Scapula, External Approach
PW5X7Z Revision of Autologous Tissue Substitute in Right Scapula, External Approach
PW5XJZ Revision of Synthetic Substitute in Right Scapula, External Approach
PW5XKZ Revision of Nonautologous Tissue Substitute in Right Scapula, External Approach
PW604Z Revision of Internal Fixation Device in Left Scapula, Open Approach
PW607Z Revision of Autologous Tissue Substitute in Left Scapula, Open Approach
PW60JZ Revision of Synthetic Substitute in Left Scapula, Open Approach
0PW60KZ Revision of Nonautologous Tissue Substitute in Left Scapula, Open Approach
0PW634Z Revision of Internal Fixation Device in Left Scapula, Percutaneous Approach
0PW637Z Revision of Autologous Tissue Substitute in Left Scapula, Percutaneous Approach
0PW63JZ Revision of Synthetic Substitute in Left Scapula, Percutaneous Approach
0PW63KZ Revision of Nonautologous Tissue Substitute in Left Scapula, Percutaneous Approach
0PW644Z Revision of Internal Fixation Device in Left Scapula, Percutaneous Endoscopic Approach
0PW647Z Revision of Autologous Tissue Substitute in Left Scapula, Percutaneous Endoscopic Approach
0PW64JZ Revision of Synthetic Substitute in Left Scapula, Percutaneous Endoscopic Approach
0PW64KZ Revision of Nonautologous Tissue Substitute in Left Scapula, Percutaneous Endoscopic Approach
0PW6X4Z Revision of Internal Fixation Device in Left Scapula, External Approach
0PW6X7Z Revision of Autologous Tissue Substitute in Left Scapula, External Approach
0PW6XJZ Revision of Synthetic Substitute in Left Scapula, External Approach
0PW6XKZ Revision of Nonautologous Tissue Substitute in Left Scapula, External Approach
0PW704Z Revision of Internal Fixation Device in Right Glenoid Cavity, Open Approach
0PW707Z Revision of Autologous Tissue Substitute in Right Glenoid Cavity, Open Approach
0PW70JZ Revision of Synthetic Substitute in Right Glenoid Cavity, Open Approach
0PW70KZ Revision of Nonautologous Tissue Substitute in Right Glenoid Cavity, Open Approach
0PW734Z Revision of Internal Fixation Device in Right Glenoid Cavity, Percutaneous Approach
0PW737Z Revision of Autologous Tissue Substitute in Right Glenoid Cavity, Percutaneous Approach
0PW73JZ Revision of Synthetic Substitute in Right Glenoid Cavity, Percutaneous Approach
0PW73KZ Revision of Nonautologous Tissue Substitute in Right Glenoid Cavity, Percutaneous Approach
0PW744Z Revision of Internal Fixation Device in Right Glenoid Cavity, Percutaneous Endoscopic Approach
0PW747Z Revision of Autologous Tissue Substitute in Right Glenoid Cavity, Percutaneous Endoscopic Approach
0PW74JZ Revision of Synthetic Substitute in Right Glenoid Cavity, Percutaneous Endoscopic Approach
0PW74KZ Revision of Nonautologous Tissue Substitute in Right Glenoid Cavity, Percutaneous Endoscopic Approach
0PW7X4Z Revision of Internal Fixation Device in Right Glenoid Cavity, External Approach
0PW7X7Z Revision of Autologous Tissue Substitute in Right Glenoid Cavity, External Approach
0PW7XJZ Revision of Synthetic Substitute in Right Glenoid Cavity, External Approach
0PW7XKZ Revision of Nonautologous Tissue Substitute in Right Glenoid Cavity, External Approach
0PW804Z Revision of Internal Fixation Device in Left Glenoid Cavity, Open Approach
0PW807Z Revision of Autologous Tissue Substitute in Left Glenoid Cavity, Open Approach
0PW80JZ Revision of Synthetic Substitute in Left Glenoid Cavity, Open Approach
0PW80KZ Revision of Nonautologous Tissue Substitute in Left Glenoid Cavity, Open Approach
0PW834Z Revision of Internal Fixation Device in Left Glenoid Cavity, Percutaneous Approach
0PW837Z Revision of Autologous Tissue Substitute in Left Glenoid Cavity, Percutaneous Approach
0PW83JZ Revision of Synthetic Substitute in Left Glenoid Cavity, Percutaneous Approach
0PW83KZ Revision of Nonautologous Tissue Substitute in Left Glenoid Cavity, Percutaneous Approach
0PW844Z Revision of Internal Fixation Device in Left Glenoid Cavity, Percutaneous Endoscopic Approach
0PW847Z Revision of Autologous Tissue Substitute in Left Glenoid Cavity, Percutaneous Endoscopic Approach
0PW84JZ Revision of Synthetic Substitute in Left Glenoid Cavity, Percutaneous Endoscopic Approach
0PW84KZ Revision of Nonautologous Tissue Substitute in Left Glenoid Cavity, Percutaneous Endoscopic Approach
0PW8X4Z Revision of Internal Fixation Device in Left Glenoid Cavity, External Approach
0PW8X7Z Revision of Autologous Tissue Substitute in Left Glenoid Cavity, External Approach
0PW8XJZ Revision of Synthetic Substitute in Left Glenoid Cavity, External Approach
0PW8XKZ Revision of Nonautologous Tissue Substitute in Left Glenoid Cavity, External Approach
0PW904Z Revision of Internal Fixation Device in Right Clavicle, Open Approach
0PW907Z Revision of Autologous Tissue Substitute in Right Clavicle, Open Approach
0PW90JZ Revision of Synthetic Substitute in Right Clavicle, Open Approach
0PW90KZ Revision of Nonautologous Tissue Substitute in Right Clavicle, Open Approach
0PW934Z Revision of Internal Fixation Device in Right Clavicle, Percutaneous Approach
0PW937Z Revision of Autologous Tissue Substitute in Right Clavicle, Percutaneous Approach
0PW93JZ Revision of Synthetic Substitute in Right Clavicle, Percutaneous Approach
0PW93KZ Revision of Nonautologous Tissue Substitute in Right Clavicle, Percutaneous Approach
0PW944Z Revision of Internal Fixation Device in Right Clavicle, Percutaneous Endoscopic Approach
0PW947Z Revision of Autologous Tissue Substitute in Right Clavicle, Percutaneous Endoscopic Approach
0PW94JZ Revision of Synthetic Substitute in Right Clavicle, Percutaneous Endoscopic Approach
0PW94KZ Revision of Nonautologous Tissue Substitute in Right Clavicle, Percutaneous Endoscopic Approach
0PW9X4Z Revision of Internal Fixation Device in Right Clavicle, External Approach
0PW9X7Z Revision of Autologous Tissue Substitute in Right Clavicle, External Approach

0PW9XJZ Revision of Synthetic Substitute in Right Clavicle, External Approach

0PW9XKZ Revision of Nonautologous Tissue Substitute in Right Clavicle, External Approach

0PWB04Z Revision of Internal Fixation Device in Left Clavicle, Open Approach

0PWB07Z Revision of Autologous Tissue Substitute in Left Clavicle, Open Approach

0PWB0JZ Revision of Synthetic Substitute in Left Clavicle, Open Approach

0PWB0KZ Revision of Nonautologous Tissue Substitute in Left Clavicle, Open Approach

0PWB34Z Revision of Internal Fixation Device in Left Clavicle, Percutaneous Approach

0PWB37Z Revision of Autologous Tissue Substitute in Left Clavicle, Percutaneous Approach

0PWB3JZ Revision of Synthetic Substitute in Left Clavicle, Percutaneous Approach

0PWB3KZ Revision of Nonautologous Tissue Substitute in Left Clavicle, Percutaneous Approach

0PWB44Z Revision of Internal Fixation Device in Left Clavicle, Percutaneous Endoscopic Approach

0PWB47Z Revision of Autologous Tissue Substitute in Left Clavicle, Percutaneous Endoscopic Approach

0PWB4JZ Revision of Synthetic Substitute in Left Clavicle, Percutaneous Endoscopic Approach

0PWB4KZ Revision of Nonautologous Tissue Substitute in Left Clavicle, Percutaneous Endoscopic Approach

0PWBX4Z Revision of Internal Fixation Device in Left Clavicle, External Approach

0PWBX7Z Revision of Autologous Tissue Substitute in Left Clavicle, External Approach

0PWBXJZ Revision of Synthetic Substitute in Left Clavicle, External Approach

0PWBXKZ Revision of Nonautologous Tissue Substitute in Left Clavicle, External Approach

0PWC04Z Revision of Internal Fixation Device in Right Humeral Head, Open Approach

0PWC05Z Revision of External Fixation Device in Right Humeral Head, Open Approach

0PWC07Z Revision of Autologous Tissue Substitute in Right Humeral Head, Open Approach

0PWC0JZ Revision of Synthetic Substitute in Right Humeral Head, Open Approach

0PWC0KZ Revision of Nonautologous Tissue Substitute in Right Humeral Head, Open Approach

0PWC34Z Revision of Internal Fixation Device in Right Humeral Head, Percutaneous Approach

0PWC35Z Revision of External Fixation Device in Right Humeral Head, Percutaneous Approach

0PWC37Z Revision of Autologous Tissue Substitute in Right Humeral Head, Percutaneous Approach

0PWC3JZ Revision of Synthetic Substitute in Right Humeral Head, Percutaneous Approach

0PWC3KZ Revision of Nonautologous Tissue Substitute in Right Humeral Head, Percutaneous Approach

0PWC44Z Revision of Internal Fixation Device in Right Humeral Head, Percutaneous Endoscopic Approach

0PWC45Z Revision of External Fixation Device in Right Humeral Head, Percutaneous Endoscopic Approach

0PWC47Z Revision of Autologous Tissue Substitute in Right Humeral Head, Percutaneous Endoscopic Approach

0PWC4JZ Revision of Synthetic Substitute in Right Humeral Head, Percutaneous Endoscopic Approach

0PWC4KZ Revision of Nonautologous Tissue Substitute in Right Humeral Head, Percutaneous Endoscopic Approach

0PWCX4Z Revision of Internal Fixation Device in Right Humeral Head, External Approach

0PWCX5Z Revision of External Fixation Device in Right Humeral Head, External Approach

0PWCX7Z Revision of Autologous Tissue Substitute in Right Humeral Head, External Approach

0PWCXJZ Revision of Synthetic Substitute in Right Humeral Head, External Approach

0PWCXKZ Revision of Nonautologous Tissue Substitute in Right Humeral Head, External Approach

0PWD04Z Revision of Internal Fixation Device in Left Humeral Head, Open Approach

0PWD05Z Revision of External Fixation Device in Left Humeral Head, Open Approach

0PWD07Z Revision of Autologous Tissue Substitute in Left Humeral Head, Open Approach

0PWD0JZ Revision of Synthetic Substitute in Left Humeral Head, Open Approach

0PWD0KZ Revision of Nonautologous Tissue Substitute in Left Humeral Head, Open Approach

0PWD34Z Revision of Internal Fixation Device in Left Humeral Head, Percutaneous Approach

0PWD35Z Revision of External Fixation Device in Left Humeral Head, Percutaneous Approach

0PWD37Z Revision of Autologous Tissue Substitute in Left Humeral Head, Percutaneous Approach

0PWD3JZ Revision of Synthetic Substitute in Left Humeral Head, Percutaneous Approach

0PWD3KZ Revision of Nonautologous Tissue Substitute in Left Humeral Head, Percutaneous Approach

0PWD44Z Revision of Internal Fixation Device in Left Humeral Head, Percutaneous Endoscopic Approach

0PWD45Z Revision of External Fixation Device in Left Humeral Head, Percutaneous Endoscopic Approach

0PWD47Z Revision of Autologous Tissue Substitute in Left Humeral Head, Percutaneous Endoscopic Approach

0PWD4JZ Revision of Synthetic Substitute in Left Humeral Head, Percutaneous Endoscopic Approach

0PWD4KZ Revision of Nonautologous Tissue Substitute in Left Humeral Head, Percutaneous Endoscopic Approach

0PWDX4Z Revision of Internal Fixation Device in Left Humeral Head, External Approach

0PWDX5Z Revision of External Fixation Device in Left Humeral Head, External Approach

0PWDX7Z Revision of Autologous Tissue Substitute in Left Humeral Head, External Approach

0PWDXJZ Revision of Synthetic Substitute in Left Humeral Head, External Approach

0PWDXKZ Revision of Nonautologous Tissue Substitute in Left Humeral Head, External Approach

0PWF04Z Revision of Internal Fixation Device in Right Humeral Shaft, Open Approach

0PWF05Z Revision of External Fixation Device i Right Humeral Shaft, Open Approach

0PWF07Z Revision of Autologous Tissue Substit in Right Humeral Shaft, Open Approac

0PWF0JZ Revision of Synthetic Substitute in Rig Humeral Shaft, Open Approach

0PWF0KZ Revision of Nonautologous Tissue Substitute in Right Humeral Shaft, Ope Approach

0PWF34Z Revision of Internal Fixation Device in Right Humeral Shaft, Percutaneous Approach

0PWF35Z Revision of External Fixation Device in Right Humeral Shaft, Percutaneous Approach

0PWF37Z Revision of Autologous Tissue Substitu in Right Humeral Shaft, Percutaneous Approach

0PWF3JZ Revision of Synthetic Substitute in Rig Humeral Shaft, Percutaneous Approach

0PWF3KZ Revision of Nonautologous Tissue Substitute in Right Humeral Shaft, Percutaneous Approach

0PWF44Z Revision of Internal Fixation Device in Right Humeral Shaft, Percutaneous Endoscopic Approach

0PWF45Z Revision of External Fixation Device in Right Humeral Shaft, Percutaneous Endoscopic Approach

0PWF47Z Revision of Autologous Tissue Substitu in Right Humeral Shaft, Percutaneous Endoscopic Approach

0PWF4JZ Revision of Synthetic Substitute in Righ Humeral Shaft, Percutaneous Endoscop Approach

0PWF4KZ Revision of Nonautologous Tissue Substitute in Right Humeral Shaft, Percutaneous Endoscopic Approach

0PWFX4Z Revision of Internal Fixation Device in Right Humeral Shaft, External Approac

0PWFX5Z Revision of External Fixation Device in Right Humeral Shaft, External Approac

0PWFX7Z Revision of Autologous Tissue Substitut in Right Humeral Shaft, External Approach

0PWFXJZ Revision of Synthetic Substitute in Right Humeral Shaft, External Approach

0PWFXKZ Revision of Nonautologous Tissue Substitute in Right Humeral Shaft, External Approach

0PWG04Z Revision of Internal Fixation Device in Left Humeral Shaft, Open Approach

0PWG05Z Revision of External Fixation Device in Left Humeral Shaft, Open Approach

0PWG07Z Revision of Autologous Tissue Substitute in Left Humeral Shaft, Open Approach

0PWG0JZ Revision of Synthetic Substitute in Left Humeral Shaft, Open Approach

0PWG0KZ Revision of Nonautologous Tissue Substitute in Left Humeral Shaft, Open Approach

0PWG34Z Revision of Internal Fixation Device in Left Humeral Shaft, Percutaneous Approach

0PWG35Z Revision of External Fixation Device in Left Humeral Shaft, Percutaneous Approach

0PWG37Z Revision of Autologous Tissue Substitute in Left Humeral Shaft, Percutaneous Approach

0PWG3JZ Revision of Synthetic Substitute in Left Humeral Shaft, Percutaneous Approach

0PWG3KZ Revision of Nonautologous Tissue Substitute in Left Humeral Shaft, Percutaneous Approach

WG44Z Revision of Internal Fixation Device in Left Humeral Shaft, Percutaneous Endoscopic Approach

WG45Z Revision of External Fixation Device in Left Humeral Shaft, Percutaneous Endoscopic Approach

WG47Z Revision of Autologous Tissue Substitute in Left Humeral Shaft, Percutaneous Endoscopic Approach

WG4JZ Revision of Synthetic Substitute in Left Humeral Shaft, Percutaneous Endoscopic Approach

WG4KZ Revision of Nonautologous Tissue Substitute in Left Humeral Shaft, Percutaneous Endoscopic Approach

•WGX4Z Revision of Internal Fixation Device in Left Humeral Shaft, External Approach

•WGX5Z Revision of External Fixation Device in Left Humeral Shaft, External Approach

•WGX7Z Revision of Autologous Tissue Substitute in Left Humeral Shaft, External Approach

•WGXJZ Revision of Synthetic Substitute in Left Humeral Shaft, External Approach

•WGXKZ Revision of Nonautologous Tissue Substitute in Left Humeral Shaft, External Approach

•WH04Z Revision of Internal Fixation Device in Right Radius, Open Approach

•WH05Z Revision of External Fixation Device in Right Radius, Open Approach

•WH07Z Revision of Autologous Tissue Substitute in Right Radius, Open Approach

PWH0JZ Revision of Synthetic Substitute in Right Radius, Open Approach

PWH0KZ Revision of Nonautologous Tissue Substitute in Right Radius, Open Approach

PWH34Z Revision of Internal Fixation Device in Right Radius, Percutaneous Approach

PWH35Z Revision of External Fixation Device in Right Radius, Percutaneous Approach

PWH37Z Revision of Autologous Tissue Substitute in Right Radius, Percutaneous Approach

PWH3JZ Revision of Synthetic Substitute in Right Radius, Percutaneous Approach

PWH3KZ Revision of Nonautologous Tissue Substitute in Right Radius, Percutaneous Approach

PWH44Z Revision of Internal Fixation Device in Right Radius, Percutaneous Endoscopic Approach

PWH45Z Revision of External Fixation Device in Right Radius, Percutaneous Endoscopic Approach

PWH47Z Revision of Autologous Tissue Substitute in Right Radius, Percutaneous Endoscopic Approach

PWH4JZ Revision of Synthetic Substitute in Right Radius, Percutaneous Endoscopic Approach

PWH4KZ Revision of Nonautologous Tissue Substitute in Right Radius, Percutaneous Endoscopic Approach

•PWHX4Z Revision of Internal Fixation Device in Right Radius, External Approach

•PWHX5Z Revision of External Fixation Device in Right Radius, External Approach

•PWHX7Z Revision of Autologous Tissue Substitute in Right Radius, External Approach

•PWHXJZ Revision of Synthetic Substitute in Right Radius, External Approach

•PWHXKZ Revision of Nonautologous Tissue Substitute in Right Radius, External Approach

0PWJ04Z Revision of Internal Fixation Device in Left Radius, Open Approach

0PWJ05Z Revision of External Fixation Device in Left Radius, Open Approach

0PWJ07Z Revision of Autologous Tissue Substitute in Left Radius, Open Approach

0PWJ0JZ Revision of Synthetic Substitute in Left Radius, Open Approach

0PWJ0KZ Revision of Nonautologous Tissue Substitute in Left Radius, Open Approach

0PWJ34Z Revision of Internal Fixation Device in Left Radius, Percutaneous Approach

0PWJ35Z Revision of External Fixation Device in Left Radius, Percutaneous Approach

0PWJ37Z Revision of Autologous Tissue Substitute in Left Radius, Percutaneous Approach

0PWJ3JZ Revision of Synthetic Substitute in Left Radius, Percutaneous Approach

0PWJ3KZ Revision of Nonautologous Tissue Substitute in Left Radius, Percutaneous Approach

0PWJ44Z Revision of Internal Fixation Device in Left Radius, Percutaneous Endoscopic Approach

0PWJ45Z Revision of External Fixation Device in Left Radius, Percutaneous Endoscopic Approach

0PWJ47Z Revision of Autologous Tissue Substitute in Left Radius, Percutaneous Endoscopic Approach

0PWJ4JZ Revision of Synthetic Substitute in Left Radius, Percutaneous Endoscopic Approach

0PWJ4KZ Revision of Nonautologous Tissue Substitute in Left Radius, Percutaneous Endoscopic Approach

0PWJX4Z Revision of Internal Fixation Device in Left Radius, External Approach

0PWJX5Z Revision of External Fixation Device in Left Radius, External Approach

0PWJX7Z Revision of Autologous Tissue Substitute in Left Radius, External Approach

0PWJXJZ Revision of Synthetic Substitute in Left Radius, External Approach

0PWJXKZ Revision of Nonautologous Tissue Substitute in Left Radius, External Approach

0PWK04Z Revision of Internal Fixation Device in Right Ulna, Open Approach

0PWK05Z Revision of External Fixation Device in Right Ulna, Open Approach

0PWK07Z Revision of Autologous Tissue Substitute in Right Ulna, Open Approach

0PWK0JZ Revision of Synthetic Substitute in Right Ulna, Open Approach

0PWK0KZ Revision of Nonautologous Tissue Substitute in Right Ulna, Open Approach

0PWK34Z Revision of Internal Fixation Device in Right Ulna, Percutaneous Approach

0PWK35Z Revision of External Fixation Device in Right Ulna, Percutaneous Approach

0PWK37Z Revision of Autologous Tissue Substitute in Right Ulna, Percutaneous Approach

0PWK3JZ Revision of Synthetic Substitute in Right Ulna, Percutaneous Approach

0PWK3KZ Revision of Nonautologous Tissue Substitute in Right Ulna, Percutaneous Approach

0PWK44Z Revision of Internal Fixation Device in Right Ulna, Percutaneous Endoscopic Approach

0PWK45Z Revision of External Fixation Device in Right Ulna, Percutaneous Endoscopic Approach

0PWK47Z Revision of Autologous Tissue Substitute in Right Ulna, Percutaneous Endoscopic Approach

0PWK4JZ Revision of Synthetic Substitute in Right Ulna, Percutaneous Endoscopic Approach

0PWK4KZ Revision of Nonautologous Tissue Substitute in Right Ulna, Percutaneous Endoscopic Approach

0PWKX4Z Revision of Internal Fixation Device in Right Ulna, External Approach

0PWKX5Z Revision of External Fixation Device in Right Ulna, External Approach

0PWKX7Z Revision of Autologous Tissue Substitute in Right Ulna, External Approach

0PWKXJZ Revision of Synthetic Substitute in Right Ulna, External Approach

0PWKXKZ Revision of Nonautologous Tissue Substitute in Right Ulna, External Approach

0PWL04Z Revision of Internal Fixation Device in Left Ulna, Open Approach

0PWL05Z Revision of External Fixation Device in Left Ulna, Open Approach

0PWL07Z Revision of Autologous Tissue Substitute in Left Ulna, Open Approach

0PWL0JZ Revision of Synthetic Substitute in Left Ulna, Open Approach

0PWL0KZ Revision of Nonautologous Tissue Substitute in Left Ulna, Open Approach

0PWL34Z Revision of Internal Fixation Device in Left Ulna, Percutaneous Approach

0PWL35Z Revision of External Fixation Device in Left Ulna, Percutaneous Approach

0PWL37Z Revision of Autologous Tissue Substitute in Left Ulna, Percutaneous Approach

0PWL3JZ Revision of Synthetic Substitute in Left Ulna, Percutaneous Approach

0PWL3KZ Revision of Nonautologous Tissue Substitute in Left Ulna, Percutaneous Approach

0PWL44Z Revision of Internal Fixation Device in Left Ulna, Percutaneous Endoscopic Approach

0PWL45Z Revision of External Fixation Device in Left Ulna, Percutaneous Endoscopic Approach

0PWL47Z Revision of Autologous Tissue Substitute in Left Ulna, Percutaneous Endoscopic Approach

0PWL4JZ Revision of Synthetic Substitute in Left Ulna, Percutaneous Endoscopic Approach

0PWL4KZ Revision of Nonautologous Tissue Substitute in Left Ulna, Percutaneous Endoscopic Approach

0PWLX4Z Revision of Internal Fixation Device in Left Ulna, External Approach

0PWLX5Z Revision of External Fixation Device in Left Ulna, External Approach

0PWLX7Z Revision of Autologous Tissue Substitute in Left Ulna, External Approach

0PWLXJZ Revision of Synthetic Substitute in Left Ulna, External Approach

0PWLXKZ Revision of Nonautologous Tissue Substitute in Left Ulna, External Approach

0PWM04Z Revision of Internal Fixation Device in Right Carpal, Open Approach

0PWM05Z Revision of External Fixation Device in Right Carpal, Open Approach

0PWM07Z Revision of Autologous Tissue Substitute in Right Carpal, Open Approach

0PWM0JZ Revision of Synthetic Substitute in Right Carpal, Open Approach

0PWM0KZ Revision of Nonautologous Tissue Substitute in Right Carpal, Open Approach
0PWM34Z Revision of Internal Fixation Device in Right Carpal, Percutaneous Approach
0PWM35Z Revision of External Fixation Device in Right Carpal, Percutaneous Approach
0PWM37Z Revision of Autologous Tissue Substitute in Right Carpal, Percutaneous Approach
0PWM3JZ Revision of Synthetic Substitute in Right Carpal, Percutaneous Approach
0PWM3KZ Revision of Nonautologous Tissue Substitute in Right Carpal, Percutaneous Approach
0PWM44Z Revision of Internal Fixation Device in Right Carpal, Percutaneous Endoscopic Approach
0PWM45Z Revision of External Fixation Device in Right Carpal, Percutaneous Endoscopic Approach
0PWM47Z Revision of Autologous Tissue Substitute in Right Carpal, Percutaneous Endoscopic Approach
0PWM4JZ Revision of Synthetic Substitute in Right Carpal, Percutaneous Endoscopic Approach
0PWM4KZ Revision of Nonautologous Tissue Substitute in Right Carpal, Percutaneous Endoscopic Approach
0PWMX4Z Revision of Internal Fixation Device in Right Carpal, External Approach
0PWMX5Z Revision of External Fixation Device in Right Carpal, External Approach
0PWMX7Z Revision of Autologous Tissue Substitute in Right Carpal, External Approach
0PWMXJZ Revision of Synthetic Substitute in Right Carpal, External Approach
0PWMXKZ Revision of Nonautologous Tissue Substitute in Right Carpal, External Approach
0PWN04Z Revision of Internal Fixation Device in Left Carpal, Open Approach
0PWN05Z Revision of External Fixation Device in Left Carpal, Open Approach
0PWN07Z Revision of Autologous Tissue Substitute in Left Carpal, Open Approach
0PWN0JZ Revision of Synthetic Substitute in Left Carpal, Open Approach
0PWN0KZ Revision of Nonautologous Tissue Substitute in Left Carpal, Open Approach
0PWN34Z Revision of Internal Fixation Device in Left Carpal, Percutaneous Approach
0PWN35Z Revision of External Fixation Device in Left Carpal, Percutaneous Approach
0PWN37Z Revision of Autologous Tissue Substitute in Left Carpal, Percutaneous Approach
0PWN3JZ Revision of Synthetic Substitute in Left Carpal, Percutaneous Approach
0PWN3KZ Revision of Nonautologous Tissue Substitute in Left Carpal, Percutaneous Approach
0PWN44Z Revision of Internal Fixation Device in Left Carpal, Percutaneous Endoscopic Approach
0PWN45Z Revision of External Fixation Device in Left Carpal, Percutaneous Endoscopic Approach
0PWN47Z Revision of Autologous Tissue Substitute in Left Carpal, Percutaneous Endoscopic Approach
0PWN4JZ Revision of Synthetic Substitute in Left Carpal, Percutaneous Endoscopic Approach
0PWN4KZ Revision of Nonautologous Tissue Substitute in Left Carpal, Percutaneous Endoscopic Approach
0PWNX4Z Revision of Internal Fixation Device in Left Carpal, External Approach
0PWNX5Z Revision of External Fixation Device in Left Carpal, External Approach
0PWNX7Z Revision of Autologous Tissue Substitute in Left Carpal, External Approach
0PWNXJZ Revision of Synthetic Substitute in Left Carpal, External Approach
0PWNXKZ Revision of Nonautologous Tissue Substitute in Left Carpal, External Approach
0PWP04Z Revision of Internal Fixation Device in Right Metacarpal, Open Approach
0PWP05Z Revision of External Fixation Device in Right Metacarpal, Open Approach
0PWP07Z Revision of Autologous Tissue Substitute in Right Metacarpal, Open Approach
0PWP0JZ Revision of Synthetic Substitute in Right Metacarpal, Open Approach
0PWP0KZ Revision of Nonautologous Tissue Substitute in Right Metacarpal, Open Approach
0PWP34Z Revision of Internal Fixation Device in Right Metacarpal, Percutaneous Approach
0PWP35Z Revision of External Fixation Device in Right Metacarpal, Percutaneous Approach
0PWP37Z Revision of Autologous Tissue Substitute in Right Metacarpal, Percutaneous Approach
0PWP3JZ Revision of Synthetic Substitute in Right Metacarpal, Percutaneous Approach
0PWP3KZ Revision of Nonautologous Tissue Substitute in Right Metacarpal, Percutaneous Approach
0PWP44Z Revision of Internal Fixation Device in Right Metacarpal, Percutaneous Endoscopic Approach
0PWP45Z Revision of External Fixation Device in Right Metacarpal, Percutaneous Endoscopic Approach
0PWP47Z Revision of Autologous Tissue Substitute in Right Metacarpal, Percutaneous Endoscopic Approach
0PWP4JZ Revision of Synthetic Substitute in Right Metacarpal, Percutaneous Endoscopic Approach
0PWP4KZ Revision of Nonautologous Tissue Substitute in Right Metacarpal, Percutaneous Endoscopic Approach
0PWPX4Z Revision of Internal Fixation Device in Right Metacarpal, External Approach
0PWPX5Z Revision of External Fixation Device in Right Metacarpal, External Approach
0PWPX7Z Revision of Autologous Tissue Substitute in Right Metacarpal, External Approach
0PWPXJZ Revision of Synthetic Substitute in Right Metacarpal, External Approach
0PWPXKZ Revision of Nonautologous Tissue Substitute in Right Metacarpal, External Approach
0PWQ04Z Revision of Internal Fixation Device in Left Metacarpal, Open Approach
0PWQ05Z Revision of External Fixation Device in Left Metacarpal, Open Approach
0PWQ07Z Revision of Autologous Tissue Substitute in Left Metacarpal, Open Approach
0PWQ0JZ Revision of Synthetic Substitute in Left Metacarpal, Open Approach
0PWQ0KZ Revision of Nonautologous Tissue Substitute in Left Metacarpal, Open Approach
0PWQ34Z Revision of Internal Fixation Device in Left Metacarpal, Percutaneous Approach
0PWQ35Z Revision of External Fixation Device in Left Metacarpal, Percutaneous Approach
0PWQ37Z Revision of Autologous Tissue Substitute in Left Metacarpal, Percutaneous Approach
0PWQ3JZ Revision of Synthetic Substitute in Left Metacarpal, Percutaneous Approach
0PWQ3KZ Revision of Nonautologous Tissue Substitute in Left Metacarpal, Percutaneous Approach
0PWQ44Z Revision of Internal Fixation Device in Left Metacarpal, Percutaneous Endoscopic Approach
0PWQ45Z Revision of External Fixation Device in Left Metacarpal, Percutaneous Endoscopic Approach
0PWQ47Z Revision of Autologous Tissue Substitute in Left Metacarpal, Percutaneous Endoscopic Approach
0PWQ4JZ Revision of Synthetic Substitute in Left Metacarpal, Percutaneous Endoscopic Approach
0PWQ4KZ Revision of Nonautologous Tissue Substitute in Left Metacarpal, Percutaneous Endoscopic Approach
0PWQX4Z Revision of Internal Fixation Device in Left Metacarpal, External Approach
0PWQX5Z Revision of External Fixation Device in Left Metacarpal, External Approach
0PWQX7Z Revision of Autologous Tissue Substitute in Left Metacarpal, External Approach
0PWQXJZ Revision of Synthetic Substitute in Left Metacarpal, External Approach
0PWQXKZ Revision of Nonautologous Tissue Substitute in Left Metacarpal, External Approach
0PWR04Z Revision of Internal Fixation Device in Right Thumb Phalanx, Open Approach
0PWR05Z Revision of External Fixation Device in Right Thumb Phalanx, Open Approach
0PWR07Z Revision of Autologous Tissue Substitute in Right Thumb Phalanx, Open Approach
0PWR0JZ Revision of Synthetic Substitute in Right Thumb Phalanx, Open Approach
0PWR0KZ Revision of Nonautologous Tissue Substitute in Right Thumb Phalanx, Open Approach
0PWR34Z Revision of Internal Fixation Device in Right Thumb Phalanx, Percutaneous Approach
0PWR35Z Revision of External Fixation Device in Right Thumb Phalanx, Percutaneous Approach
0PWR37Z Revision of Autologous Tissue Substitute in Right Thumb Phalanx, Percutaneous Approach
0PWR3JZ Revision of Synthetic Substitute in Right Thumb Phalanx, Percutaneous Approach
0PWR3KZ Revision of Nonautologous Tissue Substitute in Right Thumb Phalanx, Percutaneous Approach
0PWR44Z Revision of Internal Fixation Device in Right Thumb Phalanx, Percutaneous Endoscopic Approach
0PWR45Z Revision of External Fixation Device in Right Thumb Phalanx, Percutaneous Endoscopic Approach
0PWR47Z Revision of Autologous Tissue Substitute in Right Thumb Phalanx, Percutaneous Endoscopic Approach
0PWR4JZ Revision of Synthetic Substitute in Right Thumb Phalanx, Percutaneous Endoscopic Approach
0PWR4KZ Revision of Nonautologous Tissue Substitute in Right Thumb Phalanx, Percutaneous Endoscopic Approach

WRX4Z Revision of Internal Fixation Device in Right Thumb Phalanx, External Approach

WRX5Z Revision of External Fixation Device in Right Thumb Phalanx, External Approach

WRX7Z Revision of Autologous Tissue Substitute in Right Thumb Phalanx, External Approach

WRXJZ Revision of Synthetic Substitute in Right Thumb Phalanx, External Approach

WRXKZ Revision of Nonautologous Tissue Substitute in Right Thumb Phalanx, External Approach

WS04Z Revision of Internal Fixation Device in Left Thumb Phalanx, Open Approach

WS05Z Revision of External Fixation Device in Left Thumb Phalanx, Open Approach

WS07Z Revision of Autologous Tissue Substitute in Left Thumb Phalanx, Open Approach

WS0JZ Revision of Synthetic Substitute in Left Thumb Phalanx, Open Approach

WS0KZ Revision of Nonautologous Tissue Substitute in Left Thumb Phalanx, Open Approach

PWS34Z Revision of Internal Fixation Device in Left Thumb Phalanx, Percutaneous Approach

PWS35Z Revision of External Fixation Device in Left Thumb Phalanx, Percutaneous Approach

PWS37Z Revision of Autologous Tissue Substitute in Left Thumb Phalanx, Percutaneous Approach

PWS3JZ Revision of Synthetic Substitute in Left Thumb Phalanx, Percutaneous Approach

PWS3KZ Revision of Nonautologous Tissue Substitute in Left Thumb Phalanx, Percutaneous Approach

PWS44Z Revision of Internal Fixation Device in Left Thumb Phalanx, Percutaneous Endoscopic Approach

PWS45Z Revision of External Fixation Device in Left Thumb Phalanx, Percutaneous Endoscopic Approach

PWS47Z Revision of Autologous Tissue Substitute in Left Thumb Phalanx, Percutaneous Endoscopic Approach

PWS4JZ Revision of Synthetic Substitute in Left Thumb Phalanx, Percutaneous Endoscopic Approach

PWS4KZ Revision of Nonautologous Tissue Substitute in Left Thumb Phalanx, Percutaneous Endoscopic Approach

PWSX4Z Revision of Internal Fixation Device in Left Thumb Phalanx, External Approach

PWSX5Z Revision of External Fixation Device in Left Thumb Phalanx, External Approach

PWSX7Z Revision of Autologous Tissue Substitute in Left Thumb Phalanx, External Approach

PWSXJZ Revision of Synthetic Substitute in Left Thumb Phalanx, External Approach

0PWSXKZ Revision of Nonautologous Tissue Substitute in Left Thumb Phalanx, External Approach

0PWT04Z Revision of Internal Fixation Device in Right Finger Phalanx, Open Approach

0PWT05Z Revision of External Fixation Device in Right Finger Phalanx, Open Approach

0PWT07Z Revision of Autologous Tissue Substitute in Right Finger Phalanx, Open Approach

0PWT0JZ Revision of Synthetic Substitute in Right Finger Phalanx, Open Approach

0PWT0KZ Revision of Nonautologous Tissue Substitute in Right Finger Phalanx, Open Approach

0PWT34Z Revision of Internal Fixation Device in Right Finger Phalanx, Percutaneous Approach

0PWT35Z Revision of External Fixation Device in Right Finger Phalanx, Percutaneous Approach

0PWT37Z Revision of Autologous Tissue Substitute in Right Finger Phalanx, Percutaneous Approach

0PWT3JZ Revision of Synthetic Substitute in Right Finger Phalanx, Percutaneous Approach

0PWT3KZ Revision of Nonautologous Tissue Substitute in Right Finger Phalanx, Percutaneous Approach

0PWT44Z Revision of Internal Fixation Device in Right Finger Phalanx, Percutaneous Endoscopic Approach

0PWT45Z Revision of External Fixation Device in Right Finger Phalanx, Percutaneous Endoscopic Approach

0PWT47Z Revision of Autologous Tissue Substitute in Right Finger Phalanx, Percutaneous Endoscopic Approach

0PWT4JZ Revision of Synthetic Substitute in Right Finger Phalanx, Percutaneous Endoscopic Approach

0PWT4KZ Revision of Nonautologous Tissue Substitute in Right Finger Phalanx, Percutaneous Endoscopic Approach

0PWTX4Z Revision of Internal Fixation Device in Right Finger Phalanx, External Approach

0PWTX5Z Revision of External Fixation Device in Right Finger Phalanx, External Approach

0PWTX7Z Revision of Autologous Tissue Substitute in Right Finger Phalanx, External Approach

0PWTXJZ Revision of Synthetic Substitute in Right Finger Phalanx, External Approach

0PWTXKZ Revision of Nonautologous Tissue Substitute in Right Finger Phalanx, External Approach

0PWV04Z Revision of Internal Fixation Device in Left Finger Phalanx, Open Approach

0PWV05Z Revision of External Fixation Device in Left Finger Phalanx, Open Approach

0PWV07Z Revision of Autologous Tissue Substitute in Left Finger Phalanx, Open Approach

0PWV0JZ Revision of Synthetic Substitute in Left Finger Phalanx, Open Approach

0PWV0KZ Revision of Nonautologous Tissue Substitute in Left Finger Phalanx, Open Approach

0PWV34Z Revision of Internal Fixation Device in Left Finger Phalanx, Percutaneous Approach

0PWV35Z Revision of External Fixation Device in Left Finger Phalanx, Percutaneous Approach

0PWV37Z Revision of Autologous Tissue Substitute in Left Finger Phalanx, Percutaneous Approach

0PWV3JZ Revision of Synthetic Substitute in Left Finger Phalanx, Percutaneous Approach

0PWV3KZ Revision of Nonautologous Tissue Substitute in Left Finger Phalanx, Percutaneous Approach

0PWV44Z Revision of Internal Fixation Device in Left Finger Phalanx, Percutaneous Endoscopic Approach

0PWV45Z Revision of External Fixation Device in Left Finger Phalanx, Percutaneous Endoscopic Approach

0PWV47Z Revision of Autologous Tissue Substitute in Left Finger Phalanx, Percutaneous Endoscopic Approach

0PWV4JZ Revision of Synthetic Substitute in Left Finger Phalanx, Percutaneous Endoscopic Approach

0PWV4KZ Revision of Nonautologous Tissue Substitute in Left Finger Phalanx, Percutaneous Endoscopic Approach

0PWVX4Z Revision of Internal Fixation Device in Left Finger Phalanx, External Approach

0PWVX5Z Revision of External Fixation Device in Left Finger Phalanx, External Approach

0PWVX7Z Revision of Autologous Tissue Substitute in Left Finger Phalanx, External Approach

0PWVXJZ Revision of Synthetic Substitute in Left Finger Phalanx, External Approach

0PWVXKZ Revision of Nonautologous Tissue Substitute in Left Finger Phalanx, External Approach

0PWY00Z Revision of Drainage Device in Upper Bone, Open Approach

0PWY0MZ Revision of Bone Growth Stimulator in Upper Bone, Open Approach

0PWY30Z Revision of Drainage Device in Upper Bone, Percutaneous Approach

0PWY3MZ Revision of Bone Growth Stimulator in Upper Bone, Percutaneous Approach

0PWY40Z Revision of Drainage Device in Upper Bone, Percutaneous Endoscopic Approach

0PWY4MZ Revision of Bone Growth Stimulator in Upper Bone, Percutaneous Endoscopic Approach

0PWYX0Z Revision of Drainage Device in Upper Bone, External Approach

0PWYXMZ Revision of Bone Growth Stimulator in Upper Bone, External Approach

Bones - Front and Back Views

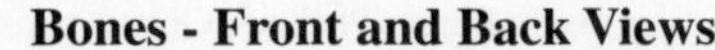

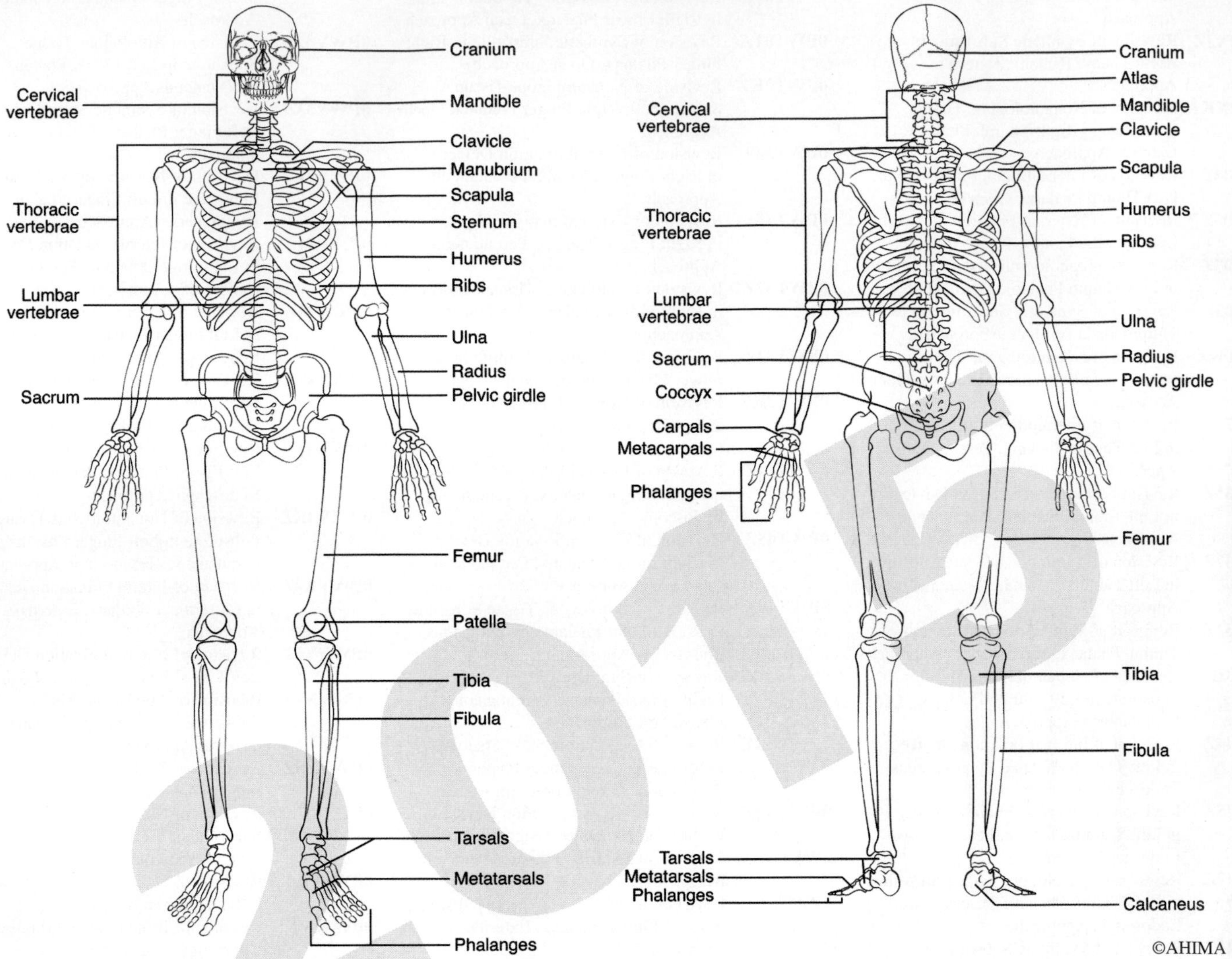

Vertebrae

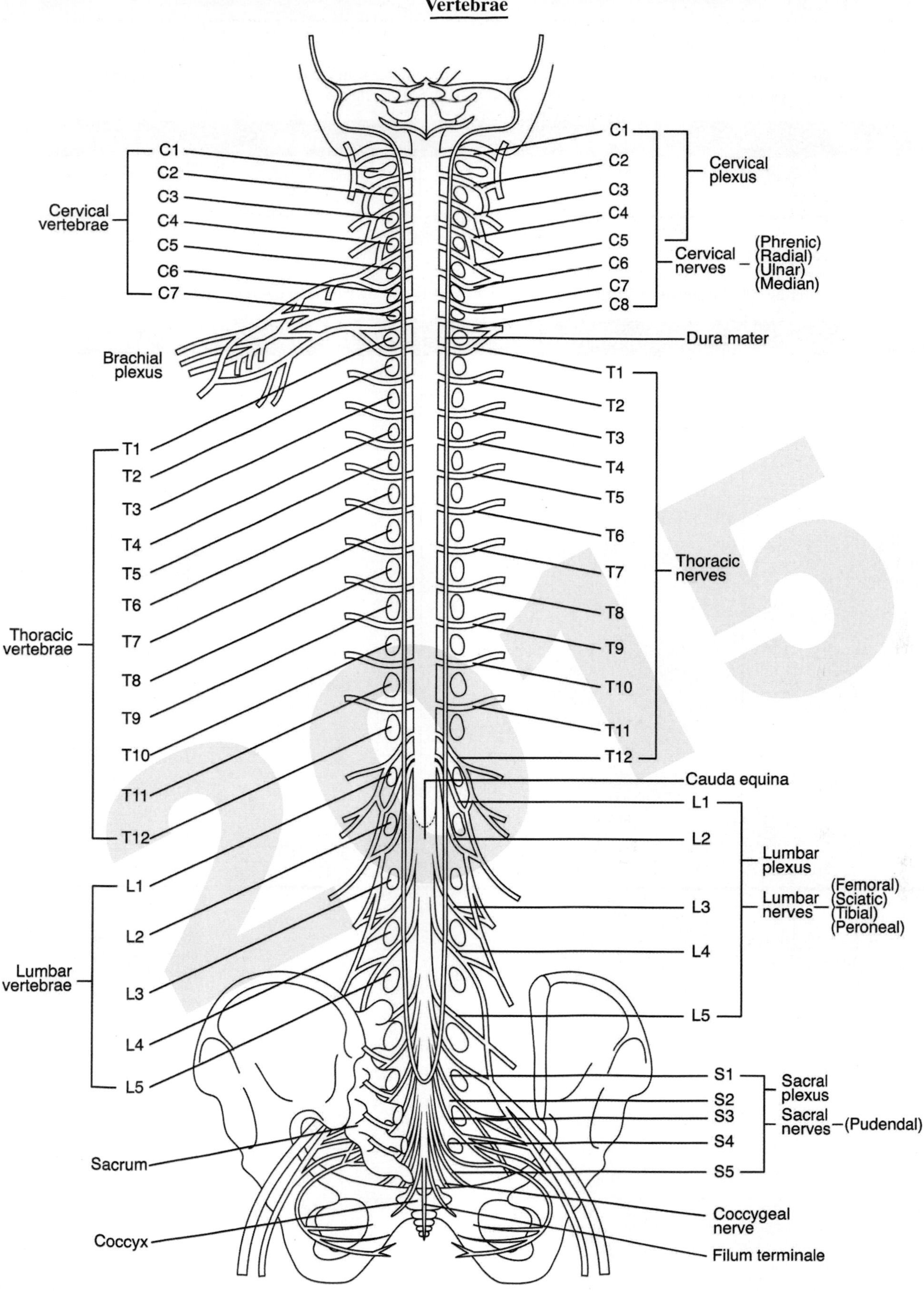
C1
C2
C3
C4
C5
C6
C7
Cervical vertebrae
Brachial plexus
T1
T2
T3
T4
T5
T6
T7
T8
T9
T10
T11
T12
Thoracic vertebrae
L1
L2
L3
L4
L5
Lumbar vertebrae
Sacrum
Coccyx
C1
C2
C3
C4
Cervical plexus
C5
C6
C7
C8
Cervical nerves – (Phrenic) (Radial) (Ulnar) (Median)
Dura mater
T1
T2
T3
T4
T5
T6
T7
T8
T9
T10
T11
T12
Thoracic nerves
Cauda equina
L1
L2
L3
L4
L5
Lumbar plexus
Lumbar nerves – (Femoral) (Sciatic) (Tibial) (Peroneal)
S1
S2
S3
S4
S5
Sacral plexus
Sacral nerves – (Pudendal)
Coccygeal nerve
Filum terminale

Lower Bones Tables 0Q2–0QW

Section 0 **Medical and Surgical**
Body System Q **Lower Bones**
Operation 2 **Change:** Taking out or off a device from a body part and putting back an identical or similar device in or on the same body part without cutting or puncturing the skin or a mucous membrane

Body Part (4th)	Approach (5th)	Device (6th)	Qualifier (7th)
Y Lower Bone	**X** External	**0** Drainage Device **Y** Other Device	**Z** No Qualifier

Section 0 **Medical and Surgical**
Body System Q **Lower Bones**
Operation 5 **Destruction:** Physical eradication of all or a portion of a body part by the direct use of energy, force, or a destructive agent

Body Part (4th)	Approach (5th)	Device (6th)	Qualifier (7th)
0 Lumbar Vertebra **1** Sacrum **2** Pelvic Bone, Right **3** Pelvic Bone, Left **4** Acetabulum, Right **5** Acetabulum, Left **6** Upper Femur, Right **7** Upper Femur, Left **8** Femoral Shaft, Right **9** Femoral Shaft, Left **B** Lower Femur, Right **C** Lower Femur, Left **D** Patella, Right **F** Patella, Left **G** Tibia, Right **H** Tibia, Left **J** Fibula, Right **K** Fibula, Left **L** Tarsal, Right **M** Tarsal, Left **N** Metatarsal, Right **P** Metatarsal, Left **Q** Toe Phalanx, Right **R** Toe Phalanx, Left **S** Coccyx	**0** Open **3** Percutaneous **4** Percutaneous Endoscopic	**Z** No Device	**Z** No Qualifier

Section 0 **Medical and Surgical**
Body System Q **Lower Bones**
Operation 8 **Division:** Cutting into a body part, without draining fluids and/or gases from the body part, in order to separate or transect a body part

Body Part (4th)	Approach (5th)	Device (6th)	Qualifier (7th)
0 Lumbar Vertebra **1** Sacrum **2** Pelvic Bone, Right **3** Pelvic Bone, Left **4** Acetabulum, Right **5** Acetabulum, Left **6** Upper Femur, Right **7** Upper Femur, Left **8** Femoral Shaft, Right **9** Femoral Shaft, Left **B** Lower Femur, Right **C** Lower Femur, Left **D** Patella, Right **F** Patella, Left **G** Tibia, Right **H** Tibia, Left **J** Fibula, Right **K** Fibula, Left **L** Tarsal, Right **M** Tarsal, Left **N** Metatarsal, Right **P** Metatarsal, Left **Q** Toe Phalanx, Right **R** Toe Phalanx, Left **S** Coccyx	**0** Open **3** Percutaneous **4** Percutaneous Endoscopic	**Z** No Device	**Z** No Qualifier

Section 0 **Medical and Surgical**
Body System Q **Lower Bones**
Operation 9 **Drainage:** Taking or letting out fluids and/or gases from a body part

Body Part (4th)	Approach (5th)	Device (6th)	Qualifier (7th)
0 Lumbar Vertebra **1** Sacrum **2** Pelvic Bone, Right **3** Pelvic Bone, Left **4** Acetabulum, Right **5** Acetabulum, Left **6** Upper Femur, Right **7** Upper Femur, Left **8** Femoral Shaft, Right **9** Femoral Shaft, Left **B** Lower Femur, Right **C** Lower Femur, Left **D** Patella, Right **F** Patella, Left **G** Tibia, Right **H** Tibia, Left **J** Fibula, Right **K** Fibula, Left **L** Tarsal, Right **M** Tarsal, Left **N** Metatarsal, Right **P** Metatarsal, Left **Q** Toe Phalanx, Right **R** Toe Phalanx, Left **S** Coccyx	**0** Open **3** Percutaneous **4** Percutaneous Endoscopic	**0** Drainage Device	**Z** No Qualifier

Continued →

0Q9 Continue

Section 0 **Medical and Surgical**
Body System Q **Lower Bones**
Operation 9 **Drainage:** Taking or letting out fluids and/or gases from a body part

Body Part (4th)	Approach (5th)	Device (6th)	Qualifier (7th)
0 Lumbar Vertebra **1** Sacrum **2** Pelvic Bone, Right **3** Pelvic Bone, Left **4** Acetabulum, Right **5** Acetabulum, Left **6** Upper Femur, Right **7** Upper Femur, Left **8** Femoral Shaft, Right **9** Femoral Shaft, Left **B** Lower Femur, Right **C** Lower Femur, Left **D** Patella, Right **F** Patella, Left **G** Tibia, Right **H** Tibia, Left **J** Fibula, Right **K** Fibula, Left **L** Tarsal, Right **M** Tarsal, Left **N** Metatarsal, Right **P** Metatarsal, Left **Q** Toe Phalanx, Right **R** Toe Phalanx, Left **S** Coccyx	**0** Open **3** Percutaneous **4** Percutaneous Endoscopic	**Z** No Device	**X** Diagnostic **Z** No Qualifier

Section 0 **Medical and Surgical**
Body System Q **Lower Bones**
Operation B **Excision:** Cutting out or off, without replacement, a portion of a body part

Body Part (4th)	Approach (5th)	Device (6th)	Qualifier (7th)
0 Lumbar Vertebra **1** Sacrum **2** Pelvic Bone, Right **3** Pelvic Bone, Left **4** Acetabulum, Right **5** Acetabulum, Left **6** Upper Femur, Right **7** Upper Femur, Left **8** Femoral Shaft, Right **9** Femoral Shaft, Left **B** Lower Femur, Right **C** Lower Femur, Left **D** Patella, Right **F** Patella, Left **G** Tibia, Right **H** Tibia, Left **J** Fibula, Right **K** Fibula, Left **L** Tarsal, Right **M** Tarsal, Left **N** Metatarsal, Right **P** Metatarsal, Left **Q** Toe Phalanx, Right **R** Toe Phalanx, Left **S** Coccyx	**0** Open **3** Percutaneous **4** Percutaneous Endoscopic	**Z** No Device	**X** Diagnostic **Z** No Qualifier

Section 0 **Medical and Surgical**
Body System Q **Lower Bones**
Operation C **Extirpation:** Taking or cutting out solid matter from a body part

Body Part (4th)	Approach (5th)	Device (6th)	Qualifier (7th)
0 Lumbar Vertebra **1** Sacrum **2** Pelvic Bone, Right **3** Pelvic Bone, Left **4** Acetabulum, Right **5** Acetabulum, Left **6** Upper Femur, Right **7** Upper Femur, Left **8** Femoral Shaft, Right **9** Femoral Shaft, Left **B** Lower Femur, Right **C** Lower Femur, Left **D** Patella, Right **F** Patella, Left **G** Tibia, Right **H** Tibia, Left **J** Fibula, Right **K** Fibula, Left **L** Tarsal, Right **M** Tarsal, Left **N** Metatarsal, Right **P** Metatarsal, Left **Q** Toe Phalanx, Right **R** Toe Phalanx, Left **S** Coccyx	**0** Open **3** Percutaneous **4** Percutaneous Endoscopic	**Z** No Device	**Z** No Qualifier

Section 0 **Medical and Surgical**
Body System Q **Lower Bones**
Operation H **Insertion:** Putting in a nonbiological appliance that monitors, assists, performs, or prevents a physiological function but does not physically take the place of a body part

Body Part (4th)	Approach (5th)	Device (6th)	Qualifier (7th)
0 Lumbar Vertebra **1** Sacrum **2** Pelvic Bone, Right **3** Pelvic Bone, Left **4** Acetabulum, Right **5** Acetabulum, Left **D** Patella, Right **F** Patella, Left **L** Tarsal, Right **M** Tarsal, Left **N** Metatarsal, Right **P** Metatarsal, Left **Q** Toe Phalanx, Right **R** Toe Phalanx, Left **S** Coccyx	**0** Open **3** Percutaneous **4** Percutaneous Endoscopic	**4** Internal Fixation Device **5** External Fixation Device	**Z** No Qualifier
6 Upper Femur, Right **7** Upper Femur, Left **8** Femoral Shaft, Right **9** Femoral Shaft, Left **B** Lower Femur, Right **C** Lower Femur, Left **G** Tibia, Right **H** Tibia, Left **J** Fibula, Right **K** Fibula, Left	**0** Open **3** Percutaneous **4** Percutaneous Endoscopic	**4** Internal Fixation Device **5** External Fixation Device **6** Internal Fixation Device, Intramedullary **8** External Fixation Device, Limb Lengthening **B** External Fixation Device, Monoplanar **C** External Fixation Device, Ring **D** External Fixation Device, Hybrid	**Z** No Qualifier

Continued →

0QH Continued

Section 0 **Medical and Surgical**
Body System Q **Lower Bones**
Operation H **Insertion:** Putting in a nonbiological appliance that monitors, assists, performs, or prevents a physiological function but does not physically take the place of a body part

Body Part (4th)	Approach (5th)	Device (6th)	Qualifier (7th)
Y Lower Bone	0 Open 3 Percutaneous 4 Percutaneous Endoscopic	M Bone Growth Stimulator	Z No Qualifier

Section 0 **Medical and Surgical**
Body System Q **Lower Bones**
Operation J **Inspection:** Visually and/or manually exploring a body part

Body Part (4th)	Approach (5th)	Device (6th)	Qualifier (7th)
Y Lower Bone	0 Open 3 Percutaneous 4 Percutaneous Endoscopic X External	Z No Device	Z No Qualifier

Section 0 **Medical and Surgical**
Body System Q **Lower Bones**
Operation N **Release:** Freeing a body part from an abnormal physical constraint by cutting or by the use of force

Body Part (4th)	Approach (5th)	Device (6th)	Qualifier (7th)
0 Lumbar Vertebra 1 Sacrum 2 Pelvic Bone, Right 3 Pelvic Bone, Left 4 Acetabulum, Right 5 Acetabulum, Left 6 Upper Femur, Right 7 Upper Femur, Left 8 Femoral Shaft, Right 9 Femoral Shaft, Left B Lower Femur, Right C Lower Femur, Left D Patella, Right F Patella, Left G Tibia, Right H Tibia, Left J Fibula, Right K Fibula, Left L Tarsal, Right M Tarsal, Left N Metatarsal, Right P Metatarsal, Left Q Toe Phalanx, Right R Toe Phalanx, Left S Coccyx	0 Open 3 Percutaneous 4 Percutaneous Endoscopic	Z No Device	Z No Qualifier

Section 0 **Medical and Surgical**
Body System Q **Lower Bones**
Operation P **Removal:** Taking out or off a device from a body part

Body Part (4th)	Approach (5th)	Device (6th)	Qualifier (7th)
0 Lumbar Vertebra 1 Sacrum 4 Acetabulum, Right 5 Acetabulum, Left S Coccyx	0 Open 3 Percutaneous 4 Percutaneous Endoscopic	4 Internal Fixation Device 7 Autologous Tissue Substitute J Synthetic Substitute K Nonautologous Tissue Substitute	Z No Qualifier

Continued →

Section	0	**Medical and Surgical**
Body System	Q	**Lower Bones**
Operation	P	**Removal:** Taking out or off a device from a body part

Body Part (4th)	Approach (5th)	Device (6th)	Qualifier (7th)
0 Lumbar Vertebra **1** Sacrum **4** Acetabulum, Right **5** Acetabulum, Left **S** Coccyx	**X** External	**4** Internal Fixation Device	**Z** No Qualifier
2 Pelvic Bone, Right **3** Pelvic Bone, Left **6** Upper Femur, Right **7** Upper Femur, Left **8** Femoral Shaft, Right **9** Femoral Shaft, Left **B** Lower Femur, Right **C** Lower Femur, Left **D** Patella, Right **F** Patella, Left **G** Tibia, Right **H** Tibia, Left **J** Fibula, Right **K** Fibula, Left **L** Tarsal, Right **M** Tarsal, Left **N** Metatarsal, Right **P** Metatarsal, Left **Q** Toe Phalanx, Right **R** Toe Phalanx, Left	**0** Open **3** Percutaneous **4** Percutaneous Endoscopic	**4** Internal Fixation Device **5** External Fixation Device **7** Autologous Tissue Substitute **J** Synthetic Substitute **K** Nonautologous Tissue Substitute	**Z** No Qualifier
2 Pelvic Bone, Right **3** Pelvic Bone, Left **6** Upper Femur, Right **7** Upper Femur, Left **8** Femoral Shaft, Right **9** Femoral Shaft, Left **B** Lower Femur, Right **C** Lower Femur, Left **D** Patella, Right **F** Patella, Left **G** Tibia, Right **H** Tibia, Left **J** Fibula, Right **K** Fibula, Left **L** Tarsal, Right **M** Tarsal, Left **N** Metatarsal, Right **P** Metatarsal, Left **Q** Toe Phalanx, Right **R** Toe Phalanx, Left	**X** External	**4** Internal Fixation Device **5** External Fixation Device	**Z** No Qualifier
Y Lower Bone	**0** Open **3** Percutaneous **4** Percutaneous Endoscopic **X** External	**0** Drainage Device **M** Bone Growth Stimulator	**Z** No Qualifier

Section 0 **Medical and Surgical**
Body System Q **Lower Bones**
Operation Q **Repair:** Restoring, to the extent possible, a body part to its normal anatomic structure and function

Body Part (4th)	Approach (5th)	Device (6th)	Qualifier (7th)
0 Lumbar Vertebra **1** Sacrum **2** Pelvic Bone, Right **3** Pelvic Bone, Left **4** Acetabulum, Right **5** Acetabulum, Left **6** Upper Femur, Right **7** Upper Femur, Left **8** Femoral Shaft, Right **9** Femoral Shaft, Left **B** Lower Femur, Right **C** Lower Femur, Left **D** Patella, Right **F** Patella, Left **G** Tibia, Right **H** Tibia, Left **J** Fibula, Right **K** Fibula, Left **L** Tarsal, Right **M** Tarsal, Left **N** Metatarsal, Right **P** Metatarsal, Left **Q** Toe Phalanx, Right **R** Toe Phalanx, Left **S** Coccyx	**0** Open **3** Percutaneous **4** Percutaneous Endoscopic **X** External	**Z** No Device	**Z** No Qualifier

Section 0 **Medical and Surgical**
Body System Q **Lower Bones**
Operation R **Replacement:** Putting in or on biological or synthetic material that physically takes the place and/or function of all or a portion of a body part

Body Part (4th)	Approach (5th)	Device (6th)	Qualifier (7th)
0 Lumbar Vertebra **1** Sacrum **2** Pelvic Bone, Right **3** Pelvic Bone, Left **4** Acetabulum, Right **5** Acetabulum, Left **6** Upper Femur, Right **7** Upper Femur, Left **8** Femoral Shaft, Right **9** Femoral Shaft, Left **B** Lower Femur, Right **C** Lower Femur, Left **D** Patella, Right **F** Patella, Left **G** Tibia, Right **H** Tibia, Left **J** Fibula, Right **K** Fibula, Left **L** Tarsal, Right **M** Tarsal, Left **N** Metatarsal, Right **P** Metatarsal, Left **Q** Toe Phalanx, Right **R** Toe Phalanx, Left **S** Coccyx	**0** Open **3** Percutaneous **4** Percutaneous Endoscopic	**7** Autologous Tissue Substitute **J** Synthetic Substitute **K** Nonautologous Tissue Substitute	**Z** No Qualifier

Section 0 **Medical and Surgical**
Body System Q **Lower Bones**
Operation S **Reposition:** Moving to its normal location, or other suitable location, all or a portion of a body part

Body Part (4th)	Approach (5th)	Device (6th)	Qualifier (7th)
0 Lumbar Vertebra **1** Sacrum **4** Acetabulum, Right **5** Acetabulum, Left **S** Coccyx	**0** Open **3** Percutaneous **4** Percutaneous Endoscopic	**4** Internal Fixation Device **Z** No Device	**Z** No Qualifier
0 Lumbar Vertebra **1** Sacrum **4** Acetabulum, Right **5** Acetabulum, Left **S** Coccyx	**X** External	**Z** No Device	**Z** No Qualifier
2 Pelvic Bone, Right **3** Pelvic Bone, Left **D** Patella, Right **F** Patella, Left **L** Tarsal, Right **M** Tarsal, Left **N** Metatarsal, Right **P** Metatarsal, Left **Q** Toe Phalanx, Right **R** Toe Phalanx, Left	**0** Open **3** Percutaneous **4** Percutaneous Endoscopic	**4** Internal Fixation Device **5** External Fixation Device **Z** No Device	**Z** No Qualifier
2 Pelvic Bone, Right **3** Pelvic Bone, Left **D** Patella, Right **F** Patella, Left **L** Tarsal, Right **M** Tarsal, Left **N** Metatarsal, Right **P** Metatarsal, Left **Q** Toe Phalanx, Right **R** Toe Phalanx, Left	**X** External	**Z** No Device	**Z** No Qualifier
6 Upper Femur, Right **7** Upper Femur, Left **8** Femoral Shaft, Right **9** Femoral Shaft, Left **B** Lower Femur, Right **C** Lower Femur, Left **G** Tibia, Right **H** Tibia, Left **J** Fibula, Right **K** Fibula, Left	**0** Open **3** Percutaneous **4** Percutaneous Endoscopic	**4** Internal Fixation Device **5** External Fixation Device **6** Internal Fixation Device, Intramedullary **B** External Fixation Device, Monoplanar **C** External Fixation Device, Ring **D** External Fixation Device, Hybrid **Z** No Device	**Z** No Qualifier
6 Upper Femur, Right **7** Upper Femur, Left **8** Femoral Shaft, Right **9** Femoral Shaft, Left **B** Lower Femur, Right **C** Lower Femur, Left **G** Tibia, Right **H** Tibia, Left **J** Fibula, Right **K** Fibula, Left	**X** External	**Z** No Device	**Z** No Qualifier

Section 0 **Medical and Surgical**
Body System Q **Lower Bones**
Operation T **Resection:** Cutting out or off, without replacement, all of a body part

Body Part (4th)	Approach (5th)	Device (6th)	Qualifier (7th)
2 Pelvic Bone, Right **3** Pelvic Bone, Left **4** Acetabulum, Right **5** Acetabulum, Left **6** Upper Femur, Right **7** Upper Femur, Left **8** Femoral Shaft, Right **9** Femoral Shaft, Left **B** Lower Femur, Right **C** Lower Femur, Left **D** Patella, Right **F** Patella, Left **G** Tibia, Right **H** Tibia, Left **J** Fibula, Right **K** Fibula, Left **L** Tarsal, Right **M** Tarsal, Left **N** Metatarsal, Right **P** Metatarsal, Left **Q** Toe Phalanx, Right **R** Toe Phalanx, Left **S** Coccyx	**0** Open	**Z** No Device	**Z** No Qualifier

Section 0 **Medical and Surgical**
Body System Q **Lower Bones**
Operation U **Supplement:** Putting in or on biological or synthetic material that physically reinforces and/or augments the function of a portion of a body part

Body Part (4th)	Approach (5th)	Device (6th)	Qualifier (7th)
0 Lumbar Vertebra **1** Sacrum **2** Pelvic Bone, Right **3** Pelvic Bone, Left **4** Acetabulum, Right **5** Acetabulum, Left **6** Upper Femur, Right **7** Upper Femur, Left **8** Femoral Shaft, Right **9** Femoral Shaft, Left **B** Lower Femur, Right **C** Lower Femur, Left **D** Patella, Right **F** Patella, Left **G** Tibia, Right **H** Tibia, Left **J** Fibula, Right **K** Fibula, Left **L** Tarsal, Right **M** Tarsal, Left **N** Metatarsal, Right **P** Metatarsal, Left **Q** Toe Phalanx, Right **R** Toe Phalanx, Left **S** Coccyx	**0** Open **3** Percutaneous **4** Percutaneous Endoscopic	**7** Autologous Tissue Substitute **J** Synthetic Substitute **K** Nonautologous Tissue Substitute	**Z** No Qualifier

ction 0 **Medical and Surgical**
ody System Q **Lower Bones**
peration W **Revision:** Correcting, to the extent possible, a portion of a malfunctioning device or the position of a displaced device

Body Part (4th)	Approach (5th)	Device (6th)	Qualifier (7th)
0 Lumbar Vertebra **1** Sacrum **4** Acetabulum, Right **5** Acetabulum, Left **S** Coccyx	**0** Open **3** Percutaneous **4** Percutaneous Endoscopic **X** External	**4** Internal Fixation Device **7** Autologous Tissue Substitute **J** Synthetic Substitute **K** Nonautologous Tissue Substitute	**Z** No Qualifier
2 Pelvic Bone, Right **3** Pelvic Bone, Left **6** Upper Femur, Right **7** Upper Femur, Left **8** Femoral Shaft, Right **9** Femoral Shaft, Left **B** Lower Femur, Right **C** Lower Femur, Left **D** Patella, Right **F** Patella, Left **G** Tibia, Right **H** Tibia, Left **J** Fibula, Right **K** Fibula, Left **L** Tarsal, Right **M** Tarsal, Left **N** Metatarsal, Right **P** Metatarsal, Left **Q** Toe Phalanx, Right **R** Toe Phalanx, Left	**0** Open **3** Percutaneous **4** Percutaneous Endoscopic **X** External	**4** Internal Fixation Device **5** External Fixation Device **7** Autologous Tissue Substitute **J** Synthetic Substitute **K** Nonautologous Tissue Substitute	**Z** No Qualifier
Y Lower Bone	**0** Open **3** Percutaneous **4** Percutaneous Endoscopic **X** External	**0** Drainage Device **M** Bone Growth Stimulator	**Z** No Qualifier

ower Bones Code Listing 0Q2–0QW

Q2 – Lower Bones, Change

eview Coding Guideline B6.1c

Q2YX0Z Change Drainage Device in Lower Bone, External Approach

0Q2YXYZ Change Other Device in Lower Bone, External Approach

Q5 – Lower Bones, Destruction

Q500ZZ Destruction of Lumbar Vertebra, Open Approach
Q503ZZ Destruction of Lumbar Vertebra, Percutaneous Approach
Q504ZZ Destruction of Lumbar Vertebra, Percutaneous Endoscopic Approach
0Q510ZZ Destruction of Sacrum, Open Approach
0Q513ZZ Destruction of Sacrum, Percutaneous Approach
0Q514ZZ Destruction of Sacrum, Percutaneous Endoscopic Approach
0Q520ZZ Destruction of Right Pelvic Bone, Open Approach
0Q523ZZ Destruction of Right Pelvic Bone, Percutaneous Approach
0Q524ZZ Destruction of Right Pelvic Bone, Percutaneous Endoscopic Approach
0Q530ZZ Destruction of Left Pelvic Bone, Open Approach
0Q533ZZ Destruction of Left Pelvic Bone, Percutaneous Approach
0Q534ZZ Destruction of Left Pelvic Bone, Percutaneous Endoscopic Approach
0Q540ZZ Destruction of Right Acetabulum, Open Approach
0Q543ZZ Destruction of Right Acetabulum, Percutaneous Approach
0Q544ZZ Destruction of Right Acetabulum, Percutaneous Endoscopic Approach
0Q550ZZ Destruction of Left Acetabulum, Open Approach
0Q553ZZ Destruction of Left Acetabulum, Percutaneous Approach
0Q554ZZ Destruction of Left Acetabulum, Percutaneous Endoscopic Approach
0Q560ZZ Destruction of Right Upper Femur, Open Approach
0Q563ZZ Destruction of Right Upper Femur, Percutaneous Approach
0Q564ZZ Destruction of Right Upper Femur, Percutaneous Endoscopic Approach
0Q570ZZ Destruction of Left Upper Femur, Open Approach
0Q573ZZ Destruction of Left Upper Femur, Percutaneous Approach
0Q574ZZ Destruction of Left Upper Femur, Percutaneous Endoscopic Approach
0Q580ZZ Destruction of Right Femoral Shaft, Open Approach
0Q583ZZ Destruction of Right Femoral Shaft, Percutaneous Approach
0Q584ZZ Destruction of Right Femoral Shaft, Percutaneous Endoscopic Approach
0Q590ZZ Destruction of Left Femoral Shaft, Open Approach
0Q593ZZ Destruction of Left Femoral Shaft, Percutaneous Approach
0Q594ZZ Destruction of Left Femoral Shaft, Percutaneous Endoscopic Approach
0Q5B0ZZ Destruction of Right Lower Femur, Open Approach
0Q5B3ZZ Destruction of Right Lower Femur, Percutaneous Approach
0Q5B4ZZ Destruction of Right Lower Femur, Percutaneous Endoscopic Approach
0Q5C0ZZ Destruction of Left Lower Femur, Open Approach

0Q5C3ZZ Destruction of Left Lower Femur, Percutaneous Approach
0Q5C4ZZ Destruction of Left Lower Femur, Percutaneous Endoscopic Approach
0Q5D0ZZ Destruction of Right Patella, Open Approach
0Q5D3ZZ Destruction of Right Patella, Percutaneous Approach
0Q5D4ZZ Destruction of Right Patella, Percutaneous Endoscopic Approach
0Q5F0ZZ Destruction of Left Patella, Open Approach
0Q5F3ZZ Destruction of Left Patella, Percutaneous Approach
0Q5F4ZZ Destruction of Left Patella, Percutaneous Endoscopic Approach
0Q5G0ZZ Destruction of Right Tibia, Open Approach
0Q5G3ZZ Destruction of Right Tibia, Percutaneous Approach
0Q5G4ZZ Destruction of Right Tibia, Percutaneous Endoscopic Approach
0Q5H0ZZ Destruction of Left Tibia, Open Approach
0Q5H3ZZ Destruction of Left Tibia, Percutaneous Approach
0Q5H4ZZ Destruction of Left Tibia, Percutaneous Endoscopic Approach
0Q5J0ZZ Destruction of Right Fibula, Open Approach
0Q5J3ZZ Destruction of Right Fibula, Percutaneous Approach
0Q5J4ZZ Destruction of Right Fibula, Percutaneous Endoscopic Approach
0Q5K0ZZ Destruction of Left Fibula, Open Approach
0Q5K3ZZ Destruction of Left Fibula, Percutaneous Approach
0Q5K4ZZ Destruction of Left Fibula, Percutaneous Endoscopic Approach
0Q5L0ZZ Destruction of Right Tarsal, Open Approach
0Q5L3ZZ Destruction of Right Tarsal, Percutaneous Approach
0Q5L4ZZ Destruction of Right Tarsal, Percutaneous Endoscopic Approach
0Q5M0ZZ Destruction of Left Tarsal, Open Approach
0Q5M3ZZ Destruction of Left Tarsal, Percutaneous Approach
0Q5M4ZZ Destruction of Left Tarsal, Percutaneous Endoscopic Approach
0Q5N0ZZ Destruction of Right Metatarsal, Open Approach
0Q5N3ZZ Destruction of Right Metatarsal, Percutaneous Approach
0Q5N4ZZ Destruction of Right Metatarsal, Percutaneous Endoscopic Approach
0Q5P0ZZ Destruction of Left Metatarsal, Open Approach
0Q5P3ZZ Destruction of Left Metatarsal, Percutaneous Approach
0Q5P4ZZ Destruction of Left Metatarsal, Percutaneous Endoscopic Approach
0Q5Q0ZZ Destruction of Right Toe Phalanx, Open Approach
0Q5Q3ZZ Destruction of Right Toe Phalanx, Percutaneous Approach
0Q5Q4ZZ Destruction of Right Toe Phalanx, Percutaneous Endoscopic Approach
0Q5R0ZZ Destruction of Left Toe Phalanx, Open Approach
0Q5R3ZZ Destruction of Left Toe Phalanx, Percutaneous Approach
0Q5R4ZZ Destruction of Left Toe Phalanx, Percutaneous Endoscopic Approach
0Q5S0ZZ Destruction of Coccyx, Open Approach
0Q5S3ZZ Destruction of Coccyx, Percutaneous Approach
0Q5S4ZZ Destruction of Coccyx, Percutaneous Endoscopic Approach

0Q8 – Lower Bones, Division

Review Coding Guideline B3.14

0Q800ZZ Division of Lumbar Vertebra, Open Approach
0Q803ZZ Division of Lumbar Vertebra, Percutaneous Approach
0Q804ZZ Division of Lumbar Vertebra, Percutaneous Endoscopic Approach
0Q810ZZ Division of Sacrum, Open Approach
0Q813ZZ Division of Sacrum, Percutaneous Approach
0Q814ZZ Division of Sacrum, Percutaneous Endoscopic Approach
0Q820ZZ Division of Right Pelvic Bone, Open Approach
0Q823ZZ Division of Right Pelvic Bone, Percutaneous Approach
0Q824ZZ Division of Right Pelvic Bone, Percutaneous Endoscopic Approach
0Q830ZZ Division of Left Pelvic Bone, Open Approach
0Q833ZZ Division of Left Pelvic Bone, Percutaneous Approach
0Q834ZZ Division of Left Pelvic Bone, Percutaneous Endoscopic Approach
0Q840ZZ Division of Right Acetabulum, Open Approach
0Q843ZZ Division of Right Acetabulum, Percutaneous Approach
0Q844ZZ Division of Right Acetabulum, Percutaneous Endoscopic Approach
0Q850ZZ Division of Left Acetabulum, Open Approach
0Q853ZZ Division of Left Acetabulum, Percutaneous Approach
0Q854ZZ Division of Left Acetabulum, Percutaneous Endoscopic Approach
0Q860ZZ Division of Right Upper Femur, Open Approach
0Q863ZZ Division of Right Upper Femur, Percutaneous Approach
0Q864ZZ Division of Right Upper Femur, Percutaneous Endoscopic Approach
0Q870ZZ Division of Left Upper Femur, Open Approach
0Q873ZZ Division of Left Upper Femur, Percutaneous Approach
0Q874ZZ Division of Left Upper Femur, Percutaneous Endoscopic Approach
0Q880ZZ Division of Right Femoral Shaft, Open Approach
0Q883ZZ Division of Right Femoral Shaft, Percutaneous Approach
0Q884ZZ Division of Right Femoral Shaft, Percutaneous Endoscopic Approach
0Q890ZZ Division of Left Femoral Shaft, Open Approach
0Q893ZZ Division of Left Femoral Shaft, Percutaneous Approach
0Q894ZZ Division of Left Femoral Shaft, Percutaneous Endoscopic Approach
0Q8B0ZZ Division of Right Lower Femur, Open Approach
0Q8B3ZZ Division of Right Lower Femur, Percutaneous Approach
0Q8B4ZZ Division of Right Lower Femur, Percutaneous Endoscopic Approach
0Q8C0ZZ Division of Left Lower Femur, Open Approach
0Q8C3ZZ Division of Left Lower Femur, Percutaneous Approach
0Q8C4ZZ Division of Left Lower Femur, Percutaneous Endoscopic Approach
0Q8D0ZZ Division of Right Patella, Open Approach
0Q8D3ZZ Division of Right Patella, Percutaneous Approach
0Q8D4ZZ Division of Right Patella, Percutaneous Endoscopic Approach
0Q8F0ZZ Division of Left Patella, Open Approach
0Q8F3ZZ Division of Left Patella, Percutaneous Approach
0Q8F4ZZ Division of Left Patella, Percutaneous Endoscopic Approach
0Q8G0ZZ Division of Right Tibia, Open Approach
0Q8G3ZZ Division of Right Tibia, Percutaneous Approach
0Q8G4ZZ Division of Right Tibia, Percutaneous Endoscopic Approach
0Q8H0ZZ Division of Left Tibia, Open Approach
0Q8H3ZZ Division of Left Tibia, Percutaneous Approach
0Q8H4ZZ Division of Left Tibia, Percutaneous Endoscopic Approach
0Q8J0ZZ Division of Right Fibula, Open Approach
0Q8J3ZZ Division of Right Fibula, Percutaneous Approach
0Q8J4ZZ Division of Right Fibula, Percutaneous Endoscopic Approach
0Q8K0ZZ Division of Left Fibula, Open Approach
0Q8K3ZZ Division of Left Fibula, Percutaneous Approach
0Q8K4ZZ Division of Left Fibula, Percutaneous Endoscopic Approach
0Q8L0ZZ Division of Right Tarsal, Open Approach
0Q8L3ZZ Division of Right Tarsal, Percutaneous Approach
0Q8L4ZZ Division of Right Tarsal, Percutaneous Endoscopic Approach
0Q8M0ZZ Division of Left Tarsal, Open Approach
0Q8M3ZZ Division of Left Tarsal, Percutaneous Approach
0Q8M4ZZ Division of Left Tarsal, Percutaneous Endoscopic Approach
0Q8N0ZZ Division of Right Metatarsal, Open Approach
0Q8N3ZZ Division of Right Metatarsal, Percutaneous Approach
0Q8N4ZZ Division of Right Metatarsal, Percutaneous Endoscopic Approach
0Q8P0ZZ Division of Left Metatarsal, Open Approach
0Q8P3ZZ Division of Left Metatarsal, Percutaneous Approach
0Q8P4ZZ Division of Left Metatarsal, Percutaneous Endoscopic Approach
0Q8Q0ZZ Division of Right Toe Phalanx, Open Approach
0Q8Q3ZZ Division of Right Toe Phalanx, Percutaneous Approach
0Q8Q4ZZ Division of Right Toe Phalanx, Percutaneous Endoscopic Approach
0Q8R0ZZ Division of Left Toe Phalanx, Open Approach
0Q8R3ZZ Division of Left Toe Phalanx, Percutaneous Approach

Q8R4ZZ Division of Left Toe Phalanx, Percutaneous Endoscopic Approach
Q8S0ZZ Division of Coccyx, Open Approach
0Q8S3ZZ Division of Coccyx, Percutaneous Approach
0Q8S4ZZ Division of Coccyx, Percutaneous Endoscopic Approach

Q9 – Lower Bones, Drainage

eview Coding Guidelines B3.4a and B3.4b

eview Coding Guideline B6.2

Q9000Z Drainage of Lumbar Vertebra with Drainage Device, Open Approach
Q900ZX Drainage of Lumbar Vertebra, Open Approach, Diagnostic
Q900ZZ Drainage of Lumbar Vertebra, Open Approach
Q9030Z Drainage of Lumbar Vertebra with Drainage Device, Percutaneous Approach
Q903ZX Drainage of Lumbar Vertebra, Percutaneous Approach, Diagnostic
Q903ZZ Drainage of Lumbar Vertebra, Percutaneous Approach
Q9040Z Drainage of Lumbar Vertebra with Drainage Device, Percutaneous Endoscopic Approach
Q904ZX Drainage of Lumbar Vertebra, Percutaneous Endoscopic Approach, Diagnostic
Q904ZZ Drainage of Lumbar Vertebra, Percutaneous Endoscopic Approach
Q9100Z Drainage of Sacrum with Drainage Device, Open Approach
Q910ZX Drainage of Sacrum, Open Approach, Diagnostic
Q910ZZ Drainage of Sacrum, Open Approach
Q9130Z Drainage of Sacrum with Drainage Device, Percutaneous Approach
Q913ZX Drainage of Sacrum, Percutaneous Approach, Diagnostic
Q913ZZ Drainage of Sacrum, Percutaneous Approach
Q9140Z Drainage of Sacrum with Drainage Device, Percutaneous Endoscopic Approach
Q914ZX Drainage of Sacrum, Percutaneous Endoscopic Approach, Diagnostic
Q914ZZ Drainage of Sacrum, Percutaneous Endoscopic Approach
0Q9200Z Drainage of Right Pelvic Bone with Drainage Device, Open Approach
0Q920ZX Drainage of Right Pelvic Bone, Open Approach, Diagnostic
0Q920ZZ Drainage of Right Pelvic Bone, Open Approach
0Q9230Z Drainage of Right Pelvic Bone with Drainage Device, Percutaneous Approach
0Q923ZX Drainage of Right Pelvic Bone, Percutaneous Approach, Diagnostic
0Q923ZZ Drainage of Right Pelvic Bone, Percutaneous Approach
0Q9240Z Drainage of Right Pelvic Bone with Drainage Device, Percutaneous Endoscopic Approach
0Q924ZX Drainage of Right Pelvic Bone, Percutaneous Endoscopic Approach, Diagnostic
0Q924ZZ Drainage of Right Pelvic Bone, Percutaneous Endoscopic Approach
0Q9300Z Drainage of Left Pelvic Bone with Drainage Device, Open Approach
0Q930ZX Drainage of Left Pelvic Bone, Open Approach, Diagnostic
0Q930ZZ Drainage of Left Pelvic Bone, Open Approach
0Q9330Z Drainage of Left Pelvic Bone with Drainage Device, Percutaneous Approach
0Q933ZX Drainage of Left Pelvic Bone, Percutaneous Approach, Diagnostic
0Q933ZZ Drainage of Left Pelvic Bone, Percutaneous Approach
0Q9340Z Drainage of Left Pelvic Bone with Drainage Device, Percutaneous Endoscopic Approach
0Q934ZX Drainage of Left Pelvic Bone, Percutaneous Endoscopic Approach, Diagnostic
0Q934ZZ Drainage of Left Pelvic Bone, Percutaneous Endoscopic Approach
0Q9400Z Drainage of Right Acetabulum with Drainage Device, Open Approach
0Q940ZX Drainage of Right Acetabulum, Open Approach, Diagnostic
0Q940ZZ Drainage of Right Acetabulum, Open Approach
0Q9430Z Drainage of Right Acetabulum with Drainage Device, Percutaneous Approach
0Q943ZX Drainage of Right Acetabulum, Percutaneous Approach, Diagnostic
0Q943ZZ Drainage of Right Acetabulum, Percutaneous Approach
0Q9440Z Drainage of Right Acetabulum with Drainage Device, Percutaneous Endoscopic Approach
0Q944ZX Drainage of Right Acetabulum, Percutaneous Endoscopic Approach, Diagnostic
0Q944ZZ Drainage of Right Acetabulum, Percutaneous Endoscopic Approach
0Q9500Z Drainage of Left Acetabulum with Drainage Device, Open Approach
0Q950ZX Drainage of Left Acetabulum, Open Approach, Diagnostic
0Q950ZZ Drainage of Left Acetabulum, Open Approach
0Q9530Z Drainage of Left Acetabulum with Drainage Device, Percutaneous Approach
0Q953ZX Drainage of Left Acetabulum, Percutaneous Approach, Diagnostic
0Q953ZZ Drainage of Left Acetabulum, Percutaneous Approach
0Q9540Z Drainage of Left Acetabulum with Drainage Device, Percutaneous Endoscopic Approach
0Q954ZX Drainage of Left Acetabulum, Percutaneous Endoscopic Approach, Diagnostic
0Q954ZZ Drainage of Left Acetabulum, Percutaneous Endoscopic Approach
0Q9600Z Drainage of Right Upper Femur with Drainage Device, Open Approach
0Q960ZX Drainage of Right Upper Femur, Open Approach, Diagnostic
0Q960ZZ Drainage of Right Upper Femur, Open Approach
0Q9630Z Drainage of Right Upper Femur with Drainage Device, Percutaneous Approach
0Q963ZX Drainage of Right Upper Femur, Percutaneous Approach, Diagnostic
0Q963ZZ Drainage of Right Upper Femur, Percutaneous Approach
0Q9640Z Drainage of Right Upper Femur with Drainage Device, Percutaneous Endoscopic Approach
0Q964ZX Drainage of Right Upper Femur, Percutaneous Endoscopic Approach, Diagnostic
0Q964ZZ Drainage of Right Upper Femur, Percutaneous Endoscopic Approach
0Q9700Z Drainage of Left Upper Femur with Drainage Device, Open Approach
0Q970ZX Drainage of Left Upper Femur, Open Approach, Diagnostic
0Q970ZZ Drainage of Left Upper Femur, Open Approach
0Q9730Z Drainage of Left Upper Femur with Drainage Device, Percutaneous Approach
0Q973ZX Drainage of Left Upper Femur, Percutaneous Approach, Diagnostic
0Q973ZZ Drainage of Left Upper Femur, Percutaneous Approach
0Q9740Z Drainage of Left Upper Femur with Drainage Device, Percutaneous Endoscopic Approach
0Q974ZX Drainage of Left Upper Femur, Percutaneous Endoscopic Approach, Diagnostic
0Q974ZZ Drainage of Left Upper Femur, Percutaneous Endoscopic Approach
0Q9800Z Drainage of Right Femoral Shaft with Drainage Device, Open Approach
0Q980ZX Drainage of Right Femoral Shaft, Open Approach, Diagnostic
0Q980ZZ Drainage of Right Femoral Shaft, Open Approach
0Q9830Z Drainage of Right Femoral Shaft with Drainage Device, Percutaneous Approach
0Q983ZX Drainage of Right Femoral Shaft, Percutaneous Approach, Diagnostic
0Q983ZZ Drainage of Right Femoral Shaft, Percutaneous Approach
0Q9840Z Drainage of Right Femoral Shaft with Drainage Device, Percutaneous Endoscopic Approach
0Q984ZX Drainage of Right Femoral Shaft, Percutaneous Endoscopic Approach, Diagnostic
0Q984ZZ Drainage of Right Femoral Shaft, Percutaneous Endoscopic Approach
0Q9900Z Drainage of Left Femoral Shaft with Drainage Device, Open Approach
0Q990ZX Drainage of Left Femoral Shaft, Open Approach, Diagnostic
0Q990ZZ Drainage of Left Femoral Shaft, Open Approach
0Q9930Z Drainage of Left Femoral Shaft with Drainage Device, Percutaneous Approach
0Q993ZX Drainage of Left Femoral Shaft, Percutaneous Approach, Diagnostic
0Q993ZZ Drainage of Left Femoral Shaft, Percutaneous Approach
0Q9940Z Drainage of Left Femoral Shaft with Drainage Device, Percutaneous Endoscopic Approach
0Q994ZX Drainage of Left Femoral Shaft, Percutaneous Endoscopic Approach, Diagnostic
0Q994ZZ Drainage of Left Femoral Shaft, Percutaneous Endoscopic Approach
0Q9B00Z Drainage of Right Lower Femur with Drainage Device, Open Approach

0Q9B0ZX Drainage of Right Lower Femur, Open Approach, Diagnostic
0Q9B0ZZ Drainage of Right Lower Femur, Open Approach
0Q9B30Z Drainage of Right Lower Femur with Drainage Device, Percutaneous Approach
0Q9B3ZX Drainage of Right Lower Femur, Percutaneous Approach, Diagnostic
0Q9B3ZZ Drainage of Right Lower Femur, Percutaneous Approach
0Q9B40Z Drainage of Right Lower Femur with Drainage Device, Percutaneous Endoscopic Approach
0Q9B4ZX Drainage of Right Lower Femur, Percutaneous Endoscopic Approach, Diagnostic
0Q9B4ZZ Drainage of Right Lower Femur, Percutaneous Endoscopic Approach
0Q9C00Z Drainage of Left Lower Femur with Drainage Device, Open Approach
0Q9C0ZX Drainage of Left Lower Femur, Open Approach, Diagnostic
0Q9C0ZZ Drainage of Left Lower Femur, Open Approach
0Q9C30Z Drainage of Left Lower Femur with Drainage Device, Percutaneous Approach
0Q9C3ZX Drainage of Left Lower Femur, Percutaneous Approach, Diagnostic
0Q9C3ZZ Drainage of Left Lower Femur, Percutaneous Approach
0Q9C40Z Drainage of Left Lower Femur with Drainage Device, Percutaneous Endoscopic Approach
0Q9C4ZX Drainage of Left Lower Femur, Percutaneous Endoscopic Approach, Diagnostic
0Q9C4ZZ Drainage of Left Lower Femur, Percutaneous Endoscopic Approach
0Q9D00Z Drainage of Right Patella with Drainage Device, Open Approach
0Q9D0ZX Drainage of Right Patella, Open Approach, Diagnostic
0Q9D0ZZ Drainage of Right Patella, Open Approach
0Q9D30Z Drainage of Right Patella with Drainage Device, Percutaneous Approach
0Q9D3ZX Drainage of Right Patella, Percutaneous Approach, Diagnostic
0Q9D3ZZ Drainage of Right Patella, Percutaneous Approach
0Q9D40Z Drainage of Right Patella with Drainage Device, Percutaneous Endoscopic Approach
0Q9D4ZX Drainage of Right Patella, Percutaneous Endoscopic Approach, Diagnostic
0Q9D4ZZ Drainage of Right Patella, Percutaneous Endoscopic Approach
0Q9F00Z Drainage of Left Patella with Drainage Device, Open Approach
0Q9F0ZX Drainage of Left Patella, Open Approach, Diagnostic
0Q9F0ZZ Drainage of Left Patella, Open Approach
0Q9F30Z Drainage of Left Patella with Drainage Device, Percutaneous Approach
0Q9F3ZX Drainage of Left Patella, Percutaneous Approach, Diagnostic
0Q9F3ZZ Drainage of Left Patella, Percutaneous Approach
0Q9F40Z Drainage of Left Patella with Drainage Device, Percutaneous Endoscopic Approach
0Q9F4ZX Drainage of Left Patella, Percutaneous Endoscopic Approach, Diagnostic
0Q9F4ZZ Drainage of Left Patella, Percutaneous Endoscopic Approach
0Q9G00Z Drainage of Right Tibia with Drainage Device, Open Approach
0Q9G0ZX Drainage of Right Tibia, Open Approach, Diagnostic
0Q9G0ZZ Drainage of Right Tibia, Open Approach
0Q9G30Z Drainage of Right Tibia with Drainage Device, Percutaneous Approach
0Q9G3ZX Drainage of Right Tibia, Percutaneous Approach, Diagnostic
0Q9G3ZZ Drainage of Right Tibia, Percutaneous Approach
0Q9G40Z Drainage of Right Tibia with Drainage Device, Percutaneous Endoscopic Approach
0Q9G4ZX Drainage of Right Tibia, Percutaneous Endoscopic Approach, Diagnostic
0Q9G4ZZ Drainage of Right Tibia, Percutaneous Endoscopic Approach
0Q9H00Z Drainage of Left Tibia with Drainage Device, Open Approach
0Q9H0ZX Drainage of Left Tibia, Open Approach, Diagnostic
0Q9H0ZZ Drainage of Left Tibia, Open Approach
0Q9H30Z Drainage of Left Tibia with Drainage Device, Percutaneous Approach
0Q9H3ZX Drainage of Left Tibia, Percutaneous Approach, Diagnostic
0Q9H3ZZ Drainage of Left Tibia, Percutaneous Approach
0Q9H40Z Drainage of Left Tibia with Drainage Device, Percutaneous Endoscopic Approach
0Q9H4ZX Drainage of Left Tibia, Percutaneous Endoscopic Approach, Diagnostic
0Q9H4ZZ Drainage of Left Tibia, Percutaneous Endoscopic Approach
0Q9J00Z Drainage of Right Fibula with Drainage Device, Open Approach
0Q9J0ZX Drainage of Right Fibula, Open Approach, Diagnostic
0Q9J0ZZ Drainage of Right Fibula, Open Approach
0Q9J30Z Drainage of Right Fibula with Drainage Device, Percutaneous Approach
0Q9J3ZX Drainage of Right Fibula, Percutaneous Approach, Diagnostic
0Q9J3ZZ Drainage of Right Fibula, Percutaneous Approach
0Q9J40Z Drainage of Right Fibula with Drainage Device, Percutaneous Endoscopic Approach
0Q9J4ZX Drainage of Right Fibula, Percutaneous Endoscopic Approach, Diagnostic
0Q9J4ZZ Drainage of Right Fibula, Percutaneous Endoscopic Approach
0Q9K00Z Drainage of Left Fibula with Drainage Device, Open Approach
0Q9K0ZX Drainage of Left Fibula, Open Approach, Diagnostic
0Q9K0ZZ Drainage of Left Fibula, Open Approach
0Q9K30Z Drainage of Left Fibula with Drainage Device, Percutaneous Approach
0Q9K3ZX Drainage of Left Fibula, Percutaneous Approach, Diagnostic
0Q9K3ZZ Drainage of Left Fibula, Percutaneous Approach
0Q9K40Z Drainage of Left Fibula with Drainage Device, Percutaneous Endoscopic Approach
0Q9K4ZX Drainage of Left Fibula, Percutaneous Endoscopic Approach, Diagnostic
0Q9K4ZZ Drainage of Left Fibula, Percutaneous Endoscopic Approach
0Q9L00Z Drainage of Right Tarsal with Drainage Device, Open Approach
0Q9L0ZX Drainage of Right Tarsal, Open Approach, Diagnostic
0Q9L0ZZ Drainage of Right Tarsal, Open Approach
0Q9L30Z Drainage of Right Tarsal with Drainage Device, Percutaneous Approach
0Q9L3ZX Drainage of Right Tarsal, Percutaneous Approach, Diagnostic
0Q9L3ZZ Drainage of Right Tarsal, Percutaneous Approach
0Q9L40Z Drainage of Right Tarsal with Drainage Device, Percutaneous Endoscopic Approach
0Q9L4ZX Drainage of Right Tarsal, Percutaneous Endoscopic Approach, Diagnostic
0Q9L4ZZ Drainage of Right Tarsal, Percutaneous Endoscopic Approach
0Q9M00Z Drainage of Left Tarsal with Drainage Device, Open Approach
0Q9M0ZX Drainage of Left Tarsal, Open Approach, Diagnostic
0Q9M0ZZ Drainage of Left Tarsal, Open Approach
0Q9M30Z Drainage of Left Tarsal with Drainage Device, Percutaneous Approach
0Q9M3ZX Drainage of Left Tarsal, Percutaneous Approach, Diagnostic
0Q9M3ZZ Drainage of Left Tarsal, Percutaneous Approach
0Q9M40Z Drainage of Left Tarsal with Drainage Device, Percutaneous Endoscopic Approach
0Q9M4ZX Drainage of Left Tarsal, Percutaneous Endoscopic Approach, Diagnostic
0Q9M4ZZ Drainage of Left Tarsal, Percutaneous Endoscopic Approach
0Q9N00Z Drainage of Right Metatarsal with Drainage Device, Open Approach
0Q9N0ZX Drainage of Right Metatarsal, Open Approach, Diagnostic
0Q9N0ZZ Drainage of Right Metatarsal, Open Approach
0Q9N30Z Drainage of Right Metatarsal with Drainage Device, Percutaneous Approach
0Q9N3ZX Drainage of Right Metatarsal, Percutaneous Approach, Diagnostic
0Q9N3ZZ Drainage of Right Metatarsal, Percutaneous Approach
0Q9N40Z Drainage of Right Metatarsal with Drainage Device, Percutaneous Endoscopic Approach
0Q9N4ZX Drainage of Right Metatarsal, Percutaneous Endoscopic Approach, Diagnostic
0Q9N4ZZ Drainage of Right Metatarsal, Percutaneous Endoscopic Approach
0Q9P00Z Drainage of Left Metatarsal with Drainage Device, Open Approach
0Q9P0ZX Drainage of Left Metatarsal, Open Approach, Diagnostic
0Q9P0ZZ Drainage of Left Metatarsal, Open Approach
0Q9P30Z Drainage of Left Metatarsal with Drainage Device, Percutaneous Approach
0Q9P3ZX Drainage of Left Metatarsal, Percutaneous Approach, Diagnostic
0Q9P3ZZ Drainage of Left Metatarsal, Percutaneous Approach
0Q9P40Z Drainage of Left Metatarsal with Drainage Device, Percutaneous Endoscopic Approach
0Q9P4ZX Drainage of Left Metatarsal, Percutaneous Endoscopic Approach, Diagnostic
0Q9P4ZZ Drainage of Left Metatarsal, Percutaneous Endoscopic Approach
0Q9Q00Z Drainage of Right Toe Phalanx with Drainage Device, Open Approach
0Q9Q0ZX Drainage of Right Toe Phalanx, Open Approach, Diagnostic
0Q9Q0ZZ Drainage of Right Toe Phalanx, Open Approach
0Q9Q30Z Drainage of Right Toe Phalanx with Drainage Device, Percutaneous Approach

0Q9Q3ZX Drainage of Right Toe Phalanx, Percutaneous Approach, Diagnostic
0Q9Q3ZZ Drainage of Right Toe Phalanx, Percutaneous Approach
0Q9Q40Z Drainage of Right Toe Phalanx with Drainage Device, Percutaneous Endoscopic Approach
0Q9Q4ZX Drainage of Right Toe Phalanx, Percutaneous Endoscopic Approach, Diagnostic
0Q9Q4ZZ Drainage of Right Toe Phalanx, Percutaneous Endoscopic Approach
0Q9R00Z Drainage of Left Toe Phalanx with Drainage Device, Open Approach
0Q9R0ZX Drainage of Left Toe Phalanx, Open Approach, Diagnostic
0Q9R0ZZ Drainage of Left Toe Phalanx, Open Approach
0Q9R30Z Drainage of Left Toe Phalanx with Drainage Device, Percutaneous Approach
0Q9R3ZX Drainage of Left Toe Phalanx, Percutaneous Approach, Diagnostic
0Q9R3ZZ Drainage of Left Toe Phalanx, Percutaneous Approach
0Q9R40Z Drainage of Left Toe Phalanx with Drainage Device, Percutaneous Endoscopic Approach
0Q9R4ZX Drainage of Left Toe Phalanx, Percutaneous Endoscopic Approach, Diagnostic
0Q9R4ZZ Drainage of Left Toe Phalanx, Percutaneous Endoscopic Approach
0Q9S00Z Drainage of Coccyx with Drainage Device, Open Approach
0Q9S0ZX Drainage of Coccyx, Open Approach, Diagnostic
0Q9S0ZZ Drainage of Coccyx, Open Approach
0Q9S30Z Drainage of Coccyx with Drainage Device, Percutaneous Approach
0Q9S3ZX Drainage of Coccyx, Percutaneous Approach, Diagnostic
0Q9S3ZZ Drainage of Coccyx, Percutaneous Approach
0Q9S40Z Drainage of Coccyx with Drainage Device, Percutaneous Endoscopic Approach
0Q9S4ZX Drainage of Coccyx, Percutaneous Endoscopic Approach, Diagnostic
0Q9S4ZZ Drainage of Coccyx, Percutaneous Endoscopic Approach

0QB – Lower Bones, Excision

Review Coding Guidelines B3.4a and B3.4b

Review Coding Guideline B3.5

Review Coding Guideline B3.8

0QB00ZX Excision of Lumbar Vertebra, Open Approach, Diagnostic
0QB00ZZ Excision of Lumbar Vertebra, Open Approach
0QB03ZX Excision of Lumbar Vertebra, Percutaneous Approach, Diagnostic
0QB03ZZ Excision of Lumbar Vertebra, Percutaneous Approach
0QB04ZX Excision of Lumbar Vertebra, Percutaneous Endoscopic Approach, Diagnostic
0QB04ZZ Excision of Lumbar Vertebra, Percutaneous Endoscopic Approach
0QB10ZX Excision of Sacrum, Open Approach, Diagnostic
0QB10ZZ Excision of Sacrum, Open Approach
0QB13ZX Excision of Sacrum, Percutaneous Approach, Diagnostic
0QB13ZZ Excision of Sacrum, Percutaneous Approach
0QB14ZX Excision of Sacrum, Percutaneous Endoscopic Approach, Diagnostic
0QB14ZZ Excision of Sacrum, Percutaneous Endoscopic Approach
0QB20ZX Excision of Right Pelvic Bone, Open Approach, Diagnostic
0QB20ZZ Excision of Right Pelvic Bone, Open Approach
AHA CC: 2Q, 2014, 6-7
0QB23ZX Excision of Right Pelvic Bone, Percutaneous Approach, Diagnostic
0QB23ZZ Excision of Right Pelvic Bone, Percutaneous Approach
0QB24ZX Excision of Right Pelvic Bone, Percutaneous Endoscopic Approach, Diagnostic
0QB24ZZ Excision of Right Pelvic Bone, Percutaneous Endoscopic Approach
0QB30ZX Excision of Left Pelvic Bone, Open Approach, Diagnostic
0QB30ZZ Excision of Left Pelvic Bone, Open Approach
0QB33ZX Excision of Left Pelvic Bone, Percutaneous Approach, Diagnostic
0QB33ZZ Excision of Left Pelvic Bone, Percutaneous Approach
0QB34ZX Excision of Left Pelvic Bone, Percutaneous Endoscopic Approach, Diagnostic
0QB34ZZ Excision of Left Pelvic Bone, Percutaneous Endoscopic Approach
0QB40ZX Excision of Right Acetabulum, Open Approach, Diagnostic
0QB40ZZ Excision of Right Acetabulum, Open Approach
0QB43ZX Excision of Right Acetabulum, Percutaneous Approach, Diagnostic
0QB43ZZ Excision of Right Acetabulum, Percutaneous Approach
0QB44ZX Excision of Right Acetabulum, Percutaneous Endoscopic Approach, Diagnostic
0QB44ZZ Excision of Right Acetabulum, Percutaneous Endoscopic Approach
0QB50ZX Excision of Left Acetabulum, Open Approach, Diagnostic
0QB50ZZ Excision of Left Acetabulum, Open Approach
0QB53ZX Excision of Left Acetabulum, Percutaneous Approach, Diagnostic
0QB53ZZ Excision of Left Acetabulum, Percutaneous Approach
0QB54ZX Excision of Left Acetabulum, Percutaneous Endoscopic Approach, Diagnostic
0QB54ZZ Excision of Left Acetabulum, Percutaneous Endoscopic Approach
0QB60ZX Excision of Right Upper Femur, Open Approach, Diagnostic
0QB60ZZ Excision of Right Upper Femur, Open Approach
0QB63ZX Excision of Right Upper Femur, Percutaneous Approach, Diagnostic
0QB63ZZ Excision of Right Upper Femur, Percutaneous Approach
0QB64ZX Excision of Right Upper Femur, Percutaneous Endoscopic Approach, Diagnostic
0QB64ZZ Excision of Right Upper Femur, Percutaneous Endoscopic Approach
0QB70ZX Excision of Left Upper Femur, Open Approach, Diagnostic
0QB70ZZ Excision of Left Upper Femur, Open Approach
0QB73ZX Excision of Left Upper Femur, Percutaneous Approach, Diagnostic
0QB73ZZ Excision of Left Upper Femur, Percutaneous Approach
0QB74ZX Excision of Left Upper Femur, Percutaneous Endoscopic Approach, Diagnostic
0QB74ZZ Excision of Left Upper Femur, Percutaneous Endoscopic Approach
0QB80ZX Excision of Right Femoral Shaft, Open Approach, Diagnostic
0QB80ZZ Excision of Right Femoral Shaft, Open Approach
0QB83ZX Excision of Right Femoral Shaft, Percutaneous Approach, Diagnostic
0QB83ZZ Excision of Right Femoral Shaft, Percutaneous Approach
0QB84ZX Excision of Right Femoral Shaft, Percutaneous Endoscopic Approach, Diagnostic
0QB84ZZ Excision of Right Femoral Shaft, Percutaneous Endoscopic Approach
0QB90ZX Excision of Left Femoral Shaft, Open Approach, Diagnostic
0QB90ZZ Excision of Left Femoral Shaft, Open Approach
0QB93ZX Excision of Left Femoral Shaft, Percutaneous Approach, Diagnostic
0QB93ZZ Excision of Left Femoral Shaft, Percutaneous Approach
0QB94ZX Excision of Left Femoral Shaft, Percutaneous Endoscopic Approach, Diagnostic
0QB94ZZ Excision of Left Femoral Shaft, Percutaneous Endoscopic Approach
0QBB0ZX Excision of Right Lower Femur, Open Approach, Diagnostic
0QBB0ZZ Excision of Right Lower Femur, Open Approach
0QBB3ZX Excision of Right Lower Femur, Percutaneous Approach, Diagnostic
0QBB3ZZ Excision of Right Lower Femur, Percutaneous Approach
0QBB4ZX Excision of Right Lower Femur, Percutaneous Endoscopic Approach, Diagnostic
0QBB4ZZ Excision of Right Lower Femur, Percutaneous Endoscopic Approach
0QBC0ZX Excision of Left Lower Femur, Open Approach, Diagnostic
0QBC0ZZ Excision of Left Lower Femur, Open Approach
0QBC3ZX Excision of Left Lower Femur, Percutaneous Approach, Diagnostic
0QBC3ZZ Excision of Left Lower Femur, Percutaneous Approach

0QBC4ZX Excision of Left Lower Femur, Percutaneous Endoscopic Approach, Diagnostic

0QBC4ZZ Excision of Left Lower Femur, Percutaneous Endoscopic Approach

0QBD0ZX Excision of Right Patella, Open Approach, Diagnostic

0QBD0ZZ Excision of Right Patella, Open Approach

0QBD3ZX Excision of Right Patella, Percutaneous Approach, Diagnostic

0QBD3ZZ Excision of Right Patella, Percutaneous Approach

0QBD4ZX Excision of Right Patella, Percutaneous Endoscopic Approach, Diagnostic

0QBD4ZZ Excision of Right Patella, Percutaneous Endoscopic Approach

0QBF0ZX Excision of Left Patella, Open Approach, Diagnostic

0QBF0ZZ Excision of Left Patella, Open Approach

0QBF3ZX Excision of Left Patella, Percutaneous Approach, Diagnostic

0QBF3ZZ Excision of Left Patella, Percutaneous Approach

0QBF4ZX Excision of Left Patella, Percutaneous Endoscopic Approach, Diagnostic

0QBF4ZZ Excision of Left Patella, Percutaneous Endoscopic Approach

0QBG0ZX Excision of Right Tibia, Open Approach, Diagnostic

0QBG0ZZ Excision of Right Tibia, Open Approach

0QBG3ZX Excision of Right Tibia, Percutaneous Approach, Diagnostic

0QBG3ZZ Excision of Right Tibia, Percutaneous Approach

0QBG4ZX Excision of Right Tibia, Percutaneous Endoscopic Approach, Diagnostic

0QBG4ZZ Excision of Right Tibia, Percutaneous Endoscopic Approach

0QBH0ZX Excision of Left Tibia, Open Approach, Diagnostic

0QBH0ZZ Excision of Left Tibia, Open Approach

0QBH3ZX Excision of Left Tibia, Percutaneous Approach, Diagnostic

0QBH3ZZ Excision of Left Tibia, Percutaneous Approach

0QBH4ZX Excision of Left Tibia, Percutaneous Endoscopic Approach, Diagnostic

0QBH4ZZ Excision of Left Tibia, Percutaneous Endoscopic Approach

0QBJ0ZX Excision of Right Fibula, Open Approach, Diagnostic

0QBJ0ZZ Excision of Right Fibula, Open Approach

0QBJ3ZX Excision of Right Fibula, Percutaneous Approach, Diagnostic

0QBJ3ZZ Excision of Right Fibula, Percutaneous Approach

0QBJ4ZX Excision of Right Fibula, Percutaneous Endoscopic Approach, Diagnostic

0QBJ4ZZ Excision of Right Fibula, Percutaneous Endoscopic Approach

0QBK0ZX Excision of Left Fibula, Open Approach, Diagnostic

0QBK0ZZ Excision of Left Fibula, Open Approach
AHA CC: 2Q, 2013, 39-40

0QBK3ZX Excision of Left Fibula, Percutaneous Approach, Diagnostic

0QBK3ZZ Excision of Left Fibula, Percutaneous Approach

0QBK4ZX Excision of Left Fibula, Percutaneous Endoscopic Approach, Diagnostic

0QBK4ZZ Excision of Left Fibula, Percutaneous Endoscopic Approach

0QBL0ZX Excision of Right Tarsal, Open Approach, Diagnostic

0QBL0ZZ Excision of Right Tarsal, Open Approach

0QBL3ZX Excision of Right Tarsal, Percutaneous Approach, Diagnostic

0QBL3ZZ Excision of Right Tarsal, Percutaneous Approach

0QBL4ZX Excision of Right Tarsal, Percutaneous Endoscopic Approach, Diagnostic

0QBL4ZZ Excision of Right Tarsal, Percutaneous Endoscopic Approach

0QBM0ZX Excision of Left Tarsal, Open Approach, Diagnostic

0QBM0ZZ Excision of Left Tarsal, Open Approach

0QBM3ZX Excision of Left Tarsal, Percutaneous Approach, Diagnostic

0QBM3ZZ Excision of Left Tarsal, Percutaneous Approach

0QBM4ZX Excision of Left Tarsal, Percutaneous Endoscopic Approach, Diagnostic

0QBM4ZZ Excision of Left Tarsal, Percutaneous Endoscopic Approach

0QBN0ZX Excision of Right Metatarsal, Open Approach, Diagnostic

0QBN0ZZ Excision of Right Metatarsal, Open Approach

0QBN3ZX Excision of Right Metatarsal, Percutaneous Approach, Diagnostic

0QBN3ZZ Excision of Right Metatarsal, Percutaneous Approach

0QBN4ZX Excision of Right Metatarsal, Percutaneous Endoscopic Approach, Diagnostic

0QBN4ZZ Excision of Right Metatarsal, Percutaneous Endoscopic Approach

0QBP0ZX Excision of Left Metatarsal, Open Approach, Diagnostic

0QBP0ZZ Excision of Left Metatarsal, Open Approach

0QBP3ZX Excision of Left Metatarsal, Percutaneous Approach, Diagnostic

0QBP3ZZ Excision of Left Metatarsal, Percutaneous Approach

0QBP4ZX Excision of Left Metatarsal, Percutaneous Endoscopic Approach, Diagnostic

0QBP4ZZ Excision of Left Metatarsal, Percutaneous Endoscopic Approach

0QBQ0ZX Excision of Right Toe Phalanx, Open Approach, Diagnostic

0QBQ0ZZ Excision of Right Toe Phalanx, Open Approach

0QBQ3ZX Excision of Right Toe Phalanx, Percutaneous Approach, Diagnostic

0QBQ3ZZ Excision of Right Toe Phalanx, Percutaneous Approach

0QBQ4ZX Excision of Right Toe Phalanx, Percutaneous Endoscopic Approach, Diagnostic

0QBQ4ZZ Excision of Right Toe Phalanx, Percutaneous Endoscopic Approach

0QBR0ZX Excision of Left Toe Phalanx, Open Approach, Diagnostic

0QBR0ZZ Excision of Left Toe Phalanx, Open Approach

0QBR3ZX Excision of Left Toe Phalanx, Percutaneous Approach, Diagnostic

0QBR3ZZ Excision of Left Toe Phalanx, Percutaneous Approach

0QBR4ZX Excision of Left Toe Phalanx, Percutaneous Endoscopic Approach, Diagnostic

0QBR4ZZ Excision of Left Toe Phalanx, Percutaneous Endoscopic Approach

0QBS0ZX Excision of Coccyx, Open Approach, Diagnostic

0QBS0ZZ Excision of Coccyx, Open Approach

0QBS3ZX Excision of Coccyx, Percutaneous Approach, Diagnostic

0QBS3ZZ Excision of Coccyx, Percutaneous Approach

0QBS4ZX Excision of Coccyx, Percutaneous Endoscopic Approach, Diagnostic

0QBS4ZZ Excision of Coccyx, Percutaneous Endoscopic Approach

0QC – Lower Bones, Extirpation

0QC00ZZ Extirpation of Matter from Lumbar Vertebra, Open Approach

0QC03ZZ Extirpation of Matter from Lumbar Vertebra, Percutaneous Approach

0QC04ZZ Extirpation of Matter from Lumbar Vertebra, Percutaneous Endoscopic Approach

0QC10ZZ Extirpation of Matter from Sacrum, Open Approach

0QC13ZZ Extirpation of Matter from Sacrum, Percutaneous Approach

0QC14ZZ Extirpation of Matter from Sacrum, Percutaneous Endoscopic Approach

0QC20ZZ Extirpation of Matter from Right Pelvic Bone, Open Approach

0QC23ZZ Extirpation of Matter from Right Pelvic Bone, Percutaneous Approach

0QC24ZZ Extirpation of Matter from Right Pelvic Bone, Percutaneous Endoscopic Approach

0QC30ZZ Extirpation of Matter from Left Pelvic Bone, Open Approach

0QC33ZZ Extirpation of Matter from Left Pelvic Bone, Percutaneous Approach

0QC34ZZ Extirpation of Matter from Left Pelvic Bone, Percutaneous Endoscopic Approach

0QC40ZZ Extirpation of Matter from Right Acetabulum, Open Approach

0QC43ZZ Extirpation of Matter from Right Acetabulum, Percutaneous Approach

0QC44ZZ Extirpation of Matter from Right Acetabulum, Percutaneous Endoscopic Approach

0QC50ZZ Extirpation of Matter from Left Acetabulum, Open Approach

0QC53ZZ Extirpation of Matter from Left Acetabulum, Percutaneous Approach

0QC54ZZ Extirpation of Matter from Left Acetabulum, Percutaneous Endoscopic Approach

0QC60ZZ Extirpation of Matter from Right Upper Femur, Open Approach

0QC63ZZ Extirpation of Matter from Right Upper Femur, Percutaneous Approach

0QC64ZZ Extirpation of Matter from Right Upper Femur, Percutaneous Endoscopic Approach

0QC70ZZ Extirpation of Matter from Left Upper Femur, Open Approach

0QC73ZZ Extirpation of Matter from Left Upper Femur, Percutaneous Approach

0QC74ZZ Extirpation of Matter from Left Upper Femur, Percutaneous Endoscopic Approach

0QC80ZZ Extirpation of Matter from Right Femoral Shaft, Open Approach

0QC83ZZ Extirpation of Matter from Right Femoral Shaft, Percutaneous Approach

0QC84ZZ Extirpation of Matter from Right Femoral Shaft, Percutaneous Endoscopic Approach

C90ZZ Extirpation of Matter from Left Femoral Shaft, Open Approach
C93ZZ Extirpation of Matter from Left Femoral Shaft, Percutaneous Approach
C94ZZ Extirpation of Matter from Left Femoral Shaft, Percutaneous Endoscopic Approach
CB0ZZ Extirpation of Matter from Right Lower Femur, Open Approach
CB3ZZ Extirpation of Matter from Right Lower Femur, Percutaneous Approach
CB4ZZ Extirpation of Matter from Right Lower Femur, Percutaneous Endoscopic Approach
CC0ZZ Extirpation of Matter from Left Lower Femur, Open Approach
CC3ZZ Extirpation of Matter from Left Lower Femur, Percutaneous Approach
CC4ZZ Extirpation of Matter from Left Lower Femur, Percutaneous Endoscopic Approach
CD0ZZ Extirpation of Matter from Right Patella, Open Approach
CD3ZZ Extirpation of Matter from Right Patella, Percutaneous Approach
CD4ZZ Extirpation of Matter from Right Patella, Percutaneous Endoscopic Approach
QCF0ZZ Extirpation of Matter from Left Patella, Open Approach
QCF3ZZ Extirpation of Matter from Left Patella, Percutaneous Approach
QCF4ZZ Extirpation of Matter from Left Patella, Percutaneous Endoscopic Approach
QCG0ZZ Extirpation of Matter from Right Tibia, Open Approach
0QCG3ZZ Extirpation of Matter from Right Tibia, Percutaneous Approach
0QCG4ZZ Extirpation of Matter from Right Tibia, Percutaneous Endoscopic Approach
0QCH0ZZ Extirpation of Matter from Left Tibia, Open Approach
0QCH3ZZ Extirpation of Matter from Left Tibia, Percutaneous Approach
0QCH4ZZ Extirpation of Matter from Left Tibia, Percutaneous Endoscopic Approach
0QCJ0ZZ Extirpation of Matter from Right Fibula, Open Approach
0QCJ3ZZ Extirpation of Matter from Right Fibula, Percutaneous Approach
0QCJ4ZZ Extirpation of Matter from Right Fibula, Percutaneous Endoscopic Approach
0QCK0ZZ Extirpation of Matter from Left Fibula, Open Approach
0QCK3ZZ Extirpation of Matter from Left Fibula, Percutaneous Approach
0QCK4ZZ Extirpation of Matter from Left Fibula, Percutaneous Endoscopic Approach
0QCL0ZZ Extirpation of Matter from Right Tarsal, Open Approach
0QCL3ZZ Extirpation of Matter from Right Tarsal, Percutaneous Approach
0QCL4ZZ Extirpation of Matter from Right Tarsal, Percutaneous Endoscopic Approach
0QCM0ZZ Extirpation of Matter from Left Tarsal, Open Approach
0QCM3ZZ Extirpation of Matter from Left Tarsal, Percutaneous Approach
0QCM4ZZ Extirpation of Matter from Left Tarsal, Percutaneous Endoscopic Approach
0QCN0ZZ Extirpation of Matter from Right Metatarsal, Open Approach
0QCN3ZZ Extirpation of Matter from Right Metatarsal, Percutaneous Approach
0QCN4ZZ Extirpation of Matter from Right Metatarsal, Percutaneous Endoscopic Approach
0QCP0ZZ Extirpation of Matter from Left Metatarsal, Open Approach
0QCP3ZZ Extirpation of Matter from Left Metatarsal, Percutaneous Approach
0QCP4ZZ Extirpation of Matter from Left Metatarsal, Percutaneous Endoscopic Approach
0QCQ0ZZ Extirpation of Matter from Right Toe Phalanx, Open Approach
0QCQ3ZZ Extirpation of Matter from Right Toe Phalanx, Percutaneous Approach
0QCQ4ZZ Extirpation of Matter from Right Toe Phalanx, Percutaneous Endoscopic Approach
0QCR0ZZ Extirpation of Matter from Left Toe Phalanx, Open Approach
0QCR3ZZ Extirpation of Matter from Left Toe Phalanx, Percutaneous Approach
0QCR4ZZ Extirpation of Matter from Left Toe Phalanx, Percutaneous Endoscopic Approach
0QCS0ZZ Extirpation of Matter from Coccyx, Open Approach
0QCS3ZZ Extirpation of Matter from Coccyx, Percutaneous Approach
0QCS4ZZ Extirpation of Matter from Coccyx, Percutaneous Endoscopic Approach

QH – Lower Bones, Insertion

QH004Z Insertion of Internal Fixation Device into Lumbar Vertebra, Open Approach
QH005Z Insertion of External Fixation Device into Lumbar Vertebra, Open Approach
QH034Z Insertion of Internal Fixation Device into Lumbar Vertebra, Percutaneous Approach
QH035Z Insertion of External Fixation Device into Lumbar Vertebra, Percutaneous Approach
QH044Z Insertion of Internal Fixation Device into Lumbar Vertebra, Percutaneous Endoscopic Approach
QH045Z Insertion of External Fixation Device into Lumbar Vertebra, Percutaneous Endoscopic Approach
QH104Z Insertion of Internal Fixation Device into Sacrum, Open Approach
QH105Z Insertion of External Fixation Device into Sacrum, Open Approach
QH134Z Insertion of Internal Fixation Device into Sacrum, Percutaneous Approach
QH135Z Insertion of External Fixation Device into Sacrum, Percutaneous Approach
QH144Z Insertion of Internal Fixation Device into Sacrum, Percutaneous Endoscopic Approach
0QH145Z Insertion of External Fixation Device into Sacrum, Percutaneous Endoscopic Approach
0QH204Z Insertion of Internal Fixation Device into Right Pelvic Bone, Open Approach
0QH205Z Insertion of External Fixation Device into Right Pelvic Bone, Open Approach
0QH234Z Insertion of Internal Fixation Device into Right Pelvic Bone, Percutaneous Approach
0QH235Z Insertion of External Fixation Device into Right Pelvic Bone, Percutaneous Approach
0QH244Z Insertion of Internal Fixation Device into Right Pelvic Bone, Percutaneous Endoscopic Approach
0QH245Z Insertion of External Fixation Device into Right Pelvic Bone, Percutaneous Endoscopic Approach
0QH304Z Insertion of Internal Fixation Device into Left Pelvic Bone, Open Approach
0QH305Z Insertion of External Fixation Device into Left Pelvic Bone, Open Approach
0QH334Z Insertion of Internal Fixation Device into Left Pelvic Bone, Percutaneous Approach
0QH335Z Insertion of External Fixation Device into Left Pelvic Bone, Percutaneous Approach
0QH344Z Insertion of Internal Fixation Device into Left Pelvic Bone, Percutaneous Endoscopic Approach
0QH345Z Insertion of External Fixation Device into Left Pelvic Bone, Percutaneous Endoscopic Approach
0QH404Z Insertion of Internal Fixation Device into Right Acetabulum, Open Approach
0QH405Z Insertion of External Fixation Device into Right Acetabulum, Open Approach
0QH434Z Insertion of Internal Fixation Device into Right Acetabulum, Percutaneous Approach
0QH435Z Insertion of External Fixation Device into Right Acetabulum, Percutaneous Approach
0QH444Z Insertion of Internal Fixation Device into Right Acetabulum, Percutaneous Endoscopic Approach
0QH445Z Insertion of External Fixation Device into Right Acetabulum, Percutaneous Endoscopic Approach
0QH504Z Insertion of Internal Fixation Device into Left Acetabulum, Open Approach
0QH505Z Insertion of External Fixation Device into Left Acetabulum, Open Approach
0QH534Z Insertion of Internal Fixation Device into Left Acetabulum, Percutaneous Approach
0QH535Z Insertion of External Fixation Device into Left Acetabulum, Percutaneous Approach
0QH544Z Insertion of Internal Fixation Device into Left Acetabulum, Percutaneous Endoscopic Approach
0QH545Z Insertion of External Fixation Device into Left Acetabulum, Percutaneous Endoscopic Approach
0QH604Z Insertion of Internal Fixation Device into Right Upper Femur, Open Approach
0QH605Z Insertion of External Fixation Device into Right Upper Femur, Open Approach
0QH606Z Insertion of Intramedullary Internal Fixation Device into Right Upper Femur, Open Approach
0QH608Z Insertion of Limb Lengthening External Fixation Device into Right Upper Femur, Open Approach
0QH60BZ Insertion of Monoplanar External Fixation Device into Right Upper Femur, Open Approach
0QH60CZ Insertion of Ring External Fixation Device into Right Upper Femur, Open Approach
0QH60DZ Insertion of Hybrid External Fixation Device into Right Upper Femur, Open Approach
0QH634Z Insertion of Internal Fixation Device into Right Upper Femur, Percutaneous Approach

0QH635Z Insertion of External Fixation Device into Right Upper Femur, Percutaneous Approach

0QH636Z Insertion of Intramedullary Internal Fixation Device into Right Upper Femur, Percutaneous Approach

0QH638Z Insertion of Limb Lengthening External Fixation Device into Right Upper Femur, Percutaneous Approach

0QH63BZ Insertion of Monoplanar External Fixation Device into Right Upper Femur, Percutaneous Approach

0QH63CZ Insertion of Ring External Fixation Device into Right Upper Femur, Percutaneous Approach

0QH63DZ Insertion of Hybrid External Fixation Device into Right Upper Femur, Percutaneous Approach

0QH644Z Insertion of Internal Fixation Device into Right Upper Femur, Percutaneous Endoscopic Approach

0QH645Z Insertion of External Fixation Device into Right Upper Femur, Percutaneous Endoscopic Approach

0QH646Z Insertion of Intramedullary Internal Fixation Device into Right Upper Femur, Percutaneous Endoscopic Approach

0QH648Z Insertion of Limb Lengthening External Fixation Device into Right Upper Femur, Percutaneous Endoscopic Approach

0QH64BZ Insertion of Monoplanar External Fixation Device into Right Upper Femur, Percutaneous Endoscopic Approach

0QH64CZ Insertion of Ring External Fixation Device into Right Upper Femur, Percutaneous Endoscopic Approach

0QH64DZ Insertion of Hybrid External Fixation Device into Right Upper Femur, Percutaneous Endoscopic Approach

0QH704Z Insertion of Internal Fixation Device into Left Upper Femur, Open Approach

0QH705Z Insertion of External Fixation Device into Left Upper Femur, Open Approach

0QH706Z Insertion of Intramedullary Internal Fixation Device into Left Upper Femur, Open Approach

0QH708Z Insertion of Limb Lengthening External Fixation Device into Left Upper Femur, Open Approach

0QH70BZ Insertion of Monoplanar External Fixation Device into Left Upper Femur, Open Approach

0QH70CZ Insertion of Ring External Fixation Device into Left Upper Femur, Open Approach

0QH70DZ Insertion of Hybrid External Fixation Device into Left Upper Femur, Open Approach

0QH734Z Insertion of Internal Fixation Device into Left Upper Femur, Percutaneous Approach

0QH735Z Insertion of External Fixation Device into Left Upper Femur, Percutaneous Approach

0QH736Z Insertion of Intramedullary Internal Fixation Device into Left Upper Femur, Percutaneous Approach

0QH738Z Insertion of Limb Lengthening External Fixation Device into Left Upper Femur, Percutaneous Approach

0QH73BZ Insertion of Monoplanar External Fixation Device into Left Upper Femur, Percutaneous Approach

0QH73CZ Insertion of Ring External Fixation Device into Left Upper Femur, Percutaneous Approach

0QH73DZ Insertion of Hybrid External Fixation Device into Left Upper Femur, Percutaneous Approach

0QH744Z Insertion of Internal Fixation Device into Left Upper Femur, Percutaneous Endoscopic Approach

0QH745Z Insertion of External Fixation Device into Left Upper Femur, Percutaneous Endoscopic Approach

0QH746Z Insertion of Intramedullary Internal Fixation Device into Left Upper Femur, Percutaneous Endoscopic Approach

0QH748Z Insertion of Limb Lengthening External Fixation Device into Left Upper Femur, Percutaneous Endoscopic Approach

0QH74BZ Insertion of Monoplanar External Fixation Device into Left Upper Femur, Percutaneous Endoscopic Approach

0QH74CZ Insertion of Ring External Fixation Device into Left Upper Femur, Percutaneous Endoscopic Approach

0QH74DZ Insertion of Hybrid External Fixation Device into Left Upper Femur, Percutaneous Endoscopic Approach

0QH804Z Insertion of Internal Fixation Device into Right Femoral Shaft, Open Approach

0QH805Z Insertion of External Fixation Device into Right Femoral Shaft, Open Approach

0QH806Z Insertion of Intramedullary Internal Fixation Device into Right Femoral Shaft, Open Approach

0QH808Z Insertion of Limb Lengthening External Fixation Device into Right Femoral Shaft, Open Approach

0QH80BZ Insertion of Monoplanar External Fixation Device into Right Femoral Shaft, Open Approach

0QH80CZ Insertion of Ring External Fixation Device into Right Femoral Shaft, Open Approach

0QH80DZ Insertion of Hybrid External Fixation Device into Right Femoral Shaft, Open Approach

0QH834Z Insertion of Internal Fixation Device into Right Femoral Shaft, Percutaneous Approach

0QH835Z Insertion of External Fixation Device into Right Femoral Shaft, Percutaneous Approach

0QH836Z Insertion of Intramedullary Internal Fixation Device into Right Femoral Shaft, Percutaneous Approach

0QH838Z Insertion of Limb Lengthening External Fixation Device into Right Femoral Shaft, Percutaneous Approach

0QH83BZ Insertion of Monoplanar External Fixation Device into Right Femoral Shaft, Percutaneous Approach

0QH83CZ Insertion of Ring External Fixation Device into Right Femoral Shaft, Percutaneous Approach

0QH83DZ Insertion of Hybrid External Fixation Device into Right Femoral Shaft, Percutaneous Approach

0QH844Z Insertion of Internal Fixation Device into Right Femoral Shaft, Percutaneous Endoscopic Approach

0QH845Z Insertion of External Fixation Device into Right Femoral Shaft, Percutaneous Endoscopic Approach

0QH846Z Insertion of Intramedullary Internal Fixation Device into Right Femoral Shaft, Percutaneous Endoscopic Approach

0QH848Z Insertion of Limb Lengthening External Fixation Device into Right Femoral Shaft, Percutaneous Endoscopic Approach

0QH84BZ Insertion of Monoplanar External Fixation Device into Right Femoral Shaft, Percutaneous Endoscopic Approach

0QH84CZ Insertion of Ring External Fixation Dev[illegible] into Right Femoral Shaft, Percutaneous Endoscopic Approach

0QH84DZ Insertion of Hybrid External Fixation Device into Right Femoral Shaft, Percutaneous Endoscopic Approach

0QH904Z Insertion of Internal Fixation Device int[illegible] Left Femoral Shaft, Open Approach

0QH905Z Insertion of External Fixation Device int[illegible] Left Femoral Shaft, Open Approach

0QH906Z Insertion of Intramedullary Internal Fixation Device into Left Femoral Shaft, Open Approach

0QH908Z Insertion of Limb Lengthening External Fixation Device into Left Femoral Shaft, Open Approach

0QH90BZ Insertion of Monoplanar External Fixatic[illegible] Device into Left Femoral Shaft, Open Approach

0QH90CZ Insertion of Ring External Fixation Device into Left Femoral Shaft, Open Approach

0QH90DZ Insertion of Hybrid External Fixation Device into Left Femoral Shaft, Open Approach

0QH934Z Insertion of Internal Fixation Device into Left Femoral Shaft, Percutaneous Approach

0QH935Z Insertion of External Fixation Device into Left Femoral Shaft, Percutaneous Approach

0QH936Z Insertion of Intramedullary Internal Fixation Device into Left Femoral Shaft, Percutaneous Approach

0QH938Z Insertion of Limb Lengthening External Fixation Device into Left Femoral Shaft, Percutaneous Approach

0QH93BZ Insertion of Monoplanar External Fixation Device into Left Femoral Shaft, Percutaneous Approach

0QH93CZ Insertion of Ring External Fixation Devic[illegible] into Left Femoral Shaft, Percutaneous Approach

0QH93DZ Insertion of Hybrid External Fixation Device into Left Femoral Shaft, Percutaneous Approach

0QH944Z Insertion of Internal Fixation Device into Left Femoral Shaft, Percutaneous Endoscopic Approach

0QH945Z Insertion of External Fixation Device into Left Femoral Shaft, Percutaneous Endoscopic Approach

0QH946Z Insertion of Intramedullary Internal Fixation Device into Left Femoral Shaft, Percutaneous Endoscopic Approach

0QH948Z Insertion of Limb Lengthening External Fixation Device into Left Femoral Shaft, Percutaneous Endoscopic Approach

0QH94BZ Insertion of Monoplanar External Fixation Device into Left Femoral Shaft, Percutaneous Endoscopic Approach

0QH94CZ Insertion of Ring External Fixation Device into Left Femoral Shaft, Percutaneous Endoscopic Approach

0QH94DZ Insertion of Hybrid External Fixation Device into Left Femoral Shaft, Percutaneous Endoscopic Approach

0QHB04Z Insertion of Internal Fixation Device into Right Lower Femur, Open Approach

0QHB05Z Insertion of External Fixation Device into Right Lower Femur, Open Approach

0QHB06Z Insertion of Intramedullary Internal Fixation Device into Right Lower Femur, Open Approach

0QHB08Z Insertion of Limb Lengthening External Fixation Device into Right Lower Femur, Open Approach

HB0BZ Insertion of Monoplanar External Fixation Device into Right Lower Femur, Open Approach

HB0CZ Insertion of Ring External Fixation Device into Right Lower Femur, Open Approach

HB0DZ Insertion of Hybrid External Fixation Device into Right Lower Femur, Open Approach

QHB34Z Insertion of Internal Fixation Device into Right Lower Femur, Percutaneous Approach

QHB35Z Insertion of External Fixation Device into Right Lower Femur, Percutaneous Approach

QHB36Z Insertion of Intramedullary Internal Fixation Device into Right Lower Femur, Percutaneous Approach

QHB38Z Insertion of Limb Lengthening External Fixation Device into Right Lower Femur, Percutaneous Approach

QHB3BZ Insertion of Monoplanar External Fixation Device into Right Lower Femur, Percutaneous Approach

QHB3CZ Insertion of Ring External Fixation Device into Right Lower Femur, Percutaneous Approach

QHB3DZ Insertion of Hybrid External Fixation Device into Right Lower Femur, Percutaneous Approach

QHB44Z Insertion of Internal Fixation Device into Right Lower Femur, Percutaneous Endoscopic Approach

QHB45Z Insertion of External Fixation Device into Right Lower Femur, Percutaneous Endoscopic Approach

QHB46Z Insertion of Intramedullary Internal Fixation Device into Right Lower Femur, Percutaneous Endoscopic Approach

QHB48Z Insertion of Limb Lengthening External Fixation Device into Right Lower Femur, Percutaneous Endoscopic Approach

QHB4BZ Insertion of Monoplanar External Fixation Device into Right Lower Femur, Percutaneous Endoscopic Approach

QHB4CZ Insertion of Ring External Fixation Device into Right Lower Femur, Percutaneous Endoscopic Approach

QHB4DZ Insertion of Hybrid External Fixation Device into Right Lower Femur, Percutaneous Endoscopic Approach

QHC04Z Insertion of Internal Fixation Device into Left Lower Femur, Open Approach

QHC05Z Insertion of External Fixation Device into Left Lower Femur, Open Approach

QHC06Z Insertion of Intramedullary Internal Fixation Device into Left Lower Femur, Open Approach

QHC08Z Insertion of Limb Lengthening External Fixation Device into Left Lower Femur, Open Approach

QHC0BZ Insertion of Monoplanar External Fixation Device into Left Lower Femur, Open Approach

QHC0CZ Insertion of Ring External Fixation Device into Left Lower Femur, Open Approach

0QHC0DZ Insertion of Hybrid External Fixation Device into Left Lower Femur, Open Approach

0QHC34Z Insertion of Internal Fixation Device into Left Lower Femur, Percutaneous Approach

0QHC35Z Insertion of External Fixation Device into Left Lower Femur, Percutaneous Approach

0QHC36Z Insertion of Intramedullary Internal Fixation Device into Left Lower Femur, Percutaneous Approach

0QHC38Z Insertion of Limb Lengthening External Fixation Device into Left Lower Femur, Percutaneous Approach

0QHC3BZ Insertion of Monoplanar External Fixation Device into Left Lower Femur, Percutaneous Approach

0QHC3CZ Insertion of Ring External Fixation Device into Left Lower Femur, Percutaneous Approach

0QHC3DZ Insertion of Hybrid External Fixation Device into Left Lower Femur, Percutaneous Approach

0QHC44Z Insertion of Internal Fixation Device into Left Lower Femur, Percutaneous Endoscopic Approach

0QHC45Z Insertion of External Fixation Device into Left Lower Femur, Percutaneous Endoscopic Approach

0QHC46Z Insertion of Intramedullary Internal Fixation Device into Left Lower Femur, Percutaneous Endoscopic Approach

0QHC48Z Insertion of Limb Lengthening External Fixation Device into Left Lower Femur, Percutaneous Endoscopic Approach

0QHC4BZ Insertion of Monoplanar External Fixation Device into Left Lower Femur, Percutaneous Endoscopic Approach

0QHC4CZ Insertion of Ring External Fixation Device into Left Lower Femur, Percutaneous Endoscopic Approach

0QHC4DZ Insertion of Hybrid External Fixation Device into Left Lower Femur, Percutaneous Endoscopic Approach

0QHD04Z Insertion of Internal Fixation Device into Right Patella, Open Approach

0QHD05Z Insertion of External Fixation Device into Right Patella, Open Approach

0QHD34Z Insertion of Internal Fixation Device into Right Patella, Percutaneous Approach

0QHD35Z Insertion of External Fixation Device into Right Patella, Percutaneous Approach

0QHD44Z Insertion of Internal Fixation Device into Right Patella, Percutaneous Endoscopic Approach

0QHD45Z Insertion of External Fixation Device into Right Patella, Percutaneous Endoscopic Approach

0QHF04Z Insertion of Internal Fixation Device into Left Patella, Open Approach

0QHF05Z Insertion of External Fixation Device into Left Patella, Open Approach

0QHF34Z Insertion of Internal Fixation Device into Left Patella, Percutaneous Approach

0QHF35Z Insertion of External Fixation Device into Left Patella, Percutaneous Approach

0QHF44Z Insertion of Internal Fixation Device into Left Patella, Percutaneous Endoscopic Approach

0QHF45Z Insertion of External Fixation Device into Left Patella, Percutaneous Endoscopic Approach

0QHG04Z Insertion of Internal Fixation Device into Right Tibia, Open Approach

0QHG05Z Insertion of External Fixation Device into Right Tibia, Open Approach

0QHG06Z Insertion of Intramedullary Internal Fixation Device into Right Tibia, Open Approach

0QHG08Z Insertion of Limb Lengthening External Fixation Device into Right Tibia, Open Approach

0QHG0BZ Insertion of Monoplanar External Fixation Device into Right Tibia, Open Approach

0QHG0CZ Insertion of Ring External Fixation Device into Right Tibia, Open Approach

0QHG0DZ Insertion of Hybrid External Fixation Device into Right Tibia, Open Approach

0QHG34Z Insertion of Internal Fixation Device into Right Tibia, Percutaneous Approach

0QHG35Z Insertion of External Fixation Device into Right Tibia, Percutaneous Approach

0QHG36Z Insertion of Intramedullary Internal Fixation Device into Right Tibia, Percutaneous Approach

0QHG38Z Insertion of Limb Lengthening External Fixation Device into Right Tibia, Percutaneous Approach

0QHG3BZ Insertion of Monoplanar External Fixation Device into Right Tibia, Percutaneous Approach

0QHG3CZ Insertion of Ring External Fixation Device into Right Tibia, Percutaneous Approach

0QHG3DZ Insertion of Hybrid External Fixation Device into Right Tibia, Percutaneous Approach

0QHG44Z Insertion of Internal Fixation Device into Right Tibia, Percutaneous Endoscopic Approach

0QHG45Z Insertion of External Fixation Device into Right Tibia, Percutaneous Endoscopic Approach

0QHG46Z Insertion of Intramedullary Internal Fixation Device into Right Tibia, Percutaneous Endoscopic Approach

0QHG48Z Insertion of Limb Lengthening External Fixation Device into Right Tibia, Percutaneous Endoscopic Approach

0QHG4BZ Insertion of Monoplanar External Fixation Device into Right Tibia, Percutaneous Endoscopic Approach

0QHG4CZ Insertion of Ring External Fixation Device into Right Tibia, Percutaneous Endoscopic Approach

0QHG4DZ Insertion of Hybrid External Fixation Device into Right Tibia, Percutaneous Endoscopic Approach

0QHH04Z Insertion of Internal Fixation Device into Left Tibia, Open Approach

0QHH05Z Insertion of External Fixation Device into Left Tibia, Open Approach

0QHH06Z Insertion of Intramedullary Internal Fixation Device into Left Tibia, Open Approach

0QHH08Z Insertion of Limb Lengthening External Fixation Device into Left Tibia, Open Approach

0QHH0BZ Insertion of Monoplanar External Fixation Device into Left Tibia, Open Approach

0QHH0CZ Insertion of Ring External Fixation Device into Left Tibia, Open Approach

0QHH0DZ Insertion of Hybrid External Fixation Device into Left Tibia, Open Approach

0QHH34Z Insertion of Internal Fixation Device into Left Tibia, Percutaneous Approach

0QHH35Z Insertion of External Fixation Device into Left Tibia, Percutaneous Approach

0QHH36Z Insertion of Intramedullary Internal Fixation Device into Left Tibia, Percutaneous Approach

0QHH38Z Insertion of Limb Lengthening External Fixation Device into Left Tibia, Percutaneous Approach

0QHH3BZ Insertion of Monoplanar External Fixation Device into Left Tibia, Percutaneous Approach

0QHH3CZ Insertion of Ring External Fixation Device into Left Tibia, Percutaneous Approach
0QHH3DZ Insertion of Hybrid External Fixation Device into Left Tibia, Percutaneous Approach
0QHH44Z Insertion of Internal Fixation Device into Left Tibia, Percutaneous Endoscopic Approach
0QHH45Z Insertion of External Fixation Device into Left Tibia, Percutaneous Endoscopic Approach
0QHH46Z Insertion of Intramedullary Internal Fixation Device into Left Tibia, Percutaneous Endoscopic Approach
0QHH48Z Insertion of Limb Lengthening External Fixation Device into Left Tibia, Percutaneous Endoscopic Approach
0QHH4BZ Insertion of Monoplanar External Fixation Device into Left Tibia, Percutaneous Endoscopic Approach
0QHH4CZ Insertion of Ring External Fixation Device into Left Tibia, Percutaneous Endoscopic Approach
0QHH4DZ Insertion of Hybrid External Fixation Device into Left Tibia, Percutaneous Endoscopic Approach
0QHJ04Z Insertion of Internal Fixation Device into Right Fibula, Open Approach
0QHJ05Z Insertion of External Fixation Device into Right Fibula, Open Approach
0QHJ06Z Insertion of Intramedullary Internal Fixation Device into Right Fibula, Open Approach
0QHJ08Z Insertion of Limb Lengthening External Fixation Device into Right Fibula, Open Approach
0QHJ0BZ Insertion of Monoplanar External Fixation Device into Right Fibula, Open Approach
0QHJ0CZ Insertion of Ring External Fixation Device into Right Fibula, Open Approach
0QHJ0DZ Insertion of Hybrid External Fixation Device into Right Fibula, Open Approach
0QHJ34Z Insertion of Internal Fixation Device into Right Fibula, Percutaneous Approach
0QHJ35Z Insertion of External Fixation Device into Right Fibula, Percutaneous Approach
0QHJ36Z Insertion of Intramedullary Internal Fixation Device into Right Fibula, Percutaneous Approach
0QHJ38Z Insertion of Limb Lengthening External Fixation Device into Right Fibula, Percutaneous Approach
0QHJ3BZ Insertion of Monoplanar External Fixation Device into Right Fibula, Percutaneous Approach
0QHJ3CZ Insertion of Ring External Fixation Device into Right Fibula, Percutaneous Approach
0QHJ3DZ Insertion of Hybrid External Fixation Device into Right Fibula, Percutaneous Approach
0QHJ44Z Insertion of Internal Fixation Device into Right Fibula, Percutaneous Endoscopic Approach
0QHJ45Z Insertion of External Fixation Device into Right Fibula, Percutaneous Endoscopic Approach
0QHJ46Z Insertion of Intramedullary Internal Fixation Device into Right Fibula, Percutaneous Endoscopic Approach
0QHJ48Z Insertion of Limb Lengthening External Fixation Device into Right Fibula, Percutaneous Endoscopic Approach
0QHJ4BZ Insertion of Monoplanar External Fixation Device into Right Fibula, Percutaneous Endoscopic Approach
0QHJ4CZ Insertion of Ring External Fixation Device into Right Fibula, Percutaneous Endoscopic Approach
0QHJ4DZ Insertion of Hybrid External Fixation Device into Right Fibula, Percutaneous Endoscopic Approach
0QHK04Z Insertion of Internal Fixation Device into Left Fibula, Open Approach
0QHK05Z Insertion of External Fixation Device into Left Fibula, Open Approach
0QHK06Z Insertion of Intramedullary Internal Fixation Device into Left Fibula, Open Approach
0QHK08Z Insertion of Limb Lengthening External Fixation Device into Left Fibula, Open Approach
0QHK0BZ Insertion of Monoplanar External Fixation Device into Left Fibula, Open Approach
0QHK0CZ Insertion of Ring External Fixation Device into Left Fibula, Open Approach
0QHK0DZ Insertion of Hybrid External Fixation Device into Left Fibula, Open Approach
0QHK34Z Insertion of Internal Fixation Device into Left Fibula, Percutaneous Approach
0QHK35Z Insertion of External Fixation Device into Left Fibula, Percutaneous Approach
0QHK36Z Insertion of Intramedullary Internal Fixation Device into Left Fibula, Percutaneous Approach
0QHK38Z Insertion of Limb Lengthening External Fixation Device into Left Fibula, Percutaneous Approach
0QHK3BZ Insertion of Monoplanar External Fixation Device into Left Fibula, Percutaneous Approach
0QHK3CZ Insertion of Ring External Fixation Device into Left Fibula, Percutaneous Approach
0QHK3DZ Insertion of Hybrid External Fixation Device into Left Fibula, Percutaneous Approach
0QHK44Z Insertion of Internal Fixation Device into Left Fibula, Percutaneous Endoscopic Approach
0QHK45Z Insertion of External Fixation Device into Left Fibula, Percutaneous Endoscopic Approach
0QHK46Z Insertion of Intramedullary Internal Fixation Device into Left Fibula, Percutaneous Endoscopic Approach
0QHK48Z Insertion of Limb Lengthening External Fixation Device into Left Fibula, Percutaneous Endoscopic Approach
0QHK4BZ Insertion of Monoplanar External Fixation Device into Left Fibula, Percutaneous Endoscopic Approach
0QHK4CZ Insertion of Ring External Fixation Device into Left Fibula, Percutaneous Endoscopic Approach
0QHK4DZ Insertion of Hybrid External Fixation Device into Left Fibula, Percutaneous Endoscopic Approach
0QHL04Z Insertion of Internal Fixation Device into Right Tarsal, Open Approach
0QHL05Z Insertion of External Fixation Device into Right Tarsal, Open Approach
0QHL34Z Insertion of Internal Fixation Device into Right Tarsal, Percutaneous Approach
0QHL35Z Insertion of External Fixation Device into Right Tarsal, Percutaneous Approach
0QHL44Z Insertion of Internal Fixation Device into Right Tarsal, Percutaneous Endoscopic Approach
0QHL45Z Insertion of External Fixation Device in Right Tarsal, Percutaneous Endoscopic Approach
0QHM04Z Insertion of Internal Fixation Device in Left Tarsal, Open Approach
0QHM05Z Insertion of External Fixation Device in Left Tarsal, Open Approach
0QHM34Z Insertion of Internal Fixation Device in Left Tarsal, Percutaneous Approach
0QHM35Z Insertion of External Fixation Device in Left Tarsal, Percutaneous Approach
0QHM44Z Insertion of Internal Fixation Device in Left Tarsal, Percutaneous Endoscopic Approach
0QHM45Z Insertion of External Fixation Device in Left Tarsal, Percutaneous Endoscopic Approach
0QHN04Z Insertion of Internal Fixation Device int Right Metatarsal, Open Approach
0QHN05Z Insertion of External Fixation Device in Right Metatarsal, Open Approach
0QHN34Z Insertion of Internal Fixation Device int Right Metatarsal, Percutaneous Approa
0QHN35Z Insertion of External Fixation Device in Right Metatarsal, Percutaneous Approa
0QHN44Z Insertion of Internal Fixation Device into Right Metatarsal, Percutaneous Endoscopic Approach
0QHN45Z Insertion of External Fixation Device into Right Metatarsal, Percutaneous Endoscopic Approach
0QHP04Z Insertion of Internal Fixation Device int Left Metatarsal, Open Approach
0QHP05Z Insertion of External Fixation Device in Left Metatarsal, Open Approach
0QHP34Z Insertion of Internal Fixation Device int Left Metatarsal, Percutaneous Approach
0QHP35Z Insertion of External Fixation Device int Left Metatarsal, Percutaneous Approach
0QHP44Z Insertion of Internal Fixation Device into Left Metatarsal, Percutaneous Endoscopic Approach
0QHP45Z Insertion of External Fixation Device into Left Metatarsal, Percutaneous Endoscopic Approach
0QHQ04Z Insertion of Internal Fixation Device int Right Toe Phalanx, Open Approach
0QHQ05Z Insertion of External Fixation Device int Right Toe Phalanx, Open Approach
0QHQ34Z Insertion of Internal Fixation Device into Right Toe Phalanx, Percutaneous Approach
0QHQ35Z Insertion of External Fixation Device into Right Toe Phalanx, Percutaneous Approach
0QHQ44Z Insertion of Internal Fixation Device into Right Toe Phalanx, Percutaneous Endoscopic Approach
0QHQ45Z Insertion of External Fixation Device into Right Toe Phalanx, Percutaneous Endoscopic Approach
0QHR04Z Insertion of Internal Fixation Device into Left Toe Phalanx, Open Approach
0QHR05Z Insertion of External Fixation Device into Left Toe Phalanx, Open Approach
0QHR34Z Insertion of Internal Fixation Device into Left Toe Phalanx, Percutaneous Approach
0QHR35Z Insertion of External Fixation Device into Left Toe Phalanx, Percutaneous Approach
0QHR44Z Insertion of Internal Fixation Device into Left Toe Phalanx, Percutaneous Endoscopic Approach
0QHR45Z Insertion of External Fixation Device into Left Toe Phalanx, Percutaneous Endoscopic Approach

HS04Z Insertion of Internal Fixation Device into Coccyx, Open Approach
HS05Z Insertion of External Fixation Device into Coccyx, Open Approach
HS34Z Insertion of Internal Fixation Device into Coccyx, Percutaneous Approach
HS35Z Insertion of External Fixation Device into Coccyx, Percutaneous Approach
0QHS44Z Insertion of Internal Fixation Device into Coccyx, Percutaneous Endoscopic Approach
0QHS45Z Insertion of External Fixation Device into Coccyx, Percutaneous Endoscopic Approach
0QHY0MZ Insertion of Bone Growth Stimulator into Lower Bone, Open Approach
0QHY3MZ Insertion of Bone Growth Stimulator into Lower Bone, Percutaneous Approach
0QHY4MZ Insertion of Bone Growth Stimulator into Lower Bone, Percutaneous Endoscopic Approach

ՋJ – Lower Bones, Inspection

eview Coding Guideline B3.5

eview Coding Guidelines B3.11a, B3.11b and B3.11c

JY0ZZ Inspection of Lower Bone, Open Approach
JY3ZZ Inspection of Lower Bone, Percutaneous Approach
0QJY4ZZ Inspection of Lower Bone, Percutaneous Endoscopic Approach
0QJYXZZ Inspection of Lower Bone, External Approach

QN – Lower Bones, Release

eview Coding Guideline B3.13

eview Coding Guideline B3.14

N00ZZ Release Lumbar Vertebra, Open Approach
N03ZZ Release Lumbar Vertebra, Percutaneous Approach
N04ZZ Release Lumbar Vertebra, Percutaneous Endoscopic Approach
N10ZZ Release Sacrum, Open Approach
N13ZZ Release Sacrum, Percutaneous Approach
N14ZZ Release Sacrum, Percutaneous Endoscopic Approach
N20ZZ Release Right Pelvic Bone, Open Approach
QN23ZZ Release Right Pelvic Bone, Percutaneous Approach
QN24ZZ Release Right Pelvic Bone, Percutaneous Endoscopic Approach
QN30ZZ Release Left Pelvic Bone, Open Approach
QN33ZZ Release Left Pelvic Bone, Percutaneous Approach
QN34ZZ Release Left Pelvic Bone, Percutaneous Endoscopic Approach
QN40ZZ Release Right Acetabulum, Open Approach
QN43ZZ Release Right Acetabulum, Percutaneous Approach
QN44ZZ Release Right Acetabulum, Percutaneous Endoscopic Approach
QN50ZZ Release Left Acetabulum, Open Approach
QN53ZZ Release Left Acetabulum, Percutaneous Approach
QN54ZZ Release Left Acetabulum, Percutaneous Endoscopic Approach
QN60ZZ Release Right Upper Femur, Open Approach
QN63ZZ Release Right Upper Femur, Percutaneous Approach
QN64ZZ Release Right Upper Femur, Percutaneous Endoscopic Approach
QN70ZZ Release Left Upper Femur, Open Approach
QN73ZZ Release Left Upper Femur, Percutaneous Approach
QN74ZZ Release Left Upper Femur, Percutaneous Endoscopic Approach
QN80ZZ Release Right Femoral Shaft, Open Approach
0QN83ZZ Release Right Femoral Shaft, Percutaneous Approach
0QN84ZZ Release Right Femoral Shaft, Percutaneous Endoscopic Approach
0QN90ZZ Release Left Femoral Shaft, Open Approach
0QN93ZZ Release Left Femoral Shaft, Percutaneous Approach
0QN94ZZ Release Left Femoral Shaft, Percutaneous Endoscopic Approach
0QNB0ZZ Release Right Lower Femur, Open Approach
0QNB3ZZ Release Right Lower Femur, Percutaneous Approach
0QNB4ZZ Release Right Lower Femur, Percutaneous Endoscopic Approach
0QNC0ZZ Release Left Lower Femur, Open Approach
0QNC3ZZ Release Left Lower Femur, Percutaneous Approach
0QNC4ZZ Release Left Lower Femur, Percutaneous Endoscopic Approach
0QND0ZZ Release Right Patella, Open Approach
0QND3ZZ Release Right Patella, Percutaneous Approach
0QND4ZZ Release Right Patella, Percutaneous Endoscopic Approach
0QNF0ZZ Release Left Patella, Open Approach
0QNF3ZZ Release Left Patella, Percutaneous Approach
0QNF4ZZ Release Left Patella, Percutaneous Endoscopic Approach
0QNG0ZZ Release Right Tibia, Open Approach
0QNG3ZZ Release Right Tibia, Percutaneous Approach
0QNG4ZZ Release Right Tibia, Percutaneous Endoscopic Approach
0QNH0ZZ Release Left Tibia, Open Approach
0QNH3ZZ Release Left Tibia, Percutaneous Approach
0QNH4ZZ Release Left Tibia, Percutaneous Endoscopic Approach
0QNJ0ZZ Release Right Fibula, Open Approach
0QNJ3ZZ Release Right Fibula, Percutaneous Approach
0QNJ4ZZ Release Right Fibula, Percutaneous Endoscopic Approach
0QNK0ZZ Release Left Fibula, Open Approach
0QNK3ZZ Release Left Fibula, Percutaneous Approach
0QNK4ZZ Release Left Fibula, Percutaneous Endoscopic Approach
0QNL0ZZ Release Right Tarsal, Open Approach
0QNL3ZZ Release Right Tarsal, Percutaneous Approach
0QNL4ZZ Release Right Tarsal, Percutaneous Endoscopic Approach
0QNM0ZZ Release Left Tarsal, Open Approach
0QNM3ZZ Release Left Tarsal, Percutaneous Approach
0QNM4ZZ Release Left Tarsal, Percutaneous Endoscopic Approach
0QNN0ZZ Release Right Metatarsal, Open Approach
0QNN3ZZ Release Right Metatarsal, Percutaneous Approach
0QNN4ZZ Release Right Metatarsal, Percutaneous Endoscopic Approach
0QNP0ZZ Release Left Metatarsal, Open Approach
0QNP3ZZ Release Left Metatarsal, Percutaneous Approach
0QNP4ZZ Release Left Metatarsal, Percutaneous Endoscopic Approach
0QNQ0ZZ Release Right Toe Phalanx, Open Approach
0QNQ3ZZ Release Right Toe Phalanx, Percutaneous Approach
0QNQ4ZZ Release Right Toe Phalanx, Percutaneous Endoscopic Approach
0QNR0ZZ Release Left Toe Phalanx, Open Approach
0QNR3ZZ Release Left Toe Phalanx, Percutaneous Approach
0QNR4ZZ Release Left Toe Phalanx, Percutaneous Endoscopic Approach
0QNS0ZZ Release Coccyx, Open Approach
0QNS3ZZ Release Coccyx, Percutaneous Approach
0QNS4ZZ Release Coccyx, Percutaneous Endoscopic Approach

QP – Lower Bones, Removal

Review Coding Guideline B6.1c

QP004Z Removal of Internal Fixation Device from Lumbar Vertebra, Open Approach
0QP007Z Removal of Autologous Tissue Substitute from Lumbar Vertebra, Open Approach
0QP00JZ Removal of Synthetic Substitute from Lumbar Vertebra, Open Approach

0QP00KZ Removal of Nonautologous Tissue Substitute from Lumbar Vertebra, Open Approach
0QP034Z Removal of Internal Fixation Device from Lumbar Vertebra, Percutaneous Approach
0QP037Z Removal of Autologous Tissue Substitute from Lumbar Vertebra, Percutaneous Approach
0QP03JZ Removal of Synthetic Substitute from Lumbar Vertebra, Percutaneous Approach
0QP03KZ Removal of Nonautologous Tissue Substitute from Lumbar Vertebra, Percutaneous Approach
0QP044Z Removal of Internal Fixation Device from Lumbar Vertebra, Percutaneous Endoscopic Approach
0QP047Z Removal of Autologous Tissue Substitute from Lumbar Vertebra, Percutaneous Endoscopic Approach
0QP04JZ Removal of Synthetic Substitute from Lumbar Vertebra, Percutaneous Endoscopic Approach
0QP04KZ Removal of Nonautologous Tissue Substitute from Lumbar Vertebra, Percutaneous Endoscopic Approach
0QP0X4Z Removal of Internal Fixation Device from Lumbar Vertebra, External Approach
0QP104Z Removal of Internal Fixation Device from Sacrum, Open Approach
0QP107Z Removal of Autologous Tissue Substitute from Sacrum, Open Approach
0QP10JZ Removal of Synthetic Substitute from Sacrum, Open Approach
0QP10KZ Removal of Nonautologous Tissue Substitute from Sacrum, Open Approach
0QP134Z Removal of Internal Fixation Device from Sacrum, Percutaneous Approach
0QP137Z Removal of Autologous Tissue Substitute from Sacrum, Percutaneous Approach
0QP13JZ Removal of Synthetic Substitute from Sacrum, Percutaneous Approach
0QP13KZ Removal of Nonautologous Tissue Substitute from Sacrum, Percutaneous Approach
0QP144Z Removal of Internal Fixation Device from Sacrum, Percutaneous Endoscopic Approach
0QP147Z Removal of Autologous Tissue Substitute from Sacrum, Percutaneous Endoscopic Approach
0QP14JZ Removal of Synthetic Substitute from Sacrum, Percutaneous Endoscopic Approach
0QP14KZ Removal of Nonautologous Tissue Substitute from Sacrum, Percutaneous Endoscopic Approach
0QP1X4Z Removal of Internal Fixation Device from Sacrum, External Approach
0QP204Z Removal of Internal Fixation Device from Right Pelvic Bone, Open Approach
0QP205Z Removal of External Fixation Device from Right Pelvic Bone, Open Approach
0QP207Z Removal of Autologous Tissue Substitute from Right Pelvic Bone, Open Approach
0QP20JZ Removal of Synthetic Substitute from Right Pelvic Bone, Open Approach
0QP20KZ Removal of Nonautologous Tissue Substitute from Right Pelvic Bone, Open Approach
0QP234Z Removal of Internal Fixation Device from Right Pelvic Bone, Percutaneous Approach
0QP235Z Removal of External Fixation Device from Right Pelvic Bone, Percutaneous Approach
0QP237Z Removal of Autologous Tissue Substitute from Right Pelvic Bone, Percutaneous Approach
0QP23JZ Removal of Synthetic Substitute from Right Pelvic Bone, Percutaneous Approach
0QP23KZ Removal of Nonautologous Tissue Substitute from Right Pelvic Bone, Percutaneous Approach
0QP244Z Removal of Internal Fixation Device from Right Pelvic Bone, Percutaneous Endoscopic Approach
0QP245Z Removal of External Fixation Device from Right Pelvic Bone, Percutaneous Endoscopic Approach
0QP247Z Removal of Autologous Tissue Substitute from Right Pelvic Bone, Percutaneous Endoscopic Approach
0QP24JZ Removal of Synthetic Substitute from Right Pelvic Bone, Percutaneous Endoscopic Approach
0QP24KZ Removal of Nonautologous Tissue Substitute from Right Pelvic Bone, Percutaneous Endoscopic Approach
0QP2X4Z Removal of Internal Fixation Device from Right Pelvic Bone, External Approach
0QP2X5Z Removal of External Fixation Device from Right Pelvic Bone, External Approach
0QP304Z Removal of Internal Fixation Device from Left Pelvic Bone, Open Approach
0QP305Z Removal of External Fixation Device from Left Pelvic Bone, Open Approach
0QP307Z Removal of Autologous Tissue Substitute from Left Pelvic Bone, Open Approach
0QP30JZ Removal of Synthetic Substitute from Left Pelvic Bone, Open Approach
0QP30KZ Removal of Nonautologous Tissue Substitute from Left Pelvic Bone, Open Approach
0QP334Z Removal of Internal Fixation Device from Left Pelvic Bone, Percutaneous Approach
0QP335Z Removal of External Fixation Device from Left Pelvic Bone, Percutaneous Approach
0QP337Z Removal of Autologous Tissue Substitute from Left Pelvic Bone, Percutaneous Approach
0QP33JZ Removal of Synthetic Substitute from Left Pelvic Bone, Percutaneous Approach
0QP33KZ Removal of Nonautologous Tissue Substitute from Left Pelvic Bone, Percutaneous Approach
0QP344Z Removal of Internal Fixation Device from Left Pelvic Bone, Percutaneous Endoscopic Approach
0QP345Z Removal of External Fixation Device from Left Pelvic Bone, Percutaneous Endoscopic Approach
0QP347Z Removal of Autologous Tissue Substitute from Left Pelvic Bone, Percutaneous Endoscopic Approach
0QP34JZ Removal of Synthetic Substitute from Left Pelvic Bone, Percutaneous Endoscopic Approach
0QP34KZ Removal of Nonautologous Tissue Substitute from Left Pelvic Bone, Percutaneous Endoscopic Approach
0QP3X4Z Removal of Internal Fixation Device from Left Pelvic Bone, External Approach
0QP3X5Z Removal of External Fixation Device from Left Pelvic Bone, External Approach
0QP404Z Removal of Internal Fixation Device from Right Acetabulum, Open Approach
0QP407Z Removal of Autologous Tissue Substitute from Right Acetabulum, Open Approach
0QP40JZ Removal of Synthetic Substitute from Right Acetabulum, Open Approach
0QP40KZ Removal of Nonautologous Tissue Substitute from Right Acetabulum, Open Approach
0QP434Z Removal of Internal Fixation Device from Right Acetabulum, Percutaneous Approach
0QP437Z Removal of Autologous Tissue Substitute from Right Acetabulum, Percutaneous Approach
0QP43JZ Removal of Synthetic Substitute from Right Acetabulum, Percutaneous Approach
0QP43KZ Removal of Nonautologous Tissue Substitute from Right Acetabulum, Percutaneous Approach
0QP444Z Removal of Internal Fixation Device from Right Acetabulum, Percutaneous Endoscopic Approach
0QP447Z Removal of Autologous Tissue Substitute from Right Acetabulum, Percutaneous Endoscopic Approach
0QP44JZ Removal of Synthetic Substitute from Right Acetabulum, Percutaneous Endoscopic Approach
0QP44KZ Removal of Nonautologous Tissue Substitute from Right Acetabulum, Percutaneous Endoscopic Approach
0QP4X4Z Removal of Internal Fixation Device from Right Acetabulum, External Approach
0QP504Z Removal of Internal Fixation Device from Left Acetabulum, Open Approach
0QP507Z Removal of Autologous Tissue Substitute from Left Acetabulum, Open Approach
0QP50JZ Removal of Synthetic Substitute from Left Acetabulum, Open Approach
0QP50KZ Removal of Nonautologous Tissue Substitute from Left Acetabulum, Open Approach
0QP534Z Removal of Internal Fixation Device from Left Acetabulum, Percutaneous Approach
0QP537Z Removal of Autologous Tissue Substitute from Left Acetabulum, Percutaneous Approach
0QP53JZ Removal of Synthetic Substitute from Left Acetabulum, Percutaneous Approach
0QP53KZ Removal of Nonautologous Tissue Substitute from Left Acetabulum, Percutaneous Approach
0QP544Z Removal of Internal Fixation Device from Left Acetabulum, Percutaneous Endoscopic Approach
0QP547Z Removal of Autologous Tissue Substitute from Left Acetabulum, Percutaneous Endoscopic Approach
0QP54JZ Removal of Synthetic Substitute from Left Acetabulum, Percutaneous Endoscopic Approach
0QP54KZ Removal of Nonautologous Tissue Substitute from Left Acetabulum, Percutaneous Endoscopic Approach
0QP5X4Z Removal of Internal Fixation Device from Left Acetabulum, External Approach
0QP604Z Removal of Internal Fixation Device from Right Upper Femur, Open Approach
0QP605Z Removal of External Fixation Device from Right Upper Femur, Open Approach
0QP607Z Removal of Autologous Tissue Substitute from Right Upper Femur, Open Approach
0QP60JZ Removal of Synthetic Substitute from Right Upper Femur, Open Approach
0QP60KZ Removal of Nonautologous Tissue Substitute from Right Upper Femur, Open Approach
0QP634Z Removal of Internal Fixation Device from Right Upper Femur, Percutaneous Approach

P635Z Removal of External Fixation Device from Right Upper Femur, Percutaneous Approach
P637Z Removal of Autologous Tissue Substitute from Right Upper Femur, Percutaneous Approach
P63JZ Removal of Synthetic Substitute from Right Upper Femur, Percutaneous Approach
P63KZ Removal of Nonautologous Tissue Substitute from Right Upper Femur, Percutaneous Approach
P644Z Removal of Internal Fixation Device from Right Upper Femur, Percutaneous Endoscopic Approach
P645Z Removal of External Fixation Device from Right Upper Femur, Percutaneous Endoscopic Approach
P647Z Removal of Autologous Tissue Substitute from Right Upper Femur, Percutaneous Endoscopic Approach
QP64JZ Removal of Synthetic Substitute from Right Upper Femur, Percutaneous Endoscopic Approach
QP64KZ Removal of Nonautologous Tissue Substitute from Right Upper Femur, Percutaneous Endoscopic Approach
QP6X4Z Removal of Internal Fixation Device from Right Upper Femur, External Approach
QP6X5Z Removal of External Fixation Device from Right Upper Femur, External Approach
QP704Z Removal of Internal Fixation Device from Left Upper Femur, Open Approach
QP705Z Removal of External Fixation Device from Left Upper Femur, Open Approach
QP707Z Removal of Autologous Tissue Substitute from Left Upper Femur, Open Approach
QP70JZ Removal of Synthetic Substitute from Left Upper Femur, Open Approach
QP70KZ Removal of Nonautologous Tissue Substitute from Left Upper Femur, Open Approach
QP734Z Removal of Internal Fixation Device from Left Upper Femur, Percutaneous Approach
QP735Z Removal of External Fixation Device from Left Upper Femur, Percutaneous Approach
QP737Z Removal of Autologous Tissue Substitute from Left Upper Femur, Percutaneous Approach
QP73JZ Removal of Synthetic Substitute from Left Upper Femur, Percutaneous Approach
QP73KZ Removal of Nonautologous Tissue Substitute from Left Upper Femur, Percutaneous Approach
QP744Z Removal of Internal Fixation Device from Left Upper Femur, Percutaneous Endoscopic Approach
QP745Z Removal of External Fixation Device from Left Upper Femur, Percutaneous Endoscopic Approach
QP747Z Removal of Autologous Tissue Substitute from Left Upper Femur, Percutaneous Endoscopic Approach
QP74JZ Removal of Synthetic Substitute from Left Upper Femur, Percutaneous Endoscopic Approach
QP74KZ Removal of Nonautologous Tissue Substitute from Left Upper Femur, Percutaneous Endoscopic Approach
QP7X4Z Removal of Internal Fixation Device from Left Upper Femur, External Approach
QP7X5Z Removal of External Fixation Device from Left Upper Femur, External Approach
QP804Z Removal of Internal Fixation Device from Right Femoral Shaft, Open Approach

0QP805Z Removal of External Fixation Device from Right Femoral Shaft, Open Approach
0QP807Z Removal of Autologous Tissue Substitute from Right Femoral Shaft, Open Approach
0QP80JZ Removal of Synthetic Substitute from Right Femoral Shaft, Open Approach
0QP80KZ Removal of Nonautologous Tissue Substitute from Right Femoral Shaft, Open Approach
0QP834Z Removal of Internal Fixation Device from Right Femoral Shaft, Percutaneous Approach
0QP835Z Removal of External Fixation Device from Right Femoral Shaft, Percutaneous Approach
0QP837Z Removal of Autologous Tissue Substitute from Right Femoral Shaft, Percutaneous Approach
0QP83JZ Removal of Synthetic Substitute from Right Femoral Shaft, Percutaneous Approach
0QP83KZ Removal of Nonautologous Tissue Substitute from Right Femoral Shaft, Percutaneous Approach
0QP844Z Removal of Internal Fixation Device from Right Femoral Shaft, Percutaneous Endoscopic Approach
0QP845Z Removal of External Fixation Device from Right Femoral Shaft, Percutaneous Endoscopic Approach
0QP847Z Removal of Autologous Tissue Substitute from Right Femoral Shaft, Percutaneous Endoscopic Approach
0QP84JZ Removal of Synthetic Substitute from Right Femoral Shaft, Percutaneous Endoscopic Approach
0QP84KZ Removal of Nonautologous Tissue Substitute from Right Femoral Shaft, Percutaneous Endoscopic Approach
0QP8X4Z Removal of Internal Fixation Device from Right Femoral Shaft, External Approach
0QP8X5Z Removal of External Fixation Device from Right Femoral Shaft, External Approach
0QP904Z Removal of Internal Fixation Device from Left Femoral Shaft, Open Approach
0QP905Z Removal of External Fixation Device from Left Femoral Shaft, Open Approach
0QP907Z Removal of Autologous Tissue Substitute from Left Femoral Shaft, Open Approach
0QP90JZ Removal of Synthetic Substitute from Left Femoral Shaft, Open Approach
0QP90KZ Removal of Nonautologous Tissue Substitute from Left Femoral Shaft, Open Approach
0QP934Z Removal of Internal Fixation Device from Left Femoral Shaft, Percutaneous Approach
0QP935Z Removal of External Fixation Device from Left Femoral Shaft, Percutaneous Approach
0QP937Z Removal of Autologous Tissue Substitute from Left Femoral Shaft, Percutaneous Approach
0QP93JZ Removal of Synthetic Substitute from Left Femoral Shaft, Percutaneous Approach
0QP93KZ Removal of Nonautologous Tissue Substitute from Left Femoral Shaft, Percutaneous Approach
0QP944Z Removal of Internal Fixation Device from Left Femoral Shaft, Percutaneous Endoscopic Approach
0QP945Z Removal of External Fixation Device from Left Femoral Shaft, Percutaneous Endoscopic Approach
0QP947Z Removal of Autologous Tissue Substitute from Left Femoral Shaft, Percutaneous Endoscopic Approach

0QP94JZ Removal of Synthetic Substitute from Left Femoral Shaft, Percutaneous Endoscopic Approach
0QP94KZ Removal of Nonautologous Tissue Substitute from Left Femoral Shaft, Percutaneous Endoscopic Approach
0QP9X4Z Removal of Internal Fixation Device from Left Femoral Shaft, External Approach
0QP9X5Z Removal of External Fixation Device from Left Femoral Shaft, External Approach
0QPB04Z Removal of Internal Fixation Device from Right Lower Femur, Open Approach
0QPB05Z Removal of External Fixation Device from Right Lower Femur, Open Approach
0QPB07Z Removal of Autologous Tissue Substitute from Right Lower Femur, Open Approach
0QPB0JZ Removal of Synthetic Substitute from Right Lower Femur, Open Approach
0QPB0KZ Removal of Nonautologous Tissue Substitute from Right Lower Femur, Open Approach
0QPB34Z Removal of Internal Fixation Device from Right Lower Femur, Percutaneous Approach
0QPB35Z Removal of External Fixation Device from Right Lower Femur, Percutaneous Approach
0QPB37Z Removal of Autologous Tissue Substitute from Right Lower Femur, Percutaneous Approach
0QPB3JZ Removal of Synthetic Substitute from Right Lower Femur, Percutaneous Approach
0QPB3KZ Removal of Nonautologous Tissue Substitute from Right Lower Femur, Percutaneous Approach
0QPB44Z Removal of Internal Fixation Device from Right Lower Femur, Percutaneous Endoscopic Approach
0QPB45Z Removal of External Fixation Device from Right Lower Femur, Percutaneous Endoscopic Approach
0QPB47Z Removal of Autologous Tissue Substitute from Right Lower Femur, Percutaneous Endoscopic Approach
0QPB4JZ Removal of Synthetic Substitute from Right Lower Femur, Percutaneous Endoscopic Approach
0QPB4KZ Removal of Nonautologous Tissue Substitute from Right Lower Femur, Percutaneous Endoscopic Approach
0QPBX4Z Removal of Internal Fixation Device from Right Lower Femur, External Approach
0QPBX5Z Removal of External Fixation Device from Right Lower Femur, External Approach
0QPC04Z Removal of Internal Fixation Device from Left Lower Femur, Open Approach
0QPC05Z Removal of External Fixation Device from Left Lower Femur, Open Approach
0QPC07Z Removal of Autologous Tissue Substitute from Left Lower Femur, Open Approach
0QPC0JZ Removal of Synthetic Substitute from Left Lower Femur, Open Approach
0QPC0KZ Removal of Nonautologous Tissue Substitute from Left Lower Femur, Open Approach
0QPC34Z Removal of Internal Fixation Device from Left Lower Femur, Percutaneous Approach
0QPC35Z Removal of External Fixation Device from Left Lower Femur, Percutaneous Approach
0QPC37Z Removal of Autologous Tissue Substitute from Left Lower Femur, Percutaneous Approach

0QPC3JZ Removal of Synthetic Substitute from Left Lower Femur, Percutaneous Approach

0QPC3KZ Removal of Nonautologous Tissue Substitute from Left Lower Femur, Percutaneous Approach

0QPC44Z Removal of Internal Fixation Device from Left Lower Femur, Percutaneous Endoscopic Approach

0QPC45Z Removal of External Fixation Device from Left Lower Femur, Percutaneous Endoscopic Approach

0QPC47Z Removal of Autologous Tissue Substitute from Left Lower Femur, Percutaneous Endoscopic Approach

0QPC4JZ Removal of Synthetic Substitute from Left Lower Femur, Percutaneous Endoscopic Approach

0QPC4KZ Removal of Nonautologous Tissue Substitute from Left Lower Femur, Percutaneous Endoscopic Approach

0QPCX4Z Removal of Internal Fixation Device from Left Lower Femur, External Approach

0QPCX5Z Removal of External Fixation Device from Left Lower Femur, External Approach

0QPD04Z Removal of Internal Fixation Device from Right Patella, Open Approach

0QPD05Z Removal of External Fixation Device from Right Patella, Open Approach

0QPD07Z Removal of Autologous Tissue Substitute from Right Patella, Open Approach

0QPD0JZ Removal of Synthetic Substitute from Right Patella, Open Approach

0QPD0KZ Removal of Nonautologous Tissue Substitute from Right Patella, Open Approach

0QPD34Z Removal of Internal Fixation Device from Right Patella, Percutaneous Approach

0QPD35Z Removal of External Fixation Device from Right Patella, Percutaneous Approach

0QPD37Z Removal of Autologous Tissue Substitute from Right Patella, Percutaneous Approach

0QPD3JZ Removal of Synthetic Substitute from Right Patella, Percutaneous Approach

0QPD3KZ Removal of Nonautologous Tissue Substitute from Right Patella, Percutaneous Approach

0QPD44Z Removal of Internal Fixation Device from Right Patella, Percutaneous Endoscopic Approach

0QPD45Z Removal of External Fixation Device from Right Patella, Percutaneous Endoscopic Approach

0QPD47Z Removal of Autologous Tissue Substitute from Right Patella, Percutaneous Endoscopic Approach

0QPD4JZ Removal of Synthetic Substitute from Right Patella, Percutaneous Endoscopic Approach

0QPD4KZ Removal of Nonautologous Tissue Substitute from Right Patella, Percutaneous Endoscopic Approach

0QPDX4Z Removal of Internal Fixation Device from Right Patella, External Approach

0QPDX5Z Removal of External Fixation Device from Right Patella, External Approach

0QPF04Z Removal of Internal Fixation Device from Left Patella, Open Approach

0QPF05Z Removal of External Fixation Device from Left Patella, Open Approach

0QPF07Z Removal of Autologous Tissue Substitute from Left Patella, Open Approach

0QPF0JZ Removal of Synthetic Substitute from Left Patella, Open Approach

0QPF0KZ Removal of Nonautologous Tissue Substitute from Left Patella, Open Approach

0QPF34Z Removal of Internal Fixation Device from Left Patella, Percutaneous Approach

0QPF35Z Removal of External Fixation Device from Left Patella, Percutaneous Approach

0QPF37Z Removal of Autologous Tissue Substitute from Left Patella, Percutaneous Approach

0QPF3JZ Removal of Synthetic Substitute from Left Patella, Percutaneous Approach

0QPF3KZ Removal of Nonautologous Tissue Substitute from Left Patella, Percutaneous Approach

0QPF44Z Removal of Internal Fixation Device from Left Patella, Percutaneous Endoscopic Approach

0QPF45Z Removal of External Fixation Device from Left Patella, Percutaneous Endoscopic Approach

0QPF47Z Removal of Autologous Tissue Substitute from Left Patella, Percutaneous Endoscopic Approach

0QPF4JZ Removal of Synthetic Substitute from Left Patella, Percutaneous Endoscopic Approach

0QPF4KZ Removal of Nonautologous Tissue Substitute from Left Patella, Percutaneous Endoscopic Approach

0QPFX4Z Removal of Internal Fixation Device from Left Patella, External Approach

0QPFX5Z Removal of External Fixation Device from Left Patella, External Approach

0QPG04Z Removal of Internal Fixation Device from Right Tibia, Open Approach

0QPG05Z Removal of External Fixation Device from Right Tibia, Open Approach

0QPG07Z Removal of Autologous Tissue Substitute from Right Tibia, Open Approach

0QPG0JZ Removal of Synthetic Substitute from Right Tibia, Open Approach

0QPG0KZ Removal of Nonautologous Tissue Substitute from Right Tibia, Open Approach

0QPG34Z Removal of Internal Fixation Device from Right Tibia, Percutaneous Approach

0QPG35Z Removal of External Fixation Device from Right Tibia, Percutaneous Approach

0QPG37Z Removal of Autologous Tissue Substitute from Right Tibia, Percutaneous Approach

0QPG3JZ Removal of Synthetic Substitute from Right Tibia, Percutaneous Approach

0QPG3KZ Removal of Nonautologous Tissue Substitute from Right Tibia, Percutaneous Approach

0QPG44Z Removal of Internal Fixation Device from Right Tibia, Percutaneous Endoscopic Approach

0QPG45Z Removal of External Fixation Device from Right Tibia, Percutaneous Endoscopic Approach

0QPG47Z Removal of Autologous Tissue Substitute from Right Tibia, Percutaneous Endoscopic Approach

0QPG4JZ Removal of Synthetic Substitute from Right Tibia, Percutaneous Endoscopic Approach

0QPG4KZ Removal of Nonautologous Tissue Substitute from Right Tibia, Percutaneous Endoscopic Approach

0QPGX4Z Removal of Internal Fixation Device from Right Tibia, External Approach

0QPGX5Z Removal of External Fixation Device from Right Tibia, External Approach

0QPH04Z Removal of Internal Fixation Device fro Left Tibia, Open Approach

0QPH05Z Removal of External Fixation Device from Left Tibia, Open Approach

0QPH07Z Removal of Autologous Tissue Substitu from Left Tibia, Open Approach

0QPH0JZ Removal of Synthetic Substitute from Left Tibia, Open Approach

0QPH0KZ Removal of Nonautologous Tissue Substitute from Left Tibia, Open Approach

0QPH34Z Removal of Internal Fixation Device fro Left Tibia, Percutaneous Approach

0QPH35Z Removal of External Fixation Device from Left Tibia, Percutaneous Approach

0QPH37Z Removal of Autologous Tissue Substitut from Left Tibia, Percutaneous Approach

0QPH3JZ Removal of Synthetic Substitute from Left Tibia, Percutaneous Approach

0QPH3KZ Removal of Nonautologous Tissue Substitute from Left Tibia, Percutaneous Approach

0QPH44Z Removal of Internal Fixation Device fro Left Tibia, Percutaneous Endoscopic Approach

0QPH45Z Removal of External Fixation Device from Left Tibia, Percutaneous Endoscop Approach

0QPH47Z Removal of Autologous Tissue Substitut from Left Tibia, Percutaneous Endoscop Approach

0QPH4JZ Removal of Synthetic Substitute from Left Tibia, Percutaneous Endoscopic Approach

0QPH4KZ Removal of Nonautologous Tissue Substitute from Left Tibia, Percutaneous Endoscopic Approach

0QPHX4Z Removal of Internal Fixation Device fro Left Tibia, External Approach

0QPHX5Z Removal of External Fixation Device from Left Tibia, External Approach

0QPJ04Z Removal of Internal Fixation Device fro Right Fibula, Open Approach

0QPJ05Z Removal of External Fixation Device from Right Fibula, Open Approach

0QPJ07Z Removal of Autologous Tissue Substitute from Right Fibula, Open Approach

0QPJ0JZ Removal of Synthetic Substitute from Right Fibula, Open Approach

0QPJ0KZ Removal of Nonautologous Tissue Substitute from Right Fibula, Open Approach

0QPJ34Z Removal of Internal Fixation Device fron Right Fibula, Percutaneous Approach

0QPJ35Z Removal of External Fixation Device from Right Fibula, Percutaneous Approach

0QPJ37Z Removal of Autologous Tissue Substitute from Right Fibula, Percutaneous Approach

0QPJ3JZ Removal of Synthetic Substitute from Right Fibula, Percutaneous Approach

0QPJ3KZ Removal of Nonautologous Tissue Substitute from Right Fibula, Percutaneous Approach

0QPJ44Z Removal of Internal Fixation Device fron Right Fibula, Percutaneous Endoscopic Approach

0QPJ45Z Removal of External Fixation Device from Right Fibula, Percutaneous Endoscopic Approach

0QPJ47Z Removal of Autologous Tissue Substitute from Right Fibula, Percutaneous Endoscopic Approach

0QPJ4JZ Removal of Synthetic Substitute from Right Fibula, Percutaneous Endoscopic Approach
0QPJ4KZ Removal of Nonautologous Tissue Substitute from Right Fibula, Percutaneous Endoscopic Approach
0QPJX4Z Removal of Internal Fixation Device from Right Fibula, External Approach
0QPJX5Z Removal of External Fixation Device from Right Fibula, External Approach
0QPK04Z Removal of Internal Fixation Device from Left Fibula, Open Approach
0QPK05Z Removal of External Fixation Device from Left Fibula, Open Approach
0QPK07Z Removal of Autologous Tissue Substitute from Left Fibula, Open Approach
0QPK0JZ Removal of Synthetic Substitute from Left Fibula, Open Approach
0QPK0KZ Removal of Nonautologous Tissue Substitute from Left Fibula, Open Approach
0QPK34Z Removal of Internal Fixation Device from Left Fibula, Percutaneous Approach
0QPK35Z Removal of External Fixation Device from Left Fibula, Percutaneous Approach
0QPK37Z Removal of Autologous Tissue Substitute from Left Fibula, Percutaneous Approach
0QPK3JZ Removal of Synthetic Substitute from Left Fibula, Percutaneous Approach
0QPK3KZ Removal of Nonautologous Tissue Substitute from Left Fibula, Percutaneous Approach
0QPK44Z Removal of Internal Fixation Device from Left Fibula, Percutaneous Endoscopic Approach
0QPK45Z Removal of External Fixation Device from Left Fibula, Percutaneous Endoscopic Approach
0QPK47Z Removal of Autologous Tissue Substitute from Left Fibula, Percutaneous Endoscopic Approach
0QPK4JZ Removal of Synthetic Substitute from Left Fibula, Percutaneous Endoscopic Approach
0QPK4KZ Removal of Nonautologous Tissue Substitute from Left Fibula, Percutaneous Endoscopic Approach
0QPKX4Z Removal of Internal Fixation Device from Left Fibula, External Approach
0QPKX5Z Removal of External Fixation Device from Left Fibula, External Approach
0QPL04Z Removal of Internal Fixation Device from Right Tarsal, Open Approach
0QPL05Z Removal of External Fixation Device from Right Tarsal, Open Approach
0QPL07Z Removal of Autologous Tissue Substitute from Right Tarsal, Open Approach
0QPL0JZ Removal of Synthetic Substitute from Right Tarsal, Open Approach
0QPL0KZ Removal of Nonautologous Tissue Substitute from Right Tarsal, Open Approach
0QPL34Z Removal of Internal Fixation Device from Right Tarsal, Percutaneous Approach
0QPL35Z Removal of External Fixation Device from Right Tarsal, Percutaneous Approach
0QPL37Z Removal of Autologous Tissue Substitute from Right Tarsal, Percutaneous Approach
0QPL3JZ Removal of Synthetic Substitute from Right Tarsal, Percutaneous Approach
0QPL3KZ Removal of Nonautologous Tissue Substitute from Right Tarsal, Percutaneous Approach
0QPL44Z Removal of Internal Fixation Device from Right Tarsal, Percutaneous Endoscopic Approach
0QPL45Z Removal of External Fixation Device from Right Tarsal, Percutaneous Endoscopic Approach
0QPL47Z Removal of Autologous Tissue Substitute from Right Tarsal, Percutaneous Endoscopic Approach
0QPL4JZ Removal of Synthetic Substitute from Right Tarsal, Percutaneous Endoscopic Approach
0QPL4KZ Removal of Nonautologous Tissue Substitute from Right Tarsal, Percutaneous Endoscopic Approach
0QPLX4Z Removal of Internal Fixation Device from Right Tarsal, External Approach
0QPLX5Z Removal of External Fixation Device from Right Tarsal, External Approach
0QPM04Z Removal of Internal Fixation Device from Left Tarsal, Open Approach
0QPM05Z Removal of External Fixation Device from Left Tarsal, Open Approach
0QPM07Z Removal of Autologous Tissue Substitute from Left Tarsal, Open Approach
0QPM0JZ Removal of Synthetic Substitute from Left Tarsal, Open Approach
0QPM0KZ Removal of Nonautologous Tissue Substitute from Left Tarsal, Open Approach
0QPM34Z Removal of Internal Fixation Device from Left Tarsal, Percutaneous Approach
0QPM35Z Removal of External Fixation Device from Left Tarsal, Percutaneous Approach
0QPM37Z Removal of Autologous Tissue Substitute from Left Tarsal, Percutaneous Approach
0QPM3JZ Removal of Synthetic Substitute from Left Tarsal, Percutaneous Approach
0QPM3KZ Removal of Nonautologous Tissue Substitute from Left Tarsal, Percutaneous Approach
0QPM44Z Removal of Internal Fixation Device from Left Tarsal, Percutaneous Endoscopic Approach
0QPM45Z Removal of External Fixation Device from Left Tarsal, Percutaneous Endoscopic Approach
0QPM47Z Removal of Autologous Tissue Substitute from Left Tarsal, Percutaneous Endoscopic Approach
0QPM4JZ Removal of Synthetic Substitute from Left Tarsal, Percutaneous Endoscopic Approach
0QPM4KZ Removal of Nonautologous Tissue Substitute from Left Tarsal, Percutaneous Endoscopic Approach
0QPMX4Z Removal of Internal Fixation Device from Left Tarsal, External Approach
0QPMX5Z Removal of External Fixation Device from Left Tarsal, External Approach
0QPN04Z Removal of Internal Fixation Device from Right Metatarsal, Open Approach
0QPN05Z Removal of External Fixation Device from Right Metatarsal, Open Approach
0QPN07Z Removal of Autologous Tissue Substitute from Right Metatarsal, Open Approach
0QPN0JZ Removal of Synthetic Substitute from Right Metatarsal, Open Approach
0QPN0KZ Removal of Nonautologous Tissue Substitute from Right Metatarsal, Open Approach
0QPN34Z Removal of Internal Fixation Device from Right Metatarsal, Percutaneous Approach
0QPN35Z Removal of External Fixation Device from Right Metatarsal, Percutaneous Approach
0QPN37Z Removal of Autologous Tissue Substitute from Right Metatarsal, Percutaneous Approach
0QPN3JZ Removal of Synthetic Substitute from Right Metatarsal, Percutaneous Approach
0QPN3KZ Removal of Nonautologous Tissue Substitute from Right Metatarsal, Percutaneous Approach
0QPN44Z Removal of Internal Fixation Device from Right Metatarsal, Percutaneous Endoscopic Approach
0QPN45Z Removal of External Fixation Device from Right Metatarsal, Percutaneous Endoscopic Approach
0QPN47Z Removal of Autologous Tissue Substitute from Right Metatarsal, Percutaneous Endoscopic Approach
0QPN4JZ Removal of Synthetic Substitute from Right Metatarsal, Percutaneous Endoscopic Approach
0QPN4KZ Removal of Nonautologous Tissue Substitute from Right Metatarsal, Percutaneous Endoscopic Approach
0QPNX4Z Removal of Internal Fixation Device from Right Metatarsal, External Approach
0QPNX5Z Removal of External Fixation Device from Right Metatarsal, External Approach
0QPP04Z Removal of Internal Fixation Device from Left Metatarsal, Open Approach
0QPP05Z Removal of External Fixation Device from Left Metatarsal, Open Approach
0QPP07Z Removal of Autologous Tissue Substitute from Left Metatarsal, Open Approach
0QPP0JZ Removal of Synthetic Substitute from Left Metatarsal, Open Approach
0QPP0KZ Removal of Nonautologous Tissue Substitute from Left Metatarsal, Open Approach
0QPP34Z Removal of Internal Fixation Device from Left Metatarsal, Percutaneous Approach
0QPP35Z Removal of External Fixation Device from Left Metatarsal, Percutaneous Approach
0QPP37Z Removal of Autologous Tissue Substitute from Left Metatarsal, Percutaneous Approach
0QPP3JZ Removal of Synthetic Substitute from Left Metatarsal, Percutaneous Approach
0QPP3KZ Removal of Nonautologous Tissue Substitute from Left Metatarsal, Percutaneous Approach
0QPP44Z Removal of Internal Fixation Device from Left Metatarsal, Percutaneous Endoscopic Approach
0QPP45Z Removal of External Fixation Device from Left Metatarsal, Percutaneous Endoscopic Approach
0QPP47Z Removal of Autologous Tissue Substitute from Left Metatarsal, Percutaneous Endoscopic Approach
0QPP4JZ Removal of Synthetic Substitute from Left Metatarsal, Percutaneous Endoscopic Approach
0QPP4KZ Removal of Nonautologous Tissue Substitute from Left Metatarsal, Percutaneous Endoscopic Approach
0QPPX4Z Removal of Internal Fixation Device from Left Metatarsal, External Approach
0QPPX5Z Removal of External Fixation Device from Left Metatarsal, External Approach
0QPQ04Z Removal of Internal Fixation Device from Right Toe Phalanx, Open Approach
0QPQ05Z Removal of External Fixation Device from Right Toe Phalanx, Open Approach
0QPQ07Z Removal of Autologous Tissue Substitute from Right Toe Phalanx, Open Approach

0QPQ0JZ Removal of Synthetic Substitute from Right Toe Phalanx, Open Approach
0QPQ0KZ Removal of Nonautologous Tissue Substitute from Right Toe Phalanx, Open Approach
0QPQ34Z Removal of Internal Fixation Device from Right Toe Phalanx, Percutaneous Approach
0QPQ35Z Removal of External Fixation Device from Right Toe Phalanx, Percutaneous Approach
0QPQ37Z Removal of Autologous Tissue Substitute from Right Toe Phalanx, Percutaneous Approach
0QPQ3JZ Removal of Synthetic Substitute from Right Toe Phalanx, Percutaneous Approach
0QPQ3KZ Removal of Nonautologous Tissue Substitute from Right Toe Phalanx, Percutaneous Approach
0QPQ44Z Removal of Internal Fixation Device from Right Toe Phalanx, Percutaneous Endoscopic Approach
0QPQ45Z Removal of External Fixation Device from Right Toe Phalanx, Percutaneous Endoscopic Approach
0QPQ47Z Removal of Autologous Tissue Substitute from Right Toe Phalanx, Percutaneous Endoscopic Approach
0QPQ4JZ Removal of Synthetic Substitute from Right Toe Phalanx, Percutaneous Endoscopic Approach
0QPQ4KZ Removal of Nonautologous Tissue Substitute from Right Toe Phalanx, Percutaneous Endoscopic Approach
0QPQX4Z Removal of Internal Fixation Device from Right Toe Phalanx, External Approach
0QPQX5Z Removal of External Fixation Device from Right Toe Phalanx, External Approach
0QPR04Z Removal of Internal Fixation Device from Left Toe Phalanx, Open Approach
0QPR05Z Removal of External Fixation Device from Left Toe Phalanx, Open Approach
0QPR07Z Removal of Autologous Tissue Substitute from Left Toe Phalanx, Open Approach
0QPR0JZ Removal of Synthetic Substitute from Left Toe Phalanx, Open Approach
0QPR0KZ Removal of Nonautologous Tissue Substitute from Left Toe Phalanx, Open Approach
0QPR34Z Removal of Internal Fixation Device from Left Toe Phalanx, Percutaneous Approach
0QPR35Z Removal of External Fixation Device from Left Toe Phalanx, Percutaneous Approach
0QPR37Z Removal of Autologous Tissue Substitute from Left Toe Phalanx, Percutaneous Approach
0QPR3JZ Removal of Synthetic Substitute from Left Toe Phalanx, Percutaneous Approach
0QPR3KZ Removal of Nonautologous Tissue Substitute from Left Toe Phalanx, Percutaneous Approach
0QPR44Z Removal of Internal Fixation Device from Left Toe Phalanx, Percutaneous Endoscopic Approach
0QPR45Z Removal of External Fixation Device from Left Toe Phalanx, Percutaneous Endoscopic Approach
0QPR47Z Removal of Autologous Tissue Substitute from Left Toe Phalanx, Percutaneous Endoscopic Approach
0QPR4JZ Removal of Synthetic Substitute from Left Toe Phalanx, Percutaneous Endoscopic Approach
0QPR4KZ Removal of Nonautologous Tissue Substitute from Left Toe Phalanx, Percutaneous Endoscopic Approach
0QPRX4Z Removal of Internal Fixation Device from Left Toe Phalanx, External Approach
0QPRX5Z Removal of External Fixation Device from Left Toe Phalanx, External Approach
0QPS04Z Removal of Internal Fixation Device from Coccyx, Open Approach
0QPS07Z Removal of Autologous Tissue Substitute from Coccyx, Open Approach
0QPS0JZ Removal of Synthetic Substitute from Coccyx, Open Approach
0QPS0KZ Removal of Nonautologous Tissue Substitute from Coccyx, Open Approach
0QPS34Z Removal of Internal Fixation Device fro Coccyx, Percutaneous Approach
0QPS37Z Removal of Autologous Tissue Substitu from Coccyx, Percutaneous Approach
0QPS3JZ Removal of Synthetic Substitute from Coccyx, Percutaneous Approach
0QPS3KZ Removal of Nonautologous Tissue Substitute from Coccyx, Percutaneous Approach
0QPS44Z Removal of Internal Fixation Device from Coccyx, Percutaneous Endoscopic Approach
0QPS47Z Removal of Autologous Tissue Substitu from Coccyx, Percutaneous Endoscopic Approach
0QPS4JZ Removal of Synthetic Substitute from Coccyx, Percutaneous Endoscopic Approach
0QPS4KZ Removal of Nonautologous Tissue Substitute from Coccyx, Percutaneous Endoscopic Approach
0QPSX4Z Removal of Internal Fixation Device from Coccyx, External Approach
0QPY00Z Removal of Drainage Device from Low Bone, Open Approach
0QPY0MZ Removal of Bone Growth Stimulator from Lower Bone, Open Approach
0QPY30Z Removal of Drainage Device from Low Bone, Percutaneous Approach
0QPY3MZ Removal of Bone Growth Stimulator from Lower Bone, Percutaneous Approach
0QPY40Z Removal of Drainage Device from Lower Bone, Percutaneous Endoscopic Approach
0QPY4MZ Removal of Bone Growth Stimulator from Lower Bone, Percutaneous Endoscopic Approach
0QPYX0Z Removal of Drainage Device from Low Bone, External Approach
0QPYXMZ Removal of Bone Growth Stimulator from Lower Bone, External Approach

0QQ – Lower Bones, Repair

Review Coding Guideline B3.5

0QQ00ZZ Repair Lumbar Vertebra, Open Approach
0QQ03ZZ Repair Lumbar Vertebra, Percutaneous Approach
0QQ04ZZ Repair Lumbar Vertebra, Percutaneous Endoscopic Approach
0QQ0XZZ Repair Lumbar Vertebra, External Approach
0QQ10ZZ Repair Sacrum, Open Approach
0QQ13ZZ Repair Sacrum, Percutaneous Approach
0QQ14ZZ Repair Sacrum, Percutaneous Endoscopic Approach
0QQ1XZZ Repair Sacrum, External Approach
0QQ20ZZ Repair Right Pelvic Bone, Open Approach
0QQ23ZZ Repair Right Pelvic Bone, Percutaneous Approach
0QQ24ZZ Repair Right Pelvic Bone, Percutaneous Endoscopic Approach
0QQ2XZZ Repair Right Pelvic Bone, External Approach
0QQ30ZZ Repair Left Pelvic Bone, Open Approach
0QQ33ZZ Repair Left Pelvic Bone, Percutaneous Approach
0QQ34ZZ Repair Left Pelvic Bone, Percutaneous Endoscopic Approach
0QQ3XZZ Repair Left Pelvic Bone, External Approach
0QQ40ZZ Repair Right Acetabulum, Open Approach
0QQ43ZZ Repair Right Acetabulum, Percutaneous Approach
0QQ44ZZ Repair Right Acetabulum, Percutaneous Endoscopic Approach
0QQ4XZZ Repair Right Acetabulum, External Approach
0QQ50ZZ Repair Left Acetabulum, Open Approach
0QQ53ZZ Repair Left Acetabulum, Percutaneous Approach
0QQ54ZZ Repair Left Acetabulum, Percutaneous Endoscopic Approach
0QQ5XZZ Repair Left Acetabulum, External Approach
0QQ60ZZ Repair Right Upper Femur, Open Approach
0QQ63ZZ Repair Right Upper Femur, Percutaneous Approach
0QQ64ZZ Repair Right Upper Femur, Percutaneous Endoscopic Approach
0QQ6XZZ Repair Right Upper Femur, External Approach
0QQ70ZZ Repair Left Upper Femur, Open Approach
0QQ73ZZ Repair Left Upper Femur, Percutaneous Approach
0QQ74ZZ Repair Left Upper Femur, Percutaneous Endoscopic Approach
0QQ7XZZ Repair Left Upper Femur, External Approach
0QQ80ZZ Repair Right Femoral Shaft, Open Approach
0QQ83ZZ Repair Right Femoral Shaft, Percutaneou Approach
0QQ84ZZ Repair Right Femoral Shaft, Percutaneou Endoscopic Approach
0QQ8XZZ Repair Right Femoral Shaft, External Approach
0QQ90ZZ Repair Left Femoral Shaft, Open Approach
0QQ93ZZ Repair Left Femoral Shaft, Percutaneous Approach
0QQ94ZZ Repair Left Femoral Shaft, Percutaneous Endoscopic Approach
0QQ9XZZ Repair Left Femoral Shaft, External Approach
0QQB0ZZ Repair Right Lower Femur, Open Approach
0QQB3ZZ Repair Right Lower Femur, Percutaneous Approach

QB4ZZ Repair Right Lower Femur, Percutaneous Endoscopic Approach
QBXZZ Repair Right Lower Femur, External Approach
QC0ZZ Repair Left Lower Femur, Open Approach
QC3ZZ Repair Left Lower Femur, Percutaneous Approach
QC4ZZ Repair Left Lower Femur, Percutaneous Endoscopic Approach
QCXZZ Repair Left Lower Femur, External Approach
QD0ZZ Repair Right Patella, Open Approach
QD3ZZ Repair Right Patella, Percutaneous Approach
QD4ZZ Repair Right Patella, Percutaneous Endoscopic Approach
QDXZZ Repair Right Patella, External Approach
QF0ZZ Repair Left Patella, Open Approach
QF3ZZ Repair Left Patella, Percutaneous Approach
QF4ZZ Repair Left Patella, Percutaneous Endoscopic Approach
QFXZZ Repair Left Patella, External Approach
QG0ZZ Repair Right Tibia, Open Approach
QG3ZZ Repair Right Tibia, Percutaneous Approach
QG4ZZ Repair Right Tibia, Percutaneous Endoscopic Approach
QGXZZ Repair Right Tibia, External Approach
QH0ZZ Repair Left Tibia, Open Approach
0QQH3ZZ Repair Left Tibia, Percutaneous Approach
0QQH4ZZ Repair Left Tibia, Percutaneous Endoscopic Approach
0QQHXZZ Repair Left Tibia, External Approach
0QQJ0ZZ Repair Right Fibula, Open Approach
0QQJ3ZZ Repair Right Fibula, Percutaneous Approach
0QQJ4ZZ Repair Right Fibula, Percutaneous Endoscopic Approach
0QQJXZZ Repair Right Fibula, External Approach
0QQK0ZZ Repair Left Fibula, Open Approach
0QQK3ZZ Repair Left Fibula, Percutaneous Approach
0QQK4ZZ Repair Left Fibula, Percutaneous Endoscopic Approach
0QQKXZZ Repair Left Fibula, External Approach
0QQL0ZZ Repair Right Tarsal, Open Approach
0QQL3ZZ Repair Right Tarsal, Percutaneous Approach
0QQL4ZZ Repair Right Tarsal, Percutaneous Endoscopic Approach
0QQLXZZ Repair Right Tarsal, External Approach
0QQM0ZZ Repair Left Tarsal, Open Approach
0QQM3ZZ Repair Left Tarsal, Percutaneous Approach
0QQM4ZZ Repair Left Tarsal, Percutaneous Endoscopic Approach
0QQMXZZ Repair Left Tarsal, External Approach
0QQN0ZZ Repair Right Metatarsal, Open Approach
0QQN3ZZ Repair Right Metatarsal, Percutaneous Approach
0QQN4ZZ Repair Right Metatarsal, Percutaneous Endoscopic Approach
0QQNXZZ Repair Right Metatarsal, External Approach
0QQP0ZZ Repair Left Metatarsal, Open Approach
0QQP3ZZ Repair Left Metatarsal, Percutaneous Approach
0QQP4ZZ Repair Left Metatarsal, Percutaneous Endoscopic Approach
0QQPXZZ Repair Left Metatarsal, External Approach
0QQQ0ZZ Repair Right Toe Phalanx, Open Approach
0QQQ3ZZ Repair Right Toe Phalanx, Percutaneous Approach
0QQQ4ZZ Repair Right Toe Phalanx, Percutaneous Endoscopic Approach
0QQQXZZ Repair Right Toe Phalanx, External Approach
0QQR0ZZ Repair Left Toe Phalanx, Open Approach
0QQR3ZZ Repair Left Toe Phalanx, Percutaneous Approach
0QQR4ZZ Repair Left Toe Phalanx, Percutaneous Endoscopic Approach
0QQRXZZ Repair Left Toe Phalanx, External Approach
0QQS0ZZ Repair Coccyx, Open Approach
0QQS3ZZ Repair Coccyx, Percutaneous Approach
0QQS4ZZ Repair Coccyx, Percutaneous Endoscopic Approach
0QQSXZZ Repair Coccyx, External Approach

QR – Lower Bones, Replacement

QR007Z Replacement of Lumbar Vertebra with Autologous Tissue Substitute, Open Approach
QR00JZ Replacement of Lumbar Vertebra with Synthetic Substitute, Open Approach
QR00KZ Replacement of Lumbar Vertebra with Nonautologous Tissue Substitute, Open Approach
QR037Z Replacement of Lumbar Vertebra with Autologous Tissue Substitute, Percutaneous Approach
QR03JZ Replacement of Lumbar Vertebra with Synthetic Substitute, Percutaneous Approach
QR03KZ Replacement of Lumbar Vertebra with Nonautologous Tissue Substitute, Percutaneous Approach
QR047Z Replacement of Lumbar Vertebra with Autologous Tissue Substitute, Percutaneous Endoscopic Approach
QR04JZ Replacement of Lumbar Vertebra with Synthetic Substitute, Percutaneous Endoscopic Approach
QR04KZ Replacement of Lumbar Vertebra with Nonautologous Tissue Substitute, Percutaneous Endoscopic Approach
QR107Z Replacement of Sacrum with Autologous Tissue Substitute, Open Approach
QR10JZ Replacement of Sacrum with Synthetic Substitute, Open Approach
QR10KZ Replacement of Sacrum with Nonautologous Tissue Substitute, Open Approach
QR137Z Replacement of Sacrum with Autologous Tissue Substitute, Percutaneous Approach
QR13JZ Replacement of Sacrum with Synthetic Substitute, Percutaneous Approach
QR13KZ Replacement of Sacrum with Nonautologous Tissue Substitute, Percutaneous Approach
0QR147Z Replacement of Sacrum with Autologous Tissue Substitute, Percutaneous Endoscopic Approach
0QR14JZ Replacement of Sacrum with Synthetic Substitute, Percutaneous Endoscopic Approach
0QR14KZ Replacement of Sacrum with Nonautologous Tissue Substitute, Percutaneous Endoscopic Approach
0QR207Z Replacement of Right Pelvic Bone with Autologous Tissue Substitute, Open Approach
0QR20JZ Replacement of Right Pelvic Bone with Synthetic Substitute, Open Approach
0QR20KZ Replacement of Right Pelvic Bone with Nonautologous Tissue Substitute, Open Approach
0QR237Z Replacement of Right Pelvic Bone with Autologous Tissue Substitute, Percutaneous Approach
0QR23JZ Replacement of Right Pelvic Bone with Synthetic Substitute, Percutaneous Approach
0QR23KZ Replacement of Right Pelvic Bone with Nonautologous Tissue Substitute, Percutaneous Approach
0QR247Z Replacement of Right Pelvic Bone with Autologous Tissue Substitute, Percutaneous Endoscopic Approach
0QR24JZ Replacement of Right Pelvic Bone with Synthetic Substitute, Percutaneous Endoscopic Approach
0QR24KZ Replacement of Right Pelvic Bone with Nonautologous Tissue Substitute, Percutaneous Endoscopic Approach
0QR307Z Replacement of Left Pelvic Bone with Autologous Tissue Substitute, Open Approach
0QR30JZ Replacement of Left Pelvic Bone with Synthetic Substitute, Open Approach
0QR30KZ Replacement of Left Pelvic Bone with Nonautologous Tissue Substitute, Open Approach
0QR337Z Replacement of Left Pelvic Bone with Autologous Tissue Substitute, Percutaneous Approach
0QR33JZ Replacement of Left Pelvic Bone with Synthetic Substitute, Percutaneous Approach
0QR33KZ Replacement of Left Pelvic Bone with Nonautologous Tissue Substitute, Percutaneous Approach
0QR347Z Replacement of Left Pelvic Bone with Autologous Tissue Substitute, Percutaneous Endoscopic Approach
0QR34JZ Replacement of Left Pelvic Bone with Synthetic Substitute, Percutaneous Endoscopic Approach
0QR34KZ Replacement of Left Pelvic Bone with Nonautologous Tissue Substitute, Percutaneous Endoscopic Approach
0QR407Z Replacement of Right Acetabulum with Autologous Tissue Substitute, Open Approach
0QR40JZ Replacement of Right Acetabulum with Synthetic Substitute, Open Approach
0QR40KZ Replacement of Right Acetabulum with Nonautologous Tissue Substitute, Open Approach
0QR437Z Replacement of Right Acetabulum with Autologous Tissue Substitute, Percutaneous Approach
0QR43JZ Replacement of Right Acetabulum with Synthetic Substitute, Percutaneous Approach
0QR43KZ Replacement of Right Acetabulum with Nonautologous Tissue Substitute, Percutaneous Approach
0QR447Z Replacement of Right Acetabulum with Autologous Tissue Substitute, Percutaneous Endoscopic Approach

0QR44JZ Replacement of Right Acetabulum with Synthetic Substitute, Percutaneous Endoscopic Approach
0QR44KZ Replacement of Right Acetabulum with Nonautologous Tissue Substitute, Percutaneous Endoscopic Approach
0QR507Z Replacement of Left Acetabulum with Autologous Tissue Substitute, Open Approach
0QR50JZ Replacement of Left Acetabulum with Synthetic Substitute, Open Approach
0QR50KZ Replacement of Left Acetabulum with Nonautologous Tissue Substitute, Open Approach
0QR537Z Replacement of Left Acetabulum with Autologous Tissue Substitute, Percutaneous Approach
0QR53JZ Replacement of Left Acetabulum with Synthetic Substitute, Percutaneous Approach
0QR53KZ Replacement of Left Acetabulum with Nonautologous Tissue Substitute, Percutaneous Approach
0QR547Z Replacement of Left Acetabulum with Autologous Tissue Substitute, Percutaneous Endoscopic Approach
0QR54JZ Replacement of Left Acetabulum with Synthetic Substitute, Percutaneous Endoscopic Approach
0QR54KZ Replacement of Left Acetabulum with Nonautologous Tissue Substitute, Percutaneous Endoscopic Approach
0QR607Z Replacement of Right Upper Femur with Autologous Tissue Substitute, Open Approach
0QR60JZ Replacement of Right Upper Femur with Synthetic Substitute, Open Approach
0QR60KZ Replacement of Right Upper Femur with Nonautologous Tissue Substitute, Open Approach
0QR637Z Replacement of Right Upper Femur with Autologous Tissue Substitute, Percutaneous Approach
0QR63JZ Replacement of Right Upper Femur with Synthetic Substitute, Percutaneous Approach
0QR63KZ Replacement of Right Upper Femur with Nonautologous Tissue Substitute, Percutaneous Approach
0QR647Z Replacement of Right Upper Femur with Autologous Tissue Substitute, Percutaneous Endoscopic Approach
0QR64JZ Replacement of Right Upper Femur with Synthetic Substitute, Percutaneous Endoscopic Approach
0QR64KZ Replacement of Right Upper Femur with Nonautologous Tissue Substitute, Percutaneous Endoscopic Approach
0QR707Z Replacement of Left Upper Femur with Autologous Tissue Substitute, Open Approach
0QR70JZ Replacement of Left Upper Femur with Synthetic Substitute, Open Approach
0QR70KZ Replacement of Left Upper Femur with Nonautologous Tissue Substitute, Open Approach
0QR737Z Replacement of Left Upper Femur with Autologous Tissue Substitute, Percutaneous Approach
0QR73JZ Replacement of Left Upper Femur with Synthetic Substitute, Percutaneous Approach
0QR73KZ Replacement of Left Upper Femur with Nonautologous Tissue Substitute, Percutaneous Approach
0QR747Z Replacement of Left Upper Femur with Autologous Tissue Substitute, Percutaneous Endoscopic Approach
0QR74JZ Replacement of Left Upper Femur with Synthetic Substitute, Percutaneous Endoscopic Approach
0QR74KZ Replacement of Left Upper Femur with Nonautologous Tissue Substitute, Percutaneous Endoscopic Approach
0QR807Z Replacement of Right Femoral Shaft with Autologous Tissue Substitute, Open Approach
0QR80JZ Replacement of Right Femoral Shaft with Synthetic Substitute, Open Approach
0QR80KZ Replacement of Right Femoral Shaft with Nonautologous Tissue Substitute, Open Approach
0QR837Z Replacement of Right Femoral Shaft with Autologous Tissue Substitute, Percutaneous Approach
0QR83JZ Replacement of Right Femoral Shaft with Synthetic Substitute, Percutaneous Approach
0QR83KZ Replacement of Right Femoral Shaft with Nonautologous Tissue Substitute, Percutaneous Approach
0QR847Z Replacement of Right Femoral Shaft with Autologous Tissue Substitute, Percutaneous Endoscopic Approach
0QR84JZ Replacement of Right Femoral Shaft with Synthetic Substitute, Percutaneous Endoscopic Approach
0QR84KZ Replacement of Right Femoral Shaft with Nonautologous Tissue Substitute, Percutaneous Endoscopic Approach
0QR907Z Replacement of Left Femoral Shaft with Autologous Tissue Substitute, Open Approach
0QR90JZ Replacement of Left Femoral Shaft with Synthetic Substitute, Open Approach
0QR90KZ Replacement of Left Femoral Shaft with Nonautologous Tissue Substitute, Open Approach
0QR937Z Replacement of Left Femoral Shaft with Autologous Tissue Substitute, Percutaneous Approach
0QR93JZ Replacement of Left Femoral Shaft with Synthetic Substitute, Percutaneous Approach
0QR93KZ Replacement of Left Femoral Shaft with Nonautologous Tissue Substitute, Percutaneous Approach
0QR947Z Replacement of Left Femoral Shaft with Autologous Tissue Substitute, Percutaneous Endoscopic Approach
0QR94JZ Replacement of Left Femoral Shaft with Synthetic Substitute, Percutaneous Endoscopic Approach
0QR94KZ Replacement of Left Femoral Shaft with Nonautologous Tissue Substitute, Percutaneous Endoscopic Approach
0QRB07Z Replacement of Right Lower Femur with Autologous Tissue Substitute, Open Approach
0QRB0JZ Replacement of Right Lower Femur with Synthetic Substitute, Open Approach
0QRB0KZ Replacement of Right Lower Femur with Nonautologous Tissue Substitute, Open Approach
0QRB37Z Replacement of Right Lower Femur with Autologous Tissue Substitute, Percutaneous Approach
0QRB3JZ Replacement of Right Lower Femur with Synthetic Substitute, Percutaneous Approach
0QRB3KZ Replacement of Right Lower Femur with Nonautologous Tissue Substitute, Percutaneous Approach
0QRB47Z Replacement of Right Lower Femur with Autologous Tissue Substitute, Percutaneous Endoscopic Approach
0QRB4JZ Replacement of Right Lower Femur with Synthetic Substitute, Percutaneous Endoscopic Approach
0QRB4KZ Replacement of Right Lower Femur with Nonautologous Tissue Substitute, Percutaneous Endoscopic Approach
0QRC07Z Replacement of Left Lower Femur with Autologous Tissue Substitute, Open Approach
0QRC0JZ Replacement of Left Lower Femur with Synthetic Substitute, Open Approach
0QRC0KZ Replacement of Left Lower Femur with Nonautologous Tissue Substitute, Open Approach
0QRC37Z Replacement of Left Lower Femur with Autologous Tissue Substitute, Percutaneous Approach
0QRC3JZ Replacement of Left Lower Femur with Synthetic Substitute, Percutaneous Approach
0QRC3KZ Replacement of Left Lower Femur with Nonautologous Tissue Substitute, Percutaneous Approach
0QRC47Z Replacement of Left Lower Femur with Autologous Tissue Substitute, Percutaneous Endoscopic Approach
0QRC4JZ Replacement of Left Lower Femur with Synthetic Substitute, Percutaneous Endoscopic Approach
0QRC4KZ Replacement of Left Lower Femur with Nonautologous Tissue Substitute, Percutaneous Endoscopic Approach
0QRD07Z Replacement of Right Patella with Autologous Tissue Substitute, Open Approach
0QRD0JZ Replacement of Right Patella with Synthetic Substitute, Open Approach
0QRD0KZ Replacement of Right Patella with Nonautologous Tissue Substitute, Open Approach
0QRD37Z Replacement of Right Patella with Autologous Tissue Substitute, Percutaneous Approach
0QRD3JZ Replacement of Right Patella with Synthetic Substitute, Percutaneous Approach
0QRD3KZ Replacement of Right Patella with Nonautologous Tissue Substitute, Percutaneous Approach
0QRD47Z Replacement of Right Patella with Autologous Tissue Substitute, Percutaneous Endoscopic Approach
0QRD4JZ Replacement of Right Patella with Synthetic Substitute, Percutaneous Endoscopic Approach
0QRD4KZ Replacement of Right Patella with Nonautologous Tissue Substitute, Percutaneous Endoscopic Approach
0QRF07Z Replacement of Left Patella with Autologous Tissue Substitute, Open Approach
0QRF0JZ Replacement of Left Patella with Synthetic Substitute, Open Approach
0QRF0KZ Replacement of Left Patella with Nonautologous Tissue Substitute, Open Approach
0QRF37Z Replacement of Left Patella with Autologous Tissue Substitute, Percutaneous Approach

QRF3JZ Replacement of Left Patella with Synthetic Substitute, Percutaneous Approach

QRF3KZ Replacement of Left Patella with Nonautologous Tissue Substitute, Percutaneous Approach

QRF47Z Replacement of Left Patella with Autologous Tissue Substitute, Percutaneous Endoscopic Approach

QRF4JZ Replacement of Left Patella with Synthetic Substitute, Percutaneous Endoscopic Approach

QRF4KZ Replacement of Left Patella with Nonautologous Tissue Substitute, Percutaneous Endoscopic Approach

QRG07Z Replacement of Right Tibia with Autologous Tissue Substitute, Open Approach

QRG0JZ Replacement of Right Tibia with Synthetic Substitute, Open Approach

QRG0KZ Replacement of Right Tibia with Nonautologous Tissue Substitute, Open Approach

QRG37Z Replacement of Right Tibia with Autologous Tissue Substitute, Percutaneous Approach

QRG3JZ Replacement of Right Tibia with Synthetic Substitute, Percutaneous Approach

QRG3KZ Replacement of Right Tibia with Nonautologous Tissue Substitute, Percutaneous Approach

QRG47Z Replacement of Right Tibia with Autologous Tissue Substitute, Percutaneous Endoscopic Approach

QRG4JZ Replacement of Right Tibia with Synthetic Substitute, Percutaneous Endoscopic Approach

QRG4KZ Replacement of Right Tibia with Nonautologous Tissue Substitute, Percutaneous Endoscopic Approach

QRH07Z Replacement of Left Tibia with Autologous Tissue Substitute, Open Approach

QRH0JZ Replacement of Left Tibia with Synthetic Substitute, Open Approach

QRH0KZ Replacement of Left Tibia with Nonautologous Tissue Substitute, Open Approach

QRH37Z Replacement of Left Tibia with Autologous Tissue Substitute, Percutaneous Approach

QRH3JZ Replacement of Left Tibia with Synthetic Substitute, Percutaneous Approach

QRH3KZ Replacement of Left Tibia with Nonautologous Tissue Substitute, Percutaneous Approach

QRH47Z Replacement of Left Tibia with Autologous Tissue Substitute, Percutaneous Endoscopic Approach

QRH4JZ Replacement of Left Tibia with Synthetic Substitute, Percutaneous Endoscopic Approach

0QRH4KZ Replacement of Left Tibia with Nonautologous Tissue Substitute, Percutaneous Endoscopic Approach

0QRJ07Z Replacement of Right Fibula with Autologous Tissue Substitute, Open Approach

0QRJ0JZ Replacement of Right Fibula with Synthetic Substitute, Open Approach

0QRJ0KZ Replacement of Right Fibula with Nonautologous Tissue Substitute, Open Approach

0QRJ37Z Replacement of Right Fibula with Autologous Tissue Substitute, Percutaneous Approach

0QRJ3JZ Replacement of Right Fibula with Synthetic Substitute, Percutaneous Approach

0QRJ3KZ Replacement of Right Fibula with Nonautologous Tissue Substitute, Percutaneous Approach

0QRJ47Z Replacement of Right Fibula with Autologous Tissue Substitute, Percutaneous Endoscopic Approach

0QRJ4JZ Replacement of Right Fibula with Synthetic Substitute, Percutaneous Endoscopic Approach

0QRJ4KZ Replacement of Right Fibula with Nonautologous Tissue Substitute, Percutaneous Endoscopic Approach

0QRK07Z Replacement of Left Fibula with Autologous Tissue Substitute, Open Approach

0QRK0JZ Replacement of Left Fibula with Synthetic Substitute, Open Approach

0QRK0KZ Replacement of Left Fibula with Nonautologous Tissue Substitute, Open Approach

0QRK37Z Replacement of Left Fibula with Autologous Tissue Substitute, Percutaneous Approach

0QRK3JZ Replacement of Left Fibula with Synthetic Substitute, Percutaneous Approach

0QRK3KZ Replacement of Left Fibula with Nonautologous Tissue Substitute, Percutaneous Approach

0QRK47Z Replacement of Left Fibula with Autologous Tissue Substitute, Percutaneous Endoscopic Approach

0QRK4JZ Replacement of Left Fibula with Synthetic Substitute, Percutaneous Endoscopic Approach

0QRK4KZ Replacement of Left Fibula with Nonautologous Tissue Substitute, Percutaneous Endoscopic Approach

0QRL07Z Replacement of Right Tarsal with Autologous Tissue Substitute, Open Approach

0QRL0JZ Replacement of Right Tarsal with Synthetic Substitute, Open Approach

0QRL0KZ Replacement of Right Tarsal with Nonautologous Tissue Substitute, Open Approach

0QRL37Z Replacement of Right Tarsal with Autologous Tissue Substitute, Percutaneous Approach

0QRL3JZ Replacement of Right Tarsal with Synthetic Substitute, Percutaneous Approach

0QRL3KZ Replacement of Right Tarsal with Nonautologous Tissue Substitute, Percutaneous Approach

0QRL47Z Replacement of Right Tarsal with Autologous Tissue Substitute, Percutaneous Endoscopic Approach

0QRL4JZ Replacement of Right Tarsal with Synthetic Substitute, Percutaneous Endoscopic Approach

0QRL4KZ Replacement of Right Tarsal with Nonautologous Tissue Substitute, Percutaneous Endoscopic Approach

0QRM07Z Replacement of Left Tarsal with Autologous Tissue Substitute, Open Approach

0QRM0JZ Replacement of Left Tarsal with Synthetic Substitute, Open Approach

0QRM0KZ Replacement of Left Tarsal with Nonautologous Tissue Substitute, Open Approach

0QRM37Z Replacement of Left Tarsal with Autologous Tissue Substitute, Percutaneous Approach

0QRM3JZ Replacement of Left Tarsal with Synthetic Substitute, Percutaneous Approach

0QRM3KZ Replacement of Left Tarsal with Nonautologous Tissue Substitute, Percutaneous Approach

0QRM47Z Replacement of Left Tarsal with Autologous Tissue Substitute, Percutaneous Endoscopic Approach

0QRM4JZ Replacement of Left Tarsal with Synthetic Substitute, Percutaneous Endoscopic Approach

0QRM4KZ Replacement of Left Tarsal with Nonautologous Tissue Substitute, Percutaneous Endoscopic Approach

0QRN07Z Replacement of Right Metatarsal with Autologous Tissue Substitute, Open Approach

0QRN0JZ Replacement of Right Metatarsal with Synthetic Substitute, Open Approach

0QRN0KZ Replacement of Right Metatarsal with Nonautologous Tissue Substitute, Open Approach

0QRN37Z Replacement of Right Metatarsal with Autologous Tissue Substitute, Percutaneous Approach

0QRN3JZ Replacement of Right Metatarsal with Synthetic Substitute, Percutaneous Approach

0QRN3KZ Replacement of Right Metatarsal with Nonautologous Tissue Substitute, Percutaneous Approach

0QRN47Z Replacement of Right Metatarsal with Autologous Tissue Substitute, Percutaneous Endoscopic Approach

0QRN4JZ Replacement of Right Metatarsal with Synthetic Substitute, Percutaneous Endoscopic Approach

0QRN4KZ Replacement of Right Metatarsal with Nonautologous Tissue Substitute, Percutaneous Endoscopic Approach

0QRP07Z Replacement of Left Metatarsal with Autologous Tissue Substitute, Open Approach

0QRP0JZ Replacement of Left Metatarsal with Synthetic Substitute, Open Approach

0QRP0KZ Replacement of Left Metatarsal with Nonautologous Tissue Substitute, Open Approach

0QRP37Z Replacement of Left Metatarsal with Autologous Tissue Substitute, Percutaneous Approach

0QRP3JZ Replacement of Left Metatarsal with Synthetic Substitute, Percutaneous Approach

0QRP3KZ Replacement of Left Metatarsal with Nonautologous Tissue Substitute, Percutaneous Approach

0QRP47Z Replacement of Left Metatarsal with Autologous Tissue Substitute, Percutaneous Endoscopic Approach

0QRP4JZ Replacement of Left Metatarsal with Synthetic Substitute, Percutaneous Endoscopic Approach

0QRP4KZ Replacement of Left Metatarsal with Nonautologous Tissue Substitute, Percutaneous Endoscopic Approach

0QRQ07Z Replacement of Right Toe Phalanx with Autologous Tissue Substitute, Open Approach

0QRQ0JZ Replacement of Right Toe Phalanx with Synthetic Substitute, Open Approach

0QRQ0KZ Replacement of Right Toe Phalanx with Nonautologous Tissue Substitute, Open Approach

0QSR05Z Reposition Left Toe Phalanx with External Fixation Device, Open Approach
0QSR0ZZ Reposition Left Toe Phalanx, Open Approach
0QSR34Z Reposition Left Toe Phalanx with Internal Fixation Device, Percutaneous Approach
0QSR35Z Reposition Left Toe Phalanx with External Fixation Device, Percutaneous Approach
0QSR3ZZ Reposition Left Toe Phalanx, Percutaneous Approach
0QSR44Z Reposition Left Toe Phalanx with Internal Fixation Device, Percutaneous Endoscopic Approach
0QSR45Z Reposition Left Toe Phalanx with External Fixation Device, Percutaneous Endoscopic Approach
0QSR4ZZ Reposition Left Toe Phalanx, Percutaneous Endoscopic Approach
0QSRXZZ Reposition Left Toe Phalanx, External Approach
0QSS04Z Reposition Coccyx with Internal Fixation Device, Open Approach
0QSS0ZZ Reposition Coccyx, Open Approach
0QSS34Z Reposition Coccyx with Internal Fixation Device, Percutaneous Approach
0QSS3ZZ Reposition Coccyx, Percutaneous Approach
+ *See table 0QU to construct a code for Supplement of with synthetic substitute.*
0QSS44Z Reposition Coccyx with Internal Fixation Device, Percutaneous Endoscopic Approach
0QSS4ZZ Reposition Coccyx, Percutaneous Endoscopic Approach
0QSSXZZ Reposition Coccyx, External Approach

0QT – Lower Bones, Resection

Review Coding Guideline B3.8

0QT20ZZ Resection of Right Pelvic Bone, Open Approach
0QT30ZZ Resection of Left Pelvic Bone, Open Approach
0QT40ZZ Resection of Right Acetabulum, Open Approach
0QT50ZZ Resection of Left Acetabulum, Open Approach
0QT60ZZ Resection of Right Upper Femur, Open Approach
0QT70ZZ Resection of Left Upper Femur, Open Approach
0QT80ZZ Resection of Right Femoral Shaft, Open Approach
0QT90ZZ Resection of Left Femoral Shaft, Open Approach
0QTB0ZZ Resection of Right Lower Femur, Open Approach
0QTC0ZZ Resection of Left Lower Femur, Open Approach
0QTD0ZZ Resection of Right Patella, Open Approach
0QTF0ZZ Resection of Left Patella, Open Approach
0QTG0ZZ Resection of Right Tibia, Open Approach
0QTH0ZZ Resection of Left Tibia, Open Approach
0QTJ0ZZ Resection of Right Fibula, Open Approach
0QTK0ZZ Resection of Left Fibula, Open Approach
0QTL0ZZ Resection of Right Tarsal, Open Approach
0QTM0ZZ Resection of Left Tarsal, Open Approach
0QTN0ZZ Resection of Right Metatarsal, Open Approach
0QTP0ZZ Resection of Left Metatarsal, Open Approach
0QTQ0ZZ Resection of Right Toe Phalanx, Open Approach
0QTR0ZZ Resection of Left Toe Phalanx, Open Approach
0QTS0ZZ Resection of Coccyx, Open Approach

0QU – Lower Bones, Supplement

0QU007Z Supplement Lumbar Vertebra with Autologous Tissue Substitute, Open Approach
0QU00JZ Supplement Lumbar Vertebra with Synthetic Substitute, Open Approach
0QU00KZ Supplement Lumbar Vertebra with Nonautologous Tissue Substitute, Open Approach
0QU037Z Supplement Lumbar Vertebra with Autologous Tissue Substitute, Percutaneous Approach
0QU03JZ Supplement Lumbar Vertebra with Synthetic Substitute, Percutaneous Approach
AHA CC: 2Q, 2014, 12-13
0QU03KZ Supplement Lumbar Vertebra with Nonautologous Tissue Substitute, Percutaneous Approach
0QU047Z Supplement Lumbar Vertebra with Autologous Tissue Substitute, Percutaneous Endoscopic Approach
0QU04JZ Supplement Lumbar Vertebra with Synthetic Substitute, Percutaneous Endoscopic Approach
0QU04KZ Supplement Lumbar Vertebra with Nonautologous Tissue Substitute, Percutaneous Endoscopic Approach
0QU107Z Supplement Sacrum with Autologous Tissue Substitute, Open Approach
0QU10JZ Supplement Sacrum with Synthetic Substitute, Open Approach
0QU10KZ Supplement Sacrum with Nonautologous Tissue Substitute, Open Approach
0QU137Z Supplement Sacrum with Autologous Tissue Substitute, Percutaneous Approach
0QU13JZ Supplement Sacrum with Synthetic Substitute, Percutaneous Approach
0QU13KZ Supplement Sacrum with Nonautologous Tissue Substitute, Percutaneous Approach
0QU147Z Supplement Sacrum with Autologous Tissue Substitute, Percutaneous Endoscopic Approach
0QU14JZ Supplement Sacrum with Synthetic Substitute, Percutaneous Endoscopic Approach
0QU14KZ Supplement Sacrum with Nonautologous Tissue Substitute, Percutaneous Endoscopic Approach
0QU207Z Supplement Right Pelvic Bone with Autologous Tissue Substitute, Open Approach
0QU20JZ Supplement Right Pelvic Bone with Synthetic Substitute, Open Approach
AHA CC: 2Q, 2013, 35-36
0QU20KZ Supplement Right Pelvic Bone with Nonautologous Tissue Substitute, Open Approach
0QU237Z Supplement Right Pelvic Bone with Autologous Tissue Substitute, Percutaneous Approach
0QU23JZ Supplement Right Pelvic Bone with Synthetic Substitute, Percutaneous Approach
0QU23KZ Supplement Right Pelvic Bone with Nonautologous Tissue Substitute, Percutaneous Approach
0QU247Z Supplement Right Pelvic Bone with Autologous Tissue Substitute, Percutaneous Endoscopic Approach
0QU24JZ Supplement Right Pelvic Bone with Synthetic Substitute, Percutaneous Endoscopic Approach
0QU24KZ Supplement Right Pelvic Bone with Nonautologous Tissue Substitute, Percutaneous Endoscopic Approach
0QU307Z Supplement Left Pelvic Bone with Autologous Tissue Substitute, Open Approach
0QU30JZ Supplement Left Pelvic Bone with Synthetic Substitute, Open Approach
0QU30KZ Supplement Left Pelvic Bone with Nonautologous Tissue Substitute, Open Approach
0QU337Z Supplement Left Pelvic Bone with Autologous Tissue Substitute, Percutaneous Approach
0QU33JZ Supplement Left Pelvic Bone with Synthetic Substitute, Percutaneous Approach
0QU33KZ Supplement Left Pelvic Bone with Nonautologous Tissue Substitute, Percutaneous Approach
0QU347Z Supplement Left Pelvic Bone with Autologous Tissue Substitute, Percutaneous Endoscopic Approach
0QU34JZ Supplement Left Pelvic Bone with Synthetic Substitute, Percutaneous Endoscopic Approach
0QU34KZ Supplement Left Pelvic Bone with Nonautologous Tissue Substitute, Percutaneous Endoscopic Approach
0QU407Z Supplement Right Acetabulum with Autologous Tissue Substitute, Open Approach
0QU40JZ Supplement Right Acetabulum with Synthetic Substitute, Open Approach
0QU40KZ Supplement Right Acetabulum with Nonautologous Tissue Substitute, Open Approach
0QU437Z Supplement Right Acetabulum with Autologous Tissue Substitute, Percutaneous Approach
0QU43JZ Supplement Right Acetabulum with Synthetic Substitute, Percutaneous Approach
0QU43KZ Supplement Right Acetabulum with Nonautologous Tissue Substitute, Percutaneous Approach
0QU447Z Supplement Right Acetabulum with Autologous Tissue Substitute, Percutaneous Endoscopic Approach

U44JZ Supplement Right Acetabulum with Synthetic Substitute, Percutaneous Endoscopic Approach

U44KZ Supplement Right Acetabulum with Nonautologous Tissue Substitute, Percutaneous Endoscopic Approach

U507Z Supplement Left Acetabulum with Autologous Tissue Substitute, Open Approach

U50JZ Supplement Left Acetabulum with Synthetic Substitute, Open Approach

U50KZ Supplement Left Acetabulum with Nonautologous Tissue Substitute, Open Approach

U537Z Supplement Left Acetabulum with Autologous Tissue Substitute, Percutaneous Approach

U53JZ Supplement Left Acetabulum with Synthetic Substitute, Percutaneous Approach

U53KZ Supplement Left Acetabulum with Nonautologous Tissue Substitute, Percutaneous Approach

U547Z Supplement Left Acetabulum with Autologous Tissue Substitute, Percutaneous Endoscopic Approach

U54JZ Supplement Left Acetabulum with Synthetic Substitute, Percutaneous Endoscopic Approach

QU54KZ Supplement Left Acetabulum with Nonautologous Tissue Substitute, Percutaneous Endoscopic Approach

QU607Z Supplement Right Upper Femur with Autologous Tissue Substitute, Open Approach

QU60JZ Supplement Right Upper Femur with Synthetic Substitute, Open Approach

QU60KZ Supplement Right Upper Femur with Nonautologous Tissue Substitute, Open Approach

QU637Z Supplement Right Upper Femur with Autologous Tissue Substitute, Percutaneous Approach

QU63JZ Supplement Right Upper Femur with Synthetic Substitute, Percutaneous Approach

QU63KZ Supplement Right Upper Femur with Nonautologous Tissue Substitute, Percutaneous Approach

QU647Z Supplement Right Upper Femur with Autologous Tissue Substitute, Percutaneous Endoscopic Approach

QU64JZ Supplement Right Upper Femur with Synthetic Substitute, Percutaneous Endoscopic Approach

QU64KZ Supplement Right Upper Femur with Nonautologous Tissue Substitute, Percutaneous Endoscopic Approach

QU707Z Supplement Left Upper Femur with Autologous Tissue Substitute, Open Approach

QU70JZ Supplement Left Upper Femur with Synthetic Substitute, Open Approach

QU70KZ Supplement Left Upper Femur with Nonautologous Tissue Substitute, Open Approach

0QU737Z Supplement Left Upper Femur with Autologous Tissue Substitute, Percutaneous Approach

0QU73JZ Supplement Left Upper Femur with Synthetic Substitute, Percutaneous Approach

0QU73KZ Supplement Left Upper Femur with Nonautologous Tissue Substitute, Percutaneous Approach

0QU747Z Supplement Left Upper Femur with Autologous Tissue Substitute, Percutaneous Endoscopic Approach

0QU74JZ Supplement Left Upper Femur with Synthetic Substitute, Percutaneous Endoscopic Approach

0QU74KZ Supplement Left Upper Femur with Nonautologous Tissue Substitute, Percutaneous Endoscopic Approach

0QU807Z Supplement Right Femoral Shaft with Autologous Tissue Substitute, Open Approach

0QU80JZ Supplement Right Femoral Shaft with Synthetic Substitute, Open Approach

0QU80KZ Supplement Right Femoral Shaft with Nonautologous Tissue Substitute, Open Approach

0QU837Z Supplement Right Femoral Shaft with Autologous Tissue Substitute, Percutaneous Approach

0QU83JZ Supplement Right Femoral Shaft with Synthetic Substitute, Percutaneous Approach

0QU83KZ Supplement Right Femoral Shaft with Nonautologous Tissue Substitute, Percutaneous Approach

0QU847Z Supplement Right Femoral Shaft with Autologous Tissue Substitute, Percutaneous Endoscopic Approach

0QU84JZ Supplement Right Femoral Shaft with Synthetic Substitute, Percutaneous Endoscopic Approach

0QU84KZ Supplement Right Femoral Shaft with Nonautologous Tissue Substitute, Percutaneous Endoscopic Approach

0QU907Z Supplement Left Femoral Shaft with Autologous Tissue Substitute, Open Approach

0QU90JZ Supplement Left Femoral Shaft with Synthetic Substitute, Open Approach

0QU90KZ Supplement Left Femoral Shaft with Nonautologous Tissue Substitute, Open Approach

0QU937Z Supplement Left Femoral Shaft with Autologous Tissue Substitute, Percutaneous Approach

0QU93JZ Supplement Left Femoral Shaft with Synthetic Substitute, Percutaneous Approach

0QU93KZ Supplement Left Femoral Shaft with Nonautologous Tissue Substitute, Percutaneous Approach

0QU947Z Supplement Left Femoral Shaft with Autologous Tissue Substitute, Percutaneous Endoscopic Approach

0QU94JZ Supplement Left Femoral Shaft with Synthetic Substitute, Percutaneous Endoscopic Approach

0QU94KZ Supplement Left Femoral Shaft with Nonautologous Tissue Substitute, Percutaneous Endoscopic Approach

0QUB07Z Supplement Right Lower Femur with Autologous Tissue Substitute, Open Approach

0QUB0JZ Supplement Right Lower Femur with Synthetic Substitute, Open Approach

0QUB0KZ Supplement Right Lower Femur with Nonautologous Tissue Substitute, Open Approach

0QUB37Z Supplement Right Lower Femur with Autologous Tissue Substitute, Percutaneous Approach

0QUB3JZ Supplement Right Lower Femur with Synthetic Substitute, Percutaneous Approach

0QUB3KZ Supplement Right Lower Femur with Nonautologous Tissue Substitute, Percutaneous Approach

0QUB47Z Supplement Right Lower Femur with Autologous Tissue Substitute, Percutaneous Endoscopic Approach

0QUB4JZ Supplement Right Lower Femur with Synthetic Substitute, Percutaneous Endoscopic Approach

0QUB4KZ Supplement Right Lower Femur with Nonautologous Tissue Substitute, Percutaneous Endoscopic Approach

0QUC07Z Supplement Left Lower Femur with Autologous Tissue Substitute, Open Approach

0QUC0JZ Supplement Left Lower Femur with Synthetic Substitute, Open Approach

0QUC0KZ Supplement Left Lower Femur with Nonautologous Tissue Substitute, Open Approach

0QUC37Z Supplement Left Lower Femur with Autologous Tissue Substitute, Percutaneous Approach

0QUC3JZ Supplement Left Lower Femur with Synthetic Substitute, Percutaneous Approach

0QUC3KZ Supplement Left Lower Femur with Nonautologous Tissue Substitute, Percutaneous Approach

0QUC47Z Supplement Left Lower Femur with Autologous Tissue Substitute, Percutaneous Endoscopic Approach

0QUC4JZ Supplement Left Lower Femur with Synthetic Substitute, Percutaneous Endoscopic Approach

0QUC4KZ Supplement Left Lower Femur with Nonautologous Tissue Substitute, Percutaneous Endoscopic Approach

0QUD07Z Supplement Right Patella with Autologous Tissue Substitute, Open Approach

0QUD0JZ Supplement Right Patella with Synthetic Substitute, Open Approach

0QUD0KZ Supplement Right Patella with Nonautologous Tissue Substitute, Open Approach

0QUD37Z Supplement Right Patella with Autologous Tissue Substitute, Percutaneous Approach

0QUD3JZ Supplement Right Patella with Synthetic Substitute, Percutaneous Approach

0QUD3KZ Supplement Right Patella with Nonautologous Tissue Substitute, Percutaneous Approach

0QUD47Z Supplement Right Patella with Autologous Tissue Substitute, Percutaneous Endoscopic Approach

0QUD4JZ Supplement Right Patella with Synthetic Substitute, Percutaneous Endoscopic Approach

0QUD4KZ Supplement Right Patella with Nonautologous Tissue Substitute, Percutaneous Endoscopic Approach

0QUF07Z Supplement Left Patella with Autologous Tissue Substitute, Open Approach

0QUF0JZ Supplement Left Patella with Synthetic Substitute, Open Approach

0QUF0KZ Supplement Left Patella with Nonautologous Tissue Substitute, Open Approach

0QUF37Z Supplement Left Patella with Autologous Tissue Substitute, Percutaneous Approach

0QUF3JZ Supplement Left Patella with Synthetic Substitute, Percutaneous Approach

0QUF3KZ Supplement Left Patella with Nonautologous Tissue Substitute, Percutaneous Approach

0QUF47Z Supplement Left Patella with Autologous Tissue Substitute, Percutaneous Endoscopic Approach

0QUF4JZ Supplement Left Patella with Synthetic Substitute, Percutaneous Endoscopic Approach

0QUF4KZ Supplement Left Patella with Nonautologous Tissue Substitute, Percutaneous Endoscopic Approach
0QUG07Z Supplement Right Tibia with Autologous Tissue Substitute, Open Approach
0QUG0JZ Supplement Right Tibia with Synthetic Substitute, Open Approach
0QUG0KZ Supplement Right Tibia with Nonautologous Tissue Substitute, Open Approach
0QUG37Z Supplement Right Tibia with Autologous Tissue Substitute, Percutaneous Approach
0QUG3JZ Supplement Right Tibia with Synthetic Substitute, Percutaneous Approach
0QUG3KZ Supplement Right Tibia with Nonautologous Tissue Substitute, Percutaneous Approach
0QUG47Z Supplement Right Tibia with Autologous Tissue Substitute, Percutaneous Endoscopic Approach
0QUG4JZ Supplement Right Tibia with Synthetic Substitute, Percutaneous Endoscopic Approach
0QUG4KZ Supplement Right Tibia with Nonautologous Tissue Substitute, Percutaneous Endoscopic Approach
0QUH07Z Supplement Left Tibia with Autologous Tissue Substitute, Open Approach
0QUH0JZ Supplement Left Tibia with Synthetic Substitute, Open Approach
0QUH0KZ Supplement Left Tibia with Nonautologous Tissue Substitute, Open Approach
0QUH37Z Supplement Left Tibia with Autologous Tissue Substitute, Percutaneous Approach
0QUH3JZ Supplement Left Tibia with Synthetic Substitute, Percutaneous Approach
0QUH3KZ Supplement Left Tibia with Nonautologous Tissue Substitute, Percutaneous Approach
0QUH47Z Supplement Left Tibia with Autologous Tissue Substitute, Percutaneous Endoscopic Approach
0QUH4JZ Supplement Left Tibia with Synthetic Substitute, Percutaneous Endoscopic Approach
0QUH4KZ Supplement Left Tibia with Nonautologous Tissue Substitute, Percutaneous Endoscopic Approach
0QUJ07Z Supplement Right Fibula with Autologous Tissue Substitute, Open Approach
0QUJ0JZ Supplement Right Fibula with Synthetic Substitute, Open Approach
0QUJ0KZ Supplement Right Fibula with Nonautologous Tissue Substitute, Open Approach
0QUJ37Z Supplement Right Fibula with Autologous Tissue Substitute, Percutaneous Approach
0QUJ3JZ Supplement Right Fibula with Synthetic Substitute, Percutaneous Approach
0QUJ3KZ Supplement Right Fibula with Nonautologous Tissue Substitute, Percutaneous Approach
0QUJ47Z Supplement Right Fibula with Autologous Tissue Substitute, Percutaneous Endoscopic Approach
0QUJ4JZ Supplement Right Fibula with Synthetic Substitute, Percutaneous Endoscopic Approach
0QUJ4KZ Supplement Right Fibula with Nonautologous Tissue Substitute, Percutaneous Endoscopic Approach
0QUK07Z Supplement Left Fibula with Autologous Tissue Substitute, Open Approach
0QUK0JZ Supplement Left Fibula with Synthetic Substitute, Open Approach
0QUK0KZ Supplement Left Fibula with Nonautologous Tissue Substitute, Open Approach
0QUK37Z Supplement Left Fibula with Autologous Tissue Substitute, Percutaneous Approach
0QUK3JZ Supplement Left Fibula with Synthetic Substitute, Percutaneous Approach
0QUK3KZ Supplement Left Fibula with Nonautologous Tissue Substitute, Percutaneous Approach
0QUK47Z Supplement Left Fibula with Autologous Tissue Substitute, Percutaneous Endoscopic Approach
0QUK4JZ Supplement Left Fibula with Synthetic Substitute, Percutaneous Endoscopic Approach
0QUK4KZ Supplement Left Fibula with Nonautologous Tissue Substitute, Percutaneous Endoscopic Approach
0QUL07Z Supplement Right Tarsal with Autologous Tissue Substitute, Open Approach
0QUL0JZ Supplement Right Tarsal with Synthetic Substitute, Open Approach
0QUL0KZ Supplement Right Tarsal with Nonautologous Tissue Substitute, Open Approach
0QUL37Z Supplement Right Tarsal with Autologous Tissue Substitute, Percutaneous Approach
0QUL3JZ Supplement Right Tarsal with Synthetic Substitute, Percutaneous Approach
0QUL3KZ Supplement Right Tarsal with Nonautologous Tissue Substitute, Percutaneous Approach
0QUL47Z Supplement Right Tarsal with Autologous Tissue Substitute, Percutaneous Endoscopic Approach
0QUL4JZ Supplement Right Tarsal with Synthetic Substitute, Percutaneous Endoscopic Approach
0QUL4KZ Supplement Right Tarsal with Nonautologous Tissue Substitute, Percutaneous Endoscopic Approach
0QUM07Z Supplement Left Tarsal with Autologous Tissue Substitute, Open Approach
0QUM0JZ Supplement Left Tarsal with Synthetic Substitute, Open Approach
0QUM0KZ Supplement Left Tarsal with Nonautologous Tissue Substitute, Open Approach
0QUM37Z Supplement Left Tarsal with Autologous Tissue Substitute, Percutaneous Approach
0QUM3JZ Supplement Left Tarsal with Synthetic Substitute, Percutaneous Approach
0QUM3KZ Supplement Left Tarsal with Nonautologous Tissue Substitute, Percutaneous Approach
0QUM47Z Supplement Left Tarsal with Autologous Tissue Substitute, Percutaneous Endoscopic Approach
0QUM4JZ Supplement Left Tarsal with Synthetic Substitute, Percutaneous Endoscopic Approach
0QUM4KZ Supplement Left Tarsal with Nonautologous Tissue Substitute, Percutaneous Endoscopic Approach
0QUN07Z Supplement Right Metatarsal with Autologous Tissue Substitute, Open Approach
0QUN0JZ Supplement Right Metatarsal with Synthetic Substitute, Open Approach
0QUN0KZ Supplement Right Metatarsal with Nonautologous Tissue Substitute, Open Approach
0QUN37Z Supplement Right Metatarsal with Autologous Tissue Substitute, Percutaneous Approach
0QUN3JZ Supplement Right Metatarsal with Synthetic Substitute, Percutaneous Approach
0QUN3KZ Supplement Right Metatarsal with Nonautologous Tissue Substitute, Percutaneous Approach
0QUN47Z Supplement Right Metatarsal with Autologous Tissue Substitute, Percutaneous Endoscopic Approach
0QUN4JZ Supplement Right Metatarsal with Synthetic Substitute, Percutaneous Endoscopic Approach
0QUN4KZ Supplement Right Metatarsal with Nonautologous Tissue Substitute, Percutaneous Endoscopic Approach
0QUP07Z Supplement Left Metatarsal with Autologous Tissue Substitute, Open Approach
0QUP0JZ Supplement Left Metatarsal with Synthetic Substitute, Open Approach
0QUP0KZ Supplement Left Metatarsal with Nonautologous Tissue Substitute, Open Approach
0QUP37Z Supplement Left Metatarsal with Autologous Tissue Substitute, Percutaneous Approach
0QUP3JZ Supplement Left Metatarsal with Synthetic Substitute, Percutaneous Approach
0QUP3KZ Supplement Left Metatarsal with Nonautologous Tissue Substitute, Percutaneous Approach
0QUP47Z Supplement Left Metatarsal with Autologous Tissue Substitute, Percutaneous Endoscopic Approach
0QUP4JZ Supplement Left Metatarsal with Synthetic Substitute, Percutaneous Endoscopic Approach
0QUP4KZ Supplement Left Metatarsal with Nonautologous Tissue Substitute, Percutaneous Endoscopic Approach
0QUQ07Z Supplement Right Toe Phalanx with Autologous Tissue Substitute, Open Approach
0QUQ0JZ Supplement Right Toe Phalanx with Synthetic Substitute, Open Approach
0QUQ0KZ Supplement Right Toe Phalanx with Nonautologous Tissue Substitute, Open Approach
0QUQ37Z Supplement Right Toe Phalanx with Autologous Tissue Substitute, Percutaneous Approach
0QUQ3JZ Supplement Right Toe Phalanx with Synthetic Substitute, Percutaneous Approach
0QUQ3KZ Supplement Right Toe Phalanx with Nonautologous Tissue Substitute, Percutaneous Approach
0QUQ47Z Supplement Right Toe Phalanx with Autologous Tissue Substitute, Percutaneous Endoscopic Approach
0QUQ4JZ Supplement Right Toe Phalanx with Synthetic Substitute, Percutaneous Endoscopic Approach
0QUQ4KZ Supplement Right Toe Phalanx with Nonautologous Tissue Substitute, Percutaneous Endoscopic Approach
0QUR07Z Supplement Left Toe Phalanx with Autologous Tissue Substitute, Open Approach
0QUR0JZ Supplement Left Toe Phalanx with Synthetic Substitute, Open Approach

QUR0KZ Supplement Left Toe Phalanx with Nonautologous Tissue Substitute, Open Approach

QUR37Z Supplement Left Toe Phalanx with Autologous Tissue Substitute, Percutaneous Approach

QUR3JZ Supplement Left Toe Phalanx with Synthetic Substitute, Percutaneous Approach

QUR3KZ Supplement Left Toe Phalanx with Nonautologous Tissue Substitute, Percutaneous Approach

QUR47Z Supplement Left Toe Phalanx with Autologous Tissue Substitute, Percutaneous Endoscopic Approach

0QUR4JZ Supplement Left Toe Phalanx with Synthetic Substitute, Percutaneous Endoscopic Approach

0QUR4KZ Supplement Left Toe Phalanx with Nonautologous Tissue Substitute, Percutaneous Endoscopic Approach

0QUS07Z Supplement Coccyx with Autologous Tissue Substitute, Open Approach

0QUS0JZ Supplement Coccyx with Synthetic Substitute, Open Approach

0QUS0KZ Supplement Coccyx with Nonautologous Tissue Substitute, Open Approach

0QUS37Z Supplement Coccyx with Autologous Tissue Substitute, Percutaneous Approach

0QUS3JZ Supplement Coccyx with Synthetic Substitute, Percutaneous Approach

0QUS3KZ Supplement Coccyx with Nonautologous Tissue Substitute, Percutaneous Approach

0QUS47Z Supplement Coccyx with Autologous Tissue Substitute, Percutaneous Endoscopic Approach

0QUS4JZ Supplement Coccyx with Synthetic Substitute, Percutaneous Endoscopic Approach

0QUS4KZ Supplement Coccyx with Nonautologous Tissue Substitute, Percutaneous Endoscopic Approach

QW – Lower Bones, Revision

eview Coding Guideline B6.1c

QW004Z Revision of Internal Fixation Device in Lumbar Vertebra, Open Approach

QW007Z Revision of Autologous Tissue Substitute in Lumbar Vertebra, Open Approach

QW00JZ Revision of Synthetic Substitute in Lumbar Vertebra, Open Approach

QW00KZ Revision of Nonautologous Tissue Substitute in Lumbar Vertebra, Open Approach

QW034Z Revision of Internal Fixation Device in Lumbar Vertebra, Percutaneous Approach

QW037Z Revision of Autologous Tissue Substitute in Lumbar Vertebra, Percutaneous Approach

QW03JZ Revision of Synthetic Substitute in Lumbar Vertebra, Percutaneous Approach

QW03KZ Revision of Nonautologous Tissue Substitute in Lumbar Vertebra, Percutaneous Approach

QW044Z Revision of Internal Fixation Device in Lumbar Vertebra, Percutaneous Endoscopic Approach

QW047Z Revision of Autologous Tissue Substitute in Lumbar Vertebra, Percutaneous Endoscopic Approach

QW04JZ Revision of Synthetic Substitute in Lumbar Vertebra, Percutaneous Endoscopic Approach

QW04KZ Revision of Nonautologous Tissue Substitute in Lumbar Vertebra, Percutaneous Endoscopic Approach

QW0X4Z Revision of Internal Fixation Device in Lumbar Vertebra, External Approach

QW0X7Z Revision of Autologous Tissue Substitute in Lumbar Vertebra, External Approach

QW0XJZ Revision of Synthetic Substitute in Lumbar Vertebra, External Approach

QW0XKZ Revision of Nonautologous Tissue Substitute in Lumbar Vertebra, External Approach

QW104Z Revision of Internal Fixation Device in Sacrum, Open Approach

QW107Z Revision of Autologous Tissue Substitute in Sacrum, Open Approach

0QW10JZ Revision of Synthetic Substitute in Sacrum, Open Approach

0QW10KZ Revision of Nonautologous Tissue Substitute in Sacrum, Open Approach

0QW134Z Revision of Internal Fixation Device in Sacrum, Percutaneous Approach

0QW137Z Revision of Autologous Tissue Substitute in Sacrum, Percutaneous Approach

0QW13JZ Revision of Synthetic Substitute in Sacrum, Percutaneous Approach

0QW13KZ Revision of Nonautologous Tissue Substitute in Sacrum, Percutaneous Approach

0QW144Z Revision of Internal Fixation Device in Sacrum, Percutaneous Endoscopic Approach

0QW147Z Revision of Autologous Tissue Substitute in Sacrum, Percutaneous Endoscopic Approach

0QW14JZ Revision of Synthetic Substitute in Sacrum, Percutaneous Endoscopic Approach

0QW14KZ Revision of Nonautologous Tissue Substitute in Sacrum, Percutaneous Endoscopic Approach

0QW1X4Z Revision of Internal Fixation Device in Sacrum, External Approach

0QW1X7Z Revision of Autologous Tissue Substitute in Sacrum, External Approach

0QW1XJZ Revision of Synthetic Substitute in Sacrum, External Approach

0QW1XKZ Revision of Nonautologous Tissue Substitute in Sacrum, External Approach

0QW204Z Revision of Internal Fixation Device in Right Pelvic Bone, Open Approach

0QW205Z Revision of External Fixation Device in Right Pelvic Bone, Open Approach

0QW207Z Revision of Autologous Tissue Substitute in Right Pelvic Bone, Open Approach

0QW20JZ Revision of Synthetic Substitute in Right Pelvic Bone, Open Approach

0QW20KZ Revision of Nonautologous Tissue Substitute in Right Pelvic Bone, Open Approach

0QW234Z Revision of Internal Fixation Device in Right Pelvic Bone, Percutaneous Approach

0QW235Z Revision of External Fixation Device in Right Pelvic Bone, Percutaneous Approach

0QW237Z Revision of Autologous Tissue Substitute in Right Pelvic Bone, Percutaneous Approach

0QW23JZ Revision of Synthetic Substitute in Right Pelvic Bone, Percutaneous Approach

0QW23KZ Revision of Nonautologous Tissue Substitute in Right Pelvic Bone, Percutaneous Approach

0QW244Z Revision of Internal Fixation Device in Right Pelvic Bone, Percutaneous Endoscopic Approach

0QW245Z Revision of External Fixation Device in Right Pelvic Bone, Percutaneous Endoscopic Approach

0QW247Z Revision of Autologous Tissue Substitute in Right Pelvic Bone, Percutaneous Endoscopic Approach

0QW24JZ Revision of Synthetic Substitute in Right Pelvic Bone, Percutaneous Endoscopic Approach

0QW24KZ Revision of Nonautologous Tissue Substitute in Right Pelvic Bone, Percutaneous Endoscopic Approach

0QW2X4Z Revision of Internal Fixation Device in Right Pelvic Bone, External Approach

0QW2X5Z Revision of External Fixation Device in Right Pelvic Bone, External Approach

0QW2X7Z Revision of Autologous Tissue Substitute in Right Pelvic Bone, External Approach

0QW2XJZ Revision of Synthetic Substitute in Right Pelvic Bone, External Approach

0QW2XKZ Revision of Nonautologous Tissue Substitute in Right Pelvic Bone, External Approach

0QW304Z Revision of Internal Fixation Device in Left Pelvic Bone, Open Approach

0QW305Z Revision of External Fixation Device in Left Pelvic Bone, Open Approach

0QW307Z Revision of Autologous Tissue Substitute in Left Pelvic Bone, Open Approach

0QW30JZ Revision of Synthetic Substitute in Left Pelvic Bone, Open Approach

0QW30KZ Revision of Nonautologous Tissue Substitute in Left Pelvic Bone, Open Approach

0QW334Z Revision of Internal Fixation Device in Left Pelvic Bone, Percutaneous Approach

0QW335Z Revision of External Fixation Device in Left Pelvic Bone, Percutaneous Approach

0QW337Z Revision of Autologous Tissue Substitute in Left Pelvic Bone, Percutaneous Approach

0QW33JZ Revision of Synthetic Substitute in Left Pelvic Bone, Percutaneous Approach

0QW33KZ Revision of Nonautologous Tissue Substitute in Left Pelvic Bone, Percutaneous Approach

0QW344Z Revision of Internal Fixation Device in Left Pelvic Bone, Percutaneous Endoscopic Approach

0QW345Z Revision of External Fixation Device in Left Pelvic Bone, Percutaneous Endoscopic Approach

0QW347Z Revision of Autologous Tissue Substitute in Left Pelvic Bone, Percutaneous Endoscopic Approach

0QW34JZ Revision of Synthetic Substitute in Left Pelvic Bone, Percutaneous Endoscopic Approach

0QW34KZ Revision of Nonautologous Tissue Substitute in Left Pelvic Bone, Percutaneous Endoscopic Approach

0QW3X4Z Revision of Internal Fixation Device in Left Pelvic Bone, External Approach

0QW3X5Z Revision of External Fixation Device in Left Pelvic Bone, External Approach
0QW3X7Z Revision of Autologous Tissue Substitute in Left Pelvic Bone, External Approach
0QW3XJZ Revision of Synthetic Substitute in Left Pelvic Bone, External Approach
0QW3XKZ Revision of Nonautologous Tissue Substitute in Left Pelvic Bone, External Approach
0QW404Z Revision of Internal Fixation Device in Right Acetabulum, Open Approach
0QW407Z Revision of Autologous Tissue Substitute in Right Acetabulum, Open Approach
0QW40JZ Revision of Synthetic Substitute in Right Acetabulum, Open Approach
0QW40KZ Revision of Nonautologous Tissue Substitute in Right Acetabulum, Open Approach
0QW434Z Revision of Internal Fixation Device in Right Acetabulum, Percutaneous Approach
0QW437Z Revision of Autologous Tissue Substitute in Right Acetabulum, Percutaneous Approach
0QW43JZ Revision of Synthetic Substitute in Right Acetabulum, Percutaneous Approach
0QW43KZ Revision of Nonautologous Tissue Substitute in Right Acetabulum, Percutaneous Approach
0QW444Z Revision of Internal Fixation Device in Right Acetabulum, Percutaneous Endoscopic Approach
0QW447Z Revision of Autologous Tissue Substitute in Right Acetabulum, Percutaneous Endoscopic Approach
0QW44JZ Revision of Synthetic Substitute in Right Acetabulum, Percutaneous Endoscopic Approach
0QW44KZ Revision of Nonautologous Tissue Substitute in Right Acetabulum, Percutaneous Endoscopic Approach
0QW4X4Z Revision of Internal Fixation Device in Right Acetabulum, External Approach
0QW4X7Z Revision of Autologous Tissue Substitute in Right Acetabulum, External Approach
0QW4XJZ Revision of Synthetic Substitute in Right Acetabulum, External Approach
0QW4XKZ Revision of Nonautologous Tissue Substitute in Right Acetabulum, External Approach
0QW504Z Revision of Internal Fixation Device in Left Acetabulum, Open Approach
0QW507Z Revision of Autologous Tissue Substitute in Left Acetabulum, Open Approach
0QW50JZ Revision of Synthetic Substitute in Left Acetabulum, Open Approach
0QW50KZ Revision of Nonautologous Tissue Substitute in Left Acetabulum, Open Approach
0QW534Z Revision of Internal Fixation Device in Left Acetabulum, Percutaneous Approach
0QW537Z Revision of Autologous Tissue Substitute in Left Acetabulum, Percutaneous Approach
0QW53JZ Revision of Synthetic Substitute in Left Acetabulum, Percutaneous Approach
0QW53KZ Revision of Nonautologous Tissue Substitute in Left Acetabulum, Percutaneous Approach
0QW544Z Revision of Internal Fixation Device in Left Acetabulum, Percutaneous Endoscopic Approach
0QW547Z Revision of Autologous Tissue Substitute in Left Acetabulum, Percutaneous Endoscopic Approach
0QW54JZ Revision of Synthetic Substitute in Left Acetabulum, Percutaneous Endoscopic Approach
0QW54KZ Revision of Nonautologous Tissue Substitute in Left Acetabulum, Percutaneous Endoscopic Approach
0QW5X4Z Revision of Internal Fixation Device in Left Acetabulum, External Approach
0QW5X7Z Revision of Autologous Tissue Substitute in Left Acetabulum, External Approach
0QW5XJZ Revision of Synthetic Substitute in Left Acetabulum, External Approach
0QW5XKZ Revision of Nonautologous Tissue Substitute in Left Acetabulum, External Approach
0QW604Z Revision of Internal Fixation Device in Right Upper Femur, Open Approach
0QW605Z Revision of External Fixation Device in Right Upper Femur, Open Approach
0QW607Z Revision of Autologous Tissue Substitute in Right Upper Femur, Open Approach
0QW60JZ Revision of Synthetic Substitute in Right Upper Femur, Open Approach
0QW60KZ Revision of Nonautologous Tissue Substitute in Right Upper Femur, Open Approach
0QW634Z Revision of Internal Fixation Device in Right Upper Femur, Percutaneous Approach
0QW635Z Revision of External Fixation Device in Right Upper Femur, Percutaneous Approach
0QW637Z Revision of Autologous Tissue Substitute in Right Upper Femur, Percutaneous Approach
0QW63JZ Revision of Synthetic Substitute in Right Upper Femur, Percutaneous Approach
0QW63KZ Revision of Nonautologous Tissue Substitute in Right Upper Femur, Percutaneous Approach
0QW644Z Revision of Internal Fixation Device in Right Upper Femur, Percutaneous Endoscopic Approach
0QW645Z Revision of External Fixation Device in Right Upper Femur, Percutaneous Endoscopic Approach
0QW647Z Revision of Autologous Tissue Substitute in Right Upper Femur, Percutaneous Endoscopic Approach
0QW64JZ Revision of Synthetic Substitute in Right Upper Femur, Percutaneous Endoscopic Approach
0QW64KZ Revision of Nonautologous Tissue Substitute in Right Upper Femur, Percutaneous Endoscopic Approach
0QW6X4Z Revision of Internal Fixation Device in Right Upper Femur, External Approach
0QW6X5Z Revision of External Fixation Device in Right Upper Femur, External Approach
0QW6X7Z Revision of Autologous Tissue Substitute in Right Upper Femur, External Approach
0QW6XJZ Revision of Synthetic Substitute in Right Upper Femur, External Approach
0QW6XKZ Revision of Nonautologous Tissue Substitute in Right Upper Femur, External Approach
0QW704Z Revision of Internal Fixation Device in Left Upper Femur, Open Approach
0QW705Z Revision of External Fixation Device in Left Upper Femur, Open Approach
0QW707Z Revision of Autologous Tissue Substitute in Left Upper Femur, Open Approach
0QW70JZ Revision of Synthetic Substitute in Left Upper Femur, Open Approach
0QW70KZ Revision of Nonautologous Tissue Substitute in Left Upper Femur, Open Approach
0QW734Z Revision of Internal Fixation Device in Left Upper Femur, Percutaneous Approach
0QW735Z Revision of External Fixation Device in Left Upper Femur, Percutaneous Approach
0QW737Z Revision of Autologous Tissue Substitute in Left Upper Femur, Percutaneous Approach
0QW73JZ Revision of Synthetic Substitute in Left Upper Femur, Percutaneous Approach
0QW73KZ Revision of Nonautologous Tissue Substitute in Left Upper Femur, Percutaneous Approach
0QW744Z Revision of Internal Fixation Device in Left Upper Femur, Percutaneous Endoscopic Approach
0QW745Z Revision of External Fixation Device in Left Upper Femur, Percutaneous Endoscopic Approach
0QW747Z Revision of Autologous Tissue Substitute in Left Upper Femur, Percutaneous Endoscopic Approach
0QW74JZ Revision of Synthetic Substitute in Left Upper Femur, Percutaneous Endoscopic Approach
0QW74KZ Revision of Nonautologous Tissue Substitute in Left Upper Femur, Percutaneous Endoscopic Approach
0QW7X4Z Revision of Internal Fixation Device in Left Upper Femur, External Approach
0QW7X5Z Revision of External Fixation Device in Left Upper Femur, External Approach
0QW7X7Z Revision of Autologous Tissue Substitute in Left Upper Femur, External Approach
0QW7XJZ Revision of Synthetic Substitute in Left Upper Femur, External Approach
0QW7XKZ Revision of Nonautologous Tissue Substitute in Left Upper Femur, External Approach
0QW804Z Revision of Internal Fixation Device in Right Femoral Shaft, Open Approach
0QW805Z Revision of External Fixation Device in Right Femoral Shaft, Open Approach
0QW807Z Revision of Autologous Tissue Substitute in Right Femoral Shaft, Open Approach
0QW80JZ Revision of Synthetic Substitute in Right Femoral Shaft, Open Approach
0QW80KZ Revision of Nonautologous Tissue Substitute in Right Femoral Shaft, Open Approach
0QW834Z Revision of Internal Fixation Device in Right Femoral Shaft, Percutaneous Approach
0QW835Z Revision of External Fixation Device in Right Femoral Shaft, Percutaneous Approach
0QW837Z Revision of Autologous Tissue Substitute in Right Femoral Shaft, Percutaneous Approach
0QW83JZ Revision of Synthetic Substitute in Right Femoral Shaft, Percutaneous Approach
0QW83KZ Revision of Nonautologous Tissue Substitute in Right Femoral Shaft, Percutaneous Approach
0QW844Z Revision of Internal Fixation Device in Right Femoral Shaft, Percutaneous Endoscopic Approach
0QW845Z Revision of External Fixation Device in Right Femoral Shaft, Percutaneous Endoscopic Approach
0QW847Z Revision of Autologous Tissue Substitute in Right Femoral Shaft, Percutaneous Endoscopic Approach

QW84JZ Revision of Synthetic Substitute in Right Femoral Shaft, Percutaneous Endoscopic Approach

QW84KZ Revision of Nonautologous Tissue Substitute in Right Femoral Shaft, Percutaneous Endoscopic Approach

QW8X4Z Revision of Internal Fixation Device in Right Femoral Shaft, External Approach

QW8X5Z Revision of External Fixation Device in Right Femoral Shaft, External Approach

QW8X7Z Revision of Autologous Tissue Substitute in Right Femoral Shaft, External Approach

QW8XJZ Revision of Synthetic Substitute in Right Femoral Shaft, External Approach

QW8XKZ Revision of Nonautologous Tissue Substitute in Right Femoral Shaft, External Approach

QW904Z Revision of Internal Fixation Device in Left Femoral Shaft, Open Approach

QW905Z Revision of External Fixation Device in Left Femoral Shaft, Open Approach

QW907Z Revision of Autologous Tissue Substitute in Left Femoral Shaft, Open Approach

QW90JZ Revision of Synthetic Substitute in Left Femoral Shaft, Open Approach

QW90KZ Revision of Nonautologous Tissue Substitute in Left Femoral Shaft, Open Approach

QW934Z Revision of Internal Fixation Device in Left Femoral Shaft, Percutaneous Approach

QW935Z Revision of External Fixation Device in Left Femoral Shaft, Percutaneous Approach

QW937Z Revision of Autologous Tissue Substitute in Left Femoral Shaft, Percutaneous Approach

QW93JZ Revision of Synthetic Substitute in Left Femoral Shaft, Percutaneous Approach

QW93KZ Revision of Nonautologous Tissue Substitute in Left Femoral Shaft, Percutaneous Approach

QW944Z Revision of Internal Fixation Device in Left Femoral Shaft, Percutaneous Endoscopic Approach

QW945Z Revision of External Fixation Device in Left Femoral Shaft, Percutaneous Endoscopic Approach

0QW947Z Revision of Autologous Tissue Substitute in Left Femoral Shaft, Percutaneous Endoscopic Approach

0QW94JZ Revision of Synthetic Substitute in Left Femoral Shaft, Percutaneous Endoscopic Approach

0QW94KZ Revision of Nonautologous Tissue Substitute in Left Femoral Shaft, Percutaneous Endoscopic Approach

0QW9X4Z Revision of Internal Fixation Device in Left Femoral Shaft, External Approach

0QW9X5Z Revision of External Fixation Device in Left Femoral Shaft, External Approach

0QW9X7Z Revision of Autologous Tissue Substitute in Left Femoral Shaft, External Approach

0QW9XJZ Revision of Synthetic Substitute in Left Femoral Shaft, External Approach

0QW9XKZ Revision of Nonautologous Tissue Substitute in Left Femoral Shaft, External Approach

0QWB04Z Revision of Internal Fixation Device in Right Lower Femur, Open Approach

0QWB05Z Revision of External Fixation Device in Right Lower Femur, Open Approach

0QWB07Z Revision of Autologous Tissue Substitute in Right Lower Femur, Open Approach

0QWB0JZ Revision of Synthetic Substitute in Right Lower Femur, Open Approach

0QWB0KZ Revision of Nonautologous Tissue Substitute in Right Lower Femur, Open Approach

0QWB34Z Revision of Internal Fixation Device in Right Lower Femur, Percutaneous Approach

0QWB35Z Revision of External Fixation Device in Right Lower Femur, Percutaneous Approach

0QWB37Z Revision of Autologous Tissue Substitute in Right Lower Femur, Percutaneous Approach

0QWB3JZ Revision of Synthetic Substitute in Right Lower Femur, Percutaneous Approach

0QWB3KZ Revision of Nonautologous Tissue Substitute in Right Lower Femur, Percutaneous Approach

0QWB44Z Revision of Internal Fixation Device in Right Lower Femur, Percutaneous Endoscopic Approach

0QWB45Z Revision of External Fixation Device in Right Lower Femur, Percutaneous Endoscopic Approach

0QWB47Z Revision of Autologous Tissue Substitute in Right Lower Femur, Percutaneous Endoscopic Approach

0QWB4JZ Revision of Synthetic Substitute in Right Lower Femur, Percutaneous Endoscopic Approach

0QWB4KZ Revision of Nonautologous Tissue Substitute in Right Lower Femur, Percutaneous Endoscopic Approach

0QWBX4Z Revision of Internal Fixation Device in Right Lower Femur, External Approach

0QWBX5Z Revision of External Fixation Device in Right Lower Femur, External Approach

0QWBX7Z Revision of Autologous Tissue Substitute in Right Lower Femur, External Approach

0QWBXJZ Revision of Synthetic Substitute in Right Lower Femur, External Approach

0QWBXKZ Revision of Nonautologous Tissue Substitute in Right Lower Femur, External Approach

0QWC04Z Revision of Internal Fixation Device in Left Lower Femur, Open Approach

0QWC05Z Revision of External Fixation Device in Left Lower Femur, Open Approach

0QWC07Z Revision of Autologous Tissue Substitute in Left Lower Femur, Open Approach

0QWC0JZ Revision of Synthetic Substitute in Left Lower Femur, Open Approach

0QWC0KZ Revision of Nonautologous Tissue Substitute in Left Lower Femur, Open Approach

0QWC34Z Revision of Internal Fixation Device in Left Lower Femur, Percutaneous Approach

0QWC35Z Revision of External Fixation Device in Left Lower Femur, Percutaneous Approach

0QWC37Z Revision of Autologous Tissue Substitute in Left Lower Femur, Percutaneous Approach

0QWC3JZ Revision of Synthetic Substitute in Left Lower Femur, Percutaneous Approach

0QWC3KZ Revision of Nonautologous Tissue Substitute in Left Lower Femur, Percutaneous Approach

0QWC44Z Revision of Internal Fixation Device in Left Lower Femur, Percutaneous Endoscopic Approach

0QWC45Z Revision of External Fixation Device in Left Lower Femur, Percutaneous Endoscopic Approach

0QWC47Z Revision of Autologous Tissue Substitute in Left Lower Femur, Percutaneous Endoscopic Approach

0QWC4JZ Revision of Synthetic Substitute in Left Lower Femur, Percutaneous Endoscopic Approach

0QWC4KZ Revision of Nonautologous Tissue Substitute in Left Lower Femur, Percutaneous Endoscopic Approach

0QWCX4Z Revision of Internal Fixation Device in Left Lower Femur, External Approach

0QWCX5Z Revision of External Fixation Device in Left Lower Femur, External Approach

0QWCX7Z Revision of Autologous Tissue Substitute in Left Lower Femur, External Approach

0QWCXJZ Revision of Synthetic Substitute in Left Lower Femur, External Approach

0QWCXKZ Revision of Nonautologous Tissue Substitute in Left Lower Femur, External Approach

0QWD04Z Revision of Internal Fixation Device in Right Patella, Open Approach

0QWD05Z Revision of External Fixation Device in Right Patella, Open Approach

0QWD07Z Revision of Autologous Tissue Substitute in Right Patella, Open Approach

0QWD0JZ Revision of Synthetic Substitute in Right Patella, Open Approach

0QWD0KZ Revision of Nonautologous Tissue Substitute in Right Patella, Open Approach

0QWD34Z Revision of Internal Fixation Device in Right Patella, Percutaneous Approach

0QWD35Z Revision of External Fixation Device in Right Patella, Percutaneous Approach

0QWD37Z Revision of Autologous Tissue Substitute in Right Patella, Percutaneous Approach

0QWD3JZ Revision of Synthetic Substitute in Right Patella, Percutaneous Approach

0QWD3KZ Revision of Nonautologous Tissue Substitute in Right Patella, Percutaneous Approach

0QWD44Z Revision of Internal Fixation Device in Right Patella, Percutaneous Endoscopic Approach

0QWD45Z Revision of External Fixation Device in Right Patella, Percutaneous Endoscopic Approach

0QWD47Z Revision of Autologous Tissue Substitute in Right Patella, Percutaneous Endoscopic Approach

0QWD4JZ Revision of Synthetic Substitute in Right Patella, Percutaneous Endoscopic Approach

0QWD4KZ Revision of Nonautologous Tissue Substitute in Right Patella, Percutaneous Endoscopic Approach

0QWDX4Z Revision of Internal Fixation Device in Right Patella, External Approach

0QWDX5Z Revision of External Fixation Device in Right Patella, External Approach

0QWDX7Z Revision of Autologous Tissue Substitute in Right Patella, External Approach

0QWDXJZ Revision of Synthetic Substitute in Right Patella, External Approach

0QWDXKZ Revision of Nonautologous Tissue Substitute in Right Patella, External Approach

0QWF04Z Revision of Internal Fixation Device in Left Patella, Open Approach

0QWF05Z Revision of External Fixation Device in Left Patella, Open Approach

0QWF07Z Revision of Autologous Tissue Substitute in Left Patella, Open Approach

0QWF0JZ Revision of Synthetic Substitute in Left Patella, Open Approach

0QWF0KZ Revision of Nonautologous Tissue Substitute in Left Patella, Open Approach

0QWF34Z Revision of Internal Fixation Device in Left Patella, Percutaneous Approach

0QWF35Z Revision of External Fixation Device in Left Patella, Percutaneous Approach

0QWF37Z Revision of Autologous Tissue Substitute in Left Patella, Percutaneous Approach

0QWF3JZ Revision of Synthetic Substitute in Left Patella, Percutaneous Approach

0QWF3KZ Revision of Nonautologous Tissue Substitute in Left Patella, Percutaneous Approach

0QWF44Z Revision of Internal Fixation Device in Left Patella, Percutaneous Endoscopic Approach

0QWF45Z Revision of External Fixation Device in Left Patella, Percutaneous Endoscopic Approach

0QWF47Z Revision of Autologous Tissue Substitute in Left Patella, Percutaneous Endoscopic Approach

0QWF4JZ Revision of Synthetic Substitute in Left Patella, Percutaneous Endoscopic Approach

0QWF4KZ Revision of Nonautologous Tissue Substitute in Left Patella, Percutaneous Endoscopic Approach

0QWFX4Z Revision of Internal Fixation Device in Left Patella, External Approach

0QWFX5Z Revision of External Fixation Device in Left Patella, External Approach

0QWFX7Z Revision of Autologous Tissue Substitute in Left Patella, External Approach

0QWFXJZ Revision of Synthetic Substitute in Left Patella, External Approach

0QWFXKZ Revision of Nonautologous Tissue Substitute in Left Patella, External Approach

0QWG04Z Revision of Internal Fixation Device in Right Tibia, Open Approach

0QWG05Z Revision of External Fixation Device in Right Tibia, Open Approach

0QWG07Z Revision of Autologous Tissue Substitute in Right Tibia, Open Approach

0QWG0JZ Revision of Synthetic Substitute in Right Tibia, Open Approach

0QWG0KZ Revision of Nonautologous Tissue Substitute in Right Tibia, Open Approach

0QWG34Z Revision of Internal Fixation Device in Right Tibia, Percutaneous Approach

0QWG35Z Revision of External Fixation Device in Right Tibia, Percutaneous Approach

0QWG37Z Revision of Autologous Tissue Substitute in Right Tibia, Percutaneous Approach

0QWG3JZ Revision of Synthetic Substitute in Right Tibia, Percutaneous Approach

0QWG3KZ Revision of Nonautologous Tissue Substitute in Right Tibia, Percutaneous Approach

0QWG44Z Revision of Internal Fixation Device in Right Tibia, Percutaneous Endoscopic Approach

0QWG45Z Revision of External Fixation Device in Right Tibia, Percutaneous Endoscopic Approach

0QWG47Z Revision of Autologous Tissue Substitute in Right Tibia, Percutaneous Endoscopic Approach

0QWG4JZ Revision of Synthetic Substitute in Right Tibia, Percutaneous Endoscopic Approach

0QWG4KZ Revision of Nonautologous Tissue Substitute in Right Tibia, Percutaneous Endoscopic Approach

0QWGX4Z Revision of Internal Fixation Device in Right Tibia, External Approach

0QWGX5Z Revision of External Fixation Device in Right Tibia, External Approach

0QWGX7Z Revision of Autologous Tissue Substitute in Right Tibia, External Approach

0QWGXJZ Revision of Synthetic Substitute in Right Tibia, External Approach

0QWGXKZ Revision of Nonautologous Tissue Substitute in Right Tibia, External Approach

0QWH04Z Revision of Internal Fixation Device in Left Tibia, Open Approach

0QWH05Z Revision of External Fixation Device in Left Tibia, Open Approach

0QWH07Z Revision of Autologous Tissue Substitute in Left Tibia, Open Approach

0QWH0JZ Revision of Synthetic Substitute in Left Tibia, Open Approach

0QWH0KZ Revision of Nonautologous Tissue Substitute in Left Tibia, Open Approach

0QWH34Z Revision of Internal Fixation Device in Left Tibia, Percutaneous Approach

0QWH35Z Revision of External Fixation Device in Left Tibia, Percutaneous Approach

0QWH37Z Revision of Autologous Tissue Substitute in Left Tibia, Percutaneous Approach

0QWH3JZ Revision of Synthetic Substitute in Left Tibia, Percutaneous Approach

0QWH3KZ Revision of Nonautologous Tissue Substitute in Left Tibia, Percutaneous Approach

0QWH44Z Revision of Internal Fixation Device in Left Tibia, Percutaneous Endoscopic Approach

0QWH45Z Revision of External Fixation Device in Left Tibia, Percutaneous Endoscopic Approach

0QWH47Z Revision of Autologous Tissue Substitute in Left Tibia, Percutaneous Endoscopic Approach

0QWH4JZ Revision of Synthetic Substitute in Left Tibia, Percutaneous Endoscopic Approach

0QWH4KZ Revision of Nonautologous Tissue Substitute in Left Tibia, Percutaneous Endoscopic Approach

0QWHX4Z Revision of Internal Fixation Device in Left Tibia, External Approach

0QWHX5Z Revision of External Fixation Device in Left Tibia, External Approach

0QWHX7Z Revision of Autologous Tissue Substitute in Left Tibia, External Approach

0QWHXJZ Revision of Synthetic Substitute in Left Tibia, External Approach

0QWHXKZ Revision of Nonautologous Tissue Substitute in Left Tibia, External Approach

0QWJ04Z Revision of Internal Fixation Device in Right Fibula, Open Approach

0QWJ05Z Revision of External Fixation Device in Right Fibula, Open Approach

0QWJ07Z Revision of Autologous Tissue Substitute in Right Fibula, Open Approach

0QWJ0JZ Revision of Synthetic Substitute in Rig Fibula, Open Approach

0QWJ0KZ Revision of Nonautologous Tissue Substitute in Right Fibula, Open Approach

0QWJ34Z Revision of Internal Fixation Device in Right Fibula, Percutaneous Approach

0QWJ35Z Revision of External Fixation Device ir Right Fibula, Percutaneous Approach

0QWJ37Z Revision of Autologous Tissue Substitute in Right Fibula, Percutaneou Approach

0QWJ3JZ Revision of Synthetic Substitute in Rig Fibula, Percutaneous Approach

0QWJ3KZ Revision of Nonautologous Tissue Substitute in Right Fibula, Percutaneou Approach

0QWJ44Z Revision of Internal Fixation Device in Right Fibula, Percutaneous Endoscopic Approach

0QWJ45Z Revision of External Fixation Device in Right Fibula, Percutaneous Endoscopic Approach

0QWJ47Z Revision of Autologous Tissue Substitute in Right Fibula, Percutaneous Endoscopic Approach

0QWJ4JZ Revision of Synthetic Substitute in Right Fibula, Percutaneous Endoscopic Approach

0QWJ4KZ Revision of Nonautologous Tissue Substitute in Right Fibula, Percutaneous Endoscopic Approach

0QWJX4Z Revision of Internal Fixation Device in Right Fibula, External Approach

0QWJX5Z Revision of External Fixation Device in Right Fibula, External Approach

0QWJX7Z Revision of Autologous Tissue Substitute in Right Fibula, External Approach

0QWJXJZ Revision of Synthetic Substitute in Righ Fibula, External Approach

0QWJXKZ Revision of Nonautologous Tissue Substitute in Right Fibula, External Approach

0QWK04Z Revision of Internal Fixation Device in Left Fibula, Open Approach

0QWK05Z Revision of External Fixation Device in Left Fibula, Open Approach

0QWK07Z Revision of Autologous Tissue Substitute in Left Fibula, Open Approach

0QWK0JZ Revision of Synthetic Substitute in Left Fibula, Open Approach

0QWK0KZ Revision of Nonautologous Tissue Substitute in Left Fibula, Open Approach

0QWK34Z Revision of Internal Fixation Device in Left Fibula, Percutaneous Approach

0QWK35Z Revision of External Fixation Device in Left Fibula, Percutaneous Approach

0QWK37Z Revision of Autologous Tissue Substitute in Left Fibula, Percutaneous Approach

0QWK3JZ Revision of Synthetic Substitute in Left Fibula, Percutaneous Approach

0QWK3KZ Revision of Nonautologous Tissue Substitute in Left Fibula, Percutaneous Approach

0QWK44Z Revision of Internal Fixation Device in Left Fibula, Percutaneous Endoscopic Approach

0QWK45Z Revision of External Fixation Device in Left Fibula, Percutaneous Endoscopic Approach

0QWK47Z Revision of Autologous Tissue Substitute in Left Fibula, Percutaneous Endoscopic Approach

0QWK4JZ Revision of Synthetic Substitute in Left Fibula, Percutaneous Endoscopic Approach

0QWK4KZ Revision of Nonautologous Tissue Substitute in Left Fibula, Percutaneous Endoscopic Approach

0QWKX4Z Revision of Internal Fixation Device in Left Fibula, External Approach

0QWKX5Z Revision of External Fixation Device in Left Fibula, External Approach

0QWKX7Z Revision of Autologous Tissue Substitute in Left Fibula, External Approach

0QWKXJZ Revision of Synthetic Substitute in Left Fibula, External Approach

0QWKXKZ Revision of Nonautologous Tissue Substitute in Left Fibula, External Approach

0QWL04Z Revision of Internal Fixation Device in Right Tarsal, Open Approach

0QWL05Z Revision of External Fixation Device in Right Tarsal, Open Approach

0QWL07Z Revision of Autologous Tissue Substitute in Right Tarsal, Open Approach

0QWL0JZ Revision of Synthetic Substitute in Right Tarsal, Open Approach

0QWL0KZ Revision of Nonautologous Tissue Substitute in Right Tarsal, Open Approach

0QWL34Z Revision of Internal Fixation Device in Right Tarsal, Percutaneous Approach

0QWL35Z Revision of External Fixation Device in Right Tarsal, Percutaneous Approach

0QWL37Z Revision of Autologous Tissue Substitute in Right Tarsal, Percutaneous Approach

0QWL3JZ Revision of Synthetic Substitute in Right Tarsal, Percutaneous Approach

0QWL3KZ Revision of Nonautologous Tissue Substitute in Right Tarsal, Percutaneous Approach

0QWL44Z Revision of Internal Fixation Device in Right Tarsal, Percutaneous Endoscopic Approach

0QWL45Z Revision of External Fixation Device in Right Tarsal, Percutaneous Endoscopic Approach

0QWL47Z Revision of Autologous Tissue Substitute in Right Tarsal, Percutaneous Endoscopic Approach

0QWL4JZ Revision of Synthetic Substitute in Right Tarsal, Percutaneous Endoscopic Approach

0QWL4KZ Revision of Nonautologous Tissue Substitute in Right Tarsal, Percutaneous Endoscopic Approach

0QWLX4Z Revision of Internal Fixation Device in Right Tarsal, External Approach

0QWLX5Z Revision of External Fixation Device in Right Tarsal, External Approach

0QWLX7Z Revision of Autologous Tissue Substitute in Right Tarsal, External Approach

0QWLXJZ Revision of Synthetic Substitute in Right Tarsal, External Approach

0QWLXKZ Revision of Nonautologous Tissue Substitute in Right Tarsal, External Approach

0QWM04Z Revision of Internal Fixation Device in Left Tarsal, Open Approach

0QWM05Z Revision of External Fixation Device in Left Tarsal, Open Approach

0QWM07Z Revision of Autologous Tissue Substitute in Left Tarsal, Open Approach

0QWM0JZ Revision of Synthetic Substitute in Left Tarsal, Open Approach

0QWM0KZ Revision of Nonautologous Tissue Substitute in Left Tarsal, Open Approach

0QWM34Z Revision of Internal Fixation Device in Left Tarsal, Percutaneous Approach

0QWM35Z Revision of External Fixation Device in Left Tarsal, Percutaneous Approach

0QWM37Z Revision of Autologous Tissue Substitute in Left Tarsal, Percutaneous Approach

0QWM3JZ Revision of Synthetic Substitute in Left Tarsal, Percutaneous Approach

0QWM3KZ Revision of Nonautologous Tissue Substitute in Left Tarsal, Percutaneous Approach

0QWM44Z Revision of Internal Fixation Device in Left Tarsal, Percutaneous Endoscopic Approach

0QWM45Z Revision of External Fixation Device in Left Tarsal, Percutaneous Endoscopic Approach

0QWM47Z Revision of Autologous Tissue Substitute in Left Tarsal, Percutaneous Endoscopic Approach

0QWM4JZ Revision of Synthetic Substitute in Left Tarsal, Percutaneous Endoscopic Approach

0QWM4KZ Revision of Nonautologous Tissue Substitute in Left Tarsal, Percutaneous Endoscopic Approach

0QWMX4Z Revision of Internal Fixation Device in Left Tarsal, External Approach

0QWMX5Z Revision of External Fixation Device in Left Tarsal, External Approach

0QWMX7Z Revision of Autologous Tissue Substitute in Left Tarsal, External Approach

0QWMXJZ Revision of Synthetic Substitute in Left Tarsal, External Approach

0QWMXKZ Revision of Nonautologous Tissue Substitute in Left Tarsal, External Approach

0QWN04Z Revision of Internal Fixation Device in Right Metatarsal, Open Approach

0QWN05Z Revision of External Fixation Device in Right Metatarsal, Open Approach

0QWN07Z Revision of Autologous Tissue Substitute in Right Metatarsal, Open Approach

0QWN0JZ Revision of Synthetic Substitute in Right Metatarsal, Open Approach

0QWN0KZ Revision of Nonautologous Tissue Substitute in Right Metatarsal, Open Approach

0QWN34Z Revision of Internal Fixation Device in Right Metatarsal, Percutaneous Approach

0QWN35Z Revision of External Fixation Device in Right Metatarsal, Percutaneous Approach

0QWN37Z Revision of Autologous Tissue Substitute in Right Metatarsal, Percutaneous Approach

0QWN3JZ Revision of Synthetic Substitute in Right Metatarsal, Percutaneous Approach

0QWN3KZ Revision of Nonautologous Tissue Substitute in Right Metatarsal, Percutaneous Approach

0QWN44Z Revision of Internal Fixation Device in Right Metatarsal, Percutaneous Endoscopic Approach

0QWN45Z Revision of External Fixation Device in Right Metatarsal, Percutaneous Endoscopic Approach

0QWN47Z Revision of Autologous Tissue Substitute in Right Metatarsal, Percutaneous Endoscopic Approach

0QWN4JZ Revision of Synthetic Substitute in Right Metatarsal, Percutaneous Endoscopic Approach

0QWN4KZ Revision of Nonautologous Tissue Substitute in Right Metatarsal, Percutaneous Endoscopic Approach

0QWNX4Z Revision of Internal Fixation Device in Right Metatarsal, External Approach

0QWNX5Z Revision of External Fixation Device in Right Metatarsal, External Approach

0QWNX7Z Revision of Autologous Tissue Substitute in Right Metatarsal, External Approach

0QWNXJZ Revision of Synthetic Substitute in Right Metatarsal, External Approach

0QWNXKZ Revision of Nonautologous Tissue Substitute in Right Metatarsal, External Approach

0QWP04Z Revision of Internal Fixation Device in Left Metatarsal, Open Approach

0QWP05Z Revision of External Fixation Device in Left Metatarsal, Open Approach

0QWP07Z Revision of Autologous Tissue Substitute in Left Metatarsal, Open Approach

0QWP0JZ Revision of Synthetic Substitute in Left Metatarsal, Open Approach

0QWP0KZ Revision of Nonautologous Tissue Substitute in Left Metatarsal, Open Approach

0QWP34Z Revision of Internal Fixation Device in Left Metatarsal, Percutaneous Approach

0QWP35Z Revision of External Fixation Device in Left Metatarsal, Percutaneous Approach

0QWP37Z Revision of Autologous Tissue Substitute in Left Metatarsal, Percutaneous Approach

0QWP3JZ Revision of Synthetic Substitute in Left Metatarsal, Percutaneous Approach

0QWP3KZ Revision of Nonautologous Tissue Substitute in Left Metatarsal, Percutaneous Approach

0QWP44Z Revision of Internal Fixation Device in Left Metatarsal, Percutaneous Endoscopic Approach

0QWP45Z Revision of External Fixation Device in Left Metatarsal, Percutaneous Endoscopic Approach

0QWP47Z Revision of Autologous Tissue Substitute in Left Metatarsal, Percutaneous Endoscopic Approach

0QWP4JZ Revision of Synthetic Substitute in Left Metatarsal, Percutaneous Endoscopic Approach

0QWP4KZ Revision of Nonautologous Tissue Substitute in Left Metatarsal, Percutaneous Endoscopic Approach

0QWPX4Z Revision of Internal Fixation Device in Left Metatarsal, External Approach

0QWPX5Z Revision of External Fixation Device in Left Metatarsal, External Approach

0QWPX7Z Revision of Autologous Tissue Substitute in Left Metatarsal, External Approach

0QWPXJZ Revision of Synthetic Substitute in Left Metatarsal, External Approach

0QWPXKZ Revision of Nonautologous Tissue Substitute in Left Metatarsal, External Approach

0QWQ04Z Revision of Internal Fixation Device in Right Toe Phalanx, Open Approach

0QWQ05Z Revision of External Fixation Device in Right Toe Phalanx, Open Approach

0QWQ07Z Revision of Autologous Tissue Substitute in Right Toe Phalanx, Open Approach
0QWQ0JZ Revision of Synthetic Substitute in Right Toe Phalanx, Open Approach
0QWQ0KZ Revision of Nonautologous Tissue Substitute in Right Toe Phalanx, Open Approach
0QWQ34Z Revision of Internal Fixation Device in Right Toe Phalanx, Percutaneous Approach
0QWQ35Z Revision of External Fixation Device in Right Toe Phalanx, Percutaneous Approach
0QWQ37Z Revision of Autologous Tissue Substitute in Right Toe Phalanx, Percutaneous Approach
0QWQ3JZ Revision of Synthetic Substitute in Right Toe Phalanx, Percutaneous Approach
0QWQ3KZ Revision of Nonautologous Tissue Substitute in Right Toe Phalanx, Percutaneous Approach
0QWQ44Z Revision of Internal Fixation Device in Right Toe Phalanx, Percutaneous Endoscopic Approach
0QWQ45Z Revision of External Fixation Device in Right Toe Phalanx, Percutaneous Endoscopic Approach
0QWQ47Z Revision of Autologous Tissue Substitute in Right Toe Phalanx, Percutaneous Endoscopic Approach
0QWQ4JZ Revision of Synthetic Substitute in Right Toe Phalanx, Percutaneous Endoscopic Approach
0QWQ4KZ Revision of Nonautologous Tissue Substitute in Right Toe Phalanx, Percutaneous Endoscopic Approach
0QWQX4Z Revision of Internal Fixation Device in Right Toe Phalanx, External Approach
0QWQX5Z Revision of External Fixation Device in Right Toe Phalanx, External Approach
0QWQX7Z Revision of Autologous Tissue Substitute in Right Toe Phalanx, External Approach
0QWQXJZ Revision of Synthetic Substitute in Right Toe Phalanx, External Approach
0QWQXKZ Revision of Nonautologous Tissue Substitute in Right Toe Phalanx, External Approach
0QWR04Z Revision of Internal Fixation Device in Left Toe Phalanx, Open Approach
0QWR05Z Revision of External Fixation Device in Left Toe Phalanx, Open Approach
0QWR07Z Revision of Autologous Tissue Substitute in Left Toe Phalanx, Open Approach
0QWR0JZ Revision of Synthetic Substitute in Left Toe Phalanx, Open Approach
0QWR0KZ Revision of Nonautologous Tissue Substitute in Left Toe Phalanx, Open Approach
0QWR34Z Revision of Internal Fixation Device in Left Toe Phalanx, Percutaneous Approach
0QWR35Z Revision of External Fixation Device in Left Toe Phalanx, Percutaneous Approach
0QWR37Z Revision of Autologous Tissue Substitute in Left Toe Phalanx, Percutaneous Approach
0QWR3JZ Revision of Synthetic Substitute in Left Toe Phalanx, Percutaneous Approach
0QWR3KZ Revision of Nonautologous Tissue Substitute in Left Toe Phalanx, Percutaneous Approach
0QWR44Z Revision of Internal Fixation Device in Left Toe Phalanx, Percutaneous Endoscopic Approach
0QWR45Z Revision of External Fixation Device in Left Toe Phalanx, Percutaneous Endoscopic Approach
0QWR47Z Revision of Autologous Tissue Substitute in Left Toe Phalanx, Percutaneous Endoscopic Approach
0QWR4JZ Revision of Synthetic Substitute in Left Toe Phalanx, Percutaneous Endoscopic Approach
0QWR4KZ Revision of Nonautologous Tissue Substitute in Left Toe Phalanx, Percutaneous Endoscopic Approach
0QWRX4Z Revision of Internal Fixation Device in Left Toe Phalanx, External Approach
0QWRX5Z Revision of External Fixation Device in Left Toe Phalanx, External Approach
0QWRX7Z Revision of Autologous Tissue Substitute in Left Toe Phalanx, External Approach
0QWRXJZ Revision of Synthetic Substitute in Left Toe Phalanx, External Approach
0QWRXKZ Revision of Nonautologous Tissue Substitute in Left Toe Phalanx, External Approach
0QWS04Z Revision of Internal Fixation Device in Coccyx, Open Approach
0QWS07Z Revision of Autologous Tissue Substitute in Coccyx, Open Approach
0QWS0JZ Revision of Synthetic Substitute in Coccyx, Open Approach
0QWS0KZ Revision of Nonautologous Tissue Substitute in Coccyx, Open Approach
0QWS34Z Revision of Internal Fixation Device in Coccyx, Percutaneous Approach
0QWS37Z Revision of Autologous Tissue Substitute in Coccyx, Percutaneous Approach
0QWS3JZ Revision of Synthetic Substitute in Coccyx, Percutaneous Approach
0QWS3KZ Revision of Nonautologous Tissue Substitute in Coccyx, Percutaneous Approach
0QWS44Z Revision of Internal Fixation Device in Coccyx, Percutaneous Endoscopic Approach
0QWS47Z Revision of Autologous Tissue Substitute in Coccyx, Percutaneous Endoscopic Approach
0QWS4JZ Revision of Synthetic Substitute in Coccyx, Percutaneous Endoscopic Approach
0QWS4KZ Revision of Nonautologous Tissue Substitute in Coccyx, Percutaneous Endoscopic Approach
0QWSX4Z Revision of Internal Fixation Device in Coccyx, External Approach
0QWSX7Z Revision of Autologous Tissue Substitute in Coccyx, External Approach
0QWSXJZ Revision of Synthetic Substitute in Coccyx, External Approach
0QWSXKZ Revision of Nonautologous Tissue Substitute in Coccyx, External Approach
0QWY00Z Revision of Drainage Device in Lower Bone, Open Approach
0QWY0MZ Revision of Bone Growth Stimulator in Lower Bone, Open Approach
0QWY30Z Revision of Drainage Device in Lower Bone, Percutaneous Approach
0QWY3MZ Revision of Bone Growth Stimulator in Lower Bone, Percutaneous Approach
0QWY40Z Revision of Drainage Device in Lower Bone, Percutaneous Endoscopic Approach
0QWY4MZ Revision of Bone Growth Stimulator in Lower Bone, Percutaneous Endoscopic Approach
0QWYX0Z Revision of Drainage Device in Lower Bone, External Approach
0QWYXMZ Revision of Bone Growth Stimulator in Lower Bone, External Approach

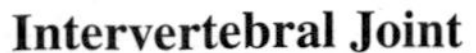

Intervertebral Joint

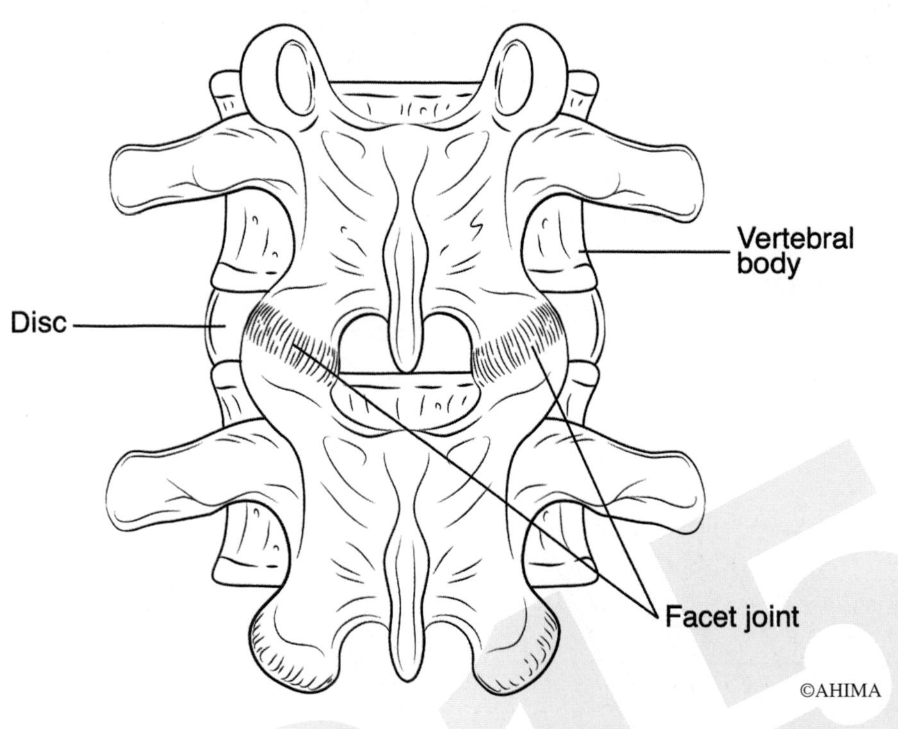

Shoulder

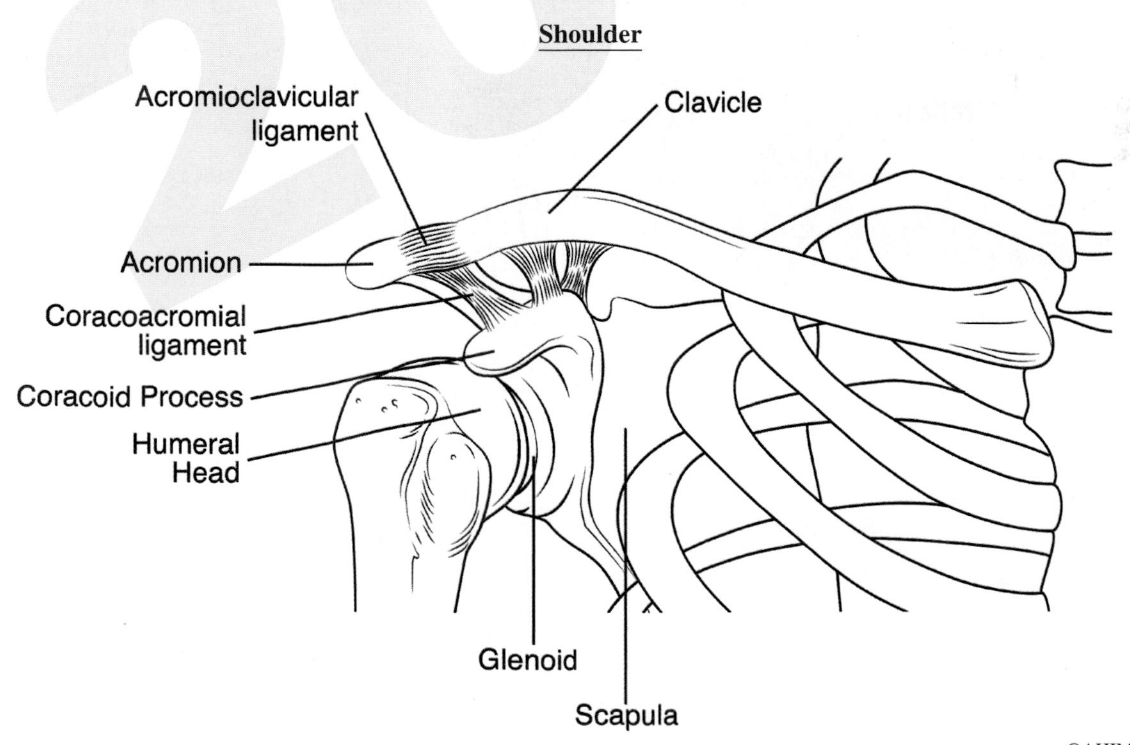

Elbow

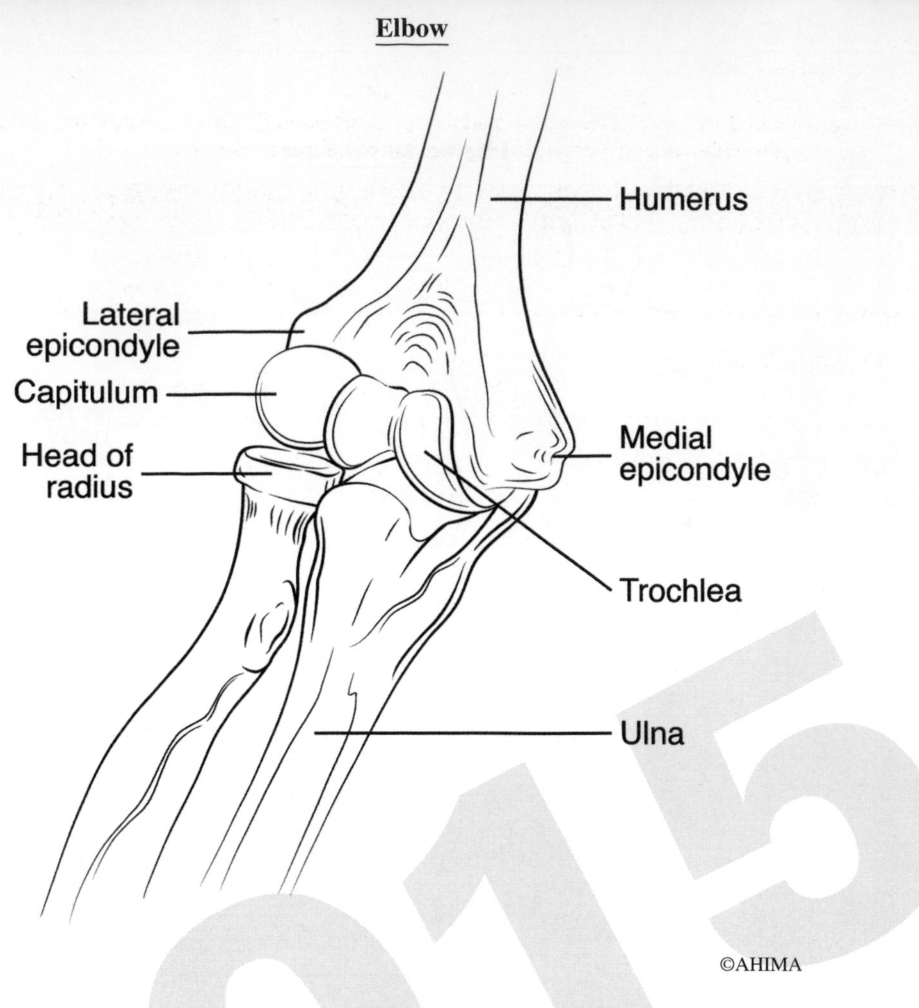
Humerus
Lateral epicondyle
Capitulum
Head of radius
Medial epicondyle
Trochlea
Ulna
©AHIMA

Wrist

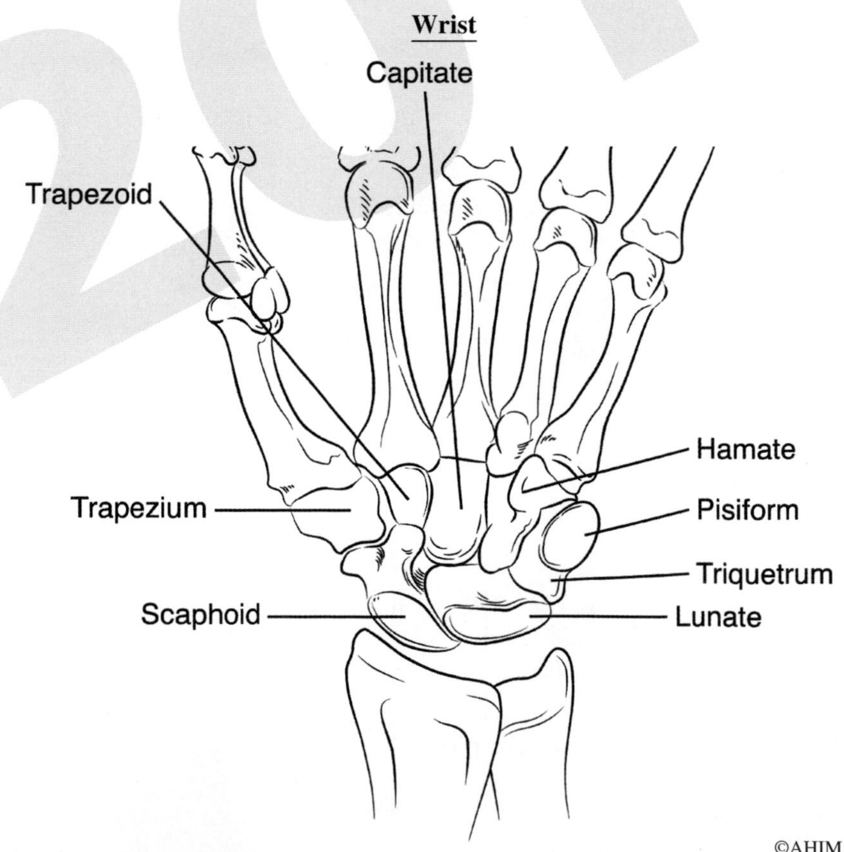
Capitate
Trapezoid
Hamate
Trapezium
Pisiform
Triquetrum
Scaphoid
Lunate
©AHIMA

ection 0 **Medical and Surgical**
ody System R **Upper Joints**
peration 2 **Change:** Taking out or off a device from a body part and putting back an identical or similar device in or on the same body part without cutting or puncturing the skin or a mucous membrane

Body Part (4th)	Approach (5th)	Device (6th)	Qualifier (7th)
Y Upper Joint	**X** External	**0** Drainage Device **Y** Other Device	**Z** No Qualifier

ection 0 **Medical and Surgical**
ody System R **Upper Joints**
peration 5 **Destruction:** Physical eradication of all or a portion of a body part by the direct use of energy, force, or a destructive agent

Body Part (4th)	Approach (5th)	Device (6th)	Qualifier (7th)
0 Occipital-cervical Joint **1** Cervical Vertebral Joint **3** Cervical Vertebral Disc **4** Cervicothoracic Vertebral Joint **5** Cervicothoracic Vertebral Disc **6** Thoracic Vertebral Joint **9** Thoracic Vertebral Disc **A** Thoracolumbar Vertebral Joint **B** Thoracolumbar Vertebral Disc **C** Temporomandibular Joint, Right **D** Temporomandibular Joint, Left **E** Sternoclavicular Joint, Right **F** Sternoclavicular Joint, Left **G** Acromioclavicular Joint, Right **H** Acromioclavicular Joint, Left **J** Shoulder Joint, Right **K** Shoulder Joint, Left **L** Elbow Joint, Right **M** Elbow Joint, Left **N** Wrist Joint, Right **P** Wrist Joint, Left **Q** Carpal Joint, Right **R** Carpal Joint, Left **S** Metacarpocarpal Joint, Right **T** Metacarpocarpal Joint, Left **U** Metacarpophalangeal Joint, Right **V** Metacarpophalangeal Joint, Left **W** Finger Phalangeal Joint, Right **X** Finger Phalangeal Joint, Left	**0** Open **3** Percutaneous **4** Percutaneous Endoscopic	**Z** No Device	**Z** No Qualifier

Section **0** **Medical and Surgical**
Body System **R** **Upper Joints**
Operation **9** **Drainage:** Taking or letting out fluids and/or gases from a body part

Body Part (4th)	Approach (5th)	Device (6th)	Qualifier (7th)
0 Occipital-cervical Joint **1** Cervical Vertebral Joint **3** Cervical Vertebral Disc **4** Cervicothoracic Vertebral Joint **5** Cervicothoracic Vertebral Disc **6** Thoracic Vertebral Joint **9** Thoracic Vertebral Disc **A** Thoracolumbar Vertebral Joint **B** Thoracolumbar Vertebral Disc **C** Temporomandibular Joint, Right **D** Temporomandibular Joint, Left **E** Sternoclavicular Joint, Right **F** Sternoclavicular Joint, Left **G** Acromioclavicular Joint, Right **H** Acromioclavicular Joint, Left **J** Shoulder Joint, Right **K** Shoulder Joint, Left **L** Elbow Joint, Right **M** Elbow Joint, Left **N** Wrist Joint, Right **P** Wrist Joint, Left **Q** Carpal Joint, Right **R** Carpal Joint, Left **S** Metacarpocarpal Joint, Right **T** Metacarpocarpal Joint, Left **U** Metacarpophalangeal Joint, Right **V** Metacarpophalangeal Joint, Left **W** Finger Phalangeal Joint, Right **X** Finger Phalangeal Joint, Left	**0** Open **3** Percutaneous **4** Percutaneous Endoscopic	**0** Drainage Device	**Z** No Qualifier
0 Occipital-cervical Joint **1** Cervical Vertebral Joint **3** Cervical Vertebral Disc **4** Cervicothoracic Vertebral Joint **5** Cervicothoracic Vertebral Disc **6** Thoracic Vertebral Joint **9** Thoracic Vertebral Disc **A** Thoracolumbar Vertebral Joint **B** Thoracolumbar Vertebral Disc **C** Temporomandibular Joint, Right **D** Temporomandibular Joint, Left **E** Sternoclavicular Joint, Right **F** Sternoclavicular Joint, Left **G** Acromioclavicular Joint, Right **H** Acromioclavicular Joint, Left **J** Shoulder Joint, Right **K** Shoulder Joint, Left **L** Elbow Joint, Right **M** Elbow Joint, Left **N** Wrist Joint, Right **P** Wrist Joint, Left **Q** Carpal Joint, Right **R** Carpal Joint, Left **S** Metacarpocarpal Joint, Right **T** Metacarpocarpal Joint, Left **U** Metacarpophalangeal Joint, Right **V** Metacarpophalangeal Joint, Left **W** Finger Phalangeal Joint, Right **X** Finger Phalangeal Joint, Left	**0** Open **3** Percutaneous **4** Percutaneous Endoscopic	**Z** No Device	**X** Diagnostic **Z** No Qualifier

Section 0 Medical and Surgical
Body System R Upper Joints
Operation B **Excision:** Cutting out or off, without replacement, a portion of a body part

Body Part (4th)	Approach (5th)	Device (6th)	Qualifier (7th)
0 Occipital-cervical Joint **1** Cervical Vertebral Joint **3** Cervical Vertebral Disc **4** Cervicothoracic Vertebral Joint **5** Cervicothoracic Vertebral Disc **6** Thoracic Vertebral Joint **9** Thoracic Vertebral Disc **A** Thoracolumbar Vertebral Joint **B** Thoracolumbar Vertebral Disc **C** Temporomandibular Joint, Right **D** Temporomandibular Joint, Left **E** Sternoclavicular Joint, Right **F** Sternoclavicular Joint, Left **G** Acromioclavicular Joint, Right **H** Acromioclavicular Joint, Left **J** Shoulder Joint, Right **K** Shoulder Joint, Left **L** Elbow Joint, Right **M** Elbow Joint, Left **N** Wrist Joint, Right **P** Wrist Joint, Left **Q** Carpal Joint, Right **R** Carpal Joint, Left **S** Metacarpocarpal Joint, Right **T** Metacarpocarpal Joint, Left **U** Metacarpophalangeal Joint, Right **V** Metacarpophalangeal Joint, Left **W** Finger Phalangeal Joint, Right **X** Finger Phalangeal Joint, Left	**0** Open **3** Percutaneous **4** Percutaneous Endoscopic	**Z** No Device	**X** Diagnostic **Z** No Qualifier

Section 0 **Medical and Surgical**
Body System R **Upper Joints**
Operation C **Extirpation:** Taking or cutting out solid matter from a body part

Body Part (4th)	Approach (5th)	Device (6th)	Qualifier (7th)
0 Occipital-cervical Joint **1** Cervical Vertebral Joint **3** Cervical Vertebral Disc **4** Cervicothoracic Vertebral Joint **5** Cervicothoracic Vertebral Disc **6** Thoracic Vertebral Joint **9** Thoracic Vertebral Disc **A** Thoracolumbar Vertebral Joint **B** Thoracolumbar Vertebral Disc **C** Temporomandibular Joint, Right **D** Temporomandibular Joint, Left **E** Sternoclavicular Joint, Right **F** Sternoclavicular Joint, Left **G** Acromioclavicular Joint, Right **H** Acromioclavicular Joint, Left **J** Shoulder Joint, Right **K** Shoulder Joint, Left **L** Elbow Joint, Right **M** Elbow Joint, Left **N** Wrist Joint, Right **P** Wrist Joint, Left **Q** Carpal Joint, Right **R** Carpal Joint, Left **S** Metacarpocarpal Joint, Right **T** Metacarpocarpal Joint, Left **U** Metacarpophalangeal Joint, Right **V** Metacarpophalangeal Joint, Left **W** Finger Phalangeal Joint, Right **X** Finger Phalangeal Joint, Left	**0** Open **3** Percutaneous **4** Percutaneous Endoscopic	**Z** No Device	**Z** No Qualifier

Section 0 **Medical and Surgical**
Body System R **Upper Joints**
Operation G **Fusion:** Joining together portions of an articular body part rendering the articular body part immobile

Body Part (4th)	Approach (5th)	Device (6th)	Qualifier (7th)
0 Occipital-cervical Joint **1** Cervical Vertebral Joint **2** Cervical Vertebral Joints, 2 or more **4** Cervicothoracic Vertebral Joint **6** Thoracic Vertebral Joint **7** Thoracic Vertebral Joints, 2 to 7 **8** Thoracic Vertebral Joints, 8 or more **A** Thoracolumbar Vertebral Joint	**0** Open **3** Percutaneous **4** Percutaneous Endoscopic	**7** Autologous Tissue Substitute **A** Interbody Fusion Device **J** Synthetic Substitute **K** Nonautologous Tissue Substitute **Z** No Device	**0** Anterior Approach, Anterior Column **1** Posterior Approach, Posterior Column **J** Posterior Approach, Anterior Column
C Temporomandibular Joint, Right **D** Temporomandibular Joint, Left **E** Sternoclavicular Joint, Right **F** Sternoclavicular Joint, Left **G** Acromioclavicular Joint, Right **H** Acromioclavicular Joint, Left **J** Shoulder Joint, Right **K** Shoulder Joint, Left	**0** Open **3** Percutaneous **4** Percutaneous Endoscopic	**4** Internal Fixation Device **7** Autologous Tissue Substitute **J** Synthetic Substitute **K** Nonautologous Tissue Substitute **Z** No Device	**Z** No Qualifier

Continued →

Section 0 Medical and Surgical
Body System R Upper Joints
Operation G **Fusion:** Joining together portions of an articular body part rendering the articular body part immobile

Body Part (4th)	Approach (5th)	Device (6th)	Qualifier (7th)
L Elbow Joint, Right **M** Elbow Joint, Left **N** Wrist Joint, Right **P** Wrist Joint, Left **Q** Carpal Joint, Right **R** Carpal Joint, Left **S** Metacarpocarpal Joint, Right **T** Metacarpocarpal Joint, Left **U** Metacarpophalangeal Joint, Right **V** Metacarpophalangeal Joint, Left **W** Finger Phalangeal Joint, Right **X** Finger Phalangeal Joint, Left	**0** Open **3** Percutaneous **4** Percutaneous Endoscopic	**4** Internal Fixation Device **5** External Fixation Device **7** Autologous Tissue Substitute **J** Synthetic Substitute **K** Nonautologous Tissue Substitute **Z** No Device	**Z** No Qualifier

Section 0 Medical and Surgical
Body System R Upper Joints
Operation H **Insertion:** Putting in a nonbiological appliance that monitors, assists, performs, or prevents a physiological function but does not physically take the place of a body part

Body Part (4th)	Approach (5th)	Device (6th)	Qualifier (7th)
0 Occipital-cervical Joint **1** Cervical Vertebral Joint **4** Cervicothoracic Vertebral Joint **6** Thoracic Vertebral Joint **A** Thoracolumbar Vertebral Joint	**0** Open **3** Percutaneous **4** Percutaneous Endoscopic	**3** Infusion Device **4** Internal Fixation Device **8** Spacer **B** Spinal Stabilization Device, Interspinous Process **C** Spinal Stabilization Device, Pedicle-Based **D** Spinal Stabilization Device, Facet Replacement	**Z** No Qualifier
3 Cervical Vertebral Disc **5** Cervicothoracic Vertebral Disc **9** Thoracic Vertebral Disc **B** Thoracolumbar Vertebral Disc	**0** Open **3** Percutaneous **4** Percutaneous Endoscopic	**3** Infusion Device	**Z** No Qualifier
C Temporomandibular Joint, Right **D** Temporomandibular Joint, Left **E** Sternoclavicular Joint, Right **F** Sternoclavicular Joint, Left **G** Acromioclavicular Joint, Right **H** Acromioclavicular Joint, Left **J** Shoulder Joint, Right **K** Shoulder Joint, Left	**0** Open **3** Percutaneous **4** Percutaneous Endoscopic	**3** Infusion Device **4** Internal Fixation Device **8** Spacer	**Z** No Qualifier
L Elbow Joint, Right **M** Elbow Joint, Left **N** Wrist Joint, Right **P** Wrist Joint, Left **Q** Carpal Joint, Right **R** Carpal Joint, Left **S** Metacarpocarpal Joint, Right **T** Metacarpocarpal Joint, Left **U** Metacarpophalangeal Joint, Right **V** Metacarpophalangeal Joint, Left **W** Finger Phalangeal Joint, Right **X** Finger Phalangeal Joint, Left	**0** Open **3** Percutaneous **4** Percutaneous Endoscopic	**3** Infusion Device **4** Internal Fixation Device **5** External Fixation Device **8** Spacer	**Z** No Qualifier

Section 0 **Medical and Surgical**
Body System R **Upper Joints**
Operation J **Inspection:** Visually and/or manually exploring a body part

Body Part (4th)	Approach (5th)	Device (6th)	Qualifier (7th)
0 Occipital-cervical Joint **1** Cervical Vertebral Joint **3** Cervical Vertebral Disc **4** Cervicothoracic Vertebral Joint **5** Cervicothoracic Vertebral Disc **6** Thoracic Vertebral Joint **9** Thoracic Vertebral Disc **A** Thoracolumbar Vertebral Joint **B** Thoracolumbar Vertebral Disc **C** Temporomandibular Joint, Right **D** Temporomandibular Joint, Left **E** Sternoclavicular Joint, Right **F** Sternoclavicular Joint, Left **G** Acromioclavicular Joint, Right **H** Acromioclavicular Joint, Left **J** Shoulder Joint, Right **K** Shoulder Joint, Left **L** Elbow Joint, Right **M** Elbow Joint, Left **N** Wrist Joint, Right **P** Wrist Joint, Left **Q** Carpal Joint, Right **R** Carpal Joint, Left **S** Metacarpocarpal Joint, Right **T** Metacarpocarpal Joint, Left **U** Metacarpophalangeal Joint, Right **V** Metacarpophalangeal Joint, Left **W** Finger Phalangeal Joint, Right **X** Finger Phalangeal Joint, Left	**0** Open **3** Percutaneous **4** Percutaneous Endoscopic **X** External	**Z** No Device	**Z** No Qualifier

Section 0 **Medical and Surgical**
Body System R **Upper Joints**
Operation N **Release:** Freeing a body part from an abnormal physical constraint by cutting or by the use of force

Body Part (4th)	Approach (5th)	Device (6th)	Qualifier (7th)
0 Occipital-cervical Joint **1** Cervical Vertebral Joint **3** Cervical Vertebral Disc **4** Cervicothoracic Vertebral Joint **5** Cervicothoracic Vertebral Disc **6** Thoracic Vertebral Joint **9** Thoracic Vertebral Disc **A** Thoracolumbar Vertebral Joint **B** Thoracolumbar Vertebral Disc **C** Temporomandibular Joint, Right **D** Temporomandibular Joint, Left **E** Sternoclavicular Joint, Right **F** Sternoclavicular Joint, Left **G** Acromioclavicular Joint, Right **H** Acromioclavicular Joint, Left **J** Shoulder Joint, Right **K** Shoulder Joint, Left **L** Elbow Joint, Right **M** Elbow Joint, Left **N** Wrist Joint, Right **P** Wrist Joint, Left **Q** Carpal Joint, Right **R** Carpal Joint, Left **S** Metacarpocarpal Joint, Right **T** Metacarpocarpal Joint, Left **U** Metacarpophalangeal Joint, Right **V** Metacarpophalangeal Joint, Left **W** Finger Phalangeal Joint, Right **X** Finger Phalangeal Joint, Left	**0** Open **3** Percutaneous **4** Percutaneous Endoscopic **X** External	**Z** No Device	**Z** No Qualifier

ection	0	**Medical and Surgical**
ody System	R	**Upper Joints**
peration	P	**Removal:** Taking out or off a device from a body part

Body Part (4th)	Approach (5th)	Device (6th)	Qualifier (7th)
0 Occipital-cervical Joint **1** Cervical Vertebral Joint **4** Cervicothoracic Vertebral Joint **6** Thoracic Vertebral Joint **A** Thoracolumbar Vertebral Joint	**0** Open **3** Percutaneous **4** Percutaneous Endoscopic	**0** Drainage Device **3** Infusion Device **4** Internal Fixation Device **7** Autologous Tissue Substitute **8** Spacer **A** Interbody Fusion Device **J** Synthetic Substitute **K** Nonautologous Tissue Substitute	**Z** No Qualifier
0 Occipital-cervical Joint **1** Cervical Vertebral Joint **4** Cervicothoracic Vertebral Joint **6** Thoracic Vertebral Joint **A** Thoracolumbar Vertebral Joint	**X** External	**0** Drainage Device **3** Infusion Device **4** Internal Fixation Device	**Z** No Qualifier
3 Cervical Vertebral Disc **5** Cervicothoracic Vertebral Disc **9** Thoracic Vertebral Disc **B** Thoracolumbar Vertebral Disc	**0** Open **3** Percutaneous **4** Percutaneous Endoscopic	**0** Drainage Device **3** Infusion Device **7** Autologous Tissue Substitute **J** Synthetic Substitute **K** Nonautologous Tissue Substitute	**Z** No Qualifier
3 Cervical Vertebral Disc **5** Cervicothoracic Vertebral Disc **9** Thoracic Vertebral Disc **B** Thoracolumbar Vertebral Disc	**X** External	**0** Drainage Device **3** Infusion Device	**Z** No Qualifier
C Temporomandibular Joint, Right **D** Temporomandibular Joint, Left **E** Sternoclavicular Joint, Right **F** Sternoclavicular Joint, Left **G** Acromioclavicular Joint, Right **H** Acromioclavicular Joint, Left **J** Shoulder Joint, Right **K** Shoulder Joint, Left	**0** Open **3** Percutaneous **4** Percutaneous Endoscopic	**0** Drainage Device **3** Infusion Device **4** Internal Fixation Device **7** Autologous Tissue Substitute **8** Spacer **J** Synthetic Substitute **K** Nonautologous Tissue Substitute	**Z** No Qualifier
C Temporomandibular Joint, Right **D** Temporomandibular Joint, Left **E** Sternoclavicular Joint, Right **F** Sternoclavicular Joint, Left **G** Acromioclavicular Joint, Right **H** Acromioclavicular Joint, Left **J** Shoulder Joint, Right **K** Shoulder Joint, Left	**X** External	**0** Drainage Device **3** Infusion Device **4** Internal Fixation Device	**Z** No Qualifier
L Elbow Joint, Right **M** Elbow Joint, Left **N** Wrist Joint, Right **P** Wrist Joint, Left **Q** Carpal Joint, Right **R** Carpal Joint, Left **S** Metacarpocarpal Joint, Right **T** Metacarpocarpal Joint, Left **U** Metacarpophalangeal Joint, Right **V** Metacarpophalangeal Joint, Left **W** Finger Phalangeal Joint, Right **X** Finger Phalangeal Joint, Left	**0** Open **3** Percutaneous **4** Percutaneous Endoscopic	**0** Drainage Device **3** Infusion Device **4** Internal Fixation Device **5** External Fixation Device **7** Autologous Tissue Substitute **8** Spacer **J** Synthetic Substitute **K** Nonautologous Tissue Substitute	**Z** No Qualifier

Continued →

Section **0** **Medical and Surgical**
Body System **R** **Upper Joints**
Operation **P** **Removal:** Taking out or off a device from a body part

Body Part (4th)	Approach (5th)	Device (6th)	Qualifier (7th)
L Elbow Joint, Right **M** Elbow Joint, Left **N** Wrist Joint, Right **P** Wrist Joint, Left **Q** Carpal Joint, Right **R** Carpal Joint, Left **S** Metacarpocarpal Joint, Right **T** Metacarpocarpal Joint, Left **U** Metacarpophalangeal Joint, Right **V** Metacarpophalangeal Joint, Left **W** Finger Phalangeal Joint, Right **X** Finger Phalangeal Joint, Left	**X** External	**0** Drainage Device **3** Infusion Device **4** Internal Fixation Device **5** External Fixation Device	**Z** No Qualifier

Section **0** **Medical and Surgical**
Body System **R** **Upper Joints**
Operation **Q** **Repair:** Restoring, to the extent possible, a body part to its normal anatomic structure and function

Body Part (4th)	Approach (5th)	Device (6th)	Qualifier (7th)
0 Occipital-cervical Joint **1** Cervical Vertebral Joint **3** Cervical Vertebral Disc **4** Cervicothoracic Vertebral Joint **5** Cervicothoracic Vertebral Disc **6** Thoracic Vertebral Joint **9** Thoracic Vertebral Disc **A** Thoracolumbar Vertebral Joint **B** Thoracolumbar Vertebral Disc **C** Temporomandibular Joint, Right **D** Temporomandibular Joint, Left **E** Sternoclavicular Joint, Right **F** Sternoclavicular Joint, Left **G** Acromioclavicular Joint, Right **H** Acromioclavicular Joint, Left **J** Shoulder Joint, Right **K** Shoulder Joint, Left **L** Elbow Joint, Right **M** Elbow Joint, Left **N** Wrist Joint, Right **P** Wrist Joint, Left **Q** Carpal Joint, Right **R** Carpal Joint, Left **S** Metacarpocarpal Joint, Right **T** Metacarpocarpal Joint, Left **U** Metacarpophalangeal Joint, Right **V** Metacarpophalangeal Joint, Left **W** Finger Phalangeal Joint, Right **X** Finger Phalangeal Joint, Left	**0** Open **3** Percutaneous **4** Percutaneous Endoscopic **X** External	**Z** No Device	**Z** No Qualifier

Section 0 **Medical and Surgical**
Body System R **Upper Joints**
Operation R **Replacement:** Putting in or on biological or synthetic material that physically takes the place and/or function of all or a portion of a body part

Body Part (4th)	Approach (5th)	Device (6th)	Qualifier (7th)
0 Occipital-cervical Joint **1** Cervical Vertebral Joint **3** Cervical Vertebral Disc **4** Cervicothoracic Vertebral Joint **5** Cervicothoracic Vertebral Disc **6** Thoracic Vertebral Joint **9** Thoracic Vertebral Disc **A** Thoracolumbar Vertebral Joint **B** Thoracolumbar Vertebral Disc **C** Temporomandibular Joint, Right **D** Temporomandibular Joint, Left **E** Sternoclavicular Joint, Right **F** Sternoclavicular Joint, Left **G** Acromioclavicular Joint, Right **H** Acromioclavicular Joint, Left **L** Elbow Joint, Right **M** Elbow Joint, Left **N** Wrist Joint, Right **P** Wrist Joint, Left **Q** Carpal Joint, Right **R** Carpal Joint, Left **S** Metacarpocarpal Joint, Right **T** Metacarpocarpal Joint, Left **U** Metacarpophalangeal Joint, Right **V** Metacarpophalangeal Joint, Left **W** Finger Phalangeal Joint, Right **X** Finger Phalangeal Joint, Left	**0** Open	**7** Autologous Tissue Substitute **J** Synthetic Substitute **K** Nonautologous Tissue Substitute	**Z** No Qualifier
J Shoulder Joint, Right **K** Shoulder Joint, Left	**0** Open	**0** Synthetic Substitute, Reverse Ball and Socket **7** Autologous Tissue Substitute **K** Nonautologous Tissue Substitute	**Z** No Qualifier
J Shoulder Joint, Right **K** Shoulder Joint, Left	**0** Open	**J** Synthetic Substitute	**6** Humeral Surface **7** Glenoid Surface **Z** No Qualifier

Section 0 **Medical and Surgical**
Body System R **Upper Joints**
Operation S **Reposition:** Moving to its normal location, or other suitable location, all or a portion of a body part

Body Part (4th)	Approach (5th)	Device (6th)	Qualifier (7th)
0 Occipital-cervical Joint **1** Cervical Vertebral Joint **4** Cervicothoracic Vertebral Joint **6** Thoracic Vertebral Joint **A** Thoracolumbar Vertebral Joint **C** Temporomandibular Joint, Right **D** Temporomandibular Joint, Left **E** Sternoclavicular Joint, Right **F** Sternoclavicular Joint, Left **G** Acromioclavicular Joint, Right **H** Acromioclavicular Joint, Left **J** Shoulder Joint, Right **K** Shoulder Joint, Left	**0** Open **3** Percutaneous **4** Percutaneous Endoscopic **X** External	**4** Internal Fixation Device **Z** No Device	**Z** No Qualifier

Continued →

Section 0 **Medical and Surgical**
Body System R **Upper Joints**
Operation S **Reposition:** Moving to its normal location, or other suitable location, all or a portion of a body part

Body Part (4th)	Approach (5th)	Device (6th)	Qualifier (7th)
L Elbow Joint, Right **M** Elbow Joint, Left **N** Wrist Joint, Right **P** Wrist Joint, Left **Q** Carpal Joint, Right **R** Carpal Joint, Left **S** Metacarpocarpal Joint, Right **T** Metacarpocarpal Joint, Left **U** Metacarpophalangeal Joint, Right **V** Metacarpophalangeal Joint, Left **W** Finger Phalangeal Joint, Right **X** Finger Phalangeal Joint, Left	**0** Open **3** Percutaneous **4** Percutaneous Endoscopic **X** External	**4** Internal Fixation Device **5** External Fixation Device **Z** No Device	**Z** No Qualifier

Section 0 **Medical and Surgical**
Body System R **Upper Joints**
Operation T **Resection:** Cutting out or off, without replacement, all of a body part

Body Part (4th)	Approach (5th)	Device (6th)	Qualifier (7th)
3 Cervical Vertebral Disc **4** Cervicothoracic Vertebral Joint **5** Cervicothoracic Vertebral Disc **9** Thoracic Vertebral Disc **B** Thoracolumbar Vertebral Disc **C** Temporomandibular Joint, Right **D** Temporomandibular Joint, Left **E** Sternoclavicular Joint, Right **F** Sternoclavicular Joint, Left **G** Acromioclavicular Joint, Right **H** Acromioclavicular Joint, Left **J** Shoulder Joint, Right **K** Shoulder Joint, Left **L** Elbow Joint, Right **M** Elbow Joint, Left **N** Wrist Joint, Right **P** Wrist Joint, Left **Q** Carpal Joint, Right **R** Carpal Joint, Left **S** Metacarpocarpal Joint, Right **T** Metacarpocarpal Joint, Left **U** Metacarpophalangeal Joint, Right **V** Metacarpophalangeal Joint, Left **W** Finger Phalangeal Joint, Right **X** Finger Phalangeal Joint, Left	**0** Open	**Z** No Device	**Z** No Qualifier

Section 0 **Medical and Surgical**
Body System R **Upper Joints**
Operation U **Supplement:** Putting in or on biological or synthetic material that physically reinforces and/or augments the function of a portion of a body part

Body Part (4th)	Approach (5th)	Device (6th)	Qualifier (7th)
0 Occipital-cervical Joint **1** Cervical Vertebral Joint **3** Cervical Vertebral Disc **4** Cervicothoracic Vertebral Joint **5** Cervicothoracic Vertebral Disc **6** Thoracic Vertebral Joint **9** Thoracic Vertebral Disc **A** Thoracolumbar Vertebral Joint **B** Thoracolumbar Vertebral Disc **C** Temporomandibular Joint, Right **D** Temporomandibular Joint, Left **E** Sternoclavicular Joint, Right **F** Sternoclavicular Joint, Left **G** Acromioclavicular Joint, Right **H** Acromioclavicular Joint, Left **J** Shoulder Joint, Right **K** Shoulder Joint, Left **L** Elbow Joint, Right **M** Elbow Joint, Left **N** Wrist Joint, Right **P** Wrist Joint, Left **Q** Carpal Joint, Right **R** Carpal Joint, Left **S** Metacarpocarpal Joint, Right **T** Metacarpocarpal Joint, Left **U** Metacarpophalangeal Joint, Right **V** Metacarpophalangeal Joint, Left **W** Finger Phalangeal Joint, Right **X** Finger Phalangeal Joint, Left	**0** Open **3** Percutaneous **4** Percutaneous Endoscopic	**7** Autologous Tissue Substitute **J** Synthetic Substitute **K** Nonautologous Tissue Substitute	**Z** No Qualifier

Section 0 **Medical and Surgical**
Body System R **Upper Joints**
Operation W **Revision:** Correcting, to the extent possible, a portion of a malfunctioning device or the position of a displaced device

Body Part (4th)	Approach (5th)	Device (6th)	Qualifier (7th)
0 Occipital-cervical Joint **1** Cervical Vertebral Joint **4** Cervicothoracic Vertebral Joint **6** Thoracic Vertebral Joint **A** Thoracolumbar Vertebral Joint	**0** Open **3** Percutaneous **4** Percutaneous Endoscopic **X** External	**0** Drainage Device **3** Infusion Device **4** Internal Fixation Device **7** Autologous Tissue Substitute **8** Spacer **A** Interbody Fusion Device **J** Synthetic Substitute **K** Nonautologous Tissue Substitute	**Z** No Qualifier
3 Cervical Vertebral Disc **5** Cervicothoracic Vertebral Disc **9** Thoracic Vertebral Disc **B** Thoracolumbar Vertebral Disc	**0** Open **3** Percutaneous **4** Percutaneous Endoscopic **X** External	**0** Drainage Device **3** Infusion Device **7** Autologous Tissue Substitute **J** Synthetic Substitute **K** Nonautologous Tissue Substitute	**Z** No Qualifier
C Temporomandibular Joint, Right **D** Temporomandibular Joint, Left **E** Sternoclavicular Joint, Right **F** Sternoclavicular Joint, Left **G** Acromioclavicular Joint, Right **H** Acromioclavicular Joint, Left **J** Shoulder Joint, Right **K** Shoulder Joint, Left	**0** Open **3** Percutaneous **4** Percutaneous Endoscopic **X** External	**0** Drainage Device **3** Infusion Device **4** Internal Fixation Device **7** Autologous Tissue Substitute **8** Spacer **J** Synthetic Substitute **K** Nonautologous Tissue Substitute	**Z** No Qualifier

Continued →

Section 0 **Medical and Surgical**
Body System R **Upper Joints**
Operation W **Revision:** Correcting, to the extent possible, a portion of a malfunctioning device or the position of a displaced device

Body Part (4th)	Approach (5th)	Device (6th)	Qualifier (7th)
L Elbow Joint, Right **M** Elbow Joint, Left **N** Wrist Joint, Right **P** Wrist Joint, Left **Q** Carpal Joint, Right **R** Carpal Joint, Left **S** Metacarpocarpal Joint, Right **T** Metacarpocarpal Joint, Left **U** Metacarpophalangeal Joint, Right **V** Metacarpophalangeal Joint, Left **W** Finger Phalangeal Joint, Right **X** Finger Phalangeal Joint, Left	**0** Open **3** Percutaneous **4** Percutaneous Endoscopic **X** External	**0** Drainage Device **3** Infusion Device **4** Internal Fixation Device **5** External Fixation Device **7** Autologous Tissue Substitute **8** Spacer **J** Synthetic Substitute **K** Nonautologous Tissue Substitute	**Z** No Qualifier

Upper Joints Code Listing 0R2–0RW

Review Coding Guideline B4.5

0R2 – Upper Joints, Change

Review Coding Guideline B6.1c

0R2YX0Z Change Drainage Device in Upper Joint, External Approach

0R2YXYZ Change Other Device in Upper Joint, External Approach

0R5 – Upper Joints, Destruction

0R500ZZ Destruction of Occipital-cervical Joint, Open Approach
0R503ZZ Destruction of Occipital-cervical Joint, Percutaneous Approach
0R504ZZ Destruction of Occipital-cervical Joint, Percutaneous Endoscopic Approach
0R510ZZ Destruction of Cervical Vertebral Joint, Open Approach
0R513ZZ Destruction of Cervical Vertebral Joint, Percutaneous Approach
0R514ZZ Destruction of Cervical Vertebral Joint, Percutaneous Endoscopic Approach
0R530ZZ Destruction of Cervical Vertebral Disc, Open Approach
0R533ZZ Destruction of Cervical Vertebral Disc, Percutaneous Approach
0R534ZZ Destruction of Cervical Vertebral Disc, Percutaneous Endoscopic Approach
0R540ZZ Destruction of Cervicothoracic Vertebral Joint, Open Approach
0R543ZZ Destruction of Cervicothoracic Vertebral Joint, Percutaneous Approach
0R544ZZ Destruction of Cervicothoracic Vertebral Joint, Percutaneous Endoscopic Approach
0R550ZZ Destruction of Cervicothoracic Vertebral Disc, Open Approach
0R553ZZ Destruction of Cervicothoracic Vertebral Disc, Percutaneous Approach
0R554ZZ Destruction of Cervicothoracic Vertebral Disc, Percutaneous Endoscopic Approach
0R560ZZ Destruction of Thoracic Vertebral Joint, Open Approach
0R563ZZ Destruction of Thoracic Vertebral Joint, Percutaneous Approach
0R564ZZ Destruction of Thoracic Vertebral Joint, Percutaneous Endoscopic Approach
0R590ZZ Destruction of Thoracic Vertebral Disc, Open Approach
0R593ZZ Destruction of Thoracic Vertebral Disc, Percutaneous Approach
0R594ZZ Destruction of Thoracic Vertebral Disc, Percutaneous Endoscopic Approach
0R5A0ZZ Destruction of Thoracolumbar Vertebral Joint, Open Approach
0R5A3ZZ Destruction of Thoracolumbar Vertebral Joint, Percutaneous Approach
0R5A4ZZ Destruction of Thoracolumbar Vertebral Joint, Percutaneous Endoscopic Approach
0R5B0ZZ Destruction of Thoracolumbar Vertebral Disc, Open Approach
0R5B3ZZ Destruction of Thoracolumbar Vertebral Disc, Percutaneous Approach
0R5B4ZZ Destruction of Thoracolumbar Vertebral Disc, Percutaneous Endoscopic Approach
0R5C0ZZ Destruction of Right Temporomandibular Joint, Open Approach
0R5C3ZZ Destruction of Right Temporomandibular Joint, Percutaneous Approach
0R5C4ZZ Destruction of Right Temporomandibular Joint, Percutaneous Endoscopic Approach
0R5D0ZZ Destruction of Left Temporomandibular Joint, Open Approach
0R5D3ZZ Destruction of Left Temporomandibular Joint, Percutaneous Approach
0R5D4ZZ Destruction of Left Temporomandibular Joint, Percutaneous Endoscopic Approach
0R5E0ZZ Destruction of Right Sternoclavicular Joint, Open Approach
0R5E3ZZ Destruction of Right Sternoclavicular Joint, Percutaneous Approach
0R5E4ZZ Destruction of Right Sternoclavicular Joint, Percutaneous Endoscopic Approach
0R5F0ZZ Destruction of Left Sternoclavicular Joint, Open Approach
0R5F3ZZ Destruction of Left Sternoclavicular Joint, Percutaneous Approach
0R5F4ZZ Destruction of Left Sternoclavicular Joint, Percutaneous Endoscopic Approach
0R5G0ZZ Destruction of Right Acromioclavicular Joint, Open Approach
0R5G3ZZ Destruction of Right Acromioclavicular Joint, Percutaneous Approach
0R5G4ZZ Destruction of Right Acromioclavicular Joint, Percutaneous Endoscopic Approach
0R5H0ZZ Destruction of Left Acromioclavicular Joint, Open Approach
0R5H3ZZ Destruction of Left Acromioclavicular Joint, Percutaneous Approach
0R5H4ZZ Destruction of Left Acromioclavicular Joint, Percutaneous Endoscopic Approach
0R5J0ZZ Destruction of Right Shoulder Joint, Open Approach
0R5J3ZZ Destruction of Right Shoulder Joint, Percutaneous Approach
0R5J4ZZ Destruction of Right Shoulder Joint, Percutaneous Endoscopic Approach
0R5K0ZZ Destruction of Left Shoulder Joint, Open Approach
0R5K3ZZ Destruction of Left Shoulder Joint, Percutaneous Approach
0R5K4ZZ Destruction of Left Shoulder Joint, Percutaneous Endoscopic Approach
0R5L0ZZ Destruction of Right Elbow Joint, Open Approach
0R5L3ZZ Destruction of Right Elbow Joint, Percutaneous Approach
0R5L4ZZ Destruction of Right Elbow Joint, Percutaneous Endoscopic Approach
0R5M0ZZ Destruction of Left Elbow Joint, Open Approach
0R5M3ZZ Destruction of Left Elbow Joint, Percutaneous Approach
0R5M4ZZ Destruction of Left Elbow Joint, Percutaneous Endoscopic Approach
0R5N0ZZ Destruction of Right Wrist Joint, Open Approach
0R5N3ZZ Destruction of Right Wrist Joint, Percutaneous Approach
0R5N4ZZ Destruction of Right Wrist Joint, Percutaneous Endoscopic Approach

R5P0ZZ Destruction of Left Wrist Joint, Open Approach
R5P3ZZ Destruction of Left Wrist Joint, Percutaneous Approach
R5P4ZZ Destruction of Left Wrist Joint, Percutaneous Endoscopic Approach
R5Q0ZZ Destruction of Right Carpal Joint, Open Approach
R5Q3ZZ Destruction of Right Carpal Joint, Percutaneous Approach
R5Q4ZZ Destruction of Right Carpal Joint, Percutaneous Endoscopic Approach
R5R0ZZ Destruction of Left Carpal Joint, Open Approach
R5R3ZZ Destruction of Left Carpal Joint, Percutaneous Approach
R5R4ZZ Destruction of Left Carpal Joint, Percutaneous Endoscopic Approach
0R5S0ZZ Destruction of Right Metacarpocarpal Joint, Open Approach
0R5S3ZZ Destruction of Right Metacarpocarpal Joint, Percutaneous Approach
0R5S4ZZ Destruction of Right Metacarpocarpal Joint, Percutaneous Endoscopic Approach
0R5T0ZZ Destruction of Left Metacarpocarpal Joint, Open Approach
0R5T3ZZ Destruction of Left Metacarpocarpal Joint, Percutaneous Approach
0R5T4ZZ Destruction of Left Metacarpocarpal Joint, Percutaneous Endoscopic Approach
0R5U0ZZ Destruction of Right Metacarpophalangeal Joint, Open Approach
0R5U3ZZ Destruction of Right Metacarpophalangeal Joint, Percutaneous Approach
0R5U4ZZ Destruction of Right Metacarpophalangeal Joint, Percutaneous Endoscopic Approach
0R5V0ZZ Destruction of Left Metacarpophalangeal Joint, Open Approach
0R5V3ZZ Destruction of Left Metacarpophalangeal Joint, Percutaneous Approach
0R5V4ZZ Destruction of Left Metacarpophalangeal Joint, Percutaneous Endoscopic Approach
0R5W0ZZ Destruction of Right Finger Phalangeal Joint, Open Approach
0R5W3ZZ Destruction of Right Finger Phalangeal Joint, Percutaneous Approach
0R5W4ZZ Destruction of Right Finger Phalangeal Joint, Percutaneous Endoscopic Approach
0R5X0ZZ Destruction of Left Finger Phalangeal Joint, Open Approach
0R5X3ZZ Destruction of Left Finger Phalangeal Joint, Percutaneous Approach
0R5X4ZZ Destruction of Left Finger Phalangeal Joint, Percutaneous Endoscopic Approach

R9 – Upper Joints, Drainage

eview Coding Guidelines B3.4a and B3.4b

eview Coding Guideline B6.2

R9000Z Drainage of Occipital-cervical Joint with Drainage Device, Open Approach
R900ZX Drainage of Occipital-cervical Joint, Open Approach, Diagnostic
R900ZZ Drainage of Occipital-cervical Joint, Open Approach
R9030Z Drainage of Occipital-cervical Joint with Drainage Device, Percutaneous Approach
R903ZX Drainage of Occipital-cervical Joint, Percutaneous Approach, Diagnostic
R903ZZ Drainage of Occipital-cervical Joint, Percutaneous Approach
R9040Z Drainage of Occipital-cervical Joint with Drainage Device, Percutaneous Endoscopic Approach
R904ZX Drainage of Occipital-cervical Joint, Percutaneous Endoscopic Approach, Diagnostic
R904ZZ Drainage of Occipital-cervical Joint, Percutaneous Endoscopic Approach
R9100Z Drainage of Cervical Vertebral Joint with Drainage Device, Open Approach
R910ZX Drainage of Cervical Vertebral Joint, Open Approach, Diagnostic
R910ZZ Drainage of Cervical Vertebral Joint, Open Approach
R9130Z Drainage of Cervical Vertebral Joint with Drainage Device, Percutaneous Approach
R913ZX Drainage of Cervical Vertebral Joint, Percutaneous Approach, Diagnostic
R913ZZ Drainage of Cervical Vertebral Joint, Percutaneous Approach
R9140Z Drainage of Cervical Vertebral Joint with Drainage Device, Percutaneous Endoscopic Approach
R914ZX Drainage of Cervical Vertebral Joint, Percutaneous Endoscopic Approach, Diagnostic
0R914ZZ Drainage of Cervical Vertebral Joint, Percutaneous Endoscopic Approach
0R9300Z Drainage of Cervical Vertebral Disc with Drainage Device, Open Approach
0R930ZX Drainage of Cervical Vertebral Disc, Open Approach, Diagnostic
0R930ZZ Drainage of Cervical Vertebral Disc, Open Approach
0R9330Z Drainage of Cervical Vertebral Disc with Drainage Device, Percutaneous Approach
0R933ZX Drainage of Cervical Vertebral Disc, Percutaneous Approach, Diagnostic
0R933ZZ Drainage of Cervical Vertebral Disc, Percutaneous Approach
0R9340Z Drainage of Cervical Vertebral Disc with Drainage Device, Percutaneous Endoscopic Approach
0R934ZX Drainage of Cervical Vertebral Disc, Percutaneous Endoscopic Approach, Diagnostic
0R934ZZ Drainage of Cervical Vertebral Disc, Percutaneous Endoscopic Approach
0R9400Z Drainage of Cervicothoracic Vertebral Joint with Drainage Device, Open Approach
0R940ZX Drainage of Cervicothoracic Vertebral Joint, Open Approach, Diagnostic
0R940ZZ Drainage of Cervicothoracic Vertebral Joint, Open Approach
0R9430Z Drainage of Cervicothoracic Vertebral Joint with Drainage Device, Percutaneous Approach
0R943ZX Drainage of Cervicothoracic Vertebral Joint, Percutaneous Approach, Diagnostic
0R943ZZ Drainage of Cervicothoracic Vertebral Joint, Percutaneous Approach
0R9440Z Drainage of Cervicothoracic Vertebral Joint with Drainage Device, Percutaneous Endoscopic Approach
0R944ZX Drainage of Cervicothoracic Vertebral Joint, Percutaneous Endoscopic Approach, Diagnostic
0R944ZZ Drainage of Cervicothoracic Vertebral Joint, Percutaneous Endoscopic Approach
0R9500Z Drainage of Cervicothoracic Vertebral Disc with Drainage Device, Open Approach
0R950ZX Drainage of Cervicothoracic Vertebral Disc, Open Approach, Diagnostic
0R950ZZ Drainage of Cervicothoracic Vertebral Disc, Open Approach
0R9530Z Drainage of Cervicothoracic Vertebral Disc with Drainage Device, Percutaneous Approach
0R953ZX Drainage of Cervicothoracic Vertebral Disc, Percutaneous Approach, Diagnostic
0R953ZZ Drainage of Cervicothoracic Vertebral Disc, Percutaneous Approach
0R9540Z Drainage of Cervicothoracic Vertebral Disc with Drainage Device, Percutaneous Endoscopic Approach
0R954ZX Drainage of Cervicothoracic Vertebral Disc, Percutaneous Endoscopic Approach, Diagnostic
0R954ZZ Drainage of Cervicothoracic Vertebral Disc, Percutaneous Endoscopic Approach
0R9600Z Drainage of Thoracic Vertebral Joint with Drainage Device, Open Approach
0R960ZX Drainage of Thoracic Vertebral Joint, Open Approach, Diagnostic
0R960ZZ Drainage of Thoracic Vertebral Joint, Open Approach
0R9630Z Drainage of Thoracic Vertebral Joint with Drainage Device, Percutaneous Approach
0R963ZX Drainage of Thoracic Vertebral Joint, Percutaneous Approach, Diagnostic
0R963ZZ Drainage of Thoracic Vertebral Joint, Percutaneous Approach
0R9640Z Drainage of Thoracic Vertebral Joint with Drainage Device, Percutaneous Endoscopic Approach
0R964ZX Drainage of Thoracic Vertebral Joint, Percutaneous Endoscopic Approach, Diagnostic
0R964ZZ Drainage of Thoracic Vertebral Joint, Percutaneous Endoscopic Approach
0R9900Z Drainage of Thoracic Vertebral Disc with Drainage Device, Open Approach
0R990ZX Drainage of Thoracic Vertebral Disc, Open Approach, Diagnostic
0R990ZZ Drainage of Thoracic Vertebral Disc, Open Approach
0R9930Z Drainage of Thoracic Vertebral Disc with Drainage Device, Percutaneous Approach
0R993ZX Drainage of Thoracic Vertebral Disc, Percutaneous Approach, Diagnostic
0R993ZZ Drainage of Thoracic Vertebral Disc, Percutaneous Approach
0R9940Z Drainage of Thoracic Vertebral Disc with Drainage Device, Percutaneous Endoscopic Approach
0R994ZX Drainage of Thoracic Vertebral Disc, Percutaneous Endoscopic Approach, Diagnostic
0R994ZZ Drainage of Thoracic Vertebral Disc, Percutaneous Endoscopic Approach
0R9A00Z Drainage of Thoracolumbar Vertebral Joint with Drainage Device, Open Approach
0R9A0ZX Drainage of Thoracolumbar Vertebral Joint, Open Approach, Diagnostic
0R9A0ZZ Drainage of Thoracolumbar Vertebral Joint, Open Approach
0R9A30Z Drainage of Thoracolumbar Vertebral Joint with Drainage Device, Percutaneous Approach
0R9A3ZX Drainage of Thoracolumbar Vertebral Joint, Percutaneous Approach, Diagnostic

0R9A3ZZ Drainage of Thoracolumbar Vertebral Joint, Percutaneous Approach
0R9A40Z Drainage of Thoracolumbar Vertebral Joint with Drainage Device, Percutaneous Endoscopic Approach
0R9A4ZX Drainage of Thoracolumbar Vertebral Joint, Percutaneous Endoscopic Approach, Diagnostic
0R9A4ZZ Drainage of Thoracolumbar Vertebral Joint, Percutaneous Endoscopic Approach
0R9B00Z Drainage of Thoracolumbar Vertebral Disc with Drainage Device, Open Approach
0R9B0ZX Drainage of Thoracolumbar Vertebral Disc, Open Approach, Diagnostic
0R9B0ZZ Drainage of Thoracolumbar Vertebral Disc, Open Approach
0R9B30Z Drainage of Thoracolumbar Vertebral Disc with Drainage Device, Percutaneous Approach
0R9B3ZX Drainage of Thoracolumbar Vertebral Disc, Percutaneous Approach, Diagnostic
0R9B3ZZ Drainage of Thoracolumbar Vertebral Disc, Percutaneous Approach
0R9B40Z Drainage of Thoracolumbar Vertebral Disc with Drainage Device, Percutaneous Endoscopic Approach
0R9B4ZX Drainage of Thoracolumbar Vertebral Disc, Percutaneous Endoscopic Approach, Diagnostic
0R9B4ZZ Drainage of Thoracolumbar Vertebral Disc, Percutaneous Endoscopic Approach
0R9C00Z Drainage of Right Temporomandibular Joint with Drainage Device, Open Approach
0R9C0ZX Drainage of Right Temporomandibular Joint, Open Approach, Diagnostic
0R9C0ZZ Drainage of Right Temporomandibular Joint, Open Approach
0R9C30Z Drainage of Right Temporomandibular Joint with Drainage Device, Percutaneous Approach
0R9C3ZX Drainage of Right Temporomandibular Joint, Percutaneous Approach, Diagnostic
0R9C3ZZ Drainage of Right Temporomandibular Joint, Percutaneous Approach
0R9C40Z Drainage of Right Temporomandibular Joint with Drainage Device, Percutaneous Endoscopic Approach
0R9C4ZX Drainage of Right Temporomandibular Joint, Percutaneous Endoscopic Approach, Diagnostic
0R9C4ZZ Drainage of Right Temporomandibular Joint, Percutaneous Endoscopic Approach
0R9D00Z Drainage of Left Temporomandibular Joint with Drainage Device, Open Approach
0R9D0ZX Drainage of Left Temporomandibular Joint, Open Approach, Diagnostic
0R9D0ZZ Drainage of Left Temporomandibular Joint, Open Approach
0R9D30Z Drainage of Left Temporomandibular Joint with Drainage Device, Percutaneous Approach
0R9D3ZX Drainage of Left Temporomandibular Joint, Percutaneous Approach, Diagnostic
0R9D3ZZ Drainage of Left Temporomandibular Joint, Percutaneous Approach
0R9D40Z Drainage of Left Temporomandibular Joint with Drainage Device, Percutaneous Endoscopic Approach
0R9D4ZX Drainage of Left Temporomandibular Joint, Percutaneous Endoscopic Approach, Diagnostic
0R9D4ZZ Drainage of Left Temporomandibular Joint, Percutaneous Endoscopic Approach
0R9E00Z Drainage of Right Sternoclavicular Joint with Drainage Device, Open Approach
0R9E0ZX Drainage of Right Sternoclavicular Joint, Open Approach, Diagnostic
0R9E0ZZ Drainage of Right Sternoclavicular Joint, Open Approach
0R9E30Z Drainage of Right Sternoclavicular Joint with Drainage Device, Percutaneous Approach
0R9E3ZX Drainage of Right Sternoclavicular Joint, Percutaneous Approach, Diagnostic
0R9E3ZZ Drainage of Right Sternoclavicular Joint, Percutaneous Approach
0R9E40Z Drainage of Right Sternoclavicular Joint with Drainage Device, Percutaneous Endoscopic Approach
0R9E4ZX Drainage of Right Sternoclavicular Joint, Percutaneous Endoscopic Approach, Diagnostic
0R9E4ZZ Drainage of Right Sternoclavicular Joint, Percutaneous Endoscopic Approach
0R9F00Z Drainage of Left Sternoclavicular Joint with Drainage Device, Open Approach
0R9F0ZX Drainage of Left Sternoclavicular Joint, Open Approach, Diagnostic
0R9F0ZZ Drainage of Left Sternoclavicular Joint, Open Approach
0R9F30Z Drainage of Left Sternoclavicular Joint with Drainage Device, Percutaneous Approach
0R9F3ZX Drainage of Left Sternoclavicular Joint, Percutaneous Approach, Diagnostic
0R9F3ZZ Drainage of Left Sternoclavicular Joint, Percutaneous Approach
0R9F40Z Drainage of Left Sternoclavicular Joint with Drainage Device, Percutaneous Endoscopic Approach
0R9F4ZX Drainage of Left Sternoclavicular Joint, Percutaneous Endoscopic Approach, Diagnostic
0R9F4ZZ Drainage of Left Sternoclavicular Joint, Percutaneous Endoscopic Approach
0R9G00Z Drainage of Right Acromioclavicular Joint with Drainage Device, Open Approach
0R9G0ZX Drainage of Right Acromioclavicular Joint, Open Approach, Diagnostic
0R9G0ZZ Drainage of Right Acromioclavicular Joint, Open Approach
0R9G30Z Drainage of Right Acromioclavicular Joint with Drainage Device, Percutaneous Approach
0R9G3ZX Drainage of Right Acromioclavicular Joint, Percutaneous Approach, Diagnostic
0R9G3ZZ Drainage of Right Acromioclavicular Joint, Percutaneous Approach
0R9G40Z Drainage of Right Acromioclavicular Joint with Drainage Device, Percutaneous Endoscopic Approach
0R9G4ZX Drainage of Right Acromioclavicular Joint, Percutaneous Endoscopic Approach, Diagnostic
0R9G4ZZ Drainage of Right Acromioclavicular Joint, Percutaneous Endoscopic Approach
0R9H00Z Drainage of Left Acromioclavicular Joint with Drainage Device, Open Approach
0R9H0ZX Drainage of Left Acromioclavicular Joint, Open Approach, Diagnostic
0R9H0ZZ Drainage of Left Acromioclavicular Joint, Open Approach
0R9H30Z Drainage of Left Acromioclavicular Joint with Drainage Device, Percutaneous Approach
0R9H3ZX Drainage of Left Acromioclavicular Joint, Percutaneous Approach, Diagnostic
0R9H3ZZ Drainage of Left Acromioclavicular Joint, Percutaneous Approach
0R9H40Z Drainage of Left Acromioclavicular Joint with Drainage Device, Percutaneous Endoscopic Approach
0R9H4ZX Drainage of Left Acromioclavicular Joint, Percutaneous Endoscopic Approach, Diagnostic
0R9H4ZZ Drainage of Left Acromioclavicular Joint, Percutaneous Endoscopic Approach
0R9J00Z Drainage of Right Shoulder Joint with Drainage Device, Open Approach
0R9J0ZX Drainage of Right Shoulder Joint, Open Approach, Diagnostic
0R9J0ZZ Drainage of Right Shoulder Joint, Open Approach
0R9J30Z Drainage of Right Shoulder Joint with Drainage Device, Percutaneous Approach
0R9J3ZX Drainage of Right Shoulder Joint, Percutaneous Approach, Diagnostic
0R9J3ZZ Drainage of Right Shoulder Joint, Percutaneous Approach
0R9J40Z Drainage of Right Shoulder Joint with Drainage Device, Percutaneous Endoscopic Approach
0R9J4ZX Drainage of Right Shoulder Joint, Percutaneous Endoscopic Approach, Diagnostic
0R9J4ZZ Drainage of Right Shoulder Joint, Percutaneous Endoscopic Approach
0R9K00Z Drainage of Left Shoulder Joint with Drainage Device, Open Approach
0R9K0ZX Drainage of Left Shoulder Joint, Open Approach, Diagnostic
0R9K0ZZ Drainage of Left Shoulder Joint, Open Approach
0R9K30Z Drainage of Left Shoulder Joint with Drainage Device, Percutaneous Approach
0R9K3ZX Drainage of Left Shoulder Joint, Percutaneous Approach, Diagnostic
0R9K3ZZ Drainage of Left Shoulder Joint, Percutaneous Approach
0R9K40Z Drainage of Left Shoulder Joint with Drainage Device, Percutaneous Endoscopic Approach
0R9K4ZX Drainage of Left Shoulder Joint, Percutaneous Endoscopic Approach, Diagnostic
0R9K4ZZ Drainage of Left Shoulder Joint, Percutaneous Endoscopic Approach
0R9L00Z Drainage of Right Elbow Joint with Drainage Device, Open Approach
0R9L0ZX Drainage of Right Elbow Joint, Open Approach, Diagnostic
0R9L0ZZ Drainage of Right Elbow Joint, Open Approach
0R9L30Z Drainage of Right Elbow Joint with Drainage Device, Percutaneous Approach
0R9L3ZX Drainage of Right Elbow Joint, Percutaneous Approach, Diagnostic
0R9L3ZZ Drainage of Right Elbow Joint, Percutaneous Approach
0R9L40Z Drainage of Right Elbow Joint with Drainage Device, Percutaneous Endoscopic Approach
0R9L4ZX Drainage of Right Elbow Joint, Percutaneous Endoscopic Approach, Diagnostic
0R9L4ZZ Drainage of Right Elbow Joint, Percutaneous Endoscopic Approach
0R9M00Z Drainage of Left Elbow Joint with Drainage Device, Open Approach
0R9M0ZX Drainage of Left Elbow Joint, Open Approach, Diagnostic
0R9M0ZZ Drainage of Left Elbow Joint, Open Approach

R9M30Z Drainage of Left Elbow Joint with Drainage Device, Percutaneous Approach
R9M3ZX Drainage of Left Elbow Joint, Percutaneous Approach, Diagnostic
R9M3ZZ Drainage of Left Elbow Joint, Percutaneous Approach
R9M40Z Drainage of Left Elbow Joint with Drainage Device, Percutaneous Endoscopic Approach
R9M4ZX Drainage of Left Elbow Joint, Percutaneous Endoscopic Approach, Diagnostic
R9M4ZZ Drainage of Left Elbow Joint, Percutaneous Endoscopic Approach
R9N00Z Drainage of Right Wrist Joint with Drainage Device, Open Approach
R9N0ZX Drainage of Right Wrist Joint, Open Approach, Diagnostic
R9N0ZZ Drainage of Right Wrist Joint, Open Approach
R9N30Z Drainage of Right Wrist Joint with Drainage Device, Percutaneous Approach
R9N3ZX Drainage of Right Wrist Joint, Percutaneous Approach, Diagnostic
R9N3ZZ Drainage of Right Wrist Joint, Percutaneous Approach
R9N40Z Drainage of Right Wrist Joint with Drainage Device, Percutaneous Endoscopic Approach
R9N4ZX Drainage of Right Wrist Joint, Percutaneous Endoscopic Approach, Diagnostic
R9N4ZZ Drainage of Right Wrist Joint, Percutaneous Endoscopic Approach
R9P00Z Drainage of Left Wrist Joint with Drainage Device, Open Approach
R9P0ZX Drainage of Left Wrist Joint, Open Approach, Diagnostic
R9P0ZZ Drainage of Left Wrist Joint, Open Approach
R9P30Z Drainage of Left Wrist Joint with Drainage Device, Percutaneous Approach
R9P3ZX Drainage of Left Wrist Joint, Percutaneous Approach, Diagnostic
R9P3ZZ Drainage of Left Wrist Joint, Percutaneous Approach
R9P40Z Drainage of Left Wrist Joint with Drainage Device, Percutaneous Endoscopic Approach
R9P4ZX Drainage of Left Wrist Joint, Percutaneous Endoscopic Approach, Diagnostic
R9P4ZZ Drainage of Left Wrist Joint, Percutaneous Endoscopic Approach
R9Q00Z Drainage of Right Carpal Joint with Drainage Device, Open Approach
R9Q0ZX Drainage of Right Carpal Joint, Open Approach, Diagnostic
R9Q0ZZ Drainage of Right Carpal Joint, Open Approach
R9Q30Z Drainage of Right Carpal Joint with Drainage Device, Percutaneous Approach
R9Q3ZX Drainage of Right Carpal Joint, Percutaneous Approach, Diagnostic
R9Q3ZZ Drainage of Right Carpal Joint, Percutaneous Approach
R9Q40Z Drainage of Right Carpal Joint with Drainage Device, Percutaneous Endoscopic Approach
0R9Q4ZX Drainage of Right Carpal Joint, Percutaneous Endoscopic Approach, Diagnostic
0R9Q4ZZ Drainage of Right Carpal Joint, Percutaneous Endoscopic Approach
0R9R00Z Drainage of Left Carpal Joint with Drainage Device, Open Approach
0R9R0ZX Drainage of Left Carpal Joint, Open Approach, Diagnostic
0R9R0ZZ Drainage of Left Carpal Joint, Open Approach
0R9R30Z Drainage of Left Carpal Joint with Drainage Device, Percutaneous Approach
0R9R3ZX Drainage of Left Carpal Joint, Percutaneous Approach, Diagnostic
0R9R3ZZ Drainage of Left Carpal Joint, Percutaneous Approach
0R9R40Z Drainage of Left Carpal Joint with Drainage Device, Percutaneous Endoscopic Approach
0R9R4ZX Drainage of Left Carpal Joint, Percutaneous Endoscopic Approach, Diagnostic
0R9R4ZZ Drainage of Left Carpal Joint, Percutaneous Endoscopic Approach
0R9S00Z Drainage of Right Metacarpocarpal Joint with Drainage Device, Open Approach
0R9S0ZX Drainage of Right Metacarpocarpal Joint, Open Approach, Diagnostic
0R9S0ZZ Drainage of Right Metacarpocarpal Joint, Open Approach
0R9S30Z Drainage of Right Metacarpocarpal Joint with Drainage Device, Percutaneous Approach
0R9S3ZX Drainage of Right Metacarpocarpal Joint, Percutaneous Approach, Diagnostic
0R9S3ZZ Drainage of Right Metacarpocarpal Joint, Percutaneous Approach
0R9S40Z Drainage of Right Metacarpocarpal Joint with Drainage Device, Percutaneous Endoscopic Approach
0R9S4ZX Drainage of Right Metacarpocarpal Joint, Percutaneous Endoscopic Approach, Diagnostic
0R9S4ZZ Drainage of Right Metacarpocarpal Joint, Percutaneous Endoscopic Approach
0R9T00Z Drainage of Left Metacarpocarpal Joint with Drainage Device, Open Approach
0R9T0ZX Drainage of Left Metacarpocarpal Joint, Open Approach, Diagnostic
0R9T0ZZ Drainage of Left Metacarpocarpal Joint, Open Approach
0R9T30Z Drainage of Left Metacarpocarpal Joint with Drainage Device, Percutaneous Approach
0R9T3ZX Drainage of Left Metacarpocarpal Joint, Percutaneous Approach, Diagnostic
0R9T3ZZ Drainage of Left Metacarpocarpal Joint, Percutaneous Approach
0R9T40Z Drainage of Left Metacarpocarpal Joint with Drainage Device, Percutaneous Endoscopic Approach
0R9T4ZX Drainage of Left Metacarpocarpal Joint, Percutaneous Endoscopic Approach, Diagnostic
0R9T4ZZ Drainage of Left Metacarpocarpal Joint, Percutaneous Endoscopic Approach
0R9U00Z Drainage of Right Metacarpophalangeal Joint with Drainage Device, Open Approach
0R9U0ZX Drainage of Right Metacarpophalangeal Joint, Open Approach, Diagnostic
0R9U0ZZ Drainage of Right Metacarpophalangeal Joint, Open Approach
0R9U30Z Drainage of Right Metacarpophalangeal Joint with Drainage Device, Percutaneous Approach
0R9U3ZX Drainage of Right Metacarpophalangeal Joint, Percutaneous Approach, Diagnostic
0R9U3ZZ Drainage of Right Metacarpophalangeal Joint, Percutaneous Approach
0R9U40Z Drainage of Right Metacarpophalangeal Joint with Drainage Device, Percutaneous Endoscopic Approach
0R9U4ZX Drainage of Right Metacarpophalangeal Joint, Percutaneous Endoscopic Approach, Diagnostic
0R9U4ZZ Drainage of Right Metacarpophalangeal Joint, Percutaneous Endoscopic Approach
0R9V00Z Drainage of Left Metacarpophalangeal Joint with Drainage Device, Open Approach
0R9V0ZX Drainage of Left Metacarpophalangeal Joint, Open Approach, Diagnostic
0R9V0ZZ Drainage of Left Metacarpophalangeal Joint, Open Approach
0R9V30Z Drainage of Left Metacarpophalangeal Joint with Drainage Device, Percutaneous Approach
0R9V3ZX Drainage of Left Metacarpophalangeal Joint, Percutaneous Approach, Diagnostic
0R9V3ZZ Drainage of Left Metacarpophalangeal Joint, Percutaneous Approach
0R9V40Z Drainage of Left Metacarpophalangeal Joint with Drainage Device, Percutaneous Endoscopic Approach
0R9V4ZX Drainage of Left Metacarpophalangeal Joint, Percutaneous Endoscopic Approach, Diagnostic
0R9V4ZZ Drainage of Left Metacarpophalangeal Joint, Percutaneous Endoscopic Approach
0R9W00Z Drainage of Right Finger Phalangeal Joint with Drainage Device, Open Approach
0R9W0ZX Drainage of Right Finger Phalangeal Joint, Open Approach, Diagnostic
0R9W0ZZ Drainage of Right Finger Phalangeal Joint, Open Approach
0R9W30Z Drainage of Right Finger Phalangeal Joint with Drainage Device, Percutaneous Approach
0R9W3ZX Drainage of Right Finger Phalangeal Joint, Percutaneous Approach, Diagnostic
0R9W3ZZ Drainage of Right Finger Phalangeal Joint, Percutaneous Approach
0R9W40Z Drainage of Right Finger Phalangeal Joint with Drainage Device, Percutaneous Endoscopic Approach
0R9W4ZX Drainage of Right Finger Phalangeal Joint, Percutaneous Endoscopic Approach, Diagnostic
0R9W4ZZ Drainage of Right Finger Phalangeal Joint, Percutaneous Endoscopic Approach
0R9X00Z Drainage of Left Finger Phalangeal Joint with Drainage Device, Open Approach
0R9X0ZX Drainage of Left Finger Phalangeal Joint, Open Approach, Diagnostic
0R9X0ZZ Drainage of Left Finger Phalangeal Joint, Open Approach
0R9X30Z Drainage of Left Finger Phalangeal Joint with Drainage Device, Percutaneous Approach
0R9X3ZX Drainage of Left Finger Phalangeal Joint, Percutaneous Approach, Diagnostic
0R9X3ZZ Drainage of Left Finger Phalangeal Joint, Percutaneous Approach
0R9X40Z Drainage of Left Finger Phalangeal Joint with Drainage Device, Percutaneous Endoscopic Approach
0R9X4ZX Drainage of Left Finger Phalangeal Joint, Percutaneous Endoscopic Approach, Diagnostic
0R9X4ZZ Drainage of Left Finger Phalangeal Joint, Percutaneous Endoscopic Approach

0RB – Upper Joints, Excision

Review Coding Guidelines B3.4a and B3.4b

Review Coding Guideline B3.5

Review Coding Guideline B3.8

0RB00ZX Excision of Occipital-cervical Joint, Open Approach, Diagnostic
0RB00ZZ Excision of Occipital-cervical Joint, Open Approach
0RB03ZX Excision of Occipital-cervical Joint, Percutaneous Approach, Diagnostic
0RB03ZZ Excision of Occipital-cervical Joint, Percutaneous Approach
0RB04ZX Excision of Occipital-cervical Joint, Percutaneous Endoscopic Approach, Diagnostic
0RB04ZZ Excision of Occipital-cervical Joint, Percutaneous Endoscopic Approach
0RB10ZX Excision of Cervical Vertebral Joint, Open Approach, Diagnostic
0RB10ZZ Excision of Cervical Vertebral Joint, Open Approach
0RB13ZX Excision of Cervical Vertebral Joint, Percutaneous Approach, Diagnostic
0RB13ZZ Excision of Cervical Vertebral Joint, Percutaneous Approach
0RB14ZX Excision of Cervical Vertebral Joint, Percutaneous Endoscopic Approach, Diagnostic
0RB14ZZ Excision of Cervical Vertebral Joint, Percutaneous Endoscopic Approach
0RB30ZX Excision of Cervical Vertebral Disc, Open Approach, Diagnostic
0RB30ZZ Excision of Cervical Vertebral Disc, Open Approach
0RB33ZX Excision of Cervical Vertebral Disc, Percutaneous Approach, Diagnostic
0RB33ZZ Excision of Cervical Vertebral Disc, Percutaneous Approach
0RB34ZX Excision of Cervical Vertebral Disc, Percutaneous Endoscopic Approach, Diagnostic
0RB34ZZ Excision of Cervical Vertebral Disc, Percutaneous Endoscopic Approach
0RB40ZX Excision of Cervicothoracic Vertebral Joint, Open Approach, Diagnostic
0RB40ZZ Excision of Cervicothoracic Vertebral Joint, Open Approach
0RB43ZX Excision of Cervicothoracic Vertebral Joint, Percutaneous Approach, Diagnostic
0RB43ZZ Excision of Cervicothoracic Vertebral Joint, Percutaneous Approach
0RB44ZX Excision of Cervicothoracic Vertebral Joint, Percutaneous Endoscopic Approach, Diagnostic
0RB44ZZ Excision of Cervicothoracic Vertebral Joint, Percutaneous Endoscopic Approach
0RB50ZX Excision of Cervicothoracic Vertebral Disc, Open Approach, Diagnostic
0RB50ZZ Excision of Cervicothoracic Vertebral Disc, Open Approach
0RB53ZX Excision of Cervicothoracic Vertebral Disc, Percutaneous Approach, Diagnostic
0RB53ZZ Excision of Cervicothoracic Vertebral Disc, Percutaneous Approach
0RB54ZX Excision of Cervicothoracic Vertebral Disc, Percutaneous Endoscopic Approach, Diagnostic
0RB54ZZ Excision of Cervicothoracic Vertebral Disc, Percutaneous Endoscopic Approach
0RB60ZX Excision of Thoracic Vertebral Joint, Open Approach, Diagnostic
0RB60ZZ Excision of Thoracic Vertebral Joint, Open Approach
0RB63ZX Excision of Thoracic Vertebral Joint, Percutaneous Approach, Diagnostic
0RB63ZZ Excision of Thoracic Vertebral Joint, Percutaneous Approach
0RB64ZX Excision of Thoracic Vertebral Joint, Percutaneous Endoscopic Approach, Diagnostic
0RB64ZZ Excision of Thoracic Vertebral Joint, Percutaneous Endoscopic Approach
0RB90ZX Excision of Thoracic Vertebral Disc, Open Approach, Diagnostic
0RB90ZZ Excision of Thoracic Vertebral Disc, Open Approach
0RB93ZX Excision of Thoracic Vertebral Disc, Percutaneous Approach, Diagnostic
0RB93ZZ Excision of Thoracic Vertebral Disc, Percutaneous Approach
0RB94ZX Excision of Thoracic Vertebral Disc, Percutaneous Endoscopic Approach, Diagnostic
0RB94ZZ Excision of Thoracic Vertebral Disc, Percutaneous Endoscopic Approach
0RBA0ZX Excision of Thoracolumbar Vertebral Joint, Open Approach, Diagnostic
0RBA0ZZ Excision of Thoracolumbar Vertebral Joint, Open Approach
0RBA3ZX Excision of Thoracolumbar Vertebral Joint, Percutaneous Approach, Diagnostic
0RBA3ZZ Excision of Thoracolumbar Vertebral Joint, Percutaneous Approach
0RBA4ZX Excision of Thoracolumbar Vertebral Joint, Percutaneous Endoscopic Approach, Diagnostic
0RBA4ZZ Excision of Thoracolumbar Vertebral Joint, Percutaneous Endoscopic Approach
0RBB0ZX Excision of Thoracolumbar Vertebral Disc, Open Approach, Diagnostic
0RBB0ZZ Excision of Thoracolumbar Vertebral Disc, Open Approach
0RBB3ZX Excision of Thoracolumbar Vertebral Disc, Percutaneous Approach, Diagnostic
0RBB3ZZ Excision of Thoracolumbar Vertebral Disc, Percutaneous Approach
0RBB4ZX Excision of Thoracolumbar Vertebral Disc, Percutaneous Endoscopic Approach, Diagnostic
0RBB4ZZ Excision of Thoracolumbar Vertebral Disc, Percutaneous Endoscopic Approach
0RBC0ZX Excision of Right Temporomandibular Joint, Open Approach, Diagnostic
0RBC0ZZ Excision of Right Temporomandibular Joint, Open Approach
0RBC3ZX Excision of Right Temporomandibular Joint, Percutaneous Approach, Diagnostic
0RBC3ZZ Excision of Right Temporomandibular Joint, Percutaneous Approach
0RBC4ZX Excision of Right Temporomandibular Joint, Percutaneous Endoscopic Approach, Diagnostic
0RBC4ZZ Excision of Right Temporomandibular Joint, Percutaneous Endoscopic Approach
0RBD0ZX Excision of Left Temporomandibular Joint, Open Approach, Diagnostic
0RBD0ZZ Excision of Left Temporomandibular Joint, Open Approach
0RBD3ZX Excision of Left Temporomandibular Joint, Percutaneous Approach, Diagnostic
0RBD3ZZ Excision of Left Temporomandibular Joint, Percutaneous Approach
0RBD4ZX Excision of Left Temporomandibular Joint, Percutaneous Endoscopic Approach, Diagnostic
0RBD4ZZ Excision of Left Temporomandibular Joint, Percutaneous Endoscopic Approac
0RBE0ZX Excision of Right Sternoclavicular Joint Open Approach, Diagnostic
0RBE0ZZ Excision of Right Sternoclavicular Joint Open Approach
0RBE3ZX Excision of Right Sternoclavicular Joint, Percutaneous Approach, Diagnostic
0RBE3ZZ Excision of Right Sternoclavicular Joint, Percutaneous Approach
0RBE4ZX Excision of Right Sternoclavicular Joint, Percutaneous Endoscopic Approach, Diagnostic
0RBE4ZZ Excision of Right Sternoclavicular Joint, Percutaneous Endoscopic Approach
0RBF0ZX Excision of Left Sternoclavicular Joint, Open Approach, Diagnostic
0RBF0ZZ Excision of Left Sternoclavicular Joint, Open Approach
0RBF3ZX Excision of Left Sternoclavicular Joint, Percutaneous Approach, Diagnostic
0RBF3ZZ Excision of Left Sternoclavicular Joint, Percutaneous Approach
0RBF4ZX Excision of Left Sternoclavicular Joint, Percutaneous Endoscopic Approach, Diagnostic
0RBF4ZZ Excision of Left Sternoclavicular Joint, Percutaneous Endoscopic Approach
0RBG0ZX Excision of Right Acromioclavicular Joint, Open Approach, Diagnostic
0RBG0ZZ Excision of Right Acromioclavicular Joint, Open Approach
0RBG3ZX Excision of Right Acromioclavicular Joint, Percutaneous Approach, Diagnosti
0RBG3ZZ Excision of Right Acromioclavicular Joint, Percutaneous Approach
0RBG4ZX Excision of Right Acromioclavicular Joint, Percutaneous Endoscopic Approach, Diagnostic
0RBG4ZZ Excision of Right Acromioclavicular Joint, Percutaneous Endoscopic Approach
0RBH0ZX Excision of Left Acromioclavicular Joint, Open Approach, Diagnostic
0RBH0ZZ Excision of Left Acromioclavicular Joint, Open Approach
0RBH3ZX Excision of Left Acromioclavicular Joint, Percutaneous Approach, Diagnostic
0RBII3ZZ Excision of Lcft Acromioclavicular Joint, Percutaneous Approach
0RBH4ZX Excision of Left Acromioclavicular Joint, Percutaneous Endoscopic Approach, Diagnostic
0RBH4ZZ Excision of Left Acromioclavicular Joint, Percutaneous Endoscopic Approach
0RBJ0ZX Excision of Right Shoulder Joint, Open Approach, Diagnostic
0RBJ0ZZ Excision of Right Shoulder Joint, Open Approach
0RBJ3ZX Excision of Right Shoulder Joint, Percutaneous Approach, Diagnostic
0RBJ3ZZ Excision of Right Shoulder Joint, Percutaneous Approach
0RBJ4ZX Excision of Right Shoulder Joint, Percutaneous Endoscopic Approach, Diagnostic
0RBJ4ZZ Excision of Right Shoulder Joint, Percutaneous Endoscopic Approach

RBK0ZX Excision of Left Shoulder Joint, Open Approach, Diagnostic
RBK0ZZ Excision of Left Shoulder Joint, Open Approach
RBK3ZX Excision of Left Shoulder Joint, Percutaneous Approach, Diagnostic
RBK3ZZ Excision of Left Shoulder Joint, Percutaneous Approach
RBK4ZX Excision of Left Shoulder Joint, Percutaneous Endoscopic Approach, Diagnostic
RBK4ZZ Excision of Left Shoulder Joint, Percutaneous Endoscopic Approach
RBL0ZX Excision of Right Elbow Joint, Open Approach, Diagnostic
RBL0ZZ Excision of Right Elbow Joint, Open Approach
RBL3ZX Excision of Right Elbow Joint, Percutaneous Approach, Diagnostic
RBL3ZZ Excision of Right Elbow Joint, Percutaneous Approach
RBL4ZX Excision of Right Elbow Joint, Percutaneous Endoscopic Approach, Diagnostic
RBL4ZZ Excision of Right Elbow Joint, Percutaneous Endoscopic Approach
RBM0ZX Excision of Left Elbow Joint, Open Approach, Diagnostic
RBM0ZZ Excision of Left Elbow Joint, Open Approach
RBM3ZX Excision of Left Elbow Joint, Percutaneous Approach, Diagnostic
RBM3ZZ Excision of Left Elbow Joint, Percutaneous Approach
RBM4ZX Excision of Left Elbow Joint, Percutaneous Endoscopic Approach, Diagnostic
RBM4ZZ Excision of Left Elbow Joint, Percutaneous Endoscopic Approach
RBN0ZX Excision of Right Wrist Joint, Open Approach, Diagnostic
RBN0ZZ Excision of Right Wrist Joint, Open Approach
RBN3ZX Excision of Right Wrist Joint, Percutaneous Approach, Diagnostic
RBN3ZZ Excision of Right Wrist Joint, Percutaneous Approach
RBN4ZX Excision of Right Wrist Joint, Percutaneous Endoscopic Approach, Diagnostic
RBN4ZZ Excision of Right Wrist Joint, Percutaneous Endoscopic Approach
RBP0ZX Excision of Left Wrist Joint, Open Approach, Diagnostic
RBP0ZZ Excision of Left Wrist Joint, Open Approach
RBP3ZX Excision of Left Wrist Joint, Percutaneous Approach, Diagnostic
0RBP3ZZ Excision of Left Wrist Joint, Percutaneous Approach
0RBP4ZX Excision of Left Wrist Joint, Percutaneous Endoscopic Approach, Diagnostic
0RBP4ZZ Excision of Left Wrist Joint, Percutaneous Endoscopic Approach
0RBQ0ZX Excision of Right Carpal Joint, Open Approach, Diagnostic
0RBQ0ZZ Excision of Right Carpal Joint, Open Approach
0RBQ3ZX Excision of Right Carpal Joint, Percutaneous Approach, Diagnostic
0RBQ3ZZ Excision of Right Carpal Joint, Percutaneous Approach
0RBQ4ZX Excision of Right Carpal Joint, Percutaneous Endoscopic Approach, Diagnostic
0RBQ4ZZ Excision of Right Carpal Joint, Percutaneous Endoscopic Approach
0RBR0ZX Excision of Left Carpal Joint, Open Approach, Diagnostic
0RBR0ZZ Excision of Left Carpal Joint, Open Approach
0RBR3ZX Excision of Left Carpal Joint, Percutaneous Approach, Diagnostic
0RBR3ZZ Excision of Left Carpal Joint, Percutaneous Approach
0RBR4ZX Excision of Left Carpal Joint, Percutaneous Endoscopic Approach, Diagnostic
0RBR4ZZ Excision of Left Carpal Joint, Percutaneous Endoscopic Approach
0RBS0ZX Excision of Right Metacarpocarpal Joint, Open Approach, Diagnostic
0RBS0ZZ Excision of Right Metacarpocarpal Joint, Open Approach
0RBS3ZX Excision of Right Metacarpocarpal Joint, Percutaneous Approach, Diagnostic
0RBS3ZZ Excision of Right Metacarpocarpal Joint, Percutaneous Approach
0RBS4ZX Excision of Right Metacarpocarpal Joint, Percutaneous Endoscopic Approach, Diagnostic
0RBS4ZZ Excision of Right Metacarpocarpal Joint, Percutaneous Endoscopic Approach
0RBT0ZX Excision of Left Metacarpocarpal Joint, Open Approach, Diagnostic
0RBT0ZZ Excision of Left Metacarpocarpal Joint, Open Approach
0RBT3ZX Excision of Left Metacarpocarpal Joint, Percutaneous Approach, Diagnostic
0RBT3ZZ Excision of Left Metacarpocarpal Joint, Percutaneous Approach
0RBT4ZX Excision of Left Metacarpocarpal Joint, Percutaneous Endoscopic Approach, Diagnostic
0RBT4ZZ Excision of Left Metacarpocarpal Joint, Percutaneous Endoscopic Approach
0RBU0ZX Excision of Right Metacarpophalangeal Joint, Open Approach, Diagnostic
0RBU0ZZ Excision of Right Metacarpophalangeal Joint, Open Approach
0RBU3ZX Excision of Right Metacarpophalangeal Joint, Percutaneous Approach, Diagnostic
0RBU3ZZ Excision of Right Metacarpophalangeal Joint, Percutaneous Approach
0RBU4ZX Excision of Right Metacarpophalangeal Joint, Percutaneous Endoscopic Approach, Diagnostic
0RBU4ZZ Excision of Right Metacarpophalangeal Joint, Percutaneous Endoscopic Approach
0RBV0ZX Excision of Left Metacarpophalangeal Joint, Open Approach, Diagnostic
0RBV0ZZ Excision of Left Metacarpophalangeal Joint, Open Approach
0RBV3ZX Excision of Left Metacarpophalangeal Joint, Percutaneous Approach, Diagnostic
0RBV3ZZ Excision of Left Metacarpophalangeal Joint, Percutaneous Approach
0RBV4ZX Excision of Left Metacarpophalangeal Joint, Percutaneous Endoscopic Approach, Diagnostic
0RBV4ZZ Excision of Left Metacarpophalangeal Joint, Percutaneous Endoscopic Approach
0RBW0ZX Excision of Right Finger Phalangeal Joint, Open Approach, Diagnostic
0RBW0ZZ Excision of Right Finger Phalangeal Joint, Open Approach
0RBW3ZX Excision of Right Finger Phalangeal Joint, Percutaneous Approach, Diagnostic
0RBW3ZZ Excision of Right Finger Phalangeal Joint, Percutaneous Approach
0RBW4ZX Excision of Right Finger Phalangeal Joint, Percutaneous Endoscopic Approach, Diagnostic
0RBW4ZZ Excision of Right Finger Phalangeal Joint, Percutaneous Endoscopic Approach
0RBX0ZX Excision of Left Finger Phalangeal Joint, Open Approach, Diagnostic
0RBX0ZZ Excision of Left Finger Phalangeal Joint, Open Approach
0RBX3ZX Excision of Left Finger Phalangeal Joint, Percutaneous Approach, Diagnostic
0RBX3ZZ Excision of Left Finger Phalangeal Joint, Percutaneous Approach
0RBX4ZX Excision of Left Finger Phalangeal Joint, Percutaneous Endoscopic Approach, Diagnostic
0RBX4ZZ Excision of Left Finger Phalangeal Joint, Percutaneous Endoscopic Approach

RC – Upper Joints, Extirpation

RC00ZZ Extirpation of Matter from Occipital-cervical Joint, Open Approach
RC03ZZ Extirpation of Matter from Occipital-cervical Joint, Percutaneous Approach
RC04ZZ Extirpation of Matter from Occipital-cervical Joint, Percutaneous Endoscopic Approach
RC10ZZ Extirpation of Matter from Cervical Vertebral Joint, Open Approach
RC13ZZ Extirpation of Matter from Cervical Vertebral Joint, Percutaneous Approach
0RC14ZZ Extirpation of Matter from Cervical Vertebral Joint, Percutaneous Endoscopic Approach
RC30ZZ Extirpation of Matter from Cervical Vertebral Disc, Open Approach
0RC33ZZ Extirpation of Matter from Cervical Vertebral Disc, Percutaneous Approach
0RC34ZZ Extirpation of Matter from Cervical Vertebral Disc, Percutaneous Endoscopic Approach
0RC40ZZ Extirpation of Matter from Cervicothoracic Vertebral Joint, Open Approach
0RC43ZZ Extirpation of Matter from Cervicothoracic Vertebral Joint, Percutaneous Approach
0RC44ZZ Extirpation of Matter from Cervicothoracic Vertebral Joint, Percutaneous Endoscopic Approach
0RC50ZZ Extirpation of Matter from Cervicothoracic Vertebral Disc, Open Approach
0RC53ZZ Extirpation of Matter from Cervicothoracic Vertebral Disc, Percutaneous Approach
0RC54ZZ Extirpation of Matter from Cervicothoracic Vertebral Disc, Percutaneous Endoscopic Approach
0RC60ZZ Extirpation of Matter from Thoracic Vertebral Joint, Open Approach
0RC63ZZ Extirpation of Matter from Thoracic Vertebral Joint, Percutaneous Approach
0RC64ZZ Extirpation of Matter from Thoracic Vertebral Joint, Percutaneous Endoscopic Approach
0RC90ZZ Extirpation of Matter from Thoracic Vertebral Disc, Open Approach
0RC93ZZ Extirpation of Matter from Thoracic Vertebral Disc, Percutaneous Approach

0RC94ZZ Extirpation of Matter from Thoracic Vertebral Disc, Percutaneous Endoscopic Approach

0RCA0ZZ Extirpation of Matter from Thoracolumbar Vertebral Joint, Open Approach

0RCA3ZZ Extirpation of Matter from Thoracolumbar Vertebral Joint, Percutaneous Approach

0RCA4ZZ Extirpation of Matter from Thoracolumbar Vertebral Joint, Percutaneous Endoscopic Approach

0RCB0ZZ Extirpation of Matter from Thoracolumbar Vertebral Disc, Open Approach

0RCB3ZZ Extirpation of Matter from Thoracolumbar Vertebral Disc, Percutaneous Approach

0RCB4ZZ Extirpation of Matter from Thoracolumbar Vertebral Disc, Percutaneous Endoscopic Approach

0RCC0ZZ Extirpation of Matter from Right Temporomandibular Joint, Open Approach

0RCC3ZZ Extirpation of Matter from Right Temporomandibular Joint, Percutaneous Approach

0RCC4ZZ Extirpation of Matter from Right Temporomandibular Joint, Percutaneous Endoscopic Approach

0RCD0ZZ Extirpation of Matter from Left Temporomandibular Joint, Open Approach

0RCD3ZZ Extirpation of Matter from Left Temporomandibular Joint, Percutaneous Approach

0RCD4ZZ Extirpation of Matter from Left Temporomandibular Joint, Percutaneous Endoscopic Approach

0RCE0ZZ Extirpation of Matter from Right Sternoclavicular Joint, Open Approach

0RCE3ZZ Extirpation of Matter from Right Sternoclavicular Joint, Percutaneous Approach

0RCE4ZZ Extirpation of Matter from Right Sternoclavicular Joint, Percutaneous Endoscopic Approach

0RCF0ZZ Extirpation of Matter from Left Sternoclavicular Joint, Open Approach

0RCF3ZZ Extirpation of Matter from Left Sternoclavicular Joint, Percutaneous Approach

0RCF4ZZ Extirpation of Matter from Left Sternoclavicular Joint, Percutaneous Endoscopic Approach

0RCG0ZZ Extirpation of Matter from Right Acromioclavicular Joint, Open Approach

0RCG3ZZ Extirpation of Matter from Right Acromioclavicular Joint, Percutaneous Approach

0RCG4ZZ Extirpation of Matter from Right Acromioclavicular Joint, Percutaneous Endoscopic Approach

0RCH0ZZ Extirpation of Matter from Left Acromioclavicular Joint, Open Approach

0RCH3ZZ Extirpation of Matter from Left Acromioclavicular Joint, Percutaneous Approach

0RCH4ZZ Extirpation of Matter from Left Acromioclavicular Joint, Percutaneous Endoscopic Approach

0RCJ0ZZ Extirpation of Matter from Right Shoulder Joint, Open Approach

0RCJ3ZZ Extirpation of Matter from Right Shoulder Joint, Percutaneous Approach

0RCJ4ZZ Extirpation of Matter from Right Shoulder Joint, Percutaneous Endoscopic Approach

0RCK0ZZ Extirpation of Matter from Left Shoulder Joint, Open Approach

0RCK3ZZ Extirpation of Matter from Left Shoulder Joint, Percutaneous Approach

0RCK4ZZ Extirpation of Matter from Left Shoulder Joint, Percutaneous Endoscopic Approach

0RCL0ZZ Extirpation of Matter from Right Elbow Joint, Open Approach

0RCL3ZZ Extirpation of Matter from Right Elbow Joint, Percutaneous Approach

0RCL4ZZ Extirpation of Matter from Right Elbow Joint, Percutaneous Endoscopic Approach

0RCM0ZZ Extirpation of Matter from Left Elbow Joint, Open Approach

0RCM3ZZ Extirpation of Matter from Left Elbow Joint, Percutaneous Approach

0RCM4ZZ Extirpation of Matter from Left Elbow Joint, Percutaneous Endoscopic Approach

0RCN0ZZ Extirpation of Matter from Right Wrist Joint, Open Approach

0RCN3ZZ Extirpation of Matter from Right Wrist Joint, Percutaneous Approach

0RCN4ZZ Extirpation of Matter from Right Wrist Joint, Percutaneous Endoscopic Approach

0RCP0ZZ Extirpation of Matter from Left Wrist Joint, Open Approach

0RCP3ZZ Extirpation of Matter from Left Wrist Joint, Percutaneous Approach

0RCP4ZZ Extirpation of Matter from Left Wrist Joint, Percutaneous Endoscopic Approach

0RCQ0ZZ Extirpation of Matter from Right Carpal Joint, Open Approach

0RCQ3ZZ Extirpation of Matter from Right Carpal Joint, Percutaneous Approach

0RCQ4ZZ Extirpation of Matter from Right Carpal Joint, Percutaneous Endoscopic Approach

0RCR0ZZ Extirpation of Matter from Left Carpal Joint, Open Approach

0RCR3ZZ Extirpation of Matter from Left Carpal Joint, Percutaneous Approach

0RCR4ZZ Extirpation of Matter from Left Carpal Joint, Percutaneous Endoscopic Approach

0RCS0ZZ Extirpation of Matter from Right Metacarpocarpal Joint, Open Approach

0RCS3ZZ Extirpation of Matter from Right Metacarpocarpal Joint, Percutaneous Approach

0RCS4ZZ Extirpation of Matter from Right Metacarpocarpal Joint, Percutaneous Endoscopic Approach

0RCT0ZZ Extirpation of Matter from Left Metacarpocarpal Joint, Open Approach

0RCT3ZZ Extirpation of Matter from Left Metacarpocarpal Joint, Percutaneous Approach

0RCT4ZZ Extirpation of Matter from Left Metacarpocarpal Joint, Percutaneous Endoscopic Approach

0RCU0ZZ Extirpation of Matter from Right Metacarpophalangeal Joint, Open Approach

0RCU3ZZ Extirpation of Matter from Right Metacarpophalangeal Joint, Percutaneou[s] Approach

0RCU4ZZ Extirpation of Matter from Right Metacarpophalangeal Joint, Percutaneou[s] Endoscopic Approach

0RCV0ZZ Extirpation of Matter from Left Metacarpophalangeal Joint, Open Approach

0RCV3ZZ Extirpation of Matter from Left Metacarpophalangeal Joint, Percutaneou[s] Approach

0RCV4ZZ Extirpation of Matter from Left Metacarpophalangeal Joint, Percutaneou[s] Endoscopic Approach

0RCW0ZZ Extirpation of Matter from Right Finger Phalangeal Joint, Open Approach

0RCW3ZZ Extirpation of Matter from Right Finger Phalangeal Joint, Percutaneous Approach

0RCW4ZZ Extirpation of Matter from Right Finger Phalangeal Joint, Percutaneous Endoscopic Approach

0RCX0ZZ Extirpation of Matter from Left Finger Phalangeal Joint, Open Approach

0RCX3ZZ Extirpation of Matter from Left Finger Phalangeal Joint, Percutaneous Approach

0RCX4ZZ Extirpation of Matter from Left Finger Phalangeal Joint, Percutaneous Endoscopic Approach

0RG – Upper Joints, Fusion

For Fusion procedures involving the vertebral joints

Review Coding Guidelines B3.10a, B3.10b and B3.10c

0RG0070 Fusion of Occipital-cervical Joint with Autologous Tissue Substitute, Anterior Approach, Anterior Column, Open Approach

HAC When reported with secondary diagnosis code T84.60XA, T84.610A, T84.611A, T84.612A, T84.613A, T84.614A, T84.615A, T84.619A, T84.63XA, T84.69XA, T84.7XXA

0RG0071 Fusion of Occipital-cervical Joint with Autologous Tissue Substitute, Posterior Approach, Posterior Column, Open Approach

HAC When reported with secondary diagnosis code T84.60XA, T84.610A, T84.611A, T84.612A, T84.613A, T84.614A, T84.615A, T84.619A, T84.63XA, T84.69XA, T84.7XXA

0RG007J Fusion of Occipital-cervical Joint with Autologous Tissue Substitute, Posterior Approach, Anterior Column, Open Approach

HAC When reported with secondary diagnosis code T84.60XA, T84.610A, T84.611A, T84.612A, T84.613A, T84.614A, T84.615A, T84.619A, T84.63XA, T84.69XA, T84.7XXA

0RG00A0 Fusion of Occipital-cervical Joint with Interbody Fusion Device, Anterior Approach, Anterior Column, Open Approach

HAC When reported with secondary diagnosis code T84.60XA, T84.610A, T84.611A, T84.612A, T84.613A, T84.614A, T84.615A, T84.619A, T84.63XA, T84.69XA, T84.7XXA

0RG00A1 Fusion of Occipital-cervical Joint with Interbody Fusion Device, Posterior Approach, Posterior Column, Open Approach

Note Continued

RG00A1 Continued Note

HAC When reported with secondary diagnosis code T84.60XA, T84.610A, T84.611A, T84.612A, T84.613A, T84.614A, T84.615A, T84.619A, T84.63XA, T84.69XA, T84.7XXA

RG00AJ Fusion of Occipital-cervical Joint with Interbody Fusion Device, Posterior Approach, Anterior Column, Open Approach

HAC When reported with secondary diagnosis code T84.60XA, T84.610A, T84.611A, T84.612A, T84.613A, T84.614A, T84.615A, T84.619A, T84.63XA, T84.69XA, T84.7XXA

RG00J0 Fusion of Occipital-cervical Joint with Synthetic Substitute, Anterior Approach, Anterior Column, Open Approach

HAC When reported with secondary diagnosis code T84.60XA, T84.610A, T84.611A, T84.612A, T84.613A, T84.614A, T84.615A, T84.619A, T84.63XA, T84.69XA, T84.7XXA

RG00J1 Fusion of Occipital-cervical Joint with Synthetic Substitute, Posterior Approach, Posterior Column, Open Approach

HAC When reported with secondary diagnosis code T84.60XA, T84.610A, T84.611A, T84.612A, T84.613A, T84.614A, T84.615A, T84.619A, T84.63XA, T84.69XA, T84.7XXA

RG00JJ Fusion of Occipital-cervical Joint with Synthetic Substitute, Posterior Approach, Anterior Column, Open Approach

HAC When reported with secondary diagnosis code T84.60XA, T84.610A, T84.611A, T84.612A, T84.613A, T84.614A, T84.615A, T84.619A, T84.63XA, T84.69XA, T84.7XXA

RG00K0 Fusion of Occipital-cervical Joint with Nonautologous Tissue Substitute, Anterior Approach, Anterior Column, Open Approach

HAC When reported with secondary diagnosis code T84.60XA, T84.610A, T84.611A, T84.612A, T84.613A, T84.614A, T84.615A, T84.619A, T84.63XA, T84.69XA, T84.7XXA

RG00K1 Fusion of Occipital-cervical Joint with Nonautologous Tissue Substitute, Posterior Approach, Posterior Column, Open Approach

HAC When reported with secondary diagnosis code T84.60XA, T84.610A, T84.611A, T84.612A, T84.613A, T84.614A, T84.615A, T84.619A, T84.63XA, T84.69XA, T84.7XXA

RG00KJ Fusion of Occipital-cervical Joint with Nonautologous Tissue Substitute, Posterior Approach, Anterior Column, Open Approach

HAC When reported with secondary diagnosis code T84.60XA, T84.610A, T84.611A, T84.612A, T84.613A, T84.614A, T84.615A, T84.619A, T84.63XA, T84.69XA, T84.7XXA

RG00Z0 Fusion of Occipital-cervical Joint, Anterior Approach, Anterior Column, Open Approach

HAC When reported with secondary diagnosis code T84.60XA, T84.610A, T84.611A, T84.612A, T84.613A, T84.614A, T84.615A, T84.619A, T84.63XA, T84.69XA, T84.7XXA

RG00Z1 Fusion of Occipital-cervical Joint, Posterior Approach, Posterior Column, Open Approach

HAC When reported with secondary diagnosis code T84.60XA, T84.610A, T84.611A, T84.612A, T84.613A, T84.614A, T84.615A, T84.619A, T84.63XA, T84.69XA, T84.7XXA

0RG00ZJ Fusion of Occipital-cervical Joint, Posterior Approach, Anterior Column, Open Approach

HAC When reported with secondary diagnosis code T84.60XA, T84.610A, T84.611A, T84.612A, T84.613A, T84.614A, T84.615A, T84.619A, T84.63XA, T84.69XA, T84.7XXA

0RG0370 Fusion of Occipital-cervical Joint with Autologous Tissue Substitute, Anterior Approach, Anterior Column, Percutaneous Approach

HAC When reported with secondary diagnosis code T84.60XA, T84.610A, T84.611A, T84.612A, T84.613A, T84.614A, T84.615A, T84.619A, T84.63XA, T84.69XA, T84.7XXA

0RG0371 Fusion of Occipital-cervical Joint with Autologous Tissue Substitute, Posterior Approach, Posterior Column, Percutaneous Approach

HAC When reported with secondary diagnosis code T84.60XA, T84.610A, T84.611A, T84.612A, T84.613A, T84.614A, T84.615A, T84.619A, T84.63XA, T84.69XA, T84.7XXA

0RG037J Fusion of Occipital-cervical Joint with Autologous Tissue Substitute, Posterior Approach, Anterior Column, Percutaneous Approach

HAC When reported with secondary diagnosis code T84.60XA, T84.610A, T84.611A, T84.612A, T84.613A, T84.614A, T84.615A, T84.619A, T84.63XA, T84.69XA, T84.7XXA

0RG03A0 Fusion of Occipital-cervical Joint with Interbody Fusion Device, Anterior Approach, Anterior Column, Percutaneous Approach

HAC When reported with secondary diagnosis code T84.60XA, T84.610A, T84.611A, T84.612A, T84.613A, T84.614A, T84.615A, T84.619A, T84.63XA, T84.69XA, T84.7XXA

0RG03A1 Fusion of Occipital-cervical Joint with Interbody Fusion Device, Posterior Approach, Posterior Column, Percutaneous Approach

HAC When reported with secondary diagnosis code T84.60XA, T84.610A, T84.611A, T84.612A, T84.613A, T84.614A, T84.615A, T84.619A, T84.63XA, T84.69XA, T84.7XXA

0RG03AJ Fusion of Occipital-cervical Joint with Interbody Fusion Device, Posterior Approach, Anterior Column, Percutaneous Approach

HAC When reported with secondary diagnosis code T84.60XA, T84.610A, T84.611A, T84.612A, T84.613A, T84.614A, T84.615A, T84.619A, T84.63XA, T84.69XA, T84.7XXA

0RG03J0 Fusion of Occipital-cervical Joint with Synthetic Substitute, Anterior Approach, Anterior Column, Percutaneous Approach

HAC When reported with secondary diagnosis code T84.60XA, T84.610A, T84.611A, T84.612A, T84.613A, T84.614A, T84.615A, T84.619A, T84.63XA, T84.69XA, T84.7XXA

0RG03J1 Fusion of Occipital-cervical Joint with Synthetic Substitute, Posterior Approach, Posterior Column, Percutaneous Approach

HAC When reported with secondary diagnosis code T84.60XA, T84.610A, T84.611A, T84.612A, T84.613A, T84.614A, T84.615A, T84.619A, T84.63XA, T84.69XA, T84.7XXA

0RG03JJ Fusion of Occipital-cervical Joint with Synthetic Substitute, Posterior Approach, Anterior Column, Percutaneous Approach

HAC When reported with secondary diagnosis code T84.60XA, T84.610A, T84.611A, T84.612A, T84.613A, T84.614A, T84.615A, T84.619A, T84.63XA, T84.69XA, T84.7XXA

0RG03K0 Fusion of Occipital-cervical Joint with Nonautologous Tissue Substitute, Anterior Approach, Anterior Column, Percutaneous Approach

HAC When reported with secondary diagnosis code T84.60XA, T84.610A, T84.611A, T84.612A, T84.613A, T84.614A, T84.615A, T84.619A, T84.63XA, T84.69XA, T84.7XXA

0RG03K1 Fusion of Occipital-cervical Joint with Nonautologous Tissue Substitute, Posterior Approach, Posterior Column, Percutaneous Approach

HAC When reported with secondary diagnosis code T84.60XA, T84.610A, T84.611A, T84.612A, T84.613A, T84.614A, T84.615A, T84.619A, T84.63XA, T84.69XA, T84.7XXA

0RG03KJ Fusion of Occipital-cervical Joint with Nonautologous Tissue Substitute, Posterior Approach, Anterior Column, Percutaneous Approach

HAC When reported with secondary diagnosis code T84.60XA, T84.610A, T84.611A, T84.612A, T84.613A, T84.614A, T84.615A, T84.619A, T84.63XA, T84.69XA, T84.7XXA

0RG03Z0 Fusion of Occipital-cervical Joint, Anterior Approach, Anterior Column, Percutaneous Approach

HAC When reported with secondary diagnosis code T84.60XA, T84.610A, T84.611A, T84.612A, T84.613A, T84.614A, T84.615A, T84.619A, T84.63XA, T84.69XA, T84.7XXA

0RG03Z1 Fusion of Occipital-cervical Joint, Posterior Approach, Posterior Column, Percutaneous Approach

HAC When reported with secondary diagnosis code T84.60XA, T84.610A, T84.611A, T84.612A, T84.613A, T84.614A, T84.615A, T84.619A, T84.63XA, T84.69XA, T84.7XXA

0RG03ZJ Fusion of Occipital-cervical Joint, Posterior Approach, Anterior Column, Percutaneous Approach

HAC When reported with secondary diagnosis code T84.60XA, T84.610A, T84.611A, T84.612A, T84.613A, T84.614A, T84.615A, T84.619A, T84.63XA, T84.69XA, T84.7XXA

0RG0470 Fusion of Occipital-cervical Joint with Autologous Tissue Substitute, Anterior Approach, Anterior Column, Percutaneous Endoscopic Approach

HAC When reported with secondary diagnosis code T84.60XA, T84.610A, T84.611A, T84.612A, T84.613A, T84.614A, T84.615A, T84.619A, T84.63XA, T84.69XA, T84.7XXA

0RG0471 Fusion of Occipital-cervical Joint with Autologous Tissue Substitute, Posterior Approach, Posterior Column, Percutaneous Endoscopic Approach

Note Continued

0RG0471 Continued Note

HAC When reported with secondary diagnosis code T84.60XA, T84.610A, T84.611A, T84.612A, T84.613A, T84.614A, T84.615A, T84.619A, T84.63XA, T84.69XA, T84.7XXA

0RG047J Fusion of Occipital-cervical Joint with Autologous Tissue Substitute, Posterior Approach, Anterior Column, Percutaneous Endoscopic Approach

HAC When reported with secondary diagnosis code T84.60XA, T84.610A, T84.611A, T84.612A, T84.613A, T84.614A, T84.615A, T84.619A, T84.63XA, T84.69XA, T84.7XXA

0RG04A0 Fusion of Occipital-cervical Joint with Interbody Fusion Device, Anterior Approach, Anterior Column, Percutaneous Endoscopic Approach

HAC When reported with secondary diagnosis code T84.60XA, T84.610A, T84.611A, T84.612A, T84.613A, T84.614A, T84.615A, T84.619A, T84.63XA, T84.69XA, T84.7XXA

0RG04A1 Fusion of Occipital-cervical Joint with Interbody Fusion Device, Posterior Approach, Posterior Column, Percutaneous Endoscopic Approach

HAC When reported with secondary diagnosis code T84.60XA, T84.610A, T84.611A, T84.612A, T84.613A, T84.614A, T84.615A, T84.619A, T84.63XA, T84.69XA, T84.7XXA

0RG04AJ Fusion of Occipital-cervical Joint with Interbody Fusion Device, Posterior Approach, Anterior Column, Percutaneous Endoscopic Approach

HAC When reported with secondary diagnosis code T84.60XA, T84.610A, T84.611A, T84.612A, T84.613A, T84.614A, T84.615A, T84.619A, T84.63XA, T84.69XA, T84.7XXA

0RG04J0 Fusion of Occipital-cervical Joint with Synthetic Substitute, Anterior Approach, Anterior Column, Percutaneous Endoscopic Approach

HAC When reported with secondary diagnosis code T84.60XA, T84.610A, T84.611A, T84.612A, T84.613A, T84.614A, T84.615A, T84.619A, T84.63XA, T84.69XA, T84.7XXA

0RG04J1 Fusion of Occipital-cervical Joint with Synthetic Substitute, Posterior Approach, Posterior Column, Percutaneous Endoscopic Approach

HAC When reported with secondary diagnosis code T84.60XA, T84.610A, T84.611A, T84.612A, T84.613A, T84.614A, T84.615A, T84.619A, T84.63XA, T84.69XA, T84.7XXA

0RG04JJ Fusion of Occipital-cervical Joint with Synthetic Substitute, Posterior Approach, Anterior Column, Percutaneous Endoscopic Approach

HAC When reported with secondary diagnosis code T84.60XA, T84.610A, T84.611A, T84.612A, T84.613A, T84.614A, T84.615A, T84.619A, T84.63XA, T84.69XA, T84.7XXA

0RG04K0 Fusion of Occipital-cervical Joint with Nonautologous Tissue Substitute, Anterior Approach, Anterior Column, Percutaneous Endoscopic Approach

HAC When reported with secondary diagnosis code T84.60XA, T84.610A, T84.611A, T84.612A, T84.613A, T84.614A, T84.615A, T84.619A, T84.63XA, T84.69XA, T84.7XXA

0RG04K1 Fusion of Occipital-cervical Joint with Nonautologous Tissue Substitute, Posterior Approach, Posterior Column, Percutaneous Endoscopic Approach

HAC When reported with secondary diagnosis code T84.60XA, T84.610A, T84.611A, T84.612A, T84.613A, T84.614A, T84.615A, T84.619A, T84.63XA, T84.69XA, T84.7XXA

0RG04KJ Fusion of Occipital-cervical Joint with Nonautologous Tissue Substitute, Posterior Approach, Anterior Column, Percutaneous Endoscopic Approach

HAC When reported with secondary diagnosis code T84.60XA, T84.610A, T84.611A, T84.612A, T84.613A, T84.614A, T84.615A, T84.619A, T84.63XA, T84.69XA, T84.7XXA

0RG04Z0 Fusion of Occipital-cervical Joint, Anterior Approach, Anterior Column, Percutaneous Endoscopic Approach

HAC When reported with secondary diagnosis code T84.60XA, T84.610A, T84.611A, T84.612A, T84.613A, T84.614A, T84.615A, T84.619A, T84.63XA, T84.69XA, T84.7XXA

0RG04Z1 Fusion of Occipital-cervical Joint, Posterior Approach, Posterior Column, Percutaneous Endoscopic Approach

HAC When reported with secondary diagnosis code T84.60XA, T84.610A, T84.611A, T84.612A, T84.613A, T84.614A, T84.615A, T84.619A, T84.63XA, T84.69XA, T84.7XXA

0RG04ZJ Fusion of Occipital-cervical Joint, Posterior Approach, Anterior Column, Percutaneous Endoscopic Approach

HAC When reported with secondary diagnosis code T84.60XA, T84.610A, T84.611A, T84.612A, T84.613A, T84.614A, T84.615A, T84.619A, T84.63XA, T84.69XA, T84.7XXA

0RG1070 Fusion of Cervical Vertebral Joint with Autologous Tissue Substitute, Anterior Approach, Anterior Column, Open Approach

HAC When reported with secondary diagnosis code T84.60XA, T84.610A, T84.611A, T84.612A, T84.613A, T84.614A, T84.615A, T84.619A, T84.63XA, T84.69XA, T84.7XXA

0RG1071 Fusion of Cervical Vertebral Joint with Autologous Tissue Substitute, Posterior Approach, Posterior Column, Open Approach

HAC When reported with secondary diagnosis code T84.60XA, T84.610A, T84.611A, T84.612A, T84.613A, T84.614A, T84.615A, T84.619A, T84.63XA, T84.69XA, T84.7XXA

0RG107J Fusion of Cervical Vertebral Joint with Autologous Tissue Substitute, Posterior Approach, Anterior Column, Open Approach

HAC When reported with secondary diagnosis code T84.60XA, T84.610A, T84.611A, T84.612A, T84.613A, T84.614A, T84.615A, T84.619A, T84.63XA, T84.69XA, T84.7XXA

0RG10A0 Fusion of Cervical Vertebral Joint with Interbody Fusion Device, Anterior Approach, Anterior Column, Open Approach

HAC When reported with secondary diagnosis code T84.60XA, T84.610A, T84.611A, T84.612A, T84.613A, T84.614A, T84.615A, T84.619A, T84.63XA, T84.69XA, T84.7XXA

0RG10A1 Fusion of Cervical Vertebral Joint with Interbody Fusion Device, Posterior Approach, Posterior Column, Open Approach

HAC When reported with secondary diagnosis code T84.60XA, T84.610A, T84.611A, T84.612A, T84.613A, T84.614A, T84.615A, T84.619A, T84.63XA, T84.69XA, T84.7XXA

0RG10AJ Fusion of Cervical Vertebral Joint with Interbody Fusion Device, Posterior Approach, Anterior Column, Open Approach

HAC When reported with secondary diagnosis code T84.60XA, T84.610A, T84.611A, T84.612A, T84.613A, T84.614A, T84.615A, T84.619A, T84.63XA, T84.69XA, T84.7XXA

0RG10J0 Fusion of Cervical Vertebral Joint with Synthetic Substitute, Anterior Approach, Anterior Column, Open Approach

HAC When reported with secondary diagnosis code T84.60XA, T84.610A, T84.611A, T84.612A, T84.613A, T84.614A, T84.615A, T84.619A, T84.63XA, T84.69XA, T84.7XXA

0RG10J1 Fusion of Cervical Vertebral Joint with Synthetic Substitute, Posterior Approach, Posterior Column, Open Approach

HAC When reported with secondary diagnosis code T84.60XA, T84.610A, T84.611A, T84.612A, T84.613A, T84.614A, T84.615A, T84.619A, T84.63XA, T84.69XA, T84.7XXA

0RG10JJ Fusion of Cervical Vertebral Joint with Synthetic Substitute, Posterior Approach, Anterior Column, Open Approach

HAC When reported with secondary diagnosis code T84.60XA, T84.610A, T84.611A, T84.612A, T84.613A, T84.614A, T84.615A, T84.619A, T84.63XA, T84.69XA, T84.7XXA

0RG10K0 Fusion of Cervical Vertebral Joint with Nonautologous Tissue Substitute, Anterior Approach, Anterior Column, Open Approach

HAC When reported with secondary diagnosis code T84.60XA, T84.610A, T84.611A, T84.612A, T84.613A, T84.614A, T84.615A, T84.619A, T84.63XA, T84.69XA, T84.7XXA

0RG10K1 Fusion of Cervical Vertebral Joint with Nonautologous Tissue Substitute, Posterior Approach, Posterior Column, Open Approach

HAC When reported with secondary diagnosis code T84.60XA, T84.610A, T84.611A, T84.612A, T84.613A, T84.614A, T84.615A, T84.619A, T84.63XA, T84.69XA, T84.7XXA

0RG10KJ Fusion of Cervical Vertebral Joint with Nonautologous Tissue Substitute, Posterior Approach, Anterior Column, Open Approach

HAC When reported with secondary diagnosis code T84.60XA, T84.610A, T84.611A, T84.612A, T84.613A, T84.614A, T84.615A, T84.619A, T84.63XA, T84.69XA, T84.7XXA

0RG10Z0 Fusion of Cervical Vertebral Joint, Anterior Approach, Anterior Column, Open Approach

HAC When reported with secondary diagnosis code T84.60XA, T84.610A, T84.611A, T84.612A, T84.613A, T84.614A, T84.615A, T84.619A, T84.63XA, T84.69XA, T84.7XXA

RG10Z1 Fusion of Cervical Vertebral Joint, Posterior Approach, Posterior Column, Open Approach

HAC When reported with secondary diagnosis code T84.60XA, T84.610A, T84.611A, T84.612A, T84.613A, T84.614A, T84.615A, T84.619A, T84.63XA, T84.69XA, T84.7XXA

RG10ZJ Fusion of Cervical Vertebral Joint, Posterior Approach, Anterior Column, Open Approach

HAC When reported with secondary diagnosis code T84.60XA, T84.610A, T84.611A, T84.612A, T84.613A, T84.614A, T84.615A, T84.619A, T84.63XA, T84.69XA, T84.7XXA

RG1370 Fusion of Cervical Vertebral Joint with Autologous Tissue Substitute, Anterior Approach, Anterior Column, Percutaneous Approach

HAC When reported with secondary diagnosis code T84.60XA, T84.610A, T84.611A, T84.612A, T84.613A, T84.614A, T84.615A, T84.619A, T84.63XA, T84.69XA, T84.7XXA

RG1371 Fusion of Cervical Vertebral Joint with Autologous Tissue Substitute, Posterior Approach, Posterior Column, Percutaneous Approach

HAC When reported with secondary diagnosis code T84.60XA, T84.610A, T84.611A, T84.612A, T84.613A, T84.614A, T84.615A, T84.619A, T84.63XA, T84.69XA, T84.7XXA

RG137J Fusion of Cervical Vertebral Joint with Autologous Tissue Substitute, Posterior Approach, Anterior Column, Percutaneous Approach

HAC When reported with secondary diagnosis code T84.60XA, T84.610A, T84.611A, T84.612A, T84.613A, T84.614A, T84.615A, T84.619A, T84.63XA, T84.69XA, T84.7XXA

RG13A0 Fusion of Cervical Vertebral Joint with Interbody Fusion Device, Anterior Approach, Anterior Column, Percutaneous Approach

HAC When reported with secondary diagnosis code T84.60XA, T84.610A, T84.611A, T84.612A, T84.613A, T84.614A, T84.615A, T84.619A, T84.63XA, T84.69XA, T84.7XXA

0RG13A1 Fusion of Cervical Vertebral Joint with Interbody Fusion Device, Posterior Approach, Posterior Column, Percutaneous Approach

HAC When reported with secondary diagnosis code T84.60XA, T84.610A, T84.611A, T84.612A, T84.613A, T84.614A, T84.615A, T84.619A, T84.63XA, T84.69XA, T84.7XXA

0RG13AJ Fusion of Cervical Vertebral Joint with Interbody Fusion Device, Posterior Approach, Anterior Column, Percutaneous Approach

HAC When reported with secondary diagnosis code T84.60XA, T84.610A, T84.611A, T84.612A, T84.613A, T84.614A, T84.615A, T84.619A, T84.63XA, T84.69XA, T84.7XXA

0RG13J0 Fusion of Cervical Vertebral Joint with Synthetic Substitute, Anterior Approach, Anterior Column, Percutaneous Approach

HAC When reported with secondary diagnosis code T84.60XA, T84.610A, T84.611A, T84.612A, T84.613A, T84.614A, T84.615A, T84.619A, T84.63XA, T84.69XA, T84.7XXA

0RG13J1 Fusion of Cervical Vertebral Joint with Synthetic Substitute, Posterior Approach, Posterior Column, Percutaneous Approach

HAC When reported with secondary diagnosis code T84.60XA, T84.610A, T84.611A, T84.612A, T84.613A, T84.614A, T84.615A, T84.619A, T84.63XA, T84.69XA, T84.7XXA

0RG13JJ Fusion of Cervical Vertebral Joint with Synthetic Substitute, Posterior Approach, Anterior Column, Percutaneous Approach

HAC When reported with secondary diagnosis code T84.60XA, T84.610A, T84.611A, T84.612A, T84.613A, T84.614A, T84.615A, T84.619A, T84.63XA, T84.69XA, T84.7XXA

0RG13K0 Fusion of Cervical Vertebral Joint with Nonautologous Tissue Substitute, Anterior Approach, Anterior Column, Percutaneous Approach

HAC When reported with secondary diagnosis code T84.60XA, T84.610A, T84.611A, T84.612A, T84.613A, T84.614A, T84.615A, T84.619A, T84.63XA, T84.69XA, T84.7XXA

0RG13K1 Fusion of Cervical Vertebral Joint with Nonautologous Tissue Substitute, Posterior Approach, Posterior Column, Percutaneous Approach

HAC When reported with secondary diagnosis code T84.60XA, T84.610A, T84.611A, T84.612A, T84.613A, T84.614A, T84.615A, T84.619A, T84.63XA, T84.69XA, T84.7XXA

0RG13KJ Fusion of Cervical Vertebral Joint with Nonautologous Tissue Substitute, Posterior Approach, Anterior Column, Percutaneous Approach

HAC When reported with secondary diagnosis code T84.60XA, T84.610A, T84.611A, T84.612A, T84.613A, T84.614A, T84.615A, T84.619A, T84.63XA, T84.69XA, T84.7XXA

0RG13Z0 Fusion of Cervical Vertebral Joint, Anterior Approach, Anterior Column, Percutaneous Approach

HAC When reported with secondary diagnosis code T84.60XA, T84.610A, T84.611A, T84.612A, T84.613A, T84.614A, T84.615A, T84.619A, T84.63XA, T84.69XA, T84.7XXA

0RG13Z1 Fusion of Cervical Vertebral Joint, Posterior Approach, Posterior Column, Percutaneous Approach

HAC When reported with secondary diagnosis code T84.60XA, T84.610A, T84.611A, T84.612A, T84.613A, T84.614A, T84.615A, T84.619A, T84.63XA, T84.69XA, T84.7XXA

0RG13ZJ Fusion of Cervical Vertebral Joint, Posterior Approach, Anterior Column, Percutaneous Approach

HAC When reported with secondary diagnosis code T84.60XA, T84.610A, T84.611A, T84.612A, T84.613A, T84.614A, T84.615A, T84.619A, T84.63XA, T84.69XA, T84.7XXA

0RG1470 Fusion of Cervical Vertebral Joint with Autologous Tissue Substitute, Anterior Approach, Anterior Column, Percutaneous Endoscopic Approach

HAC When reported with secondary diagnosis code T84.60XA, T84.610A, T84.611A, T84.612A, T84.613A, T84.614A, T84.615A, T84.619A, T84.63XA, T84.69XA, T84.7XXA

0RG1471 Fusion of Cervical Vertebral Joint with Autologous Tissue Substitute, Posterior Approach, Posterior Column, Percutaneous Endoscopic Approach

HAC When reported with secondary diagnosis code T84.60XA, T84.610A, T84.611A, T84.612A, T84.613A, T84.614A, T84.615A, T84.619A, T84.63XA, T84.69XA, T84.7XXA

0RG147J Fusion of Cervical Vertebral Joint with Autologous Tissue Substitute, Posterior Approach, Anterior Column, Percutaneous Endoscopic Approach

HAC When reported with secondary diagnosis code T84.60XA, T84.610A, T84.611A, T84.612A, T84.613A, T84.614A, T84.615A, T84.619A, T84.63XA, T84.69XA, T84.7XXA

0RG14A0 Fusion of Cervical Vertebral Joint with Interbody Fusion Device, Anterior Approach, Anterior Column, Percutaneous Endoscopic Approach

HAC When reported with secondary diagnosis code T84.60XA, T84.610A, T84.611A, T84.612A, T84.613A, T84.614A, T84.615A, T84.619A, T84.63XA, T84.69XA, T84.7XXA

0RG14A1 Fusion of Cervical Vertebral Joint with Interbody Fusion Device, Posterior Approach, Posterior Column, Percutaneous Endoscopic Approach

HAC When reported with secondary diagnosis code T84.60XA, T84.610A, T84.611A, T84.612A, T84.613A, T84.614A, T84.615A, T84.619A, T84.63XA, T84.69XA, T84.7XXA

0RG14AJ Fusion of Cervical Vertebral Joint with Interbody Fusion Device, Posterior Approach, Anterior Column, Percutaneous Endoscopic Approach

HAC When reported with secondary diagnosis code T84.60XA, T84.610A, T84.611A, T84.612A, T84.613A, T84.614A, T84.615A, T84.619A, T84.63XA, T84.69XA, T84.7XXA

0RG14J0 Fusion of Cervical Vertebral Joint with Synthetic Substitute, Anterior Approach, Anterior Column, Percutaneous Endoscopic Approach

HAC When reported with secondary diagnosis code T84.60XA, T84.610A, T84.611A, T84.612A, T84.613A, T84.614A, T84.615A, T84.619A, T84.63XA, T84.69XA, T84.7XXA

0RG14J1 Fusion of Cervical Vertebral Joint with Synthetic Substitute, Posterior Approach, Posterior Column, Percutaneous Endoscopic Approach

HAC When reported with secondary diagnosis code T84.60XA, T84.610A, T84.611A, T84.612A, T84.613A, T84.614A, T84.615A, T84.619A, T84.63XA, T84.69XA, T84.7XXA

0RG14JJ Fusion of Cervical Vertebral Joint with Synthetic Substitute, Posterior Approach, Anterior Column, Percutaneous Endoscopic Approach

HAC When reported with secondary diagnosis code T84.60XA, T84.610A, T84.611A, T84.612A, T84.613A, T84.614A, T84.615A, T84.619A, T84.63XA, T84.69XA, T84.7XXA

0RG14K0 Fusion of Cervical Vertebral Joint with Nonautologous Tissue Substitute, Anterior Approach, Anterior Column, Percutaneous Endoscopic Approach

Note Continued

0RG14K0 Continued Note

HAC When reported with secondary diagnosis code T84.60XA, T84.610A, T84.611A, T84.612A, T84.613A, T84.614A, T84.615A, T84.619A, T84.63XA, T84.69XA, T84.7XXA

0RG14K1 Fusion of Cervical Vertebral Joint with Nonautologous Tissue Substitute, Posterior Approach, Posterior Column, Percutaneous Endoscopic Approach

HAC When reported with secondary diagnosis code T84.60XA, T84.610A, T84.611A, T84.612A, T84.613A, T84.614A, T84.615A, T84.619A, T84.63XA, T84.69XA, T84.7XXA

0RG14KJ Fusion of Cervical Vertebral Joint with Nonautologous Tissue Substitute, Posterior Approach, Anterior Column, Percutaneous Endoscopic Approach

HAC When reported with secondary diagnosis code T84.60XA, T84.610A, T84.611A, T84.612A, T84.613A, T84.614A, T84.615A, T84.619A, T84.63XA, T84.69XA, T84.7XXA

0RG14Z0 Fusion of Cervical Vertebral Joint, Anterior Approach, Anterior Column, Percutaneous Endoscopic Approach

HAC When reported with secondary diagnosis code T84.60XA, T84.610A, T84.611A, T84.612A, T84.613A, T84.614A, T84.615A, T84.619A, T84.63XA, T84.69XA, T84.7XXA

0RG14Z1 Fusion of Cervical Vertebral Joint, Posterior Approach, Posterior Column, Percutaneous Endoscopic Approach

HAC When reported with secondary diagnosis code T84.60XA, T84.610A, T84.611A, T84.612A, T84.613A, T84.614A, T84.615A, T84.619A, T84.63XA, T84.69XA, T84.7XXA

0RG14ZJ Fusion of Cervical Vertebral Joint, Posterior Approach, Anterior Column, Percutaneous Endoscopic Approach

HAC When reported with secondary diagnosis code T84.60XA, T84.610A, T84.611A, T84.612A, T84.613A, T84.614A, T84.615A, T84.619A, T84.63XA, T84.69XA, T84.7XXA

0RG2070 Fusion of 2 or more Cervical Vertebral Joints with Autologous Tissue Substitute, Anterior Approach, Anterior Column, Open Approach

HAC When reported with secondary diagnosis code T84.60XA, T84.610A, T84.611A, T84.612A, T84.613A, T84.614A, T84.615A, T84.619A, T84.63XA, T84.69XA, T84.7XXA

0RG2071 Fusion of 2 or more Cervical Vertebral Joints with Autologous Tissue Substitute, Posterior Approach, Posterior Column, Open Approach

HAC When reported with secondary diagnosis code T84.60XA, T84.610A, T84.611A, T84.612A, T84.613A, T84.614A, T84.615A, T84.619A, T84.63XA, T84.69XA, T84.7XXA

0RG207J Fusion of 2 or more Cervical Vertebral Joints with Autologous Tissue Substitute, Posterior Approach, Anterior Column, Open Approach

HAC When reported with secondary diagnosis code T84.60XA, T84.610A, T84.611A, T84.612A, T84.613A, T84.614A, T84.615A, T84.619A, T84.63XA, T84.69XA, T84.7XXA

0RG20A0 Fusion of 2 or more Cervical Vertebral Joints with Interbody Fusion Device, Anterior Approach, Anterior Column, Open Approach

HAC When reported with secondary diagnosis code T84.60XA, T84.610A, T84.611A, T84.612A, T84.613A, T84.614A, T84.615A, T84.619A, T84.63XA, T84.69XA, T84.7XXA

0RG20A1 Fusion of 2 or more Cervical Vertebral Joints with Interbody Fusion Device, Posterior Approach, Posterior Column, Open Approach

HAC When reported with secondary diagnosis code T84.60XA, T84.610A, T84.611A, T84.612A, T84.613A, T84.614A, T84.615A, T84.619A, T84.63XA, T84.69XA, T84.7XXA

0RG20AJ Fusion of 2 or more Cervical Vertebral Joints with Interbody Fusion Device, Posterior Approach, Anterior Column, Open Approach

HAC When reported with secondary diagnosis code T84.60XA, T84.610A, T84.611A, T84.612A, T84.613A, T84.614A, T84.615A, T84.619A, T84.63XA, T84.69XA, T84.7XXA

0RG20J0 Fusion of 2 or more Cervical Vertebral Joints with Synthetic Substitute, Anterior Approach, Anterior Column, Open Approach

HAC When reported with secondary diagnosis code T84.60XA, T84.610A, T84.611A, T84.612A, T84.613A, T84.614A, T84.615A, T84.619A, T84.63XA, T84.69XA, T84.7XXA

0RG20J1 Fusion of 2 or more Cervical Vertebral Joints with Synthetic Substitute, Posterior Approach, Posterior Column, Open Approach

HAC When reported with secondary diagnosis code T84.60XA, T84.610A, T84.611A, T84.612A, T84.613A, T84.614A, T84.615A, T84.619A, T84.63XA, T84.69XA, T84.7XXA

0RG20JJ Fusion of 2 or more Cervical Vertebral Joints with Synthetic Substitute, Posterior Approach, Anterior Column, Open Approach

HAC When reported with secondary diagnosis code T84.60XA, T84.610A, T84.611A, T84.612A, T84.613A, T84.614A, T84.615A, T84.619A, T84.63XA, T84.69XA, T84.7XXA

0RG20K0 Fusion of 2 or more Cervical Vertebral Joints with Nonautologous Tissue Substitute, Anterior Approach, Anterior Column, Open Approach

HAC When reported with secondary diagnosis code T84.60XA, T84.610A, T84.611A, T84.612A, T84.613A, T84.614A, T84.615A, T84.619A, T84.63XA, T84.69XA, T84.7XXA

0RG20K1 Fusion of 2 or more Cervical Vertebral Joints with Nonautologous Tissue Substitute, Posterior Approach, Posterior Column, Open Approach

HAC When reported with secondary diagnosis code T84.60XA, T84.610A, T84.611A, T84.612A, T84.613A, T84.614A, T84.615A, T84.619A, T84.63XA, T84.69XA, T84.7XXA

0RG20KJ Fusion of 2 or more Cervical Vertebral Joints with Nonautologous Tissue Substitute, Posterior Approach, Anterior Column, Open Approach

HAC When reported with secondary diagnosis code T84.60XA, T84.610A, T84.611A, T84.612A, T84.613A, T84.614A, T84.615A, T84.619A, T84.63XA, T84.69XA, T84.7XXA

0RG20Z0 Fusion of 2 or more Cervical Vertebral Joints, Anterior Approach, Anterior Column, Open Approach

HAC When reported with secondary diagnosis code T84.60XA, T84.610A, T84.611A, T84.612A, T84.613A, T84.614A, T84.615A, T84.619A, T84.63XA, T84.69XA, T84.7XXA

0RG20Z1 Fusion of 2 or more Cervical Vertebral Joints, Posterior Approach, Posterior Column, Open Approach

HAC When reported with secondary diagnosis code T84.60XA, T84.610A, T84.611A, T84.612A, T84.613A, T84.614A, T84.615A, T84.619A, T84.63XA, T84.69XA, T84.7XXA

0RG20ZJ Fusion of 2 or more Cervical Vertebral Joints, Posterior Approach, Anterior Column, Open Approach

HAC When reported with secondary diagnosis code T84.60XA, T84.610A, T84.611A, T84.612A, T84.613A, T84.614A, T84.615A, T84.619A, T84.63XA, T84.69XA, T84.7XXA

0RG2370 Fusion of 2 or more Cervical Vertebral Joints with Autologous Tissue Substitute, Anterior Approach, Anterior Column, Percutaneous Approach

HAC When reported with secondary diagnosis code T84.60XA, T84.610A, T84.611A, T84.612A, T84.613A, T84.614A, T84.615A, T84.619A, T84.63XA, T84.69XA, T84.7XXA

0RG2371 Fusion of 2 or more Cervical Vertebral Joints with Autologous Tissue Substitute, Posterior Approach, Posterior Column, Percutaneous Approach

HAC When reported with secondary diagnosis code T84.60XA, T84.610A, T84.611A, T84.612A, T84.613A, T84.614A, T84.615A, T84.619A, T84.63XA, T84.69XA, T84.7XXA

0RG237J Fusion of 2 or more Cervical Vertebral Joints with Autologous Tissue Substitute, Posterior Approach, Anterior Column, Percutaneous Approach

HAC When reported with secondary diagnosis code T84.60XA, T84.610A, T84.611A, T84.612A, T84.613A, T84.614A, T84.615A, T84.619A, T84.63XA, T84.69XA, T84.7XXA

0RG23A0 Fusion of 2 or more Cervical Vertebral Joints with Interbody Fusion Device, Anterior Approach, Anterior Column, Percutaneous Approach

HAC When reported with secondary diagnosis code T84.60XA, T84.610A, T84.611A, T84.612A, T84.613A, T84.614A, T84.615A, T84.619A, T84.63XA, T84.69XA, T84.7XXA

0RG23A1 Fusion of 2 or more Cervical Vertebral Joints with Interbody Fusion Device, Posterior Approach, Posterior Column, Percutaneous Approach

HAC When reported with secondary diagnosis code T84.60XA, T84.610A, T84.611A, T84.612A, T84.613A, T84.614A, T84.615A, T84.619A, T84.63XA, T84.69XA, T84.7XXA

0RG23AJ Fusion of 2 or more Cervical Vertebral Joints with Interbody Fusion Device, Posterior Approach, Anterior Column, Percutaneous Approach

Note Continued

RG23AJ Continued Note

HAC When reported with secondary diagnosis code T84.60XA, T84.610A, T84.611A, T84.612A, T84.613A, T84.614A, T84.615A, T84.619A, T84.63XA, T84.69XA, T84.7XXA

RG23J0 Fusion of 2 or more Cervical Vertebral Joints with Synthetic Substitute, Anterior Approach, Anterior Column, Percutaneous Approach

HAC When reported with secondary diagnosis code T84.60XA, T84.610A, T84.611A, T84.612A, T84.613A, T84.614A, T84.615A, T84.619A, T84.63XA, T84.69XA, T84.7XXA

RG23J1 Fusion of 2 or more Cervical Vertebral Joints with Synthetic Substitute, Posterior Approach, Posterior Column, Percutaneous Approach

HAC When reported with secondary diagnosis code T84.60XA, T84.610A, T84.611A, T84.612A, T84.613A, T84.614A, T84.615A, T84.619A, T84.63XA, T84.69XA, T84.7XXA

RG23JJ Fusion of 2 or more Cervical Vertebral Joints with Synthetic Substitute, Posterior Approach, Anterior Column, Percutaneous Approach

HAC When reported with secondary diagnosis code T84.60XA, T84.610A, T84.611A, T84.612A, T84.613A, T84.614A, T84.615A, T84.619A, T84.63XA, T84.69XA, T84.7XXA

RG23K0 Fusion of 2 or more Cervical Vertebral Joints with Nonautologous Tissue Substitute, Anterior Approach, Anterior Column, Percutaneous Approach

HAC When reported with secondary diagnosis code T84.60XA, T84.610A, T84.611A, T84.612A, T84.613A, T84.614A, T84.615A, T84.619A, T84.63XA, T84.69XA, T84.7XXA

RG23K1 Fusion of 2 or more Cervical Vertebral Joints with Nonautologous Tissue Substitute, Posterior Approach, Posterior Column, Percutaneous Approach

HAC When reported with secondary diagnosis code T84.60XA, T84.610A, T84.611A, T84.612A, T84.613A, T84.614A, T84.615A, T84.619A, T84.63XA, T84.69XA, T84.7XXA

RG23KJ Fusion of 2 or more Cervical Vertebral Joints with Nonautologous Tissue Substitute, Posterior Approach, Anterior Column, Percutaneous Approach

HAC When reported with secondary diagnosis code T84.60XA, T84.610A, T84.611A, T84.612A, T84.613A, T84.614A, T84.615A, T84.619A, T84.63XA, T84.69XA, T84.7XXA

RG23Z0 Fusion of 2 or more Cervical Vertebral Joints, Anterior Approach, Anterior Column, Percutaneous Approach

HAC When reported with secondary diagnosis code T84.60XA, T84.610A, T84.611A, T84.612A, T84.613A, T84.614A, T84.615A, T84.619A, T84.63XA, T84.69XA, T84.7XXA

RG23Z1 Fusion of 2 or more Cervical Vertebral Joints, Posterior Approach, Posterior Column, Percutaneous Approach

HAC When reported with secondary diagnosis code T84.60XA, T84.610A, T84.611A, T84.612A, T84.613A, T84.614A, T84.615A, T84.619A, T84.63XA, T84.69XA, T84.7XXA

0RG23ZJ Fusion of 2 or more Cervical Vertebral Joints, Posterior Approach, Anterior Column, Percutaneous Approach

HAC When reported with secondary diagnosis code T84.60XA, T84.610A, T84.611A, T84.612A, T84.613A, T84.614A, T84.615A, T84.619A, T84.63XA, T84.69XA, T84.7XXA

0RG2470 Fusion of 2 or more Cervical Vertebral Joints with Autologous Tissue Substitute, Anterior Approach, Anterior Column, Percutaneous Endoscopic Approach

HAC When reported with secondary diagnosis code T84.60XA, T84.610A, T84.611A, T84.612A, T84.613A, T84.614A, T84.615A, T84.619A, T84.63XA, T84.69XA, T84.7XXA

0RG2471 Fusion of 2 or more Cervical Vertebral Joints with Autologous Tissue Substitute, Posterior Approach, Posterior Column, Percutaneous Endoscopic Approach

HAC When reported with secondary diagnosis code T84.60XA, T84.610A, T84.611A, T84.612A, T84.613A, T84.614A, T84.615A, T84.619A, T84.63XA, T84.69XA, T84.7XXA

0RG247J Fusion of 2 or more Cervical Vertebral Joints with Autologous Tissue Substitute, Posterior Approach, Anterior Column, Percutaneous Endoscopic Approach

HAC When reported with secondary diagnosis code T84.60XA, T84.610A, T84.611A, T84.612A, T84.613A, T84.614A, T84.615A, T84.619A, T84.63XA, T84.69XA, T84.7XXA

0RG24A0 Fusion of 2 or more Cervical Vertebral Joints with Interbody Fusion Device, Anterior Approach, Anterior Column, Percutaneous Endoscopic Approach

HAC When reported with secondary diagnosis code T84.60XA, T84.610A, T84.611A, T84.612A, T84.613A, T84.614A, T84.615A, T84.619A, T84.63XA, T84.69XA, T84.7XXA

0RG24A1 Fusion of 2 or more Cervical Vertebral Joints with Interbody Fusion Device, Posterior Approach, Posterior Column, Percutaneous Endoscopic Approach

HAC When reported with secondary diagnosis code T84.60XA, T84.610A, T84.611A, T84.612A, T84.613A, T84.614A, T84.615A, T84.619A, T84.63XA, T84.69XA, T84.7XXA

0RG24AJ Fusion of 2 or more Cervical Vertebral Joints with Interbody Fusion Device, Posterior Approach, Anterior Column, Percutaneous Endoscopic Approach

HAC When reported with secondary diagnosis code T84.60XA, T84.610A, T84.611A, T84.612A, T84.613A, T84.614A, T84.615A, T84.619A, T84.63XA, T84.69XA, T84.7XXA

0RG24J0 Fusion of 2 or more Cervical Vertebral Joints with Synthetic Substitute, Anterior Approach, Anterior Column, Percutaneous Endoscopic Approach

HAC When reported with secondary diagnosis code T84.60XA, T84.610A, T84.611A, T84.612A, T84.613A, T84.614A, T84.615A, T84.619A, T84.63XA, T84.69XA, T84.7XXA

0RG24J1 Fusion of 2 or more Cervical Vertebral Joints with Synthetic Substitute, Posterior Approach, Posterior Column, Percutaneous Endoscopic Approach

HAC When reported with secondary diagnosis code T84.60XA, T84.610A, T84.611A, T84.612A, T84.613A, T84.614A, T84.615A, T84.619A, T84.63XA, T84.69XA, T84.7XXA

0RG24JJ Fusion of 2 or more Cervical Vertebral Joints with Synthetic Substitute, Posterior Approach, Anterior Column, Percutaneous Endoscopic Approach

HAC When reported with secondary diagnosis code T84.60XA, T84.610A, T84.611A, T84.612A, T84.613A, T84.614A, T84.615A, T84.619A, T84.63XA, T84.69XA, T84.7XXA

0RG24K0 Fusion of 2 or more Cervical Vertebral Joints with Nonautologous Tissue Substitute, Anterior Approach, Anterior Column, Percutaneous Endoscopic Approach

HAC When reported with secondary diagnosis code T84.60XA, T84.610A, T84.611A, T84.612A, T84.613A, T84.614A, T84.615A, T84.619A, T84.63XA, T84.69XA, T84.7XXA

0RG24K1 Fusion of 2 or more Cervical Vertebral Joints with Nonautologous Tissue Substitute, Posterior Approach, Posterior Column, Percutaneous Endoscopic Approach

HAC When reported with secondary diagnosis code T84.60XA, T84.610A, T84.611A, T84.612A, T84.613A, T84.614A, T84.615A, T84.619A, T84.63XA, T84.69XA, T84.7XXA

0RG24KJ Fusion of 2 or more Cervical Vertebral Joints with Nonautologous Tissue Substitute, Posterior Approach, Anterior Column, Percutaneous Endoscopic Approach

HAC When reported with secondary diagnosis code T84.60XA, T84.610A, T84.611A, T84.612A, T84.613A, T84.614A, T84.615A, T84.619A, T84.63XA, T84.69XA, T84.7XXA

0RG24Z0 Fusion of 2 or more Cervical Vertebral Joints, Anterior Approach, Anterior Column, Percutaneous Endoscopic Approach

HAC When reported with secondary diagnosis code T84.60XA, T84.610A, T84.611A, T84.612A, T84.613A, T84.614A, T84.615A, T84.619A, T84.63XA, T84.69XA, T84.7XXA

0RG24Z1 Fusion of 2 or more Cervical Vertebral Joints, Posterior Approach, Posterior Column, Percutaneous Endoscopic Approach

HAC When reported with secondary diagnosis code T84.60XA, T84.610A, T84.611A, T84.612A, T84.613A, T84.614A, T84.615A, T84.619A, T84.63XA, T84.69XA, T84.7XXA

0RG24ZJ Fusion of 2 or more Cervical Vertebral Joints, Posterior Approach, Anterior Column, Percutaneous Endoscopic Approach

HAC When reported with secondary diagnosis code T84.60XA, T84.610A, T84.611A, T84.612A, T84.613A, T84.614A, T84.615A, T84.619A, T84.63XA, T84.69XA, T84.7XXA

0RG4070 Fusion of Cervicothoracic Vertebral Joint with Autologous Tissue Substitute, Anterior Approach, Anterior Column, Open Approach

HAC When reported with secondary diagnosis code T84.60XA, T84.610A, T84.611A, T84.612A, T84.613A, T84.614A, T84.615A, T84.619A, T84.63XA, T84.69XA, T84.7XXA

0RG4071 Fusion of Cervicothoracic Vertebral Joint with Autologous Tissue Substitute, Posterior Approach, Posterior Column, Open Approach

HAC When reported with secondary diagnosis code T84.60XA, T84.610A, T84.611A, T84.612A, T84.613A, T84.614A, T84.615A, T84.619A, T84.63XA, T84.69XA, T84.7XXA

0RG407J Fusion of Cervicothoracic Vertebral Joint with Autologous Tissue Substitute, Posterior Approach, Anterior Column, Open Approach

HAC When reported with secondary diagnosis code T84.60XA, T84.610A, T84.611A, T84.612A, T84.613A, T84.614A, T84.615A, T84.619A, T84.63XA, T84.69XA, T84.7XXA

0RG40A0 Fusion of Cervicothoracic Vertebral Joint with Interbody Fusion Device, Anterior Approach, Anterior Column, Open Approach

AHA CC: 1Q, 2013, 29-30; 2Q, 2014, 7-8

HAC When reported with secondary diagnosis code T84.60XA, T84.610A, T84.611A, T84.612A, T84.613A, T84.614A, T84.615A, T84.619A, T84.63XA, T84.69XA, T84.7XXA

0RG40A1 Fusion of Cervicothoracic Vertebral Joint with Interbody Fusion Device, Posterior Approach, Posterior Column, Open Approach

HAC When reported with secondary diagnosis code T84.60XA, T84.610A, T84.611A, T84.612A, T84.613A, T84.614A, T84.615A, T84.619A, T84.63XA, T84.69XA, T84.7XXA

0RG40AJ Fusion of Cervicothoracic Vertebral Joint with Interbody Fusion Device, Posterior Approach, Anterior Column, Open Approach

HAC When reported with secondary diagnosis code T84.60XA, T84.610A, T84.611A, T84.612A, T84.613A, T84.614A, T84.615A, T84.619A, T84.63XA, T84.69XA, T84.7XXA

0RG40J0 Fusion of Cervicothoracic Vertebral Joint with Synthetic Substitute, Anterior Approach, Anterior Column, Open Approach

HAC When reported with secondary diagnosis code T84.60XA, T84.610A, T84.611A, T84.612A, T84.613A, T84.614A, T84.615A, T84.619A, T84.63XA, T84.69XA, T84.7XXA

0RG40J1 Fusion of Cervicothoracic Vertebral Joint with Synthetic Substitute, Posterior Approach, Posterior Column, Open Approach

HAC When reported with secondary diagnosis code T84.60XA, T84.610A, T84.611A, T84.612A, T84.613A, T84.614A, T84.615A, T84.619A, T84.63XA, T84.69XA, T84.7XXA

0RG40JJ Fusion of Cervicothoracic Vertebral Joint with Synthetic Substitute, Posterior Approach, Anterior Column, Open Approach

HAC When reported with secondary diagnosis code T84.60XA, T84.610A, T84.611A, T84.612A, T84.613A, T84.614A, T84.615A, T84.619A, T84.63XA, T84.69XA, T84.7XXA

0RG40K0 Fusion of Cervicothoracic Vertebral Joint with Nonautologous Tissue Substitute, Anterior Approach, Anterior Column, Open Approach

HAC When reported with secondary diagnosis code T84.60XA, T84.610A, T84.611A, T84.612A, T84.613A, T84.614A, T84.615A, T84.619A, T84.63XA, T84.69XA, T84.7XXA

0RG40K1 Fusion of Cervicothoracic Vertebral Joint with Nonautologous Tissue Substitute, Posterior Approach, Posterior Column, Open Approach

HAC When reported with secondary diagnosis code T84.60XA, T84.610A, T84.611A, T84.612A, T84.613A, T84.614A, T84.615A, T84.619A, T84.63XA, T84.69XA, T84.7XXA

0RG40KJ Fusion of Cervicothoracic Vertebral Joint with Nonautologous Tissue Substitute, Posterior Approach, Anterior Column, Open Approach

HAC When reported with secondary diagnosis code T84.60XA, T84.610A, T84.611A, T84.612A, T84.613A, T84.614A, T84.615A, T84.619A, T84.63XA, T84.69XA, T84.7XXA

0RG40Z0 Fusion of Cervicothoracic Vertebral Joint, Anterior Approach, Anterior Column, Open Approach

HAC When reported with secondary diagnosis code T84.60XA, T84.610A, T84.611A, T84.612A, T84.613A, T84.614A, T84.615A, T84.619A, T84.63XA, T84.69XA, T84.7XXA

0RG40Z1 Fusion of Cervicothoracic Vertebral Joint, Posterior Approach, Posterior Column, Open Approach

HAC When reported with secondary diagnosis code T84.60XA, T84.610A, T84.611A, T84.612A, T84.613A, T84.614A, T84.615A, T84.619A, T84.63XA, T84.69XA, T84.7XXA

0RG40ZJ Fusion of Cervicothoracic Vertebral Joint, Posterior Approach, Anterior Column, Open Approach

HAC When reported with secondary diagnosis code T84.60XA, T84.610A, T84.611A, T84.612A, T84.613A, T84.614A, T84.615A, T84.619A, T84.63XA, T84.69XA, T84.7XXA

0RG4370 Fusion of Cervicothoracic Vertebral Joint with Autologous Tissue Substitute, Anterior Approach, Anterior Column, Percutaneous Approach

HAC When reported with secondary diagnosis code T84.60XA, T84.610A, T84.611A, T84.612A, T84.613A, T84.614A, T84.615A, T84.619A, T84.63XA, T84.69XA, T84.7XXA

0RG4371 Fusion of Cervicothoracic Vertebral Joint with Autologous Tissue Substitute, Posterior Approach, Posterior Column, Percutaneous Approach

HAC When reported with secondary diagnosis code T84.60XA, T84.610A, T84.611A, T84.612A, T84.613A, T84.614A, T84.615A, T84.619A, T84.63XA, T84.69XA, T84.7XXA

0RG437J Fusion of Cervicothoracic Vertebral Joint with Autologous Tissue Substitute, Posterior Approach, Anterior Column, Percutaneous Approach

HAC When reported with secondary diagnosis code T84.60XA, T84.610A, T84.611A, T84.612A, T84.613A, T84.614A, T84.615A, T84.619A, T84.63XA, T84.69XA, T84.7XXA

0RG43A0 Fusion of Cervicothoracic Vertebral Joint with Interbody Fusion Device, Anterior Approach, Anterior Column, Percutaneous Approach

HAC When reported with secondary diagnosis code T84.60XA, T84.610A, T84.611A, T84.612A, T84.613A, T84.614A, T84.615A, T84.619A, T84.63XA, T84.69XA, T84.7XXA

0RG43A1 Fusion of Cervicothoracic Vertebral Joint with Interbody Fusion Device, Posterior Approach, Posterior Column, Percutaneous Approach

HAC When reported with secondary diagnosis code T84.60XA, T84.610A, T84.611A, T84.612A, T84.613A, T84.614A, T84.615A, T84.619A, T84.63XA, T84.69XA, T84.7XXA

0RG43AJ Fusion of Cervicothoracic Vertebral Joint with Interbody Fusion Device, Posterior Approach, Anterior Column, Percutaneous Approach

HAC When reported with secondary diagnosis code T84.60XA, T84.610A, T84.611A, T84.612A, T84.613A, T84.614A, T84.615A, T84.619A, T84.63XA, T84.69XA, T84.7XXA

0RG43J0 Fusion of Cervicothoracic Vertebral Joint with Synthetic Substitute, Anterior Approach, Anterior Column, Percutaneous Approach

HAC When reported with secondary diagnosis code T84.60XA, T84.610A, T84.611A, T84.612A, T84.613A, T84.614A, T84.615A, T84.619A, T84.63XA, T84.69XA, T84.7XXA

0RG43J1 Fusion of Cervicothoracic Vertebral Joint with Synthetic Substitute, Posterior Approach, Posterior Column, Percutaneous Approach

HAC When reported with secondary diagnosis code T84.60XA, T84.610A, T84.611A, T84.612A, T84.613A, T84.614A, T84.615A, T84.619A, T84.63XA, T84.69XA, T84.7XXA

0RG43JJ Fusion of Cervicothoracic Vertebral Joint with Synthetic Substitute, Posterior Approach, Anterior Column, Percutaneous Approach

HAC When reported with secondary diagnosis code T84.60XA, T84.610A, T84.611A, T84.612A, T84.613A, T84.614A, T84.615A, T84.619A, T84.63XA, T84.69XA, T84.7XXA

0RG43K0 Fusion of Cervicothoracic Vertebral Joint with Nonautologous Tissue Substitute, Anterior Approach, Anterior Column, Percutaneous Approach

HAC When reported with secondary diagnosis code T84.60XA, T84.610A, T84.611A, T84.612A, T84.613A, T84.614A, T84.615A, T84.619A, T84.63XA, T84.69XA, T84.7XXA

0RG43K1 Fusion of Cervicothoracic Vertebral Joint with Nonautologous Tissue Substitute, Posterior Approach, Posterior Column, Percutaneous Approach

HAC When reported with secondary diagnosis code T84.60XA, T84.610A, T84.611A, T84.612A, T84.613A, T84.614A, T84.615A, T84.619A, T84.63XA, T84.69XA, T84.7XXA

0RG43KJ Fusion of Cervicothoracic Vertebral Joint with Nonautologous Tissue Substitute, Posterior Approach, Anterior Column, Percutaneous Approach

HAC When reported with secondary diagnosis code T84.60XA, T84.610A, T84.611A, T84.612A, T84.613A, T84.614A, T84.615A, T84.619A, T84.63XA, T84.69XA, T84.7XXA

RG43Z0 Fusion of Cervicothoracic Vertebral Joint, Anterior Approach, Anterior Column, Percutaneous Approach
HAC When reported with secondary diagnosis code T84.60XA, T84.610A, T84.611A, T84.612A, T84.613A, T84.614A, T84.615A, T84.619A, T84.63XA, T84.69XA, T84.7XXA

RG43Z1 Fusion of Cervicothoracic Vertebral Joint, Posterior Approach, Posterior Column, Percutaneous Approach
HAC When reported with secondary diagnosis code T84.60XA, T84.610A, T84.611A, T84.612A, T84.613A, T84.614A, T84.615A, T84.619A, T84.63XA, T84.69XA, T84.7XXA

RG43ZJ Fusion of Cervicothoracic Vertebral Joint, Posterior Approach, Anterior Column, Percutaneous Approach
HAC When reported with secondary diagnosis code T84.60XA, T84.610A, T84.611A, T84.612A, T84.613A, T84.614A, T84.615A, T84.619A, T84.63XA, T84.69XA, T84.7XXA

RG4470 Fusion of Cervicothoracic Vertebral Joint with Autologous Tissue Substitute, Anterior Approach, Anterior Column, Percutaneous Endoscopic Approach
HAC When reported with secondary diagnosis code T84.60XA, T84.610A, T84.611A, T84.612A, T84.613A, T84.614A, T84.615A, T84.619A, T84.63XA, T84.69XA, T84.7XXA

RG4471 Fusion of Cervicothoracic Vertebral Joint with Autologous Tissue Substitute, Posterior Approach, Posterior Column, Percutaneous Endoscopic Approach
HAC When reported with secondary diagnosis code T84.60XA, T84.610A, T84.611A, T84.612A, T84.613A, T84.614A, T84.615A, T84.619A, T84.63XA, T84.69XA, T84.7XXA

RG447J Fusion of Cervicothoracic Vertebral Joint with Autologous Tissue Substitute, Posterior Approach, Anterior Column, Percutaneous Endoscopic Approach
HAC When reported with secondary diagnosis code T84.60XA, T84.610A, T84.611A, T84.612A, T84.613A, T84.614A, T84.615A, T84.619A, T84.63XA, T84.69XA, T84.7XXA

RG44A0 Fusion of Cervicothoracic Vertebral Joint with Interbody Fusion Device, Anterior Approach, Anterior Column, Percutaneous Endoscopic Approach
HAC When reported with secondary diagnosis code T84.60XA, T84.610A, T84.611A, T84.612A, T84.613A, T84.614A, T84.615A, T84.619A, T84.63XA, T84.69XA, T84.7XXA

0RG44A1 Fusion of Cervicothoracic Vertebral Joint with Interbody Fusion Device, Posterior Approach, Posterior Column, Percutaneous Endoscopic Approach
HAC When reported with secondary diagnosis code T84.60XA, T84.610A, T84.611A, T84.612A, T84.613A, T84.614A, T84.615A, T84.619A, T84.63XA, T84.69XA, T84.7XXA

0RG44AJ Fusion of Cervicothoracic Vertebral Joint with Interbody Fusion Device, Posterior Approach, Anterior Column, Percutaneous Endoscopic Approach
HAC When reported with secondary diagnosis code T84.60XA, T84.610A, T84.611A, T84.612A, T84.613A, T84.614A, T84.615A, T84.619A, T84.63XA, T84.69XA, T84.7XXA

0RG44J0 Fusion of Cervicothoracic Vertebral Joint with Synthetic Substitute, Anterior Approach, Anterior Column, Percutaneous Endoscopic Approach
HAC When reported with secondary diagnosis code T84.60XA, T84.610A, T84.611A, T84.612A, T84.613A, T84.614A, T84.615A, T84.619A, T84.63XA, T84.69XA, T84.7XXA

0RG44J1 Fusion of Cervicothoracic Vertebral Joint with Synthetic Substitute, Posterior Approach, Posterior Column, Percutaneous Endoscopic Approach
HAC When reported with secondary diagnosis code T84.60XA, T84.610A, T84.611A, T84.612A, T84.613A, T84.614A, T84.615A, T84.619A, T84.63XA, T84.69XA, T84.7XXA

0RG44JJ Fusion of Cervicothoracic Vertebral Joint with Synthetic Substitute, Posterior Approach, Anterior Column, Percutaneous Endoscopic Approach
HAC When reported with secondary diagnosis code T84.60XA, T84.610A, T84.611A, T84.612A, T84.613A, T84.614A, T84.615A, T84.619A, T84.63XA, T84.69XA, T84.7XXA

0RG44K0 Fusion of Cervicothoracic Vertebral Joint with Nonautologous Tissue Substitute, Anterior Approach, Anterior Column, Percutaneous Endoscopic Approach
HAC When reported with secondary diagnosis code T84.60XA, T84.610A, T84.611A, T84.612A, T84.613A, T84.614A, T84.615A, T84.619A, T84.63XA, T84.69XA, T84.7XXA

0RG44K1 Fusion of Cervicothoracic Vertebral Joint with Nonautologous Tissue Substitute, Posterior Approach, Posterior Column, Percutaneous Endoscopic Approach
HAC When reported with secondary diagnosis code T84.60XA, T84.610A, T84.611A, T84.612A, T84.613A, T84.614A, T84.615A, T84.619A, T84.63XA, T84.69XA, T84.7XXA

0RG44KJ Fusion of Cervicothoracic Vertebral Joint with Nonautologous Tissue Substitute, Posterior Approach, Anterior Column, Percutaneous Endoscopic Approach
HAC When reported with secondary diagnosis code T84.60XA, T84.610A, T84.611A, T84.612A, T84.613A, T84.614A, T84.615A, T84.619A, T84.63XA, T84.69XA, T84.7XXA

0RG44Z0 Fusion of Cervicothoracic Vertebral Joint, Anterior Approach, Anterior Column, Percutaneous Endoscopic Approach
HAC When reported with secondary diagnosis code T84.60XA, T84.610A, T84.611A, T84.612A, T84.613A, T84.614A, T84.615A, T84.619A, T84.63XA, T84.69XA, T84.7XXA

0RG44Z1 Fusion of Cervicothoracic Vertebral Joint, Posterior Approach, Posterior Column, Percutaneous Endoscopic Approach
HAC When reported with secondary diagnosis code T84.60XA, T84.610A, T84.611A, T84.612A, T84.613A, T84.614A, T84.615A, T84.619A, T84.63XA, T84.69XA, T84.7XXA

0RG44ZJ Fusion of Cervicothoracic Vertebral Joint, Posterior Approach, Anterior Column, Percutaneous Endoscopic Approach
HAC When reported with secondary diagnosis code T84.60XA, T84.610A, T84.611A, T84.612A, T84.613A, T84.614A, T84.615A, T84.619A, T84.63XA, T84.69XA, T84.7XXA

0RG6070 Fusion of Thoracic Vertebral Joint with Autologous Tissue Substitute, Anterior Approach, Anterior Column, Open Approach
HAC When reported with secondary diagnosis code T84.60XA, T84.610A, T84.611A, T84.612A, T84.613A, T84.614A, T84.615A, T84.619A, T84.63XA, T84.69XA, T84.7XXA

0RG6071 Fusion of Thoracic Vertebral Joint with Autologous Tissue Substitute, Posterior Approach, Posterior Column, Open Approach
HAC When reported with secondary diagnosis code T84.60XA, T84.610A, T84.611A, T84.612A, T84.613A, T84.614A, T84.615A, T84.619A, T84.63XA, T84.69XA, T84.7XXA

0RG607J Fusion of Thoracic Vertebral Joint with Autologous Tissue Substitute, Posterior Approach, Anterior Column, Open Approach
HAC When reported with secondary diagnosis code T84.60XA, T84.610A, T84.611A, T84.612A, T84.613A, T84.614A, T84.615A, T84.619A, T84.63XA, T84.69XA, T84.7XXA

0RG60A0 Fusion of Thoracic Vertebral Joint with Interbody Fusion Device, Anterior Approach, Anterior Column, Open Approach
HAC When reported with secondary diagnosis code T84.60XA, T84.610A, T84.611A, T84.612A, T84.613A, T84.614A, T84.615A, T84.619A, T84.63XA, T84.69XA, T84.7XXA

0RG60A1 Fusion of Thoracic Vertebral Joint with Interbody Fusion Device, Posterior Approach, Posterior Column, Open Approach
HAC When reported with secondary diagnosis code T84.60XA, T84.610A, T84.611A, T84.612A, T84.613A, T84.614A, T84.615A, T84.619A, T84.63XA, T84.69XA, T84.7XXA

0RG60AJ Fusion of Thoracic Vertebral Joint with Interbody Fusion Device, Posterior Approach, Anterior Column, Open Approach
HAC When reported with secondary diagnosis code T84.60XA, T84.610A, T84.611A, T84.612A, T84.613A, T84.614A, T84.615A, T84.619A, T84.63XA, T84.69XA, T84.7XXA

0RG60J0 Fusion of Thoracic Vertebral Joint with Synthetic Substitute, Anterior Approach, Anterior Column, Open Approach
HAC When reported with secondary diagnosis code T84.60XA, T84.610A, T84.611A, T84.612A, T84.613A, T84.614A, T84.615A, T84.619A, T84.63XA, T84.69XA, T84.7XXA

0RG60J1 Fusion of Thoracic Vertebral Joint with Synthetic Substitute, Posterior Approach, Posterior Column, Open Approach
HAC When reported with secondary diagnosis code T84.60XA, T84.610A, T84.611A, T84.612A, T84.613A, T84.614A, T84.615A, T84.619A, T84.63XA, T84.69XA, T84.7XXA

0RG60JJ Fusion of Thoracic Vertebral Joint with Synthetic Substitute, Posterior Approach, Anterior Column, Open Approach
HAC When reported with secondary diagnosis code T84.60XA, T84.610A, T84.611A, T84.612A, T84.613A, T84.614A, T84.615A, T84.619A, T84.63XA, T84.69XA, T84.7XXA

0RG60K0 Fusion of Thoracic Vertebral Joint with Nonautologous Tissue Substitute, Anterior Approach, Anterior Column, Open Approach
HAC When reported with secondary diagnosis code T84.60XA, T84.610A, T84.611A, T84.612A, T84.613A, T84.614A, T84.615A, T84.619A, T84.63XA, T84.69XA, T84.7XXA

0RG60K1 Fusion of Thoracic Vertebral Joint with Nonautologous Tissue Substitute, Posterior Approach, Posterior Column, Open Approach
HAC When reported with secondary diagnosis code T84.60XA, T84.610A, T84.611A, T84.612A, T84.613A, T84.614A, T84.615A, T84.619A, T84.63XA, T84.69XA, T84.7XXA

0RG60KJ Fusion of Thoracic Vertebral Joint with Nonautologous Tissue Substitute, Posterior Approach, Anterior Column, Open Approach
HAC When reported with secondary diagnosis code T84.60XA, T84.610A, T84.611A, T84.612A, T84.613A, T84.614A, T84.615A, T84.619A, T84.63XA, T84.69XA, T84.7XXA

0RG60Z0 Fusion of Thoracic Vertebral Joint, Anterior Approach, Anterior Column, Open Approach
HAC When reported with secondary diagnosis code T84.60XA, T84.610A, T84.611A, T84.612A, T84.613A, T84.614A, T84.615A, T84.619A, T84.63XA, T84.69XA, T84.7XXA

0RG60Z1 Fusion of Thoracic Vertebral Joint, Posterior Approach, Posterior Column, Open Approach
HAC When reported with secondary diagnosis code T84.60XA, T84.610A, T84.611A, T84.612A, T84.613A, T84.614A, T84.615A, T84.619A, T84.63XA, T84.69XA, T84.7XXA

0RG60ZJ Fusion of Thoracic Vertebral Joint, Posterior Approach, Anterior Column, Open Approach
HAC When reported with secondary diagnosis code T84.60XA, T84.610A, T84.611A, T84.612A, T84.613A, T84.614A, T84.615A, T84.619A, T84.63XA, T84.69XA, T84.7XXA

0RG6370 Fusion of Thoracic Vertebral Joint with Autologous Tissue Substitute, Anterior Approach, Anterior Column, Percutaneous Approach
HAC When reported with secondary diagnosis code T84.60XA, T84.610A, T84.611A, T84.612A, T84.613A, T84.614A, T84.615A, T84.619A, T84.63XA, T84.69XA, T84.7XXA

0RG6371 Fusion of Thoracic Vertebral Joint with Autologous Tissue Substitute, Posterior Approach, Posterior Column, Percutaneous Approach
HAC When reported with secondary diagnosis code T84.60XA, T84.610A, T84.611A, T84.612A, T84.613A, T84.614A, T84.615A, T84.619A, T84.63XA, T84.69XA, T84.7XXA

0RG637J Fusion of Thoracic Vertebral Joint with Autologous Tissue Substitute, Posterior Approach, Anterior Column, Percutaneous Approach
HAC When reported with secondary diagnosis code T84.60XA, T84.610A, T84.611A, T84.612A, T84.613A, T84.614A, T84.615A, T84.619A, T84.63XA, T84.69XA, T84.7XXA

0RG63A0 Fusion of Thoracic Vertebral Joint with Interbody Fusion Device, Anterior Approach, Anterior Column, Percutaneous Approach
HAC When reported with secondary diagnosis code T84.60XA, T84.610A, T84.611A, T84.612A, T84.613A, T84.614A, T84.615A, T84.619A, T84.63XA, T84.69XA, T84.7XXA

0RG63A1 Fusion of Thoracic Vertebral Joint with Interbody Fusion Device, Posterior Approach, Posterior Column, Percutaneous Approach
HAC When reported with secondary diagnosis code T84.60XA, T84.610A, T84.611A, T84.612A, T84.613A, T84.614A, T84.615A, T84.619A, T84.63XA, T84.69XA, T84.7XXA

0RG63AJ Fusion of Thoracic Vertebral Joint with Interbody Fusion Device, Posterior Approach, Anterior Column, Percutaneous Approach
HAC When reported with secondary diagnosis code T84.60XA, T84.610A, T84.611A, T84.612A, T84.613A, T84.614A, T84.615A, T84.619A, T84.63XA, T84.69XA, T84.7XXA

0RG63J0 Fusion of Thoracic Vertebral Joint with Synthetic Substitute, Anterior Approach, Anterior Column, Percutaneous Approach
HAC When reported with secondary diagnosis code T84.60XA, T84.610A, T84.611A, T84.612A, T84.613A, T84.614A, T84.615A, T84.619A, T84.63XA, T84.69XA, T84.7XXA

0RG63J1 Fusion of Thoracic Vertebral Joint with Synthetic Substitute, Posterior Approach, Posterior Column, Percutaneous Approach
HAC When reported with secondary diagnosis code T84.60XA, T84.610A, T84.611A, T84.612A, T84.613A, T84.614A, T84.615A, T84.619A, T84.63XA, T84.69XA, T84.7XXA

0RG63JJ Fusion of Thoracic Vertebral Joint with Synthetic Substitute, Posterior Approach, Anterior Column, Percutaneous Approach
HAC When reported with secondary diagnosis code T84.60XA, T84.610A, T84.611A, T84.612A, T84.613A, T84.614A, T84.615A, T84.619A, T84.63XA, T84.69XA, T84.7XXA

0RG63K0 Fusion of Thoracic Vertebral Joint with Nonautologous Tissue Substitute, Anterior Approach, Anterior Column, Percutaneous Approach
HAC When reported with secondary diagnosis code T84.60XA, T84.610A, T84.611A, T84.612A, T84.613A, T84.614A, T84.615A, T84.619A, T84.63XA, T84.69XA, T84.7XXA

0RG63K1 Fusion of Thoracic Vertebral Joint with Nonautologous Tissue Substitute, Posterior Approach, Posterior Column, Percutaneous Approach
HAC When reported with secondary diagnosis code T84.60XA, T84.610A, T84.611A, T84.612A, T84.613A, T84.614A, T84.615A, T84.619A, T84.63XA, T84.69XA, T84.7XXA

0RG63KJ Fusion of Thoracic Vertebral Joint with Nonautologous Tissue Substitute, Posterior Approach, Anterior Column, Percutaneous Approach
HAC When reported with secondary diagnosis code T84.60XA, T84.610A, T84.611A, T84.612A, T84.613A, T84.614A, T84.615A, T84.619A, T84.63XA, T84.69XA, T84.7XXA

0RG63Z0 Fusion of Thoracic Vertebral Joint, Anterior Approach, Anterior Column, Percutaneous Approach
HAC When reported with secondary diagnosis code T84.60XA, T84.610A, T84.611A, T84.612A, T84.613A, T84.614A, T84.615A, T84.619A, T84.63XA, T84.69XA, T84.7XXA

0RG63Z1 Fusion of Thoracic Vertebral Joint, Posterior Approach, Posterior Column, Percutaneous Approach
HAC When reported with secondary diagnosis code T84.60XA, T84.610A, T84.611A, T84.612A, T84.613A, T84.614A, T84.615A, T84.619A, T84.63XA, T84.69XA, T84.7XXA

0RG63ZJ Fusion of Thoracic Vertebral Joint, Posterior Approach, Anterior Column, Percutaneous Approach
HAC When reported with secondary diagnosis code T84.60XA, T84.610A, T84.611A, T84.612A, T84.613A, T84.614A, T84.615A, T84.619A, T84.63XA, T84.69XA, T84.7XXA

0RG6470 Fusion of Thoracic Vertebral Joint with Autologous Tissue Substitute, Anterior Approach, Anterior Column, Percutaneou Endoscopic Approach
HAC When reported with secondary diagnosis code T84.60XA, T84.610A, T84.611A, T84.612A, T84.613A, T84.614A, T84.615A, T84.619A, T84.63XA, T84.69XA, T84.7XXA

0RG6471 Fusion of Thoracic Vertebral Joint with Autologous Tissue Substitute, Posterior Approach, Posterior Column, Percutaneous Endoscopic Approach
HAC When reported with secondary diagnosis code T84.60XA, T84.610A, T84.611A, T84.612A, T84.613A, T84.614A, T84.615A, T84.619A, T84.63XA, T84.69XA, T84.7XXA

0RG647J Fusion of Thoracic Vertebral Joint with Autologous Tissue Substitute, Posterior Approach, Anterior Column, Percutaneous Endoscopic Approach
HAC When reported with secondary diagnosis code T84.60XA, T84.610A, T84.611A, T84.612A, T84.613A, T84.614A, T84.615A, T84.619A, T84.63XA, T84.69XA, T84.7XXA

0RG64A0 Fusion of Thoracic Vertebral Joint with Interbody Fusion Device, Anterior Approach, Anterior Column, Percutaneous Endoscopic Approach
HAC When reported with secondary diagnosis code T84.60XA, T84.610A, T84.611A, T84.612A, T84.613A, T84.614A, T84.615A, T84.619A, T84.63XA, T84.69XA, T84.7XXA

0RG64A1 Fusion of Thoracic Vertebral Joint with Interbody Fusion Device, Posterior Approach, Posterior Column, Percutaneous Endoscopic Approach
HAC When reported with secondary diagnosis code T84.60XA, T84.610A, T84.611A, T84.612A, T84.613A, T84.614A, T84.615A, T84.619A, T84.63XA, T84.69XA, T84.7XXA

0RG64AJ Fusion of Thoracic Vertebral Joint with Interbody Fusion Device, Posterior Approach, Anterior Column, Percutaneous Endoscopic Approach
HAC When reported with secondary diagnosis code T84.60XA, T84.610A, T84.611A, T84.612A, T84.613A, T84.614A, T84.615A, T84.619A, T84.63XA, T84.69XA, T84.7XXA

0RG64J0 Fusion of Thoracic Vertebral Joint with Synthetic Substitute, Anterior Approach, Anterior Column, Percutaneous Endoscopic Approach
HAC When reported with secondary diagnosis code T84.60XA, T84.610A, T84.611A, T84.612A, T84.613A, T84.614A, T84.615A, T84.619A, T84.63XA, T84.69XA, T84.7XXA

0RG64J1 Fusion of Thoracic Vertebral Joint with Synthetic Substitute, Posterior Approach, Posterior Column, Percutaneous Endoscopic Approach
HAC When reported with secondary diagnosis code T84.60XA, T84.610A, T84.611A, T84.612A, T84.613A, T84.614A, T84.615A, T84.619A, T84.63XA, T84.69XA, T84.7XXA

0RG64JJ Fusion of Thoracic Vertebral Joint with Synthetic Substitute, Posterior Approach, Anterior Column, Percutaneous Endoscopic Approach
HAC When reported with secondary diagnosis code T84.60XA, T84.610A, T84.611A, T84.612A, T84.613A, T84.614A, T84.615A, T84.619A, T84.63XA, T84.69XA, T84.7XXA

0RG64K0 Fusion of Thoracic Vertebral Joint with Nonautologous Tissue Substitute, Anterior Approach, Anterior Column, Percutaneous Endoscopic Approach
HAC When reported with secondary diagnosis code T84.60XA, T84.610A, T84.611A, T84.612A, T84.613A, T84.614A, T84.615A, T84.619A, T84.63XA, T84.69XA, T84.7XXA

0RG64K1 Fusion of Thoracic Vertebral Joint with Nonautologous Tissue Substitute, Posterior Approach, Posterior Column, Percutaneous Endoscopic Approach
HAC When reported with secondary diagnosis code T84.60XA, T84.610A, T84.611A, T84.612A, T84.613A, T84.614A, T84.615A, T84.619A, T84.63XA, T84.69XA, T84.7XXA

0RG64KJ Fusion of Thoracic Vertebral Joint with Nonautologous Tissue Substitute, Posterior Approach, Anterior Column, Percutaneous Endoscopic Approach
HAC When reported with secondary diagnosis code T84.60XA, T84.610A, T84.611A, T84.612A, T84.613A, T84.614A, T84.615A, T84.619A, T84.63XA, T84.69XA, T84.7XXA

0RG64Z0 Fusion of Thoracic Vertebral Joint, Anterior Approach, Anterior Column, Percutaneous Endoscopic Approach
HAC When reported with secondary diagnosis code T84.60XA, T84.610A, T84.611A, T84.612A, T84.613A, T84.614A, T84.615A, T84.619A, T84.63XA, T84.69XA, T84.7XXA

0RG64Z1 Fusion of Thoracic Vertebral Joint, Posterior Approach, Posterior Column, Percutaneous Endoscopic Approach
HAC When reported with secondary diagnosis code T84.60XA, T84.610A, T84.611A, T84.612A, T84.613A, T84.614A, T84.615A, T84.619A, T84.63XA, T84.69XA, T84.7XXA

0RG64ZJ Fusion of Thoracic Vertebral Joint, Posterior Approach, Anterior Column, Percutaneous Endoscopic Approach
HAC When reported with secondary diagnosis code T84.60XA, T84.610A, T84.611A, T84.612A, T84.613A, T84.614A, T84.615A, T84.619A, T84.63XA, T84.69XA, T84.7XXA

0RG7070 Fusion of 2 to 7 Thoracic Vertebral Joints with Autologous Tissue Substitute, Anterior Approach, Anterior Column, Open Approach
HAC When reported with secondary diagnosis code T84.60XA, T84.610A, T84.611A, T84.612A, T84.613A, T84.614A, T84.615A, T84.619A, T84.63XA, T84.69XA, T84.7XXA
\+ Fusion of nine or more joints when reported with Fusion of two or more lumbar vertebral joints. *See table 0SG to construct Fusion code.*

0RG7071 Fusion of 2 to 7 Thoracic Vertebral Joints with Autologous Tissue Substitute, Posterior Approach, Posterior Column, Open Approach
AHA CC: 1Q, 2013, 21-23
HAC When reported with secondary diagnosis code T84.60XA, T84.610A, T84.611A, T84.612A, T84.613A, T84.614A, T84.615A, T84.619A, T84.63XA, T84.69XA, T84.7XXA
\+ Fusion of nine or more joints when reported with Fusion of two or more lumbar vertebral joints. *See table 0SG to construct Fusion code.*

0RG707J Fusion of 2 to 7 Thoracic Vertebral Joints with Autologous Tissue Substitute, Posterior Approach, Anterior Column, Open Approach
HAC When reported with secondary diagnosis code T84.60XA, T84.610A, T84.611A, T84.612A, T84.613A, T84.614A, T84.615A, T84.619A, T84.63XA, T84.69XA, T84.7XXA
\+ Fusion of nine or more joints when reported with Fusion of two or more lumbar vertebral joints. *See table 0SG to construct Fusion code.*

0RG70A0 Fusion of 2 to 7 Thoracic Vertebral Joints with Interbody Fusion Device, Anterior Approach, Anterior Column, Open Approach
HAC When reported with secondary diagnosis code T84.60XA, T84.610A, T84.611A, T84.612A, T84.613A, T84.614A, T84.615A, T84.619A, T84.63XA, T84.69XA, T84.7XXA
\+ Fusion of nine or more joints when reported with Fusion of two or more lumbar vertebral joints. *See table 0SG to construct Fusion code.*

0RG70A1 Fusion of 2 to 7 Thoracic Vertebral Joints with Interbody Fusion Device, Posterior Approach, Posterior Column, Open Approach
HAC When reported with secondary diagnosis code T84.60XA, T84.610A, T84.611A, T84.612A, T84.613A, T84.614A, T84.615A, T84.619A, T84.63XA, T84.69XA, T84.7XXA
\+ Fusion of nine or more joints when reported with Fusion of two or more lumbar vertebral joints. *See table 0SG to construct Fusion code.*

0RG70AJ Fusion of 2 to 7 Thoracic Vertebral Joints with Interbody Fusion Device, Posterior Approach, Anterior Column, Open Approach
HAC When reported with secondary diagnosis code T84.60XA, T84.610A, T84.611A, T84.612A, T84.613A, T84.614A, T84.615A, T84.619A, T84.63XA, T84.69XA, T84.7XXA
\+ Fusion of nine or more joints when reported with Fusion of two or more lumbar vertebral joints. *See table 0SG to construct Fusion code.*

0RG70J0 Fusion of 2 to 7 Thoracic Vertebral Joints with Synthetic Substitute, Anterior Approach, Anterior Column, Open Approach
HAC When reported with secondary diagnosis code T84.60XA, T84.610A, T84.611A, T84.612A, T84.613A, T84.614A, T84.615A, T84.619A, T84.63XA, T84.69XA, T84.7XXA
\+ Fusion of nine or more joints when reported with Fusion of two or more lumbar vertebral joints. *See table 0SG to construct Fusion code.*

0RG70J1 Fusion of 2 to 7 Thoracic Vertebral Joints with Synthetic Substitute, Posterior Approach, Posterior Column, Open Approach
HAC When reported with secondary diagnosis code T84.60XA, T84.610A, T84.611A, T84.612A, T84.613A, T84.614A, T84.615A, T84.619A, T84.63XA, T84.69XA, T84.7XXA
\+ Fusion of nine or more joints when reported with Fusion of two or more lumbar vertebral joints. *See table 0SG to construct Fusion code.*

0RG70JJ Fusion of 2 to 7 Thoracic Vertebral Joints with Synthetic Substitute, Posterior Approach, Anterior Column, Open Approach
HAC When reported with secondary diagnosis code T84.60XA, T84.610A, T84.611A, T84.612A, T84.613A, T84.614A, T84.615A, T84.619A, T84.63XA, T84.69XA, T84.7XXA
\+ Fusion of nine or more joints when reported with Fusion of two or more lumbar vertebral joints. *See table 0SG to construct Fusion code.*

0RG70K0 Fusion of 2 to 7 Thoracic Vertebral Joints with Nonautologous Tissue Substitute, Anterior Approach, Anterior Column, Open Approach
HAC When reported with secondary diagnosis code T84.60XA, T84.610A, T84.611A, T84.612A, T84.613A, T84.614A, T84.615A, T84.619A, T84.63XA, T84.69XA, T84.7XXA
\+ Fusion of nine or more joints when reported with Fusion of two or more lumbar vertebral joints. *See table 0SG to construct Fusion code.*

0RG70K1 Fusion of 2 to 7 Thoracic Vertebral Joints with Nonautologous Tissue Substitute, Posterior Approach, Posterior Column, Open Approach
HAC When reported with secondary diagnosis code T84.60XA, T84.610A, T84.611A, T84.612A, T84.613A, T84.614A, T84.615A, T84.619A, T84.63XA, T84.69XA, T84.7XXA
\+ Fusion of nine or more joints when reported with Fusion of two or more lumbar vertebral joints. *See table 0SG to construct Fusion code.*

0RG70KJ Fusion of 2 to 7 Thoracic Vertebral Joints with Nonautologous Tissue Substitute, Posterior Approach, Anterior Column, Open Approach
HAC When reported with secondary diagnosis code T84.60XA, T84.610A, T84.611A, T84.612A, T84.613A, T84.614A, T84.615A, T84.619A, T84.63XA, T84.69XA, T84.7XXA
\+ Fusion of nine or more joints when reported with Fusion of two or more lumbar vertebral joints. *See table 0SG to construct Fusion code.*

0RG70Z0 Fusion of 2 to 7 Thoracic Vertebral Joints, Anterior Approach, Anterior Column, Open Approach

HAC When reported with secondary diagnosis code T84.60XA, T84.610A, T84.611A, T84.612A, T84.613A, T84.614A, T84.615A, T84.619A, T84.63XA, T84.69XA, T84.7XXA

+ Fusion of nine or more joints when reported with Fusion of two or more lumbar vertebral joints. *See table 0SG to construct Fusion code.*

0RG70Z1 Fusion of 2 to 7 Thoracic Vertebral Joints, Posterior Approach, Posterior Column, Open Approach

HAC When reported with secondary diagnosis code T84.60XA, T84.610A, T84.611A, T84.612A, T84.613A, T84.614A, T84.615A, T84.619A, T84.63XA, T84.69XA, T84.7XXA

+ Fusion of nine or more joints when reported with Fusion of two or more lumbar vertebral joints. *See table 0SG to construct Fusion code.*

0RG70ZJ Fusion of 2 to 7 Thoracic Vertebral Joints, Posterior Approach, Anterior Column, Open Approach

HAC When reported with secondary diagnosis code T84.60XA, T84.610A, T84.611A, T84.612A, T84.613A, T84.614A, T84.615A, T84.619A, T84.63XA, T84.69XA, T84.7XXA

+ Fusion of nine or more joints when reported with Fusion of two or more lumbar vertebral joints. *See table 0SG to construct Fusion code.*

0RG7370 Fusion of 2 to 7 Thoracic Vertebral Joints with Autologous Tissue Substitute, Anterior Approach, Anterior Column, Percutaneous Approach

HAC When reported with secondary diagnosis code T84.60XA, T84.610A, T84.611A, T84.612A, T84.613A, T84.614A, T84.615A, T84.619A, T84.63XA, T84.69XA, T84.7XXA

+ Fusion of nine or more joints when reported with Fusion of two or more lumbar vertebral joints. *See table 0SG to construct Fusion code.*

0RG7371 Fusion of 2 to 7 Thoracic Vertebral Joints with Autologous Tissue Substitute, Posterior Approach, Posterior Column, Percutaneous Approach

HAC When reported with secondary diagnosis code T84.60XA, T84.610A, T84.611A, T84.612A, T84.613A, T84.614A, T84.615A, T84.619A, T84.63XA, T84.69XA, T84.7XXA

+ Fusion of nine or more joints when reported with Fusion of two or more lumbar vertebral joints. *See table 0SG to construct Fusion code.*

0RG737J Fusion of 2 to 7 Thoracic Vertebral Joints with Autologous Tissue Substitute, Posterior Approach, Anterior Column, Percutaneous Approach

HAC When reported with secondary diagnosis code T84.60XA, T84.610A, T84.611A, T84.612A, T84.613A, T84.614A, T84.615A, T84.619A, T84.63XA, T84.69XA, T84.7XXA

+ Fusion of nine or more joints when reported with Fusion of two or more lumbar vertebral joints. *See table 0SG to construct Fusion code.*

0RG73A0 Fusion of 2 to 7 Thoracic Vertebral Joints with Interbody Fusion Device, Anterior Approach, Anterior Column, Percutaneous Approach

HAC When reported with secondary diagnosis code T84.60XA, T84.610A, T84.611A, T84.612A, T84.613A, T84.614A, T84.615A, T84.619A, T84.63XA, T84.69XA, T84.7XXA

+ Fusion of nine or more joints when reported with Fusion of two or more lumbar vertebral joints. *See table 0SG to construct Fusion code.*

0RG73A1 Fusion of 2 to 7 Thoracic Vertebral Joints with Interbody Fusion Device, Posterior Approach, Posterior Column, Percutaneous Approach

HAC When reported with secondary diagnosis code T84.60XA, T84.610A, T84.611A, T84.612A, T84.613A, T84.614A, T84.615A, T84.619A, T84.63XA, T84.69XA, T84.7XXA

+ Fusion of nine or more joints when reported with Fusion of two or more lumbar vertebral joints. *See table 0SG to construct Fusion code.*

0RG73AJ Fusion of 2 to 7 Thoracic Vertebral Joints with Interbody Fusion Device, Posterior Approach, Anterior Column, Percutaneous Approach

HAC When reported with secondary diagnosis code T84.60XA, T84.610A, T84.611A, T84.612A, T84.613A, T84.614A, T84.615A, T84.619A, T84.63XA, T84.69XA, T84.7XXA

+ Fusion of nine or more joints when reported with Fusion of two or more lumbar vertebral joints. *See table 0SG to construct Fusion code.*

0RG73J0 Fusion of 2 to 7 Thoracic Vertebral Joints with Synthetic Substitute, Anterior Approach, Anterior Column, Percutaneous Approach

HAC When reported with secondary diagnosis code T84.60XA, T84.610A, T84.611A, T84.612A, T84.613A, T84.614A, T84.615A, T84.619A, T84.63XA, T84.69XA, T84.7XXA

+ Fusion of nine or more joints when reported with Fusion of two or more lumbar vertebral joints. *See table 0SG to construct Fusion code.*

0RG73J1 Fusion of 2 to 7 Thoracic Vertebral Joints with Synthetic Substitute, Posterior Approach, Posterior Column, Percutaneous Approach

HAC When reported with secondary diagnosis code T84.60XA, T84.610A, T84.611A, T84.612A, T84.613A, T84.614A, T84.615A, T84.619A, T84.63XA, T84.69XA, T84.7XXA

+ Fusion of nine or more joints when reported with Fusion of two or more lumbar vertebral joints. *See table 0SG to construct Fusion code.*

0RG73JJ Fusion of 2 to 7 Thoracic Vertebral Joints with Synthetic Substitute, Posterior Approach, Anterior Column, Percutaneous Approach

HAC When reported with secondary diagnosis code T84.60XA, T84.610A, T84.611A, T84.612A, T84.613A, T84.614A, T84.615A, T84.619A, T84.63XA, T84.69XA, T84.7XXA

+ Fusion of nine or more joints when reported with Fusion of two or more lumbar vertebral joints. *See table 0SG to construct Fusion code.*

0RG73K0 Fusion of 2 to 7 Thoracic Vertebral Joints with Nonautologous Tissue Substitute, Anterior Approach, Anterior Column, Percutaneous Approach

HAC When reported with secondary diagnosis code T84.60XA, T84.610A, T84.611A, T84.612A, T84.613A, T84.614A, T84.615A, T84.619A, T84.63XA, T84.69XA, T84.7XXA

+ Fusion of nine or more joints when reported with Fusion of two or more lumbar vertebral joints. *See table 0SG to construct Fusion code.*

0RG73K1 Fusion of 2 to 7 Thoracic Vertebral Joints with Nonautologous Tissue Substitute, Posterior Approach, Posterior Column, Percutaneous Approach

HAC When reported with secondary diagnosis code T84.60XA, T84.610A, T84.611A, T84.612A, T84.613A, T84.614A, T84.615A, T84.619A, T84.63XA, T84.69XA, T84.7XXA

+ Fusion of nine or more joints when reported with Fusion of two or more lumbar vertebral joints. *See table 0SG to construct Fusion code.*

0RG73KJ Fusion of 2 to 7 Thoracic Vertebral Joints with Nonautologous Tissue Substitute, Posterior Approach, Anterior Column, Percutaneous Approach

HAC When reported with secondary diagnosis code T84.60XA, T84.610A, T84.611A, T84.612A, T84.613A, T84.614A, T84.615A, T84.619A, T84.63XA, T84.69XA, T84.7XXA

+ Fusion of nine or more joints when reported with Fusion of two or more lumbar vertebral joints. *See table 0SG to construct Fusion code.*

0RG73Z0 Fusion of 2 to 7 Thoracic Vertebral Joints, Anterior Approach, Anterior Column, Percutaneous Approach

HAC When reported with secondary diagnosis code T84.60XA, T84.610A, T84.611A, T84.612A, T84.613A, T84.614A, T84.615A, T84.619A, T84.63XA, T84.69XA, T84.7XXA

+ Fusion of nine or more joints when reported with Fusion of two or more lumbar vertebral joints. *See table 0SG to construct Fusion code.*

0RG73Z1 Fusion of 2 to 7 Thoracic Vertebral Joints, Posterior Approach, Posterior Column, Percutaneous Approach

HAC When reported with secondary diagnosis code T84.60XA, T84.610A, T84.611A, T84.612A, T84.613A, T84.614A, T84.615A, T84.619A, T84.63XA, T84.69XA, T84.7XXA

+ Fusion of nine or more joints when reported with Fusion of two or more lumbar vertebral joints. *See table 0SG to construct Fusion code.*

0RG73ZJ Fusion of 2 to 7 Thoracic Vertebral Joints, Posterior Approach, Anterior Column, Percutaneous Approach

HAC When reported with secondary diagnosis code T84.60XA, T84.610A, T84.611A, T84.612A, T84.613A, T84.614A, T84.615A, T84.619A, T84.63XA, T84.69XA, T84.7XXA

+ Fusion of nine or more joints when reported with Fusion of two or more lumbar vertebral joints. *See table 0SG to construct Fusion code.*

0RG7470 Fusion of 2 to 7 Thoracic Vertebral Joints with Autologous Tissue Substitute, Anterior Approach, Anterior Column, Percutaneous Endoscopic Approach

Note Continued

RG7470 Continued Note

HAC When reported with secondary diagnosis code T84.60XA, T84.610A, T84.611A, T84.612A, T84.613A, T84.614A, T84.615A, T84.619A, T84.63XA, T84.69XA, T84.7XXA

+ Fusion of nine or more joints when reported with Fusion of two or more lumbar vertebral joints. *See table 0SG to construct Fusion code.*

RG7471 Fusion of 2 to 7 Thoracic Vertebral Joints with Autologous Tissue Substitute, Posterior Approach, Posterior Column, Percutaneous Endoscopic Approach

HAC When reported with secondary diagnosis code T84.60XA, T84.610A, T84.611A, T84.612A, T84.613A, T84.614A, T84.615A, T84.619A, T84.63XA, T84.69XA, T84.7XXA

+ Fusion of nine or more joints when reported with Fusion of two or more lumbar vertebral joints. *See table 0SG to construct Fusion code.*

RG747J Fusion of 2 to 7 Thoracic Vertebral Joints with Autologous Tissue Substitute, Posterior Approach, Anterior Column, Percutaneous Endoscopic Approach

HAC When reported with secondary diagnosis code T84.60XA, T84.610A, T84.611A, T84.612A, T84.613A, T84.614A, T84.615A, T84.619A, T84.63XA, T84.69XA, T84.7XXA

+ Fusion of nine or more joints when reported with Fusion of two or more lumbar vertebral joints. *See table 0SG to construct Fusion code.*

0RG74A0 Fusion of 2 to 7 Thoracic Vertebral Joints with Interbody Fusion Device, Anterior Approach, Anterior Column, Percutaneous Endoscopic Approach

HAC When reported with secondary diagnosis code T84.60XA, T84.610A, T84.611A, T84.612A, T84.613A, T84.614A, T84.615A, T84.619A, T84.63XA, T84.69XA, T84.7XXA

+ Fusion of nine or more joints when reported with Fusion of two or more lumbar vertebral joints. *See table 0SG to construct Fusion code.*

0RG74A1 Fusion of 2 to 7 Thoracic Vertebral Joints with Interbody Fusion Device, Posterior Approach, Posterior Column, Percutaneous Endoscopic Approach

HAC When reported with secondary diagnosis code T84.60XA, T84.610A, T84.611A, T84.612A, T84.613A, T84.614A, T84.615A, T84.619A, T84.63XA, T84.69XA, T84.7XXA

+ Fusion of nine or more joints when reported with Fusion of two or more lumbar vertebral joints. *See table 0SG to construct Fusion code.*

0RG74AJ Fusion of 2 to 7 Thoracic Vertebral Joints with Interbody Fusion Device, Posterior Approach, Anterior Column, Percutaneous Endoscopic Approach

HAC When reported with secondary diagnosis code T84.60XA, T84.610A, T84.611A, T84.612A, T84.613A, T84.614A, T84.615A, T84.619A, T84.63XA, T84.69XA, T84.7XXA

+ Fusion of nine or more joints when reported with Fusion of two or more lumbar vertebral joints. *See table 0SG to construct Fusion code.*

0RG74J0 Fusion of 2 to 7 Thoracic Vertebral Joints with Synthetic Substitute, Anterior Approach, Anterior Column, Percutaneous Endoscopic Approach

HAC When reported with secondary diagnosis code T84.60XA, T84.610A, T84.611A, T84.612A, T84.613A, T84.614A, T84.615A, T84.619A, T84.63XA, T84.69XA, T84.7XXA

+ Fusion of nine or more joints when reported with Fusion of two or more lumbar vertebral joints. *See table 0SG to construct Fusion code.*

0RG74J1 Fusion of 2 to 7 Thoracic Vertebral Joints with Synthetic Substitute, Posterior Approach, Posterior Column, Percutaneous Endoscopic Approach

HAC When reported with secondary diagnosis code T84.60XA, T84.610A, T84.611A, T84.612A, T84.613A, T84.614A, T84.615A, T84.619A, T84.63XA, T84.69XA, T84.7XXA

+ Fusion of nine or more joints when reported with Fusion of two or more lumbar vertebral joints. *See table 0SG to construct Fusion code.*

0RG74JJ Fusion of 2 to 7 Thoracic Vertebral Joints with Synthetic Substitute, Posterior Approach, Anterior Column, Percutaneous Endoscopic Approach

HAC When reported with secondary diagnosis code T84.60XA, T84.610A, T84.611A, T84.612A, T84.613A, T84.614A, T84.615A, T84.619A, T84.63XA, T84.69XA, T84.7XXA

+ Fusion of nine or more joints when reported with Fusion of two or more lumbar vertebral joints. *See table 0SG to construct Fusion code.*

0RG74K0 Fusion of 2 to 7 Thoracic Vertebral Joints with Nonautologous Tissue Substitute, Anterior Approach, Anterior Column, Percutaneous Endoscopic Approach

HAC When reported with secondary diagnosis code T84.60XA, T84.610A, T84.611A, T84.612A, T84.613A, T84.614A, T84.615A, T84.619A, T84.63XA, T84.69XA, T84.7XXA

+ Fusion of nine or more joints when reported with Fusion of two or more lumbar vertebral joints. *See table 0SG to construct Fusion code.*

0RG74K1 Fusion of 2 to 7 Thoracic Vertebral Joints with Nonautologous Tissue Substitute, Posterior Approach, Posterior Column, Percutaneous Endoscopic Approach

HAC When reported with secondary diagnosis code T84.60XA, T84.610A, T84.611A, T84.612A, T84.613A, T84.614A, T84.615A, T84.619A, T84.63XA, T84.69XA, T84.7XXA

+ Fusion of nine or more joints when reported with Fusion of two or more lumbar vertebral joints. *See table 0SG to construct Fusion code.*

0RG74KJ Fusion of 2 to 7 Thoracic Vertebral Joints with Nonautologous Tissue Substitute, Posterior Approach, Anterior Column, Percutaneous Endoscopic Approach

HAC When reported with secondary diagnosis code T84.60XA, T84.610A, T84.611A, T84.612A, T84.613A, T84.614A, T84.615A, T84.619A, T84.63XA, T84.69XA, T84.7XXA

+ Fusion of nine or more joints when reported with Fusion of two or more lumbar vertebral joints. *See table 0SG to construct Fusion code.*

0RG74Z0 Fusion of 2 to 7 Thoracic Vertebral Joints, Anterior Approach, Anterior Column, Percutaneous Endoscopic Approach

HAC When reported with secondary diagnosis code T84.60XA, T84.610A, T84.611A, T84.612A, T84.613A, T84.614A, T84.615A, T84.619A, T84.63XA, T84.69XA, T84.7XXA

+ Fusion of nine or more joints when reported with Fusion of two or more lumbar vertebral joints. *See table 0SG to construct Fusion code.*

0RG74Z1 Fusion of 2 to 7 Thoracic Vertebral Joints, Posterior Approach, Posterior Column, Percutaneous Endoscopic Approach

HAC When reported with secondary diagnosis code T84.60XA, T84.610A, T84.611A, T84.612A, T84.613A, T84.614A, T84.615A, T84.619A, T84.63XA, T84.69XA, T84.7XXA

+ Fusion of nine or more joints when reported with Fusion of two or more lumbar vertebral joints. *See table 0SG to construct Fusion code.*

0RG74ZJ Fusion of 2 to 7 Thoracic Vertebral Joints, Posterior Approach, Anterior Column, Percutaneous Endoscopic Approach

HAC When reported with secondary diagnosis code T84.60XA, T84.610A, T84.611A, T84.612A, T84.613A, T84.614A, T84.615A, T84.619A, T84.63XA, T84.69XA, T84.7XXA

+ Fusion of nine or more joints when reported with Fusion of two or more lumbar vertebral joints. *See table 0SG to construct Fusion code.*

0RG8070 Fusion of 8 or more Thoracic Vertebral Joints with Autologous Tissue Substitute, Anterior Approach, Anterior Column, Open Approach

HAC When reported with secondary diagnosis code T84.60XA, T84.610A, T84.611A, T84.612A, T84.613A, T84.614A, T84.615A, T84.619A, T84.63XA, T84.69XA, T84.7XXA

0RG8071 Fusion of 8 or more Thoracic Vertebral Joints with Autologous Tissue Substitute, Posterior Approach, Posterior Column, Open Approach

HAC When reported with secondary diagnosis code T84.60XA, T84.610A, T84.611A, T84.612A, T84.613A, T84.614A, T84.615A, T84.619A, T84.63XA, T84.69XA, T84.7XXA

0RG807J Fusion of 8 or more Thoracic Vertebral Joints with Autologous Tissue Substitute, Posterior Approach, Anterior Column, Open Approach

HAC When reported with secondary diagnosis code T84.60XA, T84.610A, T84.611A, T84.612A, T84.613A, T84.614A, T84.615A, T84.619A, T84.63XA, T84.69XA, T84.7XXA

0RG80A0 Fusion of 8 or more Thoracic Vertebral Joints with Interbody Fusion Device, Anterior Approach, Anterior Column, Open Approach

HAC When reported with secondary diagnosis code T84.60XA, T84.610A, T84.611A, T84.612A, T84.613A, T84.614A, T84.615A, T84.619A, T84.63XA, T84.69XA, T84.7XXA

0RG80A1 Fusion of 8 or more Thoracic Vertebral Joints with Interbody Fusion Device, Posterior Approach, Posterior Column, Open Approach

Note Continued

0RG80A1 Continued Note

HAC When reported with secondary diagnosis code T84.60XA, T84.610A, T84.611A, T84.612A, T84.613A, T84.614A, T84.615A, T84.619A, T84.63XA, T84.69XA, T84.7XXA

0RG80AJ Fusion of 8 or more Thoracic Vertebral Joints with Interbody Fusion Device, Posterior Approach, Anterior Column, Open Approach

HAC When reported with secondary diagnosis code T84.60XA, T84.610A, T84.611A, T84.612A, T84.613A, T84.614A, T84.615A, T84.619A, T84.63XA, T84.69XA, T84.7XXA

0RG80J0 Fusion of 8 or more Thoracic Vertebral Joints with Synthetic Substitute, Anterior Approach, Anterior Column, Open Approach

HAC When reported with secondary diagnosis code T84.60XA, T84.610A, T84.611A, T84.612A, T84.613A, T84.614A, T84.615A, T84.619A, T84.63XA, T84.69XA, T84.7XXA

0RG80J1 Fusion of 8 or more Thoracic Vertebral Joints with Synthetic Substitute, Posterior Approach, Posterior Column, Open Approach

HAC When reported with secondary diagnosis code T84.60XA, T84.610A, T84.611A, T84.612A, T84.613A, T84.614A, T84.615A, T84.619A, T84.63XA, T84.69XA, T84.7XXA

0RG80JJ Fusion of 8 or more Thoracic Vertebral Joints with Synthetic Substitute, Posterior Approach, Anterior Column, Open Approach

HAC When reported with secondary diagnosis code T84.60XA, T84.610A, T84.611A, T84.612A, T84.613A, T84.614A, T84.615A, T84.619A, T84.63XA, T84.69XA, T84.7XXA

0RG80K0 Fusion of 8 or more Thoracic Vertebral Joints with Nonautologous Tissue Substitute, Anterior Approach, Anterior Column, Open Approach

HAC When reported with secondary diagnosis code T84.60XA, T84.610A, T84.611A, T84.612A, T84.613A, T84.614A, T84.615A, T84.619A, T84.63XA, T84.69XA, T84.7XXA

0RG80K1 Fusion of 8 or more Thoracic Vertebral Joints with Nonautologous Tissue Substitute, Posterior Approach, Posterior Column, Open Approach

HAC When reported with secondary diagnosis code T84.60XA, T84.610A, T84.611A, T84.612A, T84.613A, T84.614A, T84.615A, T84.619A, T84.63XA, T84.69XA, T84.7XXA

0RG80KJ Fusion of 8 or more Thoracic Vertebral Joints with Nonautologous Tissue Substitute, Posterior Approach, Anterior Column, Open Approach

HAC When reported with secondary diagnosis code T84.60XA, T84.610A, T84.611A, T84.612A, T84.613A, T84.614A, T84.615A, T84.619A, T84.63XA, T84.69XA, T84.7XXA

0RG80Z0 Fusion of 8 or more Thoracic Vertebral Joints, Anterior Approach, Anterior Column, Open Approach

HAC When reported with secondary diagnosis code T84.60XA, T84.610A, T84.611A, T84.612A, T84.613A, T84.614A, T84.615A, T84.619A, T84.63XA, T84.69XA, T84.7XXA

0RG80Z1 Fusion of 8 or more Thoracic Vertebral Joints, Posterior Approach, Posterior Column, Open Approach

HAC When reported with secondary diagnosis code T84.60XA, T84.610A, T84.611A, T84.612A, T84.613A, T84.614A, T84.615A, T84.619A, T84.63XA, T84.69XA, T84.7XXA

0RG80ZJ Fusion of 8 or more Thoracic Vertebral Joints, Posterior Approach, Anterior Column, Open Approach

HAC When reported with secondary diagnosis code T84.60XA, T84.610A, T84.611A, T84.612A, T84.613A, T84.614A, T84.615A, T84.619A, T84.63XA, T84.69XA, T84.7XXA

0RG8370 Fusion of 8 or more Thoracic Vertebral Joints with Autologous Tissue Substitute, Anterior Approach, Anterior Column, Percutaneous Approach

HAC When reported with secondary diagnosis code T84.60XA, T84.610A, T84.611A, T84.612A, T84.613A, T84.614A, T84.615A, T84.619A, T84.63XA, T84.69XA, T84.7XXA

0RG8371 Fusion of 8 or more Thoracic Vertebral Joints with Autologous Tissue Substitute, Posterior Approach, Posterior Column, Percutaneous Approach

HAC When reported with secondary diagnosis code T84.60XA, T84.610A, T84.611A, T84.612A, T84.613A, T84.614A, T84.615A, T84.619A, T84.63XA, T84.69XA, T84.7XXA

0RG837J Fusion of 8 or more Thoracic Vertebral Joints with Autologous Tissue Substitute, Posterior Approach, Anterior Column, Percutaneous Approach

HAC When reported with secondary diagnosis code T84.60XA, T84.610A, T84.611A, T84.612A, T84.613A, T84.614A, T84.615A, T84.619A, T84.63XA, T84.69XA, T84.7XXA

0RG83A0 Fusion of 8 or more Thoracic Vertebral Joints with Interbody Fusion Device, Anterior Approach, Anterior Column, Percutaneous Approach

HAC When reported with secondary diagnosis code T84.60XA, T84.610A, T84.611A, T84.612A, T84.613A, T84.614A, T84.615A, T84.619A, T84.63XA, T84.69XA, T84.7XXA

0RG83A1 Fusion of 8 or more Thoracic Vertebral Joints with Interbody Fusion Device, Posterior Approach, Posterior Column, Percutaneous Approach

HAC When reported with secondary diagnosis code T84.60XA, T84.610A, T84.611A, T84.612A, T84.613A, T84.614A, T84.615A, T84.619A, T84.63XA, T84.69XA, T84.7XXA

0RG83AJ Fusion of 8 or more Thoracic Vertebral Joints with Interbody Fusion Device, Posterior Approach, Anterior Column, Percutaneous Approach

HAC When reported with secondary diagnosis code T84.60XA, T84.610A, T84.611A, T84.612A, T84.613A, T84.614A, T84.615A, T84.619A, T84.63XA, T84.69XA, T84.7XXA

0RG83J0 Fusion of 8 or more Thoracic Vertebral Joints with Synthetic Substitute, Anterior Approach, Anterior Column, Percutaneous Approach

HAC When reported with secondary diagnosis code T84.60XA, T84.610A, T84.611A, T84.612A, T84.613A, T84.614A, T84.615A, T84.619A, T84.63XA, T84.69XA, T84.7XXA

0RG83J1 Fusion of 8 or more Thoracic Vertebral Joints with Synthetic Substitute, Posterior Approach, Posterior Column, Percutaneous Approach

HAC When reported with secondary diagnosis code T84.60XA, T84.610A, T84.611A, T84.612A, T84.613A, T84.614A, T84.615A, T84.619A, T84.63XA, T84.69XA, T84.7XXA

0RG83JJ Fusion of 8 or more Thoracic Vertebral Joints with Synthetic Substitute, Posterior Approach, Anterior Column, Percutaneous Approach

HAC When reported with secondary diagnosis code T84.60XA, T84.610A, T84.611A, T84.612A, T84.613A, T84.614A, T84.615A, T84.619A, T84.63XA, T84.69XA, T84.7XXA

0RG83K0 Fusion of 8 or more Thoracic Vertebral Joints with Nonautologous Tissue Substitute, Anterior Approach, Anterior Column, Percutaneous Approach

HAC When reported with secondary diagnosis code T84.60XA, T84.610A, T84.611A, T84.612A, T84.613A, T84.614A, T84.615A, T84.619A, T84.63XA, T84.69XA, T84.7XXA

0RG83K1 Fusion of 8 or more Thoracic Vertebral Joints with Nonautologous Tissue Substitute, Posterior Approach, Posterior Column, Percutaneous Approach

HAC When reported with secondary diagnosis code T84.60XA, T84.610A, T84.611A, T84.612A, T84.613A, T84.614A, T84.615A, T84.619A, T84.63XA, T84.69XA, T84.7XXA

0RG83KJ Fusion of 8 or more Thoracic Vertebral Joints with Nonautologous Tissue Substitute, Posterior Approach, Anterior Column, Percutaneous Approach

HAC When reported with secondary diagnosis code T84.60XA, T84.610A, T84.611A, T84.612A, T84.613A, T84.614A, T84.615A, T84.619A, T84.63XA, T84.69XA, T84.7XXA

0RG83Z0 Fusion of 8 or more Thoracic Vertebral Joints, Anterior Approach, Anterior Column, Percutaneous Approach

HAC When reported with secondary diagnosis code T84.60XA, T84.610A, T84.611A, T84.612A, T84.613A, T84.614A, T84.615A, T84.619A, T84.63XA, T84.69XA, T84.7XXA

0RG83Z1 Fusion of 8 or more Thoracic Vertebral Joints, Posterior Approach, Posterior Column, Percutaneous Approach

HAC When reported with secondary diagnosis code T84.60XA, T84.610A, T84.611A, T84.612A, T84.613A, T84.614A, T84.615A, T84.619A, T84.63XA, T84.69XA, T84.7XXA

0RG83ZJ Fusion of 8 or more Thoracic Vertebral Joints, Posterior Approach, Anterior Column, Percutaneous Approach

HAC When reported with secondary diagnosis code T84.60XA, T84.610A, T84.611A, T84.612A, T84.613A, T84.614A, T84.615A, T84.619A, T84.63XA, T84.69XA, T84.7XXA

0RG8470 Fusion of 8 or more Thoracic Vertebral Joints with Autologous Tissue Substitute, Anterior Approach, Anterior Column, Percutaneous Endoscopic Approach

Note Continued

0RG8470 Continued Note

HAC When reported with secondary diagnosis code T84.60XA, T84.610A, T84.611A, T84.612A, T84.613A, T84.614A, T84.615A, T84.619A, T84.63XA, T84.69XA, T84.7XXA

0RG8471 Fusion of 8 or more Thoracic Vertebral Joints with Autologous Tissue Substitute, Posterior Approach, Posterior Column, Percutaneous Endoscopic Approach

HAC When reported with secondary diagnosis code T84.60XA, T84.610A, T84.611A, T84.612A, T84.613A, T84.614A, T84.615A, T84.619A, T84.63XA, T84.69XA, T84.7XXA

0RG847J Fusion of 8 or more Thoracic Vertebral Joints with Autologous Tissue Substitute, Posterior Approach, Anterior Column, Percutaneous Endoscopic Approach

HAC When reported with secondary diagnosis code T84.60XA, T84.610A, T84.611A, T84.612A, T84.613A, T84.614A, T84.615A, T84.619A, T84.63XA, T84.69XA, T84.7XXA

0RG84A0 Fusion of 8 or more Thoracic Vertebral Joints with Interbody Fusion Device, Anterior Approach, Anterior Column, Percutaneous Endoscopic Approach

HAC When reported with secondary diagnosis code T84.60XA, T84.610A, T84.611A, T84.612A, T84.613A, T84.614A, T84.615A, T84.619A, T84.63XA, T84.69XA, T84.7XXA

0RG84A1 Fusion of 8 or more Thoracic Vertebral Joints with Interbody Fusion Device, Posterior Approach, Posterior Column, Percutaneous Endoscopic Approach

HAC When reported with secondary diagnosis code T84.60XA, T84.610A, T84.611A, T84.612A, T84.613A, T84.614A, T84.615A, T84.619A, T84.63XA, T84.69XA, T84.7XXA

0RG84AJ Fusion of 8 or more Thoracic Vertebral Joints with Interbody Fusion Device, Posterior Approach, Anterior Column, Percutaneous Endoscopic Approach

HAC When reported with secondary diagnosis code T84.60XA, T84.610A, T84.611A, T84.612A, T84.613A, T84.614A, T84.615A, T84.619A, T84.63XA, T84.69XA, T84.7XXA

0RG84J0 Fusion of 8 or more Thoracic Vertebral Joints with Synthetic Substitute, Anterior Approach, Anterior Column, Percutaneous Endoscopic Approach

HAC When reported with secondary diagnosis code T84.60XA, T84.610A, T84.611A, T84.612A, T84.613A, T84.614A, T84.615A, T84.619A, T84.63XA, T84.69XA, T84.7XXA

0RG84J1 Fusion of 8 or more Thoracic Vertebral Joints with Synthetic Substitute, Posterior Approach, Posterior Column, Percutaneous Endoscopic Approach

HAC When reported with secondary diagnosis code T84.60XA, T84.610A, T84.611A, T84.612A, T84.613A, T84.614A, T84.615A, T84.619A, T84.63XA, T84.69XA, T84.7XXA

0RG84JJ Fusion of 8 or more Thoracic Vertebral Joints with Synthetic Substitute, Posterior Approach, Anterior Column, Percutaneous Endoscopic Approach

HAC When reported with secondary diagnosis code T84.60XA, T84.610A, T84.611A, T84.612A, T84.613A, T84.614A, T84.615A, T84.619A, T84.63XA, T84.69XA, T84.7XXA

0RG84K0 Fusion of 8 or more Thoracic Vertebral Joints with Nonautologous Tissue Substitute, Anterior Approach, Anterior Column, Percutaneous Endoscopic Approach

HAC When reported with secondary diagnosis code T84.60XA, T84.610A, T84.611A, T84.612A, T84.613A, T84.614A, T84.615A, T84.619A, T84.63XA, T84.69XA, T84.7XXA

0RG84K1 Fusion of 8 or more Thoracic Vertebral Joints with Nonautologous Tissue Substitute, Posterior Approach, Posterior Column, Percutaneous Endoscopic Approach

HAC When reported with secondary diagnosis code T84.60XA, T84.610A, T84.611A, T84.612A, T84.613A, T84.614A, T84.615A, T84.619A, T84.63XA, T84.69XA, T84.7XXA

0RG84KJ Fusion of 8 or more Thoracic Vertebral Joints with Nonautologous Tissue Substitute, Posterior Approach, Anterior Column, Percutaneous Endoscopic Approach

HAC When reported with secondary diagnosis code T84.60XA, T84.610A, T84.611A, T84.612A, T84.613A, T84.614A, T84.615A, T84.619A, T84.63XA, T84.69XA, T84.7XXA

0RG84Z0 Fusion of 8 or more Thoracic Vertebral Joints, Anterior Approach, Anterior Column, Percutaneous Endoscopic Approach

HAC When reported with secondary diagnosis code T84.60XA, T84.610A, T84.611A, T84.612A, T84.613A, T84.614A, T84.615A, T84.619A, T84.63XA, T84.69XA, T84.7XXA

0RG84Z1 Fusion of 8 or more Thoracic Vertebral Joints, Posterior Approach, Posterior Column, Percutaneous Endoscopic Approach

HAC When reported with secondary diagnosis code T84.60XA, T84.610A, T84.611A, T84.612A, T84.613A, T84.614A, T84.615A, T84.619A, T84.63XA, T84.69XA, T84.7XXA

0RG84ZJ Fusion of 8 or more Thoracic Vertebral Joints, Posterior Approach, Anterior Column, Percutaneous Endoscopic Approach

HAC When reported with secondary diagnosis code T84.60XA, T84.610A, T84.611A, T84.612A, T84.613A, T84.614A, T84.615A, T84.619A, T84.63XA, T84.69XA, T84.7XXA

0RGA070 Fusion of Thoracolumbar Vertebral Joint with Autologous Tissue Substitute, Anterior Approach, Anterior Column, Open Approach

HAC When reported with secondary diagnosis code T84.60XA, T84.610A, T84.611A, T84.612A, T84.613A, T84.614A, T84.615A, T84.619A, T84.63XA, T84.69XA, T84.7XXA

0RGA071 Fusion of Thoracolumbar Vertebral Joint with Autologous Tissue Substitute, Posterior Approach, Posterior Column, Open Approach

AHA CC: 1Q, 2013, 21-23

HAC When reported with secondary diagnosis code T84.60XA, T84.610A, T84.611A, T84.612A, T84.613A, T84.614A, T84.615A, T84.619A, T84.63XA, T84.69XA, T84.7XXA

0RGA07J Fusion of Thoracolumbar Vertebral Joint with Autologous Tissue Substitute, Posterior Approach, Anterior Column, Open Approach

HAC When reported with secondary diagnosis code T84.60XA, T84.610A, T84.611A, T84.612A, T84.613A, T84.614A, T84.615A, T84.619A, T84.63XA, T84.69XA, T84.7XXA

0RGA0A0 Fusion of Thoracolumbar Vertebral Joint with Interbody Fusion Device, Anterior Approach, Anterior Column, Open Approach

HAC When reported with secondary diagnosis code T84.60XA, T84.610A, T84.611A, T84.612A, T84.613A, T84.614A, T84.615A, T84.619A, T84.63XA, T84.69XA, T84.7XXA

0RGA0A1 Fusion of Thoracolumbar Vertebral Joint with Interbody Fusion Device, Posterior Approach, Posterior Column, Open Approach

HAC When reported with secondary diagnosis code T84.60XA, T84.610A, T84.611A, T84.612A, T84.613A, T84.614A, T84.615A, T84.619A, T84.63XA, T84.69XA, T84.7XXA

0RGA0AJ Fusion of Thoracolumbar Vertebral Joint with Interbody Fusion Device, Posterior Approach, Anterior Column, Open Approach

HAC When reported with secondary diagnosis code T84.60XA, T84.610A, T84.611A, T84.612A, T84.613A, T84.614A, T84.615A, T84.619A, T84.63XA, T84.69XA, T84.7XXA

0RGA0J0 Fusion of Thoracolumbar Vertebral Joint with Synthetic Substitute, Anterior Approach, Anterior Column, Open Approach

HAC When reported with secondary diagnosis code T84.60XA, T84.610A, T84.611A, T84.612A, T84.613A, T84.614A, T84.615A, T84.619A, T84.63XA, T84.69XA, T84.7XXA

0RGA0J1 Fusion of Thoracolumbar Vertebral Joint with Synthetic Substitute, Posterior Approach, Posterior Column, Open Approach

HAC When reported with secondary diagnosis code T84.60XA, T84.610A, T84.611A, T84.612A, T84.613A, T84.614A, T84.615A, T84.619A, T84.63XA, T84.69XA, T84.7XXA

0RGA0JJ Fusion of Thoracolumbar Vertebral Joint with Synthetic Substitute, Posterior Approach, Anterior Column, Open Approach

HAC When reported with secondary diagnosis code T84.60XA, T84.610A, T84.611A, T84.612A, T84.613A, T84.614A, T84.615A, T84.619A, T84.63XA, T84.69XA, T84.7XXA

0RGA0K0 Fusion of Thoracolumbar Vertebral Joint with Nonautologous Tissue Substitute, Anterior Approach, Anterior Column, Open Approach

HAC When reported with secondary diagnosis code T84.60XA, T84.610A, T84.611A, T84.612A, T84.613A, T84.614A, T84.615A, T84.619A, T84.63XA, T84.69XA, T84.7XXA

0RGA0K1 Fusion of Thoracolumbar Vertebral Joint with Nonautologous Tissue Substitute, Posterior Approach, Posterior Column, Open Approach

Note Continued

0RGA0K1 Continued Note

HAC When reported with secondary diagnosis code T84.60XA, T84.610A, T84.611A, T84.612A, T84.613A, T84.614A, T84.615A, T84.619A, T84.63XA, T84.69XA, T84.7XXA

0RGA0KJ Fusion of Thoracolumbar Vertebral Joint with Nonautologous Tissue Substitute, Posterior Approach, Anterior Column, Open Approach

HAC When reported with secondary diagnosis code T84.60XA, T84.610A, T84.611A, T84.612A, T84.613A, T84.614A, T84.615A, T84.619A, T84.63XA, T84.69XA, T84.7XXA

0RGA0Z0 Fusion of Thoracolumbar Vertebral Joint, Anterior Approach, Anterior Column, Open Approach

HAC When reported with secondary diagnosis code T84.60XA, T84.610A, T84.611A, T84.612A, T84.613A, T84.614A, T84.615A, T84.619A, T84.63XA, T84.69XA, T84.7XXA

0RGA0Z1 Fusion of Thoracolumbar Vertebral Joint, Posterior Approach, Posterior Column, Open Approach

HAC When reported with secondary diagnosis code T84.60XA, T84.610A, T84.611A, T84.612A, T84.613A, T84.614A, T84.615A, T84.619A, T84.63XA, T84.69XA, T84.7XXA

0RGA0ZJ Fusion of Thoracolumbar Vertebral Joint, Posterior Approach, Anterior Column, Open Approach

HAC When reported with secondary diagnosis code T84.60XA, T84.610A, T84.611A, T84.612A, T84.613A, T84.614A, T84.615A, T84.619A, T84.63XA, T84.69XA, T84.7XXA

0RGA370 Fusion of Thoracolumbar Vertebral Joint with Autologous Tissue Substitute, Anterior Approach, Anterior Column, Percutaneous Approach

HAC When reported with secondary diagnosis code T84.60XA, T84.610A, T84.611A, T84.612A, T84.613A, T84.614A, T84.615A, T84.619A, T84.63XA, T84.69XA, T84.7XXA

0RGA371 Fusion of Thoracolumbar Vertebral Joint with Autologous Tissue Substitute, Posterior Approach, Posterior Column, Percutaneous Approach

HAC When reported with secondary diagnosis code T84.60XA, T84.610A, T84.611A, T84.612A, T84.613A, T84.614A, T84.615A, T84.619A, T84.63XA, T84.69XA, T84.7XXA

0RGA37J Fusion of Thoracolumbar Vertebral Joint with Autologous Tissue Substitute, Posterior Approach, Anterior Column, Percutaneous Approach

HAC When reported with secondary diagnosis code T84.60XA, T84.610A, T84.611A, T84.612A, T84.613A, T84.614A, T84.615A, T84.619A, T84.63XA, T84.69XA, T84.7XXA

0RGA3A0 Fusion of Thoracolumbar Vertebral Joint with Interbody Fusion Device, Anterior Approach, Anterior Column, Percutaneous Approach

HAC When reported with secondary diagnosis code T84.60XA, T84.610A, T84.611A, T84.612A, T84.613A, T84.614A, T84.615A, T84.619A, T84.63XA, T84.69XA, T84.7XXA

0RGA3A1 Fusion of Thoracolumbar Vertebral Joint with Interbody Fusion Device, Posterior Approach, Posterior Column, Percutaneous Approach

HAC When reported with secondary diagnosis code T84.60XA, T84.610A, T84.611A, T84.612A, T84.613A, T84.614A, T84.615A, T84.619A, T84.63XA, T84.69XA, T84.7XXA

0RGA3AJ Fusion of Thoracolumbar Vertebral Joint with Interbody Fusion Device, Posterior Approach, Anterior Column, Percutaneous Approach

HAC When reported with secondary diagnosis code T84.60XA, T84.610A, T84.611A, T84.612A, T84.613A, T84.614A, T84.615A, T84.619A, T84.63XA, T84.69XA, T84.7XXA

0RGA3J0 Fusion of Thoracolumbar Vertebral Joint with Synthetic Substitute, Anterior Approach, Anterior Column, Percutaneous Approach

HAC When reported with secondary diagnosis code T84.60XA, T84.610A, T84.611A, T84.612A, T84.613A, T84.614A, T84.615A, T84.619A, T84.63XA, T84.69XA, T84.7XXA

0RGA3J1 Fusion of Thoracolumbar Vertebral Joint with Synthetic Substitute, Posterior Approach, Posterior Column, Percutaneous Approach

HAC When reported with secondary diagnosis code T84.60XA, T84.610A, T84.611A, T84.612A, T84.613A, T84.614A, T84.615A, T84.619A, T84.63XA, T84.69XA, T84.7XXA

0RGA3JJ Fusion of Thoracolumbar Vertebral Joint with Synthetic Substitute, Posterior Approach, Anterior Column, Percutaneous Approach

HAC When reported with secondary diagnosis code T84.60XA, T84.610A, T84.611A, T84.612A, T84.613A, T84.614A, T84.615A, T84.619A, T84.63XA, T84.69XA, T84.7XXA

0RGA3K0 Fusion of Thoracolumbar Vertebral Joint with Nonautologous Tissue Substitute, Anterior Approach, Anterior Column, Percutaneous Approach

HAC When reported with secondary diagnosis code T84.60XA, T84.610A, T84.611A, T84.612A, T84.613A, T84.614A, T84.615A, T84.619A, T84.63XA, T84.69XA, T84.7XXA

0RGA3K1 Fusion of Thoracolumbar Vertebral Joint with Nonautologous Tissue Substitute, Posterior Approach, Posterior Column, Percutaneous Approach

HAC When reported with secondary diagnosis code T84.60XA, T84.610A, T84.611A, T84.612A, T84.613A, T84.614A, T84.615A, T84.619A, T84.63XA, T84.69XA, T84.7XXA

0RGA3KJ Fusion of Thoracolumbar Vertebral Joint with Nonautologous Tissue Substitute, Posterior Approach, Anterior Column, Percutaneous Approach

HAC When reported with secondary diagnosis code T84.60XA, T84.610A, T84.611A, T84.612A, T84.613A, T84.614A, T84.615A, T84.619A, T84.63XA, T84.69XA, T84.7XXA

0RGA3Z0 Fusion of Thoracolumbar Vertebral Joint, Anterior Approach, Anterior Column, Percutaneous Approach

HAC When reported with secondary diagnosis code T84.60XA, T84.610A, T84.611A, T84.612A, T84.613A, T84.614A, T84.615A, T84.619A, T84.63XA, T84.69XA, T84.7XXA

0RGA3Z1 Fusion of Thoracolumbar Vertebral Joint, Posterior Approach, Posterior Column, Percutaneous Approach

HAC When reported with secondary diagnosis code T84.60XA, T84.610A, T84.611A, T84.612A, T84.613A, T84.614A, T84.615A, T84.619A, T84.63XA, T84.69XA, T84.7XXA

0RGA3ZJ Fusion of Thoracolumbar Vertebral Joint, Posterior Approach, Anterior Column, Percutaneous Approach

HAC When reported with secondary diagnosis code T84.60XA, T84.610A, T84.611A, T84.612A, T84.613A, T84.614A, T84.615A, T84.619A, T84.63XA, T84.69XA, T84.7XXA

0RGA470 Fusion of Thoracolumbar Vertebral Joint with Autologous Tissue Substitute, Anterior Approach, Anterior Column, Percutaneous Endoscopic Approach

HAC When reported with secondary diagnosis code T84.60XA, T84.610A, T84.611A, T84.612A, T84.613A, T84.614A, T84.615A, T84.619A, T84.63XA, T84.69XA, T84.7XXA

0RGA471 Fusion of Thoracolumbar Vertebral Joint with Autologous Tissue Substitute, Posterior Approach, Posterior Column, Percutaneous Endoscopic Approach

HAC When reported with secondary diagnosis code T84.60XA, T84.610A, T84.611A, T84.612A, T84.613A, T84.614A, T84.615A, T84.619A, T84.63XA, T84.69XA, T84.7XXA

0RGA47J Fusion of Thoracolumbar Vertebral Joint with Autologous Tissue Substitute, Posterior Approach, Anterior Column, Percutaneous Endoscopic Approach

HAC When reported with secondary diagnosis code T84.60XA, T84.610A, T84.611A, T84.612A, T84.613A, T84.614A, T84.615A, T84.619A, T84.63XA, T84.69XA, T84.7XXA

0RGA4A0 Fusion of Thoracolumbar Vertebral Joint with Interbody Fusion Device, Anterior Approach, Anterior Column, Percutaneous Endoscopic Approach

HAC When reported with secondary diagnosis code T84.60XA, T84.610A, T84.611A, T84.612A, T84.613A, T84.614A, T84.615A, T84.619A, T84.63XA, T84.69XA, T84.7XXA

0RGA4A1 Fusion of Thoracolumbar Vertebral Joint with Interbody Fusion Device, Posterior Approach, Posterior Column, Percutaneous Endoscopic Approach

HAC When reported with secondary diagnosis code T84.60XA, T84.610A, T84.611A, T84.612A, T84.613A, T84.614A, T84.615A, T84.619A, T84.63XA, T84.69XA, T84.7XXA

0RGA4AJ Fusion of Thoracolumbar Vertebral Joint with Interbody Fusion Device, Posterior Approach, Anterior Column, Percutaneous Endoscopic Approach

HAC When reported with secondary diagnosis code T84.60XA, T84.610A, T84.611A, T84.612A, T84.613A, T84.614A, T84.615A, T84.619A, T84.63XA, T84.69XA, T84.7XXA

0RGA4J0 Fusion of Thoracolumbar Vertebral Joint with Synthetic Substitute, Anterior Approach, Anterior Column, Percutaneous Endoscopic Approach

Note Continued

RGA4J0 Continued Note

HAC When reported with secondary diagnosis code T84.60XA, T84.610A, T84.611A, T84.612A, T84.613A, T84.614A, T84.615A, T84.619A, T84.63XA, T84.69XA, T84.7XXA

RGA4J1 Fusion of Thoracolumbar Vertebral Joint with Synthetic Substitute, Posterior Approach, Posterior Column, Percutaneous Endoscopic Approach

HAC When reported with secondary diagnosis code T84.60XA, T84.610A, T84.611A, T84.612A, T84.613A, T84.614A, T84.615A, T84.619A, T84.63XA, T84.69XA, T84.7XXA

RGA4JJ Fusion of Thoracolumbar Vertebral Joint with Synthetic Substitute, Posterior Approach, Anterior Column, Percutaneous Endoscopic Approach

HAC When reported with secondary diagnosis code T84.60XA, T84.610A, T84.611A, T84.612A, T84.613A, T84.614A, T84.615A, T84.619A, T84.63XA, T84.69XA, T84.7XXA

RGA4K0 Fusion of Thoracolumbar Vertebral Joint with Nonautologous Tissue Substitute, Anterior Approach, Anterior Column, Percutaneous Endoscopic Approach

HAC When reported with secondary diagnosis code T84.60XA, T84.610A, T84.611A, T84.612A, T84.613A, T84.614A, T84.615A, T84.619A, T84.63XA, T84.69XA, T84.7XXA

RGA4K1 Fusion of Thoracolumbar Vertebral Joint with Nonautologous Tissue Substitute, Posterior Approach, Posterior Column, Percutaneous Endoscopic Approach

HAC When reported with secondary diagnosis code T84.60XA, T84.610A, T84.611A, T84.612A, T84.613A, T84.614A, T84.615A, T84.619A, T84.63XA, T84.69XA, T84.7XXA

0RGA4KJ Fusion of Thoracolumbar Vertebral Joint with Nonautologous Tissue Substitute, Posterior Approach, Anterior Column, Percutaneous Endoscopic Approach

HAC When reported with secondary diagnosis code T84.60XA, T84.610A, T84.611A, T84.612A, T84.613A, T84.614A, T84.615A, T84.619A, T84.63XA, T84.69XA, T84.7XXA

0RGA4Z0 Fusion of Thoracolumbar Vertebral Joint, Anterior Approach, Anterior Column, Percutaneous Endoscopic Approach

HAC When reported with secondary diagnosis code T84.60XA, T84.610A, T84.611A, T84.612A, T84.613A, T84.614A, T84.615A, T84.619A, T84.63XA, T84.69XA, T84.7XXA

0RGA4Z1 Fusion of Thoracolumbar Vertebral Joint, Posterior Approach, Posterior Column, Percutaneous Endoscopic Approach

HAC When reported with secondary diagnosis code T84.60XA, T84.610A, T84.611A, T84.612A, T84.613A, T84.614A, T84.615A, T84.619A, T84.63XA, T84.69XA, T84.7XXA

0RGA4ZJ Fusion of Thoracolumbar Vertebral Joint, Posterior Approach, Anterior Column, Percutaneous Endoscopic Approach

HAC When reported with secondary diagnosis code T84.60XA, T84.610A, T84.611A, T84.612A, T84.613A, T84.614A, T84.615A, T84.619A, T84.63XA, T84.69XA, T84.7XXA

0RGC04Z Fusion of Right Temporomandibular Joint with Internal Fixation Device, Open Approach

0RGC07Z Fusion of Right Temporomandibular Joint with Autologous Tissue Substitute, Open Approach

0RGC0JZ Fusion of Right Temporomandibular Joint with Synthetic Substitute, Open Approach

0RGC0KZ Fusion of Right Temporomandibular Joint with Nonautologous Tissue Substitute, Open Approach

0RGC0ZZ Fusion of Right Temporomandibular Joint, Open Approach

0RGC34Z Fusion of Right Temporomandibular Joint with Internal Fixation Device, Percutaneous Approach

0RGC37Z Fusion of Right Temporomandibular Joint with Autologous Tissue Substitute, Percutaneous Approach

0RGC3JZ Fusion of Right Temporomandibular Joint with Synthetic Substitute, Percutaneous Approach

0RGC3KZ Fusion of Right Temporomandibular Joint with Nonautologous Tissue Substitute, Percutaneous Approach

0RGC3ZZ Fusion of Right Temporomandibular Joint, Percutaneous Approach

0RGC44Z Fusion of Right Temporomandibular Joint with Internal Fixation Device, Percutaneous Endoscopic Approach

0RGC47Z Fusion of Right Temporomandibular Joint with Autologous Tissue Substitute, Percutaneous Endoscopic Approach

0RGC4JZ Fusion of Right Temporomandibular Joint with Synthetic Substitute, Percutaneous Endoscopic Approach

0RGC4KZ Fusion of Right Temporomandibular Joint with Nonautologous Tissue Substitute, Percutaneous Endoscopic Approach

0RGC4ZZ Fusion of Right Temporomandibular Joint, Percutaneous Endoscopic Approach

0RGD04Z Fusion of Left Temporomandibular Joint with Internal Fixation Device, Open Approach

0RGD07Z Fusion of Left Temporomandibular Joint with Autologous Tissue Substitute, Open Approach

0RGD0JZ Fusion of Left Temporomandibular Joint with Synthetic Substitute, Open Approach

0RGD0KZ Fusion of Left Temporomandibular Joint with Nonautologous Tissue Substitute, Open Approach

0RGD0ZZ Fusion of Left Temporomandibular Joint, Open Approach

0RGD34Z Fusion of Left Temporomandibular Joint with Internal Fixation Device, Percutaneous Approach

0RGD37Z Fusion of Left Temporomandibular Joint with Autologous Tissue Substitute, Percutaneous Approach

0RGD3JZ Fusion of Left Temporomandibular Joint with Synthetic Substitute, Percutaneous Approach

0RGD3KZ Fusion of Left Temporomandibular Joint with Nonautologous Tissue Substitute, Percutaneous Approach

0RGD3ZZ Fusion of Left Temporomandibular Joint, Percutaneous Approach

0RGD44Z Fusion of Left Temporomandibular Joint with Internal Fixation Device, Percutaneous Endoscopic Approach

0RGD47Z Fusion of Left Temporomandibular Joint with Autologous Tissue Substitute, Percutaneous Endoscopic Approach

0RGD4JZ Fusion of Left Temporomandibular Joint with Synthetic Substitute, Percutaneous Endoscopic Approach

0RGD4KZ Fusion of Left Temporomandibular Joint with Nonautologous Tissue Substitute, Percutaneous Endoscopic Approach

0RGD4ZZ Fusion of Left Temporomandibular Joint, Percutaneous Endoscopic Approach

0RGE04Z Fusion of Right Sternoclavicular Joint with Internal Fixation Device, Open Approach

HAC When reported with secondary diagnosis code T84.60XA, T84.610A, T84.611A, T84.612A, T84.613A, T84.614A, T84.615A, T84.619A, T84.63XA, T84.69XA, T84.7XXA

0RGE07Z Fusion of Right Sternoclavicular Joint with Autologous Tissue Substitute, Open Approach

HAC When reported with secondary diagnosis code T84.60XA, T84.610A, T84.611A, T84.612A, T84.613A, T84.614A, T84.615A, T84.619A, T84.63XA, T84.69XA, T84.7XXA

0RGE0JZ Fusion of Right Sternoclavicular Joint with Synthetic Substitute, Open Approach

HAC When reported with secondary diagnosis code T84.60XA, T84.610A, T84.611A, T84.612A, T84.613A, T84.614A, T84.615A, T84.619A, T84.63XA, T84.69XA, T84.7XXA

0RGE0KZ Fusion of Right Sternoclavicular Joint with Nonautologous Tissue Substitute, Open Approach

HAC When reported with secondary diagnosis code T84.60XA, T84.610A, T84.611A, T84.612A, T84.613A, T84.614A, T84.615A, T84.619A, T84.63XA, T84.69XA, T84.7XXA

0RGE0ZZ Fusion of Right Sternoclavicular Joint, Open Approach

HAC When reported with secondary diagnosis code T84.60XA, T84.610A, T84.611A, T84.612A, T84.613A, T84.614A, T84.615A, T84.619A, T84.63XA, T84.69XA, T84.7XXA

0RGE34Z Fusion of Right Sternoclavicular Joint with Internal Fixation Device, Percutaneous Approach

HAC When reported with secondary diagnosis code T84.60XA, T84.610A, T84.611A, T84.612A, T84.613A, T84.614A, T84.615A, T84.619A, T84.63XA, T84.69XA, T84.7XXA

0RGE37Z Fusion of Right Sternoclavicular Joint with Autologous Tissue Substitute, Percutaneous Approach

HAC When reported with secondary diagnosis code T84.60XA, T84.610A, T84.611A, T84.612A, T84.613A, T84.614A, T84.615A, T84.619A, T84.63XA, T84.69XA, T84.7XXA

0RGE3JZ Fusion of Right Sternoclavicular Joint with Synthetic Substitute, Percutaneous Approach

HAC When reported with secondary diagnosis code T84.60XA, T84.610A, T84.611A, T84.612A, T84.613A, T84.614A, T84.615A, T84.619A, T84.63XA, T84.69XA, T84.7XXA

0RGE3KZ Fusion of Right Sternoclavicular Joint with Nonautologous Tissue Substitute, Percutaneous Approach

HAC When reported with secondary diagnosis code T84.60XA, T84.610A, T84.611A, T84.612A, T84.613A, T84.614A, T84.615A, T84.619A, T84.63XA, T84.69XA, T84.7XXA

0RGE3ZZ Fusion of Right Sternoclavicular Joint, Percutaneous Approach
HAC When reported with secondary diagnosis code T84.60XA, T84.610A, T84.611A, T84.612A, T84.613A, T84.614A, T84.615A, T84.619A, T84.63XA, T84.69XA, T84.7XXA

0RGE44Z Fusion of Right Sternoclavicular Joint with Internal Fixation Device, Percutaneous Endoscopic Approach
HAC When reported with secondary diagnosis code T84.60XA, T84.610A, T84.611A, T84.612A, T84.613A, T84.614A, T84.615A, T84.619A, T84.63XA, T84.69XA, T84.7XXA

0RGE47Z Fusion of Right Sternoclavicular Joint with Autologous Tissue Substitute, Percutaneous Endoscopic Approach
HAC When reported with secondary diagnosis code T84.60XA, T84.610A, T84.611A, T84.612A, T84.613A, T84.614A, T84.615A, T84.619A, T84.63XA, T84.69XA, T84.7XXA

0RGE4JZ Fusion of Right Sternoclavicular Joint with Synthetic Substitute, Percutaneous Endoscopic Approach
HAC When reported with secondary diagnosis code T84.60XA, T84.610A, T84.611A, T84.612A, T84.613A, T84.614A, T84.615A, T84.619A, T84.63XA, T84.69XA, T84.7XXA

0RGE4KZ Fusion of Right Sternoclavicular Joint with Nonautologous Tissue Substitute, Percutaneous Endoscopic Approach
HAC When reported with secondary diagnosis code T84.60XA, T84.610A, T84.611A, T84.612A, T84.613A, T84.614A, T84.615A, T84.619A, T84.63XA, T84.69XA, T84.7XXA

0RGE4ZZ Fusion of Right Sternoclavicular Joint, Percutaneous Endoscopic Approach
HAC When reported with secondary diagnosis code T84.60XA, T84.610A, T84.611A, T84.612A, T84.613A, T84.614A, T84.615A, T84.619A, T84.63XA, T84.69XA, T84.7XXA

0RGF04Z Fusion of Left Sternoclavicular Joint with Internal Fixation Device, Open Approach
HAC When reported with secondary diagnosis code T84.60XA, T84.610A, T84.611A, T84.612A, T84.613A, T84.614A, T84.615A, T84.619A, T84.63XA, T84.69XA, T84.7XXA

0RGF07Z Fusion of Left Sternoclavicular Joint with Autologous Tissue Substitute, Open Approach
HAC When reported with secondary diagnosis code T84.60XA, T84.610A, T84.611A, T84.612A, T84.613A, T84.614A, T84.615A, T84.619A, T84.63XA, T84.69XA, T84.7XXA

0RGF0JZ Fusion of Left Sternoclavicular Joint with Synthetic Substitute, Open Approach
HAC When reported with secondary diagnosis code T84.60XA, T84.610A, T84.611A, T84.612A, T84.613A, T84.614A, T84.615A, T84.619A, T84.63XA, T84.69XA, T84.7XXA

0RGF0KZ Fusion of Left Sternoclavicular Joint with Nonautologous Tissue Substitute, Open Approach
HAC When reported with secondary diagnosis code T84.60XA, T84.610A, T84.611A, T84.612A, T84.613A, T84.614A, T84.615A, T84.619A, T84.63XA, T84.69XA, T84.7XXA

0RGF0ZZ Fusion of Left Sternoclavicular Joint, Open Approach
HAC When reported with secondary diagnosis code T84.60XA, T84.610A, T84.611A, T84.612A, T84.613A, T84.614A, T84.615A, T84.619A, T84.63XA, T84.69XA, T84.7XXA

0RGF34Z Fusion of Left Sternoclavicular Joint with Internal Fixation Device, Percutaneous Approach
HAC When reported with secondary diagnosis code T84.60XA, T84.610A, T84.611A, T84.612A, T84.613A, T84.614A, T84.615A, T84.619A, T84.63XA, T84.69XA, T84.7XXA

0RGF37Z Fusion of Left Sternoclavicular Joint with Autologous Tissue Substitute, Percutaneous Approach
HAC When reported with secondary diagnosis code T84.60XA, T84.610A, T84.611A, T84.612A, T84.613A, T84.614A, T84.615A, T84.619A, T84.63XA, T84.69XA, T84.7XXA

0RGF3JZ Fusion of Left Sternoclavicular Joint with Synthetic Substitute, Percutaneous Approach
HAC When reported with secondary diagnosis code T84.60XA, T84.610A, T84.611A, T84.612A, T84.613A, T84.614A, T84.615A, T84.619A, T84.63XA, T84.69XA, T84.7XXA

0RGF3KZ Fusion of Left Sternoclavicular Joint with Nonautologous Tissue Substitute, Percutaneous Approach
HAC When reported with secondary diagnosis code T84.60XA, T84.610A, T84.611A, T84.612A, T84.613A, T84.614A, T84.615A, T84.619A, T84.63XA, T84.69XA, T84.7XXA

0RGF3ZZ Fusion of Left Sternoclavicular Joint, Percutaneous Approach
HAC When reported with secondary diagnosis code T84.60XA, T84.610A, T84.611A, T84.612A, T84.613A, T84.614A, T84.615A, T84.619A, T84.63XA, T84.69XA, T84.7XXA

0RGF44Z Fusion of Left Sternoclavicular Joint with Internal Fixation Device, Percutaneous Endoscopic Approach
HAC When reported with secondary diagnosis code T84.60XA, T84.610A, T84.611A, T84.612A, T84.613A, T84.614A, T84.615A, T84.619A, T84.63XA, T84.69XA, T84.7XXA

0RGF47Z Fusion of Left Sternoclavicular Joint with Autologous Tissue Substitute, Percutaneous Endoscopic Approach
HAC When reported with secondary diagnosis code T84.60XA, T84.610A, T84.611A, T84.612A, T84.613A, T84.614A, T84.615A, T84.619A, T84.63XA, T84.69XA, T84.7XXA

0RGF4JZ Fusion of Left Sternoclavicular Joint with Synthetic Substitute, Percutaneous Endoscopic Approach
HAC When reported with secondary diagnosis code T84.60XA, T84.610A, T84.611A, T84.612A, T84.613A, T84.614A, T84.615A, T84.619A, T84.63XA, T84.69XA, T84.7XXA

0RGF4KZ Fusion of Left Sternoclavicular Joint with Nonautologous Tissue Substitute, Percutaneous Endoscopic Approach
HAC When reported with secondary diagnosis code T84.60XA, T84.610A, T84.611A, T84.612A, T84.613A, T84.614A, T84.615A, T84.619A, T84.63XA, T84.69XA, T84.7XXA

0RGF4ZZ Fusion of Left Sternoclavicular Joint, Percutaneous Endoscopic Approach
HAC When reported with secondary diagnosis code T84.60XA, T84.610A, T84.611A, T84.612A, T84.613A, T84.614A, T84.615A, T84.619A, T84.63XA, T84.69XA, T84.7XXA

0RGG04Z Fusion of Right Acromioclavicular Joint with Internal Fixation Device, Open Approach
HAC When reported with secondary diagnosis code T84.60XA, T84.610A, T84.611A, T84.612A, T84.613A, T84.614A, T84.615A, T84.619A, T84.63XA, T84.69XA, T84.7XXA

0RGG07Z Fusion of Right Acromioclavicular Joint with Autologous Tissue Substitute, Open Approach
HAC When reported with secondary diagnosis code T84.60XA, T84.610A, T84.611A, T84.612A, T84.613A, T84.614A, T84.615A, T84.619A, T84.63XA, T84.69XA, T84.7XXA

0RGG0JZ Fusion of Right Acromioclavicular Joint with Synthetic Substitute, Open Approach
HAC When reported with secondary diagnosis code T84.60XA, T84.610A, T84.611A, T84.612A, T84.613A, T84.614A, T84.615A, T84.619A, T84.63XA, T84.69XA, T84.7XXA

0RGG0KZ Fusion of Right Acromioclavicular Joint with Nonautologous Tissue Substitute, Open Approach
HAC When reported with secondary diagnosis code T84.60XA, T84.610A, T84.611A, T84.612A, T84.613A, T84.614A, T84.615A, T84.619A, T84.63XA, T84.69XA, T84.7XXA

0RGG0ZZ Fusion of Right Acromioclavicular Joint, Open Approach
HAC When reported with secondary diagnosis code T84.60XA, T84.610A, T84.611A, T84.612A, T84.613A, T84.614A, T84.615A, T84.619A, T84.63XA, T84.69XA, T84.7XXA

0RGG34Z Fusion of Right Acromioclavicular Joint with Internal Fixation Device, Percutaneous Approach
HAC When reported with secondary diagnosis code T84.60XA, T84.610A, T84.611A, T84.612A, T84.613A, T84.614A, T84.615A, T84.619A, T84.63XA, T84.69XA, T84.7XXA

0RGG37Z Fusion of Right Acromioclavicular Joint with Autologous Tissue Substitute, Percutaneous Approach
HAC When reported with secondary diagnosis code T84.60XA, T84.610A, T84.611A, T84.612A, T84.613A, T84.614A, T84.615A, T84.619A, T84.63XA, T84.69XA, T84.7XXA

0RGG3JZ Fusion of Right Acromioclavicular Joint with Synthetic Substitute, Percutaneous Approach
HAC When reported with secondary diagnosis code T84.60XA, T84.610A, T84.611A, T84.612A, T84.613A, T84.614A, T84.615A, T84.619A, T84.63XA, T84.69XA, T84.7XXA

0RGG3KZ Fusion of Right Acromioclavicular Joint with Nonautologous Tissue Substitute, Percutaneous Approach
HAC When reported with secondary diagnosis code T84.60XA, T84.610A, T84.611A, T84.612A, T84.613A, T84.614A, T84.615A, T84.619A, T84.63XA, T84.69XA, T84.7XXA

RGG3ZZ Fusion of Right Acromioclavicular Joint, Percutaneous Approach
HAC When reported with secondary diagnosis code T84.60XA, T84.610A, T84.611A, T84.612A, T84.613A, T84.614A, T84.615A, T84.619A, T84.63XA, T84.69XA, T84.7XXA

RGG44Z Fusion of Right Acromioclavicular Joint with Internal Fixation Device, Percutaneous Endoscopic Approach
HAC When reported with secondary diagnosis code T84.60XA, T84.610A, T84.611A, T84.612A, T84.613A, T84.614A, T84.615A, T84.619A, T84.63XA, T84.69XA, T84.7XXA

RGG47Z Fusion of Right Acromioclavicular Joint with Autologous Tissue Substitute, Percutaneous Endoscopic Approach
HAC When reported with secondary diagnosis code T84.60XA, T84.610A, T84.611A, T84.612A, T84.613A, T84.614A, T84.615A, T84.619A, T84.63XA, T84.69XA, T84.7XXA

RGG4JZ Fusion of Right Acromioclavicular Joint with Synthetic Substitute, Percutaneous Endoscopic Approach
HAC When reported with secondary diagnosis code T84.60XA, T84.610A, T84.611A, T84.612A, T84.613A, T84.614A, T84.615A, T84.619A, T84.63XA, T84.69XA, T84.7XXA

RGG4KZ Fusion of Right Acromioclavicular Joint with Nonautologous Tissue Substitute, Percutaneous Endoscopic Approach
HAC When reported with secondary diagnosis code T84.60XA, T84.610A, T84.611A, T84.612A, T84.613A, T84.614A, T84.615A, T84.619A, T84.63XA, T84.69XA, T84.7XXA

RGG4ZZ Fusion of Right Acromioclavicular Joint, Percutaneous Endoscopic Approach
HAC When reported with secondary diagnosis code T84.60XA, T84.610A, T84.611A, T84.612A, T84.613A, T84.614A, T84.615A, T84.619A, T84.63XA, T84.69XA, T84.7XXA

0RGH04Z Fusion of Left Acromioclavicular Joint with Internal Fixation Device, Open Approach
HAC When reported with secondary diagnosis code T84.60XA, T84.610A, T84.611A, T84.612A, T84.613A, T84.614A, T84.615A, T84.619A, T84.63XA, T84.69XA, T84.7XXA

0RGH07Z Fusion of Left Acromioclavicular Joint with Autologous Tissue Substitute, Open Approach
HAC When reported with secondary diagnosis code T84.60XA, T84.610A, T84.611A, T84.612A, T84.613A, T84.614A, T84.615A, T84.619A, T84.63XA, T84.69XA, T84.7XXA

0RGH0JZ Fusion of Left Acromioclavicular Joint with Synthetic Substitute, Open Approach
HAC When reported with secondary diagnosis code T84.60XA, T84.610A, T84.611A, T84.612A, T84.613A, T84.614A, T84.615A, T84.619A, T84.63XA, T84.69XA, T84.7XXA

0RGH0KZ Fusion of Left Acromioclavicular Joint with Nonautologous Tissue Substitute, Open Approach
HAC When reported with secondary diagnosis code T84.60XA, T84.610A, T84.611A, T84.612A, T84.613A, T84.614A, T84.615A, T84.619A, T84.63XA, T84.69XA, T84.7XXA

0RGH0ZZ Fusion of Left Acromioclavicular Joint, Open Approach
HAC When reported with secondary diagnosis code T84.60XA, T84.610A, T84.611A, T84.612A, T84.613A, T84.614A, T84.615A, T84.619A, T84.63XA, T84.69XA, T84.7XXA

0RGH34Z Fusion of Left Acromioclavicular Joint with Internal Fixation Device, Percutaneous Approach
HAC When reported with secondary diagnosis code T84.60XA, T84.610A, T84.611A, T84.612A, T84.613A, T84.614A, T84.615A, T84.619A, T84.63XA, T84.69XA, T84.7XXA

0RGH37Z Fusion of Left Acromioclavicular Joint with Autologous Tissue Substitute, Percutaneous Approach
HAC When reported with secondary diagnosis code T84.60XA, T84.610A, T84.611A, T84.612A, T84.613A, T84.614A, T84.615A, T84.619A, T84.63XA, T84.69XA, T84.7XXA

0RGH3JZ Fusion of Left Acromioclavicular Joint with Synthetic Substitute, Percutaneous Approach
HAC When reported with secondary diagnosis code T84.60XA, T84.610A, T84.611A, T84.612A, T84.613A, T84.614A, T84.615A, T84.619A, T84.63XA, T84.69XA, T84.7XXA

0RGH3KZ Fusion of Left Acromioclavicular Joint with Nonautologous Tissue Substitute, Percutaneous Approach
HAC When reported with secondary diagnosis code T84.60XA, T84.610A, T84.611A, T84.612A, T84.613A, T84.614A, T84.615A, T84.619A, T84.63XA, T84.69XA, T84.7XXA

0RGH3ZZ Fusion of Left Acromioclavicular Joint, Percutaneous Approach
HAC When reported with secondary diagnosis code T84.60XA, T84.610A, T84.611A, T84.612A, T84.613A, T84.614A, T84.615A, T84.619A, T84.63XA, T84.69XA, T84.7XXA

0RGH44Z Fusion of Left Acromioclavicular Joint with Internal Fixation Device, Percutaneous Endoscopic Approach
HAC When reported with secondary diagnosis code T84.60XA, T84.610A, T84.611A, T84.612A, T84.613A, T84.614A, T84.615A, T84.619A, T84.63XA, T84.69XA, T84.7XXA

0RGH47Z Fusion of Left Acromioclavicular Joint with Autologous Tissue Substitute, Percutaneous Endoscopic Approach
HAC When reported with secondary diagnosis code T84.60XA, T84.610A, T84.611A, T84.612A, T84.613A, T84.614A, T84.615A, T84.619A, T84.63XA, T84.69XA, T84.7XXA

0RGH4JZ Fusion of Left Acromioclavicular Joint with Synthetic Substitute, Percutaneous Endoscopic Approach
HAC When reported with secondary diagnosis code T84.60XA, T84.610A, T84.611A, T84.612A, T84.613A, T84.614A, T84.615A, T84.619A, T84.63XA, T84.69XA, T84.7XXA

0RGH4KZ Fusion of Left Acromioclavicular Joint with Nonautologous Tissue Substitute, Percutaneous Endoscopic Approach
HAC When reported with secondary diagnosis code T84.60XA, T84.610A, T84.611A, T84.612A, T84.613A, T84.614A, T84.615A, T84.619A, T84.63XA, T84.69XA, T84.7XXA

0RGH4ZZ Fusion of Left Acromioclavicular Joint, Percutaneous Endoscopic Approach
HAC When reported with secondary diagnosis code T84.60XA, T84.610A, T84.611A, T84.612A, T84.613A, T84.614A, T84.615A, T84.619A, T84.63XA, T84.69XA, T84.7XXA

0RGJ04Z Fusion of Right Shoulder Joint with Internal Fixation Device, Open Approach
HAC When reported with secondary diagnosis code T84.60XA, T84.610A, T84.611A, T84.612A, T84.613A, T84.614A, T84.615A, T84.619A, T84.63XA, T84.69XA, T84.7XXA

0RGJ07Z Fusion of Right Shoulder Joint with Autologous Tissue Substitute, Open Approach
HAC When reported with secondary diagnosis code T84.60XA, T84.610A, T84.611A, T84.612A, T84.613A, T84.614A, T84.615A, T84.619A, T84.63XA, T84.69XA, T84.7XXA

0RGJ0JZ Fusion of Right Shoulder Joint with Synthetic Substitute, Open Approach
HAC When reported with secondary diagnosis code T84.60XA, T84.610A, T84.611A, T84.612A, T84.613A, T84.614A, T84.615A, T84.619A, T84.63XA, T84.69XA, T84.7XXA

0RGJ0KZ Fusion of Right Shoulder Joint with Nonautologous Tissue Substitute, Open Approach
HAC When reported with secondary diagnosis code T84.60XA, T84.610A, T84.611A, T84.612A, T84.613A, T84.614A, T84.615A, T84.619A, T84.63XA, T84.69XA, T84.7XXA

0RGJ0ZZ Fusion of Right Shoulder Joint, Open Approach
HAC When reported with secondary diagnosis code T84.60XA, T84.610A, T84.611A, T84.612A, T84.613A, T84.614A, T84.615A, T84.619A, T84.63XA, T84.69XA, T84.7XXA

0RGJ34Z Fusion of Right Shoulder Joint with Internal Fixation Device, Percutaneous Approach
HAC When reported with secondary diagnosis code T84.60XA, T84.610A, T84.611A, T84.612A, T84.613A, T84.614A, T84.615A, T84.619A, T84.63XA, T84.69XA, T84.7XXA

0RGJ37Z Fusion of Right Shoulder Joint with Autologous Tissue Substitute, Percutaneous Approach
HAC When reported with secondary diagnosis code T84.60XA, T84.610A, T84.611A, T84.612A, T84.613A, T84.614A, T84.615A, T84.619A, T84.63XA, T84.69XA, T84.7XXA

0RGJ3JZ Fusion of Right Shoulder Joint with Synthetic Substitute, Percutaneous Approach
HAC When reported with secondary diagnosis code T84.60XA, T84.610A, T84.611A, T84.612A, T84.613A, T84.614A, T84.615A, T84.619A, T84.63XA, T84.69XA, T84.7XXA

0RGJ3KZ Fusion of Right Shoulder Joint with Nonautologous Tissue Substitute, Percutaneous Approach
HAC When reported with secondary diagnosis code T84.60XA, T84.610A, T84.611A, T84.612A, T84.613A, T84.614A, T84.615A, T84.619A, T84.63XA, T84.69XA, T84.7XXA

0RGJ3ZZ Fusion of Right Shoulder Joint, Percutaneous Approach
HAC When reported with secondary diagnosis code T84.60XA, T84.610A, T84.611A, T84.612A, T84.613A, T84.614A, T84.615A, T84.619A, T84.63XA, T84.69XA, T84.7XXA

0RGJ44Z Fusion of Right Shoulder Joint with Internal Fixation Device, Percutaneous Endoscopic Approach
HAC When reported with secondary diagnosis code T84.60XA, T84.610A, T84.611A, T84.612A, T84.613A, T84.614A, T84.615A, T84.619A, T84.63XA, T84.69XA, T84.7XXA

0RGJ47Z Fusion of Right Shoulder Joint with Autologous Tissue Substitute, Percutaneous Endoscopic Approach
HAC When reported with secondary diagnosis code T84.60XA, T84.610A, T84.611A, T84.612A, T84.613A, T84.614A, T84.615A, T84.619A, T84.63XA, T84.69XA, T84.7XXA

0RGJ4JZ Fusion of Right Shoulder Joint with Synthetic Substitute, Percutaneous Endoscopic Approach
HAC When reported with secondary diagnosis code T84.60XA, T84.610A, T84.611A, T84.612A, T84.613A, T84.614A, T84.615A, T84.619A, T84.63XA, T84.69XA, T84.7XXA

0RGJ4KZ Fusion of Right Shoulder Joint with Nonautologous Tissue Substitute, Percutaneous Endoscopic Approach
HAC When reported with secondary diagnosis code T84.60XA, T84.610A, T84.611A, T84.612A, T84.613A, T84.614A, T84.615A, T84.619A, T84.63XA, T84.69XA, T84.7XXA

0RGJ4ZZ Fusion of Right Shoulder Joint, Percutaneous Endoscopic Approach
HAC When reported with secondary diagnosis code T84.60XA, T84.610A, T84.611A, T84.612A, T84.613A, T84.614A, T84.615A, T84.619A, T84.63XA, T84.69XA, T84.7XXA

0RGK04Z Fusion of Left Shoulder Joint with Internal Fixation Device, Open Approach
HAC When reported with secondary diagnosis code T84.60XA, T84.610A, T84.611A, T84.612A, T84.613A, T84.614A, T84.615A, T84.619A, T84.63XA, T84.69XA, T84.7XXA

0RGK07Z Fusion of Left Shoulder Joint with Autologous Tissue Substitute, Open Approach
HAC When reported with secondary diagnosis code T84.60XA, T84.610A, T84.611A, T84.612A, T84.613A, T84.614A, T84.615A, T84.619A, T84.63XA, T84.69XA, T84.7XXA

0RGK0JZ Fusion of Left Shoulder Joint with Synthetic Substitute, Open Approach
HAC When reported with secondary diagnosis code T84.60XA, T84.610A, T84.611A, T84.612A, T84.613A, T84.614A, T84.615A, T84.619A, T84.63XA, T84.69XA, T84.7XXA

0RGK0KZ Fusion of Left Shoulder Joint with Nonautologous Tissue Substitute, Open Approach
HAC When reported with secondary diagnosis code T84.60XA, T84.610A, T84.611A, T84.612A, T84.613A, T84.614A, T84.615A, T84.619A, T84.63XA, T84.69XA, T84.7XXA

0RGK0ZZ Fusion of Left Shoulder Joint, Open Approach
HAC When reported with secondary diagnosis code T84.60XA, T84.610A, T84.611A, T84.612A, T84.613A, T84.614A, T84.615A, T84.619A, T84.63XA, T84.69XA, T84.7XXA

0RGK34Z Fusion of Left Shoulder Joint with Internal Fixation Device, Percutaneous Approach
HAC When reported with secondary diagnosis code T84.60XA, T84.610A, T84.611A, T84.612A, T84.613A, T84.614A, T84.615A, T84.619A, T84.63XA, T84.69XA, T84.7XXA

0RGK37Z Fusion of Left Shoulder Joint with Autologous Tissue Substitute, Percutaneous Approach
HAC When reported with secondary diagnosis code T84.60XA, T84.610A, T84.611A, T84.612A, T84.613A, T84.614A, T84.615A, T84.619A, T84.63XA, T84.69XA, T84.7XXA

0RGK3JZ Fusion of Left Shoulder Joint with Synthetic Substitute, Percutaneous Approach
HAC When reported with secondary diagnosis code T84.60XA, T84.610A, T84.611A, T84.612A, T84.613A, T84.614A, T84.615A, T84.619A, T84.63XA, T84.69XA, T84.7XXA

0RGK3KZ Fusion of Left Shoulder Joint with Nonautologous Tissue Substitute, Percutaneous Approach
HAC When reported with secondary diagnosis code T84.60XA, T84.610A, T84.611A, T84.612A, T84.613A, T84.614A, T84.615A, T84.619A, T84.63XA, T84.69XA, T84.7XXA

0RGK3ZZ Fusion of Left Shoulder Joint, Percutaneous Approach
HAC When reported with secondary diagnosis code T84.60XA, T84.610A, T84.611A, T84.612A, T84.613A, T84.614A, T84.615A, T84.619A, T84.63XA, T84.69XA, T84.7XXA

0RGK44Z Fusion of Left Shoulder Joint with Internal Fixation Device, Percutaneous Endoscopic Approach
HAC When reported with secondary diagnosis code T84.60XA, T84.610A, T84.611A, T84.612A, T84.613A, T84.614A, T84.615A, T84.619A, T84.63XA, T84.69XA, T84.7XXA

0RGK47Z Fusion of Left Shoulder Joint with Autologous Tissue Substitute, Percutaneous Endoscopic Approach
HAC When reported with secondary diagnosis code T84.60XA, T84.610A, T84.611A, T84.612A, T84.613A, T84.614A, T84.615A, T84.619A, T84.63XA, T84.69XA, T84.7XXA

0RGK4JZ Fusion of Left Shoulder Joint with Synthetic Substitute, Percutaneous Endoscopic Approach
HAC When reported with secondary diagnosis code T84.60XA, T84.610A, T84.611A, T84.612A, T84.613A, T84.614A, T84.615A, T84.619A, T84.63XA, T84.69XA, T84.7XXA

0RGK4KZ Fusion of Left Shoulder Joint with Nonautologous Tissue Substitute, Percutaneous Endoscopic Approach
HAC When reported with secondary diagnosis code T84.60XA, T84.610A, T84.611A, T84.612A, T84.613A, T84.614A, T84.615A, T84.619A, T84.63XA, T84.69XA, T84.7XXA

0RGK4ZZ Fusion of Left Shoulder Joint, Percutaneous Endoscopic Approach
HAC When reported with secondary diagnosis code T84.60XA, T84.610A, T84.611A, T84.612A, T84.613A, T84.614A, T84.615A, T84.619A, T84.63XA, T84.69XA, T84.7XXA

0RGL04Z Fusion of Right Elbow Joint with Internal Fixation Device, Open Approach
HAC When reported with secondary diagnosis code T84.60XA, T84.610A, T84.611A, T84.612A, T84.613A, T84.614A, T84.615A, T84.619A, T84.63XA, T84.69XA, T84.7XXA

0RGL05Z Fusion of Right Elbow Joint with External Fixation Device, Open Approach
HAC When reported with secondary diagnosis code T84.60XA, T84.610A, T84.611A, T84.612A, T84.613A, T84.614A, T84.615A, T84.619A, T84.63XA, T84.69XA, T84.7XXA

0RGL07Z Fusion of Right Elbow Joint with Autologous Tissue Substitute, Open Approach
HAC When reported with secondary diagnosis code T84.60XA, T84.610A, T84.611A, T84.612A, T84.613A, T84.614A, T84.615A, T84.619A, T84.63XA, T84.69XA, T84.7XXA

0RGL0JZ Fusion of Right Elbow Joint with Synthetic Substitute, Open Approach
HAC When reported with secondary diagnosis code T84.60XA, T84.610A, T84.611A, T84.612A, T84.613A, T84.614A, T84.615A, T84.619A, T84.63XA, T84.69XA, T84.7XXA

0RGL0KZ Fusion of Right Elbow Joint with Nonautologous Tissue Substitute, Open Approach
HAC When reported with secondary diagnosis code T84.60XA, T84.610A, T84.611A, T84.612A, T84.613A, T84.614A, T84.615A, T84.619A, T84.63XA, T84.69XA, T84.7XXA

0RGL0ZZ Fusion of Right Elbow Joint, Open Approach
HAC When reported with secondary diagnosis code T84.60XA, T84.610A, T84.611A, T84.612A, T84.613A, T84.614A, T84.615A, T84.619A, T84.63XA, T84.69XA, T84.7XXA

0RGL34Z Fusion of Right Elbow Joint with Internal Fixation Device, Percutaneous Approach
HAC When reported with secondary diagnosis code T84.60XA, T84.610A, T84.611A, T84.612A, T84.613A, T84.614A, T84.615A, T84.619A, T84.63XA, T84.69XA, T84.7XXA

0RGL35Z Fusion of Right Elbow Joint with External Fixation Device, Percutaneous Approach
HAC When reported with secondary diagnosis code T84.60XA, T84.610A, T84.611A, T84.612A, T84.613A, T84.614A, T84.615A, T84.619A, T84.63XA, T84.69XA, T84.7XXA

0RGL37Z Fusion of Right Elbow Joint with Autologous Tissue Substitute, Percutaneous Approach
HAC When reported with secondary diagnosis code T84.60XA, T84.610A, T84.611A, T84.612A, T84.613A, T84.614A, T84.615A, T84.619A, T84.63XA, T84.69XA, T84.7XXA

0RGL3JZ Fusion of Right Elbow Joint with Synthetic Substitute, Percutaneous Approach

Note Continued

RGL3JZ Continued Note

HAC When reported with secondary diagnosis code T84.60XA, T84.610A, T84.611A, T84.612A, T84.613A, T84.614A, T84.615A, T84.619A, T84.63XA, T84.69XA, T84.7XXA

RGL3KZ Fusion of Right Elbow Joint with Nonautologous Tissue Substitute, Percutaneous Approach

HAC When reported with secondary diagnosis code T84.60XA, T84.610A, T84.611A, T84.612A, T84.613A, T84.614A, T84.615A, T84.619A, T84.63XA, T84.69XA, T84.7XXA

RGL3ZZ Fusion of Right Elbow Joint, Percutaneous Approach

HAC When reported with secondary diagnosis code T84.60XA, T84.610A, T84.611A, T84.612A, T84.613A, T84.614A, T84.615A, T84.619A, T84.63XA, T84.69XA, T84.7XXA

RGL44Z Fusion of Right Elbow Joint with Internal Fixation Device, Percutaneous Endoscopic Approach

HAC When reported with secondary diagnosis code T84.60XA, T84.610A, T84.611A, T84.612A, T84.613A, T84.614A, T84.615A, T84.619A, T84.63XA, T84.69XA, T84.7XXA

RGL45Z Fusion of Right Elbow Joint with External Fixation Device, Percutaneous Endoscopic Approach

HAC When reported with secondary diagnosis code T84.60XA, T84.610A, T84.611A, T84.612A, T84.613A, T84.614A, T84.615A, T84.619A, T84.63XA, T84.69XA, T84.7XXA

RGL47Z Fusion of Right Elbow Joint with Autologous Tissue Substitute, Percutaneous Endoscopic Approach

HAC When reported with secondary diagnosis code T84.60XA, T84.610A, T84.611A, T84.612A, T84.613A, T84.614A, T84.615A, T84.619A, T84.63XA, T84.69XA, T84.7XXA

RGL4JZ Fusion of Right Elbow Joint with Synthetic Substitute, Percutaneous Endoscopic Approach

HAC When reported with secondary diagnosis code T84.60XA, T84.610A, T84.611A, T84.612A, T84.613A, T84.614A, T84.615A, T84.619A, T84.63XA, T84.69XA, T84.7XXA

RGL4KZ Fusion of Right Elbow Joint with Nonautologous Tissue Substitute, Percutaneous Endoscopic Approach

HAC When reported with secondary diagnosis code T84.60XA, T84.610A, T84.611A, T84.612A, T84.613A, T84.614A, T84.615A, T84.619A, T84.63XA, T84.69XA, T84.7XXA

0RGL4ZZ Fusion of Right Elbow Joint, Percutaneous Endoscopic Approach

HAC When reported with secondary diagnosis code T84.60XA, T84.610A, T84.611A, T84.612A, T84.613A, T84.614A, T84.615A, T84.619A, T84.63XA, T84.69XA, T84.7XXA

0RGM04Z Fusion of Left Elbow Joint with Internal Fixation Device, Open Approach

HAC When reported with secondary diagnosis code T84.60XA, T84.610A, T84.611A, T84.612A, T84.613A, T84.614A, T84.615A, T84.619A, T84.63XA, T84.69XA, T84.7XXA

0RGM05Z Fusion of Left Elbow Joint with External Fixation Device, Open Approach

HAC When reported with secondary diagnosis code T84.60XA, T84.610A, T84.611A, T84.612A, T84.613A, T84.614A, T84.615A, T84.619A, T84.63XA, T84.69XA, T84.7XXA

0RGM07Z Fusion of Left Elbow Joint with Autologous Tissue Substitute, Open Approach

HAC When reported with secondary diagnosis code T84.60XA, T84.610A, T84.611A, T84.612A, T84.613A, T84.614A, T84.615A, T84.619A, T84.63XA, T84.69XA, T84.7XXA

0RGM0JZ Fusion of Left Elbow Joint with Synthetic Substitute, Open Approach

HAC When reported with secondary diagnosis code T84.60XA, T84.610A, T84.611A, T84.612A, T84.613A, T84.614A, T84.615A, T84.619A, T84.63XA, T84.69XA, T84.7XXA

0RGM0KZ Fusion of Left Elbow Joint with Nonautologous Tissue Substitute, Open Approach

HAC When reported with secondary diagnosis code T84.60XA, T84.610A, T84.611A, T84.612A, T84.613A, T84.614A, T84.615A, T84.619A, T84.63XA, T84.69XA, T84.7XXA

0RGM0ZZ Fusion of Left Elbow Joint, Open Approach

HAC When reported with secondary diagnosis code T84.60XA, T84.610A, T84.611A, T84.612A, T84.613A, T84.614A, T84.615A, T84.619A, T84.63XA, T84.69XA, T84.7XXA

0RGM34Z Fusion of Left Elbow Joint with Internal Fixation Device, Percutaneous Approach

HAC When reported with secondary diagnosis code T84.60XA, T84.610A, T84.611A, T84.612A, T84.613A, T84.614A, T84.615A, T84.619A, T84.63XA, T84.69XA, T84.7XXA

0RGM35Z Fusion of Left Elbow Joint with External Fixation Device, Percutaneous Approach

HAC When reported with secondary diagnosis code T84.60XA, T84.610A, T84.611A, T84.612A, T84.613A, T84.614A, T84.615A, T84.619A, T84.63XA, T84.69XA, T84.7XXA

0RGM37Z Fusion of Left Elbow Joint with Autologous Tissue Substitute, Percutaneous Approach

HAC When reported with secondary diagnosis code T84.60XA, T84.610A, T84.611A, T84.612A, T84.613A, T84.614A, T84.615A, T84.619A, T84.63XA, T84.69XA, T84.7XXA

0RGM3JZ Fusion of Left Elbow Joint with Synthetic Substitute, Percutaneous Approach

HAC When reported with secondary diagnosis code T84.60XA, T84.610A, T84.611A, T84.612A, T84.613A, T84.614A, T84.615A, T84.619A, T84.63XA, T84.69XA, T84.7XXA

0RGM3KZ Fusion of Left Elbow Joint with Nonautologous Tissue Substitute, Percutaneous Approach

HAC When reported with secondary diagnosis code T84.60XA, T84.610A, T84.611A, T84.612A, T84.613A, T84.614A, T84.615A, T84.619A, T84.63XA, T84.69XA, T84.7XXA

0RGM3ZZ Fusion of Left Elbow Joint, Percutaneous Approach

HAC When reported with secondary diagnosis code T84.60XA, T84.610A, T84.611A, T84.612A, T84.613A, T84.614A, T84.615A, T84.619A, T84.63XA, T84.69XA, T84.7XXA

0RGM44Z Fusion of Left Elbow Joint with Internal Fixation Device, Percutaneous Endoscopic Approach

HAC When reported with secondary diagnosis code T84.60XA, T84.610A, T84.611A, T84.612A, T84.613A, T84.614A, T84.615A, T84.619A, T84.63XA, T84.69XA, T84.7XXA

0RGM45Z Fusion of Left Elbow Joint with External Fixation Device, Percutaneous Endoscopic Approach

HAC When reported with secondary diagnosis code T84.60XA, T84.610A, T84.611A, T84.612A, T84.613A, T84.614A, T84.615A, T84.619A, T84.63XA, T84.69XA, T84.7XXA

0RGM47Z Fusion of Left Elbow Joint with Autologous Tissue Substitute, Percutaneous Endoscopic Approach

HAC When reported with secondary diagnosis code T84.60XA, T84.610A, T84.611A, T84.612A, T84.613A, T84.614A, T84.615A, T84.619A, T84.63XA, T84.69XA, T84.7XXA

0RGM4JZ Fusion of Left Elbow Joint with Synthetic Substitute, Percutaneous Endoscopic Approach

HAC When reported with secondary diagnosis code T84.60XA, T84.610A, T84.611A, T84.612A, T84.613A, T84.614A, T84.615A, T84.619A, T84.63XA, T84.69XA, T84.7XXA

0RGM4KZ Fusion of Left Elbow Joint with Nonautologous Tissue Substitute, Percutaneous Endoscopic Approach

HAC When reported with secondary diagnosis code T84.60XA, T84.610A, T84.611A, T84.612A, T84.613A, T84.614A, T84.615A, T84.619A, T84.63XA, T84.69XA, T84.7XXA

0RGM4ZZ Fusion of Left Elbow Joint, Percutaneous Endoscopic Approach

HAC When reported with secondary diagnosis code T84.60XA, T84.610A, T84.611A, T84.612A, T84.613A, T84.614A, T84.615A, T84.619A, T84.63XA, T84.69XA, T84.7XXA

0RGN04Z Fusion of Right Wrist Joint with Internal Fixation Device, Open Approach

0RGN05Z Fusion of Right Wrist Joint with External Fixation Device, Open Approach

0RGN07Z Fusion of Right Wrist Joint with Autologous Tissue Substitute, Open Approach

0RGN0JZ Fusion of Right Wrist Joint with Synthetic Substitute, Open Approach

0RGN0KZ Fusion of Right Wrist Joint with Nonautologous Tissue Substitute, Open Approach

0RGN0ZZ Fusion of Right Wrist Joint, Open Approach

0RGN34Z Fusion of Right Wrist Joint with Internal Fixation Device, Percutaneous Approach

0RGN35Z Fusion of Right Wrist Joint with External Fixation Device, Percutaneous Approach

0RGN37Z Fusion of Right Wrist Joint with Autologous Tissue Substitute, Percutaneous Approach

0RGN3JZ Fusion of Right Wrist Joint with Synthetic Substitute, Percutaneous Approach

0RGN3KZ Fusion of Right Wrist Joint with Nonautologous Tissue Substitute, Percutaneous Approach

0RGN3ZZ Fusion of Right Wrist Joint, Percutaneous Approach

0RGN44Z Fusion of Right Wrist Joint with Internal Fixation Device, Percutaneous Endoscopic Approach

0RGN45Z Fusion of Right Wrist Joint with External Fixation Device, Percutaneous Endoscopic Approach

0RGN47Z Fusion of Right Wrist Joint with Autologous Tissue Substitute, Percutaneous Endoscopic Approach

0RGN4JZ Fusion of Right Wrist Joint with Synthetic Substitute, Percutaneous Endoscopic Approach

0RGN4KZ Fusion of Right Wrist Joint with Nonautologous Tissue Substitute, Percutaneous Endoscopic Approach

0RGN4ZZ Fusion of Right Wrist Joint, Percutaneous Endoscopic Approach

0RGP04Z Fusion of Left Wrist Joint with Internal Fixation Device, Open Approach

0RGP05Z Fusion of Left Wrist Joint with External Fixation Device, Open Approach

0RGP07Z Fusion of Left Wrist Joint with Autologous Tissue Substitute, Open Approach

0RGP0JZ Fusion of Left Wrist Joint with Synthetic Substitute, Open Approach

0RGP0KZ Fusion of Left Wrist Joint with Nonautologous Tissue Substitute, Open Approach

0RGP0ZZ Fusion of Left Wrist Joint, Open Approach

0RGP34Z Fusion of Left Wrist Joint with Internal Fixation Device, Percutaneous Approach

0RGP35Z Fusion of Left Wrist Joint with External Fixation Device, Percutaneous Approach

0RGP37Z Fusion of Left Wrist Joint with Autologous Tissue Substitute, Percutaneous Approach

0RGP3JZ Fusion of Left Wrist Joint with Synthetic Substitute, Percutaneous Approach

0RGP3KZ Fusion of Left Wrist Joint with Nonautologous Tissue Substitute, Percutaneous Approach

0RGP3ZZ Fusion of Left Wrist Joint, Percutaneous Approach

0RGP44Z Fusion of Left Wrist Joint with Internal Fixation Device, Percutaneous Endoscopic Approach

0RGP45Z Fusion of Left Wrist Joint with External Fixation Device, Percutaneous Endoscopic Approach

0RGP47Z Fusion of Left Wrist Joint with Autologous Tissue Substitute, Percutaneous Endoscopic Approach

0RGP4JZ Fusion of Left Wrist Joint with Synthetic Substitute, Percutaneous Endoscopic Approach

0RGP4KZ Fusion of Left Wrist Joint with Nonautologous Tissue Substitute, Percutaneous Endoscopic Approach

0RGP4ZZ Fusion of Left Wrist Joint, Percutaneous Endoscopic Approach

0RGQ04Z Fusion of Right Carpal Joint with Internal Fixation Device, Open Approach

0RGQ05Z Fusion of Right Carpal Joint with External Fixation Device, Open Approach

0RGQ07Z Fusion of Right Carpal Joint with Autologous Tissue Substitute, Open Approach

0RGQ0JZ Fusion of Right Carpal Joint with Synthetic Substitute, Open Approach

0RGQ0KZ Fusion of Right Carpal Joint with Nonautologous Tissue Substitute, Open Approach

0RGQ0ZZ Fusion of Right Carpal Joint, Open Approach

0RGQ34Z Fusion of Right Carpal Joint with Internal Fixation Device, Percutaneous Approach

0RGQ35Z Fusion of Right Carpal Joint with External Fixation Device, Percutaneous Approach

0RGQ37Z Fusion of Right Carpal Joint with Autologous Tissue Substitute, Percutaneous Approach

0RGQ3JZ Fusion of Right Carpal Joint with Synthetic Substitute, Percutaneous Approach

0RGQ3KZ Fusion of Right Carpal Joint with Nonautologous Tissue Substitute, Percutaneous Approach

0RGQ3ZZ Fusion of Right Carpal Joint, Percutaneous Approach

0RGQ44Z Fusion of Right Carpal Joint with Internal Fixation Device, Percutaneous Endoscopic Approach

0RGQ45Z Fusion of Right Carpal Joint with External Fixation Device, Percutaneous Endoscopic Approach

0RGQ47Z Fusion of Right Carpal Joint with Autologous Tissue Substitute, Percutaneous Endoscopic Approach

0RGQ4JZ Fusion of Right Carpal Joint with Synthetic Substitute, Percutaneous Endoscopic Approach

0RGQ4KZ Fusion of Right Carpal Joint with Nonautologous Tissue Substitute, Percutaneous Endoscopic Approach

0RGQ4ZZ Fusion of Right Carpal Joint, Percutaneous Endoscopic Approach

0RGR04Z Fusion of Left Carpal Joint with Internal Fixation Device, Open Approach

0RGR05Z Fusion of Left Carpal Joint with External Fixation Device, Open Approach

0RGR07Z Fusion of Left Carpal Joint with Autologous Tissue Substitute, Open Approach

0RGR0JZ Fusion of Left Carpal Joint with Synthetic Substitute, Open Approach

0RGR0KZ Fusion of Left Carpal Joint with Nonautologous Tissue Substitute, Open Approach

0RGR0ZZ Fusion of Left Carpal Joint, Open Approach

0RGR34Z Fusion of Left Carpal Joint with Internal Fixation Device, Percutaneous Approach

0RGR35Z Fusion of Left Carpal Joint with External Fixation Device, Percutaneous Approach

0RGR37Z Fusion of Left Carpal Joint with Autologous Tissue Substitute, Percutaneous Approach

0RGR3JZ Fusion of Left Carpal Joint with Synthetic Substitute, Percutaneous Approach

0RGR3KZ Fusion of Left Carpal Joint with Nonautologous Tissue Substitute, Percutaneous Approach

0RGR3ZZ Fusion of Left Carpal Joint, Percutaneous Approach

0RGR44Z Fusion of Left Carpal Joint with Internal Fixation Device, Percutaneous Endoscopic Approach

0RGR45Z Fusion of Left Carpal Joint with External Fixation Device, Percutaneous Endoscopic Approach

0RGR47Z Fusion of Left Carpal Joint with Autologous Tissue Substitute, Percutaneous Endoscopic Approach

0RGR4JZ Fusion of Left Carpal Joint with Synthetic Substitute, Percutaneous Endoscopic Approach

0RGR4KZ Fusion of Left Carpal Joint with Nonautologous Tissue Substitute, Percutaneous Endoscopic Approach

0RGR4ZZ Fusion of Left Carpal Joint, Percutaneo Endoscopic Approach

0RGS04Z Fusion of Right Metacarpocarpal Joint with Internal Fixation Device, Open Approach

0RGS05Z Fusion of Right Metacarpocarpal Joint with External Fixation Device, Open Approach

0RGS07Z Fusion of Right Metacarpocarpal Joint with Autologous Tissue Substitute, Oper Approach

0RGS0JZ Fusion of Right Metacarpocarpal Joint with Synthetic Substitute, Open Approa

0RGS0KZ Fusion of Right Metacarpocarpal Joint with Nonautologous Tissue Substitute, Open Approach

0RGS0ZZ Fusion of Right Metacarpocarpal Joint, Open Approach

0RGS34Z Fusion of Right Metacarpocarpal Joint with Internal Fixation Device, Percutaneous Approach

0RGS35Z Fusion of Right Metacarpocarpal Joint with External Fixation Device, Percutaneous Approach

0RGS37Z Fusion of Right Metacarpocarpal Joint with Autologous Tissue Substitute, Percutaneous Approach

0RGS3JZ Fusion of Right Metacarpocarpal Joint with Synthetic Substitute, Percutaneous Approach

0RGS3KZ Fusion of Right Metacarpocarpal Joint with Nonautologous Tissue Substitute, Percutaneous Approach

0RGS3ZZ Fusion of Right Metacarpocarpal Joint, Percutaneous Approach

0RGS44Z Fusion of Right Metacarpocarpal Joint with Internal Fixation Device, Percutaneous Endoscopic Approach

0RGS45Z Fusion of Right Metacarpocarpal Joint with External Fixation Device, Percutaneous Endoscopic Approach

0RGS47Z Fusion of Right Metacarpocarpal Joint with Autologous Tissue Substitute, Percutaneous Endoscopic Approach

0RGS4JZ Fusion of Right Metacarpocarpal Joint with Synthetic Substitute, Percutaneous Endoscopic Approach

0RGS4KZ Fusion of Right Metacarpocarpal Joint with Nonautologous Tissue Substitute, Percutaneous Endoscopic Approach

0RGS4ZZ Fusion of Right Metacarpocarpal Joint, Percutaneous Endoscopic Approach

0RGT04Z Fusion of Left Metacarpocarpal Joint with Internal Fixation Device, Open Approach

0RGT05Z Fusion of Left Metacarpocarpal Joint with External Fixation Device, Open Approach

0RGT07Z Fusion of Left Metacarpocarpal Joint with Autologous Tissue Substitute, Open Approach

0RGT0JZ Fusion of Left Metacarpocarpal Joint with Synthetic Substitute, Open Approach

0RGT0KZ Fusion of Left Metacarpocarpal Joint with Nonautologous Tissue Substitute, Open Approach

0RGT0ZZ Fusion of Left Metacarpocarpal Joint, Open Approach

0RGT34Z Fusion of Left Metacarpocarpal Joint with Internal Fixation Device, Percutaneous Approach

0RGT35Z Fusion of Left Metacarpocarpal Joint with External Fixation Device, Percutaneous Approach

0RGT37Z Fusion of Left Metacarpocarpal Joint with Autologous Tissue Substitute, Percutaneous Approach

0RGT3JZ Fusion of Left Metacarpocarpal Joint with Synthetic Substitute, Percutaneous Approach

0RGT3KZ Fusion of Left Metacarpocarpal Joint with Nonautologous Tissue Substitute, Percutaneous Approach
0RGT3ZZ Fusion of Left Metacarpocarpal Joint, Percutaneous Approach
0RGT44Z Fusion of Left Metacarpocarpal Joint with Internal Fixation Device, Percutaneous Endoscopic Approach
0RGT45Z Fusion of Left Metacarpocarpal Joint with External Fixation Device, Percutaneous Endoscopic Approach
0RGT47Z Fusion of Left Metacarpocarpal Joint with Autologous Tissue Substitute, Percutaneous Endoscopic Approach
0RGT4JZ Fusion of Left Metacarpocarpal Joint with Synthetic Substitute, Percutaneous Endoscopic Approach
0RGT4KZ Fusion of Left Metacarpocarpal Joint with Nonautologous Tissue Substitute, Percutaneous Endoscopic Approach
0RGT4ZZ Fusion of Left Metacarpocarpal Joint, Percutaneous Endoscopic Approach
0RGU04Z Fusion of Right Metacarpophalangeal Joint with Internal Fixation Device, Open Approach
0RGU05Z Fusion of Right Metacarpophalangeal Joint with External Fixation Device, Open Approach
0RGU07Z Fusion of Right Metacarpophalangeal Joint with Autologous Tissue Substitute, Open Approach
0RGU0JZ Fusion of Right Metacarpophalangeal Joint with Synthetic Substitute, Open Approach
0RGU0KZ Fusion of Right Metacarpophalangeal Joint with Nonautologous Tissue Substitute, Open Approach
0RGU0ZZ Fusion of Right Metacarpophalangeal Joint, Open Approach
0RGU34Z Fusion of Right Metacarpophalangeal Joint with Internal Fixation Device, Percutaneous Approach
0RGU35Z Fusion of Right Metacarpophalangeal Joint with External Fixation Device, Percutaneous Approach
0RGU37Z Fusion of Right Metacarpophalangeal Joint with Autologous Tissue Substitute, Percutaneous Approach
0RGU3JZ Fusion of Right Metacarpophalangeal Joint with Synthetic Substitute, Percutaneous Approach
0RGU3KZ Fusion of Right Metacarpophalangeal Joint with Nonautologous Tissue Substitute, Percutaneous Approach
0RGU3ZZ Fusion of Right Metacarpophalangeal Joint, Percutaneous Approach
0RGU44Z Fusion of Right Metacarpophalangeal Joint with Internal Fixation Device, Percutaneous Endoscopic Approach
0RGU45Z Fusion of Right Metacarpophalangeal Joint with External Fixation Device, Percutaneous Endoscopic Approach
0RGU47Z Fusion of Right Metacarpophalangeal Joint with Autologous Tissue Substitute, Percutaneous Endoscopic Approach
0RGU4JZ Fusion of Right Metacarpophalangeal Joint with Synthetic Substitute, Percutaneous Endoscopic Approach
0RGU4KZ Fusion of Right Metacarpophalangeal Joint with Nonautologous Tissue Substitute, Percutaneous Endoscopic Approach
0RGU4ZZ Fusion of Right Metacarpophalangeal Joint, Percutaneous Endoscopic Approach
0RGV04Z Fusion of Left Metacarpophalangeal Joint with Internal Fixation Device, Open Approach
0RGV05Z Fusion of Left Metacarpophalangeal Joint with External Fixation Device, Open Approach
0RGV07Z Fusion of Left Metacarpophalangeal Joint with Autologous Tissue Substitute, Open Approach
0RGV0JZ Fusion of Left Metacarpophalangeal Joint with Synthetic Substitute, Open Approach
0RGV0KZ Fusion of Left Metacarpophalangeal Joint with Nonautologous Tissue Substitute, Open Approach
0RGV0ZZ Fusion of Left Metacarpophalangeal Joint, Open Approach
0RGV34Z Fusion of Left Metacarpophalangeal Joint with Internal Fixation Device, Percutaneous Approach
0RGV35Z Fusion of Left Metacarpophalangeal Joint with External Fixation Device, Percutaneous Approach
0RGV37Z Fusion of Left Metacarpophalangeal Joint with Autologous Tissue Substitute, Percutaneous Approach
0RGV3JZ Fusion of Left Metacarpophalangeal Joint with Synthetic Substitute, Percutaneous Approach
0RGV3KZ Fusion of Left Metacarpophalangeal Joint with Nonautologous Tissue Substitute, Percutaneous Approach
0RGV3ZZ Fusion of Left Metacarpophalangeal Joint, Percutaneous Approach
0RGV44Z Fusion of Left Metacarpophalangeal Joint with Internal Fixation Device, Percutaneous Endoscopic Approach
0RGV45Z Fusion of Left Metacarpophalangeal Joint with External Fixation Device, Percutaneous Endoscopic Approach
0RGV47Z Fusion of Left Metacarpophalangeal Joint with Autologous Tissue Substitute, Percutaneous Endoscopic Approach
0RGV4JZ Fusion of Left Metacarpophalangeal Joint with Synthetic Substitute, Percutaneous Endoscopic Approach
0RGV4KZ Fusion of Left Metacarpophalangeal Joint with Nonautologous Tissue Substitute, Percutaneous Endoscopic Approach
0RGV4ZZ Fusion of Left Metacarpophalangeal Joint, Percutaneous Endoscopic Approach
0RGW04Z Fusion of Right Finger Phalangeal Joint with Internal Fixation Device, Open Approach
0RGW05Z Fusion of Right Finger Phalangeal Joint with External Fixation Device, Open Approach
0RGW07Z Fusion of Right Finger Phalangeal Joint with Autologous Tissue Substitute, Open Approach
0RGW0JZ Fusion of Right Finger Phalangeal Joint with Synthetic Substitute, Open Approach
0RGW0KZ Fusion of Right Finger Phalangeal Joint with Nonautologous Tissue Substitute, Open Approach
0RGW0ZZ Fusion of Right Finger Phalangeal Joint, Open Approach
0RGW34Z Fusion of Right Finger Phalangeal Joint with Internal Fixation Device, Percutaneous Approach
0RGW35Z Fusion of Right Finger Phalangeal Joint with External Fixation Device, Percutaneous Approach
0RGW37Z Fusion of Right Finger Phalangeal Joint with Autologous Tissue Substitute, Percutaneous Approach
0RGW3JZ Fusion of Right Finger Phalangeal Joint with Synthetic Substitute, Percutaneous Approach
0RGW3KZ Fusion of Right Finger Phalangeal Joint with Nonautologous Tissue Substitute, Percutaneous Approach
0RGW3ZZ Fusion of Right Finger Phalangeal Joint, Percutaneous Approach
0RGW44Z Fusion of Right Finger Phalangeal Joint with Internal Fixation Device, Percutaneous Endoscopic Approach
0RGW45Z Fusion of Right Finger Phalangeal Joint with External Fixation Device, Percutaneous Endoscopic Approach
0RGW47Z Fusion of Right Finger Phalangeal Joint with Autologous Tissue Substitute, Percutaneous Endoscopic Approach
0RGW4JZ Fusion of Right Finger Phalangeal Joint with Synthetic Substitute, Percutaneous Endoscopic Approach
0RGW4KZ Fusion of Right Finger Phalangeal Joint with Nonautologous Tissue Substitute, Percutaneous Endoscopic Approach
0RGW4ZZ Fusion of Right Finger Phalangeal Joint, Percutaneous Endoscopic Approach
0RGX04Z Fusion of Left Finger Phalangeal Joint with Internal Fixation Device, Open Approach
0RGX05Z Fusion of Left Finger Phalangeal Joint with External Fixation Device, Open Approach
0RGX07Z Fusion of Left Finger Phalangeal Joint with Autologous Tissue Substitute, Open Approach
0RGX0JZ Fusion of Left Finger Phalangeal Joint with Synthetic Substitute, Open Approach
0RGX0KZ Fusion of Left Finger Phalangeal Joint with Nonautologous Tissue Substitute, Open Approach
0RGX0ZZ Fusion of Left Finger Phalangeal Joint, Open Approach
0RGX34Z Fusion of Left Finger Phalangeal Joint with Internal Fixation Device, Percutaneous Approach
0RGX35Z Fusion of Left Finger Phalangeal Joint with External Fixation Device, Percutaneous Approach
0RGX37Z Fusion of Left Finger Phalangeal Joint with Autologous Tissue Substitute, Percutaneous Approach
0RGX3JZ Fusion of Left Finger Phalangeal Joint with Synthetic Substitute, Percutaneous Approach
0RGX3KZ Fusion of Left Finger Phalangeal Joint with Nonautologous Tissue Substitute, Percutaneous Approach
0RGX3ZZ Fusion of Left Finger Phalangeal Joint, Percutaneous Approach
0RGX44Z Fusion of Left Finger Phalangeal Joint with Internal Fixation Device, Percutaneous Endoscopic Approach
0RGX45Z Fusion of Left Finger Phalangeal Joint with External Fixation Device, Percutaneous Endoscopic Approach
0RGX47Z Fusion of Left Finger Phalangeal Joint with Autologous Tissue Substitute, Percutaneous Endoscopic Approach
0RGX4JZ Fusion of Left Finger Phalangeal Joint with Synthetic Substitute, Percutaneous Endoscopic Approach
0RGX4KZ Fusion of Left Finger Phalangeal Joint with Nonautologous Tissue Substitute, Percutaneous Endoscopic Approach
0RGX4ZZ Fusion of Left Finger Phalangeal Joint, Percutaneous Endoscopic Approach

0RH – Upper Joints, Insertion

0RH003Z Insertion of Infusion Device into Occipital-cervical Joint, Open Approach
0RH004Z Insertion of Internal Fixation Device into Occipital-cervical Joint, Open Approach
0RH008Z Insertion of Spacer into Occipital-cervical Joint, Open Approach
0RH00BZ Insertion of Interspinous Process Spinal Stabilization Device into Occipital-cervical Joint, Open Approach
0RH00CZ Insertion of Pedicle-Based Spinal Stabilization Device into Occipital-cervical Joint, Open Approach
0RH00DZ Insertion of Facet Replacement Spinal Stabilization Device into Occipital-cervical Joint, Open Approach
0RH033Z Insertion of Infusion Device into Occipital-cervical Joint, Percutaneous Approach
0RH034Z Insertion of Internal Fixation Device into Occipital-cervical Joint, Percutaneous Approach
0RH038Z Insertion of Spacer into Occipital-cervical Joint, Percutaneous Approach
0RH03BZ Insertion of Interspinous Process Spinal Stabilization Device into Occipital-cervical Joint, Percutaneous Approach
0RH03CZ Insertion of Pedicle-Based Spinal Stabilization Device into Occipital-cervical Joint, Percutaneous Approach
0RH03DZ Insertion of Facet Replacement Spinal Stabilization Device into Occipital-cervical Joint, Percutaneous Approach
0RH043Z Insertion of Infusion Device into Occipital-cervical Joint, Percutaneous Endoscopic Approach
0RH044Z Insertion of Internal Fixation Device into Occipital-cervical Joint, Percutaneous Endoscopic Approach
0RH048Z Insertion of Spacer into Occipital-cervical Joint, Percutaneous Endoscopic Approach
0RH04BZ Insertion of Interspinous Process Spinal Stabilization Device into Occipital-cervical Joint, Percutaneous Endoscopic Approach
0RH04CZ Insertion of Pedicle-Based Spinal Stabilization Device into Occipital-cervical Joint, Percutaneous Endoscopic Approach
0RH04DZ Insertion of Facet Replacement Spinal Stabilization Device into Occipital-cervical Joint, Percutaneous Endoscopic Approach
0RH103Z Insertion of Infusion Device into Cervical Vertebral Joint, Open Approach
0RH104Z Insertion of Internal Fixation Device into Cervical Vertebral Joint, Open Approach
0RH108Z Insertion of Spacer into Cervical Vertebral Joint, Open Approach
0RH10BZ Insertion of Interspinous Process Spinal Stabilization Device into Cervical Vertebral Joint, Open Approach
0RH10CZ Insertion of Pedicle-Based Spinal Stabilization Device into Cervical Vertebral Joint, Open Approach
0RH10DZ Insertion of Facet Replacement Spinal Stabilization Device into Cervical Vertebral Joint, Open Approach
0RH133Z Insertion of Infusion Device into Cervical Vertebral Joint, Percutaneous Approach
0RH134Z Insertion of Internal Fixation Device into Cervical Vertebral Joint, Percutaneous Approach
0RH138Z Insertion of Spacer into Cervical Vertebral Joint, Percutaneous Approach
0RH13BZ Insertion of Interspinous Process Spinal Stabilization Device into Cervical Vertebral Joint, Percutaneous Approach
0RH13CZ Insertion of Pedicle-Based Spinal Stabilization Device into Cervical Vertebral Joint, Percutaneous Approach
0RH13DZ Insertion of Facet Replacement Spinal Stabilization Device into Cervical Vertebral Joint, Percutaneous Approach
0RH143Z Insertion of Infusion Device into Cervical Vertebral Joint, Percutaneous Endoscopic Approach
0RH144Z Insertion of Internal Fixation Device into Cervical Vertebral Joint, Percutaneous Endoscopic Approach
0RH148Z Insertion of Spacer into Cervical Vertebral Joint, Percutaneous Endoscopic Approach
0RH14BZ Insertion of Interspinous Process Spinal Stabilization Device into Cervical Vertebral Joint, Percutaneous Endoscopic Approach
0RH14CZ Insertion of Pedicle-Based Spinal Stabilization Device into Cervical Vertebral Joint, Percutaneous Endoscopic Approach
0RH14DZ Insertion of Facet Replacement Spinal Stabilization Device into Cervical Vertebral Joint, Percutaneous Endoscopic Approach
0RH303Z Insertion of Infusion Device into Cervical Vertebral Disc, Open Approach
0RH333Z Insertion of Infusion Device into Cervical Vertebral Disc, Percutaneous Approach
0RH343Z Insertion of Infusion Device into Cervical Vertebral Disc, Percutaneous Endoscopic Approach
0RH403Z Insertion of Infusion Device into Cervicothoracic Vertebral Joint, Open Approach
0RH404Z Insertion of Internal Fixation Device into Cervicothoracic Vertebral Joint, Open Approach
0RH408Z Insertion of Spacer into Cervicothoracic Vertebral Joint, Open Approach
0RH40BZ Insertion of Interspinous Process Spinal Stabilization Device into Cervicothoracic Vertebral Joint, Open Approach
0RH40CZ Insertion of Pedicle-Based Spinal Stabilization Device into Cervicothoracic Vertebral Joint, Open Approach
0RH40DZ Insertion of Facet Replacement Spinal Stabilization Device into Cervicothoracic Vertebral Joint, Open Approach
0RH433Z Insertion of Infusion Device into Cervicothoracic Vertebral Joint, Percutaneous Approach
0RH434Z Insertion of Internal Fixation Device into Cervicothoracic Vertebral Joint, Percutaneous Approach
0RH438Z Insertion of Spacer into Cervicothoracic Vertebral Joint, Percutaneous Approach
0RH43BZ Insertion of Interspinous Process Spinal Stabilization Device into Cervicothoracic Vertebral Joint, Percutaneous Approach
0RH43CZ Insertion of Pedicle-Based Spinal Stabilization Device into Cervicothoracic Vertebral Joint, Percutaneous Approach
0RH43DZ Insertion of Facet Replacement Spinal Stabilization Device into Cervicothoracic Vertebral Joint, Percutaneous Approach
0RH443Z Insertion of Infusion Device into Cervicothoracic Vertebral Joint, Percutaneous Endoscopic Approach
0RH444Z Insertion of Internal Fixation Device into Cervicothoracic Vertebral Joint, Percutaneous Endoscopic Approach
0RH448Z Insertion of Spacer into Cervicothoracic Vertebral Joint, Percutaneous Endoscopic Approach
0RH44BZ Insertion of Interspinous Process Spinal Stabilization Device into Cervicothoracic Vertebral Joint, Percutaneous Endoscopic Approach
0RH44CZ Insertion of Pedicle-Based Spinal Stabilization Device into Cervicothoracic Vertebral Joint, Percutaneous Endoscopic Approach
0RH44DZ Insertion of Facet Replacement Spinal Stabilization Device into Cervicothoracic Vertebral Joint, Percutaneous Endoscopic Approach
0RH503Z Insertion of Infusion Device into Cervicothoracic Vertebral Disc, Open Approach
0RH533Z Insertion of Infusion Device into Cervicothoracic Vertebral Disc, Percutaneous Approach
0RH543Z Insertion of Infusion Device into Cervicothoracic Vertebral Disc, Percutaneous Endoscopic Approach
0RH603Z Insertion of Infusion Device into Thoracic Vertebral Joint, Open Approach
0RH604Z Insertion of Internal Fixation Device into Thoracic Vertebral Joint, Open Approach
0RH608Z Insertion of Spacer into Thoracic Vertebral Joint, Open Approach
0RH60BZ Insertion of Interspinous Process Spinal Stabilization Device into Thoracic Vertebral Joint, Open Approach
0RH60CZ Insertion of Pedicle-Based Spinal Stabilization Device into Thoracic Vertebral Joint, Open Approach
0RH60DZ Insertion of Facet Replacement Spinal Stabilization Device into Thoracic Vertebral Joint, Open Approach
0RH633Z Insertion of Infusion Device into Thoracic Vertebral Joint, Percutaneous Approach
0RH634Z Insertion of Internal Fixation Device into Thoracic Vertebral Joint, Percutaneous Approach
0RH638Z Insertion of Spacer into Thoracic Vertebral Joint, Percutaneous Approach
0RH63BZ Insertion of Interspinous Process Spinal Stabilization Device into Thoracic Vertebral Joint, Percutaneous Approach
0RH63CZ Insertion of Pedicle-Based Spinal Stabilization Device into Thoracic Vertebral Joint, Percutaneous Approach
0RH63DZ Insertion of Facet Replacement Spinal Stabilization Device into Thoracic Vertebral Joint, Percutaneous Approach
0RH643Z Insertion of Infusion Device into Thoracic Vertebral Joint, Percutaneous Endoscopic Approach
0RH644Z Insertion of Internal Fixation Device into Thoracic Vertebral Joint, Percutaneous Endoscopic Approach
0RH648Z Insertion of Spacer into Thoracic Vertebral Joint, Percutaneous Endoscopic Approach
0RH64BZ Insertion of Interspinous Process Spinal Stabilization Device into Thoracic Vertebral Joint, Percutaneous Endoscopic Approach
0RH64CZ Insertion of Pedicle-Based Spinal Stabilization Device into Thoracic Vertebral Joint, Percutaneous Endoscopic Approach
0RH64DZ Insertion of Facet Replacement Spinal Stabilization Device into Thoracic Vertebral Joint, Percutaneous Endoscopic Approach

RH903Z Insertion of Infusion Device into Thoracic Vertebral Disc, Open Approach

RH933Z Insertion of Infusion Device into Thoracic Vertebral Disc, Percutaneous Approach

RH943Z Insertion of Infusion Device into Thoracic Vertebral Disc, Percutaneous Endoscopic Approach

RHA03Z Insertion of Infusion Device into Thoracolumbar Vertebral Joint, Open Approach

RHA04Z Insertion of Internal Fixation Device into Thoracolumbar Vertebral Joint, Open Approach

RHA08Z Insertion of Spacer into Thoracolumbar Vertebral Joint, Open Approach

RHA0BZ Insertion of Interspinous Process Spinal Stabilization Device into Thoracolumbar Vertebral Joint, Open Approach

RHA0CZ Insertion of Pedicle-Based Spinal Stabilization Device into Thoracolumbar Vertebral Joint, Open Approach

RHA0DZ Insertion of Facet Replacement Spinal Stabilization Device into Thoracolumbar Vertebral Joint, Open Approach

RHA33Z Insertion of Infusion Device into Thoracolumbar Vertebral Joint, Percutaneous Approach

RHA34Z Insertion of Internal Fixation Device into Thoracolumbar Vertebral Joint, Percutaneous Approach

RHA38Z Insertion of Spacer into Thoracolumbar Vertebral Joint, Percutaneous Approach

RHA3BZ Insertion of Interspinous Process Spinal Stabilization Device into Thoracolumbar Vertebral Joint, Percutaneous Approach

RHA3CZ Insertion of Pedicle-Based Spinal Stabilization Device into Thoracolumbar Vertebral Joint, Percutaneous Approach

RHA3DZ Insertion of Facet Replacement Spinal Stabilization Device into Thoracolumbar Vertebral Joint, Percutaneous Approach

0RHA43Z Insertion of Infusion Device into Thoracolumbar Vertebral Joint, Percutaneous Endoscopic Approach

0RHA44Z Insertion of Internal Fixation Device into Thoracolumbar Vertebral Joint, Percutaneous Endoscopic Approach

0RHA48Z Insertion of Spacer into Thoracolumbar Vertebral Joint, Percutaneous Endoscopic Approach

0RHA4BZ Insertion of Interspinous Process Spinal Stabilization Device into Thoracolumbar Vertebral Joint, Percutaneous Endoscopic Approach

0RHA4CZ Insertion of Pedicle-Based Spinal Stabilization Device into Thoracolumbar Vertebral Joint, Percutaneous Endoscopic Approach

0RHA4DZ Insertion of Facet Replacement Spinal Stabilization Device into Thoracolumbar Vertebral Joint, Percutaneous Endoscopic Approach

0RHB03Z Insertion of Infusion Device into Thoracolumbar Vertebral Disc, Open Approach

0RHB33Z Insertion of Infusion Device into Thoracolumbar Vertebral Disc, Percutaneous Approach

0RHB43Z Insertion of Infusion Device into Thoracolumbar Vertebral Disc, Percutaneous Endoscopic Approach

0RHC03Z Insertion of Infusion Device into Right Temporomandibular Joint, Open Approach

0RHC04Z Insertion of Internal Fixation Device into Right Temporomandibular Joint, Open Approach

0RHC08Z Insertion of Spacer into Right Temporomandibular Joint, Open Approach

0RHC33Z Insertion of Infusion Device into Right Temporomandibular Joint, Percutaneous Approach

0RHC34Z Insertion of Internal Fixation Device into Right Temporomandibular Joint, Percutaneous Approach

0RHC38Z Insertion of Spacer into Right Temporomandibular Joint, Percutaneous Approach

0RHC43Z Insertion of Infusion Device into Right Temporomandibular Joint, Percutaneous Endoscopic Approach

0RHC44Z Insertion of Internal Fixation Device into Right Temporomandibular Joint, Percutaneous Endoscopic Approach

0RHC48Z Insertion of Spacer into Right Temporomandibular Joint, Percutaneous Endoscopic Approach

0RHD03Z Insertion of Infusion Device into Left Temporomandibular Joint, Open Approach

0RHD04Z Insertion of Internal Fixation Device into Left Temporomandibular Joint, Open Approach

0RHD08Z Insertion of Spacer into Left Temporomandibular Joint, Open Approach

0RHD33Z Insertion of Infusion Device into Left Temporomandibular Joint, Percutaneous Approach

0RHD34Z Insertion of Internal Fixation Device into Left Temporomandibular Joint, Percutaneous Approach

0RHD38Z Insertion of Spacer into Left Temporomandibular Joint, Percutaneous Approach

0RHD43Z Insertion of Infusion Device into Left Temporomandibular Joint, Percutaneous Endoscopic Approach

0RHD44Z Insertion of Internal Fixation Device into Left Temporomandibular Joint, Percutaneous Endoscopic Approach

0RHD48Z Insertion of Spacer into Left Temporomandibular Joint, Percutaneous Endoscopic Approach

0RHE03Z Insertion of Infusion Device into Right Sternoclavicular Joint, Open Approach

0RHE04Z Insertion of Internal Fixation Device into Right Sternoclavicular Joint, Open Approach

0RHE08Z Insertion of Spacer into Right Sternoclavicular Joint, Open Approach

0RHE33Z Insertion of Infusion Device into Right Sternoclavicular Joint, Percutaneous Approach

0RHE34Z Insertion of Internal Fixation Device into Right Sternoclavicular Joint, Percutaneous Approach

0RHE38Z Insertion of Spacer into Right Sternoclavicular Joint, Percutaneous Approach

0RHE43Z Insertion of Infusion Device into Right Sternoclavicular Joint, Percutaneous Endoscopic Approach

0RHE44Z Insertion of Internal Fixation Device into Right Sternoclavicular Joint, Percutaneous Endoscopic Approach

0RHE48Z Insertion of Spacer into Right Sternoclavicular Joint, Percutaneous Endoscopic Approach

0RHF03Z Insertion of Infusion Device into Left Sternoclavicular Joint, Open Approach

0RHF04Z Insertion of Internal Fixation Device into Left Sternoclavicular Joint, Open Approach

0RHF08Z Insertion of Spacer into Left Sternoclavicular Joint, Open Approach

0RHF33Z Insertion of Infusion Device into Left Sternoclavicular Joint, Percutaneous Approach

0RHF34Z Insertion of Internal Fixation Device into Left Sternoclavicular Joint, Percutaneous Approach

0RHF38Z Insertion of Spacer into Left Sternoclavicular Joint, Percutaneous Approach

0RHF43Z Insertion of Infusion Device into Left Sternoclavicular Joint, Percutaneous Endoscopic Approach

0RHF44Z Insertion of Internal Fixation Device into Left Sternoclavicular Joint, Percutaneous Endoscopic Approach

0RHF48Z Insertion of Spacer into Left Sternoclavicular Joint, Percutaneous Endoscopic Approach

0RHG03Z Insertion of Infusion Device into Right Acromioclavicular Joint, Open Approach

0RHG04Z Insertion of Internal Fixation Device into Right Acromioclavicular Joint, Open Approach

0RHG08Z Insertion of Spacer into Right Acromioclavicular Joint, Open Approach

0RHG33Z Insertion of Infusion Device into Right Acromioclavicular Joint, Percutaneous Approach

0RHG34Z Insertion of Internal Fixation Device into Right Acromioclavicular Joint, Percutaneous Approach

0RHG38Z Insertion of Spacer into Right Acromioclavicular Joint, Percutaneous Approach

0RHG43Z Insertion of Infusion Device into Right Acromioclavicular Joint, Percutaneous Endoscopic Approach

0RHG44Z Insertion of Internal Fixation Device into Right Acromioclavicular Joint, Percutaneous Endoscopic Approach

0RHG48Z Insertion of Spacer into Right Acromioclavicular Joint, Percutaneous Endoscopic Approach

0RHH03Z Insertion of Infusion Device into Left Acromioclavicular Joint, Open Approach

0RHH04Z Insertion of Internal Fixation Device into Left Acromioclavicular Joint, Open Approach

0RHH08Z Insertion of Spacer into Left Acromioclavicular Joint, Open Approach

0RHH33Z Insertion of Infusion Device into Left Acromioclavicular Joint, Percutaneous Approach

0RHH34Z Insertion of Internal Fixation Device into Left Acromioclavicular Joint, Percutaneous Approach

0RHH38Z Insertion of Spacer into Left Acromioclavicular Joint, Percutaneous Approach

0RHH43Z Insertion of Infusion Device into Left Acromioclavicular Joint, Percutaneous Endoscopic Approach

0RHH44Z Insertion of Internal Fixation Device into Left Acromioclavicular Joint, Percutaneous Endoscopic Approach

0RHH48Z Insertion of Spacer into Left Acromioclavicular Joint, Percutaneous Endoscopic Approach

0RHJ03Z Insertion of Infusion Device into Right Shoulder Joint, Open Approach

0RHJ04Z Insertion of Internal Fixation Device into Right Shoulder Joint, Open Approach

0RHJ08Z Insertion of Spacer into Right Shoulder Joint, Open Approach

0RHJ33Z Insertion of Infusion Device into Right Shoulder Joint, Percutaneous Approach

0RHJ34Z Insertion of Internal Fixation Device into Right Shoulder Joint, Percutaneous Approach
0RHJ38Z Insertion of Spacer into Right Shoulder Joint, Percutaneous Approach
0RHJ43Z Insertion of Infusion Device into Right Shoulder Joint, Percutaneous Endoscopic Approach
0RHJ44Z Insertion of Internal Fixation Device into Right Shoulder Joint, Percutaneous Endoscopic Approach
0RHJ48Z Insertion of Spacer into Right Shoulder Joint, Percutaneous Endoscopic Approach
0RHK03Z Insertion of Infusion Device into Left Shoulder Joint, Open Approach
0RHK04Z Insertion of Internal Fixation Device into Left Shoulder Joint, Open Approach
0RHK08Z Insertion of Spacer into Left Shoulder Joint, Open Approach
0RHK33Z Insertion of Infusion Device into Left Shoulder Joint, Percutaneous Approach
0RHK34Z Insertion of Internal Fixation Device into Left Shoulder Joint, Percutaneous Approach
0RHK38Z Insertion of Spacer into Left Shoulder Joint, Percutaneous Approach
0RHK43Z Insertion of Infusion Device into Left Shoulder Joint, Percutaneous Endoscopic Approach
0RHK44Z Insertion of Internal Fixation Device into Left Shoulder Joint, Percutaneous Endoscopic Approach
0RHK48Z Insertion of Spacer into Left Shoulder Joint, Percutaneous Endoscopic Approach
0RHL03Z Insertion of Infusion Device into Right Elbow Joint, Open Approach
0RHL04Z Insertion of Internal Fixation Device into Right Elbow Joint, Open Approach
0RHL05Z Insertion of External Fixation Device into Right Elbow Joint, Open Approach
0RHL08Z Insertion of Spacer into Right Elbow Joint, Open Approach
0RHL33Z Insertion of Infusion Device into Right Elbow Joint, Percutaneous Approach
0RHL34Z Insertion of Internal Fixation Device into Right Elbow Joint, Percutaneous Approach
0RHL35Z Insertion of External Fixation Device into Right Elbow Joint, Percutaneous Approach
0RHL38Z Insertion of Spacer into Right Elbow Joint, Percutaneous Approach
0RHL43Z Insertion of Infusion Device into Right Elbow Joint, Percutaneous Endoscopic Approach
0RHL44Z Insertion of Internal Fixation Device into Right Elbow Joint, Percutaneous Endoscopic Approach
0RHL45Z Insertion of External Fixation Device into Right Elbow Joint, Percutaneous Endoscopic Approach
0RHL48Z Insertion of Spacer into Right Elbow Joint, Percutaneous Endoscopic Approach
0RHM03Z Insertion of Infusion Device into Left Elbow Joint, Open Approach
0RHM04Z Insertion of Internal Fixation Device into Left Elbow Joint, Open Approach
0RHM05Z Insertion of External Fixation Device into Left Elbow Joint, Open Approach
0RHM08Z Insertion of Spacer into Left Elbow Joint, Open Approach
0RHM33Z Insertion of Infusion Device into Left Elbow Joint, Percutaneous Approach
0RHM34Z Insertion of Internal Fixation Device into Left Elbow Joint, Percutaneous Approach
0RHM35Z Insertion of External Fixation Device into Left Elbow Joint, Percutaneous Approach
0RHM38Z Insertion of Spacer into Left Elbow Joint, Percutaneous Approach
0RHM43Z Insertion of Infusion Device into Left Elbow Joint, Percutaneous Endoscopic Approach
0RHM44Z Insertion of Internal Fixation Device into Left Elbow Joint, Percutaneous Endoscopic Approach
0RHM45Z Insertion of External Fixation Device into Left Elbow Joint, Percutaneous Endoscopic Approach
0RHM48Z Insertion of Spacer into Left Elbow Joint, Percutaneous Endoscopic Approach
0RHN03Z Insertion of Infusion Device into Right Wrist Joint, Open Approach
0RHN04Z Insertion of Internal Fixation Device into Right Wrist Joint, Open Approach
0RHN05Z Insertion of External Fixation Device into Right Wrist Joint, Open Approach
0RHN08Z Insertion of Spacer into Right Wrist Joint, Open Approach
0RHN33Z Insertion of Infusion Device into Right Wrist Joint, Percutaneous Approach
0RHN34Z Insertion of Internal Fixation Device into Right Wrist Joint, Percutaneous Approach
0RHN35Z Insertion of External Fixation Device into Right Wrist Joint, Percutaneous Approach
0RHN38Z Insertion of Spacer into Right Wrist Joint, Percutaneous Approach
0RHN43Z Insertion of Infusion Device into Right Wrist Joint, Percutaneous Endoscopic Approach
0RHN44Z Insertion of Internal Fixation Device into Right Wrist Joint, Percutaneous Endoscopic Approach
0RHN45Z Insertion of External Fixation Device into Right Wrist Joint, Percutaneous Endoscopic Approach
0RHN48Z Insertion of Spacer into Right Wrist Joint, Percutaneous Endoscopic Approach
0RHP03Z Insertion of Infusion Device into Left Wrist Joint, Open Approach
0RHP04Z Insertion of Internal Fixation Device into Left Wrist Joint, Open Approach
0RHP05Z Insertion of External Fixation Device into Left Wrist Joint, Open Approach
0RHP08Z Insertion of Spacer into Left Wrist Joint, Open Approach
0RHP33Z Insertion of Infusion Device into Left Wrist Joint, Percutaneous Approach
0RHP34Z Insertion of Internal Fixation Device into Left Wrist Joint, Percutaneous Approach
0RHP35Z Insertion of External Fixation Device into Left Wrist Joint, Percutaneous Approach
0RHP38Z Insertion of Spacer into Left Wrist Joint, Percutaneous Approach
0RHP43Z Insertion of Infusion Device into Left Wrist Joint, Percutaneous Endoscopic Approach
0RHP44Z Insertion of Internal Fixation Device into Left Wrist Joint, Percutaneous Endoscopic Approach
0RHP45Z Insertion of External Fixation Device into Left Wrist Joint, Percutaneous Endoscopic Approach
0RHP48Z Insertion of Spacer into Left Wrist Joint, Percutaneous Endoscopic Approach
0RHQ03Z Insertion of Infusion Device into Right Carpal Joint, Open Approach
0RHQ04Z Insertion of Internal Fixation Device into Right Carpal Joint, Open Approach
0RHQ05Z Insertion of External Fixation Device into Right Carpal Joint, Open Approach
0RHQ08Z Insertion of Spacer into Right Carpal Joint, Open Approach
0RHQ33Z Insertion of Infusion Device into Right Carpal Joint, Percutaneous Approach
0RHQ34Z Insertion of Internal Fixation Device into Right Carpal Joint, Percutaneous Approach
0RHQ35Z Insertion of External Fixation Device into Right Carpal Joint, Percutaneous Approach
0RHQ38Z Insertion of Spacer into Right Carpal Joint, Percutaneous Approach
0RHQ43Z Insertion of Infusion Device into Right Carpal Joint, Percutaneous Endoscopic Approach
0RHQ44Z Insertion of Internal Fixation Device into Right Carpal Joint, Percutaneous Endoscopic Approach
0RHQ45Z Insertion of External Fixation Device into Right Carpal Joint, Percutaneous Endoscopic Approach
0RHQ48Z Insertion of Spacer into Right Carpal Joint, Percutaneous Endoscopic Approach
0RHR03Z Insertion of Infusion Device into Left Carpal Joint, Open Approach
0RHR04Z Insertion of Internal Fixation Device into Left Carpal Joint, Open Approach
0RHR05Z Insertion of External Fixation Device into Left Carpal Joint, Open Approach
0RHR08Z Insertion of Spacer into Left Carpal Joint, Open Approach
0RHR33Z Insertion of Infusion Device into Left Carpal Joint, Percutaneous Approach
0RHR34Z Insertion of Internal Fixation Device into Left Carpal Joint, Percutaneous Approach
0RHR35Z Insertion of External Fixation Device into Left Carpal Joint, Percutaneous Approach
0RHR38Z Insertion of Spacer into Left Carpal Joint, Percutaneous Approach
0RHR43Z Insertion of Infusion Device into Left Carpal Joint, Percutaneous Endoscopic Approach
0RHR44Z Insertion of Internal Fixation Device into Left Carpal Joint, Percutaneous Endoscopic Approach
0RHR45Z Insertion of External Fixation Device into Left Carpal Joint, Percutaneous Endoscopic Approach
0RHR48Z Insertion of Spacer into Left Carpal Joint, Percutaneous Endoscopic Approach
0RHS03Z Insertion of Infusion Device into Right Metacarpocarpal Joint, Open Approach
0RHS04Z Insertion of Internal Fixation Device into Right Metacarpocarpal Joint, Open Approach
0RHS05Z Insertion of External Fixation Device into Right Metacarpocarpal Joint, Open Approach
0RHS08Z Insertion of Spacer into Right Metacarpocarpal Joint, Open Approach
0RHS33Z Insertion of Infusion Device into Right Metacarpocarpal Joint, Percutaneous Approach
0RHS34Z Insertion of Internal Fixation Device into Right Metacarpocarpal Joint, Percutaneous Approach
0RHS35Z Insertion of External Fixation Device into Right Metacarpocarpal Joint, Percutaneous Approach
0RHS38Z Insertion of Spacer into Right Metacarpocarpal Joint, Percutaneous Approach
0RHS43Z Insertion of Infusion Device into Right Metacarpocarpal Joint, Percutaneous Endoscopic Approach
0RHS44Z Insertion of Internal Fixation Device into Right Metacarpocarpal Joint, Percutaneous Endoscopic Approach
0RHS45Z Insertion of External Fixation Device into Right Metacarpocarpal Joint, Percutaneous Endoscopic Approach

RHS48Z Insertion of Spacer into Right Metacarpocarpal Joint, Percutaneous Endoscopic Approach

RHT03Z Insertion of Infusion Device into Left Metacarpocarpal Joint, Open Approach

RHT04Z Insertion of Internal Fixation Device into Left Metacarpocarpal Joint, Open Approach

RHT05Z Insertion of External Fixation Device into Left Metacarpocarpal Joint, Open Approach

RHT08Z Insertion of Spacer into Left Metacarpocarpal Joint, Open Approach

RHT33Z Insertion of Infusion Device into Left Metacarpocarpal Joint, Percutaneous Approach

RHT34Z Insertion of Internal Fixation Device into Left Metacarpocarpal Joint, Percutaneous Approach

RHT35Z Insertion of External Fixation Device into Left Metacarpocarpal Joint, Percutaneous Approach

RHT38Z Insertion of Spacer into Left Metacarpocarpal Joint, Percutaneous Approach

RHT43Z Insertion of Infusion Device into Left Metacarpocarpal Joint, Percutaneous Endoscopic Approach

RHT44Z Insertion of Internal Fixation Device into Left Metacarpocarpal Joint, Percutaneous Endoscopic Approach

RHT45Z Insertion of External Fixation Device into Left Metacarpocarpal Joint, Percutaneous Endoscopic Approach

RHT48Z Insertion of Spacer into Left Metacarpocarpal Joint, Percutaneous Endoscopic Approach

RHU03Z Insertion of Infusion Device into Right Metacarpophalangeal Joint, Open Approach

RHU04Z Insertion of Internal Fixation Device into Right Metacarpophalangeal Joint, Open Approach

RHU05Z Insertion of External Fixation Device into Right Metacarpophalangeal Joint, Open Approach

RHU08Z Insertion of Spacer into Right Metacarpophalangeal Joint, Open Approach

RHU33Z Insertion of Infusion Device into Right Metacarpophalangeal Joint, Percutaneous Approach

RHU34Z Insertion of Internal Fixation Device into Right Metacarpophalangeal Joint, Percutaneous Approach

RHU35Z Insertion of External Fixation Device into Right Metacarpophalangeal Joint, Percutaneous Approach

0RHU38Z Insertion of Spacer into Right Metacarpophalangeal Joint, Percutaneous Approach

0RHU43Z Insertion of Infusion Device into Right Metacarpophalangeal Joint, Percutaneous Endoscopic Approach

0RHU44Z Insertion of Internal Fixation Device into Right Metacarpophalangeal Joint, Percutaneous Endoscopic Approach

0RHU45Z Insertion of External Fixation Device into Right Metacarpophalangeal Joint, Percutaneous Endoscopic Approach

0RHU48Z Insertion of Spacer into Right Metacarpophalangeal Joint, Percutaneous Endoscopic Approach

0RHV03Z Insertion of Infusion Device into Left Metacarpophalangeal Joint, Open Approach

0RHV04Z Insertion of Internal Fixation Device into Left Metacarpophalangeal Joint, Open Approach

0RHV05Z Insertion of External Fixation Device into Left Metacarpophalangeal Joint, Open Approach

0RHV08Z Insertion of Spacer into Left Metacarpophalangeal Joint, Open Approach

0RHV33Z Insertion of Infusion Device into Left Metacarpophalangeal Joint, Percutaneous Approach

0RHV34Z Insertion of Internal Fixation Device into Left Metacarpophalangeal Joint, Percutaneous Approach

0RHV35Z Insertion of External Fixation Device into Left Metacarpophalangeal Joint, Percutaneous Approach

0RHV38Z Insertion of Spacer into Left Metacarpophalangeal Joint, Percutaneous Approach

0RHV43Z Insertion of Infusion Device into Left Metacarpophalangeal Joint, Percutaneous Endoscopic Approach

0RHV44Z Insertion of Internal Fixation Device into Left Metacarpophalangeal Joint, Percutaneous Endoscopic Approach

0RHV45Z Insertion of External Fixation Device into Left Metacarpophalangeal Joint, Percutaneous Endoscopic Approach

0RHV48Z Insertion of Spacer into Left Metacarpophalangeal Joint, Percutaneous Endoscopic Approach

0RHW03Z Insertion of Infusion Device into Right Finger Phalangeal Joint, Open Approach

0RHW04Z Insertion of Internal Fixation Device into Right Finger Phalangeal Joint, Open Approach

0RHW05Z Insertion of External Fixation Device into Right Finger Phalangeal Joint, Open Approach

0RHW08Z Insertion of Spacer into Right Finger Phalangeal Joint, Open Approach

0RHW33Z Insertion of Infusion Device into Right Finger Phalangeal Joint, Percutaneous Approach

0RHW34Z Insertion of Internal Fixation Device into Right Finger Phalangeal Joint, Percutaneous Approach

0RHW35Z Insertion of External Fixation Device into Right Finger Phalangeal Joint, Percutaneous Approach

0RHW38Z Insertion of Spacer into Right Finger Phalangeal Joint, Percutaneous Approach

0RHW43Z Insertion of Infusion Device into Right Finger Phalangeal Joint, Percutaneous Endoscopic Approach

0RHW44Z Insertion of Internal Fixation Device into Right Finger Phalangeal Joint, Percutaneous Endoscopic Approach

0RHW45Z Insertion of External Fixation Device into Right Finger Phalangeal Joint, Percutaneous Endoscopic Approach

0RHW48Z Insertion of Spacer into Right Finger Phalangeal Joint, Percutaneous Endoscopic Approach

0RHX03Z Insertion of Infusion Device into Left Finger Phalangeal Joint, Open Approach

0RHX04Z Insertion of Internal Fixation Device into Left Finger Phalangeal Joint, Open Approach

0RHX05Z Insertion of External Fixation Device into Left Finger Phalangeal Joint, Open Approach

0RHX08Z Insertion of Spacer into Left Finger Phalangeal Joint, Open Approach

0RHX33Z Insertion of Infusion Device into Left Finger Phalangeal Joint, Percutaneous Approach

0RHX34Z Insertion of Internal Fixation Device into Left Finger Phalangeal Joint, Percutaneous Approach

0RHX35Z Insertion of External Fixation Device into Left Finger Phalangeal Joint, Percutaneous Approach

0RHX38Z Insertion of Spacer into Left Finger Phalangeal Joint, Percutaneous Approach

0RHX43Z Insertion of Infusion Device into Left Finger Phalangeal Joint, Percutaneous Endoscopic Approach

0RHX44Z Insertion of Internal Fixation Device into Left Finger Phalangeal Joint, Percutaneous Endoscopic Approach

0RHX45Z Insertion of External Fixation Device into Left Finger Phalangeal Joint, Percutaneous Endoscopic Approach

0RHX48Z Insertion of Spacer into Left Finger Phalangeal Joint, Percutaneous Endoscopic Approach

RJ – Upper Joints, Inspection

Review Coding Guideline B3.5

Review Coding Guidelines B3.11a, B3.11b and B3.11c

0RJ00ZZ Inspection of Occipital-cervical Joint, Open Approach

0RJ03ZZ Inspection of Occipital-cervical Joint, Percutaneous Approach

0RJ04ZZ Inspection of Occipital-cervical Joint, Percutaneous Endoscopic Approach

0RJ0XZZ Inspection of Occipital-cervical Joint, External Approach

0RJ10ZZ Inspection of Cervical Vertebral Joint, Open Approach

0RJ13ZZ Inspection of Cervical Vertebral Joint, Percutaneous Approach

0RJ14ZZ Inspection of Cervical Vertebral Joint, Percutaneous Endoscopic Approach

0RJ1XZZ Inspection of Cervical Vertebral Joint, External Approach

0RJ30ZZ Inspection of Cervical Vertebral Disc, Open Approach

0RJ33ZZ Inspection of Cervical Vertebral Disc, Percutaneous Approach

0RJ34ZZ Inspection of Cervical Vertebral Disc, Percutaneous Endoscopic Approach

0RJ3XZZ Inspection of Cervical Vertebral Disc, External Approach

0RJ40ZZ Inspection of Cervicothoracic Vertebral Joint, Open Approach

0RJ43ZZ Inspection of Cervicothoracic Vertebral Joint, Percutaneous Approach

0RJ44ZZ Inspection of Cervicothoracic Vertebral Joint, Percutaneous Endoscopic Approach

0RJ4XZZ Inspection of Cervicothoracic Vertebral Joint, External Approach

0RJ50ZZ Inspection of Cervicothoracic Vertebral Disc, Open Approach

0RJ53ZZ Inspection of Cervicothoracic Vertebral Disc, Percutaneous Approach

0RJ54ZZ Inspection of Cervicothoracic Vertebral Disc, Percutaneous Endoscopic Approach

0RJ5XZZ Inspection of Cervicothoracic Vertebral Disc, External Approach

0RJ60ZZ Inspection of Thoracic Vertebral Joint, Open Approach

0RJ63ZZ Inspection of Thoracic Vertebral Joint, Percutaneous Approach

0RJ64ZZ Inspection of Thoracic Vertebral Joint, Percutaneous Endoscopic Approach

0RJ6XZZ Inspection of Thoracic Vertebral Joint, External Approach

0RJ90ZZ Inspection of Thoracic Vertebral Disc, Open Approach

0RJ93ZZ Inspection of Thoracic Vertebral Disc, Percutaneous Approach

0RJ94ZZ Inspection of Thoracic Vertebral Disc, Percutaneous Endoscopic Approach

0RJ9XZZ Inspection of Thoracic Vertebral Disc, External Approach

0RJA0ZZ Inspection of Thoracolumbar Vertebral Joint, Open Approach

0RJA3ZZ Inspection of Thoracolumbar Vertebral Joint, Percutaneous Approach

0RJA4ZZ Inspection of Thoracolumbar Vertebral Joint, Percutaneous Endoscopic Approach

0RJAXZZ Inspection of Thoracolumbar Vertebral Joint, External Approach

0RJB0ZZ Inspection of Thoracolumbar Vertebral Disc, Open Approach

0RJB3ZZ Inspection of Thoracolumbar Vertebral Disc, Percutaneous Approach

0RJB4ZZ Inspection of Thoracolumbar Vertebral Disc, Percutaneous Endoscopic Approach

0RJBXZZ Inspection of Thoracolumbar Vertebral Disc, External Approach

0RJC0ZZ Inspection of Right Temporomandibular Joint, Open Approach

0RJC3ZZ Inspection of Right Temporomandibular Joint, Percutaneous Approach

0RJC4ZZ Inspection of Right Temporomandibular Joint, Percutaneous Endoscopic Approach

0RJCXZZ Inspection of Right Temporomandibular Joint, External Approach

0RJD0ZZ Inspection of Left Temporomandibular Joint, Open Approach

0RJD3ZZ Inspection of Left Temporomandibular Joint, Percutaneous Approach

0RJD4ZZ Inspection of Left Temporomandibular Joint, Percutaneous Endoscopic Approach

0RJDXZZ Inspection of Left Temporomandibular Joint, External Approach

0RJE0ZZ Inspection of Right Sternoclavicular Joint, Open Approach

0RJE3ZZ Inspection of Right Sternoclavicular Joint, Percutaneous Approach

0RJE4ZZ Inspection of Right Sternoclavicular Joint, Percutaneous Endoscopic Approach

0RJEXZZ Inspection of Right Sternoclavicular Joint, External Approach

0RJF0ZZ Inspection of Left Sternoclavicular Joint, Open Approach

0RJF3ZZ Inspection of Left Sternoclavicular Joint, Percutaneous Approach

0RJF4ZZ Inspection of Left Sternoclavicular Joint, Percutaneous Endoscopic Approach

0RJFXZZ Inspection of Left Sternoclavicular Joint, External Approach

0RJG0ZZ Inspection of Right Acromioclavicular Joint, Open Approach

0RJG3ZZ Inspection of Right Acromioclavicular Joint, Percutaneous Approach

0RJG4ZZ Inspection of Right Acromioclavicular Joint, Percutaneous Endoscopic Approach

0RJGXZZ Inspection of Right Acromioclavicular Joint, External Approach

0RJH0ZZ Inspection of Left Acromioclavicular Joint, Open Approach

0RJH3ZZ Inspection of Left Acromioclavicular Joint, Percutaneous Approach

0RJH4ZZ Inspection of Left Acromioclavicular Joint, Percutaneous Endoscopic Approach

0RJHXZZ Inspection of Left Acromioclavicular Joint, External Approach

0RJJ0ZZ Inspection of Right Shoulder Joint, Open Approach

0RJJ3ZZ Inspection of Right Shoulder Joint, Percutaneous Approach

0RJJ4ZZ Inspection of Right Shoulder Joint, Percutaneous Endoscopic Approach

0RJJXZZ Inspection of Right Shoulder Joint, External Approach

0RJK0ZZ Inspection of Left Shoulder Joint, Open Approach

0RJK3ZZ Inspection of Left Shoulder Joint, Percutaneous Approach

0RJK4ZZ Inspection of Left Shoulder Joint, Percutaneous Endoscopic Approach

0RJKXZZ Inspection of Left Shoulder Joint, External Approach

0RJL0ZZ Inspection of Right Elbow Joint, Open Approach

0RJL3ZZ Inspection of Right Elbow Joint, Percutaneous Approach

0RJL4ZZ Inspection of Right Elbow Joint, Percutaneous Endoscopic Approach

0RJLXZZ Inspection of Right Elbow Joint, External Approach

0RJM0ZZ Inspection of Left Elbow Joint, Open Approach

0RJM3ZZ Inspection of Left Elbow Joint, Percutaneous Approach

0RJM4ZZ Inspection of Left Elbow Joint, Percutaneous Endoscopic Approach

0RJMXZZ Inspection of Left Elbow Joint, External Approach

0RJN0ZZ Inspection of Right Wrist Joint, Open Approach

0RJN3ZZ Inspection of Right Wrist Joint, Percutaneous Approach

0RJN4ZZ Inspection of Right Wrist Joint, Percutaneous Endoscopic Approach

0RJNXZZ Inspection of Right Wrist Joint, External Approach

0RJP0ZZ Inspection of Left Wrist Joint, Open Approach

0RJP3ZZ Inspection of Left Wrist Joint, Percutaneous Approach

0RJP4ZZ Inspection of Left Wrist Joint, Percutaneous Endoscopic Approach

0RJPXZZ Inspection of Left Wrist Joint, External Approach

0RJQ0ZZ Inspection of Right Carpal Joint, Open Approach

0RJQ3ZZ Inspection of Right Carpal Joint, Percutaneous Approach

0RJQ4ZZ Inspection of Right Carpal Joint, Percutaneous Endoscopic Approach

0RJQXZZ Inspection of Right Carpal Joint, Extern Approach

0RJR0ZZ Inspection of Left Carpal Joint, Open Approach

0RJR3ZZ Inspection of Left Carpal Joint, Percutaneous Approach

0RJR4ZZ Inspection of Left Carpal Joint, Percutaneous Endoscopic Approach

0RJRXZZ Inspection of Left Carpal Joint, External Approach

0RJS0ZZ Inspection of Right Metacarpocarpal Joint, Open Approach

0RJS3ZZ Inspection of Right Metacarpocarpal Joint, Percutaneous Approach

0RJS4ZZ Inspection of Right Metacarpocarpal Joint, Percutaneous Endoscopic Approac

0RJSXZZ Inspection of Right Metacarpocarpal Joint, External Approach

0RJT0ZZ Inspection of Left Metacarpocarpal Joint Open Approach

0RJT3ZZ Inspection of Left Metacarpocarpal Joint Percutaneous Approach

0RJT4ZZ Inspection of Left Metacarpocarpal Joint Percutaneous Endoscopic Approach

0RJTXZZ Inspection of Left Metacarpocarpal Joint External Approach

0RJU0ZZ Inspection of Right Metacarpophalangeal Joint, Open Approach

0RJU3ZZ Inspection of Right Metacarpophalangeal Joint, Percutaneous Approach

0RJU4ZZ Inspection of Right Metacarpophalangeal Joint, Percutaneous Endoscopic Approach

0RJUXZZ Inspection of Right Metacarpophalangeal Joint, External Approach

0RJV0ZZ Inspection of Left Metacarpophalangeal Joint, Open Approach

0RJV3ZZ Inspection of Left Metacarpophalangeal Joint, Percutaneous Approach

0RJV4ZZ Inspection of Left Metacarpophalangeal Joint, Percutaneous Endoscopic Approach

0RJVXZZ Inspection of Left Metacarpophalangeal Joint, External Approach

0RJW0ZZ Inspection of Right Finger Phalangeal Joint, Open Approach

0RJW3ZZ Inspection of Right Finger Phalangeal Joint, Percutaneous Approach

0RJW4ZZ Inspection of Right Finger Phalangeal Joint, Percutaneous Endoscopic Approach

0RJWXZZ Inspection of Right Finger Phalangeal Joint, External Approach

0RJX0ZZ Inspection of Left Finger Phalangeal Joint, Open Approach

0RJX3ZZ Inspection of Left Finger Phalangeal Joint, Percutaneous Approach

0RJX4ZZ Inspection of Left Finger Phalangeal Joint, Percutaneous Endoscopic Approach

0RJXXZZ Inspection of Left Finger Phalangeal Joint, External Approach

0RN – Upper Joints, Release

Review Coding Guideline B3.13

0RN00ZZ Release Occipital-cervical Joint, Open Approach

0RN03ZZ Release Occipital-cervical Joint, Percutaneous Approach

0RN04ZZ Release Occipital-cervical Joint, Percutaneous Endoscopic Approach

0RN0XZZ Release Occipital-cervical Joint, External Approach

0RN10ZZ Release Cervical Vertebral Joint, Open Approach

0RN13ZZ Release Cervical Vertebral Joint, Percutaneous Approach

0RN14ZZ Release Cervical Vertebral Joint, Percutaneous Endoscopic Approach

0RN1XZZ Release Cervical Vertebral Joint, External Approach

0RN30ZZ Release Cervical Vertebral Disc, Open Approach

RN33ZZ Release Cervical Vertebral Disc, Percutaneous Approach
RN34ZZ Release Cervical Vertebral Disc, Percutaneous Endoscopic Approach
RN3XZZ Release Cervical Vertebral Disc, External Approach
RN40ZZ Release Cervicothoracic Vertebral Joint, Open Approach
RN43ZZ Release Cervicothoracic Vertebral Joint, Percutaneous Approach
RN44ZZ Release Cervicothoracic Vertebral Joint, Percutaneous Endoscopic Approach
RN4XZZ Release Cervicothoracic Vertebral Joint, External Approach
RN50ZZ Release Cervicothoracic Vertebral Disc, Open Approach
RN53ZZ Release Cervicothoracic Vertebral Disc, Percutaneous Approach
RN54ZZ Release Cervicothoracic Vertebral Disc, Percutaneous Endoscopic Approach
RN5XZZ Release Cervicothoracic Vertebral Disc, External Approach
RN60ZZ Release Thoracic Vertebral Joint, Open Approach
RN63ZZ Release Thoracic Vertebral Joint, Percutaneous Approach
RN64ZZ Release Thoracic Vertebral Joint, Percutaneous Endoscopic Approach
RN6XZZ Release Thoracic Vertebral Joint, External Approach
RN90ZZ Release Thoracic Vertebral Disc, Open Approach
RN93ZZ Release Thoracic Vertebral Disc, Percutaneous Approach
RN94ZZ Release Thoracic Vertebral Disc, Percutaneous Endoscopic Approach
RN9XZZ Release Thoracic Vertebral Disc, External Approach
RNA0ZZ Release Thoracolumbar Vertebral Joint, Open Approach
RNA3ZZ Release Thoracolumbar Vertebral Joint, Percutaneous Approach
RNA4ZZ Release Thoracolumbar Vertebral Joint, Percutaneous Endoscopic Approach
RNAXZZ Release Thoracolumbar Vertebral Joint, External Approach
RNB0ZZ Release Thoracolumbar Vertebral Disc, Open Approach
RNB3ZZ Release Thoracolumbar Vertebral Disc, Percutaneous Approach
RNB4ZZ Release Thoracolumbar Vertebral Disc, Percutaneous Endoscopic Approach
RNBXZZ Release Thoracolumbar Vertebral Disc, External Approach
0RNC0ZZ Release Right Temporomandibular Joint, Open Approach
0RNC3ZZ Release Right Temporomandibular Joint, Percutaneous Approach
0RNC4ZZ Release Right Temporomandibular Joint, Percutaneous Endoscopic Approach
0RNCXZZ Release Right Temporomandibular Joint, External Approach
0RND0ZZ Release Left Temporomandibular Joint, Open Approach
0RND3ZZ Release Left Temporomandibular Joint, Percutaneous Approach
0RND4ZZ Release Left Temporomandibular Joint, Percutaneous Endoscopic Approach
0RNDXZZ Release Left Temporomandibular Joint, External Approach
0RNE0ZZ Release Right Sternoclavicular Joint, Open Approach
0RNE3ZZ Release Right Sternoclavicular Joint, Percutaneous Approach
0RNE4ZZ Release Right Sternoclavicular Joint, Percutaneous Endoscopic Approach
0RNEXZZ Release Right Sternoclavicular Joint, External Approach
0RNF0ZZ Release Left Sternoclavicular Joint, Open Approach
0RNF3ZZ Release Left Sternoclavicular Joint, Percutaneous Approach
0RNF4ZZ Release Left Sternoclavicular Joint, Percutaneous Endoscopic Approach
0RNFXZZ Release Left Sternoclavicular Joint, External Approach
0RNG0ZZ Release Right Acromioclavicular Joint, Open Approach
0RNG3ZZ Release Right Acromioclavicular Joint, Percutaneous Approach
0RNG4ZZ Release Right Acromioclavicular Joint, Percutaneous Endoscopic Approach
0RNGXZZ Release Right Acromioclavicular Joint, External Approach
0RNH0ZZ Release Left Acromioclavicular Joint, Open Approach
0RNH3ZZ Release Left Acromioclavicular Joint, Percutaneous Approach
0RNH4ZZ Release Left Acromioclavicular Joint, Percutaneous Endoscopic Approach
0RNHXZZ Release Left Acromioclavicular Joint, External Approach
0RNJ0ZZ Release Right Shoulder Joint, Open Approach
0RNJ3ZZ Release Right Shoulder Joint, Percutaneous Approach
0RNJ4ZZ Release Right Shoulder Joint, Percutaneous Endoscopic Approach
0RNJXZZ Release Right Shoulder Joint, External Approach
0RNK0ZZ Release Left Shoulder Joint, Open Approach
0RNK3ZZ Release Left Shoulder Joint, Percutaneous Approach
0RNK4ZZ Release Left Shoulder Joint, Percutaneous Endoscopic Approach
0RNKXZZ Release Left Shoulder Joint, External Approach
0RNL0ZZ Release Right Elbow Joint, Open Approach
0RNL3ZZ Release Right Elbow Joint, Percutaneous Approach
0RNL4ZZ Release Right Elbow Joint, Percutaneous Endoscopic Approach
0RNLXZZ Release Right Elbow Joint, External Approach
0RNM0ZZ Release Left Elbow Joint, Open Approach
0RNM3ZZ Release Left Elbow Joint, Percutaneous Approach
0RNM4ZZ Release Left Elbow Joint, Percutaneous Endoscopic Approach
0RNMXZZ Release Left Elbow Joint, External Approach
0RNN0ZZ Release Right Wrist Joint, Open Approach
0RNN3ZZ Release Right Wrist Joint, Percutaneous Approach
0RNN4ZZ Release Right Wrist Joint, Percutaneous Endoscopic Approach
0RNNXZZ Release Right Wrist Joint, External Approach
0RNP0ZZ Release Left Wrist Joint, Open Approach
0RNP3ZZ Release Left Wrist Joint, Percutaneous Approach
0RNP4ZZ Release Left Wrist Joint, Percutaneous Endoscopic Approach
0RNPXZZ Release Left Wrist Joint, External Approach
0RNQ0ZZ Release Right Carpal Joint, Open Approach
0RNQ3ZZ Release Right Carpal Joint, Percutaneous Approach
0RNQ4ZZ Release Right Carpal Joint, Percutaneous Endoscopic Approach
0RNQXZZ Release Right Carpal Joint, External Approach
0RNR0ZZ Release Left Carpal Joint, Open Approach
0RNR3ZZ Release Left Carpal Joint, Percutaneous Approach
0RNR4ZZ Release Left Carpal Joint, Percutaneous Endoscopic Approach
0RNRXZZ Release Left Carpal Joint, External Approach
0RNS0ZZ Release Right Metacarpocarpal Joint, Open Approach
0RNS3ZZ Release Right Metacarpocarpal Joint, Percutaneous Approach
0RNS4ZZ Release Right Metacarpocarpal Joint, Percutaneous Endoscopic Approach
0RNSXZZ Release Right Metacarpocarpal Joint, External Approach
0RNT0ZZ Release Left Metacarpocarpal Joint, Open Approach
0RNT3ZZ Release Left Metacarpocarpal Joint, Percutaneous Approach
0RNT4ZZ Release Left Metacarpocarpal Joint, Percutaneous Endoscopic Approach
0RNTXZZ Release Left Metacarpocarpal Joint, External Approach
0RNU0ZZ Release Right Metacarpophalangeal Joint, Open Approach
0RNU3ZZ Release Right Metacarpophalangeal Joint, Percutaneous Approach
0RNU4ZZ Release Right Metacarpophalangeal Joint, Percutaneous Endoscopic Approach
0RNUXZZ Release Right Metacarpophalangeal Joint, External Approach
0RNV0ZZ Release Left Metacarpophalangeal Joint, Open Approach
0RNV3ZZ Release Left Metacarpophalangeal Joint, Percutaneous Approach
0RNV4ZZ Release Left Metacarpophalangeal Joint, Percutaneous Endoscopic Approach
0RNVXZZ Release Left Metacarpophalangeal Joint, External Approach
0RNW0ZZ Release Right Finger Phalangeal Joint, Open Approach
0RNW3ZZ Release Right Finger Phalangeal Joint, Percutaneous Approach
0RNW4ZZ Release Right Finger Phalangeal Joint, Percutaneous Endoscopic Approach
0RNWXZZ Release Right Finger Phalangeal Joint, External Approach
0RNX0ZZ Release Left Finger Phalangeal Joint, Open Approach
0RNX3ZZ Release Left Finger Phalangeal Joint, Percutaneous Approach
0RNX4ZZ Release Left Finger Phalangeal Joint, Percutaneous Endoscopic Approach
0RNXXZZ Release Left Finger Phalangeal Joint, External Approach

0RP – Upper Joints, Removal

Review Coding Guideline B6.1c

0RP000Z Removal of Drainage Device from Occipital-cervical Joint, Open Approach
0RP003Z Removal of Infusion Device from Occipital-cervical Joint, Open Approach
0RP004Z Removal of Internal Fixation Device from Occipital-cervical Joint, Open Approach

0RP007Z Removal of Autologous Tissue Substitute from Occipital-cervical Joint, Open Approach
0RP008Z Removal of Spacer from Occipital-cervical Joint, Open Approach
0RP00AZ Removal of Interbody Fusion Device from Occipital-cervical Joint, Open Approach
0RP00JZ Removal of Synthetic Substitute from Occipital-cervical Joint, Open Approach
0RP00KZ Removal of Nonautologous Tissue Substitute from Occipital-cervical Joint, Open Approach
0RP030Z Removal of Drainage Device from Occipital-cervical Joint, Percutaneous Approach
0RP033Z Removal of Infusion Device from Occipital-cervical Joint, Percutaneous Approach
0RP034Z Removal of Internal Fixation Device from Occipital-cervical Joint, Percutaneous Approach
0RP037Z Removal of Autologous Tissue Substitute from Occipital-cervical Joint, Percutaneous Approach
0RP038Z Removal of Spacer from Occipital-cervical Joint, Percutaneous Approach
0RP03AZ Removal of Interbody Fusion Device from Occipital-cervical Joint, Percutaneous Approach
0RP03JZ Removal of Synthetic Substitute from Occipital-cervical Joint, Percutaneous Approach
0RP03KZ Removal of Nonautologous Tissue Substitute from Occipital-cervical Joint, Percutaneous Approach
0RP040Z Removal of Drainage Device from Occipital-cervical Joint, Percutaneous Endoscopic Approach
0RP043Z Removal of Infusion Device from Occipital-cervical Joint, Percutaneous Endoscopic Approach
0RP044Z Removal of Internal Fixation Device from Occipital-cervical Joint, Percutaneous Endoscopic Approach
0RP047Z Removal of Autologous Tissue Substitute from Occipital-cervical Joint, Percutaneous Endoscopic Approach
0RP048Z Removal of Spacer from Occipital-cervical Joint, Percutaneous Endoscopic Approach
0RP04AZ Removal of Interbody Fusion Device from Occipital-cervical Joint, Percutaneous Endoscopic Approach
0RP04JZ Removal of Synthetic Substitute from Occipital-cervical Joint, Percutaneous Endoscopic Approach
0RP04KZ Removal of Nonautologous Tissue Substitute from Occipital-cervical Joint, Percutaneous Endoscopic Approach
0RP0X0Z Removal of Drainage Device from Occipital-cervical Joint, External Approach
0RP0X3Z Removal of Infusion Device from Occipital-cervical Joint, External Approach
0RP0X4Z Removal of Internal Fixation Device from Occipital-cervical Joint, External Approach
0RP100Z Removal of Drainage Device from Cervical Vertebral Joint, Open Approach
0RP103Z Removal of Infusion Device from Cervical Vertebral Joint, Open Approach
0RP104Z Removal of Internal Fixation Device from Cervical Vertebral Joint, Open Approach
0RP107Z Removal of Autologous Tissue Substitute from Cervical Vertebral Joint, Open Approach
0RP108Z Removal of Spacer from Cervical Vertebral Joint, Open Approach
0RP10AZ Removal of Interbody Fusion Device from Cervical Vertebral Joint, Open Approach
0RP10JZ Removal of Synthetic Substitute from Cervical Vertebral Joint, Open Approach
0RP10KZ Removal of Nonautologous Tissue Substitute from Cervical Vertebral Joint, Open Approach
0RP130Z Removal of Drainage Device from Cervical Vertebral Joint, Percutaneous Approach
0RP133Z Removal of Infusion Device from Cervical Vertebral Joint, Percutaneous Approach
0RP134Z Removal of Internal Fixation Device from Cervical Vertebral Joint, Percutaneous Approach
0RP137Z Removal of Autologous Tissue Substitute from Cervical Vertebral Joint, Percutaneous Approach
0RP138Z Removal of Spacer from Cervical Vertebral Joint, Percutaneous Approach
0RP13AZ Removal of Interbody Fusion Device from Cervical Vertebral Joint, Percutaneous Approach
0RP13JZ Removal of Synthetic Substitute from Cervical Vertebral Joint, Percutaneous Approach
0RP13KZ Removal of Nonautologous Tissue Substitute from Cervical Vertebral Joint, Percutaneous Approach
0RP140Z Removal of Drainage Device from Cervical Vertebral Joint, Percutaneous Endoscopic Approach
0RP143Z Removal of Infusion Device from Cervical Vertebral Joint, Percutaneous Endoscopic Approach
0RP144Z Removal of Internal Fixation Device from Cervical Vertebral Joint, Percutaneous Endoscopic Approach
0RP147Z Removal of Autologous Tissue Substitute from Cervical Vertebral Joint, Percutaneous Endoscopic Approach
0RP148Z Removal of Spacer from Cervical Vertebral Joint, Percutaneous Endoscopic Approach
0RP14AZ Removal of Interbody Fusion Device from Cervical Vertebral Joint, Percutaneous Endoscopic Approach
0RP14JZ Removal of Synthetic Substitute from Cervical Vertebral Joint, Percutaneous Endoscopic Approach
0RP14KZ Removal of Nonautologous Tissue Substitute from Cervical Vertebral Joint, Percutaneous Endoscopic Approach
0RP1X0Z Removal of Drainage Device from Cervical Vertebral Joint, External Approach
0RP1X3Z Removal of Infusion Device from Cervical Vertebral Joint, External Approach
0RP1X4Z Removal of Internal Fixation Device from Cervical Vertebral Joint, External Approach
0RP300Z Removal of Drainage Device from Cervical Vertebral Disc, Open Approach
0RP303Z Removal of Infusion Device from Cervical Vertebral Disc, Open Approach
0RP307Z Removal of Autologous Tissue Substitute from Cervical Vertebral Disc, Open Approach
0RP30JZ Removal of Synthetic Substitute from Cervical Vertebral Disc, Open Approach
0RP30KZ Removal of Nonautologous Tissue Substitute from Cervical Vertebral Disc, Open Approach
0RP330Z Removal of Drainage Device from Cervical Vertebral Disc, Percutaneous Approach
0RP333Z Removal of Infusion Device from Cervic Vertebral Disc, Percutaneous Approach
0RP337Z Removal of Autologous Tissue Substitute from Cervical Vertebral Disc, Percutaneous Approach
0RP33JZ Removal of Synthetic Substitute from Cervical Vertebral Disc, Percutaneous Approach
0RP33KZ Removal of Nonautologous Tissue Substitute from Cervical Vertebral Disc, Percutaneous Approach
0RP340Z Removal of Drainage Device from Cervical Vertebral Disc, Percutaneous Endoscopic Approach
0RP343Z Removal of Infusion Device from Cervica Vertebral Disc, Percutaneous Endoscopic Approach
0RP347Z Removal of Autologous Tissue Substitute from Cervical Vertebral Disc, Percutaneous Endoscopic Approach
0RP34JZ Removal of Synthetic Substitute from Cervical Vertebral Disc, Percutaneous Endoscopic Approach
0RP34KZ Removal of Nonautologous Tissue Substitute from Cervical Vertebral Disc, Percutaneous Endoscopic Approach
0RP3X0Z Removal of Drainage Device from Cervical Vertebral Disc, External Approach
0RP3X3Z Removal of Infusion Device from Cervical Vertebral Disc, External Approach
0RP400Z Removal of Drainage Device from Cervicothoracic Vertebral Joint, Open Approach
0RP403Z Removal of Infusion Device from Cervicothoracic Vertebral Joint, Open Approach
0RP404Z Removal of Internal Fixation Device from Cervicothoracic Vertebral Joint, Open Approach
0RP407Z Removal of Autologous Tissue Substitute from Cervicothoracic Vertebral Joint, Open Approach
0RP408Z Removal of Spacer from Cervicothoracic Vertebral Joint, Open Approach
0RP40AZ Removal of Interbody Fusion Device from Cervicothoracic Vertebral Joint, Open Approach
0RP40JZ Removal of Synthetic Substitute from Cervicothoracic Vertebral Joint, Open Approach
0RP40KZ Removal of Nonautologous Tissue Substitute from Cervicothoracic Vertebral Joint, Open Approach
0RP430Z Removal of Drainage Device from Cervicothoracic Vertebral Joint, Percutaneous Approach
0RP433Z Removal of Infusion Device from Cervicothoracic Vertebral Joint, Percutaneous Approach
0RP434Z Removal of Internal Fixation Device from Cervicothoracic Vertebral Joint, Percutaneous Approach
0RP437Z Removal of Autologous Tissue Substitute from Cervicothoracic Vertebral Joint, Percutaneous Approach
0RP438Z Removal of Spacer from Cervicothoracic Vertebral Joint, Percutaneous Approach
0RP43AZ Removal of Interbody Fusion Device from Cervicothoracic Vertebral Joint, Percutaneous Approach
0RP43JZ Removal of Synthetic Substitute from Cervicothoracic Vertebral Joint, Percutaneous Approach
0RP43KZ Removal of Nonautologous Tissue Substitute from Cervicothoracic Vertebral Joint, Percutaneous Approach

RP440Z Removal of Drainage Device from Cervicothoracic Vertebral Joint, Percutaneous Endoscopic Approach

RP443Z Removal of Infusion Device from Cervicothoracic Vertebral Joint, Percutaneous Endoscopic Approach

RP444Z Removal of Internal Fixation Device from Cervicothoracic Vertebral Joint, Percutaneous Endoscopic Approach

RP447Z Removal of Autologous Tissue Substitute from Cervicothoracic Vertebral Joint, Percutaneous Endoscopic Approach

RP448Z Removal of Spacer from Cervicothoracic Vertebral Joint, Percutaneous Endoscopic Approach

RP44AZ Removal of Interbody Fusion Device from Cervicothoracic Vertebral Joint, Percutaneous Endoscopic Approach

RP44JZ Removal of Synthetic Substitute from Cervicothoracic Vertebral Joint, Percutaneous Endoscopic Approach

RP44KZ Removal of Nonautologous Tissue Substitute from Cervicothoracic Vertebral Joint, Percutaneous Endoscopic Approach

RP4X0Z Removal of Drainage Device from Cervicothoracic Vertebral Joint, External Approach

RP4X3Z Removal of Infusion Device from Cervicothoracic Vertebral Joint, External Approach

RP4X4Z Removal of Internal Fixation Device from Cervicothoracic Vertebral Joint, External Approach

RP500Z Removal of Drainage Device from Cervicothoracic Vertebral Disc, Open Approach

RP503Z Removal of Infusion Device from Cervicothoracic Vertebral Disc, Open Approach

RP507Z Removal of Autologous Tissue Substitute from Cervicothoracic Vertebral Disc, Open Approach

RP50JZ Removal of Synthetic Substitute from Cervicothoracic Vertebral Disc, Open Approach

RP50KZ Removal of Nonautologous Tissue Substitute from Cervicothoracic Vertebral Disc, Open Approach

RP530Z Removal of Drainage Device from Cervicothoracic Vertebral Disc, Percutaneous Approach

RP533Z Removal of Infusion Device from Cervicothoracic Vertebral Disc, Percutaneous Approach

RP537Z Removal of Autologous Tissue Substitute from Cervicothoracic Vertebral Disc, Percutaneous Approach

RP53JZ Removal of Synthetic Substitute from Cervicothoracic Vertebral Disc, Percutaneous Approach

RP53KZ Removal of Nonautologous Tissue Substitute from Cervicothoracic Vertebral Disc, Percutaneous Approach

RP540Z Removal of Drainage Device from Cervicothoracic Vertebral Disc, Percutaneous Endoscopic Approach

RP543Z Removal of Infusion Device from Cervicothoracic Vertebral Disc, Percutaneous Endoscopic Approach

0RP547Z Removal of Autologous Tissue Substitute from Cervicothoracic Vertebral Disc, Percutaneous Endoscopic Approach

0RP54JZ Removal of Synthetic Substitute from Cervicothoracic Vertebral Disc, Percutaneous Endoscopic Approach

0RP54KZ Removal of Nonautologous Tissue Substitute from Cervicothoracic Vertebral Disc, Percutaneous Endoscopic Approach

0RP5X0Z Removal of Drainage Device from Cervicothoracic Vertebral Disc, External Approach

0RP5X3Z Removal of Infusion Device from Cervicothoracic Vertebral Disc, External Approach

0RP600Z Removal of Drainage Device from Thoracic Vertebral Joint, Open Approach

0RP603Z Removal of Infusion Device from Thoracic Vertebral Joint, Open Approach

0RP604Z Removal of Internal Fixation Device from Thoracic Vertebral Joint, Open Approach

0RP607Z Removal of Autologous Tissue Substitute from Thoracic Vertebral Joint, Open Approach

0RP608Z Removal of Spacer from Thoracic Vertebral Joint, Open Approach

0RP60AZ Removal of Interbody Fusion Device from Thoracic Vertebral Joint, Open Approach

0RP60JZ Removal of Synthetic Substitute from Thoracic Vertebral Joint, Open Approach

0RP60KZ Removal of Nonautologous Tissue Substitute from Thoracic Vertebral Joint, Open Approach

0RP630Z Removal of Drainage Device from Thoracic Vertebral Joint, Percutaneous Approach

0RP633Z Removal of Infusion Device from Thoracic Vertebral Joint, Percutaneous Approach

0RP634Z Removal of Internal Fixation Device from Thoracic Vertebral Joint, Percutaneous Approach

0RP637Z Removal of Autologous Tissue Substitute from Thoracic Vertebral Joint, Percutaneous Approach

0RP638Z Removal of Spacer from Thoracic Vertebral Joint, Percutaneous Approach

0RP63AZ Removal of Interbody Fusion Device from Thoracic Vertebral Joint, Percutaneous Approach

0RP63JZ Removal of Synthetic Substitute from Thoracic Vertebral Joint, Percutaneous Approach

0RP63KZ Removal of Nonautologous Tissue Substitute from Thoracic Vertebral Joint, Percutaneous Approach

0RP640Z Removal of Drainage Device from Thoracic Vertebral Joint, Percutaneous Endoscopic Approach

0RP643Z Removal of Infusion Device from Thoracic Vertebral Joint, Percutaneous Endoscopic Approach

0RP644Z Removal of Internal Fixation Device from Thoracic Vertebral Joint, Percutaneous Endoscopic Approach

0RP647Z Removal of Autologous Tissue Substitute from Thoracic Vertebral Joint, Percutaneous Endoscopic Approach

0RP648Z Removal of Spacer from Thoracic Vertebral Joint, Percutaneous Endoscopic Approach

0RP64AZ Removal of Interbody Fusion Device from Thoracic Vertebral Joint, Percutaneous Endoscopic Approach

0RP64JZ Removal of Synthetic Substitute from Thoracic Vertebral Joint, Percutaneous Endoscopic Approach

0RP64KZ Removal of Nonautologous Tissue Substitute from Thoracic Vertebral Joint, Percutaneous Endoscopic Approach

0RP6X0Z Removal of Drainage Device from Thoracic Vertebral Joint, External Approach

0RP6X3Z Removal of Infusion Device from Thoracic Vertebral Joint, External Approach

0RP6X4Z Removal of Internal Fixation Device from Thoracic Vertebral Joint, External Approach

0RP900Z Removal of Drainage Device from Thoracic Vertebral Disc, Open Approach

0RP903Z Removal of Infusion Device from Thoracic Vertebral Disc, Open Approach

0RP907Z Removal of Autologous Tissue Substitute from Thoracic Vertebral Disc, Open Approach

0RP90JZ Removal of Synthetic Substitute from Thoracic Vertebral Disc, Open Approach

0RP90KZ Removal of Nonautologous Tissue Substitute from Thoracic Vertebral Disc, Open Approach

0RP930Z Removal of Drainage Device from Thoracic Vertebral Disc, Percutaneous Approach

0RP933Z Removal of Infusion Device from Thoracic Vertebral Disc, Percutaneous Approach

0RP937Z Removal of Autologous Tissue Substitute from Thoracic Vertebral Disc, Percutaneous Approach

0RP93JZ Removal of Synthetic Substitute from Thoracic Vertebral Disc, Percutaneous Approach

0RP93KZ Removal of Nonautologous Tissue Substitute from Thoracic Vertebral Disc, Percutaneous Approach

0RP940Z Removal of Drainage Device from Thoracic Vertebral Disc, Percutaneous Endoscopic Approach

0RP943Z Removal of Infusion Device from Thoracic Vertebral Disc, Percutaneous Endoscopic Approach

0RP947Z Removal of Autologous Tissue Substitute from Thoracic Vertebral Disc, Percutaneous Endoscopic Approach

0RP94JZ Removal of Synthetic Substitute from Thoracic Vertebral Disc, Percutaneous Endoscopic Approach

0RP94KZ Removal of Nonautologous Tissue Substitute from Thoracic Vertebral Disc, Percutaneous Endoscopic Approach

0RP9X0Z Removal of Drainage Device from Thoracic Vertebral Disc, External Approach

0RP9X3Z Removal of Infusion Device from Thoracic Vertebral Disc, External Approach

0RPA00Z Removal of Drainage Device from Thoracolumbar Vertebral Joint, Open Approach

0RPA03Z Removal of Infusion Device from Thoracolumbar Vertebral Joint, Open Approach

0RPA04Z Removal of Internal Fixation Device from Thoracolumbar Vertebral Joint, Open Approach

0RPA07Z Removal of Autologous Tissue Substitute from Thoracolumbar Vertebral Joint, Open Approach

0RPA08Z Removal of Spacer from Thoracolumbar Vertebral Joint, Open Approach

0RPA0AZ Removal of Interbody Fusion Device from Thoracolumbar Vertebral Joint, Open Approach

0RPA0JZ Removal of Synthetic Substitute from Thoracolumbar Vertebral Joint, Open Approach

0RPA0KZ Removal of Nonautologous Tissue Substitute from Thoracolumbar Vertebral Joint, Open Approach

0RPA30Z Removal of Drainage Device from Thoracolumbar Vertebral Joint, Percutaneous Approach

0RPA33Z Removal of Infusion Device from Thoracolumbar Vertebral Joint, Percutaneous Approach
0RPA34Z Removal of Internal Fixation Device from Thoracolumbar Vertebral Joint, Percutaneous Approach
0RPA37Z Removal of Autologous Tissue Substitute from Thoracolumbar Vertebral Joint, Percutaneous Approach
0RPA38Z Removal of Spacer from Thoracolumbar Vertebral Joint, Percutaneous Approach
0RPA3AZ Removal of Interbody Fusion Device from Thoracolumbar Vertebral Joint, Percutaneous Approach
0RPA3JZ Removal of Synthetic Substitute from Thoracolumbar Vertebral Joint, Percutaneous Approach
0RPA3KZ Removal of Nonautologous Tissue Substitute from Thoracolumbar Vertebral Joint, Percutaneous Approach
0RPA40Z Removal of Drainage Device from Thoracolumbar Vertebral Joint, Percutaneous Endoscopic Approach
0RPA43Z Removal of Infusion Device from Thoracolumbar Vertebral Joint, Percutaneous Endoscopic Approach
0RPA44Z Removal of Internal Fixation Device from Thoracolumbar Vertebral Joint, Percutaneous Endoscopic Approach
0RPA47Z Removal of Autologous Tissue Substitute from Thoracolumbar Vertebral Joint, Percutaneous Endoscopic Approach
0RPA48Z Removal of Spacer from Thoracolumbar Vertebral Joint, Percutaneous Endoscopic Approach
0RPA4AZ Removal of Interbody Fusion Device from Thoracolumbar Vertebral Joint, Percutaneous Endoscopic Approach
0RPA4JZ Removal of Synthetic Substitute from Thoracolumbar Vertebral Joint, Percutaneous Endoscopic Approach
0RPA4KZ Removal of Nonautologous Tissue Substitute from Thoracolumbar Vertebral Joint, Percutaneous Endoscopic Approach
0RPAX0Z Removal of Drainage Device from Thoracolumbar Vertebral Joint, External Approach
0RPAX3Z Removal of Infusion Device from Thoracolumbar Vertebral Joint, External Approach
0RPAX4Z Removal of Internal Fixation Device from Thoracolumbar Vertebral Joint, External Approach
0RPB00Z Removal of Drainage Device from Thoracolumbar Vertebral Disc, Open Approach
0RPB03Z Removal of Infusion Device from Thoracolumbar Vertebral Disc, Open Approach
0RPB07Z Removal of Autologous Tissue Substitute from Thoracolumbar Vertebral Disc, Open Approach
0RPB0JZ Removal of Synthetic Substitute from Thoracolumbar Vertebral Disc, Open Approach
0RPB0KZ Removal of Nonautologous Tissue Substitute from Thoracolumbar Vertebral Disc, Open Approach
0RPB30Z Removal of Drainage Device from Thoracolumbar Vertebral Disc, Percutaneous Approach
0RPB33Z Removal of Infusion Device from Thoracolumbar Vertebral Disc, Percutaneous Approach
0RPB37Z Removal of Autologous Tissue Substitute from Thoracolumbar Vertebral Disc, Percutaneous Approach
0RPB3JZ Removal of Synthetic Substitute from Thoracolumbar Vertebral Disc, Percutaneous Approach
0RPB3KZ Removal of Nonautologous Tissue Substitute from Thoracolumbar Vertebral Disc, Percutaneous Approach
0RPB40Z Removal of Drainage Device from Thoracolumbar Vertebral Disc, Percutaneous Endoscopic Approach
0RPB43Z Removal of Infusion Device from Thoracolumbar Vertebral Disc, Percutaneous Endoscopic Approach
0RPB47Z Removal of Autologous Tissue Substitute from Thoracolumbar Vertebral Disc, Percutaneous Endoscopic Approach
0RPB4JZ Removal of Synthetic Substitute from Thoracolumbar Vertebral Disc, Percutaneous Endoscopic Approach
0RPB4KZ Removal of Nonautologous Tissue Substitute from Thoracolumbar Vertebral Disc, Percutaneous Endoscopic Approach
0RPBX0Z Removal of Drainage Device from Thoracolumbar Vertebral Disc, External Approach
0RPBX3Z Removal of Infusion Device from Thoracolumbar Vertebral Disc, External Approach
0RPC00Z Removal of Drainage Device from Right Temporomandibular Joint, Open Approach
0RPC03Z Removal of Infusion Device from Right Temporomandibular Joint, Open Approach
0RPC04Z Removal of Internal Fixation Device from Right Temporomandibular Joint, Open Approach
0RPC07Z Removal of Autologous Tissue Substitute from Right Temporomandibular Joint, Open Approach
0RPC08Z Removal of Spacer from Right Temporomandibular Joint, Open Approach
0RPC0JZ Removal of Synthetic Substitute from Right Temporomandibular Joint, Open Approach
0RPC0KZ Removal of Nonautologous Tissue Substitute from Right Temporomandibular Joint, Open Approach
0RPC30Z Removal of Drainage Device from Right Temporomandibular Joint, Percutaneous Approach
0RPC33Z Removal of Infusion Device from Right Temporomandibular Joint, Percutaneous Approach
0RPC34Z Removal of Internal Fixation Device from Right Temporomandibular Joint, Percutaneous Approach
0RPC37Z Removal of Autologous Tissue Substitute from Right Temporomandibular Joint, Percutaneous Approach
0RPC38Z Removal of Spacer from Right Temporomandibular Joint, Percutaneous Approach
0RPC3JZ Removal of Synthetic Substitute from Right Temporomandibular Joint, Percutaneous Approach
0RPC3KZ Removal of Nonautologous Tissue Substitute from Right Temporomandibular Joint, Percutaneous Approach
0RPC40Z Removal of Drainage Device from Right Temporomandibular Joint, Percutaneous Endoscopic Approach
0RPC43Z Removal of Infusion Device from Right Temporomandibular Joint, Percutaneous Endoscopic Approach
0RPC44Z Removal of Internal Fixation Device from Right Temporomandibular Joint, Percutaneous Endoscopic Approach
0RPC47Z Removal of Autologous Tissue Substitu from Right Temporomandibular Joint, Percutaneous Endoscopic Approach
0RPC48Z Removal of Spacer from Right Temporomandibular Joint, Percutaneous Endoscopic Approach
0RPC4JZ Removal of Synthetic Substitute from Right Temporomandibular Joint, Percutaneous Endoscopic Approach
0RPC4KZ Removal of Nonautologous Tissue Substitute from Right Temporomandibul Joint, Percutaneous Endoscopic Approac
0RPCX0Z Removal of Drainage Device from Righ Temporomandibular Joint, External Approach
0RPCX3Z Removal of Infusion Device from Right Temporomandibular Joint, External Approach
0RPCX4Z Removal of Internal Fixation Device fro Right Temporomandibular Joint, Externa Approach
0RPD00Z Removal of Drainage Device from Left Temporomandibular Joint, Open Approach
0RPD03Z Removal of Infusion Device from Left Temporomandibular Joint, Open Approach
0RPD04Z Removal of Internal Fixation Device fror Left Temporomandibular Joint, Open Approach
0RPD07Z Removal of Autologous Tissue Substitute from Left Temporomandibular Joint, Open Approach
0RPD08Z Removal of Spacer from Left Temporomandibular Joint, Open Approach
0RPD0JZ Removal of Synthetic Substitute from Left Temporomandibular Joint, Open Approach
0RPD0KZ Removal of Nonautologous Tissue Substitute from Left Temporomandibular Joint, Open Approach
0RPD30Z Removal of Drainage Device from Left Temporomandibular Joint, Percutaneous Approach
0RPD33Z Removal of Infusion Device from Left Temporomandibular Joint, Percutaneous Approach
0RPD34Z Removal of Internal Fixation Device from Left Temporomandibular Joint, Percutaneous Approach
0RPD37Z Removal of Autologous Tissue Substitute from Left Temporomandibular Joint, Percutaneous Approach
0RPD38Z Removal of Spacer from Left Temporomandibular Joint, Percutaneous Approach
0RPD3JZ Removal of Synthetic Substitute from Left Temporomandibular Joint, Percutaneous Approach
0RPD3KZ Removal of Nonautologous Tissue Substitute from Left Temporomandibular Joint, Percutaneous Approach
0RPD40Z Removal of Drainage Device from Left Temporomandibular Joint, Percutaneous Endoscopic Approach
0RPD43Z Removal of Infusion Device from Left Temporomandibular Joint, Percutaneous Endoscopic Approach
0RPD44Z Removal of Internal Fixation Device from Left Temporomandibular Joint, Percutaneous Endoscopic Approach
0RPD47Z Removal of Autologous Tissue Substitute from Left Temporomandibular Joint, Percutaneous Endoscopic Approach
0RPD48Z Removal of Spacer from Left Temporomandibular Joint, Percutaneous Endoscopic Approach

RPD4JZ Removal of Synthetic Substitute from Left Temporomandibular Joint, Percutaneous Endoscopic Approach

RPD4KZ Removal of Nonautologous Tissue Substitute from Left Temporomandibular Joint, Percutaneous Endoscopic Approach

RPDX0Z Removal of Drainage Device from Left Temporomandibular Joint, External Approach

RPDX3Z Removal of Infusion Device from Left Temporomandibular Joint, External Approach

RPDX4Z Removal of Internal Fixation Device from Left Temporomandibular Joint, External Approach

RPE00Z Removal of Drainage Device from Right Sternoclavicular Joint, Open Approach

RPE03Z Removal of Infusion Device from Right Sternoclavicular Joint, Open Approach

RPE04Z Removal of Internal Fixation Device from Right Sternoclavicular Joint, Open Approach

RPE07Z Removal of Autologous Tissue Substitute from Right Sternoclavicular Joint, Open Approach

RPE08Z Removal of Spacer from Right Sternoclavicular Joint, Open Approach

RPE0JZ Removal of Synthetic Substitute from Right Sternoclavicular Joint, Open Approach

RPE0KZ Removal of Nonautologous Tissue Substitute from Right Sternoclavicular Joint, Open Approach

RPE30Z Removal of Drainage Device from Right Sternoclavicular Joint, Percutaneous Approach

RPE33Z Removal of Infusion Device from Right Sternoclavicular Joint, Percutaneous Approach

RPE34Z Removal of Internal Fixation Device from Right Sternoclavicular Joint, Percutaneous Approach

RPE37Z Removal of Autologous Tissue Substitute from Right Sternoclavicular Joint, Percutaneous Approach

RPE38Z Removal of Spacer from Right Sternoclavicular Joint, Percutaneous Approach

RPE3JZ Removal of Synthetic Substitute from Right Sternoclavicular Joint, Percutaneous Approach

RPE3KZ Removal of Nonautologous Tissue Substitute from Right Sternoclavicular Joint, Percutaneous Approach

RPE40Z Removal of Drainage Device from Right Sternoclavicular Joint, Percutaneous Endoscopic Approach

RPE43Z Removal of Infusion Device from Right Sternoclavicular Joint, Percutaneous Endoscopic Approach

RPE44Z Removal of Internal Fixation Device from Right Sternoclavicular Joint, Percutaneous Endoscopic Approach

RPE47Z Removal of Autologous Tissue Substitute from Right Sternoclavicular Joint, Percutaneous Endoscopic Approach

RPE48Z Removal of Spacer from Right Sternoclavicular Joint, Percutaneous Endoscopic Approach

RPE4JZ Removal of Synthetic Substitute from Right Sternoclavicular Joint, Percutaneous Endoscopic Approach

0RPE4KZ Removal of Nonautologous Tissue Substitute from Right Sternoclavicular Joint, Percutaneous Endoscopic Approach

0RPEX0Z Removal of Drainage Device from Right Sternoclavicular Joint, External Approach

0RPEX3Z Removal of Infusion Device from Right Sternoclavicular Joint, External Approach

0RPEX4Z Removal of Internal Fixation Device from Right Sternoclavicular Joint, External Approach

0RPF00Z Removal of Drainage Device from Left Sternoclavicular Joint, Open Approach

0RPF03Z Removal of Infusion Device from Left Sternoclavicular Joint, Open Approach

0RPF04Z Removal of Internal Fixation Device from Left Sternoclavicular Joint, Open Approach

0RPF07Z Removal of Autologous Tissue Substitute from Left Sternoclavicular Joint, Open Approach

0RPF08Z Removal of Spacer from Left Sternoclavicular Joint, Open Approach

0RPF0JZ Removal of Synthetic Substitute from Left Sternoclavicular Joint, Open Approach

0RPF0KZ Removal of Nonautologous Tissue Substitute from Left Sternoclavicular Joint, Open Approach

0RPF30Z Removal of Drainage Device from Left Sternoclavicular Joint, Percutaneous Approach

0RPF33Z Removal of Infusion Device from Left Sternoclavicular Joint, Percutaneous Approach

0RPF34Z Removal of Internal Fixation Device from Left Sternoclavicular Joint, Percutaneous Approach

0RPF37Z Removal of Autologous Tissue Substitute from Left Sternoclavicular Joint, Percutaneous Approach

0RPF38Z Removal of Spacer from Left Sternoclavicular Joint, Percutaneous Approach

0RPF3JZ Removal of Synthetic Substitute from Left Sternoclavicular Joint, Percutaneous Approach

0RPF3KZ Removal of Nonautologous Tissue Substitute from Left Sternoclavicular Joint, Percutaneous Approach

0RPF40Z Removal of Drainage Device from Left Sternoclavicular Joint, Percutaneous Endoscopic Approach

0RPF43Z Removal of Infusion Device from Left Sternoclavicular Joint, Percutaneous Endoscopic Approach

0RPF44Z Removal of Internal Fixation Device from Left Sternoclavicular Joint, Percutaneous Endoscopic Approach

0RPF47Z Removal of Autologous Tissue Substitute from Left Sternoclavicular Joint, Percutaneous Endoscopic Approach

0RPF48Z Removal of Spacer from Left Sternoclavicular Joint, Percutaneous Endoscopic Approach

0RPF4JZ Removal of Synthetic Substitute from Left Sternoclavicular Joint, Percutaneous Endoscopic Approach

0RPF4KZ Removal of Nonautologous Tissue Substitute from Left Sternoclavicular Joint, Percutaneous Endoscopic Approach

0RPFX0Z Removal of Drainage Device from Left Sternoclavicular Joint, External Approach

0RPFX3Z Removal of Infusion Device from Left Sternoclavicular Joint, External Approach

0RPFX4Z Removal of Internal Fixation Device from Left Sternoclavicular Joint, External Approach

0RPG00Z Removal of Drainage Device from Right Acromioclavicular Joint, Open Approach

0RPG03Z Removal of Infusion Device from Right Acromioclavicular Joint, Open Approach

0RPG04Z Removal of Internal Fixation Device from Right Acromioclavicular Joint, Open Approach

0RPG07Z Removal of Autologous Tissue Substitute from Right Acromioclavicular Joint, Open Approach

0RPG08Z Removal of Spacer from Right Acromioclavicular Joint, Open Approach

0RPG0JZ Removal of Synthetic Substitute from Right Acromioclavicular Joint, Open Approach

0RPG0KZ Removal of Nonautologous Tissue Substitute from Right Acromioclavicular Joint, Open Approach

0RPG30Z Removal of Drainage Device from Right Acromioclavicular Joint, Percutaneous Approach

0RPG33Z Removal of Infusion Device from Right Acromioclavicular Joint, Percutaneous Approach

0RPG34Z Removal of Internal Fixation Device from Right Acromioclavicular Joint, Percutaneous Approach

0RPG37Z Removal of Autologous Tissue Substitute from Right Acromioclavicular Joint, Percutaneous Approach

0RPG38Z Removal of Spacer from Right Acromioclavicular Joint, Percutaneous Approach

0RPG3JZ Removal of Synthetic Substitute from Right Acromioclavicular Joint, Percutaneous Approach

0RPG3KZ Removal of Nonautologous Tissue Substitute from Right Acromioclavicular Joint, Percutaneous Approach

0RPG40Z Removal of Drainage Device from Right Acromioclavicular Joint, Percutaneous Endoscopic Approach

0RPG43Z Removal of Infusion Device from Right Acromioclavicular Joint, Percutaneous Endoscopic Approach

0RPG44Z Removal of Internal Fixation Device from Right Acromioclavicular Joint, Percutaneous Endoscopic Approach

0RPG47Z Removal of Autologous Tissue Substitute from Right Acromioclavicular Joint, Percutaneous Endoscopic Approach

0RPG48Z Removal of Spacer from Right Acromioclavicular Joint, Percutaneous Endoscopic Approach

0RPG4JZ Removal of Synthetic Substitute from Right Acromioclavicular Joint, Percutaneous Endoscopic Approach

0RPG4KZ Removal of Nonautologous Tissue Substitute from Right Acromioclavicular Joint, Percutaneous Endoscopic Approach

0RPGX0Z Removal of Drainage Device from Right Acromioclavicular Joint, External Approach

0RPGX3Z Removal of Infusion Device from Right Acromioclavicular Joint, External Approach

0RPGX4Z Removal of Internal Fixation Device from Right Acromioclavicular Joint, External Approach

0RPH00Z Removal of Drainage Device from Left Acromioclavicular Joint, Open Approach

0RPH03Z Removal of Infusion Device from Left Acromioclavicular Joint, Open Approach

0RPH04Z Removal of Internal Fixation Device from Left Acromioclavicular Joint, Open Approach

0RPH07Z Removal of Autologous Tissue Substitute from Left Acromioclavicular Joint, Open Approach

0RPH08Z Removal of Spacer from Left Acromioclavicular Joint, Open Approach

0RPH0JZ Removal of Synthetic Substitute from Left Acromioclavicular Joint, Open Approach
0RPH0KZ Removal of Nonautologous Tissue Substitute from Left Acromioclavicular Joint, Open Approach
0RPH30Z Removal of Drainage Device from Left Acromioclavicular Joint, Percutaneous Approach
0RPH33Z Removal of Infusion Device from Left Acromioclavicular Joint, Percutaneous Approach
0RPH34Z Removal of Internal Fixation Device from Left Acromioclavicular Joint, Percutaneous Approach
0RPH37Z Removal of Autologous Tissue Substitute from Left Acromioclavicular Joint, Percutaneous Approach
0RPH38Z Removal of Spacer from Left Acromioclavicular Joint, Percutaneous Approach
0RPH3JZ Removal of Synthetic Substitute from Left Acromioclavicular Joint, Percutaneous Approach
0RPH3KZ Removal of Nonautologous Tissue Substitute from Left Acromioclavicular Joint, Percutaneous Approach
0RPH40Z Removal of Drainage Device from Left Acromioclavicular Joint, Percutaneous Endoscopic Approach
0RPH43Z Removal of Infusion Device from Left Acromioclavicular Joint, Percutaneous Endoscopic Approach
0RPH44Z Removal of Internal Fixation Device from Left Acromioclavicular Joint, Percutaneous Endoscopic Approach
0RPH47Z Removal of Autologous Tissue Substitute from Left Acromioclavicular Joint, Percutaneous Endoscopic Approach
0RPH48Z Removal of Spacer from Left Acromioclavicular Joint, Percutaneous Endoscopic Approach
0RPH4JZ Removal of Synthetic Substitute from Left Acromioclavicular Joint, Percutaneous Endoscopic Approach
0RPH4KZ Removal of Nonautologous Tissue Substitute from Left Acromioclavicular Joint, Percutaneous Endoscopic Approach
0RPHX0Z Removal of Drainage Device from Left Acromioclavicular Joint, External Approach
0RPHX3Z Removal of Infusion Device from Left Acromioclavicular Joint, External Approach
0RPHX4Z Removal of Internal Fixation Device from Left Acromioclavicular Joint, External Approach
0RPJ00Z Removal of Drainage Device from Right Shoulder Joint, Open Approach
0RPJ03Z Removal of Infusion Device from Right Shoulder Joint, Open Approach
0RPJ04Z Removal of Internal Fixation Device from Right Shoulder Joint, Open Approach
0RPJ07Z Removal of Autologous Tissue Substitute from Right Shoulder Joint, Open Approach
0RPJ08Z Removal of Spacer from Right Shoulder Joint, Open Approach
0RPJ0JZ Removal of Synthetic Substitute from Right Shoulder Joint, Open Approach
0RPJ0KZ Removal of Nonautologous Tissue Substitute from Right Shoulder Joint, Open Approach
0RPJ30Z Removal of Drainage Device from Right Shoulder Joint, Percutaneous Approach
0RPJ33Z Removal of Infusion Device from Right Shoulder Joint, Percutaneous Approach
0RPJ34Z Removal of Internal Fixation Device from Right Shoulder Joint, Percutaneous Approach
0RPJ37Z Removal of Autologous Tissue Substitute from Right Shoulder Joint, Percutaneous Approach
0RPJ38Z Removal of Spacer from Right Shoulder Joint, Percutaneous Approach
0RPJ3JZ Removal of Synthetic Substitute from Right Shoulder Joint, Percutaneous Approach
0RPJ3KZ Removal of Nonautologous Tissue Substitute from Right Shoulder Joint, Percutaneous Approach
0RPJ40Z Removal of Drainage Device from Right Shoulder Joint, Percutaneous Endoscopic Approach
0RPJ43Z Removal of Infusion Device from Right Shoulder Joint, Percutaneous Endoscopic Approach
0RPJ44Z Removal of Internal Fixation Device from Right Shoulder Joint, Percutaneous Endoscopic Approach
0RPJ47Z Removal of Autologous Tissue Substitute from Right Shoulder Joint, Percutaneous Endoscopic Approach
0RPJ48Z Removal of Spacer from Right Shoulder Joint, Percutaneous Endoscopic Approach
0RPJ4JZ Removal of Synthetic Substitute from Right Shoulder Joint, Percutaneous Endoscopic Approach
0RPJ4KZ Removal of Nonautologous Tissue Substitute from Right Shoulder Joint, Percutaneous Endoscopic Approach
0RPJX0Z Removal of Drainage Device from Right Shoulder Joint, External Approach
0RPJX3Z Removal of Infusion Device from Right Shoulder Joint, External Approach
0RPJX4Z Removal of Internal Fixation Device from Right Shoulder Joint, External Approach
0RPK00Z Removal of Drainage Device from Left Shoulder Joint, Open Approach
0RPK03Z Removal of Infusion Device from Left Shoulder Joint, Open Approach
0RPK04Z Removal of Internal Fixation Device from Left Shoulder Joint, Open Approach
0RPK07Z Removal of Autologous Tissue Substitute from Left Shoulder Joint, Open Approach
0RPK08Z Removal of Spacer from Left Shoulder Joint, Open Approach
0RPK0JZ Removal of Synthetic Substitute from Left Shoulder Joint, Open Approach
0RPK0KZ Removal of Nonautologous Tissue Substitute from Left Shoulder Joint, Open Approach
0RPK30Z Removal of Drainage Device from Left Shoulder Joint, Percutaneous Approach
0RPK33Z Removal of Infusion Device from Left Shoulder Joint, Percutaneous Approach
0RPK34Z Removal of Internal Fixation Device from Left Shoulder Joint, Percutaneous Approach
0RPK37Z Removal of Autologous Tissue Substitute from Left Shoulder Joint, Percutaneous Approach
0RPK38Z Removal of Spacer from Left Shoulder Joint, Percutaneous Approach
0RPK3JZ Removal of Synthetic Substitute from Left Shoulder Joint, Percutaneous Approach
0RPK3KZ Removal of Nonautologous Tissue Substitute from Left Shoulder Joint, Percutaneous Approach
0RPK40Z Removal of Drainage Device from Left Shoulder Joint, Percutaneous Endoscopic Approach
0RPK43Z Removal of Infusion Device from Left Shoulder Joint, Percutaneous Endoscopic Approach
0RPK44Z Removal of Internal Fixation Device from Left Shoulder Joint, Percutaneous Endoscopic Approach
0RPK47Z Removal of Autologous Tissue Substitute from Left Shoulder Joint, Percutaneous Endoscopic Approach
0RPK48Z Removal of Spacer from Left Shoulder Joint, Percutaneous Endoscopic Approach
0RPK4JZ Removal of Synthetic Substitute from Left Shoulder Joint, Percutaneous Endoscopic Approach
0RPK4KZ Removal of Nonautologous Tissue Substitute from Left Shoulder Joint, Percutaneous Endoscopic Approach
0RPKX0Z Removal of Drainage Device from Left Shoulder Joint, External Approach
0RPKX3Z Removal of Infusion Device from Left Shoulder Joint, External Approach
0RPKX4Z Removal of Internal Fixation Device from Left Shoulder Joint, External Approach
0RPL00Z Removal of Drainage Device from Right Elbow Joint, Open Approach
0RPL03Z Removal of Infusion Device from Right Elbow Joint, Open Approach
0RPL04Z Removal of Internal Fixation Device from Right Elbow Joint, Open Approach
0RPL05Z Removal of External Fixation Device from Right Elbow Joint, Open Approach
0RPL07Z Removal of Autologous Tissue Substitute from Right Elbow Joint, Open Approach
0RPL08Z Removal of Spacer from Right Elbow Joint, Open Approach
0RPL0JZ Removal of Synthetic Substitute from Right Elbow Joint, Open Approach
0RPL0KZ Removal of Nonautologous Tissue Substitute from Right Elbow Joint, Open Approach
0RPL30Z Removal of Drainage Device from Right Elbow Joint, Percutaneous Approach
0RPL33Z Removal of Infusion Device from Right Elbow Joint, Percutaneous Approach
0RPL34Z Removal of Internal Fixation Device from Right Elbow Joint, Percutaneous Approach
0RPL35Z Removal of External Fixation Device from Right Elbow Joint, Percutaneous Approach
0RPL37Z Removal of Autologous Tissue Substitute from Right Elbow Joint, Percutaneous Approach
0RPL38Z Removal of Spacer from Right Elbow Joint, Percutaneous Approach
0RPL3JZ Removal of Synthetic Substitute from Right Elbow Joint, Percutaneous Approach
0RPL3KZ Removal of Nonautologous Tissue Substitute from Right Elbow Joint, Percutaneous Approach
0RPL40Z Removal of Drainage Device from Right Elbow Joint, Percutaneous Endoscopic Approach
0RPL43Z Removal of Infusion Device from Right Elbow Joint, Percutaneous Endoscopic Approach
0RPL44Z Removal of Internal Fixation Device from Right Elbow Joint, Percutaneous Endoscopic Approach
0RPL45Z Removal of External Fixation Device from Right Elbow Joint, Percutaneous Endoscopic Approach
0RPL47Z Removal of Autologous Tissue Substitute from Right Elbow Joint, Percutaneous Endoscopic Approach

RPL48Z Removal of Spacer from Right Elbow Joint, Percutaneous Endoscopic Approach

RPL4JZ Removal of Synthetic Substitute from Right Elbow Joint, Percutaneous Endoscopic Approach

RPL4KZ Removal of Nonautologous Tissue Substitute from Right Elbow Joint, Percutaneous Endoscopic Approach

RPLX0Z Removal of Drainage Device from Right Elbow Joint, External Approach

RPLX3Z Removal of Infusion Device from Right Elbow Joint, External Approach

RPLX4Z Removal of Internal Fixation Device from Right Elbow Joint, External Approach

RPLX5Z Removal of External Fixation Device from Right Elbow Joint, External Approach

RPM00Z Removal of Drainage Device from Left Elbow Joint, Open Approach

RPM03Z Removal of Infusion Device from Left Elbow Joint, Open Approach

RPM04Z Removal of Internal Fixation Device from Left Elbow Joint, Open Approach

RPM05Z Removal of External Fixation Device from Left Elbow Joint, Open Approach

RPM07Z Removal of Autologous Tissue Substitute from Left Elbow Joint, Open Approach

RPM08Z Removal of Spacer from Left Elbow Joint, Open Approach

RPM0JZ Removal of Synthetic Substitute from Left Elbow Joint, Open Approach

RPM0KZ Removal of Nonautologous Tissue Substitute from Left Elbow Joint, Open Approach

RPM30Z Removal of Drainage Device from Left Elbow Joint, Percutaneous Approach

RPM33Z Removal of Infusion Device from Left Elbow Joint, Percutaneous Approach

RPM34Z Removal of Internal Fixation Device from Left Elbow Joint, Percutaneous Approach

RPM35Z Removal of External Fixation Device from Left Elbow Joint, Percutaneous Approach

RPM37Z Removal of Autologous Tissue Substitute from Left Elbow Joint, Percutaneous Approach

RPM38Z Removal of Spacer from Left Elbow Joint, Percutaneous Approach

RPM3JZ Removal of Synthetic Substitute from Left Elbow Joint, Percutaneous Approach

RPM3KZ Removal of Nonautologous Tissue Substitute from Left Elbow Joint, Percutaneous Approach

RPM40Z Removal of Drainage Device from Left Elbow Joint, Percutaneous Endoscopic Approach

RPM43Z Removal of Infusion Device from Left Elbow Joint, Percutaneous Endoscopic Approach

RPM44Z Removal of Internal Fixation Device from Left Elbow Joint, Percutaneous Endoscopic Approach

RPM45Z Removal of External Fixation Device from Left Elbow Joint, Percutaneous Endoscopic Approach

0RPM47Z Removal of Autologous Tissue Substitute from Left Elbow Joint, Percutaneous Endoscopic Approach

0RPM48Z Removal of Spacer from Left Elbow Joint, Percutaneous Endoscopic Approach

0RPM4JZ Removal of Synthetic Substitute from Left Elbow Joint, Percutaneous Endoscopic Approach

0RPM4KZ Removal of Nonautologous Tissue Substitute from Left Elbow Joint, Percutaneous Endoscopic Approach

0RPMX0Z Removal of Drainage Device from Left Elbow Joint, External Approach

0RPMX3Z Removal of Infusion Device from Left Elbow Joint, External Approach

0RPMX4Z Removal of Internal Fixation Device from Left Elbow Joint, External Approach

0RPMX5Z Removal of External Fixation Device from Left Elbow Joint, External Approach

0RPN00Z Removal of Drainage Device from Right Wrist Joint, Open Approach

0RPN03Z Removal of Infusion Device from Right Wrist Joint, Open Approach

0RPN04Z Removal of Internal Fixation Device from Right Wrist Joint, Open Approach

0RPN05Z Removal of External Fixation Device from Right Wrist Joint, Open Approach

0RPN07Z Removal of Autologous Tissue Substitute from Right Wrist Joint, Open Approach

0RPN08Z Removal of Spacer from Right Wrist Joint, Open Approach

0RPN0JZ Removal of Synthetic Substitute from Right Wrist Joint, Open Approach

0RPN0KZ Removal of Nonautologous Tissue Substitute from Right Wrist Joint, Open Approach

0RPN30Z Removal of Drainage Device from Right Wrist Joint, Percutaneous Approach

0RPN33Z Removal of Infusion Device from Right Wrist Joint, Percutaneous Approach

0RPN34Z Removal of Internal Fixation Device from Right Wrist Joint, Percutaneous Approach

0RPN35Z Removal of External Fixation Device from Right Wrist Joint, Percutaneous Approach

0RPN37Z Removal of Autologous Tissue Substitute from Right Wrist Joint, Percutaneous Approach

0RPN38Z Removal of Spacer from Right Wrist Joint, Percutaneous Approach

0RPN3JZ Removal of Synthetic Substitute from Right Wrist Joint, Percutaneous Approach

0RPN3KZ Removal of Nonautologous Tissue Substitute from Right Wrist Joint, Percutaneous Approach

0RPN40Z Removal of Drainage Device from Right Wrist Joint, Percutaneous Endoscopic Approach

0RPN43Z Removal of Infusion Device from Right Wrist Joint, Percutaneous Endoscopic Approach

0RPN44Z Removal of Internal Fixation Device from Right Wrist Joint, Percutaneous Endoscopic Approach

0RPN45Z Removal of External Fixation Device from Right Wrist Joint, Percutaneous Endoscopic Approach

0RPN47Z Removal of Autologous Tissue Substitute from Right Wrist Joint, Percutaneous Endoscopic Approach

0RPN48Z Removal of Spacer from Right Wrist Joint, Percutaneous Endoscopic Approach

0RPN4JZ Removal of Synthetic Substitute from Right Wrist Joint, Percutaneous Endoscopic Approach

0RPN4KZ Removal of Nonautologous Tissue Substitute from Right Wrist Joint, Percutaneous Endoscopic Approach

0RPNX0Z Removal of Drainage Device from Right Wrist Joint, External Approach

0RPNX3Z Removal of Infusion Device from Right Wrist Joint, External Approach

0RPNX4Z Removal of Internal Fixation Device from Right Wrist Joint, External Approach

0RPNX5Z Removal of External Fixation Device from Right Wrist Joint, External Approach

0RPP00Z Removal of Drainage Device from Left Wrist Joint, Open Approach

0RPP03Z Removal of Infusion Device from Left Wrist Joint, Open Approach

0RPP04Z Removal of Internal Fixation Device from Left Wrist Joint, Open Approach

0RPP05Z Removal of External Fixation Device from Left Wrist Joint, Open Approach

0RPP07Z Removal of Autologous Tissue Substitute from Left Wrist Joint, Open Approach

0RPP08Z Removal of Spacer from Left Wrist Joint, Open Approach

0RPP0JZ Removal of Synthetic Substitute from Left Wrist Joint, Open Approach

0RPP0KZ Removal of Nonautologous Tissue Substitute from Left Wrist Joint, Open Approach

0RPP30Z Removal of Drainage Device from Left Wrist Joint, Percutaneous Approach

0RPP33Z Removal of Infusion Device from Left Wrist Joint, Percutaneous Approach

0RPP34Z Removal of Internal Fixation Device from Left Wrist Joint, Percutaneous Approach

0RPP35Z Removal of External Fixation Device from Left Wrist Joint, Percutaneous Approach

0RPP37Z Removal of Autologous Tissue Substitute from Left Wrist Joint, Percutaneous Approach

0RPP38Z Removal of Spacer from Left Wrist Joint, Percutaneous Approach

0RPP3JZ Removal of Synthetic Substitute from Left Wrist Joint, Percutaneous Approach

0RPP3KZ Removal of Nonautologous Tissue Substitute from Left Wrist Joint, Percutaneous Approach

0RPP40Z Removal of Drainage Device from Left Wrist Joint, Percutaneous Endoscopic Approach

0RPP43Z Removal of Infusion Device from Left Wrist Joint, Percutaneous Endoscopic Approach

0RPP44Z Removal of Internal Fixation Device from Left Wrist Joint, Percutaneous Endoscopic Approach

0RPP45Z Removal of External Fixation Device from Left Wrist Joint, Percutaneous Endoscopic Approach

0RPP47Z Removal of Autologous Tissue Substitute from Left Wrist Joint, Percutaneous Endoscopic Approach

0RPP48Z Removal of Spacer from Left Wrist Joint, Percutaneous Endoscopic Approach

0RPP4JZ Removal of Synthetic Substitute from Left Wrist Joint, Percutaneous Endoscopic Approach

0RPP4KZ Removal of Nonautologous Tissue Substitute from Left Wrist Joint, Percutaneous Endoscopic Approach

0RPPX0Z Removal of Drainage Device from Left Wrist Joint, External Approach

0RPPX3Z Removal of Infusion Device from Left Wrist Joint, External Approach

0RPPX4Z Removal of Internal Fixation Device from Left Wrist Joint, External Approach

0RPPX5Z Removal of External Fixation Device from Left Wrist Joint, External Approach

0RPQ00Z Removal of Drainage Device from Right Carpal Joint, Open Approach

0RPQ03Z Removal of Infusion Device from Right Carpal Joint, Open Approach
0RPQ04Z Removal of Internal Fixation Device from Right Carpal Joint, Open Approach
0RPQ05Z Removal of External Fixation Device from Right Carpal Joint, Open Approach
0RPQ07Z Removal of Autologous Tissue Substitute from Right Carpal Joint, Open Approach
0RPQ08Z Removal of Spacer from Right Carpal Joint, Open Approach
0RPQ0JZ Removal of Synthetic Substitute from Right Carpal Joint, Open Approach
0RPQ0KZ Removal of Nonautologous Tissue Substitute from Right Carpal Joint, Open Approach
0RPQ30Z Removal of Drainage Device from Right Carpal Joint, Percutaneous Approach
0RPQ33Z Removal of Infusion Device from Right Carpal Joint, Percutaneous Approach
0RPQ34Z Removal of Internal Fixation Device from Right Carpal Joint, Percutaneous Approach
0RPQ35Z Removal of External Fixation Device from Right Carpal Joint, Percutaneous Approach
0RPQ37Z Removal of Autologous Tissue Substitute from Right Carpal Joint, Percutaneous Approach
0RPQ38Z Removal of Spacer from Right Carpal Joint, Percutaneous Approach
0RPQ3JZ Removal of Synthetic Substitute from Right Carpal Joint, Percutaneous Approach
0RPQ3KZ Removal of Nonautologous Tissue Substitute from Right Carpal Joint, Percutaneous Approach
0RPQ40Z Removal of Drainage Device from Right Carpal Joint, Percutaneous Endoscopic Approach
0RPQ43Z Removal of Infusion Device from Right Carpal Joint, Percutaneous Endoscopic Approach
0RPQ44Z Removal of Internal Fixation Device from Right Carpal Joint, Percutaneous Endoscopic Approach
0RPQ45Z Removal of External Fixation Device from Right Carpal Joint, Percutaneous Endoscopic Approach
0RPQ47Z Removal of Autologous Tissue Substitute from Right Carpal Joint, Percutaneous Endoscopic Approach
0RPQ48Z Removal of Spacer from Right Carpal Joint, Percutaneous Endoscopic Approach
0RPQ4JZ Removal of Synthetic Substitute from Right Carpal Joint, Percutaneous Endoscopic Approach
0RPQ4KZ Removal of Nonautologous Tissue Substitute from Right Carpal Joint, Percutaneous Endoscopic Approach
0RPQX0Z Removal of Drainage Device from Right Carpal Joint, External Approach
0RPQX3Z Removal of Infusion Device from Right Carpal Joint, External Approach
0RPQX4Z Removal of Internal Fixation Device from Right Carpal Joint, External Approach
0RPQX5Z Removal of External Fixation Device from Right Carpal Joint, External Approach
0RPR00Z Removal of Drainage Device from Left Carpal Joint, Open Approach
0RPR03Z Removal of Infusion Device from Left Carpal Joint, Open Approach
0RPR04Z Removal of Internal Fixation Device from Left Carpal Joint, Open Approach
0RPR05Z Removal of External Fixation Device from Left Carpal Joint, Open Approach
0RPR07Z Removal of Autologous Tissue Substitute from Left Carpal Joint, Open Approach
0RPR08Z Removal of Spacer from Left Carpal Joint, Open Approach
0RPR0JZ Removal of Synthetic Substitute from Left Carpal Joint, Open Approach
0RPR0KZ Removal of Nonautologous Tissue Substitute from Left Carpal Joint, Open Approach
0RPR30Z Removal of Drainage Device from Left Carpal Joint, Percutaneous Approach
0RPR33Z Removal of Infusion Device from Left Carpal Joint, Percutaneous Approach
0RPR34Z Removal of Internal Fixation Device from Left Carpal Joint, Percutaneous Approach
0RPR35Z Removal of External Fixation Device from Left Carpal Joint, Percutaneous Approach
0RPR37Z Removal of Autologous Tissue Substitute from Left Carpal Joint, Percutaneous Approach
0RPR38Z Removal of Spacer from Left Carpal Joint, Percutaneous Approach
0RPR3JZ Removal of Synthetic Substitute from Left Carpal Joint, Percutaneous Approach
0RPR3KZ Removal of Nonautologous Tissue Substitute from Left Carpal Joint, Percutaneous Approach
0RPR40Z Removal of Drainage Device from Left Carpal Joint, Percutaneous Endoscopic Approach
0RPR43Z Removal of Infusion Device from Left Carpal Joint, Percutaneous Endoscopic Approach
0RPR44Z Removal of Internal Fixation Device from Left Carpal Joint, Percutaneous Endoscopic Approach
0RPR45Z Removal of External Fixation Device from Left Carpal Joint, Percutaneous Endoscopic Approach
0RPR47Z Removal of Autologous Tissue Substitute from Left Carpal Joint, Percutaneous Endoscopic Approach
0RPR48Z Removal of Spacer from Left Carpal Joint, Percutaneous Endoscopic Approach
0RPR4JZ Removal of Synthetic Substitute from Left Carpal Joint, Percutaneous Endoscopic Approach
0RPR4KZ Removal of Nonautologous Tissue Substitute from Left Carpal Joint, Percutaneous Endoscopic Approach
0RPRX0Z Removal of Drainage Device from Left Carpal Joint, External Approach
0RPRX3Z Removal of Infusion Device from Left Carpal Joint, External Approach
0RPRX4Z Removal of Internal Fixation Device from Left Carpal Joint, External Approach
0RPRX5Z Removal of External Fixation Device from Left Carpal Joint, External Approach
0RPS00Z Removal of Drainage Device from Right Metacarpocarpal Joint, Open Approach
0RPS03Z Removal of Infusion Device from Right Metacarpocarpal Joint, Open Approach
0RPS04Z Removal of Internal Fixation Device from Right Metacarpocarpal Joint, Open Approach
0RPS05Z Removal of External Fixation Device from Right Metacarpocarpal Joint, Open Approach
0RPS07Z Removal of Autologous Tissue Substitute from Right Metacarpocarpal Joint, Open Approach
0RPS08Z Removal of Spacer from Right Metacarpocarpal Joint, Open Approach
0RPS0JZ Removal of Synthetic Substitute from Right Metacarpocarpal Joint, Open Approach
0RPS0KZ Removal of Nonautologous Tissue Substitute from Right Metacarpocarpal Joint, Open Approach
0RPS30Z Removal of Drainage Device from Right Metacarpocarpal Joint, Percutaneous Approach
0RPS33Z Removal of Infusion Device from Right Metacarpocarpal Joint, Percutaneous Approach
0RPS34Z Removal of Internal Fixation Device from Right Metacarpocarpal Joint, Percutaneous Approach
0RPS35Z Removal of External Fixation Device from Right Metacarpocarpal Joint, Percutaneous Approach
0RPS37Z Removal of Autologous Tissue Substitute from Right Metacarpocarpal Joint, Percutaneous Approach
0RPS38Z Removal of Spacer from Right Metacarpocarpal Joint, Percutaneous Approach
0RPS3JZ Removal of Synthetic Substitute from Right Metacarpocarpal Joint, Percutaneous Approach
0RPS3KZ Removal of Nonautologous Tissue Substitute from Right Metacarpocarpal Joint, Percutaneous Approach
0RPS40Z Removal of Drainage Device from Right Metacarpocarpal Joint, Percutaneous Endoscopic Approach
0RPS43Z Removal of Infusion Device from Right Metacarpocarpal Joint, Percutaneous Endoscopic Approach
0RPS44Z Removal of Internal Fixation Device from Right Metacarpocarpal Joint, Percutaneous Endoscopic Approach
0RPS45Z Removal of External Fixation Device from Right Metacarpocarpal Joint, Percutaneous Endoscopic Approach
0RPS47Z Removal of Autologous Tissue Substitute from Right Metacarpocarpal Joint, Percutaneous Endoscopic Approach
0RPS48Z Removal of Spacer from Right Metacarpocarpal Joint, Percutaneous Endoscopic Approach
0RPS4JZ Removal of Synthetic Substitute from Right Metacarpocarpal Joint, Percutaneous Endoscopic Approach
0RPS4KZ Removal of Nonautologous Tissue Substitute from Right Metacarpocarpal Joint, Percutaneous Endoscopic Approach
0RPSX0Z Removal of Drainage Device from Right Metacarpocarpal Joint, External Approach
0RPSX3Z Removal of Infusion Device from Right Metacarpocarpal Joint, External Approach
0RPSX4Z Removal of Internal Fixation Device from Right Metacarpocarpal Joint, External Approach
0RPSX5Z Removal of External Fixation Device from Right Metacarpocarpal Joint, External Approach
0RPT00Z Removal of Drainage Device from Left Metacarpocarpal Joint, Open Approach
0RPT03Z Removal of Infusion Device from Left Metacarpocarpal Joint, Open Approach
0RPT04Z Removal of Internal Fixation Device from Left Metacarpocarpal Joint, Open Approach
0RPT05Z Removal of External Fixation Device from Left Metacarpocarpal Joint, Open Approach
0RPT07Z Removal of Autologous Tissue Substitute from Left Metacarpocarpal Joint, Open Approach
0RPT08Z Removal of Spacer from Left Metacarpocarpal Joint, Open Approach
0RPT0JZ Removal of Synthetic Substitute from Left Metacarpocarpal Joint, Open Approach
0RPT0KZ Removal of Nonautologous Tissue Substitute from Left Metacarpocarpal Joint, Open Approach

RPT30Z Removal of Drainage Device from Left Metacarpocarpal Joint, Percutaneous Approach

RPT33Z Removal of Infusion Device from Left Metacarpocarpal Joint, Percutaneous Approach

RPT34Z Removal of Internal Fixation Device from Left Metacarpocarpal Joint, Percutaneous Approach

RPT35Z Removal of External Fixation Device from Left Metacarpocarpal Joint, Percutaneous Approach

RPT37Z Removal of Autologous Tissue Substitute from Left Metacarpocarpal Joint, Percutaneous Approach

RPT38Z Removal of Spacer from Left Metacarpocarpal Joint, Percutaneous Approach

RPT3JZ Removal of Synthetic Substitute from Left Metacarpocarpal Joint, Percutaneous Approach

RPT3KZ Removal of Nonautologous Tissue Substitute from Left Metacarpocarpal Joint, Percutaneous Approach

RPT40Z Removal of Drainage Device from Left Metacarpocarpal Joint, Percutaneous Endoscopic Approach

RPT43Z Removal of Infusion Device from Left Metacarpocarpal Joint, Percutaneous Endoscopic Approach

RPT44Z Removal of Internal Fixation Device from Left Metacarpocarpal Joint, Percutaneous Endoscopic Approach

RPT45Z Removal of External Fixation Device from Left Metacarpocarpal Joint, Percutaneous Endoscopic Approach

0RPT47Z Removal of Autologous Tissue Substitute from Left Metacarpocarpal Joint, Percutaneous Endoscopic Approach

0RPT48Z Removal of Spacer from Left Metacarpocarpal Joint, Percutaneous Endoscopic Approach

0RPT4JZ Removal of Synthetic Substitute from Left Metacarpocarpal Joint, Percutaneous Endoscopic Approach

0RPT4KZ Removal of Nonautologous Tissue Substitute from Left Metacarpocarpal Joint, Percutaneous Endoscopic Approach

0RPTX0Z Removal of Drainage Device from Left Metacarpocarpal Joint, External Approach

0RPTX3Z Removal of Infusion Device from Left Metacarpocarpal Joint, External Approach

0RPTX4Z Removal of Internal Fixation Device from Left Metacarpocarpal Joint, External Approach

0RPTX5Z Removal of External Fixation Device from Left Metacarpocarpal Joint, External Approach

0RPU00Z Removal of Drainage Device from Right Metacarpophalangeal Joint, Open Approach

0RPU03Z Removal of Infusion Device from Right Metacarpophalangeal Joint, Open Approach

0RPU04Z Removal of Internal Fixation Device from Right Metacarpophalangeal Joint, Open Approach

0RPU05Z Removal of External Fixation Device from Right Metacarpophalangeal Joint, Open Approach

0RPU07Z Removal of Autologous Tissue Substitute from Right Metacarpophalangeal Joint, Open Approach

0RPU08Z Removal of Spacer from Right Metacarpophalangeal Joint, Open Approach

0RPU0JZ Removal of Synthetic Substitute from Right Metacarpophalangeal Joint, Open Approach

0RPU0KZ Removal of Nonautologous Tissue Substitute from Right Metacarpophalangeal Joint, Open Approach

0RPU30Z Removal of Drainage Device from Right Metacarpophalangeal Joint, Percutaneous Approach

0RPU33Z Removal of Infusion Device from Right Metacarpophalangeal Joint, Percutaneous Approach

0RPU34Z Removal of Internal Fixation Device from Right Metacarpophalangeal Joint, Percutaneous Approach

0RPU35Z Removal of External Fixation Device from Right Metacarpophalangeal Joint, Percutaneous Approach

0RPU37Z Removal of Autologous Tissue Substitute from Right Metacarpophalangeal Joint, Percutaneous Approach

0RPU38Z Removal of Spacer from Right Metacarpophalangeal Joint, Percutaneous Approach

0RPU3JZ Removal of Synthetic Substitute from Right Metacarpophalangeal Joint, Percutaneous Approach

0RPU3KZ Removal of Nonautologous Tissue Substitute from Right Metacarpophalangeal Joint, Percutaneous Approach

0RPU40Z Removal of Drainage Device from Right Metacarpophalangeal Joint, Percutaneous Endoscopic Approach

0RPU43Z Removal of Infusion Device from Right Metacarpophalangeal Joint, Percutaneous Endoscopic Approach

0RPU44Z Removal of Internal Fixation Device from Right Metacarpophalangeal Joint, Percutaneous Endoscopic Approach

0RPU45Z Removal of External Fixation Device from Right Metacarpophalangeal Joint, Percutaneous Endoscopic Approach

0RPU47Z Removal of Autologous Tissue Substitute from Right Metacarpophalangeal Joint, Percutaneous Endoscopic Approach

0RPU48Z Removal of Spacer from Right Metacarpophalangeal Joint, Percutaneous Endoscopic Approach

0RPU4JZ Removal of Synthetic Substitute from Right Metacarpophalangeal Joint, Percutaneous Endoscopic Approach

0RPU4KZ Removal of Nonautologous Tissue Substitute from Right Metacarpophalangeal Joint, Percutaneous Endoscopic Approach

0RPUX0Z Removal of Drainage Device from Right Metacarpophalangeal Joint, External Approach

0RPUX3Z Removal of Infusion Device from Right Metacarpophalangeal Joint, External Approach

0RPUX4Z Removal of Internal Fixation Device from Right Metacarpophalangeal Joint, External Approach

0RPUX5Z Removal of External Fixation Device from Right Metacarpophalangeal Joint, External Approach

0RPV00Z Removal of Drainage Device from Left Metacarpophalangeal Joint, Open Approach

0RPV03Z Removal of Infusion Device from Left Metacarpophalangeal Joint, Open Approach

0RPV04Z Removal of Internal Fixation Device from Left Metacarpophalangeal Joint, Open Approach

0RPV05Z Removal of External Fixation Device from Left Metacarpophalangeal Joint, Open Approach

0RPV07Z Removal of Autologous Tissue Substitute from Left Metacarpophalangeal Joint, Open Approach

0RPV08Z Removal of Spacer from Left Metacarpophalangeal Joint, Open Approach

0RPV0JZ Removal of Synthetic Substitute from Left Metacarpophalangeal Joint, Open Approach

0RPV0KZ Removal of Nonautologous Tissue Substitute from Left Metacarpophalangeal Joint, Open Approach

0RPV30Z Removal of Drainage Device from Left Metacarpophalangeal Joint, Percutaneous Approach

0RPV33Z Removal of Infusion Device from Left Metacarpophalangeal Joint, Percutaneous Approach

0RPV34Z Removal of Internal Fixation Device from Left Metacarpophalangeal Joint, Percutaneous Approach

0RPV35Z Removal of External Fixation Device from Left Metacarpophalangeal Joint, Percutaneous Approach

0RPV37Z Removal of Autologous Tissue Substitute from Left Metacarpophalangeal Joint, Percutaneous Approach

0RPV38Z Removal of Spacer from Left Metacarpophalangeal Joint, Percutaneous Approach

0RPV3JZ Removal of Synthetic Substitute from Left Metacarpophalangeal Joint, Percutaneous Approach

0RPV3KZ Removal of Nonautologous Tissue Substitute from Left Metacarpophalangeal Joint, Percutaneous Approach

0RPV40Z Removal of Drainage Device from Left Metacarpophalangeal Joint, Percutaneous Endoscopic Approach

0RPV43Z Removal of Infusion Device from Left Metacarpophalangeal Joint, Percutaneous Endoscopic Approach

0RPV44Z Removal of Internal Fixation Device from Left Metacarpophalangeal Joint, Percutaneous Endoscopic Approach

0RPV45Z Removal of External Fixation Device from Left Metacarpophalangeal Joint, Percutaneous Endoscopic Approach

0RPV47Z Removal of Autologous Tissue Substitute from Left Metacarpophalangeal Joint, Percutaneous Endoscopic Approach

0RPV48Z Removal of Spacer from Left Metacarpophalangeal Joint, Percutaneous Endoscopic Approach

0RPV4JZ Removal of Synthetic Substitute from Left Metacarpophalangeal Joint, Percutaneous Endoscopic Approach

0RPV4KZ Removal of Nonautologous Tissue Substitute from Left Metacarpophalangeal Joint, Percutaneous Endoscopic Approach

0RPVX0Z Removal of Drainage Device from Left Metacarpophalangeal Joint, External Approach

0RPVX3Z Removal of Infusion Device from Left Metacarpophalangeal Joint, External Approach

0RPVX4Z Removal of Internal Fixation Device from Left Metacarpophalangeal Joint, External Approach

0RPVX5Z Removal of External Fixation Device from Left Metacarpophalangeal Joint, External Approach

0RPW00Z Removal of Drainage Device from Right Finger Phalangeal Joint, Open Approach
0RPW03Z Removal of Infusion Device from Right Finger Phalangeal Joint, Open Approach
0RPW04Z Removal of Internal Fixation Device from Right Finger Phalangeal Joint, Open Approach
0RPW05Z Removal of External Fixation Device from Right Finger Phalangeal Joint, Open Approach
0RPW07Z Removal of Autologous Tissue Substitute from Right Finger Phalangeal Joint, Open Approach
0RPW08Z Removal of Spacer from Right Finger Phalangeal Joint, Open Approach
0RPW0JZ Removal of Synthetic Substitute from Right Finger Phalangeal Joint, Open Approach
0RPW0KZ Removal of Nonautologous Tissue Substitute from Right Finger Phalangeal Joint, Open Approach
0RPW30Z Removal of Drainage Device from Right Finger Phalangeal Joint, Percutaneous Approach
0RPW33Z Removal of Infusion Device from Right Finger Phalangeal Joint, Percutaneous Approach
0RPW34Z Removal of Internal Fixation Device from Right Finger Phalangeal Joint, Percutaneous Approach
0RPW35Z Removal of External Fixation Device from Right Finger Phalangeal Joint, Percutaneous Approach
0RPW37Z Removal of Autologous Tissue Substitute from Right Finger Phalangeal Joint, Percutaneous Approach
0RPW38Z Removal of Spacer from Right Finger Phalangeal Joint, Percutaneous Approach
0RPW3JZ Removal of Synthetic Substitute from Right Finger Phalangeal Joint, Percutaneous Approach
0RPW3KZ Removal of Nonautologous Tissue Substitute from Right Finger Phalangeal Joint, Percutaneous Approach
0RPW40Z Removal of Drainage Device from Right Finger Phalangeal Joint, Percutaneous Endoscopic Approach
0RPW43Z Removal of Infusion Device from Right Finger Phalangeal Joint, Percutaneous Endoscopic Approach
0RPW44Z Removal of Internal Fixation Device from Right Finger Phalangeal Joint, Percutaneous Endoscopic Approach
0RPW45Z Removal of External Fixation Device from Right Finger Phalangeal Joint, Percutaneous Endoscopic Approach
0RPW47Z Removal of Autologous Tissue Substitute from Right Finger Phalangeal Joint, Percutaneous Endoscopic Approach
0RPW48Z Removal of Spacer from Right Finger Phalangeal Joint, Percutaneous Endoscopic Approach
0RPW4JZ Removal of Synthetic Substitute from Right Finger Phalangeal Joint, Percutaneous Endoscopic Approach
0RPW4KZ Removal of Nonautologous Tissue Substitute from Right Finger Phalangeal Joint, Percutaneous Endoscopic Approach
0RPWX0Z Removal of Drainage Device from Right Finger Phalangeal Joint, External Approach
0RPWX3Z Removal of Infusion Device from Right Finger Phalangeal Joint, External Approach
0RPWX4Z Removal of Internal Fixation Device from Right Finger Phalangeal Joint, External Approach
0RPWX5Z Removal of External Fixation Device from Right Finger Phalangeal Joint, External Approach
0RPX00Z Removal of Drainage Device from Left Finger Phalangeal Joint, Open Approach
0RPX03Z Removal of Infusion Device from Left Finger Phalangeal Joint, Open Approach
0RPX04Z Removal of Internal Fixation Device from Left Finger Phalangeal Joint, Open Approach
0RPX05Z Removal of External Fixation Device from Left Finger Phalangeal Joint, Open Approach
0RPX07Z Removal of Autologous Tissue Substitute from Left Finger Phalangeal Joint, Open Approach
0RPX08Z Removal of Spacer from Left Finger Phalangeal Joint, Open Approach
0RPX0JZ Removal of Synthetic Substitute from Left Finger Phalangeal Joint, Open Approach
0RPX0KZ Removal of Nonautologous Tissue Substitute from Left Finger Phalangeal Joint, Open Approach
0RPX30Z Removal of Drainage Device from Left Finger Phalangeal Joint, Percutaneous Approach
0RPX33Z Removal of Infusion Device from Left Finger Phalangeal Joint, Percutaneous Approach
0RPX34Z Removal of Internal Fixation Device from Left Finger Phalangeal Joint, Percutaneous Approach
0RPX35Z Removal of External Fixation Device from Left Finger Phalangeal Joint, Percutaneous Approach
0RPX37Z Removal of Autologous Tissue Substitute from Left Finger Phalangeal Joint, Percutaneous Approach
0RPX38Z Removal of Spacer from Left Finger Phalangeal Joint, Percutaneous Approach
0RPX3JZ Removal of Synthetic Substitute from Left Finger Phalangeal Joint, Percutaneous Approach
0RPX3KZ Removal of Nonautologous Tissue Substitute from Left Finger Phalangeal Joint, Percutaneous Approach
0RPX40Z Removal of Drainage Device from Left Finger Phalangeal Joint, Percutaneous Endoscopic Approach
0RPX43Z Removal of Infusion Device from Left Finger Phalangeal Joint, Percutaneous Endoscopic Approach
0RPX44Z Removal of Internal Fixation Device from Left Finger Phalangeal Joint, Percutaneous Endoscopic Approach
0RPX45Z Removal of External Fixation Device from Left Finger Phalangeal Joint, Percutaneous Endoscopic Approach
0RPX47Z Removal of Autologous Tissue Substitute from Left Finger Phalangeal Joint, Percutaneous Endoscopic Approach
0RPX48Z Removal of Spacer from Left Finger Phalangeal Joint, Percutaneous Endoscopic Approach
0RPX4JZ Removal of Synthetic Substitute from Left Finger Phalangeal Joint, Percutaneous Endoscopic Approach
0RPX4KZ Removal of Nonautologous Tissue Substitute from Left Finger Phalangeal Joint, Percutaneous Endoscopic Approach
0RPXX0Z Removal of Drainage Device from Left Finger Phalangeal Joint, External Approach
0RPXX3Z Removal of Infusion Device from Left Finger Phalangeal Joint, External Approach
0RPXX4Z Removal of Internal Fixation Device from Left Finger Phalangeal Joint, External Approach
0RPXX5Z Removal of External Fixation Device from Left Finger Phalangeal Joint, External Approach

0RQ – Upper Joints, Repair

Review Coding Guideline B3.5

0RQ00ZZ Repair Occipital-cervical Joint, Open Approach
0RQ03ZZ Repair Occipital-cervical Joint, Percutaneous Approach
0RQ04ZZ Repair Occipital-cervical Joint, Percutaneous Endoscopic Approach
0RQ0XZZ Repair Occipital-cervical Joint, External Approach
0RQ10ZZ Repair Cervical Vertebral Joint, Open Approach
0RQ13ZZ Repair Cervical Vertebral Joint, Percutaneous Approach
0RQ14ZZ Repair Cervical Vertebral Joint, Percutaneous Endoscopic Approach
0RQ1XZZ Repair Cervical Vertebral Joint, External Approach
0RQ30ZZ Repair Cervical Vertebral Disc, Open Approach
0RQ33ZZ Repair Cervical Vertebral Disc, Percutaneous Approach
0RQ34ZZ Repair Cervical Vertebral Disc, Percutaneous Endoscopic Approach
0RQ3XZZ Repair Cervical Vertebral Disc, External Approach
0RQ40ZZ Repair Cervicothoracic Vertebral Joint, Open Approach
0RQ43ZZ Repair Cervicothoracic Vertebral Joint, Percutaneous Approach
0RQ44ZZ Repair Cervicothoracic Vertebral Joint, Percutaneous Endoscopic Approach
0RQ4XZZ Repair Cervicothoracic Vertebral Joint, External Approach
0RQ50ZZ Repair Cervicothoracic Vertebral Disc, Open Approach
0RQ53ZZ Repair Cervicothoracic Vertebral Disc, Percutaneous Approach
0RQ54ZZ Repair Cervicothoracic Vertebral Disc, Percutaneous Endoscopic Approach
0RQ5XZZ Repair Cervicothoracic Vertebral Disc, External Approach
0RQ60ZZ Repair Thoracic Vertebral Joint, Open Approach
0RQ63ZZ Repair Thoracic Vertebral Joint, Percutaneous Approach
0RQ64ZZ Repair Thoracic Vertebral Joint, Percutaneous Endoscopic Approach
0RQ6XZZ Repair Thoracic Vertebral Joint, External Approach

RQ90ZZ Repair Thoracic Vertebral Disc, Open Approach

RQ93ZZ Repair Thoracic Vertebral Disc, Percutaneous Approach

RQ94ZZ Repair Thoracic Vertebral Disc, Percutaneous Endoscopic Approach

RQ9XZZ Repair Thoracic Vertebral Disc, External Approach

RQA0ZZ Repair Thoracolumbar Vertebral Joint, Open Approach

RQA3ZZ Repair Thoracolumbar Vertebral Joint, Percutaneous Approach

RQA4ZZ Repair Thoracolumbar Vertebral Joint, Percutaneous Endoscopic Approach

RQAXZZ Repair Thoracolumbar Vertebral Joint, External Approach

RQB0ZZ Repair Thoracolumbar Vertebral Disc, Open Approach

RQB3ZZ Repair Thoracolumbar Vertebral Disc, Percutaneous Approach

RQB4ZZ Repair Thoracolumbar Vertebral Disc, Percutaneous Endoscopic Approach

RQBXZZ Repair Thoracolumbar Vertebral Disc, External Approach

RQC0ZZ Repair Right Temporomandibular Joint, Open Approach

RQC3ZZ Repair Right Temporomandibular Joint, Percutaneous Approach

RQC4ZZ Repair Right Temporomandibular Joint, Percutaneous Endoscopic Approach

RQCXZZ Repair Right Temporomandibular Joint, External Approach

RQD0ZZ Repair Left Temporomandibular Joint, Open Approach

RQD3ZZ Repair Left Temporomandibular Joint, Percutaneous Approach

RQD4ZZ Repair Left Temporomandibular Joint, Percutaneous Endoscopic Approach

RQDXZZ Repair Left Temporomandibular Joint, External Approach

RQE0ZZ Repair Right Sternoclavicular Joint, Open Approach

HAC When reported with secondary diagnosis code T84.60XA, T84.610A, T84.611A, T84.612A, T84.613A, T84.614A, T84.615A, T84.619A, T84.63XA, T84.69XA, T84.7XXA

RQE3ZZ Repair Right Sternoclavicular Joint, Percutaneous Approach

HAC When reported with secondary diagnosis code T84.60XA, T84.610A, T84.611A, T84.612A, T84.613A, T84.614A, T84.615A, T84.619A, T84.63XA, T84.69XA, T84.7XXA

RQE4ZZ Repair Right Sternoclavicular Joint, Percutaneous Endoscopic Approach

HAC When reported with secondary diagnosis code T84.60XA, T84.610A, T84.611A, T84.612A, T84.613A, T84.614A, T84.615A, T84.619A, T84.63XA, T84.69XA, T84.7XXA

RQEXZZ Repair Right Sternoclavicular Joint, External Approach

HAC When reported with secondary diagnosis code T84.60XA, T84.610A, T84.611A, T84.612A, T84.613A, T84.614A, T84.615A, T84.619A, T84.63XA, T84.69XA, T84.7XXA

RQF0ZZ Repair Left Sternoclavicular Joint, Open Approach

HAC When reported with secondary diagnosis code T84.60XA, T84.610A, T84.611A, T84.612A, T84.613A, T84.614A, T84.615A, T84.619A, T84.63XA, T84.69XA, T84.7XXA

0RQF3ZZ Repair Left Sternoclavicular Joint, Percutaneous Approach

HAC When reported with secondary diagnosis code T84.60XA, T84.610A, T84.611A, T84.612A, T84.613A, T84.614A, T84.615A, T84.619A, T84.63XA, T84.69XA, T84.7XXA

0RQF4ZZ Repair Left Sternoclavicular Joint, Percutaneous Endoscopic Approach

HAC When reported with secondary diagnosis code T84.60XA, T84.610A, T84.611A, T84.612A, T84.613A, T84.614A, T84.615A, T84.619A, T84.63XA, T84.69XA, T84.7XXA

0RQFXZZ Repair Left Sternoclavicular Joint, External Approach

HAC When reported with secondary diagnosis code T84.60XA, T84.610A, T84.611A, T84.612A, T84.613A, T84.614A, T84.615A, T84.619A, T84.63XA, T84.69XA, T84.7XXA

0RQG0ZZ Repair Right Acromioclavicular Joint, Open Approach

HAC When reported with secondary diagnosis code T84.60XA, T84.610A, T84.611A, T84.612A, T84.613A, T84.614A, T84.615A, T84.619A, T84.63XA, T84.69XA, T84.7XXA

0RQG3ZZ Repair Right Acromioclavicular Joint, Percutaneous Approach

HAC When reported with secondary diagnosis code T84.60XA, T84.610A, T84.611A, T84.612A, T84.613A, T84.614A, T84.615A, T84.619A, T84.63XA, T84.69XA, T84.7XXA

0RQG4ZZ Repair Right Acromioclavicular Joint, Percutaneous Endoscopic Approach

HAC When reported with secondary diagnosis code T84.60XA, T84.610A, T84.611A, T84.612A, T84.613A, T84.614A, T84.615A, T84.619A, T84.63XA, T84.69XA, T84.7XXA

0RQGXZZ Repair Right Acromioclavicular Joint, External Approach

HAC When reported with secondary diagnosis code T84.60XA, T84.610A, T84.611A, T84.612A, T84.613A, T84.614A, T84.615A, T84.619A, T84.63XA, T84.69XA, T84.7XXA

0RQH0ZZ Repair Left Acromioclavicular Joint, Open Approach

HAC When reported with secondary diagnosis code T84.60XA, T84.610A, T84.611A, T84.612A, T84.613A, T84.614A, T84.615A, T84.619A, T84.63XA, T84.69XA, T84.7XXA

0RQH3ZZ Repair Left Acromioclavicular Joint, Percutaneous Approach

HAC When reported with secondary diagnosis code T84.60XA, T84.610A, T84.611A, T84.612A, T84.613A, T84.614A, T84.615A, T84.619A, T84.63XA, T84.69XA, T84.7XXA

0RQH4ZZ Repair Left Acromioclavicular Joint, Percutaneous Endoscopic Approach

HAC When reported with secondary diagnosis code T84.60XA, T84.610A, T84.611A, T84.612A, T84.613A, T84.614A, T84.615A, T84.619A, T84.63XA, T84.69XA, T84.7XXA

0RQHXZZ Repair Left Acromioclavicular Joint, External Approach

HAC When reported with secondary diagnosis code T84.60XA, T84.610A, T84.611A, T84.612A, T84.613A, T84.614A, T84.615A, T84.619A, T84.63XA, T84.69XA, T84.7XXA

0RQJ0ZZ Repair Right Shoulder Joint, Open Approach

HAC When reported with secondary diagnosis code T84.60XA, T84.610A, T84.611A, T84.612A, T84.613A, T84.614A, T84.615A, T84.619A, T84.63XA, T84.69XA, T84.7XXA

0RQJ3ZZ Repair Right Shoulder Joint, Percutaneous Approach

HAC When reported with secondary diagnosis code T84.60XA, T84.610A, T84.611A, T84.612A, T84.613A, T84.614A, T84.615A, T84.619A, T84.63XA, T84.69XA, T84.7XXA

0RQJ4ZZ Repair Right Shoulder Joint, Percutaneous Endoscopic Approach

HAC When reported with secondary diagnosis code T84.60XA, T84.610A, T84.611A, T84.612A, T84.613A, T84.614A, T84.615A, T84.619A, T84.63XA, T84.69XA, T84.7XXA

0RQJXZZ Repair Right Shoulder Joint, External Approach

HAC When reported with secondary diagnosis code T84.60XA, T84.610A, T84.611A, T84.612A, T84.613A, T84.614A, T84.615A, T84.619A, T84.63XA, T84.69XA, T84.7XXA

0RQK0ZZ Repair Left Shoulder Joint, Open Approach

HAC When reported with secondary diagnosis code T84.60XA, T84.610A, T84.611A, T84.612A, T84.613A, T84.614A, T84.615A, T84.619A, T84.63XA, T84.69XA, T84.7XXA

0RQK3ZZ Repair Left Shoulder Joint, Percutaneous Approach

HAC When reported with secondary diagnosis code T84.60XA, T84.610A, T84.611A, T84.612A, T84.613A, T84.614A, T84.615A, T84.619A, T84.63XA, T84.69XA, T84.7XXA

0RQK4ZZ Repair Left Shoulder Joint, Percutaneous Endoscopic Approach

HAC When reported with secondary diagnosis code T84.60XA, T84.610A, T84.611A, T84.612A, T84.613A, T84.614A, T84.615A, T84.619A, T84.63XA, T84.69XA, T84.7XXA

0RQKXZZ Repair Left Shoulder Joint, External Approach

HAC When reported with secondary diagnosis code T84.60XA, T84.610A, T84.611A, T84.612A, T84.613A, T84.614A, T84.615A, T84.619A, T84.63XA, T84.69XA, T84.7XXA

0RQL0ZZ Repair Right Elbow Joint, Open Approach

HAC When reported with secondary diagnosis code T84.60XA, T84.610A, T84.611A, T84.612A, T84.613A, T84.614A, T84.615A, T84.619A, T84.63XA, T84.69XA, T84.7XXA

0RQL3ZZ Repair Right Elbow Joint, Percutaneous Approach

HAC When reported with secondary diagnosis code T84.60XA, T84.610A, T84.611A, T84.612A, T84.613A, T84.614A, T84.615A, T84.619A, T84.63XA, T84.69XA, T84.7XXA

0RQL4ZZ Repair Right Elbow Joint, Percutaneous Endoscopic Approach

HAC When reported with secondary diagnosis code T84.60XA, T84.610A, T84.611A, T84.612A, T84.613A, T84.614A, T84.615A, T84.619A, T84.63XA, T84.69XA, T84.7XXA

0RQLXZZ Repair Right Elbow Joint, External Approach
HAC When reported with secondary diagnosis code T84.60XA, T84.610A, T84.611A, T84.612A, T84.613A, T84.614A, T84.615A, T84.619A, T84.63XA, T84.69XA, T84.7XXA
0RQM0ZZ Repair Left Elbow Joint, Open Approach
HAC When reported with secondary diagnosis code T84.60XA, T84.610A, T84.611A, T84.612A, T84.613A, T84.614A, T84.615A, T84.619A, T84.63XA, T84.69XA, T84.7XXA
0RQM3ZZ Repair Left Elbow Joint, Percutaneous Approach
HAC When reported with secondary diagnosis code T84.60XA, T84.610A, T84.611A, T84.612A, T84.613A, T84.614A, T84.615A, T84.619A, T84.63XA, T84.69XA, T84.7XXA
0RQM4ZZ Repair Left Elbow Joint, Percutaneous Endoscopic Approach
HAC When reported with secondary diagnosis code T84.60XA, T84.610A, T84.611A, T84.612A, T84.613A, T84.614A, T84.615A, T84.619A, T84.63XA, T84.69XA, T84.7XXA
0RQMXZZ Repair Left Elbow Joint, External Approach
HAC When reported with secondary diagnosis code T84.60XA, T84.610A, T84.611A, T84.612A, T84.613A, T84.614A, T84.615A, T84.619A, T84.63XA, T84.69XA, T84.7XXA
0RQN0ZZ Repair Right Wrist Joint, Open Approach
0RQN3ZZ Repair Right Wrist Joint, Percutaneous Approach
0RQN4ZZ Repair Right Wrist Joint, Percutaneous Endoscopic Approach
0RQNXZZ Repair Right Wrist Joint, External Approach
0RQP0ZZ Repair Left Wrist Joint, Open Approach
0RQP3ZZ Repair Left Wrist Joint, Percutaneous Approach
0RQP4ZZ Repair Left Wrist Joint, Percutaneous Endoscopic Approach
0RQPXZZ Repair Left Wrist Joint, External Approach
0RQQ0ZZ Repair Right Carpal Joint, Open Approach
0RQQ3ZZ Repair Right Carpal Joint, Percutaneous Approach
0RQQ4ZZ Repair Right Carpal Joint, Percutaneous Endoscopic Approach
0RQQXZZ Repair Right Carpal Joint, External Approach
0RQR0ZZ Repair Left Carpal Joint, Open Approach
0RQR3ZZ Repair Left Carpal Joint, Percutaneous Approach
0RQR4ZZ Repair Left Carpal Joint, Percutaneous Endoscopic Approach
0RQRXZZ Repair Left Carpal Joint, External Approach
0RQS0ZZ Repair Right Metacarpocarpal Joint, Open Approach
0RQS3ZZ Repair Right Metacarpocarpal Joint, Percutaneous Approach
0RQS4ZZ Repair Right Metacarpocarpal Joint, Percutaneous Endoscopic Approach
0RQSXZZ Repair Right Metacarpocarpal Joint, External Approach
0RQT0ZZ Repair Left Metacarpocarpal Joint, Open Approach
0RQT3ZZ Repair Left Metacarpocarpal Joint, Percutaneous Approach
0RQT4ZZ Repair Left Metacarpocarpal Joint, Percutaneous Endoscopic Approach
0RQTXZZ Repair Left Metacarpocarpal Joint, External Approach
0RQU0ZZ Repair Right Metacarpophalangeal Joint, Open Approach
0RQU3ZZ Repair Right Metacarpophalangeal Joint, Percutaneous Approach
0RQU4ZZ Repair Right Metacarpophalangeal Joint, Percutaneous Endoscopic Approach
0RQUXZZ Repair Right Metacarpophalangeal Joint, External Approach
0RQV0ZZ Repair Left Metacarpophalangeal Joint, Open Approach
0RQV3ZZ Repair Left Metacarpophalangeal Joint, Percutaneous Approach
0RQV4ZZ Repair Left Metacarpophalangeal Joint, Percutaneous Endoscopic Approach
0RQVXZZ Repair Left Metacarpophalangeal Joint, External Approach
0RQW0ZZ Repair Right Finger Phalangeal Joint, Open Approach
0RQW3ZZ Repair Right Finger Phalangeal Joint, Percutaneous Approach
0RQW4ZZ Repair Right Finger Phalangeal Joint, Percutaneous Endoscopic Approach
0RQWXZZ Repair Right Finger Phalangeal Joint, External Approach
0RQX0ZZ Repair Left Finger Phalangeal Joint, Open Approach
0RQX3ZZ Repair Left Finger Phalangeal Joint, Percutaneous Approach
0RQX4ZZ Repair Left Finger Phalangeal Joint, Percutaneous Endoscopic Approach
0RQXXZZ Repair Left Finger Phalangeal Joint, External Approach

0RR – Upper Joints, Replacement

0RR007Z Replacement of Occipital-cervical Joint with Autologous Tissue Substitute, Open Approach
0RR00JZ Replacement of Occipital-cervical Joint with Synthetic Substitute, Open Approach
0RR00KZ Replacement of Occipital-cervical Joint with Nonautologous Tissue Substitute, Open Approach
0RR107Z Replacement of Cervical Vertebral Joint with Autologous Tissue Substitute, Open Approach
0RR10JZ Replacement of Cervical Vertebral Joint with Synthetic Substitute, Open Approach
0RR10KZ Replacement of Cervical Vertebral Joint with Nonautologous Tissue Substitute, Open Approach
0RR307Z Replacement of Cervical Vertebral Disc with Autologous Tissue Substitute, Open Approach
0RR30JZ Replacement of Cervical Vertebral Disc with Synthetic Substitute, Open Approach
0RR30KZ Replacement of Cervical Vertebral Disc with Nonautologous Tissue Substitute, Open Approach
0RR407Z Replacement of Cervicothoracic Vertebral Joint with Autologous Tissue Substitute, Open Approach
0RR40JZ Replacement of Cervicothoracic Vertebral Joint with Synthetic Substitute, Open Approach
0RR40KZ Replacement of Cervicothoracic Vertebral Joint with Nonautologous Tissue Substitute, Open Approach
0RR507Z Replacement of Cervicothoracic Vertebral Disc with Autologous Tissue Substitute, Open Approach
0RR50JZ Replacement of Cervicothoracic Vertebral Disc with Synthetic Substitute, Open Approach
0RR50KZ Replacement of Cervicothoracic Vertebral Disc with Nonautologous Tissue Substitute, Open Approach
0RR607Z Replacement of Thoracic Vertebral Joint with Autologous Tissue Substitute, Open Approach
0RR60JZ Replacement of Thoracic Vertebral Joint with Synthetic Substitute, Open Approach
0RR60KZ Replacement of Thoracic Vertebral Joint with Nonautologous Tissue Substitute, Open Approach
0RR907Z Replacement of Thoracic Vertebral Disc with Autologous Tissue Substitute, Open Approach
0RR90JZ Replacement of Thoracic Vertebral Disc with Synthetic Substitute, Open Approach
0RR90KZ Replacement of Thoracic Vertebral Disc with Nonautologous Tissue Substitute, Open Approach
0RRA07Z Replacement of Thoracolumbar Vertebral Joint with Autologous Tissue Substitute, Open Approach
0RRA0JZ Replacement of Thoracolumbar Vertebral Joint with Synthetic Substitute, Open Approach
0RRA0KZ Replacement of Thoracolumbar Vertebral Joint with Nonautologous Tissue Substitute, Open Approach
0RRB07Z Replacement of Thoracolumbar Vertebral Disc with Autologous Tissue Substitute, Open Approach
0RRB0JZ Replacement of Thoracolumbar Vertebral Disc with Synthetic Substitute, Open Approach
0RRB0KZ Replacement of Thoracolumbar Vertebral Disc with Nonautologous Tissue Substitute, Open Approach
0RRC07Z Replacement of Right Temporomandibular Joint with Autologous Tissue Substitute, Open Approach
0RRC0JZ Replacement of Right Temporomandibular Joint with Synthetic Substitute, Open Approach
0RRC0KZ Replacement of Right Temporomandibular Joint with Nonautologous Tissue Substitute, Open Approach
0RRD07Z Replacement of Left Temporomandibular Joint with Autologous Tissue Substitute, Open Approach
0RRD0JZ Replacement of Left Temporomandibular Joint with Synthetic Substitute, Open Approach
0RRD0KZ Replacement of Left Temporomandibular Joint with Nonautologous Tissue Substitute, Open Approach
0RRE07Z Replacement of Right Sternoclavicular Joint with Autologous Tissue Substitute, Open Approach
0RRE0JZ Replacement of Right Sternoclavicular Joint with Synthetic Substitute, Open Approach
0RRE0KZ Replacement of Right Sternoclavicular Joint with Nonautologous Tissue Substitute, Open Approach
0RRF07Z Replacement of Left Sternoclavicular Joint with Autologous Tissue Substitute, Open Approach
0RRF0JZ Replacement of Left Sternoclavicular Joint with Synthetic Substitute, Open Approach

RRF0KZ Replacement of Left Sternoclavicular Joint with Nonautologous Tissue Substitute, Open Approach
RRG07Z Replacement of Right Acromioclavicular Joint with Autologous Tissue Substitute, Open Approach
RRG0JZ Replacement of Right Acromioclavicular Joint with Synthetic Substitute, Open Approach
RRG0KZ Replacement of Right Acromioclavicular Joint with Nonautologous Tissue Substitute, Open Approach
RRH07Z Replacement of Left Acromioclavicular Joint with Autologous Tissue Substitute, Open Approach
0RRH0JZ Replacement of Left Acromioclavicular Joint with Synthetic Substitute, Open Approach
0RRH0KZ Replacement of Left Acromioclavicular Joint with Nonautologous Tissue Substitute, Open Approach
0RRJ00Z Replacement of Right Shoulder Joint with Reverse Ball and Socket Synthetic Substitute, Open Approach
0RRJ07Z Replacement of Right Shoulder Joint with Autologous Tissue Substitute, Open Approach
0RRJ0J6 Replacement of Right Shoulder Joint with Synthetic Substitute, Humeral Surface, Open Approach
0RRJ0J7 Replacement of Right Shoulder Joint with Synthetic Substitute, Glenoid Surface, Open Approach
0RRJ0JZ Replacement of Right Shoulder Joint with Synthetic Substitute, Open Approach
0RRJ0KZ Replacement of Right Shoulder Joint with Nonautologous Tissue Substitute, Open Approach
0RRK00Z Replacement of Left Shoulder Joint with Reverse Ball and Socket Synthetic Substitute, Open Approach
0RRK07Z Replacement of Left Shoulder Joint with Autologous Tissue Substitute, Open Approach
0RRK0J6 Replacement of Left Shoulder Joint with Synthetic Substitute, Humeral Surface, Open Approach
0RRK0J7 Replacement of Left Shoulder Joint with Synthetic Substitute, Glenoid Surface, Open Approach
0RRK0JZ Replacement of Left Shoulder Joint with Synthetic Substitute, Open Approach
0RRK0KZ Replacement of Left Shoulder Joint with Nonautologous Tissue Substitute, Open Approach
0RRL07Z Replacement of Right Elbow Joint with Autologous Tissue Substitute, Open Approach
0RRL0JZ Replacement of Right Elbow Joint with Synthetic Substitute, Open Approach
0RRL0KZ Replacement of Right Elbow Joint with Nonautologous Tissue Substitute, Open Approach
0RRM07Z Replacement of Left Elbow Joint with Autologous Tissue Substitute, Open Approach
0RRM0JZ Replacement of Left Elbow Joint with Synthetic Substitute, Open Approach
0RRM0KZ Replacement of Left Elbow Joint with Nonautologous Tissue Substitute, Open Approach
0RRN07Z Replacement of Right Wrist Joint with Autologous Tissue Substitute, Open Approach
0RRN0JZ Replacement of Right Wrist Joint with Synthetic Substitute, Open Approach
0RRN0KZ Replacement of Right Wrist Joint with Nonautologous Tissue Substitute, Open Approach
0RRP07Z Replacement of Left Wrist Joint with Autologous Tissue Substitute, Open Approach
0RRP0JZ Replacement of Left Wrist Joint with Synthetic Substitute, Open Approach
0RRP0KZ Replacement of Left Wrist Joint with Nonautologous Tissue Substitute, Open Approach
0RRQ07Z Replacement of Right Carpal Joint with Autologous Tissue Substitute, Open Approach
0RRQ0JZ Replacement of Right Carpal Joint with Synthetic Substitute, Open Approach
0RRQ0KZ Replacement of Right Carpal Joint with Nonautologous Tissue Substitute, Open Approach
0RRR07Z Replacement of Left Carpal Joint with Autologous Tissue Substitute, Open Approach
0RRR0JZ Replacement of Left Carpal Joint with Synthetic Substitute, Open Approach
0RRR0KZ Replacement of Left Carpal Joint with Nonautologous Tissue Substitute, Open Approach
0RRS07Z Replacement of Right Metacarpocarpal Joint with Autologous Tissue Substitute, Open Approach
0RRS0JZ Replacement of Right Metacarpocarpal Joint with Synthetic Substitute, Open Approach
0RRS0KZ Replacement of Right Metacarpocarpal Joint with Nonautologous Tissue Substitute, Open Approach
0RRT07Z Replacement of Left Metacarpocarpal Joint with Autologous Tissue Substitute, Open Approach
0RRT0JZ Replacement of Left Metacarpocarpal Joint with Synthetic Substitute, Open Approach
0RRT0KZ Replacement of Left Metacarpocarpal Joint with Nonautologous Tissue Substitute, Open Approach
0RRU07Z Replacement of Right Metacarpophalangeal Joint with Autologous Tissue Substitute, Open Approach
0RRU0JZ Replacement of Right Metacarpophalangeal Joint with Synthetic Substitute, Open Approach
0RRU0KZ Replacement of Right Metacarpophalangeal Joint with Nonautologous Tissue Substitute, Open Approach
0RRV07Z Replacement of Left Metacarpophalangeal Joint with Autologous Tissue Substitute, Open Approach
0RRV0JZ Replacement of Left Metacarpophalangeal Joint with Synthetic Substitute, Open Approach
0RRV0KZ Replacement of Left Metacarpophalangeal Joint with Nonautologous Tissue Substitute, Open Approach
0RRW07Z Replacement of Right Finger Phalangeal Joint with Autologous Tissue Substitute, Open Approach
0RRW0JZ Replacement of Right Finger Phalangeal Joint with Synthetic Substitute, Open Approach
0RRW0KZ Replacement of Right Finger Phalangeal Joint with Nonautologous Tissue Substitute, Open Approach
0RRX07Z Replacement of Left Finger Phalangeal Joint with Autologous Tissue Substitute, Open Approach
0RRX0JZ Replacement of Left Finger Phalangeal Joint with Synthetic Substitute, Open Approach
0RRX0KZ Replacement of Left Finger Phalangeal Joint with Nonautologous Tissue Substitute, Open Approach

0RS – Upper Joints, Reposition

0RS004Z Reposition Occipital-cervical Joint with Internal Fixation Device, Open Approach
0RS00ZZ Reposition Occipital-cervical Joint, Open Approach
0RS034Z Reposition Occipital-cervical Joint with Internal Fixation Device, Percutaneous Approach
0RS03ZZ Reposition Occipital-cervical Joint, Percutaneous Approach
0RS044Z Reposition Occipital-cervical Joint with Internal Fixation Device, Percutaneous Endoscopic Approach
0RS04ZZ Reposition Occipital-cervical Joint, Percutaneous Endoscopic Approach
0RS0X4Z Reposition Occipital-cervical Joint with Internal Fixation Device, External Approach
0RS0XZZ Reposition Occipital-cervical Joint, External Approach
0RS104Z Reposition Cervical Vertebral Joint with Internal Fixation Device, Open Approach
0RS10ZZ Reposition Cervical Vertebral Joint, Open Approach
0RS134Z Reposition Cervical Vertebral Joint with Internal Fixation Device, Percutaneous Approach
0RS13ZZ Reposition Cervical Vertebral Joint, Percutaneous Approach
0RS144Z Reposition Cervical Vertebral Joint with Internal Fixation Device, Percutaneous Endoscopic Approach
0RS14ZZ Reposition Cervical Vertebral Joint, Percutaneous Endoscopic Approach
0RS1X4Z Reposition Cervical Vertebral Joint with Internal Fixation Device, External Approach
0RS1XZZ Reposition Cervical Vertebral Joint, External Approach
AHA CC: 2Q, 2013, 39
0RS404Z Reposition Cervicothoracic Vertebral Joint with Internal Fixation Device, Open Approach
0RS40ZZ Reposition Cervicothoracic Vertebral Joint, Open Approach
0RS434Z Reposition Cervicothoracic Vertebral Joint with Internal Fixation Device, Percutaneous Approach
0RS43ZZ Reposition Cervicothoracic Vertebral Joint, Percutaneous Approach
0RS444Z Reposition Cervicothoracic Vertebral Joint with Internal Fixation Device, Percutaneous Endoscopic Approach
0RS44ZZ Reposition Cervicothoracic Vertebral Joint, Percutaneous Endoscopic Approach
0RS4X4Z Reposition Cervicothoracic Vertebral Joint with Internal Fixation Device, External Approach
0RS4XZZ Reposition Cervicothoracic Vertebral Joint, External Approach

0RS604Z Reposition Thoracic Vertebral Joint with Internal Fixation Device, Open Approach
0RS60ZZ Reposition Thoracic Vertebral Joint, Open Approach
0RS634Z Reposition Thoracic Vertebral Joint with Internal Fixation Device, Percutaneous Approach
0RS63ZZ Reposition Thoracic Vertebral Joint, Percutaneous Approach
0RS644Z Reposition Thoracic Vertebral Joint with Internal Fixation Device, Percutaneous Endoscopic Approach
0RS64ZZ Reposition Thoracic Vertebral Joint, Percutaneous Endoscopic Approach
0RS6X4Z Reposition Thoracic Vertebral Joint with Internal Fixation Device, External Approach
0RS6XZZ Reposition Thoracic Vertebral Joint, External Approach
0RSA04Z Reposition Thoracolumbar Vertebral Joint with Internal Fixation Device, Open Approach
0RSA0ZZ Reposition Thoracolumbar Vertebral Joint, Open Approach
0RSA34Z Reposition Thoracolumbar Vertebral Joint with Internal Fixation Device, Percutaneous Approach
0RSA3ZZ Reposition Thoracolumbar Vertebral Joint, Percutaneous Approach
0RSA44Z Reposition Thoracolumbar Vertebral Joint with Internal Fixation Device, Percutaneous Endoscopic Approach
0RSA4ZZ Reposition Thoracolumbar Vertebral Joint, Percutaneous Endoscopic Approach
0RSAX4Z Reposition Thoracolumbar Vertebral Joint with Internal Fixation Device, External Approach
0RSAXZZ Reposition Thoracolumbar Vertebral Joint, External Approach
0RSC04Z Reposition Right Temporomandibular Joint with Internal Fixation Device, Open Approach
0RSC0ZZ Reposition Right Temporomandibular Joint, Open Approach
0RSC34Z Reposition Right Temporomandibular Joint with Internal Fixation Device, Percutaneous Approach
0RSC3ZZ Reposition Right Temporomandibular Joint, Percutaneous Approach
0RSC44Z Reposition Right Temporomandibular Joint with Internal Fixation Device, Percutaneous Endoscopic Approach
0RSC4ZZ Reposition Right Temporomandibular Joint, Percutaneous Endoscopic Approach
0RSCX4Z Reposition Right Temporomandibular Joint with Internal Fixation Device, External Approach
0RSCXZZ Reposition Right Temporomandibular Joint, External Approach
0RSD04Z Reposition Left Temporomandibular Joint with Internal Fixation Device, Open Approach
0RSD0ZZ Reposition Left Temporomandibular Joint, Open Approach
0RSD34Z Reposition Left Temporomandibular Joint with Internal Fixation Device, Percutaneous Approach
0RSD3ZZ Reposition Left Temporomandibular Joint, Percutaneous Approach
0RSD44Z Reposition Left Temporomandibular Joint with Internal Fixation Device, Percutaneous Endoscopic Approach
0RSD4ZZ Reposition Left Temporomandibular Joint, Percutaneous Endoscopic Approach
0RSDX4Z Reposition Left Temporomandibular Joint with Internal Fixation Device, External Approach
0RSDXZZ Reposition Left Temporomandibular Joint, External Approach
0RSE04Z Reposition Right Sternoclavicular Joint with Internal Fixation Device, Open Approach
0RSE0ZZ Reposition Right Sternoclavicular Joint, Open Approach
0RSE34Z Reposition Right Sternoclavicular Joint with Internal Fixation Device, Percutaneous Approach
0RSE3ZZ Reposition Right Sternoclavicular Joint, Percutaneous Approach
0RSE44Z Reposition Right Sternoclavicular Joint with Internal Fixation Device, Percutaneous Endoscopic Approach
0RSE4ZZ Reposition Right Sternoclavicular Joint, Percutaneous Endoscopic Approach
0RSEX4Z Reposition Right Sternoclavicular Joint with Internal Fixation Device, External Approach
0RSEXZZ Reposition Right Sternoclavicular Joint, External Approach
0RSF04Z Reposition Left Sternoclavicular Joint with Internal Fixation Device, Open Approach
0RSF0ZZ Reposition Left Sternoclavicular Joint, Open Approach
0RSF34Z Reposition Left Sternoclavicular Joint with Internal Fixation Device, Percutaneous Approach
0RSF3ZZ Reposition Left Sternoclavicular Joint, Percutaneous Approach
0RSF44Z Reposition Left Sternoclavicular Joint with Internal Fixation Device, Percutaneous Endoscopic Approach
0RSF4ZZ Reposition Left Sternoclavicular Joint, Percutaneous Endoscopic Approach
0RSFX4Z Reposition Left Sternoclavicular Joint with Internal Fixation Device, External Approach
0RSFXZZ Reposition Left Sternoclavicular Joint, External Approach
0RSG04Z Reposition Right Acromioclavicular Joint with Internal Fixation Device, Open Approach
0RSG0ZZ Reposition Right Acromioclavicular Joint, Open Approach
0RSG34Z Reposition Right Acromioclavicular Joint with Internal Fixation Device, Percutaneous Approach
0RSG3ZZ Reposition Right Acromioclavicular Joint, Percutaneous Approach
0RSG44Z Reposition Right Acromioclavicular Joint with Internal Fixation Device, Percutaneous Endoscopic Approach
0RSG4ZZ Reposition Right Acromioclavicular Joint, Percutaneous Endoscopic Approach
0RSGX4Z Reposition Right Acromioclavicular Joint with Internal Fixation Device, External Approach
0RSGXZZ Reposition Right Acromioclavicular Joint, External Approach
0RSH04Z Reposition Left Acromioclavicular Joint with Internal Fixation Device, Open Approach
0RSH0ZZ Reposition Left Acromioclavicular Joint, Open Approach
0RSH34Z Reposition Left Acromioclavicular Joint with Internal Fixation Device, Percutaneous Approach
0RSH3ZZ Reposition Left Acromioclavicular Joint, Percutaneous Approach
0RSH44Z Reposition Left Acromioclavicular Joint with Internal Fixation Device, Percutaneous Endoscopic Approach
0RSH4ZZ Reposition Left Acromioclavicular Joint, Percutaneous Endoscopic Approach
0RSHX4Z Reposition Left Acromioclavicular Joint with Internal Fixation Device, External Approach
0RSHXZZ Reposition Left Acromioclavicular Joint, External Approach
0RSJ04Z Reposition Right Shoulder Joint with Internal Fixation Device, Open Approach
0RSJ0ZZ Reposition Right Shoulder Joint, Open Approach
0RSJ34Z Reposition Right Shoulder Joint with Internal Fixation Device, Percutaneous Approach
0RSJ3ZZ Reposition Right Shoulder Joint, Percutaneous Approach
0RSJ44Z Reposition Right Shoulder Joint with Internal Fixation Device, Percutaneous Endoscopic Approach
0RSJ4ZZ Reposition Right Shoulder Joint, Percutaneous Endoscopic Approach
0RSJX4Z Reposition Right Shoulder Joint with Internal Fixation Device, External Approach
0RSJXZZ Reposition Right Shoulder Joint, External Approach
0RSK04Z Reposition Left Shoulder Joint with Internal Fixation Device, Open Approach
0RSK0ZZ Reposition Left Shoulder Joint, Open Approach
0RSK34Z Reposition Left Shoulder Joint with Internal Fixation Device, Percutaneous Approach
0RSK3ZZ Reposition Left Shoulder Joint, Percutaneous Approach
0RSK44Z Reposition Left Shoulder Joint with Internal Fixation Device, Percutaneous Endoscopic Approach
0RSK4ZZ Reposition Left Shoulder Joint, Percutaneous Endoscopic Approach
0RSKX4Z Reposition Left Shoulder Joint with Internal Fixation Device, External Approach
0RSKXZZ Reposition Left Shoulder Joint, External Approach
0RSL04Z Reposition Right Elbow Joint with Internal Fixation Device, Open Approach
0RSL05Z Reposition Right Elbow Joint with External Fixation Device, Open Approach
0RSL0ZZ Reposition Right Elbow Joint, Open Approach
0RSL34Z Reposition Right Elbow Joint with Internal Fixation Device, Percutaneous Approach
0RSL35Z Reposition Right Elbow Joint with External Fixation Device, Percutaneous Approach
0RSL3ZZ Reposition Right Elbow Joint, Percutaneous Approach
0RSL44Z Reposition Right Elbow Joint with Internal Fixation Device, Percutaneous Endoscopic Approach
0RSL45Z Reposition Right Elbow Joint with External Fixation Device, Percutaneous Endoscopic Approach
0RSL4ZZ Reposition Right Elbow Joint, Percutaneous Endoscopic Approach
0RSLX4Z Reposition Right Elbow Joint with Internal Fixation Device, External Approach
0RSLX5Z Reposition Right Elbow Joint with External Fixation Device, External Approach
0RSLXZZ Reposition Right Elbow Joint, External Approach
0RSM04Z Reposition Left Elbow Joint with Internal Fixation Device, Open Approach
0RSM05Z Reposition Left Elbow Joint with External Fixation Device, Open Approach
0RSM0ZZ Reposition Left Elbow Joint, Open Approach

0RSM34Z Reposition Left Elbow Joint with Internal Fixation Device, Percutaneous Approach
0RSM35Z Reposition Left Elbow Joint with External Fixation Device, Percutaneous Approach
0RSM3ZZ Reposition Left Elbow Joint, Percutaneous Approach
0RSM44Z Reposition Left Elbow Joint with Internal Fixation Device, Percutaneous Endoscopic Approach
0RSM45Z Reposition Left Elbow Joint with External Fixation Device, Percutaneous Endoscopic Approach
0RSM4ZZ Reposition Left Elbow Joint, Percutaneous Endoscopic Approach
0RSMX4Z Reposition Left Elbow Joint with Internal Fixation Device, External Approach
0RSMX5Z Reposition Left Elbow Joint with External Fixation Device, External Approach
0RSMXZZ Reposition Left Elbow Joint, External Approach
0RSN04Z Reposition Right Wrist Joint with Internal Fixation Device, Open Approach
0RSN05Z Reposition Right Wrist Joint with External Fixation Device, Open Approach
0RSN0ZZ Reposition Right Wrist Joint, Open Approach
0RSN34Z Reposition Right Wrist Joint with Internal Fixation Device, Percutaneous Approach
0RSN35Z Reposition Right Wrist Joint with External Fixation Device, Percutaneous Approach
0RSN3ZZ Reposition Right Wrist Joint, Percutaneous Approach
0RSN44Z Reposition Right Wrist Joint with Internal Fixation Device, Percutaneous Endoscopic Approach
0RSN45Z Reposition Right Wrist Joint with External Fixation Device, Percutaneous Endoscopic Approach
0RSN4ZZ Reposition Right Wrist Joint, Percutaneous Endoscopic Approach
0RSNX4Z Reposition Right Wrist Joint with Internal Fixation Device, External Approach
0RSNX5Z Reposition Right Wrist Joint with External Fixation Device, External Approach
0RSNXZZ Reposition Right Wrist Joint, External Approach
0RSP04Z Reposition Left Wrist Joint with Internal Fixation Device, Open Approach
0RSP05Z Reposition Left Wrist Joint with External Fixation Device, Open Approach
0RSP0ZZ Reposition Left Wrist Joint, Open Approach
0RSP34Z Reposition Left Wrist Joint with Internal Fixation Device, Percutaneous Approach
0RSP35Z Reposition Left Wrist Joint with External Fixation Device, Percutaneous Approach
0RSP3ZZ Reposition Left Wrist Joint, Percutaneous Approach
0RSP44Z Reposition Left Wrist Joint with Internal Fixation Device, Percutaneous Endoscopic Approach
0RSP45Z Reposition Left Wrist Joint with External Fixation Device, Percutaneous Endoscopic Approach
0RSP4ZZ Reposition Left Wrist Joint, Percutaneous Endoscopic Approach
0RSPX4Z Reposition Left Wrist Joint with Internal Fixation Device, External Approach
0RSPX5Z Reposition Left Wrist Joint with External Fixation Device, External Approach
0RSPXZZ Reposition Left Wrist Joint, External Approach
0RSQ04Z Reposition Right Carpal Joint with Internal Fixation Device, Open Approach
0RSQ05Z Reposition Right Carpal Joint with External Fixation Device, Open Approach
0RSQ0ZZ Reposition Right Carpal Joint, Open Approach
0RSQ34Z Reposition Right Carpal Joint with Internal Fixation Device, Percutaneous Approach
0RSQ35Z Reposition Right Carpal Joint with External Fixation Device, Percutaneous Approach
0RSQ3ZZ Reposition Right Carpal Joint, Percutaneous Approach
0RSQ44Z Reposition Right Carpal Joint with Internal Fixation Device, Percutaneous Endoscopic Approach
0RSQ45Z Reposition Right Carpal Joint with External Fixation Device, Percutaneous Endoscopic Approach
0RSQ4ZZ Reposition Right Carpal Joint, Percutaneous Endoscopic Approach
0RSQX4Z Reposition Right Carpal Joint with Internal Fixation Device, External Approach
0RSQX5Z Reposition Right Carpal Joint with External Fixation Device, External Approach
0RSQXZZ Reposition Right Carpal Joint, External Approach
0RSR04Z Reposition Left Carpal Joint with Internal Fixation Device, Open Approach
0RSR05Z Reposition Left Carpal Joint with External Fixation Device, Open Approach
0RSR0ZZ Reposition Left Carpal Joint, Open Approach
0RSR34Z Reposition Left Carpal Joint with Internal Fixation Device, Percutaneous Approach
0RSR35Z Reposition Left Carpal Joint with External Fixation Device, Percutaneous Approach
0RSR3ZZ Reposition Left Carpal Joint, Percutaneous Approach
0RSR44Z Reposition Left Carpal Joint with Internal Fixation Device, Percutaneous Endoscopic Approach
0RSR45Z Reposition Left Carpal Joint with External Fixation Device, Percutaneous Endoscopic Approach
0RSR4ZZ Reposition Left Carpal Joint, Percutaneous Endoscopic Approach
0RSRX4Z Reposition Left Carpal Joint with Internal Fixation Device, External Approach
0RSRX5Z Reposition Left Carpal Joint with External Fixation Device, External Approach
0RSRXZZ Reposition Left Carpal Joint, External Approach
0RSS04Z Reposition Right Metacarpocarpal Joint with Internal Fixation Device, Open Approach
0RSS05Z Reposition Right Metacarpocarpal Joint with External Fixation Device, Open Approach
0RSS0ZZ Reposition Right Metacarpocarpal Joint, Open Approach
0RSS34Z Reposition Right Metacarpocarpal Joint with Internal Fixation Device, Percutaneous Approach
0RSS35Z Reposition Right Metacarpocarpal Joint with External Fixation Device, Percutaneous Approach
0RSS3ZZ Reposition Right Metacarpocarpal Joint, Percutaneous Approach
0RSS44Z Reposition Right Metacarpocarpal Joint with Internal Fixation Device, Percutaneous Endoscopic Approach
0RSS45Z Reposition Right Metacarpocarpal Joint with External Fixation Device, Percutaneous Endoscopic Approach
0RSS4ZZ Reposition Right Metacarpocarpal Joint, Percutaneous Endoscopic Approach
0RSSX4Z Reposition Right Metacarpocarpal Joint with Internal Fixation Device, External Approach
0RSSX5Z Reposition Right Metacarpocarpal Joint with External Fixation Device, External Approach
0RSSXZZ Reposition Right Metacarpocarpal Joint, External Approach
0RST04Z Reposition Left Metacarpocarpal Joint with Internal Fixation Device, Open Approach
0RST05Z Reposition Left Metacarpocarpal Joint with External Fixation Device, Open Approach
0RST0ZZ Reposition Left Metacarpocarpal Joint, Open Approach
0RST34Z Reposition Left Metacarpocarpal Joint with Internal Fixation Device, Percutaneous Approach
0RST35Z Reposition Left Metacarpocarpal Joint with External Fixation Device, Percutaneous Approach
0RST3ZZ Reposition Left Metacarpocarpal Joint, Percutaneous Approach
0RST44Z Reposition Left Metacarpocarpal Joint with Internal Fixation Device, Percutaneous Endoscopic Approach
0RST45Z Reposition Left Metacarpocarpal Joint with External Fixation Device, Percutaneous Endoscopic Approach
0RST4ZZ Reposition Left Metacarpocarpal Joint, Percutaneous Endoscopic Approach
0RSTX4Z Reposition Left Metacarpocarpal Joint with Internal Fixation Device, External Approach
0RSTX5Z Reposition Left Metacarpocarpal Joint with External Fixation Device, External Approach
0RSTXZZ Reposition Left Metacarpocarpal Joint, External Approach
0RSU04Z Reposition Right Metacarpophalangeal Joint with Internal Fixation Device, Open Approach
0RSU05Z Reposition Right Metacarpophalangeal Joint with External Fixation Device, Open Approach
0RSU0ZZ Reposition Right Metacarpophalangeal Joint, Open Approach
0RSU34Z Reposition Right Metacarpophalangeal Joint with Internal Fixation Device, Percutaneous Approach
0RSU35Z Reposition Right Metacarpophalangeal Joint with External Fixation Device, Percutaneous Approach
0RSU3ZZ Reposition Right Metacarpophalangeal Joint, Percutaneous Approach
0RSU44Z Reposition Right Metacarpophalangeal Joint with Internal Fixation Device, Percutaneous Endoscopic Approach
0RSU45Z Reposition Right Metacarpophalangeal Joint with External Fixation Device, Percutaneous Endoscopic Approach
0RSU4ZZ Reposition Right Metacarpophalangeal Joint, Percutaneous Endoscopic Approach
0RSUX4Z Reposition Right Metacarpophalangeal Joint with Internal Fixation Device, External Approach
0RSUX5Z Reposition Right Metacarpophalangeal Joint with External Fixation Device, External Approach
0RSUXZZ Reposition Right Metacarpophalangeal Joint, External Approach
0RSV04Z Reposition Left Metacarpophalangeal Joint with Internal Fixation Device, Open Approach
0RSV05Z Reposition Left Metacarpophalangeal Joint with External Fixation Device, Open Approach

0RSV0ZZ Reposition Left Metacarpophalangeal Joint, Open Approach
0RSV34Z Reposition Left Metacarpophalangeal Joint with Internal Fixation Device, Percutaneous Approach
0RSV35Z Reposition Left Metacarpophalangeal Joint with External Fixation Device, Percutaneous Approach
0RSV3ZZ Reposition Left Metacarpophalangeal Joint, Percutaneous Approach
0RSV44Z Reposition Left Metacarpophalangeal Joint with Internal Fixation Device, Percutaneous Endoscopic Approach
0RSV45Z Reposition Left Metacarpophalangeal Joint with External Fixation Device, Percutaneous Endoscopic Approach
0RSV4ZZ Reposition Left Metacarpophalangeal Joint, Percutaneous Endoscopic Approach
0RSVX4Z Reposition Left Metacarpophalangeal Joint with Internal Fixation Device, External Approach
0RSVX5Z Reposition Left Metacarpophalangeal Joint with External Fixation Device, External Approach
0RSVXZZ Reposition Left Metacarpophalangeal Joint, External Approach
0RSW04Z Reposition Right Finger Phalangeal Joint with Internal Fixation Device, Open Approach
0RSW05Z Reposition Right Finger Phalangeal Joint with External Fixation Device, Open Approach
0RSW0ZZ Reposition Right Finger Phalangeal Joint, Open Approach
0RSW34Z Reposition Right Finger Phalangeal Joint with Internal Fixation Device, Percutaneous Approach
0RSW35Z Reposition Right Finger Phalangeal Joint with External Fixation Device, Percutaneous Approach
0RSW3ZZ Reposition Right Finger Phalangeal Joint, Percutaneous Approach
0RSW44Z Reposition Right Finger Phalangeal Joint with Internal Fixation Device, Percutaneous Endoscopic Approach
0RSW45Z Reposition Right Finger Phalangeal Joint with External Fixation Device, Percutaneous Endoscopic Approach
0RSW4ZZ Reposition Right Finger Phalangeal Joint, Percutaneous Endoscopic Approach
0RSWX4Z Reposition Right Finger Phalangeal Joint with Internal Fixation Device, External Approach
0RSWX5Z Reposition Right Finger Phalangeal Joint with External Fixation Device, External Approach
0RSWXZZ Reposition Right Finger Phalangeal Joint, External Approach
0RSX04Z Reposition Left Finger Phalangeal Joint with Internal Fixation Device, Open Approach
0RSX05Z Reposition Left Finger Phalangeal Joint with External Fixation Device, Open Approach
0RSX0ZZ Reposition Left Finger Phalangeal Joint, Open Approach
0RSX34Z Reposition Left Finger Phalangeal Joint with Internal Fixation Device, Percutaneous Approach
0RSX35Z Reposition Left Finger Phalangeal Joint with External Fixation Device, Percutaneous Approach
0RSX3ZZ Reposition Left Finger Phalangeal Joint, Percutaneous Approach
0RSX44Z Reposition Left Finger Phalangeal Joint with Internal Fixation Device, Percutaneous Endoscopic Approach
0RSX45Z Reposition Left Finger Phalangeal Joint with External Fixation Device, Percutaneous Endoscopic Approach
0RSX4ZZ Reposition Left Finger Phalangeal Joint, Percutaneous Endoscopic Approach
0RSXX4Z Reposition Left Finger Phalangeal Joint with Internal Fixation Device, External Approach
0RSXX5Z Reposition Left Finger Phalangeal Joint with External Fixation Device, External Approach
0RSXXZZ Reposition Left Finger Phalangeal Joint, External Approach

0RT – Upper Joints, Resection

Review Coding Guideline B3.8

0RT30ZZ Resection of Cervical Vertebral Disc, Open Approach
0RT40ZZ Resection of Cervicothoracic Vertebral Joint, Open Approach
0RT50ZZ Resection of Cervicothoracic Vertebral Disc, Open Approach
AHA CC: 2Q, 2014, 7-8
0RT90ZZ Resection of Thoracic Vertebral Disc, Open Approach
0RTB0ZZ Resection of Thoracolumbar Vertebral Disc, Open Approach
0RTC0ZZ Resection of Right Temporomandibular Joint, Open Approach
0RTD0ZZ Resection of Left Temporomandibular Joint, Open Approach
0RTE0ZZ Resection of Right Sternoclavicular Joint, Open Approach
0RTF0ZZ Resection of Left Sternoclavicular Joint, Open Approach
0RTG0ZZ Resection of Right Acromioclavicular Joint, Open Approach
0RTH0ZZ Resection of Left Acromioclavicular Joint, Open Approach
0RTJ0ZZ Resection of Right Shoulder Joint, Open Approach
0RTK0ZZ Resection of Left Shoulder Joint, Open Approach
0RTL0ZZ Resection of Right Elbow Joint, Open Approach
0RTM0ZZ Resection of Left Elbow Joint, Open Approach
0RTN0ZZ Resection of Right Wrist Joint, Open Approach
0RTP0ZZ Resection of Left Wrist Joint, Open Approach
0RTQ0ZZ Resection of Right Carpal Joint, Open Approach
0RTR0ZZ Resection of Left Carpal Joint, Open Approach
0RTS0ZZ Resection of Right Metacarpocarpal Joint, Open Approach
0RTT0ZZ Resection of Left Metacarpocarpal Joint, Open Approach
0RTU0ZZ Resection of Right Metacarpophalangeal Joint, Open Approach
0RTV0ZZ Resection of Left Metacarpophalangeal Joint, Open Approach
0RTW0ZZ Resection of Right Finger Phalangeal Joint, Open Approach
0RTX0ZZ Resection of Left Finger Phalangeal Joint, Open Approach

0RU – Upper Joints, Supplement

0RU007Z Supplement Occipital-cervical Joint with Autologous Tissue Substitute, Open Approach
0RU00JZ Supplement Occipital-cervical Joint with Synthetic Substitute, Open Approach
0RU00KZ Supplement Occipital-cervical Joint with Nonautologous Tissue Substitute, Open Approach
0RU037Z Supplement Occipital-cervical Joint with Autologous Tissue Substitute, Percutaneous Approach
0RU03JZ Supplement Occipital-cervical Joint with Synthetic Substitute, Percutaneous Approach
0RU03KZ Supplement Occipital-cervical Joint with Nonautologous Tissue Substitute, Percutaneous Approach
0RU047Z Supplement Occipital-cervical Joint with Autologous Tissue Substitute, Percutaneous Endoscopic Approach
0RU04JZ Supplement Occipital-cervical Joint with Synthetic Substitute, Percutaneous Endoscopic Approach
0RU04KZ Supplement Occipital-cervical Joint with Nonautologous Tissue Substitute, Percutaneous Endoscopic Approach
0RU107Z Supplement Cervical Vertebral Joint with Autologous Tissue Substitute, Open Approach
0RU10JZ Supplement Cervical Vertebral Joint with Synthetic Substitute, Open Approach
0RU10KZ Supplement Cervical Vertebral Joint with Nonautologous Tissue Substitute, Open Approach
0RU137Z Supplement Cervical Vertebral Joint with Autologous Tissue Substitute, Percutaneous Approach
0RU13JZ Supplement Cervical Vertebral Joint with Synthetic Substitute, Percutaneous Approach
0RU13KZ Supplement Cervical Vertebral Joint with Nonautologous Tissue Substitute, Percutaneous Approach
0RU147Z Supplement Cervical Vertebral Joint with Autologous Tissue Substitute, Percutaneous Endoscopic Approach
0RU14JZ Supplement Cervical Vertebral Joint with Synthetic Substitute, Percutaneous Endoscopic Approach
0RU14KZ Supplement Cervical Vertebral Joint with Nonautologous Tissue Substitute, Percutaneous Endoscopic Approach
0RU307Z Supplement Cervical Vertebral Disc with Autologous Tissue Substitute, Open Approach
0RU30JZ Supplement Cervical Vertebral Disc with Synthetic Substitute, Open Approach
0RU30KZ Supplement Cervical Vertebral Disc with Nonautologous Tissue Substitute, Open Approach

0RU337Z Supplement Cervical Vertebral Disc with Autologous Tissue Substitute, Percutaneous Approach

0RU33JZ Supplement Cervical Vertebral Disc with Synthetic Substitute, Percutaneous Approach

0RU33KZ Supplement Cervical Vertebral Disc with Nonautologous Tissue Substitute, Percutaneous Approach

0RU347Z Supplement Cervical Vertebral Disc with Autologous Tissue Substitute, Percutaneous Endoscopic Approach

0RU34JZ Supplement Cervical Vertebral Disc with Synthetic Substitute, Percutaneous Endoscopic Approach

0RU34KZ Supplement Cervical Vertebral Disc with Nonautologous Tissue Substitute, Percutaneous Endoscopic Approach

0RU407Z Supplement Cervicothoracic Vertebral Joint with Autologous Tissue Substitute, Open Approach

0RU40JZ Supplement Cervicothoracic Vertebral Joint with Synthetic Substitute, Open Approach

0RU40KZ Supplement Cervicothoracic Vertebral Joint with Nonautologous Tissue Substitute, Open Approach

0RU437Z Supplement Cervicothoracic Vertebral Joint with Autologous Tissue Substitute, Percutaneous Approach

0RU43JZ Supplement Cervicothoracic Vertebral Joint with Synthetic Substitute, Percutaneous Approach

0RU43KZ Supplement Cervicothoracic Vertebral Joint with Nonautologous Tissue Substitute, Percutaneous Approach

0RU447Z Supplement Cervicothoracic Vertebral Joint with Autologous Tissue Substitute, Percutaneous Endoscopic Approach

0RU44JZ Supplement Cervicothoracic Vertebral Joint with Synthetic Substitute, Percutaneous Endoscopic Approach

0RU44KZ Supplement Cervicothoracic Vertebral Joint with Nonautologous Tissue Substitute, Percutaneous Endoscopic Approach

0RU507Z Supplement Cervicothoracic Vertebral Disc with Autologous Tissue Substitute, Open Approach

0RU50JZ Supplement Cervicothoracic Vertebral Disc with Synthetic Substitute, Open Approach

0RU50KZ Supplement Cervicothoracic Vertebral Disc with Nonautologous Tissue Substitute, Open Approach

0RU537Z Supplement Cervicothoracic Vertebral Disc with Autologous Tissue Substitute, Percutaneous Approach

0RU53JZ Supplement Cervicothoracic Vertebral Disc with Synthetic Substitute, Percutaneous Approach

0RU53KZ Supplement Cervicothoracic Vertebral Disc with Nonautologous Tissue Substitute, Percutaneous Approach

0RU547Z Supplement Cervicothoracic Vertebral Disc with Autologous Tissue Substitute, Percutaneous Endoscopic Approach

0RU54JZ Supplement Cervicothoracic Vertebral Disc with Synthetic Substitute, Percutaneous Endoscopic Approach

0RU54KZ Supplement Cervicothoracic Vertebral Disc with Nonautologous Tissue Substitute, Percutaneous Endoscopic Approach

0RU607Z Supplement Thoracic Vertebral Joint with Autologous Tissue Substitute, Open Approach

0RU60JZ Supplement Thoracic Vertebral Joint with Synthetic Substitute, Open Approach

0RU60KZ Supplement Thoracic Vertebral Joint with Nonautologous Tissue Substitute, Open Approach

0RU637Z Supplement Thoracic Vertebral Joint with Autologous Tissue Substitute, Percutaneous Approach

0RU63JZ Supplement Thoracic Vertebral Joint with Synthetic Substitute, Percutaneous Approach

0RU63KZ Supplement Thoracic Vertebral Joint with Nonautologous Tissue Substitute, Percutaneous Approach

0RU647Z Supplement Thoracic Vertebral Joint with Autologous Tissue Substitute, Percutaneous Endoscopic Approach

0RU64JZ Supplement Thoracic Vertebral Joint with Synthetic Substitute, Percutaneous Endoscopic Approach

0RU64KZ Supplement Thoracic Vertebral Joint with Nonautologous Tissue Substitute, Percutaneous Endoscopic Approach

0RU907Z Supplement Thoracic Vertebral Disc with Autologous Tissue Substitute, Open Approach

0RU90JZ Supplement Thoracic Vertebral Disc with Synthetic Substitute, Open Approach

0RU90KZ Supplement Thoracic Vertebral Disc with Nonautologous Tissue Substitute, Open Approach

0RU937Z Supplement Thoracic Vertebral Disc with Autologous Tissue Substitute, Percutaneous Approach

0RU93JZ Supplement Thoracic Vertebral Disc with Synthetic Substitute, Percutaneous Approach

0RU93KZ Supplement Thoracic Vertebral Disc with Nonautologous Tissue Substitute, Percutaneous Approach

0RU947Z Supplement Thoracic Vertebral Disc with Autologous Tissue Substitute, Percutaneous Endoscopic Approach

0RU94JZ Supplement Thoracic Vertebral Disc with Synthetic Substitute, Percutaneous Endoscopic Approach

0RU94KZ Supplement Thoracic Vertebral Disc with Nonautologous Tissue Substitute, Percutaneous Endoscopic Approach

0RUA07Z Supplement Thoracolumbar Vertebral Joint with Autologous Tissue Substitute, Open Approach

0RUA0JZ Supplement Thoracolumbar Vertebral Joint with Synthetic Substitute, Open Approach

0RUA0KZ Supplement Thoracolumbar Vertebral Joint with Nonautologous Tissue Substitute, Open Approach

0RUA37Z Supplement Thoracolumbar Vertebral Joint with Autologous Tissue Substitute, Percutaneous Approach

0RUA3JZ Supplement Thoracolumbar Vertebral Joint with Synthetic Substitute, Percutaneous Approach

0RUA3KZ Supplement Thoracolumbar Vertebral Joint with Nonautologous Tissue Substitute, Percutaneous Approach

0RUA47Z Supplement Thoracolumbar Vertebral Joint with Autologous Tissue Substitute, Percutaneous Endoscopic Approach

0RUA4JZ Supplement Thoracolumbar Vertebral Joint with Synthetic Substitute, Percutaneous Endoscopic Approach

0RUA4KZ Supplement Thoracolumbar Vertebral Joint with Nonautologous Tissue Substitute, Percutaneous Endoscopic Approach

0RUB07Z Supplement Thoracolumbar Vertebral Disc with Autologous Tissue Substitute, Open Approach

0RUB0JZ Supplement Thoracolumbar Vertebral Disc with Synthetic Substitute, Open Approach

0RUB0KZ Supplement Thoracolumbar Vertebral Disc with Nonautologous Tissue Substitute, Open Approach

0RUB37Z Supplement Thoracolumbar Vertebral Disc with Autologous Tissue Substitute, Percutaneous Approach

0RUB3JZ Supplement Thoracolumbar Vertebral Disc with Synthetic Substitute, Percutaneous Approach

0RUB3KZ Supplement Thoracolumbar Vertebral Disc with Nonautologous Tissue Substitute, Percutaneous Approach

0RUB47Z Supplement Thoracolumbar Vertebral Disc with Autologous Tissue Substitute, Percutaneous Endoscopic Approach

0RUB4JZ Supplement Thoracolumbar Vertebral Disc with Synthetic Substitute, Percutaneous Endoscopic Approach

0RUB4KZ Supplement Thoracolumbar Vertebral Disc with Nonautologous Tissue Substitute, Percutaneous Endoscopic Approach

0RUC07Z Supplement Right Temporomandibular Joint with Autologous Tissue Substitute, Open Approach

0RUC0JZ Supplement Right Temporomandibular Joint with Synthetic Substitute, Open Approach

0RUC0KZ Supplement Right Temporomandibular Joint with Nonautologous Tissue Substitute, Open Approach

0RUC37Z Supplement Right Temporomandibular Joint with Autologous Tissue Substitute, Percutaneous Approach

0RUC3JZ Supplement Right Temporomandibular Joint with Synthetic Substitute, Percutaneous Approach

0RUC3KZ Supplement Right Temporomandibular Joint with Nonautologous Tissue Substitute, Percutaneous Approach

0RUC47Z Supplement Right Temporomandibular Joint with Autologous Tissue Substitute, Percutaneous Endoscopic Approach

0RUC4JZ Supplement Right Temporomandibular Joint with Synthetic Substitute, Percutaneous Endoscopic Approach

0RUC4KZ Supplement Right Temporomandibular Joint with Nonautologous Tissue Substitute, Percutaneous Endoscopic Approach

0RUD07Z Supplement Left Temporomandibular Joint with Autologous Tissue Substitute, Open Approach

0RUD0JZ Supplement Left Temporomandibular Joint with Synthetic Substitute, Open Approach

0RUD0KZ Supplement Left Temporomandibular Joint with Nonautologous Tissue Substitute, Open Approach

0RUD37Z Supplement Left Temporomandibular Joint with Autologous Tissue Substitute, Percutaneous Approach

0RUD3JZ Supplement Left Temporomandibular Joint with Synthetic Substitute, Percutaneous Approach

0RUD3KZ Supplement Left Temporomandibular Joint with Nonautologous Tissue Substitute, Percutaneous Approach

0RUD47Z Supplement Left Temporomandibular Joint with Autologous Tissue Substitute, Percutaneous Endoscopic Approach

0RUD4JZ Supplement Left Temporomandibular Joint with Synthetic Substitute, Percutaneous Endoscopic Approach

0RUD4KZ Supplement Left Temporomandibular Joint with Nonautologous Tissue Substitute, Percutaneous Endoscopic Approach

0RUE07Z Supplement Right Sternoclavicular Joint with Autologous Tissue Substitute, Open Approach
- HAC When reported with secondary diagnosis code T84.60XA, T84.610A, T84.611A, T84.612A, T84.613A, T84.614A, T84.615A, T84.619A, T84.63XA, T84.69XA, T84.7XXA

0RUE0JZ Supplement Right Sternoclavicular Joint with Synthetic Substitute, Open Approach
- HAC When reported with secondary diagnosis code T84.60XA, T84.610A, T84.611A, T84.612A, T84.613A, T84.614A, T84.615A, T84.619A, T84.63XA, T84.69XA, T84.7XXA

0RUE0KZ Supplement Right Sternoclavicular Joint with Nonautologous Tissue Substitute, Open Approach
- HAC When reported with secondary diagnosis code T84.60XA, T84.610A, T84.611A, T84.612A, T84.613A, T84.614A, T84.615A, T84.619A, T84.63XA, T84.69XA, T84.7XXA

0RUE37Z Supplement Right Sternoclavicular Joint with Autologous Tissue Substitute, Percutaneous Approach
- HAC When reported with secondary diagnosis code T84.60XA, T84.610A, T84.611A, T84.612A, T84.613A, T84.614A, T84.615A, T84.619A, T84.63XA, T84.69XA, T84.7XXA

0RUE3JZ Supplement Right Sternoclavicular Joint with Synthetic Substitute, Percutaneous Approach
- HAC When reported with secondary diagnosis code T84.60XA, T84.610A, T84.611A, T84.612A, T84.613A, T84.614A, T84.615A, T84.619A, T84.63XA, T84.69XA, T84.7XXA

0RUE3KZ Supplement Right Sternoclavicular Joint with Nonautologous Tissue Substitute, Percutaneous Approach
- HAC When reported with secondary diagnosis code T84.60XA, T84.610A, T84.611A, T84.612A, T84.613A, T84.614A, T84.615A, T84.619A, T84.63XA, T84.69XA, T84.7XXA

0RUE47Z Supplement Right Sternoclavicular Joint with Autologous Tissue Substitute, Percutaneous Endoscopic Approach
- HAC When reported with secondary diagnosis code T84.60XA, T84.610A, T84.611A, T84.612A, T84.613A, T84.614A, T84.615A, T84.619A, T84.63XA, T84.69XA, T84.7XXA

0RUE4JZ Supplement Right Sternoclavicular Joint with Synthetic Substitute, Percutaneous Endoscopic Approach
- HAC When reported with secondary diagnosis code T84.60XA, T84.610A, T84.611A, T84.612A, T84.613A, T84.614A, T84.615A, T84.619A, T84.63XA, T84.69XA, T84.7XXA

0RUE4KZ Supplement Right Sternoclavicular Joint with Nonautologous Tissue Substitute, Percutaneous Endoscopic Approach
- HAC When reported with secondary diagnosis code T84.60XA, T84.610A, T84.611A, T84.612A, T84.613A, T84.614A, T84.615A, T84.619A, T84.63XA, T84.69XA, T84.7XXA

0RUF07Z Supplement Left Sternoclavicular Joint with Autologous Tissue Substitute, Open Approach
- HAC When reported with secondary diagnosis code T84.60XA, T84.610A, T84.611A, T84.612A, T84.613A, T84.614A, T84.615A, T84.619A, T84.63XA, T84.69XA, T84.7XXA

0RUF0JZ Supplement Left Sternoclavicular Joint with Synthetic Substitute, Open Approach
- HAC When reported with secondary diagnosis code T84.60XA, T84.610A, T84.611A, T84.612A, T84.613A, T84.614A, T84.615A, T84.619A, T84.63XA, T84.69XA, T84.7XXA

0RUF0KZ Supplement Left Sternoclavicular Joint with Nonautologous Tissue Substitute, Open Approach
- HAC When reported with secondary diagnosis code T84.60XA, T84.610A, T84.611A, T84.612A, T84.613A, T84.614A, T84.615A, T84.619A, T84.63XA, T84.69XA, T84.7XXA

0RUF37Z Supplement Left Sternoclavicular Joint with Autologous Tissue Substitute, Percutaneous Approach
- HAC When reported with secondary diagnosis code T84.60XA, T84.610A, T84.611A, T84.612A, T84.613A, T84.614A, T84.615A, T84.619A, T84.63XA, T84.69XA, T84.7XXA

0RUF3JZ Supplement Left Sternoclavicular Joint with Synthetic Substitute, Percutaneous Approach
- HAC When reported with secondary diagnosis code T84.60XA, T84.610A, T84.611A, T84.612A, T84.613A, T84.614A, T84.615A, T84.619A, T84.63XA, T84.69XA, T84.7XXA

0RUF3KZ Supplement Left Sternoclavicular Joint with Nonautologous Tissue Substitute, Percutaneous Approach
- HAC When reported with secondary diagnosis code T84.60XA, T84.610A, T84.611A, T84.612A, T84.613A, T84.614A, T84.615A, T84.619A, T84.63XA, T84.69XA, T84.7XXA

0RUF47Z Supplement Left Sternoclavicular Joint with Autologous Tissue Substitute, Percutaneous Endoscopic Approach
- HAC When reported with secondary diagnosis code T84.60XA, T84.610A, T84.611A, T84.612A, T84.613A, T84.614A, T84.615A, T84.619A, T84.63XA, T84.69XA, T84.7XXA

0RUF4JZ Supplement Left Sternoclavicular Joint with Synthetic Substitute, Percutaneous Endoscopic Approach
- HAC When reported with secondary diagnosis code T84.60XA, T84.610A, T84.611A, T84.612A, T84.613A, T84.614A, T84.615A, T84.619A, T84.63XA, T84.69XA, T84.7XXA

0RUF4KZ Supplement Left Sternoclavicular Joint with Nonautologous Tissue Substitute, Percutaneous Endoscopic Approach
- HAC When reported with secondary diagnosis code T84.60XA, T84.610A, T84.611A, T84.612A, T84.613A, T84.614A, T84.615A, T84.619A, T84.63XA, T84.69XA, T84.7XXA

0RUG07Z Supplement Right Acromioclavicular Joint with Autologous Tissue Substitute, Open Approach
- HAC When reported with secondary diagnosis code T84.60XA, T84.610A, T84.611A, T84.612A, T84.613A, T84.614A, T84.615A, T84.619A, T84.63XA, T84.69XA, T84.7XXA

0RUG0JZ Supplement Right Acromioclavicular Joint with Synthetic Substitute, Open Approach
- HAC When reported with secondary diagnosis code T84.60XA, T84.610A, T84.611A, T84.612A, T84.613A, T84.614A, T84.615A, T84.619A, T84.63XA, T84.69XA, T84.7XXA

0RUG0KZ Supplement Right Acromioclavicular Joint with Nonautologous Tissue Substitute, Open Approach
- HAC When reported with secondary diagnosis code T84.60XA, T84.610A, T84.611A, T84.612A, T84.613A, T84.614A, T84.615A, T84.619A, T84.63XA, T84.69XA, T84.7XXA

0RUG37Z Supplement Right Acromioclavicular Joint with Autologous Tissue Substitute, Percutaneous Approach
- HAC When reported with secondary diagnosis code T84.60XA, T84.610A, T84.611A, T84.612A, T84.613A, T84.614A, T84.615A, T84.619A, T84.63XA, T84.69XA, T84.7XXA

0RUG3JZ Supplement Right Acromioclavicular Joint with Synthetic Substitute, Percutaneous Approach
- HAC When reported with secondary diagnosis code T84.60XA, T84.610A, T84.611A, T84.612A, T84.613A, T84.614A, T84.615A, T84.619A, T84.63XA, T84.69XA, T84.7XXA

0RUG3KZ Supplement Right Acromioclavicular Joint with Nonautologous Tissue Substitute, Percutaneous Approach
- HAC When reported with secondary diagnosis code T84.60XA, T84.610A, T84.611A, T84.612A, T84.613A, T84.614A, T84.615A, T84.619A, T84.63XA, T84.69XA, T84.7XXA

0RUG47Z Supplement Right Acromioclavicular Joint with Autologous Tissue Substitute, Percutaneous Endoscopic Approach
- HAC When reported with secondary diagnosis code T84.60XA, T84.610A, T84.611A, T84.612A, T84.613A, T84.614A, T84.615A, T84.619A, T84.63XA, T84.69XA, T84.7XXA

0RUG4JZ Supplement Right Acromioclavicular Joint with Synthetic Substitute, Percutaneous Endoscopic Approach
- HAC When reported with secondary diagnosis code T84.60XA, T84.610A, T84.611A, T84.612A, T84.613A, T84.614A, T84.615A, T84.619A, T84.63XA, T84.69XA, T84.7XXA

0RUG4KZ Supplement Right Acromioclavicular Joint with Nonautologous Tissue Substitute, Percutaneous Endoscopic Approach
- HAC When reported with secondary diagnosis code T84.60XA, T84.610A, T84.611A, T84.612A, T84.613A, T84.614A, T84.615A, T84.619A, T84.63XA, T84.69XA, T84.7XXA

0RUH07Z Supplement Left Acromioclavicular Joint with Autologous Tissue Substitute, Open Approach
- HAC When reported with secondary diagnosis code T84.60XA, T84.610A, T84.611A, T84.612A, T84.613A, T84.614A, T84.615A, T84.619A, T84.63XA, T84.69XA, T84.7XXA

0RUH0JZ Supplement Left Acromioclavicular Joint with Synthetic Substitute, Open Approach
HAC When reported with secondary diagnosis code T84.60XA, T84.610A, T84.611A, T84.612A, T84.613A, T84.614A, T84.615A, T84.619A, T84.63XA, T84.69XA, T84.7XXA

0RUH0KZ Supplement Left Acromioclavicular Joint with Nonautologous Tissue Substitute, Open Approach
HAC When reported with secondary diagnosis code T84.60XA, T84.610A, T84.611A, T84.612A, T84.613A, T84.614A, T84.615A, T84.619A, T84.63XA, T84.69XA, T84.7XXA

0RUH37Z Supplement Left Acromioclavicular Joint with Autologous Tissue Substitute, Percutaneous Approach
HAC When reported with secondary diagnosis code T84.60XA, T84.610A, T84.611A, T84.612A, T84.613A, T84.614A, T84.615A, T84.619A, T84.63XA, T84.69XA, T84.7XXA

0RUH3JZ Supplement Left Acromioclavicular Joint with Synthetic Substitute, Percutaneous Approach
HAC When reported with secondary diagnosis code T84.60XA, T84.610A, T84.611A, T84.612A, T84.613A, T84.614A, T84.615A, T84.619A, T84.63XA, T84.69XA, T84.7XXA

0RUH3KZ Supplement Left Acromioclavicular Joint with Nonautologous Tissue Substitute, Percutaneous Approach
HAC When reported with secondary diagnosis code T84.60XA, T84.610A, T84.611A, T84.612A, T84.613A, T84.614A, T84.615A, T84.619A, T84.63XA, T84.69XA, T84.7XXA

0RUH47Z Supplement Left Acromioclavicular Joint with Autologous Tissue Substitute, Percutaneous Endoscopic Approach
HAC When reported with secondary diagnosis code T84.60XA, T84.610A, T84.611A, T84.612A, T84.613A, T84.614A, T84.615A, T84.619A, T84.63XA, T84.69XA, T84.7XXA

0RUH4JZ Supplement Left Acromioclavicular Joint with Synthetic Substitute, Percutaneous Endoscopic Approach
HAC When reported with secondary diagnosis code T84.60XA, T84.610A, T84.611A, T84.612A, T84.613A, T84.614A, T84.615A, T84.619A, T84.63XA, T84.69XA, T84.7XXA

0RUH4KZ Supplement Left Acromioclavicular Joint with Nonautologous Tissue Substitute, Percutaneous Endoscopic Approach
HAC When reported with secondary diagnosis code T84.60XA, T84.610A, T84.611A, T84.612A, T84.613A, T84.614A, T84.615A, T84.619A, T84.63XA, T84.69XA, T84.7XXA

0RUJ07Z Supplement Right Shoulder Joint with Autologous Tissue Substitute, Open Approach
HAC When reported with secondary diagnosis code T84.60XA, T84.610A, T84.611A, T84.612A, T84.613A, T84.614A, T84.615A, T84.619A, T84.63XA, T84.69XA, T84.7XXA

0RUJ0JZ Supplement Right Shoulder Joint with Synthetic Substitute, Open Approach
HAC When reported with secondary diagnosis code T84.60XA, T84.610A, T84.611A, T84.612A, T84.613A, T84.614A, T84.615A, T84.619A, T84.63XA, T84.69XA, T84.7XXA

0RUJ0KZ Supplement Right Shoulder Joint with Nonautologous Tissue Substitute, Open Approach
HAC When reported with secondary diagnosis code T84.60XA, T84.610A, T84.611A, T84.612A, T84.613A, T84.614A, T84.615A, T84.619A, T84.63XA, T84.69XA, T84.7XXA

0RUJ37Z Supplement Right Shoulder Joint with Autologous Tissue Substitute, Percutaneous Approach
HAC When reported with secondary diagnosis code T84.60XA, T84.610A, T84.611A, T84.612A, T84.613A, T84.614A, T84.615A, T84.619A, T84.63XA, T84.69XA, T84.7XXA

0RUJ3JZ Supplement Right Shoulder Joint with Synthetic Substitute, Percutaneous Approach
HAC When reported with secondary diagnosis code T84.60XA, T84.610A, T84.611A, T84.612A, T84.613A, T84.614A, T84.615A, T84.619A, T84.63XA, T84.69XA, T84.7XXA

0RUJ3KZ Supplement Right Shoulder Joint with Nonautologous Tissue Substitute, Percutaneous Approach
HAC When reported with secondary diagnosis code T84.60XA, T84.610A, T84.611A, T84.612A, T84.613A, T84.614A, T84.615A, T84.619A, T84.63XA, T84.69XA, T84.7XXA

0RUJ47Z Supplement Right Shoulder Joint with Autologous Tissue Substitute, Percutaneous Endoscopic Approach
HAC When reported with secondary diagnosis code T84.60XA, T84.610A, T84.611A, T84.612A, T84.613A, T84.614A, T84.615A, T84.619A, T84.63XA, T84.69XA, T84.7XXA

0RUJ4JZ Supplement Right Shoulder Joint with Synthetic Substitute, Percutaneous Endoscopic Approach
HAC When reported with secondary diagnosis code T84.60XA, T84.610A, T84.611A, T84.612A, T84.613A, T84.614A, T84.615A, T84.619A, T84.63XA, T84.69XA, T84.7XXA

0RUJ4KZ Supplement Right Shoulder Joint with Nonautologous Tissue Substitute, Percutaneous Endoscopic Approach
HAC When reported with secondary diagnosis code T84.60XA, T84.610A, T84.611A, T84.612A, T84.613A, T84.614A, T84.615A, T84.619A, T84.63XA, T84.69XA, T84.7XXA

0RUK07Z Supplement Left Shoulder Joint with Autologous Tissue Substitute, Open Approach
HAC When reported with secondary diagnosis code T84.60XA, T84.610A, T84.611A, T84.612A, T84.613A, T84.614A, T84.615A, T84.619A, T84.63XA, T84.69XA, T84.7XXA

0RUK0JZ Supplement Left Shoulder Joint with Synthetic Substitute, Open Approach
HAC When reported with secondary diagnosis code T84.60XA, T84.610A, T84.611A, T84.612A, T84.613A, T84.614A, T84.615A, T84.619A, T84.63XA, T84.69XA, T84.7XXA

0RUK0KZ Supplement Left Shoulder Joint with Nonautologous Tissue Substitute, Open Approach
HAC When reported with secondary diagnosis code T84.60XA, T84.610A, T84.611A, T84.612A, T84.613A, T84.614A, T84.615A, T84.619A, T84.63XA, T84.69XA, T84.7XXA

0RUK37Z Supplement Left Shoulder Joint with Autologous Tissue Substitute, Percutaneous Approach
HAC When reported with secondary diagnosis code T84.60XA, T84.610A, T84.611A, T84.612A, T84.613A, T84.614A, T84.615A, T84.619A, T84.63XA, T84.69XA, T84.7XXA

0RUK3JZ Supplement Left Shoulder Joint with Synthetic Substitute, Percutaneous Approach
HAC When reported with secondary diagnosis code T84.60XA, T84.610A, T84.611A, T84.612A, T84.613A, T84.614A, T84.615A, T84.619A, T84.63XA, T84.69XA, T84.7XXA

0RUK3KZ Supplement Left Shoulder Joint with Nonautologous Tissue Substitute, Percutaneous Approach
HAC When reported with secondary diagnosis code T84.60XA, T84.610A, T84.611A, T84.612A, T84.613A, T84.614A, T84.615A, T84.619A, T84.63XA, T84.69XA, T84.7XXA

0RUK47Z Supplement Left Shoulder Joint with Autologous Tissue Substitute, Percutaneous Endoscopic Approach
HAC When reported with secondary diagnosis code T84.60XA, T84.610A, T84.611A, T84.612A, T84.613A, T84.614A, T84.615A, T84.619A, T84.63XA, T84.69XA, T84.7XXA

0RUK4JZ Supplement Left Shoulder Joint with Synthetic Substitute, Percutaneous Endoscopic Approach
HAC When reported with secondary diagnosis code T84.60XA, T84.610A, T84.611A, T84.612A, T84.613A, T84.614A, T84.615A, T84.619A, T84.63XA, T84.69XA, T84.7XXA

0RUK4KZ Supplement Left Shoulder Joint with Nonautologous Tissue Substitute, Percutaneous Endoscopic Approach
HAC When reported with secondary diagnosis code T84.60XA, T84.610A, T84.611A, T84.612A, T84.613A, T84.614A, T84.615A, T84.619A, T84.63XA, T84.69XA, T84.7XXA

0RUL07Z Supplement Right Elbow Joint with Autologous Tissue Substitute, Open Approach
HAC When reported with secondary diagnosis code T84.60XA, T84.610A, T84.611A, T84.612A, T84.613A, T84.614A, T84.615A, T84.619A, T84.63XA, T84.69XA, T84.7XXA

0RUL0JZ Supplement Right Elbow Joint with Synthetic Substitute, Open Approach
HAC When reported with secondary diagnosis code T84.60XA, T84.610A, T84.611A, T84.612A, T84.613A, T84.614A, T84.615A, T84.619A, T84.63XA, T84.69XA, T84.7XXA

0RUL0KZ Supplement Right Elbow Joint with Nonautologous Tissue Substitute, Open Approach
HAC When reported with secondary diagnosis code T84.60XA, T84.610A, T84.611A, T84.612A, T84.613A, T84.614A, T84.615A, T84.619A, T84.63XA, T84.69XA, T84.7XXA

0RUL37Z Supplement Right Elbow Joint with Autologous Tissue Substitute, Percutaneous Approach
HAC When reported with secondary diagnosis code T84.60XA, T84.610A, T84.611A, T84.612A, T84.613A, T84.614A, T84.615A, T84.619A, T84.63XA, T84.69XA, T84.7XXA

0RUL3JZ Supplement Right Elbow Joint with Synthetic Substitute, Percutaneous Approach
HAC When reported with secondary diagnosis code T84.60XA, T84.610A, T84.611A, T84.612A, T84.613A, T84.614A, T84.615A, T84.619A, T84.63XA, T84.69XA, T84.7XXA

0RUL3KZ Supplement Right Elbow Joint with Nonautologous Tissue Substitute, Percutaneous Approach
HAC When reported with secondary diagnosis code T84.60XA, T84.610A, T84.611A, T84.612A, T84.613A, T84.614A, T84.615A, T84.619A, T84.63XA, T84.69XA, T84.7XXA

0RUL47Z Supplement Right Elbow Joint with Autologous Tissue Substitute, Percutaneous Endoscopic Approach
HAC When reported with secondary diagnosis code T84.60XA, T84.610A, T84.611A, T84.612A, T84.613A, T84.614A, T84.615A, T84.619A, T84.63XA, T84.69XA, T84.7XXA

0RUL4JZ Supplement Right Elbow Joint with Synthetic Substitute, Percutaneous Endoscopic Approach
HAC When reported with secondary diagnosis code T84.60XA, T84.610A, T84.611A, T84.612A, T84.613A, T84.614A, T84.615A, T84.619A, T84.63XA, T84.69XA, T84.7XXA

0RUL4KZ Supplement Right Elbow Joint with Nonautologous Tissue Substitute, Percutaneous Endoscopic Approach
HAC When reported with secondary diagnosis code T84.60XA, T84.610A, T84.611A, T84.612A, T84.613A, T84.614A, T84.615A, T84.619A, T84.63XA, T84.69XA, T84.7XXA

0RUM07Z Supplement Left Elbow Joint with Autologous Tissue Substitute, Open Approach
HAC When reported with secondary diagnosis code T84.60XA, T84.610A, T84.611A, T84.612A, T84.613A, T84.614A, T84.615A, T84.619A, T84.63XA, T84.69XA, T84.7XXA

0RUM0JZ Supplement Left Elbow Joint with Synthetic Substitute, Open Approach
HAC When reported with secondary diagnosis code T84.60XA, T84.610A, T84.611A, T84.612A, T84.613A, T84.614A, T84.615A, T84.619A, T84.63XA, T84.69XA, T84.7XXA

0RUM0KZ Supplement Left Elbow Joint with Nonautologous Tissue Substitute, Open Approach
HAC When reported with secondary diagnosis code T84.60XA, T84.610A, T84.611A, T84.612A, T84.613A, T84.614A, T84.615A, T84.619A, T84.63XA, T84.69XA, T84.7XXA

0RUM37Z Supplement Left Elbow Joint with Autologous Tissue Substitute, Percutaneous Approach
HAC When reported with secondary diagnosis code T84.60XA, T84.610A, T84.611A, T84.612A, T84.613A, T84.614A, T84.615A, T84.619A, T84.63XA, T84.69XA, T84.7XXA

0RUM3JZ Supplement Left Elbow Joint with Synthetic Substitute, Percutaneous Approach
HAC When reported with secondary diagnosis code T84.60XA, T84.610A, T84.611A, T84.612A, T84.613A, T84.614A, T84.615A, T84.619A, T84.63XA, T84.69XA, T84.7XXA

0RUM3KZ Supplement Left Elbow Joint with Nonautologous Tissue Substitute, Percutaneous Approach
HAC When reported with secondary diagnosis code T84.60XA, T84.610A, T84.611A, T84.612A, T84.613A, T84.614A, T84.615A, T84.619A, T84.63XA, T84.69XA, T84.7XXA

0RUM47Z Supplement Left Elbow Joint with Autologous Tissue Substitute, Percutaneous Endoscopic Approach
HAC When reported with secondary diagnosis code T84.60XA, T84.610A, T84.611A, T84.612A, T84.613A, T84.614A, T84.615A, T84.619A, T84.63XA, T84.69XA, T84.7XXA

0RUM4JZ Supplement Left Elbow Joint with Synthetic Substitute, Percutaneous Endoscopic Approach
HAC When reported with secondary diagnosis code T84.60XA, T84.610A, T84.611A, T84.612A, T84.613A, T84.614A, T84.615A, T84.619A, T84.63XA, T84.69XA, T84.7XXA

0RUM4KZ Supplement Left Elbow Joint with Nonautologous Tissue Substitute, Percutaneous Endoscopic Approach
HAC When reported with secondary diagnosis code T84.60XA, T84.610A, T84.611A, T84.612A, T84.613A, T84.614A, T84.615A, T84.619A, T84.63XA, T84.69XA, T84.7XXA

0RUN07Z Supplement Right Wrist Joint with Autologous Tissue Substitute, Open Approach

0RUN0JZ Supplement Right Wrist Joint with Synthetic Substitute, Open Approach

0RUN0KZ Supplement Right Wrist Joint with Nonautologous Tissue Substitute, Open Approach

0RUN37Z Supplement Right Wrist Joint with Autologous Tissue Substitute, Percutaneous Approach

0RUN3JZ Supplement Right Wrist Joint with Synthetic Substitute, Percutaneous Approach

0RUN3KZ Supplement Right Wrist Joint with Nonautologous Tissue Substitute, Percutaneous Approach

0RUN47Z Supplement Right Wrist Joint with Autologous Tissue Substitute, Percutaneous Endoscopic Approach

0RUN4JZ Supplement Right Wrist Joint with Synthetic Substitute, Percutaneous Endoscopic Approach

0RUN4KZ Supplement Right Wrist Joint with Nonautologous Tissue Substitute, Percutaneous Endoscopic Approach

0RUP07Z Supplement Left Wrist Joint with Autologous Tissue Substitute, Open Approach

0RUP0JZ Supplement Left Wrist Joint with Syntheti Substitute, Open Approach

0RUP0KZ Supplement Left Wrist Joint with Nonautologous Tissue Substitute, Open Approach

0RUP37Z Supplement Left Wrist Joint with Autologous Tissue Substitute, Percutaneous Approach

0RUP3JZ Supplement Left Wrist Joint with Synthetic Substitute, Percutaneous Approach

0RUP3KZ Supplement Left Wrist Joint with Nonautologous Tissue Substitute, Percutaneous Approach

0RUP47Z Supplement Left Wrist Joint with Autologous Tissue Substitute, Percutaneous Endoscopic Approach

0RUP4JZ Supplement Left Wrist Joint with Synthetic Substitute, Percutaneous Endoscopic Approach

0RUP4KZ Supplement Left Wrist Joint with Nonautologous Tissue Substitute, Percutaneous Endoscopic Approach

0RUQ07Z Supplement Right Carpal Joint with Autologous Tissue Substitute, Open Approach

0RUQ0JZ Supplement Right Carpal Joint with Synthetic Substitute, Open Approach

0RUQ0KZ Supplement Right Carpal Joint with Nonautologous Tissue Substitute, Open Approach

0RUQ37Z Supplement Right Carpal Joint with Autologous Tissue Substitute, Percutaneous Approach

0RUQ3JZ Supplement Right Carpal Joint with Synthetic Substitute, Percutaneous Approach

0RUQ3KZ Supplement Right Carpal Joint with Nonautologous Tissue Substitute, Percutaneous Approach

0RUQ47Z Supplement Right Carpal Joint with Autologous Tissue Substitute, Percutaneous Endoscopic Approach

0RUQ4JZ Supplement Right Carpal Joint with Synthetic Substitute, Percutaneous Endoscopic Approach

0RUQ4KZ Supplement Right Carpal Joint with Nonautologous Tissue Substitute, Percutaneous Endoscopic Approach

0RUR07Z Supplement Left Carpal Joint with Autologous Tissue Substitute, Open Approach

0RUR0JZ Supplement Left Carpal Joint with Synthetic Substitute, Open Approach

0RUR0KZ Supplement Left Carpal Joint with Nonautologous Tissue Substitute, Open Approach

0RUR37Z Supplement Left Carpal Joint with Autologous Tissue Substitute, Percutaneous Approach

0RUR3JZ Supplement Left Carpal Joint with Synthetic Substitute, Percutaneous Approach

0RUR3KZ Supplement Left Carpal Joint with Nonautologous Tissue Substitute, Percutaneous Approach

0RUR47Z Supplement Left Carpal Joint with Autologous Tissue Substitute, Percutaneous Endoscopic Approach

0RUR4JZ Supplement Left Carpal Joint with Synthetic Substitute, Percutaneous Endoscopic Approach

0RUR4KZ Supplement Left Carpal Joint with Nonautologous Tissue Substitute, Percutaneous Endoscopic Approach

0RUS07Z Supplement Right Metacarpocarpal Joint with Autologous Tissue Substitute, Open Approach

0RUS0JZ Supplement Right Metacarpocarpal Joint with Synthetic Substitute, Open Approach
0RUS0KZ Supplement Right Metacarpocarpal Joint with Nonautologous Tissue Substitute, Open Approach
0RUS37Z Supplement Right Metacarpocarpal Joint with Autologous Tissue Substitute, Percutaneous Approach
0RUS3JZ Supplement Right Metacarpocarpal Joint with Synthetic Substitute, Percutaneous Approach
0RUS3KZ Supplement Right Metacarpocarpal Joint with Nonautologous Tissue Substitute, Percutaneous Approach
0RUS47Z Supplement Right Metacarpocarpal Joint with Autologous Tissue Substitute, Percutaneous Endoscopic Approach
0RUS4JZ Supplement Right Metacarpocarpal Joint with Synthetic Substitute, Percutaneous Endoscopic Approach
0RUS4KZ Supplement Right Metacarpocarpal Joint with Nonautologous Tissue Substitute, Percutaneous Endoscopic Approach
0RUT07Z Supplement Left Metacarpocarpal Joint with Autologous Tissue Substitute, Open Approach
0RUT0JZ Supplement Left Metacarpocarpal Joint with Synthetic Substitute, Open Approach
0RUT0KZ Supplement Left Metacarpocarpal Joint with Nonautologous Tissue Substitute, Open Approach
0RUT37Z Supplement Left Metacarpocarpal Joint with Autologous Tissue Substitute, Percutaneous Approach
0RUT3JZ Supplement Left Metacarpocarpal Joint with Synthetic Substitute, Percutaneous Approach
0RUT3KZ Supplement Left Metacarpocarpal Joint with Nonautologous Tissue Substitute, Percutaneous Approach
0RUT47Z Supplement Left Metacarpocarpal Joint with Autologous Tissue Substitute, Percutaneous Endoscopic Approach
0RUT4JZ Supplement Left Metacarpocarpal Joint with Synthetic Substitute, Percutaneous Endoscopic Approach
0RUT4KZ Supplement Left Metacarpocarpal Joint with Nonautologous Tissue Substitute, Percutaneous Endoscopic Approach
0RUU07Z Supplement Right Metacarpophalangeal Joint with Autologous Tissue Substitute, Open Approach
0RUU0JZ Supplement Right Metacarpophalangeal Joint with Synthetic Substitute, Open Approach
0RUU0KZ Supplement Right Metacarpophalangeal Joint with Nonautologous Tissue Substitute, Open Approach
0RUU37Z Supplement Right Metacarpophalangeal Joint with Autologous Tissue Substitute, Percutaneous Approach
0RUU3JZ Supplement Right Metacarpophalangeal Joint with Synthetic Substitute, Percutaneous Approach
0RUU3KZ Supplement Right Metacarpophalangeal Joint with Nonautologous Tissue Substitute, Percutaneous Approach
0RUU47Z Supplement Right Metacarpophalangeal Joint with Autologous Tissue Substitute, Percutaneous Endoscopic Approach
0RUU4JZ Supplement Right Metacarpophalangeal Joint with Synthetic Substitute, Percutaneous Endoscopic Approach
0RUU4KZ Supplement Right Metacarpophalangeal Joint with Nonautologous Tissue Substitute, Percutaneous Endoscopic Approach
0RUV07Z Supplement Left Metacarpophalangeal Joint with Autologous Tissue Substitute, Open Approach
0RUV0JZ Supplement Left Metacarpophalangeal Joint with Synthetic Substitute, Open Approach
0RUV0KZ Supplement Left Metacarpophalangeal Joint with Nonautologous Tissue Substitute, Open Approach
0RUV37Z Supplement Left Metacarpophalangeal Joint with Autologous Tissue Substitute, Percutaneous Approach
0RUV3JZ Supplement Left Metacarpophalangeal Joint with Synthetic Substitute, Percutaneous Approach
0RUV3KZ Supplement Left Metacarpophalangeal Joint with Nonautologous Tissue Substitute, Percutaneous Approach
0RUV47Z Supplement Left Metacarpophalangeal Joint with Autologous Tissue Substitute, Percutaneous Endoscopic Approach
0RUV4JZ Supplement Left Metacarpophalangeal Joint with Synthetic Substitute, Percutaneous Endoscopic Approach
0RUV4KZ Supplement Left Metacarpophalangeal Joint with Nonautologous Tissue Substitute, Percutaneous Endoscopic Approach
0RUW07Z Supplement Right Finger Phalangeal Joint with Autologous Tissue Substitute, Open Approach
0RUW0JZ Supplement Right Finger Phalangeal Joint with Synthetic Substitute, Open Approach
0RUW0KZ Supplement Right Finger Phalangeal Joint with Nonautologous Tissue Substitute, Open Approach
0RUW37Z Supplement Right Finger Phalangeal Joint with Autologous Tissue Substitute, Percutaneous Approach
0RUW3JZ Supplement Right Finger Phalangeal Joint with Synthetic Substitute, Percutaneous Approach
0RUW3KZ Supplement Right Finger Phalangeal Joint with Nonautologous Tissue Substitute, Percutaneous Approach
0RUW47Z Supplement Right Finger Phalangeal Joint with Autologous Tissue Substitute, Percutaneous Endoscopic Approach
0RUW4JZ Supplement Right Finger Phalangeal Joint with Synthetic Substitute, Percutaneous Endoscopic Approach
0RUW4KZ Supplement Right Finger Phalangeal Joint with Nonautologous Tissue Substitute, Percutaneous Endoscopic Approach
0RUX07Z Supplement Left Finger Phalangeal Joint with Autologous Tissue Substitute, Open Approach
0RUX0JZ Supplement Left Finger Phalangeal Joint with Synthetic Substitute, Open Approach
0RUX0KZ Supplement Left Finger Phalangeal Joint with Nonautologous Tissue Substitute, Open Approach
0RUX37Z Supplement Left Finger Phalangeal Joint with Autologous Tissue Substitute, Percutaneous Approach
0RUX3JZ Supplement Left Finger Phalangeal Joint with Synthetic Substitute, Percutaneous Approach
0RUX3KZ Supplement Left Finger Phalangeal Joint with Nonautologous Tissue Substitute, Percutaneous Approach
0RUX47Z Supplement Left Finger Phalangeal Joint with Autologous Tissue Substitute, Percutaneous Endoscopic Approach
0RUX4JZ Supplement Left Finger Phalangeal Joint with Synthetic Substitute, Percutaneous Endoscopic Approach
0RUX4KZ Supplement Left Finger Phalangeal Joint with Nonautologous Tissue Substitute, Percutaneous Endoscopic Approach

0RW – Upper Joints, Revision

Review Coding Guideline B6.1c

0RW000Z Revision of Drainage Device in Occipital-cervical Joint, Open Approach
0RW003Z Revision of Infusion Device in Occipital-cervical Joint, Open Approach
0RW004Z Revision of Internal Fixation Device in Occipital-cervical Joint, Open Approach
0RW007Z Revision of Autologous Tissue Substitute in Occipital-cervical Joint, Open Approach
0RW008Z Revision of Spacer in Occipital-cervical Joint, Open Approach
0RW00AZ Revision of Interbody Fusion Device in Occipital-cervical Joint, Open Approach
0RW00JZ Revision of Synthetic Substitute in Occipital-cervical Joint, Open Approach
0RW00KZ Revision of Nonautologous Tissue Substitute in Occipital-cervical Joint, Open Approach
0RW030Z Revision of Drainage Device in Occipital-cervical Joint, Percutaneous Approach
0RW033Z Revision of Infusion Device in Occipital-cervical Joint, Percutaneous Approach
0RW034Z Revision of Internal Fixation Device in Occipital-cervical Joint, Percutaneous Approach
0RW037Z Revision of Autologous Tissue Substitute in Occipital-cervical Joint, Percutaneous Approach
0RW038Z Revision of Spacer in Occipital-cervical Joint, Percutaneous Approach
0RW03AZ Revision of Interbody Fusion Device in Occipital-cervical Joint, Percutaneous Approach
0RW03JZ Revision of Synthetic Substitute in Occipital-cervical Joint, Percutaneous Approach
0RW03KZ Revision of Nonautologous Tissue Substitute in Occipital-cervical Joint, Percutaneous Approach
0RW040Z Revision of Drainage Device in Occipital-cervical Joint, Percutaneous Endoscopic Approach
0RW043Z Revision of Infusion Device in Occipital-cervical Joint, Percutaneous Endoscopic Approach
0RW044Z Revision of Internal Fixation Device in Occipital-cervical Joint, Percutaneous Endoscopic Approach
0RW047Z Revision of Autologous Tissue Substitute in Occipital-cervical Joint, Percutaneous Endoscopic Approach
0RW048Z Revision of Spacer in Occipital-cervical Joint, Percutaneous Endoscopic Approach

0RW04AZ Revision of Interbody Fusion Device in Occipital-cervical Joint, Percutaneous Endoscopic Approach
0RW04JZ Revision of Synthetic Substitute in Occipital-cervical Joint, Percutaneous Endoscopic Approach
0RW04KZ Revision of Nonautologous Tissue Substitute in Occipital-cervical Joint, Percutaneous Endoscopic Approach
0RW0X0Z Revision of Drainage Device in Occipital-cervical Joint, External Approach
0RW0X3Z Revision of Infusion Device in Occipital-cervical Joint, External Approach
0RW0X4Z Revision of Internal Fixation Device in Occipital-cervical Joint, External Approach
0RW0X7Z Revision of Autologous Tissue Substitute in Occipital-cervical Joint, External Approach
0RW0X8Z Revision of Spacer in Occipital-cervical Joint, External Approach
0RW0XAZ Revision of Interbody Fusion Device in Occipital-cervical Joint, External Approach
0RW0XJZ Revision of Synthetic Substitute in Occipital-cervical Joint, External Approach
0RW0XKZ Revision of Nonautologous Tissue Substitute in Occipital-cervical Joint, External Approach
0RW100Z Revision of Drainage Device in Cervical Vertebral Joint, Open Approach
0RW103Z Revision of Infusion Device in Cervical Vertebral Joint, Open Approach
0RW104Z Revision of Internal Fixation Device in Cervical Vertebral Joint, Open Approach
0RW107Z Revision of Autologous Tissue Substitute in Cervical Vertebral Joint, Open Approach
0RW108Z Revision of Spacer in Cervical Vertebral Joint, Open Approach
0RW10AZ Revision of Interbody Fusion Device in Cervical Vertebral Joint, Open Approach
0RW10JZ Revision of Synthetic Substitute in Cervical Vertebral Joint, Open Approach
0RW10KZ Revision of Nonautologous Tissue Substitute in Cervical Vertebral Joint, Open Approach
0RW130Z Revision of Drainage Device in Cervical Vertebral Joint, Percutaneous Approach
0RW133Z Revision of Infusion Device in Cervical Vertebral Joint, Percutaneous Approach
0RW134Z Revision of Internal Fixation Device in Cervical Vertebral Joint, Percutaneous Approach
0RW137Z Revision of Autologous Tissue Substitute in Cervical Vertebral Joint, Percutaneous Approach
0RW138Z Revision of Spacer in Cervical Vertebral Joint, Percutaneous Approach
0RW13AZ Revision of Interbody Fusion Device in Cervical Vertebral Joint, Percutaneous Approach
0RW13JZ Revision of Synthetic Substitute in Cervical Vertebral Joint, Percutaneous Approach
0RW13KZ Revision of Nonautologous Tissue Substitute in Cervical Vertebral Joint, Percutaneous Approach
0RW140Z Revision of Drainage Device in Cervical Vertebral Joint, Percutaneous Endoscopic Approach
0RW143Z Revision of Infusion Device in Cervical Vertebral Joint, Percutaneous Endoscopic Approach
0RW144Z Revision of Internal Fixation Device in Cervical Vertebral Joint, Percutaneous Endoscopic Approach
0RW147Z Revision of Autologous Tissue Substitute in Cervical Vertebral Joint, Percutaneous Endoscopic Approach
0RW148Z Revision of Spacer in Cervical Vertebral Joint, Percutaneous Endoscopic Approach
0RW14AZ Revision of Interbody Fusion Device in Cervical Vertebral Joint, Percutaneous Endoscopic Approach
0RW14JZ Revision of Synthetic Substitute in Cervical Vertebral Joint, Percutaneous Endoscopic Approach
0RW14KZ Revision of Nonautologous Tissue Substitute in Cervical Vertebral Joint, Percutaneous Endoscopic Approach
0RW1X0Z Revision of Drainage Device in Cervical Vertebral Joint, External Approach
0RW1X3Z Revision of Infusion Device in Cervical Vertebral Joint, External Approach
0RW1X4Z Revision of Internal Fixation Device in Cervical Vertebral Joint, External Approach
0RW1X7Z Revision of Autologous Tissue Substitute in Cervical Vertebral Joint, External Approach
0RW1X8Z Revision of Spacer in Cervical Vertebral Joint, External Approach
0RW1XAZ Revision of Interbody Fusion Device in Cervical Vertebral Joint, External Approach
0RW1XJZ Revision of Synthetic Substitute in Cervical Vertebral Joint, External Approach
0RW1XKZ Revision of Nonautologous Tissue Substitute in Cervical Vertebral Joint, External Approach
0RW300Z Revision of Drainage Device in Cervical Vertebral Disc, Open Approach
0RW303Z Revision of Infusion Device in Cervical Vertebral Disc, Open Approach
0RW307Z Revision of Autologous Tissue Substitute in Cervical Vertebral Disc, Open Approach
0RW30JZ Revision of Synthetic Substitute in Cervical Vertebral Disc, Open Approach
0RW30KZ Revision of Nonautologous Tissue Substitute in Cervical Vertebral Disc, Open Approach
0RW330Z Revision of Drainage Device in Cervical Vertebral Disc, Percutaneous Approach
0RW333Z Revision of Infusion Device in Cervical Vertebral Disc, Percutaneous Approach
0RW337Z Revision of Autologous Tissue Substitute in Cervical Vertebral Disc, Percutaneous Approach
0RW33JZ Revision of Synthetic Substitute in Cervical Vertebral Disc, Percutaneous Approach
0RW33KZ Revision of Nonautologous Tissue Substitute in Cervical Vertebral Disc, Percutaneous Approach
0RW340Z Revision of Drainage Device in Cervical Vertebral Disc, Percutaneous Endoscopic Approach
0RW343Z Revision of Infusion Device in Cervical Vertebral Disc, Percutaneous Endoscopic Approach
0RW347Z Revision of Autologous Tissue Substitute in Cervical Vertebral Disc, Percutaneous Endoscopic Approach
0RW34JZ Revision of Synthetic Substitute in Cervical Vertebral Disc, Percutaneous Endoscopic Approach
0RW34KZ Revision of Nonautologous Tissue Substitute in Cervical Vertebral Disc, Percutaneous Endoscopic Approach
0RW3X0Z Revision of Drainage Device in Cervical Vertebral Disc, External Approach
0RW3X3Z Revision of Infusion Device in Cervical Vertebral Disc, External Approach
0RW3X7Z Revision of Autologous Tissue Substitute in Cervical Vertebral Disc, External Approach
0RW3XJZ Revision of Synthetic Substitute in Cervical Vertebral Disc, External Approach
0RW3XKZ Revision of Nonautologous Tissue Substitute in Cervical Vertebral Disc, External Approach
0RW400Z Revision of Drainage Device in Cervicothoracic Vertebral Joint, Open Approach
0RW403Z Revision of Infusion Device in Cervicothoracic Vertebral Joint, Open Approach
0RW404Z Revision of Internal Fixation Device in Cervicothoracic Vertebral Joint, Open Approach
0RW407Z Revision of Autologous Tissue Substitute in Cervicothoracic Vertebral Joint, Open Approach
0RW408Z Revision of Spacer in Cervicothoracic Vertebral Joint, Open Approach
0RW40AZ Revision of Interbody Fusion Device in Cervicothoracic Vertebral Joint, Open Approach
0RW40JZ Revision of Synthetic Substitute in Cervicothoracic Vertebral Joint, Open Approach
0RW40KZ Revision of Nonautologous Tissue Substitute in Cervicothoracic Vertebral Joint, Open Approach
0RW430Z Revision of Drainage Device in Cervicothoracic Vertebral Joint, Percutaneous Approach
0RW433Z Revision of Infusion Device in Cervicothoracic Vertebral Joint, Percutaneous Approach
0RW434Z Revision of Internal Fixation Device in Cervicothoracic Vertebral Joint, Percutaneous Approach
0RW437Z Revision of Autologous Tissue Substitute in Cervicothoracic Vertebral Joint, Percutaneous Approach
0RW438Z Revision of Spacer in Cervicothoracic Vertebral Joint, Percutaneous Approach
0RW43AZ Revision of Interbody Fusion Device in Cervicothoracic Vertebral Joint, Percutaneous Approach
0RW43JZ Revision of Synthetic Substitute in Cervicothoracic Vertebral Joint, Percutaneous Approach
0RW43KZ Revision of Nonautologous Tissue Substitute in Cervicothoracic Vertebral Joint, Percutaneous Approach
0RW440Z Revision of Drainage Device in Cervicothoracic Vertebral Joint, Percutaneous Endoscopic Approach
0RW443Z Revision of Infusion Device in Cervicothoracic Vertebral Joint, Percutaneous Endoscopic Approach
0RW444Z Revision of Internal Fixation Device in Cervicothoracic Vertebral Joint, Percutaneous Endoscopic Approach
0RW447Z Revision of Autologous Tissue Substitute in Cervicothoracic Vertebral Joint, Percutaneous Endoscopic Approach
0RW448Z Revision of Spacer in Cervicothoracic Vertebral Joint, Percutaneous Endoscopic Approach
0RW44AZ Revision of Interbody Fusion Device in Cervicothoracic Vertebral Joint, Percutaneous Endoscopic Approach

0RW44JZ Revision of Synthetic Substitute in Cervicothoracic Vertebral Joint, Percutaneous Endoscopic Approach
0RW44KZ Revision of Nonautologous Tissue Substitute in Cervicothoracic Vertebral Joint, Percutaneous Endoscopic Approach
0RW4X0Z Revision of Drainage Device in Cervicothoracic Vertebral Joint, External Approach
0RW4X3Z Revision of Infusion Device in Cervicothoracic Vertebral Joint, External Approach
0RW4X4Z Revision of Internal Fixation Device in Cervicothoracic Vertebral Joint, External Approach
0RW4X7Z Revision of Autologous Tissue Substitute in Cervicothoracic Vertebral Joint, External Approach
0RW4X8Z Revision of Spacer in Cervicothoracic Vertebral Joint, External Approach
0RW4XAZ Revision of Interbody Fusion Device in Cervicothoracic Vertebral Joint, External Approach
0RW4XJZ Revision of Synthetic Substitute in Cervicothoracic Vertebral Joint, External Approach
0RW4XKZ Revision of Nonautologous Tissue Substitute in Cervicothoracic Vertebral Joint, External Approach
0RW500Z Revision of Drainage Device in Cervicothoracic Vertebral Disc, Open Approach
0RW503Z Revision of Infusion Device in Cervicothoracic Vertebral Disc, Open Approach
0RW507Z Revision of Autologous Tissue Substitute in Cervicothoracic Vertebral Disc, Open Approach
0RW50JZ Revision of Synthetic Substitute in Cervicothoracic Vertebral Disc, Open Approach
0RW50KZ Revision of Nonautologous Tissue Substitute in Cervicothoracic Vertebral Disc, Open Approach
0RW530Z Revision of Drainage Device in Cervicothoracic Vertebral Disc, Percutaneous Approach
0RW533Z Revision of Infusion Device in Cervicothoracic Vertebral Disc, Percutaneous Approach
0RW537Z Revision of Autologous Tissue Substitute in Cervicothoracic Vertebral Disc, Percutaneous Approach
0RW53JZ Revision of Synthetic Substitute in Cervicothoracic Vertebral Disc, Percutaneous Approach
0RW53KZ Revision of Nonautologous Tissue Substitute in Cervicothoracic Vertebral Disc, Percutaneous Approach
0RW540Z Revision of Drainage Device in Cervicothoracic Vertebral Disc, Percutaneous Endoscopic Approach
0RW543Z Revision of Infusion Device in Cervicothoracic Vertebral Disc, Percutaneous Endoscopic Approach
0RW547Z Revision of Autologous Tissue Substitute in Cervicothoracic Vertebral Disc, Percutaneous Endoscopic Approach
0RW54JZ Revision of Synthetic Substitute in Cervicothoracic Vertebral Disc, Percutaneous Endoscopic Approach
0RW54KZ Revision of Nonautologous Tissue Substitute in Cervicothoracic Vertebral Disc, Percutaneous Endoscopic Approach
0RW5X0Z Revision of Drainage Device in Cervicothoracic Vertebral Disc, External Approach
0RW5X3Z Revision of Infusion Device in Cervicothoracic Vertebral Disc, External Approach
0RW5X7Z Revision of Autologous Tissue Substitute in Cervicothoracic Vertebral Disc, External Approach
0RW5XJZ Revision of Synthetic Substitute in Cervicothoracic Vertebral Disc, External Approach
0RW5XKZ Revision of Nonautologous Tissue Substitute in Cervicothoracic Vertebral Disc, External Approach
0RW600Z Revision of Drainage Device in Thoracic Vertebral Joint, Open Approach
0RW603Z Revision of Infusion Device in Thoracic Vertebral Joint, Open Approach
0RW604Z Revision of Internal Fixation Device in Thoracic Vertebral Joint, Open Approach
0RW607Z Revision of Autologous Tissue Substitute in Thoracic Vertebral Joint, Open Approach
0RW608Z Revision of Spacer in Thoracic Vertebral Joint, Open Approach
0RW60AZ Revision of Interbody Fusion Device in Thoracic Vertebral Joint, Open Approach
0RW60JZ Revision of Synthetic Substitute in Thoracic Vertebral Joint, Open Approach
0RW60KZ Revision of Nonautologous Tissue Substitute in Thoracic Vertebral Joint, Open Approach
0RW630Z Revision of Drainage Device in Thoracic Vertebral Joint, Percutaneous Approach
0RW633Z Revision of Infusion Device in Thoracic Vertebral Joint, Percutaneous Approach
0RW634Z Revision of Internal Fixation Device in Thoracic Vertebral Joint, Percutaneous Approach
0RW637Z Revision of Autologous Tissue Substitute in Thoracic Vertebral Joint, Percutaneous Approach
0RW638Z Revision of Spacer in Thoracic Vertebral Joint, Percutaneous Approach
0RW63AZ Revision of Interbody Fusion Device in Thoracic Vertebral Joint, Percutaneous Approach
0RW63JZ Revision of Synthetic Substitute in Thoracic Vertebral Joint, Percutaneous Approach
0RW63KZ Revision of Nonautologous Tissue Substitute in Thoracic Vertebral Joint, Percutaneous Approach
0RW640Z Revision of Drainage Device in Thoracic Vertebral Joint, Percutaneous Endoscopic Approach
0RW643Z Revision of Infusion Device in Thoracic Vertebral Joint, Percutaneous Endoscopic Approach
0RW644Z Revision of Internal Fixation Device in Thoracic Vertebral Joint, Percutaneous Endoscopic Approach
0RW647Z Revision of Autologous Tissue Substitute in Thoracic Vertebral Joint, Percutaneous Endoscopic Approach
0RW648Z Revision of Spacer in Thoracic Vertebral Joint, Percutaneous Endoscopic Approach
0RW64AZ Revision of Interbody Fusion Device in Thoracic Vertebral Joint, Percutaneous Endoscopic Approach
0RW64JZ Revision of Synthetic Substitute in Thoracic Vertebral Joint, Percutaneous Endoscopic Approach
0RW64KZ Revision of Nonautologous Tissue Substitute in Thoracic Vertebral Joint, Percutaneous Endoscopic Approach
0RW6X0Z Revision of Drainage Device in Thoracic Vertebral Joint, External Approach
0RW6X3Z Revision of Infusion Device in Thoracic Vertebral Joint, External Approach
0RW6X4Z Revision of Internal Fixation Device in Thoracic Vertebral Joint, External Approach
0RW6X7Z Revision of Autologous Tissue Substitute in Thoracic Vertebral Joint, External Approach
0RW6X8Z Revision of Spacer in Thoracic Vertebral Joint, External Approach
0RW6XAZ Revision of Interbody Fusion Device in Thoracic Vertebral Joint, External Approach
0RW6XJZ Revision of Synthetic Substitute in Thoracic Vertebral Joint, External Approach
0RW6XKZ Revision of Nonautologous Tissue Substitute in Thoracic Vertebral Joint, External Approach
0RW900Z Revision of Drainage Device in Thoracic Vertebral Disc, Open Approach
0RW903Z Revision of Infusion Device in Thoracic Vertebral Disc, Open Approach
0RW907Z Revision of Autologous Tissue Substitute in Thoracic Vertebral Disc, Open Approach
0RW90JZ Revision of Synthetic Substitute in Thoracic Vertebral Disc, Open Approach
0RW90KZ Revision of Nonautologous Tissue Substitute in Thoracic Vertebral Disc, Open Approach
0RW930Z Revision of Drainage Device in Thoracic Vertebral Disc, Percutaneous Approach
0RW933Z Revision of Infusion Device in Thoracic Vertebral Disc, Percutaneous Approach
0RW937Z Revision of Autologous Tissue Substitute in Thoracic Vertebral Disc, Percutaneous Approach
0RW93JZ Revision of Synthetic Substitute in Thoracic Vertebral Disc, Percutaneous Approach
0RW93KZ Revision of Nonautologous Tissue Substitute in Thoracic Vertebral Disc, Percutaneous Approach
0RW940Z Revision of Drainage Device in Thoracic Vertebral Disc, Percutaneous Endoscopic Approach
0RW943Z Revision of Infusion Device in Thoracic Vertebral Disc, Percutaneous Endoscopic Approach
0RW947Z Revision of Autologous Tissue Substitute in Thoracic Vertebral Disc, Percutaneous Endoscopic Approach
0RW94JZ Revision of Synthetic Substitute in Thoracic Vertebral Disc, Percutaneous Endoscopic Approach
0RW94KZ Revision of Nonautologous Tissue Substitute in Thoracic Vertebral Disc, Percutaneous Endoscopic Approach
0RW9X0Z Revision of Drainage Device in Thoracic Vertebral Disc, External Approach
0RW9X3Z Revision of Infusion Device in Thoracic Vertebral Disc, External Approach
0RW9X7Z Revision of Autologous Tissue Substitute in Thoracic Vertebral Disc, External Approach
0RW9XJZ Revision of Synthetic Substitute in Thoracic Vertebral Disc, External Approach
0RW9XKZ Revision of Nonautologous Tissue Substitute in Thoracic Vertebral Disc, External Approach

0RWA00Z Revision of Drainage Device in Thoracolumbar Vertebral Joint, Open Approach
0RWA03Z Revision of Infusion Device in Thoracolumbar Vertebral Joint, Open Approach
0RWA04Z Revision of Internal Fixation Device in Thoracolumbar Vertebral Joint, Open Approach
0RWA07Z Revision of Autologous Tissue Substitute in Thoracolumbar Vertebral Joint, Open Approach
0RWA08Z Revision of Spacer in Thoracolumbar Vertebral Joint, Open Approach
0RWA0AZ Revision of Interbody Fusion Device in Thoracolumbar Vertebral Joint, Open Approach
0RWA0JZ Revision of Synthetic Substitute in Thoracolumbar Vertebral Joint, Open Approach
0RWA0KZ Revision of Nonautologous Tissue Substitute in Thoracolumbar Vertebral Joint, Open Approach
0RWA30Z Revision of Drainage Device in Thoracolumbar Vertebral Joint, Percutaneous Approach
0RWA33Z Revision of Infusion Device in Thoracolumbar Vertebral Joint, Percutaneous Approach
0RWA34Z Revision of Internal Fixation Device in Thoracolumbar Vertebral Joint, Percutaneous Approach
0RWA37Z Revision of Autologous Tissue Substitute in Thoracolumbar Vertebral Joint, Percutaneous Approach
0RWA38Z Revision of Spacer in Thoracolumbar Vertebral Joint, Percutaneous Approach
0RWA3AZ Revision of Interbody Fusion Device in Thoracolumbar Vertebral Joint, Percutaneous Approach
0RWA3JZ Revision of Synthetic Substitute in Thoracolumbar Vertebral Joint, Percutaneous Approach
0RWA3KZ Revision of Nonautologous Tissue Substitute in Thoracolumbar Vertebral Joint, Percutaneous Approach
0RWA40Z Revision of Drainage Device in Thoracolumbar Vertebral Joint, Percutaneous Endoscopic Approach
0RWA43Z Revision of Infusion Device in Thoracolumbar Vertebral Joint, Percutaneous Endoscopic Approach
0RWA44Z Revision of Internal Fixation Device in Thoracolumbar Vertebral Joint, Percutaneous Endoscopic Approach
0RWA47Z Revision of Autologous Tissue Substitute in Thoracolumbar Vertebral Joint, Percutaneous Endoscopic Approach
0RWA48Z Revision of Spacer in Thoracolumbar Vertebral Joint, Percutaneous Endoscopic Approach
0RWA4AZ Revision of Interbody Fusion Device in Thoracolumbar Vertebral Joint, Percutaneous Endoscopic Approach
0RWA4JZ Revision of Synthetic Substitute in Thoracolumbar Vertebral Joint, Percutaneous Endoscopic Approach
0RWA4KZ Revision of Nonautologous Tissue Substitute in Thoracolumbar Vertebral Joint, Percutaneous Endoscopic Approach
0RWAX0Z Revision of Drainage Device in Thoracolumbar Vertebral Joint, External Approach
0RWAX3Z Revision of Infusion Device in Thoracolumbar Vertebral Joint, External Approach
0RWAX4Z Revision of Internal Fixation Device in Thoracolumbar Vertebral Joint, External Approach
0RWAX7Z Revision of Autologous Tissue Substitute in Thoracolumbar Vertebral Joint, External Approach
0RWAX8Z Revision of Spacer in Thoracolumbar Vertebral Joint, External Approach
0RWAXAZ Revision of Interbody Fusion Device in Thoracolumbar Vertebral Joint, External Approach
0RWAXJZ Revision of Synthetic Substitute in Thoracolumbar Vertebral Joint, External Approach
0RWAXKZ Revision of Nonautologous Tissue Substitute in Thoracolumbar Vertebral Joint, External Approach
0RWB00Z Revision of Drainage Device in Thoracolumbar Vertebral Disc, Open Approach
0RWB03Z Revision of Infusion Device in Thoracolumbar Vertebral Disc, Open Approach
0RWB07Z Revision of Autologous Tissue Substitute in Thoracolumbar Vertebral Disc, Open Approach
0RWB0JZ Revision of Synthetic Substitute in Thoracolumbar Vertebral Disc, Open Approach
0RWB0KZ Revision of Nonautologous Tissue Substitute in Thoracolumbar Vertebral Disc, Open Approach
0RWB30Z Revision of Drainage Device in Thoracolumbar Vertebral Disc, Percutaneous Approach
0RWB33Z Revision of Infusion Device in Thoracolumbar Vertebral Disc, Percutaneous Approach
0RWB37Z Revision of Autologous Tissue Substitute in Thoracolumbar Vertebral Disc, Percutaneous Approach
0RWB3JZ Revision of Synthetic Substitute in Thoracolumbar Vertebral Disc, Percutaneous Approach
0RWB3KZ Revision of Nonautologous Tissue Substitute in Thoracolumbar Vertebral Disc, Percutaneous Approach
0RWB40Z Revision of Drainage Device in Thoracolumbar Vertebral Disc, Percutaneous Endoscopic Approach
0RWB43Z Revision of Infusion Device in Thoracolumbar Vertebral Disc, Percutaneous Endoscopic Approach
0RWB47Z Revision of Autologous Tissue Substitute in Thoracolumbar Vertebral Disc, Percutaneous Endoscopic Approach
0RWB4JZ Revision of Synthetic Substitute in Thoracolumbar Vertebral Disc, Percutaneous Endoscopic Approach
0RWB4KZ Revision of Nonautologous Tissue Substitute in Thoracolumbar Vertebral Disc, Percutaneous Endoscopic Approach
0RWBX0Z Revision of Drainage Device in Thoracolumbar Vertebral Disc, External Approach
0RWBX3Z Revision of Infusion Device in Thoracolumbar Vertebral Disc, External Approach
0RWBX7Z Revision of Autologous Tissue Substitute in Thoracolumbar Vertebral Disc, External Approach
0RWBXJZ Revision of Synthetic Substitute in Thoracolumbar Vertebral Disc, External Approach
0RWBXKZ Revision of Nonautologous Tissue Substitute in Thoracolumbar Vertebral Disc, External Approach
0RWC00Z Revision of Drainage Device in Right Temporomandibular Joint, Open Approach
0RWC03Z Revision of Infusion Device in Right Temporomandibular Joint, Open Approach
0RWC04Z Revision of Internal Fixation Device in Right Temporomandibular Joint, Open Approach
0RWC07Z Revision of Autologous Tissue Substitute in Right Temporomandibular Joint, Open Approach
0RWC08Z Revision of Spacer in Right Temporomandibular Joint, Open Approach
0RWC0JZ Revision of Synthetic Substitute in Right Temporomandibular Joint, Open Approach
0RWC0KZ Revision of Nonautologous Tissue Substitute in Right Temporomandibular Joint, Open Approach
0RWC30Z Revision of Drainage Device in Right Temporomandibular Joint, Percutaneous Approach
0RWC33Z Revision of Infusion Device in Right Temporomandibular Joint, Percutaneous Approach
0RWC34Z Revision of Internal Fixation Device in Right Temporomandibular Joint, Percutaneous Approach
0RWC37Z Revision of Autologous Tissue Substitute in Right Temporomandibular Joint, Percutaneous Approach
0RWC38Z Revision of Spacer in Right Temporomandibular Joint, Percutaneous Approach
0RWC3JZ Revision of Synthetic Substitute in Right Temporomandibular Joint, Percutaneous Approach
0RWC3KZ Revision of Nonautologous Tissue Substitute in Right Temporomandibular Joint, Percutaneous Approach
0RWC40Z Revision of Drainage Device in Right Temporomandibular Joint, Percutaneous Endoscopic Approach
0RWC43Z Revision of Infusion Device in Right Temporomandibular Joint, Percutaneous Endoscopic Approach
0RWC44Z Revision of Internal Fixation Device in Right Temporomandibular Joint, Percutaneous Endoscopic Approach
0RWC47Z Revision of Autologous Tissue Substitute in Right Temporomandibular Joint, Percutaneous Endoscopic Approach
0RWC48Z Revision of Spacer in Right Temporomandibular Joint, Percutaneous Endoscopic Approach
0RWC4JZ Revision of Synthetic Substitute in Right Temporomandibular Joint, Percutaneous Endoscopic Approach
0RWC4KZ Revision of Nonautologous Tissue Substitute in Right Temporomandibular Joint, Percutaneous Endoscopic Approach
0RWCX0Z Revision of Drainage Device in Right Temporomandibular Joint, External Approach
0RWCX3Z Revision of Infusion Device in Right Temporomandibular Joint, External Approach
0RWCX4Z Revision of Internal Fixation Device in Right Temporomandibular Joint, External Approach

0RWCX7Z Revision of Autologous Tissue Substitute in Right Temporomandibular Joint, External Approach
0RWCX8Z Revision of Spacer in Right Temporomandibular Joint, External Approach
0RWCXJZ Revision of Synthetic Substitute in Right Temporomandibular Joint, External Approach
0RWCXKZ Revision of Nonautologous Tissue Substitute in Right Temporomandibular Joint, External Approach
0RWD00Z Revision of Drainage Device in Left Temporomandibular Joint, Open Approach
0RWD03Z Revision of Infusion Device in Left Temporomandibular Joint, Open Approach
0RWD04Z Revision of Internal Fixation Device in Left Temporomandibular Joint, Open Approach
0RWD07Z Revision of Autologous Tissue Substitute in Left Temporomandibular Joint, Open Approach
0RWD08Z Revision of Spacer in Left Temporomandibular Joint, Open Approach
0RWD0JZ Revision of Synthetic Substitute in Left Temporomandibular Joint, Open Approach
0RWD0KZ Revision of Nonautologous Tissue Substitute in Left Temporomandibular Joint, Open Approach
0RWD30Z Revision of Drainage Device in Left Temporomandibular Joint, Percutaneous Approach
0RWD33Z Revision of Infusion Device in Left Temporomandibular Joint, Percutaneous Approach
0RWD34Z Revision of Internal Fixation Device in Left Temporomandibular Joint, Percutaneous Approach
0RWD37Z Revision of Autologous Tissue Substitute in Left Temporomandibular Joint, Percutaneous Approach
0RWD38Z Revision of Spacer in Left Temporomandibular Joint, Percutaneous Approach
0RWD3JZ Revision of Synthetic Substitute in Left Temporomandibular Joint, Percutaneous Approach
0RWD3KZ Revision of Nonautologous Tissue Substitute in Left Temporomandibular Joint, Percutaneous Approach
0RWD40Z Revision of Drainage Device in Left Temporomandibular Joint, Percutaneous Endoscopic Approach
0RWD43Z Revision of Infusion Device in Left Temporomandibular Joint, Percutaneous Endoscopic Approach
0RWD44Z Revision of Internal Fixation Device in Left Temporomandibular Joint, Percutaneous Endoscopic Approach
0RWD47Z Revision of Autologous Tissue Substitute in Left Temporomandibular Joint, Percutaneous Endoscopic Approach
0RWD48Z Revision of Spacer in Left Temporomandibular Joint, Percutaneous Endoscopic Approach
0RWD4JZ Revision of Synthetic Substitute in Left Temporomandibular Joint, Percutaneous Endoscopic Approach
0RWD4KZ Revision of Nonautologous Tissue Substitute in Left Temporomandibular Joint, Percutaneous Endoscopic Approach
0RWDX0Z Revision of Drainage Device in Left Temporomandibular Joint, External Approach
0RWDX3Z Revision of Infusion Device in Left Temporomandibular Joint, External Approach
0RWDX4Z Revision of Internal Fixation Device in Left Temporomandibular Joint, External Approach
0RWDX7Z Revision of Autologous Tissue Substitute in Left Temporomandibular Joint, External Approach
0RWDX8Z Revision of Spacer in Left Temporomandibular Joint, External Approach
0RWDXJZ Revision of Synthetic Substitute in Left Temporomandibular Joint, External Approach
0RWDXKZ Revision of Nonautologous Tissue Substitute in Left Temporomandibular Joint, External Approach
0RWE00Z Revision of Drainage Device in Right Sternoclavicular Joint, Open Approach
0RWE03Z Revision of Infusion Device in Right Sternoclavicular Joint, Open Approach
0RWE04Z Revision of Internal Fixation Device in Right Sternoclavicular Joint, Open Approach
0RWE07Z Revision of Autologous Tissue Substitute in Right Sternoclavicular Joint, Open Approach
0RWE08Z Revision of Spacer in Right Sternoclavicular Joint, Open Approach
0RWE0JZ Revision of Synthetic Substitute in Right Sternoclavicular Joint, Open Approach
0RWE0KZ Revision of Nonautologous Tissue Substitute in Right Sternoclavicular Joint, Open Approach
0RWE30Z Revision of Drainage Device in Right Sternoclavicular Joint, Percutaneous Approach
0RWE33Z Revision of Infusion Device in Right Sternoclavicular Joint, Percutaneous Approach
0RWE34Z Revision of Internal Fixation Device in Right Sternoclavicular Joint, Percutaneous Approach
0RWE37Z Revision of Autologous Tissue Substitute in Right Sternoclavicular Joint, Percutaneous Approach
0RWE38Z Revision of Spacer in Right Sternoclavicular Joint, Percutaneous Approach
0RWE3JZ Revision of Synthetic Substitute in Right Sternoclavicular Joint, Percutaneous Approach
0RWE3KZ Revision of Nonautologous Tissue Substitute in Right Sternoclavicular Joint, Percutaneous Approach
0RWE40Z Revision of Drainage Device in Right Sternoclavicular Joint, Percutaneous Endoscopic Approach
0RWE43Z Revision of Infusion Device in Right Sternoclavicular Joint, Percutaneous Endoscopic Approach
0RWE44Z Revision of Internal Fixation Device in Right Sternoclavicular Joint, Percutaneous Endoscopic Approach
0RWE47Z Revision of Autologous Tissue Substitute in Right Sternoclavicular Joint, Percutaneous Endoscopic Approach
0RWE48Z Revision of Spacer in Right Sternoclavicular Joint, Percutaneous Endoscopic Approach
0RWE4JZ Revision of Synthetic Substitute in Right Sternoclavicular Joint, Percutaneous Endoscopic Approach
0RWE4KZ Revision of Nonautologous Tissue Substitute in Right Sternoclavicular Joint, Percutaneous Endoscopic Approach
0RWEX0Z Revision of Drainage Device in Right Sternoclavicular Joint, External Approach
0RWEX3Z Revision of Infusion Device in Right Sternoclavicular Joint, External Approach
0RWEX4Z Revision of Internal Fixation Device in Right Sternoclavicular Joint, External Approach
0RWEX7Z Revision of Autologous Tissue Substitute in Right Sternoclavicular Joint, External Approach
0RWEX8Z Revision of Spacer in Right Sternoclavicular Joint, External Approach
0RWEXJZ Revision of Synthetic Substitute in Right Sternoclavicular Joint, External Approach
0RWEXKZ Revision of Nonautologous Tissue Substitute in Right Sternoclavicular Joint, External Approach
0RWF00Z Revision of Drainage Device in Left Sternoclavicular Joint, Open Approach
0RWF03Z Revision of Infusion Device in Left Sternoclavicular Joint, Open Approach
0RWF04Z Revision of Internal Fixation Device in Left Sternoclavicular Joint, Open Approach
0RWF07Z Revision of Autologous Tissue Substitute in Left Sternoclavicular Joint, Open Approach
0RWF08Z Revision of Spacer in Left Sternoclavicular Joint, Open Approach
0RWF0JZ Revision of Synthetic Substitute in Left Sternoclavicular Joint, Open Approach
0RWF0KZ Revision of Nonautologous Tissue Substitute in Left Sternoclavicular Joint, Open Approach
0RWF30Z Revision of Drainage Device in Left Sternoclavicular Joint, Percutaneous Approach
0RWF33Z Revision of Infusion Device in Left Sternoclavicular Joint, Percutaneous Approach
0RWF34Z Revision of Internal Fixation Device in Left Sternoclavicular Joint, Percutaneous Approach
0RWF37Z Revision of Autologous Tissue Substitute in Left Sternoclavicular Joint, Percutaneous Approach
0RWF38Z Revision of Spacer in Left Sternoclavicular Joint, Percutaneous Approach
0RWF3JZ Revision of Synthetic Substitute in Left Sternoclavicular Joint, Percutaneous Approach
0RWF3KZ Revision of Nonautologous Tissue Substitute in Left Sternoclavicular Joint, Percutaneous Approach
0RWF40Z Revision of Drainage Device in Left Sternoclavicular Joint, Percutaneous Endoscopic Approach
0RWF43Z Revision of Infusion Device in Left Sternoclavicular Joint, Percutaneous Endoscopic Approach
0RWF44Z Revision of Internal Fixation Device in Left Sternoclavicular Joint, Percutaneous Endoscopic Approach
0RWF47Z Revision of Autologous Tissue Substitute in Left Sternoclavicular Joint, Percutaneous Endoscopic Approach
0RWF48Z Revision of Spacer in Left Sternoclavicular Joint, Percutaneous Endoscopic Approach
0RWF4JZ Revision of Synthetic Substitute in Left Sternoclavicular Joint, Percutaneous Endoscopic Approach

0RWF4KZ Revision of Nonautologous Tissue Substitute in Left Sternoclavicular Joint, Percutaneous Endoscopic Approach
0RWFX0Z Revision of Drainage Device in Left Sternoclavicular Joint, External Approach
0RWFX3Z Revision of Infusion Device in Left Sternoclavicular Joint, External Approach
0RWFX4Z Revision of Internal Fixation Device in Left Sternoclavicular Joint, External Approach
0RWFX7Z Revision of Autologous Tissue Substitute in Left Sternoclavicular Joint, External Approach
0RWFX8Z Revision of Spacer in Left Sternoclavicular Joint, External Approach
0RWFXJZ Revision of Synthetic Substitute in Left Sternoclavicular Joint, External Approach
0RWFXKZ Revision of Nonautologous Tissue Substitute in Left Sternoclavicular Joint, External Approach
0RWG00Z Revision of Drainage Device in Right Acromioclavicular Joint, Open Approach
0RWG03Z Revision of Infusion Device in Right Acromioclavicular Joint, Open Approach
0RWG04Z Revision of Internal Fixation Device in Right Acromioclavicular Joint, Open Approach
0RWG07Z Revision of Autologous Tissue Substitute in Right Acromioclavicular Joint, Open Approach
0RWG08Z Revision of Spacer in Right Acromioclavicular Joint, Open Approach
0RWG0JZ Revision of Synthetic Substitute in Right Acromioclavicular Joint, Open Approach
0RWG0KZ Revision of Nonautologous Tissue Substitute in Right Acromioclavicular Joint, Open Approach
0RWG30Z Revision of Drainage Device in Right Acromioclavicular Joint, Percutaneous Approach
0RWG33Z Revision of Infusion Device in Right Acromioclavicular Joint, Percutaneous Approach
0RWG34Z Revision of Internal Fixation Device in Right Acromioclavicular Joint, Percutaneous Approach
0RWG37Z Revision of Autologous Tissue Substitute in Right Acromioclavicular Joint, Percutaneous Approach
0RWG38Z Revision of Spacer in Right Acromioclavicular Joint, Percutaneous Approach
0RWG3JZ Revision of Synthetic Substitute in Right Acromioclavicular Joint, Percutaneous Approach
0RWG3KZ Revision of Nonautologous Tissue Substitute in Right Acromioclavicular Joint, Percutaneous Approach
0RWG40Z Revision of Drainage Device in Right Acromioclavicular Joint, Percutaneous Endoscopic Approach
0RWG43Z Revision of Infusion Device in Right Acromioclavicular Joint, Percutaneous Endoscopic Approach
0RWG44Z Revision of Internal Fixation Device in Right Acromioclavicular Joint, Percutaneous Endoscopic Approach
0RWG47Z Revision of Autologous Tissue Substitute in Right Acromioclavicular Joint, Percutaneous Endoscopic Approach
0RWG48Z Revision of Spacer in Right Acromioclavicular Joint, Percutaneous Endoscopic Approach
0RWG4JZ Revision of Synthetic Substitute in Right Acromioclavicular Joint, Percutaneous Endoscopic Approach
0RWG4KZ Revision of Nonautologous Tissue Substitute in Right Acromioclavicular Joint, Percutaneous Endoscopic Approach
0RWGX0Z Revision of Drainage Device in Right Acromioclavicular Joint, External Approach
0RWGX3Z Revision of Infusion Device in Right Acromioclavicular Joint, External Approach
0RWGX4Z Revision of Internal Fixation Device in Right Acromioclavicular Joint, External Approach
0RWGX7Z Revision of Autologous Tissue Substitute in Right Acromioclavicular Joint, External Approach
0RWGX8Z Revision of Spacer in Right Acromioclavicular Joint, External Approach
0RWGXJZ Revision of Synthetic Substitute in Right Acromioclavicular Joint, External Approach
0RWGXKZ Revision of Nonautologous Tissue Substitute in Right Acromioclavicular Joint, External Approach
0RWH00Z Revision of Drainage Device in Left Acromioclavicular Joint, Open Approach
0RWH03Z Revision of Infusion Device in Left Acromioclavicular Joint, Open Approach
0RWH04Z Revision of Internal Fixation Device in Left Acromioclavicular Joint, Open Approach
0RWH07Z Revision of Autologous Tissue Substitute in Left Acromioclavicular Joint, Open Approach
0RWH08Z Revision of Spacer in Left Acromioclavicular Joint, Open Approach
0RWH0JZ Revision of Synthetic Substitute in Left Acromioclavicular Joint, Open Approach
0RWH0KZ Revision of Nonautologous Tissue Substitute in Left Acromioclavicular Joint, Open Approach
0RWH30Z Revision of Drainage Device in Left Acromioclavicular Joint, Percutaneous Approach
0RWH33Z Revision of Infusion Device in Left Acromioclavicular Joint, Percutaneous Approach
0RWH34Z Revision of Internal Fixation Device in Left Acromioclavicular Joint, Percutaneous Approach
0RWH37Z Revision of Autologous Tissue Substitute in Left Acromioclavicular Joint, Percutaneous Approach
0RWH38Z Revision of Spacer in Left Acromioclavicular Joint, Percutaneous Approach
0RWH3JZ Revision of Synthetic Substitute in Left Acromioclavicular Joint, Percutaneous Approach
0RWH3KZ Revision of Nonautologous Tissue Substitute in Left Acromioclavicular Joint, Percutaneous Approach
0RWH40Z Revision of Drainage Device in Left Acromioclavicular Joint, Percutaneous Endoscopic Approach
0RWH43Z Revision of Infusion Device in Left Acromioclavicular Joint, Percutaneous Endoscopic Approach
0RWH44Z Revision of Internal Fixation Device in Left Acromioclavicular Joint, Percutaneous Endoscopic Approach
0RWH47Z Revision of Autologous Tissue Substitute in Left Acromioclavicular Joint, Percutaneous Endoscopic Approach
0RWH48Z Revision of Spacer in Left Acromioclavicular Joint, Percutaneous Endoscopic Approach
0RWH4JZ Revision of Synthetic Substitute in Left Acromioclavicular Joint, Percutaneous Endoscopic Approach
0RWH4KZ Revision of Nonautologous Tissue Substitute in Left Acromioclavicular Joint, Percutaneous Endoscopic Approach
0RWHX0Z Revision of Drainage Device in Left Acromioclavicular Joint, External Approach
0RWHX3Z Revision of Infusion Device in Left Acromioclavicular Joint, External Approach
0RWHX4Z Revision of Internal Fixation Device in Left Acromioclavicular Joint, External Approach
0RWHX7Z Revision of Autologous Tissue Substitute in Left Acromioclavicular Joint, External Approach
0RWHX8Z Revision of Spacer in Left Acromioclavicular Joint, External Approach
0RWHXJZ Revision of Synthetic Substitute in Left Acromioclavicular Joint, External Approach
0RWHXKZ Revision of Nonautologous Tissue Substitute in Left Acromioclavicular Joint, External Approach
0RWJ00Z Revision of Drainage Device in Right Shoulder Joint, Open Approach
0RWJ03Z Revision of Infusion Device in Right Shoulder Joint, Open Approach
0RWJ04Z Revision of Internal Fixation Device in Right Shoulder Joint, Open Approach
0RWJ07Z Revision of Autologous Tissue Substitute in Right Shoulder Joint, Open Approach
0RWJ08Z Revision of Spacer in Right Shoulder Joint, Open Approach
0RWJ0JZ Revision of Synthetic Substitute in Right Shoulder Joint, Open Approach
0RWJ0KZ Revision of Nonautologous Tissue Substitute in Right Shoulder Joint, Open Approach
0RWJ30Z Revision of Drainage Device in Right Shoulder Joint, Percutaneous Approach
0RWJ33Z Revision of Infusion Device in Right Shoulder Joint, Percutaneous Approach
0RWJ34Z Revision of Internal Fixation Device in Right Shoulder Joint, Percutaneous Approach
0RWJ37Z Revision of Autologous Tissue Substitute in Right Shoulder Joint, Percutaneous Approach
0RWJ38Z Revision of Spacer in Right Shoulder Joint, Percutaneous Approach
0RWJ3JZ Revision of Synthetic Substitute in Right Shoulder Joint, Percutaneous Approach
0RWJ3KZ Revision of Nonautologous Tissue Substitute in Right Shoulder Joint, Percutaneous Approach
0RWJ40Z Revision of Drainage Device in Right Shoulder Joint, Percutaneous Endoscopic Approach
0RWJ43Z Revision of Infusion Device in Right Shoulder Joint, Percutaneous Endoscopic Approach
0RWJ44Z Revision of Internal Fixation Device in Right Shoulder Joint, Percutaneous Endoscopic Approach
0RWJ47Z Revision of Autologous Tissue Substitute in Right Shoulder Joint, Percutaneous Endoscopic Approach
0RWJ48Z Revision of Spacer in Right Shoulder Joint, Percutaneous Endoscopic Approach
0RWJ4JZ Revision of Synthetic Substitute in Right Shoulder Joint, Percutaneous Endoscopic Approach

0RWJ4KZ Revision of Nonautologous Tissue Substitute in Right Shoulder Joint, Percutaneous Endoscopic Approach
0RWJX0Z Revision of Drainage Device in Right Shoulder Joint, External Approach
0RWJX3Z Revision of Infusion Device in Right Shoulder Joint, External Approach
0RWJX4Z Revision of Internal Fixation Device in Right Shoulder Joint, External Approach
0RWJX7Z Revision of Autologous Tissue Substitute in Right Shoulder Joint, External Approach
0RWJX8Z Revision of Spacer in Right Shoulder Joint, External Approach
0RWJXJZ Revision of Synthetic Substitute in Right Shoulder Joint, External Approach
0RWJXKZ Revision of Nonautologous Tissue Substitute in Right Shoulder Joint, External Approach
0RWK00Z Revision of Drainage Device in Left Shoulder Joint, Open Approach
0RWK03Z Revision of Infusion Device in Left Shoulder Joint, Open Approach
0RWK04Z Revision of Internal Fixation Device in Left Shoulder Joint, Open Approach
0RWK07Z Revision of Autologous Tissue Substitute in Left Shoulder Joint, Open Approach
0RWK08Z Revision of Spacer in Left Shoulder Joint, Open Approach
0RWK0JZ Revision of Synthetic Substitute in Left Shoulder Joint, Open Approach
0RWK0KZ Revision of Nonautologous Tissue Substitute in Left Shoulder Joint, Open Approach
0RWK30Z Revision of Drainage Device in Left Shoulder Joint, Percutaneous Approach
0RWK33Z Revision of Infusion Device in Left Shoulder Joint, Percutaneous Approach
0RWK34Z Revision of Internal Fixation Device in Left Shoulder Joint, Percutaneous Approach
0RWK37Z Revision of Autologous Tissue Substitute in Left Shoulder Joint, Percutaneous Approach
0RWK38Z Revision of Spacer in Left Shoulder Joint, Percutaneous Approach
0RWK3JZ Revision of Synthetic Substitute in Left Shoulder Joint, Percutaneous Approach
0RWK3KZ Revision of Nonautologous Tissue Substitute in Left Shoulder Joint, Percutaneous Approach
0RWK40Z Revision of Drainage Device in Left Shoulder Joint, Percutaneous Endoscopic Approach
0RWK43Z Revision of Infusion Device in Left Shoulder Joint, Percutaneous Endoscopic Approach
0RWK44Z Revision of Internal Fixation Device in Left Shoulder Joint, Percutaneous Endoscopic Approach
0RWK47Z Revision of Autologous Tissue Substitute in Left Shoulder Joint, Percutaneous Endoscopic Approach
0RWK48Z Revision of Spacer in Left Shoulder Joint, Percutaneous Endoscopic Approach
0RWK4JZ Revision of Synthetic Substitute in Left Shoulder Joint, Percutaneous Endoscopic Approach
0RWK4KZ Revision of Nonautologous Tissue Substitute in Left Shoulder Joint, Percutaneous Endoscopic Approach
0RWKX0Z Revision of Drainage Device in Left Shoulder Joint, External Approach
0RWKX3Z Revision of Infusion Device in Left Shoulder Joint, External Approach
0RWKX4Z Revision of Internal Fixation Device in Left Shoulder Joint, External Approach
0RWKX7Z Revision of Autologous Tissue Substitute in Left Shoulder Joint, External Approach
0RWKX8Z Revision of Spacer in Left Shoulder Joint, External Approach
0RWKXJZ Revision of Synthetic Substitute in Left Shoulder Joint, External Approach
0RWKXKZ Revision of Nonautologous Tissue Substitute in Left Shoulder Joint, External Approach
0RWL00Z Revision of Drainage Device in Right Elbow Joint, Open Approach
0RWL03Z Revision of Infusion Device in Right Elbow Joint, Open Approach
0RWL04Z Revision of Internal Fixation Device in Right Elbow Joint, Open Approach
0RWL05Z Revision of External Fixation Device in Right Elbow Joint, Open Approach
0RWL07Z Revision of Autologous Tissue Substitute in Right Elbow Joint, Open Approach
0RWL08Z Revision of Spacer in Right Elbow Joint, Open Approach
0RWL0JZ Revision of Synthetic Substitute in Right Elbow Joint, Open Approach
0RWL0KZ Revision of Nonautologous Tissue Substitute in Right Elbow Joint, Open Approach
0RWL30Z Revision of Drainage Device in Right Elbow Joint, Percutaneous Approach
0RWL33Z Revision of Infusion Device in Right Elbow Joint, Percutaneous Approach
0RWL34Z Revision of Internal Fixation Device in Right Elbow Joint, Percutaneous Approach
0RWL35Z Revision of External Fixation Device in Right Elbow Joint, Percutaneous Approach
0RWL37Z Revision of Autologous Tissue Substitute in Right Elbow Joint, Percutaneous Approach
0RWL38Z Revision of Spacer in Right Elbow Joint, Percutaneous Approach
0RWL3JZ Revision of Synthetic Substitute in Right Elbow Joint, Percutaneous Approach
0RWL3KZ Revision of Nonautologous Tissue Substitute in Right Elbow Joint, Percutaneous Approach
0RWL40Z Revision of Drainage Device in Right Elbow Joint, Percutaneous Endoscopic Approach
0RWL43Z Revision of Infusion Device in Right Elbow Joint, Percutaneous Endoscopic Approach
0RWL44Z Revision of Internal Fixation Device in Right Elbow Joint, Percutaneous Endoscopic Approach
0RWL45Z Revision of External Fixation Device in Right Elbow Joint, Percutaneous Endoscopic Approach
0RWL47Z Revision of Autologous Tissue Substitute in Right Elbow Joint, Percutaneous Endoscopic Approach
0RWL48Z Revision of Spacer in Right Elbow Joint, Percutaneous Endoscopic Approach
0RWL4JZ Revision of Synthetic Substitute in Right Elbow Joint, Percutaneous Endoscopic Approach
0RWL4KZ Revision of Nonautologous Tissue Substitute in Right Elbow Joint, Percutaneous Endoscopic Approach
0RWLX0Z Revision of Drainage Device in Right Elbow Joint, External Approach
0RWLX3Z Revision of Infusion Device in Right Elbow Joint, External Approach
0RWLX4Z Revision of Internal Fixation Device in Right Elbow Joint, External Approach
0RWLX5Z Revision of External Fixation Device in Right Elbow Joint, External Approach
0RWLX7Z Revision of Autologous Tissue Substitute in Right Elbow Joint, External Approach
0RWLX8Z Revision of Spacer in Right Elbow Joint, External Approach
0RWLXJZ Revision of Synthetic Substitute in Right Elbow Joint, External Approach
0RWLXKZ Revision of Nonautologous Tissue Substitute in Right Elbow Joint, External Approach
0RWM00Z Revision of Drainage Device in Left Elbow Joint, Open Approach
0RWM03Z Revision of Infusion Device in Left Elbow Joint, Open Approach
0RWM04Z Revision of Internal Fixation Device in Left Elbow Joint, Open Approach
0RWM05Z Revision of External Fixation Device in Left Elbow Joint, Open Approach
0RWM07Z Revision of Autologous Tissue Substitute in Left Elbow Joint, Open Approach
0RWM08Z Revision of Spacer in Left Elbow Joint, Open Approach
0RWM0JZ Revision of Synthetic Substitute in Left Elbow Joint, Open Approach
0RWM0KZ Revision of Nonautologous Tissue Substitute in Left Elbow Joint, Open Approach
0RWM30Z Revision of Drainage Device in Left Elbow Joint, Percutaneous Approach
0RWM33Z Revision of Infusion Device in Left Elbow Joint, Percutaneous Approach
0RWM34Z Revision of Internal Fixation Device in Left Elbow Joint, Percutaneous Approach
0RWM35Z Revision of External Fixation Device in Left Elbow Joint, Percutaneous Approach
0RWM37Z Revision of Autologous Tissue Substitute in Left Elbow Joint, Percutaneous Approach
0RWM38Z Revision of Spacer in Left Elbow Joint, Percutaneous Approach
0RWM3JZ Revision of Synthetic Substitute in Left Elbow Joint, Percutaneous Approach
0RWM3KZ Revision of Nonautologous Tissue Substitute in Left Elbow Joint, Percutaneous Approach
0RWM40Z Revision of Drainage Device in Left Elbow Joint, Percutaneous Endoscopic Approach
0RWM43Z Revision of Infusion Device in Left Elbow Joint, Percutaneous Endoscopic Approach
0RWM44Z Revision of Internal Fixation Device in Left Elbow Joint, Percutaneous Endoscopic Approach
0RWM45Z Revision of External Fixation Device in Left Elbow Joint, Percutaneous Endoscopic Approach
0RWM47Z Revision of Autologous Tissue Substitute in Left Elbow Joint, Percutaneous Endoscopic Approach
0RWM48Z Revision of Spacer in Left Elbow Joint, Percutaneous Endoscopic Approach
0RWM4JZ Revision of Synthetic Substitute in Left Elbow Joint, Percutaneous Endoscopic Approach
0RWM4KZ Revision of Nonautologous Tissue Substitute in Left Elbow Joint, Percutaneous Endoscopic Approach
0RWMX0Z Revision of Drainage Device in Left Elbow Joint, External Approach

0RWMX3Z Revision of Infusion Device in Left Elbow Joint, External Approach
0RWMX4Z Revision of Internal Fixation Device in Left Elbow Joint, External Approach
0RWMX5Z Revision of External Fixation Device in Left Elbow Joint, External Approach
0RWMX7Z Revision of Autologous Tissue Substitute in Left Elbow Joint, External Approach
0RWMX8Z Revision of Spacer in Left Elbow Joint, External Approach
0RWMXJZ Revision of Synthetic Substitute in Left Elbow Joint, External Approach
0RWMXKZ Revision of Nonautologous Tissue Substitute in Left Elbow Joint, External Approach
0RWN00Z Revision of Drainage Device in Right Wrist Joint, Open Approach
0RWN03Z Revision of Infusion Device in Right Wrist Joint, Open Approach
0RWN04Z Revision of Internal Fixation Device in Right Wrist Joint, Open Approach
0RWN05Z Revision of External Fixation Device in Right Wrist Joint, Open Approach
0RWN07Z Revision of Autologous Tissue Substitute in Right Wrist Joint, Open Approach
0RWN08Z Revision of Spacer in Right Wrist Joint, Open Approach
0RWN0JZ Revision of Synthetic Substitute in Right Wrist Joint, Open Approach
0RWN0KZ Revision of Nonautologous Tissue Substitute in Right Wrist Joint, Open Approach
0RWN30Z Revision of Drainage Device in Right Wrist Joint, Percutaneous Approach
0RWN33Z Revision of Infusion Device in Right Wrist Joint, Percutaneous Approach
0RWN34Z Revision of Internal Fixation Device in Right Wrist Joint, Percutaneous Approach
0RWN35Z Revision of External Fixation Device in Right Wrist Joint, Percutaneous Approach
0RWN37Z Revision of Autologous Tissue Substitute in Right Wrist Joint, Percutaneous Approach
0RWN38Z Revision of Spacer in Right Wrist Joint, Percutaneous Approach
0RWN3JZ Revision of Synthetic Substitute in Right Wrist Joint, Percutaneous Approach
0RWN3KZ Revision of Nonautologous Tissue Substitute in Right Wrist Joint, Percutaneous Approach
0RWN40Z Revision of Drainage Device in Right Wrist Joint, Percutaneous Endoscopic Approach
0RWN43Z Revision of Infusion Device in Right Wrist Joint, Percutaneous Endoscopic Approach
0RWN44Z Revision of Internal Fixation Device in Right Wrist Joint, Percutaneous Endoscopic Approach
0RWN45Z Revision of External Fixation Device in Right Wrist Joint, Percutaneous Endoscopic Approach
0RWN47Z Revision of Autologous Tissue Substitute in Right Wrist Joint, Percutaneous Endoscopic Approach
0RWN48Z Revision of Spacer in Right Wrist Joint, Percutaneous Endoscopic Approach
0RWN4JZ Revision of Synthetic Substitute in Right Wrist Joint, Percutaneous Endoscopic Approach
0RWN4KZ Revision of Nonautologous Tissue Substitute in Right Wrist Joint, Percutaneous Endoscopic Approach
0RWNX0Z Revision of Drainage Device in Right Wrist Joint, External Approach
0RWNX3Z Revision of Infusion Device in Right Wrist Joint, External Approach
0RWNX4Z Revision of Internal Fixation Device in Right Wrist Joint, External Approach
0RWNX5Z Revision of External Fixation Device in Right Wrist Joint, External Approach
0RWNX7Z Revision of Autologous Tissue Substitute in Right Wrist Joint, External Approach
0RWNX8Z Revision of Spacer in Right Wrist Joint, External Approach
0RWNXJZ Revision of Synthetic Substitute in Right Wrist Joint, External Approach
0RWNXKZ Revision of Nonautologous Tissue Substitute in Right Wrist Joint, External Approach
0RWP00Z Revision of Drainage Device in Left Wrist Joint, Open Approach
0RWP03Z Revision of Infusion Device in Left Wrist Joint, Open Approach
0RWP04Z Revision of Internal Fixation Device in Left Wrist Joint, Open Approach
0RWP05Z Revision of External Fixation Device in Left Wrist Joint, Open Approach
0RWP07Z Revision of Autologous Tissue Substitute in Left Wrist Joint, Open Approach
0RWP08Z Revision of Spacer in Left Wrist Joint, Open Approach
0RWP0JZ Revision of Synthetic Substitute in Left Wrist Joint, Open Approach
0RWP0KZ Revision of Nonautologous Tissue Substitute in Left Wrist Joint, Open Approach
0RWP30Z Revision of Drainage Device in Left Wrist Joint, Percutaneous Approach
0RWP33Z Revision of Infusion Device in Left Wrist Joint, Percutaneous Approach
0RWP34Z Revision of Internal Fixation Device in Left Wrist Joint, Percutaneous Approach
0RWP35Z Revision of External Fixation Device in Left Wrist Joint, Percutaneous Approach
0RWP37Z Revision of Autologous Tissue Substitute in Left Wrist Joint, Percutaneous Approach
0RWP38Z Revision of Spacer in Left Wrist Joint, Percutaneous Approach
0RWP3JZ Revision of Synthetic Substitute in Left Wrist Joint, Percutaneous Approach
0RWP3KZ Revision of Nonautologous Tissue Substitute in Left Wrist Joint, Percutaneous Approach
0RWP40Z Revision of Drainage Device in Left Wrist Joint, Percutaneous Endoscopic Approach
0RWP43Z Revision of Infusion Device in Left Wrist Joint, Percutaneous Endoscopic Approach
0RWP44Z Revision of Internal Fixation Device in Left Wrist Joint, Percutaneous Endoscopic Approach
0RWP45Z Revision of External Fixation Device in Left Wrist Joint, Percutaneous Endoscopic Approach
0RWP47Z Revision of Autologous Tissue Substitute in Left Wrist Joint, Percutaneous Endoscopic Approach
0RWP48Z Revision of Spacer in Left Wrist Joint, Percutaneous Endoscopic Approach
0RWP4JZ Revision of Synthetic Substitute in Left Wrist Joint, Percutaneous Endoscopic Approach
0RWP4KZ Revision of Nonautologous Tissue Substitute in Left Wrist Joint, Percutaneous Endoscopic Approach
0RWPX0Z Revision of Drainage Device in Left Wrist Joint, External Approach
0RWPX3Z Revision of Infusion Device in Left Wrist Joint, External Approach
0RWPX4Z Revision of Internal Fixation Device in Left Wrist Joint, External Approach
0RWPX5Z Revision of External Fixation Device in Left Wrist Joint, External Approach
0RWPX7Z Revision of Autologous Tissue Substitute in Left Wrist Joint, External Approach
0RWPX8Z Revision of Spacer in Left Wrist Joint, External Approach
0RWPXJZ Revision of Synthetic Substitute in Left Wrist Joint, External Approach
0RWPXKZ Revision of Nonautologous Tissue Substitute in Left Wrist Joint, External Approach
0RWQ00Z Revision of Drainage Device in Right Carpal Joint, Open Approach
0RWQ03Z Revision of Infusion Device in Right Carpal Joint, Open Approach
0RWQ04Z Revision of Internal Fixation Device in Right Carpal Joint, Open Approach
0RWQ05Z Revision of External Fixation Device in Right Carpal Joint, Open Approach
0RWQ07Z Revision of Autologous Tissue Substitute in Right Carpal Joint, Open Approach
0RWQ08Z Revision of Spacer in Right Carpal Joint, Open Approach
0RWQ0JZ Revision of Synthetic Substitute in Right Carpal Joint, Open Approach
0RWQ0KZ Revision of Nonautologous Tissue Substitute in Right Carpal Joint, Open Approach
0RWQ30Z Revision of Drainage Device in Right Carpal Joint, Percutaneous Approach
0RWQ33Z Revision of Infusion Device in Right Carpal Joint, Percutaneous Approach
0RWQ34Z Revision of Internal Fixation Device in Right Carpal Joint, Percutaneous Approach
0RWQ35Z Revision of External Fixation Device in Right Carpal Joint, Percutaneous Approach
0RWQ37Z Revision of Autologous Tissue Substitute in Right Carpal Joint, Percutaneous Approach
0RWQ38Z Revision of Spacer in Right Carpal Joint, Percutaneous Approach
0RWQ3JZ Revision of Synthetic Substitute in Right Carpal Joint, Percutaneous Approach
0RWQ3KZ Revision of Nonautologous Tissue Substitute in Right Carpal Joint, Percutaneous Approach
0RWQ40Z Revision of Drainage Device in Right Carpal Joint, Percutaneous Endoscopic Approach
0RWQ43Z Revision of Infusion Device in Right Carpal Joint, Percutaneous Endoscopic Approach
0RWQ44Z Revision of Internal Fixation Device in Right Carpal Joint, Percutaneous Endoscopic Approach
0RWQ45Z Revision of External Fixation Device in Right Carpal Joint, Percutaneous Endoscopic Approach
0RWQ47Z Revision of Autologous Tissue Substitute in Right Carpal Joint, Percutaneous Endoscopic Approach
0RWQ48Z Revision of Spacer in Right Carpal Joint, Percutaneous Endoscopic Approach
0RWQ4JZ Revision of Synthetic Substitute in Right Carpal Joint, Percutaneous Endoscopic Approach

0RWQ4KZ Revision of Nonautologous Tissue Substitute in Right Carpal Joint, Percutaneous Endoscopic Approach
0RWQX0Z Revision of Drainage Device in Right Carpal Joint, External Approach
0RWQX3Z Revision of Infusion Device in Right Carpal Joint, External Approach
0RWQX4Z Revision of Internal Fixation Device in Right Carpal Joint, External Approach
0RWQX5Z Revision of External Fixation Device in Right Carpal Joint, External Approach
0RWQX7Z Revision of Autologous Tissue Substitute in Right Carpal Joint, External Approach
0RWQX8Z Revision of Spacer in Right Carpal Joint, External Approach
0RWQXJZ Revision of Synthetic Substitute in Right Carpal Joint, External Approach
0RWQXKZ Revision of Nonautologous Tissue Substitute in Right Carpal Joint, External Approach
0RWR00Z Revision of Drainage Device in Left Carpal Joint, Open Approach
0RWR03Z Revision of Infusion Device in Left Carpal Joint, Open Approach
0RWR04Z Revision of Internal Fixation Device in Left Carpal Joint, Open Approach
0RWR05Z Revision of External Fixation Device in Left Carpal Joint, Open Approach
0RWR07Z Revision of Autologous Tissue Substitute in Left Carpal Joint, Open Approach
0RWR08Z Revision of Spacer in Left Carpal Joint, Open Approach
0RWR0JZ Revision of Synthetic Substitute in Left Carpal Joint, Open Approach
0RWR0KZ Revision of Nonautologous Tissue Substitute in Left Carpal Joint, Open Approach
0RWR30Z Revision of Drainage Device in Left Carpal Joint, Percutaneous Approach
0RWR33Z Revision of Infusion Device in Left Carpal Joint, Percutaneous Approach
0RWR34Z Revision of Internal Fixation Device in Left Carpal Joint, Percutaneous Approach
0RWR35Z Revision of External Fixation Device in Left Carpal Joint, Percutaneous Approach
0RWR37Z Revision of Autologous Tissue Substitute in Left Carpal Joint, Percutaneous Approach
0RWR38Z Revision of Spacer in Left Carpal Joint, Percutaneous Approach
0RWR3JZ Revision of Synthetic Substitute in Left Carpal Joint, Percutaneous Approach
0RWR3KZ Revision of Nonautologous Tissue Substitute in Left Carpal Joint, Percutaneous Approach
0RWR40Z Revision of Drainage Device in Left Carpal Joint, Percutaneous Endoscopic Approach
0RWR43Z Revision of Infusion Device in Left Carpal Joint, Percutaneous Endoscopic Approach
0RWR44Z Revision of Internal Fixation Device in Left Carpal Joint, Percutaneous Endoscopic Approach
0RWR45Z Revision of External Fixation Device in Left Carpal Joint, Percutaneous Endoscopic Approach
0RWR47Z Revision of Autologous Tissue Substitute in Left Carpal Joint, Percutaneous Endoscopic Approach
0RWR48Z Revision of Spacer in Left Carpal Joint, Percutaneous Endoscopic Approach
0RWR4JZ Revision of Synthetic Substitute in Left Carpal Joint, Percutaneous Endoscopic Approach
0RWR4KZ Revision of Nonautologous Tissue Substitute in Left Carpal Joint, Percutaneous Endoscopic Approach
0RWRX0Z Revision of Drainage Device in Left Carpal Joint, External Approach
0RWRX3Z Revision of Infusion Device in Left Carpal Joint, External Approach
0RWRX4Z Revision of Internal Fixation Device in Left Carpal Joint, External Approach
0RWRX5Z Revision of External Fixation Device in Left Carpal Joint, External Approach
0RWRX7Z Revision of Autologous Tissue Substitute in Left Carpal Joint, External Approach
0RWRX8Z Revision of Spacer in Left Carpal Joint, External Approach
0RWRXJZ Revision of Synthetic Substitute in Left Carpal Joint, External Approach
0RWRXKZ Revision of Nonautologous Tissue Substitute in Left Carpal Joint, External Approach
0RWS00Z Revision of Drainage Device in Right Metacarpocarpal Joint, Open Approach
0RWS03Z Revision of Infusion Device in Right Metacarpocarpal Joint, Open Approach
0RWS04Z Revision of Internal Fixation Device in Right Metacarpocarpal Joint, Open Approach
0RWS05Z Revision of External Fixation Device in Right Metacarpocarpal Joint, Open Approach
0RWS07Z Revision of Autologous Tissue Substitute in Right Metacarpocarpal Joint, Open Approach
0RWS08Z Revision of Spacer in Right Metacarpocarpal Joint, Open Approach
0RWS0JZ Revision of Synthetic Substitute in Right Metacarpocarpal Joint, Open Approach
0RWS0KZ Revision of Nonautologous Tissue Substitute in Right Metacarpocarpal Joint, Open Approach
0RWS30Z Revision of Drainage Device in Right Metacarpocarpal Joint, Percutaneous Approach
0RWS33Z Revision of Infusion Device in Right Metacarpocarpal Joint, Percutaneous Approach
0RWS34Z Revision of Internal Fixation Device in Right Metacarpocarpal Joint, Percutaneous Approach
0RWS35Z Revision of External Fixation Device in Right Metacarpocarpal Joint, Percutaneous Approach
0RWS37Z Revision of Autologous Tissue Substitute in Right Metacarpocarpal Joint, Percutaneous Approach
0RWS38Z Revision of Spacer in Right Metacarpocarpal Joint, Percutaneous Approach
0RWS3JZ Revision of Synthetic Substitute in Right Metacarpocarpal Joint, Percutaneous Approach
0RWS3KZ Revision of Nonautologous Tissue Substitute in Right Metacarpocarpal Joint, Percutaneous Approach
0RWS40Z Revision of Drainage Device in Right Metacarpocarpal Joint, Percutaneous Endoscopic Approach
0RWS43Z Revision of Infusion Device in Right Metacarpocarpal Joint, Percutaneous Endoscopic Approach
0RWS44Z Revision of Internal Fixation Device in Right Metacarpocarpal Joint, Percutaneous Endoscopic Approach
0RWS45Z Revision of External Fixation Device in Right Metacarpocarpal Joint, Percutaneous Endoscopic Approach
0RWS47Z Revision of Autologous Tissue Substitute in Right Metacarpocarpal Joint, Percutaneous Endoscopic Approach
0RWS48Z Revision of Spacer in Right Metacarpocarpal Joint, Percutaneous Endoscopic Approach
0RWS4JZ Revision of Synthetic Substitute in Right Metacarpocarpal Joint, Percutaneous Endoscopic Approach
0RWS4KZ Revision of Nonautologous Tissue Substitute in Right Metacarpocarpal Joint, Percutaneous Endoscopic Approach
0RWSX0Z Revision of Drainage Device in Right Metacarpocarpal Joint, External Approach
0RWSX3Z Revision of Infusion Device in Right Metacarpocarpal Joint, External Approach
0RWSX4Z Revision of Internal Fixation Device in Right Metacarpocarpal Joint, External Approach
0RWSX5Z Revision of External Fixation Device in Right Metacarpocarpal Joint, External Approach
0RWSX7Z Revision of Autologous Tissue Substitute in Right Metacarpocarpal Joint, External Approach
0RWSX8Z Revision of Spacer in Right Metacarpocarpal Joint, External Approach
0RWSXJZ Revision of Synthetic Substitute in Right Metacarpocarpal Joint, External Approach
0RWSXKZ Revision of Nonautologous Tissue Substitute in Right Metacarpocarpal Joint, External Approach
0RWT00Z Revision of Drainage Device in Left Metacarpocarpal Joint, Open Approach
0RWT03Z Revision of Infusion Device in Left Metacarpocarpal Joint, Open Approach
0RWT04Z Revision of Internal Fixation Device in Left Metacarpocarpal Joint, Open Approach
0RWT05Z Revision of External Fixation Device in Left Metacarpocarpal Joint, Open Approach
0RWT07Z Revision of Autologous Tissue Substitute in Left Metacarpocarpal Joint, Open Approach
0RWT08Z Revision of Spacer in Left Metacarpocarpal Joint, Open Approach
0RWT0JZ Revision of Synthetic Substitute in Left Metacarpocarpal Joint, Open Approach
0RWT0KZ Revision of Nonautologous Tissue Substitute in Left Metacarpocarpal Joint, Open Approach
0RWT30Z Revision of Drainage Device in Left Metacarpocarpal Joint, Percutaneous Approach
0RWT33Z Revision of Infusion Device in Left Metacarpocarpal Joint, Percutaneous Approach
0RWT34Z Revision of Internal Fixation Device in Left Metacarpocarpal Joint, Percutaneous Approach
0RWT35Z Revision of External Fixation Device in Left Metacarpocarpal Joint, Percutaneous Approach
0RWT37Z Revision of Autologous Tissue Substitute in Left Metacarpocarpal Joint, Percutaneous Approach

0RWT38Z Revision of Spacer in Left Metacarpocarpal Joint, Percutaneous Approach

0RWT3JZ Revision of Synthetic Substitute in Left Metacarpocarpal Joint, Percutaneous Approach

0RWT3KZ Revision of Nonautologous Tissue Substitute in Left Metacarpocarpal Joint, Percutaneous Approach

0RWT40Z Revision of Drainage Device in Left Metacarpocarpal Joint, Percutaneous Endoscopic Approach

0RWT43Z Revision of Infusion Device in Left Metacarpocarpal Joint, Percutaneous Endoscopic Approach

0RWT44Z Revision of Internal Fixation Device in Left Metacarpocarpal Joint, Percutaneous Endoscopic Approach

0RWT45Z Revision of External Fixation Device in Left Metacarpocarpal Joint, Percutaneous Endoscopic Approach

0RWT47Z Revision of Autologous Tissue Substitute in Left Metacarpocarpal Joint, Percutaneous Endoscopic Approach

0RWT48Z Revision of Spacer in Left Metacarpocarpal Joint, Percutaneous Endoscopic Approach

0RWT4JZ Revision of Synthetic Substitute in Left Metacarpocarpal Joint, Percutaneous Endoscopic Approach

0RWT4KZ Revision of Nonautologous Tissue Substitute in Left Metacarpocarpal Joint, Percutaneous Endoscopic Approach

0RWTX0Z Revision of Drainage Device in Left Metacarpocarpal Joint, External Approach

0RWTX3Z Revision of Infusion Device in Left Metacarpocarpal Joint, External Approach

0RWTX4Z Revision of Internal Fixation Device in Left Metacarpocarpal Joint, External Approach

0RWTX5Z Revision of External Fixation Device in Left Metacarpocarpal Joint, External Approach

0RWTX7Z Revision of Autologous Tissue Substitute in Left Metacarpocarpal Joint, External Approach

0RWTX8Z Revision of Spacer in Left Metacarpocarpal Joint, External Approach

0RWTXJZ Revision of Synthetic Substitute in Left Metacarpocarpal Joint, External Approach

0RWTXKZ Revision of Nonautologous Tissue Substitute in Left Metacarpocarpal Joint, External Approach

0RWU00Z Revision of Drainage Device in Right Metacarpophalangeal Joint, Open Approach

0RWU03Z Revision of Infusion Device in Right Metacarpophalangeal Joint, Open Approach

0RWU04Z Revision of Internal Fixation Device in Right Metacarpophalangeal Joint, Open Approach

0RWU05Z Revision of External Fixation Device in Right Metacarpophalangeal Joint, Open Approach

0RWU07Z Revision of Autologous Tissue Substitute in Right Metacarpophalangeal Joint, Open Approach

0RWU08Z Revision of Spacer in Right Metacarpophalangeal Joint, Open Approach

0RWU0JZ Revision of Synthetic Substitute in Right Metacarpophalangeal Joint, Open Approach

0RWU0KZ Revision of Nonautologous Tissue Substitute in Right Metacarpophalangeal Joint, Open Approach

0RWU30Z Revision of Drainage Device in Right Metacarpophalangeal Joint, Percutaneous Approach

0RWU33Z Revision of Infusion Device in Right Metacarpophalangeal Joint, Percutaneous Approach

0RWU34Z Revision of Internal Fixation Device in Right Metacarpophalangeal Joint, Percutaneous Approach

0RWU35Z Revision of External Fixation Device in Right Metacarpophalangeal Joint, Percutaneous Approach

0RWU37Z Revision of Autologous Tissue Substitute in Right Metacarpophalangeal Joint, Percutaneous Approach

0RWU38Z Revision of Spacer in Right Metacarpophalangeal Joint, Percutaneous Approach

0RWU3JZ Revision of Synthetic Substitute in Right Metacarpophalangeal Joint, Percutaneous Approach

0RWU3KZ Revision of Nonautologous Tissue Substitute in Right Metacarpophalangeal Joint, Percutaneous Approach

0RWU40Z Revision of Drainage Device in Right Metacarpophalangeal Joint, Percutaneous Endoscopic Approach

0RWU43Z Revision of Infusion Device in Right Metacarpophalangeal Joint, Percutaneous Endoscopic Approach

0RWU44Z Revision of Internal Fixation Device in Right Metacarpophalangeal Joint, Percutaneous Endoscopic Approach

0RWU45Z Revision of External Fixation Device in Right Metacarpophalangeal Joint, Percutaneous Endoscopic Approach

0RWU47Z Revision of Autologous Tissue Substitute in Right Metacarpophalangeal Joint, Percutaneous Endoscopic Approach

0RWU48Z Revision of Spacer in Right Metacarpophalangeal Joint, Percutaneous Endoscopic Approach

0RWU4JZ Revision of Synthetic Substitute in Right Metacarpophalangeal Joint, Percutaneous Endoscopic Approach

0RWU4KZ Revision of Nonautologous Tissue Substitute in Right Metacarpophalangeal Joint, Percutaneous Endoscopic Approach

0RWUX0Z Revision of Drainage Device in Right Metacarpophalangeal Joint, External Approach

0RWUX3Z Revision of Infusion Device in Right Metacarpophalangeal Joint, External Approach

0RWUX4Z Revision of Internal Fixation Device in Right Metacarpophalangeal Joint, External Approach

0RWUX5Z Revision of External Fixation Device in Right Metacarpophalangeal Joint, External Approach

0RWUX7Z Revision of Autologous Tissue Substitute in Right Metacarpophalangeal Joint, External Approach

0RWUX8Z Revision of Spacer in Right Metacarpophalangeal Joint, External Approach

0RWUXJZ Revision of Synthetic Substitute in Right Metacarpophalangeal Joint, External Approach

0RWUXKZ Revision of Nonautologous Tissue Substitute in Right Metacarpophalangeal Joint, External Approach

0RWV00Z Revision of Drainage Device in Left Metacarpophalangeal Joint, Open Approach

0RWV03Z Revision of Infusion Device in Left Metacarpophalangeal Joint, Open Approach

0RWV04Z Revision of Internal Fixation Device in Left Metacarpophalangeal Joint, Open Approach

0RWV05Z Revision of External Fixation Device in Left Metacarpophalangeal Joint, Open Approach

0RWV07Z Revision of Autologous Tissue Substitute in Left Metacarpophalangeal Joint, Open Approach

0RWV08Z Revision of Spacer in Left Metacarpophalangeal Joint, Open Approach

0RWV0JZ Revision of Synthetic Substitute in Left Metacarpophalangeal Joint, Open Approach

0RWV0KZ Revision of Nonautologous Tissue Substitute in Left Metacarpophalangeal Joint, Open Approach

0RWV30Z Revision of Drainage Device in Left Metacarpophalangeal Joint, Percutaneous Approach

0RWV33Z Revision of Infusion Device in Left Metacarpophalangeal Joint, Percutaneous Approach

0RWV34Z Revision of Internal Fixation Device in Left Metacarpophalangeal Joint, Percutaneous Approach

0RWV35Z Revision of External Fixation Device in Left Metacarpophalangeal Joint, Percutaneous Approach

0RWV37Z Revision of Autologous Tissue Substitute in Left Metacarpophalangeal Joint, Percutaneous Approach

0RWV38Z Revision of Spacer in Left Metacarpophalangeal Joint, Percutaneous Approach

0RWV3JZ Revision of Synthetic Substitute in Left Metacarpophalangeal Joint, Percutaneous Approach

0RWV3KZ Revision of Nonautologous Tissue Substitute in Left Metacarpophalangeal Joint, Percutaneous Approach

0RWV40Z Revision of Drainage Device in Left Metacarpophalangeal Joint, Percutaneous Endoscopic Approach

0RWV43Z Revision of Infusion Device in Left Metacarpophalangeal Joint, Percutaneous Endoscopic Approach

0RWV44Z Revision of Internal Fixation Device in Left Metacarpophalangeal Joint, Percutaneous Endoscopic Approach

0RWV45Z Revision of External Fixation Device in Left Metacarpophalangeal Joint, Percutaneous Endoscopic Approach

0RWV47Z Revision of Autologous Tissue Substitute in Left Metacarpophalangeal Joint, Percutaneous Endoscopic Approach

0RWV48Z Revision of Spacer in Left Metacarpophalangeal Joint, Percutaneous Endoscopic Approach

0RWV4JZ Revision of Synthetic Substitute in Left Metacarpophalangeal Joint, Percutaneous Endoscopic Approach

0RWV4KZ Revision of Nonautologous Tissue Substitute in Left Metacarpophalangeal Joint, Percutaneous Endoscopic Approach

0RWVX0Z Revision of Drainage Device in Left Metacarpophalangeal Joint, External Approach

RWVX3Z Revision of Infusion Device in Left Metacarpophalangeal Joint, External Approach
RWVX4Z Revision of Internal Fixation Device in Left Metacarpophalangeal Joint, External Approach
RWVX5Z Revision of External Fixation Device in Left Metacarpophalangeal Joint, External Approach
RWVX7Z Revision of Autologous Tissue Substitute in Left Metacarpophalangeal Joint, External Approach
RWVX8Z Revision of Spacer in Left Metacarpophalangeal Joint, External Approach
RWVXJZ Revision of Synthetic Substitute in Left Metacarpophalangeal Joint, External Approach
RWVXKZ Revision of Nonautologous Tissue Substitute in Left Metacarpophalangeal Joint, External Approach
RWW00Z Revision of Drainage Device in Right Finger Phalangeal Joint, Open Approach
RWW03Z Revision of Infusion Device in Right Finger Phalangeal Joint, Open Approach
RWW04Z Revision of Internal Fixation Device in Right Finger Phalangeal Joint, Open Approach
RWW05Z Revision of External Fixation Device in Right Finger Phalangeal Joint, Open Approach
RWW07Z Revision of Autologous Tissue Substitute in Right Finger Phalangeal Joint, Open Approach
RWW08Z Revision of Spacer in Right Finger Phalangeal Joint, Open Approach
RWW0JZ Revision of Synthetic Substitute in Right Finger Phalangeal Joint, Open Approach
RWW0KZ Revision of Nonautologous Tissue Substitute in Right Finger Phalangeal Joint, Open Approach
RWW30Z Revision of Drainage Device in Right Finger Phalangeal Joint, Percutaneous Approach
RWW33Z Revision of Infusion Device in Right Finger Phalangeal Joint, Percutaneous Approach
RWW34Z Revision of Internal Fixation Device in Right Finger Phalangeal Joint, Percutaneous Approach
RWW35Z Revision of External Fixation Device in Right Finger Phalangeal Joint, Percutaneous Approach
0RWW37Z Revision of Autologous Tissue Substitute in Right Finger Phalangeal Joint, Percutaneous Approach
0RWW38Z Revision of Spacer in Right Finger Phalangeal Joint, Percutaneous Approach
0RWW3JZ Revision of Synthetic Substitute in Right Finger Phalangeal Joint, Percutaneous Approach
0RWW3KZ Revision of Nonautologous Tissue Substitute in Right Finger Phalangeal Joint, Percutaneous Approach
0RWW40Z Revision of Drainage Device in Right Finger Phalangeal Joint, Percutaneous Endoscopic Approach
0RWW43Z Revision of Infusion Device in Right Finger Phalangeal Joint, Percutaneous Endoscopic Approach
0RWW44Z Revision of Internal Fixation Device in Right Finger Phalangeal Joint, Percutaneous Endoscopic Approach
0RWW45Z Revision of External Fixation Device in Right Finger Phalangeal Joint, Percutaneous Endoscopic Approach
0RWW47Z Revision of Autologous Tissue Substitute in Right Finger Phalangeal Joint, Percutaneous Endoscopic Approach
0RWW48Z Revision of Spacer in Right Finger Phalangeal Joint, Percutaneous Endoscopic Approach
0RWW4JZ Revision of Synthetic Substitute in Right Finger Phalangeal Joint, Percutaneous Endoscopic Approach
0RWW4KZ Revision of Nonautologous Tissue Substitute in Right Finger Phalangeal Joint, Percutaneous Endoscopic Approach
0RWWX0Z Revision of Drainage Device in Right Finger Phalangeal Joint, External Approach
0RWWX3Z Revision of Infusion Device in Right Finger Phalangeal Joint, External Approach
0RWWX4Z Revision of Internal Fixation Device in Right Finger Phalangeal Joint, External Approach
0RWWX5Z Revision of External Fixation Device in Right Finger Phalangeal Joint, External Approach
0RWWX7Z Revision of Autologous Tissue Substitute in Right Finger Phalangeal Joint, External Approach
0RWWX8Z Revision of Spacer in Right Finger Phalangeal Joint, External Approach
0RWWXJZ Revision of Synthetic Substitute in Right Finger Phalangeal Joint, External Approach
0RWWXKZ Revision of Nonautologous Tissue Substitute in Right Finger Phalangeal Joint, External Approach
0RWX00Z Revision of Drainage Device in Left Finger Phalangeal Joint, Open Approach
0RWX03Z Revision of Infusion Device in Left Finger Phalangeal Joint, Open Approach
0RWX04Z Revision of Internal Fixation Device in Left Finger Phalangeal Joint, Open Approach
0RWX05Z Revision of External Fixation Device in Left Finger Phalangeal Joint, Open Approach
0RWX07Z Revision of Autologous Tissue Substitute in Left Finger Phalangeal Joint, Open Approach
0RWX08Z Revision of Spacer in Left Finger Phalangeal Joint, Open Approach
0RWX0JZ Revision of Synthetic Substitute in Left Finger Phalangeal Joint, Open Approach
0RWX0KZ Revision of Nonautologous Tissue Substitute in Left Finger Phalangeal Joint, Open Approach
0RWX30Z Revision of Drainage Device in Left Finger Phalangeal Joint, Percutaneous Approach
0RWX33Z Revision of Infusion Device in Left Finger Phalangeal Joint, Percutaneous Approach
0RWX34Z Revision of Internal Fixation Device in Left Finger Phalangeal Joint, Percutaneous Approach
0RWX35Z Revision of External Fixation Device in Left Finger Phalangeal Joint, Percutaneous Approach
0RWX37Z Revision of Autologous Tissue Substitute in Left Finger Phalangeal Joint, Percutaneous Approach
0RWX38Z Revision of Spacer in Left Finger Phalangeal Joint, Percutaneous Approach
0RWX3JZ Revision of Synthetic Substitute in Left Finger Phalangeal Joint, Percutaneous Approach
0RWX3KZ Revision of Nonautologous Tissue Substitute in Left Finger Phalangeal Joint, Percutaneous Approach
0RWX40Z Revision of Drainage Device in Left Finger Phalangeal Joint, Percutaneous Endoscopic Approach
0RWX43Z Revision of Infusion Device in Left Finger Phalangeal Joint, Percutaneous Endoscopic Approach
0RWX44Z Revision of Internal Fixation Device in Left Finger Phalangeal Joint, Percutaneous Endoscopic Approach
0RWX45Z Revision of External Fixation Device in Left Finger Phalangeal Joint, Percutaneous Endoscopic Approach
0RWX47Z Revision of Autologous Tissue Substitute in Left Finger Phalangeal Joint, Percutaneous Endoscopic Approach
0RWX48Z Revision of Spacer in Left Finger Phalangeal Joint, Percutaneous Endoscopic Approach
0RWX4JZ Revision of Synthetic Substitute in Left Finger Phalangeal Joint, Percutaneous Endoscopic Approach
0RWX4KZ Revision of Nonautologous Tissue Substitute in Left Finger Phalangeal Joint, Percutaneous Endoscopic Approach
0RWXX0Z Revision of Drainage Device in Left Finger Phalangeal Joint, External Approach
0RWXX3Z Revision of Infusion Device in Left Finger Phalangeal Joint, External Approach
0RWXX4Z Revision of Internal Fixation Device in Left Finger Phalangeal Joint, External Approach
0RWXX5Z Revision of External Fixation Device in Left Finger Phalangeal Joint, External Approach
0RWXX7Z Revision of Autologous Tissue Substitute in Left Finger Phalangeal Joint, External Approach
0RWXX8Z Revision of Spacer in Left Finger Phalangeal Joint, External Approach
0RWXXJZ Revision of Synthetic Substitute in Left Finger Phalangeal Joint, External Approach
0RWXXKZ Revision of Nonautologous Tissue Substitute in Left Finger Phalangeal Joint, External Approach

Intervertebral Joint

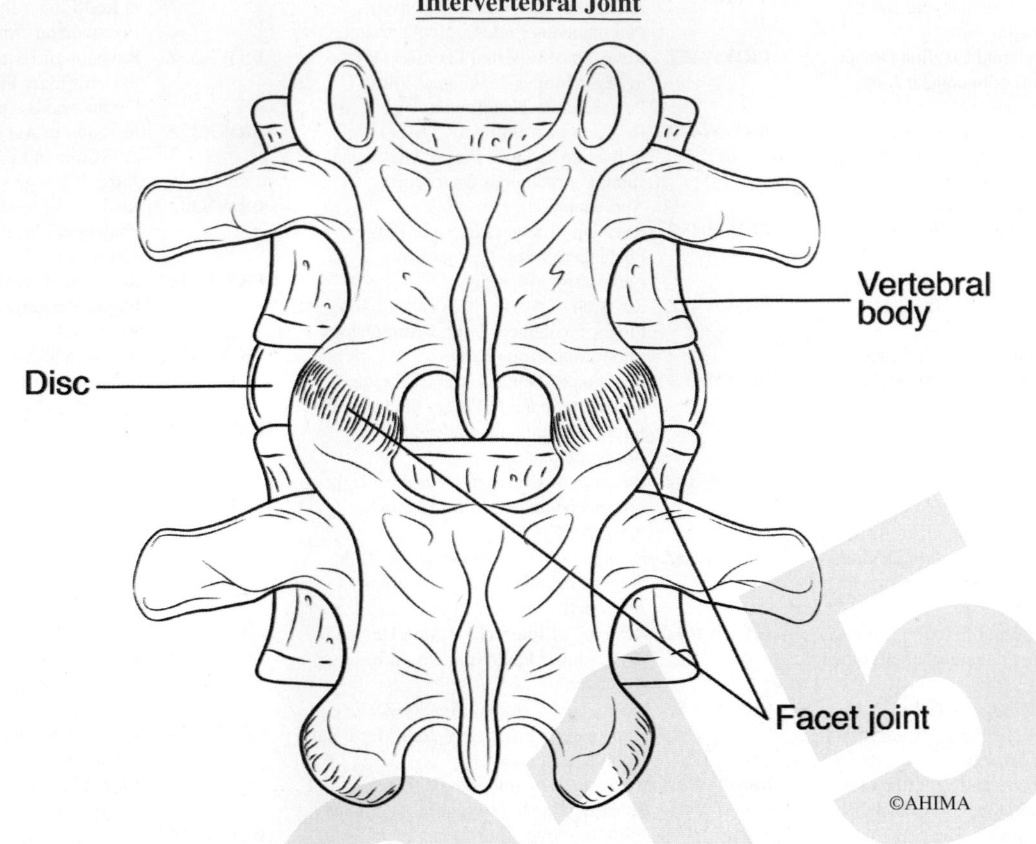

Hip

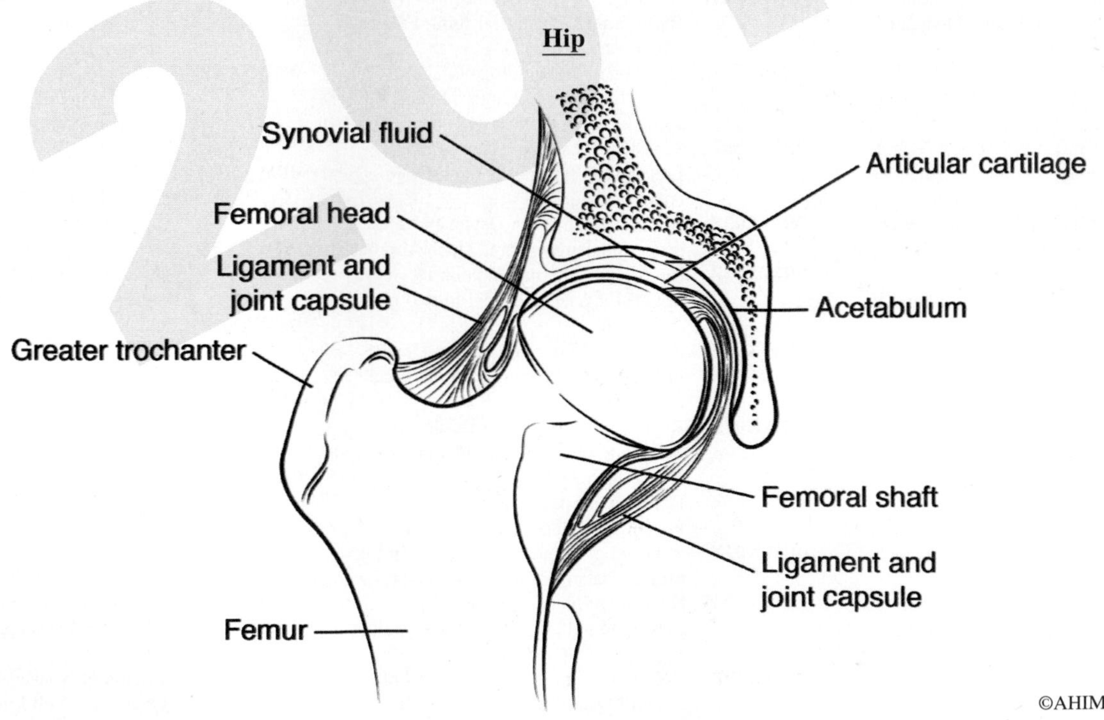

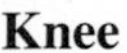

Knee

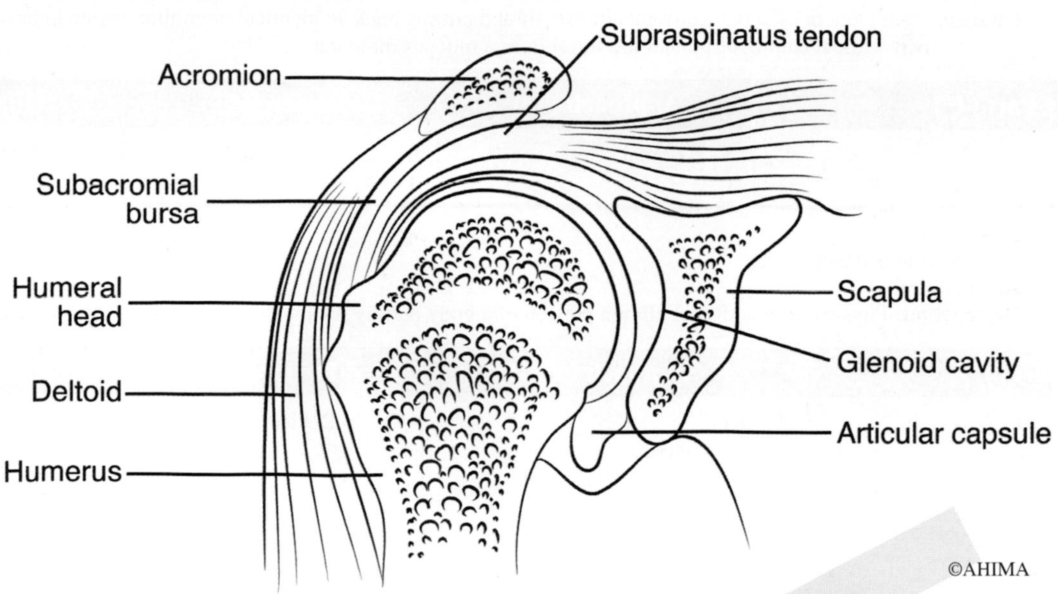
Supraspinatus tendon
Acromion
Subacromial bursa
Humeral head
Deltoid
Humerus
Scapula
Glenoid cavity
Articular capsule
©AHIMA

Ankle

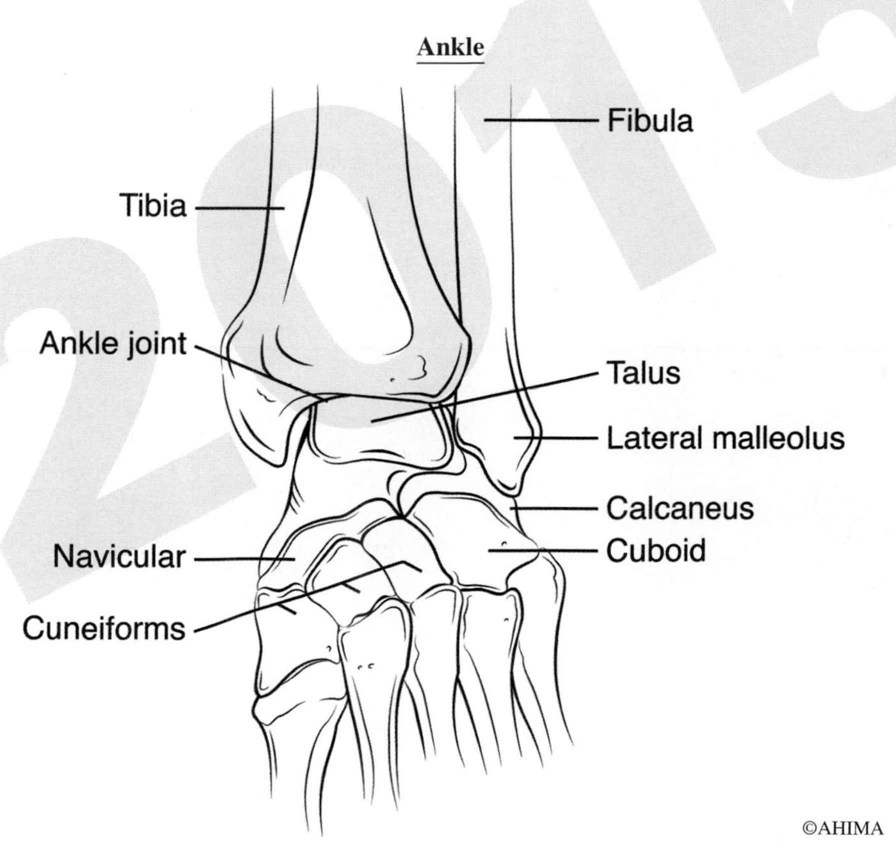
Fibula
Tibia
Ankle joint
Talus
Lateral malleolus
Calcaneus
Navicular
Cuboid
Cuneiforms
©AHIMA

Lower Joints Tables 0S2–0SW

Section 0 **Medical and Surgical**
Body System S **Lower Joints**
Operation 2 **Change:** Taking out or off a device from a body part and putting back an identical or similar device in or on the same body part without cutting or puncturing the skin or a mucous membrane

Body Part (4th)	Approach (5th)	Device (6th)	Qualifier (7th)
Y Lower Joint	**X** External	**0** Drainage Device **Y** Other Device	**Z** No Qualifier

Section 0 **Medical and Surgical**
Body System S **Lower Joints**
Operation 5 **Destruction:** Physical eradication of all or a portion of a body part by the direct use of energy, force, or a destructive agent

Body Part (4th)	Approach (5th)	Device (6th)	Qualifier (7th)
0 Lumbar Vertebral Joint **2** Lumbar Vertebral Disc **3** Lumbosacral Joint **4** Lumbosacral Disc **5** Sacrococcygeal Joint **6** Coccygeal Joint **7** Sacroiliac Joint, Right **8** Sacroiliac Joint, Left **9** Hip Joint, Right **B** Hip Joint, Left **C** Knee Joint, Right **D** Knee Joint, Left **F** Ankle Joint, Right **G** Ankle Joint, Left **H** Tarsal Joint, Right **J** Tarsal Joint, Left **K** Metatarsal-Tarsal Joint, Right **L** Metatarsal-Tarsal Joint, Left **M** Metatarsal-Phalangeal Joint, Right **N** Metatarsal-Phalangeal Joint, Left **P** Toe Phalangeal Joint, Right **Q** Toe Phalangeal Joint, Left	**0** Open **3** Percutaneous **4** Percutaneous Endoscopic	**Z** No Device	**Z** No Qualifier

ection **0** **Medical and Surgical**
ody System **S** **Lower Joints**
peration **9** **Drainage:** Taking or letting out fluids and/or gases from a body part

Body Part (4th)	Approach (5th)	Device (6th)	Qualifier (7th)
0 Lumbar Vertebral Joint **2** Lumbar Vertebral Disc **3** Lumbosacral Joint **4** Lumbosacral Disc **5** Sacrococcygeal Joint **6** Coccygeal Joint **7** Sacroiliac Joint, Right **8** Sacroiliac Joint, Left **9** Hip Joint, Right **B** Hip Joint, Left **C** Knee Joint, Right **D** Knee Joint, Left **F** Ankle Joint, Right **G** Ankle Joint, Left **H** Tarsal Joint, Right **J** Tarsal Joint, Left **K** Metatarsal-Tarsal Joint, Right **L** Metatarsal-Tarsal Joint, Left **L** Metatarsal-Tarsal Joint, Left **M** Metatarsal-Phalangeal Joint, Right **N** Metatarsal-Phalangeal Joint, Left **P** Toe Phalangeal Joint, Right **Q** Toe Phalangeal Joint, Left	**0** Open **3** Percutaneous **4** Percutaneous Endoscopic	**0** Drainage Device	**Z** No Qualifier
0 Lumbar Vertebral Joint **2** Lumbar Vertebral Disc **3** Lumbosacral Joint **4** Lumbosacral Disc **5** Sacrococcygeal Joint **6** Coccygeal Joint **7** Sacroiliac Joint, Right **8** Sacroiliac Joint, Left **9** Hip Joint, Right **B** Hip Joint, Left **C** Knee Joint, Right **D** Knee Joint, Left **F** Ankle Joint, Right **G** Ankle Joint, Left **H** Tarsal Joint, Right **J** Tarsal Joint, Left **K** Metatarsal-Tarsal Joint, Right **L** Metatarsal-Tarsal Joint, Left **M** Metatarsal-Phalangeal Joint, Right **N** Metatarsal-Phalangeal Joint, Left **P** Toe Phalangeal Joint, Right **Q** Toe Phalangeal Joint, Left	**0** Open **3** Percutaneous **4** Percutaneous Endoscopic	**Z** No Device	**X** Diagnostic **Z** No Qualifier

Section 0 **Medical and Surgical**
Body System S **Lower Joints**
Operation B **Excision:** Cutting out or off, without replacement, a portion of a body part

Body Part (4th)	Approach (5th)	Device (6th)	Qualifier (7th)
0 Lumbar Vertebral Joint **2** Lumbar Vertebral Disc **3** Lumbosacral Joint **4** Lumbosacral Disc **5** Sacrococcygeal Joint **6** Coccygeal Joint **7** Sacroiliac Joint, Right **8** Sacroiliac Joint, Left **9** Hip Joint, Right **B** Hip Joint, Left **C** Knee Joint, Right **D** Knee Joint, Left **F** Ankle Joint, Right **G** Ankle Joint, Left **H** Tarsal Joint, Right **J** Tarsal Joint, Left **K** Metatarsal-Tarsal Joint, Right **L** Metatarsal-Tarsal Joint, Left **M** Metatarsal-Phalangeal Joint, Right **N** Metatarsal-Phalangeal Joint, Left **P** Toe Phalangeal Joint, Right **Q** Toe Phalangeal Joint, Left	**0** Open **3** Percutaneous **4** Percutaneous Endoscopic	**Z** No Device	**X** Diagnostic **Z** No Qualifier

Section 0 **Medical and Surgical**
Body System S **Lower Joints**
Operation C **Extirpation:** Taking or cutting out solid matter from a body part

Body Part (4th)	Approach (5th)	Device (6th)	Qualifier (7th)
0 Lumbar Vertebral Joint **2** Lumbar Vertebral Disc **3** Lumbosacral Joint **4** Lumbosacral Disc **5** Sacrococcygeal Joint **6** Coccygeal Joint **7** Sacroiliac Joint, Right **8** Sacroiliac Joint, Left **9** Hip Joint, Right **B** Hip Joint, Left **C** Knee Joint, Right **D** Knee Joint, Left **F** Ankle Joint, Right **G** Ankle Joint, Left **H** Tarsal Joint, Right **J** Tarsal Joint, Left **K** Metatarsal-Tarsal Joint, Right **L** Metatarsal-Tarsal Joint, Left **M** Metatarsal-Phalangeal Joint, Right **N** Metatarsal-Phalangeal Joint, Left **P** Toe Phalangeal Joint, Right **Q** Toe Phalangeal Joint, Left	**0** Open **3** Percutaneous **4** Percutaneous Endoscopic	**Z** No Device	**Z** No Qualifier

Section 0 Medical and Surgical
Body System S Lower Joints
Operation G **Fusion:** Joining together portions of an articular body part rendering the articular body part immobile

Body Part (4th)	Approach (5th)	Device (6th)	Qualifier (7th)
0 Lumbar Vertebral Joint 1 Lumbar Vertebral Joints, 2 or more 3 Lumbosacral Joint	0 Open 3 Percutaneous 4 Percutaneous Endoscopic	7 Autologous Tissue Substitute A Interbody Fusion Device J Synthetic Substitute K Nonautologous Tissue Substitute Z No Device	0 Anterior Approach, Anterior Column 1 Posterior Approach, Posterior Column J Posterior Approach, Anterior Column
5 Sacrococcygeal Joint 6 Coccygeal Joint 7 Sacroiliac Joint, Right 8 Sacroiliac Joint, Left	0 Open 3 Percutaneous 4 Percutaneous Endoscopic	4 Internal Fixation Device 7 Autologous Tissue Substitute J Synthetic Substitute K Nonautologous Tissue Substitute Z No Device	Z No Qualifier
9 Hip Joint, Right B Hip Joint, Left C Knee Joint, Right D Knee Joint, Left F Ankle Joint, Right G Ankle Joint, Left H Tarsal Joint, Right J Tarsal Joint, Left K Metatarsal-Tarsal Joint, Right L Metatarsal-Tarsal Joint, Left M Metatarsal-Phalangeal Joint, Right N Metatarsal-Phalangeal Joint, Left P Toe Phalangeal Joint, Right Q Toe Phalangeal Joint, Left	0 Open 3 Percutaneous 4 Percutaneous Endoscopic	4 Internal Fixation Device 5 External Fixation Device 7 Autologous Tissue Substitute J Synthetic Substitute K Nonautologous Tissue Substitute Z No Device	Z No Qualifier

Section 0 Medical and Surgical
Body System S Lower Joints
Operation H **Insertion:** Putting in a nonbiological appliance that monitors, assists, performs, or prevents a physiological function but does not physically take the place of a body part

Body Part (4th)	Approach (5th)	Device (6th)	Qualifier (7th)
0 Lumbar Vertebral Joint 3 Lumbosacral Joint	0 Open 3 Percutaneous 4 Percutaneous Endoscopic	3 Infusion Device 4 Internal Fixation Device 8 Spacer B Spinal Stabilization Device, Interspinous Process C Spinal Stabilization Device, Pedicle-Based D Spinal Stabilization Device, Facet Replacement	Z No Qualifier
2 Lumbar Vertebral Disc 4 Lumbosacral Disc	0 Open 3 Percutaneous 4 Percutaneous Endoscopic	3 Infusion Device 8 Spacer	Z No Qualifier
5 Sacrococcygeal Joint 6 Coccygeal Joint 7 Sacroiliac Joint, Right 8 Sacroiliac Joint, Left	0 Open 3 Percutaneous 4 Percutaneous Endoscopic	3 Infusion Device 4 Internal Fixation Device 8 Spacer	Z No Qualifier

Continued →

Section 0 **Medical and Surgical**
Body System S **Lower Joints**
Operation H **Insertion:** Putting in a nonbiological appliance that monitors, assists, performs, or prevents a physiological function but does not physically take the place of a body part

Body Part (4th)	Approach (5th)	Device (6th)	Qualifier (7th)
9 Hip Joint, Right **B** Hip Joint, Left **C** Knee Joint, Right **D** Knee Joint, Left **F** Ankle Joint, Right **G** Ankle Joint, Left **H** Tarsal Joint, Right **J** Tarsal Joint, Left **K** Metatarsal-Tarsal Joint, Right **L** Metatarsal-Tarsal Joint, Left **M** Metatarsal-Phalangeal Joint, Right **N** Metatarsal-Phalangeal Joint, Left **P** Toe Phalangeal Joint, Right **Q** Toe Phalangeal Joint, Left	**0** Open **3** Percutaneous **4** Percutaneous Endoscopic	**3** Infusion Device **4** Internal Fixation Device **5** External Fixation Device **8** Spacer	**Z** No Qualifier

Section 0 **Medical and Surgical**
Body System S **Lower Joints**
Operation J **Inspection:** Visually and/or manually exploring a body part

Body Part (4th)	Approach (5th)	Device (6th)	Qualifier (7th)
0 Lumbar Vertebral Joint **2** Lumbar Vertebral Disc **3** Lumbosacral Joint **4** Lumbosacral Disc **5** Sacrococcygeal Joint **6** Coccygeal Joint **7** Sacroiliac Joint, Right **8** Sacroiliac Joint, Left **9** Hip Joint, Right **B** Hip Joint, Left **C** Knee Joint, Right **D** Knee Joint, Left **F** Ankle Joint, Right **G** Ankle Joint, Left **H** Tarsal Joint, Right **J** Tarsal Joint, Left **K** Metatarsal-Tarsal Joint, Right **L** Metatarsal-Tarsal Joint, Left **M** Metatarsal-Phalangeal Joint, Right **N** Metatarsal-Phalangeal Joint, Left **P** Toe Phalangeal Joint, Right **Q** Toe Phalangeal Joint, Left	**0** Open **3** Percutaneous **4** Percutaneous Endoscopic **X** External	**Z** No Device	**Z** No Qualifier

Section 0 Medical and Surgical
Body System S Lower Joints
Operation N **Release:** Freeing a body part from an abnormal physical constraint by cutting or by the use of force

Body Part (4th)	Approach (5th)	Device (6th)	Qualifier (7th)
0 Lumbar Vertebral Joint **2** Lumbar Vertebral Disc **3** Lumbosacral Joint **4** Lumbosacral Disc **5** Sacrococcygeal Joint **6** Coccygeal Joint **7** Sacroiliac Joint, Right **8** Sacroiliac Joint, Left **9** Hip Joint, Right **B** Hip Joint, Left **C** Knee Joint, Right **D** Knee Joint, Left **F** Ankle Joint, Right **G** Ankle Joint, Left **H** Tarsal Joint, Right **J** Tarsal Joint, Left **K** Metatarsal-Tarsal Joint, Right **L** Metatarsal-Tarsal Joint, Left **M** Metatarsal-Phalangeal Joint, Right **N** Metatarsal-Phalangeal Joint, Left **P** Toe Phalangeal Joint, Right **Q** Toe Phalangeal Joint, Left	**0** Open **3** Percutaneous **4** Percutaneous Endoscopic **X** External	**Z** No Device	**Z** No Qualifier

Section 0 Medical and Surgical
Body System S Lower Joints
Operation P **Removal:** Taking out or off a device from a body part

Body Part (4th)	Approach (5th)	Device (6th)	Qualifier (7th)
0 Lumbar Vertebral Joint **3** Lumbosacral Joint	**0** Open **3** Percutaneous **4** Percutaneous Endoscopic	**0** Drainage Device **3** Infusion Device **4** Internal Fixation Device **7** Autologous Tissue Substitute **8** Spacer **A** Interbody Fusion Device **J** Synthetic Substitute **K** Nonautologous Tissue Substitute	**Z** No Qualifier
0 Lumbar Vertebral Joint **3** Lumbosacral Joint	**X** External	**0** Drainage Device **3** Infusion Device **4** Internal Fixation Device	**Z** No Qualifier
2 Lumbar Vertebral Disc **4** Lumbosacral Disc	**0** Open **3** Percutaneous **4** Percutaneous Endoscopic	**0** Drainage Device **3** Infusion Device **7** Autologous Tissue Substitute **J** Synthetic Substitute **K** Nonautologous Tissue Substitute	**Z** No Qualifier
2 Lumbar Vertebral Disc **4** Lumbosacral Disc	**X** External	**0** Drainage Device **3** Infusion Device	**Z** No Qualifier
5 Sacrococcygeal Joint **6** Coccygeal Joint **7** Sacroiliac Joint, Right **8** Sacroiliac Joint, Left	**0** Open **3** Percutaneous **4** Percutaneous Endoscopic	**0** Drainage Device **3** Infusion Device **4** Internal Fixation Device **7** Autologous Tissue Substitute **8** Spacer **J** Synthetic Substitute **K** Nonautologous Tissue Substitute	**Z** No Qualifier

Continued →

Section 0 **Medical and Surgical**
Body System S **Lower Joints**
Operation P **Removal:** Taking out or off a device from a body part

Body Part (4th)	Approach (5th)	Device (6th)	Qualifier (7th)
5 Sacrococcygeal Joint **6** Coccygeal Joint **7** Sacroiliac Joint, Right **8** Sacroiliac Joint, Left	**X** External	**0** Drainage Device **3** Infusion Device **4** Internal Fixation Device	**Z** No Qualifier
9 Hip Joint, Right **B** Hip Joint, Left	**0** Open	**0** Drainage Device **3** Infusion Device **4** Internal Fixation Device **5** External Fixation Device **7** Autologous Tissue Substitute **8** Spacer **9** Liner **B** Resurfacing Device **J** Synthetic Substitute **K** Nonautologous Tissue Substitute	**Z** No Qualifier
9 Hip Joint, Right **B** Hip Joint, Left	**3** Percutaneous **4** Percutaneous Endoscopic	**0** Drainage Device **3** Infusion Device **4** Internal Fixation Device **5** External Fixation Device **7** Autologous Tissue Substitute **8** Spacer **J** Synthetic Substitute **K** Nonautologous Tissue Substitute	**Z** No Qualifier
9 Hip Joint, Right **B** Hip Joint, Left	**X** External	**0** Drainage Device **3** Infusion Device **4** Internal Fixation Device **5** External Fixation Device	**Z** No Qualifier
C Knee Joint, Right **D** Knee Joint, Left	**0** Open	**0** Drainage Device **3** Infusion Device **4** Internal Fixation Device **5** External Fixation Device **7** Autologous Tissue Substitute **8** Spacer **9** Liner **J** Synthetic Substitute **K** Nonautologous Tissue Substitute	**Z** No Qualifier
C Knee Joint, Right **D** Knee Joint, Left	**3** Percutaneous **4** Percutaneous Endoscopic	**0** Drainage Device **3** Infusion Device **4** Internal Fixation Device **5** External Fixation Device **7** Autologous Tissue Substitute **8** Spacer **J** Synthetic Substitute **K** Nonautologous Tissue Substitute	**Z** No Qualifier
C Knee Joint, Right **D** Knee Joint, Left	**X** External	**0** Drainage Device **3** Infusion Device **4** Internal Fixation Device **5** External Fixation Device	**Z** No Qualifier
F Ankle Joint, Right **G** Ankle Joint, Left **H** Tarsal Joint, Right **J** Tarsal Joint, Left **K** Metatarsal-Tarsal Joint, Right **L** Metatarsal-Tarsal Joint, Left **M** Metatarsal-Phalangeal Joint, Right **N** Metatarsal-Phalangeal Joint, Left **P** Toe Phalangeal Joint, Right **Q** Toe Phalangeal Joint, Left	**0** Open **3** Percutaneous **4** Percutaneous Endoscopic	**0** Drainage Device **3** Infusion Device **4** Internal Fixation Device **5** External Fixation Device **7** Autologous Tissue Substitute **8** Spacer **J** Synthetic Substitute **K** Nonautologous Tissue Substitute	**Z** No Qualifier

Continued →

Section 0 Medical and Surgical
Body System S Lower Joints
Operation P **Removal:** Taking out or off a device from a body part

Body Part (4th)	Approach (5th)	Device (6th)	Qualifier (7th)
F Ankle Joint, Right G Ankle Joint, Left H Tarsal Joint, Right J Tarsal Joint, Left K Metatarsal-Tarsal Joint, Right L Metatarsal-Tarsal Joint, Left M Metatarsal-Phalangeal Joint, Right N Metatarsal-Phalangeal Joint, Left P Toe Phalangeal Joint, Right Q Toe Phalangeal Joint, Left	X External	0 Drainage Device 3 Infusion Device 4 Internal Fixation Device 5 External Fixation Device	Z No Qualifier

Section 0 Medical and Surgical
Body System S Lower Joints
Operation Q **Repair:** Restoring, to the extent possible, a body part to its normal anatomic structure and function

Body Part (4th)	Approach (5th)	Device (6th)	Qualifier (7th)
0 Lumbar Vertebral Joint 2 Lumbar Vertebral Disc 3 Lumbosacral Joint 4 Lumbosacral Disc 5 Sacrococcygeal Joint 6 Coccygeal Joint 7 Sacroiliac Joint, Right 8 Sacroiliac Joint, Left 9 Hip Joint, Right B Hip Joint, Left C Knee Joint, Right D Knee Joint, Left F Ankle Joint, Right G Ankle Joint, Left H Tarsal Joint, Right J Tarsal Joint, Left K Metatarsal-Tarsal Joint, Right L Metatarsal-Tarsal Joint, Left M Metatarsal-Phalangeal Joint, Right N Metatarsal-Phalangeal Joint, Left P Toe Phalangeal Joint, Right Q Toe Phalangeal Joint, Left	0 Open 3 Percutaneous 4 Percutaneous Endoscopic X External	Z No Device	Z No Qualifier

Section 0 Medical and Surgical
Body System S Lower Joints
Operation R **Replacement:** Putting in or on biological or synthetic material that physically takes the place and/or function of all or a portion of a body part

Body Part (4th)	Approach (5th)	Device (6th)	Qualifier (7th)
0 Lumbar Vertebral Joint 2 Lumbar Vertebral Disc 3 Lumbosacral Joint 4 Lumbosacral Disc 5 Sacrococcygeal Joint 6 Coccygeal Joint 7 Sacroiliac Joint, Right 8 Sacroiliac Joint, Left H Tarsal Joint, Right J Tarsal Joint, Left K Metatarsal-Tarsal Joint, Right L Metatarsal-Tarsal Joint, Left M Metatarsal-Phalangeal Joint, Right N Metatarsal-Phalangeal Joint, Left P Toe Phalangeal Joint, Right Q Toe Phalangeal Joint, Left	0 Open	7 Autologous Tissue Substitute J Synthetic Substitute K Nonautologous Tissue Substitute	Z No Qualifier

Continued →

Section 0 **Medical and Surgical**
Body System S **Lower Joints**
Operation R **Replacement:** Putting in or on biological or synthetic material that physically takes the place and/or function of all or a portion of a body part

Body Part (4th)	Approach (5th)	Device (6th)	Qualifier (7th)
9 Hip Joint, Right **B** Hip Joint, Left	**0** Open	**1** Synthetic Substitute, Metal **2** Synthetic Substitute, Metal on Polyethylene **3** Synthetic Substitute, Ceramic **4** Synthetic Substitute, Ceramic on Polyethylene **J** Synthetic Substitute	**9** Cemented **A** Uncemented **Z** No Qualifier
9 Hip Joint, Right **B** Hip Joint, Left	**0** Open	**7** Autologous Tissue Substitute **K** Nonautologous Tissue Substitute	**Z** No Qualifier
A Hip Joint, Acetabular Surface, Right **E** Hip Joint, Acetabular Surface, Left	**0** Open	**0** Synthetic Substitute, Polyethylene **1** Synthetic Substitute, Metal **3** Synthetic Substitute, Ceramic **J** Synthetic Substitute	**9** Cemented **A** Uncemented **Z** No Qualifier
A Hip Joint, Acetabular Surface, Right **E** Hip Joint, Acetabular Surface, Left	**0** Open	**7** Autologous Tissue Substitute **K** Nonautologous Tissue Substitute	**Z** No Qualifier
C Knee Joint, Right **D** Knee Joint, Left **F** Ankle Joint, Right **G** Ankle Joint, Left **T** Knee Joint, Femoral Surface, Right **U** Knee Joint, Femoral Surface, Left **V** Knee Joint, Tibial Surface, Right **W** Knee Joint, Tibial Surface, Left	**0** Open	**7** Autologous Tissue Substitute **K** Nonautologous Tissue Substitute	**Z** No Qualifier
C Knee Joint, Right **D** Knee Joint, Left **F** Ankle Joint, Right **G** Ankle Joint, Left **T** Knee Joint, Femoral Surface, Right **U** Knee Joint, Femoral Surface, Left **V** Knee Joint, Tibial Surface, Right **W** Knee Joint, Tibial Surface, Left	**0** Open	**J** Synthetic Substitute	**9** Cemented **A** Uncemented **Z** No Qualifier
R Hip Joint, Femoral Surface, Right **S** Hip Joint, Femoral Surface, Left	**0** Open	**1** Synthetic Substitute, Metal **3** Synthetic Substitute, Ceramic **J** Synthetic Substitute	**9** Cemented **A** Uncemented **Z** No Qualifier
R Hip Joint, Femoral Surface, Right **S** Hip Joint, Femoral Surface, Left	**0** Open	**7** Autologous Tissue Substitute **K** Nonautologous Tissue Substitute	**Z** No Qualifier

Section 0 **Medical and Surgical**
Body System S **Lower Joints**
Operation S **Reposition:** Moving to its normal location, or other suitable location, all or a portion of a body part

Body Part (4th)	Approach (5th)	Device (6th)	Qualifier (7th)
0 Lumbar Vertebral Joint **3** Lumbosacral Joint **5** Sacrococcygeal Joint **6** Coccygeal Joint **7** Sacroiliac Joint, Right **8** Sacroiliac Joint, Left	**0** Open **3** Percutaneous **4** Percutaneous Endoscopic **X** External	**4** Internal Fixation Device **Z** No Device	**Z** No Qualifier

Continued →

Section 0 **Medical and Surgical**
Body System S **Lower Joints**
Operation S **Reposition:** Moving to its normal location, or other suitable location, all or a portion of a body part

Body Part (4th)	Approach (5th)	Device (6th)	Qualifier (7th)
9 Hip Joint, Right **B** Hip Joint, Left **C** Knee Joint, Right **D** Knee Joint, Left **F** Ankle Joint, Right **G** Ankle Joint, Left **H** Tarsal Joint, Right **J** Tarsal Joint, Left **K** Metatarsal-Tarsal Joint, Right **L** Metatarsal-Tarsal Joint, Left **M** Metatarsal-Phalangeal Joint, Right **N** Metatarsal-Phalangeal Joint, Left **P** Toe Phalangeal Joint, Right **Q** Toe Phalangeal Joint, Left	**0** Open **3** Percutaneous **4** Percutaneous Endoscopic **X** External	**4** Internal Fixation Device **5** External Fixation Device **Z** No Device	**Z** No Qualifier

Section 0 **Medical and Surgical**
Body System S **Lower Joints**
Operation T **Resection:** Cutting out or off, without replacement, all of a body part

Body Part (4th)	Approach (5th)	Device (6th)	Qualifier (7th)
2 Lumbar Vertebral Disc **4** Lumbosacral Disc **5** Sacrococcygeal Joint **6** Coccygeal Joint **7** Sacroiliac Joint, Right **8** Sacroiliac Joint, Left **9** Hip Joint, Right **B** Hip Joint, Left **C** Knee Joint, Right **D** Knee Joint, Left **F** Ankle Joint, Right **G** Ankle Joint, Left **H** Tarsal Joint, Right **J** Tarsal Joint, Left **K** Metatarsal-Tarsal Joint, Right **L** Metatarsal-Tarsal Joint, Left **M** Metatarsal-Phalangeal Joint, Right **N** Metatarsal-Phalangeal Joint, Left **P** Toe Phalangeal Joint, Right **Q** Toe Phalangeal Joint, Left	**0** Open	**Z** No Device	**Z** No Qualifier

Section 0 **Medical and Surgical**
Body System S **Lower Joints**
Operation U **Supplement:** Putting in or on biological or synthetic material that physically reinforces and/or augments the function of a portion of a body part

Body Part (4th)	Approach (5th)	Device (6th)	Qualifier (7th)
0 Lumbar Vertebral Joint **2** Lumbar Vertebral Disc **3** Lumbosacral Joint **4** Lumbosacral Disc **5** Sacrococcygeal Joint **6** Coccygeal Joint **7** Sacroiliac Joint, Right **8** Sacroiliac Joint, Left **F** Ankle Joint, Right **G** Ankle Joint, Left **H** Tarsal Joint, Right **J** Tarsal Joint, Left **K** Metatarsal-Tarsal Joint, Right **L** Metatarsal-Tarsal Joint, Left **M** Metatarsal-Phalangeal Joint, Right **N** Metatarsal-Phalangeal Joint, Left **P** Toe Phalangeal Joint, Right **Q** Toe Phalangeal Joint, Left	**0** Open **3** Percutaneous **4** Percutaneous Endoscopic	**7** Autologous Tissue Substitute **J** Synthetic Substitute **K** Nonautologous Tissue Substitute	**Z** No Qualifier
9 Hip Joint, Right **B** Hip Joint, Left	**0** Open	**7** Autologous Tissue Substitute **9** Liner **B** Resurfacing Device **J** Synthetic Substitute **K** Nonautologous Tissue Substitute	**Z** No Qualifier
9 Hip Joint, Right **B** Hip Joint, Left	**3** Percutaneous **4** Percutaneous Endoscopic	**7** Autologous Tissue Substitute **J** Synthetic Substitute **K** Nonautologous Tissue Substitute	**Z** No Qualifier
A Hip Joint, Acetabular Surface, Right **E** Hip Joint, Acetabular Surface, Left **R** Hip Joint, Femoral Surface, Right **S** Hip Joint, Femoral Surface, Left	**0** Open	**9** Liner **B** Resurfacing Device	**Z** No Qualifier
C Knee Joint, Right **D** Knee Joint, Left	**0** Open	**7** Autologous Tissue Substitute **J** Synthetic Substitute **K** Nonautologous Tissue Substitute	**Z** No Qualifier
C Knee Joint, Right **D** Knee Joint, Left	**0** Open	**9** Liner	**C** Patellar Surface **Z** No Qualifier
C Knee Joint, Right **D** Knee Joint, Left	**3** Percutaneous **4** Percutaneous Endoscopic	**7** Autologous Tissue Substitute **J** Synthetic Substitute **K** Nonautologous Tissue Substitute	**Z** No Qualifier
T Knee Joint, Femoral Surface, Right **U** Knee Joint, Femoral Surface, Left **V** Knee Joint, Tibial Surface, Right **W** Knee Joint, Tibial Surface, Left	**0** Open	**9** Liner	**Z** No Qualifier

Section 0 Medical and Surgical
Body System S Lower Joints
Operation W **Revision:** Correcting, to the extent possible, a portion of a malfunctioning device or the position of a displaced device

Body Part (4th)	Approach (5th)	Device (6th)	Qualifier (7th)
0 Lumbar Vertebral Joint **3** Lumbosacral Joint	**0** Open **3** Percutaneous **4** Percutaneous Endoscopic **X** External	**0** Drainage Device **3** Infusion Device **4** Internal Fixation Device **7** Autologous Tissue Substitute **8** Spacer **A** Interbody Fusion Device **J** Synthetic Substitute **K** Nonautologous Tissue Substitute	**Z** No Qualifier
2 Lumbar Vertebral Disc **4** Lumbosacral Disc	**0** Open **3** Percutaneous **4** Percutaneous Endoscopic **X** External	**0** Drainage Device **3** Infusion Device **7** Autologous Tissue Substitute **J** Synthetic Substitute **K** Nonautologous Tissue Substitute	**Z** No Qualifier
5 Sacrococcygeal Joint **6** Coccygeal Joint **7** Sacroiliac Joint, Right **8** Sacroiliac Joint, Left	**0** Open **3** Percutaneous **4** Percutaneous Endoscopic **X** External	**0** Drainage Device **3** Infusion Device **4** Internal Fixation Device **7** Autologous Tissue Substitute **8** Spacer **J** Synthetic Substitute **K** Nonautologous Tissue Substitute	**Z** No Qualifier
9 Hip Joint, Right **B** Hip Joint, Left	**0** Open	**0** Drainage Device **3** Infusion Device **4** Internal Fixation Device **5** External Fixation Device **7** Autologous Tissue Substitute **8** Spacer **9** Liner **B** Resurfacing Device **J** Synthetic Substitute **K** Nonautologous Tissue Substitute	**Z** No Qualifier
9 Hip Joint, Right **B** Hip Joint, Left	**3** Percutaneous **4** Percutaneous Endoscopic **X** External	**0** Drainage Device **3** Infusion Device **4** Internal Fixation Device **5** External Fixation Device **7** Autologous Tissue Substitute **8** Spacer **J** Synthetic Substitute **K** Nonautologous Tissue Substitute	**Z** No Qualifier
C Knee Joint, Right **D** Knee Joint, Left	**0** Open	**0** Drainage Device **3** Infusion Device **4** Internal Fixation Device **5** External Fixation Device **7** Autologous Tissue Substitute **8** Spacer **9** Liner **J** Synthetic Substitute **K** Nonautologous Tissue Substitute	**Z** No Qualifier
C Knee Joint, Right **D** Knee Joint, Left	**3** Percutaneous **4** Percutaneous Endoscopic **X** External	**0** Drainage Device **3** Infusion Device **4** Internal Fixation Device **5** External Fixation Device **7** Autologous Tissue Substitute **8** Spacer **J** Synthetic Substitute **K** Nonautologous Tissue Substitute	**Z** No Qualifier

Continued →

Section	**0**	**Medical and Surgical**
Body System	**S**	**Lower Joints**
Operation	**W**	**Revision:** Correcting, to the extent possible, a portion of a malfunctioning device or the position of a displaced device

0SW Continue

Body Part (4th)	Approach (5th)	Device (6th)	Qualifier (7th)
F Ankle Joint, Right **G** Ankle Joint, Left **H** Tarsal Joint, Right **J** Tarsal Joint, Left **K** Metatarsal-Tarsal Joint, Right **L** Metatarsal-Tarsal Joint, Left **M** Metatarsal-Phalangeal Joint, Right **N** Metatarsal-Phalangeal Joint, Left **P** Toe Phalangeal Joint, Right **Q** Toe Phalangeal Joint, Left	**0** Open **3** Percutaneous **4** Percutaneous Endoscopic **X** External	**0** Drainage Device **3** Infusion Device **4** Internal Fixation Device **5** External Fixation Device **7** Autologous Tissue Substitute **8** Spacer **J** Synthetic Substitute **K** Nonautologous Tissue Substitute	**Z** No Qualifier

Lower Joints Code Listing 0S2–0SW

Review Coding Guideline B4.5

0S2 – Lower Joints, Change

Review Coding Guideline B6.1c

0S2YX0Z Change Drainage Device in Lower Joint, External Approach

0S2YXYZ Change Other Device in Lower Joint, External Approach

0S5 – Lower Joints, Destruction

0S500ZZ Destruction of Lumbar Vertebral Joint, Open Approach

0S503ZZ Destruction of Lumbar Vertebral Joint, Percutaneous Approach

0S504ZZ Destruction of Lumbar Vertebral Joint, Percutaneous Endoscopic Approach

0S520ZZ Destruction of Lumbar Vertebral Disc, Open Approach

0S523ZZ Destruction of Lumbar Vertebral Disc, Percutaneous Approach

0S524ZZ Destruction of Lumbar Vertebral Disc, Percutaneous Endoscopic Approach

0S530ZZ Destruction of Lumbosacral Joint, Open Approach

0S533ZZ Destruction of Lumbosacral Joint, Percutaneous Approach

0S534ZZ Destruction of Lumbosacral Joint, Percutaneous Endoscopic Approach

0S540ZZ Destruction of Lumbosacral Disc, Open Approach

0S543ZZ Destruction of Lumbosacral Disc, Percutaneous Approach

0S544ZZ Destruction of Lumbosacral Disc, Percutaneous Endoscopic Approach

0S550ZZ Destruction of Sacrococcygeal Joint, Open Approach

0S553ZZ Destruction of Sacrococcygeal Joint, Percutaneous Approach

0S554ZZ Destruction of Sacrococcygeal Joint, Percutaneous Endoscopic Approach

0S560ZZ Destruction of Coccygeal Joint, Open Approach

0S563ZZ Destruction of Coccygeal Joint, Percutaneous Approach

0S564ZZ Destruction of Coccygeal Joint, Percutaneous Endoscopic Approach

0S570ZZ Destruction of Right Sacroiliac Joint, Open Approach

0S573ZZ Destruction of Right Sacroiliac Joint, Percutaneous Approach

0S574ZZ Destruction of Right Sacroiliac Joint, Percutaneous Endoscopic Approach

0S580ZZ Destruction of Left Sacroiliac Joint, Open Approach

0S583ZZ Destruction of Left Sacroiliac Joint, Percutaneous Approach

0S584ZZ Destruction of Left Sacroiliac Joint, Percutaneous Endoscopic Approach

0S590ZZ Destruction of Right Hip Joint, Open Approach

0S593ZZ Destruction of Right Hip Joint, Percutaneous Approach

0S594ZZ Destruction of Right Hip Joint, Percutaneous Endoscopic Approach

0S5B0ZZ Destruction of Left Hip Joint, Open Approach

0S5B3ZZ Destruction of Left Hip Joint, Percutaneous Approach

0S5B4ZZ Destruction of Left Hip Joint, Percutaneous Endoscopic Approach

0S5C0ZZ Destruction of Right Knee Joint, Open Approach

0S5C3ZZ Destruction of Right Knee Joint, Percutaneous Approach

0S5C4ZZ Destruction of Right Knee Joint, Percutaneous Endoscopic Approach

0S5D0ZZ Destruction of Left Knee Joint, Open Approach

0S5D3ZZ Destruction of Left Knee Joint, Percutaneous Approach

0S5D4ZZ Destruction of Left Knee Joint, Percutaneous Endoscopic Approach

0S5F0ZZ Destruction of Right Ankle Joint, Open Approach

0S5F3ZZ Destruction of Right Ankle Joint, Percutaneous Approach

0S5F4ZZ Destruction of Right Ankle Joint, Percutaneous Endoscopic Approach

0S5G0ZZ Destruction of Left Ankle Joint, Open Approach

0S5G3ZZ Destruction of Left Ankle Joint, Percutaneous Approach

0S5G4ZZ Destruction of Left Ankle Joint, Percutaneous Endoscopic Approach

0S5H0ZZ Destruction of Right Tarsal Joint, Open Approach

0S5H3ZZ Destruction of Right Tarsal Joint, Percutaneous Approach

0S5H4ZZ Destruction of Right Tarsal Joint, Percutaneous Endoscopic Approach

0S5J0ZZ Destruction of Left Tarsal Joint, Open Approach

0S5J3ZZ Destruction of Left Tarsal Joint, Percutaneous Approach

0S5J4ZZ Destruction of Left Tarsal Joint, Percutaneous Endoscopic Approach

0S5K0ZZ Destruction of Right Metatarsal-Tarsal Joint, Open Approach

0S5K3ZZ Destruction of Right Metatarsal-Tarsal Joint, Percutaneous Approach

0S5K4ZZ Destruction of Right Metatarsal-Tarsal Joint, Percutaneous Endoscopic Approach

0S5L0ZZ Destruction of Left Metatarsal-Tarsal Joint, Open Approach

0S5L3ZZ Destruction of Left Metatarsal-Tarsal Joint, Percutaneous Approach

0S5L4ZZ Destruction of Left Metatarsal-Tarsal Joint, Percutaneous Endoscopic Approach

0S5M0ZZ Destruction of Right Metatarsal-Phalangeal Joint, Open Approach

0S5M3ZZ Destruction of Right Metatarsal-Phalangeal Joint, Percutaneous Approach

0S5M4ZZ Destruction of Right Metatarsal-Phalangeal Joint, Percutaneous Endoscopic Approach

0S5N0ZZ Destruction of Left Metatarsal-Phalangeal Joint, Open Approach

0S5N3ZZ Destruction of Left Metatarsal-Phalangeal Joint, Percutaneous Approach

0S5N4ZZ Destruction of Left Metatarsal-Phalangeal Joint, Percutaneous Endoscopic Approach

0S5P0ZZ Destruction of Right Toe Phalangeal Joint, Open Approach
0S5P3ZZ Destruction of Right Toe Phalangeal Joint, Percutaneous Approach
0S5P4ZZ Destruction of Right Toe Phalangeal Joint, Percutaneous Endoscopic Approach
0S5Q0ZZ Destruction of Left Toe Phalangeal Joint, Open Approach
0S5Q3ZZ Destruction of Left Toe Phalangeal Joint, Percutaneous Approach
0S5Q4ZZ Destruction of Left Toe Phalangeal Joint, Percutaneous Endoscopic Approach

0S9 – Lower Joints, Drainage

Review Coding Guidelines B3.4a and B3.4b

Review Coding Guideline B6.2

0S9000Z Drainage of Lumbar Vertebral Joint with Drainage Device, Open Approach
0S900ZX Drainage of Lumbar Vertebral Joint, Open Approach, Diagnostic
0S900ZZ Drainage of Lumbar Vertebral Joint, Open Approach
0S9030Z Drainage of Lumbar Vertebral Joint with Drainage Device, Percutaneous Approach
0S903ZX Drainage of Lumbar Vertebral Joint, Percutaneous Approach, Diagnostic
0S903ZZ Drainage of Lumbar Vertebral Joint, Percutaneous Approach
0S9040Z Drainage of Lumbar Vertebral Joint with Drainage Device, Percutaneous Endoscopic Approach
0S904ZX Drainage of Lumbar Vertebral Joint, Percutaneous Endoscopic Approach, Diagnostic
0S904ZZ Drainage of Lumbar Vertebral Joint, Percutaneous Endoscopic Approach
0S9200Z Drainage of Lumbar Vertebral Disc with Drainage Device, Open Approach
0S920ZX Drainage of Lumbar Vertebral Disc, Open Approach, Diagnostic
0S920ZZ Drainage of Lumbar Vertebral Disc, Open Approach
0S9230Z Drainage of Lumbar Vertebral Disc with Drainage Device, Percutaneous Approach
0S923ZX Drainage of Lumbar Vertebral Disc, Percutaneous Approach, Diagnostic
0S923ZZ Drainage of Lumbar Vertebral Disc, Percutaneous Approach
0S9240Z Drainage of Lumbar Vertebral Disc with Drainage Device, Percutaneous Endoscopic Approach
0S924ZX Drainage of Lumbar Vertebral Disc, Percutaneous Endoscopic Approach, Diagnostic
0S924ZZ Drainage of Lumbar Vertebral Disc, Percutaneous Endoscopic Approach
0S9300Z Drainage of Lumbosacral Joint with Drainage Device, Open Approach
0S930ZX Drainage of Lumbosacral Joint, Open Approach, Diagnostic
0S930ZZ Drainage of Lumbosacral Joint, Open Approach
0S9330Z Drainage of Lumbosacral Joint with Drainage Device, Percutaneous Approach
0S933ZX Drainage of Lumbosacral Joint, Percutaneous Approach, Diagnostic
0S933ZZ Drainage of Lumbosacral Joint, Percutaneous Approach
0S9340Z Drainage of Lumbosacral Joint with Drainage Device, Percutaneous Endoscopic Approach
0S934ZX Drainage of Lumbosacral Joint, Percutaneous Endoscopic Approach, Diagnostic
0S934ZZ Drainage of Lumbosacral Joint, Percutaneous Endoscopic Approach
0S9400Z Drainage of Lumbosacral Disc with Drainage Device, Open Approach
0S940ZX Drainage of Lumbosacral Disc, Open Approach, Diagnostic
0S940ZZ Drainage of Lumbosacral Disc, Open Approach
0S9430Z Drainage of Lumbosacral Disc with Drainage Device, Percutaneous Approach
0S943ZX Drainage of Lumbosacral Disc, Percutaneous Approach, Diagnostic
0S943ZZ Drainage of Lumbosacral Disc, Percutaneous Approach
0S9440Z Drainage of Lumbosacral Disc with Drainage Device, Percutaneous Endoscopic Approach
0S944ZX Drainage of Lumbosacral Disc, Percutaneous Endoscopic Approach, Diagnostic
0S944ZZ Drainage of Lumbosacral Disc, Percutaneous Endoscopic Approach
0S9500Z Drainage of Sacrococcygeal Joint with Drainage Device, Open Approach
0S950ZX Drainage of Sacrococcygeal Joint, Open Approach, Diagnostic
0S950ZZ Drainage of Sacrococcygeal Joint, Open Approach
0S9530Z Drainage of Sacrococcygeal Joint with Drainage Device, Percutaneous Approach
0S953ZX Drainage of Sacrococcygeal Joint, Percutaneous Approach, Diagnostic
0S953ZZ Drainage of Sacrococcygeal Joint, Percutaneous Approach
0S9540Z Drainage of Sacrococcygeal Joint with Drainage Device, Percutaneous Endoscopic Approach
0S954ZX Drainage of Sacrococcygeal Joint, Percutaneous Endoscopic Approach, Diagnostic
0S954ZZ Drainage of Sacrococcygeal Joint, Percutaneous Endoscopic Approach
0S9600Z Drainage of Coccygeal Joint with Drainage Device, Open Approach
0S960ZX Drainage of Coccygeal Joint, Open Approach, Diagnostic
0S960ZZ Drainage of Coccygeal Joint, Open Approach
0S9630Z Drainage of Coccygeal Joint with Drainage Device, Percutaneous Approach
0S963ZX Drainage of Coccygeal Joint, Percutaneous Approach, Diagnostic
0S963ZZ Drainage of Coccygeal Joint, Percutaneous Approach
0S9640Z Drainage of Coccygeal Joint with Drainage Device, Percutaneous Endoscopic Approach
0S964ZX Drainage of Coccygeal Joint, Percutaneous Endoscopic Approach, Diagnostic
0S964ZZ Drainage of Coccygeal Joint, Percutaneous Endoscopic Approach
0S9700Z Drainage of Right Sacroiliac Joint with Drainage Device, Open Approach
0S970ZX Drainage of Right Sacroiliac Joint, Open Approach, Diagnostic
0S970ZZ Drainage of Right Sacroiliac Joint, Open Approach
0S9730Z Drainage of Right Sacroiliac Joint with Drainage Device, Percutaneous Approach
0S973ZX Drainage of Right Sacroiliac Joint, Percutaneous Approach, Diagnostic
0S973ZZ Drainage of Right Sacroiliac Joint, Percutaneous Approach
0S9740Z Drainage of Right Sacroiliac Joint with Drainage Device, Percutaneous Endoscopic Approach
0S974ZX Drainage of Right Sacroiliac Joint, Percutaneous Endoscopic Approach, Diagnostic
0S974ZZ Drainage of Right Sacroiliac Joint, Percutaneous Endoscopic Approach
0S9800Z Drainage of Left Sacroiliac Joint with Drainage Device, Open Approach
0S980ZX Drainage of Left Sacroiliac Joint, Open Approach, Diagnostic
0S980ZZ Drainage of Left Sacroiliac Joint, Open Approach
0S9830Z Drainage of Left Sacroiliac Joint with Drainage Device, Percutaneous Approach
0S983ZX Drainage of Left Sacroiliac Joint, Percutaneous Approach, Diagnostic
0S983ZZ Drainage of Left Sacroiliac Joint, Percutaneous Approach
0S9840Z Drainage of Left Sacroiliac Joint with Drainage Device, Percutaneous Endoscopic Approach
0S984ZX Drainage of Left Sacroiliac Joint, Percutaneous Endoscopic Approach, Diagnostic
0S984ZZ Drainage of Left Sacroiliac Joint, Percutaneous Endoscopic Approach
0S9900Z Drainage of Right Hip Joint with Drainage Device, Open Approach
0S990ZX Drainage of Right Hip Joint, Open Approach, Diagnostic
0S990ZZ Drainage of Right Hip Joint, Open Approach
0S9930Z Drainage of Right Hip Joint with Drainage Device, Percutaneous Approach
0S993ZX Drainage of Right Hip Joint, Percutaneous Approach, Diagnostic
0S993ZZ Drainage of Right Hip Joint, Percutaneous Approach
0S9940Z Drainage of Right Hip Joint with Drainage Device, Percutaneous Endoscopic Approach
0S994ZX Drainage of Right Hip Joint, Percutaneous Endoscopic Approach, Diagnostic
0S994ZZ Drainage of Right Hip Joint, Percutaneous Endoscopic Approach
0S9B00Z Drainage of Left Hip Joint with Drainage Device, Open Approach
0S9B0ZX Drainage of Left Hip Joint, Open Approach, Diagnostic
0S9B0ZZ Drainage of Left Hip Joint, Open Approach
0S9B30Z Drainage of Left Hip Joint with Drainage Device, Percutaneous Approach
0S9B3ZX Drainage of Left Hip Joint, Percutaneous Approach, Diagnostic
0S9B3ZZ Drainage of Left Hip Joint, Percutaneous Approach
0S9B40Z Drainage of Left Hip Joint with Drainage Device, Percutaneous Endoscopic Approach
0S9B4ZX Drainage of Left Hip Joint, Percutaneous Endoscopic Approach, Diagnostic
0S9B4ZZ Drainage of Left Hip Joint, Percutaneous Endoscopic Approach

0S9C00Z Drainage of Right Knee Joint with Drainage Device, Open Approach
0S9C0ZX Drainage of Right Knee Joint, Open Approach, Diagnostic
0S9C0ZZ Drainage of Right Knee Joint, Open Approach
0S9C30Z Drainage of Right Knee Joint with Drainage Device, Percutaneous Approach
0S9C3ZX Drainage of Right Knee Joint, Percutaneous Approach, Diagnostic
0S9C3ZZ Drainage of Right Knee Joint, Percutaneous Approach
0S9C40Z Drainage of Right Knee Joint with Drainage Device, Percutaneous Endoscopic Approach
0S9C4ZX Drainage of Right Knee Joint, Percutaneous Endoscopic Approach, Diagnostic
0S9C4ZZ Drainage of Right Knee Joint, Percutaneous Endoscopic Approach
0S9D00Z Drainage of Left Knee Joint with Drainage Device, Open Approach
0S9D0ZX Drainage of Left Knee Joint, Open Approach, Diagnostic
0S9D0ZZ Drainage of Left Knee Joint, Open Approach
0S9D30Z Drainage of Left Knee Joint with Drainage Device, Percutaneous Approach
0S9D3ZX Drainage of Left Knee Joint, Percutaneous Approach, Diagnostic
0S9D3ZZ Drainage of Left Knee Joint, Percutaneous Approach
0S9D40Z Drainage of Left Knee Joint with Drainage Device, Percutaneous Endoscopic Approach
0S9D4ZX Drainage of Left Knee Joint, Percutaneous Endoscopic Approach, Diagnostic
0S9D4ZZ Drainage of Left Knee Joint, Percutaneous Endoscopic Approach
0S9F00Z Drainage of Right Ankle Joint with Drainage Device, Open Approach
0S9F0ZX Drainage of Right Ankle Joint, Open Approach, Diagnostic
0S9F0ZZ Drainage of Right Ankle Joint, Open Approach
0S9F30Z Drainage of Right Ankle Joint with Drainage Device, Percutaneous Approach
0S9F3ZX Drainage of Right Ankle Joint, Percutaneous Approach, Diagnostic
0S9F3ZZ Drainage of Right Ankle Joint, Percutaneous Approach
0S9F40Z Drainage of Right Ankle Joint with Drainage Device, Percutaneous Endoscopic Approach
0S9F4ZX Drainage of Right Ankle Joint, Percutaneous Endoscopic Approach, Diagnostic
0S9F4ZZ Drainage of Right Ankle Joint, Percutaneous Endoscopic Approach
0S9G00Z Drainage of Left Ankle Joint with Drainage Device, Open Approach
0S9G0ZX Drainage of Left Ankle Joint, Open Approach, Diagnostic
0S9G0ZZ Drainage of Left Ankle Joint, Open Approach
0S9G30Z Drainage of Left Ankle Joint with Drainage Device, Percutaneous Approach
0S9G3ZX Drainage of Left Ankle Joint, Percutaneous Approach, Diagnostic
0S9G3ZZ Drainage of Left Ankle Joint, Percutaneous Approach
0S9G40Z Drainage of Left Ankle Joint with Drainage Device, Percutaneous Endoscopic Approach
0S9G4ZX Drainage of Left Ankle Joint, Percutaneous Endoscopic Approach, Diagnostic
0S9G4ZZ Drainage of Left Ankle Joint, Percutaneous Endoscopic Approach
0S9H00Z Drainage of Right Tarsal Joint with Drainage Device, Open Approach
0S9H0ZX Drainage of Right Tarsal Joint, Open Approach, Diagnostic
0S9H0ZZ Drainage of Right Tarsal Joint, Open Approach
0S9H30Z Drainage of Right Tarsal Joint with Drainage Device, Percutaneous Approach
0S9H3ZX Drainage of Right Tarsal Joint, Percutaneous Approach, Diagnostic
0S9H3ZZ Drainage of Right Tarsal Joint, Percutaneous Approach
0S9H40Z Drainage of Right Tarsal Joint with Drainage Device, Percutaneous Endoscopic Approach
0S9H4ZX Drainage of Right Tarsal Joint, Percutaneous Endoscopic Approach, Diagnostic
0S9H4ZZ Drainage of Right Tarsal Joint, Percutaneous Endoscopic Approach
0S9J00Z Drainage of Left Tarsal Joint with Drainage Device, Open Approach
0S9J0ZX Drainage of Left Tarsal Joint, Open Approach, Diagnostic
0S9J0ZZ Drainage of Left Tarsal Joint, Open Approach
0S9J30Z Drainage of Left Tarsal Joint with Drainage Device, Percutaneous Approach
0S9J3ZX Drainage of Left Tarsal Joint, Percutaneous Approach, Diagnostic
0S9J3ZZ Drainage of Left Tarsal Joint, Percutaneous Approach
0S9J40Z Drainage of Left Tarsal Joint with Drainage Device, Percutaneous Endoscopic Approach
0S9J4ZX Drainage of Left Tarsal Joint, Percutaneous Endoscopic Approach, Diagnostic
0S9J4ZZ Drainage of Left Tarsal Joint, Percutaneous Endoscopic Approach
0S9K00Z Drainage of Right Metatarsal-Tarsal Joint with Drainage Device, Open Approach
0S9K0ZX Drainage of Right Metatarsal-Tarsal Joint, Open Approach, Diagnostic
0S9K0ZZ Drainage of Right Metatarsal-Tarsal Joint, Open Approach
0S9K30Z Drainage of Right Metatarsal-Tarsal Joint with Drainage Device, Percutaneous Approach
0S9K3ZX Drainage of Right Metatarsal-Tarsal Joint, Percutaneous Approach, Diagnostic
0S9K3ZZ Drainage of Right Metatarsal-Tarsal Joint, Percutaneous Approach
0S9K40Z Drainage of Right Metatarsal-Tarsal Joint with Drainage Device, Percutaneous Endoscopic Approach
0S9K4ZX Drainage of Right Metatarsal-Tarsal Joint, Percutaneous Endoscopic Approach, Diagnostic
0S9K4ZZ Drainage of Right Metatarsal-Tarsal Joint, Percutaneous Endoscopic Approach
0S9L00Z Drainage of Left Metatarsal-Tarsal Joint with Drainage Device, Open Approach
0.0S9L0ZZ Drainage of Left Metatarsal-Tarsal Joint, Open Approach
0S9L30Z Drainage of Left Metatarsal-Tarsal Joint with Drainage Device, Percutaneous Approach
0S9L3ZX Drainage of Left Metatarsal-Tarsal Joint, Percutaneous Approach, Diagnostic
0S9L3ZZ Drainage of Left Metatarsal-Tarsal Joint, Percutaneous Approach
0S9L40Z Drainage of Left Metatarsal-Tarsal Joint with Drainage Device, Percutaneous Endoscopic Approach
0S9L4ZX Drainage of Left Metatarsal-Tarsal Joint, Percutaneous Endoscopic Approach, Diagnostic
0S9L4ZZ Drainage of Left Metatarsal-Tarsal Joint, Percutaneous Endoscopic Approach
0S9M00Z Drainage of Right Metatarsal-Phalangeal Joint with Drainage Device, Open Approach
0S9M0ZX Drainage of Right Metatarsal-Phalangeal Joint, Open Approach, Diagnostic
0S9M0ZZ Drainage of Right Metatarsal-Phalangeal Joint, Open Approach
0S9M30Z Drainage of Right Metatarsal-Phalangeal Joint with Drainage Device, Percutaneous Approach
0S9M3ZX Drainage of Right Metatarsal-Phalangeal Joint, Percutaneous Approach, Diagnostic
0S9M3ZZ Drainage of Right Metatarsal-Phalangeal Joint, Percutaneous Approach
0S9M40Z Drainage of Right Metatarsal-Phalangeal Joint with Drainage Device, Percutaneous Endoscopic Approach
0S9M4ZX Drainage of Right Metatarsal-Phalangeal Joint, Percutaneous Endoscopic Approach, Diagnostic
0S9M4ZZ Drainage of Right Metatarsal-Phalangeal Joint, Percutaneous Endoscopic Approach
0S9N00Z Drainage of Left Metatarsal-Phalangeal Joint with Drainage Device, Open Approach
0S9N0ZX Drainage of Left Metatarsal-Phalangeal Joint, Open Approach, Diagnostic
0S9N0ZZ Drainage of Left Metatarsal-Phalangeal Joint, Open Approach
0S9N30Z Drainage of Left Metatarsal-Phalangeal Joint with Drainage Device, Percutaneous Approach
0S9N3ZX Drainage of Left Metatarsal-Phalangeal Joint, Percutaneous Approach, Diagnostic
0S9N3ZZ Drainage of Left Metatarsal-Phalangeal Joint, Percutaneous Approach
0S9N40Z Drainage of Left Metatarsal-Phalangeal Joint with Drainage Device, Percutaneous Endoscopic Approach
0S9N4ZX Drainage of Left Metatarsal-Phalangeal Joint, Percutaneous Endoscopic Approach, Diagnostic
0S9N4ZZ Drainage of Left Metatarsal-Phalangeal Joint, Percutaneous Endoscopic Approach
0S9P00Z Drainage of Right Toe Phalangeal Joint with Drainage Device, Open Approach
0S9P0ZX Drainage of Right Toe Phalangeal Joint, Open Approach, Diagnostic
0S9P0ZZ Drainage of Right Toe Phalangeal Joint, Open Approach
0S9P30Z Drainage of Right Toe Phalangeal Joint with Drainage Device, Percutaneous Approach
0S9P3ZX Drainage of Right Toe Phalangeal Joint, Percutaneous Approach, Diagnostic
0S9P3ZZ Drainage of Right Toe Phalangeal Joint, Percutaneous Approach
0S9P40Z Drainage of Right Toe Phalangeal Joint with Drainage Device, Percutaneous Endoscopic Approach
0S9P4ZX Drainage of Right Toe Phalangeal Joint, Percutaneous Endoscopic Approach, Diagnostic
0S9P4ZZ Drainage of Right Toe Phalangeal Joint, Percutaneous Endoscopic Approach
0S9Q00Z Drainage of Left Toe Phalangeal Joint with Drainage Device, Open Approach
0S9Q0ZX Drainage of Left Toe Phalangeal Joint, Open Approach, Diagnostic
0S9Q0ZZ Drainage of Left Toe Phalangeal Joint, Open Approach

0S9Q30Z Drainage of Left Toe Phalangeal Joint with Drainage Device, Percutaneous Approach
0S9Q3ZX Drainage of Left Toe Phalangeal Joint, Percutaneous Approach, Diagnostic
0S9Q3ZZ Drainage of Left Toe Phalangeal Joint, Percutaneous Approach
0S9Q40Z Drainage of Left Toe Phalangeal Joint with Drainage Device, Percutaneous Endoscopic Approach
0S9Q4ZX Drainage of Left Toe Phalangeal Joint, Percutaneous Endoscopic Approach, Diagnostic
0S9Q4ZZ Drainage of Left Toe Phalangeal Joint, Percutaneous Endoscopic Approach

0SB – Lower Joints, Excision

Review Coding Guidelines B3.4a and B3.4b

Review Coding Guideline B3.5

Review Coding Guideline B3.8

0SB00ZX Excision of Lumbar Vertebral Joint, Open Approach, Diagnostic
0SB00ZZ Excision of Lumbar Vertebral Joint, Open Approach
0SB03ZX Excision of Lumbar Vertebral Joint, Percutaneous Approach, Diagnostic
0SB03ZZ Excision of Lumbar Vertebral Joint, Percutaneous Approach
0SB04ZX Excision of Lumbar Vertebral Joint, Percutaneous Endoscopic Approach, Diagnostic
0SB04ZZ Excision of Lumbar Vertebral Joint, Percutaneous Endoscopic Approach
0SB20ZX Excision of Lumbar Vertebral Disc, Open Approach, Diagnostic
0SB20ZZ Excision of Lumbar Vertebral Disc, Open Approach
AHA CC: 2Q, 2014, 6-7
0SB23ZX Excision of Lumbar Vertebral Disc, Percutaneous Approach, Diagnostic
0SB23ZZ Excision of Lumbar Vertebral Disc, Percutaneous Approach
0SB24ZX Excision of Lumbar Vertebral Disc, Percutaneous Endoscopic Approach, Diagnostic
0SB24ZZ Excision of Lumbar Vertebral Disc, Percutaneous Endoscopic Approach
0SB30ZX Excision of Lumbosacral Joint, Open Approach, Diagnostic
0SB30ZZ Excision of Lumbosacral Joint, Open Approach
0SB33ZX Excision of Lumbosacral Joint, Percutaneous Approach, Diagnostic
0SB33ZZ Excision of Lumbosacral Joint, Percutaneous Approach
0SB34ZX Excision of Lumbosacral Joint, Percutaneous Endoscopic Approach, Diagnostic
0SB34ZZ Excision of Lumbosacral Joint, Percutaneous Endoscopic Approach
0SB40ZX Excision of Lumbosacral Disc, Open Approach, Diagnostic
0SB40ZZ Excision of Lumbosacral Disc, Open Approach
0SB43ZX Excision of Lumbosacral Disc, Percutaneous Approach, Diagnostic
0SB43ZZ Excision of Lumbosacral Disc, Percutaneous Approach
0SB44ZX Excision of Lumbosacral Disc, Percutaneous Endoscopic Approach, Diagnostic
0SB44ZZ Excision of Lumbosacral Disc, Percutaneous Endoscopic Approach
0SB50ZX Excision of Sacrococcygeal Joint, Open Approach, Diagnostic
0SB50ZZ Excision of Sacrococcygeal Joint, Open Approach
0SB53ZX Excision of Sacrococcygeal Joint, Percutaneous Approach, Diagnostic
0SB53ZZ Excision of Sacrococcygeal Joint, Percutaneous Approach
0SB54ZX Excision of Sacrococcygeal Joint, Percutaneous Endoscopic Approach, Diagnostic
0SB54ZZ Excision of Sacrococcygeal Joint, Percutaneous Endoscopic Approach
0SB60ZX Excision of Coccygeal Joint, Open Approach, Diagnostic
0SB60ZZ Excision of Coccygeal Joint, Open Approach
0SB63ZX Excision of Coccygeal Joint, Percutaneous Approach, Diagnostic
0SB63ZZ Excision of Coccygeal Joint, Percutaneous Approach
0SB64ZX Excision of Coccygeal Joint, Percutaneous Endoscopic Approach, Diagnostic
0SB64ZZ Excision of Coccygeal Joint, Percutaneous Endoscopic Approach
0SB70ZX Excision of Right Sacroiliac Joint, Open Approach, Diagnostic
0SB70ZZ Excision of Right Sacroiliac Joint, Open Approach
0SB73ZX Excision of Right Sacroiliac Joint, Percutaneous Approach, Diagnostic
0SB73ZZ Excision of Right Sacroiliac Joint, Percutaneous Approach
0SB74ZX Excision of Right Sacroiliac Joint, Percutaneous Endoscopic Approach, Diagnostic
0SB74ZZ Excision of Right Sacroiliac Joint, Percutaneous Endoscopic Approach
0SB80ZX Excision of Left Sacroiliac Joint, Open Approach, Diagnostic
0SB80ZZ Excision of Left Sacroiliac Joint, Open Approach
0SB83ZX Excision of Left Sacroiliac Joint, Percutaneous Approach, Diagnostic
0SB83ZZ Excision of Left Sacroiliac Joint, Percutaneous Approach
0SB84ZX Excision of Left Sacroiliac Joint, Percutaneous Endoscopic Approach, Diagnostic
0SB84ZZ Excision of Left Sacroiliac Joint, Percutaneous Endoscopic Approach
0SB90ZX Excision of Right Hip Joint, Open Approach, Diagnostic
0SB90ZZ Excision of Right Hip Joint, Open Approach
0SB93ZX Excision of Right Hip Joint, Percutaneous Approach, Diagnostic
0SB93ZZ Excision of Right Hip Joint, Percutaneous Approach
0SB94ZX Excision of Right Hip Joint, Percutaneous Endoscopic Approach, Diagnostic
0SB94ZZ Excision of Right Hip Joint, Percutaneous Endoscopic Approach
0SBB0ZX Excision of Left Hip Joint, Open Approach, Diagnostic
0SBB0ZZ Excision of Left Hip Joint, Open Approach
0SBB3ZX Excision of Left Hip Joint, Percutaneous Approach, Diagnostic
0SBB3ZZ Excision of Left Hip Joint, Percutaneous Approach
0SBB4ZX Excision of Left Hip Joint, Percutaneous Endoscopic Approach, Diagnostic
0SBB4ZZ Excision of Left Hip Joint, Percutaneous Endoscopic Approach
0SBC0ZX Excision of Right Knee Joint, Open Approach, Diagnostic
0SBC0ZZ Excision of Right Knee Joint, Open Approach
0SBC3ZX Excision of Right Knee Joint, Percutaneous Approach, Diagnostic
0SBC3ZZ Excision of Right Knee Joint, Percutaneous Approach
0SBC4ZX Excision of Right Knee Joint, Percutaneous Endoscopic Approach, Diagnostic
0SBC4ZZ Excision of Right Knee Joint, Percutaneous Endoscopic Approach
0SBD0ZX Excision of Left Knee Joint, Open Approach, Diagnostic
0SBD0ZZ Excision of Left Knee Joint, Open Approach
0SBD3ZX Excision of Left Knee Joint, Percutaneous Approach, Diagnostic
0SBD3ZZ Excision of Left Knee Joint, Percutaneous Approach
0SBD4ZX Excision of Left Knee Joint, Percutaneous Endoscopic Approach, Diagnostic
0SBD4ZZ Excision of Left Knee Joint, Percutaneous Endoscopic Approach
0SBF0ZX Excision of Right Ankle Joint, Open Approach, Diagnostic
0SBF0ZZ Excision of Right Ankle Joint, Open Approach
0SBF3ZX Excision of Right Ankle Joint, Percutaneous Approach, Diagnostic
0SBF3ZZ Excision of Right Ankle Joint, Percutaneous Approach
0SBF4ZX Excision of Right Ankle Joint, Percutaneous Endoscopic Approach, Diagnostic
0SBF4ZZ Excision of Right Ankle Joint, Percutaneous Endoscopic Approach
0SBG0ZX Excision of Left Ankle Joint, Open Approach, Diagnostic
0SBG0ZZ Excision of Left Ankle Joint, Open Approach
0SBG3ZX Excision of Left Ankle Joint, Percutaneous Approach, Diagnostic
0SBG3ZZ Excision of Left Ankle Joint, Percutaneous Approach
0SBG4ZX Excision of Left Ankle Joint, Percutaneous Endoscopic Approach, Diagnostic
0SBG4ZZ Excision of Left Ankle Joint, Percutaneous Endoscopic Approach
0SBH0ZX Excision of Right Tarsal Joint, Open Approach, Diagnostic
0SBH0ZZ Excision of Right Tarsal Joint, Open Approach
0SBH3ZX Excision of Right Tarsal Joint, Percutaneous Approach, Diagnostic
0SBH3ZZ Excision of Right Tarsal Joint, Percutaneous Approach
0SBH4ZX Excision of Right Tarsal Joint, Percutaneous Endoscopic Approach, Diagnostic
0SBH4ZZ Excision of Right Tarsal Joint, Percutaneous Endoscopic Approach
0SBJ0ZX Excision of Left Tarsal Joint, Open Approach, Diagnostic

0SBJ0ZZ Excision of Left Tarsal Joint, Open Approach
0SBJ3ZX Excision of Left Tarsal Joint, Percutaneous Approach, Diagnostic
0SBJ3ZZ Excision of Left Tarsal Joint, Percutaneous Approach
0SBJ4ZX Excision of Left Tarsal Joint, Percutaneous Endoscopic Approach, Diagnostic
0SBJ4ZZ Excision of Left Tarsal Joint, Percutaneous Endoscopic Approach
0SBK0ZX Excision of Right Metatarsal-Tarsal Joint, Open Approach, Diagnostic
0SBK0ZZ Excision of Right Metatarsal-Tarsal Joint, Open Approach
0SBK3ZX Excision of Right Metatarsal-Tarsal Joint, Percutaneous Approach, Diagnostic
0SBK3ZZ Excision of Right Metatarsal-Tarsal Joint, Percutaneous Approach
0SBK4ZX Excision of Right Metatarsal-Tarsal Joint, Percutaneous Endoscopic Approach, Diagnostic
0SBK4ZZ Excision of Right Metatarsal-Tarsal Joint, Percutaneous Endoscopic Approach
0SBL0ZX Excision of Left Metatarsal-Tarsal Joint, Open Approach, Diagnostic
0SBL0ZZ Excision of Left Metatarsal-Tarsal Joint, Open Approach
0SBL3ZX Excision of Left Metatarsal-Tarsal Joint, Percutaneous Approach, Diagnostic
0SBL3ZZ Excision of Left Metatarsal-Tarsal Joint, Percutaneous Approach
0SBL4ZX Excision of Left Metatarsal-Tarsal Joint, Percutaneous Endoscopic Approach, Diagnostic
0SBL4ZZ Excision of Left Metatarsal-Tarsal Joint, Percutaneous Endoscopic Approach
0SBM0ZX Excision of Right Metatarsal-Phalangeal Joint, Open Approach, Diagnostic
0SBM0ZZ Excision of Right Metatarsal-Phalangeal Joint, Open Approach
0SBM3ZX Excision of Right Metatarsal-Phalangeal Joint, Percutaneous Approach, Diagnostic
0SBM3ZZ Excision of Right Metatarsal-Phalangeal Joint, Percutaneous Approach
0SBM4ZX Excision of Right Metatarsal-Phalangeal Joint, Percutaneous Endoscopic Approach, Diagnostic
0SBM4ZZ Excision of Right Metatarsal-Phalangeal Joint, Percutaneous Endoscopic Approach
0SBN0ZX Excision of Left Metatarsal-Phalangeal Joint, Open Approach, Diagnostic
0SBN0ZZ Excision of Left Metatarsal-Phalangeal Joint, Open Approach
0SBN3ZX Excision of Left Metatarsal-Phalangeal Joint, Percutaneous Approach, Diagnostic
0SBN3ZZ Excision of Left Metatarsal-Phalangeal Joint, Percutaneous Approach
0SBN4ZX Excision of Left Metatarsal-Phalangeal Joint, Percutaneous Endoscopic Approach, Diagnostic
0SBN4ZZ Excision of Left Metatarsal-Phalangeal Joint, Percutaneous Endoscopic Approach
0SBP0ZX Excision of Right Toe Phalangeal Joint, Open Approach, Diagnostic
0SBP0ZZ Excision of Right Toe Phalangeal Joint, Open Approach
0SBP3ZX Excision of Right Toe Phalangeal Joint, Percutaneous Approach, Diagnostic
0SBP3ZZ Excision of Right Toe Phalangeal Joint, Percutaneous Approach
0SBP4ZX Excision of Right Toe Phalangeal Joint, Percutaneous Endoscopic Approach, Diagnostic
0SBP4ZZ Excision of Right Toe Phalangeal Joint, Percutaneous Endoscopic Approach
0SBQ0ZX Excision of Left Toe Phalangeal Joint, Open Approach, Diagnostic
0SBQ0ZZ Excision of Left Toe Phalangeal Joint, Open Approach
0SBQ3ZX Excision of Left Toe Phalangeal Joint, Percutaneous Approach, Diagnostic
0SBQ3ZZ Excision of Left Toe Phalangeal Joint, Percutaneous Approach
0SBQ4ZX Excision of Left Toe Phalangeal Joint, Percutaneous Endoscopic Approach, Diagnostic
0SBQ4ZZ Excision of Left Toe Phalangeal Joint, Percutaneous Endoscopic Approach

0SC – Lower Joints, Extirpation

0SC00ZZ Extirpation of Matter from Lumbar Vertebral Joint, Open Approach
0SC03ZZ Extirpation of Matter from Lumbar Vertebral Joint, Percutaneous Approach
0SC04ZZ Extirpation of Matter from Lumbar Vertebral Joint, Percutaneous Endoscopic Approach
0SC20ZZ Extirpation of Matter from Lumbar Vertebral Disc, Open Approach
0SC23ZZ Extirpation of Matter from Lumbar Vertebral Disc, Percutaneous Approach
0SC24ZZ Extirpation of Matter from Lumbar Vertebral Disc, Percutaneous Endoscopic Approach
0SC30ZZ Extirpation of Matter from Lumbosacral Joint, Open Approach
0SC33ZZ Extirpation of Matter from Lumbosacral Joint, Percutaneous Approach
0SC34ZZ Extirpation of Matter from Lumbosacral Joint, Percutaneous Endoscopic Approach
0SC40ZZ Extirpation of Matter from Lumbosacral Disc, Open Approach
0SC43ZZ Extirpation of Matter from Lumbosacral Disc, Percutaneous Approach
0SC44ZZ Extirpation of Matter from Lumbosacral Disc, Percutaneous Endoscopic Approach
0SC50ZZ Extirpation of Matter from Sacrococcygeal Joint, Open Approach
0SC53ZZ Extirpation of Matter from Sacrococcygeal Joint, Percutaneous Approach
0SC54ZZ Extirpation of Matter from Sacrococcygeal Joint, Percutaneous Endoscopic Approach
0SC60ZZ Extirpation of Matter from Coccygeal Joint, Open Approach
0SC63ZZ Extirpation of Matter from Coccygeal Joint, Percutaneous Approach
0SC64ZZ Extirpation of Matter from Coccygeal Joint, Percutaneous Endoscopic Approach
0SC70ZZ Extirpation of Matter from Right Sacroiliac Joint, Open Approach
0SC73ZZ Extirpation of Matter from Right Sacroiliac Joint, Percutaneous Approach
0SC74ZZ Extirpation of Matter from Right Sacroiliac Joint, Percutaneous Endoscopic Approach
0SC80ZZ Extirpation of Matter from Left Sacroiliac Joint, Open Approach
0SC83ZZ Extirpation of Matter from Left Sacroiliac Joint, Percutaneous Approach
0SC84ZZ Extirpation of Matter from Left Sacroiliac Joint, Percutaneous Endoscopic Approach
0SC90ZZ Extirpation of Matter from Right Hip Joint, Open Approach
0SC93ZZ Extirpation of Matter from Right Hip Joint, Percutaneous Approach
0SC94ZZ Extirpation of Matter from Right Hip Joint, Percutaneous Endoscopic Approach
0SCB0ZZ Extirpation of Matter from Left Hip Joint, Open Approach
0SCB3ZZ Extirpation of Matter from Left Hip Joint, Percutaneous Approach
0SCB4ZZ Extirpation of Matter from Left Hip Joint, Percutaneous Endoscopic Approach
0SCC0ZZ Extirpation of Matter from Right Knee Joint, Open Approach
0SCC3ZZ Extirpation of Matter from Right Knee Joint, Percutaneous Approach
0SCC4ZZ Extirpation of Matter from Right Knee Joint, Percutaneous Endoscopic Approach
0SCD0ZZ Extirpation of Matter from Left Knee Joint, Open Approach
0SCD3ZZ Extirpation of Matter from Left Knee Joint, Percutaneous Approach
0SCD4ZZ Extirpation of Matter from Left Knee Joint, Percutaneous Endoscopic Approach
0SCF0ZZ Extirpation of Matter from Right Ankle Joint, Open Approach
0SCF3ZZ Extirpation of Matter from Right Ankle Joint, Percutaneous Approach
0SCF4ZZ Extirpation of Matter from Right Ankle Joint, Percutaneous Endoscopic Approach
0SCG0ZZ Extirpation of Matter from Left Ankle Joint, Open Approach
0SCG3ZZ Extirpation of Matter from Left Ankle Joint, Percutaneous Approach
0SCG4ZZ Extirpation of Matter from Left Ankle Joint, Percutaneous Endoscopic Approach
0SCH0ZZ Extirpation of Matter from Right Tarsal Joint, Open Approach
0SCH3ZZ Extirpation of Matter from Right Tarsal Joint, Percutaneous Approach
0SCH4ZZ Extirpation of Matter from Right Tarsal Joint, Percutaneous Endoscopic Approach
0SCJ0ZZ Extirpation of Matter from Left Tarsal Joint, Open Approach
0SCJ3ZZ Extirpation of Matter from Left Tarsal Joint, Percutaneous Approach
0SCJ4ZZ Extirpation of Matter from Left Tarsal Joint, Percutaneous Endoscopic Approach
0SCK0ZZ Extirpation of Matter from Right Metatarsal-Tarsal Joint, Open Approach
0SCK3ZZ Extirpation of Matter from Right Metatarsal-Tarsal Joint, Percutaneous Approach
0SCK4ZZ Extirpation of Matter from Right Metatarsal-Tarsal Joint, Percutaneous Endoscopic Approach
0SCL0ZZ Extirpation of Matter from Left Metatarsal-Tarsal Joint, Open Approach
0SCL3ZZ Extirpation of Matter from Left Metatarsal-Tarsal Joint, Percutaneous Approach
0SCL4ZZ Extirpation of Matter from Left Metatarsal-Tarsal Joint, Percutaneous Endoscopic Approach
0SCM0ZZ Extirpation of Matter from Right Metatarsal-Phalangeal Joint, Open Approach
0SCM3ZZ Extirpation of Matter from Right Metatarsal-Phalangeal Joint, Percutaneous Approach
0SCM4ZZ Extirpation of Matter from Right Metatarsal-Phalangeal Joint, Percutaneous Endoscopic Approach
0SCN0ZZ Extirpation of Matter from Left Metatarsal-Phalangeal Joint, Open Approach

0SCN3ZZ Extirpation of Matter from Left Metatarsal-Phalangeal Joint, Percutaneous Approach

0SCN4ZZ Extirpation of Matter from Left Metatarsal-Phalangeal Joint, Percutaneous Endoscopic Approach

0SCP0ZZ Extirpation of Matter from Right Toe Phalangeal Joint, Open Approach

0SCP3ZZ Extirpation of Matter from Right Toe Phalangeal Joint, Percutaneous Approach

0SCP4ZZ Extirpation of Matter from Right Toe Phalangeal Joint, Percutaneous Endoscopic Approach

0SCQ0ZZ Extirpation of Matter from Left Toe Phalangeal Joint, Open Approach

0SCQ3ZZ Extirpation of Matter from Left Toe Phalangeal Joint, Percutaneous Approach

0SCQ4ZZ Extirpation of Matter from Left Toe Phalangeal Joint, Percutaneous Endoscopic Approach

0SG – Lower Joints, Fusion

For Fusion procedures involving the vertebral joints

Review Coding Guidelines B3.10a, B3.10b and B3.10c

0SG0070 Fusion of Lumbar Vertebral Joint with Autologous Tissue Substitute, Anterior Approach, Anterior Column, Open Approach

HAC When reported with secondary diagnosis code T84.60XA, T84.610A, T84.611A, T84.612A, T84.613A, T84.614A, T84.615A, T84.619A, T84.63XA, T84.69XA, T84.7XXA

0SG0071 Fusion of Lumbar Vertebral Joint with Autologous Tissue Substitute, Posterior Approach, Posterior Column, Open Approach

AHA CC: 1Q, 2013, 21-23; 3Q, 2013, 25-26

HAC When reported with secondary diagnosis code T84.60XA, T84.610A, T84.611A, T84.612A, T84.613A, T84.614A, T84.615A, T84.619A, T84.63XA, T84.69XA, T84.7XXA

0SG007J Fusion of Lumbar Vertebral Joint with Autologous Tissue Substitute, Posterior Approach, Anterior Column, Open Approach

AHA CC: 2Q, 2014, 6-7

HAC When reported with secondary diagnosis code T84.60XA, T84.610A, T84.611A, T84.612A, T84.613A, T84.614A, T84.615A, T84.619A, T84.63XA, T84.69XA, T84.7XXA

0SG00A0 Fusion of Lumbar Vertebral Joint with Interbody Fusion Device, Anterior Approach, Anterior Column, Open Approach

HAC When reported with secondary diagnosis code T84.60XA, T84.610A, T84.611A, T84.612A, T84.613A, T84.614A, T84.615A, T84.619A, T84.63XA, T84.69XA, T84.7XXA

0SG00A1 Fusion of Lumbar Vertebral Joint with Interbody Fusion Device, Posterior Approach, Posterior Column, Open Approach

HAC When reported with secondary diagnosis code T84.60XA, T84.610A, T84.611A, T84.612A, T84.613A, T84.614A, T84.615A, T84.619A, T84.63XA, T84.69XA, T84.7XXA

0SG00AJ Fusion of Lumbar Vertebral Joint with Interbody Fusion Device, Posterior Approach, Anterior Column, Open Approach

AHA CC: 3Q, 2013, 25-26

HAC When reported with secondary diagnosis code T84.60XA, T84.610A, T84.611A, T84.612A, T84.613A, T84.614A, T84.615A, T84.619A, T84.63XA, T84.69XA, T84.7XXA

0SG00J0 Fusion of Lumbar Vertebral Joint with Synthetic Substitute, Anterior Approach, Anterior Column, Open Approach

HAC When reported with secondary diagnosis code T84.60XA, T84.610A, T84.611A, T84.612A, T84.613A, T84.614A, T84.615A, T84.619A, T84.63XA, T84.69XA, T84.7XXA

0SG00J1 Fusion of Lumbar Vertebral Joint with Synthetic Substitute, Posterior Approach, Posterior Column, Open Approach

HAC When reported with secondary diagnosis code T84.60XA, T84.610A, T84.611A, T84.612A, T84.613A, T84.614A, T84.615A, T84.619A, T84.63XA, T84.69XA, T84.7XXA

0SG00JJ Fusion of Lumbar Vertebral Joint with Synthetic Substitute, Posterior Approach, Anterior Column, Open Approach

HAC When reported with secondary diagnosis code T84.60XA, T84.610A, T84.611A, T84.612A, T84.613A, T84.614A, T84.615A, T84.619A, T84.63XA, T84.69XA, T84.7XXA

0SG00K0 Fusion of Lumbar Vertebral Joint with Nonautologous Tissue Substitute, Anterior Approach, Anterior Column, Open Approach

HAC When reported with secondary diagnosis code T84.60XA, T84.610A, T84.611A, T84.612A, T84.613A, T84.614A, T84.615A, T84.619A, T84.63XA, T84.69XA, T84.7XXA

0SG00K1 Fusion of Lumbar Vertebral Joint with Nonautologous Tissue Substitute, Posterior Approach, Posterior Column, Open Approach

HAC When reported with secondary diagnosis code T84.60XA, T84.610A, T84.611A, T84.612A, T84.613A, T84.614A, T84.615A, T84.619A, T84.63XA, T84.69XA, T84.7XXA

0SG00KJ Fusion of Lumbar Vertebral Joint with Nonautologous Tissue Substitute, Posterior Approach, Anterior Column, Open Approach

HAC When reported with secondary diagnosis code T84.60XA, T84.610A, T84.611A, T84.612A, T84.613A, T84.614A, T84.615A, T84.619A, T84.63XA, T84.69XA, T84.7XXA

0SG00Z0 Fusion of Lumbar Vertebral Joint, Anterior Approach, Anterior Column, Open Approach

HAC When reported with secondary diagnosis code T84.60XA, T84.610A, T84.611A, T84.612A, T84.613A, T84.614A, T84.615A, T84.619A, T84.63XA, T84.69XA, T84.7XXA

0SG00Z1 Fusion of Lumbar Vertebral Joint, Posterior Approach, Posterior Column, Open Approach

HAC When reported with secondary diagnosis code T84.60XA, T84.610A, T84.611A, T84.612A, T84.613A, T84.614A, T84.615A, T84.619A, T84.63XA, T84.69XA, T84.7XXA

0SG00ZJ Fusion of Lumbar Vertebral Joint, Posterior Approach, Anterior Column, Open Approach

HAC When reported with secondary diagnosis code T84.60XA, T84.610A, T84.611A, T84.612A, T84.613A, T84.614A, T84.615A, T84.619A, T84.63XA, T84.69XA, T84.7XXA

0SG0370 Fusion of Lumbar Vertebral Joint with Autologous Tissue Substitute, Anterior Approach, Anterior Column, Percutaneous Approach

HAC When reported with secondary diagnosis code T84.60XA, T84.610A, T84.611A, T84.612A, T84.613A, T84.614A, T84.615A, T84.619A, T84.63XA, T84.69XA, T84.7XXA

0SG0371 Fusion of Lumbar Vertebral Joint with Autologous Tissue Substitute, Posterior Approach, Posterior Column, Percutaneous Approach

HAC When reported with secondary diagnosis code T84.60XA, T84.610A, T84.611A, T84.612A, T84.613A, T84.614A, T84.615A, T84.619A, T84.63XA, T84.69XA, T84.7XXA

0SG037J Fusion of Lumbar Vertebral Joint with Autologous Tissue Substitute, Posterior Approach, Anterior Column, Percutaneous Approach

HAC When reported with secondary diagnosis code T84.60XA, T84.610A, T84.611A, T84.612A, T84.613A, T84.614A, T84.615A, T84.619A, T84.63XA, T84.69XA, T84.7XXA

0SG03A0 Fusion of Lumbar Vertebral Joint with Interbody Fusion Device, Anterior Approach, Anterior Column, Percutaneous Approach

HAC When reported with secondary diagnosis code T84.60XA, T84.610A, T84.611A, T84.612A, T84.613A, T84.614A, T84.615A, T84.619A, T84.63XA, T84.69XA, T84.7XXA

0SG03A1 Fusion of Lumbar Vertebral Joint with Interbody Fusion Device, Posterior Approach, Posterior Column, Percutaneous Approach

HAC When reported with secondary diagnosis code T84.60XA, T84.610A, T84.611A, T84.612A, T84.613A, T84.614A, T84.615A, T84.619A, T84.63XA, T84.69XA, T84.7XXA

0SG03AJ Fusion of Lumbar Vertebral Joint with Interbody Fusion Device, Posterior Approach, Anterior Column, Percutaneous Approach

HAC When reported with secondary diagnosis code T84.60XA, T84.610A, T84.611A, T84.612A, T84.613A, T84.614A, T84.615A, T84.619A, T84.63XA, T84.69XA, T84.7XXA

0SG03J0 Fusion of Lumbar Vertebral Joint with Synthetic Substitute, Anterior Approach, Anterior Column, Percutaneous Approach

HAC When reported with secondary diagnosis code T84.60XA, T84.610A, T84.611A, T84.612A, T84.613A, T84.614A, T84.615A, T84.619A, T84.63XA, T84.69XA, T84.7XXA

0SG03J1 Fusion of Lumbar Vertebral Joint with Synthetic Substitute, Posterior Approach, Posterior Column, Percutaneous Approach

HAC When reported with secondary diagnosis code T84.60XA, T84.610A, T84.611A, T84.612A, T84.613A, T84.614A, T84.615A, T84.619A, T84.63XA, T84.69XA, T84.7XXA

0SG03JJ Fusion of Lumbar Vertebral Joint with Synthetic Substitute, Posterior Approach, Anterior Column, Percutaneous Approach

HAC When reported with secondary diagnosis code T84.60XA, T84.610A, T84.611A, T84.612A, T84.613A, T84.614A, T84.615A, T84.619A, T84.63XA, T84.69XA, T84.7XXA

0SG03K0 Fusion of Lumbar Vertebral Joint with Nonautologous Tissue Substitute, Anterior Approach, Anterior Column, Percutaneous Approach

HAC When reported with secondary diagnosis code T84.60XA, T84.610A, T84.611A, T84.612A, T84.613A, T84.614A, T84.615A, T84.619A, T84.63XA, T84.69XA, T84.7XXA

0SG03K1 Fusion of Lumbar Vertebral Joint with Nonautologous Tissue Substitute, Posterior Approach, Posterior Column, Percutaneous Approach

HAC When reported with secondary diagnosis code T84.60XA, T84.610A, T84.611A, T84.612A, T84.613A, T84.614A, T84.615A, T84.619A, T84.63XA, T84.69XA, T84.7XXA

0SG03KJ Fusion of Lumbar Vertebral Joint with Nonautologous Tissue Substitute, Posterior Approach, Anterior Column, Percutaneous Approach

HAC When reported with secondary diagnosis code T84.60XA, T84.610A, T84.611A, T84.612A, T84.613A, T84.614A, T84.615A, T84.619A, T84.63XA, T84.69XA, T84.7XXA

0SG03Z0 Fusion of Lumbar Vertebral Joint, Anterior Approach, Anterior Column, Percutaneous Approach

HAC When reported with secondary diagnosis code T84.60XA, T84.610A, T84.611A, T84.612A, T84.613A, T84.614A, T84.615A, T84.619A, T84.63XA, T84.69XA, T84.7XXA

0SG03Z1 Fusion of Lumbar Vertebral Joint, Posterior Approach, Posterior Column, Percutaneous Approach

HAC When reported with secondary diagnosis code T84.60XA, T84.610A, T84.611A, T84.612A, T84.613A, T84.614A, T84.615A, T84.619A, T84.63XA, T84.69XA, T84.7XXA

0SG03ZJ Fusion of Lumbar Vertebral Joint, Posterior Approach, Anterior Column, Percutaneous Approach

HAC When reported with secondary diagnosis code T84.60XA, T84.610A, T84.611A, T84.612A, T84.613A, T84.614A, T84.615A, T84.619A, T84.63XA, T84.69XA, T84.7XXA

0SG0470 Fusion of Lumbar Vertebral Joint with Autologous Tissue Substitute, Anterior Approach, Anterior Column, Percutaneous Endoscopic Approach

HAC When reported with secondary diagnosis code T84.60XA, T84.610A, T84.611A, T84.612A, T84.613A, T84.614A, T84.615A, T84.619A, T84.63XA, T84.69XA, T84.7XXA

0SG0471 Fusion of Lumbar Vertebral Joint with Autologous Tissue Substitute, Posterior Approach, Posterior Column, Percutaneous Endoscopic Approach

HAC When reported with secondary diagnosis code T84.60XA, T84.610A, T84.611A, T84.612A, T84.613A, T84.614A, T84.615A, T84.619A, T84.63XA, T84.69XA, T84.7XXA

0SG047J Fusion of Lumbar Vertebral Joint with Autologous Tissue Substitute, Posterior Approach, Anterior Column, Percutaneous Endoscopic Approach

HAC When reported with secondary diagnosis code T84.60XA, T84.610A, T84.611A, T84.612A, T84.613A, T84.614A, T84.615A, T84.619A, T84.63XA, T84.69XA, T84.7XXA

0SG04A0 Fusion of Lumbar Vertebral Joint with Interbody Fusion Device, Anterior Approach, Anterior Column, Percutaneous Endoscopic Approach

HAC When reported with secondary diagnosis code T84.60XA, T84.610A, T84.611A, T84.612A, T84.613A, T84.614A, T84.615A, T84.619A, T84.63XA, T84.69XA, T84.7XXA

0SG04A1 Fusion of Lumbar Vertebral Joint with Interbody Fusion Device, Posterior Approach, Posterior Column, Percutaneous Endoscopic Approach

HAC When reported with secondary diagnosis code T84.60XA, T84.610A, T84.611A, T84.612A, T84.613A, T84.614A, T84.615A, T84.619A, T84.63XA, T84.69XA, T84.7XXA

0SG04AJ Fusion of Lumbar Vertebral Joint with Interbody Fusion Device, Posterior Approach, Anterior Column, Percutaneous Endoscopic Approach

HAC When reported with secondary diagnosis code T84.60XA, T84.610A, T84.611A, T84.612A, T84.613A, T84.614A, T84.615A, T84.619A, T84.63XA, T84.69XA, T84.7XXA

0SG04J0 Fusion of Lumbar Vertebral Joint with Synthetic Substitute, Anterior Approach, Anterior Column, Percutaneous Endoscopic Approach

HAC When reported with secondary diagnosis code T84.60XA, T84.610A, T84.611A, T84.612A, T84.613A, T84.614A, T84.615A, T84.619A, T84.63XA, T84.69XA, T84.7XXA

0SG04J1 Fusion of Lumbar Vertebral Joint with Synthetic Substitute, Posterior Approach, Posterior Column, Percutaneous Endoscopic Approach

HAC When reported with secondary diagnosis code T84.60XA, T84.610A, T84.611A, T84.612A, T84.613A, T84.614A, T84.615A, T84.619A, T84.63XA, T84.69XA, T84.7XXA

0SG04JJ Fusion of Lumbar Vertebral Joint with Synthetic Substitute, Posterior Approach, Anterior Column, Percutaneous Endoscopic Approach

HAC When reported with secondary diagnosis code T84.60XA, T84.610A, T84.611A, T84.612A, T84.613A, T84.614A, T84.615A, T84.619A, T84.63XA, T84.69XA, T84.7XXA

0SG04K0 Fusion of Lumbar Vertebral Joint with Nonautologous Tissue Substitute, Anterior Approach, Anterior Column, Percutaneous Endoscopic Approach

HAC When reported with secondary diagnosis code T84.60XA, T84.610A, T84.611A, T84.612A, T84.613A, T84.614A, T84.615A, T84.619A, T84.63XA, T84.69XA, T84.7XXA

0SG04K1 Fusion of Lumbar Vertebral Joint with Nonautologous Tissue Substitute, Posterior Approach, Posterior Column, Percutaneous Endoscopic Approach

HAC When reported with secondary diagnosis code T84.60XA, T84.610A, T84.611A, T84.612A, T84.613A, T84.614A, T84.615A, T84.619A, T84.63XA, T84.69XA, T84.7XXA

0SG04KJ Fusion of Lumbar Vertebral Joint with Nonautologous Tissue Substitute, Posterior Approach, Anterior Column, Percutaneous Endoscopic Approach

HAC When reported with secondary diagnosis code T84.60XA, T84.610A, T84.611A, T84.612A, T84.613A, T84.614A, T84.615A, T84.619A, T84.63XA, T84.69XA, T84.7XXA

0SG04Z0 Fusion of Lumbar Vertebral Joint, Anterior Approach, Anterior Column, Percutaneous Endoscopic Approach

HAC When reported with secondary diagnosis code T84.60XA, T84.610A, T84.611A, T84.612A, T84.613A, T84.614A, T84.615A, T84.619A, T84.63XA, T84.69XA, T84.7XXA

0SG04Z1 Fusion of Lumbar Vertebral Joint, Posterior Approach, Posterior Column, Percutaneous Endoscopic Approach

HAC When reported with secondary diagnosis code T84.60XA, T84.610A, T84.611A, T84.612A, T84.613A, T84.614A, T84.615A, T84.619A, T84.63XA, T84.69XA, T84.7XXA

0SG04ZJ Fusion of Lumbar Vertebral Joint, Posterior Approach, Anterior Column, Percutaneous Endoscopic Approach

HAC When reported with secondary diagnosis code T84.60XA, T84.610A, T84.611A, T84.612A, T84.613A, T84.614A, T84.615A, T84.619A, T84.63XA, T84.69XA, T84.7XXA

0SG1070 Fusion of 2 or more Lumbar Vertebral Joints with Autologous Tissue Substitute, Anterior Approach, Anterior Column, Open Approach

HAC When reported with secondary diagnosis code T84.60XA, T84.610A, T84.611A, T84.612A, T84.613A, T84.614A, T84.615A, T84.619A, T84.63XA, T84.69XA, T84.7XXA

0SG1071 Fusion of 2 or more Lumbar Vertebral Joints with Autologous Tissue Substitute, Posterior Approach, Posterior Column, Open Approach

HAC When reported with secondary diagnosis code T84.60XA, T84.610A, T84.611A, T84.612A, T84.613A, T84.614A, T84.615A, T84.619A, T84.63XA, T84.69XA, T84.7XXA

0SG107J Fusion of 2 or more Lumbar Vertebral Joints with Autologous Tissue Substitute, Posterior Approach, Anterior Column, Open Approach

Note Continued

0SG107J Continued Note

HAC When reported with secondary diagnosis code T84.60XA, T84.610A, T84.611A, T84.612A, T84.613A, T84.614A, T84.615A, T84.619A, T84.63XA, T84.69XA, T84.7XXA

0SG10A0 Fusion of 2 or more Lumbar Vertebral Joints with Interbody Fusion Device, Anterior Approach, Anterior Column, Open Approach

HAC When reported with secondary diagnosis code T84.60XA, T84.610A, T84.611A, T84.612A, T84.613A, T84.614A, T84.615A, T84.619A, T84.63XA, T84.69XA, T84.7XXA

0SG10A1 Fusion of 2 or more Lumbar Vertebral Joints with Interbody Fusion Device, Posterior Approach, Posterior Column, Open Approach

HAC When reported with secondary diagnosis code T84.60XA, T84.610A, T84.611A, T84.612A, T84.613A, T84.614A, T84.615A, T84.619A, T84.63XA, T84.69XA, T84.7XXA

0SG10AJ Fusion of 2 or more Lumbar Vertebral Joints with Interbody Fusion Device, Posterior Approach, Anterior Column, Open Approach

HAC When reported with secondary diagnosis code T84.60XA, T84.610A, T84.611A, T84.612A, T84.613A, T84.614A, T84.615A, T84.619A, T84.63XA, T84.69XA, T84.7XXA

0SG10J0 Fusion of 2 or more Lumbar Vertebral Joints with Synthetic Substitute, Anterior Approach, Anterior Column, Open Approach

HAC When reported with secondary diagnosis code T84.60XA, T84.610A, T84.611A, T84.612A, T84.613A, T84.614A, T84.615A, T84.619A, T84.63XA, T84.69XA, T84.7XXA

0SG10J1 Fusion of 2 or more Lumbar Vertebral Joints with Synthetic Substitute, Posterior Approach, Posterior Column, Open Approach

HAC When reported with secondary diagnosis code T84.60XA, T84.610A, T84.611A, T84.612A, T84.613A, T84.614A, T84.615A, T84.619A, T84.63XA, T84.69XA, T84.7XXA

0SG10JJ Fusion of 2 or more Lumbar Vertebral Joints with Synthetic Substitute, Posterior Approach, Anterior Column, Open Approach

HAC When reported with secondary diagnosis code T84.60XA, T84.610A, T84.611A, T84.612A, T84.613A, T84.614A, T84.615A, T84.619A, T84.63XA, T84.69XA, T84.7XXA

0SG10K0 Fusion of 2 or more Lumbar Vertebral Joints with Nonautologous Tissue Substitute, Anterior Approach, Anterior Column, Open Approach

HAC When reported with secondary diagnosis code T84.60XA, T84.610A, T84.611A, T84.612A, T84.613A, T84.614A, T84.615A, T84.619A, T84.63XA, T84.69XA, T84.7XXA

0SG10K1 Fusion of 2 or more Lumbar Vertebral Joints with Nonautologous Tissue Substitute, Posterior Approach, Posterior Column, Open Approach

HAC When reported with secondary diagnosis code T84.60XA, T84.610A, T84.611A, T84.612A, T84.613A, T84.614A, T84.615A, T84.619A, T84.63XA, T84.69XA, T84.7XXA

0SG10KJ Fusion of 2 or more Lumbar Vertebral Joints with Nonautologous Tissue Substitute, Posterior Approach, Anterior Column, Open Approach

HAC When reported with secondary diagnosis code T84.60XA, T84.610A, T84.611A, T84.612A, T84.613A, T84.614A, T84.615A, T84.619A, T84.63XA, T84.69XA, T84.7XXA

0SG10Z0 Fusion of 2 or more Lumbar Vertebral Joints, Anterior Approach, Anterior Column, Open Approach

HAC When reported with secondary diagnosis code T84.60XA, T84.610A, T84.611A, T84.612A, T84.613A, T84.614A, T84.615A, T84.619A, T84.63XA, T84.69XA, T84.7XXA

0SG10Z1 Fusion of 2 or more Lumbar Vertebral Joints, Posterior Approach, Posterior Column, Open Approach

HAC When reported with secondary diagnosis code T84.60XA, T84.610A, T84.611A, T84.612A, T84.613A, T84.614A, T84.615A, T84.619A, T84.63XA, T84.69XA, T84.7XXA

0SG10ZJ Fusion of 2 or more Lumbar Vertebral Joints, Posterior Approach, Anterior Column, Open Approach

HAC When reported with secondary diagnosis code T84.60XA, T84.610A, T84.611A, T84.612A, T84.613A, T84.614A, T84.615A, T84.619A, T84.63XA, T84.69XA, T84.7XXA

0SG1370 Fusion of 2 or more Lumbar Vertebral Joints with Autologous Tissue Substitute, Anterior Approach, Anterior Column, Percutaneous Approach

HAC When reported with secondary diagnosis code T84.60XA, T84.610A, T84.611A, T84.612A, T84.613A, T84.614A, T84.615A, T84.619A, T84.63XA, T84.69XA, T84.7XXA

0SG1371 Fusion of 2 or more Lumbar Vertebral Joints with Autologous Tissue Substitute, Posterior Approach, Posterior Column, Percutaneous Approach

HAC When reported with secondary diagnosis code T84.60XA, T84.610A, T84.611A, T84.612A, T84.613A, T84.614A, T84.615A, T84.619A, T84.63XA, T84.69XA, T84.7XXA

0SG137J Fusion of 2 or more Lumbar Vertebral Joints with Autologous Tissue Substitute, Posterior Approach, Anterior Column, Percutaneous Approach

HAC When reported with secondary diagnosis code T84.60XA, T84.610A, T84.611A, T84.612A, T84.613A, T84.614A, T84.615A, T84.619A, T84.63XA, T84.69XA, T84.7XXA

0SG13A0 Fusion of 2 or more Lumbar Vertebral Joints with Interbody Fusion Device, Anterior Approach, Anterior Column, Percutaneous Approach

HAC When reported with secondary diagnosis code T84.60XA, T84.610A, T84.611A, T84.612A, T84.613A, T84.614A, T84.615A, T84.619A, T84.63XA, T84.69XA, T84.7XXA

0SG13A1 Fusion of 2 or more Lumbar Vertebral Joints with Interbody Fusion Device, Posterior Approach, Posterior Column, Percutaneous Approach

HAC When reported with secondary diagnosis code T84.60XA, T84.610A, T84.611A, T84.612A, T84.613A, T84.614A, T84.615A, T84.619A, T84.63XA, T84.69XA, T84.7XXA

0SG13AJ Fusion of 2 or more Lumbar Vertebral Joints with Interbody Fusion Device, Posterior Approach, Anterior Column, Percutaneous Approach

HAC When reported with secondary diagnosis code T84.60XA, T84.610A, T84.611A, T84.612A, T84.613A, T84.614A, T84.615A, T84.619A, T84.63XA, T84.69XA, T84.7XXA

0SG13J0 Fusion of 2 or more Lumbar Vertebral Joints with Synthetic Substitute, Anterior Approach, Anterior Column, Percutaneous Approach

HAC When reported with secondary diagnosis code T84.60XA, T84.610A, T84.611A, T84.612A, T84.613A, T84.614A, T84.615A, T84.619A, T84.63XA, T84.69XA, T84.7XXA

0SG13J1 Fusion of 2 or more Lumbar Vertebral Joints with Synthetic Substitute, Posterior Approach, Posterior Column, Percutaneous Approach

HAC When reported with secondary diagnosis code T84.60XA, T84.610A, T84.611A, T84.612A, T84.613A, T84.614A, T84.615A, T84.619A, T84.63XA, T84.69XA, T84.7XXA

0SG13JJ Fusion of 2 or more Lumbar Vertebral Joints with Synthetic Substitute, Posterior Approach, Anterior Column, Percutaneous Approach

HAC When reported with secondary diagnosis code T84.60XA, T84.610A, T84.611A, T84.612A, T84.613A, T84.614A, T84.615A, T84.619A, T84.63XA, T84.69XA, T84.7XXA

0SG13K0 Fusion of 2 or more Lumbar Vertebral Joints with Nonautologous Tissue Substitute, Anterior Approach, Anterior Column, Percutaneous Approach

HAC When reported with secondary diagnosis code T84.60XA, T84.610A, T84.611A, T84.612A, T84.613A, T84.614A, T84.615A, T84.619A, T84.63XA, T84.69XA, T84.7XXA

0SG13K1 Fusion of 2 or more Lumbar Vertebral Joints with Nonautologous Tissue Substitute, Posterior Approach, Posterior Column, Percutaneous Approach

HAC When reported with secondary diagnosis code T84.60XA, T84.610A, T84.611A, T84.612A, T84.613A, T84.614A, T84.615A, T84.619A, T84.63XA, T84.69XA, T84.7XXA

0SG13KJ Fusion of 2 or more Lumbar Vertebral Joints with Nonautologous Tissue Substitute, Posterior Approach, Anterior Column, Percutaneous Approach

HAC When reported with secondary diagnosis code T84.60XA, T84.610A, T84.611A, T84.612A, T84.613A, T84.614A, T84.615A, T84.619A, T84.63XA, T84.69XA, T84.7XXA

0SG13Z0 Fusion of 2 or more Lumbar Vertebral Joints, Anterior Approach, Anterior Column, Percutaneous Approach

HAC When reported with secondary diagnosis code T84.60XA, T84.610A, T84.611A, T84.612A, T84.613A, T84.614A, T84.615A, T84.619A, T84.63XA, T84.69XA, T84.7XXA

0SG13Z1 Fusion of 2 or more Lumbar Vertebral Joints, Posterior Approach, Posterior Column, Percutaneous Approach

Note Continued

0SG13Z1 Continued Note

HAC When reported with secondary diagnosis code T84.60XA, T84.610A, T84.611A, T84.612A, T84.613A, T84.614A, T84.615A, T84.619A, T84.63XA, T84.69XA, T84.7XXA

0SG13ZJ Fusion of 2 or more Lumbar Vertebral Joints, Posterior Approach, Anterior Column, Percutaneous Approach

HAC When reported with secondary diagnosis code T84.60XA, T84.610A, T84.611A, T84.612A, T84.613A, T84.614A, T84.615A, T84.619A, T84.63XA, T84.69XA, T84.7XXA

0SG1470 Fusion of 2 or more Lumbar Vertebral Joints with Autologous Tissue Substitute, Anterior Approach, Anterior Column, Percutaneous Endoscopic Approach

HAC When reported with secondary diagnosis code T84.60XA, T84.610A, T84.611A, T84.612A, T84.613A, T84.614A, T84.615A, T84.619A, T84.63XA, T84.69XA, T84.7XXA

0SG1471 Fusion of 2 or more Lumbar Vertebral Joints with Autologous Tissue Substitute, Posterior Approach, Posterior Column, Percutaneous Endoscopic Approach

HAC When reported with secondary diagnosis code T84.60XA, T84.610A, T84.611A, T84.612A, T84.613A, T84.614A, T84.615A, T84.619A, T84.63XA, T84.69XA, T84.7XXA

0SG147J Fusion of 2 or more Lumbar Vertebral Joints with Autologous Tissue Substitute, Posterior Approach, Anterior Column, Percutaneous Endoscopic Approach

HAC When reported with secondary diagnosis code T84.60XA, T84.610A, T84.611A, T84.612A, T84.613A, T84.614A, T84.615A, T84.619A, T84.63XA, T84.69XA, T84.7XXA

0SG14A0 Fusion of 2 or more Lumbar Vertebral Joints with Interbody Fusion Device, Anterior Approach, Anterior Column, Percutaneous Endoscopic Approach

HAC When reported with secondary diagnosis code T84.60XA, T84.610A, T84.611A, T84.612A, T84.613A, T84.614A, T84.615A, T84.619A, T84.63XA, T84.69XA, T84.7XXA

0SG14A1 Fusion of 2 or more Lumbar Vertebral Joints with Interbody Fusion Device, Posterior Approach, Posterior Column, Percutaneous Endoscopic Approach

HAC When reported with secondary diagnosis code T84.60XA, T84.610A, T84.611A, T84.612A, T84.613A, T84.614A, T84.615A, T84.619A, T84.63XA, T84.69XA, T84.7XXA

0SG14AJ Fusion of 2 or more Lumbar Vertebral Joints with Interbody Fusion Device, Posterior Approach, Anterior Column, Percutaneous Endoscopic Approach

HAC When reported with secondary diagnosis code T84.60XA, T84.610A, T84.611A, T84.612A, T84.613A, T84.614A, T84.615A, T84.619A, T84.63XA, T84.69XA, T84.7XXA

0SG14J0 Fusion of 2 or more Lumbar Vertebral Joints with Synthetic Substitute, Anterior Approach, Anterior Column, Percutaneous Endoscopic Approach

HAC When reported with secondary diagnosis code T84.60XA, T84.610A, T84.611A, T84.612A, T84.613A, T84.614A, T84.615A, T84.619A, T84.63XA, T84.69XA, T84.7XXA

0SG14J1 Fusion of 2 or more Lumbar Vertebral Joints with Synthetic Substitute, Posterior Approach, Posterior Column, Percutaneous Endoscopic Approach

HAC When reported with secondary diagnosis code T84.60XA, T84.610A, T84.611A, T84.612A, T84.613A, T84.614A, T84.615A, T84.619A, T84.63XA, T84.69XA, T84.7XXA

0SG14JJ Fusion of 2 or more Lumbar Vertebral Joints with Synthetic Substitute, Posterior Approach, Anterior Column, Percutaneous Endoscopic Approach

HAC When reported with secondary diagnosis code T84.60XA, T84.610A, T84.611A, T84.612A, T84.613A, T84.614A, T84.615A, T84.619A, T84.63XA, T84.69XA, T84.7XXA

0SG14K0 Fusion of 2 or more Lumbar Vertebral Joints with Nonautologous Tissue Substitute, Anterior Approach, Anterior Column, Percutaneous Endoscopic Approach

HAC When reported with secondary diagnosis code T84.60XA, T84.610A, T84.611A, T84.612A, T84.613A, T84.614A, T84.615A, T84.619A, T84.63XA, T84.69XA, T84.7XXA

0SG14K1 Fusion of 2 or more Lumbar Vertebral Joints with Nonautologous Tissue Substitute, Posterior Approach, Posterior Column, Percutaneous Endoscopic Approach

HAC When reported with secondary diagnosis code T84.60XA, T84.610A, T84.611A, T84.612A, T84.613A, T84.614A, T84.615A, T84.619A, T84.63XA, T84.69XA, T84.7XXA

0SG14KJ Fusion of 2 or more Lumbar Vertebral Joints with Nonautologous Tissue Substitute, Posterior Approach, Anterior Column, Percutaneous Endoscopic Approach

HAC When reported with secondary diagnosis code T84.60XA, T84.610A, T84.611A, T84.612A, T84.613A, T84.614A, T84.615A, T84.619A, T84.63XA, T84.69XA, T84.7XXA

0SG14Z0 Fusion of 2 or more Lumbar Vertebral Joints, Anterior Approach, Anterior Column, Percutaneous Endoscopic Approach

HAC When reported with secondary diagnosis code T84.60XA, T84.610A, T84.611A, T84.612A, T84.613A, T84.614A, T84.615A, T84.619A, T84.63XA, T84.69XA, T84.7XXA

0SG14Z1 Fusion of 2 or more Lumbar Vertebral Joints, Posterior Approach, Posterior Column, Percutaneous Endoscopic Approach

HAC When reported with secondary diagnosis code T84.60XA, T84.610A, T84.611A, T84.612A, T84.613A, T84.614A, T84.615A, T84.619A, T84.63XA, T84.69XA, T84.7XXA

0SG14ZJ Fusion of 2 or more Lumbar Vertebral Joints, Posterior Approach, Anterior Column, Percutaneous Endoscopic Approach

HAC When reported with secondary diagnosis code T84.60XA, T84.610A, T84.611A, T84.612A, T84.613A, T84.614A, T84.615A, T84.619A, T84.63XA, T84.69XA, T84.7XXA

0SG3070 Fusion of Lumbosacral Joint with Autologous Tissue Substitute, Anterior Approach, Anterior Column, Open Approach

HAC When reported with secondary diagnosis code T84.60XA, T84.610A, T84.611A, T84.612A, T84.613A, T84.614A, T84.615A, T84.619A, T84.63XA, T84.69XA, T84.7XXA

0SG3071 Fusion of Lumbosacral Joint with Autologous Tissue Substitute, Posterior Approach, Posterior Column, Open Approach

HAC When reported with secondary diagnosis code T84.60XA, T84.610A, T84.611A, T84.612A, T84.613A, T84.614A, T84.615A, T84.619A, T84.63XA, T84.69XA, T84.7XXA

0SG307J Fusion of Lumbosacral Joint with Autologous Tissue Substitute, Posterior Approach, Anterior Column, Open Approach

HAC When reported with secondary diagnosis code T84.60XA, T84.610A, T84.611A, T84.612A, T84.613A, T84.614A, T84.615A, T84.619A, T84.63XA, T84.69XA, T84.7XXA

0SG30A0 Fusion of Lumbosacral Joint with Interbody Fusion Device, Anterior Approach, Anterior Column, Open Approach

HAC When reported with secondary diagnosis code T84.60XA, T84.610A, T84.611A, T84.612A, T84.613A, T84.614A, T84.615A, T84.619A, T84.63XA, T84.69XA, T84.7XXA

0SG30A1 Fusion of Lumbosacral Joint with Interbody Fusion Device, Posterior Approach, Posterior Column, Open Approach

HAC When reported with secondary diagnosis code T84.60XA, T84.610A, T84.611A, T84.612A, T84.613A, T84.614A, T84.615A, T84.619A, T84.63XA, T84.69XA, T84.7XXA

0SG30AJ Fusion of Lumbosacral Joint with Interbody Fusion Device, Posterior Approach, Anterior Column, Open Approach

HAC When reported with secondary diagnosis code T84.60XA, T84.610A, T84.611A, T84.612A, T84.613A, T84.614A, T84.615A, T84.619A, T84.63XA, T84.69XA, T84.7XXA

0SG30J0 Fusion of Lumbosacral Joint with Synthetic Substitute, Anterior Approach, Anterior Column, Open Approach

HAC When reported with secondary diagnosis code T84.60XA, T84.610A, T84.611A, T84.612A, T84.613A, T84.614A, T84.615A, T84.619A, T84.63XA, T84.69XA, T84.7XXA

0SG30J1 Fusion of Lumbosacral Joint with Synthetic Substitute, Posterior Approach, Posterior Column, Open Approach

HAC When reported with secondary diagnosis code T84.60XA, T84.610A, T84.611A, T84.612A, T84.613A, T84.614A, T84.615A, T84.619A, T84.63XA, T84.69XA, T84.7XXA

0SG30JJ Fusion of Lumbosacral Joint with Synthetic Substitute, Posterior Approach, Anterior Column, Open Approach

HAC When reported with secondary diagnosis code T84.60XA, T84.610A, T84.611A, T84.612A, T84.613A, T84.614A, T84.615A, T84.619A, T84.63XA, T84.69XA, T84.7XXA

0SG30K0 Fusion of Lumbosacral Joint with Nonautologous Tissue Substitute, Anterior Approach, Anterior Column, Open Approach

Note Continued

0SG30K0 Continued Note

HAC When reported with secondary diagnosis code T84.60XA, T84.610A, T84.611A, T84.612A, T84.613A, T84.614A, T84.615A, T84.619A, T84.63XA, T84.69XA, T84.7XXA

0SG30K1 Fusion of Lumbosacral Joint with Nonautologous Tissue Substitute, Posterior Approach, Posterior Column, Open Approach

HAC When reported with secondary diagnosis code T84.60XA, T84.610A, T84.611A, T84.612A, T84.613A, T84.614A, T84.615A, T84.619A, T84.63XA, T84.69XA, T84.7XXA

0SG30KJ Fusion of Lumbosacral Joint with Nonautologous Tissue Substitute, Posterior Approach, Anterior Column, Open Approach

HAC When reported with secondary diagnosis code T84.60XA, T84.610A, T84.611A, T84.612A, T84.613A, T84.614A, T84.615A, T84.619A, T84.63XA, T84.69XA, T84.7XXA

0SG30Z0 Fusion of Lumbosacral Joint, Anterior Approach, Anterior Column, Open Approach

HAC When reported with secondary diagnosis code T84.60XA, T84.610A, T84.611A, T84.612A, T84.613A, T84.614A, T84.615A, T84.619A, T84.63XA, T84.69XA, T84.7XXA

0SG30Z1 Fusion of Lumbosacral Joint, Posterior Approach, Posterior Column, Open Approach

HAC When reported with secondary diagnosis code T84.60XA, T84.610A, T84.611A, T84.612A, T84.613A, T84.614A, T84.615A, T84.619A, T84.63XA, T84.69XA, T84.7XXA

0SG30ZJ Fusion of Lumbosacral Joint, Posterior Approach, Anterior Column, Open Approach

HAC When reported with secondary diagnosis code T84.60XA, T84.610A, T84.611A, T84.612A, T84.613A, T84.614A, T84.615A, T84.619A, T84.63XA, T84.69XA, T84.7XXA

0SG3370 Fusion of Lumbosacral Joint with Autologous Tissue Substitute, Anterior Approach, Anterior Column, Percutaneous Approach

HAC When reported with secondary diagnosis code T84.60XA, T84.610A, T84.611A, T84.612A, T84.613A, T84.614A, T84.615A, T84.619A, T84.63XA, T84.69XA, T84.7XXA

0SG3371 Fusion of Lumbosacral Joint with Autologous Tissue Substitute, Posterior Approach, Posterior Column, Percutaneous Approach

HAC When reported with secondary diagnosis code T84.60XA, T84.610A, T84.611A, T84.612A, T84.613A, T84.614A, T84.615A, T84.619A, T84.63XA, T84.69XA, T84.7XXA

0SG337J Fusion of Lumbosacral Joint with Autologous Tissue Substitute, Posterior Approach, Anterior Column, Percutaneous Approach

HAC When reported with secondary diagnosis code T84.60XA, T84.610A, T84.611A, T84.612A, T84.613A, T84.614A, T84.615A, T84.619A, T84.63XA, T84.69XA, T84.7XXA

0SG33A0 Fusion of Lumbosacral Joint with Interbody Fusion Device, Anterior Approach, Anterior Column, Percutaneous Approach

HAC When reported with secondary diagnosis code T84.60XA, T84.610A, T84.611A, T84.612A, T84.613A, T84.614A, T84.615A, T84.619A, T84.63XA, T84.69XA, T84.7XXA

0SG33A1 Fusion of Lumbosacral Joint with Interbody Fusion Device, Posterior Approach, Posterior Column, Percutaneous Approach

HAC When reported with secondary diagnosis code T84.60XA, T84.610A, T84.611A, T84.612A, T84.613A, T84.614A, T84.615A, T84.619A, T84.63XA, T84.69XA, T84.7XXA

0SG33AJ Fusion of Lumbosacral Joint with Interbody Fusion Device, Posterior Approach, Anterior Column, Percutaneous Approach

HAC When reported with secondary diagnosis code T84.60XA, T84.610A, T84.611A, T84.612A, T84.613A, T84.614A, T84.615A, T84.619A, T84.63XA, T84.69XA, T84.7XXA

0SG33J0 Fusion of Lumbosacral Joint with Synthetic Substitute, Anterior Approach, Anterior Column, Percutaneous Approach

HAC When reported with secondary diagnosis code T84.60XA, T84.610A, T84.611A, T84.612A, T84.613A, T84.614A, T84.615A, T84.619A, T84.63XA, T84.69XA, T84.7XXA

0SG33J1 Fusion of Lumbosacral Joint with Synthetic Substitute, Posterior Approach, Posterior Column, Percutaneous Approach

HAC When reported with secondary diagnosis code T84.60XA, T84.610A, T84.611A, T84.612A, T84.613A, T84.614A, T84.615A, T84.619A, T84.63XA, T84.69XA, T84.7XXA

0SG33JJ Fusion of Lumbosacral Joint with Synthetic Substitute, Posterior Approach, Anterior Column, Percutaneous Approach

HAC When reported with secondary diagnosis code T84.60XA, T84.610A, T84.611A, T84.612A, T84.613A, T84.614A, T84.615A, T84.619A, T84.63XA, T84.69XA, T84.7XXA

0SG33K0 Fusion of Lumbosacral Joint with Nonautologous Tissue Substitute, Anterior Approach, Anterior Column, Percutaneous Approach

HAC When reported with secondary diagnosis code T84.60XA, T84.610A, T84.611A, T84.612A, T84.613A, T84.614A, T84.615A, T84.619A, T84.63XA, T84.69XA, T84.7XXA

0SG33K1 Fusion of Lumbosacral Joint with Nonautologous Tissue Substitute, Posterior Approach, Posterior Column, Percutaneous Approach

HAC When reported with secondary diagnosis code T84.60XA, T84.610A, T84.611A, T84.612A, T84.613A, T84.614A, T84.615A, T84.619A, T84.63XA, T84.69XA, T84.7XXA

0SG33KJ Fusion of Lumbosacral Joint with Nonautologous Tissue Substitute, Posterior Approach, Anterior Column, Percutaneous Approach

HAC When reported with secondary diagnosis code T84.60XA, T84.610A, T84.611A, T84.612A, T84.613A, T84.614A, T84.615A, T84.619A, T84.63XA, T84.69XA, T84.7XXA

0SG33Z0 Fusion of Lumbosacral Joint, Anterior Approach, Anterior Column, Percutaneous Approach

HAC When reported with secondary diagnosis code T84.60XA, T84.610A, T84.611A, T84.612A, T84.613A, T84.614A, T84.615A, T84.619A, T84.63XA, T84.69XA, T84.7XXA

0SG33Z1 Fusion of Lumbosacral Joint, Posterior Approach, Posterior Column, Percutaneous Approach

HAC When reported with secondary diagnosis code T84.60XA, T84.610A, T84.611A, T84.612A, T84.613A, T84.614A, T84.615A, T84.619A, T84.63XA, T84.69XA, T84.7XXA

0SG33ZJ Fusion of Lumbosacral Joint, Posterior Approach, Anterior Column, Percutaneous Approach

HAC When reported with secondary diagnosis code T84.60XA, T84.610A, T84.611A, T84.612A, T84.613A, T84.614A, T84.615A, T84.619A, T84.63XA, T84.69XA, T84.7XXA

0SG3470 Fusion of Lumbosacral Joint with Autologous Tissue Substitute, Anterior Approach, Anterior Column, Percutaneous Endoscopic Approach

HAC When reported with secondary diagnosis code T84.60XA, T84.610A, T84.611A, T84.612A, T84.613A, T84.614A, T84.615A, T84.619A, T84.63XA, T84.69XA, T84.7XXA

0SG3471 Fusion of Lumbosacral Joint with Autologous Tissue Substitute, Posterior Approach, Posterior Column, Percutaneous Endoscopic Approach

HAC When reported with secondary diagnosis code T84.60XA, T84.610A, T84.611A, T84.612A, T84.613A, T84.614A, T84.615A, T84.619A, T84.63XA, T84.69XA, T84.7XXA

0SG347J Fusion of Lumbosacral Joint with Autologous Tissue Substitute, Posterior Approach, Anterior Column, Percutaneous Endoscopic Approach

HAC When reported with secondary diagnosis code T84.60XA, T84.610A, T84.611A, T84.612A, T84.613A, T84.614A, T84.615A, T84.619A, T84.63XA, T84.69XA, T84.7XXA

0SG34A0 Fusion of Lumbosacral Joint with Interbody Fusion Device, Anterior Approach, Anterior Column, Percutaneous Endoscopic Approach

HAC When reported with secondary diagnosis code T84.60XA, T84.610A, T84.611A, T84.612A, T84.613A, T84.614A, T84.615A, T84.619A, T84.63XA, T84.69XA, T84.7XXA

0SG34A1 Fusion of Lumbosacral Joint with Interbody Fusion Device, Posterior Approach, Posterior Column, Percutaneous Endoscopic Approach

HAC When reported with secondary diagnosis code T84.60XA, T84.610A, T84.611A, T84.612A, T84.613A, T84.614A, T84.615A, T84.619A, T84.63XA, T84.69XA, T84.7XXA

0SG34AJ Fusion of Lumbosacral Joint with Interbody Fusion Device, Posterior Approach, Anterior Column, Percutaneous Endoscopic Approach

HAC When reported with secondary diagnosis code T84.60XA, T84.610A, T84.611A, T84.612A, T84.613A, T84.614A, T84.615A, T84.619A, T84.63XA, T84.69XA, T84.7XXA

0SG34J0 Fusion of Lumbosacral Joint with Synthetic Substitute, Anterior Approach, Anterior Column, Percutaneous Endoscopic Approach

Note Continued

0SG34J0 Continued Note

HAC When reported with secondary diagnosis code T84.60XA, T84.610A, T84.611A, T84.612A, T84.613A, T84.614A, T84.615A, T84.619A, T84.63XA, T84.69XA, T84.7XXA

0SG34J1 Fusion of Lumbosacral Joint with Synthetic Substitute, Posterior Approach, Posterior Column, Percutaneous Endoscopic Approach

HAC When reported with secondary diagnosis code T84.60XA, T84.610A, T84.611A, T84.612A, T84.613A, T84.614A, T84.615A, T84.619A, T84.63XA, T84.69XA, T84.7XXA

0SG34JJ Fusion of Lumbosacral Joint with Synthetic Substitute, Posterior Approach, Anterior Column, Percutaneous Endoscopic Approach

HAC When reported with secondary diagnosis code T84.60XA, T84.610A, T84.611A, T84.612A, T84.613A, T84.614A, T84.615A, T84.619A, T84.63XA, T84.69XA, T84.7XXA

0SG34K0 Fusion of Lumbosacral Joint with Nonautologous Tissue Substitute, Anterior Approach, Anterior Column, Percutaneous Endoscopic Approach

HAC When reported with secondary diagnosis code T84.60XA, T84.610A, T84.611A, T84.612A, T84.613A, T84.614A, T84.615A, T84.619A, T84.63XA, T84.69XA, T84.7XXA

0SG34K1 Fusion of Lumbosacral Joint with Nonautologous Tissue Substitute, Posterior Approach, Posterior Column, Percutaneous Endoscopic Approach

HAC When reported with secondary diagnosis code T84.60XA, T84.610A, T84.611A, T84.612A, T84.613A, T84.614A, T84.615A, T84.619A, T84.63XA, T84.69XA, T84.7XXA

0SG34KJ Fusion of Lumbosacral Joint with Nonautologous Tissue Substitute, Posterior Approach, Anterior Column, Percutaneous Endoscopic Approach

HAC When reported with secondary diagnosis code T84.60XA, T84.610A, T84.611A, T84.612A, T84.613A, T84.614A, T84.615A, T84.619A, T84.63XA, T84.69XA, T84.7XXA

0SG34Z0 Fusion of Lumbosacral Joint, Anterior Approach, Anterior Column, Percutaneous Endoscopic Approach

HAC When reported with secondary diagnosis code T84.60XA, T84.610A, T84.611A, T84.612A, T84.613A, T84.614A, T84.615A, T84.619A, T84.63XA, T84.69XA, T84.7XXA

0SG34Z1 Fusion of Lumbosacral Joint, Posterior Approach, Posterior Column, Percutaneous Endoscopic Approach

HAC When reported with secondary diagnosis code T84.60XA, T84.610A, T84.611A, T84.612A, T84.613A, T84.614A, T84.615A, T84.619A, T84.63XA, T84.69XA, T84.7XXA

0SG34ZJ Fusion of Lumbosacral Joint, Posterior Approach, Anterior Column, Percutaneous Endoscopic Approach

HAC When reported with secondary diagnosis code T84.60XA, T84.610A, T84.611A, T84.612A, T84.613A, T84.614A, T84.615A, T84.619A, T84.63XA, T84.69XA, T84.7XXA

0SG504Z Fusion of Sacrococcygeal Joint with Internal Fixation Device, Open Approach

0SG507Z Fusion of Sacrococcygeal Joint with Autologous Tissue Substitute, Open Approach

0SG50JZ Fusion of Sacrococcygeal Joint with Synthetic Substitute, Open Approach

0SG50KZ Fusion of Sacrococcygeal Joint with Nonautologous Tissue Substitute, Open Approach

0SG50ZZ Fusion of Sacrococcygeal Joint, Open Approach

0SG534Z Fusion of Sacrococcygeal Joint with Internal Fixation Device, Percutaneous Approach

0SG537Z Fusion of Sacrococcygeal Joint with Autologous Tissue Substitute, Percutaneous Approach

0SG53JZ Fusion of Sacrococcygeal Joint with Synthetic Substitute, Percutaneous Approach

0SG53KZ Fusion of Sacrococcygeal Joint with Nonautologous Tissue Substitute, Percutaneous Approach

0SG53ZZ Fusion of Sacrococcygeal Joint, Percutaneous Approach

0SG544Z Fusion of Sacrococcygeal Joint with Internal Fixation Device, Percutaneous Endoscopic Approach

0SG547Z Fusion of Sacrococcygeal Joint with Autologous Tissue Substitute, Percutaneous Endoscopic Approach

0SG54JZ Fusion of Sacrococcygeal Joint with Synthetic Substitute, Percutaneous Endoscopic Approach

0SG54KZ Fusion of Sacrococcygeal Joint with Nonautologous Tissue Substitute, Percutaneous Endoscopic Approach

0SG54ZZ Fusion of Sacrococcygeal Joint, Percutaneous Endoscopic Approach

0SG604Z Fusion of Coccygeal Joint with Internal Fixation Device, Open Approach

0SG607Z Fusion of Coccygeal Joint with Autologous Tissue Substitute, Open Approach

0SG60JZ Fusion of Coccygeal Joint with Synthetic Substitute, Open Approach

0SG60KZ Fusion of Coccygeal Joint with Nonautologous Tissue Substitute, Open Approach

0SG60ZZ Fusion of Coccygeal Joint, Open Approach

0SG634Z Fusion of Coccygeal Joint with Internal Fixation Device, Percutaneous Approach

0SG637Z Fusion of Coccygeal Joint with Autologous Tissue Substitute, Percutaneous Approach

0SG63JZ Fusion of Coccygeal Joint with Synthetic Substitute, Percutaneous Approach

0SG63KZ Fusion of Coccygeal Joint with Nonautologous Tissue Substitute, Percutaneous Approach

0SG63ZZ Fusion of Coccygeal Joint, Percutaneous Approach

0SG644Z Fusion of Coccygeal Joint with Internal Fixation Device, Percutaneous Endoscopic Approach

0SG647Z Fusion of Coccygeal Joint with Autologous Tissue Substitute, Percutaneous Endoscopic Approach

0SG64JZ Fusion of Coccygeal Joint with Synthetic Substitute, Percutaneous Endoscopic Approach

0SG64KZ Fusion of Coccygeal Joint with Nonautologous Tissue Substitute, Percutaneous Endoscopic Approach

0SG64ZZ Fusion of Coccygeal Joint, Percutaneous Endoscopic Approach

0SG704Z Fusion of Right Sacroiliac Joint with Internal Fixation Device, Open Approach

HAC When reported with secondary diagnosis code T84.60XA, T84.610A, T84.611A, T84.612A, T84.613A, T84.614A, T84.615A, T84.619A, T84.63XA, T84.69XA, T84.7XXA

0SG707Z Fusion of Right Sacroiliac Joint with Autologous Tissue Substitute, Open Approach

HAC When reported with secondary diagnosis code T84.60XA, T84.610A, T84.611A, T84.612A, T84.613A, T84.614A, T84.615A, T84.619A, T84.63XA, T84.69XA, T84.7XXA

0SG70JZ Fusion of Right Sacroiliac Joint with Synthetic Substitute, Open Approach

HAC When reported with secondary diagnosis code T84.60XA, T84.610A, T84.611A, T84.612A, T84.613A, T84.614A, T84.615A, T84.619A, T84.63XA, T84.69XA, T84.7XXA

0SG70KZ Fusion of Right Sacroiliac Joint with Nonautologous Tissue Substitute, Open Approach

HAC When reported with secondary diagnosis code T84.60XA, T84.610A, T84.611A, T84.612A, T84.613A, T84.614A, T84.615A, T84.619A, T84.63XA, T84.69XA, T84.7XXA

0SG70ZZ Fusion of Right Sacroiliac Joint, Open Approach

HAC When reported with secondary diagnosis code T84.60XA, T84.610A, T84.611A, T84.612A, T84.613A, T84.614A, T84.615A, T84.619A, T84.63XA, T84.69XA, T84.7XXA

0SG734Z Fusion of Right Sacroiliac Joint with Internal Fixation Device, Percutaneous Approach

HAC When reported with secondary diagnosis code T84.60XA, T84.610A, T84.611A, T84.612A, T84.613A, T84.614A, T84.615A, T84.619A, T84.63XA, T84.69XA, T84.7XXA

0SG737Z Fusion of Right Sacroiliac Joint with Autologous Tissue Substitute, Percutaneous Approach

HAC When reported with secondary diagnosis code T84.60XA, T84.610A, T84.611A, T84.612A, T84.613A, T84.614A, T84.615A, T84.619A, T84.63XA, T84.69XA, T84.7XXA

0SG73JZ Fusion of Right Sacroiliac Joint with Synthetic Substitute, Percutaneous Approach

HAC When reported with secondary diagnosis code T84.60XA, T84.610A, T84.611A, T84.612A, T84.613A, T84.614A, T84.615A, T84.619A, T84.63XA, T84.69XA, T84.7XXA

0SG73KZ Fusion of Right Sacroiliac Joint with Nonautologous Tissue Substitute, Percutaneous Approach

HAC When reported with secondary diagnosis code T84.60XA, T84.610A, T84.611A, T84.612A, T84.613A, T84.614A, T84.615A, T84.619A, T84.63XA, T84.69XA, T84.7XXA

0SG73ZZ Fusion of Right Sacroiliac Joint, Percutaneous Approach

HAC When reported with secondary diagnosis code T84.60XA, T84.610A, T84.611A, T84.612A, T84.613A, T84.614A, T84.615A, T84.619A, T84.63XA, T84.69XA, T84.7XXA

0SG744Z Fusion of Right Sacroiliac Joint with Internal Fixation Device, Percutaneous Endoscopic Approach

Note Continued

0SG744Z Continued Note

HAC When reported with secondary diagnosis code T84.60XA, T84.610A, T84.611A, T84.612A, T84.613A, T84.614A, T84.615A, T84.619A, T84.63XA, T84.69XA, T84.7XXA

0SG747Z Fusion of Right Sacroiliac Joint with Autologous Tissue Substitute, Percutaneous Endoscopic Approach

HAC When reported with secondary diagnosis code T84.60XA, T84.610A, T84.611A, T84.612A, T84.613A, T84.614A, T84.615A, T84.619A, T84.63XA, T84.69XA, T84.7XXA

0SG74JZ Fusion of Right Sacroiliac Joint with Synthetic Substitute, Percutaneous Endoscopic Approach

HAC When reported with secondary diagnosis code T84.60XA, T84.610A, T84.611A, T84.612A, T84.613A, T84.614A, T84.615A, T84.619A, T84.63XA, T84.69XA, T84.7XXA

0SG74KZ Fusion of Right Sacroiliac Joint with Nonautologous Tissue Substitute, Percutaneous Endoscopic Approach

HAC When reported with secondary diagnosis code T84.60XA, T84.610A, T84.611A, T84.612A, T84.613A, T84.614A, T84.615A, T84.619A, T84.63XA, T84.69XA, T84.7XXA

0SG74ZZ Fusion of Right Sacroiliac Joint, Percutaneous Endoscopic Approach

HAC When reported with secondary diagnosis code T84.60XA, T84.610A, T84.611A, T84.612A, T84.613A, T84.614A, T84.615A, T84.619A, T84.63XA, T84.69XA, T84.7XXA

0SG804Z Fusion of Left Sacroiliac Joint with Internal Fixation Device, Open Approach

HAC When reported with secondary diagnosis code T84.60XA, T84.610A, T84.611A, T84.612A, T84.613A, T84.614A, T84.615A, T84.619A, T84.63XA, T84.69XA, T84.7XXA

0SG807Z Fusion of Left Sacroiliac Joint with Autologous Tissue Substitute, Open Approach

HAC When reported with secondary diagnosis code T84.60XA, T84.610A, T84.611A, T84.612A, T84.613A, T84.614A, T84.615A, T84.619A, T84.63XA, T84.69XA, T84.7XXA

0SG80JZ Fusion of Left Sacroiliac Joint with Synthetic Substitute, Open Approach

HAC When reported with secondary diagnosis code T84.60XA, T84.610A, T84.611A, T84.612A, T84.613A, T84.614A, T84.615A, T84.619A, T84.63XA, T84.69XA, T84.7XXA

0SG80KZ Fusion of Left Sacroiliac Joint with Nonautologous Tissue Substitute, Open Approach

HAC When reported with secondary diagnosis code T84.60XA, T84.610A, T84.611A, T84.612A, T84.613A, T84.614A, T84.615A, T84.619A, T84.63XA, T84.69XA, T84.7XXA

0SG80ZZ Fusion of Left Sacroiliac Joint, Open Approach

HAC When reported with secondary diagnosis code T84.60XA, T84.610A, T84.611A, T84.612A, T84.613A, T84.614A, T84.615A, T84.619A, T84.63XA, T84.69XA, T84.7XXA

0SG834Z Fusion of Left Sacroiliac Joint with Internal Fixation Device, Percutaneous Approach

HAC When reported with secondary diagnosis code T84.60XA, T84.610A, T84.611A, T84.612A, T84.613A, T84.614A, T84.615A, T84.619A, T84.63XA, T84.69XA, T84.7XXA

0SG837Z Fusion of Left Sacroiliac Joint with Autologous Tissue Substitute, Percutaneous Approach

HAC When reported with secondary diagnosis code T84.60XA, T84.610A, T84.611A, T84.612A, T84.613A, T84.614A, T84.615A, T84.619A, T84.63XA, T84.69XA, T84.7XXA

0SG83JZ Fusion of Left Sacroiliac Joint with Synthetic Substitute, Percutaneous Approach

HAC When reported with secondary diagnosis code T84.60XA, T84.610A, T84.611A, T84.612A, T84.613A, T84.614A, T84.615A, T84.619A, T84.63XA, T84.69XA, T84.7XXA

0SG83KZ Fusion of Left Sacroiliac Joint with Nonautologous Tissue Substitute, Percutaneous Approach

HAC When reported with secondary diagnosis code T84.60XA, T84.610A, T84.611A, T84.612A, T84.613A, T84.614A, T84.615A, T84.619A, T84.63XA, T84.69XA, T84.7XXA

0SG83ZZ Fusion of Left Sacroiliac Joint, Percutaneous Approach

HAC When reported with secondary diagnosis code T84.60XA, T84.610A, T84.611A, T84.612A, T84.613A, T84.614A, T84.615A, T84.619A, T84.63XA, T84.69XA, T84.7XXA

0SG844Z Fusion of Left Sacroiliac Joint with Internal Fixation Device, Percutaneous Endoscopic Approach

HAC When reported with secondary diagnosis code T84.60XA, T84.610A, T84.611A, T84.612A, T84.613A, T84.614A, T84.615A, T84.619A, T84.63XA, T84.69XA, T84.7XXA

0SG847Z Fusion of Left Sacroiliac Joint with Autologous Tissue Substitute, Percutaneous Endoscopic Approach

HAC When reported with secondary diagnosis code T84.60XA, T84.610A, T84.611A, T84.612A, T84.613A, T84.614A, T84.615A, T84.619A, T84.63XA, T84.69XA, T84.7XXA

0SG84JZ Fusion of Left Sacroiliac Joint with Synthetic Substitute, Percutaneous Endoscopic Approach

HAC When reported with secondary diagnosis code T84.60XA, T84.610A, T84.611A, T84.612A, T84.613A, T84.614A, T84.615A, T84.619A, T84.63XA, T84.69XA, T84.7XXA

0SG84KZ Fusion of Left Sacroiliac Joint with Nonautologous Tissue Substitute, Percutaneous Endoscopic Approach

HAC When reported with secondary diagnosis code T84.60XA, T84.610A, T84.611A, T84.612A, T84.613A, T84.614A, T84.615A, T84.619A, T84.63XA, T84.69XA, T84.7XXA

0SG84ZZ Fusion of Left Sacroiliac Joint, Percutaneous Endoscopic Approach

HAC When reported with secondary diagnosis code T84.60XA, T84.610A, T84.611A, T84.612A, T84.613A, T84.614A, T84.615A, T84.619A, T84.63XA, T84.69XA, T84.7XXA

0SG904Z Fusion of Right Hip Joint with Internal Fixation Device, Open Approach

0SG905Z Fusion of Right Hip Joint with External Fixation Device, Open Approach

0SG907Z Fusion of Right Hip Joint with Autologous Tissue Substitute, Open Approach

0SG90JZ Fusion of Right Hip Joint with Synthetic Substitute, Open Approach

0SG90KZ Fusion of Right Hip Joint with Nonautologous Tissue Substitute, Open Approach

0SG90ZZ Fusion of Right Hip Joint, Open Approach

0SG934Z Fusion of Right Hip Joint with Internal Fixation Device, Percutaneous Approach

0SG935Z Fusion of Right Hip Joint with External Fixation Device, Percutaneous Approach

0SG937Z Fusion of Right Hip Joint with Autologous Tissue Substitute, Percutaneous Approach

0SG93JZ Fusion of Right Hip Joint with Synthetic Substitute, Percutaneous Approach

0SG93KZ Fusion of Right Hip Joint with Nonautologous Tissue Substitute, Percutaneous Approach

0SG93ZZ Fusion of Right Hip Joint, Percutaneous Approach

0SG944Z Fusion of Right Hip Joint with Internal Fixation Device, Percutaneous Endoscopic Approach

0SG945Z Fusion of Right Hip Joint with External Fixation Device, Percutaneous Endoscopic Approach

0SG947Z Fusion of Right Hip Joint with Autologous Tissue Substitute, Percutaneous Endoscopic Approach

0SG94JZ Fusion of Right Hip Joint with Synthetic Substitute, Percutaneous Endoscopic Approach

0SG94KZ Fusion of Right Hip Joint with Nonautologous Tissue Substitute, Percutaneous Endoscopic Approach

0SG94ZZ Fusion of Right Hip Joint, Percutaneous Endoscopic Approach

0SGB04Z Fusion of Left Hip Joint with Internal Fixation Device, Open Approach

0SGB05Z Fusion of Left Hip Joint with External Fixation Device, Open Approach

0SGB07Z Fusion of Left Hip Joint with Autologous Tissue Substitute, Open Approach

0SGB0JZ Fusion of Left Hip Joint with Synthetic Substitute, Open Approach

0SGB0KZ Fusion of Left Hip Joint with Nonautologous Tissue Substitute, Open Approach

0SGB0ZZ Fusion of Left Hip Joint, Open Approach

0SGB34Z Fusion of Left Hip Joint with Internal Fixation Device, Percutaneous Approach

0SGB35Z Fusion of Left Hip Joint with External Fixation Device, Percutaneous Approach

0SGB37Z Fusion of Left Hip Joint with Autologous Tissue Substitute, Percutaneous Approach

0SGB3JZ Fusion of Left Hip Joint with Synthetic Substitute, Percutaneous Approach

0SGB3KZ Fusion of Left Hip Joint with Nonautologous Tissue Substitute, Percutaneous Approach

0SGB3ZZ Fusion of Left Hip Joint, Percutaneous Approach

0SGB44Z Fusion of Left Hip Joint with Internal Fixation Device, Percutaneous Endoscopic Approach

0SGB45Z Fusion of Left Hip Joint with External Fixation Device, Percutaneous Endoscopic Approach

0SGB47Z Fusion of Left Hip Joint with Autologous Tissue Substitute, Percutaneous Endoscopic Approach

0SGB4JZ Fusion of Left Hip Joint with Synthetic Substitute, Percutaneous Endoscopic Approach
0SGB4KZ Fusion of Left Hip Joint with Nonautologous Tissue Substitute, Percutaneous Endoscopic Approach
0SGB4ZZ Fusion of Left Hip Joint, Percutaneous Endoscopic Approach
0SGC04Z Fusion of Right Knee Joint with Internal Fixation Device, Open Approach
0SGC05Z Fusion of Right Knee Joint with External Fixation Device, Open Approach
0SGC07Z Fusion of Right Knee Joint with Autologous Tissue Substitute, Open Approach
0SGC0JZ Fusion of Right Knee Joint with Synthetic Substitute, Open Approach
0SGC0KZ Fusion of Right Knee Joint with Nonautologous Tissue Substitute, Open Approach
0SGC0ZZ Fusion of Right Knee Joint, Open Approach
0SGC34Z Fusion of Right Knee Joint with Internal Fixation Device, Percutaneous Approach
0SGC35Z Fusion of Right Knee Joint with External Fixation Device, Percutaneous Approach
0SGC37Z Fusion of Right Knee Joint with Autologous Tissue Substitute, Percutaneous Approach
0SGC3JZ Fusion of Right Knee Joint with Synthetic Substitute, Percutaneous Approach
0SGC3KZ Fusion of Right Knee Joint with Nonautologous Tissue Substitute, Percutaneous Approach
0SGC3ZZ Fusion of Right Knee Joint, Percutaneous Approach
0SGC44Z Fusion of Right Knee Joint with Internal Fixation Device, Percutaneous Endoscopic Approach
0SGC45Z Fusion of Right Knee Joint with External Fixation Device, Percutaneous Endoscopic Approach
0SGC47Z Fusion of Right Knee Joint with Autologous Tissue Substitute, Percutaneous Endoscopic Approach
0SGC4JZ Fusion of Right Knee Joint with Synthetic Substitute, Percutaneous Endoscopic Approach
0SGC4KZ Fusion of Right Knee Joint with Nonautologous Tissue Substitute, Percutaneous Endoscopic Approach
0SGC4ZZ Fusion of Right Knee Joint, Percutaneous Endoscopic Approach
0SGD04Z Fusion of Left Knee Joint with Internal Fixation Device, Open Approach
0SGD05Z Fusion of Left Knee Joint with External Fixation Device, Open Approach
0SGD07Z Fusion of Left Knee Joint with Autologous Tissue Substitute, Open Approach
0SGD0JZ Fusion of Left Knee Joint with Synthetic Substitute, Open Approach
0SGD0KZ Fusion of Left Knee Joint with Nonautologous Tissue Substitute, Open Approach
0SGD0ZZ Fusion of Left Knee Joint, Open Approach
0SGD34Z Fusion of Left Knee Joint with Internal Fixation Device, Percutaneous Approach
0SGD35Z Fusion of Left Knee Joint with External Fixation Device, Percutaneous Approach
0SGD37Z Fusion of Left Knee Joint with Autologous Tissue Substitute, Percutaneous Approach
0SGD3JZ Fusion of Left Knee Joint with Synthetic Substitute, Percutaneous Approach
0SGD3KZ Fusion of Left Knee Joint with Nonautologous Tissue Substitute, Percutaneous Approach
0SGD3ZZ Fusion of Left Knee Joint, Percutaneous Approach
0SGD44Z Fusion of Left Knee Joint with Internal Fixation Device, Percutaneous Endoscopic Approach
0SGD45Z Fusion of Left Knee Joint with External Fixation Device, Percutaneous Endoscopic Approach
0SGD47Z Fusion of Left Knee Joint with Autologous Tissue Substitute, Percutaneous Endoscopic Approach
0SGD4JZ Fusion of Left Knee Joint with Synthetic Substitute, Percutaneous Endoscopic Approach
0SGD4KZ Fusion of Left Knee Joint with Nonautologous Tissue Substitute, Percutaneous Endoscopic Approach
0SGD4ZZ Fusion of Left Knee Joint, Percutaneous Endoscopic Approach
0SGF04Z Fusion of Right Ankle Joint with Internal Fixation Device, Open Approach
0SGF05Z Fusion of Right Ankle Joint with External Fixation Device, Open Approach
0SGF07Z Fusion of Right Ankle Joint with Autologous Tissue Substitute, Open Approach
0SGF0JZ Fusion of Right Ankle Joint with Synthetic Substitute, Open Approach
0SGF0KZ Fusion of Right Ankle Joint with Nonautologous Tissue Substitute, Open Approach
0SGF0ZZ Fusion of Right Ankle Joint, Open Approach
0SGF34Z Fusion of Right Ankle Joint with Internal Fixation Device, Percutaneous Approach
0SGF35Z Fusion of Right Ankle Joint with External Fixation Device, Percutaneous Approach
0SGF37Z Fusion of Right Ankle Joint with Autologous Tissue Substitute, Percutaneous Approach
0SGF3JZ Fusion of Right Ankle Joint with Synthetic Substitute, Percutaneous Approach
0SGF3KZ Fusion of Right Ankle Joint with Nonautologous Tissue Substitute, Percutaneous Approach
0SGF3ZZ Fusion of Right Ankle Joint, Percutaneous Approach
0SGF44Z Fusion of Right Ankle Joint with Internal Fixation Device, Percutaneous Endoscopic Approach
0SGF45Z Fusion of Right Ankle Joint with External Fixation Device, Percutaneous Endoscopic Approach
0SGF47Z Fusion of Right Ankle Joint with Autologous Tissue Substitute, Percutaneous Endoscopic Approach
0SGF4JZ Fusion of Right Ankle Joint with Synthetic Substitute, Percutaneous Endoscopic Approach
0SGF4KZ Fusion of Right Ankle Joint with Nonautologous Tissue Substitute, Percutaneous Endoscopic Approach
0SGF4ZZ Fusion of Right Ankle Joint, Percutaneous Endoscopic Approach
0SGG04Z Fusion of Left Ankle Joint with Internal Fixation Device, Open Approach
AHA CC: 2Q, 2013, 39-40
0SGG05Z Fusion of Left Ankle Joint with External Fixation Device, Open Approach
0SGG07Z Fusion of Left Ankle Joint with Autologous Tissue Substitute, Open Approach
AHA CC: 2Q, 2013, 39-40
0SGG0JZ Fusion of Left Ankle Joint with Synthetic Substitute, Open Approach
0SGG0KZ Fusion of Left Ankle Joint with Nonautologous Tissue Substitute, Open Approach
0SGG0ZZ Fusion of Left Ankle Joint, Open Approach
0SGG34Z Fusion of Left Ankle Joint with Internal Fixation Device, Percutaneous Approach
0SGG35Z Fusion of Left Ankle Joint with External Fixation Device, Percutaneous Approach
0SGG37Z Fusion of Left Ankle Joint with Autologous Tissue Substitute, Percutaneous Approach
0SGG3JZ Fusion of Left Ankle Joint with Synthetic Substitute, Percutaneous Approach
0SGG3KZ Fusion of Left Ankle Joint with Nonautologous Tissue Substitute, Percutaneous Approach
0SGG3ZZ Fusion of Left Ankle Joint, Percutaneous Approach
0SGG44Z Fusion of Left Ankle Joint with Internal Fixation Device, Percutaneous Endoscopic Approach
0SGG45Z Fusion of Left Ankle Joint with External Fixation Device, Percutaneous Endoscopic Approach
0SGG47Z Fusion of Left Ankle Joint with Autologous Tissue Substitute, Percutaneous Endoscopic Approach
0SGG4JZ Fusion of Left Ankle Joint with Synthetic Substitute, Percutaneous Endoscopic Approach
0SGG4KZ Fusion of Left Ankle Joint with Nonautologous Tissue Substitute, Percutaneous Endoscopic Approach
0SGG4ZZ Fusion of Left Ankle Joint, Percutaneous Endoscopic Approach
0SGH04Z Fusion of Right Tarsal Joint with Internal Fixation Device, Open Approach
0SGH05Z Fusion of Right Tarsal Joint with External Fixation Device, Open Approach
0SGH07Z Fusion of Right Tarsal Joint with Autologous Tissue Substitute, Open Approach
0SGH0JZ Fusion of Right Tarsal Joint with Synthetic Substitute, Open Approach
0SGH0KZ Fusion of Right Tarsal Joint with Nonautologous Tissue Substitute, Open Approach
0SGH0ZZ Fusion of Right Tarsal Joint, Open Approach
0SGH34Z Fusion of Right Tarsal Joint with Internal Fixation Device, Percutaneous Approach
0SGH35Z Fusion of Right Tarsal Joint with External Fixation Device, Percutaneous Approach
0SGH37Z Fusion of Right Tarsal Joint with Autologous Tissue Substitute, Percutaneous Approach
0SGH3JZ Fusion of Right Tarsal Joint with Synthetic Substitute, Percutaneous Approach
0SGH3KZ Fusion of Right Tarsal Joint with Nonautologous Tissue Substitute, Percutaneous Approach
0SGH3ZZ Fusion of Right Tarsal Joint, Percutaneous Approach
0SGH44Z Fusion of Right Tarsal Joint with Internal Fixation Device, Percutaneous Endoscopic Approach
0SGH45Z Fusion of Right Tarsal Joint with External Fixation Device, Percutaneous Endoscopic Approach
0SGH47Z Fusion of Right Tarsal Joint with Autologous Tissue Substitute, Percutaneous Endoscopic Approach
0SGH4JZ Fusion of Right Tarsal Joint with Synthetic Substitute, Percutaneous Endoscopic Approach
0SGH4KZ Fusion of Right Tarsal Joint with Nonautologous Tissue Substitute, Percutaneous Endoscopic Approach
0SGH4ZZ Fusion of Right Tarsal Joint, Percutaneous Endoscopic Approach

0SGJ04Z Fusion of Left Tarsal Joint with Internal Fixation Device, Open Approach
0SGJ05Z Fusion of Left Tarsal Joint with External Fixation Device, Open Approach
0SGJ07Z Fusion of Left Tarsal Joint with Autologous Tissue Substitute, Open Approach
0SGJ0JZ Fusion of Left Tarsal Joint with Synthetic Substitute, Open Approach
0SGJ0KZ Fusion of Left Tarsal Joint with Nonautologous Tissue Substitute, Open Approach
0SGJ0ZZ Fusion of Left Tarsal Joint, Open Approach
0SGJ34Z Fusion of Left Tarsal Joint with Internal Fixation Device, Percutaneous Approach
0SGJ35Z Fusion of Left Tarsal Joint with External Fixation Device, Percutaneous Approach
0SGJ37Z Fusion of Left Tarsal Joint with Autologous Tissue Substitute, Percutaneous Approach
0SGJ3JZ Fusion of Left Tarsal Joint with Synthetic Substitute, Percutaneous Approach
0SGJ3KZ Fusion of Left Tarsal Joint with Nonautologous Tissue Substitute, Percutaneous Approach
0SGJ3ZZ Fusion of Left Tarsal Joint, Percutaneous Approach
0SGJ44Z Fusion of Left Tarsal Joint with Internal Fixation Device, Percutaneous Endoscopic Approach
0SGJ45Z Fusion of Left Tarsal Joint with External Fixation Device, Percutaneous Endoscopic Approach
0SGJ47Z Fusion of Left Tarsal Joint with Autologous Tissue Substitute, Percutaneous Endoscopic Approach
0SGJ4JZ Fusion of Left Tarsal Joint with Synthetic Substitute, Percutaneous Endoscopic Approach
0SGJ4KZ Fusion of Left Tarsal Joint with Nonautologous Tissue Substitute, Percutaneous Endoscopic Approach
0SGJ4ZZ Fusion of Left Tarsal Joint, Percutaneous Endoscopic Approach
0SGK04Z Fusion of Right Metatarsal-Tarsal Joint with Internal Fixation Device, Open Approach
0SGK05Z Fusion of Right Metatarsal-Tarsal Joint with External Fixation Device, Open Approach
0SGK07Z Fusion of Right Metatarsal-Tarsal Joint with Autologous Tissue Substitute, Open Approach
0SGK0JZ Fusion of Right Metatarsal-Tarsal Joint with Synthetic Substitute, Open Approach
0SGK0KZ Fusion of Right Metatarsal-Tarsal Joint with Nonautologous Tissue Substitute, Open Approach
0SGK0ZZ Fusion of Right Metatarsal-Tarsal Joint, Open Approach
0SGK34Z Fusion of Right Metatarsal-Tarsal Joint with Internal Fixation Device, Percutaneous Approach
0SGK35Z Fusion of Right Metatarsal-Tarsal Joint with External Fixation Device, Percutaneous Approach
0SGK37Z Fusion of Right Metatarsal-Tarsal Joint with Autologous Tissue Substitute, Percutaneous Approach
0SGK3JZ Fusion of Right Metatarsal-Tarsal Joint with Synthetic Substitute, Percutaneous Approach
0SGK3KZ Fusion of Right Metatarsal-Tarsal Joint with Nonautologous Tissue Substitute, Percutaneous Approach
0SGK3ZZ Fusion of Right Metatarsal-Tarsal Joint, Percutaneous Approach
0SGK44Z Fusion of Right Metatarsal-Tarsal Joint with Internal Fixation Device, Percutaneous Endoscopic Approach
0SGK45Z Fusion of Right Metatarsal-Tarsal Joint with External Fixation Device, Percutaneous Endoscopic Approach
0SGK47Z Fusion of Right Metatarsal-Tarsal Joint with Autologous Tissue Substitute, Percutaneous Endoscopic Approach
0SGK4JZ Fusion of Right Metatarsal-Tarsal Joint with Synthetic Substitute, Percutaneous Endoscopic Approach
0SGK4KZ Fusion of Right Metatarsal-Tarsal Joint with Nonautologous Tissue Substitute, Percutaneous Endoscopic Approach
0SGK4ZZ Fusion of Right Metatarsal-Tarsal Joint, Percutaneous Endoscopic Approach
0SGL04Z Fusion of Left Metatarsal-Tarsal Joint with Internal Fixation Device, Open Approach
0SGL05Z Fusion of Left Metatarsal-Tarsal Joint with External Fixation Device, Open Approach
0SGL07Z Fusion of Left Metatarsal-Tarsal Joint with Autologous Tissue Substitute, Open Approach
0SGL0JZ Fusion of Left Metatarsal-Tarsal Joint with Synthetic Substitute, Open Approach
0SGL0KZ Fusion of Left Metatarsal-Tarsal Joint with Nonautologous Tissue Substitute, Open Approach
0SGL0ZZ Fusion of Left Metatarsal-Tarsal Joint, Open Approach
0SGL34Z Fusion of Left Metatarsal-Tarsal Joint with Internal Fixation Device, Percutaneous Approach
0SGL35Z Fusion of Left Metatarsal-Tarsal Joint with External Fixation Device, Percutaneous Approach
0SGL37Z Fusion of Left Metatarsal-Tarsal Joint with Autologous Tissue Substitute, Percutaneous Approach
0SGL3JZ Fusion of Left Metatarsal-Tarsal Joint with Synthetic Substitute, Percutaneous Approach
0SGL3KZ Fusion of Left Metatarsal-Tarsal Joint with Nonautologous Tissue Substitute, Percutaneous Approach
0SGL3ZZ Fusion of Left Metatarsal-Tarsal Joint, Percutaneous Approach
0SGL44Z Fusion of Left Metatarsal-Tarsal Joint with Internal Fixation Device, Percutaneous Endoscopic Approach
0SGL45Z Fusion of Left Metatarsal-Tarsal Joint with External Fixation Device, Percutaneous Endoscopic Approach
0SGL47Z Fusion of Left Metatarsal-Tarsal Joint with Autologous Tissue Substitute, Percutaneous Endoscopic Approach
0SGL4JZ Fusion of Left Metatarsal-Tarsal Joint with Synthetic Substitute, Percutaneous Endoscopic Approach
0SGL4KZ Fusion of Left Metatarsal-Tarsal Joint with Nonautologous Tissue Substitute, Percutaneous Endoscopic Approach
0SGL4ZZ Fusion of Left Metatarsal-Tarsal Joint, Percutaneous Endoscopic Approach
0SGM04Z Fusion of Right Metatarsal-Phalangeal Joint with Internal Fixation Device, Open Approach
0SGM05Z Fusion of Right Metatarsal-Phalangeal Joint with External Fixation Device, Open Approach
0SGM07Z Fusion of Right Metatarsal-Phalangeal Joint with Autologous Tissue Substitute, Open Approach
0SGM0JZ Fusion of Right Metatarsal-Phalangeal Joint with Synthetic Substitute, Open Approach
0SGM0KZ Fusion of Right Metatarsal-Phalangeal Joint with Nonautologous Tissue Substitute, Open Approach
0SGM0ZZ Fusion of Right Metatarsal-Phalangeal Joint, Open Approach
0SGM34Z Fusion of Right Metatarsal-Phalangeal Joint with Internal Fixation Device, Percutaneous Approach
0SGM35Z Fusion of Right Metatarsal-Phalangeal Joint with External Fixation Device, Percutaneous Approach
0SGM37Z Fusion of Right Metatarsal-Phalangeal Joint with Autologous Tissue Substitute, Percutaneous Approach
0SGM3JZ Fusion of Right Metatarsal-Phalangeal Joint with Synthetic Substitute, Percutaneous Approach
0SGM3KZ Fusion of Right Metatarsal-Phalangeal Joint with Nonautologous Tissue Substitute, Percutaneous Approach
0SGM3ZZ Fusion of Right Metatarsal-Phalangeal Joint, Percutaneous Approach
0SGM44Z Fusion of Right Metatarsal-Phalangeal Joint with Internal Fixation Device, Percutaneous Endoscopic Approach
0SGM45Z Fusion of Right Metatarsal-Phalangeal Joint with External Fixation Device, Percutaneous Endoscopic Approach
0SGM47Z Fusion of Right Metatarsal-Phalangeal Joint with Autologous Tissue Substitute, Percutaneous Endoscopic Approach
0SGM4JZ Fusion of Right Metatarsal-Phalangeal Joint with Synthetic Substitute, Percutaneous Endoscopic Approach
0SGM4KZ Fusion of Right Metatarsal-Phalangeal Joint with Nonautologous Tissue Substitute, Percutaneous Endoscopic Approach
0SGM4ZZ Fusion of Right Metatarsal-Phalangeal Joint, Percutaneous Endoscopic Approach
0SGN04Z Fusion of Left Metatarsal-Phalangeal Joint with Internal Fixation Device, Open Approach
0SGN05Z Fusion of Left Metatarsal-Phalangeal Joint with External Fixation Device, Open Approach
0SGN07Z Fusion of Left Metatarsal-Phalangeal Joint with Autologous Tissue Substitute, Open Approach
0SGN0JZ Fusion of Left Metatarsal-Phalangeal Joint with Synthetic Substitute, Open Approach
0SGN0KZ Fusion of Left Metatarsal-Phalangeal Joint with Nonautologous Tissue Substitute, Open Approach
0SGN0ZZ Fusion of Left Metatarsal-Phalangeal Joint, Open Approach
0SGN34Z Fusion of Left Metatarsal-Phalangeal Joint with Internal Fixation Device, Percutaneous Approach
0SGN35Z Fusion of Left Metatarsal-Phalangeal Joint with External Fixation Device, Percutaneous Approach
0SGN37Z Fusion of Left Metatarsal-Phalangeal Joint with Autologous Tissue Substitute, Percutaneous Approach
0SGN3JZ Fusion of Left Metatarsal-Phalangeal Joint with Synthetic Substitute, Percutaneous Approach
0SGN3KZ Fusion of Left Metatarsal-Phalangeal Joint with Nonautologous Tissue Substitute, Percutaneous Approach
0SGN3ZZ Fusion of Left Metatarsal-Phalangeal Joint, Percutaneous Approach
0SGN44Z Fusion of Left Metatarsal-Phalangeal Joint with Internal Fixation Device, Percutaneous Endoscopic Approach

0SGN45Z Fusion of Left Metatarsal-Phalangeal Joint with External Fixation Device, Percutaneous Endoscopic Approach
0SGN47Z Fusion of Left Metatarsal-Phalangeal Joint with Autologous Tissue Substitute, Percutaneous Endoscopic Approach
0SGN4JZ Fusion of Left Metatarsal-Phalangeal Joint with Synthetic Substitute, Percutaneous Endoscopic Approach
0SGN4KZ Fusion of Left Metatarsal-Phalangeal Joint with Nonautologous Tissue Substitute, Percutaneous Endoscopic Approach
0SGN4ZZ Fusion of Left Metatarsal-Phalangeal Joint, Percutaneous Endoscopic Approach
0SGP04Z Fusion of Right Toe Phalangeal Joint with Internal Fixation Device, Open Approach
0SGP05Z Fusion of Right Toe Phalangeal Joint with External Fixation Device, Open Approach
0SGP07Z Fusion of Right Toe Phalangeal Joint with Autologous Tissue Substitute, Open Approach
0SGP0JZ Fusion of Right Toe Phalangeal Joint with Synthetic Substitute, Open Approach
0SGP0KZ Fusion of Right Toe Phalangeal Joint with Nonautologous Tissue Substitute, Open Approach
0SGP0ZZ Fusion of Right Toe Phalangeal Joint, Open Approach
0SGP34Z Fusion of Right Toe Phalangeal Joint with Internal Fixation Device, Percutaneous Approach
0SGP35Z Fusion of Right Toe Phalangeal Joint with External Fixation Device, Percutaneous Approach
0SGP37Z Fusion of Right Toe Phalangeal Joint with Autologous Tissue Substitute, Percutaneous Approach
0SGP3JZ Fusion of Right Toe Phalangeal Joint with Synthetic Substitute, Percutaneous Approach
0SGP3KZ Fusion of Right Toe Phalangeal Joint with Nonautologous Tissue Substitute, Percutaneous Approach
0SGP3ZZ Fusion of Right Toe Phalangeal Joint, Percutaneous Approach
0SGP44Z Fusion of Right Toe Phalangeal Joint with Internal Fixation Device, Percutaneous Endoscopic Approach
0SGP45Z Fusion of Right Toe Phalangeal Joint with External Fixation Device, Percutaneous Endoscopic Approach
0SGP47Z Fusion of Right Toe Phalangeal Joint with Autologous Tissue Substitute, Percutaneous Endoscopic Approach
0SGP4JZ Fusion of Right Toe Phalangeal Joint with Synthetic Substitute, Percutaneous Endoscopic Approach
0SGP4KZ Fusion of Right Toe Phalangeal Joint with Nonautologous Tissue Substitute, Percutaneous Endoscopic Approach
0SGP4ZZ Fusion of Right Toe Phalangeal Joint, Percutaneous Endoscopic Approach
0SGQ04Z Fusion of Left Toe Phalangeal Joint with Internal Fixation Device, Open Approach
0SGQ05Z Fusion of Left Toe Phalangeal Joint with External Fixation Device, Open Approach
0SGQ07Z Fusion of Left Toe Phalangeal Joint with Autologous Tissue Substitute, Open Approach
0SGQ0JZ Fusion of Left Toe Phalangeal Joint with Synthetic Substitute, Open Approach
0SGQ0KZ Fusion of Left Toe Phalangeal Joint with Nonautologous Tissue Substitute, Open Approach
0SGQ0ZZ Fusion of Left Toe Phalangeal Joint, Open Approach
0SGQ34Z Fusion of Left Toe Phalangeal Joint with Internal Fixation Device, Percutaneous Approach
0SGQ35Z Fusion of Left Toe Phalangeal Joint with External Fixation Device, Percutaneous Approach
0SGQ37Z Fusion of Left Toe Phalangeal Joint with Autologous Tissue Substitute, Percutaneous Approach
0SGQ3JZ Fusion of Left Toe Phalangeal Joint with Synthetic Substitute, Percutaneous Approach
0SGQ3KZ Fusion of Left Toe Phalangeal Joint with Nonautologous Tissue Substitute, Percutaneous Approach
0SGQ3ZZ Fusion of Left Toe Phalangeal Joint, Percutaneous Approach
0SGQ44Z Fusion of Left Toe Phalangeal Joint with Internal Fixation Device, Percutaneous Endoscopic Approach
0SGQ45Z Fusion of Left Toe Phalangeal Joint with External Fixation Device, Percutaneous Endoscopic Approach
0SGQ47Z Fusion of Left Toe Phalangeal Joint with Autologous Tissue Substitute, Percutaneous Endoscopic Approach
0SGQ4JZ Fusion of Left Toe Phalangeal Joint with Synthetic Substitute, Percutaneous Endoscopic Approach
0SGQ4KZ Fusion of Left Toe Phalangeal Joint with Nonautologous Tissue Substitute, Percutaneous Endoscopic Approach
0SGQ4ZZ Fusion of Left Toe Phalangeal Joint, Percutaneous Endoscopic Approach

0SH – Lower Joints, Insertion

0SH003Z Insertion of Infusion Device into Lumbar Vertebral Joint, Open Approach
0SH004Z Insertion of Internal Fixation Device into Lumbar Vertebral Joint, Open Approach
0SH008Z Insertion of Spacer into Lumbar Vertebral Joint, Open Approach
0SH00BZ Insertion of Interspinous Process Spinal Stabilization Device into Lumbar Vertebral Joint, Open Approach
0SH00CZ Insertion of Pedicle-Based Spinal Stabilization Device into Lumbar Vertebral Joint, Open Approach
0SH00DZ Insertion of Facet Replacement Spinal Stabilization Device into Lumbar Vertebral Joint, Open Approach
0SH033Z Insertion of Infusion Device into Lumbar Vertebral Joint, Percutaneous Approach
0SH034Z Insertion of Internal Fixation Device into Lumbar Vertebral Joint, Percutaneous Approach
0SH038Z Insertion of Spacer into Lumbar Vertebral Joint, Percutaneous Approach
0SH03BZ Insertion of Interspinous Process Spinal Stabilization Device into Lumbar Vertebral Joint, Percutaneous Approach
0SH03CZ Insertion of Pedicle-Based Spinal Stabilization Device into Lumbar Vertebral Joint, Percutaneous Approach
0SH03DZ Insertion of Facet Replacement Spinal Stabilization Device into Lumbar Vertebral Joint, Percutaneous Approach
0SH043Z Insertion of Infusion Device into Lumbar Vertebral Joint, Percutaneous Endoscopic Approach
0SH044Z Insertion of Internal Fixation Device into Lumbar Vertebral Joint, Percutaneous Endoscopic Approach
0SH048Z Insertion of Spacer into Lumbar Vertebral Joint, Percutaneous Endoscopic Approach
0SH04BZ Insertion of Interspinous Process Spinal Stabilization Device into Lumbar Vertebral Joint, Percutaneous Endoscopic Approach
0SH04CZ Insertion of Pedicle-Based Spinal Stabilization Device into Lumbar Vertebral Joint, Percutaneous Endoscopic Approach
0SH04DZ Insertion of Facet Replacement Spinal Stabilization Device into Lumbar Vertebral Joint, Percutaneous Endoscopic Approach
0SH203Z Insertion of Infusion Device into Lumbar Vertebral Disc, Open Approach
0SH208Z Insertion of Spacer into Lumbar Vertebral Disc, Open Approach
0SH233Z Insertion of Infusion Device into Lumbar Vertebral Disc, Percutaneous Approach
0SH238Z Insertion of Spacer into Lumbar Vertebral Disc, Percutaneous Approach
0SH243Z Insertion of Infusion Device into Lumbar Vertebral Disc, Percutaneous Endoscopic Approach
0SH248Z Insertion of Spacer into Lumbar Vertebral Disc, Percutaneous Endoscopic Approach
0SH303Z Insertion of Infusion Device into Lumbosacral Joint, Open Approach
0SH304Z Insertion of Internal Fixation Device into Lumbosacral Joint, Open Approach
0SH308Z Insertion of Spacer into Lumbosacral Joint, Open Approach
0SH30BZ Insertion of Interspinous Process Spinal Stabilization Device into Lumbosacral Joint, Open Approach
0SH30CZ Insertion of Pedicle-Based Spinal Stabilization Device into Lumbosacral Joint, Open Approach
0SH30DZ Insertion of Facet Replacement Spinal Stabilization Device into Lumbosacral Joint, Open Approach
0SH333Z Insertion of Infusion Device into Lumbosacral Joint, Percutaneous Approach
0SH334Z Insertion of Internal Fixation Device into Lumbosacral Joint, Percutaneous Approach
0SH338Z Insertion of Spacer into Lumbosacral Joint, Percutaneous Approach
0SH33BZ Insertion of Interspinous Process Spinal Stabilization Device into Lumbosacral Joint, Percutaneous Approach
0SH33CZ Insertion of Pedicle-Based Spinal Stabilization Device into Lumbosacral Joint, Percutaneous Approach
0SH33DZ Insertion of Facet Replacement Spinal Stabilization Device into Lumbosacral Joint, Percutaneous Approach
0SH343Z Insertion of Infusion Device into Lumbosacral Joint, Percutaneous Endoscopic Approach
0SH344Z Insertion of Internal Fixation Device into Lumbosacral Joint, Percutaneous Endoscopic Approach
0SH348Z Insertion of Spacer into Lumbosacral Joint, Percutaneous Endoscopic Approach
0SH34BZ Insertion of Interspinous Process Spinal Stabilization Device into Lumbosacral Joint, Percutaneous Endoscopic Approach
0SH34CZ Insertion of Pedicle-Based Spinal Stabilization Device into Lumbosacral Joint, Percutaneous Endoscopic Approach

0SH34DZ Insertion of Facet Replacement Spinal Stabilization Device into Lumbosacral Joint, Percutaneous Endoscopic Approach
0SH403Z Insertion of Infusion Device into Lumbosacral Disc, Open Approach
0SH408Z Insertion of Spacer into Lumbosacral Disc, Open Approach
0SH433Z Insertion of Infusion Device into Lumbosacral Disc, Percutaneous Approach
0SH438Z Insertion of Spacer into Lumbosacral Disc, Percutaneous Approach
0SH443Z Insertion of Infusion Device into Lumbosacral Disc, Percutaneous Endoscopic Approach
0SH448Z Insertion of Spacer into Lumbosacral Disc, Percutaneous Endoscopic Approach
0SH503Z Insertion of Infusion Device into Sacrococcygeal Joint, Open Approach
0SH504Z Insertion of Internal Fixation Device into Sacrococcygeal Joint, Open Approach
0SH508Z Insertion of Spacer into Sacrococcygeal Joint, Open Approach
0SH533Z Insertion of Infusion Device into Sacrococcygeal Joint, Percutaneous Approach
0SH534Z Insertion of Internal Fixation Device into Sacrococcygeal Joint, Percutaneous Approach
0SH538Z Insertion of Spacer into Sacrococcygeal Joint, Percutaneous Approach
0SH543Z Insertion of Infusion Device into Sacrococcygeal Joint, Percutaneous Endoscopic Approach
0SH544Z Insertion of Internal Fixation Device into Sacrococcygeal Joint, Percutaneous Endoscopic Approach
0SH548Z Insertion of Spacer into Sacrococcygeal Joint, Percutaneous Endoscopic Approach
0SH603Z Insertion of Infusion Device into Coccygeal Joint, Open Approach
0SH604Z Insertion of Internal Fixation Device into Coccygeal Joint, Open Approach
0SH608Z Insertion of Spacer into Coccygeal Joint, Open Approach
0SH633Z Insertion of Infusion Device into Coccygeal Joint, Percutaneous Approach
0SH634Z Insertion of Internal Fixation Device into Coccygeal Joint, Percutaneous Approach
0SH638Z Insertion of Spacer into Coccygeal Joint, Percutaneous Approach
0SH643Z Insertion of Infusion Device into Coccygeal Joint, Percutaneous Endoscopic Approach
0SH644Z Insertion of Internal Fixation Device into Coccygeal Joint, Percutaneous Endoscopic Approach
0SH648Z Insertion of Spacer into Coccygeal Joint, Percutaneous Endoscopic Approach
0SH703Z Insertion of Infusion Device into Right Sacroiliac Joint, Open Approach
0SH704Z Insertion of Internal Fixation Device into Right Sacroiliac Joint, Open Approach
0SH708Z Insertion of Spacer into Right Sacroiliac Joint, Open Approach
0SH733Z Insertion of Infusion Device into Right Sacroiliac Joint, Percutaneous Approach
0SH734Z Insertion of Internal Fixation Device into Right Sacroiliac Joint, Percutaneous Approach
0SH738Z Insertion of Spacer into Right Sacroiliac Joint, Percutaneous Approach
0SH743Z Insertion of Infusion Device into Right Sacroiliac Joint, Percutaneous Endoscopic Approach
0SH744Z Insertion of Internal Fixation Device into Right Sacroiliac Joint, Percutaneous Endoscopic Approach
0SH748Z Insertion of Spacer into Right Sacroiliac Joint, Percutaneous Endoscopic Approach
0SH803Z Insertion of Infusion Device into Left Sacroiliac Joint, Open Approach
0SH804Z Insertion of Internal Fixation Device into Left Sacroiliac Joint, Open Approach
0SH808Z Insertion of Spacer into Left Sacroiliac Joint, Open Approach
0SH833Z Insertion of Infusion Device into Left Sacroiliac Joint, Percutaneous Approach
0SH834Z Insertion of Internal Fixation Device into Left Sacroiliac Joint, Percutaneous Approach
0SH838Z Insertion of Spacer into Left Sacroiliac Joint, Percutaneous Approach
0SH843Z Insertion of Infusion Device into Left Sacroiliac Joint, Percutaneous Endoscopic Approach
0SH844Z Insertion of Internal Fixation Device into Left Sacroiliac Joint, Percutaneous Endoscopic Approach
0SH848Z Insertion of Spacer into Left Sacroiliac Joint, Percutaneous Endoscopic Approach
0SH903Z Insertion of Infusion Device into Right Hip Joint, Open Approach
0SH904Z Insertion of Internal Fixation Device into Right Hip Joint, Open Approach
0SH905Z Insertion of External Fixation Device into Right Hip Joint, Open Approach
0SH908Z Insertion of Spacer into Right Hip Joint, Open Approach
0SH933Z Insertion of Infusion Device into Right Hip Joint, Percutaneous Approach
0SH934Z Insertion of Internal Fixation Device into Right Hip Joint, Percutaneous Approach
0SH935Z Insertion of External Fixation Device into Right Hip Joint, Percutaneous Approach
0SH938Z Insertion of Spacer into Right Hip Joint, Percutaneous Approach
0SH943Z Insertion of Infusion Device into Right Hip Joint, Percutaneous Endoscopic Approach
0SH944Z Insertion of Internal Fixation Device into Right Hip Joint, Percutaneous Endoscopic Approach
0SH945Z Insertion of External Fixation Device into Right Hip Joint, Percutaneous Endoscopic Approach
0SH948Z Insertion of Spacer into Right Hip Joint, Percutaneous Endoscopic Approach
0SHB03Z Insertion of Infusion Device into Left Hip Joint, Open Approach
0SHB04Z Insertion of Internal Fixation Device into Left Hip Joint, Open Approach
0SHB05Z Insertion of External Fixation Device into Left Hip Joint, Open Approach
0SHB08Z Insertion of Spacer into Left Hip Joint, Open Approach
0SHB33Z Insertion of Infusion Device into Left Hip Joint, Percutaneous Approach
0SHB34Z Insertion of Internal Fixation Device into Left Hip Joint, Percutaneous Approach
0SHB35Z Insertion of External Fixation Device into Left Hip Joint, Percutaneous Approach
0SHB38Z Insertion of Spacer into Left Hip Joint, Percutaneous Approach
0SHB43Z Insertion of Infusion Device into Left Hip Joint, Percutaneous Endoscopic Approach
0SHB44Z Insertion of Internal Fixation Device into Left Hip Joint, Percutaneous Endoscopic Approach
0SHB45Z Insertion of External Fixation Device into Left Hip Joint, Percutaneous Endoscopic Approach
0SHB48Z Insertion of Spacer into Left Hip Joint, Percutaneous Endoscopic Approach
0SHC03Z Insertion of Infusion Device into Right Knee Joint, Open Approach
0SHC04Z Insertion of Internal Fixation Device into Right Knee Joint, Open Approach
0SHC05Z Insertion of External Fixation Device into Right Knee Joint, Open Approach
0SHC08Z Insertion of Spacer into Right Knee Joint, Open Approach
0SHC33Z Insertion of Infusion Device into Right Knee Joint, Percutaneous Approach
0SHC34Z Insertion of Internal Fixation Device into Right Knee Joint, Percutaneous Approach
0SHC35Z Insertion of External Fixation Device into Right Knee Joint, Percutaneous Approach
0SHC38Z Insertion of Spacer into Right Knee Joint, Percutaneous Approach
0SHC43Z Insertion of Infusion Device into Right Knee Joint, Percutaneous Endoscopic Approach
0SHC44Z Insertion of Internal Fixation Device into Right Knee Joint, Percutaneous Endoscopic Approach
0SHC45Z Insertion of External Fixation Device into Right Knee Joint, Percutaneous Endoscopic Approach
0SHC48Z Insertion of Spacer into Right Knee Joint, Percutaneous Endoscopic Approach
0SHD03Z Insertion of Infusion Device into Left Knee Joint, Open Approach
0SHD04Z Insertion of Internal Fixation Device into Left Knee Joint, Open Approach
0SHD05Z Insertion of External Fixation Device into Left Knee Joint, Open Approach
0SHD08Z Insertion of Spacer into Left Knee Joint, Open Approach
0SHD33Z Insertion of Infusion Device into Left Knee Joint, Percutaneous Approach
0SHD34Z Insertion of Internal Fixation Device into Left Knee Joint, Percutaneous Approach
0SHD35Z Insertion of External Fixation Device into Left Knee Joint, Percutaneous Approach
0SHD38Z Insertion of Spacer into Left Knee Joint, Percutaneous Approach
0SHD43Z Insertion of Infusion Device into Left Knee Joint, Percutaneous Endoscopic Approach
0SHD44Z Insertion of Internal Fixation Device into Left Knee Joint, Percutaneous Endoscopic Approach
0SHD45Z Insertion of External Fixation Device into Left Knee Joint, Percutaneous Endoscopic Approach
0SHD48Z Insertion of Spacer into Left Knee Joint, Percutaneous Endoscopic Approach
0SHF03Z Insertion of Infusion Device into Right Ankle Joint, Open Approach
0SHF04Z Insertion of Internal Fixation Device into Right Ankle Joint, Open Approach
0SHF05Z Insertion of External Fixation Device into Right Ankle Joint, Open Approach
0SHF08Z Insertion of Spacer into Right Ankle Joint, Open Approach
0SHF33Z Insertion of Infusion Device into Right Ankle Joint, Percutaneous Approach
0SHF34Z Insertion of Internal Fixation Device into Right Ankle Joint, Percutaneous Approach
0SHF35Z Insertion of External Fixation Device into Right Ankle Joint, Percutaneous Approach
0SHF38Z Insertion of Spacer into Right Ankle Joint, Percutaneous Approach
0SHF43Z Insertion of Infusion Device into Right Ankle Joint, Percutaneous Endoscopic Approach
0SHF44Z Insertion of Internal Fixation Device into Right Ankle Joint, Percutaneous Endoscopic Approach
0SHF45Z Insertion of External Fixation Device into Right Ankle Joint, Percutaneous Endoscopic Approach
0SHF48Z Insertion of Spacer into Right Ankle Joint, Percutaneous Endoscopic Approach

0SHG03Z Insertion of Infusion Device into Left Ankle Joint, Open Approach
0SHG04Z Insertion of Internal Fixation Device into Left Ankle Joint, Open Approach
0SHG05Z Insertion of External Fixation Device into Left Ankle Joint, Open Approach
0SHG08Z Insertion of Spacer into Left Ankle Joint, Open Approach
0SHG33Z Insertion of Infusion Device into Left Ankle Joint, Percutaneous Approach
0SHG34Z Insertion of Internal Fixation Device into Left Ankle Joint, Percutaneous Approach
0SHG35Z Insertion of External Fixation Device into Left Ankle Joint, Percutaneous Approach
0SHG38Z Insertion of Spacer into Left Ankle Joint, Percutaneous Approach
0SHG43Z Insertion of Infusion Device into Left Ankle Joint, Percutaneous Endoscopic Approach
0SHG44Z Insertion of Internal Fixation Device into Left Ankle Joint, Percutaneous Endoscopic Approach
0SHG45Z Insertion of External Fixation Device into Left Ankle Joint, Percutaneous Endoscopic Approach
0SHG48Z Insertion of Spacer into Left Ankle Joint, Percutaneous Endoscopic Approach
0SHH03Z Insertion of Infusion Device into Right Tarsal Joint, Open Approach
0SHH04Z Insertion of Internal Fixation Device into Right Tarsal Joint, Open Approach
0SHH05Z Insertion of External Fixation Device into Right Tarsal Joint, Open Approach
0SHH08Z Insertion of Spacer into Right Tarsal Joint, Open Approach
0SHH33Z Insertion of Infusion Device into Right Tarsal Joint, Percutaneous Approach
0SHH34Z Insertion of Internal Fixation Device into Right Tarsal Joint, Percutaneous Approach
0SHH35Z Insertion of External Fixation Device into Right Tarsal Joint, Percutaneous Approach
0SHH38Z Insertion of Spacer into Right Tarsal Joint, Percutaneous Approach
0SHH43Z Insertion of Infusion Device into Right Tarsal Joint, Percutaneous Endoscopic Approach
0SHH44Z Insertion of Internal Fixation Device into Right Tarsal Joint, Percutaneous Endoscopic Approach
0SHH45Z Insertion of External Fixation Device into Right Tarsal Joint, Percutaneous Endoscopic Approach
0SHH48Z Insertion of Spacer into Right Tarsal Joint, Percutaneous Endoscopic Approach
0SHJ03Z Insertion of Infusion Device into Left Tarsal Joint, Open Approach
0SHJ04Z Insertion of Internal Fixation Device into Left Tarsal Joint, Open Approach
0SHJ05Z Insertion of External Fixation Device into Left Tarsal Joint, Open Approach
0SHJ08Z Insertion of Spacer into Left Tarsal Joint, Open Approach
0SHJ33Z Insertion of Infusion Device into Left Tarsal Joint, Percutaneous Approach
0SHJ34Z Insertion of Internal Fixation Device into Left Tarsal Joint, Percutaneous Approach
0SHJ35Z Insertion of External Fixation Device into Left Tarsal Joint, Percutaneous Approach
0SHJ38Z Insertion of Spacer into Left Tarsal Joint, Percutaneous Approach
0SHJ43Z Insertion of Infusion Device into Left Tarsal Joint, Percutaneous Endoscopic Approach
0SHJ44Z Insertion of Internal Fixation Device into Left Tarsal Joint, Percutaneous Endoscopic Approach
0SHJ45Z Insertion of External Fixation Device into Left Tarsal Joint, Percutaneous Endoscopic Approach
0SHJ48Z Insertion of Spacer into Left Tarsal Joint, Percutaneous Endoscopic Approach
0SHK03Z Insertion of Infusion Device into Right Metatarsal-Tarsal Joint, Open Approach
0SHK04Z Insertion of Internal Fixation Device into Right Metatarsal-Tarsal Joint, Open Approach
0SHK05Z Insertion of External Fixation Device into Right Metatarsal-Tarsal Joint, Open Approach
0SHK08Z Insertion of Spacer into Right Metatarsal-Tarsal Joint, Open Approach
0SHK33Z Insertion of Infusion Device into Right Metatarsal-Tarsal Joint, Percutaneous Approach
0SHK34Z Insertion of Internal Fixation Device into Right Metatarsal-Tarsal Joint, Percutaneous Approach
0SHK35Z Insertion of External Fixation Device into Right Metatarsal-Tarsal Joint, Percutaneous Approach
0SHK38Z Insertion of Spacer into Right Metatarsal-Tarsal Joint, Percutaneous Approach
0SHK43Z Insertion of Infusion Device into Right Metatarsal-Tarsal Joint, Percutaneous Endoscopic Approach
0SHK44Z Insertion of Internal Fixation Device into Right Metatarsal-Tarsal Joint, Percutaneous Endoscopic Approach
0SHK45Z Insertion of External Fixation Device into Right Metatarsal-Tarsal Joint, Percutaneous Endoscopic Approach
0SHK48Z Insertion of Spacer into Right Metatarsal-Tarsal Joint, Percutaneous Endoscopic Approach
0SHL03Z Insertion of Infusion Device into Left Metatarsal-Tarsal Joint, Open Approach
0SHL04Z Insertion of Internal Fixation Device into Left Metatarsal-Tarsal Joint, Open Approach
0SHL05Z Insertion of External Fixation Device into Left Metatarsal-Tarsal Joint, Open Approach
0SHL08Z Insertion of Spacer into Left Metatarsal-Tarsal Joint, Open Approach
0SHL33Z Insertion of Infusion Device into Left Metatarsal-Tarsal Joint, Percutaneous Approach
0SHL34Z Insertion of Internal Fixation Device into Left Metatarsal-Tarsal Joint, Percutaneous Approach
0SHL35Z Insertion of External Fixation Device into Left Metatarsal-Tarsal Joint, Percutaneous Approach
0SHL38Z Insertion of Spacer into Left Metatarsal-Tarsal Joint, Percutaneous Approach
0SHL43Z Insertion of Infusion Device into Left Metatarsal-Tarsal Joint, Percutaneous Endoscopic Approach
0SHL44Z Insertion of Internal Fixation Device into Left Metatarsal-Tarsal Joint, Percutaneous Endoscopic Approach
0SHL45Z Insertion of External Fixation Device into Left Metatarsal-Tarsal Joint, Percutaneous Endoscopic Approach
0SHL48Z Insertion of Spacer into Left Metatarsal-Tarsal Joint, Percutaneous Endoscopic Approach
0SHM03Z Insertion of Infusion Device into Right Metatarsal-Phalangeal Joint, Open Approach
0SHM04Z Insertion of Internal Fixation Device into Right Metatarsal-Phalangeal Joint, Open Approach
0SHM05Z Insertion of External Fixation Device into Right Metatarsal-Phalangeal Joint, Open Approach
0SHM08Z Insertion of Spacer into Right Metatarsal-Phalangeal Joint, Open Approach
0SHM33Z Insertion of Infusion Device into Right Metatarsal-Phalangeal Joint, Percutaneous Approach
0SHM34Z Insertion of Internal Fixation Device into Right Metatarsal-Phalangeal Joint, Percutaneous Approach
0SHM35Z Insertion of External Fixation Device into Right Metatarsal-Phalangeal Joint, Percutaneous Approach
0SHM38Z Insertion of Spacer into Right Metatarsal-Phalangeal Joint, Percutaneous Approach
0SHM43Z Insertion of Infusion Device into Right Metatarsal-Phalangeal Joint, Percutaneous Endoscopic Approach
0SHM44Z Insertion of Internal Fixation Device into Right Metatarsal-Phalangeal Joint, Percutaneous Endoscopic Approach
0SHM45Z Insertion of External Fixation Device into Right Metatarsal-Phalangeal Joint, Percutaneous Endoscopic Approach
0SHM48Z Insertion of Spacer into Right Metatarsal-Phalangeal Joint, Percutaneous Endoscopic Approach
0SHN03Z Insertion of Infusion Device into Left Metatarsal-Phalangeal Joint, Open Approach
0SHN04Z Insertion of Internal Fixation Device into Left Metatarsal-Phalangeal Joint, Open Approach
0SHN05Z Insertion of External Fixation Device into Left Metatarsal-Phalangeal Joint, Open Approach
0SHN08Z Insertion of Spacer into Left Metatarsal-Phalangeal Joint, Open Approach
0SHN33Z Insertion of Infusion Device into Left Metatarsal-Phalangeal Joint, Percutaneous Approach
0SHN34Z Insertion of Internal Fixation Device into Left Metatarsal-Phalangeal Joint, Percutaneous Approach
0SHN35Z Insertion of External Fixation Device into Left Metatarsal-Phalangeal Joint, Percutaneous Approach
0SHN38Z Insertion of Spacer into Left Metatarsal-Phalangeal Joint, Percutaneous Approach
0SHN43Z Insertion of Infusion Device into Left Metatarsal-Phalangeal Joint, Percutaneous Endoscopic Approach
0SHN44Z Insertion of Internal Fixation Device into Left Metatarsal-Phalangeal Joint, Percutaneous Endoscopic Approach
0SHN45Z Insertion of External Fixation Device into Left Metatarsal-Phalangeal Joint, Percutaneous Endoscopic Approach
0SHN48Z Insertion of Spacer into Left Metatarsal-Phalangeal Joint, Percutaneous Endoscopic Approach
0SHP03Z Insertion of Infusion Device into Right Toe Phalangeal Joint, Open Approach
0SHP04Z Insertion of Internal Fixation Device into Right Toe Phalangeal Joint, Open Approach
0SHP05Z Insertion of External Fixation Device into Right Toe Phalangeal Joint, Open Approach
0SHP08Z Insertion of Spacer into Right Toe Phalangeal Joint, Open Approach
0SHP33Z Insertion of Infusion Device into Right Toe Phalangeal Joint, Percutaneous Approach
0SHP34Z Insertion of Internal Fixation Device into Right Toe Phalangeal Joint, Percutaneous Approach

0SHP35Z Insertion of External Fixation Device into Right Toe Phalangeal Joint, Percutaneous Approach
0SHP38Z Insertion of Spacer into Right Toe Phalangeal Joint, Percutaneous Approach
0SHP43Z Insertion of Infusion Device into Right Toe Phalangeal Joint, Percutaneous Endoscopic Approach
0SHP44Z Insertion of Internal Fixation Device into Right Toe Phalangeal Joint, Percutaneous Endoscopic Approach
0SHP45Z Insertion of External Fixation Device into Right Toe Phalangeal Joint, Percutaneous Endoscopic Approach
0SHP48Z Insertion of Spacer into Right Toe Phalangeal Joint, Percutaneous Endoscopic Approach
0SHQ03Z Insertion of Infusion Device into Left Toe Phalangeal Joint, Open Approach
0SHQ04Z Insertion of Internal Fixation Device into Left Toe Phalangeal Joint, Open Approach
0SHQ05Z Insertion of External Fixation Device into Left Toe Phalangeal Joint, Open Approach
0SHQ08Z Insertion of Spacer into Left Toe Phalangeal Joint, Open Approach
0SHQ33Z Insertion of Infusion Device into Left Toe Phalangeal Joint, Percutaneous Approach
0SHQ34Z Insertion of Internal Fixation Device into Left Toe Phalangeal Joint, Percutaneous Approach
0SHQ35Z Insertion of External Fixation Device into Left Toe Phalangeal Joint, Percutaneous Approach
0SHQ38Z Insertion of Spacer into Left Toe Phalangeal Joint, Percutaneous Approach
0SHQ43Z Insertion of Infusion Device into Left Toe Phalangeal Joint, Percutaneous Endoscopic Approach
0SHQ44Z Insertion of Internal Fixation Device into Left Toe Phalangeal Joint, Percutaneous Endoscopic Approach
0SHQ45Z Insertion of External Fixation Device into Left Toe Phalangeal Joint, Percutaneous Endoscopic Approach
0SHQ48Z Insertion of Spacer into Left Toe Phalangeal Joint, Percutaneous Endoscopic Approach

0SJ – Lower Joints, Inspection

Review Coding Guideline B3.5

Review Coding Guidelines B3.11a, B3.11b and B3.11c

0SJ00ZZ Inspection of Lumbar Vertebral Joint, Open Approach
0SJ03ZZ Inspection of Lumbar Vertebral Joint, Percutaneous Approach
0SJ04ZZ Inspection of Lumbar Vertebral Joint, Percutaneous Endoscopic Approach
0SJ0XZZ Inspection of Lumbar Vertebral Joint, External Approach
0SJ20ZZ Inspection of Lumbar Vertebral Disc, Open Approach
0SJ23ZZ Inspection of Lumbar Vertebral Disc, Percutaneous Approach
0SJ24ZZ Inspection of Lumbar Vertebral Disc, Percutaneous Endoscopic Approach
0SJ2XZZ Inspection of Lumbar Vertebral Disc, External Approach
0SJ30ZZ Inspection of Lumbosacral Joint, Open Approach
0SJ33ZZ Inspection of Lumbosacral Joint, Percutaneous Approach
0SJ34ZZ Inspection of Lumbosacral Joint, Percutaneous Endoscopic Approach
0SJ3XZZ Inspection of Lumbosacral Joint, External Approach
0SJ40ZZ Inspection of Lumbosacral Disc, Open Approach
0SJ43ZZ Inspection of Lumbosacral Disc, Percutaneous Approach
0SJ44ZZ Inspection of Lumbosacral Disc, Percutaneous Endoscopic Approach
0SJ4XZZ Inspection of Lumbosacral Disc, External Approach
0SJ50ZZ Inspection of Sacrococcygeal Joint, Open Approach
0SJ53ZZ Inspection of Sacrococcygeal Joint, Percutaneous Approach
0SJ54ZZ Inspection of Sacrococcygeal Joint, Percutaneous Endoscopic Approach
0SJ5XZZ Inspection of Sacrococcygeal Joint, External Approach
0SJ60ZZ Inspection of Coccygeal Joint, Open Approach
0SJ63ZZ Inspection of Coccygeal Joint, Percutaneous Approach
0SJ64ZZ Inspection of Coccygeal Joint, Percutaneous Endoscopic Approach
0SJ6XZZ Inspection of Coccygeal Joint, External Approach
0SJ70ZZ Inspection of Right Sacroiliac Joint, Open Approach
0SJ73ZZ Inspection of Right Sacroiliac Joint, Percutaneous Approach
0SJ74ZZ Inspection of Right Sacroiliac Joint, Percutaneous Endoscopic Approach
0SJ7XZZ Inspection of Right Sacroiliac Joint, External Approach
0SJ80ZZ Inspection of Left Sacroiliac Joint, Open Approach
0SJ83ZZ Inspection of Left Sacroiliac Joint, Percutaneous Approach
0SJ84ZZ Inspection of Left Sacroiliac Joint, Percutaneous Endoscopic Approach
0SJ8XZZ Inspection of Left Sacroiliac Joint, External Approach
0SJ90ZZ Inspection of Right Hip Joint, Open Approach
0SJ93ZZ Inspection of Right Hip Joint, Percutaneous Approach
0SJ94ZZ Inspection of Right Hip Joint, Percutaneous Endoscopic Approach
0SJ9XZZ Inspection of Right Hip Joint, External Approach
0SJB0ZZ Inspection of Left Hip Joint, Open Approach
0SJB3ZZ Inspection of Left Hip Joint, Percutaneous Approach
0SJB4ZZ Inspection of Left Hip Joint, Percutaneous Endoscopic Approach
0SJBXZZ Inspection of Left Hip Joint, External Approach
0SJC0ZZ Inspection of Right Knee Joint, Open Approach
0SJC3ZZ Inspection of Right Knee Joint, Percutaneous Approach
0SJC4ZZ Inspection of Right Knee Joint, Percutaneous Endoscopic Approach
0SJCXZZ Inspection of Right Knee Joint, External Approach
0SJD0ZZ Inspection of Left Knee Joint, Open Approach
0SJD3ZZ Inspection of Left Knee Joint, Percutaneous Approach
0SJD4ZZ Inspection of Left Knee Joint, Percutaneous Endoscopic Approach
0SJDXZZ Inspection of Left Knee Joint, External Approach
0SJF0ZZ Inspection of Right Ankle Joint, Open Approach
0SJF3ZZ Inspection of Right Ankle Joint, Percutaneous Approach
0SJF4ZZ Inspection of Right Ankle Joint, Percutaneous Endoscopic Approach
0SJFXZZ Inspection of Right Ankle Joint, External Approach
0SJG0ZZ Inspection of Left Ankle Joint, Open Approach
0SJG3ZZ Inspection of Left Ankle Joint, Percutaneous Approach
0SJG4ZZ Inspection of Left Ankle Joint, Percutaneous Endoscopic Approach
0SJGXZZ Inspection of Left Ankle Joint, External Approach
0SJH0ZZ Inspection of Right Tarsal Joint, Open Approach
0SJH3ZZ Inspection of Right Tarsal Joint, Percutaneous Approach
0SJH4ZZ Inspection of Right Tarsal Joint, Percutaneous Endoscopic Approach
0SJHXZZ Inspection of Right Tarsal Joint, External Approach
0SJJ0ZZ Inspection of Left Tarsal Joint, Open Approach
0SJJ3ZZ Inspection of Left Tarsal Joint, Percutaneous Approach
0SJJ4ZZ Inspection of Left Tarsal Joint, Percutaneous Endoscopic Approach
0SJJXZZ Inspection of Left Tarsal Joint, External Approach
0SJK0ZZ Inspection of Right Metatarsal-Tarsal Joint, Open Approach
0SJK3ZZ Inspection of Right Metatarsal-Tarsal Joint, Percutaneous Approach
0SJK4ZZ Inspection of Right Metatarsal-Tarsal Joint, Percutaneous Endoscopic Approach
0SJKXZZ Inspection of Right Metatarsal-Tarsal Joint, External Approach
0SJL0ZZ Inspection of Left Metatarsal-Tarsal Joint, Open Approach
0SJL3ZZ Inspection of Left Metatarsal-Tarsal Joint, Percutaneous Approach
0SJL4ZZ Inspection of Left Metatarsal-Tarsal Joint, Percutaneous Endoscopic Approach
0SJLXZZ Inspection of Left Metatarsal-Tarsal Joint, External Approach
0SJM0ZZ Inspection of Right Metatarsal-Phalangeal Joint, Open Approach
0SJM3ZZ Inspection of Right Metatarsal-Phalangeal Joint, Percutaneous Approach
0SJM4ZZ Inspection of Right Metatarsal-Phalangeal Joint, Percutaneous Endoscopic Approach
0SJMXZZ Inspection of Right Metatarsal-Phalangeal Joint, External Approach
0SJN0ZZ Inspection of Left Metatarsal-Phalangeal Joint, Open Approach
0SJN3ZZ Inspection of Left Metatarsal-Phalangeal Joint, Percutaneous Approach
0SJN4ZZ Inspection of Left Metatarsal-Phalangeal Joint, Percutaneous Endoscopic Approach
0SJNXZZ Inspection of Left Metatarsal-Phalangeal Joint, External Approach

0SJP0ZZ Inspection of Right Toe Phalangeal Joint, Open Approach
0SJP3ZZ Inspection of Right Toe Phalangeal Joint, Percutaneous Approach
0SJP4ZZ Inspection of Right Toe Phalangeal Joint, Percutaneous Endoscopic Approach
0SJPXZZ Inspection of Right Toe Phalangeal Joint, External Approach
0SJQ0ZZ Inspection of Left Toe Phalangeal Joint, Open Approach
0SJQ3ZZ Inspection of Left Toe Phalangeal Joint, Percutaneous Approach
0SJQ4ZZ Inspection of Left Toe Phalangeal Joint, Percutaneous Endoscopic Approach
0SJQXZZ Inspection of Left Toe Phalangeal Joint, External Approach

0SN – Lower Joints, Release

Review Coding Guideline B3.13

0SN00ZZ Release Lumbar Vertebral Joint, Open Approach
0SN03ZZ Release Lumbar Vertebral Joint, Percutaneous Approach
0SN04ZZ Release Lumbar Vertebral Joint, Percutaneous Endoscopic Approach
0SN0XZZ Release Lumbar Vertebral Joint, External Approach
0SN20ZZ Release Lumbar Vertebral Disc, Open Approach
0SN23ZZ Release Lumbar Vertebral Disc, Percutaneous Approach
0SN24ZZ Release Lumbar Vertebral Disc, Percutaneous Endoscopic Approach
0SN2XZZ Release Lumbar Vertebral Disc, External Approach
0SN30ZZ Release Lumbosacral Joint, Open Approach
0SN33ZZ Release Lumbosacral Joint, Percutaneous Approach
0SN34ZZ Release Lumbosacral Joint, Percutaneous Endoscopic Approach
0SN3XZZ Release Lumbosacral Joint, External Approach
0SN40ZZ Release Lumbosacral Disc, Open Approach
0SN43ZZ Release Lumbosacral Disc, Percutaneous Approach
0SN44ZZ Release Lumbosacral Disc, Percutaneous Endoscopic Approach
0SN4XZZ Release Lumbosacral Disc, External Approach
0SN50ZZ Release Sacrococcygeal Joint, Open Approach
0SN53ZZ Release Sacrococcygeal Joint, Percutaneous Approach
0SN54ZZ Release Sacrococcygeal Joint, Percutaneous Endoscopic Approach
0SN5XZZ Release Sacrococcygeal Joint, External Approach
0SN60ZZ Release Coccygeal Joint, Open Approach
0SN63ZZ Release Coccygeal Joint, Percutaneous Approach
0SN64ZZ Release Coccygeal Joint, Percutaneous Endoscopic Approach
0SN6XZZ Release Coccygeal Joint, External Approach
0SN70ZZ Release Right Sacroiliac Joint, Open Approach
0SN73ZZ Release Right Sacroiliac Joint, Percutaneous Approach
0SN74ZZ Release Right Sacroiliac Joint, Percutaneous Endoscopic Approach
0SN7XZZ Release Right Sacroiliac Joint, External Approach
0SN80ZZ Release Left Sacroiliac Joint, Open Approach
0SN83ZZ Release Left Sacroiliac Joint, Percutaneous Approach
0SN84ZZ Release Left Sacroiliac Joint, Percutaneous Endoscopic Approach
0SN8XZZ Release Left Sacroiliac Joint, External Approach
0SN90ZZ Release Right Hip Joint, Open Approach
0SN93ZZ Release Right Hip Joint, Percutaneous Approach
0SN94ZZ Release Right Hip Joint, Percutaneous Endoscopic Approach
0SN9XZZ Release Right Hip Joint, External Approach
0SNB0ZZ Release Left Hip Joint, Open Approach
0SNB3ZZ Release Left Hip Joint, Percutaneous Approach
0SNB4ZZ Release Left Hip Joint, Percutaneous Endoscopic Approach
0SNBXZZ Release Left Hip Joint, External Approach
0SNC0ZZ Release Right Knee Joint, Open Approach
0SNC3ZZ Release Right Knee Joint, Percutaneous Approach
0SNC4ZZ Release Right Knee Joint, Percutaneous Endoscopic Approach
0SNCXZZ Release Right Knee Joint, External Approach
0SND0ZZ Release Left Knee Joint, Open Approach
0SND3ZZ Release Left Knee Joint, Percutaneous Approach
0SND4ZZ Release Left Knee Joint, Percutaneous Endoscopic Approach
0SNDXZZ Release Left Knee Joint, External Approach
0SNF0ZZ Release Right Ankle Joint, Open Approach
0SNF3ZZ Release Right Ankle Joint, Percutaneous Approach
0SNF4ZZ Release Right Ankle Joint, Percutaneous Endoscopic Approach
0SNFXZZ Release Right Ankle Joint, External Approach
0SNG0ZZ Release Left Ankle Joint, Open Approach
0SNG3ZZ Release Left Ankle Joint, Percutaneous Approach
0SNG4ZZ Release Left Ankle Joint, Percutaneous Endoscopic Approach
0SNGXZZ Release Left Ankle Joint, External Approach
0SNH0ZZ Release Right Tarsal Joint, Open Approach
0SNH3ZZ Release Right Tarsal Joint, Percutaneous Approach
0SNH4ZZ Release Right Tarsal Joint, Percutaneous Endoscopic Approach
0SNHXZZ Release Right Tarsal Joint, External Approach
0SNJ0ZZ Release Left Tarsal Joint, Open Approach
0SNJ3ZZ Release Left Tarsal Joint, Percutaneous Approach
0SNJ4ZZ Release Left Tarsal Joint, Percutaneous Endoscopic Approach
0SNJXZZ Release Left Tarsal Joint, External Approach
0SNK0ZZ Release Right Metatarsal-Tarsal Joint, Open Approach
0SNK3ZZ Release Right Metatarsal-Tarsal Joint, Percutaneous Approach
0SNK4ZZ Release Right Metatarsal-Tarsal Joint, Percutaneous Endoscopic Approach
0SNKXZZ Release Right Metatarsal-Tarsal Joint, External Approach
0SNL0ZZ Release Left Metatarsal-Tarsal Joint, Open Approach
0SNL3ZZ Release Left Metatarsal-Tarsal Joint, Percutaneous Approach
0SNL4ZZ Release Left Metatarsal-Tarsal Joint, Percutaneous Endoscopic Approach
0SNLXZZ Release Left Metatarsal-Tarsal Joint, External Approach
0SNM0ZZ Release Right Metatarsal-Phalangeal Joint, Open Approach
0SNM3ZZ Release Right Metatarsal-Phalangeal Joint, Percutaneous Approach
0SNM4ZZ Release Right Metatarsal-Phalangeal Joint, Percutaneous Endoscopic Approach
0SNMXZZ Release Right Metatarsal-Phalangeal Joint, External Approach
0SNN0ZZ Release Left Metatarsal-Phalangeal Joint, Open Approach
0SNN3ZZ Release Left Metatarsal-Phalangeal Joint, Percutaneous Approach
0SNN4ZZ Release Left Metatarsal-Phalangeal Joint, Percutaneous Endoscopic Approach
0SNNXZZ Release Left Metatarsal-Phalangeal Joint, External Approach
0SNP0ZZ Release Right Toe Phalangeal Joint, Open Approach
0SNP3ZZ Release Right Toe Phalangeal Joint, Percutaneous Approach
0SNP4ZZ Release Right Toe Phalangeal Joint, Percutaneous Endoscopic Approach
0SNPXZZ Release Right Toe Phalangeal Joint, External Approach
0SNQ0ZZ Release Left Toe Phalangeal Joint, Open Approach
0SNQ3ZZ Release Left Toe Phalangeal Joint, Percutaneous Approach
0SNQ4ZZ Release Left Toe Phalangeal Joint, Percutaneous Endoscopic Approach
0SNQXZZ Release Left Toe Phalangeal Joint, External Approach

0SP – Lower Joints, Removal

Review Coding Guideline B6.1c

0SP000Z Removal of Drainage Device from Lumbar Vertebral Joint, Open Approach
0SP003Z Removal of Infusion Device from Lumbar Vertebral Joint, Open Approach
0SP004Z Removal of Internal Fixation Device from Lumbar Vertebral Joint, Open Approach
0SP007Z Removal of Autologous Tissue Substitute from Lumbar Vertebral Joint, Open Approach
0SP008Z Removal of Spacer from Lumbar Vertebral Joint, Open Approach
0SP00AZ Removal of Interbody Fusion Device from Lumbar Vertebral Joint, Open Approach
0SP00JZ Removal of Synthetic Substitute from Lumbar Vertebral Joint, Open Approach
0SP00KZ Removal of Nonautologous Tissue Substitute from Lumbar Vertebral Joint, Open Approach
0SP030Z Removal of Drainage Device from Lumbar Vertebral Joint, Percutaneous Approach

0SP033Z Removal of Infusion Device from Lumbar Vertebral Joint, Percutaneous Approach
0SP034Z Removal of Internal Fixation Device from Lumbar Vertebral Joint, Percutaneous Approach
0SP037Z Removal of Autologous Tissue Substitute from Lumbar Vertebral Joint, Percutaneous Approach
0SP038Z Removal of Spacer from Lumbar Vertebral Joint, Percutaneous Approach
0SP03AZ Removal of Interbody Fusion Device from Lumbar Vertebral Joint, Percutaneous Approach
0SP03JZ Removal of Synthetic Substitute from Lumbar Vertebral Joint, Percutaneous Approach
0SP03KZ Removal of Nonautologous Tissue Substitute from Lumbar Vertebral Joint, Percutaneous Approach
0SP040Z Removal of Drainage Device from Lumbar Vertebral Joint, Percutaneous Endoscopic Approach
0SP043Z Removal of Infusion Device from Lumbar Vertebral Joint, Percutaneous Endoscopic Approach
0SP044Z Removal of Internal Fixation Device from Lumbar Vertebral Joint, Percutaneous Endoscopic Approach
0SP047Z Removal of Autologous Tissue Substitute from Lumbar Vertebral Joint, Percutaneous Endoscopic Approach
0SP048Z Removal of Spacer from Lumbar Vertebral Joint, Percutaneous Endoscopic Approach
0SP04AZ Removal of Interbody Fusion Device from Lumbar Vertebral Joint, Percutaneous Endoscopic Approach
0SP04JZ Removal of Synthetic Substitute from Lumbar Vertebral Joint, Percutaneous Endoscopic Approach
0SP04KZ Removal of Nonautologous Tissue Substitute from Lumbar Vertebral Joint, Percutaneous Endoscopic Approach
0SP0X0Z Removal of Drainage Device from Lumbar Vertebral Joint, External Approach
0SP0X3Z Removal of Infusion Device from Lumbar Vertebral Joint, External Approach
0SP0X4Z Removal of Internal Fixation Device from Lumbar Vertebral Joint, External Approach
0SP200Z Removal of Drainage Device from Lumbar Vertebral Disc, Open Approach
0SP203Z Removal of Infusion Device from Lumbar Vertebral Disc, Open Approach
0SP207Z Removal of Autologous Tissue Substitute from Lumbar Vertebral Disc, Open Approach
0SP20JZ Removal of Synthetic Substitute from Lumbar Vertebral Disc, Open Approach
0SP20KZ Removal of Nonautologous Tissue Substitute from Lumbar Vertebral Disc, Open Approach
0SP230Z Removal of Drainage Device from Lumbar Vertebral Disc, Percutaneous Approach
0SP233Z Removal of Infusion Device from Lumbar Vertebral Disc, Percutaneous Approach
0SP237Z Removal of Autologous Tissue Substitute from Lumbar Vertebral Disc, Percutaneous Approach
0SP23JZ Removal of Synthetic Substitute from Lumbar Vertebral Disc, Percutaneous Approach
0SP23KZ Removal of Nonautologous Tissue Substitute from Lumbar Vertebral Disc, Percutaneous Approach
0SP240Z Removal of Drainage Device from Lumbar Vertebral Disc, Percutaneous Endoscopic Approach
0SP243Z Removal of Infusion Device from Lumbar Vertebral Disc, Percutaneous Endoscopic Approach
0SP247Z Removal of Autologous Tissue Substitute from Lumbar Vertebral Disc, Percutaneous Endoscopic Approach
0SP24JZ Removal of Synthetic Substitute from Lumbar Vertebral Disc, Percutaneous Endoscopic Approach
0SP24KZ Removal of Nonautologous Tissue Substitute from Lumbar Vertebral Disc, Percutaneous Endoscopic Approach
0SP2X0Z Removal of Drainage Device from Lumbar Vertebral Disc, External Approach
0SP2X3Z Removal of Infusion Device from Lumbar Vertebral Disc, External Approach
0SP300Z Removal of Drainage Device from Lumbosacral Joint, Open Approach
0SP303Z Removal of Infusion Device from Lumbosacral Joint, Open Approach
0SP304Z Removal of Internal Fixation Device from Lumbosacral Joint, Open Approach
0SP307Z Removal of Autologous Tissue Substitute from Lumbosacral Joint, Open Approach
0SP308Z Removal of Spacer from Lumbosacral Joint, Open Approach
0SP30AZ Removal of Interbody Fusion Device from Lumbosacral Joint, Open Approach
0SP30JZ Removal of Synthetic Substitute from Lumbosacral Joint, Open Approach
0SP30KZ Removal of Nonautologous Tissue Substitute from Lumbosacral Joint, Open Approach
0SP330Z Removal of Drainage Device from Lumbosacral Joint, Percutaneous Approach
0SP333Z Removal of Infusion Device from Lumbosacral Joint, Percutaneous Approach
0SP334Z Removal of Internal Fixation Device from Lumbosacral Joint, Percutaneous Approach
0SP337Z Removal of Autologous Tissue Substitute from Lumbosacral Joint, Percutaneous Approach
0SP338Z Removal of Spacer from Lumbosacral Joint, Percutaneous Approach
0SP33AZ Removal of Interbody Fusion Device from Lumbosacral Joint, Percutaneous Approach
0SP33JZ Removal of Synthetic Substitute from Lumbosacral Joint, Percutaneous Approach
0SP33KZ Removal of Nonautologous Tissue Substitute from Lumbosacral Joint, Percutaneous Approach
0SP340Z Removal of Drainage Device from Lumbosacral Joint, Percutaneous Endoscopic Approach
0SP343Z Removal of Infusion Device from Lumbosacral Joint, Percutaneous Endoscopic Approach
0SP344Z Removal of Internal Fixation Device from Lumbosacral Joint, Percutaneous Endoscopic Approach
0SP347Z Removal of Autologous Tissue Substitute from Lumbosacral Joint, Percutaneous Endoscopic Approach
0SP348Z Removal of Spacer from Lumbosacral Joint, Percutaneous Endoscopic Approach
0SP34AZ Removal of Interbody Fusion Device from Lumbosacral Joint, Percutaneous Endoscopic Approach
0SP34JZ Removal of Synthetic Substitute from Lumbosacral Joint, Percutaneous Endoscopic Approach
0SP34KZ Removal of Nonautologous Tissue Substitute from Lumbosacral Joint, Percutaneous Endoscopic Approach
0SP3X0Z Removal of Drainage Device from Lumbosacral Joint, External Approach
0SP3X3Z Removal of Infusion Device from Lumbosacral Joint, External Approach
0SP3X4Z Removal of Internal Fixation Device from Lumbosacral Joint, External Approach
0SP400Z Removal of Drainage Device from Lumbosacral Disc, Open Approach
0SP403Z Removal of Infusion Device from Lumbosacral Disc, Open Approach
0SP407Z Removal of Autologous Tissue Substitute from Lumbosacral Disc, Open Approach
0SP40JZ Removal of Synthetic Substitute from Lumbosacral Disc, Open Approach
0SP40KZ Removal of Nonautologous Tissue Substitute from Lumbosacral Disc, Open Approach
0SP430Z Removal of Drainage Device from Lumbosacral Disc, Percutaneous Approach
0SP433Z Removal of Infusion Device from Lumbosacral Disc, Percutaneous Approach
0SP437Z Removal of Autologous Tissue Substitute from Lumbosacral Disc, Percutaneous Approach
0SP43JZ Removal of Synthetic Substitute from Lumbosacral Disc, Percutaneous Approach
0SP43KZ Removal of Nonautologous Tissue Substitute from Lumbosacral Disc, Percutaneous Approach
0SP440Z Removal of Drainage Device from Lumbosacral Disc, Percutaneous Endoscopic Approach
0SP443Z Removal of Infusion Device from Lumbosacral Disc, Percutaneous Endoscopic Approach
0SP447Z Removal of Autologous Tissue Substitute from Lumbosacral Disc, Percutaneous Endoscopic Approach
0SP44JZ Removal of Synthetic Substitute from Lumbosacral Disc, Percutaneous Endoscopic Approach
0SP44KZ Removal of Nonautologous Tissue Substitute from Lumbosacral Disc, Percutaneous Endoscopic Approach
0SP4X0Z Removal of Drainage Device from Lumbosacral Disc, External Approach
0SP4X3Z Removal of Infusion Device from Lumbosacral Disc, External Approach
0SP500Z Removal of Drainage Device from Sacrococcygeal Joint, Open Approach
0SP503Z Removal of Infusion Device from Sacrococcygeal Joint, Open Approach
0SP504Z Removal of Internal Fixation Device from Sacrococcygeal Joint, Open Approach
0SP507Z Removal of Autologous Tissue Substitute from Sacrococcygeal Joint, Open Approach
0SP508Z Removal of Spacer from Sacrococcygeal Joint, Open Approach
0SP50JZ Removal of Synthetic Substitute from Sacrococcygeal Joint, Open Approach
0SP50KZ Removal of Nonautologous Tissue Substitute from Sacrococcygeal Joint, Open Approach
0SP530Z Removal of Drainage Device from Sacrococcygeal Joint, Percutaneous Approach
0SP533Z Removal of Infusion Device from Sacrococcygeal Joint, Percutaneous Approach
0SP534Z Removal of Internal Fixation Device from Sacrococcygeal Joint, Percutaneous Approach
0SP537Z Removal of Autologous Tissue Substitute from Sacrococcygeal Joint, Percutaneous Approach

0SP538Z Removal of Spacer from Sacrococcygeal Joint, Percutaneous Approach
0SP53JZ Removal of Synthetic Substitute from Sacrococcygeal Joint, Percutaneous Approach
0SP53KZ Removal of Nonautologous Tissue Substitute from Sacrococcygeal Joint, Percutaneous Approach
0SP540Z Removal of Drainage Device from Sacrococcygeal Joint, Percutaneous Endoscopic Approach
0SP543Z Removal of Infusion Device from Sacrococcygeal Joint, Percutaneous Endoscopic Approach
0SP544Z Removal of Internal Fixation Device from Sacrococcygeal Joint, Percutaneous Endoscopic Approach
0SP547Z Removal of Autologous Tissue Substitute from Sacrococcygeal Joint, Percutaneous Endoscopic Approach
0SP548Z Removal of Spacer from Sacrococcygeal Joint, Percutaneous Endoscopic Approach
0SP54JZ Removal of Synthetic Substitute from Sacrococcygeal Joint, Percutaneous Endoscopic Approach
0SP54KZ Removal of Nonautologous Tissue Substitute from Sacrococcygeal Joint, Percutaneous Endoscopic Approach
0SP5X0Z Removal of Drainage Device from Sacrococcygeal Joint, External Approach
0SP5X3Z Removal of Infusion Device from Sacrococcygeal Joint, External Approach
0SP5X4Z Removal of Internal Fixation Device from Sacrococcygeal Joint, External Approach
0SP600Z Removal of Drainage Device from Coccygeal Joint, Open Approach
0SP603Z Removal of Infusion Device from Coccygeal Joint, Open Approach
0SP604Z Removal of Internal Fixation Device from Coccygeal Joint, Open Approach
0SP607Z Removal of Autologous Tissue Substitute from Coccygeal Joint, Open Approach
0SP608Z Removal of Spacer from Coccygeal Joint, Open Approach
0SP60JZ Removal of Synthetic Substitute from Coccygeal Joint, Open Approach
0SP60KZ Removal of Nonautologous Tissue Substitute from Coccygeal Joint, Open Approach
0SP630Z Removal of Drainage Device from Coccygeal Joint, Percutaneous Approach
0SP633Z Removal of Infusion Device from Coccygeal Joint, Percutaneous Approach
0SP634Z Removal of Internal Fixation Device from Coccygeal Joint, Percutaneous Approach
0SP637Z Removal of Autologous Tissue Substitute from Coccygeal Joint, Percutaneous Approach
0SP638Z Removal of Spacer from Coccygeal Joint, Percutaneous Approach
0SP63JZ Removal of Synthetic Substitute from Coccygeal Joint, Percutaneous Approach
0SP63KZ Removal of Nonautologous Tissue Substitute from Coccygeal Joint, Percutaneous Approach
0SP640Z Removal of Drainage Device from Coccygeal Joint, Percutaneous Endoscopic Approach
0SP643Z Removal of Infusion Device from Coccygeal Joint, Percutaneous Endoscopic Approach
0SP644Z Removal of Internal Fixation Device from Coccygeal Joint, Percutaneous Endoscopic Approach
0SP647Z Removal of Autologous Tissue Substitute from Coccygeal Joint, Percutaneous Endoscopic Approach
0SP648Z Removal of Spacer from Coccygeal Joint, Percutaneous Endoscopic Approach
0SP64JZ Removal of Synthetic Substitute from Coccygeal Joint, Percutaneous Endoscopic Approach
0SP64KZ Removal of Nonautologous Tissue Substitute from Coccygeal Joint, Percutaneous Endoscopic Approach
0SP6X0Z Removal of Drainage Device from Coccygeal Joint, External Approach
0SP6X3Z Removal of Infusion Device from Coccygeal Joint, External Approach
0SP6X4Z Removal of Internal Fixation Device from Coccygeal Joint, External Approach
0SP700Z Removal of Drainage Device from Right Sacroiliac Joint, Open Approach
0SP703Z Removal of Infusion Device from Right Sacroiliac Joint, Open Approach
0SP704Z Removal of Internal Fixation Device from Right Sacroiliac Joint, Open Approach
0SP707Z Removal of Autologous Tissue Substitute from Right Sacroiliac Joint, Open Approach
0SP708Z Removal of Spacer from Right Sacroiliac Joint, Open Approach
0SP70JZ Removal of Synthetic Substitute from Right Sacroiliac Joint, Open Approach
0SP70KZ Removal of Nonautologous Tissue Substitute from Right Sacroiliac Joint, Open Approach
0SP730Z Removal of Drainage Device from Right Sacroiliac Joint, Percutaneous Approach
0SP733Z Removal of Infusion Device from Right Sacroiliac Joint, Percutaneous Approach
0SP734Z Removal of Internal Fixation Device from Right Sacroiliac Joint, Percutaneous Approach
0SP737Z Removal of Autologous Tissue Substitute from Right Sacroiliac Joint, Percutaneous Approach
0SP738Z Removal of Spacer from Right Sacroiliac Joint, Percutaneous Approach
0SP73JZ Removal of Synthetic Substitute from Right Sacroiliac Joint, Percutaneous Approach
0SP73KZ Removal of Nonautologous Tissue Substitute from Right Sacroiliac Joint, Percutaneous Approach
0SP740Z Removal of Drainage Device from Right Sacroiliac Joint, Percutaneous Endoscopic Approach
0SP743Z Removal of Infusion Device from Right Sacroiliac Joint, Percutaneous Endoscopic Approach
0SP744Z Removal of Internal Fixation Device from Right Sacroiliac Joint, Percutaneous Endoscopic Approach
0SP747Z Removal of Autologous Tissue Substitute from Right Sacroiliac Joint, Percutaneous Endoscopic Approach
0SP748Z Removal of Spacer from Right Sacroiliac Joint, Percutaneous Endoscopic Approach
0SP74JZ Removal of Synthetic Substitute from Right Sacroiliac Joint, Percutaneous Endoscopic Approach
0SP74KZ Removal of Nonautologous Tissue Substitute from Right Sacroiliac Joint, Percutaneous Endoscopic Approach
0SP7X0Z Removal of Drainage Device from Right Sacroiliac Joint, External Approach
0SP7X3Z Removal of Infusion Device from Right Sacroiliac Joint, External Approach
0SP7X4Z Removal of Internal Fixation Device from Right Sacroiliac Joint, External Approach
0SP800Z Removal of Drainage Device from Left Sacroiliac Joint, Open Approach
0SP803Z Removal of Infusion Device from Left Sacroiliac Joint, Open Approach
0SP804Z Removal of Internal Fixation Device from Left Sacroiliac Joint, Open Approach
0SP807Z Removal of Autologous Tissue Substitute from Left Sacroiliac Joint, Open Approach
0SP808Z Removal of Spacer from Left Sacroiliac Joint, Open Approach
0SP80JZ Removal of Synthetic Substitute from Left Sacroiliac Joint, Open Approach
0SP80KZ Removal of Nonautologous Tissue Substitute from Left Sacroiliac Joint, Open Approach
0SP830Z Removal of Drainage Device from Left Sacroiliac Joint, Percutaneous Approach
0SP833Z Removal of Infusion Device from Left Sacroiliac Joint, Percutaneous Approach
0SP834Z Removal of Internal Fixation Device from Left Sacroiliac Joint, Percutaneous Approach
0SP837Z Removal of Autologous Tissue Substitute from Left Sacroiliac Joint, Percutaneous Approach
0SP838Z Removal of Spacer from Left Sacroiliac Joint, Percutaneous Approach
0SP83JZ Removal of Synthetic Substitute from Left Sacroiliac Joint, Percutaneous Approach
0SP83KZ Removal of Nonautologous Tissue Substitute from Left Sacroiliac Joint, Percutaneous Approach
0SP840Z Removal of Drainage Device from Left Sacroiliac Joint, Percutaneous Endoscopic Approach
0SP843Z Removal of Infusion Device from Left Sacroiliac Joint, Percutaneous Endoscopic Approach
0SP844Z Removal of Internal Fixation Device from Left Sacroiliac Joint, Percutaneous Endoscopic Approach
0SP847Z Removal of Autologous Tissue Substitute from Left Sacroiliac Joint, Percutaneous Endoscopic Approach
0SP848Z Removal of Spacer from Left Sacroiliac Joint, Percutaneous Endoscopic Approach
0SP84JZ Removal of Synthetic Substitute from Left Sacroiliac Joint, Percutaneous Endoscopic Approach
0SP84KZ Removal of Nonautologous Tissue Substitute from Left Sacroiliac Joint, Percutaneous Endoscopic Approach
0SP8X0Z Removal of Drainage Device from Left Sacroiliac Joint, External Approach
0SP8X3Z Removal of Infusion Device from Left Sacroiliac Joint, External Approach
0SP8X4Z Removal of Internal Fixation Device from Left Sacroiliac Joint, External Approach
0SP900Z Removal of Drainage Device from Right Hip Joint, Open Approach
0SP903Z Removal of Infusion Device from Right Hip Joint, Open Approach
0SP904Z Removal of Internal Fixation Device from Right Hip Joint, Open Approach
0SP905Z Removal of External Fixation Device from Right Hip Joint, Open Approach
0SP907Z Removal of Autologous Tissue Substitute from Right Hip Joint, Open Approach
0SP908Z Removal of Spacer from Right Hip Joint, Open Approach
0SP909Z Removal of Liner from Right Hip Joint, Open Approach
+ *If replacement, see table 0SU to construct a code for Supplement with liner.*
0SP90BZ Removal of Resurfacing Device from Right Hip Joint, Open Approach
0SP90JZ Removal of Synthetic Substitute from Right Hip Joint, Open Approach
+ *If replacement see table 0SR to construct a code for the Replacement of the device.*
0SP90KZ Removal of Nonautologous Tissue Substitute from Right Hip Joint, Open Approach

0SP930Z Removal of Drainage Device from Right Hip Joint, Percutaneous Approach
0SP933Z Removal of Infusion Device from Right Hip Joint, Percutaneous Approach
0SP934Z Removal of Internal Fixation Device from Right Hip Joint, Percutaneous Approach
0SP935Z Removal of External Fixation Device from Right Hip Joint, Percutaneous Approach
0SP937Z Removal of Autologous Tissue Substitute from Right Hip Joint, Percutaneous Approach
0SP938Z Removal of Spacer from Right Hip Joint, Percutaneous Approach
0SP93JZ Removal of Synthetic Substitute from Right Hip Joint, Percutaneous Approach
0SP93KZ Removal of Nonautologous Tissue Substitute from Right Hip Joint, Percutaneous Approach
0SP940Z Removal of Drainage Device from Right Hip Joint, Percutaneous Endoscopic Approach
0SP943Z Removal of Infusion Device from Right Hip Joint, Percutaneous Endoscopic Approach
0SP944Z Removal of Internal Fixation Device from Right Hip Joint, Percutaneous Endoscopic Approach
0SP945Z Removal of External Fixation Device from Right Hip Joint, Percutaneous Endoscopic Approach
0SP947Z Removal of Autologous Tissue Substitute from Right Hip Joint, Percutaneous Endoscopic Approach
0SP948Z Removal of Spacer from Right Hip Joint, Percutaneous Endoscopic Approach
0SP94JZ Removal of Synthetic Substitute from Right Hip Joint, Percutaneous Endoscopic Approach
0SP94KZ Removal of Nonautologous Tissue Substitute from Right Hip Joint, Percutaneous Endoscopic Approach
0SP9X0Z Removal of Drainage Device from Right Hip Joint, External Approach
0SP9X3Z Removal of Infusion Device from Right Hip Joint, External Approach
0SP9X4Z Removal of Internal Fixation Device from Right Hip Joint, External Approach
0SP9X5Z Removal of External Fixation Device from Right Hip Joint, External Approach
0SPB00Z Removal of Drainage Device from Left Hip Joint, Open Approach
0SPB03Z Removal of Infusion Device from Left Hip Joint, Open Approach
0SPB04Z Removal of Internal Fixation Device from Left Hip Joint, Open Approach
0SPB05Z Removal of External Fixation Device from Left Hip Joint, Open Approach
0SPB07Z Removal of Autologous Tissue Substitute from Left Hip Joint, Open Approach
0SPB08Z Removal of Spacer from Left Hip Joint, Open Approach
0SPB09Z Removal of Liner from Left Hip Joint, Open Approach
+ *If replacement, see table 0SU to construct a code for Supplement with liner.*
0SPB0BZ Removal of Resurfacing Device from Left Hip Joint, Open Approach
0SPB0JZ Removal of Synthetic Substitute from Left Hip Joint, Open Approach
+ *If replacement see table 0SR to construct a code for the Replacement of the device.*
0SPB0KZ Removal of Nonautologous Tissue Substitute from Left Hip Joint, Open Approach
0SPB30Z Removal of Drainage Device from Left Hip Joint, Percutaneous Approach
0SPB33Z Removal of Infusion Device from Left Hip Joint, Percutaneous Approach
0SPB34Z Removal of Internal Fixation Device from Left Hip Joint, Percutaneous Approach
0SPB35Z Removal of External Fixation Device from Left Hip Joint, Percutaneous Approach
0SPB37Z Removal of Autologous Tissue Substitute from Left Hip Joint, Percutaneous Approach
0SPB38Z Removal of Spacer from Left Hip Joint, Percutaneous Approach
0SPB3JZ Removal of Synthetic Substitute from Left Hip Joint, Percutaneous Approach
0SPB3KZ Removal of Nonautologous Tissue Substitute from Left Hip Joint, Percutaneous Approach
0SPB40Z Removal of Drainage Device from Left Hip Joint, Percutaneous Endoscopic Approach
0SPB43Z Removal of Infusion Device from Left Hip Joint, Percutaneous Endoscopic Approach
0SPB44Z Removal of Internal Fixation Device from Left Hip Joint, Percutaneous Endoscopic Approach
0SPB45Z Removal of External Fixation Device from Left Hip Joint, Percutaneous Endoscopic Approach
0SPB47Z Removal of Autologous Tissue Substitute from Left Hip Joint, Percutaneous Endoscopic Approach
0SPB48Z Removal of Spacer from Left Hip Joint, Percutaneous Endoscopic Approach
0SPB4JZ Removal of Synthetic Substitute from Left Hip Joint, Percutaneous Endoscopic Approach
0SPB4KZ Removal of Nonautologous Tissue Substitute from Left Hip Joint, Percutaneous Endoscopic Approach
0SPBX0Z Removal of Drainage Device from Left Hip Joint, External Approach
0SPBX3Z Removal of Infusion Device from Left Hip Joint, External Approach
0SPBX4Z Removal of Internal Fixation Device from Left Hip Joint, External Approach
0SPBX5Z Removal of External Fixation Device from Left Hip Joint, External Approach
0SPC00Z Removal of Drainage Device from Right Knee Joint, Open Approach
0SPC03Z Removal of Infusion Device from Right Knee Joint, Open Approach
0SPC04Z Removal of Internal Fixation Device from Right Knee Joint, Open Approach
0SPC05Z Removal of External Fixation Device from Right Knee Joint, Open Approach
0SPC07Z Removal of Autologous Tissue Substitute from Right Knee Joint, Open Approach
0SPC08Z Removal of Spacer from Right Knee Joint, Open Approach
0SPC09Z Removal of Liner from Right Knee Joint, Open Approach
+ *If replacement, see table 0SU to construct a code for Supplement with liner.*
0SPC0JZ Removal of Synthetic Substitute from Right Knee Joint, Open Approach
+ *If replacement see table 0SR to construct a code for the Replacement of the device.*
0SPC0KZ Removal of Nonautologous Tissue Substitute from Right Knee Joint, Open Approach
0SPC30Z Removal of Drainage Device from Right Knee Joint, Percutaneous Approach
0SPC33Z Removal of Infusion Device from Right Knee Joint, Percutaneous Approach
0SPC34Z Removal of Internal Fixation Device from Right Knee Joint, Percutaneous Approach
0SPC35Z Removal of External Fixation Device from Right Knee Joint, Percutaneous Approach
0SPC37Z Removal of Autologous Tissue Substitute from Right Knee Joint, Percutaneous Approach
0SPC38Z Removal of Spacer from Right Knee Joint, Percutaneous Approach
0SPC3JZ Removal of Synthetic Substitute from Right Knee Joint, Percutaneous Approach
0SPC3KZ Removal of Nonautologous Tissue Substitute from Right Knee Joint, Percutaneous Approach
0SPC40Z Removal of Drainage Device from Right Knee Joint, Percutaneous Endoscopic Approach
0SPC43Z Removal of Infusion Device from Right Knee Joint, Percutaneous Endoscopic Approach
0SPC44Z Removal of Internal Fixation Device from Right Knee Joint, Percutaneous Endoscopic Approach
0SPC45Z Removal of External Fixation Device from Right Knee Joint, Percutaneous Endoscopic Approach
0SPC47Z Removal of Autologous Tissue Substitute from Right Knee Joint, Percutaneous Endoscopic Approach
0SPC48Z Removal of Spacer from Right Knee Joint, Percutaneous Endoscopic Approach
0SPC4JZ Removal of Synthetic Substitute from Right Knee Joint, Percutaneous Endoscopic Approach
+ *If replacement see table 0SR to construct a code for the Replacement of the device.*
0SPC4KZ Removal of Nonautologous Tissue Substitute from Right Knee Joint, Percutaneous Endoscopic Approach
0SPCX0Z Removal of Drainage Device from Right Knee Joint, External Approach
0SPCX3Z Removal of Infusion Device from Right Knee Joint, External Approach
0SPCX4Z Removal of Internal Fixation Device from Right Knee Joint, External Approach
0SPCX5Z Removal of External Fixation Device from Right Knee Joint, External Approach
0SPD00Z Removal of Drainage Device from Left Knee Joint, Open Approach
0SPD03Z Removal of Infusion Device from Left Knee Joint, Open Approach
0SPD04Z Removal of Internal Fixation Device from Left Knee Joint, Open Approach
0SPD05Z Removal of External Fixation Device from Left Knee Joint, Open Approach
0SPD07Z Removal of Autologous Tissue Substitute from Left Knee Joint, Open Approach
0SPD08Z Removal of Spacer from Left Knee Joint, Open Approach
0SPD09Z Removal of Liner from Left Knee Joint, Open Approach
+ *If replacement, see table 0SU to construct a code for Supplement with liner.*
0SPD0JZ Removal of Synthetic Substitute from Left Knee Joint, Open Approach
+ *If replacement see table 0SR to construct a code for the Replacement of the device.*
0SPD0KZ Removal of Nonautologous Tissue Substitute from Left Knee Joint, Open Approach
0SPD30Z Removal of Drainage Device from Left Knee Joint, Percutaneous Approach
0SPD33Z Removal of Infusion Device from Left Knee Joint, Percutaneous Approach
0SPD34Z Removal of Internal Fixation Device from Left Knee Joint, Percutaneous Approach
0SPD35Z Removal of External Fixation Device from Left Knee Joint, Percutaneous Approach
0SPD37Z Removal of Autologous Tissue Substitute from Left Knee Joint, Percutaneous Approach
0SPD38Z Removal of Spacer from Left Knee Joint, Percutaneous Approach
0SPD3JZ Removal of Synthetic Substitute from Left Knee Joint, Percutaneous Approach

0SPD3KZ Removal of Nonautologous Tissue Substitute from Left Knee Joint, Percutaneous Approach

0SPD40Z Removal of Drainage Device from Left Knee Joint, Percutaneous Endoscopic Approach

0SPD43Z Removal of Infusion Device from Left Knee Joint, Percutaneous Endoscopic Approach

0SPD44Z Removal of Internal Fixation Device from Left Knee Joint, Percutaneous Endoscopic Approach

0SPD45Z Removal of External Fixation Device from Left Knee Joint, Percutaneous Endoscopic Approach

0SPD47Z Removal of Autologous Tissue Substitute from Left Knee Joint, Percutaneous Endoscopic Approach

0SPD48Z Removal of Spacer from Left Knee Joint, Percutaneous Endoscopic Approach

0SPD4JZ Removal of Synthetic Substitute from Left Knee Joint, Percutaneous Endoscopic Approach

+ *If replacement see table 0SR to construct a code for the Replacement of the device.*

0SPD4KZ Removal of Nonautologous Tissue Substitute from Left Knee Joint, Percutaneous Endoscopic Approach

0SPDX0Z Removal of Drainage Device from Left Knee Joint, External Approach

0SPDX3Z Removal of Infusion Device from Left Knee Joint, External Approach

0SPDX4Z Removal of Internal Fixation Device from Left Knee Joint, External Approach

0SPDX5Z Removal of External Fixation Device from Left Knee Joint, External Approach

0SPF00Z Removal of Drainage Device from Right Ankle Joint, Open Approach

0SPF03Z Removal of Infusion Device from Right Ankle Joint, Open Approach

0SPF04Z Removal of Internal Fixation Device from Right Ankle Joint, Open Approach

0SPF05Z Removal of External Fixation Device from Right Ankle Joint, Open Approach

0SPF07Z Removal of Autologous Tissue Substitute from Right Ankle Joint, Open Approach

0SPF08Z Removal of Spacer from Right Ankle Joint, Open Approach

0SPF0JZ Removal of Synthetic Substitute from Right Ankle Joint, Open Approach

0SPF0KZ Removal of Nonautologous Tissue Substitute from Right Ankle Joint, Open Approach

0SPF30Z Removal of Drainage Device from Right Ankle Joint, Percutaneous Approach

0SPF33Z Removal of Infusion Device from Right Ankle Joint, Percutaneous Approach

0SPF34Z Removal of Internal Fixation Device from Right Ankle Joint, Percutaneous Approach

0SPF35Z Removal of External Fixation Device from Right Ankle Joint, Percutaneous Approach

0SPF37Z Removal of Autologous Tissue Substitute from Right Ankle Joint, Percutaneous Approach

0SPF38Z Removal of Spacer from Right Ankle Joint, Percutaneous Approach

0SPF3JZ Removal of Synthetic Substitute from Right Ankle Joint, Percutaneous Approach

0SPF3KZ Removal of Nonautologous Tissue Substitute from Right Ankle Joint, Percutaneous Approach

0SPF40Z Removal of Drainage Device from Right Ankle Joint, Percutaneous Endoscopic Approach

0SPF43Z Removal of Infusion Device from Right Ankle Joint, Percutaneous Endoscopic Approach

0SPF44Z Removal of Internal Fixation Device from Right Ankle Joint, Percutaneous Endoscopic Approach

0SPF45Z Removal of External Fixation Device from Right Ankle Joint, Percutaneous Endoscopic Approach

0SPF47Z Removal of Autologous Tissue Substitute from Right Ankle Joint, Percutaneous Endoscopic Approach

0SPF48Z Removal of Spacer from Right Ankle Joint, Percutaneous Endoscopic Approach

0SPF4JZ Removal of Synthetic Substitute from Right Ankle Joint, Percutaneous Endoscopic Approach

0SPF4KZ Removal of Nonautologous Tissue Substitute from Right Ankle Joint, Percutaneous Endoscopic Approach

0SPFX0Z Removal of Drainage Device from Right Ankle Joint, External Approach

0SPFX3Z Removal of Infusion Device from Right Ankle Joint, External Approach

0SPFX4Z Removal of Internal Fixation Device from Right Ankle Joint, External Approach

0SPFX5Z Removal of External Fixation Device from Right Ankle Joint, External Approach

0SPG00Z Removal of Drainage Device from Left Ankle Joint, Open Approach

0SPG03Z Removal of Infusion Device from Left Ankle Joint, Open Approach

0SPG04Z Removal of Internal Fixation Device from Left Ankle Joint, Open Approach

AHA CC: 2Q, 2013, 39-40

0SPG05Z Removal of External Fixation Device from Left Ankle Joint, Open Approach

0SPG07Z Removal of Autologous Tissue Substitute from Left Ankle Joint, Open Approach

0SPG08Z Removal of Spacer from Left Ankle Joint, Open Approach

0SPG0JZ Removal of Synthetic Substitute from Left Ankle Joint, Open Approach

0SPG0KZ Removal of Nonautologous Tissue Substitute from Left Ankle Joint, Open Approach

0SPG30Z Removal of Drainage Device from Left Ankle Joint, Percutaneous Approach

0SPG33Z Removal of Infusion Device from Left Ankle Joint, Percutaneous Approach

0SPG34Z Removal of Internal Fixation Device from Left Ankle Joint, Percutaneous Approach

0SPG35Z Removal of External Fixation Device from Left Ankle Joint, Percutaneous Approach

0SPG37Z Removal of Autologous Tissue Substitute from Left Ankle Joint, Percutaneous Approach

0SPG38Z Removal of Spacer from Left Ankle Joint, Percutaneous Approach

0SPG3JZ Removal of Synthetic Substitute from Left Ankle Joint, Percutaneous Approach

0SPG3KZ Removal of Nonautologous Tissue Substitute from Left Ankle Joint, Percutaneous Approach

0SPG40Z Removal of Drainage Device from Left Ankle Joint, Percutaneous Endoscopic Approach

0SPG43Z Removal of Infusion Device from Left Ankle Joint, Percutaneous Endoscopic Approach

0SPG44Z Removal of Internal Fixation Device from Left Ankle Joint, Percutaneous Endoscopic Approach

0SPG45Z Removal of External Fixation Device from Left Ankle Joint, Percutaneous Endoscopic Approach

0SPG47Z Removal of Autologous Tissue Substitute from Left Ankle Joint, Percutaneous Endoscopic Approach

0SPG48Z Removal of Spacer from Left Ankle Joint, Percutaneous Endoscopic Approach

0SPG4JZ Removal of Synthetic Substitute from Left Ankle Joint, Percutaneous Endoscopic Approach

0SPG4KZ Removal of Nonautologous Tissue Substitute from Left Ankle Joint, Percutaneous Endoscopic Approach

0SPGX0Z Removal of Drainage Device from Left Ankle Joint, External Approach

0SPGX3Z Removal of Infusion Device from Left Ankle Joint, External Approach

0SPGX4Z Removal of Internal Fixation Device from Left Ankle Joint, External Approach

0SPGX5Z Removal of External Fixation Device from Left Ankle Joint, External Approach

0SPH00Z Removal of Drainage Device from Right Tarsal Joint, Open Approach

0SPH03Z Removal of Infusion Device from Right Tarsal Joint, Open Approach

0SPH04Z Removal of Internal Fixation Device from Right Tarsal Joint, Open Approach

0SPH05Z Removal of External Fixation Device from Right Tarsal Joint, Open Approach

0SPH07Z Removal of Autologous Tissue Substitute from Right Tarsal Joint, Open Approach

0SPH08Z Removal of Spacer from Right Tarsal Joint, Open Approach

0SPH0JZ Removal of Synthetic Substitute from Right Tarsal Joint, Open Approach

0SPH0KZ Removal of Nonautologous Tissue Substitute from Right Tarsal Joint, Open Approach

0SPH30Z Removal of Drainage Device from Right Tarsal Joint, Percutaneous Approach

0SPH33Z Removal of Infusion Device from Right Tarsal Joint, Percutaneous Approach

0SPH34Z Removal of Internal Fixation Device from Right Tarsal Joint, Percutaneous Approach

0SPH35Z Removal of External Fixation Device from Right Tarsal Joint, Percutaneous Approach

0SPH37Z Removal of Autologous Tissue Substitute from Right Tarsal Joint, Percutaneous Approach

0SPH38Z Removal of Spacer from Right Tarsal Joint, Percutaneous Approach

0SPH3JZ Removal of Synthetic Substitute from Right Tarsal Joint, Percutaneous Approach

0SPH3KZ Removal of Nonautologous Tissue Substitute from Right Tarsal Joint, Percutaneous Approach

0SPH40Z Removal of Drainage Device from Right Tarsal Joint, Percutaneous Endoscopic Approach

0SPH43Z Removal of Infusion Device from Right Tarsal Joint, Percutaneous Endoscopic Approach

0SPH44Z Removal of Internal Fixation Device from Right Tarsal Joint, Percutaneous Endoscopic Approach

0SPH45Z Removal of External Fixation Device from Right Tarsal Joint, Percutaneous Endoscopic Approach

0SPH47Z Removal of Autologous Tissue Substitute from Right Tarsal Joint, Percutaneous Endoscopic Approach

0SPH48Z Removal of Spacer from Right Tarsal Joint, Percutaneous Endoscopic Approach

0SPH4JZ Removal of Synthetic Substitute from Right Tarsal Joint, Percutaneous Endoscopic Approach

0SPH4KZ Removal of Nonautologous Tissue Substitute from Right Tarsal Joint, Percutaneous Endoscopic Approach

0SPHX0Z Removal of Drainage Device from Right Tarsal Joint, External Approach

0SPHX3Z Removal of Infusion Device from Right Tarsal Joint, External Approach

0SPHX4Z Removal of Internal Fixation Device from Right Tarsal Joint, External Approach
0SPHX5Z Removal of External Fixation Device from Right Tarsal Joint, External Approach
0SPJ00Z Removal of Drainage Device from Left Tarsal Joint, Open Approach
0SPJ03Z Removal of Infusion Device from Left Tarsal Joint, Open Approach
0SPJ04Z Removal of Internal Fixation Device from Left Tarsal Joint, Open Approach
0SPJ05Z Removal of External Fixation Device from Left Tarsal Joint, Open Approach
0SPJ07Z Removal of Autologous Tissue Substitute from Left Tarsal Joint, Open Approach
0SPJ08Z Removal of Spacer from Left Tarsal Joint, Open Approach
0SPJ0JZ Removal of Synthetic Substitute from Left Tarsal Joint, Open Approach
0SPJ0KZ Removal of Nonautologous Tissue Substitute from Left Tarsal Joint, Open Approach
0SPJ30Z Removal of Drainage Device from Left Tarsal Joint, Percutaneous Approach
0SPJ33Z Removal of Infusion Device from Left Tarsal Joint, Percutaneous Approach
0SPJ34Z Removal of Internal Fixation Device from Left Tarsal Joint, Percutaneous Approach
0SPJ35Z Removal of External Fixation Device from Left Tarsal Joint, Percutaneous Approach
0SPJ37Z Removal of Autologous Tissue Substitute from Left Tarsal Joint, Percutaneous Approach
0SPJ38Z Removal of Spacer from Left Tarsal Joint, Percutaneous Approach
0SPJ3JZ Removal of Synthetic Substitute from Left Tarsal Joint, Percutaneous Approach
0SPJ3KZ Removal of Nonautologous Tissue Substitute from Left Tarsal Joint, Percutaneous Approach
0SPJ40Z Removal of Drainage Device from Left Tarsal Joint, Percutaneous Endoscopic Approach
0SPJ43Z Removal of Infusion Device from Left Tarsal Joint, Percutaneous Endoscopic Approach
0SPJ44Z Removal of Internal Fixation Device from Left Tarsal Joint, Percutaneous Endoscopic Approach
0SPJ45Z Removal of External Fixation Device from Left Tarsal Joint, Percutaneous Endoscopic Approach
0SPJ47Z Removal of Autologous Tissue Substitute from Left Tarsal Joint, Percutaneous Endoscopic Approach
0SPJ48Z Removal of Spacer from Left Tarsal Joint, Percutaneous Endoscopic Approach
0SPJ4JZ Removal of Synthetic Substitute from Left Tarsal Joint, Percutaneous Endoscopic Approach
0SPJ4KZ Removal of Nonautologous Tissue Substitute from Left Tarsal Joint, Percutaneous Endoscopic Approach
0SPJX0Z Removal of Drainage Device from Left Tarsal Joint, External Approach
0SPJX3Z Removal of Infusion Device from Left Tarsal Joint, External Approach
0SPJX4Z Removal of Internal Fixation Device from Left Tarsal Joint, External Approach
0SPJX5Z Removal of External Fixation Device from Left Tarsal Joint, External Approach
0SPK00Z Removal of Drainage Device from Right Metatarsal-Tarsal Joint, Open Approach
0SPK03Z Removal of Infusion Device from Right Metatarsal-Tarsal Joint, Open Approach
0SPK04Z Removal of Internal Fixation Device from Right Metatarsal-Tarsal Joint, Open Approach
0SPK05Z Removal of External Fixation Device from Right Metatarsal-Tarsal Joint, Open Approach
0SPK07Z Removal of Autologous Tissue Substitute from Right Metatarsal-Tarsal Joint, Open Approach
0SPK08Z Removal of Spacer from Right Metatarsal-Tarsal Joint, Open Approach
0SPK0JZ Removal of Synthetic Substitute from Right Metatarsal-Tarsal Joint, Open Approach
0SPK0KZ Removal of Nonautologous Tissue Substitute from Right Metatarsal-Tarsal Joint, Open Approach
0SPK30Z Removal of Drainage Device from Right Metatarsal-Tarsal Joint, Percutaneous Approach
0SPK33Z Removal of Infusion Device from Right Metatarsal-Tarsal Joint, Percutaneous Approach
0SPK34Z Removal of Internal Fixation Device from Right Metatarsal-Tarsal Joint, Percutaneous Approach
0SPK35Z Removal of External Fixation Device from Right Metatarsal-Tarsal Joint, Percutaneous Approach
0SPK37Z Removal of Autologous Tissue Substitute from Right Metatarsal-Tarsal Joint, Percutaneous Approach
0SPK38Z Removal of Spacer from Right Metatarsal-Tarsal Joint, Percutaneous Approach
0SPK3JZ Removal of Synthetic Substitute from Right Metatarsal-Tarsal Joint, Percutaneous Approach
0SPK3KZ Removal of Nonautologous Tissue Substitute from Right Metatarsal-Tarsal Joint, Percutaneous Approach
0SPK40Z Removal of Drainage Device from Right Metatarsal-Tarsal Joint, Percutaneous Endoscopic Approach
0SPK43Z Removal of Infusion Device from Right Metatarsal-Tarsal Joint, Percutaneous Endoscopic Approach
0SPK44Z Removal of Internal Fixation Device from Right Metatarsal-Tarsal Joint, Percutaneous Endoscopic Approach
0SPK45Z Removal of External Fixation Device from Right Metatarsal-Tarsal Joint, Percutaneous Endoscopic Approach
0SPK47Z Removal of Autologous Tissue Substitute from Right Metatarsal-Tarsal Joint, Percutaneous Endoscopic Approach
0SPK48Z Removal of Spacer from Right Metatarsal-Tarsal Joint, Percutaneous Endoscopic Approach
0SPK4JZ Removal of Synthetic Substitute from Right Metatarsal-Tarsal Joint, Percutaneous Endoscopic Approach
0SPK4KZ Removal of Nonautologous Tissue Substitute from Right Metatarsal-Tarsal Joint, Percutaneous Endoscopic Approach
0SPKX0Z Removal of Drainage Device from Right Metatarsal-Tarsal Joint, External Approach
0SPKX3Z Removal of Infusion Device from Right Metatarsal-Tarsal Joint, External Approach
0SPKX4Z Removal of Internal Fixation Device from Right Metatarsal-Tarsal Joint, External Approach
0SPKX5Z Removal of External Fixation Device from Right Metatarsal-Tarsal Joint, External Approach
0SPL00Z Removal of Drainage Device from Left Metatarsal-Tarsal Joint, Open Approach
0SPL03Z Removal of Infusion Device from Left Metatarsal-Tarsal Joint, Open Approach
0SPL04Z Removal of Internal Fixation Device from Left Metatarsal-Tarsal Joint, Open Approach
0SPL05Z Removal of External Fixation Device from Left Metatarsal-Tarsal Joint, Open Approach
0SPL07Z Removal of Autologous Tissue Substitute from Left Metatarsal-Tarsal Joint, Open Approach
0SPL08Z Removal of Spacer from Left Metatarsal-Tarsal Joint, Open Approach
0SPL0JZ Removal of Synthetic Substitute from Left Metatarsal-Tarsal Joint, Open Approach
0SPL0KZ Removal of Nonautologous Tissue Substitute from Left Metatarsal-Tarsal Joint, Open Approach
0SPL30Z Removal of Drainage Device from Left Metatarsal-Tarsal Joint, Percutaneous Approach
0SPL33Z Removal of Infusion Device from Left Metatarsal-Tarsal Joint, Percutaneous Approach
0SPL34Z Removal of Internal Fixation Device from Left Metatarsal-Tarsal Joint, Percutaneous Approach
0SPL35Z Removal of External Fixation Device from Left Metatarsal-Tarsal Joint, Percutaneous Approach
0SPL37Z Removal of Autologous Tissue Substitute from Left Metatarsal-Tarsal Joint, Percutaneous Approach
0SPL38Z Removal of Spacer from Left Metatarsal-Tarsal Joint, Percutaneous Approach
0SPL3JZ Removal of Synthetic Substitute from Left Metatarsal-Tarsal Joint, Percutaneous Approach
0SPL3KZ Removal of Nonautologous Tissue Substitute from Left Metatarsal-Tarsal Joint, Percutaneous Approach
0SPL40Z Removal of Drainage Device from Left Metatarsal-Tarsal Joint, Percutaneous Endoscopic Approach
0SPL43Z Removal of Infusion Device from Left Metatarsal-Tarsal Joint, Percutaneous Endoscopic Approach
0SPL44Z Removal of Internal Fixation Device from Left Metatarsal-Tarsal Joint, Percutaneous Endoscopic Approach
0SPL45Z Removal of External Fixation Device from Left Metatarsal-Tarsal Joint, Percutaneous Endoscopic Approach
0SPL47Z Removal of Autologous Tissue Substitute from Left Metatarsal-Tarsal Joint, Percutaneous Endoscopic Approach
0SPL48Z Removal of Spacer from Left Metatarsal-Tarsal Joint, Percutaneous Endoscopic Approach
0SPL4JZ Removal of Synthetic Substitute from Left Metatarsal-Tarsal Joint, Percutaneous Endoscopic Approach
0SPL4KZ Removal of Nonautologous Tissue Substitute from Left Metatarsal-Tarsal Joint, Percutaneous Endoscopic Approach
0SPLX0Z Removal of Drainage Device from Left Metatarsal-Tarsal Joint, External Approach
0SPLX3Z Removal of Infusion Device from Left Metatarsal-Tarsal Joint, External Approach
0SPLX4Z Removal of Internal Fixation Device from Left Metatarsal-Tarsal Joint, External Approach
0SPLX5Z Removal of External Fixation Device from Left Metatarsal-Tarsal Joint, External Approach
0SPM00Z Removal of Drainage Device from Right Metatarsal-Phalangeal Joint, Open Approach
0SPM03Z Removal of Infusion Device from Right Metatarsal-Phalangeal Joint, Open Approach
0SPM04Z Removal of Internal Fixation Device from Right Metatarsal-Phalangeal Joint, Open Approach

0SPM05Z Removal of External Fixation Device from Right Metatarsal-Phalangeal Joint, Open Approach
0SPM07Z Removal of Autologous Tissue Substitute from Right Metatarsal-Phalangeal Joint, Open Approach
0SPM08Z Removal of Spacer from Right Metatarsal-Phalangeal Joint, Open Approach
0SPM0JZ Removal of Synthetic Substitute from Right Metatarsal-Phalangeal Joint, Open Approach
0SPM0KZ Removal of Nonautologous Tissue Substitute from Right Metatarsal-Phalangeal Joint, Open Approach
0SPM30Z Removal of Drainage Device from Right Metatarsal-Phalangeal Joint, Percutaneous Approach
0SPM33Z Removal of Infusion Device from Right Metatarsal-Phalangeal Joint, Percutaneous Approach
0SPM34Z Removal of Internal Fixation Device from Right Metatarsal-Phalangeal Joint, Percutaneous Approach
0SPM35Z Removal of External Fixation Device from Right Metatarsal-Phalangeal Joint, Percutaneous Approach
0SPM37Z Removal of Autologous Tissue Substitute from Right Metatarsal-Phalangeal Joint, Percutaneous Approach
0SPM38Z Removal of Spacer from Right Metatarsal-Phalangeal Joint, Percutaneous Approach
0SPM3JZ Removal of Synthetic Substitute from Right Metatarsal-Phalangeal Joint, Percutaneous Approach
0SPM3KZ Removal of Nonautologous Tissue Substitute from Right Metatarsal-Phalangeal Joint, Percutaneous Approach
0SPM40Z Removal of Drainage Device from Right Metatarsal-Phalangeal Joint, Percutaneous Endoscopic Approach
0SPM43Z Removal of Infusion Device from Right Metatarsal-Phalangeal Joint, Percutaneous Endoscopic Approach
0SPM44Z Removal of Internal Fixation Device from Right Metatarsal-Phalangeal Joint, Percutaneous Endoscopic Approach
0SPM45Z Removal of External Fixation Device from Right Metatarsal-Phalangeal Joint, Percutaneous Endoscopic Approach
0SPM47Z Removal of Autologous Tissue Substitute from Right Metatarsal-Phalangeal Joint, Percutaneous Endoscopic Approach
0SPM48Z Removal of Spacer from Right Metatarsal-Phalangeal Joint, Percutaneous Endoscopic Approach
0SPM4JZ Removal of Synthetic Substitute from Right Metatarsal-Phalangeal Joint, Percutaneous Endoscopic Approach
0SPM4KZ Removal of Nonautologous Tissue Substitute from Right Metatarsal-Phalangeal Joint, Percutaneous Endoscopic Approach
0SPMX0Z Removal of Drainage Device from Right Metatarsal-Phalangeal Joint, External Approach
0SPMX3Z Removal of Infusion Device from Right Metatarsal-Phalangeal Joint, External Approach
0SPMX4Z Removal of Internal Fixation Device from Right Metatarsal-Phalangeal Joint, External Approach
0SPMX5Z Removal of External Fixation Device from Right Metatarsal-Phalangeal Joint, External Approach
0SPN00Z Removal of Drainage Device from Left Metatarsal-Phalangeal Joint, Open Approach
0SPN03Z Removal of Infusion Device from Left Metatarsal-Phalangeal Joint, Open Approach
0SPN04Z Removal of Internal Fixation Device from Left Metatarsal-Phalangeal Joint, Open Approach
0SPN05Z Removal of External Fixation Device from Left Metatarsal-Phalangeal Joint, Open Approach
0SPN07Z Removal of Autologous Tissue Substitute from Left Metatarsal-Phalangeal Joint, Open Approach
0SPN08Z Removal of Spacer from Left Metatarsal-Phalangeal Joint, Open Approach
0SPN0JZ Removal of Synthetic Substitute from Left Metatarsal-Phalangeal Joint, Open Approach
0SPN0KZ Removal of Nonautologous Tissue Substitute from Left Metatarsal-Phalangeal Joint, Open Approach
0SPN30Z Removal of Drainage Device from Left Metatarsal-Phalangeal Joint, Percutaneous Approach
0SPN33Z Removal of Infusion Device from Left Metatarsal-Phalangeal Joint, Percutaneous Approach
0SPN34Z Removal of Internal Fixation Device from Left Metatarsal-Phalangeal Joint, Percutaneous Approach
0SPN35Z Removal of External Fixation Device from Left Metatarsal-Phalangeal Joint, Percutaneous Approach
0SPN37Z Removal of Autologous Tissue Substitute from Left Metatarsal-Phalangeal Joint, Percutaneous Approach
0SPN38Z Removal of Spacer from Left Metatarsal-Phalangeal Joint, Percutaneous Approach
0SPN3JZ Removal of Synthetic Substitute from Left Metatarsal-Phalangeal Joint, Percutaneous Approach
0SPN3KZ Removal of Nonautologous Tissue Substitute from Left Metatarsal-Phalangeal Joint, Percutaneous Approach
0SPN40Z Removal of Drainage Device from Left Metatarsal-Phalangeal Joint, Percutaneous Endoscopic Approach
0SPN43Z Removal of Infusion Device from Left Metatarsal-Phalangeal Joint, Percutaneous Endoscopic Approach
0SPN44Z Removal of Internal Fixation Device from Left Metatarsal-Phalangeal Joint, Percutaneous Endoscopic Approach
0SPN45Z Removal of External Fixation Device from Left Metatarsal-Phalangeal Joint, Percutaneous Endoscopic Approach
0SPN47Z Removal of Autologous Tissue Substitute from Left Metatarsal-Phalangeal Joint, Percutaneous Endoscopic Approach
0SPN48Z Removal of Spacer from Left Metatarsal-Phalangeal Joint, Percutaneous Endoscopic Approach
0SPN4JZ Removal of Synthetic Substitute from Left Metatarsal-Phalangeal Joint, Percutaneous Endoscopic Approach
0SPN4KZ Removal of Nonautologous Tissue Substitute from Left Metatarsal-Phalangeal Joint, Percutaneous Endoscopic Approach
0SPNX0Z Removal of Drainage Device from Left Metatarsal-Phalangeal Joint, External Approach
0SPNX3Z Removal of Infusion Device from Left Metatarsal-Phalangeal Joint, External Approach
0SPNX4Z Removal of Internal Fixation Device from Left Metatarsal-Phalangeal Joint, External Approach
0SPNX5Z Removal of External Fixation Device from Left Metatarsal-Phalangeal Joint, External Approach
0SPP00Z Removal of Drainage Device from Right Toe Phalangeal Joint, Open Approach
0SPP03Z Removal of Infusion Device from Right Toe Phalangeal Joint, Open Approach
0SPP04Z Removal of Internal Fixation Device from Right Toe Phalangeal Joint, Open Approach
0SPP05Z Removal of External Fixation Device from Right Toe Phalangeal Joint, Open Approach
0SPP07Z Removal of Autologous Tissue Substitute from Right Toe Phalangeal Joint, Open Approach
0SPP08Z Removal of Spacer from Right Toe Phalangeal Joint, Open Approach
0SPP0JZ Removal of Synthetic Substitute from Right Toe Phalangeal Joint, Open Approach
0SPP0KZ Removal of Nonautologous Tissue Substitute from Right Toe Phalangeal Joint, Open Approach
0SPP30Z Removal of Drainage Device from Right Toe Phalangeal Joint, Percutaneous Approach
0SPP33Z Removal of Infusion Device from Right Toe Phalangeal Joint, Percutaneous Approach
0SPP34Z Removal of Internal Fixation Device from Right Toe Phalangeal Joint, Percutaneous Approach
0SPP35Z Removal of External Fixation Device from Right Toe Phalangeal Joint, Percutaneous Approach
0SPP37Z Removal of Autologous Tissue Substitute from Right Toe Phalangeal Joint, Percutaneous Approach
0SPP38Z Removal of Spacer from Right Toe Phalangeal Joint, Percutaneous Approach
0SPP3JZ Removal of Synthetic Substitute from Right Toe Phalangeal Joint, Percutaneous Approach
0SPP3KZ Removal of Nonautologous Tissue Substitute from Right Toe Phalangeal Joint, Percutaneous Approach
0SPP40Z Removal of Drainage Device from Right Toe Phalangeal Joint, Percutaneous Endoscopic Approach
0SPP43Z Removal of Infusion Device from Right Toe Phalangeal Joint, Percutaneous Endoscopic Approach
0SPP44Z Removal of Internal Fixation Device from Right Toe Phalangeal Joint, Percutaneous Endoscopic Approach
0SPP45Z Removal of External Fixation Device from Right Toe Phalangeal Joint, Percutaneous Endoscopic Approach
0SPP47Z Removal of Autologous Tissue Substitute from Right Toe Phalangeal Joint, Percutaneous Endoscopic Approach
0SPP48Z Removal of Spacer from Right Toe Phalangeal Joint, Percutaneous Endoscopic Approach
0SPP4JZ Removal of Synthetic Substitute from Right Toe Phalangeal Joint, Percutaneous Endoscopic Approach
0SPP4KZ Removal of Nonautologous Tissue Substitute from Right Toe Phalangeal Joint, Percutaneous Endoscopic Approach
0SPPX0Z Removal of Drainage Device from Right Toe Phalangeal Joint, External Approach
0SPPX3Z Removal of Infusion Device from Right Toe Phalangeal Joint, External Approach
0SPPX4Z Removal of Internal Fixation Device from Right Toe Phalangeal Joint, External Approach

0SPPX5Z Removal of External Fixation Device from Right Toe Phalangeal Joint, External Approach
0SPQ00Z Removal of Drainage Device from Left Toe Phalangeal Joint, Open Approach
0SPQ03Z Removal of Infusion Device from Left Toe Phalangeal Joint, Open Approach
0SPQ04Z Removal of Internal Fixation Device from Left Toe Phalangeal Joint, Open Approach
0SPQ05Z Removal of External Fixation Device from Left Toe Phalangeal Joint, Open Approach
0SPQ07Z Removal of Autologous Tissue Substitute from Left Toe Phalangeal Joint, Open Approach
0SPQ08Z Removal of Spacer from Left Toe Phalangeal Joint, Open Approach
0SPQ0JZ Removal of Synthetic Substitute from Left Toe Phalangeal Joint, Open Approach
0SPQ0KZ Removal of Nonautologous Tissue Substitute from Left Toe Phalangeal Joint, Open Approach
0SPQ30Z Removal of Drainage Device from Left Toe Phalangeal Joint, Percutaneous Approach
0SPQ33Z Removal of Infusion Device from Left Toe Phalangeal Joint, Percutaneous Approach
0SPQ34Z Removal of Internal Fixation Device from Left Toe Phalangeal Joint, Percutaneous Approach
0SPQ35Z Removal of External Fixation Device from Left Toe Phalangeal Joint, Percutaneous Approach
0SPQ37Z Removal of Autologous Tissue Substitute from Left Toe Phalangeal Joint, Percutaneous Approach
0SPQ38Z Removal of Spacer from Left Toe Phalangeal Joint, Percutaneous Approach
0SPQ3JZ Removal of Synthetic Substitute from Left Toe Phalangeal Joint, Percutaneous Approach
0SPQ3KZ Removal of Nonautologous Tissue Substitute from Left Toe Phalangeal Joint, Percutaneous Approach
0SPQ40Z Removal of Drainage Device from Left Toe Phalangeal Joint, Percutaneous Endoscopic Approach
0SPQ43Z Removal of Infusion Device from Left Toe Phalangeal Joint, Percutaneous Endoscopic Approach
0SPQ44Z Removal of Internal Fixation Device from Left Toe Phalangeal Joint, Percutaneous Endoscopic Approach
0SPQ45Z Removal of External Fixation Device from Left Toe Phalangeal Joint, Percutaneous Endoscopic Approach
0SPQ47Z Removal of Autologous Tissue Substitute from Left Toe Phalangeal Joint, Percutaneous Endoscopic Approach
0SPQ48Z Removal of Spacer from Left Toe Phalangeal Joint, Percutaneous Endoscopic Approach
0SPQ4JZ Removal of Synthetic Substitute from Left Toe Phalangeal Joint, Percutaneous Endoscopic Approach
0SPQ4KZ Removal of Nonautologous Tissue Substitute from Left Toe Phalangeal Joint, Percutaneous Endoscopic Approach
0SPQX0Z Removal of Drainage Device from Left Toe Phalangeal Joint, External Approach
0SPQX3Z Removal of Infusion Device from Left Toe Phalangeal Joint, External Approach
0SPQX4Z Removal of Internal Fixation Device from Left Toe Phalangeal Joint, External Approach
0SPQX5Z Removal of External Fixation Device from Left Toe Phalangeal Joint, External Approach

0SQ – Lower Joints, Repair

Review Coding Guideline B3.5

0SQ00ZZ Repair Lumbar Vertebral Joint, Open Approach
0SQ03ZZ Repair Lumbar Vertebral Joint, Percutaneous Approach
0SQ04ZZ Repair Lumbar Vertebral Joint, Percutaneous Endoscopic Approach
0SQ0XZZ Repair Lumbar Vertebral Joint, External Approach
0SQ20ZZ Repair Lumbar Vertebral Disc, Open Approach
0SQ23ZZ Repair Lumbar Vertebral Disc, Percutaneous Approach
0SQ24ZZ Repair Lumbar Vertebral Disc, Percutaneous Endoscopic Approach
0SQ2XZZ Repair Lumbar Vertebral Disc, External Approach
0SQ30ZZ Repair Lumbosacral Joint, Open Approach
0SQ33ZZ Repair Lumbosacral Joint, Percutaneous Approach
0SQ34ZZ Repair Lumbosacral Joint, Percutaneous Endoscopic Approach
0SQ3XZZ Repair Lumbosacral Joint, External Approach
0SQ40ZZ Repair Lumbosacral Disc, Open Approach
0SQ43ZZ Repair Lumbosacral Disc, Percutaneous Approach
0SQ44ZZ Repair Lumbosacral Disc, Percutaneous Endoscopic Approach
0SQ4XZZ Repair Lumbosacral Disc, External Approach
0SQ50ZZ Repair Sacrococcygeal Joint, Open Approach
0SQ53ZZ Repair Sacrococcygeal Joint, Percutaneous Approach
0SQ54ZZ Repair Sacrococcygeal Joint, Percutaneous Endoscopic Approach
0SQ5XZZ Repair Sacrococcygeal Joint, External Approach
0SQ60ZZ Repair Coccygeal Joint, Open Approach
0SQ63ZZ Repair Coccygeal Joint, Percutaneous Approach
0SQ64ZZ Repair Coccygeal Joint, Percutaneous Endoscopic Approach
0SQ6XZZ Repair Coccygeal Joint, External Approach
0SQ70ZZ Repair Right Sacroiliac Joint, Open Approach
0SQ73ZZ Repair Right Sacroiliac Joint, Percutaneous Approach
0SQ74ZZ Repair Right Sacroiliac Joint, Percutaneous Endoscopic Approach
0SQ7XZZ Repair Right Sacroiliac Joint, External Approach
0SQ80ZZ Repair Left Sacroiliac Joint, Open Approach
0SQ83ZZ Repair Left Sacroiliac Joint, Percutaneous Approach
0SQ84ZZ Repair Left Sacroiliac Joint, Percutaneous Endoscopic Approach
0SQ8XZZ Repair Left Sacroiliac Joint, External Approach
0SQ90ZZ Repair Right Hip Joint, Open Approach
0SQ93ZZ Repair Right Hip Joint, Percutaneous Approach
0SQ94ZZ Repair Right Hip Joint, Percutaneous Endoscopic Approach
0SQ9XZZ Repair Right Hip Joint, External Approach
0SQB0ZZ Repair Left Hip Joint, Open Approach
0SQB3ZZ Repair Left Hip Joint, Percutaneous Approach
0SQB4ZZ Repair Left Hip Joint, Percutaneous Endoscopic Approach
0SQBXZZ Repair Left Hip Joint, External Approach
0SQC0ZZ Repair Right Knee Joint, Open Approach
0SQC3ZZ Repair Right Knee Joint, Percutaneous Approach
0SQC4ZZ Repair Right Knee Joint, Percutaneous Endoscopic Approach
0SQCXZZ Repair Right Knee Joint, External Approach
0SQD0ZZ Repair Left Knee Joint, Open Approach
0SQD3ZZ Repair Left Knee Joint, Percutaneous Approach
0SQD4ZZ Repair Left Knee Joint, Percutaneous Endoscopic Approach
0SQDXZZ Repair Left Knee Joint, External Approach
0SQF0ZZ Repair Right Ankle Joint, Open Approach
0SQF3ZZ Repair Right Ankle Joint, Percutaneous Approach
0SQF4ZZ Repair Right Ankle Joint, Percutaneous Endoscopic Approach
0SQFXZZ Repair Right Ankle Joint, External Approach
0SQG0ZZ Repair Left Ankle Joint, Open Approach
0SQG3ZZ Repair Left Ankle Joint, Percutaneous Approach
0SQG4ZZ Repair Left Ankle Joint, Percutaneous Endoscopic Approach
0SQGXZZ Repair Left Ankle Joint, External Approach
0SQH0ZZ Repair Right Tarsal Joint, Open Approach
0SQH3ZZ Repair Right Tarsal Joint, Percutaneous Approach
0SQH4ZZ Repair Right Tarsal Joint, Percutaneous Endoscopic Approach
0SQHXZZ Repair Right Tarsal Joint, External Approach
0SQJ0ZZ Repair Left Tarsal Joint, Open Approach
0SQJ3ZZ Repair Left Tarsal Joint, Percutaneous Approach
0SQJ4ZZ Repair Left Tarsal Joint, Percutaneous Endoscopic Approach
0SQJXZZ Repair Left Tarsal Joint, External Approach
0SQK0ZZ Repair Right Metatarsal-Tarsal Joint, Open Approach
0SQK3ZZ Repair Right Metatarsal-Tarsal Joint, Percutaneous Approach
0SQK4ZZ Repair Right Metatarsal-Tarsal Joint, Percutaneous Endoscopic Approach
0SQKXZZ Repair Right Metatarsal-Tarsal Joint, External Approach
0SQL0ZZ Repair Left Metatarsal-Tarsal Joint, Open Approach
0SQL3ZZ Repair Left Metatarsal-Tarsal Joint, Percutaneous Approach
0SQL4ZZ Repair Left Metatarsal-Tarsal Joint, Percutaneous Endoscopic Approach
0SQLXZZ Repair Left Metatarsal-Tarsal Joint, External Approach
0SQM0ZZ Repair Right Metatarsal-Phalangeal Joint, Open Approach
0SQM3ZZ Repair Right Metatarsal-Phalangeal Joint, Percutaneous Approach
0SQM4ZZ Repair Right Metatarsal-Phalangeal Joint, Percutaneous Endoscopic Approach
0SQMXZZ Repair Right Metatarsal-Phalangeal Joint, External Approach

0SQN0ZZ Repair Left Metatarsal-Phalangeal Joint, Open Approach
0SQN3ZZ Repair Left Metatarsal-Phalangeal Joint, Percutaneous Approach
0SQN4ZZ Repair Left Metatarsal-Phalangeal Joint, Percutaneous Endoscopic Approach
0SQNXZZ Repair Left Metatarsal-Phalangeal Joint, External Approach
0SQP0ZZ Repair Right Toe Phalangeal Joint, Open Approach
0SQP3ZZ Repair Right Toe Phalangeal Joint, Percutaneous Approach
0SQP4ZZ Repair Right Toe Phalangeal Joint, Percutaneous Endoscopic Approach
0SQPXZZ Repair Right Toe Phalangeal Joint, External Approach
0SQQ0ZZ Repair Left Toe Phalangeal Joint, Open Approach
0SQQ3ZZ Repair Left Toe Phalangeal Joint, Percutaneous Approach
0SQQ4ZZ Repair Left Toe Phalangeal Joint, Percutaneous Endoscopic Approach
0SQQXZZ Repair Left Toe Phalangeal Joint, External Approach

0SR – Lower Joints, Replacement

0SR007Z Replacement of Lumbar Vertebral Joint with Autologous Tissue Substitute, Open Approach
0SR00JZ Replacement of Lumbar Vertebral Joint with Synthetic Substitute, Open Approach
0SR00KZ Replacement of Lumbar Vertebral Joint with Nonautologous Tissue Substitute, Open Approach
0SR207Z Replacement of Lumbar Vertebral Disc with Autologous Tissue Substitute, Open Approach
0SR20JZ Replacement of Lumbar Vertebral Disc with Synthetic Substitute, Open Approach
▲ *When the patients age is greater than 60 years old*
0SR20KZ Replacement of Lumbar Vertebral Disc with Nonautologous Tissue Substitute, Open Approach
0SR307Z Replacement of Lumbosacral Joint with Autologous Tissue Substitute, Open Approach
0SR30JZ Replacement of Lumbosacral Joint with Synthetic Substitute, Open Approach
0SR30KZ Replacement of Lumbosacral Joint with Nonautologous Tissue Substitute, Open Approach
0SR407Z Replacement of Lumbosacral Disc with Autologous Tissue Substitute, Open Approach
0SR40JZ Replacement of Lumbosacral Disc with Synthetic Substitute, Open Approach
▲ *When the patients age is greater than 60 years old*
0SR40KZ Replacement of Lumbosacral Disc with Nonautologous Tissue Substitute, Open Approach
0SR507Z Replacement of Sacrococcygeal Joint with Autologous Tissue Substitute, Open Approach
0SR50JZ Replacement of Sacrococcygeal Joint with Synthetic Substitute, Open Approach
0SR50KZ Replacement of Sacrococcygeal Joint with Nonautologous Tissue Substitute, Open Approach
0SR607Z Replacement of Coccygeal Joint with Autologous Tissue Substitute, Open Approach
0SR60JZ Replacement of Coccygeal Joint with Synthetic Substitute, Open Approach
0SR60KZ Replacement of Coccygeal Joint with Nonautologous Tissue Substitute, Open Approach
0SR707Z Replacement of Right Sacroiliac Joint with Autologous Tissue Substitute, Open Approach
0SR70JZ Replacement of Right Sacroiliac Joint with Synthetic Substitute, Open Approach
0SR70KZ Replacement of Right Sacroiliac Joint with Nonautologous Tissue Substitute, Open Approach
0SR807Z Replacement of Left Sacroiliac Joint with Autologous Tissue Substitute, Open Approach
0SR80JZ Replacement of Left Sacroiliac Joint with Synthetic Substitute, Open Approach
0SR80KZ Replacement of Left Sacroiliac Joint with Nonautologous Tissue Substitute, Open Approach
0SR9019 Replacement of Right Hip Joint with Metal Synthetic Substitute, Cemented, Open Approach
0SR901A Replacement of Right Hip Joint with Metal Synthetic Substitute, Uncemented, Open Approach
0SR901Z Replacement of Right Hip Joint with Metal Synthetic Substitute, Open Approach
0SR9029 Replacement of Right Hip Joint with Metal on Polyethylene Synthetic Substitute, Cemented, Open Approach
0SR902A Replacement of Right Hip Joint with Metal on Polyethylene Synthetic Substitute, Uncemented, Open Approach
0SR902Z Replacement of Right Hip Joint with Metal on Polyethylene Synthetic Substitute, Open Approach
0SR9039 Replacement of Right Hip Joint with Ceramic Synthetic Substitute, Cemented, Open Approach
0SR903A Replacement of Right Hip Joint with Ceramic Synthetic Substitute, Uncemented, Open Approach
0SR903Z Replacement of Right Hip Joint with Ceramic Synthetic Substitute, Open Approach
0SR9049 Replacement of Right Hip Joint with Ceramic on Polyethylene Synthetic Substitute, Cemented, Open Approach
0SR904A Replacement of Right Hip Joint with Ceramic on Polyethylene Synthetic Substitute, Uncemented, Open Approach
0SR904Z Replacement of Right Hip Joint with Ceramic on Polyethylene Synthetic Substitute, Open Approach
0SR907Z Replacement of Right Hip Joint with Autologous Tissue Substitute, Open Approach
0SR90J9 Replacement of Right Hip Joint with Synthetic Substitute, Cemented, Open Approach
0SR90JA Replacement of Right Hip Joint with Synthetic Substitute, Uncemented, Open Approach
0SR90JZ Replacement of Right Hip Joint with Synthetic Substitute, Open Approach
0SR90KZ Replacement of Right Hip Joint with Nonautologous Tissue Substitute, Open Approach
0SRA009 Replacement of Right Hip Joint, Acetabular Surface with Polyethylene Synthetic Substitute, Cemented, Open Approach
0SRA00A Replacement of Right Hip Joint, Acetabular Surface with Polyethylene Synthetic Substitute, Uncemented, Open Approach
0SRA00Z Replacement of Right Hip Joint, Acetabular Surface with Polyethylene Synthetic Substitute, Open Approach
0SRA019 Replacement of Right Hip Joint, Acetabular Surface with Metal Synthetic Substitute, Cemented, Open Approach
0SRA01A Replacement of Right Hip Joint, Acetabular Surface with Metal Synthetic Substitute, Uncemented, Open Approach
0SRA01Z Replacement of Right Hip Joint, Acetabular Surface with Metal Synthetic Substitute, Open Approach
0SRA039 Replacement of Right Hip Joint, Acetabular Surface with Ceramic Synthetic Substitute, Cemented, Open Approach
0SRA03A Replacement of Right Hip Joint, Acetabular Surface with Ceramic Synthetic Substitute, Uncemented, Open Approach
0SRA03Z Replacement of Right Hip Joint, Acetabular Surface with Ceramic Synthetic Substitute, Open Approach
0SRA07Z Replacement of Right Hip Joint, Acetabular Surface with Autologous Tissue Substitute, Open Approach
0SRA0J9 Replacement of Right Hip Joint, Acetabular Surface with Synthetic Substitute, Cemented, Open Approach
0SRA0JA Replacement of Right Hip Joint, Acetabular Surface with Synthetic Substitute, Uncemented, Open Approach
0SRA0JZ Replacement of Right Hip Joint, Acetabular Surface with Synthetic Substitute, Open Approach
0SRA0KZ Replacement of Right Hip Joint, Acetabular Surface with Nonautologous Tissue Substitute, Open Approach
0SRB019 Replacement of Left Hip Joint with Metal Synthetic Substitute, Cemented, Open Approach
0SRB01A Replacement of Left Hip Joint with Metal Synthetic Substitute, Uncemented, Open Approach
0SRB01Z Replacement of Left Hip Joint with Metal Synthetic Substitute, Open Approach
0SRB029 Replacement of Left Hip Joint with Metal on Polyethylene Synthetic Substitute, Cemented, Open Approach
0SRB02A Replacement of Left Hip Joint with Metal on Polyethylene Synthetic Substitute, Uncemented, Open Approach
0SRB02Z Replacement of Left Hip Joint with Metal on Polyethylene Synthetic Substitute, Open Approach
0SRB039 Replacement of Left Hip Joint with Ceramic Synthetic Substitute, Cemented, Open Approach
0SRB03A Replacement of Left Hip Joint with Ceramic Synthetic Substitute, Uncemented, Open Approach
0SRB03Z Replacement of Left Hip Joint with Ceramic Synthetic Substitute, Open Approach
0SRB049 Replacement of Left Hip Joint with Ceramic on Polyethylene Synthetic Substitute, Cemented, Open Approach
0SRB04A Replacement of Left Hip Joint with Ceramic on Polyethylene Synthetic Substitute, Uncemented, Open Approach

0SRB04Z	Replacement of Left Hip Joint with Ceramic on Polyethylene Synthetic Substitute, Open Approach
0SRB07Z	Replacement of Left Hip Joint with Autologous Tissue Substitute, Open Approach
0SRB0J9	Replacement of Left Hip Joint with Synthetic Substitute, Cemented, Open Approach
0SRB0JA	Replacement of Left Hip Joint with Synthetic Substitute, Uncemented, Open Approach
0SRB0JZ	Replacement of Left Hip Joint with Synthetic Substitute, Open Approach
0SRB0KZ	Replacement of Left Hip Joint with Nonautologous Tissue Substitute, Open Approach
0SRC07Z	Replacement of Right Knee Joint with Autologous Tissue Substitute, Open Approach
0SRC0J9	Replacement of Right Knee Joint with Synthetic Substitute, Cemented, Open Approach
0SRC0JA	Replacement of Right Knee Joint with Synthetic Substitute, Uncemented, Open Approach
0SRC0JZ	Replacement of Right Knee Joint with Synthetic Substitute, Open Approach
0SRC0KZ	Replacement of Right Knee Joint with Nonautologous Tissue Substitute, Open Approach
0SRD07Z	Replacement of Left Knee Joint with Autologous Tissue Substitute, Open Approach
0SRD0J9	Replacement of Left Knee Joint with Synthetic Substitute, Cemented, Open Approach
0SRD0JA	Replacement of Left Knee Joint with Synthetic Substitute, Uncemented, Open Approach
0SRD0JZ	Replacement of Left Knee Joint with Synthetic Substitute, Open Approach
0SRD0KZ	Replacement of Left Knee Joint with Nonautologous Tissue Substitute, Open Approach
0SRE009	Replacement of Left Hip Joint, Acetabular Surface with Polyethylene Synthetic Substitute, Cemented, Open Approach
0SRE00A	Replacement of Left Hip Joint, Acetabular Surface with Polyethylene Synthetic Substitute, Uncemented, Open Approach
0SRE00Z	Replacement of Left Hip Joint, Acetabular Surface with Polyethylene Synthetic Substitute, Open Approach
0SRE019	Replacement of Left Hip Joint, Acetabular Surface with Metal Synthetic Substitute, Cemented, Open Approach
0SRE01A	Replacement of Left Hip Joint, Acetabular Surface with Metal Synthetic Substitute, Uncemented, Open Approach
0SRE01Z	Replacement of Left Hip Joint, Acetabular Surface with Metal Synthetic Substitute, Open Approach
0SRE039	Replacement of Left Hip Joint, Acetabular Surface with Ceramic Synthetic Substitute, Cemented, Open Approach
0SRE03A	Replacement of Left Hip Joint, Acetabular Surface with Ceramic Synthetic Substitute, Uncemented, Open Approach
0SRE03Z	Replacement of Left Hip Joint, Acetabular Surface with Ceramic Synthetic Substitute, Open Approach
0SRE07Z	Replacement of Left Hip Joint, Acetabular Surface with Autologous Tissue Substitute, Open Approach
0SRE0J9	Replacement of Left Hip Joint, Acetabular Surface with Synthetic Substitute, Cemented, Open Approach
0SRE0JA	Replacement of Left Hip Joint, Acetabular Surface with Synthetic Substitute, Uncemented, Open Approach
0SRE0JZ	Replacement of Left Hip Joint, Acetabular Surface with Synthetic Substitute, Open Approach
0SRE0KZ	Replacement of Left Hip Joint, Acetabular Surface with Nonautologous Tissue Substitute, Open Approach
0SRF07Z	Replacement of Right Ankle Joint with Autologous Tissue Substitute, Open Approach
0SRF0J9	Replacement of Right Ankle Joint with Synthetic Substitute, Cemented, Open Approach
0SRF0JA	Replacement of Right Ankle Joint with Synthetic Substitute, Uncemented, Open Approach
0SRF0JZ	Replacement of Right Ankle Joint with Synthetic Substitute, Open Approach
0SRF0KZ	Replacement of Right Ankle Joint with Nonautologous Tissue Substitute, Open Approach
0SRG07Z	Replacement of Left Ankle Joint with Autologous Tissue Substitute, Open Approach
0SRG0J9	Replacement of Left Ankle Joint with Synthetic Substitute, Cemented, Open Approach
0SRG0JA	Replacement of Left Ankle Joint with Synthetic Substitute, Uncemented, Open Approach
0SRG0JZ	Replacement of Left Ankle Joint with Synthetic Substitute, Open Approach
0SRG0KZ	Replacement of Left Ankle Joint with Nonautologous Tissue Substitute, Open Approach
0SRH07Z	Replacement of Right Tarsal Joint with Autologous Tissue Substitute, Open Approach
0SRH0JZ	Replacement of Right Tarsal Joint with Synthetic Substitute, Open Approach
0SRH0KZ	Replacement of Right Tarsal Joint with Nonautologous Tissue Substitute, Open Approach
0SRJ07Z	Replacement of Left Tarsal Joint with Autologous Tissue Substitute, Open Approach
0SRJ0JZ	Replacement of Left Tarsal Joint with Synthetic Substitute, Open Approach
0SRJ0KZ	Replacement of Left Tarsal Joint with Nonautologous Tissue Substitute, Open Approach
0SRK07Z	Replacement of Right Metatarsal-Tarsal Joint with Autologous Tissue Substitute, Open Approach
0SRK0JZ	Replacement of Right Metatarsal-Tarsal Joint with Synthetic Substitute, Open Approach
0SRK0KZ	Replacement of Right Metatarsal-Tarsal Joint with Nonautologous Tissue Substitute, Open Approach
0SRL07Z	Replacement of Left Metatarsal-Tarsal Joint with Autologous Tissue Substitute, Open Approach
0SRL0JZ	Replacement of Left Metatarsal-Tarsal Joint with Synthetic Substitute, Open Approach
0SRL0KZ	Replacement of Left Metatarsal-Tarsal Joint with Nonautologous Tissue Substitute, Open Approach
0SRM07Z	Replacement of Right Metatarsal-Phalangeal Joint with Autologous Tissue Substitute, Open Approach
0SRM0JZ	Replacement of Right Metatarsal-Phalangeal Joint with Synthetic Substitute, Open Approach
0SRM0KZ	Replacement of Right Metatarsal-Phalangeal Joint with Nonautologous Tissue Substitute, Open Approach
0SRN07Z	Replacement of Left Metatarsal-Phalangeal Joint with Autologous Tissue Substitute, Open Approach
0SRN0JZ	Replacement of Left Metatarsal-Phalangeal Joint with Synthetic Substitute, Open Approach
0SRN0KZ	Replacement of Left Metatarsal-Phalangeal Joint with Nonautologous Tissue Substitute, Open Approach
0SRP07Z	Replacement of Right Toe Phalangeal Joint with Autologous Tissue Substitute, Open Approach
0SRP0JZ	Replacement of Right Toe Phalangeal Joint with Synthetic Substitute, Open Approach
0SRP0KZ	Replacement of Right Toe Phalangeal Joint with Nonautologous Tissue Substitute, Open Approach
0SRQ07Z	Replacement of Left Toe Phalangeal Joint with Autologous Tissue Substitute, Open Approach
0SRQ0JZ	Replacement of Left Toe Phalangeal Joint with Synthetic Substitute, Open Approach
0SRQ0KZ	Replacement of Left Toe Phalangeal Joint with Nonautologous Tissue Substitute, Open Approach
0SRR019	Replacement of Right Hip Joint, Femoral Surface with Metal Synthetic Substitute, Cemented, Open Approach
0SRR01A	Replacement of Right Hip Joint, Femoral Surface with Metal Synthetic Substitute, Uncemented, Open Approach
0SRR01Z	Replacement of Right Hip Joint, Femoral Surface with Metal Synthetic Substitute, Open Approach
0SRR039	Replacement of Right Hip Joint, Femoral Surface with Ceramic Synthetic Substitute, Cemented, Open Approach
0SRR03A	Replacement of Right Hip Joint, Femoral Surface with Ceramic Synthetic Substitute, Uncemented, Open Approach
0SRR03Z	Replacement of Right Hip Joint, Femoral Surface with Ceramic Synthetic Substitute, Open Approach
0SRR07Z	Replacement of Right Hip Joint, Femoral Surface with Autologous Tissue Substitute, Open Approach
0SRR0J9	Replacement of Right Hip Joint, Femoral Surface with Synthetic Substitute, Cemented, Open Approach
0SRR0JA	Replacement of Right Hip Joint, Femoral Surface with Synthetic Substitute, Uncemented, Open Approach
0SRR0JZ	Replacement of Right Hip Joint, Femoral Surface with Synthetic Substitute, Open Approach
0SRR0KZ	Replacement of Right Hip Joint, Femoral Surface with Nonautologous Tissue Substitute, Open Approach
0SRS019	Replacement of Left Hip Joint, Femoral Surface with Metal Synthetic Substitute, Cemented, Open Approach
0SRS01A	Replacement of Left Hip Joint, Femoral Surface with Metal Synthetic Substitute, Uncemented, Open Approach
0SRS01Z	Replacement of Left Hip Joint, Femoral Surface with Metal Synthetic Substitute, Open Approach
0SRS039	Replacement of Left Hip Joint, Femoral Surface with Ceramic Synthetic Substitute, Cemented, Open Approach
0SRS03A	Replacement of Left Hip Joint, Femoral Surface with Ceramic Synthetic Substitute, Uncemented, Open Approach

0SRS03Z Replacement of Left Hip Joint, Femoral Surface with Ceramic Synthetic Substitute, Open Approach

0SRS07Z Replacement of Left Hip Joint, Femoral Surface with Autologous Tissue Substitute, Open Approach

0SRS0J9 Replacement of Left Hip Joint, Femoral Surface with Synthetic Substitute, Cemented, Open Approach

0SRS0JA Replacement of Left Hip Joint, Femoral Surface with Synthetic Substitute, Uncemented, Open Approach

0SRS0JZ Replacement of Left Hip Joint, Femoral Surface with Synthetic Substitute, Open Approach

0SRS0KZ Replacement of Left Hip Joint, Femoral Surface with Nonautologous Tissue Substitute, Open Approach

0SRT07Z Replacement of Right Knee Joint, Femoral Surface with Autologous Tissue Substitute, Open Approach

0SRT0J9 Replacement of Right Knee Joint, Femoral Surface with Synthetic Substitute, Cemented, Open Approach

0SRT0JA Replacement of Right Knee Joint, Femoral Surface with Synthetic Substitute, Uncemented, Open Approach

0SRT0JZ Replacement of Right Knee Joint, Femoral Surface with Synthetic Substitute, Open Approach

0SRT0KZ Replacement of Right Knee Joint, Femoral Surface with Nonautologous Tissue Substitute, Open Approach

0SRU07Z Replacement of Left Knee Joint, Femoral Surface with Autologous Tissue Substitute, Open Approach

0SRU0J9 Replacement of Left Knee Joint, Femoral Surface with Synthetic Substitute, Cemented, Open Approach

0SRU0JA Replacement of Left Knee Joint, Femoral Surface with Synthetic Substitute, Uncemented, Open Approach

0SRU0JZ Replacement of Left Knee Joint, Femoral Surface with Synthetic Substitute, Open Approach

0SRU0KZ Replacement of Left Knee Joint, Femoral Surface with Nonautologous Tissue Substitute, Open Approach

0SRV07Z Replacement of Right Knee Joint, Tibial Surface with Autologous Tissue Substitute, Open Approach

0SRV0J9 Replacement of Right Knee Joint, Tibial Surface with Synthetic Substitute, Cemented, Open Approach

0SRV0JA Replacement of Right Knee Joint, Tibial Surface with Synthetic Substitute, Uncemented, Open Approach

0SRV0JZ Replacement of Right Knee Joint, Tibial Surface with Synthetic Substitute, Open Approach

0SRV0KZ Replacement of Right Knee Joint, Tibial Surface with Nonautologous Tissue Substitute, Open Approach

0SRW07Z Replacement of Left Knee Joint, Tibial Surface with Autologous Tissue Substitute, Open Approach

0SRW0J9 Replacement of Left Knee Joint, Tibial Surface with Synthetic Substitute, Cemented, Open Approach

0SRW0JA Replacement of Left Knee Joint, Tibial Surface with Synthetic Substitute, Uncemented, Open Approach

0SRW0JZ Replacement of Left Knee Joint, Tibial Surface with Synthetic Substitute, Open Approach

0SRW0KZ Replacement of Left Knee Joint, Tibial Surface with Nonautologous Tissue Substitute, Open Approach

0SS – Lower Joints, Reposition

0SS004Z Reposition Lumbar Vertebral Joint with Internal Fixation Device, Open Approach

0SS00ZZ Reposition Lumbar Vertebral Joint, Open Approach

0SS034Z Reposition Lumbar Vertebral Joint with Internal Fixation Device, Percutaneous Approach

0SS03ZZ Reposition Lumbar Vertebral Joint, Percutaneous Approach

0SS044Z Reposition Lumbar Vertebral Joint with Internal Fixation Device, Percutaneous Endoscopic Approach

0SS04ZZ Reposition Lumbar Vertebral Joint, Percutaneous Endoscopic Approach

0SS0X4Z Reposition Lumbar Vertebral Joint with Internal Fixation Device, External Approach

0SS0XZZ Reposition Lumbar Vertebral Joint, External Approach

0SS304Z Reposition Lumbosacral Joint with Internal Fixation Device, Open Approach

0SS30ZZ Reposition Lumbosacral Joint, Open Approach

0SS334Z Reposition Lumbosacral Joint with Internal Fixation Device, Percutaneous Approach

0SS33ZZ Reposition Lumbosacral Joint, Percutaneous Approach

0SS344Z Reposition Lumbosacral Joint with Internal Fixation Device, Percutaneous Endoscopic Approach

0SS34ZZ Reposition Lumbosacral Joint, Percutaneous Endoscopic Approach

0SS3X4Z Reposition Lumbosacral Joint with Internal Fixation Device, External Approach

0SS3XZZ Reposition Lumbosacral Joint, External Approach

0SS504Z Reposition Sacrococcygeal Joint with Internal Fixation Device, Open Approach

0SS50ZZ Reposition Sacrococcygeal Joint, Open Approach

0SS534Z Reposition Sacrococcygeal Joint with Internal Fixation Device, Percutaneous Approach

0SS53ZZ Reposition Sacrococcygeal Joint, Percutaneous Approach

0SS544Z Reposition Sacrococcygeal Joint with Internal Fixation Device, Percutaneous Endoscopic Approach

0SS54ZZ Reposition Sacrococcygeal Joint, Percutaneous Endoscopic Approach

0SS5X4Z Reposition Sacrococcygeal Joint with Internal Fixation Device, External Approach

0SS5XZZ Reposition Sacrococcygeal Joint, External Approach

0SS604Z Reposition Coccygeal Joint with Internal Fixation Device, Open Approach

0SS60ZZ Reposition Coccygeal Joint, Open Approach

0SS634Z Reposition Coccygeal Joint with Internal Fixation Device, Percutaneous Approach

0SS63ZZ Reposition Coccygeal Joint, Percutaneous Approach

0SS644Z Reposition Coccygeal Joint with Internal Fixation Device, Percutaneous Endoscopic Approach

0SS64ZZ Reposition Coccygeal Joint, Percutaneous Endoscopic Approach

0SS6X4Z Reposition Coccygeal Joint with Internal Fixation Device, External Approach

0SS6XZZ Reposition Coccygeal Joint, External Approach

0SS704Z Reposition Right Sacroiliac Joint with Internal Fixation Device, Open Approach

0SS70ZZ Reposition Right Sacroiliac Joint, Open Approach

0SS734Z Reposition Right Sacroiliac Joint with Internal Fixation Device, Percutaneous Approach

0SS73ZZ Reposition Right Sacroiliac Joint, Percutaneous Approach

0SS744Z Reposition Right Sacroiliac Joint with Internal Fixation Device, Percutaneous Endoscopic Approach

0SS74ZZ Reposition Right Sacroiliac Joint, Percutaneous Endoscopic Approach

0SS7X4Z Reposition Right Sacroiliac Joint with Internal Fixation Device, External Approach

0SS7XZZ Reposition Right Sacroiliac Joint, External Approach

0SS804Z Reposition Left Sacroiliac Joint with Internal Fixation Device, Open Approach

0SS80ZZ Reposition Left Sacroiliac Joint, Open Approach

0SS834Z Reposition Left Sacroiliac Joint with Internal Fixation Device, Percutaneous Approach

0SS83ZZ Reposition Left Sacroiliac Joint, Percutaneous Approach

0SS844Z Reposition Left Sacroiliac Joint with Internal Fixation Device, Percutaneous Endoscopic Approach

0SS84ZZ Reposition Left Sacroiliac Joint, Percutaneous Endoscopic Approach

0SS8X4Z Reposition Left Sacroiliac Joint with Internal Fixation Device, External Approach

0SS8XZZ Reposition Left Sacroiliac Joint, External Approach

0SS904Z Reposition Right Hip Joint with Internal Fixation Device, Open Approach

0SS905Z Reposition Right Hip Joint with External Fixation Device, Open Approach

0SS90ZZ Reposition Right Hip Joint, Open Approach

0SS934Z Reposition Right Hip Joint with Internal Fixation Device, Percutaneous Approach

0SS935Z Reposition Right Hip Joint with External Fixation Device, Percutaneous Approach

0SS93ZZ Reposition Right Hip Joint, Percutaneous Approach

0SS944Z Reposition Right Hip Joint with Internal Fixation Device, Percutaneous Endoscopic Approach

0SS945Z Reposition Right Hip Joint with External Fixation Device, Percutaneous Endoscopic Approach

0SS94ZZ Reposition Right Hip Joint, Percutaneous Endoscopic Approach

0SS9X4Z Reposition Right Hip Joint with Internal Fixation Device, External Approach

0SS9X5Z Reposition Right Hip Joint with External Fixation Device, External Approach

0SS9XZZ Reposition Right Hip Joint, External Approach

0SSB04Z Reposition Left Hip Joint with Internal Fixation Device, Open Approach

0SSB05Z Reposition Left Hip Joint with External Fixation Device, Open Approach

0SSB0ZZ Reposition Left Hip Joint, Open Approach

0SSB34Z Reposition Left Hip Joint with Internal Fixation Device, Percutaneous Approach
0SSB35Z Reposition Left Hip Joint with External Fixation Device, Percutaneous Approach
0SSB3ZZ Reposition Left Hip Joint, Percutaneous Approach
0SSB44Z Reposition Left Hip Joint with Internal Fixation Device, Percutaneous Endoscopic Approach
0SSB45Z Reposition Left Hip Joint with External Fixation Device, Percutaneous Endoscopic Approach
0SSB4ZZ Reposition Left Hip Joint, Percutaneous Endoscopic Approach
0SSBX4Z Reposition Left Hip Joint with Internal Fixation Device, External Approach
0SSBX5Z Reposition Left Hip Joint with External Fixation Device, External Approach
0SSBXZZ Reposition Left Hip Joint, External Approach
0SSC04Z Reposition Right Knee Joint with Internal Fixation Device, Open Approach
0SSC05Z Reposition Right Knee Joint with External Fixation Device, Open Approach
0SSC0ZZ Reposition Right Knee Joint, Open Approach
0SSC34Z Reposition Right Knee Joint with Internal Fixation Device, Percutaneous Approach
0SSC35Z Reposition Right Knee Joint with External Fixation Device, Percutaneous Approach
0SSC3ZZ Reposition Right Knee Joint, Percutaneous Approach
0SSC44Z Reposition Right Knee Joint with Internal Fixation Device, Percutaneous Endoscopic Approach
0SSC45Z Reposition Right Knee Joint with External Fixation Device, Percutaneous Endoscopic Approach
0SSC4ZZ Reposition Right Knee Joint, Percutaneous Endoscopic Approach
0SSCX4Z Reposition Right Knee Joint with Internal Fixation Device, External Approach
0SSCX5Z Reposition Right Knee Joint with External Fixation Device, External Approach
0SSCXZZ Reposition Right Knee Joint, External Approach
0SSD04Z Reposition Left Knee Joint with Internal Fixation Device, Open Approach
0SSD05Z Reposition Left Knee Joint with External Fixation Device, Open Approach
0SSD0ZZ Reposition Left Knee Joint, Open Approach
0SSD34Z Reposition Left Knee Joint with Internal Fixation Device, Percutaneous Approach
0SSD35Z Reposition Left Knee Joint with External Fixation Device, Percutaneous Approach
0SSD3ZZ Reposition Left Knee Joint, Percutaneous Approach
0SSD44Z Reposition Left Knee Joint with Internal Fixation Device, Percutaneous Endoscopic Approach
0SSD45Z Reposition Left Knee Joint with External Fixation Device, Percutaneous Endoscopic Approach
0SSD4ZZ Reposition Left Knee Joint, Percutaneous Endoscopic Approach
0SSDX4Z Reposition Left Knee Joint with Internal Fixation Device, External Approach
0SSDX5Z Reposition Left Knee Joint with External Fixation Device, External Approach
0SSDXZZ Reposition Left Knee Joint, External Approach
0SSF04Z Reposition Right Ankle Joint with Internal Fixation Device, Open Approach
0SSF05Z Reposition Right Ankle Joint with External Fixation Device, Open Approach
0SSF0ZZ Reposition Right Ankle Joint, Open Approach
0SSF34Z Reposition Right Ankle Joint with Internal Fixation Device, Percutaneous Approach
0SSF35Z Reposition Right Ankle Joint with External Fixation Device, Percutaneous Approach
0SSF3ZZ Reposition Right Ankle Joint, Percutaneous Approach
0SSF44Z Reposition Right Ankle Joint with Internal Fixation Device, Percutaneous Endoscopic Approach
0SSF45Z Reposition Right Ankle Joint with External Fixation Device, Percutaneous Endoscopic Approach
0SSF4ZZ Reposition Right Ankle Joint, Percutaneous Endoscopic Approach
0SSFX4Z Reposition Right Ankle Joint with Internal Fixation Device, External Approach
0SSFX5Z Reposition Right Ankle Joint with External Fixation Device, External Approach
0SSFXZZ Reposition Right Ankle Joint, External Approach
0SSG04Z Reposition Left Ankle Joint with Internal Fixation Device, Open Approach
0SSG05Z Reposition Left Ankle Joint with External Fixation Device, Open Approach
0SSG0ZZ Reposition Left Ankle Joint, Open Approach
0SSG34Z Reposition Left Ankle Joint with Internal Fixation Device, Percutaneous Approach
0SSG35Z Reposition Left Ankle Joint with External Fixation Device, Percutaneous Approach
0SSG3ZZ Reposition Left Ankle Joint, Percutaneous Approach
0SSG44Z Reposition Left Ankle Joint with Internal Fixation Device, Percutaneous Endoscopic Approach
0SSG45Z Reposition Left Ankle Joint with External Fixation Device, Percutaneous Endoscopic Approach
0SSG4ZZ Reposition Left Ankle Joint, Percutaneous Endoscopic Approach
0SSGX4Z Reposition Left Ankle Joint with Internal Fixation Device, External Approach
0SSGX5Z Reposition Left Ankle Joint with External Fixation Device, External Approach
0SSGXZZ Reposition Left Ankle Joint, External Approach
0SSH04Z Reposition Right Tarsal Joint with Internal Fixation Device, Open Approach
0SSH05Z Reposition Right Tarsal Joint with External Fixation Device, Open Approach
0SSH0ZZ Reposition Right Tarsal Joint, Open Approach
0SSH34Z Reposition Right Tarsal Joint with Internal Fixation Device, Percutaneous Approach
0SSH35Z Reposition Right Tarsal Joint with External Fixation Device, Percutaneous Approach
0SSH3ZZ Reposition Right Tarsal Joint, Percutaneous Approach
0SSH44Z Reposition Right Tarsal Joint with Internal Fixation Device, Percutaneous Endoscopic Approach
0SSH45Z Reposition Right Tarsal Joint with External Fixation Device, Percutaneous Endoscopic Approach
0SSH4ZZ Reposition Right Tarsal Joint, Percutaneous Endoscopic Approach
0SSHX4Z Reposition Right Tarsal Joint with Internal Fixation Device, External Approach
0SSHX5Z Reposition Right Tarsal Joint with External Fixation Device, External Approach
0SSHXZZ Reposition Right Tarsal Joint, External Approach
0SSJ04Z Reposition Left Tarsal Joint with Internal Fixation Device, Open Approach
0SSJ05Z Reposition Left Tarsal Joint with External Fixation Device, Open Approach
0SSJ0ZZ Reposition Left Tarsal Joint, Open Approach
0SSJ34Z Reposition Left Tarsal Joint with Internal Fixation Device, Percutaneous Approach
0SSJ35Z Reposition Left Tarsal Joint with External Fixation Device, Percutaneous Approach
0SSJ3ZZ Reposition Left Tarsal Joint, Percutaneous Approach
0SSJ44Z Reposition Left Tarsal Joint with Internal Fixation Device, Percutaneous Endoscopic Approach
0SSJ45Z Reposition Left Tarsal Joint with External Fixation Device, Percutaneous Endoscopic Approach
0SSJ4ZZ Reposition Left Tarsal Joint, Percutaneous Endoscopic Approach
0SSJX4Z Reposition Left Tarsal Joint with Internal Fixation Device, External Approach
0SSJX5Z Reposition Left Tarsal Joint with External Fixation Device, External Approach
0SSJXZZ Reposition Left Tarsal Joint, External Approach
0SSK04Z Reposition Right Metatarsal-Tarsal Joint with Internal Fixation Device, Open Approach
0SSK05Z Reposition Right Metatarsal-Tarsal Joint with External Fixation Device, Open Approach
0SSK0ZZ Reposition Right Metatarsal-Tarsal Joint, Open Approach
0SSK34Z Reposition Right Metatarsal-Tarsal Joint with Internal Fixation Device, Percutaneous Approach
0SSK35Z Reposition Right Metatarsal-Tarsal Joint with External Fixation Device, Percutaneous Approach
0SSK3ZZ Reposition Right Metatarsal-Tarsal Joint, Percutaneous Approach
0SSK44Z Reposition Right Metatarsal-Tarsal Joint with Internal Fixation Device, Percutaneous Endoscopic Approach
0SSK45Z Reposition Right Metatarsal-Tarsal Joint with External Fixation Device, Percutaneous Endoscopic Approach
0SSK4ZZ Reposition Right Metatarsal-Tarsal Joint, Percutaneous Endoscopic Approach
0SSKX4Z Reposition Right Metatarsal-Tarsal Joint with Internal Fixation Device, External Approach
0SSKX5Z Reposition Right Metatarsal-Tarsal Joint with External Fixation Device, External Approach
0SSKXZZ Reposition Right Metatarsal-Tarsal Joint, External Approach
0SSL04Z Reposition Left Metatarsal-Tarsal Joint with Internal Fixation Device, Open Approach
0SSL05Z Reposition Left Metatarsal-Tarsal Joint with External Fixation Device, Open Approach
0SSL0ZZ Reposition Left Metatarsal-Tarsal Joint, Open Approach
0SSL34Z Reposition Left Metatarsal-Tarsal Joint with Internal Fixation Device, Percutaneous Approach
0SSL35Z Reposition Left Metatarsal-Tarsal Joint with External Fixation Device, Percutaneous Approach
0SSL3ZZ Reposition Left Metatarsal-Tarsal Joint, Percutaneous Approach

0SSL44Z Reposition Left Metatarsal-Tarsal Joint with Internal Fixation Device, Percutaneous Endoscopic Approach
0SSL45Z Reposition Left Metatarsal-Tarsal Joint with External Fixation Device, Percutaneous Endoscopic Approach
0SSL4ZZ Reposition Left Metatarsal-Tarsal Joint, Percutaneous Endoscopic Approach
0SSLX4Z Reposition Left Metatarsal-Tarsal Joint with Internal Fixation Device, External Approach
0SSLX5Z Reposition Left Metatarsal-Tarsal Joint with External Fixation Device, External Approach
0SSLXZZ Reposition Left Metatarsal-Tarsal Joint, External Approach
0SSM04Z Reposition Right Metatarsal-Phalangeal Joint with Internal Fixation Device, Open Approach
0SSM05Z Reposition Right Metatarsal-Phalangeal Joint with External Fixation Device, Open Approach
0SSM0ZZ Reposition Right Metatarsal-Phalangeal Joint, Open Approach
0SSM34Z Reposition Right Metatarsal-Phalangeal Joint with Internal Fixation Device, Percutaneous Approach
0SSM35Z Reposition Right Metatarsal-Phalangeal Joint with External Fixation Device, Percutaneous Approach
0SSM3ZZ Reposition Right Metatarsal-Phalangeal Joint, Percutaneous Approach
0SSM44Z Reposition Right Metatarsal-Phalangeal Joint with Internal Fixation Device, Percutaneous Endoscopic Approach
0SSM45Z Reposition Right Metatarsal-Phalangeal Joint with External Fixation Device, Percutaneous Endoscopic Approach
0SSM4ZZ Reposition Right Metatarsal-Phalangeal Joint, Percutaneous Endoscopic Approach
0SSMX4Z Reposition Right Metatarsal-Phalangeal Joint with Internal Fixation Device, External Approach
0SSMX5Z Reposition Right Metatarsal-Phalangeal Joint with External Fixation Device, External Approach
0SSMXZZ Reposition Right Metatarsal-Phalangeal Joint, External Approach
0SSN04Z Reposition Left Metatarsal-Phalangeal Joint with Internal Fixation Device, Open Approach
0SSN05Z Reposition Left Metatarsal-Phalangeal Joint with External Fixation Device, Open Approach
0SSN0ZZ Reposition Left Metatarsal-Phalangeal Joint, Open Approach
0SSN34Z Reposition Left Metatarsal-Phalangeal Joint with Internal Fixation Device, Percutaneous Approach
0SSN35Z Reposition Left Metatarsal-Phalangeal Joint with External Fixation Device, Percutaneous Approach
0SSN3ZZ Reposition Left Metatarsal-Phalangeal Joint, Percutaneous Approach
0SSN44Z Reposition Left Metatarsal-Phalangeal Joint with Internal Fixation Device, Percutaneous Endoscopic Approach
0SSN45Z Reposition Left Metatarsal-Phalangeal Joint with External Fixation Device, Percutaneous Endoscopic Approach
0SSN4ZZ Reposition Left Metatarsal-Phalangeal Joint, Percutaneous Endoscopic Approach
0SSNX4Z Reposition Left Metatarsal-Phalangeal Joint with Internal Fixation Device, External Approach
0SSNX5Z Reposition Left Metatarsal-Phalangeal Joint with External Fixation Device, External Approach
0SSNXZZ Reposition Left Metatarsal-Phalangeal Joint, External Approach
0SSP04Z Reposition Right Toe Phalangeal Joint with Internal Fixation Device, Open Approach
0SSP05Z Reposition Right Toe Phalangeal Joint with External Fixation Device, Open Approach
0SSP0ZZ Reposition Right Toe Phalangeal Joint, Open Approach
0SSP34Z Reposition Right Toe Phalangeal Joint with Internal Fixation Device, Percutaneous Approach
0SSP35Z Reposition Right Toe Phalangeal Joint with External Fixation Device, Percutaneous Approach
0SSP3ZZ Reposition Right Toe Phalangeal Joint, Percutaneous Approach
0SSP44Z Reposition Right Toe Phalangeal Joint with Internal Fixation Device, Percutaneous Endoscopic Approach
0SSP45Z Reposition Right Toe Phalangeal Joint with External Fixation Device, Percutaneous Endoscopic Approach
0SSP4ZZ Reposition Right Toe Phalangeal Joint, Percutaneous Endoscopic Approach
0SSPX4Z Reposition Right Toe Phalangeal Joint with Internal Fixation Device, External Approach
0SSPX5Z Reposition Right Toe Phalangeal Joint with External Fixation Device, External Approach
0SSPXZZ Reposition Right Toe Phalangeal Joint, External Approach
0SSQ04Z Reposition Left Toe Phalangeal Joint with Internal Fixation Device, Open Approach
0SSQ05Z Reposition Left Toe Phalangeal Joint with External Fixation Device, Open Approach
0SSQ0ZZ Reposition Left Toe Phalangeal Joint, Open Approach
0SSQ34Z Reposition Left Toe Phalangeal Joint with Internal Fixation Device, Percutaneous Approach
0SSQ35Z Reposition Left Toe Phalangeal Joint with External Fixation Device, Percutaneous Approach
0SSQ3ZZ Reposition Left Toe Phalangeal Joint, Percutaneous Approach
0SSQ44Z Reposition Left Toe Phalangeal Joint with Internal Fixation Device, Percutaneous Endoscopic Approach
0SSQ45Z Reposition Left Toe Phalangeal Joint with External Fixation Device, Percutaneous Endoscopic Approach
0SSQ4ZZ Reposition Left Toe Phalangeal Joint, Percutaneous Endoscopic Approach
0SSQX4Z Reposition Left Toe Phalangeal Joint with Internal Fixation Device, External Approach
0SSQX5Z Reposition Left Toe Phalangeal Joint with External Fixation Device, External Approach
0SSQXZZ Reposition Left Toe Phalangeal Joint, External Approach

0ST – Lower Joints, Resection

Review Coding Guideline B3.8

0ST20ZZ Resection of Lumbar Vertebral Disc, Open Approach
0ST40ZZ Resection of Lumbosacral Disc, Open Approach
0ST50ZZ Resection of Sacrococcygeal Joint, Open Approach
0ST60ZZ Resection of Coccygeal Joint, Open Approach
0ST70ZZ Resection of Right Sacroiliac Joint, Open Approach
0ST80ZZ Resection of Left Sacroiliac Joint, Open Approach
0ST90ZZ Resection of Right Hip Joint, Open Approach
0STB0ZZ Resection of Left Hip Joint, Open Approach
0STC0ZZ Resection of Right Knee Joint, Open Approach
0STD0ZZ Resection of Left Knee Joint, Open Approach
0STF0ZZ Resection of Right Ankle Joint, Open Approach
0STG0ZZ Resection of Left Ankle Joint, Open Approach
0STH0ZZ Resection of Right Tarsal Joint, Open Approach
0STJ0ZZ Resection of Left Tarsal Joint, Open Approach
0STK0ZZ Resection of Right Metatarsal-Tarsal Joint, Open Approach
0STL0ZZ Resection of Left Metatarsal-Tarsal Joint, Open Approach
0STM0ZZ Resection of Right Metatarsal-Phalangeal Joint, Open Approach
0STN0ZZ Resection of Left Metatarsal-Phalangeal Joint, Open Approach
0STP0ZZ Resection of Right Toe Phalangeal Joint, Open Approach
0STQ0ZZ Resection of Left Toe Phalangeal Joint, Open Approach

0SU – Lower Joints, Supplement

0SU007Z Supplement Lumbar Vertebral Joint with Autologous Tissue Substitute, Open Approach
0SU00JZ Supplement Lumbar Vertebral Joint with Synthetic Substitute, Open Approach
0SU00KZ Supplement Lumbar Vertebral Joint with Nonautologous Tissue Substitute, Open Approach
0SU037Z Supplement Lumbar Vertebral Joint with Autologous Tissue Substitute, Percutaneous Approach
0SU03JZ Supplement Lumbar Vertebral Joint with Synthetic Substitute, Percutaneous Approach
0SU03KZ Supplement Lumbar Vertebral Joint with Nonautologous Tissue Substitute, Percutaneous Approach
0SU047Z Supplement Lumbar Vertebral Joint with Autologous Tissue Substitute, Percutaneous Endoscopic Approach
0SU04JZ Supplement Lumbar Vertebral Joint with Synthetic Substitute, Percutaneous Endoscopic Approach
0SU04KZ Supplement Lumbar Vertebral Joint with Nonautologous Tissue Substitute, Percutaneous Endoscopic Approach

0SU207Z Supplement Lumbar Vertebral Disc with Autologous Tissue Substitute, Open Approach
0SU20JZ Supplement Lumbar Vertebral Disc with Synthetic Substitute, Open Approach
0SU20KZ Supplement Lumbar Vertebral Disc with Nonautologous Tissue Substitute, Open Approach
0SU237Z Supplement Lumbar Vertebral Disc with Autologous Tissue Substitute, Percutaneous Approach
0SU23JZ Supplement Lumbar Vertebral Disc with Synthetic Substitute, Percutaneous Approach
0SU23KZ Supplement Lumbar Vertebral Disc with Nonautologous Tissue Substitute, Percutaneous Approach
0SU247Z Supplement Lumbar Vertebral Disc with Autologous Tissue Substitute, Percutaneous Endoscopic Approach
0SU24JZ Supplement Lumbar Vertebral Disc with Synthetic Substitute, Percutaneous Endoscopic Approach
0SU24KZ Supplement Lumbar Vertebral Disc with Nonautologous Tissue Substitute, Percutaneous Endoscopic Approach
0SU307Z Supplement Lumbosacral Joint with Autologous Tissue Substitute, Open Approach
0SU30JZ Supplement Lumbosacral Joint with Synthetic Substitute, Open Approach
0SU30KZ Supplement Lumbosacral Joint with Nonautologous Tissue Substitute, Open Approach
0SU337Z Supplement Lumbosacral Joint with Autologous Tissue Substitute, Percutaneous Approach
0SU33JZ Supplement Lumbosacral Joint with Synthetic Substitute, Percutaneous Approach
0SU33KZ Supplement Lumbosacral Joint with Nonautologous Tissue Substitute, Percutaneous Approach
0SU347Z Supplement Lumbosacral Joint with Autologous Tissue Substitute, Percutaneous Endoscopic Approach
0SU34JZ Supplement Lumbosacral Joint with Synthetic Substitute, Percutaneous Endoscopic Approach
0SU34KZ Supplement Lumbosacral Joint with Nonautologous Tissue Substitute, Percutaneous Endoscopic Approach
0SU407Z Supplement Lumbosacral Disc with Autologous Tissue Substitute, Open Approach
0SU40JZ Supplement Lumbosacral Disc with Synthetic Substitute, Open Approach
0SU40KZ Supplement Lumbosacral Disc with Nonautologous Tissue Substitute, Open Approach
0SU437Z Supplement Lumbosacral Disc with Autologous Tissue Substitute, Percutaneous Approach
0SU43JZ Supplement Lumbosacral Disc with Synthetic Substitute, Percutaneous Approach
0SU43KZ Supplement Lumbosacral Disc with Nonautologous Tissue Substitute, Percutaneous Approach
0SU447Z Supplement Lumbosacral Disc with Autologous Tissue Substitute, Percutaneous Endoscopic Approach
0SU44JZ Supplement Lumbosacral Disc with Synthetic Substitute, Percutaneous Endoscopic Approach
0SU44KZ Supplement Lumbosacral Disc with Nonautologous Tissue Substitute, Percutaneous Endoscopic Approach
0SU507Z Supplement Sacrococcygeal Joint with Autologous Tissue Substitute, Open Approach
0SU50JZ Supplement Sacrococcygeal Joint with Synthetic Substitute, Open Approach
0SU50KZ Supplement Sacrococcygeal Joint with Nonautologous Tissue Substitute, Open Approach
0SU537Z Supplement Sacrococcygeal Joint with Autologous Tissue Substitute, Percutaneous Approach
0SU53JZ Supplement Sacrococcygeal Joint with Synthetic Substitute, Percutaneous Approach
0SU53KZ Supplement Sacrococcygeal Joint with Nonautologous Tissue Substitute, Percutaneous Approach
0SU547Z Supplement Sacrococcygeal Joint with Autologous Tissue Substitute, Percutaneous Endoscopic Approach
0SU54JZ Supplement Sacrococcygeal Joint with Synthetic Substitute, Percutaneous Endoscopic Approach
0SU54KZ Supplement Sacrococcygeal Joint with Nonautologous Tissue Substitute, Percutaneous Endoscopic Approach
0SU607Z Supplement Coccygeal Joint with Autologous Tissue Substitute, Open Approach
0SU60JZ Supplement Coccygeal Joint with Synthetic Substitute, Open Approach
0SU60KZ Supplement Coccygeal Joint with Nonautologous Tissue Substitute, Open Approach
0SU637Z Supplement Coccygeal Joint with Autologous Tissue Substitute, Percutaneous Approach
0SU63JZ Supplement Coccygeal Joint with Synthetic Substitute, Percutaneous Approach
0SU63KZ Supplement Coccygeal Joint with Nonautologous Tissue Substitute, Percutaneous Approach
0SU647Z Supplement Coccygeal Joint with Autologous Tissue Substitute, Percutaneous Endoscopic Approach
0SU64JZ Supplement Coccygeal Joint with Synthetic Substitute, Percutaneous Endoscopic Approach
0SU64KZ Supplement Coccygeal Joint with Nonautologous Tissue Substitute, Percutaneous Endoscopic Approach
0SU707Z Supplement Right Sacroiliac Joint with Autologous Tissue Substitute, Open Approach
0SU70JZ Supplement Right Sacroiliac Joint with Synthetic Substitute, Open Approach
0SU70KZ Supplement Right Sacroiliac Joint with Nonautologous Tissue Substitute, Open Approach
0SU737Z Supplement Right Sacroiliac Joint with Autologous Tissue Substitute, Percutaneous Approach
0SU73JZ Supplement Right Sacroiliac Joint with Synthetic Substitute, Percutaneous Approach
0SU73KZ Supplement Right Sacroiliac Joint with Nonautologous Tissue Substitute, Percutaneous Approach
0SU747Z Supplement Right Sacroiliac Joint with Autologous Tissue Substitute, Percutaneous Endoscopic Approach
0SU74JZ Supplement Right Sacroiliac Joint with Synthetic Substitute, Percutaneous Endoscopic Approach
0SU74KZ Supplement Right Sacroiliac Joint with Nonautologous Tissue Substitute, Percutaneous Endoscopic Approach
0SU807Z Supplement Left Sacroiliac Joint with Autologous Tissue Substitute, Open Approach
0SU80JZ Supplement Left Sacroiliac Joint with Synthetic Substitute, Open Approach
0SU80KZ Supplement Left Sacroiliac Joint with Nonautologous Tissue Substitute, Open Approach
0SU837Z Supplement Left Sacroiliac Joint with Autologous Tissue Substitute, Percutaneous Approach
0SU83JZ Supplement Left Sacroiliac Joint with Synthetic Substitute, Percutaneous Approach
0SU83KZ Supplement Left Sacroiliac Joint with Nonautologous Tissue Substitute, Percutaneous Approach
0SU847Z Supplement Left Sacroiliac Joint with Autologous Tissue Substitute, Percutaneous Endoscopic Approach
0SU84JZ Supplement Left Sacroiliac Joint with Synthetic Substitute, Percutaneous Endoscopic Approach
0SU84KZ Supplement Left Sacroiliac Joint with Nonautologous Tissue Substitute, Percutaneous Endoscopic Approach
0SU907Z Supplement Right Hip Joint with Autologous Tissue Substitute, Open Approach
0SU909Z Supplement Right Hip Joint with Liner, Open Approach
0SU90BZ Supplement Right Hip Joint with Resurfacing Device, Open Approach
HAC When reported with secondary diagnosis code I26.02, I26.09, I26.92, I26.99, I82.401-I82.4Z9
0SU90JZ Supplement Right Hip Joint with Synthetic Substitute, Open Approach
0SU90KZ Supplement Right Hip Joint with Nonautologous Tissue Substitute, Open Approach
0SU937Z Supplement Right Hip Joint with Autologous Tissue Substitute, Percutaneous Approach
0SU93JZ Supplement Right Hip Joint with Synthetic Substitute, Percutaneous Approach
0SU93KZ Supplement Right Hip Joint with Nonautologous Tissue Substitute, Percutaneous Approach
0SU947Z Supplement Right Hip Joint with Autologous Tissue Substitute, Percutaneous Endoscopic Approach
0SU94JZ Supplement Right Hip Joint with Synthetic Substitute, Percutaneous Endoscopic Approach
0SU94KZ Supplement Right Hip Joint with Nonautologous Tissue Substitute, Percutaneous Endoscopic Approach
0SUA09Z Supplement Right Hip Joint, Acetabular Surface with Liner, Open Approach
0SUA0BZ Supplement Right Hip Joint, Acetabular Surface with Resurfacing Device, Open Approach
HAC When reported with secondary diagnosis code I26.02, I26.09, I26.92, I26.99, I82.401-I82.4Z9
0SUB07Z Supplement Left Hip Joint with Autologous Tissue Substitute, Open Approach
0SUB09Z Supplement Left Hip Joint with Liner, Open Approach
0SUB0BZ Supplement Left Hip Joint with Resurfacing Device, Open Approach
HAC When reported with secondary diagnosis code I26.02, I26.09, I26.92, I26.99, I82.401-I82.4Z9
0SUB0JZ Supplement Left Hip Joint with Synthetic Substitute, Open Approach

0SUB0KZ Supplement Left Hip Joint with Nonautologous Tissue Substitute, Open Approach
0SUB37Z Supplement Left Hip Joint with Autologous Tissue Substitute, Percutaneous Approach
0SUB3JZ Supplement Left Hip Joint with Synthetic Substitute, Percutaneous Approach
0SUB3KZ Supplement Left Hip Joint with Nonautologous Tissue Substitute, Percutaneous Approach
0SUB47Z Supplement Left Hip Joint with Autologous Tissue Substitute, Percutaneous Endoscopic Approach
0SUB4JZ Supplement Left Hip Joint with Synthetic Substitute, Percutaneous Endoscopic Approach
0SUB4KZ Supplement Left Hip Joint with Nonautologous Tissue Substitute, Percutaneous Endoscopic Approach
0SUC07Z Supplement Right Knee Joint with Autologous Tissue Substitute, Open Approach
0SUC09C Supplement Right Knee Joint with Liner, Patellar Surface, Open Approach
0SUC09Z Supplement Right Knee Joint with Liner, Open Approach
0SUC0JZ Supplement Right Knee Joint with Synthetic Substitute, Open Approach
0SUC0KZ Supplement Right Knee Joint with Nonautologous Tissue Substitute, Open Approach
0SUC37Z Supplement Right Knee Joint with Autologous Tissue Substitute, Percutaneous Approach
0SUC3JZ Supplement Right Knee Joint with Synthetic Substitute, Percutaneous Approach
0SUC3KZ Supplement Right Knee Joint with Nonautologous Tissue Substitute, Percutaneous Approach
0SUC47Z Supplement Right Knee Joint with Autologous Tissue Substitute, Percutaneous Endoscopic Approach
0SUC4JZ Supplement Right Knee Joint with Synthetic Substitute, Percutaneous Endoscopic Approach
0SUC4KZ Supplement Right Knee Joint with Nonautologous Tissue Substitute, Percutaneous Endoscopic Approach
0SUD07Z Supplement Left Knee Joint with Autologous Tissue Substitute, Open Approach
0SUD09C Supplement Left Knee Joint with Liner, Patellar Surface, Open Approach
0SUD09Z Supplement Left Knee Joint with Liner, Open Approach
0SUD0JZ Supplement Left Knee Joint with Synthetic Substitute, Open Approach
0SUD0KZ Supplement Left Knee Joint with Nonautologous Tissue Substitute, Open Approach
0SUD37Z Supplement Left Knee Joint with Autologous Tissue Substitute, Percutaneous Approach
0SUD3JZ Supplement Left Knee Joint with Synthetic Substitute, Percutaneous Approach
0SUD3KZ Supplement Left Knee Joint with Nonautologous Tissue Substitute, Percutaneous Approach
0SUD47Z Supplement Left Knee Joint with Autologous Tissue Substitute, Percutaneous Endoscopic Approach
0SUD4JZ Supplement Left Knee Joint with Synthetic Substitute, Percutaneous Endoscopic Approach
0SUD4KZ Supplement Left Knee Joint with Nonautologous Tissue Substitute, Percutaneous Endoscopic Approach
0SUE09Z Supplement Left Hip Joint, Acetabular Surface with Liner, Open Approach
0SUE0BZ Supplement Left Hip Joint, Acetabular Surface with Resurfacing Device, Open Approach
HAC When reported with secondary diagnosis code I26.02, I26.09, I26.92, I26.99, I82.401-I82.4Z9
0SUF07Z Supplement Right Ankle Joint with Autologous Tissue Substitute, Open Approach
0SUF0JZ Supplement Right Ankle Joint with Synthetic Substitute, Open Approach
0SUF0KZ Supplement Right Ankle Joint with Nonautologous Tissue Substitute, Open Approach
0SUF37Z Supplement Right Ankle Joint with Autologous Tissue Substitute, Percutaneous Approach
0SUF3JZ Supplement Right Ankle Joint with Synthetic Substitute, Percutaneous Approach
0SUF3KZ Supplement Right Ankle Joint with Nonautologous Tissue Substitute, Percutaneous Approach
0SUF47Z Supplement Right Ankle Joint with Autologous Tissue Substitute, Percutaneous Endoscopic Approach
0SUF4JZ Supplement Right Ankle Joint with Synthetic Substitute, Percutaneous Endoscopic Approach
0SUF4KZ Supplement Right Ankle Joint with Nonautologous Tissue Substitute, Percutaneous Endoscopic Approach
0SUG07Z Supplement Left Ankle Joint with Autologous Tissue Substitute, Open Approach
0SUG0JZ Supplement Left Ankle Joint with Synthetic Substitute, Open Approach
0SUG0KZ Supplement Left Ankle Joint with Nonautologous Tissue Substitute, Open Approach
0SUG37Z Supplement Left Ankle Joint with Autologous Tissue Substitute, Percutaneous Approach
0SUG3JZ Supplement Left Ankle Joint with Synthetic Substitute, Percutaneous Approach
0SUG3KZ Supplement Left Ankle Joint with Nonautologous Tissue Substitute, Percutaneous Approach
0SUG47Z Supplement Left Ankle Joint with Autologous Tissue Substitute, Percutaneous Endoscopic Approach
0SUG4JZ Supplement Left Ankle Joint with Synthetic Substitute, Percutaneous Endoscopic Approach
0SUG4KZ Supplement Left Ankle Joint with Nonautologous Tissue Substitute, Percutaneous Endoscopic Approach
0SUH07Z Supplement Right Tarsal Joint with Autologous Tissue Substitute, Open Approach
0SUH0JZ Supplement Right Tarsal Joint with Synthetic Substitute, Open Approach
0SUH0KZ Supplement Right Tarsal Joint with Nonautologous Tissue Substitute, Open Approach
0SUH37Z Supplement Right Tarsal Joint with Autologous Tissue Substitute, Percutaneous Approach
0SUH3JZ Supplement Right Tarsal Joint with Synthetic Substitute, Percutaneous Approach
0SUH3KZ Supplement Right Tarsal Joint with Nonautologous Tissue Substitute, Percutaneous Approach
0SUH47Z Supplement Right Tarsal Joint with Autologous Tissue Substitute, Percutaneous Endoscopic Approach
0SUH4JZ Supplement Right Tarsal Joint with Synthetic Substitute, Percutaneous Endoscopic Approach
0SUH4KZ Supplement Right Tarsal Joint with Nonautologous Tissue Substitute, Percutaneous Endoscopic Approach
0SUJ07Z Supplement Left Tarsal Joint with Autologous Tissue Substitute, Open Approach
0SUJ0JZ Supplement Left Tarsal Joint with Synthetic Substitute, Open Approach
0SUJ0KZ Supplement Left Tarsal Joint with Nonautologous Tissue Substitute, Open Approach
0SUJ37Z Supplement Left Tarsal Joint with Autologous Tissue Substitute, Percutaneous Approach
0SUJ3JZ Supplement Left Tarsal Joint with Synthetic Substitute, Percutaneous Approach
0SUJ3KZ Supplement Left Tarsal Joint with Nonautologous Tissue Substitute, Percutaneous Approach
0SUJ47Z Supplement Left Tarsal Joint with Autologous Tissue Substitute, Percutaneous Endoscopic Approach
0SUJ4JZ Supplement Left Tarsal Joint with Synthetic Substitute, Percutaneous Endoscopic Approach
0SUJ4KZ Supplement Left Tarsal Joint with Nonautologous Tissue Substitute, Percutaneous Endoscopic Approach
0SUK07Z Supplement Right Metatarsal-Tarsal Joint with Autologous Tissue Substitute, Open Approach
0SUK0JZ Supplement Right Metatarsal-Tarsal Joint with Synthetic Substitute, Open Approach
0SUK0KZ Supplement Right Metatarsal-Tarsal Joint with Nonautologous Tissue Substitute, Open Approach
0SUK37Z Supplement Right Metatarsal-Tarsal Joint with Autologous Tissue Substitute, Percutaneous Approach
0SUK3JZ Supplement Right Metatarsal-Tarsal Joint with Synthetic Substitute, Percutaneous Approach
0SUK3KZ Supplement Right Metatarsal-Tarsal Joint with Nonautologous Tissue Substitute, Percutaneous Approach
0SUK47Z Supplement Right Metatarsal-Tarsal Joint with Autologous Tissue Substitute, Percutaneous Endoscopic Approach
0SUK4JZ Supplement Right Metatarsal-Tarsal Joint with Synthetic Substitute, Percutaneous Endoscopic Approach
0SUK4KZ Supplement Right Metatarsal-Tarsal Joint with Nonautologous Tissue Substitute, Percutaneous Endoscopic Approach
0SUL07Z Supplement Left Metatarsal-Tarsal Joint with Autologous Tissue Substitute, Open Approach
0SUL0JZ Supplement Left Metatarsal-Tarsal Joint with Synthetic Substitute, Open Approach
0SUL0KZ Supplement Left Metatarsal-Tarsal Joint with Nonautologous Tissue Substitute, Open Approach
0SUL37Z Supplement Left Metatarsal-Tarsal Joint with Autologous Tissue Substitute, Percutaneous Approach
0SUL3JZ Supplement Left Metatarsal-Tarsal Joint with Synthetic Substitute, Percutaneous Approach

0SUL3KZ Supplement Left Metatarsal-Tarsal Joint with Nonautologous Tissue Substitute, Percutaneous Approach
0SUL47Z Supplement Left Metatarsal-Tarsal Joint with Autologous Tissue Substitute, Percutaneous Endoscopic Approach
0SUL4JZ Supplement Left Metatarsal-Tarsal Joint with Synthetic Substitute, Percutaneous Endoscopic Approach
0SUL4KZ Supplement Left Metatarsal-Tarsal Joint with Nonautologous Tissue Substitute, Percutaneous Endoscopic Approach
0SUM07Z Supplement Right Metatarsal-Phalangeal Joint with Autologous Tissue Substitute, Open Approach
0SUM0JZ Supplement Right Metatarsal-Phalangeal Joint with Synthetic Substitute, Open Approach
0SUM0KZ Supplement Right Metatarsal-Phalangeal Joint with Nonautologous Tissue Substitute, Open Approach
0SUM37Z Supplement Right Metatarsal-Phalangeal Joint with Autologous Tissue Substitute, Percutaneous Approach
0SUM3JZ Supplement Right Metatarsal-Phalangeal Joint with Synthetic Substitute, Percutaneous Approach
0SUM3KZ Supplement Right Metatarsal-Phalangeal Joint with Nonautologous Tissue Substitute, Percutaneous Approach
0SUM47Z Supplement Right Metatarsal-Phalangeal Joint with Autologous Tissue Substitute, Percutaneous Endoscopic Approach
0SUM4JZ Supplement Right Metatarsal-Phalangeal Joint with Synthetic Substitute, Percutaneous Endoscopic Approach
0SUM4KZ Supplement Right Metatarsal-Phalangeal Joint with Nonautologous Tissue Substitute, Percutaneous Endoscopic Approach
0SUN07Z Supplement Left Metatarsal-Phalangeal Joint with Autologous Tissue Substitute, Open Approach
0SUN0JZ Supplement Left Metatarsal-Phalangeal Joint with Synthetic Substitute, Open Approach
0SUN0KZ Supplement Left Metatarsal-Phalangeal Joint with Nonautologous Tissue Substitute, Open Approach
0SUN37Z Supplement Left Metatarsal-Phalangeal Joint with Autologous Tissue Substitute, Percutaneous Approach
0SUN3JZ Supplement Left Metatarsal-Phalangeal Joint with Synthetic Substitute, Percutaneous Approach
0SUN3KZ Supplement Left Metatarsal-Phalangeal Joint with Nonautologous Tissue Substitute, Percutaneous Approach
0SUN47Z Supplement Left Metatarsal-Phalangeal Joint with Autologous Tissue Substitute, Percutaneous Endoscopic Approach
0SUN4JZ Supplement Left Metatarsal-Phalangeal Joint with Synthetic Substitute, Percutaneous Endoscopic Approach
0SUN4KZ Supplement Left Metatarsal-Phalangeal Joint with Nonautologous Tissue Substitute, Percutaneous Endoscopic Approach
0SUP07Z Supplement Right Toe Phalangeal Joint with Autologous Tissue Substitute, Open Approach
0SUP0JZ Supplement Right Toe Phalangeal Joint with Synthetic Substitute, Open Approach
0SUP0KZ Supplement Right Toe Phalangeal Joint with Nonautologous Tissue Substitute, Open Approach
0SUP37Z Supplement Right Toe Phalangeal Joint with Autologous Tissue Substitute, Percutaneous Approach
0SUP3JZ Supplement Right Toe Phalangeal Joint with Synthetic Substitute, Percutaneous Approach
0SUP3KZ Supplement Right Toe Phalangeal Joint with Nonautologous Tissue Substitute, Percutaneous Approach
0SUP47Z Supplement Right Toe Phalangeal Joint with Autologous Tissue Substitute, Percutaneous Endoscopic Approach
0SUP4JZ Supplement Right Toe Phalangeal Joint with Synthetic Substitute, Percutaneous Endoscopic Approach
0SUP4KZ Supplement Right Toe Phalangeal Joint with Nonautologous Tissue Substitute, Percutaneous Endoscopic Approach
0SUQ07Z Supplement Left Toe Phalangeal Joint with Autologous Tissue Substitute, Open Approach
0SUQ0JZ Supplement Left Toe Phalangeal Joint with Synthetic Substitute, Open Approach
0SUQ0KZ Supplement Left Toe Phalangeal Joint with Nonautologous Tissue Substitute, Open Approach
0SUQ37Z Supplement Left Toe Phalangeal Joint with Autologous Tissue Substitute, Percutaneous Approach
0SUQ3JZ Supplement Left Toe Phalangeal Joint with Synthetic Substitute, Percutaneous Approach
0SUQ3KZ Supplement Left Toe Phalangeal Joint with Nonautologous Tissue Substitute, Percutaneous Approach
0SUQ47Z Supplement Left Toe Phalangeal Joint with Autologous Tissue Substitute, Percutaneous Endoscopic Approach
0SUQ4JZ Supplement Left Toe Phalangeal Joint with Synthetic Substitute, Percutaneous Endoscopic Approach
0SUQ4KZ Supplement Left Toe Phalangeal Joint with Nonautologous Tissue Substitute, Percutaneous Endoscopic Approach
0SUR09Z Supplement Right Hip Joint, Femoral Surface with Liner, Open Approach
0SUR0BZ Supplement Right Hip Joint, Femoral Surface with Resurfacing Device, Open Approach
HAC When reported with secondary diagnosis code I26.02, I26.09, I26.92, I26.99, I82.401-I82.4Z9
0SUS09Z Supplement Left Hip Joint, Femoral Surface with Liner, Open Approach
0SUS0BZ Supplement Left Hip Joint, Femoral Surface with Resurfacing Device, Open Approach
HAC When reported with secondary diagnosis code I26.02, I26.09, I26.92, I26.99, I82.401-I82.4Z9
0SUT09Z Supplement Right Knee Joint, Femoral Surface with Liner, Open Approach
0SUU09Z Supplement Left Knee Joint, Femoral Surface with Liner, Open Approach
0SUV09Z Supplement Right Knee Joint, Tibial Surface with Liner, Open Approach
0SUW09Z Supplement Left Knee Joint, Tibial Surface with Liner, Open Approach

0SW – Lower Joints, Revision

Review Coding Guideline B6.1c

0SW000Z Revision of Drainage Device in Lumbar Vertebral Joint, Open Approach
0SW003Z Revision of Infusion Device in Lumbar Vertebral Joint, Open Approach
0SW004Z Revision of Internal Fixation Device in Lumbar Vertebral Joint, Open Approach
0SW007Z Revision of Autologous Tissue Substitute in Lumbar Vertebral Joint, Open Approach
0SW008Z Revision of Spacer in Lumbar Vertebral Joint, Open Approach
0SW00AZ Revision of Interbody Fusion Device in Lumbar Vertebral Joint, Open Approach
0SW00JZ Revision of Synthetic Substitute in Lumbar Vertebral Joint, Open Approach
0SW00KZ Revision of Nonautologous Tissue Substitute in Lumbar Vertebral Joint, Open Approach
0SW030Z Revision of Drainage Device in Lumbar Vertebral Joint, Percutaneous Approach
0SW033Z Revision of Infusion Device in Lumbar Vertebral Joint, Percutaneous Approach
0SW034Z Revision of Internal Fixation Device in Lumbar Vertebral Joint, Percutaneous Approach
0SW037Z Revision of Autologous Tissue Substitute in Lumbar Vertebral Joint, Percutaneous Approach
0SW038Z Revision of Spacer in Lumbar Vertebral Joint, Percutaneous Approach
0SW03AZ Revision of Interbody Fusion Device in Lumbar Vertebral Joint, Percutaneous Approach
0SW03JZ Revision of Synthetic Substitute in Lumbar Vertebral Joint, Percutaneous Approach
0SW03KZ Revision of Nonautologous Tissue Substitute in Lumbar Vertebral Joint, Percutaneous Approach
0SW040Z Revision of Drainage Device in Lumbar Vertebral Joint, Percutaneous Endoscopic Approach
0SW043Z Revision of Infusion Device in Lumbar Vertebral Joint, Percutaneous Endoscopic Approach
0SW044Z Revision of Internal Fixation Device in Lumbar Vertebral Joint, Percutaneous Endoscopic Approach
0SW047Z Revision of Autologous Tissue Substitute in Lumbar Vertebral Joint, Percutaneous Endoscopic Approach
0SW048Z Revision of Spacer in Lumbar Vertebral Joint, Percutaneous Endoscopic Approach
0SW04AZ Revision of Interbody Fusion Device in Lumbar Vertebral Joint, Percutaneous Endoscopic Approach
0SW04JZ Revision of Synthetic Substitute in Lumbar Vertebral Joint, Percutaneous Endoscopic Approach
0SW04KZ Revision of Nonautologous Tissue Substitute in Lumbar Vertebral Joint, Percutaneous Endoscopic Approach
0SW0X0Z Revision of Drainage Device in Lumbar Vertebral Joint, External Approach
0SW0X3Z Revision of Infusion Device in Lumbar Vertebral Joint, External Approach
0SW0X4Z Revision of Internal Fixation Device in Lumbar Vertebral Joint, External Approach
0SW0X7Z Revision of Autologous Tissue Substitute in Lumbar Vertebral Joint, External Approach

0SW0X8Z Revision of Spacer in Lumbar Vertebral Joint, External Approach
0SW0XAZ Revision of Interbody Fusion Device in Lumbar Vertebral Joint, External Approach
0SW0XJZ Revision of Synthetic Substitute in Lumbar Vertebral Joint, External Approach
0SW0XKZ Revision of Nonautologous Tissue Substitute in Lumbar Vertebral Joint, External Approach
0SW200Z Revision of Drainage Device in Lumbar Vertebral Disc, Open Approach
0SW203Z Revision of Infusion Device in Lumbar Vertebral Disc, Open Approach
0SW207Z Revision of Autologous Tissue Substitute in Lumbar Vertebral Disc, Open Approach
0SW20JZ Revision of Synthetic Substitute in Lumbar Vertebral Disc, Open Approach
0SW20KZ Revision of Nonautologous Tissue Substitute in Lumbar Vertebral Disc, Open Approach
0SW230Z Revision of Drainage Device in Lumbar Vertebral Disc, Percutaneous Approach
0SW233Z Revision of Infusion Device in Lumbar Vertebral Disc, Percutaneous Approach
0SW237Z Revision of Autologous Tissue Substitute in Lumbar Vertebral Disc, Percutaneous Approach
0SW23JZ Revision of Synthetic Substitute in Lumbar Vertebral Disc, Percutaneous Approach
0SW23KZ Revision of Nonautologous Tissue Substitute in Lumbar Vertebral Disc, Percutaneous Approach
0SW240Z Revision of Drainage Device in Lumbar Vertebral Disc, Percutaneous Endoscopic Approach
0SW243Z Revision of Infusion Device in Lumbar Vertebral Disc, Percutaneous Endoscopic Approach
0SW247Z Revision of Autologous Tissue Substitute in Lumbar Vertebral Disc, Percutaneous Endoscopic Approach
0SW24JZ Revision of Synthetic Substitute in Lumbar Vertebral Disc, Percutaneous Endoscopic Approach
0SW24KZ Revision of Nonautologous Tissue Substitute in Lumbar Vertebral Disc, Percutaneous Endoscopic Approach
0SW2X0Z Revision of Drainage Device in Lumbar Vertebral Disc, External Approach
0SW2X3Z Revision of Infusion Device in Lumbar Vertebral Disc, External Approach
0SW2X7Z Revision of Autologous Tissue Substitute in Lumbar Vertebral Disc, External Approach
0SW2XJZ Revision of Synthetic Substitute in Lumbar Vertebral Disc, External Approach
0SW2XKZ Revision of Nonautologous Tissue Substitute in Lumbar Vertebral Disc, External Approach
0SW300Z Revision of Drainage Device in Lumbosacral Joint, Open Approach
0SW303Z Revision of Infusion Device in Lumbosacral Joint, Open Approach
0SW304Z Revision of Internal Fixation Device in Lumbosacral Joint, Open Approach
0SW307Z Revision of Autologous Tissue Substitute in Lumbosacral Joint, Open Approach
0SW308Z Revision of Spacer in Lumbosacral Joint, Open Approach
0SW30AZ Revision of Interbody Fusion Device in Lumbosacral Joint, Open Approach
0SW30JZ Revision of Synthetic Substitute in Lumbosacral Joint, Open Approach
0SW30KZ Revision of Nonautologous Tissue Substitute in Lumbosacral Joint, Open Approach
0SW330Z Revision of Drainage Device in Lumbosacral Joint, Percutaneous Approach
0SW333Z Revision of Infusion Device in Lumbosacral Joint, Percutaneous Approach
0SW334Z Revision of Internal Fixation Device in Lumbosacral Joint, Percutaneous Approach
0SW337Z Revision of Autologous Tissue Substitute in Lumbosacral Joint, Percutaneous Approach
0SW338Z Revision of Spacer in Lumbosacral Joint, Percutaneous Approach
0SW33AZ Revision of Interbody Fusion Device in Lumbosacral Joint, Percutaneous Approach
0SW33JZ Revision of Synthetic Substitute in Lumbosacral Joint, Percutaneous Approach
0SW33KZ Revision of Nonautologous Tissue Substitute in Lumbosacral Joint, Percutaneous Approach
0SW340Z Revision of Drainage Device in Lumbosacral Joint, Percutaneous Endoscopic Approach
0SW343Z Revision of Infusion Device in Lumbosacral Joint, Percutaneous Endoscopic Approach
0SW344Z Revision of Internal Fixation Device in Lumbosacral Joint, Percutaneous Endoscopic Approach
0SW347Z Revision of Autologous Tissue Substitute in Lumbosacral Joint, Percutaneous Endoscopic Approach
0SW348Z Revision of Spacer in Lumbosacral Joint, Percutaneous Endoscopic Approach
0SW34AZ Revision of Interbody Fusion Device in Lumbosacral Joint, Percutaneous Endoscopic Approach
0SW34JZ Revision of Synthetic Substitute in Lumbosacral Joint, Percutaneous Endoscopic Approach
0SW34KZ Revision of Nonautologous Tissue Substitute in Lumbosacral Joint, Percutaneous Endoscopic Approach
0SW3X0Z Revision of Drainage Device in Lumbosacral Joint, External Approach
0SW3X3Z Revision of Infusion Device in Lumbosacral Joint, External Approach
0SW3X4Z Revision of Internal Fixation Device in Lumbosacral Joint, External Approach
0SW3X7Z Revision of Autologous Tissue Substitute in Lumbosacral Joint, External Approach
0SW3X8Z Revision of Spacer in Lumbosacral Joint, External Approach
0SW3XAZ Revision of Interbody Fusion Device in Lumbosacral Joint, External Approach
0SW3XJZ Revision of Synthetic Substitute in Lumbosacral Joint, External Approach
0SW3XKZ Revision of Nonautologous Tissue Substitute in Lumbosacral Joint, External Approach
0SW400Z Revision of Drainage Device in Lumbosacral Disc, Open Approach
0SW403Z Revision of Infusion Device in Lumbosacral Disc, Open Approach
0SW407Z Revision of Autologous Tissue Substitute in Lumbosacral Disc, Open Approach
0SW40JZ Revision of Synthetic Substitute in Lumbosacral Disc, Open Approach
0SW40KZ Revision of Nonautologous Tissue Substitute in Lumbosacral Disc, Open Approach
0SW430Z Revision of Drainage Device in Lumbosacral Disc, Percutaneous Approach
0SW433Z Revision of Infusion Device in Lumbosacral Disc, Percutaneous Approach
0SW437Z Revision of Autologous Tissue Substitute in Lumbosacral Disc, Percutaneous Approach
0SW43JZ Revision of Synthetic Substitute in Lumbosacral Disc, Percutaneous Approach
0SW43KZ Revision of Nonautologous Tissue Substitute in Lumbosacral Disc, Percutaneous Approach
0SW440Z Revision of Drainage Device in Lumbosacral Disc, Percutaneous Endoscopic Approach
0SW443Z Revision of Infusion Device in Lumbosacral Disc, Percutaneous Endoscopic Approach
0SW447Z Revision of Autologous Tissue Substitute in Lumbosacral Disc, Percutaneous Endoscopic Approach
0SW44JZ Revision of Synthetic Substitute in Lumbosacral Disc, Percutaneous Endoscopic Approach
0SW44KZ Revision of Nonautologous Tissue Substitute in Lumbosacral Disc, Percutaneous Endoscopic Approach
0SW4X0Z Revision of Drainage Device in Lumbosacral Disc, External Approach
0SW4X3Z Revision of Infusion Device in Lumbosacral Disc, External Approach
0SW4X7Z Revision of Autologous Tissue Substitute in Lumbosacral Disc, External Approach
0SW4XJZ Revision of Synthetic Substitute in Lumbosacral Disc, External Approach
0SW4XKZ Revision of Nonautologous Tissue Substitute in Lumbosacral Disc, External Approach
0SW500Z Revision of Drainage Device in Sacrococcygeal Joint, Open Approach
0SW503Z Revision of Infusion Device in Sacrococcygeal Joint, Open Approach
0SW504Z Revision of Internal Fixation Device in Sacrococcygeal Joint, Open Approach
0SW507Z Revision of Autologous Tissue Substitute in Sacrococcygeal Joint, Open Approach
0SW508Z Revision of Spacer in Sacrococcygeal Joint, Open Approach
0SW50JZ Revision of Synthetic Substitute in Sacrococcygeal Joint, Open Approach
0SW50KZ Revision of Nonautologous Tissue Substitute in Sacrococcygeal Joint, Open Approach
0SW530Z Revision of Drainage Device in Sacrococcygeal Joint, Percutaneous Approach
0SW533Z Revision of Infusion Device in Sacrococcygeal Joint, Percutaneous Approach
0SW534Z Revision of Internal Fixation Device in Sacrococcygeal Joint, Percutaneous Approach
0SW537Z Revision of Autologous Tissue Substitute in Sacrococcygeal Joint, Percutaneous Approach
0SW538Z Revision of Spacer in Sacrococcygeal Joint, Percutaneous Approach
0SW53JZ Revision of Synthetic Substitute in Sacrococcygeal Joint, Percutaneous Approach
0SW53KZ Revision of Nonautologous Tissue Substitute in Sacrococcygeal Joint, Percutaneous Approach

0SW540Z Revision of Drainage Device in Sacrococcygeal Joint, Percutaneous Endoscopic Approach
0SW543Z Revision of Infusion Device in Sacrococcygeal Joint, Percutaneous Endoscopic Approach
0SW544Z Revision of Internal Fixation Device in Sacrococcygeal Joint, Percutaneous Endoscopic Approach
0SW547Z Revision of Autologous Tissue Substitute in Sacrococcygeal Joint, Percutaneous Endoscopic Approach
0SW548Z Revision of Spacer in Sacrococcygeal Joint, Percutaneous Endoscopic Approach
0SW54JZ Revision of Synthetic Substitute in Sacrococcygeal Joint, Percutaneous Endoscopic Approach
0SW54KZ Revision of Nonautologous Tissue Substitute in Sacrococcygeal Joint, Percutaneous Endoscopic Approach
0SW5X0Z Revision of Drainage Device in Sacrococcygeal Joint, External Approach
0SW5X3Z Revision of Infusion Device in Sacrococcygeal Joint, External Approach
0SW5X4Z Revision of Internal Fixation Device in Sacrococcygeal Joint, External Approach
0SW5X7Z Revision of Autologous Tissue Substitute in Sacrococcygeal Joint, External Approach
0SW5X8Z Revision of Spacer in Sacrococcygeal Joint, External Approach
0SW5XJZ Revision of Synthetic Substitute in Sacrococcygeal Joint, External Approach
0SW5XKZ Revision of Nonautologous Tissue Substitute in Sacrococcygeal Joint, External Approach
0SW600Z Revision of Drainage Device in Coccygeal Joint, Open Approach
0SW603Z Revision of Infusion Device in Coccygeal Joint, Open Approach
0SW604Z Revision of Internal Fixation Device in Coccygeal Joint, Open Approach
0SW607Z Revision of Autologous Tissue Substitute in Coccygeal Joint, Open Approach
0SW608Z Revision of Spacer in Coccygeal Joint, Open Approach
0SW60JZ Revision of Synthetic Substitute in Coccygeal Joint, Open Approach
0SW60KZ Revision of Nonautologous Tissue Substitute in Coccygeal Joint, Open Approach
0SW630Z Revision of Drainage Device in Coccygeal Joint, Percutaneous Approach
0SW633Z Revision of Infusion Device in Coccygeal Joint, Percutaneous Approach
0SW634Z Revision of Internal Fixation Device in Coccygeal Joint, Percutaneous Approach
0SW637Z Revision of Autologous Tissue Substitute in Coccygeal Joint, Percutaneous Approach
0SW638Z Revision of Spacer in Coccygeal Joint, Percutaneous Approach
0SW63JZ Revision of Synthetic Substitute in Coccygeal Joint, Percutaneous Approach
0SW63KZ Revision of Nonautologous Tissue Substitute in Coccygeal Joint, Percutaneous Approach
0SW640Z Revision of Drainage Device in Coccygeal Joint, Percutaneous Endoscopic Approach
0SW643Z Revision of Infusion Device in Coccygeal Joint, Percutaneous Endoscopic Approach
0SW644Z Revision of Internal Fixation Device in Coccygeal Joint, Percutaneous Endoscopic Approach
0SW647Z Revision of Autologous Tissue Substitute in Coccygeal Joint, Percutaneous Endoscopic Approach
0SW648Z Revision of Spacer in Coccygeal Joint, Percutaneous Endoscopic Approach
0SW64JZ Revision of Synthetic Substitute in Coccygeal Joint, Percutaneous Endoscopic Approach
0SW64KZ Revision of Nonautologous Tissue Substitute in Coccygeal Joint, Percutaneous Endoscopic Approach
0SW6X0Z Revision of Drainage Device in Coccygeal Joint, External Approach
0SW6X3Z Revision of Infusion Device in Coccygeal Joint, External Approach
0SW6X4Z Revision of Internal Fixation Device in Coccygeal Joint, External Approach
0SW6X7Z Revision of Autologous Tissue Substitute in Coccygeal Joint, External Approach
0SW6X8Z Revision of Spacer in Coccygeal Joint, External Approach
0SW6XJZ Revision of Synthetic Substitute in Coccygeal Joint, External Approach
0SW6XKZ Revision of Nonautologous Tissue Substitute in Coccygeal Joint, External Approach
0SW700Z Revision of Drainage Device in Right Sacroiliac Joint, Open Approach
0SW703Z Revision of Infusion Device in Right Sacroiliac Joint, Open Approach
0SW704Z Revision of Internal Fixation Device in Right Sacroiliac Joint, Open Approach
0SW707Z Revision of Autologous Tissue Substitute in Right Sacroiliac Joint, Open Approach
0SW708Z Revision of Spacer in Right Sacroiliac Joint, Open Approach
0SW70JZ Revision of Synthetic Substitute in Right Sacroiliac Joint, Open Approach
0SW70KZ Revision of Nonautologous Tissue Substitute in Right Sacroiliac Joint, Open Approach
0SW730Z Revision of Drainage Device in Right Sacroiliac Joint, Percutaneous Approach
0SW733Z Revision of Infusion Device in Right Sacroiliac Joint, Percutaneous Approach
0SW734Z Revision of Internal Fixation Device in Right Sacroiliac Joint, Percutaneous Approach
0SW737Z Revision of Autologous Tissue Substitute in Right Sacroiliac Joint, Percutaneous Approach
0SW738Z Revision of Spacer in Right Sacroiliac Joint, Percutaneous Approach
0SW73JZ Revision of Synthetic Substitute in Right Sacroiliac Joint, Percutaneous Approach
0SW73KZ Revision of Nonautologous Tissue Substitute in Right Sacroiliac Joint, Percutaneous Approach
0SW740Z Revision of Drainage Device in Right Sacroiliac Joint, Percutaneous Endoscopic Approach
0SW743Z Revision of Infusion Device in Right Sacroiliac Joint, Percutaneous Endoscopic Approach
0SW744Z Revision of Internal Fixation Device in Right Sacroiliac Joint, Percutaneous Endoscopic Approach
0SW747Z Revision of Autologous Tissue Substitute in Right Sacroiliac Joint, Percutaneous Endoscopic Approach
0SW748Z Revision of Spacer in Right Sacroiliac Joint, Percutaneous Endoscopic Approach
0SW74JZ Revision of Synthetic Substitute in Right Sacroiliac Joint, Percutaneous Endoscopic Approach
0SW74KZ Revision of Nonautologous Tissue Substitute in Right Sacroiliac Joint, Percutaneous Endoscopic Approach
0SW7X0Z Revision of Drainage Device in Right Sacroiliac Joint, External Approach
0SW7X3Z Revision of Infusion Device in Right Sacroiliac Joint, External Approach
0SW7X4Z Revision of Internal Fixation Device in Right Sacroiliac Joint, External Approach
0SW7X7Z Revision of Autologous Tissue Substitute in Right Sacroiliac Joint, External Approach
0SW7X8Z Revision of Spacer in Right Sacroiliac Joint, External Approach
0SW7XJZ Revision of Synthetic Substitute in Right Sacroiliac Joint, External Approach
0SW7XKZ Revision of Nonautologous Tissue Substitute in Right Sacroiliac Joint, External Approach
0SW800Z Revision of Drainage Device in Left Sacroiliac Joint, Open Approach
0SW803Z Revision of Infusion Device in Left Sacroiliac Joint, Open Approach
0SW804Z Revision of Internal Fixation Device in Left Sacroiliac Joint, Open Approach
0SW807Z Revision of Autologous Tissue Substitute in Left Sacroiliac Joint, Open Approach
0SW808Z Revision of Spacer in Left Sacroiliac Joint, Open Approach
0SW80JZ Revision of Synthetic Substitute in Left Sacroiliac Joint, Open Approach
0SW80KZ Revision of Nonautologous Tissue Substitute in Left Sacroiliac Joint, Open Approach
0SW830Z Revision of Drainage Device in Left Sacroiliac Joint, Percutaneous Approach
0SW833Z Revision of Infusion Device in Left Sacroiliac Joint, Percutaneous Approach
0SW834Z Revision of Internal Fixation Device in Left Sacroiliac Joint, Percutaneous Approach
0SW837Z Revision of Autologous Tissue Substitute in Left Sacroiliac Joint, Percutaneous Approach
0SW838Z Revision of Spacer in Left Sacroiliac Joint, Percutaneous Approach
0SW83JZ Revision of Synthetic Substitute in Left Sacroiliac Joint, Percutaneous Approach
0SW83KZ Revision of Nonautologous Tissue Substitute in Left Sacroiliac Joint, Percutaneous Approach
0SW840Z Revision of Drainage Device in Left Sacroiliac Joint, Percutaneous Endoscopic Approach
0SW843Z Revision of Infusion Device in Left Sacroiliac Joint, Percutaneous Endoscopic Approach
0SW844Z Revision of Internal Fixation Device in Left Sacroiliac Joint, Percutaneous Endoscopic Approach
0SW847Z Revision of Autologous Tissue Substitute in Left Sacroiliac Joint, Percutaneous Endoscopic Approach
0SW848Z Revision of Spacer in Left Sacroiliac Joint, Percutaneous Endoscopic Approach
0SW84JZ Revision of Synthetic Substitute in Left Sacroiliac Joint, Percutaneous Endoscopic Approach
0SW84KZ Revision of Nonautologous Tissue Substitute in Left Sacroiliac Joint, Percutaneous Endoscopic Approach
0SW8X0Z Revision of Drainage Device in Left Sacroiliac Joint, External Approach
0SW8X3Z Revision of Infusion Device in Left Sacroiliac Joint, External Approach
0SW8X4Z Revision of Internal Fixation Device in Left Sacroiliac Joint, External Approach
0SW8X7Z Revision of Autologous Tissue Substitute in Left Sacroiliac Joint, External Approach
0SW8X8Z Revision of Spacer in Left Sacroiliac Joint, External Approach

0SW8XJZ Revision of Synthetic Substitute in Left Sacroiliac Joint, External Approach
0SW8XKZ Revision of Nonautologous Tissue Substitute in Left Sacroiliac Joint, External Approach
0SW900Z Revision of Drainage Device in Right Hip Joint, Open Approach
0SW903Z Revision of Infusion Device in Right Hip Joint, Open Approach
0SW904Z Revision of Internal Fixation Device in Right Hip Joint, Open Approach
0SW905Z Revision of External Fixation Device in Right Hip Joint, Open Approach
0SW907Z Revision of Autologous Tissue Substitute in Right Hip Joint, Open Approach
0SW908Z Revision of Spacer in Right Hip Joint, Open Approach
0SW909Z Revision of Liner in Right Hip Joint, Open Approach
0SW90BZ Revision of Resurfacing Device in Right Hip Joint, Open Approach
0SW90JZ Revision of Synthetic Substitute in Right Hip Joint, Open Approach
0SW90KZ Revision of Nonautologous Tissue Substitute in Right Hip Joint, Open Approach
0SW930Z Revision of Drainage Device in Right Hip Joint, Percutaneous Approach
0SW933Z Revision of Infusion Device in Right Hip Joint, Percutaneous Approach
0SW934Z Revision of Internal Fixation Device in Right Hip Joint, Percutaneous Approach
0SW935Z Revision of External Fixation Device in Right Hip Joint, Percutaneous Approach
0SW937Z Revision of Autologous Tissue Substitute in Right Hip Joint, Percutaneous Approach
0SW938Z Revision of Spacer in Right Hip Joint, Percutaneous Approach
0SW93JZ Revision of Synthetic Substitute in Right Hip Joint, Percutaneous Approach
0SW93KZ Revision of Nonautologous Tissue Substitute in Right Hip Joint, Percutaneous Approach
0SW940Z Revision of Drainage Device in Right Hip Joint, Percutaneous Endoscopic Approach
0SW943Z Revision of Infusion Device in Right Hip Joint, Percutaneous Endoscopic Approach
0SW944Z Revision of Internal Fixation Device in Right Hip Joint, Percutaneous Endoscopic Approach
0SW945Z Revision of External Fixation Device in Right Hip Joint, Percutaneous Endoscopic Approach
0SW947Z Revision of Autologous Tissue Substitute in Right Hip Joint, Percutaneous Endoscopic Approach
0SW948Z Revision of Spacer in Right Hip Joint, Percutaneous Endoscopic Approach
0SW94JZ Revision of Synthetic Substitute in Right Hip Joint, Percutaneous Endoscopic Approach
0SW94KZ Revision of Nonautologous Tissue Substitute in Right Hip Joint, Percutaneous Endoscopic Approach
0SW9X0Z Revision of Drainage Device in Right Hip Joint, External Approach
0SW9X3Z Revision of Infusion Device in Right Hip Joint, External Approach
0SW9X4Z Revision of Internal Fixation Device in Right Hip Joint, External Approach
0SW9X5Z Revision of External Fixation Device in Right Hip Joint, External Approach
0SW9X7Z Revision of Autologous Tissue Substitute in Right Hip Joint, External Approach
0SW9X8Z Revision of Spacer in Right Hip Joint, External Approach
0SW9XJZ Revision of Synthetic Substitute in Right Hip Joint, External Approach
0SW9XKZ Revision of Nonautologous Tissue Substitute in Right Hip Joint, External Approach
0SWB00Z Revision of Drainage Device in Left Hip Joint, Open Approach
0SWB03Z Revision of Infusion Device in Left Hip Joint, Open Approach
0SWB04Z Revision of Internal Fixation Device in Left Hip Joint, Open Approach
0SWB05Z Revision of External Fixation Device in Left Hip Joint, Open Approach
0SWB07Z Revision of Autologous Tissue Substitute in Left Hip Joint, Open Approach
0SWB08Z Revision of Spacer in Left Hip Joint, Open Approach
0SWB09Z Revision of Liner in Left Hip Joint, Open Approach
0SWB0BZ Revision of Resurfacing Device in Left Hip Joint, Open Approach
0SWB0JZ Revision of Synthetic Substitute in Left Hip Joint, Open Approach
0SWB0KZ Revision of Nonautologous Tissue Substitute in Left Hip Joint, Open Approach
0SWB30Z Revision of Drainage Device in Left Hip Joint, Percutaneous Approach
0SWB33Z Revision of Infusion Device in Left Hip Joint, Percutaneous Approach
0SWB34Z Revision of Internal Fixation Device in Left Hip Joint, Percutaneous Approach
0SWB35Z Revision of External Fixation Device in Left Hip Joint, Percutaneous Approach
0SWB37Z Revision of Autologous Tissue Substitute in Left Hip Joint, Percutaneous Approach
0SWB38Z Revision of Spacer in Left Hip Joint, Percutaneous Approach
0SWB3JZ Revision of Synthetic Substitute in Left Hip Joint, Percutaneous Approach
0SWB3KZ Revision of Nonautologous Tissue Substitute in Left Hip Joint, Percutaneous Approach
0SWB40Z Revision of Drainage Device in Left Hip Joint, Percutaneous Endoscopic Approach
0SWB43Z Revision of Infusion Device in Left Hip Joint, Percutaneous Endoscopic Approach
0SWB44Z Revision of Internal Fixation Device in Left Hip Joint, Percutaneous Endoscopic Approach
0SWB45Z Revision of External Fixation Device in Left Hip Joint, Percutaneous Endoscopic Approach
0SWB47Z Revision of Autologous Tissue Substitute in Left Hip Joint, Percutaneous Endoscopic Approach
0SWB48Z Revision of Spacer in Left Hip Joint, Percutaneous Endoscopic Approach
0SWB4JZ Revision of Synthetic Substitute in Left Hip Joint, Percutaneous Endoscopic Approach
0SWB4KZ Revision of Nonautologous Tissue Substitute in Left Hip Joint, Percutaneous Endoscopic Approach
0SWBX0Z Revision of Drainage Device in Left Hip Joint, External Approach
0SWBX3Z Revision of Infusion Device in Left Hip Joint, External Approach
0SWBX4Z Revision of Internal Fixation Device in Left Hip Joint, External Approach
0SWBX5Z Revision of External Fixation Device in Left Hip Joint, External Approach
0SWBX7Z Revision of Autologous Tissue Substitute in Left Hip Joint, External Approach
0SWBX8Z Revision of Spacer in Left Hip Joint, External Approach
0SWBXJZ Revision of Synthetic Substitute in Left Hip Joint, External Approach
0SWBXKZ Revision of Nonautologous Tissue Substitute in Left Hip Joint, External Approach
0SWC00Z Revision of Drainage Device in Right Knee Joint, Open Approach
0SWC03Z Revision of Infusion Device in Right Knee Joint, Open Approach
0SWC04Z Revision of Internal Fixation Device in Right Knee Joint, Open Approach
0SWC05Z Revision of External Fixation Device in Right Knee Joint, Open Approach
0SWC07Z Revision of Autologous Tissue Substitute in Right Knee Joint, Open Approach
0SWC08Z Revision of Spacer in Right Knee Joint, Open Approach
0SWC09Z Revision of Liner in Right Knee Joint, Open Approach
0SWC0JZ Revision of Synthetic Substitute in Right Knee Joint, Open Approach
0SWC0KZ Revision of Nonautologous Tissue Substitute in Right Knee Joint, Open Approach
0SWC30Z Revision of Drainage Device in Right Knee Joint, Percutaneous Approach
0SWC33Z Revision of Infusion Device in Right Knee Joint, Percutaneous Approach
0SWC34Z Revision of Internal Fixation Device in Right Knee Joint, Percutaneous Approach
0SWC35Z Revision of External Fixation Device in Right Knee Joint, Percutaneous Approach
0SWC37Z Revision of Autologous Tissue Substitute in Right Knee Joint, Percutaneous Approach
0SWC38Z Revision of Spacer in Right Knee Joint, Percutaneous Approach
0SWC3JZ Revision of Synthetic Substitute in Right Knee Joint, Percutaneous Approach
0SWC3KZ Revision of Nonautologous Tissue Substitute in Right Knee Joint, Percutaneous Approach
0SWC40Z Revision of Drainage Device in Right Knee Joint, Percutaneous Endoscopic Approach
0SWC43Z Revision of Infusion Device in Right Knee Joint, Percutaneous Endoscopic Approach
0SWC44Z Revision of Internal Fixation Device in Right Knee Joint, Percutaneous Endoscopic Approach
0SWC45Z Revision of External Fixation Device in Right Knee Joint, Percutaneous Endoscopic Approach
0SWC47Z Revision of Autologous Tissue Substitute in Right Knee Joint, Percutaneous Endoscopic Approach
0SWC48Z Revision of Spacer in Right Knee Joint, Percutaneous Endoscopic Approach
0SWC4JZ Revision of Synthetic Substitute in Right Knee Joint, Percutaneous Endoscopic Approach
0SWC4KZ Revision of Nonautologous Tissue Substitute in Right Knee Joint, Percutaneous Endoscopic Approach
0SWCX0Z Revision of Drainage Device in Right Knee Joint, External Approach
0SWCX3Z Revision of Infusion Device in Right Knee Joint, External Approach
0SWCX4Z Revision of Internal Fixation Device in Right Knee Joint, External Approach
0SWCX5Z Revision of External Fixation Device in Right Knee Joint, External Approach
0SWCX7Z Revision of Autologous Tissue Substitute in Right Knee Joint, External Approach
0SWCX8Z Revision of Spacer in Right Knee Joint, External Approach
0SWCXJZ Revision of Synthetic Substitute in Right Knee Joint, External Approach

0SWCXKZ Revision of Nonautologous Tissue Substitute in Right Knee Joint, External Approach
0SWD00Z Revision of Drainage Device in Left Knee Joint, Open Approach
0SWD03Z Revision of Infusion Device in Left Knee Joint, Open Approach
0SWD04Z Revision of Internal Fixation Device in Left Knee Joint, Open Approach
0SWD05Z Revision of External Fixation Device in Left Knee Joint, Open Approach
0SWD07Z Revision of Autologous Tissue Substitute in Left Knee Joint, Open Approach
0SWD08Z Revision of Spacer in Left Knee Joint, Open Approach
0SWD09Z Revision of Liner in Left Knee Joint, Open Approach
0SWD0JZ Revision of Synthetic Substitute in Left Knee Joint, Open Approach
0SWD0KZ Revision of Nonautologous Tissue Substitute in Left Knee Joint, Open Approach
0SWD30Z Revision of Drainage Device in Left Knee Joint, Percutaneous Approach
0SWD33Z Revision of Infusion Device in Left Knee Joint, Percutaneous Approach
0SWD34Z Revision of Internal Fixation Device in Left Knee Joint, Percutaneous Approach
0SWD35Z Revision of External Fixation Device in Left Knee Joint, Percutaneous Approach
0SWD37Z Revision of Autologous Tissue Substitute in Left Knee Joint, Percutaneous Approach
0SWD38Z Revision of Spacer in Left Knee Joint, Percutaneous Approach
0SWD3JZ Revision of Synthetic Substitute in Left Knee Joint, Percutaneous Approach
0SWD3KZ Revision of Nonautologous Tissue Substitute in Left Knee Joint, Percutaneous Approach
0SWD40Z Revision of Drainage Device in Left Knee Joint, Percutaneous Endoscopic Approach
0SWD43Z Revision of Infusion Device in Left Knee Joint, Percutaneous Endoscopic Approach
0SWD44Z Revision of Internal Fixation Device in Left Knee Joint, Percutaneous Endoscopic Approach
0SWD45Z Revision of External Fixation Device in Left Knee Joint, Percutaneous Endoscopic Approach
0SWD47Z Revision of Autologous Tissue Substitute in Left Knee Joint, Percutaneous Endoscopic Approach
0SWD48Z Revision of Spacer in Left Knee Joint, Percutaneous Endoscopic Approach
0SWD4JZ Revision of Synthetic Substitute in Left Knee Joint, Percutaneous Endoscopic Approach
0SWD4KZ Revision of Nonautologous Tissue Substitute in Left Knee Joint, Percutaneous Endoscopic Approach
0SWDX0Z Revision of Drainage Device in Left Knee Joint, External Approach
0SWDX3Z Revision of Infusion Device in Left Knee Joint, External Approach
0SWDX4Z Revision of Internal Fixation Device in Left Knee Joint, External Approach
0SWDX5Z Revision of External Fixation Device in Left Knee Joint, External Approach
0SWDX7Z Revision of Autologous Tissue Substitute in Left Knee Joint, External Approach
0SWDX8Z Revision of Spacer in Left Knee Joint, External Approach
0SWDXJZ Revision of Synthetic Substitute in Left Knee Joint, External Approach
0SWDXKZ Revision of Nonautologous Tissue Substitute in Left Knee Joint, External Approach
0SWF00Z Revision of Drainage Device in Right Ankle Joint, Open Approach
0SWF03Z Revision of Infusion Device in Right Ankle Joint, Open Approach
0SWF04Z Revision of Internal Fixation Device in Right Ankle Joint, Open Approach
0SWF05Z Revision of External Fixation Device in Right Ankle Joint, Open Approach
0SWF07Z Revision of Autologous Tissue Substitute in Right Ankle Joint, Open Approach
0SWF08Z Revision of Spacer in Right Ankle Joint, Open Approach
0SWF0JZ Revision of Synthetic Substitute in Right Ankle Joint, Open Approach
0SWF0KZ Revision of Nonautologous Tissue Substitute in Right Ankle Joint, Open Approach
0SWF30Z Revision of Drainage Device in Right Ankle Joint, Percutaneous Approach
0SWF33Z Revision of Infusion Device in Right Ankle Joint, Percutaneous Approach
0SWF34Z Revision of Internal Fixation Device in Right Ankle Joint, Percutaneous Approach
0SWF35Z Revision of External Fixation Device in Right Ankle Joint, Percutaneous Approach
0SWF37Z Revision of Autologous Tissue Substitute in Right Ankle Joint, Percutaneous Approach
0SWF38Z Revision of Spacer in Right Ankle Joint, Percutaneous Approach
0SWF3JZ Revision of Synthetic Substitute in Right Ankle Joint, Percutaneous Approach
0SWF3KZ Revision of Nonautologous Tissue Substitute in Right Ankle Joint, Percutaneous Approach
0SWF40Z Revision of Drainage Device in Right Ankle Joint, Percutaneous Endoscopic Approach
0SWF43Z Revision of Infusion Device in Right Ankle Joint, Percutaneous Endoscopic Approach
0SWF44Z Revision of Internal Fixation Device in Right Ankle Joint, Percutaneous Endoscopic Approach
0SWF45Z Revision of External Fixation Device in Right Ankle Joint, Percutaneous Endoscopic Approach
0SWF47Z Revision of Autologous Tissue Substitute in Right Ankle Joint, Percutaneous Endoscopic Approach
0SWF48Z Revision of Spacer in Right Ankle Joint, Percutaneous Endoscopic Approach
0SWF4JZ Revision of Synthetic Substitute in Right Ankle Joint, Percutaneous Endoscopic Approach
0SWF4KZ Revision of Nonautologous Tissue Substitute in Right Ankle Joint, Percutaneous Endoscopic Approach
0SWFX0Z Revision of Drainage Device in Right Ankle Joint, External Approach
0SWFX3Z Revision of Infusion Device in Right Ankle Joint, External Approach
0SWFX4Z Revision of Internal Fixation Device in Right Ankle Joint, External Approach
0SWFX5Z Revision of External Fixation Device in Right Ankle Joint, External Approach
0SWFX7Z Revision of Autologous Tissue Substitute in Right Ankle Joint, External Approach
0SWFX8Z Revision of Spacer in Right Ankle Joint, External Approach
0SWFXJZ Revision of Synthetic Substitute in Right Ankle Joint, External Approach
0SWFXKZ Revision of Nonautologous Tissue Substitute in Right Ankle Joint, External Approach
0SWG00Z Revision of Drainage Device in Left Ankle Joint, Open Approach
0SWG03Z Revision of Infusion Device in Left Ankle Joint, Open Approach
0SWG04Z Revision of Internal Fixation Device in Left Ankle Joint, Open Approach
0SWG05Z Revision of External Fixation Device in Left Ankle Joint, Open Approach
0SWG07Z Revision of Autologous Tissue Substitute in Left Ankle Joint, Open Approach
0SWG08Z Revision of Spacer in Left Ankle Joint, Open Approach
0SWG0JZ Revision of Synthetic Substitute in Left Ankle Joint, Open Approach
0SWG0KZ Revision of Nonautologous Tissue Substitute in Left Ankle Joint, Open Approach
0SWG30Z Revision of Drainage Device in Left Ankle Joint, Percutaneous Approach
0SWG33Z Revision of Infusion Device in Left Ankle Joint, Percutaneous Approach
0SWG34Z Revision of Internal Fixation Device in Left Ankle Joint, Percutaneous Approach
0SWG35Z Revision of External Fixation Device in Left Ankle Joint, Percutaneous Approach
0SWG37Z Revision of Autologous Tissue Substitute in Left Ankle Joint, Percutaneous Approach
0SWG38Z Revision of Spacer in Left Ankle Joint, Percutaneous Approach
0SWG3JZ Revision of Synthetic Substitute in Left Ankle Joint, Percutaneous Approach
0SWG3KZ Revision of Nonautologous Tissue Substitute in Left Ankle Joint, Percutaneous Approach
0SWG40Z Revision of Drainage Device in Left Ankle Joint, Percutaneous Endoscopic Approach
0SWG43Z Revision of Infusion Device in Left Ankle Joint, Percutaneous Endoscopic Approach
0SWG44Z Revision of Internal Fixation Device in Left Ankle Joint, Percutaneous Endoscopic Approach
0SWG45Z Revision of External Fixation Device in Left Ankle Joint, Percutaneous Endoscopic Approach
0SWG47Z Revision of Autologous Tissue Substitute in Left Ankle Joint, Percutaneous Endoscopic Approach
0SWG48Z Revision of Spacer in Left Ankle Joint, Percutaneous Endoscopic Approach
0SWG4JZ Revision of Synthetic Substitute in Left Ankle Joint, Percutaneous Endoscopic Approach
0SWG4KZ Revision of Nonautologous Tissue Substitute in Left Ankle Joint, Percutaneous Endoscopic Approach
0SWGX0Z Revision of Drainage Device in Left Ankle Joint, External Approach
0SWGX3Z Revision of Infusion Device in Left Ankle Joint, External Approach
0SWGX4Z Revision of Internal Fixation Device in Left Ankle Joint, External Approach
0SWGX5Z Revision of External Fixation Device in Left Ankle Joint, External Approach
0SWGX7Z Revision of Autologous Tissue Substitute in Left Ankle Joint, External Approach
0SWGX8Z Revision of Spacer in Left Ankle Joint, External Approach
0SWGXJZ Revision of Synthetic Substitute in Left Ankle Joint, External Approach
0SWGXKZ Revision of Nonautologous Tissue Substitute in Left Ankle Joint, External Approach
0SWH00Z Revision of Drainage Device in Right Tarsal Joint, Open Approach
0SWH03Z Revision of Infusion Device in Right Tarsal Joint, Open Approach

0SWH04Z Revision of Internal Fixation Device in Right Tarsal Joint, Open Approach
0SWH05Z Revision of External Fixation Device in Right Tarsal Joint, Open Approach
0SWH07Z Revision of Autologous Tissue Substitute in Right Tarsal Joint, Open Approach
0SWH08Z Revision of Spacer in Right Tarsal Joint, Open Approach
0SWH0JZ Revision of Synthetic Substitute in Right Tarsal Joint, Open Approach
0SWH0KZ Revision of Nonautologous Tissue Substitute in Right Tarsal Joint, Open Approach
0SWH30Z Revision of Drainage Device in Right Tarsal Joint, Percutaneous Approach
0SWH33Z Revision of Infusion Device in Right Tarsal Joint, Percutaneous Approach
0SWH34Z Revision of Internal Fixation Device in Right Tarsal Joint, Percutaneous Approach
0SWH35Z Revision of External Fixation Device in Right Tarsal Joint, Percutaneous Approach
0SWH37Z Revision of Autologous Tissue Substitute in Right Tarsal Joint, Percutaneous Approach
0SWH38Z Revision of Spacer in Right Tarsal Joint, Percutaneous Approach
0SWH3JZ Revision of Synthetic Substitute in Right Tarsal Joint, Percutaneous Approach
0SWH3KZ Revision of Nonautologous Tissue Substitute in Right Tarsal Joint, Percutaneous Approach
0SWH40Z Revision of Drainage Device in Right Tarsal Joint, Percutaneous Endoscopic Approach
0SWH43Z Revision of Infusion Device in Right Tarsal Joint, Percutaneous Endoscopic Approach
0SWH44Z Revision of Internal Fixation Device in Right Tarsal Joint, Percutaneous Endoscopic Approach
0SWH45Z Revision of External Fixation Device in Right Tarsal Joint, Percutaneous Endoscopic Approach
0SWH47Z Revision of Autologous Tissue Substitute in Right Tarsal Joint, Percutaneous Endoscopic Approach
0SWH48Z Revision of Spacer in Right Tarsal Joint, Percutaneous Endoscopic Approach
0SWH4JZ Revision of Synthetic Substitute in Right Tarsal Joint, Percutaneous Endoscopic Approach
0SWH4KZ Revision of Nonautologous Tissue Substitute in Right Tarsal Joint, Percutaneous Endoscopic Approach
0SWHX0Z Revision of Drainage Device in Right Tarsal Joint, External Approach
0SWHX3Z Revision of Infusion Device in Right Tarsal Joint, External Approach
0SWHX4Z Revision of Internal Fixation Device in Right Tarsal Joint, External Approach
0SWHX5Z Revision of External Fixation Device in Right Tarsal Joint, External Approach
0SWHX7Z Revision of Autologous Tissue Substitute in Right Tarsal Joint, External Approach
0SWHX8Z Revision of Spacer in Right Tarsal Joint, External Approach
0SWHXJZ Revision of Synthetic Substitute in Right Tarsal Joint, External Approach
0SWHXKZ Revision of Nonautologous Tissue Substitute in Right Tarsal Joint, External Approach
0SWJ00Z Revision of Drainage Device in Left Tarsal Joint, Open Approach
0SWJ03Z Revision of Infusion Device in Left Tarsal Joint, Open Approach
0SWJ04Z Revision of Internal Fixation Device in Left Tarsal Joint, Open Approach
0SWJ05Z Revision of External Fixation Device in Left Tarsal Joint, Open Approach
0SWJ07Z Revision of Autologous Tissue Substitute in Left Tarsal Joint, Open Approach
0SWJ08Z Revision of Spacer in Left Tarsal Joint, Open Approach
0SWJ0JZ Revision of Synthetic Substitute in Left Tarsal Joint, Open Approach
0SWJ0KZ Revision of Nonautologous Tissue Substitute in Left Tarsal Joint, Open Approach
0SWJ30Z Revision of Drainage Device in Left Tarsal Joint, Percutaneous Approach
0SWJ33Z Revision of Infusion Device in Left Tarsal Joint, Percutaneous Approach
0SWJ34Z Revision of Internal Fixation Device in Left Tarsal Joint, Percutaneous Approach
0SWJ35Z Revision of External Fixation Device in Left Tarsal Joint, Percutaneous Approach
0SWJ37Z Revision of Autologous Tissue Substitute in Left Tarsal Joint, Percutaneous Approach
0SWJ38Z Revision of Spacer in Left Tarsal Joint, Percutaneous Approach
0SWJ3JZ Revision of Synthetic Substitute in Left Tarsal Joint, Percutaneous Approach
0SWJ3KZ Revision of Nonautologous Tissue Substitute in Left Tarsal Joint, Percutaneous Approach
0SWJ40Z Revision of Drainage Device in Left Tarsal Joint, Percutaneous Endoscopic Approach
0SWJ43Z Revision of Infusion Device in Left Tarsal Joint, Percutaneous Endoscopic Approach
0SWJ44Z Revision of Internal Fixation Device in Left Tarsal Joint, Percutaneous Endoscopic Approach
0SWJ45Z Revision of External Fixation Device in Left Tarsal Joint, Percutaneous Endoscopic Approach
0SWJ47Z Revision of Autologous Tissue Substitute in Left Tarsal Joint, Percutaneous Endoscopic Approach
0SWJ48Z Revision of Spacer in Left Tarsal Joint, Percutaneous Endoscopic Approach
0SWJ4JZ Revision of Synthetic Substitute in Left Tarsal Joint, Percutaneous Endoscopic Approach
0SWJ4KZ Revision of Nonautologous Tissue Substitute in Left Tarsal Joint, Percutaneous Endoscopic Approach
0SWJX0Z Revision of Drainage Device in Left Tarsal Joint, External Approach
0SWJX3Z Revision of Infusion Device in Left Tarsal Joint, External Approach
0SWJX4Z Revision of Internal Fixation Device in Left Tarsal Joint, External Approach
0SWJX5Z Revision of External Fixation Device in Left Tarsal Joint, External Approach
0SWJX7Z Revision of Autologous Tissue Substitute in Left Tarsal Joint, External Approach
0SWJX8Z Revision of Spacer in Left Tarsal Joint, External Approach
0SWJXJZ Revision of Synthetic Substitute in Left Tarsal Joint, External Approach
0SWJXKZ Revision of Nonautologous Tissue Substitute in Left Tarsal Joint, External Approach
0SWK00Z Revision of Drainage Device in Right Metatarsal-Tarsal Joint, Open Approach
0SWK03Z Revision of Infusion Device in Right Metatarsal-Tarsal Joint, Open Approach
0SWK04Z Revision of Internal Fixation Device in Right Metatarsal-Tarsal Joint, Open Approach
0SWK05Z Revision of External Fixation Device in Right Metatarsal-Tarsal Joint, Open Approach
0SWK07Z Revision of Autologous Tissue Substitute in Right Metatarsal-Tarsal Joint, Open Approach
0SWK08Z Revision of Spacer in Right Metatarsal-Tarsal Joint, Open Approach
0SWK0JZ Revision of Synthetic Substitute in Right Metatarsal-Tarsal Joint, Open Approach
0SWK0KZ Revision of Nonautologous Tissue Substitute in Right Metatarsal-Tarsal Joint, Open Approach
0SWK30Z Revision of Drainage Device in Right Metatarsal-Tarsal Joint, Percutaneous Approach
0SWK33Z Revision of Infusion Device in Right Metatarsal-Tarsal Joint, Percutaneous Approach
0SWK34Z Revision of Internal Fixation Device in Right Metatarsal-Tarsal Joint, Percutaneous Approach
0SWK35Z Revision of External Fixation Device in Right Metatarsal-Tarsal Joint, Percutaneous Approach
0SWK37Z Revision of Autologous Tissue Substitute in Right Metatarsal-Tarsal Joint, Percutaneous Approach
0SWK38Z Revision of Spacer in Right Metatarsal-Tarsal Joint, Percutaneous Approach
0SWK3JZ Revision of Synthetic Substitute in Right Metatarsal-Tarsal Joint, Percutaneous Approach
0SWK3KZ Revision of Nonautologous Tissue Substitute in Right Metatarsal-Tarsal Joint, Percutaneous Approach
0SWK40Z Revision of Drainage Device in Right Metatarsal-Tarsal Joint, Percutaneous Endoscopic Approach
0SWK43Z Revision of Infusion Device in Right Metatarsal-Tarsal Joint, Percutaneous Endoscopic Approach
0SWK44Z Revision of Internal Fixation Device in Right Metatarsal-Tarsal Joint, Percutaneous Endoscopic Approach
0SWK45Z Revision of External Fixation Device in Right Metatarsal-Tarsal Joint, Percutaneous Endoscopic Approach
0SWK47Z Revision of Autologous Tissue Substitute in Right Metatarsal-Tarsal Joint, Percutaneous Endoscopic Approach
0SWK48Z Revision of Spacer in Right Metatarsal-Tarsal Joint, Percutaneous Endoscopic Approach
0SWK4JZ Revision of Synthetic Substitute in Right Metatarsal-Tarsal Joint, Percutaneous Endoscopic Approach
0SWK4KZ Revision of Nonautologous Tissue Substitute in Right Metatarsal-Tarsal Joint, Percutaneous Endoscopic Approach
0SWKX0Z Revision of Drainage Device in Right Metatarsal-Tarsal Joint, External Approach
0SWKX3Z Revision of Infusion Device in Right Metatarsal-Tarsal Joint, External Approach
0SWKX4Z Revision of Internal Fixation Device in Right Metatarsal-Tarsal Joint, External Approach
0SWKX5Z Revision of External Fixation Device in Right Metatarsal-Tarsal Joint, External Approach

0SWKX7Z Revision of Autologous Tissue Substitute in Right Metatarsal-Tarsal Joint, External Approach
0SWKX8Z Revision of Spacer in Right Metatarsal-Tarsal Joint, External Approach
0SWKXJZ Revision of Synthetic Substitute in Right Metatarsal-Tarsal Joint, External Approach
0SWKXKZ Revision of Nonautologous Tissue Substitute in Right Metatarsal-Tarsal Joint, External Approach
0SWL00Z Revision of Drainage Device in Left Metatarsal-Tarsal Joint, Open Approach
0SWL03Z Revision of Infusion Device in Left Metatarsal-Tarsal Joint, Open Approach
0SWL04Z Revision of Internal Fixation Device in Left Metatarsal-Tarsal Joint, Open Approach
0SWL05Z Revision of External Fixation Device in Left Metatarsal-Tarsal Joint, Open Approach
0SWL07Z Revision of Autologous Tissue Substitute in Left Metatarsal-Tarsal Joint, Open Approach
0SWL08Z Revision of Spacer in Left Metatarsal-Tarsal Joint, Open Approach
0SWL0JZ Revision of Synthetic Substitute in Left Metatarsal-Tarsal Joint, Open Approach
0SWL0KZ Revision of Nonautologous Tissue Substitute in Left Metatarsal-Tarsal Joint, Open Approach
0SWL30Z Revision of Drainage Device in Left Metatarsal-Tarsal Joint, Percutaneous Approach
0SWL33Z Revision of Infusion Device in Left Metatarsal-Tarsal Joint, Percutaneous Approach
0SWL34Z Revision of Internal Fixation Device in Left Metatarsal-Tarsal Joint, Percutaneous Approach
0SWL35Z Revision of External Fixation Device in Left Metatarsal-Tarsal Joint, Percutaneous Approach
0SWL37Z Revision of Autologous Tissue Substitute in Left Metatarsal-Tarsal Joint, Percutaneous Approach
0SWL38Z Revision of Spacer in Left Metatarsal-Tarsal Joint, Percutaneous Approach
0SWL3JZ Revision of Synthetic Substitute in Left Metatarsal-Tarsal Joint, Percutaneous Approach
0SWL3KZ Revision of Nonautologous Tissue Substitute in Left Metatarsal-Tarsal Joint, Percutaneous Approach
0SWL40Z Revision of Drainage Device in Left Metatarsal-Tarsal Joint, Percutaneous Endoscopic Approach
0SWL43Z Revision of Infusion Device in Left Metatarsal-Tarsal Joint, Percutaneous Endoscopic Approach
0SWL44Z Revision of Internal Fixation Device in Left Metatarsal-Tarsal Joint, Percutaneous Endoscopic Approach
0SWL45Z Revision of External Fixation Device in Left Metatarsal-Tarsal Joint, Percutaneous Endoscopic Approach
0SWL47Z Revision of Autologous Tissue Substitute in Left Metatarsal-Tarsal Joint, Percutaneous Endoscopic Approach
0SWL48Z Revision of Spacer in Left Metatarsal-Tarsal Joint, Percutaneous Endoscopic Approach
0SWL4JZ Revision of Synthetic Substitute in Left Metatarsal-Tarsal Joint, Percutaneous Endoscopic Approach
0SWL4KZ Revision of Nonautologous Tissue Substitute in Left Metatarsal-Tarsal Joint, Percutaneous Endoscopic Approach
0SWLX0Z Revision of Drainage Device in Left Metatarsal-Tarsal Joint, External Approach
0SWLX3Z Revision of Infusion Device in Left Metatarsal-Tarsal Joint, External Approach
0SWLX4Z Revision of Internal Fixation Device in Left Metatarsal-Tarsal Joint, External Approach
0SWLX5Z Revision of External Fixation Device in Left Metatarsal-Tarsal Joint, External Approach
0SWLX7Z Revision of Autologous Tissue Substitute in Left Metatarsal-Tarsal Joint, External Approach
0SWLX8Z Revision of Spacer in Left Metatarsal-Tarsal Joint, External Approach
0SWLXJZ Revision of Synthetic Substitute in Left Metatarsal-Tarsal Joint, External Approach
0SWLXKZ Revision of Nonautologous Tissue Substitute in Left Metatarsal-Tarsal Joint, External Approach
0SWM00Z Revision of Drainage Device in Right Metatarsal-Phalangeal Joint, Open Approach
0SWM03Z Revision of Infusion Device in Right Metatarsal-Phalangeal Joint, Open Approach
0SWM04Z Revision of Internal Fixation Device in Right Metatarsal-Phalangeal Joint, Open Approach
0SWM05Z Revision of External Fixation Device in Right Metatarsal-Phalangeal Joint, Open Approach
0SWM07Z Revision of Autologous Tissue Substitute in Right Metatarsal-Phalangeal Joint, Open Approach
0SWM08Z Revision of Spacer in Right Metatarsal-Phalangeal Joint, Open Approach
0SWM0JZ Revision of Synthetic Substitute in Right Metatarsal-Phalangeal Joint, Open Approach
0SWM0KZ Revision of Nonautologous Tissue Substitute in Right Metatarsal-Phalangeal Joint, Open Approach
0SWM30Z Revision of Drainage Device in Right Metatarsal-Phalangeal Joint, Percutaneous Approach
0SWM33Z Revision of Infusion Device in Right Metatarsal-Phalangeal Joint, Percutaneous Approach
0SWM34Z Revision of Internal Fixation Device in Right Metatarsal-Phalangeal Joint, Percutaneous Approach
0SWM35Z Revision of External Fixation Device in Right Metatarsal-Phalangeal Joint, Percutaneous Approach
0SWM37Z Revision of Autologous Tissue Substitute in Right Metatarsal-Phalangeal Joint, Percutaneous Approach
0SWM38Z Revision of Spacer in Right Metatarsal-Phalangeal Joint, Percutaneous Approach
0SWM3JZ Revision of Synthetic Substitute in Right Metatarsal-Phalangeal Joint, Percutaneous Approach
0SWM3KZ Revision of Nonautologous Tissue Substitute in Right Metatarsal-Phalangeal Joint, Percutaneous Approach
0SWM40Z Revision of Drainage Device in Right Metatarsal-Phalangeal Joint, Percutaneous Endoscopic Approach
0SWM43Z Revision of Infusion Device in Right Metatarsal-Phalangeal Joint, Percutaneous Endoscopic Approach
0SWM44Z Revision of Internal Fixation Device in Right Metatarsal-Phalangeal Joint, Percutaneous Endoscopic Approach
0SWM45Z Revision of External Fixation Device in Right Metatarsal-Phalangeal Joint, Percutaneous Endoscopic Approach
0SWM47Z Revision of Autologous Tissue Substitute in Right Metatarsal-Phalangeal Joint, Percutaneous Endoscopic Approach
0SWM48Z Revision of Spacer in Right Metatarsal-Phalangeal Joint, Percutaneous Endoscopic Approach
0SWM4JZ Revision of Synthetic Substitute in Right Metatarsal-Phalangeal Joint, Percutaneous Endoscopic Approach
0SWM4KZ Revision of Nonautologous Tissue Substitute in Right Metatarsal-Phalangeal Joint, Percutaneous Endoscopic Approach
0SWMX0Z Revision of Drainage Device in Right Metatarsal-Phalangeal Joint, External Approach
0SWMX3Z Revision of Infusion Device in Right Metatarsal-Phalangeal Joint, External Approach
0SWMX4Z Revision of Internal Fixation Device in Right Metatarsal-Phalangeal Joint, External Approach
0SWMX5Z Revision of External Fixation Device in Right Metatarsal-Phalangeal Joint, External Approach
0SWMX7Z Revision of Autologous Tissue Substitute in Right Metatarsal-Phalangeal Joint, External Approach
0SWMX8Z Revision of Spacer in Right Metatarsal-Phalangeal Joint, External Approach
0SWMXJZ Revision of Synthetic Substitute in Right Metatarsal-Phalangeal Joint, External Approach
0SWMXKZ Revision of Nonautologous Tissue Substitute in Right Metatarsal-Phalangeal Joint, External Approach
0SWN00Z Revision of Drainage Device in Left Metatarsal-Phalangeal Joint, Open Approach
0SWN03Z Revision of Infusion Device in Left Metatarsal-Phalangeal Joint, Open Approach
0SWN04Z Revision of Internal Fixation Device in Left Metatarsal-Phalangeal Joint, Open Approach
0SWN05Z Revision of External Fixation Device in Left Metatarsal-Phalangeal Joint, Open Approach
0SWN07Z Revision of Autologous Tissue Substitute in Left Metatarsal-Phalangeal Joint, Open Approach
0SWN08Z Revision of Spacer in Left Metatarsal-Phalangeal Joint, Open Approach
0SWN0JZ Revision of Synthetic Substitute in Left Metatarsal-Phalangeal Joint, Open Approach
0SWN0KZ Revision of Nonautologous Tissue Substitute in Left Metatarsal-Phalangeal Joint, Open Approach
0SWN30Z Revision of Drainage Device in Left Metatarsal-Phalangeal Joint, Percutaneous Approach
0SWN33Z Revision of Infusion Device in Left Metatarsal-Phalangeal Joint, Percutaneous Approach
0SWN34Z Revision of Internal Fixation Device in Left Metatarsal-Phalangeal Joint, Percutaneous Approach
0SWN35Z Revision of External Fixation Device in Left Metatarsal-Phalangeal Joint, Percutaneous Approach
0SWN37Z Revision of Autologous Tissue Substitute in Left Metatarsal-Phalangeal Joint, Percutaneous Approach

Lower Urinary Tract

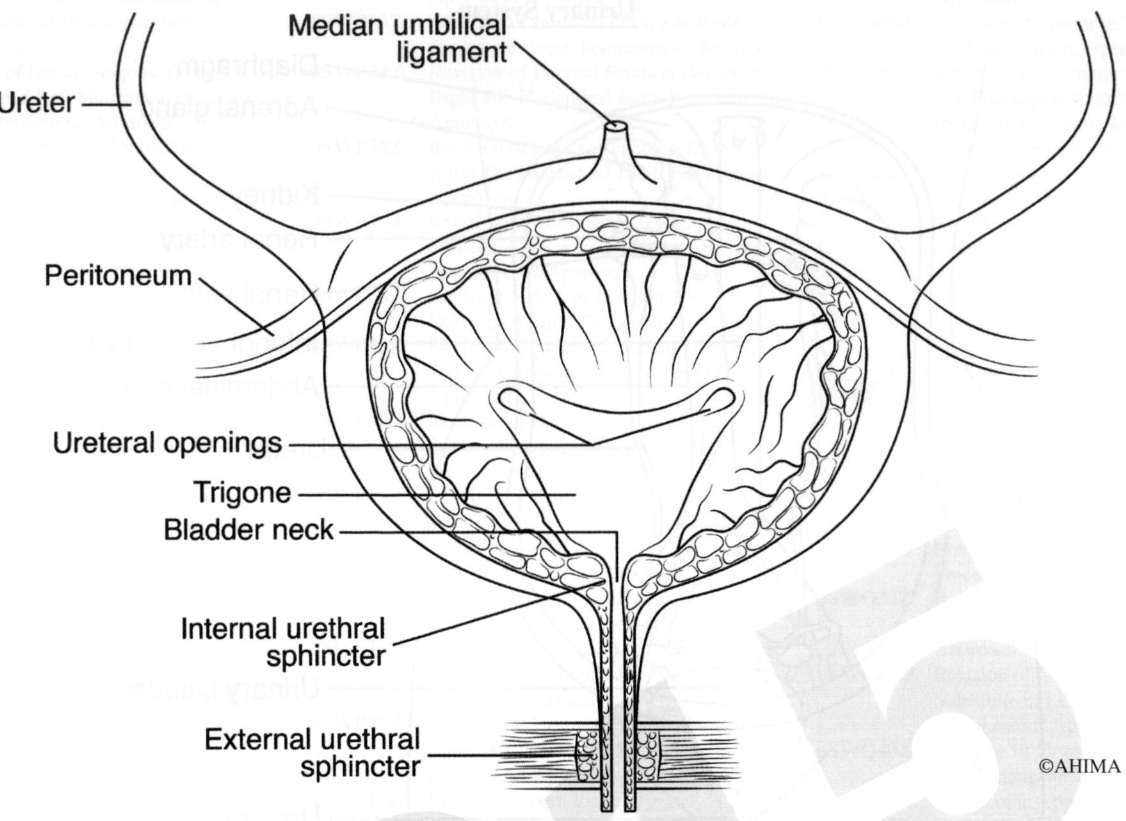

Kidney

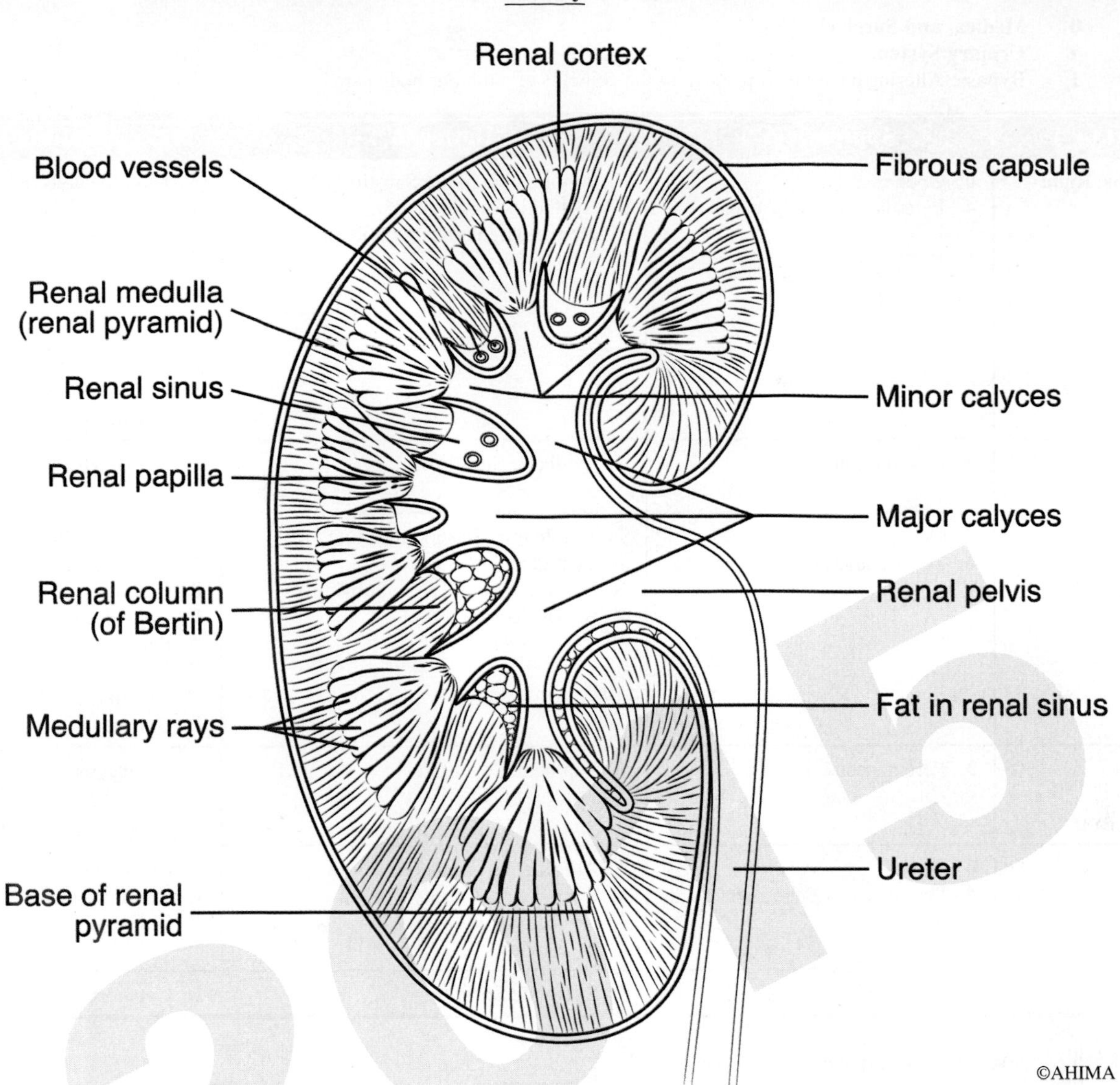
Renal cortex
Blood vessels
Fibrous capsule
Renal medulla (renal pyramid)
Renal sinus
Minor calyces
Renal papilla
Major calyces
Renal column (of Bertin)
Renal pelvis
Fat in renal sinus
Medullary rays
Ureter
Base of renal pyramid
©AHIMA

Urinary System Tables 0T1–0TY

Section 0 **Medical and Surgical**
Body System T **Urinary System**
Operation 1 **Bypass:** Altering the route of passage of the contents of a tubular body part

Body Part (4th)	Approach (5th)	Device (6th)	Qualifier (7th)
3 Kidney Pelvis, Right **4** Kidney Pelvis, Left	**0** Open **4** Percutaneous Endoscopic	**7** Autologous Tissue Substitute **J** Synthetic Substitute **K** Nonautologous Tissue Substitute **Z** No Device	**3** Kidney Pelvis, Right **4** Kidney Pelvis, Left **6** Ureter, Right **7** Ureter, Left **8** Colon **9** Colocutaneous **A** Ileum **B** Bladder **C** Ileocutaneous **D** Cutaneous
3 Kidney Pelvis, Right **4** Kidney Pelvis, Left	**3** Percutaneous	**J** Synthetic Substitute	**D** Cutaneous
6 Ureter, Right **7** Ureter, Left **8** Ureters, Bilateral	**0** Open **4** Percutaneous Endoscopic	**7** Autologous Tissue Substitute **J** Synthetic Substitute **K** Nonautologous Tissue Substitute **Z** No Device	**6** Ureter, Right **7** Ureter, Left **8** Colon **9** Colocutaneous **A** Ileum **B** Bladder **C** Ileocutaneous **D** Cutaneous
6 Ureter, Right **7** Ureter, Left **8** Ureters, Bilateral	**3** Percutaneous	**J** Synthetic Substitute	**D** Cutaneous
B Bladder	**0** Open **4** Percutaneous Endoscopic	**7** Autologous Tissue Substitute **J** Synthetic Substitute **K** Nonautologous Tissue Substitute **Z** No Device	**9** Colocutaneous **C** Ileocutaneous **D** Cutaneous
B Bladder	**3** Percutaneous	**J** Synthetic Substitute	**D** Cutaneous

Section 0 **Medical and Surgical**
Body System T **Urinary System**
Operation 2 **Change:** Taking out or off a device from a body part and putting back an identical or similar device in or on the same body part without cutting or puncturing the skin or a mucous membrane

Body Part (4th)	Approach (5th)	Device (6th)	Qualifier (7th)
5 Kidney **9** Ureter **B** Bladder **D** Urethra	**X** External	**0** Drainage Device **Y** Other Device	**Z** No Qualifier

Section 0 **Medical and Surgical**
Body System T **Urinary System**
Operation 5 **Destruction:** Physical eradication of all or a portion of a body part by the direct use of energy, force, or a destructive agent

Body Part (4th)	Approach (5th)	Device (6th)	Qualifier (7th)
0 Kidney, Right **1** Kidney, Left **3** Kidney Pelvis, Right **4** Kidney Pelvis, Left **6** Ureter, Right **7** Ureter, Left **B** Bladder **C** Bladder Neck	**0** Open **3** Percutaneous **4** Percutaneous Endoscopic **7** Via Natural or Artificial Opening **8** Via Natural or Artificial Opening Endoscopic	**Z** No Device	**Z** No Qualifier

Continued →

Section 0 **Medical and Surgical**
Body System T **Urinary System**
Operation 5 **Destruction:** Physical eradication of all or a portion of a body part by the direct use of energy, force, or a destructive agent

Body Part (4th)	Approach (5th)	Device (6th)	Qualifier (7th)
D Urethra	**0** Open **3** Percutaneous **4** Percutaneous Endoscopic **7** Via Natural or Artificial Opening **8** Via Natural or Artificial Opening Endoscopic **X** External	**Z** No Device	**Z** No Qualifier

Section 0 **Medical and Surgical**
Body System T **Urinary System**
Operation 7 **Dilation:** Expanding an orifice or the lumen of a tubular body part

Body Part (4th)	Approach (5th)	Device (6th)	Qualifier (7th)
3 Kidney Pelvis, Right **4** Kidney Pelvis, Left **6** Ureter, Right **7** Ureter, Left **8** Ureters, Bilateral **B** Bladder **C** Bladder Neck **D** Urethra	**0** Open **3** Percutaneous **4** Percutaneous Endoscopic **7** Via Natural or Artificial Opening **8** Via Natural or Artificial Opening Endoscopic	**D** Intraluminal Device **Z** No Device	**Z** No Qualifier

Section 0 **Medical and Surgical**
Body System T **Urinary System**
Operation 8 **Division:** Cutting into a body part, without draining fluids and/or gases from the body part, in order to separate or transect a body part

Body Part (4th)	Approach (5th)	Device (6th)	Qualifier (7th)
2 Kidneys, Bilateral **C** Bladder Neck	**0** Open **3** Percutaneous **4** Percutaneous Endoscopic	**Z** No Device	**Z** No Qualifier

Section 0 **Medical and Surgical**
Body System T **Urinary System**
Operation 9 **Drainage:** Taking or letting out fluids and/or gases from a body part

Body Part (4th)	Approach (5th)	Device (6th)	Qualifier (7th)
0 Kidney, Right **1** Kidney, Left **3** Kidney Pelvis, Right **4** Kidney Pelvis, Left **6** Ureter, Right **7** Ureter, Left **8** Ureters, Bilateral **B** Bladder **C** Bladder Neck	**0** Open **3** Percutaneous **4** Percutaneous Endoscopic **7** Via Natural or Artificial Opening **8** Via Natural or Artificial Opening Endoscopic	**0** Drainage Device	**Z** No Qualifier
0 Kidney, Right **1** Kidney, Left **3** Kidney Pelvis, Right **4** Kidney Pelvis, Left **6** Ureter, Right **7** Ureter, Left **8** Ureters, Bilateral **B** Bladder **C** Bladder Neck	**0** Open **3** Percutaneous **4** Percutaneous Endoscopic **7** Via Natural or Artificial Opening **8** Via Natural or Artificial Opening Endoscopic	**Z** No Device	**X** Diagnostic **Z** No Qualifier

Continued →

Section 0 **Medical and Surgical**
Body System T **Urinary System**
Operation 9 **Drainage:** Taking or letting out fluids and/or gases from a body part

Body Part (4th)	Approach (5th)	Device (6th)	Qualifier (7th)
D Urethra	**0** Open **3** Percutaneous **4** Percutaneous Endoscopic **7** Via Natural or Artificial Opening **8** Via Natural or Artificial Opening Endoscopic **X** External	**0** Drainage Device	**Z** No Qualifier
D Urethra	**0** Open **3** Percutaneous **4** Percutaneous Endoscopic **7** Via Natural or Artificial Opening **8** Via Natural or Artificial Opening Endoscopic **X** External	**Z** No Device	**X** Diagnostic **Z** No Qualifier

Section 0 **Medical and Surgical**
Body System T **Urinary System**
Operation B **Excision:** Cutting out or off, without replacement, a portion of a body part

Body Part (4th)	Approach (5th)	Device (6th)	Qualifier (7th)
0 Kidney, Right **1** Kidney, Left **3** Kidney Pelvis, Right **4** Kidney Pelvis, Left **6** Ureter, Right **7** Ureter, Left **B** Bladder **C** Bladder Neck	**0** Open **3** Percutaneous **4** Percutaneous Endoscopic **7** Via Natural or Artificial Opening **8** Via Natural or Artificial Opening Endoscopic	**Z** No Device	**X** Diagnostic **Z** No Qualifier
D Urethra	**0** Open **3** Percutaneous **4** Percutaneous Endoscopic **7** Via Natural or Artificial Opening **8** Via Natural or Artificial Opening Endoscopic **X** External	**Z** No Device	**X** Diagnostic **Z** No Qualifier

Section 0 **Medical and Surgical**
Body System T **Urinary System**
Operation C **Extirpation:** Taking or cutting out solid matter from a body part

Body Part (4th)	Approach (5th)	Device (6th)	Qualifier (7th)
0 Kidney, Right **1** Kidney, Left **3** Kidney Pelvis, Right **4** Kidney Pelvis, Left **6** Ureter, Right **7** Ureter, Left **B** Bladder **C** Bladder Neck	**0** Open **3** Percutaneous **4** Percutaneous Endoscopic **7** Via Natural or Artificial Opening **8** Via Natural or Artificial Opening Endoscopic	**Z** No Device	**Z** No Qualifier
D Urethra	**0** Open **3** Percutaneous **4** Percutaneous Endoscopic **7** Via Natural or Artificial Opening **8** Via Natural or Artificial Opening Endoscopic **X** External	**Z** No Device	**Z** No Qualifier

Section 0 **Medical and Surgical**
Body System T **Urinary System**
Operation D **Extraction:** Pulling or stripping out or off all or a portion of a body part by the use of force

Body Part (4th)	Approach (5th)	Device (6th)	Qualifier (7th)
0 Kidney, Right **1** Kidney, Left	**0** Open **3** Percutaneous **4** Percutaneous Endoscopic	**Z** No Device	**Z** No Qualifier

Section 0 **Medical and Surgical**
Body System T **Urinary System**
Operation F **Fragmentation:** Breaking solid matter in a body part into pieces

Body Part (4th)	Approach (5th)	Device (6th)	Qualifier (7th)
3 Kidney Pelvis, Right **4** Kidney Pelvis, Left **6** Ureter, Right **7** Ureter, Left **B** Bladder **C** Bladder Neck **D** Urethra	**0** Open **3** Percutaneous **4** Percutaneous Endoscopic **7** Via Natural or Artificial Opening **8** Via Natural or Artificial Opening Endoscopic **X** External	**Z** No Device	**Z** No Qualifier

Section 0 **Medical and Surgical**
Body System T **Urinary System**
Operation H **Insertion:** Putting in a nonbiological appliance that monitors, assists, performs, or prevents a physiological function but does not physically take the place of a body part

Body Part (4th)	Approach (5th)	Device (6th)	Qualifier (7th)
5 Kidney	**0** Open **3** Percutaneous **4** Percutaneous Endoscopic **7** Via Natural or Artificial Opening **8** Via Natural or Artificial Opening Endoscopic	**2** Monitoring Device **3** Infusion Device	**Z** No Qualifier
9 Ureter	**0** Open **3** Percutaneous **4** Percutaneous Endoscopic **7** Via Natural or Artificial Opening **8** Via Natural or Artificial Opening Endoscopic	**2** Monitoring Device **3** Infusion Device **M** Stimulator Lead	**Z** No Qualifier
B Bladder	**0** Open **3** Percutaneous **4** Percutaneous Endoscopic **7** Via Natural or Artificial Opening **8** Via Natural or Artificial Opening Endoscopic	**2** Monitoring Device **3** Infusion Device **L** Artificial Sphincter **M** Stimulator Lead	**Z** No Qualifier
C Bladder Neck	**0** Open **3** Percutaneous **4** Percutaneous Endoscopic **7** Via Natural or Artificial Opening **8** Via Natural or Artificial Opening Endoscopic	**L** Artificial Sphincter	**Z** No Qualifier
D Urethra	**0** Open **3** Percutaneous **4** Percutaneous Endoscopic **7** Via Natural or Artificial Opening **8** Via Natural or Artificial Opening Endoscopic **X** External	**2** Monitoring Device **3** Infusion Device **L** Artificial Sphincter	**Z** No Qualifier

Section 0 **Medical and Surgical**
Body System T **Urinary System**
Operation J **Inspection:** Visually and/or manually exploring a body part

Body Part (4th)	Approach (5th)	Device (6th)	Qualifier (7th)
5 Kidney **9** Ureter **B** Bladder **D** Urethra	**0** Open **3** Percutaneous **4** Percutaneous Endoscopic **7** Via Natural or Artificial Opening **8** Via Natural or Artificial Opening Endoscopic **X** External	**Z** No Device	**Z** No Qualifier

Section 0 **Medical and Surgical**
Body System T **Urinary System**
Operation L **Occlusion:** Completely closing an orifice or the lumen of a tubular body part

Body Part (4th)	Approach (5th)	Device (6th)	Qualifier (7th)
3 Kidney Pelvis, Right **4** Kidney Pelvis, Left **6** Ureter, Right **7** Ureter, Left **B** Bladder **C** Bladder Neck	**0** Open **3** Percutaneous **4** Percutaneous Endoscopic	**C** Extraluminal Device **D** Intraluminal Device **Z** No Device	**Z** No Qualifier
3 Kidney Pelvis, Right **4** Kidney Pelvis, Left **6** Ureter, Right **7** Ureter, Left **B** Bladder **C** Bladder Neck	**7** Via Natural or Artificial Opening **8** Via Natural or Artificial Opening Endoscopic	**D** Intraluminal Device **Z** No Device	**Z** No Qualifier
D Urethra	**0** Open **3** Percutaneous **4** Percutaneous Endoscopic **X** External	**C** Extraluminal Device **D** Intraluminal Device **Z** No Device	**Z** No Qualifier
D Urethra	**7** Via Natural or Artificial Opening **8** Via Natural or Artificial Opening Endoscopic	**D** Intraluminal Device **Z** No Device	**Z** No Qualifier

Section 0 **Medical and Surgical**
Body System T **Urinary System**
Operation M **Reattachment:** Putting back in or on all or a portion of a separated body part to its normal location or other suitable location

Body Part (4th)	Approach (5th)	Device (6th)	Qualifier (7th)
0 Kidney, Right **1** Kidney, Left **2** Kidneys, Bilateral **3** Kidney Pelvis, Right **4** Kidney Pelvis, Left **6** Ureter, Right **7** Ureter, Left **8** Ureters, Bilateral **B** Bladder **C** Bladder Neck **D** Urethra	**0** Open **4** Percutaneous Endoscopic	**Z** No Device	**Z** No Qualifier

Section 0 **Medical and Surgical**
Body System T **Urinary System**
Operation N **Release:** Freeing a body part from an abnormal physical constraint by cutting or by the use of force

Body Part (4th)	Approach (5th)	Device (6th)	Qualifier (7th)
0 Kidney, Right **1** Kidney, Left **3** Kidney Pelvis, Right **4** Kidney Pelvis, Left **6** Ureter, Right **7** Ureter, Left **B** Bladder **C** Bladder Neck	**0** Open **3** Percutaneous **4** Percutaneous Endoscopic **7** Via Natural or Artificial Opening **8** Via Natural or Artificial Opening Endoscopic	**Z** No Device	**Z** No Qualifier
D Urethra	**0** Open **3** Percutaneous **4** Percutaneous Endoscopic **7** Via Natural or Artificial Opening **8** Via Natural or Artificial Opening Endoscopic **X** External	**Z** No Device	**Z** No Qualifier

Section 0 **Medical and Surgical**
Body System T **Urinary System**
Operation P **Removal:** Taking out or off a device from a body part

Body Part (4th)	Approach (5th)	Device (6th)	Qualifier (7th)
5 Kidney	**0** Open **3** Percutaneous **4** Percutaneous Endoscopic **7** Via Natural or Artificial Opening **8** Via Natural or Artificial Opening Endoscopic	**0** Drainage Device **2** Monitoring Device **3** Infusion Device **7** Autologous Tissue Substitute **C** Extraluminal Device **D** Intraluminal Device **J** Synthetic Substitute **K** Nonautologous Tissue Substitute	**Z** No Qualifier
5 Kidney	**X** External	**0** Drainage Device **2** Monitoring Device **3** Infusion Device **D** Intraluminal Device	**Z** No Qualifier
9 Ureter	**0** Open **3** Percutaneous **4** Percutaneous Endoscopic **7** Via Natural or Artificial Opening **8** Via Natural or Artificial Opening Endoscopic	**0** Drainage Device **2** Monitoring Device **3** Infusion Device **7** Autologous Tissue Substitute **C** Extraluminal Device **D** Intraluminal Device **J** Synthetic Substitute **K** Nonautologous Tissue Substitute **M** Stimulator Lead	**Z** No Qualifier
9 Ureter	**X** External	**0** Drainage Device **2** Monitoring Device **3** Infusion Device **D** Intraluminal Device **M** Stimulator Lead	**Z** No Qualifier
B Bladder	**0** Open **3** Percutaneous **4** Percutaneous Endoscopic **7** Via Natural or Artificial Opening **8** Via Natural or Artificial Opening Endoscopic	**0** Drainage Device **2** Monitoring Device **3** Infusion Device **7** Autologous Tissue Substitute **C** Extraluminal Device **D** Intraluminal Device **J** Synthetic Substitute **K** Nonautologous Tissue Substitute **L** Artificial Sphincter **M** Stimulator Lead	**Z** No Qualifier

Continued →

Section 0 **Medical and Surgical**
Body System T **Urinary System**
Operation P **Removal:** Taking out or off a device from a body part

Body Part (4th)	Approach (5th)	Device (6th)	Qualifier (7th)
B Bladder	**X** External	**0** Drainage Device **2** Monitoring Device **3** Infusion Device **D** Intraluminal Device **L** Artificial Sphincter **M** Stimulator Lead	**Z** No Qualifier
D Urethra	**0** Open **3** Percutaneous **4** Percutaneous Endoscopic **7** Via Natural or Artificial Opening **8** Via Natural or Artificial Opening Endoscopic	**0** Drainage Device **2** Monitoring Device **3** Infusion Device **7** Autologous Tissue Substitute **C** Extraluminal Device **D** Intraluminal Device **J** Synthetic Substitute **K** Nonautologous Tissue Substitute **L** Artificial Sphincter	**Z** No Qualifier
D Urethra	**X** External	**0** Drainage Device **2** Monitoring Device **3** Infusion Device **D** Intraluminal Device **L** Artificial Sphincter	**Z** No Qualifier

Section 0 **Medical and Surgical**
Body System T **Urinary System**
Operation Q **Repair:** Restoring, to the extent possible, a body part to its normal anatomic structure and function

Body Part (4th)	Approach (5th)	Device (6th)	Qualifier (7th)
0 Kidney, Right **1** Kidney, Left **3** Kidney Pelvis, Right **4** Kidney Pelvis, Left **6** Ureter, Right **7** Ureter, Left **B** Bladder **C** Bladder Neck	**0** Open **3** Percutaneous **4** Percutaneous Endoscopic **7** Via Natural or Artificial Opening **8** Via Natural or Artificial Opening Endoscopic	**Z** No Device	**Z** No Qualifier
D Urethra	**0** Open **3** Percutaneous **4** Percutaneous Endoscopic **7** Via Natural or Artificial Opening **8** Via Natural or Artificial Opening Endoscopic **X** External	**Z** No Device	**Z** No Qualifier

Section 0 **Medical and Surgical**
Body System T **Urinary System**
Operation R **Replacement:** Putting in or on biological or synthetic material that physically takes the place and/or function of all or a portion of a body part

Body Part (4th)	Approach (5th)	Device (6th)	Qualifier (7th)
3 Kidney Pelvis, Right **4** Kidney Pelvis, Left **6** Ureter, Right **7** Ureter, Left **B** Bladder **C** Bladder Neck	**0** Open **4** Percutaneous Endoscopic **7** Via Natural or Artificial Opening **8** Via Natural or Artificial Opening Endoscopic	**7** Autologous Tissue Substitute **J** Synthetic Substitute **K** Nonautologous Tissue Substitute	**Z** No Qualifier
D Urethra	**0** Open **4** Percutaneous Endoscopic **7** Via Natural or Artificial Opening **8** Via Natural or Artificial Opening Endoscopic **X** External	**7** Autologous Tissue Substitute **J** Synthetic Substitute **K** Nonautologous Tissue Substitute	**Z** No Qualifier

Section 0 Medical and Surgical
Body System T Urinary System
Operation S **Reposition:** Moving to its normal location, or other suitable location, all or a portion of a body part

Body Part (4th)	Approach (5th)	Device (6th)	Qualifier (7th)
0 Kidney, Right 1 Kidney, Left 2 Kidneys, Bilateral 3 Kidney Pelvis, Right 4 Kidney Pelvis, Left 6 Ureter, Right 7 Ureter, Left 8 Ureters, Bilateral B Bladder C Bladder Neck D Urethra	0 Open 4 Percutaneous Endoscopic	Z No Device	Z No Qualifier

Section 0 Medical and Surgical
Body System T Urinary System
Operation T **Resection:** Cutting out or off, without replacement, all of a body part

Body Part (4th)	Approach (5th)	Device (6th)	Qualifier (7th)
0 Kidney, Right 1 Kidney, Left 2 Kidneys, Bilateral	0 Open 4 Percutaneous Endoscopic	Z No Device	Z No Qualifier
3 Kidney Pelvis, Right 4 Kidney Pelvis, Left 6 Ureter, Right 7 Ureter, Left B Bladder C Bladder Neck D Urethra	0 Open 4 Percutaneous Endoscopic 7 Via Natural or Artificial Opening 8 Via Natural or Artificial Opening Endoscopic	Z No Device	Z No Qualifier

Section 0 Medical and Surgical
Body System T Urinary System
Operation U **Supplement:** Putting in or on biological or synthetic material that physically reinforces and/or augments the function of a portion of a body part

Body Part (4th)	Approach (5th)	Device (6th)	Qualifier (7th)
3 Kidney Pelvis, Right 4 Kidney Pelvis, Left 6 Ureter, Right 7 Ureter, Left B Bladder C Bladder Neck	0 Open 4 Percutaneous Endoscopic 7 Via Natural or Artificial Opening 8 Via Natural or Artificial Opening Endoscopic	7 Autologous Tissue Substitute J Synthetic Substitute K Nonautologous Tissue Substitute	Z No Qualifier
D Urethra	0 Open 4 Percutaneous Endoscopic 7 Via Natural or Artificial Opening 8 Via Natural or Artificial Opening Endoscopic X External	7 Autologous Tissue Substitute J Synthetic Substitute K Nonautologous Tissue Substitute	Z No Qualifier

Section 0 Medical and Surgical
Body System T Urinary System
Operation V **Restriction:** Partially closing an orifice or the lumen of a tubular body part

Body Part (4th)	Approach (5th)	Device (6th)	Qualifier (7th)
3 Kidney Pelvis, Right 4 Kidney Pelvis, Left 6 Ureter, Right 7 Ureter, Left B Bladder C Bladder Neck	0 Open 3 Percutaneous 4 Percutaneous Endoscopic	C Extraluminal Device D Intraluminal Device Z No Device	Z No Qualifier

Continued →

Section 0 **Medical and Surgical**
Body System T **Urinary System**
Operation V **Restriction:** Partially closing an orifice or the lumen of a tubular body part

Body Part (4th)	Approach (5th)	Device (6th)	Qualifier (7th)
3 Kidney Pelvis, Right **4** Kidney Pelvis, Left **6** Ureter, Right **7** Ureter, Left **B** Bladder **C** Bladder Neck	**7** Via Natural or Artificial Opening **8** Via Natural or Artificial Opening Endoscopic	**D** Intraluminal Device **Z** No Device	**Z** No Qualifier
D Urethra	**0** Open **3** Percutaneous **4** Percutaneous Endoscopic	**C** Extraluminal Device **D** Intraluminal Device **Z** No Device	**Z** No Qualifier
D Urethra	**7** Via Natural or Artificial Opening **8** Via Natural or Artificial Opening Endoscopic	**D** Intraluminal Device **Z** No Device	**Z** No Qualifier
D Urethra	**X** External	**Z** No Device	**Z** No Qualifier

Section 0 **Medical and Surgical**
Body System T **Urinary System**
Operation W **Revision:** Correcting, to the extent possible, a portion of a malfunctioning device or the position of a displaced device

Body Part (4th)	Approach (5th)	Device (6th)	Qualifier (7th)
5 Kidney	**0** Open **3** Percutaneous **4** Percutaneous Endoscopic **7** Via Natural or Artificial Opening **8** Via Natural or Artificial Opening Endoscopic **X** External	**0** Drainage Device **2** Monitoring Device **3** Infusion Device **7** Autologous Tissue Substitute **C** Extraluminal Device **D** Intraluminal Device **J** Synthetic Substitute **K** Nonautologous Tissue Substitute	**Z** No Qualifier
9 Ureter	**0** Open **3** Percutaneous **4** Percutaneous Endoscopic **7** Via Natural or Artificial Opening **8** Via Natural or Artificial Opening Endoscopic **X** External	**0** Drainage Device **2** Monitoring Device **3** Infusion Device **7** Autologous Tissue Substitute **C** Extraluminal Device **D** Intraluminal Device **J** Synthetic Substitute **K** Nonautologous Tissue Substitute **M** Stimulator Lead	**Z** No Qualifier
B Bladder	**0** Open **3** Percutaneous **4** Percutaneous Endoscopic **7** Via Natural or Artificial Opening **8** Via Natural or Artificial Opening Endoscopic **X** External	**0** Drainage Device **2** Monitoring Device **3** Infusion Device **7** Autologous Tissue Substitute **C** Extraluminal Device **D** Intraluminal Device **J** Synthetic Substitute **K** Nonautologous Tissue Substitute **L** Artificial Sphincter **M** Stimulator Lead	**Z** No Qualifier
D Urethra	**0** Open **3** Percutaneous **4** Percutaneous Endoscopic **7** Via Natural or Artificial Opening **8** Via Natural or Artificial Opening Endoscopic **X** External	**0** Drainage Device **2** Monitoring Device **3** Infusion Device **7** Autologous Tissue Substitute **C** Extraluminal Device **D** Intraluminal Device **J** Synthetic Substitute **K** Nonautologous Tissue Substitute **L** Artificial Sphincter	**Z** No Qualifier

Section 0 Medical and Surgical
Body System T Urinary System
Operation Y **Transplantation:** Putting in or on all or a portion of a living body part taken from another individual or animal to physically take the place and/or function of all or a portion of a similar body part

Body Part (4th)	Approach (5th)	Device (6th)	Qualifier (7th)
0 Kidney, Right **1** Kidney, Left	**0** Open	**Z** No Device	**0** Allogeneic **1** Syngeneic **2** Zooplastic

Urinary System Code Listing 0T1–0TY

0T1 – Urinary System, Bypass

Review Coding Guideline B3.6a

0T13073 Bypass Right Kidney Pelvis to Right Kidney Pelvis with Autologous Tissue Substitute, Open Approach
0T13074 Bypass Right Kidney Pelvis to Left Kidney Pelvis with Autologous Tissue Substitute, Open Approach
0T13076 Bypass Right Kidney Pelvis to Right Ureter with Autologous Tissue Substitute, Open Approach
0T13077 Bypass Right Kidney Pelvis to Left Ureter with Autologous Tissue Substitute, Open Approach
0T13078 Bypass Right Kidney Pelvis to Colon with Autologous Tissue Substitute, Open Approach
0T13079 Bypass Right Kidney Pelvis to Colocutaneous with Autologous Tissue Substitute, Open Approach
0T1307A Bypass Right Kidney Pelvis to Ileum with Autologous Tissue Substitute, Open Approach
0T1307B Bypass Right Kidney Pelvis to Bladder with Autologous Tissue Substitute, Open Approach
0T1307C Bypass Right Kidney Pelvis to Ileocutaneous with Autologous Tissue Substitute, Open Approach
0T1307D Bypass Right Kidney Pelvis to Cutaneous with Autologous Tissue Substitute, Open Approach
0T130J3 Bypass Right Kidney Pelvis to Right Kidney Pelvis with Synthetic Substitute, Open Approach
0T130J4 Bypass Right Kidney Pelvis to Left Kidney Pelvis with Synthetic Substitute, Open Approach
0T130J6 Bypass Right Kidney Pelvis to Right Ureter with Synthetic Substitute, Open Approach
0T130J7 Bypass Right Kidney Pelvis to Left Ureter with Synthetic Substitute, Open Approach
0T130J8 Bypass Right Kidney Pelvis to Colon with Synthetic Substitute, Open Approach
0T130J9 Bypass Right Kidney Pelvis to Colocutaneous with Synthetic Substitute, Open Approach
0T130JA Bypass Right Kidney Pelvis to Ileum with Synthetic Substitute, Open Approach
0T130JB Bypass Right Kidney Pelvis to Bladder with Synthetic Substitute, Open Approach
0T130JC Bypass Right Kidney Pelvis to Ileocutaneous with Synthetic Substitute, Open Approach
0T130JD Bypass Right Kidney Pelvis to Cutaneous with Synthetic Substitute, Open Approach
0T130K3 Bypass Right Kidney Pelvis to Right Kidney Pelvis with Nonautologous Tissue Substitute, Open Approach
0T130K4 Bypass Right Kidney Pelvis to Left Kidney Pelvis with Nonautologous Tissue Substitute, Open Approach
0T130K6 Bypass Right Kidney Pelvis to Right Ureter with Nonautologous Tissue Substitute, Open Approach
0T130K7 Bypass Right Kidney Pelvis to Left Ureter with Nonautologous Tissue Substitute, Open Approach
0T130K8 Bypass Right Kidney Pelvis to Colon with Nonautologous Tissue Substitute, Open Approach
0T130K9 Bypass Right Kidney Pelvis to Colocutaneous with Nonautologous Tissue Substitute, Open Approach
0T130KA Bypass Right Kidney Pelvis to Ileum with Nonautologous Tissue Substitute, Open Approach
0T130KB Bypass Right Kidney Pelvis to Bladder with Nonautologous Tissue Substitute, Open Approach
0T130KC Bypass Right Kidney Pelvis to Ileocutaneous with Nonautologous Tissue Substitute, Open Approach
0T130KD Bypass Right Kidney Pelvis to Cutaneous with Nonautologous Tissue Substitute, Open Approach
0T130Z3 Bypass Right Kidney Pelvis to Right Kidney Pelvis, Open Approach
0T130Z4 Bypass Right Kidney Pelvis to Left Kidney Pelvis, Open Approach
0T130Z6 Bypass Right Kidney Pelvis to Right Ureter, Open Approach
0T130Z7 Bypass Right Kidney Pelvis to Left Ureter, Open Approach
0T130Z8 Bypass Right Kidney Pelvis to Colon, Open Approach
0T130Z9 Bypass Right Kidney Pelvis to Colocutaneous, Open Approach
0T130ZA Bypass Right Kidney Pelvis to Ileum, Open Approach
0T130ZB Bypass Right Kidney Pelvis to Bladder, Open Approach
0T130ZC Bypass Right Kidney Pelvis to Ileocutaneous, Open Approach
0T130ZD Bypass Right Kidney Pelvis to Cutaneous, Open Approach
0T133JD Bypass Right Kidney Pelvis to Cutaneous with Synthetic Substitute, Percutaneous Approach
0T13473 Bypass Right Kidney Pelvis to Right Kidney Pelvis with Autologous Tissue Substitute, Percutaneous Endoscopic Approach
0T13474 Bypass Right Kidney Pelvis to Left Kidney Pelvis with Autologous Tissue Substitute, Percutaneous Endoscopic Approach
0T13476 Bypass Right Kidney Pelvis to Right Ureter with Autologous Tissue Substitute, Percutaneous Endoscopic Approach
0T13477 Bypass Right Kidney Pelvis to Left Ureter with Autologous Tissue Substitute, Percutaneous Endoscopic Approach
0T13478 Bypass Right Kidney Pelvis to Colon with Autologous Tissue Substitute, Percutaneous Endoscopic Approach
0T13479 Bypass Right Kidney Pelvis to Colocutaneous with Autologous Tissue Substitute, Percutaneous Endoscopic Approach
0T1347A Bypass Right Kidney Pelvis to Ileum with Autologous Tissue Substitute, Percutaneous Endoscopic Approach
0T1347B Bypass Right Kidney Pelvis to Bladder with Autologous Tissue Substitute, Percutaneous Endoscopic Approach
0T1347C Bypass Right Kidney Pelvis to Ileocutaneous with Autologous Tissue Substitute, Percutaneous Endoscopic Approach
0T1347D Bypass Right Kidney Pelvis to Cutaneous with Autologous Tissue Substitute, Percutaneous Endoscopic Approach
0T134J3 Bypass Right Kidney Pelvis to Right Kidney Pelvis with Synthetic Substitute, Percutaneous Endoscopic Approach
0T134J4 Bypass Right Kidney Pelvis to Left Kidney Pelvis with Synthetic Substitute, Percutaneous Endoscopic Approach
0T134J6 Bypass Right Kidney Pelvis to Right Ureter with Synthetic Substitute, Percutaneous Endoscopic Approach
0T134J7 Bypass Right Kidney Pelvis to Left Ureter with Synthetic Substitute, Percutaneous Endoscopic Approach
0T134J8 Bypass Right Kidney Pelvis to Colon with Synthetic Substitute, Percutaneous Endoscopic Approach
0T134J9 Bypass Right Kidney Pelvis to Colocutaneous with Synthetic Substitute, Percutaneous Endoscopic Approach
0T134JA Bypass Right Kidney Pelvis to Ileum with Synthetic Substitute, Percutaneous Endoscopic Approach
0T134JB Bypass Right Kidney Pelvis to Bladder with Synthetic Substitute, Percutaneous Endoscopic Approach
0T134JC Bypass Right Kidney Pelvis to Ileocutaneous with Synthetic Substitute, Percutaneous Endoscopic Approach
0T134JD Bypass Right Kidney Pelvis to Cutaneous with Synthetic Substitute, Percutaneous Endoscopic Approach
0T134K3 Bypass Right Kidney Pelvis to Right Kidney Pelvis with Nonautologous Tissue Substitute, Percutaneous Endoscopic Approach

0T134K4 Bypass Right Kidney Pelvis to Left Kidney Pelvis with Nonautologous Tissue Substitute, Percutaneous Endoscopic Approach
0T134K6 Bypass Right Kidney Pelvis to Right Ureter with Nonautologous Tissue Substitute, Percutaneous Endoscopic Approach
0T134K7 Bypass Right Kidney Pelvis to Left Ureter with Nonautologous Tissue Substitute, Percutaneous Endoscopic Approach
0T134K8 Bypass Right Kidney Pelvis to Colon with Nonautologous Tissue Substitute, Percutaneous Endoscopic Approach
0T134K9 Bypass Right Kidney Pelvis to Colocutaneous with Nonautologous Tissue Substitute, Percutaneous Endoscopic Approach
0T134KA Bypass Right Kidney Pelvis to Ileum with Nonautologous Tissue Substitute, Percutaneous Endoscopic Approach
0T134KB Bypass Right Kidney Pelvis to Bladder with Nonautologous Tissue Substitute, Percutaneous Endoscopic Approach
0T134KC Bypass Right Kidney Pelvis to Ileocutaneous with Nonautologous Tissue Substitute, Percutaneous Endoscopic Approach
0T134KD Bypass Right Kidney Pelvis to Cutaneous with Nonautologous Tissue Substitute, Percutaneous Endoscopic Approach
0T134Z3 Bypass Right Kidney Pelvis to Right Kidney Pelvis, Percutaneous Endoscopic Approach
0T134Z4 Bypass Right Kidney Pelvis to Left Kidney Pelvis, Percutaneous Endoscopic Approach
0T134Z6 Bypass Right Kidney Pelvis to Right Ureter, Percutaneous Endoscopic Approach
0T134Z7 Bypass Right Kidney Pelvis to Left Ureter, Percutaneous Endoscopic Approach
0T134Z8 Bypass Right Kidney Pelvis to Colon, Percutaneous Endoscopic Approach
0T134Z9 Bypass Right Kidney Pelvis to Colocutaneous, Percutaneous Endoscopic Approach
0T134ZA Bypass Right Kidney Pelvis to Ileum, Percutaneous Endoscopic Approach
0T134ZB Bypass Right Kidney Pelvis to Bladder, Percutaneous Endoscopic Approach
0T134ZC Bypass Right Kidney Pelvis to Ileocutaneous, Percutaneous Endoscopic Approach
0T134ZD Bypass Right Kidney Pelvis to Cutaneous, Percutaneous Endoscopic Approach
0T14073 Bypass Left Kidney Pelvis to Right Kidney Pelvis with Autologous Tissue Substitute, Open Approach
0T14074 Bypass Left Kidney Pelvis to Left Kidney Pelvis with Autologous Tissue Substitute, Open Approach
0T14076 Bypass Left Kidney Pelvis to Right Ureter with Autologous Tissue Substitute, Open Approach
0T14077 Bypass Left Kidney Pelvis to Left Ureter with Autologous Tissue Substitute, Open Approach
0T14078 Bypass Left Kidney Pelvis to Colon with Autologous Tissue Substitute, Open Approach
0T14079 Bypass Left Kidney Pelvis to Colocutaneous with Autologous Tissue Substitute, Open Approach
0T1407A Bypass Left Kidney Pelvis to Ileum with Autologous Tissue Substitute, Open Approach
0T1407B Bypass Left Kidney Pelvis to Bladder with Autologous Tissue Substitute, Open Approach
0T1407C Bypass Left Kidney Pelvis to Ileocutaneous with Autologous Tissue Substitute, Open Approach
0T1407D Bypass Left Kidney Pelvis to Cutaneous with Autologous Tissue Substitute, Open Approach
0T140J3 Bypass Left Kidney Pelvis to Right Kidney Pelvis with Synthetic Substitute, Open Approach
0T140J4 Bypass Left Kidney Pelvis to Left Kidney Pelvis with Synthetic Substitute, Open Approach
0T140J6 Bypass Left Kidney Pelvis to Right Ureter with Synthetic Substitute, Open Approach
0T140J7 Bypass Left Kidney Pelvis to Left Ureter with Synthetic Substitute, Open Approach
0T140J8 Bypass Left Kidney Pelvis to Colon with Synthetic Substitute, Open Approach
0T140J9 Bypass Left Kidney Pelvis to Colocutaneous with Synthetic Substitute, Open Approach
0T140JA Bypass Left Kidney Pelvis to Ileum with Synthetic Substitute, Open Approach
0T140JB Bypass Left Kidney Pelvis to Bladder with Synthetic Substitute, Open Approach
0T140JC Bypass Left Kidney Pelvis to Ileocutaneous with Synthetic Substitute, Open Approach
0T140JD Bypass Left Kidney Pelvis to Cutaneous with Synthetic Substitute, Open Approach
0T140K3 Bypass Left Kidney Pelvis to Right Kidney Pelvis with Nonautologous Tissue Substitute, Open Approach
0T140K4 Bypass Left Kidney Pelvis to Left Kidney Pelvis with Nonautologous Tissue Substitute, Open Approach
0T140K6 Bypass Left Kidney Pelvis to Right Ureter with Nonautologous Tissue Substitute, Open Approach
0T140K7 Bypass Left Kidney Pelvis to Left Ureter with Nonautologous Tissue Substitute, Open Approach
0T140K8 Bypass Left Kidney Pelvis to Colon with Nonautologous Tissue Substitute, Open Approach
0T140K9 Bypass Left Kidney Pelvis to Colocutaneous with Nonautologous Tissue Substitute, Open Approach
0T140KA Bypass Left Kidney Pelvis to Ileum with Nonautologous Tissue Substitute, Open Approach
0T140KB Bypass Left Kidney Pelvis to Bladder with Nonautologous Tissue Substitute, Open Approach
0T140KC Bypass Left Kidney Pelvis to Ileocutaneous with Nonautologous Tissue Substitute, Open Approach
0T140KD Bypass Left Kidney Pelvis to Cutaneous with Nonautologous Tissue Substitute, Open Approach
0T140Z3 Bypass Left Kidney Pelvis to Right Kidney Pelvis, Open Approach
0T140Z4 Bypass Left Kidney Pelvis to Left Kidney Pelvis, Open Approach
0T140Z6 Bypass Left Kidney Pelvis to Right Ureter, Open Approach
0T140Z7 Bypass Left Kidney Pelvis to Left Ureter, Open Approach
0T140Z8 Bypass Left Kidney Pelvis to Colon, Open Approach
0T140Z9 Bypass Left Kidney Pelvis to Colocutaneous, Open Approach
0T140ZA Bypass Left Kidney Pelvis to Ileum, Open Approach
0T140ZB Bypass Left Kidney Pelvis to Bladder, Open Approach
0T140ZC Bypass Left Kidney Pelvis to Ileocutaneous, Open Approach
0T140ZD Bypass Left Kidney Pelvis to Cutaneous, Open Approach
0T143JD Bypass Left Kidney Pelvis to Cutaneous with Synthetic Substitute, Percutaneous Approach
0T14473 Bypass Left Kidney Pelvis to Right Kidney Pelvis with Autologous Tissue Substitute, Percutaneous Endoscopic Approach
0T14474 Bypass Left Kidney Pelvis to Left Kidney Pelvis with Autologous Tissue Substitute, Percutaneous Endoscopic Approach
0T14476 Bypass Left Kidney Pelvis to Right Ureter with Autologous Tissue Substitute, Percutaneous Endoscopic Approach
0T14477 Bypass Left Kidney Pelvis to Left Ureter with Autologous Tissue Substitute, Percutaneous Endoscopic Approach
0T14478 Bypass Left Kidney Pelvis to Colon with Autologous Tissue Substitute, Percutaneous Endoscopic Approach
0T14479 Bypass Left Kidney Pelvis to Colocutaneous with Autologous Tissue Substitute, Percutaneous Endoscopic Approach
0T1447A Bypass Left Kidney Pelvis to Ileum with Autologous Tissue Substitute, Percutaneous Endoscopic Approach
0T1447B Bypass Left Kidney Pelvis to Bladder with Autologous Tissue Substitute, Percutaneous Endoscopic Approach
0T1447C Bypass Left Kidney Pelvis to Ileocutaneous with Autologous Tissue Substitute, Percutaneous Endoscopic Approach
0T1447D Bypass Left Kidney Pelvis to Cutaneous with Autologous Tissue Substitute, Percutaneous Endoscopic Approach
0T144J3 Bypass Left Kidney Pelvis to Right Kidney Pelvis with Synthetic Substitute, Percutaneous Endoscopic Approach
0T144J4 Bypass Left Kidney Pelvis to Left Kidney Pelvis with Synthetic Substitute, Percutaneous Endoscopic Approach
0T144J6 Bypass Left Kidney Pelvis to Right Ureter with Synthetic Substitute, Percutaneous Endoscopic Approach
0T144J7 Bypass Left Kidney Pelvis to Left Ureter with Synthetic Substitute, Percutaneous Endoscopic Approach
0T144J8 Bypass Left Kidney Pelvis to Colon with Synthetic Substitute, Percutaneous Endoscopic Approach
0T144J9 Bypass Left Kidney Pelvis to Colocutaneous with Synthetic Substitute, Percutaneous Endoscopic Approach
0T144JA Bypass Left Kidney Pelvis to Ileum with Synthetic Substitute, Percutaneous Endoscopic Approach
0T144JB Bypass Left Kidney Pelvis to Bladder with Synthetic Substitute, Percutaneous Endoscopic Approach
0T144JC Bypass Left Kidney Pelvis to Ileocutaneous with Synthetic Substitute, Percutaneous Endoscopic Approach
0T144JD Bypass Left Kidney Pelvis to Cutaneous with Synthetic Substitute, Percutaneous Endoscopic Approach
0T144K3 Bypass Left Kidney Pelvis to Right Kidney Pelvis with Nonautologous Tissue Substitute, Percutaneous Endoscopic Approach

0T144K4 Bypass Left Kidney Pelvis to Left Kidney Pelvis with Nonautologous Tissue Substitute, Percutaneous Endoscopic Approach
0T144K6 Bypass Left Kidney Pelvis to Right Ureter with Nonautologous Tissue Substitute, Percutaneous Endoscopic Approach
0T144K7 Bypass Left Kidney Pelvis to Left Ureter with Nonautologous Tissue Substitute, Percutaneous Endoscopic Approach
0T144K8 Bypass Left Kidney Pelvis to Colon with Nonautologous Tissue Substitute, Percutaneous Endoscopic Approach
0T144K9 Bypass Left Kidney Pelvis to Colocutaneous with Nonautologous Tissue Substitute, Percutaneous Endoscopic Approach
0T144KA Bypass Left Kidney Pelvis to Ileum with Nonautologous Tissue Substitute, Percutaneous Endoscopic Approach
0T144KB Bypass Left Kidney Pelvis to Bladder with Nonautologous Tissue Substitute, Percutaneous Endoscopic Approach
0T144KC Bypass Left Kidney Pelvis to Ileocutaneous with Nonautologous Tissue Substitute, Percutaneous Endoscopic Approach
0T144KD Bypass Left Kidney Pelvis to Cutaneous with Nonautologous Tissue Substitute, Percutaneous Endoscopic Approach
0T144Z3 Bypass Left Kidney Pelvis to Right Kidney Pelvis, Percutaneous Endoscopic Approach
0T144Z4 Bypass Left Kidney Pelvis to Left Kidney Pelvis, Percutaneous Endoscopic Approach
0T144Z6 Bypass Left Kidney Pelvis to Right Ureter, Percutaneous Endoscopic Approach
0T144Z7 Bypass Left Kidney Pelvis to Left Ureter, Percutaneous Endoscopic Approach
0T144Z8 Bypass Left Kidney Pelvis to Colon, Percutaneous Endoscopic Approach
0T144Z9 Bypass Left Kidney Pelvis to Colocutaneous, Percutaneous Endoscopic Approach
0T144ZA Bypass Left Kidney Pelvis to Ileum, Percutaneous Endoscopic Approach
0T144ZB Bypass Left Kidney Pelvis to Bladder, Percutaneous Endoscopic Approach
0T144ZC Bypass Left Kidney Pelvis to Ileocutaneous, Percutaneous Endoscopic Approach
0T144ZD Bypass Left Kidney Pelvis to Cutaneous, Percutaneous Endoscopic Approach
0T16076 Bypass Right Ureter to Right Ureter with Autologous Tissue Substitute, Open Approach
0T16077 Bypass Right Ureter to Left Ureter with Autologous Tissue Substitute, Open Approach
0T16078 Bypass Right Ureter to Colon with Autologous Tissue Substitute, Open Approach
0T16079 Bypass Right Ureter to Colocutaneous with Autologous Tissue Substitute, Open Approach
0T1607A Bypass Right Ureter to Ileum with Autologous Tissue Substitute, Open Approach
0T1607B Bypass Right Ureter to Bladder with Autologous Tissue Substitute, Open Approach
0T1607C Bypass Right Ureter to Ileocutaneous with Autologous Tissue Substitute, Open Approach
0T1607D Bypass Right Ureter to Cutaneous with Autologous Tissue Substitute, Open Approach
0T160J6 Bypass Right Ureter to Right Ureter with Synthetic Substitute, Open Approach
0T160J7 Bypass Right Ureter to Left Ureter with Synthetic Substitute, Open Approach
0T160J8 Bypass Right Ureter to Colon with Synthetic Substitute, Open Approach
0T160J9 Bypass Right Ureter to Colocutaneous with Synthetic Substitute, Open Approach
0T160JA Bypass Right Ureter to Ileum with Synthetic Substitute, Open Approach
0T160JB Bypass Right Ureter to Bladder with Synthetic Substitute, Open Approach
0T160JC Bypass Right Ureter to Ileocutaneous with Synthetic Substitute, Open Approach
0T160JD Bypass Right Ureter to Cutaneous with Synthetic Substitute, Open Approach
0T160K6 Bypass Right Ureter to Right Ureter with Nonautologous Tissue Substitute, Open Approach
0T160K7 Bypass Right Ureter to Left Ureter with Nonautologous Tissue Substitute, Open Approach
0T160K8 Bypass Right Ureter to Colon with Nonautologous Tissue Substitute, Open Approach
0T160K9 Bypass Right Ureter to Colocutaneous with Nonautologous Tissue Substitute, Open Approach
0T160KA Bypass Right Ureter to Ileum with Nonautologous Tissue Substitute, Open Approach
0T160KB Bypass Right Ureter to Bladder with Nonautologous Tissue Substitute, Open Approach
0T160KC Bypass Right Ureter to Ileocutaneous with Nonautologous Tissue Substitute, Open Approach
0T160KD Bypass Right Ureter to Cutaneous with Nonautologous Tissue Substitute, Open Approach
0T160Z6 Bypass Right Ureter to Right Ureter, Open Approach
0T160Z7 Bypass Right Ureter to Left Ureter, Open Approach
0T160Z8 Bypass Right Ureter to Colon, Open Approach
0T160Z9 Bypass Right Ureter to Colocutaneous, Open Approach
0T160ZA Bypass Right Ureter to Ileum, Open Approach
0T160ZB Bypass Right Ureter to Bladder, Open Approach
0T160ZC Bypass Right Ureter to Ileocutaneous, Open Approach
0T160ZD Bypass Right Ureter to Cutaneous, Open Approach
0T163JD Bypass Right Ureter to Cutaneous with Synthetic Substitute, Percutaneous Approach
0T16476 Bypass Right Ureter to Right Ureter with Autologous Tissue Substitute, Percutaneous Endoscopic Approach
0T16477 Bypass Right Ureter to Left Ureter with Autologous Tissue Substitute, Percutaneous Endoscopic Approach
0T16478 Bypass Right Ureter to Colon with Autologous Tissue Substitute, Percutaneous Endoscopic Approach
0T16479 Bypass Right Ureter to Colocutaneous with Autologous Tissue Substitute, Percutaneous Endoscopic Approach
0T1647A Bypass Right Ureter to Ileum with Autologous Tissue Substitute, Percutaneous Endoscopic Approach
0T1647B Bypass Right Ureter to Bladder with Autologous Tissue Substitute, Percutaneous Endoscopic Approach
0T1647C Bypass Right Ureter to Ileocutaneous with Autologous Tissue Substitute, Percutaneous Endoscopic Approach
0T1647D Bypass Right Ureter to Cutaneous with Autologous Tissue Substitute, Percutaneous Endoscopic Approach
0T164J6 Bypass Right Ureter to Right Ureter with Synthetic Substitute, Percutaneous Endoscopic Approach
0T164J7 Bypass Right Ureter to Left Ureter with Synthetic Substitute, Percutaneous Endoscopic Approach
0T164J8 Bypass Right Ureter to Colon with Synthetic Substitute, Percutaneous Endoscopic Approach
0T164J9 Bypass Right Ureter to Colocutaneous with Synthetic Substitute, Percutaneous Endoscopic Approach
0T164JA Bypass Right Ureter to Ileum with Synthetic Substitute, Percutaneous Endoscopic Approach
0T164JB Bypass Right Ureter to Bladder with Synthetic Substitute, Percutaneous Endoscopic Approach
0T164JC Bypass Right Ureter to Ileocutaneous with Synthetic Substitute, Percutaneous Endoscopic Approach
0T164JD Bypass Right Ureter to Cutaneous with Synthetic Substitute, Percutaneous Endoscopic Approach
0T164K6 Bypass Right Ureter to Right Ureter with Nonautologous Tissue Substitute, Percutaneous Endoscopic Approach
0T164K7 Bypass Right Ureter to Left Ureter with Nonautologous Tissue Substitute, Percutaneous Endoscopic Approach
0T164K8 Bypass Right Ureter to Colon with Nonautologous Tissue Substitute, Percutaneous Endoscopic Approach
0T164K9 Bypass Right Ureter to Colocutaneous with Nonautologous Tissue Substitute, Percutaneous Endoscopic Approach
0T164KA Bypass Right Ureter to Ileum with Nonautologous Tissue Substitute, Percutaneous Endoscopic Approach
0T164KB Bypass Right Ureter to Bladder with Nonautologous Tissue Substitute, Percutaneous Endoscopic Approach
0T164KC Bypass Right Ureter to Ileocutaneous with Nonautologous Tissue Substitute, Percutaneous Endoscopic Approach
0T164KD Bypass Right Ureter to Cutaneous with Nonautologous Tissue Substitute, Percutaneous Endoscopic Approach
0T164Z6 Bypass Right Ureter to Right Ureter, Percutaneous Endoscopic Approach
0T164Z7 Bypass Right Ureter to Left Ureter, Percutaneous Endoscopic Approach
0T164Z8 Bypass Right Ureter to Colon, Percutaneous Endoscopic Approach
0T164Z9 Bypass Right Ureter to Colocutaneous, Percutaneous Endoscopic Approach
0T164ZA Bypass Right Ureter to Ileum, Percutaneous Endoscopic Approach
0T164ZB Bypass Right Ureter to Bladder, Percutaneous Endoscopic Approach
0T164ZC Bypass Right Ureter to Ileocutaneous, Percutaneous Endoscopic Approach
0T164ZD Bypass Right Ureter to Cutaneous, Percutaneous Endoscopic Approach
0T17076 Bypass Left Ureter to Right Ureter with Autologous Tissue Substitute, Open Approach
0T17077 Bypass Left Ureter to Left Ureter with Autologous Tissue Substitute, Open Approach

0T17078 Bypass Left Ureter to Colon with Autologous Tissue Substitute, Open Approach
0T17079 Bypass Left Ureter to Colocutaneous with Autologous Tissue Substitute, Open Approach
0T1707A Bypass Left Ureter to Ileum with Autologous Tissue Substitute, Open Approach
0T1707B Bypass Left Ureter to Bladder with Autologous Tissue Substitute, Open Approach
0T1707C Bypass Left Ureter to Ileocutaneous with Autologous Tissue Substitute, Open Approach
0T1707D Bypass Left Ureter to Cutaneous with Autologous Tissue Substitute, Open Approach
0T170J6 Bypass Left Ureter to Right Ureter with Synthetic Substitute, Open Approach
0T170J7 Bypass Left Ureter to Left Ureter with Synthetic Substitute, Open Approach
0T170J8 Bypass Left Ureter to Colon with Synthetic Substitute, Open Approach
0T170J9 Bypass Left Ureter to Colocutaneous with Synthetic Substitute, Open Approach
0T170JA Bypass Left Ureter to Ileum with Synthetic Substitute, Open Approach
0T170JB Bypass Left Ureter to Bladder with Synthetic Substitute, Open Approach
0T170JC Bypass Left Ureter to Ileocutaneous with Synthetic Substitute, Open Approach
0T170JD Bypass Left Ureter to Cutaneous with Synthetic Substitute, Open Approach
0T170K6 Bypass Left Ureter to Right Ureter with Nonautologous Tissue Substitute, Open Approach
0T170K7 Bypass Left Ureter to Left Ureter with Nonautologous Tissue Substitute, Open Approach
0T170K8 Bypass Left Ureter to Colon with Nonautologous Tissue Substitute, Open Approach
0T170K9 Bypass Left Ureter to Colocutaneous with Nonautologous Tissue Substitute, Open Approach
0T170KA Bypass Left Ureter to Ileum with Nonautologous Tissue Substitute, Open Approach
0T170KB Bypass Left Ureter to Bladder with Nonautologous Tissue Substitute, Open Approach
0T170KC Bypass Left Ureter to Ileocutaneous with Nonautologous Tissue Substitute, Open Approach
0T170KD Bypass Left Ureter to Cutaneous with Nonautologous Tissue Substitute, Open Approach
0T170Z6 Bypass Left Ureter to Right Ureter, Open Approach
0T170Z7 Bypass Left Ureter to Left Ureter, Open Approach
0T170Z8 Bypass Left Ureter to Colon, Open Approach
0T170Z9 Bypass Left Ureter to Colocutaneous, Open Approach
0T170ZA Bypass Left Ureter to Ileum, Open Approach
0T170ZB Bypass Left Ureter to Bladder, Open Approach
0T170ZC Bypass Left Ureter to Ileocutaneous, Open Approach
0T170ZD Bypass Left Ureter to Cutaneous, Open Approach
0T173JD Bypass Left Ureter to Cutaneous with Synthetic Substitute, Percutaneous Approach
0T17476 Bypass Left Ureter to Right Ureter with Autologous Tissue Substitute, Percutaneous Endoscopic Approach
0T17477 Bypass Left Ureter to Left Ureter with Autologous Tissue Substitute, Percutaneous Endoscopic Approach
0T17478 Bypass Left Ureter to Colon with Autologous Tissue Substitute, Percutaneous Endoscopic Approach
0T17479 Bypass Left Ureter to Colocutaneous with Autologous Tissue Substitute, Percutaneous Endoscopic Approach
0T1747A Bypass Left Ureter to Ileum with Autologous Tissue Substitute, Percutaneous Endoscopic Approach
0T1747B Bypass Left Ureter to Bladder with Autologous Tissue Substitute, Percutaneous Endoscopic Approach
0T1747C Bypass Left Ureter to Ileocutaneous with Autologous Tissue Substitute, Percutaneous Endoscopic Approach
0T1747D Bypass Left Ureter to Cutaneous with Autologous Tissue Substitute, Percutaneous Endoscopic Approach
0T174J6 Bypass Left Ureter to Right Ureter with Synthetic Substitute, Percutaneous Endoscopic Approach
0T174J7 Bypass Left Ureter to Left Ureter with Synthetic Substitute, Percutaneous Endoscopic Approach
0T174J8 Bypass Left Ureter to Colon with Synthetic Substitute, Percutaneous Endoscopic Approach
0T174J9 Bypass Left Ureter to Colocutaneous with Synthetic Substitute, Percutaneous Endoscopic Approach
0T174JA Bypass Left Ureter to Ileum with Synthetic Substitute, Percutaneous Endoscopic Approach
0T174JB Bypass Left Ureter to Bladder with Synthetic Substitute, Percutaneous Endoscopic Approach
0T174JC Bypass Left Ureter to Ileocutaneous with Synthetic Substitute, Percutaneous Endoscopic Approach
0T174JD Bypass Left Ureter to Cutaneous with Synthetic Substitute, Percutaneous Endoscopic Approach
0T174K6 Bypass Left Ureter to Right Ureter with Nonautologous Tissue Substitute, Percutaneous Endoscopic Approach
0T174K7 Bypass Left Ureter to Left Ureter with Nonautologous Tissue Substitute, Percutaneous Endoscopic Approach
0T174K8 Bypass Left Ureter to Colon with Nonautologous Tissue Substitute, Percutaneous Endoscopic Approach
0T174K9 Bypass Left Ureter to Colocutaneous with Nonautologous Tissue Substitute, Percutaneous Endoscopic Approach
0T174KA Bypass Left Ureter to Ileum with Nonautologous Tissue Substitute, Percutaneous Endoscopic Approach
0T174KB Bypass Left Ureter to Bladder with Nonautologous Tissue Substitute, Percutaneous Endoscopic Approach
0T174KC Bypass Left Ureter to Ileocutaneous with Nonautologous Tissue Substitute, Percutaneous Endoscopic Approach
0T174KD Bypass Left Ureter to Cutaneous with Nonautologous Tissue Substitute, Percutaneous Endoscopic Approach
0T174Z6 Bypass Left Ureter to Right Ureter, Percutaneous Endoscopic Approach
0T174Z7 Bypass Left Ureter to Left Ureter, Percutaneous Endoscopic Approach
0T174Z8 Bypass Left Ureter to Colon, Percutaneous Endoscopic Approach
0T174Z9 Bypass Left Ureter to Colocutaneous, Percutaneous Endoscopic Approach
0T174ZA Bypass Left Ureter to Ileum, Percutaneous Endoscopic Approach
0T174ZB Bypass Left Ureter to Bladder, Percutaneous Endoscopic Approach
0T174ZC Bypass Left Ureter to Ileocutaneous, Percutaneous Endoscopic Approach
0T174ZD Bypass Left Ureter to Cutaneous, Percutaneous Endoscopic Approach
0T18076 Bypass Bilateral Ureters to Right Ureter with Autologous Tissue Substitute, Open Approach
0T18077 Bypass Bilateral Ureters to Left Ureter with Autologous Tissue Substitute, Open Approach
0T18078 Bypass Bilateral Ureters to Colon with Autologous Tissue Substitute, Open Approach
0T18079 Bypass Bilateral Ureters to Colocutaneous with Autologous Tissue Substitute, Open Approach
0T1807A Bypass Bilateral Ureters to Ileum with Autologous Tissue Substitute, Open Approach
0T1807B Bypass Bilateral Ureters to Bladder with Autologous Tissue Substitute, Open Approach
0T1807C Bypass Bilateral Ureters to Ileocutaneous with Autologous Tissue Substitute, Open Approach
0T1807D Bypass Bilateral Ureters to Cutaneous with Autologous Tissue Substitute, Open Approach
0T180J6 Bypass Bilateral Ureters to Right Ureter with Synthetic Substitute, Open Approach
0T180J7 Bypass Bilateral Ureters to Left Ureter with Synthetic Substitute, Open Approach
0T180J8 Bypass Bilateral Ureters to Colon with Synthetic Substitute, Open Approach
0T180J9 Bypass Bilateral Ureters to Colocutaneous with Synthetic Substitute, Open Approach
0T180JA Bypass Bilateral Ureters to Ileum with Synthetic Substitute, Open Approach
0T180JB Bypass Bilateral Ureters to Bladder with Synthetic Substitute, Open Approach
0T180JC Bypass Bilateral Ureters to Ileocutaneous with Synthetic Substitute, Open Approach
0T180JD Bypass Bilateral Ureters to Cutaneous with Synthetic Substitute, Open Approach
0T180K6 Bypass Bilateral Ureters to Right Ureter with Nonautologous Tissue Substitute, Open Approach
0T180K7 Bypass Bilateral Ureters to Left Ureter with Nonautologous Tissue Substitute, Open Approach
0T180K8 Bypass Bilateral Ureters to Colon with Nonautologous Tissue Substitute, Open Approach
0T180K9 Bypass Bilateral Ureters to Colocutaneous with Nonautologous Tissue Substitute, Open Approach
0T180KA Bypass Bilateral Ureters to Ileum with Nonautologous Tissue Substitute, Open Approach
0T180KB Bypass Bilateral Ureters to Bladder with Nonautologous Tissue Substitute, Open Approach
0T180KC Bypass Bilateral Ureters to Ileocutaneous with Nonautologous Tissue Substitute, Open Approach
0T180KD Bypass Bilateral Ureters to Cutaneous with Nonautologous Tissue Substitute, Open Approach
0T180Z6 Bypass Bilateral Ureters to Right Ureter, Open Approach
0T180Z7 Bypass Bilateral Ureters to Left Ureter, Open Approach

0T180Z8 Bypass Bilateral Ureters to Colon, Open Approach
0T180Z9 Bypass Bilateral Ureters to Colocutaneous, Open Approach
0T180ZA Bypass Bilateral Ureters to Ileum, Open Approach
0T180ZB Bypass Bilateral Ureters to Bladder, Open Approach
0T180ZC Bypass Bilateral Ureters to Ileocutaneous, Open Approach
0T180ZD Bypass Bilateral Ureters to Cutaneous, Open Approach
0T183JD Bypass Bilateral Ureters to Cutaneous with Synthetic Substitute, Percutaneous Approach
0T18476 Bypass Bilateral Ureters to Right Ureter with Autologous Tissue Substitute, Percutaneous Endoscopic Approach
0T18477 Bypass Bilateral Ureters to Left Ureter with Autologous Tissue Substitute, Percutaneous Endoscopic Approach
0T18478 Bypass Bilateral Ureters to Colon with Autologous Tissue Substitute, Percutaneous Endoscopic Approach
0T18479 Bypass Bilateral Ureters to Colocutaneous with Autologous Tissue Substitute, Percutaneous Endoscopic Approach
0T1847A Bypass Bilateral Ureters to Ileum with Autologous Tissue Substitute, Percutaneous Endoscopic Approach
0T1847B Bypass Bilateral Ureters to Bladder with Autologous Tissue Substitute, Percutaneous Endoscopic Approach
0T1847C Bypass Bilateral Ureters to Ileocutaneous with Autologous Tissue Substitute, Percutaneous Endoscopic Approach
0T1847D Bypass Bilateral Ureters to Cutaneous with Autologous Tissue Substitute, Percutaneous Endoscopic Approach
0T184J6 Bypass Bilateral Ureters to Right Ureter with Synthetic Substitute, Percutaneous Endoscopic Approach
0T184J7 Bypass Bilateral Ureters to Left Ureter with Synthetic Substitute, Percutaneous Endoscopic Approach
0T184J8 Bypass Bilateral Ureters to Colon with Synthetic Substitute, Percutaneous Endoscopic Approach
0T184J9 Bypass Bilateral Ureters to Colocutaneous with Synthetic Substitute, Percutaneous Endoscopic Approach
0T184JA Bypass Bilateral Ureters to Ileum with Synthetic Substitute, Percutaneous Endoscopic Approach
0T184JB Bypass Bilateral Ureters to Bladder with Synthetic Substitute, Percutaneous Endoscopic Approach
0T184JC Bypass Bilateral Ureters to Ileocutaneous with Synthetic Substitute, Percutaneous Endoscopic Approach
0T184JD Bypass Bilateral Ureters to Cutaneous with Synthetic Substitute, Percutaneous Endoscopic Approach
0T184K6 Bypass Bilateral Ureters to Right Ureter with Nonautologous Tissue Substitute, Percutaneous Endoscopic Approach
0T184K7 Bypass Bilateral Ureters to Left Ureter with Nonautologous Tissue Substitute, Percutaneous Endoscopic Approach
0T184K8 Bypass Bilateral Ureters to Colon with Nonautologous Tissue Substitute, Percutaneous Endoscopic Approach
0T184K9 Bypass Bilateral Ureters to Colocutaneous with Nonautologous Tissue Substitute, Percutaneous Endoscopic Approach
0T184KA Bypass Bilateral Ureters to Ileum with Nonautologous Tissue Substitute, Percutaneous Endoscopic Approach
0T184KB Bypass Bilateral Ureters to Bladder with Nonautologous Tissue Substitute, Percutaneous Endoscopic Approach
0T184KC Bypass Bilateral Ureters to Ileocutaneous with Nonautologous Tissue Substitute, Percutaneous Endoscopic Approach
0T184KD Bypass Bilateral Ureters to Cutaneous with Nonautologous Tissue Substitute, Percutaneous Endoscopic Approach
0T184Z6 Bypass Bilateral Ureters to Right Ureter, Percutaneous Endoscopic Approach
0T184Z7 Bypass Bilateral Ureters to Left Ureter, Percutaneous Endoscopic Approach
0T184Z8 Bypass Bilateral Ureters to Colon, Percutaneous Endoscopic Approach
0T184Z9 Bypass Bilateral Ureters to Colocutaneous, Percutaneous Endoscopic Approach
0T184ZA Bypass Bilateral Ureters to Ileum, Percutaneous Endoscopic Approach
0T184ZB Bypass Bilateral Ureters to Bladder, Percutaneous Endoscopic Approach
0T184ZC Bypass Bilateral Ureters to Ileocutaneous, Percutaneous Endoscopic Approach
0T184ZD Bypass Bilateral Ureters to Cutaneous, Percutaneous Endoscopic Approach
0T1B079 Bypass Bladder to Colocutaneous with Autologous Tissue Substitute, Open Approach
0T1B07C Bypass Bladder to Ileocutaneous with Autologous Tissue Substitute, Open Approach
0T1B07D Bypass Bladder to Cutaneous with Autologous Tissue Substitute, Open Approach
0T1B0J9 Bypass Bladder to Colocutaneous with Synthetic Substitute, Open Approach
0T1B0JC Bypass Bladder to Ileocutaneous with Synthetic Substitute, Open Approach
0T1B0JD Bypass Bladder to Cutaneous with Synthetic Substitute, Open Approach
0T1B0K9 Bypass Bladder to Colocutaneous with Nonautologous Tissue Substitute, Open Approach
0T1B0KC Bypass Bladder to Ileocutaneous with Nonautologous Tissue Substitute, Open Approach
0T1B0KD Bypass Bladder to Cutaneous with Nonautologous Tissue Substitute, Open Approach
0T1B0Z9 Bypass Bladder to Colocutaneous, Open Approach
0T1B0ZC Bypass Bladder to Ileocutaneous, Open Approach
0T1B0ZD Bypass Bladder to Cutaneous, Open Approach
0T1B3JD Bypass Bladder to Cutaneous with Synthetic Substitute, Percutaneous Approach
0T1B479 Bypass Bladder to Colocutaneous with Autologous Tissue Substitute, Percutaneous Endoscopic Approach
0T1B47C Bypass Bladder to Ileocutaneous with Autologous Tissue Substitute, Percutaneous Endoscopic Approach
0T1B47D Bypass Bladder to Cutaneous with Autologous Tissue Substitute, Percutaneous Endoscopic Approach
0T1B4J9 Bypass Bladder to Colocutaneous with Synthetic Substitute, Percutaneous Endoscopic Approach
0T1B4JC Bypass Bladder to Ileocutaneous with Synthetic Substitute, Percutaneous Endoscopic Approach
0T1B4JD Bypass Bladder to Cutaneous with Synthetic Substitute, Percutaneous Endoscopic Approach
0T1B4K9 Bypass Bladder to Colocutaneous with Nonautologous Tissue Substitute, Percutaneous Endoscopic Approach
0T1B4KC Bypass Bladder to Ileocutaneous with Nonautologous Tissue Substitute, Percutaneous Endoscopic Approach
0T1B4KD Bypass Bladder to Cutaneous with Nonautologous Tissue Substitute, Percutaneous Endoscopic Approach
0T1B4Z9 Bypass Bladder to Colocutaneous, Percutaneous Endoscopic Approach
0T1B4ZC Bypass Bladder to Ileocutaneous, Percutaneous Endoscopic Approach
0T1B4ZD Bypass Bladder to Cutaneous, Percutaneous Endoscopic Approach

0T2 – Urinary System, Change

Review Coding Guideline B6.1c

0T25X0Z Change Drainage Device in Kidney, External Approach
0T25XYZ Change Other Device in Kidney, External Approach
0T29X0Z Change Drainage Device in Ureter, External Approach
0T29XYZ Change Other Device in Ureter, External Approach
0T2BX0Z Change Drainage Device in Bladder, External Approach
0T2BXYZ Change Other Device in Bladder, External Approach
0T2DX0Z Change Drainage Device in Urethra, External Approach
0T2DXYZ Change Other Device in Urethra, External Approach

0T5 – Urinary System, Destruction

0T500ZZ Destruction of Right Kidney, Open Approach
0T503ZZ Destruction of Right Kidney, Percutaneous Approach
0T504ZZ Destruction of Right Kidney, Percutaneous Endoscopic Approach
0T507ZZ Destruction of Right Kidney, Via Natural or Artificial Opening
0T508ZZ Destruction of Right Kidney, Via Natural or Artificial Opening Endoscopic
0T510ZZ Destruction of Left Kidney, Open Approach
0T513ZZ Destruction of Left Kidney, Percutaneous Approach
0T514ZZ Destruction of Left Kidney, Percutaneous Endoscopic Approach
0T517ZZ Destruction of Left Kidney, Via Natural or Artificial Opening

0T518ZZ Destruction of Left Kidney, Via Natural or Artificial Opening Endoscopic
0T530ZZ Destruction of Right Kidney Pelvis, Open Approach
0T533ZZ Destruction of Right Kidney Pelvis, Percutaneous Approach
0T534ZZ Destruction of Right Kidney Pelvis, Percutaneous Endoscopic Approach
0T537ZZ Destruction of Right Kidney Pelvis, Via Natural or Artificial Opening
0T538ZZ Destruction of Right Kidney Pelvis, Via Natural or Artificial Opening Endoscopic
0T540ZZ Destruction of Left Kidney Pelvis, Open Approach
0T543ZZ Destruction of Left Kidney Pelvis, Percutaneous Approach
0T544ZZ Destruction of Left Kidney Pelvis, Percutaneous Endoscopic Approach
0T547ZZ Destruction of Left Kidney Pelvis, Via Natural or Artificial Opening
0T548ZZ Destruction of Left Kidney Pelvis, Via Natural or Artificial Opening Endoscopic
0T560ZZ Destruction of Right Ureter, Open Approach
0T563ZZ Destruction of Right Ureter, Percutaneous Approach
0T564ZZ Destruction of Right Ureter, Percutaneous Endoscopic Approach
0T567ZZ Destruction of Right Ureter, Via Natural or Artificial Opening
0T568ZZ Destruction of Right Ureter, Via Natural or Artificial Opening Endoscopic
0T570ZZ Destruction of Left Ureter, Open Approach
0T573ZZ Destruction of Left Ureter, Percutaneous Approach
0T574ZZ Destruction of Left Ureter, Percutaneous Endoscopic Approach
0T577ZZ Destruction of Left Ureter, Via Natural or Artificial Opening
0T578ZZ Destruction of Left Ureter, Via Natural or Artificial Opening Endoscopic
0T5B0ZZ Destruction of Bladder, Open Approach
0T5B3ZZ Destruction of Bladder, Percutaneous Approach
0T5B4ZZ Destruction of Bladder, Percutaneous Endoscopic Approach
0T5B7ZZ Destruction of Bladder, Via Natural or Artificial Opening
0T5B8ZZ Destruction of Bladder, Via Natural or Artificial Opening Endoscopic
0T5C0ZZ Destruction of Bladder Neck, Open Approach
0T5C3ZZ Destruction of Bladder Neck, Percutaneous Approach
0T5C4ZZ Destruction of Bladder Neck, Percutaneous Endoscopic Approach
0T5C7ZZ Destruction of Bladder Neck, Via Natural or Artificial Opening
0T5C8ZZ Destruction of Bladder Neck, Via Natural or Artificial Opening Endoscopic
0T5D0ZZ Destruction of Urethra, Open Approach
0T5D3ZZ Destruction of Urethra, Percutaneous Approach
0T5D4ZZ Destruction of Urethra, Percutaneous Endoscopic Approach
0T5D7ZZ Destruction of Urethra, Via Natural or Artificial Opening
0T5D8ZZ Destruction of Urethra, Via Natural or Artificial Opening Endoscopic
0T5DXZZ Destruction of Urethra, External Approach

0T7 – Urinary System, Dilation

0T730DZ Dilation of Right Kidney Pelvis with Intraluminal Device, Open Approach
0T730ZZ Dilation of Right Kidney Pelvis, Open Approach
0T733DZ Dilation of Right Kidney Pelvis with Intraluminal Device, Percutaneous Approach
0T733ZZ Dilation of Right Kidney Pelvis, Percutaneous Approach
0T734DZ Dilation of Right Kidney Pelvis with Intraluminal Device, Percutaneous Endoscopic Approach
0T734ZZ Dilation of Right Kidney Pelvis, Percutaneous Endoscopic Approach
0T737DZ Dilation of Right Kidney Pelvis with Intraluminal Device, Via Natural or Artificial Opening
0T737ZZ Dilation of Right Kidney Pelvis, Via Natural or Artificial Opening
0T738DZ Dilation of Right Kidney Pelvis with Intraluminal Device, Via Natural or Artificial Opening Endoscopic
0T738ZZ Dilation of Right Kidney Pelvis, Via Natural or Artificial Opening Endoscopic
0T740DZ Dilation of Left Kidney Pelvis with Intraluminal Device, Open Approach
0T740ZZ Dilation of Left Kidney Pelvis, Open Approach
0T743DZ Dilation of Left Kidney Pelvis with Intraluminal Device, Percutaneous Approach
0T743ZZ Dilation of Left Kidney Pelvis, Percutaneous Approach
0T744DZ Dilation of Left Kidney Pelvis with Intraluminal Device, Percutaneous Endoscopic Approach
0T744ZZ Dilation of Left Kidney Pelvis, Percutaneous Endoscopic Approach
0T747DZ Dilation of Left Kidney Pelvis with Intraluminal Device, Via Natural or Artificial Opening
0T747ZZ Dilation of Left Kidney Pelvis, Via Natural or Artificial Opening
0T748DZ Dilation of Left Kidney Pelvis with Intraluminal Device, Via Natural or Artificial Opening Endoscopic
0T748ZZ Dilation of Left Kidney Pelvis, Via Natural or Artificial Opening Endoscopic
0T760DZ Dilation of Right Ureter with Intraluminal Device, Open Approach
0T760ZZ Dilation of Right Ureter, Open Approach
0T763DZ Dilation of Right Ureter with Intraluminal Device, Percutaneous Approach
0T763ZZ Dilation of Right Ureter, Percutaneous Approach
0T764DZ Dilation of Right Ureter with Intraluminal Device, Percutaneous Endoscopic Approach
0T764ZZ Dilation of Right Ureter, Percutaneous Endoscopic Approach
0T767DZ Dilation of Right Ureter with Intraluminal Device, Via Natural or Artificial Opening
0T767ZZ Dilation of Right Ureter, Via Natural or Artificial Opening
0T768DZ Dilation of Right Ureter with Intraluminal Device, Via Natural or Artificial Opening Endoscopic
0T768ZZ Dilation of Right Ureter, Via Natural or Artificial Opening Endoscopic
0T770DZ Dilation of Left Ureter with Intraluminal Device, Open Approach
0T770ZZ Dilation of Left Ureter, Open Approach
0T773DZ Dilation of Left Ureter with Intraluminal Device, Percutaneous Approach
0T773ZZ Dilation of Left Ureter, Percutaneous Approach
0T774DZ Dilation of Left Ureter with Intraluminal Device, Percutaneous Endoscopic Approach
0T774ZZ Dilation of Left Ureter, Percutaneous Endoscopic Approach
0T777DZ Dilation of Left Ureter with Intraluminal Device, Via Natural or Artificial Opening
0T777ZZ Dilation of Left Ureter, Via Natural or Artificial Opening
0T778DZ Dilation of Left Ureter with Intraluminal Device, Via Natural or Artificial Opening Endoscopic
0T778ZZ Dilation of Left Ureter, Via Natural or Artificial Opening Endoscopic
0T780DZ Dilation of Bilateral Ureters with Intraluminal Device, Open Approach
0T780ZZ Dilation of Bilateral Ureters, Open Approach
0T783DZ Dilation of Bilateral Ureters with Intraluminal Device, Percutaneous Approach
0T783ZZ Dilation of Bilateral Ureters, Percutaneous Approach
0T784DZ Dilation of Bilateral Ureters with Intraluminal Device, Percutaneous Endoscopic Approach
0T784ZZ Dilation of Bilateral Ureters, Percutaneous Endoscopic Approach
0T787DZ Dilation of Bilateral Ureters with Intraluminal Device, Via Natural or Artificial Opening
0T787ZZ Dilation of Bilateral Ureters, Via Natural or Artificial Opening
0T788DZ Dilation of Bilateral Ureters with Intraluminal Device, Via Natural or Artificial Opening Endoscopic
0T788ZZ Dilation of Bilateral Ureters, Via Natural or Artificial Opening Endoscopic
0T7B0DZ Dilation of Bladder with Intraluminal Device, Open Approach
0T7B0ZZ Dilation of Bladder, Open Approach
0T7B3DZ Dilation of Bladder with Intraluminal Device, Percutaneous Approach
0T7B3ZZ Dilation of Bladder, Percutaneous Approach
0T7B4DZ Dilation of Bladder with Intraluminal Device, Percutaneous Endoscopic Approach
0T7B4ZZ Dilation of Bladder, Percutaneous Endoscopic Approach
0T7B7DZ Dilation of Bladder with Intraluminal Device, Via Natural or Artificial Opening
0T7B7ZZ Dilation of Bladder, Via Natural or Artificial Opening
0T7B8DZ Dilation of Bladder with Intraluminal Device, Via Natural or Artificial Opening Endoscopic
0T7B8ZZ Dilation of Bladder, Via Natural or Artificial Opening Endoscopic
0T7C0DZ Dilation of Bladder Neck with Intraluminal Device, Open Approach
0T7C0ZZ Dilation of Bladder Neck, Open Approach
0T7C3DZ Dilation of Bladder Neck with Intraluminal Device, Percutaneous Approach
0T7C3ZZ Dilation of Bladder Neck, Percutaneous Approach
0T7C4DZ Dilation of Bladder Neck with Intraluminal Device, Percutaneous Endoscopic Approach
0T7C4ZZ Dilation of Bladder Neck, Percutaneous Endoscopic Approach
0T7C7DZ Dilation of Bladder Neck with Intraluminal Device, Via Natural or Artificial Opening
0T7C7ZZ Dilation of Bladder Neck, Via Natural or Artificial Opening

0T7C8DZ Dilation of Bladder Neck with Intraluminal Device, Via Natural or Artificial Opening Endoscopic
0T7C8ZZ Dilation of Bladder Neck, Via Natural or Artificial Opening Endoscopic
0T7D0DZ Dilation of Urethra with Intraluminal Device, Open Approach
0T7D0ZZ Dilation of Urethra, Open Approach
0T7D3DZ Dilation of Urethra with Intraluminal Device, Percutaneous Approach
0T7D3ZZ Dilation of Urethra, Percutaneous Approach
0T7D4DZ Dilation of Urethra with Intraluminal Device, Percutaneous Endoscopic Approach
0T7D4ZZ Dilation of Urethra, Percutaneous Endoscopic Approach
0T7D7DZ Dilation of Urethra with Intraluminal Device, Via Natural or Artificial Opening
0T7D7ZZ Dilation of Urethra, Via Natural or Artificial Opening
0T7D8DZ Dilation of Urethra with Intraluminal Device, Via Natural or Artificial Opening Endoscopic
AHA CC: 4Q, 2013, 123
0T7D8ZZ Dilation of Urethra, Via Natural or Artificial Opening Endoscopic

0T8 – Urinary System, Division

Review Coding Guideline B3.14

0T820ZZ Division of Bilateral Kidneys, Open Approach
0T823ZZ Division of Bilateral Kidneys, Percutaneous Approach
0T824ZZ Division of Bilateral Kidneys, Percutaneous Endoscopic Approach
0T8C0ZZ Division of Bladder Neck, Open Approach
0T8C3ZZ Division of Bladder Neck, Percutaneous Approach
0T8C4ZZ Division of Bladder Neck, Percutaneous Endoscopic Approach

0T9 – Urinary System, Drainage

Review Coding Guidelines B3.4a and B3.4b

Review Coding Guideline B6.2

0T9000Z Drainage of Right Kidney with Drainage Device, Open Approach
0T900ZX Drainage of Right Kidney, Open Approach, Diagnostic
0T900ZZ Drainage of Right Kidney, Open Approach
0T9030Z Drainage of Right Kidney with Drainage Device, Percutaneous Approach
0T903ZX Drainage of Right Kidney, Percutaneous Approach, Diagnostic
0T903ZZ Drainage of Right Kidney, Percutaneous Approach
0T9040Z Drainage of Right Kidney with Drainage Device, Percutaneous Endoscopic Approach
0T904ZX Drainage of Right Kidney, Percutaneous Endoscopic Approach, Diagnostic
0T904ZZ Drainage of Right Kidney, Percutaneous Endoscopic Approach
0T9070Z Drainage of Right Kidney with Drainage Device, Via Natural or Artificial Opening
0T907ZX Drainage of Right Kidney, Via Natural or Artificial Opening, Diagnostic
0T907ZZ Drainage of Right Kidney, Via Natural or Artificial Opening
0T9080Z Drainage of Right Kidney with Drainage Device, Via Natural or Artificial Opening Endoscopic
0T908ZX Drainage of Right Kidney, Via Natural or Artificial Opening Endoscopic, Diagnostic
0T908ZZ Drainage of Right Kidney, Via Natural or Artificial Opening Endoscopic
0T9100Z Drainage of Left Kidney with Drainage Device, Open Approach
0T910ZX Drainage of Left Kidney, Open Approach, Diagnostic
0T910ZZ Drainage of Left Kidney, Open Approach
0T9130Z Drainage of Left Kidney with Drainage Device, Percutaneous Approach
0T913ZX Drainage of Left Kidney, Percutaneous Approach, Diagnostic
0T913ZZ Drainage of Left Kidney, Percutaneous Approach
0T9140Z Drainage of Left Kidney with Drainage Device, Percutaneous Endoscopic Approach
0T914ZX Drainage of Left Kidney, Percutaneous Endoscopic Approach, Diagnostic
0T914ZZ Drainage of Left Kidney, Percutaneous Endoscopic Approach
0T9170Z Drainage of Left Kidney with Drainage Device, Via Natural or Artificial Opening
0T917ZX Drainage of Left Kidney, Via Natural or Artificial Opening, Diagnostic
0T917ZZ Drainage of Left Kidney, Via Natural or Artificial Opening
0T9180Z Drainage of Left Kidney with Drainage Device, Via Natural or Artificial Opening Endoscopic
0T918ZX Drainage of Left Kidney, Via Natural or Artificial Opening Endoscopic, Diagnostic
0T918ZZ Drainage of Left Kidney, Via Natural or Artificial Opening Endoscopic
0T9300Z Drainage of Right Kidney Pelvis with Drainage Device, Open Approach
0T930ZX Drainage of Right Kidney Pelvis, Open Approach, Diagnostic
0T930ZZ Drainage of Right Kidney Pelvis, Open Approach
0T9330Z Drainage of Right Kidney Pelvis with Drainage Device, Percutaneous Approach
0T933ZX Drainage of Right Kidney Pelvis, Percutaneous Approach, Diagnostic
0T933ZZ Drainage of Right Kidney Pelvis, Percutaneous Approach
0T9340Z Drainage of Right Kidney Pelvis with Drainage Device, Percutaneous Endoscopic Approach
0T934ZX Drainage of Right Kidney Pelvis, Percutaneous Endoscopic Approach, Diagnostic
0T934ZZ Drainage of Right Kidney Pelvis, Percutaneous Endoscopic Approach
0T9370Z Drainage of Right Kidney Pelvis with Drainage Device, Via Natural or Artificial Opening
0T937ZX Drainage of Right Kidney Pelvis, Via Natural or Artificial Opening, Diagnostic
0T937ZZ Drainage of Right Kidney Pelvis, Via Natural or Artificial Opening
0T9380Z Drainage of Right Kidney Pelvis with Drainage Device, Via Natural or Artificial Opening Endoscopic
0T938ZX Drainage of Right Kidney Pelvis, Via Natural or Artificial Opening Endoscopic, Diagnostic
0T938ZZ Drainage of Right Kidney Pelvis, Via Natural or Artificial Opening Endoscopic
0T9400Z Drainage of Left Kidney Pelvis with Drainage Device, Open Approach
0T940ZX Drainage of Left Kidney Pelvis, Open Approach, Diagnostic
0T940ZZ Drainage of Left Kidney Pelvis, Open Approach
0T9430Z Drainage of Left Kidney Pelvis with Drainage Device, Percutaneous Approach
0T943ZX Drainage of Left Kidney Pelvis, Percutaneous Approach, Diagnostic
0T943ZZ Drainage of Left Kidney Pelvis, Percutaneous Approach
0T9440Z Drainage of Left Kidney Pelvis with Drainage Device, Percutaneous Endoscopic Approach
0T944ZX Drainage of Left Kidney Pelvis, Percutaneous Endoscopic Approach, Diagnostic
0T944ZZ Drainage of Left Kidney Pelvis, Percutaneous Endoscopic Approach
0T9470Z Drainage of Left Kidney Pelvis with Drainage Device, Via Natural or Artificial Opening
0T947ZX Drainage of Left Kidney Pelvis, Via Natural or Artificial Opening, Diagnostic
0T947ZZ Drainage of Left Kidney Pelvis, Via Natural or Artificial Opening
0T9480Z Drainage of Left Kidney Pelvis with Drainage Device, Via Natural or Artificial Opening Endoscopic
0T948ZX Drainage of Left Kidney Pelvis, Via Natural or Artificial Opening Endoscopic, Diagnostic
0T948ZZ Drainage of Left Kidney Pelvis, Via Natural or Artificial Opening Endoscopic
0T9600Z Drainage of Right Ureter with Drainage Device, Open Approach
0T960ZX Drainage of Right Ureter, Open Approach, Diagnostic
0T960ZZ Drainage of Right Ureter, Open Approach
0T9630Z Drainage of Right Ureter with Drainage Device, Percutaneous Approach
0T963ZX Drainage of Right Ureter, Percutaneous Approach, Diagnostic
0T963ZZ Drainage of Right Ureter, Percutaneous Approach
0T9640Z Drainage of Right Ureter with Drainage Device, Percutaneous Endoscopic Approach
0T964ZX Drainage of Right Ureter, Percutaneous Endoscopic Approach, Diagnostic
0T964ZZ Drainage of Right Ureter, Percutaneous Endoscopic Approach
0T9670Z Drainage of Right Ureter with Drainage Device, Via Natural or Artificial Opening
0T967ZX Drainage of Right Ureter, Via Natural or Artificial Opening, Diagnostic

0T967ZZ Drainage of Right Ureter, Via Natural or Artificial Opening
0T9680Z Drainage of Right Ureter with Drainage Device, Via Natural or Artificial Opening Endoscopic
0T968ZX Drainage of Right Ureter, Via Natural or Artificial Opening Endoscopic, Diagnostic
0T968ZZ Drainage of Right Ureter, Via Natural or Artificial Opening Endoscopic
0T9700Z Drainage of Left Ureter with Drainage Device, Open Approach
0T970ZX Drainage of Left Ureter, Open Approach, Diagnostic
0T970ZZ Drainage of Left Ureter, Open Approach
0T9730Z Drainage of Left Ureter with Drainage Device, Percutaneous Approach
0T973ZX Drainage of Left Ureter, Percutaneous Approach, Diagnostic
0T973ZZ Drainage of Left Ureter, Percutaneous Approach
0T9740Z Drainage of Left Ureter with Drainage Device, Percutaneous Endoscopic Approach
0T974ZX Drainage of Left Ureter, Percutaneous Endoscopic Approach, Diagnostic
0T974ZZ Drainage of Left Ureter, Percutaneous Endoscopic Approach
0T9770Z Drainage of Left Ureter with Drainage Device, Via Natural or Artificial Opening
0T977ZX Drainage of Left Ureter, Via Natural or Artificial Opening, Diagnostic
0T977ZZ Drainage of Left Ureter, Via Natural or Artificial Opening
0T9780Z Drainage of Left Ureter with Drainage Device, Via Natural or Artificial Opening Endoscopic
0T978ZX Drainage of Left Ureter, Via Natural or Artificial Opening Endoscopic, Diagnostic
0T978ZZ Drainage of Left Ureter, Via Natural or Artificial Opening Endoscopic
0T9800Z Drainage of Bilateral Ureters with Drainage Device, Open Approach
0T980ZX Drainage of Bilateral Ureters, Open Approach, Diagnostic
0T980ZZ Drainage of Bilateral Ureters, Open Approach
0T9830Z Drainage of Bilateral Ureters with Drainage Device, Percutaneous Approach
0T983ZX Drainage of Bilateral Ureters, Percutaneous Approach, Diagnostic
0T983ZZ Drainage of Bilateral Ureters, Percutaneous Approach
0T9840Z Drainage of Bilateral Ureters with Drainage Device, Percutaneous Endoscopic Approach
0T984ZX Drainage of Bilateral Ureters, Percutaneous Endoscopic Approach, Diagnostic
0T984ZZ Drainage of Bilateral Ureters, Percutaneous Endoscopic Approach
0T9870Z Drainage of Bilateral Ureters with Drainage Device, Via Natural or Artificial Opening
0T987ZX Drainage of Bilateral Ureters, Via Natural or Artificial Opening, Diagnostic
0T987ZZ Drainage of Bilateral Ureters, Via Natural or Artificial Opening
0T9880Z Drainage of Bilateral Ureters with Drainage Device, Via Natural or Artificial Opening Endoscopic
0T988ZX Drainage of Bilateral Ureters, Via Natural or Artificial Opening Endoscopic, Diagnostic
0T988ZZ Drainage of Bilateral Ureters, Via Natural or Artificial Opening Endoscopic
0T9B00Z Drainage of Bladder with Drainage Device, Open Approach
0T9B0ZX Drainage of Bladder, Open Approach, Diagnostic
0T9B0ZZ Drainage of Bladder, Open Approach
0T9B30Z Drainage of Bladder with Drainage Device, Percutaneous Approach
0T9B3ZX Drainage of Bladder, Percutaneous Approach, Diagnostic
0T9B3ZZ Drainage of Bladder, Percutaneous Approach
0T9B40Z Drainage of Bladder with Drainage Device, Percutaneous Endoscopic Approach
0T9B4ZX Drainage of Bladder, Percutaneous Endoscopic Approach, Diagnostic
0T9B4ZZ Drainage of Bladder, Percutaneous Endoscopic Approach
0T9B70Z Drainage of Bladder with Drainage Device, Via Natural or Artificial Opening
0T9B7ZX Drainage of Bladder, Via Natural or Artificial Opening, Diagnostic
0T9B7ZZ Drainage of Bladder, Via Natural or Artificial Opening
0T9B80Z Drainage of Bladder with Drainage Device, Via Natural or Artificial Opening Endoscopic
0T9B8ZX Drainage of Bladder, Via Natural or Artificial Opening Endoscopic, Diagnostic
0T9B8ZZ Drainage of Bladder, Via Natural or Artificial Opening Endoscopic
0T9C00Z Drainage of Bladder Neck with Drainage Device, Open Approach
0T9C0ZX Drainage of Bladder Neck, Open Approach, Diagnostic
0T9C0ZZ Drainage of Bladder Neck, Open Approach
0T9C30Z Drainage of Bladder Neck with Drainage Device, Percutaneous Approach
0T9C3ZX Drainage of Bladder Neck, Percutaneous Approach, Diagnostic
0T9C3ZZ Drainage of Bladder Neck, Percutaneous Approach
0T9C40Z Drainage of Bladder Neck with Drainage Device, Percutaneous Endoscopic Approach
0T9C4ZX Drainage of Bladder Neck, Percutaneous Endoscopic Approach, Diagnostic
0T9C4ZZ Drainage of Bladder Neck, Percutaneous Endoscopic Approach
0T9C70Z Drainage of Bladder Neck with Drainage Device, Via Natural or Artificial Opening
0T9C7ZX Drainage of Bladder Neck, Via Natural or Artificial Opening, Diagnostic
0T9C7ZZ Drainage of Bladder Neck, Via Natural or Artificial Opening
0T9C80Z Drainage of Bladder Neck with Drainage Device, Via Natural or Artificial Opening Endoscopic
0T9C8ZX Drainage of Bladder Neck, Via Natural or Artificial Opening Endoscopic, Diagnostic
0T9C8ZZ Drainage of Bladder Neck, Via Natural or Artificial Opening Endoscopic
0T9D00Z Drainage of Urethra with Drainage Device, Open Approach
0T9D0ZX Drainage of Urethra, Open Approach, Diagnostic
0T9D0ZZ Drainage of Urethra, Open Approach
0T9D30Z Drainage of Urethra with Drainage Device, Percutaneous Approach
0T9D3ZX Drainage of Urethra, Percutaneous Approach, Diagnostic
0T9D3ZZ Drainage of Urethra, Percutaneous Approach
0T9D40Z Drainage of Urethra with Drainage Device, Percutaneous Endoscopic Approach
0T9D4ZX Drainage of Urethra, Percutaneous Endoscopic Approach, Diagnostic
0T9D4ZZ Drainage of Urethra, Percutaneous Endoscopic Approach
0T9D70Z Drainage of Urethra with Drainage Device, Via Natural or Artificial Opening
0T9D7ZX Drainage of Urethra, Via Natural or Artificial Opening, Diagnostic
0T9D7ZZ Drainage of Urethra, Via Natural or Artificial Opening
0T9D80Z Drainage of Urethra with Drainage Device, Via Natural or Artificial Opening Endoscopic
0T9D8ZX Drainage of Urethra, Via Natural or Artificial Opening Endoscopic, Diagnostic
0T9D8ZZ Drainage of Urethra, Via Natural or Artificial Opening Endoscopic
0T9DX0Z Drainage of Urethra with Drainage Device, External Approach
0T9DXZX Drainage of Urethra, External Approach, Diagnostic
0T9DXZZ Drainage of Urethra, External Approach

0TB – Urinary System, Excision

Review Coding Guidelines B3.4a and B3.4b

Review Coding Guideline B3.8

0TB00ZX Excision of Right Kidney, Open Approach, Diagnostic
0TB00ZZ Excision of Right Kidney, Open Approach
0TB03ZX Excision of Right Kidney, Percutaneous Approach, Diagnostic
0TB03ZZ Excision of Right Kidney, Percutaneous Approach
0TB04ZX Excision of Right Kidney, Percutaneous Endoscopic Approach, Diagnostic
0TB04ZZ Excision of Right Kidney, Percutaneous Endoscopic Approach
0TB07ZX Excision of Right Kidney, Via Natural or Artificial Opening, Diagnostic
0TB07ZZ Excision of Right Kidney, Via Natural or Artificial Opening
0TB08ZX Excision of Right Kidney, Via Natural or Artificial Opening Endoscopic, Diagnostic
0TB08ZZ Excision of Right Kidney, Via Natural or Artificial Opening Endoscopic
0TB10ZX Excision of Left Kidney, Open Approach, Diagnostic
0TB10ZZ Excision of Left Kidney, Open Approach
0TB13ZX Excision of Left Kidney, Percutaneous Approach, Diagnostic
0TB13ZZ Excision of Left Kidney, Percutaneous Approach
0TB14ZX Excision of Left Kidney, Percutaneous Endoscopic Approach, Diagnostic
0TB14ZZ Excision of Left Kidney, Percutaneous Endoscopic Approach
0TB17ZX Excision of Left Kidney, Via Natural or Artificial Opening, Diagnostic
0TB17ZZ Excision of Left Kidney, Via Natural or Artificial Opening
0TB18ZX Excision of Left Kidney, Via Natural or Artificial Opening Endoscopic, Diagnostic
0TB18ZZ Excision of Left Kidney, Via Natural or Artificial Opening Endoscopic

0TB30ZX Excision of Right Kidney Pelvis, Open Approach, Diagnostic
0TB30ZZ Excision of Right Kidney Pelvis, Open Approach
0TB33ZX Excision of Right Kidney Pelvis, Percutaneous Approach, Diagnostic
0TB33ZZ Excision of Right Kidney Pelvis, Percutaneous Approach
0TB34ZX Excision of Right Kidney Pelvis, Percutaneous Endoscopic Approach, Diagnostic
0TB34ZZ Excision of Right Kidney Pelvis, Percutaneous Endoscopic Approach
0TB37ZX Excision of Right Kidney Pelvis, Via Natural or Artificial Opening, Diagnostic
0TB37ZZ Excision of Right Kidney Pelvis, Via Natural or Artificial Opening
0TB38ZX Excision of Right Kidney Pelvis, Via Natural or Artificial Opening Endoscopic, Diagnostic
0TB38ZZ Excision of Right Kidney Pelvis, Via Natural or Artificial Opening Endoscopic
0TB40ZX Excision of Left Kidney Pelvis, Open Approach, Diagnostic
0TB40ZZ Excision of Left Kidney Pelvis, Open Approach
0TB43ZX Excision of Left Kidney Pelvis, Percutaneous Approach, Diagnostic
0TB43ZZ Excision of Left Kidney Pelvis, Percutaneous Approach
0TB44ZX Excision of Left Kidney Pelvis, Percutaneous Endoscopic Approach, Diagnostic
0TB44ZZ Excision of Left Kidney Pelvis, Percutaneous Endoscopic Approach
0TB47ZX Excision of Left Kidney Pelvis, Via Natural or Artificial Opening, Diagnostic
0TB47ZZ Excision of Left Kidney Pelvis, Via Natural or Artificial Opening
0TB48ZX Excision of Left Kidney Pelvis, Via Natural or Artificial Opening Endoscopic, Diagnostic
0TB48ZZ Excision of Left Kidney Pelvis, Via Natural or Artificial Opening Endoscopic
0TB60ZX Excision of Right Ureter, Open Approach, Diagnostic
0TB60ZZ Excision of Right Ureter, Open Approach
0TB63ZX Excision of Right Ureter, Percutaneous Approach, Diagnostic
0TB63ZZ Excision of Right Ureter, Percutaneous Approach
0TB64ZX Excision of Right Ureter, Percutaneous Endoscopic Approach, Diagnostic
0TB64ZZ Excision of Right Ureter, Percutaneous Endoscopic Approach
0TB67ZX Excision of Right Ureter, Via Natural or Artificial Opening, Diagnostic
0TB67ZZ Excision of Right Ureter, Via Natural or Artificial Opening
0TB68ZX Excision of Right Ureter, Via Natural or Artificial Opening Endoscopic, Diagnostic
0TB68ZZ Excision of Right Ureter, Via Natural or Artificial Opening Endoscopic
0TB70ZX Excision of Left Ureter, Open Approach, Diagnostic
0TB70ZZ Excision of Left Ureter, Open Approach
0TB73ZX Excision of Left Ureter, Percutaneous Approach, Diagnostic
0TB73ZZ Excision of Left Ureter, Percutaneous Approach
0TB74ZX Excision of Left Ureter, Percutaneous Endoscopic Approach, Diagnostic
0TB74ZZ Excision of Left Ureter, Percutaneous Endoscopic Approach
0TB77ZX Excision of Left Ureter, Via Natural or Artificial Opening, Diagnostic
0TB77ZZ Excision of Left Ureter, Via Natural or Artificial Opening
0TB78ZX Excision of Left Ureter, Via Natural or Artificial Opening Endoscopic, Diagnostic
0TB78ZZ Excision of Left Ureter, Via Natural or Artificial Opening Endoscopic
0TBB0ZX Excision of Bladder, Open Approach, Diagnostic
0TBB0ZZ Excision of Bladder, Open Approach
0TBB3ZX Excision of Bladder, Percutaneous Approach, Diagnostic
0TBB3ZZ Excision of Bladder, Percutaneous Approach
0TBB4ZX Excision of Bladder, Percutaneous Endoscopic Approach, Diagnostic
0TBB4ZZ Excision of Bladder, Percutaneous Endoscopic Approach
0TBB7ZX Excision of Bladder, Via Natural or Artificial Opening, Diagnostic
0TBB7ZZ Excision of Bladder, Via Natural or Artificial Opening
0TBB8ZX Excision of Bladder, Via Natural or Artificial Opening Endoscopic, Diagnostic
0TBB8ZZ Excision of Bladder, Via Natural or Artificial Opening Endoscopic
AHA CC: 2Q, 2014, 8
0TBC0ZX Excision of Bladder Neck, Open Approach, Diagnostic
0TBC0ZZ Excision of Bladder Neck, Open Approach
0TBC3ZX Excision of Bladder Neck, Percutaneous Approach, Diagnostic
0TBC3ZZ Excision of Bladder Neck, Percutaneous Approach
0TBC4ZX Excision of Bladder Neck, Percutaneous Endoscopic Approach, Diagnostic
0TBC4ZZ Excision of Bladder Neck, Percutaneous Endoscopic Approach
0TBC7ZX Excision of Bladder Neck, Via Natural or Artificial Opening, Diagnostic
0TBC7ZZ Excision of Bladder Neck, Via Natural or Artificial Opening
0TBC8ZX Excision of Bladder Neck, Via Natural or Artificial Opening Endoscopic, Diagnostic
0TBC8ZZ Excision of Bladder Neck, Via Natural or Artificial Opening Endoscopic
0TBD0ZX Excision of Urethra, Open Approach, Diagnostic
0TBD0ZZ Excision of Urethra, Open Approach
0TBD3ZX Excision of Urethra, Percutaneous Approach, Diagnostic
0TBD3ZZ Excision of Urethra, Percutaneous Approach
0TBD4ZX Excision of Urethra, Percutaneous Endoscopic Approach, Diagnostic
0TBD4ZZ Excision of Urethra, Percutaneous Endoscopic Approach
0TBD7ZX Excision of Urethra, Via Natural or Artificial Opening, Diagnostic
0TBD7ZZ Excision of Urethra, Via Natural or Artificial Opening
0TBD8ZX Excision of Urethra, Via Natural or Artificial Opening Endoscopic, Diagnostic
0TBD8ZZ Excision of Urethra, Via Natural or Artificial Opening Endoscopic
0TBDXZX Excision of Urethra, External Approach, Diagnostic
0TBDXZZ Excision of Urethra, External Approach

0TC – Urinary System, Extirpation

0TC00ZZ Extirpation of Matter from Right Kidney, Open Approach
0TC03ZZ Extirpation of Matter from Right Kidney, Percutaneous Approach
0TC04ZZ Extirpation of Matter from Right Kidney, Percutaneous Endoscopic Approach
0TC07ZZ Extirpation of Matter from Right Kidney, Via Natural or Artificial Opening
0TC08ZZ Extirpation of Matter from Right Kidney, Via Natural or Artificial Opening Endoscopic
0TC10ZZ Extirpation of Matter from Left Kidney, Open Approach
0TC13ZZ Extirpation of Matter from Left Kidney, Percutaneous Approach
0TC14ZZ Extirpation of Matter from Left Kidney, Percutaneous Endoscopic Approach
0TC17ZZ Extirpation of Matter from Left Kidney, Via Natural or Artificial Opening
0TC18ZZ Extirpation of Matter from Left Kidney, Via Natural or Artificial Opening Endoscopic
0TC30ZZ Extirpation of Matter from Right Kidney Pelvis, Open Approach
0TC33ZZ Extirpation of Matter from Right Kidney Pelvis, Percutaneous Approach
0TC34ZZ Extirpation of Matter from Right Kidney Pelvis, Percutaneous Endoscopic Approach
0TC37ZZ Extirpation of Matter from Right Kidney Pelvis, Via Natural or Artificial Opening
0TC38ZZ Extirpation of Matter from Right Kidney Pelvis, Via Natural or Artificial Opening Endoscopic
0TC40ZZ Extirpation of Matter from Left Kidney Pelvis, Open Approach
0TC43ZZ Extirpation of Matter from Left Kidney Pelvis, Percutaneous Approach
0TC44ZZ Extirpation of Matter from Left Kidney Pelvis, Percutaneous Endoscopic Approach
0TC47ZZ Extirpation of Matter from Left Kidney Pelvis, Via Natural or Artificial Opening
0TC48ZZ Extirpation of Matter from Left Kidney Pelvis, Via Natural or Artificial Opening Endoscopic
0TC60ZZ Extirpation of Matter from Right Ureter, Open Approach
0TC63ZZ Extirpation of Matter from Right Ureter, Percutaneous Approach
0TC64ZZ Extirpation of Matter from Right Ureter, Percutaneous Endoscopic Approach
0TC67ZZ Extirpation of Matter from Right Ureter, Via Natural or Artificial Opening
0TC68ZZ Extirpation of Matter from Right Ureter, Via Natural or Artificial Opening Endoscopic
AHA CC: 4Q, 2013, 122-123
0TC70ZZ Extirpation of Matter from Left Ureter, Open Approach
0TC73ZZ Extirpation of Matter from Left Ureter, Percutaneous Approach
0TC74ZZ Extirpation of Matter from Left Ureter, Percutaneous Endoscopic Approach
0TC77ZZ Extirpation of Matter from Left Ureter, Via Natural or Artificial Opening
0TC78ZZ Extirpation of Matter from Left Ureter, Via Natural or Artificial Opening Endoscopic
0TCB0ZZ Extirpation of Matter from Bladder, Open Approach

0TCB3ZZ Extirpation of Matter from Bladder, Percutaneous Approach
0TCB4ZZ Extirpation of Matter from Bladder, Percutaneous Endoscopic Approach
0TCB7ZZ Extirpation of Matter from Bladder, Via Natural or Artificial Opening
0TCB8ZZ Extirpation of Matter from Bladder, Via Natural or Artificial Opening Endoscopic
0TCC0ZZ Extirpation of Matter from Bladder Neck, Open Approach
0TCC3ZZ Extirpation of Matter from Bladder Neck, Percutaneous Approach
0TCC4ZZ Extirpation of Matter from Bladder Neck, Percutaneous Endoscopic Approach
0TCC7ZZ Extirpation of Matter from Bladder Neck, Via Natural or Artificial Opening
0TCC8ZZ Extirpation of Matter from Bladder Neck, Via Natural or Artificial Opening Endoscopic
0TCD0ZZ Extirpation of Matter from Urethra, Open Approach
0TCD3ZZ Extirpation of Matter from Urethra, Percutaneous Approach
0TCD4ZZ Extirpation of Matter from Urethra, Percutaneous Endoscopic Approach
0TCD7ZZ Extirpation of Matter from Urethra, Via Natural or Artificial Opening
0TCD8ZZ Extirpation of Matter from Urethra, Via Natural or Artificial Opening Endoscopic
0TCDXZZ Extirpation of Matter from Urethra, External Approach

0TD – Urinary System, Extraction

0TD00ZZ Extraction of Right Kidney, Open Approach
0TD03ZZ Extraction of Right Kidney, Percutaneous Approach
0TD04ZZ Extraction of Right Kidney, Percutaneous Endoscopic Approach
0TD10ZZ Extraction of Left Kidney, Open Approach
0TD13ZZ Extraction of Left Kidney, Percutaneous Approach
0TD14ZZ Extraction of Left Kidney, Percutaneous Endoscopic Approach

0TF – Urinary System, Fragmentation

0TF30ZZ Fragmentation in Right Kidney Pelvis, Open Approach
0TF33ZZ Fragmentation in Right Kidney Pelvis, Percutaneous Approach
0TF34ZZ Fragmentation in Right Kidney Pelvis, Percutaneous Endoscopic Approach
0TF37ZZ Fragmentation in Right Kidney Pelvis, Via Natural or Artificial Opening
0TF38ZZ Fragmentation in Right Kidney Pelvis, Via Natural or Artificial Opening Endoscopic
● **0TF3XZZ** Fragmentation in Right Kidney Pelvis, External Approach
AHA CC: 4Q, 2013, 122
0TF40ZZ Fragmentation in Left Kidney Pelvis, Open Approach
0TF43ZZ Fragmentation in Left Kidney Pelvis, Percutaneous Approach
0TF44ZZ Fragmentation in Left Kidney Pelvis, Percutaneous Endoscopic Approach
0TF47ZZ Fragmentation in Left Kidney Pelvis, Via Natural or Artificial Opening
0TF48ZZ Fragmentation in Left Kidney Pelvis, Via Natural or Artificial Opening Endoscopic
● **0TF4XZZ** Fragmentation in Left Kidney Pelvis, External Approach
0TF60ZZ Fragmentation in Right Ureter, Open Approach
0TF63ZZ Fragmentation in Right Ureter, Percutaneous Approach
0TF64ZZ Fragmentation in Right Ureter, Percutaneous Endoscopic Approach
0TF67ZZ Fragmentation in Right Ureter, Via Natural or Artificial Opening
0TF68ZZ Fragmentation in Right Ureter, Via Natural or Artificial Opening Endoscopic
● **0TF6XZZ** Fragmentation in Right Ureter, External Approach
0TF70ZZ Fragmentation in Left Ureter, Open Approach
0TF73ZZ Fragmentation in Left Ureter, Percutaneous Approach
0TF74ZZ Fragmentation in Left Ureter, Percutaneous Endoscopic Approach
0TF77ZZ Fragmentation in Left Ureter, Via Natural or Artificial Opening
0TF78ZZ Fragmentation in Left Ureter, Via Natural or Artificial Opening Endoscopic
● **0TF7XZZ** Fragmentation in Left Ureter, External Approach
0TFB0ZZ Fragmentation in Bladder, Open Approach
0TFB3ZZ Fragmentation in Bladder, Percutaneous Approach
0TFB4ZZ Fragmentation in Bladder, Percutaneous Endoscopic Approach
0TFB7ZZ Fragmentation in Bladder, Via Natural or Artificial Opening
0TFB8ZZ Fragmentation in Bladder, Via Natural or Artificial Opening Endoscopic
● **0TFBXZZ** Fragmentation in Bladder, External Approach
0TFC0ZZ Fragmentation in Bladder Neck, Open Approach
0TFC3ZZ Fragmentation in Bladder Neck, Percutaneous Approach
0TFC4ZZ Fragmentation in Bladder Neck, Percutaneous Endoscopic Approach
0TFC7ZZ Fragmentation in Bladder Neck, Via Natural or Artificial Opening
0TFC8ZZ Fragmentation in Bladder Neck, Via Natural or Artificial Opening Endoscopic
● **0TFCXZZ** Fragmentation in Bladder Neck, External Approach
0TFD0ZZ Fragmentation in Urethra, Open Approach
0TFD3ZZ Fragmentation in Urethra, Percutaneous Approach
0TFD4ZZ Fragmentation in Urethra, Percutaneous Endoscopic Approach
0TFD7ZZ Fragmentation in Urethra, Via Natural or Artificial Opening
▲ **0TFD8ZZ** Fragmentation in Urethra, Via Natural or Artificial Opening Endoscopic
0TFDXZZ Fragmentation in Urethra, External Approach

0TH – Urinary System, Insertion

0TH502Z Insertion of Monitoring Device into Kidney, Open Approach
0TH503Z Insertion of Infusion Device into Kidney, Open Approach
0TH532Z Insertion of Monitoring Device into Kidney, Percutaneous Approach
0TH533Z Insertion of Infusion Device into Kidney, Percutaneous Approach
0TH542Z Insertion of Monitoring Device into Kidney, Percutaneous Endoscopic Approach
0TH543Z Insertion of Infusion Device into Kidney, Percutaneous Endoscopic Approach
0TH572Z Insertion of Monitoring Device into Kidney, Via Natural or Artificial Opening
0TH573Z Insertion of Infusion Device into Kidney, Via Natural or Artificial Opening
0TH582Z Insertion of Monitoring Device into Kidney, Via Natural or Artificial Opening Endoscopic
0TH583Z Insertion of Infusion Device into Kidney, Via Natural or Artificial Opening Endoscopic
0TH902Z Insertion of Monitoring Device into Ureter, Open Approach
0TH903Z Insertion of Infusion Device into Ureter, Open Approach
0TH90MZ Insertion of Stimulator Lead into Ureter, Open Approach
0TH932Z Insertion of Monitoring Device into Ureter, Percutaneous Approach
0TH933Z Insertion of Infusion Device into Ureter, Percutaneous Approach
0TH93MZ Insertion of Stimulator Lead into Ureter, Percutaneous Approach
0TH942Z Insertion of Monitoring Device into Ureter, Percutaneous Endoscopic Approach
0TH943Z Insertion of Infusion Device into Ureter, Percutaneous Endoscopic Approach
0TH94MZ Insertion of Stimulator Lead into Ureter, Percutaneous Endoscopic Approach
0TH972Z Insertion of Monitoring Device into Ureter, Via Natural or Artificial Opening
0TH973Z Insertion of Infusion Device into Ureter, Via Natural or Artificial Opening
0TH97MZ Insertion of Stimulator Lead into Ureter, Via Natural or Artificial Opening
0TH982Z Insertion of Monitoring Device into Ureter, Via Natural or Artificial Opening Endoscopic
0TH983Z Insertion of Infusion Device into Ureter, Via Natural or Artificial Opening Endoscopic
0TH98MZ Insertion of Stimulator Lead into Ureter, Via Natural or Artificial Opening Endoscopic
0THB02Z Insertion of Monitoring Device into Bladder, Open Approach
0THB03Z Insertion of Infusion Device into Bladder, Open Approach
0THB0LZ Insertion of Artificial Sphincter into Bladder, Open Approach
▲ **0THB0MZ** Insertion of Stimulator Lead into Bladder, Open Approach
0THB32Z Insertion of Monitoring Device into Bladder, Percutaneous Approach
0THB33Z Insertion of Infusion Device into Bladder, Percutaneous Approach

0THB3LZ Insertion of Artificial Sphincter into Bladder, Percutaneous Approach
▲**0THB3MZ** Insertion of Stimulator Lead into Bladder, Percutaneous Approach
0THB42Z Insertion of Monitoring Device into Bladder, Percutaneous Endoscopic Approach
0THB43Z Insertion of Infusion Device into Bladder, Percutaneous Endoscopic Approach
0THB4LZ Insertion of Artificial Sphincter into Bladder, Percutaneous Endoscopic Approach
▲**0THB4MZ** Insertion of Stimulator Lead into Bladder, Percutaneous Endoscopic Approach
0THB72Z Insertion of Monitoring Device into Bladder, Via Natural or Artificial Opening
0THB73Z Insertion of Infusion Device into Bladder, Via Natural or Artificial Opening
0THB7LZ Insertion of Artificial Sphincter into Bladder, Via Natural or Artificial Opening
▲**0THB7MZ** Insertion of Stimulator Lead into Bladder, Via Natural or Artificial Opening
0THB82Z Insertion of Monitoring Device into Bladder, Via Natural or Artificial Opening Endoscopic
0THB83Z Insertion of Infusion Device into Bladder, Via Natural or Artificial Opening Endoscopic
0THB8LZ Insertion of Artificial Sphincter into Bladder, Via Natural or Artificial Opening Endoscopic
▲ **0THB8MZ** Insertion of Stimulator Lead into Bladder, Via Natural or Artificial Opening Endoscopic
0THC0LZ Insertion of Artificial Sphincter into Bladder Neck, Open Approach
0THC3LZ Insertion of Artificial Sphincter into Bladder Neck, Percutaneous Approach
0THC4LZ Insertion of Artificial Sphincter into Bladder Neck, Percutaneous Endoscopic Approach
0THC7LZ Insertion of Artificial Sphincter into Bladder Neck, Via Natural or Artificial Opening
0THC8LZ Insertion of Artificial Sphincter into Bladder Neck, Via Natural or Artificial Opening Endoscopic
0THD02Z Insertion of Monitoring Device into Urethra, Open Approach
0THD03Z Insertion of Infusion Device into Urethra, Open Approach
0THD0LZ Insertion of Artificial Sphincter into Urethra, Open Approach
0THD32Z Insertion of Monitoring Device into Urethra, Percutaneous Approach
0THD33Z Insertion of Infusion Device into Urethra, Percutaneous Approach
0THD3LZ Insertion of Artificial Sphincter into Urethra, Percutaneous Approach
0THD42Z Insertion of Monitoring Device into Urethra, Percutaneous Endoscopic Approach
0THD43Z Insertion of Infusion Device into Urethra, Percutaneous Endoscopic Approach
0THD4LZ Insertion of Artificial Sphincter into Urethra, Percutaneous Endoscopic Approach
0THD72Z Insertion of Monitoring Device into Urethra, Via Natural or Artificial Opening
0THD73Z Insertion of Infusion Device into Urethra, Via Natural or Artificial Opening
0THD7LZ Insertion of Artificial Sphincter into Urethra, Via Natural or Artificial Opening
0THD82Z Insertion of Monitoring Device into Urethra, Via Natural or Artificial Opening Endoscopic
0THD83Z Insertion of Infusion Device into Urethra, Via Natural or Artificial Opening Endoscopic
0THD8LZ Insertion of Artificial Sphincter into Urethra, Via Natural or Artificial Opening Endoscopic
0THDX2Z Insertion of Monitoring Device into Urethra, External Approach
0THDX3Z Insertion of Infusion Device into Urethra, External Approach
0THDXLZ Insertion of Artificial Sphincter into Urethra, External Approach

0TJ – Urinary System, Inspection

Review Coding Guidelines B3.11a, B3.11b and B3.11c

0TJ50ZZ Inspection of Kidney, Open Approach
0TJ53ZZ Inspection of Kidney, Percutaneous Approach
0TJ54ZZ Inspection of Kidney, Percutaneous Endoscopic Approach
0TJ57ZZ Inspection of Kidney, Via Natural or Artificial Opening
0TJ58ZZ Inspection of Kidney, Via Natural or Artificial Opening Endoscopic
0TJ5XZZ Inspection of Kidney, External Approach
0TJ90ZZ Inspection of Ureter, Open Approach
0TJ93ZZ Inspection of Ureter, Percutaneous Approach
0TJ94ZZ Inspection of Ureter, Percutaneous Endoscopic Approach
0TJ97ZZ Inspection of Ureter, Via Natural or Artificial Opening
0TJ98ZZ Inspection of Ureter, Via Natural or Artificial Opening Endoscopic
0TJ9XZZ Inspection of Ureter, External Approach
0TJB0ZZ Inspection of Bladder, Open Approach
0TJB3ZZ Inspection of Bladder, Percutaneous Approach
0TJB4ZZ Inspection of Bladder, Percutaneous Endoscopic Approach
0TJB7ZZ Inspection of Bladder, Via Natural or Artificial Opening
0TJB8ZZ Inspection of Bladder, Via Natural or Artificial Opening Endoscopic
0TJBXZZ Inspection of Bladder, External Approach
0TJD0ZZ Inspection of Urethra, Open Approach
0TJD3ZZ Inspection of Urethra, Percutaneous Approach
0TJD4ZZ Inspection of Urethra, Percutaneous Endoscopic Approach
0TJD7ZZ Inspection of Urethra, Via Natural or Artificial Opening
0TJD8ZZ Inspection of Urethra, Via Natural or Artificial Opening Endoscopic
0TJDXZZ Inspection of Urethra, External Approach

0TL – Urinary System, Occlusion

0TL30CZ Occlusion of Right Kidney Pelvis with Extraluminal Device, Open Approach
0TL30DZ Occlusion of Right Kidney Pelvis with Intraluminal Device, Open Approach
0TL30ZZ Occlusion of Right Kidney Pelvis, Open Approach
0TL33CZ Occlusion of Right Kidney Pelvis with Extraluminal Device, Percutaneous Approach
0TL33DZ Occlusion of Right Kidney Pelvis with Intraluminal Device, Percutaneous Approach
0TL33ZZ Occlusion of Right Kidney Pelvis, Percutaneous Approach
0TL34CZ Occlusion of Right Kidney Pelvis with Extraluminal Device, Percutaneous Endoscopic Approach
0TL34DZ Occlusion of Right Kidney Pelvis with Intraluminal Device, Percutaneous Endoscopic Approach
0TL34ZZ Occlusion of Right Kidney Pelvis, Percutaneous Endoscopic Approach
0TL37DZ Occlusion of Right Kidney Pelvis with Intraluminal Device, Via Natural or Artificial Opening
0TL37ZZ Occlusion of Right Kidney Pelvis, Via Natural or Artificial Opening
0TL38DZ Occlusion of Right Kidney Pelvis with Intraluminal Device, Via Natural or Artificial Opening Endoscopic
0TL38ZZ Occlusion of Right Kidney Pelvis, Via Natural or Artificial Opening Endoscopic
0TL40CZ Occlusion of Left Kidney Pelvis with Extraluminal Device, Open Approach
0TL40DZ Occlusion of Left Kidney Pelvis with Intraluminal Device, Open Approach
0TL40ZZ Occlusion of Left Kidney Pelvis, Open Approach
0TL43CZ Occlusion of Left Kidney Pelvis with Extraluminal Device, Percutaneous Approach
0TL43DZ Occlusion of Left Kidney Pelvis with Intraluminal Device, Percutaneous Approach
0TL43ZZ Occlusion of Left Kidney Pelvis, Percutaneous Approach
0TL44CZ Occlusion of Left Kidney Pelvis with Extraluminal Device, Percutaneous Endoscopic Approach
0TL44DZ Occlusion of Left Kidney Pelvis with Intraluminal Device, Percutaneous Endoscopic Approach
0TL44ZZ Occlusion of Left Kidney Pelvis, Percutaneous Endoscopic Approach
0TL47DZ Occlusion of Left Kidney Pelvis with Intraluminal Device, Via Natural or Artificial Opening
0TL47ZZ Occlusion of Left Kidney Pelvis, Via Natural or Artificial Opening
0TL48DZ Occlusion of Left Kidney Pelvis with Intraluminal Device, Via Natural or Artificial Opening Endoscopic
0TL48ZZ Occlusion of Left Kidney Pelvis, Via Natural or Artificial Opening Endoscopic
0TL60CZ Occlusion of Right Ureter with Extraluminal Device, Open Approach

0TL60DZ Occlusion of Right Ureter with Intraluminal Device, Open Approach
0TL60ZZ Occlusion of Right Ureter, Open Approach
0TL63CZ Occlusion of Right Ureter with Extraluminal Device, Percutaneous Approach
0TL63DZ Occlusion of Right Ureter with Intraluminal Device, Percutaneous Approach
0TL63ZZ Occlusion of Right Ureter, Percutaneous Approach
0TL64CZ Occlusion of Right Ureter with Extraluminal Device, Percutaneous Endoscopic Approach
0TL64DZ Occlusion of Right Ureter with Intraluminal Device, Percutaneous Endoscopic Approach
0TL64ZZ Occlusion of Right Ureter, Percutaneous Endoscopic Approach
0TL67DZ Occlusion of Right Ureter with Intraluminal Device, Via Natural or Artificial Opening
0TL67ZZ Occlusion of Right Ureter, Via Natural or Artificial Opening
0TL68DZ Occlusion of Right Ureter with Intraluminal Device, Via Natural or Artificial Opening Endoscopic
0TL68ZZ Occlusion of Right Ureter, Via Natural or Artificial Opening Endoscopic
0TL70CZ Occlusion of Left Ureter with Extraluminal Device, Open Approach
0TL70DZ Occlusion of Left Ureter with Intraluminal Device, Open Approach
0TL70ZZ Occlusion of Left Ureter, Open Approach
0TL73CZ Occlusion of Left Ureter with Extraluminal Device, Percutaneous Approach
0TL73DZ Occlusion of Left Ureter with Intraluminal Device, Percutaneous Approach
0TL73ZZ Occlusion of Left Ureter, Percutaneous Approach
0TL74CZ Occlusion of Left Ureter with Extraluminal Device, Percutaneous Endoscopic Approach
0TL74DZ Occlusion of Left Ureter with Intraluminal Device, Percutaneous Endoscopic Approach
0TL74ZZ Occlusion of Left Ureter, Percutaneous Endoscopic Approach
0TL77DZ Occlusion of Left Ureter with Intraluminal Device, Via Natural or Artificial Opening
0TL77ZZ Occlusion of Left Ureter, Via Natural or Artificial Opening
0TL78DZ Occlusion of Left Ureter with Intraluminal Device, Via Natural or Artificial Opening Endoscopic
0TL78ZZ Occlusion of Left Ureter, Via Natural or Artificial Opening Endoscopic
0TLB0CZ Occlusion of Bladder with Extraluminal Device, Open Approach
0TLB0DZ Occlusion of Bladder with Intraluminal Device, Open Approach
0TLB0ZZ Occlusion of Bladder, Open Approach
0TLB3CZ Occlusion of Bladder with Extraluminal Device, Percutaneous Approach
0TLB3DZ Occlusion of Bladder with Intraluminal Device, Percutaneous Approach
0TLB3ZZ Occlusion of Bladder, Percutaneous Approach
0TLB4CZ Occlusion of Bladder with Extraluminal Device, Percutaneous Endoscopic Approach
0TLB4DZ Occlusion of Bladder with Intraluminal Device, Percutaneous Endoscopic Approach
0TLB4ZZ Occlusion of Bladder, Percutaneous Endoscopic Approach
0TLB7DZ Occlusion of Bladder with Intraluminal Device, Via Natural or Artificial Opening
0TLB7ZZ Occlusion of Bladder, Via Natural or Artificial Opening
0TLB8DZ Occlusion of Bladder with Intraluminal Device, Via Natural or Artificial Opening Endoscopic
0TLB8ZZ Occlusion of Bladder, Via Natural or Artificial Opening Endoscopic
0TLC0CZ Occlusion of Bladder Neck with Extraluminal Device, Open Approach
0TLC0DZ Occlusion of Bladder Neck with Intraluminal Device, Open Approach
0TLC0ZZ Occlusion of Bladder Neck, Open Approach
0TLC3CZ Occlusion of Bladder Neck with Extraluminal Device, Percutaneous Approach
0TLC3DZ Occlusion of Bladder Neck with Intraluminal Device, Percutaneous Approach
0TLC3ZZ Occlusion of Bladder Neck, Percutaneous Approach
0TLC4CZ Occlusion of Bladder Neck with Extraluminal Device, Percutaneous Endoscopic Approach
0TLC4DZ Occlusion of Bladder Neck with Intraluminal Device, Percutaneous Endoscopic Approach
0TLC4ZZ Occlusion of Bladder Neck, Percutaneous Endoscopic Approach
0TLC7DZ Occlusion of Bladder Neck with Intraluminal Device, Via Natural or Artificial Opening
0TLC7ZZ Occlusion of Bladder Neck, Via Natural or Artificial Opening
0TLC8DZ Occlusion of Bladder Neck with Intraluminal Device, Via Natural or Artificial Opening Endoscopic
0TLC8ZZ Occlusion of Bladder Neck, Via Natural or Artificial Opening Endoscopic
0TLD0CZ Occlusion of Urethra with Extraluminal Device, Open Approach
0TLD0DZ Occlusion of Urethra with Intraluminal Device, Open Approach
0TLD0ZZ Occlusion of Urethra, Open Approach
0TLD3CZ Occlusion of Urethra with Extraluminal Device, Percutaneous Approach
0TLD3DZ Occlusion of Urethra with Intraluminal Device, Percutaneous Approach
0TLD3ZZ Occlusion of Urethra, Percutaneous Approach
0TLD4CZ Occlusion of Urethra with Extraluminal Device, Percutaneous Endoscopic Approach
0TLD4DZ Occlusion of Urethra with Intraluminal Device, Percutaneous Endoscopic Approach
0TLD4ZZ Occlusion of Urethra, Percutaneous Endoscopic Approach
0TLD7DZ Occlusion of Urethra with Intraluminal Device, Via Natural or Artificial Opening
0TLD7ZZ Occlusion of Urethra, Via Natural or Artificial Opening
0TLD8DZ Occlusion of Urethra with Intraluminal Device, Via Natural or Artificial Opening Endoscopic
0TLD8ZZ Occlusion of Urethra, Via Natural or Artificial Opening Endoscopic
0TLDXCZ Occlusion of Urethra with Extraluminal Device, External Approach
0TLDXDZ Occlusion of Urethra with Intraluminal Device, External Approach
0TLDXZZ Occlusion of Urethra, External Approach

0TM – Urinary System, Reattachment

0TM00ZZ Reattachment of Right Kidney, Open Approach
0TM04ZZ Reattachment of Right Kidney, Percutaneous Endoscopic Approach
0TM10ZZ Reattachment of Left Kidney, Open Approach
0TM14ZZ Reattachment of Left Kidney, Percutaneous Endoscopic Approach
0TM20ZZ Reattachment of Bilateral Kidneys, Open Approach
0TM24ZZ Reattachment of Bilateral Kidneys, Percutaneous Endoscopic Approach
0TM30ZZ Reattachment of Right Kidney Pelvis, Open Approach
0TM34ZZ Reattachment of Right Kidney Pelvis, Percutaneous Endoscopic Approach
0TM40ZZ Reattachment of Left Kidney Pelvis, Open Approach
0TM44ZZ Reattachment of Left Kidney Pelvis, Percutaneous Endoscopic Approach
0TM60ZZ Reattachment of Right Ureter, Open Approach
0TM64ZZ Reattachment of Right Ureter, Percutaneous Endoscopic Approach
0TM70ZZ Reattachment of Left Ureter, Open Approach
0TM74ZZ Reattachment of Left Ureter, Percutaneous Endoscopic Approach
0TM80ZZ Reattachment of Bilateral Ureters, Open Approach
0TM84ZZ Reattachment of Bilateral Ureters, Percutaneous Endoscopic Approach
0TMB0ZZ Reattachment of Bladder, Open Approach
0TMB4ZZ Reattachment of Bladder, Percutaneous Endoscopic Approach
0TMC0ZZ Reattachment of Bladder Neck, Open Approach
0TMC4ZZ Reattachment of Bladder Neck, Percutaneous Endoscopic Approach
0TMD0ZZ Reattachment of Urethra, Open Approach
0TMD4ZZ Reattachment of Urethra, Percutaneous Endoscopic Approach

0TN – Urinary System, Release

Review Coding Guideline B3.13

Review Coding Guideline B3.14

0TN00ZZ Release Right Kidney, Open Approach
0TN03ZZ Release Right Kidney, Percutaneous Approach
0TN04ZZ Release Right Kidney, Percutaneous Endoscopic Approach

0TN07ZZ Release Right Kidney, Via Natural or Artificial Opening
0TN08ZZ Release Right Kidney, Via Natural or Artificial Opening Endoscopic
0TN10ZZ Release Left Kidney, Open Approach
0TN13ZZ Release Left Kidney, Percutaneous Approach
0TN14ZZ Release Left Kidney, Percutaneous Endoscopic Approach
0TN17ZZ Release Left Kidney, Via Natural or Artificial Opening
0TN18ZZ Release Left Kidney, Via Natural or Artificial Opening Endoscopic
0TN30ZZ Release Right Kidney Pelvis, Open Approach
0TN33ZZ Release Right Kidney Pelvis, Percutaneous Approach
0TN34ZZ Release Right Kidney Pelvis, Percutaneous Endoscopic Approach
0TN37ZZ Release Right Kidney Pelvis, Via Natural or Artificial Opening
0TN38ZZ Release Right Kidney Pelvis, Via Natural or Artificial Opening Endoscopic
0TN40ZZ Release Left Kidney Pelvis, Open Approach
0TN43ZZ Release Left Kidney Pelvis, Percutaneous Approach
0TN44ZZ Release Left Kidney Pelvis, Percutaneous Endoscopic Approach
0TN47ZZ Release Left Kidney Pelvis, Via Natural or Artificial Opening
0TN48ZZ Release Left Kidney Pelvis, Via Natural or Artificial Opening Endoscopic
0TN60ZZ Release Right Ureter, Open Approach
0TN63ZZ Release Right Ureter, Percutaneous Approach
0TN64ZZ Release Right Ureter, Percutaneous Endoscopic Approach
0TN67ZZ Release Right Ureter, Via Natural or Artificial Opening
0TN68ZZ Release Right Ureter, Via Natural or Artificial Opening Endoscopic
0TN70ZZ Release Left Ureter, Open Approach
0TN73ZZ Release Left Ureter, Percutaneous Approach
0TN74ZZ Release Left Ureter, Percutaneous Endoscopic Approach
0TN77ZZ Release Left Ureter, Via Natural or Artificial Opening
0TN78ZZ Release Left Ureter, Via Natural or Artificial Opening Endoscopic
0TNB0ZZ Release Bladder, Open Approach
0TNB3ZZ Release Bladder, Percutaneous Approach
0TNB4ZZ Release Bladder, Percutaneous Endoscopic Approach
0TNB7ZZ Release Bladder, Via Natural or Artificial Opening
0TNB8ZZ Release Bladder, Via Natural or Artificial Opening Endoscopic
0TNC0ZZ Release Bladder Neck, Open Approach
0TNC3ZZ Release Bladder Neck, Percutaneous Approach
0TNC4ZZ Release Bladder Neck, Percutaneous Endoscopic Approach
0TNC7ZZ Release Bladder Neck, Via Natural or Artificial Opening
0TNC8ZZ Release Bladder Neck, Via Natural or Artificial Opening Endoscopic
0TND0ZZ Release Urethra, Open Approach
0TND3ZZ Release Urethra, Percutaneous Approach
0TND4ZZ Release Urethra, Percutaneous Endoscopic Approach
0TND7ZZ Release Urethra, Via Natural or Artificial Opening
0TND8ZZ Release Urethra, Via Natural or Artificial Opening Endoscopic
0TNDXZZ Release Urethra, External Approach

0TP – Urinary System, Removal

Review Coding Guideline B6.1c

0TP500Z Removal of Drainage Device from Kidney, Open Approach
0TP502Z Removal of Monitoring Device from Kidney, Open Approach
0TP503Z Removal of Infusion Device from Kidney, Open Approach
0TP507Z Removal of Autologous Tissue Substitute from Kidney, Open Approach
0TP50CZ Removal of Extraluminal Device from Kidney, Open Approach
0TP50DZ Removal of Intraluminal Device from Kidney, Open Approach
0TP50JZ Removal of Synthetic Substitute from Kidney, Open Approach
0TP50KZ Removal of Nonautologous Tissue Substitute from Kidney, Open Approach
0TP530Z Removal of Drainage Device from Kidney, Percutaneous Approach
0TP532Z Removal of Monitoring Device from Kidney, Percutaneous Approach
0TP533Z Removal of Infusion Device from Kidney, Percutaneous Approach
0TP537Z Removal of Autologous Tissue Substitute from Kidney, Percutaneous Approach
0TP53CZ Removal of Extraluminal Device from Kidney, Percutaneous Approach
0TP53DZ Removal of Intraluminal Device from Kidney, Percutaneous Approach
0TP53JZ Removal of Synthetic Substitute from Kidney, Percutaneous Approach
0TP53KZ Removal of Nonautologous Tissue Substitute from Kidney, Percutaneous Approach
0TP540Z Removal of Drainage Device from Kidney, Percutaneous Endoscopic Approach
0TP542Z Removal of Monitoring Device from Kidney, Percutaneous Endoscopic Approach
0TP543Z Removal of Infusion Device from Kidney, Percutaneous Endoscopic Approach
0TP547Z Removal of Autologous Tissue Substitute from Kidney, Percutaneous Endoscopic Approach
0TP54CZ Removal of Extraluminal Device from Kidney, Percutaneous Endoscopic Approach
0TP54DZ Removal of Intraluminal Device from Kidney, Percutaneous Endoscopic Approach
0TP54JZ Removal of Synthetic Substitute from Kidney, Percutaneous Endoscopic Approach
0TP54KZ Removal of Nonautologous Tissue Substitute from Kidney, Percutaneous Endoscopic Approach
0TP570Z Removal of Drainage Device from Kidney, Via Natural or Artificial Opening
0TP572Z Removal of Monitoring Device from Kidney, Via Natural or Artificial Opening
0TP573Z Removal of Infusion Device from Kidney, Via Natural or Artificial Opening
0TP577Z Removal of Autologous Tissue Substitute from Kidney, Via Natural or Artificial Opening
0TP57CZ Removal of Extraluminal Device from Kidney, Via Natural or Artificial Opening
0TP57DZ Removal of Intraluminal Device from Kidney, Via Natural or Artificial Opening
0TP57JZ Removal of Synthetic Substitute from Kidney, Via Natural or Artificial Opening
0TP57KZ Removal of Nonautologous Tissue Substitute from Kidney, Via Natural or Artificial Opening
0TP580Z Removal of Drainage Device from Kidney, Via Natural or Artificial Opening Endoscopic
0TP582Z Removal of Monitoring Device from Kidney, Via Natural or Artificial Opening Endoscopic
0TP583Z Removal of Infusion Device from Kidney, Via Natural or Artificial Opening Endoscopic
0TP587Z Removal of Autologous Tissue Substitute from Kidney, Via Natural or Artificial Opening Endoscopic
0TP58CZ Removal of Extraluminal Device from Kidney, Via Natural or Artificial Opening Endoscopic
0TP58DZ Removal of Intraluminal Device from Kidney, Via Natural or Artificial Opening Endoscopic
0TP58JZ Removal of Synthetic Substitute from Kidney, Via Natural or Artificial Opening Endoscopic
0TP58KZ Removal of Nonautologous Tissue Substitute from Kidney, Via Natural or Artificial Opening Endoscopic
0TP5X0Z Removal of Drainage Device from Kidney, External Approach
0TP5X2Z Removal of Monitoring Device from Kidney, External Approach
0TP5X3Z Removal of Infusion Device from Kidney, External Approach
0TP5XDZ Removal of Intraluminal Device from Kidney, External Approach
0TP900Z Removal of Drainage Device from Ureter, Open Approach
0TP902Z Removal of Monitoring Device from Ureter, Open Approach
0TP903Z Removal of Infusion Device from Ureter, Open Approach
0TP907Z Removal of Autologous Tissue Substitute from Ureter, Open Approach
0TP90CZ Removal of Extraluminal Device from Ureter, Open Approach
0TP90DZ Removal of Intraluminal Device from Ureter, Open Approach
0TP90JZ Removal of Synthetic Substitute from Ureter, Open Approach
0TP90KZ Removal of Nonautologous Tissue Substitute from Ureter, Open Approach
0TP90MZ Removal of Stimulator Lead from Ureter, Open Approach
0TP930Z Removal of Drainage Device from Ureter, Percutaneous Approach
0TP932Z Removal of Monitoring Device from Ureter, Percutaneous Approach
0TP933Z Removal of Infusion Device from Ureter, Percutaneous Approach
0TP937Z Removal of Autologous Tissue Substitute from Ureter, Percutaneous Approach
0TP93CZ Removal of Extraluminal Device from Ureter, Percutaneous Approach
0TP93DZ Removal of Intraluminal Device from Ureter, Percutaneous Approach
0TP93JZ Removal of Synthetic Substitute from Ureter, Percutaneous Approach

0TP93KZ Removal of Nonautologous Tissue Substitute from Ureter, Percutaneous Approach
0TP93MZ Removal of Stimulator Lead from Ureter, Percutaneous Approach
0TP940Z Removal of Drainage Device from Ureter, Percutaneous Endoscopic Approach
0TP942Z Removal of Monitoring Device from Ureter, Percutaneous Endoscopic Approach
0TP943Z Removal of Infusion Device from Ureter, Percutaneous Endoscopic Approach
0TP947Z Removal of Autologous Tissue Substitute from Ureter, Percutaneous Endoscopic Approach
0TP94CZ Removal of Extraluminal Device from Ureter, Percutaneous Endoscopic Approach
0TP94DZ Removal of Intraluminal Device from Ureter, Percutaneous Endoscopic Approach
0TP94JZ Removal of Synthetic Substitute from Ureter, Percutaneous Endoscopic Approach
0TP94KZ Removal of Nonautologous Tissue Substitute from Ureter, Percutaneous Endoscopic Approach
0TP94MZ Removal of Stimulator Lead from Ureter, Percutaneous Endoscopic Approach
0TP970Z Removal of Drainage Device from Ureter, Via Natural or Artificial Opening
0TP972Z Removal of Monitoring Device from Ureter, Via Natural or Artificial Opening
0TP973Z Removal of Infusion Device from Ureter, Via Natural or Artificial Opening
0TP977Z Removal of Autologous Tissue Substitute from Ureter, Via Natural or Artificial Opening
0TP97CZ Removal of Extraluminal Device from Ureter, Via Natural or Artificial Opening
0TP97DZ Removal of Intraluminal Device from Ureter, Via Natural or Artificial Opening
0TP97JZ Removal of Synthetic Substitute from Ureter, Via Natural or Artificial Opening
0TP97KZ Removal of Nonautologous Tissue Substitute from Ureter, Via Natural or Artificial Opening
0TP97MZ Removal of Stimulator Lead from Ureter, Via Natural or Artificial Opening
0TP980Z Removal of Drainage Device from Ureter, Via Natural or Artificial Opening Endoscopic
0TP982Z Removal of Monitoring Device from Ureter, Via Natural or Artificial Opening Endoscopic
0TP983Z Removal of Infusion Device from Ureter, Via Natural or Artificial Opening Endoscopic
0TP987Z Removal of Autologous Tissue Substitute from Ureter, Via Natural or Artificial Opening Endoscopic
0TP98CZ Removal of Extraluminal Device from Ureter, Via Natural or Artificial Opening Endoscopic
0TP98DZ Removal of Intraluminal Device from Ureter, Via Natural or Artificial Opening Endoscopic
0TP98JZ Removal of Synthetic Substitute from Ureter, Via Natural or Artificial Opening Endoscopic
0TP98KZ Removal of Nonautologous Tissue Substitute from Ureter, Via Natural or Artificial Opening Endoscopic
0TP98MZ Removal of Stimulator Lead from Ureter, Via Natural or Artificial Opening Endoscopic
0TP9X0Z Removal of Drainage Device from Ureter, External Approach
0TP9X2Z Removal of Monitoring Device from Ureter, External Approach
0TP9X3Z Removal of Infusion Device from Ureter, External Approach
0TP9XDZ Removal of Intraluminal Device from Ureter, External Approach
0TP9XMZ Removal of Stimulator Lead from Ureter, External Approach
0TPB00Z Removal of Drainage Device from Bladder, Open Approach
0TPB02Z Removal of Monitoring Device from Bladder, Open Approach
0TPB03Z Removal of Infusion Device from Bladder, Open Approach
0TPB07Z Removal of Autologous Tissue Substitute from Bladder, Open Approach
0TPB0CZ Removal of Extraluminal Device from Bladder, Open Approach
0TPB0DZ Removal of Intraluminal Device from Bladder, Open Approach
0TPB0JZ Removal of Synthetic Substitute from Bladder, Open Approach
0TPB0KZ Removal of Nonautologous Tissue Substitute from Bladder, Open Approach
0TPB0LZ Removal of Artificial Sphincter from Bladder, Open Approach
▲ **0TPB0MZ** Removal of Stimulator Lead from Bladder, Open Approach
0TPB30Z Removal of Drainage Device from Bladder, Percutaneous Approach
0TPB32Z Removal of Monitoring Device from Bladder, Percutaneous Approach
0TPB33Z Removal of Infusion Device from Bladder, Percutaneous Approach
0TPB37Z Removal of Autologous Tissue Substitute from Bladder, Percutaneous Approach
0TPB3CZ Removal of Extraluminal Device from Bladder, Percutaneous Approach
0TPB3DZ Removal of Intraluminal Device from Bladder, Percutaneous Approach
0TPB3JZ Removal of Synthetic Substitute from Bladder, Percutaneous Approach
0TPB3KZ Removal of Nonautologous Tissue Substitute from Bladder, Percutaneous Approach
0TPB3LZ Removal of Artificial Sphincter from Bladder, Percutaneous Approach
▲ **0TPB3MZ** Removal of Stimulator Lead from Bladder, Percutaneous Approach
0TPB40Z Removal of Drainage Device from Bladder, Percutaneous Endoscopic Approach
0TPB42Z Removal of Monitoring Device from Bladder, Percutaneous Endoscopic Approach
0TPB43Z Removal of Infusion Device from Bladder, Percutaneous Endoscopic Approach
0TPB47Z Removal of Autologous Tissue Substitute from Bladder, Percutaneous Endoscopic Approach
0TPB4CZ Removal of Extraluminal Device from Bladder, Percutaneous Endoscopic Approach
0TPB4DZ Removal of Intraluminal Device from Bladder, Percutaneous Endoscopic Approach
0TPB4JZ Removal of Synthetic Substitute from Bladder, Percutaneous Endoscopic Approach
0TPB4KZ Removal of Nonautologous Tissue Substitute from Bladder, Percutaneous Endoscopic Approach
0TPB4LZ Removal of Artificial Sphincter from Bladder, Percutaneous Endoscopic Approach
▲ **0TPB4MZ** Removal of Stimulator Lead from Bladder, Percutaneous Endoscopic Approach
0TPB70Z Removal of Drainage Device from Bladder, Via Natural or Artificial Opening
0TPB72Z Removal of Monitoring Device from Bladder, Via Natural or Artificial Opening
0TPB73Z Removal of Infusion Device from Bladder, Via Natural or Artificial Opening
0TPB77Z Removal of Autologous Tissue Substitute from Bladder, Via Natural or Artificial Opening
0TPB7CZ Removal of Extraluminal Device from Bladder, Via Natural or Artificial Opening
0TPB7DZ Removal of Intraluminal Device from Bladder, Via Natural or Artificial Opening
0TPB7JZ Removal of Synthetic Substitute from Bladder, Via Natural or Artificial Opening
0TPB7KZ Removal of Nonautologous Tissue Substitute from Bladder, Via Natural or Artificial Opening
0TPB7LZ Removal of Artificial Sphincter from Bladder, Via Natural or Artificial Opening
▲ **0TPB7MZ** Removal of Stimulator Lead from Bladder, Via Natural or Artificial Opening
0TPB80Z Removal of Drainage Device from Bladder, Via Natural or Artificial Opening Endoscopic
0TPB82Z Removal of Monitoring Device from Bladder, Via Natural or Artificial Opening Endoscopic
0TPB83Z Removal of Infusion Device from Bladder, Via Natural or Artificial Opening Endoscopic
0TPB87Z Removal of Autologous Tissue Substitute from Bladder, Via Natural or Artificial Opening Endoscopic
0TPB8CZ Removal of Extraluminal Device from Bladder, Via Natural or Artificial Opening Endoscopic
0TPB8DZ Removal of Intraluminal Device from Bladder, Via Natural or Artificial Opening Endoscopic
0TPB8JZ Removal of Synthetic Substitute from Bladder, Via Natural or Artificial Opening Endoscopic
0TPB8KZ Removal of Nonautologous Tissue Substitute from Bladder, Via Natural or Artificial Opening Endoscopic
0TPB8LZ Removal of Artificial Sphincter from Bladder, Via Natural or Artificial Opening Endoscopic
▲ **0TPB8MZ** Removal of Stimulator Lead from Bladder, Via Natural or Artificial Opening Endoscopic
0TPBX0Z Removal of Drainage Device from Bladder, External Approach
0TPBX2Z Removal of Monitoring Device from Bladder, External Approach
0TPBX3Z Removal of Infusion Device from Bladder, External Approach
0TPBXDZ Removal of Intraluminal Device from Bladder, External Approach
0TPBXLZ Removal of Artificial Sphincter from Bladder, External Approach
0TPBXMZ Removal of Stimulator Lead from Bladder, External Approach

0TPD00Z Removal of Drainage Device from Urethra, Open Approach
0TPD02Z Removal of Monitoring Device from Urethra, Open Approach
0TPD03Z Removal of Infusion Device from Urethra, Open Approach
0TPD07Z Removal of Autologous Tissue Substitute from Urethra, Open Approach
0TPD0CZ Removal of Extraluminal Device from Urethra, Open Approach
0TPD0DZ Removal of Intraluminal Device from Urethra, Open Approach
0TPD0JZ Removal of Synthetic Substitute from Urethra, Open Approach
0TPD0KZ Removal of Nonautologous Tissue Substitute from Urethra, Open Approach
0TPD0LZ Removal of Artificial Sphincter from Urethra, Open Approach
0TPD30Z Removal of Drainage Device from Urethra, Percutaneous Approach
0TPD32Z Removal of Monitoring Device from Urethra, Percutaneous Approach
0TPD33Z Removal of Infusion Device from Urethra, Percutaneous Approach
0TPD37Z Removal of Autologous Tissue Substitute from Urethra, Percutaneous Approach
0TPD3CZ Removal of Extraluminal Device from Urethra, Percutaneous Approach
0TPD3DZ Removal of Intraluminal Device from Urethra, Percutaneous Approach
0TPD3JZ Removal of Synthetic Substitute from Urethra, Percutaneous Approach
0TPD3KZ Removal of Nonautologous Tissue Substitute from Urethra, Percutaneous Approach
0TPD3LZ Removal of Artificial Sphincter from Urethra, Percutaneous Approach
0TPD40Z Removal of Drainage Device from Urethra, Percutaneous Endoscopic Approach
0TPD42Z Removal of Monitoring Device from Urethra, Percutaneous Endoscopic Approach
0TPD43Z Removal of Infusion Device from Urethra, Percutaneous Endoscopic Approach
0TPD47Z Removal of Autologous Tissue Substitute from Urethra, Percutaneous Endoscopic Approach
0TPD4CZ Removal of Extraluminal Device from Urethra, Percutaneous Endoscopic Approach
0TPD4DZ Removal of Intraluminal Device from Urethra, Percutaneous Endoscopic Approach
0TPD4JZ Removal of Synthetic Substitute from Urethra, Percutaneous Endoscopic Approach
0TPD4KZ Removal of Nonautologous Tissue Substitute from Urethra, Percutaneous Endoscopic Approach
0TPD4LZ Removal of Artificial Sphincter from Urethra, Percutaneous Endoscopic Approach
0TPD70Z Removal of Drainage Device from Urethra, Via Natural or Artificial Opening
0TPD72Z Removal of Monitoring Device from Urethra, Via Natural or Artificial Opening
0TPD73Z Removal of Infusion Device from Urethra, Via Natural or Artificial Opening
0TPD77Z Removal of Autologous Tissue Substitute from Urethra, Via Natural or Artificial Opening
0TPD7CZ Removal of Extraluminal Device from Urethra, Via Natural or Artificial Opening
0TPD7DZ Removal of Intraluminal Device from Urethra, Via Natural or Artificial Opening
0TPD7JZ Removal of Synthetic Substitute from Urethra, Via Natural or Artificial Opening
0TPD7KZ Removal of Nonautologous Tissue Substitute from Urethra, Via Natural or Artificial Opening
0TPD7LZ Removal of Artificial Sphincter from Urethra, Via Natural or Artificial Opening
0TPD80Z Removal of Drainage Device from Urethra, Via Natural or Artificial Opening Endoscopic
0TPD82Z Removal of Monitoring Device from Urethra, Via Natural or Artificial Opening Endoscopic
0TPD83Z Removal of Infusion Device from Urethra, Via Natural or Artificial Opening Endoscopic
0TPD87Z Removal of Autologous Tissue Substitute from Urethra, Via Natural or Artificial Opening Endoscopic
0TPD8CZ Removal of Extraluminal Device from Urethra, Via Natural or Artificial Opening Endoscopic
0TPD8DZ Removal of Intraluminal Device from Urethra, Via Natural or Artificial Opening Endoscopic
0TPD8JZ Removal of Synthetic Substitute from Urethra, Via Natural or Artificial Opening Endoscopic
0TPD8KZ Removal of Nonautologous Tissue Substitute from Urethra, Via Natural or Artificial Opening Endoscopic
0TPD8LZ Removal of Artificial Sphincter from Urethra, Via Natural or Artificial Opening Endoscopic
0TPDX0Z Removal of Drainage Device from Urethra, External Approach
0TPDX2Z Removal of Monitoring Device from Urethra, External Approach
0TPDX3Z Removal of Infusion Device from Urethra, External Approach
0TPDXDZ Removal of Intraluminal Device from Urethra, External Approach
0TPDXLZ Removal of Artificial Sphincter from Urethra, External Approach

0TQ – Urinary System, Repair

0TQ00ZZ Repair Right Kidney, Open Approach
0TQ03ZZ Repair Right Kidney, Percutaneous Approach
0TQ04ZZ Repair Right Kidney, Percutaneous Endoscopic Approach
0TQ07ZZ Repair Right Kidney, Via Natural or Artificial Opening
0TQ08ZZ Repair Right Kidney, Via Natural or Artificial Opening Endoscopic
0TQ10ZZ Repair Left Kidney, Open Approach
0TQ13ZZ Repair Left Kidney, Percutaneous Approach
0TQ14ZZ Repair Left Kidney, Percutaneous Endoscopic Approach
0TQ17ZZ Repair Left Kidney, Via Natural or Artificial Opening
0TQ18ZZ Repair Left Kidney, Via Natural or Artificial Opening Endoscopic
0TQ30ZZ Repair Right Kidney Pelvis, Open Approach
0TQ33ZZ Repair Right Kidney Pelvis, Percutaneous Approach
0TQ34ZZ Repair Right Kidney Pelvis, Percutaneous Endoscopic Approach
0TQ37ZZ Repair Right Kidney Pelvis, Via Natural or Artificial Opening
0TQ38ZZ Repair Right Kidney Pelvis, Via Natural or Artificial Opening Endoscopic
0TQ40ZZ Repair Left Kidney Pelvis, Open Approach
0TQ43ZZ Repair Left Kidney Pelvis, Percutaneous Approach
0TQ44ZZ Repair Left Kidney Pelvis, Percutaneous Endoscopic Approach
0TQ47ZZ Repair Left Kidney Pelvis, Via Natural or Artificial Opening
0TQ48ZZ Repair Left Kidney Pelvis, Via Natural or Artificial Opening Endoscopic
0TQ60ZZ Repair Right Ureter, Open Approach
0TQ63ZZ Repair Right Ureter, Percutaneous Approach
0TQ64ZZ Repair Right Ureter, Percutaneous Endoscopic Approach
0TQ67ZZ Repair Right Ureter, Via Natural or Artificial Opening
0TQ68ZZ Repair Right Ureter, Via Natural or Artificial Opening Endoscopic
0TQ70ZZ Repair Left Ureter, Open Approach
0TQ73ZZ Repair Left Ureter, Percutaneous Approach
0TQ74ZZ Repair Left Ureter, Percutaneous Endoscopic Approach
0TQ77ZZ Repair Left Ureter, Via Natural or Artificial Opening
0TQ78ZZ Repair Left Ureter, Via Natural or Artificial Opening Endoscopic
0TQB0ZZ Repair Bladder, Open Approach
+ Urostomy takedown when performed with code 0WQFXZ2, Repair of abdominal wall, stoma, external approach or 0WQFXZZ, Repair of abdominal wall, external approach.
0TQB3ZZ Repair Bladder, Percutaneous Approach
+ Urostomy takedown when performed with code 0WQFXZ2, Repair of abdominal wall, stoma, external approach or 0WQFXZZ, Repair of abdominal wall, external approach.
0TQB4ZZ Repair Bladder, Percutaneous Endoscopic Approach
+ Urostomy takedown when performed with code 0WQFXZ2, Repair of abdominal wall, stoma, external approach or 0WQFXZZ, Repair of abdominal wall, external approach.
0TQB7ZZ Repair Bladder, Via Natural or Artificial Opening
0TQB8ZZ Repair Bladder, Via Natural or Artificial Opening Endoscopic
0TQC0ZZ Repair Bladder Neck, Open Approach
0TQC3ZZ Repair Bladder Neck, Percutaneous Approach
0TQC4ZZ Repair Bladder Neck, Percutaneous Endoscopic Approach
0TQC7ZZ Repair Bladder Neck, Via Natural or Artificial Opening
0TQC8ZZ Repair Bladder Neck, Via Natural or Artificial Opening Endoscopic
0TQD0ZZ Repair Urethra, Open Approach
0TQD3ZZ Repair Urethra, Percutaneous Approach
0TQD4ZZ Repair Urethra, Percutaneous Endoscopic Approach
0TQD7ZZ Repair Urethra, Via Natural or Artificial Opening
0TQD8ZZ Repair Urethra, Via Natural or Artificial Opening Endoscopic
0TQDXZZ Repair Urethra, External Approach

0TR – Urinary System, Replacement

0TR307Z Replacement of Right Kidney Pelvis with Autologous Tissue Substitute, Open Approach
0TR30JZ Replacement of Right Kidney Pelvis with Synthetic Substitute, Open Approach
0TR30KZ Replacement of Right Kidney Pelvis with Nonautologous Tissue Substitute, Open Approach
0TR347Z Replacement of Right Kidney Pelvis with Autologous Tissue Substitute, Percutaneous Endoscopic Approach
0TR34JZ Replacement of Right Kidney Pelvis with Synthetic Substitute, Percutaneous Endoscopic Approach
0TR34KZ Replacement of Right Kidney Pelvis with Nonautologous Tissue Substitute, Percutaneous Endoscopic Approach
0TR377Z Replacement of Right Kidney Pelvis with Autologous Tissue Substitute, Via Natural or Artificial Opening
0TR37JZ Replacement of Right Kidney Pelvis with Synthetic Substitute, Via Natural or Artificial Opening
0TR37KZ Replacement of Right Kidney Pelvis with Nonautologous Tissue Substitute, Via Natural or Artificial Opening
0TR387Z Replacement of Right Kidney Pelvis with Autologous Tissue Substitute, Via Natural or Artificial Opening Endoscopic
0TR38JZ Replacement of Right Kidney Pelvis with Synthetic Substitute, Via Natural or Artificial Opening Endoscopic
0TR38KZ Replacement of Right Kidney Pelvis with Nonautologous Tissue Substitute, Via Natural or Artificial Opening Endoscopic
0TR407Z Replacement of Left Kidney Pelvis with Autologous Tissue Substitute, Open Approach
0TR40JZ Replacement of Left Kidney Pelvis with Synthetic Substitute, Open Approach
0TR40KZ Replacement of Left Kidney Pelvis with Nonautologous Tissue Substitute, Open Approach
0TR447Z Replacement of Left Kidney Pelvis with Autologous Tissue Substitute, Percutaneous Endoscopic Approach
0TR44JZ Replacement of Left Kidney Pelvis with Synthetic Substitute, Percutaneous Endoscopic Approach
0TR44KZ Replacement of Left Kidney Pelvis with Nonautologous Tissue Substitute, Percutaneous Endoscopic Approach
0TR477Z Replacement of Left Kidney Pelvis with Autologous Tissue Substitute, Via Natural or Artificial Opening
0TR47JZ Replacement of Left Kidney Pelvis with Synthetic Substitute, Via Natural or Artificial Opening
0TR47KZ Replacement of Left Kidney Pelvis with Nonautologous Tissue Substitute, Via Natural or Artificial Opening
0TR487Z Replacement of Left Kidney Pelvis with Autologous Tissue Substitute, Via Natural or Artificial Opening Endoscopic
0TR48JZ Replacement of Left Kidney Pelvis with Synthetic Substitute, Via Natural or Artificial Opening Endoscopic
0TR48KZ Replacement of Left Kidney Pelvis with Nonautologous Tissue Substitute, Via Natural or Artificial Opening Endoscopic
0TR607Z Replacement of Right Ureter with Autologous Tissue Substitute, Open Approach
0TR60JZ Replacement of Right Ureter with Synthetic Substitute, Open Approach
0TR60KZ Replacement of Right Ureter with Nonautologous Tissue Substitute, Open Approach
0TR647Z Replacement of Right Ureter with Autologous Tissue Substitute, Percutaneous Endoscopic Approach
0TR64JZ Replacement of Right Ureter with Synthetic Substitute, Percutaneous Endoscopic Approach
0TR64KZ Replacement of Right Ureter with Nonautologous Tissue Substitute, Percutaneous Endoscopic Approach
0TR677Z Replacement of Right Ureter with Autologous Tissue Substitute, Via Natural or Artificial Opening
0TR67JZ Replacement of Right Ureter with Synthetic Substitute, Via Natural or Artificial Opening
0TR67KZ Replacement of Right Ureter with Nonautologous Tissue Substitute, Via Natural or Artificial Opening
0TR687Z Replacement of Right Ureter with Autologous Tissue Substitute, Via Natural or Artificial Opening Endoscopic
0TR68JZ Replacement of Right Ureter with Synthetic Substitute, Via Natural or Artificial Opening Endoscopic
0TR68KZ Replacement of Right Ureter with Nonautologous Tissue Substitute, Via Natural or Artificial Opening Endoscopic
0TR707Z Replacement of Left Ureter with Autologous Tissue Substitute, Open Approach
0TR70JZ Replacement of Left Ureter with Synthetic Substitute, Open Approach
0TR70KZ Replacement of Left Ureter with Nonautologous Tissue Substitute, Open Approach
0TR747Z Replacement of Left Ureter with Autologous Tissue Substitute, Percutaneous Endoscopic Approach
0TR74JZ Replacement of Left Ureter with Synthetic Substitute, Percutaneous Endoscopic Approach
0TR74KZ Replacement of Left Ureter with Nonautologous Tissue Substitute, Percutaneous Endoscopic Approach
0TR777Z Replacement of Left Ureter with Autologous Tissue Substitute, Via Natural or Artificial Opening
0TR77JZ Replacement of Left Ureter with Synthetic Substitute, Via Natural or Artificial Opening
0TR77KZ Replacement of Left Ureter with Nonautologous Tissue Substitute, Via Natural or Artificial Opening
0TR787Z Replacement of Left Ureter with Autologous Tissue Substitute, Via Natural or Artificial Opening Endoscopic
0TR78JZ Replacement of Left Ureter with Synthetic Substitute, Via Natural or Artificial Opening Endoscopic
0TR78KZ Replacement of Left Ureter with Nonautologous Tissue Substitute, Via Natural or Artificial Opening Endoscopic
0TRB07Z Replacement of Bladder with Autologous Tissue Substitute, Open Approach
0TRB0JZ Replacement of Bladder with Synthetic Substitute, Open Approach
0TRB0KZ Replacement of Bladder with Nonautologous Tissue Substitute, Open Approach
0TRB47Z Replacement of Bladder with Autologous Tissue Substitute, Percutaneous Endoscopic Approach
0TRB4JZ Replacement of Bladder with Synthetic Substitute, Percutaneous Endoscopic Approach
0TRB4KZ Replacement of Bladder with Nonautologous Tissue Substitute, Percutaneous Endoscopic Approach
0TRB77Z Replacement of Bladder with Autologous Tissue Substitute, Via Natural or Artificial Opening
0TRB7JZ Replacement of Bladder with Synthetic Substitute, Via Natural or Artificial Opening
0TRB7KZ Replacement of Bladder with Nonautologous Tissue Substitute, Via Natural or Artificial Opening
0TRB87Z Replacement of Bladder with Autologous Tissue Substitute, Via Natural or Artificial Opening Endoscopic
0TRB8JZ Replacement of Bladder with Synthetic Substitute, Via Natural or Artificial Opening Endoscopic
0TRB8KZ Replacement of Bladder with Nonautologous Tissue Substitute, Via Natural or Artificial Opening Endoscopic
0TRC07Z Replacement of Bladder Neck with Autologous Tissue Substitute, Open Approach
0TRC0JZ Replacement of Bladder Neck with Synthetic Substitute, Open Approach
0TRC0KZ Replacement of Bladder Neck with Nonautologous Tissue Substitute, Open Approach
0TRC47Z Replacement of Bladder Neck with Autologous Tissue Substitute, Percutaneous Endoscopic Approach
0TRC4JZ Replacement of Bladder Neck with Synthetic Substitute, Percutaneous Endoscopic Approach
0TRC4KZ Replacement of Bladder Neck with Nonautologous Tissue Substitute, Percutaneous Endoscopic Approach
0TRC77Z Replacement of Bladder Neck with Autologous Tissue Substitute, Via Natural or Artificial Opening
0TRC7JZ Replacement of Bladder Neck with Synthetic Substitute, Via Natural or Artificial Opening
0TRC7KZ Replacement of Bladder Neck with Nonautologous Tissue Substitute, Via Natural or Artificial Opening
0TRC87Z Replacement of Bladder Neck with Autologous Tissue Substitute, Via Natural or Artificial Opening Endoscopic
0TRC8JZ Replacement of Bladder Neck with Synthetic Substitute, Via Natural or Artificial Opening Endoscopic
0TRC8KZ Replacement of Bladder Neck with Nonautologous Tissue Substitute, Via Natural or Artificial Opening Endoscopic
0TRD07Z Replacement of Urethra with Autologous Tissue Substitute, Open Approach
0TRD0JZ Replacement of Urethra with Synthetic Substitute, Open Approach
0TRD0KZ Replacement of Urethra with Nonautologous Tissue Substitute, Open Approach
0TRD47Z Replacement of Urethra with Autologous Tissue Substitute, Percutaneous Endoscopic Approach
0TRD4JZ Replacement of Urethra with Synthetic Substitute, Percutaneous Endoscopic Approach

0TRD4KZ Replacement of Urethra with Nonautologous Tissue Substitute, Percutaneous Endoscopic Approach
0TRD77Z Replacement of Urethra with Autologous Tissue Substitute, Via Natural or Artificial Opening
0TRD7JZ Replacement of Urethra with Synthetic Substitute, Via Natural or Artificial Opening
0TRD7KZ Replacement of Urethra with Nonautologous Tissue Substitute, Via Natural or Artificial Opening
0TRD87Z Replacement of Urethra with Autologous Tissue Substitute, Via Natural or Artificial Opening Endoscopic
0TRD8JZ Replacement of Urethra with Synthetic Substitute, Via Natural or Artificial Opening Endoscopic
0TRD8KZ Replacement of Urethra with Nonautologous Tissue Substitute, Via Natural or Artificial Opening Endoscopic
0TRDX7Z Replacement of Urethra with Autologous Tissue Substitute, External Approach
0TRDXJZ Replacement of Urethra with Synthetic Substitute, External Approach
0TRDXKZ Replacement of Urethra with Nonautologous Tissue Substitute, External Approach

0TS – Urinary System, Reposition

0TS00ZZ Reposition Right Kidney, Open Approach
0TS04ZZ Reposition Right Kidney, Percutaneous Endoscopic Approach
0TS10ZZ Reposition Left Kidney, Open Approach
0TS14ZZ Reposition Left Kidney, Percutaneous Endoscopic Approach
0TS20ZZ Reposition Bilateral Kidneys, Open Approach
0TS24ZZ Reposition Bilateral Kidneys, Percutaneous Endoscopic Approach
0TS30ZZ Reposition Right Kidney Pelvis, Open Approach
0TS34ZZ Reposition Right Kidney Pelvis, Percutaneous Endoscopic Approach
0TS40ZZ Reposition Left Kidney Pelvis, Open Approach
0TS44ZZ Reposition Left Kidney Pelvis, Percutaneous Endoscopic Approach
0TS60ZZ Reposition Right Ureter, Open Approach
0TS64ZZ Reposition Right Ureter, Percutaneous Endoscopic Approach
0TS70ZZ Reposition Left Ureter, Open Approach
0TS74ZZ Reposition Left Ureter, Percutaneous Endoscopic Approach
0TS80ZZ Reposition Bilateral Ureters, Open Approach
0TS84ZZ Reposition Bilateral Ureters, Percutaneous Endoscopic Approach
0TSB0ZZ Reposition Bladder, Open Approach
0TSB4ZZ Reposition Bladder, Percutaneous Endoscopic Approach
0TSC0ZZ Reposition Bladder Neck, Open Approach
0TSC4ZZ Reposition Bladder Neck, Percutaneous Endoscopic Approach
0TSD0ZZ Reposition Urethra, Open Approach
0TSD4ZZ Reposition Urethra, Percutaneous Endoscopic Approach

0TT – Urinary System, Resection

Review Coding Guideline B3.8

0TT00ZZ Resection of Right Kidney, Open Approach
0TT04ZZ Resection of Right Kidney, Percutaneous Endoscopic Approach
0TT10ZZ Resection of Left Kidney, Open Approach
0TT14ZZ Resection of Left Kidney, Percutaneous Endoscopic Approach
0TT20ZZ Resection of Bilateral Kidneys, Open Approach
0TT24ZZ Resection of Bilateral Kidneys, Percutaneous Endoscopic Approach
0TT30ZZ Resection of Right Kidney Pelvis, Open Approach
0TT34ZZ Resection of Right Kidney Pelvis, Percutaneous Endoscopic Approach
0TT37ZZ Resection of Right Kidney Pelvis, Via Natural or Artificial Opening
0TT38ZZ Resection of Right Kidney Pelvis, Via Natural or Artificial Opening Endoscopic
0TT40ZZ Resection of Left Kidney Pelvis, Open Approach
0TT44ZZ Resection of Left Kidney Pelvis, Percutaneous Endoscopic Approach
0TT47ZZ Resection of Left Kidney Pelvis, Via Natural or Artificial Opening
0TT48ZZ Resection of Left Kidney Pelvis, Via Natural or Artificial Opening Endoscopic
0TT60ZZ Resection of Right Ureter, Open Approach
0TT64ZZ Resection of Right Ureter, Percutaneous Endoscopic Approach
0TT67ZZ Resection of Right Ureter, Via Natural or Artificial Opening
0TT68ZZ Resection of Right Ureter, Via Natural or Artificial Opening Endoscopic
0TT70ZZ Resection of Left Ureter, Open Approach
0TT74ZZ Resection of Left Ureter, Percutaneous Endoscopic Approach
0TT77ZZ Resection of Left Ureter, Via Natural or Artificial Opening
0TT78ZZ Resection of Left Ureter, Via Natural or Artificial Opening Endoscopic
0TTB0ZZ Resection of Bladder, Open Approach
+ Pelvic evisceration when reported with Resection of urethra, bilateral ovaries, bilateral fallopian tubes, uterus, cervix and vagina. *See tables 0TT and 0UT to construct the Resection codes.*
0TTB4ZZ Resection of Bladder, Percutaneous Endoscopic Approach
0TTB7ZZ Resection of Bladder, Via Natural or Artificial Opening
0TTB8ZZ Resection of Bladder, Via Natural or Artificial Opening Endoscopic
0TTC0ZZ Resection of Bladder Neck, Open Approach
0TTC4ZZ Resection of Bladder Neck, Percutaneous Endoscopic Approach
0TTC7ZZ Resection of Bladder Neck, Via Natural or Artificial Opening
0TTC8ZZ Resection of Bladder Neck, Via Natural or Artificial Opening Endoscopic
● **0TTD0ZZ** Resection of Urethra, Open Approach
0TTD4ZZ Resection of Urethra, Percutaneous Endoscopic Approach
0TTD7ZZ Resection of Urethra, Via Natural or Artificial Opening
0TTD8ZZ Resection of Urethra, Via Natural or Artificial Opening Endoscopic

0TU – Urinary System, Supplement

0TU307Z Supplement Right Kidney Pelvis with Autologous Tissue Substitute, Open Approach
0TU30JZ Supplement Right Kidney Pelvis with Synthetic Substitute, Open Approach
0TU30KZ Supplement Right Kidney Pelvis with Nonautologous Tissue Substitute, Open Approach
0TU347Z Supplement Right Kidney Pelvis with Autologous Tissue Substitute, Percutaneous Endoscopic Approach
0TU34JZ Supplement Right Kidney Pelvis with Synthetic Substitute, Percutaneous Endoscopic Approach
0TU34KZ Supplement Right Kidney Pelvis with Nonautologous Tissue Substitute, Percutaneous Endoscopic Approach
0TU377Z Supplement Right Kidney Pelvis with Autologous Tissue Substitute, Via Natural or Artificial Opening
0TU37JZ Supplement Right Kidney Pelvis with Synthetic Substitute, Via Natural or Artificial Opening
0TU37KZ Supplement Right Kidney Pelvis with Nonautologous Tissue Substitute, Via Natural or Artificial Opening
0TU387Z Supplement Right Kidney Pelvis with Autologous Tissue Substitute, Via Natural or Artificial Opening Endoscopic
0TU38JZ Supplement Right Kidney Pelvis with Synthetic Substitute, Via Natural or Artificial Opening Endoscopic
0TU38KZ Supplement Right Kidney Pelvis with Nonautologous Tissue Substitute, Via Natural or Artificial Opening Endoscopic
0TU407Z Supplement Left Kidney Pelvis with Autologous Tissue Substitute, Open Approach
0TU40JZ Supplement Left Kidney Pelvis with Synthetic Substitute, Open Approach
0TU40KZ Supplement Left Kidney Pelvis with Nonautologous Tissue Substitute, Open Approach
0TU447Z Supplement Left Kidney Pelvis with Autologous Tissue Substitute, Percutaneous Endoscopic Approach
0TU44JZ Supplement Left Kidney Pelvis with Synthetic Substitute, Percutaneous Endoscopic Approach
0TU44KZ Supplement Left Kidney Pelvis with Nonautologous Tissue Substitute, Percutaneous Endoscopic Approach

0TU477Z Supplement Left Kidney Pelvis with Autologous Tissue Substitute, Via Natural or Artificial Opening

0TU47JZ Supplement Left Kidney Pelvis with Synthetic Substitute, Via Natural or Artificial Opening

0TU47KZ Supplement Left Kidney Pelvis with Nonautologous Tissue Substitute, Via Natural or Artificial Opening

0TU487Z Supplement Left Kidney Pelvis with Autologous Tissue Substitute, Via Natural or Artificial Opening Endoscopic

0TU48JZ Supplement Left Kidney Pelvis with Synthetic Substitute, Via Natural or Artificial Opening Endoscopic

0TU48KZ Supplement Left Kidney Pelvis with Nonautologous Tissue Substitute, Via Natural or Artificial Opening Endoscopic

0TU607Z Supplement Right Ureter with Autologous Tissue Substitute, Open Approach

0TU60JZ Supplement Right Ureter with Synthetic Substitute, Open Approach

0TU60KZ Supplement Right Ureter with Nonautologous Tissue Substitute, Open Approach

0TU647Z Supplement Right Ureter with Autologous Tissue Substitute, Percutaneous Endoscopic Approach

0TU64JZ Supplement Right Ureter with Synthetic Substitute, Percutaneous Endoscopic Approach

0TU64KZ Supplement Right Ureter with Nonautologous Tissue Substitute, Percutaneous Endoscopic Approach

0TU677Z Supplement Right Ureter with Autologous Tissue Substitute, Via Natural or Artificial Opening

0TU67JZ Supplement Right Ureter with Synthetic Substitute, Via Natural or Artificial Opening

0TU67KZ Supplement Right Ureter with Nonautologous Tissue Substitute, Via Natural or Artificial Opening

0TU687Z Supplement Right Ureter with Autologous Tissue Substitute, Via Natural or Artificial Opening Endoscopic

0TU68JZ Supplement Right Ureter with Synthetic Substitute, Via Natural or Artificial Opening Endoscopic

0TU68KZ Supplement Right Ureter with Nonautologous Tissue Substitute, Via Natural or Artificial Opening Endoscopic

0TU707Z Supplement Left Ureter with Autologous Tissue Substitute, Open Approach

0TU70JZ Supplement Left Ureter with Synthetic Substitute, Open Approach

0TU70KZ Supplement Left Ureter with Nonautologous Tissue Substitute, Open Approach

0TU747Z Supplement Left Ureter with Autologous Tissue Substitute, Percutaneous Endoscopic Approach

0TU74JZ Supplement Left Ureter with Synthetic Substitute, Percutaneous Endoscopic Approach

0TU74KZ Supplement Left Ureter with Nonautologous Tissue Substitute, Percutaneous Endoscopic Approach

0TU777Z Supplement Left Ureter with Autologous Tissue Substitute, Via Natural or Artificial Opening

0TU77JZ Supplement Left Ureter with Synthetic Substitute, Via Natural or Artificial Opening

0TU77KZ Supplement Left Ureter with Nonautologous Tissue Substitute, Via Natural or Artificial Opening

0TU787Z Supplement Left Ureter with Autologous Tissue Substitute, Via Natural or Artificial Opening Endoscopic

0TU78JZ Supplement Left Ureter with Synthetic Substitute, Via Natural or Artificial Opening Endoscopic

0TU78KZ Supplement Left Ureter with Nonautologous Tissue Substitute, Via Natural or Artificial Opening Endoscopic

0TUB07Z Supplement Bladder with Autologous Tissue Substitute, Open Approach

0TUB0JZ Supplement Bladder with Synthetic Substitute, Open Approach

0TUB0KZ Supplement Bladder with Nonautologous Tissue Substitute, Open Approach

0TUB47Z Supplement Bladder with Autologous Tissue Substitute, Percutaneous Endoscopic Approach

0TUB4JZ Supplement Bladder with Synthetic Substitute, Percutaneous Endoscopic Approach

0TUB4KZ Supplement Bladder with Nonautologous Tissue Substitute, Percutaneous Endoscopic Approach

0TUB77Z Supplement Bladder with Autologous Tissue Substitute, Via Natural or Artificial Opening

0TUB7JZ Supplement Bladder with Synthetic Substitute, Via Natural or Artificial Opening

0TUB7KZ Supplement Bladder with Nonautologous Tissue Substitute, Via Natural or Artificial Opening

0TUB87Z Supplement Bladder with Autologous Tissue Substitute, Via Natural or Artificial Opening Endoscopic

0TUB8JZ Supplement Bladder with Synthetic Substitute, Via Natural or Artificial Opening Endoscopic

0TUB8KZ Supplement Bladder with Nonautologous Tissue Substitute, Via Natural or Artificial Opening Endoscopic

0TUC07Z Supplement Bladder Neck with Autologous Tissue Substitute, Open Approach

0TUC0JZ Supplement Bladder Neck with Synthetic Substitute, Open Approach

0TUC0KZ Supplement Bladder Neck with Nonautologous Tissue Substitute, Open Approach

0TUC47Z Supplement Bladder Neck with Autologous Tissue Substitute, Percutaneous Endoscopic Approach

0TUC4JZ Supplement Bladder Neck with Synthetic Substitute, Percutaneous Endoscopic Approach

0TUC4KZ Supplement Bladder Neck with Nonautologous Tissue Substitute, Percutaneous Endoscopic Approach

0TUC77Z Supplement Bladder Neck with Autologous Tissue Substitute, Via Natural or Artificial Opening

0TUC7JZ Supplement Bladder Neck with Synthetic Substitute, Via Natural or Artificial Opening

0TUC7KZ Supplement Bladder Neck with Nonautologous Tissue Substitute, Via Natural or Artificial Opening

0TUC87Z Supplement Bladder Neck with Autologous Tissue Substitute, Via Natural or Artificial Opening Endoscopic

0TUC8JZ Supplement Bladder Neck with Synthetic Substitute, Via Natural or Artificial Opening Endoscopic

0TUC8KZ Supplement Bladder Neck with Nonautologous Tissue Substitute, Via Natural or Artificial Opening Endoscopic

0TUD07Z Supplement Urethra with Autologous Tissue Substitute, Open Approach

0TUD0JZ Supplement Urethra with Synthetic Substitute, Open Approach

0TUD0KZ Supplement Urethra with Nonautologous Tissue Substitute, Open Approach

0TUD47Z Supplement Urethra with Autologous Tissue Substitute, Percutaneous Endoscopic Approach

0TUD4JZ Supplement Urethra with Synthetic Substitute, Percutaneous Endoscopic Approach

0TUD4KZ Supplement Urethra with Nonautologous Tissue Substitute, Percutaneous Endoscopic Approach

0TUD77Z Supplement Urethra with Autologous Tissue Substitute, Via Natural or Artificial Opening

0TUD7JZ Supplement Urethra with Synthetic Substitute, Via Natural or Artificial Opening

0TUD7KZ Supplement Urethra with Nonautologous Tissue Substitute, Via Natural or Artificial Opening

0TUD87Z Supplement Urethra with Autologous Tissue Substitute, Via Natural or Artificial Opening Endoscopic

0TUD8JZ Supplement Urethra with Synthetic Substitute, Via Natural or Artificial Opening Endoscopic

0TUD8KZ Supplement Urethra with Nonautologous Tissue Substitute, Via Natural or Artificial Opening Endoscopic

0TUDX7Z Supplement Urethra with Autologous Tissue Substitute, External Approach

0TUDXJZ Supplement Urethra with Synthetic Substitute, External Approach

0TUDXKZ Supplement Urethra with Nonautologous Tissue Substitute, External Approach

0TV – Urinary System, Restriction

0TV30CZ Restriction of Right Kidney Pelvis with Extraluminal Device, Open Approach

0TV30DZ Restriction of Right Kidney Pelvis with Intraluminal Device, Open Approach

0TV30ZZ Restriction of Right Kidney Pelvis, Open Approach

0TV33CZ Restriction of Right Kidney Pelvis with Extraluminal Device, Percutaneous Approach

0TV33DZ Restriction of Right Kidney Pelvis with Intraluminal Device, Percutaneous Approach

0TV33ZZ Restriction of Right Kidney Pelvis, Percutaneous Approach

0TV34CZ Restriction of Right Kidney Pelvis with Extraluminal Device, Percutaneous Endoscopic Approach

0TV34DZ Restriction of Right Kidney Pelvis with Intraluminal Device, Percutaneous Endoscopic Approach

0TV34ZZ Restriction of Right Kidney Pelvis, Percutaneous Endoscopic Approach

0TV37DZ Restriction of Right Kidney Pelvis with Intraluminal Device, Via Natural or Artificial Opening
0TV37ZZ Restriction of Right Kidney Pelvis, Via Natural or Artificial Opening
0TV38DZ Restriction of Right Kidney Pelvis with Intraluminal Device, Via Natural or Artificial Opening Endoscopic
0TV38ZZ Restriction of Right Kidney Pelvis, Via Natural or Artificial Opening Endoscopic
0TV40CZ Restriction of Left Kidney Pelvis with Extraluminal Device, Open Approach
0TV40DZ Restriction of Left Kidney Pelvis with Intraluminal Device, Open Approach
0TV40ZZ Restriction of Left Kidney Pelvis, Open Approach
0TV43CZ Restriction of Left Kidney Pelvis with Extraluminal Device, Percutaneous Approach
0TV43DZ Restriction of Left Kidney Pelvis with Intraluminal Device, Percutaneous Approach
0TV43ZZ Restriction of Left Kidney Pelvis, Percutaneous Approach
0TV44CZ Restriction of Left Kidney Pelvis with Extraluminal Device, Percutaneous Endoscopic Approach
0TV44DZ Restriction of Left Kidney Pelvis with Intraluminal Device, Percutaneous Endoscopic Approach
0TV44ZZ Restriction of Left Kidney Pelvis, Percutaneous Endoscopic Approach
0TV47DZ Restriction of Left Kidney Pelvis with Intraluminal Device, Via Natural or Artificial Opening
0TV47ZZ Restriction of Left Kidney Pelvis, Via Natural or Artificial Opening
0TV48DZ Restriction of Left Kidney Pelvis with Intraluminal Device, Via Natural or Artificial Opening Endoscopic
0TV48ZZ Restriction of Left Kidney Pelvis, Via Natural or Artificial Opening Endoscopic
0TV60CZ Restriction of Right Ureter with Extraluminal Device, Open Approach
0TV60DZ Restriction of Right Ureter with Intraluminal Device, Open Approach
0TV60ZZ Restriction of Right Ureter, Open Approach
0TV63CZ Restriction of Right Ureter with Extraluminal Device, Percutaneous Approach
0TV63DZ Restriction of Right Ureter with Intraluminal Device, Percutaneous Approach
0TV63ZZ Restriction of Right Ureter, Percutaneous Approach
0TV64CZ Restriction of Right Ureter with Extraluminal Device, Percutaneous Endoscopic Approach
0TV64DZ Restriction of Right Ureter with Intraluminal Device, Percutaneous Endoscopic Approach
0TV64ZZ Restriction of Right Ureter, Percutaneous Endoscopic Approach
0TV67DZ Restriction of Right Ureter with Intraluminal Device, Via Natural or Artificial Opening
0TV67ZZ Restriction of Right Ureter, Via Natural or Artificial Opening
0TV68DZ Restriction of Right Ureter with Intraluminal Device, Via Natural or Artificial Opening Endoscopic
0TV68ZZ Restriction of Right Ureter, Via Natural or Artificial Opening Endoscopic
0TV70CZ Restriction of Left Ureter with Extraluminal Device, Open Approach
0TV70DZ Restriction of Left Ureter with Intraluminal Device, Open Approach
0TV70ZZ Restriction of Left Ureter, Open Approach
0TV73CZ Restriction of Left Ureter with Extraluminal Device, Percutaneous Approach
0TV73DZ Restriction of Left Ureter with Intraluminal Device, Percutaneous Approach
0TV73ZZ Restriction of Left Ureter, Percutaneous Approach
0TV74CZ Restriction of Left Ureter with Extraluminal Device, Percutaneous Endoscopic Approach
0TV74DZ Restriction of Left Ureter with Intraluminal Device, Percutaneous Endoscopic Approach
0TV74ZZ Restriction of Left Ureter, Percutaneous Endoscopic Approach
0TV77DZ Restriction of Left Ureter with Intraluminal Device, Via Natural or Artificial Opening
0TV77ZZ Restriction of Left Ureter, Via Natural or Artificial Opening
0TV78DZ Restriction of Left Ureter with Intraluminal Device, Via Natural or Artificial Opening Endoscopic
0TV78ZZ Restriction of Left Ureter, Via Natural or Artificial Opening Endoscopic
0TVB0CZ Restriction of Bladder with Extraluminal Device, Open Approach
0TVB0DZ Restriction of Bladder with Intraluminal Device, Open Approach
0TVB0ZZ Restriction of Bladder, Open Approach
0TVB3CZ Restriction of Bladder with Extraluminal Device, Percutaneous Approach
0TVB3DZ Restriction of Bladder with Intraluminal Device, Percutaneous Approach
0TVB3ZZ Restriction of Bladder, Percutaneous Approach
0TVB4CZ Restriction of Bladder with Extraluminal Device, Percutaneous Endoscopic Approach
0TVB4DZ Restriction of Bladder with Intraluminal Device, Percutaneous Endoscopic Approach
0TVB4ZZ Restriction of Bladder, Percutaneous Endoscopic Approach
0TVB7DZ Restriction of Bladder with Intraluminal Device, Via Natural or Artificial Opening
0TVB7ZZ Restriction of Bladder, Via Natural or Artificial Opening
0TVB8DZ Restriction of Bladder with Intraluminal Device, Via Natural or Artificial Opening Endoscopic
0TVB8ZZ Restriction of Bladder, Via Natural or Artificial Opening Endoscopic
0TVC0CZ Restriction of Bladder Neck with Extraluminal Device, Open Approach
0TVC0DZ Restriction of Bladder Neck with Intraluminal Device, Open Approach
0TVC0ZZ Restriction of Bladder Neck, Open Approach
0TVC3CZ Restriction of Bladder Neck with Extraluminal Device, Percutaneous Approach
0TVC3DZ Restriction of Bladder Neck with Intraluminal Device, Percutaneous Approach
0TVC3ZZ Restriction of Bladder Neck, Percutaneous Approach
0TVC4CZ Restriction of Bladder Neck with Extraluminal Device, Percutaneous Endoscopic Approach
0TVC4DZ Restriction of Bladder Neck with Intraluminal Device, Percutaneous Endoscopic Approach
0TVC4ZZ Restriction of Bladder Neck, Percutaneous Endoscopic Approach
0TVC7DZ Restriction of Bladder Neck with Intraluminal Device, Via Natural or Artificial Opening
0TVC7ZZ Restriction of Bladder Neck, Via Natural or Artificial Opening
0TVC8DZ Restriction of Bladder Neck with Intraluminal Device, Via Natural or Artificial Opening Endoscopic
0TVC8ZZ Restriction of Bladder Neck, Via Natural or Artificial Opening Endoscopic
0TVD0CZ Restriction of Urethra with Extraluminal Device, Open Approach
0TVD0DZ Restriction of Urethra with Intraluminal Device, Open Approach
0TVD0ZZ Restriction of Urethra, Open Approach
0TVD3CZ Restriction of Urethra with Extraluminal Device, Percutaneous Approach
0TVD3DZ Restriction of Urethra with Intraluminal Device, Percutaneous Approach
0TVD3ZZ Restriction of Urethra, Percutaneous Approach
0TVD4CZ Restriction of Urethra with Extraluminal Device, Percutaneous Endoscopic Approach
0TVD4DZ Restriction of Urethra with Intraluminal Device, Percutaneous Endoscopic Approach
0TVD4ZZ Restriction of Urethra, Percutaneous Endoscopic Approach
0TVD7DZ Restriction of Urethra with Intraluminal Device, Via Natural or Artificial Opening
0TVD7ZZ Restriction of Urethra, Via Natural or Artificial Opening
0TVD8DZ Restriction of Urethra with Intraluminal Device, Via Natural or Artificial Opening Endoscopic
0TVD8ZZ Restriction of Urethra, Via Natural or Artificial Opening Endoscopic
0TVDXZZ Restriction of Urethra, External Approach

0TW – Urinary System, Revision

Review Coding Guideline B6.1c

0TW500Z Revision of Drainage Device in Kidney, Open Approach
0TW502Z Revision of Monitoring Device in Kidney, Open Approach
0TW503Z Revision of Infusion Device in Kidney, Open Approach
0TW507Z Revision of Autologous Tissue Substitute in Kidney, Open Approach
0TW50CZ Revision of Extraluminal Device in Kidney, Open Approach
0TW50DZ Revision of Intraluminal Device in Kidney, Open Approach
0TW50JZ Revision of Synthetic Substitute in Kidney, Open Approach
0TW50KZ Revision of Nonautologous Tissue Substitute in Kidney, Open Approach
0TW530Z Revision of Drainage Device in Kidney, Percutaneous Approach

0TW532Z Revision of Monitoring Device in Kidney, Percutaneous Approach

0TW533Z Revision of Infusion Device in Kidney, Percutaneous Approach

0TW537Z Revision of Autologous Tissue Substitute in Kidney, Percutaneous Approach

0TW53CZ Revision of Extraluminal Device in Kidney, Percutaneous Approach

0TW53DZ Revision of Intraluminal Device in Kidney, Percutaneous Approach

0TW53JZ Revision of Synthetic Substitute in Kidney, Percutaneous Approach

0TW53KZ Revision of Nonautologous Tissue Substitute in Kidney, Percutaneous Approach

0TW540Z Revision of Drainage Device in Kidney, Percutaneous Endoscopic Approach

0TW542Z Revision of Monitoring Device in Kidney, Percutaneous Endoscopic Approach

0TW543Z Revision of Infusion Device in Kidney, Percutaneous Endoscopic Approach

0TW547Z Revision of Autologous Tissue Substitute in Kidney, Percutaneous Endoscopic Approach

0TW54CZ Revision of Extraluminal Device in Kidney, Percutaneous Endoscopic Approach

0TW54DZ Revision of Intraluminal Device in Kidney, Percutaneous Endoscopic Approach

0TW54JZ Revision of Synthetic Substitute in Kidney, Percutaneous Endoscopic Approach

0TW54KZ Revision of Nonautologous Tissue Substitute in Kidney, Percutaneous Endoscopic Approach

0TW570Z Revision of Drainage Device in Kidney, Via Natural or Artificial Opening

0TW570Z Revision of Monitoring Device in Kidney, Via Natural or Artificial Opening

0TW573Z Revision of Infusion Device in Kidney, Via Natural or Artificial Opening

0TW577Z Revision of Autologous Tissue Substitute in Kidney, Via Natural or Artificial Opening

0TW57CZ Revision of Extraluminal Device in Kidney, Via Natural or Artificial Opening

0TW57DZ Revision of Intraluminal Device in Kidney, Via Natural or Artificial Opening

0TW57JZ Revision of Synthetic Substitute in Kidney, Via Natural or Artificial Opening

0TW57KZ Revision of Nonautologous Tissue Substitute in Kidney, Via Natural or Artificial Opening

0TW580Z Revision of Drainage Device in Kidney, Via Natural or Artificial Opening Endoscopic

0TW582Z Revision of Monitoring Device in Kidney, Via Natural or Artificial Opening Endoscopic

0TW583Z Revision of Infusion Device in Kidney, Via Natural or Artificial Opening Endoscopic

0TW587Z Revision of Autologous Tissue Substitute in Kidney, Via Natural or Artificial Opening Endoscopic

0TW58CZ Revision of Extraluminal Device in Kidney, Via Natural or Artificial Opening Endoscopic

0TW58DZ Revision of Intraluminal Device in Kidney, Via Natural or Artificial Opening Endoscopic

0TW58JZ Revision of Synthetic Substitute in Kidney, Via Natural or Artificial Opening Endoscopic

0TW58KZ Revision of Nonautologous Tissue Substitute in Kidney, Via Natural or Artificial Opening Endoscopic

0TW5X0Z Revision of Drainage Device in Kidney, External Approach

0TW5X2Z Revision of Monitoring Device in Kidney, External Approach

0TW5X3Z Revision of Infusion Device in Kidney, External Approach

0TW5X7Z Revision of Autologous Tissue Substitute in Kidney, External Approach

0TW5XCZ Revision of Extraluminal Device in Kidney, External Approach

0TW5XDZ Revision of Intraluminal Device in Kidney, External Approach

0TW5XJZ Revision of Synthetic Substitute in Kidney, External Approach

0TW5XKZ Revision of Nonautologous Tissue Substitute in Kidney, External Approach

0TW900Z Revision of Drainage Device in Ureter, Open Approach

0TW902Z Revision of Monitoring Device in Ureter, Open Approach

0TW903Z Revision of Infusion Device in Ureter, Open Approach

0TW907Z Revision of Autologous Tissue Substitute in Ureter, Open Approach

0TW90CZ Revision of Extraluminal Device in Ureter, Open Approach

0TW90DZ Revision of Intraluminal Device in Ureter, Open Approach

0TW90JZ Revision of Synthetic Substitute in Ureter, Open Approach

0TW90KZ Revision of Nonautologous Tissue Substitute in Ureter, Open Approach

0TW90MZ Revision of Stimulator Lead in Ureter, Open Approach

0TW930Z Revision of Drainage Device in Ureter, Percutaneous Approach

0TW932Z Revision of Monitoring Device in Ureter, Percutaneous Approach

0TW933Z Revision of Infusion Device in Ureter, Percutaneous Approach

0TW937Z Revision of Autologous Tissue Substitute in Ureter, Percutaneous Approach

0TW93CZ Revision of Extraluminal Device in Ureter, Percutaneous Approach

0TW93DZ Revision of Intraluminal Device in Ureter, Percutaneous Approach

0TW93JZ Revision of Synthetic Substitute in Ureter, Percutaneous Approach

0TW93KZ Revision of Nonautologous Tissue Substitute in Ureter, Percutaneous Approach

0TW93MZ Revision of Stimulator Lead in Ureter, Percutaneous Approach

0TW940Z Revision of Drainage Device in Ureter, Percutaneous Endoscopic Approach

0TW942Z Revision of Monitoring Device in Ureter, Percutaneous Endoscopic Approach

0TW943Z Revision of Infusion Device in Ureter, Percutaneous Endoscopic Approach

0TW947Z Revision of Autologous Tissue Substitute in Ureter, Percutaneous Endoscopic Approach

0TW94CZ Revision of Extraluminal Device in Ureter, Percutaneous Endoscopic Approach

0TW94DZ Revision of Intraluminal Device in Ureter, Percutaneous Endoscopic Approach

0TW94JZ Revision of Synthetic Substitute in Ureter, Percutaneous Endoscopic Approach

0TW94KZ Revision of Nonautologous Tissue Substitute in Ureter, Percutaneous Endoscopic Approach

0TW94MZ Revision of Stimulator Lead in Ureter, Percutaneous Endoscopic Approach

0TW970Z Revision of Drainage Device in Ureter, Via Natural or Artificial Opening

0TW972Z Revision of Monitoring Device in Ureter, Via Natural or Artificial Opening

0TW973Z Revision of Infusion Device in Ureter, Via Natural or Artificial Opening

0TW977Z Revision of Autologous Tissue Substitute in Ureter, Via Natural or Artificial Opening

0TW97CZ Revision of Extraluminal Device in Ureter, Via Natural or Artificial Opening

0TW97DZ Revision of Intraluminal Device in Ureter, Via Natural or Artificial Opening

0TW97JZ Revision of Synthetic Substitute in Ureter, Via Natural or Artificial Opening

0TW97KZ Revision of Nonautologous Tissue Substitute in Ureter, Via Natural or Artificial Opening

0TW97MZ Revision of Stimulator Lead in Ureter, Via Natural or Artificial Opening

0TW980Z Revision of Drainage Device in Ureter, Via Natural or Artificial Opening Endoscopic

0TW982Z Revision of Monitoring Device in Ureter, Via Natural or Artificial Opening Endoscopic

0TW983Z Revision of Infusion Device in Ureter, Via Natural or Artificial Opening Endoscopic

0TW987Z Revision of Autologous Tissue Substitute in Ureter, Via Natural or Artificial Opening Endoscopic

0TW98CZ Revision of Extraluminal Device in Ureter, Via Natural or Artificial Opening Endoscopic

0TW98DZ Revision of Intraluminal Device in Ureter, Via Natural or Artificial Opening Endoscopic

0TW98JZ Revision of Synthetic Substitute in Ureter, Via Natural or Artificial Opening Endoscopic

0TW98KZ Revision of Nonautologous Tissue Substitute in Ureter, Via Natural or Artificial Opening Endoscopic

0TW98MZ Revision of Stimulator Lead in Ureter, Via Natural or Artificial Opening Endoscopic

0TW9X0Z Revision of Drainage Device in Ureter, External Approach

0TW9X2Z Revision of Monitoring Device in Ureter, External Approach

0TW9X3Z Revision of Infusion Device in Ureter, External Approach

0TW9X7Z Revision of Autologous Tissue Substitute in Ureter, External Approach

0TW9XCZ Revision of Extraluminal Device in Ureter, External Approach

0TW9XDZ Revision of Intraluminal Device in Ureter, External Approach

0TW9XJZ Revision of Synthetic Substitute in Ureter, External Approach

0TW9XKZ Revision of Nonautologous Tissue Substitute in Ureter, External Approach

0TW9XMZ Revision of Stimulator Lead in Ureter, External Approach

0TWB00Z Revision of Drainage Device in Bladder, Open Approach

0TWB02Z Revision of Monitoring Device in Bladder, Open Approach

0TWB03Z Revision of Infusion Device in Bladder, Open Approach

0TWB07Z Revision of Autologous Tissue Substitute in Bladder, Open Approach

0TWB0CZ Revision of Extraluminal Device in Bladder, Open Approach

0TWB0DZ Revision of Intraluminal Device in Bladder, Open Approach

0TWB0JZ Revision of Synthetic Substitute in Bladder, Open Approach

0TWB0KZ Revision of Nonautologous Tissue Substitute in Bladder, Open Approach
0TWB0LZ Revision of Artificial Sphincter in Bladder, Open Approach
0TWB0MZ Revision of Stimulator Lead in Bladder, Open Approach
0TWB30Z Revision of Drainage Device in Bladder, Percutaneous Approach
0TWB32Z Revision of Monitoring Device in Bladder, Percutaneous Approach
0TWB33Z Revision of Infusion Device in Bladder, Percutaneous Approach
0TWB37Z Revision of Autologous Tissue Substitute in Bladder, Percutaneous Approach
0TWB3CZ Revision of Extraluminal Device in Bladder, Percutaneous Approach
0TWB3DZ Revision of Intraluminal Device in Bladder, Percutaneous Approach
0TWB3JZ Revision of Synthetic Substitute in Bladder, Percutaneous Approach
0TWB3KZ Revision of Nonautologous Tissue Substitute in Bladder, Percutaneous Approach
0TWB3LZ Revision of Artificial Sphincter in Bladder, Percutaneous Approach
0TWB3MZ Revision of Stimulator Lead in Bladder, Percutaneous Approach
0TWB40Z Revision of Drainage Device in Bladder, Percutaneous Endoscopic Approach
0TWB42Z Revision of Monitoring Device in Bladder, Percutaneous Endoscopic Approach
0TWB43Z Revision of Infusion Device in Bladder, Percutaneous Endoscopic Approach
0TWB47Z Revision of Autologous Tissue Substitute in Bladder, Percutaneous Endoscopic Approach
0TWB4CZ Revision of Extraluminal Device in Bladder, Percutaneous Endoscopic Approach
0TWB4DZ Revision of Intraluminal Device in Bladder, Percutaneous Endoscopic Approach
0TWB4JZ Revision of Synthetic Substitute in Bladder, Percutaneous Endoscopic Approach
0TWB4KZ Revision of Nonautologous Tissue Substitute in Bladder, Percutaneous Endoscopic Approach
0TWB4LZ Revision of Artificial Sphincter in Bladder, Percutaneous Endoscopic Approach
0TWB4MZ Revision of Stimulator Lead in Bladder, Percutaneous Endoscopic Approach
0TWB70Z Revision of Drainage Device in Bladder, Via Natural or Artificial Opening
0TWB72Z Revision of Monitoring Device in Bladder, Via Natural or Artificial Opening
0TWB73Z Revision of Infusion Device in Bladder, Via Natural or Artificial Opening
0TWB77Z Revision of Autologous Tissue Substitute in Bladder, Via Natural or Artificial Opening
0TWB7CZ Revision of Extraluminal Device in Bladder, Via Natural or Artificial Opening
0TWB7DZ Revision of Intraluminal Device in Bladder, Via Natural or Artificial Opening
0TWB7JZ Revision of Synthetic Substitute in Bladder, Via Natural or Artificial Opening
0TWB7KZ Revision of Nonautologous Tissue Substitute in Bladder, Via Natural or Artificial Opening
0TWB7LZ Revision of Artificial Sphincter in Bladder, Via Natural or Artificial Opening
0TWB7MZ Revision of Stimulator Lead in Bladder, Via Natural or Artificial Opening
0TWB80Z Revision of Drainage Device in Bladder, Via Natural or Artificial Opening Endoscopic
0TWB82Z Revision of Monitoring Device in Bladder, Via Natural or Artificial Opening Endoscopic
0TWB83Z Revision of Infusion Device in Bladder, Via Natural or Artificial Opening Endoscopic
0TWB87Z Revision of Autologous Tissue Substitute in Bladder, Via Natural or Artificial Opening Endoscopic
0TWB8CZ Revision of Extraluminal Device in Bladder, Via Natural or Artificial Opening Endoscopic
0TWB8DZ Revision of Intraluminal Device in Bladder, Via Natural or Artificial Opening Endoscopic
0TWB8JZ Revision of Synthetic Substitute in Bladder, Via Natural or Artificial Opening Endoscopic
0TWB8KZ Revision of Nonautologous Tissue Substitute in Bladder, Via Natural or Artificial Opening Endoscopic
0TWB8LZ Revision of Artificial Sphincter in Bladder, Via Natural or Artificial Opening Endoscopic
0TWB8MZ Revision of Stimulator Lead in Bladder, Via Natural or Artificial Opening Endoscopic
0TWBX0Z Revision of Drainage Device in Bladder, External Approach
0TWBX2Z Revision of Monitoring Device in Bladder, External Approach
0TWBX3Z Revision of Infusion Device in Bladder, External Approach
0TWBX7Z Revision of Autologous Tissue Substitute in Bladder, External Approach
0TWBXCZ Revision of Extraluminal Device in Bladder, External Approach
0TWBXDZ Revision of Intraluminal Device in Bladder, External Approach
0TWBXJZ Revision of Synthetic Substitute in Bladder, External Approach
0TWBXKZ Revision of Nonautologous Tissue Substitute in Bladder, External Approach
0TWBXLZ Revision of Artificial Sphincter in Bladder, External Approach
0TWBXMZ Revision of Stimulator Lead in Bladder, External Approach
0TWD00Z Revision of Drainage Device in Urethra, Open Approach
0TWD02Z Revision of Monitoring Device in Urethra, Open Approach
0TWD03Z Revision of Infusion Device in Urethra, Open Approach
0TWD07Z Revision of Autologous Tissue Substitute in Urethra, Open Approach
0TWD0CZ Revision of Extraluminal Device in Urethra, Open Approach
0TWD0DZ Revision of Intraluminal Device in Urethra, Open Approach
0TWD0JZ Revision of Synthetic Substitute in Urethra, Open Approach
0TWD0KZ Revision of Nonautologous Tissue Substitute in Urethra, Open Approach
0TWD0LZ Revision of Artificial Sphincter in Urethra, Open Approach
0TWD30Z Revision of Drainage Device in Urethra, Percutaneous Approach
0TWD32Z Revision of Monitoring Device in Urethra, Percutaneous Approach
0TWD33Z Revision of Infusion Device in Urethra, Percutaneous Approach
0TWD37Z Revision of Autologous Tissue Substitute in Urethra, Percutaneous Approach
0TWD3CZ Revision of Extraluminal Device in Urethra, Percutaneous Approach
0TWD3DZ Revision of Intraluminal Device in Urethra, Percutaneous Approach
0TWD3JZ Revision of Synthetic Substitute in Urethra, Percutaneous Approach
0TWD3KZ Revision of Nonautologous Tissue Substitute in Urethra, Percutaneous Approach
0TWD3LZ Revision of Artificial Sphincter in Urethra, Percutaneous Approach
0TWD40Z Revision of Drainage Device in Urethra, Percutaneous Endoscopic Approach
0TWD42Z Revision of Monitoring Device in Urethra, Percutaneous Endoscopic Approach
0TWD43Z Revision of Infusion Device in Urethra, Percutaneous Endoscopic Approach
0TWD47Z Revision of Autologous Tissue Substitute in Urethra, Percutaneous Endoscopic Approach
0TWD4CZ Revision of Extraluminal Device in Urethra, Percutaneous Endoscopic Approach
0TWD4DZ Revision of Intraluminal Device in Urethra, Percutaneous Endoscopic Approach
0TWD4JZ Revision of Synthetic Substitute in Urethra, Percutaneous Endoscopic Approach
0TWD4KZ Revision of Nonautologous Tissue Substitute in Urethra, Percutaneous Endoscopic Approach
0TWD4LZ Revision of Artificial Sphincter in Urethra, Percutaneous Endoscopic Approach
0TWD70Z Revision of Drainage Device in Urethra, Via Natural or Artificial Opening
0TWD72Z Revision of Monitoring Device in Urethra, Via Natural or Artificial Opening
0TWD73Z Revision of Infusion Device in Urethra, Via Natural or Artificial Opening
0TWD77Z Revision of Autologous Tissue Substitute in Urethra, Via Natural or Artificial Opening
0TWD7CZ Revision of Extraluminal Device in Urethra, Via Natural or Artificial Opening
0TWD7DZ Revision of Intraluminal Device in Urethra, Via Natural or Artificial Opening
0TWD7JZ Revision of Synthetic Substitute in Urethra, Via Natural or Artificial Opening
0TWD7KZ Revision of Nonautologous Tissue Substitute in Urethra, Via Natural or Artificial Opening
0TWD7LZ Revision of Artificial Sphincter in Urethra, Via Natural or Artificial Opening
0TWD80Z Revision of Drainage Device in Urethra, Via Natural or Artificial Opening Endoscopic
0TWD82Z Revision of Monitoring Device in Urethra, Via Natural or Artificial Opening Endoscopic
0TWD83Z Revision of Infusion Device in Urethra, Via Natural or Artificial Opening Endoscopic
0TWD87Z Revision of Autologous Tissue Substitute in Urethra, Via Natural or Artificial Opening Endoscopic

0TWD8CZ Revision of Extraluminal Device in Urethra, Via Natural or Artificial Opening Endoscopic

0TWD8DZ Revision of Intraluminal Device in Urethra, Via Natural or Artificial Opening Endoscopic

0TWD8JZ Revision of Synthetic Substitute in Urethra, Via Natural or Artificial Opening Endoscopic

0TWD8KZ Revision of Nonautologous Tissue Substitute in Urethra, Via Natural or Artificial Opening Endoscopic

0TWD8LZ Revision of Artificial Sphincter in Urethra, Via Natural or Artificial Opening Endoscopic

0TWDX0Z Revision of Drainage Device in Urethra, External Approach

0TWDX2Z Revision of Monitoring Device in Urethra, External Approach

0TWDX3Z Revision of Infusion Device in Urethra, External Approach

0TWDX7Z Revision of Autologous Tissue Substitute in Urethra, External Approach

0TWDXCZ Revision of Extraluminal Device in Urethra, External Approach

0TWDXDZ Revision of Intraluminal Device in Urethra, External Approach

0TWDXJZ Revision of Synthetic Substitute in Urethra, External Approach

0TWDXKZ Revision of Nonautologous Tissue Substitute in Urethra, External Approach

0TWDXLZ Revision of Artificial Sphincter in Urethra, External Approach

0TY – Urinary System, Transplantation

Review Coding Guideline B3.16

0TY00Z0 Transplantation of Right Kidney, Allogeneic, Open Approach
+ Kidney/Pancreas transplant when reported with Transplant of the Pancreas. *See table 0FY to construct the Transplantation code.*

0TY00Z1 Transplantation of Right Kidney, Syngeneic, Open Approach
+ Kidney/Pancreas transplant when reported with Transplant of the Pancreas. *See table 0FY to construct the Transplantation code.*

0TY00Z2 Transplantation of Right Kidney, Zooplastic, Open Approach
+ Kidney/Pancreas transplant when reported with Transplant of the Pancreas. *See table 0FY to construct the Transplantation code.*

0TY10Z0 Transplantation of Left Kidney, Allogeneic, Open Approach
+ Kidney/Pancreas transplant when reported with Transplant of the Pancreas. *See table 0FY to construct the Transplantation code.*

0TY10Z1 Transplantation of Left Kidney, Syngeneic, Open Approach
+ Kidney/Pancreas transplant when reported with Transplant of the Pancreas. *See table 0FY to construct the Transplantation code.*

0TY10Z2 Transplantation of Left Kidney, Zooplastic, Open Approach
+ Kidney/Pancreas transplant when reported with Transplant of the Pancreas. *See table 0FY to construct the Transplantation code.*

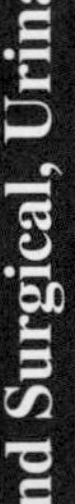

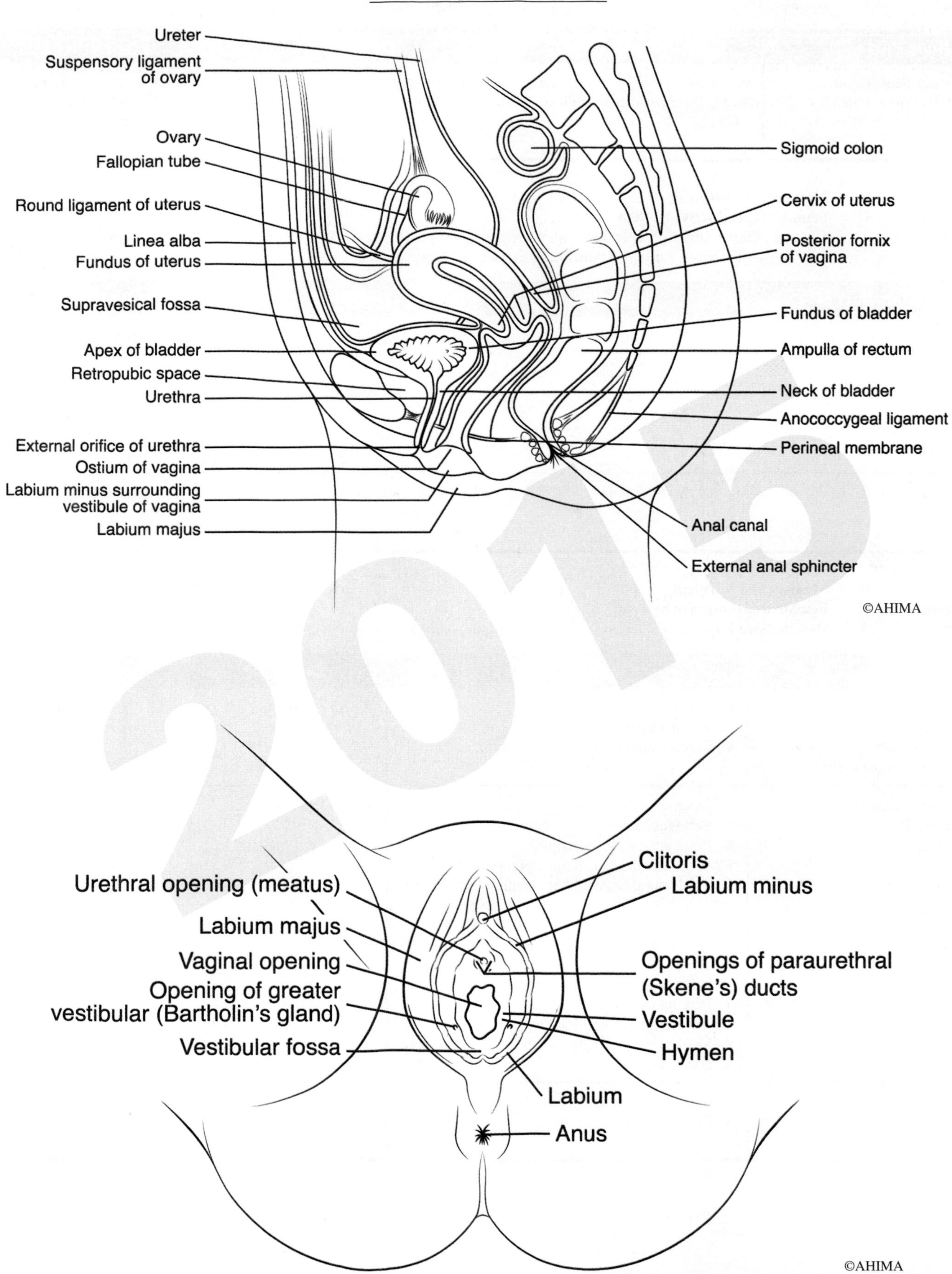
Female Reproductive System
Ureter
Suspensory ligament of ovary
Ovary
Fallopian tube
Round ligament of uterus
Linea alba
Fundus of uterus
Supravesical fossa
Apex of bladder
Retropubic space
Urethra
External orifice of urethra
Ostium of vagina
Labium minus surrounding vestibule of vagina
Labium majus
Sigmoid colon
Cervix of uterus
Posterior fornix of vagina
Fundus of bladder
Ampulla of rectum
Neck of bladder
Anococcygeal ligament
Perineal membrane
Anal canal
External anal sphincter
©AHIMA
Urethral opening (meatus)
Labium majus
Vaginal opening
Opening of greater vestibular (Bartholin's gland)
Vestibular fossa
Clitoris
Labium minus
Openings of paraurethral (Skene's) ducts
Vestibule
Hymen
Labium
Anus
©AHIMA

Female Reproductive System Tables 0U1–0UY

Section 0 **Medical and Surgical**
Body System U **Female Reproductive System**
Operation 1 **Bypass:** Altering the route of passage of the contents of a tubular body part

Body Part (4th)	Approach (5th)	Device (6th)	Qualifier (7th)
5 Fallopian Tube, Right **6** Fallopian Tube, Left	**0** Open **4** Percutaneous Endoscopic	**7** Autologous Tissue Substitute **J** Synthetic Substitute **K** Nonautologous Tissue Substitute **Z** No Device	**5** Fallopian Tube, Right **6** Fallopian Tube, Left **9** Uterus

Section 0 **Medical and Surgical**
Body System U **Female Reproductive System**
Operation 2 **Change:** Taking out or off a device from a body part and putting back an identical or similar device in or on the same body part without cutting or puncturing the skin or a mucous membrane

Body Part (4th)	Approach (5th)	Device (6th)	Qualifier (7th)
3 Ovary **8** Fallopian Tube **M** Vulva	**X** External	**0** Drainage Device **Y** Other Device	**Z** No Qualifier
D Uterus and Cervix	**X** External	**0** Drainage Device **H** Contraceptive Device **Y** Other Device	**Z** No Qualifier
H Vagina and Cul-de-sac	**X** External	**0** Drainage Device **G** Intraluminal Device, Pessary **Y** Other Device	**Z** No Qualifier

Section 0 **Medical and Surgical**
Body System U **Female Reproductive System**
Operation 5 **Destruction:** Physical eradication of all or a portion of a body part by the direct use of energy, force, or a destructive agent

Body Part (4th)	Approach (5th)	Device (6th)	Qualifier (7th)
0 Ovary, Right **1** Ovary, Left **2** Ovaries, Bilateral **4** Uterine Supporting Structure	**0** Open **3** Percutaneous **4** Percutaneous Endoscopic	**Z** No Device	**Z** No Qualifier
5 Fallopian Tube, Right **6** Fallopian Tube, Left **7** Fallopian Tubes, Bilateral **9** Uterus **B** Endometrium **C** Cervix **F** Cul-de-sac	**0** Open **3** Percutaneous **4** Percutaneous Endoscopic **7** Via Natural or Artificial Opening **8** Via Natural or Artificial Opening Endoscopic	**Z** No Device	**Z** No Qualifier
G Vagina **K** Hymen	**0** Open **3** Percutaneous **4** Percutaneous Endoscopic **7** Via Natural or Artificial Opening **8** Via Natural or Artificial Opening Endoscopic **X** External	**Z** No Device	**Z** No Qualifier
J Clitoris **L** Vestibular Gland **M** Vulva	**0** Open **X** External	**Z** No Device	**Z** No Qualifier

Section 0 Medical and Surgical
Body System U Female Reproductive System
Operation 7 **Dilation:** Expanding an orifice or the lumen of a tubular body part

Body Part (4th)	Approach (5th)	Device (6th)	Qualifier (7th)
5 Fallopian Tube, Right 6 Fallopian Tube, Left 7 Fallopian Tubes, Bilateral 9 Uterus C Cervix G Vagina	0 Open 3 Percutaneous 4 Percutaneous Endoscopic 7 Via Natural or Artificial Opening 8 Via Natural or Artificial Opening Endoscopic	D Intraluminal Device Z No Device	Z No Qualifier
K Hymen	0 Open 3 Percutaneous 4 Percutaneous Endoscopic 7 Via Natural or Artificial Opening 8 Via Natural or Artificial Opening Endoscopic X External	D Intraluminal Device Z No Device	Z No Qualifier

Section 0 Medical and Surgical
Body System U Female Reproductive System
Operation 8 **Division:** Cutting into a body part, without draining fluids and/or gases from the body part, in order to separate or transect a body part

Body Part (4th)	Approach (5th)	Device (6th)	Qualifier (7th)
0 Ovary, Right 1 Ovary, Left 2 Ovaries, Bilateral 4 Uterine Supporting Structure	0 Open 3 Percutaneous 4 Percutaneous Endoscopic	Z No Device	Z No Qualifier
K Hymen	7 Via Natural or Artificial Opening 8 Via Natural or Artificial Opening Endoscopic X External	Z No Device	Z No Qualifier

Section 0 Medical and Surgical
Body System U Female Reproductive System
Operation 9 **Drainage:** Taking or letting out fluids and/or gases from a body part

Body Part (4th)	Approach (5th)	Device (6th)	Qualifier (7th)
0 Ovary, Right 1 Ovary, Left 2 Ovaries, Bilateral	0 Open 3 Percutaneous 4 Percutaneous Endoscopic	0 Drainage Device	Z No Qualifier
0 Ovary, Right 1 Ovary, Left 2 Ovaries, Bilateral	0 Open 3 Percutaneous 4 Percutaneous Endoscopic	Z No Device	X Diagnostic Z No Qualifier
0 Ovary, Right 1 Ovary, Left 2 Ovaries, Bilateral	X External	Z No Device	Z No Qualifier
4 Uterine Supporting Structure	0 Open 3 Percutaneous 4 Percutaneous Endoscopic	0 Drainage Device	Z No Qualifier
4 Uterine Supporting Structure	0 Open 3 Percutaneous 4 Percutaneous Endoscopic	Z No Device	X Diagnostic Z No Qualifier
5 Fallopian Tube, Right 6 Fallopian Tube, Left 7 Fallopian Tubes, Bilateral 9 Uterus C Cervix F Cul-de-sac	0 Open 3 Percutaneous 4 Percutaneous Endoscopic 7 Via Natural or Artificial Opening 8 Via Natural or Artificial Opening Endoscopic	0 Drainage Device	Z No Qualifier

Continued →

Section 0 **Medical and Surgical**
Body System U **Female Reproductive System**
Operation 9 **Drainage:** Taking or letting out fluids and/or gases from a body part

Body Part (4th)	Approach (5th)	Device (6th)	Qualifier (7th)
5 Fallopian Tube, Right **6** Fallopian Tube, Left **7** Fallopian Tubes, Bilateral **9** Uterus **C** Cervix **F** Cul-de-sac	**0** Open **3** Percutaneous **4** Percutaneous Endoscopic **7** Via Natural or Artificial Opening **8** Via Natural or Artificial Opening Endoscopic	**Z** No Device	**X** Diagnostic **Z** No Qualifier
G Vagina **K** Hymen	**0** Open **3** Percutaneous **4** Percutaneous Endoscopic **7** Via Natural or Artificial Opening **8** Via Natural or Artificial Opening Endoscopic **X** External	**0** Drainage Device	**Z** No Qualifier
G Vagina **K** Hymen	**0** Open **3** Percutaneous **4** Percutaneous Endoscopic **7** Via Natural or Artificial Opening **8** Via Natural or Artificial Opening Endoscopic **X** External	**Z** No Device	**X** Diagnostic **Z** No Qualifier
J Clitoris **L** Vestibular Gland **M** Vulva	**0** Open **X** External	**0** Drainage Device	**Z** No Qualifier
J Clitoris **L** Vestibular Gland **M** Vulva	**0** Open **X** External	**Z** No Device	**X** Diagnostic **Z** No Qualifier

Section 0 **Medical and Surgical**
Body System U **Female Reproductive System**
Operation B **Excision:** Cutting out or off, without replacement, a portion of a body part

Body Part (4th)	Approach (5th)	Device (6th)	Qualifier (7th)
0 Ovary, Right **1** Ovary, Left **2** Ovaries, Bilateral **4** Uterine Supporting Structure **5** Fallopian Tube, Right **6** Fallopian Tube, Left **7** Fallopian Tubes, Bilateral **9** Uterus **C** Cervix **F** Cul-de-sac	**0** Open **3** Percutaneous **4** Percutaneous Endoscopic **7** Via Natural or Artificial Opening **8** Via Natural or Artificial Opening Endoscopic	**Z** No Device	**X** Diagnostic **Z** No Qualifier
G Vagina **K** Hymen	**0** Open **3** Percutaneous **4** Percutaneous Endoscopic **7** Via Natural or Artificial Opening **8** Via Natural or Artificial Opening Endoscopic **X** External	**Z** No Device	**X** Diagnostic **Z** No Qualifier
J Clitoris **L** Vestibular Gland **M** Vulva	**0** Open **X** External	**Z** No Device	**X** Diagnostic **Z** No Qualifier

Section 0 **Medical and Surgical**
Body System U **Female Reproductive System**
Operation C **Extirpation:** Taking or cutting out solid matter from a body part

Body Part (4th)	Approach (5th)	Device (6th)	Qualifier (7th)
0 Ovary, Right **1** Ovary, Left **2** Ovaries, Bilateral **4** Uterine Supporting Structure	**0** Open **3** Percutaneous **4** Percutaneous Endoscopic	**Z** No Device	**Z** No Qualifier
5 Fallopian Tube, Right **6** Fallopian Tube, Left **7** Fallopian Tubes, Bilateral **9** Uterus **B** Endometrium **C** Cervix **F** Cul-de-sac	**0** Open **3** Percutaneous **4** Percutaneous Endoscopic **7** Via Natural or Artificial Opening **8** Via Natural or Artificial Opening Endoscopic	**Z** No Device	**Z** No Qualifier
G Vagina **K** Hymen	**0** Open **3** Percutaneous **4** Percutaneous Endoscopic **7** Via Natural or Artificial Opening **8** Via Natural or Artificial Opening Endoscopic **X** External	**Z** No Device	**Z** No Qualifier
J Clitoris **L** Vestibular Gland **M** Vulva	**0** Open **X** External	**Z** No Device	**Z** No Qualifier

Section 0 **Medical and Surgical**
Body System U **Female Reproductive System**
Operation D **Extraction:** Pulling or stripping out or off all or a portion of a body part by the use of force

Body Part (4th)	Approach (5th)	Device (6th)	Qualifier (7th)
B Endometrium	**7** Via Natural or Artificial Opening **8** Via Natural or Artificial Opening Endoscopic	**Z** No Device	**X** Diagnostic **Z** No Qualifier
N Ova	**0** Open **3** Percutaneous **4** Percutaneous Endoscopic	**Z** No Device	**Z** No Qualifier

Section 0 **Medical and Surgical**
Body System U **Female Reproductive System**
Operation F **Fragmentation:** Breaking solid matter in a body part into pieces

Body Part (4th)	Approach (5th)	Device (6th)	Qualifier (7th)
5 Fallopian Tube, Right **6** Fallopian Tube, Left **7** Fallopian Tubes, Bilateral **9** Uterus	**0** Open **3** Percutaneous **4** Percutaneous Endoscopic **7** Via Natural or Artificial Opening **8** Via Natural or Artificial Opening Endoscopic **X** External	**Z** No Device	**Z** No Qualifier

Section 0 **Medical and Surgical**
Body System U **Female Reproductive System**
Operation H **Insertion:** Putting in a nonbiological appliance that monitors, assists, performs, or prevents a physiological function but does not physically take the place of a body part

Body Part (4th)	Approach (5th)	Device (6th)	Qualifier (7th)
3 Ovary	0 Open 3 Percutaneous 4 Percutaneous Endoscopic	3 Infusion Device	Z No Qualifier
8 Fallopian Tube D Uterus and Cervix H Vagina and Cul-de-sac	0 Open 3 Percutaneous 4 Percutaneous Endoscopic 7 Via Natural or Artificial Opening 8 Via Natural or Artificial Opening Endoscopic	3 Infusion Device	Z No Qualifier
9 Uterus	7 Via Natural or Artificial Opening 8 Via Natural or Artificial Opening Endoscopic	H Contraceptive Device	Z No Qualifier
C Cervix	0 Open 3 Percutaneous 4 Percutaneous Endoscopic	1 Radioactive Element	Z No Qualifier
C Cervix	7 Via Natural or Artificial Opening 8 Via Natural or Artificial Opening Endoscopic	1 Radioactive Element H Contraceptive Device	Z No Qualifier
F Cul-de-sac	7 Via Natural or Artificial Opening 8 Via Natural or Artificial Opening Endoscopic	G Intraluminal Device, Pessary	Z No Qualifier
G Vagina	0 Open 3 Percutaneous 4 Percutaneous Endoscopic X External	1 Radioactive Element	Z No Qualifier
G Vagina	7 Via Natural or Artificial Opening 8 Via Natural or Artificial Opening Endoscopic	1 Radioactive Element G Intraluminal Device, Pessary	Z No Qualifier

Section 0 **Medical and Surgical**
Body System U **Female Reproductive System**
Operation J **Inspection:** Visually and/or manually exploring a body part

Body Part (4th)	Approach (5th)	Device (6th)	Qualifier (7th)
3 Ovary	0 Open 3 Percutaneous 4 Percutaneous Endoscopic X External	Z No Device	Z No Qualifier
8 Fallopian Tube D Uterus and Cervix H Vagina and Cul-de-sac	0 Open 3 Percutaneous 4 Percutaneous Endoscopic 7 Via Natural or Artificial Opening 8 Via Natural or Artificial Opening Endoscopic X External	Z No Device	Z No Qualifier
M Vulva	0 Open X External	Z No Device	Z No Qualifier

Section 0 **Medical and Surgical**
Body System U **Female Reproductive System**
Operation L **Occlusion:** Completely closing an orifice or the lumen of a tubular body part

Body Part (4th)	Approach (5th)	Device (6th)	Qualifier (7th)
5 Fallopian Tube, Right 6 Fallopian Tube, Left 7 Fallopian Tubes, Bilateral	0 Open 3 Percutaneous 4 Percutaneous Endoscopic	C Extraluminal Device D Intraluminal Device Z No Device	Z No Qualifier

Continued →

0UL Continued

Section 0 **Medical and Surgical**
Body System U **Female Reproductive System**
Operation L **Occlusion:** Completely closing an orifice or the lumen of a tubular body part

Body Part (4th)	Approach (5th)	Device (6th)	Qualifier (7th)
5 Fallopian Tube, Right **6** Fallopian Tube, Left **7** Fallopian Tubes, Bilateral	**7** Via Natural or Artificial Opening **8** Via Natural or Artificial Opening Endoscopic	**D** Intraluminal Device **Z** No Device	**Z** No Qualifier
F Cul-de-sac **G** Vagina	**7** Via Natural or Artificial Opening **8** Via Natural or Artificial Opening Endoscopic	**D** Intraluminal Device **Z** No Device	**Z** No Qualifier

Section 0 **Medical and Surgical**
Body System U **Female Reproductive System**
Operation M **Reattachment:** Putting back in or on all or a portion of a separated body part to its normal location or other suitable location

Body Part (4th)	Approach (5th)	Device (6th)	Qualifier (7th)
0 Ovary, Right **1** Ovary, Left **2** Ovaries, Bilateral **4** Uterine Supporting Structure **5** Fallopian Tube, Right **6** Fallopian Tube, Left **7** Fallopian Tubes, Bilateral **9** Uterus **C** Cervix **F** Cul-de-sac **G** Vagina	**0** Open **4** Percutaneous Endoscopic	**Z** No Device	**Z** No Qualifier
J Clitoris **M** Vulva	**X** External	**Z** No Device	**Z** No Qualifier
K Hymen	**0** Open **4** Percutaneous Endoscopic **X** External	**Z** No Device	**Z** No Qualifier

Section 0 **Medical and Surgical**
Body System U **Female Reproductive System**
Operation N **Release:** Freeing a body part from an abnormal physical constraint by cutting or by the use of force

Body Part (4th)	Approach (5th)	Device (6th)	Qualifier (7th)
0 Ovary, Right **1** Ovary, Left **2** Ovaries, Bilateral **4** Uterine Supporting Structure	**0** Open **3** Percutaneous **4** Percutaneous Endoscopic	**Z** No Device	**Z** No Qualifier
5 Fallopian Tube, Right **6** Fallopian Tube, Left **7** Fallopian Tubes, Bilateral **9** Uterus **C** Cervix **F** Cul-de-sac	**0** Open **3** Percutaneous **4** Percutaneous Endoscopic **7** Via Natural or Artificial Opening **8** Via Natural or Artificial Opening Endoscopic	**Z** No Device	**Z** No Qualifier
G Vagina **K** Hymen	**0** Open **3** Percutaneous **4** Percutaneous Endoscopic **7** Via Natural or Artificial Opening **8** Via Natural or Artificial Opening Endoscopic **X** External	**Z** No Device	**Z** No Qualifier
J Clitoris **L** Vestibular Gland **M** Vulva	**0** Open **X** External	**Z** No Device	**Z** No Qualifier

Section 0 **Medical and Surgical**
Body System U **Female Reproductive System**
Operation P **Removal:** Taking out or off a device from a body part

Body Part (4th)	Approach (5th)	Device (6th)	Qualifier (7th)
3 Ovary	**0** Open **3** Percutaneous **4** Percutaneous Endoscopic **X** External	**0** Drainage Device **3** Infusion Device	**Z** No Qualifier
8 Fallopian Tube	**0** Open **3** Percutaneous **4** Percutaneous Endoscopic **7** Via Natural or Artificial Opening **8** Via Natural or Artificial Opening Endoscopic	**0** Drainage Device **3** Infusion Device **7** Autologous Tissue Substitute **C** Extraluminal Device **D** Intraluminal Device **J** Synthetic Substitute **K** Nonautologous Tissue Substitute	**Z** No Qualifier
8 Fallopian Tube	**X** External	**0** Drainage Device **3** Infusion Device **D** Intraluminal Device	**Z** No Qualifier
D Uterus and Cervix	**0** Open **3** Percutaneous **4** Percutaneous Endoscopic **7** Via Natural or Artificial Opening **8** Via Natural or Artificial Opening Endoscopic	**0** Drainage Device **1** Radioactive Element **3** Infusion Device **7** Autologous Tissue Substitute **C** Extraluminal Device **D** Intraluminal Device **H** Contraceptive Device **J** Synthetic Substitute **K** Nonautologous Tissue Substitute	**Z** No Qualifier
D Uterus and Cervix	**X** External	**0** Drainage Device **3** Infusion Device **D** Intraluminal Device **H** Contraceptive Device	**Z** No Qualifier
H Vagina and Cul-de-sac	**0** Open **3** Percutaneous **4** Percutaneous Endoscopic **7** Via Natural or Artificial Opening **8** Via Natural or Artificial Opening Endoscopic	**0** Drainage Device **1** Radioactive Element **3** Infusion Device **7** Autologous Tissue Substitute **D** Intraluminal Device **J** Synthetic Substitute **K** Nonautologous Tissue Substitute	**Z** No Qualifier
H Vagina and Cul-de-sac	**X** External	**0** Drainage Device **1** Radioactive Element **3** Infusion Device **D** Intraluminal Device	**Z** No Qualifier
M Vulva	**0** Open	**0** Drainage Device **7** Autologous Tissue Substitute **J** Synthetic Substitute **K** Nonautologous Tissue Substitute	**Z** No Qualifier
M Vulva	**X** External	**0** Drainage Device	**Z** No Qualifier

Section 0 **Medical and Surgical**
Body System U **Female Reproductive System**
Operation Q **Repair:** Restoring, to the extent possible, a body part to its normal anatomic structure and function

Body Part (4th)	Approach (5th)	Device (6th)	Qualifier (7th)
0 Ovary, Right **1** Ovary, Left **2** Ovaries, Bilateral **4** Uterine Supporting Structure	**0** Open **3** Percutaneous **4** Percutaneous Endoscopic	**Z** No Device	**Z** No Qualifier

Continued →

Section	0	Medical and Surgical
Body System	U	Female Reproductive System
Operation	Q	**Repair:** Restoring, to the extent possible, a body part to its normal anatomic structure and function

0UQ Continued

Body Part (4th)	Approach (5th)	Device (6th)	Qualifier (7th)
5 Fallopian Tube, Right **6** Fallopian Tube, Left **7** Fallopian Tubes, Bilateral **9** Uterus **C** Cervix **F** Cul-de-sac	**0** Open **3** Percutaneous **4** Percutaneous Endoscopic **7** Via Natural or Artificial Opening **8** Via Natural or Artificial Opening Endoscopic	**Z** No Device	**Z** No Qualifier
G Vagina **K** Hymen	**0** Open **3** Percutaneous **4** Percutaneous Endoscopic **7** Via Natural or Artificial Opening **8** Via Natural or Artificial Opening Endoscopic **X** External	**Z** No Device	**Z** No Qualifier
J Clitoris **L** Vestibular Gland **M** Vulva	**0** Open **X** External	**Z** No Device	**Z** No Qualifier

Section	0	Medical and Surgical
Body System	U	Female Reproductive System
Operation	S	**Reposition:** Moving to its normal location, or other suitable location, all or a portion of a body part

Body Part (4th)	Approach (5th)	Device (6th)	Qualifier (7th)
0 Ovary, Right **1** Ovary, Left **2** Ovaries, Bilateral **4** Uterine Supporting Structure **5** Fallopian Tube, Right **6** Fallopian Tube, Left **7** Fallopian Tubes, Bilateral **C** Cervix **F** Cul-de-sac	**0** Open **4** Percutaneous Endoscopic	**Z** No Device	**Z** No Qualifier
9 Uterus **G** Vagina	**0** Open **4** Percutaneous Endoscopic **X** External	**Z** No Device	**Z** No Qualifier

Section	0	Medical and Surgical
Body System	U	Female Reproductive System
Operation	T	**Resection:** Cutting out or off, without replacement, all of a body part

Body Part (4th)	Approach (5th)	Device (6th)	Qualifier (7th)
0 Ovary, Right **1** Ovary, Left **2** Ovaries, Bilateral **5** Fallopian Tube, Right **6** Fallopian Tube, Left **7** Fallopian Tubes, Bilateral **9** Uterus	**0** Open **4** Percutaneous Endoscopic **7** Via Natural or Artificial Opening **8** Via Natural or Artificial Opening Endoscopic **F** Via Natural or Artificial Opening With Percutaneous Endoscopic Assistance	**Z** No Device	**Z** No Qualifier
4 Uterine Supporting Structure **C** Cervix **F** Cul-de-sac **G** Vagina	**0** Open **4** Percutaneous Endoscopic **7** Via Natural or Artificial Opening **8** Via Natural or Artificial Opening Endoscopic	**Z** No Device	**Z** No Qualifier
J Clitoris **L** Vestibular Gland **M** Vulva	**0** Open **X** External	**Z** No Device	**Z** No Qualifier

Continued →

Section 0 **Medical and Surgical**
Body System U **Female Reproductive System**
Operation T **Resection:** Cutting out or off, without replacement, all of a body part

Body Part (4th)	Approach (5th)	Device (6th)	Qualifier (7th)
K Hymen	**0** Open **4** Percutaneous Endoscopic **7** Via Natural or Artificial Opening **8** Via Natural or Artificial Opening Endoscopic **X** External	**Z** No Device	**Z** No Qualifier

Section 0 **Medical and Surgical**
Body System U **Female Reproductive System**
Operation U **Supplement:** Putting in or on biological or synthetic material that physically reinforces and/or augments the function of a portion of a body part

Body Part (4th)	Approach (5th)	Device (6th)	Qualifier (7th)
4 Uterine Supporting Structure	**0** Open **4** Percutaneous Endoscopic	**7** Autologous Tissue Substitute **J** Synthetic Substitute **K** Nonautologous Tissue Substitute	**Z** No Qualifier
5 Fallopian Tube, Right **6** Fallopian Tube, Left **7** Fallopian Tubes, Bilateral **F** Cul-de-sac	**0** Open **4** Percutaneous Endoscopic **7** Via Natural or Artificial Opening **8** Via Natural or Artificial Opening Endoscopic	**7** Autologous Tissue Substitute **J** Synthetic Substitute **K** Nonautologous Tissue Substitute	**Z** No Qualifier
G Vagina **K** Hymen	**0** Open **4** Percutaneous Endoscopic **7** Via Natural or Artificial Opening **8** Via Natural or Artificial Opening Endoscopic **X** External	**7** Autologous Tissue Substitute **J** Synthetic Substitute **K** Nonautologous Tissue Substitute	**Z** No Qualifier
J Clitoris **M** Vulva	**0** Open **X** External	**7** Autologous Tissue Substitute **J** Synthetic Substitute **K** Nonautologous Tissue Substitute	**Z** No Qualifier

Section 0 **Medical and Surgical**
Body System U **Female Reproductive System**
Operation V **Restriction:** Partially closing an orifice or the lumen of a tubular body part

Body Part (4th)	Approach (5th)	Device (6th)	Qualifier (7th)
C Cervix	**0** Open **3** Percutaneous **4** Percutaneous Endoscopic	**C** Extraluminal Device **D** Intraluminal Device **Z** No Device	**Z** No Qualifier
C Cervix	**7** Via Natural or Artificial Opening **8** Via Natural or Artificial Opening Endoscopic	**D** Intraluminal Device **Z** No Device	**Z** No Qualifier

Section 0 **Medical and Surgical**
Body System U **Female Reproductive System**
Operation W **Revision:** Correcting, to the extent possible, a portion of a malfunctioning device or the position of a displaced device

Body Part (4th)	Approach (5th)	Device (6th)	Qualifier (7th)
3 Ovary	**0** Open **3** Percutaneous **4** Percutaneous Endoscopic **X** External	**0** Drainage Device **3** Infusion Device	**Z** No Qualifier

Continued →

Section	**0**	**Medical and Surgical**
Body System	**U**	**Female Reproductive System**
Operation	**W**	**Revision:** Correcting, to the extent possible, a portion of a malfunctioning device or the position of a displaced device

Body Part (4th)	Approach (5th)	Device (6th)	Qualifier (7th)
8 Fallopian Tube	**0** Open **3** Percutaneous **4** Percutaneous Endoscopic **7** Via Natural or Artificial Opening **8** Via Natural or Artificial Opening Endoscopic **X** External	**0** Drainage Device **3** Infusion Device **7** Autologous Tissue Substitute **C** Extraluminal Device **D** Intraluminal Device **J** Synthetic Substitute **K** Nonautologous Tissue Substitute	**Z** No Qualifier
D Uterus and Cervix	**0** Open **3** Percutaneous **4** Percutaneous Endoscopic **7** Via Natural or Artificial Opening **8** Via Natural or Artificial Opening Endoscopic	**0** Drainage Device **1** Radioactive Element **3** Infusion Device **7** Autologous Tissue Substitute **C** Extraluminal Device **D** Intraluminal Device **H** Contraceptive Device **J** Synthetic Substitute **K** Nonautologous Tissue Substitute	**Z** No Qualifier
D Uterus and Cervix	**X** External	**0** Drainage Device **3** Infusion Device **7** Autologous Tissue Substitute **C** Extraluminal Device **D** Intraluminal Device **H** Contraceptive Device **J** Synthetic Substitute **K** Nonautologous Tissue Substitute	**Z** No Qualifier
H Vagina and Cul-de-sac	**0** Open **3** Percutaneous **4** Percutaneous Endoscopic **7** Via Natural or Artificial Opening **8** Via Natural or Artificial Opening Endoscopic	**0** Drainage Device **1** Radioactive Element **3** Infusion Device **7** Autologous Tissue Substitute **D** Intraluminal Device **J** Synthetic Substitute **K** Nonautologous Tissue Substitute	**Z** No Qualifier
H Vagina and Cul-de-sac	**X** External	**0** Drainage Device **3** Infusion Device **7** Autologous Tissue Substitute **D** Intraluminal Device **J** Synthetic Substitute **K** Nonautologous Tissue Substitute	**Z** No Qualifier
M Vulva	**0** Open **X** External	**0** Drainage Device **7** Autologous Tissue Substitute **J** Synthetic Substitute **K** Nonautologous Tissue Substitute	**Z** No Qualifier

Section	**0**	**Medical and Surgical**
Body System	**U**	**Female Reproductive System**
Operation	**Y**	**Transplantation:** Putting in or on all or a portion of a living body part taken from another individual or animal to physically take the place and/or function of all or a portion of a similar body part

Body Part (4th)	Approach (5th)	Device (6th)	Qualifier (7th)
0 Ovary, Right **1** Ovary, Left	**0** Open	**Z** No Device	**0** Allogeneic **1** Syngeneic **2** Zooplastic

Female Reproductive System Code Listing 0U1–0UY

0U1 – Female Reproductive System, Bypass

Review Coding Guideline B3.6a

♀ **0U15075** Bypass Right Fallopian Tube to Right Fallopian Tube with Autologous Tissue Substitute, Open Approach
♀ **0U15076** Bypass Right Fallopian Tube to Left Fallopian Tube with Autologous Tissue Substitute, Open Approach
♀ **0U15079** Bypass Right Fallopian Tube to Uterus with Autologous Tissue Substitute, Open Approach
♀ **0U150J5** Bypass Right Fallopian Tube to Right Fallopian Tube with Synthetic Substitute, Open Approach
♀ **0U150J6** Bypass Right Fallopian Tube to Left Fallopian Tube with Synthetic Substitute, Open Approach
♀ **0U150J9** Bypass Right Fallopian Tube to Uterus with Synthetic Substitute, Open Approach
♀ **0U150K5** Bypass Right Fallopian Tube to Right Fallopian Tube with Nonautologous Tissue Substitute, Open Approach
♀ **0U150K6** Bypass Right Fallopian Tube to Left Fallopian Tube with Nonautologous Tissue Substitute, Open Approach
♀ **0U150K9** Bypass Right Fallopian Tube to Uterus with Nonautologous Tissue Substitute, Open Approach
♀ **0U150Z5** Bypass Right Fallopian Tube to Right Fallopian Tube, Open Approach
♀ **0U150Z6** Bypass Right Fallopian Tube to Left Fallopian Tube, Open Approach
♀ **0U150Z9** Bypass Right Fallopian Tube to Uterus, Open Approach
♀ **0U15475** Bypass Right Fallopian Tube to Right Fallopian Tube with Autologous Tissue Substitute, Percutaneous Endoscopic Approach
♀ **0U15476** Bypass Right Fallopian Tube to Left Fallopian Tube with Autologous Tissue Substitute, Percutaneous Endoscopic Approach
♀ **0U15479** Bypass Right Fallopian Tube to Uterus with Autologous Tissue Substitute, Percutaneous Endoscopic Approach
♀ **0U154J5** Bypass Right Fallopian Tube to Right Fallopian Tube with Synthetic Substitute, Percutaneous Endoscopic Approach
♀ **0U154J6** Bypass Right Fallopian Tube to Left Fallopian Tube with Synthetic Substitute, Percutaneous Endoscopic Approach
♀ **0U154J9** Bypass Right Fallopian Tube to Uterus with Synthetic Substitute, Percutaneous Endoscopic Approach
♀ **0U154K5** Bypass Right Fallopian Tube to Right Fallopian Tube with Nonautologous Tissue Substitute, Percutaneous Endoscopic Approach
♀ **0U154K6** Bypass Right Fallopian Tube to Left Fallopian Tube with Nonautologous Tissue Substitute, Percutaneous Endoscopic Approach
♀ **0U154K9** Bypass Right Fallopian Tube to Uterus with Nonautologous Tissue Substitute, Percutaneous Endoscopic Approach
♀ **0U154Z5** Bypass Right Fallopian Tube to Right Fallopian Tube, Percutaneous Endoscopic Approach
♀ **0U154Z6** Bypass Right Fallopian Tube to Left Fallopian Tube, Percutaneous Endoscopic Approach
♀ **0U154Z9** Bypass Right Fallopian Tube to Uterus, Percutaneous Endoscopic Approach
♀ **0U16075** Bypass Left Fallopian Tube to Right Fallopian Tube with Autologous Tissue Substitute, Open Approach
♀ **0U16076** Bypass Left Fallopian Tube to Left Fallopian Tube with Autologous Tissue Substitute, Open Approach
♀ **0U16079** Bypass Left Fallopian Tube to Uterus with Autologous Tissue Substitute, Open Approach
♀ **0U160J5** Bypass Left Fallopian Tube to Right Fallopian Tube with Synthetic Substitute, Open Approach
♀ **0U160J6** Bypass Left Fallopian Tube to Left Fallopian Tube with Synthetic Substitute, Open Approach
♀ **0U160J9** Bypass Left Fallopian Tube to Uterus with Synthetic Substitute, Open Approach
♀ **0U160K5** Bypass Left Fallopian Tube to Right Fallopian Tube with Nonautologous Tissue Substitute, Open Approach
♀ **0U160K6** Bypass Left Fallopian Tube to Left Fallopian Tube with Nonautologous Tissue Substitute, Open Approach
♀ **0U160K9** Bypass Left Fallopian Tube to Uterus with Nonautologous Tissue Substitute, Open Approach
♀ **0U160Z5** Bypass Left Fallopian Tube to Right Fallopian Tube, Open Approach
♀ **0U160Z6** Bypass Left Fallopian Tube to Left Fallopian Tube, Open Approach
♀ **0U160Z9** Bypass Left Fallopian Tube to Uterus, Open Approach
♀ **0U16475** Bypass Left Fallopian Tube to Right Fallopian Tube with Autologous Tissue Substitute, Percutaneous Endoscopic Approach
♀ **0U16476** Bypass Left Fallopian Tube to Left Fallopian Tube with Autologous Tissue Substitute, Percutaneous Endoscopic Approach
♀ **0U16479** Bypass Left Fallopian Tube to Uterus with Autologous Tissue Substitute, Percutaneous Endoscopic Approach
♀ **0U164J5** Bypass Left Fallopian Tube to Right Fallopian Tube with Synthetic Substitute, Percutaneous Endoscopic Approach
♀ **0U164J6** Bypass Left Fallopian Tube to Left Fallopian Tube with Synthetic Substitute, Percutaneous Endoscopic Approach
♀ **0U164J9** Bypass Left Fallopian Tube to Uterus with Synthetic Substitute, Percutaneous Endoscopic Approach
♀ **0U164K5** Bypass Left Fallopian Tube to Right Fallopian Tube with Nonautologous Tissue Substitute, Percutaneous Endoscopic Approach
♀ **0U164K6** Bypass Left Fallopian Tube to Left Fallopian Tube with Nonautologous Tissue Substitute, Percutaneous Endoscopic Approach
♀ **0U164K9** Bypass Left Fallopian Tube to Uterus with Nonautologous Tissue Substitute, Percutaneous Endoscopic Approach
♀ **0U164Z5** Bypass Left Fallopian Tube to Right Fallopian Tube, Percutaneous Endoscopic Approach
♀ **0U164Z6** Bypass Left Fallopian Tube to Left Fallopian Tube, Percutaneous Endoscopic Approach
♀ **0U164Z9** Bypass Left Fallopian Tube to Uterus, Percutaneous Endoscopic Approach

0U2 – Female Reproductive System, Change

Review Coding Guideline B6.1c

♀ **0U23X0Z** Change Drainage Device in Ovary, External Approach
♀ **0U23XYZ** Change Other Device in Ovary, External Approach
♀ **0U28X0Z** Change Drainage Device in Fallopian Tube, External Approach
♀ **0U28XYZ** Change Other Device in Fallopian Tube, External Approach
♀ **0U2DX0Z** Change Drainage Device in Uterus and Cervix, External Approach
♀ **0U2DXHZ** Change Contraceptive Device in Uterus and Cervix, External Approach
♀ **0U2DXYZ** Change Other Device in Uterus and Cervix, External Approach
♀ **0U2HX0Z** Change Drainage Device in Vagina and Cul-de-sac, External Approach
♀ **0U2HXGZ** Change Pessary in Vagina and Cul-de-sac, External Approach
♀ **0U2HXYZ** Change Other Device in Vagina and Cul-de-sac, External Approach
♀ **0U2MX0Z** Change Drainage Device in Vulva, External Approach
♀ **0U2MXYZ** Change Other Device in Vulva, External Approach

0U5 – Female Reproductive System, Destruction

♀ **0U500ZZ** Destruction of Right Ovary, Open Approach
♀ **0U503ZZ** Destruction of Right Ovary, Percutaneous Approach
♀ **0U504ZZ** Destruction of Right Ovary, Percutaneous Endoscopic Approach
♀ **0U510ZZ** Destruction of Left Ovary, Open Approach
♀ **0U513ZZ** Destruction of Left Ovary, Percutaneous Approach
♀ **0U514ZZ** Destruction of Left Ovary, Percutaneous Endoscopic Approach
♀ **0U520ZZ** Destruction of Bilateral Ovaries, Open Approach
♀ **0U523ZZ** Destruction of Bilateral Ovaries, Percutaneous Approach
♀ **0U524ZZ** Destruction of Bilateral Ovaries, Percutaneous Endoscopic Approach
♀ **0U540ZZ** Destruction of Uterine Supporting Structure, Open Approach
♀ **0U543ZZ** Destruction of Uterine Supporting Structure, Percutaneous Approach

♀ Female-only ♂ Male-only Limited Coverage ● Non-OR HAC-associated procedure ▲ Non-covered procedures + Combination

♀0U544ZZ Destruction of Uterine Supporting Structure, Percutaneous Endoscopic Approach
♀0U550ZZ Destruction of Right Fallopian Tube, Open Approach
♀0U553ZZ Destruction of Right Fallopian Tube, Percutaneous Approach
♀0U554ZZ Destruction of Right Fallopian Tube, Percutaneous Endoscopic Approach
♀0U557ZZ Destruction of Right Fallopian Tube, Via Natural or Artificial Opening
♀0U558ZZ Destruction of Right Fallopian Tube, Via Natural or Artificial Opening Endoscopic
♀0U560ZZ Destruction of Left Fallopian Tube, Open Approach
♀0U563ZZ Destruction of Left Fallopian Tube, Percutaneous Approach
♀0U564ZZ Destruction of Left Fallopian Tube, Percutaneous Endoscopic Approach
♀0U567ZZ Destruction of Left Fallopian Tube, Via Natural or Artificial Opening
♀0U568ZZ Destruction of Left Fallopian Tube, Via Natural or Artificial Opening Endoscopic
♀▲0U570ZZ Destruction of Bilateral Fallopian Tubes, Open Approach
♀▲0U573ZZ Destruction of Bilateral Fallopian Tubes, Percutaneous Approach
♀▲0U574ZZ Destruction of Bilateral Fallopian Tubes, Percutaneous Endoscopic Approach
♀▲0U577ZZ Destruction of Bilateral Fallopian Tubes, Via Natural or Artificial Opening
♀▲0U578ZZ Destruction of Bilateral Fallopian Tubes, Via Natural or Artificial Opening Endoscopic
♀ 0U590ZZ Destruction of Uterus, Open Approach
♀ 0U593ZZ Destruction of Uterus, Percutaneous Approach
♀ 0U594ZZ Destruction of Uterus, Percutaneous Endoscopic Approach
♀ 0U597ZZ Destruction of Uterus, Via Natural or Artificial Opening
♀ 0U598ZZ Destruction of Uterus, Via Natural or Artificial Opening Endoscopic
♀ 0U5B0ZZ Destruction of Endometrium, Open Approach
♀ 0U5B3ZZ Destruction of Endometrium, Percutaneous Approach
♀ 0U5B4ZZ Destruction of Endometrium, Percutaneous Endoscopic Approach
♀ 0U5B7ZZ Destruction of Endometrium, Via Natural or Artificial Opening
♀ 0U5B8ZZ Destruction of Endometrium, Via Natural or Artificial Opening Endoscopic
♀ 0U5C0ZZ Destruction of Cervix, Open Approach
♀ 0U5C3ZZ Destruction of Cervix, Percutaneous Approach
♀ 0U5C4ZZ Destruction of Cervix, Percutaneous Endoscopic Approach
♀ 0U5C7ZZ Destruction of Cervix, Via Natural or Artificial Opening
♀ 0U5C8ZZ Destruction of Cervix, Via Natural or Artificial Opening Endoscopic
♀ 0U5F0ZZ Destruction of Cul-de-sac, Open Approach
♀ 0U5F3ZZ Destruction of Cul-de-sac, Percutaneous Approach
♀ 0U5F4ZZ Destruction of Cul-de-sac, Percutaneous Endoscopic Approach
♀ 0U5F7ZZ Destruction of Cul-de-sac, Via Natural or Artificial Opening
♀ 0U5F8ZZ Destruction of Cul-de-sac, Via Natural or Artificial Opening Endoscopic
♀ 0U5G0ZZ Destruction of Vagina, Open Approach
♀ 0U5G3ZZ Destruction of Vagina, Percutaneous Approach
♀ 0U5G4ZZ Destruction of Vagina, Percutaneous Endoscopic Approach
♀ 0U5G7ZZ Destruction of Vagina, Via Natural or Artificial Opening
♀ 0U5G8ZZ Destruction of Vagina, Via Natural or Artificial Opening Endoscopic
♀ 0U5GXZZ Destruction of Vagina, External Approach
♀ 0U5J0ZZ Destruction of Clitoris, Open Approach
♀ 0U5JXZZ Destruction of Clitoris, External Approach
♀ 0U5K0ZZ Destruction of Hymen, Open Approach
♀ 0U5K3ZZ Destruction of Hymen, Percutaneous Approach
♀ 0U5K4ZZ Destruction of Hymen, Percutaneous Endoscopic Approach
♀ 0U5K7ZZ Destruction of Hymen, Via Natural or Artificial Opening
♀▲ 0U5K8ZZ Destruction of Hymen, Via Natural or Artificial Opening Endoscopic
♀ 0U5KXZZ Destruction of Hymen, External Approach
♀ 0U5L0ZZ Destruction of Vestibular Gland, Open Approach
♀ 0U5LXZZ Destruction of Vestibular Gland, External Approach
♀ 0U5M0ZZ Destruction of Vulva, Open Approach
♀ 0U5MXZZ Destruction of Vulva, External Approach

0U7 – Female Reproductive System, Dilation

♀0U750DZ Dilation of Right Fallopian Tube with Intraluminal Device, Open Approach
♀0U750ZZ Dilation of Right Fallopian Tube, Open Approach
♀0U753DZ Dilation of Right Fallopian Tube with Intraluminal Device, Percutaneous Approach
♀0U753ZZ Dilation of Right Fallopian Tube, Percutaneous Approach
♀0U754DZ Dilation of Right Fallopian Tube with Intraluminal Device, Percutaneous Endoscopic Approach
♀0U754ZZ Dilation of Right Fallopian Tube, Percutaneous Endoscopic Approach
♀0U757DZ Dilation of Right Fallopian Tube with Intraluminal Device, Via Natural or Artificial Opening
♀0U757ZZ Dilation of Right Fallopian Tube, Via Natural or Artificial Opening
♀0U758DZ Dilation of Right Fallopian Tube with Intraluminal Device, Via Natural or Artificial Opening Endoscopic
♀0U758ZZ Dilation of Right Fallopian Tube, Via Natural or Artificial Opening Endoscopic
♀0U760DZ Dilation of Left Fallopian Tube with Intraluminal Device, Open Approach
♀0U760ZZ Dilation of Left Fallopian Tube, Open Approach
♀0U763DZ Dilation of Left Fallopian Tube with Intraluminal Device, Percutaneous Approach
♀0U763ZZ Dilation of Left Fallopian Tube, Percutaneous Approach
♀0U764DZ Dilation of Left Fallopian Tube with Intraluminal Device, Percutaneous Endoscopic Approach
♀0U764ZZ Dilation of Left Fallopian Tube, Percutaneous Endoscopic Approach
♀ 0U767DZ Dilation of Left Fallopian Tube with Intraluminal Device, Via Natural or Artificial Opening
♀ 0U767ZZ Dilation of Left Fallopian Tube, Via Natural or Artificial Opening
♀ 0U768DZ Dilation of Left Fallopian Tube with Intraluminal Device, Via Natural or Artificial Opening Endoscopic
♀ 0U768ZZ Dilation of Left Fallopian Tube, Via Natural or Artificial Opening Endoscopic
♀ 0U770DZ Dilation of Bilateral Fallopian Tubes with Intraluminal Device, Open Approach
♀ 0U770ZZ Dilation of Bilateral Fallopian Tubes, Open Approach
♀ 0U773DZ Dilation of Bilateral Fallopian Tubes with Intraluminal Device, Percutaneous Approach
♀ 0U773ZZ Dilation of Bilateral Fallopian Tubes, Percutaneous Approach
♀ 0U774DZ Dilation of Bilateral Fallopian Tubes with Intraluminal Device, Percutaneous Endoscopic Approach
♀ 0U774ZZ Dilation of Bilateral Fallopian Tubes, Percutaneous Endoscopic Approach
♀ 0U777DZ Dilation of Bilateral Fallopian Tubes with Intraluminal Device, Via Natural or Artificial Opening
♀ 0U777ZZ Dilation of Bilateral Fallopian Tubes, Via Natural or Artificial Opening
♀ 0U778DZ Dilation of Bilateral Fallopian Tubes with Intraluminal Device, Via Natural or Artificial Opening Endoscopic
♀ 0U778ZZ Dilation of Bilateral Fallopian Tubes, Via Natural or Artificial Opening Endoscopic
♀ 0U790DZ Dilation of Uterus with Intraluminal Device, Open Approach
♀ 0U790ZZ Dilation of Uterus, Open Approach
♀ 0U793DZ Dilation of Uterus with Intraluminal Device, Percutaneous Approach
♀ 0U793ZZ Dilation of Uterus, Percutaneous Approach
♀ 0U794DZ Dilation of Uterus with Intraluminal Device, Percutaneous Endoscopic Approach
♀ 0U794ZZ Dilation of Uterus, Percutaneous Endoscopic Approach
♀ 0U797DZ Dilation of Uterus with Intraluminal Device, Via Natural or Artificial Opening
♀ 0U797ZZ Dilation of Uterus, Via Natural or Artificial Opening
♀ 0U798DZ Dilation of Uterus with Intraluminal Device, Via Natural or Artificial Opening Endoscopic
♀ 0U798ZZ Dilation of Uterus, Via Natural or Artificial Opening Endoscopic
♀ 0U7C0DZ Dilation of Cervix with Intraluminal Device, Open Approach
♀ 0U7C0ZZ Dilation of Cervix, Open Approach
♀ 0U7C3DZ Dilation of Cervix with Intraluminal Device, Percutaneous Approach
♀ 0U7C3ZZ Dilation of Cervix, Percutaneous Approach
♀ 0U7C4DZ Dilation of Cervix with Intraluminal Device, Percutaneous Endoscopic Approach
♀ 0U7C4ZZ Dilation of Cervix, Percutaneous Endoscopic Approach
♀ 0U7C7DZ Dilation of Cervix with Intraluminal Device, Via Natural or Artificial Opening
♀ 0U7C7ZZ Dilation of Cervix, Via Natural or Artificial Opening
♀ 0U7C8DZ Dilation of Cervix with Intraluminal Device, Via Natural or Artificial Opening Endoscopic
♀ 0U7C8ZZ Dilation of Cervix, Via Natural or Artificial Opening Endoscopic
♀ 0U7G0DZ Dilation of Vagina with Intraluminal Device, Open Approach
♀ 0U7G0ZZ Dilation of Vagina, Open Approach
♀ 0U7G3DZ Dilation of Vagina with Intraluminal Device, Percutaneous Approach

♀ **0U7G3ZZ** Dilation of Vagina, Percutaneous Approach
♀ **0U7G4DZ** Dilation of Vagina with Intraluminal Device, Percutaneous Endoscopic Approach
♀ **0U7G4ZZ** Dilation of Vagina, Percutaneous Endoscopic Approach
♀ **0U7G7DZ** Dilation of Vagina with Intraluminal Device, Via Natural or Artificial Opening
♀ **0U7G7ZZ** Dilation of Vagina, Via Natural or Artificial Opening
♀ **0U7G8DZ** Dilation of Vagina with Intraluminal Device, Via Natural or Artificial Opening Endoscopic
♀ **0U7G8ZZ** Dilation of Vagina, Via Natural or Artificial Opening Endoscopic
♀ **0U7K0DZ** Dilation of Hymen with Intraluminal Device, Open Approach
♀ **0U7K0ZZ** Dilation of Hymen, Open Approach
♀ **0U7K3DZ** Dilation of Hymen with Intraluminal Device, Percutaneous Approach
♀ **0U7K3ZZ** Dilation of Hymen, Percutaneous Approach
♀ **0U7K4DZ** Dilation of Hymen with Intraluminal Device, Percutaneous Endoscopic Approach
♀ **0U7K4ZZ** Dilation of Hymen, Percutaneous Endoscopic Approach
♀ **0U7K7DZ** Dilation of Hymen with Intraluminal Device, Via Natural or Artificial Opening
♀ **0U7K7ZZ** Dilation of Hymen, Via Natural or Artificial Opening
♀ **0U7K8DZ** Dilation of Hymen with Intraluminal Device, Via Natural or Artificial Opening Endoscopic
♀ **0U7K8ZZ** Dilation of Hymen, Via Natural or Artificial Opening Endoscopic
♀ **0U7KXDZ** Dilation of Hymen with Intraluminal Device, External Approach
♀ **0U7KXZZ** Dilation of Hymen, External Approach

0U8 – Female Reproductive System, Division

Review Coding Guideline B3.14

♀ **0U800ZZ** Division of Right Ovary, Open Approach
♀ **0U803ZZ** Division of Right Ovary, Percutaneous Approach
♀ **0U804ZZ** Division of Right Ovary, Percutaneous Endoscopic Approach
♀ **0U810ZZ** Division of Left Ovary, Open Approach
♀ **0U813ZZ** Division of Left Ovary, Percutaneous Approach
♀ **0U814ZZ** Division of Left Ovary, Percutaneous Endoscopic Approach
♀ **0U820ZZ** Division of Bilateral Ovaries, Open Approach
♀ **0U823ZZ** Division of Bilateral Ovaries, Percutaneous Approach
♀ **0U824ZZ** Division of Bilateral Ovaries, Percutaneous Endoscopic Approach
♀ **0U840ZZ** Division of Uterine Supporting Structure, Open Approach
♀ **0U843ZZ** Division of Uterine Supporting Structure, Percutaneous Approach
♀ **0U844ZZ** Division of Uterine Supporting Structure, Percutaneous Endoscopic Approach
♀ **0U8K7ZZ** Division of Hymen, Via Natural or Artificial Opening
♀ **0U8K8ZZ** Division of Hymen, Via Natural or Artificial Opening Endoscopic
♀ **0U8KXZZ** Division of Hymen, External Approach

0U9 – Female Reproductive System, Drainage

Review Coding Guidelines B3.4a and B3.4b

Review Coding Guideline B6.2

♀ **0U9000Z** Drainage of Right Ovary with Drainage Device, Open Approach
♀ **0U900ZX** Drainage of Right Ovary, Open Approach, Diagnostic
♀ **0U900ZZ** Drainage of Right Ovary, Open Approach
♀ **0U9030Z** Drainage of Right Ovary with Drainage Device, Percutaneous Approach
♀ **0U903ZX** Drainage of Right Ovary, Percutaneous Approach, Diagnostic
♀ **0U903ZZ** Drainage of Right Ovary, Percutaneous Approach
♀ **0U9040Z** Drainage of Right Ovary with Drainage Device, Percutaneous Endoscopic Approach
♀ **0U904ZX** Drainage of Right Ovary, Percutaneous Endoscopic Approach, Diagnostic
♀ **0U904ZZ** Drainage of Right Ovary, Percutaneous Endoscopic Approach
♀ **0U90XZZ** Drainage of Right Ovary, External Approach
♀ **0U9100Z** Drainage of Left Ovary with Drainage Device, Open Approach
♀ **0U910ZX** Drainage of Left Ovary, Open Approach, Diagnostic
♀ **0U910ZZ** Drainage of Left Ovary, Open Approach
♀ **0U9130Z** Drainage of Left Ovary with Drainage Device, Percutaneous Approach
♀ **0U913ZX** Drainage of Left Ovary, Percutaneous Approach, Diagnostic
♀ **0U913ZZ** Drainage of Left Ovary, Percutaneous Approach
♀ **0U9140Z** Drainage of Left Ovary with Drainage Device, Percutaneous Endoscopic Approach
♀ **0U914ZX** Drainage of Left Ovary, Percutaneous Endoscopic Approach, Diagnostic
♀ **0U914ZZ** Drainage of Left Ovary, Percutaneous Endoscopic Approach
♀ **0U91XZZ** Drainage of Left Ovary, External Approach
♀ **0U9200Z** Drainage of Bilateral Ovaries with Drainage Device, Open Approach
♀ **0U920ZX** Drainage of Bilateral Ovaries, Open Approach, Diagnostic
♀ **0U920ZZ** Drainage of Bilateral Ovaries, Open Approach
♀ **0U9230Z** Drainage of Bilateral Ovaries with Drainage Device, Percutaneous Approach
♀ **0U923ZX** Drainage of Bilateral Ovaries, Percutaneous Approach, Diagnostic
♀ **0U923ZZ** Drainage of Bilateral Ovaries, Percutaneous Approach
♀ **0U9240Z** Drainage of Bilateral Ovaries with Drainage Device, Percutaneous Endoscopic Approach
♀ **0U924ZX** Drainage of Bilateral Ovaries, Percutaneous Endoscopic Approach, Diagnostic
♀ **0U924ZZ** Drainage of Bilateral Ovaries, Percutaneous Endoscopic Approach
♀ **0U92XZZ** Drainage of Bilateral Ovaries, External Approach
♀ **0U9400Z** Drainage of Uterine Supporting Structure with Drainage Device, Open Approach
♀ **0U940ZX** Drainage of Uterine Supporting Structure, Open Approach, Diagnostic
♀ **0U940ZZ** Drainage of Uterine Supporting Structure, Open Approach
♀ **0U9430Z** Drainage of Uterine Supporting Structure with Drainage Device, Percutaneous Approach
♀ **0U943ZX** Drainage of Uterine Supporting Structure, Percutaneous Approach, Diagnostic
♀ **0U943ZZ** Drainage of Uterine Supporting Structure, Percutaneous Approach
♀ **0U9440Z** Drainage of Uterine Supporting Structure with Drainage Device, Percutaneous Endoscopic Approach
♀ **0U944ZX** Drainage of Uterine Supporting Structure, Percutaneous Endoscopic Approach, Diagnostic
♀ **0U944ZZ** Drainage of Uterine Supporting Structure, Percutaneous Endoscopic Approach
♀ **0U9500Z** Drainage of Right Fallopian Tube with Drainage Device, Open Approach
♀ **0U950ZX** Drainage of Right Fallopian Tube, Open Approach, Diagnostic
♀ **0U950ZZ** Drainage of Right Fallopian Tube, Open Approach
♀ **0U9530Z** Drainage of Right Fallopian Tube with Drainage Device, Percutaneous Approach
♀ **0U953ZX** Drainage of Right Fallopian Tube, Percutaneous Approach, Diagnostic
♀ **0U953ZZ** Drainage of Right Fallopian Tube, Percutaneous Approach
♀ **0U9540Z** Drainage of Right Fallopian Tube with Drainage Device, Percutaneous Endoscopic Approach
♀ **0U954ZX** Drainage of Right Fallopian Tube, Percutaneous Endoscopic Approach, Diagnostic
♀ **0U954ZZ** Drainage of Right Fallopian Tube, Percutaneous Endoscopic Approach
♀ **0U9570Z** Drainage of Right Fallopian Tube with Drainage Device, Via Natural or Artificial Opening
♀ **0U957ZX** Drainage of Right Fallopian Tube, Via Natural or Artificial Opening, Diagnostic
♀ **0U957ZZ** Drainage of Right Fallopian Tube, Via Natural or Artificial Opening
♀ **0U9580Z** Drainage of Right Fallopian Tube with Drainage Device, Via Natural or Artificial Opening Endoscopic
♀ **0U958ZX** Drainage of Right Fallopian Tube, Via Natural or Artificial Opening Endoscopic, Diagnostic
♀ **0U958ZZ** Drainage of Right Fallopian Tube, Via Natural or Artificial Opening Endoscopic
♀ **0U9600Z** Drainage of Left Fallopian Tube with Drainage Device, Open Approach
♀ **0U960ZX** Drainage of Left Fallopian Tube, Open Approach, Diagnostic
♀ **0U960ZZ** Drainage of Left Fallopian Tube, Open Approach

♀0U9630Z Drainage of Left Fallopian Tube with Drainage Device, Percutaneous Approach
♀0U963ZX Drainage of Left Fallopian Tube, Percutaneous Approach, Diagnostic
♀0U963ZZ Drainage of Left Fallopian Tube, Percutaneous Approach
♀0U9640Z Drainage of Left Fallopian Tube with Drainage Device, Percutaneous Endoscopic Approach
♀0U964ZX Drainage of Left Fallopian Tube, Percutaneous Endoscopic Approach, Diagnostic
♀0U964ZZ Drainage of Left Fallopian Tube, Percutaneous Endoscopic Approach
♀0U9670Z Drainage of Left Fallopian Tube with Drainage Device, Via Natural or Artificial Opening
♀0U967ZX Drainage of Left Fallopian Tube, Via Natural or Artificial Opening, Diagnostic
♀0U967ZZ Drainage of Left Fallopian Tube, Via Natural or Artificial Opening
♀0U9680Z Drainage of Left Fallopian Tube with Drainage Device, Via Natural or Artificial Opening Endoscopic
♀0U968ZX Drainage of Left Fallopian Tube, Via Natural or Artificial Opening Endoscopic, Diagnostic
♀0U968ZZ Drainage of Left Fallopian Tube, Via Natural or Artificial Opening Endoscopic
♀0U9700Z Drainage of Bilateral Fallopian Tubes with Drainage Device, Open Approach
♀0U970ZX Drainage of Bilateral Fallopian Tubes, Open Approach, Diagnostic
♀0U970ZZ Drainage of Bilateral Fallopian Tubes, Open Approach
♀0U9730Z Drainage of Bilateral Fallopian Tubes with Drainage Device, Percutaneous Approach
♀0U973ZX Drainage of Bilateral Fallopian Tubes, Percutaneous Approach, Diagnostic
♀0U973ZZ Drainage of Bilateral Fallopian Tubes, Percutaneous Approach
♀0U9740Z Drainage of Bilateral Fallopian Tubes with Drainage Device, Percutaneous Endoscopic Approach
♀0U974ZX Drainage of Bilateral Fallopian Tubes, Percutaneous Endoscopic Approach, Diagnostic
♀0U974ZZ Drainage of Bilateral Fallopian Tubes, Percutaneous Endoscopic Approach
♀0U9770Z Drainage of Bilateral Fallopian Tubes with Drainage Device, Via Natural or Artificial Opening
♀0U977ZX Drainage of Bilateral Fallopian Tubes, Via Natural or Artificial Opening, Diagnostic
♀0U977ZZ Drainage of Bilateral Fallopian Tubes, Via Natural or Artificial Opening
♀0U9780Z Drainage of Bilateral Fallopian Tubes with Drainage Device, Via Natural or Artificial Opening Endoscopic
♀0U978ZX Drainage of Bilateral Fallopian Tubes, Via Natural or Artificial Opening Endoscopic, Diagnostic
♀0U978ZZ Drainage of Bilateral Fallopian Tubes, Via Natural or Artificial Opening Endoscopic
♀0U9900Z Drainage of Uterus with Drainage Device, Open Approach
♀0U990ZX Drainage of Uterus, Open Approach, Diagnostic
♀0U990ZZ Drainage of Uterus, Open Approach
♀0U9930Z Drainage of Uterus with Drainage Device, Percutaneous Approach
♀0U993ZX Drainage of Uterus, Percutaneous Approach, Diagnostic
♀0U993ZZ Drainage of Uterus, Percutaneous Approach
♀0U9940Z Drainage of Uterus with Drainage Device, Percutaneous Endoscopic Approach
♀ 0U994ZX Drainage of Uterus, Percutaneous Endoscopic Approach, Diagnostic
♀ 0U994ZZ Drainage of Uterus, Percutaneous Endoscopic Approach
♀ 0U9970Z Drainage of Uterus with Drainage Device, Via Natural or Artificial Opening
♀ 0U997ZX Drainage of Uterus, Via Natural or Artificial Opening, Diagnostic
♀ 0U997ZZ Drainage of Uterus, Via Natural or Artificial Opening
♀ 0U9980Z Drainage of Uterus with Drainage Device, Via Natural or Artificial Opening Endoscopic
♀ 0U998ZX Drainage of Uterus, Via Natural or Artificial Opening Endoscopic, Diagnostic
♀ 0U998ZZ Drainage of Uterus, Via Natural or Artificial Opening Endoscopic
♀ 0U9C00Z Drainage of Cervix with Drainage Device, Open Approach
♀ 0U9C0ZX Drainage of Cervix, Open Approach, Diagnostic
♀ 0U9C0ZZ Drainage of Cervix, Open Approach
♀ 0U9C30Z Drainage of Cervix with Drainage Device, Percutaneous Approach
♀ 0U9C3ZX Drainage of Cervix, Percutaneous Approach, Diagnostic
♀ 0U9C3ZZ Drainage of Cervix, Percutaneous Approach
♀ 0U9C40Z Drainage of Cervix with Drainage Device, Percutaneous Endoscopic Approach
♀ 0U9C4ZX Drainage of Cervix, Percutaneous Endoscopic Approach, Diagnostic
♀ 0U9C4ZZ Drainage of Cervix, Percutaneous Endoscopic Approach
♀ 0U9C70Z Drainage of Cervix with Drainage Device, Via Natural or Artificial Opening
♀ 0U9C7ZX Drainage of Cervix, Via Natural or Artificial Opening, Diagnostic
♀ 0U9C7ZZ Drainage of Cervix, Via Natural or Artificial Opening
♀ 0U9C80Z Drainage of Cervix with Drainage Device, Via Natural or Artificial Opening Endoscopic
♀ 0U9C8ZX Drainage of Cervix, Via Natural or Artificial Opening Endoscopic, Diagnostic
♀ 0U9C8ZZ Drainage of Cervix, Via Natural or Artificial Opening Endoscopic
♀ 0U9F00Z Drainage of Cul-de-sac with Drainage Device, Open Approach
♀ 0U9F0ZX Drainage of Cul-de-sac, Open Approach, Diagnostic
♀ 0U9F0ZZ Drainage of Cul-de-sac, Open Approach
♀ 0U9F30Z Drainage of Cul-de-sac with Drainage Device, Percutaneous Approach
♀ 0U9F3ZX Drainage of Cul-de-sac, Percutaneous Approach, Diagnostic
♀ 0U9F3ZZ Drainage of Cul-de-sac, Percutaneous Approach
♀ 0U9F40Z Drainage of Cul-de-sac with Drainage Device, Percutaneous Endoscopic Approach
♀ 0U9F4ZX Drainage of Cul-de-sac, Percutaneous Endoscopic Approach, Diagnostic
♀ 0U9F4ZZ Drainage of Cul-de-sac, Percutaneous Endoscopic Approach
♀ 0U9F70Z Drainage of Cul-de-sac with Drainage Device, Via Natural or Artificial Opening
♀ 0U9F7ZX Drainage of Cul-de-sac, Via Natural or Artificial Opening, Diagnostic
♀ 0U9F7ZZ Drainage of Cul-de-sac, Via Natural or Artificial Opening
♀ 0U9F80Z Drainage of Cul-de-sac with Drainage Device, Via Natural or Artificial Opening Endoscopic
♀ 0U9F8ZX Drainage of Cul-de-sac, Via Natural or Artificial Opening Endoscopic, Diagnostic
♀ 0U9F8ZZ Drainage of Cul-de-sac, Via Natural or Artificial Opening Endoscopic
♀ 0U9G00Z Drainage of Vagina with Drainage Device, Open Approach
♀ 0U9G0ZX Drainage of Vagina, Open Approach, Diagnostic
♀ 0U9G0ZZ Drainage of Vagina, Open Approach
♀ 0U9G30Z Drainage of Vagina with Drainage Device, Percutaneous Approach
♀ 0U9G3ZX Drainage of Vagina, Percutaneous Approach, Diagnostic
♀ 0U9G3ZZ Drainage of Vagina, Percutaneous Approach
♀ 0U9G40Z Drainage of Vagina with Drainage Device, Percutaneous Endoscopic Approach
♀ 0U9G4ZX Drainage of Vagina, Percutaneous Endoscopic Approach, Diagnostic
♀ 0U9G4ZZ Drainage of Vagina, Percutaneous Endoscopic Approach
♀ 0U9G70Z Drainage of Vagina with Drainage Device, Via Natural or Artificial Opening
♀ 0U9G7ZX Drainage of Vagina, Via Natural or Artificial Opening, Diagnostic
♀ 0U9G7ZZ Drainage of Vagina, Via Natural or Artificial Opening
♀ 0U9G80Z Drainage of Vagina with Drainage Device, Via Natural or Artificial Opening Endoscopic
♀ 0U9G8ZX Drainage of Vagina, Via Natural or Artificial Opening Endoscopic, Diagnostic
♀ 0U9G8ZZ Drainage of Vagina, Via Natural or Artificial Opening Endoscopic
♀ 0U9GX0Z Drainage of Vagina with Drainage Device, External Approach
♀ 0U9GXZX Drainage of Vagina, External Approach, Diagnostic
♀ 0U9GXZZ Drainage of Vagina, External Approach
♀ 0U9J00Z Drainage of Clitoris with Drainage Device, Open Approach
♀ 0U9J0ZX Drainage of Clitoris, Open Approach, Diagnostic
♀ 0U9J0ZZ Drainage of Clitoris, Open Approach
♀ 0U9JX0Z Drainage of Clitoris with Drainage Device, External Approach
♀ 0U9JXZX Drainage of Clitoris, External Approach, Diagnostic
♀ 0U9JXZZ Drainage of Clitoris, External Approach
♀ 0U9K00Z Drainage of Hymen with Drainage Device, Open Approach
♀ 0U9K0ZX Drainage of Hymen, Open Approach, Diagnostic
♀ 0U9K0ZZ Drainage of Hymen, Open Approach
♀ 0U9K30Z Drainage of Hymen with Drainage Device, Percutaneous Approach
♀ 0U9K3ZX Drainage of Hymen, Percutaneous Approach, Diagnostic
♀ 0U9K3ZZ Drainage of Hymen, Percutaneous Approach
♀ 0U9K40Z Drainage of Hymen with Drainage Device, Percutaneous Endoscopic Approach
♀ 0U9K4ZX Drainage of Hymen, Percutaneous Endoscopic Approach, Diagnostic
♀ 0U9K4ZZ Drainage of Hymen, Percutaneous Endoscopic Approach
♀ 0U9K70Z Drainage of Hymen with Drainage Device, Via Natural or Artificial Opening
♀ 0U9K7ZX Drainage of Hymen, Via Natural or Artificial Opening, Diagnostic
♀ 0U9K7ZZ Drainage of Hymen, Via Natural or Artificial Opening
♀ 0U9K80Z Drainage of Hymen with Drainage Device, Via Natural or Artificial Opening Endoscopic
♀ 0U9K8ZX Drainage of Hymen, Via Natural or Artificial Opening Endoscopic, Diagnostic
♀ 0U9K8ZZ Drainage of Hymen, Via Natural or Artificial Opening Endoscopic

♀ **0U9KX0Z** Drainage of Hymen with Drainage Device, External Approach
♀ **0U9KXZX** Drainage of Hymen, External Approach, Diagnostic
♀ **0U9KXZZ** Drainage of Hymen, External Approach
♀ **0U9L00Z** Drainage of Vestibular Gland with Drainage Device, Open Approach
♀ **0U9L0ZX** Drainage of Vestibular Gland, Open Approach, Diagnostic
♀ **0U9L0ZZ** Drainage of Vestibular Gland, Open Approach
♀ **0U9LX0Z** Drainage of Vestibular Gland with Drainage Device, External Approach
♀ **0U9LXZX** Drainage of Vestibular Gland, External Approach, Diagnostic
♀ **0U9LXZZ** Drainage of Vestibular Gland, External Approach
♀ **0U9M00Z** Drainage of Vulva with Drainage Device, Open Approach
♀ **0U9M0ZX** Drainage of Vulva, Open Approach, Diagnostic
♀ **0U9M0ZZ** Drainage of Vulva, Open Approach
♀ **0U9MX0Z** Drainage of Vulva with Drainage Device, External Approach
♀ **0U9MXZX** Drainage of Vulva, External Approach, Diagnostic
♀ **0U9MXZZ** Drainage of Vulva, External Approach

0UB – Female Reproductive System, Excision

Review Coding Guidelines B3.4a and B3.4b

Review Coding Guideline B3.8

♀ **0UB00ZX** Excision of Right Ovary, Open Approach, Diagnostic
♀ **0UB00ZZ** Excision of Right Ovary, Open Approach
♀ **0UB03ZX** Excision of Right Ovary, Percutaneous Approach, Diagnostic
♀ **0UB03ZZ** Excision of Right Ovary, Percutaneous Approach
♀ **0UB04ZX** Excision of Right Ovary, Percutaneous Endoscopic Approach, Diagnostic
♀ **0UB04ZZ** Excision of Right Ovary, Percutaneous Endoscopic Approach
♀ **0UB07ZX** Excision of Right Ovary, Via Natural or Artificial Opening, Diagnostic
♀ **0UB07ZZ** Excision of Right Ovary, Via Natural or Artificial Opening
♀ **0UB08ZX** Excision of Right Ovary, Via Natural or Artificial Opening Endoscopic, Diagnostic
♀ **0UB08ZZ** Excision of Right Ovary, Via Natural or Artificial Opening Endoscopic
♀ **0UB10ZX** Excision of Left Ovary, Open Approach, Diagnostic
♀ **0UB10ZZ** Excision of Left Ovary, Open Approach
♀ **0UB13ZX** Excision of Left Ovary, Percutaneous Approach, Diagnostic
♀ **0UB13ZZ** Excision of Left Ovary, Percutaneous Approach
♀ **0UB14ZX** Excision of Left Ovary, Percutaneous Endoscopic Approach, Diagnostic
♀ **0UB14ZZ** Excision of Left Ovary, Percutaneous Endoscopic Approach
♀ **0UB17ZX** Excision of Left Ovary, Via Natural or Artificial Opening, Diagnostic
♀ **0UB17ZZ** Excision of Left Ovary, Via Natural or Artificial Opening
♀ **0UB18ZX** Excision of Left Ovary, Via Natural or Artificial Opening Endoscopic, Diagnostic
♀ **0UB18ZZ** Excision of Left Ovary, Via Natural or Artificial Opening Endoscopic
♀ **0UB20ZX** Excision of Bilateral Ovaries, Open Approach, Diagnostic
♀ **0UB20ZZ** Excision of Bilateral Ovaries, Open Approach
♀ **0UB23ZX** Excision of Bilateral Ovaries, Percutaneous Approach, Diagnostic
♀ **0UB23ZZ** Excision of Bilateral Ovaries, Percutaneous Approach
♀ **0UB24ZX** Excision of Bilateral Ovaries, Percutaneous Endoscopic Approach, Diagnostic
♀ **0UB24ZZ** Excision of Bilateral Ovaries, Percutaneous Endoscopic Approach
♀ **0UB27ZX** Excision of Bilateral Ovaries, Via Natural or Artificial Opening, Diagnostic
♀ **0UB27ZZ** Excision of Bilateral Ovaries, Via Natural or Artificial Opening
♀ **0UB28ZX** Excision of Bilateral Ovaries, Via Natural or Artificial Opening Endoscopic, Diagnostic
♀ **0UB28ZZ** Excision of Bilateral Ovaries, Via Natural or Artificial Opening Endoscopic
♀ **0UB40ZX** Excision of Uterine Supporting Structure, Open Approach, Diagnostic
♀ **0UB40ZZ** Excision of Uterine Supporting Structure, Open Approach
♀ **0UB43ZX** Excision of Uterine Supporting Structure, Percutaneous Approach, Diagnostic
♀ **0UB43ZZ** Excision of Uterine Supporting Structure, Percutaneous Approach
♀ **0UB44ZX** Excision of Uterine Supporting Structure, Percutaneous Endoscopic Approach, Diagnostic
♀ **0UB44ZZ** Excision of Uterine Supporting Structure, Percutaneous Endoscopic Approach
♀ **0UB47ZX** Excision of Uterine Supporting Structure, Via Natural or Artificial Opening, Diagnostic
♀ **0UB47ZZ** Excision of Uterine Supporting Structure, Via Natural or Artificial Opening
♀ **0UB48ZX** Excision of Uterine Supporting Structure, Via Natural or Artificial Opening Endoscopic, Diagnostic
♀ **0UB48ZZ** Excision of Uterine Supporting Structure, Via Natural or Artificial Opening Endoscopic
♀ **0UB50ZX** Excision of Right Fallopian Tube, Open Approach, Diagnostic
♀ **0UB50ZZ** Excision of Right Fallopian Tube, Open Approach
♀ **0UB53ZX** Excision of Right Fallopian Tube, Percutaneous Approach, Diagnostic
♀ **0UB53ZZ** Excision of Right Fallopian Tube, Percutaneous Approach
♀ **0UB54ZX** Excision of Right Fallopian Tube, Percutaneous Endoscopic Approach, Diagnostic
♀ **0UB54ZZ** Excision of Right Fallopian Tube, Percutaneous Endoscopic Approach
♀ **0UB57ZX** Excision of Right Fallopian Tube, Via Natural or Artificial Opening, Diagnostic
♀ **0UB57ZZ** Excision of Right Fallopian Tube, Via Natural or Artificial Opening
♀ **0UB58ZX** Excision of Right Fallopian Tube, Via Natural or Artificial Opening Endoscopic, Diagnostic
♀ **0UB58ZZ** Excision of Right Fallopian Tube, Via Natural or Artificial Opening Endoscopic
♀ **0UB60ZX** Excision of Left Fallopian Tube, Open Approach, Diagnostic
♀ **0UB60ZZ** Excision of Left Fallopian Tube, Open Approach
♀ **0UB63ZX** Excision of Left Fallopian Tube, Percutaneous Approach, Diagnostic
♀ **0UB63ZZ** Excision of Left Fallopian Tube, Percutaneous Approach
♀ **0UB64ZX** Excision of Left Fallopian Tube, Percutaneous Endoscopic Approach, Diagnostic
♀ **0UB64ZZ** Excision of Left Fallopian Tube, Percutaneous Endoscopic Approach
♀ **0UB67ZX** Excision of Left Fallopian Tube, Via Natural or Artificial Opening, Diagnostic
♀ **0UB67ZZ** Excision of Left Fallopian Tube, Via Natural or Artificial Opening
♀ **0UB68ZX** Excision of Left Fallopian Tube, Via Natural or Artificial Opening Endoscopic, Diagnostic
♀ **0UB68ZZ** Excision of Left Fallopian Tube, Via Natural or Artificial Opening Endoscopic
♀ **0UB70ZX** Excision of Bilateral Fallopian Tubes, Open Approach, Diagnostic
♀ **0UB70ZZ** Excision of Bilateral Fallopian Tubes, Open Approach
♀ **0UB73ZX** Excision of Bilateral Fallopian Tubes, Percutaneous Approach, Diagnostic
♀ **0UB73ZZ** Excision of Bilateral Fallopian Tubes, Percutaneous Approach
♀ **0UB74ZX** Excision of Bilateral Fallopian Tubes, Percutaneous Endoscopic Approach, Diagnostic
♀ **0UB74ZZ** Excision of Bilateral Fallopian Tubes, Percutaneous Endoscopic Approach
♀ **0UB77ZX** Excision of Bilateral Fallopian Tubes, Via Natural or Artificial Opening, Diagnostic
♀ **0UB77ZZ** Excision of Bilateral Fallopian Tubes, Via Natural or Artificial Opening
♀ **0UB78ZX** Excision of Bilateral Fallopian Tubes, Via Natural or Artificial Opening Endoscopic, Diagnostic
♀ **0UB78ZZ** Excision of Bilateral Fallopian Tubes, Via Natural or Artificial Opening Endoscopic
♀ **0UB90ZX** Excision of Uterus, Open Approach, Diagnostic
♀ **0UB90ZZ** Excision of Uterus, Open Approach
♀ **0UB93ZX** Excision of Uterus, Percutaneous Approach, Diagnostic
♀ **0UB93ZZ** Excision of Uterus, Percutaneous Approach
♀ **0UB94ZX** Excision of Uterus, Percutaneous Endoscopic Approach, Diagnostic
♀ **0UB94ZZ** Excision of Uterus, Percutaneous Endoscopic Approach
♀ **0UB97ZX** Excision of Uterus, Via Natural or Artificial Opening, Diagnostic
♀ **0UB97ZZ** Excision of Uterus, Via Natural or Artificial Opening
♀ **0UB98ZX** Excision of Uterus, Via Natural or Artificial Opening Endoscopic, Diagnostic
♀ **0UB98ZZ** Excision of Uterus, Via Natural or Artificial Opening Endoscopic
♀ **0UBC0ZX** Excision of Cervix, Open Approach, Diagnostic
♀ **0UBC0ZZ** Excision of Cervix, Open Approach
♀ **0UBC3ZX** Excision of Cervix, Percutaneous Approach, Diagnostic
♀ **0UBC3ZZ** Excision of Cervix, Percutaneous Approach
♀ **0UBC4ZX** Excision of Cervix, Percutaneous Endoscopic Approach, Diagnostic

♀0UBC4ZZ Excision of Cervix, Percutaneous Endoscopic Approach
♀0UBC7ZX Excision of Cervix, Via Natural or Artificial Opening, Diagnostic
♀0UBC7ZZ Excision of Cervix, Via Natural or Artificial Opening
♀0UBC8ZX Excision of Cervix, Via Natural or Artificial Opening Endoscopic, Diagnostic
♀0UBC8ZZ Excision of Cervix, Via Natural or Artificial Opening Endoscopic
♀0UBF0ZX Excision of Cul-de-sac, Open Approach, Diagnostic
♀0UBF0ZZ Excision of Cul-de-sac, Open Approach
♀0UBF3ZX Excision of Cul-de-sac, Percutaneous Approach, Diagnostic
♀0UBF3ZZ Excision of Cul-de-sac, Percutaneous Approach
♀0UBF4ZX Excision of Cul-de-sac, Percutaneous Endoscopic Approach, Diagnostic
♀0UBF4ZZ Excision of Cul-de-sac, Percutaneous Endoscopic Approach
♀0UBF7ZX Excision of Cul-de-sac, Via Natural or Artificial Opening, Diagnostic
♀0UBF7ZZ Excision of Cul-de-sac, Via Natural or Artificial Opening
♀0UBF8ZX Excision of Cul-de-sac, Via Natural or Artificial Opening Endoscopic, Diagnostic
♀0UBF8ZZ Excision of Cul-de-sac, Via Natural or Artificial Opening Endoscopic
♀0UBG0ZX Excision of Vagina, Open Approach, Diagnostic
♀ 0UBG0ZZ Excision of Vagina, Open Approach
♀ 0UBG3ZX Excision of Vagina, Percutaneous Approach, Diagnostic
♀ 0UBG3ZZ Excision of Vagina, Percutaneous Approach
♀ 0UBG4ZX Excision of Vagina, Percutaneous Endoscopic Approach, Diagnostic
♀ 0UBG4ZZ Excision of Vagina, Percutaneous Endoscopic Approach
♀ 0UBG7ZX Excision of Vagina, Via Natural or Artificial Opening, Diagnostic
♀ 0UBG7ZZ Excision of Vagina, Via Natural or Artificial Opening
♀ 0UBG8ZX Excision of Vagina, Via Natural or Artificial Opening Endoscopic, Diagnostic
♀ 0UBG8ZZ Excision of Vagina, Via Natural or Artificial Opening Endoscopic
♀ 0UBGXZX Excision of Vagina, External Approach, Diagnostic
♀ 0UBGXZZ Excision of Vagina, External Approach
♀ 0UBJ0ZX Excision of Clitoris, Open Approach, Diagnostic
♀ 0UBJ0ZZ Excision of Clitoris, Open Approach
♀ 0UBJXZX Excision of Clitoris, External Approach, Diagnostic
♀ 0UBJXZZ Excision of Clitoris, External Approach
♀ 0UBK0ZX Excision of Hymen, Open Approach, Diagnostic
♀ 0UBK0ZZ Excision of Hymen, Open Approach
♀ 0UBK3ZX Excision of Hymen, Percutaneous Approach, Diagnostic
♀ 0UBK3ZZ Excision of Hymen, Percutaneous Approach
♀ 0UBK4ZX Excision of Hymen, Percutaneous Endoscopic Approach, Diagnostic
♀ 0UBK4ZZ Excision of Hymen, Percutaneous Endoscopic Approach
♀ 0UBK7ZX Excision of Hymen, Via Natural or Artificial Opening, Diagnostic
♀ 0UBK7ZZ Excision of Hymen, Via Natural or Artificial Opening
♀ 0UBK8ZX Excision of Hymen, Via Natural or Artificial Opening Endoscopic, Diagnostic
♀ 0UBK8ZZ Excision of Hymen, Via Natural or Artificial Opening Endoscopic
♀ 0UBKXZX Excision of Hymen, External Approach, Diagnostic
♀ 0UBKXZZ Excision of Hymen, External Approach
♀ 0UBL0ZX Excision of Vestibular Gland, Open Approach, Diagnostic
♀ 0UBL0ZZ Excision of Vestibular Gland, Open Approach
♀ 0UBLXZX Excision of Vestibular Gland, External Approach, Diagnostic
♀ 0UBLXZZ Excision of Vestibular Gland, External Approach
♀ 0UBM0ZX Excision of Vulva, Open Approach, Diagnostic
♀ 0UBM0ZZ Excision of Vulva, Open Approach
♀ 0UBMXZX Excision of Vulva, External Approach, Diagnostic
♀ 0UBMXZZ Excision of Vulva, External Approach

0UC – Female Reproductive System, Extirpation

♀0UC00ZZ Extirpation of Matter from Right Ovary, Open Approach
♀0UC03ZZ Extirpation of Matter from Right Ovary, Percutaneous Approach
♀0UC04ZZ Extirpation of Matter from Right Ovary, Percutaneous Endoscopic Approach
♀0UC10ZZ Extirpation of Matter from Left Ovary, Open Approach
♀0UC13ZZ Extirpation of Matter from Left Ovary, Percutaneous Approach
♀0UC14ZZ Extirpation of Matter from Left Ovary, Percutaneous Endoscopic Approach
♀0UC20ZZ Extirpation of Matter from Bilateral Ovaries, Open Approach
♀0UC23ZZ Extirpation of Matter from Bilateral Ovaries, Percutaneous Approach
♀0UC24ZZ Extirpation of Matter from Bilateral Ovaries, Percutaneous Endoscopic Approach
♀0UC40ZZ Extirpation of Matter from Uterine Supporting Structure, Open Approach
♀0UC43ZZ Extirpation of Matter from Uterine Supporting Structure, Percutaneous Approach
♀0UC44ZZ Extirpation of Matter from Uterine Supporting Structure, Percutaneous Endoscopic Approach
♀0UC50ZZ Extirpation of Matter from Right Fallopian Tube, Open Approach
♀0UC53ZZ Extirpation of Matter from Right Fallopian Tube, Percutaneous Approach
♀0UC54ZZ Extirpation of Matter from Right Fallopian Tube, Percutaneous Endoscopic Approach
♀0UC57ZZ Extirpation of Matter from Right Fallopian Tube, Via Natural or Artificial Opening
♀0UC58ZZ Extirpation of Matter from Right Fallopian Tube, Via Natural or Artificial Opening Endoscopic
♀0UC60ZZ Extirpation of Matter from Left Fallopian Tube, Open Approach
♀ 0UC63ZZ Extirpation of Matter from Left Fallopian Tube, Percutaneous Approach
♀ 0UC64ZZ Extirpation of Matter from Left Fallopian Tube, Percutaneous Endoscopic Approach
♀ 0UC67ZZ Extirpation of Matter from Left Fallopian Tube, Via Natural or Artificial Opening
♀ 0UC68ZZ Extirpation of Matter from Left Fallopian Tube, Via Natural or Artificial Opening Endoscopic
♀ 0UC70ZZ Extirpation of Matter from Bilateral Fallopian Tubes, Open Approach
♀ 0UC73ZZ Extirpation of Matter from Bilateral Fallopian Tubes, Percutaneous Approach
♀ 0UC74ZZ Extirpation of Matter from Bilateral Fallopian Tubes, Percutaneous Endoscopic Approach
♀ 0UC77ZZ Extirpation of Matter from Bilateral Fallopian Tubes, Via Natural or Artificial Opening
♀ 0UC78ZZ Extirpation of Matter from Bilateral Fallopian Tubes, Via Natural or Artificial Opening Endoscopic
♀ 0UC90ZZ Extirpation of Matter from Uterus, Open Approach
♀ 0UC93ZZ Extirpation of Matter from Uterus, Percutaneous Approach
♀ 0UC94ZZ Extirpation of Matter from Uterus, Percutaneous Endoscopic Approach
♀ 0UC97ZZ Extirpation of Matter from Uterus, Via Natural or Artificial Opening
AHA CC: 2Q, 2013, 38
♀ 0UC98ZZ Extirpation of Matter from Uterus, Via Natural or Artificial Opening Endoscopic
♀ 0UCB0ZZ Extirpation of Matter from Endometrium, Open Approach
♀ 0UCB3ZZ Extirpation of Matter from Endometrium, Percutaneous Approach
♀ 0UCB4ZZ Extirpation of Matter from Endometrium, Percutaneous Endoscopic Approach
♀ 0UCB7ZZ Extirpation of Matter from Endometrium, Via Natural or Artificial Opening
♀ 0UCB8ZZ Extirpation of Matter from Endometrium, Via Natural or Artificial Opening Endoscopic
♀ 0UCC0ZZ Extirpation of Matter from Cervix, Open Approach
♀ 0UCC3ZZ Extirpation of Matter from Cervix, Percutaneous Approach
♀ 0UCC4ZZ Extirpation of Matter from Cervix, Percutaneous Endoscopic Approach
♀ 0UCC7ZZ Extirpation of Matter from Cervix, Via Natural or Artificial Opening
♀ 0UCC8ZZ Extirpation of Matter from Cervix, Via Natural or Artificial Opening Endoscopic
♀ 0UCF0ZZ Extirpation of Matter from Cul-de-sac, Open Approach
♀ 0UCF3ZZ Extirpation of Matter from Cul-de-sac, Percutaneous Approach
♀ 0UCF4ZZ Extirpation of Matter from Cul-de-sac, Percutaneous Endoscopic Approach
♀ 0UCF7ZZ Extirpation of Matter from Cul-de-sac, Via Natural or Artificial Opening
♀ 0UCF8ZZ Extirpation of Matter from Cul-de-sac, Via Natural or Artificial Opening Endoscopic
♀ 0UCG0ZZ Extirpation of Matter from Vagina, Open Approach
♀ 0UCG3ZZ Extirpation of Matter from Vagina, Percutaneous Approach
♀ 0UCG4ZZ Extirpation of Matter from Vagina, Percutaneous Endoscopic Approach
♀ 0UCG7ZZ Extirpation of Matter from Vagina, Via Natural or Artificial Opening
♀ 0UCG8ZZ Extirpation of Matter from Vagina, Via Natural or Artificial Opening Endoscopic
♀ 0UCGXZZ Extirpation of Matter from Vagina, External Approach
♀ 0UCJ0ZZ Extirpation of Matter from Clitoris, Open Approach

♀ **0UCJXZZ** Extirpation of Matter from Clitoris, External Approach
♀ **0UCK0ZZ** Extirpation of Matter from Hymen, Open Approach
♀ **0UCK3ZZ** Extirpation of Matter from Hymen, Percutaneous Approach
♀ **0UCK4ZZ** Extirpation of Matter from Hymen, Percutaneous Endoscopic Approach
♀ **0UCK7ZZ** Extirpation of Matter from Hymen, Via Natural or Artificial Opening
♀ **0UCK8ZZ** Extirpation of Matter from Hymen, Via Natural or Artificial Opening Endoscopic
♀ **0UCKXZZ** Extirpation of Matter from Hymen, External Approach
♀ **0UCL0ZZ** Extirpation of Matter from Vestibular Gland, Open Approach
♀ **0UCLXZZ** Extirpation of Matter from Vestibular Gland, External Approach
♀ **0UCM0ZZ** Extirpation of Matter from Vulva, Open Approach
♀ **0UCMXZZ** Extirpation of Matter from Vulva, External Approach

0UD – Female Reproductive System, Extraction

Review Coding Guidelines B3.4a and B3.4b

Review Coding Guideline C2

♀ **0UDB7ZX** Extraction of Endometrium, Via Natural or Artificial Opening, Diagnostic
♀ **0UDB7ZZ** Extraction of Endometrium, Via Natural or Artificial Opening
♀ **0UDB8ZX** Extraction of Endometrium, Via Natural or Artificial Opening Endoscopic, Diagnostic
♀ **0UDB8ZZ** Extraction of Endometrium, Via Natural or Artificial Opening Endoscopic
♀ **0UDN0ZZ** Extraction of Ova, Open
♀ **0UDN3ZZ** Extraction of Ova, Percutaneous
♀ **0UDN4ZZ** Extraction of Ova, Percutaneous Endoscopic

0UF – Female Reproductive System, Fragmentation

♀ **0UF50ZZ** Fragmentation in Right Fallopian Tube, Open Approach
♀ **0UF53ZZ** Fragmentation in Right Fallopian Tube, Percutaneous Approach
♀ **0UF54ZZ** Fragmentation in Right Fallopian Tube, Percutaneous Endoscopic Approach
♀ **0UF57ZZ** Fragmentation in Right Fallopian Tube, Via Natural or Artificial Opening
♀ **0UF58ZZ** Fragmentation in Right Fallopian Tube, Via Natural or Artificial Opening Endoscopic
♀ ▲ **0UF5XZZ** Fragmentation in Right Fallopian Tube, External Approach
♀ **0UF60ZZ** Fragmentation in Left Fallopian Tube, Open Approach
♀ **0UF63ZZ** Fragmentation in Left Fallopian Tube, Percutaneous Approach
♀ **0UF64ZZ** Fragmentation in Left Fallopian Tube, Percutaneous Endoscopic Approach
♀ **0UF67ZZ** Fragmentation in Left Fallopian Tube, Via Natural or Artificial Opening
♀ **0UF68ZZ** Fragmentation in Left Fallopian Tube, Via Natural or Artificial Opening Endoscopic
♀ ▲ **0UF6XZZ** Fragmentation in Left Fallopian Tube, External Approach
♀ **0UF70ZZ** Fragmentation in Bilateral Fallopian Tubes, Open Approach
♀ **0UF73ZZ** Fragmentation in Bilateral Fallopian Tubes, Percutaneous Approach
♀ **0UF74ZZ** Fragmentation in Bilateral Fallopian Tubes, Percutaneous Endoscopic Approach
♀ **0UF77ZZ** Fragmentation in Bilateral Fallopian Tubes, Via Natural or Artificial Opening
♀ **0UF78ZZ** Fragmentation in Bilateral Fallopian Tubes, Via Natural or Artificial Opening Endoscopic
♀ ▲ **0UF7XZZ** Fragmentation in Bilateral Fallopian Tubes, External Approach
♀ **0UF90ZZ** Fragmentation in Uterus, Open Approach
♀ **0UF93ZZ** Fragmentation in Uterus, Percutaneous Approach
♀ **0UF94ZZ** Fragmentation in Uterus, Percutaneous Endoscopic Approach
♀ **0UF97ZZ** Fragmentation in Uterus, Via Natural or Artificial Opening
♀ **0UF98ZZ** Fragmentation in Uterus, Via Natural or Artificial Opening Endoscopic
♀ ▲ **0UF9XZZ** Fragmentation in Uterus, External Approach

0UH – Female Reproductive System, Insertion

♀ **0UH303Z** Insertion of Infusion Device into Ovary, Open Approach
♀ **0UH333Z** Insertion of Infusion Device into Ovary, Percutaneous Approach
♀ **0UH343Z** Insertion of Infusion Device into Ovary, Percutaneous Endoscopic Approach
♀ **0UH803Z** Insertion of Infusion Device into Fallopian Tube, Open Approach
♀ **0UH833Z** Insertion of Infusion Device into Fallopian Tube, Percutaneous Approach
♀ **0UH843Z** Insertion of Infusion Device into Fallopian Tube, Percutaneous Endoscopic Approach
♀ **0UH873Z** Insertion of Infusion Device into Fallopian Tube, Via Natural or Artificial Opening
♀ **0UH883Z** Insertion of Infusion Device into Fallopian Tube, Via Natural or Artificial Opening Endoscopic
♀ **0UH97HZ** Insertion of Contraceptive Device into Uterus, Via Natural or Artificial Opening
AHA CC: 2Q, 2013, 34
♀ **0UH98HZ** Insertion of Contraceptive Device into Uterus, Via Natural or Artificial Opening Endoscopic
♀ **0UHC01Z** Insertion of Radioactive Element into Cervix, Open Approach
♀ **0UHC31Z** Insertion of Radioactive Element into Cervix, Percutaneous Approach
♀ **0UHC41Z** Insertion of Radioactive Element into Cervix, Percutaneous Endoscopic Approach
♀ **0UHC71Z** Insertion of Radioactive Element into Cervix, Via Natural or Artificial Opening
♀ **0UHC7HZ** Insertion of Contraceptive Device into Cervix, Via Natural or Artificial Opening
♀ **0UHC81Z** Insertion of Radioactive Element into Cervix, Via Natural or Artificial Opening Endoscopic
♀ **0UHC8HZ** Insertion of Contraceptive Device into Cervix, Via Natural or Artificial Opening Endoscopic
♀ **0UHD03Z** Insertion of Infusion Device into Uterus and Cervix, Open Approach
♀ **0UHD33Z** Insertion of Infusion Device into Uterus and Cervix, Percutaneous Approach
♀ **0UHD43Z** Insertion of Infusion Device into Uterus and Cervix, Percutaneous Endoscopic Approach
♀ **0UHD73Z** Insertion of Infusion Device into Uterus and Cervix, Via Natural or Artificial Opening
♀ **0UHD83Z** Insertion of Infusion Device into Uterus and Cervix, Via Natural or Artificial Opening Endoscopic
♀ **0UHF7GZ** Insertion of Pessary into Cul-de-sac, Via Natural or Artificial Opening
♀ **0UHF8GZ** Insertion of Pessary into Cul-de-sac, Via Natural or Artificial Opening Endoscopic
♀ **0UHG01Z** Insertion of Radioactive Element into Vagina, Open Approach
♀ **0UHG31Z** Insertion of Radioactive Element into Vagina, Percutaneous Approach
♀ **0UHG41Z** Insertion of Radioactive Element into Vagina, Percutaneous Endoscopic Approach
♀ **0UHG71Z** Insertion of Radioactive Element into Vagina, Via Natural or Artificial Opening
♀ **0UHG7GZ** Insertion of Pessary into Vagina, Via Natural or Artificial Opening
♀ **0UHG81Z** Insertion of Radioactive Element into Vagina, Via Natural or Artificial Opening Endoscopic
♀ **0UHG8GZ** Insertion of Pessary into Vagina, Via Natural or Artificial Opening Endoscopic
♀ **0UHGX1Z** Insertion of Radioactive Element into Vagina, External Approach
♀ **0UHH03Z** Insertion of Infusion Device into Vagina and Cul-de-sac, Open Approach
♀ **0UHH33Z** Insertion of Infusion Device into Vagina and Cul-de-sac, Percutaneous Approach
♀ **0UHH43Z** Insertion of Infusion Device into Vagina and Cul-de-sac, Percutaneous Endoscopic Approach
♀ **0UHH73Z** Insertion of Infusion Device into Vagina and Cul-de-sac, Via Natural or Artificial Opening
♀ **0UHH83Z** Insertion of Infusion Device into Vagina and Cul-de-sac, Via Natural or Artificial Opening Endoscopic

0UJ – Female Reproductive System, Inspection

Review Coding Guidelines B3.11a, B3.11b and B3.11c

♀ **0UJ30ZZ** Inspection of Ovary, Open Approach
♀ **0UJ33ZZ** Inspection of Ovary, Percutaneous Approach
♀ **0UJ34ZZ** Inspection of Ovary, Percutaneous Endoscopic Approach

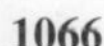

♀0UJ3XZZ Inspection of Ovary, External Approach
♀0UJ80ZZ Inspection of Fallopian Tube, Open Approach
♀0UJ83ZZ Inspection of Fallopian Tube, Percutaneous Approach
♀0UJ84ZZ Inspection of Fallopian Tube, Percutaneous Endoscopic Approach
♀0UJ87ZZ Inspection of Fallopian Tube, Via Natural or Artificial Opening
♀0UJ88ZZ Inspection of Fallopian Tube, Via Natural or Artificial Opening Endoscopic
♀0UJ8XZZ Inspection of Fallopian Tube, External Approach
♀ 0UJD0ZZ Inspection of Uterus and Cervix, Open Approach
♀ 0UJD3ZZ Inspection of Uterus and Cervix, Percutaneous Approach
♀ 0UJD4ZZ Inspection of Uterus and Cervix, Percutaneous Endoscopic Approach
♀ 0UJD7ZZ Inspection of Uterus and Cervix, Via Natural or Artificial Opening
♀ 0UJD8ZZ Inspection of Uterus and Cervix, Via Natural or Artificial Opening Endoscopic
♀ 0UJDXZZ Inspection of Uterus and Cervix, External Approach
♀ 0UJH0ZZ Inspection of Vagina and Cul-de-sac, Open Approach
♀ 0UJH3ZZ Inspection of Vagina and Cul-de-sac, Percutaneous Approach
♀ 0UJH4ZZ Inspection of Vagina and Cul-de-sac, Percutaneous Endoscopic Approach
♀ 0UJH7ZZ Inspection of Vagina and Cul-de-sac, Via Natural or Artificial Opening
♀ 0UJH8ZZ Inspection of Vagina and Cul-de-sac, Via Natural or Artificial Opening Endoscopic
♀ 0UJHXZZ Inspection of Vagina and Cul-de-sac, External Approach
♀ 0UJM0ZZ Inspection of Vulva, Open Approach
♀ 0UJMXZZ Inspection of Vulva, External Approach

0UL – Female Reproductive System, Occlusion

♀0UL50CZ Occlusion of Right Fallopian Tube with Extraluminal Device, Open Approach
♀0UL50DZ Occlusion of Right Fallopian Tube with Intraluminal Device, Open Approach
♀0UL50ZZ Occlusion of Right Fallopian Tube, Open Approach
♀0UL53CZ Occlusion of Right Fallopian Tube with Extraluminal Device, Percutaneous Approach
♀0UL53DZ Occlusion of Right Fallopian Tube with Intraluminal Device, Percutaneous Approach
♀0UL53ZZ Occlusion of Right Fallopian Tube, Percutaneous Approach
♀0UL54CZ Occlusion of Right Fallopian Tube with Extraluminal Device, Percutaneous Endoscopic Approach
♀0UL54DZ Occlusion of Right Fallopian Tube with Intraluminal Device, Percutaneous Endoscopic Approach
♀0UL54ZZ Occlusion of Right Fallopian Tube, Percutaneous Endoscopic Approach
♀0UL57DZ Occlusion of Right Fallopian Tube with Intraluminal Device, Via Natural or Artificial Opening
♀0UL57ZZ Occlusion of Right Fallopian Tube, Via Natural or Artificial Opening
♀0UL58DZ Occlusion of Right Fallopian Tube with Intraluminal Device, Via Natural or Artificial Opening Endoscopic
♀0UL58ZZ Occlusion of Right Fallopian Tube, Via Natural or Artificial Opening Endoscopic
♀0UL60CZ Occlusion of Left Fallopian Tube with Extraluminal Device, Open Approach
♀0UL60DZ Occlusion of Left Fallopian Tube with Intraluminal Device, Open Approach
♀0UL60ZZ Occlusion of Left Fallopian Tube, Open Approach
♀ 0UL63CZ Occlusion of Left Fallopian Tube with Extraluminal Device, Percutaneous Approach
♀ 0UL63DZ Occlusion of Left Fallopian Tube with Intraluminal Device, Percutaneous Approach
♀ 0UL63ZZ Occlusion of Left Fallopian Tube, Percutaneous Approach
♀ 0UL64CZ Occlusion of Left Fallopian Tube with Extraluminal Device, Percutaneous Endoscopic Approach
♀ 0UL64DZ Occlusion of Left Fallopian Tube with Intraluminal Device, Percutaneous Endoscopic Approach
♀ 0UL64ZZ Occlusion of Left Fallopian Tube, Percutaneous Endoscopic Approach
♀ 0UL67DZ Occlusion of Left Fallopian Tube with Intraluminal Device, Via Natural or Artificial Opening
♀ 0UL67ZZ Occlusion of Left Fallopian Tube, Via Natural or Artificial Opening
♀ 0UL68DZ Occlusion of Left Fallopian Tube with Intraluminal Device, Via Natural or Artificial Opening Endoscopic
♀ 0UL68ZZ Occlusion of Left Fallopian Tube, Via Natural or Artificial Opening Endoscopic
♀ ▲ 0UL70CZ Occlusion of Bilateral Fallopian Tubes with Extraluminal Device, Open Approach
♀ ▲ 0UL70DZ Occlusion of Bilateral Fallopian Tubes with Intraluminal Device, Open Approach
♀ ▲ 0UL70ZZ Occlusion of Bilateral Fallopian Tubes, Open Approach
♀ ▲ 0UL73CZ Occlusion of Bilateral Fallopian Tubes with Extraluminal Device, Percutaneous Approach
♀ ▲ 0UL73DZ Occlusion of Bilateral Fallopian Tubes with Intraluminal Device, Percutaneous Approach
♀ ▲ 0UL73ZZ Occlusion of Bilateral Fallopian Tubes, Percutaneous Approach
♀ ▲ 0UL74CZ Occlusion of Bilateral Fallopian Tubes with Extraluminal Device, Percutaneous Endoscopic Approach
♀ ▲ 0UL74DZ Occlusion of Bilateral Fallopian Tubes with Intraluminal Device, Percutaneous Endoscopic Approach
♀ ▲ 0UL74ZZ Occlusion of Bilateral Fallopian Tubes, Percutaneous Endoscopic Approach
♀ ▲ 0UL77DZ Occlusion of Bilateral Fallopian Tubes with Intraluminal Device, Via Natural or Artificial Opening
♀ ▲ 0UL77ZZ Occlusion of Bilateral Fallopian Tubes, Via Natural or Artificial Opening
♀ ▲ 0UL78DZ Occlusion of Bilateral Fallopian Tubes with Intraluminal Device, Via Natural or Artificial Opening Endoscopic
♀ ▲ 0UL78ZZ Occlusion of Bilateral Fallopian Tubes, Via Natural or Artificial Opening Endoscopic
♀ 0ULF7DZ Occlusion of Cul-de-sac with Intraluminal Device, Via Natural or Artificial Opening
♀ 0ULF7ZZ Occlusion of Cul-de-sac, Via Natural or Artificial Opening
♀ 0ULF8DZ Occlusion of Cul-de-sac with Intraluminal Device, Via Natural or Artificial Opening Endoscopic
♀ 0ULF8ZZ Occlusion of Cul-de-sac, Via Natural or Artificial Opening Endoscopic
♀ 0ULG7DZ Occlusion of Vagina with Intraluminal Device, Via Natural or Artificial Opening
♀ 0ULG7ZZ Occlusion of Vagina, Via Natural or Artificial Opening
♀ 0ULG8DZ Occlusion of Vagina with Intraluminal Device, Via Natural or Artificial Opening Endoscopic
♀ 0ULG8ZZ Occlusion of Vagina, Via Natural or Artificial Opening Endoscopic

0UM – Female Reproductive System, Reattachment

♀0UM00ZZ Reattachment of Right Ovary, Open Approach
♀0UM04ZZ Reattachment of Right Ovary, Percutaneous Endoscopic Approach
♀0UM10ZZ Reattachment of Left Ovary, Open Approach
♀0UM14ZZ Reattachment of Left Ovary, Percutaneous Endoscopic Approach
♀0UM20ZZ Reattachment of Bilateral Ovaries, Open Approach
♀0UM24ZZ Reattachment of Bilateral Ovaries, Percutaneous Endoscopic Approach
♀0UM40ZZ Reattachment of Uterine Supporting Structure, Open Approach
♀0UM44ZZ Reattachment of Uterine Supporting Structure, Percutaneous Endoscopic Approach
♀ 0UM50ZZ Reattachment of Right Fallopian Tube, Open Approach
♀ 0UM54ZZ Reattachment of Right Fallopian Tube, Percutaneous Endoscopic Approach
♀ 0UM60ZZ Reattachment of Left Fallopian Tube, Open Approach
♀ 0UM64ZZ Reattachment of Left Fallopian Tube, Percutaneous Endoscopic Approach
♀ 0UM70ZZ Reattachment of Bilateral Fallopian Tubes, Open Approach
♀ 0UM74ZZ Reattachment of Bilateral Fallopian Tubes, Percutaneous Endoscopic Approach
♀ 0UM90ZZ Reattachment of Uterus, Open Approach
♀ 0UM94ZZ Reattachment of Uterus, Percutaneous Endoscopic Approach
♀ 0UMC0ZZ Reattachment of Cervix, Open Approach
♀ 0UMC4ZZ Reattachment of Cervix, Percutaneous Endoscopic Approach
♀ 0UMF0ZZ Reattachment of Cul-de-sac, Open Approach
♀ 0UMF4ZZ Reattachment of Cul-de-sac, Percutaneous Endoscopic Approach
♀ 0UMG0ZZ Reattachment of Vagina, Open Approach
♀ 0UMG4ZZ Reattachment of Vagina, Percutaneous Endoscopic Approach
♀ 0UMJXZZ Reattachment of Clitoris, External Approach
♀ 0UMK0ZZ Reattachment of Hymen, Open Approach
♀ 0UMK4ZZ Reattachment of Hymen, Percutaneous Endoscopic Approach
♀ 0UMKXZZ Reattachment of Hymen, External Approach
♀ 0UMMXZZ Reattachment of Vulva, External Approach

0UN – Female Reproductive System, Release

Review Coding Guideline B3.13

Review Coding Guideline B3.14

♀ **0UN00ZZ** Release Right Ovary, Open Approach
♀ **0UN03ZZ** Release Right Ovary, Percutaneous Approach
♀ **0UN04ZZ** Release Right Ovary, Percutaneous Endoscopic Approach
♀ **0UN10ZZ** Release Left Ovary, Open Approach
♀ **0UN13ZZ** Release Left Ovary, Percutaneous Approach
♀ **0UN14ZZ** Release Left Ovary, Percutaneous Endoscopic Approach
♀ **0UN20ZZ** Release Bilateral Ovaries, Open Approach
♀ **0UN23ZZ** Release Bilateral Ovaries, Percutaneous Approach
♀ **0UN24ZZ** Release Bilateral Ovaries, Percutaneous Endoscopic Approach
♀ **0UN40ZZ** Release Uterine Supporting Structure, Open Approach
♀ **0UN43ZZ** Release Uterine Supporting Structure, Percutaneous Approach
♀ **0UN44ZZ** Release Uterine Supporting Structure, Percutaneous Endoscopic Approach
♀ **0UN50ZZ** Release Right Fallopian Tube, Open Approach
♀ **0UN53ZZ** Release Right Fallopian Tube, Percutaneous Approach
♀ **0UN54ZZ** Release Right Fallopian Tube, Percutaneous Endoscopic Approach
♀ **0UN57ZZ** Release Right Fallopian Tube, Via Natural or Artificial Opening
♀ **0UN58ZZ** Release Right Fallopian Tube, Via Natural or Artificial Opening Endoscopic
♀ **0UN60ZZ** Release Left Fallopian Tube, Open Approach
♀ **0UN63ZZ** Release Left Fallopian Tube, Percutaneous Approach
♀ **0UN64ZZ** Release Left Fallopian Tube, Percutaneous Endoscopic Approach
♀ **0UN67ZZ** Release Left Fallopian Tube, Via Natural or Artificial Opening
♀ **0UN68ZZ** Release Left Fallopian Tube, Via Natural or Artificial Opening Endoscopic
♀ **0UN70ZZ** Release Bilateral Fallopian Tubes, Open Approach
♀ **0UN73ZZ** Release Bilateral Fallopian Tubes, Percutaneous Approach
♀ **0UN74ZZ** Release Bilateral Fallopian Tubes, Percutaneous Endoscopic Approach
♀ **0UN77ZZ** Release Bilateral Fallopian Tubes, Via Natural or Artificial Opening
♀ **0UN78ZZ** Release Bilateral Fallopian Tubes, Via Natural or Artificial Opening Endoscopic
♀ **0UN90ZZ** Release Uterus, Open Approach
♀ **0UN93ZZ** Release Uterus, Percutaneous Approach
♀ **0UN94ZZ** Release Uterus, Percutaneous Endoscopic Approach
♀ **0UN97ZZ** Release Uterus, Via Natural or Artificial Opening
♀ **0UN98ZZ** Release Uterus, Via Natural or Artificial Opening Endoscopic
♀ **0UNC0ZZ** Release Cervix, Open Approach
♀ **0UNC3ZZ** Release Cervix, Percutaneous Approach
♀ **0UNC4ZZ** Release Cervix, Percutaneous Endoscopic Approach
♀ **0UNC7ZZ** Release Cervix, Via Natural or Artificial Opening
♀ **0UNC8ZZ** Release Cervix, Via Natural or Artificial Opening Endoscopic
♀ **0UNF0ZZ** Release Cul-de-sac, Open Approach
♀ **0UNF3ZZ** Release Cul-de-sac, Percutaneous Approach
♀ **0UNF4ZZ** Release Cul-de-sac, Percutaneous Endoscopic Approach
♀ **0UNF7ZZ** Release Cul-de-sac, Via Natural or Artificial Opening
♀ **0UNF8ZZ** Release Cul-de-sac, Via Natural or Artificial Opening Endoscopic
♀ **0UNG0ZZ** Release Vagina, Open Approach
♀ **0UNG3ZZ** Release Vagina, Percutaneous Approach
♀ **0UNG4ZZ** Release Vagina, Percutaneous Endoscopic Approach
♀ **0UNG7ZZ** Release Vagina, Via Natural or Artificial Opening
♀ **0UNG8ZZ** Release Vagina, Via Natural or Artificial Opening Endoscopic
♀ **0UNGXZZ** Release Vagina, External Approach
♀ **0UNJ0ZZ** Release Clitoris, Open Approach
♀ **0UNJXZZ** Release Clitoris, External Approach
♀ **0UNK0ZZ** Release Hymen, Open Approach
♀ **0UNK3ZZ** Release Hymen, Percutaneous Approach
♀ **0UNK4ZZ** Release Hymen, Percutaneous Endoscopic Approach
♀ **0UNK7ZZ** Release Hymen, Via Natural or Artificial Opening
♀ **0UNK8ZZ** Release Hymen, Via Natural or Artificial Opening Endoscopic
♀ **0UNKXZZ** Release Hymen, External Approach
♀ **0UNL0ZZ** Release Vestibular Gland, Open Approach
♀ **0UNLXZZ** Release Vestibular Gland, External Approach
♀ **0UNM0ZZ** Release Vulva, Open Approach
♀ **0UNMXZZ** Release Vulva, External Approach

0UP – Female Reproductive System, Removal

Review Coding Guideline B6.1c

♀ **0UP300Z** Removal of Drainage Device from Ovary, Open Approach
♀ **0UP303Z** Removal of Infusion Device from Ovary, Open Approach
♀ **0UP330Z** Removal of Drainage Device from Ovary, Percutaneous Approach
♀ **0UP333Z** Removal of Infusion Device from Ovary, Percutaneous Approach
♀ **0UP340Z** Removal of Drainage Device from Ovary, Percutaneous Endoscopic Approach
♀ **0UP343Z** Removal of Infusion Device from Ovary, Percutaneous Endoscopic Approach
♀ **0UP3X0Z** Removal of Drainage Device from Ovary, External Approach
♀ **0UP3X3Z** Removal of Infusion Device from Ovary, External Approach
♀ **0UP800Z** Removal of Drainage Device from Fallopian Tube, Open Approach
♀ **0UP803Z** Removal of Infusion Device from Fallopian Tube, Open Approach
♀ **0UP807Z** Removal of Autologous Tissue Substitute from Fallopian Tube, Open Approach
♀ **0UP80CZ** Removal of Extraluminal Device from Fallopian Tube, Open Approach
♀ **0UP80DZ** Removal of Intraluminal Device from Fallopian Tube, Open Approach
♀ **0UP80JZ** Removal of Synthetic Substitute from Fallopian Tube, Open Approach
♀ **0UP80KZ** Removal of Nonautologous Tissue Substitute from Fallopian Tube, Open Approach
♀ **0UP830Z** Removal of Drainage Device from Fallopian Tube, Percutaneous Approach
♀ **0UP833Z** Removal of Infusion Device from Fallopian Tube, Percutaneous Approach
♀ **0UP837Z** Removal of Autologous Tissue Substitute from Fallopian Tube, Percutaneous Approach
♀ **0UP83CZ** Removal of Extraluminal Device from Fallopian Tube, Percutaneous Approach
♀ **0UP83DZ** Removal of Intraluminal Device from Fallopian Tube, Percutaneous Approach
♀ **0UP83JZ** Removal of Synthetic Substitute from Fallopian Tube, Percutaneous Approach
♀ **0UP83KZ** Removal of Nonautologous Tissue Substitute from Fallopian Tube, Percutaneous Approach
♀ **0UP840Z** Removal of Drainage Device from Fallopian Tube, Percutaneous Endoscopic Approach
♀ **0UP843Z** Removal of Infusion Device from Fallopian Tube, Percutaneous Endoscopic Approach
♀ **0UP847Z** Removal of Autologous Tissue Substitute from Fallopian Tube, Percutaneous Endoscopic Approach
♀ **0UP84CZ** Removal of Extraluminal Device from Fallopian Tube, Percutaneous Endoscopic Approach
♀ **0UP84DZ** Removal of Intraluminal Device from Fallopian Tube, Percutaneous Endoscopic Approach
♀ **0UP84JZ** Removal of Synthetic Substitute from Fallopian Tube, Percutaneous Endoscopic Approach
♀ **0UP84KZ** Removal of Nonautologous Tissue Substitute from Fallopian Tube, Percutaneous Endoscopic Approach
♀ **0UP870Z** Removal of Drainage Device from Fallopian Tube, Via Natural or Artificial Opening
♀ **0UP873Z** Removal of Infusion Device from Fallopian Tube, Via Natural or Artificial Opening
♀ **0UP877Z** Removal of Autologous Tissue Substitute from Fallopian Tube, Via Natural or Artificial Opening
♀ **0UP87CZ** Removal of Extraluminal Device from Fallopian Tube, Via Natural or Artificial Opening
♀ **0UP87DZ** Removal of Intraluminal Device from Fallopian Tube, Via Natural or Artificial Opening
♀ **0UP87JZ** Removal of Synthetic Substitute from Fallopian Tube, Via Natural or Artificial Opening
♀ **0UP87KZ** Removal of Nonautologous Tissue Substitute from Fallopian Tube, Via Natural or Artificial Opening
♀ **0UP880Z** Removal of Drainage Device from Fallopian Tube, Via Natural or Artificial Opening Endoscopic

♀0UP883Z Removal of Infusion Device from Fallopian Tube, Via Natural or Artificial Opening Endoscopic
♀0UP887Z Removal of Autologous Tissue Substitute from Fallopian Tube, Via Natural or Artificial Opening Endoscopic
♀0UP88CZ Removal of Extraluminal Device from Fallopian Tube, Via Natural or Artificial Opening Endoscopic
♀0UP88DZ Removal of Intraluminal Device from Fallopian Tube, Via Natural or Artificial Opening Endoscopic
♀0UP88JZ Removal of Synthetic Substitute from Fallopian Tube, Via Natural or Artificial Opening Endoscopic
♀0UP88KZ Removal of Nonautologous Tissue Substitute from Fallopian Tube, Via Natural or Artificial Opening Endoscopic
♀0UP8X0Z Removal of Drainage Device from Fallopian Tube, External Approach
♀0UP8X3Z Removal of Infusion Device from Fallopian Tube, External Approach
♀0UP8XDZ Removal of Intraluminal Device from Fallopian Tube, External Approach
♀0UPD00Z Removal of Drainage Device from Uterus and Cervix, Open Approach
♀0UPD01Z Removal of Radioactive Element from Uterus and Cervix, Open Approach
♀0UPD03Z Removal of Infusion Device from Uterus and Cervix, Open Approach
♀0UPD07Z Removal of Autologous Tissue Substitute from Uterus and Cervix, Open Approach
♀0UPD0CZ Removal of Extraluminal Device from Uterus and Cervix, Open Approach
♀0UPD0DZ Removal of Intraluminal Device from Uterus and Cervix, Open Approach
♀0UPD0HZ Removal of Contraceptive Device from Uterus and Cervix, Open Approach
♀0UPD0JZ Removal of Synthetic Substitute from Uterus and Cervix, Open Approach
♀0UPD0KZ Removal of Nonautologous Tissue Substitute from Uterus and Cervix, Open Approach
♀0UPD30Z Removal of Drainage Device from Uterus and Cervix, Percutaneous Approach
♀0UPD31Z Removal of Radioactive Element from Uterus and Cervix, Percutaneous Approach
♀0UPD33Z Removal of Infusion Device from Uterus and Cervix, Percutaneous Approach
♀0UPD37Z Removal of Autologous Tissue Substitute from Uterus and Cervix, Percutaneous Approach
♀0UPD3CZ Removal of Extraluminal Device from Uterus and Cervix, Percutaneous Approach
♀0UPD3DZ Removal of Intraluminal Device from Uterus and Cervix, Percutaneous Approach
♀0UPD3HZ Removal of Contraceptive Device from Uterus and Cervix, Percutaneous Approach
♀0UPD3JZ Removal of Synthetic Substitute from Uterus and Cervix, Percutaneous Approach
♀0UPD3KZ Removal of Nonautologous Tissue Substitute from Uterus and Cervix, Percutaneous Approach
♀0UPD40Z Removal of Drainage Device from Uterus and Cervix, Percutaneous Endoscopic Approach
♀0UPD41Z Removal of Radioactive Element from Uterus and Cervix, Percutaneous Endoscopic Approach
♀0UPD43Z Removal of Infusion Device from Uterus and Cervix, Percutaneous Endoscopic Approach
♀ 0UPD47Z Removal of Autologous Tissue Substitute from Uterus and Cervix, Percutaneous Endoscopic Approach
♀ 0UPD4CZ Removal of Extraluminal Device from Uterus and Cervix, Percutaneous Endoscopic Approach
♀ 0UPD4DZ Removal of Intraluminal Device from Uterus and Cervix, Percutaneous Endoscopic Approach
♀ 0UPD4HZ Removal of Contraceptive Device from Uterus and Cervix, Percutaneous Endoscopic Approach
♀ 0UPD4JZ Removal of Synthetic Substitute from Uterus and Cervix, Percutaneous Endoscopic Approach
♀ 0UPD4KZ Removal of Nonautologous Tissue Substitute from Uterus and Cervix, Percutaneous Endoscopic Approach
♀ 0UPD70Z Removal of Drainage Device from Uterus and Cervix, Via Natural or Artificial Opening
♀ 0UPD71Z Removal of Radioactive Element from Uterus and Cervix, Via Natural or Artificial Opening
♀ 0UPD73Z Removal of Infusion Device from Uterus and Cervix, Via Natural or Artificial Opening
♀ 0UPD77Z Removal of Autologous Tissue Substitute from Uterus and Cervix, Via Natural or Artificial Opening
♀ 0UPD7CZ Removal of Extraluminal Device from Uterus and Cervix, Via Natural or Artificial Opening
♀ 0UPD7DZ Removal of Intraluminal Device from Uterus and Cervix, Via Natural or Artificial Opening
♀ 0UPD7HZ Removal of Contraceptive Device from Uterus and Cervix, Via Natural or Artificial Opening
♀ 0UPD7JZ Removal of Synthetic Substitute from Uterus and Cervix, Via Natural or Artificial Opening
♀ 0UPD7KZ Removal of Nonautologous Tissue Substitute from Uterus and Cervix, Via Natural or Artificial Opening
♀ 0UPD80Z Removal of Drainage Device from Uterus and Cervix, Via Natural or Artificial Opening Endoscopic
♀ 0UPD81Z Removal of Radioactive Element from Uterus and Cervix, Via Natural or Artificial Opening Endoscopic
♀ 0UPD83Z Removal of Infusion Device from Uterus and Cervix, Via Natural or Artificial Opening Endoscopic
♀ 0UPD87Z Removal of Autologous Tissue Substitute from Uterus and Cervix, Via Natural or Artificial Opening Endoscopic
♀ 0UPD8CZ Removal of Extraluminal Device from Uterus and Cervix, Via Natural or Artificial Opening Endoscopic
♀ 0UPD8DZ Removal of Intraluminal Device from Uterus and Cervix, Via Natural or Artificial Opening Endoscopic
♀ 0UPD8HZ Removal of Contraceptive Device from Uterus and Cervix, Via Natural or Artificial Opening Endoscopic
♀ 0UPD8JZ Removal of Synthetic Substitute from Uterus and Cervix, Via Natural or Artificial Opening Endoscopic
♀ 0UPD8KZ Removal of Nonautologous Tissue Substitute from Uterus and Cervix, Via Natural or Artificial Opening Endoscopic
♀ 0UPDX0Z Removal of Drainage Device from Uterus and Cervix, External Approach
♀ 0UPDX3Z Removal of Infusion Device from Uterus and Cervix, External Approach
♀ 0UPDXDZ Removal of Intraluminal Device from Uterus and Cervix, External Approach
♀ 0UPDXHZ Removal of Contraceptive Device from Uterus and Cervix, External Approach
♀ 0UPH00Z Removal of Drainage Device from Vagina and Cul-de-sac, Open Approach
♀ 0UPH01Z Removal of Radioactive Element from Vagina and Cul-de-sac, Open Approach
♀ 0UPH03Z Removal of Infusion Device from Vagina and Cul-de-sac, Open Approach
♀ 0UPH07Z Removal of Autologous Tissue Substitute from Vagina and Cul-de-sac, Open Approach
♀ 0UPH0DZ Removal of Intraluminal Device from Vagina and Cul-de-sac, Open Approach
♀ 0UPH0JZ Removal of Synthetic Substitute from Vagina and Cul-de-sac, OpenApproach
♀ 0UPH0KZ Removal of Nonautologous Tissue Substitute from Vagina and Cul-de-sac, Open Approach
♀ 0UPH30Z Removal of Drainage Device from Vagina and Cul-de-sac, Percutaneous Approach
♀ 0UPH31Z Removal of Radioactive Element from Vagina and Cul-de-sac, Percutaneous Approach
♀ 0UPH33Z Removal of Infusion Device from Vagina and Cul-de-sac, Percutaneous Approach
♀ 0UPH37Z Removal of Autologous Tissue Substitute from Vagina and Cul-de-sac, Percutaneous Approach
♀ 0UPH3DZ Removal of Intraluminal Device from Vagina and Cul-de-sac, Percutaneous Approach
♀ 0UPH3JZ Removal of Synthetic Substitute from Vagina and Cul-de-sac, Percutaneous Approach
♀ 0UPH3KZ Removal of Nonautologous Tissue Substitute from Vagina and Cul-de-sac, Percutaneous Approach
♀ 0UPH40Z Removal of Drainage Device from Vagina and Cul-de-sac, Percutaneous Endoscopic Approach
♀ 0UPH41Z Removal of Radioactive Element from Vagina and Cul-de-sac, Percutaneous Endoscopic Approach
♀ 0UPH43Z Removal of Infusion Device from Vagina and Cul-de-sac, Percutaneous Endoscopic Approach
♀ 0UPH47Z Removal of Autologous Tissue Substitute from Vagina and Cul-de-sac, Percutaneous Endoscopic Approach
♀ 0UPH4DZ Removal of Intraluminal Device from Vagina and Cul-de-sac, Percutaneous Endoscopic Approach
♀ 0UPH4JZ Removal of Synthetic Substitute from Vagina and Cul-de-sac, Percutaneous Endoscopic Approach
♀ 0UPH4KZ Removal of Nonautologous Tissue Substitute from Vagina and Cul-de-sac, Percutaneous Endoscopic Approach
♀ 0UPH70Z Removal of Drainage Device from Vagina and Cul-de-sac, Via Natural or Artificial Opening
♀ 0UPH71Z Removal of Radioactive Element from Vagina and Cul-de-sac, Via Natural or Artificial Opening
♀ 0UPH73Z Removal of Infusion Device from Vagina and Cul-de-sac, Via Natural or Artificial Opening
♀ 0UPH77Z Removal of Autologous Tissue Substitute from Vagina and Cul-de-sac, Via Natural or Artificial Opening
♀ 0UPH7DZ Removal of Intraluminal Device from Vagina and Cul-de-sac, Via Natural or Artificial Opening

♀ **0UPH7JZ** Removal of Synthetic Substitute from Vagina and Cul-de-sac, Via Natural or Artificial Opening
♀ **0UPH7KZ** Removal of Nonautologous Tissue Substitute from Vagina and Cul-de-sac, Via Natural or Artificial Opening
♀ **0UPH80Z** Removal of Drainage Device from Vagina and Cul-de-sac, Via Natural or Artificial Opening Endoscopic
♀ **0UPH81Z** Removal of Radioactive Element from Vagina and Cul-de-sac, Via Natural or Artificial Opening Endoscopic
♀ **0UPH83Z** Removal of Infusion Device from Vagina and Cul-de-sac, Via Natural or Artificial Opening Endoscopic
♀ **0UPH87Z** Removal of Autologous Tissue Substitute from Vagina and Cul-de-sac, Via Natural or Artificial Opening Endoscopic
♀ **0UPH8DZ** Removal of Intraluminal Device from Vagina and Cul-de-sac, Via Natural or Artificial Opening Endoscopic
♀ **0UPH8JZ** Removal of Synthetic Substitute from Vagina and Cul-de-sac, Via Natural or Artificial Opening Endoscopic
♀ **0UPH8KZ** Removal of Nonautologous Tissue Substitute from Vagina and Cul-de-sac, Via Natural or Artificial Opening Endoscopic
♀ **0UPHX0Z** Removal of Drainage Device from Vagina and Cul-de-sac, External Approach
♀ **0UPHX1Z** Removal of Radioactive Element from Vagina and Cul-de-sac, External Approach
♀ **0UPHX3Z** Removal of Infusion Device from Vagina and Cul-de-sac, External Approach
♀ **0UPHXDZ** Removal of Intraluminal Device from Vagina and Cul-de-sac, External Approach
♀ **0UPM00Z** Removal of Drainage Device from Vulva, Open Approach
♀ **0UPM07Z** Removal of Autologous Tissue Substitute from Vulva, Open Approach
♀ **0UPM0JZ** Removal of Synthetic Substitute from Vulva, Open Approach
♀ **0UPM0KZ** Removal of Nonautologous Tissue Substitute from Vulva, Open Approach
♀ **0UPMX0Z** Removal of Drainage Device from Vulva, External Approach

0UQ – Female Reproductive System, Repair

♀ **0UQ00ZZ** Repair Right Ovary, Open Approach
♀ **0UQ03ZZ** Repair Right Ovary, Percutaneous Approach
♀ **0UQ04ZZ** Repair Right Ovary, Percutaneous Endoscopic Approach
♀ **0UQ10ZZ** Repair Left Ovary, Open Approach
♀ **0UQ13ZZ** Repair Left Ovary, Percutaneous Approach
♀ **0UQ14ZZ** Repair Left Ovary, Percutaneous Endoscopic Approach
♀ **0UQ20ZZ** Repair Bilateral Ovaries, Open Approach
♀ **0UQ23ZZ** Repair Bilateral Ovaries, Percutaneous Approach
♀ **0UQ24ZZ** Repair Bilateral Ovaries, Percutaneous Endoscopic Approach
♀ **0UQ40ZZ** Repair Uterine Supporting Structure, Open Approach
♀ **0UQ43ZZ** Repair Uterine Supporting Structure, Percutaneous Approach
♀ **0UQ44ZZ** Repair Uterine Supporting Structure, Percutaneous Endoscopic Approach
♀ **0UQ50ZZ** Repair Right Fallopian Tube, Open Approach
♀ **0UQ53ZZ** Repair Right Fallopian Tube, Percutaneous Approach
♀ **0UQ54ZZ** Repair Right Fallopian Tube, Percutaneous Endoscopic Approach
♀ **0UQ57ZZ** Repair Right Fallopian Tube, Via Natural or Artificial Opening
♀ **0UQ58ZZ** Repair Right Fallopian Tube, Via Natural or Artificial Opening Endoscopic
♀ **0UQ60ZZ** Repair Left Fallopian Tube, Open Approach
♀ **0UQ63ZZ** Repair Left Fallopian Tube, Percutaneous Approach
♀ **0UQ64ZZ** Repair Left Fallopian Tube, Percutaneous Endoscopic Approach
♀ **0UQ67ZZ** Repair Left Fallopian Tube, Via Natural or Artificial Opening
♀ **0UQ68ZZ** Repair Left Fallopian Tube, Via Natural or Artificial Opening Endoscopic
♀ **0UQ70ZZ** Repair Bilateral Fallopian Tubes, Open Approach
♀ **0UQ73ZZ** Repair Bilateral Fallopian Tubes, Percutaneous Approach
♀ **0UQ74ZZ** Repair Bilateral Fallopian Tubes, Percutaneous Endoscopic Approach
♀ **0UQ77ZZ** Repair Bilateral Fallopian Tubes, Via Natural or Artificial Opening
♀ **0UQ78ZZ** Repair Bilateral Fallopian Tubes, Via Natural or Artificial Opening Endoscopic
♀ **0UQ90ZZ** Repair Uterus, Open Approach
♀ **0UQ93ZZ** Repair Uterus, Percutaneous Approach
♀ **0UQ94ZZ** Repair Uterus, Percutaneous Endoscopic Approach
♀ **0UQ97ZZ** Repair Uterus, Via Natural or Artificial Opening
♀ **0UQ98ZZ** Repair Uterus, Via Natural or Artificial Opening Endoscopic
♀ **0UQC0ZZ** Repair Cervix, Open Approach
♀ **0UQC3ZZ** Repair Cervix, Percutaneous Approach
♀ **0UQC4ZZ** Repair Cervix, Percutaneous Endoscopic Approach
♀ **0UQC7ZZ** Repair Cervix, Via Natural or Artificial Opening
♀ **0UQC8ZZ** Repair Cervix, Via Natural or Artificial Opening Endoscopic
♀ **0UQF0ZZ** Repair Cul-de-sac, Open Approach
♀ **0UQF3ZZ** Repair Cul-de-sac, Percutaneous Approach
♀ **0UQF4ZZ** Repair Cul-de-sac, Percutaneous Endoscopic Approach
♀ **0UQF7ZZ** Repair Cul-de-sac, Via Natural or Artificial Opening
♀ **0UQF8ZZ** Repair Cul-de-sac, Via Natural or Artificial Opening Endoscopic
♀ **0UQG0ZZ** Repair Vagina, Open Approach
♀ **0UQG3ZZ** Repair Vagina, Percutaneous Approach
♀ **0UQG4ZZ** Repair Vagina, Percutaneous Endoscopic Approach
♀ ● **0UQG7ZZ** Repair Vagina, Via Natural or Artificial Opening
♀ ● **0UQG8ZZ** Repair Vagina, Via Natural or Artificial Opening Endoscopic
♀ ● **0UQGXZZ** Repair Vagina, External Approach
♀ **0UQJ0ZZ** Repair Clitoris, Open Approach
♀ **0UQJXZZ** Repair Clitoris, External Approach
AHA CC: 4Q, 2013, 120-121
♀ **0UQK0ZZ** Repair Hymen, Open Approach
♀ **0UQK3ZZ** Repair Hymen, Percutaneous Approach
♀ **0UQK4ZZ** Repair Hymen, Percutaneous Endoscopic Approach
♀ **0UQK7ZZ** Repair Hymen, Via Natural or Artificial Opening
♀ **0UQK8ZZ** Repair Hymen, Via Natural or Artificial Opening Endoscopic
♀ **0UQKXZZ** Repair Hymen, External Approach
♀ **0UQL0ZZ** Repair Vestibular Gland, Open Approach
♀ **0UQLXZZ** Repair Vestibular Gland, External Approach
♀ ● **0UQM0ZZ** Repair Vulva, Open Approach
♀ ● **0UQMXZZ** Repair Vulva, External Approach

0US – Female Reproductive System, Reposition

♀ **0US00ZZ** Reposition Right Ovary, Open Approach
♀ **0US04ZZ** Reposition Right Ovary, Percutaneous Endoscopic Approach
♀ **0US10ZZ** Reposition Left Ovary, Open Approach
♀ **0US14ZZ** Reposition Left Ovary, Percutaneous Endoscopic Approach
♀ **0US20ZZ** Reposition Bilateral Ovaries, Open Approach
♀ **0US24ZZ** Reposition Bilateral Ovaries, Percutaneous Endoscopic Approach
♀ **0US40ZZ** Reposition Uterine Supporting Structure, Open Approach
♀ **0US44ZZ** Reposition Uterine Supporting Structure, Percutaneous Endoscopic Approach
♀ **0US50ZZ** Reposition Right Fallopian Tube, Open Approach
♀ **0US54ZZ** Reposition Right Fallopian Tube, Percutaneous Endoscopic Approach
♀ **0US60ZZ** Reposition Left Fallopian Tube, Open Approach
♀ **0US64ZZ** Reposition Left Fallopian Tube, Percutaneous Endoscopic Approach
♀ **0US70ZZ** Reposition Bilateral Fallopian Tubes, Open Approach
♀ **0US74ZZ** Reposition Bilateral Fallopian Tubes, Percutaneous Endoscopic Approach
♀ **0US90ZZ** Reposition Uterus, Open Approach
♀ **0US94ZZ** Reposition Uterus, Percutaneous Endoscopic Approach
♀ **0US9XZZ** Reposition Uterus, External Approach
♀ **0USC0ZZ** Reposition Cervix, Open Approach
♀ **0USC4ZZ** Reposition Cervix, Percutaneous Endoscopic Approach
♀ **0USF0ZZ** Reposition Cul-de-sac, Open Approach
♀ **0USF4ZZ** Reposition Cul-de-sac, Percutaneous Endoscopic Approach
♀ **0USG0ZZ** Reposition Vagina, Open Approach
♀ **0USG4ZZ** Reposition Vagina, Percutaneous Endoscopic Approach
♀ **0USGXZZ** Reposition Vagina, External Approach

0UT – Female Reproductive System, Resection

Review Coding Guideline B3.8

♀ **0UT00ZZ** Resection of Right Ovary, Open Approach
AHA CC: 1Q, 2013, 24
♀ **0UT04ZZ** Resection of Right Ovary, Percutaneous Endoscopic Approach
♀ **0UT07ZZ** Resection of Right Ovary, Via Natural or Artificial Opening

♀0UT08ZZ Resection of Right Ovary, Via Natural or Artificial Opening Endoscopic
♀0UT0FZZ Resection of Right Ovary, Via Natural or Artificial Opening With Percutaneous Endoscopic Assistance
♀0UT10ZZ Resection of Left Ovary, Open Approach
♀0UT14ZZ Resection of Left Ovary, Percutaneous Endoscopic Approach
♀0UT17ZZ Resection of Left Ovary, Via Natural or Artificial Opening
♀0UT18ZZ Resection of Left Ovary, Via Natural or Artificial Opening Endoscopic
♀0UT1FZZ Resection of Left Ovary, Via Natural or Artificial Opening With Percutaneous Endoscopic Assistance
♀0UT20ZZ Resection of Bilateral Ovaries, Open Approach
♀0UT24ZZ Resection of Bilateral Ovaries, Percutaneous Endoscopic Approach
♀0UT27ZZ Resection of Bilateral Ovaries, Via Natural or Artificial Opening
♀0UT28ZZ Resection of Bilateral Ovaries, Via Natural or Artificial Opening Endoscopic
♀0UT2FZZ Resection of Bilateral Ovaries, Via Natural or Artificial Opening With Percutaneous Endoscopic Assistance
♀0UT40ZZ Resection of Uterine Supporting Structure, Open Approach
+ Radical hysterectomy when reported with resection of the uterus and cervix. *See table 0UT to construct the Resection codes.*
♀0UT44ZZ Resection of Uterine Supporting Structure, Percutaneous Endoscopic Approach
+ Radical hysterectomy when reported with resection of the uterus and cervix. *See table 0UT to construct the Resection codes.*
♀0UT47ZZ Resection of Uterine Supporting Structure, Via Natural or Artificial Opening
+ Radical hysterectomy when reported with resection of the uterus and cervix. *See table 0UT to construct the Resection codes.*
♀ 0UT48ZZ Resection of Uterine Supporting Structure, Via Natural or Artificial Opening Endoscopic
+ Radical hysterectomy when reported with resection of the uterus and cervix. *See table 0UT to construct the Resection codes.*
♀ 0UT50ZZ Resection of Right Fallopian Tube, Open Approach
♀ 0UT54ZZ Resection of Right Fallopian Tube, Percutaneous Endoscopic Approach
♀ 0UT57ZZ Resection of Right Fallopian Tube, Via Natural or Artificial Opening
♀ 0UT58ZZ Resection of Right Fallopian Tube, Via Natural or Artificial Opening Endoscopic
♀ 0UT5FZZ Resection of Right Fallopian Tube, Via Natural or Artificial Opening With Percutaneous Endoscopic Assistance
♀ 0UT60ZZ Resection of Left Fallopian Tube, Open Approach
♀ 0UT64ZZ Resection of Left Fallopian Tube, Percutaneous Endoscopic Approach
♀ 0UT67ZZ Resection of Left Fallopian Tube, Via Natural or Artificial Opening
♀ 0UT68ZZ Resection of Left Fallopian Tube, Via Natural or Artificial Opening Endoscopic
♀ 0UT6FZZ Resection of Left Fallopian Tube, Via Natural or Artificial Opening With Percutaneous Endoscopic Assistance
♀ 0UT70ZZ Resection of Bilateral Fallopian Tubes, Open Approach
♀ 0UT74ZZ Resection of Bilateral Fallopian Tubes, Percutaneous Endoscopic Approach
♀ 0UT77ZZ Resection of Bilateral Fallopian Tubes, Via Natural or Artificial Opening
♀ 0UT78ZZ Resection of Bilateral Fallopian Tubes, Via Natural or Artificial Opening Endoscopic
♀ 0UT7FZZ Resection of Bilateral Fallopian Tubes, Via Natural or Artificial Opening With Percutaneous Endoscopic Assistance
♀ 0UT90ZZ Resection of Uterus, Open Approach
AHA CC: 3Q, 2013, 28
♀ 0UT94ZZ Resection of Uterus, Percutaneous Endoscopic Approach
♀ 0UT97ZZ Resection of Uterus, Via Natural or Artificial Opening
♀ 0UT98ZZ Resection of Uterus, Via Natural or Artificial Opening Endoscopic
♀ 0UT9FZZ Resection of Uterus, Via Natural or Artificial Opening With Percutaneous Endoscopic Assistance
♀ 0UTC0ZZ Resection of Cervix, Open Approach
AHA CC: 3Q, 2013, 28
♀ 0UTC4ZZ Resection of Cervix, Percutaneous Endoscopic Approach
♀ 0UTC7ZZ Resection of Cervix, Via Natural or Artificial Opening
♀ 0UTC8ZZ Resection of Cervix, Via Natural or Artificial Opening Endoscopic
♀ 0UTF0ZZ Resection of Cul-de-sac, Open Approach
♀ 0UTF4ZZ Resection of Cul-de-sac, Percutaneous Endoscopic Approach
♀ 0UTF7ZZ Resection of Cul-de-sac, Via Natural or Artificial Opening
♀ 0UTF8ZZ Resection of Cul-de-sac, Via Natural or Artificial Opening Endoscopic
♀ 0UTG0ZZ Resection of Vagina, Open Approach
♀ 0UTG4ZZ Resection of Vagina, Percutaneous Endoscopic Approach
♀ 0UTG7ZZ Resection of Vagina, Via Natural or Artificial Opening
♀ 0UTG8ZZ Resection of Vagina, Via Natural or Artificial Opening Endoscopic
♀ 0UTJ0ZZ Resection of Clitoris, Open Approach
♀ 0UTJXZZ Resection of Clitoris, External Approach
♀ 0UTK0ZZ Resection of Hymen, Open Approach
♀ 0UTK4ZZ Resection of Hymen, Percutaneous Endoscopic Approach
♀ 0UTK7ZZ Resection of Hymen, Via Natural or Artificial Opening
♀ 0UTK8ZZ Resection of Hymen, Via Natural or Artificial Opening Endoscopic
♀ 0UTKXZZ Resection of Hymen, External Approach
♀ 0UTL0ZZ Resection of Vestibular Gland, Open Approach
♀ 0UTLXZZ Resection of Vestibular Gland, External Approach
♀ 0UTM0ZZ Resection of Vulva, Open Approach
♀ 0UTMXZZ Resection of Vulva, External Approach

0UU – Female Reproductive System, Supplement

♀0UU407Z Supplement Uterine Supporting Structure with Autologous Tissue Substitute, Open Approach
♀0UU40JZ Supplement Uterine Supporting Structure with Synthetic Substitute, Open Approach
♀0UU40KZ Supplement Uterine Supporting Structure with Nonautologous Tissue Substitute, Open Approach
♀0UU447Z Supplement Uterine Supporting Structure with Autologous Tissue Substitute, Percutaneous Endoscopic Approach
♀0UU44JZ Supplement Uterine Supporting Structure with Synthetic Substitute, Percutaneous Endoscopic Approach
♀0UU44KZ Supplement Uterine Supporting Structure with Nonautologous Tissue Substitute, Percutaneous Endoscopic Approach
♀0UU507Z Supplement Right Fallopian Tube with Autologous Tissue Substitute, Open Approach
♀0UU50JZ Supplement Right Fallopian Tube with Synthetic Substitute, Open Approach
♀0UU50KZ Supplement Right Fallopian Tube with Nonautologous Tissue Substitute, Open Approach
♀0UU547Z Supplement Right Fallopian Tube with Autologous Tissue Substitute, Percutaneous Endoscopic Approach
♀ 0UU54JZ Supplement Right Fallopian Tube with Synthetic Substitute, Percutaneous Endoscopic Approach
♀ 0UU54KZ Supplement Right Fallopian Tube with Nonautologous Tissue Substitute, Percutaneous Endoscopic Approach
♀ 0UU577Z Supplement Right Fallopian Tube with Autologous Tissue Substitute, Via Natural or Artificial Opening
♀ 0UU57JZ Supplement Right Fallopian Tube with Synthetic Substitute, Via Natural or Artificial Opening
♀ 0UU57KZ Supplement Right Fallopian Tube with Nonautologous Tissue Substitute, Via Natural or Artificial Opening
♀ 0UU587Z Supplement Right Fallopian Tube with Autologous Tissue Substitute, Via Natural or Artificial Opening Endoscopic
♀ 0UU58JZ Supplement Right Fallopian Tube with Synthetic Substitute, Via Natural or Artificial Opening Endoscopic
♀ 0UU58KZ Supplement Right Fallopian Tube with Nonautologous Tissue Substitute, Via Natural or Artificial Opening Endoscopic
♀ 0UU607Z Supplement Left Fallopian Tube with Autologous Tissue Substitute, Open Approach
♀ 0UU60JZ Supplement Left Fallopian Tube with Synthetic Substitute, Open Approach
♀ 0UU60KZ Supplement Left Fallopian Tube with Nonautologous Tissue Substitute, Open Approach
♀ 0UU647Z Supplement Left Fallopian Tube with Autologous Tissue Substitute, Percutaneous Endoscopic Approach
♀ 0UU64JZ Supplement Left Fallopian Tube with Synthetic Substitute, Percutaneous Endoscopic Approach
♀ 0UU64KZ Supplement Left Fallopian Tube with Nonautologous Tissue Substitute, Percutaneous Endoscopic Approach
♀ 0UU677Z Supplement Left Fallopian Tube with Autologous Tissue Substitute, Via Natural or Artificial Opening
♀ 0UU67JZ Supplement Left Fallopian Tube with Synthetic Substitute, Via Natural or Artificial Opening
♀ 0UU67KZ Supplement Left Fallopian Tube with Nonautologous Tissue Substitute, Via Natural or Artificial Opening
♀ 0UU687Z Supplement Left Fallopian Tube with Autologous Tissue Substitute, Via Natural or Artificial Opening Endoscopic
♀ 0UU68JZ Supplement Left Fallopian Tube with Synthetic Substitute, Via Natural or Artificial Opening Endoscopic
♀ 0UU68KZ Supplement Left Fallopian Tube with Nonautologous Tissue Substitute, Via Natural or Artificial Opening Endoscopic

♀ **0UU707Z** Supplement Bilateral Fallopian Tubes with Autologous Tissue Substitute, Open Approach
♀ **0UU70JZ** Supplement Bilateral Fallopian Tubes with Synthetic Substitute, Open Approach
♀ **0UU70KZ** Supplement Bilateral Fallopian Tubes with Nonautologous Tissue Substitute, Open Approach
♀ **0UU747Z** Supplement Bilateral Fallopian Tubes with Autologous Tissue Substitute, Percutaneous Endoscopic Approach
♀ **0UU74JZ** Supplement Bilateral Fallopian Tubes with Synthetic Substitute, Percutaneous Endoscopic Approach
♀ **0UU74KZ** Supplement Bilateral Fallopian Tubes with Nonautologous Tissue Substitute, Percutaneous Endoscopic Approach
♀ **0UU777Z** Supplement Bilateral Fallopian Tubes with Autologous Tissue Substitute, Via Natural or Artificial Opening
♀ **0UU77JZ** Supplement Bilateral Fallopian Tubes with Synthetic Substitute, Via Natural or Artificial Opening
♀ **0UU77KZ** Supplement Bilateral Fallopian Tubes with Nonautologous Tissue Substitute, Via Natural or Artificial Opening
♀ **0UU787Z** Supplement Bilateral Fallopian Tubes with Autologous Tissue Substitute, Via Natural or Artificial Opening Endoscopic
♀ **0UU78JZ** Supplement Bilateral Fallopian Tubes with Synthetic Substitute, Via Natural or Artificial Opening Endoscopic
♀ **0UU78KZ** Supplement Bilateral Fallopian Tubes with Nonautologous Tissue Substitute, Via Natural or Artificial Opening Endoscopic
♀ **0UUF07Z** Supplement Cul-de-sac with Autologous Tissue Substitute, Open Approach
♀ **0UUF0JZ** Supplement Cul-de-sac with Synthetic Substitute, Open Approach
♀ **0UUF0KZ** Supplement Cul-de-sac with Nonautologous Tissue Substitute, Open Approach
♀ **0UUF47Z** Supplement Cul-de-sac with Autologous Tissue Substitute, Percutaneous Endoscopic Approach
♀ **0UUF4JZ** Supplement Cul-de-sac with Synthetic Substitute, Percutaneous Endoscopic Approach
♀ **0UUF4KZ** Supplement Cul-de-sac with Nonautologous Tissue Substitute, Percutaneous Endoscopic Approach
♀ **0UUF77Z** Supplement Cul-de-sac with Autologous Tissue Substitute, Via Natural or Artificial Opening
♀ **0UUF7JZ** Supplement Cul-de-sac with Synthetic Substitute, Via Natural or Artificial Opening
♀ **0UUF7KZ** Supplement Cul-de-sac with Nonautologous Tissue Substitute, Via Natural or Artificial Opening
♀ **0UUF87Z** Supplement Cul-de-sac with Autologous Tissue Substitute, Via Natural or Artificial Opening Endoscopic
♀ **0UUF8JZ** Supplement Cul-de-sac with Synthetic Substitute, Via Natural or Artificial Opening Endoscopic
♀ **0UUF8KZ** Supplement Cul-de-sac with Nonautologous Tissue Substitute, Via Natural or Artificial Opening Endoscopic
♀ **0UUG07Z** Supplement Vagina with Autologous Tissue Substitute, Open Approach
♀ **0UUG0JZ** Supplement Vagina with Synthetic Substitute, Open Approach
♀ **0UUG0KZ** Supplement Vagina with Nonautologous Tissue Substitute, Open Approach
♀ **0UUG47Z** Supplement Vagina with Autologous Tissue Substitute, Percutaneous Endoscopic Approach
♀ **0UUG4JZ** Supplement Vagina with Synthetic Substitute, Percutaneous Endoscopic Approach
♀ **0UUG4KZ** Supplement Vagina with Nonautologous Tissue Substitute, Percutaneous Endoscopic Approach
♀ **0UUG77Z** Supplement Vagina with Autologous Tissue Substitute, Via Natural or Artificial Opening
♀ **0UUG7JZ** Supplement Vagina with Synthetic Substitute, Via Natural or Artificial Opening
♀ **0UUG7KZ** Supplement Vagina with Nonautologous Tissue Substitute, Via Natural or Artificial Opening
♀ **0UUG87Z** Supplement Vagina with Autologous Tissue Substitute, Via Natural or Artificial Opening Endoscopic
♀ **0UUG8JZ** Supplement Vagina with Synthetic Substitute, Via Natural or Artificial Opening Endoscopic
♀ **0UUG8KZ** Supplement Vagina with Nonautologous Tissue Substitute, Via Natural or Artificial Opening Endoscopic
♀ **0UUGX7Z** Supplement Vagina with Autologous Tissue Substitute, External Approach
♀ **0UUGXJZ** Supplement Vagina with Synthetic Substitute, External Approach
♀ **0UUGXKZ** Supplement Vagina with Nonautologous Tissue Substitute, External Approach
♀ **0UUJ07Z** Supplement Clitoris with Autologous Tissue Substitute, Open Approach
♀ **0UUJ0JZ** Supplement Clitoris with Synthetic Substitute, Open Approach
♀ **0UUJ0KZ** Supplement Clitoris with Nonautologous Tissue Substitute, Open Approach
♀ **0UUJX7Z** Supplement Clitoris with Autologous Tissue Substitute, External Approach
♀ **0UUJXJZ** Supplement Clitoris with Synthetic Substitute, External Approach
♀ **0UUJXKZ** Supplement Clitoris with Nonautologous Tissue Substitute, External Approach
♀ **0UUK07Z** Supplement Hymen with Autologous Tissue Substitute, Open Approach
♀ **0UUK0JZ** Supplement Hymen with Synthetic Substitute, Open Approach
♀ **0UUK0KZ** Supplement Hymen with Nonautologous Tissue Substitute, Open Approach
♀ **0UUK47Z** Supplement Hymen with Autologous Tissue Substitute, Percutaneous Endoscopic Approach
♀ **0UUK4JZ** Supplement Hymen with Synthetic Substitute, Percutaneous Endoscopic Approach
♀ **0UUK4KZ** Supplement Hymen with Nonautologous Tissue Substitute, Percutaneous Endoscopic Approach
♀ **0UUK77Z** Supplement Hymen with Autologous Tissue Substitute, Via Natural or Artificial Opening
♀ **0UUK7JZ** Supplement Hymen with Synthetic Substitute, Via Natural or Artificial Opening
♀ **0UUK7KZ** Supplement Hymen with Nonautologous Tissue Substitute, Via Natural or Artificial Opening
♀ **0UUK87Z** Supplement Hymen with Autologous Tissue Substitute, Via Natural or Artificial Opening Endoscopic
♀ **0UUK8JZ** Supplement Hymen with Synthetic Substitute, Via Natural or Artificial Opening Endoscopic
♀ **0UUK8KZ** Supplement Hymen with Nonautologous Tissue Substitute, Via Natural or Artificial Opening Endoscopic
♀ **0UUKX7Z** Supplement Hymen with Autologous Tissue Substitute, External Approach
♀ **0UUKXJZ** Supplement Hymen with Synthetic Substitute, External Approach
♀ **0UUKXKZ** Supplement Hymen with Nonautologous Tissue Substitute, External Approach
♀ **0UUM07Z** Supplement Vulva with Autologous Tissue Substitute, Open Approach
♀ **0UUM0JZ** Supplement Vulva with Synthetic Substitute, Open Approach
♀ **0UUM0KZ** Supplement Vulva with Nonautologous Tissue Substitute, Open Approach
♀ **0UUMX7Z** Supplement Vulva with Autologous Tissue Substitute, External Approach
♀ **0UUMXJZ** Supplement Vulva with Synthetic Substitute, External Approach
♀ **0UUMXKZ** Supplement Vulva with Nonautologous Tissue Substitute, External Approach

0UV – Female Reproductive System, Restriction

♀ **0UVC0CZ** Restriction of Cervix with Extraluminal Device, Open Approach
♀ **0UVC0DZ** Restriction of Cervix with Intraluminal Device, Open Approach
♀ **0UVC0ZZ** Restriction of Cervix, Open Approach
♀ **0UVC3CZ** Restriction of Cervix with Extraluminal Device, Percutaneous Approach
♀ **0UVC3DZ** Restriction of Cervix with Intraluminal Device, Percutaneous Approach
♀ **0UVC3ZZ** Restriction of Cervix, Percutaneous Approach
♀ **0UVC4CZ** Restriction of Cervix with Extraluminal Device, Percutaneous Endoscopic Approach
♀ **0UVC4DZ** Restriction of Cervix with Intraluminal Device, Percutaneous Endoscopic Approach
♀ **0UVC4ZZ** Restriction of Cervix, Percutaneous Endoscopic Approach
♀ **0UVC7DZ** Restriction of Cervix with Intraluminal Device, Via Natural or Artificial Opening
♀ **0UVC7ZZ** Restriction of Cervix, Via Natural or Artificial Opening
♀ **0UVC8DZ** Restriction of Cervix with Intraluminal Device, Via Natural or Artificial Opening Endoscopic
♀ **0UVC8ZZ** Restriction of Cervix, Via Natural or Artificial Opening Endoscopic

0UW – Female Reproductive System, Revision

Review Coding Guideline B6.1c

♀ **0UW300Z** Revision of Drainage Device in Ovary, Open Approach
♀ **0UW303Z** Revision of Infusion Device in Ovary, Open Approach
♀ **0UW330Z** Revision of Drainage Device in Ovary, Percutaneous Approach

♀0UW333Z Revision of Infusion Device in Ovary, Percutaneous Approach
♀0UW340Z Revision of Drainage Device in Ovary, Percutaneous Endoscopic Approach
♀0UW343Z Revision of Infusion Device in Ovary, Percutaneous Endoscopic Approach
♀0UW3X0Z Revision of Drainage Device in Ovary, External Approach
♀0UW3X3Z Revision of Infusion Device in Ovary, External Approach
♀0UW800Z Revision of Drainage Device in Fallopian Tube, Open Approach
♀0UW803Z Revision of Infusion Device in Fallopian Tube, Open Approach
♀0UW807Z Revision of Autologous Tissue Substitute in Fallopian Tube, Open Approach
♀0UW80CZ Revision of Extraluminal Device in Fallopian Tube, Open Approach
♀0UW80DZ Revision of Intraluminal Device in Fallopian Tube, Open Approach
♀0UW80JZ Revision of Synthetic Substitute in Fallopian Tube, Open Approach
♀0UW80KZ Revision of Nonautologous Tissue Substitute in Fallopian Tube, Open Approach
♀0UW830Z Revision of Drainage Device in Fallopian Tube, Percutaneous Approach
♀0UW833Z Revision of Infusion Device in Fallopian Tube, Percutaneous Approach
♀0UW837Z Revision of Autologous Tissue Substitute in Fallopian Tube, Percutaneous Approach
♀0UW83CZ Revision of Extraluminal Device in Fallopian Tube, Percutaneous Approach
♀0UW83DZ Revision of Intraluminal Device in Fallopian Tube, Percutaneous Approach
♀0UW83JZ Revision of Synthetic Substitute in Fallopian Tube, Percutaneous Approach
♀0UW83KZ Revision of Nonautologous Tissue Substitute in Fallopian Tube, Percutaneous Approach
♀0UW840Z Revision of Drainage Device in Fallopian Tube, Percutaneous Endoscopic Approach
♀0UW843Z Revision of Infusion Device in Fallopian Tube, Percutaneous Endoscopic Approach
♀0UW847Z Revision of Autologous Tissue Substitute in Fallopian Tube, Percutaneous Endoscopic Approach
♀0UW84CZ Revision of Extraluminal Device in Fallopian Tube, Percutaneous Endoscopic Approach
♀0UW84DZ Revision of Intraluminal Device in Fallopian Tube, Percutaneous Endoscopic Approach
♀0UW84JZ Revision of Synthetic Substitute in Fallopian Tube, Percutaneous Endoscopic Approach
♀0UW84KZ Revision of Nonautologous Tissue Substitute in Fallopian Tube, Percutaneous Endoscopic Approach
♀0UW870Z Revision of Drainage Device in Fallopian Tube, Via Natural or Artificial Opening
♀0UW873Z Revision of Infusion Device in Fallopian Tube, Via Natural or Artificial Opening
♀0UW877Z Revision of Autologous Tissue Substitute in Fallopian Tube, Via Natural or Artificial Opening
♀0UW87CZ Revision of Extraluminal Device in Fallopian Tube, Via Natural or Artificial Opening
♀0UW87DZ Revision of Intraluminal Device in Fallopian Tube, Via Natural or Artificial Opening
♀0UW87JZ Revision of Synthetic Substitute in Fallopian Tube, Via Natural or Artificial Opening
♀0UW87KZ Revision of Nonautologous Tissue Substitute in Fallopian Tube, Via Natural or Artificial Opening
♀ 0UW880Z Revision of Drainage Device in Fallopian Tube, Via Natural or Artificial Opening Endoscopic
♀ 0UW883Z Revision of Infusion Device in Fallopian Tube, Via Natural or Artificial Opening Endoscopic
♀ 0UW887Z Revision of Autologous Tissue Substitute in Fallopian Tube, Via Natural or Artificial Opening Endoscopic
♀ 0UW88CZ Revision of Extraluminal Device in Fallopian Tube, Via Natural or Artificial Opening Endoscopic
♀ 0UW88DZ Revision of Intraluminal Device in Fallopian Tube, Via Natural or Artificial Opening Endoscopic
♀ 0UW88JZ Revision of Synthetic Substitute in Fallopian Tube, Via Natural or Artificial Opening Endoscopic
♀ 0UW88KZ Revision of Nonautologous Tissue Substitute in Fallopian Tube, Via Natural or Artificial Opening Endoscopic
♀ 0UW8X0Z Revision of Drainage Device in Fallopian Tube, External Approach
♀ 0UW8X3Z Revision of Infusion Device in Fallopian Tube, External Approach
♀ 0UW8X7Z Revision of Autologous Tissue Substitute in Fallopian Tube, External Approach
♀ 0UW8XCZ Revision of Extraluminal Device in Fallopian Tube, External Approach
♀ 0UW8XDZ Revision of Intraluminal Device in Fallopian Tube, External Approach
♀ 0UW8XJZ Revision of Synthetic Substitute in Fallopian Tube, External Approach
♀ 0UW8XKZ Revision of Nonautologous Tissue Substitute in Fallopian Tube, External Approach
♀ 0UWD00Z Revision of Drainage Device in Uterus and Cervix, Open Approach
♀ 0UWD01Z Revision of Radioactive Element in Uterus and Cervix, Open Approach
♀ 0UWD03Z Revision of Infusion Device in Uterus and Cervix, Open Approach
♀ 0UWD07Z Revision of Autologous Tissue Substitute in Uterus and Cervix, Open Approach
♀ 0UWD0CZ Revision of Extraluminal Device in Uterus and Cervix, Open Approach
♀ 0UWD0DZ Revision of Intraluminal Device in Uterus and Cervix, Open Approach
♀ 0UWD0HZ Revision of Contraceptive Device in Uterus and Cervix, Open Approach
♀ 0UWD0JZ Revision of Synthetic Substitute in Uterus and Cervix, Open Approach
♀ 0UWD0KZ Revision of Nonautologous Tissue Substitute in Uterus and Cervix, Open Approach
♀ 0UWD30Z Revision of Drainage Device in Uterus and Cervix, Percutaneous Approach
♀ 0UWD31Z Revision of Radioactive Element in Uterus and Cervix, Percutaneous Approach
♀ 0UWD33Z Revision of Infusion Device in Uterus and Cervix, Percutaneous Approach
♀ 0UWD37Z Revision of Autologous Tissue Substitute in Uterus and Cervix, Percutaneous Approach
♀ 0UWD3CZ Revision of Extraluminal Device in Uterus and Cervix, Percutaneous Approach
♀ 0UWD3DZ Revision of Intraluminal Device in Uterus and Cervix, Percutaneous Approach
♀ 0UWD3HZ Revision of Contraceptive Device in Uterus and Cervix, Percutaneous Approach
♀ 0UWD3JZ Revision of Synthetic Substitute in Uterus and Cervix, Percutaneous Approach
♀ 0UWD3KZ Revision of Nonautologous Tissue Substitute in Uterus and Cervix, Percutaneous Approach
♀ 0UWD40Z Revision of Drainage Device in Uterus and Cervix, Percutaneous Endoscopic Approach
♀ 0UWD41Z Revision of Radioactive Element in Uterus and Cervix, Percutaneous Endoscopic Approach
♀ 0UWD43Z Revision of Infusion Device in Uterus and Cervix, Percutaneous Endoscopic Approach
♀ 0UWD47Z Revision of Autologous Tissue Substitute in Uterus and Cervix, Percutaneous Endoscopic Approach
♀ 0UWD4CZ Revision of Extraluminal Device in Uterus and Cervix, Percutaneous Endoscopic Approach
♀ 0UWD4DZ Revision of Intraluminal Device in Uterus and Cervix, Percutaneous Endoscopic Approach
♀ 0UWD4HZ Revision of Contraceptive Device in Uterus and Cervix, Percutaneous Endoscopic Approach
♀ 0UWD4JZ Revision of Synthetic Substitute in Uterus and Cervix, Percutaneous Endoscopic Approach
♀ 0UWD4KZ Revision of Nonautologous Tissue Substitute in Uterus and Cervix, Percutaneous Endoscopic Approach
♀ 0UWD70Z Revision of Drainage Device in Uterus and Cervix, Via Natural or Artificial Opening
♀ 0UWD71Z Revision of Radioactive Element in Uterus and Cervix, Via Natural or Artificial Opening
♀ 0UWD73Z Revision of Infusion Device in Uterus and Cervix, Via Natural or Artificial Opening
♀ 0UWD77Z Revision of Autologous Tissue Substitute in Uterus and Cervix, Via Natural or Artificial Opening
♀ 0UWD7CZ Revision of Extraluminal Device in Uterus and Cervix, Via Natural or Artificial Opening
♀ 0UWD7DZ Revision of Intraluminal Device in Uterus and Cervix, Via Natural or Artificial Opening
♀ 0UWD7HZ Revision of Contraceptive Device in Uterus and Cervix, Via Natural or Artificial Opening
♀ 0UWD7JZ Revision of Synthetic Substitute in Uterus and Cervix, Via Natural or Artificial Opening
♀ 0UWD7KZ Revision of Nonautologous Tissue Substitute in Uterus and Cervix, Via Natural or Artificial Opening
♀ 0UWD80Z Revision of Drainage Device in Uterus and Cervix, Via Natural or Artificial Opening Endoscopic
♀ 0UWD81Z Revision of Radioactive Element in Uterus and Cervix, Via Natural or Artificial Opening Endoscopic
♀ 0UWD83Z Revision of Infusion Device in Uterus and Cervix, Via Natural or Artificial Opening Endoscopic
♀ 0UWD87Z Revision of Autologous Tissue Substitute in Uterus and Cervix, Via Natural or Artificial Opening Endoscopic
♀ 0UWD8CZ Revision of Extraluminal Device in Uterus and Cervix, Via Natural or Artificial Opening Endoscopic
♀ 0UWD8DZ Revision of Intraluminal Device in Uterus and Cervix, Via Natural or Artificial Opening Endoscopic
♀ 0UWD8HZ Revision of Contraceptive Device in Uterus and Cervix, Via Natural or Artificial Opening Endoscopic

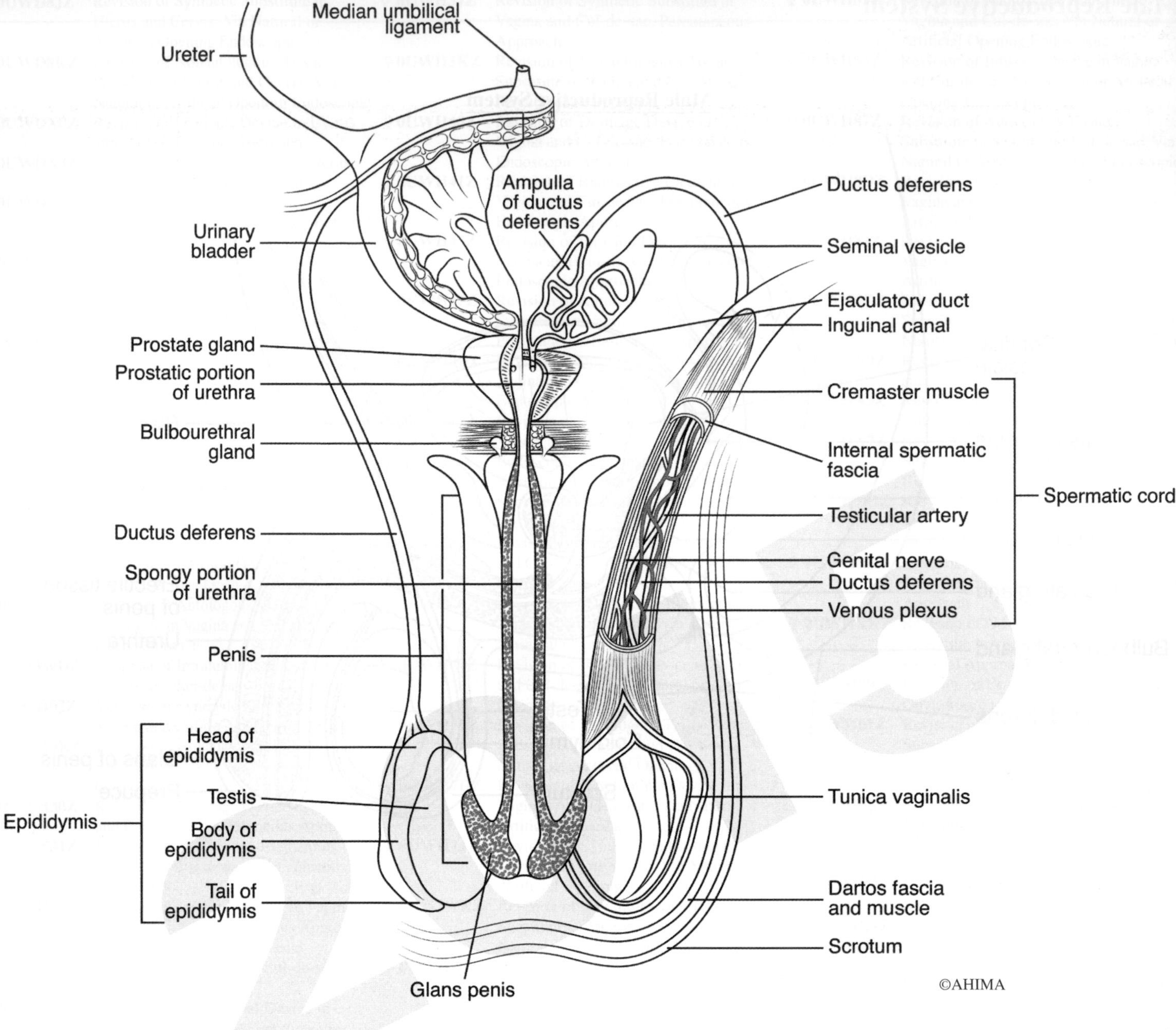
Median umbilical ligament
Ureter
Urinary bladder
Ampulla of ductus deferens
Ductus deferens
Seminal vesicle
Ejaculatory duct
Inguinal canal
Prostate gland
Prostatic portion of urethra
Cremaster muscle
Bulbourethral gland
Internal spermatic fascia
Spermatic cord
Testicular artery
Ductus deferens
Genital nerve
Spongy portion of urethra
Ductus deferens
Venous plexus
Penis
Head of epididymis
Testis
Tunica vaginalis
Epididymis
Body of epididymis
Tail of epididymis
Dartos fascia and muscle
Scrotum
Glans penis
©AHIMA

Section 0 **Medical and Surgical**
Body System V **Male Reproductive System**
Operation 1 **Bypass:** Altering the route of passage of the contents of a tubular body part

Body Part (4th)	Approach (5th)	Device (6th)	Qualifier (7th)
N Vas Deferens, Right P Vas Deferens, Left Q Vas Deferens, Bilateral	0 Open 4 Percutaneous Endoscopic	7 Autologous Tissue Substitute J Synthetic Substitute K Nonautologous Tissue Substitute Z No Device	J Epididymis, Right K Epididymis, Left N Vas Deferens, Right P Vas Deferens, Left

Section 0 **Medical and Surgical**
Body System V **Male Reproductive System**
Operation 2 **Change:** Taking out or off a device from a body part and putting back an identical or similar device in or on the same body part without cutting or puncturing the skin or a mucous membrane

Body Part (4th)	Approach (5th)	Device (6th)	Qualifier (7th)
4 Prostate and Seminal Vesicles 8 Scrotum and Tunica Vaginalis D Testis M Epididymis and Spermatic Cord R Vas Deferens S Penis	X External	0 Drainage Device Y Other Device	Z No Qualifier

Section 0 **Medical and Surgical**
Body System V **Male Reproductive System**
Operation 5 **Destruction:** Physical eradication of all or a portion of a body part by the direct use of energy, force, or a destructive agent

Body Part (4th)	Approach (5th)	Device (6th)	Qualifier (7th)
0 Prostate	0 Open 3 Percutaneous 4 Percutaneous Endoscopic 7 Via Natural or Artificial Opening 8 Via Natural or Artificial Opening Endoscopic	Z No Device	Z No Qualifier
1 Seminal Vesicle, Right 2 Seminal Vesicle, Left 3 Seminal Vesicles, Bilateral 6 Tunica Vaginalis, Right 7 Tunica Vaginalis, Left 9 Testis, Right B Testis, Left C Testes, Bilateral F Spermatic Cord, Right G Spermatic Cord, Left H Spermatic Cords, Bilateral J Epididymis, Right K Epididymis, Left L Epididymis, Bilateral N Vas Deferens, Right P Vas Deferens, Left Q Vas Deferens, Bilateral	0 Open 3 Percutaneous 4 Percutaneous Endoscopic	Z No Device	Z No Qualifier
5 Scrotum S Penis T Prepuce	0 Open 3 Percutaneous 4 Percutaneous Endoscopic X External	Z No Device	Z No Qualifier

Section 0 **Medical and Surgical**
Body System V **Male Reproductive System**
Operation 7 **Dilation:** Expanding an orifice or the lumen of a tubular body part

Body Part (4th)	Approach (5th)	Device (6th)	Qualifier (7th)
N Vas Deferens, Right **P** Vas Deferens, Left **Q** Vas Deferens, Bilateral	**0** Open **3** Percutaneous **4** Percutaneous Endoscopic	**D** Intraluminal Device **Z** No Device	**Z** No Qualifier

Section 0 **Medical and Surgical**
Body System V **Male Reproductive System**
Operation 9 **Drainage:** Taking or letting out fluids and/or gases from a body part

Body Part (4th)	Approach (5th)	Device (6th)	Qualifier (7th)
0 Prostate	**0** Open **3** Percutaneous **4** Percutaneous Endoscopic **7** Via Natural or Artificial Opening **8** Via Natural or Artificial Opening Endoscopic	**0** Drainage Device	**Z** No Qualifier
0 Prostate	**0** Open **3** Percutaneous **4** Percutaneous Endoscopic **7** Via Natural or Artificial Opening **8** Via Natural or Artificial Opening Endoscopic	**Z** No Device	**X** Diagnostic **Z** No Qualifier
1 Seminal Vesicle, Right **2** Seminal Vesicle, Left **3** Seminal Vesicles, Bilateral **6** Tunica Vaginalis, Right **7** Tunica Vaginalis, Left **9** Testis, Right **B** Testis, Left **C** Testes, Bilateral **F** Spermatic Cord, Right **G** Spermatic Cord, Left **H** Spermatic Cords, Bilateral **J** Epididymis, Right **K** Epididymis, Left **L** Epididymis, Bilateral **N** Vas Deferens, Right **P** Vas Deferens, Left **Q** Vas Deferens, Bilateral	**0** Open **3** Percutaneous **4** Percutaneous Endoscopic	**0** Drainage Device	**Z** No Qualifier
1 Seminal Vesicle, Right **2** Seminal Vesicle, Left **3** Seminal Vesicles, Bilateral **6** Tunica Vaginalis, Right **7** Tunica Vaginalis, Left **9** Testis, Right **B** Testis, Left **C** Testes, Bilateral **F** Spermatic Cord, Right **G** Spermatic Cord, Left **H** Spermatic Cords, Bilateral **J** Epididymis, Right **K** Epididymis, Left **L** Epididymis, Bilateral **N** Vas Deferens, Right **P** Vas Deferens, Left **Q** Vas Deferens, Bilateral	**0** Open **3** Percutaneous **4** Percutaneous Endoscopic	**Z** No Device	**X** Diagnostic **Z** No Qualifier
5 Scrotum **S** Penis **T** Prepuce	**0** Open **3** Percutaneous **4** Percutaneous Endoscopic **X** External	**0** Drainage Device	**Z** No Qualifier

Continued →

Section 0 Medical and Surgical
Body System V Male Reproductive System
Operation 9 **Drainage:** Taking or letting out fluids and/or gases from a body part

Body Part (4th)	Approach (5th)	Device (6th)	Qualifier (7th)
5 Scrotum S Penis T Prepuce	0 Open 3 Percutaneous 4 Percutaneous Endoscopic X External	Z No Device	X Diagnostic Z No Qualifier

Section 0 Medical and Surgical
Body System V Male Reproductive System
Operation B **Excision:** Cutting out or off, without replacement, a portion of a body part

Body Part (4th)	Approach (5th)	Device (6th)	Qualifier (7th)
0 Prostate	0 Open 3 Percutaneous 4 Percutaneous Endoscopic 7 Via Natural or Artificial Opening 8 Via Natural or Artificial Opening Endoscopic	Z No Device	X Diagnostic Z No Qualifier
1 Seminal Vesicle, Right 2 Seminal Vesicle, Left 3 Seminal Vesicles, Bilateral 6 Tunica Vaginalis, Right 7 Tunica Vaginalis, Left 9 Testis, Right B Testis, Left C Testes, Bilateral F Spermatic Cord, Right G Spermatic Cord, Left H Spermatic Cords, Bilateral J Epididymis, Right K Epididymis, Left L Epididymis, Bilateral N Vas Deferens, Right P Vas Deferens, Left Q Vas Deferens, Bilateral	0 Open 3 Percutaneous 4 Percutaneous Endoscopic	Z No Device	X Diagnostic Z No Qualifier
5 Scrotum S Penis T Prepuce	0 Open 3 Percutaneous 4 Percutaneous Endoscopic X External	Z No Device	X Diagnostic Z No Qualifier

Section 0 Medical and Surgical
Body System V Male Reproductive System
Operation C **Extirpation:** Taking or cutting out solid matter from a body part

Body Part (4th)	Approach (5th)	Device (6th)	Qualifier (7th)
0 Prostate	0 Open 3 Percutaneous 4 Percutaneous Endoscopic 7 Via Natural or Artificial Opening 8 Via Natural or Artificial Opening Endoscopic	Z No Device	Z No Qualifier

Continued →

Section 0 **Medical and Surgical**
Body System V **Male Reproductive System**
Operation C **Extirpation:** Taking or cutting out solid matter from a body part

Body Part (4th)	Approach (5th)	Device (6th)	Qualifier (7th)
1 Seminal Vesicle, Right **2** Seminal Vesicle, Left **3** Seminal Vesicles, Bilateral **6** Tunica Vaginalis, Right **7** Tunica Vaginalis, Left **9** Testis, Right **B** Testis, Left **C** Testes, Bilateral **F** Spermatic Cord, Right **G** Spermatic Cord, Left **H** Spermatic Cords, Bilateral **J** Epididymis, Right **K** Epididymis, Left **L** Epididymis, Bilateral **N** Vas Deferens, Right **P** Vas Deferens, Left **Q** Vas Deferens, Bilateral	**0** Open **3** Percutaneous **4** Percutaneous Endoscopic	**Z** No Device	**Z** No Qualifier
5 Scrotum **S** Penis **T** Prepuce	**0** Open **3** Percutaneous **4** Percutaneous Endoscopic **X** External	**Z** No Device	**Z** No Qualifier

Section 0 **Medical and Surgical**
Body System V **Male Reproductive System**
Operation H **Insertion:** Putting in a nonbiological appliance that monitors, assists, performs, or prevents a physiological function but does not physically take the place of a body part

Body Part (4th)	Approach (5th)	Device (6th)	Qualifier (7th)
0 Prostate	**0** Open **3** Percutaneous **4** Percutaneous Endoscopic **7** Via Natural or Artificial Opening **8** Via Natural or Artificial Opening Endoscopic	**1** Radioactive Element	**Z** No Qualifier
4 Prostate and Seminal Vesicles **8** Scrotum and Tunica Vaginalis **D** Testis **M** Epididymis and Spermatic Cord **R** Vas Deferens	**0** Open **3** Percutaneous **4** Percutaneous Endoscopic **7** Via Natural or Artificial Opening **8** Via Natural or Artificial Opening Endoscopic	**3** Infusion Device	**Z** No Qualifier
S Penis	**0** Open **3** Percutaneous **4** Percutaneous Endoscopic **X** External	**3** Infusion Device	**Z** No Qualifier

Section 0 **Medical and Surgical**
Body System V **Male Reproductive System**
Operation J **Inspection:** Visually and/or manually exploring a body part

Body Part (4th)	Approach (5th)	Device (6th)	Qualifier (7th)
4 Prostate and Seminal Vesicles **8** Scrotum and Tunica Vaginalis **D** Testis **M** Epididymis and Spermatic Cord **R** Vas Deferens **S** Penis	**0** Open **3** Percutaneous **4** Percutaneous Endoscopic **X** External	**Z** No Device	**Z** No Qualifier

Section 0 **Medical and Surgical**
Body System V **Male Reproductive System**
Operation L **Occlusion:** Completely closing an orifice or the lumen of a tubular body part

Body Part (4th)	Approach (5th)	Device (6th)	Qualifier (7th)
F Spermatic Cord, Right **G** Spermatic Cord, Left **H** Spermatic Cords, Bilateral **N** Vas Deferens, Right **P** Vas Deferens, Left **Q** Vas Deferens, Bilateral	**0** Open **3** Percutaneous **4** Percutaneous Endoscopic	**C** Extraluminal Device **D** Intraluminal Device **Z** No Device	**Z** No Qualifier

Section 0 **Medical and Surgical**
Body System V **Male Reproductive System**
Operation M **Reattachment:** Putting back in or on all or a portion of a separated body part to its normal location or other suitable location

Body Part (4th)	Approach (5th)	Device (6th)	Qualifier (7th)
5 Scrotum **S** Penis	**X** External	**Z** No Device	**Z** No Qualifier
6 Tunica Vaginalis, Right **7** Tunica Vaginalis, Left **9** Testis, Right **B** Testis, Left **C** Testes, Bilateral **F** Spermatic Cord, Right **G** Spermatic Cord, Left **H** Spermatic Cords, Bilateral	**0** Open **4** Percutaneous Endoscopic	**Z** No Device	**Z** No Qualifier

Section 0 **Medical and Surgical**
Body System V **Male Reproductive System**
Operation N **Release:** Freeing a body part from an abnormal physical constraint by cutting or by the use of force

Body Part (4th)	Approach (5th)	Device (6th)	Qualifier (7th)
0 Prostate	**0** Open **3** Percutaneous **4** Percutaneous Endoscopic **7** Via Natural or Artificial Opening **8** Via Natural or Artificial Opening Endoscopic	**Z** No Device	**Z** No Qualifier
1 Seminal Vesicle, Right **2** Seminal Vesicle, Left **3** Seminal Vesicles, Bilateral **6** Tunica Vaginalis, Right **7** Tunica Vaginalis, Left **9** Testis, Right **B** Testis, Left **C** Testes, Bilateral **F** Spermatic Cord, Right **G** Spermatic Cord, Left **H** Spermatic Cords, Bilateral **J** Epididymis, Right **K** Epididymis, Left **L** Epididymis, Bilateral **N** Vas Deferens, Right **P** Vas Deferens, Left **Q** Vas Deferens, Bilateral	**0** Open **3** Percutaneous **4** Percutaneous Endoscopic	**Z** No Device	**Z** No Qualifier
5 Scrotum **S** Penis **T** Prepuce	**0** Open **3** Percutaneous **4** Percutaneous Endoscopic **X** External	**Z** No Device	**Z** No Qualifier

Section 0 **Medical and Surgical**
Body System V **Male Reproductive System**
Operation P **Removal:** Taking out or off a device from a body part

Body Part (4th)	Approach (5th)	Device (6th)	Qualifier (7th)
4 Prostate and Seminal Vesicles	**0** Open **3** Percutaneous **4** Percutaneous Endoscopic **7** Via Natural or Artificial Opening **8** Via Natural or Artificial Opening Endoscopic	**0** Drainage Device **1** Radioactive Element **3** Infusion Device **7** Autologous Tissue Substitute **J** Synthetic Substitute **K** Nonautologous Tissue Substitute	**Z** No Qualifier
4 Prostate and Seminal Vesicles	**X** External	**0** Drainage Device **1** Radioactive Element **3** Infusion Device	**Z** No Qualifier
8 Scrotum and Tunica Vaginalis **D** Testis **S** Penis	**0** Open **3** Percutaneous **4** Percutaneous Endoscopic **7** Via Natural or Artificial Opening **8** Via Natural or Artificial Opening Endoscopic	**0** Drainage Device **3** Infusion Device **7** Autologous Tissue Substitute **J** Synthetic Substitute **K** Nonautologous Tissue Substitute	**Z** No Qualifier
8 Scrotum and Tunica Vaginalis **D** Testis **S** Penis	**X** External	**0** Drainage Device **3** Infusion Device	**Z** No Qualifier
M Epididymis and Spermatic Cord	**0** Open **3** Percutaneous **4** Percutaneous Endoscopic **7** Via Natural or Artificial Opening **8** Via Natural or Artificial Opening Endoscopic	**0** Drainage Device **3** Infusion Device **7** Autologous Tissue Substitute **C** Extraluminal Device **J** Synthetic Substitute **K** Nonautologous Tissue Substitute	**Z** No Qualifier
M Epididymis and Spermatic Cord	**X** External	**0** Drainage Device **3** Infusion Device	**Z** No Qualifier
R Vas Deferens	**0** Open **3** Percutaneous **4** Percutaneous Endoscopic **7** Via Natural or Artificial Opening **8** Via Natural or Artificial Opening Endoscopic	**0** Drainage Device **3** Infusion Device **7** Autologous Tissue Substitute **C** Extraluminal Device **D** Intraluminal Device **J** Synthetic Substitute **K** Nonautologous Tissue Substitute	**Z** No Qualifier
R Vas Deferens	**X** External	**0** Drainage Device **3** Infusion Device **D** Intraluminal Device	**Z** No Qualifier

Section 0 **Medical and Surgical**
Body System V **Male Reproductive System**
Operation Q **Repair:** Restoring, to the extent possible, a body part to its normal anatomic structure and function

Body Part (4th)	Approach (5th)	Device (6th)	Qualifier (7th)
0 Prostate	**0** Open **3** Percutaneous **4** Percutaneous Endoscopic **7** Via Natural or Artificial Opening **8** Via Natural or Artificial Opening Endoscopic	**Z** No Device	**Z** No Qualifier

Continued →

Section 0 **Medical and Surgical**
Body System V **Male Reproductive System**
Operation Q **Repair:** Restoring, to the extent possible, a body part to its normal anatomic structure and function

Body Part (4th)	Approach (5th)	Device (6th)	Qualifier (7th)
1 Seminal Vesicle, Right **2** Seminal Vesicle, Left **3** Seminal Vesicles, Bilateral **6** Tunica Vaginalis, Right **7** Tunica Vaginalis, Left **9** Testis, Right **B** Testis, Left **C** Testes, Bilateral **F** Spermatic Cord, Right **G** Spermatic Cord, Left **H** Spermatic Cords, Bilateral **J** Epididymis, Right **K** Epididymis, Left **L** Epididymis, Bilateral **N** Vas Deferens, Right **P** Vas Deferens, Left **Q** Vas Deferens, Bilateral	**0** Open **3** Percutaneous **4** Percutaneous Endoscopic	**Z** No Device	**Z** No Qualifier
5 Scrotum **S** Penis **T** Prepuce	**0** Open **3** Percutaneous **4** Percutaneous Endoscopic **X** External	**Z** No Device	**Z** No Qualifier

Section 0 **Medical and Surgical**
Body System V **Male Reproductive System**
Operation R **Replacement:** Putting in or on biological or synthetic material that physically takes the place and/or function of all or a portion of a body part

Body Part (4th)	Approach (5th)	Device (6th)	Qualifier (7th)
9 Testis, Right **B** Testis, Left **C** Testes, Bilateral	**0** Open	**J** Synthetic Substitute	**Z** No Qualifier

Section 0 **Medical and Surgical**
Body System V **Male Reproductive System**
Operation S **Reposition:** Moving to its normal location, or other suitable location, all or a portion of a body part

Body Part (4th)	Approach (5th)	Device (6th)	Qualifier (7th)
9 Testis, Right **B** Testis, Left **C** Testes, Bilateral **F** Spermatic Cord, Right **G** Spermatic Cord, Left **H** Spermatic Cords, Bilateral	**0** Open **3** Percutaneous **4** Percutaneous Endoscopic	**Z** No Device	**Z** No Qualifier

Section 0 **Medical and Surgical**
Body System V **Male Reproductive System**
Operation T **Resection:** Cutting out or off, without replacement, all of a body part

Body Part (4th)	Approach (5th)	Device (6th)	Qualifier (7th)
0 Prostate	**0** Open **4** Percutaneous Endoscopic **7** Via Natural or Artificial Opening **8** Via Natural or Artificial Opening Endoscopic	**Z** No Device	**Z** No Qualifier

Continued →

Section 0 **Medical and Surgical**
Body System V **Male Reproductive System**
Operation T **Resection:** Cutting out or off, without replacement, all of a body part

Body Part (4th)	Approach (5th)	Device (6th)	Qualifier (7th)
1 Seminal Vesicle, Right **2** Seminal Vesicle, Left **3** Seminal Vesicles, Bilateral **6** Tunica Vaginalis, Right **7** Tunica Vaginalis, Left **9** Testis, Right **B** Testis, Left **C** Testes, Bilateral **F** Spermatic Cord, Right **G** Spermatic Cord, Left **H** Spermatic Cords, Bilateral **J** Epididymis, Right **K** Epididymis, Left **L** Epididymis, Bilateral **N** Vas Deferens, Right **P** Vas Deferens, Left **Q** Vas Deferens, Bilateral	**0** Open **4** Percutaneous Endoscopic	**Z** No Device	**Z** No Qualifier
5 Scrotum **S** Penis **T** Prepuce	**0** Open **4** Percutaneous Endoscopic **X** External	**Z** No Device	**Z** No Qualifier

Section 0 **Medical and Surgical**
Body System V **Male Reproductive System**
Operation U **Supplement:** Putting in or on biological or synthetic material that physically reinforces and/or augments the function of a portion of a body part

Body Part (4th)	Approach (5th)	Device (6th)	Qualifier (7th)
1 Seminal Vesicle, Right **2** Seminal Vesicle, Left **3** Seminal Vesicles, Bilateral **6** Tunica Vaginalis, Right **7** Tunica Vaginalis, Left **F** Spermatic Cord, Right **G** Spermatic Cord, Left **H** Spermatic Cords, Bilateral **J** Epididymis, Right **K** Epididymis, Left **L** Epididymis, Bilateral **N** Vas Deferens, Right **P** Vas Deferens, Left **Q** Vas Deferens, Bilateral	**0** Open **4** Percutaneous Endoscopic	**7** Autologous Tissue Substitute **J** Synthetic Substitute **K** Nonautologous Tissue Substitute	**Z** No Qualifier
5 Scrotum **S** Penis **T** Prepuce	**0** Open **4** Percutaneous Endoscopic **X** External	**7** Autologous Tissue Substitute **J** Synthetic Substitute **K** Nonautologous Tissue Substitute	**Z** No Qualifier
9 Testis, Right **B** Testis, Left **C** Testes, Bilateral	**0** Open	**7** Autologous Tissue Substitute **J** Synthetic Substitute **K** Nonautologous Tissue Substitute	**Z** No Qualifier

Section	**0**	**Medical and Surgical**
Body System	**V**	**Male Reproductive System**
Operation	**W**	**Revision:** Correcting, to the extent possible, a portion of a malfunctioning device or the position of a displaced device

Body Part (4th)	Approach (5th)	Device (6th)	Qualifier (7th)
4 Prostate and Seminal Vesicles **8** Scrotum and Tunica Vaginalis **D** Testis **S** Penis	**0** Open **3** Percutaneous **4** Percutaneous Endoscopic **7** Via Natural or Artificial Opening **8** Via Natural or Artificial Opening Endoscopic **X** External	**0** Drainage Device **3** Infusion Device **7** Autologous Tissue Substitute **J** Synthetic Substitute **K** Nonautologous Tissue Substitute	**Z** No Qualifier
M Epididymis and Spermatic Cord	**0** Open **3** Percutaneous **4** Percutaneous Endoscopic **7** Via Natural or Artificial Opening **8** Via Natural or Artificial Opening Endoscopic **X** External	**0** Drainage Device **3** Infusion Device **7** Autologous Tissue Substitute **C** Extraluminal Device **J** Synthetic Substitute **K** Nonautologous Tissue Substitute	**Z** No Qualifier
R Vas Deferens	**0** Open **3** Percutaneous **4** Percutaneous Endoscopic **7** Via Natural or Artificial Opening **8** Via Natural or Artificial Opening Endoscopic **X** External	**0** Drainage Device **3** Infusion Device **7** Autologous Tissue Substitute **C** Extraluminal Device **D** Intraluminal Device **J** Synthetic Substitute **K** Nonautologous Tissue Substitute	**Z** No Qualifier

Male Reproductive System Code Listing 0V1–0VW

0V1 – Male Reproductive System, Bypass

Review Coding Guideline B3.6a

♂**0V1N07J** Bypass Right Vas Deferens to Right Epididymis with Autologous Tissue Substitute, Open Approach
♂**0V1N07K** Bypass Right Vas Deferens to Left Epididymis with Autologous Tissue Substitute, Open Approach
♂**0V1N07N** Bypass Right Vas Deferens to Right Vas Deferens with Autologous Tissue Substitute, Open Approach
♂**0V1N07P** Bypass Right Vas Deferens to Left Vas Deferens with Autologous Tissue Substitute, Open Approach
♂**0V1N0JJ** Bypass Right Vas Deferens to Right Epididymis with Synthetic Substitute, Open Approach
♂**0V1N0JK** Bypass Right Vas Deferens to Left Epididymis with Synthetic Substitute, Open Approach
♂**0V1N0JN** Bypass Right Vas Deferens to Right Vas Deferens with Synthetic Substitute, Open Approach
♂**0V1N0JP** Bypass Right Vas Deferens to Left Vas Deferens with Synthetic Substitute, Open Approach
♂**0V1N0KJ** Bypass Right Vas Deferens to Right Epididymis with Nonautologous Tissue Substitute, Open Approach
♂**0V1N0KK** Bypass Right Vas Deferens to Left Epididymis with Nonautologous Tissue Substitute, Open Approach
♂**0V1N0KN** Bypass Right Vas Deferens to Right Vas Deferens with Nonautologous Tissue Substitute, Open Approach
♂**0V1N0KP** Bypass Right Vas Deferens to Left Vas Deferens with Nonautologous Tissue Substitute, Open Approach
♂**0V1N0ZJ** Bypass Right Vas Deferens to Right Epididymis, Open Approach
♂ **0V1N0ZK** Bypass Right Vas Deferens to Left Epididymis, Open Approach
♂ **0V1N0ZN** Bypass Right Vas Deferens to Right Vas Deferens, Open Approach
♂ **0V1N0ZP** Bypass Right Vas Deferens to Left Vas Deferens, Open Approach
♂ **0V1N47J** Bypass Right Vas Deferens to Right Epididymis with Autologous Tissue Substitute, Percutaneous Endoscopic Approach
♂ **0V1N47K** Bypass Right Vas Deferens to Left Epididymis with Autologous Tissue Substitute, Percutaneous Endoscopic Approach
♂ **0V1N47N** Bypass Right Vas Deferens to Right Vas Deferens with Autologous Tissue Substitute, Percutaneous Endoscopic Approach
♂ **0V1N47P** Bypass Right Vas Deferens to Left Vas Deferens with Autologous Tissue Substitute, Percutaneous Endoscopic Approach
♂ **0V1N4JJ** Bypass Right Vas Deferens to Right Epididymis with Synthetic Substitute, Percutaneous Endoscopic Approach
♂ **0V1N4JK** Bypass Right Vas Deferens to Left Epididymis with Synthetic Substitute, Percutaneous Endoscopic Approach
♂ **0V1N4JN** Bypass Right Vas Deferens to Right Vas Deferens with Synthetic Substitute, Percutaneous Endoscopic Approach
♂ **0V1N4JP** Bypass Right Vas Deferens to Left Vas Deferens with Synthetic Substitute, Percutaneous Endoscopic Approach
♂ **0V1N4KJ** Bypass Right Vas Deferens to Right Epididymis with Nonautologous Tissue Substitute, Percutaneous Endoscopic Approach
♂ **0V1N4KK** Bypass Right Vas Deferens to Left Epididymis with Nonautologous Tissue Substitute, Percutaneous Endoscopic Approach
♂ **0V1N4KN** Bypass Right Vas Deferens to Right Vas Deferens with Nonautologous Tissue Substitute, Percutaneous Endoscopic Approach
♂ **0V1N4KP** Bypass Right Vas Deferens to Left Vas Deferens with Nonautologous Tissue Substitute, Percutaneous Endoscopic Approach
♂ **0V1N4ZJ** Bypass Right Vas Deferens to Right Epididymis, Percutaneous Endoscopic Approach
♂ **0V1N4ZK** Bypass Right Vas Deferens to Left Epididymis, Percutaneous Endoscopic Approach
♂ **0V1N4ZN** Bypass Right Vas Deferens to Right Vas Deferens, Percutaneous Endoscopic Approach
♂ **0V1N4ZP** Bypass Right Vas Deferens to Left Vas Deferens, Percutaneous Endoscopic Approach
♂ **0V1P07J** Bypass Left Vas Deferens to Right Epididymis with Autologous Tissue Substitute, Open Approach
♂ **0V1P07K** Bypass Left Vas Deferens to Left Epididymis with Autologous Tissue Substitute, Open Approach
♂ **0V1P07N** Bypass Left Vas Deferens to Right Vas Deferens with Autologous Tissue Substitute, Open Approach
♂ **0V1P07P** Bypass Left Vas Deferens to Left Vas Deferens with Autologous Tissue Substitute, Open Approach

♂ **0V1P0JJ** Bypass Left Vas Deferens to Right Epididymis with Synthetic Substitute, Open Approach
♂ **0V1P0JK** Bypass Left Vas Deferens to Left Epididymis with Synthetic Substitute, Open Approach
♂ **0V1P0JN** Bypass Left Vas Deferens to Right Vas Deferens with Synthetic Substitute, Open Approach
♂ **0V1P0JP** Bypass Left Vas Deferens to Left Vas Deferens with Synthetic Substitute, Open Approach
♂ **0V1P0KJ** Bypass Left Vas Deferens to Right Epididymis with Nonautologous Tissue Substitute, Open Approach
♂ **0V1P0KK** Bypass Left Vas Deferens to Left Epididymis with Nonautologous Tissue Substitute, Open Approach
♂ **0V1P0KN** Bypass Left Vas Deferens to Right Vas Deferens with Nonautologous Tissue Substitute, Open Approach
♂ **0V1P0KP** Bypass Left Vas Deferens to Left Vas Deferens with Nonautologous Tissue Substitute, Open Approach
♂ **0V1P0ZJ** Bypass Left Vas Deferens to Right Epididymis, Open Approach
♂ **0V1P0ZK** Bypass Left Vas Deferens to Left Epididymis, Open Approach
♂ **0V1P0ZN** Bypass Left Vas Deferens to Right Vas Deferens, Open Approach
♂ **0V1P0ZP** Bypass Left Vas Deferens to Left Vas Deferens, Open Approach
♂ **0V1P47J** Bypass Left Vas Deferens to Right Epididymis with Autologous Tissue Substitute, Percutaneous Endoscopic Approach
♂ **0V1P47K** Bypass Left Vas Deferens to Left Epididymis with Autologous Tissue Substitute, Percutaneous Endoscopic Approach
♂ **0V1P47N** Bypass Left Vas Deferens to Right Vas Deferens with Autologous Tissue Substitute, Percutaneous Endoscopic Approach
♂ **0V1P47P** Bypass Left Vas Deferens to Left Vas Deferens with Autologous Tissue Substitute, Percutaneous Endoscopic Approach
♂ **0V1P4JJ** Bypass Left Vas Deferens to Right Epididymis with Synthetic Substitute, Percutaneous Endoscopic Approach
♂ **0V1P4JK** Bypass Left Vas Deferens to Left Epididymis with Synthetic Substitute, Percutaneous Endoscopic Approach
♂ **0V1P4JN** Bypass Left Vas Deferens to Right Vas Deferens with Synthetic Substitute, Percutaneous Endoscopic Approach
♂ **0V1P4JP** Bypass Left Vas Deferens to Left Vas Deferens with Synthetic Substitute, Percutaneous Endoscopic Approach
♂ **0V1P4KJ** Bypass Left Vas Deferens to Right Epididymis with Nonautologous Tissue Substitute, Percutaneous Endoscopic Approach
♂ **0V1P4KK** Bypass Left Vas Deferens to Left Epididymis with Nonautologous Tissue Substitute, Percutaneous Endoscopic Approach
♂ **0V1P4KN** Bypass Left Vas Deferens to Right Vas Deferens with Nonautologous Tissue Substitute, Percutaneous Endoscopic Approach
♂ **0V1P4KP** Bypass Left Vas Deferens to Left Vas Deferens with Nonautologous Tissue Substitute, Percutaneous Endoscopic Approach
♂ **0V1P4ZJ** Bypass Left Vas Deferens to Right Epididymis, Percutaneous Endoscopic Approach
♂ **0V1P4ZK** Bypass Left Vas Deferens to Left Epididymis, Percutaneous Endoscopic Approach
♂ **0V1P4ZN** Bypass Left Vas Deferens to Right Vas Deferens, Percutaneous Endoscopic Approach
♂ **0V1P4ZP** Bypass Left Vas Deferens to Left Vas Deferens, Percutaneous Endoscopic Approach
♂ **0V1Q07J** Bypass Bilateral Vas Deferens to Right Epididymis with Autologous Tissue Substitute, Open Approach
♂ **0V1Q07K** Bypass Bilateral Vas Deferens to Left Epididymis with Autologous Tissue Substitute, Open Approach
♂ **0V1Q07N** Bypass Bilateral Vas Deferens to Right Vas Deferens with Autologous Tissue Substitute, Open Approach
♂ **0V1Q07P** Bypass Bilateral Vas Deferens to Left Vas Deferens with Autologous Tissue Substitute, Open Approach
♂ **0V1Q0JJ** Bypass Bilateral Vas Deferens to Right Epididymis with Synthetic Substitute, Open Approach
♂ **0V1Q0JK** Bypass Bilateral Vas Deferens to Left Epididymis with Synthetic Substitute, Open Approach
♂ **0V1Q0JN** Bypass Bilateral Vas Deferens to Right Vas Deferens with Synthetic Substitute, Open Approach
♂ **0V1Q0JP** Bypass Bilateral Vas Deferens to Left Vas Deferens with Synthetic Substitute, Open Approach
♂ **0V1Q0KJ** Bypass Bilateral Vas Deferens to Right Epididymis with Nonautologous Tissue Substitute, Open Approach
♂ **0V1Q0KK** Bypass Bilateral Vas Deferens to Left Epididymis with Nonautologous Tissue Substitute, Open Approach
♂ **0V1Q0KN** Bypass Bilateral Vas Deferens to Right Vas Deferens with Nonautologous Tissue Substitute, Open Approach
♂ **0V1Q0KP** Bypass Bilateral Vas Deferens to Left Vas Deferens with Nonautologous Tissue Substitute, Open Approach
♂ **0V1Q0ZJ** Bypass Bilateral Vas Deferens to Right Epididymis, Open Approach
♂ **0V1Q0ZK** Bypass Bilateral Vas Deferens to Left Epididymis, Open Approach
♂ **0V1Q0ZN** Bypass Bilateral Vas Deferens to Right Vas Deferens, Open Approach
♂ **0V1Q0ZP** Bypass Bilateral Vas Deferens to Left Vas Deferens, Open Approach
♂ **0V1Q47J** Bypass Bilateral Vas Deferens to Right Epididymis with Autologous Tissue Substitute, Percutaneous Endoscopic Approach
♂ **0V1Q47K** Bypass Bilateral Vas Deferens to Left Epididymis with Autologous Tissue Substitute, Percutaneous Endoscopic Approach
♂ **0V1Q47N** Bypass Bilateral Vas Deferens to Right Vas Deferens with Autologous Tissue Substitute, Percutaneous Endoscopic Approach
♂ **0V1Q47P** Bypass Bilateral Vas Deferens to Left Vas Deferens with Autologous Tissue Substitute, Percutaneous Endoscopic Approach
♂ **0V1Q4JJ** Bypass Bilateral Vas Deferens to Right Epididymis with Synthetic Substitute, Percutaneous Endoscopic Approach
♂ **0V1Q4JK** Bypass Bilateral Vas Deferens to Left Epididymis with Synthetic Substitute, Percutaneous Endoscopic Approach
♂ **0V1Q4JN** Bypass Bilateral Vas Deferens to Right Vas Deferens with Synthetic Substitute, Percutaneous Endoscopic Approach
♂ **0V1Q4JP** Bypass Bilateral Vas Deferens to Left Vas Deferens with Synthetic Substitute, Percutaneous Endoscopic Approach
♂ **0V1Q4KJ** Bypass Bilateral Vas Deferens to Right Epididymis with Nonautologous Tissue Substitute, Percutaneous Endoscopic Approach
♂ **0V1Q4KK** Bypass Bilateral Vas Deferens to Left Epididymis with Nonautologous Tissue Substitute, Percutaneous Endoscopic Approach
♂ **0V1Q4KN** Bypass Bilateral Vas Deferens to Right Vas Deferens with Nonautologous Tissue Substitute, Percutaneous Endoscopic Approach
♂ **0V1Q4KP** Bypass Bilateral Vas Deferens to Left Vas Deferens with Nonautologous Tissue Substitute, Percutaneous Endoscopic Approach
♂ **0V1Q4ZJ** Bypass Bilateral Vas Deferens to Right Epididymis, Percutaneous Endoscopic Approach
♂ **0V1Q4ZK** Bypass Bilateral Vas Deferens to Left Epididymis, Percutaneous Endoscopic Approach
♂ **0V1Q4ZN** Bypass Bilateral Vas Deferens to Right Vas Deferens, Percutaneous Endoscopic Approach
♂ **0V1Q4ZP** Bypass Bilateral Vas Deferens to Left Vas Deferens, Percutaneous Endoscopic Approach

0V2 – Male Reproductive System, Change

Review Coding Guideline B6.1c

♂ **0V24X0Z** Change Drainage Device in Prostate and Seminal Vesicles, External Approach
♂ **0V24XYZ** Change Other Device in Prostate and Seminal Vesicles, External Approach
♂ **0V28X0Z** Change Drainage Device in Scrotum and Tunica Vaginalis, External Approach
♂ **0V28XYZ** Change Other Device in Scrotum and Tunica Vaginalis, External Approach
♂ **0V2DX0Z** Change Drainage Device in Testis, External Approach
♂ **0V2DXYZ** Change Other Device in Testis, External Approach
♂ **0V2MX0Z** Change Drainage Device in Epididymis and Spermatic Cord, External Approach
♂ **0V2MXYZ** Change Other Device in Epididymis and Spermatic Cord, External Approach
♂ **0V2RX0Z** Change Drainage Device in Vas Deferens, External Approach
♂ **0V2RXYZ** Change Other Device in Vas Deferens, External Approach
♂ **0V2SX0Z** Change Drainage Device in Penis, External Approach
♂ **0V2SXYZ** Change Other Device in Penis, External Approach

0V5 – Male Reproductive System, Destruction

♂ **0V500ZZ** Destruction of Prostate, Open Approach
♂ **0V503ZZ** Destruction of Prostate, Percutaneous Approach
♂ **0V504ZZ** Destruction of Prostate, Percutaneous Endoscopic Approach
♂ **0V507ZZ** Destruction of Prostate, Via Natural or Artificial Opening
♂ **0V508ZZ** Destruction of Prostate, Via Natural or Artificial Opening Endoscopic
♂ **0V510ZZ** Destruction of Right Seminal Vesicle, Open Approach
♂ **0V513ZZ** Destruction of Right Seminal Vesicle, Percutaneous Approach
♂ **0V514ZZ** Destruction of Right Seminal Vesicle, Percutaneous Endoscopic Approach
♂ **0V520ZZ** Destruction of Left Seminal Vesicle, Open Approach
♂ **0V523ZZ** Destruction of Left Seminal Vesicle, Percutaneous Approach
♂ **0V524ZZ** Destruction of Left Seminal Vesicle, Percutaneous Endoscopic Approach
♂ **0V530ZZ** Destruction of Bilateral Seminal Vesicles, Open Approach
♂ **0V533ZZ** Destruction of Bilateral Seminal Vesicles, Percutaneous Approach
♂ **0V534ZZ** Destruction of Bilateral Seminal Vesicles, Percutaneous Endoscopic Approach
♂ **0V550ZZ** Destruction of Scrotum, Open Approach
♂ **0V553ZZ** Destruction of Scrotum, Percutaneous Approach
♂ **0V554ZZ** Destruction of Scrotum, Percutaneous Endoscopic Approach
♂ **0V55XZZ** Destruction of Scrotum, External Approach
♂ **0V560ZZ** Destruction of Right Tunica Vaginalis, Open Approach
♂ **0V563ZZ** Destruction of Right Tunica Vaginalis, Percutaneous Approach
♂ **0V564ZZ** Destruction of Right Tunica Vaginalis, Percutaneous Endoscopic Approach
♂ **0V570ZZ** Destruction of Left Tunica Vaginalis, Open Approach
♂ **0V573ZZ** Destruction of Left Tunica Vaginalis, Percutaneous Approach
♂ **0V574ZZ** Destruction of Left Tunica Vaginalis, Percutaneous Endoscopic Approach
♂ **0V590ZZ** Destruction of Right Testis, Open Approach
♂ **0V593ZZ** Destruction of Right Testis, Percutaneous Approach
♂ **0V594ZZ** Destruction of Right Testis, Percutaneous Endoscopic Approach
♂ **0V5B0ZZ** Destruction of Left Testis, Open Approach
♂ **0V5B3ZZ** Destruction of Left Testis, Percutaneous Approach
♂ **0V5B4ZZ** Destruction of Left Testis, Percutaneous Endoscopic Approach
♂ **0V5C0ZZ** Destruction of Bilateral Testes, Open Approach
♂ **0V5C3ZZ** Destruction of Bilateral Testes, Percutaneous Approach
♂ **0V5C4ZZ** Destruction of Bilateral Testes, Percutaneous Endoscopic Approach
♂ **0V5F0ZZ** Destruction of Right Spermatic Cord, Open Approach
♂ **0V5F3ZZ** Destruction of Right Spermatic Cord, Percutaneous Approach
♂ **0V5F4ZZ** Destruction of Right Spermatic Cord, Percutaneous Endoscopic Approach
♂ **0V5G0ZZ** Destruction of Left Spermatic Cord, Open Approach
♂ **0V5G3ZZ** Destruction of Left Spermatic Cord, Percutaneous Approach
♂ **0V5G4ZZ** Destruction of Left Spermatic Cord, Percutaneous Endoscopic Approach
♂ **0V5H0ZZ** Destruction of Bilateral Spermatic Cords, Open Approach
♂ **0V5H3ZZ** Destruction of Bilateral Spermatic Cords, Percutaneous Approach
♂ **0V5H4ZZ** Destruction of Bilateral Spermatic Cords, Percutaneous Endoscopic Approach
♂ **0V5J0ZZ** Destruction of Right Epididymis, Open Approach
♂ **0V5J3ZZ** Destruction of Right Epididymis, Percutaneous Approach
♂ **0V5J4ZZ** Destruction of Right Epididymis, Percutaneous Endoscopic Approach
♂ **0V5K0ZZ** Destruction of Left Epididymis, Open Approach
♂ **0V5K3ZZ** Destruction of Left Epididymis, Percutaneous Approach
♂ **0V5K4ZZ** Destruction of Left Epididymis, Percutaneous Endoscopic Approach
♂ **0V5L0ZZ** Destruction of Bilateral Epididymis, Open Approach
♂ **0V5L3ZZ** Destruction of Bilateral Epididymis, Percutaneous Approach
♂ **0V5L4ZZ** Destruction of Bilateral Epididymis, Percutaneous Endoscopic Approach
♂ ▲ **0V5N0ZZ** Destruction of Right Vas Deferens, Open Approach
♂ ▲ **0V5N3ZZ** Destruction of Right Vas Deferens, Percutaneous Approach
♂ ▲ **0V5N4ZZ** Destruction of Right Vas Deferens, Percutaneous Endoscopic Approach
♂ ▲ **0V5P0ZZ** Destruction of Left Vas Deferens, Open Approach
♂ ▲ **0V5P3ZZ** Destruction of Left Vas Deferens, Percutaneous Approach
♂ ▲ **0V5P4ZZ** Destruction of Left Vas Deferens, Percutaneous Endoscopic Approach
♂ **0V5Q0ZZ** Destruction of Bilateral Vas Deferens, Open Approach
♂ **0V5Q3ZZ** Destruction of Bilateral Vas Deferens, Percutaneous Approach
♂ **0V5Q4ZZ** Destruction of Bilateral Vas Deferens, Percutaneous Endoscopic Approach
♂ **0V5S0ZZ** Destruction of Penis, Open Approach
♂ **0V5S3ZZ** Destruction of Penis, Percutaneous Approach
♂ **0V5S4ZZ** Destruction of Penis, Percutaneous Endoscopic Approach
♂ **0V5SXZZ** Destruction of Penis, External Approach
♂ **0V5T0ZZ** Destruction of Prepuce, Open Approach
♂ **0V5T3ZZ** Destruction of Prepuce, Percutaneous Approach
♂ **0V5T4ZZ** Destruction of Prepuce, Percutaneous Endoscopic Approach
♂ **0V5TXZZ** Destruction of Prepuce, External Approach

0V7 – Male Reproductive System, Dilation

♂ **0V7N0DZ** Dilation of Right Vas Deferens with Intraluminal Device, Open Approach
♂ **0V7N0ZZ** Dilation of Right Vas Deferens, Open Approach
♂ **0V7N3DZ** Dilation of Right Vas Deferens with Intraluminal Device, Percutaneous Approach
♂ **0V7N3ZZ** Dilation of Right Vas Deferens, Percutaneous Approach
♂ **0V7N4DZ** Dilation of Right Vas Deferens with Intraluminal Device, Percutaneous Endoscopic Approach
♂ **0V7N4ZZ** Dilation of Right Vas Deferens, Percutaneous Endoscopic Approach
♂ **0V7P0DZ** Dilation of Left Vas Deferens with Intraluminal Device, Open Approach
♂ **0V7P0ZZ** Dilation of Left Vas Deferens, Open Approach
♂ **0V7P3DZ** Dilation of Left Vas Deferens with Intraluminal Device, Percutaneous Approach
♂ **0V7P3ZZ** Dilation of Left Vas Deferens, Percutaneous Approach
♂ **0V7P4DZ** Dilation of Left Vas Deferens with Intraluminal Device, Percutaneous Endoscopic Approach
♂ **0V7P4ZZ** Dilation of Left Vas Deferens, Percutaneous Endoscopic Approach
♂ **0V7Q0DZ** Dilation of Bilateral Vas Deferens with Intraluminal Device, Open Approach
♂ **0V7Q0ZZ** Dilation of Bilateral Vas Deferens, Open Approach
♂ **0V7Q3DZ** Dilation of Bilateral Vas Deferens with Intraluminal Device, Percutaneous Approach
♂ **0V7Q3ZZ** Dilation of Bilateral Vas Deferens, Percutaneous Approach
♂ **0V7Q4DZ** Dilation of Bilateral Vas Deferens with Intraluminal Device, Percutaneous Endoscopic Approach
♂ **0V7Q4ZZ** Dilation of Bilateral Vas Deferens, Percutaneous Endoscopic Approach

0V9 – Male Reproductive System, Drainage

Review Coding Guidelines B3.4a and B3.4b

Review Coding Guideline B6.2

♂ **0V9000Z** Drainage of Prostate with Drainage Device, Open Approach
♂ **0V900ZX** Drainage of Prostate, Open Approach, Diagnostic
♂ **0V900ZZ** Drainage of Prostate, Open Approach
♂ **0V9030Z** Drainage of Prostate with Drainage Device, Percutaneous Approach
♂ **0V903ZX** Drainage of Prostate, Percutaneous Approach, Diagnostic
♂ **0V903ZZ** Drainage of Prostate, Percutaneous Approach
♂ **0V9040Z** Drainage of Prostate with Drainage Device, Percutaneous Endoscopic Approach
♂ **0V904ZX** Drainage of Prostate, Percutaneous Endoscopic Approach, Diagnostic
♂ **0V904ZZ** Drainage of Prostate, Percutaneous Endoscopic Approach
♂ **0V9070Z** Drainage of Prostate with Drainage Device, Via Natural or Artificial Opening
♂ **0V907ZX** Drainage of Prostate, Via Natural or Artificial Opening, Diagnostic
♂ **0V907ZZ** Drainage of Prostate, Via Natural or Artificial Opening
♂ **0V9080Z** Drainage of Prostate with Drainage Device, Via Natural or Artificial Opening Endoscopic

♂ **0V908ZX** Drainage of Prostate, Via Natural or Artificial Opening Endoscopic, Diagnostic
♂ **0V908ZZ** Drainage of Prostate, Via Natural or Artificial Opening Endoscopic
♂ **0V9100Z** Drainage of Right Seminal Vesicle with Drainage Device, Open Approach
♂ **0V910ZX** Drainage of Right Seminal Vesicle, Open Approach, Diagnostic
♂ **0V910ZZ** Drainage of Right Seminal Vesicle, Open Approach
♂ **0V9130Z** Drainage of Right Seminal Vesicle with Drainage Device, Percutaneous Approach
♂ **0V913ZX** Drainage of Right Seminal Vesicle, Percutaneous Approach, Diagnostic
♂ **0V913ZZ** Drainage of Right Seminal Vesicle, Percutaneous Approach
♂ **0V9140Z** Drainage of Right Seminal Vesicle with Drainage Device, Percutaneous Endoscopic Approach
♂ **0V914ZX** Drainage of Right Seminal Vesicle, Percutaneous Endoscopic Approach, Diagnostic
♂ **0V914ZZ** Drainage of Right Seminal Vesicle, Percutaneous Endoscopic Approach
♂ **0V9200Z** Drainage of Left Seminal Vesicle with Drainage Device, Open Approach
♂ **0V920ZX** Drainage of Left Seminal Vesicle, Open Approach, Diagnostic
♂ **0V920ZZ** Drainage of Left Seminal Vesicle, Open Approach
♂ **0V9230Z** Drainage of Left Seminal Vesicle with Drainage Device, Percutaneous Approach
♂ **0V923ZX** Drainage of Left Seminal Vesicle, Percutaneous Approach, Diagnostic
♂ **0V923ZZ** Drainage of Left Seminal Vesicle, Percutaneous Approach
♂ **0V9240Z** Drainage of Left Seminal Vesicle with Drainage Device, Percutaneous Endoscopic Approach
♂ **0V924ZX** Drainage of Left Seminal Vesicle, Percutaneous Endoscopic Approach, Diagnostic
♂ **0V924ZZ** Drainage of Left Seminal Vesicle, Percutaneous Endoscopic Approach
♂ **0V9300Z** Drainage of Bilateral Seminal Vesicles with Drainage Device, Open Approach
♂ **0V930ZX** Drainage of Bilateral Seminal Vesicles, Open Approach, Diagnostic
♂ **0V930ZZ** Drainage of Bilateral Seminal Vesicles, Open Approach
♂ **0V9330Z** Drainage of Bilateral Seminal Vesicles with Drainage Device, Percutaneous Approach
♂ **0V933ZX** Drainage of Bilateral Seminal Vesicles, Percutaneous Approach, Diagnostic
♂ **0V933ZZ** Drainage of Bilateral Seminal Vesicles, Percutaneous Approach
♂ **0V9340Z** Drainage of Bilateral Seminal Vesicles with Drainage Device, Percutaneous Endoscopic Approach
♂ **0V934ZX** Drainage of Bilateral Seminal Vesicles, Percutaneous Endoscopic Approach, Diagnostic
♂ **0V934ZZ** Drainage of Bilateral Seminal Vesicles, Percutaneous Endoscopic Approach
♂ **0V9500Z** Drainage of Scrotum with Drainage Device, Open Approach
♂ **0V950ZX** Drainage of Scrotum, Open Approach, Diagnostic
♂ **0V950ZZ** Drainage of Scrotum, Open Approach
♂ **0V9530Z** Drainage of Scrotum with Drainage Device, Percutaneous Approach
♂ **0V953ZX** Drainage of Scrotum, Percutaneous Approach, Diagnostic
♂ **0V953ZZ** Drainage of Scrotum, Percutaneous Approach
♂ **0V9540Z** Drainage of Scrotum with Drainage Device, Percutaneous Endoscopic Approach
♂ **0V954ZX** Drainage of Scrotum, Percutaneous Endoscopic Approach, Diagnostic
♂ **0V954ZZ** Drainage of Scrotum, Percutaneous Endoscopic Approach
♂ **0V95X0Z** Drainage of Scrotum with Drainage Device, External Approach
♂ **0V95XZX** Drainage of Scrotum, External Approach, Diagnostic
♂ **0V95XZZ** Drainage of Scrotum, External Approach
♂ **0V9600Z** Drainage of Right Tunica Vaginalis with Drainage Device, Open Approach
♂ **0V960ZX** Drainage of Right Tunica Vaginalis, Open Approach, Diagnostic
♂ **0V960ZZ** Drainage of Right Tunica Vaginalis, Open Approach
♂ **0V9630Z** Drainage of Right Tunica Vaginalis with Drainage Device, Percutaneous Approach
♂ **0V963ZX** Drainage of Right Tunica Vaginalis, Percutaneous Approach, Diagnostic
♂ **0V963ZZ** Drainage of Right Tunica Vaginalis, Percutaneous Approach
♂ **0V9640Z** Drainage of Right Tunica Vaginalis with Drainage Device, Percutaneous Endoscopic Approach
♂ **0V964ZX** Drainage of Right Tunica Vaginalis, Percutaneous Endoscopic Approach, Diagnostic
♂ **0V964ZZ** Drainage of Right Tunica Vaginalis, Percutaneous Endoscopic Approach
♂ **0V9700Z** Drainage of Left Tunica Vaginalis with Drainage Device, Open Approach
♂ **0V970ZX** Drainage of Left Tunica Vaginalis, Open Approach, Diagnostic
♂ **0V970ZZ** Drainage of Left Tunica Vaginalis, Open Approach
♂ **0V9730Z** Drainage of Left Tunica Vaginalis with Drainage Device, Percutaneous Approach
♂ **0V973ZX** Drainage of Left Tunica Vaginalis, Percutaneous Approach, Diagnostic
♂ **0V973ZZ** Drainage of Left Tunica Vaginalis, Percutaneous Approach
♂ **0V9740Z** Drainage of Left Tunica Vaginalis with Drainage Device, Percutaneous Endoscopic Approach
♂ **0V974ZX** Drainage of Left Tunica Vaginalis, Percutaneous Endoscopic Approach, Diagnostic
♂ **0V974ZZ** Drainage of Left Tunica Vaginalis, Percutaneous Endoscopic Approach
♂ **0V9900Z** Drainage of Right Testis with Drainage Device, Open Approach
♂ **0V990ZX** Drainage of Right Testis, Open Approach, Diagnostic
♂ **0V990ZZ** Drainage of Right Testis, Open Approach
♂ **0V9930Z** Drainage of Right Testis with Drainage Device, Percutaneous Approach
♂ **0V993ZX** Drainage of Right Testis, Percutaneous Approach, Diagnostic
♂ **0V993ZZ** Drainage of Right Testis, Percutaneous Approach
♂ **0V9940Z** Drainage of Right Testis with Drainage Device, Percutaneous Endoscopic Approach
♂ **0V994ZX** Drainage of Right Testis, Percutaneous Endoscopic Approach, Diagnostic
♂ **0V994ZZ** Drainage of Right Testis, Percutaneous Endoscopic Approach
♂ **0V9B00Z** Drainage of Left Testis with Drainage Device, Open Approach
♂ **0V9B0ZX** Drainage of Left Testis, Open Approach, Diagnostic
♂ **0V9B0ZZ** Drainage of Left Testis, Open Approach
♂ **0V9B30Z** Drainage of Left Testis with Drainage Device, Percutaneous Approach
♂ **0V9B3ZX** Drainage of Left Testis, Percutaneous Approach, Diagnostic
♂ **0V9B3ZZ** Drainage of Left Testis, Percutaneous Approach
♂ **0V9B40Z** Drainage of Left Testis with Drainage Device, Percutaneous Endoscopic Approach
♂ **0V9B4ZX** Drainage of Left Testis, Percutaneous Endoscopic Approach, Diagnostic
♂ **0V9B4ZZ** Drainage of Left Testis, Percutaneous Endoscopic Approach
♂ **0V9C00Z** Drainage of Bilateral Testes with Drainage Device, Open Approach
♂ **0V9C0ZX** Drainage of Bilateral Testes, Open Approach, Diagnostic
♂ **0V9C0ZZ** Drainage of Bilateral Testes, Open Approach
♂ **0V9C30Z** Drainage of Bilateral Testes with Drainage Device, Percutaneous Approach
♂ **0V9C3ZX** Drainage of Bilateral Testes, Percutaneous Approach, Diagnostic
♂ **0V9C3ZZ** Drainage of Bilateral Testes, Percutaneous Approach
♂ **0V9C40Z** Drainage of Bilateral Testes with Drainage Device, Percutaneous Endoscopic Approach
♂ **0V9C4ZX** Drainage of Bilateral Testes, Percutaneous Endoscopic Approach, Diagnostic
♂ **0V9C4ZZ** Drainage of Bilateral Testes, Percutaneous Endoscopic Approach
♂ **0V9F00Z** Drainage of Right Spermatic Cord with Drainage Device, Open Approach
♂ **0V9F0ZX** Drainage of Right Spermatic Cord, Open Approach, Diagnostic
♂ **0V9F0ZZ** Drainage of Right Spermatic Cord, Open Approach
♂ **0V9F30Z** Drainage of Right Spermatic Cord with Drainage Device, Percutaneous Approach
♂ **0V9F3ZX** Drainage of Right Spermatic Cord, Percutaneous Approach, Diagnostic
♂ **0V9F3ZZ** Drainage of Right Spermatic Cord, Percutaneous Approach
♂ **0V9F40Z** Drainage of Right Spermatic Cord with Drainage Device, Percutaneous Endoscopic Approach
♂ **0V9F4ZX** Drainage of Right Spermatic Cord, Percutaneous Endoscopic Approach, Diagnostic
♂ **0V9F4ZZ** Drainage of Right Spermatic Cord, Percutaneous Endoscopic Approach
♂ **0V9G00Z** Drainage of Left Spermatic Cord with Drainage Device, Open Approach
♂ **0V9G0ZX** Drainage of Left Spermatic Cord, Open Approach, Diagnostic
♂ **0V9G0ZZ** Drainage of Left Spermatic Cord, Open Approach
♂ **0V9G30Z** Drainage of Left Spermatic Cord with Drainage Device, Percutaneous Approach
♂ **0V9G3ZX** Drainage of Left Spermatic Cord, Percutaneous Approach, Diagnostic
♂ **0V9G3ZZ** Drainage of Left Spermatic Cord, Percutaneous Approach
♂ **0V9G40Z** Drainage of Left Spermatic Cord with Drainage Device, Percutaneous Endoscopic Approach
♂ **0V9G4ZX** Drainage of Left Spermatic Cord, Percutaneous Endoscopic Approach, Diagnostic
♂ **0V9G4ZZ** Drainage of Left Spermatic Cord, Percutaneous Endoscopic Approach
♂ **0V9H00Z** Drainage of Bilateral Spermatic Cords with Drainage Device, Open Approach
♂ **0V9H0ZX** Drainage of Bilateral Spermatic Cords, Open Approach, Diagnostic
♂ **0V9H0ZZ** Drainage of Bilateral Spermatic Cords, Open Approach

♂0V9H30Z Drainage of Bilateral Spermatic Cords with Drainage Device, Percutaneous Approach
♂0V9H3ZX Drainage of Bilateral Spermatic Cords, Percutaneous Approach, Diagnostic
♂0V9H3ZZ Drainage of Bilateral Spermatic Cords, Percutaneous Approach
♂0V9H40Z Drainage of Bilateral Spermatic Cords with Drainage Device, Percutaneous Endoscopic Approach
♂0V9H4ZX Drainage of Bilateral Spermatic Cords, Percutaneous Endoscopic Approach, Diagnostic
♂0V9H4ZZ Drainage of Bilateral Spermatic Cords, Percutaneous Endoscopic Approach
♂0V9J00Z Drainage of Right Epididymis with Drainage Device, Open Approach
♂0V9J0ZX Drainage of Right Epididymis, Open Approach, Diagnostic
♂0V9J0ZZ Drainage of Right Epididymis, Open Approach
♂0V9J30Z Drainage of Right Epididymis with Drainage Device, Percutaneous Approach
♂0V9J3ZX Drainage of Right Epididymis, Percutaneous Approach, Diagnostic
♂0V9J3ZZ Drainage of Right Epididymis, Percutaneous Approach
♂0V9J40Z Drainage of Right Epididymis with Drainage Device, Percutaneous Endoscopic Approach
♂0V9J4ZX Drainage of Right Epididymis, Percutaneous Endoscopic Approach, Diagnostic
♂0V9J4ZZ Drainage of Right Epididymis, Percutaneous Endoscopic Approach
♂0V9K00Z Drainage of Left Epididymis with Drainage Device, Open Approach
♂0V9K0ZX Drainage of Left Epididymis, Open Approach, Diagnostic
♂0V9K0ZZ Drainage of Left Epididymis, Open Approach
♂0V9K30Z Drainage of Left Epididymis with Drainage Device, Percutaneous Approach
♂0V9K3ZX Drainage of Left Epididymis, Percutaneous Approach, Diagnostic
♂0V9K3ZZ Drainage of Left Epididymis, Percutaneous Approach
♂0V9K40Z Drainage of Left Epididymis with Drainage Device, Percutaneous Endoscopic Approach
♂0V9K4ZX Drainage of Left Epididymis, Percutaneous Endoscopic Approach, Diagnostic
♂0V9K4ZZ Drainage of Left Epididymis, Percutaneous Endoscopic Approach
♂0V9L00Z Drainage of Bilateral Epididymis with Drainage Device, Open Approach
♂0V9L0ZX Drainage of Bilateral Epididymis, Open Approach, Diagnostic
♂0V9L0ZZ Drainage of Bilateral Epididymis, Open Approach
♂0V9L30Z Drainage of Bilateral Epididymis with Drainage Device, Percutaneous Approach
♂0V9L3ZX Drainage of Bilateral Epididymis, Percutaneous Approach, Diagnostic
♂0V9L3ZZ Drainage of Bilateral Epididymis, Percutaneous Approach
♂0V9L40Z Drainage of Bilateral Epididymis with Drainage Device, Percutaneous Endoscopic Approach
♂0V9L4ZX Drainage of Bilateral Epididymis, Percutaneous Endoscopic Approach, Diagnostic
♂0V9L4ZZ Drainage of Bilateral Epididymis, Percutaneous Endoscopic Approach
♂0V9N00Z Drainage of Right Vas Deferens with Drainage Device, Open Approach
♂0V9N0ZX Drainage of Right Vas Deferens, Open Approach, Diagnostic
♂0V9N0ZZ Drainage of Right Vas Deferens, Open Approach
♂0V9N30Z Drainage of Right Vas Deferens with Drainage Device, Percutaneous Approach
♂0V9N3ZX Drainage of Right Vas Deferens, Percutaneous Approach, Diagnostic
♂0V9N3ZZ Drainage of Right Vas Deferens, Percutaneous Approach
♂0V9N40Z Drainage of Right Vas Deferens with Drainage Device, Percutaneous Endoscopic Approach
♂0V9N4ZX Drainage of Right Vas Deferens, Percutaneous Endoscopic Approach, Diagnostic
♂0V9N4ZZ Drainage of Right Vas Deferens, Percutaneous Endoscopic Approach
♂0V9P00Z Drainage of Left Vas Deferens with Drainage Device, Open Approach
♂0V9P0ZX Drainage of Left Vas Deferens, Open Approach, Diagnostic
♂0V9P0ZZ Drainage of Left Vas Deferens, Open Approach
♂0V9P30Z Drainage of Left Vas Deferens with Drainage Device, Percutaneous Approach
♂0V9P3ZX Drainage of Left Vas Deferens, Percutaneous Approach, Diagnostic
♂0V9P3ZZ Drainage of Left Vas Deferens, Percutaneous Approach
♂0V9P40Z Drainage of Left Vas Deferens with Drainage Device, Percutaneous Endoscopic Approach
♂0V9P4ZX Drainage of Left Vas Deferens, Percutaneous Endoscopic Approach, Diagnostic
♂0V9P4ZZ Drainage of Left Vas Deferens, Percutaneous Endoscopic Approach
♂0V9Q00Z Drainage of Bilateral Vas Deferens with Drainage Device, Open Approach
♂0V9Q0ZX Drainage of Bilateral Vas Deferens, Open Approach, Diagnostic
♂0V9Q0ZZ Drainage of Bilateral Vas Deferens, Open Approach
♂0V9Q30Z Drainage of Bilateral Vas Deferens with Drainage Device, Percutaneous Approach
♂0V9Q3ZX Drainage of Bilateral Vas Deferens, Percutaneous Approach, Diagnostic
♂0V9Q3ZZ Drainage of Bilateral Vas Deferens, Percutaneous Approach
♂0V9Q40Z Drainage of Bilateral Vas Deferens with Drainage Device, Percutaneous Endoscopic Approach
♂0V9Q4ZX Drainage of Bilateral Vas Deferens, Percutaneous Endoscopic Approach, Diagnostic
♂0V9Q4ZZ Drainage of Bilateral Vas Deferens, Percutaneous Endoscopic Approach
♂0V9S00Z Drainage of Penis with Drainage Device, Open Approach
♂0V9S0ZX Drainage of Penis, Open Approach, Diagnostic
♂0V9S0ZZ Drainage of Penis, Open Approach
♂0V9S30Z Drainage of Penis with Drainage Device, Percutaneous Approach
♂0V9S3ZX Drainage of Penis, Percutaneous Approach, Diagnostic
♂0V9S3ZZ Drainage of Penis, Percutaneous Approach
♂0V9S40Z Drainage of Penis with Drainage Device, Percutaneous Endoscopic Approach
♂0V9S4ZX Drainage of Penis, Percutaneous Endoscopic Approach, Diagnostic
♂0V9S4ZZ Drainage of Penis, Percutaneous Endoscopic Approach
♂0V9SX0Z Drainage of Penis with Drainage Device, External Approach
♂0V9SXZX Drainage of Penis, External Approach, Diagnostic
♂0V9SXZZ Drainage of Penis, External Approach
♂0V9T00Z Drainage of Prepuce with Drainage Device, Open Approach
♂0V9T0ZX Drainage of Prepuce, Open Approach, Diagnostic
♂0V9T0ZZ Drainage of Prepuce, Open Approach
♂0V9T30Z Drainage of Prepuce with Drainage Device, Percutaneous Approach
♂0V9T3ZX Drainage of Prepuce, Percutaneous Approach, Diagnostic
♂0V9T3ZZ Drainage of Prepuce, Percutaneous Approach
♂0V9T40Z Drainage of Prepuce with Drainage Device, Percutaneous Endoscopic Approach
♂0V9T4ZX Drainage of Prepuce, Percutaneous Endoscopic Approach, Diagnostic
♂0V9T4ZZ Drainage of Prepuce, Percutaneous Endoscopic Approach
♂0V9TX0Z Drainage of Prepuce with Drainage Device, External Approach
♂0V9TXZX Drainage of Prepuce, External Approach, Diagnostic
♂0V9TXZZ Drainage of Prepuce, External Approach

0VB – Male Reproductive System, Excision

Review Coding Guidelines B3.4a and B3.4b

Review Coding Guideline B3.8

♂0VB00ZX Excision of Prostate, Open Approach, Diagnostic
♂0VB00ZZ Excision of Prostate, Open Approach
♂0VB03ZX Excision of Prostate, Percutaneous Approach, Diagnostic
♂0VB03ZZ Excision of Prostate, Percutaneous Approach
♂0VB04ZX Excision of Prostate, Percutaneous Endoscopic Approach, Diagnostic
♂0VB04ZZ Excision of Prostate, Percutaneous Endoscopic Approach
♂0VB07ZX Excision of Prostate, Via Natural or Artificial Opening, Diagnostic
♂0VB07ZZ Excision of Prostate, Via Natural or Artificial Opening
♂0VB08ZX Excision of Prostate, Via Natural or Artificial Opening Endoscopic, Diagnostic
♂0VB08ZZ Excision of Prostate, Via Natural or Artificial Opening Endoscopic
♂0VB10ZX Excision of Right Seminal Vesicle, Open Approach, Diagnostic
♂0VB10ZZ Excision of Right Seminal Vesicle, Open Approach
♂0VB13ZX Excision of Right Seminal Vesicle, Percutaneous Approach, Diagnostic
♂0VB13ZZ Excision of Right Seminal Vesicle, Percutaneous Approach
♂0VB14ZX Excision of Right Seminal Vesicle, Percutaneous Endoscopic Approach, Diagnostic
♂0VB14ZZ Excision of Right Seminal Vesicle, Percutaneous Endoscopic Approach

♂ **0VB20ZX** Excision of Left Seminal Vesicle, Open Approach, Diagnostic
♂ **0VB20ZZ** Excision of Left Seminal Vesicle, Open Approach
♂ **0VB23ZX** Excision of Left Seminal Vesicle, Percutaneous Approach, Diagnostic
♂ **0VB23ZZ** Excision of Left Seminal Vesicle, Percutaneous Approach
♂ **0VB24ZX** Excision of Left Seminal Vesicle, Percutaneous Endoscopic Approach, Diagnostic
♂ **0VB24ZZ** Excision of Left Seminal Vesicle, Percutaneous Endoscopic Approach
♂ **0VB30ZX** Excision of Bilateral Seminal Vesicles, Open Approach, Diagnostic
♂ **0VB30ZZ** Excision of Bilateral Seminal Vesicles, Open Approach
♂ **0VB33ZX** Excision of Bilateral Seminal Vesicles, Percutaneous Approach, Diagnostic
♂ **0VB33ZZ** Excision of Bilateral Seminal Vesicles, Percutaneous Approach
♂ **0VB34ZX** Excision of Bilateral Seminal Vesicles, Percutaneous Endoscopic Approach, Diagnostic
♂ **0VB34ZZ** Excision of Bilateral Seminal Vesicles, Percutaneous Endoscopic Approach
♂ **0VB50ZX** Excision of Scrotum, Open Approach, Diagnostic
♂ **0VB50ZZ** Excision of Scrotum, Open Approach
♂ **0VB53ZX** Excision of Scrotum, Percutaneous Approach, Diagnostic
♂ **0VB53ZZ** Excision of Scrotum, Percutaneous Approach
♂ **0VB54ZX** Excision of Scrotum, Percutaneous Endoscopic Approach, Diagnostic
♂ **0VB54ZZ** Excision of Scrotum, Percutaneous Endoscopic Approach
♂ **0VB5XZX** Excision of Scrotum, External Approach, Diagnostic
♂ **0VB5XZZ** Excision of Scrotum, External Approach
♂ **0VB60ZX** Excision of Right Tunica Vaginalis, Open Approach, Diagnostic
♂ **0VB60ZZ** Excision of Right Tunica Vaginalis, Open Approach
♂ **0VB63ZX** Excision of Right Tunica Vaginalis, Percutaneous Approach, Diagnostic
♂ **0VB63ZZ** Excision of Right Tunica Vaginalis, Percutaneous Approach
♂ **0VB64ZX** Excision of Right Tunica Vaginalis, Percutaneous Endoscopic Approach, Diagnostic
♂ **0VB64ZZ** Excision of Right Tunica Vaginalis, Percutaneous Endoscopic Approach
♂ **0VB70ZX** Excision of Left Tunica Vaginalis, Open Approach, Diagnostic
♂ **0VB70ZZ** Excision of Left Tunica Vaginalis, Open Approach
♂ **0VB73ZX** Excision of Left Tunica Vaginalis, Percutaneous Approach, Diagnostic
♂ **0VB73ZZ** Excision of Left Tunica Vaginalis, Percutaneous Approach
♂ **0VB74ZX** Excision of Left Tunica Vaginalis, Percutaneous Endoscopic Approach, Diagnostic
♂ **0VB74ZZ** Excision of Left Tunica Vaginalis, Percutaneous Endoscopic Approach
♂ **0VB90ZX** Excision of Right Testis, Open Approach, Diagnostic
♂ **0VB90ZZ** Excision of Right Testis, Open Approach
♂ **0VB93ZX** Excision of Right Testis, Percutaneous Approach, Diagnostic
♂ **0VB93ZZ** Excision of Right Testis, Percutaneous Approach
♂ **0VB94ZX** Excision of Right Testis, Percutaneous Endoscopic Approach, Diagnostic
♂ **0VB94ZZ** Excision of Right Testis, Percutaneous Endoscopic Approach
♂ **0VBB0ZX** Excision of Left Testis, Open Approach, Diagnostic
♂ **0VBB0ZZ** Excision of Left Testis, Open Approach
♂ **0VBB3ZX** Excision of Left Testis, Percutaneous Approach, Diagnostic
♂ **0VBB3ZZ** Excision of Left Testis, Percutaneous Approach
♂ **0VBB4ZX** Excision of Left Testis, Percutaneous Endoscopic Approach, Diagnostic
♂ **0VBB4ZZ** Excision of Left Testis, Percutaneous Endoscopic Approach
♂ **0VBC0ZX** Excision of Bilateral Testes, Open Approach, Diagnostic
♂ **0VBC0ZZ** Excision of Bilateral Testes, Open Approach
♂ **0VBC3ZX** Excision of Bilateral Testes, Percutaneous Approach, Diagnostic
♂ **0VBC3ZZ** Excision of Bilateral Testes, Percutaneous Approach
♂ **0VBC4ZX** Excision of Bilateral Testes, Percutaneous Endoscopic Approach, Diagnostic
♂ **0VBC4ZZ** Excision of Bilateral Testes, Percutaneous Endoscopic Approach
♂ **0VBF0ZX** Excision of Right Spermatic Cord, Open Approach, Diagnostic
♂ **0VBF0ZZ** Excision of Right Spermatic Cord, Open Approach
♂ **0VBF3ZX** Excision of Right Spermatic Cord, Percutaneous Approach, Diagnostic
♂ **0VBF3ZZ** Excision of Right Spermatic Cord, Percutaneous Approach
♂ **0VBF4ZX** Excision of Right Spermatic Cord, Percutaneous Endoscopic Approach, Diagnostic
♂ **0VBF4ZZ** Excision of Right Spermatic Cord, Percutaneous Endoscopic Approach
♂ **0VBG0ZX** Excision of Left Spermatic Cord, Open Approach, Diagnostic
♂ **0VBG0ZZ** Excision of Left Spermatic Cord, Open Approach
♂ **0VBG3ZX** Excision of Left Spermatic Cord, Percutaneous Approach, Diagnostic
♂ **0VBG3ZZ** Excision of Left Spermatic Cord, Percutaneous Approach
♂ **0VBG4ZX** Excision of Left Spermatic Cord, Percutaneous Endoscopic Approach, Diagnostic
♂ **0VBG4ZZ** Excision of Left Spermatic Cord, Percutaneous Endoscopic Approach
♂ **0VBH0ZX** Excision of Bilateral Spermatic Cords, Open Approach, vDiagnostic
♂ **0VBH0ZZ** Excision of Bilateral Spermatic Cords, Open Approach
♂ **0VBH3ZX** Excision of Bilateral Spermatic Cords, Percutaneous Approach, Diagnostic
♂ **0VBH3ZZ** Excision of Bilateral Spermatic Cords, Percutaneous Approach
♂ **0VBH4ZX** Excision of Bilateral Spermatic Cords, Percutaneous Endoscopic Approach, Diagnostic
♂ **0VBH4ZZ** Excision of Bilateral Spermatic Cords, Percutaneous Endoscopic Approach
♂ **0VBJ0ZX** Excision of Right Epididymis, Open Approach, Diagnostic
♂ **0VBJ0ZZ** Excision of Right Epididymis, Open Approach
♂ **0VBJ3ZX** Excision of Right Epididymis, Percutaneous Approach, Diagnostic
♂ **0VBJ3ZZ** Excision of Right Epididymis, Percutaneous Approach
♂ **0VBJ4ZX** Excision of Right Epididymis, Percutaneous Endoscopic Approach, Diagnostic
♂ **0VBJ4ZZ** Excision of Right Epididymis, Percutaneous Endoscopic Approach
♂ **0VBK0ZX** Excision of Left Epididymis, Open Approach, Diagnostic
♂ **0VBK0ZZ** Excision of Left Epididymis, Open Approach
♂ **0VBK3ZX** Excision of Left Epididymis, Percutaneous Approach, Diagnostic
♂ **0VBK3ZZ** Excision of Left Epididymis, Percutaneous Approach
♂ **0VBK4ZX** Excision of Left Epididymis, Percutaneous Endoscopic Approach, Diagnostic
♂ **0VBK4ZZ** Excision of Left Epididymis, Percutaneous Endoscopic Approach
♂ **0VBL0ZX** Excision of Bilateral Epididymis, Open Approach, Diagnostic
♂ **0VBL0ZZ** Excision of Bilateral Epididymis, Open Approach
♂ **0VBL3ZX** Excision of Bilateral Epididymis, Percutaneous Approach, Diagnostic
♂ **0VBL3ZZ** Excision of Bilateral Epididymis, Percutaneous Approach
♂ **0VBL4ZX** Excision of Bilateral Epididymis, Percutaneous Endoscopic Approach, Diagnostic
♂ **0VBL4ZZ** Excision of Bilateral Epididymis, Percutaneous Endoscopic Approach
♂ **0VBN0ZX** Excision of Right Vas Deferens, Open Approach, Diagnostic
♂ ▲ **0VBN0ZZ** Excision of Right Vas Deferens, Open Approach
♂ **0VBN3ZX** Excision of Right Vas Deferens, Percutaneous Approach, Diagnostic
♂ ▲ **0VBN3ZZ** Excision of Right Vas Deferens, Percutaneous Approach
♂ **0VBN4ZX** Excision of Right Vas Deferens, Percutaneous Endoscopic Approach, Diagnostic
♂ ▲ **0VBN4ZZ** Excision of Right Vas Deferens, Percutaneous Endoscopic Approach
♂ **0VBP0ZX** Excision of Left Vas Deferens, Open Approach, Diagnostic
♂ **0VBP0ZZ** Excision of Left Vas Deferens, Open Approach
♂ **0VBP3ZX** Excision of Left Vas Deferens, Percutaneous Approach, Diagnostic
♂ ▲ **0VBP3ZZ** Excision of Left Vas Deferens, Percutaneous Approach
♂ **0VBP4ZX** Excision of Left Vas Deferens, Percutaneous Endoscopic Approach, Diagnostic
♂ ▲ **0VBP4ZZ** Excision of Left Vas Deferens, Percutaneous Endoscopic Approach
♂ **0VBQ0ZX** Excision of Bilateral Vas Deferens, Open Approach, Diagnostic
♂ ▲ **0VBQ0ZZ** Excision of Bilateral Vas Deferens, Open Approach
♂ **0VBQ3ZX** Excision of Bilateral Vas Deferens, Percutaneous Approach, Diagnostic
♂ ▲ **0VBQ3ZZ** Excision of Bilateral Vas Deferens, Percutaneous Approach
♂ **0VBQ4ZX** Excision of Bilateral Vas Deferens, Percutaneous Endoscopic Approach, Diagnostic
♂ ▲ **0VBQ4ZZ** Excision of Bilateral Vas Deferens, Percutaneous Endoscopic Approach
♂ **0VBS0ZX** Excision of Penis, Open Approach, Diagnostic
♂ **0VBS0ZZ** Excision of Penis, Open Approach
♂ **0VBS3ZX** Excision of Penis, Percutaneous Approach, Diagnostic
♂ **0VBS3ZZ** Excision of Penis, Percutaneous Approach
♂ **0VBS4ZX** Excision of Penis, Percutaneous Endoscopic Approach, Diagnostic
♂ **0VBS4ZZ** Excision of Penis, Percutaneous Endoscopic Approach
♂ **0VBSXZX** Excision of Penis, External Approach, Diagnostic
♂ **0VBSXZZ** Excision of Penis, External Approach
♂ **0VBT0ZX** Excision of Prepuce, Open Approach, Diagnostic

♂0VBT0ZZ Excision of Prepuce, Open Approach
♂0VBT3ZX Excision of Prepuce, Percutaneous Approach, Diagnostic
♂0VBT3ZZ Excision of Prepuce, Percutaneous Approach
♂ 0VBT4ZX Excision of Prepuce, Percutaneous Endoscopic Approach, Diagnostic
♂ 0VBT4ZZ Excision of Prepuce, Percutaneous Endoscopic Approach
♂ 0VBTXZX Excision of Prepuce, External Approach, Diagnostic
♂ 0VBTXZZ Excision of Prepuce, External Approach

0VC – Male Reproductive System, Extirpation

♂0VC00ZZ Extirpation of Matter from Prostate, Open Approach
♂0VC03ZZ Extirpation of Matter from Prostate, Percutaneous Approach
♂0VC04ZZ Extirpation of Matter from Prostate, Percutaneous Endoscopic Approach
♂0VC07ZZ Extirpation of Matter from Prostate, Via Natural or Artificial Opening
♂0VC08ZZ Extirpation of Matter from Prostate, Via Natural or Artificial Opening Endoscopic
♂0VC10ZZ Extirpation of Matter from Right Seminal Vesicle, Open Approach
♂0VC13ZZ Extirpation of Matter from Right Seminal Vesicle, Percutaneous Approach
♂0VC14ZZ Extirpation of Matter from Right Seminal Vesicle, Percutaneous Endoscopic Approach
♂0VC20ZZ Extirpation of Matter from Left Seminal Vesicle, Open Approach
♂0VC23ZZ Extirpation of Matter from Left Seminal Vesicle, Percutaneous Approach
♂0VC24ZZ Extirpation of Matter from Left Seminal Vesicle, Percutaneous Endoscopic Approach
♂0VC30ZZ Extirpation of Matter from Bilateral Seminal Vesicles, Open Approach
♂0VC33ZZ Extirpation of Matter from Bilateral Seminal Vesicles, Percutaneous Approach
♂0VC34ZZ Extirpation of Matter from Bilateral Seminal Vesicles, Percutaneous Endoscopic Approach
♂0VC50ZZ Extirpation of Matter from Scrotum, Open Approach
♂0VC53ZZ Extirpation of Matter from Scrotum, Percutaneous Approach
♂0VC54ZZ Extirpation of Matter from Scrotum, Percutaneous Endoscopic Approach
♂0VC5XZZ Extirpation of Matter from Scrotum, External Approach
♂0VC60ZZ Extirpation of Matter from Right Tunica Vaginalis, Open Approach
♂0VC63ZZ Extirpation of Matter from Right Tunica Vaginalis, Percutaneous Approach
♂0VC64ZZ Extirpation of Matter from Right Tunica Vaginalis, Percutaneous Endoscopic Approach
♂0VC70ZZ Extirpation of Matter from Left Tunica Vaginalis, Open Approach
♂0VC73ZZ Extirpation of Matter from Left Tunica Vaginalis, Percutaneous Approach
♂ 0VC74ZZ Extirpation of Matter from Left Tunica Vaginalis, Percutaneous Endoscopic Approach
♂ 0VC90ZZ Extirpation of Matter from Right Testis, Open Approach
♂ 0VC93ZZ Extirpation of Matter from Right Testis, Percutaneous Approach
♂ 0VC94ZZ Extirpation of Matter from Right Testis, Percutaneous Endoscopic Approach
♂ 0VCB0ZZ Extirpation of Matter from Left Testis, Open Approach
♂ 0VCB3ZZ Extirpation of Matter from Left Testis, Percutaneous Approach
♂ 0VCB4ZZ Extirpation of Matter from Left Testis, Percutaneous Endoscopic Approach
♂ 0VCC0ZZ Extirpation of Matter from Bilateral Testes, Open Approach
♂ 0VCC3ZZ Extirpation of Matter from Bilateral Testes, Percutaneous Approach
♂ 0VCC4ZZ Extirpation of Matter from Bilateral Testes, Percutaneous Endoscopic Approach
♂ 0VCF0ZZ Extirpation of Matter from Right Spermatic Cord, Open Approach
♂ 0VCF3ZZ Extirpation of Matter from Right Spermatic Cord, Percutaneous Approach
♂ 0VCF4ZZ Extirpation of Matter from Right Spermatic Cord, Percutaneous Endoscopic Approach
♂ 0VCG0ZZ Extirpation of Matter from Left Spermatic Cord, Open Approach
♂ 0VCG3ZZ Extirpation of Matter from Left Spermatic Cord, Percutaneous Approach
♂ 0VCG4ZZ Extirpation of Matter from Left Spermatic Cord, Percutaneous Endoscopic Approach
♂ 0VCH0ZZ Extirpation of Matter from Bilateral Spermatic Cords, Open Approach
♂ 0VCH3ZZ Extirpation of Matter from Bilateral Spermatic Cords, Percutaneous Approach
♂ 0VCH4ZZ Extirpation of Matter from Bilateral Spermatic Cords, Percutaneous Endoscopic Approach
♂ 0VCJ0ZZ Extirpation of Matter from Right Epididymis, Open Approach
♂ 0VCJ3ZZ Extirpation of Matter from Right Epididymis, Percutaneous Approach
♂ 0VCJ4ZZ Extirpation of Matter from Right Epididymis, Percutaneous Endoscopic Approach
♂ 0VCK0ZZ Extirpation of Matter from Left Epididymis, Open Approach
♂ 0VCK3ZZ Extirpation of Matter from Left Epididymis, Percutaneous Approach
♂ 0VCK4ZZ Extirpation of Matter from Left Epididymis, Percutaneous Endoscopic Approach
♂ 0VCL0ZZ Extirpation of Matter from Bilateral Epididymis, Open Approach
♂ 0VCL3ZZ Extirpation of Matter from Bilateral Epididymis, Percutaneous Approach
♂ 0VCL4ZZ Extirpation of Matter from Bilateral Epididymis, Percutaneous Endoscopic Approach
♂ 0VCN0ZZ Extirpation of Matter from Right Vas Deferens, Open Approach
♂ 0VCN3ZZ Extirpation of Matter from Right Vas Deferens, Percutaneous Approach
♂ 0VCN4ZZ Extirpation of Matter from Right Vas Deferens, Percutaneous Endoscopic Approach
♂ 0VCP0ZZ Extirpation of Matter from Left Vas Deferens, Open Approach
♂ 0VCP3ZZ Extirpation of Matter from Left Vas Deferens, Percutaneous Approach
♂ 0VCP4ZZ Extirpation of Matter from Left Vas Deferens, Percutaneous Endoscopic Approach
♂ 0VCQ0ZZ Extirpation of Matter from Bilateral Vas Deferens, Open Approach
♂ 0VCQ3ZZ Extirpation of Matter from Bilateral Vas Deferens, Percutaneous Approach
♂ 0VCQ4ZZ Extirpation of Matter from Bilateral Vas Deferens, Percutaneous Endoscopic Approach
♂ 0VCS0ZZ Extirpation of Matter from Penis, Open Approach
♂ 0VCS3ZZ Extirpation of Matter from Penis, Percutaneous Approach
♂ 0VCS4ZZ Extirpation of Matter from Penis, Percutaneous Endoscopic Approach
♂ 0VCSXZZ Extirpation of Matter from Penis, External Approach
♂ 0VCT0ZZ Extirpation of Matter from Prepuce, Open Approach
♂ 0VCT3ZZ Extirpation of Matter from Prepuce, Percutaneous Approach
♂ 0VCT4ZZ Extirpation of Matter from Prepuce, Percutaneous Endoscopic Approach
♂ 0VCTXZZ Extirpation of Matter from Prepuce, External Approach

0VH – Male Reproductive System, Insertion

♂0VH001Z Insertion of Radioactive Element into Prostate, Open Approach
♂0VH031Z Insertion of Radioactive Element into Prostate, Percutaneous Approach
♂0VH041Z Insertion of Radioactive Element into Prostate, Percutaneous Endoscopic Approach
♂0VH071Z Insertion of Radioactive Element into Prostate, Via Natural or Artificial Opening
♂0VH081Z Insertion of Radioactive Element into Prostate, Via Natural or Artificial Opening Endoscopic
♂0VH403Z Insertion of Infusion Device into Prostate and Seminal Vesicles, Open Approach
♂0VH433Z Insertion of Infusion Device into Prostate and Seminal Vesicles, Percutaneous Approach
♂ 0VH443Z Insertion of Infusion Device into Prostate and Seminal Vesicles, Percutaneous Endoscopic Approach
♂ 0VH473Z Insertion of Infusion Device into Prostate and Seminal Vesicles, Via Natural or Artificial Opening
♂ 0VH483Z Insertion of Infusion Device into Prostate and Seminal Vesicles, Via Natural or Artificial Opening Endoscopic
♂ 0VH803Z Insertion of Infusion Device into Scrotum and Tunica Vaginalis, Open Approach
♂ 0VH833Z Insertion of Infusion Device into Scrotum and Tunica Vaginalis, Percutaneous Approach
♂ 0VH843Z Insertion of Infusion Device into Scrotum and Tunica Vaginalis, Percutaneous Endoscopic Approach
♂ 0VH873Z Insertion of Infusion Device into Scrotum and Tunica Vaginalis, Via Natural or Artificial Opening
♂ 0VH883Z Insertion of Infusion Device into Scrotum and Tunica Vaginalis, Via Natural or Artificial Opening Endoscopic
♂ 0VHD03Z Insertion of Infusion Device into Testis, Open Approach
♂ 0VHD33Z Insertion of Infusion Device into Testis, Percutaneous Approach
♂ 0VHD43Z Insertion of Infusion Device into Testis, Percutaneous Endoscopic Approach
♂ 0VHD73Z Insertion of Infusion Device into Testis, Via Natural or Artificial Opening
♂ 0VHD83Z Insertion of Infusion Device into Testis, Via Natural or Artificial Opening Endoscopic

♂ 0VHM03Z Insertion of Infusion Device into Epididymis and Spermatic Cord, Open Approach
♂ 0VHM33Z Insertion of Infusion Device into Epididymis and Spermatic Cord, Percutaneous Approach
♂ 0VHM43Z Insertion of Infusion Device into Epididymis and Spermatic Cord, Percutaneous Endoscopic Approach
♂ 0VHM73Z Insertion of Infusion Device into Epididymis and Spermatic Cord, Via Natural or Artificial Opening
♂ 0VHM83Z Insertion of Infusion Device into Epididymis and Spermatic Cord, Via Natural or Artificial Opening Endoscopic
♂ 0VHR03Z Insertion of Infusion Device into Vas Deferens, Open Approach
♂ 0VHR33Z Insertion of Infusion Device into Vas Deferens, Percutaneous Approach
♂ 0VHR43Z Insertion of Infusion Device into Vas Deferens, Percutaneous Endoscopic Approach
♂ 0VHR73Z Insertion of Infusion Device into Vas Deferens, Via Natural or Artificial Opening
♂ 0VHR83Z Insertion of Infusion Device into Vas Deferens, Via Natural or Artificial Opening Endoscopic
♂ 0VHS03Z Insertion of Infusion Device into Penis, Open Approach
♂ 0VHS33Z Insertion of Infusion Device into Penis, Percutaneous Approach
♂ 0VHS43Z Insertion of Infusion Device into Penis, Percutaneous Endoscopic Approach
♂ 0VHSX3Z Insertion of Infusion Device into Penis, External Approach

0VJ – Male Reproductive System, Inspection

Review Coding Guidelines B3.11a, B3.11b and B3.11c

♂ 0VJ40ZZ Inspection of Prostate and Seminal Vesicles, Open Approach
♂ 0VJ43ZZ Inspection of Prostate and Seminal Vesicles, Percutaneous Approach
♂ 0VJ44ZZ Inspection of Prostate and Seminal Vesicles, Percutaneous Endoscopic Approach
♂ 0VJ4XZZ Inspection of Prostate and Seminal Vesicles, External Approach
♂ 0VJ80ZZ Inspection of Scrotum and Tunica Vaginalis, Open Approach
♂ 0VJ83ZZ Inspection of Scrotum and Tunica Vaginalis, Percutaneous Approach
♂ 0VJ84ZZ Inspection of Scrotum and Tunica Vaginalis, Percutaneous Endoscopic Approach
♂ 0VJ8XZZ Inspection of Scrotum and Tunica Vaginalis, External Approach
♂ 0VJD0ZZ Inspection of Testis, Open Approach
♂ 0VJD3ZZ Inspection of Testis, Percutaneous Approach
♂ 0VJD4ZZ Inspection of Testis, Percutaneous Endoscopic Approach
♂ 0VJDXZZ Inspection of Testis, External Approach
♂ 0VJM0ZZ Inspection of Epididymis and Spermatic Cord, Open Approach
♂ 0VJM3ZZ Inspection of Epididymis and Spermatic Cord, Percutaneous Approach
♂ 0VJM4ZZ Inspection of Epididymis and Spermatic Cord, Percutaneous Endoscopic Approach
♂ 0VJMXZZ Inspection of Epididymis and Spermatic Cord, External Approach
♂ 0VJR0ZZ Inspection of Vas Deferens, Open Approach
♂ 0VJR3ZZ Inspection of Vas Deferens, Percutaneous Approach
♂ 0VJR4ZZ Inspection of Vas Deferens, Percutaneous Endoscopic Approach
♂ 0VJRXZZ Inspection of Vas Deferens, External Approach
♂ 0VJS0ZZ Inspection of Penis, Open Approach
♂ 0VJS3ZZ Inspection of Penis, Percutaneous Approach
♂ 0VJS4ZZ Inspection of Penis, Percutaneous Endoscopic Approach
♂ 0VJSXZZ Inspection of Penis, External Approach

0VL – Male Reproductive System, Occlusion

♂ ▲ 0VLF0CZ Occlusion of Right Spermatic Cord with Extraluminal Device, Open Approach
♂ ▲ 0VLF0DZ Occlusion of Right Spermatic Cord with Intraluminal Device, Open Approach
♂ 0VLF0ZZ Occlusion of Right Spermatic Cord, Open Approach
♂ ▲ 0VLF3CZ Occlusion of Right Spermatic Cord with Extraluminal Device, Percutaneous Approach
♂ ▲ 0VLF3DZ Occlusion of Right Spermatic Cord with Intraluminal Device, Percutaneous Approach
♂ ▲ 0VLF3ZZ Occlusion of Right Spermatic Cord, Percutaneous Approach
♂ ▲ 0VLF4CZ Occlusion of Right Spermatic Cord with Extraluminal Device, Percutaneous Endoscopic Approach
♂ ▲ 0VLF4DZ Occlusion of Right Spermatic Cord with Intraluminal Device, Percutaneous Endoscopic Approach
♂ 0VLF4ZZ Occlusion of Right Spermatic Cord, Percutaneous Endoscopic Approach
♂ ▲ 0VLG0CZ Occlusion of Left Spermatic Cord with Extraluminal Device, Open Approach
♂ ▲ 0VLG0DZ Occlusion of Left Spermatic Cord with Intraluminal Device, Open Approach
♂ ▲ 0VLG0ZZ Occlusion of Left Spermatic Cord, Open Approach
♂ ▲ 0VLG3CZ Occlusion of Left Spermatic Cord with Extraluminal Device, Percutaneous Approach
♂ ▲ 0VLG3DZ Occlusion of Left Spermatic Cord with Intraluminal Device, Percutaneous Approach
♂ ▲ 0VLG3ZZ Occlusion of Left Spermatic Cord, Percutaneous Approach
♂ ▲ 0VLG4CZ Occlusion of Left Spermatic Cord with Extraluminal Device, Percutaneous Endoscopic Approach
♂ ▲ 0VLG4DZ Occlusion of Left Spermatic Cord with Intraluminal Device, Percutaneous Endoscopic Approach
♂ ▲ 0VLG4ZZ Occlusion of Left Spermatic Cord, Percutaneous Endoscopic Approach
♂ ▲ 0VLH0CZ Occlusion of Bilateral Spermatic Cords with Extraluminal Device, Open Approach
♂ ▲ 0VLH0DZ Occlusion of Bilateral Spermatic Cords with Intraluminal Device, Open Approach
♂ ▲ 0VLH0ZZ Occlusion of Bilateral Spermatic Cords, Open Approach
♂ ▲ 0VLH3CZ Occlusion of Bilateral Spermatic Cords with Extraluminal Device, Percutaneous Approach
♂ ▲ 0VLH3DZ Occlusion of Bilateral Spermatic Cords with Intraluminal Device, Percutaneous Approach
♂ ▲ 0VLH3ZZ Occlusion of Bilateral Spermatic Cords, Percutaneous Approach
♂ ▲ 0VLH4CZ Occlusion of Bilateral Spermatic Cords with Extraluminal Device, Percutaneous Endoscopic Approach
♂ ▲ 0VLH4DZ Occlusion of Bilateral Spermatic Cords with Intraluminal Device, Percutaneous Endoscopic Approach
♂ ▲ 0VLH4ZZ Occlusion of Bilateral Spermatic Cords, Percutaneous Endoscopic Approach
♂ ▲ 0VLN0CZ Occlusion of Right Vas Deferens with Extraluminal Device, Open Approach
♂ 0VLN0DZ Occlusion of Right Vas Deferens with Intraluminal Device, Open Approach
♂ ▲ 0VLN0ZZ Occlusion of Right Vas Deferens, Open Approach
♂ ▲ 0VLN3CZ Occlusion of Right Vas Deferens with Extraluminal Device, Percutaneous Approach
♂ ▲ 0VLN3DZ Occlusion of Right Vas Deferens with Intraluminal Device, Percutaneous Approach
♂ ▲ 0VLN3ZZ Occlusion of Right Vas Deferens, Percutaneous Approach
♂ ▲ 0VLN4CZ Occlusion of Right Vas Deferens with Extraluminal Device, Percutaneous Endoscopic Approach
♂ 0VLN4DZ Occlusion of Right Vas Deferens with Intraluminal Device, Percutaneous Endoscopic Approach
♂ ▲ 0VLN4ZZ Occlusion of Right Vas Deferens, Percutaneous Endoscopic Approach
♂ ▲ 0VLP0CZ Occlusion of Left Vas Deferens with Extraluminal Device, Open Approach
♂ ▲ 0VLP0DZ Occlusion of Left Vas Deferens with Intraluminal Device, Open Approach
♂ ▲ 0VLP0ZZ Occlusion of Left Vas Deferens, Open Approach
♂ ▲ 0VLP3CZ Occlusion of Left Vas Deferens with Extraluminal Device, Percutaneous Approach
♂ ▲ 0VLP3DZ Occlusion of Left Vas Deferens with Intraluminal Device, Percutaneous Approach
♂ ▲ 0VLP3ZZ Occlusion of Left Vas Deferens, Percutaneous Approach
♂ ▲ 0VLP4CZ Occlusion of Left Vas Deferens with Extraluminal Device, Percutaneous Endoscopic Approach
♂ ▲ 0VLP4DZ Occlusion of Left Vas Deferens with Intraluminal Device, Percutaneous Endoscopic Approach
♂ ▲ 0VLP4ZZ Occlusion of Left Vas Deferens, Percutaneous Endoscopic Approach
♂ ▲ 0VLQ0CZ Occlusion of Bilateral Vas Deferens with Extraluminal Device, Open Approach
♂ ▲ 0VLQ0DZ Occlusion of Bilateral Vas Deferens with Intraluminal Device, Open Approach
♂ ▲ 0VLQ0ZZ Occlusion of Bilateral Vas Deferens, Open Approach
♂ ▲ 0VLQ3CZ Occlusion of Bilateral Vas Deferens with Extraluminal Device, Percutaneous Approach

♂▲ **0VLQ3DZ** Occlusion of Bilateral Vas Deferens with Intraluminal Device, Percutaneous Approach
♂▲ **0VLQ3ZZ** Occlusion of Bilateral Vas Deferens, Percutaneous Approach
♂▲ **0VLQ4CZ** Occlusion of Bilateral Vas Deferens with Extraluminal Device, Percutaneous Endoscopic Approach
♂ **0VLQ4DZ** Occlusion of Bilateral Vas Deferens with Intraluminal Device, Percutaneous Endoscopic Approach
♂▲ **0VLQ4ZZ** Occlusion of Bilateral Vas Deferens, Percutaneous Endoscopic Approach

0VM – Male Reproductive System, Reattachment

♂ **0VM5XZZ** Reattachment of Scrotum, External Approach
♂ **0VM60ZZ** Reattachment of Right Tunica Vaginalis, Open Approach
♂ **0VM64ZZ** Reattachment of Right Tunica Vaginalis, Percutaneous Endoscopic Approach
♂ **0VM70ZZ** Reattachment of Left Tunica Vaginalis, Open Approach
♂ **0VM74ZZ** Reattachment of Left Tunica Vaginalis, Percutaneous Endoscopic Approach
♂ **0VM90ZZ** Reattachment of Right Testis, Open Approach
♂ **0VM94ZZ** Reattachment of Right Testis, Percutaneous Endoscopic Approach
♂ **0VMB0ZZ** Reattachment of Left Testis, Open Approach
♂ **0VMB4ZZ** Reattachment of Left Testis, Percutaneous Endoscopic Approach
♂ **0VMC0ZZ** Reattachment of Bilateral Testes, Open Approach
♂ **0VMC4ZZ** Reattachment of Bilateral Testes, Percutaneous Endoscopic Approach
♂ **0VMF0ZZ** Reattachment of Right Spermatic Cord, Open Approach
♂ **0VMF4ZZ** Reattachment of Right Spermatic Cord, Percutaneous Endoscopic Approach
♂ **0VMG0ZZ** Reattachment of Left Spermatic Cord, Open Approach
♂ **0VMG4ZZ** Reattachment of Left Spermatic Cord, Percutaneous Endoscopic Approach
♂ **0VMH0ZZ** Reattachment of Bilateral Spermatic Cords, Open Approach
♂ **0VMH4ZZ** Reattachment of Bilateral Spermatic Cords, Percutaneous Endoscopic Approach
♂ **0VMSXZZ** Reattachment of Penis, External Approach

0VN – Male Reproductive System, Release

Review Coding Guideline B3.13

♂ **0VN00ZZ** Release Prostate, Open Approach
♂ **0VN03ZZ** Release Prostate, Percutaneous Approach
♂ **0VN04ZZ** Release Prostate, Percutaneous Endoscopic Approach
♂ **0VN07ZZ** Release Prostate, Via Natural or Artificial Opening
♂ **0VN08ZZ** Release Prostate, Via Natural or Artificial Opening Endoscopic
♂ **0VN10ZZ** Release Right Seminal Vesicle, Open Approach
♂ **0VN13ZZ** Release Right Seminal Vesicle, Percutaneous Approach
♂ **0VN14ZZ** Release Right Seminal Vesicle, Percutaneous Endoscopic Approach
♂ **0VN20ZZ** Release Left Seminal Vesicle, Open Approach
♂ **0VN23ZZ** Release Left Seminal Vesicle, Percutaneous Approach
♂ **0VN24ZZ** Release Left Seminal Vesicle, Percutaneous Endoscopic Approach
♂ **0VN30ZZ** Release Bilateral Seminal Vesicles, Open Approach
♂ **0VN33ZZ** Release Bilateral Seminal Vesicles, Percutaneous Approach
♂ **0VN34ZZ** Release Bilateral Seminal Vesicles, Percutaneous Endoscopic Approach
♂ **0VN50ZZ** Release Scrotum, Open Approach
♂ **0VN53ZZ** Release Scrotum, Percutaneous Approach
♂ **0VN54ZZ** Release Scrotum, Percutaneous Endoscopic Approach
♂ **0VN5XZZ** Release Scrotum, External Approach
♂ **0VN60ZZ** Release Right Tunica Vaginalis, Open Approach
♂ **0VN63ZZ** Release Right Tunica Vaginalis, Percutaneous Approach
♂ **0VN64ZZ** Release Right Tunica Vaginalis, Percutaneous Endoscopic Approach
♂ **0VN70ZZ** Release Left Tunica Vaginalis, Open Approach
♂ **0VN73ZZ** Release Left Tunica Vaginalis, Percutaneous Approach
♂ **0VN74ZZ** Release Left Tunica Vaginalis, Percutaneous Endoscopic Approach
♂ **0VN90ZZ** Release Right Testis, Open Approach
♂ **0VN93ZZ** Release Right Testis, Percutaneous Approach
♂ **0VN94ZZ** Release Right Testis, Percutaneous Endoscopic Approach
♂ **0VNB0ZZ** Release Left Testis, Open Approach
♂ **0VNB3ZZ** Release Left Testis, Percutaneous Approach
♂ **0VNB4ZZ** Release Left Testis, Percutaneous Endoscopic Approach
♂ **0VNC0ZZ** Release Bilateral Testes, Open Approach
♂ **0VNC3ZZ** Release Bilateral Testes, Percutaneous Approach
♂ **0VNC4ZZ** Release Bilateral Testes, Percutaneous Endoscopic Approach
♂ **0VNF0ZZ** Release Right Spermatic Cord, Open Approach
♂ **0VNF3ZZ** Release Right Spermatic Cord, Percutaneous Approach
♂ **0VNF4ZZ** Release Right Spermatic Cord, Percutaneous Endoscopic Approach
♂ **0VNG0ZZ** Release Left Spermatic Cord, Open Approach
♂ **0VNG3ZZ** Release Left Spermatic Cord, Percutaneous Approach
♂ **0VNG4ZZ** Release Left Spermatic Cord, Percutaneous Endoscopic Approach
♂ **0VNH0ZZ** Release Bilateral Spermatic Cords, Open Approach
♂ **0VNH3ZZ** Release Bilateral Spermatic Cords, Percutaneous Approach
♂ **0VNH4ZZ** Release Bilateral Spermatic Cords, Percutaneous Endoscopic Approach
♂ **0VNJ0ZZ** Release Right Epididymis, Open Approach
♂ **0VNJ3ZZ** Release Right Epididymis, Percutaneous Approach
♂ **0VNJ4ZZ** Release Right Epididymis, Percutaneous Endoscopic Approach
♂ **0VNK0ZZ** Release Left Epididymis, Open Approach
♂ **0VNK3ZZ** Release Left Epididymis, Percutaneous Approach
♂ **0VNK4ZZ** Release Left Epididymis, Percutaneous Endoscopic Approach
♂ **0VNL0ZZ** Release Bilateral Epididymis, Open Approach
♂ **0VNL3ZZ** Release Bilateral Epididymis, Percutaneous Approach
♂ **0VNL4ZZ** Release Bilateral Epididymis, Percutaneous Endoscopic Approach
♂ **0VNN0ZZ** Release Right Vas Deferens, Open Approach
♂ **0VNN3ZZ** Release Right Vas Deferens, Percutaneous Approach
♂ **0VNN4ZZ** Release Right Vas Deferens, Percutaneous Endoscopic Approach
♂ **0VNP0ZZ** Release Left Vas Deferens, Open Approach
♂ **0VNP3ZZ** Release Left Vas Deferens, Percutaneous Approach
♂ **0VNP4ZZ** Release Left Vas Deferens, Percutaneous Endoscopic Approach
♂ **0VNQ0ZZ** Release Bilateral Vas Deferens, Open Approach
♂ **0VNQ3ZZ** Release Bilateral Vas Deferens, Percutaneous Approach
♂ **0VNQ4ZZ** Release Bilateral Vas Deferens, Percutaneous Endoscopic Approach
♂ **0VNS0ZZ** Release Penis, Open Approach
♂ **0VNS3ZZ** Release Penis, Percutaneous Approach
♂ **0VNS4ZZ** Release Penis, Percutaneous Endoscopic Approach
♂ **0VNSXZZ** Release Penis, External Approach
♂ **0VNT0ZZ** Release Prepuce, Open Approach
♂ **0VNT3ZZ** Release Prepuce, Percutaneous Approach
♂ **0VNT4ZZ** Release Prepuce, Percutaneous Endoscopic Approach
♂ **0VNTXZZ** Release Prepuce, External Approach

0VP – Male Reproductive System, Removal

Review Coding Guideline B6.1c

♂ **0VP400Z** Removal of Drainage Device from Prostate and Seminal Vesicles, Open Approach
♂ **0VP401Z** Removal of Radioactive Element from Prostate and Seminal Vesicles, Open Approach
♂ **0VP403Z** Removal of Infusion Device from Prostate and Seminal Vesicles, Open Approach
♂ **0VP407Z** Removal of Autologous Tissue Substitute from Prostate and Seminal Vesicles, Open Approach
♂ **0VP40JZ** Removal of Synthetic Substitute from Prostate and Seminal Vesicles, Open Approach

♂ **0VP40KZ** Removal of Nonautologous Tissue Substitute from Prostate and Seminal Vesicles, Open Approach
♂ **0VP430Z** Removal of Drainage Device from Prostate and Seminal Vesicles, Percutaneous Approach
♂ **0VP431Z** Removal of Radioactive Element from Prostate and Seminal Vesicles, Percutaneous Approach
♂ **0VP433Z** Removal of Infusion Device from Prostate and Seminal Vesicles, Percutaneous Approach
♂ **0VP437Z** Removal of Autologous Tissue Substitute from Prostate and Seminal Vesicles, Percutaneous Approach
♂ **0VP43JZ** Removal of Synthetic Substitute from Prostate and Seminal Vesicles, Percutaneous Approach
♂ **0VP43KZ** Removal of Nonautologous Tissue Substitute from Prostate and Seminal Vesicles, Percutaneous Approach
♂ **0VP440Z** Removal of Drainage Device from Prostate and Seminal Vesicles, Percutaneous Endoscopic Approach
♂ **0VP441Z** Removal of Radioactive Element from Prostate and Seminal Vesicles, Percutaneous Endoscopic Approach
♂ **0VP443Z** Removal of Infusion Device from Prostate and Seminal Vesicles, Percutaneous Endoscopic Approach
♂ **0VP447Z** Removal of Autologous Tissue Substitute from Prostate and Seminal Vesicles, Percutaneous Endoscopic Approach
♂ **0VP44JZ** Removal of Synthetic Substitute from Prostate and Seminal Vesicles, Percutaneous Endoscopic Approach
♂ **0VP44KZ** Removal of Nonautologous Tissue Substitute from Prostate and Seminal Vesicles, Percutaneous Endoscopic Approach
♂ **0VP470Z** Removal of Drainage Device from Prostate and Seminal Vesicles, Via Natural or Artificial Opening
♂ **0VP471Z** Removal of Radioactive Element from Prostate and Seminal Vesicles, Via Natural or Artificial Opening
♂ **0VP473Z** Removal of Infusion Device from Prostate and Seminal Vesicles, Via Natural or Artificial Opening
♂ **0VP477Z** Removal of Autologous Tissue Substitute from Prostate and Seminal Vesicles, Via Natural or Artificial Opening
♂ **0VP47JZ** Removal of Synthetic Substitute from Prostate and Seminal Vesicles, Via Natural or Artificial Opening
♂ **0VP47KZ** Removal of Nonautologous Tissue Substitute from Prostate and Seminal Vesicles, Via Natural or Artificial Opening
♂ **0VP480Z** Removal of Drainage Device from Prostate and Seminal Vesicles, Via Natural or Artificial Opening Endoscopic
♂ **0VP481Z** Removal of Radioactive Element from Prostate and Seminal Vesicles, Via Natural or Artificial Opening Endoscopic
♂ **0VP483Z** Removal of Infusion Device from Prostate and Seminal Vesicles, Via Natural or Artificial Opening Endoscopic
♂ **0VP487Z** Removal of Autologous Tissue Substitute from Prostate and Seminal Vesicles, Via Natural or Artificial Opening Endoscopic
♂ **0VP48JZ** Removal of Synthetic Substitute from Prostate and Seminal Vesicles, Via Natural or Artificial Opening Endoscopic
♂ **0VP48KZ** Removal of Nonautologous Tissue Substitute from Prostate and Seminal Vesicles, Via Natural or Artificial Opening Endoscopic
♂ **0VP4X0Z** Removal of Drainage Device from Prostate and Seminal Vesicles, External Approach
♂ **0VP4X1Z** Removal of Radioactive Element from Prostate and Seminal Vesicles, External Approach
♂ **0VP4X3Z** Removal of Infusion Device from Prostate and Seminal Vesicles, External Approach
♂ **0VP800Z** Removal of Drainage Device from Scrotum and Tunica Vaginalis, Open Approach
♂ **0VP803Z** Removal of Infusion Device from Scrotum and Tunica Vaginalis, Open Approach
♂ **0VP807Z** Removal of Autologous Tissue Substitute from Scrotum and Tunica Vaginalis, Open Approach
♂ **0VP80JZ** Removal of Synthetic Substitute from Scrotum and Tunica Vaginalis, Open Approach
♂ **0VP80KZ** Removal of Nonautologous Tissue Substitute from Scrotum and Tunica Vaginalis, Open Approach
♂ **0VP830Z** Removal of Drainage Device from Scrotum and Tunica Vaginalis, Percutaneous Approach
♂ **0VP833Z** Removal of Infusion Device from Scrotum and Tunica Vaginalis, Percutaneous Approach
♂ **0VP837Z** Removal of Autologous Tissue Substitute from Scrotum and Tunica Vaginalis, Percutaneous Approach
♂ **0VP83JZ** Removal of Synthetic Substitute from Scrotum and Tunica Vaginalis, Percutaneous Approach
♂ **0VP83KZ** Removal of Nonautologous Tissue Substitute from Scrotum and Tunica Vaginalis, Percutaneous Approach
♂ **0VP840Z** Removal of Drainage Device from Scrotum and Tunica Vaginalis, Percutaneous Endoscopic Approach
♂ **0VP843Z** Removal of Infusion Device from Scrotum and Tunica Vaginalis, Percutaneous Endoscopic Approach
♂ **0VP847Z** Removal of Autologous Tissue Substitute from Scrotum and Tunica Vaginalis, Percutaneous Endoscopic Approach
♂ **0VP84JZ** Removal of Synthetic Substitute from Scrotum and Tunica Vaginalis, Percutaneous Endoscopic Approach
♂ **0VP84KZ** Removal of Nonautologous Tissue Substitute from Scrotum and Tunica Vaginalis, Percutaneous Endoscopic Approach
♂ **0VP870Z** Removal of Drainage Device from Scrotum and Tunica Vaginalis, Via Natural or Artificial Opening
♂ **0VP873Z** Removal of Infusion Device from Scrotum and Tunica Vaginalis, Via Natural or Artificial Opening
♂ **0VP877Z** Removal of Autologous Tissue Substitute from Scrotum and Tunica Vaginalis, Via Natural or Artificial Opening
♂ **0VP87JZ** Removal of Synthetic Substitute from Scrotum and Tunica Vaginalis, Via Natural or Artificial Opening
♂ **0VP87KZ** Removal of Nonautologous Tissue Substitute from Scrotum and Tunica Vaginalis, Via Natural or Artificial Opening
♂ **0VP880Z** Removal of Drainage Device from Scrotum and Tunica Vaginalis, Via Natural or Artificial Opening Endoscopic
♂ **0VP883Z** Removal of Infusion Device from Scrotum and Tunica Vaginalis, Via Natural or Artificial Opening Endoscopic
♂ **0VP887Z** Removal of Autologous Tissue Substitute from Scrotum and Tunica Vaginalis, Via Natural or Artificial Opening Endoscopic
♂ **0VP88JZ** Removal of Synthetic Substitute from Scrotum and Tunica Vaginalis, Via Natural or Artificial Opening Endoscopic
♂ **0VP88KZ** Removal of Nonautologous Tissue Substitute from Scrotum and Tunica Vaginalis, Via Natural or Artificial Opening Endoscopic
♂ **0VP8X0Z** Removal of Drainage Device from Scrotum and Tunica Vaginalis, External Approach
♂ **0VP8X3Z** Removal of Infusion Device from Scrotum and Tunica Vaginalis, External Approach
♂ **0VPD00Z** Removal of Drainage Device from Testis, Open Approach
♂ **0VPD03Z** Removal of Infusion Device from Testis, Open Approach
♂ **0VPD07Z** Removal of Autologous Tissue Substitute from Testis, Open Approach
♂ **0VPD0JZ** Removal of Synthetic Substitute from Testis, Open Approach
♂ **0VPD0KZ** Removal of Nonautologous Tissue Substitute from Testis, Open Approach
♂ **0VPD30Z** Removal of Drainage Device from Testis, Percutaneous Approach
♂ **0VPD33Z** Removal of Infusion Device from Testis, Percutaneous Approach
♂ **0VPD37Z** Removal of Autologous Tissue Substitute from Testis, Percutaneous Approach
♂ **0VPD3JZ** Removal of Synthetic Substitute from Testis, Percutaneous Approach
♂ **0VPD3KZ** Removal of Nonautologous Tissue Substitute from Testis, Percutaneous Approach
♂ **0VPD40Z** Removal of Drainage Device from Testis, Percutaneous Endoscopic Approach
♂ **0VPD43Z** Removal of Infusion Device from Testis, Percutaneous Endoscopic Approach
♂ **0VPD47Z** Removal of Autologous Tissue Substitute from Testis, Percutaneous Endoscopic Approach
♂ **0VPD4JZ** Removal of Synthetic Substitute from Testis, Percutaneous Endoscopic Approach
♂ **0VPD4KZ** Removal of Nonautologous Tissue Substitute from Testis, Percutaneous Endoscopic Approach
♂ **0VPD70Z** Removal of Drainage Device from Testis, Via Natural or Artificial Opening
♂ **0VPD73Z** Removal of Infusion Device from Testis, Via Natural or Artificial Opening
♂ **0VPD77Z** Removal of Autologous Tissue Substitute from Testis, Via Natural or Artificial Opening
♂ **0VPD7JZ** Removal of Synthetic Substitute from Testis, Via Natural or Artificial Opening
♂ **0VPD7KZ** Removal of Nonautologous Tissue Substitute from Testis, Via Natural or Artificial Opening
♂ **0VPD80Z** Removal of Drainage Device from Testis, Via Natural or Artificial Opening Endoscopic
♂ **0VPD83Z** Removal of Infusion Device from Testis, Via Natural or Artificial Opening Endoscopic
♂ **0VPD87Z** Removal of Autologous Tissue Substitute from Testis, Via Natural or Artificial Opening Endoscopic
♂ **0VPD8JZ** Removal of Synthetic Substitute from Testis, Via Natural or Artificial Opening Endoscopic
♂ **0VPD8KZ** Removal of Nonautologous Tissue Substitute from Testis, Via Natural or Artificial Opening Endoscopic
♂ **0VPDX0Z** Removal of Drainage Device from Testis, External Approach
♂ **0VPDX3Z** Removal of Infusion Device from Testis, External Approach

♂0VPM00Z Removal of Drainage Device from Epididymis and Spermatic Cord, Open Approach
♂0VPM03Z Removal of Infusion Device from Epididymis and Spermatic Cord, Open Approach
♂0VPM07Z Removal of Autologous Tissue Substitute from Epididymis and Spermatic Cord, Open Approach
♂0VPM0CZ Removal of Extraluminal Device from Epididymis and Spermatic Cord, Open Approach
♂0VPM0JZ Removal of Synthetic Substitute from Epididymis and Spermatic Cord, Open Approach
♂0VPM0KZ Removal of Nonautologous Tissue Substitute from Epididymis and Spermatic Cord, Open Approach
♂0VPM30Z Removal of Drainage Device from Epididymis and Spermatic Cord, Percutaneous Approach
♂0VPM33Z Removal of Infusion Device from Epididymis and Spermatic Cord, Percutaneous Approach
♂0VPM37Z Removal of Autologous Tissue Substitute from Epididymis and Spermatic Cord, Percutaneous Approach
♂0VPM3CZ Removal of Extraluminal Device from Epididymis and Spermatic Cord, Percutaneous Approach
♂0VPM3JZ Removal of Synthetic Substitute from Epididymis and Spermatic Cord, Percutaneous Approach
♂0VPM3KZ Removal of Nonautologous Tissue Substitute from Epididymis and Spermatic Cord, Percutaneous Approach
♂0VPM40Z Removal of Drainage Device from Epididymis and Spermatic Cord, Percutaneous Endoscopic Approach
♂0VPM43Z Removal of Infusion Device from Epididymis and Spermatic Cord, Percutaneous Endoscopic Approach
♂0VPM47Z Removal of Autologous Tissue Substitute from Epididymis and Spermatic Cord, Percutaneous Endoscopic Approach
♂0VPM4CZ Removal of Extraluminal Device from Epididymis and Spermatic Cord, Percutaneous Endoscopic Approach
♂0VPM4JZ Removal of Synthetic Substitute from Epididymis and Spermatic Cord, Percutaneous Endoscopic Approach
♂0VPM4KZ Removal of Nonautologous Tissue Substitute from Epididymis and Spermatic Cord, Percutaneous Endoscopic Approach
♂0VPM70Z Removal of Drainage Device from Epididymis and Spermatic Cord, Via Natural or Artificial Opening
♂0VPM73Z Removal of Infusion Device from Epididymis and Spermatic Cord, Via Natural or Artificial Opening
♂0VPM77Z Removal of Autologous Tissue Substitute from Epididymis and Spermatic Cord, Via Natural or Artificial Opening
♂0VPM7CZ Removal of Extraluminal Device from Epididymis and Spermatic Cord, Via Natural or Artificial Opening
♂0VPM7JZ Removal of Synthetic Substitute from Epididymis and Spermatic Cord, Via Natural or Artificial Opening
♂0VPM7KZ Removal of Nonautologous Tissue Substitute from Epididymis and Spermatic Cord, Via Natural or Artificial Opening
♂0VPM80Z Removal of Drainage Device from Epididymis and Spermatic Cord, Via Natural or Artificial Opening Endoscopic
♂ 0VPM83Z Removal of Infusion Device from Epididymis and Spermatic Cord, Via Natural or Artificial Opening Endoscopic
♂ 0VPM87Z Removal of Autologous Tissue Substitute from Epididymis and Spermatic Cord, Via Natural or Artificial Opening Endoscopic
♂ 0VPM8CZ Removal of Extraluminal Device from Epididymis and Spermatic Cord, Via Natural or Artificial Opening Endoscopic
♂ 0VPM8JZ Removal of Synthetic Substitute from Epididymis and Spermatic Cord, Via Natural or Artificial Opening Endoscopic
♂ 0VPM8KZ Removal of Nonautologous Tissue Substitute from Epididymis and Spermatic Cord, Via Natural or Artificial Opening Endoscopic
♂ 0VPMX0Z Removal of Drainage Device from Epididymis and Spermatic Cord, External Approach
♂ 0VPMX3Z Removal of Infusion Device from Epididymis and Spermatic Cord, External Approach
♂ 0VPR00Z Removal of Drainage Device from Vas Deferens, Open Approach
♂ 0VPR03Z Removal of Infusion Device from Vas Deferens, Open Approach
♂ 0VPR07Z Removal of Autologous Tissue Substitute from Vas Deferens, Open Approach
♂ 0VPR0CZ Removal of Extraluminal Device from Vas Deferens, Open Approach
♂ 0VPR0DZ Removal of Intraluminal Device from Vas Deferens, Open Approach
♂ 0VPR0JZ Removal of Synthetic Substitute from Vas Deferens, Open Approach
♂ 0VPR0KZ Removal of Nonautologous Tissue Substitute from Vas Deferens, Open Approach
♂ 0VPR30Z Removal of Drainage Device from Vas Deferens, Percutaneous Approach
♂ 0VPR33Z Removal of Infusion Device from Vas Deferens, Percutaneous Approach
♂ 0VPR37Z Removal of Autologous Tissue Substitute from Vas Deferens, Percutaneous Approach
♂ 0VPR3CZ Removal of Extraluminal Device from Vas Deferens, Percutaneous Approach
♂ 0VPR3DZ Removal of Intraluminal Device from Vas Deferens, Percutaneous Approach
♂ 0VPR3JZ Removal of Synthetic Substitute from Vas Deferens, Percutaneous Approach
♂ 0VPR3KZ Removal of Nonautologous Tissue Substitute from Vas Deferens, Percutaneous Approach
♂ 0VPR40Z Removal of Drainage Device from Vas Deferens, Percutaneous Endoscopic Approach
♂ 0VPR43Z Removal of Infusion Device from Vas Deferens, Percutaneous Endoscopic Approach
♂ 0VPR47Z Removal of Autologous Tissue Substitute from Vas Deferens, Percutaneous Endoscopic Approach
♂ 0VPR4CZ Removal of Extraluminal Device from Vas Deferens, Percutaneous Endoscopic Approach
♂ 0VPR4DZ Removal of Intraluminal Device from Vas Deferens, Percutaneous Endoscopic Approach
♂ 0VPR4JZ Removal of Synthetic Substitute from Vas Deferens, Percutaneous Endoscopic Approach
♂ 0VPR4KZ Removal of Nonautologous Tissue Substitute from Vas Deferens, Percutaneous Endoscopic Approach
♂ 0VPR70Z Removal of Drainage Device from Vas Deferens, Via Natural or Artificial Opening
♂ 0VPR73Z Removal of Infusion Device from Vas Deferens, Via Natural or Artificial Opening
♂ 0VPR77Z Removal of Autologous Tissue Substitute from Vas Deferens, Via Natural or Artificial Opening
♂ 0VPR7CZ Removal of Extraluminal Device from Vas Deferens, Via Natural or Artificial Opening
♂ 0VPR7DZ Removal of Intraluminal Device from Vas Deferens, Via Natural or Artificial Opening
♂ 0VPR7JZ Removal of Synthetic Substitute from Vas Deferens, Via Natural or Artificial Opening
♂ 0VPR7KZ Removal of Nonautologous Tissue Substitute from Vas Deferens, Via Natural or Artificial Opening
♂ 0VPR80Z Removal of Drainage Device from Vas Deferens, Via Natural or Artificial Opening Endoscopic
♂ 0VPR83Z Removal of Infusion Device from Vas Deferens, Via Natural or Artificial Opening Endoscopic
♂ 0VPR87Z Removal of Autologous Tissue Substitute from Vas Deferens, Via Natural or Artificial Opening Endoscopic
♂ 0VPR8CZ Removal of Extraluminal Device from Vas Deferens, Via Natural or Artificial Opening Endoscopic
♂ 0VPR8DZ Removal of Intraluminal Device from Vas Deferens, Via Natural or Artificial Opening Endoscopic
♂ 0VPR8JZ Removal of Synthetic Substitute from Vas Deferens, Via Natural or Artificial Opening Endoscopic
♂ 0VPR8KZ Removal of Nonautologous Tissue Substitute from Vas Deferens, Via Natural or Artificial Opening Endoscopic
♂ 0VPRX0Z Removal of Drainage Device from Vas Deferens, External Approach
♂ 0VPRX3Z Removal of Infusion Device from Vas Deferens, External Approach
♂ 0VPRXDZ Removal of Intraluminal Device from Vas Deferens, External Approach
♂ 0VPS00Z Removal of Drainage Device from Penis, Open Approach
♂ 0VPS03Z Removal of Infusion Device from Penis, Open Approach
♂ 0VPS07Z Removal of Autologous Tissue Substitute from Penis, Open Approach
♂ 0VPS0JZ Removal of Synthetic Substitute from Penis, Open Approach
♂ 0VPS0KZ Removal of Nonautologous Tissue Substitute from Penis, Open Approach
♂ 0VPS30Z Removal of Drainage Device from Penis, Percutaneous Approach
♂ 0VPS33Z Removal of Infusion Device from Penis, Percutaneous Approach
♂ 0VPS37Z Removal of Autologous Tissue Substitute from Penis, Percutaneous Approach
♂ 0VPS3JZ Removal of Synthetic Substitute from Penis, Percutaneous Approach
♂ 0VPS3KZ Removal of Nonautologous Tissue Substitute from Penis, Percutaneous Approach
♂ 0VPS40Z Removal of Drainage Device from Penis, Percutaneous Endoscopic Approach
♂ 0VPS43Z Removal of Infusion Device from Penis, Percutaneous Endoscopic Approach

♂ **0VPS47Z** Removal of Autologous Tissue Substitute from Penis, Percutaneous Endoscopic Approach
♂ **0VPS4JZ** Removal of Synthetic Substitute from Penis, Percutaneous Endoscopic Approach
♂ **0VPS4KZ** Removal of Nonautologous Tissue Substitute from Penis, Percutaneous Endoscopic Approach
♂ **0VPS70Z** Removal of Drainage Device from Penis, Via Natural or Artificial Opening
♂ **0VPS73Z** Removal of Infusion Device from Penis, Via Natural or Artificial Opening
♂ **0VPS77Z** Removal of Autologous Tissue Substitute from Penis, Via Natural or Artificial Opening
♂ **0VPS7JZ** Removal of Synthetic Substitute from Penis, Via Natural or Artificial Opening
♂ **0VPS7KZ** Removal of Nonautologous Tissue Substitute from Penis, Via Natural or Artificial Opening
♂ **0VPS80Z** Removal of Drainage Device from Penis, Via Natural or Artificial Opening Endoscopic
♂ **0VPS83Z** Removal of Infusion Device from Penis, Via Natural or Artificial Opening Endoscopic
♂ **0VPS87Z** Removal of Autologous Tissue Substitute from Penis, Via Natural or Artificial Opening Endoscopic
♂ **0VPS8JZ** Removal of Synthetic Substitute from Penis, Via Natural or Artificial Opening Endoscopic
♂ **0VPS8KZ** Removal of Nonautologous Tissue Substitute from Penis, Via Natural or Artificial Opening Endoscopic
♂ **0VPSX0Z** Removal of Drainage Device from Penis, External Approach
♂ **0VPSX3Z** Removal of Infusion Device from Penis, External Approach

0VQ – Male Reproductive System, Repair

♂ **0VQ00ZZ** Repair Prostate, Open Approach
♂ **0VQ03ZZ** Repair Prostate, Percutaneous Approach
♂ **0VQ04ZZ** Repair Prostate, Percutaneous Endoscopic Approach
♂ **0VQ07ZZ** Repair Prostate, Via Natural or Artificial Opening
♂ **0VQ08ZZ** Repair Prostate, Via Natural or Artificial Opening Endoscopic
♂ **0VQ10ZZ** Repair Right Seminal Vesicle, Open Approach
♂ **0VQ13ZZ** Repair Right Seminal Vesicle, Percutaneous Approach
♂ **0VQ14ZZ** Repair Right Seminal Vesicle, Percutaneous Endoscopic Approach
♂ **0VQ20ZZ** Repair Left Seminal Vesicle, Open Approach
♂ **0VQ23ZZ** Repair Left Seminal Vesicle, Percutaneous Approach
♂ **0VQ24ZZ** Repair Left Seminal Vesicle, Percutaneous Endoscopic Approach
♂ **0VQ30ZZ** Repair Bilateral Seminal Vesicles, Open Approach
♂ **0VQ33ZZ** Repair Bilateral Seminal Vesicles, Percutaneous Approach
♂ **0VQ34ZZ** Repair Bilateral Seminal Vesicles, Percutaneous Endoscopic Approach
♂ **0VQ50ZZ** Repair Scrotum, Open Approach
♂ **0VQ53ZZ** Repair Scrotum, Percutaneous Approach
♂ **0VQ54ZZ** Repair Scrotum, Percutaneous Endoscopic Approach
♂ **0VQ5XZZ** Repair Scrotum, External Approach
♂ **0VQ60ZZ** Repair Right Tunica Vaginalis, Open Approach
♂ **0VQ63ZZ** Repair Right Tunica Vaginalis, Percutaneous Approach
♂ **0VQ64ZZ** Repair Right Tunica Vaginalis, Percutaneous Endoscopic Approach
♂ **0VQ70ZZ** Repair Left Tunica Vaginalis, Open Approach
♂ **0VQ73ZZ** Repair Left Tunica Vaginalis, Percutaneous Approach
♂ **0VQ74ZZ** Repair Left Tunica Vaginalis, Percutaneous Endoscopic Approach
♂ **0VQ90ZZ** Repair Right Testis, Open Approach
♂ **0VQ93ZZ** Repair Right Testis, Percutaneous Approach
♂ **0VQ94ZZ** Repair Right Testis, Percutaneous Endoscopic Approach
♂ **0VQB0ZZ** Repair Left Testis, Open Approach
♂ **0VQB3ZZ** Repair Left Testis, Percutaneous Approach
♂ **0VQB4ZZ** Repair Left Testis, Percutaneous Endoscopic Approach
♂ **0VQC0ZZ** Repair Bilateral Testes, Open Approach
♂ **0VQC3ZZ** Repair Bilateral Testes, Percutaneous Approach
♂ **0VQC4ZZ** Repair Bilateral Testes, Percutaneous Endoscopic Approach
♂ **0VQF0ZZ** Repair Right Spermatic Cord, Open Approach
♂ **0VQF3ZZ** Repair Right Spermatic Cord, Percutaneous Approach
♂ **0VQF4ZZ** Repair Right Spermatic Cord, Percutaneous Endoscopic Approach
♂ **0VQG0ZZ** Repair Left Spermatic Cord, Open Approach
♂ **0VQG3ZZ** Repair Left Spermatic Cord, Percutaneous Approach
♂ **0VQG4ZZ** Repair Left Spermatic Cord, Percutaneous Endoscopic Approach
♂ **0VQH0ZZ** Repair Bilateral Spermatic Cords, Open Approach
♂ **0VQH3ZZ** Repair Bilateral Spermatic Cords, Percutaneous Approach
♂ **0VQH4ZZ** Repair Bilateral Spermatic Cords, Percutaneous Endoscopic Approach
♂ **0VQJ0ZZ** Repair Right Epididymis, Open Approach
♂ **0VQJ3ZZ** Repair Right Epididymis, Percutaneous Approach
♂ **0VQJ4ZZ** Repair Right Epididymis, Percutaneous Endoscopic Approach
♂ **0VQK0ZZ** Repair Left Epididymis, Open Approach
♂ **0VQK3ZZ** Repair Left Epididymis, Percutaneous Approach
♂ **0VQK4ZZ** Repair Left Epididymis, Percutaneous Endoscopic Approach
♂ **0VQL0ZZ** Repair Bilateral Epididymis, Open Approach
♂ **0VQL3ZZ** Repair Bilateral Epididymis, Percutaneous Approach
♂ **0VQL4ZZ** Repair Bilateral Epididymis, Percutaneous Endoscopic Approach
♂ **0VQN0ZZ** Repair Right Vas Deferens, Open Approach
♂ **0VQN3ZZ** Repair Right Vas Deferens, Percutaneous Approach
♂ **0VQN4ZZ** Repair Right Vas Deferens, Percutaneous Endoscopic Approach
♂ **0VQP0ZZ** Repair Left Vas Deferens, Open Approach
♂ **0VQP3ZZ** Repair Left Vas Deferens, Percutaneous Approach
♂ **0VQP4ZZ** Repair Left Vas Deferens, Percutaneous Endoscopic Approach
♂ **0VQQ0ZZ** Repair Bilateral Vas Deferens, Open Approach
♂ **0VQQ3ZZ** Repair Bilateral Vas Deferens, Percutaneous Approach
♂ **0VQQ4ZZ** Repair Bilateral Vas Deferens, Percutaneous Endoscopic Approach
♂ **0VQS0ZZ** Repair Penis, Open Approach
♂ **0VQS3ZZ** Repair Penis, Percutaneous Approach
♂ **0VQS4ZZ** Repair Penis, Percutaneous Endoscopic Approach
♂ **0VQSXZZ** Repair Penis, External Approach
♂ **0VQT0ZZ** Repair Prepuce, Open Approach
♂ **0VQT3ZZ** Repair Prepuce, Percutaneous Approach
♂ **0VQT4ZZ** Repair Prepuce, Percutaneous Endoscopic Approach
♂ **0VQTXZZ** Repair Prepuce, External Approach

0VR – Male Reproductive System, Replacement

♂ **0VR90JZ** Replacement of Right Testis with Synthetic Substitute, Open Approach
♂ **0VRB0JZ** Replacement of Left Testis with Synthetic Substitute, Open Approach
♂ **0VRC0JZ** Replacement of Bilateral Testes with Synthetic Substitute, Open Approach

0VS – Male Reproductive System, Reposition

♂ **0VS90ZZ** Reposition Right Testis, Open Approach
♂ **0VS93ZZ** Reposition Right Testis, Percutaneous Approach
♂ **0VS94ZZ** Reposition Right Testis, Percutaneous Endoscopic Approach
♂ **0VSB0ZZ** Reposition Left Testis, Open Approach
♂ **0VSB3ZZ** Reposition Left Testis, Percutaneous Approach
♂ **0VSB4ZZ** Reposition Left Testis, Percutaneous Endoscopic Approach
♂ **0VSC0ZZ** Reposition Bilateral Testes, Open Approach
♂ **0VSC3ZZ** Reposition Bilateral Testes, Percutaneous Approach
♂ **0VSC4ZZ** Reposition Bilateral Testes, Percutaneous Endoscopic Approach
♂ **0VSF0ZZ** Reposition Right Spermatic Cord, Open Approach
♂ **0VSF3ZZ** Reposition Right Spermatic Cord, Percutaneous Approach
♂ **0VSF4ZZ** Reposition Right Spermatic Cord, Percutaneous Endoscopic Approach
♂ **0VSG0ZZ** Reposition Left Spermatic Cord, Open Approach
♂ **0VSG3ZZ** Reposition Left Spermatic Cord, Percutaneous Approach
♂ **0VSG4ZZ** Reposition Left Spermatic Cord, Percutaneous Endoscopic Approach
♂ **0VSH0ZZ** Reposition Bilateral Spermatic Cords, Open Approach
♂ **0VSH3ZZ** Reposition Bilateral Spermatic Cords, Percutaneous Approach
♂ **0VSH4ZZ** Reposition Bilateral Spermatic Cords, Percutaneous Endoscopic Approach

0VT – Male Reproductive System, Resection

Review Coding Guideline B3.8

♂ **0VT00ZZ** Resection of Prostate, Open Approach
+ Radical prostatectomy when reported with Resection of bilateral seminal vesicles. *See table 0VT to construct the Resection code.*

♂ **0VT04ZZ** Resection of Prostate, Percutaneous Endoscopic Approach
+ Radical prostatectomy when reported with Resection of bilateral seminal vesicles. *See table 0VT to construct the Resection code.*

♂ **0VT07ZZ** Resection of Prostate, Via Natural or Artificial Opening
+ Radical prostatectomy when reported with Resection of bilateral seminal vesicles. *See table 0VT to construct the Resection code.*

♂ **0VT08ZZ** Resection of Prostate, Via Natural or Artificial Opening Endoscopic
+ Radical prostatectomy when reported with Resection of bilateral seminal vesicles. *See table 0VT to construct the Resection code.*

♂ **0VT10ZZ** Resection of Right Seminal Vesicle, Open Approach
♂ **0VT14ZZ** Resection of Right Seminal Vesicle, Percutaneous Endoscopic Approach
♂ **0VT20ZZ** Resection of Left Seminal Vesicle, Open Approach
♂ **0VT24ZZ** Resection of Left Seminal Vesicle, Percutaneous Endoscopic Approach
♂ **0VT30ZZ** Resection of Bilateral Seminal Vesicles, Open Approach
♂ **0VT34ZZ** Resection of Bilateral Seminal Vesicles, Percutaneous Endoscopic Approach
♂ **0VT50ZZ** Resection of Scrotum, Open Approach
♂ **0VT54ZZ** Resection of Scrotum, Percutaneous Endoscopic Approach
♂ **0VT5XZZ** Resection of Scrotum, External Approach
♂ **0VT60ZZ** Resection of Right Tunica Vaginalis, Open Approach
♂ **0VT64ZZ** Resection of Right Tunica Vaginalis, Percutaneous Endoscopic Approach
♂ **0VT70ZZ** Resection of Left Tunica Vaginalis, Open Approach
♂ **0VT74ZZ** Resection of Left Tunica Vaginalis, Percutaneous Endoscopic Approach
♂ **0VT90ZZ** Resection of Right Testis, Open Approach
♂ **0VT94ZZ** Resection of Right Testis, Percutaneous Endoscopic Approach
♂ **0VTB0ZZ** Resection of Left Testis, Open Approach
♂ **0VTB4ZZ** Resection of Left Testis, Percutaneous Endoscopic Approach
♂ **0VTC0ZZ** Resection of Bilateral Testes, Open Approach
♂ **0VTC4ZZ** Resection of Bilateral Testes, Percutaneous Endoscopic Approach
♂ **0VTF0ZZ** Resection of Right Spermatic Cord, Open Approach
♂ **0VTF4ZZ** Resection of Right Spermatic Cord, Percutaneous Endoscopic Approach
♂ **0VTG0ZZ** Resection of Left Spermatic Cord, Open Approach
♂ **0VTG4ZZ** Resection of Left Spermatic Cord, Percutaneous Endoscopic Approach
♂ **0VTH0ZZ** Resection of Bilateral Spermatic Cords, Open Approach
♂ **0VTH4ZZ** Resection of Bilateral Spermatic Cords, Percutaneous Endoscopic Approach
♂ **0VTJ0ZZ** Resection of Right Epididymis, Open Approach
♂ **0VTJ4ZZ** Resection of Right Epididymis, Percutaneous Endoscopic Approach
♂ **0VTK0ZZ** Resection of Left Epididymis, Open Approach
♂ **0VTK4ZZ** Resection of Left Epididymis, Percutaneous Endoscopic Approach
♂ **0VTL0ZZ** Resection of Bilateral Epididymis, Open Approach
♂ **0VTL4ZZ** Resection of Bilateral Epididymis, Percutaneous Endoscopic Approach
♂ ▲ **0VTN0ZZ** Resection of Right Vas Deferens, Open Approach
♂ ▲ **0VTN4ZZ** Resection of Right Vas Deferens, Percutaneous Endoscopic Approach
♂ ▲ **0VTP0ZZ** Resection of Left Vas Deferens, Open Approach
♂ ▲ **0VTP4ZZ** Resection of Left Vas Deferens, Percutaneous Endoscopic Approach
♂ ▲ **0VTQ0ZZ** Resection of Bilateral Vas Deferens, Open Approach
♂ ▲ **0VTQ4ZZ** Resection of Bilateral Vas Deferens, Percutaneous Endoscopic Approach
♂ **0VTS0ZZ** Resection of Penis, Open Approach
♂ **0VTS4ZZ** Resection of Penis, Percutaneous Endoscopic Approach
♂ **0VTSXZZ** Resection of Penis, External Approach
♂ **0VTT0ZZ** Resection of Prepuce, Open Approach
♂ **0VTT4ZZ** Resection of Prepuce, Percutaneous Endoscopic Approach
♂ **0VTTXZZ** Resection of Prepuce, External Approach

0VU – Male Reproductive System, Supplement

♂ **0VU107Z** Supplement Right Seminal Vesicle with Autologous Tissue Substitute, Open Approach
♂ **0VU10JZ** Supplement Right Seminal Vesicle with Synthetic Substitute, Open Approach
♂ **0VU10KZ** Supplement Right Seminal Vesicle with Nonautologous Tissue Substitute, Open Approach
♂ **0VU147Z** Supplement Right Seminal Vesicle with Autologous Tissue Substitute, Percutaneous Endoscopic Approach
♂ **0VU14JZ** Supplement Right Seminal Vesicle with Synthetic Substitute, Percutaneous Endoscopic Approach
♂ **0VU14KZ** Supplement Right Seminal Vesicle with Nonautologous Tissue Substitute, Percutaneous Endoscopic Approach
♂ **0VU207Z** Supplement Left Seminal Vesicle with Autologous Tissue Substitute, Open Approach
♂ **0VU20JZ** Supplement Left Seminal Vesicle with Synthetic Substitute, Open Approach
♂ **0VU20KZ** Supplement Left Seminal Vesicle with Nonautologous Tissue Substitute, Open Approach
♂ **0VU247Z** Supplement Left Seminal Vesicle with Autologous Tissue Substitute, Percutaneous Endoscopic Approach
♂ **0VU24JZ** Supplement Left Seminal Vesicle with Synthetic Substitute, Percutaneous Endoscopic Approach
♂ **0VU24KZ** Supplement Left Seminal Vesicle with Nonautologous Tissue Substitute, Percutaneous Endoscopic Approach
♂ **0VU307Z** Supplement Bilateral Seminal Vesicles with Autologous Tissue Substitute, Open Approach
♂ **0VU30JZ** Supplement Bilateral Seminal Vesicles with Synthetic Substitute, Open Approach
♂ **0VU30KZ** Supplement Bilateral Seminal Vesicles with Nonautologous Tissue Substitute, Open Approach
♂ **0VU347Z** Supplement Bilateral Seminal Vesicles with Autologous Tissue Substitute, Percutaneous Endoscopic Approach
♂ **0VU34JZ** Supplement Bilateral Seminal Vesicles with Synthetic Substitute, Percutaneous Endoscopic Approach
♂ **0VU34KZ** Supplement Bilateral Seminal Vesicles with Nonautologous Tissue Substitute, Percutaneous Endoscopic Approach
♂ **0VU507Z** Supplement Scrotum with Autologous Tissue Substitute, Open Approach
♂ **0VU50JZ** Supplement Scrotum with Synthetic Substitute, Open Approach
♂ **0VU50KZ** Supplement Scrotum with Nonautologous Tissue Substitute, Open Approach
♂ **0VU547Z** Supplement Scrotum with Autologous Tissue Substitute, Percutaneous Endoscopic Approach
♂ **0VU54JZ** Supplement Scrotum with Synthetic Substitute, Percutaneous Endoscopic Approach
♂ **0VU54KZ** Supplement Scrotum with Nonautologous Tissue Substitute, Percutaneous Endoscopic Approach
♂ **0VU5X7Z** Supplement Scrotum with Autologous Tissue Substitute, External Approach
♂ **0VU5XJZ** Supplement Scrotum with Synthetic Substitute, External Approach
♂ **0VU5XKZ** Supplement Scrotum with Nonautologous Tissue Substitute, External Approach
♂ **0VU607Z** Supplement Right Tunica Vaginalis with Autologous Tissue Substitute, Open Approach
♂ **0VU60JZ** Supplement Right Tunica Vaginalis with Synthetic Substitute, Open Approach
♂ **0VU60KZ** Supplement Right Tunica Vaginalis with Nonautologous Tissue Substitute, Open Approach
♂ **0VU647Z** Supplement Right Tunica Vaginalis with Autologous Tissue Substitute, Percutaneous Endoscopic Approach
♂ **0VU64JZ** Supplement Right Tunica Vaginalis with Synthetic Substitute, Percutaneous Endoscopic Approach
♂ **0VU64KZ** Supplement Right Tunica Vaginalis with Nonautologous Tissue Substitute, Percutaneous Endoscopic Approach
♂ **0VU707Z** Supplement Left Tunica Vaginalis with Autologous Tissue Substitute, Open Approach
♂ **0VU70JZ** Supplement Left Tunica Vaginalis with Synthetic Substitute, Open Approach
♂ **0VU70KZ** Supplement Left Tunica Vaginalis with Nonautologous Tissue Substitute, Open Approach
♂ **0VU747Z** Supplement Left Tunica Vaginalis with Autologous Tissue Substitute, Percutaneous Endoscopic Approach
♂ **0VU74JZ** Supplement Left Tunica Vaginalis with Synthetic Substitute, Percutaneous Endoscopic Approach
♂ **0VU74KZ** Supplement Left Tunica Vaginalis with Nonautologous Tissue Substitute, Percutaneous Endoscopic Approach
♂ **0VU907Z** Supplement Right Testis with Autologous Tissue Substitute, Open Approach
♂ **0VU90JZ** Supplement Right Testis with Synthetic Substitute, Open Approach

♂ **0VU90KZ** Supplement Right Testis with Nonautologous Tissue Substitute, Open Approach
♂ **0VUB07Z** Supplement Left Testis with Autologous Tissue Substitute, Open Approach
♂ **0VUB0JZ** Supplement Left Testis with Synthetic Substitute, Open Approach
♂ **0VUB0KZ** Supplement Left Testis with Nonautologous Tissue Substitute, Open Approach
♂ **0VUC07Z** Supplement Bilateral Testes with Autologous Tissue Substitute, Open Approach
♂ **0VUC0JZ** Supplement Bilateral Testes with Synthetic Substitute, Open Approach
♂ **0VUC0KZ** Supplement Bilateral Testes with Nonautologous Tissue Substitute, Open Approach
♂ **0VUF07Z** Supplement Right Spermatic Cord with Autologous Tissue Substitute, Open Approach
♂ **0VUF0JZ** Supplement Right Spermatic Cord with Synthetic Substitute, Open Approach
♂ **0VUF0KZ** Supplement Right Spermatic Cord with Nonautologous Tissue Substitute, Open Approach
♂ **0VUF47Z** Supplement Right Spermatic Cord with Autologous Tissue Substitute, Percutaneous Endoscopic Approach
♂ **0VUF4JZ** Supplement Right Spermatic Cord with Synthetic Substitute, Percutaneous Endoscopic Approach
♂ **0VUF4KZ** Supplement Right Spermatic Cord with Nonautologous Tissue Substitute, Percutaneous Endoscopic Approach
♂ **0VUG07Z** Supplement Left Spermatic Cord with Autologous Tissue Substitute, Open Approach
♂ **0VUG0JZ** Supplement Left Spermatic Cord with Synthetic Substitute, Open Approach
♂ **0VUG0KZ** Supplement Left Spermatic Cord with Nonautologous Tissue Substitute, Open Approach
♂ **0VUG47Z** Supplement Left Spermatic Cord with Autologous Tissue Substitute, Percutaneous Endoscopic Approach
♂ **0VUG4JZ** Supplement Left Spermatic Cord with Synthetic Substitute, Percutaneous Endoscopic Approach
♂ **0VUG4KZ** Supplement Left Spermatic Cord with Nonautologous Tissue Substitute, Percutaneous Endoscopic Approach
♂ **0VUH07Z** Supplement Bilateral Spermatic Cords with Autologous Tissue Substitute, Open Approach
♂ **0VUH0JZ** Supplement Bilateral Spermatic Cords with Synthetic Substitute, Open Approach
♂ **0VUH0KZ** Supplement Bilateral Spermatic Cords with Nonautologous Tissue Substitute, Open Approach
♂ **0VUH47Z** Supplement Bilateral Spermatic Cords with Autologous Tissue Substitute, Percutaneous Endoscopic Approach
♂ **0VUH4JZ** Supplement Bilateral Spermatic Cords with Synthetic Substitute, Percutaneous Endoscopic Approach
♂ **0VUH4KZ** Supplement Bilateral Spermatic Cords with Nonautologous Tissue Substitute, Percutaneous Endoscopic Approach
♂ **0VUJ07Z** Supplement Right Epididymis with Autologous Tissue Substitute, Open Approach
♂ **0VUJ0JZ** Supplement Right Epididymis with Synthetic Substitute, Open Approach
♂ **0VUJ0KZ** Supplement Right Epididymis with Nonautologous Tissue Substitute, Open Approach
♂ **0VUJ47Z** Supplement Right Epididymis with Autologous Tissue Substitute, Percutaneous Endoscopic Approach
♂ **0VUJ4JZ** Supplement Right Epididymis with Synthetic Substitute, Percutaneous Endoscopic Approach
♂ **0VUJ4KZ** Supplement Right Epididymis with Nonautologous Tissue Substitute, Percutaneous Endoscopic Approach
♂ **0VUK07Z** Supplement Left Epididymis with Autologous Tissue Substitute, Open Approach
♂ **0VUK0JZ** Supplement Left Epididymis with Synthetic Substitute, Open Approach
♂ **0VUK0KZ** Supplement Left Epididymis with Nonautologous Tissue Substitute, Open Approach
♂ **0VUK47Z** Supplement Left Epididymis with Autologous Tissue Substitute, Percutaneous Endoscopic Approach
♂ **0VUK4JZ** Supplement Left Epididymis with Synthetic Substitute, Percutaneous Endoscopic Approach
♂ **0VUK4KZ** Supplement Left Epididymis with Nonautologous Tissue Substitute, Percutaneous Endoscopic Approach
♂ **0VUL07Z** Supplement Bilateral Epididymis with Autologous Tissue Substitute, Open Approach
♂ **0VUL0JZ** Supplement Bilateral Epididymis with Synthetic Substitute, Open Approach
♂ **0VUL0KZ** Supplement Bilateral Epididymis with Nonautologous Tissue Substitute, Open Approach
♂ **0VUL47Z** Supplement Bilateral Epididymis with Autologous Tissue Substitute, Percutaneous Endoscopic Approach
♂ **0VUL4JZ** Supplement Bilateral Epididymis with Synthetic Substitute, Percutaneous Endoscopic Approach
♂ **0VUL4KZ** Supplement Bilateral Epididymis with Nonautologous Tissue Substitute, Percutaneous Endoscopic Approach
♂ **0VUN07Z** Supplement Right Vas Deferens with Autologous Tissue Substitute, Open Approach
♂ **0VUN0JZ** Supplement Right Vas Deferens with Synthetic Substitute, Open Approach
♂ **0VUN0KZ** Supplement Right Vas Deferens with Nonautologous Tissuc Substitute, Open Approach
♂ **0VUN47Z** Supplement Right Vas Deferens with Autologous Tissue Substitute, Percutaneous Endoscopic Approach
♂ **0VUN4JZ** Supplement Right Vas Deferens with Synthetic Substitute, Percutaneous Endoscopic Approach
♂ **0VUN4KZ** Supplement Right Vas Deferens with Nonautologous Tissue Substitute, Percutaneous Endoscopic Approach
♂ **0VUP07Z** Supplement Left Vas Deferens with Autologous Tissue Substitute, Open Approach
♂ **0VUP0JZ** Supplement Left Vas Deferens with Synthetic Substitute, Open Approach
♂ **0VUP0KZ** Supplement Left Vas Deferens with Nonautologous Tissue Substitute, Open Approach
♂ **0VUP47Z** Supplement Left Vas Deferens with Autologous Tissue Substitute, Percutaneous Endoscopic Approach
♂ **0VUP4JZ** Supplement Left Vas Deferens with Synthetic Substitute, Percutaneous Endoscopic Approach
♂ **0VUP4KZ** Supplement Left Vas Deferens with Nonautologous Tissue Substitute, Percutaneous Endoscopic Approach
♂ **0VUQ07Z** Supplement Bilateral Vas Deferens with Autologous Tissue Substitute, Open Approach
♂ **0VUQ0JZ** Supplement Bilateral Vas Deferens with Synthetic Substitute, Open Approach
♂ **0VUQ0KZ** Supplement Bilateral Vas Deferens with Nonautologous Tissue Substitute, Open Approach
♂ **0VUQ47Z** Supplement Bilateral Vas Deferens with Autologous Tissue Substitute, Percutaneous Endoscopic Approach
♂ **0VUQ4JZ** Supplement Bilateral Vas Deferens with Synthetic Substitute, Percutaneous Endoscopic Approach
♂ **0VUQ4KZ** Supplement Bilateral Vas Deferens with Nonautologous Tissue Substitute, Percutaneous Endoscopic Approach
♂ **0VUS07Z** Supplement Penis with Autologous Tissue Substitute, Open Approach
♂ **0VUS0JZ** Supplement Penis with Synthetic Substitute, Open Approach
♂ **0VUS0KZ** Supplement Penis with Nonautologous Tissue Substitute, Open Approach
♂ **0VUS47Z** Supplement Penis with Autologous Tissue Substitute, Percutaneous Endoscopic Approach
♂ **0VUS4JZ** Supplement Penis with Synthetic Substitute, Percutaneous Endoscopic Approach
♂ **0VUS4KZ** Supplement Penis with Nonautologous Tissue Substitute, Percutaneous Endoscopic Approach
♂ **0VUSX7Z** Supplement Penis with Autologous Tissue Substitute, External Approach
♂ **0VUSXJZ** Supplement Penis with Synthetic Substitute, External Approach
♂ **0VUSXKZ** Supplement Penis with Nonautologous Tissue Substitute, External Approach
♂ **0VUT07Z** Supplement Prepuce with Autologous Tissue Substitute, Open Approach
♂ **0VUT0JZ** Supplement Prepuce with Synthetic Substitute, Open Approach
♂ **0VUT0KZ** Supplement Prepuce with Nonautologous Tissue Substitute, Open Approach
♂ **0VUT47Z** Supplement Prepuce with Autologous Tissue Substitute, Percutaneous Endoscopic Approach
♂ **0VUT4JZ** Supplement Prepuce with Synthetic Substitute, Percutaneous Endoscopic Approach
♂ **0VUT4KZ** Supplement Prepuce with Nonautologous Tissue Substitute, Percutaneous Endoscopic Approach
♂ **0VUTX7Z** Supplement Prepuce with Autologous Tissue Substitute, External Approach
♂ **0VUTXJZ** Supplement Prepuce with Synthetic Substitute, External Approach
♂ **0VUTXKZ** Supplement Prepuce with Nonautologous Tissue Substitute, External Approach

Review Coding Guideline B6.1c

♂**0VW400Z** Revision of Drainage Device in Prostate and Seminal Vesicles, Open Approach
♂**0VW403Z** Revision of Infusion Device in Prostate and Seminal Vesicles, Open Approach
♂**0VW407Z** Revision of Autologous Tissue Substitute in Prostate and Seminal Vesicles, Open Approach
♂**0VW40JZ** Revision of Synthetic Substitute in Prostate and Seminal Vesicles, Open Approach
♂**0VW40KZ** Revision of Nonautologous Tissue Substitute in Prostate and Seminal Vesicles, Open Approach
♂**0VW430Z** Revision of Drainage Device in Prostate and Seminal Vesicles, Percutaneous Approach
♂**0VW433Z** Revision of Infusion Device in Prostate and Seminal Vesicles, Percutaneous Approach
♂**0VW437Z** Revision of Autologous Tissue Substitute in Prostate and Seminal Vesicles, Percutaneous Approach
♂**0VW43JZ** Revision of Synthetic Substitute in Prostate and Seminal Vesicles, Percutaneous Approach
♂**0VW43KZ** Revision of Nonautologous Tissue Substitute in Prostate and Seminal Vesicles, Percutaneous Approach
♂**0VW440Z** Revision of Drainage Device in Prostate and Seminal Vesicles, Percutaneous Endoscopic Approach
♂**0VW443Z** Revision of Infusion Device in Prostate and Seminal Vesicles, Percutaneous Endoscopic Approach
♂**0VW447Z** Revision of Autologous Tissue Substitute in Prostate and Seminal Vesicles, Percutaneous Endoscopic Approach
♂**0VW44JZ** Revision of Synthetic Substitute in Prostate and Seminal Vesicles, Percutaneous Endoscopic Approach
♂**0VW44KZ** Revision of Nonautologous Tissue Substitute in Prostate and Seminal Vesicles, Percutaneous Endoscopic Approach
♂**0VW470Z** Revision of Drainage Device in Prostate and Seminal Vesicles, Via Natural or Artificial Opening
♂**0VW473Z** Revision of Infusion Device in Prostate and Seminal Vesicles, Via Natural or Artificial Opening
♂**0VW477Z** Revision of Autologous Tissue Substitute in Prostate and Seminal Vesicles, Via Natural or Artificial Opening
♂**0VW47JZ** Revision of Synthetic Substitute in Prostate and Seminal Vesicles, Via Natural or Artificial Opening
♂**0VW47KZ** Revision of Nonautologous Tissue Substitute in Prostate and Seminal Vesicles, Via Natural or Artificial Opening
♂**0VW480Z** Revision of Drainage Device in Prostate and Seminal Vesicles, Via Natural or Artificial Opening Endoscopic
♂**0VW483Z** Revision of Infusion Device in Prostate and Seminal Vesicles, Via Natural or Artificial Opening Endoscopic
♂**0VW487Z** Revision of Autologous Tissue Substitute in Prostate and Seminal Vesicles, Via Natural or Artificial Opening Endoscopic
♂**0VW48JZ** Revision of Synthetic Substitute in Prostate and Seminal Vesicles, Via Natural or Artificial Opening Endoscopic
♂ **0VW48KZ** Revision of Nonautologous Tissue Substitute in Prostate and Seminal Vesicles, Via Natural or Artificial Opening Endoscopic
♂ **0VW4X0Z** Revision of Drainage Device in Prostate and Seminal Vesicles, External Approach
♂ **0VW4X3Z** Revision of Infusion Device in Prostate and Seminal Vesicles, External Approach
♂ **0VW4X7Z** Revision of Autologous Tissue Substitute in Prostate and Seminal Vesicles, External Approach
♂ **0VW4XJZ** Revision of Synthetic Substitute in Prostate and Seminal Vesicles, External Approach
♂ **0VW4XKZ** Revision of Nonautologous Tissue Substitute in Prostate and Seminal Vesicles, External Approach
♂ **0VW800Z** Revision of Drainage Device in Scrotum and Tunica Vaginalis, Open Approach
♂ **0VW803Z** Revision of Infusion Device in Scrotum and Tunica Vaginalis, Open Approach
♂ **0VW807Z** Revision of Autologous Tissue Substitute in Scrotum and Tunica Vaginalis, Open Approach
♂ **0VW80JZ** Revision of Synthetic Substitute in Scrotum and Tunica Vaginalis, Open Approach
♂ **0VW80KZ** Revision of Nonautologous Tissue Substitute in Scrotum and Tunica Vaginalis, Open Approach
♂ **0VW830Z** Revision of Drainage Device in Scrotum and Tunica Vaginalis, Percutaneous Approach
♂ **0VW833Z** Revision of Infusion Device in Scrotum and Tunica Vaginalis, Percutaneous Approach
♂ **0VW837Z** Revision of Autologous Tissue Substitute in Scrotum and Tunica Vaginalis, Percutaneous Approach
♂ **0VW83JZ** Revision of Synthetic Substitute in Scrotum and Tunica Vaginalis, Percutaneous Approach
♂ **0VW83KZ** Revision of Nonautologous Tissue Substitute in Scrotum and Tunica Vaginalis, Percutaneous Approach
♂ **0VW840Z** Revision of Drainage Device in Scrotum and Tunica Vaginalis, Percutaneous Endoscopic Approach
♂ **0VW843Z** Revision of Infusion Device in Scrotum and Tunica Vaginalis, Percutaneous Endoscopic Approach
♂ **0VW847Z** Revision of Autologous Tissue Substitute in Scrotum and Tunica Vaginalis, Percutaneous Endoscopic Approach
♂ **0VW84JZ** Revision of Synthetic Substitute in Scrotum and Tunica Vaginalis, Percutaneous Endoscopic Approach
♂ **0VW84KZ** Revision of Nonautologous Tissue Substitute in Scrotum and Tunica Vaginalis, Percutaneous Endoscopic Approach
♂ **0VW870Z** Revision of Drainage Device in Scrotum and Tunica Vaginalis, Via Natural or Artificial Opening
♂ **0VW873Z** Revision of Infusion Device in Scrotum and Tunica Vaginalis, Via Natural or Artificial Opening
♂ **0VW877Z** Revision of Autologous Tissue Substitute in Scrotum and Tunica Vaginalis, Via Natural or Artificial Opening
♂ **0VW87JZ** Revision of Synthetic Substitute in Scrotum and Tunica Vaginalis, Via Natural or Artificial Opening
♂ **0VW87KZ** Revision of Nonautologous Tissue Substitute in Scrotum and Tunica Vaginalis, Via Natural or Artificial Opening
♂ **0VW880Z** Revision of Drainage Device in Scrotum and Tunica Vaginalis, Via Natural or Artificial Opening Endoscopic
♂ **0VW883Z** Revision of Infusion Device in Scrotum and Tunica Vaginalis, Via Natural or Artificial Opening Endoscopic
♂ **0VW887Z** Revision of Autologous Tissue Substitute in Scrotum and Tunica Vaginalis, Via Natural or Artificial Opening Endoscopic
♂ **0VW88JZ** Revision of Synthetic Substitute in Scrotum and Tunica Vaginalis, Via Natural or Artificial Opening Endoscopic
♂ **0VW88KZ** Revision of Nonautologous Tissue Substitute in Scrotum and Tunica Vaginalis, Via Natural or Artificial Opening Endoscopic
♂ **0VW8X0Z** Revision of Drainage Device in Scrotum and Tunica Vaginalis, External Approach
♂ **0VW8X3Z** Revision of Infusion Device in Scrotum and Tunica Vaginalis, External Approach
♂ **0VW8X7Z** Revision of Autologous Tissue Substitute in Scrotum and Tunica Vaginalis, External Approach
♂ **0VW8XJZ** Revision of Synthetic Substitute in Scrotum and Tunica Vaginalis, External Approach
♂ **0VW8XKZ** Revision of Nonautologous Tissue Substitute in Scrotum and Tunica Vaginalis, External Approach
♂ **0VWD00Z** Revision of Drainage Device in Testis, Open Approach
♂ **0VWD03Z** Revision of Infusion Device in Testis, Open Approach
♂ **0VWD07Z** Revision of Autologous Tissue Substitute in Testis, Open Approach
♂ **0VWD0JZ** Revision of Synthetic Substitute in Testis, Open Approach
♂ **0VWD0KZ** Revision of Nonautologous Tissue Substitute in Testis, Open Approach
♂ **0VWD30Z** Revision of Drainage Device in Testis, Percutaneous Approach
♂ **0VWD33Z** Revision of Infusion Device in Testis, Percutaneous Approach
♂ **0VWD37Z** Revision of Autologous Tissue Substitute in Testis, Percutaneous Approach
♂ **0VWD3JZ** Revision of Synthetic Substitute in Testis, Percutaneous Approach
♂ **0VWD3KZ** Revision of Nonautologous Tissue Substitute in Testis, Percutaneous Approach
♂ **0VWD40Z** Revision of Drainage Device in Testis, Percutaneous Endoscopic Approach
♂ **0VWD43Z** Revision of Infusion Device in Testis, Percutaneous Endoscopic Approach
♂ **0VWD47Z** Revision of Autologous Tissue Substitute in Testis, Percutaneous Endoscopic Approach
♂ **0VWD4JZ** Revision of Synthetic Substitute in Testis, Percutaneous Endoscopic Approach
♂ **0VWD4KZ** Revision of Nonautologous Tissue Substitute in Testis, Percutaneous Endoscopic Approach
♂ **0VWD70Z** Revision of Drainage Device in Testis, Via Natural or Artificial Opening
♂ **0VWD73Z** Revision of Infusion Device in Testis, Via Natural or Artificial Opening
♂ **0VWD77Z** Revision of Autologous Tissue Substitute in Testis, Via Natural or Artificial Opening

♂ **0VWD7JZ** Revision of Synthetic Substitute in Testis, Via Natural or Artificial Opening

♂ **0VWD7KZ** Revision of Nonautologous Tissue Substitute in Testis, Via Natural or Artificial Opening

♂ **0VWD80Z** Revision of Drainage Device in Testis, Via Natural or Artificial Opening Endoscopic

♂ **0VWD83Z** Revision of Infusion Device in Testis, Via Natural or Artificial Opening Endoscopic

♂ **0VWD87Z** Revision of Autologous Tissue Substitute in Testis, Via Natural or Artificial Opening Endoscopic

♂ **0VWD8JZ** Revision of Synthetic Substitute in Testis, Via Natural or Artificial Opening Endoscopic

♂ **0VWD8KZ** Revision of Nonautologous Tissue Substitute in Testis, Via Natural or Artificial Opening Endoscopic

♂ **0VWDX0Z** Revision of Drainage Device in Testis, External Approach

♂ **0VWDX3Z** Revision of Infusion Device in Testis, External Approach

♂ **0VWDX7Z** Revision of Autologous Tissue Substitute in Testis, External Approach

♂ **0VWDXJZ** Revision of Synthetic Substitute in Testis, External Approach

♂ **0VWDXKZ** Revision of Nonautologous Tissue Substitute in Testis, External Approach

♂ **0VWM00Z** Revision of Drainage Device in Epididymis and Spermatic Cord, Open Approach

♂ **0VWM03Z** Revision of Infusion Device in Epididymis and Spermatic Cord, Open Approach

♂ **0VWM07Z** Revision of Autologous Tissue Substitute in Epididymis and Spermatic Cord, Open Approach

♂ **0VWM0CZ** Revision of Extraluminal Device in Epididymis and Spermatic Cord, Open Approach

♂ **0VWM0JZ** Revision of Synthetic Substitute in Epididymis and Spermatic Cord, Open Approach

♂ **0VWM0KZ** Revision of Nonautologous Tissue Substitute in Epididymis and Spermatic Cord, Open Approach

♂ **0VWM30Z** Revision of Drainage Device in Epididymis and Spermatic Cord, Percutaneous Approach

♂ **0VWM33Z** Revision of Infusion Device in Epididymis and Spermatic Cord, Percutaneous Approach

♂ **0VWM37Z** Revision of Autologous Tissue Substitute in Epididymis and Spermatic Cord, Percutaneous Approach

♂ **0VWM3CZ** Revision of Extraluminal Device in Epididymis and Spermatic Cord, Percutaneous Approach

♂ **0VWM3JZ** Revision of Synthetic Substitute in Epididymis and Spermatic Cord, Percutaneous Approach

♂ **0VWM3KZ** Revision of Nonautologous Tissue Substitute in Epididymis and Spermatic Cord, Percutaneous Approach

♂ **0VWM40Z** Revision of Drainage Device in Epididymis and Spermatic Cord, Percutaneous Endoscopic Approach

♂ **0VWM43Z** Revision of Infusion Device in Epididymis and Spermatic Cord, Percutaneous Endoscopic Approach

♂ **0VWM47Z** Revision of Autologous Tissue Substitute in Epididymis and Spermatic Cord, Percutaneous Endoscopic Approach

♂ **0VWM4CZ** Revision of Extraluminal Device in Epididymis and Spermatic Cord, Percutaneous Endoscopic Approach

♂ **0VWM4JZ** Revision of Synthetic Substitute in Epididymis and Spermatic Cord, Percutaneous Endoscopic Approach

♂ **0VWM4KZ** Revision of Nonautologous Tissue Substitute in Epididymis and Spermatic Cord, Percutaneous Endoscopic Approach

♂ **0VWM70Z** Revision of Drainage Device in Epididymis and Spermatic Cord, Via Natural or Artificial Opening

♂ **0VWM73Z** Revision of Infusion Device in Epididymis and Spermatic Cord, Via Natural or Artificial Opening

♂ **0VWM77Z** Revision of Autologous Tissue Substitute in Epididymis and Spermatic Cord, Via Natural or Artificial Opening

♂ **0VWM7CZ** Revision of Extraluminal Device in Epididymis and Spermatic Cord, Via Natural or Artificial Opening

♂ **0VWM7JZ** Revision of Synthetic Substitute in Epididymis and Spermatic Cord, Via Natural or Artificial Opening

♂ **0VWM7KZ** Revision of Nonautologous Tissue Substitute in Epididymis and Spermatic Cord, Via Natural or Artificial Opening

♂ **0VWM80Z** Revision of Drainage Device in Epididymis and Spermatic Cord, Via Natural or Artificial Opening Endoscopic

♂ **0VWM83Z** Revision of Infusion Device in Epididymis and Spermatic Cord, Via Natural or Artificial Opening Endoscopic

♂ **0VWM87Z** Revision of Autologous Tissue Substitute in Epididymis and Spermatic Cord, Via Natural or Artificial Opening Endoscopic

♂ **0VWM8CZ** Revision of Extraluminal Device in Epididymis and Spermatic Cord, Via Natural or Artificial Opening Endoscopic

♂ **0VWM8JZ** Revision of Synthetic Substitute in Epididymis and Spermatic Cord, Via Natural or Artificial Opening Endoscopic

♂ **0VWM8KZ** Revision of Nonautologous Tissue Substitute in Epididymis and Spermatic Cord, Via Natural or Artificial Opening Endoscopic

♂ **0VWMX0Z** Revision of Drainage Device in Epididymis and Spermatic Cord, External Approach

♂ **0VWMX3Z** Revision of Infusion Device in Epididymis and Spermatic Cord, External Approach

♂ **0VWMX7Z** Revision of Autologous Tissue Substitute in Epididymis and Spermatic Cord, External Approach

♂ **0VWMXCZ** Revision of Extraluminal Device in Epididymis and Spermatic Cord, External Approach

♂ **0VWMXJZ** Revision of Synthetic Substitute in Epididymis and Spermatic Cord, External Approach

♂ **0VWMXKZ** Revision of Nonautologous Tissue Substitute in Epididymis and Spermatic Cord, External Approach

♂ **0VWR00Z** Revision of Drainage Device in Vas Deferens, Open Approach

♂ **0VWR03Z** Revision of Infusion Device in Vas Deferens, Open Approach

♂ **0VWR07Z** Revision of Autologous Tissue Substitute in Vas Deferens, Open Approach

♂ **0VWR0CZ** Revision of Extraluminal Device in Vas Deferens, Open Approach

♂ **0VWR0DZ** Revision of Intraluminal Device in Vas Deferens, Open Approach

♂ **0VWR0JZ** Revision of Synthetic Substitute in Vas Deferens, Open Approach

♂ **0VWR0KZ** Revision of Nonautologous Tissue Substitute in Vas Deferens, Open Approach

♂ **0VWR30Z** Revision of Drainage Device in Vas Deferens, Percutaneous Approach

♂ **0VWR33Z** Revision of Infusion Device in Vas Deferens, Percutaneous Approach

♂ **0VWR37Z** Revision of Autologous Tissue Substitute in Vas Deferens, Percutaneous Approach

♂ **0VWR3CZ** Revision of Extraluminal Device in Vas Deferens, Percutaneous Approach

♂ **0VWR3DZ** Revision of Intraluminal Device in Vas Deferens, Percutaneous Approach

♂ **0VWR3JZ** Revision of Synthetic Substitute in Vas Deferens, Percutaneous Approach

♂ **0VWR3KZ** Revision of Nonautologous Tissue Substitute in Vas Deferens, Percutaneous Approach

♂ **0VWR40Z** Revision of Drainage Device in Vas Deferens, Percutaneous Endoscopic Approach

♂ **0VWR43Z** Revision of Infusion Device in Vas Deferens, Percutaneous Endoscopic Approach

♂ **0VWR47Z** Revision of Autologous Tissue Substitute in Vas Deferens, Percutaneous Endoscopic Approach

♂ **0VWR4CZ** Revision of Extraluminal Device in Vas Deferens, Percutaneous Endoscopic Approach

♂ **0VWR4DZ** Revision of Intraluminal Device in Vas Deferens, Percutaneous Endoscopic Approach

♂ **0VWR4JZ** Revision of Synthetic Substitute in Vas Deferens, Percutaneous Endoscopic Approach

♂ **0VWR4KZ** Revision of Nonautologous Tissue Substitute in Vas Deferens, Percutaneous Endoscopic Approach

♂ **0VWR70Z** Revision of Drainage Device in Vas Deferens, Via Natural or Artificial Opening

♂ **0VWR73Z** Revision of Infusion Device in Vas Deferens, Via Natural or Artificial Opening

♂ **0VWR77Z** Revision of Autologous Tissue Substitute in Vas Deferens, Via Natural or Artificial Opening

♂ **0VWR7CZ** Revision of Extraluminal Device in Vas Deferens, Via Natural or Artificial Opening

♂ **0VWR7DZ** Revision of Intraluminal Device in Vas Deferens, Via Natural or Artificial Opening

♂ **0VWR7JZ** Revision of Synthetic Substitute in Vas Deferens, Via Natural or Artificial Opening

♂ **0VWR7KZ** Revision of Nonautologous Tissue Substitute in Vas Deferens, Via Natural or Artificial Opening

♂ **0VWR80Z** Revision of Drainage Device in Vas Deferens, Via Natural or Artificial Opening Endoscopic

♂ **0VWR83Z** Revision of Infusion Device in Vas Deferens, Via Natural or Artificial Opening Endoscopic

♂ **0VWR87Z** Revision of Autologous Tissue Substitute in Vas Deferens, Via Natural or Artificial Opening Endoscopic

♂ **0VWR8CZ** Revision of Extraluminal Device in Vas Deferens, Via Natural or Artificial Opening Endoscopic

♂ **0VWR8DZ** Revision of Intraluminal Device in Vas Deferens, Via Natural or Artificial Opening Endoscopic

♂0VWR8JZ Revision of Synthetic Substitute in Vas Deferens, Via Natural or Artificial Opening Endoscopic

♂0VWR8KZ Revision of Nonautologous Tissue Substitute in Vas Deferens, Via Natural or Artificial Opening Endoscopic

♂0VWRX0Z Revision of Drainage Device in Vas Deferens, External Approach

♂0VWRX3Z Revision of Infusion Device in Vas Deferens, External Approach

♂0VWRX7Z Revision of Autologous Tissue Substitute in Vas Deferens, External Approach

♂0VWRXCZ Revision of Extraluminal Device in Vas Deferens, External Approach

♂0VWRXDZ Revision of Intraluminal Device in Vas Deferens, External Approach

♂0VWRXJZ Revision of Synthetic Substitute in Vas Deferens, External Approach

♂0VWRXKZ Revision of Nonautologous Tissue Substitute in Vas Deferens, External Approach

♂0VWS00Z Revision of Drainage Device in Penis, Open Approach

♂0VWS03Z Revision of Infusion Device in Penis, Open Approach

♂0VWS07Z Revision of Autologous Tissue Substitute in Penis, Open Approach

♂0VWS0JZ Revision of Synthetic Substitute in Penis, Open Approach

♂ 0VWS0KZ Revision of Nonautologous Tissue Substitute in Penis, Open Approach

♂ 0VWS30Z Revision of Drainage Device in Penis, Percutaneous Approach

♂ 0VWS33Z Revision of Infusion Device in Penis, Percutaneous Approach

♂ 0VWS37Z Revision of Autologous Tissue Substitute in Penis, Percutaneous Approach

♂ 0VWS3JZ Revision of Synthetic Substitute in Penis, Percutaneous Approach

♂ 0VWS3KZ Revision of Nonautologous Tissue Substitute in Penis, Percutaneous Approach

♂ 0VWS40Z Revision of Drainage Device in Penis, Percutaneous Endoscopic Approach

♂ 0VWS43Z Revision of Infusion Device in Penis, Percutaneous Endoscopic Approach

♂ 0VWS47Z Revision of Autologous Tissue Substitute in Penis, Percutaneous Endoscopic Approach

♂ 0VWS4JZ Revision of Synthetic Substitute in Penis, Percutaneous Endoscopic Approach

♂ 0VWS4KZ Revision of Nonautologous Tissue Substitute in Penis, Percutaneous Endoscopic Approach

♂ 0VWS70Z Revision of Drainage Device in Penis, Via Natural or Artificial Opening

♂ 0VWS73Z Revision of Infusion Device in Penis, Via Natural or Artificial Opening

♂ 0VWS77Z Revision of Autologous Tissue Substitute in Penis, Via Natural or Artificial Opening

♂ 0VWS7JZ Revision of Synthetic Substitute in Penis, Via Natural or Artificial Opening

♂ 0VWS7KZ Revision of Nonautologous Tissue Substitute in Penis, Via Natural or Artificial Opening

♂ 0VWS80Z Revision of Drainage Device in Penis, Via Natural or Artificial Opening Endoscopic

♂ 0VWS83Z Revision of Infusion Device in Penis, Via Natural or Artificial Opening Endoscopic

♂ 0VWS87Z Revision of Autologous Tissue Substitute in Penis, Via Natural or Artificial Opening Endoscopic

♂ 0VWS8JZ Revision of Synthetic Substitute in Penis, Via Natural or Artificial Opening Endoscopic

♂ 0VWS8KZ Revision of Nonautologous Tissue Substitute in Penis, Via Natural or Artificial Opening Endoscopic

♂ 0VWSX0Z Revision of Drainage Device in Penis, External Approach

♂ 0VWSX3Z Revision of Infusion Device in Penis, External Approach

♂ 0VWSX7Z Revision of Autologous Tissue Substitute in Penis, External Approach

♂ 0VWSXJZ Revision of Synthetic Substitute in Penis, External Approach

♂ 0VWSXKZ Revision of Nonautologous Tissue Substitute in Penis, External Approach

Anatomical Regions, General Tables 0W0–0WW

Section 0 **Medical and Surgical**
Body System W **Anatomical Regions, General**
Operation 0 **Alteration:** Modifying the anatomic structure of a body part without affecting the function of the body part

Body Part (4th)	Approach (5th)	Device (6th)	Qualifier (7th)
0 Head **2** Face **4** Upper Jaw **5** Lower Jaw **6** Neck **8** Chest Wall **F** Abdominal Wall **K** Upper Back **L** Lower Back **M** Perineum, Male **N** Perineum, Female	**0** Open **3** Percutaneous **4** Percutaneous Endoscopic	**7** Autologous Tissue Substitute **J** Synthetic Substitute **K** Nonautologous Tissue Substitute **Z** No Device	**Z** No Qualifier

Section 0 **Medical and Surgical**
Body System W **Anatomical Regions, General**
Operation 1 **Bypass:** Altering the route of passage of the contents of a tubular body part

Body Part (4th)	Approach (5th)	Device (6th)	Qualifier (7th)
1 Cranial Cavity	**0** Open	**J** Synthetic Substitute	**9** Pleural Cavity, Right **B** Pleural Cavity, Left **G** Peritoneal Cavity **J** Pelvic Cavity
9 Pleural Cavity, Right **B** Pleural Cavity, Left **G** Peritoneal Cavity **J** Pelvic Cavity	**0** Open **4** Percutaneous Endoscopic	**J** Synthetic Substitute	**4** Cutaneous **9** Pleural Cavity, Right **B** Pleural Cavity, Left **G** Peritoneal Cavity **J** Pelvic Cavity **Y** Lower Vein
9 Pleural Cavity, Right **B** Pleural Cavity, Left **G** Peritoneal Cavity **J** Pelvic Cavity	**3** Percutaneous	**J** Synthetic Substitute	**4** Cutaneous

Section 0 **Medical and Surgical**
Body System W **Anatomical Regions, General**
Operation 2 **Change:** Taking out or off a device from a body part and putting back an identical or similar device in or on the same body part without cutting or puncturing the skin or a mucous membrane

Body Part (4th)	Approach (5th)	Device (6th)	Qualifier (7th)
0 Head **1** Cranial Cavity **2** Face **4** Upper Jaw **5** Lower Jaw **6** Neck **8** Chest Wall **9** Pleural Cavity, Right **B** Pleural Cavity, Left **C** Mediastinum **D** Pericardial Cavity **F** Abdominal Wall **G** Peritoneal Cavity **H** Retroperitoneum **J** Pelvic Cavity **K** Upper Back **L** Lower Back **M** Perineum, Male **N** Perineum, Female	**X** External	**0** Drainage Device **Y** Other Device	**Z** No Qualifier

Section 0 **Medical and Surgical**
Body System W **Anatomical Regions, General**
Operation 3 **Control:** Stopping, or attempting to stop, postprocedural bleeding

Body Part (4th)	Approach (5th)	Device (6th)	Qualifier (7th)
0 Head **1** Cranial Cavity **2** Face **4** Upper Jaw **5** Lower Jaw **6** Neck **8** Chest Wall **9** Pleural Cavity, Right **B** Pleural Cavity, Left **C** Mediastinum **D** Pericardial Cavity **F** Abdominal Wall **G** Peritoneal Cavity **H** Retroperitoneum **J** Pelvic Cavity **K** Upper Back **L** Lower Back **M** Perineum, Male **N** Perineum, Female	**0** Open **3** Percutaneous **4** Percutaneous Endoscopic	**Z** No Device	**Z** No Qualifier
3 Oral Cavity and Throat	**0** Open **3** Percutaneous **4** Percutaneous Endoscopic **7** Via Natural or Artificial Opening **8** Via Natural or Artificial Opening Endoscopic **X** External	**Z** No Device	**Z** No Qualifier
P Gastrointestinal Tract **Q** Respiratory Tract **R** Genitourinary Tract	**0** Open **3** Percutaneous **4** Percutaneous Endoscopic **7** Via Natural or Artificial Opening **8** Via Natural or Artificial Opening Endoscopic	**Z** No Device	**Z** No Qualifier

Section 0 **Medical and Surgical**
Body System W **Anatomical Regions, General**
Operation 4 **Creation:** Making a new genital structure that does not take over the function of a body part

Body Part (4th)	Approach (5th)	Device (6th)	Qualifier (7th)
M Perineum, Male	**0** Open	**7** Autologous Tissue Substitute **J** Synthetic Substitute **K** Nonautologous Tissue Substitute **Z** No Device	**0** Vagina
N Perineum, Female	**0** Open	**7** Autologous Tissue Substitute **J** Synthetic Substitute **K** Nonautologous Tissue Substitute **Z** No Device	**1** Penis

Section 0 **Medical and Surgical**
Body System W **Anatomical Regions, General**
Operation 8 **Division:** Cutting into a body part, without draining fluids and/or gases from the body part, in order to separate or transect a body part

Body Part (4th)	Approach (5th)	Device (6th)	Qualifier (7th)
N Perineum, Female	**X** External	**Z** No Device	**Z** No Qualifier

Section 0 **Medical and Surgical**
Body System W **Anatomical Regions, General**
Operation 9 **Drainage:** Taking or letting out fluids and/or gases from a body part

Body Part (4th)	Approach (5th)	Device (6th)	Qualifier (7th)
0 Head **1** Cranial Cavity **2** Face **3** Oral Cavity and Throat **4** Upper Jaw **5** Lower Jaw **6** Neck **8** Chest Wall **9** Pleural Cavity, Right **B** Pleural Cavity, Left **C** Mediastinum **D** Pericardial Cavity **F** Abdominal Wall **G** Peritoneal Cavity **H** Retroperitoneum **J** Pelvic Cavity **K** Upper Back **L** Lower Back **M** Perineum, Male **N** Perineum, Female	**0** Open **3** Percutaneous **4** Percutaneous Endoscopic	**0** Drainage Device	**Z** No Qualifier
0 Head **1** Cranial Cavity **2** Face **3** Oral Cavity and Throat **4** Upper Jaw **5** Lower Jaw **6** Neck **8** Chest Wall **9** Pleural Cavity, Right **B** Pleural Cavity, Left **C** Mediastinum **D** Pericardial Cavity **F** Abdominal Wall **G** Peritoneal Cavity **H** Retroperitoneum **J** Pelvic Cavity **K** Upper Back **L** Lower Back **M** Perineum, Male **N** Perineum, Female	**0** Open **3** Percutaneous **4** Percutaneous Endoscopic	**Z** No Device	**X** Diagnostic **Z** No Qualifier

Section 0 **Medical and Surgical**
Body System W **Anatomical Regions, General**
Operation B **Excision:** Cutting out or off, without replacement, a portion of a body part

Body Part (4th)	Approach (5th)	Device (6th)	Qualifier (7th)
0 Head **2** Face **4** Upper Jaw **5** Lower Jaw **8** Chest Wall **K** Upper Back **L** Lower Back **M** Perineum, Male **N** Perineum, Female	**0** Open **3** Percutaneous **4** Percutaneous Endoscopic **X** External	**Z** No Device	**X** Diagnostic **Z** No Qualifier
6 Neck **F** Abdominal Wall	**0** Open **3** Percutaneous **4** Percutaneous Endoscopic	**Z** No Device	**X** Diagnostic **Z** No Qualifier

Continued →

Section 0 **Medical and Surgical**
Body System W **Anatomical Regions, General**
Operation B **Excision:** Cutting out or off, without replacement, a portion of a body part

Body Part (4th)	Approach (5th)	Device (6th)	Qualifier (7th)
6 Neck **F** Abdominal Wall	**X** External	**Z** No Device	**2** Stoma **X** Diagnostic **Z** No Qualifier
C Mediastinum **H** Retroperitoneum	**0** Open **3** Percutaneous **4** Percutaneous Endoscopic	**Z** No Device	**X** Diagnostic **Z** No Qualifier

Section 0 **Medical and Surgical**
Body System W **Anatomical Regions, General**
Operation C **Extirpation:** Taking or cutting out solid matter from a body part

Body Part (4th)	Approach (5th)	Device (6th)	Qualifier (7th)
1 Cranial Cavity **3** Oral Cavity and Throat **9** Pleural Cavity, Right **B** Pleural Cavity, Left **C** Mediastinum **D** Pericardial Cavity **G** Peritoneal Cavity **J** Pelvic Cavity	**0** Open **3** Percutaneous **4** Percutaneous Endoscopic **X** External	**Z** No Device	**Z** No Qualifier
P Gastrointestinal Tract **Q** Respiratory Tract **R** Genitourinary Tract	**0** Open **3** Percutaneous **4** Percutaneous Endoscopic **7** Via Natural or Artificial Opening **8** Via Natural or Artificial Opening Endoscopic **X** External	**Z** No Device	**Z** No Qualifier

Section 0 **Medical and Surgical**
Body System W **Anatomical Regions, General**
Operation F **Fragmentation:** Breaking solid matter in a body part into pieces

Body Part (4th)	Approach (5th)	Device (6th)	Qualifier (7th)
1 Cranial Cavity **3** Oral Cavity and Throat **9** Pleural Cavity, Right **B** Pleural Cavity, Left **C** Mediastinum **D** Pericardial Cavity **G** Peritoneal Cavity **J** Pelvic Cavity	**0** Open **3** Percutaneous **4** Percutaneous Endoscopic **X** External	**Z** No Device	**Z** No Qualifier
P Gastrointestinal Tract **Q** Respiratory Tract **R** Genitourinary Tract	**0** Open **3** Percutaneous **4** Percutaneous Endoscopic **7** Via Natural or Artificial Opening **8** Via Natural or Artificial Opening Endoscopic **X** External	**Z** No Device	**Z** No Qualifier

Section 0 **Medical and Surgical**
Body System W **Anatomical Regions, General**
Operation H **Insertion:** Putting in a nonbiological appliance that monitors, assists, performs, or prevents a physiological function but does not physically take the place of a body part

Body Part (4th)	Approach (5th)	Device (6th)	Qualifier (7th)
0 Head **1** Cranial Cavity **2** Face **3** Oral Cavity and Throat **4** Upper Jaw **5** Lower Jaw **6** Neck **8** Chest Wall **9** Pleural Cavity, Right **B** Pleural Cavity, Left **C** Mediastinum **D** Pericardial Cavity **F** Abdominal Wall **G** Peritoneal Cavity **H** Retroperitoneum **J** Pelvic Cavity **K** Upper Back **L** Lower Back **M** Perineum, Male **N** Perineum, Female	**0** Open **3** Percutaneous **4** Percutaneous Endoscopic	**1** Radioactive Element **3** Infusion Device **Y** Other Device	**Z** No Qualifier
P Gastrointestinal Tract **Q** Respiratory Tract **R** Genitourinary Tract	**0** Open **3** Percutaneous **4** Percutaneous Endoscopic **7** Via Natural or Artificial Opening **8** Via Natural or Artificial Opening Endoscopic	**1** Radioactive Element **3** Infusion Device **Y** Other Device	**Z** No Qualifier

Section 0 **Medical and Surgical**
Body System W **Anatomical Regions, General**
Operation J **Inspection:** Visually and/or manually exploring a body part

Body Part (4th)	Approach (5th)	Device (6th)	Qualifier (7th)
0 Head **2** Face **3** Oral Cavity and Throat **4** Upper Jaw **5** Lower Jaw **6** Neck **8** Chest Wall **F** Abdominal Wall **K** Upper Back **L** Lower Back **M** Perineum, Male **N** Perineum, Female	**0** Open **3** Percutaneous **4** Percutaneous Endoscopic **X** External	**Z** No Device	**Z** No Qualifier
1 Cranial Cavity **9** Pleural Cavity, Right **B** Pleural Cavity, Left **C** Mediastinum **D** Pericardial Cavity **G** Peritoneal Cavity **H** Retroperitoneum **J** Pelvic Cavity	**0** Open **3** Percutaneous **4** Percutaneous Endoscopic	**Z** No Device	**Z** No Qualifier
P Gastrointestinal Tract **Q** Respiratory Tract **R** Genitourinary Tract	**0** Open **3** Percutaneous **4** Percutaneous Endoscopic **7** Via Natural or Artificial Opening **8** Via Natural or Artificial Opening Endoscopic	**Z** No Device	**Z** No Qualifier

Section 0 **Medical and Surgical**
Body System W **Anatomical Regions, General**
Operation M **Reattachment:** Putting back in or on all or a portion of a separated body part to its normal location or other suitable location

Body Part (4th)	Approach (5th)	Device (6th)	Qualifier (7th)
2 Face **4** Upper Jaw **5** Lower Jaw **6** Neck **8** Chest Wall **F** Abdominal Wall **K** Upper Back **L** Lower Back **M** Perineum, Male **N** Perineum, Female	**0** Open	**Z** No Device	**Z** No Qualifier

Section 0 **Medical and Surgical**
Body System W **Anatomical Regions, General**
Operation P **Removal:** Taking out or off a device from a body part

Body Part (4th)	Approach (5th)	Device (6th)	Qualifier (7th)
0 Head **2** Face **4** Upper Jaw **5** Lower Jaw **6** Neck **8** Chest Wall **C** Mediastinum **F** Abdominal Wall **K** Upper Back **L** Lower Back **M** Perineum, Male **N** Perineum, Female	**0** Open **3** Percutaneous **4** Percutaneous Endoscopic **X** External	**0** Drainage Device **1** Radioactive Element **3** Infusion Device **7** Autologous Tissue Substitute **J** Synthetic Substitute **K** Nonautologous Tissue Substitute **Y** Other Device	**Z** No Qualifier
1 Cranial Cavity **9** Pleural Cavity, Right **B** Pleural Cavity, Left **G** Peritoneal Cavity **J** Pelvic Cavity	**0** Open **3** Percutaneous **4** Percutaneous Endoscopic	**0** Drainage Device **1** Radioactive Element **3** Infusion Device **J** Synthetic Substitute **Y** Other Device	**Z** No Qualifier
1 Cranial Cavity **9** Pleural Cavity, Right **B** Pleural Cavity, Left **G** Peritoneal Cavity **J** Pelvic Cavity	**X** External	**0** Drainage Device **1** Radioactive Element **3** Infusion Device	**Z** No Qualifier
D Pericardial Cavity **H** Retroperitoneum	**0** Open **3** Percutaneous **4** Percutaneous Endoscopic	**0** Drainage Device **1** Radioactive Element **3** Infusion Device **Y** Other Device	**Z** No Qualifier
D Pericardial Cavity **H** Retroperitoneum	**X** External	**0** Drainage Device **1** Radioactive Element **3** Infusion Device	**Z** No Qualifier
P Gastrointestinal Tract **Q** Respiratory Tract **R** Genitourinary Tract	**0** Open **3** Percutaneous **4** Percutaneous Endoscopic **7** Via Natural or Artificial Opening **8** Via Natural or Artificial Opening Endoscopic **X** External	**1** Radioactive Element **3** Infusion Device **Y** Other Device	**Z** No Qualifier

Section 0 Medical and Surgical
Body System W Anatomical Regions, General
Operation Q **Repair:** Restoring, to the extent possible, a body part to its normal anatomic structure and function

Body Part (4th)	Approach (5th)	Device (6th)	Qualifier (7th)
0 Head **2** Face **4** Upper Jaw **5** Lower Jaw **8** Chest Wall **K** Upper Back **L** Lower Back **M** Perineum, Male **N** Perineum, Female	**0** Open **3** Percutaneous **4** Percutaneous Endoscopic **X** External	**Z** No Device	**Z** No Qualifier
6 Neck **F** Abdominal Wall	**0** Open **3** Percutaneous **4** Percutaneous Endoscopic	**Z** No Device	**Z** No Qualifier
6 Neck **F** Abdominal Wall	**X** External	**Z** No Device	**2** Stoma **Z** No Qualifier
C Mediastinum	**0** Open **3** Percutaneous **4** Percutaneous Endoscopic	**Z** No Device	**Z** No Qualifier

Section 0 Medical and Surgical
Body System W Anatomical Regions, General
Operation U **Supplement:** Putting in or on biological or synthetic material that physically reinforces and/or augments the function of a portion of a body part

Body Part (4th)	Approach (5th)	Device (6th)	Qualifier (7th)
0 Head **2** Face **4** Upper Jaw **5** Lower Jaw **6** Neck **8** Chest Wall **C** Mediastinum **F** Abdominal Wall **K** Upper Back **L** Lower Back **M** Perineum, Male **N** Perineum, Female	**0** Open **4** Percutaneous Endoscopic	**7** Autologous Tissue Substitute **J** Synthetic Substitute **K** Nonautologous Tissue Substitute	**Z** No Qualifier

Section 0 Medical and Surgical
Body System W Anatomical Regions, General
Operation W **Revision:** Correcting, to the extent possible, a portion of a malfunctioning device or the position of a displaced device

Body Part (4th)	Approach (5th)	Device (6th)	Qualifier (7th)
0 Head **2** Face **4** Upper Jaw **5** Lower Jaw **6** Neck **8** Chest Wall **C** Mediastinum **F** Abdominal Wall **K** Upper Back **L** Lower Back **M** Perineum, Male **N** Perineum, Female	**0** Open **3** Percutaneous **4** Percutaneous Endoscopic **X** External	**0** Drainage Device **1** Radioactive Element **3** Infusion Device **7** Autologous Tissue Substitute **J** Synthetic Substitute **K** Nonautologous Tissue Substitute **Y** Other Device	**Z** No Qualifier

Continued →

Body Part (4th)	Approach (5th)	Device (6th)	Qualifier (7th)
1 Cranial Cavity 9 Pleural Cavity, Right B Pleural Cavity, Left G Peritoneal Cavity J Pelvic Cavity	0 Open 3 Percutaneous 4 Percutaneous Endoscopic X External	0 Drainage Device 1 Radioactive Element 3 Infusion Device J Synthetic Substitute Y Other Device	Z No Qualifier
D Pericardial Cavity H Retroperitoneum	0 Open 3 Percutaneous 4 Percutaneous Endoscopic X External	0 Drainage Device 1 Radioactive Element 3 Infusion Device Y Other Device	Z No Qualifier
P Gastrointestinal Tract Q Respiratory Tract R Genitourinary Tract	0 Open 3 Percutaneous 4 Percutaneous Endoscopic 7 Via Natural or Artificial Opening 8 Via Natural or Artificial Opening Endoscopic X External	1 Radioactive Element 3 Infusion Device Y Other Device	Z No Qualifier

Anatomical Regions, General Code Listing 0W0–0WW

0W0 – Anatomical Regions, General, Alteration

0W0007Z Alteration of Head with Autologous Tissue Substitute, Open Approach
0W000JZ Alteration of Head with Synthetic Substitute, Open Approach
0W000KZ Alteration of Head with Nonautologous Tissue Substitute, Open Approach
0W000ZZ Alteration of Head, Open Approach
0W0037Z Alteration of Head with Autologous Tissue Substitute, Percutaneous Approach
0W003JZ Alteration of Head with Synthetic Substitute, Percutaneous Approach
0W003KZ Alteration of Head with Nonautologous Tissue Substitute, Percutaneous Approach
0W003ZZ Alteration of Head, Percutaneous Approach
0W0047Z Alteration of Head with Autologous Tissue Substitute, Percutaneous Endoscopic Approach
0W004JZ Alteration of Head with Synthetic Substitute, Percutaneous Endoscopic Approach
0W004KZ Alteration of Head with Nonautologous Tissue Substitute, Percutaneous Endoscopic Approach
0W004ZZ Alteration of Head, Percutaneous Endoscopic Approach
0W0207Z Alteration of Face with Autologous Tissue Substitute, Open Approach
0W020JZ Alteration of Face with Synthetic Substitute, Open Approach
0W020KZ Alteration of Face with Nonautologous Tissue Substitute, Open Approach
0W020ZZ Alteration of Face, Open Approach
0W0237Z Alteration of Face with Autologous Tissue Substitute, Percutaneous Approach
0W023JZ Alteration of Face with Synthetic Substitute, Percutaneous Approach
0W023KZ Alteration of Face with Nonautologous Tissue Substitute, Percutaneous Approach
0W023ZZ Alteration of Face, Percutaneous Approach
0W0247Z Alteration of Face with Autologous Tissue Substitute, Percutaneous Endoscopic Approach
0W024JZ Alteration of Face with Synthetic Substitute, Percutaneous Endoscopic Approach
0W024KZ Alteration of Face with Nonautologous Tissue Substitute, Percutaneous Endoscopic Approach
0W024ZZ Alteration of Face, Percutaneous Endoscopic Approach
0W0407Z Alteration of Upper Jaw with Autologous Tissue Substitute, Open Approach
0W040JZ Alteration of Upper Jaw with Synthetic Substitute, Open Approach
0W040KZ Alteration of Upper Jaw with Nonautologous Tissue Substitute, Open Approach
0W040ZZ Alteration of Upper Jaw, Open Approach
0W0437Z Alteration of Upper Jaw with Autologous Tissue Substitute, Percutaneous Approach
0W043JZ Alteration of Upper Jaw with Synthetic Substitute, Percutaneous Approach
0W043KZ Alteration of Upper Jaw with Nonautologous Tissue Substitute, Percutaneous Approach
0W043ZZ Alteration of Upper Jaw, Percutaneous Approach
0W0447Z Alteration of Upper Jaw with Autologous Tissue Substitute, Percutaneous Endoscopic Approach
0W044JZ Alteration of Upper Jaw with Synthetic Substitute, Percutaneous Endoscopic Approach
0W044KZ Alteration of Upper Jaw with Nonautologous Tissue Substitute, Percutaneous Endoscopic Approach
0W044ZZ Alteration of Upper Jaw, Percutaneous Endoscopic Approach
0W0507Z Alteration of Lower Jaw with Autologous Tissue Substitute, Open Approach
0W050JZ Alteration of Lower Jaw with Synthetic Substitute, Open Approach
0W050KZ Alteration of Lower Jaw with Nonautologous Tissue Substitute, Open Approach
0W050ZZ Alteration of Lower Jaw, Open Approach
0W0537Z Alteration of Lower Jaw with Autologous Tissue Substitute, Percutaneous Approach
0W053JZ Alteration of Lower Jaw with Synthetic Substitute, Percutaneous Approach
0W053KZ Alteration of Lower Jaw with Nonautologous Tissue Substitute, Percutaneous Approach
0W053ZZ Alteration of Lower Jaw, Percutaneous Approach
0W0547Z Alteration of Lower Jaw with Autologous Tissue Substitute, Percutaneous Endoscopic Approach
0W054JZ Alteration of Lower Jaw with Synthetic Substitute, Percutaneous Endoscopic Approach
0W054KZ Alteration of Lower Jaw with Nonautologous Tissue Substitute, Percutaneous Endoscopic Approach
0W054ZZ Alteration of Lower Jaw, Percutaneous Endoscopic Approach
0W0607Z Alteration of Neck with Autologous Tissue Substitute, Open Approach
0W060JZ Alteration of Neck with Synthetic Substitute, Open Approach
0W060KZ Alteration of Neck with Nonautologous Tissue Substitute, Open Approach
0W060ZZ Alteration of Neck, Open Approach
0W0637Z Alteration of Neck with Autologous Tissue Substitute, Percutaneous Approach
0W063JZ Alteration of Neck with Synthetic Substitute, Percutaneous Approach
0W063KZ Alteration of Neck with Nonautologous Tissue Substitute, Percutaneous Approach
0W063ZZ Alteration of Neck, Percutaneous Approach
0W0647Z Alteration of Neck with Autologous Tissue Substitute, Percutaneous Endoscopic Approach
0W064JZ Alteration of Neck with Synthetic Substitute, Percutaneous Endoscopic Approach
0W064KZ Alteration of Neck with Nonautologous Tissue Substitute, Percutaneous Endoscopic Approach

0W064ZZ Alteration of Neck, Percutaneous Endoscopic Approach
0W0807Z Alteration of Chest Wall with Autologous Tissue Substitute, Open Approach
0W080JZ Alteration of Chest Wall with Synthetic Substitute, Open Approach
0W080KZ Alteration of Chest Wall with Nonautologous Tissue Substitute, Open Approach
0W080ZZ Alteration of Chest Wall, Open Approach
0W0837Z Alteration of Chest Wall with Autologous Tissue Substitute, Percutaneous Approach
0W083JZ Alteration of Chest Wall with Synthetic Substitute, Percutaneous Approach
0W083KZ Alteration of Chest Wall with Nonautologous Tissue Substitute, Percutaneous Approach
0W083ZZ Alteration of Chest Wall, Percutaneous Approach
0W0847Z Alteration of Chest Wall with Autologous Tissue Substitute, Percutaneous Endoscopic Approach
0W084JZ Alteration of Chest Wall with Synthetic Substitute, Percutaneous Endoscopic Approach
0W084KZ Alteration of Chest Wall with Nonautologous Tissue Substitute, Percutaneous Endoscopic Approach
0W084ZZ Alteration of Chest Wall, Percutaneous Endoscopic Approach
0W0F07Z Alteration of Abdominal Wall with Autologous Tissue Substitute, Open Approach
0W0F0JZ Alteration of Abdominal Wall with Synthetic Substitute, Open Approach
0W0F0KZ Alteration of Abdominal Wall with Nonautologous Tissue Substitute, Open Approach
0W0F0ZZ Alteration of Abdominal Wall, Open Approach
0W0F37Z Alteration of Abdominal Wall with Autologous Tissue Substitute, Percutaneous Approach
0W0F3JZ Alteration of Abdominal Wall with Synthetic Substitute, Percutaneous Approach
0W0F3KZ Alteration of Abdominal Wall with Nonautologous Tissue Substitute, Percutaneous Approach
0W0F3ZZ Alteration of Abdominal Wall, Percutaneous Approach
0W0F47Z Alteration of Abdominal Wall with Autologous Tissue Substitute, Percutaneous Endoscopic Approach
0W0F4JZ Alteration of Abdominal Wall with Synthetic Substitute, Percutaneous Endoscopic Approach
0W0F4KZ Alteration of Abdominal Wall with Nonautologous Tissue Substitute, Percutaneous Endoscopic Approach
0W0F4ZZ Alteration of Abdominal Wall, Percutaneous Endoscopic Approach
0W0K07Z Alteration of Upper Back with Autologous Tissue Substitute, Open Approach
0W0K0JZ Alteration of Upper Back with Synthetic Substitute, Open Approach
0W0K0KZ Alteration of Upper Back with Nonautologous Tissue Substitute, Open Approach
0W0K0ZZ Alteration of Upper Back, Open Approach
0W0K37Z Alteration of Upper Back with Autologous Tissue Substitute, Percutaneous Approach
0W0K3JZ Alteration of Upper Back with Synthetic Substitute, Percutaneous Approach
0W0K3KZ Alteration of Upper Back with Nonautologous Tissue Substitute, Percutaneous Approach
0W0K3ZZ Alteration of Upper Back, Percutaneous Approach
0W0K47Z Alteration of Upper Back with Autologous Tissue Substitute, Percutaneous Endoscopic Approach
0W0K4JZ Alteration of Upper Back with Synthetic Substitute, Percutaneous Endoscopic Approach
0W0K4KZ Alteration of Upper Back with Nonautologous Tissue Substitute, Percutaneous Endoscopic Approach
0W0K4ZZ Alteration of Upper Back, Percutaneous Endoscopic Approach
0W0L07Z Alteration of Lower Back with Autologous Tissue Substitute, Open Approach
0W0L0JZ Alteration of Lower Back with Synthetic Substitute, Open Approach
0W0L0KZ Alteration of Lower Back with Nonautologous Tissue Substitute, Open Approach
0W0L0ZZ Alteration of Lower Back, Open Approach
0W0L37Z Alteration of Lower Back with Autologous Tissue Substitute, Percutaneous Approach
0W0L3JZ Alteration of Lower Back with Synthetic Substitute, Percutaneous Approach
0W0L3KZ Alteration of Lower Back with Nonautologous Tissue Substitute, Percutaneous Approach
0W0L3ZZ Alteration of Lower Back, Percutaneous Approach
0W0L47Z Alteration of Lower Back with Autologous Tissue Substitute, Percutaneous Endoscopic Approach
0W0L4JZ Alteration of Lower Back with Synthetic Substitute, Percutaneous Endoscopic Approach
0W0L4KZ Alteration of Lower Back with Nonautologous Tissue Substitute, Percutaneous Endoscopic Approach
0W0L4ZZ Alteration of Lower Back, Percutaneous Endoscopic Approach
♂ **0W0M07Z** Alteration of Male Perineum with Autologous Tissue Substitute, Open Approach
♂ **0W0M0JZ** Alteration of Male Perineum with Synthetic Substitute, Open Approach
♂ **0W0M0KZ** Alteration of Male Perineum with Nonautologous Tissue Substitute, Open Approach
♂ **0W0M0ZZ** Alteration of Male Perineum, Open Approach
♂ **0W0M37Z** Alteration of Male Perineum with Autologous Tissue Substitute, Percutaneous Approach
♂ **0W0M3JZ** Alteration of Male Perineum with Synthetic Substitute, Percutaneous Approach
♂ **0W0M3KZ** Alteration of Male Perineum with Nonautologous Tissue Substitute, Percutaneous Approach
♂ **0W0M3ZZ** Alteration of Male Perineum, Percutaneous Approach
♂ **0W0M47Z** Alteration of Male Perineum with Autologous Tissue Substitute, Percutaneous Endoscopic Approach
♂ **0W0M4JZ** Alteration of Male Perineum with Synthetic Substitute, Percutaneous Endoscopic Approach
♂ **0W0M4KZ** Alteration of Male Perineum with Nonautologous Tissue Substitute, Percutaneous Endoscopic Approach
♂ **0W0M4ZZ** Alteration of Male Perineum, Percutaneous Endoscopic Approach
♀ **0W0N07Z** Alteration of Female Perineum with Autologous Tissue Substitute, Open Approach
♀ **0W0N0JZ** Alteration of Female Perineum with Synthetic Substitute, Open Approach
♀ **0W0N0KZ** Alteration of Female Perineum with Nonautologous Tissue Substitute, Open Approach
♀ **0W0N0ZZ** Alteration of Female Perineum, Open Approach
♀ **0W0N37Z** Alteration of Female Perineum with Autologous Tissue Substitute, Percutaneous Approach
♀ **0W0N3JZ** Alteration of Female Perineum with Synthetic Substitute, Percutaneous Approach
♀ **0W0N3KZ** Alteration of Female Perineum with Nonautologous Tissue Substitute, Percutaneous Approach
♀ **0W0N3ZZ** Alteration of Female Perineum, Percutaneous Approach
♀ **0W0N47Z** Alteration of Female Perineum with Autologous Tissue Substitute, Percutaneous Endoscopic Approach
♀ **0W0N4JZ** Alteration of Female Perineum with Synthetic Substitute, Percutaneous Endoscopic Approach
♀ **0W0N4KZ** Alteration of Female Perineum with Nonautologous Tissue Substitute, Percutaneous Endoscopic Approach
♀ **0W0N4ZZ** Alteration of Female Perineum, Percutaneous Endoscopic Approach

0W1 – Anatomical Regions, General, Bypass

Review Coding Guideline B3.6a

0W110J9 Bypass Cranial Cavity to Right Pleural Cavity with Synthetic Substitute, Open Approach
0W110JB Bypass Cranial Cavity to Left Pleural Cavity with Synthetic Substitute, Open Approach
0W110JG Bypass Cranial Cavity to Peritoneal Cavity with Synthetic Substitute, Open Approach
0W110JJ Bypass Cranial Cavity to Pelvic Cavity with Synthetic Substitute, Open Approach
0W190J4 Bypass Right Pleural Cavity to Cutaneous with Synthetic Substitute, Open Approach
0W190J9 Bypass Right Pleural Cavity to Right Pleural Cavity with Synthetic Substitute, Open Approach
0W190JB Bypass Right Pleural Cavity to Left Pleural Cavity with Synthetic Substitute, Open Approach
0W190JG Bypass Right Pleural Cavity to Peritoneal Cavity with Synthetic Substitute, Open Approach
0W190JJ Bypass Right Pleural Cavity to Pelvic Cavity with Synthetic Substitute, Open Approach
0W190JY Bypass Right Pleural Cavity to Lower Vein with Synthetic Substitute, Open Approach
0W193J4 Bypass Right Pleural Cavity to Cutaneous with Synthetic Substitute, Percutaneous Approach
0W194J4 Bypass Right Pleural Cavity to Cutaneous with Synthetic Substitute, Percutaneous Endoscopic Approach

0W194J9 Bypass Right Pleural Cavity to Right Pleural Cavity with Synthetic Substitute, Percutaneous Endoscopic Approach
0W194JB Bypass Right Pleural Cavity to Left Pleural Cavity with Synthetic Substitute, Percutaneous Endoscopic Approach
0W194JG Bypass Right Pleural Cavity to Peritoneal Cavity with Synthetic Substitute, Percutaneous Endoscopic Approach
0W194JJ Bypass Right Pleural Cavity to Pelvic Cavity with Synthetic Substitute, Percutaneous Endoscopic Approach
0W194JY Bypass Right Pleural Cavity to Lower Vein with Synthetic Substitute, Percutaneous Endoscopic Approach
0W1B0J4 Bypass Left Pleural Cavity to Cutaneous with Synthetic Substitute, Open Approach
0W1B0J9 Bypass Left Pleural Cavity to Right Pleural Cavity with Synthetic Substitute, Open Approach
0W1B0JB Bypass Left Pleural Cavity to Left Pleural Cavity with Synthetic Substitute, Open Approach
0W1B0JG Bypass Left Pleural Cavity to Peritoneal Cavity with Synthetic Substitute, Open Approach
0W1B0JJ Bypass Left Pleural Cavity to Pelvic Cavity with Synthetic Substitute, Open Approach
0W1B0JY Bypass Left Pleural Cavity to Lower Vein with Synthetic Substitute, Open Approach
0W1B3J4 Bypass Left Pleural Cavity to Cutaneous with Synthetic Substitute, Percutaneous Approach
0W1B4J4 Bypass Left Pleural Cavity to Cutaneous with Synthetic Substitute, Percutaneous Endoscopic Approach
0W1B4J9 Bypass Left Pleural Cavity to Right Pleural Cavity with Synthetic Substitute, Percutaneous Endoscopic Approach
0W1B4JB Bypass Left Pleural Cavity to Left Pleural Cavity with Synthetic Substitute, Percutaneous Endoscopic Approach
0W1B4JG Bypass Left Pleural Cavity to Peritoneal Cavity with Synthetic Substitute, Percutaneous Endoscopic Approach
0W1B4JJ Bypass Left Pleural Cavity to Pelvic Cavity with Synthetic Substitute, Percutaneous Endoscopic Approach
0W1B4JY Bypass Left Pleural Cavity to Lower Vein with Synthetic Substitute, Percutaneous Endoscopic Approach
0W1G0J4 Bypass Peritoneal Cavity to Cutaneous with Synthetic Substitute, Open Approach
0W1G0J9 Bypass Peritoneal Cavity to Right Pleural Cavity with Synthetic Substitute, Open Approach
0W1G0JB Bypass Peritoneal Cavity to Left Pleural Cavity with Synthetic Substitute, Open Approach
0W1G0JG Bypass Peritoneal Cavity to Peritoneal Cavity with Synthetic Substitute, Open Approach
0W1G0JJ Bypass Peritoneal Cavity to Pelvic Cavity with Synthetic Substitute, Open Approach
0W1G0JY Bypass Peritoneal Cavity to Lower Vein with Synthetic Substitute, Open Approach
0W1G3J4 Bypass Peritoneal Cavity to Cutaneous with Synthetic Substitute, Percutaneous Approach
AHA CC: 4Q, 2013, 126-127
0W1G4J4 Bypass Peritoneal Cavity to Cutaneous with Synthetic Substitute, Percutaneous Endoscopic Approach
0W1G4J9 Bypass Peritoneal Cavity to Right Pleural Cavity with Synthetic Substitute, Percutaneous Endoscopic Approach
0W1G4JB Bypass Peritoneal Cavity to Left Pleural Cavity with Synthetic Substitute, Percutaneous Endoscopic Approach
0W1G4JG Bypass Peritoneal Cavity to Peritoneal Cavity with Synthetic Substitute, Percutaneous Endoscopic Approach
0W1G4JJ Bypass Peritoneal Cavity to Pelvic Cavity with Synthetic Substitute, Percutaneous Endoscopic Approach
0W1G4JY Bypass Peritoneal Cavity to Lower Vein with Synthetic Substitute, Percutaneous Endoscopic Approach
♀ **0W1J0J4** Bypass Pelvic Cavity to Cutaneous with Synthetic Substitute, Open Approach
♀ **0W1J0J9** Bypass Pelvic Cavity to Right Pleural Cavity with Synthetic Substitute, Open Approach
♀ **0W1J0JB** Bypass Pelvic Cavity to Left Pleural Cavity with Synthetic Substitute, Open Approach
♀ **0W1J0JG** Bypass Pelvic Cavity to Peritoneal Cavity with Synthetic Substitute, Open Approach
♀ **0W1J0JJ** Bypass Pelvic Cavity to Pelvic Cavity with Synthetic Substitute, Open Approach
♀ **0W1J0JY** Bypass Pelvic Cavity to Lower Vein with Synthetic Substitute, Open Approach
♀ **0W1J3J4** Bypass Pelvic Cavity to Cutaneous with Synthetic Substitute, Percutaneous Approach
♀ **0W1J4J4** Bypass Pelvic Cavity to Cutaneous with Synthetic Substitute, Percutaneous Endoscopic Approach
♀ **0W1J4J9** Bypass Pelvic Cavity to Right Pleural Cavity with Synthetic Substitute, Percutaneous Endoscopic Approach
♀ **0W1J4JB** Bypass Pelvic Cavity to Left Pleural Cavity with Synthetic Substitute, Percutaneous Endoscopic Approach
♀ **0W1J4JG** Bypass Pelvic Cavity to Peritoneal Cavity with Synthetic Substitute, Percutaneous Endoscopic Approach
♀ **0W1J4JJ** Bypass Pelvic Cavity to Pelvic Cavity with Synthetic Substitute, Percutaneous Endoscopic Approach
♀ **0W1J4JY** Bypass Pelvic Cavity to Lower Vein with Synthetic Substitute, Percutaneous Endoscopic Approach
This is a female-only service, however, it is not included in the female-only edit logic for MCE V30

0W2 – Anatomical Regions, General, Change

Review Coding Guideline B6.1c

0W20X0Z Change Drainage Device in Head, External Approach
0W20XYZ Change Other Device in Head, External Approach
0W21X0Z Change Drainage Device in Cranial Cavity, External Approach
0W21XYZ Change Other Device in Cranial Cavity, External Approach
0W22X0Z Change Drainage Device in Face, External Approach
0W22XYZ Change Other Device in Face, External Approach
0W24X0Z Change Drainage Device in Upper Jaw, External Approach
0W24XYZ Change Other Device in Upper Jaw, External Approach
0W25X0Z Change Drainage Device in Lower Jaw, External Approach
0W25XYZ Change Other Device in Lower Jaw, External Approach
0W26X0Z Change Drainage Device in Neck, External Approach
0W26XYZ Change Other Device in Neck, External Approach
0W28X0Z Change Drainage Device in Chest Wall, External Approach
0W28XYZ Change Other Device in Chest Wall, External Approach
0W29X0Z Change Drainage Device in Right Pleural Cavity, External Approach
0W29XYZ Change Other Device in Right Pleural Cavity, External Approach
0W2BX0Z Change Drainage Device in Left Pleural Cavity, External Approach
0W2BXYZ Change Other Device in Left Pleural Cavity, External Approach
0W2CX0Z Change Drainage Device in Mediastinum, External Approach
0W2CXYZ Change Other Device in Mediastinum, External Approach
0W2DX0Z Change Drainage Device in Pericardial Cavity, External Approach
0W2DXYZ Change Other Device in Pericardial Cavity, External Approach
0W2FX0Z Change Drainage Device in Abdominal Wall, External Approach
0W2FXYZ Change Other Device in Abdominal Wall, External Approach
0W2GX0Z Change Drainage Device in Peritoneal Cavity, External Approach
0W2GXYZ Change Other Device in Peritoneal Cavity, External Approach
0W2HX0Z Change Drainage Device in Retroperitoneum, External Approach
0W2HXYZ Change Other Device in Retroperitoneum, External Approach
0W2JX0Z Change Drainage Device in Pelvic Cavity, External Approach
0W2JXYZ Change Other Device in Pelvic Cavity, External Approach
0W2KX0Z Change Drainage Device in Upper Back, External Approach
0W2KXYZ Change Other Device in Upper Back, External Approach
0W2LX0Z Change Drainage Device in Lower Back, External Approach
0W2LXYZ Change Other Device in Lower Back, External Approach
0W2MX0Z Change Drainage Device in Male Perineum, External Approach
0W2MXYZ Change Other Device in Male Perineum, External Approach
0W2NX0Z Change Drainage Device in Female Perineum, External Approach
0W2NXYZ Change Other Device in Female Perineum, External Approach

0W3 – Anatomical Regions, General, Control

Review Coding Guideline B3.7

0W300ZZ Control Bleeding in Head, Open Approach
0W303ZZ Control Bleeding in Head, Percutaneous Approach
0W304ZZ Control Bleeding in Head, Percutaneous Endoscopic Approach
0W310ZZ Control Bleeding in Cranial Cavity, Open Approach
0W313ZZ Control Bleeding in Cranial Cavity, Percutaneous Approach
0W314ZZ Control Bleeding in Cranial Cavity, Percutaneous Endoscopic Approach
0W320ZZ Control Bleeding in Face, Open Approach
0W323ZZ Control Bleeding in Face, Percutaneous Approach
0W324ZZ Control Bleeding in Face, Percutaneous Endoscopic Approach
0W330ZZ Control Bleeding in Oral Cavity and Throat, Open Approach
0W333ZZ Control Bleeding in Oral Cavity and Throat, Percutaneous Approach
0W334ZZ Control Bleeding in Oral Cavity and Throat, Percutaneous Endoscopic Approach
0W337ZZ Control Bleeding in Oral Cavity and Throat, Via Natural or Artificial Opening
0W338ZZ Control Bleeding in Oral Cavity and Throat, Via Natural or Artificial Opening Endoscopic
0W33XZZ Control Bleeding in Oral Cavity and Throat, External Approach
0W340ZZ Control Bleeding in Upper Jaw, Open Approach
0W343ZZ Control Bleeding in Upper Jaw, Percutaneous Approach
0W344ZZ Control Bleeding in Upper Jaw, Percutaneous Endoscopic Approach
0W350ZZ Control Bleeding in Lower Jaw, Open Approach
0W353ZZ Control Bleeding in Lower Jaw, Percutaneous Approach
0W354ZZ Control Bleeding in Lower Jaw, Percutaneous Endoscopic Approach
0W360ZZ Control Bleeding in Neck, Open Approach
0W363ZZ Control Bleeding in Neck, Percutaneous Approach
0W364ZZ Control Bleeding in Neck, Percutaneous Endoscopic Approach
0W380ZZ Control Bleeding in Chest Wall, Open Approach
0W383ZZ Control Bleeding in Chest Wall, Percutaneous Approach
0W384ZZ Control Bleeding in Chest Wall, Percutaneous Endoscopic Approach
0W390ZZ Control Bleeding in Right Pleural Cavity, Open Approach
0W393ZZ Control Bleeding in Right Pleural Cavity, Percutaneous Approach
0W394ZZ Control Bleeding in Right Pleural Cavity, Percutaneous Endoscopic Approach
0W3B0ZZ Control Bleeding in Left Pleural Cavity, Open Approach
0W3B3ZZ Control Bleeding in Left Pleural Cavity, Percutaneous Approach
0W3B4ZZ Control Bleeding in Left Pleural Cavity, Percutaneous Endoscopic Approach
0W3C0ZZ Control Bleeding in Mediastinum, Open Approach
0W3C3ZZ Control Bleeding in Mediastinum, Percutaneous Approach
0W3C4ZZ Control Bleeding in Mediastinum, Percutaneous Endoscopic Approach
0W3D0ZZ Control Bleeding in Pericardial Cavity, Open Approach
0W3D3ZZ Control Bleeding in Pericardial Cavity, Percutaneous Approach
0W3D4ZZ Control Bleeding in Pericardial Cavity, Percutaneous Endoscopic Approach
0W3F0ZZ Control Bleeding in Abdominal Wall, Open Approach
0W3F3ZZ Control Bleeding in Abdominal Wall, Percutaneous Approach
0W3F4ZZ Control Bleeding in Abdominal Wall, Percutaneous Endoscopic Approach
0W3G0ZZ Control Bleeding in Peritoneal Cavity, Open Approach
0W3G3ZZ Control Bleeding in Peritoneal Cavity, Percutaneous Approach
0W3G4ZZ Control Bleeding in Peritoneal Cavity, Percutaneous Endoscopic Approach
0W3H0ZZ Control Bleeding in Retroperitoneum, Open Approach
0W3H3ZZ Control Bleeding in Retroperitoneum, Percutaneous Approach
0W3H4ZZ Control Bleeding in Retroperitoneum, Percutaneous Endoscopic Approach
0W3J0ZZ Control Bleeding in Pelvic Cavity, Open Approach
0W3J3ZZ Control Bleeding in Pelvic Cavity, Percutaneous Approach
0W3J4ZZ Control Bleeding in Pelvic Cavity, Percutaneous Endoscopic Approach
0W3K0ZZ Control Bleeding in Upper Back, Open Approach
0W3K3ZZ Control Bleeding in Upper Back, Percutaneous Approach
0W3K4ZZ Control Bleeding in Upper Back, Percutaneous Endoscopic Approach
0W3L0ZZ Control Bleeding in Lower Back, Open Approach
0W3L3ZZ Control Bleeding in Lower Back, Percutaneous Approach
0W3L4ZZ Control Bleeding in Lower Back, Percutaneous Endoscopic Approach
0W3M0ZZ Control Bleeding in Male Perineum, Open Approach
0W3M3ZZ Control Bleeding in Male Perineum, Percutaneous Approach
0W3M4ZZ Control Bleeding in Male Perineum, Percutaneous Endoscopic Approach
0W3N0ZZ Control Bleeding in Female Perineum, Open Approach
0W3N3ZZ Control Bleeding in Female Perineum, Percutaneous Approach
0W3N4ZZ Control Bleeding in Female Perineum, Percutaneous Endoscopic Approach
0W3P0ZZ Control Bleeding in Gastrointestinal Tract, Open Approach
0W3P3ZZ Control Bleeding in Gastrointestinal Tract, Percutaneous Approach
0W3P4ZZ Control Bleeding in Gastrointestinal Tract, Percutaneous Endoscopic Approach
0W3P7ZZ Control Bleeding in Gastrointestinal Tract, Via Natural or Artificial Opening
0W3P8ZZ Control Bleeding in Gastrointestinal Tract, Via Natural or Artificial Opening Endoscopic
0W3Q0ZZ Control Bleeding in Respiratory Tract, Open Approach
0W3Q3ZZ Control Bleeding in Respiratory Tract, Percutaneous Approach
0W3Q4ZZ Control Bleeding in Respiratory Tract, Percutaneous Endoscopic Approach
0W3Q7ZZ Control Bleeding in Respiratory Tract, Via Natural or Artificial Opening
0W3Q8ZZ Control Bleeding in Respiratory Tract, Via Natural or Artificial Opening Endoscopic
0W3R0ZZ Control Bleeding in Genitourinary Tract, Open Approach
0W3R3ZZ Control Bleeding in Genitourinary Tract, Percutaneous Approach
0W3R4ZZ Control Bleeding in Genitourinary Tract, Percutaneous Endoscopic Approach
0W3R7ZZ Control Bleeding in Genitourinary Tract, Via Natural or Artificial Opening
0W3R8ZZ Control Bleeding in Genitourinary Tract, Via Natural or Artificial Opening Endoscopic

0W4 – Anatomical Regions, General, Creation

♂ ▲ **0W4M070** Creation of Vagina in Male Perineum with Autologous Tissue Substitute, Open Approach
♂ ▲ **0W4M0J0** Creation of Vagina in Male Perineum with Synthetic Substitute, Open Approach
♂ ▲ **0W4M0K0** Creation of Vagina in Male Perineum with Nonautologous Tissue Substitute, Open Approach
♂ ▲ **0W4M0Z0** Creation of Vagina in Male Perineum, Open Approach
♀ ▲ **0W4N071** Creation of Penis in Female Perineum with Autologous Tissue Substitute, Open Approach
♀ ▲ **0W4N0J1** Creation of Penis in Female Perineum with Synthetic Substitute, Open Approach
♀ ▲ **0W4N0K1** Creation of Penis in Female Perineum with Nonautologous Tissue Substitute, Open Approach
♀ ▲ **0W4N0Z1** Creation of Penis in Female Perineum, Open Approach

0W8 – Anatomical Regions, General, Division

♀ **0W8NXZZ** Division of Female Perineum, External Approach

0W9 – Anatomical Regions, General, Drainage

Review Coding Guidelines B3.4a and B3.4b

Review Coding Guideline B6.2

0W9000Z Drainage of Head with Drainage Device, Open Approach
0W900ZX Drainage of Head, Open Approach, Diagnostic
0W900ZZ Drainage of Head, Open Approach
0W9030Z Drainage of Head with Drainage Device, Percutaneous Approach
0W903ZX Drainage of Head, Percutaneous Approach, Diagnostic
0W903ZZ Drainage of Head, Percutaneous Approach
0W9040Z Drainage of Head with Drainage Device, Percutaneous Endoscopic Approach
0W904ZX Drainage of Head, Percutaneous Endoscopic Approach, Diagnostic
0W904ZZ Drainage of Head, Percutaneous Endoscopic Approach
0W9100Z Drainage of Cranial Cavity with Drainage Device, Open Approach
0W910ZX Drainage of Cranial Cavity, Open Approach, Diagnostic
0W910ZZ Drainage of Cranial Cavity, Open Approach
0W9130Z Drainage of Cranial Cavity with Drainage Device, Percutaneous Approach
0W913ZX Drainage of Cranial Cavity, Percutaneous Approach, Diagnostic
0W913ZZ Drainage of Cranial Cavity, Percutaneous Approach
0W9140Z Drainage of Cranial Cavity with Drainage Device, Percutaneous Endoscopic Approach
0W914ZX Drainage of Cranial Cavity, Percutaneous Endoscopic Approach, Diagnostic
0W914ZZ Drainage of Cranial Cavity, Percutaneous Endoscopic Approach
0W9200Z Drainage of Face with Drainage Device, Open Approach
0W920ZX Drainage of Face, Open Approach, Diagnostic
0W920ZZ Drainage of Face, Open Approach
0W9230Z Drainage of Face with Drainage Device, Percutaneous Approach
0W923ZX Drainage of Face, Percutaneous Approach, Diagnostic
0W923ZZ Drainage of Face, Percutaneous Approach
0W9240Z Drainage of Face with Drainage Device, Percutaneous Endoscopic Approach
0W924ZX Drainage of Face, Percutaneous Endoscopic Approach, Diagnostic
0W924ZZ Drainage of Face, Percutaneous Endoscopic Approach
0W9300Z Drainage of Oral Cavity and Throat with Drainage Device, Open Approach
0W930ZX Drainage of Oral Cavity and Throat, Open Approach, Diagnostic
0W930ZZ Drainage of Oral Cavity and Throat, Open Approach
0W9330Z Drainage of Oral Cavity and Throat with Drainage Device, Percutaneous Approach
0W933ZX Drainage of Oral Cavity and Throat, Percutaneous Approach, Diagnostic
0W933ZZ Drainage of Oral Cavity and Throat, Percutaneous Approach
0W9340Z Drainage of Oral Cavity and Throat with Drainage Device, Percutaneous Endoscopic Approach
0W934ZX Drainage of Oral Cavity and Throat, Percutaneous Endoscopic Approach, Diagnostic
0W934ZZ Drainage of Oral Cavity and Throat, Percutaneous Endoscopic Approach
0W9400Z Drainage of Upper Jaw with Drainage Device, Open Approach
0W940ZX Drainage of Upper Jaw, Open Approach, Diagnostic
0W940ZZ Drainage of Upper Jaw, Open Approach
0W9430Z Drainage of Upper Jaw with Drainage Device, Percutaneous Approach
0W943ZX Drainage of Upper Jaw, Percutaneous Approach, Diagnostic
0W943ZZ Drainage of Upper Jaw, Percutaneous Approach
0W9440Z Drainage of Upper Jaw with Drainage Device, Percutaneous Endoscopic Approach
0W944ZX Drainage of Upper Jaw, Percutaneous Endoscopic Approach, Diagnostic
0W944ZZ Drainage of Upper Jaw, Percutaneous Endoscopic Approach
0W9500Z Drainage of Lower Jaw with Drainage Device, Open Approach
0W950ZX Drainage of Lower Jaw, Open Approach, Diagnostic
0W950ZZ Drainage of Lower Jaw, Open Approach
0W9530Z Drainage of Lower Jaw with Drainage Device, Percutaneous Approach
0W953ZX Drainage of Lower Jaw, Percutaneous Approach, Diagnostic
0W953ZZ Drainage of Lower Jaw, Percutaneous Approach
0W9540Z Drainage of Lower Jaw with Drainage Device, Percutaneous Endoscopic Approach
0W954ZX Drainage of Lower Jaw, Percutaneous Endoscopic Approach, Diagnostic
0W954ZZ Drainage of Lower Jaw, Percutaneous Endoscopic Approach
0W9600Z Drainage of Neck with Drainage Device, Open Approach
0W960ZX Drainage of Neck, Open Approach, Diagnostic
0W960ZZ Drainage of Neck, Open Approach
0W9630Z Drainage of Neck with Drainage Device, Percutaneous Approach
0W963ZX Drainage of Neck, Percutaneous Approach, Diagnostic
0W963ZZ Drainage of Neck, Percutaneous Approach
0W9640Z Drainage of Neck with Drainage Device, Percutaneous Endoscopic Approach
0W964ZX Drainage of Neck, Percutaneous Endoscopic Approach, Diagnostic
0W964ZZ Drainage of Neck, Percutaneous Endoscopic Approach
0W9800Z Drainage of Chest Wall with Drainage Device, Open Approach
0W980ZX Drainage of Chest Wall, Open Approach, Diagnostic
0W980ZZ Drainage of Chest Wall, Open Approach
0W9830Z Drainage of Chest Wall with Drainage Device, Percutaneous Approach
0W983ZX Drainage of Chest Wall, Percutaneous Approach, Diagnostic
0W983ZZ Drainage of Chest Wall, Percutaneous Approach
0W9840Z Drainage of Chest Wall with Drainage Device, Percutaneous Endoscopic Approach
0W984ZX Drainage of Chest Wall, Percutaneous Endoscopic Approach, Diagnostic
0W984ZZ Drainage of Chest Wall, Percutaneous Endoscopic Approach
0W9900Z Drainage of Right Pleural Cavity with Drainage Device, Open Approach
0W990ZX Drainage of Right Pleural Cavity, Open Approach, Diagnostic
0W990ZZ Drainage of Right Pleural Cavity, Open Approach
0W9930Z Drainage of Right Pleural Cavity with Drainage Device, Percutaneous Approach
0W993ZX Drainage of Right Pleural Cavity, Percutaneous Approach, Diagnostic
0W993ZZ Drainage of Right Pleural Cavity, Percutaneous Approach
0W9940Z Drainage of Right Pleural Cavity with Drainage Device, Percutaneous Endoscopic Approach
0W994ZX Drainage of Right Pleural Cavity, Percutaneous Endoscopic Approach, Diagnostic
0W994ZZ Drainage of Right Pleural Cavity, Percutaneous Endoscopic Approach
0W9B00Z Drainage of Left Pleural Cavity with Drainage Device, Open Approach
0W9B0ZX Drainage of Left Pleural Cavity, Open Approach, Diagnostic
0W9B0ZZ Drainage of Left Pleural Cavity, Open Approach
0W9B30Z Drainage of Left Pleural Cavity with Drainage Device, Percutaneous Approach
0W9B3ZX Drainage of Left Pleural Cavity, Percutaneous Approach, Diagnostic
0W9B3ZZ Drainage of Left Pleural Cavity, Percutaneous Approach
0W9B40Z Drainage of Left Pleural Cavity with Drainage Device, Percutaneous Endoscopic Approach
0W9B4ZX Drainage of Left Pleural Cavity, Percutaneous Endoscopic Approach, Diagnostic
0W9B4ZZ Drainage of Left Pleural Cavity, Percutaneous Endoscopic Approach
0W9C00Z Drainage of Mediastinum with Drainage Device, Open Approach
0W9C0ZX Drainage of Mediastinum, Open Approach, Diagnostic
0W9C0ZZ Drainage of Mediastinum, Open Approach
0W9C30Z Drainage of Mediastinum with Drainage Device, Percutaneous Approach
0W9C3ZX Drainage of Mediastinum, Percutaneous Approach, Diagnostic
0W9C3ZZ Drainage of Mediastinum, Percutaneous Approach
0W9C40Z Drainage of Mediastinum with Drainage Device, Percutaneous Endoscopic Approach
0W9C4ZX Drainage of Mediastinum, Percutaneous Endoscopic Approach, Diagnostic
0W9C4ZZ Drainage of Mediastinum, Percutaneous Endoscopic Approach
0W9D00Z Drainage of Pericardial Cavity with Drainage Device, Open Approach
0W9D0ZX Drainage of Pericardial Cavity, Open Approach, Diagnostic
0W9D0ZZ Drainage of Pericardial Cavity, Open Approach
0W9D30Z Drainage of Pericardial Cavity with Drainage Device, Percutaneous Approach
0W9D3ZX Drainage of Pericardial Cavity, Percutaneous Approach, Diagnostic
0W9D3ZZ Drainage of Pericardial Cavity, Percutaneous Approach
0W9D40Z Drainage of Pericardial Cavity with Drainage Device, Percutaneous Endoscopic Approach

0W9D4ZX Drainage of Pericardial Cavity, Percutaneous Endoscopic Approach, Diagnostic
0W9D4ZZ Drainage of Pericardial Cavity, Percutaneous Endoscopic Approach
0W9F00Z Drainage of Abdominal Wall with Drainage Device, Open Approach
0W9F0ZX Drainage of Abdominal Wall, Open Approach, Diagnostic
0W9F0ZZ Drainage of Abdominal Wall, Open Approach
0W9F30Z Drainage of Abdominal Wall with Drainage Device, Percutaneous Approach
0W9F3ZX Drainage of Abdominal Wall, Percutaneous Approach, Diagnostic
0W9F3ZZ Drainage of Abdominal Wall, Percutaneous Approach
0W9F40Z Drainage of Abdominal Wall with Drainage Device, Percutaneous Endoscopic Approach
0W9F4ZX Drainage of Abdominal Wall, Percutaneous Endoscopic Approach, Diagnostic
0W9F4ZZ Drainage of Abdominal Wall, Percutaneous Endoscopic Approach
0W9G00Z Drainage of Peritoneal Cavity with Drainage Device, Open Approach
0W9G0ZX Drainage of Peritoneal Cavity, Open Approach, Diagnostic
0W9G0ZZ Drainage of Peritoneal Cavity, Open Approach
0W9G30Z Drainage of Peritoneal Cavity with Drainage Device, Percutaneous Approach
0W9G3ZX Drainage of Peritoneal Cavity, Percutaneous Approach, Diagnostic
0W9G3ZZ Drainage of Peritoneal Cavity, Percutaneous Approach
0W9G40Z Drainage of Peritoneal Cavity with Drainage Device, Percutaneous Endoscopic Approach
0W9G4ZX Drainage of Peritoneal Cavity, Percutaneous Endoscopic Approach, Diagnostic
0W9G4ZZ Drainage of Peritoneal Cavity, Percutaneous Endoscopic Approach
0W9H00Z Drainage of Retroperitoneum with Drainage Device, Open Approach
0W9H0ZX Drainage of Retroperitoneum, Open Approach, Diagnostic
0W9H0ZZ Drainage of Retroperitoneum, Open Approach
0W9H30Z Drainage of Retroperitoneum with Drainage Device, Percutaneous Approach
0W9H3ZX Drainage of Retroperitoneum, Percutaneous Approach, Diagnostic
0W9H3ZZ Drainage of Retroperitoneum, Percutaneous Approach
0W9H40Z Drainage of Retroperitoneum with Drainage Device, Percutaneous Endoscopic Approach
0W9H4ZX Drainage of Retroperitoneum, Percutaneous Endoscopic Approach, Diagnostic
0W9H4ZZ Drainage of Retroperitoneum, Percutaneous Endoscopic Approach
0W9J00Z Drainage of Pelvic Cavity with Drainage Device, Open Approach
0W9J0ZX Drainage of Pelvic Cavity, Open Approach, Diagnostic
0W9J0ZZ Drainage of Pelvic Cavity, Open Approach
0W9J30Z Drainage of Pelvic Cavity with Drainage Device, Percutaneous Approach
0W9J3ZX Drainage of Pelvic Cavity, Percutaneous Approach, Diagnostic
0W9J3ZZ Drainage of Pelvic Cavity, Percutaneous Approach
0W9J40Z Drainage of Pelvic Cavity with Drainage Device, Percutaneous Endoscopic Approach
0W9J4ZX Drainage of Pelvic Cavity, Percutaneous Endoscopic Approach, Diagnostic
0W9J4ZZ Drainage of Pelvic Cavity, Percutaneous Endoscopic Approach
0W9K00Z Drainage of Upper Back with Drainage Device, Open Approach
0W9K0ZX Drainage of Upper Back, Open Approach, Diagnostic
0W9K0ZZ Drainage of Upper Back, Open Approach
0W9K30Z Drainage of Upper Back with Drainage Device, Percutaneous Approach
0W9K3ZX Drainage of Upper Back, Percutaneous Approach, Diagnostic
0W9K3ZZ Drainage of Upper Back, Percutaneous Approach
0W9K40Z Drainage of Upper Back with Drainage Device, Percutaneous Endoscopic Approach
0W9K4ZX Drainage of Upper Back, Percutaneous Endoscopic Approach, Diagnostic
0W9K4ZZ Drainage of Upper Back, Percutaneous Endoscopic Approach
0W9L00Z Drainage of Lower Back with Drainage Device, Open Approach
0W9L0ZX Drainage of Lower Back, Open Approach, Diagnostic
0W9L0ZZ Drainage of Lower Back, Open Approach
0W9L30Z Drainage of Lower Back with Drainage Device, Percutaneous Approach
0W9L3ZX Drainage of Lower Back, Percutaneous Approach, Diagnostic
0W9L3ZZ Drainage of Lower Back, Percutaneous Approach
0W9L40Z Drainage of Lower Back with Drainage Device, Percutaneous Endoscopic Approach
0W9L4ZX Drainage of Lower Back, Percutaneous Endoscopic Approach, Diagnostic
0W9L4ZZ Drainage of Lower Back, Percutaneous Endoscopic Approach
♂ **0W9M00Z** Drainage of Male Perineum with Drainage Device, Open Approach
♂ **0W9M0ZX** Drainage of Male Perineum, Open Approach, Diagnostic
♂ **0W9M0ZZ** Drainage of Male Perineum, Open Approach
♂ **0W9M30Z** Drainage of Male Perineum with Drainage Device, Percutaneous Approach
♂ **0W9M3ZX** Drainage of Male Perineum, Percutaneous Approach, Diagnostic
♂ **0W9M3ZZ** Drainage of Male Perineum, Percutaneous Approach
♂ **0W9M40Z** Drainage of Male Perineum with Drainage Device, Percutaneous Endoscopic Approach
♂ **0W9M4ZX** Drainage of Male Perineum, Percutaneous Endoscopic Approach, Diagnostic
♂ **0W9M4ZZ** Drainage of Male Perineum, Percutaneous Endoscopic Approach
♀ **0W9N00Z** Drainage of Female Perineum with Drainage Device, Open Approach
♀ **0W9N0ZX** Drainage of Female Perineum, Open Approach, Diagnostic
♀ **0W9N0ZZ** Drainage of Female Perineum, Open Approach
♀ **0W9N30Z** Drainage of Female Perineum with Drainage Device, Percutaneous Approach
♀ **0W9N3ZX** Drainage of Female Perineum, Percutaneous Approach, Diagnostic
♀ **0W9N3ZZ** Drainage of Female Perineum, Percutaneous Approach
♀ **0W9N40Z** Drainage of Female Perineum with Drainage Device, Percutaneous Endoscopic Approach
♀ **0W9N4ZX** Drainage of Female Perineum, Percutaneous Endoscopic Approach, Diagnostic
This is a female-only service, however, it is not included in the female-only edit logic for MCE V30
♀ **0W9N4ZZ** Drainage of Female Perineum, Percutaneous Endoscopic Approach

0WB – Anatomical Regions, General, Excision

Review Coding Guidelines B3.4a and B3.4b

0WB00ZX Excision of Head, Open Approach, Diagnostic
0WB00ZZ Excision of Head, Open Approach
0WB03ZX Excision of Head, Percutaneous Approach, Diagnostic
0WB03ZZ Excision of Head, Percutaneous Approach
0WB04ZX Excision of Head, Percutaneous Endoscopic Approach, Diagnostic
0WB04ZZ Excision of Head, Percutaneous Endoscopic Approach
0WB0XZX Excision of Head, External Approach, Diagnostic
0WB0XZZ Excision of Head, External Approach
0WB20ZX Excision of Face, Open Approach, Diagnostic
0WB20ZZ Excision of Face, Open Approach
0WB23ZX Excision of Face, Percutaneous Approach, Diagnostic
0WB23ZZ Excision of Face, Percutaneous Approach
0WB24ZX Excision of Face, Percutaneous Endoscopic Approach, Diagnostic
0WB24ZZ Excision of Face, Percutaneous Endoscopic Approach
0WB2XZX Excision of Face, External Approach, Diagnostic
0WB2XZZ Excision of Face, External Approach
0WB40ZX Excision of Upper Jaw, Open Approach, Diagnostic
0WB40ZZ Excision of Upper Jaw, Open Approach
0WB43ZX Excision of Upper Jaw, Percutaneous Approach, Diagnostic
0WB43ZZ Excision of Upper Jaw, Percutaneous Approach
0WB44ZX Excision of Upper Jaw, Percutaneous Endoscopic Approach, Diagnostic
0WB44ZZ Excision of Upper Jaw, Percutaneous Endoscopic Approach
0WB4XZX Excision of Upper Jaw, External Approach, Diagnostic
0WB4XZZ Excision of Upper Jaw, External Approach
0WB50ZX Excision of Lower Jaw, Open Approach, Diagnostic
0WB50ZZ Excision of Lower Jaw, Open Approach
0WB53ZX Excision of Lower Jaw, Percutaneous Approach, Diagnostic
0WB53ZZ Excision of Lower Jaw, Percutaneous Approach
0WB54ZX Excision of Lower Jaw, Percutaneous Endoscopic Approach, Diagnostic

0WB54ZZ Excision of Lower Jaw, Percutaneous Endoscopic Approach
0WB5XZX Excision of Lower Jaw, External Approach, Diagnostic
0WB5XZZ Excision of Lower Jaw, External Approach
0WB60ZX Excision of Neck, Open Approach, Diagnostic
0WB60ZZ Excision of Neck, Open Approach
0WB63ZX Excision of Neck, Percutaneous Approach, Diagnostic
0WB63ZZ Excision of Neck, Percutaneous Approach
0WB64ZX Excision of Neck, Percutaneous Endoscopic Approach, Diagnostic
0WB64ZZ Excision of Neck, Percutaneous Endoscopic Approach
0WB6XZ2 Excision of Neck, Stoma, External Approach
0WB6XZX Excision of Neck, External Approach, Diagnostic
0WB6XZZ Excision of Neck, External Approach
0WB80ZX Excision of Chest Wall, Open Approach, Diagnostic
0WB80ZZ Excision of Chest Wall, Open Approach
0WB83ZX Excision of Chest Wall, Percutaneous Approach, Diagnostic
0WB83ZZ Excision of Chest Wall, Percutaneous Approach
0WB84ZX Excision of Chest Wall, Percutaneous Endoscopic Approach, Diagnostic
0WB84ZZ Excision of Chest Wall, Percutaneous Endoscopic Approach
0WB8XZX Excision of Chest Wall, External Approach, Diagnostic
0WB8XZZ Excision of Chest Wall, External Approach
0WBC0ZX Excision of Mediastinum, Open Approach, Diagnostic
0WBC0ZZ Excision of Mediastinum, Open Approach
0WBC3ZX Excision of Mediastinum, Percutaneous Approach, Diagnostic
0WBC3ZZ Excision of Mediastinum, Percutaneous Approach
0WBC4ZX Excision of Mediastinum, Percutaneous Endoscopic Approach, Diagnostic
0WBC4ZZ Excision of Mediastinum, Percutaneous Endoscopic Approach
0WBF0ZX Excision of Abdominal Wall, Open Approach, Diagnostic
0WBF0ZZ Excision of Abdominal Wall, Open Approach
0WBF3ZX Excision of Abdominal Wall, Percutaneous Approach, Diagnostic
0WBF3ZZ Excision of Abdominal Wall, Percutaneous Approach
0WBF4ZX Excision of Abdominal Wall, Percutaneous Endoscopic Approach, Diagnostic
0WBF4ZZ Excision of Abdominal Wall, Percutaneous Endoscopic Approach
0WBFXZ2 Excision of Abdominal Wall, Stoma, External Approach
0WBFXZX Excision of Abdominal Wall, External Approach, Diagnostic
0WBFXZZ Excision of Abdominal Wall, External Approach
0WBH0ZX Excision of Retroperitoneum, Open Approach, Diagnostic
0WBH0ZZ Excision of Retroperitoneum, Open Approach
0WBH3ZX Excision of Retroperitoneum, Percutaneous Approach, Diagnostic
0WBH3ZZ Excision of Retroperitoneum, Percutaneous Approach
0WBH4ZX Excision of Retroperitoneum, Percutaneous Endoscopic Approach, Diagnostic
0WBH4ZZ Excision of Retroperitoneum, Percutaneous Endoscopic Approach
0WBK0ZX Excision of Upper Back, Open Approach, Diagnostic
0WBK0ZZ Excision of Upper Back, Open Approach
0WBK3ZX Excision of Upper Back, Percutaneous Approach, Diagnostic
0WBK3ZZ Excision of Upper Back, Percutaneous Approach
0WBK4ZX Excision of Upper Back, Percutaneous Endoscopic Approach, Diagnostic
0WBK4ZZ Excision of Upper Back, Percutaneous Endoscopic Approach
0WBKXZX Excision of Upper Back, External Approach, Diagnostic
0WBKXZZ Excision of Upper Back, External Approach
0WBL0ZX Excision of Lower Back, Open Approach, Diagnostic
0WBL0ZZ Excision of Lower Back, Open Approach
0WBL3ZX Excision of Lower Back, Percutaneous Approach, Diagnostic
0WBL3ZZ Excision of Lower Back, Percutaneous Approach
0WBL4ZX Excision of Lower Back, Percutaneous Endoscopic Approach, Diagnostic
0WBL4ZZ Excision of Lower Back, Percutaneous Endoscopic Approach
0WBLXZX Excision of Lower Back, External Approach, Diagnostic
0WBLXZZ Excision of Lower Back, External Approach
♂ 0WBM0ZX Excision of Male Perineum, Open Approach, Diagnostic
♂ 0WBM0ZZ Excision of Male Perineum, Open Approach
♂ 0WBM3ZX Excision of Male Perineum, Percutaneous Approach, Diagnostic
♂ 0WBM3ZZ Excision of Male Perineum, Percutaneous Approach
♂ 0WBM4ZX Excision of Male Perineum, Percutaneous Endoscopic Approach, Diagnostic
♂ 0WBM4ZZ Excision of Male Perineum, Percutaneous Endoscopic Approach
♂ 0WBMXZX Excision of Male Perineum, External Approach, Diagnostic
♂ 0WBMXZZ Excision of Male Perineum, External Approach
♀ 0WBN0ZX Excision of Female Perineum, Open Approach, Diagnostic
♀ 0WBN0ZZ Excision of Female Perineum, Open Approach
♀ 0WBN3ZX Excision of Female Perineum, Percutaneous Approach, Diagnostic
♀ 0WBN3ZZ Excision of Female Perineum, Percutaneous Approach
♀ 0WBN4ZX Excision of Female Perineum, Percutaneous Endoscopic Approach, Diagnostic
♀ 0WBN4ZZ Excision of Female Perineum, Percutaneous Endoscopic Approach
♀ 0WBNXZX Excision of Female Perineum, External Approach, Diagnostic
♀ 0WBNXZZ Excision of Female Perineum, External Approach
AHA CC: 4Q, 2013, 119-120

0WC – Anatomical Regions, General, Extirpation

0WC10ZZ Extirpation of Matter from Cranial Cavity, Open Approach
0WC13ZZ Extirpation of Matter from Cranial Cavity, Percutaneous Approach
0WC14ZZ Extirpation of Matter from Cranial Cavity, Percutaneous Endoscopic Approach
0WC1XZZ Extirpation of Matter from Cranial Cavity, External Approach
0WC30ZZ Extirpation of Matter from Oral Cavity and Throat, Open Approach
0WC33ZZ Extirpation of Matter from Oral Cavity and Throat, Percutaneous Approach
0WC34ZZ Extirpation of Matter from Oral Cavity and Throat, Percutaneous Endoscopic Approach
0WC3XZZ Extirpation of Matter from Oral Cavity and Throat, External Approach
0WC90ZZ Extirpation of Matter from Right Pleural Cavity, Open Approach
0WC93ZZ Extirpation of Matter from Right Pleural Cavity, Percutaneous Approach
0WC94ZZ Extirpation of Matter from Right Pleural Cavity, Percutaneous Endoscopic Approach
0WC9XZZ Extirpation of Matter from Right Pleural Cavity, External Approach
0WCB0ZZ Extirpation of Matter from Left Pleural Cavity, Open Approach
0WCB3ZZ Extirpation of Matter from Left Pleural Cavity, Percutaneous Approach
0WCB4ZZ Extirpation of Matter from Left Pleural Cavity, Percutaneous Endoscopic Approach
0WCBXZZ Extirpation of Matter from Left Pleural Cavity, External Approach
0WCC0ZZ Extirpation of Matter from Mediastinum, Open Approach
0WCC3ZZ Extirpation of Matter from Mediastinum, Percutaneous Approach
0WCC4ZZ Extirpation of Matter from Mediastinum, Percutaneous Endoscopic Approach
0WCCXZZ Extirpation of Matter from Mediastinum, External Approach
0WCD0ZZ Extirpation of Matter from Pericardial Cavity, Open Approach
0WCD3ZZ Extirpation of Matter from Pericardial Cavity, Percutaneous Approach
0WCD4ZZ Extirpation of Matter from Pericardial Cavity, Percutaneous Endoscopic Approach
0WCDXZZ Extirpation of Matter from Pericardial Cavity, External Approach
0WCG0ZZ Extirpation of Matter from Peritoneal Cavity, Open Approach
0WCG3ZZ Extirpation of Matter from Peritoneal Cavity, Percutaneous Approach
0WCG4ZZ Extirpation of Matter from Peritoneal Cavity, Percutaneous Endoscopic Approach
0WCGXZZ Extirpation of Matter from Peritoneal Cavity, External Approach
0WCJ0ZZ Extirpation of Matter from Pelvic Cavity, Open Approach
0WCJ3ZZ Extirpation of Matter from Pelvic Cavity, Percutaneous Approach
0WCJ4ZZ Extirpation of Matter from Pelvic Cavity, Percutaneous Endoscopic Approach
0WCJXZZ Extirpation of Matter from Pelvic Cavity, External Approach
0WCP0ZZ Extirpation of Matter from Gastrointestinal Tract, Open Approach
0WCP3ZZ Extirpation of Matter from Gastrointestinal Tract, Percutaneous Approach
0WCP4ZZ Extirpation of Matter from Gastrointestinal Tract, Percutaneous Endoscopic Approach
0WCP7ZZ Extirpation of Matter from Gastrointestinal Tract, Via Natural or Artificial Opening

0WCP8ZZ Extirpation of Matter from Gastrointestinal Tract, Via Natural or Artificial Opening Endoscopic

0WCPXZZ Extirpation of Matter from Gastrointestinal Tract, External Approach

0WCQ0ZZ Extirpation of Matter from Respiratory Tract, Open Approach

0WCQ3ZZ Extirpation of Matter from Respiratory Tract, Percutaneous Approach

0WCQ4ZZ Extirpation of Matter from Respiratory Tract, Percutaneous Endoscopic Approach

0WCQ7ZZ Extirpation of Matter from Respiratory Tract, Via Natural or Artificial Opening

0WCQ8ZZ Extirpation of Matter from Respiratory Tract, Via Natural or Artificial Opening Endoscopic

0WCQXZZ Extirpation of Matter from Respiratory Tract, External Approach

0WCR0ZZ Extirpation of Matter from Genitourinary Tract, Open Approach

0WCR3ZZ Extirpation of Matter from Genitourinary Tract, Percutaneous Approach

0WCR4ZZ Extirpation of Matter from Genitourinary Tract, Percutaneous Endoscopic Approach

0WCR7ZZ Extirpation of Matter from Genitourinary Tract, Via Natural or Artificial Opening

0WCR8ZZ Extirpation of Matter from Genitourinary Tract, Via Natural or Artificial Opening Endoscopic

0WCRXZZ Extirpation of Matter from Genitourinary Tract, External Approach

0WF – Anatomical Regions, General, Fragmentation

0WF10ZZ Fragmentation in Cranial Cavity, Open Approach

0WF13ZZ Fragmentation in Cranial Cavity, Percutaneous Approach

0WF14ZZ Fragmentation in Cranial Cavity, Percutaneous Endoscopic Approach

▲ **0WF1XZZ** Fragmentation in Cranial Cavity, External Approach

0WF30ZZ Fragmentation in Oral Cavity and Throat, Open Approach

0WF33ZZ Fragmentation in Oral Cavity and Throat, Percutaneous Approach

0WF34ZZ Fragmentation in Oral Cavity and Throat, Percutaneous Endoscopic Approach

▲ **0WF3XZZ** Fragmentation in Oral Cavity and Throat, External Approach

0WF90ZZ Fragmentation in Right Pleural Cavity, Open Approach

0WF93ZZ Fragmentation in Right Pleural Cavity, Percutaneous Approach

0WF94ZZ Fragmentation in Right Pleural Cavity, Percutaneous Endoscopic Approach

▲ **0WF9XZZ** Fragmentation in Right Pleural Cavity, External Approach

0WFB0ZZ Fragmentation in Left Pleural Cavity, Open Approach

0WFB3ZZ Fragmentation in Left Pleural Cavity, Percutaneous Approach

0WFB4ZZ Fragmentation in Left Pleural Cavity, Percutaneous Endoscopic Approach

▲ **0WFBXZZ** Fragmentation in Left Pleural Cavity, External Approach

0WFC0ZZ Fragmentation in Mediastinum, Open Approach

0WFC3ZZ Fragmentation in Mediastinum, Percutaneous Approach

0WFC4ZZ Fragmentation in Mediastinum, Percutaneous Endoscopic Approach

▲ **0WFCXZZ** Fragmentation in Mediastinum, External Approach

0WFD0ZZ Fragmentation in Pericardial Cavity, Open Approach

0WFD3ZZ Fragmentation in Pericardial Cavity, Percutaneous Approach

0WFD4ZZ Fragmentation in Pericardial Cavity, Percutaneous Endoscopic Approach

0WFDXZZ Fragmentation in Pericardial Cavity, External Approach

0WFG0ZZ Fragmentation in Peritoneal Cavity, Open Approach

0WFG3ZZ Fragmentation in Peritoneal Cavity, Percutaneous Approach

0WFG4ZZ Fragmentation in Peritoneal Cavity, Percutaneous Endoscopic Approach

▲ **0WFGXZZ** Fragmentation in Peritoneal Cavity, External Approach

0WFJ0ZZ Fragmentation in Pelvic Cavity, Open Approach

0WFJ3ZZ Fragmentation in Pelvic Cavity, Percutaneous Approach

0WFJ4ZZ Fragmentation in Pelvic Cavity, Percutaneous Endoscopic Approach

▲ **0WFJXZZ** Fragmentation in Pelvic Cavity, External Approach

0WFP0ZZ Fragmentation in Gastrointestinal Tract, Open Approach

0WFP3ZZ Fragmentation in Gastrointestinal Tract, Percutaneous Approach

0WFP4ZZ Fragmentation in Gastrointestinal Tract, Percutaneous Endoscopic Approach

0WFP7ZZ Fragmentation in Gastrointestinal Tract, Via Natural or Artificial Opening

0WFP8ZZ Fragmentation in Gastrointestinal Tract, Via Natural or Artificial Opening Endoscopic

▲ **0WFPXZZ** Fragmentation in Gastrointestinal Tract, External Approach

0WFQ0ZZ Fragmentation in Respiratory Tract, Open Approach

0WFQ3ZZ Fragmentation in Respiratory Tract, Percutaneous Approach

0WFQ4ZZ Fragmentation in Respiratory Tract, Percutaneous Endoscopic Approach

0WFQ7ZZ Fragmentation in Respiratory Tract, Via Natural or Artificial Opening

0WFQ8ZZ Fragmentation in Respiratory Tract, Via Natural or Artificial Opening Endoscopic

▲ **0WFQXZZ** Fragmentation in Respiratory Tract, External Approach

0WFR0ZZ Fragmentation in Genitourinary Tract, Open Approach

0WFR3ZZ Fragmentation in Genitourinary Tract, Percutaneous Approach

0WFR4ZZ Fragmentation in Genitourinary Tract, Percutaneous Endoscopic Approach

0WFR7ZZ Fragmentation in Genitourinary Tract, Via Natural or Artificial Opening

0WFR8ZZ Fragmentation in Genitourinary Tract, Via Natural or Artificial Opening Endoscopic

● **0WFRXZZ** Fragmentation in Genitourinary Tract, External Approach

0WH – Anatomical Regions, General, Insertion

0WH001Z Insertion of Radioactive Element into Head, Open Approach

● **0WH003Z** Insertion of Infusion Device into Head, Open Approach

● **0WH00YZ** Insertion of Other Device into Head, Open Approach

0WH031Z Insertion of Radioactive Element into Head, Percutaneous Approach

● **0WH033Z** Insertion of Infusion Device into Head, Percutaneous Approach

● **0WH03YZ** Insertion of Other Device into Head, Percutaneous Approach

0WH041Z Insertion of Radioactive Element into Head, Percutaneous Endoscopic Approach

● **0WH043Z** Insertion of Infusion Device into Head, Percutaneous Endoscopic Approach

● **0WH04YZ** Insertion of Other Device into Head, Percutaneous Endoscopic Approach

0WH101Z Insertion of Radioactive Element into Cranial Cavity, Open Approach

0WH103Z Insertion of Infusion Device into Cranial Cavity, Open Approach

0WH10YZ Insertion of Other Device into Cranial Cavity, Open Approach

0WH131Z Insertion of Radioactive Element into Cranial Cavity, Percutaneous Approach

0WH133Z Insertion of Infusion Device into Cranial Cavity, Percutaneous Approach

0WH13YZ Insertion of Other Device into Cranial Cavity, Percutaneous Approach

0WH141Z Insertion of Radioactive Element into Cranial Cavity, Percutaneous Endoscopic Approach

0WH143Z Insertion of Infusion Device into Cranial Cavity, Percutaneous Endoscopic Approach

0WH14YZ Insertion of Other Device into Cranial Cavity, Percutaneous Endoscopic Approach

0WH201Z Insertion of Radioactive Element into Face, Open Approach

● **0WH203Z** Insertion of Infusion Device into Face, Open Approach

● **0WH20YZ** Insertion of Other Device into Face, Open Approach

0WH231Z Insertion of Radioactive Element into Face, Percutaneous Approach

● **0WH233Z** Insertion of Infusion Device into Face, Percutaneous Approach

● **0WH23YZ** Insertion of Other Device into Face, Percutaneous Approach

0WH241Z Insertion of Radioactive Element into Face, Percutaneous Endoscopic Approach

● **0WH243Z** Insertion of Infusion Device into Face, Percutaneous Endoscopic Approach

● **0WH24YZ** Insertion of Other Device into Face, Percutaneous Endoscopic Approach

0WH301Z Insertion of Radioactive Element into Oral Cavity and Throat, Open Approach

0WH303Z Insertion of Infusion Device into Oral Cavity and Throat, Open Approach

0WH30YZ Insertion of Other Device into Oral Cavity and Throat, Open Approach

0WH331Z Insertion of Radioactive Element into Oral Cavity and Throat, Percutaneous Approach

0WH333Z Insertion of Infusion Device into Oral Cavity and Throat, Percutaneous Approach

0WH33YZ Insertion of Other Device into Oral Cavity and Throat, Percutaneous Approach

0WH341Z Insertion of Radioactive Element into Oral Cavity and Throat, Percutaneous Endoscopic Approach
0WH343Z Insertion of Infusion Device into Oral Cavity and Throat, Percutaneous Endoscopic Approach
0WH34YZ Insertion of Other Device into Oral Cavity and Throat, Percutaneous Endoscopic Approach
0WH401Z Insertion of Radioactive Element into Upper Jaw, Open Approach
●**0WH403Z** Insertion of Infusion Device into Upper Jaw, Open Approach
●**0WH40YZ** Insertion of Other Device into Upper Jaw, Open Approach
0WH431Z Insertion of Radioactive Element into Upper Jaw, Percutaneous Approach
●**0WH433Z** Insertion of Infusion Device into Upper Jaw, Percutaneous Approach
●**0WH43YZ** Insertion of Other Device into Upper Jaw, Percutaneous Approach
0WH441Z Insertion of Radioactive Element into Upper Jaw, Percutaneous Endoscopic Approach
●**0WH443Z** Insertion of Infusion Device into Upper Jaw, Percutaneous Endoscopic Approach
●**0WH44YZ** Insertion of Other Device into Upper Jaw, Percutaneous Endoscopic Approach
0WH501Z Insertion of Radioactive Element into Lower Jaw, Open Approach
●**0WH503Z** Insertion of Infusion Device into Lower Jaw, Open Approach
●**0WH50YZ** Insertion of Other Device into Lower Jaw, Open Approach
0WH531Z Insertion of Radioactive Element into Lower Jaw, Percutaneous Approach
●**0WH533Z** Insertion of Infusion Device into Lower Jaw, Percutaneous Approach
●**0WH53YZ** Insertion of Other Device into Lower Jaw, Percutaneous Approach
0WH541Z Insertion of Radioactive Element into Lower Jaw, Percutaneous Endoscopic Approach
●**0WH543Z** Insertion of Infusion Device into Lower Jaw, Percutaneous Endoscopic Approach
●**0WH54YZ** Insertion of Other Device into Lower Jaw, Percutaneous Endoscopic Approach
0WH601Z Insertion of Radioactive Element into Neck, Open Approach
●**0WH603Z** Insertion of Infusion Device into Neck, Open Approach
●**0WH60YZ** Insertion of Other Device into Neck, Open Approach
0WH631Z Insertion of Radioactive Element into Neck, Percutaneous Approach
●**0WH633Z** Insertion of Infusion Device into Neck, Percutaneous Approach
●**0WH63YZ** Insertion of Other Device into Neck, Percutaneous Approach
0WH641Z Insertion of Radioactive Element into Neck, Percutaneous Endoscopic Approach
●**0WH643Z** Insertion of Infusion Device into Neck, Percutaneous Endoscopic Approach
●**0WH64YZ** Insertion of Other Device into Neck, Percutaneous Endoscopic Approach
0WH801Z Insertion of Radioactive Element into Chest Wall, Open Approach
0WH803Z Insertion of Infusion Device into Chest Wall, Open Approach
0WH80YZ Insertion of Other Device into Chest Wall, Open Approach
0WH831Z Insertion of Radioactive Element into Chest Wall, Percutaneous Approach
0WH833Z Insertion of Infusion Device into Chest Wall, Percutaneous Approach
0WH83YZ Insertion of Other Device into Chest Wall, Percutaneous Approach
0WH841Z Insertion of Radioactive Element into Chest Wall, Percutaneous Endoscopic Approach
0WH843Z Insertion of Infusion Device into Chest Wall, Percutaneous Endoscopic Approach
0WH84YZ Insertion of Other Device into Chest Wall, Percutaneous Endoscopic Approach
0WH901Z Insertion of Radioactive Element into Right Pleural Cavity, Open Approach
0WH903Z Insertion of Infusion Device into Right Pleural Cavity, Open Approach
0WH90YZ Insertion of Other Device into Right Pleural Cavity, Open Approach
0WH931Z Insertion of Radioactive Element into Right Pleural Cavity, Percutaneous Approach
0WH933Z Insertion of Infusion Device into Right Pleural Cavity, Percutaneous Approach
0WH93YZ Insertion of Other Device into Right Pleural Cavity, Percutaneous Approach
0WH941Z Insertion of Radioactive Element into Right Pleural Cavity, Percutaneous Endoscopic Approach
0WH943Z Insertion of Infusion Device into Right Pleural Cavity, Percutaneous Endoscopic Approach
0WH94YZ Insertion of Other Device into Right Pleural Cavity, Percutaneous Endoscopic Approach
0WHB01Z Insertion of Radioactive Element into Left Pleural Cavity, Open Approach
0WHB03Z Insertion of Infusion Device into Left Pleural Cavity, Open Approach
0WHB0YZ Insertion of Other Device into Left Pleural Cavity, Open Approach
0WHB31Z Insertion of Radioactive Element into Left Pleural Cavity, Percutaneous Approach
0WHB33Z Insertion of Infusion Device into Left Pleural Cavity, Percutaneous Approach
0WHB3YZ Insertion of Other Device into Left Pleural Cavity, Percutaneous Approach
0WHB41Z Insertion of Radioactive Element into Left Pleural Cavity, Percutaneous Endoscopic Approach
0WHB43Z Insertion of Infusion Device into Left Pleural Cavity, Percutaneous Endoscopic Approach
0WHB4YZ Insertion of Other Device into Left Pleural Cavity, Percutaneous Endoscopic Approach
0WHC01Z Insertion of Radioactive Element into Mediastinum, Open Approach
0WHC03Z Insertion of Infusion Device into Mediastinum, Open Approach
0WHC0YZ Insertion of Other Device into Mediastinum, Open Approach
0WHC31Z Insertion of Radioactive Element into Mediastinum, Percutaneous Approach
0WHC33Z Insertion of Infusion Device into Mediastinum, Percutaneous Approach
0WHC3YZ Insertion of Other Device into Mediastinum, Percutaneous Approach
0WHC41Z Insertion of Radioactive Element into Mediastinum, Percutaneous Endoscopic Approach
0WHC43Z Insertion of Infusion Device into Mediastinum, Percutaneous Endoscopic Approach
0WHC4YZ Insertion of Other Device into Mediastinum, Percutaneous Endoscopic Approach
0WHD01Z Insertion of Radioactive Element into Pericardial Cavity, Open Approach
0WHD03Z Insertion of Infusion Device into Pericardial Cavity, Open Approach
0WHD0YZ Insertion of Other Device into Pericardial Cavity, Open Approach
0WHD31Z Insertion of Radioactive Element into Pericardial Cavity, Percutaneous Approach
0WHD33Z Insertion of Infusion Device into Pericardial Cavity, Percutaneous Approach
0WHD3YZ Insertion of Other Device into Pericardial Cavity, Percutaneous Approach
0WHD41Z Insertion of Radioactive Element into Pericardial Cavity, Percutaneous Endoscopic Approach
0WHD43Z Insertion of Infusion Device into Pericardial Cavity, Percutaneous Endoscopic Approach
0WHD4YZ Insertion of Other Device into Pericardial Cavity, Percutaneous Endoscopic Approach
0WHF01Z Insertion of Radioactive Element into Abdominal Wall, Open Approach
0WHF03Z Insertion of Infusion Device into Abdominal Wall, Open Approach
0WHF0YZ Insertion of Other Device into Abdominal Wall, Open Approach
0WHF31Z Insertion of Radioactive Element into Abdominal Wall, Percutaneous Approach
0WHF33Z Insertion of Infusion Device into Abdominal Wall, Percutaneous Approach
0WHF3YZ Insertion of Other Device into Abdominal Wall, Percutaneous Approach
0WHF41Z Insertion of Radioactive Element into Abdominal Wall, Percutaneous Endoscopic Approach
0WHF43Z Insertion of Infusion Device into Abdominal Wall, Percutaneous Endoscopic Approach
0WHF4YZ Insertion of Other Device into Abdominal Wall, Percutaneous Endoscopic Approach
0WHG01Z Insertion of Radioactive Element into Peritoneal Cavity, Open Approach
0WHG03Z Insertion of Infusion Device into Peritoneal Cavity, Open Approach
0WHG0YZ Insertion of Other Device into Peritoneal Cavity, Open Approach
0WHG31Z Insertion of Radioactive Element into Peritoneal Cavity, Percutaneous Approach
0WHG33Z Insertion of Infusion Device into Peritoneal Cavity, Percutaneous Approach
0WHG3YZ Insertion of Other Device into Peritoneal Cavity, Percutaneous Approach
0WHG41Z Insertion of Radioactive Element into Peritoneal Cavity, Percutaneous Endoscopic Approach
0WHG43Z Insertion of Infusion Device into Peritoneal Cavity, Percutaneous Endoscopic Approach
0WHG4YZ Insertion of Other Device into Peritoneal Cavity, Percutaneous Endoscopic Approach
0WHH01Z Insertion of Radioactive Element into Retroperitoneum, Open Approach
0WHH03Z Insertion of Infusion Device into Retroperitoneum, Open Approach
0WHH0YZ Insertion of Other Device into Retroperitoneum, Open Approach
0WHH31Z Insertion of Radioactive Element into Retroperitoneum, Percutaneous Approach
0WHH33Z Insertion of Infusion Device into Retroperitoneum, Percutaneous Approach
0WHH3YZ Insertion of Other Device into Retroperitoneum, Percutaneous Approach
0WHH41Z Insertion of Radioactive Element into Retroperitoneum, Percutaneous Endoscopic Approach
0WHH43Z Insertion of Infusion Device into Retroperitoneum, Percutaneous Endoscopic Approach
0WHH4YZ Insertion of Other Device into Retroperitoneum, Percutaneous Endoscopic Approach

0WHJ01Z Insertion of Radioactive Element into Pelvic Cavity, Open Approach
0WHJ03Z Insertion of Infusion Device into Pelvic Cavity, Open Approach
0WHJ0YZ Insertion of Other Device into Pelvic Cavity, Open Approach
0WHJ31Z Insertion of Radioactive Element into Pelvic Cavity, Percutaneous Approach
0WHJ33Z Insertion of Infusion Device into Pelvic Cavity, Percutaneous Approach
0WHJ3YZ Insertion of Other Device into Pelvic Cavity, Percutaneous Approach
0WHJ41Z Insertion of Radioactive Element into Pelvic Cavity, Percutaneous Endoscopic Approach
0WHJ43Z Insertion of Infusion Device into Pelvic Cavity, Percutaneous Endoscopic Approach
0WHJ4YZ Insertion of Other Device into Pelvic Cavity, Percutaneous Endoscopic Approach
0WHK01Z Insertion of Radioactive Element into Upper Back, Open Approach
● **0WHK03Z** Insertion of Infusion Device into Upper Back, Open Approach
● **0WHK0YZ** Insertion of Other Device into Upper Back, Open Approach
0WHK31Z Insertion of Radioactive Element into Upper Back, Percutaneous Approach
● **0WHK33Z** Insertion of Infusion Device into Upper Back, Percutaneous Approach
● **0WHK3YZ** Insertion of Other Device into Upper Back, Percutaneous Approach
0WHK41Z Insertion of Radioactive Element into Upper Back, Percutaneous Endoscopic Approach
● **0WHK43Z** Insertion of Infusion Device into Upper Back, Percutaneous Endoscopic Approach
● **0WHK4YZ** Insertion of Other Device into Upper Back, Percutaneous Endoscopic Approach
0WHL01Z Insertion of Radioactive Element into Lower Back, Open Approach
● **0WHL03Z** Insertion of Infusion Device into Lower Back, Open Approach
● **0WHL0YZ** Insertion of Other Device into Lower Back, Open Approach
0WHL31Z Insertion of Radioactive Element into Lower Back, Percutaneous Approach
● **0WHL33Z** Insertion of Infusion Device into Lower Back, Percutaneous Approach
● **0WHL3YZ** Insertion of Other Device into Lower Back, Percutaneous Approach
0WHL41Z Insertion of Radioactive Element into Lower Back, Percutaneous Endoscopic Approach
● **0WHL43Z** Insertion of Infusion Device into Lower Back, Percutaneous Endoscopic Approach
● **0WHL4YZ** Insertion of Other Device into Lower Back, Percutaneous Endoscopic Approach
♂ **0WHM01Z** Insertion of Radioactive Element into Male Perineum, Open Approach
This is a male-only service, however, it is not included in the male-only edit logic for MCE V30
♂● **0WHM03Z** Insertion of Infusion Device into Male Perineum, Open Approach
This is a male-only service, however, it is not included in the male-only edit logic for MCE V30
♂● **0WHM0YZ** Insertion of Other Device into Male Perineum, Open Approach
This is a male-only service, however, it is not included in the male-only edit logic for MCE V30
♂ **0WHM31Z** Insertion of Radioactive Element into Male Perineum, Percutaneous Approach
This is a male-only service, however, it is not included in the male-only edit logic for MCE V30
♂● **0WHM33Z** Insertion of Infusion Device into Male Perineum, Percutaneous Approach
This is a male-only service, however, it is not included in the male-only edit logic for MCE V30
♂● **0WHM3YZ** Insertion of Other Device into Male Perineum, Percutaneous Approach
This is a male-only service, however, it is not included in the male-only edit logic for MCE V30
♂ **0WHM41Z** Insertion of Radioactive Element into Male Perineum, Percutaneous Endoscopic Approach
This is a male-only service, however, it is not included in the male-only edit logic for MCE V30
♂● **0WHM43Z** Insertion of Infusion Device into Male Perineum, Percutaneous Endoscopic Approach
This is a male-only service, however, it is not included in the male-only edit logic for MCE V30
♂● **0WHM4YZ** Insertion of Other Device into Male Perineum, Percutaneous Endoscopic Approach
This is a male-only service, however, it is not included in the male-only edit logic for MCE V30
♀ **0WHN01Z** Insertion of Radioactive Element into Female Perineum, Open Approach
This is a female-only service, however, it is not included in the female-only edit logic for MCE V30
♀ **0WHN03Z** Insertion of Infusion Device into Female Perineum, Open Approach
♀ **0WHN0YZ** Insertion of Other Device into Female Perineum, Open Approach
♀ **0WHN31Z** Insertion of Radioactive Element into Female Perineum, Percutaneous Approach
This is a female-only service, however, it is not included in the female-only edit logic for MCE V30
♀ **0WHN33Z** Insertion of Infusion Device into Female Perineum, Percutaneous Approach
♀ **0WHN3YZ** Insertion of Other Device into Female Perineum, Percutaneous Approach
♀ **0WHN41Z** Insertion of Radioactive Element into Female Perineum, Percutaneous Endoscopic Approach
This is a female-only service, however, it is not included in the female-only edit logic for MCE V30
♀ **0WHN43Z** Insertion of Infusion Device into Female Perineum, Percutaneous Endoscopic Approach
♀ **0WHN4YZ** Insertion of Other Device into Female Perineum, Percutaneous Endoscopic Approach
0WHP01Z Insertion of Radioactive Element into Gastrointestinal Tract, Open Approach
0WHP03Z Insertion of Infusion Device into Gastrointestinal Tract, Open Approach
0WHP0YZ Insertion of Other Device into Gastrointestinal Tract, Open Approach
0WHP31Z Insertion of Radioactive Element into Gastrointestinal Tract, Percutaneous Approach
0WHP33Z Insertion of Infusion Device into Gastrointestinal Tract, Percutaneous Approach
0WHP3YZ Insertion of Other Device into Gastrointestinal Tract, Percutaneous Approach
0WHP41Z Insertion of Radioactive Element into Gastrointestinal Tract, Percutaneous Endoscopic Approach
0WHP43Z Insertion of Infusion Device into Gastrointestinal Tract, Percutaneous Endoscopic Approach
0WHP4YZ Insertion of Other Device into Gastrointestinal Tract, Percutaneous Endoscopic Approach
0WHP71Z Insertion of Radioactive Element into Gastrointestinal Tract, Via Natural or Artificial Opening
0WHP73Z Insertion of Infusion Device into Gastrointestinal Tract, Via Natural or Artificial Opening
0WHP7YZ Insertion of Other Device into Gastrointestinal Tract, Via Natural or Artificial Opening
0WHP81Z Insertion of Radioactive Element into Gastrointestinal Tract, Via Natural or Artificial Opening Endoscopic
0WHP83Z Insertion of Infusion Device into Gastrointestinal Tract, Via Natural or Artificial Opening Endoscopic
0WHP8YZ Insertion of Other Device into Gastrointestinal Tract, Via Natural or Artificial Opening Endoscopic
0WHQ01Z Insertion of Radioactive Element into Respiratory Tract, Open Approach
0WHQ03Z Insertion of Infusion Device into Respiratory Tract, Open Approach
0WHQ0YZ Insertion of Other Device into Respiratory Tract, Open Approach
0WHQ31Z Insertion of Radioactive Element into Respiratory Tract, Percutaneous Approach
0WHQ33Z Insertion of Infusion Device into Respiratory Tract, Percutaneous Approach
0WHQ3YZ Insertion of Other Device into Respiratory Tract, Percutaneous Approach
0WHQ41Z Insertion of Radioactive Element into Respiratory Tract, Percutaneous Endoscopic Approach
0WHQ43Z Insertion of Infusion Device into Respiratory Tract, Percutaneous Endoscopic Approach
0WHQ4YZ Insertion of Other Device into Respiratory Tract, Percutaneous Endoscopic Approach
0WHQ71Z Insertion of Radioactive Element into Respiratory Tract, Via Natural or Artificial Opening
0WHQ73Z Insertion of Infusion Device into Respiratory Tract, Via Natural or Artificial Opening
0WHQ7YZ Insertion of Other Device into Respiratory Tract, Via Natural or Artificial Opening
0WHQ81Z Insertion of Radioactive Element into Respiratory Tract, Via Natural or Artificial Opening Endoscopic
0WHQ83Z Insertion of Infusion Device into Respiratory Tract, Via Natural or Artificial Opening Endoscopic
0WHQ8YZ Insertion of Other Device into Respiratory Tract, Via Natural or Artificial Opening Endoscopic
0WHR01Z Insertion of Radioactive Element into Genitourinary Tract, Open Approach
0WHR03Z Insertion of Infusion Device into Genitourinary Tract, Open Approach
0WHR0YZ Insertion of Other Device into Genitourinary Tract, Open Approach
0WHR31Z Insertion of Radioactive Element into Genitourinary Tract, Percutaneous Approach
0WHR33Z Insertion of Infusion Device into Genitourinary Tract, Percutaneous Approach

0WHR3YZ Insertion of Other Device into Genitourinary Tract, Percutaneous Approach
0WHR41Z Insertion of Radioactive Element into Genitourinary Tract, Percutaneous Endoscopic Approach
0WHR43Z Insertion of Infusion Device into Genitourinary Tract, Percutaneous Endoscopic Approach
0WHR4YZ Insertion of Other Device into Genitourinary Tract, Percutaneous Endoscopic Approach
0WHR71Z Insertion of Radioactive Element into Genitourinary Tract, Via Natural or Artificial Opening
0WHR73Z Insertion of Infusion Device into Genitourinary Tract, Via Natural or Artificial Opening
0WHR7YZ Insertion of Other Device into Genitourinary Tract, Via Natural or Artificial Opening
0WHR81Z Insertion of Radioactive Element into Genitourinary Tract, Via Natural or Artificial Opening Endoscopic
0WHR83Z Insertion of Infusion Device into Genitourinary Tract, Via Natural or Artificial Opening Endoscopic
0WHR8YZ Insertion of Other Device into Genitourinary Tract, Via Natural or Artificial Opening Endoscopic

0WJ – Anatomical Regions, General, Inspection

Review Coding Guidelines B3.11a, B3.11b and B3.11c

●**0WJ00ZZ** Inspection of Head, Open Approach
0WJ03ZZ Inspection of Head, Percutaneous Approach
0WJ04ZZ Inspection of Head, Percutaneous Endoscopic Approach
0WJ0XZZ Inspection of Head, External Approach
0WJ10ZZ Inspection of Cranial Cavity, Open Approach
0WJ13ZZ Inspection of Cranial Cavity, Percutaneous Approach
0WJ14ZZ Inspection of Cranial Cavity, Percutaneous Endoscopic Approach
●**0WJ20ZZ** Inspection of Face, Open Approach
0WJ23ZZ Inspection of Face, Percutaneous Approach
0WJ24ZZ Inspection of Face, Percutaneous Endoscopic Approach
0WJ2XZZ Inspection of Face, External Approach
0WJ30ZZ Inspection of Oral Cavity and Throat, Open Approach
0WJ33ZZ Inspection of Oral Cavity and Throat, Percutaneous Approach
0WJ34ZZ Inspection of Oral Cavity and Throat, Percutaneous Endoscopic Approach
0WJ3XZZ Inspection of Oral Cavity and Throat, External Approach
●**0WJ40ZZ** Inspection of Upper Jaw, Open Approach
0WJ43ZZ Inspection of Upper Jaw, Percutaneous Approach
0WJ44ZZ Inspection of Upper Jaw, Percutaneous Endoscopic Approach
0WJ4XZZ Inspection of Upper Jaw, External Approach
●**0WJ50ZZ** Inspection of Lower Jaw, Open Approach
0WJ53ZZ Inspection of Lower Jaw, Percutaneous Approach
0WJ54ZZ Inspection of Lower Jaw, Percutaneous Endoscopic Approach
0WJ5XZZ Inspection of Lower Jaw, External Approach
0WJ60ZZ Inspection of Neck, Open Approach
0WJ63ZZ Inspection of Neck, Percutaneous Approach
0WJ64ZZ Inspection of Neck, Percutaneous Endoscopic Approach
0WJ6XZZ Inspection of Neck, External Approach
0WJ80ZZ Inspection of Chest Wall, Open Approach
0WJ83ZZ Inspection of Chest Wall, Percutaneous Approach
0WJ84ZZ Inspection of Chest Wall, Percutaneous Endoscopic Approach
0WJ8XZZ Inspection of Chest Wall, External Approach
0WJ90ZZ Inspection of Right Pleural Cavity, Open Approach
0WJ93ZZ Inspection of Right Pleural Cavity, Percutaneous Approach
0WJ94ZZ Inspection of Right Pleural Cavity, Percutaneous Endoscopic Approach
0WJB0ZZ Inspection of Left Pleural Cavity, Open Approach
0WJB3ZZ Inspection of Left Pleural Cavity, Percutaneous Approach
0WJB4ZZ Inspection of Left Pleural Cavity, Percutaneous Endoscopic Approach
0WJC0ZZ Inspection of Mediastinum, Open Approach
0WJC3ZZ Inspection of Mediastinum, Percutaneous Approach
0WJC4ZZ Inspection of Mediastinum, Percutaneous Endoscopic Approach
0WJD0ZZ Inspection of Pericardial Cavity, Open Approach
0WJD3ZZ Inspection of Pericardial Cavity, Percutaneous Approach
0WJD4ZZ Inspection of Pericardial Cavity, Percutaneous Endoscopic Approach
0WJF0ZZ Inspection of Abdominal Wall, Open Approach
0WJF3ZZ Inspection of Abdominal Wall, Percutaneous Approach
0WJF4ZZ Inspection of Abdominal Wall, Percutaneous Endoscopic Approach
0WJFXZZ Inspection of Abdominal Wall, External Approach
0WJG0ZZ Inspection of Peritoneal Cavity, Open Approach
0WJG3ZZ Inspection of Peritoneal Cavity, Percutaneous Approach
0WJG4ZZ Inspection of Peritoneal Cavity, Percutaneous Endoscopic Approach
AHA CC: 2Q, 2013, 36-37
0WJH0ZZ Inspection of Retroperitoneum, Open Approach
0WJH3ZZ Inspection of Retroperitoneum, Percutaneous Approach
0WJH4ZZ Inspection of Retroperitoneum, Percutaneous Endoscopic Approach
0WJJ0ZZ Inspection of Pelvic Cavity, Open Approach
0WJJ3ZZ Inspection of Pelvic Cavity, Percutaneous Approach
0WJJ4ZZ Inspection of Pelvic Cavity, Percutaneous Endoscopic Approach
● **0WJK0ZZ** Inspection of Upper Back, Open Approach
0WJK3ZZ Inspection of Upper Back, Percutaneous Approach
0WJK4ZZ Inspection of Upper Back, Percutaneous Endoscopic Approach
0WJKXZZ Inspection of Upper Back, External Approach
● **0WJL0ZZ** Inspection of Lower Back, Open Approach
0WJL3ZZ Inspection of Lower Back, Percutaneous Approach
0WJL4ZZ Inspection of Lower Back, Percutaneous Endoscopic Approach
0WJLXZZ Inspection of Lower Back, External Approach
♂ **0WJM0ZZ** Inspection of Male Perineum, Open Approach
♂ **0WJM3ZZ** Inspection of Male Perineum, Percutaneous Approach
♂ **0WJM4ZZ** Inspection of Male Perineum, Percutaneous Endoscopic Approach
♂ **0WJMXZZ** Inspection of Male Perineum, External Approach
♀ **0WJN0ZZ** Inspection of Female Perineum, Open Approach
♀ **0WJN3ZZ** Inspection of Female Perineum, Percutaneous Approach
♀ **0WJN4ZZ** Inspection of Female Perineum, Percutaneous Endoscopic Approach
♀ **0WJNXZZ** Inspection of Female Perineum, External Approach
0WJP0ZZ Inspection of Gastrointestinal Tract, Open Approach
0WJP3ZZ Inspection of Gastrointestinal Tract, Percutaneous Approach
0WJP4ZZ Inspection of Gastrointestinal Tract, Percutaneous Endoscopic Approach
0WJP7ZZ Inspection of Gastrointestinal Tract, Via Natural or Artificial Opening Approach
0WJP8ZZ Inspection of Gastrointestinal Tract, Via Natural or Artificial Opening Endoscopic Approach
0WJQ0ZZ Inspection of Respiratory Tract, Open Approach
0WJQ3ZZ Inspection of Respiratory Tract, Percutaneous Approach
0WJQ4ZZ Inspection of Respiratory Tract, Percutaneous Endoscopic Approach
0WJQ7ZZ Inspection of Respiratory Tract, Via Natural or Artificial Opening Approach
0WJQ8ZZ Inspection of Respiratory Tract, Via Natural or Artificial Opening Endoscopic Approach
0WJR0ZZ Inspection of Genitourinary Tract, Open Approach
0WJR3ZZ Inspection of Genitourinary Tract, Percutaneous Approach
0WJR4ZZ Inspection of Genitourinary Tract, Percutaneous Endoscopic Approach
0WJR7ZZ Inspection of Genitourinary Tract, Via Natural or Artificial Opening Approach
0WJR8ZZ Inspection of Genitourinary Tract, Via Natural or Artificial Opening Endoscopic Approach

0WM – Anatomical Regions, General, Reattachment

0WM20ZZ Reattachment of Face, Open Approach
0WM40ZZ Reattachment of Upper Jaw, Open Approach
0WM50ZZ Reattachment of Lower Jaw, Open Approach
0WM60ZZ Reattachment of Neck, Open Approach
0WM80ZZ Reattachment of Chest Wall, Open Approach
0WMF0ZZ Reattachment of Abdominal Wall, Open Approach
0WMK0ZZ Reattachment of Upper Back, Open Approach
0WML0ZZ Reattachment of Lower Back, Open Approach
♂ **0WMM0ZZ** Reattachment of Male Perineum, Open Approach
♀ **0WMN0ZZ** Reattachment of Female Perineum, Open Approach

0WP – Anatomical Regions, General, Removal

Review Coding Guideline B6.1c

0WP000Z Removal of Drainage Device from Head, Open Approach
0WP001Z Removal of Radioactive Element from Head, Open Approach
0WP003Z Removal of Infusion Device from Head, Open Approach
0WP007Z Removal of Autologous Tissue Substitute from Head, Open Approach
0WP00JZ Removal of Synthetic Substitute from Head, Open Approach
0WP00KZ Removal of Nonautologous Tissue Substitute from Head, Open Approach
0WP00YZ Removal of Other Device from Head, Open Approach
0WP030Z Removal of Drainage Device from Head, Percutaneous Approach
0WP031Z Removal of Radioactive Element from Head, Percutaneous Approach
0WP033Z Removal of Infusion Device from Head, Percutaneous Approach
0WP037Z Removal of Autologous Tissue Substitute from Head, Percutaneous Approach
0WP03JZ Removal of Synthetic Substitute from Head, Percutaneous Approach
0WP03KZ Removal of Nonautologous Tissue Substitute from Head, Percutaneous Approach
0WP03YZ Removal of Other Device from Head, Percutaneous Approach
0WP040Z Removal of Drainage Device from Head, Percutaneous Endoscopic Approach
0WP041Z Removal of Radioactive Element from Head, Percutaneous Endoscopic Approach
0WP043Z Removal of Infusion Device from Head, Percutaneous Endoscopic Approach
0WP047Z Removal of Autologous Tissue Substitute from Head, Percutaneous Endoscopic Approach
0WP04JZ Removal of Synthetic Substitute from Head, Percutaneous Endoscopic Approach
0WP04KZ Removal of Nonautologous Tissue Substitute from Head, Percutaneous Endoscopic Approach
0WP04YZ Removal of Other Device from Head, Percutaneous Endoscopic Approach
0WP0X0Z Removal of Drainage Device from Head, External Approach
0WP0X1Z Removal of Radioactive Element from Head, External Approach
0WP0X3Z Removal of Infusion Device from Head, External Approach
0WP0X7Z Removal of Autologous Tissue Substitute from Head, External Approach
0WP0XJZ Removal of Synthetic Substitute from Head, External Approach
0WP0XKZ Removal of Nonautologous Tissue Substitute from Head, External Approach
0WP0XYZ Removal of Other Device from Head, External Approach
0WP100Z Removal of Drainage Device from Cranial Cavity, Open Approach
0WP101Z Removal of Radioactive Element from Cranial Cavity, Open Approach
0WP103Z Removal of Infusion Device from Cranial Cavity, Open Approach
0WP10JZ Removal of Synthetic Substitute from Cranial Cavity, Open Approach
0WP10YZ Removal of Other Device from Cranial Cavity, Open Approach
0WP130Z Removal of Drainage Device from Cranial Cavity, Percutaneous Approach
0WP131Z Removal of Radioactive Element from Cranial Cavity, Percutaneous Approach
0WP133Z Removal of Infusion Device from Cranial Cavity, Percutaneous Approach
0WP13JZ Removal of Synthetic Substitute from Cranial Cavity, Percutaneous Approach
0WP13YZ Removal of Other Device from Cranial Cavity, Percutaneous Approach
0WP140Z Removal of Drainage Device from Cranial Cavity, Percutaneous Endoscopic Approach
0WP141Z Removal of Radioactive Element from Cranial Cavity, Percutaneous Endoscopic Approach
0WP143Z Removal of Infusion Device from Cranial Cavity, Percutaneous Endoscopic Approach
0WP14JZ Removal of Synthetic Substitute from Cranial Cavity, Percutaneous Endoscopic Approach
0WP14YZ Removal of Other Device from Cranial Cavity, Percutaneous Endoscopic Approach
0WP1X0Z Removal of Drainage Device from Cranial Cavity, External Approach
0WP1X1Z Removal of Radioactive Element from Cranial Cavity, External Approach
0WP1X3Z Removal of Infusion Device from Cranial Cavity, External Approach
0WP200Z Removal of Drainage Device from Face, Open Approach
0WP201Z Removal of Radioactive Element from Face, Open Approach
0WP203Z Removal of Infusion Device from Face, Open Approach
0WP207Z Removal of Autologous Tissue Substitute from Face, Open Approach
0WP20JZ Removal of Synthetic Substitute from Face, Open Approach
0WP20KZ Removal of Nonautologous Tissue Substitute from Face, Open Approach
0WP20YZ Removal of Other Device from Face, Open Approach
0WP230Z Removal of Drainage Device from Face, Percutaneous Approach
0WP231Z Removal of Radioactive Element from Face, Percutaneous Approach
0WP233Z Removal of Infusion Device from Face, Percutaneous Approach
0WP237Z Removal of Autologous Tissue Substitute from Face, Percutaneous Approach
0WP23JZ Removal of Synthetic Substitute from Face, Percutaneous Approach
0WP23KZ Removal of Nonautologous Tissue Substitute from Face, Percutaneous Approach
0WP23YZ Removal of Other Device from Face, Percutaneous Approach
0WP240Z Removal of Drainage Device from Face, Percutaneous Endoscopic Approach
0WP241Z Removal of Radioactive Element from Face, Percutaneous Endoscopic Approach
0WP243Z Removal of Infusion Device from Face, Percutaneous Endoscopic Approach
0WP247Z Removal of Autologous Tissue Substitute from Face, Percutaneous Endoscopic Approach
0WP24JZ Removal of Synthetic Substitute from Face, Percutaneous Endoscopic Approach
0WP24KZ Removal of Nonautologous Tissue Substitute from Face, Percutaneous Endoscopic Approach
0WP24YZ Removal of Other Device from Face, Percutaneous Endoscopic Approach
0WP2X0Z Removal of Drainage Device from Face, External Approach
0WP2X1Z Removal of Radioactive Element from Face, External Approach
0WP2X3Z Removal of Infusion Device from Face, External Approach
0WP2X7Z Removal of Autologous Tissue Substitute from Face, External Approach
0WP2XJZ Removal of Synthetic Substitute from Face, External Approach
0WP2XKZ Removal of Nonautologous Tissue Substitute from Face, External Approach
0WP2XYZ Removal of Other Device from Face, External Approach
0WP400Z Removal of Drainage Device from Upper Jaw, Open Approach
0WP401Z Removal of Radioactive Element from Upper Jaw, Open Approach
0WP403Z Removal of Infusion Device from Upper Jaw, Open Approach
0WP407Z Removal of Autologous Tissue Substitute from Upper Jaw, Open Approach
0WP40JZ Removal of Synthetic Substitute from Upper Jaw, Open Approach
0WP40KZ Removal of Nonautologous Tissue Substitute from Upper Jaw, Open Approach
0WP40YZ Removal of Other Device from Upper Jaw, Open Approach
0WP430Z Removal of Drainage Device from Upper Jaw, Percutaneous Approach
0WP431Z Removal of Radioactive Element from Upper Jaw, Percutaneous Approach
0WP433Z Removal of Infusion Device from Upper Jaw, Percutaneous Approach
0WP437Z Removal of Autologous Tissue Substitute from Upper Jaw, Percutaneous Approach
0WP43JZ Removal of Synthetic Substitute from Upper Jaw, Percutaneous Approach
0WP43KZ Removal of Nonautologous Tissue Substitute from Upper Jaw, Percutaneous Approach
0WP43YZ Removal of Other Device from Upper Jaw, Percutaneous Approach
0WP440Z Removal of Drainage Device from Upper Jaw, Percutaneous Endoscopic Approach

0WP441Z Removal of Radioactive Element from Upper Jaw, Percutaneous Endoscopic Approach
0WP443Z Removal of Infusion Device from Upper Jaw, Percutaneous Endoscopic Approach
0WP447Z Removal of Autologous Tissue Substitute from Upper Jaw, Percutaneous Endoscopic Approach
0WP44JZ Removal of Synthetic Substitute from Upper Jaw, Percutaneous Endoscopic Approach
0WP44KZ Removal of Nonautologous Tissue Substitute from Upper Jaw, Percutaneous Endoscopic Approach
0WP44YZ Removal of Other Device from Upper Jaw, Percutaneous Endoscopic Approach
0WP4X0Z Removal of Drainage Device from Upper Jaw, External Approach
0WP4X1Z Removal of Radioactive Element from Upper Jaw, External Approach
0WP4X3Z Removal of Infusion Device from Upper Jaw, External Approach
0WP4X7Z Removal of Autologous Tissue Substitute from Upper Jaw, External Approach
0WP4XJZ Removal of Synthetic Substitute from Upper Jaw, External Approach
0WP4XKZ Removal of Nonautologous Tissue Substitute from Upper Jaw, External Approach
0WP4XYZ Removal of Other Device from Upper Jaw, External Approach
0WP500Z Removal of Drainage Device from Lower Jaw, Open Approach
0WP501Z Removal of Radioactive Element from Lower Jaw, Open Approach
0WP503Z Removal of Infusion Device from Lower Jaw, Open Approach
0WP507Z Removal of Autologous Tissue Substitute from Lower Jaw, Open Approach
0WP50JZ Removal of Synthetic Substitute from Lower Jaw, Open Approach
0WP50KZ Removal of Nonautologous Tissue Substitute from Lower Jaw, Open Approach
0WP50YZ Removal of Other Device from Lower Jaw, Open Approach
0WP530Z Removal of Drainage Device from Lower Jaw, Percutaneous Approach
0WP531Z Removal of Radioactive Element from Lower Jaw, Percutaneous Approach
0WP533Z Removal of Infusion Device from Lower Jaw, Percutaneous Approach
0WP537Z Removal of Autologous Tissue Substitute from Lower Jaw, Percutaneous Approach
0WP53JZ Removal of Synthetic Substitute from Lower Jaw, Percutaneous Approach
0WP53KZ Removal of Nonautologous Tissue Substitute from Lower Jaw, Percutaneous Approach
0WP53YZ Removal of Other Device from Lower Jaw, Percutaneous Approach
0WP540Z Removal of Drainage Device from Lower Jaw, Percutaneous Endoscopic Approach
0WP541Z Removal of Radioactive Element from Lower Jaw, Percutaneous Endoscopic Approach
0WP543Z Removal of Infusion Device from Lower Jaw, Percutaneous Endoscopic Approach
0WP547Z Removal of Autologous Tissue Substitute from Lower Jaw, Percutaneous Endoscopic Approach
0WP54JZ Removal of Synthetic Substitute from Lower Jaw, Percutaneous Endoscopic Approach
0WP54KZ Removal of Nonautologous Tissue Substitute from Lower Jaw, Percutaneous Endoscopic Approach
0WP54YZ Removal of Other Device from Lower Jaw, Percutaneous Endoscopic Approach
0WP5X0Z Removal of Drainage Device from Lower Jaw, External Approach
0WP5X1Z Removal of Radioactive Element from Lower Jaw, External Approach
0WP5X3Z Removal of Infusion Device from Lower Jaw, External Approach
0WP5X7Z Removal of Autologous Tissue Substitute from Lower Jaw, External Approach
0WP5XJZ Removal of Synthetic Substitute from Lower Jaw, External Approach
0WP5XKZ Removal of Nonautologous Tissue Substitute from Lower Jaw, External Approach
0WP5XYZ Removal of Other Device from Lower Jaw, External Approach
0WP600Z Removal of Drainage Device from Neck, Open Approach
0WP601Z Removal of Radioactive Element from Neck, Open Approach
0WP603Z Removal of Infusion Device from Neck, Open Approach
0WP607Z Removal of Autologous Tissue Substitute from Neck, Open Approach
0WP60JZ Removal of Synthetic Substitute from Neck, Open Approach
0WP60KZ Removal of Nonautologous Tissue Substitute from Neck, Open Approach
0WP60YZ Removal of Other Device from Neck, Open Approach
0WP630Z Removal of Drainage Device from Neck, Percutaneous Approach
0WP631Z Removal of Radioactive Element from Neck, Percutaneous Approach
0WP633Z Removal of Infusion Device from Neck, Percutaneous Approach
0WP637Z Removal of Autologous Tissue Substitute from Neck, Percutaneous Approach
0WP63JZ Removal of Synthetic Substitute from Neck, Percutaneous Approach
0WP63KZ Removal of Nonautologous Tissue Substitute from Neck, Percutaneous Approach
0WP63YZ Removal of Other Device from Neck, Percutaneous Approach
0WP640Z Removal of Drainage Device from Neck, Percutaneous Endoscopic Approach
0WP641Z Removal of Radioactive Element from Neck, Percutaneous Endoscopic Approach
0WP643Z Removal of Infusion Device from Neck, Percutaneous Endoscopic Approach
0WP647Z Removal of Autologous Tissue Substitute from Neck, Percutaneous Endoscopic Approach
0WP64JZ Removal of Synthetic Substitute from Neck, Percutaneous Endoscopic Approach
0WP64KZ Removal of Nonautologous Tissue Substitute from Neck, Percutaneous Endoscopic Approach
0WP64YZ Removal of Other Device from Neck, Percutaneous Endoscopic Approach
0WP6X0Z Removal of Drainage Device from Neck, External Approach
0WP6X1Z Removal of Radioactive Element from Neck, External Approach
0WP6X3Z Removal of Infusion Device from Neck, External Approach
0WP6X7Z Removal of Autologous Tissue Substitute from Neck, External Approach
0WP6XJZ Removal of Synthetic Substitute from Neck, External Approach
0WP6XKZ Removal of Nonautologous Tissue Substitute from Neck, External Approach
0WP6XYZ Removal of Other Device from Neck, External Approach
0WP800Z Removal of Drainage Device from Chest Wall, Open Approach
0WP801Z Removal of Radioactive Element from Chest Wall, Open Approach
0WP803Z Removal of Infusion Device from Chest Wall, Open Approach
0WP807Z Removal of Autologous Tissue Substitute from Chest Wall, Open Approach
0WP80JZ Removal of Synthetic Substitute from Chest Wall, Open Approach
0WP80KZ Removal of Nonautologous Tissue Substitute from Chest Wall, Open Approach
0WP80YZ Removal of Other Device from Chest Wall, Open Approach
0WP830Z Removal of Drainage Device from Chest Wall, Percutaneous Approach
0WP831Z Removal of Radioactive Element from Chest Wall, Percutaneous Approach
0WP833Z Removal of Infusion Device from Chest Wall, Percutaneous Approach
0WP837Z Removal of Autologous Tissue Substitute from Chest Wall, Percutaneous Approach
0WP83JZ Removal of Synthetic Substitute from Chest Wall, Percutaneous Approach
0WP83KZ Removal of Nonautologous Tissue Substitute from Chest Wall, Percutaneous Approach
0WP83YZ Removal of Other Device from Chest Wall, Percutaneous Approach
0WP840Z Removal of Drainage Device from Chest Wall, Percutaneous Endoscopic Approach
0WP841Z Removal of Radioactive Element from Chest Wall, Percutaneous Endoscopic Approach
0WP843Z Removal of Infusion Device from Chest Wall, Percutaneous Endoscopic Approach
0WP847Z Removal of Autologous Tissue Substitute from Chest Wall, Percutaneous Endoscopic Approach
0WP84JZ Removal of Synthetic Substitute from Chest Wall, Percutaneous Endoscopic Approach
0WP84KZ Removal of Nonautologous Tissue Substitute from Chest Wall, Percutaneous Endoscopic Approach
0WP84YZ Removal of Other Device from Chest Wall, Percutaneous Endoscopic Approach
0WP8X0Z Removal of Drainage Device from Chest Wall, External Approach
0WP8X1Z Removal of Radioactive Element from Chest Wall, External Approach
0WP8X3Z Removal of Infusion Device from Chest Wall, External Approach
0WP8X7Z Removal of Autologous Tissue Substitute from Chest Wall, External Approach
0WP8XJZ Removal of Synthetic Substitute from Chest Wall, External Approach
0WP8XKZ Removal of Nonautologous Tissue Substitute from Chest Wall, External Approach
0WP8XYZ Removal of Other Device from Chest Wall, External Approach
0WP900Z Removal of Drainage Device from Right Pleural Cavity, Open Approach
0WP901Z Removal of Radioactive Element from Right Pleural Cavity, Open Approach
0WP903Z Removal of Infusion Device from Right Pleural Cavity, Open Approach
0WP90JZ Removal of Synthetic Substitute from Right Pleural Cavity, Open Approach
0WP90YZ Removal of Other Device from Right Pleural Cavity, Open Approach
0WP930Z Removal of Drainage Device from Right Pleural Cavity, Percutaneous Approach

0WP931Z Removal of Radioactive Element from Right Pleural Cavity, Percutaneous Approach
0WP933Z Removal of Infusion Device from Right Pleural Cavity, Percutaneous Approach
0WP93JZ Removal of Synthetic Substitute from Right Pleural Cavity, Percutaneous Approach
0WP93YZ Removal of Other Device from Right Pleural Cavity, Percutaneous Approach
0WP940Z Removal of Drainage Device from Right Pleural Cavity, Percutaneous Endoscopic Approach
0WP941Z Removal of Radioactive Element from Right Pleural Cavity, Percutaneous Endoscopic Approach
0WP943Z Removal of Infusion Device from Right Pleural Cavity, Percutaneous Endoscopic Approach
0WP94JZ Removal of Synthetic Substitute from Right Pleural Cavity, Percutaneous Endoscopic Approach
0WP94YZ Removal of Other Device from Right Pleural Cavity, Percutaneous Endoscopic Approach
0WP9X0Z Removal of Drainage Device from Right Pleural Cavity, External Approach
0WP9X1Z Removal of Radioactive Element from Right Pleural Cavity, External Approach
0WP9X3Z Removal of Infusion Device from Right Pleural Cavity, External Approach
0WPB00Z Removal of Drainage Device from Left Pleural Cavity, Open Approach
0WPB01Z Removal of Radioactive Element from Left Pleural Cavity, Open Approach
0WPB03Z Removal of Infusion Device from Left Pleural Cavity, Open Approach
0WPB0JZ Removal of Synthetic Substitute from Left Pleural Cavity, Open Approach
0WPB0YZ Removal of Other Device from Left Pleural Cavity, Open Approach
0WPB30Z Removal of Drainage Device from Left Pleural Cavity, Percutaneous Approach
0WPB31Z Removal of Radioactive Element from Left Pleural Cavity, Percutaneous Approach
0WPB33Z Removal of Infusion Device from Left Pleural Cavity, Percutaneous Approach
0WPB3JZ Removal of Synthetic Substitute from Left Pleural Cavity, Percutaneous Approach
0WPB3YZ Removal of Other Device from Left Pleural Cavity, Percutaneous Approach
0WPB40Z Removal of Drainage Device from Left Pleural Cavity, Percutaneous Endoscopic Approach
0WPB41Z Removal of Radioactive Element from Left Pleural Cavity, Percutaneous Endoscopic Approach
0WPB43Z Removal of Infusion Device from Left Pleural Cavity, Percutaneous Endoscopic Approach
0WPB4JZ Removal of Synthetic Substitute from Left Pleural Cavity, Percutaneous Endoscopic Approach
0WPB4YZ Removal of Other Device from Left Pleural Cavity, Percutaneous Endoscopic Approach
0WPBX0Z Removal of Drainage Device from Left Pleural Cavity, External Approach
0WPBX1Z Removal of Radioactive Element from Left Pleural Cavity, External Approach
0WPBX3Z Removal of Infusion Device from Left Pleural Cavity, External Approach
0WPC00Z Removal of Drainage Device from Mediastinum, Open Approach
0WPC01Z Removal of Radioactive Element from Mediastinum, Open Approach
0WPC03Z Removal of Infusion Device from Mediastinum, Open Approach
0WPC07Z Removal of Autologous Tissue Substitute from Mediastinum, Open Approach
0WPC0JZ Removal of Synthetic Substitute from Mediastinum, Open Approach
0WPC0KZ Removal of Nonautologous Tissue Substitute from Mediastinum, Open Approach
0WPC0YZ Removal of Other Device from Mediastinum, Open Approach
0WPC30Z Removal of Drainage Device from Mediastinum, Percutaneous Approach
0WPC31Z Removal of Radioactive Element from Mediastinum, Percutaneous Approach
0WPC33Z Removal of Infusion Device from Mediastinum, Percutaneous Approach
0WPC37Z Removal of Autologous Tissue Substitute from Mediastinum, Percutaneous Approach
0WPC3JZ Removal of Synthetic Substitute from Mediastinum, Percutaneous Approach
0WPC3KZ Removal of Nonautologous Tissue Substitute from Mediastinum, Percutaneous Approach
0WPC3YZ Removal of Other Device from Mediastinum, Percutaneous Approach
0WPC40Z Removal of Drainage Device from Mediastinum, Percutaneous Endoscopic Approach
0WPC41Z Removal of Radioactive Element from Mediastinum, Percutaneous Endoscopic Approach
0WPC43Z Removal of Infusion Device from Mediastinum, Percutaneous Endoscopic Approach
0WPC47Z Removal of Autologous Tissue Substitute from Mediastinum, Percutaneous Endoscopic Approach
0WPC4JZ Removal of Synthetic Substitute from Mediastinum, Percutaneous Endoscopic Approach
0WPC4KZ Removal of Nonautologous Tissue Substitute from Mediastinum, Percutaneous Endoscopic Approach
0WPC4YZ Removal of Other Device from Mediastinum, Percutaneous Endoscopic Approach
0WPCX0Z Removal of Drainage Device from Mediastinum, External Approach
0WPCX1Z Removal of Radioactive Element from Mediastinum, External Approach
0WPCX3Z Removal of Infusion Device from Mediastinum, External Approach
0WPCX7Z Removal of Autologous Tissue Substitute from Mediastinum, External Approach
0WPCXJZ Removal of Synthetic Substitute from Mediastinum, External Approach
0WPCXKZ Removal of Nonautologous Tissue Substitute from Mediastinum, External Approach
0WPCXYZ Removal of Other Device from Mediastinum, External Approach
0WPD00Z Removal of Drainage Device from Pericardial Cavity, Open Approach
0WPD01Z Removal of Radioactive Element from Pericardial Cavity, Open Approach
0WPD03Z Removal of Infusion Device from Pericardial Cavity, Open Approach
0WPD0YZ Removal of Other Device from Pericardial Cavity, Open Approach
0WPD30Z Removal of Drainage Device from Pericardial Cavity, Percutaneous Approach
0WPD31Z Removal of Radioactive Element from Pericardial Cavity, Percutaneous Approach
0WPD33Z Removal of Infusion Device from Pericardial Cavity, Percutaneous Approach
0WPD3YZ Removal of Other Device from Pericardial Cavity, Percutaneous Approach
0WPD40Z Removal of Drainage Device from Pericardial Cavity, Percutaneous Endoscopic Approach
0WPD41Z Removal of Radioactive Element from Pericardial Cavity, Percutaneous Endoscopic Approach
0WPD43Z Removal of Infusion Device from Pericardial Cavity, Percutaneous Endoscopic Approach
0WPD4YZ Removal of Other Device from Pericardial Cavity, Percutaneous Endoscopic Approach
0WPDX0Z Removal of Drainage Device from Pericardial Cavity, External Approach
0WPDX1Z Removal of Radioactive Element from Pericardial Cavity, External Approach
0WPDX3Z Removal of Infusion Device from Pericardial Cavity, External Approach
0WPF00Z Removal of Drainage Device from Abdominal Wall, Open Approach
0WPF01Z Removal of Radioactive Element from Abdominal Wall, Open Approach
0WPF03Z Removal of Infusion Device from Abdominal Wall, Open Approach
0WPF07Z Removal of Autologous Tissue Substitute from Abdominal Wall, Open Approach
0WPF0JZ Removal of Synthetic Substitute from Abdominal Wall, Open Approach
0WPF0KZ Removal of Nonautologous Tissue Substitute from Abdominal Wall, Open Approach
0WPF0YZ Removal of Other Device from Abdominal Wall, Open Approach
0WPF30Z Removal of Drainage Device from Abdominal Wall, Percutaneous Approach
0WPF31Z Removal of Radioactive Element from Abdominal Wall, Percutaneous Approach
0WPF33Z Removal of Infusion Device from Abdominal Wall, Percutaneous Approach
0WPF37Z Removal of Autologous Tissue Substitute from Abdominal Wall, Percutaneous Approach
0WPF3JZ Removal of Synthetic Substitute from Abdominal Wall, Percutaneous Approach
0WPF3KZ Removal of Nonautologous Tissue Substitute from Abdominal Wall, Percutaneous Approach
0WPF3YZ Removal of Other Device from Abdominal Wall, Percutaneous Approach
0WPF40Z Removal of Drainage Device from Abdominal Wall, Percutaneous Endoscopic Approach
0WPF41Z Removal of Radioactive Element from Abdominal Wall, Percutaneous Endoscopic Approach
0WPF43Z Removal of Infusion Device from Abdominal Wall, Percutaneous Endoscopic Approach
0WPF47Z Removal of Autologous Tissue Substitute from Abdominal Wall, Percutaneous Endoscopic Approach
0WPF4JZ Removal of Synthetic Substitute from Abdominal Wall, Percutaneous Endoscopic Approach
0WPF4KZ Removal of Nonautologous Tissue Substitute from Abdominal Wall, Percutaneous Endoscopic Approach
0WPF4YZ Removal of Other Device from Abdominal Wall, Percutaneous Endoscopic Approach
0WPFX0Z Removal of Drainage Device from Abdominal Wall, External Approach

0WPFX1Z Removal of Radioactive Element from Abdominal Wall, External Approach
0WPFX3Z Removal of Infusion Device from Abdominal Wall, External Approach
0WPFX7Z Removal of Autologous Tissue Substitute from Abdominal Wall, External Approach
0WPFXJZ Removal of Synthetic Substitute from Abdominal Wall, External Approach
0WPFXKZ Removal of Nonautologous Tissue Substitute from Abdominal Wall, External Approach
0WPFXYZ Removal of Other Device from Abdominal Wall, External Approach
0WPG00Z Removal of Drainage Device from Peritoneal Cavity, Open Approach
0WPG01Z Removal of Radioactive Element from Peritoneal Cavity, Open Approach
0WPG03Z Removal of Infusion Device from Peritoneal Cavity, Open Approach
0WPG0JZ Removal of Synthetic Substitute from Peritoneal Cavity, Open Approach
0WPG0YZ Removal of Other Device from Peritoneal Cavity, Open Approach
0WPG30Z Removal of Drainage Device from Peritoneal Cavity, Percutaneous Approach
0WPG31Z Removal of Radioactive Element from Peritoneal Cavity, Percutaneous Approach
0WPG33Z Removal of Infusion Device from Peritoneal Cavity, Percutaneous Approach
0WPG3JZ Removal of Synthetic Substitute from Peritoneal Cavity, Percutaneous Approach
0WPG3YZ Removal of Other Device from Peritoneal Cavity, Percutaneous Approach
0WPG40Z Removal of Drainage Device from Peritoneal Cavity, Percutaneous Endoscopic Approach
0WPG41Z Removal of Radioactive Element from Peritoneal Cavity, Percutaneous Endoscopic Approach
0WPG43Z Removal of Infusion Device from Peritoneal Cavity, Percutaneous Endoscopic Approach
0WPG4JZ Removal of Synthetic Substitute from Peritoneal Cavity, Percutaneous Endoscopic Approach
0WPG4YZ Removal of Other Device from Peritoneal Cavity, Percutaneous Endoscopic Approach
0WPGX0Z Removal of Drainage Device from Peritoneal Cavity, External Approach
0WPGX1Z Removal of Radioactive Element from Peritoneal Cavity, External Approach
0WPGX3Z Removal of Infusion Device from Peritoneal Cavity, External Approach
0WPH00Z Removal of Drainage Device from Retroperitoneum, Open Approach
0WPH01Z Removal of Radioactive Element from Retroperitoneum, Open Approach
0WPH03Z Removal of Infusion Device from Retroperitoneum, Open Approach
0WPH0YZ Removal of Other Device from Retroperitoneum, Open Approach
0WPH30Z Removal of Drainage Device from Retroperitoneum, Percutaneous Approach
0WPH31Z Removal of Radioactive Element from Retroperitoneum, Percutaneous Approach
0WPH33Z Removal of Infusion Device from Retroperitoneum, Percutaneous Approach
0WPH3YZ Removal of Other Device from Retroperitoneum, Percutaneous Approach
0WPH40Z Removal of Drainage Device from Retroperitoneum, Percutaneous Endoscopic Approach
0WPH41Z Removal of Radioactive Element from Retroperitoneum, Percutaneous Endoscopic Approach
0WPH43Z Removal of Infusion Device from Retroperitoneum, Percutaneous Endoscopic Approach
0WPH4YZ Removal of Other Device from Retroperitoneum, Percutaneous Endoscopic Approach
0WPHX0Z Removal of Drainage Device from Retroperitoneum, External Approach
0WPHX1Z Removal of Radioactive Element from Retroperitoneum, External Approach
0WPHX3Z Removal of Infusion Device from Retroperitoneum, External Approach
0WPJ00Z Removal of Drainage Device from Pelvic Cavity, Open Approach
0WPJ01Z Removal of Radioactive Element from Pelvic Cavity, Open Approach
0WPJ03Z Removal of Infusion Device from Pelvic Cavity, Open Approach
0WPJ0JZ Removal of Synthetic Substitute from Pelvic Cavity, Open Approach
0WPJ0YZ Removal of Other Device from Pelvic Cavity, Open Approach
0WPJ30Z Removal of Drainage Device from Pelvic Cavity, Percutaneous Approach
0WPJ31Z Removal of Radioactive Element from Pelvic Cavity, Percutaneous Approach
0WPJ33Z Removal of Infusion Device from Pelvic Cavity, Percutaneous Approach
0WPJ3JZ Removal of Synthetic Substitute from Pelvic Cavity, Percutaneous Approach
0WPJ3YZ Removal of Other Device from Pelvic Cavity, Percutaneous Approach
0WPJ40Z Removal of Drainage Device from Pelvic Cavity, Percutaneous Endoscopic Approach
0WPJ41Z Removal of Radioactive Element from Pelvic Cavity, Percutaneous Endoscopic Approach
0WPJ43Z Removal of Infusion Device from Pelvic Cavity, Percutaneous Endoscopic Approach
0WPJ4JZ Removal of Synthetic Substitute from Pelvic Cavity, Percutaneous Endoscopic Approach
0WPJ4YZ Removal of Other Device from Pelvic Cavity, Percutaneous Endoscopic Approach
0WPJX0Z Removal of Drainage Device from Pelvic Cavity, External Approach
0WPJX1Z Removal of Radioactive Element from Pelvic Cavity, External Approach
0WPJX3Z Removal of Infusion Device from Pelvic Cavity, External Approach
0WPK00Z Removal of Drainage Device from Upper Back, Open Approach
0WPK01Z Removal of Radioactive Element from Upper Back, Open Approach
0WPK03Z Removal of Infusion Device from Upper Back, Open Approach
0WPK07Z Removal of Autologous Tissue Substitute from Upper Back, Open Approach
0WPK0JZ Removal of Synthetic Substitute from Upper Back, Open Approach
0WPK0KZ Removal of Nonautologous Tissue Substitute from Upper Back, Open Approach
0WPK0YZ Removal of Other Device from Upper Back, Open Approach
0WPK30Z Removal of Drainage Device from Upper Back, Percutaneous Approach
0WPK31Z Removal of Radioactive Element from Upper Back, Percutaneous Approach
0WPK33Z Removal of Infusion Device from Upper Back, Percutaneous Approach
0WPK37Z Removal of Autologous Tissue Substitute from Upper Back, Percutaneous Approach
0WPK3JZ Removal of Synthetic Substitute from Upper Back, Percutaneous Approach
0WPK3KZ Removal of Nonautologous Tissue Substitute from Upper Back, Percutaneous Approach
0WPK3YZ Removal of Other Device from Upper Back, Percutaneous Approach
0WPK40Z Removal of Drainage Device from Upper Back, Percutaneous Endoscopic Approach
0WPK41Z Removal of Radioactive Element from Upper Back, Percutaneous Endoscopic Approach
0WPK43Z Removal of Infusion Device from Upper Back, Percutaneous Endoscopic Approach
0WPK47Z Removal of Autologous Tissue Substitute from Upper Back, Percutaneous Endoscopic Approach
0WPK4JZ Removal of Synthetic Substitute from Upper Back, Percutaneous Endoscopic Approach
0WPK4KZ Removal of Nonautologous Tissue Substitute from Upper Back, Percutaneous Endoscopic Approach
0WPK4YZ Removal of Other Device from Upper Back, Percutaneous Endoscopic Approach
0WPKX0Z Removal of Drainage Device from Upper Back, External Approach
0WPKX1Z Removal of Radioactive Element from Upper Back, External Approach
0WPKX3Z Removal of Infusion Device from Upper Back, External Approach
0WPKX7Z Removal of Autologous Tissue Substitute from Upper Back, External Approach
0WPKXJZ Removal of Synthetic Substitute from Upper Back, External Approach
0WPKXKZ Removal of Nonautologous Tissue Substitute from Upper Back, External Approach
0WPKXYZ Removal of Other Device from Upper Back, External Approach
0WPL00Z Removal of Drainage Device from Lower Back, Open Approach
0WPL01Z Removal of Radioactive Element from Lower Back, Open Approach
0WPL03Z Removal of Infusion Device from Lower Back, Open Approach
0WPL07Z Removal of Autologous Tissue Substitute from Lower Back, Open Approach
0WPL0JZ Removal of Synthetic Substitute from Lower Back, Open Approach
0WPL0KZ Removal of Nonautologous Tissue Substitute from Lower Back, Open Approach
0WPL0YZ Removal of Other Device from Lower Back, Open Approach
0WPL30Z Removal of Drainage Device from Lower Back, Percutaneous Approach
0WPL31Z Removal of Radioactive Element from Lower Back, Percutaneous Approach
0WPL33Z Removal of Infusion Device from Lower Back, Percutaneous Approach
0WPL37Z Removal of Autologous Tissue Substitute from Lower Back, Percutaneous Approach
0WPL3JZ Removal of Synthetic Substitute from Lower Back, Percutaneous Approach
0WPL3KZ Removal of Nonautologous Tissue Substitute from Lower Back, Percutaneous Approach
0WPL3YZ Removal of Other Device from Lower Back, Percutaneous Approach

0WPL40Z Removal of Drainage Device from Lower Back, Percutaneous Endoscopic Approach
0WPL41Z Removal of Radioactive Element from Lower Back, Percutaneous Endoscopic Approach
0WPL43Z Removal of Infusion Device from Lower Back, Percutaneous Endoscopic Approach
0WPL47Z Removal of Autologous Tissue Substitute from Lower Back, Percutaneous Endoscopic Approach
0WPL4JZ Removal of Synthetic Substitute from Lower Back, Percutaneous Endoscopic Approach
0WPL4KZ Removal of Nonautologous Tissue Substitute from Lower Back, Percutaneous Endoscopic Approach
0WPL4YZ Removal of Other Device from Lower Back, Percutaneous Endoscopic Approach
0WPLX0Z Removal of Drainage Device from Lower Back, External Approach
0WPLX1Z Removal of Radioactive Element from Lower Back, External Approach
0WPLX3Z Removal of Infusion Device from Lower Back, External Approach
0WPLX7Z Removal of Autologous Tissue Substitute from Lower Back, External Approach
0WPLXJZ Removal of Synthetic Substitute from Lower Back, External Approach
0WPLXKZ Removal of Nonautologous Tissue Substitute from Lower Back, External Approach
0WPLXYZ Removal of Other Device from Lower Back, External Approach
♂ **0WPM00Z** Removal of Drainage Device from Male Perineum, Open Approach
♂ **0WPM01Z** Removal of Radioactive Element from Male Perineum, Open Approach
♂ **0WPM03Z** Removal of Infusion Device from Male Perineum, Open Approach
♂ **0WPM07Z** Removal of Autologous Tissue Substitute from Male Perineum, Open Approach
♂ **0WPM0JZ** Removal of Synthetic Substitute from Male Perineum, Open Approach
♂ **0WPM0KZ** Removal of Nonautologous Tissue Substitute from Male Perineum, Open Approach
♂ **0WPM0YZ** Removal of Other Device from Male Perineum, Open Approach
♂ **0WPM30Z** Removal of Drainage Device from Male Perineum, Percutaneous Approach
♂ **0WPM31Z** Removal of Radioactive Element from Male Perineum, Percutaneous Approach
♂ **0WPM33Z** Removal of Infusion Device from Male Perineum, Percutaneous Approach
♂ **0WPM37Z** Removal of Autologous Tissue Substitute from Male Perineum, Percutaneous Approach
♂ **0WPM3JZ** Removal of Synthetic Substitute from Male Perineum, Percutaneous Approach
♂ **0WPM3KZ** Removal of Nonautologous Tissue Substitute from Male Perineum, Percutaneous Approach
♂ **0WPM3YZ** Removal of Other Device from Male Perineum, Percutaneous Approach
♂ **0WPM40Z** Removal of Drainage Device from Male Perineum, Percutaneous Endoscopic Approach
♂ **0WPM41Z** Removal of Radioactive Element from Male Perineum, Percutaneous Endoscopic Approach
♂ **0WPM43Z** Removal of Infusion Device from Male Perineum, Percutaneous Endoscopic Approach
♂ **0WPM47Z** Removal of Autologous Tissue Substitute from Male Perineum, Percutaneous Endoscopic Approach
♂ **0WPM4JZ** Removal of Synthetic Substitute from Male Perineum, Percutaneous Endoscopic Approach
♂ **0WPM4KZ** Removal of Nonautologous Tissue Substitute from Male Perineum, Percutaneous Endoscopic Approach
♂ **0WPM4YZ** Removal of Other Device from Male Perineum, Percutaneous Endoscopic Approach
♂ **0WPMX0Z** Removal of Drainage Device from Male Perineum, External Approach
♂ **0WPMX1Z** Removal of Radioactive Element from Male Perineum, External Approach
♂ **0WPMX3Z** Removal of Infusion Device from Male Perineum, External Approach
♂ **0WPMX7Z** Removal of Autologous Tissue Substitute from Male Perineum, External Approach
♂ **0WPMXJZ** Removal of Synthetic Substitute from Male Perineum, External Approach
♂ **0WPMXKZ** Removal of Nonautologous Tissue Substitute from Male Perineum, External Approach
♂ **0WPMXYZ** Removal of Other Device from Male Perineum, External Approach
♀ **0WPN00Z** Removal of Drainage Device from Female Perineum, Open Approach
♀ **0WPN01Z** Removal of Radioactive Element from Female Perineum, Open Approach
♀ **0WPN03Z** Removal of Infusion Device from Female Perineum, Open Approach
♀ **0WPN07Z** Removal of Autologous Tissue Substitute from Female Perineum, Open Approach
♀ **0WPN0JZ** Removal of Synthetic Substitute from Female Perineum, Open Approach
♀ **0WPN0KZ** Removal of Nonautologous Tissue Substitute from Female Perineum, Open Approach
♀ **0WPN0YZ** Removal of Other Device from Female Perineum, Open Approach
♀ **0WPN30Z** Removal of Drainage Device from Female Perineum, Percutaneous Approach
♀ **0WPN31Z** Removal of Radioactive Element from Female Perineum, Percutaneous Approach
♀ **0WPN33Z** Removal of Infusion Device from Female Perineum, Percutaneous Approach
♀ **0WPN37Z** Removal of Autologous Tissue Substitute from Female Perineum, Percutaneous Approach
♀ **0WPN3JZ** Removal of Synthetic Substitute from Female Perineum, Percutaneous Approach
♀ **0WPN3KZ** Removal of Nonautologous Tissue Substitute from Female Perineum, Percutaneous Approach
♀ **0WPN3YZ** Removal of Other Device from Female Perineum, Percutaneous Approach
♀ **0WPN40Z** Removal of Drainage Device from Female Perineum, Percutaneous Endoscopic Approach
♀ **0WPN41Z** Removal of Radioactive Element from Female Perineum, Percutaneous Endoscopic Approach
♀ **0WPN43Z** Removal of Infusion Device from Female Perineum, Percutaneous Endoscopic Approach
♀ **0WPN47Z** Removal of Autologous Tissue Substitute from Female Perineum, Percutaneous Endoscopic Approach
♀ **0WPN4JZ** Removal of Synthetic Substitute from Female Perineum, Percutaneous Endoscopic Approach
♀ **0WPN4KZ** Removal of Nonautologous Tissue Substitute from Female Perineum, Percutaneous Endoscopic Approach
♀ **0WPN4YZ** Removal of Other Device from Female Perineum, Percutaneous Endoscopic Approach
♀ **0WPNX0Z** Removal of Drainage Device from Female Perineum, External Approach
♀ **0WPNX1Z** Removal of Radioactive Element from Female Perineum, External Approach
♀ **0WPNX3Z** Removal of Infusion Device from Female Perineum, External Approach
♀ **0WPNX7Z** Removal of Autologous Tissue Substitute from Female Perineum, External Approach
♀ **0WPNXJZ** Removal of Synthetic Substitute from Female Perineum, External Approach
♀ **0WPNXKZ** Removal of Nonautologous Tissue Substitute from Female Perineum, External Approach
♀ **0WPNXYZ** Removal of Other Device from Female Perineum, External Approach
0WPP01Z Removal of Radioactive Element from Gastrointestinal Tract, Open Approach
0WPP03Z Removal of Infusion Device from Gastrointestinal Tract, Open Approach
0WPP0YZ Removal of Other Device from Gastrointestinal Tract, Open Approach
0WPP31Z Removal of Radioactive Element from Gastrointestinal Tract, Percutaneous Approach
0WPP33Z Removal of Infusion Device from Gastrointestinal Tract, Percutaneous Approach
0WPP3YZ Removal of Other Device from Gastrointestinal Tract, Percutaneous Approach
0WPP41Z Removal of Radioactive Element from Gastrointestinal Tract, Percutaneous Endoscopic Approach
0WPP43Z Removal of Infusion Device from Gastrointestinal Tract, Percutaneous Endoscopic Approach
0WPP4YZ Removal of Other Device from Gastrointestinal Tract, Percutaneous Endoscopic Approach
0WPP71Z Removal of Radioactive Element from Gastrointestinal Tract, Via Natural or Artificial Opening
0WPP73Z Removal of Infusion Device from Gastrointestinal Tract, Via Natural or Artificial Opening
0WPP7YZ Removal of Other Device from Gastrointestinal Tract, Via Natural or Artificial Opening
0WPP81Z Removal of Radioactive Element from Gastrointestinal Tract, Via Natural or Artificial Opening Endoscopic
0WPP83Z Removal of Infusion Device from Gastrointestinal Tract, Via Natural or Artificial Opening Endoscopic
0WPP8YZ Removal of Other Device from Gastrointestinal Tract, Via Natural or Artificial Opening Endoscopic
0WPPX1Z Removal of Radioactive Element from Gastrointestinal Tract, External Approach
0WPPX3Z Removal of Infusion Device from Gastrointestinal Tract, External Approach
0WPPXYZ Removal of Other Device from Gastrointestinal Tract, External Approach
0WPQ01Z Removal of Radioactive Element from Respiratory Tract, Open Approach
0WPQ03Z Removal of Infusion Device from Respiratory Tract, Open Approach
0WPQ0YZ Removal of Other Device from Respiratory Tract, Open Approach

0WPQ31Z Removal of Radioactive Element from Respiratory Tract, Percutaneous Approach
0WPQ33Z Removal of Infusion Device from Respiratory Tract, Percutaneous Approach
0WPQ3YZ Removal of Other Device from Respiratory Tract, Percutaneous Approach
0WPQ41Z Removal of Radioactive Element from Respiratory Tract, Percutaneous Endoscopic Approach
0WPQ43Z Removal of Infusion Device from Respiratory Tract, Percutaneous Endoscopic Approach
0WPQ4YZ Removal of Other Device from Respiratory Tract, Percutaneous Endoscopic Approach
0WPQ71Z Removal of Radioactive Element from Respiratory Tract, Via Natural or Artificial Opening
0WPQ73Z Removal of Infusion Device from Respiratory Tract, Via Natural or Artificial Opening
0WPQ7YZ Removal of Other Device from Respiratory Tract, Via Natural or Artificial Opening
0WPQ81Z Removal of Radioactive Element from Respiratory Tract, Via Natural or Artificial Opening Endoscopic
0WPQ83Z Removal of Infusion Device from Respiratory Tract, Via Natural or Artificial Opening Endoscopic
0WPQ8YZ Removal of Other Device from Respiratory Tract, Via Natural or Artificial Opening Endoscopic
0WPQX1Z Removal of Radioactive Element from Respiratory Tract, External Approach
0WPQX3Z Removal of Infusion Device from Respiratory Tract, External Approach
0WPQXYZ Removal of Other Device from Respiratory Tract, External Approach
0WPR01Z Removal of Radioactive Element from Genitourinary Tract, Open Approach
0WPR03Z Removal of Infusion Device from Genitourinary Tract, Open Approach
0WPR0YZ Removal of Other Device from Genitourinary Tract, Open Approach
0WPR31Z Removal of Radioactive Element from Genitourinary Tract, Percutaneous Approach
0WPR33Z Removal of Infusion Device from Genitourinary Tract, Percutaneous Approach
0WPR3YZ Removal of Other Device from Genitourinary Tract, Percutaneous Approach
0WPR41Z Removal of Radioactive Element from Genitourinary Tract, Percutaneous Endoscopic Approach
0WPR43Z Removal of Infusion Device from Genitourinary Tract, Percutaneous Endoscopic Approach
0WPR4YZ Removal of Other Device from Genitourinary Tract, Percutaneous Endoscopic Approach
0WPR71Z Removal of Radioactive Element from Genitourinary Tract, Via Natural or Artificial Opening
0WPR73Z Removal of Infusion Device from Genitourinary Tract, Via Natural or Artificial Opening
0WPR7YZ Removal of Other Device from Genitourinary Tract, Via Natural or Artificial Opening
0WPR81Z Removal of Radioactive Element from Genitourinary Tract, Via Natural or Artificial Opening Endoscopic
0WPR83Z Removal of Infusion Device from Genitourinary Tract, Via Natural or Artificial Opening Endoscopic
0WPR8YZ Removal of Other Device from Genitourinary Tract, Via Natural or Artificial Opening Endoscopic
0WPRX1Z Removal of Radioactive Element from Genitourinary Tract, External Approach
0WPRX3Z Removal of Infusion Device from Genitourinary Tract, External Approach
0WPRXYZ Removal of Other Device from Genitourinary Tract, External Approach

0WQ – Anatomical Regions, General, Repair

0WQ00ZZ Repair Head, Open Approach
0WQ03ZZ Repair Head, Percutaneous Approach
0WQ04ZZ Repair Head, Percutaneous Endoscopic Approach
0WQ0XZZ Repair Head, External Approach
0WQ20ZZ Repair Face, Open Approach
0WQ23ZZ Repair Face, Percutaneous Approach
0WQ24ZZ Repair Face, Percutaneous Endoscopic Approach
0WQ2XZZ Repair Face, External Approach
0WQ40ZZ Repair Upper Jaw, Open Approach
0WQ43ZZ Repair Upper Jaw, Percutaneous Approach
0WQ44ZZ Repair Upper Jaw, Percutaneous Endoscopic Approach
0WQ4XZZ Repair Upper Jaw, External Approach
0WQ50ZZ Repair Lower Jaw, Open Approach
0WQ53ZZ Repair Lower Jaw, Percutaneous Approach
0WQ54ZZ Repair Lower Jaw, Percutaneous Endoscopic Approach
0WQ5XZZ Repair Lower Jaw, External Approach
0WQ60ZZ Repair Neck, Open Approach
0WQ63ZZ Repair Neck, Percutaneous Approach
0WQ64ZZ Repair Neck, Percutaneous Endoscopic Approach
0WQ6XZ2 Repair Neck, Stoma, External Approach
0WQ6XZZ Repair Neck, External Approach
0WQ80ZZ Repair Chest Wall, Open Approach
0WQ83ZZ Repair Chest Wall, Percutaneous Approach
0WQ84ZZ Repair Chest Wall, Percutaneous Endoscopic Approach
0WQ8XZZ Repair Chest Wall, External Approach
0WQC0ZZ Repair Mediastinum, Open Approach
0WQC3ZZ Repair Mediastinum, Percutaneous Approach
0WQC4ZZ Repair Mediastinum, Percutaneous Endoscopic Approach
0WQF0ZZ Repair Abdominal Wall, Open Approach
0WQF3ZZ Repair Abdominal Wall, Percutaneous Approach
0WQF4ZZ Repair Abdominal Wall, Percutaneous Endoscopic Approach
0WQFXZ2 Repair Abdominal Wall, Stoma, External Approach
0WQFXZZ Repair Abdominal Wall, External Approach
0WQK0ZZ Repair Upper Back, Open Approach
0WQK3ZZ Repair Upper Back, Percutaneous Approach
0WQK4ZZ Repair Upper Back, Percutaneous Endoscopic Approach
0WQKXZZ Repair Upper Back, External Approach
0WQL0ZZ Repair Lower Back, Open Approach
0WQL3ZZ Repair Lower Back, Percutaneous Approach
0WQL4ZZ Repair Lower Back, Percutaneous Endoscopic Approach
0WQLXZZ Repair Lower Back, External Approach
♂ **0WQM0ZZ** Repair Male Perineum, Open Approach
This is a male-only service, however, it is not included in the male-only edit logic for MCE V30
♂ **0WQM3ZZ** Repair Male Perineum, Percutaneous Approach
This is a male-only service, however, it is not included in the male-only edit logic for MCE V30
♂ **0WQM4ZZ** Repair Male Perineum, Percutaneous Endoscopic Approach
This is a male-only service, however, it is not included in the male-only edit logic for MCE V30
♂ **0WQMXZZ** Repair Male Perineum, External Approach
This is a male-only service, however, it is not included in the male-only edit logic for MCE V30
♀ **0WQN0ZZ** Repair Female Perineum, Open Approach
♀ **0WQN3ZZ** Repair Female Perineum, Percutaneous Approach
♀ **0WQN4ZZ** Repair Female Perineum, Percutaneous Endoscopic Approach
♀ **0WQNXZZ** Repair Female Perineum, External Approach

0WU – Anatomical Regions, General, Supplement

0WU007Z Supplement Head with Autologous Tissue Substitute, Open Approach
0WU00JZ Supplement Head with Synthetic Substitute, Open Approach
0WU00KZ Supplement Head with Nonautologous Tissue Substitute, Open Approach
0WU047Z Supplement Head with Autologous Tissue Substitute, Percutaneous Endoscopic Approach
0WU04JZ Supplement Head with Synthetic Substitute, Percutaneous Endoscopic Approach
0WU04KZ Supplement Head with Nonautologous Tissue Substitute, Percutaneous Endoscopic Approach
0WU207Z Supplement Face with Autologous Tissue Substitute, Open Approach
0WU20JZ Supplement Face with Synthetic Substitute, Open Approach
0WU20KZ Supplement Face with Nonautologous Tissue Substitute, Open Approach
0WU247Z Supplement Face with Autologous Tissue Substitute, Percutaneous Endoscopic Approach
0WU24JZ Supplement Face with Synthetic Substitute, Percutaneous Endoscopic Approach
0WU24KZ Supplement Face with Nonautologous Tissue Substitute, Percutaneous Endoscopic Approach
0WU407Z Supplement Upper Jaw with Autologous Tissue Substitute, Open Approach
0WU40JZ Supplement Upper Jaw with Synthetic Substitute, Open Approach
0WU40KZ Supplement Upper Jaw with Nonautologous Tissue Substitute, Open Approach

0WU447Z Supplement Upper Jaw with Autologous Tissue Substitute, Percutaneous Endoscopic Approach
0WU44JZ Supplement Upper Jaw with Synthetic Substitute, Percutaneous Endoscopic Approach
0WU44KZ Supplement Upper Jaw with Nonautologous Tissue Substitute, Percutaneous Endoscopic Approach
0WU507Z Supplement Lower Jaw with Autologous Tissue Substitute, Open Approach
0WU50JZ Supplement Lower Jaw with Synthetic Substitute, Open Approach
0WU50KZ Supplement Lower Jaw with Nonautologous Tissue Substitute, Open Approach
0WU547Z Supplement Lower Jaw with Autologous Tissue Substitute, Percutaneous Endoscopic Approach
0WU54JZ Supplement Lower Jaw with Synthetic Substitute, Percutaneous Endoscopic Approach
0WU54KZ Supplement Lower Jaw with Nonautologous Tissue Substitute, Percutaneous Endoscopic Approach
0WU607Z Supplement Neck with Autologous Tissue Substitute, Open Approach
0WU60JZ Supplement Neck with Synthetic Substitute, Open Approach
0WU60KZ Supplement Neck with Nonautologous Tissue Substitute, Open Approach
0WU647Z Supplement Neck with Autologous Tissue Substitute, Percutaneous Endoscopic Approach
0WU64JZ Supplement Neck with Synthetic Substitute, Percutaneous Endoscopic Approach
0WU64KZ Supplement Neck with Nonautologous Tissue Substitute, Percutaneous Endoscopic Approach
0WU807Z Supplement Chest Wall with Autologous Tissue Substitute, Open Approach
0WU80JZ Supplement Chest Wall with Synthetic Substitute, Open Approach
AHA CC: 4Q, 2012, 101-102
0WU80KZ Supplement Chest Wall with Nonautologous Tissue Substitute, Open Approach
0WU847Z Supplement Chest Wall with Autologous Tissue Substitute, Percutaneous Endoscopic Approach
0WU84JZ Supplement Chest Wall with Synthetic Substitute, Percutaneous Endoscopic Approach
0WU84KZ Supplement Chest Wall with Nonautologous Tissue Substitute, Percutaneous Endoscopic Approach
0WUC07Z Supplement Mediastinum with Autologous Tissue Substitute, Open Approach
0WUC0JZ Supplement Mediastinum with Synthetic Substitute, Open Approach
0WUC0KZ Supplement Mediastinum with Nonautologous Tissue Substitute, Open Approach
0WUC47Z Supplement Mediastinum with Autologous Tissue Substitute, Percutaneous Endoscopic Approach
0WUC4JZ Supplement Mediastinum with Synthetic Substitute, Percutaneous Endoscopic Approach
0WUC4KZ Supplement Mediastinum with Nonautologous Tissue Substitute, Percutaneous Endoscopic Approach
0WUF07Z Supplement Abdominal Wall with Autologous Tissue Substitute, Open Approach
0WUF0JZ Supplement Abdominal Wall with Synthetic Substitute, Open Approach
0WUF0KZ Supplement Abdominal Wall with Nonautologous Tissue Substitute, Open Approach
0WUF47Z Supplement Abdominal Wall with Autologous Tissue Substitute, Percutaneous Endoscopic Approach
0WUF4JZ Supplement Abdominal Wall with Synthetic Substitute, Percutaneous Endoscopic Approach
0WUF4KZ Supplement Abdominal Wall with Nonautologous Tissue Substitute, Percutaneous Endoscopic Approach
0WUK07Z Supplement Upper Back with Autologous Tissue Substitute, Open Approach
0WUK0JZ Supplement Upper Back with Synthetic Substitute, Open Approach
0WUK0KZ Supplement Upper Back with Nonautologous Tissue Substitute, Open Approach
0WUK47Z Supplement Upper Back with Autologous Tissue Substitute, Percutaneous Endoscopic Approach
0WUK4JZ Supplement Upper Back with Synthetic Substitute, Percutaneous Endoscopic Approach
0WUK4KZ Supplement Upper Back with Nonautologous Tissue Substitute, Percutaneous Endoscopic Approach
0WUL07Z Supplement Lower Back with Autologous Tissue Substitute, Open Approach
0WUL0JZ Supplement Lower Back with Synthetic Substitute, Open Approach
0WUL0KZ Supplement Lower Back with Nonautologous Tissue Substitute, Open Approach
0WUL47Z Supplement Lower Back with Autologous Tissue Substitute, Percutaneous Endoscopic Approach
0WUL4JZ Supplement Lower Back with Synthetic Substitute, Percutaneous Endoscopic Approach
0WUL4KZ Supplement Lower Back with Nonautologous Tissue Substitute, Percutaneous Endoscopic Approach
♂ **0WUM07Z** Supplement Male Perineum with Autologous Tissue Substitute, Open Approach
♂ **0WUM0JZ** Supplement Male Perineum with Synthetic Substitute, Open Approach
♂ **0WUM0KZ** Supplement Male Perineum with Nonautologous Tissue Substitute, Open Approach
♂ **0WUM47Z** Supplement Male Perineum with Autologous Tissue Substitute, Percutaneous Endoscopic Approach
♂ **0WUM4JZ** Supplement Male Perineum with Synthetic Substitute, Percutaneous Endoscopic Approach
♂ **0WUM4KZ** Supplement Male Perineum with Nonautologous Tissue Substitute, Percutaneous Endoscopic Approach
♀ **0WUN07Z** Supplement Female Perineum with Autologous Tissue Substitute, Open Approach
♀ **0WUN0JZ** Supplement Female Perineum with Synthetic Substitute, Open Approach
♀ **0WUN0KZ** Supplement Female Perineum with Nonautologous Tissue Substitute, Open Approach
♀ **0WUN47Z** Supplement Female Perineum with Autologous Tissue Substitute, Percutaneous Endoscopic Approach
♀ **0WUN4JZ** Supplement Female Perineum with Synthetic Substitute, Percutaneous Endoscopic Approach
♀ **0WUN4KZ** Supplement Female Perineum with Nonautologous Tissue Substitute, Percutaneous Endoscopic Approach

0WW – Anatomical Regions, General, Revision

Review Coding Guideline B6.1c

● **0WW000Z** Revision of Drainage Device in Head, Open Approach
● **0WW001Z** Revision of Radioactive Element in Head, Open Approach
● **0WW003Z** Revision of Infusion Device in Head, Open Approach
● **0WW007Z** Revision of Autologous Tissue Substitute in Head, Open Approach
● **0WW00JZ** Revision of Synthetic Substitute in Head, Open Approach
● **0WW00KZ** Revision of Nonautologous Tissue Substitute in Head, Open Approach
● **0WW00YZ** Revision of Other Device in Head, Open Approach
● **0WW030Z** Revision of Drainage Device in Head, Percutaneous Approach
● **0WW031Z** Revision of Radioactive Element in Head, Percutaneous Approach
● **0WW033Z** Revision of Infusion Device in Head, Percutaneous Approach
● **0WW037Z** Revision of Autologous Tissue Substitute in Head, Percutaneous Approach
● **0WW03JZ** Revision of Synthetic Substitute in Head, Percutaneous Approach
● **0WW03KZ** Revision of Nonautologous Tissue Substitute in Head, Percutaneous Approach
● **0WW03YZ** Revision of Other Device in Head, Percutaneous Approach
● **0WW040Z** Revision of Drainage Device in Head, Percutaneous Endoscopic Approach
● **0WW041Z** Revision of Radioactive Element in Head, Percutaneous Endoscopic Approach
● **0WW043Z** Revision of Infusion Device in Head, Percutaneous Endoscopic Approach
● **0WW047Z** Revision of Autologous Tissue Substitute in Head, Percutaneous Endoscopic Approach
● **0WW04JZ** Revision of Synthetic Substitute in Head, Percutaneous Endoscopic Approach
● **0WW04KZ** Revision of Nonautologous Tissue Substitute in Head, Percutaneous Endoscopic Approach
● **0WW04YZ** Revision of Other Device in Head, Percutaneous Endoscopic Approach
0WW0X0Z Revision of Drainage Device in Head, External Approach
0WW0X1Z Revision of Radioactive Element in Head, External Approach
0WW0X3Z Revision of Infusion Device in Head, External Approach
0WW0X7Z Revision of Autologous Tissue Substitute in Head, External Approach

0WW0XJZ Revision of Synthetic Substitute in Head, External Approach
0WW0XKZ Revision of Nonautologous Tissue Substitute in Head, External Approach
0WW0XYZ Revision of Other Device in Head, External Approach
0WW100Z Revision of Drainage Device in Cranial Cavity, Open Approach
0WW101Z Revision of Radioactive Element in Cranial Cavity, Open Approach
0WW103Z Revision of Infusion Device in Cranial Cavity, Open Approach
0WW10JZ Revision of Synthetic Substitute in Cranial Cavity, Open Approach
0WW10YZ Revision of Other Device in Cranial Cavity, Open Approach
0WW130Z Revision of Drainage Device in Cranial Cavity, Percutaneous Approach
0WW131Z Revision of Radioactive Element in Cranial Cavity, Percutaneous Approach
0WW133Z Revision of Infusion Device in Cranial Cavity, Percutaneous Approach
0WW13JZ Revision of Synthetic Substitute in Cranial Cavity, Percutaneous Approach
0WW13YZ Revision of Other Device in Cranial Cavity, Percutaneous Approach
0WW140Z Revision of Drainage Device in Cranial Cavity, Percutaneous Endoscopic Approach
0WW141Z Revision of Radioactive Element in Cranial Cavity, Percutaneous Endoscopic Approach
0WW143Z Revision of Infusion Device in Cranial Cavity, Percutaneous Endoscopic Approach
0WW14JZ Revision of Synthetic Substitute in Cranial Cavity, Percutaneous Endoscopic Approach
0WW14YZ Revision of Other Device in Cranial Cavity, Percutaneous Endoscopic Approach
0WW1X0Z Revision of Drainage Device in Cranial Cavity, External Approach
0WW1X1Z Revision of Radioactive Element in Cranial Cavity, External Approach
0WW1X3Z Revision of Infusion Device in Cranial Cavity, External Approach
0WW1XJZ Revision of Synthetic Substitute in Cranial Cavity, External Approach
0WW1XYZ Revision of Other Device in Cranial Cavity, External Approach
● 0WW200Z Revision of Drainage Device in Face, Open Approach
● 0WW201Z Revision of Radioactive Element in Face, Open Approach
● 0WW203Z Revision of Infusion Device in Face, Open Approach
● 0WW207Z Revision of Autologous Tissue Substitute in Face, Open Approach
● 0WW20JZ Revision of Synthetic Substitute in Face, Open Approach
● 0WW20KZ Revision of Nonautologous Tissue Substitute in Face, Open Approach
● 0WW20YZ Revision of Other Device in Face, Open Approach
● 0WW230Z Revision of Drainage Device in Face, Percutaneous Approach
● 0WW231Z Revision of Radioactive Element in Face, Percutaneous Approach
● 0WW233Z Revision of Infusion Device in Face, Percutaneous Approach
● 0WW237Z Revision of Autologous Tissue Substitute in Face, Percutaneous Approach
● 0WW23JZ Revision of Synthetic Substitute in Face, Percutaneous Approach
● 0WW23KZ Revision of Nonautologous Tissue Substitute in Face, Percutaneous Approach
● 0WW23YZ Revision of Other Device in Face, Percutaneous Approach
● 0WW240Z Revision of Drainage Device in Face, Percutaneous Endoscopic Approach
● 0WW241Z Revision of Radioactive Element in Face, Percutaneous Endoscopic Approach
● 0WW243Z Revision of Infusion Device in Face, Percutaneous Endoscopic Approach
● 0WW247Z Revision of Autologous Tissue Substitute in Face, Percutaneous Endoscopic Approach
● 0WW24JZ Revision of Synthetic Substitute in Face, Percutaneous Endoscopic Approach
● 0WW24KZ Revision of Nonautologous Tissue Substitute in Face, Percutaneous Endoscopic Approach
● 0WW24YZ Revision of Other Device in Face, Percutaneous Endoscopic Approach
0WW2X0Z Revision of Drainage Device in Face, External Approach
0WW2X1Z Revision of Radioactive Element in Face, External Approach
0WW2X3Z Revision of Infusion Device in Face, External Approach
0WW2X7Z Revision of Autologous Tissue Substitute in Face, External Approach
0WW2XJZ Revision of Synthetic Substitute in Face, External Approach
0WW2XKZ Revision of Nonautologous Tissue Substitute in Face, External Approach
0WW2XYZ Revision of Other Device in Face, External Approach
● 0WW400Z Revision of Drainage Device in Upper Jaw, Open Approach
● 0WW401Z Revision of Radioactive Element in Upper Jaw, Open Approach
● 0WW403Z Revision of Infusion Device in Upper Jaw, Open Approach
● 0WW407Z Revision of Autologous Tissue Substitute in Upper Jaw, Open Approach
● 0WW40JZ Revision of Synthetic Substitute in Upper Jaw, Open Approach
● 0WW40KZ Revision of Nonautologous Tissue Substitute in Upper Jaw, Open Approach
● 0WW40YZ Revision of Other Device in Upper Jaw, Open Approach
● 0WW430Z Revision of Drainage Device in Upper Jaw, Percutaneous Approach
● 0WW431Z Revision of Radioactive Element in Upper Jaw, Percutaneous Approach
● 0WW433Z Revision of Infusion Device in Upper Jaw, Percutaneous Approach
● 0WW437Z Revision of Autologous Tissue Substitute in Upper Jaw, Percutaneous Approach
● 0WW43JZ Revision of Synthetic Substitute in Upper Jaw, Percutaneous Approach
● 0WW43KZ Revision of Nonautologous Tissue Substitute in Upper Jaw, Percutaneous Approach
● 0WW43YZ Revision of Other Device in Upper Jaw, Percutaneous Approach
● 0WW440Z Revision of Drainage Device in Upper Jaw, Percutaneous Endoscopic Approach
● 0WW441Z Revision of Radioactive Element in Upper Jaw, Percutaneous Endoscopic Approach
● 0WW443Z Revision of Infusion Device in Upper Jaw, Percutaneous Endoscopic Approach
● 0WW447Z Revision of Autologous Tissue Substitute in Upper Jaw, Percutaneous Endoscopic Approach
● 0WW44JZ Revision of Synthetic Substitute in Upper Jaw, Percutaneous Endoscopic Approach
● 0WW44KZ Revision of Nonautologous Tissue Substitute in Upper Jaw, Percutaneous Endoscopic Approach
● 0WW44YZ Revision of Other Device in Upper Jaw, Percutaneous Endoscopic Approach
0WW4X0Z Revision of Drainage Device in Upper Jaw, External Approach
0WW4X1Z Revision of Radioactive Element in Upper Jaw, External Approach
0WW4X3Z Revision of Infusion Device in Upper Jaw, External Approach
0WW4X7Z Revision of Autologous Tissue Substitute in Upper Jaw, External Approach
0WW4XJZ Revision of Synthetic Substitute in Upper Jaw, External Approach
0WW4XKZ Revision of Nonautologous Tissue Substitute in Upper Jaw, External Approach
0WW4XYZ Revision of Other Device in Upper Jaw, External Approach
● 0WW500Z Revision of Drainage Device in Lower Jaw, Open Approach
● 0WW501Z Revision of Radioactive Element in Lower Jaw, Open Approach
● 0WW503Z Revision of Infusion Device in Lower Jaw, Open Approach
● 0WW507Z Revision of Autologous Tissue Substitute in Lower Jaw, Open Approach
● 0WW50JZ Revision of Synthetic Substitute in Lower Jaw, Open Approach
● 0WW50KZ Revision of Nonautologous Tissue Substitute in Lower Jaw, Open Approach
● 0WW50YZ Revision of Other Device in Lower Jaw, Open Approach
● 0WW530Z Revision of Drainage Device in Lower Jaw, Percutaneous Approach
● 0WW531Z Revision of Radioactive Element in Lower Jaw, Percutaneous Approach
● 0WW533Z Revision of Infusion Device in Lower Jaw, Percutaneous Approach
● 0WW537Z Revision of Autologous Tissue Substitute in Lower Jaw, Percutaneous Approach
● 0WW53JZ Revision of Synthetic Substitute in Lower Jaw, Percutaneous Approach
● 0WW53KZ Revision of Nonautologous Tissue Substitute in Lower Jaw, Percutaneous Approach
● 0WW53YZ Revision of Other Device in Lower Jaw, Percutaneous Approach
● 0WW540Z Revision of Drainage Device in Lower Jaw, Percutaneous Endoscopic Approach
● 0WW541Z Revision of Radioactive Element in Lower Jaw, Percutaneous Endoscopic Approach
● 0WW543Z Revision of Infusion Device in Lower Jaw, Percutaneous Endoscopic Approach
● 0WW547Z Revision of Autologous Tissue Substitute in Lower Jaw, Percutaneous Endoscopic Approach
● 0WW54JZ Revision of Synthetic Substitute in Lower Jaw, Percutaneous Endoscopic Approach
● 0WW54KZ Revision of Nonautologous Tissue Substitute in Lower Jaw, Percutaneous Endoscopic Approach
● 0WW54YZ Revision of Other Device in Lower Jaw, Percutaneous Endoscopic Approach
0WW5X0Z Revision of Drainage Device in Lower Jaw, External Approach
0WW5X1Z Revision of Radioactive Element in Lower Jaw, External Approach
0WW5X3Z Revision of Infusion Device in Lower Jaw, External Approach
0WW5X7Z Revision of Autologous Tissue Substitute in Lower Jaw, External Approach
0WW5XJZ Revision of Synthetic Substitute in Lower Jaw, External Approach

0WW5XKZ Revision of Nonautologous Tissue Substitute in Lower Jaw, External Approach
0WW5XYZ Revision of Other Device in Lower Jaw, External Approach
● **0WW600Z** Revision of Drainage Device in Neck, Open Approach
● **0WW601Z** Revision of Radioactive Element in Neck, Open Approach
● **0WW603Z** Revision of Infusion Device in Neck, Open Approach
● **0WW607Z** Revision of Autologous Tissue Substitute in Neck, Open Approach
● **0WW60JZ** Revision of Synthetic Substitute in Neck, Open Approach
● **0WW60KZ** Revision of Nonautologous Tissue Substitute in Neck, Open Approach
● **0WW60YZ** Revision of Other Device in Neck, Open Approach
● **0WW630Z** Revision of Drainage Device in Neck, Percutaneous Approach
● **0WW631Z** Revision of Radioactive Element in Neck, Percutaneous Approach
● **0WW633Z** Revision of Infusion Device in Neck, Percutaneous Approach
● **0WW637Z** Revision of Autologous Tissue Substitute in Neck, Percutaneous Approach
● **0WW63JZ** Revision of Synthetic Substitute in Neck, Percutaneous Approach
● **0WW63KZ** Revision of Nonautologous Tissue Substitute in Neck, Percutaneous Approach
● **0WW63YZ** Revision of Other Device in Neck, Percutaneous Approach
● **0WW640Z** Revision of Drainage Device in Neck, Percutaneous Endoscopic Approach
● **0WW641Z** Revision of Radioactive Element in Neck, Percutaneous Endoscopic Approach
● **0WW643Z** Revision of Infusion Device in Neck, Percutaneous Endoscopic Approach
● **0WW647Z** Revision of Autologous Tissue Substitute in Neck, Percutaneous Endoscopic Approach
● **0WW64JZ** Revision of Synthetic Substitute in Neck, Percutaneous Endoscopic Approach
● **0WW64KZ** Revision of Nonautologous Tissue Substitute in Neck, Percutaneous Endoscopic Approach
● **0WW64YZ** Revision of Other Device in Neck, Percutaneous Endoscopic Approach
0WW6X0Z Revision of Drainage Device in Neck, External Approach
0WW6X1Z Revision of Radioactive Element in Neck, External Approach
0WW6X3Z Revision of Infusion Device in Neck, External Approach
0WW6X7Z Revision of Autologous Tissue Substitute in Neck, External Approach
0WW6XJZ Revision of Synthetic Substitute in Neck, External Approach
0WW6XKZ Revision of Nonautologous Tissue Substitute in Neck, External Approach
0WW6XYZ Revision of Other Device in Neck, External Approach
0WW800Z Revision of Drainage Device in Chest Wall, Open Approach
0WW801Z Revision of Radioactive Element in Chest Wall, Open Approach
0WW803Z Revision of Infusion Device in Chest Wall, Open Approach
0WW807Z Revision of Autologous Tissue Substitute in Chest Wall, Open Approach
0WW80JZ Revision of Synthetic Substitute in Chest Wall, Open Approach
0WW80KZ Revision of Nonautologous Tissue Substitute in Chest Wall, Open Approach
0WW80YZ Revision of Other Device in Chest Wall, Open Approach
0WW830Z Revision of Drainage Device in Chest Wall, Percutaneous Approach
0WW831Z Revision of Radioactive Element in Chest Wall, Percutaneous Approach
0WW833Z Revision of Infusion Device in Chest Wall, Percutaneous Approach
0WW837Z Revision of Autologous Tissue Substitute in Chest Wall, Percutaneous Approach
0WW83JZ Revision of Synthetic Substitute in Chest Wall, Percutaneous Approach
0WW83KZ Revision of Nonautologous Tissue Substitute in Chest Wall, Percutaneous Approach
0WW83YZ Revision of Other Device in Chest Wall, Percutaneous Approach
0WW840Z Revision of Drainage Device in Chest Wall, Percutaneous Endoscopic Approach
0WW841Z Revision of Radioactive Element in Chest Wall, Percutaneous Endoscopic Approach
0WW843Z Revision of Infusion Device in Chest Wall, Percutaneous Endoscopic Approach
0WW847Z Revision of Autologous Tissue Substitute in Chest Wall, Percutaneous Endoscopic Approach
0WW84JZ Revision of Synthetic Substitute in Chest Wall, Percutaneous Endoscopic Approach
0WW84KZ Revision of Nonautologous Tissue Substitute in Chest Wall, Percutaneous Endoscopic Approach
0WW84YZ Revision of Other Device in Chest Wall, Percutaneous Endoscopic Approach
0WW8X0Z Revision of Drainage Device in Chest Wall, External Approach
0WW8X1Z Revision of Radioactive Element in Chest Wall, External Approach
0WW8X3Z Revision of Infusion Device in Chest Wall, External Approach
0WW8X7Z Revision of Autologous Tissue Substitute in Chest Wall, External Approach
0WW8XJZ Revision of Synthetic Substitute in Chest Wall, External Approach
0WW8XKZ Revision of Nonautologous Tissue Substitute in Chest Wall, External Approach
0WW8XYZ Revision of Other Device in Chest Wall, External Approach
0WW900Z Revision of Drainage Device in Right Pleural Cavity, Open Approach
0WW901Z Revision of Radioactive Element in Right Pleural Cavity, Open Approach
0WW903Z Revision of Infusion Device in Right Pleural Cavity, Open Approach
0WW90JZ Revision of Synthetic Substitute in Right Pleural Cavity, Open Approach
0WW90YZ Revision of Other Device in Right Pleural Cavity, Open Approach
0WW930Z Revision of Drainage Device in Right Pleural Cavity, Percutaneous Approach
0WW931Z Revision of Radioactive Element in Right Pleural Cavity, Percutaneous Approach
0WW933Z Revision of Infusion Device in Right Pleural Cavity, Percutaneous Approach
0WW93JZ Revision of Synthetic Substitute in Right Pleural Cavity, Percutaneous Approach
0WW93YZ Revision of Other Device in Right Pleural Cavity, Percutaneous Approach
0WW940Z Revision of Drainage Device in Right Pleural Cavity, Percutaneous Endoscopic Approach
0WW941Z Revision of Radioactive Element in Right Pleural Cavity, Percutaneous Endoscopic Approach
0WW943Z Revision of Infusion Device in Right Pleural Cavity, Percutaneous Endoscopic Approach
0WW94JZ Revision of Synthetic Substitute in Right Pleural Cavity, Percutaneous Endoscopic Approach
0WW94YZ Revision of Other Device in Right Pleural Cavity, Percutaneous Endoscopic Approach
0WW9X0Z Revision of Drainage Device in Right Pleural Cavity, External Approach
0WW9X1Z Revision of Radioactive Element in Right Pleural Cavity, External Approach
0WW9X3Z Revision of Infusion Device in Right Pleural Cavity, External Approach
0WW9XJZ Revision of Synthetic Substitute in Right Pleural Cavity, External Approach
0WW9XYZ Revision of Other Device in Right Pleural Cavity, External Approach
0WWB00Z Revision of Drainage Device in Left Pleural Cavity, Open Approach
0WWB01Z Revision of Radioactive Element in Left Pleural Cavity, Open Approach
0WWB03Z Revision of Infusion Device in Left Pleural Cavity, Open Approach
0WWB0JZ Revision of Synthetic Substitute in Left Pleural Cavity, Open Approach
0WWB0YZ Revision of Other Device in Left Pleural Cavity, Open Approach
0WWB30Z Revision of Drainage Device in Left Pleural Cavity, Percutaneous Approach
0WWB31Z Revision of Radioactive Element in Left Pleural Cavity, Percutaneous Approach
0WWB33Z Revision of Infusion Device in Left Pleural Cavity, Percutaneous Approach
0WWB3JZ Revision of Synthetic Substitute in Left Pleural Cavity, Percutaneous Approach
0WWB3YZ Revision of Other Device in Left Pleural Cavity, Percutaneous Approach
0WWB40Z Revision of Drainage Device in Left Pleural Cavity, Percutaneous Endoscopic Approach
0WWB41Z Revision of Radioactive Element in Left Pleural Cavity, Percutaneous Endoscopic Approach
0WWB43Z Revision of Infusion Device in Left Pleural Cavity, Percutaneous Endoscopic Approach
0WWB4JZ Revision of Synthetic Substitute in Left Pleural Cavity, Percutaneous Endoscopic Approach
0WWB4YZ Revision of Other Device in Left Pleural Cavity, Percutaneous Endoscopic Approach
0WWBX0Z Revision of Drainage Device in Left Pleural Cavity, External Approach
0WWBX1Z Revision of Radioactive Element in Left Pleural Cavity, External Approach
0WWBX3Z Revision of Infusion Device in Left Pleural Cavity, External Approach
0WWBXJZ Revision of Synthetic Substitute in Left Pleural Cavity, External Approach
0WWBXYZ Revision of Other Device in Left Pleural Cavity, External Approach
0WWC00Z Revision of Drainage Device in Mediastinum, Open Approach
0WWC01Z Revision of Radioactive Element in Mediastinum, Open Approach
0WWC03Z Revision of Infusion Device in Mediastinum, Open Approach
0WWC07Z Revision of Autologous Tissue Substitute in Mediastinum, Open Approach
0WWC0JZ Revision of Synthetic Substitute in Mediastinum, Open Approach

0WWC0KZ Revision of Nonautologous Tissue Substitute in Mediastinum, Open Approach
0WWC0YZ Revision of Other Device in Mediastinum, Open Approach
0WWC30Z Revision of Drainage Device in Mediastinum, Percutaneous Approach
0WWC31Z Revision of Radioactive Element in Mediastinum, Percutaneous Approach
0WWC33Z Revision of Infusion Device in Mediastinum, Percutaneous Approach
0WWC37Z Revision of Autologous Tissue Substitute in Mediastinum, Percutaneous Approach
0WWC3JZ Revision of Synthetic Substitute in Mediastinum, Percutaneous Approach
0WWC3KZ Revision of Nonautologous Tissue Substitute in Mediastinum, Percutaneous Approach
0WWC3YZ Revision of Other Device in Mediastinum, Percutaneous Approach
0WWC40Z Revision of Drainage Device in Mediastinum, Percutaneous Endoscopic Approach
0WWC41Z Revision of Radioactive Element in Mediastinum, Percutaneous Endoscopic Approach
0WWC43Z Revision of Infusion Device in Mediastinum, Percutaneous Endoscopic Approach
0WWC47Z Revision of Autologous Tissue Substitute in Mediastinum, Percutaneous Endoscopic Approach
0WWC4JZ Revision of Synthetic Substitute in Mediastinum, Percutaneous Endoscopic Approach
0WWC4KZ Revision of Nonautologous Tissue Substitute in Mediastinum, Percutaneous Endoscopic Approach
0WWC4YZ Revision of Other Device in Mediastinum, Percutaneous Endoscopic Approach
0WWCX0Z Revision of Drainage Device in Mediastinum, External Approach
0WWCX1Z Revision of Radioactive Element in Mediastinum, External Approach
0WWCX3Z Revision of Infusion Device in Mediastinum, External Approach
0WWCX7Z Revision of Autologous Tissue Substitute in Mediastinum, External Approach
0WWCXJZ Revision of Synthetic Substitute in Mediastinum, External Approach
0WWCXKZ Revision of Nonautologous Tissue Substitute in Mediastinum, External Approach
0WWCXYZ Revision of Other Device in Mediastinum, External Approach
0WWD00Z Revision of Drainage Device in Pericardial Cavity, Open Approach
0WWD01Z Revision of Radioactive Element in Pericardial Cavity, Open Approach
0WWD03Z Revision of Infusion Device in Pericardial Cavity, Open Approach
0WWD0YZ Revision of Other Device in Pericardial Cavity, Open Approach
0WWD30Z Revision of Drainage Device in Pericardial Cavity, Percutaneous Approach
0WWD31Z Revision of Radioactive Element in Pericardial Cavity, Percutaneous Approach
0WWD33Z Revision of Infusion Device in Pericardial Cavity, Percutaneous Approach
0WWD3YZ Revision of Other Device in Pericardial Cavity, Percutaneous Approach
0WWD40Z Revision of Drainage Device in Pericardial Cavity, Percutaneous Endoscopic Approach
0WWD41Z Revision of Radioactive Element in Pericardial Cavity, Percutaneous Endoscopic Approach
0WWD43Z Revision of Infusion Device in Pericardial Cavity, Percutaneous Endoscopic Approach
0WWD4YZ Revision of Other Device in Pericardial Cavity, Percutaneous Endoscopic Approach
0WWDX0Z Revision of Drainage Device in Pericardial Cavity, External Approach
0WWDX1Z Revision of Radioactive Element in Pericardial Cavity, External Approach
0WWDX3Z Revision of Infusion Device in Pericardial Cavity, External Approach
0WWDXYZ Revision of Other Device in Pericardial Cavity, External Approach
0WWF00Z Revision of Drainage Device in Abdominal Wall, Open Approach
0WWF01Z Revision of Radioactive Element in Abdominal Wall, Open Approach
0WWF03Z Revision of Infusion Device in Abdominal Wall, Open Approach
0WWF07Z Revision of Autologous Tissue Substitute in Abdominal Wall, Open Approach
0WWF0JZ Revision of Synthetic Substitute in Abdominal Wall, Open Approach
0WWF0KZ Revision of Nonautologous Tissue Substitute in Abdominal Wall, Open Approach
0WWF0YZ Revision of Other Device in Abdominal Wall, Open Approach
0WWF30Z Revision of Drainage Device in Abdominal Wall, Percutaneous Approach
0WWF31Z Revision of Radioactive Element in Abdominal Wall, Percutaneous Approach
0WWF33Z Revision of Infusion Device in Abdominal Wall, Percutaneous Approach
0WWF37Z Revision of Autologous Tissue Substitute in Abdominal Wall, Percutaneous Approach
0WWF3JZ Revision of Synthetic Substitute in Abdominal Wall, Percutaneous Approach
0WWF3KZ Revision of Nonautologous Tissue Substitute in Abdominal Wall, Percutaneous Approach
0WWF3YZ Revision of Other Device in Abdominal Wall, Percutaneous Approach
0WWF40Z Revision of Drainage Device in Abdominal Wall, Percutaneous Endoscopic Approach
0WWF41Z Revision of Radioactive Element in Abdominal Wall, Percutaneous Endoscopic Approach
0WWF43Z Revision of Infusion Device in Abdominal Wall, Percutaneous Endoscopic Approach
0WWF47Z Revision of Autologous Tissue Substitute in Abdominal Wall, Percutaneous Endoscopic Approach
0WWF4JZ Revision of Synthetic Substitute in Abdominal Wall, Percutaneous Endoscopic Approach
0WWF4KZ Revision of Nonautologous Tissue Substitute in Abdominal Wall, Percutaneous Endoscopic Approach
0WWF4YZ Revision of Other Device in Abdominal Wall, Percutaneous Endoscopic Approach
0WWFX0Z Revision of Drainage Device in Abdominal Wall, External Approach
0WWFX1Z Revision of Radioactive Element in Abdominal Wall, External Approach
0WWFX3Z Revision of Infusion Device in Abdominal Wall, External Approach
0WWFX7Z Revision of Autologous Tissue Substitute in Abdominal Wall, External Approach
0WWFXJZ Revision of Synthetic Substitute in Abdominal Wall, External Approach
0WWFXKZ Revision of Nonautologous Tissue Substitute in Abdominal Wall, External Approach
0WWFXYZ Revision of Other Device in Abdominal Wall, External Approach
0WWG00Z Revision of Drainage Device in Peritoneal Cavity, Open Approach
0WWG01Z Revision of Radioactive Element in Peritoneal Cavity, Open Approach
0WWG03Z Revision of Infusion Device in Peritoneal Cavity, Open Approach
0WWG0JZ Revision of Synthetic Substitute in Peritoneal Cavity, Open Approach
0WWG0YZ Revision of Other Device in Peritoneal Cavity, Open Approach
0WWG30Z Revision of Drainage Device in Peritoneal Cavity, Percutaneous Approach
0WWG31Z Revision of Radioactive Element in Peritoneal Cavity, Percutaneous Approach
0WWG33Z Revision of Infusion Device in Peritoneal Cavity, Percutaneous Approach
0WWG3JZ Revision of Synthetic Substitute in Peritoneal Cavity, Percutaneous Approach
0WWG3YZ Revision of Other Device in Peritoneal Cavity, Percutaneous Approach
0WWG40Z Revision of Drainage Device in Peritoneal Cavity, Percutaneous Endoscopic Approach
0WWG41Z Revision of Radioactive Element in Peritoneal Cavity, Percutaneous Endoscopic Approach
0WWG43Z Revision of Infusion Device in Peritoneal Cavity, Percutaneous Endoscopic Approach
0WWG4JZ Revision of Synthetic Substitute in Peritoneal Cavity, Percutaneous Endoscopic Approach
0WWG4YZ Revision of Other Device in Peritoneal Cavity, Percutaneous Endoscopic Approach
0WWGX0Z Revision of Drainage Device in Peritoneal Cavity, External Approach
0WWGX1Z Revision of Radioactive Element in Peritoneal Cavity, External Approach
0WWGX3Z Revision of Infusion Device in Peritoneal Cavity, External Approach
0WWGXJZ Revision of Synthetic Substitute in Peritoneal Cavity, External Approach
0WWGXYZ Revision of Other Device in Peritoneal Cavity, External Approach
0WWH00Z Revision of Drainage Device in Retroperitoneum, Open Approach
0WWH01Z Revision of Radioactive Element in Retroperitoneum, Open Approach
0WWH03Z Revision of Infusion Device in Retroperitoneum, Open Approach
0WWH0YZ Revision of Other Device in Retroperitoneum, Open Approach
0WWH30Z Revision of Drainage Device in Retroperitoneum, Percutaneous Approach
0WWH31Z Revision of Radioactive Element in Retroperitoneum, Percutaneous Approach
0WWH33Z Revision of Infusion Device in Retroperitoneum, Percutaneous Approach
0WWH3YZ Revision of Other Device in Retroperitoneum, Percutaneous Approach
0WWH40Z Revision of Drainage Device in Retroperitoneum, Percutaneous Endoscopic Approach
0WWH41Z Revision of Radioactive Element in Retroperitoneum, Percutaneous Endoscopic Approach
0WWH43Z Revision of Infusion Device in Retroperitoneum, Percutaneous Endoscopic Approach

0WWH4YZ Revision of Other Device in Retroperitoneum, Percutaneous Endoscopic Approach
0WWHX0Z Revision of Drainage Device in Retroperitoneum, External Approach
0WWHX1Z Revision of Radioactive Element in Retroperitoneum, External Approach
0WWHX3Z Revision of Infusion Device in Retroperitoneum, External Approach
0WWHXYZ Revision of Other Device in Retroperitoneum, External Approach
0WWJ00Z Revision of Drainage Device in Pelvic Cavity, Open Approach
0WWJ01Z Revision of Radioactive Element in Pelvic Cavity, Open Approach
0WWJ03Z Revision of Infusion Device in Pelvic Cavity, Open Approach
0WWJ0JZ Revision of Synthetic Substitute in Pelvic Cavity, Open Approach
0WWJ0YZ Revision of Other Device in Pelvic Cavity, Open Approach
0WWJ30Z Revision of Drainage Device in Pelvic Cavity, Percutaneous Approach
0WWJ31Z Revision of Radioactive Element in Pelvic Cavity, Percutaneous Approach
0WWJ33Z Revision of Infusion Device in Pelvic Cavity, Percutaneous Approach
0WWJ3JZ Revision of Synthetic Substitute in Pelvic Cavity, Percutaneous Approach
0WWJ3YZ Revision of Other Device in Pelvic Cavity, Percutaneous Approach
0WWJ40Z Revision of Drainage Device in Pelvic Cavity, Percutaneous Endoscopic Approach
0WWJ41Z Revision of Radioactive Element in Pelvic Cavity, Percutaneous Endoscopic Approach
0WWJ43Z Revision of Infusion Device in Pelvic Cavity, Percutaneous Endoscopic Approach
0WWJ4JZ Revision of Synthetic Substitute in Pelvic Cavity, Percutaneous Endoscopic Approach
0WWJ4YZ Revision of Other Device in Pelvic Cavity, Percutaneous Endoscopic Approach
0WWJX0Z Revision of Drainage Device in Pelvic Cavity, External Approach
0WWJX1Z Revision of Radioactive Element in Pelvic Cavity, External Approach
0WWJX3Z Revision of Infusion Device in Pelvic Cavity, External Approach
0WWJXJZ Revision of Synthetic Substitute in Pelvic Cavity, External Approach
0WWJXYZ Revision of Other Device in Pelvic Cavity, External Approach
● **0WWK00Z** Revision of Drainage Device in Upper Back, Open Approach
● **0WWK01Z** Revision of Radioactive Element in Upper Back, Open Approach
● **0WWK03Z** Revision of Infusion Device in Upper Back, Open Approach
● **0WWK07Z** Revision of Autologous Tissue Substitute in Upper Back, Open Approach
● **0WWK0JZ** Revision of Synthetic Substitute in Upper Back, Open Approach
● **0WWK0KZ** Revision of Nonautologous Tissue Substitute in Upper Back, Open Approach
● **0WWK0YZ** Revision of Other Device in Upper Back, Open Approach
● **0WWK30Z** Revision of Drainage Device in Upper Back, Percutaneous Approach
● **0WWK31Z** Revision of Radioactive Element in Upper Back, Percutaneous Approach
● **0WWK33Z** Revision of Infusion Device in Upper Back, Percutaneous Approach
● **0WWK37Z** Revision of Autologous Tissue Substitute in Upper Back, Percutaneous Approach
● **0WWK3JZ** Revision of Synthetic Substitute in Upper Back, Percutaneous Approach
● **0WWK3KZ** Revision of Nonautologous Tissue Substitute in Upper Back, Percutaneous Approach
● **0WWK3YZ** Revision of Other Device in Upper Back, Percutaneous Approach
● **0WWK40Z** Revision of Drainage Device in Upper Back, Percutaneous Endoscopic Approach
● **0WWK41Z** Revision of Radioactive Element in Upper Back, Percutaneous Endoscopic Approach
● **0WWK43Z** Revision of Infusion Device in Upper Back, Percutaneous Endoscopic Approach
● **0WWK47Z** Revision of Autologous Tissue Substitute in Upper Back, Percutaneous Endoscopic Approach
● **0WWK4JZ** Revision of Synthetic Substitute in Upper Back, Percutaneous Endoscopic Approach
● **0WWK4KZ** Revision of Nonautologous Tissue Substitute in Upper Back, Percutaneous Endoscopic Approach
● **0WWK4YZ** Revision of Other Device in Upper Back, Percutaneous Endoscopic Approach
0WWKX0Z Revision of Drainage Device in Upper Back, External Approach
0WWKX1Z Revision of Radioactive Element in Upper Back, External Approach
0WWKX3Z Revision of Infusion Device in Upper Back, External Approach
0WWKX7Z Revision of Autologous Tissue Substitute in Upper Back, External Approach
0WWKXJZ Revision of Synthetic Substitute in Upper Back, External Approach
0WWKXKZ Revision of Nonautologous Tissue Substitute in Upper Back, External Approach
0WWKXYZ Revision of Other Device in Upper Back, External Approach
● **0WWL00Z** Revision of Drainage Device in Lower Back, Open Approach
● **0WWL01Z** Revision of Radioactive Element in Lower Back, Open Approach
● **0WWL03Z** Revision of Infusion Device in Lower Back, Open Approach
● **0WWL07Z** Revision of Autologous Tissue Substitute in Lower Back, Open Approach
● **0WWL0JZ** Revision of Synthetic Substitute in Lower Back, Open Approach
● **0WWL0KZ** Revision of Nonautologous Tissue Substitute in Lower Back, Open Approach
● **0WWL0YZ** Revision of Other Device in Lower Back, Open Approach
● **0WWL30Z** Revision of Drainage Device in Lower Back, Percutaneous Approach
● **0WWL31Z** Revision of Radioactive Element in Lower Back, Percutaneous Approach
● **0WWL33Z** Revision of Infusion Device in Lower Back, Percutaneous Approach
● **0WWL37Z** Revision of Autologous Tissue Substitute in Lower Back, Percutaneous Approach
● **0WWL3JZ** Revision of Synthetic Substitute in Lower Back, Percutaneous Approach
● **0WWL3KZ** Revision of Nonautologous Tissue Substitute in Lower Back, Percutaneous Approach
● **0WWL3YZ** Revision of Other Device in Lower Back, Percutaneous Approach
● **0WWL40Z** Revision of Drainage Device in Lower Back, Percutaneous Endoscopic Approach
● **0WWL41Z** Revision of Radioactive Element in Lower Back, Percutaneous Endoscopic Approach
● **0WWL43Z** Revision of Infusion Device in Lower Back, Percutaneous Endoscopic Approach
● **0WWL47Z** Revision of Autologous Tissue Substitute in Lower Back, Percutaneous Endoscopic Approach
● **0WWL4JZ** Revision of Synthetic Substitute in Lower Back, Percutaneous Endoscopic Approach
● **0WWL4KZ** Revision of Nonautologous Tissue Substitute in Lower Back, Percutaneous Endoscopic Approach
● **0WWL4YZ** Revision of Other Device in Lower Back, Percutaneous Endoscopic Approach
0WWLX0Z Revision of Drainage Device in Lower Back, External Approach
0WWLX1Z Revision of Radioactive Element in Lower Back, External Approach
0WWLX3Z Revision of Infusion Device in Lower Back, External Approach
0WWLX7Z Revision of Autologous Tissue Substitute in Lower Back, External Approach
0WWLXJZ Revision of Synthetic Substitute in Lower Back, External Approach
0WWLXKZ Revision of Nonautologous Tissue Substitute in Lower Back, External Approach
0WWLXYZ Revision of Other Device in Lower Back, External Approach
♂ ● **0WWM00Z** Revision of Drainage Device in Male Perineum, Open Approach
♂ ● **0WWM01Z** Revision of Radioactive Element in Male Perineum, Open Approach
♂ ● **0WWM03Z** Revision of Infusion Device in Male Perineum, Open Approach
♂ **0WWM07Z** Revision of Autologous Tissue Substitute in Male Perineum, Open Approach
♂ ● **0WWM0JZ** Revision of Synthetic Substitute in Male Perineum, Open Approach
♂ **0WWM0KZ** Revision of Nonautologous Tissue Substitute in Male Perineum, Open Approach
♂ ● **0WWM0YZ** Revision of Other Device in Male Perineum, Open Approach
♂ ● **0WWM30Z** Revision of Drainage Device in Male Perineum, Percutaneous Approach
♂ ● **0WWM31Z** Revision of Radioactive Element in Male Perineum, Percutaneous Approach
♂ ● **0WWM33Z** Revision of Infusion Device in Male Perineum, Percutaneous Approach
♂ **0WWM37Z** Revision of Autologous Tissue Substitute in Male Perineum, Percutaneous Approach
♂ ● **0WWM3JZ** Revision of Synthetic Substitute in Male Perineum, Percutaneous Approach
♂ **0WWM3KZ** Revision of Nonautologous Tissue Substitute in Male Perineum, Percutaneous Approach
♂ ● **0WWM3YZ** Revision of Other Device in Male Perineum, Percutaneous Approach
♂ ● **0WWM40Z** Revision of Drainage Device in Male Perineum, Percutaneous Endoscopic Approach
♂ ● **0WWM41Z** Revision of Radioactive Element in Male Perineum, Percutaneous Endoscopic Approach
♂ ● **0WWM43Z** Revision of Infusion Device in Male Perineum, Percutaneous Endoscopic Approach
♂ **0WWM47Z** Revision of Autologous Tissue Substitute in Male Perineum, Percutaneous Endoscopic Approach
♂ ● **0WWM4JZ** Revision of Synthetic Substitute in Male Perineum, Percutaneous Endoscopic Approach

♂0WWM4KZ Revision of Nonautologous Tissue Substitute in Male Perineum, Percutaneous Endoscopic Approach
♂●0WWM4YZ Revision of Other Device in Male Perineum, Percutaneous Endoscopic Approach
♂0WWMX0Z Revision of Drainage Device in Male Perineum, External Approach
♂0WWMX1Z Revision of Radioactive Element in Male Perineum, External Approach
♂0WWMX3Z Revision of Infusion Device in Male Perineum, External Approach
♂0WWMX7Z Revision of Autologous Tissue Substitute in Male Perineum, External Approach
♂0WWMXJZ Revision of Synthetic Substitute in Male Perineum, External Approach
♂0WWMXKZ Revision of Nonautologous Tissue Substitute in Male Perineum, External Approach
This is a male-only service, however, it is not included in the male-only edit logic for MCE V30
♂0WWMXYZ Revision of Other Device in Male Perineum, External Approach
This is a male-only service, however, it is not included in the male-only edit logic for MCE V30
♀0WWN00Z Revision of Drainage Device in Female Perineum, Open Approach
♀0WWN01Z Revision of Radioactive Element in Female Perineum, Open Approach
♀0WWN03Z Revision of Infusion Device in Female Perineum, Open Approach
♀0WWN07Z Revision of Autologous Tissue Substitute in Female Perineum, Open Approach
♀0WWN0JZ Revision of Synthetic Substitute in Female Perineum, Open Approach
♀0WWN0KZ Revision of Nonautologous Tissue Substitute in Female Perineum, Open Approach
♀0WWN0YZ Revision of Other Device in Female Perineum, Open Approach
♀0WWN30Z Revision of Drainage Device in Female Perineum, Percutaneous Approach
♀0WWN31Z Revision of Radioactive Element in Female Perineum, Percutaneous Approach
♀0WWN33Z Revision of Infusion Device in Female Perineum, Percutaneous Approach
♀0WWN37Z Revision of Autologous Tissue Substitute in Female Perineum, Percutaneous Approach
♀0WWN3JZ Revision of Synthetic Substitute in Female Perineum, Percutaneous Approach
♀0WWN3KZ Revision of Nonautologous Tissue Substitute in Female Perineum, Percutaneous Approach
♀0WWN3YZ Revision of Other Device in Female Perineum, Percutaneous Approach
♀0WWN40Z Revision of Drainage Device in Female Perineum, Percutaneous Endoscopic Approach
♀0WWN41Z Revision of Radioactive Element in Female Perineum, Percutaneous Endoscopic Approach
♀0WWN43Z Revision of Infusion Device in Female Perineum, Percutaneous Endoscopic Approach
♀0WWN47Z Revision of Autologous Tissue Substitute in Female Perineum, Percutaneous Endoscopic Approach
♀0WWN4JZ Revision of Synthetic Substitute in Female Perineum, Percutaneous Endoscopic Approach
♀ 0WWN4KZ Revision of Nonautologous Tissue Substitute in Female Perineum, Percutaneous Endoscopic Approach
♀ 0WWN4YZ Revision of Other Device in Female Perineum, Percutaneous Endoscopic Approach
♀ 0WWNX0Z Revision of Drainage Device in Female Perineum, External Approach
♀ 0WWNX1Z Revision of Radioactive Element in Female Perineum, External Approach
♀ 0WWNX3Z Revision of Infusion Device in Female Perineum, External Approach
♀ 0WWNX7Z Revision of Autologous Tissue Substitute in Female Perineum, External Approach
♀ 0WWNXJZ Revision of Synthetic Substitute in Female Perineum, External Approach
♀ 0WWNXKZ Revision of Nonautologous Tissue Substitute in Female Perineum, External Approach
♀ 0WWNXYZ Revision of Other Device in Female Perineum, External Approach
0WWP01Z Revision of Radioactive Element in Gastrointestinal Tract, Open Approach
0WWP03Z Revision of Infusion Device in Gastrointestinal Tract, Open Approach
0WWP0YZ Revision of Other Device in Gastrointestinal Tract, Open Approach
0WWP31Z Revision of Radioactive Element in Gastrointestinal Tract, Percutaneous Approach
0WWP33Z Revision of Infusion Device in Gastrointestinal Tract, Percutaneous Approach
0WWP3YZ Revision of Other Device in Gastrointestinal Tract, Percutaneous Approach
0WWP41Z Revision of Radioactive Element in Gastrointestinal Tract, Percutaneous Endoscopic Approach
0WWP43Z Revision of Infusion Device in Gastrointestinal Tract, Percutaneous Endoscopic Approach
0WWP4YZ Revision of Other Device in Gastrointestinal Tract, Percutaneous Endoscopic Approach
0WWP71Z Revision of Radioactive Element in Gastrointestinal Tract, Via Natural or Artificial Opening
0WWP73Z Revision of Infusion Device in Gastrointestinal Tract, Via Natural or Artificial Opening
0WWP7YZ Revision of Other Device in Gastrointestinal Tract, Via Natural or Artificial Opening
0WWP81Z Revision of Radioactive Element in Gastrointestinal Tract, Via Natural or Artificial Opening Endoscopic
0WWP83Z Revision of Infusion Device in Gastrointestinal Tract, Via Natural or Artificial Opening Endoscopic
0WWP8YZ Revision of Other Device in Gastrointestinal Tract, Via Natural or Artificial Opening Endoscopic
0WWPX1Z Revision of Radioactive Element in Gastrointestinal Tract, External Approach
0WWPX3Z Revision of Infusion Device in Gastrointestinal Tract, External Approach
0WWPXYZ Revision of Other Device in Gastrointestinal Tract, External Approach
0WWQ01Z Revision of Radioactive Element in Respiratory Tract, Open Approach
0WWQ03Z Revision of Infusion Device in Respiratory Tract, Open Approach
0WWQ0YZ Revision of Other Device in Respiratory Tract, Open Approach
0WWQ31Z Revision of Radioactive Element in Respiratory Tract, Percutaneous Approach
0WWQ33Z Revision of Infusion Device in Respiratory Tract, Percutaneous Approach
0WWQ3YZ Revision of Other Device in Respiratory Tract, Percutaneous Approach
0WWQ41Z Revision of Radioactive Element in Respiratory Tract, Percutaneous Endoscopic Approach
0WWQ43Z Revision of Infusion Device in Respiratory Tract, Percutaneous Endoscopic Approach
0WWQ4YZ Revision of Other Device in Respiratory Tract, Percutaneous Endoscopic Approach
0WWQ71Z Revision of Radioactive Element in Respiratory Tract, Via Natural or Artificial Opening
0WWQ73Z Revision of Infusion Device in Respiratory Tract, Via Natural or Artificial Opening
0WWQ7YZ Revision of Other Device in Respiratory Tract, Via Natural or Artificial Opening
0WWQ81Z Revision of Radioactive Element in Respiratory Tract, Via Natural or Artificial Opening Endoscopic
0WWQ83Z Revision of Infusion Device in Respiratory Tract, Via Natural or Artificial Opening Endoscopic
0WWQ8YZ Revision of Other Device in Respiratory Tract, Via Natural or Artificial Opening Endoscopic
0WWQX1Z Revision of Radioactive Element in Respiratory Tract, External Approach
0WWQX3Z Revision of Infusion Device in Respiratory Tract, External Approach
0WWQXYZ Revision of Other Device in Respiratory Tract, External Approach
0WWR01Z Revision of Radioactive Element in Genitourinary Tract, Open Approach
0WWR03Z Revision of Infusion Device in Genitourinary Tract, Open Approach
0WWR0YZ Revision of Other Device in Genitourinary Tract, Open Approach
0WWR31Z Revision of Radioactive Element in Genitourinary Tract, Percutaneous Approach
0WWR33Z Revision of Infusion Device in Genitourinary Tract, Percutaneous Approach
0WWR3YZ Revision of Other Device in Genitourinary Tract, Percutaneous Approach
0WWR41Z Revision of Radioactive Element in Genitourinary Tract, Percutaneous Endoscopic Approach
0WWR43Z Revision of Infusion Device in Genitourinary Tract, Percutaneous Endoscopic Approach
0WWR4YZ Revision of Other Device in Genitourinary Tract, Percutaneous Endoscopic Approach
0WWR71Z Revision of Radioactive Element in Genitourinary Tract, Via Natural or Artificial Opening
0WWR73Z Revision of Infusion Device in Genitourinary Tract, Via Natural or Artificial Opening
0WWR7YZ Revision of Other Device in Genitourinary Tract, Via Natural or Artificial Opening

0WWR81Z Revision of Radioactive Element in Genitourinary Tract, Via Natural or Artificial Opening Endoscopic

0WWR83Z Revision of Infusion Device in Genitourinary Tract, Via Natural or Artificial Opening Endoscopic

0WWR8YZ Revision of Other Device in Genitourinary Tract, Via Natural or Artificial Opening Endoscopic

0WWRX1Z Revision of Radioactive Element in Genitourinary Tract, External Approach

0WWRX3Z Revision of Infusion Device in Genitourinary Tract, External Approach

0WWRXYZ Revision of Other Device in Genitourinary Tract, External Approach

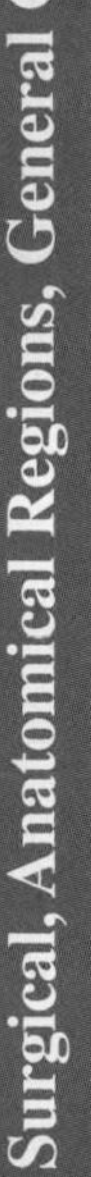

Anatomical Regions, Upper Extremities Tables 0X0–0XX

Section 0 **Medical and Surgical**
Body System X **Anatomical Regions, Upper Extremities**
Operation 0 **Alteration:** Modifying the anatomic structure of a body part without affecting the function of the body part

Body Part (4th)	Approach (5th)	Device (6th)	Qualifier (7th)
2 Shoulder Region, Right **3** Shoulder Region, Left **4** Axilla, Right **5** Axilla, Left **6** Upper Extremity, Right **7** Upper Extremity, Left **8** Upper Arm, Right **9** Upper Arm, Left **B** Elbow Region, Right **C** Elbow Region, Left **D** Lower Arm, Right **F** Lower Arm, Left **G** Wrist Region, Right **H** Wrist Region, Left	**0** Open **3** Percutaneous **4** Percutaneous Endoscopic	**7** Autologous Tissue Substitute **J** Synthetic Substitute **K** Nonautologous Tissue Substitute **Z** No Device	**Z** No Qualifier

Section 0 **Medical and Surgical**
Body System X **Anatomical Regions, Upper Extremities**
Operation 2 **Change:** Taking out or off a device from a body part and putting back an identical or similar device in or on the same body part without cutting or puncturing the skin or a mucous membrane

Body Part (4th)	Approach (5th)	Device (6th)	Qualifier (7th)
6 Upper Extremity, Right **7** Upper Extremity, Left	**X** External	**0** Drainage Device **Y** Other Device	**Z** No Qualifier

Section 0 **Medical and Surgical**
Body System X **Anatomical Regions, Upper Extremities**
Operation 3 **Control:** Stopping, or attempting to stop, postprocedural bleeding

Body Part (4th)	Approach (5th)	Device (6th)	Qualifier (7th)
2 Shoulder Region, Right **3** Shoulder Region, Left **4** Axilla, Right **5** Axilla, Left **6** Upper Extremity, Right **7** Upper Extremity, Left **8** Upper Arm, Right **9** Upper Arm, Left **B** Elbow Region, Right **C** Elbow Region, Left **D** Lower Arm, Right **F** Lower Arm, Left **G** Wrist Region, Right **H** Wrist Region, Left **J** Hand, Right **K** Hand, Left	**0** Open **3** Percutaneous **4** Percutaneous Endoscopic	**Z** No Device	**Z** No Qualifier

Section 0 **Medical and Surgical**
Body System X **Anatomical Regions, Upper Extremities**
Operation 6 **Detachment:** Cutting off all or a portion of the upper or lower extremities

Body Part (4th)	Approach (5th)	Device (6th)	Qualifier (7th)
0 Forequarter, Right **1** Forequarter, Left **2** Shoulder Region, Right **3** Shoulder Region, Left **B** Elbow Region, Right **C** Elbow Region, Left	**0** Open	**Z** No Device	**Z** No Qualifier
8 Upper Arm, Right **9** Upper Arm, Left **D** Lower Arm, Right **F** Lower Arm, Left	**0** Open	**Z** No Device	**1** High **2** Mid **3** Low
J Hand, Right **K** Hand, Left	**0** Open	**Z** No Device	**0** Complete **4** Complete 1st Ray **5** Complete 2nd Ray **6** Complete 3rd Ray **7** Complete 4th Ray **8** Complete 5th Ray **9** Partial 1st Ray **B** Partial 2nd Ray **C** Partial 3rd Ray **D** Partial 4th Ray **F** Partial 5th Ray
L Thumb, Right **M** Thumb, Left **N** Index Finger, Right **P** Index Finger, Left **Q** Middle Finger, Right **R** Middle Finger, Left **S** Ring Finger, Right **T** Ring Finger, Left **V** Little Finger, Right **W** Little Finger, Left	**0** Open	**Z** No Device	**0** Complete **1** High **2** Mid **3** Low

Section 0 **Medical and Surgical**
Body System X **Anatomical Regions, Upper Extremities**
Operation 9 **Drainage:** Taking or letting out fluids and/or gases from a body part

Body Part (4th)	Approach (5th)	Device (6th)	Qualifier (7th)
2 Shoulder Region, Right **3** Shoulder Region, Left **4** Axilla, Right **5** Axilla, Left **6** Upper Extremity, Right **7** Upper Extremity, Left **8** Upper Arm, Right **9** Upper Arm, Left **B** Elbow Region, Right **C** Elbow Region, Left **D** Lower Arm, Right **F** Lower Arm, Left **G** Wrist Region, Right **H** Wrist Region, Left **J** Hand, Right **K** Hand, Left	**0** Open **3** Percutaneous **4** Percutaneous Endoscopic	**0** Drainage Device	**Z** No Qualifier

Continued →

Section 0 Medical and Surgical
Body System X Anatomical Regions, Upper Extremities
Operation 9 **Drainage:** Taking or letting out fluids and/or gases from a body part

Body Part (4th)	Approach (5th)	Device (6th)	Qualifier (7th)
2 Shoulder Region, Right 3 Shoulder Region, Left 4 Axilla, Right 5 Axilla, Left 6 Upper Extremity, Right 7 Upper Extremity, Left 8 Upper Arm, Right 9 Upper Arm, Left B Elbow Region, Right C Elbow Region, Left D Lower Arm, Right F Lower Arm, Left G Wrist Region, Right H Wrist Region, Left J Hand, Right K Hand, Left	0 Open 3 Percutaneous 4 Percutaneous Endoscopic	Z No Device	X Diagnostic Z No Qualifier

Section 0 Medical and Surgical
Body System X Anatomical Regions, Upper Extremities
Operation B **Excision:** Cutting out or off, without replacement, a portion of a body part

Body Part (4th)	Approach (5th)	Device (6th)	Qualifier (7th)
2 Shoulder Region, Right 3 Shoulder Region, Left 4 Axilla, Right 5 Axilla, Left 6 Upper Extremity, Right 7 Upper Extremity, Left 8 Upper Arm, Right 9 Upper Arm, Left B Elbow Region, Right C Elbow Region, Left D Lower Arm, Right F Lower Arm, Left G Wrist Region, Right H Wrist Region, Left J Hand, Right K Hand, Left	0 Open 3 Percutaneous 4 Percutaneous Endoscopic	Z No Device	X Diagnostic Z No Qualifier

Section 0 Medical and Surgical
Body System X Anatomical Regions, Upper Extremities
Operation H **Insertion:** Putting in a nonbiological appliance that monitors, assists, performs, or prevents a physiological function but does not physically take the place of a body part

Body Part (4th)	Approach (5th)	Device (6th)	Qualifier (7th)
2 Shoulder Region, Right 3 Shoulder Region, Left 4 Axilla, Right 5 Axilla, Left 6 Upper Extremity, Right 7 Upper Extremity, Left 8 Upper Arm, Right 9 Upper Arm, Left B Elbow Region, Right C Elbow Region, Left D Lower Arm, Right F Lower Arm, Left G Wrist Region, Right H Wrist Region, Left J Hand, Right K Hand, Left	0 Open 3 Percutaneous 4 Percutaneous Endoscopic	1 Radioactive Element 3 Infusion Device Y Other Device	Z No Qualifier

Section 0 **Medical and Surgical**
Body System X **Anatomical Regions, Upper Extremities**
Operation J **Inspection:** Visually and/or manually exploring a body part

Body Part (4th)	Approach (5th)	Device (6th)	Qualifier (7th)
2 Shoulder Region, Right **3** Shoulder Region, Left **4** Axilla, Right **5** Axilla, Left **6** Upper Extremity, Right **7** Upper Extremity, Left **8** Upper Arm, Right **9** Upper Arm, Left **B** Elbow Region, Right **C** Elbow Region, Left **D** Lower Arm, Right **F** Lower Arm, Left **G** Wrist Region, Right **H** Wrist Region, Left **J** Hand, Right **K** Hand, Left	**0** Open **3** Percutaneous **4** Percutaneous Endoscopic **X** External	**Z** No Device	**Z** No Qualifier

Section 0 **Medical and Surgical**
Body System X **Anatomical Regions, Upper Extremities**
Operation M **Reattachment:** Putting back in or on all or a portion of a separated body part to its normal location or other suitable location

Body Part (4th)	Approach (5th)	Device (6th)	Qualifier (7th)
0 Forequarter, Right **1** Forequarter, Left **2** Shoulder Region, Right **3** Shoulder Region, Left **4** Axilla, Right **5** Axilla, Left **6** Upper Extremity, Right **7** Upper Extremity, Left **8** Upper Arm, Right **9** Upper Arm, Left **B** Elbow Region, Right **C** Elbow Region, Left **D** Lower Arm, Right **F** Lower Arm, Left **G** Wrist Region, Right **H** Wrist Region, Left **J** Hand, Right **K** Hand, Left **L** Thumb, Right **M** Thumb, Left **N** Index Finger, Right **P** Index Finger, Left **Q** Middle Finger, Right **R** Middle Finger, Left **S** Ring Finger, Right **T** Ring Finger, Left **V** Little Finger, Right **W** Little Finger, Left	**0** Open	**Z** No Device	**Z** No Qualifier

Section 0 **Medical and Surgical**
Body System X **Anatomical Regions, Upper Extremities**
Operation P **Removal:** Taking out or off a device from a body part

Body Part (4th)	Approach (5th)	Device (6th)	Qualifier (7th)
6 Upper Extremity, Right **7** Upper Extremity, Left	**0** Open **3** Percutaneous **4** Percutaneous Endoscopic **X** External	**0** Drainage Device **1** Radioactive Element **3** Infusion Device **7** Autologous Tissue Substitute **J** Synthetic Substitute **K** Nonautologous Tissue Substitute **Y** Other Device	**Z** No Qualifier

Section 0 **Medical and Surgical**
Body System X **Anatomical Regions, Upper Extremities**
Operation Q **Repair:** Restoring, to the extent possible, a body part to its normal anatomic structure and function

Body Part (4th)	Approach (5th)	Device (6th)	Qualifier (7th)
2 Shoulder Region, Right **3** Shoulder Region, Left **4** Axilla, Right **5** Axilla, Left **6** Upper Extremity, Right **7** Upper Extremity, Left **8** Upper Arm, Right **9** Upper Arm, Left **B** Elbow Region, Right **C** Elbow Region, Left **D** Lower Arm, Right **F** Lower Arm, Left **G** Wrist Region, Right **H** Wrist Region, Left **J** Hand, Right **K** Hand, Left **L** Thumb, Right **M** Thumb, Left **N** Index Finger, Right **P** Index Finger, Left **Q** Middle Finger, Right **R** Middle Finger, Left **S** Ring Finger, Right **T** Ring Finger, Left **V** Little Finger, Right **W** Little Finger, Left	**0** Open **3** Percutaneous **4** Percutaneous Endoscopic **X** External	**Z** No Device	**Z** No Qualifier

Section 0 **Medical and Surgical**
Body System X **Anatomical Regions, Upper Extremities**
Operation R **Replacement:** Putting in or on biological or synthetic material that physically takes the place and/or function of all or a portion of a body part

Body Part (4th)	Approach (5th)	Device (6th)	Qualifier (7th)
L Thumb, Right **M** Thumb, Left	**0** Open **4** Percutaneous Endoscopic	**7** Autologous Tissue Substitute	**N** Toe, Right **P** Toe, Left

Section 0 **Medical and Surgical**
Body System X **Anatomical Regions, Upper Extremities**
Operation U **Supplement:** Putting in or on biological or synthetic material that physically reinforces and/or augments the function of a portion of a body part

Body Part (4th)	Approach (5th)	Device (6th)	Qualifier (7th)
2 Shoulder Region, Right **3** Shoulder Region, Left **4** Axilla, Right **5** Axilla, Left **6** Upper Extremity, Right **7** Upper Extremity, Left **8** Upper Arm, Right **9** Upper Arm, Left **B** Elbow Region, Right **C** Elbow Region, Left **D** Lower Arm, Right **F** Lower Arm, Left **G** Wrist Region, Right **H** Wrist Region, Left **J** Hand, Right **K** Hand, Left **L** Thumb, Right **M** Thumb, Left **N** Index Finger, Right **P** Index Finger, Left **Q** Middle Finger, Right **R** Middle Finger, Left **S** Ring Finger, Right **T** Ring Finger, Left **V** Little Finger, Right **W** Little Finger, Left	**0** Open **4** Percutaneous Endoscopic	**7** Autologous Tissue Substitute **J** Synthetic Substitute **K** Nonautologous Tissue Substitute	**Z** No Qualifier

Section 0 **Medical and Surgical**
Body System X **Anatomical Regions, Upper Extremities**
Operation W **Revision:** Correcting, to the extent possible, a portion of a malfunctioning device or the position of a displaced device

Body Part (4th)	Approach (5th)	Device (6th)	Qualifier (7th)
6 Upper Extremity, Right **7** Upper Extremity, Left	**0** Open **3** Percutaneous **4** Percutaneous Endoscopic **X** External	**0** Drainage Device **3** Infusion Device **7** Autologous Tissue Substitute **J** Synthetic Substitute **K** Nonautologous Tissue Substitute **Y** Other Device	**Z** No Qualifier

Section 0 **Medical and Surgical**
Body System X **Anatomical Regions, Upper Extremities**
Operation X **Transfer:** Moving, without taking out, all or a portion of a body part to another location to take over the function of all or a portion of a body part

Body Part (4th)	Approach (5th)	Device (6th)	Qualifier (7th)
N Index Finger, Right	**0** Open	**Z** No Device	**L** Thumb, Right
P Index Finger, Left	**0** Open	**Z** No Device	**M** Thumb, Left

Anatomical Regions, Upper Extremities Code Listing 0X0–0XX

0X0 – Anatomical Regions, Upper Extremities, Alteration

0X0207Z Alteration of Right Shoulder Region with Autologous Tissue Substitute, Open Approach
0X020JZ Alteration of Right Shoulder Region with Synthetic Substitute, Open Approach
0X020KZ Alteration of Right Shoulder Region with Nonautologous Tissue Substitute, Open Approach
0X020ZZ Alteration of Right Shoulder Region, Open Approach
0X0237Z Alteration of Right Shoulder Region with Autologous Tissue Substitute, Percutaneous Approach
0X023JZ Alteration of Right Shoulder Region with Synthetic Substitute, Percutaneous Approach
0X023KZ Alteration of Right Shoulder Region with Nonautologous Tissue Substitute, Percutaneous Approach
0X023ZZ Alteration of Right Shoulder Region, Percutaneous Approach
0X0247Z Alteration of Right Shoulder Region with Autologous Tissue Substitute, Percutaneous Endoscopic Approach
0X024JZ Alteration of Right Shoulder Region with Synthetic Substitute, Percutaneous Endoscopic Approach
0X024KZ Alteration of Right Shoulder Region with Nonautologous Tissue Substitute, Percutaneous Endoscopic Approach
0X024ZZ Alteration of Right Shoulder Region, Percutaneous Endoscopic Approach
0X0307Z Alteration of Left Shoulder Region with Autologous Tissue Substitute, Open Approach
0X030JZ Alteration of Left Shoulder Region with Synthetic Substitute, Open Approach
0X030KZ Alteration of Left Shoulder Region with Nonautologous Tissue Substitute, Open Approach
0X030ZZ Alteration of Left Shoulder Region, Open Approach
0X0337Z Alteration of Left Shoulder Region with Autologous Tissue Substitute, Percutaneous Approach
0X033JZ Alteration of Left Shoulder Region with Synthetic Substitute, Percutaneous Approach
0X033KZ Alteration of Left Shoulder Region with Nonautologous Tissue Substitute, Percutaneous Approach
0X033ZZ Alteration of Left Shoulder Region, Percutaneous Approach
0X0347Z Alteration of Left Shoulder Region with Autologous Tissue Substitute, Percutaneous Endoscopic Approach
0X034JZ Alteration of Left Shoulder Region with Synthetic Substitute, Percutaneous Endoscopic Approach
0X034KZ Alteration of Left Shoulder Region with Nonautologous Tissue Substitute, Percutaneous Endoscopic Approach
0X034ZZ Alteration of Left Shoulder Region, Percutaneous Endoscopic Approach
0X0407Z Alteration of Right Axilla with Autologous Tissue Substitute, Open Approach
0X040JZ Alteration of Right Axilla with Synthetic Substitute, Open Approach
0X040KZ Alteration of Right Axilla with Nonautologous Tissue Substitute, Open Approach
0X040ZZ Alteration of Right Axilla, Open Approach
0X0437Z Alteration of Right Axilla with Autologous Tissue Substitute, Percutaneous Approach
0X043JZ Alteration of Right Axilla with Synthetic Substitute, Percutaneous Approach
0X043KZ Alteration of Right Axilla with Nonautologous Tissue Substitute, Percutaneous Approach
0X043ZZ Alteration of Right Axilla, Percutaneous Approach
0X0447Z Alteration of Right Axilla with Autologous Tissue Substitute, Percutaneous Endoscopic Approach
0X044JZ Alteration of Right Axilla with Synthetic Substitute, Percutaneous Endoscopic Approach
0X044KZ Alteration of Right Axilla with Nonautologous Tissue Substitute, Percutaneous Endoscopic Approach
0X044ZZ Alteration of Right Axilla, Percutaneous Endoscopic Approach
0X0507Z Alteration of Left Axilla with Autologous Tissue Substitute, Open Approach
0X050JZ Alteration of Left Axilla with Synthetic Substitute, Open Approach
0X050KZ Alteration of Left Axilla with Nonautologous Tissue Substitute, Open Approach
0X050ZZ Alteration of Left Axilla, Open Approach
0X0537Z Alteration of Left Axilla with Autologous Tissue Substitute, Percutaneous Approach
0X053JZ Alteration of Left Axilla with Synthetic Substitute, Percutaneous Approach
0X053KZ Alteration of Left Axilla with Nonautologous Tissue Substitute, Percutaneous Approach
0X053ZZ Alteration of Left Axilla, Percutaneous Approach
0X0547Z Alteration of Left Axilla with Autologous Tissue Substitute, Percutaneous Endoscopic Approach
0X054JZ Alteration of Left Axilla with Synthetic Substitute, Percutaneous Endoscopic Approach
0X054KZ Alteration of Left Axilla with Nonautologous Tissue Substitute, Percutaneous Endoscopic Approach
0X054ZZ Alteration of Left Axilla, Percutaneous Endoscopic Approach
0X0607Z Alteration of Right Upper Extremity with Autologous Tissue Substitute, Open Approach
0X060JZ Alteration of Right Upper Extremity with Synthetic Substitute, Open Approach
0X060KZ Alteration of Right Upper Extremity with Nonautologous Tissue Substitute, Open Approach
0X060ZZ Alteration of Right Upper Extremity, Open Approach
0X0637Z Alteration of Right Upper Extremity with Autologous Tissue Substitute, Percutaneous Approach
0X063JZ Alteration of Right Upper Extremity with Synthetic Substitute, Percutaneous Approach
0X063KZ Alteration of Right Upper Extremity with Nonautologous Tissue Substitute, Percutaneous Approach
0X063ZZ Alteration of Right Upper Extremity, Percutaneous Approach
0X0647Z Alteration of Right Upper Extremity with Autologous Tissue Substitute, Percutaneous Endoscopic Approach
0X064JZ Alteration of Right Upper Extremity with Synthetic Substitute, Percutaneous Endoscopic Approach
0X064KZ Alteration of Right Upper Extremity with Nonautologous Tissue Substitute, Percutaneous Endoscopic Approach
0X064ZZ Alteration of Right Upper Extremity, Percutaneous Endoscopic Approach
0X0707Z Alteration of Left Upper Extremity with Autologous Tissue Substitute, Open Approach
0X070JZ Alteration of Left Upper Extremity with Synthetic Substitute, Open Approach
0X070KZ Alteration of Left Upper Extremity with Nonautologous Tissue Substitute, Open Approach
0X070ZZ Alteration of Left Upper Extremity, Open Approach
0X0737Z Alteration of Left Upper Extremity with Autologous Tissue Substitute, Percutaneous Approach
0X073JZ Alteration of Left Upper Extremity with Synthetic Substitute, Percutaneous Approach
0X073KZ Alteration of Left Upper Extremity with Nonautologous Tissue Substitute, Percutaneous Approach
0X073ZZ Alteration of Left Upper Extremity, Percutaneous Approach
0X0747Z Alteration of Left Upper Extremity with Autologous Tissue Substitute, Percutaneous Endoscopic Approach
0X074JZ Alteration of Left Upper Extremity with Synthetic Substitute, Percutaneous Endoscopic Approach
0X074KZ Alteration of Left Upper Extremity with Nonautologous Tissue Substitute, Percutaneous Endoscopic Approach
0X074ZZ Alteration of Left Upper Extremity, Percutaneous Endoscopic Approach
0X0807Z Alteration of Right Upper Arm with Autologous Tissue Substitute, Open Approach
0X080JZ Alteration of Right Upper Arm with Synthetic Substitute, Open Approach
0X080KZ Alteration of Right Upper Arm with Nonautologous Tissue Substitute, Open Approach
0X080ZZ Alteration of Right Upper Arm, Open Approach
0X0837Z Alteration of Right Upper Arm with Autologous Tissue Substitute, Percutaneous Approach
0X083JZ Alteration of Right Upper Arm with Synthetic Substitute, Percutaneous Approach
0X083KZ Alteration of Right Upper Arm with Nonautologous Tissue Substitute, Percutaneous Approach
0X083ZZ Alteration of Right Upper Arm, Percutaneous Approach
0X0847Z Alteration of Right Upper Arm with Autologous Tissue Substitute, Percutaneous Endoscopic Approach
0X084JZ Alteration of Right Upper Arm with Synthetic Substitute, Percutaneous Endoscopic Approach
0X084KZ Alteration of Right Upper Arm with Nonautologous Tissue Substitute, Percutaneous Endoscopic Approach
0X084ZZ Alteration of Right Upper Arm, Percutaneous Endoscopic Approach

0X0907Z Alteration of Left Upper Arm with Autologous Tissue Substitute, Open Approach
0X090JZ Alteration of Left Upper Arm with Synthetic Substitute, Open Approach
0X090KZ Alteration of Left Upper Arm with Nonautologous Tissue Substitute, Open Approach
0X090ZZ Alteration of Left Upper Arm, Open Approach
0X0937Z Alteration of Left Upper Arm with Autologous Tissue Substitute, Percutaneous Approach
0X093JZ Alteration of Left Upper Arm with Synthetic Substitute, Percutaneous Approach
0X093KZ Alteration of Left Upper Arm with Nonautologous Tissue Substitute, Percutaneous Approach
0X093ZZ Alteration of Left Upper Arm, Percutaneous Approach
0X0947Z Alteration of Left Upper Arm with Autologous Tissue Substitute, Percutaneous Endoscopic Approach
0X094JZ Alteration of Left Upper Arm with Synthetic Substitute, Percutaneous Endoscopic Approach
0X094KZ Alteration of Left Upper Arm with Nonautologous Tissue Substitute, Percutaneous Endoscopic Approach
0X094ZZ Alteration of Left Upper Arm, Percutaneous Endoscopic Approach
0X0B07Z Alteration of Right Elbow Region with Autologous Tissue Substitute, Open Approach
0X0B0JZ Alteration of Right Elbow Region with Synthetic Substitute, Open Approach
0X0B0KZ Alteration of Right Elbow Region with Nonautologous Tissue Substitute, Open Approach
0X0B0ZZ Alteration of Right Elbow Region, Open Approach
0X0B37Z Alteration of Right Elbow Region with Autologous Tissue Substitute, Percutaneous Approach
0X0B3JZ Alteration of Right Elbow Region with Synthetic Substitute, Percutaneous Approach
0X0B3KZ Alteration of Right Elbow Region with Nonautologous Tissue Substitute, Percutaneous Approach
0X0B3ZZ Alteration of Right Elbow Region, Percutaneous Approach
0X0B47Z Alteration of Right Elbow Region with Autologous Tissue Substitute, Percutaneous Endoscopic Approach
0X0B4JZ Alteration of Right Elbow Region with Synthetic Substitute, Percutaneous Endoscopic Approach
0X0B4KZ Alteration of Right Elbow Region with Nonautologous Tissue Substitute, Percutaneous Endoscopic Approach
0X0B4ZZ Alteration of Right Elbow Region, Percutaneous Endoscopic Approach
0X0C07Z Alteration of Left Elbow Region with Autologous Tissue Substitute, Open Approach
0X0C0JZ Alteration of Left Elbow Region with Synthetic Substitute, Open Approach
0X0C0KZ Alteration of Left Elbow Region with Nonautologous Tissue Substitute, Open Approach
0X0C0ZZ Alteration of Left Elbow Region, Open Approach
0X0C37Z Alteration of Left Elbow Region with Autologous Tissue Substitute, Percutaneous Approach
0X0C3JZ Alteration of Left Elbow Region with Synthetic Substitute, Percutaneous Approach
0X0C3KZ Alteration of Left Elbow Region with Nonautologous Tissue Substitute, Percutaneous Approach
0X0C3ZZ Alteration of Left Elbow Region, Percutaneous Approach
0X0C47Z Alteration of Left Elbow Region with Autologous Tissue Substitute, Percutaneous Endoscopic Approach
0X0C4JZ Alteration of Left Elbow Region with Synthetic Substitute, Percutaneous Endoscopic Approach
0X0C4KZ Alteration of Left Elbow Region with Nonautologous Tissue Substitute, Percutaneous Endoscopic Approach
0X0C4ZZ Alteration of Left Elbow Region, Percutaneous Endoscopic Approach
0X0D07Z Alteration of Right Lower Arm with Autologous Tissue Substitute, Open Approach
0X0D0JZ Alteration of Right Lower Arm with Synthetic Substitute, Open Approach
0X0D0KZ Alteration of Right Lower Arm with Nonautologous Tissue Substitute, Open Approach
0X0D0ZZ Alteration of Right Lower Arm, Open Approach
0X0D37Z Alteration of Right Lower Arm with Autologous Tissue Substitute, Percutaneous Approach
0X0D3JZ Alteration of Right Lower Arm with Synthetic Substitute, Percutaneous Approach
0X0D3KZ Alteration of Right Lower Arm with Nonautologous Tissue Substitute, Percutaneous Approach
0X0D3ZZ Alteration of Right Lower Arm, Percutaneous Approach
0X0D47Z Alteration of Right Lower Arm with Autologous Tissue Substitute, Percutaneous Endoscopic Approach
0X0D4JZ Alteration of Right Lower Arm with Synthetic Substitute, Percutaneous Endoscopic Approach
0X0D4KZ Alteration of Right Lower Arm with Nonautologous Tissue Substitute, Percutaneous Endoscopic Approach
0X0D4ZZ Alteration of Right Lower Arm, Percutaneous Endoscopic Approach
0X0F07Z Alteration of Left Lower Arm with Autologous Tissue Substitute, Open Approach
0X0F0JZ Alteration of Left Lower Arm with Synthetic Substitute, Open Approach
0X0F0KZ Alteration of Left Lower Arm with Nonautologous Tissue Substitute, Open Approach
0X0F0ZZ Alteration of Left Lower Arm, Open Approach
0X0F37Z Alteration of Left Lower Arm with Autologous Tissue Substitute, Percutaneous Approach
0X0F3JZ Alteration of Left Lower Arm with Synthetic Substitute, Percutaneous Approach
0X0F3KZ Alteration of Left Lower Arm with Nonautologous Tissue Substitute, Percutaneous Approach
0X0F3ZZ Alteration of Left Lower Arm, Percutaneous Approach
0X0F47Z Alteration of Left Lower Arm with Autologous Tissue Substitute, Percutaneous Endoscopic Approach
0X0F4JZ Alteration of Left Lower Arm with Synthetic Substitute, Percutaneous Endoscopic Approach
0X0F4KZ Alteration of Left Lower Arm with Nonautologous Tissue Substitute, Percutaneous Endoscopic Approach
0X0F4ZZ Alteration of Left Lower Arm, Percutaneous Endoscopic Approach
0X0G07Z Alteration of Right Wrist Region with Autologous Tissue Substitute, Open Approach
0X0G0JZ Alteration of Right Wrist Region with Synthetic Substitute, Open Approach
0X0G0KZ Alteration of Right Wrist Region with Nonautologous Tissue Substitute, Open Approach
0X0G0ZZ Alteration of Right Wrist Region, Open Approach
0X0G37Z Alteration of Right Wrist Region with Autologous Tissue Substitute, Percutaneous Approach
0X0G3JZ Alteration of Right Wrist Region with Synthetic Substitute, Percutaneous Approach
0X0G3KZ Alteration of Right Wrist Region with Nonautologous Tissue Substitute, Percutaneous Approach
0X0G3ZZ Alteration of Right Wrist Region, Percutaneous Approach
0X0G47Z Alteration of Right Wrist Region with Autologous Tissue Substitute, Percutaneous Endoscopic Approach
0X0G4JZ Alteration of Right Wrist Region with Synthetic Substitute, Percutaneous Endoscopic Approach
0X0G4KZ Alteration of Right Wrist Region with Nonautologous Tissue Substitute, Percutaneous Endoscopic Approach
0X0G4ZZ Alteration of Right Wrist Region, Percutaneous Endoscopic Approach
0X0H07Z Alteration of Left Wrist Region with Autologous Tissue Substitute, Open Approach
0X0H0JZ Alteration of Left Wrist Region with Synthetic Substitute, Open Approach
0X0H0KZ Alteration of Left Wrist Region with Nonautologous Tissue Substitute, Open Approach
0X0H0ZZ Alteration of Left Wrist Region, Open Approach
0X0H37Z Alteration of Left Wrist Region with Autologous Tissue Substitute, Percutaneous Approach
0X0H3JZ Alteration of Left Wrist Region with Synthetic Substitute, Percutaneous Approach
0X0H3KZ Alteration of Left Wrist Region with Nonautologous Tissue Substitute, Percutaneous Approach
0X0H3ZZ Alteration of Left Wrist Region, Percutaneous Approach
0X0H47Z Alteration of Left Wrist Region with Autologous Tissue Substitute, Percutaneous Endoscopic Approach
0X0H4JZ Alteration of Left Wrist Region with Synthetic Substitute, Percutaneous Endoscopic Approach
0X0H4KZ Alteration of Left Wrist Region with Nonautologous Tissue Substitute, Percutaneous Endoscopic Approach
0X0H4ZZ Alteration of Left Wrist Region, Percutaneous Endoscopic Approach

0X2 – Anatomical Regions, Upper Extremities, Change

Review Coding Guideline B6.1c

0X26X0Z Change Drainage Device in Right Upper Extremity, External Approach
0X26XYZ Change Other Device in Right Upper Extremity, External Approach
0X27X0Z Change Drainage Device in Left Upper Extremity, External Approach
0X27XYZ Change Other Device in Left Upper Extremity, External Approach

0X3 – Anatomical Regions, Upper Extremities, Control

Review Coding Guideline B3.7

0X320ZZ Control Bleeding in Right Shoulder Region, Open Approach
0X323ZZ Control Bleeding in Right Shoulder Region, Percutaneous Approach
0X324ZZ Control Bleeding in Right Shoulder Region, Percutaneous Endoscopic Approach
0X330ZZ Control Bleeding in Left Shoulder Region, Open Approach
0X333ZZ Control Bleeding in Left Shoulder Region, Percutaneous Approach
0X334ZZ Control Bleeding in Left Shoulder Region, Percutaneous Endoscopic Approach
0X340ZZ Control Bleeding in Right Axilla, Open Approach
0X343ZZ Control Bleeding in Right Axilla, Percutaneous Approach
0X344ZZ Control Bleeding in Right Axilla, Percutaneous Endoscopic Approach
0X350ZZ Control Bleeding in Left Axilla, Open Approach
0X353ZZ Control Bleeding in Left Axilla, Percutaneous Approach
0X354ZZ Control Bleeding in Left Axilla, Percutaneous Endoscopic Approach
0X360ZZ Control Bleeding in Right Upper Extremity, Open Approach
0X363ZZ Control Bleeding in Right Upper Extremity, Percutaneous Approach
0X364ZZ Control Bleeding in Right Upper Extremity, Percutaneous Endoscopic Approach
0X370ZZ Control Bleeding in Left Upper Extremity, Open Approach
0X373ZZ Control Bleeding in Left Upper Extremity, Percutaneous Approach
0X374ZZ Control Bleeding in Left Upper Extremity, Percutaneous Endoscopic Approach
0X380ZZ Control Bleeding in Right Upper Arm, Open Approach
0X383ZZ Control Bleeding in Right Upper Arm, Percutaneous Approach
0X384ZZ Control Bleeding in Right Upper Arm, Percutaneous Endoscopic Approach
0X390ZZ Control Bleeding in Left Upper Arm, Open Approach
0X393ZZ Control Bleeding in Left Upper Arm, Percutaneous Approach
0X394ZZ Control Bleeding in Left Upper Arm, Percutaneous Endoscopic Approach
0X3B0ZZ Control Bleeding in Right Elbow Region, Open Approach
0X3B3ZZ Control Bleeding in Right Elbow Region, Percutaneous Approach
0X3B4ZZ Control Bleeding in Right Elbow Region, Percutaneous Endoscopic Approach
0X3C0ZZ Control Bleeding in Left Elbow Region, Open Approach
0X3C3ZZ Control Bleeding in Left Elbow Region, Percutaneous Approach
0X3C4ZZ Control Bleeding in Left Elbow Region, Percutaneous Endoscopic Approach
0X3D0ZZ Control Bleeding in Right Lower Arm, Open Approach
0X3D3ZZ Control Bleeding in Right Lower Arm, Percutaneous Approach
0X3D4ZZ Control Bleeding in Right Lower Arm, Percutaneous Endoscopic Approach
0X3F0ZZ Control Bleeding in Left Lower Arm, Open Approach
0X3F3ZZ Control Bleeding in Left Lower Arm, Percutaneous Approach
0X3F4ZZ Control Bleeding in Left Lower Arm, Percutaneous Endoscopic Approach
0X3G0ZZ Control Bleeding in Right Wrist Region, Open Approach
0X3G3ZZ Control Bleeding in Right Wrist Region, Percutaneous Approach
0X3G4ZZ Control Bleeding in Right Wrist Region, Percutaneous Endoscopic Approach
0X3H0ZZ Control Bleeding in Left Wrist Region, Open Approach
0X3H3ZZ Control Bleeding in Left Wrist Region, Percutaneous Approach
0X3H4ZZ Control Bleeding in Left Wrist Region, Percutaneous Endoscopic Approach
0X3J0ZZ Control Bleeding in Right Hand, Open Approach
0X3J3ZZ Control Bleeding in Right Hand, Percutaneous Approach
0X3J4ZZ Control Bleeding in Right Hand, Percutaneous Endoscopic Approach
0X3K0ZZ Control Bleeding in Left Hand, Open Approach
0X3K3ZZ Control Bleeding in Left Hand, Percutaneous Approach
0X3K4ZZ Control Bleeding in Left Hand, Percutaneous Endoscopic Approach

0X6 – Anatomical Regions, Upper Extremities, Detachment

0X600ZZ Detachment at Right Forequarter, Open Approach
0X610ZZ Detachment at Left Forequarter, Open Approach
0X620ZZ Detachment at Right Shoulder Region, Open Approach
0X630ZZ Detachment at Left Shoulder Region, Open Approach
0X680Z1 Detachment at Right Upper Arm, High, Open Approach
0X680Z2 Detachment at Right Upper Arm, Mid, Open Approach
0X680Z3 Detachment at Right Upper Arm, Low, Open Approach
0X690Z1 Detachment at Left Upper Arm, High, Open Approach
0X690Z2 Detachment at Left Upper Arm, Mid, Open Approach
0X690Z3 Detachment at Left Upper Arm, Low, Open Approach
0X6B0ZZ Detachment at Right Elbow Region, Open Approach
0X6C0ZZ Detachment at Left Elbow Region, Open Approach
0X6D0Z1 Detachment at Right Lower Arm, High, Open Approach
0X6D0Z2 Detachment at Right Lower Arm, Mid, Open Approach
0X6D0Z3 Detachment at Right Lower Arm, Low, Open Approach
0X6F0Z1 Detachment at Left Lower Arm, High, Open Approach
0X6F0Z2 Detachment at Left Lower Arm, Mid, Open Approach
0X6F0Z3 Detachment at Left Lower Arm, Low, Open Approach
0X6J0Z0 Detachment at Right Hand, Complete, Open Approach
0X6J0Z4 Detachment at Right Hand, Complete 1st Ray, Open Approach
0X6J0Z5 Detachment at Right Hand, Complete 2nd Ray, Open Approach
0X6J0Z6 Detachment at Right Hand, Complete 3rd Ray, Open Approach
0X6J0Z7 Detachment at Right Hand, Complete 4th Ray, Open Approach
0X6J0Z8 Detachment at Right Hand, Complete 5th Ray, Open Approach
0X6J0Z9 Detachment at Right Hand, Partial 1st Ray, Open Approach
0X6J0ZB Detachment at Right Hand, Partial 2nd Ray, Open Approach
0X6J0ZC Detachment at Right Hand, Partial 3rd Ray, Open Approach
0X6J0ZD Detachment at Right Hand, Partial 4th Ray, Open Approach
0X6J0ZF Detachment at Right Hand, Partial 5th Ray, Open Approach
0X6K0Z0 Detachment at Left Hand, Complete, Open Approach
0X6K0Z4 Detachment at Left Hand, Complete 1st Ray, Open Approach
0X6K0Z5 Detachment at Left Hand, Complete 2nd Ray, Open Approach
0X6K0Z6 Detachment at Left Hand, Complete 3rd Ray, Open Approach
0X6K0Z7 Detachment at Left Hand, Complete 4th Ray, Open Approach
0X6K0Z8 Detachment at Left Hand, Complete 5th Ray, Open Approach
0X6K0Z9 Detachment at Left Hand, Partial 1st Ray, Open Approach
0X6K0ZB Detachment at Left Hand, Partial 2nd Ray, Open Approach
0X6K0ZC Detachment at Left Hand, Partial 3rd Ray, Open Approach
0X6K0ZD Detachment at Left Hand, Partial 4th Ray, Open Approach

0X6K0ZF Detachment at Left Hand, Partial 5th Ray, Open Approach
0X6L0Z0 Detachment at Right Thumb, Complete, Open Approach
0X6L0Z1 Detachment at Right Thumb, High, Open Approach
0X6L0Z2 Detachment at Right Thumb, Mid, Open Approach
0X6L0Z3 Detachment at Right Thumb, Low, Open Approach
0X6M0Z0 Detachment at Left Thumb, Complete, Open Approach
0X6M0Z1 Detachment at Left Thumb, High, Open Approach
0X6M0Z2 Detachment at Left Thumb, Mid, Open Approach
0X6M0Z3 Detachment at Left Thumb, Low, Open Approach
0X6N0Z0 Detachment at Right Index Finger, Complete, Open Approach
0X6N0Z1 Detachment at Right Index Finger, High, Open Approach
0X6N0Z2 Detachment at Right Index Finger, Mid, Open Approach
0X6N0Z3 Detachment at Right Index Finger, Low, Open Approach
0X6P0Z0 Detachment at Left Index Finger, Complete, Open Approach
0X6P0Z1 Detachment at Left Index Finger, High, Open Approach
0X6P0Z2 Detachment at Left Index Finger, Mid, Open Approach
0X6P0Z3 Detachment at Left Index Finger, Low, Open Approach
0X6Q0Z0 Detachment at Right Middle Finger, Complete, Open Approach
0X6Q0Z1 Detachment at Right Middle Finger, High, Open Approach
0X6Q0Z2 Detachment at Right Middle Finger, Mid, Open Approach
0X6Q0Z3 Detachment at Right Middle Finger, Low, Open Approach
0X6R0Z0 Detachment at Left Middle Finger, Complete, Open Approach
0X6R0Z1 Detachment at Left Middle Finger, High, Open Approach
0X6R0Z2 Detachment at Left Middle Finger, Mid, Open Approach
0X6R0Z3 Detachment at Left Middle Finger, Low, Open Approach
0X6S0Z0 Detachment at Right Ring Finger, Complete, Open Approach
0X6S0Z1 Detachment at Right Ring Finger, High, Open Approach
0X6S0Z2 Detachment at Right Ring Finger, Mid, Open Approach
0X6S0Z3 Detachment at Right Ring Finger, Low, Open Approach
0X6T0Z0 Detachment at Left Ring Finger, Complete, Open Approach
0X6T0Z1 Detachment at Left Ring Finger, High, Open Approach
0X6T0Z2 Detachment at Left Ring Finger, Mid, Open Approach
0X6T0Z3 Detachment at Left Ring Finger, Low, Open Approach
0X6V0Z0 Detachment at Right Little Finger, Complete, Open Approach
0X6V0Z1 Detachment at Right Little Finger, High, Open Approach
0X6V0Z2 Detachment at Right Little Finger, Mid, Open Approach
0X6V0Z3 Detachment at Right Little Finger, Low, Open Approach
0X6W0Z0 Detachment at Left Little Finger, Complete, Open Approach
0X6W0Z1 Detachment at Left Little Finger, High, Open Approach
0X6W0Z2 Detachment at Left Little Finger, Mid, Open Approach
0X6W0Z3 Detachment at Left Little Finger, Low, Open Approach

0X9 – Anatomical Regions, Upper Extremities, Drainage

Review Coding Guidelines B3.4a and B3.4b

Review Coding Guideline B6.2

0X9200Z Drainage of Right Shoulder Region with Drainage Device, Open Approach
0X920ZX Drainage of Right Shoulder Region, Open Approach, Diagnostic
0X920ZZ Drainage of Right Shoulder Region, Open Approach
0X9230Z Drainage of Right Shoulder Region with Drainage Device, Percutaneous Approach
0X923ZX Drainage of Right Shoulder Region, Percutaneous Approach, Diagnostic
0X923ZZ Drainage of Right Shoulder Region, Percutaneous Approach
0X9240Z Drainage of Right Shoulder Region with Drainage Device, Percutaneous Endoscopic Approach
0X924ZX Drainage of Right Shoulder Region, Percutaneous Endoscopic Approach, Diagnostic
0X924ZZ Drainage of Right Shoulder Region, Percutaneous Endoscopic Approach
0X9300Z Drainage of Left Shoulder Region with Drainage Device, Open Approach
0X930ZX Drainage of Left Shoulder Region, Open Approach, Diagnostic
0X930ZZ Drainage of Left Shoulder Region, Open Approach
0X9330Z Drainage of Left Shoulder Region with Drainage Device, Percutaneous Approach
0X933ZX Drainage of Left Shoulder Region, Percutaneous Approach, Diagnostic
0X933ZZ Drainage of Left Shoulder Region, Percutaneous Approach
0X9340Z Drainage of Left Shoulder Region with Drainage Device, Percutaneous Endoscopic Approach
0X934ZX Drainage of Left Shoulder Region, Percutaneous Endoscopic Approach, Diagnostic
0X934ZZ Drainage of Left Shoulder Region, Percutaneous Endoscopic Approach
0X9400Z Drainage of Right Axilla with Drainage Device, Open Approach
0X940ZX Drainage of Right Axilla, Open Approach, Diagnostic
0X940ZZ Drainage of Right Axilla, Open Approach
0X9430Z Drainage of Right Axilla with Drainage Device, Percutaneous Approach
0X943ZX Drainage of Right Axilla, Percutaneous Approach, Diagnostic
0X943ZZ Drainage of Right Axilla, Percutaneous Approach
0X9440Z Drainage of Right Axilla with Drainage Device, Percutaneous Endoscopic Approach
0X944ZX Drainage of Right Axilla, Percutaneous Endoscopic Approach, Diagnostic
0X944ZZ Drainage of Right Axilla, Percutaneous Endoscopic Approach
0X9500Z Drainage of Left Axilla with Drainage Device, Open Approach
0X950ZX Drainage of Left Axilla, Open Approach, Diagnostic
0X950ZZ Drainage of Left Axilla, Open Approach
0X9530Z Drainage of Left Axilla with Drainage Device, Percutaneous Approach
0X953ZX Drainage of Left Axilla, Percutaneous Approach, Diagnostic
0X953ZZ Drainage of Left Axilla, Percutaneous Approach
0X9540Z Drainage of Left Axilla with Drainage Device, Percutaneous Endoscopic Approach
0X954ZX Drainage of Left Axilla, Percutaneous Endoscopic Approach, Diagnostic
0X954ZZ Drainage of Left Axilla, Percutaneous Endoscopic Approach
0X9600Z Drainage of Right Upper Extremity with Drainage Device, Open Approach
0X960ZX Drainage of Right Upper Extremity, Open Approach, Diagnostic
0X960ZZ Drainage of Right Upper Extremity, Open Approach
0X9630Z Drainage of Right Upper Extremity with Drainage Device, Percutaneous Approach
0X963ZX Drainage of Right Upper Extremity, Percutaneous Approach, Diagnostic
0X963ZZ Drainage of Right Upper Extremity, Percutaneous Approach
0X9640Z Drainage of Right Upper Extremity with Drainage Device, Percutaneous Endoscopic Approach
0X964ZX Drainage of Right Upper Extremity, Percutaneous Endoscopic Approach, Diagnostic
0X964ZZ Drainage of Right Upper Extremity, Percutaneous Endoscopic Approach
0X9700Z Drainage of Left Upper Extremity with Drainage Device, Open Approach
0X970ZX Drainage of Left Upper Extremity, Open Approach, Diagnostic
0X970ZZ Drainage of Left Upper Extremity, Open Approach
0X9730Z Drainage of Left Upper Extremity with Drainage Device, Percutaneous Approach
0X973ZX Drainage of Left Upper Extremity, Percutaneous Approach, Diagnostic
0X973ZZ Drainage of Left Upper Extremity, Percutaneous Approach
0X9740Z Drainage of Left Upper Extremity with Drainage Device, Percutaneous Endoscopic Approach
0X974ZX Drainage of Left Upper Extremity, Percutaneous Endoscopic Approach, Diagnostic
0X974ZZ Drainage of Left Upper Extremity, Percutaneous Endoscopic Approach
0X9800Z Drainage of Right Upper Arm with Drainage Device, Open Approach
0X980ZX Drainage of Right Upper Arm, Open Approach, Diagnostic
0X980ZZ Drainage of Right Upper Arm, Open Approach
0X9830Z Drainage of Right Upper Arm with Drainage Device, Percutaneous Approach
0X983ZX Drainage of Right Upper Arm, Percutaneous Approach, Diagnostic

0X983ZZ Drainage of Right Upper Arm, Percutaneous Approach
0X9840Z Drainage of Right Upper Arm with Drainage Device, Percutaneous Endoscopic Approach
0X984ZX Drainage of Right Upper Arm, Percutaneous Endoscopic Approach, Diagnostic
0X984ZZ Drainage of Right Upper Arm, Percutaneous Endoscopic Approach
0X9900Z Drainage of Left Upper Arm with Drainage Device, Open Approach
0X990ZX Drainage of Left Upper Arm, Open Approach, Diagnostic
0X990ZZ Drainage of Left Upper Arm, Open Approach
0X9930Z Drainage of Left Upper Arm with Drainage Device, Percutaneous Approach
0X993ZX Drainage of Left Upper Arm, Percutaneous Approach, Diagnostic
0X993ZZ Drainage of Left Upper Arm, Percutaneous Approach
0X9940Z Drainage of Left Upper Arm with Drainage Device, Percutaneous Endoscopic Approach
0X994ZX Drainage of Left Upper Arm, Percutaneous Endoscopic Approach, Diagnostic
0X994ZZ Drainage of Left Upper Arm, Percutaneous Endoscopic Approach
0X9B00Z Drainage of Right Elbow Region with Drainage Device, Open Approach
0X9B0ZX Drainage of Right Elbow Region, Open Approach, Diagnostic
0X9B0ZZ Drainage of Right Elbow Region, Open Approach
0X9B30Z Drainage of Right Elbow Region with Drainage Device, Percutaneous Approach
0X9B3ZX Drainage of Right Elbow Region, Percutaneous Approach, Diagnostic
0X9B3ZZ Drainage of Right Elbow Region, Percutaneous Approach
0X9B40Z Drainage of Right Elbow Region with Drainage Device, Percutaneous Endoscopic Approach
0X9B4ZX Drainage of Right Elbow Region, Percutaneous Endoscopic Approach, Diagnostic
0X9B4ZZ Drainage of Right Elbow Region, Percutaneous Endoscopic Approach
0X9C00Z Drainage of Left Elbow Region with Drainage Device, Open Approach
0X9C0ZX Drainage of Left Elbow Region, Open Approach, Diagnostic
0X9C0ZZ Drainage of Left Elbow Region, Open Approach
0X9C30Z Drainage of Left Elbow Region with Drainage Device, Percutaneous Approach
0X9C3ZX Drainage of Left Elbow Region, Percutaneous Approach, Diagnostic
0X9C3ZZ Drainage of Left Elbow Region, Percutaneous Approach
0X9C40Z Drainage of Left Elbow Region with Drainage Device, Percutaneous Endoscopic Approach
0X9C4ZX Drainage of Left Elbow Region, Percutaneous Endoscopic Approach, Diagnostic
0X9C4ZZ Drainage of Left Elbow Region, Percutaneous Endoscopic Approach
0X9D00Z Drainage of Right Lower Arm with Drainage Device, Open Approach
0X9D0ZX Drainage of Right Lower Arm, Open Approach, Diagnostic
0X9D0ZZ Drainage of Right Lower Arm, Open Approach
0X9D30Z Drainage of Right Lower Arm with Drainage Device, Percutaneous Approach
0X9D3ZX Drainage of Right Lower Arm, Percutaneous Approach, Diagnostic
0X9D3ZZ Drainage of Right Lower Arm, Percutaneous Approach
0X9D40Z Drainage of Right Lower Arm with Drainage Device, Percutaneous Endoscopic Approach
0X9D4ZX Drainage of Right Lower Arm, Percutaneous Endoscopic Approach, Diagnostic
0X9D4ZZ Drainage of Right Lower Arm, Percutaneous Endoscopic Approach
0X9F00Z Drainage of Left Lower Arm with Drainage Device, Open Approach
0X9F0ZX Drainage of Left Lower Arm, Open Approach, Diagnostic
0X9F0ZZ Drainage of Left Lower Arm, Open Approach
0X9F30Z Drainage of Left Lower Arm with Drainage Device, Percutaneous Approach
0X9F3ZX Drainage of Left Lower Arm, Percutaneous Approach, Diagnostic
0X9F3ZZ Drainage of Left Lower Arm, Percutaneous Approach
0X9F40Z Drainage of Left Lower Arm with Drainage Device, Percutaneous Endoscopic Approach
0X9F4ZX Drainage of Left Lower Arm, Percutaneous Endoscopic Approach, Diagnostic
0X9F4ZZ Drainage of Left Lower Arm, Percutaneous Endoscopic Approach
0X9G00Z Drainage of Right Wrist Region with Drainage Device, Open Approach
0X9G0ZX Drainage of Right Wrist Region, Open Approach, Diagnostic
0X9G0ZZ Drainage of Right Wrist Region, Open Approach
0X9G30Z Drainage of Right Wrist Region with Drainage Device, Percutaneous Approach
0X9G3ZX Drainage of Right Wrist Region, Percutaneous Approach, Diagnostic
0X9G3ZZ Drainage of Right Wrist Region, Percutaneous Approach
0X9G40Z Drainage of Right Wrist Region with Drainage Device, Percutaneous Endoscopic Approach
0X9G4ZX Drainage of Right Wrist Region, Percutaneous Endoscopic Approach, Diagnostic
0X9G4ZZ Drainage of Right Wrist Region, Percutaneous Endoscopic Approach
0X9H00Z Drainage of Left Wrist Region with Drainage Device, Open Approach
0X9H0ZX Drainage of Left Wrist Region, Open Approach, Diagnostic
0X9H0ZZ Drainage of Left Wrist Region, Open Approach
0X9H30Z Drainage of Left Wrist Region with Drainage Device, Percutaneous Approach
0X9H3ZX Drainage of Left Wrist Region, Percutaneous Approach, Diagnostic
0X9H3ZZ Drainage of Left Wrist Region, Percutaneous Approach
0X9H40Z Drainage of Left Wrist Region with Drainage Device, Percutaneous Endoscopic Approach
0X9H4ZX Drainage of Left Wrist Region, Percutaneous Endoscopic Approach, Diagnostic
0X9H4ZZ Drainage of Left Wrist Region, Percutaneous Endoscopic Approach
0X9J00Z Drainage of Right Hand with Drainage Device, Open Approach
0X9J0ZX Drainage of Right Hand, Open Approach, Diagnostic
0X9J0ZZ Drainage of Right Hand, Open Approach
0X9J30Z Drainage of Right Hand with Drainage Device, Percutaneous Approach
0X9J3ZX Drainage of Right Hand, Percutaneous Approach, Diagnostic
0X9J3ZZ Drainage of Right Hand, Percutaneous Approach
0X9J40Z Drainage of Right Hand with Drainage Device, Percutaneous Endoscopic Approach
0X9J4ZX Drainage of Right Hand, Percutaneous Endoscopic Approach, Diagnostic
0X9J4ZZ Drainage of Right Hand, Percutaneous Endoscopic Approach
0X9K00Z Drainage of Left Hand with Drainage Device, Open Approach
0X9K0ZX Drainage of Left Hand, Open Approach, Diagnostic
0X9K0ZZ Drainage of Left Hand, Open Approach
0X9K30Z Drainage of Left Hand with Drainage Device, Percutaneous Approach
0X9K3ZX Drainage of Left Hand, Percutaneous Approach, Diagnostic
0X9K3ZZ Drainage of Left Hand, Percutaneous Approach
0X9K40Z Drainage of Left Hand with Drainage Device, Percutaneous Endoscopic Approach
0X9K4ZX Drainage of Left Hand, Percutaneous Endoscopic Approach, Diagnostic
0X9K4ZZ Drainage of Left Hand, Percutaneous Endoscopic Approach

0XB – Anatomical Regions, Upper Extremities, Excision

Review Coding Guidelines B3.4a and B3.4b

0XB20ZX Excision of Right Shoulder Region, Open Approach, Diagnostic
0XB20ZZ Excision of Right Shoulder Region, Open Approach
0XB23ZX Excision of Right Shoulder Region, Percutaneous Approach, Diagnostic
0XB23ZZ Excision of Right Shoulder Region, Percutaneous Approach
0XB24ZX Excision of Right Shoulder Region, Percutaneous Endoscopic Approach, Diagnostic
0XB24ZZ Excision of Right Shoulder Region, Percutaneous Endoscopic Approach
0XB30ZX Excision of Left Shoulder Region, Open Approach, Diagnostic
0XB30ZZ Excision of Left Shoulder Region, Open Approach
0XB33ZX Excision of Left Shoulder Region, Percutaneous Approach, Diagnostic
0XB33ZZ Excision of Left Shoulder Region, Percutaneous Approach
0XB34ZX Excision of Left Shoulder Region, Percutaneous Endoscopic Approach, Diagnostic
0XB34ZZ Excision of Left Shoulder Region, Percutaneous Endoscopic Approach

0XB40ZX Excision of Right Axilla, Open Approach, Diagnostic
0XB40ZZ Excision of Right Axilla, Open Approach
0XB43ZX Excision of Right Axilla, Percutaneous Approach, Diagnostic
0XB43ZZ Excision of Right Axilla, Percutaneous Approach
0XB44ZX Excision of Right Axilla, Percutaneous Endoscopic Approach, Diagnostic
0XB44ZZ Excision of Right Axilla, Percutaneous Endoscopic Approach
0XB50ZX Excision of Left Axilla, Open Approach, Diagnostic
0XB50ZZ Excision of Left Axilla, Open Approach
0XB53ZX Excision of Left Axilla, Percutaneous Approach, Diagnostic
0XB53ZZ Excision of Left Axilla, Percutaneous Approach
0XB54ZX Excision of Left Axilla, Percutaneous Endoscopic Approach, Diagnostic
0XB54ZZ Excision of Left Axilla, Percutaneous Endoscopic Approach
0XB60ZX Excision of Right Upper Extremity, Open Approach, Diagnostic
0XB60ZZ Excision of Right Upper Extremity, Open Approach
0XB63ZX Excision of Right Upper Extremity, Percutaneous Approach, Diagnostic
0XB63ZZ Excision of Right Upper Extremity, Percutaneous Approach
0XB64ZX Excision of Right Upper Extremity, Percutaneous Endoscopic Approach, Diagnostic
0XB64ZZ Excision of Right Upper Extremity, Percutaneous Endoscopic Approach
0XB70ZX Excision of Left Upper Extremity, Open Approach, Diagnostic
0XB70ZZ Excision of Left Upper Extremity, Open Approach
0XB73ZX Excision of Left Upper Extremity, Percutaneous Approach, Diagnostic
0XB73ZZ Excision of Left Upper Extremity, Percutaneous Approach
0XB74ZX Excision of Left Upper Extremity, Percutaneous Endoscopic Approach, Diagnostic
0XB74ZZ Excision of Left Upper Extremity, Percutaneous Endoscopic Approach
0XB80ZX Excision of Right Upper Arm, Open Approach, Diagnostic
0XB80ZZ Excision of Right Upper Arm, Open Approach
0XB83ZX Excision of Right Upper Arm, Percutaneous Approach, Diagnostic
0XB83ZZ Excision of Right Upper Arm, Percutaneous Approach
0XB84ZX Excision of Right Upper Arm, Percutaneous Endoscopic Approach, Diagnostic
0XB84ZZ Excision of Right Upper Arm, Percutaneous Endoscopic Approach
0XB90ZX Excision of Left Upper Arm, Open Approach, Diagnostic
0XB90ZZ Excision of Left Upper Arm, Open Approach
0XB93ZX Excision of Left Upper Arm, Percutaneous Approach, Diagnostic
0XB93ZZ Excision of Left Upper Arm, Percutaneous Approach
0XB94ZX Excision of Left Upper Arm, Percutaneous Endoscopic Approach, Diagnostic
0XB94ZZ Excision of Left Upper Arm, Percutaneous Endoscopic Approach
0XBB0ZX Excision of Right Elbow Region, Open Approach, Diagnostic
0XBB0ZZ Excision of Right Elbow Region, Open Approach
0XBB3ZX Excision of Right Elbow Region, Percutaneous Approach, Diagnostic
0XBB3ZZ Excision of Right Elbow Region, Percutaneous Approach
0XBB4ZX Excision of Right Elbow Region, Percutaneous Endoscopic Approach, Diagnostic
0XBB4ZZ Excision of Right Elbow Region, Percutaneous Endoscopic Approach
0XBC0ZX Excision of Left Elbow Region, Open Approach, Diagnostic
0XBC0ZZ Excision of Left Elbow Region, Open Approach
0XBC3ZX Excision of Left Elbow Region, Percutaneous Approach, Diagnostic
0XBC3ZZ Excision of Left Elbow Region, Percutaneous Approach
0XBC4ZX Excision of Left Elbow Region, Percutaneous Endoscopic Approach, Diagnostic
0XBC4ZZ Excision of Left Elbow Region, Percutaneous Endoscopic Approach
0XBD0ZX Excision of Right Lower Arm, Open Approach, Diagnostic
0XBD0ZZ Excision of Right Lower Arm, Open Approach
0XBD3ZX Excision of Right Lower Arm, Percutaneous Approach, Diagnostic
0XBD3ZZ Excision of Right Lower Arm, Percutaneous Approach
0XBD4ZX Excision of Right Lower Arm, Percutaneous Endoscopic Approach, Diagnostic
0XBD4ZZ Excision of Right Lower Arm, Percutaneous Endoscopic Approach
0XBF0ZX Excision of Left Lower Arm, Open Approach, Diagnostic
0XBF0ZZ Excision of Left Lower Arm, Open Approach
0XBF3ZX Excision of Left Lower Arm, Percutaneous Approach, Diagnostic
0XBF3ZZ Excision of Left Lower Arm, Percutaneous Approach
0XBF4ZX Excision of Left Lower Arm, Percutaneous Endoscopic Approach, Diagnostic
0XBF4ZZ Excision of Left Lower Arm, Percutaneous Endoscopic Approach
0XBG0ZX Excision of Right Wrist Region, Open Approach, Diagnostic
0XBG0ZZ Excision of Right Wrist Region, Open Approach
0XBG3ZX Excision of Right Wrist Region, Percutaneous Approach, Diagnostic
0XBG3ZZ Excision of Right Wrist Region, Percutaneous Approach
0XBG4ZX Excision of Right Wrist Region, Percutaneous Endoscopic Approach, Diagnostic
0XBG4ZZ Excision of Right Wrist Region, Percutaneous Endoscopic Approach
0XBH0ZX Excision of Left Wrist Region, Open Approach, Diagnostic
0XBH0ZZ Excision of Left Wrist Region, Open Approach
0XBH3ZX Excision of Left Wrist Region, Percutaneous Approach, Diagnostic
0XBH3ZZ Excision of Left Wrist Region, Percutaneous Approach
0XBH4ZX Excision of Left Wrist Region, Percutaneous Endoscopic Approach, Diagnostic
0XBH4ZZ Excision of Left Wrist Region, Percutaneous Endoscopic Approach
0XBJ0ZX Excision of Right Hand, Open Approach, Diagnostic
0XBJ0ZZ Excision of Right Hand, Open Approach
0XBJ3ZX Excision of Right Hand, Percutaneous Approach, Diagnostic
0XBJ3ZZ Excision of Right Hand, Percutaneous Approach
0XBJ4ZX Excision of Right Hand, Percutaneous Endoscopic Approach, Diagnostic
0XBJ4ZZ Excision of Right Hand, Percutaneous Endoscopic Approach
0XBK0ZX Excision of Left Hand, Open Approach, Diagnostic
0XBK0ZZ Excision of Left Hand, Open Approach
0XBK3ZX Excision of Left Hand, Percutaneous Approach, Diagnostic
0XBK3ZZ Excision of Left Hand, Percutaneous Approach
0XBK4ZX Excision of Left Hand, Percutaneous Endoscopic Approach, Diagnostic
0XBK4ZZ Excision of Left Hand, Percutaneous Endoscopic Approach

0XH – Anatomical Regions, Upper Extremities, Insertion

0XH201Z Insertion of Radioactive Element into Right Shoulder Region, Open Approach
● **0XH203Z** Insertion of Infusion Device into Right Shoulder Region, Open Approach
● **0XH20YZ** Insertion of Other Device into Right Shoulder Region, Open Approach
0XH231Z Insertion of Radioactive Element into Right Shoulder Region, Percutaneous Approach
● **0XH233Z** Insertion of Infusion Device into Right Shoulder Region, Percutaneous Approach
● **0XH23YZ** Insertion of Other Device into Right Shoulder Region, Percutaneous Approach
0XH241Z Insertion of Radioactive Element into Right Shoulder Region, Percutaneous Endoscopic Approach
● **0XH243Z** Insertion of Infusion Device into Right Shoulder Region, Percutaneous Endoscopic Approach
● **0XH24YZ** Insertion of Other Device into Right Shoulder Region, Percutaneous Endoscopic Approach
0XH301Z Insertion of Radioactive Element into Left Shoulder Region, Open Approach
● **0XH303Z** Insertion of Infusion Device into Left Shoulder Region, Open Approach
● **0XH30YZ** Insertion of Other Device into Left Shoulder Region, Open Approach
0XH331Z Insertion of Radioactive Element into Left Shoulder Region, Percutaneous Approach
● **0XH333Z** Insertion of Infusion Device into Left Shoulder Region, Percutaneous Approach
● **0XH33YZ** Insertion of Other Device into Left Shoulder Region, Percutaneous Approach
0XH341Z Insertion of Radioactive Element into Left Shoulder Region, Percutaneous Endoscopic Approach
● **0XH343Z** Insertion of Infusion Device into Left Shoulder Region, Percutaneous Endoscopic Approach
● **0XH34YZ** Insertion of Other Device into Left Shoulder Region, Percutaneous Endoscopic Approach
0XH401Z Insertion of Radioactive Element into Right Axilla, Open Approach
● **0XH403Z** Insertion of Infusion Device into Right Axilla, Open Approach

●0XH40YZ Insertion of Other Device into Right Axilla, Open Approach
0XH431Z Insertion of Radioactive Element into Right Axilla, Percutaneous Approach
●0XH433Z Insertion of Infusion Device into Right Axilla, Percutaneous Approach
●0XH43YZ Insertion of Other Device into Right Axilla, Percutaneous Approach
0XH441Z Insertion of Radioactive Element into Right Axilla, Percutaneous Endoscopic Approach
●0XH443Z Insertion of Infusion Device into Right Axilla, Percutaneous Endoscopic Approach
●0XH44YZ Insertion of Other Device into Right Axilla, Percutaneous Endoscopic Approach
0XH501Z Insertion of Radioactive Element into Left Axilla, Open Approach
●0XH503Z Insertion of Infusion Device into Left Axilla, Open Approach
●0XH50YZ Insertion of Other Device into Left Axilla, Open Approach
0XH531Z Insertion of Radioactive Element into Left Axilla, Percutaneous Approach
●0XH533Z Insertion of Infusion Device into Left Axilla, Percutaneous Approach
●0XH53YZ Insertion of Other Device into Left Axilla, Percutaneous Approach
0XH541Z Insertion of Radioactive Element into Left Axilla, Percutaneous Endoscopic Approach
●0XH543Z Insertion of Infusion Device into Left Axilla, Percutaneous Endoscopic Approach
●0XH54YZ Insertion of Other Device into Left Axilla, Percutaneous Endoscopic Approach
0XH601Z Insertion of Radioactive Element into Right Upper Extremity, Open Approach
●0XH603Z Insertion of Infusion Device into Right Upper Extremity, Open Approach
●0XH60YZ Insertion of Other Device into Right Upper Extremity, Open Approach
0XH631Z Insertion of Radioactive Element into Right Upper Extremity, Percutaneous Approach
●0XH633Z Insertion of Infusion Device into Right Upper Extremity, Percutaneous Approach
●0XH63YZ Insertion of Other Device into Right Upper Extremity, Percutaneous Approach
0XH641Z Insertion of Radioactive Element into Right Upper Extremity, Percutaneous Endoscopic Approach
●0XH643Z Insertion of Infusion Device into Right Upper Extremity, Percutaneous Endoscopic Approach
●0XH64YZ Insertion of Other Device into Right Upper Extremity, Percutaneous Endoscopic Approach
0XH701Z Insertion of Radioactive Element into Left Upper Extremity, Open Approach
●0XH703Z Insertion of Infusion Device into Left Upper Extremity, Open Approach
●0XH70YZ Insertion of Other Device into Left Upper Extremity, Open Approach
0XH731Z Insertion of Radioactive Element into Left Upper Extremity, Percutaneous Approach
●0XH733Z Insertion of Infusion Device into Left Upper Extremity, Percutaneous Approach
●0XH73YZ Insertion of Other Device into Left Upper Extremity, Percutaneous Approach
0XH741Z Insertion of Radioactive Element into Left Upper Extremity, Percutaneous Endoscopic Approach
●0XH743Z Insertion of Infusion Device into Left Upper Extremity, Percutaneous Endoscopic Approach
●0XH74YZ Insertion of Other Device into Left Upper Extremity, Percutaneous Endoscopic Approach
0XH801Z Insertion of Radioactive Element into Right Upper Arm, Open Approach
● 0XH803Z Insertion of Infusion Device into Right Upper Arm, Open Approach
● 0XH80YZ Insertion of Other Device into Right Upper Arm, Open Approach
0XH831Z Insertion of Radioactive Element into Right Upper Arm, Percutaneous Approach
● 0XH833Z Insertion of Infusion Device into Right Upper Arm, Percutaneous Approach
● 0XH83YZ Insertion of Other Device into Right Upper Arm, Percutaneous Approach
0XH841Z Insertion of Radioactive Element into Right Upper Arm, Percutaneous Endoscopic Approach
● 0XH843Z Insertion of Infusion Device into Right Upper Arm, Percutaneous Endoscopic Approach
● 0XH84YZ Insertion of Other Device into Right Upper Arm, Percutaneous Endoscopic Approach
0XH901Z Insertion of Radioactive Element into Left Upper Arm, Open Approach
● 0XH903Z Insertion of Infusion Device into Left Upper Arm, Open Approach
● 0XH90YZ Insertion of Other Device into Left Upper Arm, Open Approach
0XH931Z Insertion of Radioactive Element into Left Upper Arm, Percutaneous Approach
● 0XH933Z Insertion of Infusion Device into Left Upper Arm, Percutaneous Approach
● 0XH93YZ Insertion of Other Device into Left Upper Arm, Percutaneous Approach
0XH941Z Insertion of Radioactive Element into Left Upper Arm, Percutaneous Endoscopic Approach
● 0XH943Z Insertion of Infusion Device into Left Upper Arm, Percutaneous Endoscopic Approach
● 0XH94YZ Insertion of Other Device into Left Upper Arm, Percutaneous Endoscopic Approach
0XHB01Z Insertion of Radioactive Element into Right Elbow Region, Open Approach
● 0XHB03Z Insertion of Infusion Device into Right Elbow Region, Open Approach
● 0XHB0YZ Insertion of Other Device into Right Elbow Region, Open Approach
0XHB31Z Insertion of Radioactive Element into Right Elbow Region, Percutaneous Approach
● 0XHB33Z Insertion of Infusion Device into Right Elbow Region, Percutaneous Approach
● 0XHB3YZ Insertion of Other Device into Right Elbow Region, Percutaneous Approach
0XHB41Z Insertion of Radioactive Element into Right Elbow Region, Percutaneous Endoscopic Approach
● 0XHB43Z Insertion of Infusion Device into Right Elbow Region, Percutaneous Endoscopic Approach
● 0XHB4YZ Insertion of Other Device into Right Elbow Region, Percutaneous Endoscopic Approach
0XHC01Z Insertion of Radioactive Element into Left Elbow Region, Open Approach
● 0XHC03Z Insertion of Infusion Device into Left Elbow Region, Open Approach
● 0XHC0YZ Insertion of Other Device into Left Elbow Region, Open Approach
0XHC31Z Insertion of Radioactive Element into Left Elbow Region, Percutaneous Approach
● 0XHC33Z Insertion of Infusion Device into Left Elbow Region, Percutaneous Approach
● 0XHC3YZ Insertion of Other Device into Left Elbow Region, Percutaneous Approach
0XHC41Z Insertion of Radioactive Element into Left Elbow Region, Percutaneous Endoscopic Approach
● 0XHC43Z Insertion of Infusion Device into Left Elbow Region, Percutaneous Endoscopic Approach
● 0XHC4YZ Insertion of Other Device into Left Elbow Region, Percutaneous Endoscopic Approach
0XHD01Z Insertion of Radioactive Element into Right Lower Arm, Open Approach
● 0XHD03Z Insertion of Infusion Device into Right Lower Arm, Open Approach
● 0XHD0YZ Insertion of Other Device into Right Lower Arm, Open Approach
0XHD31Z Insertion of Radioactive Element into Right Lower Arm, Percutaneous Approach
● 0XHD33Z Insertion of Infusion Device into Right Lower Arm, Percutaneous Approach
● 0XHD3YZ Insertion of Other Device into Right Lower Arm, Percutaneous Approach
0XHD41Z Insertion of Radioactive Element into Right Lower Arm, Percutaneous Endoscopic Approach
● 0XHD43Z Insertion of Infusion Device into Right Lower Arm, Percutaneous Endoscopic Approach
● 0XHD4YZ Insertion of Other Device into Right Lower Arm, Percutaneous Endoscopic Approach
0XHF01Z Insertion of Radioactive Element into Left Lower Arm, Open Approach
● 0XHF03Z Insertion of Infusion Device into Left Lower Arm, Open Approach
● 0XHF0YZ Insertion of Other Device into Left Lower Arm, Open Approach
0XHF31Z Insertion of Radioactive Element into Left Lower Arm, Percutaneous Approach
● 0XHF33Z Insertion of Infusion Device into Left Lower Arm, Percutaneous Approach
● 0XHF3YZ Insertion of Other Device into Left Lower Arm, Percutaneous Approach
0XHF41Z Insertion of Radioactive Element into Left Lower Arm, Percutaneous Endoscopic Approach
● 0XHF43Z Insertion of Infusion Device into Left Lower Arm, Percutaneous Endoscopic Approach
● 0XHF4YZ Insertion of Other Device into Left Lower Arm, Percutaneous Endoscopic Approach
0XHG01Z Insertion of Radioactive Element into Right Wrist Region, Open Approach
● 0XHG03Z Insertion of Infusion Device into Right Wrist Region, Open Approach
● 0XHG0YZ Insertion of Other Device into Right Wrist Region, Open Approach
0XHG31Z Insertion of Radioactive Element into Right Wrist Region, Percutaneous Approach
● 0XHG33Z Insertion of Infusion Device into Right Wrist Region, Percutaneous Approach
● 0XHG3YZ Insertion of Other Device into Right Wrist Region, Percutaneous Approach
0XHG41Z Insertion of Radioactive Element into Right Wrist Region, Percutaneous Endoscopic Approach
● 0XHG43Z Insertion of Infusion Device into Right Wrist Region, Percutaneous Endoscopic Approach
● 0XHG4YZ Insertion of Other Device into Right Wrist Region, Percutaneous Endoscopic Approach
0XHH01Z Insertion of Radioactive Element into Left Wrist Region, Open Approach
● 0XHH03Z Insertion of Infusion Device into Left Wrist Region, Open Approach
● 0XHH0YZ Insertion of Other Device into Left Wrist Region, Open Approach
0XHH31Z Insertion of Radioactive Element into Left Wrist Region, Percutaneous Approach

● **0XHH33Z** Insertion of Infusion Device into Left Wrist Region, Percutaneous Approach
● **0XHH3YZ** Insertion of Other Device into Left Wrist Region, Percutaneous Approach
0XHH41Z Insertion of Radioactive Element into Left Wrist Region, Percutaneous Endoscopic Approach
● **0XHH43Z** Insertion of Infusion Device into Left Wrist Region, Percutaneous Endoscopic Approach
● **0XHH4YZ** Insertion of Other Device into Left Wrist Region, Percutaneous Endoscopic Approach
0XHJ01Z Insertion of Radioactive Element into Right Hand, Open Approach
● **0XHJ03Z** Insertion of Infusion Device into Right Hand, Open Approach
● **0XHJ0YZ** Insertion of Other Device into Right Hand, Open Approach
0XHJ31Z Insertion of Radioactive Element into Right Hand, Percutaneous Approach
● **0XHJ33Z** Insertion of Infusion Device into Right Hand, Percutaneous Approach
● **0XHJ3YZ** Insertion of Other Device into Right Hand, Percutaneous Approach
0XHJ41Z Insertion of Radioactive Element into Right Hand, Percutaneous Endoscopic Approach
● **0XHJ43Z** Insertion of Infusion Device into Right Hand, Percutaneous Endoscopic Approach
● **0XHJ4YZ** Insertion of Other Device into Right Hand, Percutaneous Endoscopic Approach
0XHK01Z Insertion of Radioactive Element into Left Hand, Open Approach
● **0XHK03Z** Insertion of Infusion Device into Left Hand, Open Approach
● **0XHK0YZ** Insertion of Other Device into Left Hand, Open Approach
0XHK31Z Insertion of Radioactive Element into Left Hand, Percutaneous Approach
● **0XHK33Z** Insertion of Infusion Device into Left Hand, Percutaneous Approach
● **0XHK3YZ** Insertion of Other Device into Left Hand, Percutaneous Approach
0XHK41Z Insertion of Radioactive Element into Left Hand, Percutaneous Endoscopic Approach
● **0XHK43Z** Insertion of Infusion Device into Left Hand, Percutaneous Endoscopic Approach
● **0XHK4YZ** Insertion of Other Device into Left Hand, Percutaneous Endoscopic Approach

0XJ – Anatomical Regions, Upper Extremities, Inspection

Review Coding Guidelines B3.11a, B3.11b and B3.11c

● **0XJ20ZZ** Inspection of Right Shoulder Region, Open Approach
0XJ23ZZ Inspection of Right Shoulder Region, Percutaneous Approach
0XJ24ZZ Inspection of Right Shoulder Region, Percutaneous Endoscopic Approach
0XJ2XZZ Inspection of Right Shoulder Region, External Approach
● **0XJ30ZZ** Inspection of Left Shoulder Region, Open Approach
0XJ33ZZ Inspection of Left Shoulder Region, Percutaneous Approach
0XJ34ZZ Inspection of Left Shoulder Region, Percutaneous Endoscopic Approach
0XJ3XZZ Inspection of Left Shoulder Region, External Approach
● **0XJ40ZZ** Inspection of Right Axilla, Open Approach
0XJ43ZZ Inspection of Right Axilla, Percutaneous Approach
0XJ44ZZ Inspection of Right Axilla, Percutaneous Endoscopic Approach
0XJ4XZZ Inspection of Right Axilla, External Approach
● **0XJ50ZZ** Inspection of Left Axilla, Open Approach
0XJ53ZZ Inspection of Left Axilla, Percutaneous Approach
0XJ54ZZ Inspection of Left Axilla, Percutaneous Endoscopic Approach
0XJ5XZZ Inspection of Left Axilla, External Approach
● **0XJ60ZZ** Inspection of Right Upper Extremity, Open Approach
0XJ63ZZ Inspection of Right Upper Extremity, Percutaneous Approach
0XJ64ZZ Inspection of Right Upper Extremity, Percutaneous Endoscopic Approach
0XJ6XZZ Inspection of Right Upper Extremity, External Approach
● **0XJ70ZZ** Inspection of Left Upper Extremity, Open Approach
0XJ73ZZ Inspection of Left Upper Extremity, Percutaneous Approach
0XJ74ZZ Inspection of Left Upper Extremity, Percutaneous Endoscopic Approach
0XJ7XZZ Inspection of Left Upper Extremity, External Approach
● **0XJ80ZZ** Inspection of Right Upper Arm, Open Approach
0XJ83ZZ Inspection of Right Upper Arm, Percutaneous Approach
0XJ84ZZ Inspection of Right Upper Arm, Percutaneous Endoscopic Approach
0XJ8XZZ Inspection of Right Upper Arm, External Approach
● **0XJ90ZZ** Inspection of Left Upper Arm, Open Approach
0XJ93ZZ Inspection of Left Upper Arm, Percutaneous Approach
0XJ94ZZ Inspection of Left Upper Arm, Percutaneous Endoscopic Approach
0XJ9XZZ Inspection of Left Upper Arm, External Approach
● **0XJB0ZZ** Inspection of Right Elbow Region, Open Approach
0XJB3ZZ Inspection of Right Elbow Region, Percutaneous Approach
0XJB4ZZ Inspection of Right Elbow Region, Percutaneous Endoscopic Approach
0XJBXZZ Inspection of Right Elbow Region, External Approach
● **0XJC0ZZ** Inspection of Left Elbow Region, Open Approach
0XJC3ZZ Inspection of Left Elbow Region, Percutaneous Approach
0XJC4ZZ Inspection of Left Elbow Region, Percutaneous Endoscopic Approach
0XJCXZZ Inspection of Left Elbow Region, External Approach
● **0XJD0ZZ** Inspection of Right Lower Arm, Open Approach
0XJD3ZZ Inspection of Right Lower Arm, Percutaneous Approach
0XJD4ZZ Inspection of Right Lower Arm, Percutaneous Endoscopic Approach
0XJDXZZ Inspection of Right Lower Arm, External Approach
● **0XJF0ZZ** Inspection of Left Lower Arm, Open Approach
0XJF3ZZ Inspection of Left Lower Arm, Percutaneous Approach
0XJF4ZZ Inspection of Left Lower Arm, Percutaneous Endoscopic Approach
0XJFXZZ Inspection of Left Lower Arm, External Approach
● **0XJG0ZZ** Inspection of Right Wrist Region, Open Approach
0XJG3ZZ Inspection of Right Wrist Region, Percutaneous Approach
0XJG4ZZ Inspection of Right Wrist Region, Percutaneous Endoscopic Approach
0XJGXZZ Inspection of Right Wrist Region, External Approach
● **0XJH0ZZ** Inspection of Left Wrist Region, Open Approach
0XJH3ZZ Inspection of Left Wrist Region, Percutaneous Approach
0XJH4ZZ Inspection of Left Wrist Region, Percutaneous Endoscopic Approach
0XJHXZZ Inspection of Left Wrist Region, External Approach
● **0XJJ0ZZ** Inspection of Right Hand, Open Approach
0XJJ3ZZ Inspection of Right Hand, Percutaneous Approach
0XJJ4ZZ Inspection of Right Hand, Percutaneous Endoscopic Approach
0XJJXZZ Inspection of Right Hand, External Approach
● **0XJK0ZZ** Inspection of Left Hand, Open Approach
0XJK3ZZ Inspection of Left Hand, Percutaneous Approach
0XJK4ZZ Inspection of Left Hand, Percutaneous Endoscopic Approach
0XJKXZZ Inspection of Left Hand, External Approach

0XM – Anatomical Regions, Upper Extremities, Reattachment

0XM00ZZ Reattachment of Right Forequarter, Open Approach
0XM10ZZ Reattachment of Left Forequarter, Open Approach
0XM20ZZ Reattachment of Right Shoulder Region, Open Approach
0XM30ZZ Reattachment of Left Shoulder Region, Open Approach
0XM40ZZ Reattachment of Right Axilla, Open Approach
0XM50ZZ Reattachment of Left Axilla, Open Approach
0XM60ZZ Reattachment of Right Upper Extremity, Open Approach
0XM70ZZ Reattachment of Left Upper Extremity, Open Approach
0XM80ZZ Reattachment of Right Upper Arm, Open Approach
0XM90ZZ Reattachment of Left Upper Arm, Open Approach
0XMB0ZZ Reattachment of Right Elbow Region, Open Approach
0XMC0ZZ Reattachment of Left Elbow Region, Open Approach
0XMD0ZZ Reattachment of Right Lower Arm, Open Approach
0XMF0ZZ Reattachment of Left Lower Arm, Open Approach
0XMG0ZZ Reattachment of Right Wrist Region, Open Approach

0XMH0ZZ Reattachment of Left Wrist Region, Open Approach
0XMJ0ZZ Reattachment of Right Hand, Open Approach
0XMK0ZZ Reattachment of Left Hand, Open Approach
0XML0ZZ Reattachment of Right Thumb, Open Approach
0XMM0ZZ Reattachment of Left Thumb, Open Approach
0XMN0ZZ Reattachment of Right Index Finger, Open Approach
0XMP0ZZ Reattachment of Left Index Finger, Open Approach
0XMQ0ZZ Reattachment of Right Middle Finger, Open Approach
0XMR0ZZ Reattachment of Left Middle Finger, Open Approach
0XMS0ZZ Reattachment of Right Ring Finger, Open Approach
0XMT0ZZ Reattachment of Left Ring Finger, Open Approach
0XMV0ZZ Reattachment of Right Little Finger, Open Approach
0XMW0ZZ Reattachment of Left Little Finger, Open Approach

0XP – Anatomical Regions, Upper Extremities, Removal

Review Coding Guideline B6.1c

0XP600Z Removal of Drainage Device from Right Upper Extremity, Open Approach
0XP601Z Removal of Radioactive Element from Right Upper Extremity, Open Approach
0XP603Z Removal of Infusion Device from Right Upper Extremity, Open Approach
0XP607Z Removal of Autologous Tissue Substitute from Right Upper Extremity, Open Approach
0XP60JZ Removal of Synthetic Substitute from Right Upper Extremity, Open Approach
0XP60KZ Removal of Nonautologous Tissue Substitute from Right Upper Extremity, Open Approach
0XP60YZ Removal of Other Device from Right Upper Extremity, Open Approach
0XP630Z Removal of Drainage Device from Right Upper Extremity, Percutaneous Approach
0XP631Z Removal of Radioactive Element from Right Upper Extremity, Percutaneous Approach
0XP633Z Removal of Infusion Device from Right Upper Extremity, Percutaneous Approach
0XP637Z Removal of Autologous Tissue Substitute from Right Upper Extremity, Percutaneous Approach
0XP63JZ Removal of Synthetic Substitute from Right Upper Extremity, Percutaneous Approach
0XP63KZ Removal of Nonautologous Tissue Substitute from Right Upper Extremity, Percutaneous Approach
0XP63YZ Removal of Other Device from Right Upper Extremity, Percutaneous Approach
0XP640Z Removal of Drainage Device from Right Upper Extremity, Percutaneous Endoscopic Approach
0XP641Z Removal of Radioactive Element from Right Upper Extremity, Percutaneous Endoscopic Approach
0XP643Z Removal of Infusion Device from Right Upper Extremity, Percutaneous Endoscopic Approach
0XP647Z Removal of Autologous Tissue Substitute from Right Upper Extremity, Percutaneous Endoscopic Approach
0XP64JZ Removal of Synthetic Substitute from Right Upper Extremity, Percutaneous Endoscopic Approach
0XP64KZ Removal of Nonautologous Tissue Substitute from Right Upper Extremity, Percutaneous Endoscopic Approach
0XP64YZ Removal of Other Device from Right Upper Extremity, Percutaneous Endoscopic Approach
0XP6X0Z Removal of Drainage Device from Right Upper Extremity, External Approach
0XP6X1Z Removal of Radioactive Element from Right Upper Extremity, External Approach
0XP6X3Z Removal of Infusion Device from Right Upper Extremity, External Approach
0XP6X7Z Removal of Autologous Tissue Substitute from Right Upper Extremity, External Approach
0XP6XJZ Removal of Synthetic Substitute from Right Upper Extremity, External Approach
0XP6XKZ Removal of Nonautologous Tissue Substitute from Right Upper Extremity, External Approach
0XP6XYZ Removal of Other Device from Right Upper Extremity, External Approach
0XP700Z Removal of Drainage Device from Left Upper Extremity, Open Approach
0XP701Z Removal of Radioactive Element from Left Upper Extremity, Open Approach
0XP703Z Removal of Infusion Device from Left Upper Extremity, Open Approach
0XP707Z Removal of Autologous Tissue Substitute from Left Upper Extremity, Open Approach
0XP70JZ Removal of Synthetic Substitute from Left Upper Extremity, Open Approach
0XP70KZ Removal of Nonautologous Tissue Substitute from Left Upper Extremity, Open Approach
0XP70YZ Removal of Other Device from Left Upper Extremity, Open Approach
0XP730Z Removal of Drainage Device from Left Upper Extremity, Percutaneous Approach
0XP731Z Removal of Radioactive Element from Left Upper Extremity, Percutaneous Approach
0XP733Z Removal of Infusion Device from Left Upper Extremity, Percutaneous Approach
0XP737Z Removal of Autologous Tissue Substitute from Left Upper Extremity, Percutaneous Approach
0XP73JZ Removal of Synthetic Substitute from Left Upper Extremity, Percutaneous Approach
0XP73KZ Removal of Nonautologous Tissue Substitute from Left Upper Extremity, Percutaneous Approach
0XP73YZ Removal of Other Device from Left Upper Extremity, Percutaneous Approach
0XP740Z Removal of Drainage Device from Left Upper Extremity, Percutaneous Endoscopic Approach
0XP741Z Removal of Radioactive Element from Left Upper Extremity, Percutaneous Endoscopic Approach
0XP743Z Removal of Infusion Device from Left Upper Extremity, Percutaneous Endoscopic Approach
0XP747Z Removal of Autologous Tissue Substitute from Left Upper Extremity, Percutaneous Endoscopic Approach
0XP74JZ Removal of Synthetic Substitute from Left Upper Extremity, Percutaneous Endoscopic Approach
0XP74KZ Removal of Nonautologous Tissue Substitute from Left Upper Extremity, Percutaneous Endoscopic Approach
0XP74YZ Removal of Other Device from Left Upper Extremity, Percutaneous Endoscopic Approach
0XP7X0Z Removal of Drainage Device from Left Upper Extremity, External Approach
0XP7X1Z Removal of Radioactive Element from Left Upper Extremity, External Approach
0XP7X3Z Removal of Infusion Device from Left Upper Extremity, External Approach
0XP7X7Z Removal of Autologous Tissue Substitute from Left Upper Extremity, External Approach
0XP7XJZ Removal of Synthetic Substitute from Left Upper Extremity, External Approach
0XP7XKZ Removal of Nonautologous Tissue Substitute from Left Upper Extremity, External Approach
0XP7XYZ Removal of Other Device from Left Upper Extremity, External Approach

0XQ – Anatomical Regions, Upper Extremities, Repair

0XQ20ZZ Repair Right Shoulder Region, Open Approach
0XQ23ZZ Repair Right Shoulder Region, Percutaneous Approach
0XQ24ZZ Repair Right Shoulder Region, Percutaneous Endoscopic Approach
0XQ2XZZ Repair Right Shoulder Region, External Approach
0XQ30ZZ Repair Left Shoulder Region, Open Approach
0XQ33ZZ Repair Left Shoulder Region, Percutaneous Approach
0XQ34ZZ Repair Left Shoulder Region, Percutaneous Endoscopic Approach
0XQ3XZZ Repair Left Shoulder Region, External Approach
0XQ40ZZ Repair Right Axilla, Open Approach
0XQ43ZZ Repair Right Axilla, Percutaneous Approach
0XQ44ZZ Repair Right Axilla, Percutaneous Endoscopic Approach
0XQ4XZZ Repair Right Axilla, External Approach
0XQ50ZZ Repair Left Axilla, Open Approach
0XQ53ZZ Repair Left Axilla, Percutaneous Approach
0XQ54ZZ Repair Left Axilla, Percutaneous Endoscopic Approach
0XQ5XZZ Repair Left Axilla, External Approach
0XQ60ZZ Repair Right Upper Extremity, Open Approach
0XQ63ZZ Repair Right Upper Extremity, Percutaneous Approach

0XQ64ZZ Repair Right Upper Extremity, Percutaneous Endoscopic Approach
0XQ6XZZ Repair Right Upper Extremity, External Approach
0XQ70ZZ Repair Left Upper Extremity, Open Approach
0XQ73ZZ Repair Left Upper Extremity, Percutaneous Approach
0XQ74ZZ Repair Left Upper Extremity, Percutaneous Endoscopic Approach
0XQ7XZZ Repair Left Upper Extremity, External Approach
0XQ80ZZ Repair Right Upper Arm, Open Approach
0XQ83ZZ Repair Right Upper Arm, Percutaneous Approach
0XQ84ZZ Repair Right Upper Arm, Percutaneous Endoscopic Approach
0XQ8XZZ Repair Right Upper Arm, External Approach
0XQ90ZZ Repair Left Upper Arm, Open Approach
0XQ93ZZ Repair Left Upper Arm, Percutaneous Approach
0XQ94ZZ Repair Left Upper Arm, Percutaneous Endoscopic Approach
0XQ9XZZ Repair Left Upper Arm, External Approach
0XQB0ZZ Repair Right Elbow Region, Open Approach
0XQB3ZZ Repair Right Elbow Region, Percutaneous Approach
0XQB4ZZ Repair Right Elbow Region, Percutaneous Endoscopic Approach
0XQBXZZ Repair Right Elbow Region, External Approach
0XQC0ZZ Repair Left Elbow Region, Open Approach
0XQC3ZZ Repair Left Elbow Region, Percutaneous Approach
0XQC4ZZ Repair Left Elbow Region, Percutaneous Endoscopic Approach
0XQCXZZ Repair Left Elbow Region, External Approach
0XQD0ZZ Repair Right Lower Arm, Open Approach
0XQD3ZZ Repair Right Lower Arm, Percutaneous Approach
0XQD4ZZ Repair Right Lower Arm, Percutaneous Endoscopic Approach
0XQDXZZ Repair Right Lower Arm, External Approach
0XQF0ZZ Repair Left Lower Arm, Open Approach
0XQF3ZZ Repair Left Lower Arm, Percutaneous Approach
0XQF4ZZ Repair Left Lower Arm, Percutaneous Endoscopic Approach
0XQFXZZ Repair Left Lower Arm, External Approach
0XQG0ZZ Repair Right Wrist Region, Open Approach
0XQG3ZZ Repair Right Wrist Region, Percutaneous Approach
0XQG4ZZ Repair Right Wrist Region, Percutaneous Endoscopic Approach
0XQGXZZ Repair Right Wrist Region, External Approach
0XQH0ZZ Repair Left Wrist Region, Open Approach
0XQH3ZZ Repair Left Wrist Region, Percutaneous Approach
0XQH4ZZ Repair Left Wrist Region, Percutaneous Endoscopic Approach
0XQHXZZ Repair Left Wrist Region, External Approach
0XQJ0ZZ Repair Right Hand, Open Approach
0XQJ3ZZ Repair Right Hand, Percutaneous Approach
0XQJ4ZZ Repair Right Hand, Percutaneous Endoscopic Approach
0XQJXZZ Repair Right Hand, External Approach
0XQK0ZZ Repair Left Hand, Open Approach
0XQK3ZZ Repair Left Hand, Percutaneous Approach
0XQK4ZZ Repair Left Hand, Percutaneous Endoscopic Approach
0XQKXZZ Repair Left Hand, External Approach
0XQL0ZZ Repair Right Thumb, Open Approach
0XQL3ZZ Repair Right Thumb, Percutaneous Approach
0XQL4ZZ Repair Right Thumb, Percutaneous Endoscopic Approach
0XQLXZZ Repair Right Thumb, External Approach
0XQM0ZZ Repair Left Thumb, Open Approach
0XQM3ZZ Repair Left Thumb, Percutaneous Approach
0XQM4ZZ Repair Left Thumb, Percutaneous Endoscopic Approach
0XQMXZZ Repair Left Thumb, External Approach
0XQN0ZZ Repair Right Index Finger, Open Approach
0XQN3ZZ Repair Right Index Finger, Percutaneous Approach
0XQN4ZZ Repair Right Index Finger, Percutaneous Endoscopic Approach
0XQNXZZ Repair Right Index Finger, External Approach
0XQP0ZZ Repair Left Index Finger, Open Approach
0XQP3ZZ Repair Left Index Finger, Percutaneous Approach
0XQP4ZZ Repair Left Index Finger, Percutaneous Endoscopic Approach
0XQPXZZ Repair Left Index Finger, External Approach
0XQQ0ZZ Repair Right Middle Finger, Open Approach
0XQQ3ZZ Repair Right Middle Finger, Percutaneous Approach
0XQQ4ZZ Repair Right Middle Finger, Percutaneous Endoscopic Approach
0XQQXZZ Repair Right Middle Finger, External Approach
0XQR0ZZ Repair Left Middle Finger, Open Approach
0XQR3ZZ Repair Left Middle Finger, Percutaneous Approach
0XQR4ZZ Repair Left Middle Finger, Percutaneous Endoscopic Approach
0XQRXZZ Repair Left Middle Finger, External Approach
0XQS0ZZ Repair Right Ring Finger, Open Approach
0XQS3ZZ Repair Right Ring Finger, Percutaneous Approach
0XQS4ZZ Repair Right Ring Finger, Percutaneous Endoscopic Approach
0XQSXZZ Repair Right Ring Finger, External Approach
0XQT0ZZ Repair Left Ring Finger, Open Approach
0XQT3ZZ Repair Left Ring Finger, Percutaneous Approach
0XQT4ZZ Repair Left Ring Finger, Percutaneous Endoscopic Approach
0XQTXZZ Repair Left Ring Finger, External Approach
0XQV0ZZ Repair Right Little Finger, Open Approach
0XQV3ZZ Repair Right Little Finger, Percutaneous Approach
0XQV4ZZ Repair Right Little Finger, Percutaneous Endoscopic Approach
0XQVXZZ Repair Right Little Finger, External Approach
0XQW0ZZ Repair Left Little Finger, Open Approach
0XQW3ZZ Repair Left Little Finger, Percutaneous Approach
0XQW4ZZ Repair Left Little Finger, Percutaneous Endoscopic Approach
0XQWXZZ Repair Left Little Finger, External Approach

0XR – Anatomical Regions, Upper Extremities, Replacement

0XRL07N Replacement of Right Thumb with Right Toe, Autologous Tissue Substitute, Open Approach
0XRL07P Replacement of Right Thumb with Left Toe, Autologous Tissue Substitute, Open Approach
0XRL47N Replacement of Right Thumb with Right Toe, Autologous Tissue Substitute, Percutaneous Endoscopic Approach
0XRL47P Replacement of Right Thumb with Left Toe, Autologous Tissue Substitute, Percutaneous Endoscopic Approach
0XRM07N Replacement of Left Thumb with Right Toe, Autologous Tissue Substitute, Open Approach
0XRM07P Replacement of Left Thumb with Left Toe, Autologous Tissue Substitute, Open Approach
0XRM47N Replacement of Left Thumb with Right Toe, Autologous Tissue Substitute, Percutaneous Endoscopic Approach
0XRM47P Replacement of Left Thumb with Left Toe, Autologous Tissue Substitute, Percutaneous Endoscopic Approach

0XU – Anatomical Regions, Upper Extremities, Supplement

0XU207Z Supplement Right Shoulder Region with Autologous Tissue Substitute, Open Approach
0XU20JZ Supplement Right Shoulder Region with Synthetic Substitute, Open Approach
0XU20KZ Supplement Right Shoulder Region with Nonautologous Tissue Substitute, Open Approach
0XU247Z Supplement Right Shoulder Region with Autologous Tissue Substitute, Percutaneous Endoscopic Approach
0XU24JZ Supplement Right Shoulder Region with Synthetic Substitute, Percutaneous Endoscopic Approach
0XU24KZ Supplement Right Shoulder Region with Nonautologous Tissue Substitute, Percutaneous Endoscopic Approach
0XU307Z Supplement Left Shoulder Region with Autologous Tissue Substitute, Open Approach
0XU30JZ Supplement Left Shoulder Region with Synthetic Substitute, Open Approach
0XU30KZ Supplement Left Shoulder Region with Nonautologous Tissue Substitute, Open Approach

0XU347Z Supplement Left Shoulder Region with Autologous Tissue Substitute, Percutaneous Endoscopic Approach
0XU34JZ Supplement Left Shoulder Region with Synthetic Substitute, Percutaneous Endoscopic Approach
0XU34KZ Supplement Left Shoulder Region with Nonautologous Tissue Substitute, Percutaneous Endoscopic Approach
0XU407Z Supplement Right Axilla with Autologous Tissue Substitute, Open Approach
0XU40JZ Supplement Right Axilla with Synthetic Substitute, Open Approach
0XU40KZ Supplement Right Axilla with Nonautologous Tissue Substitute, Open Approach
0XU447Z Supplement Right Axilla with Autologous Tissue Substitute, Percutaneous Endoscopic Approach
0XU44JZ Supplement Right Axilla with Synthetic Substitute, Percutaneous Endoscopic Approach
0XU44KZ Supplement Right Axilla with Nonautologous Tissue Substitute, Percutaneous Endoscopic Approach
0XU507Z Supplement Left Axilla with Autologous Tissue Substitute, Open Approach
0XU50JZ Supplement Left Axilla with Synthetic Substitute, Open Approach
0XU50KZ Supplement Left Axilla with Nonautologous Tissue Substitute, Open Approach
0XU547Z Supplement Left Axilla with Autologous Tissue Substitute, Percutaneous Endoscopic Approach
0XU54JZ Supplement Left Axilla with Synthetic Substitute, Percutaneous Endoscopic Approach
0XU54KZ Supplement Left Axilla with Nonautologous Tissue Substitute, Percutaneous Endoscopic Approach
0XU607Z Supplement Right Upper Extremity with Autologous Tissue Substitute, Open Approach
0XU60JZ Supplement Right Upper Extremity with Synthetic Substitute, Open Approach
0XU60KZ Supplement Right Upper Extremity with Nonautologous Tissue Substitute, Open Approach
0XU647Z Supplement Right Upper Extremity with Autologous Tissue Substitute, Percutaneous Endoscopic Approach
0XU64JZ Supplement Right Upper Extremity with Synthetic Substitute, Percutaneous Endoscopic Approach
0XU64KZ Supplement Right Upper Extremity with Nonautologous Tissue Substitute, Percutaneous Endoscopic Approach
0XU707Z Supplement Left Upper Extremity with Autologous Tissue Substitute, Open Approach
0XU70JZ Supplement Left Upper Extremity with Synthetic Substitute, Open Approach
0XU70KZ Supplement Left Upper Extremity with Nonautologous Tissue Substitute, Open Approach
0XU747Z Supplement Left Upper Extremity with Autologous Tissue Substitute, Percutaneous Endoscopic Approach
0XU74JZ Supplement Left Upper Extremity with Synthetic Substitute, Percutaneous Endoscopic Approach
0XU74KZ Supplement Left Upper Extremity with Nonautologous Tissue Substitute, Percutaneous Endoscopic Approach
0XU807Z Supplement Right Upper Arm with Autologous Tissue Substitute, Open Approach
0XU80JZ Supplement Right Upper Arm with Synthetic Substitute, Open Approach
0XU80KZ Supplement Right Upper Arm with Nonautologous Tissue Substitute, Open Approach
0XU847Z Supplement Right Upper Arm with Autologous Tissue Substitute, Percutaneous Endoscopic Approach
0XU84JZ Supplement Right Upper Arm with Synthetic Substitute, Percutaneous Endoscopic Approach
0XU84KZ Supplement Right Upper Arm with Nonautologous Tissue Substitute, Percutaneous Endoscopic Approach
0XU907Z Supplement Left Upper Arm with Autologous Tissue Substitute, Open Approach
0XU90JZ Supplement Left Upper Arm with Synthetic Substitute, Open Approach
0XU90KZ Supplement Left Upper Arm with Nonautologous Tissue Substitute, Open Approach
0XU947Z Supplement Left Upper Arm with Autologous Tissue Substitute, Percutaneous Endoscopic Approach
0XU94JZ Supplement Left Upper Arm with Synthetic Substitute, Percutaneous Endoscopic Approach
0XU94KZ Supplement Left Upper Arm with Nonautologous Tissue Substitute, Percutaneous Endoscopic Approach
0XUB07Z Supplement Right Elbow Region with Autologous Tissue Substitute, Open Approach
0XUB0JZ Supplement Right Elbow Region with Synthetic Substitute, Open Approach
0XUB0KZ Supplement Right Elbow Region with Nonautologous Tissue Substitute, Open Approach
0XUB47Z Supplement Right Elbow Region with Autologous Tissue Substitute, Percutaneous Endoscopic Approach
0XUB4JZ Supplement Right Elbow Region with Synthetic Substitute, Percutaneous Endoscopic Approach
0XUB4KZ Supplement Right Elbow Region with Nonautologous Tissue Substitute, Percutaneous Endoscopic Approach
0XUC07Z Supplement Left Elbow Region with Autologous Tissue Substitute, Open Approach
0XUC0JZ Supplement Left Elbow Region with Synthetic Substitute, Open Approach
0XUC0KZ Supplement Left Elbow Region with Nonautologous Tissue Substitute, Open Approach
0XUC47Z Supplement Left Elbow Region with Autologous Tissue Substitute, Percutaneous Endoscopic Approach
0XUC4JZ Supplement Left Elbow Region with Synthetic Substitute, Percutaneous Endoscopic Approach
0XUC4KZ Supplement Left Elbow Region with Nonautologous Tissue Substitute, Percutaneous Endoscopic Approach
0XUD07Z Supplement Right Lower Arm with Autologous Tissue Substitute, Open Approach
0XUD0JZ Supplement Right Lower Arm with Synthetic Substitute, Open Approach
0XUD0KZ Supplement Right Lower Arm with Nonautologous Tissue Substitute, Open Approach
0XUD47Z Supplement Right Lower Arm with Autologous Tissue Substitute, Percutaneous Endoscopic Approach
0XUD4JZ Supplement Right Lower Arm with Synthetic Substitute, Percutaneous Endoscopic Approach
0XUD4KZ Supplement Right Lower Arm with Nonautologous Tissue Substitute, Percutaneous Endoscopic Approach
0XUF07Z Supplement Left Lower Arm with Autologous Tissue Substitute, Open Approach
0XUF0JZ Supplement Left Lower Arm with Synthetic Substitute, Open Approach
0XUF0KZ Supplement Left Lower Arm with Nonautologous Tissue Substitute, Open Approach
0XUF47Z Supplement Left Lower Arm with Autologous Tissue Substitute, Percutaneous Endoscopic Approach
0XUF4JZ Supplement Left Lower Arm with Synthetic Substitute, Percutaneous Endoscopic Approach
0XUF4KZ Supplement Left Lower Arm with Nonautologous Tissue Substitute, Percutaneous Endoscopic Approach
0XUG07Z Supplement Right Wrist Region with Autologous Tissue Substitute, Open Approach
0XUG0JZ Supplement Right Wrist Region with Synthetic Substitute, Open Approach
0XUG0KZ Supplement Right Wrist Region with Nonautologous Tissue Substitute, Open Approach
0XUG47Z Supplement Right Wrist Region with Autologous Tissue Substitute, Percutaneous Endoscopic Approach
0XUG4JZ Supplement Right Wrist Region with Synthetic Substitute, Percutaneous Endoscopic Approach
0XUG4KZ Supplement Right Wrist Region with Nonautologous Tissue Substitute, Percutaneous Endoscopic Approach
0XUH07Z Supplement Left Wrist Region with Autologous Tissue Substitute, Open Approach
0XUH0JZ Supplement Left Wrist Region with Synthetic Substitute, Open Approach
0XUH0KZ Supplement Left Wrist Region with Nonautologous Tissue Substitute, Open Approach
0XUH47Z Supplement Left Wrist Region with Autologous Tissue Substitute, Percutaneous Endoscopic Approach
0XUH4JZ Supplement Left Wrist Region with Synthetic Substitute, Percutaneous Endoscopic Approach
0XUH4KZ Supplement Left Wrist Region with Nonautologous Tissue Substitute, Percutaneous Endoscopic Approach
0XUJ07Z Supplement Right Hand with Autologous Tissue Substitute, Open Approach
0XUJ0JZ Supplement Right Hand with Synthetic Substitute, Open Approach
0XUJ0KZ Supplement Right Hand with Nonautologous Tissue Substitute, Open Approach
0XUJ47Z Supplement Right Hand with Autologous Tissue Substitute, Percutaneous Endoscopic Approach
0XUJ4JZ Supplement Right Hand with Synthetic Substitute, Percutaneous Endoscopic Approach
0XUJ4KZ Supplement Right Hand with Nonautologous Tissue Substitute, Percutaneous Endoscopic Approach
0XUK07Z Supplement Left Hand with Autologous Tissue Substitute, Open Approach
0XUK0JZ Supplement Left Hand with Synthetic Substitute, Open Approach

0XUK0KZ Supplement Left Hand with Nonautologous Tissue Substitute, Open Approach
0XUK47Z Supplement Left Hand with Autologous Tissue Substitute, Percutaneous Endoscopic Approach
0XUK4JZ Supplement Left Hand with Synthetic Substitute, Percutaneous Endoscopic Approach
0XUK4KZ Supplement Left Hand with Nonautologous Tissue Substitute, Percutaneous Endoscopic Approach
0XUL07Z Supplement Right Thumb with Autologous Tissue Substitute, Open Approach
0XUL0JZ Supplement Right Thumb with Synthetic Substitute, Open Approach
0XUL0KZ Supplement Right Thumb with Nonautologous Tissue Substitute, Open Approach
0XUL47Z Supplement Right Thumb with Autologous Tissue Substitute, Percutaneous Endoscopic Approach
0XUL4JZ Supplement Right Thumb with Synthetic Substitute, Percutaneous Endoscopic Approach
0XUL4KZ Supplement Right Thumb with Nonautologous Tissue Substitute, Percutaneous Endoscopic Approach
0XUM07Z Supplement Left Thumb with Autologous Tissue Substitute, Open Approach
0XUM0JZ Supplement Left Thumb with Synthetic Substitute, Open Approach
0XUM0KZ Supplement Left Thumb with Nonautologous Tissue Substitute, Open Approach
0XUM47Z Supplement Left Thumb with Autologous Tissue Substitute, Percutaneous Endoscopic Approach
0XUM4JZ Supplement Left Thumb with Synthetic Substitute, Percutaneous Endoscopic Approach
0XUM4KZ Supplement Left Thumb with Nonautologous Tissue Substitute, Percutaneous Endoscopic Approach
0XUN07Z Supplement Right Index Finger with Autologous Tissue Substitute, Open Approach
0XUN0JZ Supplement Right Index Finger with Synthetic Substitute, Open Approach
0XUN0KZ Supplement Right Index Finger with Nonautologous Tissue Substitute, Open Approach
0XUN47Z Supplement Right Index Finger with Autologous Tissue Substitute, Percutaneous Endoscopic Approach
0XUN4JZ Supplement Right Index Finger with Synthetic Substitute, Percutaneous Endoscopic Approach
0XUN4KZ Supplement Right Index Finger with Nonautologous Tissue Substitute, Percutaneous Endoscopic Approach
0XUP07Z Supplement Left Index Finger with Autologous Tissue Substitute, Open Approach
0XUP0JZ Supplement Left Index Finger with Synthetic Substitute, Open Approach
0XUP0KZ Supplement Left Index Finger with Nonautologous Tissue Substitute, Open Approach
0XUP47Z Supplement Left Index Finger with Autologous Tissue Substitute, Percutaneous Endoscopic Approach
0XUP4JZ Supplement Left Index Finger with Synthetic Substitute, Percutaneous Endoscopic Approach
0XUP4KZ Supplement Left Index Finger with Nonautologous Tissue Substitute, Percutaneous Endoscopic Approach
0XUQ07Z Supplement Right Middle Finger with Autologous Tissue Substitute, Open Approach
0XUQ0JZ Supplement Right Middle Finger with Synthetic Substitute, Open Approach
0XUQ0KZ Supplement Right Middle Finger with Nonautologous Tissue Substitute, Open Approach
0XUQ47Z Supplement Right Middle Finger with Autologous Tissue Substitute, Percutaneous Endoscopic Approach
0XUQ4JZ Supplement Right Middle Finger with Synthetic Substitute, Percutaneous Endoscopic Approach
0XUQ4KZ Supplement Right Middle Finger with Nonautologous Tissue Substitute, Percutaneous Endoscopic Approach
0XUR07Z Supplement Left Middle Finger with Autologous Tissue Substitute, Open Approach
0XUR0JZ Supplement Left Middle Finger with Synthetic Substitute, Open Approach
0XUR0KZ Supplement Left Middle Finger with Nonautologous Tissue Substitute, Open Approach
0XUR47Z Supplement Left Middle Finger with Autologous Tissue Substitute, Percutaneous Endoscopic Approach
0XUR4JZ Supplement Left Middle Finger with Synthetic Substitute, Percutaneous Endoscopic Approach
0XUR4KZ Supplement Left Middle Finger with Nonautologous Tissue Substitute, Percutaneous Endoscopic Approach
0XUS07Z Supplement Right Ring Finger with Autologous Tissue Substitute, Open Approach
0XUS0JZ Supplement Right Ring Finger with Synthetic Substitute, Open Approach
0XUS0KZ Supplement Right Ring Finger with Nonautologous Tissue Substitute, Open Approach
0XUS47Z Supplement Right Ring Finger with Autologous Tissue Substitute, Percutaneous Endoscopic Approach
0XUS4JZ Supplement Right Ring Finger with Synthetic Substitute, Percutaneous Endoscopic Approach
0XUS4KZ Supplement Right Ring Finger with Nonautologous Tissue Substitute, Percutaneous Endoscopic Approach
0XUT07Z Supplement Left Ring Finger with Autologous Tissue Substitute, Open Approach
0XUT0JZ Supplement Left Ring Finger with Synthetic Substitute, Open Approach
0XUT0KZ Supplement Left Ring Finger with Nonautologous Tissue Substitute, Open Approach
0XUT47Z Supplement Left Ring Finger with Autologous Tissue Substitute, Percutaneous Endoscopic Approach
0XUT4JZ Supplement Left Ring Finger with Synthetic Substitute, Percutaneous Endoscopic Approach
0XUT4KZ Supplement Left Ring Finger with Nonautologous Tissue Substitute, Percutaneous Endoscopic Approach
0XUV07Z Supplement Right Little Finger with Autologous Tissue Substitute, Open Approach
0XUV0JZ Supplement Right Little Finger with Synthetic Substitute, Open Approach
0XUV0KZ Supplement Right Little Finger with Nonautologous Tissue Substitute, Open Approach
0XUV47Z Supplement Right Little Finger with Autologous Tissue Substitute, Percutaneous Endoscopic Approach
0XUV4JZ Supplement Right Little Finger with Synthetic Substitute, Percutaneous Endoscopic Approach
0XUV4KZ Supplement Right Little Finger with Nonautologous Tissue Substitute, Percutaneous Endoscopic Approach
0XUW07Z Supplement Left Little Finger with Autologous Tissue Substitute, Open Approach
0XUW0JZ Supplement Left Little Finger with Synthetic Substitute, Open Approach
0XUW0KZ Supplement Left Little Finger with Nonautologous Tissue Substitute, Open Approach
0XUW47Z Supplement Left Little Finger with Autologous Tissue Substitute, Percutaneous Endoscopic Approach
0XUW4JZ Supplement Left Little Finger with Synthetic Substitute, Percutaneous Endoscopic Approach
0XUW4KZ Supplement Left Little Finger with Nonautologous Tissue Substitute, Percutaneous Endoscopic Approach

0XW – Anatomical Regions, Upper Extremities, Revision

Review Coding Guideline B6.1c

● **0XW600Z** Revision of Drainage Device in Right Upper Extremity, Open Approach
● **0XW603Z** Revision of Infusion Device in Right Upper Extremity, Open Approach
● **0XW607Z** Revision of Autologous Tissue Substitute in Right Upper Extremity, Open Approach
● **0XW60JZ** Revision of Synthetic Substitute in Right Upper Extremity, Open Approach
● **0XW60KZ** Revision of Nonautologous Tissue Substitute in Right Upper Extremity, Open Approach
● **0XW60YZ** Revision of Other Device in Right Upper Extremity, Open Approach
● **0XW630Z** Revision of Drainage Device in Right Upper Extremity, Percutaneous Approach
● **0XW633Z** Revision of Infusion Device in Right Upper Extremity, Percutaneous Approach
● **0XW637Z** Revision of Autologous Tissue Substitute in Right Upper Extremity, Percutaneous Approach
● **0XW63JZ** Revision of Synthetic Substitute in Right Upper Extremity, Percutaneous Approach
● **0XW63KZ** Revision of Nonautologous Tissue Substitute in Right Upper Extremity, Percutaneous Approach
● **0XW63YZ** Revision of Other Device in Right Upper Extremity, Percutaneous Approach

- ● 0XW640Z Revision of Drainage Device in Right Upper Extremity, Percutaneous Endoscopic Approach
- ● 0XW643Z Revision of Infusion Device in Right Upper Extremity, Percutaneous Endoscopic Approach
- ● 0XW647Z Revision of Autologous Tissue Substitute in Right Upper Extremity, Percutaneous Endoscopic Approach
- ● 0XW64JZ Revision of Synthetic Substitute in Right Upper Extremity, Percutaneous Endoscopic Approach
- ● 0XW64KZ Revision of Nonautologous Tissue Substitute in Right Upper Extremity, Percutaneous Endoscopic Approach
- ● 0XW64YZ Revision of Other Device in Right Upper Extremity, Percutaneous Endoscopic Approach
- 0XW6X0Z Revision of Drainage Device in Right Upper Extremity, External Approach
- 0XW6X3Z Revision of Infusion Device in Right Upper Extremity, External Approach
- 0XW6X7Z Revision of Autologous Tissue Substitute in Right Upper Extremity, External Approach
- 0XW6XJZ Revision of Synthetic Substitute in Right Upper Extremity, External Approach
- 0XW6XKZ Revision of Nonautologous Tissue Substitute in Right Upper Extremity, External Approach
- 0XW6XYZ Revision of Other Device in Right Upper Extremity, External Approach
- ● 0XW700Z Revision of Drainage Device in Left Upper Extremity, Open Approach
- ● 0XW703Z Revision of Infusion Device in Left Upper Extremity, Open Approach
- ● 0XW707Z Revision of Autologous Tissue Substitute in Left Upper Extremity, Open Approach
- ● 0XW70JZ Revision of Synthetic Substitute in Left Upper Extremity, Open Approach
- ● 0XW70KZ Revision of Nonautologous Tissue Substitute in Left Upper Extremity, Open Approach
- ● 0XW70YZ Revision of Other Device in Left Upper Extremity, Open Approach
- ● 0XW730Z Revision of Drainage Device in Left Upper Extremity, Percutaneous Approach
- ● 0XW733Z Revision of Infusion Device in Left Upper Extremity, Percutaneous Approach
- ● 0XW737Z Revision of Autologous Tissue Substitute in Left Upper Extremity, Percutaneous Approach
- ● 0XW73JZ Revision of Synthetic Substitute in Left Upper Extremity, Percutaneous Approach
- ● 0XW73KZ Revision of Nonautologous Tissue Substitute in Left Upper Extremity, Percutaneous Approach
- ● 0XW73YZ Revision of Other Device in Left Upper Extremity, Percutaneous Approach
- ● 0XW740Z Revision of Drainage Device in Left Upper Extremity, Percutaneous Endoscopic Approach
- ● 0XW743Z Revision of Infusion Device in Left Upper Extremity, Percutaneous Endoscopic Approach
- ● 0XW747Z Revision of Autologous Tissue Substitute in Left Upper Extremity, Percutaneous Endoscopic Approach
- ● 0XW74JZ Revision of Synthetic Substitute in Left Upper Extremity, Percutaneous Endoscopic Approach
- ● 0XW74KZ Revision of Nonautologous Tissue Substitute in Left Upper Extremity, Percutaneous Endoscopic Approach
- ● 0XW74YZ Revision of Other Device in Left Upper Extremity, Percutaneous Endoscopic Approach
- 0XW7X0Z Revision of Drainage Device in Left Upper Extremity, External Approach
- 0XW7X3Z Revision of Infusion Device in Left Upper Extremity, External Approach
- 0XW7X7Z Revision of Autologous Tissue Substitute in Left Upper Extremity, External Approach
- 0XW7XJZ Revision of Synthetic Substitute in Left Upper Extremity, External Approach
- 0XW7XKZ Revision of Nonautologous Tissue Substitute in Left Upper Extremity, External Approach
- 0XW7XYZ Revision of Other Device in Left Upper Extremity, External Approach

0XX – Anatomical Regions, Upper Extremities, Transfer

- 0XXN0ZL Transfer Right Index Finger to Right Thumb, Open Approach
- 0XXP0ZM Transfer Left Index Finger to Left Thumb, Open Approach

Anatomical Regions, Lower Extremities

Anatomical Regions, Lower Extremities 0Y0–0YW

Section 0 **Medical and Surgical**
Body System Y **Anatomical Regions, Lower Extremities**
Operation 0 **Alteration:** Modifying the anatomic structure of a body part without affecting the function of the body part

Body Part (4th)	Approach (5th)	Device (6th)	Qualifier (7th)
0 Buttock, Right **1** Buttock, Left **9** Lower Extremity, Right **B** Lower Extremity, Left **C** Upper Leg, Right **D** Upper Leg, Left **F** Knee Region, Right **G** Knee Region, Left **H** Lower Leg, Right **J** Lower Leg, Left **K** Ankle Region, Right **L** Ankle Region, Left	**0** Open **3** Percutaneous **4** Percutaneous Endoscopic	**7** Autologous Tissue Substitute **J** Synthetic Substitute **K** Nonautologous Tissue Substitute **Z** No Device	**Z** No Qualifier

Section 0 **Medical and Surgical**
Body System Y **Anatomical Regions, Lower Extremities**
Operation 2 **Change:** Taking out or off a device from a body part and putting back an identical or similar device in or on the same body part without cutting or puncturing the skin or a mucous membrane

Body Part (4th)	Approach (5th)	Device (6th)	Qualifier (7th)
9 Lower Extremity, Right **B** Lower Extremity, Left	**X** External	**0** Drainage Device **Y** Other Device	**Z** No Qualifier

Section 0 **Medical and Surgical**
Body System Y **Anatomical Regions, Lower Extremities**
Operation 3 **Control:** Stopping, or attempting to stop, postprocedural bleeding

Body Part (4th)	Approach (5th)	Device (6th)	Qualifier (7th)
0 Buttock, Right **1** Buttock, Left **5** Inguinal Region, Right **6** Inguinal Region, Left **7** Femoral Region, Right **8** Femoral Region, Left **9** Lower Extremity, Right **B** Lower Extremity, Left **C** Upper Leg, Right **D** Upper Leg, Left **F** Knee Region, Right **G** Knee Region, Left **H** Lower Leg, Right **J** Lower Leg, Left **K** Ankle Region, Right **L** Ankle Region, Left **M** Foot, Right **N** Foot, Left	**0** Open **3** Percutaneous **4** Percutaneous Endoscopic	**Z** No Device	**Z** No Qualifier

Section 0 **Medical and Surgical**
Body System Y **Anatomical Regions, Lower Extremities**
Operation 6 **Detachment:** Cutting off all or a portion of the upper or lower extremities

Body Part (4th)	Approach (5th)	Device (6th)	Qualifier (7th)
2 Hindquarter, Right **3** Hindquarter, Left **4** Hindquarter, Bilateral **7** Femoral Region, Right **8** Femoral Region, Left **F** Knee Region, Right **G** Knee Region, Left	**0** Open	**Z** No Device	**Z** No Qualifier
C Upper Leg, Right **D** Upper Leg, Left **H** Lower Leg, Right **J** Lower Leg, Left	**0** Open	**Z** No Device	**1** High **2** Mid **3** Low
M Foot, Right **N** Foot, Left	**0** Open	**Z** No Device	**0** Complete **4** Complete 1st Ray **5** Complete 2nd Ray **6** Complete 3rd Ray **7** Complete 4th Ray **8** Complete 5th Ray **9** Partial 1st Ray **B** Partial 2nd Ray **C** Partial 3rd Ray **D** Partial 4th Ray **F** Partial 5th Ray
P 1st Toe, Right **Q** 1st Toe, Left **R** 2nd Toe, Right **S** 2nd Toe, Left **T** 3rd Toe, Right **U** 3rd Toe, Left **V** 4th Toe, Right **W** 4th Toe, Left **X** 5th Toe, Right **Y** 5th Toe, Left	**0** Open	**Z** No Device	**0** Complete **1** High **2** Mid **3** Low

Section 0 **Medical and Surgical**
Body System Y **Anatomical Regions, Lower Extremities**
Operation 9 **Drainage:** Taking or letting out fluids and/or gases from a body part

Body Part (4th)	Approach (5th)	Device (6th)	Qualifier (7th)
0 Buttock, Right **1** Buttock, Left **5** Inguinal Region, Right **6** Inguinal Region, Left **7** Femoral Region, Right **8** Femoral Region, Left **9** Lower Extremity, Right **B** Lower Extremity, Left **C** Upper Leg, Right **D** Upper Leg, Left **F** Knee Region, Right **G** Knee Region, Left **H** Lower Leg, Right **J** Lower Leg, Left **K** Ankle Region, Right **L** Ankle Region, Left **M** Foot, Right **N** Foot, Left	**0** Open **3** Percutaneous **4** Percutaneous Endoscopic	**0** Drainage Device	**Z** No Qualifier

Continued →

Section 0 **Medical and Surgical**
Body System Y **Anatomical Regions, Lower Extremities**
Operation 9 **Drainage:** Taking or letting out fluids and/or gases from a body part

Body Part (4th)	Approach (5th)	Device (6th)	Qualifier (7th)
0 Buttock, Right **1** Buttock, Left **5** Inguinal Region, Right **6** Inguinal Region, Left **7** Femoral Region, Right **8** Femoral Region, Left **9** Lower Extremity, Right **B** Lower Extremity, Left **C** Upper Leg, Right **D** Upper Leg, Left **F** Knee Region, Right **G** Knee Region, Left **H** Lower Leg, Right **J** Lower Leg, Left **K** Ankle Region, Right **L** Ankle Region, Left **M** Foot, Right **N** Foot, Left	**0** Open **3** Percutaneous **4** Percutaneous Endoscopic	**Z** No Device	**X** Diagnostic **Z** No Qualifier

Section 0 **Medical and Surgical**
Body System Y **Anatomical Regions, Lower Extremities**
Operation B **Excision:** Cutting out or off, without replacement, a portion of a body part

Body Part (4th)	Approach (5th)	Device (6th)	Qualifier (7th)
0 Buttock, Right **1** Buttock, Left **5** Inguinal Region, Right **6** Inguinal Region, Left **7** Femoral Region, Right **8** Femoral Region, Left **9** Lower Extremity, Right **B** Lower Extremity, Left **C** Upper Leg, Right **D** Upper Leg, Left **F** Knee Region, Right **G** Knee Region, Left **H** Lower Leg, Right **J** Lower Leg, Left **K** Ankle Region, Right **L** Ankle Region, Left **M** Foot, Right **N** Foot, Left	**0** Open **3** Percutaneous **4** Percutaneous Endoscopic	**Z** No Device	**X** Diagnostic **Z** No Qualifier

Section 0 **Medical and Surgical**
Body System Y **Anatomical Regions, Lower Extremities**
Operation H **Insertion:** Putting in a nonbiological appliance that monitors, assists, performs, or prevents a physiological function but does not physically take the place of a body part

Body Part (4th)	Approach (5th)	Device (6th)	Qualifier (7th)
0 Buttock, Right **1** Buttock, Left **5** Inguinal Region, Right **6** Inguinal Region, Left **7** Femoral Region, Right **8** Femoral Region, Left **9** Lower Extremity, Right **B** Lower Extremity, Left **C** Upper Leg, Right **D** Upper Leg, Left **F** Knee Region, Right **G** Knee Region, Left **H** Lower Leg, Right **J** Lower Leg, Left **K** Ankle Region, Right **L** Ankle Region, Left **M** Foot, Right **N** Foot, Left	**0** Open **3** Percutaneous **4** Percutaneous Endoscopic	**1** Radioactive Element **3** Infusion Device **Y** Other Device	**Z** No Qualifier

Section 0 **Medical and Surgical**
Body System Y **Anatomical Regions, Lower Extremities**
Operation J **Inspection:** Visually and/or manually exploring a body part

Body Part (4th)	Approach (5th)	Device (6th)	Qualifier (7th)
0 Buttock, Right **1** Buttock, Left **5** Inguinal Region, Right **6** Inguinal Region, Left **7** Femoral Region, Right **8** Femoral Region, Left **9** Lower Extremity, Right **A** Inguinal Region, Bilateral **B** Lower Extremity, Left **C** Upper Leg, Right **D** Upper Leg, Left **E** Femoral Region, Bilateral **F** Knee Region, Right **G** Knee Region, Left **H** Lower Leg, Right **J** Lower Leg, Left **K** Ankle Region, Right **L** Ankle Region, Left **M** Foot, Right **N** Foot, Left	**0** Open **3** Percutaneous **4** Percutaneous Endoscopic **X** External	**Z** No Device	**Z** No Qualifier

Section 0 **Medical and Surgical**
Body System Y **Anatomical Regions, Lower Extremities**
Operation M **Reattachment:** Putting back in or on all or a portion of a separated body part to its normal location or other suitable location

Body Part (4th)	Approach (5th)	Device (6th)	Qualifier (7th)
0 Buttock, Right **1** Buttock, Left **2** Hindquarter, Right **3** Hindquarter, Left **4** Hindquarter, Bilateral **5** Inguinal Region, Right **6** Inguinal Region, Left **7** Femoral Region, Right **8** Femoral Region, Left **9** Lower Extremity, Right **B** Lower Extremity, Left **C** Upper Leg, Right **D** Upper Leg, Left **F** Knee Region, Right **G** Knee Region, Left **H** Lower Leg, Right **J** Lower Leg, Left **K** Ankle Region, Right **L** Ankle Region, Left **M** Foot, Right **N** Foot, Left **P** 1st Toe, Right **Q** 1st Toe, Left **R** 2nd Toe, Right **S** 2nd Toe, Left **T** 3rd Toe, Right **U** 3rd Toe, Left **V** 4th Toe, Right **W** 4th Toe, Left **X** 5th Toe, Right **Y** 5th Toe, Left	**0** Open	**Z** No Device	**Z** No Qualifier

Section 0 **Medical and Surgical**
Body System Y **Anatomical Regions, Lower Extremities**
Operation P **Removal:** Taking out or off a device from a body part

Body Part (4th)	Approach (5th)	Device (6th)	Qualifier (7th)
9 Lower Extremity, Right **B** Lower Extremity, Left	**0** Open **3** Percutaneous **4** Percutaneous Endoscopic **X** External	**0** Drainage Device **1** Radioactive Element **3** Infusion Device **7** Autologous Tissue Substitute **J** Synthetic Substitute **K** Nonautologous Tissue Substitute **Y** Other Device	**Z** No Qualifier

Section 0 **Medical and Surgical**
Body System Y **Anatomical Regions, Lower Extremities**
Operation Q **Repair:** Restoring, to the extent possible, a body part to its normal anatomic structure and function

Body Part (4th)	Approach (5th)	Device (6th)	Qualifier (7th)
0 Buttock, Right **1** Buttock, Left **5** Inguinal Region, Right **6** Inguinal Region, Left **7** Femoral Region, Right **8** Femoral Region, Left **9** Lower Extremity, Right **A** Inguinal Region, Bilateral **B** Lower Extremity, Left **C** Upper Leg, Right **D** Upper Leg, Left **E** Femoral Region, Bilateral **F** Knee Region, Right **G** Knee Region, Left **H** Lower Leg, Right **J** Lower Leg, Left **K** Ankle Region, Right **L** Ankle Region, Left **M** Foot, Right **N** Foot, Left **P** 1st Toe, Right **Q** 1st Toe, Left **R** 2nd Toe, Right **S** 2nd Toe, Left **T** 3rd Toe, Right **U** 3rd Toe, Left **V** 4th Toe, Right **W** 4th Toe, Left **X** 5th Toe, Right **Y** 5th Toe, Left	**0** Open **3** Percutaneous **4** Percutaneous Endoscopic **X** External	**Z** No Device	**Z** No Qualifier

Section 0 **Medical and Surgical**
Body System Y **Anatomical Regions, Lower Extremities**
Operation U **Supplement:** Putting in or on biological or synthetic material that physically reinforces and/or augments the function of a portion of a body part

Body Part (4th)	Approach (5th)	Device (6th)	Qualifier (7th)
0 Buttock, Right **1** Buttock, Left **5** Inguinal Region, Right **6** Inguinal Region, Left **7** Femoral Region, Right **8** Femoral Region, Left **9** Lower Extremity, Right **A** Inguinal Region, Bilateral **B** Lower Extremity, Left **C** Upper Leg, Right **D** Upper Leg, Left **E** Femoral Region, Bilateral **F** Knee Region, Right **G** Knee Region, Left **H** Lower Leg, Right **J** Lower Leg, Left **K** Ankle Region, Right **L** Ankle Region, Left **M** Foot, Right **N** Foot, Left **P** 1st Toe, Right **Q** 1st Toe, Left **R** 2nd Toe, Right **S** 2nd Toe, Left **T** 3rd Toe, Right **U** 3rd Toe, Left **V** 4th Toe, Right **W** 4th Toe, Left **X** 5th Toe, Right **Y** 5th Toe, Left	**0** Open **4** Percutaneous Endoscopic	**7** Autologous Tissue Substitute **J** Synthetic Substitute **K** Nonautologous Tissue Substitute	**Z** No Qualifier

Section 0 **Medical and Surgical**
Body System Y **Anatomical Regions, Lower Extremities**
Operation W **Revision:** Correcting, to the extent possible, a portion of a malfunctioning device or the position of a displaced device

Body Part (4th)	Approach (5th)	Device (6th)	Qualifier (7th)
9 Lower Extremity, Right **B** Lower Extremity, Left	**0** Open **3** Percutaneous **4** Percutaneous Endoscopic **X** External	**0** Drainage Device **3** Infusion Device **7** Autologous Tissue Substitute **J** Synthetic Substitute **K** Nonautologous Tissue Substitute **Y** Other Device	**Z** No Qualifier

Anatomical Regions, Lower Extremities Code Listing 0Y0–0YW

0Y0 – Anatomical Regions, Lower Extremities, Alteration

0Y0007Z Alteration of Right Buttock with Autologous Tissue Substitute, Open Approach
0Y000JZ Alteration of Right Buttock with Synthetic Substitute, Open Approach
0Y000KZ Alteration of Right Buttock with Nonautologous Tissue Substitute, Open Approach
0Y000ZZ Alteration of Right Buttock, Open Approach
0Y0037Z Alteration of Right Buttock with Autologous Tissue Substitute, Percutaneous Approach
0Y003JZ Alteration of Right Buttock with Synthetic Substitute, Percutaneous Approach
0Y003KZ Alteration of Right Buttock with Nonautologous Tissue Substitute, Percutaneous Approach
0Y003ZZ Alteration of Right Buttock, Percutaneous Approach
0Y0047Z Alteration of Right Buttock with Autologous Tissue Substitute, Percutaneous Endoscopic Approach
0Y004JZ Alteration of Right Buttock with Synthetic Substitute, Percutaneous Endoscopic Approach
0Y004KZ Alteration of Right Buttock with Nonautologous Tissue Substitute, Percutaneous Endoscopic Approach
0Y004ZZ Alteration of Right Buttock, Percutaneous Endoscopic Approach
0Y0107Z Alteration of Left Buttock with Autologous Tissue Substitute, Open Approach
0Y010JZ Alteration of Left Buttock with Synthetic Substitute, Open Approach
0Y010KZ Alteration of Left Buttock with Nonautologous Tissue Substitute, Open Approach
0Y010ZZ Alteration of Left Buttock, Open Approach
0Y0137Z Alteration of Left Buttock with Autologous Tissue Substitute, Percutaneous Approach
0Y013JZ Alteration of Left Buttock with Synthetic Substitute, Percutaneous Approach
0Y013KZ Alteration of Left Buttock with Nonautologous Tissue Substitute, Percutaneous Approach

0Y013ZZ Alteration of Left Buttock, Percutaneous Approach
0Y0147Z Alteration of Left Buttock with Autologous Tissue Substitute, Percutaneous Endoscopic Approach
0Y014JZ Alteration of Left Buttock with Synthetic Substitute, Percutaneous Endoscopic Approach
0Y014KZ Alteration of Left Buttock with Nonautologous Tissue Substitute, Percutaneous Endoscopic Approach
0Y014ZZ Alteration of Left Buttock, Percutaneous Endoscopic Approach
0Y0907Z Alteration of Right Lower Extremity with Autologous Tissue Substitute, Open Approach
0Y090JZ Alteration of Right Lower Extremity with Synthetic Substitute, Open Approach
0Y090KZ Alteration of Right Lower Extremity with Nonautologous Tissue Substitute, Open Approach
0Y090ZZ Alteration of Right Lower Extremity, Open Approach
0Y0937Z Alteration of Right Lower Extremity with Autologous Tissue Substitute, Percutaneous Approach
0Y093JZ Alteration of Right Lower Extremity with Synthetic Substitute, Percutaneous Approach
0Y093KZ Alteration of Right Lower Extremity with Nonautologous Tissue Substitute, Percutaneous Approach
0Y093ZZ Alteration of Right Lower Extremity, Percutaneous Approach
0Y0947Z Alteration of Right Lower Extremity with Autologous Tissue Substitute, Percutaneous Endoscopic Approach
0Y094JZ Alteration of Right Lower Extremity with Synthetic Substitute, Percutaneous Endoscopic Approach
0Y094KZ Alteration of Right Lower Extremity with Nonautologous Tissue Substitute, Percutaneous Endoscopic Approach
0Y094ZZ Alteration of Right Lower Extremity, Percutaneous Endoscopic Approach
0Y0B07Z Alteration of Left Lower Extremity with Autologous Tissue Substitute, Open Approach
0Y0B0JZ Alteration of Left Lower Extremity with Synthetic Substitute, Open Approach
0Y0B0KZ Alteration of Left Lower Extremity with Nonautologous Tissue Substitute, Open Approach
0Y0B0ZZ Alteration of Left Lower Extremity, Open Approach
0Y0B37Z Alteration of Left Lower Extremity with Autologous Tissue Substitute, Percutaneous Approach
0Y0B3JZ Alteration of Left Lower Extremity with Synthetic Substitute, Percutaneous Approach
0Y0B3KZ Alteration of Left Lower Extremity with Nonautologous Tissue Substitute, Percutaneous Approach
0Y0B3ZZ Alteration of Left Lower Extremity, Percutaneous Approach
0Y0B47Z Alteration of Left Lower Extremity with Autologous Tissue Substitute, Percutaneous Endoscopic Approach
0Y0B4JZ Alteration of Left Lower Extremity with Synthetic Substitute, Percutaneous Endoscopic Approach
0Y0B4KZ Alteration of Left Lower Extremity with Nonautologous Tissue Substitute, Percutaneous Endoscopic Approach
0Y0B4ZZ Alteration of Left Lower Extremity, Percutaneous Endoscopic Approach
0Y0C07Z Alteration of Right Upper Leg with Autologous Tissue Substitute, Open Approach
0Y0C0JZ Alteration of Right Upper Leg with Synthetic Substitute, Open Approach
0Y0C0KZ Alteration of Right Upper Leg with Nonautologous Tissue Substitute, Open Approach
0Y0C0ZZ Alteration of Right Upper Leg, Open Approach
0Y0C37Z Alteration of Right Upper Leg with Autologous Tissue Substitute, Percutaneous Approach
0Y0C3JZ Alteration of Right Upper Leg with Synthetic Substitute, Percutaneous Approach
0Y0C3KZ Alteration of Right Upper Leg with Nonautologous Tissue Substitute, Percutaneous Approach
0Y0C3ZZ Alteration of Right Upper Leg, Percutaneous Approach
0Y0C47Z Alteration of Right Upper Leg with Autologous Tissue Substitute, Percutaneous Endoscopic Approach
0Y0C4JZ Alteration of Right Upper Leg with Synthetic Substitute, Percutaneous Endoscopic Approach
0Y0C4KZ Alteration of Right Upper Leg with Nonautologous Tissue Substitute, Percutaneous Endoscopic Approach
0Y0C4ZZ Alteration of Right Upper Leg, Percutaneous Endoscopic Approach
0Y0D07Z Alteration of Left Upper Leg with Autologous Tissue Substitute, Open Approach
0Y0D0JZ Alteration of Left Upper Leg with Synthetic Substitute, Open Approach
0Y0D0KZ Alteration of Left Upper Leg with Nonautologous Tissue Substitute, Open Approach
0Y0D0ZZ Alteration of Left Upper Leg, Open Approach
0Y0D37Z Alteration of Left Upper Leg with Autologous Tissue Substitute, Percutaneous Approach
0Y0D3JZ Alteration of Left Upper Leg with Synthetic Substitute, Percutaneous Approach
0Y0D3KZ Alteration of Left Upper Leg with Nonautologous Tissue Substitute, Percutaneous Approach
0Y0D3ZZ Alteration of Left Upper Leg, Percutaneous Approach
0Y0D47Z Alteration of Left Upper Leg with Autologous Tissue Substitute, Percutaneous Endoscopic Approach
0Y0D4JZ Alteration of Left Upper Leg with Synthetic Substitute, Percutaneous Endoscopic Approach
0Y0D4KZ Alteration of Left Upper Leg with Nonautologous Tissue Substitute, Percutaneous Endoscopic Approach
0Y0D4ZZ Alteration of Left Upper Leg, Percutaneous Endoscopic Approach
0Y0F07Z Alteration of Right Knee Region with Autologous Tissue Substitute, Open Approach
0Y0F0JZ Alteration of Right Knee Region with Synthetic Substitute, Open Approach
0Y0F0KZ Alteration of Right Knee Region with Nonautologous Tissue Substitute, Open Approach
0Y0F0ZZ Alteration of Right Knee Region, Open Approach
0Y0F37Z Alteration of Right Knee Region with Autologous Tissue Substitute, Percutaneous Approach
0Y0F3JZ Alteration of Right Knee Region with Synthetic Substitute, Percutaneous Approach
0Y0F3KZ Alteration of Right Knee Region with Nonautologous Tissue Substitute, Percutaneous Approach
0Y0F3ZZ Alteration of Right Knee Region, Percutaneous Approach
0Y0F47Z Alteration of Right Knee Region with Autologous Tissue Substitute, Percutaneous Endoscopic Approach
0Y0F4JZ Alteration of Right Knee Region with Synthetic Substitute, Percutaneous Endoscopic Approach
0Y0F4KZ Alteration of Right Knee Region with Nonautologous Tissue Substitute, Percutaneous Endoscopic Approach
0Y0F4ZZ Alteration of Right Knee Region, Percutaneous Endoscopic Approach
0Y0G07Z Alteration of Left Knee Region with Autologous Tissue Substitute, Open Approach
0Y0G0JZ Alteration of Left Knee Region with Synthetic Substitute, Open Approach
0Y0G0KZ Alteration of Left Knee Region with Nonautologous Tissue Substitute, Open Approach
0Y0G0ZZ Alteration of Left Knee Region, Open Approach
0Y0G37Z Alteration of Left Knee Region with Autologous Tissue Substitute, Percutaneous Approach
0Y0G3JZ Alteration of Left Knee Region with Synthetic Substitute, Percutaneous Approach
0Y0G3KZ Alteration of Left Knee Region with Nonautologous Tissue Substitute, Percutaneous Approach
0Y0G3ZZ Alteration of Left Knee Region, Percutaneous Approach
0Y0G47Z Alteration of Left Knee Region with Autologous Tissue Substitute, Percutaneous Endoscopic Approach
0Y0G4JZ Alteration of Left Knee Region with Synthetic Substitute, Percutaneous Endoscopic Approach
0Y0G4KZ Alteration of Left Knee Region with Nonautologous Tissue Substitute, Percutaneous Endoscopic Approach
0Y0G4ZZ Alteration of Left Knee Region, Percutaneous Endoscopic Approach
0Y0H07Z Alteration of Right Lower Leg with Autologous Tissue Substitute, Open Approach
0Y0H0JZ Alteration of Right Lower Leg with Synthetic Substitute, Open Approach
0Y0H0KZ Alteration of Right Lower Leg with Nonautologous Tissue Substitute, Open Approach
0Y0H0ZZ Alteration of Right Lower Leg, Open Approach
0Y0H37Z Alteration of Right Lower Leg with Autologous Tissue Substitute, Percutaneous Approach
0Y0H3JZ Alteration of Right Lower Leg with Synthetic Substitute, Percutaneous Approach
0Y0H3KZ Alteration of Right Lower Leg with Nonautologous Tissue Substitute, Percutaneous Approach
0Y0H3ZZ Alteration of Right Lower Leg, Percutaneous Approach
0Y0H47Z Alteration of Right Lower Leg with Autologous Tissue Substitute, Percutaneous Endoscopic Approach
0Y0H4JZ Alteration of Right Lower Leg with Synthetic Substitute, Percutaneous Endoscopic Approach

0Y0H4KZ Alteration of Right Lower Leg with Nonautologous Tissue Substitute, Percutaneous Endoscopic Approach
0Y0H4ZZ Alteration of Right Lower Leg, Percutaneous Endoscopic Approach
0Y0J07Z Alteration of Left Lower Leg with Autologous Tissue Substitute, Open Approach
0Y0J0JZ Alteration of Left Lower Leg with Synthetic Substitute, Open Approach
0Y0J0KZ Alteration of Left Lower Leg with Nonautologous Tissue Substitute, Open Approach
0Y0J0ZZ Alteration of Left Lower Leg, Open Approach
0Y0J37Z Alteration of Left Lower Leg with Autologous Tissue Substitute, Percutaneous Approach
0Y0J3JZ Alteration of Left Lower Leg with Synthetic Substitute, Percutaneous Approach
0Y0J3KZ Alteration of Left Lower Leg with Nonautologous Tissue Substitute, Percutaneous Approach
0Y0J3ZZ Alteration of Left Lower Leg, Percutaneous Approach
0Y0J47Z Alteration of Left Lower Leg with Autologous Tissue Substitute, Percutaneous Endoscopic Approach
0Y0J4JZ Alteration of Left Lower Leg with Synthetic Substitute, Percutaneous Endoscopic Approach
0Y0J4KZ Alteration of Left Lower Leg with Nonautologous Tissue Substitute, Percutaneous Endoscopic Approach
0Y0J4ZZ Alteration of Left Lower Leg, Percutaneous Endoscopic Approach
0Y0K07Z Alteration of Right Ankle Region with Autologous Tissue Substitute, Open Approach
0Y0K0JZ Alteration of Right Ankle Region with Synthetic Substitute, Open Approach
0Y0K0KZ Alteration of Right Ankle Region with Nonautologous Tissue Substitute, Open Approach
0Y0K0ZZ Alteration of Right Ankle Region, Open Approach
0Y0K37Z Alteration of Right Ankle Region with Autologous Tissue Substitute, Percutaneous Approach
0Y0K3JZ Alteration of Right Ankle Region with Synthetic Substitute, Percutaneous Approach
0Y0K3KZ Alteration of Right Ankle Region with Nonautologous Tissue Substitute, Percutaneous Approach
0Y0K3ZZ Alteration of Right Ankle Region, Percutaneous Approach
0Y0K47Z Alteration of Right Ankle Region with Autologous Tissue Substitute, Percutaneous Endoscopic Approach
0Y0K4JZ Alteration of Right Ankle Region with Synthetic Substitute, Percutaneous Endoscopic Approach
0Y0K4KZ Alteration of Right Ankle Region with Nonautologous Tissue Substitute, Percutaneous Endoscopic Approach
0Y0K4ZZ Alteration of Right Ankle Region, Percutaneous Endoscopic Approach
0Y0L07Z Alteration of Left Ankle Region with Autologous Tissue Substitute, Open Approach
0Y0L0JZ Alteration of Left Ankle Region with Synthetic Substitute, Open Approach
0Y0L0KZ Alteration of Left Ankle Region with Nonautologous Tissue Substitute, Open Approach
0Y0L0ZZ Alteration of Left Ankle Region, Open Approach
0Y0L37Z Alteration of Left Ankle Region with Autologous Tissue Substitute, Percutaneous Approach
0Y0L3JZ Alteration of Left Ankle Region with Synthetic Substitute, Percutaneous Approach
0Y0L3KZ Alteration of Left Ankle Region with Nonautologous Tissue Substitute, Percutaneous Approach
0Y0L3ZZ Alteration of Left Ankle Region, Percutaneous Approach
0Y0L47Z Alteration of Left Ankle Region with Autologous Tissue Substitute, Percutaneous Endoscopic Approach
0Y0L4JZ Alteration of Left Ankle Region with Synthetic Substitute, Percutaneous Endoscopic Approach
0Y0L4KZ Alteration of Left Ankle Region with Nonautologous Tissue Substitute, Percutaneous Endoscopic Approach
0Y0L4ZZ Alteration of Left Ankle Region, Percutaneous Endoscopic Approach

0Y2 – Anatomical Regions, Lower Extremities, Change

Review Coding Guideline B6.1c

0Y29X0Z Change Drainage Device in Right Lower Extremity, External Approach
0Y29XYZ Change Other Device in Right Lower Extremity, External Approach
0Y2BX0Z Change Drainage Device in Left Lower Extremity, External Approach
0Y2BXYZ Change Other Device in Left Lower Extremity, External Approach

0Y3 – Anatomical Regions, Lower Extremities, Control

Review Coding Guideline B3.7

0Y300ZZ Control Bleeding in Right Buttock, Open Approach
0Y303ZZ Control Bleeding in Right Buttock, Percutaneous Approach
0Y304ZZ Control Bleeding in Right Buttock, Percutaneous Endoscopic Approach
0Y310ZZ Control Bleeding in Left Buttock, Open Approach
0Y313ZZ Control Bleeding in Left Buttock, Percutaneous Approach
0Y314ZZ Control Bleeding in Left Buttock, Percutaneous Endoscopic Approach
0Y350ZZ Control Bleeding in Right Inguinal Region, Open Approach
0Y353ZZ Control Bleeding in Right Inguinal Region, Percutaneous Approach
0Y354ZZ Control Bleeding in Right Inguinal Region, Percutaneous Endoscopic Approach
0Y360ZZ Control Bleeding in Left Inguinal Region, Open Approach
0Y363ZZ Control Bleeding in Left Inguinal Region, Percutaneous Approach
0Y364ZZ Control Bleeding in Left Inguinal Region, Percutaneous Endoscopic Approach
0Y370ZZ Control Bleeding in Right Femoral Region, Open Approach
0Y373ZZ Control Bleeding in Right Femoral Region, Percutaneous Approach
0Y374ZZ Control Bleeding in Right Femoral Region, Percutaneous Endoscopic Approach
0Y380ZZ Control Bleeding in Left Femoral Region, Open Approach
0Y383ZZ Control Bleeding in Left Femoral Region, Percutaneous Approach
0Y384ZZ Control Bleeding in Left Femoral Region, Percutaneous Endoscopic Approach
0Y390ZZ Control Bleeding in Right Lower Extremity, Open Approach
0Y393ZZ Control Bleeding in Right Lower Extremity, Percutaneous Approach
0Y394ZZ Control Bleeding in Right Lower Extremity, Percutaneous Endoscopic Approach
0Y3B0ZZ Control Bleeding in Left Lower Extremity, Open Approach
0Y3B3ZZ Control Bleeding in Left Lower Extremity, Percutaneous Approach
0Y3B4ZZ Control Bleeding in Left Lower Extremity, Percutaneous Endoscopic Approach
0Y3C0ZZ Control Bleeding in Right Upper Leg, Open Approach
0Y3C3ZZ Control Bleeding in Right Upper Leg, Percutaneous Approach
0Y3C4ZZ Control Bleeding in Right Upper Leg, Percutaneous Endoscopic Approach
0Y3D0ZZ Control Bleeding in Left Upper Leg, Open Approach
0Y3D3ZZ Control Bleeding in Left Upper Leg, Percutaneous Approach
0Y3D4ZZ Control Bleeding in Left Upper Leg, Percutaneous Endoscopic Approach
0Y3F0ZZ Control Bleeding in Right Knee Region, Open Approach
0Y3F3ZZ Control Bleeding in Right Knee Region, Percutaneous Approach
0Y3F4ZZ Control Bleeding in Right Knee Region, Percutaneous Endoscopic Approach
0Y3G0ZZ Control Bleeding in Left Knee Region, Open Approach
0Y3G3ZZ Control Bleeding in Left Knee Region, Percutaneous Approach
0Y3G4ZZ Control Bleeding in Left Knee Region, Percutaneous Endoscopic Approach
0Y3H0ZZ Control Bleeding in Right Lower Leg, Open Approach
0Y3H3ZZ Control Bleeding in Right Lower Leg, Percutaneous Approach
0Y3H4ZZ Control Bleeding in Right Lower Leg, Percutaneous Endoscopic Approach
0Y3J0ZZ Control Bleeding in Left Lower Leg, Open Approach
0Y3J3ZZ Control Bleeding in Left Lower Leg, Percutaneous Approach

0Y3J4ZZ Control Bleeding in Left Lower Leg, Percutaneous Endoscopic Approach
0Y3K0ZZ Control Bleeding in Right Ankle Region, Open Approach
0Y3K3ZZ Control Bleeding in Right Ankle Region, Percutaneous Approach
0Y3K4ZZ Control Bleeding in Right Ankle Region, Percutaneous Endoscopic Approach
0Y3L0ZZ Control Bleeding in Left Ankle Region, Open Approach
0Y3L3ZZ Control Bleeding in Left Ankle Region, Percutaneous Approach
0Y3L4ZZ Control Bleeding in Left Ankle Region, Percutaneous Endoscopic Approach
0Y3M0ZZ Control Bleeding in Right Foot, Open Approach
0Y3M3ZZ Control Bleeding in Right Foot, Percutaneous Approach
0Y3M4ZZ Control Bleeding in Right Foot, Percutaneous Endoscopic Approach
0Y3N0ZZ Control Bleeding in Left Foot, Open Approach
0Y3N3ZZ Control Bleeding in Left Foot, Percutaneous Approach
0Y3N4ZZ Control Bleeding in Left Foot, Percutaneous Endoscopic Approach

0Y6 – Anatomical Regions, Lower Extremities, Detachment

0Y620ZZ Detachment at Right Hindquarter, Open Approach
0Y630ZZ Detachment at Left Hindquarter, Open Approach
0Y640ZZ Detachment at Bilateral Hindquarter, Open Approach
0Y670ZZ Detachment at Right Femoral Region, Open Approach
0Y680ZZ Detachment at Left Femoral Region, Open Approach
0Y6C0Z1 Detachment at Right Upper Leg, High, Open Approach
0Y6C0Z2 Detachment at Right Upper Leg, Mid, Open Approach
0Y6C0Z3 Detachment at Right Upper Leg, Low, Open Approach
0Y6D0Z1 Detachment at Left Upper Leg, High, Open Approach
0Y6D0Z2 Detachment at Left Upper Leg, Mid, Open Approach
0Y6D0Z3 Detachment at Left Upper Leg, Low, Open Approach
0Y6F0ZZ Detachment at Right Knee Region, Open Approach
0Y6G0ZZ Detachment at Left Knee Region, Open Approach
0Y6H0Z1 Detachment at Right Lower Leg, High, Open Approach
0Y6H0Z2 Detachment at Right Lower Leg, Mid, Open Approach
0Y6H0Z3 Detachment at Right Lower Leg, Low, Open Approach
0Y6J0Z1 Detachment at Left Lower Leg, High, Open Approach
0Y6J0Z2 Detachment at Left Lower Leg, Mid, Open Approach
0Y6J0Z3 Detachment at Left Lower Leg, Low, Open Approach
0Y6M0Z0 Detachment at Right Foot, Complete, Open Approach
0Y6M0Z4 Detachment at Right Foot, Complete 1st Ray, Open Approach
0Y6M0Z5 Detachment at Right Foot, Complete 2nd Ray, Open Approach
0Y6M0Z6 Detachment at Right Foot, Complete 3rd Ray, Open Approach
0Y6M0Z7 Detachment at Right Foot, Complete 4th Ray, Open Approach
0Y6M0Z8 Detachment at Right Foot, Complete 5th Ray, Open Approach
0Y6M0Z9 Detachment at Right Foot, Partial 1st Ray, Open Approach
0Y6M0ZB Detachment at Right Foot, Partial 2nd Ray, Open Approach
0Y6M0ZC Detachment at Right Foot, Partial 3rd Ray, Open Approach
0Y6M0ZD Detachment at Right Foot, Partial 4th Ray, Open Approach
0Y6M0ZF Detachment at Right Foot, Partial 5th Ray, Open Approach
0Y6N0Z0 Detachment at Left Foot, Complete, Open Approach
0Y6N0Z4 Detachment at Left Foot, Complete 1st Ray, Open Approach
0Y6N0Z5 Detachment at Left Foot, Complete 2nd Ray, Open Approach
0Y6N0Z6 Detachment at Left Foot, Complete 3rd Ray, Open Approach
0Y6N0Z7 Detachment at Left Foot, Complete 4th Ray, Open Approach
0Y6N0Z8 Detachment at Left Foot, Complete 5th Ray, Open Approach
0Y6N0Z9 Detachment at Left Foot, Partial 1st Ray, Open Approach
0Y6N0ZB Detachment at Left Foot, Partial 2nd Ray, Open Approach
0Y6N0ZC Detachment at Left Foot, Partial 3rd Ray, Open Approach
0Y6N0ZD Detachment at Left Foot, Partial 4th Ray, Open Approach
0Y6N0ZF Detachment at Left Foot, Partial 5th Ray, Open Approach
0Y6P0Z0 Detachment at Right 1st Toe, Complete, Open Approach
0Y6P0Z1 Detachment at Right 1st Toe, High, Open Approach
0Y6P0Z2 Detachment at Right 1st Toe, Mid, Open Approach
0Y6P0Z3 Detachment at Right 1st Toe, Low, Open Approach
0Y6Q0Z0 Detachment at Left 1st Toe, Complete, Open Approach
0Y6Q0Z1 Detachment at Left 1st Toe, High, Open Approach
0Y6Q0Z2 Detachment at Left 1st Toe, Mid, Open Approach
0Y6Q0Z3 Detachment at Left 1st Toe, Low, Open Approach
0Y6R0Z0 Detachment at Right 2nd Toe, Complete, Open Approach
0Y6R0Z1 Detachment at Right 2nd Toe, High, Open Approach
0Y6R0Z2 Detachment at Right 2nd Toe, Mid, Open Approach
0Y6R0Z3 Detachment at Right 2nd Toe, Low, Open Approach
0Y6S0Z0 Detachment at Left 2nd Toe, Complete, Open Approach
0Y6S0Z1 Detachment at Left 2nd Toe, High, Open Approach
0Y6S0Z2 Detachment at Left 2nd Toe, Mid, Open Approach
0Y6S0Z3 Detachment at Left 2nd Toe, Low, Open Approach
0Y6T0Z0 Detachment at Right 3rd Toe, Complete, Open Approach
0Y6T0Z1 Detachment at Right 3rd Toe, High, Open Approach
0Y6T0Z2 Detachment at Right 3rd Toe, Mid, Open Approach
0Y6T0Z3 Detachment at Right 3rd Toe, Low, Open Approach
0Y6U0Z0 Detachment at Left 3rd Toe, Complete, Open Approach
0Y6U0Z1 Detachment at Left 3rd Toe, High, Open Approach
0Y6U0Z2 Detachment at Left 3rd Toe, Mid, Open Approach
0Y6U0Z3 Detachment at Left 3rd Toe, Low, Open Approach
0Y6V0Z0 Detachment at Right 4th Toe, Complete, Open Approach
0Y6V0Z1 Detachment at Right 4th Toe, High, Open Approach
0Y6V0Z2 Detachment at Right 4th Toe, Mid, Open Approach
0Y6V0Z3 Detachment at Right 4th Toe, Low, Open Approach
0Y6W0Z0 Detachment at Left 4th Toe, Complete, Open Approach
0Y6W0Z1 Detachment at Left 4th Toe, High, Open Approach
0Y6W0Z2 Detachment at Left 4th Toe, Mid, Open Approach
0Y6W0Z3 Detachment at Left 4th Toe, Low, Open Approach
0Y6X0Z0 Detachment at Right 5th Toe, Complete, Open Approach
0Y6X0Z1 Detachment at Right 5th Toe, High, Open Approach
0Y6X0Z2 Detachment at Right 5th Toe, Mid, Open Approach
0Y6X0Z3 Detachment at Right 5th Toe, Low, Open Approach
0Y6Y0Z0 Detachment at Left 5th Toe, Complete, Open Approach
0Y6Y0Z1 Detachment at Left 5th Toe, High, Open Approach
0Y6Y0Z2 Detachment at Left 5th Toe, Mid, Open Approach
0Y6Y0Z3 Detachment at Left 5th Toe, Low, Open Approach

0Y9 – Anatomical Regions, Lower Extremities, Drainage

Review Coding Guidelines B3.4a and B3.4b

Review Coding Guideline B6.2

0Y9000Z Drainage of Right Buttock with Drainage Device, Open Approach
0Y900ZX Drainage of Right Buttock, Open Approach, Diagnostic
0Y900ZZ Drainage of Right Buttock, Open Approach

0Y9030Z Drainage of Right Buttock with Drainage Device, Percutaneous Approach
0Y903ZX Drainage of Right Buttock, Percutaneous Approach, Diagnostic
0Y903ZZ Drainage of Right Buttock, Percutaneous Approach
0Y9040Z Drainage of Right Buttock with Drainage Device, Percutaneous Endoscopic Approach
0Y904ZX Drainage of Right Buttock, Percutaneous Endoscopic Approach, Diagnostic
0Y904ZZ Drainage of Right Buttock, Percutaneous Endoscopic Approach
0Y9100Z Drainage of Left Buttock with Drainage Device, Open Approach
0Y910ZX Drainage of Left Buttock, Open Approach, Diagnostic
0Y910ZZ Drainage of Left Buttock, Open Approach
0Y9130Z Drainage of Left Buttock with Drainage Device, Percutaneous Approach
0Y913ZX Drainage of Left Buttock, Percutaneous Approach, Diagnostic
0Y913ZZ Drainage of Left Buttock, Percutaneous Approach
0Y9140Z Drainage of Left Buttock with Drainage Device, Percutaneous Endoscopic Approach
0Y914ZX Drainage of Left Buttock, Percutaneous Endoscopic Approach, Diagnostic
0Y914ZZ Drainage of Left Buttock, Percutaneous Endoscopic Approach
0Y9500Z Drainage of Right Inguinal Region with Drainage Device, Open Approach
0Y950ZX Drainage of Right Inguinal Region, Open Approach, Diagnostic
0Y950ZZ Drainage of Right Inguinal Region, Open Approach
0Y9530Z Drainage of Right Inguinal Region w ith Drainage Device, Percutaneous Approach
0Y953ZX Drainage of Right Inguinal Region, Percutaneous Approach, Diagnostic
0Y953ZZ Drainage of Right Inguinal Region, Percutaneous Approach
0Y9540Z Drainage of Right Inguinal Region with Drainage Device, Percutaneous Endoscopic Approach
0Y954ZX Drainage of Right Inguinal Region, Percutaneous Endoscopic Approach, Diagnostic
0Y954ZZ Drainage of Right Inguinal Region, Percutaneous Endoscopic Approach
0Y9600Z Drainage of Left Inguinal Region with Drainage Device, Open Approach
0Y960ZX Drainage of Left Inguinal Region, Open Approach, Diagnostic
0Y960ZZ Drainage of Left Inguinal Region, Open Approach
0Y9630Z Drainage of Left Inguinal Region with Drainage Device, Percutaneous Approach
0Y963ZX Drainage of Left Inguinal Region, Percutaneous Approach, Diagnostic
0Y963ZZ Drainage of Left Inguinal Region, Percutaneous Approach
0Y9640Z Drainage of Left Inguinal Region with Drainage Device, Percutaneous Endoscopic Approach
0Y964ZX Drainage of Left Inguinal Region, Percutaneous Endoscopic Approach, Diagnostic
0Y964ZZ Drainage of Left Inguinal Region, Percutaneous Endoscopic Approach
0Y9700Z Drainage of Right Femoral Region with Drainage Device, Open Approach
0Y970ZX Drainage of Right Femoral Region, Open Approach, Diagnostic
0Y970ZZ Drainage of Right Femoral Region, Open Approach
0Y9730Z Drainage of Right Femoral Region with Drainage Device, Percutaneous Approach
0Y973ZX Drainage of Right Femoral Region, Percutaneous Approach, Diagnostic
0Y973ZZ Drainage of Right Femoral Region, Percutaneous Approach
0Y9740Z Drainage of Right Femoral Region with Drainage Device, Percutaneous Endoscopic Approach
0Y974ZX Drainage of Right Femoral Region, Percutaneous Endoscopic Approach, Diagnostic
0Y974ZZ Drainage of Right Femoral Region, Percutaneous Endoscopic Approach
0Y9800Z Drainage of Left Femoral Region with Drainage Device, Open Approach
0Y980ZX Drainage of Left Femoral Region, Open Approach, Diagnostic
0Y980ZZ Drainage of Left Femoral Region, Open Approach
0Y9830Z Drainage of Left Femoral Region with Drainage Device, Percutaneous Approach
0Y983ZX Drainage of Left Femoral Region, Percutaneous Approach, Diagnostic
0Y983ZZ Drainage of Left Femoral Region, Percutaneous Approach
0Y9840Z Drainage of Left Femoral Region with Drainage Device, Percutaneous Endoscopic Approach
0Y984ZX Drainage of Left Femoral Region, Percutaneous Endoscopic Approach, Diagnostic
0Y984ZZ Drainage of Left Femoral Region, Percutaneous Endoscopic Approach
0Y9900Z Drainage of Right Lower Extremity with Drainage Device, Open Approach
0Y990ZX Drainage of Right Lower Extremity, Open Approach, Diagnostic
0Y990ZZ Drainage of Right Lower Extremity, Open Approach
0Y9930Z Drainage of Right Lower Extremity with Drainage Device, Percutaneous Approach
0Y993ZX Drainage of Right Lower Extremity, Percutaneous Approach, Diagnostic
0Y993ZZ Drainage of Right Lower Extremity, Percutaneous Approach
0Y9940Z Drainage of Right Lower Extremity with Drainage Device, Percutaneous Endoscopic Approach
0Y994ZX Drainage of Right Lower Extremity, Percutaneous Endoscopic Approach, Diagnostic
0Y994ZZ Drainage of Right Lower Extremity, Percutaneous Endoscopic Approach
0Y9B00Z Drainage of Left Lower Extremity with Drainage Device, Open Approach
0Y9B0ZX Drainage of Left Lower Extremity, Open Approach, Diagnostic
0Y9B0ZZ Drainage of Left Lower Extremity, Open Approach
0Y9B30Z Drainage of Left Lower Extremity with Drainage Device, Percutaneous Approach
0Y9B3ZX Drainage of Left Lower Extremity, Percutaneous Approach, Diagnostic
0Y9B3ZZ Drainage of Left Lower Extremity, Percutaneous Approach
0Y9B40Z Drainage of Left Lower Extremity with Drainage Device, Percutaneous Endoscopic Approach
0Y9B4ZX Drainage of Left Lower Extremity, Percutaneous Endoscopic Approach, Diagnostic
0Y9B4ZZ Drainage of Left Lower Extremity, Percutaneous Endoscopic Approach
0Y9C00Z Drainage of Right Upper Leg with Drainage Device, Open Approach
0Y9C0ZX Drainage of Right Upper Leg, Open Approach, Diagnostic
0Y9C0ZZ Drainage of Right Upper Leg, Open Approach
0Y9C30Z Drainage of Right Upper Leg with Drainage Device, Percutaneous Approach
0Y9C3ZX Drainage of Right Upper Leg, Percutaneous Approach, Diagnostic
0Y9C3ZZ Drainage of Right Upper Leg, Percutaneous Approach
0Y9C40Z Drainage of Right Upper Leg with Drainage Device, Percutaneous Endoscopic Approach
0Y9C4ZX Drainage of Right Upper Leg, Percutaneous Endoscopic Approach, Diagnostic
0Y9C4ZZ Drainage of Right Upper Leg, Percutaneous Endoscopic Approach
0Y9D00Z Drainage of Left Upper Leg with Drainage Device, Open Approach
0Y9D0ZX Drainage of Left Upper Leg, Open Approach, Diagnostic
0Y9D0ZZ Drainage of Left Upper Leg, Open Approach
0Y9D30Z Drainage of Left Upper Leg with Drainage Device, Percutaneous Approach
0Y9D3ZX Drainage of Left Upper Leg, Percutaneous Approach, Diagnostic
0Y9D3ZZ Drainage of Left Upper Leg, Percutaneous Approach
0Y9D40Z Drainage of Left Upper Leg with Drainage Device, Percutaneous Endoscopic Approach
0Y9D4ZX Drainage of Left Upper Leg, Percutaneous Endoscopic Approach, Diagnostic
0Y9D4ZZ Drainage of Left Upper Leg, Percutaneous Endoscopic Approach
0Y9F00Z Drainage of Right Knee Region with Drainage Device, Open Approach
0Y9F0ZX Drainage of Right Knee Region, Open Approach, Diagnostic
0Y9F0ZZ Drainage of Right Knee Region, Open Approach
0Y9F30Z Drainage of Right Knee Region with Drainage Device, Percutaneous Approach
0Y9F3ZX Drainage of Right Knee Region, Percutaneous Approach, Diagnostic
0Y9F3ZZ Drainage of Right Knee Region, Percutaneous Approach
0Y9F40Z Drainage of Right Knee Region with Drainage Device, Percutaneous Endoscopic Approach
0Y9F4ZX Drainage of Right Knee Region, Percutaneous Endoscopic Approach, Diagnostic
0Y9F4ZZ Drainage of Right Knee Region, Percutaneous Endoscopic Approach
0Y9G00Z Drainage of Left Knee Region with Drainage Device, Open Approach
0Y9G0ZX Drainage of Left Knee Region, Open Approach, Diagnostic
0Y9G0ZZ Drainage of Left Knee Region, Open Approach
0Y9G30Z Drainage of Left Knee Region with Drainage Device, Percutaneous Approach
0Y9G3ZX Drainage of Left Knee Region, Percutaneous Approach, Diagnostic
0Y9G3ZZ Drainage of Left Knee Region, Percutaneous Approach
0Y9G40Z Drainage of Left Knee Region with Drainage Device, Percutaneous Endoscopic Approach
0Y9G4ZX Drainage of Left Knee Region, Percutaneous Endoscopic Approach, Diagnostic
0Y9G4ZZ Drainage of Left Knee Region, Percutaneous Endoscopic Approach

0Y9H00Z Drainage of Right Lower Leg with Drainage Device, Open Approach
0Y9H0ZX Drainage of Right Lower Leg, Open Approach, Diagnostic
0Y9H0ZZ Drainage of Right Lower Leg, Open Approach
0Y9H30Z Drainage of Right Lower Leg with Drainage Device, Percutaneous Approach
0Y9H3ZX Drainage of Right Lower Leg, Percutaneous Approach, Diagnostic
0Y9H3ZZ Drainage of Right Lower Leg, Percutaneous Approach
0Y9H40Z Drainage of Right Lower Leg with Drainage Device, Percutaneous Endoscopic Approach
0Y9H4ZX Drainage of Right Lower Leg, Percutaneous Endoscopic Approach, Diagnostic
0Y9H4ZZ Drainage of Right Lower Leg, Percutaneous Endoscopic Approach
0Y9J00Z Drainage of Left Lower Leg with Drainage Device, Open Approach
0Y9J0ZX Drainage of Left Lower Leg, Open Approach, Diagnostic
0Y9J0ZZ Drainage of Left Lower Leg, Open Approach
0Y9J30Z Drainage of Left Lower Leg with Drainage Device, Percutaneous Approach
0Y9J3ZX Drainage of Left Lower Leg, Percutaneous Approach, Diagnostic
0Y9J3ZZ Drainage of Left Lower Leg, Percutaneous Approach
0Y9J40Z Drainage of Left Lower Leg with Drainage Device, Percutaneous Endoscopic Approach
0Y9J4ZX Drainage of Left Lower Leg, Percutaneous Endoscopic Approach, Diagnostic
0Y9J4ZZ Drainage of Left Lower Leg, Percutaneous Endoscopic Approach
0Y9K00Z Drainage of Right Ankle Region with Drainage Device, Open Approach
0Y9K0ZX Drainage of Right Ankle Region, Open Approach, Diagnostic
0Y9K0ZZ Drainage of Right Ankle Region, Open Approach
0Y9K30Z Drainage of Right Ankle Region with Drainage Device, Percutaneous Approach
0Y9K3ZX Drainage of Right Ankle Region, Percutaneous Approach, Diagnostic
0Y9K3ZZ Drainage of Right Ankle Region, Percutaneous Approach
0Y9K40Z Drainage of Right Ankle Region with Drainage Device, Percutaneous Endoscopic Approach
0Y9K4ZX Drainage of Right Ankle Region, Percutaneous Endoscopic Approach, Diagnostic
0Y9K4ZZ Drainage of Right Ankle Region, Percutaneous Endoscopic Approach
0Y9L00Z Drainage of Left Ankle Region with Drainage Device, Open Approach
0Y9L0ZX Drainage of Left Ankle Region, Open Approach, Diagnostic
0Y9L0ZZ Drainage of Left Ankle Region, Open Approach
0Y9L30Z Drainage of Left Ankle Region with Drainage Device, Percutaneous Approach
0Y9L3ZX Drainage of Left Ankle Region, Percutaneous Approach, Diagnostic
0Y9L3ZZ Drainage of Left Ankle Region, Percutaneous Approach
0Y9L40Z Drainage of Left Ankle Region with Drainage Device, Percutaneous Endoscopic Approach
0Y9L4ZX Drainage of Left Ankle Region, Percutaneous Endoscopic Approach, Diagnostic
0Y9L4ZZ Drainage of Left Ankle Region, Percutaneous Endoscopic Approach
0Y9M00Z Drainage of Right Foot with Drainage Device, Open Approach
0Y9M0ZX Drainage of Right Foot, Open Approach, Diagnostic
0Y9M0ZZ Drainage of Right Foot, Open Approach
0Y9M30Z Drainage of Right Foot with Drainage Device, Percutaneous Approach
0Y9M3ZX Drainage of Right Foot, Percutaneous Approach, Diagnostic
0Y9M3ZZ Drainage of Right Foot, Percutaneous Approach
0Y9M40Z Drainage of Right Foot with Drainage Device, Percutaneous Endoscopic Approach
0Y9M4ZX Drainage of Right Foot, Percutaneous Endoscopic Approach, Diagnostic
0Y9M4ZZ Drainage of Right Foot, Percutaneous Endoscopic Approach
0Y9N00Z Drainage of Left Foot with Drainage Device, Open Approach
0Y9N0ZX Drainage of Left Foot, Open Approach, Diagnostic
0Y9N0ZZ Drainage of Left Foot, Open Approach
0Y9N30Z Drainage of Left Foot with Drainage Device, Percutaneous Approach
0Y9N3ZX Drainage of Left Foot, Percutaneous Approach, Diagnostic
0Y9N3ZZ Drainage of Left Foot, Percutaneous Approach
0Y9N40Z Drainage of Left Foot with Drainage Device, Percutaneous Endoscopic Approach
0Y9N4ZX Drainage of Left Foot, Percutaneous Endoscopic Approach, Diagnostic
0Y9N4ZZ Drainage of Left Foot, Percutaneous Endoscopic Approach

0YB – Anatomical Regions, Lower Extremities, Excision

Review Coding Guidelines B3.4a and B3.4b

0YB00ZX Excision of Right Buttock, Open Approach, Diagnostic
0YB00ZZ Excision of Right Buttock, Open Approach
0YB03ZX Excision of Right Buttock, Percutaneous Approach, Diagnostic
0YB03ZZ Excision of Right Buttock, Percutaneous Approach
0YB04ZX Excision of Right Buttock, Percutaneous Endoscopic Approach, Diagnostic
0YB04ZZ Excision of Right Buttock, Percutaneous Endoscopic Approach
0YB10ZX Excision of Left Buttock, Open Approach, Diagnostic
0YB10ZZ Excision of Left Buttock, Open Approach
0YB13ZX Excision of Left Buttock, Percutaneous Approach, Diagnostic
0YB13ZZ Excision of Left Buttock, Percutaneous Approach
0YB14ZX Excision of Left Buttock, Percutaneous Endoscopic Approach, Diagnostic
0YB14ZZ Excision of Left Buttock, Percutaneous Endoscopic Approach
0YB50ZX Excision of Right Inguinal Region, Open Approach, Diagnostic
0YB50ZZ Excision of Right Inguinal Region, Open Approach
0YB53ZX Excision of Right Inguinal Region, Percutaneous Approach, Diagnostic
0YB53ZZ Excision of Right Inguinal Region, Percutaneous Approach
0YB54ZX Excision of Right Inguinal Region, Percutaneous Endoscopic Approach, Diagnostic
0YB54ZZ Excision of Right Inguinal Region, Percutaneous Endoscopic Approach
0YB60ZX Excision of Left Inguinal Region, Open Approach, Diagnostic
0YB60ZZ Excision of Left Inguinal Region, Open Approach
0YB63ZX Excision of Left Inguinal Region, Percutaneous Approach, Diagnostic
0YB63ZZ Excision of Left Inguinal Region, Percutaneous Approach
0YB64ZX Excision of Left Inguinal Region, Percutaneous Endoscopic Approach, Diagnostic
0YB64ZZ Excision of Left Inguinal Region, Percutaneous Endoscopic Approach
0YB70ZX Excision of Right Femoral Region, Open Approach, Diagnostic
0YB70ZZ Excision of Right Femoral Region, Open Approach
0YB73ZX Excision of Right Femoral Region, Percutaneous Approach, Diagnostic
0YB73ZZ Excision of Right Femoral Region, Percutaneous Approach
0YB74ZX Excision of Right Femoral Region, Percutaneous Endoscopic Approach, Diagnostic
0YB74ZZ Excision of Right Femoral Region, Percutaneous Endoscopic Approach
0YB80ZX Excision of Left Femoral Region, Open Approach, Diagnostic
0YB80ZZ Excision of Left Femoral Region, Open Approach
0YB83ZX Excision of Left Femoral Region, Percutaneous Approach, Diagnostic
0YB83ZZ Excision of Left Femoral Region, Percutaneous Approach
0YB84ZX Excision of Left Femoral Region, Percutaneous Endoscopic Approach, Diagnostic
0YB84ZZ Excision of Left Femoral Region, Percutaneous Endoscopic Approach
0YB90ZX Excision of Right Lower Extremity, Open Approach, Diagnostic
0YB90ZZ Excision of Right Lower Extremity, Open Approach
0YB93ZX Excision of Right Lower Extremity, Percutaneous Approach, Diagnostic
0YB93ZZ Excision of Right Lower Extremity, Percutaneous Approach
0YB94ZX Excision of Right Lower Extremity, Percutaneous Endoscopic Approach, Diagnostic
0YB94ZZ Excision of Right Lower Extremity, Percutaneous Endoscopic Approach
0YBB0ZX Excision of Left Lower Extremity, Open Approach, Diagnostic
0YBB0ZZ Excision of Left Lower Extremity, Open Approach
0YBB3ZX Excision of Left Lower Extremity, Percutaneous Approach, Diagnostic
0YBB3ZZ Excision of Left Lower Extremity, Percutaneous Approach

0YBB4ZX Excision of Left Lower Extremity, Percutaneous Endoscopic Approach, Diagnostic
0YBB4ZZ Excision of Left Lower Extremity, Percutaneous Endoscopic Approach
0YBC0ZX Excision of Right Upper Leg, Open Approach, Diagnostic
0YBC0ZZ Excision of Right Upper Leg, Open Approach
0YBC3ZX Excision of Right Upper Leg, Percutaneous Approach, Diagnostic
0YBC3ZZ Excision of Right Upper Leg, Percutaneous Approach
0YBC4ZX Excision of Right Upper Leg, Percutaneous Endoscopic Approach, Diagnostic
0YBC4ZZ Excision of Right Upper Leg, Percutaneous Endoscopic Approach
0YBD0ZX Excision of Left Upper Leg, Open Approach, Diagnostic
0YBD0ZZ Excision of Left Upper Leg, Open Approach
0YBD3ZX Excision of Left Upper Leg, Percutaneous Approach, Diagnostic
0YBD3ZZ Excision of Left Upper Leg, Percutaneous Approach
0YBD4ZX Excision of Left Upper Leg, Percutaneous Endoscopic Approach, Diagnostic
0YBD4ZZ Excision of Left Upper Leg, Percutaneous Endoscopic Approach
0YBF0ZX Excision of Right Knee Region, Open Approach, Diagnostic
0YBF0ZZ Excision of Right Knee Region, Open Approach
0YBF3ZX Excision of Right Knee Region, Percutaneous Approach, Diagnostic
0YBF3ZZ Excision of Right Knee Region, Percutaneous Approach
0YBF4ZX Excision of Right Knee Region, Percutaneous Endoscopic Approach, Diagnostic
0YBF4ZZ Excision of Right Knee Region, Percutaneous Endoscopic Approach
0YBG0ZX Excision of Left Knee Region, Open Approach, Diagnostic
0YBG0ZZ Excision of Left Knee Region, Open Approach
0YBG3ZX Excision of Left Knee Region, Percutaneous Approach, Diagnostic
0YBG3ZZ Excision of Left Knee Region, Percutaneous Approach
0YBG4ZX Excision of Left Knee Region, Percutaneous Endoscopic Approach, Diagnostic
0YBG4ZZ Excision of Left Knee Region, Percutaneous Endoscopic Approach
0YBH0ZX Excision of Right Lower Leg, Open Approach, Diagnostic
0YBH0ZZ Excision of Right Lower Leg, Open Approach
0YBH3ZX Excision of Right Lower Leg, Percutaneous Approach, Diagnostic
0YBH3ZZ Excision of Right Lower Leg, Percutaneous Approach
0YBH4ZX Excision of Right Lower Leg, Percutaneous Endoscopic Approach, Diagnostic
0YBH4ZZ Excision of Right Lower Leg, Percutaneous Endoscopic Approach
0YBJ0ZX Excision of Left Lower Leg, Open Approach, Diagnostic
0YBJ0ZZ Excision of Left Lower Leg, Open Approach
0YBJ3ZX Excision of Left Lower Leg, Percutaneous Approach, Diagnostic
0YBJ3ZZ Excision of Left Lower Leg, Percutaneous Approach
0YBJ4ZX Excision of Left Lower Leg, Percutaneous Endoscopic Approach, Diagnostic
0YBJ4ZZ Excision of Left Lower Leg, Percutaneous Endoscopic Approach
0YBK0ZX Excision of Right Ankle Region, Open Approach, Diagnostic
0YBK0ZZ Excision of Right Ankle Region, Open Approach
0YBK3ZX Excision of Right Ankle Region, Percutaneous Approach, Diagnostic
0YBK3ZZ Excision of Right Ankle Region, Percutaneous Approach
0YBK4ZX Excision of Right Ankle Region, Percutaneous Endoscopic Approach, Diagnostic
0YBK4ZZ Excision of Right Ankle Region, Percutaneous Endoscopic Approach
0YBL0ZX Excision of Left Ankle Region, Open Approach, Diagnostic
0YBL0ZZ Excision of Left Ankle Region, Open Approach
0YBL3ZX Excision of Left Ankle Region, Percutaneous Approach, Diagnostic
0YBL3ZZ Excision of Left Ankle Region, Percutaneous Approach
0YBL4ZX Excision of Left Ankle Region, Percutaneous Endoscopic Approach, Diagnostic
0YBL4ZZ Excision of Left Ankle Region, Percutaneous Endoscopic Approach
0YBM0ZX Excision of Right Foot, Open Approach, Diagnostic
0YBM0ZZ Excision of Right Foot, Open Approach
0YBM3ZX Excision of Right Foot, Percutaneous Approach, Diagnostic
0YBM3ZZ Excision of Right Foot, Percutaneous Approach
0YBM4ZX Excision of Right Foot, Percutaneous Endoscopic Approach, Diagnostic
0YBM4ZZ Excision of Right Foot, Percutaneous Endoscopic Approach
0YBN0ZX Excision of Left Foot, Open Approach, Diagnostic
0YBN0ZZ Excision of Left Foot, Open Approach
0YBN3ZX Excision of Left Foot, Percutaneous Approach, Diagnostic
0YBN3ZZ Excision of Left Foot, Percutaneous Approach
0YBN4ZX Excision of Left Foot, Percutaneous Endoscopic Approach, Diagnostic
0YBN4ZZ Excision of Left Foot, Percutaneous Endoscopic Approach

0YH – Anatomical Regions, Lower Extremities, Insertion

0YH001Z Insertion of Radioactive Element into Right Buttock, Open Approach
● **0YH003Z** Insertion of Infusion Device into Right Buttock, Open Approach
● **0YH00YZ** Insertion of Other Device into Right Buttock, Open Approach
0YH031Z Insertion of Radioactive Element into Right Buttock, Percutaneous Approach
● **0YH033Z** Insertion of Infusion Device into Right Buttock, Percutaneous Approach
● **0YH03YZ** Insertion of Other Device into Right Buttock, Percutaneous Approach
0YH041Z Insertion of Radioactive Element into Right Buttock, Percutaneous Endoscopic Approach
● **0YH043Z** Insertion of Infusion Device into Right Buttock, Percutaneous Endoscopic Approach
● **0YH04YZ** Insertion of Other Device into Right Buttock, Percutaneous Endoscopic Approach
0YH101Z Insertion of Radioactive Element into Left Buttock, Open Approach
● **0YH103Z** Insertion of Infusion Device into Left Buttock, Open Approach
● **0YH10YZ** Insertion of Other Device into Left Buttock, Open Approach
0YH131Z Insertion of Radioactive Element into Left Buttock, Percutaneous Approach
● **0YH133Z** Insertion of Infusion Device into Left Buttock, Percutaneous Approach
● **0YH13YZ** Insertion of Other Device into Left Buttock, Percutaneous Approach
0YH141Z Insertion of Radioactive Element into Left Buttock, Percutaneous Endoscopic Approach
● **0YH143Z** Insertion of Infusion Device into Left Buttock, Percutaneous Endoscopic Approach
● **0YH14YZ** Insertion of Other Device into Left Buttock, Percutaneous Endoscopic Approach
0YH501Z Insertion of Radioactive Element into Right Inguinal Region, Open Approach
● **0YH503Z** Insertion of Infusion Device into Right Inguinal Region, Open Approach
● **0YH50YZ** Insertion of Other Device into Right Inguinal Region, Open Approach
0YH531Z Insertion of Radioactive Element into Right Inguinal Region, Percutaneous Approach
● **0YH533Z** Insertion of Infusion Device into Right Inguinal Region, Percutaneous Approach
● **0YH53YZ** Insertion of Other Device into Right Inguinal Region, Percutaneous Approach
0YH541Z Insertion of Radioactive Element into Right Inguinal Region, Percutaneous Endoscopic Approach
● **0YH543Z** Insertion of Infusion Device into Right Inguinal Region, Percutaneous Endoscopic Approach
● **0YH54YZ** Insertion of Other Device into Right Inguinal Region, Percutaneous Endoscopic Approach
0YH601Z Insertion of Radioactive Element into Left Inguinal Region, Open Approach
● **0YH603Z** Insertion of Infusion Device into Left Inguinal Region, Open Approach
● **0YH60YZ** Insertion of Other Device into Left Inguinal Region, Open Approach
0YH631Z Insertion of Radioactive Element into Left Inguinal Region, Percutaneous Approach
● **0YH633Z** Insertion of Infusion Device into Left Inguinal Region, Percutaneous Approach
● **0YH63YZ** Insertion of Other Device into Left Inguinal Region, Percutaneous Approach
0YH641Z Insertion of Radioactive Element into Left Inguinal Region, Percutaneous Endoscopic Approach
● **0YH643Z** Insertion of Infusion Device into Left Inguinal Region, Percutaneous Endoscopic Approach
● **0YH64YZ** Insertion of Other Device into Left Inguinal Region, Percutaneous Endoscopic Approach
0YH701Z Insertion of Radioactive Element into Right Femoral Region, Open Approach
● **0YH703Z** Insertion of Infusion Device into Right Femoral Region, Open Approach
● **0YH70YZ** Insertion of Other Device into Right Femoral Region, Open Approach

0YH731Z Insertion of Radioactive Element into Right Femoral Region, Percutaneous Approach
●**0YH733Z** Insertion of Infusion Device into Right Femoral Region, Percutaneous Approach
●**0YH73YZ** Insertion of Other Device into Right Femoral Region, Percutaneous Approach
0YH741Z Insertion of Radioactive Element into Right Femoral Region, Percutaneous Endoscopic Approach
●**0YH743Z** Insertion of Infusion Device into Right Femoral Region, Percutaneous Endoscopic Approach
●**0YH74YZ** Insertion of Other Device into Right Femoral Region, Percutaneous Endoscopic Approach
0YH801Z Insertion of Radioactive Element into Left Femoral Region, Open Approach
●**0YH803Z** Insertion of Infusion Device into Left Femoral Region, Open Approach
●**0YH80YZ** Insertion of Other Device into Left Femoral Region, Open Approach
0YH831Z Insertion of Radioactive Element into Left Femoral Region, Percutaneous Approach
●**0YH833Z** Insertion of Infusion Device into Left Femoral Region, Percutaneous Approach
●**0YH83YZ** Insertion of Other Device into Left Femoral Region, Percutaneous Approach
0YH841Z Insertion of Radioactive Element into Left Femoral Region, Percutaneous Endoscopic Approach
●**0YH843Z** Insertion of Infusion Device into Left Femoral Region, Percutaneous Endoscopic Approach
●**0YH84YZ** Insertion of Other Device into Left Femoral Region, Percutaneous Endoscopic Approach
0YH901Z Insertion of Radioactive Element into Right Lower Extremity, Open Approach
●**0YH903Z** Insertion of Infusion Device into Right Lower Extremity, Open Approach
●**0YH90YZ** Insertion of Other Device into Right Lower Extremity, Open Approach
0YH931Z Insertion of Radioactive Element into Right Lower Extremity, Percutaneous Approach
●**0YH933Z** Insertion of Infusion Device into Right Lower Extremity, Percutaneous Approach
●**0YH93YZ** Insertion of Other Device into Right Lower Extremity, Percutaneous Approach
0YH941Z Insertion of Radioactive Element into Right Lower Extremity, Percutaneous Endoscopic Approach
●**0YH943Z** Insertion of Infusion Device into Right Lower Extremity, Percutaneous Endoscopic Approach
●**0YH94YZ** Insertion of Other Device into Right Lower Extremity, Percutaneous Endoscopic Approach
0YHB01Z Insertion of Radioactive Element into Left Lower Extremity, Open Approach
●**0YHB03Z** Insertion of Infusion Device into Left Lower Extremity, Open Approach
●**0YHB0YZ** Insertion of Other Device into Left Lower Extremity, Open Approach
0YHB31Z Insertion of Radioactive Element into Left Lower Extremity, Percutaneous Approach
●**0YHB33Z** Insertion of Infusion Device into Left Lower Extremity, Percutaneous Approach
●**0YHB3YZ** Insertion of Other Device into Left Lower Extremity, Percutaneous Approach
0YHB41Z Insertion of Radioactive Element into Left Lower Extremity, Percutaneous Endoscopic Approach
●**0YHB43Z** Insertion of Infusion Device into Left Lower Extremity, Percutaneous Endoscopic Approach
● **0YHB4YZ** Insertion of Other Device into Left Lower Extremity, Percutaneous Endoscopic Approach
0YHC01Z Insertion of Radioactive Element into Right Upper Leg, Open Approach
● **0YHC03Z** Insertion of Infusion Device into Right Upper Leg, Open Approach
● **0YHC0YZ** Insertion of Other Device into Right Upper Leg, Open Approach
0YHC31Z Insertion of Radioactive Element into Right Upper Leg, Percutaneous Approach
● **0YHC33Z** Insertion of Infusion Device into Right Upper Leg, Percutaneous Approach
● **0YHC3YZ** Insertion of Other Device into Right Upper Leg, Percutaneous Approach
0YHC41Z Insertion of Radioactive Element into Right Upper Leg, Percutaneous Endoscopic Approach
● **0YHC43Z** Insertion of Infusion Device into Right Upper Leg, Percutaneous Endoscopic Approach
● **0YHC4YZ** Insertion of Other Device into Right Upper Leg, Percutaneous Endoscopic Approach
0YHD01Z Insertion of Radioactive Element into Left Upper Leg, Open Approach
● **0YHD03Z** Insertion of Infusion Device into Left Upper Leg, Open Approach
● **0YHD0YZ** Insertion of Other Device into Left Upper Leg, Open Approach
0YHD31Z Insertion of Radioactive Element into Left Upper Leg, Percutaneous Approach
● **0YHD33Z** Insertion of Infusion Device into Left Upper Leg, Percutaneous Approach
● **0YHD3YZ** Insertion of Other Device into Left Upper Leg, Percutaneous Approach
0YHD41Z Insertion of Radioactive Element into Left Upper Leg, Percutaneous Endoscopic Approach
● **0YHD43Z** Insertion of Infusion Device into Left Upper Leg, Percutaneous Endoscopic Approach
● **0YHD4YZ** Insertion of Other Device into Left Upper Leg, Percutaneous Endoscopic Approach
0YHF01Z Insertion of Radioactive Element into Right Knee Region, Open Approach
● **0YHF03Z** Insertion of Infusion Device into Right Knee Region, Open Approach
● **0YHF0YZ** Insertion of Other Device into Right Knee Region, Open Approach
0YHF31Z Insertion of Radioactive Element into Right Knee Region, Percutaneous Approach
● **0YHF33Z** Insertion of Infusion Device into Right Knee Region, Percutaneous Approach
● **0YHF3YZ** Insertion of Other Device into Right Knee Region, Percutaneous Approach
0YHF41Z Insertion of Radioactive Element into Right Knee Region, Percutaneous Endoscopic Approach
● **0YHF43Z** Insertion of Infusion Device into Right Knee Region, Percutaneous Endoscopic Approach
● **0YHF4YZ** Insertion of Other Device into Right Knee Region, Percutaneous Endoscopic Approach
0YHG01Z Insertion of Radioactive Element into Left Knee Region, Open Approach
● **0YHG03Z** Insertion of Infusion Device into Left Knee Region, Open Approach
● **0YHG0YZ** Insertion of Other Device into Left Knee Region, Open Approach
0YHG31Z Insertion of Radioactive Element into Left Knee Region, Percutaneous Approach
● **0YHG33Z** Insertion of Infusion Device into Left Knee Region, Percutaneous Approach
● **0YHG3YZ** Insertion of Other Device into Left Knee Region, Percutaneous Approach
0YHG41Z Insertion of Radioactive Element into Left Knee Region, Percutaneous Endoscopic Approach
● **0YHG43Z** Insertion of Infusion Device into Left Knee Region, Percutaneous Endoscopic Approach
● **0YHG4YZ** Insertion of Other Device into Left Knee Region, Percutaneous Endoscopic Approach
0YHH01Z Insertion of Radioactive Element into Right Lower Leg, Open Approach
● **0YHH03Z** Insertion of Infusion Device into Right Lower Leg, Open Approach
● **0YHH0YZ** Insertion of Other Device into Right Lower Leg, Open Approach
0YHH31Z Insertion of Radioactive Element into Right Lower Leg, Percutaneous Approach
● **0YHH33Z** Insertion of Infusion Device into Right Lower Leg, Percutaneous Approach
● **0YHH3YZ** Insertion of Other Device into Right Lower Leg, Percutaneous Approach
0YHH41Z Insertion of Radioactive Element into Right Lower Leg, Percutaneous Endoscopic Approach
● **0YHH43Z** Insertion of Infusion Device into Right Lower Leg, Percutaneous Endoscopic Approach
● **0YHH4YZ** Insertion of Other Device into Right Lower Leg, Percutaneous Endoscopic Approach
0YHJ01Z Insertion of Radioactive Element into Left Lower Leg, Open Approach
● **0YHJ03Z** Insertion of Infusion Device into Left Lower Leg, Open Approach
● **0YHJ0YZ** Insertion of Other Device into Left Lower Leg, Open Approach
0YHJ31Z Insertion of Radioactive Element into Left Lower Leg, Percutaneous Approach
● **0YHJ33Z** Insertion of Infusion Device into Left Lower Leg, Percutaneous Approach
● **0YHJ3YZ** Insertion of Other Device into Left Lower Leg, Percutaneous Approach
0YHJ41Z Insertion of Radioactive Element into Left Lower Leg, Percutaneous Endoscopic Approach
● **0YHJ43Z** Insertion of Infusion Device into Left Lower Leg, Percutaneous Endoscopic Approach
● **0YHJ4YZ** Insertion of Other Device into Left Lower Leg, Percutaneous Endoscopic Approach
0YHK01Z Insertion of Radioactive Element into Right Ankle Region, Open Approach
● **0YHK03Z** Insertion of Infusion Device into Right Ankle Region, Open Approach
● **0YHK0YZ** Insertion of Other Device into Right Ankle Region, Open Approach
0YHK31Z Insertion of Radioactive Element into Right Ankle Region, Percutaneous Approach
● **0YHK33Z** Insertion of Infusion Device into Right Ankle Region, Percutaneous Approach
● **0YHK3YZ** Insertion of Other Device into Right Ankle Region, Percutaneous Approach
0YHK41Z Insertion of Radioactive Element into Right Ankle Region, Percutaneous Endoscopic Approach
● **0YHK43Z** Insertion of Infusion Device into Right Ankle Region, Percutaneous Endoscopic Approach
● **0YHK4YZ** Insertion of Other Device into Right Ankle Region, Percutaneous Endoscopic Approach

0YHL01Z Insertion of Radioactive Element into Left Ankle Region, Open Approach
● **0YHL03Z** Insertion of Infusion Device into Left Ankle Region, Open Approach
● **0YHL0YZ** Insertion of Other Device into Left Ankle Region, Open Approach
0YHL31Z Insertion of Radioactive Element into Left Ankle Region, Percutaneous Approach
● **0YHL33Z** Insertion of Infusion Device into Left Ankle Region, Percutaneous Approach
● **0YHL3YZ** Insertion of Other Device into Left Ankle Region, Percutaneous Approach
0YHL41Z Insertion of Radioactive Element into Left Ankle Region, Percutaneous Endoscopic Approach
● **0YHL43Z** Insertion of Infusion Device into Left Ankle Region, Percutaneous Endoscopic Approach
● **0YHL4YZ** Insertion of Other Device into Left Ankle Region, Percutaneous Endoscopic Approach
0YHM01Z Insertion of Radioactive Element into Right Foot, Open Approach
● **0YHM03Z** Insertion of Infusion Device into Right Foot, Open Approach
● **0YHM0YZ** Insertion of Other Device into Right Foot, Open Approach
0YHM31Z Insertion of Radioactive Element into Right Foot, Percutaneous Approach
● **0YHM33Z** Insertion of Infusion Device into Right Foot, Percutaneous Approach
● **0YHM3YZ** Insertion of Other Device into Right Foot, Percutaneous Approach
0YHM41Z Insertion of Radioactive Element into Right Foot, Percutaneous Endoscopic Approach
● **0YHM43Z** Insertion of Infusion Device into Right Foot, Percutaneous Endoscopic Approach
● **0YHM4YZ** Insertion of Other Device into Right Foot, Percutaneous Endoscopic Approach
0YHN01Z Insertion of Radioactive Element into Left Foot, Open Approach
● **0YHN03Z** Insertion of Infusion Device into Left Foot, Open Approach
● **0YHN0YZ** Insertion of Other Device into Left Foot, Open Approach
0YHN31Z Insertion of Radioactive Element into Left Foot, Percutaneous Approach
● **0YHN33Z** Insertion of Infusion Device into Left Foot, Percutaneous Approach
● **0YHN3YZ** Insertion of Other Device into Left Foot, Percutaneous Approach
0YHN41Z Insertion of Radioactive Element into Left Foot, Percutaneous Endoscopic Approach
● **0YHN43Z** Insertion of Infusion Device into Left Foot, Percutaneous Endoscopic Approach
● **0YHN4YZ** Insertion of Other Device into Left Foot, Percutaneous Endoscopic Approach

0YJ – Anatomical Regions, Lower Extremities, Inspection

Review Coding Guidelines B3.11a, B3.11b and B3.11c

● **0YJ00ZZ** Inspection of Right Buttock, Open Approach
0YJ03ZZ Inspection of Right Buttock, Percutaneous Approach
0YJ04ZZ Inspection of Right Buttock, Percutaneous Endoscopic Approach
0YJ0XZZ Inspection of Right Buttock, External Approach
● **0YJ10ZZ** Inspection of Left Buttock, Open Approach
0YJ13ZZ Inspection of Left Buttock, Percutaneous Approach
0YJ14ZZ Inspection of Left Buttock, Percutaneous Endoscopic Approach
0YJ1XZZ Inspection of Left Buttock, External Approach
0YJ50ZZ Inspection of Right Inguinal Region, Open Approach
0YJ53ZZ Inspection of Right Inguinal Region, Percutaneous Approach
0YJ54ZZ Inspection of Right Inguinal Region, Percutaneous Endoscopic Approach
0YJ5XZZ Inspection of Right Inguinal Region, External Approach
0YJ60ZZ Inspection of Left Inguinal Region, Open Approach
0YJ63ZZ Inspection of Left Inguinal Region, Percutaneous Approach
0YJ64ZZ Inspection of Left Inguinal Region, Percutaneous Endoscopic Approach
0YJ6XZZ Inspection of Left Inguinal Region, External Approach
0YJ70ZZ Inspection of Right Femoral Region, Open Approach
0YJ73ZZ Inspection of Right Femoral Region, Percutaneous Approach
0YJ74ZZ Inspection of Right Femoral Region, Percutaneous Endoscopic Approach
0YJ7XZZ Inspection of Right Femoral Region, External Approach
● **0YJ80ZZ** Inspection of Left Femoral Region, Open Approach
0YJ83ZZ Inspection of Left Femoral Region, Percutaneous Approach
0YJ84ZZ Inspection of Left Femoral Region, Percutaneous Endoscopic Approach
0YJ8XZZ Inspection of Left Femoral Region, External Approach
● **0YJ90ZZ** Inspection of Right Lower Extremity, Open Approach
0YJ93ZZ Inspection of Right Lower Extremity, Percutaneous Approach
0YJ94ZZ Inspection of Right Lower Extremity, Percutaneous Endoscopic Approach
0YJ9XZZ Inspection of Right Lower Extremity, External Approach
0YJA0ZZ Inspection of Bilateral Inguinal Region, Open Approach
0YJA3ZZ Inspection of Bilateral Inguinal Region, Percutaneous Approach
0YJA4ZZ Inspection of Bilateral Inguinal Region, Percutaneous Endoscopic Approach
0YJAXZZ Inspection of Bilateral Inguinal Region, External Approach
● **0YJB0ZZ** Inspection of Left Lower Extremity, Open Approach
0YJB3ZZ Inspection of Left Lower Extremity, Percutaneous Approach
0YJB4ZZ Inspection of Left Lower Extremity, Percutaneous Endoscopic Approach
0YJBXZZ Inspection of Left Lower Extremity, External Approach
● **0YJC0ZZ** Inspection of Right Upper Leg, Open Approach
0YJC3ZZ Inspection of Right Upper Leg, Percutaneous Approach
0YJC4ZZ Inspection of Right Upper Leg, Percutaneous Endoscopic Approach
0YJCXZZ Inspection of Right Upper Leg, External Approach
● **0YJD0ZZ** Inspection of Left Upper Leg, Open Approach
0YJD3ZZ Inspection of Left Upper Leg, Percutaneous Approach
0YJD4ZZ Inspection of Left Upper Leg, Percutaneous Endoscopic Approach
0YJDXZZ Inspection of Left Upper Leg, External Approach
● **0YJE0ZZ** Inspection of Bilateral Femoral Region, Open Approach
0YJE3ZZ Inspection of Bilateral Femoral Region, Percutaneous Approach
0YJE4ZZ Inspection of Bilateral Femoral Region, Percutaneous Endoscopic Approach
0YJEXZZ Inspection of Bilateral Femoral Region, External Approach
● **0YJF0ZZ** Inspection of Right Knee Region, Open Approach
0YJF3ZZ Inspection of Right Knee Region, Percutaneous Approach
0YJF4ZZ Inspection of Right Knee Region, Percutaneous Endoscopic Approach
0YJFXZZ Inspection of Right Knee Region, External Approach
● **0YJG0ZZ** Inspection of Left Knee Region, Open Approach
0YJG3ZZ Inspection of Left Knee Region, Percutaneous Approach
0YJG4ZZ Inspection of Left Knee Region, Percutaneous Endoscopic Approach
0YJGXZZ Inspection of Left Knee Region, External Approach
● **0YJH0ZZ** Inspection of Right Lower Leg, Open Approach
0YJH3ZZ Inspection of Right Lower Leg, Percutaneous Approach
0YJH4ZZ Inspection of Right Lower Leg, Percutaneous Endoscopic Approach
0YJHXZZ Inspection of Right Lower Leg, External Approach
● **0YJJ0ZZ** Inspection of Left Lower Leg, Open Approach
0YJJ3ZZ Inspection of Left Lower Leg, Percutaneous Approach
0YJJ4ZZ Inspection of Left Lower Leg, Percutaneous Endoscopic Approach
0YJJXZZ Inspection of Left Lower Leg, External Approach
● **0YJK0ZZ** Inspection of Right Ankle Region, Open Approach
0YJK3ZZ Inspection of Right Ankle Region, Percutaneous Approach
0YJK4ZZ Inspection of Right Ankle Region, Percutaneous Endoscopic Approach
0YJKXZZ Inspection of Right Ankle Region, External Approach
● **0YJL0ZZ** Inspection of Left Ankle Region, Open Approach
0YJL3ZZ Inspection of Left Ankle Region, Percutaneous Approach
0YJL4ZZ Inspection of Left Ankle Region, Percutaneous Endoscopic Approach
0YJLXZZ Inspection of Left Ankle Region, External Approach
● **0YJM0ZZ** Inspection of Right Foot, Open Approach
0YJM3ZZ Inspection of Right Foot, Percutaneous Approach
0YJM4ZZ Inspection of Right Foot, Percutaneous Endoscopic Approach
0YJMXZZ Inspection of Right Foot, External Approach

●0YJN0ZZ Inspection of Left Foot, Open Approach
0YJN3ZZ Inspection of Left Foot, Percutaneous Approach
0YJN4ZZ Inspection of Left Foot, Percutaneous Endoscopic Approach
0YJNXZZ Inspection of Left Foot, External Approach

0YM – Anatomical Regions, Lower Extremities, Reattachment

0YM00ZZ Reattachment of Right Buttock, Open Approach
0YM10ZZ Reattachment of Left Buttock, Open Approach
0YM20ZZ Reattachment of Right Hindquarter, Open Approach
0YM30ZZ Reattachment of Left Hindquarter, Open Approach
0YM40ZZ Reattachment of Bilateral Hindquarter, Open Approach
0YM50ZZ Reattachment of Right Inguinal Region, Open Approach
0YM60ZZ Reattachment of Left Inguinal Region, Open Approach
0YM70ZZ Reattachment of Right Femoral Region, Open Approach
0YM80ZZ Reattachment of Left Femoral Region, Open Approach
0YM90ZZ Reattachment of Right Lower Extremity, Open Approach
0YMB0ZZ Reattachment of Left Lower Extremity, Open Approach
0YMC0ZZ Reattachment of Right Upper Leg, Open Approach
0YMD0ZZ Reattachment of Left Upper Leg, Open Approach
0YMF0ZZ Reattachment of Right Knee Region, Open Approach
0YMG0ZZ Reattachment of Left Knee Region, Open Approach
0YMH0ZZ Reattachment of Right Lower Leg, Open Approach
0YMJ0ZZ Reattachment of Left Lower Leg, Open Approach
0YMK0ZZ Reattachment of Right Ankle Region, Open Approach
0YML0ZZ Reattachment of Left Ankle Region, Open Approach
0YMM0ZZ Reattachment of Right Foot, Open Approach
0YMN0ZZ Reattachment of Left Foot, Open Approach
0YMP0ZZ Reattachment of Right 1st Toe, Open Approach
0YMQ0ZZ Reattachment of Left 1st Toe, Open Approach
0YMR0ZZ Reattachment of Right 2nd Toe, Open Approach
0YMS0ZZ Reattachment of Left 2nd Toe, Open Approach
0YMT0ZZ Reattachment of Right 3rd Toe, Open Approach
0YMU0ZZ Reattachment of Left 3rd Toe, Open Approach
0YMV0ZZ Reattachment of Right 4th Toe, Open Approach
0YMW0ZZ Reattachment of Left 4th Toe, Open Approach
0YMX0ZZ Reattachment of Right 5th Toe, Open Approach
0YMY0ZZ Reattachment of Left 5th Toe, Open Approach

0YP – Anatomical Regions, Lower Extremities, Removal

Review Coding Guideline B6.1c

0YP900Z Removal of Drainage Device from Right Lower Extremity, Open Approach
0YP901Z Removal of Radioactive Element from Right Lower Extremity, Open Approach
0YP903Z Removal of Infusion Device from Right Lower Extremity, Open Approach
0YP907Z Removal of Autologous Tissue Substitute from Right Lower Extremity, Open Approach
0YP90JZ Removal of Synthetic Substitute from Right Lower Extremity, Open Approach
0YP90KZ Removal of Nonautologous Tissue Substitute from Right Lower Extremity, Open Approach
0YP90YZ Removal of Other Device from Right Lower Extremity, Open Approach
0YP930Z Removal of Drainage Device from Right Lower Extremity, Percutaneous Approach
0YP931Z Removal of Radioactive Element from Right Lower Extremity, Percutaneous Approach
0YP933Z Removal of Infusion Device from Right Lower Extremity, Percutaneous Approach
0YP937Z Removal of Autologous Tissue Substitute from Right Lower Extremity, Percutaneous Approach
0YP93JZ Removal of Synthetic Substitute from Right Lower Extremity, Percutaneous Approach
0YP93KZ Removal of Nonautologous Tissue Substitute from Right Lower Extremity, Percutaneous Approach
0YP93YZ Removal of Other Device from Right Lower Extremity, Percutaneous Approach
0YP940Z Removal of Drainage Device from Right Lower Extremity, Percutaneous Endoscopic Approach
0YP941Z Removal of Radioactive Element from Right Lower Extremity, Percutaneous Endoscopic Approach
0YP943Z Removal of Infusion Device from Right Lower Extremity, Percutaneous Endoscopic Approach
0YP947Z Removal of Autologous Tissue Substitute from Right Lower Extremity, Percutaneous Endoscopic Approach
0YP94JZ Removal of Synthetic Substitute from Right Lower Extremity, Percutaneous Endoscopic Approach
0YP94KZ Removal of Nonautologous Tissue Substitute from Right Lower Extremity, Percutaneous Endoscopic Approach
0YP94YZ Removal of Other Device from Right Lower Extremity, Percutaneous Endoscopic Approach
0YP9X0Z Removal of Drainage Device from Right Lower Extremity, External Approach
0YP9X1Z Removal of Radioactive Element from Right Lower Extremity, External Approach
0YP9X3Z Removal of Infusion Device from Right Lower Extremity, External Approach
0YP9X7Z Removal of Autologous Tissue Substitute from Right Lower Extremity, External Approach
0YP9XJZ Removal of Synthetic Substitute from Right Lower Extremity, External Approach
0YP9XKZ Removal of Nonautologous Tissue Substitute from Right Lower Extremity, External Approach
0YP9XYZ Removal of Other Device from Right Lower Extremity, External Approach
0YPB00Z Removal of Drainage Device from Left Lower Extremity, Open Approach
0YPB01Z Removal of Radioactive Element from Left Lower Extremity, Open Approach
0YPB03Z Removal of Infusion Device from Left Lower Extremity, Open Approach
0YPB07Z Removal of Autologous Tissue Substitute from Left Lower Extremity, Open Approach
0YPB0JZ Removal of Synthetic Substitute from Left Lower Extremity, Open Approach
0YPB0KZ Removal of Nonautologous Tissue Substitute from Left Lower Extremity, Open Approach
0YPB0YZ Removal of Other Device from Left Lower Extremity, Open Approach
0YPB30Z Removal of Drainage Device from Left Lower Extremity, Percutaneous Approach
0YPB31Z Removal of Radioactive Element from Left Lower Extremity, Percutaneous Approach
0YPB33Z Removal of Infusion Device from Left Lower Extremity, Percutaneous Approach
0YPB37Z Removal of Autologous Tissue Substitute from Left Lower Extremity, Percutaneous Approach
0YPB3JZ Removal of Synthetic Substitute from Left Lower Extremity, Percutaneous Approach
0YPB3KZ Removal of Nonautologous Tissue Substitute from Left Lower Extremity, Percutaneous Approach
0YPB3YZ Removal of Other Device from Left Lower Extremity, Percutaneous Approach
0YPB40Z Removal of Drainage Device from Left Lower Extremity, Percutaneous Endoscopic Approach
0YPB41Z Removal of Radioactive Element from Left Lower Extremity, Percutaneous Endoscopic Approach
0YPB43Z Removal of Infusion Device from Left Lower Extremity, Percutaneous Endoscopic Approach
0YPB47Z Removal of Autologous Tissue Substitute from Left Lower Extremity, Percutaneous Endoscopic Approach
0YPB4JZ Removal of Synthetic Substitute from Left Lower Extremity, Percutaneous Endoscopic Approach
0YPB4KZ Removal of Nonautologous Tissue Substitute from Left Lower Extremity, Percutaneous Endoscopic Approach
0YPB4YZ Removal of Other Device from Left Lower Extremity, Percutaneous Endoscopic Approach
0YPBX0Z Removal of Drainage Device from Left Lower Extremity, External Approach
0YPBX1Z Removal of Radioactive Element from Left Lower Extremity, External Approach

0YPBX3Z Removal of Infusion Device from Left Lower Extremity, External Approach
0YPBX7Z Removal of Autologous Tissue Substitute from Left Lower Extremity, External Approach
0YPBXJZ Removal of Synthetic Substitute from Left Lower Extremity, External Approach
0YPBXKZ Removal of Nonautologous Tissue Substitute from Left Lower Extremity, External Approach
0YPBXYZ Removal of Other Device from Left Lower Extremity, External Approach

0YQ – Anatomical Regions, Lower Extremities, Repair

0YQ00ZZ Repair Right Buttock, Open Approach
0YQ03ZZ Repair Right Buttock, Percutaneous Approach
0YQ04ZZ Repair Right Buttock, Percutaneous Endoscopic Approach
0YQ0XZZ Repair Right Buttock, External Approach
0YQ10ZZ Repair Left Buttock, Open Approach
0YQ13ZZ Repair Left Buttock, Percutaneous Approach
0YQ14ZZ Repair Left Buttock, Percutaneous Endoscopic Approach
0YQ1XZZ Repair Left Buttock, External Approach
0YQ50ZZ Repair Right Inguinal Region, Open Approach
0YQ53ZZ Repair Right Inguinal Region, Percutaneous Approach
0YQ54ZZ Repair Right Inguinal Region, Percutaneous Endoscopic Approach
0YQ5XZZ Repair Right Inguinal Region, External Approach
0YQ60ZZ Repair Left Inguinal Region, Open Approach
0YQ63ZZ Repair Left Inguinal Region, Percutaneous Approach
0YQ64ZZ Repair Left Inguinal Region, Percutaneous Endoscopic Approach
0YQ6XZZ Repair Left Inguinal Region, External Approach
0YQ70ZZ Repair Right Femoral Region, Open Approach
0YQ73ZZ Repair Right Femoral Region, Percutaneous Approach
0YQ74ZZ Repair Right Femoral Region, Percutaneous Endoscopic Approach
0YQ7XZZ Repair Right Femoral Region, External Approach
0YQ80ZZ Repair Left Femoral Region, Open Approach
0YQ83ZZ Repair Left Femoral Region, Percutaneous Approach
0YQ84ZZ Repair Left Femoral Region, Percutaneous Endoscopic Approach
0YQ8XZZ Repair Left Femoral Region, External Approach
0YQ90ZZ Repair Right Lower Extremity, Open Approach
0YQ93ZZ Repair Right Lower Extremity, Percutaneous Approach
0YQ94ZZ Repair Right Lower Extremity, Percutaneous Endoscopic Approach
0YQ9XZZ Repair Right Lower Extremity, External Approach
0YQA0ZZ Repair Bilateral Inguinal Region, Open Approach
0YQA3ZZ Repair Bilateral Inguinal Region, Percutaneous Approach
0YQA4ZZ Repair Bilateral Inguinal Region, Percutaneous Endoscopic Approach
0YQAXZZ Repair Bilateral Inguinal Region, External Approach
0YQB0ZZ Repair Left Lower Extremity, Open Approach
0YQB3ZZ Repair Left Lower Extremity, Percutaneous Approach
0YQB4ZZ Repair Left Lower Extremity, Percutaneous Endoscopic Approach
0YQBXZZ Repair Left Lower Extremity, External Approach
0YQC0ZZ Repair Right Upper Leg, Open Approach
0YQC3ZZ Repair Right Upper Leg, Percutaneous Approach
0YQC4ZZ Repair Right Upper Leg, Percutaneous Endoscopic Approach
0YQCXZZ Repair Right Upper Leg, External Approach
0YQD0ZZ Repair Left Upper Leg, Open Approach
0YQD3ZZ Repair Left Upper Leg, Percutaneous Approach
0YQD4ZZ Repair Left Upper Leg, Percutaneous Endoscopic Approach
0YQDXZZ Repair Left Upper Leg, External Approach
0YQE0ZZ Repair Bilateral Femoral Region, Open Approach
0YQE3ZZ Repair Bilateral Femoral Region, Percutaneous Approach
0YQE4ZZ Repair Bilateral Femoral Region, Percutaneous Endoscopic Approach
0YQEXZZ Repair Bilateral Femoral Region, External Approach
0YQF0ZZ Repair Right Knee Region, Open Approach
0YQF3ZZ Repair Right Knee Region, Percutaneous Approach
0YQF4ZZ Repair Right Knee Region, Percutaneous Endoscopic Approach
0YQFXZZ Repair Right Knee Region, External Approach
0YQG0ZZ Repair Left Knee Region, Open Approach
0YQG3ZZ Repair Left Knee Region, Percutaneous Approach
0YQG4ZZ Repair Left Knee Region, Percutaneous Endoscopic Approach
0YQGXZZ Repair Left Knee Region, External Approach
0YQH0ZZ Repair Right Lower Leg, Open Approach
0YQH3ZZ Repair Right Lower Leg, Percutaneous Approach
0YQH4ZZ Repair Right Lower Leg, Percutaneous Endoscopic Approach
0YQHXZZ Repair Right Lower Leg, External Approach
0YQJ0ZZ Repair Left Lower Leg, Open Approach
0YQJ3ZZ Repair Left Lower Leg, Percutaneous Approach
0YQJ4ZZ Repair Left Lower Leg, Percutaneous Endoscopic Approach
0YQJXZZ Repair Left Lower Leg, External Approach
0YQK0ZZ Repair Right Ankle Region, Open Approach
0YQK3ZZ Repair Right Ankle Region, Percutaneous Approach
0YQK4ZZ Repair Right Ankle Region, Percutaneous Endoscopic Approach
0YQKXZZ Repair Right Ankle Region, External Approach
0YQL0ZZ Repair Left Ankle Region, Open Approach
0YQL3ZZ Repair Left Ankle Region, Percutaneous Approach
0YQL4ZZ Repair Left Ankle Region, Percutaneous Endoscopic Approach
0YQLXZZ Repair Left Ankle Region, External Approach
0YQM0ZZ Repair Right Foot, Open Approach
0YQM3ZZ Repair Right Foot, Percutaneous Approach
0YQM4ZZ Repair Right Foot, Percutaneous Endoscopic Approach
0YQMXZZ Repair Right Foot, External Approach
0YQN0ZZ Repair Left Foot, Open Approach
0YQN3ZZ Repair Left Foot, Percutaneous Approach
0YQN4ZZ Repair Left Foot, Percutaneous Endoscopic Approach
0YQNXZZ Repair Left Foot, External Approach
0YQP0ZZ Repair Right 1st Toe, Open Approach
0YQP3ZZ Repair Right 1st Toe, Percutaneous Approach
0YQP4ZZ Repair Right 1st Toe, Percutaneous Endoscopic Approach
0YQPXZZ Repair Right 1st Toe, External Approach
0YQQ0ZZ Repair Left 1st Toe, Open Approach
0YQQ3ZZ Repair Left 1st Toe, Percutaneous Approach
0YQQ4ZZ Repair Left 1st Toe, Percutaneous Endoscopic Approach
0YQQXZZ Repair Left 1st Toe, External Approach
0YQR0ZZ Repair Right 2nd Toe, Open Approach
0YQR3ZZ Repair Right 2nd Toe, Percutaneous Approach
0YQR4ZZ Repair Right 2nd Toe, Percutaneous Endoscopic Approach
0YQRXZZ Repair Right 2nd Toe, External Approach
0YQS0ZZ Repair Left 2nd Toe, Open Approach
0YQS3ZZ Repair Left 2nd Toe, Percutaneous Approach
0YQS4ZZ Repair Left 2nd Toe, Percutaneous Endoscopic Approach
0YQSXZZ Repair Left 2nd Toe, External Approach
0YQT0ZZ Repair Right 3rd Toe, Open Approach
0YQT3ZZ Repair Right 3rd Toe, Percutaneous Approach
0YQT4ZZ Repair Right 3rd Toe, Percutaneous Endoscopic Approach
0YQTXZZ Repair Right 3rd Toe, External Approach
0YQU0ZZ Repair Left 3rd Toe, Open Approach
0YQU3ZZ Repair Left 3rd Toe, Percutaneous Approach
0YQU4ZZ Repair Left 3rd Toe, Percutaneous Endoscopic Approach
0YQUXZZ Repair Left 3rd Toe, External Approach
0YQV0ZZ Repair Right 4th Toe, Open Approach
0YQV3ZZ Repair Right 4th Toe, Percutaneous Approach
0YQV4ZZ Repair Right 4th Toe, Percutaneous Endoscopic Approach
0YQVXZZ Repair Right 4th Toe, External Approach
0YQW0ZZ Repair Left 4th Toe, Open Approach
0YQW3ZZ Repair Left 4th Toe, Percutaneous Approach
0YQW4ZZ Repair Left 4th Toe, Percutaneous Endoscopic Approach
0YQWXZZ Repair Left 4th Toe, External Approach
0YQX0ZZ Repair Right 5th Toe, Open Approach
0YQX3ZZ Repair Right 5th Toe, Percutaneous Approach
0YQX4ZZ Repair Right 5th Toe, Percutaneous Endoscopic Approach
0YQXXZZ Repair Right 5th Toe, External Approach
0YQY0ZZ Repair Left 5th Toe, Open Approach
0YQY3ZZ Repair Left 5th Toe, Percutaneous Approach
0YQY4ZZ Repair Left 5th Toe, Percutaneous Endoscopic Approach
0YQYXZZ Repair Left 5th Toe, External Approach

0YU007Z Supplement Right Buttock with Autologous Tissue Substitute, Open Approach
0YU00JZ Supplement Right Buttock with Synthetic Substitute, Open Approach
0YU00KZ Supplement Right Buttock with Nonautologous Tissue Substitute, Open Approach
0YU047Z Supplement Right Buttock with Autologous Tissue Substitute, Percutaneous Endoscopic Approach
0YU04JZ Supplement Right Buttock with Synthetic Substitute, Percutaneous Endoscopic Approach
0YU04KZ Supplement Right Buttock with Nonautologous Tissue Substitute, Percutaneous Endoscopic Approach
0YU107Z Supplement Left Buttock with Autologous Tissue Substitute, Open Approach
0YU10JZ Supplement Left Buttock with Synthetic Substitute, Open Approach
0YU10KZ Supplement Left Buttock with Nonautologous Tissue Substitute, Open Approach
0YU147Z Supplement Left Buttock with Autologous Tissue Substitute, Percutaneous Endoscopic Approach
0YU14JZ Supplement Left Buttock with Synthetic Substitute, Percutaneous Endoscopic Approach
0YU14KZ Supplement Left Buttock with Nonautologous Tissue Substitute, Percutaneous Endoscopic Approach
0YU507Z Supplement Right Inguinal Region with Autologous Tissue Substitute, Open Approach
0YU50JZ Supplement Right Inguinal Region with Synthetic Substitute, Open Approach
0YU50KZ Supplement Right Inguinal Region with Nonautologous Tissue Substitute, Open Approach
0YU547Z Supplement Right Inguinal Region with Autologous Tissue Substitute, Percutaneous Endoscopic Approach
0YU54JZ Supplement Right Inguinal Region with Synthetic Substitute, Percutaneous Endoscopic Approach
0YU54KZ Supplement Right Inguinal Region with Nonautologous Tissue Substitute, Percutaneous Endoscopic Approach
0YU607Z Supplement Left Inguinal Region with Autologous Tissue Substitute, Open Approach
0YU60JZ Supplement Left Inguinal Region with Synthetic Substitute, Open Approach
0YU60KZ Supplement Left Inguinal Region with Nonautologous Tissue Substitute, Open Approach
0YU647Z Supplement Left Inguinal Region with Autologous Tissue Substitute, Percutaneous Endoscopic Approach
0YU64JZ Supplement Left Inguinal Region with Synthetic Substitute, Percutaneous Endoscopic Approach
0YU64KZ Supplement Left Inguinal Region with Nonautologous Tissue Substitute, Percutaneous Endoscopic Approach
0YU707Z Supplement Right Femoral Region with Autologous Tissue Substitute, Open Approach
0YU70JZ Supplement Right Femoral Region with Synthetic Substitute, Open Approach
0YU70KZ Supplement Right Femoral Region with Nonautologous Tissue Substitute, Open Approach
0YU747Z Supplement Right Femoral Region with Autologous Tissue Substitute, Percutaneous Endoscopic Approach
0YU74JZ Supplement Right Femoral Region with Synthetic Substitute, Percutaneous Endoscopic Approach
0YU74KZ Supplement Right Femoral Region with Nonautologous Tissue Substitute, Percutaneous Endoscopic Approach
0YU807Z Supplement Left Femoral Region with Autologous Tissue Substitute, Open Approach
0YU80JZ Supplement Left Femoral Region with Synthetic Substitute, Open Approach
0YU80KZ Supplement Left Femoral Region with Nonautologous Tissue Substitute, Open Approach
0YU847Z Supplement Left Femoral Region with Autologous Tissue Substitute, Percutaneous Endoscopic Approach
0YU84JZ Supplement Left Femoral Region with Synthetic Substitute, Percutaneous Endoscopic Approach
0YU84KZ Supplement Left Femoral Region with Nonautologous Tissue Substitute, Percutaneous Endoscopic Approach
0YU907Z Supplement Right Lower Extremity with Autologous Tissue Substitute, Open Approach
0YU90JZ Supplement Right Lower Extremity with Synthetic Substitute, Open Approach
0YU90KZ Supplement Right Lower Extremity with Nonautologous Tissue Substitute, Open Approach
0YU947Z Supplement Right Lower Extremity with Autologous Tissue Substitute, Percutaneous Endoscopic Approach
0YU94JZ Supplement Right Lower Extremity with Synthetic Substitute, Percutaneous Endoscopic Approach
0YU94KZ Supplement Right Lower Extremity with Nonautologous Tissue Substitute, Percutaneous Endoscopic Approach
0YUA07Z Supplement Bilateral Inguinal Region with Autologous Tissue Substitute, Open Approach
0YUA0JZ Supplement Bilateral Inguinal Region with Synthetic Substitute, Open Approach
0YUA0KZ Supplement Bilateral Inguinal Region with Nonautologous Tissue Substitute, Open Approach
0YUA47Z Supplement Bilateral Inguinal Region with Autologous Tissue Substitute, Percutaneous Endoscopic Approach
0YUA4JZ Supplement Bilateral Inguinal Region with Synthetic Substitute, Percutaneous Endoscopic Approach
0YUA4KZ Supplement Bilateral Inguinal Region with Nonautologous Tissue Substitute, Percutaneous Endoscopic Approach
0YUB07Z Supplement Left Lower Extremity with Autologous Tissue Substitute, Open Approach
0YUB0JZ Supplement Left Lower Extremity with Synthetic Substitute, Open Approach
0YUB0KZ Supplement Left Lower Extremity with Nonautologous Tissue Substitute, Open Approach
0YUB47Z Supplement Left Lower Extremity with Autologous Tissue Substitute, Percutaneous Endoscopic Approach
0YUB4JZ Supplement Left Lower Extremity with Synthetic Substitute, Percutaneous Endoscopic Approach
0YUB4KZ Supplement Left Lower Extremity with Nonautologous Tissue Substitute, Percutaneous Endoscopic Approach
0YUC07Z Supplement Right Upper Leg with Autologous Tissue Substitute, Open Approach
0YUC0JZ Supplement Right Upper Leg with Synthetic Substitute, Open Approach
0YUC0KZ Supplement Right Upper Leg with Nonautologous Tissue Substitute, Open Approach
0YUC47Z Supplement Right Upper Leg with Autologous Tissue Substitute, Percutaneous Endoscopic Approach
0YUC4JZ Supplement Right Upper Leg with Synthetic Substitute, Percutaneous Endoscopic Approach
0YUC4KZ Supplement Right Upper Leg with Nonautologous Tissue Substitute, Percutaneous Endoscopic Approach
0YUD07Z Supplement Left Upper Leg with Autologous Tissue Substitute, Open Approach
0YUD0JZ Supplement Left Upper Leg with Synthetic Substitute, Open Approach
0YUD0KZ Supplement Left Upper Leg with Nonautologous Tissue Substitute, Open Approach
0YUD47Z Supplement Left Upper Leg with Autologous Tissue Substitute, Percutaneous Endoscopic Approach
0YUD4JZ Supplement Left Upper Leg with Synthetic Substitute, Percutaneous Endoscopic Approach
0YUD4KZ Supplement Left Upper Leg with Nonautologous Tissue Substitute, Percutaneous Endoscopic Approach
0YUE07Z Supplement Bilateral Femoral Region with Autologous Tissue Substitute, Open Approach
0YUE0JZ Supplement Bilateral Femoral Region with Synthetic Substitute, Open Approach
0YUE0KZ Supplement Bilateral Femoral Region with Nonautologous Tissue Substitute, Open Approach
0YUE47Z Supplement Bilateral Femoral Region with Autologous Tissue Substitute, Percutaneous Endoscopic Approach
0YUE4JZ Supplement Bilateral Femoral Region with Synthetic Substitute, Percutaneous Endoscopic Approach
0YUE4KZ Supplement Bilateral Femoral Region with Nonautologous Tissue Substitute, Percutaneous Endoscopic Approach
0YUF07Z Supplement Right Knee Region with Autologous Tissue Substitute, Open Approach
0YUF0JZ Supplement Right Knee Region with Synthetic Substitute, Open Approach
0YUF0KZ Supplement Right Knee Region with Nonautologous Tissue Substitute, Open Approach
0YUF47Z Supplement Right Knee Region with Autologous Tissue Substitute, Percutaneous Endoscopic Approach
0YUF4JZ Supplement Right Knee Region with Synthetic Substitute, Percutaneous Endoscopic Approach
0YUF4KZ Supplement Right Knee Region with Nonautologous Tissue Substitute, Percutaneous Endoscopic Approach
0YUG07Z Supplement Left Knee Region with Autologous Tissue Substitute, Open Approach
0YUG0JZ Supplement Left Knee Region with Synthetic Substitute, Open Approach

0YUG0KZ Supplement Left Knee Region with Nonautologous Tissue Substitute, Open Approach
0YUG47Z Supplement Left Knee Region with Autologous Tissue Substitute, Percutaneous Endoscopic Approach
0YUG4JZ Supplement Left Knee Region with Synthetic Substitute, Percutaneous Endoscopic Approach
0YUG4KZ Supplement Left Knee Region with Nonautologous Tissue Substitute, Percutaneous Endoscopic Approach
0YUH07Z Supplement Right Lower Leg with Autologous Tissue Substitute, Open Approach
0YUH0JZ Supplement Right Lower Leg with Synthetic Substitute, Open Approach
0YUH0KZ Supplement Right Lower Leg with Nonautologous Tissue Substitute, Open Approach
0YUH47Z Supplement Right Lower Leg with Autologous Tissue Substitute, Percutaneous Endoscopic Approach
0YUH4JZ Supplement Right Lower Leg with Synthetic Substitute, Percutaneous Endoscopic Approach
0YUH4KZ Supplement Right Lower Leg with Nonautologous Tissue Substitute, Percutaneous Endoscopic Approach
0YUJ07Z Supplement Left Lower Leg with Autologous Tissue Substitute, Open Approach
0YUJ0JZ Supplement Left Lower Leg with Synthetic Substitute, Open Approach
0YUJ0KZ Supplement Left Lower Leg with Nonautologous Tissue Substitute, Open Approach
0YUJ47Z Supplement Left Lower Leg with Autologous Tissue Substitute, Percutaneous Endoscopic Approach
0YUJ4JZ Supplement Left Lower Leg with Synthetic Substitute, Percutaneous Endoscopic Approach
0YUJ4KZ Supplement Left Lower Leg with Nonautologous Tissue Substitute, Percutaneous Endoscopic Approach
0YUK07Z Supplement Right Ankle Region with Autologous Tissue Substitute, Open Approach
0YUK0JZ Supplement Right Ankle Region with Synthetic Substitute, Open Approach
0YUK0KZ Supplement Right Ankle Region with Nonautologous Tissue Substitute, Open Approach
0YUK47Z Supplement Right Ankle Region with Autologous Tissue Substitute, Percutaneous Endoscopic Approach
0YUK4JZ Supplement Right Ankle Region with Synthetic Substitute, Percutaneous Endoscopic Approach
0YUK4KZ Supplement Right Ankle Region with Nonautologous Tissue Substitute, Percutaneous Endoscopic Approach
0YUL07Z Supplement Left Ankle Region with Autologous Tissue Substitute, Open Approach
0YUL0JZ Supplement Left Ankle Region with Synthetic Substitute, Open Approach
0YUL0KZ Supplement Left Ankle Region with Nonautologous Tissue Substitute, Open Approach
0YUL47Z Supplement Left Ankle Region with Autologous Tissue Substitute, Percutaneous Endoscopic Approach
0YUL4JZ Supplement Left Ankle Region with Synthetic Substitute, Percutaneous Endoscopic Approach
0YUL4KZ Supplement Left Ankle Region with Nonautologous Tissue Substitute, Percutaneous Endoscopic Approach
0YUM07Z Supplement Right Foot with Autologous Tissue Substitute, Open Approach
0YUM0JZ Supplement Right Foot with Synthetic Substitute, Open Approach
0YUM0KZ Supplement Right Foot with Nonautologous Tissue Substitute, Open Approach
0YUM47Z Supplement Right Foot with Autologous Tissue Substitute, Percutaneous Endoscopic Approach
0YUM4JZ Supplement Right Foot with Synthetic Substitute, Percutaneous Endoscopic Approach
0YUM4KZ Supplement Right Foot with Nonautologous Tissue Substitute, Percutaneous Endoscopic Approach
0YUN07Z Supplement Left Foot with Autologous Tissue Substitute, Open Approach
0YUN0JZ Supplement Left Foot with Synthetic Substitute, Open Approach
0YUN0KZ Supplement Left Foot with Nonautologous Tissue Substitute, Open Approach
0YUN47Z Supplement Left Foot with Autologous Tissue Substitute, Percutaneous Endoscopic Approach
0YUN4JZ Supplement Left Foot with Synthetic Substitute, Percutaneous Endoscopic Approach
0YUN4KZ Supplement Left Foot with Nonautologous Tissue Substitute, Percutaneous Endoscopic Approach
0YUP07Z Supplement Right 1st Toe with Autologous Tissue Substitute, Open Approach
0YUP0JZ Supplement Right 1st Toe with Synthetic Substitute, Open Approach
0YUP0KZ Supplement Right 1st Toe with Nonautologous Tissue Substitute, Open Approach
0YUP47Z Supplement Right 1st Toe with Autologous Tissue Substitute, Percutaneous Endoscopic Approach
0YUP4JZ Supplement Right 1st Toe with Synthetic Substitute, Percutaneous Endoscopic Approach
0YUP4KZ Supplement Right 1st Toe with Nonautologous Tissue Substitute, Percutaneous Endoscopic Approach
0YUQ07Z Supplement Left 1st Toe with Autologous Tissue Substitute, Open Approach
0YUQ0JZ Supplement Left 1st Toe with Synthetic Substitute, Open Approach
0YUQ0KZ Supplement Left 1st Toe with Nonautologous Tissue Substitute, Open Approach
0YUQ47Z Supplement Left 1st Toe with Autologous Tissue Substitute, Percutaneous Endoscopic Approach
0YUQ4JZ Supplement Left 1st Toe with Synthetic Substitute, Percutaneous Endoscopic Approach
0YUQ4KZ Supplement Left 1st Toe with Nonautologous Tissue Substitute, Percutaneous Endoscopic Approach
0YUR07Z Supplement Right 2nd Toe with Autologous Tissue Substitute, Open Approach
0YUR0JZ Supplement Right 2nd Toe with Synthetic Substitute, Open Approach
0YUR0KZ Supplement Right 2nd Toe with Nonautologous Tissue Substitute, Open Approach
0YUR47Z Supplement Right 2nd Toe with Autologous Tissue Substitute, Percutaneous Endoscopic Approach
0YUR4JZ Supplement Right 2nd Toe with Synthetic Substitute, Percutaneous Endoscopic Approach
0YUR4KZ Supplement Right 2nd Toe with Nonautologous Tissue Substitute, Percutaneous Endoscopic Approach
0YUS07Z Supplement Left 2nd Toe with Autologous Tissue Substitute, Open Approach
0YUS0JZ Supplement Left 2nd Toe with Synthetic Substitute, Open Approach
0YUS0KZ Supplement Left 2nd Toe with Nonautologous Tissue Substitute, Open Approach
0YUS47Z Supplement Left 2nd Toe with Autologous Tissue Substitute, Percutaneous Endoscopic Approach
0YUS4JZ Supplement Left 2nd Toe with Synthetic Substitute, Percutaneous Endoscopic Approach
0YUS4KZ Supplement Left 2nd Toe with Nonautologous Tissue Substitute, Percutaneous Endoscopic Approach
0YUT07Z Supplement Right 3rd Toe with Autologous Tissue Substitute, Open Approach
0YUT0JZ Supplement Right 3rd Toe with Synthetic Substitute, Open Approach
0YUT0KZ Supplement Right 3rd Toe with Nonautologous Tissue Substitute, Open Approach
0YUT47Z Supplement Right 3rd Toe with Autologous Tissue Substitute, Percutaneous Endoscopic Approach
0YUT4JZ Supplement Right 3rd Toe with Synthetic Substitute, Percutaneous Endoscopic Approach
0YUT4KZ Supplement Right 3rd Toe with Nonautologous Tissue Substitute, Percutaneous Endoscopic Approach
0YUU07Z Supplement Left 3rd Toe with Autologous Tissue Substitute, Open Approach
0YUU0JZ Supplement Left 3rd Toe with Synthetic Substitute, Open Approach
0YUU0KZ Supplement Left 3rd Toe with Nonautologous Tissue Substitute, Open Approach
0YUU47Z Supplement Left 3rd Toe with Autologous Tissue Substitute, Percutaneous Endoscopic Approach
0YUU4JZ Supplement Left 3rd Toe with Synthetic Substitute, Percutaneous Endoscopic Approach
0YUU4KZ Supplement Left 3rd Toe with Nonautologous Tissue Substitute, Percutaneous Endoscopic Approach
0YUV07Z Supplement Right 4th Toe with Autologous Tissue Substitute, Open Approach
0YUV0JZ Supplement Right 4th Toe with Synthetic Substitute, Open Approach
0YUV0KZ Supplement Right 4th Toe with Nonautologous Tissue Substitute, Open Approach
0YUV47Z Supplement Right 4th Toe with Autologous Tissue Substitute, Percutaneous Endoscopic Approach
0YUV4JZ Supplement Right 4th Toe with Synthetic Substitute, Percutaneous Endoscopic Approach
0YUV4KZ Supplement Right 4th Toe with Nonautologous Tissue Substitute, Percutaneous Endoscopic Approach

0YUW07Z Supplement Left 4th Toe with Autologous Tissue Substitute, Open Approach
0YUW0JZ Supplement Left 4th Toe with Synthetic Substitute, Open Approach
0YUW0KZ Supplement Left 4th Toe with Nonautologous Tissue Substitute, Open Approach
0YUW47Z Supplement Left 4th Toe with Autologous Tissue Substitute, Percutaneous Endoscopic Approach
0YUW4JZ Supplement Left 4th Toe with Synthetic Substitute, Percutaneous Endoscopic Approach
0YUW4KZ Supplement Left 4th Toe with Nonautologous Tissue Substitute, Percutaneous Endoscopic Approach
0YUX07Z Supplement Right 5th Toe with Autologous Tissue Substitute, Open Approach
0YUX0JZ Supplement Right 5th Toe with Synthetic Substitute, Open Approach
0YUX0KZ Supplement Right 5th Toe with Nonautologous Tissue Substitute, Open Approach
0YUX47Z Supplement Right 5th Toe with Autologous Tissue Substitute, Percutaneous Endoscopic Approach
0YUX4JZ Supplement Right 5th Toe with Synthetic Substitute, Percutaneous Endoscopic Approach
0YUX4KZ Supplement Right 5th Toe with Nonautologous Tissue Substitute, Percutaneous Endoscopic Approach
0YUY07Z Supplement Left 5th Toe with Autologous Tissue Substitute, Open Approach
0YUY0JZ Supplement Left 5th Toe with Synthetic Substitute, Open Approach
0YUY0KZ Supplement Left 5th Toe with Nonautologous Tissue Substitute, Open Approach
0YUY47Z Supplement Left 5th Toe with Autologous Tissue Substitute, Percutaneous Endoscopic Approach
0YUY4JZ Supplement Left 5th Toe with Synthetic Substitute, Percutaneous Endoscopic Approach
0YUY4KZ Supplement Left 5th Toe with Nonautologous Tissue Substitute, Percutaneous Endoscopic Approach

0YW – Anatomical Regions, Lower Extremities, Revision

Review Coding Guideline B6.1c

● **0YW900Z** Revision of Drainage Device in Right Lower Extremity, Open Approach
● **0YW903Z** Revision of Infusion Device in Right Lower Extremity, Open Approach
● **0YW907Z** Revision of Autologous Tissue Substitute in Right Lower Extremity, Open Approach
● **0YW90JZ** Revision of Synthetic Substitute in Right Lower Extremity, Open Approach
● **0YW90KZ** Revision of Nonautologous Tissue Substitute in Right Lower Extremity, Open Approach
● **0YW90YZ** Revision of Other Device in Right Lower Extremity, Open Approach
● **0YW930Z** Revision of Drainage Device in Right Lower Extremity, Percutaneous Approach
● **0YW933Z** Revision of Infusion Device in Right Lower Extremity, Percutaneous Approach
● **0YW937Z** Revision of Autologous Tissue Substitute in Right Lower Extremity, Percutaneous Approach
● **0YW93JZ** Revision of Synthetic Substitute in Right Lower Extremity, Percutaneous Approach
● **0YW93KZ** Revision of Nonautologous Tissue Substitute in Right Lower Extremity, Percutaneous Approach
● **0YW93YZ** Revision of Other Device in Right Lower Extremity, Percutaneous Approach
● **0YW940Z** Revision of Drainage Device in Right Lower Extremity, Percutaneous Endoscopic Approach
● **0YW943Z** Revision of Infusion Device in Right Lower Extremity, Percutaneous Endoscopic Approach
● **0YW947Z** Revision of Autologous Tissue Substitute in Right Lower Extremity, Percutaneous Endoscopic Approach
● **0YW94JZ** Revision of Synthetic Substitute in Right Lower Extremity, Percutaneous Endoscopic Approach
● **0YW94KZ** Revision of Nonautologous Tissue Substitute in Right Lower Extremity, Percutaneous Endoscopic Approach
● **0YW94YZ** Revision of Other Device in Right Lower Extremity, Percutaneous Endoscopic Approach
0YW9X0Z Revision of Drainage Device in Right Lower Extremity, External Approach
0YW9X3Z Revision of Infusion Device in Right Lower Extremity, External Approach
0YW9X7Z Revision of Autologous Tissue Substitute in Right Lower Extremity, External Approach
0YW9XJZ Revision of Synthetic Substitute in Right Lower Extremity, External Approach
0YW9XKZ Revision of Nonautologous Tissue Substitute in Right Lower Extremity, External Approach
0YW9XYZ Revision of Other Device in Right Lower Extremity, External Approach
● **0YWB00Z** Revision of Drainage Device in Left Lower Extremity, Open Approach
● **0YWB03Z** Revision of Infusion Device in Left Lower Extremity, Open Approach
● **0YWB07Z** Revision of Autologous Tissue Substitute in Left Lower Extremity, Open Approach
● **0YWB0JZ** Revision of Synthetic Substitute in Left Lower Extremity, Open Approach
● **0YWB0KZ** Revision of Nonautologous Tissue Substitute in Left Lower Extremity, Open Approach
● **0YWB0YZ** Revision of Other Device in Left Lower Extremity, Open Approach
● **0YWB30Z** Revision of Drainage Device in Left Lower Extremity, Percutaneous Approach
● **0YWB33Z** Revision of Infusion Device in Left Lower Extremity, Percutaneous Approach
● **0YWB37Z** Revision of Autologous Tissue Substitute in Left Lower Extremity, Percutaneous Approach
● **0YWB3JZ** Revision of Synthetic Substitute in Left Lower Extremity, Percutaneous Approach
● **0YWB3KZ** Revision of Nonautologous Tissue Substitute in Left Lower Extremity, Percutaneous Approach
● **0YWB3YZ** Revision of Other Device in Left Lower Extremity, Percutaneous Approach
● **0YWB40Z** Revision of Drainage Device in Left Lower Extremity, Percutaneous Endoscopic Approach
● **0YWB43Z** Revision of Infusion Device in Left Lower Extremity, Percutaneous Endoscopic Approach
● **0YWB47Z** Revision of Autologous Tissue Substitute in Left Lower Extremity, Percutaneous Endoscopic Approach
● **0YWB4JZ** Revision of Synthetic Substitute in Left Lower Extremity, Percutaneous Endoscopic Approach
● **0YWB4KZ** Revision of Nonautologous Tissue Substitute in Left Lower Extremity, Percutaneous Endoscopic Approach
● **0YWB4YZ** Revision of Other Device in Left Lower Extremity, Percutaneous Endoscopic Approach
0YWBX0Z Revision of Drainage Device in Left Lower Extremity, External Approach
0YWBX3Z Revision of Infusion Device in Left Lower Extremity, External Approach
0YWBX7Z Revision of Autologous Tissue Substitute in Left Lower Extremity, External Approach
0YWBXJZ Revision of Synthetic Substitute in Left Lower Extremity, External Approach
0YWBXKZ Revision of Nonautologous Tissue Substitute in Left Lower Extremity, External Approach
0YWBXYZ Revision of Other Device in Left Lower Extremity, External Approach

Section 1 **Obstetrics**
Body System 0 **Pregnancy**
Operation 9 **Drainage:** Taking or letting out fluids and/or gases from a body part

Body Part (4th)	Approach (5th)	Device (6th)	Qualifier (7th)
0 Products of Conception	**0** Open **3** Percutaneous **4** Percutaneous Endoscopic **7** Via Natural or Artificial Opening **8** Via Natural or Artificial Opening Endoscopic	**Z** No Device	**9** Fetal Blood **A** Fetal Cerebrospinal Fluid **B** Fetal Fluid, Other **C** Amniotic Fluid, Therapeutic **D** Fluid, Other **U** Amniotic Fluid, Diagnostic

Section 1 **Obstetrics**
Body System 0 **Pregnancy**
Operation A **Abortion:** Artificially terminating a pregnancy

Body Part (4th)	Approach (5th)	Device (6th)	Qualifier (7th)
0 Products of Conception	**0** Open **3** Percutaneous **4** Percutaneous Endoscopic **8** Via Natural or Artificial Opening Endoscopic	**Z** No Device	**Z** No Qualifier
0 Products of Conception	**7** Via Natural or Artificial Opening	**Z** No Device	**6** Vacuum **W** Laminaria **X** Abortifacient **Z** No Qualifier

Section 1 **Obstetrics**
Body System 0 **Pregnancy**
Operation D **Extraction:** Pulling or stripping out or off all or a portion of a body part by the use of force

Body Part (4th)	Approach (5th)	Device (6th)	Qualifier (7th)
0 Products of Conception	**0** Open	**Z** No Device	**0** Classical **1** Low Cervical **2** Extraperitoneal
0 Products of Conception	**7** Via Natural or Artificial Opening	**Z** No Device	**3** Low Forceps **4** Mid Forceps **5** High Forceps **6** Vacuum **7** Internal Version **8** Other
1 Products of Conception, Retained **2** Products of Conception, Ectopic	**7** Via Natural or Artificial Opening **8** Via Natural or Artificial Opening Endoscopic	**Z** No Device	**Z** No Qualifier

Section 1 **Obstetrics**
Body System 0 **Pregnancy**
Operation E **Delivery:** Assisting the passage of the products of conception from the genital canal

Body Part (4th)	Approach (5th)	Device (6th)	Qualifier (7th)
0 Products of Conception	**X** External	**Z** No Device	**Z** No Qualifier

Section 1 **Obstetrics**
Body System 0 **Pregnancy**
Operation H **Insertion:** Putting in a nonbiological appliance that monitors, assists, performs, or prevents a physiological function but does not physically take the place of a body part

Body Part (4th)	Approach (5th)	Device (6th)	Qualifier (7th)
0 Products of Conception	**0** Open **7** Via Natural or Artificial Opening	**3** Monitoring Electrode **Y** Other Device	**Z** No Qualifier

Section 1 **Obstetrics**
Body System 0 **Pregnancy**
Operation J **Inspection:** Visually and/or manually exploring a body part

Body Part (4th)	Approach (5th)	Device (6th)	Qualifier (7th)
0 Products of Conception **1** Products of Conception, Retained **2** Products of Conception, Ectopic	**0** Open **3** Percutaneous **4** Percutaneous Endoscopic **7** Via Natural or Artificial Opening **8** Via Natural or Artificial Opening Endoscopic **X** External	**Z** No Device	**Z** No Qualifier

Section 1 **Obstetrics**
Body System 0 **Pregnancy**
Operation P **Removal:** Taking out or off a device from a body part, region or orifice

Body Part (4th)	Approach (5th)	Device (6th)	Qualifier (7th)
0 Products of Conception	**0** Open **7** Via Natural or Artificial Opening	**3** Monitoring Electrode **Y** Other Device	**Z** No Qualifier

Section 1 **Obstetrics**
Body System 0 **Pregnancy**
Operation Q **Repair:** Restoring, to the extent possible, a body part to its normal anatomic structure and function

Body Part (4th)	Approach (5th)	Device (6th)	Qualifier (7th)
0 Products of Conception	**0** Open **3** Percutaneous **4** Percutaneous Endoscopic **7** Via Natural or Artificial Opening **8** Via Natural or Artificial Opening Endoscopic	**Y** Other Device **Z** No Device	**E** Nervous System **F** Cardiovascular System **G** Lymphatics and Hemic **H** Eye **J** Ear, Nose and Sinus **K** Respiratory System **L** Mouth and Throat **M** Gastrointestinal System **N** Hepatobiliary and Pancreas **P** Endocrine System **Q** Skin **R** Musculoskeletal System **S** Urinary System **T** Female Reproductive System **V** Male Reproductive System **Y** Other Body System

Section 1 **Obstetrics**
Body System 0 **Pregnancy**
Operation S **Reposition:** Moving to its normal location, or other suitable location, all or a portion of a body part

Body Part (4th)	Approach (5th)	Device (6th)	Qualifier (7th)
0 Products of Conception	**7** Via Natural or Artificial Opening **X** External	**Z** No Device	**Z** No Qualifier
2 Products of Conception, Ectopic	**0** Open **3** Percutaneous **4** Percutaneous Endoscopic **7** Via Natural or Artificial Opening **8** Via Natural or Artificial Opening Endoscopic	**Z** No Device	**Z** No Qualifier

Section 1 **Obstetrics**
Body System 0 **Pregnancy**
Operation T **Resection:** Cutting out or off, without replacement, all of a body part

Body Part (4th)	Approach (5th)	Device (6th)	Qualifier (7th)
2 Products of Conception, Ectopic	**0** Open **3** Percutaneous **4** Percutaneous Endoscopic **7** Via Natural or Artificial Opening **8** Via Natural or Artificial Opening Endoscopic	**Z** No Device	**Z** No Qualifier

Section 1 **Obstetrics**
Body System 0 **Pregnancy**
Operation Y **Transplantation:** Putting in or on all or a portion of a living body part taken from another individual or animal to physically take the place and/or function of all or a portion of a similar body part

Body Part (4th)	Approach (5th)	Device (6th)	Qualifier (7th)
0 Products of Conception	**3** Percutaneous **4** Percutaneous Endoscopic **7** Via Natural or Artificial Opening	**Z** No Device	**E** Nervous System **F** Cardiovascular System **G** Lymphatics and Hemic **H** Eye **J** Ear, Nose and Sinus **K** Respiratory System **L** Mouth and Throat **M** Gastrointestinal System **N** Hepatobiliary and Pancreas **P** Endocrine System **Q** Skin **R** Musculoskeletal System **S** Urinary System **T** Female Reproductive System **V** Male Reproductive System **Y** Other Body System

102 – Obstetrics, Pregnancy, Change

Review Coding Guideline C1

♀**102073Z** Change Monitoring Electrode in Products of Conception, Via Natural or Artificial Opening

♀**10207YZ** Change Other Device in Products of Conception, Via Natural or Artificial Opening

109 – Obstetrics, Pregnancy, Drainage

♀**10900Z9** Drainage of Fetal Blood from Products of Conception, Open Approach

♀**10900ZA** Drainage of Fetal Cerebrospinal Fluid from Products of Conception, Open Approach

♀**10900ZB** Drainage of Other Fetal Fluid from Products of Conception, Open Approach

♀**10900ZC** Drainage of Amniotic Fluid, Therapeutic from Products of Conception, Open Approach

♀**10900ZD** Drainage of Other Fluid from Products of Conception, Open Approach

♀**10900ZU** Drainage of Amniotic Fluid, Diagnostic from Products of Conception, Open Approach

♀**10903Z9** Drainage of Fetal Blood from Products of Conception, Percutaneous Approach

♀**10903ZA** Drainage of Fetal Cerebrospinal Fluid from Products of Conception, Percutaneous Approach

♀**10903ZB** Drainage of Other Fetal Fluid from Products of Conception, Percutaneous Approach

♀**10903ZC** Drainage of Amniotic Fluid, Therapeutic from Products of Conception, Percutaneous Approach

♀**10903ZD** Drainage of Other Fluid from Products of Conception, Percutaneous Approach

♀**10903ZU** Drainage of Amniotic Fluid, Diagnostic from Products of Conception, Percutaneous Approach

♀**10904Z9** Drainage of Fetal Blood from Products of Conception, Percutaneous Endoscopic Approach

♀**10904ZA** Drainage of Fetal Cerebrospinal Fluid from Products of Conception, Percutaneous Endoscopic Approach

♀**10904ZB** Drainage of Other Fetal Fluid from Products of Conception, Percutaneous Endoscopic Approach

♀**10904ZC** Drainage of Amniotic Fluid, Therapeutic from Products of Conception, Percutaneous Endoscopic Approach

♀**10904ZD** Drainage of Other Fluid from Products of Conception, Percutaneous Endoscopic Approach

♀**10904ZU** Drainage of Amniotic Fluid, Diagnostic from Products of Conception, Percutaneous Endoscopic Approach

♀**10907Z9** Drainage of Fetal Blood from Products of Conception, Via Natural or Artificial Opening

♀**10907ZA** Drainage of Fetal Cerebrospinal Fluid from Products of Conception, Via Natural or Artificial Opening

♀**10907ZB** Drainage of Other Fetal Fluid from Products of Conception, Via Natural or Artificial Opening

♀**10907ZC** Drainage of Amniotic Fluid, Therapeutic from Products of Conception, Via Natural or Artificial Opening
AHA CC: 2Q, 2014, 9-10

♀**10907ZD** Drainage of Other Fluid from Products of Conception, Via Natural or Artificial Opening

♀**10907ZU** Drainage of Amniotic Fluid, Diagnostic from Products of Conception, Via Natural or Artificial Opening

♀**10908Z9** Drainage of Fetal Blood from Products of Conception, Via Natural or Artificial Opening Endoscopic

♀**10908ZA** Drainage of Fetal Cerebrospinal Fluid from Products of Conception, Via Natural or Artificial Opening Endoscopic

♀**10908ZB** Drainage of Other Fetal Fluid from Products of Conception, Via Natural or Artificial Opening Endoscopic

♀**10908ZC** Drainage of Amniotic Fluid, Therapeutic from Products of Conception, Via Natural or Artificial Opening Endoscopic

♀**10908ZD** Drainage of Other Fluid from Products of Conception, Via Natural or Artificial Opening Endoscopic

♀**10908ZU** Drainage of Amniotic Fluid, Diagnostic from Products of Conception, Via Natural or Artificial Opening Endoscopic

10A – Obstetrics, Pregnancy, Abortion

♀**10A00ZZ** Abortion of Products of Conception, Open Approach

♀**10A03ZZ** Abortion of Products of Conception, Percutaneous Approach

♀**10A04ZZ** Abortion of Products of Conception, Percutaneous Endoscopic Approach

♀● **10A07Z6** Abortion of Products of Conception, Vacuum, Via Natural or Artificial Opening

♀**10A07ZW** Abortion of Products of Conception, Laminaria, Via Natural or Artificial Opening

♀**10A07ZX** Abortion of Products of Conception, Abortifacient, Via Natural or Artificial Opening

♀**10A07ZZ** Abortion of Products of Conception, Via Natural or Artificial Opening

♀**10A08ZZ** Abortion of Products of Conception, Via Natural or Artificial Opening Endoscopic

10D – Obstetrics, Pregnancy, Extraction

Review Coding Guideline C2

♀**10D00Z0** Extraction of Products of Conception, Classical, Open Approach

♀**10D00Z1** Extraction of Products of Conception, Low Cervical, Open Approach

♀**10D00Z2** Extraction of Products of Conception, Extraperitoneal, Open Approach

♀● **10D07Z3** Extraction of Products of Conception, Low Forceps, Via Natural or Artificial Opening

♀● **10D07Z4** Extraction of Products of Conception, Mid Forceps, Via Natural or Artificial Opening

♀● **10D07Z5** Extraction of Products of Conception, High Forceps, Via Natural or Artificial Opening

♀● **10D07Z6** Extraction of Products of Conception, Vacuum, Via Natural or Artificial Opening

♀● **10D07Z7** Extraction of Products of Conception, Internal Version, Via Natural or Artificial Opening

♀● **10D07Z8** Extraction of Products of Conception, Other, Via Natural or Artificial Opening

♀**10D17ZZ** Extraction of Products of Conception, Retained, Via Natural or Artificial Opening

♀**10D18ZZ** Extraction of Products of Conception, Retained, Via Natural or Artificial Opening Endoscopic

♀**10D27ZZ** Extraction of Products of Conception, Ectopic, Via Natural or Artificial Opening

♀**10D28ZZ** Extraction of Products of Conception, Ectopic, Via Natural or Artificial Opening Endoscopic

10E – Obstetrics, Pregnancy, Delivery

♀● **10E0XZZ** Delivery of Products of Conception, External Approach
AHA CC: 2Q, 2014, 9-10

10H – Obstetrics, Pregnancy, Insertion

♀ **10H003Z** Insertion of Monitoring Electrode into Products of Conception, Open Approach
♀ **10H00YZ** Insertion of Other Device into Products of Conception, Open Approach
♀ **10H073Z** Insertion of Monitoring Electrode into Products of Conception, Via Natural or Artificial Opening
♀ **10H07YZ** Insertion of Other Device into Products of Conception, Via Natural or Artificial Opening
AHA CC: 2Q, 2013, 36

10J – Obstetrics, Pregnancy, Inspection

♀ **10J00ZZ** Inspection of Products of Conception, Open Approach
♀ **10J03ZZ** Inspection of Products of Conception, Percutaneous Approach
♀ **10J04ZZ** Inspection of Products of Conception, Percutaneous Endoscopic Approach
♀ **10J07ZZ** Inspection of Products of Conception, Via Natural or Artificial Opening
♀ **10J08ZZ** Inspection of Products of Conception, Via Natural or Artificial Opening Endoscopic
♀ **10J0XZZ** Inspection of Products of Conception, External Approach
♀ **10J10ZZ** Inspection of Products of Conception, Retained, Open Approach
♀ **10J13ZZ** Inspection of Products of Conception, Retained, Percutaneous Approach
♀ **10J14ZZ** Inspection of Products of Conception, Retained, Percutaneous Endoscopic Approach
♀ **10J17ZZ** Inspection of Products of Conception, Retained, Via Natural or Artificial Opening
♀ **10J18ZZ** Inspection of Products of Conception, Retained, Via Natural or Artificial Opening Endoscopic
♀ **10J1XZZ** Inspection of Products of Conception, Retained, External Approach
♀ **10J20ZZ** Inspection of Products of Conception, Ectopic, Open Approach
♀ **10J23ZZ** Inspection of Products of Conception, Ectopic, Percutaneous Approach
♀ **10J24ZZ** Inspection of Products of Conception, Ectopic, Percutaneous Endoscopic Approach
♀ **10J27ZZ** Inspection of Products of Conception, Ectopic, Via Natural or Artificial Opening
♀ **10J28ZZ** Inspection of Products of Conception, Ectopic, Via Natural or Artificial Opening Endoscopic
♀ **10J2XZZ** Inspection of Products of Conception, Ectopic, External Approach

10P – Obstetrics, Pregnancy, Removal

♀ **10P003Z** Removal of Monitoring Electrode from Products of Conception, Open Approach
♀ **10P00YZ** Removal of Other Device from Products of Conception, Open Approach
♀ **10P073Z** Removal of Monitoring Electrode from Products of Conception, Via Natural or Artificial Opening
♀ **10P07YZ** Removal of Other Device from Products of Conception, Via Natural or Artificial Opening

10Q – Obstetrics, Pregnancy, Repair

♀ **10Q00YE** Repair Nervous System in Products of Conception with Other Device, Open Approach
♀ **10Q00YF** Repair Cardiovascular System in Products of Conception with Other Device, Open Approach
♀ **10Q00YG** Repair Lymphatics and Hemic in Products of Conception with Other Device, Open Approach
♀ **10Q00YH** Repair Eye in Products of Conception with Other Device, Open Approach
♀ **10Q00YJ** Repair Ear, Nose and Sinus in Products of Conception with Other Device, Open Approach
♀ **10Q00YK** Repair Respiratory System in Products of Conception with Other Device, Open Approach
♀ **10Q00YL** Repair Mouth and Throat in Products of Conception with Other Device, Open Approach
♀ **10Q00YM** Repair Gastrointestinal System in Products of Conception with Other Device, Open Approach
♀ **10Q00YN** Repair Hepatobiliary and Pancreas in Products of Conception with Other Device, Open Approach
♀ **10Q00YP** Repair Endocrine System in Products of Conception with Other Device, Open Approach
♀ **10Q00YQ** Repair Skin in Products of Conception with Other Device, Open Approach
♀ **10Q00YR** Repair Musculoskeletal System in Products of Conception with Other Device, Open Approach
♀ **10Q00YS** Repair Urinary System in Products of Conception with Other Device, Open Approach
♀ **10Q00YT** Repair Female Reproductive System in Products of Conception with Other Device, Open Approach
♀ **10Q00YV** Repair Male Reproductive System in Products of Conception with Other Device, Open Approach
♀ **10Q00YY** Repair Other Body System in Products of Conception with Other Device, Open Approach
♀ **10Q00ZE** Repair Nervous System in Products of Conception, Open Approach
♀ **10Q00ZF** Repair Cardiovascular System in Products of Conception, Open Approach
♀ **10Q00ZG** Repair Lymphatics and Hemic in Products of Conception, Open Approach
♀ **10Q00ZH** Repair Eye in Products of Conception, Open Approach
♀ **10Q00ZJ** Repair Ear, Nose and Sinus in Products of Conception, Open Approach
♀ **10Q00ZK** Repair Respiratory System in Products of Conception, Open Approach
♀ **10Q00ZL** Repair Mouth and Throat in Products of Conception, Open Approach
♀ **10Q00ZM** Repair Gastrointestinal System in Products of Conception, Open Approach
♀ **10Q00ZN** Repair Hepatobiliary and Pancreas in Products of Conception, Open Approach
♀ **10Q00ZP** Repair Endocrine System in Products of Conception, Open Approach
♀ **10Q00ZQ** Repair Skin in Products of Conception, Open Approach
♀ **10Q00ZR** Repair Musculoskeletal System in Products of Conception, Open Approach
♀ **10Q00ZS** Repair Urinary System in Products of Conception, Open Approach
♀ **10Q00ZT** Repair Female Reproductive System in Products of Conception, Open Approach
♀ **10Q00ZV** Repair Male Reproductive System in Products of Conception, Open Approach
♀ **10Q00ZY** Repair Other Body System in Products of Conception, Open Approach
♀ **10Q03YE** Repair Nervous System in Products of Conception with Other Device, Percutaneous Approach
♀ **10Q03YF** Repair Cardiovascular System in Products of Conception with Other Device, Percutaneous Approach
♀ **10Q03YG** Repair Lymphatics and Hemic in Products of Conception with Other Device, Percutaneous Approach
♀ **10Q03YH** Repair Eye in Products of Conception with Other Device, Percutaneous Approach
♀ **10Q03YJ** Repair Ear, Nose and Sinus in Products of Conception with Other Device, Percutaneous Approach
♀ **10Q03YK** Repair Respiratory System in Products of Conception with Other Device, Percutaneous Approach
♀ **10Q03YL** Repair Mouth and Throat in Products of Conception with Other Device, Percutaneous Approach
♀ **10Q03YM** Repair Gastrointestinal System in Products of Conception with Other Device, Percutaneous Approach
♀ **10Q03YN** Repair Hepatobiliary and Pancreas in Products of Conception with Other Device, Percutaneous Approach
♀ **10Q03YP** Repair Endocrine System in Products of Conception with Other Device, Percutaneous Approach
♀ **10Q03YQ** Repair Skin in Products of Conception with Other Device, Percutaneous Approach
♀ **10Q03YR** Repair Musculoskeletal System in Products of Conception with Other Device, Percutaneous Approach
♀ **10Q03YS** Repair Urinary System in Products of Conception with Other Device, Percutaneous Approach
♀ **10Q03YT** Repair Female Reproductive System in Products of Conception with Other Device, Percutaneous Approach
♀ **10Q03YV** Repair Male Reproductive System in Products of Conception with Other Device, Percutaneous Approach
♀ **10Q03YY** Repair Other Body System in Products of Conception with Other Device, Percutaneous Approach
♀ **10Q03ZE** Repair Nervous System in Products of Conception, Percutaneous Approach
♀ **10Q03ZF** Repair Cardiovascular System in Products of Conception, Percutaneous Approach

♀10Q03ZG Repair Lymphatics and Hemic in Products of Conception, Percutaneous Approach
♀10Q03ZH Repair Eye in Products of Conception, Percutaneous Approach
♀10Q03ZJ Repair Ear, Nose and Sinus in Products of Conception, Percutaneous Approach
♀10Q03ZK Repair Respiratory System in Products of Conception, Percutaneous Approach
♀10Q03ZL Repair Mouth and Throat in Products of Conception, Percutaneous Approach
♀10Q03ZM Repair Gastrointestinal System in Products of Conception, Percutaneous Approach
♀10Q03ZN Repair Hepatobiliary and Pancreas in Products of Conception, Percutaneous Approach
♀10Q03ZP Repair Endocrine System in Products of Conception, Percutaneous Approach
♀10Q03ZQ Repair Skin in Products of Conception, Percutaneous Approach
♀10Q03ZR Repair Musculoskeletal System in Products of Conception, Percutaneous Approach
♀10Q03ZS Repair Urinary System in Products of Conception, Percutaneous Approach
♀10Q03ZT Repair Female Reproductive System in Products of Conception, Percutaneous Approach
♀10Q03ZV Repair Male Reproductive System in Products of Conception, Percutaneous Approach
♀10Q03ZY Repair Other Body System in Products of Conception, Percutaneous Approach
♀10Q04YE Repair Nervous System in Products of Conception with Other Device, Percutaneous Endoscopic Approach
♀10Q04YF Repair Cardiovascular System in Products of Conception with Other Device, Percutaneous Endoscopic Approach
♀10Q04YG Repair Lymphatics and Hemic in Products of Conception with Other Device, Percutaneous Endoscopic Approach
♀10Q04YH Repair Eye in Products of Conception with Other Device, Percutaneous Endoscopic Approach
♀10Q04YJ Repair Ear, Nose and Sinus in Products of Conception with Other Device, Percutaneous Endoscopic Approach
♀10Q04YK Repair Respiratory System in Products of Conception with Other Device, Percutaneous Endoscopic Approach
♀10Q04YL Repair Mouth and Throat in Products of Conception with Other Device, Percutaneous Endoscopic Approach
♀10Q04YM Repair Gastrointestinal System in Products of Conception with Other Device, Percutaneous Endoscopic Approach
♀10Q04YN Repair Hepatobiliary and Pancreas in Products of Conception with Other Device, Percutaneous Endoscopic Approach
♀10Q04YP Repair Endocrine System in Products of Conception with Other Device, Percutaneous Endoscopic Approach
♀10Q04YQ Repair Skin in Products of Conception with Other Device, Percutaneous Endoscopic Approach
♀10Q04YR Repair Musculoskeletal System in Products of Conception with Other Device, Percutaneous Endoscopic Approach
♀10Q04YS Repair Urinary System in Products of Conception with Other Device, Percutaneous Endoscopic Approach
♀10Q04YT Repair Female Reproductive System in Products of Conception with Other Device, Percutaneous Endoscopic Approach
♀10Q04YV Repair Male Reproductive System in Products of Conception with Other Device, Percutaneous Endoscopic Approach
♀10Q04YY Repair Other Body System in Products of Conception with Other Device, Percutaneous Endoscopic Approach
♀10Q04ZE Repair Nervous System in Products of Conception, Percutaneous Endoscopic Approach
♀10Q04ZF Repair Cardiovascular System in Products of Conception, Percutaneous Endoscopic Approach
♀10Q04ZG Repair Lymphatics and Hemic in Products of Conception, Percutaneous Endoscopic Approach
♀10Q04ZH Repair Eye in Products of Conception, Percutaneous Endoscopic Approach
♀10Q04ZJ Repair Ear, Nose and Sinus in Products of Conception, Percutaneous Endoscopic Approach
♀10Q04ZK Repair Respiratory System in Products of Conception, Percutaneous Endoscopic Approach
♀10Q04ZL Repair Mouth and Throat in Products of Conception, Percutaneous Endoscopic Approach
♀10Q04ZM Repair Gastrointestinal System in Products of Conception, Percutaneous Endoscopic Approach
♀10Q04ZN Repair Hepatobiliary and Pancreas in Products of Conception, Percutaneous Endoscopic Approach
♀10Q04ZP Repair Endocrine System in Products of Conception, Percutaneous Endoscopic Approach
♀10Q04ZQ Repair Skin in Products of Conception, Percutaneous Endoscopic Approach
♀10Q04ZR Repair Musculoskeletal System in Products of Conception, Percutaneous Endoscopic Approach
♀10Q04ZS Repair Urinary System in Products of Conception, Percutaneous Endoscopic Approach
♀10Q04ZT Repair Female Reproductive System in Products of Conception, Percutaneous Endoscopic Approach
♀10Q04ZV Repair Male Reproductive System in Products of Conception, Percutaneous Endoscopic Approach
♀10Q04ZY Repair Other Body System in Products of Conception, Percutaneous Endoscopic Approach
♀10Q07YE Repair Nervous System in Products of Conception with Other Device, Via Natural or Artificial Opening
♀10Q07YF Repair Cardiovascular System in Products of Conception with Other Device, Via Natural or Artificial Opening
♀10Q07YG Repair Lymphatics and Hemic in Products of Conception with Other Device, Via Natural or Artificial Opening
♀10Q07YH Repair Eye in Products of Conception with Other Device, Via Natural or Artificial Opening
♀10Q07YJ Repair Ear, Nose and Sinus in Products of Conception with Other Device, Via Natural or Artificial Opening
♀10Q07YK Repair Respiratory System in Products of Conception with Other Device, Via Natural or Artificial Opening
♀10Q07YL Repair Mouth and Throat in Products of Conception with Other Device, Via Natural or Artificial Opening
♀10Q07YM Repair Gastrointestinal System in Products of Conception with Other Device, Via Natural or Artificial Opening
♀10Q07YN Repair Hepatobiliary and Pancreas in Products of Conception with Other Device, Via Natural or Artificial Opening
♀10Q07YP Repair Endocrine System in Products of Conception with Other Device, Via Natural or Artificial Opening
♀10Q07YQ Repair Skin in Products of Conception with Other Device, Via Natural or Artificial Opening
♀10Q07YR Repair Musculoskeletal System in Products of Conception with Other Device, Via Natural or Artificial Opening
♀10Q07YS Repair Urinary System in Products of Conception with Other Device, Via Natural or Artificial Opening
♀10Q07YT Repair Female Reproductive System in Products of Conception with Other Device, Via Natural or Artificial Opening
♀10Q07YV Repair Male Reproductive System in Products of Conception with Other Device, Via Natural or Artificial Opening
♀10Q07YY Repair Other Body System in Products of Conception with Other Device, Via Natural or Artificial Opening
♀10Q07ZE Repair Nervous System in Products of Conception, Via Natural or Artificial Opening
♀10Q07ZF Repair Cardiovascular System in Products of Conception, Via Natural or Artificial Opening
♀10Q07ZG Repair Lymphatics and Hemic in Products of Conception, Via Natural or Artificial Opening
♀10Q07ZH Repair Eye in Products of Conception, Via Natural or Artificial Opening
♀10Q07ZJ Repair Ear, Nose and Sinus in Products of Conception, Via Natural or Artificial Opening
♀10Q07ZK Repair Respiratory System in Products of Conception, Via Natural or Artificial Opening
♀10Q07ZL Repair Mouth and Throat in Products of Conception, Via Natural or Artificial Opening
♀10Q07ZM Repair Gastrointestinal System in Products of Conception, Via Natural or Artificial Opening
♀10Q07ZN Repair Hepatobiliary and Pancreas in Products of Conception, Via Natural or Artificial Opening
♀10Q07ZP Repair Endocrine System in Products of Conception, Via Natural or Artificial Opening
♀10Q07ZQ Repair Skin in Products of Conception, Via Natural or Artificial Opening
♀10Q07ZR Repair Musculoskeletal System in Products of Conception, Via Natural or Artificial Opening
♀10Q07ZS Repair Urinary System in Products of Conception, Via Natural or Artificial Opening
♀10Q07ZT Repair Female Reproductive System in Products of Conception, Via Natural or Artificial Opening
♀10Q07ZV Repair Male Reproductive System in Products of Conception, Via Natural or Artificial Opening
♀10Q07ZY Repair Other Body System in Products of Conception, Via Natural or Artificial Opening
♀10Q08YE Repair Nervous System in Products of Conception with Other Device, Via Natural or Artificial Opening Endoscopic
♀10Q08YF Repair Cardiovascular System in Products of Conception with Other Device, Via Natural or Artificial Opening Endoscopic

♀ **10Q08YG** Repair Lymphatics and Hemic in Products of Conception with Other Device, Via Natural or Artificial Opening Endoscopic
♀ **10Q08YH** Repair Eye in Products of Conception with Other Device, Via Natural or Artificial Opening Endoscopic
♀ **10Q08YJ** Repair Ear, Nose and Sinus in Products of Conception with Other Device, Via Natural or Artificial Opening Endoscopic
♀ **10Q08YK** Repair Respiratory System in Products of Conception with Other Device, Via Natural or Artificial Opening Endoscopic
♀ **10Q08YL** Repair Mouth and Throat in Products of Conception with Other Device, Via Natural or Artificial Opening Endoscopic
♀ **10Q08YM** Repair Gastrointestinal System in Products of Conception with Other Device, Via Natural or Artificial Opening Endoscopic
♀ **10Q08YN** Repair Hepatobiliary and Pancreas in Products of Conception with Other Device, Via Natural or Artificial Opening Endoscopic
♀ **10Q08YP** Repair Endocrine System in Products of Conception with Other Device, Via Natural or Artificial Opening Endoscopic
♀ **10Q08YQ** Repair Skin in Products of Conception with Other Device, Via Natural or Artificial Opening Endoscopic
♀ **10Q08YR** Repair Musculoskeletal System in Products of Conception with Other Device, Via Natural or Artificial Opening Endoscopic
♀ **10Q08YS** Repair Urinary System in Products of Conception with Other Device, Via Natural or Artificial Opening Endoscopic
♀ **10Q08YT** Repair Female Reproductive System in Products of Conception with Other Device, Via Natural or Artificial Opening Endoscopic
♀ **10Q08YV** Repair Male Reproductive System in Products of Conception with Other Device, Via Natural or Artificial Opening Endoscopic
♀ **10Q08YY** Repair Other Body System in Products of Conception with Other Device, Via Natural or Artificial Opening Endoscopic
♀ **10Q08ZE** Repair Nervous System in Products of Conception, Via Natural or Artificial Opening Endoscopic
♀ **10Q08ZF** Repair Cardiovascular System in Products of Conception, Via Natural or Artificial Opening Endoscopic
♀ **10Q08ZG** Repair Lymphatics and Hemic in Products of Conception, Via Natural or Artificial Opening Endoscopic
♀ **10Q08ZH** Repair Eye in Products of Conception, Via Natural or Artificial Opening Endoscopic
♀ **10Q08ZJ** Repair Ear, Nose and Sinus in Products of Conception, Via Natural or Artificial Opening Endoscopic
♀ **10Q08ZK** Repair Respiratory System in Products of Conception, Via Natural or Artificial Opening Endoscopic
♀ **10Q08ZL** Repair Mouth and Throat in Products of Conception, Via Natural or Artificial Opening Endoscopic
♀ **10Q08ZM** Repair Gastrointestinal System in Products of Conception, Via Natural or Artificial Opening Endoscopic
♀ **10Q08ZN** Repair Hepatobiliary and Pancreas in Products of Conception, Via Natural or Artificial Opening Endoscopic
♀ **10Q08ZP** Repair Endocrine System in Products of Conception, Via Natural or Artificial Opening Endoscopic
♀ **10Q08ZQ** Repair Skin in Products of Conception, Via Natural or Artificial Opening Endoscopic
♀ **10Q08ZR** Repair Musculoskeletal System in Products of Conception, Via Natural or Artificial Opening Endoscopic
♀ **10Q08ZS** Repair Urinary System in Products of Conception, Via Natural or Artificial Opening Endoscopic
♀ **10Q08ZT** Repair Female Reproductive System in Products of Conception, Via Natural or Artificial Opening Endoscopic
♀ **10Q08ZV** Repair Male Reproductive System in Products of Conception, Via Natural or Artificial Opening Endoscopic
♀ **10Q08ZY** Repair Other Body System in Products of Conception, Via Natural or Artificial Opening Endoscopic

10S – Obstetrics, Pregnancy, Reposition

♀● **10S07ZZ** Reposition Products of Conception, Via Natural or Artificial Opening
♀ **10S0XZZ** Reposition Products of Conception, External Approach
♀ **10S20ZZ** Reposition Products of Conception, Ectopic, Open Approach
♀ **10S23ZZ** Reposition Products of Conception, Ectopic, Percutaneous Approach
♀ **10S24ZZ** Reposition Products of Conception, Ectopic, Percutaneous Endoscopic Approach
♀ **10S27ZZ** Reposition Products of Conception, Ectopic, Via Natural or Artificial Opening
♀ **10S28ZZ** Reposition Products of Conception, Ectopic, Via Natural or Artificial Opening Endoscopic

10T – Obstetrics, Pregnancy, Resection

♀ **10T20ZZ** Resection of Products of Conception, Ectopic, Open Approach
♀ **10T23ZZ** Resection of Products of Conception, Ectopic, Percutaneous Approach
♀ **10T24ZZ** Resection of Products of Conception, Ectopic, Percutaneous Endoscopic Approach
♀ **10T27ZZ** Resection of Products of Conception, Ectopic, Via Natural or Artificial Opening
♀ **10T28ZZ** Resection of Products of Conception, Ectopic, Via Natural or Artificial Opening Endoscopic

10Y – Obstetrics, Pregnancy, Transplantation

♀ **10Y03ZE** Transplantation of Nervous System into Products of Conception, Percutaneous Approach
♀ **10Y03ZF** Transplantation of Cardiovascular System into Products of Conception, Percutaneous Approach
♀ **10Y03ZG** Transplantation of Lymphatics and Hemic into Products of Conception, Percutaneous Approach
♀ **10Y03ZH** Transplantation of Eye into Products of Conception, Percutaneous Approach
♀ **10Y03ZJ** Transplantation of Ear, Nose and Sinus into Products of Conception, Percutaneous Approach
♀ **10Y03ZK** Transplantation of Respiratory System into Products of Conception, Percutaneous Approach
♀ **10Y03ZL** Transplantation of Mouth and Throat into Products of Conception, Percutaneous Approach
♀ **10Y03ZM** Transplantation of Gastrointestinal System into Products of Conception, Percutaneous Approach
♀ **10Y03ZN** Transplantation of Hepatobiliary and Pancreas into Products of Conception, Percutaneous Approach
♀ **10Y03ZP** Transplantation of Endocrine System into Products of Conception, Percutaneous Approach
♀ **10Y03ZQ** Transplantation of Skin into Products of Conception, Percutaneous Approach
♀ **10Y03ZR** Transplantation of Musculoskeletal System into Products of Conception, Percutaneous Approach
♀ **10Y03ZS** Transplantation of Urinary System into Products of Conception, Percutaneous Approach
♀ **10Y03ZT** Transplantation of Female Reproductive System into Products of Conception, Percutaneous Approach
♀ **10Y03ZV** Transplantation of Male Reproductive System into Products of Conception, Percutaneous Approach
♀ **10Y03ZY** Transplantation of Other Body System into Products of Conception, Percutaneous Approach
♀ **10Y04ZE** Transplantation of Nervous System into Products of Conception, Percutaneous Endoscopic Approach
♀ **10Y04ZF** Transplantation of Cardiovascular System into Products of Conception, Percutaneous Endoscopic Approach
♀ **10Y04ZG** Transplantation of Lymphatics and Hemic into Products of Conception, Percutaneous Endoscopic Approach
♀ **10Y04ZH** Transplantation of Eye into Products of Conception, Percutaneous Endoscopic Approach
♀ **10Y04ZJ** Transplantation of Ear, Nose and Sinus into Products of Conception, Percutaneous Endoscopic Approach
♀ **10Y04ZK** Transplantation of Respiratory System into Products of Conception, Percutaneous Endoscopic Approach
♀ **10Y04ZL** Transplantation of Mouth and Throat into Products of Conception, Percutaneous Endoscopic Approach
♀ **10Y04ZM** Transplantation of Gastrointestinal System into Products of Conception, Percutaneous Endoscopic Approach
♀ **10Y04ZN** Transplantation of Hepatobiliary and Pancreas into Products of Conception, Percutaneous Endoscopic Approach
♀ **10Y04ZP** Transplantation of Endocrine System into Products of Conception, Percutaneous Endoscopic Approach

♀10Y04ZQ Transplantation of Skin into Products of Conception, Percutaneous Endoscopic Approach

♀10Y04ZR Transplantation of Musculoskeletal System into Products of Conception, Percutaneous Endoscopic Approach

♀10Y04ZS Transplantation of Urinary System into Products of Conception, Percutaneous Endoscopic Approach

♀10Y04ZT Transplantation of Female Reproductive System into Products of Conception, Percutaneous Endoscopic Approach

♀10Y04ZV Transplantation of Male Reproductive System into Products of Conception, Percutaneous Endoscopic Approach

♀10Y04ZY Transplantation of Other Body System into Products of Conception, Percutaneous Endoscopic Approach

♀10Y07ZE Transplantation of Nervous System into Products of Conception, Via Natural or Artificial Opening

♀ 10Y07ZF Transplantation of Cardiovascular System into Products of Conception, Via Natural or Artificial Opening

♀ 10Y07ZG Transplantation of Lymphatics and Hemic into Products of Conception, Via Natural or Artificial Opening

♀ 10Y07ZH Transplantation of Eye into Products of Conception, Via Natural or Artificial Opening

♀ 10Y07ZJ Transplantation of Ear, Nose and Sinus into Products of Conception, Via Natural or Artificial Opening

♀ 10Y07ZK Transplantation of Respiratory System into Products of Conception, Via Natural or Artificial Opening

♀ 10Y07ZL Transplantation of Mouth and Throat into Products of Conception, Via Natural or Artificial Opening

♀ 10Y07ZM Transplantation of Gastrointestinal System into Products of Conception, Via Natural or Artificial Opening

♀ 10Y07ZN Transplantation of Hepatobiliary and Pancreas into Products of Conception, Via Natural or Artificial Opening

♀ 10Y07ZP Transplantation of Endocrine System into Products of Conception, Via Natural or Artificial Opening

♀ 10Y07ZQ Transplantation of Skin into Products of Conception, Via Natural or Artificial Opening

♀ 10Y07ZR Transplantation of Musculoskeletal System into Products of Conception, Via Natural or Artificial Opening

♀ 10Y07ZS Transplantation of Urinary System into Products of Conception, Via Natural or Artificial Opening

♀ 10Y07ZT Transplantation of Female Reproductive System into Products of Conception, Via Natural or Artificial Opening

♀ 10Y07ZV Transplantation of Male Reproductive System into Products of Conception, Via Natural or Artificial Opening

♀ 10Y07ZY Transplantation of Other Body System into Products of Conception, Via Natural or Artificial Opening

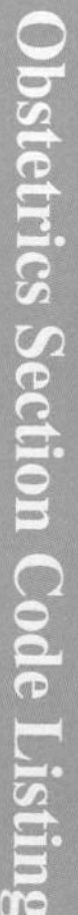

Placement Section (2W0–2Y5)

Within each section of ICD-10-PCS the characters have different meanings. The seven character meanings for the Placement section are illustrated below through the procedure example of *Placement of pressure dressing on abdominal wall.*

Section	Body System	Root Operation	Body Region	Approach	Device	Qualifier
Placement	Anatomical Regions	Compression	Abdominal Wall	External	Pressure Dressing	None
2	W	1	3	X	6	Z

Section (Character 1)

All Placement procedure codes have a first character value of 2.

Body System (Character 2)

The alphanumeric character for the body system is placed in the second position. There are two character values applicable for the Placement section. The character value of W is reported for anatomical regions. The character value Y is reported for anatomical orifices.

Root Operations (Character 3)

The alphanumeric character value for root operations is placed in the third position. The following are the root operations applicable to the Placement section with their associated meaning. Note that the root operation definitions for ICD-10-PCS may differ from the terms that coders currently use with ICD-9-CM Volume 3.

Character Value	Root Operation	Root Operation Definition
0	Change	Taking out or off a device from a body part and putting back an identical or similar device in or on the same body part without cutting or puncturing the skin or a mucous membrane
1	Compression	Putting pressure on a body region
2	Dressing	Putting material on a body region for protection
3	Immobilization	Limiting or preventing motion of a body region
4	Packing	Putting material in a body region or orifice
5	Removal	Taking out or off a device from a body part
6	Traction	Exerting a pulling force on a body region in a distal direction

Body Region (Character 4)

For each body system the applicable body part character values will be available for procedure code construction. An example of a body region is Chest Wall.

Approach (Character 5)

The only approach technique utilized for the Placement section is External approach and is reported with the character value of X.

Character Value	Approach	Approach Definition
X	External	Procedures performed directly on the skin or mucous membrane and procedures performed indirectly by the application of external force through the skin or mucous membrane

Device (Character 6)

Depending on the procedure performed there may or may not be a device used. There are several types of devices included in the Placement section. Here is a sample list of the devices included in this section:

- Cast
- Packing material
- Pressure dressing
- Traction apparatus

When a device is not utilized during the procedure, the placeholder Z is the character value that should be reported.

Qualifier (Character 7)

The qualifier represents an additional attribute for the procedure when applicable. Currently, there are no qualifiers in the Placement section; therefore, the placeholder character value of Z should be reported.

Section Notes

Before reporting Change and Removal procedures in this section users should *Review coding guideline B6.1c.*

AHA Coding Clinic®

2W60X0Z Traction of Head using Traction Apparatus - AHA CC: 2Q, 2013, 39

Placement Section Tables

Placement Tables 2W0–2Y5

Section 2 **Placement**
Body System W **Anatomical Regions**
Operation 0 **Change:** Taking out or off a device from a body part and putting back an identical or similar device in or on the same body part without cutting or puncturing the skin or a mucous membrane

Body Region (4th)	Approach (5th)	Device (6th)	Qualifier (7th)
0 Head **2** Neck **3** Abdominal Wall **4** Chest Wall **5** Back **6** Inguinal Region, Right **7** Inguinal Region, Left **8** Upper Extremity, Right **9** Upper Extremity, Left **A** Upper Arm, Right **B** Upper Arm, Left **C** Lower Arm, Right **D** Lower Arm, Left **E** Hand, Right **F** Hand, Left **G** Thumb, Right **H** Thumb, Left **J** Finger, Right **K** Finger, Left **L** Lower Extremity, Right **M** Lower Extremity, Left **N** Upper Leg, Right **P** Upper Leg, Left **Q** Lower Leg, Right **R** Lower Leg, Left **S** Foot, Right **T** Foot, Left **U** Toe, Right **V** Toe, Left	**X** External	**0** Traction Apparatus **1** Splint **2** Cast **3** Brace **4** Bandage **5** Packing Material **6** Pressure Dressing **7** Intermittent Pressure Device **Y** Other Device	**Z** No Qualifier
1 Face	**X** External	**0** Traction Apparatus **1** Splint **2** Cast **3** Brace **4** Bandage **5** Packing Material **6** Pressure Dressing **7** Intermittent Pressure Device **9** Wire **Y** Other Device	**Z** No Qualifier

Section 2 **Placement**
Body System W **Anatomical Regions**
Operation 1 **Compression:** Putting pressure on a body region

Body Region (4th)	Approach (5th)	Device (6th)	Qualifier (7th)
0 Head **1** Face **2** Neck **3** Abdominal Wall **4** Chest Wall **5** Back **6** Inguinal Region, Right **7** Inguinal Region, Left **8** Upper Extremity, Right **9** Upper Extremity, Left **A** Upper Arm, Right **B** Upper Arm, Left **C** Lower Arm, Right **D** Lower Arm, Left **E** Hand, Right **F** Hand, Left **G** Thumb, Right **H** Thumb, Left **J** Finger, Right **K** Finger, Left **L** Lower Extremity, Right **M** Lower Extremity, Left **N** Upper Leg, Right **P** Upper Leg, Left **Q** Lower Leg, Right **R** Lower Leg, Left **S** Foot, Right **T** Foot, Left **U** Toe, Right **V** Toe, Left	**X** External	**6** Pressure Dressing **7** Intermittent Pressure Device	**Z** No Qualifier

Section 2 **Placement**
Body System W **Anatomical Regions**
Operation 2 **Dressing:** Putting material on a body region for protection

Body Region (4th)	Approach (5th)	Device (6th)	Qualifier (7th)
0 Head **1** Face **2** Neck **3** Abdominal Wall **4** Chest Wall **5** Back **6** Inguinal Region, Right **7** Inguinal Region, Left **8** Upper Extremity, Right **9** Upper Extremity, Left **A** Upper Arm, Right **B** Upper Arm, Left **C** Lower Arm, Right **D** Lower Arm, Left **E** Hand, Right **F** Hand, Left **G** Thumb, Right **H** Thumb, Left **J** Finger, Right **K** Finger, Left **L** Lower Extremity, Right **M** Lower Extremity, Left **N** Upper Leg, Right **P** Upper Leg, Left **Q** Lower Leg, Right **R** Lower Leg, Left **S** Foot, Right **T** Foot, Left **U** Toe, Right **V** Toe, Left	**X** External	**4** Bandage	**Z** No Qualifier

Section **2** **Placement**
Body System **W** **Anatomical Regions**
Operation **3** **Immobilization:** Limiting or preventing motion of a body region

Body Region (4th)	Approach (5th)	Device (6th)	Qualifier (7th)
0 Head **2** Neck **3** Abdominal Wall **4** Chest Wall **5** Back **6** Inguinal Region, Right **7** Inguinal Region, Left **8** Upper Extremity, Right **9** Upper Extremity, Left **A** Upper Arm, Right **B** Upper Arm, Left **C** Lower Arm, Right **D** Lower Arm, Left **E** Hand, Right **F** Hand, Left **G** Thumb, Right **H** Thumb, Left **J** Finger, Right **K** Finger, Left **L** Lower Extremity, Right **M** Lower Extremity, Left **N** Upper Leg, Right **P** Upper Leg, Left **Q** Lower Leg, Right **R** Lower Leg, Left **S** Foot, Right **T** Foot, Left **U** Toe, Right **V** Toe, Left	**X** External	**1** Splint **2** Cast **3** Brace **Y** Other Device	**Z** No Qualifier
1 Face	**X** External	**1** Splint **2** Cast **3** Brace **9** Wire **Y** Other Device	**Z** No Qualifier

Section 2 **Placement**
Body System W **Anatomical Regions**
Operation 4 **Packing:** Putting material in a body region or orifice

Body Region (4th)	Approach (5th)	Device (6th)	Qualifier (7th)
0 Head **1** Face **2** Neck **3** Abdominal Wall **4** Chest Wall **5** Back **6** Inguinal Region, Right **7** Inguinal Region, Left **8** Upper Extremity, Right **9** Upper Extremity, Left **A** Upper Arm, Right **B** Upper Arm, Left **C** Lower Arm, Right **D** Lower Arm, Left **E** Hand, Right **F** Hand, Left **G** Thumb, Right **H** Thumb, Left **J** Finger, Right **K** Finger, Left **L** Lower Extremity, Right **M** Lower Extremity, Left **N** Upper Leg, Right **P** Upper Leg, Left **Q** Lower Leg, Right **R** Lower Leg, Left **S** Foot, Right **T** Foot, Left **U** Toe, Right **V** Toe, Left	**X** External	**5** Packing Material	**Z** No Qualifier

Section 2 **Placement**
Body System W **Anatomical Regions**
Operation 5 **Removal:** Taking out or off a device from a body part

Body Region (4th)	Approach (5th)	Device (6th)	Qualifier (7th)
0 Head **2** Neck **3** Abdominal Wall **4** Chest Wall **5** Back **6** Inguinal Region, Right **7** Inguinal Region, Left **8** Upper Extremity, Right **9** Upper Extremity, Left **A** Upper Arm, Right **B** Upper Arm, Left **C** Lower Arm, Right **D** Lower Arm, Left **E** Hand, Right **F** Hand, Left **G** Thumb, Right **H** Thumb, Left **J** Finger, Right **K** Finger, Left **L** Lower Extremity, Right **M** Lower Extremity, Left **N** Upper Leg, Right **P** Upper Leg, Left **Q** Lower Leg, Right **R** Lower Leg, Left **S** Foot, Right **T** Foot, Left **U** Toe, Right **V** Toe, Left	**X** External	**0** Traction Apparatus **1** Splint **2** Cast **3** Brace **4** Bandage **5** Packing Material **6** Pressure Dressing **7** Intermittent Pressure Device **Y** Other Device	**Z** No Qualifier
1 Face	**X** External	**0** Traction Apparatus **1** Splint **2** Cast **3** Brace **4** Bandage **5** Packing Material **6** Pressure Dressing **7** Intermittent Pressure Device **9** Wire **Y** Other Device	**Z** No Qualifier

Section 2 **Placement**
Body System W **Anatomical Regions**
Operation 6 **Traction:** Exerting a pulling force on a body region in a distal direction

Body Region (4th)	Approach (5th)	Device (6th)	Qualifier (7th)
0 Head 1 Face 2 Neck 3 Abdominal Wall 4 Chest Wall 5 Back 6 Inguinal Region, Right 7 Inguinal Region, Left 8 Upper Extremity, Right 9 Upper Extremity, Left A Upper Arm, Right B Upper Arm, Left C Lower Arm, Right D Lower Arm, Left E Hand, Right F Hand, Left G Thumb, Right H Thumb, Left J Finger, Right K Finger, Left L Lower Extremity, Right M Lower Extremity, Left N Upper Leg, Right P Upper Leg, Left Q Lower Leg, Right R Lower Leg, Left S Foot, Right T Foot, Left U Toe, Right V Toe, Left	X External	0 Traction Apparatus Z No Device	Z No Qualifier

Section 2 **Placement**
Body System Y **Anatomical Orifices**
Operation 0 **Change:** Taking out or off a device from a body part and putting back an identical or similar device in or on the same body part without cutting or puncturing the skin or a mucous membrane

Body Region (4th)	Approach (5th)	Device (6th)	Qualifier (7th)
0 Mouth and Pharynx 1 Nasal 2 Ear 3 Anorectal 4 Female Genital Tract 5 Urethra	X External	5 Packing Material	Z No Qualifier

Section 2 **Placement**
Body System Y **Anatomical Orifices**
Operation 4 **Packing:** Putting material in a body region or orifice

Body Region (4th)	Approach (5th)	Device (6th)	Qualifier (7th)
0 Mouth and Pharynx 1 Nasal 2 Ear 3 Anorectal 4 Female Genital Tract 5 Urethra	X External	5 Packing Material	Z No Qualifier

Section 2 **Placement**
Body System Y **Anatomical Orifices**
Operation 5 **Removal:** Taking out or off a device from a body part

Body Region (4th)	Approach (5th)	Device (6th)	Qualifier (7th)
0 Mouth and Pharynx **1** Nasal **2** Ear **3** Anorectal **4** Female Genital Tract **5** Urethra	**X** External	**5** Packing Material	**Z** No Qualifier

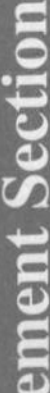

Within each section of ICD-10-PCS, the characters have different meanings. The seven character meanings for the Administration section are illustrated here through the procedure example of *Nerve block injection to median nerve*.

Section	Body System	Root Operation	Body System/ Region	Approach	Substance	Qualifier
Administration	Physiological System and Anatomical Region	Introduction	Peripheral Nerves and Plexi	Percutaneous	Regional Anesthetic	None
3	E	0	T	3	C	Z

Section (Character 1)

All Administration procedure codes have a first character value of 3.

Body System (Character 2)

The alphanumeric character for the body system is placed in the second position. There are three character values applicable for the Administration section.

Character Value	Character Value Description
0	Circulatory
C	Indwelling Device
E	Physiological System and Anatomical Region

Root Operations (Character 3)

The alphanumeric character value for root operations is placed in the third position. Listed here are the root operations applicable to the Administration section with their associated meaning. Note that the root operation definitions for ICD-10-PCS may differ from the terms that coders currently use with ICD-9-CM Volume 3.

Character Value	Root Operation	Root Operation Definition
0	Introduction	Putting in or on a therapeutic, diagnostic, nutritional, physiological, or prophylactic substance except blood or blood products
1	Irrigation	Putting in or on a cleansing substance
2	Transfusion	Putting in blood or blood products

Body System/Region (Character 4)

For each body system the applicable body part character values will be available for procedure code construction. An example of a body region is upper GI.

Approach (Character 5)

The approach is the technique used to reach the procedure site. Listed here are the approach character values for the Administration with the associated definitions.

Character Value	Approach	Approach Definition
0	Open	Cutting through the skin or mucous membrane and any other body layers necessary to expose the site of the procedure
3	Percutaneous	Entry, by puncture or minor incision, of instrumentation through the skin or mucous membrane and any other body layers necessary to reach the site of the procedure
7	Via Natural or Artificial Opening	Entry of instrumentation through a natural or artificial external opening to reach the site of the procedure
8	Via Natural or Artificial Opening Endoscopic	Entry of instrumentation through a natural or artificial external opening to reach and visualize the site of the procedure
X	External	Procedures performed directly on the skin or mucous membrane and procedures performed indirectly by the application of external force through the skin or mucous membrane

Substance (Character 6)

In the Administration section a substance is always utilized. The substance is reported in the sixth character position by the type of substance utilized. The following is a sample list of the substances included in this section:

- Anti-inflammatory
- Antineoplastic
- Bone marrow
- Platelet inhibitor
- Whole blood

Qualifier (Character 7)

The qualifier represents an additional attribute for the procedure when applicable. There are several qualifiers included in the Administration section. For example, transfusion procedures in this section include qualifiers including Autologous and Nonautologous that are reported with the character values of 0 and 1, respectively. If there is no qualifier for a procedure, the placeholder Z is the character value that should be reported.

If a coder is unsure of which option to select for the substance qualifier utilized during the procedure, Appendix F can be used to guide the selection. It is important to note that not all substance qualifier categories are provided by CMS in Appendix F. However, for example, the coding scenario indicates that Clolar was introduced percutaneously via the peripheral vein. The coder references Table 3E0 (Introduction in Physiological Systems and Anatomical Regions) under the peripheral vein, percutaneous approach, anti-neoplastic. Clolar is not a substance qualifier choice. However, the coder can then locate the substance qualifier categories in Appendix F. The category Clofarabine includes Clolar. Therefore, the coder should select P - Clofarabine for the 7th character.

Important Definitions for the Administration Section

Administration Root Operation	Qualifier	Definition
Transfusion (302)	0 - Autologous	Derived or transferred from the same individual's body*
	1 - Nonautologous	Derived or transferred from another individual's body

*Taken from The Free Dictionary by Farlex at www.thefreedictionary.com

Section Notes

Before reporting Transfusion procedures for embryonic stem cells (6th character A), bone marrow (6th character G), cord blood stem cells (6th character X) or hematopoietic stem cells (6th character Y) users should *Review coding guideline B3.16.*

Before reporting Administration codes for all Biliary and Pancreatic Tract (4th character value of J) procedures with a 6th character value of U (Pancreatic Islet Cells), users should *Review coding guideline B3.16.*

Before reporting Irrigation procedures in this section, users should *Review coding guideline B6.1c.*

Medicare Non-Covered Administration Codes

Non-Covered with pdx or sdx C91.00, C92.00, C92.10, C92.11, C92.40, C92.50, C92.60, C92.A0, C93.00, C94.00 or C95.00

30230AZ	30233AZ	30240AZ	30243AZ	30250G0	30253Y0	30263G0
30230G0	30233G0	30240G0	30243G0	30250Y0	30260G0	30263Y0
30230Y0	30233Y0	30240Y0	30243Y0	30253G0	30260Y0	

Non-Covered with pdx or sdx C90.00 or C90.01

30230G1	30233Y1	30243G1	30250Y1	30260G1	30263G1	
30230Y1	30240G1	30243Y1	30253G1	30260Y1	30263Y1	
30233G1	30240Y1	30250G1	30253Y1	30263G1		

AHA Coding Clinic®

3E013GC Introduction of Other Therapeutic Substance into Subcutaneous Tissue, Percutaneous Approach - AHA CC 2Q, 2014, 10

3E03317 Introduction of Other Thrombolytic into Peripheral Vein, Percutaneous Approach - AHA CC 4Q, 2013, 124

3E0G8TZ Introduction of Destructive Agent into Upper GI, Via Natural or Artificial Opening Endoscopic - AHA CC 1Q, 2013, 27

3E0P7GC Introduction of Other Therapeutic Substance into Female Reproductive, Via Natural or Artificial Opening - AHA CC 2Q, 2014, 8-9

Administration Tables 302–3E1

Section **3** **Administration**
Body System **0** **Circulatory**
Operation **2** **Transfusion:** Putting in blood or blood products

Body System / Region (4th)	Approach (5th)	Substance (6th)	Qualifier (7th)
3 Peripheral Vein **4** Central Vein	**0** Open **3** Percutaneous	**A** Stem Cells, Embryonic	**Z** No Qualifier
3 Peripheral Vein **4** Central Vein	**0** Open **3** Percutaneous	**G** Bone Marrow **H** Whole Blood **J** Serum Albumin **K** Frozen Plasma **L** Fresh Plasma **M** Plasma Cryoprecipitate **N** Red Blood Cells **P** Frozen Red Cells **Q** White Cells **R** Platelets **S** Globulin **T** Fibrinogen **V** Antihemophilic Factors **W** Factor IX **X** Stem Cells, Cord Blood **Y** Stem Cells, Hematopoietic	**0** Autologous **1** Nonautologous
5 Peripheral Artery **6** Central Artery	**0** Open **3** Percutaneous	**G** Bone Marrow **H** Whole Blood **J** Serum Albumin **K** Frozen Plasma **L** Fresh Plasma **M** Plasma Cryoprecipitate **N** Red Blood Cells **P** Frozen Red Cells **Q** White Cells **R** Platelets **S** Globulin **T** Fibrinogen **V** Antihemophilic Factors **W** Factor IX **X** Stem Cells, Cord Blood **Y** Stem Cells, Hematopoietic	**0** Autologous **1** Nonautologous
7 Products of Conception, Circulatory	**3** Percutaneous **7** Via Natural or Artificial Opening	**H** Whole Blood **J** Serum Albumin **K** Frozen Plasma **L** Fresh Plasma **M** Plasma Cryoprecipitate **N** Red Blood Cells **P** Frozen Red Cells **Q** White Cells **R** Platelets **S** Globulin **T** Fibrinogen **V** Antihemophilic Factors **W** Factor IX	**1** Nonautologous
8 Vein	**0** Open **3** Percutaneous	**B** 4-Factor Prothrombin Complex Concentrate	**1** Nonautologous

Section 3 **Administration**
Body System C **Indwelling Device**
Operation 1 **Irrigation:** Putting in or on a cleansing substance

Body System / Region (4th)	Approach (5th)	Substance (6th)	Qualifier (7th)
Z None	**X** External	**8** Irrigating Substance	**Z** No Qualifier

Section 3 **Administration**
Body System E **Physiological Systems and Anatomical Regions**
Operation 0 **Introduction:** Putting in or on a therapeutic, diagnostic, nutritional, physiological, or prophylactic substance except blood or blood products

Body System / Region (4th)	Approach (5th)	Substance (6th)	Qualifier (7th)
0 Skin and Mucous Membranes	**X** External	**0** Antineoplastic	**5** Other Antineoplastic **M** Monoclonal Antibody
0 Skin and Mucous Membranes	**X** External	**2** Anti-infective	**8** Oxazolidinones **9** Other Anti-infective
0 Skin and Mucous Membranes	**X** External	**3** Anti-inflammatory **4** Serum, Toxoid and Vaccine **B** Local Anesthetic **K** Other Diagnostic Substance **M** Pigment **N** Analgesics, Hypnotics, Sedatives **T** Destructive Agent	**Z** No Qualifier
0 Skin and Mucous Membranes	**X** External	**G** Other Therapeutic Substance	**C** Other Substance
1 Subcutaneous Tissue	**0** Open	**2** Anti-infective	**A** Anti-Infective Envelope
1 Subcutaneous Tissue	**3** Percutaneous	**0** Antineoplastic	**5** Other Antineoplastic **M** Monoclonal Antibody
1 Subcutaneous Tissue	**3** Percutaneous	**2** Anti-infective	**8** Oxazolidinones **9** Other Anti-infective **A** Anti-Infective Envelope
1 Subcutaneous Tissue	**3** Percutaneous	**3** Anti-inflammatory **4** Serum, Toxoid and Vaccine **6** Nutritional Substance **7** Electrolytic and Water Balance Substance **B** Local Anesthetic **H** Radioactive Substance **K** Other Diagnostic Substance **N** Analgesics, Hypnotics, Sedatives **T** Destructive Agent	**Z** No Qualifier
1 Subcutaneous Tissue	**3** Percutaneous	**G** Other Therapeutic Substance	**C** Other Substance
1 Subcutaneous Tissue	**3** Percutaneous	**V** Hormone	**G** Insulin **J** Other Hormone
2 Muscle	**3** Percutaneous	**0** Antineoplastic	**5** Other Antineoplastic **M** Monoclonal Antibody
2 Muscle	**3** Percutaneous	**2** Anti-infective	**8** Oxazolidinones **9** Other Anti-infective

Continued →

Body System / Region (4th)	Approach (5th)	Substance (6th)	Qualifier (7th)
2 Muscle	**3** Percutaneous	**3** Anti-inflammatory **4** Serum, Toxoid and Vaccine **6** Nutritional Substance **7** Electrolytic and Water Balance Substance **B** Local Anesthetic **H** Radioactive Substance **K** Other Diagnostic Substance **N** Analgesics, Hypnotics, Sedatives **T** Destructive Agent	**Z** No Qualifier
2 Muscle	**3** Percutaneous	**G** Other Therapeutic Substance	**C** Other Substance
3 Peripheral Vein	**0** Open	**0** Antineoplastic	**2** High-dose Interleukin-2 **3** Low-dose Interleukin-2 **5** Other Antineoplastic **M** Monoclonal Antibody **P** Clofarabine
3 Peripheral Vein	**0** Open	**1** Thrombolytic	**6** Recombinant Human-activated Protein C **7** Other Thrombolytic
3 Peripheral Vein	**0** Open	**2** Anti-infective	**8** Oxazolidinones **9** Other Anti-infective
3 Peripheral Vein	**0** Open	**3** Anti-inflammatory **4** Serum, Toxoid and Vaccine **6** Nutritional Substance **7** Electrolytic and Water Balance Substance **F** Intracirculatory Anesthetic **H** Radioactive Substance **K** Other Diagnostic Substance **N** Analgesics, Hypnotics, Sedatives **P** Platelet Inhibitor **R** Antiarrhythmic **T** Destructive Agent **X** Vasopressor	**Z** No Qualifier
3 Peripheral Vein	**0** Open	**G** Other Therapeutic Substance	**C** Other Substance **N** Blood Brain Barrier Disruption
3 Peripheral Vein	**0** Open	**U** Pancreatic Islet Cells	**0** Autologous **1** Nonautologous
3 Peripheral Vein	**0** Open	**V** Hormone	**G** Insulin **H** Human B-type Natriuretic Peptide **J** Other Hormone
3 Peripheral Vein	**0** Open	**W** Immunotherapeutic	**K** Immunostimulator **L** Immunosuppressive
3 Peripheral Vein	**3** Percutaneous	**0** Antineoplastic	**2** High-dose Interleukin-2 **3** Low-dose Interleukin-2 **5** Other Antineoplastic **M** Monoclonal Antibody **P** Clofarabine
3 Peripheral Vein	**3** Percutaneous	**1** Thrombolytic	**6** Recombinant Human-activated Protein C **7** Other Thrombolytic

Continued →

Section 3 **Administration**
Body System E **Physiological Systems and Anatomical Regions**
Operation 0 **Introduction:** Putting in or on a therapeutic, diagnostic, nutritional, physiological, or prophylactic substance except blood or blood products

Body System / Region (4th)	Approach (5th)	Substance (6th)	Qualifier (7th)
3 Peripheral Vein	**3** Percutaneous	**2** Anti-infective	**8** Oxazolidinones **9** Other Anti-infective
3 Peripheral Vein	**3** Percutaneous	**3** Anti-inflammatory **4** Serum, Toxoid and Vaccine **6** Nutritional Substance **7** Electrolytic and Water Balance Substance **F** Intracirculatory Anesthetic **H** Radioactive Substance **K** Other Diagnostic Substance **N** Analgesics, Hypnotics, Sedatives **P** Platelet Inhibitor **R** Antiarrhythmic **T** Destructive Agent **X** Vasopressor	**Z** No Qualifier
3 Peripheral Vein	**3** Percutaneous	**G** Other Therapeutic Substance	**C** Other Substance **N** Blood Brain Barrier Disruption **Q** Glucarpidase
3 Peripheral Vein	**3** Percutaneous	**U** Pancreatic Islet Cells	**0** Autologous **1** Nonautologous
3 Peripheral Vein	**3** Percutaneous	**V** Hormone	**G** Insulin **H** Human B-type Natriuretic Peptide **J** Other Hormone
3 Peripheral Vein	**3** Percutaneous	**W** Immunotherapeutic	**K** Immunostimulator **L** Immunosuppressive
4 Central Vein	**0** Open	**0** Antineoplastic	**2** High-dose Interleukin-2 **3** Low-dose Interleukin-2 **5** Other Antineoplastic **M** Monoclonal Antibody **P** Clofarabine
4 Central Vein	**0** Open	**1** Thrombolytic	**6** Recombinant Human-activated Protein C **7** Other Thrombolytic
4 Central Vein	**0** Open	**2** Anti-infective	**8** Oxazolidinones **9** Other Anti-infective
4 Central Vein	**0** Open	**3** Anti-inflammatory **4** Serum, Toxoid and Vaccine **6** Nutritional Substance **7** Electrolytic and Water Balance Substance **F** Intracirculatory Anesthetic **H** Radioactive Substance **K** Other Diagnostic Substance **N** Analgesics, Hypnotics, Sedatives **P** Platelet Inhibitor **R** Antiarrhythmic **T** Destructive Agent **X** Vasopressor	**Z** No Qualifier
4 Central Vein	**0** Open	**G** Other Therapeutic Substance	**C** Other Substance **N** Blood Brain Barrier Disruption

Continued →

Body System / Region (4th)	Approach (5th)	Substance (6th)	Qualifier (7th)
4 Central Vein	**0** Open	**V** Hormone	**G** Insulin **H** Human B-type Natriuretic Peptide **J** Other Hormone
4 Central Vein	**0** Open	**W** Immunotherapeutic	**K** Immunostimulator **L** Immunosuppressive
4 Central Vein	**3** Percutaneous	**0** Antineoplastic	**2** High-dose Interleukin-2 **3** Low-dose Interleukin-2 **5** Other Antineoplastic **M** Monoclonal Antibody **P** Clofarabine
4 Central Vein	**3** Percutaneous	**1** Thrombolytic	**6** Recombinant Human-activated Protein C **7** Other Thrombolytic
4 Central Vein	**3** Percutaneous	**2** Anti-infective	**8** Oxazolidinones **9** Other Anti-infective
4 Central Vein	**3** Percutaneous	**3** Anti-inflammatory **4** Serum, Toxoid and Vaccine **6** Nutritional Substance **7** Electrolytic and Water Balance Substance **F** Intracirculatory Anesthetic **H** Radioactive Substance **K** Other Diagnostic Substance **N** Analgesics, Hypnotics, Sedatives **P** Platelet Inhibitor **R** Antiarrhythmic **T** Destructive Agent **X** Vasopressor	**Z** No Qualifier
4 Central Vein	**3** Percutaneous	**G** Other Therapeutic Substance	**C** Other Substance **N** Blood Brain Barrier Disruption **Q** Glucarpidase
4 Central Vein	**3** Percutaneous	**V** Hormone	**G** Insulin **H** Human B-type Natriuretic Peptide **J** Other Hormone
4 Central Vein	**3** Percutaneous	**W** Immunotherapeutic	**K** Immunostimulator **L** Immunosuppressive
5 Peripheral Artery **6** Central Artery	**0** Open **3** Percutaneous	**0** Antineoplastic	**2** High-dose Interleukin-2 **3** Low-dose Interleukin-2 **5** Other Antineoplastic **M** Monoclonal Antibody **P** Clofarabine
5 Peripheral Artery **6** Central Artery	**0** Open **3** Percutaneous	**1** Thrombolytic	**6** Recombinant Human-activated Protein C **7** Other Thrombolytic
5 Peripheral Artery **6** Central Artery	**0** Open **3** Percutaneous	**2** Anti-infective	**8** Oxazolidinones **9** Other Anti-infective

Continued →

Section	3	Administration
Body System	E	Physiological Systems and Anatomical Regions
Operation	0	Introduction: Putting in or on a therapeutic, diagnostic, nutritional, physiological, or prophylactic substance except blood or blood products

Body System / Region (4th)	Approach (5th)	Substance (6th)	Qualifier (7th)
5 Peripheral Artery **6** Central Artery	**0** Open **3** Percutaneous	**3** Anti-inflammatory **4** Serum, Toxoid and Vaccine **6** Nutritional Substance **7** Electrolytic and Water Balance Substance **F** Intracirculatory Anesthetic **H** Radioactive Substance **K** Other Diagnostic Substance **N** Analgesics, Hypnotics, Sedatives **P** Platelet Inhibitor **R** Antiarrhythmic **T** Destructive Agent **X** Vasopressor	**Z** No Qualifier
5 Peripheral Artery **6** Central Artery	**0** Open **3** Percutaneous	**G** Other Therapeutic Substance	**C** Other Substance **N** Blood Brain Barrier Disruption
5 Peripheral Artery **6** Central Artery	**0** Open **3** Percutaneous	**V** Hormone	**G** Insulin **H** Human B-type Natriuretic Peptide **J** Other Hormone
5 Peripheral Artery **6** Central Artery	**0** Open **3** Percutaneous	**W** Immunotherapeutic	**K** Immunostimulator **L** Immunosuppressive
7 Coronary Artery **8** Heart	**0** Open **3** Percutaneous	**1** Thrombolytic	**6** Recombinant Human-activated Protein C **7** Other Thrombolytic
7 Coronary Artery **8** Heart	**0** Open **3** Percutaneous	**G** Other Therapeutic Substance	**C** Other Substance
7 Coronary Artery **8** Heart	**0** Open **3** Percutaneous	**K** Other Diagnostic Substance **P** Platelet Inhibitor	**Z** No Qualifier
9 Nose	**3** Percutaneous **7** Via Natural or Artificial Opening **X** External	**0** Antineoplastic	**5** Other Antineoplastic **M** Monoclonal Antibody
9 Nose	**3** Percutaneous **7** Via Natural or Artificial Opening **X** External	**2** Anti-infective	**8** Oxazolidinones **9** Other Anti-infective
9 Nose	**3** Percutaneous **7** Via Natural or Artificial Opening **X** External	**3** Anti-inflammatory **4** Serum, Toxoid and Vaccine **B** Local Anesthetic **H** Radioactive Substance **K** Other Diagnostic Substance **N** Analgesics, Hypnotics, Sedatives **T** Destructive Agent	**Z** No Qualifier
9 Nose	**3** Percutaneous **7** Via Natural or Artificial Opening **X** External	**G** Other Therapeutic Substance	**C** Other Substance
A Bone Marrow	**3** Percutaneous	**0** Antineoplastic	**5** Other Antineoplastic **M** Monoclonal Antibody
A Bone Marrow	**3** Percutaneous	**G** Other Therapeutic Substance	**C** Other Substance

Continued →

Section 3 **Administration**
Body System E **Physiological Systems and Anatomical Regions**
Operation 0 **Introduction:** Putting in or on a therapeutic, diagnostic, nutritional, physiological, or prophylactic substance except blood or blood products

Body System / Region (4th)	Approach (5th)	Substance (6th)	Qualifier (7th)
B Ear	**3** Percutaneous **7** Via Natural or Artificial Opening **X** External	**0** Antineoplastic	**4** Liquid Brachytherapy Radioisotope **5** Other Antineoplastic **M** Monoclonal Antibody
B Ear	**3** Percutaneous **7** Via Natural or Artificial Opening **X** External	**2** Anti-infective	**8** Oxazolidinones **9** Other Anti-infective
B Ear	**3** Percutaneous **7** Via Natural or Artificial Opening **X** External	**3** Anti-inflammatory **B** Local Anesthetic **H** Radioactive Substance **K** Other Diagnostic Substance **N** Analgesics, Hypnotics, Sedatives **T** Destructive Agent	**Z** No Qualifier
B Ear	**3** Percutaneous **7** Via Natural or Artificial Opening **X** External	**G** Other Therapeutic Substance	**C** Other Substance
C Eye	**3** Percutaneous **7** Via Natural or Artificial Opening **X** External	**0** Antineoplastic	**4** Liquid Brachytherapy Radioisotope **5** Other Antineoplastic **M** Monoclonal Antibody
C Eye	**3** Percutaneous **7** Via Natural or Artificial Opening **X** External	**2** Anti-infective	**8** Oxazolidinones **9** Other Anti-infective
C Eye	**3** Percutaneous **7** Via Natural or Artificial Opening **X** External	**3** Anti-inflammatory **B** Local Anesthetic **H** Radioactive Substance **K** Other Diagnostic Substance **M** Pigment **N** Analgesics, Hypnotics, Sedatives **T** Destructive Agent	**Z** No Qualifier
C Eye	**3** Percutaneous **7** Via Natural or Artificial Opening **X** External	**G** Other Therapeutic Substance	**C** Other Substance
C Eye	**3** Percutaneous **7** Via Natural or Artificial Opening **X** External	**S** Gas	**F** Other Gas
D Mouth and Pharynx	**3** Percutaneous **7** Via Natural or Artificial Opening **X** External	**0** Antineoplastic	**4** Liquid Brachytherapy Radioisotope **5** Other Antineoplastic **M** Monoclonal Antibody
D Mouth and Pharynx	**3** Percutaneous **7** Via Natural or Artificial Opening **X** External	**2** Anti-infective	**8** Oxazolidinones **9** Other Anti-infective

Continued →

Body System / Region (4th)	Approach (5th)	Substance (6th)	Qualifier (7th)
D Mouth and Pharynx	**3** Percutaneous **7** Via Natural or Artificial Opening **X** External	**3** Anti-inflammatory **4** Serum, Toxoid and Vaccine **6** Nutritional Substance **7** Electrolytic and Water Balance Substance **B** Local Anesthetic **H** Radioactive Substance **K** Other Diagnostic Substance **N** Analgesics, Hypnotics, Sedatives **R** Antiarrhythmic **T** Destructive Agent	**Z** No Qualifier
D Mouth and Pharynx	**3** Percutaneous **7** Via Natural or Artificial Opening **X** External	**G** Other Therapeutic Substance	**C** Other Substance
E Products of Conception **G** Upper GI **H** Lower GI **K** Genitourinary Tract **N** Male Reproductive	**3** Percutaneous **7** Via Natural or Artificial Opening **8** Via Natural or Artificial Opening Endoscopic	**0** Antineoplastic	**4** Liquid Brachytherapy Radioisotope **5** Other Antineoplastic **M** Monoclonal Antibody
E Products of Conception **G** Upper GI **H** Lower GI **K** Genitourinary Tract **N** Male Reproductive	**3** Percutaneous **7** Via Natural or Artificial Opening **8** Via Natural or Artificial Opening Endoscopic	**2** Anti-infective	**8** Oxazolidinones **9** Other Anti-infective
E Products of Conception **G** Upper GI **H** Lower GI **K** Genitourinary Tract **N** Male Reproductive	**3** Percutaneous **7** Via Natural or Artificial Opening **8** Via Natural or Artificial Opening Endoscopic	**3** Anti-inflammatory **6** Nutritional Substance **7** Electrolytic and Water Balance Substance **B** Local Anesthetic **H** Radioactive Substance **K** Other Diagnostic Substance **N** Analgesics, Hypnotics, Sedatives **T** Destructive Agent	**Z** No Qualifier
E Products of Conception **G** Upper GI **H** Lower GI **K** Genitourinary Tract **N** Male Reproductive	**3** Percutaneous **7** Via Natural or Artificial Opening **8** Via Natural or Artificial Opening Endoscopic	**G** Other Therapeutic Substance	**C** Other Substance
E Products of Conception **G** Upper GI **H** Lower GI **K** Genitourinary Tract **N** Male Reproductive	**3** Percutaneous **7** Via Natural or Artificial Opening **8** Via Natural or Artificial Opening Endoscopic	**S** Gas	**F** Other Gas
F Respiratory Tract	**3** Percutaneous	**0** Antineoplastic	**4** Liquid Brachytherapy Radioisotope **5** Other Antineoplastic **M** Monoclonal Antibody
F Respiratory Tract	**3** Percutaneous	**2** Anti-infective	**8** Oxazolidinones **9** Other Anti-infective

Continued →

Section 3 **Administration**
Body System E **Physiological Systems and Anatomical Regions**
Operation 0 **Introduction:** Putting in or on a therapeutic, diagnostic, nutritional, physiological, or prophylactic substance except blood or blood products

Body System / Region (4th)	Approach (5th)	Substance (6th)	Qualifier (7th)
F Respiratory Tract	**3** Percutaneous	**3** Anti-inflammatory **6** Nutritional Substance **7** Electrolytic and Water Balance Substance **B** Local Anesthetic **H** Radioactive Substance **K** Other Diagnostic Substance **N** Analgesics, Hypnotics, Sedatives **T** Destructive Agent	**Z** No Qualifier
F Respiratory Tract	**3** Percutaneous	**G** Other Therapeutic Substance	**C** Other Substance
F Respiratory Tract	**3** Percutaneous	**S** Gas	**D** Nitric Oxide **F** Other Gas
F Respiratory Tract	**7** Via Natural or Artificial Opening **8** Via Natural or Artificial Opening Endoscopic	**0** Antineoplastic	**4** Liquid Brachytherapy Radioisotope **5** Other Antineoplastic **M** Monoclonal Antibody
F Respiratory Tract	**7** Via Natural or Artificial Opening **8** Via Natural or Artificial Opening Endoscopic	**2** Anti-infective	**8** Oxazolidinones **9** Other Anti-infective
F Respiratory Tract	**7** Via Natural or Artificial Opening **8** Via Natural or Artificial Opening Endoscopic	**3** Anti-inflammatory **6** Nutritional Substance **7** Electrolytic and Water Balance Substance **B** Local Anesthetic **D** Inhalation Anesthetic **H** Radioactive Substance **K** Other Diagnostic Substance **N** Analgesics, Hypnotics, Sedatives **T** Destructive Agent	**Z** No Qualifier
F Respiratory Tract	**7** Via Natural or Artificial Opening **8** Via Natural or Artificial Opening Endoscopic	**G** Other Therapeutic Substance	**C** Other Substance
F Respiratory Tract	**7** Via Natural or Artificial Opening **8** Via Natural or Artificial Opening Endoscopic	**S** Gas	**D** Nitric Oxide **F** Other Gas
J Biliary and Pancreatic Tract	**3** Percutaneous **7** Via Natural or Artificial Opening **8** Via Natural or Artificial Opening Endoscopic	**0** Antineoplastic	**4** Liquid Brachytherapy Radioisotope **5** Other Antineoplastic **M** Monoclonal Antibody
J Biliary and Pancreatic Tract	**3** Percutaneous **7** Via Natural or Artificial Opening **8** Via Natural or Artificial Opening Endoscopic	**2** Anti-infective	**8** Oxazolidinones **9** Other Anti-infective

Continued →

Section 3 Administration
Body System E Physiological Systems and Anatomical Regions
Operation 0 Introduction: Putting in or on a therapeutic, diagnostic, nutritional, physiological, or prophylactic substance except blood or blood products

Body System / Region (4th)	Approach (5th)	Substance (6th)	Qualifier (7th)
J Biliary and Pancreatic Tract	3 Percutaneous 7 Via Natural or Artificial Opening 8 Via Natural or Artificial Opening Endoscopic	3 Anti-inflammatory 6 Nutritional Substance 7 Electrolytic and Water Balance Substance B Local Anesthetic H Radioactive Substance K Other Diagnostic Substance N Analgesics, Hypnotics, Sedatives T Destructive Agent	Z No Qualifier
J Biliary and Pancreatic Tract	3 Percutaneous 7 Via Natural or Artificial Opening 8 Via Natural or Artificial Opening Endoscopic	G Other Therapeutic Substance	C Other Substance
J Biliary and Pancreatic Tract	3 Percutaneous 7 Via Natural or Artificial Opening 8 Via Natural or Artificial Opening Endoscopic	S Gas	F Other Gas
J Biliary and Pancreatic Tract	3 Percutaneous 7 Via Natural or Artificial Opening 8 Via Natural or Artificial Opening Endoscopic	U Pancreatic Islet Cells	0 Autologous 1 Nonautologous
L Pleural Cavity M Peritoneal Cavity	0 Open	5 Adhesion Barrier	Z No Qualifier
L Pleural Cavity M Peritoneal Cavity	3 Percutaneous	0 Antineoplastic	4 Liquid Brachytherapy Radioisotope 5 Other Antineoplastic M Monoclonal Antibody
L Pleural Cavity M Peritoneal Cavity	3 Percutaneous	2 Anti-infective	8 Oxazolidinones 9 Other Anti-infective
L Pleural Cavity M Peritoneal Cavity	3 Percutaneous	3 Anti-inflammatory 6 Nutritional Substance 7 Electrolytic and Water Balance Substance B Local Anesthetic H Radioactive Substance K Other Diagnostic Substance N Analgesics, Hypnotics, Sedatives T Destructive Agent	Z No Qualifier
L Pleural Cavity M Peritoneal Cavity	3 Percutaneous	G Other Therapeutic Substance	C Other Substance
L Pleural Cavity M Peritoneal Cavity	3 Percutaneous	S Gas	F Other Gas
L Pleural Cavity M Peritoneal Cavity	7 Via Natural or Artificial Opening	0 Antineoplastic	4 Liquid Brachytherapy Radioisotope 5 Other Antineoplastic M Monoclonal Antibody

Continued →

Body System / Region (4th)	Approach (5th)	Substance (6th)	Qualifier (7th)
L Pleural Cavity **M** Peritoneal Cavity	**7** Via Natural or Artificial Opening	**S** Gas	**F** Other Gas
P Female Reproductive	**0** Open	**5** Adhesion Barrier	**Z** No Qualifier
P Female Reproductive	**3** Percutaneous **7** Via Natural or Artificial Opening	**0** Antineoplastic	**4** Liquid Brachytherapy Radioisotope **5** Other Antineoplastic **M** Monoclonal Antibody
P Female Reproductive	**3** Percutaneous **7** Via Natural or Artificial Opening	**2** Anti-infective	**8** Oxazolidinones **9** Other Anti-infective
P Female Reproductive	**3** Percutaneous **7** Via Natural or Artificial Opening	**3** Anti-inflammatory **6** Nutritional Substance **7** Electrolytic and Water Balance Substance **B** Local Anesthetic **H** Radioactive Substance **K** Other Diagnostic Substance **L** Sperm **N** Analgesics, Hypnotics, Sedatives **T** Destructive Agent	**Z** No Qualifier
P Female Reproductive	**3** Percutaneous **7** Via Natural or Artificial Opening	**G** Other Therapeutic Substance	**C** Other Substance
P Female Reproductive	**3** Percutaneous **7** Via Natural or Artificial Opening	**Q** Fertilized Ovum	**0** Autologous **1** Nonautologous
P Female Reproductive	**3** Percutaneous **7** Via Natural or Artificial Opening	**S** Gas	**F** Other Gas
P Female Reproductive	**8** Via Natural or Artificial Opening Endoscopic	**0** Antineoplastic	**4** Liquid Brachytherapy Radioisotope **5** Other Antineoplastic **M** Monoclonal Antibody
P Female Reproductive	**8** Via Natural or Artificial Opening Endoscopic	**2** Anti-infective	**8** Oxazolidinones **9** Other Anti-infective
P Female Reproductive	**8** Via Natural or Artificial Opening Endoscopic	**3** Anti-inflammatory **6** Nutritional Substance **7** Electrolytic and Water Balance Substance **B** Local Anesthetic **H** Radioactive Substance **K** Other Diagnostic Substance **N** Analgesics, Hypnotics, Sedatives **T** Destructive Agent	**Z** No Qualifier
P Female Reproductive	**8** Via Natural or Artificial Opening Endoscopic	**G** Other Therapeutic Substance	**C** Other Substance
P Female Reproductive	**8** Via Natural or Artificial Opening Endoscopic	**S** Gas	**F** Other Gas
Q Cranial Cavity and Brain	**0** Open	**A** Stem Cells, Embryonic	**Z** No Qualifier

Continued →

Section 3 **Administration**
Body System E **Physiological Systems and Anatomical Regions**
Operation 0 **Introduction:** Putting in or on a therapeutic, diagnostic, nutritional, physiological, or prophylactic substance except blood or blood products

Body System / Region (4th)	Approach (5th)	Substance (6th)	Qualifier (7th)
Q Cranial Cavity and Brain	**0** Open	**E** Stem Cells, Somatic	**0** Autologous **1** Nonautologous
Q Cranial Cavity and Brain	**3** Percutaneous	**0** Antineoplastic	**4** Liquid Brachytherapy Radioisotope **5** Other Antineoplastic **M** Monoclonal Antibody
Q Cranial Cavity and Brain	**3** Percutaneous	**2** Anti-infective	**8** Oxazolidinones **9** Other Anti-infective
Q Cranial Cavity and Brain	**3** Percutaneous	**3** Anti-inflammatory **6** Nutritional Substance **7** Electrolytic and Water Balance Substance **A** Stem Cells, Embryonic **B** Local Anesthetic **H** Radioactive Substance **K** Other Diagnostic Substance **N** Analgesics, Hypnotics, Sedatives **T** Destructive Agent	**Z** No Qualifier
Q Cranial Cavity and Brain	**3** Percutaneous	**E** Stem Cells, Somatic	**0** Autologous **1** Nonautologous
Q Cranial Cavity and Brain	**3** Percutaneous	**G** Other Therapeutic Substance	**C** Other Substance
Q Cranial Cavity and Brain	**3** Percutaneous	**S** Gas	**F** Other Gas
Q Cranial Cavity and Brain	**7** Via Natural or Artificial Opening	**0** Antineoplastic	**4** Liquid Brachytherapy Radioisotope **5** Other Antineoplastic **M** Monoclonal Antibody
Q Cranial Cavity and Brain	**7** Via Natural or Artificial Opening	**S** Gas	**F** Other Gas
R Spinal Canal	**0** Open	**A** Stem Cells, Embryonic	**Z** No Qualifier
R Spinal Canal	**0** Open	**E** Stem Cells, Somatic	**0** Autologous **1** Nonautologous
R Spinal Canal	**3** Percutaneous	**0** Antineoplastic	**2** High-dose Interleukin-2 **3** Low-dose Interleukin-2 **4** Liquid Brachytherapy Radioisotope **5** Other Antineoplastic **M** Monoclonal Antibody
R Spinal Canal	**3** Percutaneous	**2** Anti-infective	**8** Oxazolidinones **9** Other Anti-infective
R Spinal Canal	**3** Percutaneous	**3** Anti-inflammatory **6** Nutritional Substance **7** Electrolytic and Water Balance Substance **A** Stem Cells, Embryonic **B** Local Anesthetic **C** Regional Anesthetic **H** Radioactive Substance **K** Other Diagnostic Substance **N** Analgesics, Hypnotics, Sedatives **T** Destructive Agent	**Z** No Qualifier

Continued →

Section 3 **Administration**
Body System E **Physiological Systems and Anatomical Regions**
Operation 0 **Introduction:** Putting in or on a therapeutic, diagnostic, nutritional, physiological, or prophylactic substance except blood or blood products

Body System / Region (4th)	Approach (5th)	Substance (6th)	Qualifier (7th)
R Spinal Canal	**3** Percutaneous	**E** Stem Cells, Somatic	**0** Autologous **1** Nonautologous
R Spinal Canal	**3** Percutaneous	**G** Other Therapeutic Substance	**C** Other Substance
R Spinal Canal	**3** Percutaneous	**S** Gas	**F** Other Gas
R Spinal Canal	**7** Via Natural or Artificial Opening	**S** Gas	**F** Other Gas
S Epidural Space	**3** Percutaneous	**0** Antineoplastic	**2** High-dose Interleukin-2 **3** Low-dose Interleukin-2 **4** Liquid Brachytherapy Radioisotope **5** Other Antineoplastic **M** Monoclonal Antibody
S Epidural Space	**3** Percutaneous	**2** Anti-infective	**8** Oxazolidinones **9** Other Anti-infective
S Epidural Space	**3** Percutaneous	**3** Anti-inflammatory **6** Nutritional Substance **7** Electrolytic and Water Balance Substance **B** Local Anesthetic **C** Regional Anesthetic **H** Radioactive Substance **K** Other Diagnostic Substance **N** Analgesics, Hypnotics, Sedatives **T** Destructive Agent	**Z** No Qualifier
S Epidural Space	**3** Percutaneous	**G** Other Therapeutic Substance	**C** Other Substance
S Epidural Space	**3** Percutaneous	**S** Gas	**F** Other Gas
S Epidural Space	**7** Via Natural or Artificial Opening	**S** Gas	**F** Other Gas
T Peripheral Nerves and Plexi **X** Cranial Nerves	**3** Percutaneous	**3** Anti-inflammatory **B** Local Anesthetic **C** Regional Anesthetic **T** Destructive Agent	**Z** No Qualifier
T Peripheral Nerves and Plexi **X** Cranial Nerves	**3** Percutaneous	**G** Other Therapeutic Substance	**C** Other Substance
U Joints	**0** Open	**2** Anti-infective	**8** Oxazolidinones **9** Other Anti-infective
U Joints	**0** Open	**G** Other Therapeutic Substance	**B** Recombinant Bone Morphogenetic Protein
U Joints	**3** Percutaneous	**0** Antineoplastic	**4** Liquid Brachytherapy Radioisotope **5** Other Antineoplastic **M** Monoclonal Antibody
U Joints	**3** Percutaneous	**2** Anti-infective	**8** Oxazolidinones **9** Other Anti-infective

Continued →

Body System / Region (4th)	Approach (5th)	Substance (6th)	Qualifier (7th)
U Joints	**3** Percutaneous	**3** Anti-inflammatory **6** Nutritional Substance **7** Electrolytic and Water Balance Substance **B** Local Anesthetic **H** Radioactive Substance **K** Other Diagnostic Substance **N** Analgesics, Hypnotics, Sedatives **T** Destructive Agent	**Z** No Qualifier
U Joints	**3** Percutaneous	**G** Other Therapeutic Substance	**B** Recombinant Bone Morphogenetic Protein **C** Other Substance
U Joints	**3** Percutaneous	**S** Gas	**F** Other Gas
V Bones	**0** Open	**G** Other Therapeutic Substance	**B** Recombinant Bone Morphogenetic Protein
V Bones	**3** Percutaneous	**0** Antineoplastic	**5** Other Antineoplastic **M** Monoclonal Antibody
V Bones	**3** Percutaneous	**2** Anti-infective	**8** Oxazolidinones **9** Other Anti-infective
V Bones	**3** Percutaneous	**3** Anti-inflammatory **6** Nutritional Substance **7** Electrolytic and Water Balance Substance **B** Local Anesthetic **H** Radioactive Substance **K** Other Diagnostic Substance **N** Analgesics, Hypnotics, Sedatives **T** Destructive Agent	**Z** No Qualifier
V Bones	**3** Percutaneous	**G** Other Therapeutic Substance	**B** Recombinant Bone Morphogenetic Protein **C** Other Substance
W Lymphatics	**3** Percutaneous	**0** Antineoplastic	**5** Other Antineoplastic **M** Monoclonal Antibody
W Lymphatics	**3** Percutaneous	**2** Anti-infective	**8** Oxazolidinones **9** Other Anti-infective
W Lymphatics	**3** Percutaneous	**3** Anti-inflammatory **6** Nutritional Substance **7** Electrolytic and Water Balance Substance **B** Local Anesthetic **H** Radioactive Substance **K** Other Diagnostic Substance **N** Analgesics, Hypnotics, Sedatives **T** Destructive Agent	**Z** No Qualifier
W Lymphatics	**3** Percutaneous	**G** Other Therapeutic Substance	**C** Other Substance
Y Pericardial Cavity	**3** Percutaneous	**0** Antineoplastic	**4** Liquid Brachytherapy Radioisotope **5** Other Antineoplastic **M** Monoclonal Antibody
Y Pericardial Cavity	**3** Percutaneous	**2** Anti-infective	**8** Oxazolidinones **9** Other Anti-infective

Continued →

Section 3 Administration
Body System E Physiological Systems and Anatomical Regions
Operation 0 **Introduction:** Putting in or on a therapeutic, diagnostic, nutritional, physiological, or prophylactic substance except blood or blood products

Body System / Region (4th)	Approach (5th)	Substance (6th)	Qualifier (7th)
Y Pericardial Cavity	**3** Percutaneous	**3** Anti-inflammatory **6** Nutritional Substance **7** Electrolytic and Water Balance Substance **B** Local Anesthetic **H** Radioactive Substance **K** Other Diagnostic Substance **N** Analgesics, Hypnotics, Sedatives **T** Destructive Agent	**Z** No Qualifier
Y Pericardial Cavity	**3** Percutaneous	**G** Other Therapeutic Substance	**C** Other Substance
Y Pericardial Cavity	**3** Percutaneous	**S** Gas	**F** Other Gas
Y Pericardial Cavity	**7** Via Natural or Artificial Opening	**0** Antineoplastic	**4** Liquid Brachytherapy Radioisotope **5** Other Antineoplastic **M** Monoclonal Antibody
Y Pericardial Cavity	**7** Via Natural or Artificial Opening	**S** Gas	**F** Other Gas

Section 3 Administration
Body System E Physiological Systems and Anatomical Regions
Operation 1 **Irrigation:** Putting in or on a cleansing substance

Body System / Region (4th)	Approach (5th)	Substance (6th)	Qualifier (7th)
0 Skin and Mucous Membranes **C** Eye	**3** Percutaneous **X** External	**8** Irrigating Substance	**X** Diagnostic **Z** No Qualifier
9 Nose **B** Ear **F** Respiratory Tract **G** Upper GI **H** Lower GI **J** Biliary and Pancreatic Tract **K** Genitourinary Tract **N** Male Reproductive **P** Female Reproductive	**3** Percutaneous **7** Via Natural or Artificial Opening **8** Via Natural or Artificial Opening Endoscopic	**8** Irrigating Substance	**X** Diagnostic **Z** No Qualifier
L Pleural Cavity **Q** Cranial Cavity and Brain **R** Spinal Canal **S** Epidural Space **U** Joints **Y** Pericardial Cavity	**3** Percutaneous	**8** Irrigating Substance	**X** Diagnostic **Z** No Qualifier
M Peritoneal Cavity	**3** Percutaneous	**8** Irrigating Substance	**X** Diagnostic **Z** No Qualifier
M Peritoneal Cavity	**3** Percutaneous	**9** Dialysate	**Z** No Qualifier

Measurement and Monitoring Section (4A0–4B0)

Within each section of ICD-10-PCS the characters have different meanings. The seven character meanings for the Measurement and Monitoring section are illustrated here through the procedure example of *External electrocardiogram (EKG), single reading*.

Section	Body System	Root Operation	Body System	Approach	Function / Device	Qualifier
Measurement and Monitoring	Physiological Systems	Measurement	Cardiac	External	Electrical Activity	None
4	A	0	2	X	4	Z

Section (Character 1)

All Measurement and Monitoring procedure codes have a first character value of 4.

Body System (Character 2)

The alphanumeric character for the body system is placed in the second position. There are two character values applicable for the Measurement and Monitoring section. The character value of A is reported for physiological systems. The character value B is reported for physiological devices.

Root Operations (Character 3)

The alphanumeric character value for root operations is placed in the third position. Listed here are the root operations applicable to the Measurement and Monitoring section with their associated meaning. Note that the root operation definitions for ICD-10-PCS may differ from the terms that coders currently use with ICD-9-CM Volume 3.

Character Value	Root Operation	Root Operation Definition
0	Measurement	Determining the level of a physiological or physical function at a point in time
1	Monitoring	Determining the level of a physiological or physical function repetitively over a period of time

Body System/Region (Character 4)

For each body system the applicable body part character values will be available for procedure code construction. An example of a body region for this section is Respiratory.

Approach (Character 5)

The approach is the technique used to reach the procedure site. The following are the approach character values for the Measurement and Monitoring section with the associated definitions.

Character Value	Approach	Approach Definition
0	Open	Cutting through the skin or mucous membrane and any other body layers necessary to expose the site of the procedure
3	Percutaneous	Entry, by puncture or minor incision, of instrumentation through the skin or mucous membrane and any other body layers necessary to reach the site of the procedure
4	Percutaneous Endoscopic	Entry, by puncture or minor incision, of instrumentation through the skin or mucous membrane and any other body layers necessary to reach and visualize the site of the procedure
7	Via Natural or Artificial Opening	Entry of instrumentation through a natural or artificial external opening to reach the site of the procedure
8	Via Natural or Artificial Opening Endoscopic	Entry of instrumentation through a natural or artificial external opening to reach and visualize the site of the procedure
X	External	Procedures performed directly on the skin or mucous membrane and procedures performed indirectly by the application of external force through the skin or mucous membrane

Function/Device (Character 6)

In the Measurement and Monitoring section a function or device is always utilized. The function or device is reported in the sixth character position by the type of function monitored or measured or by the device utilized. The following is a sample list of the functions and devices included in this section:

- Conductivity
- Flow
- Metabolism
- Pressure
- Sound

Qualifier (Character 7)

The qualifier represents an additional attribute for the procedure when applicable. There are several qualifiers included in the Measurement and Monitoring section. For example, measurement procedures in this section include several qualifiers including stress that is reported with the character value of 4. If there is no qualifier for a procedure, the placeholder Z is the character valve that should be reported.

Measurement and Monitoring Section Tables

Measurement and Monitoring Tables 4A0–4B0

Section 4 **Measurement and Monitoring**
Body System A **Physiological Systems**
Operation 0 **Measurement:** Determining the level of a physiological or physical function at a point in time

Body System (4th)	Approach (5th)	Function / Device (6th)	Qualifier (7th)
0 Central Nervous	**0** Open	**2** Conductivity **4** Electrical Activity **B** Pressure	**Z** No Qualifier
0 Central Nervous	**3** Percutaneous	**4** Electrical Activity	**Z** No Qualifier
0 Central Nervous	**3** Percutaneous	**B** Pressure **K** Temperature **R** Saturation	**D** Intracranial
0 Central Nervous	**7** Via Natural or Artificial Opening	**B** Pressure **K** Temperature **R** Saturation	**D** Intracranial
0 Central Nervous	**X** External	**2** Conductivity **4** Electrical Activity	**Z** No Qualifier
1 Peripheral Nervous	**0** Open **3** Percutaneous **X** External	**2** Conductivity	**9** Sensory **B** Motor
1 Peripheral Nervous	**0** Open **3** Percutaneous **X** External	**4** Electrical Activity	**Z** No Qualifier
2 Cardiac	**0** Open **3** Percutaneous	**4** Electrical Activity **9** Output **C** Rate **F** Rhythm **H** Sound **P** Action Currents	**Z** No Qualifier
2 Cardiac	**0** Open **3** Percutaneous	**N** Sampling and Pressure	**6** Right Heart **7** Left Heart **8** Bilateral
2 Cardiac	**X** External	**4** Electrical Activity	**A** Guidance **Z** No Qualifier

Continued →

Section 4 **Measurement and Monitoring**
Body System A **Physiological Systems**
Operation 0 **Measurement:** Determining the level of a physiological or physical function at a point in time

Body System (4th)	Approach (5th)	Function / Device (6th)	Qualifier (7th)
2 Cardiac	**X** External	**9** Output **C** Rate **F** Rhythm **H** Sound **P** Action Currents	**Z** No Qualifier
2 Cardiac	**X** External	**M** Total Activity	**4** Stress
3 Arterial	**0** Open **3** Percutaneous	**5** Flow **J** Pulse	**1** Peripheral **3** Pulmonary **C** Coronary
3 Arterial	**0** Open **3** Percutaneous	**B** Pressure	**1** Peripheral **3** Pulmonary **C** Coronary **F** Other Thoracic
3 Arterial	**0** Open **3** Percutaneous	**H** Sound **R** Saturation	**1** Peripheral
3 Arterial	**X** External	**5** Flow **B** Pressure **H** Sound **J** Pulse **R** Saturation	**1** Peripheral
4 Venous	**0** Open **3** Percutaneous	**5** Flow **B** Pressure **J** Pulse	**0** Central **1** Peripheral **2** Portal **3** Pulmonary
4 Venous	**0** Open **3** Percutaneous	**R** Saturation	**1** Peripheral
4 Venous	**X** External	**5** Flow **B** Pressure **J** Pulse **R** Saturation	**1** Peripheral
5 Circulatory	**X** External	**L** Volume	**Z** No Qualifier
6 Lymphatic	**0** Open **3** Percutaneous	**5** Flow **B** Pressure	**Z** No Qualifier
7 Visual	**X** External	**0** Acuity **7** Mobility **B** Pressure	**Z** No Qualifier
8 Olfactory	**X** External	**0** Acuity	**Z** No Qualifier
9 Respiratory	**7** Via Natural or Artificial Opening **8** Via Natural or Artificial Opening Endoscopic **X** External	**1** Capacity **5** Flow **C** Rate **D** Resistance **L** Volume **M** Total Activity	**Z** No Qualifier
B Gastrointestinal	**7** Via Natural or Artificial Opening **8** Via Natural or Artificial Opening Endoscopic	**8** Motility **B** Pressure **G** Secretion	**Z** No Qualifier
C Biliary	**3** Percutaneous **4** Percutaneous Endoscopic **7** Via Natural or Artificial Opening **8** Via Natural or Artificial Opening Endoscopic	**5** Flow **B** Pressure	**Z** No Qualifier

Continued →

Section 4 **Measurement and Monitoring**
Body System A **Physiological Systems**
Operation 0 **Measurement:** Determining the level of a physiological or physical function at a point in time

Body System (4th)	Approach (5th)	Function / Device (6th)	Qualifier (7th)
D Urinary	**7** Via Natural or Artificial Opening	**3** Contractility **5** Flow **B** Pressure **D** Resistance **L** Volume	**Z** No Qualifier
F Musculoskeletal	**3** Percutaneous **X** External	**3** Contractility	**Z** No Qualifier
H Products of Conception, Cardiac	**7** Via Natural or Artificial Opening **8** Via Natural or Artificial Opening Endoscopic **X** External	**4** Electrical Activity **C** Rate **F** Rhythm **H** Sound	**Z** No Qualifier
J Products of Conception, Nervous	**7** Via Natural or Artificial Opening **8** Via Natural or Artificial Opening Endoscopic **X** External	**2** Conductivity **4** Electrical Activity **B** Pressure	**Z** No Qualifier
Z None	**7** Via Natural or Artificial Opening	**6** Metabolism **K** Temperature	**Z** No Qualifier
Z None	**X** External	**6** Metabolism **K** Temperature **Q** Sleep	**Z** No Qualifier

Section 4 **Measurement and Monitoring**
Body System A **Physiological Systems**
Operation 1 **Monitoring:** Determining the level of a physiological or physical function repetitively over a period of time

Body System (4th)	Approach (5th)	Function / Device (6th)	Qualifier (7th)
0 Central Nervous	**0** Open	**2** Conductivity **B** Pressure	**Z** No Qualifier
0 Central Nervous	**0** Open	**4** Electrical Activity	**G** Intraoperative **Z** No Qualifier
0 Central Nervous	**3** Percutaneous	**4** Electrical Activity	**G** Intraoperative **Z** No Qualifier
0 Central Nervous	**3** Percutaneous	**B** Pressure **K** Temperature **R** Saturation	**D** Intracranial
0 Central Nervous	**7** Via Natural or Artificial Opening	**B** Pressure **K** Temperature **R** Saturation	**D** Intracranial
0 Central Nervous	**X** External	**2** Conductivity	**Z** No Qualifier
0 Central Nervous	**X** External	**4** Electrical Activity	**G** Intraoperative **Z** No Qualifier
1 Peripheral Nervous	**0** Open **3** Percutaneous **X** External	**2** Conductivity	**9** Sensory **B** Motor
1 Peripheral Nervous	**0** Open **3** Percutaneous **X** External	**4** Electrical Activity	**G** Intraoperative **Z** No Qualifier

Continued →

Section	4	**Measurement and Monitoring**
Body System	A	**Physiological Systems**
Operation	1	**Monitoring:** Determining the level of a physiological or physical function repetitively over a period of time

Body System (4th)	Approach (5th)	Function / Device (6th)	Qualifier (7th)
2 Cardiac	**0** Open **3** Percutaneous	**4** Electrical Activity **9** Output **C** Rate **F** Rhythm **H** Sound	**Z** No Qualifier
2 Cardiac	**X** External	**4** Electrical Activity	**5** Ambulatory **Z** No Qualifier
2 Cardiac	**X** External	**9** Output **C** Rate **F** Rhythm **H** Sound	**Z** No Qualifier
2 Cardiac	**X** External	**M** Total Activity	**4** Stress
3 Arterial	**0** Open **3** Percutaneous	**5** Flow **B** Pressure **J** Pulse	**1** Peripheral **3** Pulmonary **C** Coronary
3 Arterial	**0** Open **3** Percutaneous	**H** Sound **R** Saturation	**1** Peripheral
3 Arterial	**X** External	**5** Flow **B** Pressure **H** Sound **J** Pulse **R** Saturation	**1** Peripheral
4 Venous	**0** Open **3** Percutaneous	**5** Flow **B** Pressure **J** Pulse	**0** Central **1** Peripheral **2** Portal **3** Pulmonary
4 Venous	**0** Open **3** Percutaneous	**R** Saturation	**0** Central **2** Portal **3** Pulmonary
4 Venous	**X** External	**5** Flow **B** Pressure **J** Pulse	**1** Peripheral
6 Lymphatic	**0** Open **3** Percutaneous	**5** Flow **B** Pressure	**Z** No Qualifier
9 Respiratory	**7** Via Natural or Artificial Opening **X** External	**1** Capacity **5** Flow **C** Rate **D** Resistance **L** Volume	**Z** No Qualifier
B Gastrointestinal	**7** Via Natural or Artificial Opening **8** Via Natural or Artificial Opening Endoscopic	**8** Motility **B** Pressure **G** Secretion	**Z** No Qualifier
D Urinary	**7** Via Natural or Artificial Opening	**3** Contractility **5** Flow **B** Pressure **D** Resistance **L** Volume	**Z** No Qualifier

Continued →

Section 4 **Measurement and Monitoring**
Body System A **Physiological Systems**
Operation 1 **Monitoring:** Determining the level of a physiological or physical function repetitively over a period of time

Body System (4th)	Approach (5th)	Function / Device (6th)	Qualifier (7th)
H Products of Conception, Cardiac	**7** Via Natural or Artificial Opening **8** Via Natural or Artificial Opening Endoscopic **X** External	**4** Electrical Activity **C** Rate **F** Rhythm **H** Sound	**Z** No Qualifier
J Products of Conception, Nervous	**7** Via Natural or Artificial Opening **8** Via Natural or Artificial Opening Endoscopic **X** External	**2** Conductivity **4** Electrical Activity **B** Pressure	**Z** No Qualifier
Z None	**7** Via Natural or Artificial Opening	**K** Temperature	**Z** No Qualifier
Z None	**X** External	**K** Temperature **Q** Sleep	**Z** No Qualifier

Section 4 **Measurement and Monitoring**
Body System B **Physiological Devices**
Operation 0 **Measurement:** Determining the level of a physiological or physical function at a point in time

Body System (4th)	Approach (5th)	Function / Device (6th)	Qualifier (7th)
0 Central Nervous **1** Peripheral Nervous **F** Musculoskeletal	**X** External	**V** Stimulator	**Z** No Qualifier
2 Cardiac	**X** External	**S** Pacemaker **T** Defibrillator	**Z** No Qualifier
9 Respiratory	**X** External	**S** Pacemaker	**Z** No Qualifier

Extracorporeal Assistance and Performance Section (5A0–5A2)

Within each section of ICD-10-PCS the characters have different meanings. The seven character meanings for the Extracorporeal Assistance and Performance section are illustrated here through the procedure example of *Hyperbaric oxygenation of wound*.

Section	Body System	Root Operation	Body System	Duration	Function	Qualifier
Extracorporeal Assistance and Performance	Physiological Systems	Assistance	Circulatory	Intermittent	Oxygenation	Hyperbaric
5	A	0	5	1	2	1

Section (Character 1)

All Extracorporeal Assistance and Performance procedure codes have a first character value of 5.

Body System (Character 2)

The alphanumeric character for the body system is placed in the second position. There is one character value applicable for the Extracorporeal Assistance and Performance section. The character value of A is reported for physiological systems.

Root Operations (Character 3)

The alphanumeric character value for root operations is placed in the third position. Listed here are the root operations applicable to the Extracorporeal Assistance and Performance section with their associated meaning. Note that the root operation definitions for ICD-10-PCS may differ from the terms that coders currently use with ICD-9-CM Volume 3.

Character Value	Root Operation	Root Operation Definition
0	Assistance	Taking over a portion of a physiological function by extracorporeal means
1	Performance	Completely taking over a physiological function by extracorporeal means
2	Restoration	Returning, or attempting to return, a physiological function to its original state by extracorporeal means

Body System (Character 4)

For each body system, the applicable body part character values will be available for procedure code construction. An example of a body region for this section is respiratory.

Duration (Character 5)

The duration represents the length of time or frequency for which the assistance or performance is utilized. Some examples of duration are Intermittent, Continuous, or Less than 24 consecutive hours.

Function (Character 6)

In the Extracorporeal Assistance and Performance section a function is always reported. The function is reported in the sixth character position. The following is a sample list of the functions utilized in this section:

- Output
- Oxygenation
- Pacing
- Ventilation

Qualifier (Character 7)

The qualifier represents an additional attribute for the procedure when applicable. There are several qualifiers included in the Extracorporeal Assistance and Performance section. For example, assistance procedures in this section include several qualifiers including Balloon Pump, which is reported with the character value of 0. If there is no qualifier for a procedure, the placeholder Z is the character valve that should be reported.

AHA Coding Clinic®

5A02210 Assistance with Cardiac Output using Balloon Pump, Continuous - AHA CC: 3Q, 2013, 18-19

5A1221Z Performance of Cardiac Output, Continuous - AHA CC: 3Q, 2013, 18-19; 1Q, 2014, 10-11

5A1223Z Performance of Cardiac Pacing, Continuous - AHA CC: 3Q, 2013, 18-19

Extracorporeal Assistance and Performance Section Tables

Extracorporeal Assistance and Performance Tables 5A0–5A2

Section 5 **Extracorporeal Assistance and Performance**
Body System A **Physiological Systems**
Operation 0 **Assistance:** Taking over a portion of a physiological function by extracorporeal means

Body System (4th)	Duration (5th)	Function (6th)	Qualifier (7th)
2 Cardiac	1 Intermittent 2 Continuous	1 Output	0 Balloon Pump 5 Pulsatile Compression 6 Other Pump D Impeller Pump
5 Circulatory	1 Intermittent 2 Continuous	2 Oxygenation	1 Hyperbaric C Supersaturated
9 Respiratory	3 Less than 24 Consecutive Hours 4 24-96 Consecutive Hours 5 Greater than 96 Consecutive Hours	5 Ventilation	7 Continuous Positive Airway Pressure 8 Intermittent Positive Airway Pressure 9 Continuous Negative Airway Pressure B Intermittent Negative Airway Pressure Z No Qualifier

Section 5 **Extracorporeal Assistance and Performance**
Body System A **Physiological Systems**
Operation 1 **Performance:** Completely taking over a physiological function by extracorporeal means

Body System (4th)	Duration (5th)	Function (6th)	Qualifier (7th)
2 Cardiac	0 Single	1 Output	2 Manual
2 Cardiac	1 Intermittent	3 Pacing	Z No Qualifier
2 Cardiac	2 Continuous	1 Output 3 Pacing	Z No Qualifier
5 Circulatory	2 Continuous	2 Oxygenation	3 Membrane
9 Respiratory	0 Single	5 Ventilation	4 Nonmechanical
9 Respiratory	3 Less than 24 Consecutive Hours 4 24-96 Consecutive Hours 5 Greater than 96 Consecutive Hours	5 Ventilation	Z No Qualifier
C Biliary D Urinary	0 Single 6 Multiple	0 Filtration	Z No Qualifier

Section 5 **Extracorporeal Assistance and Performance**
Body System A **Physiological Systems**
Operation 2 **Restoration:** Returning, or attempting to return, a physiological function to its original state by extracorporeal means.

Body System (4th)	Duration (5th)	Function (6th)	Qualifier (7th)
2 Cardiac	0 Single	4 Rhythm	Z No Qualifier

Extracorporeal Therapies Section (6A0–6A9)

Within each section of ICD-10-PCS the characters have different meanings. The seven character meanings for the Extracorporeal Therapies section are illustrated here through the procedure example of *Ultraviolet light phototherapy, series treatment.*

Section	Body System	Root Operation	Body System	Duration	Qualifier	Qualifier
Extracorporeal Therapies	Physiological Systems	UV Light Therapy	Skin	Multiple	None	None
6	A	8	0	1	Z	Z

Section (Character 1)

All Extracorporeal Therapies procedure codes have a first character value of 6.

Body System (Character 2)

The alphanumeric character for the body system is placed in the second position. There is one character value applicable for the Extracorporeal Therapies section. The character value of A is reported for physiological systems.

Root Operations (Character 3)

The alphanumeric character value for root operations is placed in the third position. Listed below are the root operations applicable to the Extracorporeal Therapies section with their associated meaning. Note that the root operation definitions for ICD-10-PCS may differ from the terms that coders currently use with ICD-9-CM Volume 3.

Character Value	Root Operation	Root Operation Definition
0	Atmospheric Control	Extracorporeal control of atmospheric pressure and composition
1	Decompression	Extracorporeal elimination of undissolved gas from body fluids
2	Electromagnetic Therapy	Extracorporeal treatment by electromagnetic rays
3	Hyperthermia	Extracorporeal raising of body temperature
4	Hypothermia	Extracorporeal lowering of body temperature
5	Pheresis	Extracorporeal separation of blood products
6	Phototherapy	Extracorporeal treatment by light rays
7	Ultrasound Therapy	Extracorporeal treatment by ultrasound
8	Ultraviolet Light Therapy	Extracorporeal treatment by ultraviolet light
9	Shock Wave Therapy	Extracorporeal treatment by shock waves

Body System (Character 4)

For each body system the applicable body part character values will be available for procedure code construction. An example of a body region for this section is Skin.

Duration (Character 5)

The duration represents the number of therapy sessions performed. Single is reported with character value 0; Multiple is reported with character value 1.

Qualifier (Character 6)

Character 6 is the first of two qualifier characters for the Extracorporeal Therapies section. The qualifier represents an additional attribute for the procedure when applicable. There are currently no qualifier values for the sixth character position, so the character value of Z is always reported.

Qualifier (Character 7)

Character 7 is the second of two qualifier characters for the Extracorporeal Therapies section. The qualifier represents an additional attribute for the procedure when applicable. There are some qualifiers included in the Extracorporeal Therapies section. For example, pheresis procedures in this section include several qualifiers including Plasma that is reported with the character value of 3. If there is no qualifier for a procedure, the placeholder Z is the character valve that should be reported.

Extracorporeal Therapies Tables 6A0–6A9

Section 6 **Extracorporeal Therapies**
Body System A **Physiological Systems**
Operation 0 **Atmospheric Control:** Extracorporeal control of atmospheric pressure and composition

Body System (4th)	Duration (5th)	Qualifier (6th)	Qualifier (7th)
Z None	**0** Single **1** Multiple	**Z** No Qualifier	**Z** No Qualifier

Section 6 **Extracorporeal Therapies**
Body System A **Physiological Systems**
Operation 1 **Decompression:** Extracorporeal elimination of undissolved gas from body fluids

Body System (4th)	Duration (5th)	Qualifier (6th)	Qualifier (7th)
5 Circulatory	**0** Single **1** Multiple	**Z** No Qualifier	**Z** No Qualifier

Section 6 **Extracorporeal Therapies**
Body System A **Physiological Systems**
Operation 2 **Electromagnetic Therapy:** Extracorporeal treatment by electromagnetic rays

Body System (4th)	Duration (5th)	Qualifier (6th)	Qualifier (7th)
1 Urinary **2** Central Nervous	**0** Single **1** Multiple	**Z** No Qualifier	**Z** No Qualifier

Section 6 **Extracorporeal Therapies**
Body System A **Physiological Systems**
Operation 3 **Hyperthermia:** Extracorporeal raising of body temperature

Body System (4th)	Duration (5th)	Qualifier (6th)	Qualifier (7th)
Z None	**0** Single **1** Multiple	**Z** No Qualifier	**Z** No Qualifier

Section 6 **Extracorporeal Therapies**
Body System A **Physiological Systems**
Operation 4 **Hypothermia:** Extracorporeal lowering of body temperature

Body System (4th)	Duration (5th)	Qualifier (6th)	Qualifier (7th)
Z None	**0** Single **1** Multiple	**Z** No Qualifier	**Z** No Qualifier

Section 6 **Extracorporeal Therapies**
Body System A **Physiological Systems**
Operation 5 **Pheresis:** Extracorporeal separation of blood products

Body System (4th)	Duration (5th)	Qualifier (6th)	Qualifier (7th)
5 Circulatory	**0** Single **1** Multiple	**Z** No Qualifier	**0** Erythrocytes **1** Leukocytes **2** Platelets **3** Plasma **T** Stem Cells, Cord Blood **V** Stem Cells, Hematopoietic

Section 6 **Extracorporeal Therapies**
Body System A **Physiological Systems**
Operation 6 **Phototherapy:** Extracorporeal treatment by light rays

Body System (4th)	Duration (5th)	Qualifier (6th)	Qualifier (7th)
0 Skin **5** Circulatory	**0** Single **1** Multiple	**Z** No Qualifier	**Z** No Qualifier

Section 6 **Extracorporeal Therapies**
Body System A **Physiological Systems**
Operation 7 **Ultrasound Therapy:** Extracorporeal treatment by ultrasound

Body System (4th)	Duration (5th)	Qualifier (6th)	Qualifier (7th)
5 Circulatory	**0** Single **1** Multiple	**Z** No Qualifier	**4** Head and Neck Vessels **5** Heart **6** Peripheral Vessels **7** Other Vessels **Z** No Qualifier

Section 6 **Extracorporeal Therapies**
Body System A **Physiological Systems**
Operation 8 **Ultraviolet Light Therapy:** Extracorporeal treatment by ultraviolet light

Body System (4th)	Duration (5th)	Qualifier (6th)	Qualifier (7th)
0 Skin	**0** Single **1** Multiple	**Z** No Qualifier	**Z** No Qualifier

Section 6 **Extracorporeal Therapies**
Body System A **Physiological Systems**
Operation 9 **Shock Wave Therapy:** Extracorporeal treatment by shock waves

Body System (4th)	Duration (5th)	Qualifier (6th)	Qualifier (7th)
3 Musculoskeletal	**0** Single **1** Multiple	**Z** No Qualifier	**Z** No Qualifier

Within each section of ICD-10-PCS, the characters have different meanings. The seven character meanings for the Osteopathic section are illustrated below through the procedure example of Indirect osteopathic treatment of sacrum.

Section	Body System	Root Operation	Body Region	Approach	Method	Qualifier
Osteopathic	Anatomical Regions	Treatment	Sacrum	External	Indirect	None
7	W	0	4	X	4	Z

Section (Character 1)

All Osteopathic procedure codes have a first character value of 7.

Body System (Character 2)

The alphanumeric character for the body system is placed in the second position. There is one character value applicable for the Osteopathic section. The character value of W is reported for anatomical regions.

Root Operations (Character 3)

The alphanumeric character value for root operations is placed in the third position. Listed here is the root operation applicable to the Osteopathic section with its associated meaning. Note that the root operation definitions for ICD-10-PCS may differ from the terms that coders currently use with ICD-9-CM Volume 3.

Character Value	Root Operation	Root Operation Definition
0	Treatment	Manual treatment to eliminate or alleviate somatic dysfunction and related disorders

Body Region (Character 4)

For each body region the applicable body part character values will be available for procedure code construction. An example of a body region for this section is Head.

Approach (Character 5)

The approach is the technique used to reach the procedure site. The following are the approach character values for the Osteopathic section with the associated definitions.

Character Value	Approach	Approach Definition
X	External	Procedures performed directly on the skin or mucous membrane and procedures performed indirectly by the application of external force through the skin or mucous membrane

Method (Character 6)

The method identifies the treatment method used to complete the osteopathic procedure. The available methods are:

- Articulatory-Raising
- Fascial Release
- General Mobilization
- High Velocity-Low Amplitude
- Indirect
- Low Velocity-High Amplitude
- Lymphatic Pump
- Muscle Energy-Isometric
- Muscle Energy-Isotonic
- Other

Qualifier (Character 7)

The qualifier represents an additional attribute for the procedure when applicable. Currently, there are no qualifiers in the Osteopathic section; therefore, the placeholder character value of Z should be reported.

Osteopathic Section Table

Osteopathic Table 7W0

Section 7 **Osteopathic**
Body System W **Anatomical Regions**
Operation 0 **Treatment:** Manual treatment to eliminate or alleviate somatic dysfunction and related disorders

Body Region (4th)	Approach (5th)	Method (6th)	Qualifier (7th)
0 Head **1** Cervical **2** Thoracic **3** Lumbar **4** Sacrum **5** Pelvis **6** Lower Extremities **7** Upper Extremities **8** Rib Cage **9** Abdomen	**X** External	**0** Articulatory-Raising **1** Fascial Release **2** General Mobilization **3** High Velocity-Low Amplitude **4** Indirect **5** Low Velocity-High Amplitude **6** Lymphatic Pump **7** Muscle Energy-Isometric **8** Muscle Energy-Isotonic **9** Other Method	**Z** None

Other Procedures Section (8C0–8E0)

Within each section of ICD-10-PCS the characters have different meanings. The seven character meanings for the Other Procedures section are illustrated here through the procedure example of Yoga therapy.

Section	Body System	Root Operation	Body Region	Approach	Method	Qualifier
Other Procedures	Physiological Systems and Anatomical Regions	Other Procedures	None	External	Other Method	Yoga Therapy
8	E	0	Z	X	Y	4

Section (Character 1)

All Other Procedures codes have a first character value of 8.

Body System (Character 2)

The alphanumeric character for the body system is placed in the second position. There are two character values applicable for the Other Procedures section. The character value of C is reported for indwelling device. Th character value of E is reported for physiological system and anatomical regions.

Root Operations (Character 3)

The alphanumeric character value for root operations is placed in the third position. Listed here is the root operation applicable to the Other Procedures section with its associated meaning. Note that the root operation definitions for ICD-10-PCS may differ from the terms that coders currently use with ICD-9-CM Volume 3.

Character Value	Root Operation	Root Operation Definition
0	Other Procedures	Methodologies which attempt to remediate or cure a disorder or disease

Body Region (Character 4)

For each body region the applicable body part character values will be available for procedure code construction. An example of a body region for this section is Lower Extremity.

Approach (Character 5)

The approach is the technique used to reach the procedure site. The following are the approach character values for the Other Procedures section with the associated definitions.

Character Value	Approach	Approach Definition
0	Open	Cutting through the skin or mucous membrane and any other body layers necessary to expose the site of the procedure
3	Percutaneous	Entry, by puncture or minor incision, of instrumentation through the skin or mucous membrane and any other body layers necessary to reach the site of the procedure
4	Percutaneous Endoscopic	Entry, by puncture or minor incision, of instrumentation through the skin or mucous membrane and any other body layers necessary to reach and visualize the site of the procedure
7	Via Natural or Artificial Opening	Entry of instrumentation through a natural or artificial external opening to reach the site of the procedure
8	Via Natural or Artificial Opening Endoscopic	Entry of instrumentation through a natural or artificial external opening to reach and visualize the site of the procedure
X	External	Procedures performed directly on the skin or mucous membrane and procedures performed indirectly by the application of external force through the skin or mucous membrane

Chiropractic Section (9WB)

Within each section of ICD-10-PCS the characters have different meanings. The seven character meanings for the Chiropractic section are illustrated here through the procedure example of Chiropractic treatment of cervical spine, short lever specific contact.

Section	Body System	Root Operation	Body Region	Approach	Method	Qualifier
Chiropractic	Anatomical Regions	Manipulation	Cervical	External	Short Lever Specific Contact	None
9	W	B	1	X	H	Z

Section (Character 1)

All Chiropractic procedure codes have a first character value of 9.

Body System (Character 2)

The alphanumeric character for the body system is placed in the second position. There is one character value applicable for the Chiropractic section. The character value of W is reported for anatomical regions.

Root Operations (Character 3)

The alphanumeric character value for root operations is placed in the third position. The following is the root operation applicable to the Chiropractic section with its associated meaning. Note that the root operation definitions for ICD-10-PCS may differ from the terms that coders currently use with ICD-9-CM Volume 3.

Character Value	Root Operation	Root Operation Definition
B	Manipulation	Manual procedure that involves a directed thrust to move a joint past the physiological range of motion, without exceeding the anatomical limit

Body Region (Character 4)

For each body region the applicable body part character values will be available for procedure code construction. An example of a body region for this section is Rib Cage.

Approach (Character 5)

The approach is the technique used to reach the procedure site. The following are the approach character values for the Chiropractic section with the associated definitions.

Character Value	Approach	Approach Definition
X	External	Procedures performed directly on the skin or mucous membrane and procedures performed indirectly by the application of external force through the skin or mucous membrane

Method (Character 6)

The method identifies the treatment method used to complete the chiropractic procedure. The available methods are:

- Non-Manual
- Indirect Visceral
- Extra-Articular
- Direct-Visual
- Long Lever Specific Contact
- Short Lever Specific Contact
- Long and Short Lever Specific Contact
- Mechanically Assisted
- Other

Qualifier (Character 7)

The qualifier represents an additional attribute for the procedure when applicable. Currently, there are no qualifiers in the Chiropractic section; therefore, the placeholder character value of Z should be reported.

Chiropractic Section Table

Chiropractic Table 9WB

Section **9** **Chiropractic**
Body System **W** **Anatomical Regions**
Operation **B** **Manipulation:** Manual procedure that involves a directed thrust to move a joint past the physiological range of motion, without exceeding the anatomical limit

Body Region (4th)	Approach (5th)	Method (6th)	Qualifier (7th)
0 Head	**X** External	**B** Non-Manual	**Z** None
1 Cervical		**C** Indirect Visceral	
2 Thoracic		**D** Extra-Articular	
3 Lumbar		**F** Direct Visceral	
4 Sacrum		**G** Long Lever Specific Contact	
5 Pelvis		**H** Short Lever Specific Contact	
6 Lower Extremities		**J** Long and Short Lever Specific Contact	
7 Upper Extremities		**K** Mechanically Assisted	
8 Rib Cage		**L** Other Method	
9 Abdomen			

Imaging Section (B00–BY4)

Within each section of ICD-10-PCS the characters have different meanings. The seven character meanings for the Imaging section are illustrated here through the procedure example of X-ray right clavicle, limited study.

Section	Body System	Root Type	Body Part	Contrast	Qualifier	Qualifier
Imaging	Non-Axial Upper Bones	Plain Radiography	Clavicle, right	None	None	None
B	P	0	4	Z	Z	Z

Section (Character 1)

All Imaging procedure codes have a first character value of B.

Body System (Character 2)

The alphanumeric character for the body system is placed in the second position. The following are the body systems applicable to the Imaging section.

Character Value	Character Value Description
0	Central Nervous System
2	Heart
3	Upper Arteries
4	Lower Arteries
5	Veins
7	Lymphatic System
8	Eye
9	Ear, Nose, Mouth and Throat
B	Respiratory System
D	Gastrointestinal System
F	Hepatobiliary System and Pancreas
G	Endocrine System
H	Skin, Subcutaneous Tissue and Breast
L	Connective Tissue
N	Skull and Facial Bones
P	Non-Axial Upper Bones
Q	Non-Axial Lower Bones
R	Axial Skeleton, Except Skull and Facial Bones
T	Urinary System
U	Female Reproductive System
V	Male Reproductive System
W	Anatomical Regions
Y	Fetus and Obstetrical

Root Types (Character 3)

The alphanumeric character value for root types is placed in the third position. Listed here are the root types applicable to the Imaging section with their associated meaning.

Character Value	Root Type	Root Type Definition
0	Plain Radiography	Planar display of an image developed from the capture of external ionizing radiation on photographic or photoconductive plate
1	Fluoroscopy	Single plane or bi-plane real time display of an image developed from the capture of external ionizing radiation on a fluorescent screen. The image may also be stored by either digital or analog means

Continued →

Character Value	Root Type	Root Type Definition
2	Computerized Tomography (CT Scan)	Computer reformatted digital display of multiplanar images developed from the capture of multiple exposures of external ionizing radiation
3	Magnetic Resonance Imaging (MRI)	Computer reformatted digital display of multiplanar images developed from the capture of radiofrequency signals emitted by nuclei in a body site excited within a magnetic field
4	Ultrasonography	Real time display of images of anatomy or flow information developed from the capture of reflected and attenuated high frequency sound waves

Body Part (Character 4)

For each body part the applicable body part character values will be available for procedure code construction. An example of a body part for this section is Spinal Cord.

Contrast (Character 5)

When contrast is utilized during an imaging procedure, the corresponding contrast character value should be reported in the fifth character position. The following are the contrast character values for the Imaging section:

- High Osmolar
- Low Osmolar
- Other Contrast

If contrast is not utilized, the placeholder character value of Z should be reported.

Qualifier (Character 6)

This qualifier character specifies when an image taken without contrast is followed by one with contrast. The character value of 0 is reported for Unenhanced and Enhanced.

Qualifier (Character 7)

The qualifier represents an additional attribute for the procedure when applicable. For example, ultrasonography procedures in this section include the qualifier Densitometry that is reported with the character value of 1 for some body parts. If there is no qualifier for a procedure, the placeholder Z is the character valve that should be reported.

Imaging Section Tables

Imaging Tables B00–BY4

Section B **Imaging**
Body System 0 **Central Nervous System**
Type 0 **Plain Radiography:** Planar display of an image developed from the capture of external ionizing radiation on photographic or photoconductive plate

Body Part (4th)	Contrast (5th)	Qualifier (6th)	Qualifier (7th)
B Spinal Cord	**0** High Osmolar **1** Low Osmolar **Y** Other Contrast **Z** None	**Z** None	**Z** None

Section B **Imaging**
Body System 0 **Central Nervous System**
Type 1 **Fluoroscopy:** Single plane or bi-plane real time display of an image developed from the capture of external ionizing radiation on a fluorescent screen. The image may also be stored by either digital or analog means

Body Part (4th)	Contrast (5th)	Qualifier (6th)	Qualifier (7th)
B Spinal Cord	**0** High Osmolar **1** Low Osmolar **Y** Other Contrast **Z** None	**Z** None	**Z** None

Section B Imaging
Body System 0 Central Nervous System
Type 2 Computerized Tomography (CT Scan): Computer reformatted digital display of multiplanar images developed from the capture of multiple exposures of external ionizing radiation

Body Part (4th)	Contrast (5th)	Qualifier (6th)	Qualifier (7th)
0 Brain 7 Cisterna 8 Cerebral Ventricle(s) 9 Sella Turcica/Pituitary Gland B Spinal Cord	0 High Osmolar 1 Low Osmolar Y Other Contrast	0 Unenhanced and Enhanced Z None	Z None
0 Brain 7 Cisterna 8 Cerebral Ventricle(s) 9 Sella Turcica/Pituitary Gland B Spinal Cord	Z None	Z None	Z None

Section B Imaging
Body System 0 Central Nervous System
Type 3 Magnetic Resonance Imaging (MRI): Computer reformatted digital display of multiplanar images developed from the capture of radiofrequency signals emitted by nuclei in a body site excited within a magnetic field

Body Part (4th)	Contrast (5th)	Qualifier (6th)	Qualifier (7th)
0 Brain 9 Sella Turcica/Pituitary Gland B Spinal Cord C Acoustic Nerves	Y Other Contrast	0 Unenhanced and Enhanced Z None	Z None
0 Brain 9 Sella Turcica/Pituitary Gland B Spinal Cord C Acoustic Nerves	Z None	Z None	Z None

Section B Imaging
Body System 0 Central Nervous System
Type 4 Ultrasonography: Real time display of images of anatomy or flow information developed from the capture of reflected and attenuated high frequency sound waves

Body Part (4th)	Contrast (5th)	Qualifier (6th)	Qualifier (7th)
0 Brain B Spinal Cord	Z None	Z None	Z None

Section B Imaging
Body System 2 Heart
Type 0 Plain Radiography: Planar display of an image developed from the capture of external ionizing radiation on photographic or photoconductive plate

Body Part (4th)	Contrast (5th)	Qualifier (6th)	Qualifier (7th)
0 Coronary Artery, Single 1 Coronary Arteries, Multiple 2 Coronary Artery Bypass Graft, Single 3 Coronary Artery Bypass Grafts, Multiple 4 Heart, Right 5 Heart, Left 6 Heart, Right and Left 7 Internal Mammary Bypass Graft, Right 8 Internal Mammary Bypass Graft, Left F Bypass Graft, Other	0 High Osmolar 1 Low Osmolar Y Other Contrast	Z None	Z None

Section B **Imaging**
Body System 2 **Heart**
Type 1 **Fluoroscopy:** Single plane or bi-plane real time display of an image developed from the capture of external ionizing radiation on a fluorescent screen. The image may also be stored by either digital or analog means

Body Part (4th)	Contrast (5th)	Qualifier (6th)	Qualifier (7th)
0 Coronary Artery, Single **1** Coronary Arteries, Multiple **2** Coronary Artery Bypass Graft, Single **3** Coronary Artery Bypass Grafts, Multiple	**0** High Osmolar **1** Low Osmolar **Y** Other Contrast	**1** Laser	**0** Intraoperative
0 Coronary Artery, Single **1** Coronary Arteries, Multiple **2** Coronary Artery Bypass Graft, Single **3** Coronary Artery Bypass Grafts, Multiple	**0** High Osmolar **1** Low Osmolar **Y** Other Contrast	**Z** None	**Z** None
4 Heart, Right **5** Heart, Left **6** Heart, Right and Left **7** Internal Mammary Bypass Graft, Right **8** Internal Mammary Bypass Graft, Left **F** Bypass Graft, Other	**0** High Osmolar **1** Low Osmolar **Y** Other Contrast	**Z** None	**Z** None

Section B **Imaging**
Body System 2 **Heart**
Type 2 **Computerized Tomography (CT Scan):** Computer reformatted digital display of multiplanar images developed from the capture of multiple exposures of external ionizing radiation

Body Part (4th)	Contrast (5th)	Qualifier (6th)	Qualifier (7th)
1 Coronary Arteries, Multiple **3** Coronary Artery Bypass Grafts, Multiple **6** Heart, Right and Left	**0** High Osmolar **1** Low Osmolar **Y** Other Contrast	**0** Unenhanced and Enhanced **Z** None	**Z** None
1 Coronary Arteries, Multiple **3** Coronary Artery Bypass Grafts, Multiple **6** Heart, Right and Left	**Z** None	**2** Intravascular Optical Coherence **Z** None	**Z** None

Section B **Imaging**
Body System 2 **Heart**
Type 3 **Magnetic Resonance Imaging (MRI):** Computer reformatted digital display of multiplanar images developed from the capture of radiofrequency signals emitted by nuclei in a body site excited within a magnetic field

Body Part (4th)	Contrast (5th)	Qualifier (6th)	Qualifier (7th)
1 Coronary Arteries, Multiple **3** Coronary Artery Bypass Grafts, Multiple **6** Heart, Right and Left	**Y** Other Contrast	**0** Unenhanced and Enhanced **Z** None	**Z** None
1 Coronary Arteries, Multiple **3** Coronary Artery Bypass Grafts, Multiple **6** Heart, Right and Left	**Z** None	**Z** None	**Z** None

Section B **Imaging**
Body System 2 **Heart**
Type 4 **Ultrasonography:** Real time display of images of anatomy or flow information developed from the capture of reflected and attenuated high frequency sound waves

Body Part (4th)	Contrast (5th)	Qualifier (6th)	Qualifier (7th)
0 Coronary Artery, Single **1** Coronary Arteries, Multiple **4** Heart, Right **5** Heart, Left **6** Heart, Right and Left **B** Heart with Aorta **C** Pericardium **D** Pediatric Heart	**Y** Other Contrast	**Z** None	**Z** None
0 Coronary Artery, Single **1** Coronary Arteries, Multiple **4** Heart, Right **5** Heart, Left **6** Heart, Right and Left **B** Heart with Aorta **C** Pericardium **D** Pediatric Heart	**Z** None	**Z** None	**3** Intravascular **4** Transesophageal **Z** None

Section B **Imaging**
Body System 3 **Upper Arteries**
Type 0 **Plain Radiography:** Planar display of an image developed from the capture of external ionizing radiation on photographic or photoconductive plate

Body Part (4th)	Contrast (5th)	Qualifier (6th)	Qualifier (7th)
0 Thoracic Aorta **1** Brachiocephalic-Subclavian Artery, Right **2** Subclavian Artery, Left **3** Common Carotid Artery, Right **4** Common Carotid Artery, Left **5** Common Carotid Arteries, Bilateral **6** Internal Carotid Artery, Right **7** Internal Carotid Artery, Left **8** Internal Carotid Arteries, Bilateral **9** External Carotid Artery, Right **B** External Carotid Artery, Left **C** External Carotid Arteries, Bilateral **D** Vertebral Artery, Right **F** Vertebral Artery, Left **G** Vertebral Arteries, Bilateral **H** Upper Extremity Arteries, Right **J** Upper Extremity Arteries, Left **K** Upper Extremity Arteries, Bilateral **L** Intercostal and Bronchial Arteries **M** Spinal Arteries **N** Upper Arteries, Other **P** Thoraco-Abdominal Aorta **Q** Cervico-Cerebral Arch **R** Intracranial Arteries **S** Pulmonary Artery, Right **T** Pulmonary Artery, Left	**0** High Osmolar **1** Low Osmolar **Y** Other Contrast **Z** None	**Z** None	**Z** None

Section B Imaging
Body System 3 Upper Arteries
Type 1 **Fluoroscopy:** Single plane or bi-plane real time display of an image developed from the capture of external ionizing radiation on a fluorescent screen. The image may also be stored by either digital or analog means

Body Part (4th)	Contrast (5th)	Qualifier (6th)	Qualifier (7th)
0 Thoracic Aorta **1** Brachiocephalic-Subclavian Artery, Right **2** Subclavian Artery, Left **3** Common Carotid Artery, Right **4** Common Carotid Artery, Left **5** Common Carotid Arteries, Bilateral **6** Internal Carotid Artery, Right **7** Internal Carotid Artery, Left **8** Internal Carotid Arteries, Bilateral **9** External Carotid Artery, Right **B** External Carotid Artery, Left **C** External Carotid Arteries, Bilateral **D** Vertebral Artery, Right **F** Vertebral Artery, Left **G** Vertebral Arteries, Bilateral **H** Upper Extremity Arteries, Right **J** Upper Extremity Arteries, Left **K** Upper Extremity Arteries, Bilateral **L** Intercostal and Bronchial Arteries **M** Spinal Arteries **N** Upper Arteries, Other **P** Thoraco-Abdominal Aorta **Q** Cervico-Cerebral Arch **R** Intracranial Arteries **S** Pulmonary Artery, Right **T** Pulmonary Artery, Left	**0** High Osmolar **1** Low Osmolar **Y** Other Contrast	**1** Laser	**0** Intraoperative
0 Thoracic Aorta **1** Brachiocephalic-Subclavian Artery, Right **2** Subclavian Artery, Left **3** Common Carotid Artery, Right **4** Common Carotid Artery, Left **5** Common Carotid Arteries, Bilateral **6** Internal Carotid Artery, Right **7** Internal Carotid Artery, Left **8** Internal Carotid Arteries, Bilateral **9** External Carotid Artery, Right **B** External Carotid Artery, Left **C** External Carotid Arteries, Bilateral **D** Vertebral Artery, Right **F** Vertebral Artery, Left **G** Vertebral Arteries, Bilateral **H** Upper Extremity Arteries, Right **J** Upper Extremity Arteries, Left **K** Upper Extremity Arteries, Bilateral **L** Intercostal and Bronchial Arteries **M** Spinal Arteries **N** Upper Arteries, Other **P** Thoraco-Abdominal Aorta **Q** Cervico-Cerebral Arch **R** Intracranial Arteries **S** Pulmonary Artery, Right **T** Pulmonary Artery, Left	**0** High Osmolar **1** Low Osmolar **Y** Other Contrast	**Z** None	**Z** None

Continued →

Section B **Imaging**
Body System 3 **Upper Arteries**
Type 1 **Fluoroscopy:** Single plane or bi-plane real time display of an image developed from the capture of external ionizing radiation on a fluorescent screen. The image may also be stored by either digital or analog means

Body Part (4th)	Contrast (5th)	Qualifier (6th)	Qualifier (7th)
0 Thoracic Aorta **1** Brachiocephalic-Subclavian Artery, Right **2** Subclavian Artery, Left **3** Common Carotid Artery, Right **4** Common Carotid Artery, Left **5** Common Carotid Arteries, Bilateral **6** Internal Carotid Artery, Right **7** Internal Carotid Artery, Left **8** Internal Carotid Arteries, Bilateral **9** External Carotid Artery, Right **B** External Carotid Artery, Left **C** External Carotid Arteries, Bilateral **D** Vertebral Artery, Right **F** Vertebral Artery, Left **G** Vertebral Arteries, Bilateral **H** Upper Extremity Arteries, Right **J** Upper Extremity Arteries, Left **K** Upper Extremity Arteries, Bilateral **L** Intercostal and Bronchial Arteries **M** Spinal Arteries **N** Upper Arteries, Other **P** Thoraco-Abdominal Aorta **Q** Cervico-Cerebral Arch **R** Intracranial Arteries **S** Pulmonary Artery, Right **T** Pulmonary Artery, Left	**Z** None	**Z** None	**Z** None

Section B **Imaging**
Body System 3 **Upper Arteries**
Type 2 **Computerized Tomography (CT Scan):** Computer reformatted digital display of multiplanar images developed from the capture of multiple exposures of external ionizing radiation

Body Part (4th)	Contrast (5th)	Qualifier (6th)	Qualifier (7th)
0 Thoracic Aorta **5** Common Carotid Arteries, Bilateral **8** Internal Carotid Arteries, Bilateral **G** Vertebral Arteries, Bilateral **R** Intracranial Arteries **S** Pulmonary Artery, Right **T** Pulmonary Artery, Left	**0** High Osmolar **1** Low Osmolar **Y** Other Contrast	**Z** None	**Z** None
0 Thoracic Aorta **5** Common Carotid Arteries, Bilateral **8** Internal Carotid Arteries, Bilateral **G** Vertebral Arteries, Bilateral **R** Intracranial Arteries **S** Pulmonary Artery, Right **T** Pulmonary Artery, Left	**Z** None	**2** Intravascular Optical Coherence **Z** None	**Z** None

Section B **Imaging**
Body System 3 **Upper Arteries**
Type 3 **Magnetic Resonance Imaging (MRI):** Computer reformatted digital display of multiplanar images developed from the capture of radiofrequency signals emitted by nuclei in a body site excited within a magnetic field

Body Part (4th)	Contrast (5th)	Qualifier (6th)	Qualifier (7th)
0 Thoracic Aorta **5** Common Carotid Arteries, Bilateral **8** Internal Carotid Arteries, Bilateral **G** Vertebral Arteries, Bilateral **H** Upper Extremity Arteries, Right **J** Upper Extremity Arteries, Left **K** Upper Extremity Arteries, Bilateral **M** Spinal Arteries **Q** Cervico-Cerebral Arch **R** Intracranial Arteries	**Y** Other Contrast	**0** Unenhanced and Enhanced **Z** None	**Z** None
0 Thoracic Aorta **5** Common Carotid Arteries, Bilateral **8** Internal Carotid Arteries, Bilateral **G** Vertebral Arteries, Bilateral **H** Upper Extremity Arteries, Right **J** Upper Extremity Arteries, Left **K** Upper Extremity Arteries, Bilateral **M** Spinal Arteries **Q** Cervico-Cerebral Arch **R** Intracranial Arteries	**Z** None	**Z** None	**Z** None

Section B **Imaging**
Body System 3 **Upper Arteries**
Type 4 **Ultrasonography:** Real time display of images of anatomy or flow information developed from the capture of reflected and attenuated high frequency sound waves

Body Part (4th)	Contrast (5th)	Qualifier (6th)	Qualifier (7th)
0 Thoracic Aorta **1** Brachiocephalic-Subclavian Artery, Right **2** Subclavian Artery, Left **3** Common Carotid Artery, Right **4** Common Carotid Artery, Left **5** Common Carotid Arteries, Bilateral **6** Internal Carotid Artery, Right **7** Internal Carotid Artery, Left **8** Internal Carotid Arteries, Bilateral **H** Upper Extremity Arteries, Right **J** Upper Extremity Arteries, Left **K** Upper Extremity Arteries, Bilateral **R** Intracranial Arteries **S** Pulmonary Artery, Right **T** Pulmonary Artery, Left **V** Ophthalmic Arteries	**Z** None	**Z** None	**3** Intravascular **Z** None

Section B **Imaging**
Body System 4 **Lower Arteries**
Type 0 **Plain Radiography:** Planar display of an image developed from the capture of external ionizing radiation on photographic or photoconductive plate

Body Part (4th)	Contrast (5th)	Qualifier (6th)	Qualifier (7th)
0 Abdominal Aorta **2** Hepatic Artery **3** Splenic Arteries **4** Superior Mesenteric Artery **5** Inferior Mesenteric Artery **6** Renal Artery, Right **7** Renal Artery, Left **8** Renal Arteries, Bilateral **9** Lumbar Arteries **B** Intra-Abdominal Arteries, Other **C** Pelvic Arteries **D** Aorta and Bilateral Lower Extremity Arteries **F** Lower Extremity Arteries, Right **G** Lower Extremity Arteries, Left **J** Lower Arteries, Other **M** Renal Artery Transplant	**0** High Osmolar **1** Low Osmolar **Y** Other Contrast	**Z** None	**Z** None

Section B **Imaging**
Body System 4 **Lower Arteries**
Type 1 **Fluoroscopy:** Single plane or bi-plane real time display of an image developed from the capture of external ionizing radiation on a fluorescent screen. The image may also be stored by either digital or analog means

Body Part (4th)	Contrast (5th)	Qualifier (6th)	Qualifier (7th)
0 Abdominal Aorta **2** Hepatic Artery **3** Splenic Arteries **4** Superior Mesenteric Artery **5** Inferior Mesenteric Artery **6** Renal Artery, Right **7** Renal Artery, Left **8** Renal Arteries, Bilateral **9** Lumbar Arteries **B** Intra-Abdominal Arteries, Other **C** Pelvic Arteries **D** Aorta and Bilateral Lower Extremity Arteries **F** Lower Extremity Arteries, Right **G** Lower Extremity Arteries, Left **J** Lower Arteries, Other	**0** High Osmolar **1** Low Osmolar **Y** Other Contrast	**1** Laser	**0** Intraoperative
0 Abdominal Aorta **2** Hepatic Artery **3** Splenic Arteries **4** Superior Mesenteric Artery **5** Inferior Mesenteric Artery **6** Renal Artery, Right **7** Renal Artery, Left **8** Renal Arteries, Bilateral **9** Lumbar Arteries **B** Intra-Abdominal Arteries, Other **C** Pelvic Arteries **D** Aorta and Bilateral Lower Extremity Arteries **F** Lower Extremity Arteries, Right **G** Lower Extremity Arteries, Left **J** Lower Arteries, Other	**0** High Osmolar **1** Low Osmolar **Y** Other Contrast	**Z** None	**Z** None

Continued →

Section B **Imaging**
Body System 4 **Lower Arteries**
Type 1 **Fluoroscopy:** Single plane or bi-plane real time display of an image developed from the capture of external ionizing radiation on a fluorescent screen. The image may also be stored by either digital or analog means

Body Part (4th)	Contrast (5th)	Qualifier (6th)	Qualifier (7th)
0 Abdominal Aorta **2** Hepatic Artery **3** Splenic Arteries **4** Superior Mesenteric Artery **5** Inferior Mesenteric Artery **6** Renal Artery, Right **7** Renal Artery, Left **8** Renal Arteries, Bilateral **9** Lumbar Arteries **B** Intra-Abdominal Arteries, Other **C** Pelvic Arteries **D** Aorta and Bilateral Lower Extremity Arteries **F** Lower Extremity Arteries, Right **G** Lower Extremity Arteries, Left **J** Lower Arteries, Other	**Z** None	**Z** None	**Z** None

Section B **Imaging**
Body System 4 **Lower Arteries**
Type 2 **Computerized Tomography (CT Scan):** Computer reformatted digital display of multiplanar images developed from the capture of multiple exposures of external ionizing radiation

Body Part (4th)	Contrast (5th)	Qualifier (6th)	Qualifier (7th)
0 Abdominal Aorta **1** Celiac Artery **4** Superior Mesenteric Artery **8** Renal Arteries, Bilateral **C** Pelvic Arteries **F** Lower Extremity Arteries, Right **G** Lower Extremity Arteries, Left **H** Lower Extremity Arteries, Bilateral **M** Renal Artery Transplant	**0** High Osmolar **1** Low Osmolar **Y** Other Contrast	**Z** None	**Z** None
0 Abdominal Aorta **1** Celiac Artery **4** Superior Mesenteric Artery **8** Renal Arteries, Bilateral **C** Pelvic Arteries **F** Lower Extremity Arteries, Right **G** Lower Extremity Arteries, Left **H** Lower Extremity Arteries, Bilateral **M** Renal Artery Transplant	**Z** None	**2** Intravascular Optical Coherence **Z** None	**Z** None

Section B **Imaging**
Body System 4 **Lower Arteries**
Type 3 **Magnetic Resonance Imaging (MRI):** Computer reformatted digital display of multiplanar images developed from the capture of radiofrequency signals emitted by nuclei in a body site excited within a magnetic field

Body Part (4th)	Contrast (5th)	Qualifier (6th)	Qualifier (7th)
0 Abdominal Aorta **1** Celiac Artery **4** Superior Mesenteric Artery **8** Renal Arteries, Bilateral **C** Pelvic Arteries **F** Lower Extremity Arteries, Right **G** Lower Extremity Arteries, Left **H** Lower Extremity Arteries, Bilateral	**Y** Other Contrast	**0** Unenhanced and Enhanced **Z** None	**Z** None

Continued →

Section B **Imaging**
Body System 4 **Lower Arteries**
Type 3 **Magnetic Resonance Imaging (MRI):** Computer reformatted digital display of multiplanar images developed from the capture of radiofrequency signals emitted by nuclei in a body site excited within a magnetic field

Body Part (4th)	Contrast (5th)	Qualifier (6th)	Qualifier (7th)
0 Abdominal Aorta **1** Celiac Artery **4** Superior Mesenteric Artery **8** Renal Arteries, Bilateral **C** Pelvic Arteries **F** Lower Extremity Arteries, Right **G** Lower Extremity Arteries, Left **H** Lower Extremity Arteries, Bilateral	**Z** None	**Z** None	**Z** None

Section B **Imaging**
Body System 4 **Lower Arteries**
Type 4 **Ultrasonography:** Real time display of images of anatomy or flow information developed from the capture of reflected and attenuated high frequency sound waves

Body Part (4th)	Contrast (5th)	Qualifier (6th)	Qualifier (7th)
0 Abdominal Aorta **4** Superior Mesenteric Artery **5** Inferior Mesenteric Artery **6** Renal Artery, Right **7** Renal Artery, Left **8** Renal Arteries, Bilateral **B** Intra-Abdominal Arteries, Other **F** Lower Extremity Arteries, Right **G** Lower Extremity Arteries, Left **H** Lower Extremity Arteries, Bilateral **K** Celiac and Mesenteric Arteries **L** Femoral Artery **N** Penile Arteries	**Z** None	**Z** None	**3** Intravascular **Z** None

Section B **Imaging**
Body System 5 **Veins**
Type 0 **Plain Radiography:** Planar display of an image developed from the capture of external ionizing radiation on photographic or photoconductive plate

Body Part (4th)	Contrast (5th)	Qualifier (6th)	Qualifier (7th)
0 Epidural Veins **1** Cerebral and Cerebellar Veins **2** Intracranial Sinuses **3** Jugular Veins, Right **4** Jugular Veins, Left **5** Jugular Veins, Bilateral **6** Subclavian Vein, Right **7** Subclavian Vein, Left **8** Superior Vena Cava **9** Inferior Vena Cava **B** Lower Extremity Veins, Right **C** Lower Extremity Veins, Left **D** Lower Extremity Veins, Bilateral **F** Pelvic (Iliac) Veins, Right **G** Pelvic (Iliac) Veins, Left **H** Pelvic (Iliac) Veins, Bilateral **J** Renal Vein, Right **K** Renal Vein, Left **L** Renal Veins, Bilateral **M** Upper Extremity Veins, Right **N** Upper Extremity Veins, Left **P** Upper Extremity Veins, Bilateral **Q** Pulmonary Vein, Right **R** Pulmonary Vein, Left **S** Pulmonary Veins, Bilateral **T** Portal and Splanchnic Veins **V** Veins, Other **W** Dialysis Shunt/Fistula	**0** High Osmolar **1** Low Osmolar **Y** Other Contrast	**Z** None	**Z** None

Section B **Imaging**
Body System 5 **Veins**
Type 1 **Fluoroscopy:** Single plane or bi-plane real time display of an image developed from the capture of external ionizing radiation on a fluorescent screen. The image may also be stored by either digital or analog means

Body Part (4th)	Contrast (5th)	Qualifier (6th)	Qualifier (7th)
0 Epidural Veins **1** Cerebral and Cerebellar Veins **2** Intracranial Sinuses **3** Jugular Veins, Right **4** Jugular Veins, Left **5** Jugular Veins, Bilateral **6** Subclavian Vein, Right **7** Subclavian Vein, Left **8** Superior Vena Cava **9** Inferior Vena Cava **B** Lower Extremity Veins, Right **C** Lower Extremity Veins, Left **D** Lower Extremity Veins, Bilateral **F** Pelvic (Iliac) Veins, Right **G** Pelvic (Iliac) Veins, Left **H** Pelvic (Iliac) Veins, Bilateral **J** Renal Vein, Right **K** Renal Vein, Left **L** Renal Veins, Bilateral **M** Upper Extremity Veins, Right **N** Upper Extremity Veins, Left **P** Upper Extremity Veins, Bilateral **Q** Pulmonary Vein, Right **R** Pulmonary Vein, Left **S** Pulmonary Veins, Bilateral **T** Portal and Splanchnic Veins **V** Veins, Other **W** Dialysis Shunt/Fistula	**0** High Osmolar **1** Low Osmolar **Y** Other Contrast **Z** None	**Z** None	**A** Guidance **Z** None

Section B **Imaging**
Body System 5 **Veins**
Type 2 **Computerized Tomography (CT Scan):** Computer reformatted digital display of multiplanar images developed from the capture of multiple exposures of external ionizing radiation

Body Part (4th)	Contrast (5th)	Qualifier (6th)	Qualifier (7th)
2 Intracranial Sinuses **8** Superior Vena Cava **9** Inferior Vena Cava **F** Pelvic (Iliac) Veins, Right **G** Pelvic (Iliac) Veins, Left **H** Pelvic (Iliac) Veins, Bilateral **J** Renal Vein, Right **K** Renal Vein, Left **L** Renal Veins, Bilateral **Q** Pulmonary Vein, Right **R** Pulmonary Vein, Left **S** Pulmonary Veins, Bilateral **T** Portal and Splanchnic Veins	**0** High Osmolar **1** Low Osmolar **Y** Other Contrast	**0** Unenhanced and Enhanced **Z** None	**Z** None
2 Intracranial Sinuses **8** Superior Vena Cava **9** Inferior Vena Cava **F** Pelvic (Iliac) Veins, Right **G** Pelvic (Iliac) Veins, Left **H** Pelvic (Iliac) Veins, Bilateral **J** Renal Vein, Right **K** Renal Vein, Left **L** Renal Veins, Bilateral **Q** Pulmonary Vein, Right **R** Pulmonary Vein, Left **S** Pulmonary Veins, Bilateral **T** Portal and Splanchnic Veins	**Z** None	**2** Intravascular Optical Coherence **Z** None	**Z** None

Section B **Imaging**
Body System 5 **Veins**
Type 3 **Magnetic Resonance Imaging (MRI):** Computer reformatted digital display of multiplanar images developed from the capture of radiofrequency signals emitted by nuclei in a body site excited within a magnetic field

Body Part (4th)	Contrast (5th)	Qualifier (6th)	Qualifier (7th)
1 Cerebral and Cerebellar Veins **2** Intracranial Sinuses **5** Jugular Veins, Bilateral **8** Superior Vena Cava **9** Inferior Vena Cava **B** Lower Extremity Veins, Right **C** Lower Extremity Veins, Left **D** Lower Extremity Veins, Bilateral **H** Pelvic (Iliac) Veins, Bilateral **L** Renal Veins, Bilateral **M** Upper Extremity Veins, Right **N** Upper Extremity Veins, Left **P** Upper Extremity Veins, Bilateral **S** Pulmonary Veins, Bilateral **T** Portal and Splanchnic Veins **V** Veins, Other	**Y** Other Contrast	**0** Unenhanced and Enhanced **Z** None	**Z** None

Continued →

Section B **Imaging**
Body System 5 **Veins**
Type 3 **Magnetic Resonance Imaging (MRI):** Computer reformatted digital display of multiplanar images developed from the capture of radiofrequency signals emitted by nuclei in a body site excited within a magnetic field

Body Part (4th)	Contrast (5th)	Qualifier (6th)	Qualifier (7th)
1 Cerebral and Cerebellar Veins **2** Intracranial Sinuses **5** Jugular Veins, Bilateral **8** Superior Vena Cava **9** Inferior Vena Cava **B** Lower Extremity Veins, Right **C** Lower Extremity Veins, Left **D** Lower Extremity Veins, Bilateral **H** Pelvic (Iliac) Veins, Bilateral **L** Renal Veins, Bilateral **M** Upper Extremity Veins, Right **N** Upper Extremity Veins, Left **P** Upper Extremity Veins, Bilateral **S** Pulmonary Veins, Bilateral **T** Portal and Splanchnic Veins **V** Veins, Other	**Z** None	**Z** None	**Z** None

Section B **Imaging**
Body System 5 **Veins**
Type 4 **Ultrasonography:** Real time display of images of anatomy or flow information developed from the capture of reflected and attenuated high frequency sound waves

Body Part (4th)	Contrast (5th)	Qualifier (6th)	Qualifier (7th)
3 Jugular Veins, Right **4** Jugular Veins, Left **6** Subclavian Vein, Right **7** Subclavian Vein, Left **8** Superior Vena Cava **9** Inferior Vena Cava **B** Lower Extremity Veins, Right **C** Lower Extremity Veins, Left **D** Lower Extremity Veins, Bilateral **J** Renal Vein, Right **K** Renal Vein, Left **L** Renal Veins, Bilateral **M** Upper Extremity Veins, Right **N** Upper Extremity Veins, Left **P** Upper Extremity Veins, Bilateral **T** Portal and Splanchnic Veins	**Z** None	**Z** None	**3** Intravascular **A** Guidance **Z** None

Section B **Imaging**
Body System 7 **Lymphatic System**
Type 0 **Plain Radiography:** Planar display of an image developed from the capture of external ionizing radiation on photographic or photoconductive plate

Body Part (4th)	Contrast (5th)	Qualifier (6th)	Qualifier (7th)
0 Abdominal/Retroperitoneal Lymphatics, Unilateral **1** Abdominal/Retroperitoneal Lymphatics, Bilateral **4** Lymphatics, Head and Neck **5** Upper Extremity Lymphatics, Right **6** Upper Extremity Lymphatics, Left **7** Upper Extremity Lymphatics, Bilateral **8** Lower Extremity Lymphatics, Right **9** Lower Extremity Lymphatics, Left **B** Lower Extremity Lymphatics, Bilateral **C** Lymphatics, Pelvic	**0** High Osmolar **1** Low Osmolar **Y** Other Contrast	**Z** None	**Z** None

Section B **Imaging**
Body System 8 **Eye**
Type 0 **Plain Radiography:** Planar display of an image developed from the capture of external ionizing radiation on photographic or photoconductive plate

Body Part (4th)	Contrast (5th)	Qualifier (6th)	Qualifier (7th)
0 Lacrimal Duct, Right **1** Lacrimal Duct, Left **2** Lacrimal Ducts, Bilateral	**0** High Osmolar **1** Low Osmolar **Y** Other Contrast	**Z** None	**Z** None
3 Optic Foramina, Right **4** Optic Foramina, Left **5** Eye, Right **6** Eye, Left **7** Eyes, Bilateral	**Z** None	**Z** None	**Z** None

Section B **Imaging**
Body System 8 **Eye**
Type 2 **Computerized Tomography (CT Scan):** Computer reformatted digital display of multiplanar images developed from the capture of multiple exposures of external ionizing radiation

Body Part (4th)	Contrast (5th)	Qualifier (6th)	Qualifier (7th)
5 Eye, Right **6** Eye, Left **7** Eyes, Bilateral	**0** High Osmolar **1** Low Osmolar **Y** Other Contrast	**0** Unenhanced and Enhanced **Z** None	**Z** None
5 Eye, Right **6** Eye, Left **7** Eyes, Bilateral	**Z** None	**Z** None	**Z** None

Section B **Imaging**
Body System 8 **Eye**
Type 3 **Magnetic Resonance Imaging (MRI):** Computer reformatted digital display of multiplanar images developed from the capture of radiofrequency signals emitted by nuclei in a body site excited within a magnetic field

Body Part (4th)	Contrast (5th)	Qualifier (6th)	Qualifier (7th)
5 Eye, Right **6** Eye, Left **7** Eyes, Bilateral	**Y** Other Contrast	**0** Unenhanced and Enhanced **Z** None	**Z** None
5 Eye, Right **6** Eye, Left **7** Eyes, Bilateral	**Z** None	**Z** None	**Z** None

Section B **Imaging**
Body System 8 **Eye**
Type 4 **Ultrasonography:** Real time display of images of anatomy or flow information developed from the capture of reflected and attenuated high frequency sound waves

Body Part (4th)	Contrast (5th)	Qualifier (6th)	Qualifier (7th)
5 Eye, Right **6** Eye, Left **7** Eyes, Bilateral	**Z** None	**Z** None	**Z** None

Section B **Imaging**
Body System 9 **Ear, Nose, Mouth and Throat**
Type 0 **Plain Radiography:** Planar display of an image developed from the capture of external ionizing radiation on photographic or photoconductive plate

Body Part (4th)	Contrast (5th)	Qualifier (6th)	Qualifier (7th)
2 Paranasal Sinuses F Nasopharynx/Oropharynx H Mastoids	Z None	Z None	Z None
4 Parotid Gland, Right 5 Parotid Gland, Left 6 Parotid Glands, Bilateral 7 Submandibular Gland, Right 8 Submandibular Gland, Left 9 Submandibular Glands, Bilateral B Salivary Gland, Right C Salivary Gland, Left D Salivary Glands, Bilateral	0 High Osmolar 1 Low Osmolar Y Other Contrast	Z None	Z None

Section B **Imaging**
Body System 9 **Ear, Nose, Mouth and Throat**
Type 1 **Fluoroscopy:** Single plane or bi-plane real time display of an image developed from the capture of external ionizing radiation on a fluorescent screen. The image may also be stored by either digital or analog means

Body Part (4th)	Contrast (5th)	Qualifier (6th)	Qualifier (7th)
G Pharynx and Epiglottis J Larynx	Y Other Contrast Z None	Z None	Z None

Section B **Imaging**
Body System 9 **Ear, Nose, Mouth and Throat**
Type 2 **Computerized Tomography (CT Scan):** Computer reformatted digital display of multiplanar images developed from the capture of multiple exposures of external ionizing radiation

Body Part (4th)	Contrast (5th)	Qualifier (6th)	Qualifier (7th)
0 Ear 2 Paranasal Sinuses 6 Parotid Glands, Bilateral 9 Submandibular Glands, Bilateral D Salivary Glands, Bilateral F Nasopharynx/Oropharynx J Larynx	0 High Osmolar 1 Low Osmolar Y Other Contrast	0 Unenhanced and Enhanced Z None	Z None
0 Ear 2 Paranasal Sinuses 6 Parotid Glands, Bilateral 9 Submandibular Glands, Bilateral D Salivary Glands, Bilateral F Nasopharynx/Oropharynx J Larynx	Z None	Z None	Z None

Section B **Imaging**
Body System 9 **Ear, Nose, Mouth and Throat**
Type 3 **Magnetic Resonance Imaging (MRI):** Computer reformatted digital display of multiplanar images developed from the capture of radiofrequency signals emitted by nuclei in a body site excited within a magnetic field

Body Part (4th)	Contrast (5th)	Qualifier (6th)	Qualifier (7th)
0 Ear 2 Paranasal Sinuses 6 Parotid Glands, Bilateral 9 Submandibular Glands, Bilateral D Salivary Glands, Bilateral F Nasopharynx/Oropharynx J Larynx	Y Other Contrast	0 Unenhanced and Enhanced Z None	Z None

Continued →

Section B **Imaging**
Body System 9 **Ear, Nose, Mouth and Throat**
Type 3 **Magnetic Resonance Imaging (MRI):** Computer reformatted digital display of multiplanar images developed from the capture of radiofrequency signals emitted by nuclei in a body site excited within a magnetic field

Body Part (4th)	Contrast (5th)	Qualifier (6th)	Qualifier (7th)
0 Ear **2** Paranasal Sinuses **6** Parotid Glands, Bilateral **9** Submandibular Glands, Bilateral **D** Salivary Glands, Bilateral **F** Nasopharynx/Oropharynx **J** Larynx	**Z** None	**Z** None	**Z** None

Section B **Imaging**
Body System B **Respiratory System**
Type 0 **Plain Radiography:** Planar display of an image developed from the capture of external ionizing radiation on photographic or photoconductive plate

Body Part (4th)	Contrast (5th)	Qualifier (6th)	Qualifier (7th)
7 Tracheobronchial Tree, Right **8** Tracheobronchial Tree, Left **9** Tracheobronchial Trees, Bilateral	**Y** Other Contrast	**Z** None	**Z** None
D Upper Airways	**Z** None	**Z** None	**Z** None

Section B **Imaging**
Body System B **Respiratory System**
Type 1 **Fluoroscopy:** Single plane or bi-plane real time display of an image developed from the capture of external ionizing radiation on a fluorescent screen. The image may also be stored by either digital or analog means

Body Part (4th)	Contrast (5th)	Qualifier (6th)	Qualifier (7th)
2 Lung, Right **3** Lung, Left **4** Lungs, Bilateral **6** Diaphragm **C** Mediastinum **D** Upper Airways	**Z** None	**Z** None	**Z** None
7 Tracheobronchial Tree, Right **8** Tracheobronchial Tree, Left **9** Tracheobronchial Trees, Bilateral	**Y** Other Contrast	**Z** None	**Z** None

Section B **Imaging**
Body System B **Respiratory System**
Type 2 **Computerized Tomography (CT Scan):** Computer reformatted digital display of multiplanar images developed from the capture of multiple exposures of external ionizing radiation

Body Part (4th)	Contrast (5th)	Qualifier (6th)	Qualifier (7th)
4 Lungs, Bilateral **7** Tracheobronchial Tree, Right **8** Tracheobronchial Tree, Left **9** Tracheobronchial Trees, Bilateral **F** Trachea/Airways	**0** High Osmolar **1** Low Osmolar **Y** Other Contrast	**0** Unenhanced and Enhanced **Z** None	**Z** None
4 Lungs, Bilateral **7** Tracheobronchial Tree, Right **8** Tracheobronchial Tree, Left **9** Tracheobronchial Trees, Bilateral **F** Trachea/Airways	**Z** None	**Z** None	**Z** None

Section B **Imaging**
Body System B **Respiratory System**
Type 3 **Magnetic Resonance Imaging (MRI):** Computer reformatted digital display of multiplanar images developed from the capture of radiofrequency signals emitted by nuclei in a body site excited within a magnetic field

Body Part (4th)	Contrast (5th)	Qualifier (6th)	Qualifier (7th)
G Lung Apices	Y Other Contrast	0 Unenhanced and Enhanced Z None	Z None
G Lung Apices	Z None	Z None	Z None

Section B **Imaging**
Body System B **Respiratory System**
Type 4 **Ultrasonography:** Real time display of images of anatomy or flow information developed from the capture of reflected and attenuated high frequency sound waves

Body Part (4th)	Contrast (5th)	Qualifier (6th)	Qualifier (7th)
B Pleura C Mediastinum	Z None	Z None	Z None

Section B **Imaging**
Body System D **Gastrointestinal System**
Type 1 **Fluoroscopy:** Single plane or bi-plane real time display of an image developed from the capture of external ionizing radiation on a fluorescent screen. The image may also be stored by either digital or analog means

Body Part (4th)	Contrast (5th)	Qualifier (6th)	Qualifier (7th)
1 Esophagus 2 Stomach 3 Small Bowel 4 Colon 5 Upper GI 6 Upper GI and Small Bowel 9 Duodenum B Mouth/Oropharynx	Y Other Contrast Z None	Z None	Z None

Section B **Imaging**
Body System D **Gastrointestinal System**
Type 2 **Computerized Tomography (CT Scan):** Computer reformatted digital display of multiplanar images developed from the capture of multiple exposures of external ionizing radiation

Body Part (4th)	Contrast (5th)	Qualifier (6th)	Qualifier (7th)
4 Colon	0 High Osmolar 1 Low Osmolar Y Other Contrast	0 Unenhanced and Enhanced Z None	Z None
4 Colon	Z None	Z None	Z None

Section B **Imaging**
Body System D **Gastrointestinal System**
Type 4 **Ultrasonography:** Real time display of images of anatomy or flow information developed from the capture of reflected and attenuated high frequency sound waves

Body Part (4th)	Contrast (5th)	Qualifier (6th)	Qualifier (7th)
1 Esophagus 2 Stomach 7 Gastrointestinal Tract 8 Appendix 9 Duodenum C Rectum	Z None	Z None	Z None

Section B **Imaging**
Body System F **Hepatobiliary System and Pancreas**
Type 0 **Plain Radiography:** Planar display of an image developed from the capture of external ionizing radiation on photographic or photoconductive plate

Body Part (4th)	Contrast (5th)	Qualifier (6th)	Qualifier (7th)
0 Bile Ducts **3** Gallbladder and Bile Ducts **C** Hepatobiliary System, All	**0** High Osmolar **1** Low Osmolar **Y** Other Contrast	**Z** None	**Z** None

Section B **Imaging**
Body System F **Hepatobiliary System and Pancreas**
Type 1 **Fluoroscopy:** Single plane or bi-plane real time display of an image developed from the capture of external ionizing radiation on a fluorescent screen. The image may also be stored by either digital or analog means

Body Part (4th)	Contrast (5th)	Qualifier (6th)	Qualifier (7th)
0 Bile Ducts **1** Biliary and Pancreatic Ducts **2** Gallbladder **3** Gallbladder and Bile Ducts **4** Gallbladder, Bile Ducts and Pancreatic Ducts **8** Pancreatic Ducts	**0** High Osmolar **1** Low Osmolar **Y** Other Contrast	**Z** None	**Z** None

Section B **Imaging**
Body System F **Hepatobiliary System and Pancreas**
Type 2 **Computerized Tomography (CT Scan):** Computer reformatted digital display of multiplanar images developed from the capture of multiple exposures of external ionizing radiation

Body Part (4th)	Contrast (5th)	Qualifier (6th)	Qualifier (7th)
5 Liver **6** Liver and Spleen **7** Pancreas **C** Hepatobiliary System, All	**0** High Osmolar **1** Low Osmolar **Y** Other Contrast	**0** Unenhanced and Enhanced **Z** None	**Z** None
5 Liver **6** Liver and Spleen **7** Pancreas **C** Hepatobiliary System, All	**Z** None	**Z** None	**Z** None

Section B **Imaging**
Body System F **Hepatobiliary System and Pancreas**
Type 3 **Magnetic Resonance Imaging (MRI):** Computer reformatted digital display of multiplanar images developed from the capture of radiofrequency signals emitted by nuclei in a body site excited within a magnetic field

Body Part (4th)	Contrast (5th)	Qualifier (6th)	Qualifier (7th)
5 Liver **6** Liver and Spleen **7** Pancreas	**Y** Other Contrast	**0** Unenhanced and Enhanced **Z** None	**Z** None
5 Liver **6** Liver and Spleen **7** Pancreas	**Z** None	**Z** None	**Z** None

Section B **Imaging**
Body System F **Hepatobiliary System and Pancreas**
Type 4 **Ultrasonography:** Real time display of images of anatomy or flow information developed from the capture of reflected and attenuated high frequency sound waves

Body Part (4th)	Contrast (5th)	Qualifier (6th)	Qualifier (7th)
0 Bile Ducts **2** Gallbladder **3** Gallbladder and Bile Ducts **5** Liver **6** Liver and Spleen **7** Pancreas **C** Hepatobiliary System, All	**Z** None	**Z** None	**Z** None

Section B **Imaging**
Body System G **Endocrine System**
Type 2 **Computerized Tomography (CT Scan):** Computer reformatted digital display of multiplanar images developed from the capture of multiple exposures of external ionizing radiation

Body Part (4th)	Contrast (5th)	Qualifier (6th)	Qualifier (7th)
2 Adrenal Glands, Bilateral **3** Parathyroid Glands **4** Thyroid Gland	**0** High Osmolar **1** Low Osmolar **Y** Other Contrast	**0** Unenhanced and Enhanced **Z** None	**Z** None
2 Adrenal Glands, Bilateral **3** Parathyroid Glands **4** Thyroid Gland	**Z** None	**Z** None	**Z** None

Section B **Imaging**
Body System G **Endocrine System**
Type 3 **Magnetic Resonance Imaging (MRI):** Computer reformatted digital display of multiplanar images developed from the capture of radiofrequency signals emitted by nuclei in a body site excited within a magnetic field

Body Part (4th)	Contrast (5th)	Qualifier (6th)	Qualifier (7th)
2 Adrenal Glands, Bilateral **3** Parathyroid Glands **4** Thyroid Gland	**Y** Other Contrast	**0** Unenhanced and Enhanced **Z** None	**Z** None
2 Adrenal Glands, Bilateral **3** Parathyroid Glands **4** Thyroid Gland	**Z** None	**Z** None	**Z** None

Section B **Imaging**
Body System G **Endocrine System**
Type 4 **Ultrasonography:** Real time display of images of anatomy or flow information developed from the capture of reflected and attenuated high frequency sound waves

Body Part (4th)	Contrast (5th)	Qualifier (6th)	Qualifier (7th)
0 Adrenal Gland, Right **1** Adrenal Gland, Left **2** Adrenal Glands, Bilateral **3** Parathyroid Glands **4** Thyroid Gland	**Z** None	**Z** None	**Z** None

Section B **Imaging**
Body System H **Skin, Subcutaneous Tissue and Breast**
Type 0 **Plain Radiography:** Planar display of an image developed from the capture of external ionizing radiation on photographic or photoconductive plate

Body Part (4th)	Contrast (5th)	Qualifier (6th)	Qualifier (7th)
0 Breast, Right **1** Breast, Left **2** Breasts, Bilateral	**Z** None	**Z** None	**Z** None
3 Single Mammary Duct, Right **4** Single Mammary Duct, Left **5** Multiple Mammary Ducts, Right **6** Multiple Mammary Ducts, Left	**0** High Osmolar **1** Low Osmolar **Y** Other Contrast **Z** None	**Z** None	**Z** None

Section B **Imaging**
Body System H **Skin, Subcutaneous Tissue and Breast**
Type 3 **Magnetic Resonance Imaging (MRI):** Computer reformatted digital display of multiplanar images developed from the capture of radiofrequency signals emitted by nuclei in a body site excited within a magnetic field

Body Part (4th)	Contrast (5th)	Qualifier (6th)	Qualifier (7th)
0 Breast, Right **1** Breast, Left **2** Breasts, Bilateral **D** Subcutaneous Tissue, Head/Neck **F** Subcutaneous Tissue, Upper Extremity **G** Subcutaneous Tissue, Thorax **H** Subcutaneous Tissue, Abdomen and Pelvis **J** Subcutaneous Tissue, Lower Extremity	**Y** Other Contrast	**0** Unenhanced and Enhanced **Z** None	**Z** None
0 Breast, Right **1** Breast, Left **2** Breasts, Bilateral **D** Subcutaneous Tissue, Head/Neck **F** Subcutaneous Tissue, Upper Extremity **G** Subcutaneous Tissue, Thorax **H** Subcutaneous Tissue, Abdomen and Pelvis **J** Subcutaneous Tissue, Lower Extremity	**Z** None	**Z** None	**Z** None

Section B **Imaging**
Body System H **Skin, Subcutaneous Tissue and Breast**
Type 4 **Ultrasonography:** Real time display of images of anatomy or flow information developed from the capture of reflected and attenuated high frequency sound waves

Body Part (4th)	Contrast (5th)	Qualifier (6th)	Qualifier (7th)
0 Breast, Right **1** Breast, Left **2** Breasts, Bilateral **7** Extremity, Upper **8** Extremity, Lower **9** Abdominal Wall **B** Chest Wall **C** Head and Neck	**Z** None	**Z** None	**Z** None

Section B Imaging
Body System L Connective Tissue
Type 3 **Magnetic Resonance Imaging (MRI):** Computer reformatted digital display of multiplanar images developed from the capture of radiofrequency signals emitted by nuclei in a body site excited within a magnetic field

Body Part (4th)	Contrast (5th)	Qualifier (6th)	Qualifier (7th)
0 Connective Tissue, Upper Extremity 1 Connective Tissue, Lower Extremity 2 Tendons, Upper Extremity 3 Tendons, Lower Extremity	Y Other Contrast	0 Unenhanced and Enhanced Z None	Z None
0 Connective Tissue, Upper Extremity 1 Connective Tissue, Lower Extremity 2 Tendons, Upper Extremity 3 Tendons, Lower Extremity	Z None	Z None	Z None

Section B Imaging
Body System L Connective Tissue
Type 4 **Ultrasonography:** Real time display of images of anatomy or flow information developed from the capture of reflected and attenuated high frequency sound waves

Body Part (4th)	Contrast (5th)	Qualifier (6th)	Qualifier (7th)
0 Connective Tissue, Upper Extremity 1 Connective Tissue, Lower Extremity 2 Tendons, Upper Extremity 3 Tendons, Lower Extremity	Z None	Z None	Z None

Section B Imaging
Body System N Skull and Facial Bones
Type 0 **Plain Radiography:** Planar display of an image developed from the capture of external ionizing radiation on photographic or photoconductive plate

Body Part (4th)	Contrast (5th)	Qualifier (6th)	Qualifier (7th)
0 Skull 1 Orbit, Right 2 Orbit, Left 3 Orbits, Bilateral 4 Nasal Bones 5 Facial Bones 6 Mandible B Zygomatic Arch, Right C Zygomatic Arch, Left D Zygomatic Arches, Bilateral G Tooth, Single H Teeth, Multiple J Teeth, All	Z None	Z None	Z None
7 Temporomandibular Joint, Right 8 Temporomandibular Joint, Left 9 Temporomandibular Joints, Bilateral	0 High Osmolar 1 Low Osmolar Y Other Contrast Z None	Z None	Z None

Section B Imaging
Body System N Skull and Facial Bones
Type 1 **Fluoroscopy:** Single plane or bi-plane real time display of an image developed from the capture of external ionizing radiation on a fluorescent screen. The image may also be stored by either digital or analog means

Body Part (4th)	Contrast (5th)	Qualifier (6th)	Qualifier (7th)
7 Temporomandibular Joint, Right 8 Temporomandibular Joint, Left 9 Temporomandibular Joints, Bilateral	0 High Osmolar 1 Low Osmolar Y Other Contrast Z None	Z None	Z None

Section B **Imaging**
Body System N **Skull and Facial Bones**
Type 2 **Computerized Tomography (CT Scan):** Computer reformatted digital display of multiplanar images developed from the capture of multiple exposures of external ionizing radiation

Body Part (4th)	Contrast (5th)	Qualifier (6th)	Qualifier (7th)
0 Skull **3** Orbits, Bilateral **5** Facial Bones **6** Mandible **9** Temporomandibular Joints, Bilateral **F** Temporal Bones	**0** High Osmolar **1** Low Osmolar **Y** Other Contrast **Z** None	**Z** None	**Z** None

Section B **Imaging**
Body System N **Skull and Facial Bones**
Type 3 **Magnetic Resonance Imaging (MRI):** Computer reformatted digital display of multiplanar images developed from the capture of radiofrequency signals emitted by nuclei in a body site excited within a magnetic field

Body Part (4th)	Contrast (5th)	Qualifier (6th)	Qualifier (7th)
9 Temporomandibular Joints, Bilateral	**Y** Other Contrast **Z** None	**Z** None	**Z** None

Section B **Imaging**
Body System P **Non-Axial Upper Bones**
Type 0 **Plain Radiography:** Planar display of an image developed from the capture of external ionizing radiation on photographic or photoconductive plate

Body Part (4th)	Contrast (5th)	Qualifier (6th)	Qualifier (7th)
0 Sternoclavicular Joint, Right **1** Sternoclavicular Joint, Left **2** Sternoclavicular Joints, Bilateral **3** Acromioclavicular Joints, Bilateral **4** Clavicle, Right **5** Clavicle, Left **6** Scapula, Right **7** Scapula, Left **A** Humerus, Right **B** Humerus, Left **E** Upper Arm, Right **F** Upper Arm, Left **J** Forearm, Right **K** Forearm, Left **N** Hand, Right **P** Hand, Left **R** Finger(s), Right **S** Finger(s), Left **X** Ribs, Right **Y** Ribs, Left	**Z** None	**Z** None	**Z** None
8 Shoulder, Right **9** Shoulder, Left **C** Hand/Finger Joint, Right **D** Hand/Finger Joint, Left **G** Elbow, Right **H** Elbow, Left **L** Wrist, Right **M** Wrist, Left	**0** High Osmolar **1** Low Osmolar **Y** Other Contrast **Z** None	**Z** None	**Z** None

Section B **Imaging**
Body System P **Non-Axial Upper Bones**
Type 1 **Fluoroscopy:** Single plane or bi-plane real time display of an image developed from the capture of external ionizing radiation on a fluorescent screen. The image may also be stored by either digital or analog means

Body Part (4th)	Contrast (5th)	Qualifier (6th)	Qualifier (7th)
0 Sternoclavicular Joint, Right **1** Sternoclavicular Joint, Left **2** Sternoclavicular Joints, Bilateral **3** Acromioclavicular Joints, Bilateral **4** Clavicle, Right **5** Clavicle, Left **6** Scapula, Right **7** Scapula, Left **A** Humerus, Right **B** Humerus, Left **E** Upper Arm, Right **F** Upper Arm, Left **J** Forearm, Right **K** Forearm, Left **N** Hand, Right **P** Hand, Left **R** Finger(s), Right **S** Finger(s), Left **X** Ribs, Right **Y** Ribs, Left	**Z** None	**Z** None	**Z** None
8 Shoulder, Right **9** Shoulder, Left **L** Wrist, Right **M** Wrist, Left	**0** High Osmolar **1** Low Osmolar **Y** Other Contrast **Z** None	**Z** None	**Z** None
C Hand/Finger Joint, Right **D** Hand/Finger Joint, Left **G** Elbow, Right **H** Elbow, Left	**0** High Osmolar **1** Low Osmolar **Y** Other Contrast	**Z** None	**Z** None

Section B **Imaging**
Body System P **Non-Axial Upper Bones**
Type 2 **Computerized Tomography (CT Scan):** Computer reformatted digital display of multiplanar images developed from the capture of multiple exposures of external ionizing radiation

Body Part (4th)	Contrast (5th)	Qualifier (6th)	Qualifier (7th)
0 Sternoclavicular Joint, Right **1** Sternoclavicular Joint, Left **W** Thorax	**0** High Osmolar **1** Low Osmolar **Y** Other Contrast	**Z** None	**Z** None

Continued →

Section	**B**	**Imaging**
Body System	**P**	**Non-Axial Upper Bones**
Type	**2**	**Computerized Tomography (CT Scan):** Computer reformatted digital display of multiplanar images developed from the capture of multiple exposures of external ionizing radiation

Body Part (4th)	Contrast (5th)	Qualifier (6th)	Qualifier (7th)
2 Sternoclavicular Joints, Bilateral **3** Acromioclavicular Joints, Bilateral **4** Clavicle, Right **5** Clavicle, Left **6** Scapula, Right **7** Scapula, Left **8** Shoulder, Right **9** Shoulder, Left **A** Humerus, Right **B** Humerus, Left **E** Upper Arm, Right **F** Upper Arm, Left **G** Elbow, Right **H** Elbow, Left **J** Forearm, Right **K** Forearm, Left **L** Wrist, Right **M** Wrist, Left **N** Hand, Right **P** Hand, Left **Q** Hands and Wrists, Bilateral **R** Finger(s), Right **S** Finger(s), Left **T** Upper Extremity, Right **U** Upper Extremity, Left **V** Upper Extremities, Bilateral **X** Ribs, Right **Y** Ribs, Left	**0** High Osmolar **1** Low Osmolar **Y** Other Contrast **Z** None	**Z** None	**Z** None
C Hand/Finger Joint, Right **D** Hand/Finger Joint, Left	**Z** None	**Z** None	**Z** None

Section	**B**	**Imaging**
Body System	**P**	**Non-Axial Upper Bones**
Type	**3**	**Magnetic Resonance Imaging (MRI):** Computer reformatted digital display of multiplanar images developed from the capture of radiofrequency signals emitted by nuclei in a body site excited within a magnetic field

Body Part (4th)	Contrast (5th)	Qualifier (6th)	Qualifier (7th)
8 Shoulder, Right **9** Shoulder, Left **C** Hand/Finger Joint, Right **D** Hand/Finger Joint, Left **E** Upper Arm, Right **F** Upper Arm, Left **G** Elbow, Right **H** Elbow, Left **J** Forearm, Right **K** Forearm, Left **L** Wrist, Right **M** Wrist, Left	**Y** Other Contrast	**0** Unenhanced and Enhanced **Z** None	**Z** None

Continued →

Section B **Imaging**
Body System P **Non-Axial Upper Bones**
Type 3 **Magnetic Resonance Imaging (MRI):** Computer reformatted digital display of multiplanar images developed from the capture of radiofrequency signals emitted by nuclei in a body site excited within a magnetic field

Body Part (4th)	Contrast (5th)	Qualifier (6th)	Qualifier (7th)
8 Shoulder, Right **9** Shoulder, Left **C** Hand/Finger Joint, Right **D** Hand/Finger Joint, Left **E** Upper Arm, Right **F** Upper Arm, Left **G** Elbow, Right **H** Elbow, Left **J** Forearm, Right **K** Forearm, Left **L** Wrist, Right **M** Wrist, Left	**Z** None	**Z** None	**Z** None

Section B **Imaging**
Body System P **Non-Axial Upper Bones**
Type 4 **Ultrasonography:** Real time display of images of anatomy or flow information developed from the capture of reflected and attenuated high frequency sound waves

Body Part (4th)	Contrast (5th)	Qualifier (6th)	Qualifier (7th)
8 Shoulder, Right **9** Shoulder, Left **G** Elbow, Right **H** Elbow, Left **L** Wrist, Right **M** Wrist, Left **N** Hand, Right **P** Hand, Left	**Z** None	**Z** None	**1** Densitometry **Z** None

Section B **Imaging**
Body System Q **Non-Axial Lower Bones**
Type 0 **Plain Radiography:** Planar display of an image developed from the capture of external ionizing radiation on photographic or photoconductive plate

Body Part (4th)	Contrast (5th)	Qualifier (6th)	Qualifier (7th)
0 Hip, Right **1** Hip, Left	**0** High Osmolar **1** Low Osmolar **Y** Other Contrast	**Z** None	**Z** None
0 Hip, Right **1** Hip, Left	**Z** None	**Z** None	**1** Densitometry **Z** None
3 Femur, Right **4** Femur, Left	**Z** None	**Z** None	**1** Densitometry **Z** None
7 Knee, Right **8** Knee, Left **G** Ankle, Right **H** Ankle, Left	**0** High Osmolar **1** Low Osmolar **Y** Other Contrast **Z** None	**Z** None	**Z** None
D Lower Leg, Right **F** Lower Leg, Left **J** Calcaneus, Right **K** Calcaneus, Left **L** Foot, Right **M** Foot, Left **P** Toe(s), Right **Q** Toe(s), Left **V** Patella, Right **W** Patella, Left	**Z** None	**Z** None	**Z** None

Continued →

Section B **Imaging**
Body System Q **Non-Axial Lower Bones**
Type 0 **Plain Radiography:** Planar display of an image developed from the capture of external ionizing radiation on photographic or photoconductive plate

Body Part (4th)	Contrast (5th)	Qualifier (6th)	Qualifier (7th)
X Foot/Toe Joint, Right **Y** Foot/Toe Joint, Left	**0** High Osmolar **1** Low Osmolar **Y** Other Contrast	**Z** None	**Z** None

Section B **Imaging**
Body System Q **Non-Axial Lower Bones**
Type 1 **Fluoroscopy:** Single plane or bi-plane real time display of an image developed from the capture of external ionizing radiation on a fluorescent screen. The image may also be stored by either digital or analog means

Body Part (4th)	Contrast (5th)	Qualifier (6th)	Qualifier (7th)
0 Hip, Right **1** Hip, Left **7** Knee, Right **8** Knee, Left **G** Ankle, Right **H** Ankle, Left **X** Foot/Toe Joint, Right **Y** Foot/Toe Joint, Left	**0** High Osmolar **1** Low Osmolar **Y** Other Contrast **Z** None	**Z** None	**Z** None
3 Femur, Right **4** Femur, Left **D** Lower Leg, Right **F** Lower Leg, Left **J** Calcaneus, Right **K** Calcaneus, Left **L** Foot, Right **M** Foot, Left **P** Toe(s), Right **Q** Toe(s), Left **V** Patella, Right **W** Patella, Left	**Z** None	**Z** None	**Z** None

Section B **Imaging**
Body System Q **Non-Axial Lower Bones**
Type 2 **Computerized Tomography (CT Scan):** Computer reformatted digital display of multiplanar images developed from the capture of multiple exposures of external ionizing radiation

Body Part (4th)	Contrast (5th)	Qualifier (6th)	Qualifier (7th)
0 Hip, Right **1** Hip, Left **3** Femur, Right **4** Femur, Left **7** Knee, Right **8** Knee, Left **D** Lower Leg, Right **F** Lower Leg, Left **G** Ankle, Right **H** Ankle, Left **J** Calcaneus, Right **K** Calcaneus, Left **L** Foot, Right **M** Foot, Left **P** Toe(s), Right **Q** Toe(s), Left **R** Lower Extremity, Right **S** Lower Extremity, Left **V** Patella, Right **W** Patella, Left **X** Foot/Toe Joint, Right **Y** Foot/Toe Joint, Left	**0** High Osmolar **1** Low Osmolar **Y** Other Contrast **Z** None	**Z** None	**Z** None

Continued →

Section B **Imaging**
Body System Q **Non-Axial Lower Bones**
Type 2 **Computerized Tomography (CT Scan):** Computer reformatted digital display of multiplanar images developed from the capture of multiple exposures of external ionizing radiation

Body Part (4th)	Contrast (5th)	Qualifier (6th)	Qualifier (7th)
B Tibia/Fibula, Right **C** Tibia/Fibula, Left	**0** High Osmolar **1** Low Osmolar **Y** Other Contrast	**Z** None	**Z** None

Section B **Imaging**
Body System Q **Non-Axial Lower Bones**
Type 3 **Magnetic Resonance Imaging (MRI):** Computer reformatted digital display of multiplanar images developed from the capture of radiofrequency signals emitted by nuclei in a body site excited within a magnetic field

Body Part (4th)	Contrast (5th)	Qualifier (6th)	Qualifier (7th)
0 Hip, Right **1** Hip, Left **3** Femur, Right **4** Femur, Left **7** Knee, Right **8** Knee, Left **D** Lower Leg, Right **F** Lower Leg, Left **G** Ankle, Right **H** Ankle, Left **J** Calcaneus, Right **K** Calcaneus, Left **L** Foot, Right **M** Foot, Left **P** Toe(s), Right **Q** Toe(s), Left **V** Patella, Right **W** Patella, Left	**Y** Other Contrast	**0** Unenhanced and Enhanced **Z** None	**Z** None
0 Hip, Right **1** Hip, Left **3** Femur, Right **4** Femur, Left **7** Knee, Right **8** Knee, Left **D** Lower Leg, Right **F** Lower Leg, Left **G** Ankle, Right **H** Ankle, Left **J** Calcaneus, Right **K** Calcaneus, Left **L** Foot, Right **M** Foot, Left **P** Toe(s), Right **Q** Toe(s), Left **V** Patella, Right **W** Patella, Left	**Z** None	**Z** None	**Z** None

Section B **Imaging**
Body System Q **Non-Axial Lower Bones**
Type 4 **Ultrasonography:** Real time display of images of anatomy or flow information developed from the capture of reflected and attenuated high frequency sound waves

Body Part (4th)	Contrast (5th)	Qualifier (6th)	Qualifier (7th)
0 Hip, Right **1** Hip, Left **2** Hips, Bilateral **7** Knee, Right **8** Knee, Left **9** Knees, Bilateral	**Z** None	**Z** None	**Z** None

Section B **Imaging**
Body System R **Axial Skeleton, Except Skull and Facial Bones**
Type 0 **Plain Radiography:** Planar display of an image developed from the capture of external ionizing radiation on photographic or photoconductive plate

Body Part (4th)	Contrast (5th)	Qualifier (6th)	Qualifier (7th)
0 Cervical Spine **7** Thoracic Spine **9** Lumbar Spine **G** Whole Spine	**Z** None	**Z** None	**1** Densitometry **Z** None
1 Cervical Disc(s) **2** Thoracic Disc(s) **3** Lumbar Disc(s) **4** Cervical Facet Joint(s) **5** Thoracic Facet Joint(s) **6** Lumbar Facet Joint(s) **D** Sacroiliac Joints	**0** High Osmolar **1** Low Osmolar **Y** Other Contrast **Z** None	**Z** None	**Z** None
8 Thoracolumbar Joint **B** Lumbosacral Joint **C** Pelvis **F** Sacrum and Coccyx **H** Sternum	**Z** None	**Z** None	**Z** None

Section B **Imaging**
Body System R **Axial Skeleton, Except Skull and Facial Bones**
Type 1 **Fluoroscopy:** Single plane or bi-plane real time display of an image developed from the capture of external ionizing radiation on a fluorescent screen. The image may also be stored by either digital or analog means

Body Part (4th)	Contrast (5th)	Qualifier (6th)	Qualifier (7th)
0 Cervical Spine **1** Cervical Disc(s) **2** Thoracic Disc(s) **3** Lumbar Disc(s) **4** Cervical Facet Joint(s) **5** Thoracic Facet Joint(s) **6** Lumbar Facet Joint(s) **7** Thoracic Spine **8** Thoracolumbar Joint **9** Lumbar Spine **B** Lumbosacral Joint **C** Pelvis **D** Sacroiliac Joints **F** Sacrum and Coccyx **G** Whole Spine **H** Sternum	**0** High Osmolar **1** Low Osmolar **Y** Other Contrast **Z** None	**Z** None	**Z** None

Section B **Imaging**
Body System R **Axial Skeleton, Except Skull and Facial Bones**
Type 2 **Computerized Tomography (CT Scan):** Computer reformatted digital display of multiplanar images developed from the capture of multiple exposures of external ionizing radiation

Body Part (4th)	Contrast (5th)	Qualifier (6th)	Qualifier (7th)
0 Cervical Spine **7** Thoracic Spine **9** Lumbar Spine **C** Pelvis **D** Sacroiliac Joints **F** Sacrum and Coccyx	**0** High Osmolar **1** Low Osmolar **Y** Other Contrast **Z** None	**Z** None	**Z** None

Section B **Imaging**
Body System R **Axial Skeleton, Except Skull and Facial Bones**
Type 3 **Magnetic Resonance Imaging (MRI):** Computer reformatted digital display of multiplanar images developed from the capture of radiofrequency signals emitted by nuclei in a body site excited within a magnetic field

Body Part (4th)	Contrast (5th)	Qualifier (6th)	Qualifier (7th)
0 Cervical Spine **1** Cervical Disc(s) **2** Thoracic Disc(s) **3** Lumbar Disc(s) **7** Thoracic Spine **9** Lumbar Spine **C** Pelvis **F** Sacrum and Coccyx	**Y** Other Contrast	**0** Unenhanced and Enhanced **Z** None	**Z** None
0 Cervical Spine **1** Cervical Disc(s) **2** Thoracic Disc(s) **3** Lumbar Disc(s) **7** Thoracic Spine **9** Lumbar Spine **C** Pelvis **F** Sacrum and Coccyx	**Z** None	**Z** None	**Z** None

Section B **Imaging**
Body System R **Axial Skeleton, Except Skull and Facial Bones**
Type 4 **Ultrasonography:** Real time display of images of anatomy or flow information developed from the capture of reflected and attenuated high frequency sound waves

Body Part (4th)	Contrast (5th)	Qualifier (6th)	Qualifier (7th)
0 Cervical Spine **7** Thoracic Spine **9** Lumbar Spine **F** Sacrum and Coccyx	**Z** None	**Z** None	**Z** None

Section B **Imaging**
Body System T **Urinary System**
Type 0 **Plain Radiography:** Planar display of an image developed from the capture of external ionizing radiation on photographic or photoconductive plate

Body Part (4th)	Contrast (5th)	Qualifier (6th)	Qualifier (7th)
0 Bladder **1** Kidney, Right **2** Kidney, Left **3** Kidneys, Bilateral **4** Kidneys, Ureters and Bladder **5** Urethra **6** Ureter, Right **7** Ureter, Left **8** Ureters, Bilateral **B** Bladder and Urethra **C** Ileal Diversion Loop	**0** High Osmolar **1** Low Osmolar **Y** Other Contrast **Z** None	**Z** None	**Z** None

Section B **Imaging**
Body System T **Urinary System**
Type 1 **Fluoroscopy:** Single plane or bi-plane real time display of an image developed from the capture of external ionizing radiation on a fluorescent screen. The image may also be stored by either digital or analog means

Body Part (4th)	Contrast (5th)	Qualifier (6th)	Qualifier (7th)
0 Bladder **1** Kidney, Right **2** Kidney, Left **3** Kidneys, Bilateral **4** Kidneys, Ureters and Bladder **5** Urethra **6** Ureter, Right **7** Ureter, Left **B** Bladder and Urethra **C** Ileal Diversion Loop **D** Kidney, Ureter and Bladder, Right **F** Kidney, Ureter and Bladder, Left **G** Ileal Loop, Ureters and Kidneys	**0** High Osmolar **1** Low Osmolar **Y** Other Contrast **Z** None	**Z** None	**Z** None

Section B **Imaging**
Body System T **Urinary System**
Type 2 **Computerized Tomography (CT Scan):** Computer reformatted digital display of multiplanar images developed from the capture of multiple exposures of external ionizing radiation

Body Part (4th)	Contrast (5th)	Qualifier (6th)	Qualifier (7th)
0 Bladder **1** Kidney, Right **2** Kidney, Left **3** Kidneys, Bilateral **9** Kidney Transplant	**0** High Osmolar **1** Low Osmolar **Y** Other Contrast	**0** Unenhanced and Enhanced **Z** None	**Z** None
0 Bladder **1** Kidney, Right **2** Kidney, Left **3** Kidneys, Bilateral **9** Kidney Transplant	**Z** None	**Z** None	**Z** None

Section B **Imaging**
Body System T **Urinary System**
Type 3 **Magnetic Resonance Imaging (MRI):** Computer reformatted digital display of multiplanar images developed from the capture of radiofrequency signals emitted by nuclei in a body site excited within a magnetic field

Body Part (4th)	Contrast (5th)	Qualifier (6th)	Qualifier (7th)
0 Bladder **1** Kidney, Right **2** Kidney, Left **3** Kidneys, Bilateral **9** Kidney Transplant	**Y** Other Contrast	**0** Unenhanced and Enhanced **Z** None	**Z** None
0 Bladder **1** Kidney, Right **2** Kidney, Left **3** Kidneys, Bilateral **9** Kidney Transplant	**Z** None	**Z** None	**Z** None

Section B Imaging
Body System T Urinary System
Type 4 **Ultrasonography:** Real time display of images of anatomy or flow information developed from the capture of reflected and attenuated high frequency sound waves

Body Part (4th)	Contrast (5th)	Qualifier (6th)	Qualifier (7th)
0 Bladder 1 Kidney, Right 2 Kidney, Left 3 Kidneys, Bilateral 5 Urethra 6 Ureter, Right 7 Ureter, Left 8 Ureters, Bilateral 9 Kidney Transplant J Kidneys and Bladder	Z None	Z None	Z None

Section B Imaging
Body System U Female Reproductive System
Type 0 **Plain Radiography:** Planar display of an image developed from the capture of external ionizing radiation on photographic or photoconductive plate

Body Part (4th)	Contrast (5th)	Qualifier (6th)	Qualifier (7th)
0 Fallopian Tube, Right 1 Fallopian Tube, Left 2 Fallopian Tubes, Bilateral 6 Uterus 8 Uterus and Fallopian Tubes 9 Vagina	0 High Osmolar 1 Low Osmolar Y Other Contrast	Z None	Z None

Section B Imaging
Body System U Female Reproductive System
Type 1 **Fluoroscopy:** Single plane or bi-plane real time display of an image developed from the capture of external ionizing radiation on a fluorescent screen. The image may also be stored by either digital or analog means

Body Part (4th)	Contrast (5th)	Qualifier (6th)	Qualifier (7th)
0 Fallopian Tube, Right 1 Fallopian Tube, Left 2 Fallopian Tubes, Bilateral 6 Uterus 8 Uterus and Fallopian Tubes 9 Vagina	0 High Osmolar 1 Low Osmolar Y Other Contrast Z None	Z None	Z None

Section B Imaging
Body System U Female Reproductive System
Type 3 **Magnetic Resonance Imaging (MRI):** Computer reformatted digital display of multiplanar images developed from the capture of radiofrequency signals emitted by nuclei in a body site excited within a magnetic field

Body Part (4th)	Contrast (5th)	Qualifier (6th)	Qualifier (7th)
3 Ovary, Right 4 Ovary, Left 5 Ovaries, Bilateral 6 Uterus 9 Vagina B Pregnant Uterus C Uterus and Ovaries	Y Other Contrast	0 Unenhanced and Enhanced Z None	Z None
3 Ovary, Right 4 Ovary, Left 5 Ovaries, Bilateral 6 Uterus 9 Vagina B Pregnant Uterus C Uterus and Ovaries	Z None	Z None	Z None

Section B **Imaging**
Body System U **Female Reproductive System**
Type 4 **Ultrasonography:** Real time display of images of anatomy or flow information developed from the capture of reflected and attenuated high frequency sound waves

Body Part (4th)	Contrast (5th)	Qualifier (6th)	Qualifier (7th)
0 Fallopian Tube, Right **1** Fallopian Tube, Left **2** Fallopian Tubes, Bilateral **3** Ovary, Right **4** Ovary, Left **5** Ovaries, Bilateral **6** Uterus **C** Uterus and Ovaries	**Y** Other Contrast **Z** None	**Z** None	**Z** None

Section B **Imaging**
Body System V **Male Reproductive System**
Type 0 **Plain Radiography:** Planar display of an image developed from the capture of external ionizing radiation on photographic or photoconductive plate

Body Part (4th)	Contrast (5th)	Qualifier (6th)	Qualifier (7th)
0 Corpora Cavernosa **1** Epididymis, Right **2** Epididymis, Left **3** Prostate **5** Testicle, Right **6** Testicle, Left **8** Vasa Vasorum	**0** High Osmolar **1** Low Osmolar **Y** Other Contrast	**Z** None	**Z** None

Section B **Imaging**
Body System V **Male Reproductive System**
Type 1 **Fluoroscopy:** Single plane or bi-plane real time display of an image developed from the capture of external ionizing radiation on a fluorescent screen. The image may also be stored by either digital or analog means

Body Part (4th)	Contrast (5th)	Qualifier (6th)	Qualifier (7th)
0 Corpora Cavernosa **8** Vasa Vasorum	**0** High Osmolar **1** Low Osmolar **Y** Other Contrast **Z** None	**Z** None	**Z** None

Section B **Imaging**
Body System V **Male Reproductive System**
Type 2 **Computerized Tomography (CT Scan):** Computer reformatted digital display of multiplanar images developed from the capture of multiple exposures of external ionizing radiation

Body Part (4th)	Contrast (5th)	Qualifier (6th)	Qualifier (7th)
3 Prostate	**0** High Osmolar **1** Low Osmolar **Y** Other Contrast	**0** Unenhanced and Enhanced **Z** None	**Z** None
3 Prostate	**Z** None	**Z** None	**Z** None

Section B **Imaging**
Body System V **Male Reproductive System**
Type 3 **Magnetic Resonance Imaging (MRI):** Computer reformatted digital display of multiplanar images developed from the capture of radiofrequency signals emitted by nuclei in a body site excited within a magnetic field

Body Part (4th)	Contrast (5th)	Qualifier (6th)	Qualifier (7th)
0 Corpora Cavernosa **3** Prostate **4** Scrotum **5** Testicle, Right **6** Testicle, Left **7** Testicles, Bilateral	**Y** Other Contrast	**0** Unenhanced and Enhanced **Z** None	**Z** None
0 Corpora Cavernosa **3** Prostate **4** Scrotum **5** Testicle, Right **6** Testicle, Left **7** Testicles, Bilateral	**Z** None	**Z** None	**Z** None

Section B **Imaging**
Body System V **Male Reproductive System**
Type 4 **Ultrasonography:** Real time display of images of anatomy or flow information developed from the capture of reflected and attenuated high frequency sound waves

Body Part (4th)	Contrast (5th)	Qualifier (6th)	Qualifier (7th)
4 Scrotum **9** Prostate and Seminal Vesicles **B** Penis	**Z** None	**Z** None	**Z** None

Section B **Imaging**
Body System W **Anatomical Regions**
Type 0 **Plain Radiography:** Planar display of an image developed from the capture of external ionizing radiation on photographic or photoconductive plate

Body Part (4th)	Contrast (5th)	Qualifier (6th)	Qualifier (7th)
0 Abdomen **1** Abdomen and Pelvis **3** Chest **B** Long Bones, All **C** Lower Extremity **J** Upper Extremity **K** Whole Body **L** Whole Skeleton **M** Whole Body, Infant	**Z** None	**Z** None	**Z** None

Section B **Imaging**
Body System W **Anatomical Regions**
Type 1 **Fluoroscopy:** Single plane or bi-plane real time display of an image developed from the capture of external ionizing radiation on a fluorescent screen. The image may also be stored by either digital or analog means

Body Part (4th)	Contrast (5th)	Qualifier (6th)	Qualifier (7th)
1 Abdomen and Pelvis **9** Head and Neck **C** Lower Extremity **J** Upper Extremity	**0** High Osmolar **1** Low Osmolar **Y** Other Contrast **Z** None	**Z** None	**Z** None

Section B Imaging
Body System W Anatomical Regions
Type 2 Computerized Tomography (CT Scan): Computer reformatted digital display of multiplanar images developed from the capture of multiple exposures of external ionizing radiation

Body Part (4th)	Contrast (5th)	Qualifier (6th)	Qualifier (7th)
0 Abdomen 1 Abdomen and Pelvis 4 Chest and Abdomen 5 Chest, Abdomen and Pelvis 8 Head 9 Head and Neck F Neck G Pelvic Region	0 High Osmolar 1 Low Osmolar Y Other Contrast	0 Unenhanced and Enhanced Z None	Z None
0 Abdomen 1 Abdomen and Pelvis 4 Chest and Abdomen 5 Chest, Abdomen and Pelvis 8 Head 9 Head and Neck F Neck G Pelvic Region	Z None	Z None	Z None

Section B Imaging
Body System W Anatomical Regions
Type 3 Magnetic Resonance Imaging (MRI): Computer reformatted digital display of multiplanar images developed from the capture of radiofrequency signals emitted by nuclei in a body site excited within a magnetic field

Body Part (4th)	Contrast (5th)	Qualifier (6th)	Qualifier (7th)
0 Abdomen 8 Head F Neck G Pelvic Region H Retroperitoneum P Brachial Plexus	Y Other Contrast	0 Unenhanced and Enhanced Z None	Z None
0 Abdomen 8 Head F Neck G Pelvic Region H Retroperitoneum P Brachial Plexus	Z None	Z None	Z None
3 Chest	Y Other Contrast	0 Unenhanced and Enhanced Z None	Z None

Section B Imaging
Body System W Anatomical Regions
Type 4 Ultrasonography: Real time display of images of anatomy or flow information developed from the capture of reflected and attenuated high frequency sound waves

Body Part (4th)	Contrast (5th)	Qualifier (6th)	Qualifier (7th)
0 Abdomen 1 Abdomen and Pelvis F Neck G Pelvic Region	Z None	Z None	Z None

Section **B** **Imaging**
Body System **Y** **Fetus and Obstetrical**
Type **3** **Magnetic Resonance Imaging (MRI):** Computer reformatted digital display of multiplanar images developed from the capture of radiofrequency signals emitted by nuclei in a body site excited within a magnetic field

Body Part (4th)	Contrast (5th)	Qualifier (6th)	Qualifier (7th)
0 Fetal Head **1** Fetal Heart **2** Fetal Thorax **3** Fetal Abdomen **4** Fetal Spine **5** Fetal Extremities **6** Whole Fetus	**Y** Other Contrast	**0** Unenhanced and Enhanced **Z** None	**Z** None
0 Fetal Head **1** Fetal Heart **2** Fetal Thorax **3** Fetal Abdomen **4** Fetal Spine **5** Fetal Extremities **6** Whole Fetus	**Z** None	**Z** None	**Z** None

Section **B** **Imaging**
Body System **Y** **Fetus and Obstetrical**
Type **4** **Ultrasonography:** Real time display of images of anatomy or flow information developed from the capture of reflected and attenuated high frequency sound waves

Body Part (4th)	Contrast (5th)	Qualifier (6th)	Qualifier (7th)
7 Fetal Umbilical Cord **8** Placenta **9** First Trimester, Single Fetus **B** First Trimester, Multiple Gestation **C** Second Trimester, Single Fetus **D** Second Trimester, Multiple Gestation **F** Third Trimester, Single Fetus **G** Third Trimester, Multiple Gestation	**Z** None	**Z** None	**Z** None

Nuclear Medicine Section (C01–CW7)

Within each section of ICD-10-PCS the characters have different meanings. The seven character meanings for the Nuclear Medicine section are illustrated here through the procedure example of *Technetium tomo scan of liver*.

Section	Body System	Root Type	Body Part	Radionuclide	Qualifier	Qualifier
Nuclear Medicine	Hepatobiliary and Pancreas	Tomographic (Tomo)	Liver	Technetium 99m	None	None
C	F	2	5	1	Z	Z

Section (Character 1)

All Nuclear Medicine procedure codes have a first character value of C.

Body System (Character 2)

The alphanumeric character for the body system is placed in the second position. The following are the body systems applicable to the Nuclear Medicine section.

Character Value	Character Value Description
0	Central Nervous System
2	Heart
5	Veins
7	Lymphatic System
8	Eye
9	Ear, Nose, Mouth and Throat
B	Respiratory System
D	Gastrointestinal System
F	Hepatobiliary System and Pancreas
G	Endocrine System
H	Skin, Subcutaneous Tissue and Breast
P	Musculoskeletal
T	Urinary System
V	Male Reproductive System
W	Anatomical Regions

Root Types (Character 3)

The alphanumeric character value for root types is placed in the third position. The following are the root types applicable to the Nuclear Medicine section with their associated meaning.

Character Value	Root Type	Root Type Definition
1	Planar Nuclear Medicine Imaging	Introduction of radioactive materials into the body for single plane display of images developed from the capture of radioactive emissions
2	Tomographic (Tomo) Nuclear Medicine Imaging	Introduction of radioactive materials into the body for three dimensional display of images developed from the capture of radioactive emissions
3	Positron Emission Tomographic (PET) Imaging	Introduction of radioactive materials into the body for three dimensional display of images developed from the simultaneous capture, 180 degrees apart, of radioactive emissions
4	Nonimaging Nuclear Medicine Uptake	Introduction of radioactive materials into the body for measurements of organ function, from the detection of radioactive emissions
5	Nonimaging Nuclear Medicine Probe	Introduction of radioactive materials into the body for the study of distribution and fate of certain substances by the detection of radioactive emissions; or, alternatively, measurement of absorption of radioactive emissions from an external source

Continued →

Character Value	Root Type	Root Type Definition
6	Nonimaging Nuclear Medicine Assay	Introduction of radioactive materials into the body for the study of body fluids and blood elements, by the detection of radioactive emissions
7	Systemic Nuclear Medicine Therapy	Introduction of unsealed radioactive materials into the body for treatment

Body Part (Character 4)

For each body part the applicable body part character values will be available for procedure code construction. An example of a body part is Cerebrospinal Fluid.

Radionuclide (Character 5)

When radionuclide is utilized during a nuclear medicine procedure, the corresponding radionuclide character value should be reported in the fifth character position. The following are examples of the radionuclide character values available for the Nuclear Medicine section.

- Krypton (Kr-81m)
- Technetium 99m (Tc-99m)
- Xenon 127 (Xe-127)
- Xenon 133 (Xe-133)
- Other Radionuclide

If radionuclide is not utilized, the placeholder character value of Z should be reported.

Qualifier (Character 6)

The qualifier represents an additional attribute for the procedure when applicable. Currently, there are no qualifiers in the Nuclear Medicine section; therefore, the placeholder character value of Z should be reported.

Qualifier (Character 7)

The qualifier represents an additional attribute for the procedure when applicable. Currently, there are no qualifiers in the Nuclear Medicine section; therefore, the placeholder character value of Z should be reported.

Nuclear Medicine Section Tables

Nuclear Medicine Tables C01–CW7

Section C **Nuclear Medicine**
Body System 0 **Central Nervous System**
Type 1 **Planar Nuclear Medicine Imaging:** Introduction of radioactive materials into the body for single plane display of images developed from the capture of radioactive emissions

Body Part (4th)	Radionuclide (5th)	Qualifier (6th)	Qualifier (7th)
0 Brain	**1** Technetium 99m (Tc-99m) **Y** Other Radionuclide	**Z** None	**Z** None
5 Cerebrospinal Fluid	**D** Indium 111 (In-111) **Y** Other Radionuclide	**Z** None	**Z** None
Y Central Nervous System	**Y** Other Radionuclide	**Z** None	**Z** None

Section C **Nuclear Medicine**
Body System 0 **Central Nervous System**
Type 2 **Tomographic (Tomo) Nuclear Medicine Imaging:** Introduction of radioactive materials into the body for three dimensional display of images developed from the capture of radioactive emissions

Body Part (4th)	Radionuclide (5th)	Qualifier (6th)	Qualifier (7th)
0 Brain	**1** Technetium 99m (Tc-99m) **F** Iodine 123 (I-123) **S** Thallium 201 (Tl-201) **Y** Other Radionuclide	**Z** None	**Z** None
5 Cerebrospinal Fluid	**D** Indium 111 (In-111) **Y** Other Radionuclide	**Z** None	**Z** None
Y Central Nervous System	**Y** Other Radionuclide	**Z** None	**Z** None

Section C **Nuclear Medicine**
Body System 0 **Central Nervous System**
Type 3 **Positron Emission Tomographic (PET) Imaging:** Introduction of radioactive materials into the body for three dimensional display of images developed from the simultaneous capture, 180 degrees apart, of radioactive emissions

Body Part (4th)	Radionuclide (5th)	Qualifier (6th)	Qualifier (7th)
0 Brain	**B** Carbon 11 (C-11) **K** Fluorine 18 (F-18) **M** Oxygen 15 (O-15) **Y** Other Radionuclide	**Z** None	**Z** None
Y Central Nervous System	**Y** Other Radionuclide	**Z** None	**Z** None

Section C **Nuclear Medicine**
Body System 0 **Central Nervous System**
Type 5 **Nonimaging Nuclear Medicine Probe:** Introduction of radioactive materials into the body for the study of distribution and fate of certain substances by the detection of radioactive emissions; or, alternatively, measurement of absorption of radioactive emissions from an external source

Body Part (4th)	Radionuclide (5th)	Qualifier (6th)	Qualifier (7th)
0 Brain	**V** Xenon 133 (Xe-133) **Y** Other Radionuclide	**Z** None	**Z** None
Y Central Nervous System	**Y** Other Radionuclide	**Z** None	**Z** None

Section C **Nuclear Medicine**
Body System 2 **Heart**
Type 1 **Planar Nuclear Medicine Imaging:** Introduction of radioactive materials into the body for single plane display of images developed from the capture of radioactive emissions

Body Part (4th)	Radionuclide (5th)	Qualifier (6th)	Qualifier (7th)
6 Heart, Right and Left	**1** Technetium 99m (Tc-99m) **Y** Other Radionuclide	**Z** None	**Z** None
G Myocardium	**1** Technetium 99m (Tc-99m) **D** Indium 111 (In-111) **S** Thallium 201 (Tl-201) **Y** Other Radionuclide **Z** None	**Z** None	**Z** None
Y Heart	**Y** Other Radionuclide	**Z** None	**Z** None

Section C **Nuclear Medicine**
Body System 2 **Heart**
Type 2 **Tomographic (Tomo) Nuclear Medicine Imaging:** Introduction of radioactive materials into the body for three dimensional display of images developed from the capture of radioactive emissions

Body Part (4th)	Radionuclide (5th)	Qualifier (6th)	Qualifier (7th)
6 Heart, Right and Left	1 Technetium 99m (Tc-99m) Y Other Radionuclide	Z None	Z None
G Myocardium	1 Technetium 99m (Tc-99m) D Indium 111 (In-111) K Fluorine 18 (F-18) S Thallium 201 (Tl-201) Y Other Radionuclide Z None	Z None	Z None
Y Heart	Y Other Radionuclide	Z None	Z None

Section C **Nuclear Medicine**
Body System 2 **Heart**
Type 3 **Positron Emission Tomographic (PET) Imaging:** Introduction of radioactive materials into the body for three dimensional display of images developed from the simultaneous capture, 180 degrees apart, of radioactive emissions

Body Part (4th)	Radionuclide (5th)	Qualifier (6th)	Qualifier (7th)
G Myocardium	K Fluorine 18 (F-18) M Oxygen 15 (O-15) Q Rubidium 82 (Rb-82) R Nitrogen 13 (N-13) Y Other Radionuclide	Z None	Z None
Y Heart	Y Other Radionuclide	Z None	Z None

Section C **Nuclear Medicine**
Body System 2 **Heart**
Type 5 **Nonimaging Nuclear Medicine Probe:** Introduction of radioactive materials into the body for the study of distribution and fate of certain substances by the detection of radioactive emissions; or, alternatively, measurement of absorption of radioactive emissions from an external source

Body Part (4th)	Radionuclide (5th)	Qualifier (6th)	Qualifier (7th)
6 Heart, Right and Left	1 Technetium 99m (Tc-99m) Y Other Radionuclide	Z None	Z None
Y Heart	Y Other Radionuclide	Z None	Z None

Section C **Nuclear Medicine**
Body System 5 **Veins**
Type 1 **Planar Nuclear Medicine Imaging:** Introduction of radioactive materials into the body for single plane display of images developed from the capture of radioactive emissions

Body Part (4th)	Radionuclide (5th)	Qualifier (6th)	Qualifier (7th)
B Lower Extremity Veins, Right C Lower Extremity Veins, Left D Lower Extremity Veins, Bilateral N Upper Extremity Veins, Right P Upper Extremity Veins, Left Q Upper Extremity Veins, Bilateral R Central Veins	1 Technetium 99m (Tc-99m) Y Other Radionuclide	Z None	Z None
Y Veins	Y Other Radionuclide	Z None	Z None

Section C **Nuclear Medicine**
Body System 7 **Lymphatic and Hematologic System**
Type 1 **Planar Nuclear Medicine Imaging:** Introduction of radioactive materials into the body for single plane display of images developed from the capture of radioactive emissions

Body Part (4th)	Radionuclide (5th)	Qualifier (6th)	Qualifier (7th)
0 Bone Marrow	**1** Technetium 99m (Tc-99m) **D** Indium 111 (In-111) **Y** Other Radionuclide	**Z** None	**Z** None
2 Spleen **5** Lymphatics, Head and Neck **D** Lymphatics, Pelvic **J** Lymphatics, Head **K** Lymphatics, Neck **L** Lymphatics, Upper Chest **M** Lymphatics, Trunk **N** Lymphatics, Upper Extremity **P** Lymphatics, Lower Extremity	**1** Technetium 99m (Tc-99m) **Y** Other Radionuclide	**Z** None	**Z** None
3 Blood	**D** Indium 111 (In-111) **Y** Other Radionuclide	**Z** None	**Z** None
Y Lymphatic and Hematologic System	**Y** Other Radionuclide	**Z** None	**Z** None

Section C **Nuclear Medicine**
Body System 7 **Lymphatic and Hematologic System**
Type 2 **Tomographic (Tomo) Nuclear Medicine Imaging:** Introduction of radioactive materials into the body for three dimensional display of images developed from the capture of radioactive emissions

Body Part (4th)	Radionuclide (5th)	Qualifier (6th)	Qualifier (7th)
2 Spleen	**1** Technetium 99m (Tc-99m) **Y** Other Radionuclide	**Z** None	**Z** None
Y Lymphatic and Hematologic System	**Y** Other Radionuclide	**Z** None	**Z** None

Section C **Nuclear Medicine**
Body System 7 **Lymphatic and Hematologic System**
Type 5 **Nonimaging Nuclear Medicine Probe:** Introduction of radioactive materials into the body for the study of distribution and fate of certain substances by the detection of radioactive emissions; or, alternatively, measurement of absorption of radioactive emissions from an external source

Body Part (4th)	Radionuclide (5th)	Qualifier (6th)	Qualifier (7th)
5 Lymphatics, Head and Neck **D** Lymphatics, Pelvic **J** Lymphatics, Head **K** Lymphatics, Neck **L** Lymphatics, Upper Chest **M** Lymphatics, Trunk **N** Lymphatics, Upper Extremity **P** Lymphatics, Lower Extremity	**1** Technetium 99m (Tc-99m) **Y** Other Radionuclide	**Z** None	**Z** None
Y Lymphatic and Hematologic System	**Y** Other Radionuclide	**Z** None	**Z** None

Section C **Nuclear Medicine**
Body System 7 **Lymphatic and Hematologic System**
Type 6 **Nonimaging Nuclear Medicine Assay:** Introduction of radioactive materials into the body for the study of body fluids and blood elements, by the detection of radioactive emissions

Body Part (4th)	Radionuclide (5th)	Qualifier (6th)	Qualifier (7th)
3 Blood	**1** Technetium 99m (Tc-99m) **7** Cobalt 58 (Co-58) **C** Cobalt 57 (Co-57) **D** Indium 111 (In-111) **H** Iodine 125 (I-125) **W** Chromium (Cr-51) **Y** Other Radionuclide	**Z** None	**Z** None
Y Lymphatic and Hematologic System	**Y** Other Radionuclide	**Z** None	**Z** None

Section C **Nuclear Medicine**
Body System 8 **Eye**
Type 1 **Planar Nuclear Medicine Imaging:** Introduction of radioactive materials into the body for single plane display of images developed from the capture of radioactive emissions

Body Part (4th)	Radionuclide (5th)	Qualifier (6th)	Qualifier (7th)
9 Lacrimal Ducts, Bilateral	**1** Technetium 99m (Tc-99m) **Y** Other Radionuclide	**Z** None	**Z** None
Y Eye	**Y** Other Radionuclide	**Z** None	**Z** None

Section C **Nuclear Medicine**
Body System 9 **Ear, Nose, Mouth and Throat**
Type 1 **Planar Nuclear Medicine Imaging:** Introduction of radioactive materials into the body for single plane display of images developed from the capture of radioactive emissions

Body Part (4th)	Radionuclide (5th)	Qualifier (6th)	Qualifier (7th)
B Salivary Glands, Bilateral	**1** Technetium 99m (Tc-99m) **Y** Other Radionuclide	**Z** None	**Z** None
Y Ear, Nose, Mouth and Throat	**Y** Other Radionuclide	**Z** None	**Z** None

Section C **Nuclear Medicine**
Body System B **Respiratory System**
Type 1 **Planar Nuclear Medicine Imaging:** Introduction of radioactive materials into the body for single plane display of images developed from the capture of radioactive emissions

Body Part (4th)	Radionuclide (5th)	Qualifier (6th)	Qualifier (7th)
2 Lungs and Bronchi	**1** Technetium 99m (Tc-99m) **9** Krypton (Kr-81m) **T** Xenon 127 (Xe-127) **V** Xenon 133 (Xe-133) **Y** Other Radionuclide	**Z** None	**Z** None
Y Respiratory System	**Y** Other Radionuclide	**Z** None	**Z** None

Section C **Nuclear Medicine**
Body System B **Respiratory System**
Type 2 **Tomographic (Tomo) Nuclear Medicine Imaging:** Introduction of radioactive materials into the body for three dimensional display of images developed from the capture of radioactive emissions

Body Part (4th)	Radionuclide (5th)	Qualifier (6th)	Qualifier (7th)
2 Lungs and Bronchi	1 Technetium 99m (Tc-99m) 9 Krypton (Kr-81m) Y Other Radionuclide	Z None	Z None
Y Respiratory System	Y Other Radionuclide	Z None	Z None

Section C **Nuclear Medicine**
Body System B **Respiratory System**
Type 3 **Positron Emission Tomographic (PET) Imaging:** Introduction of radioactive materials into the body for three dimensional display of images developed from the simultaneous capture, 180 degrees apart, of radioactive emissions

Body Part (4th)	Radionuclide (5th)	Qualifier (6th)	Qualifier (7th)
2 Lungs and Bronchi	K Fluorine 18 (F-18) Y Other Radionuclide	Z None	Z None
Y Respiratory System	Y Other Radionuclide	Z None	Z None

Section C **Nuclear Medicine**
Body System D **Gastrointestinal System**
Type 1 **Planar Nuclear Medicine Imaging:** Introduction of radioactive materials into the body for single plane display of images developed from the capture of radioactive emissions

Body Part (4th)	Radionuclide (5th)	Qualifier (6th)	Qualifier (7th)
5 Upper Gastrointestinal Tract 7 Gastrointestinal Tract	1 Technetium 99m (Tc-99m) D Indium 111 (In-111) Y Other Radionuclide	Z None	Z None
Y Digestive System	Y Other Radionuclide	Z None	Z None

Section C **Nuclear Medicine**
Body System D **Gastrointestinal System**
Type 2 **Tomographic (Tomo) Nuclear Medicine Imaging:** Introduction of radioactive materials into the body for three dimensional display of images developed from the capture of radioactive emissions

Body Part (4th)	Radionuclide (5th)	Qualifier (6th)	Qualifier (7th)
7 Gastrointestinal Tract	1 Technetium 99m (Tc-99m) D Indium 111 (In-111) Y Other Radionuclide	Z None	Z None
Y Digestive System	Y Other Radionuclide	Z None	Z None

Section C **Nuclear Medicine**
Body System F **Hepatobiliary System and Pancreas**
Type 1 **Planar Nuclear Medicine Imaging:** Introduction of radioactive materials into the body for single plane display of images developed from the capture of radioactive emissions

Body Part (4th)	Radionuclide (5th)	Qualifier (6th)	Qualifier (7th)
4 Gallbladder 5 Liver 6 Liver and Spleen C Hepatobiliary System, All	1 Technetium 99m (Tc-99m) Y Other Radionuclide	Z None	Z None
Y Hepatobiliary System and Pancreas	Y Other Radionuclide	Z None	Z None

Section C Nuclear Medicine
Body System F Hepatobiliary System and Pancreas
Type 2 Tomographic (Tomo) Nuclear Medicine Imaging: Introduction of radioactive materials into the body for three dimensional display of images developed from the capture of radioactive emissions

Body Part (4th)	Radionuclide (5th)	Qualifier (6th)	Qualifier (7th)
4 Gallbladder 5 Liver 6 Liver and Spleen	1 Technetium 99m (Tc-99m) Y Other Radionuclide	Z None	Z None
Y Hepatobiliary System and Pancreas	Y Other Radionuclide	Z None	Z None

Section C Nuclear Medicine
Body System G Endocrine System
Type 1 Planar Nuclear Medicine Imaging: Introduction of radioactive materials into the body for single plane display of images developed from the capture of radioactive emissions

Body Part (4th)	Radionuclide (5th)	Qualifier (6th)	Qualifier (7th)
1 Parathyroid Glands	1 Technetium 99m (Tc-99m) S Thallium 201 (Tl-201) Y Other Radionuclide	Z None	Z None
2 Thyroid Gland	1 Technetium 99m (Tc-99m) F Iodine 123 (I-123) G Iodine 131 (I-131) Y Other Radionuclide	Z None	Z None
4 Adrenal Glands, Bilateral	G Iodine 131 (I-131) Y Other Radionuclide	Z None	Z None
Y Endocrine System	Y Other Radionuclide	Z None	Z None

Section C Nuclear Medicine
Body System G Endocrine System
Type 2 Tomographic (Tomo) Nuclear Medicine Imaging: Introduction of radioactive materials into the body for three dimensional display of images developed from the capture of radioactive emissions

Body Part (4th)	Radionuclide (5th)	Qualifier (6th)	Qualifier (7th)
1 Parathyroid Glands	1 Technetium 99m (Tc-99m) S Thallium 201 (Tl-201) Y Other Radionuclide	Z None	Z None
Y Endocrine System	Y Other Radionuclide	Z None	Z None

Section C Nuclear Medicine
Body System G Endocrine System
Type 4 Nonimaging Nuclear Medicine Uptake: Introduction of radioactive materials into the body for measurements of organ function, from the detection of radioactive emissions

Body Part (4th)	Radionuclide (5th)	Qualifier (6th)	Qualifier (7th)
2 Thyroid Gland	1 Technetium 99m (Tc-99m) F Iodine 123 (I-123) G Iodine 131 (I-131) Y Other Radionuclide	Z None	Z None
Y Endocrine System	Y Other Radionuclide	Z None	Z None

Section C **Nuclear Medicine**
Body System H **Skin, Subcutaneous Tissue and Breast**
Type 1 **Planar Nuclear Medicine Imaging:** Introduction of radioactive materials into the body for single plane display of images developed from the capture of radioactive emissions

Body Part (4th)	Radionuclide (5th)	Qualifier (6th)	Qualifier (7th)
0 Breast, Right **1** Breast, Left **2** Breasts, Bilateral	**1** Technetium 99m (Tc-99m) **S** Thallium 201 (Tl-201) **Y** Other Radionuclide	**Z** None	**Z** None
Y Skin, Subcutaneous Tissue and Breast	**Y** Other Radionuclide	**Z** None	**Z** None

Section C **Nuclear Medicine**
Body System H **Skin, Subcutaneous Tissue and Breast**
Type 2 **Tomographic (Tomo) Nuclear Medicine Imaging:** Introduction of radioactive materials into the body for three dimensional display of images developed from the capture of radioactive emissions

Body Part (4th)	Radionuclide (5th)	Qualifier (6th)	Qualifier (7th)
0 Breast, Right **1** Breast, Left **2** Breasts, Bilateral	**1** Technetium 99m (Tc-99m) **S** Thallium 201 (Tl-201) **Y** Other Radionuclide	**Z** None	**Z** None
Y Skin, Subcutaneous Tissue and Breast	**Y** Other Radionuclide	**Z** None	**Z** None

Section C **Nuclear Medicine**
Body System P **Musculoskeletal System**
Type 1 **Planar Nuclear Medicine Imaging:** Introduction of radioactive materials into the body for single plane display of images developed from the capture of radioactive emissions

Body Part (4th)	Radionuclide (5th)	Qualifier (6th)	Qualifier (7th)
1 Skull **4** Thorax **5** Spine **6** Pelvis **7** Spine and Pelvis **8** Upper Extremity, Right **9** Upper Extremity, Left **B** Upper Extremities, Bilateral **C** Lower Extremity, Right **D** Lower Extremity, Left **F** Lower Extremities, Bilateral **Z** Musculoskeletal System, All	**1** Technetium 99m (Tc-99m) **Y** Other Radionuclide	**Z** None	**Z** None
Y Musculoskeletal System, Other	**Y** Other Radionuclide	**Z** None	**Z** None

Section C **Nuclear Medicine**
Body System P **Musculoskeletal System**
Type 2 **Tomographic (Tomo) Nuclear Medicine Imaging:** Introduction of radioactive materials into the body for three dimensional display of images developed from the capture of radioactive emissions

Body Part (4th)	Radionuclide (5th)	Qualifier (6th)	Qualifier (7th)
1 Skull 2 Cervical Spine 3 Skull and Cervical Spine 4 Thorax 6 Pelvis 7 Spine and Pelvis 8 Upper Extremity, Right 9 Upper Extremity, Left B Upper Extremities, Bilateral C Lower Extremity, Right D Lower Extremity, Left F Lower Extremities, Bilateral G Thoracic Spine H Lumbar Spine J Thoracolumbar Spine	1 Technetium 99m (Tc-99m) Y Other Radionuclide	Z None	Z None
Y Musculoskeletal System, Other	Y Other Radionuclide	Z None	Z None

Section C **Nuclear Medicine**
Body System P **Musculoskeletal System**
Type 5 **Nonimaging Nuclear Medicine Probe:** Introduction of radioactive materials into the body for the study of distribution and fate of certain substances by the detection of radioactive emissions; or, alternatively, measurement of absorption of radioactive emissions from an external source

Body Part (4th)	Radionuclide (5th)	Qualifier (6th)	Qualifier (7th)
5 Spine N Upper Extremities P Lower Extremities	Z None	Z None	Z None
Y Musculoskeletal System, Other	Y Other Radionuclide	Z None	Z None

Section C **Nuclear Medicine**
Body System T **Urinary System**
Type 1 **Planar Nuclear Medicine Imaging:** Introduction of radioactive materials into the body for single plane display of images developed from the capture of radioactive emissions

Body Part (4th)	Radionuclide (5th)	Qualifier (6th)	Qualifier (7th)
3 Kidneys, Ureters and Bladder	1 Technetium 99m (Tc-99m) F Iodine 123 (I-123) G Iodine 131 (I-131) Y Other Radionuclide	Z None	Z None
H Bladder and Ureters	1 Technetium 99m (Tc-99m) Y Other Radionuclide	Z None	Z None
Y Urinary System	Y Other Radionuclide	Z None	Z None

Section C **Nuclear Medicine**
Body System T **Urinary System**
Type 2 **Tomographic (Tomo) Nuclear Medicine Imaging:** Introduction of radioactive materials into the body for three dimensional display of images developed from the capture of radioactive emissions

Body Part (4th)	Radionuclide (5th)	Qualifier (6th)	Qualifier (7th)
3 Kidneys, Ureters and Bladder	1 Technetium 99m (Tc-99m) Y Other Radionuclide	Z None	Z None
Y Urinary System	Y Other Radionuclide	Z None	Z None

Section C **Nuclear Medicine**
Body System T **Urinary System**
Type 6 **Nonimaging Nuclear Medicine Assay:** Introduction of radioactive materials into the body for the study of body fluids and blood elements, by the detection of radioactive emissions

Body Part (4th)	Radionuclide (5th)	Qualifier (6th)	Qualifier (7th)
3 Kidneys, Ureters and Bladder	**1** Technetium 99m (Tc-99m) **F** Iodine 123 (I-123) **G** Iodine 131 (I-131) **H** Iodine 125 (I-125) **Y** Other Radionuclide	**Z** None	**Z** None
Y Urinary System	**Y** Other Radionuclide	**Z** None	**Z** None

Section C **Nuclear Medicine**
Body System V **Male Reproductive System**
Type 1 **Planar Nuclear Medicine Imaging:** Introduction of radioactive materials into the body for single plane display of images developed from the capture of radioactive emissions

Body Part (4th)	Radionuclide (5th)	Qualifier (6th)	Qualifier (7th)
9 Testicles, Bilateral	**1** Technetium 99m (Tc-99m) **Y** Other Radionuclide	**Z** None	**Z** None
Y Male Reproductive System	**Y** Other Radionuclide	**Z** None	**Z** None

Section C **Nuclear Medicine**
Body System W **Anatomical Regions**
Type 1 **Planar Nuclear Medicine Imaging:** Introduction of radioactive materials into the body for single plane display of images developed from the capture of radioactive emissions

Body Part (4th)	Radionuclide (5th)	Qualifier (6th)	Qualifier (7th)
0 Abdomen **1** Abdomen and Pelvis **4** Chest and Abdomen **6** Chest and Neck **B** Head and Neck **D** Lower Extremity **J** Pelvic Region **M** Upper Extremity **N** Whole Body	**1** Technetium 99m (Tc-99m) **D** Indium 111 (In-111) **F** Iodine 123 (I-123) **G** Iodine 131 (I-131) **L** Gallium 67 (Ga-67) **S** Thallium 201 (Tl-201) **Y** Other Radionuclide	**Z** None	**Z** None
3 Chest	**1** Technetium 99m (Tc-99m) **D** Indium 111 (In-111) **F** Iodine 123 (I-123) **G** Iodine 131 (I-131) **K** Fluorine 18 (F-18) **L** Gallium 67 (Ga-67) **S** Thallium 201 (Tl-201) **Y** Other Radionuclide	**Z** None	**Z** None
Y Anatomical Regions, Multiple	**Y** Other Radionuclide	**Z** None	**Z** None
Z Anatomical Region, Other	**Z** None	**Z** None	**Z** None

Section C **Nuclear Medicine**
Body System W **Anatomical Regions**
Type 2 **Tomographic (Tomo) Nuclear Medicine Imaging:** Introduction of radioactive materials into the body for three dimensional display of images developed from the capture of radioactive emissions

Body Part (4th)	Radionuclide (5th)	Qualifier (6th)	Qualifier (7th)
0 Abdomen **1** Abdomen and Pelvis **3** Chest **4** Chest and Abdomen **6** Chest and Neck **B** Head and Neck **D** Lower Extremity **J** Pelvic Region **M** Upper Extremity	**1** Technetium 99m (Tc-99m) **D** Indium 111 (In-111) **F** Iodine 123 (I-123) **G** Iodine 131 (I-131) **K** Fluorine 18 (F-18) **L** Gallium 67 (Ga-67) **S** Thallium 201 (Tl-201) **Y** Other Radionuclide	**Z** None	**Z** None
Y Anatomical Regions, Multiple	**Y** Other Radionuclide	**Z** None	**Z** None

Section C **Nuclear Medicine**
Body System W **Anatomical Regions**
Type 3 **Positron Emission Tomographic (PET) Imaging:** Introduction of radioactive materials into the body for three dimensional display of images developed from the simultaneous capture, 180 degrees apart, of radioactive emissions

Body Part (4th)	Radionuclide (5th)	Qualifier (6th)	Qualifier (7th)
N Whole Body	**Y** Other Radionuclide	**Z** None	**Z** None

Section C **Nuclear Medicine**
Body System W **Anatomical Regions**
Type 5 **Nonimaging Nuclear Medicine Probe:** Introduction of radioactive materials into the body for the study of distribution and fate of certain substances by the detection of radioactive emissions; or, alternatively, measurement of absorption of radioactive emissions from an external source

Body Part (4th)	Radionuclide (5th)	Qualifier (6th)	Qualifier (7th)
0 Abdomen **1** Abdomen and Pelvis **3** Chest **4** Chest and Abdomen **6** Chest and Neck **B** Head and Neck **D** Lower Extremity **J** Pelvic Region **M** Upper Extremity	**1** Technetium 99m (Tc-99m) **D** Indium 111 (In-111) **Y** Other Radionuclide	**Z** None	**Z** None

Section C **Nuclear Medicine**
Body System W **Anatomical Regions**
Type 7 **Systemic Nuclear Medicine Therapy:** Introduction of unsealed radioactive materials into the body for treatment

Body Part (4th)	Radionuclide (5th)	Qualifier (6th)	Qualifier (7th)
0 Abdomen **3** Chest	**N** Phosphorus 32 (P-32) **Y** Other Radionuclide	**Z** None	**Z** None
G Thyroid	**G** Iodine 131 (I-131) **Y** Other Radionuclide	**Z** None	**Z** None
N Whole Body	**8** Samarium 153 (Sm-153) **G** Iodine 131 (I-131) **N** Phosphorus 32 (P-32) **P** Strontium 89 (Sr-89) **Y** Other Radionuclide	**Z** None	**Z** None
Y Anatomical Regions, Multiple	**Y** Other Radionuclide	**Z** None	**Z** None

Radiation Therapy Section (D00–DWY)

Within each section of ICD-10-PCS the characters have different meanings. The seven character meanings for the Radiation Therapy section are illustrated here through the procedure example of *HDR brachytherapy of prostate using Palladium 103*.

Section	Body System	Modality	Treatment Site	Modality Qualifier	Isotope	Qualifier
Radiation Therapy	Male Reproductive System	Brachytherapy	Prostate	High Dose Rate (HDR)	Palladium 103	None
D	V	1	0	9	B	Z

Section (Character 1)

All Radiation Therapy procedure codes have a first character value of D.

Body System (Character 2)

The alphanumeric character for the body system is placed in the second position. The following are the body systems applicable to the Radiation Therapy section.

Character Value	Character Value Description
0	Central and Peripheral Nervous System
7	Lymphatic and hematologic System
8	Eye
9	Ear, Nose, Mouth and Throat
B	Respiratory System
D	Gastrointestinal System
F	Hepatobiliary System and Pancreas
G	Endocrine System
H	Skin
M	Breast
P	Musculoskeletral
T	Urinary System
U	Female Reproductive System
V	Male Reproductive System
W	Anatomical Regions

Modality (Character 3)

The alphanumeric character value for root types is placed in the third position. The following are the root types applicable to the Radiation Therapy section with their associated meaning.

Character Value	Modality	Modality Definition
0	Beam Radiation	The external use of high-energy radiation such as x-rays, photons, electrons, or protons
1	Brachytherapy	The use of radioactive sources placed directly into a tumor bearing area to generate local regions of high intensity radiation
2	Stereotactic Radiosurgery	The use of external radiation sources either from a linear accelerator or a special Cobalt-60 irradiator to deliver many beams of radiation directly to an internal structure in a single fraction
Y	Other Radiation	Other types of radiation therapy such as hyperthermia, contact radiation and plaque radiation. *See Modality qualifier, character 5, for specified types of other radiation.*

Source: CSI Navigator for Radiation Oncology, 2010

Treatment Site (Character 4)

For each treatment site the applicable body part character values will be available for procedure code construction. An example of a treatment site for this section is Brain Stem.

Modality Qualifier (Character 5)

The modality qualifier further specifies the treatment modality. The following are examples of the modality qualifier values available for the Radiation Therapy section:

- Photons >10 MeV
- Neutrons
- Electrons
- High Dose Rate
- Hyperthermia

Isotope (Character 6)

When an isotope is utilized during a radiation oncology procedure, the corresponding isotope character value should be reported in the sixth character position. The following are examples of the isotope character values available for the Radiation Therapy section:

- Iridium 192 (Ir-192)
- Iodine 125 (I-125)
- Californium 252 (Cf-252)

Qualifier (Character 7)

The qualifier represents an additional attribute for the procedure when applicable. For example, beam radiation procedures in this section include the qualifier Intraoperative that is reported with the character value of 0 for some body parts. If there is no qualifier for a procedure, the placeholder Z is the character valve that should be reported.

Radiation Therapy Section Tables

Radiation Therapy Tables D00–DWY

Section D **Radiation Therapy**
Body System 0 **Central and Peripheral Nervous System**
Modality 0 **Beam Radiation**

Treatment Site (4th)	Modality Qualifier (5th)	Isotope (6th)	Qualifier (7th)
0 Brain **1** Brain Stem **6** Spinal Cord **7** Peripheral Nerve	**0** Photons <1 MeV **1** Photons 1 - 10 MeV **2** Photons >10 MeV **4** Heavy Particles (Protons,Ions) **5** Neutrons **6** Neutron Capture	**Z** None	**Z** None
0 Brain **1** Brain Stem **6** Spinal Cord **7** Peripheral Nerve	**3** Electrons	**Z** None	**0** Intraoperative **Z** None

Section D **Radiation Therapy**
Body System 0 **Central and Peripheral Nervous System**
Modality 1 **Brachytherapy**

Treatment Site (4th)	Modality Qualifier (5th)	Isotope (6th)	Qualifier (7th)
0 Brain **1** Brain Stem **6** Spinal Cord **7** Peripheral Nerve	**9** High Dose Rate (HDR) **B** Low Dose Rate (LDR)	**7** Cesium 137 (Cs-137) **8** Iridium 192 (Ir-192) **9** Iodine 125 (I-125) **B** Palladium 103 (Pd-103) **C** Californium 252 (Cf-252) **Y** Other Isotope	**Z** None

Section D **Radiation Therapy**
Body System 0 **Central and Peripheral Nervous System**
Modality 2 **Stereotactic Radiosurgery**

Treatment Site (4th)	Modality Qualifier (5th)	Isotope (6th)	Qualifier (7th)
0 Brain **1** Brain Stem **6** Spinal Cord **7** Peripheral Nerve	**D** Stereotactic Other Photon Radiosurgery **H** Stereotactic Particulate Radiosurgery **J** Stereotactic Gamma Beam Radiosurgery	**Z** None	**Z** None

Section D **Radiation Therapy**
Body System 0 **Central and Peripheral Nervous System**
Modality Y **Other Radiation**

Treatment Site (4th)	Modality Qualifier (5th)	Isotope (6th)	Qualifier (7th)
0 Brain **1** Brain Stem **6** Spinal Cord **7** Peripheral Nerve	**7** Contact Radiation **8** Hyperthermia **F** Plaque Radiation **K** Laser Interstitial Thermal Therapy	**Z** None	**Z** None

Section D **Radiation Therapy**
Body System 7 **Lymphatic and Hematologic System**
Modality 0 **Beam Radiation**

Treatment Site (4th)	Modality Qualifier (5th)	Isotope (6th)	Qualifier (7th)
0 Bone Marrow **1** Thymus **2** Spleen **3** Lymphatics, Neck **4** Lymphatics, Axillary **5** Lymphatics, Thorax **6** Lymphatics, Abdomen **7** Lymphatics, Pelvis **8** Lymphatics, Inguinal	**0** Photons <1 MeV **1** Photons 1 - 10 MeV **2** Photons >10 MeV **4** Heavy Particles (Protons,Ions) **5** Neutrons **6** Neutron Capture	**Z** None	**Z** None
0 Bone Marrow **1** Thymus **2** Spleen **3** Lymphatics, Neck **4** Lymphatics, Axillary **5** Lymphatics, Thorax **6** Lymphatics, Abdomen **7** Lymphatics, Pelvis **8** Lymphatics, Inguinal	**3** Electrons	**Z** None	**0** Intraoperative **Z** None

Section D **Radiation Therapy**
Body System 7 **Lymphatic and Hematologic System**
Modality 1 **Brachytherapy**

Treatment Site (4th)	Modality Qualifier (5th)	Isotope (6th)	Qualifier (7th)
0 Bone Marrow **1** Thymus **2** Spleen **3** Lymphatics, Neck **4** Lymphatics, Axillary **5** Lymphatics, Thorax **6** Lymphatics, Abdomen **7** Lymphatics, Pelvis **8** Lymphatics, Inguinal	**9** High Dose Rate (HDR) **B** Low Dose Rate (LDR)	**7** Cesium 137 (Cs-137) **8** Iridium 192 (Ir-192) **9** Iodine 125 (I-125) **B** Palladium 103 (Pd-103) **C** Californium 252 (Cf-252) **Y** Other Isotope	**Z** None

Section D **Radiation Therapy**
Body System 7 **Lymphatic and Hematologic System**
Modality 2 **Stereotactic Radiosurgery**

Treatment Site (4th)	Modality Qualifier (5th)	Isotope (6th)	Qualifier (7th)
0 Bone Marrow 1 Thymus 2 Spleen 3 Lymphatics, Neck 4 Lymphatics, Axillary 5 Lymphatics, Thorax 6 Lymphatics, Abdomen 7 Lymphatics, Pelvis 8 Lymphatics, Inguinal	D Stereotactic Other Photon Radiosurgery H Stereotactic Particulate Radiosurgery J Stereotactic Gamma Beam Radiosurgery	Z None	Z None

Section D **Radiation Therapy**
Body System 7 **Lymphatic and Hematologic System**
Modality Y **Other Radiation**

Treatment Site (4th)	Modality Qualifier (5th)	Isotope (6th)	Qualifier (7th)
0 Bone Marrow 1 Thymus 2 Spleen 3 Lymphatics, Neck 4 Lymphatics, Axillary 5 Lymphatics, Thorax 6 Lymphatics, Abdomen 7 Lymphatics, Pelvis 8 Lymphatics, Inguinal	8 Hyperthermia F Plaque Radiation	Z None	Z None

Section D **Radiation Therapy**
Body System 8 **Eye**
Modality 0 **Beam Radiation**

Treatment Site (4th)	Modality Qualifier (5th)	Isotope (6th)	Qualifier (7th)
0 Eye	0 Photons <1 MeV 1 Photons 1 - 10 MeV 2 Photons >10 MeV 4 Heavy Particles (Protons,Ions) 5 Neutrons 6 Neutron Capture	Z None	Z None
0 Eye	3 Electrons	Z None	0 Intraoperative Z None

Section D **Radiation Therapy**
Body System 8 **Eye**
Modality 1 **Brachytherapy**

Treatment Site (4th)	Modality Qualifier (5th)	Isotope (6th)	Qualifier (7th)
0 Eye	9 High Dose Rate (HDR) B Low Dose Rate (LDR)	7 Cesium 137 (Cs-137) 8 Iridium 192 (Ir-192) 9 Iodine 125 (I-125) B Palladium 103 (Pd-103) C Californium 252 (Cf-252) Y Other Isotope	Z None

Section D **Radiation Therapy**
Body System 8 **Eye**
Modality 2 **Stereotactic Radiosurgery**

Treatment Site (4th)	Modality Qualifier (5th)	Isotope (6th)	Qualifier (7th)
0 Eye	**D** Stereotactic Other Photon Radiosurgery **H** Stereotactic Particulate Radiosurgery **J** Stereotactic Gamma Beam Radiosurgery	**Z** None	**Z** None

Section D **Radiation Therapy**
Body System 8 **Eye**
Modality Y **Other Radiation**

Treatment Site (4th)	Modality Qualifier (5th)	Isotope (6th)	Qualifier (7th)
0 Eye	**7** Contact Radiation **8** Hyperthermia **F** Plaque Radiation	**Z** None	**Z** None

Section D **Radiation Therapy**
Body System 9 **Ear, Nose, Mouth and Throat**
Modality 0 **Beam Radiation**

Treatment Site (4th)	Modality Qualifier (5th)	Isotope (6th)	Qualifier (7th)
0 Ear **1** Nose **3** Hypopharynx **4** Mouth **5** Tongue **6** Salivary Glands **7** Sinuses **8** Hard Palate **9** Soft Palate **B** Larynx **D** Nasopharynx **F** Oropharynx	**0** Photons <1 MeV **1** Photons 1 - 10 MeV **2** Photons >10 MeV **4** Heavy Particles (Protons,Ions) **5** Neutrons **6** Neutron Capture	**Z** None	**Z** None
0 Ear **1** Nose **3** Hypopharynx **4** Mouth **5** Tongue **6** Salivary Glands **7** Sinuses **8** Hard Palate **9** Soft Palate **B** Larynx **D** Nasopharynx **F** Oropharynx	**3** Electrons	**Z** None	**0** Intraoperative **Z** None

Section D **Radiation Therapy**
Body System 9 **Ear, Nose, Mouth and Throat**
Modality 1 **Brachytherapy**

Treatment Site (4th)	Modality Qualifier (5th)	Isotope (6th)	Qualifier (7th)
0 Ear 1 Nose 3 Hypopharynx 4 Mouth 5 Tongue 6 Salivary Glands 7 Sinuses 8 Hard Palate 9 Soft Palate B Larynx D Nasopharynx F Oropharynx	9 High Dose Rate (HDR) B Low Dose Rate (LDR)	7 Cesium 137 (Cs-137) 8 Iridium 192 (Ir-192) 9 Iodine 125 (I-125) B Palladium 103 (Pd-103) C Californium 252 (Cf-252) Y Other Isotope	Z None

Section D **Radiation Therapy**
Body System 9 **Ear, Nose, Mouth and Throat**
Modality 2 **Stereotactic Radiosurgery**

Treatment Site (4th)	Modality Qualifier (5th)	Isotope (6th)	Qualifier (7th)
0 Ear 1 Nose 4 Mouth 5 Tongue 6 Salivary Glands 7 Sinuses 8 Hard Palate 9 Soft Palate B Larynx C Pharynx D Nasopharynx	D Stereotactic Other Photon Radiosurgery H Stereotactic Particulate Radiosurgery J Stereotactic Gamma Beam Radiosurgery	Z None	Z None

Section D **Radiation Therapy**
Body System 9 **Ear, Nose, Mouth and Throat**
Modality Y **Other Radiation**

Treatment Site (4th)	Modality Qualifier (5th)	Isotope (6th)	Qualifier (7th)
0 Ear 1 Nose 5 Tongue 6 Salivary Glands 7 Sinuses 8 Hard Palate 9 Soft Palate	7 Contact Radiation 8 Hyperthermia F Plaque Radiation	Z None	Z None
3 Hypopharynx F Oropharynx	7 Contact Radiation 8 Hyperthermia	Z None	Z None
4 Mouth B Larynx D Nasopharynx	7 Contact Radiation 8 Hyperthermia C Intraoperative Radiation Therapy (IORT) F Plaque Radiation	Z None	Z None
C Pharynx	C Intraoperative Radiation Therapy (IORT) F Plaque Radiation	Z None	Z None

Section D **Radiation Therapy**
Body System B **Respiratory System**
Modality 0 **Beam Radiation**

Treatment Site (4th)	Modality Qualifier (5th)	Isotope (6th)	Qualifier (7th)
0 Trachea **1** Bronchus **2** Lung **5** Pleura **6** Mediastinum **7** Chest Wall **8** Diaphragm	**0** Photons <1 MeV **1** Photons 1 - 10 MeV **2** Photons >10 MeV **4** Heavy Particles (Protons,Ions) **5** Neutrons **6** Neutron Capture	**Z** None	**Z** None
0 Trachea **1** Bronchus **2** Lung **5** Pleura **6** Mediastinum **7** Chest Wall **8** Diaphragm	**3** Electrons	**Z** None	**0** Intraoperative **Z** None

Section D **Radiation Therapy**
Body System B **Respiratory System**
Modality 1 **Brachytherapy**

Treatment Site (4th)	Modality Qualifier (5th)	Isotope (6th)	Qualifier (7th)
0 Trachea **1** Bronchus **2** Lung **5** Pleura **6** Mediastinum **7** Chest Wall **8** Diaphragm	**9** High Dose Rate (HDR) **B** Low Dose Rate (LDR)	**7** Cesium 137 (Cs-137) **8** Iridium 192 (Ir-192) **9** Iodine 125 (I-125) **B** Palladium 103 (Pd-103) **C** Californium 252 (Cf-252) **Y** Other Isotope	**Z** None

Section D **Radiation Therapy**
Body System B **Respiratory System**
Modality 2 **Stereotactic Radiosurgery**

Treatment Site (4th)	Modality Qualifier (5th)	Isotope (6th)	Qualifier (7th)
0 Trachea **1** Bronchus **2** Lung **5** Pleura **6** Mediastinum **7** Chest Wall **8** Diaphragm	**D** Stereotactic Other Photon Radiosurgery **H** Stereotactic Particulate Radiosurgery **J** Stereotactic Gamma Beam Radiosurgery	**Z** None	**Z** None

Section D **Radiation Therapy**
Body System B **Respiratory System**
Modality Y **Other Radiation**

Treatment Site (4th)	Modality Qualifier (5th)	Isotope (6th)	Qualifier (7th)
0 Trachea **1** Bronchus **2** Lung **5** Pleura **6** Mediastinum **7** Chest Wall **8** Diaphragm	**7** Contact Radiation **8** Hyperthermia **F** Plaque Radiation **K** Laser Interstitial Thermal Therapy	**Z** None	**Z** None

Section D **Radiation Therapy**
Body System D **Gastrointestinal System**
Modality 0 **Beam Radiation**

Treatment Site (4th)	Modality Qualifier (5th)	Isotope (6th)	Qualifier (7th)
0 Esophagus **1** Stomach **2** Duodenum **3** Jejunum **4** Ileum **5** Colon **7** Rectum	**0** Photons <1 MeV **1** Photons 1 - 10 MeV **2** Photons >10 MeV **4** Heavy Particles (Protons,Ions) **5** Neutrons **6** Neutron Capture	**Z** None	**Z** None
0 Esophagus **1** Stomach **2** Duodenum **3** Jejunum **4** Ileum **5** Colon **7** Rectum	**3** Electrons	**Z** None	**0** Intraoperative **Z** None

Section D **Radiation Therapy**
Body System D **Gastrointestinal System**
Modality 1 **Brachytherapy**

Treatment Site (4th)	Modality Qualifier (5th)	Isotope (6th)	Qualifier (7th)
0 Esophagus **1** Stomach **2** Duodenum **3** Jejunum **4** Ileum **5** Colon **7** Rectum	**9** High Dose Rate (HDR) **B** Low Dose Rate (LDR)	**7** Cesium 137 (Cs-137) **8** Iridium 192 (Ir-192) **9** Iodine 125 (I-125) **B** Palladium 103 (Pd-103) **C** Californium 252 (Cf-252) **Y** Other Isotope	**Z** None

Section D **Radiation Therapy**
Body System D **Gastrointestinal System**
Modality 2 **Stereotactic Radiosurgery**

Treatment Site (4th)	Modality Qualifier (5th)	Isotope (6th)	Qualifier (7th)
0 Esophagus **1** Stomach **2** Duodenum **3** Jejunum **4** Ileum **5** Colon **7** Rectum	**D** Stereotactic Other Photon Radiosurgery **H** Stereotactic Particulate Radiosurgery **J** Stereotactic Gamma Beam Radiosurgery	**Z** None	**Z** None

Section D **Radiation Therapy**
Body System D **Gastrointestinal System**
Modality Y **Other Radiation**

Treatment Site (4th)	Modality Qualifier (5th)	Isotope (6th)	Qualifier (7th)
0 Esophagus	**7** Contact Radiation **8** Hyperthermia **F** Plaque Radiation **K** Laser Interstitial Thermal Therapy	**Z** None	**Z** None
1 Stomach **2** Duodenum **3** Jejunum **4** Ileum **5** Colon **7** Rectum	**7** Contact Radiation **8** Hyperthermia **C** Intraoperative Radiation Therapy (IORT) **F** Plaque Radiation **K** Laser Interstitial Thermal Therapy	**Z** None	**Z** None

Continued →

Section D **Radiation Therapy**
Body System D **Gastrointestinal System**
Modality Y **Other Radiation**

Treatment Site (4th)	Modality Qualifier (5th)	Isotope (6th)	Qualifier (7th)
8 Anus	**C** Intraoperative Radiation Therapy (IORT) **F** Plaque Radiation **K** Laser Interstitial Thermal Therapy	**Z** None	**Z** None

Section D **Radiation Therapy**
Body System F **Hepatobiliary System and Pancreas**
Modality 0 **Beam Radiation**

Treatment Site (4th)	Modality Qualifier (5th)	Isotope (6th)	Qualifier (7th)
0 Liver **1** Gallbladder **2** Bile Ducts **3** Pancreas	**0** Photons <1 MeV **1** Photons 1 - 10 MeV **2** Photons >10 MeV **4** Heavy Particles (Protons,Ions) **5** Neutrons **6** Neutron Capture	**Z** None	**Z** None
0 Liver **1** Gallbladder **2** Bile Ducts **3** Pancreas	**3** Electrons	**Z** None	**0** Intraoperative **Z** None

Section D **Radiation Therapy**
Body System F **Hepatobiliary System and Pancreas**
Modality 1 **Brachytherapy**

Treatment Site (4th)	Modality Qualifier (5th)	Isotope (6th)	Qualifier (7th)
0 Liver **1** Gallbladder **2** Bile Ducts **3** Pancreas	**9** High Dose Rate (HDR) **B** Low Dose Rate (LDR)	**7** Cesium 137 (Cs-137) **8** Iridium 192 (Ir-192) **9** Iodine 125 (I-125) **B** Palladium 103 (Pd-103) **C** Californium 252 (Cf-252) **Y** Other Isotope	**Z** None

Section D **Radiation Therapy**
Body System F **Hepatobiliary System and Pancreas**
Modality 2 **Stereotactic Radiosurgery**

Treatment Site (4th)	Modality Qualifier (5th)	Isotope (6th)	Qualifier (7th)
0 Liver **1** Gallbladder **2** Bile Ducts **3** Pancreas	**D** Stereotactic Other Photon Radiosurgery **H** Stereotactic Particulate Radiosurgery **J** Stereotactic Gamma Beam Radiosurgery	**Z** None	**Z** None

Section D **Radiation Therapy**
Body System F **Hepatobiliary System and Pancreas**
Modality Y **Other Radiation**

Treatment Site (4th)	Modality Qualifier (5th)	Isotope (6th)	Qualifier (7th)
0 Liver **1** Gallbladder **2** Bile Ducts **3** Pancreas	**7** Contact Radiation **8** Hyperthermia **C** Intraoperative Radiation Therapy (IORT) **F** Plaque Radiation **K** Laser Interstitial Thermal Therapy	**Z** None	**Z** None

Section	**D**	**Radiation Therapy**
Body System	**G**	**Endocrine System**
Modality	**0**	**Beam Radiation**

Treatment Site (4th)	Modality Qualifier (5th)	Isotope (6th)	Qualifier (7th)
0 Pituitary Gland 1 Pineal Body 2 Adrenal Glands 4 Parathyroid Glands 5 Thyroid	0 Photons <1 MeV 1 Photons 1 - 10 MeV 2 Photons >10 MeV 5 Neutrons 6 Neutron Capture	Z None	Z None
0 Pituitary Gland 1 Pineal Body 2 Adrenal Glands 4 Parathyroid Glands 5 Thyroid	3 Electrons	Z None	0 Intraoperative Z None

Section	**D**	**Radiation Therapy**
Body System	**G**	**Endocrine System**
Modality	**1**	**Brachytherapy**

Treatment Site (4th)	Modality Qualifier (5th)	Isotope (6th)	Qualifier (7th)
0 Pituitary Gland 1 Pineal Body 2 Adrenal Glands 4 Parathyroid Glands 5 Thyroid	9 High Dose Rate (HDR) B Low Dose Rate (LDR)	7 Cesium 137 (Cs-137) 8 Iridium 192 (Ir-192) 9 Iodine 125 (I-125) B Palladium 103 (Pd-103) C Californium 252 (Cf-252) Y Other Isotope	Z None

Section	**D**	**Radiation Therapy**
Body System	**G**	**Endocrine System**
Modality	**2**	**Stereotactic Radiosurgery**

Treatment Site (4th)	Modality Qualifier (5th)	Isotope (6th)	Qualifier (7th)
0 Pituitary Gland 1 Pineal Body 2 Adrenal Glands 4 Parathyroid Glands 5 Thyroid	D Stereotactic Other Photon Radiosurgery H Stereotactic Particulate Radiosurgery J Stereotactic Gamma Beam Radiosurgery	Z None	Z None

Section	**D**	**Radiation Therapy**
Body System	**G**	**Endocrine System**
Modality	**Y**	**Other Radiation**

Treatment Site (4th)	Modality Qualifier (5th)	Isotope (6th)	Qualifier (7th)
0 Pituitary Gland 1 Pineal Body 2 Adrenal Glands 4 Parathyroid Glands 5 Thyroid	7 Contact Radiation 8 Hyperthermia F Plaque Radiation K Laser Interstitial Thermal Therapy	Z None	Z None

Section D **Radiation Therapy**
Body System H **Skin**
Modality 0 **Beam Radiation**

Treatment Site (4th)	Modality Qualifier (5th)	Isotope (6th)	Qualifier (7th)
2 Skin, Face **3** Skin, Neck **4** Skin, Arm **6** Skin, Chest **7** Skin, Back **8** Skin, Abdomen **9** Skin, Buttock **B** Skin, Leg	**0** Photons <1 MeV **1** Photons 1 - 10 MeV **2** Photons >10 MeV **4** Heavy Particles (Protons,Ions) **5** Neutrons **6** Neutron Capture	**Z** None	**Z** None
2 Skin, Face **3** Skin, Neck **4** Skin, Arm **6** Skin, Chest **7** Skin, Back **8** Skin, Abdomen **9** Skin, Buttock **B** Skin, Leg	**3** Electrons	**Z** None	**0** Intraoperative **Z** None

Section D **Radiation Therapy**
Body System H **Skin**
Modality Y **Other Radiation**

Treatment Site (4th)	Modality Qualifier (5th)	Isotope (6th)	Qualifier (7th)
2 Skin, Face **3** Skin, Neck **4** Skin, Arm **6** Skin, Chest **7** Skin, Back **8** Skin, Abdomen **9** Skin, Buttock **B** Skin, Leg	**7** Contact Radiation **8** Hyperthermia **F** Plaque Radiation	**Z** None	**Z** None
5 Skin, Hand **C** Skin, Foot	**F** Plaque Radiation	**Z** None	**Z** None

Section D **Radiation Therapy**
Body System M **Breast**
Modality 0 **Beam Radiation**

Treatment Site (4th)	Modality Qualifier (5th)	Isotope (6th)	Qualifier (7th)
0 Breast, Left **1** Breast, Right	**0** Photons <1 MeV **1** Photons 1 - 10 MeV **2** Photons >10 MeV **4** Heavy Particles (Protons,Ions) **5** Neutrons **6** Neutron Capture	**Z** None	**Z** None
0 Breast, Left **1** Breast, Right	**3** Electrons	**Z** None	**0** Intraoperative **Z** None

Section D **Radiation Therapy**
Body System M **Breast**
Modality 1 **Brachytherapy**

Treatment Site (4th)	Modality Qualifier (5th)	Isotope (6th)	Qualifier (7th)
0 Breast, Left **1** Breast, Right	**9** High Dose Rate (HDR) **B** Low Dose Rate (LDR)	**7** Cesium 137 (Cs-137) **8** Iridium 192 (Ir-192) **9** Iodine 125 (I-125) **B** Palladium 103 (Pd-103) **C** Californium 252 (Cf-252) **Y** Other Isotope	**Z** None

Section D **Radiation Therapy**
Body System M **Breast**
Modality 2 **Stereotactic Radiosurgery**

Treatment Site (4th)	Modality Qualifier (5th)	Isotope (6th)	Qualifier (7th)
0 Breast, Left **1** Breast, Right	**D** Stereotactic Other Photon Radiosurgery **H** Stereotactic Particulate Radiosurgery **J** Stereotactic Gamma Beam Radiosurgery	**Z** None	**Z** None

Section D **Radiation Therapy**
Body System M **Breast**
Modality Y **Other Radiation**

Treatment Site (4th)	Modality Qualifier (5th)	Isotope (6th)	Qualifier (7th)
0 Breast, Left **1** Breast, Right	**7** Contact Radiation **8** Hyperthermia **F** Plaque Radiation **K** Laser Interstitial Thermal Therapy	**Z** None	**Z** None

Section D **Radiation Therapy**
Body System P **Musculoskeletal System**
Modality 0 **Beam Radiation**

Treatment Site (4th)	Modality Qualifier (5th)	Isotope (6th)	Qualifier (7th)
0 Skull **2** Maxilla **3** Mandible **4** Sternum **5** Rib(s) **6** Humerus **7** Radius/Ulna **8** Pelvic Bones **9** Femur **B** Tibia/Fibula **C** Other Bone	**0** Photons <1 MeV **1** Photons 1 - 10 MeV **2** Photons >10 MeV **4** Heavy Particles (Protons,Ions) **5** Neutrons **6** Neutron Capture	**Z** None	**Z** None
0 Skull **2** Maxilla **3** Mandible **4** Sternum **5** Rib(s) **6** Humerus **7** Radius/Ulna **8** Pelvic Bones **9** Femur **B** Tibia/Fibula **C** Other Bone	**3** Electrons	**Z** None	**0** Intraoperative **Z** None

Section D **Radiation Therapy**
Body System P **Musculoskeletal System**
Modality Y **Other Radiation**

Treatment Site (4th)	Modality Qualifier (5th)	Isotope (6th)	Qualifier (7th)
0 Skull **2** Maxilla **3** Mandible **4** Sternum **5** Rib(s) **6** Humerus **7** Radius/Ulna **8** Pelvic Bones **9** Femur **B** Tibia/Fibula **C** Other Bone	**7** Contact Radiation **8** Hyperthermia **F** Plaque Radiation	**Z** None	**Z** None

Section D **Radiation Therapy**
Body System T **Urinary System**
Modality 0 **Beam Radiation**

Treatment Site (4th)	Modality Qualifier (5th)	Isotope (6th)	Qualifier (7th)
0 Kidney **1** Ureter **2** Bladder **3** Urethra	**0** Photons <1 MeV **1** Photons 1 - 10 MeV **2** Photons >10 MeV **4** Heavy Particles (Protons,Ions) **5** Neutrons **6** Neutron Capture	**Z** None	**Z** None
0 Kidney **1** Ureter **2** Bladder **3** Urethra	**3** Electrons	**Z** None	**0** Intraoperative **Z** None

Section D **Radiation Therapy**
Body System T **Urinary System**
Modality 1 **Brachytherapy**

Treatment Site (4th)	Modality Qualifier (5th)	Isotope (6th)	Qualifier (7th)
0 Kidney **1** Ureter **2** Bladder **3** Urethra	**9** High Dose Rate (HDR) **B** Low Dose Rate (LDR)	**7** Cesium 137 (Cs-137) **8** Iridium 192 (Ir-192) **9** Iodine 125 (I-125) **B** Palladium 103 (Pd-103) **C** Californium 252 (Cf-252) **Y** Other Isotope	**Z** None

Section D **Radiation Therapy**
Body System T **Urinary System**
Modality 2 **Stereotactic Radiosurgery**

Treatment Site (4th)	Modality Qualifier (5th)	Isotope (6th)	Qualifier (7th)
0 Kidney **1** Ureter **2** Bladder **3** Urethra	**D** Stereotactic Other Photon Radiosurgery **H** Stereotactic Particulate Radiosurgery **J** Stereotactic Gamma Beam Radiosurgery	**Z** None	**Z** None

Section D **Radiation Therapy**
Body System T **Urinary System**
Modality Y **Other Radiation**

Treatment Site (4th)	Modality Qualifier (5th)	Isotope (6th)	Qualifier (7th)
0 Kidney **1** Ureter **2** Bladder **3** Urethra	**7** Contact Radiation **8** Hyperthermia **C** Intraoperative Radiation Therapy (IORT) **F** Plaque Radiation	**Z** None	**Z** None

Section D **Radiation Therapy**
Body System U **Female Reproductive System**
Modality 0 **Beam Radiation**

Treatment Site (4th)	Modality Qualifier (5th)	Isotope (6th)	Qualifier (7th)
0 Ovary **1** Cervix **2** Uterus	**0** Photons <1 MeV **1** Photons 1 - 10 MeV **2** Photons >10 MeV **4** Heavy Particles (Protons,Ions) **5** Neutrons **6** Neutron Capture	**Z** None	**Z** None

Continued →

Section	D	Radiation Therapy
Body System	U	Female Reproductive System
Modality	0	Beam Radiation

Treatment Site (4th)	Modality Qualifier (5th)	Isotope (6th)	Qualifier (7th)
0 Ovary 1 Cervix 2 Uterus	3 Electrons	Z None	0 Intraoperative Z None

Section	D	Radiation Therapy
Body System	U	Female Reproductive System
Modality	1	Brachytherapy

Treatment Site (4th)	Modality Qualifier (5th)	Isotope (6th)	Qualifier (7th)
0 Ovary 1 Cervix 2 Uterus	9 High Dose Rate (HDR) B Low Dose Rate (LDR)	7 Cesium 137 (Cs-137) 8 Iridium 192 (Ir-192) 9 Iodine 125 (I-125) B Palladium 103 (Pd-103) C Californium 252 (Cf-252) Y Other Isotope	Z None

Section	D	Radiation Therapy
Body System	U	Female Reproductive System
Modality	2	Stereotactic Radiosurgery

Treatment Site (4th)	Modality Qualifier (5th)	Isotope (6th)	Qualifier (7th)
0 Ovary 1 Cervix 2 Uterus	D Stereotactic Other Photon Radiosurgery H Stereotactic Particulate Radiosurgery J Stereotactic Gamma Beam Radiosurgery	Z None	Z None

Section	D	Radiation Therapy
Body System	U	Female Reproductive System
Modality	Y	Other Radiation

Treatment Site (4th)	Modality Qualifier (5th)	Isotope (6th)	Qualifier (7th)
0 Ovary 1 Cervix 2 Uterus	7 Contact Radiation 8 Hyperthermia C Intraoperative Radiation Therapy (IORT) F Plaque Radiation	Z None	Z None

Section	D	Radiation Therapy
Body System	V	Male Reproductive System
Modality	0	Beam Radiation

Treatment Site (4th)	Modality Qualifier (5th)	Isotope (6th)	Qualifier (7th)
0 Prostate 1 Testis	0 Photons <1 MeV 1 Photons 1 - 10 MeV 2 Photons >10 MeV 4 Heavy Particles (Protons,Ions) 5 Neutrons 6 Neutron Capture	Z None	Z None
0 Prostate 1 Testis	3 Electrons	Z None	0 Intraoperative Z None

Section D Radiation Therapy
Body System V Male Reproductive System
Modality 1 Brachytherapy

Treatment Site (4th)	Modality Qualifier (5th)	Isotope (6th)	Qualifier (7th)
0 Prostate 1 Testis	9 High Dose Rate (HDR) B Low Dose Rate (LDR)	7 Cesium 137 (Cs-137) 8 Iridium 192 (Ir-192) 9 Iodine 125 (I-125) B Palladium 103 (Pd-103) C Californium 252 (Cf-252) Y Other Isotope	Z None

Section D Radiation Therapy
Body System V Male Reproductive System
Modality 2 Stereotactic Radiosurgery

Treatment Site (4th)	Modality Qualifier (5th)	Isotope (6th)	Qualifier (7th)
0 Prostate 1 Testis	D Stereotactic Other Photon Radiosurgery H Stereotactic Particulate Radiosurgery J Stereotactic Gamma Beam Radiosurgery	Z None	Z None

Section D Radiation Therapy
Body System V Male Reproductive System
Modality Y Other Radiation

Treatment Site (4th)	Modality Qualifier (5th)	Isotope (6th)	Qualifier (7th)
0 Prostate	7 Contact Radiation 8 Hyperthermia C Intraoperative Radiation Therapy (IORT) F Plaque Radiation K Laser Interstitial Thermal Therapy	Z None	Z None
1 Testis	7 Contact Radiation 8 Hyperthermia F Plaque Radiation	Z None	Z None

Section D Radiation Therapy
Body System W Anatomical Regions
Modality 0 Beam Radiation

Treatment Site (4th)	Modality Qualifier (5th)	Isotope (6th)	Qualifier (7th)
1 Head and Neck 2 Chest 3 Abdomen 4 Hemibody 5 Whole Body 6 Pelvic Region	0 Photons <1 MeV 1 Photons 1 - 10 MeV 2 Photons >10 MeV 4 Heavy Particles (Protons,Ions) 5 Neutrons 6 Neutron Capture	Z None	Z None
1 Head and Neck 2 Chest 3 Abdomen 4 Hemibody 5 Whole Body 6 Pelvic Region	3 Electrons	Z None	0 Intraoperative Z None

Section D **Radiation Therapy**
Body System W **Anatomical Regions**
Modality 1 **Brachytherapy**

Treatment Site (4th)	Modality Qualifier (5th)	Isotope (6th)	Qualifier (7th)
1 Head and Neck **2** Chest **3** Abdomen **6** Pelvic Region	**9** High Dose Rate (HDR) **B** Low Dose Rate (LDR)	**7** Cesium 137 (Cs-137) **8** Iridium 192 (Ir-192) **9** Iodine 125 (I-125) **B** Palladium 103 (Pd-103) **C** Californium 252 (Cf-252) **Y** Other Isotope	**Z** None

Section D **Radiation Therapy**
Body System W **Anatomical Regions**
Modality 2 **Stereotactic Radiosurgery**

Treatment Site (4th)	Modality Qualifier (5th)	Isotope (6th)	Qualifier (7th)
1 Head and Neck **2** Chest **3** Abdomen **6** Pelvic Region	**D** Stereotactic Other Photon Radiosurgery **H** Stereotactic Particulate Radiosurgery **J** Stereotactic Gamma Beam Radiosurgery	**Z** None	**Z** None

Section D **Radiation Therapy**
Body System W **Anatomical Regions**
Modality Y **Other Radiation**

Treatment Site (4th)	Modality Qualifier (5th)	Isotope (6th)	Qualifier (7th)
1 Head and Neck **2** Chest **3** Abdomen **4** Hemibody **6** Pelvic Region	**7** Contact Radiation **8** Hyperthermia **F** Plaque Radiation	**Z** None	**Z** None
5 Whole Body	**7** Contact Radiation **8** Hyperthermia **F** Plaque Radiation	**Z** None	**Z** None
5 Whole Body	**G** Isotope Administration	**D** Iodine 131 (I-131) **F** Phosphorus 32 (P-32) **G** Strontium 89 (Sr-89) **H** Strontium 90 (Sr-90) **Y** Other Isotope	**Z** None

Physical Rehabilitation and Diagnostic Audiology Section (F00–F15)

Within each section of ICD-10-PCS the characters have different meanings. The seven character meanings for the Physical Rehabilitation and Diagnostic Audiology section are illustrated below through the procedure example of *Individual fitting of moveable brace, right knee*.

Section	Section Qualifier	Root Type	Body System/ Region	Type Qualifier	Equipment	Qualifier
Physical Rehabilitation and Diagnostic Audiology	Rehabilitation	Device Fitting	None	Dynamic Orthosis	Orthosis	None
F	0	D	Z	6	E	Z

Section (Character 1)

All Physical Rehabilitation and Diagnostic Audiology procedure codes have a first character value of F.

Section Qualifier (Character 2)

The alphanumeric character in the second character position identifies if the procedure is a physical rehabilitation procedure or a diagnostic audiology procedure. Physical rehabilitation is reported with character value 0, and diagnostic audiology is reported with character value 1.

Root Type (Character 3)

The alphanumeric character value for root types is placed in the third position. The following are the root types applicable to the Physical Rehabilitation and Diagnostic Audiology section with their associated meaning.

Character Value	Root Type	Root Type Definition
0	Speech Assessment	Measurement of speech and related functions
1	Motor and/or Nerve Function Assessment	Measurement of motor, nerve, and related functions
2	Activities of Daily Living Assessment	Measurement of functional level for activities of daily living
3	Hearing Assessment	Measurement of hearing and related functions
4	Hearing Aid Assessment	Measurement of the appropriateness and/or effectiveness of a hearing device
5	Vestibular Assessment	Measurement of the vestibular system and related functions
6	Speech Treatment	Application of techniques to improve, augment, or compensate for speech and related functional impairment
7	Motor Treatment	Exercise or activities to increase or facilitate motor function
8	Activities of Daily Living Treatment	Exercise or activities to facilitate functional competence for activities of daily living
9	Hearing Treatment	Application of techniques to improve, augment, or compensate for hearing and related functional impairment
B	Cochlear Implant Treatment	Application of techniques to improve the communication abilities of individuals with cochlear implant
C	Vestibular Treatment	Application of techniques to improve, augment, or compensate for vestibular and related functional impairment
D	Device Fitting	Fitting of a device designed to facilitate or support achievement of a higher level of function
F	Caregiver Training	Training in activities to support patient's optimal level of function

Body System/Region (Character 4)

For each body system/region the applicable body part character values will be available for procedure code construction. An example of a body region for this section is Musculoskeletal System—Lower Back/Lower Extremity.

Type Qualifier (Character 5)

Type qualifier further specifies the root type procedure. For example, the type qualifier of Gait Training/Functional Ambulation is used with Motor Treatment (character value 7) when applicable.

Equipment (Character 6)

If equipment is utilized during the procedure character six is used to report the type. Some examples of equipment are

- Aerobic Endurance and Conditioning
- Electrotherapeutic
- Mechanical
- Orthosis
- Prosthesis

If equipment is not utilized, the placeholder character value of Z should be reported.

Qualifier (Character 7)

The qualifier represents an additional attribute for the procedure when applicable. Currently, there are no qualifiers in the Physical Rehabilitation and Diagnostic Audiology section; therefore, the placeholder character value of Z should be reported.

Physical Rehabilitation and Diagnostic Audiology Section Tables

Physical Rehabilitation and Diagnostic Audiology Tables F00–F15

Section	**F**	**Physical Rehabilitation and Diagnostic Audiology**
Section Qualifier	**0**	**Rehabilitation**
Type	**0**	**Speech Assessment:** Measurement of speech and related functions

Body System / Region (4th)	Type Qualifier (5th)	Equipment (6th)	Qualifier (7th)
3 Neurological System - Whole Body	**G** Communicative/Cognitive Integration Skills	**K** Audiovisual **M** Augmentative / Alternative Communication **P** Computer **Y** Other Equipment **Z** None	**Z** None
Z None	**0** Filtered Speech **3** Staggered Spondaic Word **Q** Performance Intensity Phonetically Balanced Speech Discrimination **R** Brief Tone Stimuli **S** Distorted Speech **T** Dichotic Stimuli **V** Temporal Ordering of Stimuli **W** Masking Patterns	**1** Audiometer **2** Sound Field / Booth **K** Audiovisual **Z** None	**Z** None
Z None	**1** Speech Threshold **2** Speech/Word Recognition	**1** Audiometer **2** Sound Field / Booth **9** Cochlear Implant **K** Audiovisual **Z** None	**Z** None
Z None	**4** Sensorineural Acuity Level	**1** Audiometer **2** Sound Field / Booth **Z** None	**Z** None
Z None	**5** Synthetic Sentence Identification	**1** Audiometer **2** Sound Field / Booth **9** Cochlear Implant **K** Audiovisual	**Z** None
Z None	**6** Speech and/or Language Screening **7** Nonspoken Language **8** Receptive/Expressive Language **C** Aphasia **G** Communicative/Cognitive Integration Skills **L** Augmentative/Alternative Communication System	**K** Audiovisual **M** Augmentative / Alternative Communication **P** Computer **Y** Other Equipment **Z** None	**Z** None

Continued →

Section F **Physical Rehabilitation and Diagnostic Audiology**
Section Qualifier 0 **Rehabilitation**
Type 0 **Speech Assessment:** Measurement of speech and related functions

Body System / Region (4th)	Type Qualifier (5th)	Equipment (6th)	Qualifier (7th)
Z None	**9** Articulation/Phonology	**K** Audiovisual **P** Computer **Q** Speech Analysis **Y** Other Equipment **Z** None	**Z** None
Z None	**B** Motor Speech	**K** Audiovisual **N** Biosensory Feedback **P** Computer **Q** Speech Analysis **T** Aerodynamic Function **Y** Other Equipment **Z** None	**Z** None
Z None	**D** Fluency	**K** Audiovisual **N** Biosensory Feedback **P** Computer **Q** Speech Analysis **S** Voice Analysis **T** Aerodynamic Function **Y** Other Equipment **Z** None	**Z** None
Z None	**F** Voice	**K** Audiovisual **N** Biosensory Feedback **P** Computer **S** Voice Analysis **T** Aerodynamic Function **Y** Other Equipment **Z** None	**Z** None
Z None	**H** Bedside Swallowing and Oral Function **P** Oral Peripheral Mechanism	**Y** Other Equipment **Z** None	**Z** None
Z None	**J** Instrumental Swallowing and Oral Function	**T** Aerodynamic Function **W** Swallowing **Y** Other Equipment	**Z** None
Z None	**K** Orofacial Myofunctional	**K** Audiovisual **P** Computer **Y** Other Equipment **Z** None	**Z** None
Z None	**M** Voice Prosthetic	**K** Audiovisual **P** Computer **S** Voice Analysis **V** Speech Prosthesis **Y** Other Equipment **Z** None	**Z** None
Z None	**N** Non-invasive Instrumental Status	**N** Biosensory Feedback **P** Computer **Q** Speech Analysis **S** Voice Analysis **T** Aerodynamic Function **Y** Other Equipment	**Z** None
Z None	**X** Other Specified Central Auditory Processing	**Z** None	**Z** None

Section F Physical Rehabilitation and Diagnostic Audiology
Section Qualifier 0 Rehabilitation
Type 1 **Motor and/or Nerve Function Assessment:** Measurement of motor, nerve, and related functions

Body System / Region (4th)	Type Qualifier (5th)	Equipment (6th)	Qualifier (7th)
0 Neurological System - Head and Neck **1** Neurological System - Upper Back / Upper Extremity **2** Neurological System - Lower Back / Lower Extremity **3** Neurological System - Whole Body	**0** Muscle Performance	**E** Orthosis **F** Assistive, Adaptive, Supportive or Protective **U** Prosthesis **Y** Other Equipment **Z** None	**Z** None
0 Neurological System - Head and Neck **1** Neurological System - Upper Back / Upper Extremity **2** Neurological System - Lower Back / Lower Extremity **3** Neurological System - Whole Body	**1** Integumentary Integrity **3** Coordination/Dexterity **4** Motor Function **G** Reflex Integrity	**Z** None	**Z** None
0 Neurological System - Head and Neck **1** Neurological System - Upper Back / Upper Extremity **2** Neurological System - Lower Back / Lower Extremity **3** Neurological System - Whole Body	**5** Range of Motion and Joint Integrity **6** Sensory Awareness/ Processing/Integrity	**Y** Other Equipment **Z** None	**Z** None
D Integumentary System - Head and Neck **F** Integumentary System - Upper Back / Upper Extremity **G** Integumentary System - Lower Back / Lower Extremity **H** Integumentary System - Whole Body **J** Musculoskeletal System - Head and Neck **K** Musculoskeletal System - Upper Back / Upper Extremity **L** Musculoskeletal System - Lower Back / Lower Extremity **M** Musculoskeletal System - Whole Body	**0** Muscle Performance	**E** Orthosis **F** Assistive, Adaptive, Supportive or Protective **U** Prosthesis **Y** Other Equipment **Z** None	**Z** None
D Integumentary System - Head and Neck **F** Integumentary System - Upper Back / Upper Extremity **G** Integumentary System - Lower Back / Lower Extremity **H** Integumentary System - Whole Body **J** Musculoskeletal System - Head and Neck **K** Musculoskeletal System - Upper Back / Upper Extremity **L** Musculoskeletal System - Lower Back / Lower Extremity **M** Musculoskeletal System - Whole Body	**1** Integumentary Integrity	**Z** None	**Z** None
D Integumentary System - Head and Neck **F** Integumentary System - Upper Back / Upper Extremity **G** Integumentary System - Lower Back / Lower Extremity **H** Integumentary System - Whole Body **J** Musculoskeletal System - Head and Neck **K** Musculoskeletal System - Upper Back / Upper Extremity **L** Musculoskeletal System - Lower Back / Lower Extremity **M** Musculoskeletal System - Whole Body	**5** Range of Motion and Joint Integrity **6** Sensory Awareness/ Processing/Integrity	**Y** Other Equipment **Z** None	**Z** None

Continued →

Section F **Physical Rehabilitation and Diagnostic Audiology**
Section Qualifier 0 **Rehabilitation**
Type 1 **Motor and/or Nerve Function Assessment:** Measurement of motor, nerve, and related functions

Body System / Region (4th)	Type Qualifier (5th)	Equipment (6th)	Qualifier (7th)
N Genitourinary System	**0** Muscle Performance	**E** Orthosis **F** Assistive, Adaptive, Supportive or Protective **U** Prosthesis **Y** Other Equipment **Z** None	**Z** None
Z None	**2** Visual Motor Integration	**K** Audiovisual **M** Augmentative / Alternative Communication **N** Biosensory Feedback **P** Computer **Q** Speech Analysis **S** Voice Analysis **Y** Other Equipment **Z** None	**Z** None
Z None	**7** Facial Nerve Function	**7** Electrophysiologic	**Z** None
Z None	**9** Somatosensory Evoked Potentials	**J** Somatosensory	**Z** None
Z None	**B** Bed Mobility **C** Transfer **F** Wheelchair Mobility	**E** Orthosis **F** Assistive, Adaptive, Supportive or Protective **U** Prosthesis **Z** None	**Z** None
Z None	**D** Gait and/or Balance	**E** Orthosis **F** Assistive, Adaptive, Supportive or Protective **U** Prosthesis **Y** Other Equipment **Z** None	**Z** None

Section F **Physical Rehabilitation and Diagnostic Audiology**
Section Qualifier 0 **Rehabilitation**
Type 2 **Activities of Daily Living Assessment:** Measurement of functional level for activities of daily living

Body System / Region (4th)	Type Qualifier (5th)	Equipment (6th)	Qualifier (7th)
0 Neurological System - Head and Neck	**9** Cranial Nerve Integrity **D** Neuromotor Development	**Y** Other Equipment **Z** None	**Z** None
1 Neurological System - Upper Back / Upper Extremity **2** Neurological System - Lower Back / Lower Extremity **3** Neurological System - Whole Body	**D** Neuromotor Development	**Y** Other Equipment **Z** None	**Z** None
4 Circulatory System - Head and Neck **5** Circulatory System - Upper Back / Upper Extremity **6** Circulatory System - Lower Back / Lower Extremity **8** Respiratory System - Head and Neck **9** Respiratory System - Upper Back / Upper Extremity **B** Respiratory System - Lower Back / Lower Extremity	**G** Ventilation, Respiration and Circulation	**C** Mechanical **G** Aerobic Endurance and Conditioning **Y** Other Equipment **Z** None	**Z** None

Continued →

Section F **Physical Rehabilitation and Diagnostic Audiology**
Section Qualifier 0 **Rehabilitation**
Type 2 **Activities of Daily Living Assessment:** Measurement of functional level for activities of daily living

Body System / Region (4th)	Type Qualifier (5th)	Equipment (6th)	Qualifier (7th)
7 Circulatory System - Whole Body **C** Respiratory System - Whole Body	**7** Aerobic Capacity and Endurance	**E** Orthosis **G** Aerobic Endurance and Conditioning **U** Prosthesis **Y** Other Equipment **Z** None	**Z** None
7 Circulatory System - Whole Body **C** Respiratory System - Whole Body	**G** Ventilation, Respiration and Circulation	**C** Mechanical **G** Aerobic Endurance and Conditioning **Y** Other Equipment **Z** None	**Z** None
Z None	**0** Bathing/Showering **1** Dressing **3** Grooming/Personal Hygiene **4** Home Management	**E** Orthosis **F** Assistive, Adaptive, Supportive or Protective **U** Prosthesis **Z** None	**Z** None
Z None	**2** Feeding/Eating **8** Anthropometric Characteristics **F** Pain	**Y** Other Equipment **Z** None	**Z** None
Z None	**5** Perceptual Processing	**K** Audiovisual **M** Augmentative / Alternative Communication **N** Biosensory Feedback **P** Computer **Q** Speech Analysis **S** Voice Analysis **Y** Other Equipment **Z** None	**Z** None
Z None	**6** Psychosocial Skills	**Z** None	**Z** None
Z None	**B** Environmental, Home and Work Barriers **C** Ergonomics and Body Mechanics	**E** Orthosis **F** Assistive, Adaptive, Supportive or Protective **U** Prosthesis **Y** Other Equipment **Z** None	**Z** None
Z None	**H** Vocational Activities and Functional Community or Work Reintegration Skills	**E** Orthosis **F** Assistive, Adaptive, Supportive or Protective **G** Aerobic Endurance and Conditioning **U** Prosthesis **Y** Other Equipment **Z** None	**Z** None

Section F **Physical Rehabilitation and Diagnostic Audiology**
Section Qualifier 0 **Rehabilitation**
Type 6 **Speech Treatment:** Application of techniques to improve, augment, or compensate for speech and related functional impairment

Body System / Region (4th)	Type Qualifier (5th)	Equipment (6th)	Qualifier (7th)
3 Neurological System - Whole Body	**6** Communicative/Cognitive Integration Skills	**K** Audiovisual **M** Augmentative / Alternative Communication **P** Computer **Y** Other Equipment **Z** None	**Z** None

Continued →

Section F **Physical Rehabilitation and Diagnostic Audiology**
Section Qualifier 0 **Rehabilitation**
Type 6 **Speech Treatment:** Application of techniques to improve, augment, or compensate for speech and related functional impairment

Body System / Region (4th)	Type Qualifier (5th)	Equipment (6th)	Qualifier (7th)
Z None	**0** Nonspoken Language **3** Aphasia **6** Communicative/Cognitive Integration Skills	**K** Audiovisual **M** Augmentative / Alternative Communication **P** Computer **Y** Other Equipment **Z** None	**Z** None
Z None	**1** Speech-Language Pathology and Related Disorders Counseling **2** Speech-Language Pathology and Related Disorders Prevention	**K** Audiovisual **Z** None	**Z** None
Z None	**4** Articulation/Phonology	**K** Audiovisual **P** Computer **Q** Speech Analysis **T** Aerodynamic Function **Y** Other Equipment **Z** None	**Z** None
Z None	**5** Aural Rehabilitation	**K** Audiovisual **L** Assistive Listening **M** Augmentative / Alternative Communication **N** Biosensory Feedback **P** Computer **Q** Speech Analysis **S** Voice Analysis **Y** Other Equipment **Z** None	**Z** None
Z None	**7** Fluency	**4** Electroacoustic Immitance / Acoustic Reflex **K** Audiovisual **N** Biosensory Feedback **Q** Speech Analysis **S** Voice Analysis **T** Aerodynamic Function **Y** Other Equipment **Z** None	**Z** None
Z None	**8** Motor Speech	**K** Audiovisual **N** Biosensory Feedback **P** Computer **Q** Speech Analysis **S** Voice Analysis **T** Aerodynamic Function **Y** Other Equipment **Z** None	**Z** None
Z None	**9** Orofacial Myofunctional	**K** Audiovisual **P** Computer **Y** Other Equipment **Z** None	**Z** None
Z None	**B** Receptive/Expressive Language	**K** Audiovisual **L** Assistive Listening **M** Augmentative / Alternative Communication **P** Computer **Y** Other Equipment **Z** None	**Z** None

Continued →

Section F **Physical Rehabilitation and Diagnostic Audiology**
Section Qualifier 0 **Rehabilitation**
Type 6 **Speech Treatment:** Application of techniques to improve, augment, or compensate for speech and related functional impairment

Body System / Region (4th)	Type Qualifier (5th)	Equipment (6th)	Qualifier (7th)
Z None	**C** Voice	**K** Audiovisual **N** Biosensory Feedback **P** Computer **S** Voice Analysis **T** Aerodynamic Function **V** Speech Prosthesis **Y** Other Equipment **Z** None	**Z** None
Z None	**D** Swallowing Dysfunction	**M** Augmentative / Alternative Communication **T** Aerodynamic Function **V** Speech Prosthesis **Y** Other Equipment **Z** None	**Z** None

Section F **Physical Rehabilitation and Diagnostic Audiology**
Section Qualifier 0 **Rehabilitation**
Type 7 **Motor Treatment:** Exercise or activities to increase or facilitate motor function

Body System / Region (4th)	Type Qualifier (5th)	Equipment (6th)	Qualifier (7th)
0 Neurological System - Head and Neck **1** Neurological System - Upper Back / Upper Extremity **2** Neurological System - Lower Back / Lower Extremity **3** Neurological System - Whole Body **D** Integumentary System - Head and Neck **F** Integumentary System - Upper Back / Upper Extremity **G** Integumentary System - Lower Back / Lower Extremity **H** Integumentary System - Whole Body **J** Musculoskeletal System - Head and Neck **K** Musculoskeletal System - Upper Back / Upper Extremity **L** Musculoskeletal System - Lower Back / Lower Extremity **M** Musculoskeletal System - Whole Body	**0** Range of Motion and Joint Mobility **1** Muscle Performance **2** Coordination/Dexterity **3** Motor Function	**E** Orthosis **F** Assistive, Adaptive, Supportive or Protective **U** Prosthesis **Y** Other Equipment **Z** None	**Z** None
0 Neurological System - Head and Neck **1** Neurological System - Upper Back / Upper Extremity **2** Neurological System - Lower Back / Lower Extremity **3** Neurological System - Whole Body **D** Integumentary System - Head and Neck **F** Integumentary System - Upper Back / Upper Extremity **G** Integumentary System - Lower Back / Lower Extremity **H** Integumentary System - Whole Body **J** Musculoskeletal System - Head and Neck **K** Musculoskeletal System - Upper Back / Upper Extremity **L** Musculoskeletal System - Lower Back / Lower Extremity **M** Musculoskeletal System - Whole Body	**6** Therapeutic Exercise	**B** Physical Agents **C** Mechanical **D** Electrotherapeutic **E** Orthosis **F** Assistive, Adaptive, Supportive or Protective **G** Aerobic Endurance and Conditioning **H** Mechanical or Electromechanical **U** Prosthesis **Y** Other Equipment **Z** None	**Z** None
0 Neurological System - Head and Neck **1** Neurological System - Upper Back / Upper Extremity **2** Neurological System - Lower Back / Lower Extremity **3** Neurological System - Whole Body **D** Integumentary System - Head and Neck **F** Integumentary System - Upper Back / Upper Extremity **G** Integumentary System - Lower Back / Lower Extremity **H** Integumentary System - Whole Body **J** Musculoskeletal System - Head and Neck **K** Musculoskeletal System - Upper Back / Upper Extremity **L** Musculoskeletal System - Lower Back / Lower Extremity **M** Musculoskeletal System - Whole Body	**7** Manual Therapy Techniques	**Z** None	**Z** None

Continued →

Section F **Physical Rehabilitation and Diagnostic Audiology**
Section Qualifier 0 **Rehabilitation**
Type 7 **Motor Treatment:** Exercise or activities to increase or facilitate motor function

Body System / Region (4th)	Type Qualifier (5th)	Equipment (6th)	Qualifier (7th)
4 Circulatory System - Head and Neck **5** Circulatory System - Upper Back / Upper Extremity **6** Circulatory System - Lower Back / Lower Extremity **7** Circulatory System - Whole Body **8** Respiratory System - Head and Neck **9** Respiratory System - Upper Back / Upper Extremity **B** Respiratory System - Lower Back / Lower Extremity **C** Respiratory System - Whole Body	**6** Therapeutic Exercise	**B** Physical Agents **C** Mechanical **D** Electrotherapeutic **E** Orthosis **F** Assistive, Adaptive, Supportive or Protective **G** Aerobic Endurance and Conditioning **H** Mechanical or Electromechanical **U** Prosthesis **Y** Other Equipment **Z** None	**Z** None
N Genitourinary System	**1** Muscle Performance	**E** Orthosis **F** Assistive, Adaptive, Supportive or Protective **U** Prosthesis **Y** Other Equipment **Z** None	**Z** None
N Genitourinary System	**6** Therapeutic Exercise	**B** Physical Agents **C** Mechanical **D** Electrotherapeutic **E** Orthosis **F** Assistive, Adaptive, Supportive or Protective **G** Aerobic Endurance and Conditioning **H** Mechanical or Electromechanical **U** Prosthesis **Y** Other Equipment **Z** None	**Z** None
Z None	**4** Wheelchair Mobility	**D** Electrotherapeutic **E** Orthosis **F** Assistive, Adaptive, Supportive or Protective **U** Prosthesis **Y** Other Equipment **Z** None	**Z** None
Z None	**5** Bed Mobility	**C** Mechanical **E** Orthosis **F** Assistive, Adaptive, Supportive or Protective **U** Prosthesis **Y** Other Equipment **Z** None	**Z** None
Z None	**8** Transfer Training	**C** Mechanical **D** Electrotherapeutic **E** Orthosis **F** Assistive, Adaptive, Supportive or Protective **U** Prosthesis **Y** Other Equipment **Z** None	**Z** None

Continued →

Section F **Physical Rehabilitation and Diagnostic Audiology**
Section Qualifier 0 **Rehabilitation**
Type 7 **Motor Treatment:** Exercise or activities to increase or facilitate motor function

Body System / Region (4th)	Type Qualifier (5th)	Equipment (6th)	Qualifier (7th)
Z None	**9** Gait Training/Functional Ambulation	**C** Mechanical **D** Electrotherapeutic **E** Orthosis **F** Assistive, Adaptive, Supportive or Protective **G** Aerobic Endurance and Conditioning **U** Prosthesis **Y** Other Equipment **Z** None	**Z** None

Section F **Physical Rehabilitation and Diagnostic Audiology**
Section Qualifier 0 **Rehabilitation**
Type 8 **Activities of Daily Living Treatment:** Exercise or activities to facilitate functional competence for activities of daily living

Body System / Region (4th)	Type Qualifier (5th)	Equipment (6th)	Qualifier (7th)
D Integumentary System - Head and Neck **F** Integumentary System - Upper Back / Upper Extremity **G** Integumentary System - Lower Back / Lower Extremity **H** Integumentary System - Whole Body **J** Musculoskeletal System - Head and Neck **K** Musculoskeletal System - Upper Back / Upper Extremity **L** Musculoskeletal System - Lower Back / Lower Extremity **M** Musculoskeletal System - Whole Body	**5** Wound Management	**B** Physical Agents **C** Mechanical **D** Electrotherapeutic **E** Orthosis **F** Assistive, Adaptive, Supportive or Protective **U** Prosthesis **Y** Other Equipment **Z** None	**Z** None
Z None	**0** Bathing/Showering Techniques **1** Dressing Techniques **2** Grooming/Personal Hygiene	**E** Orthosis **F** Assistive, Adaptive, Supportive or Protective **U** Prosthesis **Y** Other Equipment **Z** None	**Z** None
Z None	**3** Feeding/Eating	**C** Mechanical **D** Electrotherapeutic **E** Orthosis **F** Assistive, Adaptive, Supportive or Protective **U** Prosthesis **Y** Other Equipment **Z** None	**Z** None
Z None	**4** Home Management	**D** Electrotherapeutic **E** Orthosis **F** Assistive, Adaptive, Supportive or Protective **U** Prosthesis **Y** Other Equipment **Z** None	**Z** None
Z None	**6** Psychosocial Skills	**Z** None	**Z** None

Continued →

Section F **Physical Rehabilitation and Diagnostic Audiology**
Section Qualifier 0 **Rehabilitation**
Type 8 **Activities of Daily Living Treatment:** Exercise or activities to facilitate functional competence for activities of daily living

Body System / Region (4th)	Type Qualifier (5th)	Equipment (6th)	Qualifier (7th)
Z None	**7** Vocational Activities and Functional Community or Work Reintegration Skills	**B** Physical Agents **C** Mechanical **D** Electrotherapeutic **E** Orthosis **F** Assistive, Adaptive, Supportive or Protective **G** Aerobic Endurance and Conditioning **U** Prosthesis **Y** Other Equipment **Z** None	**Z** None

Section F **Physical Rehabilitation and Diagnostic Audiology**
Section Qualifier 0 **Rehabilitation**
Type 9 **Hearing Treatment:** Application of techniques to improve, augment, or compensate for hearing and related functional impairment

Body System / Region (4th)	Type Qualifier (5th)	Equipment (6th)	Qualifier (7th)
Z None	**0** Hearing and Related Disorders Counseling **1** Hearing and Related Disorders Prevention	**K** Audiovisual **Z** None	**Z** None
Z None	**2** Auditory Processing	**K** Audiovisual **L** Assistive Listening **P** Computer **Y** Other Equipment **Z** None	**Z** None
Z None	**3** Cerumen Management	**X** Cerumen Management **Z** None	**Z** None

Section F **Physical Rehabilitation and Diagnostic Audiology**
Section Qualifier 0 **Rehabilitation**
Type B **Cochlear Implant Treatment:** Application of techniques to improve the communication abilities of individuals with cochlear implant

Body System / Region (4th)	Type Qualifier (5th)	Equipment (6th)	Qualifier (7th)
Z None	**0** Cochlear Implant Rehabilitation	**1** Audiometer **2** Sound Field / Booth **9** Cochlear Implant **K** Audiovisual **P** Computer **Y** Other Equipment	**Z** None

Section F **Physical Rehabilitation and Diagnostic Audiology**
Section Qualifier 0 **Rehabilitation**
Type C **Vestibular Treatment:** Application of techniques to improve, augment, or compensate for vestibular and related functional impairment

Body System / Region (4th)	Type Qualifier (5th)	Equipment (6th)	Qualifier (7th)
3 Neurological System - Whole Body **H** Integumentary System - Whole Body **M** Musculoskeletal System - Whole Body	**3** Postural Control	**E** Orthosis **F** Assistive, Adaptive, Supportive or Protective **U** Prosthesis **Y** Other Equipment **Z** None	**Z** None

Continued →

Section F Physical Rehabilitation and Diagnostic Audiology
Section Qualifier 0 Rehabilitation
Type C **Vestibular Treatment:** Application of techniques to improve, augment, or compensate for vestibular and related functional impairment

Body System / Region (4th)	Type Qualifier (5th)	Equipment (6th)	Qualifier (7th)
Z None	**0** Vestibular	**8** Vestibular / Balance **Z** None	**Z** None
Z None	**1** Perceptual Processing **2** Visual Motor Integration	**K** Audiovisual **L** Assistive Listening **N** Biosensory Feedback **P** Computer **Q** Speech Analysis **S** Voice Analysis **T** Aerodynamic Function **Y** Other Equipment **Z** None	**Z** None

Section F Physical Rehabilitation and Diagnostic Audiology
Section Qualifier 0 Rehabilitation
Type D **Device Fitting:** Fitting of a device designed to facilitate or support achievement of a higher level of function

Body System / Region (4th)	Type Qualifier (5th)	Equipment (6th)	Qualifier (7th)
Z None	**0** Tinnitus Masker	**5** Hearing Aid Selection / Fitting / Test **Z** None	**Z** None
Z None	**1** Monaural Hearing Aid **2** Binaural Hearing Aid **5** Assistive Listening Device	**1** Audiometer **2** Sound Field / Booth **5** Hearing Aid Selection / Fitting / Test **K** Audiovisual **L** Assistive Listening **Z** None	**Z** None
Z None	**3** Augmentative/Alternative Communication System	**M** Augmentative / Alternative Communication	**Z** None
Z None	**4** Voice Prosthetic	**S** Voice Analysis **V** Speech Prosthesis	**Z** None
Z None	**6** Dynamic Orthosis **7** Static Orthosis **8** Prosthesis **9** Assistive, Adaptive, Supportive or Protective Devices	**E** Orthosis **F** Assistive, Adaptive, Supportive or Protective **U** Prosthesis **Z** None	**Z** None

Section F **Physical Rehabilitation and Diagnostic Audiology**
Section Qualifier 0 **Rehabilitation**
Type F **Caregiver Training:** Training in activities to support patient's optimal level of function

Body System / Region (4th)	Type Qualifier (5th)	Equipment (6th)	Qualifier (7th)
Z None	**0** Bathing/Showering Technique **1** Dressing **2** Feeding and Eating **3** Grooming/Personal Hygiene **4** Bed Mobility **5** Transfer **6** Wheelchair Mobility **7** Therapeutic Exercise **8** Airway Clearance Techniques **9** Wound Management **B** Vocational Activities and Functional Community or Work Reintegration Skills **C** Gait Training/Functional Ambulation **D** Application, Proper Use and Care of Devices **F** Application, Proper Use and Care of Orthoses **G** Application, Proper Use and Care of Prosthesis **H** Home Management	**E** Orthosis **F** Assistive, Adaptive, Supportive or Protective **U** Prosthesis **Z** None	**Z** None
Z None	**J** Communication Skills	**K** Audiovisual **L** Assistive Listening **M** Augmentative / Alternative Communication **P** Computer **Z** None	**Z** None

Section F **Physical Rehabilitation and Diagnostic Audiology**
Section Qualifier 1 **Diagnostic Audiology**
Type 3 **Hearing Assessment:** Measurement of hearing and related functions

Body System / Region (4th)	Type Qualifier (5th)	Equipment (6th)	Qualifier (7th)
Z None	**0** Hearing Screening	**0** Occupational Hearing **1** Audiometer **2** Sound Field / Booth **3** Tympanometer **8** Vestibular / Balance **9** Cochlear Implant **Z** None	**Z** None
Z None	**1** Pure Tone Audiometry, Air **2** Pure Tone Audiometry, Air and Bone	**0** Occupational Hearing **1** Audiometer **2** Sound Field / Booth **Z** None	**Z** None
Z None	**3** Bekesy Audiometry **6** Visual Reinforcement Audiometry **9** Short Increment Sensitivity Index **B** Stenger **C** Pure Tone Stenger	**1** Audiometer **2** Sound Field / Booth **Z** None	**Z** None
Z None	**4** Conditioned Play Audiometry **5** Select Picture Audiometry	**1** Audiometer **2** Sound Field / Booth **K** Audiovisual **Z** None	**Z** None
Z None	**7** Alternate Binaural or Monaural Loudness Balance	**1** Audiometer **K** Audiovisual **Z** None	**Z** None

Continued →

Section F Physical Rehabilitation and Diagnostic Audiology
Section Qualifier 1 Diagnostic Audiology
Type 3 **Hearing Assessment:** Measurement of hearing and related functions

Body System / Region (4th)	Type Qualifier (5th)	Equipment (6th)	Qualifier (7th)
Z None	**8** Tone Decay **D** Tympanometry **F** Eustachian Tube Function **G** Acoustic Reflex Patterns **H** Acoustic Reflex Threshold **J** Acoustic Reflex Decay	**3** Tympanometer **4** Electroacoustic Immitance / Acoustic Reflex **Z** None	**Z** None
Z None	**K** Electrocochleography **L** Auditory Evoked Potentials	**7** Electrophysiologic **Z** None	**Z** None
Z None	**M** Evoked Otoacoustic Emissions, Screening **N** Evoked Otoacoustic Emissions, Diagnostic	**6** Otoacoustic Emission (OAE) **Z** None	**Z** None
Z None	**P** Aural Rehabilitation Status	**1** Audiometer **2** Sound Field / Booth **4** Electroacoustic Immitance / Acoustic Reflex **9** Cochlear Implant **K** Audiovisual **L** Assistive Listening **P** Computer **Z** None	**Z** None
Z None	**Q** Auditory Processing	**K** Audiovisual **P** Computer **Y** Other Equipment **Z** None	**Z** None

Section F Physical Rehabilitation and Diagnostic Audiology
Section Qualifier 1 Diagnostic Audiology
Type 4 **Hearing Aid Assessment:** Measurement of the appropriateness and/or effectiveness of a hearing device

Body System / Region (4th)	Type Qualifier (5th)	Equipment (6th)	Qualifier (7th)
Z None	**0** Cochlear Implant	**1** Audiometer **2** Sound Field / Booth **3** Tympanometer **4** Electroacoustic Immitance / Acoustic Reflex **5** Hearing Aid Selection / Fitting / Test **7** Electrophysiologic **9** Cochlear Implant **K** Audiovisual **L** Assistive Listening **P** Computer **Y** Other Equipment **Z** None	**Z** None
Z None	**1** Ear Canal Probe Microphone **6** Binaural Electroacoustic Hearing Aid Check **8** Monaural Electroacoustic Hearing Aid Check	**5** Hearing Aid Selection / Fitting / Test **Z** None	**Z** None

Continued →

Section F **Physical Rehabilitation and Diagnostic Audiology**
Section Qualifier 1 **Diagnostic Audiology**
Type 4 **Hearing Aid Assessment:** Measurement of the appropriateness and/or effectiveness of a hearing device

Body System / Region (4th)	Type Qualifier (5th)	Equipment (6th)	Qualifier (7th)
Z None	**2** Monaural Hearing Aid **3** Binaural Hearing Aid	**1** Audiometer **2** Sound Field / Booth **3** Tympanometer **4** Electroacoustic Immitance / Acoustic Reflex **5** Hearing Aid Selection / Fitting / Test **K** Audiovisual **L** Assistive Listening **P** Computer **Z** None	**Z** None
Z None	**4** Assistive Listening System/ Device Selection	**1** Audiometer **2** Sound Field / Booth **3** Tympanometer **4** Electroacoustic Immitance / Acoustic Reflex **K** Audiovisual **L** Assistive Listening **Z** None	**Z** None
Z None	**5** Sensory Aids	**1** Audiometer **2** Sound Field / Booth **3** Tympanometer **4** Electroacoustic Immitance / Acoustic Reflex **5** Hearing Aid Selection / Fitting / Test **K** Audiovisual **L** Assistive Listening **Z** None	**Z** None
Z None	**7** Ear Protector Attentuation	**0** Occupational Hearing **Z** None	**Z** None

Section F **Physical Rehabilitation and Diagnostic Audiology**
Section Qualifier 1 **Diagnostic Audiology**
Type 5 **Vestibular Assessment:** Measurement of the vestibular system and related functions

Body System / Region (4th)	Type Qualifier (5th)	Equipment (6th)	Qualifier (7th)
Z None	**0** Bithermal, Binaural Caloric Irrigation **1** Bithermal, Monaural Caloric Irrigation **2** Unithermal Binaural Screen **3** Oscillating Tracking **4** Sinusoidal Vertical Axis Rotational **5** Dix-Hallpike Dynamic **6** Computerized Dynamic Posturography	**8** Vestibular / Balance **Z** None	**Z** None
Z None	**7** Tinnitus Masker	**5** Hearing Aid Selection / Fitting / Test **Z** None	**Z** None

Mental Health Section (GZ1–GZJ)

Within each section of ICD-10-PCS the characters have different meanings. The seven character meanings for the Mental Health section are illustrated here through the procedure example of *Crisis intervention*.

Section	Body System	Root Type	Qualifier	Qualifier	Qualifier	Qualifier
Mental Health	None	Crisis Intervention	None	None	None	None
G	Z	2	Z	Z	Z	Z

Section (Character 1)

All Mental Health procedure codes have a first character value of G.

Body System (Character 2)

The body system is not specified for mental health; therefore, the placeholder character value of Z is reported in the second character position.

Root Type (Character 3)

The alphanumeric character value for root types is placed in the third position. Listed below are the root types applicable to the Mental Health section with their associated meaning.

Character Value	Root Type	Root Type Definition
1	Psychological Tests	The administration and interpretation of standardized psychological tests and measurement instruments for the assessment of psychological function
2	Crisis Intervention	Treatment of a traumatized, acutely disturbed or distressed individual for the purpose of short-term stabilization
3	Medication Management	Monitoring and adjusting the use of medications for the treatment of a mental health disorder
5	Individual Psychotherapy	Treatment of an individual with a mental health disorder by behavioral, cognitive, psychoanalytic, psychodynamic or psychophysiological means to improve functioning or well-being
6	Counseling	The application of psychological methods to treat an individual with normal developmental issues and psychological problems in order to increase function, improve well-being, alleviate distress, maladjustment or resolve crises
7	Family Psychotherapy	Treatment that includes one or more family members of an individual with a mental health disorder by behavioral, cognitive, psychoanalytic, psychodynamic or psychophysiological means to improve functioning or well-being
B	Electroconvulsive Therapy	The application of controlled electrical voltages to treat a mental health disorder
C	Biofeedback	Provision of information from the monitoring and regulating of physiological processes in conjunction with cognitive-behavioral techniques to improve patient functioning or well-being
F	Hypnosis	Induction of a state of heightened suggestibility by auditory, visual and tactile techniques to elicit an emotional or behavioral response
G	Narcosynthesis	Administration of intravenous barbiturates in order to release suppressed or repressed thoughts
H	Group Psychotherapy	Treatment of two or more individuals with a mental health disorder by behavioral, cognitive, psychoanalytic, psychodynamic or psychophysiological means to improve functioning or well-being
J	Light Therapy	Application of specialized light treatments to improve functioning or well-being

Qualifier (Character 4)

This qualifier further specifies the root type procedure. For example, the qualifier of Development further specifies the type of Psychological Tests.

Qualifier (Character 5)

The qualifier represents an additional attribute for the procedure when applicable. Currently, there are no qualifiers in the Mental Health section; therefore, the placeholder character value of Z should be reported.

Qualifier (Character 6)

The qualifier represents an additional attribute for the procedure when applicable. Currently, there are no qualifiers in the Mental Health section; therefore, the placeholder character value of Z should be reported.

Qualifier (Character 7)

The qualifier represents an additional attribute for the procedure when applicable. Currently, there are no qualifiers in the Mental Health section; therefore, the placeholder character value of Z should be reported.

Mental Health Tables

Mental Health Tables GZ1–GZJ

Section **G** **Mental Health**
Body System **Z** **None**
Type **1** **Psychological Tests:** The administration and interpretation of standardized psychological tests and measurement instruments for the assessment of psychological function

Qualifier (4th)	Qualifier (5th)	Qualifier (6th)	Qualifier (7th)
0 Developmental **1** Personality and Behavioral **2** Intellectual and Psychoeducational **3** Neuropsychological **4** Neurobehavioral and Cognitive Status	**Z** None	**Z** None	**Z** None

Section **G** **Mental Health**
Body System **Z** **None**
Type **2** **Crisis Intervention:** Treatment of a traumatized, acutely disturbed or distressed individual for the purpose of short-term stabilization

Qualifier (4th)	Qualifier (5th)	Qualifier (6th)	Qualifier (7th)
Z None	**Z** None	**Z** None	**Z** None

Section **G** **Mental Health**
Body System **Z** **None**
Type **3** **Medication Management:** Monitoring and adjusting the use of medications for the treatment of a mental health disorder

Qualifier (4th)	Qualifier (5th)	Qualifier (6th)	Qualifier (7th)
Z None	**Z** None	**Z** None	**Z** None

Section **G** **Mental Health**
Body System **Z** **None**
Type **5** **Individual Psychotherapy:** Treatment of an individual with a mental health disorder by behavioral, cognitive, psychoanalytic, psychodynamic or psychophysiological means to improve functioning or well-being

Qualifier (4th)	Qualifier (5th)	Qualifier (6th)	Qualifier (7th)
0 Interactive **1** Behavioral **2** Cognitive **3** Interpersonal **4** Psychoanalysis **5** Psychodynamic **6** Supportive **8** Cognitive-Behavioral **9** Psychophysiological	**Z** None	**Z** None	**Z** None

Section G **Mental Health**
Body System Z **None**
Type 6 **Counseling:** The application of psychological methods to treat an individual with normal developmental issues and psychological problems in order to increase function, improve well-being, alleviate distress, maladjustment or resolve crises

Qualifier (4th)	Qualifier (5th)	Qualifier (6th)	Qualifier (7th)
0 Educational 1 Vocational 3 Other Counseling	Z None	Z None	Z None

Section G **Mental Health**
Body System Z **None**
Type 7 **Family Psychotherapy:** Treatment that includes one or more family members of an individual with a mental health disorder by behavioral, cognitive, psychoanalytic, psychodynamic or psychophysiological means to improve functioning or well-being

Qualifier (4th)	Qualifier (5th)	Qualifier (6th)	Qualifier (7th)
2 Other Family Psychotherapy	Z None	Z None	Z None

Section G **Mental Health**
Body System Z **None**
Type B **Electroconvulsive Therapy:** The application of controlled electrical voltages to treat a mental health disorder

Qualifier (4th)	Qualifier (5th)	Qualifier (6th)	Qualifier (7th)
0 Unilateral-Single Seizure 1 Unilateral-Multiple Seizure 2 Bilateral-Single Seizure 3 Bilateral-Multiple Seizure 4 Other Electroconvulsive Therapy	Z None	Z None	Z None

Section G **Mental Health**
Body System Z **None**
Type C **Biofeedback:** Provision of information from the monitoring and regulating of physiological processes in conjunction with cognitive-behavioral techniques to improve patient functioning or well-being

Qualifier (4th)	Qualifier (5th)	Qualifier (6th)	Qualifier (7th)
9 Other Biofeedback	Z None	Z None	Z None

Section G **Mental Health**
Body System Z **None**
Type F **Hypnosis:** Induction of a state of heightened suggestibility by auditory, visual and tactile techniques to elicit an emotional or behavioral response

Qualifier (4th)	Qualifier (5th)	Qualifier (6th)	Qualifier (7th)
Z None	Z None	Z None	Z None

Section G **Mental Health**
Body System Z **None**
Type G **Narcosynthesis:** Administration of intravenous barbiturates in order to release suppressed or repressed thoughts

Qualifier (4th)	Qualifier (5th)	Qualifier (6th)	Qualifier (7th)
Z None	Z None	Z None	Z None

Section G **Mental Health**
Body System Z **None**
Type H **Group Psychotherapy:** Treatment of two or more individuals with a mental health disorder by behavioral, cognitive, psychoanalytic, psychodynamic or psychophysiological means to improve functioning or well-being

Qualifier (4th)	Qualifier (5th)	Qualifier (6th)	Qualifier (7th)
Z None	Z None	Z None	Z None

Section G **Mental Health**
Body System Z **None**
Type J **Light Therapy:** Application of specialized light treatments to improve functioning or well-being

Qualifier (4th)	Qualifier (5th)	Qualifier (6th)	Qualifier (7th)
Z None	Z None	Z None	Z None

Substance Abuse Section (HZ2–HZ9)

Within each section of ICD-10-PCS the characters have different meanings. The seven character meanings for the Substance Abuse section are illustrated below through the procedure example of *Substance abuse family counseling*.

Section	Body System	Root Type	Qualifier	Qualifier	Qualifier	Qualifier
Substance Abuse	None	Family Counseling	Other Family Counseling	None	None	None
H	Z	6	3	Z	Z	Z

Section (Character 1)

All Substance Abuse procedure codes have a first character value of H.

Body System (Character 2)

The body system is not specified for substance abuse; therefore, the placeholder character value of Z is reported in the second character position.

Root Type (Character 3)

The alphanumeric character value for root types is placed in the third position. The following are the root types applicable to the Substance Abuse section with their associated meaning.

Character Value	Root Type	Root Type Definition
2	Detoxification Services	Detoxification from alcohol and/or drugs
3	Individual Counseling	The application of psychological methods to treat an individual with addictive behavior
4	Group Counseling	The application of psychological methods to treat two or more individuals with addictive behavior
5	Individual Psychotherapy	Treatment of an individual with addictive behavior by behavioral, cognitive, psychoanalytic, psychodynamic or psychophysiological means
6	Family Counseling	The application of psychological methods that includes one or more family members to treat an individual with addictive behavior
8	Medication Management	Monitoring and adjusting the use of replacement medications for the treatment of addiction
9	Pharmacotherapy	The use of replacement medications for the treatment of addiction

Qualifier (Character 4)

This qualifier further specifies the root type procedure. For example, the qualifier of Cognitive further specifies the type of Individual counseling.

Qualifier (Character 5)

The qualifier represents an additional attribute for the procedure when applicable. Currently, there are no qualifiers in the Substance Abuse section; therefore, the placeholder character value of Z should be reported.

Qualifier (Character 6)

The qualifier represents an additional attribute for the procedure when applicable. Currently, there are no qualifiers in the Substance Abuse section; therefore, the placeholder character value of Z should be reported.

Qualifier (Character 7)

The qualifier represents an additional attribute for the procedure when applicable. Currently, there are no qualifiers in the Substance Abuse section; therefore, the placeholder character value of Z should be reported.

Substance Abuse Treatment Section Tables

Substance Abuse Treatment Tables HZ2–HZ9

Section H **Substance Abuse Treatment**
Body System Z **None**
Type 2 **Detoxification Services:** Detoxification from alcohol and/or drugs

Qualifier (4th)	Qualifier (5th)	Qualifier (6th)	Qualifier (7th)
Z None	**Z** None	**Z** None	**Z** None

Section H **Substance Abuse Treatment**
Body System Z **None**
Type 3 **Individual Counseling:** The application of psychological methods to treat an individual with addictive behavior

Qualifier (4th)	Qualifier (5th)	Qualifier (6th)	Qualifier (7th)
0 Cognitive **1** Behavioral **2** Cognitive-Behavioral **3** 12-Step **4** Interpersonal **5** Vocational **6** Psychoeducation **7** Motivational Enhancement **8** Confrontational **9** Continuing Care **B** Spiritual **C** Pre/Post-Test Infectious Disease	**Z** None	**Z** None	**Z** None

Section H **Substance Abuse Treatment**
Body System Z **None**
Type 4 **Group Counseling:** The application of psychological methods to treat two or more individuals with addictive behavior

Qualifier (4th)	Qualifier (5th)	Qualifier (6th)	Qualifier (7th)
0 Cognitive **1** Behavioral **2** Cognitive-Behavioral **3** 12-Step **4** Interpersonal **5** Vocational **6** Psychoeducation **7** Motivational Enhancement **8** Confrontational **9** Continuing Care **B** Spiritual **C** Pre/Post-Test Infectious Disease	**Z** None	**Z** None	**Z** None

Section H Substance Abuse Treatment
Body System Z None
Type 5 **Individual Psychotherapy:** Treatment of an individual with addictive behavior by behavioral, cognitive, psychoanalytic, psychodynamic or psychophysiological means

Qualifier (4th)	Qualifier (5th)	Qualifier (6th)	Qualifier (7th)
0 Cognitive 1 Behavioral 2 Cognitive-Behavioral 3 12-Step 4 Interpersonal 5 Interactive 6 Psychoeducation 7 Motivational Enhancement 8 Confrontational 9 Supportive B Psychoanalysis C Psychodynamic D Psychophysiological	Z None	Z None	Z None

Section H Substance Abuse Treatment
Body System Z None
Type 6 **Family Counseling:** The application of psychological methods that includes one or more family members to treat an individual with addictive behavior

Qualifier (4th)	Qualifier (5th)	Qualifier (6th)	Qualifier (7th)
3 Other Family Counseling	Z None	Z None	Z None

Section H Substance Abuse Treatment
Body System Z None
Type 8 **Medication Management:** Monitoring and adjusting the use of replacement medications for the treatment of addiction

Qualifier (4th)	Qualifier (5th)	Qualifier (6th)	Qualifier (7th)
0 Nicotine Replacement 1 Methadone Maintenance 2 Levo-alpha-acetyl-methadol (LAAM) 3 Antabuse 4 Naltrexone 5 Naloxone 6 Clonidine 7 Bupropion 8 Psychiatric Medication 9 Other Replacement Medication	Z None	Z None	Z None

Section H Substance Abuse Treatment
Body System Z None
Type 9 **Pharmacotherapy:** The use of replacement medications for the treatment of addiction

Qualifier (4th)	Qualifier (5th)	Qualifier (6th)	Qualifier (7th)
0 Nicotine Replacement 1 Methadone Maintenance 2 Levo-alpha-acetyl-methadol (LAAM) 3 Antabuse 4 Naltrexone 5 Naloxone 6 Clonidine 7 Bupropion 8 Psychiatric Medication 9 Other Replacement Medication	Z None	Z None	Z None

Appendix A: Root Operations Definitions

Section 0 - Medical and Surgical — Character 3 - Root Operation	
Alteration (0)	**Definition:** Modifying the anatomic structure of a body part without affecting the function of the body part **Explanation:** Principal purpose is to improve appearance **Includes/Examples:** Face lift, breast augmentation
Bypass (1)	**Definition:** Altering the route of passage of the contents of a tubular body part **Explanation:** Rerouting contents of a body part to a downstream area of the normal route, to a similar route and body part, or to an abnormal route and dissimilar body part. Includes one or more anastomoses, with or without the use of a device **Includes/Examples:** Coronary artery bypass, colostomy formation
Change (2)	**Definition:** Taking out or off a device from a body part and putting back an identical or similar device in or on the same body part without cutting or puncturing the skin or a mucous membrane **Explanation:** All CHANGE procedures are coded using the approach EXTERNAL **Includes/Examples:** Urinary catheter change, gastrostomy tube change
Control (3)	**Definition:** Stopping, or attempting to stop, postprocedural bleeding **Explanation:** The site of the bleeding is coded as an anatomical region and not to a specific body part **Includes/Examples:** Control of post-prostatectomy hemorrhage, control of post-tonsillectomy hemorrhage
Creation (4)	**Definition:** Making a new genital structure that does not take over the function of a body part **Explanation:** Used only for sex change operations **Includes/Examples:** Creation of vagina in a male, creation of penis in a female
Destruction (5)	**Definition:** Physical eradication of all or a portion of a body part by the direct use of energy, force, or a destructive agent **Explanation:** None of the body part is physically taken out **Includes/Examples:** Fulguration of rectal polyp, cautery of skin lesion
Detachment (6)	**Definition:** Cutting off all or a portion of the upper or lower extremities **Explanation:** The body part value is the site of the detachment, with a qualifier if applicable to further specify the level where the extremity was detached **Includes/Examples:** Below knee amputation, disarticulation of shoulder
Dilation (7)	**Definition:** Expanding an orifice or the lumen of a tubular body part **Explanation:** The orifice can be a natural orifice or an artificially created orifice. Accomplished by stretching a tubular body part using intraluminal pressure or by cutting part of the orifice or wall of the tubular body part **Includes/Examples:** Percutaneous transluminal angioplasty, pyloromyotomy
Division (8)	**Definition:** Cutting into a body part, without draining fluids and/or gases from the body part, in order to separate or transect a body part **Explanation:** All or a portion of the body part is separated into two or more portions **Includes/Examples:** Spinal cordotomy, osteotomy
Drainage (9)	**Definition:** Taking or letting out fluids and/or gases from a body part **Explanation:** The qualifier DIAGNOSTIC is used to identify drainage procedures that are biopsies **Includes/Examples:** Thoracentesis, incision and drainage
Excision (B)	**Definition:** Cutting out or off, without replacement, a portion of a body part **Explanation:** The qualifier DIAGNOSTIC is used to identify excision procedures that are biopsies **Includes/Examples:** Partial nephrectomy, liver biopsy
Extirpation (C)	**Definition:** Taking or cutting out solid matter from a body part **Explanation:** The solid matter may be an abnormal byproduct of a biological function or a foreign body; it may be imbedded in a body part or in the lumen of a tubular body part. The solid matter may or may not have been previously broken into pieces **Includes/Examples:** Thrombectomy, choledocholithotomy
Extraction (D)	**Definition:** Pulling or stripping out or off all or a portion of a body part by the use of force **Explanation:** The qualifier DIAGNOSTIC is used to identify extraction procedures that are biopsies **Includes/Examples:** Dilation and curettage, vein stripping
Fragmentation (F)	**Definition:** Breaking solid matter in a body part into pieces **Explanation:** Physical force (e.g., manual, ultrasonic) applied directly or indirectly is used to break the solid matter into pieces. The solid matter may be an abnormal byproduct of a biological function or a foreign body. The pieces of solid matter are not taken out **Includes/Examples:** Extracorporeal shockwave lithotripsy, transurethral lithotripsy
Fusion (G)	**Definition:** Joining together portions of an articular body part rendering the articular body part immobile **Explanation:** The body part is joined together by fixation device, bone graft, or other means **Includes/Examples:** Spinal fusion, ankle arthrodesis
Insertion (H)	**Definition:** Putting in a nonbiological appliance that monitors, assists, performs, or prevents a physiological function but does not physically take the place of a body part **Includes/Examples:** Insertion of radioactive implant, insertion of central venous catheter

Continued →

Section 0 - Medical and Surgical — Character 3 - Root Operation

Inspection (J)	**Definition:** Visually and/or manually exploring a body part **Explanation:** Visual exploration may be performed with or without optical instrumentation. Manual exploration may be performed directly or through intervening body layers **Includes/Examples:** Diagnostic arthroscopy, exploratory laparotomy
Map (K)	**Definition:** Locating the route of passage of electrical impulses and/or locating functional areas in a body part **Explanation:** Applicable only to the cardiac conduction mechanism and the central nervous system **Includes/Examples:** Cardiac mapping, cortical mapping
Occlusion (L)	**Definition:** Completely closing an orifice or the lumen of a tubular body part **Explanation:** The orifice can be a natural orifice or an artificially created orifice **Includes/Examples:** Fallopian tube ligation, ligation of inferior vena cava
Reattachment (M)	**Definition:** Putting back in or on all or a portion of a separated body part to its normal location or other suitable location **Explanation:** Vascular circulation and nervous pathways may or may not be reestablished **Includes/Examples:** Reattachment of hand, reattachment of avulsed kidney
Release (N)	**Definition:** Freeing a body part from an abnormal physical constraint by cutting or by the use of force **Explanation:** Some of the restraining tissue may be taken out but none of the body part is taken out **Includes/Examples:** Adhesiolysis, carpal tunnel release
Removal (P)	**Definition:** Taking out or off a device from a body part **Explanation:** If a device is taken out and a similar device put in without cutting or puncturing the skin or mucous membrane, the procedure is coded to the root operation CHANGE. Otherwise, the procedure for taking out a device is coded to the root operation REMOVAL **Includes/Examples:** Drainage tube removal, cardiac pacemaker removal
Repair (Q)	**Definition:** Restoring, to the extent possible, a body part to its normal anatomic structure and function **Explanation:** Used only when the method to accomplish the repair is not one of the other root operations **Includes/Examples:** Colostomy takedown, suture of laceration
Replacement (R)	**Definition:** Putting in or on biological or synthetic material that physically takes the place and/or function of all or a portion of a body part **Explanation:** The body part may have been taken out or replaced, or may be taken out, physically eradicated, or rendered nonfunctional during the Replacement procedure. A Removal procedure is coded for taking out the device used in a previous replacement procedure **Includes/Examples:** Total hip replacement, bone graft, free skin graft
Reposition (S)	**Definition:** Moving to its normal location, or other suitable location, all or a portion of a body part **Explanation:** The body part is moved to a new location from an abnormal location, or from a normal location where it is not functioning correctly. The body part may or may not be cut out or off to be moved to the new location **Includes/Examples:** Reposition of undescended testicle, fracture reduction
Resection (T)	**Definition:** Cutting out or off, without replacement, all of a body part **Includes/Examples:** Total nephrectomy, total lobectomy of lung
Restriction (V)	**Definition:** Partially closing an orifice or the lumen of a tubular body part **Explanation:** The orifice can be a natural orifice or an artificially created orifice **Includes/Examples:** Esophagogastric fundoplication, cervical cerclage
Revision (W)	**Definition:** Correcting, to the extent possible, a portion of a malfunctioning device or the position of a displaced device **Explanation:** Revision can include correcting a malfunctioning or displaced device by taking out or putting in components of the device such as a screw or pin **Includes/Examples:** Adjustment of position of pacemaker lead, recementing of hip prosthesis
Supplement (U)	**Definition:** Putting in or on biological or synthetic material that physically reinforces and/or augments the function of a portion of a body part **Explanation:** The biological material is non-living, or is living and from the same individual. The body part may have been previously replaced, and the Supplement procedure is performed to physically reinforce and/or augment the function of the replaced body part **Includes/Examples:** Herniorrhaphy using mesh, free nerve graft, mitral valve ring annuloplasty, put a new acetabular liner in a previous hip replacement
Transfer (X)	**Definition:** Moving, without taking out, all or a portion of a body part to another location to take over the function of all or a portion of a body part **Explanation:** The body part transferred remains connected to its vascular and nervous supply **Includes/Examples:** Tendon transfer, skin pedicle flap transfer
Transplantation (Y)	**Definition:** Putting in or on all or a portion of a living body part taken from another individual or animal to physically take the place and/or function of all or a portion of a similar body part **Explanation:** The native body part may or may not be taken out, and the transplanted body part may take over all or a portion of its function **Includes/Examples:** Kidney transplant, heart transplant

Section 1 - Obstetrics — Character 3 - Root Operations Unique to Obstetrics

Abortion (A)	**Definition:** Artificially terminating a pregnancy **Explanation:** Subdivided according to whether an additional device such as a laminaria or abortifacient is used, or whether the abortion was performed by mechanical means **Includes/Example:** Transvaginal abortion using vacuum aspiration technique

Continued →

Section 1 - Obstetrics — Character 3 - Root Operations Unique to Obstetrics	
Delivery (E)	**Definition:** Assisting the passage of the products of conception from the genital canal **Explanation:** Applies only to manually-assisted, vaginal delivery **Includes/Example:** Manually-assisted delivery

Section 2 - Placement — Character 3 - Root Operation	
Change (0)	**Definition:** Taking out or off a device from a body part and putting back an identical or similar device in or on the same body part without cutting or puncturing the skin or a mucous membrane **Includes/Example:** Change of vaginal packing
Compression (1)	**Definition:** Putting pressure on a body region **Includes/Example:** Placement of pressure dressing on abdominal wall
Dressing (2)	**Definition:** Putting material on a body region for protection **Includes/Example:** Application of sterile dressing to head wound
Immobilization (3)	**Definition:** Limiting or preventing motion of a body region **Includes/Example:** Placement of splint on left finger
Packing (4)	**Definition:** Putting material in a body region or orifice **Includes/Example:** Placement of nasal packing
Removal (5)	**Definition:** Taking out or off a device from a body part **Includes/Example:** Removal of cast from right lower leg
Traction (6)	**Definition:** Exerting a pulling force on a body region in a distal direction **Includes/Example:** Lumbar traction using motorized split-traction table

Section 3 - Administration — Character 3 - Root Operation	
Introduction (0)	**Definition:** Putting in or on a therapeutic, diagnostic, nutritional, physiological, or prophylactic substance except blood or blood products **Includes/Example:** Nerve block injection to median nerve
Irrigation (1)	**Definition:** Putting in or on a cleansing substance **Includes/Example:** Flushing of eye
Transfusion (2)	**Definition:** Putting in blood or blood products **Includes/Example:** Transfusion of cell saver red cells into central venous line

Section 4 - Measurement and Monitoring — Character 3 - Root Operation	
Measurement (0)	**Definition:** Determining the level of a physiological or physical function at a point in time **Includes/Example:** External electrocardiogram (EKG), single reading
Monitoring (1)	**Definition:** Determining the level of a physiological or physical function repetitively over a period of time **Includes/Example:** Urinary pressure monitoring

Section 5 - Extracorporeal Assistance and Performance — Character 3 - Root Operation	
Assistance (0)	**Definition:** Taking over a portion of a physiological function by extracorporeal means **Includes/Example:** Hyperbaric oxygenation of wound
Performance (1)	**Definition:** Completely taking over a physiological function by extracorporeal means **Includes/Example:** Cardiopulmonary bypass in conjunction with CABG
Restoration (2)	**Definition:** Returning, or attempting to return, a physiological function to its original state by extracorporeal means. **Includes/Example:** Attempted cardiac defibrillation, unsuccessful

Section 6 - Extracorporeal Therapies — Character 3 - Root Operation	
Atmospheric Control (0)	**Definition:** Extracorporeal control of atmospheric pressure and composition **Includes/Example:** Atmospheric control, single treatment
Decompression (1)	**Definition:** Extracorporeal elimination of undissolved gas from body fluids **Includes/Example:** Hyperbaric decompression treatment, single
Electromagnetic Therapy (2)	**Definition:** Extracorporeal treatment by electromagnetic rays **Includes/Example:** Electromagnetic therapy, central nervous, multiple treatments
Hyperthermia (3)	**Definition:** Extracorporeal raising of body temperature **Includes/Example:** Hyperthermia, single treatment

Continued →

Section 6 - Extracorporeal Therapies — Character 3 - Root Operation	
Hypothermia (4)	**Definition:** Extracorporeal lowering of body temperature **Includes/Example:** Whole body hypothermia treatment for temperature imbalances, series treatment
Pheresis (5)	**Definition:** Extracorporeal separation of blood products **Includes/Example:** Therapeutic leukopheresis, single treatment
Phototherapy (6)	**Definition:** Extracorporeal treatment by light rays **Includes/Example:** Phototherapy of circulatory system, series treatment
Shock Wave Therapy (7)	**Definition:** Extracorporeal treatment by shock waves **Includes/Example:** Shock wave therapy, musculoskeletal, single treatment
Ultrasound Therapy (8)	**Definition:** Extracorporeal treatment by ultrasound **Includes/Example:** Ultrasound therapy of the heart, single treatment
Ultraviolet Light Therapy (9)	**Definition:** Extracorporeal treatment by ultraviolet light **Includes/Example:** Ultraviolet light phototherapy, series treatment

Section 7 - Osteopathic — Character 3 - Root Operation	
Treatment (0)	**Definition:** Manual treatment to eliminate or alleviate somatic dysfunction and related disorders **Includes/Example:** Fascial release of abdomen, osteopathic treatment

Section 8 - Other Procedures — Character 3 - Root Operation	
Other Procedures (0)	**Definition:** Methodologies which attempt to remediate or cure a disorder or disease **Includes/Example:** Acupuncture

Section 9 - Chiropractic — Character 3 - Root Operation	
Manipulation (B)	**Definition:** Manual procedure that involves a directed thrust to move a joint past the physiological range of motion, without exceeding the anatomical limit **Includes/Example:** Chiropractic treatment of cervical spine, short lever specific contact

Appendix B: Type and Qualifier Definitions

Section B - Imaging — Character 3 - Root Type	
Computerized Tomography (CT Scan)	**Definition:** Computer reformatted digital display of multiplanar images developed from the capture of multiple exposures of external ionizing radiation
Fluoroscopy	**Definition:** Single plane or bi-plane real time display of an image developed from the capture of external ionizing radiation on a fluorescent screen. The image may also be stored by either digital or analog means
Magnetic Resonance Imaging (MRI)	**Definition:** Computer reformatted digital display of multiplanar images developed from the capture of radiofrequency signals emitted by nuclei in a body site excited within a magnetic field
Plain Radiography	**Definition:** Planar display of an image developed from the capture of external ionizing radiation on photographic or photoconductive plate
Ultrasonography	**Definition:** Real time display of images of anatomy or flow information developed from the capture of reflected and attenuated high frequency sound waves

Section C - Nuclear Medicine — Character 3 - Root Type	
Nonimaging Nuclear Medicine Assay	**Definition:** Introduction of radioactive materials into the body for the study of body fluids and blood elements, by the detection of radioactive emissions
Nonimaging Nuclear Medicine Probe	**Definition:** Introduction of radioactive materials into the body for the study of distribution and fate of certain substances by the detection of radioactive emissions; or, alternatively, measurement of absorption of radioactive emissions from an external source
Nonimaging Nuclear Medicine Uptake	**Definition:** Introduction of radioactive materials into the body for measurements of organ function, from the detection of radioactive emissions
Planar Nuclear Medicine Imaging	**Definition:** Introduction of radioactive materials into the body for single plane display of images developed from the capture of radioactive emissions

Continued →

Section C - Nuclear Medicine — Character 3 - Root Type	
Positron Emission Tomographic (PET) Imaging	**Definition:** Introduction of radioactive materials into the body for three dimensional display of images developed from the simultaneous capture, 180 degrees apart, of radioactive emissions
Systemic Nuclear Medicine Therapy	**Definition:** Introduction of unsealed radioactive materials into the body for treatment
Tomographic (Tomo) Nuclear Medicine Imaging	**Definition:** Introduction of radioactive materials into the body for three dimensional display of images developed from the capture of radioactive emissions

Section F - Physical Rehabilitation and Diagnostic Audiology — Character 3 - Root Type	
Activities of Daily Living Assessment	**Definition:** Measurement of functional level for activities of daily living
Activities of Daily Living Treatment	**Definition:** Exercise or activities to facilitate functional competence for activities of daily living
Caregiver Training	**Definition:** Training in activities to support patient's optimal level of function
Cochlear Implant Treatment	**Definition:** Application of techniques to improve the communication abilities of individuals with cochlear implant
Device Fitting	**Definition:** Fitting of a device designed to facilitate or support achievement of a higher level of function
Hearing Aid Assessment	**Definition:** Measurement of the appropriateness and/or effectiveness of a hearing device
Hearing Assessment	**Definition:** Measurement of hearing and related functions
Hearing Treatment	**Definition:** Application of techniques to improve, augment, or compensate for hearing and related functional impairment
Motor and/or Nerve Function Assessment	**Definition:** Measurement of motor, nerve, and related functions
Motor Treatment	**Definition:** Exercise or activities to increase or facilitate motor function
Speech Assessment	**Definition:** Measurement of speech and related functions
Speech Treatment	**Definition:** Application of techniques to improve, augment, or compensate for speech and related functional impairment
Vestibular Assessment	**Definition:** Measurement of the vestibular system and related functions
Vestibular Treatment	**Definition:** Application of techniques to improve, augment, or compensate for vestibular and related functional impairment

Section F - Physical Rehabilitation and Diagnostic Audiology — Character 5 - Type Qualifier	
Acoustic Reflex Decay	**Definition:** Measures reduction in size/strength of acoustic reflex over time **Includes/Examples:** Includes site of lesion test
Acoustic Reflex Patterns	**Definition:** Defines site of lesion based upon presence/absence of acoustic reflexes with ipsilateral vs. contralateral stimulation
Acoustic Reflex Threshold	**Definition:** Determines minimal intensity that acoustic reflex occurs with ipsilateral and/or contralateral stimulation
Aerobic Capacity and Endurance	**Definition:** Measures autonomic responses to positional changes; perceived exertion, dyspnea or angina during activity; performance during exercise protocols; standard vital signs; and blood gas analysis or oxygen consumption
Alternate Binaural or Monaural Loudness Balance	**Definition:** Determines auditory stimulus parameter that yields the same objective sensation **Includes/Examples:** Sound intensities that yield same loudness perception
Anthropometric Characteristics	**Definition:** Measures edema, body fat composition, height, weight, length and girth
Aphasia (Assessment)	**Definition:** Measures expressive and receptive speech and language function including reading and writing
Aphasia (Treatment)	**Definition:** Applying techniques to improve, augment, or compensate for receptive/ expressive language impairments
Articulation/Phonology (Assessment)	**Definition:** Measures speech production
Articulation/Phonology (Treatment)	**Definition:** Applying techniques to correct, improve, or compensate for speech productive impairment
Assistive Listening Device	**Definition:** Assists in use of effective and appropriate assistive listening device/system
Assistive Listening System/Device Selection	**Definition:** Measures the effectiveness and appropriateness of assistive listening systems/devices
Assistive, Adaptive, Supportive or Protective Devices	**Explanation:** Devices to facilitate or support achievement of a higher level of function in wheelchair mobility; bed mobility; transfer or ambulation ability; bath and showering ability; dressing; grooming; personal hygiene; play or leisure

Continued →

Section F - Physical Rehabilitation and Diagnostic Audiology — Character 5 - Type Qualifier	
Auditory Evoked Potentials	**Definition:** Measures electric responses produced by the VIIIth cranial nerve and brainstem following auditory stimulation
Auditory Processing (Assessment)	**Definition:** Evaluates ability to receive and process auditory information and comprehension of spoken language
Auditory Processing (Treatment)	**Definition:** Applying techniques to improve the receiving and processing of auditory information and comprehension of spoken language
Augmentative/Alternative Communication System (Assessment)	**Definition:** Determines the appropriateness of aids, techniques, symbols, and/or strategies to augment or replace speech and enhance communication **Includes/Examples:** Includes the use of telephones, writing equipment, emergency equipment, and TDD
Augmentative/Alternative Communication System (Treatment)	**Includes/Examples:** Includes augmentative communication devices and aids
Aural Rehabilitation	**Definition:** Applying techniques to improve the communication abilities associated with hearing loss
Aural Rehabilitation Status	**Definition:** Measures impact of a hearing loss including evaluation of receptive and expressive communication skills
Bathing/Showering	**Includes/Examples:** Includes obtaining and using supplies; soaping, rinsing, and drying body parts; maintaining bathing position; and transferring to and from bathing positions
Bathing/Showering Techniques	**Definition:** Activities to facilitate obtaining and using supplies, soaping, rinsing and drying body parts, maintaining bathing position, and transferring to and from bathing positions
Bed Mobility (Assessment)	**Definition:** Transitional movement within bed
Bed Mobility (Treatment)	**Definition:** Exercise or activities to facilitate transitional movements within bed
Bedside Swallowing and Oral Function	**Includes/Examples:** Bedside swallowing includes assessment of sucking, masticating, coughing, and swallowing. Oral function includes assessment of musculature for controlled movements, structures and functions to determine coordination and phonation
Bekesy Audiometry	**Definition:** Uses an instrument that provides a choice of discrete or continuously varying pure tones; choice of pulsed or continuous signal
Binaural Electroacoustic Hearing Aid Check	**Definition:** Determines mechanical and electroacoustic function of bilateral hearing aids using hearing aid test box
Binaural Hearing Aid (Assessment)	**Definition:** Measures the candidacy, effectiveness, and appropriateness of a hearing aids **Explanation:** Measures bilateral fit
Binaural Hearing Aid (Treatment)	**Explanation:** Assists in achieving maximum understanding and performance
Bithermal, Binaural Caloric Irrigation	**Definition:** Measures the rhythmic eye movements stimulated by changing the temperature of the vestibular system
Bithermal, Monaural Caloric Irrigation	**Definition:** Measures the rhythmic eye movements stimulated by changing the temperature of the vestibular system in one ear
Brief Tone Stimuli	**Definition:** Measures specific central auditory process
Cerumen Management	**Definition:** Includes examination of external auditory canal and tympanic membrane and removal of cerumen from external ear canal
Cochlear Implant	**Definition:** Measures candidacy for cochlear implant
Cochlear Implant Rehabilitation	**Definition:** Applying techniques to improve the communication abilities of individuals with cochlear implant; includes programming the device, providing patients/families with information
Communicative/Cognitive Integration Skills (Assessment)	**Definition:** Measures ability to use higher cortical functions **Includes/Examples:** Includes orientation, recognition, attention span, initiation and termination of activity, memory, sequencing, categorizing, concept formation, spatial operations, judgment, problem solving, generalization and pragmatic communication
Communicative/Cognitive Integration Skills (Treatment)	**Definition:** Activities to facilitate the use of higher cortical functions **Includes/Examples:** Includes level of arousal, orientation, recognition, attention span, initiation and termination of activity, memory sequencing, judgment and problem solving, learning and generalization, and pragmatic communication
Computerized Dynamic Posturography	**Definition:** Measures the status of the peripheral and central vestibular system and the sensory/motor component of balance; evaluates the efficacy of vestibular rehabilitation
Conditioned Play Audiometry	**Definition:** Behavioral measures using nonspeech and speech stimuli to obtain frequency-specific and ear-specific information on auditory status from the patient **Explanation:** Obtains speech reception threshold by having patient point to pictures of spondaic words
Coordination/Dexterity (Assessment)	**Definition:** Measures large and small muscle groups for controlled goal- directed movements **Explanation:** Dexterity includes object manipulation

Continued →

Section F - Physical Rehabilitation and Diagnostic Audiology — Character 5 - Type Qualifier	
Coordination/Dexterity (Treatment)	**Definition:** Exercise or activities to facilitate gross coordination and fine coordination
Cranial Nerve Integrity	**Definition:** Measures cranial nerve sensory and motor functions, including tastes, smell and facial expression
Dichotic Stimuli	**Definition:** Measures specific central auditory process
Distorted Speech	**Definition:** Measures specific central auditory process
Dix-Hallpike Dynamic	**Definition:** Measures nystagmus following Dix-Hallpike maneuver
Dressing	**Includes/Examples:** Includes selecting clothing and accessories, obtaining clothing from storage, dressing and, fastening and adjusting clothing and shoes, and applying and removing personal devices, prosthesis or orthosis
Dressing Techniques	**Definition:** Activities to facilitate selecting clothing and accessories, dressing and undressing, adjusting clothing and shoes, applying and removing devices, prostheses or orthoses
Dynamic Orthosis	**Includes/Examples:** Includes customized and prefabricated splints, inhibitory casts, spinal and other braces, and protective devices; allows motion through transfer of movement from other body parts or by use of outside forces
Ear Canal Probe Microphone	**Definition:** Real ear measures
Ear Protector Attentuation	**Definition:** Measures ear protector fit and effectiveness
Electrocochleography	**Definition:** Measures the VIIIth cranial nerve action potential
Environmental, Home and Work Barriers	**Definition:** Measures current and potential barriers to optimal function, including safety hazards, access problems and home or office design
Ergonomics and Body Mechanics	**Definition:** Ergonomic measurement of job tasks, work hardening or work conditioning needs; functional capacity; and body mechanics
Eustachian Tube Function	**Definition:** Measures eustachian tube function and patency of eustachian tube
Evoked Otoacoustic Emissions, Diagnostic	**Definition:** Measures auditory evoked potentials in a diagnostic format
Evoked Otoacoustic Emissions, Screening	**Definition:** Measures auditory evoked potentials in a screening format
Facial Nerve Function	**Definition:** Measures electrical activity of the VIIth cranial nerve (facial nerve)
Feeding/Eating (Assessment)	**Includes/Examples:** Includes setting up food, selecting and using utensils and tableware, bringing food or drink to mouth, cleaning face, hands, and clothing, and management of alternative methods of nourishment
Feeding/Eating (Treatment)	**Definition:** Exercise or activities to facilitate setting up food, selecting and using utensils and tableware, bringing food or drink to mouth, cleaning face, hands, and clothing, and management of alternative methods of nourishment
Filtered Speech	**Definition:** Uses high or low pass filtered speech stimuli to assess central auditory processing disorders, site of lesion testing
Fluency (Assessment)	**Definition:** Measures speech fluency or stuttering
Fluency (Treatment)	**Definition:** Applying techniques to improve and augment fluent speech
Gait and/or Balance	**Definition:** Measures biomechanical, arthrokinematic and other spatial and temporal characteristics of gait and balance
Gait Training/Functional Ambulation	**Definition:** Exercise or activities to facilitate ambulation on a variety of surfaces and in a variety of environments
Grooming/Personal Hygiene (Assessment)	**Includes/Examples:** Includes ability to obtain and use supplies in a sequential fashion, general grooming, oral hygiene, toilet hygiene, personal care devices, including care for artificial airways
Grooming/Personal Hygiene (Treatment)	**Definition:** Activities to facilitate obtaining and using supplies in a sequential fashion: general grooming, oral hygiene, toilet hygiene, cleaning body, and personal care devices, including artificial airways
Hearing and Related Disorders Counseling	**Definition:** Provides patients/families/caregivers with information, support, referrals to facilitate recovery from a communication disorder **Includes/Examples:** Includes strategies for psychosocial adjustment to hearing loss for clients and families/caregivers
Hearing and Related Disorders Prevention	**Definition:** Provides patients/families/caregivers with information and support to prevent communication disorders
Hearing Screening	**Definition:** Pass/refer measures designed to identify need for further audiologic assessment
Home Management (Assessment)	**Definition:** Obtaining and maintaining personal and household possessions and environment **Includes/Examples:** Includes clothing care, cleaning, meal preparation and cleanup, shopping, money management, household maintenance, safety procedures, and childcare/parenting

Continued →

Section F - Physical Rehabilitation and Diagnostic Audiology — Character 5 - Type Qualifier

Home Management (Treatment)	**Definition:** Activities to facilitate obtaining and maintaining personal household possessions and environment **Includes/Examples:** Includes clothing care, cleaning, meal preparation and clean-up, shopping, money management, household maintenance, safety procedures, childcare/parenting
Instrumental Swallowing and Oral Function	**Definition:** Measures swallowing function using instrumental diagnostic procedures **Explanation:** Methods include videofluoroscopy, ultrasound, manometry, endoscopy
Integumentary Integrity	**Includes/Examples:** Includes burns, skin conditions, ecchymosis, bleeding, blisters, scar tissue, wounds and other traumas, tissue mobility, turgor and texture
Manual Therapy Techniques	**Definition:** Techniques in which the therapist uses his/her hands to administer skilled movements **Includes/Examples:** Includes connective tissue massage, joint mobilization and manipulation, manual lymph drainage, manual traction, soft tissue mobilization and manipulation
Masking Patterns	**Definition:** Measures central auditory processing status
Monaural Electroacoustic Hearing Aid Check	**Definition:** Determines mechanical and electroacoustic function of one hearing aid using hearing aid test box
Monaural Hearing Aid (Assessment)	**Definition:** Measures the candidacy, effectiveness, and appropriateness of a hearing aid **Explanation:** Measures unilateral fit
Monaural Hearing Aid (Treatment)	**Explanation:** Assists in achieving maximum understanding and performance
Motor Function (Assessment)	**Definition:** Measures the body's functional and versatile movement patterns **Includes/Examples:** Includes motor assessment scales, analysis of head, trunk and limb movement, and assessment of motor learning
Motor Function (Treatment)	**Definition:** Exercise or activities to facilitate crossing midline, laterality, bilateral integration, praxis, neuromuscular relaxation, inhibition, facilitation, motor function and motor learning
Motor Speech (Assessment)	**Definition:** Measures neurological motor aspects of speech production
Motor Speech (Treatment)	**Definition:** Applying techniques to improve and augment the impaired neurological motor aspects of speech production
Muscle Performance (Assessment)	**Definition:** Measures muscle strength, power and endurance using manual testing, dynamometry or computer-assisted electromechanical muscle test; functional muscle strength, power and endurance; muscle pain, tone, or soreness; or pelvic-floor musculature **Explanation:** Muscle endurance refers to the ability to contract a muscle repeatedly over time
Muscle Performance (Treatment)	**Definition:** Exercise or activities to increase the capacity of a muscle to do work in terms of strength, power, and/or endurance **Explanation:** Muscle strength is the force exerted to overcome resistance in one maximal effort. Muscle power is work produced per unit of time, or the product of strength and speed. Muscle endurance is the ability to contract a muscle repeatedly over time
Neuromotor Development	**Definition:** Measures motor development, righting and equilibrium reactions, and reflex and equilibrium reactions
Neurophysiologic Intraoperative	**Definition:** Monitors neural status during surgery
Non-invasive Instrumental Status	**Definition:** Instrumental measures of oral, nasal, vocal, and velopharyngeal functions as they pertain to speech production
Nonspoken Language (Assessment)	**Definition:** Measures nonspoken language (print, sign, symbols) for communication
Nonspoken Language (Treatment)	**Definition:** Applying techniques that improve, augment, or compensate spoken communication
Oral Peripheral Mechanism	**Definition:** Structural measures of face, jaw, lips, tongue, teeth, hard and soft palate, pharynx as related to speech production
Orofacial Myofunctional (Assessment)	**Definition:** Measures orofacial myofunctional patterns for speech and related functions
Orofacial Myofunctional (Treatment)	**Definition:** Applying techniques to improve, alter, or augment impaired orofacial myofunctional patterns and related speech production errors
Oscillating Tracking	**Definition:** Measures ability to visually track
Pain	**Definition:** Measures muscle soreness, pain and soreness with joint movement, and pain perception **Includes/Examples:** Includes questionnaires, graphs, symptom magnification scales or visual analog scales
Perceptual Processing (Assessment)	**Definition:** Measures stereognosis, kinesthesia, body schema, right-left discrimination, form constancy, position in space, visual closure, figure-ground, depth perception, spatial relations and topographical orientation

Continued →

Section F - Physical Rehabilitation and Diagnostic Audiology — Character 5 - Type Qualifier	
Perceptual Processing (Treatment)	**Definition:** Exercise and activities to facilitate perceptual processing **Explanation:** Includes stereognosis, kinesthesia, body schema, right-left discrimination, form constancy, position in space, visual closure, figure-ground, depth perception, spatial relations, and topographical orientation **Includes/Examples:** Includes stereognosis, kinesthesia, body schema, right-left discrimination, form constancy, position in space, visual closure, figure-ground, depth perception, spatial relations, and topographical orientation
Performance Intensity Phonetically Balanced Speech Discrimination	**Definition:** Measures word recognition over varying intensity levels
Postural Control	**Definition:** Exercise or activities to increase postural alignment and control
Prosthesis	**Explanation:** Artificial substitutes for missing body parts that augment performance or function
Psychosocial Skills (Assessment)	**Definition:** The ability to interact in society and to process emotions **Includes/Examples:** Includes psychological (values, interests, self-concept); social (role performance, social conduct, interpersonal skills, self expression); self-management (coping skills, time management, self-control)
Psychosocial Skills (Treatment)	**Definition:** The ability to interact in society and to process emotions **Includes/Examples:** Includes psychological (values, interests, self-concept); social (role performance, social conduct, interpersonal skills, self expression); self-management (coping skills, time management, self-control)
Pure Tone Audiometry, Air	**Definition:** Air-conduction pure tone threshold measures with appropriate masking
Pure Tone Audiometry, Air and Bone	**Definition:** Air-conduction and bone-conduction pure tone threshold measures with appropriate masking
Pure Tone Stenger	**Definition:** Measures unilateral nonorganic hearing loss based on simultaneous presentation of pure tones of differing volume
Range of Motion and Joint Integrity	**Definition:** Measures quantity, quality, grade, and classification of joint movement and/or mobility **Explanation:** Range of Motion is the space, distance or angle through which movement occurs at a joint or series of joints. Joint integrity is the conformance of joints to expected anatomic, biomechanical and kinematic norms
Range of Motion and Joint Mobility	**Definition:** Exercise or activities to increase muscle length and joint mobility
Receptive/Expressive Language (Assessment)	**Definition:** Measures receptive and expressive language
Receptive/Expressive Language (Treatment)	**Definition:** Applying techniques tot improve and augment receptive/expressive language
Reflex Integrity	**Definition:** Measures the presence, absence, or exaggeration of developmentally appropriate, pathologic or normal reflexes
Select Picture Audiometry	**Definition:** Establishes hearing threshold levels for speech using pictures
Sensorineural Acuity Level	**Definition:** Measures sensorineural acuity masking presented via bone conduction
Sensory Aids	**Definition:** Determines the appropriateness of a sensory prosthetic device, other than a hearing aid or assistive listening system/device
Sensory Awareness/Processing/Integrity	**Includes/Examples:** Includes light touch, pressure, temperature, pain, sharp/dull, proprioception, vestibular, visual, auditory, gustatory, and olfactory
Short Increment Sensitivity Index	**Definition:** Measures the ear's ability to detect small intensity changes; site of lesion test requiring a behavioral response
Sinusoidal Vertical Axis Rotational	**Definition:** Measures nystagmus following rotation
Somatosensory Evoked Potentials	**Definition:** Measures neural activity from sites throughout the body
Speech and/or Language Screening	**Definition:** Identifies need for further speech and/or language evaluation
Speech Threshold	**Definition:** Measures minimal intensity needed to repeat spondaic words
Speech-Language Pathology and Related Disorders Counseling	**Definition:** Provides patients/families with information, support, referrals to facilitate recovery from a communication disorder
Speech-Language Pathology and Related Disorders Prevention	**Definition:** Applying techniques to avoid or minimize onset and/or development of a communication disorder
Speech/Word Recognition	**Definition:** Measures ability to repeat/identify single syllable words; scores given as a percentage; includes word recognition/speech discrimination
Staggered Spondaic Word	**Definition:** Measures central auditory processing site of lesion based upon dichotic presentation of spondaic words
Static Orthosis	**Includes/Examples:** Includes customized and prefabricated splints, inhibitory casts, spinal and other braces, and protective devices; has no moving parts, maintains joint(s) in desired position

Continued →

Section F - Physical Rehabilitation and Diagnostic Audiology — Character 5 - Type Qualifier	
Stenger	**Definition:** Measures unilateral nonorganic hearing loss based on simultaneous presentation of signals of differing volume
Swallowing Dysfunction	**Definition:** Activities to improve swallowing function in coordination with respiratory function **Includes/Examples:** Includes function and coordination of sucking, mastication, coughing, swallowing
Synthetic Sentence Identification	**Definition:** Measures central auditory dysfunction using identification of third order approximations of sentences and competing messages
Temporal Ordering of Stimuli	**Definition:** Measures specific central auditory process
Therapeutic Exercise	**Definition:** Exercise or activities to facilitate sensory awareness, sensory processing, sensory integration, balance training, conditioning, reconditioning **Includes/Examples:** Includes developmental activities, breathing exercises, aerobic endurance activities, aquatic exercises, stretching and ventilatory muscle training
Tinnitus Masker (Assessment)	**Definition:** Determines candidacy for tinnitus masker
Tinnitus Masker (Treatment)	**Explanation:** Used to verify physical fit, acoustic appropriateness, and benefit; assists in achieving maximum benefit
Tone Decay	**Definition:** Measures decrease in hearing sensitivity to a tone; site of lesion test requiring a behavioral response
Transfer	**Definition:** Transitional movement from one surface to another
Transfer Training	**Definition:** Exercise or activities to facilitate movement from one surface to another
Tympanometry	**Definition:** Measures the integrity of the middle ear; measures ease at which sound flows through the tympanic membrane while air pressure against the membrane is varied
Unithermal Binaural Screen	**Definition:** Measures the rhythmic eye movements stimulated by changing the temperature of the vestibular system in both ears using warm water, screening format
Ventilation, Respiration and Circulation	**Definition:** Measures ventilatory muscle strength, power and endurance, pulmonary function and ventilatory mechanics **Includes/Examples:** Includes ability to clear airway, activities that aggravate or relieve edema, pain, dyspnea or other symptoms, chest wall mobility, cardiopulmonary response to performance of ADL and IAD, cough and sputum, standard vital signs
Vestibular	**Definition:** Applying techniques to compensate for balance disorders; includes habituation, exercise therapy, and balance retraining
Visual Motor Integration (Assessment)	**Definition:** Coordinating the interaction of information from the eyes with body movement during activity
Visual Motor Integration (Treatment)	**Definition:** Exercise or activities to facilitate coordinating the interaction of information from eyes with body movement during activity
Visual Reinforcement Audiometry	**Definition:** Behavioral measures using nonspeech and speech stimuli to obtain frequency/ear-specific information on auditory status **Includes/Examples:** Includes a conditioned response of looking toward a visual reinforcer (e.g., lights, animated toy) every time auditory stimuli are heard
Vocational Activities and Functional Community or Work Reintegration Skills (Assessment)	**Definition:** Measures environmental, home, work (job/school/play) barriers that keep patients from functioning optimally in their environment **Includes/Examples:** Includes assessment of vocational skill and interests, environment of work (job/school/play), injury potential and injury prevention or reduction, ergonomic stressors, transportation skills, and ability to access and use community resources
Vocational Activities and Functional Community or Work Reintegration Skills (Treatment)	**Definition:** Activities to facilitate vocational exploration, body mechanics training, job acquisition, and environmental or work (job/school/play) task adaptation **Includes/Examples:** Includes injury prevention and reduction, ergonomic stressor reduction, job coaching and simulation, work hardening and conditioning, driving training, transportation skills, and use of community resources
Voice (Assessment)	**Definition:** Measures vocal structure, function and production
Voice (Treatment)	**Definition:** Applying techniques to improve voice and vocal function
Voice Prosthetic (Assessment)	**Definition:** Determines the appropriateness of voice prosthetic/adaptive device to enhance or facilitate communication
Voice Prosthetic (Treatment)	**Includes/Examples:** Includes electrolarynx, and other assistive, adaptive, supportive devices
Wheelchair Mobility (Assessment)	**Definition:** Measures fit and functional abilities within wheelchair in a variety of environments
Wheelchair Mobility (Treatment)	**Definition:** Management, maintenance and controlled operation of a wheelchair, scooter or other device, in and on a variety of surfaces and environments
Wound Management	**Includes/Examples:** Includes non-selective and selective debridement (enzymes, autolysis, sharp debridement), dressings (wound coverings, hydrogel, vacuum-assisted closure), topical agents, etc.

Section G - Mental Health — Character 3 - Root Type	
Biofeedback	**Definition:** Provision of information from the monitoring and regulating of physiological processes in conjunction with cognitive-behavioral techniques to improve patient functioning or well-being **Includes/Examples:** Includes EEG, blood pressure, skin temperature or peripheral blood flow, ECG, electrooculogram, EMG, respirometry or capnometry, GSR/EDR, perineometry to monitor/regulate bowel/bladder activity, electrogastrogram to monitor/regulate gastric motility
Counseling	**Definition:** The application of psychological methods to treat an individual with normal developmental issues and psychological problems in order to increase function, improve well-being, alleviate distress, maladjustment or resolve crises
Crisis Intervention	**Definition:** Treatment of a traumatized, acutely disturbed or distressed individual for the purpose of short-term stabilization **Includes/Examples:** Includes defusing, debriefing, counseling, psychotherapy and/or coordination of care with other providers or agencies
Electroconvulsive Therapy	**Definition:** The application of controlled electrical voltages to treat a mental health disorder **Includes/Examples:** Includes appropriate sedation and other preparation of the individual
Family Psychotherapy	**Definition:** Treatment that includes one or more family members of an individual with a mental health disorder by behavioral, cognitive, psychoanalytic, psychodynamic or psychophysiological means to improve functioning or well-being **Explanation:** Remediation of emotional or behavioral problems presented by one or more family members in cases where psychotherapy with more than one family member is indicated
Group Psychotherapy	**Definition:** Treatment of two or more individuals with a mental health disorder by behavioral, cognitive, psychoanalytic, psychodynamic or psychophysiological means to improve functioning or well-being
Hypnosis	**Definition:** Induction of a state of heightened suggestibility by auditory, visual and tactile techniques to elicit an emotional or behavioral response
Individual Psychotherapy	**Definition:** Treatment of an individual with a mental health disorder by behavioral, cognitive, psychoanalytic, psychodynamic or psychophysiological means to improve functioning or well-being
Light Therapy	**Definition:** Application of specialized light treatments to improve functioning or well-being
Medication Management	**Definition:** Monitoring and adjusting the use of medications for the treatment of a mental health disorder
Narcosynthesis	**Definition:** Administration of intravenous barbiturates in order to release suppressed or repressed thoughts
Psychological Tests	**Definition:** The administration and interpretation of standardized psychological tests and measurement instruments for the assessment of psychological function

Section G - Mental Health — Character 4 - Type Qualifier	
Behavioral	**Definition:** Primarily to modify behavior **Includes/Examples:** Includes modeling and role playing, positive reinforcement of target behaviors, response cost, and training of self-management skills
Cognitive	**Definition:** Primarily to correct cognitive distortions and errors
Cognitive-Behavioral	**Definition:** Combining cognitive and behavioral treatment strategies to improve functioning **Explanation:** Maladaptive responses are examined to determine how cognitions relate to behavior patterns in response to an event. Uses learning principles and information-processing models
Developmental	**Definition:** Age-normed developmental status of cognitive, social and adaptive behavior skills
Intellectual and Psychoeducational	**Definition:** Intellectual abilities, academic achievement and learning capabilities (including behaviors and emotional factors affecting learning
Interactive	**Definition:** Uses primarily physical aids and other forms of non-oral interaction with a patient who is physically, psychologically or developmentally unable to use ordinary language for communication **Includes/Examples:** Includes. the use of toys in symbolic play
Interpersonal	**Definition:** Helps an individual make changes in interpersonal behaviors to reduce psychological dysfunction **Includes/Examples:** Includes exploratory techniques, encouragement of affective expression, clarification of patient statements, analysis of communication patterns, use of therapy relationship and behavior change techniques
Neurobehavioral and Cognitive Status	**Definition:** Includes neurobehavioral status exam, interview(s), and observation for the clinical assessment of thinking, reasoning and judgment, acquired knowledge, attention, memory, visual spatial abilities, language functions, and planning
Neuropsychological	**Definition:** Thinking, reasoning and judgment, acquired knowledge, attention, memory, visual spatial abilities, language functions, planning
Personality and Behavioral	**Definition:** Mood, emotion, behavior, social functioning, psychopathological conditions, personality traits and characteristics

Continued →

Section G - Mental Health — Character 4 - Type Qualifier	
Psychoanalysis	**Definition:** Methods of obtaining a detailed account of past and present mental and emotional experiences to determine the source and eliminate or diminish the undesirable effects of unconscious conflicts **Explanation:** Accomplished by making the individual aware of their existence, origin, and inappropriate expression in emotions and behavior
Psychodynamic	**Definition:** Exploration of past and present emotional experiences to understand motives and drives using insight-oriented techniques to reduce the undesirable effects of internal conflicts on emotions and behavior **Explanation:** Techniques include empathetic listening, clarifying self-defeating behavior patterns, and exploring adaptive alternatives
Psychophysiological	**Definition:** Monitoring and alteration of physiological processes to help the individual associate physiological reactions combined with cognitive and behavioral strategies to gain improved control of these processes to help the individual cope more effectively
Supportive	**Definition:** Formation of therapeutic relationship primarily for providing emotional support to prevent further deterioration in functioning during periods of particular stress **Explanation:** Often used in conjunction with other therapeutic approaches
Vocational	**Definition:** Exploration of vocational interests, aptitudes and required adaptive behavior skills to develop and carry out a plan for achieving a successful vocational placement **Includes/Examples:** Includes enhancing work related adjustment and/or pursuing viable options in training education or preparation

Section H - Substance Abuse Treatment — Character 3 - Root Type	
Detoxification Services	**Definition:** Detoxification from alcohol and/or drugs **Explanation:** Not a treatment modality, but helps the patient stabilize physically and psychologically until the body becomes free of drugs and the effects of alcohol
Family Counseling	**Definition:** The application of psychological methods that includes one or more family members to treat an individual with addictive behavior **Explanation:** Provides support and education for family members of addicted individuals. Family member participation is seen as a critical area of substance abuse treatment
Group Counseling	**Definition:** The application of psychological methods to treat two or more individuals with addictive behavior **Explanation:** Provides structured group counseling sessions and healing power through the connection with others
Individual Counseling	**Definition:** The application of psychological methods to treat an individual with addictive behavior **Explanation:** Comprised of several different techniques, which apply various strategies to address drug addiction
Individual Psychotherapy	**Definition:** Treatment of an individual with addictive behavior by behavioral, cognitive, psychoanalytic, psychodynamic or psychophysiological means
Medication Management	**Definition:** Monitoring and adjusting the use of replacement medications for the treatment of addiction
Pharmacotherapy	**Definition:** The use of replacement medications for the treatment of addiction

Appendix C: Approach Definitions

Section 0 - Medical and Surgical — Character 5 - Approach	
External (X)	**Definition:** Procedures performed directly on the skin or mucous membrane and procedures performed indirectly by the application of external force through the skin or mucous membrane
Open (0)	**Definition:** Cutting through the skin or mucous membrane and any other body layers necessary to expose the site of the procedure
Percutaneous (3)	**Definition:** Entry, by puncture or minor incision, of instrumentation through the skin or mucous membrane and any other body layers necessary to reach the site of the procedure
Percutaneous Endoscopic (4)	**Definition:** Entry, by puncture or minor incision, of instrumentation through the skin or mucous membrane and any other body layers necessary to reach and visualize the site of the procedure
Via Natural or Artificial Opening (7)	**Definition:** Entry of instrumentation through a natural or artificial external opening to reach the site of the procedure
Via Natural or Artificial Opening Endoscopic (8)	**Definition:** Entry of instrumentation through a natural or artificial external opening to reach and visualize the site of the procedure
Via Natural or Artificial Opening With Percutaneous Endoscopic Assistance (F)	**Definition:** Entry of instrumentation through a natural or artificial external opening and entry, by puncture or minor incision, of instrumentation through the skin or mucous membrane and any other body layers necessary to aid in the performance of the procedure

Section 1 - Obstetrics — Character 5 - Approach	
External (X)	**Definition:** Procedures performed directly on the skin or mucous membrane and procedures performed indirectly by the application of external force through the skin or mucous membrane
Open (0)	**Definition:** Cutting through the skin or mucous membrane and any other body layers necessary to expose the site of the procedure
Percutaneous (3)	**Definition:** Entry, by puncture or minor incision, of instrumentation through the skin or mucous membrane and any other body layers necessary to reach the site of the procedure
Percutaneous Endoscopic (4)	**Definition:** Entry, by puncture or minor incision, of instrumentation through the skin or mucous membrane and any other body layers necessary to reach and visualize the site of the procedure
Via Natural or Artificial Opening (7)	**Definition:** Entry of instrumentation through a natural or artificial external opening to reach the site of the procedure
Via Natural or Artificial Opening Endoscopic (8)	**Definition:** Entry of instrumentation through a natural or artificial external opening to reach and visualize the site of the procedure

Section 2 - Placement — Character 5 - Approach	
External (X)	**Definition:** Procedures performed directly on the skin or mucous membrane and procedures performed indirectly by the application of external force through the skin or mucous membrane

Section 3 - Administration — Character 5 - Approach	
External (X)	**Definition:** Procedures performed directly on the skin or mucous membrane and procedures performed indirectly by the application of external force through the skin or mucous membrane
Open (0)	**Definition:** Cutting through the skin or mucous membrane and any other body layers necessary to expose the site of the procedure
Percutaneous (3)	**Definition:** Entry, by puncture or minor incision, of instrumentation through the skin or mucous membrane and any other body layers necessary to reach the site of the procedure
Via Natural or Artificial Opening (7)	**Definition:** Entry of instrumentation through a natural or artificial external opening to reach the site of the procedure
Via Natural or Artificial Opening Endoscopic (8)	**Definition:** Entry of instrumentation through a natural or artificial external opening to reach and visualize the site of the procedure

Section 4 - Measurement and Monitoring — Character 5 - Approach	
External (X)	**Definition:** Procedures performed directly on the skin or mucous membrane and procedures performed indirectly by the application of external force through the skin or mucous membrane
Open (0)	**Definition:** Cutting through the skin or mucous membrane and any other body layers necessary to expose the site of the procedure
Percutaneous (3)	**Definition:** Entry, by puncture or minor incision, of instrumentation through the skin or mucous membrane and any other body layers necessary to reach the site of the procedure
Percutaneous Endoscopic (4)	**Definition:** Entry, by puncture or minor incision, of instrumentation through the skin or mucous membrane and any other body layers necessary to reach and visualize the site of the procedure
Via Natural or Artificial Opening (7)	**Definition:** Entry of instrumentation through a natural or artificial external opening to reach the site of the procedure
Via Natural or Artificial Opening Endoscopic (8)	**Definition:** Entry of instrumentation through a natural or artificial external opening to reach and visualize the site of the procedure

Section 7 - Osteopathic — Character 5 - Approach	
External (X)	**Definition:** Procedures performed directly on the skin or mucous membrane and procedures performed indirectly by the application of external force through the skin or mucous membrane

Section 8 - Other Procedures — Character 5 - Approach	
External (X)	**Definition:** Procedures performed directly on the skin or mucous membrane and procedures performed indirectly by the application of external force through the skin or mucous membrane
Open (0)	**Definition:** Cutting through the skin or mucous membrane and any other body layers necessary to expose the site of the procedure
Percutaneous (3)	**Definition:** Entry, by puncture or minor incision, of instrumentation through the skin or mucous membrane and any other body layers necessary to reach the site of the procedure

Continued →

Section 8 - Other Procedures — Character 5 - Approach	
Percutaneous Endoscopic (4)	**Definition:** Entry, by puncture or minor incision, of instrumentation through the skin or mucous membrane and any other body layers necessary to reach and visualize the site of the procedure
Via Natural or Artificial Opening (7)	**Definition:** Entry of instrumentation through a natural or artificial external opening to reach the site of the procedure
Via Natural or Artificial Opening Endoscopic (8)	**Definition:** Entry of instrumentation through a natural or artificial external opening to reach and visualize the site of the procedure

Section 9 - Chiropractic — Character 5 - Approach	
External (X)	**Definition:** Procedures performed directly on the skin or mucous membrane and procedures performed indirectly by the application of external force through the skin or mucous membrane

Appendix D: Medical and Surgical Body Parts

Appendices D–F are structured to assist coders with confirming character selections within the Tables. For example, if the coder is considering the body part of Abdomen Muscle, appendix D can be referenced to identify all of the muscles that are included in the body part Abdomen Muscle (see row 2 in the table below). After reviewing the information, the coder can determine if the body part under consideration is correct or if another body part should be reviewed. The same process can be followed for devices which are included in appendix E and substances which are included in appendix F.

Section 0 - Medical and Surgical — Character 4 - Body Part	
1st Toe, Left **1st** Toe, Right	**Includes:** Hallux
Abdomen Muscle, Left **Abdomen** Muscle, Right	**Includes:** External oblique muscle Internal oblique muscle Pyramidalis muscle Rectus abdominis muscle Transversus abdominis muscle
Abdominal Aorta	**Includes:** Inferior phrenic artery Lumbar artery Median sacral artery Middle suprarenal artery Ovarian artery Testicular artery
Abdominal Sympathetic Nerve	**Includes:** **Abdominal** aortic plexus Auerbach's (myenteric) plexus Celiac (solar) plexus Celiac ganglion Gastric plexus Hepatic plexus Inferior hypogastric plexus Inferior mesenteric ganglion Inferior mesenteric plexus Meissner's (submucous) plexus Myenteric (Auerbach's) plexus Pancreatic plexus Pelvic splanchnic nerve Renal plexus Solar (celiac) plexus Splenic plexus Submucous (Meissner's) plexus Superior hypogastric plexus Superior mesenteric ganglion Superior mesenteric plexus Suprarenal plexus

Section 0 - Medical and Surgical — Character 4 - Body Part	
Abducens Nerve	**Includes:** Sixth cranial nerve
Accessory Nerve	**Includes:** Eleventh cranial nerve
Acoustic Nerve	**Includes:** Cochlear nerve Eighth cranial nerve Scarpa's (vestibular) ganglion Spiral ganglion Vestibular (Scarpa's) ganglion Vestibular nerve Vestibulocochlear nerve
Adenoids	**Includes:** Pharyngeal tonsil
Adrenal Gland **Adrenal** Gland, Left **Adrenal** Gland, Right **Adrenal** Glands, Bilateral	**Includes:** Suprarenal gland
Ampulla of Vater	**Includes:** Duodenal ampulla Hepatopancreatic ampulla
Anal Sphincter	**Includes:** External anal sphincter Internal anal sphincter
Ankle Bursa and Ligament, Left **Ankle** Bursa and Ligament, Right	**Includes:** Calcaneofibular ligament Deltoid ligament Ligament of the lateral malleolus Talofibular ligament
Ankle Joint, Left **Ankle** Joint, Right	**Includes:** Inferior tibiofibular joint Talocrural joint

Continued →

Section 0 - Medical and Surgical — Character 4 - Body Part	
Anterior Chamber, Left **Anterior** Chamber, Right	**Includes:** Aqueous humour
Anterior Tibial Artery, Left **Anterior** Tibial Artery, Right	**Includes:** Anterior lateral malleolar artery Anterior medial malleolar artery Anterior tibial recurrent artery Dorsalis pedis artery Posterior tibial recurrent artery
Anus	**Includes:** Anal orifice
Aortic Valve	**Includes:** Aortic annulus
Appendix	**Includes:** Vermiform appendix
Ascending Colon	**Includes:** Hepatic flexure
Atrial Septum	**Includes:** Interatrial septum
Atrium, Left	**Includes:** Atrium pulmonale Left auricular appendix
Atrium, Right	**Includes:** Atrium dextrum cordis Right auricular appendix Sinus venosus
Auditory Ossicle, Left **Auditory** Ossicle, Right	**Includes:** Incus Malleus Ossicular chain Stapes
Axillary Artery, Left **Axillary** Artery, Right	**Includes:** Anterior circumflex humeral artery Lateral thoracic artery Posterior circumflex humeral artery Subscapular artery Superior thoracic artery Thoracoacromial artery
Azygos Vein	**Includes:** Right ascending lumbar vein Right subcostal vein
Basal Ganglia	**Includes:** Basal nuclei Claustrum Corpus striatum Globus pallidus Substantia nigra Subthalamic nucleus
Basilic Vein, Left **Basilic** Vein, Right	**Includes:** Median antebrachial vein Median cubital vein
Bladder	**Includes:** Trigone of bladder
Brachial Artery, Left **Brachial** Artery, Right	**Includes:** Inferior ulnar collateral artery Profunda brachii Superior ulnar collateral artery

Section 0 - Medical and Surgical — Character 4 - Body Part	
Brachial Plexus	**Includes:** Axillary nerve Dorsal scapular nerve First intercostal nerve Long thoracic nerve Musculocutaneous nerve Subclavius nerve Suprascapular nerve
Brachial Vein, Left **Brachial** Vein, Right	**Includes:** Radial vein Ulnar vein
Brain	**Includes:** Cerebrum Corpus callosum Encephalon
Breast, Bilateral **Breast,** Left **Breast,** Right	**Includes:** Mammary duct Mammary gland
Buccal Mucosa	**Includes:** Buccal gland Molar gland Palatine gland
Carotid Bodies, Bilateral **Carotid** Body, Left **Carotid** Body, Right	**Includes:** Carotid glomus
Carpal Joint, Left **Carpal** Joint, Right	**Includes:** Intercarpal joint Midcarpal joint
Carpal, Left **Carpal,** Right	**Includes:** Capitate bone Hamate bone Lunate bone Pisiform bone Scaphoid bone Trapezium bone Trapezoid bone Triquetral bone
Celiac Artery	**Includes:** Celiac trunk
Cephalic Vein, Left **Cephalic** Vein, Right	**Includes:** Accessory cephalic vein
Cerebellum	**Includes:** Culmen
Cerebral Hemisphere	**Includes:** Frontal lobe Occipital lobe Parietal lobe Temporal lobe
Cerebral Meninges	**Includes:** Arachnoid mater Leptomeninges Pia mater

Continued →

Section 0 - Medical and Surgical — Character 4 - Body Part	
Cerebral Ventricle	**Includes:** Aqueduct of Sylvius Cerebral aqueduct (Sylvius) Choroid plexus Ependyma Foramen of Monro (intraventricular) Fourth ventricle Interventricular foramen (Monro) Left lateral ventricle Right lateral ventricle Third ventricle
Cervical Nerve	**Includes:** Greater occipital nerve Spinal nerve, cervical Suboccipital nerve Third occipital nerve
Cervical Plexus	**Includes:** Ansa cervicalis Cutaneous (transverse) cervical nerve Great auricular nerve Lesser occipital nerve Supraclavicular nerve Transverse (cutaneous) cervical nerve
Cervical Vertebra	**Includes:** Spinous process Vertebral arch Vertebral foramen Vertebral lamina Vertebral pedicle
Cervical Vertebral Joint	**Includes:** Atlantoaxial joint Cervical facet joint
Cervical Vertebral Joints, 2 or more	**Includes:** Cervical facet joint
Cervicothoracic Vertebral Joint	**Includes:** Cervicothoracic facet joint
Cisterna Chyli	**Includes:** Intestinal lymphatic trunk Lumbar lymphatic trunk
Coccygeal Glomus	**Includes:** Coccygeal body
Colic Vein	**Includes:** Ileocolic vein Left colic vein Middle colic vein Right colic vein
Conduction Mechanism	**Includes:** Atrioventricular node Bundle of His Bundle of Kent Sinoatrial node
Conjunctiva, Left **Conjunctiva,** Right	**Includes:** Plica semilunaris
Dura Mater	**Includes:** Cranial dura mater Dentate ligament Diaphragma sellae Falx cerebri Spinal dura mater Tentorium cerebelli

Section 0 - Medical and Surgical — Character 4 - Body Part	
Elbow Bursa and Ligament, Left **Elbow** Bursa and Ligament, Right	**Includes:** Annular ligament Olecranon bursa Radial collateral ligament Ulnar collateral ligament
Elbow Joint, Left **Elbow** Joint, Right	**Includes:** Distal humerus, involving joint Humeroradial joint Humeroulnar joint Proximal radioulnar joint
Epidural Space	**Includes:** Cranial epidural space Extradural space Spinal epidural space
Epiglottis	**Includes:** Glossoepiglottic fold
Esophagogastric Junction	**Includes:** Cardia Cardioesophageal junction Gastroesophageal (GE) junction
Esophagus, Lower	**Includes:** Abdominal esophagus
Esophagus, Middle	**Includes:** Thoracic esophagus
Esophagus, Upper	**Includes:** Cervical esophagus
Ethmoid Bone, Left **Ethmoid** Bone, Right	**Includes:** Cribriform plate
Ethmoid Sinus, Left **Ethmoid** Sinus, Right	**Includes:** Ethmoidal air cell
Eustachian Tube, Left **Eustachian** Tube, Right	**Includes:** Auditory tube Pharyngotympanic tube
External Auditory Canal, Left **External** Auditory Canal, Right	**Includes:** External auditory meatus
External Carotid Artery, Left **External** Carotid Artery, Right	**Includes:** Ascending pharyngeal artery Internal maxillary artery Lingual artery Maxillary artery Occipital artery Posterior auricular artery Superior thyroid artery
External Ear, Bilateral **External** Ear, Left **External** Ear, Right	**Includes:** Antihelix Antitragus Auricle Earlobe Helix Pinna Tragus
External Iliac Artery, Left **External** Iliac Artery, Right	**Includes:** Deep circumflex iliac artery Inferior epigastric artery

Continued →

Section 0 - Medical and Surgical — Character 4 - Body Part	
External Jugular Vein, Left **External** Jugular Vein, Right	**Includes:** Posterior auricular vein
Extraocular Muscle, Left **Extraocular** Muscle, Right	**Includes:** Inferior oblique muscle Inferior rectus muscle Lateral rectus muscle Medial rectus muscle Superior oblique muscle Superior rectus muscle
Eye, Left **Eye,** Right	**Includes:** Ciliary body Posterior chamber
Face Artery	**Includes:** Angular artery Ascending palatine artery External maxillary artery Facial artery Inferior labial artery Submental artery Superior labial artery
Face Vein, Left **Face** Vein, Right	**Includes:** Angular vein Anterior facial vein Common facial vein Deep facial vein Frontal vein Posterior facial (retromandibular) vein Supraorbital vein
Facial Muscle	**Includes:** Buccinator muscle Corrugator supercilii muscle Depressor anguli oris muscle Depressor labii inferioris muscle Depressor septi nasi muscle Depressor supercilii muscle Levator anguli oris muscle Levator labii superioris alaeque nasi Levator labii superioris alaeque nasi Levator labii superioris alaeque nasi Levator labii superioris muscle Mentalis muscle Nasalis muscle Occipitofrontalis muscle Orbicularis oris muscle Procerus muscle Risorius muscle Zygomaticus muscle
Facial Nerve	**Includes:** Chorda tympani Geniculate ganglion Greater superficial petrosal nerve Nerve to the stapedius Parotid plexus Posterior auricular nerve Seventh cranial nerve Submandibular ganglion
Fallopian Tube, Left **Fallopian** Tube, Right	**Includes:** Oviduct Salpinx Uterine tube

Section 0 - Medical and Surgical — Character 4 - Body Part	
Femoral Artery, Left **Femoral** Artery, Right	**Includes:** Circumflex iliac artery Deep femoral artery Descending genicular artery External pudendal artery Superficial epigastric artery
Femoral Nerve	**Includes:** Anterior crural nerve Saphenous nerve
Femoral Shaft, Left **Femoral** Shaft, Right	**Includes:** Body of femur
Femoral Vein, Left **Femoral** Vein, Right	**Includes:** Deep femoral (profunda femoris) vein Popliteal vein Profunda femoris (deep femoral) vein
Fibula, Left **Fibula,** Right	**Includes:** Body of fibula Head of fibula Lateral malleolus
Finger Nail	**Includes:** Nail bed Nail plate
Finger Phalangeal Joint, Left **Finger** Phalangeal Joint, Right	**Includes:** Interphalangeal (IP) joint
Foot Artery, Left **Foot** Artery, Right	**Includes:** Arcuate artery Dorsal metatarsal artery Lateral plantar artery Lateral tarsal artery Medial plantar artery
Foot Bursa and Ligament, Left **Foot** Bursa and Ligament, Right	**Includes:** Calcaneocuboid ligament Cuneonavicular ligament Intercuneiform ligament Interphalangeal ligament Metatarsal ligament Metatarsophalangeal ligament Subtalar ligament Talocalcaneal ligament Talocalcaneonavicular ligament Tarsometatarsal ligament
Foot Muscle, Left **Foot** Muscle, Right	**Includes:** Abductor hallucis muscle Adductor hallucis muscle Extensor digitorum brevis muscle Extensor hallucis brevis muscle Flexor digitorum brevis muscle Flexor hallucis brevis muscle Quadratus plantae muscle
Foot Vein, Left **Foot** Vein, Right	**Includes:** Common digital vein Dorsal metatarsal vein Dorsal venous arch Plantar digital vein Plantar metatarsal vein Plantar venous arch

Continued →

Section 0 - Medical and Surgical — Character 4 - Body Part	
Frontal Bone, Left **Frontal** Bone, Right	**Includes:** Zygomatic process of frontal bone
Gastric Artery	**Includes:** Left gastric artery Right gastric artery
Glenoid Cavity, Left **Glenoid** Cavity, Right	**Includes:** Glenoid fossa (of scapula)
Glomus Jugulare	**Includes:** Jugular body
Glossopharyngeal Nerve	**Includes:** Carotid sinus nerve Ninth cranial nerve Tympanic nerve
Greater Omentum	**Includes:** Gastrocolic ligament Gastrocolic omentum Gastrophrenic ligament Gastrosplenic ligament
Greater Saphenous Vein, Left **Greater** Saphenous Vein, Right	**Includes:** External pudendal vein Great saphenous vein Superficial circumflex iliac vein Superficial epigastric vein
Hand Artery, Left **Hand** Artery, Right	**Includes:** Deep palmar arch Princeps pollicis artery Radialis indicis Superficial palmar arch
Hand Bursa and Ligament, Left **Hand** Bursa and Ligament, Right	**Includes:** Carpometacarpal ligament Intercarpal ligament Interphalangeal ligament Lunotriquetral ligament Metacarpal ligament Metacarpophalangeal ligament Pisohamate ligament Pisometacarpal ligament Scapholunate ligament Scaphotrapezium ligament
Hand Muscle, Left **Hand** Muscle, Right	**Includes:** Hypothenar muscle Palmar interosseous muscle Thenar muscle
Hand Vein, Left **Hand** Vein, Right	**Includes:** Dorsal metacarpal vein Palmar (volar) digital vein Palmar (volar) metacarpal vein Superficial palmar venous arch Volar (palmar) digital vein Volar (palmar) metacarpal vein
Head and Neck Bursa and Ligament	**Includes:** Alar ligament of axis Cervical interspinous ligament Cervical intertransverse ligament Cervical ligamentum flavum Lateral temporomandibular ligament Sphenomandibular ligament Stylomandibular ligament Transverse ligament of atlas
Head and Neck Sympathetic Nerve	**Includes:** Cavernous plexus Cervical ganglion Ciliary ganglion Internal carotid plexus Otic ganglion Pterygopalatine (sphenopalatine) ganglion Sphenopalatine (pterygopalatine) ganglion Stellate ganglion Submandibular ganglion Submaxillary ganglion
Head Muscle	**Includes:** Auricularis muscle Masseter muscle Pterygoid muscle Splenius capitis muscle Temporalis muscle Temporoparietalis muscle
Heart, Left	**Includes:** Left coronary sulcus Obtuse margin
Heart, Right	**Includes:** Right coronary sulcus
Hemiazygos Vein	**Includes:** Left ascending lumbar vein Left subcostal vein
Hepatic Artery	**Includes:** Common hepatic artery Gastroduodenal artery Hepatic artery proper
Hip Bursa and Ligament, Left **Hip** Bursa and Ligament, Right	**Includes:** Iliofemoral ligament Ischiofemoral ligament Pubofemoral ligament Transverse acetabular ligament Trochanteric bursa
Hip Joint, Left **Hip** Joint, Right	**Includes:** Acetabulofemoral joint
Hip Muscle, Left **Hip** Muscle, Right	**Includes:** Gemellus muscle Gluteus maximus muscle Gluteus medius muscle Gluteus minimus muscle Iliacus muscle Obturator muscle Piriformis muscle Psoas muscle Quadratus femoris muscle Tensor fasciae latae muscle
Humeral Head, Left **Humeral** Head, Right	**Includes:** Greater tuberosity Lesser tuberosity Neck of humerus (anatomical)(surgical)
Humeral Shaft, Left **Humeral** Shaft, Right	**Includes:** Distal humerus Humerus, distal Lateral epicondyle of humerus Medial epicondyle of humerus

Continued →

Section 0 - Medical and Surgical — Character 4 - Body Part

Hypogastric Vein, Left **Hypogastric** Vein, Right	**Includes:** Gluteal vein Internal iliac vein Internal pudendal vein Lateral sacral vein Middle hemorrhoidal vein Obturator vein Uterine vein Vaginal vein Vesical vein
Hypoglossal Nerve	**Includes:** Twelfth cranial nerve
Hypothalamus	**Includes:** Mammillary body
Inferior Mesenteric Artery	**Includes:** Sigmoid artery Superior rectal artery
Inferior Mesenteric Vein	**Includes:** Sigmoid vein Superior rectal vein
Inferior Vena Cava	**Includes:** Postcava Right inferior phrenic vein Right ovarian vein Right second lumbar vein Right suprarenal vein Right testicular vein
Inguinal Region, Bilateral **Inguinal** Region, Left **Inguinal** Region, Right	**Includes:** Inguinal canal Inguinal triangle
Inner Ear, Left **Inner** Ear, Right	**Includes:** Bony labyrinth Bony vestibule Cochlea Round window Semicircular canal
Innominate Artery	**Includes:** Brachiocephalic artery Brachiocephalic trunk
Innominate Vein, Left **Innominate** Vein, Right	**Includes:** Brachiocephalic vein Inferior thyroid vein
Internal Carotid Artery, Left **Internal** Carotid Artery, Right	**Includes:** Caroticotympanic artery Carotid sinus Ophthalmic artery

Section 0 - Medical and Surgical — Character 4 - Body Part

Internal Iliac Artery, Left **Internal** Iliac Artery, Right	**Includes:** Deferential artery Hypogastric artery Iliolumbar artery Inferior gluteal artery Inferior vesical artery Internal pudendal artery Lateral sacral artery Middle rectal artery Obturator artery Superior gluteal artery Umbilical artery Uterine artery Vaginal artery
Internal Mammary Artery, Left **Internal** Mammary Artery, Right	**Includes:** Anterior intercostal artery Internal thoracic artery Musculophrenic artery Pericardiophrenic artery Superior epigastric artery
Intracranial Artery	**Includes:** Anterior cerebral artery Anterior choroidal artery Anterior communicating artery Basilar artery Circle of Willis Middle cerebral artery Posterior cerebral artery Posterior communicating artery Posterior inferior cerebellar artery (PICA)
Intracranial Vein	**Includes:** Anterior cerebral vein Basal (internal) cerebral vein Dural venous sinus Great cerebral vein Inferior cerebellar vein Inferior cerebral vein Internal (basal) cerebral vein Middle cerebral vein Ophthalmic vein Superior cerebellar vein Superior cerebral vein
Jejunum	**Includes:** Duodenojejunal flexure
Kidney	**Includes:** Renal calyx Renal capsule Renal cortex Renal segment
Kidney Pelvis, Left **Kidney** Pelvis, Right	**Includes:** Ureteropelvic junction (UPJ)
Kidney, Left **Kidney,** Right **Kidneys,** Bilateral	**Includes:** Renal calyx Renal capsule Renal cortex Renal segment

Continued →

Section 0 - Medical and Surgical — Character 4 - Body Part	
Knee Bursa and Ligament, Left **Knee** Bursa and Ligament, Right	**Includes:** Anterior cruciate ligament (ACL) Lateral collateral ligament (LCL) Ligament of head of fibula Medial collateral ligament (MCL) Patellar ligament Popliteal ligament Posterior cruciate ligament (PCL) Prepatellar bursa
Knee Joint, Femoral Surface, Left **Knee** Joint, Femoral Surface, Right	**Includes:** Femoropatellar joint Patellofemoral joint
Knee Joint, Left **Knee** Joint, Right	**Includes:** Femoropatellar joint Femorotibial joint Lateral meniscus Medial meniscus Patellofemoral joint Tibiofemoral joint
Knee Joint, Tibial Surface, Left **Knee** Joint, Tibial Surface, Right	**Includes:** Femorotibial joint Tibiofemoral joint
Knee Tendon, Left **Knee** Tendon, Right	**Includes:** Patellar tendon
Lacrimal Duct, Left **Lacrimal** Duct, Right	**Includes:** Lacrimal canaliculus Lacrimal punctum Lacrimal sac Nasolacrimal duct
Larynx	**Includes:** Aryepiglottic fold Arytenoid cartilage Corniculate cartilage Cricoid cartilage Cuneiform cartilage False vocal cord Glottis Rima glottidis Thyroid cartilage Ventricular fold
Lens, Left **Lens,** Right	**Includes:** Zonule of Zinn
Lesser Omentum	**Includes:** Gastrohepatic omentum Hepatogastric ligament
Lesser Saphenous Vein, Left **Lesser** Saphenous Vein, Right	**Includes:** Small saphenous vein
Liver	**Includes:** Quadrate lobe

Section 0 - Medical and Surgical — Character 4 - Body Part	
Lower Arm and Wrist Muscle, Left **Lower** Arm and Wrist Muscle, Right	**Includes:** Anatomical snuffbox Brachioradialis muscle Extensor carpi radialis muscle Extensor carpi ulnaris muscle Flexor carpi radialis muscle Flexor carpi ulnaris muscle Flexor pollicis longus muscle Palmaris longus muscle Pronator quadratus muscle Pronator teres muscle
Lower Eyelid, Left **Lower** Eyelid, Right	**Includes:** Inferior tarsal plate Medial canthus
Lower Femur, Left **Lower** Femur, Right	**Includes:** Lateral condyle of femur Lateral epicondyle of femur Medial condyle of femur Medial epicondyle of femur
Lower Leg Muscle, Left **Lower** Leg Muscle, Right	**Includes:** Extensor digitorum longus muscle Extensor hallucis longus muscle Fibularis brevis muscle Fibularis longus muscle Flexor digitorum longus muscle Flexor hallucis longus muscle Gastrocnemius muscle Peroneus brevis muscle Peroneus longus muscle Popliteus muscle Soleus muscle Tibialis anterior muscle Tibialis posterior muscle
Lower Leg Tendon, Left **Lower** Leg Tendon, Right	**Includes:** Achilles tendon
Lower Lip	**Includes:** Frenulum labii inferioris Labial gland Vermilion border
Lumbar Nerve	**Includes:** Lumbosacral trunk Spinal nerve, lumbar Superior clunic (cluneal) nerve
Lumbar Plexus	**Includes:** Accessory obturator nerve Genitofemoral nerve Iliohypogastric nerve Ilioinguinal nerve Lateral femoral cutaneous nerve Obturator nerve Superior gluteal nerve
Lumbar Spinal Cord	**Includes:** Cauda equina Conus medullaris
Lumbar Sympathetic Nerve	**Includes:** Lumbar ganglion Lumbar splanchnic nerve

Continued →

Section 0 - Medical and Surgical — Character 4 - Body Part	
Lumbar Vertebra	**Includes:** Spinous process Vertebral arch Vertebral foramen Vertebral lamina Vertebral pedicle
Lumbar Vertebral Joint	**Includes:** Lumbar facet joint
Lumbosacral Joint	**Includes:** Lumbosacral facet joint
Lymphatic, Aortic	**Includes:** Celiac lymph node Gastric lymph node Hepatic lymph node Lumbar lymph node Pancreaticosplenic lymph node Paraaortic lymph node Retroperitoneal lymph node
Lymphatic, Head	**Includes:** Buccinator lymph node Infraauricular lymph node Infraparotid lymph node Parotid lymph node Preauricular lymph node Submandibular lymph node Submaxillary lymph node Submental lymph node Subparotid lymph node Suprahyoid lymph node
Lymphatic, Left Axillary	**Includes:** Anterior (pectoral) lymph node Apical (subclavicular) lymph node Brachial (lateral) lymph node Central axillary lymph node Lateral (brachial) lymph node Pectoral (anterior) lymph node Posterior (subscapular) lymph node Subclavicular (apical) lymph node Subscapular (posterior) lymph node
Lymphatic, Left Lower Extremity	**Includes:** Femoral lymph node Popliteal lymph node
Lymphatic, Left Neck	**Includes:** Cervical lymph node Jugular lymph node Mastoid (postauricular) lymph node Occipital lymph node Postauricular (mastoid) lymph node Retropharyngeal lymph node Supraclavicular (Virchow's) lymph node Virchow's (supraclavicular) lymph node
Lymphatic, Left Upper Extremity	**Includes:** Cubital lymph node Deltopectoral (infraclavicular) lymph node Epitrochlear lymph node Infraclavicular (deltopectoral) lymph node Supratrochlear lymph node

Section 0 - Medical and Surgical — Character 4 - Body Part

Section 0 - Medical and Surgical — Character 4 - Body Part	
Lymphatic, Mesenteric	**Includes:** Inferior mesenteric lymph node Pararectal lymph node Superior mesenteric lymph node
Lymphatic, Pelvis	**Includes:** Common iliac (subaortic) lymph node Gluteal lymph node Iliac lymph node Inferior epigastric lymph node Obturator lymph node Sacral lymph node Subaortic (common iliac) lymph node Suprainguinal lymph node
Lymphatic, Right Axillary	**Includes:** Anterior (pectoral) lymph node Apical (subclavicular) lymph node Brachial (lateral) lymph node Central axillary lymph node Lateral (brachial) lymph node Pectoral (anterior) lymph node Posterior (subscapular) lymph node Subclavicular (apical) lymph node Subscapular (posterior) lymph node
Lymphatic, Right Lower Extremity	**Includes:** Femoral lymph node Popliteal lymph node
Lymphatic, Right Neck	**Includes:** Cervical lymph node Jugular lymph node Mastoid (postauricular) lymph node Occipital lymph node Postauricular (mastoid) lymph node Retropharyngeal lymph node Right jugular trunk Right lymphatic duct Right subclavian trunk Supraclavicular (Virchow's) lymph node Virchow's (supraclavicular) lymph node
Lymphatic, Right Upper Extremity	**Includes:** Cubital lymph node Deltopectoral (infraclavicular) lymph node Epitrochlear lymph node Infraclavicular (deltopectoral) lymph node Supratrochlear lymph node
Lymphatic, Thorax	**Includes:** Intercostal lymph node Mediastinal lymph node Parasternal lymph node Paratracheal lymph node Tracheobronchial lymph node
Mandible, Left **Mandible,** Right	**Includes:** Alveolar process of mandible Condyloid process Mandibular notch Mental foramen
Mastoid Sinus, Left **Mastoid** Sinus, Right	**Includes:** Mastoid air cells

Continued →

Section 0 - Medical and Surgical — Character 4 - Body Part	
Maxilla, Left **Maxilla,** Right	**Includes:** Alveolar process of maxilla
Maxillary Sinus, Left **Maxillary** Sinus, Right	**Includes:** Antrum of Highmore
Median Nerve	**Includes:** Anterior interosseous nerve Palmar cutaneous nerve
Medulla Oblongata	**Includes:** Myelencephalon
Mesentery	**Includes:** Mesoappendix Mesocolon
Metacarpocarpal Joint, Left **Metacarpocarpal** Joint, Right	**Includes:** Carpometacarpal (CMC) joint
Metatarsal-Phalangeal Joint, Left **Metatarsal-Phalangeal** Joint, Right	**Includes:** Metatarsophalangeal (MTP) joint
Metatarsal-Tarsal Joint, Left **Metatarsal-Tarsal** Joint, Right	**Includes:** Tarsometatarsal joint
Middle Ear, Left **Middle** Ear, Right	**Includes:** Oval window Tympanic cavity
Minor Salivary Gland	**Includes:** Anterior lingual gland
Mitral Valve	**Includes:** Bicuspid valve Left atrioventricular valve Mitral annulus
Nasal Bone	**Includes:** Vomer of nasal septum
Nasal Septum	**Includes:** Quadrangular cartilage Septal cartilage Vomer bone
Nasal Turbinate	**Includes:** Inferior turbinate Middle turbinate Nasal concha Superior turbinate
Nasopharynx	**Includes:** Choana Fossa of Rosenmuller Pharyngeal recess Rhinopharynx

Section 0 - Medical and Surgical — Character 4 - Body Part	
Neck Muscle, Left **Neck** Muscle, Right	**Includes:** Anterior vertebral muscle Arytenoid muscle Cricothyroid muscle Infrahyoid muscle Levator scapulae muscle Platysma muscle Scalene muscle Splenius cervicis muscle Sternocleidomastoid muscle Suprahyoid muscle Thyroarytenoid muscle
Nipple, Left **Nipple,** Right	**Includes:** Areola
Nose	**Includes:** Columella External naris Greater alar cartilage Internal naris Lateral nasal cartilage Lesser alar cartilage Nasal cavity Nostril
Occipital Bone, Left **Occipital** Bone, Right	**Includes:** Foramen magnum
Oculomotor Nerve	**Includes:** Third cranial nerve
Olfactory Nerve	**Includes:** First cranial nerve Olfactory bulb
Optic Nerve	**Includes:** Optic chiasma Second cranial nerve
Orbit, Left **Orbit,** Right	**Includes:** Bony orbit Orbital portion of ethmoid bone Orbital portion of frontal bone Orbital portion of lacrimal bone Orbital portion of maxilla Orbital portion of palatine bone Orbital portion of sphenoid bone Orbital portion of zygomatic bone
Pancreatic Duct	**Includes:** Duct of Wirsung
Pancreatic Duct, Accessory	**Includes:** Duct of Santorini
Parotid Duct, Left **Parotid** Duct, Right	**Includes:** Stensen's duct
Pelvic Bone, Left **Pelvic** Bone, Right	**Includes:** Iliac crest Ilium Ischium Pubis
Pelvic Cavity	**Includes:** Retropubic space
Penis	**Includes:** Corpus cavernosum Corpus spongiosum

Continued →

Section 0 - Medical and Surgical — Character 4 - Body Part	
Perineum Muscle	**Includes:** Bulbospongiosus muscle Cremaster muscle Deep transverse perineal muscle Ischiocavernosus muscle Superficial transverse perineal muscle
Peritoneum	**Includes:** Epiploic foramen
Peroneal Artery, Left **Peroneal** Artery, Right	**Includes:** Fibular artery
Peroneal Nerve	**Includes:** Common fibular nerve Common peroneal nerve External popliteal nerve Lateral sural cutaneous nerve
Pharynx	**Includes:** Hypopharynx Laryngopharynx Oropharynx Piriform recess (sinus)
Phrenic Nerve	**Includes:** Accessory phrenic nerve
Pituitary Gland	**Includes:** Adenohypophysis Hypophysis Neurohypophysis
Pons	**Includes:** Apneustic center Basis pontis Locus ceruleus Pneumotaxic center Pontine tegmentum Superior olivary nucleus
Popliteal Artery, Left **Popliteal** Artery, Right	**Includes:** Inferior genicular artery Middle genicular artery Superior genicular artery Sural artery
Portal Vein	**Includes:** Hepatic portal vein
Prepuce	**Includes:** Foreskin Glans penis
Pudendal Nerve	**Includes:** Posterior labial nerve Posterior scrotal nerve
Pulmonary Artery, Left	**Includes:** Arterial canal (duct) Botallo's duct Pulmoaortic canal
Pulmonary Valve	**Includes:** Pulmonary annulus Pulmonic valve
Pulmonary Vein, Left	**Includes:** Left inferior pulmonary vein Left superior pulmonary vein

Section 0 - Medical and Surgical — Character 4 - Body Part	
Pulmonary Vein, Right	**Includes:** Right inferior pulmonary vein Right superior pulmonary vein
Radial Artery, Left **Radial** Artery, Right	**Includes:** Radial recurrent artery
Radial Nerve	**Includes:** Dorsal digital nerve Musculospiral nerve Palmar cutaneous nerve Posterior interosseous nerve
Radius, Left **Radius,** Right	**Includes:** Ulnar notch
Rectum	**Includes:** Anorectal junction
Renal Artery, Left **Renal** Artery, Right	**Includes:** Inferior suprarenal artery Renal segmental artery
Renal Vein, Left	**Includes:** Left inferior phrenic vein Left ovarian vein Left second lumbar vein Left suprarenal vein Left testicular vein
Retina, Left **Retina,** Right	**Includes:** Fovea Macula Optic disc
Retroperitoneum	**Includes:** Retroperitoneal space
Sacral Nerve	**Includes:** Spinal nerve, sacral
Sacral Plexus	**Includes:** Inferior gluteal nerve Posterior femoral cutaneous nerve Pudendal nerve
Sacral Sympathetic Nerve	**Includes:** Ganglion impar (ganglion of Walther) Pelvic splanchnic nerve Sacral ganglion Sacral splanchnic nerve
Sacrococcygeal Joint	**Includes:** Sacrococcygeal symphysis
Scapula, Left **Scapula,** Right	**Includes:** Acromion (process) Coracoid process
Sciatic Nerve	**Includes:** Ischiatic nerve

Continued →

Section 0 - Medical and Surgical — Character 4 - Body Part	
Shoulder Bursa and Ligament, Left **Shoulder** Bursa and Ligament, Right	**Includes:** Acromioclavicular ligament Coracoacromial ligament Coracoclavicular ligament Coracohumeral ligament Costoclavicular ligament Glenohumeral ligament Glenoid ligament (labrum) Interclavicular ligament Sternoclavicular ligament Subacromial bursa Transverse humeral ligament Transverse scapular ligament
Shoulder Joint, Left **Shoulder** Joint, Right	**Includes:** Glenohumeral joint
Shoulder Muscle, Left **Shoulder** Muscle, Right	**Includes:** Deltoid muscle Infraspinatus muscle Subscapularis muscle Supraspinatus muscle Teres major muscle Teres minor muscle
Sigmoid Colon	**Includes:** Rectosigmoid junction Sigmoid flexure
Skin	**Includes:** Dermis Epidermis Sebaceous gland Sweat gland
Sphenoid Bone, Left **Sphenoid** Bone, Right	**Includes:** Greater wing Lesser wing Optic foramen Pterygoid process Sella turcica
Spinal Canal	**Includes:** Vertebral canal
Spinal Meninges	**Includes:** Arachnoid mater Denticulate ligament Leptomeninges Pia mater
Spleen	**Includes:** Accessory spleen
Splenic Artery	**Includes:** Left gastroepiploic artery Pancreatic artery Short gastric artery
Splenic Vein	**Includes:** Left gastroepiploic vein Pancreatic vein
Sternum	**Includes:** Manubrium Suprasternal notch Xiphoid process
Stomach, Pylorus	**Includes:** Pyloric antrum Pyloric canal Pyloric sphincter

Section 0 - Medical and Surgical — Character 4 - Body Part	
Subarachnoid Space	**Includes:** Cranial subarachnoid space Spinal subarachnoid space
Subclavian Artery, Left **Subclavian** Artery, Right	**Includes:** Costocervical trunk Dorsal scapular artery Internal thoracic artery
Subcutaneous Tissue and Fascia, Anterior Neck	**Includes:** Deep cervical fascia Pretracheal fascia
Subcutaneous Tissue and Fascia, Chest	**Includes:** Pectoral fascia
Subcutaneous Tissue and Fascia, Face	**Includes:** Masseteric fascia Orbital fascia
Subcutaneous Tissue and Fascia, Left Foot	**Includes:** Plantar fascia (aponeurosis)
Subcutaneous Tissue and Fascia, Left Hand	**Includes:** Palmar fascia (aponeurosis)
Subcutaneous Tissue and Fascia, Left Lower Arm	**Includes:** Antebrachial fascia Bicipital aponeurosis
Subcutaneous Tissue and Fascia, Left Upper Arm	**Includes:** Axillary fascia Deltoid fascia Infraspinatus fascia Subscapular aponeurosis Supraspinatus fascia
Subcutaneous Tissue and Fascia, Left Upper Leg	**Includes:** Crural fascia Fascia lata Iliac fascia Iliotibial tract (band)
Subcutaneous Tissue and Fascia, Posterior Neck	**Includes:** Prevertebral fascia
Subcutaneous Tissue and Fascia, Right Foot	**Includes:** Plantar fascia (aponeurosis)
Subcutaneous Tissue and Fascia, Right Hand	**Includes:** Palmar fascia (aponeurosis)
Subcutaneous Tissue and Fascia, Right Lower Arm	**Includes:** Antebrachial fascia Bicipital aponeurosis
Subcutaneous Tissue and Fascia, Right Upper Arm	**Includes:** Axillary fascia Deltoid fascia Infraspinatus fascia Subscapular aponeurosis Supraspinatus fascia
Subcutaneous Tissue and Fascia, Right Upper Leg	**Includes:** Crural fascia Fascia lata Iliac fascia Iliotibial tract (band)
Subcutaneous Tissue and Fascia, Scalp	**Includes:** Galea aponeurotica

Continued →

Section 0 - Medical and Surgical — Character 4 - Body Part	
Subcutaneous Tissue and Fascia, Trunk	**Includes:** External oblique aponeurosis Transversalis fascia
Subdural Space	**Includes:** Cranial subdural space Spinal subdural space
Submaxillary Gland, Left **Submaxillary** Gland, Right	**Includes:** Submandibular gland
Superior Mesenteric Artery	**Includes:** Ileal artery Ileocolic artery Inferior pancreaticoduodenal artery Jejunal artery
Superior Mesenteric Vein	**Includes:** Right gastroepiploic vein
Superior Vena Cava	**Includes:** Precava
Tarsal Joint, Left **Tarsal** Joint, Right	**Includes:** Calcaneocuboid joint Cuboideonavicular joint Cuneonavicular joint Intercuneiform joint Subtalar (talocalcaneal) joint Talocalcaneal (subtalar) joint Talocalcaneonavicular joint
Tarsal, Left **Tarsal,** Right	**Includes:** Calcaneus Cuboid bone Intermediate cuneiform bone Lateral cuneiform bone Medial cuneiform bone Navicular bone Talus bone
Temporal Artery, Left **Temporal** Artery, Right	**Includes:** Middle temporal artery Superficial temporal artery Transverse facial artery
Temporal Bone, Left **Temporal** Bone, Right	**Includes:** Mastoid process Petrous part of temoporal bone Tympanic part of temoporal bone Zygomatic process of temporal bone
Thalamus	**Includes:** Epithalamus Geniculate nucleus Metathalamus Pulvinar
Thoracic Aorta	**Includes:** Aortic arch Aortic intercostal artery Ascending aorta Bronchial artery Esophageal artery Subcostal artery
Thoracic Duct	**Includes:** Left jugular trunk Left subclavian trunk

Section 0 - Medical and Surgical — Character 4 - Body Part	
Thoracic Nerve	**Includes:** Intercostal nerve Intercostobrachial nerve Spinal nerve, thoracic Subcostal nerve
Thoracic Sympathetic Nerve	**Includes:** Cardiac plexus Esophageal plexus Greater splanchnic nerve Inferior cardiac nerve Least splanchnic nerve Lesser splanchnic nerve Middle cardiac nerve Pulmonary plexus Superior cardiac nerve Thoracic aortic plexus Thoracic ganglion
Thoracic Vertebra	**Includes:** **Spinous** process **Vertebral** arch **Vertebral** foramen **Vertebral** lamina **Vertebral** pedicle
Thoracic Vertebral Joint	**Includes:** **Costotransverse** joint **Costovertebral** joint **Thoracic** facet joint
Thoracolumbar Vertebral Joint	**Includes:** **Thoracolumbar** facet joint
Thorax Bursa and Ligament, Left **Thorax** Bursa and Ligament, Right	**Includes:** **Costotransverse** ligament **Costoxiphoid** ligament **Sternocostal** ligament
Thorax Muscle, Left **Thorax** Muscle, Right	**Includes:** **Intercostal** muscle **Levatores** costarum muscle **Pectoralis** major muscle **Pectoralis** minor muscle **Serratus** anterior muscle **Subclavius** muscle **Subcostal** muscle **Transverse** thoracis muscle
Thymus	**Includes:** **Thymus** gland
Thyroid Artery, Left **Thyroid** Artery, Right	**Includes:** **Cricothyroid** artery **Hyoid** artery **Sternocleidomastoid** artery **Superior** laryngeal artery **Superior** thyroid artery **Thyrocervical** trunk
Tibia, Left **Tibia,** Right	**Includes:** **Lateral** condyle of tibia **Medial** condyle of tibia **Medial** malleolus
Tibial Nerve	**Includes:** **Lateral** plantar nerve **Medial** plantar nerve **Medial** popliteal nerve **Medial** sural cutaneous nerve

Continued →

Section 0 - Medical and Surgical — Character 4 - Body Part	
Toe Nail	**Includes:** Nail bed Nail plate
Toe Phalangeal Joint, Left **Toe** Phalangeal Joint, Right	**Includes:** Interphalangeal (IP) joint
Tongue	**Includes:** Frenulum linguae Lingual tonsil
Tongue, Palate, Pharynx Muscle	**Includes:** Chondroglossus muscle Genioglossus muscle Hyoglossus muscle Inferior longitudinal muscle Levator veli palatini muscle Palatoglossal muscle Palatopharyngeal muscle Pharyngeal constrictor muscle Salpingopharyngeus muscle Styloglossus muscle Stylopharyngeus muscle Superior longitudinal muscle Tensor veli palatini muscle
Tonsils	**Includes:** Palatine tonsil
Transverse Colon	**Includes:** Splenic flexure
Tricuspid Valve	**Includes:** Right atrioventricular valve Tricuspid annulus
Trigeminal Nerve	**Includes:** Fifth cranial nerve Gasserian ganglion Mandibular nerve Maxillary nerve Ophthalmic nerve Trifacial nerve
Trochlear Nerve	**Includes:** Fourth cranial nerve
Trunk Bursa and Ligament, Left **Trunk** Bursa and Ligament, Right	**Includes:** Iliolumbar ligament Interspinous ligament Intertransverse ligament Ligamentum flavum Pubic ligament Sacrococcygeal ligament Sacroiliac ligament Sacrospinous ligament Sacrotuberous ligament Supraspinous ligament
Trunk Muscle, Left **Trunk** Muscle, Right	**Includes:** Coccygeus muscle Erector spinae muscle Interspinalis muscle Intertransversarius muscle Latissimus dorsi muscle Levator ani muscle Quadratus lumborum muscle Rhomboid major muscle Rhomboid minor muscle Serratus posterior muscle Transversospinalis muscle Trapezius muscle

Section 0 - Medical and Surgical — Character 4 - Body Part	
Tympanic Membrane, Left **Tympanic** Membrane, Right	**Includes:** Pars flaccida
Ulna, Left **Ulna,** Right	**Includes:** Olecranon process Radial notch
Ulnar Artery, Left **Ulnar** Artery, Right	**Includes:** Anterior ulnar recurrent artery Common interosseous artery Posterior ulnar recurrent artery
Ulnar Nerve	**Includes:** Cubital nerve
Upper Arm Muscle, Left **Upper** Arm Muscle, Right	**Includes:** Biceps brachii muscle Brachialis muscle Coracobrachialis muscle Triceps brachii muscle
Upper Eyelid, Left **Upper** Eyelid, Right	**Includes:** Lateral canthus Levator palpebrae superioris muscle Orbicularis oculi muscle Superior tarsal plate
Upper Femur, Left **Upper** Femur, Right	**Includes:** Femoral head Greater trochanter Lesser trochanter Neck of femur
Upper Leg Muscle, Left **Upper** Leg Muscle, Right	**Includes:** Adductor brevis muscle Adductor longus muscle Adductor magnus muscle Biceps femoris muscle Gracilis muscle Pectineus muscle Quadriceps (femoris) Rectus femoris muscle Sartorius muscle Semimembranosus muscle Semitendinosus muscle Vastus intermedius muscle Vastus lateralis muscle Vastus medialis muscle
Upper Lip	**Includes:** Frenulum labii superioris Labial gland Vermilion border
Ureter **Ureter,** Left **Ureter,** Right **Ureters,** Bilateral	**Includes:** Ureteral orifice Ureterovesical orifice
Urethra	**Includes:** Bulbourethral (Cowper's) gland Cowper's (bulbourethral) gland External urethral sphincter Internal urethral sphincter Membranous urethra Penile urethra Prostatic urethra

Continued →

Section 0 - Medical and Surgical — Character 4 - Body Part	
Uterine Supporting Structure	**Includes:** Broad ligament Infundibulopelvic ligament Ovarian ligament Round ligament of uterus
Uterus	**Includes:** Fundus uteri Myometrium Perimetrium Uterine cornu
Uvula	**Includes:** Palatine uvula
Vagus Nerve	**Includes:** Anterior vagal trunk Pharyngeal plexus Pneumogastric nerve Posterior vagal trunk Pulmonary plexus Recurrent laryngeal nerve Superior laryngeal nerve Tenth cranial nerve
Vas Deferens **Vas** Deferens, Bilateral **Vas** Deferens, Left **Vas** Deferens, Right	**Includes:** Ductus deferens Ejaculatory duct
Ventricle, Right	**Includes:** Conus arteriosus
Ventricular Septum	**Includes:** Interventricular septum

Section 0 - Medical and Surgical — Character 4 - Body Part	
Vertebral Artery, Left **Vertebral** Artery, Right	**Includes:** Anterior spinal artery Posterior spinal artery
Vertebral Vein, Left **Vertebral** Vein, Right	**Includes:** Deep cervical vein Suboccipital venous plexus
Vestibular Gland	**Includes:** Bartholin's (greater vestibular) gland Greater vestibular (Bartholin's) gland Paraurethral (Skene's) gland Skene's (paraurethral) gland
Vitreous, Left **Vitreous,** Right	**Includes:** Vitreous body
Vocal Cord, Left **Vocal** Cord, Right	**Includes:** Vocal fold
Vulva	**Includes:** Labia majora Labia minora
Wrist Bursa and Ligament, Left **Wrist** Bursa and Ligament, Right	**Includes:** Palmar ulnocarpal ligament Radial collateral carpal ligament Radiocarpal ligament Radioulnar ligament Ulnar collateral carpal ligament
Wrist Joint, Left **Wrist** Joint, Right	**Includes:** Distal radioulnar joint Radiocarpal joint

Appendix E: Medical and Surgical Device Table (Device Key) and Device Aggregation Table

Section 0 - Medical and Surgical — Character 6 - Device	
Artificial Sphincter in Gastrointestinal System	**Includes:** Artificial anal sphincter (AAS) Artificial bowel sphincter (neosphincter)
Artificial Sphincter in Urinary System	**Includes:** AMS 800® Urinary Control System Artificial urinary sphincter (AUS)
Autologous Arterial Tissue in Heart and Great Vessels	**Includes:** Autologous artery graft
Autologous Arterial Tissue in Lower Arteries	**Includes:** Autologous artery graft
Autologous Arterial Tissue in Lower Veins	**Includes:** Autologous artery graft
Autologous Arterial Tissue in Upper Arteries	**Includes:** Autologous artery graft
Autologous Arterial Tissue in Upper Veins	**Includes:** Autologous artery graft

Section 0 - Medical and Surgical — Character 6 - Device	
Autologous Tissue Substitute	**Includes:** Autograft Cultured epidermal cell autograft Epicel® cultured epidermal autograft
Autologous Venous Tissue in Heart and Great Vessels	**Includes:** Autologous vein graft
Autologous Venous Tissue in Lower Arteries	**Includes:** Autologous vein graft
Autologous Venous Tissue in Lower Veins	**Includes:** Autologous vein graft
Autologous Venous Tissue in Upper Arteries	**Includes:** Autologous vein graft
Autologous Venous Tissue in Upper Veins	**Includes:** Autologous vein graft

Continued →

Section 0 - Medical and Surgical — Character 6 - Device	
Bone Growth Stimulator in Head and Facial Bones	**Includes:** Electrical bone growth stimulator (EBGS) Ultrasonic osteogenic stimulator Ultrasound bone healing system
Bone Growth Stimulator in Lower Bones	**Includes:** Electrical bone growth stimulator (EBGS) Ultrasonic osteogenic stimulator Ultrasound bone healing system
Bone Growth Stimulator in Upper Bones	**Includes:** Electrical bone growth stimulator (EBGS) Ultrasonic osteogenic stimulator Ultrasound bone healing system
Cardiac Lead in Heart and Great Vessels	**Includes:** Cardiac contractility modulation lead
Cardiac Lead, Defibrillator for Insertion in Heart and Great Vessels	**Includes:** ACUITY™ Steerable Lead Attain Ability® lead Attain StarFix® (OTW) lead Cardiac resynchronization therapy (CRT) lead Corox (OTW) Bipolar Lead Durata® Defibrillation Lead ENDOTAK RELIANCE® (G) Defibrillation Lead
Cardiac Lead, Pacemaker for Insertion in Heart and Great Vessels	**Includes:** ACUITY™ Steerable Lead Attain Ability® lead Attain StarFix® (OTW) lead Cardiac resynchronization therapy (CRT) lead Corox (OTW) Bipolar Lead
Cardiac Resynchronization Defibrillator Pulse Generator for Insertion in Subcutaneous Tissue and Fascia	**Includes:** COGNIS® CRT-D Concerto II CRT-D Consulta CRT-D CONTAK RENEWAL® 3 RF (HE) CRT-D LIVIAN™ CRT-D Maximo II DR CRT-D Ovatio™ CRT-D Protecta XT CRT-D Viva (XT)(S)
Cardiac Resynchronization Pacemaker Pulse Generator for Insertion in Subcutaneous Tissue and Fascia	**Includes:** Consulta CRT-P Stratos LV Synchra CRT-P
Contraceptive Device in Female Reproductive System	**Includes:** Intrauterine device (IUD)
Contraceptive Device in Subcutaneous Tissue and Fascia	**Includes:** Subdermal progesterone implant
Contractility Modulation Device for Insertion in Subcutaneous Tissue and Fascia	**Includes:** Optimizer™ III implantable pulse generator

Section 0 - Medical and Surgical — Character 6 - Device	
Defibrillator Generator for Insertion in Subcutaneous Tissue and Fascia	**Includes:** Evera (XT)(S)(DR/VR) Implantable cardioverter-defibrillator (ICD) Maximo II DR (VR) Protecta XT DR (XT VR) Secura (DR) (VR) Virtuoso (II) (DR) (VR)
Diaphragmatic Pacemaker Lead in Respiratory System	**Includes:** Phrenic nerve stimulator lead
Drainage Device	**Includes:** Cystostomy tube Foley catheter Percutaneous nephrostomy catheter Thoracostomy tube
Epiretinal Visual Prosthesis in Eye	**Includes:** Epiretinal visual prosthesis
External Fixation Device in Head and Facial Bones	**Includes:** External fixator
External Fixation Device in Lower Bones	**Includes:** External fixator
External Fixation Device in Lower Joints	**Includes:** External fixator
External Fixation Device in Upper Bones	**Includes:** External fixator
External Fixation Device in Upper Joints	**Includes:** External fixator
External Fixation Device, Hybrid for Insertion in Upper Bones	**Includes:** Delta frame external fixator Sheffield hybrid external fixator
External Fixation Device, Hybrid for Insertion in Lower Bones	**Includes:** Delta frame external fixator Sheffield hybrid external fixator
External Fixation Device, Hybrid for Reposition in Upper Bones	**Includes:** Delta frame external fixator Sheffield hybrid external fixator
External Fixation Device, Hybrid for Reposition in Lower Bones	**Includes:** Delta frame external fixator Sheffield hybrid external fixator
External Fixation Device, Limb Lengthening for Insertion in Upper Bones	**Includes:** Ilizarov-Vecklich device
External Fixation Device, Limb Lengthening for Insertion in Lower Bones	**Includes:** Ilizarov-Vecklich device
External Fixation Device, Monoplanar for Insertion in Upper Bones	**Includes:** Uniplanar external fixator
External Fixation Device, Monoplanar for Insertion in Lower Bones	**Includes:** Uniplanar external fixator
External Fixation Device, Monoplanar for Reposition in Upper Bones	**Includes:** Uniplanar external fixator
External Fixation Device, Monoplanar for Reposition in Lower Bones	**Includes:** Uniplanar external fixator

Continued →

Section 0 - Medical and Surgical — Character 6 - Device	
External Fixation Device, Ring for Insertion in Upper Bones	**Includes:** Ilizarov external fixator Sheffield ring external fixator
External Fixation Device, Ring for Insertion in Lower Bones	**Includes:** Ilizarov external fixator Sheffield ring external fixator
External Fixation Device, Ring for Reposition in Upper Bones	**Includes:** Ilizarov external fixator Sheffield ring external fixator
External Fixation Device, Ring for Reposition in Lower Bones	**Includes:** Ilizarov external fixator Sheffield ring external fixator
External Heart Assist System in Heart and Great Vessels	**Includes:** Biventricular external heart assist system BVS 5000 Ventricular Assist Device Centrimag(R) Blood Pump TandemHeart® System Thoratec Paracorporeal Ventricular Assist Device
Extraluminal Device	**Includes:** LAP-BAND® adjustable gastric banding system REALIZE® Adjustable Gastric Band TigerPaw® system for closure of left atrial appendage
Feeding Device in Gastrointestinal System	**Includes:** Percutaneous endoscopic gastrojejunostomy (PEG/J) tube Percutaneous endoscopic gastrostomy (PEG) tube
Hearing Device in Ear, Nose, Sinus	**Includes:** Esteem® implantable hearing system
Hearing Device in Head and Facial Bones	**Includes:** Bone anchored hearing device
Hearing Device, Bone Conduction for Insertion in Ear, Nose, Sinus	**Includes:** Bone anchored hearing device
Hearing Device, Multiple Channel Cochlear Prosthesis for Insertion in Ear, Nose, Sinus	**Includes:** Cochlear implant (CI), multiple channel (electrode)
Hearing Device, Single Channel Cochlear Prosthesis for Insertion in Ear, Nose, Sinus	**Includes:** Cochlear implant (CI), single channel (electrode)
Implantable Heart Assist System in Heart and Great Vessels	**Includes:** Berlin Heart Ventricular Assist Device DeBakey Left Ventricular Assist Device DuraHeart Left Ventricular Assist System HeartMate II® Left Ventricular Assist Device (LVAD) HeartMate XVE® Left Ventricular Assist Device (LVAD) MicroMed HeartAssist Novacor Left Ventricular Assist Device Thoratec IVAD (Implantable Ventricular Assist Device)

Section 0 - Medical and Surgical — Character 6 - Device	
Infusion Device	**Includes:** Ascenda Intrathecal Catheter InDura, intrathecal catheter (1P) (spinal) Non-tunneled central venous catheter Peripherally inserted central catheter (PICC) Tunneled spinal (intrathecal) catheter
Infusion Device, Pump in Subcutaneous Tissue and Fascia	**Includes:** Implantable drug infusion pump (anti-spasmodic)(chemotherapy)(pain) Injection reservoir, pump Pump reservoir Subcutaneous injection reservoir, pump SynchroMed pump
Interbody Fusion Device in Lower Joints	**Includes:** Axial Lumbar Interbody Fusion System AxiaLIF® System CoRoent® XL Direct Lateral Interbody Fusion (DLIF) device EXtreme Lateral Interbody Fusion (XLIF) device Interbody fusion (spine) cage XLIF® System
Interbody Fusion Device in Upper Joints	**Includes:** BAK/C® Interbody Cervical Fusion System Interbody fusion (spine) cage
Internal Fixation Device in Head and Facial Bones	**Includes:** Bone screw (interlocking)(lag)(pedicle) (recessed) Kirschner wire (K-wire) Neutralization plate
Internal Fixation Device in Lower Bones	**Includes:** Bone screw (interlocking)(lag)(pedicle) (recessed) Clamp and rod internal fixation system (CRIF) Kirschner wire (K-wire) Neutralization plate
Internal Fixation Device in Lower Joints	**Includes:** Fusion screw (compression)(lag)(locking) Joint fixation plate Kirschner wire (K-wire)
Internal Fixation Device in Upper Bones	**Includes:** Bone screw (interlocking)(lag)(pedicle) (recessed) Clamp and rod internal fixation system (CRIF) Kirschner wire (K-wire) Neutralization plate
Internal Fixation Device in Upper Joints	**Includes:** Fusion screw (compression)(lag)(locking) Joint fixation plate Kirschner wire (K-wire)
Internal Fixation Device, Intramedullary in Lower Bones	**Includes:** Intramedullary (IM) rod (nail) Intramedullary skeletal kinetic distractor (ISKD) Kuntscher nail

Continued →

Section 0 - Medical and Surgical — Character 6 - Device	
Internal Fixation Device, Intramedullary in Upper Bones	**Includes:** Intramedullary (IM) rod (nail) Intramedullary skeletal kinetic distractor (ISKD) Kuntscher nail
Internal Fixation Device, Rigid Plate for Insertion in Upper Bones	**Includes:** Titanium Sternal Fixation System (TSFS)
Internal Fixation Device, Rigid Plate for Reposition in Upper Bones	**Includes:** Titanium Sternal Fixation System (TSFS)
Intraluminal Device	**Includes:** Absolute Pro Vascular (OTW) Self-Expanding Stent System Acculink (RX) Carotid Stent System AneuRx® AAA Advantage® Assurant (Cobalt) stent Carotid WALLSTENT® Monorail® Endoprosthesis CoAxia NeuroFlo catheter Colonic Z-Stent® Complete (SE) stent Driver stent (RX) (OTW) E-Luminexx™ (Biliary)(Vascular) Stent Embolization coil(s) Endurant® Endovascular Stent Graft Express® (LD) Premounted Stent System Express® Biliary SD Monorail® Premounted Stent System Express® SD Renal Monorail® Premounted Stent System FLAIR® Endovascular Stent Graft Formula™ Balloon-Expandable Renal Stent System Herculink (RX) Elite Renal Stent System LifeStent® (Flexstar)(XL) Vascular Stent System Micro-Driver stent (RX) (OTW) MULTI-LINK (VISION)(MINI-VISION) (ULTRA) Coronary Stent System Omnilink Elite Vascular Balloon Expandable Stent System Pipeline™ Embolization device (PED) Protégé® RX Carotid Stent System Stent, intraluminal (cardiovascular) (gastrointestinal)(hepatobiliary)(urinary) Talent® Converter Talent® Occluder Talent® Stent Graft (abdominal)(thoracic) Therapeutic occlusion coil(s) Ultraflex™ Precision Colonic Stent System Valiant Thoracic Stent Graft WALLSTENT® Endoprosthesis Xact Carotid Stent System Zenith Flex® AAA Endovascular Graft Zenith® Renu™ AAA Ancillary Graft Zenith TX2® TAA Endovascular Graft
Intraluminal Device, Airway in Ear, Nose, Sinus	**Includes:** Nasopharyngeal airway (NPA)
Intraluminal Device, Airway in Gastrointestinal System	**Includes:** Esophageal obturator airway (EOA)

Section 0 - Medical and Surgical — Character 6 - Device	
Intraluminal Device, Airway in Mouth and Throat	**Includes:** Guedel airway Oropharyngeal airway (OPA)
Intraluminal Device, Bioactive in Upper Arteries	**Includes:** Bioactive embolization coil(s) Micrus CERECYTE microcoil
Intraluminal Device, Drug-eluting in Heart and Great Vessels	**Includes:** CYPHER® Stent Endeavor® (III)(IV) (Sprint) Zotarolimus-eluting Coronary Stent System Everolimus-eluting coronary stent Paclitaxel-eluting coronary stent Sirolimus-eluting coronary stent TAXUS® Liberté® Paclitaxel-eluting Coronary Stent System XIENCE Everolimus Eluting Coronary Stent System Zotarolimus-eluting coronary stent
Intraluminal Device, Drug-eluting in Lower Arteries	**Includes:** Paclitaxel-eluting peripheral stent Zilver® PTX® (paclitaxel) Drug-Eluting Peripheral Stent
Intraluminal Device, Drug-eluting in Upper Arteries	**Includes:** Paclitaxel-eluting peripheral stent Zilver® PTX® (paclitaxel) Drug-Eluting Peripheral Stent
Intraluminal Device, Endobronchial Valve in Respiratory System	**Includes:** Spiration IBV™ Valve System
Intraluminal Device, Pessary in Female Reproductive System	**Includes:** Pessary ring Vaginal pessary
Intraluminal Device, Endotracheal Airway in Respiratory System	**Includes:** Endotracheal tube (cuffed)(double-lumen)
Liner in Lower Joints	**Includes:** Hip (joint) liner Joint liner (insert) Knee (implant) insert
Monitoring Device	**Includes:** Blood glucose monitoring system Cardiac event recorder Continuous Glucose Monitoring (CGM) device Implantable glucose monitoring device Loop recorder, implantable Reveal (DX)(XT)
Monitoring Device, Hemodynamic for Insertion in Subcutaneous Tissue and Fascia	**Includes:** Implantable hemodynamic monitor (IHM) Implantable hemodynamic monitoring system (IHMS)
Monitoring Device, Pressure Sensor for Insertion in Heart and Great Vessels	**Includes:** CardioMEMS® pressure sensor EndoSure® sensor

Continued →

Section 0 - Medical and Surgical — Character 6 - Device	
Neurostimulator Lead in Central Nervous System	**Includes:** Cortical strip neurostimulator lead DBS lead Deep brain neurostimulator lead RNS System lead Spinal cord neurostimulator lead
Neurostimulator Lead in Peripheral Nervous System	**Includes:** InterStim® Therapy lead
Neurostimulator Generator in Head and Facial Bones	**Includes:** RNS system neurostimulator generator
Nonautologous Tissue Substitute	**Includes:** Acellular Hydrated Dermis Bone bank bone graft Tissue bank graft
Pacemaker, Dual Chamber for Insertion in Subcutaneous Tissue and Fascia	**Includes:** Advisa (MRI) EnRhythm Kappa Revo MRI™ SureScan® pacemaker Two lead pacemaker Versa
Pacemaker, Single Chamber for Insertion in Subcutaneous Tissue and Fascia	**Includes:** Single lead pacemaker (atrium)(ventricle)
Pacemaker, Single Chamber Rate Responsive for Insertion in Subcutaneous Tissue and Fascia	**Includes:** Single lead rate responsive pacemaker (atrium)(ventricle)
Radioactive Element	**Includes:** Brachytherapy seeds
Resurfacing Device in Lower Joints	**Includes:** CONSERVE® PLUS Total Resurfacing Hip System Cormet Hip Resurfacing System
Spacer in Lower Joints	**Includes:** Joint spacer (antibiotic)
Spacer in Upper Joints	**Includes:** Joint spacer (antibiotic)
Spinal Stabilization Device, Facet Replacement for Insertion in Upper Joints	**Includes:** Facet replacement spinal stabilization device
Spinal Stabilization Device, Facet Replacement for Insertion in Lower Joints	**Includes:** Facet replacement spinal stabilization device
Spinal Stabilization Device, Interspinous Process for Insertion in Upper Joints	**Includes:** Interspinous process spinal stabilization device X-STOP® Spacer
Spinal Stabilization Device, Interspinous Process for Insertion in Lower Joints	**Includes:** Interspinous process spinal stabilization device X-STOP® Spacer
Spinal Stabilization Device, Pedicle-Based for Insertion in Upper Joints	**Includes:** Dynesys® Dynamic Stabilization System Pedicle-based dynamic stabilization device
Spinal Stabilization Device, Pedicle-Based for Insertion in Lower Joints	**Includes:** Dynesys® Dynamic Stabilization System Pedicle-based dynamic stabilization device

Section 0 - Medical and Surgical — Character 6 - Device	
Stimulator Generator in Subcutaneous Tissue and Fascia	**Includes:** Baroreflex Activation Therapy(R) (BAT(R)) Diaphragmatic pacemaker generator Mark IV Breathing Pacemaker System Phrenic nerve stimulator generator Rheos(R) System device
Stimulator Generator, Multiple Array for Insertion in Subcutaneous Tissue and Fascia	**Includes:** Activa PC neurostimulator Enterra gastric neurostimulator Neurostimulator generator, multiple channel PrimeAdvanced neurostimulator (SureScan)(MRI Safe)
Stimulator Generator, Multiple Array Rechargeable for Insertion in Subcutaneous Tissue and Fascia	**Includes:** Activa RC neurostimulator Neurostimulator generator, multiple channel rechargeable RestoreAdvanced neurostimulator (SureScan)(MRI Safe) RestoreSensor neurostimulator (SureScan) (MRI Safe) RestoreUltra neurostimulator (SureScan) (MRI Safe)
Stimulator Generator, Single Array for Insertion in Subcutaneous Tissue and Fascia	**Includes:** Activa SC neurostimulator InterStim® Therapy neurostimulator Itrel (3)(4) neurostimulator Neurostimulator generator, single channel
Stimulator Generator, Single Array Rechargeable for Insertion in Subcutaneous Tissue and Fascia	**Includes:** Neurostimulator generator, single channel rechargeable
Stimulator Lead in Gastrointestinal System	**Includes:** Gastric electrical stimulation (GES) lead Gastric pacemaker lead
Stimulator Lead in Muscles	**Includes:** Electrical muscle stimulation (EMS) lead Electronic muscle stimulator lead Neuromuscular electrical stimulation (NEMS) lead
Stimulator Lead in Upper Arteries	**Includes:** Baroreflex Activation Therapy® (BAT®) Carotid (artery) sinus (baroreceptor) lead Rheos® System lead
Stimulator Lead in Urinary System	**Includes:** Sacral nerve modulation (SNM) lead Sacral neuromodulation lead Urinary incontinence stimulator lead

Continued →

Section 0 - Medical and Surgical — Character 6 - Device	
Synthetic Substitute	**Includes:** **AbioCor®** Total Replacement Heart **AMPLATZER®** Muscular VSD Occluder **Annuloplasty** ring **Bard®** Composix® (E/X)(LP) mesh **Bard®** Composix® Kugel® patch **Bard®** Dulex™ mesh **Bard®** Ventralex™ hernia patch **BRYAN®** Cervical Disc System **Ex-PRESS™** mini glaucoma shunt **Flexible** Composite Mesh **GORE®** DUALMESH® **Holter** valve ventricular shunt **MitraClip** valve repair system **Nitinol** framed polymer mesh **Open** Pivot Aortic Valve Graft (AVG) **Open** Pivot (mechanical) valve **Partially** absorbable mesh **PHYSIOMESH™** Flexible Composite Mesh **Polymethylmethacrylate** (PMMA) **Polypropylene** mesh **PRESTIGE®** Cervical Disc **PROCEED™** Ventral Patch **Prodisc-C** **Prodisc-L** **PROLENE** Polypropylene Hernia System (PHS) **Rebound** HRD® (Hernia Repair Device) **SynCardia** Total Artificial Heart **Total** artificial (replacement) heart **ULTRAPRO** Hernia System (UHS) **ULTRAPRO** Partially Absorbable Lightweight Mesh **ULTRAPRO** Plug **Ventrio™** Hernia Patch **Zimmer®** NexGen® LPS Mobile Bearing Knee **Zimmer®** NexGen® LPS-Flex Mobile Knee
Synthetic Substitute, Ceramic for Replacement in Lower Joints	**Includes:** **Novation®** Ceramic AHS® (Articulation Hip System)
Synthetic Substitute, Ceramic on Polyethylene for Replacement in Lower Joints	**Includes:** **Oxidized** zirconium ceramic hip bearing surface
Synthetic Substitute, Intraocular Telescope for Replacement in Eye	**Includes:** **Implantable** Miniature Telescope™ (IMT)
Synthetic Substitute, Metal for Replacement in Lower Joints	**Includes:** **Cobalt/chromium** head and socket

Section 0 - Medical and Surgical — Character 6 - Device	
Synthetic Substitute, Metal on Polyethylene for Replacement in Lower Joints	**Includes:** Cobalt/chromium head and polyethylene socket
Synthetic Substitute, Polyethylene for Replacement in Lower Joints	**Includes:** Polyethylene socket
Synthetic Substitute, Reverse Ball and Socket for Replacement in Upper Joints	**Includes:** Delta III Reverse shoulder prosthesis Reverse® Shoulder Prosthesis
Tissue Expander in Skin and Breast	**Includes:** Tissue expander (inflatable)(injectable)
Tissue Expander in Subcutaneous Tissue and Fascia	**Includes:** Tissue expander (inflatable)(injectable)
Tracheostomy Device in Respiratory System	**Includes:** Tracheostomy tube
Vascular Access Device in Subcutaneous Tissue and Fascia	**Includes:** Tunneled central venous catheter Vectra® Vascular Access Graft
Vascular Access Device, Reservoir in Subcutaneous Tissue and Fascia	**Includes:** Implanted (venous)(access) port Injection reservoir, port Subcutaneous injection reservoir, port
Zooplastic Tissue in Heart and Great Vessels	**Includes:** 3f (Aortic) Bioprosthesis valve Bovine pericardial valve Bovine pericardium graft Contegra Pulmonary Valved Conduit CoreValve transcatheter aortic valve Epic™ Stented Tissue Valve (aortic) Freestyle (Stentless) Aortic Root Bioprosthesis Hancock Bioprosthesis (aortic) (mitral) valve Hancock Bioprosthetic Valved Conduit Melody® transcatheter pulmonary valve Mitroflow® Aortic Pericardial Heart Valve Mosaic Bioprosthesis (aortic) (mitral) valve Porcine (bioprosthetic) valve SAPIEN transcatheter aortic valve SJM Biocor® Stented Valve System Stented tissue valve Trifecta™ Valve (aortic) Xenograft

Device Aggregation Table

Specific Device	for Operation	in Body System	General Device
Autologous Arterial Tissue	All applicable	Heart and Great Vessels Lower Arteries Lower Veins Upper Arteries Upper Veins	**7** Autologous Tissue Substitute
Autologous Venous Tissue	All applicable	Heart and Great Vessels Lower Arteries Lower Veins Upper Arteries Upper Veins	**7** Autologous Tissue Substitute
Cardiac Lead, Defibrillator	Insertion	Heart and Great Vessels	**M** Cardiac Lead
Cardiac Lead, Pacemaker	Insertion	Heart and Great Vessels	**M** Cardiac Lead
Cardiac Resynchronization Defibrillator Pulse Generator	Insertion	Subcutaneous Tissue and Fascia	**P** Cardiac Rhythm Related Device
Cardiac Resynchronization Pacemaker Pulse Generator	Insertion	Subcutaneous Tissue and Fascia	**P** Cardiac Rhythm Related Device
Contractility Modulation Device	Insertion	Subcutaneous Tissue and Fascia	**P** Cardiac Rhythm Related Device
Defibrillator Generator	Insertion	Subcutaneous Tissue and Fascia	**P** Cardiac Rhythm Related Device
Epiretinal Visual Prosthesis	All applicable	Eye	**J** Synthetic Substitute
External Fixation Device, Hybrid	Insertion	Lower Bones Upper Bones	**5** External Fixation Device
External Fixation Device, Hybrid	Reposition	Lower Bones Upper Bones	**5** External Fixation Device
External Fixation Device, Limb Lengthening	Insertion	Lower Bones Upper Bones	**5** External Fixation Device
External Fixation Device, Monoplanar	Insertion	Lower Bones Upper Bones	**5** External Fixation Device
External Fixation Device, Monoplanar	Reposition	Lower Bones Upper Bones	**5** External Fixation Device
External Fixation Device, Ring	Insertion	Lower Bones Upper Bones	**5** External Fixation Device
External Fixation Device, Ring	Reposition	Lower Bones Upper Bones	**5** External Fixation Device
Hearing Device, Bone Conduction	Insertion	Ear, Nose, Sinus	**S** Hearing Device
Hearing Device, Multiple Channel Cochlear Prosthesis	Insertion	Ear, Nose, Sinus	**S** Hearing Device
Hearing Device, Single Channel Cochlear Prosthesis	Insertion	Ear, Nose, Sinus	**S** Hearing Device
Internal Fixation Device, Intramedullary	All applicable	Lower Bones Upper Bones	**4** Internal Fixation Device
Internal Fixation Device, Rigid Plate	Insertion	Upper Bones	**4** Internal Fixation Device
Internal Fixation Device, Rigid Plate	Reposition	Upper Bones	**4** Internal Fixation Device
Intraluminal Device, Pessary	All applicable	Female Reproductive System	**D** Intraluminal Device